The Comparative
Guide to
American Hospitals

Volume 1

Third Edition

The Comparative
Guide to
American Hospitals

Volume 1: Eastern Region

4,693 Hospitals with Key Personnel and
49 Quality Measures Relating to Heart Attack, Heart
Failure, Pneumonia, Childhood Asthma, Surgical Care,
Medical Imaging and Patient Experience

A SEDGWICK PRESS Book

Grey House
Publishing

PUBLISHER: Leslie Mackenzie
EDITOR: David Garoogian
EDITORIAL DIRECTOR: Laura Mars
PRODUCTION MANAGER: Kristen Thatcher
MARKETING DIRECTOR: Jessica Moody

A Sedgewick Press Book
Grey House Publishing, Inc.
4919 Route 22
Amenia, NY 12501
518.789.8700
FAX 845.373.6390
www.greyhouse.com
e-mail: books @greyhouse.com

Copyright © 2011 Grey House Publishing, Inc.
Third Edition

All rights reserved
Printed in Canada

Comparative guide to American hospitals. Vol. 1, Eastern region; [ed. David Garoogian]. — 3rd ed. (2011)

v. ; cm.

Includes index.
"4,693 Hospitals with Key Personnel and 49 Quality Measures Relating to Heart Attack, Heart Failure, Pneumonia, Childhood Asthma, Surgical Care, Medical Imaging and Patient Experience."

1. Hospitals--United States--Directories. 2. Hospitals--United States--Periodicals. 3. Hospitals--Ratings--United States--Statistics--Periodicals. 4. Myocardial infarction--Hospitals--United States--Directories. 5. Heart failure--Hospitals--United States--Directories. 6. Pneumonia--Hospitals--United States--Directories. I. Garoogian, David.

RA977 .C66
610/.025

4-Volume Set	ISBN: 978-1-59237-838-8
Volume 1	**ISBN: 978-1-59237-839-5**
Volume 2	ISBN: 978-1-59237-840-1
Volume 3	ISBN: 978-1-59237-841-8
Volume 4	ISBN: 978-1-59237-842-5

Table of Contents

Introduction

This is the third edition of *The Comparative Guide to American Hospitals*. It reports on how 4,693 hospitals—**310 more than last edition**—in America measure up when caring for patients with a number of specific conditions. The second edition reported on **Heart Attacks, Heart Failure, Pneumonia** and **Surgical Care**. This third edition includes additional data on **Childhood Asthma, Medical Imaging** and **Patients' Hospital Experiences**. Also new is an appendix on **30-Day Readmission Rates**.

This work is based on a Federal study (Hospital Compare) in which short-term acute care and critical access hospitals around the country voluntarily report on quality measures to receive an incentive payment established by the Medicare Prescription Drug, Improvement and Modernization Act of 2003. Each hospital in this edition is rated on 49 recognized quality measures—**25 more than last edition**—and is compared to both state and national averages.

In *The Comparative Guide to American Hospitals,* the data is organized, sorted and ranked by our editors. It is this organization and ranking that makes *The Comparative Guide to American Hospitals* a unique and valuable tool to the health care consumer. Data is presented in such a way as to inform and educate the user, who can then put the facts into a meaningful context as hospitals are evaluated state by state.

Due to the increased data, and the regional use of such data, this edition is comprised of four regional volumes—**Eastern, Southern, Central** and **Western**. In addition to comprehensive **hospital rankings and profiles** for all states in the region, each volume includes a **State-by-State Statistical Summary**.

In addition to the data from Hospital Compare, each hospital profile in *The Comparative Guide to American Hospitals* is comprised of value-added data from Grey House's *Directory of Hospital Personnel*. This critical contact data includes fax numbers, web sites, email addresses, and number of beds plus **23,685 key contact names—2,995 more names** than last edition. In addition, each state chapter includes **State Hospital Rankings**.

Section One: State Hospital Rankings & State Profiles

The first section of each regional volume of *The Comparative Guide to American Hospitals* is arranged alphabetically by state. Each state chapter starts with a ranking section, unique to Grey House, that ranks hospitals in that state on how often they meet each of the accepted quality protocols. This first section:

- **Evaluates 49 Quality Measures:** The quality measures ranked in *The Comparative Guide to American Hospitals* are based on accepted, effective treatments supported by the Centers for Medicare & Medical Services of the US Department of Health & Human Services and the Hospital Quality Alliance (HQA)—a public/private collaboration established to promote on hospital quality of care. HQA represents consumers, hospitals, doctors, employers, accrediting organizations and Federal agencies.

- **Examines Critical Conditions: Heart Attack Care** measures include angiotensin converting enzyme inhibitor (ACE inhibitor) or angiotensin receptor blocker (ARB) for left ventricular systolic dysfunction (LVSD), aspirin at arrival and discharge, beta blocker at discharge, fibrinolytic medication timing, percutaneous coronary intervention (PCI) within 90 minutes of arrival, and smoking cessation advice or counseling; **Chest Pain/Possible Heart Attack Care** *(NEW)* measures include aspirin at arrival, median time to ECG, median time to transfer, and fibrinolytic medication timing; **Heart Failure Care** measures include angiotensin converting enzyme (ACE) inhibitor or angiotensin receptor blocker (ARB) for left ventricular systolic dysfunction (LVSD), discharge instructions given, evaluation of left ventricular systolic (LVS) function, and smoking cessation advice or counseling; **Pneumonia Care** measures include appropriate initial antibiotic, blood culture timing, influenza vaccination, initial antibiotic timing, pneumococcal vaccination, and smoking cessation advice or counseling; **Surgical Care** measures include appropriate venous thromboembolism prophylaxis (VTP) within 24 hours *(NEW)*, appropriate hair removal *(NEW)*, appropriate beta blocker usage *(NEW)*, controlled postoperative blood glucose *(NEW)*, prophylactic antibiotic timing, prophylactic antibiotic selection, prophylactic antibiotic stopped, recommended

venous thromboembolism prophylaxis (VTP) ordered *(NEW)*, and urinary catheter removal *(NEW)*; **Children's Asthma Care** *(NEW)* measures include receiving systemic corticosteroids, receiving home management plan, and receiving reliever medication.

- **Examines the Use of Medical Imaging** *(NEW)*: MRI for low back pain, follow-up mammogram/ultrasound, combination abdominal CT scan, and combination chest CT scan.

- **Summarizes the Survey of Patients' Hospital Experiences** *(NEW)*
  HCAHPS (Hospital Consumer Assessment of Healthcare Providers and Systems) is a national, standardized survey of hospital patients. HCAHPS (pronounced "H-caps") was created to publicly report the patient's perspective of hospital care. The survey asks a random sample of recently discharged patients about important aspects of their hospital experience. The HCAHPS results allow consumers to make fair and objective comparisons between hospitals, and of individual hospitals to state and national benchmarks, on ten important measures of patients' perspectives of care:
  - How do patients rate the hospital overall?
  - How often did doctors communicate well with patients?
  - How often did nurses communicate well with patients?
  - How often did patients receive help quickly from hospital staff?
  - How often did staff explain about medicines before giving them to patients?
  - How often was patients' pain well controlled?
  - How often was the area around patients' rooms kept quiet at night?
  - How often were the patients' rooms and bathrooms kept clean?
  - Were patients given information about what to do during their recovery at home?
  - Would patients recommend the hospital to friends and family?

Following the ranking section, hospital profiles are listed first by city, then alpha within city. Profiles include name, address, phone, fax, web site, hospital type and ownership, number of beds, and whether the hospital provides emergency services. Further, each profile includes an average of five key medical contacts—representing not only the facility's top administration but also the physicians specifically responsible for the care of heart, pneumonia, and asthma patients, as well as surgical care. Again, these data points are unique to *The Comparative Guide to American Hospitals*, and complete the picture for health care consumers searching for quality care.

Section Two: Statistical Summary, Appendixes & Index

The second section of *The Comparative Guide to American Hospitals* includes:

- **Regional State-by-State Statistical Summary Tables** show at a glance how hospitals in the same state score and compare with each other. Hospitals are arranged alphabetically by state.

- **Appendix A: 30-Day Mortality Charts** Unique to Grey House, the Mortality Charts again, take data and organize it in a helpful, informative way for the reader. It lists hospitals nationwide that are "better" or "worse" than the national average, plus a State Summary of Hospital Mortality Rates.

- **Appendix B: 30-Day Readmission Charts** *(another unique, NEW element)* lists hospitals nationwide that are "better" or "worse" than the national average, plus a State Summary of Hospital Readmission Rates.

- **Appendix C: Glossary of Terms** provides a list of 50 medical terms to make the best use possible of the data in this edition.

- **Regional Hospital Profile Index** lists hospitals alphabetically, including city and state.

This completely revised third edition of *The Comparative Guide to American Hospitals* is a valuable guide for the entire medical community, with more hospitals, more criteria measures and more key executives than the last edition. It offers an indispensable snapshot of how hospitals measure up, not only to established "best practices," but also to each other.

We welcome your comments to this edition.

USER'S GUIDE

The listing to the right illustrates the kind of information that is or might be included in a Hospital Profile. Each numbered item of information is described in the paragraphs following the example.

❶ Saint Claire Regional Medical Center

222 Medical Circle
Morehead, KY 40351
E-mail: mjneff@st-claire.org
URL: www.st-claire.org
Type: Acute Care Hospitals
Ownership: Voluntary Non-Profit - Church

Phone: 606-783-6500
Fax: 606-783-6503

Emergency Services: Yes
Beds: 159

❷ Key Personnel:

CEO/President	Mark J Neff
Cardiac Laboratory	Charlotte Lewis
Chief of Medical Staff	Will Mehlan, MD
Infection Control	Charlette Kinney
Operating Room	Lisa Amburgery
Pediatric In-Patient Care	Nancy Maggard
Quality Assurance	Linda Fultz
Radiology	Charles Butler

❸

Measure	Cases	This Hosp.	State Avg.	U.S. Avg.
❹ Heart Attack Care				
ACE Inhibitor or ARB for LVSD[1]	14	79%	94%	96%
Aspirin at Arrival	84	100%	98%	99%
Aspirin at Discharge	72	96%	99%	98%
Beta Blocker at Discharge	73	99%	98%	98%
Fibrinolytic Medication Timing	0	-	60%	55%
PCI Within 90 Minutes of Arrival[1]	10	100%	88%	90%
Smoking Cessation Advice	36	97%	100%	99%
❺ Chest Pain/Possible Heart Attack Care				
Aspirin at Arrival	85	99%	95%	95%
Average Time to ECG (minutes)	95	1	7	8
Average Time to Transfer (minutes)[1]	4	54	65	61
Fibrinolytic Medication Timing[1]	3	33%	62%	54%
❻ Heart Failure Care				
ACE Inhibitor or ARB for LVSD	49	96%	91%	94%
Discharge Instructions	104	88%	82%	88%
Evaluation of LVS Function	129	97%	96%	98%
Smoking Cessation Advice	30	97%	98%	98%
❼ Pneumonia Care				
Appropriate Initial Antibiotic	106	92%	90%	92%
Blood Culture Timing	216	92%	95%	96%
Influenza Vaccine	113	96%	92%	91%
Initial Antibiotic Timing	196	97%	95%	95%
Pneumococcal Vaccine	183	91%	94%	93%
Smoking Cessation Advice	108	97%	98%	97%
❽ Surgical Care Improvement Project				
Appropriate VTP Within 24 Hours[2]	92	96%	91%	92%
Appropriate Hair Removal[2]	196	99%	99%	99%
Appropriate Beta Blocker Usage[2]	78	92%	93%	93%
Controlled Postoperative Blood Glucose[2]	0	-	94%	93%
Prophylactic Antibiotic Timing[2]	118	88%	97%	97%
Prophylactic Antibiotic Timing (Outpatient)	80	91%	92%	92%
Prophylactic Antibiotic Selection[2]	119	97%	98%	97%
Prophylactic Antibiotic Select. (Outpatient)	117	91%	93%	94%
Prophylactic Antibiotic Stopped[2]	116	90%	94%	94%
Recommended VTP Ordered[2]	92	98%	94%	94%
Urinary Catheter Removal[2]	42	71%	89%	90%
❾ Children's Asthma Care				
Received Systemic Corticosteroids[1]	4	100%	-	100%
Received Home Management Plan[1]	5	80%	-	71%
Received Reliever Medication[1]	5	100%	-	100%
❿ Use of Medical Imaging				
Combination Abdominal CT Scan	700	0.616	0.160	0.191
Combination Chest CT Scan	463	0.039	0.054	0.054
Follow-up Mammogram/Ultrasound	756	7.9%	7.9%	8.4%
MRI for Low Back Pain	143	43.4%	35.6%	32.7%
⓫ Survey of Patients' Hospital Experiences				
Area Around Room 'Always' Quiet at Night	300+	49%	-	58%
Doctors 'Always' Communicated Well	300+	85%	-	80%
Home Recovery Information Given	300+	83%	-	82%
Hospital Given 9 or 10 on 10 Point Scale	300+	62%	-	67%
Meds 'Always' Explained Before Given	300+	64%	-	60%
Nurses 'Always' Communicated Well	300+	80%	-	76%
Pain 'Always' Well Controlled	300+	71%	-	69%
Room and Bathroom 'Always' Clean	300+	71%	-	71%
Timely Help 'Always' Received	300+	64%	-	64%
Would Definitely Recommend Hospital	300+	66%	-	69%

❶ **Hospital Name and Record Header:** hospital name; street address; phone; fax; e-mail; URL; hospital type; ownership; emergency services (Yes/No); and number of beds.

❷ **Key Personnel:** includes the names of key personnel primarily related to the conditions covered in this publication.

❸ **Hospital Compare Data:** each table contains data covering forty-nine measures contained in the Hospital Compare database. There are five columns:

    Measure: the forty-nine quality measures reported.

      There are eleven possible footnotes:

      1. *The number of cases is too small (<25) to reliably tell how well a hospital is performing.*
      For each measure, the rate is the percent of patients for whom the treatment is appropriate. Where these numbers are small (fewer than 25 patients), the calculated rate may not accurately predict the hospital's future performance. As the quality data base is expanded to a full rolling four quarters of data for each measure, the number of cases used to determine hospitals' rates will likely increase, thereby increasing the reliability and stability of the rates. Note: This footnote does not necessarily reflect hospital size or overall patient volume.

      2. *The hospital indicated that the data submitted for this measure were based on a sample of cases.*
      A rate may be based upon the total number of cases treated by a hospital, or for a facility with a large caseload, a rate may be based on a random sample of the cases the hospital treated. This footnote indicates that a hospital chose to submit data for a sample of its total cases (following specific rules for how to the select the cases).

      3. *Data was collected during a shorter time period (fewer quarters) than the maximum possible time for this measure (one quarter equals three months.).*
      Each rate reflects the care given over a specific time period, up to a maximum of four quarters during a 12 month period. The number of quarters of data available is determined by when hospitals first began to report data using a specific measure. For example, for the ten measures in the "Starter Set", the maximum number of quarters for which a hospital could have provided data is four quarters. For measures added more recently, the maximum will be fewer than four quarters. This footnote indicates that the hospital's rate was based on data from fewer than the maximum possible number of quarters that the measure was generally collected.

      4. *Inaccurate information submitted and suppressed for one or more quarters.*
      Hospitals are required to submit accurate, reportable data to the Centers for Medicare and Medicaid Services (CMS). The rates for these measures were calculated by excluding data that had been suppressed for one or more quarters because they were identified as inaccurate.

      5. *No data is available from the hospital for this measure.*
      Hospitals volunteer to provide data for reporting on Hospital Compare. This footnote is applied when the hospital did not submit any cases for a measure or if they suppressed their data from public reporting.

      6. *Fewer than 100 patients completed the HCAHPS survey. Use these rates with caution, as the number of surveys may be too low to reliably assess hospital performance.*
      The number of completed surveys the hospital or its vendor provided to CMS is less than 100.

      7. *Survey results are based on less than 12 months of survey data.*
      This footnote is applied when HCAHPS results are based on less than 12 months of survey data.

      8. *Survey results are not available for this period.*
      This footnote is applied when a hospital did not participate in HCAHPS, did not collect sufficient HCAHPS data for public reporting purposes, or chose to suppress their HCAHPS results.

      9. *No patients were eligible for the HCAHPS Survey.*
      This footnote is applied when a hospital has no patients eligible to participate in the HCAHPS survey.

      10. *A state average was not calculated because too few hospitals in the state submitted data.*
      This footnote is applied when too few hospitals submitted data.

      11. *There were discrepancies in the data collection process.*
      This footnote is applied when there have been deviations from HCAHPS data collection protocols. CMS is working with survey vendors and/or hospitals to correct this situation.

Cases: the size of the data sample (number of patients) for each hospital and quality measure. In addition, the notation "0" is applied when a hospital provided care to patients with a condition, such as pneumonia, but the cases that the hospital submitted did not meet the specific criteria for being included in the calculation of the measure.

This Hospital: the performance rate that the hospital achieved for each quality measure. This value is expressed as a percentage of the sample size that was measured. The performance rate is calculated by dividing the numerator by the denominator. The denominator is the sum of all eligible cases (as defined in the measure specifications) submitted to the QIO Clinical Data Warehouse for the reporting period. The numerator is the sum of all eligible cases submitted for the same reporting period where the recommended care was provided.

State Average: the average rate for all hospitals reporting data in the state the hospital is located in.

U.S. Average: the average rate for all hospitals reporting nationwide.

Note: Beginning in December 2010, state and national averages for the process of care measures are calculated by summing the cases in the state or nation that "passed" the measure (Numerator) and dividing that sum by the number of cases in the state or national Denominator. For the national and state averages, a simple average was constructed where the numerator was the sum of all non-excluded hospitals' scores and the denominator was the total number of hospitals, each calculated at either the national or individual state level. For the process and survey measures, the national and state averages are calculated before excluding suppressed rates and are not recalculated using only published rates as was done prior to September 2009. Acute Care-VA Medical Centers are not included in the calculation of the national and state comparison rates.

The children's asthma care national and state averages are calculated differently. The average rate for all healthcare organizations in the nation that provide results for a measure. The average rate is calculated by dividing the total number of patients who had the recommended care provided for a measure by the total number of patients who met the inclusion and exclusion criteria for that measure in the nation for the timeframe being reported.

❹ Heart Attack Care

Every year, about one million people suffer a heart attack (acute myocardial infarction or AMI). AMI is among the leading causes of hospital admission for Medicare beneficiaries, age 65 and older.

Scientific evidence indicates that the following process of care measures represent the best practices for the treatment of AMI. Higher scores are better.

- **ACE Inhibitor or ARB for LVSD** - AMI patients with left ventricular systolic dysfunction (LVSD) and without angiotensin converting enzyme inhibitor (ACE inhibitor) contraindications or angiotensin receptor blocker (ARB) contraindications who are prescribed an ACE inhibitor or an ARB at hospital discharge.

- **Aspirin at Arrival** - Acute myocardial infarction (AMI) patients without aspirin contraindications who received aspirin within 24 hours before or after hospital arrival.

- **Aspirin at Discharge** - AMI patients without aspirin contraindications who were prescribed aspirin at hospital discharge.

- **Beta Blocker at Discharge** - AMI patients without beta-blocker contraindications who were prescribed a beta-blocker at hospital discharge.

- **Fibrinolytic Medication Timing** - AMI patients receiving fibrinolytic therapy during the hospital stay and having a time from hospital arrival to fibrinolysis of 30 minutes or less.

- **PCI Within 90 Minutes of Arrival** - AMI patients receiving Percutaneous Coronary Intervention (PCI) during the hospital stay with a time from hospital arrival to PCI of 90 minutes or less.

- **Smoking Cessation Advice** - AMI patients with a history of smoking cigarettes, who are given smoking cessation advice or counseling during a hospital stay.

❺ Chest Pain/Possible Heart Attack Care

These are all outpatient measures. Higher scores are better.

- **Aspirin at Arrival** - Acute myocardial infarction (AMI) patients without aspirin contraindications who received aspirin within 24 hours before or after hospital arrival.

- **Median Time to ECG** - Median number of minutes before outpatients with heart attack (or with chest pain that suggest a possible heart attack) got an ECG (a lower number of minutes is better).

- **Median Time to Transfer** - Median number of minutes before outpatients with heart attack who needed specialized care were transferred to another hospital (a lower number of minutes is better).

- **Fibrinolytic Medication Timing** - AMI patients receiving fibrinolytic therapy during the hospital stay and having a time from hospital arrival to fibrinolysis of 30 minutes or less.

❻ Heart Failure Care

Heart failure is the most common hospital admission diagnosis in patients age 65 or older, accounting for more than 700,000 hospitalizations among Medicare beneficiaries every year. It is associated with severe functional impairments and high rates of mortality and morbidity.

Substantial scientific evidence indicates that the following process of care measures represent the best practices for the treatment of heart failure. Higher scores are better.

- **ACE Inhibitor or ARB for LVSD** - Heart failure patients with left ventricular systolic dysfunction (LVSD) and without angiotensin converting enzyme inhibitor (ACE inhibitor) contraindications or angiotensin receptor blocker (ARB) contraindications who are prescribed an ACE inhibitor or an ARB at hospital discharge.

- **Discharge Instructions** - Heart failure patients discharged home with written instructions or educational material given to patient or care giver at discharge or during the hospital stay addressing all of the following: activity level, diet, discharge medications, follow-up appointment, weight monitoring, and what to do if symptoms worsen.

- **Evaluation of LVS Function** - Heart failure patients with documentation in the hospital record that an evaluation of the left ventricular systolic (LVS) function was performed before arrival, during hospitalization, or is planned for after discharge.

- **Smoking Cessation Advice** - Heart failure patients with a history of smoking cigarettes, who are given smoking cessation advice or counseling during a hospital stay.

❼ Pneumonia Care

Community acquired pneumonia is a major contributor to illness and mortality in the United States, causing four million episodes of illness and nearly one million hospital admissions each year.

Scientific evidence indicates that the following process of care measures represent the best practices for the treatment of community-acquired pneumonia. Higher scores are better.

- **Appropriate Initial Antibiotic** - Immunocompetent patients with pneumonia who receive an initial antibiotic regimen that is consistent with current guidelines.

- **Blood Culture Timing** - Pneumonia patients whose initial emergency room blood culture specimen was collected prior to first hospital dose of antibiotics.

- **Influenza Vaccination** - Pneumonia patients age 50 years and older, hospitalized during October, November, December, January, or February who were screened for influenza vaccine status and were vaccinated prior to discharge, if indicated.

- **Initial Antibiotic Timing** - Pneumonia inpatients who receive antibiotics within 6 hours of hospital arrival. Evidence shows better outcomes for administration times less than four hours.

- **Pneumococcal Vaccination** - Pneumonia inpatients age 65 and older who were screened for pneumococcal vaccine status and were administered the vaccine prior to discharge, if indicated.

- **Smoking Cessation Advice** - Pneumonia patients with a history of smoking cigarettes, who are given smoking cessation advice or counseling during a hospital stay.

❽ Surgical Care Improvement Project

Hospitals can reduce the risk of complications like wound infection or blood clots in surgery patients by giving the right treatments at the right time. For example, studies show a strong association of reduced incidence of post-operative infection with administration of antibiotics within the one hour prior to surgery. After the incision is closed, however, studies show that prolonged administration of prophylaxis with antibiotics may increase the risk of certain other infections at no additional benefit to the surgical patient.

Scientific evidence indicates that the following process of care measures represent the best practices for the prevention of infections after selected surgeries (colon surgery, hip and knee arthroplasty, abdominal and vaginal hysterectomy, cardiac surgery (including coronary artery bypass grafts (CABG)) and vascular surgery). Higher scores are better.

- **Appropriate VTP Within 24 Hours** - Surgery patients who received appropriate venous thromboembolism prophylaxis (VTP) within 24 Hours prior to surgical incision time to 24 hours after surgery end time.

- **Appropriate Hair Removal** - Surgery patients with appropriate surgical site hair removal. No hair removal, or hair removal with clippers or depilatory is considered appropriate. Shaving is considered inappropriate.

- **Appropriate Beta Blocker Usage** - Surgery patients who were taking heart drugs called beta blockers before coming to the hospital, who were kept on the beta blockers during the period just before and after their surgery.

- **Controlled Postoperative Blood Glucose** - Cardiac surgery patients with controlled 6 A.M. blood glucose (= 200 mg/dL) on postoperative day one (POD 1) and postoperative day two (POD 2) with surgery end date being postoperative day zero (POD 0).

- **Prophylactic Antibiotic Timing** - Surgical inpatients who received prophylactic antibiotics within 1 hour prior to surgical incision.

- **Prophylactic Antibiotic Timing (Outpatient)** - Surgical outpatients who received prophylactic antibiotics within 1 hour prior to surgical incision.

- **Prophylactic Antibiotic Selection** - Surgical inpatients who received the recommended antibiotics for their particular type of surgery.

- **Prophylactic Antibiotic Selection (Outpatient)** - Surgical outpatients who received the recommended antibiotics for their particular type of surgery.

- **Prophylactic Antibiotic Stopped** - Surgical patients whose prophylactic antibiotics were discontinued within 24 hours after surgery end time.

- **Recommended VTP Ordered** - Surgery patients with recommended venous thromboembolism prophylaxis (VTP) ordered anytime from hospital arrival to 48 hours after surgery end time.

- **Urinary Catheters Removal** - Inpatients whose urinary catheters were removed within 2 days after surgery to reduce the risk of infections. Shows the percent of surgery patients whose urinary catheters were removed on the first or second day after surgery.

⑨ Children's Asthma Care

Asthma is the most common chronic disease in children and a major cause of morbidity and increased health care expenditures nationally (Adams, et al., 2001). For children, asthma is one of the most frequent reasons for admission to hospitals (McCormick, et al., 1999). Other researchers noted that there are approximately 200,000 admissions for childhood asthma in the United States annually, representing more than $3 billion dollars in healthcare costs (Silber, et al., 2003). Under-treatment and/or inappropriate treatment of asthma are recognized as major contributors to asthma morbidity and mortality.

- **Received Systemic Corticosteroids** - Use of systemic Corticosteroid Medication in pediatric patients admitted for inpatient treatment of asthma.

- **Received Home Management Plan** - An assessment that there is documentation in the medical record that a Home Management Plan of Care (HMPC) document was given to the pediatric asthma patient/caregiver.

- **Received Reliever Medication** - Use of relievers in pediatric patients admitted for inpatient treatment of asthma.

⑩ Use of Medical Imaging

"Medical imaging" is the name for tests that create images of various parts of the body to screen for or diagnose medical conditions. Examples of medical imaging include CT scans, MRIs, and mammograms. The measures on use of medical imaging give you information about how hospitals use medical imaging tests for outpatients based on the following: 1) Protecting patients' safety, such as keeping patients' exposure to radiation and other risks as low as possible; 2) Following up properly when screening tests such as mammograms show a possible problem; 3) Avoiding the risk, stress, and cost of doing imaging tests that patients may not need.

The measures of medical imaging are based on Medicare claims data. CMS compiles this information from claims for patients in Original (fee-for-service) Medicare. It does not include people in Medicare Advantage plans or people who do not have Medicare. The information is limited to medical imaging facilities that are part of a hospital or associated with a hospital. These facilities can be inside or near the hospital, or in a different location. The information

only includes medical imaging done on outpatients. Medical imaging tests done for patients who have been admitted to the hospital as inpatients aren't included.

- **MRI for Low Back Pain** (NQF Endorsed, October 2008) - This measure calculates the percentage of patients who had an MRI of the Lumbar Spine with a diagnosis of low back pain without Medicare claims-based evidence of antecedent conservative therapy. If a number is high, it may mean the facility is doing too many unnecessary MRIs for low back pain.

- **Follow-up Mammogram/Ultrasound** (Not NQF Endorsed at this time) - This measure calculates the percentage of patients with mammography screening studies done in the outpatient hospital setting that are followed within 45 days by a diagnostic mammography or ultrasound of the breast study in an outpatient or office setting. A number that is much lower than 8% may mean there's not enough follow-up. A number much higher than 14% may mean there's too much unnecessary follow-up.

- **Combination Abdominal CT Scan** (Not NQF Endorsed at this time) - This measure calculates the ratio of CT abdomen studies that are performed both with/without contrast out of all CT abdomen studies performed (those with contrast, those without contrast, and those with both). The range for this measure is 0 to 1. A number very close to 1 may mean that too many patients are being given a combination (double) scan when a single scan is all they need.

- **Combination Chest CT Scan** (NQF Endorsed, October 2008) - This measure calculates the ratio of CT thorax studies that are performed with and without contrast out of all CT thorax studies performed (those with contrast, those without contrast, and those with both). The range for this measure is 0 to 1. A number very close to 1 may mean that too many patients are being given a combination (double) scan when a single scan is all they need.

The National Quality Forum (NQF) is an independent organization created to develop and implement a strategy for health care quality measurement and public reporting. The NQF brings together stakeholders from throughout the healthcare industry to jointly decide which quality measures meet industry standards and are suitable for reporting on Hospital Compare. While NQF endorses the quality measures, it does not monitor or review the data that are collected from and about hospitals.

NQF considers several factors when deciding whether a quality measure should be reported: 1) Whether it addresses an aspect of care or treatment that improves people's health or well-being; 2) Whether it can be measured accurately and reliably in different hospitals; 3) Whether the information can be used to improve the quality of care or to inform patients' decisions about where to go for care.

⑪ Survey of Patients' Hospital Experiences (HCAHPS)

HCAHPS (Hospital Consumer Assessment of Healthcare Providers and Systems) is a national, standardized survey of hospital patients. HCAHPS (pronounced "H-caps") was created to publicly report the patient's perspective of hospital care. The survey asks a random sample of recently discharged patients about important aspects of their hospital experience. The HCAHPS results allow consumers to make fair and objective comparisons between hospitals, and of individual hospitals to state and national benchmarks, on ten important measures of patients' perspectives of care.

HCAHPS was developed by a partnership of public and private organizations. Development of the survey was funded by the Federal government, specifically the Centers for Medicare & Medicaid Services (CMS) and the Agency for Healthcare Research and Quality (AHRQ). For more on HCAHPS information, please visit the official HCAHPS website: www.hcahpsonline.org

What questions are on the survey?

The HCAHPS survey asks patients to give feedback about topics for which they are the best source of information. The survey asks patients to answer questions about their experiences in the hospital. To make sure the HCAHPS survey data is meaningful; patients only answer questions about topics with which they have experience. The HCAHPS survey asks patients to answer questions related to ten topics. The topics and questions are listed in the table below.

HCAHPS Topic Text	HCAHPS Answer Description
How do patients rate the hospital overall?	*Patients who gave a rating of 9 or 10 (high)*
	Patients who gave a rating of 7 or 8 (medium)
	Patients who gave a rating of 6 or lower (low)
How often did doctors communicate well with patients?	*Doctors always communicated well*
	Doctors usually communicated well
	Doctors sometimes or never communicated well

HCAHPS Topic Text	HCAHPS Answer Description
How often did nurses communicate well with patients?	*Nurses always communicated well*
	Nurses usually communicated well
	Nurses sometimes or never communicated well
How often did patients receive help quickly from hospital staff?	*Patients always received help as soon as they wanted*
	Patients usually received help as soon as they wanted
	Patients sometimes or never received help as soon as they wanted
How often did staff explain about medicines before giving them to patients?	*Staff always explained*
	Staff usually explained
	Staff sometimes or never explained
How often was patients' pain well controlled?	*Pain was always well controlled*
	Pain was usually well controlled
	Pain was sometimes or never well controlled
How often was the area around patients' rooms kept quiet at night?	*Always quiet at night*
	Usually quiet at night
	Sometimes or never quiet at night
How often were the patients' rooms and bathrooms kept clean?	*Room was always clean*
	Room was usually clean
	Room was sometimes or never clean
Were patients given information about what to do during their recovery at home?	*YES, staff did give patients this information*
	NO, staff did not give patients this information
Would patients recommend the hospital to friends and family?	*YES, patients would definitely recommend the hospital*
	YES, patients would probably recommend the hospital
	NO, patients would not recommend the hospital (they probably would not or definitely would not recommend it)

Note: Answers in italics are measures included in this book.

How many patients were surveyed for each hospital and how were they selected?

The goal is for each hospital to get at least 300 completed patient surveys per year. In general, the more patients that respond to a hospital's survey, the more the results shown on this website will reflect the experiences of all the patients who used that hospital. Patients are randomly selected to participate in the HCAHPS survey. Hospitals are not allowed to choose which patients are selected.

Which hospitals participate in the HCAHPS survey?

All short-term, acute care, non-specialty hospitals are invited to participate in the HCAHPS survey. Most hospitals choose to participate. Hospitals that treat only certain types of patients or medical problems, called specialty hospitals, are not included in the HCAHPS survey. Examples include psychiatric hospitals or children's hospitals. Children's hospitals are not included because the HCAHPS survey asks about adult care only.

How is HCAHPS survey data collected?

HCAHPS survey data must be collected by organizations that are trained by the Federal government in HCAHPS survey data collection procedures. Hospitals can choose to conduct the survey in one of four ways: by mail, by telephone, by mail and telephone, or by active interactive voice recognition (IVR). Regardless of how the survey is conducted, all patients answer the same questions. Patients complete the HCAHPS survey after they leave the hospital.

Confidence Intervals

The table below enables the user to calculate confidence intervals for each reported measure.

Confidence intervals can be used to estimate the precision of the calculated rates for an individual hospital. A confidence interval is the range of values, within which an estimated value or rate is likely to fall. A confidence interval is a statistical determination of the degree of certainty associated with an estimated value. As can be seen in the table of estimated values (below), large differences between individual hospitals' rates may be significant, and small differences between hospitals are usually not significant.

The smaller the sample size, the greater the difference in rates must be order for that difference to be statistically meaning-ful. Also, as sample size varies between hospitals, it is difficult to precisely compare their rates, without considering the confidence intervals.

Over time, as the quality data base is expanded, a full four quarters of data will ultimately be available, so the number of cases used to determine hospitals' rates will likely increase, thereby increasing the reliability and stability of the rates.

Estimating Confidence Intervals for the Quality Measures: Estimated Values for Proportion Data

Sample Size	Observed Rate								
	10%	20%	30%	40%	50%	60%	70%	80%	90%
< 25	*	*	24.9	26.6	27.2	26.6	24.9	*	*
25 - 75	8.3	11.1	12.7	13.6	13.9	13.6	12.7	11.1	8.3
76 - 125	5.9	7.8	9.0	9.6	9.8	9.6	9.0	7.8	5.9
126 - 175	4.8	6.4	7.3	7.8	8.0	7.8	7.3	6.4	4.8
176 - 225	4.2	5.5	6.4	6.8	6.9	6.8	6.4	5.5	4.2
226 -275	3.7	5.0	5.7	6.1	6.2	6.1	5.7	5.0	3.7
276+	2.9	3.9	4.5	4.8	4.9	4.8	4.5	3.9	2.9

*Source: CMS/OCSQ/QIG. The values in the table are the approximate amount to add and subtract from the observed rate to estimate a 95 percent confidence interval for the given sample size. (Interpolation between the values in the table is appropriate.) * Estimates of an interval in these cells exceed the natural limits for proportions.*

Data Sources

The statistical information in this book comes from data downloaded from www.hospitalcompare.hhs.gov, a website tool developed by the Centers for Medicare & Medicaid Services (CMS). Process of Care (Heart Attack, Chest Pain/Possible Heart Attack, Heart Failure, Pneumonia, Surgical Care Improvment Project, Children's Asthma) and HCAHPS measures cover data collected April 2009 through March 2010. Use of Medical Imaging measures cover January 2008 through December 2008. Outcome of Care measures (Mortality and Readmission Rates) covers July 2006 through June 2009. *Source: www.hospitalcompare.hhs.gov, Centers for Medicare & Medicaid Services (CMS), an agency of the U.S. Department of Health and Human Services (DHHS) along with the Hospital Quality Alliance (HQA).*

Key personnel, fax numbers, e-mail addresses, URLs, and number of beds come from *Directory of Hospital Personnel, 2011,* Grey House Publishing.

Heart Attack Care

1. ACE Inhibitor or ARB for LVSD

Hospital Name	City	Rate	Cases
Hospital of St Raphael	New Haven	100%	55
Saint Marys Hospital	Waterbury	100%	31
Hartford Hospital	Hartford	98%	140
Yale-New Haven Hospital[2]	New Haven	97%	29
Saint Vincent's Medical Center	Bridgeport	96%	74
Middlesex Hospital	Middletown	94%	31
Saint Francis Hospital & Medical Center	Hartford	93%	112
Stamford Hospital	Stamford	92%	39
Waterbury Hospital	Waterbury	91%	34
Bridgeport Hospital[2]	Bridgeport	88%	60
The Hospital of Central Connecticut	New Britain	88%	41
Danbury Hospital	Danbury	85%	66

2. Aspirin at Arrival

Hospital Name	City	Rate	Cases
Bristol Hospital	Bristol	100%	35
Charlotte Hungerford Hospital	Torrington	100%	47
John Dempsey Hospital	Farmington	100%	116
Manchester Memorial Hospital	Manchester	100%	44
Middlesex Hospital	Middletown	100%	59
Milford Hospital	Milford	100%	34
Rockville General Hospital	Rockville	100%	26
Saint Marys Hospital	Waterbury	100%	168
Waterbury Hospital	Waterbury	100%	227
Yale-New Haven Hospital[2]	New Haven	100%	127
Bridgeport Hospital[2]	Bridgeport	99%	225
Danbury Hospital	Danbury	99%	303
Greenwich Hospital Association[2]	Greenwich	99%	74
Griffin Hospital	Derby	99%	92
Hartford Hospital	Hartford	99%	337
Norwalk Hospital Association	Norwalk	99%	161
Saint Francis Hospital & Medical Center	Hartford	99%	317
Saint Vincent's Medical Center	Bridgeport	99%	261
Hospital of St Raphael	New Haven	98%	227
Lawrence & Memorial Hospital[2]	New London	98%	133
Midstate Medical Center	Meriden	98%	56
Stamford Hospital	Stamford	98%	195
The Hospital of Central Connecticut	New Britain	97%	247
William W Backus Hospital	Norwich	97%	61
Windham Hospital	Willimantic	96%	27
Day Kimball Hospital	Putnam	94%	33

3. Aspirin at Discharge

Hospital Name	City	Rate	Cases
Charlotte Hungerford Hospital	Torrington	100%	36
Greenwich Hospital Association[2]	Greenwich	100%	49
Middlesex Hospital	Middletown	100%	70
Norwalk Hospital Association	Norwalk	100%	94
Saint Marys Hospital	Waterbury	100%	164
Waterbury Hospital	Waterbury	100%	219
Danbury Hospital	Danbury	99%	356
Hartford Hospital	Hartford	99%	788
Hospital of St Raphael	New Haven	99%	351
John Dempsey Hospital	Farmington	99%	134
Lawrence & Memorial Hospital[2]	New London	99%	117
Saint Francis Hospital & Medical Center	Hartford	99%	546
Saint Vincent's Medical Center	Bridgeport	99%	309
Yale-New Haven Hospital[2]	New Haven	99%	282
Stamford Hospital	Stamford	98%	180
Manchester Memorial Hospital	Manchester	97%	31
Midstate Medical Center	Meriden	97%	38
Bridgeport Hospital[2]	Bridgeport	96%	253
Griffin Hospital	Derby	96%	53
The Hospital of Central Connecticut	New Britain	93%	175
William W Backus Hospital	Norwich	92%	39

4. Beta Blocker at Discharge

Hospital Name	City	Rate	Cases
Charlotte Hungerford Hospital	Torrington	100%	38
Greenwich Hospital Association[2]	Greenwich	100%	49
Griffin Hospital	Derby	100%	51
Lawrence & Memorial Hospital[2]	New London	100%	109
Manchester Memorial Hospital	Manchester	100%	31
Middlesex Hospital	Middletown	100%	77
Saint Marys Hospital	Waterbury	100%	155
Waterbury Hospital	Waterbury	100%	215
William W Backus Hospital	Norwich	100%	37
Hartford Hospital	Hartford	99%	781
Hospital of St Raphael	New Haven	99%	334
John Dempsey Hospital	Farmington	99%	138
Norwalk Hospital Association	Norwalk	99%	98
Danbury Hospital	Danbury	98%	333
The Hospital of Central Connecticut	New Britain	98%	185
Saint Francis Hospital & Medical Center	Hartford	98%	527
Saint Vincent's Medical Center	Bridgeport	98%	307
Stamford Hospital	Stamford	98%	179
Yale-New Haven Hospital[2]	New Haven	98%	264
Midstate Medical Center	Meriden	97%	35
Bridgeport Hospital[2]	Bridgeport	95%	258

6. PCI Within 90 Minutes of Arrival

Hospital Name	City	Rate	Cases
Saint Marys Hospital	Waterbury	98%	42
The Hospital of Central Connecticut	New Britain	97%	39
Saint Francis Hospital & Medical Center	Hartford	96%	73
Norwalk Hospital Association	Norwalk	94%	33
Danbury Hospital	Danbury	91%	56
Waterbury Hospital	Waterbury	89%	38
Saint Vincent's Medical Center	Bridgeport	88%	59
Hartford Hospital	Hartford	84%	56
Lawrence & Memorial Hospital[2]	New London	84%	31
Stamford Hospital	Stamford	81%	27
Hospital of St Raphael	New Haven	60%	53

7. Smoking Cessation Advice

Hospital Name	City	Rate	Cases
Bridgeport Hospital[2]	Bridgeport	100%	46
Danbury Hospital	Danbury	100%	82
Hartford Hospital	Hartford	100%	219
The Hospital of Central Connecticut	New Britain	100%	52
Hospital of St Raphael	New Haven	100%	93
John Dempsey Hospital	Farmington	100%	26
Lawrence & Memorial Hospital[2]	New London	100%	39
Norwalk Hospital Association	Norwalk	100%	26
Saint Francis Hospital & Medical Center	Hartford	100%	166
Stamford Hospital	Stamford	100%	36
Waterbury Hospital	Waterbury	100%	64
Yale-New Haven Hospital[2]	New Haven	100%	82
Saint Vincent's Medical Center	Bridgeport	98%	61
Saint Marys Hospital	Waterbury	96%	54

Chest Pain/Possible Heart Attack Care

8. Aspirin at Arrival

Hospital Name	City	Rate	Cases
Griffin Hospital	Derby	100%	47
Lawrence & Memorial Hospital	New London	100%	26
Windham Hospital	Willimantic	100%	46
Middlesex Hospital	Middletown	99%	311
William W Backus Hospital	Norwich	99%	220
New Milford Hospital	New Milford	98%	42
Sharon Hospital	Sharon	98%	40
Johnson Memorial Hospital	Stafford Springs	97%	65
Midstate Medical Center	Meriden	97%	123
Bristol Hospital	Bristol	96%	57
Charlotte Hungerford Hospital	Torrington	96%	118
Day Kimball Hospital	Putnam	96%	115
Manchester Memorial Hospital	Manchester	96%	50
The Hospital of Central Connecticut	New Britain	95%	40
Rockville General Hospital	Rockville	88%	40

9. Median Time to ECG (minutes)

Hospital Name	City	Min.	Cases
Rockville General Hospital	Rockville	5	42
William W Backus Hospital	Norwich	5	224
Midstate Medical Center	Meriden	6	120
Day Kimball Hospital	Putnam	8	120
Lawrence & Memorial Hospital	New London	8	28
Sharon Hospital	Sharon	8	43
Bristol Hospital	Bristol	9	57
Griffin Hospital	Derby	9	47
Middlesex Hospital	Middletown	9	321
New Milford Hospital	New Milford	10	41
Windham Hospital	Willimantic	10	48
The Hospital of Central Connecticut	New Britain	11	41
Charlotte Hungerford Hospital	Torrington	12	118
Johnson Memorial Hospital	Stafford Springs	12	68
Manchester Memorial Hospital	Manchester	14	50

10. Median Time to Transfer (minutes)

Hospital Name	City	Min.	Cases
Griffin Hospital	Derby	56	26
Bristol Hospital	Bristol	57	25
Middlesex Hospital	Middletown	76	43
William W Backus Hospital	Norwich	86	52

Heart Failure Care

12. ACE Inhibitor or ARB for LVSD

Hospital Name	City	Rate	Cases
Bristol Hospital	Bristol	100%	58
Saint Marys Hospital	Waterbury	100%	83
West Haven VA Medical Center	West Haven	100%	43
Griffin Hospital	Derby	98%	42
John Dempsey Hospital	Farmington	98%	64
Manchester Memorial Hospital	Manchester	98%	42
Middlesex Hospital	Middletown	97%	126
Milford Hospital	Milford	97%	37
Day Kimball Hospital	Putnam	96%	47
Norwalk Hospital Association[2]	Norwalk	96%	82
William W Backus Hospital	Norwich	96%	85
Danbury Hospital	Danbury	95%	131
Hartford Hospital	Hartford	94%	327
Hospital of St Raphael[2]	New Haven	94%	77
Saint Francis Hospital & Medical Center[2]	Hartford	94%	123
Stamford Hospital	Stamford	93%	149
Yale-New Haven Hospital[2]	New Haven	93%	84
Johnson Memorial Hospital	Stafford Springs	92%	26
Lawrence & Memorial Hospital[2]	New London	91%	53
Bridgeport Hospital[2]	Bridgeport	90%	84
Greenwich Hospital Association[2]	Greenwich	90%	83
Midstate Medical Center	Meriden	90%	61
Saint Vincent's Medical Center	Bridgeport	90%	186
The Hospital of Central Connecticut	New Britain	89%	186
Charlotte Hungerford Hospital	Torrington	88%	32
Waterbury Hospital[2]	Waterbury	84%	93
Windham Hospital	Willimantic	79%	43

13. Discharge Instructions

Hospital Name	City	Rate	Cases
Saint Marys Hospital	Waterbury	100%	204
West Haven VA Medical Center	West Haven	100%	161
Griffin Hospital	Derby	99%	165
Johnson Memorial Hospital	Stafford Springs	99%	77
John Dempsey Hospital	Farmington	96%	156
Hospital of St Raphael[2]	New Haven	95%	228
Milford Hospital	Milford	93%	123
Saint Vincent's Medical Center	Bridgeport	92%	391
Greenwich Hospital Association[2]	Greenwich	91%	183
The Hospital of Central Connecticut	New Britain	91%	501
Middlesex Hospital	Middletown	91%	197
Charlotte Hungerford Hospital	Torrington	90%	73
Yale-New Haven Hospital[2]	New Haven	90%	223
Rockville General Hospital	Rockville	88%	58
Stamford Hospital	Stamford	88%	216
Manchester Memorial Hospital	Manchester	87%	140
Hartford Hospital	Hartford	85%	656
William W Backus Hospital	Norwich	84%	226
New Milford Hospital	New Milford	83%	41
Bridgeport Hospital[2]	Bridgeport	82%	195
Day Kimball Hospital	Putnam	81%	78
Danbury Hospital	Danbury	80%	346
Windham Hospital	Willimantic	80%	91
Lawrence & Memorial Hospital[2]	New London	79%	194
Waterbury Hospital[2]	Waterbury	77%	203
Bristol Hospital	Bristol	76%	125
Midstate Medical Center	Meriden	72%	166
Norwalk Hospital Association[2]	Norwalk	72%	220
Saint Francis Hospital & Medical Center[2]	Hartford	64%	225

14. Evaluation of LVS Function

Hospital Name	City	Rate	Cases
Bridgeport Hospital[2]	Bridgeport	100%	291
Danbury Hospital	Danbury	100%	516
Griffin Hospital	Derby	100%	257
Hartford Hospital	Hartford	100%	925
The Hospital of Central Connecticut	New Britain	100%	689
John Dempsey Hospital	Farmington	100%	218
Manchester Memorial Hospital	Manchester	100%	195
Middlesex Hospital	Middletown	100%	329
Norwalk Hospital Association[2]	Norwalk	100%	330
Rockville General Hospital	Rockville	100%	93
Saint Francis Hospital & Medical Center[2]	Hartford	100%	317
Saint Marys Hospital	Waterbury	100%	301
William W Backus Hospital	Norwich	100%	305
Windham Hospital	Willimantic	100%	138
Yale-New Haven Hospital[2]	New Haven	100%	287
Milford Hospital	Milford	99%	187
New Milford Hospital	New Milford	99%	75
Saint Vincent's Medical Center	Bridgeport	99%	577
West Haven VA Medical Center	West Haven	99%	184
Charlotte Hungerford Hospital	Torrington	98%	129
Greenwich Hospital Association[2]	Greenwich	98%	256
Hospital of St Raphael[2]	New Haven	98%	333
Stamford Hospital	Stamford	98%	328
Waterbury Hospital[2]	Waterbury	98%	321
Bristol Hospital	Bristol	97%	187
Day Kimball Hospital	Putnam	97%	114
Johnson Memorial Hospital	Stafford Springs	97%	120
Lawrence & Memorial Hospital[2]	New London	97%	287
Midstate Medical Center	Meriden	96%	245

NOTE: Hospital profiles are in alphabetical order by state, then city, then hospital within the city; Rankings exclude hospitals with less than 25 cases except for patient surveys which excludes hospitals with less than 100 cases; (a) 100–299 cases; (1) The number of cases is too small to be sure how well a hospital is performing; (2) The hospital indicated that the data submitted for this measure were based on a sample of cases; (3) Data was collected during a shorter time period (fewer quarters) than the maximum possible time for this measure; (4) Suppressed for one or more quarters by CMS; (5) No data is available from the hospital for this measure; (6) Fewer than 100 patients completed the HCAHPS survey. Use these rates with caution, as the number of surveys may be too low to reliably assess hospital performance; (7) Survey results are based on less than 12 months of data; (8) Survey results are not available for this reporting period; (9) No or very few patients were eligible for the HCAHPS survey. The scores shown, if any, reflect a very small number of surveys; (10) A state average was not calculated because too few hospitals in the state submitted data; (11) There were discrepancies in the data collection process; Please refer to the User's Guide for a full explanation of data.

Hospital Name	City	Rate	Cases
Sharon Hospital	Sharon	95%	43
Masonic Home and Hospital	Wallingford	80%	40

15. Smoking Cessation Advice

Hospital Name	City	Rate	Cases
Bridgeport Hospital[2]	Bridgeport	100%	41
Hartford Hospital	Hartford	100%	117
The Hospital of Central Connecticut	New Britain	100%	117
Hospital of St Raphael[2]	New Haven	100%	42
Lawrence & Memorial Hospital[2]	New London	100%	28
Saint Francis Hospital & Medical Center[2]	Hartford	100%	37
Saint Marys Hospital	Waterbury	100%	27
Saint Vincent's Medical Center	Bridgeport	100%	57
Stamford Hospital	Stamford	100%	33
Waterbury Hospital[2]	Waterbury	100%	48
West Haven VA Medical Center	West Haven	100%	25
William W Backus Hospital	Norwich	100%	57
Yale-New Haven Hospital[2]	New Haven	100%	48
Middlesex Hospital	Middletown	97%	31
Midstate Medical Center	Meriden	97%	30
Norwalk Hospital Association[2]	Norwalk	97%	37
Danbury Hospital	Danbury	90%	39

Pneumonia Care

16. Appropriate Initial Antibiotic

Hospital Name	City	Rate	Cases
Griffin Hospital	Derby	98%	80
The Hospital of Central Connecticut	New Britain	98%	290
Norwalk Hospital Association[2]	Norwalk	98%	100
Bristol Hospital	Bristol	97%	118
Danbury Hospital	Danbury	97%	266
Day Kimball Hospital	Putnam	97%	86
Middlesex Hospital	Middletown	96%	130
Milford Hospital	Milford	96%	95
Saint Vincent's Medical Center	Bridgeport	96%	180
Hartford Hospital	Hartford	95%	185
Hospital of St Raphael[2]	New Haven	95%	106
Johnson Memorial Hospital	Stafford Springs	95%	74
Windham Hospital	Willimantic	95%	80
New Milford Hospital	New Milford	93%	44
West Haven VA Medical Center	West Haven	93%	46
John Dempsey Hospital[2]	Farmington	92%	76
Manchester Memorial Hospital[2]	Manchester	92%	133
Midstate Medical Center[2]	Meriden	92%	127
Saint Francis Hospital & Medical Center[2]	Hartford	92%	71
Stamford Hospital	Stamford	92%	136
William W Backus Hospital[2]	Norwich	92%	99
Bridgeport Hospital[2]	Bridgeport	91%	67
Charlotte Hungerford Hospital	Torrington	90%	68
Greenwich Hospital Association[2]	Greenwich	90%	72
Saint Marys Hospital[2]	Waterbury	90%	111
Sharon Hospital	Sharon	87%	45
Waterbury Hospital[2]	Waterbury	86%	88
Rockville General Hospital	Rockville	84%	74
Lawrence & Memorial Hospital[2]	New London	81%	73
Yale-New Haven Hospital[2]	New Haven	75%	36

17. Blood Culture Timing

Hospital Name	City	Rate	Cases
Middlesex Hospital	Middletown	100%	215
Norwalk Hospital Association[2]	Norwalk	100%	156
Stamford Hospital	Stamford	100%	208
The Hospital of Central Connecticut	New Britain	99%	518
Rockville General Hospital	Rockville	99%	128
Charlotte Hungerford Hospital	Torrington	98%	101
Griffin Hospital	Derby	98%	164
Manchester Memorial Hospital[2]	Manchester	98%	233
Saint Vincent's Medical Center	Bridgeport	98%	325
West Haven VA Medical Center	West Haven	98%	90
Windham Hospital	Willimantic	98%	131
Johnson Memorial Hospital	Stafford Springs	97%	142
Bridgeport Hospital[2]	Bridgeport	96%	106
Day Kimball Hospital	Putnam	96%	155
Hartford Hospital	Hartford	96%	397
Midstate Medical Center[2]	Meriden	96%	197
Sharon Hospital	Sharon	96%	77
Danbury Hospital	Danbury	95%	373
Lawrence & Memorial Hospital[2]	New London	95%	123
Saint Marys Hospital[2]	Waterbury	95%	175
Milford Hospital	Milford	94%	179
Saint Francis Hospital & Medical Center[2]	Hartford	94%	210
Waterbury Hospital[2]	Waterbury	94%	199
Greenwich Hospital Association[2]	Greenwich	93%	151
Yale-New Haven Hospital[2]	New Haven	93%	85
New Milford Hospital	New Milford	92%	53
William W Backus Hospital[2]	Norwich	92%	161
Hospital of St Raphael[2]	New Haven	91%	163
John Dempsey Hospital[2]	Farmington	89%	151
Bristol Hospital	Bristol	87%	236

18. Influenza Vaccine

Hospital Name	City	Rate	Cases
Hartford Hospital	Hartford	100%	255
Sharon Hospital	Sharon	100%	39
John Dempsey Hospital[2]	Farmington	99%	77
Charlotte Hungerford Hospital	Torrington	97%	117
Saint Marys Hospital[2]	Waterbury	97%	72
Bristol Hospital	Bristol	96%	142
The Hospital of Central Connecticut	New Britain	96%	318
Johnson Memorial Hospital	Stafford Springs	96%	77
Manchester Memorial Hospital[2]	Manchester	96%	150
Rockville General Hospital	Rockville	96%	92
Griffin Hospital	Derby	95%	91
Middlesex Hospital	Middletown	95%	210
Milford Hospital	Milford	95%	106
West Haven VA Medical Center	West Haven	95%	65
Lawrence & Memorial Hospital[2]	New London	93%	82
Midstate Medical Center[2]	Meriden	92%	120
Stamford Hospital	Stamford	92%	133
Danbury Hospital	Danbury	89%	338
Saint Francis Hospital & Medical Center[2]	Hartford	87%	109
Windham Hospital	Willimantic	87%	68
Saint Vincent's Medical Center	Bridgeport	86%	198
Greenwich Hospital Association[2]	Greenwich	85%	91
Hospital of St Raphael[2]	New Haven	85%	118
Norwalk Hospital Association[2]	Norwalk	85%	96
Bridgeport Hospital[2]	Bridgeport	81%	81
William W Backus Hospital[2]	Norwich	81%	120
Day Kimball Hospital	Putnam	79%	76
Waterbury Hospital[2]	Waterbury	79%	117
New Milford Hospital	New Milford	77%	35
Yale-New Haven Hospital[2]	New Haven	67%	73

19. Initial Antibiotic Timing

Hospital Name	City	Rate	Cases
Bristol Hospital	Bristol	100%	225
New Milford Hospital	New Milford	100%	57
Sharon Hospital	Sharon	100%	79
Windham Hospital	Willimantic	100%	126
Griffin Hospital	Derby	99%	165
The Hospital of Central Connecticut	New Britain	99%	442
Rockville General Hospital	Rockville	99%	106
Saint Vincent's Medical Center	Bridgeport	99%	317
Danbury Hospital	Danbury	98%	444
Greenwich Hospital Association[2]	Greenwich	98%	120
Manchester Memorial Hospital[2]	Manchester	98%	201
John Dempsey Hospital[2]	Farmington	97%	130
Milford Hospital	Milford	97%	151
William W Backus Hospital[2]	Norwich	97%	195
Day Kimball Hospital	Putnam	96%	155
Middlesex Hospital	Middletown	96%	223
Norwalk Hospital Association[2]	Norwalk	96%	182
Stamford Hospital	Stamford	96%	196
Charlotte Hungerford Hospital	Torrington	95%	123
Hartford Hospital	Hartford	95%	349
Hospital of St Raphael[2]	New Haven	95%	205
Yale-New Haven Hospital[2]	New Haven	95%	86
Johnson Memorial Hospital	Stafford Springs	94%	108
Lawrence & Memorial Hospital[2]	New London	94%	122
Waterbury Hospital[2]	Waterbury	93%	198
Midstate Medical Center[2]	Meriden	90%	204
Saint Francis Hospital & Medical Center[2]	Hartford	90%	176
Saint Marys Hospital[2]	Waterbury	87%	169
Bridgeport Hospital[2]	Bridgeport	85%	102
West Haven VA Medical Center	West Haven	77%	74

20. Pneumococcal Vaccine

Hospital Name	City	Rate	Cases
Sharon Hospital	Sharon	100%	68
John Dempsey Hospital[2]	Farmington	99%	132
Manchester Memorial Hospital[2]	Manchester	99%	230
Middlesex Hospital	Middletown	99%	352
West Haven VA Medical Center	West Haven	99%	97
Griffin Hospital	Derby	98%	180
Hartford Hospital	Hartford	98%	384
The Hospital of Central Connecticut	New Britain	98%	405
Johnson Memorial Hospital	Stafford Springs	98%	125
Milford Hospital	Milford	98%	175
Rockville General Hospital	Rockville	97%	117
Bristol Hospital	Bristol	96%	196
Charlotte Hungerford Hospital	Torrington	96%	169
Saint Vincent's Medical Center	Bridgeport	96%	292
Stamford Hospital	Stamford	96%	195
Hospital of St Raphael[2]	New Haven	94%	221
Masonic Home and Hospital	Wallingford	94%	48
Saint Francis Hospital & Medical Center[2]	Hartford	94%	181
Lawrence & Memorial Hospital[2]	New London	93%	133
Greenwich Hospital Association[2]	Greenwich	91%	159
Bridgeport Hospital[2]	Bridgeport	90%	123
Midstate Medical Center[2]	Meriden	90%	199
Waterbury Hospital[2]	Waterbury	90%	195
Danbury Hospital	Danbury	88%	496
Day Kimball Hospital	Putnam	88%	121
Norwalk Hospital Association[2]	Norwalk	88%	208
Windham Hospital	Willimantic	88%	97
William W Backus Hospital[2]	Norwich	87%	181
Saint Marys Hospital[2]	Waterbury	83%	144
New Milford Hospital	New Milford	81%	57
Yale-New Haven Hospital[2]	New Haven	74%	114

21. Smoking Cessation Advice

Hospital Name	City	Rate	Cases
Bridgeport Hospital[2]	Bridgeport	100%	31
Charlotte Hungerford Hospital	Torrington	100%	44
Day Kimball Hospital	Putnam	100%	35
Griffin Hospital	Derby	100%	41
Hartford Hospital	Hartford	100%	130
The Hospital of Central Connecticut	New Britain	100%	153
Hospital of St Raphael[2]	New Haven	100%	48
Johnson Memorial Hospital	Stafford Springs	100%	39
Lawrence & Memorial Hospital[2]	New London	100%	52
Manchester Memorial Hospital[2]	Manchester	100%	63
Norwalk Hospital Association[2]	Norwalk	100%	49
Rockville General Hospital	Rockville	100%	43
Saint Francis Hospital & Medical Center[2]	Hartford	100%	61
Stamford Hospital	Stamford	100%	48
Waterbury Hospital[2]	Waterbury	100%	79
West Haven VA Medical Center	West Haven	100%	33
William W Backus Hospital[2]	Norwich	100%	83
Windham Hospital	Willimantic	100%	41
Yale-New Haven Hospital[2]	New Haven	100%	47
Middlesex Hospital	Middletown	99%	102
Saint Vincent's Medical Center	Bridgeport	99%	82
Bristol Hospital	Bristol	97%	65
Milford Hospital	Milford	97%	37
Saint Marys Hospital[2]	Waterbury	97%	39
Midstate Medical Center[2]	Meriden	93%	55
Danbury Hospital	Danbury	89%	82

Surgical Care Improvement Project

22. Appropriate VTP Within 24 Hours

Hospital Name	City	Rate	Cases
John Dempsey Hospital[2]	Farmington	100%	85
West Haven VA Medical Center[2]	West Haven	100%	142
Windham Hospital	Willimantic	100%	88
Midstate Medical Center[2]	Meriden	99%	212
New Milford Hospital[2]	New Milford	99%	76
Stamford Hospital[2]	Stamford	99%	152
Bristol Hospital	Bristol	98%	144
Griffin Hospital	Derby	98%	130
The Hospital of Central Connecticut[2]	New Britain	98%	355
Saint Vincent's Medical Center[2]	Bridgeport	98%	149
Waterbury Hospital[2]	Waterbury	98%	155
Bridgeport Hospital[2]	Bridgeport	97%	117
Hartford Hospital[2]	Hartford	97%	175
Hospital of St Raphael[2]	New Haven	97%	178
Charlotte Hungerford Hospital[2]	Torrington	95%	101
Saint Francis Hospital & Medical Center[2]	Hartford	95%	180
Johnson Memorial Hospital	Stafford Springs	94%	96
Manchester Memorial Hospital[2]	Manchester	94%	234
Middlesex Hospital	Middletown	94%	431
Norwalk Hospital Association	Norwalk	94%	341
Saint Marys Hospital[2]	Waterbury	94%	173
Yale-New Haven Hospital[2]	New Haven	93%	180
Lawrence & Memorial Hospital[2]	New London	92%	156
William W Backus Hospital[2]	Norwich	92%	219
Day Kimball Hospital	Putnam	90%	99
Milford Hospital[2]	Milford	89%	114
Rockville General Hospital	Rockville	89%	72
Greenwich Hospital Association[2]	Greenwich	88%	137
Danbury Hospital[2]	Danbury	85%	188
Sharon Hospital	Sharon	85%	52

23. Appropriate Hair Removal

Hospital Name	City	Rate	Cases
Charlotte Hungerford Hospital[2]	Torrington	100%	312
Danbury Hospital[2]	Danbury	100%	794
Day Kimball Hospital	Putnam	100%	328
Greenwich Hospital Association[2]	Greenwich	100%	295
Griffin Hospital	Derby	100%	286
Hartford Hospital[2]	Hartford	100%	759
The Hospital of Central Connecticut[2]	New Britain	100%	975
Hospital of St Raphael[2]	New Haven	100%	888
John Dempsey Hospital[2]	Farmington	100%	302
Manchester Memorial Hospital[2]	Manchester	100%	507

NOTE: Hospital profiles are in alphabetical order by state, then city, then hospital within the city; Rankings exclude hospitals with less than 25 cases except for patient surveys which excludes hospitals with less than 100 cases; (a) 100–299 cases; (1) The number of cases is too small to be sure how well a hospital is performing; (2) The hospital indicated that the data submitted for this measure were based on a sample of cases; (3) Data was collected during a shorter time period (fewer quarters) than the maximum possible time for this measure; (4) Suppressed for one or more quarters by CMS; (5) No data is available from the hospital for this measure; (6) Fewer than 100 patients completed the HCAHPS survey. Use these rates with caution, as the number of surveys may be too low to reliably assess hospital performance; (7) Survey results are based on less than 12 months of data; (8) Survey results are not available for this reporting period; (9) No or very few patients were eligible for the HCAHPS survey. The scores shown, if any, reflect a very small number of surveys; (10) A state average was not calculated because too few hospitals in the state submitted data; (11) There were discrepancies in the data collection process; Please refer to the User's Guide for a full explanation of data.

Middlesex Hospital	Middletown	100%	1160
Milford Hospital[2]	Milford	100%	449
New Milford Hospital[2]	New Milford	100%	252
Norwalk Hospital Association	Norwalk	100%	765
Rockville General Hospital	Rockville	100%	210
Saint Vincent's Medical Center[2]	Bridgeport	100%	520
Sharon Hospital	Sharon	100%	138
Stamford Hospital[2]	Stamford	100%	439
Waterbury Hospital[2]	Waterbury	100%	635
West Haven VA Medical Center[2]	West Haven	100%	288
Bristol Hospital	Bristol	99%	351
Lawrence & Memorial Hospital[2]	New London	99%	426
Midstate Medical Center[2]	Meriden	99%	601
Saint Francis Hospital & Medical Center[2]	Hartford	99%	850
William W Backus Hospital[2]	Norwich	99%	481
Windham Hospital	Willimantic	99%	155
Yale-New Haven Hospital[2]	New Haven	99%	608
Bridgeport Hospital[2]	Bridgeport	98%	468
Saint Marys Hospital[2]	Waterbury	98%	615
Johnson Memorial Hospital	Stafford Springs	97%	182

24. Appropriate Beta Blocker Usage

Hospital Name	City	Rate	Cases
Bristol Hospital	Bristol	100%	74
John Dempsey Hospital[2]	Farmington	100%	83
New Milford Hospital[2]	New Milford	100%	73
Sharon Hospital	Sharon	100%	30
West Haven VA Medical Center[2]	West Haven	100%	165
Danbury Hospital[2]	Danbury	97%	301
The Hospital of Central Connecticut[2]	New Britain	97%	322
Manchester Memorial Hospital[2]	Manchester	97%	153
Milford Hospital[2]	Milford	97%	125
Johnson Memorial Hospital	Stafford Springs	96%	48
Saint Marys Hospital[2]	Waterbury	95%	193
Saint Vincent's Medical Center[2]	Bridgeport	95%	184
Stamford Hospital[2]	Stamford	95%	130
Lawrence & Memorial Hospital[2]	New London	94%	150
Charlotte Hungerford Hospital[2]	Torrington	93%	104
Greenwich Hospital Association[2]	Greenwich	92%	97
Griffin Hospital	Derby	92%	96
Hospital of St Raphael[2]	New Haven	92%	333
Middlesex Hospital	Middletown	92%	343
Saint Francis Hospital & Medical Center[2]	Hartford	92%	320
William W Backus Hospital[2]	Norwich	92%	143
Hartford Hospital[2]	Hartford	91%	263
Norwalk Hospital Association	Norwalk	91%	207
Bridgeport Hospital[2]	Bridgeport	90%	184
Day Kimball Hospital	Putnam	90%	100
Midstate Medical Center[2]	Meriden	90%	177
Waterbury Hospital[2]	Waterbury	90%	185
Rockville General Hospital	Rockville	89%	57
Yale-New Haven Hospital[2]	New Haven	87%	218
Windham Hospital	Willimantic	86%	49

25. Controlled Postoperative Blood Glucose

Hospital Name	City	Rate	Cases
Stamford Hospital[2]	Stamford	100%	36
West Haven VA Medical Center[2]	West Haven	98%	60
Saint Vincent's Medical Center[2]	Bridgeport	97%	125
Bridgeport Hospital[2]	Bridgeport	96%	76
Saint Marys Hospital[2]	Waterbury	96%	101
Danbury Hospital[2]	Danbury	95%	135
Hartford Hospital[2]	Hartford	92%	155
Yale-New Haven Hospital[2]	New Haven	90%	120
Saint Francis Hospital & Medical Center[2]	Hartford	89%	166
Hospital of St Raphael[2]	New Haven	85%	205
Waterbury Hospital[2]	Waterbury	83%	87

26. Prophylactic Antibiotic Timing

Hospital Name	City	Rate	Cases
Norwalk Hospital Association	Norwalk	99%	448
Rockville General Hospital	Rockville	99%	144
Stamford Hospital[2]	Stamford	99%	297
Windham Hospital	Willimantic	99%	90
Danbury Hospital[2]	Danbury	98%	563
Johnson Memorial Hospital	Stafford Springs	98%	115
Lawrence & Memorial Hospital[2]	New London	98%	301
Middlesex Hospital	Middletown	98%	700
Milford Hospital[2]	Milford	98%	298
Sharon Hospital	Sharon	98%	91
West Haven VA Medical Center	West Haven	98%	189
Bridgeport Hospital[2]	Bridgeport	97%	303
Bristol Hospital	Bristol	97%	189
Griffin Hospital	Derby	97%	166
Manchester Memorial Hospital[2]	Manchester	97%	301
New Milford Hospital[2]	New Milford	97%	187
Saint Francis Hospital & Medical Center[2]	Hartford	97%	603
Saint Vincent's Medical Center[2]	Bridgeport	97%	357
Greenwich Hospital Association[2]	Greenwich	96%	228
Hospital of St Raphael[2]	New Haven	96%	668
John Dempsey Hospital[2]	Farmington	96%	196
Midstate Medical Center[2]	Meriden	96%	402
Yale-New Haven Hospital[2]	New Haven	96%	389
Day Kimball Hospital	Putnam	95%	258
Hartford Hospital[2]	Hartford	95%	451
The Hospital of Central Connecticut[2]	New Britain	95%	723
Waterbury Hospital[2]	Waterbury	94%	449
Saint Marys Hospital[2]	Waterbury	93%	437
William W Backus Hospital[2]	Norwich	92%	323
Charlotte Hungerford Hospital[2]	Torrington	91%	199

27. Prophylactic Antibiotic Timing (Outpatient)

Hospital Name	City	Rate	Cases
Bristol Hospital	Bristol	100%	114
John Dempsey Hospital	Farmington	99%	202
Greenwich Hospital Association	Greenwich	96%	349
Johnson Memorial Hospital	Stafford Springs	96%	113
Lawrence & Memorial Hospital	New London	96%	211
Norwalk Hospital Association	Norwalk	96%	247
Rockville General Hospital	Rockville	96%	97
Stamford Hospital	Stamford	96%	428
Manchester Memorial Hospital	Manchester	95%	184
Milford Hospital	Milford	95%	39
Griffin Hospital	Derby	94%	64
Saint Francis Hospital & Medical Center	Hartford	94%	756
Danbury Hospital	Danbury	92%	577
Hartford Hospital	Hartford	92%	610
Middlesex Hospital	Middletown	92%	164
William W Backus Hospital	Norwich	92%	291
New Milford Hospital	New Milford	91%	77
Saint Vincent's Medical Center	Bridgeport	91%	229
Waterbury Hospital	Waterbury	91%	140
Day Kimball Hospital	Putnam	90%	110
Windham Hospital	Willimantic	90%	63
Hospital of St Raphael	New Haven	89%	510
Midstate Medical Center	Meriden	89%	158
Charlotte Hungerford Hospital	Torrington	88%	160
Yale-New Haven Hospital	New Haven	87%	514
Bridgeport Hospital	Bridgeport	85%	467
The Hospital of Central Connecticut	New Britain	82%	236
Saint Marys Hospital	Waterbury	77%	123

28. Prophylactic Antibiotic Selection

Hospital Name	City	Rate	Cases
Milford Hospital[2]	Milford	100%	300
Rockville General Hospital	Rockville	100%	145
Bridgeport Hospital[2]	Bridgeport	99%	307
Stamford Hospital[2]	Stamford	99%	302
West Haven VA Medical Center	West Haven	99%	203
Danbury Hospital[2]	Danbury	98%	564
Day Kimball Hospital	Putnam	98%	256
Greenwich Hospital Association[2]	Greenwich	98%	229
Norwalk Hospital Association	Norwalk	98%	450
Saint Francis Hospital & Medical Center[2]	Hartford	98%	616
Yale-New Haven Hospital[2]	New Haven	98%	395
Hartford Hospital[2]	Hartford	97%	464
The Hospital of Central Connecticut[2]	New Britain	97%	723
Lawrence & Memorial Hospital[2]	New London	97%	302
Middlesex Hospital	Middletown	97%	702
New Milford Hospital[2]	New Milford	97%	189
Saint Vincent's Medical Center[2]	Bridgeport	97%	364
Waterbury Hospital[2]	Waterbury	97%	450
William W Backus Hospital[2]	Norwich	97%	320
Windham Hospital	Willimantic	97%	90
Charlotte Hungerford Hospital[2]	Torrington	96%	199
Hospital of St Raphael[2]	New Haven	96%	675
John Dempsey Hospital[2]	Farmington	96%	199
Manchester Memorial Hospital[2]	Manchester	96%	304
Saint Marys Hospital[2]	Waterbury	96%	443
Bristol Hospital	Bristol	95%	187
Griffin Hospital	Derby	95%	172
Midstate Medical Center[2]	Meriden	95%	404
Sharon Hospital	Sharon	95%	91
Johnson Memorial Hospital	Stafford Springs	93%	114

29. Prophylactic Antibiotic Selection (Outpatient)

Hospital Name	City	Rate	Cases
Milford Hospital	Milford	100%	37
New Milford Hospital	New Milford	99%	70
Saint Francis Hospital & Medical Center	Hartford	99%	777
Hartford Hospital	Hartford	98%	604
Rockville General Hospital	Rockville	98%	94
Danbury Hospital	Danbury	97%	558
Greenwich Hospital Association	Greenwich	97%	347
Griffin Hospital	Derby	97%	73
Bristol Hospital	Bristol	96%	114
Lawrence & Memorial Hospital	New London	96%	205
Stamford Hospital	Stamford	96%	422
Charlotte Hungerford Hospital	Torrington	95%	151
Day Kimball Hospital	Putnam	94%	101
Middlesex Hospital	Middletown	94%	160
Waterbury Hospital	Waterbury	94%	137
Midstate Medical Center	Meriden	93%	157
Saint Marys Hospital	Waterbury	93%	104
William W Backus Hospital	Norwich	93%	290
The Hospital of Central Connecticut	New Britain	92%	201
Manchester Memorial Hospital	Manchester	92%	177
John Dempsey Hospital	Farmington	91%	200
Johnson Memorial Hospital	Stafford Springs	90%	110
Saint Vincent's Medical Center	Bridgeport	89%	211
Norwalk Hospital Association	Norwalk	88%	242
Bridgeport Hospital	Bridgeport	87%	427
Hospital of St Raphael	New Haven	84%	482
Windham Hospital	Willimantic	78%	58
Yale-New Haven Hospital	New Haven	65%	493

30. Prophylactic Antibiotic Stopped

Hospital Name	City	Rate	Cases
Rockville General Hospital	Rockville	99%	137
Windham Hospital	Willimantic	99%	85
John Dempsey Hospital[2]	Farmington	98%	189
Manchester Memorial Hospital[2]	Manchester	98%	283
Middlesex Hospital	Middletown	98%	683
Midstate Medical Center[2]	Meriden	98%	369
Stamford Hospital[2]	Stamford	98%	287
Bristol Hospital	Bristol	97%	180
Griffin Hospital	Derby	97%	148
The Hospital of Central Connecticut[2]	New Britain	97%	691
Hospital of St Raphael[2]	New Haven	97%	638
Norwalk Hospital Association	Norwalk	97%	412
Lawrence & Memorial Hospital[2]	New London	96%	296
New Milford Hospital[2]	New Milford	96%	185
Saint Francis Hospital & Medical Center[2]	Hartford	96%	587
William W Backus Hospital[2]	Norwich	96%	307
Yale-New Haven Hospital[2]	New Haven	96%	344
Danbury Hospital[2]	Danbury	95%	538
Milford Hospital[2]	Milford	95%	289
Sharon Hospital	Sharon	95%	87
Charlotte Hungerford Hospital[2]	Torrington	94%	190
Greenwich Hospital Association[2]	Greenwich	94%	214
Hartford Hospital[2]	Hartford	94%	437
Day Kimball Hospital	Putnam	93%	249
Johnson Memorial Hospital	Stafford Springs	93%	110
Saint Marys Hospital[2]	Waterbury	93%	431
Saint Vincent's Medical Center[2]	Bridgeport	92%	330
West Haven VA Medical Center	West Haven	92%	178
Bridgeport Hospital[2]	Bridgeport	91%	267
Waterbury Hospital[2]	Waterbury	91%	438

31. Recommended VTP Ordered

Hospital Name	City	Rate	Cases
John Dempsey Hospital[2]	Farmington	100%	85
West Haven VA Medical Center[2]	West Haven	100%	142
Windham Hospital	Willimantic	100%	88
Bristol Hospital	Bristol	99%	144
The Hospital of Central Connecticut[2]	New Britain	99%	355
New Milford Hospital[2]	New Milford	99%	76
Saint Vincent's Medical Center[2]	Bridgeport	99%	149
Waterbury Hospital[2]	Waterbury	99%	155
Griffin Hospital	Derby	98%	130
Hartford Hospital[2]	Hartford	98%	175
Manchester Memorial Hospital[2]	Manchester	98%	234
Midstate Medical Center[2]	Meriden	98%	214
Bridgeport Hospital[2]	Bridgeport	97%	117
Charlotte Hungerford Hospital[2]	Torrington	97%	101
Hospital of St Raphael[2]	New Haven	97%	178
Saint Francis Hospital & Medical Center[2]	Hartford	97%	180
Stamford Hospital[2]	Stamford	97%	154
Johnson Memorial Hospital	Stafford Springs	96%	96
Middlesex Hospital	Middletown	96%	431
Rockville General Hospital	Rockville	96%	72
William W Backus Hospital[2]	Norwich	96%	219
Lawrence & Memorial Hospital[2]	New London	94%	156
Norwalk Hospital Association	Norwalk	94%	341
Saint Marys Hospital[2]	Waterbury	94%	173
Yale-New Haven Hospital[2]	New Haven	94%	181
Day Kimball Hospital	Putnam	93%	100
Milford Hospital[2]	Milford	92%	114
Danbury Hospital[2]	Danbury	91%	188
Greenwich Hospital Association[2]	Greenwich	88%	138
Sharon Hospital	Sharon	87%	53

32. Urinary Catheter Removal

Hospital Name	City	Rate	Cases
Bristol Hospital	Bristol	100%	52
West Haven VA Medical Center[2]	West Haven	100%	118
Milford Hospital[2]	Milford	98%	149

NOTE: Hospital profiles are in alphabetical order by state, then city, then hospital within the city; Rankings exclude hospitals with less than 25 cases except for patient surveys which excludes hospitals with less than 100 cases; (a) 100–299 cases; (1) The number of cases is too small to be sure how well a hospital is performing; (2) The hospital indicated that the data submitted for this measure were based on a sample of cases; (3) Data was collected during a shorter time period (fewer quarters) than the maximum possible time for this measure; (4) Suppressed for one or more quarters by CMS; (5) No data is available from the hospital for this measure; (6) Fewer than 100 patients completed the HCAHPS survey. Use these rates with caution, as the number of surveys may be too low to reliably assess hospital performance; (7) Survey results are based on less than 12 months of data; (8) Survey results are not available for this reporting period; (9) No or very few patients were eligible for the HCAHPS survey. The scores shown, if any, reflect a very small number of surveys; (10) A state average was not calculated because too few hospitals in the state submitted data; (11) There were discrepancies in the data collection process; Please refer to the User's Guide for a full explanation of data.

John Dempsey Hospital[2]	Farmington	97%	95
Danbury Hospital[2]	Danbury	96%	198
Stamford Hospital[2]	Stamford	95%	61
Waterbury Hospital[2]	Waterbury	95%	66
Griffin Hospital	Derby	93%	60
The Hospital of Central Connecticut[2]	New Britain	93%	265
Manchester Memorial Hospital[2]	Manchester	93%	75
Saint Francis Hospital & Medical Center[2]	Hartford	93%	227
Bridgeport Hospital[2]	Bridgeport	92%	95
Hospital of St Raphael[2]	New Haven	92%	216
Lawrence & Memorial Hospital[2]	New London	92%	85
Middlesex Hospital	Middletown	92%	254
William W Backus Hospital[2]	Norwich	92%	87
Hartford Hospital[2]	Hartford	91%	186
Saint Vincent's Medical Center[2]	Bridgeport	91%	117
Midstate Medical Center[2]	Meriden	90%	113
Greenwich Hospital Association[2]	Greenwich	89%	37
Johnson Memorial Hospital	Stafford Springs	89%	45
Windham Hospital	Willimantic	85%	39
Yale-New Haven Hospital[2]	New Haven	82%	160
Saint Marys Hospital[2]	Waterbury	80%	66
Rockville General Hospital	Rockville	79%	28
Norwalk Hospital Association	Norwalk	70%	80
Charlotte Hungerford Hospital[2]	Torrington	54%	26

Children's Asthma Care

33. Received Systemic Corticosteroids

Hospital Name	City	Rate	Cases
Connecticut Childrens Medical Center	Hartford	100%	365
Yale-New Haven Hospital[2]	New Haven	100%	322

34. Received Home Management Plan of Care

Hospital Name	City	Rate	Cases
Connecticut Childrens Medical Center	Hartford	90%	365
Yale-New Haven Hospital[2]	New Haven	73%	324

35. Received Reliever Medication

Hospital Name	City	Rate	Cases
Connecticut Childrens Medical Center	Hartford	100%	365
Yale-New Haven Hospital[2]	New Haven	100%	323

Use of Medical Imaging

36. Combination Abdominal CT Scan

Hospital Name	City	Ratio	Cases
Bristol Hospital	Bristol	0.010	781
Johnson Memorial Hospital	Stafford Springs	0.024	372
Waterbury Hospital	Waterbury	0.028	825
Griffin Hospital	Derby	0.040	545
Stamford Hospital	Stamford	0.040	1708
Hartford Hospital	Hartford	0.043	490
Greenwich Hospital Association	Greenwich	0.050	1070
Day Kimball Hospital	Putnam	0.052	556
New Milford Hospital	New Milford	0.057	628
Saint Francis Hospital & Medical Center	Hartford	0.058	1474
Saint Marys Hospital	Waterbury	0.061	846
William W Backus Hospital	Norwich	0.061	1563
Middlesex Hospital	Middletown	0.064	2046
Danbury Hospital	Danbury	0.065	1360
The Hospital of Central Connecticut	New Britain	0.066	1586
Norwalk Hospital Association	Norwalk	0.066	758
Windham Hospital	Willimantic	0.079	554
Manchester Memorial Hospital	Manchester	0.081	1081
Rockville General Hospital	Rockville	0.081	546
Lawrence & Memorial Hospital	New London	0.088	1370
Hospital of St Raphael	New Haven	0.093	1177
Charlotte Hungerford Hospital	Torrington	0.101	663
Milford Hospital	Milford	0.127	425
Yale-New Haven Hospital	New Haven	0.135	2598
Saint Vincent's Medical Center	Bridgeport	0.195	527
Bridgeport Hospital	Bridgeport	0.464	308
Midstate Medical Center	Meriden	0.613	917
Sharon Hospital	Sharon	0.694	363
John Dempsey Hospital	Farmington	0.724	721

37. Combination Chest CT Scan

Hospital Name	City	Ratio	Cases
Johnson Memorial Hospital	Stafford Springs	0.000	276
Lawrence & Memorial Hospital	New London	0.000	1183
Waterbury Hospital	Waterbury	0.000	634
Bristol Hospital	Bristol	0.002	537
Danbury Hospital	Danbury	0.002	1454
Midstate Medical Center	Meriden	0.002	419
Stamford Hospital	Stamford	0.002	1200
Griffin Hospital	Derby	0.003	631
Saint Marys Hospital	Waterbury	0.003	700
Yale-New Haven Hospital	New Haven	0.003	2902
Day Kimball Hospital	Putnam	0.004	513
New Milford Hospital	New Milford	0.005	618
William W Backus Hospital	Norwich	0.006	1444
Saint Francis Hospital & Medical Center	Hartford	0.007	1265
Bridgeport Hospital	Bridgeport	0.009	106
Hospital of St Raphael	New Haven	0.009	1250
Manchester Memorial Hospital	Manchester	0.009	974
The Hospital of Central Connecticut	New Britain	0.012	1171
Saint Vincent's Medical Center	Bridgeport	0.014	218
Sharon Hospital	Sharon	0.017	290
Windham Hospital	Willimantic	0.021	434
Middlesex Hospital	Middletown	0.023	1295
Rockville General Hospital	Rockville	0.023	431
Greenwich Hospital Association	Greenwich	0.034	935
Milford Hospital	Milford	0.054	186
Norwalk Hospital Association	Norwalk	0.059	590
Charlotte Hungerford Hospital	Torrington	0.075	562
Hartford Hospital	Hartford	0.232	211
John Dempsey Hospital	Farmington	0.480	638

38. Follow-up Mammogram/Ultrasound

Hospital Name	City	Rate	Cases
New Milford Hospital	New Milford	4.7%	709
Danbury Hospital	Danbury	4.9%	1377
Day Kimball Hospital	Putnam	5.5%	1339
Lawrence & Memorial Hospital	New London	5.6%	3080
William W Backus Hospital	Norwich	6.2%	2020
Johnson Memorial Hospital	Stafford Springs	6.4%	500
Rockville General Hospital	Rockville	6.5%	415
Yale-New Haven Hospital	New Haven	7.8%	4522
Hospital of St Raphael	New Haven	8.1%	529
Bristol Hospital	Bristol	8.3%	169
John Dempsey Hospital	Farmington	8.5%	704
Sharon Hospital	Sharon	8.5%	887
Midstate Medical Center	Meriden	8.8%	712
Greenwich Hospital Association	Greenwich	8.9%	1309
Middlesex Hospital	Middletown	9.0%	2828
Windham Hospital	Willimantic	9.6%	1222
Manchester Memorial Hospital	Manchester	10.1%	543
Charlotte Hungerford Hospital	Torrington	10.3%	2202
Waterbury Hospital	Waterbury	10.4%	298
Griffin Hospital	Derby	10.5%	637
Saint Vincent's Medical Center	Bridgeport	11.0%	317
Saint Marys Hospital	Waterbury	11.5%	489
The Hospital of Central Connecticut	New Britain	13.1%	2652
Hartford Hospital	Hartford	14.0%	285
Norwalk Hospital Association	Norwalk	14.3%	294
Bridgeport Hospital	Bridgeport	14.9%	87
Saint Francis Hospital & Medical Center	Hartford	15.9%	1175
Stamford Hospital	Stamford	16.5%	2159
Milford Hospital[1]	Milford	23.5%	51

39. MRI for Low Back Pain

Hospital Name	City	Rate	Cases
Saint Vincent's Medical Center[1]	Bridgeport	16.0%	50
Milford Hospital	Milford	19.7%	71
The Hospital of Central Connecticut	New Britain	21.5%	191
Manchester Memorial Hospital	Manchester	22.7%	154
Yale-New Haven Hospital	New Haven	23.3%	460
John Dempsey Hospital	Farmington	23.6%	216
Greenwich Hospital Association	Greenwich	24.3%	263
Norwalk Hospital Association	Norwalk	24.7%	397
Middlesex Hospital	Middletown	25.1%	323
William W Backus Hospital	Norwich	25.2%	278
Day Kimball Hospital	Putnam	26.2%	84
Bristol Hospital	Bristol	27.3%	77
Danbury Hospital	Danbury	27.8%	198
Griffin Hospital	Derby	28.6%	119
Midstate Medical Center	Meriden	29.0%	169
Hartford Hospital[1]	Hartford	29.4%	51
Johnson Memorial Hospital	Stafford Springs	31.0%	58
Saint Francis Hospital & Medical Center	Hartford	31.1%	312
Stamford Hospital	Stamford	31.3%	176
Lawrence & Memorial Hospital	New London	32.0%	228
Rockville General Hospital	Rockville	32.6%	95
Sharon Hospital	Sharon	32.7%	98
Windham Hospital	Willimantic	33.1%	127
New Milford Hospital	New Milford	34.5%	84
Saint Marys Hospital[1]	Waterbury	37.8%	37

Survey of Patients' Hospital Experiences

40. Area Around Room 'Always' Quiet at Night

Hospital Name	City	Rate	Cases
Milford Hospital	Milford	61%	300+
Sharon Hospital	Sharon	60%	300+
Greenwich Hospital Association	Greenwich	58%	300+
Johnson Memorial Hospital	Stafford Springs	57%	300+
Griffin Hospital	Derby	56%	300+
Midstate Medical Center	Meriden	56%	300+
New Milford Hospital	New Milford	56%	300+
Rockville General Hospital	Rockville	55%	300+
Middlesex Hospital	Middletown	53%	300+
Stamford Hospital	Stamford	53%	300+
Day Kimball Hospital	Putnam	52%	300+
Bristol Hospital	Bristol	50%	300+
Saint Vincent's Medical Center	Bridgeport	49%	300+
Charlotte Hungerford Hospital	Torrington	48%	300+
Manchester Memorial Hospital	Manchester	48%	300+
Saint Marys Hospital	Waterbury	48%	300+
William W Backus Hospital	Norwich	48%	300+
Danbury Hospital	Danbury	47%	300+
Saint Francis Hospital & Medical Center	Hartford	47%	300+
Yale-New Haven Hospital	New Haven	47%	300+
The Hospital of Central Connecticut	New Britain	46%	300+
Lawrence & Memorial Hospital	New London	46%	300+
Hartford Hospital	Hartford	44%	300+
Waterbury Hospital	Waterbury	44%	300+
Masonic Home and Hospital	Wallingford	43%	(a)
Windham Hospital	Willimantic	43%	300+
Hospital of St Raphael	New Haven	42%	300+
Bridgeport Hospital	Bridgeport	41%	300+
Norwalk Hospital Association	Norwalk	38%	300+
John Dempsey Hospital	Farmington	37%	300+

41. Doctors 'Always' Communicated Well

Hospital Name	City	Rate	Cases
Sharon Hospital	Sharon	85%	300+
Day Kimball Hospital	Putnam	82%	300+
Greenwich Hospital Association	Greenwich	82%	300+
Bristol Hospital	Bristol	81%	300+
Midstate Medical Center	Meriden	81%	300+
Milford Hospital	Milford	81%	300+
New Milford Hospital	New Milford	81%	300+
Waterbury Hospital	Waterbury	81%	300+
Danbury Hospital	Danbury	80%	300+
Norwalk Hospital Association	Norwalk	80%	300+
Saint Vincent's Medical Center	Bridgeport	80%	300+
Charlotte Hungerford Hospital	Torrington	79%	300+
Middlesex Hospital	Middletown	79%	300+
Windham Hospital	Willimantic	79%	300+
Griffin Hospital	Derby	78%	300+
Saint Marys Hospital	Waterbury	78%	300+
Stamford Hospital	Stamford	78%	300+
Manchester Memorial Hospital	Manchester	77%	300+
Saint Francis Hospital & Medical Center	Hartford	77%	300+
Bridgeport Hospital	Bridgeport	76%	300+
Hartford Hospital	Hartford	76%	300+
The Hospital of Central Connecticut	New Britain	76%	300+
Johnson Memorial Hospital	Stafford Springs	76%	300+
Hospital of St Raphael	New Haven	75%	300+
John Dempsey Hospital	Farmington	75%	300+
Lawrence & Memorial Hospital	New London	75%	300+
Rockville General Hospital	Rockville	75%	300+
Yale-New Haven Hospital	New Haven	75%	300+
William W Backus Hospital	Norwich	74%	300+
Masonic Home and Hospital	Wallingford	60%	(a)

42. Home Recovery Information Given

Hospital Name	City	Rate	Cases
Waterbury Hospital	Waterbury	88%	300+
Hartford Hospital	Hartford	86%	300+
Bristol Hospital	Bristol	85%	300+
John Dempsey Hospital	Farmington	85%	300+
Middlesex Hospital	Middletown	85%	300+
Saint Marys Hospital	Waterbury	85%	300+
Charlotte Hungerford Hospital	Torrington	84%	300+
Griffin Hospital	Derby	84%	300+
Johnson Memorial Hospital	Stafford Springs	84%	300+
Sharon Hospital	Sharon	84%	300+
The Hospital of Central Connecticut	New Britain	82%	300+
Hospital of St Raphael	New Haven	82%	300+
Midstate Medical Center	Meriden	82%	300+
New Milford Hospital	New Milford	82%	300+
Saint Francis Hospital & Medical Center	Hartford	82%	300+
William W Backus Hospital	Norwich	82%	300+
Yale-New Haven Hospital	New Haven	82%	300+
Day Kimball Hospital	Putnam	81%	300+
Manchester Memorial Hospital	Manchester	81%	300+
Milford Hospital	Milford	81%	300+
Rockville General Hospital	Rockville	81%	300+
Windham Hospital	Willimantic	81%	300+
Greenwich Hospital Association	Greenwich	80%	300+
Lawrence & Memorial Hospital	New London	80%	300+
Danbury Hospital	Danbury	79%	300+
Norwalk Hospital Association	Norwalk	79%	300+
Saint Vincent's Medical Center	Bridgeport	78%	300+
Bridgeport Hospital	Bridgeport	77%	300+
Masonic Home and Hospital	Wallingford	77%	(a)

NOTE: Hospital profiles are in alphabetical order by state, then city, then hospital within the city; Rankings exclude hospitals with less than 25 cases except for patient surveys which excludes hospitals with less than 100 cases; (a) 100–299 cases; (1) The number of cases is too small to be sure how well a hospital is performing; (2) The hospital indicated that the data submitted for this measure were based on a sample of cases; (3) Data was collected during a shorter time period (fewer quarters) than the maximum possible time for this measure; (4) Suppressed for one or more quarters by CMS; (5) No data is available from the hospital for this measure; (6) Fewer than 100 patients completed the HCAHPS survey. Use these rates with caution, as the number of surveys may be too low to reliably assess hospital performance; (7) Survey results are based on less than 12 months of data; (8) Survey results are not available for this reporting period; (9) No or very few patients were eligible for the HCAHPS survey. The scores shown, if any, reflect a very small number of surveys; (10) A state average was not calculated because too few hospitals in the state submitted data; (11) There were discrepancies in the data collection process; Please refer to the User's Guide for a full explanation of data.

Stamford Hospital	Stamford	74%	300+

43. Hospital Given 9 or 10 on 10 Point Scale

Hospital Name	City	Rate	Cases
Greenwich Hospital Association	Greenwich	79%	300+
Middlesex Hospital	Middletown	75%	300+
Sharon Hospital	Sharon	74%	300+
Griffin Hospital	Derby	71%	300+
Midstate Medical Center	Meriden	71%	300+
Milford Hospital	Milford	71%	300+
Danbury Hospital	Danbury	70%	300+
New Milford Hospital	New Milford	70%	300+
Norwalk Hospital Association	Norwalk	67%	300+
Saint Vincent's Medical Center	Bridgeport	67%	300+
William W Backus Hospital	Norwich	67%	300+
Charlotte Hungerford Hospital	Torrington	66%	300+
Windham Hospital	Willimantic	66%	300+
The Hospital of Central Connecticut	New Britain	65%	300+
Hospital of St Raphael	New Haven	65%	300+
Rockville General Hospital	Rockville	65%	300+
Stamford Hospital	Stamford	65%	300+
Day Kimball Hospital	Putnam	64%	300+
Waterbury Hospital	Waterbury	64%	300+
Yale-New Haven Hospital	New Haven	64%	300+
Bristol Hospital	Bristol	63%	300+
Saint Marys Hospital	Waterbury	63%	300+
John Dempsey Hospital	Farmington	62%	300+
Saint Francis Hospital & Medical Center	Hartford	62%	300+
Johnson Memorial Hospital	Stafford Springs	61%	300+
Hartford Hospital	Hartford	60%	300+
Lawrence & Memorial Hospital	New London	60%	300+
Manchester Memorial Hospital	Manchester	59%	300+
Masonic Home and Hospital	Wallingford	57%	(a)
Bridgeport Hospital	Bridgeport	56%	300+

44. Meds 'Always' Explained Before Given

Hospital Name	City	Rate	Cases
Bristol Hospital	Bristol	66%	300+
Midstate Medical Center	Meriden	66%	300+
Windham Hospital	Willimantic	64%	300+
Middlesex Hospital	Middletown	63%	300+
Griffin Hospital	Derby	62%	300+
Greenwich Hospital Association	Greenwich	61%	300+
Sharon Hospital	Sharon	61%	300+
Day Kimball Hospital	Putnam	60%	300+
The Hospital of Central Connecticut	New Britain	60%	300+
Norwalk Hospital Association	Norwalk	60%	300+
Charlotte Hungerford Hospital	Torrington	59%	300+
Manchester Memorial Hospital	Manchester	59%	300+
Yale-New Haven Hospital	New Haven	59%	300+
Danbury Hospital	Danbury	58%	300+
Hospital of St Raphael	New Haven	58%	300+
John Dempsey Hospital	Farmington	58%	300+
Saint Vincent's Medical Center	Bridgeport	58%	300+
Stamford Hospital	Stamford	58%	300+
Waterbury Hospital	Waterbury	58%	300+
Milford Hospital	Milford	57%	300+
New Milford Hospital	New Milford	57%	300+
Rockville General Hospital	Rockville	57%	300+
Saint Marys Hospital	Waterbury	57%	300+
Bridgeport Hospital	Bridgeport	56%	300+
Lawrence & Memorial Hospital	New London	56%	300+
Johnson Memorial Hospital	Stafford Springs	55%	300+
William W Backus Hospital	Norwich	55%	300+
Hartford Hospital	Hartford	54%	300+
Saint Francis Hospital & Medical Center	Hartford	54%	300+
Masonic Home and Hospital	Wallingford	40%	(a)

45. Nurses 'Always' Communicated Well

Hospital Name	City	Rate	Cases
Midstate Medical Center	Meriden	81%	300+
Bristol Hospital	Bristol	80%	300+
Danbury Hospital	Danbury	80%	300+
Day Kimball Hospital	Putnam	79%	300+
Charlotte Hungerford Hospital	Torrington	78%	300+
Middlesex Hospital	Middletown	78%	300+
Milford Hospital	Milford	78%	300+
New Milford Hospital	New Milford	78%	300+
Sharon Hospital	Sharon	78%	300+
Greenwich Hospital Association	Greenwich	77%	300+
Griffin Hospital	Derby	77%	300+
Rockville General Hospital	Rockville	77%	300+
Waterbury Hospital	Waterbury	77%	300+
Windham Hospital	Willimantic	77%	300+
Saint Vincent's Medical Center	Bridgeport	76%	300+
The Hospital of Central Connecticut	New Britain	75%	300+
Hospital of St Raphael	New Haven	75%	300+
Lawrence & Memorial Hospital	New London	75%	300+
Stamford Hospital	Stamford	75%	300+
Manchester Memorial Hospital	Manchester	74%	300+
Norwalk Hospital Association	Norwalk	74%	300+
William W Backus Hospital	Norwich	74%	300+
John Dempsey Hospital	Farmington	73%	300+
Johnson Memorial Hospital	Stafford Springs	73%	300+
Saint Marys Hospital	Waterbury	73%	300+
Yale-New Haven Hospital	New Haven	73%	300+
Bridgeport Hospital	Bridgeport	72%	300+
Saint Francis Hospital & Medical Center	Hartford	72%	300+
Hartford Hospital	Hartford	71%	300+
Masonic Home and Hospital	Wallingford	64%	(a)

46. Pain 'Always' Well Controlled

Hospital Name	City	Rate	Cases
Danbury Hospital	Danbury	74%	300+
Midstate Medical Center	Meriden	73%	300+
Sharon Hospital	Sharon	73%	300+
Bristol Hospital	Bristol	72%	300+
Norwalk Hospital Association	Norwalk	72%	300+
Charlotte Hungerford Hospital	Torrington	71%	300+
Middlesex Hospital	Middletown	71%	300+
New Milford Hospital	New Milford	71%	300+
Milford Hospital	Milford	70%	300+
Rockville General Hospital	Rockville	70%	300+
Stamford Hospital	Stamford	70%	300+
Griffin Hospital	Derby	69%	300+
The Hospital of Central Connecticut	New Britain	69%	300+
Lawrence & Memorial Hospital	New London	69%	300+
Manchester Memorial Hospital	Manchester	69%	300+
Waterbury Hospital	Waterbury	69%	300+
Greenwich Hospital Association	Greenwich	68%	300+
Hospital of St Raphael	New Haven	68%	300+
Windham Hospital	Willimantic	68%	300+
Day Kimball Hospital	Putnam	67%	300+
John Dempsey Hospital	Farmington	67%	300+
Johnson Memorial Hospital	Stafford Springs	67%	300+
Saint Marys Hospital	Waterbury	67%	300+
Saint Vincent's Medical Center	Bridgeport	67%	300+
Bridgeport Hospital	Bridgeport	66%	300+
Saint Francis Hospital & Medical Center	Hartford	66%	300+
Masonic Home and Hospital	Wallingford	65%	(a)
Yale-New Haven Hospital	New Haven	65%	300+
Hartford Hospital	Hartford	64%	300+
William W Backus Hospital	Norwich	64%	300+

47. Room and Bathroom 'Always' Clean

Hospital Name	City	Rate	Cases
Milford Hospital	Milford	81%	300+
Day Kimball Hospital	Putnam	80%	300+
Middlesex Hospital	Middletown	79%	300+
Greenwich Hospital Association	Greenwich	76%	300+
Griffin Hospital	Derby	74%	300+
New Milford Hospital	New Milford	74%	300+
William W Backus Hospital	Norwich	74%	300+
Midstate Medical Center	Meriden	73%	300+
Norwalk Hospital Association	Norwalk	73%	300+
Charlotte Hungerford Hospital	Torrington	72%	300+
The Hospital of Central Connecticut	New Britain	72%	300+
Sharon Hospital	Sharon	72%	300+
Windham Hospital	Willimantic	72%	300+
Saint Marys Hospital	Waterbury	71%	300+
Johnson Memorial Hospital	Stafford Springs	69%	300+
Masonic Home and Hospital	Wallingford	69%	(a)
Rockville General Hospital	Rockville	69%	300+
Danbury Hospital	Danbury	68%	300+
Hospital of St Raphael	New Haven	68%	300+
John Dempsey Hospital	Farmington	68%	300+
Bristol Hospital	Bristol	67%	300+
Saint Francis Hospital & Medical Center	Hartford	66%	300+
Lawrence & Memorial Hospital	New London	65%	300+
Hartford Hospital	Hartford	63%	300+
Saint Vincent's Medical Center	Bridgeport	63%	300+
Stamford Hospital	Stamford	63%	300+
Manchester Memorial Hospital	Manchester	62%	300+
Waterbury Hospital	Waterbury	61%	300+
Yale-New Haven Hospital	New Haven	61%	300+
Bridgeport Hospital	Bridgeport	57%	300+

48. Timely Help 'Always' Received

Hospital Name	City	Rate	Cases
Milford Hospital	Milford	69%	300+
Day Kimball Hospital	Putnam	67%	300+
Midstate Medical Center	Meriden	67%	300+
Middlesex Hospital	Middletown	66%	300+
Danbury Hospital	Danbury	65%	300+
Charlotte Hungerford Hospital	Torrington	64%	300+
New Milford Hospital	New Milford	64%	300+
Windham Hospital	Willimantic	64%	300+
Griffin Hospital	Derby	63%	300+
Rockville General Hospital	Rockville	63%	300+
Sharon Hospital	Sharon	63%	300+
Bristol Hospital	Bristol	62%	300+
Greenwich Hospital Association	Greenwich	62%	300+
Hospital of St Raphael	New Haven	62%	300+
Norwalk Hospital Association	Norwalk	62%	300+
Saint Vincent's Medical Center	Bridgeport	61%	300+
The Hospital of Central Connecticut	New Britain	60%	300+
William W Backus Hospital	Norwich	60%	300+
Waterbury Hospital	Waterbury	59%	300+
Lawrence & Memorial Hospital	New London	58%	300+
Manchester Memorial Hospital	Manchester	57%	300+
Saint Marys Hospital	Waterbury	57%	300+
Stamford Hospital	Stamford	56%	300+
Johnson Memorial Hospital	Stafford Springs	55%	300+
Saint Francis Hospital & Medical Center	Hartford	55%	300+
Yale-New Haven Hospital	New Haven	55%	300+
Bridgeport Hospital	Bridgeport	54%	300+
John Dempsey Hospital	Farmington	52%	300+
Hartford Hospital	Hartford	50%	300+
Masonic Home and Hospital	Wallingford	42%	(a)

49. Would Definitely Recommend Hospital

Hospital Name	City	Rate	Cases
Greenwich Hospital Association	Greenwich	83%	300+
Danbury Hospital	Danbury	81%	300+
Middlesex Hospital	Middletown	79%	300+
Griffin Hospital	Derby	76%	300+
Milford Hospital	Milford	75%	300+
New Milford Hospital	New Milford	75%	300+
Norwalk Hospital Association	Norwalk	75%	300+
Sharon Hospital	Sharon	75%	300+
Midstate Medical Center	Meriden	74%	300+
Saint Vincent's Medical Center	Bridgeport	73%	300+
Hartford Hospital	Hartford	71%	300+
Hospital of St Raphael	New Haven	71%	300+
Saint Francis Hospital & Medical Center	Hartford	71%	300+
William W Backus Hospital	Norwich	71%	300+
Yale-New Haven Hospital	New Haven	71%	300+
Stamford Hospital	Stamford	70%	300+
Waterbury Hospital	Waterbury	70%	300+
The Hospital of Central Connecticut	New Britain	69%	300+
Lawrence & Memorial Hospital	New London	69%	300+
Rockville General Hospital	Rockville	69%	300+
Saint Marys Hospital	Waterbury	69%	300+
Windham Hospital	Willimantic	69%	300+
Day Kimball Hospital	Putnam	67%	300+
John Dempsey Hospital	Farmington	67%	300+
Bristol Hospital	Bristol	66%	300+
Johnson Memorial Hospital	Stafford Springs	66%	300+
Manchester Memorial Hospital	Manchester	66%	300+
Masonic Home and Hospital	Wallingford	65%	(a)
Bridgeport Hospital	Bridgeport	64%	300+
Charlotte Hungerford Hospital	Torrington	62%	300+

NOTE: Hospital profiles are in alphabetical order by state, then city, then hospital within the city; Rankings exclude hospitals with less than 25 cases except for patient surveys which excludes hospitals with less than 100 cases; (a) 100–299 cases; (1) The number of cases is too small to be sure how well a hospital is performing; (2) The hospital indicated that the data submitted for this measure were based on a sample of cases; (3) Data was collected during a shorter time period (fewer quarters) than the maximum possible time for this measure; (4) Suppressed for one or more quarters by CMS; (5) No data is available from the hospital for this measure; (6) Fewer than 100 patients completed the HCAHPS survey. Use these rates with caution, as the number of surveys may be too low to reliably assess hospital performance; (7) Survey results are based on less than 12 months of data; (8) Survey results are not available for this reporting period; (9) No or very few patients were eligible for the HCAHPS survey. The scores shown, if any, reflect a very small number of surveys; (10) A state average was not calculated because too few hospitals in the state submitted data; (11) There were discrepancies in the data collection process; Please refer to the User's Guide for a full explanation of data.

Bridgeport Hospital

267 Grant Street
Bridgeport, CT 06610
Phone: 203-384-3000
Fax: 203-384-3943
E-mail: kawise@bpthosp.org
URL: www.bridgeporthospital.com
Type: Acute Care Hospitals
Emergency Services: Yes
Ownership: Voluntary Non-Profit - Private
Beds: 425

Key Personnel:
CEO/President. . . . . William Jennings
Chief of Medical Staff . . . . Constantine Manthous, MD
Infection Control. . . . . David Baker, MD
Operating Room. . . . . Karin Hooper, RN
Pediatric In-Patient Care . . . . Thomas Kennedy, MD
Quality Assurance . . . . Michael Liebowitz
Radiology. . . . . Alan D Kaye

Measure	Cases	This Hosp.	State Avg.	U.S. Avg.
Heart Attack Care				
ACE Inhibitor or ARB for LVSD[2]	60	88%	94%	96%
Aspirin at Arrival[2]	225	99%	99%	99%
Aspirin at Discharge[2]	253	96%	99%	98%
Beta Blocker at Discharge[2]	258	95%	98%	98%
Fibrinolytic Medication Timing[2]	0	-	50%	55%
PCI Within 90 Minutes of Arrival[1,2]	22	91%	87%	90%
Smoking Cessation Advice[2]	46	100%	100%	99%
Chest Pain/Possible Heart Attack Care				
Aspirin at Arrival[5]	0	-	97%	95%
Median Time to ECG (minutes)[5]	0	-	8	8
Median Time to Transfer (minutes)[5]	0	-	73	61
Fibrinolytic Medication Timing[5]	0	-	37%	54%
Heart Failure Care				
ACE Inhibitor or ARB for LVSD[2]	84	90%	93%	94%
Discharge Instructions[2]	195	82%	86%	88%
Evaluation of LVS Function[2]	291	100%	99%	98%
Smoking Cessation Advice[2]	41	100%	99%	98%
Pneumonia Care				
Appropriate Initial Antibiotic[2]	67	91%	93%	92%
Blood Culture Timing[2]	106	96%	96%	96%
Influenza Vaccine[2]	81	81%	91%	91%
Initial Antibiotic Timing[2]	102	85%	96%	95%
Pneumococcal Vaccine[2]	123	90%	93%	93%
Smoking Cessation Advice[2]	31	100%	98%	97%
Surgical Care Improvement Project				
Appropriate VTP Within 24 Hours[2]	117	97%	95%	92%
Appropriate Hair Removal[2]	468	98%	99%	99%
Appropriate Beta Blocker Usage[2]	184	90%	93%	93%
Controlled Postoperative Blood Glucose[2]	76	96%	91%	93%
Prophylactic Antibiotic Timing[2]	303	97%	96%	97%
Prophylactic Antibiotic Timing (Outpatient)	467	85%	92%	92%
Prophylactic Antibiotic Selection[2]	307	99%	97%	97%
Prophylactic Antibiotic Select. (Outpatient)	427	87%	92%	94%
Prophylactic Antibiotic Stopped[2]	267	91%	95%	94%
Recommended VTP Ordered[2]	117	97%	96%	94%
Urinary Catheter Removal[2]	95	92%	91%	90%
Children's Asthma Care				
Received Systemic Corticosteroids	-	-	-	100%
Received Home Management Plan	-	-	-	71%
Received Reliever Medication	-	-	-	100%
Use of Medical Imaging				
Combination Abdominal CT Scan	308	0.464	0.120	0.191
Combination Chest CT Scan	106	0.009	0.026	0.054
Follow-up Mammogram/Ultrasound	87	14.9%	9.2%	8.4%
MRI for Low Back Pain[5]	0	-	26.9%	32.7%
Survey of Patients' Hospital Experiences				
Area Around Room 'Always' Quiet at Night	300+	41%	-	58%
Doctors 'Always' Communicated Well	300+	76%	-	80%
Home Recovery Information Given	300+	77%	-	82%
Hospital Given 9 or 10 on 10 Point Scale	300+	56%	-	67%
Meds 'Always' Explained Before Given	300+	56%	-	60%
Nurses 'Always' Communicated Well	300+	72%	-	76%
Pain 'Always' Well Controlled	300+	66%	-	69%
Room and Bathroom 'Always' Clean	300+	57%	-	71%
Timely Help 'Always' Received	300+	54%	-	64%
Would Definitely Recommend Hospital	300+	64%	-	69%

Saint Vincent's Medical Center

2800 Main St
Bridgeport, CT 06606
Phone: 203-576-5551
Fax: 203-576-5733
E-mail: info@svhs-ct.org
URL: www.stvincents.org
Type: Acute Care Hospitals
Emergency Services: Yes
Ownership: Voluntary Non-Profit - Church
Beds: 391

Key Personnel:
CEO/President. . . . . William J Riordan
Cardiac Laboratory. . . . . Edward Kosinski, MD
Chief of Medical Staff . . . . Patrick Carolan Jr
Infection Control. . . . . Grace Kim, MD
Operating Room. . . . . Nancy Newton
Pediatric In-Patient Care . . . . Roy Schutzengel, MD
Quality Assurance . . . . Evelyn Gowel
Radiology. . . . . Robert Russo, MD

Measure	Cases	This Hosp.	State Avg.	U.S. Avg.
Heart Attack Care				
ACE Inhibitor or ARB for LVSD	74	96%	94%	96%
Aspirin at Arrival	261	99%	99%	99%
Aspirin at Discharge	309	99%	99%	98%
Beta Blocker at Discharge	307	98%	98%	98%
Fibrinolytic Medication Timing	0	-	50%	55%
PCI Within 90 Minutes of Arrival	59	88%	87%	90%
Smoking Cessation Advice	61	98%	100%	99%
Chest Pain/Possible Heart Attack Care				
Aspirin at Arrival[5]	0	-	97%	95%
Median Time to ECG (minutes)[5]	0	-	8	8
Median Time to Transfer (minutes)[5]	0	-	73	61
Fibrinolytic Medication Timing[5]	0	-	37%	54%
Heart Failure Care				
ACE Inhibitor or ARB for LVSD	186	90%	93%	94%
Discharge Instructions	391	92%	86%	88%
Evaluation of LVS Function	577	99%	99%	98%
Smoking Cessation Advice	57	100%	99%	98%
Pneumonia Care				
Appropriate Initial Antibiotic	180	96%	93%	92%
Blood Culture Timing	325	98%	96%	96%
Influenza Vaccine	198	86%	91%	91%
Initial Antibiotic Timing	317	99%	96%	95%
Pneumococcal Vaccine	292	96%	93%	93%
Smoking Cessation Advice	82	99%	98%	97%
Surgical Care Improvement Project				
Appropriate VTP Within 24 Hours[2]	149	98%	95%	92%
Appropriate Hair Removal[2]	520	100%	99%	99%
Appropriate Beta Blocker Usage[2]	184	95%	93%	93%
Controlled Postoperative Blood Glucose[2]	125	97%	91%	93%
Prophylactic Antibiotic Timing[2]	357	97%	96%	97%
Prophylactic Antibiotic Timing (Outpatient)	229	91%	92%	92%
Prophylactic Antibiotic Selection[2]	364	97%	97%	97%
Prophylactic Antibiotic Select. (Outpatient)	211	89%	92%	94%
Prophylactic Antibiotic Stopped[2]	330	92%	95%	94%
Recommended VTP Ordered[2]	149	99%	96%	94%
Urinary Catheter Removal[2]	117	91%	91%	90%
Children's Asthma Care				
Received Systemic Corticosteroids	-	-	-	100%
Received Home Management Plan	-	-	-	71%
Received Reliever Medication	-	-	-	100%
Use of Medical Imaging				
Combination Abdominal CT Scan	527	0.195	0.120	0.191
Combination Chest CT Scan	218	0.014	0.026	0.054
Follow-up Mammogram/Ultrasound	317	11.0%	9.2%	8.4%
MRI for Low Back Pain[1]	50	16.0%	26.9%	32.7%
Survey of Patients' Hospital Experiences				
Area Around Room 'Always' Quiet at Night	300+	49%	-	58%
Doctors 'Always' Communicated Well	300+	80%	-	80%
Home Recovery Information Given	300+	78%	-	82%
Hospital Given 9 or 10 on 10 Point Scale	300+	67%	-	67%
Meds 'Always' Explained Before Given	300+	58%	-	60%
Nurses 'Always' Communicated Well	300+	76%	-	76%
Pain 'Always' Well Controlled	300+	67%	-	69%
Room and Bathroom 'Always' Clean	300+	63%	-	71%
Timely Help 'Always' Received	300+	61%	-	64%
Would Definitely Recommend Hospital	300+	73%	-	69%

Bristol Hospital

Brewster Rd
Bristol, CT 06010
Phone: 860-585-3000
Fax: 860-585-3058
E-mail: info@bristolhospital.org
URL: www.bristolhospital.org
Type: Acute Care Hospitals
Emergency Services: Yes
Ownership: Voluntary Non-Profit - Private
Beds: 152

Key Personnel:
CEO/President. . . . . Thomas D Kennedy, III
Chief of Medical Staff . . . . Richard Zweig, MD
Operating Room. . . . . Ara D Bagdasarian
Pediatric In-Patient Care . . . . Delbert Hodder, MD
Quality Assurance . . . . Karen Poole, RN
Radiology. . . . . Carlos M Badiola, MD

Measure	Cases	This Hosp.	State Avg.	U.S. Avg.
Heart Attack Care				
ACE Inhibitor or ARB for LVSD[1]	5	100%	94%	96%
Aspirin at Arrival	35	100%	99%	99%
Aspirin at Discharge[1]	24	100%	99%	98%
Beta Blocker at Discharge[1]	23	100%	98%	98%
Fibrinolytic Medication Timing	0	-	50%	55%
PCI Within 90 Minutes of Arrival	0	-	87%	90%
Smoking Cessation Advice[1]	8	88%	100%	99%
Chest Pain/Possible Heart Attack Care				
Aspirin at Arrival	57	96%	97%	95%
Median Time to ECG (minutes)	57	9	8	8
Median Time to Transfer (minutes)	25	57	73	61
Fibrinolytic Medication Timing	0	-	37%	54%
Heart Failure Care				
ACE Inhibitor or ARB for LVSD	58	100%	93%	94%
Discharge Instructions	125	76%	86%	88%
Evaluation of LVS Function	187	97%	99%	98%
Smoking Cessation Advice[1]	17	88%	99%	98%
Pneumonia Care				
Appropriate Initial Antibiotic	118	97%	93%	92%
Blood Culture Timing	236	87%	96%	96%
Influenza Vaccine	142	96%	91%	91%
Initial Antibiotic Timing	225	100%	96%	95%
Pneumococcal Vaccine	196	96%	93%	93%
Smoking Cessation Advice	65	97%	98%	97%
Surgical Care Improvement Project				
Appropriate VTP Within 24 Hours	144	98%	95%	92%
Appropriate Hair Removal	351	99%	99%	99%
Appropriate Beta Blocker Usage	74	100%	93%	93%
Controlled Postoperative Blood Glucose	0	-	91%	93%
Prophylactic Antibiotic Timing	189	97%	96%	97%
Prophylactic Antibiotic Timing (Outpatient)	114	100%	92%	92%
Prophylactic Antibiotic Selection	187	95%	97%	97%
Prophylactic Antibiotic Select. (Outpatient)	114	96%	92%	94%
Prophylactic Antibiotic Stopped	180	97%	95%	94%
Recommended VTP Ordered	144	99%	96%	94%
Urinary Catheter Removal	52	100%	91%	90%
Children's Asthma Care				
Received Systemic Corticosteroids	-	-	-	100%
Received Home Management Plan	-	-	-	71%
Received Reliever Medication	-	-	-	100%
Use of Medical Imaging				
Combination Abdominal CT Scan	781	0.010	0.120	0.191
Combination Chest CT Scan	537	0.002	0.026	0.054
Follow-up Mammogram/Ultrasound	169	8.3%	9.2%	8.4%
MRI for Low Back Pain	77	27.3%	26.9%	32.7%
Survey of Patients' Hospital Experiences				
Area Around Room 'Always' Quiet at Night	300+	50%	-	58%
Doctors 'Always' Communicated Well	300+	81%	-	80%
Home Recovery Information Given	300+	85%	-	82%
Hospital Given 9 or 10 on 10 Point Scale	300+	63%	-	67%
Meds 'Always' Explained Before Given	300+	66%	-	60%
Nurses 'Always' Communicated Well	300+	80%	-	76%
Pain 'Always' Well Controlled	300+	72%	-	69%
Room and Bathroom 'Always' Clean	300+	67%	-	71%
Timely Help 'Always' Received	300+	62%	-	64%
Would Definitely Recommend Hospital	300+	66%	-	69%

NOTE: Hospital profiles are in alphabetical order by state, then city, then hospital within the city; Rankings exclude hospitals with less than 25 cases except for patient surveys which excludes hospitals with less than 100 cases; (a) 100–299 cases; (1) The number of cases is too small to be sure how well a hospital is performing; (2) The hospital indicated that the data submitted for this measure were based on a sample of cases; (3) Data was collected during a shorter time period (fewer quarters) than the maximum possible time for this measure; (4) Suppressed for one or more quarters by CMS; (5) No data is available from the hospital for this measure; (6) Fewer than 100 patients completed the HCAHPS survey. Use these rates with caution, as the number of surveys may be too low to reliably assess hospital performance; (7) Survey results are based on less than 12 months of data; (8) Survey results are not available for this reporting period; (9) No or very few patients were eligible for the HCAHPS survey. The scores shown, if any, reflect a very small number of surveys; (10) A state average was not calculated because too few hospitals in the state submitted data; (11) There were discrepancies in the data collection process; Please refer to the User's Guide for a full explanation of data.

Danbury Hospital

24 Hospital Ave
Danbury, CT 06810
Phone: 203-797-7000
Fax: 203-797-7776
URL: www.danburyhospital.com
Type: Acute Care Hospitals
Emergency Services: Yes
Ownership: Voluntary Non-Profit - Private
Beds: 371

Key Personnel:
CEO/President.............. Frank J Kelly
Chief of Medical Staff.......... Paul Jannini, MD
Infection Control.............. Barbara Welch
Operating Room.............. Joanne Thompson, RN
Pediatric In-Patient Care .... Gregory Dworkin, MD
Quality Assurance .... Dawn Myles, RN
Radiology.................. William Goldstein, MD

Measure	Cases	This Hosp.	State Avg.	U.S. Avg.
Heart Attack Care				
ACE Inhibitor or ARB for LVSD	66	85%	94%	96%
Aspirin at Arrival	303	99%	99%	99%
Aspirin at Discharge	356	99%	99%	98%
Beta Blocker at Discharge	333	98%	98%	98%
Fibrinolytic Medication Timing	0	-	50%	55%
PCI Within 90 Minutes of Arrival	56	91%	87%	90%
Smoking Cessation Advice	82	100%	100%	99%
Chest Pain/Possible Heart Attack Care				
Aspirin at Arrival[1,3]	1	100%	97%	95%
Median Time to ECG (minutes)[1,3]	1	18	8	8
Median Time to Transfer (minutes)[5]	0	-	73	61
Fibrinolytic Medication Timing[5]	0	-	37%	54%
Heart Failure Care				
ACE Inhibitor or ARB for LVSD	131	95%	93%	94%
Discharge Instructions	346	80%	86%	88%
Evaluation of LVS Function	516	100%	99%	98%
Smoking Cessation Advice	39	90%	99%	98%
Pneumonia Care				
Appropriate Initial Antibiotic	266	97%	93%	92%
Blood Culture Timing	373	95%	96%	96%
Influenza Vaccine	338	89%	91%	91%
Initial Antibiotic Timing	444	98%	96%	95%
Pneumococcal Vaccine	496	88%	93%	93%
Smoking Cessation Advice	82	89%	98%	97%
Surgical Care Improvement Project				
Appropriate VTP Within 24 Hours[2]	188	85%	95%	92%
Appropriate Hair Removal[2]	794	100%	99%	99%
Appropriate Beta Blocker Usage[2]	301	97%	93%	93%
Controlled Postoperative Blood Glucose[2]	135	95%	91%	93%
Prophylactic Antibiotic Timing[2]	563	98%	96%	97%
Prophylactic Antibiotic Timing (Outpatient)	577	92%	92%	92%
Prophylactic Antibiotic Selection[2]	564	98%	97%	97%
Prophylactic Antibiotic Select. (Outpatient)	558	97%	92%	94%
Prophylactic Antibiotic Stopped[2]	538	95%	95%	94%
Recommended VTP Ordered[2]	188	91%	96%	94%
Urinary Catheter Removal[2]	198	96%	91%	90%
Children's Asthma Care				
Received Systemic Corticosteroids	-	-	-	100%
Received Home Management Plan	-	-	-	71%
Received Reliever Medication	-	-	-	100%
Use of Medical Imaging				
Combination Abdominal CT Scan	1,360	0.065	0.120	0.191
Combination Chest CT Scan	1,454	0.002	0.026	0.054
Follow-up Mammogram/Ultrasound	1,377	4.9%	9.2%	8.4%
MRI for Low Back Pain	198	27.8%	26.9%	32.7%
Survey of Patients' Hospital Experiences				
Area Around Room 'Always' Quiet at Night	300+	47%	-	58%
Doctors 'Always' Communicated Well	300+	80%	-	80%
Home Recovery Information Given	300+	79%	-	82%
Hospital Given 9 or 10 on 10 Point Scale	300+	70%	-	67%
Meds 'Always' Explained Before Given	300+	58%	-	60%
Nurses 'Always' Communicated Well	300+	80%	-	76%
Pain 'Always' Well Controlled	300+	74%	-	69%
Room and Bathroom 'Always' Clean	300+	68%	-	71%
Timely Help 'Always' Received	300+	65%	-	64%
Would Definitely Recommend Hospital	300+	81%	-	69%

Griffin Hospital

130 Division St
Derby, CT 06418
Phone: 203-732-7500
Fax: 203-732-7569
E-mail: griffin@griffinhealth.org
URL: www.griffinhealth.org
Type: Acute Care Hospitals
Emergency Services: Yes
Ownership: Voluntary Non-Profit - Other
Beds: 119

Key Personnel:
CEO/President.............. Patrick Charmel
Chief of Medical Staff.......... Kenneth Schwartz
Coronary Care .... Mary Ann Bertini
Operating Room.............. Kim Viadero, RN
Pediatric In-Patient Care .... Anthony Wayne, MD
Quality Assurance .... Linda Evanko
Radiology.................. Christine Cooper

Measure	Cases	This Hosp.	State Avg.	U.S. Avg.
Heart Attack Care				
ACE Inhibitor or ARB for LVSD[1]	7	100%	94%	96%
Aspirin at Arrival	92	99%	99%	99%
Aspirin at Discharge	53	96%	99%	98%
Beta Blocker at Discharge	51	100%	98%	98%
Fibrinolytic Medication Timing	0	-	50%	55%
PCI Within 90 Minutes of Arrival	0	-	87%	90%
Smoking Cessation Advice[1]	6	100%	100%	99%
Chest Pain/Possible Heart Attack Care				
Aspirin at Arrival	47	100%	97%	95%
Median Time to ECG (minutes)	47	9	8	8
Median Time to Transfer (minutes)	26	56	73	61
Fibrinolytic Medication Timing	0	-	37%	54%
Heart Failure Care				
ACE Inhibitor or ARB for LVSD	42	98%	93%	94%
Discharge Instructions	165	99%	86%	88%
Evaluation of LVS Function	257	100%	99%	98%
Smoking Cessation Advice[1]	23	100%	99%	98%
Pneumonia Care				
Appropriate Initial Antibiotic	80	98%	93%	92%
Blood Culture Timing	164	98%	96%	96%
Influenza Vaccine	91	95%	91%	91%
Initial Antibiotic Timing	165	99%	96%	95%
Pneumococcal Vaccine	180	98%	93%	93%
Smoking Cessation Advice	41	100%	98%	97%
Surgical Care Improvement Project				
Appropriate VTP Within 24 Hours	130	98%	95%	92%
Appropriate Hair Removal	286	100%	99%	99%
Appropriate Beta Blocker Usage	96	92%	93%	93%
Controlled Postoperative Blood Glucose	0	-	91%	93%
Prophylactic Antibiotic Timing	166	97%	96%	97%
Prophylactic Antibiotic Timing (Outpatient)	64	94%	92%	92%
Prophylactic Antibiotic Selection	172	95%	97%	97%
Prophylactic Antibiotic Select. (Outpatient)	73	97%	92%	94%
Prophylactic Antibiotic Stopped	148	97%	95%	94%
Recommended VTP Ordered	130	98%	96%	94%
Urinary Catheter Removal	60	93%	91%	90%
Children's Asthma Care				
Received Systemic Corticosteroids	-	-	-	100%
Received Home Management Plan	-	-	-	71%
Received Reliever Medication	-	-	-	100%
Use of Medical Imaging				
Combination Abdominal CT Scan	545	0.040	0.120	0.191
Combination Chest CT Scan	631	0.003	0.026	0.054
Follow-up Mammogram/Ultrasound	637	10.5%	9.2%	8.4%
MRI for Low Back Pain	119	28.6%	26.9%	32.7%
Survey of Patients' Hospital Experiences				
Area Around Room 'Always' Quiet at Night	300+	56%	-	58%
Doctors 'Always' Communicated Well	300+	78%	-	80%
Home Recovery Information Given	300+	84%	-	82%
Hospital Given 9 or 10 on 10 Point Scale	300+	71%	-	67%
Meds 'Always' Explained Before Given	300+	62%	-	60%
Nurses 'Always' Communicated Well	300+	77%	-	76%
Pain 'Always' Well Controlled	300+	69%	-	69%
Room and Bathroom 'Always' Clean	300+	74%	-	71%
Timely Help 'Always' Received	300+	63%	-	64%
Would Definitely Recommend Hospital	300+	76%	-	69%

John Dempsey Hospital

263 Farmington Ave
Farmington, CT 06032
Phone: 860-679-1145
Fax: 860-679-4515
E-mail: ccda@up.uchc.edu
URL: www.uconnhealth.org or www.uchc.edu
Type: Acute Care Hospitals
Emergency Services: Yes
Ownership: Government - Local
Beds: 204

Key Personnel:
Cardiac Laboratory............ Dr Bruce Liang
Chief of Medical Staff.......... Bruce Carlson
Infection Control.............. Nancy Dupont
Operating Room.............. Bruce Brenner
Quality Assurance .... Barry Kels, MD
Radiology.................. XLawrence J Briggs

Measure	Cases	This Hosp.	State Avg.	U.S. Avg.
Heart Attack Care				
ACE Inhibitor or ARB for LVSD[1]	21	95%	94%	96%
Aspirin at Arrival	116	100%	99%	99%
Aspirin at Discharge	134	99%	99%	98%
Beta Blocker at Discharge	138	99%	98%	98%
Fibrinolytic Medication Timing	0	-	50%	55%
PCI Within 90 Minutes of Arrival[1]	18	83%	87%	90%
Smoking Cessation Advice	26	100%	100%	99%
Chest Pain/Possible Heart Attack Care				
Aspirin at Arrival[5]	0	-	97%	95%
Median Time to ECG (minutes)[5]	0	-	8	8
Median Time to Transfer (minutes)[5]	0	-	73	61
Fibrinolytic Medication Timing[5]	0	-	37%	54%
Heart Failure Care				
ACE Inhibitor or ARB for LVSD	64	98%	93%	94%
Discharge Instructions	156	96%	86%	88%
Evaluation of LVS Function	218	100%	99%	98%
Smoking Cessation Advice[1]	15	100%	99%	98%
Pneumonia Care				
Appropriate Initial Antibiotic[2]	76	92%	93%	92%
Blood Culture Timing[2]	151	89%	96%	96%
Influenza Vaccine[2]	77	99%	91%	91%
Initial Antibiotic Timing[2]	130	97%	96%	95%
Pneumococcal Vaccine[2]	132	99%	93%	93%
Smoking Cessation Advice[1,2]	18	100%	98%	97%
Surgical Care Improvement Project				
Appropriate VTP Within 24 Hours[2]	85	100%	95%	92%
Appropriate Hair Removal[2]	302	100%	99%	99%
Appropriate Beta Blocker Usage[2]	83	100%	93%	93%
Controlled Postoperative Blood Glucose[1,2]	16	100%	91%	93%
Prophylactic Antibiotic Timing[2]	196	96%	96%	97%
Prophylactic Antibiotic Timing (Outpatient)	202	99%	92%	92%
Prophylactic Antibiotic Selection[2]	199	96%	97%	97%
Prophylactic Antibiotic Select. (Outpatient)	200	91%	92%	94%
Prophylactic Antibiotic Stopped[2]	189	98%	95%	94%
Recommended VTP Ordered[2]	85	100%	96%	94%
Urinary Catheter Removal[2]	95	97%	91%	90%
Children's Asthma Care				
Received Systemic Corticosteroids	-	-	-	100%
Received Home Management Plan	-	-	-	71%
Received Reliever Medication	-	-	-	100%
Use of Medical Imaging				
Combination Abdominal CT Scan	721	0.724	0.120	0.191
Combination Chest CT Scan	638	0.480	0.026	0.054
Follow-up Mammogram/Ultrasound	704	8.5%	9.2%	8.4%
MRI for Low Back Pain	216	23.6%	26.9%	32.7%
Survey of Patients' Hospital Experiences				
Area Around Room 'Always' Quiet at Night	300+	37%	-	58%
Doctors 'Always' Communicated Well	300+	75%	-	80%
Home Recovery Information Given	300+	85%	-	82%
Hospital Given 9 or 10 on 10 Point Scale	300+	62%	-	67%
Meds 'Always' Explained Before Given	300+	58%	-	60%
Nurses 'Always' Communicated Well	300+	73%	-	76%
Pain 'Always' Well Controlled	300+	67%	-	69%
Room and Bathroom 'Always' Clean	300+	68%	-	71%
Timely Help 'Always' Received	300+	52%	-	64%
Would Definitely Recommend Hospital	300+	67%	-	69%

NOTE: Hospital profiles are in alphabetical order by state, then city, then hospital within the city; Rankings exclude hospitals with less than 25 cases except for patient surveys which excludes hospitals with less than 100 cases; (a) 100–299 cases; (1) The number of cases is too small to be sure how well a hospital is performing; (2) The hospital indicated that the data submitted for this measure were based on a sample of cases; (3) Data was collected during a shorter time period (fewer quarters) than the maximum possible time for this measure; (4) Suppressed for one or more quarters by CMS; (5) No data is available from the hospital for this measure; (6) Fewer than 100 patients completed the HCAHPS survey. Use these rates with caution, as the number of surveys may be too low to reliably assess hospital performance; (7) Survey results are based on less than 12 months of data; (8) Survey results are not available for this reporting period; (9) No or very few patients were eligible for the HCAHPS survey. The scores shown, if any, reflect a very small number of surveys; (10) A state average was not calculated because too few hospitals in the state submitted data; (11) There were discrepancies in the data collection process; Please refer to the User's Guide for a full explanation of data.

Greenwich Hospital Association

5 Perryridge Rd
Greenwich, CT 06830
E-mail: robin1@greenhosp
URL: www.greenhosp.org
Type: Acute Care Hospitals
Ownership: Voluntary Non-Profit - Private

Phone: 203-863-3000
Fax: 203-863-4604

Emergency Services: Yes
Beds: 174

Key Personnel:
CEO/President . . . . Frank A Corvino
Chief of Medical Staff . . . . Frederick E Siefert, MD
Infection Control . . . . Lillian Burns
Operating Room . . . . Philip J McWhorter
Pediatric Ambulatory Care . . . . . . Arnold B Korval, MD
Quality Assurance . . . . Barbara Hughes
Radiology . . . . David J Mullen, MD

Measure	Cases	This Hosp.	State Avg.	U.S. Avg.
Heart Attack Care				
ACE Inhibitor or ARB for LVSD[1,2]	11	82%	94%	96%
Aspirin at Arrival[2]	74	99%	99%	99%
Aspirin at Discharge[2]	49	100%	99%	98%
Beta Blocker at Discharge[2]	49	100%	98%	98%
Fibrinolytic Medication Timing[2]	0	-	50%	55%
PCI Within 90 Minutes of Arrival[1,2]	18	89%	87%	90%
Smoking Cessation Advice[1,2]	4	100%	100%	99%
Chest Pain/Possible Heart Attack Care				
Aspirin at Arrival[5]	0	-	97%	95%
Median Time to ECG (minutes)[5]	0	-	8	8
Median Time to Transfer (minutes)[5]	0	-	73	61
Fibrinolytic Medication Timing[5]	0	-	37%	54%
Heart Failure Care				
ACE Inhibitor or ARB for LVSD[2]	83	90%	93%	94%
Discharge Instructions[2]	183	91%	86%	88%
Evaluation of LVS Function[2]	256	98%	99%	98%
Smoking Cessation Advice[1,2]	13	100%	99%	98%
Pneumonia Care				
Appropriate Initial Antibiotic[2]	72	90%	93%	92%
Blood Culture Timing[2]	151	93%	96%	96%
Influenza Vaccine[2]	91	85%	91%	91%
Initial Antibiotic Timing[2]	120	98%	96%	95%
Pneumococcal Vaccine[2]	159	91%	93%	93%
Smoking Cessation Advice[1,2]	11	100%	98%	97%
Surgical Care Improvement Project				
Appropriate VTP Within 24 Hours[2]	137	88%	95%	92%
Appropriate Hair Removal[2]	295	100%	99%	99%
Appropriate Beta Blocker Usage[2]	97	92%	93%	93%
Controlled Postoperative Blood Glucose[2]	0	-	91%	93%
Prophylactic Antibiotic Timing[2]	228	96%	96%	97%
Prophylactic Antibiotic Timing (Outpatient)	349	96%	92%	92%
Prophylactic Antibiotic Selection[2]	229	98%	97%	97%
Prophylactic Antibiotic Select. (Outpatient)	347	97%	92%	94%
Prophylactic Antibiotic Stopped[2]	214	94%	95%	94%
Recommended VTP Ordered[2]	138	88%	96%	94%
Urinary Catheter Removal[2]	37	89%	91%	90%
Children's Asthma Care				
Received Systemic Corticosteroids	-	-	-	100%
Received Home Management Plan	-	-	-	71%
Received Reliever Medication	-	-	-	100%
Use of Medical Imaging				
Combination Abdominal CT Scan	1,070	0.050	0.120	0.191
Combination Chest CT Scan	935	0.034	0.026	0.054
Follow-up Mammogram/Ultrasound	1,309	8.9%	9.2%	8.4%
MRI for Low Back Pain	263	24.3%	26.9%	32.7%
Survey of Patients' Hospital Experiences				
Area Around Room 'Always' Quiet at Night	300+	58%	-	58%
Doctors 'Always' Communicated Well	300+	82%	-	80%
Home Recovery Information Given	300+	80%	-	82%
Hospital Given 9 or 10 on 10 Point Scale	300+	79%	-	67%
Meds 'Always' Explained Before Given	300+	61%	-	60%
Nurses 'Always' Communicated Well	300+	77%	-	76%
Pain 'Always' Well Controlled	300+	68%	-	69%
Room and Bathroom 'Always' Clean	300+	76%	-	71%
Timely Help 'Always' Received	300+	62%	-	64%
Would Definitely Recommend Hospital	300+	83%	-	69%

Connecticut Childrens Medical Center

282 Washington Street
Hartford, CT 06106
URL: www.ccmckids.org
Type: Childrens
Ownership: Voluntary Non-Profit - Private

Phone: 860-545-9000
Fax: 860-545-8560

Emergency Services: Yes
Beds: 135

Key Personnel:
CEO/President . . . . Martin J Gavin
Cardiac Laboratory . . . . Harris Lepold, MD
Chief of Medical Staff . . . . Paul H Dworkin, MD
Infection Control . . . . Jennifer Martin
Pediatric Ambulatory Care . . . . . . Carol Benjamin
Pediatric In-Patient Care . . . . Susan Maxwell
Quality Assurance . . . . Elizabeth Gnu
Radiology . . . . Diane Jay

Measure	Cases	This Hosp.	State Avg.	U.S. Avg.
Heart Attack Care				
ACE Inhibitor or ARB for LVSD	-	-	94%	96%
Aspirin at Arrival	-	-	99%	99%
Aspirin at Discharge	-	-	99%	98%
Beta Blocker at Discharge	-	-	98%	98%
Fibrinolytic Medication Timing	-	-	50%	55%
PCI Within 90 Minutes of Arrival	-	-	87%	90%
Smoking Cessation Advice	-	-	100%	99%
Chest Pain/Possible Heart Attack Care				
Aspirin at Arrival	-	-	97%	95%
Median Time to ECG (minutes)	-	-	8	8
Median Time to Transfer (minutes)	-	-	73	61
Fibrinolytic Medication Timing	-	-	37%	54%
Heart Failure Care				
ACE Inhibitor or ARB for LVSD	-	-	93%	94%
Discharge Instructions	-	-	86%	88%
Evaluation of LVS Function	-	-	99%	98%
Smoking Cessation Advice	-	-	99%	98%
Pneumonia Care				
Appropriate Initial Antibiotic	-	-	93%	92%
Blood Culture Timing	-	-	96%	96%
Influenza Vaccine	-	-	91%	91%
Initial Antibiotic Timing	-	-	96%	95%
Pneumococcal Vaccine	-	-	93%	93%
Smoking Cessation Advice	-	-	98%	97%
Surgical Care Improvement Project				
Appropriate VTP Within 24 Hours	-	-	95%	92%
Appropriate Hair Removal	-	-	99%	99%
Appropriate Beta Blocker Usage	-	-	93%	93%
Controlled Postoperative Blood Glucose	-	-	91%	93%
Prophylactic Antibiotic Timing	-	-	96%	97%
Prophylactic Antibiotic Timing (Outpatient)	-	-	92%	92%
Prophylactic Antibiotic Selection	-	-	97%	97%
Prophylactic Antibiotic Select. (Outpatient)	-	-	92%	94%
Prophylactic Antibiotic Stopped	-	-	95%	94%
Recommended VTP Ordered	-	-	96%	94%
Urinary Catheter Removal	-	-	91%	90%
Children's Asthma Care				
Received Systemic Corticosteroids	365	100%	-	100%
Received Home Management Plan	365	90%	-	71%
Received Reliever Medication	365	100%	-	100%
Use of Medical Imaging				
Combination Abdominal CT Scan	-	-	0.120	0.191
Combination Chest CT Scan	-	-	0.026	0.054
Follow-up Mammogram/Ultrasound	-	-	9.2%	8.4%
MRI for Low Back Pain	-	-	26.9%	32.7%
Survey of Patients' Hospital Experiences				
Area Around Room 'Always' Quiet at Night	-	-	-	58%
Doctors 'Always' Communicated Well	-	-	-	80%
Home Recovery Information Given	-	-	-	82%
Hospital Given 9 or 10 on 10 Point Scale	-	-	-	67%
Meds 'Always' Explained Before Given	-	-	-	60%
Nurses 'Always' Communicated Well	-	-	-	76%
Pain 'Always' Well Controlled	-	-	-	69%
Room and Bathroom 'Always' Clean	-	-	-	71%
Timely Help 'Always' Received	-	-	-	64%
Would Definitely Recommend Hospital	-	-	-	69%

Hartford Hospital

80 Seymour Street
Hartford, CT 06102
URL: www.harthosp.org
Type: Acute Care Hospitals
Ownership: Voluntary Non-Profit - Private

Phone: 860-545-5000
Fax: 860-545-5066

Emergency Services: Yes
Beds: 796

Key Personnel:
CEO/President . . . . Elliot Joseph
Chief of Medical Staff . . . . Joseph Klimek, MD
Infection Control . . . . Brian Cooper, MD
Operating Room . . . . Barbara Rodirick
Pediatric In-Patient Care . . . . Leonard Banco
Quality Assurance . . . . Allison Reynolds
Radiology . . . . Stewart Markowitz, MD

Measure	Cases	This Hosp.	State Avg.	U.S. Avg.
Heart Attack Care				
ACE Inhibitor or ARB for LVSD	140	98%	94%	96%
Aspirin at Arrival	337	99%	99%	99%
Aspirin at Discharge	788	99%	99%	98%
Beta Blocker at Discharge	781	99%	98%	98%
Fibrinolytic Medication Timing[1]	4	50%	50%	55%
PCI Within 90 Minutes of Arrival	56	84%	87%	90%
Smoking Cessation Advice	219	100%	100%	99%
Chest Pain/Possible Heart Attack Care				
Aspirin at Arrival[1,3]	1	0%	97%	95%
Median Time to ECG (minutes)[1,3]	1	16	8	8
Median Time to Transfer (minutes)[5]	0	-	73	61
Fibrinolytic Medication Timing[5]	0	-	37%	54%
Heart Failure Care				
ACE Inhibitor or ARB for LVSD	327	94%	93%	94%
Discharge Instructions	656	85%	86%	88%
Evaluation of LVS Function	925	100%	99%	98%
Smoking Cessation Advice	117	100%	99%	98%
Pneumonia Care				
Appropriate Initial Antibiotic	185	95%	93%	92%
Blood Culture Timing	397	96%	96%	96%
Influenza Vaccine	255	100%	91%	91%
Initial Antibiotic Timing	349	95%	96%	95%
Pneumococcal Vaccine	384	98%	93%	93%
Smoking Cessation Advice	130	100%	98%	97%
Surgical Care Improvement Project				
Appropriate VTP Within 24 Hours[2]	175	97%	95%	92%
Appropriate Hair Removal[2]	759	100%	99%	99%
Appropriate Beta Blocker Usage[2]	263	91%	93%	93%
Controlled Postoperative Blood Glucose[2]	155	92%	91%	93%
Prophylactic Antibiotic Timing[2]	451	95%	96%	97%
Prophylactic Antibiotic Timing (Outpatient)	610	92%	92%	92%
Prophylactic Antibiotic Selection[2]	464	97%	97%	97%
Prophylactic Antibiotic Select. (Outpatient)	604	98%	92%	94%
Prophylactic Antibiotic Stopped[2]	437	94%	95%	94%
Recommended VTP Ordered[2]	175	98%	96%	94%
Urinary Catheter Removal[2]	186	91%	91%	90%
Children's Asthma Care				
Received Systemic Corticosteroids	-	-	-	100%
Received Home Management Plan	-	-	-	71%
Received Reliever Medication	-	-	-	100%
Use of Medical Imaging				
Combination Abdominal CT Scan	490	0.043	0.120	0.191
Combination Chest CT Scan	211	0.232	0.026	0.054
Follow-up Mammogram/Ultrasound	285	14.0%	9.2%	8.4%
MRI for Low Back Pain[1]	51	29.4%	26.9%	32.7%
Survey of Patients' Hospital Experiences				
Area Around Room 'Always' Quiet at Night	300+	44%	-	58%
Doctors 'Always' Communicated Well	300+	76%	-	80%
Home Recovery Information Given	300+	86%	-	82%
Hospital Given 9 or 10 on 10 Point Scale	300+	60%	-	67%
Meds 'Always' Explained Before Given	300+	54%	-	60%
Nurses 'Always' Communicated Well	300+	71%	-	76%
Pain 'Always' Well Controlled	300+	64%	-	69%
Room and Bathroom 'Always' Clean	300+	63%	-	71%
Timely Help 'Always' Received	300+	50%	-	64%
Would Definitely Recommend Hospital	300+	71%	-	69%

NOTE: Hospital profiles are in alphabetical order by state, then city, then hospital within the city; Rankings exclude hospitals with less than 25 cases except for patient surveys which excludes hospitals with less than 100 cases; (a) 100–299 cases; (1) The number of cases is too small to be sure how well a hospital is performing; (2) The hospital indicated that the data submitted for this measure were based on a sample of cases; (3) Data was collected during a shorter time period (fewer quarters) than the maximum possible time for this measure; (4) Suppressed for one or more quarters by CMS; (5) No data is available from the hospital for this measure; (6) Fewer than 100 patients completed the HCAHPS survey. Use these rates with caution, as the number of surveys may be too low to reliably assess hospital performance; (7) Survey results are based on less than 12 months of data; (8) Survey results are not available for this reporting period; (9) No or very few patients were eligible for the HCAHPS survey. The scores shown, if any, reflect a very small number of surveys; (10) A state average was not calculated because too few hospitals in the state submitted data; (11) There were discrepancies in the data collection process; Please refer to the User's Guide for a full explanation of data.

Saint Francis Hospital & Medical Center

114 Woodland Street   Phone: 860-714-4000
Hartford, CT 06105   Fax: 860-714-8048
E-mail: webmaster@stfranciscare.org
URL: www.saintfranciscare.com
Type: Acute Care Hospitals   Emergency Services: Yes
Ownership: Voluntary Non-Profit - Church   Beds: 617
Key Personnel:
Quality Assurance . . . . Nancy Budds
Emergency Room . . . . Judy Wiehl, RN

Measure	Cases	This Hosp.	State Avg.	U.S. Avg.
Heart Attack Care				
ACE Inhibitor or ARB for LVSD	112	93%	94%	96%
Aspirin at Arrival	317	99%	99%	99%
Aspirin at Discharge	546	99%	99%	98%
Beta Blocker at Discharge	527	98%	98%	98%
Fibrinolytic Medication Timing	0	-	50%	55%
PCI Within 90 Minutes of Arrival	73	96%	87%	90%
Smoking Cessation Advice	166	100%	100%	99%
Chest Pain/Possible Heart Attack Care				
Aspirin at Arrival[1]	2	100%	97%	95%
Median Time to ECG (minutes)[1]	2	16	8	8
Median Time to Transfer (minutes)[5]	0	-	73	61
Fibrinolytic Medication Timing[5]	0	-	37%	54%
Heart Failure Care				
ACE Inhibitor or ARB for LVSD[2]	123	94%	93%	94%
Discharge Instructions[2]	225	64%	86%	88%
Evaluation of LVS Function[2]	317	100%	99%	98%
Smoking Cessation Advice[2]	37	100%	99%	98%
Pneumonia Care				
Appropriate Initial Antibiotic[2]	71	92%	93%	92%
Blood Culture Timing[2]	210	94%	96%	96%
Influenza Vaccine[2]	109	87%	91%	91%
Initial Antibiotic Timing[2]	176	90%	96%	95%
Pneumococcal Vaccine[2]	181	94%	93%	93%
Smoking Cessation Advice[2]	61	100%	98%	97%
Surgical Care Improvement Project				
Appropriate VTP Within 24 Hours[2]	180	95%	95%	92%
Appropriate Hair Removal[2]	850	99%	99%	99%
Appropriate Beta Blocker Usage[2]	320	92%	93%	93%
Controlled Postoperative Blood Glucose[2]	166	89%	91%	93%
Prophylactic Antibiotic Timing[2]	603	97%	96%	97%
Prophylactic Antibiotic Timing (Outpatient)	756	94%	92%	92%
Prophylactic Antibiotic Selection[2]	616	98%	97%	97%
Prophylactic Antibiotic Select. (Outpatient)	777	99%	92%	94%
Prophylactic Antibiotic Stopped[2]	587	96%	95%	94%
Recommended VTP Ordered[2]	180	97%	96%	94%
Urinary Catheter Removal[2]	227	93%	91%	90%
Children's Asthma Care				
Received Systemic Corticosteroids	-	-	-	100%
Received Home Management Plan	-	-	-	71%
Received Reliever Medication	-	-	-	100%
Use of Medical Imaging				
Combination Abdominal CT Scan	1,474	0.058	0.120	0.191
Combination Chest CT Scan	1,265	0.007	0.026	0.054
Follow-up Mammogram/Ultrasound	1,175	15.9%	9.2%	8.4%
MRI for Low Back Pain	312	31.1%	26.9%	32.7%
Survey of Patients' Hospital Experiences				
Area Around Room 'Always' Quiet at Night	300+	47%	-	58%
Doctors 'Always' Communicated Well	300+	77%	-	80%
Home Recovery Information Given	300+	82%	-	82%
Hospital Given 9 or 10 on 10 Point Scale	300+	62%	-	67%
Meds 'Always' Explained Before Given	300+	54%	-	60%
Nurses 'Always' Communicated Well	300+	72%	-	76%
Pain 'Always' Well Controlled	300+	66%	-	69%
Room and Bathroom 'Always' Clean	300+	66%	-	71%
Timely Help 'Always' Received	300+	55%	-	64%
Would Definitely Recommend Hospital	300+	71%	-	69%

Manchester Memorial Hospital

71 Haynes St   Phone: 860-647-4780
Manchester, CT 06040   Fax: 860-533-3444
URL: www.echn.org
Type: Acute Care Hospitals   Emergency Services: Yes
Ownership: Voluntary Non-Profit - Private   Beds: 451
Key Personnel:
CEO/President . . . . Peter J Karl
Cardiac Laboratory . . . . Hazar Dahhan, MD
Chief of Medical Staff . . . . Joel J Reich
Pediatric In-Patient Care . . . . . . Jerome Lahman, MD
Quality Assurance . . . . Leona Mariani
Radiology . . . . Stephen Hauser
Emergency Room . . . . Robert F Carroll, MD
Patient Relations . . . . Deborah A Parker, RN

Measure	Cases	This Hosp.	State Avg.	U.S. Avg.
Heart Attack Care				
ACE Inhibitor or ARB for LVSD[1]	7	100%	94%	96%
Aspirin at Arrival	44	100%	99%	99%
Aspirin at Discharge	31	97%	99%	98%
Beta Blocker at Discharge	31	100%	98%	98%
Fibrinolytic Medication Timing	0	-	50%	55%
PCI Within 90 Minutes of Arrival	0	-	87%	90%
Smoking Cessation Advice[1]	7	100%	100%	99%
Chest Pain/Possible Heart Attack Care				
Aspirin at Arrival	50	96%	97%	95%
Median Time to ECG (minutes)	50	14	8	8
Median Time to Transfer (minutes)[1,3]	4	88	73	61
Fibrinolytic Medication Timing[1]	1	0%	37%	54%
Heart Failure Care				
ACE Inhibitor or ARB for LVSD	42	98%	93%	94%
Discharge Instructions	140	87%	86%	88%
Evaluation of LVS Function	195	100%	99%	98%
Smoking Cessation Advice[1]	21	100%	99%	98%
Pneumonia Care				
Appropriate Initial Antibiotic[2]	133	92%	93%	92%
Blood Culture Timing[2]	233	98%	96%	96%
Influenza Vaccine[2]	150	96%	91%	91%
Initial Antibiotic Timing[2]	201	98%	96%	95%
Pneumococcal Vaccine[2]	230	99%	93%	93%
Smoking Cessation Advice[2]	63	100%	98%	97%
Surgical Care Improvement Project				
Appropriate VTP Within 24 Hours[2]	234	94%	95%	92%
Appropriate Hair Removal[2]	507	100%	99%	99%
Appropriate Beta Blocker Usage[2]	153	97%	93%	93%
Controlled Postoperative Blood Glucose[2]	0	-	91%	93%
Prophylactic Antibiotic Timing[2]	301	97%	96%	97%
Prophylactic Antibiotic Timing (Outpatient)	184	95%	92%	92%
Prophylactic Antibiotic Selection[2]	304	96%	97%	97%
Prophylactic Antibiotic Select. (Outpatient)	177	92%	92%	94%
Prophylactic Antibiotic Stopped[2]	283	98%	95%	94%
Recommended VTP Ordered[2]	234	98%	96%	94%
Urinary Catheter Removal[2]	75	93%	91%	90%
Children's Asthma Care				
Received Systemic Corticosteroids	-	-	-	100%
Received Home Management Plan	-	-	-	71%
Received Reliever Medication	-	-	-	100%
Use of Medical Imaging				
Combination Abdominal CT Scan	1,081	0.081	0.120	0.191
Combination Chest CT Scan	974	0.009	0.026	0.054
Follow-up Mammogram/Ultrasound	543	10.1%	9.2%	8.4%
MRI for Low Back Pain	154	22.7%	26.9%	32.7%
Survey of Patients' Hospital Experiences				
Area Around Room 'Always' Quiet at Night	300+	48%	-	58%
Doctors 'Always' Communicated Well	300+	77%	-	80%
Home Recovery Information Given	300+	81%	-	82%
Hospital Given 9 or 10 on 10 Point Scale	300+	59%	-	67%
Meds 'Always' Explained Before Given	300+	59%	-	60%
Nurses 'Always' Communicated Well	300+	74%	-	76%
Pain 'Always' Well Controlled	300+	69%	-	69%
Room and Bathroom 'Always' Clean	300+	62%	-	71%
Timely Help 'Always' Received	300+	57%	-	64%
Would Definitely Recommend Hospital	300+	66%	-	69%

Midstate Medical Center

435 Lewis Ave   Phone: 203-694-8200
Meriden, CT 06450   Fax: 203-694-7601
URL: www.midstatemedical.org
Type: Acute Care Hospitals   Emergency Services: Yes
Ownership: Voluntary Non-Profit - Private   Beds: 130
Key Personnel:
CEO/President . . . . Lucille Janatka
Chief of Medical Staff . . . . Harold Kaplan, MD
Coronary Care . . . . Lynn Amarante, RN
Infection Control . . . . Julia Chiarizio, RN
Operating Room . . . . Peg Sherwood, RN
Pediatric In-Patient Care . . . . . . Luis Alonso, MD
Quality Assurance . . . . Elizabeth Desanto
Radiology . . . . Allen Kratzer, MD

Measure	Cases	This Hosp.	State Avg.	U.S. Avg.
Heart Attack Care				
ACE Inhibitor or ARB for LVSD[1]	6	100%	94%	96%
Aspirin at Arrival	56	98%	99%	99%
Aspirin at Discharge	38	97%	99%	98%
Beta Blocker at Discharge	35	97%	98%	98%
Fibrinolytic Medication Timing	0	-	50%	55%
PCI Within 90 Minutes of Arrival	0	-	87%	90%
Smoking Cessation Advice[1]	3	100%	100%	99%
Chest Pain/Possible Heart Attack Care				
Aspirin at Arrival	123	97%	97%	95%
Median Time to ECG (minutes)	120	6	8	8
Median Time to Transfer (minutes)[1]	18	74	73	61
Fibrinolytic Medication Timing[1]	16	50%	37%	54%
Heart Failure Care				
ACE Inhibitor or ARB for LVSD	61	90%	93%	94%
Discharge Instructions	166	72%	86%	88%
Evaluation of LVS Function	245	96%	99%	98%
Smoking Cessation Advice	30	97%	99%	98%
Pneumonia Care				
Appropriate Initial Antibiotic[2]	127	92%	93%	92%
Blood Culture Timing[2]	197	96%	96%	96%
Influenza Vaccine[2]	120	92%	91%	91%
Initial Antibiotic Timing[2]	204	90%	96%	95%
Pneumococcal Vaccine[2]	199	90%	93%	93%
Smoking Cessation Advice[2]	55	93%	98%	97%
Surgical Care Improvement Project				
Appropriate VTP Within 24 Hours[2]	212	99%	95%	92%
Appropriate Hair Removal[2]	601	99%	99%	99%
Appropriate Beta Blocker Usage[2]	177	90%	93%	93%
Controlled Postoperative Blood Glucose[2]	0	-	91%	93%
Prophylactic Antibiotic Timing[2]	402	96%	96%	97%
Prophylactic Antibiotic Timing (Outpatient)	158	89%	92%	92%
Prophylactic Antibiotic Selection[2]	404	95%	97%	97%
Prophylactic Antibiotic Select. (Outpatient)	157	93%	92%	94%
Prophylactic Antibiotic Stopped[2]	369	98%	95%	94%
Recommended VTP Ordered[2]	214	98%	96%	94%
Urinary Catheter Removal[2]	113	90%	91%	90%
Children's Asthma Care				
Received Systemic Corticosteroids	-	-	-	100%
Received Home Management Plan	-	-	-	71%
Received Reliever Medication	-	-	-	100%
Use of Medical Imaging				
Combination Abdominal CT Scan	917	0.613	0.120	0.191
Combination Chest CT Scan	419	0.002	0.026	0.054
Follow-up Mammogram/Ultrasound	712	8.8%	9.2%	8.4%
MRI for Low Back Pain	169	29.0%	26.9%	32.7%
Survey of Patients' Hospital Experiences				
Area Around Room 'Always' Quiet at Night	300+	56%	-	58%
Doctors 'Always' Communicated Well	300+	81%	-	80%
Home Recovery Information Given	300+	82%	-	82%
Hospital Given 9 or 10 on 10 Point Scale	300+	71%	-	67%
Meds 'Always' Explained Before Given	300+	66%	-	60%
Nurses 'Always' Communicated Well	300+	81%	-	76%
Pain 'Always' Well Controlled	300+	73%	-	69%
Room and Bathroom 'Always' Clean	300+	73%	-	71%
Timely Help 'Always' Received	300+	67%	-	64%
Would Definitely Recommend Hospital	300+	74%	-	69%

NOTE: Hospital profiles are in alphabetical order by state, then city, then hospital within the city; Rankings exclude hospitals with less than 25 cases except for patient surveys which excludes hospitals with less than 100 cases; (a) 100–299 cases; (1) The number of cases is too small to be sure how well a hospital is performing; (2) The hospital indicated that the data submitted for this measure were based on a sample of cases; (3) Data was collected during a shorter time period (fewer quarters) than the maximum possible time for this measure; (4) Suppressed for one or more quarters by CMS; (5) No data is available from the hospital for this measure; (6) Fewer than 100 patients completed the HCAHPS survey. Use these rates with caution, as the number of surveys may be too low to reliably assess hospital performance; (7) Survey results are based on less than 12 months of data; (8) Survey results are not available for this reporting period; (9) No or very few patients were eligible for the HCAHPS survey. The scores shown, if any, reflect a very small number of surveys; (10) A state average was not calculated because too few hospitals in the state submitted data; (11) There were discrepancies in the data collection process; Please refer to the User's Guide for a full explanation of data.

Middlesex Hospital

28 Crescent St
Middletown, CT 06457
URL: www.midhosp.org
Phone: 860-344-6000
Fax: 860-344-6568
Type: Acute Care Hospitals
Emergency Services: Yes
Ownership: Voluntary Non-Profit - Private
Beds: 193

Key Personnel:
CEO/President. . . . . Robert G Kiely
Cardiac Laboratory. . . . . Arthur V McDowell, MD
Chief of Medical Staff . . . . Arthur V McDowell
Pediatric In-Patient Care . . . . Joseph Flanagan, MD
Quality Assurance . . . . Cathleen O'Hara
Radiology. . . . . Diana M Hull, Jr, MD
Emergency Room . . . . Jacquelyn Nelson, RN

Measure	Cases	This Hosp.	State Avg.	U.S. Avg.
Heart Attack Care				
ACE Inhibitor or ARB for LVSD	31	94%	94%	96%
Aspirin at Arrival	59	100%	99%	99%
Aspirin at Discharge	70	100%	99%	98%
Beta Blocker at Discharge	77	100%	98%	98%
Fibrinolytic Medication Timing	0	-	50%	55%
PCI Within 90 Minutes of Arrival	0	-	87%	90%
Smoking Cessation Advice[1]	6	100%	100%	99%
Chest Pain/Possible Heart Attack Care				
Aspirin at Arrival	311	99%	97%	95%
Median Time to ECG (minutes)	321	9	8	8
Median Time to Transfer (minutes)	43	76	73	61
Fibrinolytic Medication Timing[1]	3	0%	37%	54%
Heart Failure Care				
ACE Inhibitor or ARB for LVSD	126	97%	93%	94%
Discharge Instructions	197	91%	86%	88%
Evaluation of LVS Function	329	100%	99%	98%
Smoking Cessation Advice	31	97%	99%	98%
Pneumonia Care				
Appropriate Initial Antibiotic	130	96%	93%	92%
Blood Culture Timing	215	100%	96%	96%
Influenza Vaccine	210	95%	91%	91%
Initial Antibiotic Timing	223	96%	96%	95%
Pneumococcal Vaccine	352	99%	93%	93%
Smoking Cessation Advice	102	99%	98%	97%
Surgical Care Improvement Project				
Appropriate VTP Within 24 Hours	431	94%	95%	92%
Appropriate Hair Removal	1,160	100%	99%	99%
Appropriate Beta Blocker Usage	343	92%	93%	93%
Controlled Postoperative Blood Glucose	0	-	91%	93%
Prophylactic Antibiotic Timing	700	98%	96%	97%
Prophylactic Antibiotic Timing (Outpatient)	164	92%	92%	92%
Prophylactic Antibiotic Selection	702	97%	97%	97%
Prophylactic Antibiotic Select. (Outpatient)	160	94%	92%	94%
Prophylactic Antibiotic Stopped	683	98%	95%	94%
Recommended VTP Ordered	431	96%	96%	94%
Urinary Catheter Removal	254	92%	91%	90%
Children's Asthma Care				
Received Systemic Corticosteroids	-	-	-	100%
Received Home Management Plan	-	-	-	71%
Received Reliever Medication	-	-	-	100%
Use of Medical Imaging				
Combination Abdominal CT Scan	2,046	0.064	0.120	0.191
Combination Chest CT Scan	1,295	0.023	0.026	0.054
Follow-up Mammogram/Ultrasound	2,828	9.0%	9.2%	8.4%
MRI for Low Back Pain	323	25.1%	26.9%	32.7%
Survey of Patients' Hospital Experiences				
Area Around Room 'Always' Quiet at Night	300+	53%	-	58%
Doctors 'Always' Communicated Well	300+	79%	-	80%
Home Recovery Information Given	300+	85%	-	82%
Hospital Given 9 or 10 on 10 Point Scale	300+	75%	-	67%
Meds 'Always' Explained Before Given	300+	63%	-	60%
Nurses 'Always' Communicated Well	300+	78%	-	76%
Pain 'Always' Well Controlled	300+	71%	-	69%
Room and Bathroom 'Always' Clean	300+	79%	-	71%
Timely Help 'Always' Received	300+	66%	-	64%
Would Definitely Recommend Hospital	300+	79%	-	69%

Milford Hospital

300 Seaside Avenue
Milford, CT 06460
URL: www.milfordhospital.org
Phone: 203-876-4000
Type: Acute Care Hospitals
Emergency Services: Yes
Ownership: Voluntary Non-Profit - Private
Beds: 106

Key Personnel:
CEO/President. . . . . Joseph Frolkis
Chief of Medical Staff . . . . Nitai Riegler, MD
Operating Room. . . . . Rosemarie Esposito
Pediatric Ambulatory Care . . . . . . Jeffrey Gruskay, MD
Pediatric In-Patient Care . . . . Jeffrey Gruskay, MD
Quality Assurance . . . . Lloyd Friedman, MD
Radiology. . . . . Paul S David, MD

Measure	Cases	This Hosp.	State Avg.	U.S. Avg.
Heart Attack Care				
ACE Inhibitor or ARB for LVSD[1]	1	100%	94%	96%
Aspirin at Arrival	34	100%	99%	99%
Aspirin at Discharge[1]	14	100%	99%	98%
Beta Blocker at Discharge[1]	14	93%	98%	98%
Fibrinolytic Medication Timing	0	-	50%	55%
PCI Within 90 Minutes of Arrival	0	-	87%	90%
Smoking Cessation Advice	0	-	100%	99%
Chest Pain/Possible Heart Attack Care				
Aspirin at Arrival[1,3]	6	100%	97%	95%
Median Time to ECG (minutes)[1,3]	6	2	8	8
Median Time to Transfer (minutes)[1,3]	2	34	73	61
Fibrinolytic Medication Timing[3]	0	-	37%	54%
Heart Failure Care				
ACE Inhibitor or ARB for LVSD	37	97%	93%	94%
Discharge Instructions	123	93%	86%	88%
Evaluation of LVS Function	187	99%	99%	98%
Smoking Cessation Advice[1]	19	95%	99%	98%
Pneumonia Care				
Appropriate Initial Antibiotic	95	96%	93%	92%
Blood Culture Timing	179	94%	96%	96%
Influenza Vaccine	106	95%	91%	91%
Initial Antibiotic Timing	151	97%	96%	95%
Pneumococcal Vaccine	175	98%	93%	93%
Smoking Cessation Advice	37	97%	98%	97%
Surgical Care Improvement Project				
Appropriate VTP Within 24 Hours[2]	114	89%	95%	92%
Appropriate Hair Removal[2]	449	100%	99%	99%
Appropriate Beta Blocker Usage[2]	125	97%	93%	93%
Controlled Postoperative Blood Glucose[2]	0	-	91%	93%
Prophylactic Antibiotic Timing[2]	298	98%	96%	97%
Prophylactic Antibiotic Timing (Outpatient)	39	95%	92%	92%
Prophylactic Antibiotic Selection[2]	300	100%	97%	97%
Prophylactic Antibiotic Select. (Outpatient)	37	100%	92%	94%
Prophylactic Antibiotic Stopped[2]	289	95%	95%	94%
Recommended VTP Ordered[2]	114	92%	96%	94%
Urinary Catheter Removal[2]	149	98%	91%	90%
Children's Asthma Care				
Received Systemic Corticosteroids	-	-	-	100%
Received Home Management Plan	-	-	-	71%
Received Reliever Medication	-	-	-	100%
Use of Medical Imaging				
Combination Abdominal CT Scan	425	0.127	0.120	0.191
Combination Chest CT Scan	186	0.054	0.026	0.054
Follow-up Mammogram/Ultrasound[1]	51	23.5%	9.2%	8.4%
MRI for Low Back Pain	71	19.7%	26.9%	32.7%
Survey of Patients' Hospital Experiences				
Area Around Room 'Always' Quiet at Night	300+	61%	-	58%
Doctors 'Always' Communicated Well	300+	81%	-	80%
Home Recovery Information Given	300+	81%	-	82%
Hospital Given 9 or 10 on 10 Point Scale	300+	71%	-	67%
Meds 'Always' Explained Before Given	300+	57%	-	60%
Nurses 'Always' Communicated Well	300+	78%	-	76%
Pain 'Always' Well Controlled	300+	70%	-	69%
Room and Bathroom 'Always' Clean	300+	81%	-	71%
Timely Help 'Always' Received	300+	69%	-	64%
Would Definitely Recommend Hospital	300+	75%	-	69%

The Hospital of Central Connecticut

100 Grand Street
New Britain, CT 06050
E-mail: moreinfo@thocc.org
URL: www.thocc.org
Phone: 860-224-5011
Fax: 860-224-5779
Type: Acute Care Hospitals
Emergency Services: Yes
Ownership: Voluntary Non-Profit - Other
Beds: 330

Key Personnel:
CEO/President. . . . . Laurence Tanner
Chief of Medical Staff . . . . James L Bernene, MD
Infection Control. . . . . Diane Dowling, RN
Quality Assurance . . . . Elizabeth Schuff
Radiology. . . . . Stephen Grund, MD
Emergency Room . . . . Jeffrey Finkelstein, MD
Intensive Care Unit. . . . . Paula Bowley, RN
Patient Relations . . . . Elaine Greene

Measure	Cases	This Hosp.	State Avg.	U.S. Avg.
Heart Attack Care				
ACE Inhibitor or ARB for LVSD	41	88%	94%	96%
Aspirin at Arrival	247	97%	99%	99%
Aspirin at Discharge	175	93%	99%	98%
Beta Blocker at Discharge	185	98%	98%	98%
Fibrinolytic Medication Timing	0	-	50%	55%
PCI Within 90 Minutes of Arrival	39	97%	87%	90%
Smoking Cessation Advice	52	100%	100%	99%
Chest Pain/Possible Heart Attack Care				
Aspirin at Arrival	40	95%	97%	95%
Median Time to ECG (minutes)	41	11	8	8
Median Time to Transfer (minutes)[1]	9	44	73	61
Fibrinolytic Medication Timing	0	-	37%	54%
Heart Failure Care				
ACE Inhibitor or ARB for LVSD	186	89%	93%	94%
Discharge Instructions	501	91%	86%	88%
Evaluation of LVS Function	689	100%	99%	98%
Smoking Cessation Advice	117	100%	99%	98%
Pneumonia Care				
Appropriate Initial Antibiotic	290	98%	93%	92%
Blood Culture Timing	518	99%	96%	96%
Influenza Vaccine	318	96%	91%	91%
Initial Antibiotic Timing	442	99%	96%	95%
Pneumococcal Vaccine	405	98%	93%	93%
Smoking Cessation Advice	153	100%	98%	97%
Surgical Care Improvement Project				
Appropriate VTP Within 24 Hours[2]	355	98%	95%	92%
Appropriate Hair Removal[2]	975	100%	99%	99%
Appropriate Beta Blocker Usage[2]	322	97%	93%	93%
Controlled Postoperative Blood Glucose[2]	0	-	91%	93%
Prophylactic Antibiotic Timing[2]	723	95%	96%	97%
Prophylactic Antibiotic Timing (Outpatient)	236	82%	92%	92%
Prophylactic Antibiotic Selection[2]	723	97%	97%	97%
Prophylactic Antibiotic Select. (Outpatient)	201	92%	92%	94%
Prophylactic Antibiotic Stopped[2]	691	97%	95%	94%
Recommended VTP Ordered[2]	355	99%	96%	94%
Urinary Catheter Removal[2]	265	93%	91%	90%
Children's Asthma Care				
Received Systemic Corticosteroids	-	-	-	100%
Received Home Management Plan	-	-	-	71%
Received Reliever Medication	-	-	-	100%
Use of Medical Imaging				
Combination Abdominal CT Scan	1,586	0.066	0.120	0.191
Combination Chest CT Scan	1,171	0.012	0.026	0.054
Follow-up Mammogram/Ultrasound	2,652	13.1%	9.2%	8.4%
MRI for Low Back Pain	191	21.5%	26.9%	32.7%
Survey of Patients' Hospital Experiences				
Area Around Room 'Always' Quiet at Night	300+	46%	-	58%
Doctors 'Always' Communicated Well	300+	76%	-	80%
Home Recovery Information Given	300+	82%	-	82%
Hospital Given 9 or 10 on 10 Point Scale	300+	65%	-	67%
Meds 'Always' Explained Before Given	300+	60%	-	60%
Nurses 'Always' Communicated Well	300+	75%	-	76%
Pain 'Always' Well Controlled	300+	69%	-	69%
Room and Bathroom 'Always' Clean	300+	72%	-	71%
Timely Help 'Always' Received	300+	60%	-	64%
Would Definitely Recommend Hospital	300+	69%	-	69%

NOTE: Hospital profiles are in alphabetical order by state, then city, then hospital within the city; Rankings exclude hospitals with less than 25 cases except for patient surveys which excludes hospitals with less than 100 cases; (a) 100–299 cases; (1) The number of cases is too small to be sure how well a hospital is performing; (2) The hospital indicated that the data submitted for this measure were based on a sample of cases; (3) Data was collected during a shorter time period (fewer quarters) than the maximum possible time for this measure; (4) Suppressed for one or more quarters by CMS; (5) No data is available from the hospital for this measure; (6) Fewer than 100 patients completed the HCAHPS survey. Use these rates with caution, as the number of surveys may be too low to reliably assess hospital performance; (7) Survey results are based on less than 12 months of data; (8) Survey results are not available for this reporting period; (9) No or very few patients were eligible for the HCAHPS survey. The scores shown, if any, reflect a very small number of surveys; (10) A state average was not calculated because too few hospitals in the state submitted data; (11) There were discrepancies in the data collection process; Please refer to the User's Guide for a full explanation of data.

Hospital of St Raphael

1450 Chapel St
New Haven, CT 06511
Phone: 203-789-3000
Fax: 203-789-4053
E-mail: webmaster@srhs.org
URL: www.srhs.org
Type: Acute Care Hospitals
Emergency Services: No
Ownership: Voluntary Non-Profit - Other
Beds: 511

Key Personnel:

CEO/President. . . . . David W Benfer
Cardiac Laboratory. . . . . Thomas Donohue MD
Infection Control. . . . . John Boyce MD
Operating Room. . . . . Letty Corrado RN
Pediatric Ambulatory Care . . . . . . Richard Young MD
Pediatric In-Patient Care . . . . Richard Young MD
Quality Assurance . . . . Janeanne Lubin Szafranski
Radiology. . . . . Diego Nunez MD

Measure	Cases	This Hosp.	State Avg.	U.S. Avg.
Heart Attack Care				
ACE Inhibitor or ARB for LVSD	55	100%	94%	96%
Aspirin at Arrival	227	98%	99%	99%
Aspirin at Discharge	351	99%	99%	98%
Beta Blocker at Discharge	334	99%	98%	98%
Fibrinolytic Medication Timing	0	-	50%	55%
PCI Within 90 Minutes of Arrival	53	60%	87%	90%
Smoking Cessation Advice	93	100%	100%	99%
Chest Pain/Possible Heart Attack Care				
Aspirin at Arrival[5]	0	-	97%	95%
Median Time to ECG (minutes)[5]	0	-	8	8
Median Time to Transfer (minutes)[5]	0	-	73	61
Fibrinolytic Medication Timing[5]	0	-	37%	54%
Heart Failure Care				
ACE Inhibitor or ARB for LVSD[2]	77	94%	93%	94%
Discharge Instructions[2]	228	95%	86%	88%
Evaluation of LVS Function[2]	333	98%	99%	98%
Smoking Cessation Advice[2]	42	100%	99%	98%
Pneumonia Care				
Appropriate Initial Antibiotic[2]	106	95%	93%	92%
Blood Culture Timing[2]	163	91%	96%	96%
Influenza Vaccine[2]	118	85%	91%	91%
Initial Antibiotic Timing[2]	205	95%	96%	95%
Pneumococcal Vaccine[2]	221	94%	93%	93%
Smoking Cessation Advice[2]	48	100%	98%	97%
Surgical Care Improvement Project				
Appropriate VTP Within 24 Hours[2]	178	97%	95%	92%
Appropriate Hair Removal[2]	888	100%	99%	99%
Appropriate Beta Blocker Usage[2]	333	92%	93%	93%
Controlled Postoperative Blood Glucose[2]	205	85%	91%	93%
Prophylactic Antibiotic Timing[2]	668	96%	96%	97%
Prophylactic Antibiotic Timing (Outpatient)	510	89%	92%	92%
Prophylactic Antibiotic Selection[2]	675	96%	97%	97%
Prophylactic Antibiotic Select. (Outpatient)	482	84%	92%	94%
Prophylactic Antibiotic Stopped[2]	638	97%	95%	94%
Recommended VTP Ordered[2]	178	97%	96%	94%
Urinary Catheter Removal[2]	216	92%	91%	90%
Children's Asthma Care				
Received Systemic Corticosteroids	-	-	-	100%
Received Home Management Plan	-	-	-	71%
Received Reliever Medication	-	-	-	100%
Use of Medical Imaging				
Combination Abdominal CT Scan	1,177	0.093	0.120	0.191
Combination Chest CT Scan	1,250	0.009	0.026	0.054
Follow-up Mammogram/Ultrasound	529	8.1%	9.2%	8.4%
MRI for Low Back Pain[1]	1	0.0%	26.9%	32.7%
Survey of Patients' Hospital Experiences				
Area Around Room 'Always' Quiet at Night	300+	42%	-	58%
Doctors 'Always' Communicated Well	300+	75%	-	80%
Home Recovery Information Given	300+	82%	-	82%
Hospital Given 9 or 10 on 10 Point Scale	300+	65%	-	67%
Meds 'Always' Explained Before Given	300+	58%	-	60%
Nurses 'Always' Communicated Well	300+	75%	-	76%
Pain 'Always' Well Controlled	300+	68%	-	69%
Room and Bathroom 'Always' Clean	300+	68%	-	71%
Timely Help 'Always' Received	300+	62%	-	64%
Would Definitely Recommend Hospital	300+	71%	-	69%

Yale-New Haven Hospital

20 York St
New Haven, CT 06504
Phone: 203-688-4242
Fax: 203-688-3203
URL: www.ynhh.org
Type: Acute Care Hospitals
Emergency Services: No
Ownership: Voluntary Non-Profit - Private
Beds: 944

Key Personnel:

CEO/President. . . . . Marna P Borgstrom
Chief of Medical Staff. . . . . Peter N Herbert MD

Measure	Cases	This Hosp.	State Avg.	U.S. Avg.
Heart Attack Care				
ACE Inhibitor or ARB for LVSD[2]	29	97%	94%	96%
Aspirin at Arrival[2]	127	100%	99%	99%
Aspirin at Discharge[2]	282	99%	99%	98%
Beta Blocker at Discharge[2]	264	98%	98%	98%
Fibrinolytic Medication Timing[2]	0	-	50%	55%
PCI Within 90 Minutes of Arrival[1,2]	21	76%	87%	90%
Smoking Cessation Advice[2]	82	100%	100%	99%
Chest Pain/Possible Heart Attack Care				
Aspirin at Arrival[5]	0	-	97%	95%
Median Time to ECG (minutes)[5]	0	-	8	8
Median Time to Transfer (minutes)[5]	0	-	73	61
Fibrinolytic Medication Timing[5]	0	-	37%	54%
Heart Failure Care				
ACE Inhibitor or ARB for LVSD[2]	84	93%	93%	94%
Discharge Instructions[2]	223	90%	86%	88%
Evaluation of LVS Function[2]	287	100%	99%	98%
Smoking Cessation Advice[2]	48	100%	99%	98%
Pneumonia Care				
Appropriate Initial Antibiotic[2]	36	75%	93%	92%
Blood Culture Timing[2]	85	93%	96%	96%
Influenza Vaccine[2]	73	67%	91%	91%
Initial Antibiotic Timing[2]	86	95%	96%	95%
Pneumococcal Vaccine[2]	114	74%	93%	93%
Smoking Cessation Advice[2]	47	100%	98%	97%
Surgical Care Improvement Project				
Appropriate VTP Within 24 Hours[2]	180	93%	95%	92%
Appropriate Hair Removal[2]	608	99%	99%	99%
Appropriate Beta Blocker Usage[2]	218	87%	93%	93%
Controlled Postoperative Blood Glucose[2]	120	90%	91%	93%
Prophylactic Antibiotic Timing[2]	389	96%	96%	97%
Prophylactic Antibiotic Timing (Outpatient)	514	87%	92%	92%
Prophylactic Antibiotic Selection[2]	395	98%	97%	97%
Prophylactic Antibiotic Select. (Outpatient)	493	65%	92%	94%
Prophylactic Antibiotic Stopped[2]	344	96%	95%	94%
Recommended VTP Ordered[2]	181	94%	96%	94%
Urinary Catheter Removal[2]	160	82%	91%	90%
Children's Asthma Care				
Received Systemic Corticosteroids[2]	322	100%	-	100%
Received Home Management Plan[2]	324	73%	-	71%
Received Reliever Medication[2]	323	100%	-	100%
Use of Medical Imaging				
Combination Abdominal CT Scan	2,598	0.135	0.120	0.191
Combination Chest CT Scan	2,902	0.003	0.026	0.054
Follow-up Mammogram/Ultrasound	4,522	7.8%	9.2%	8.4%
MRI for Low Back Pain	460	23.3%	26.9%	32.7%
Survey of Patients' Hospital Experiences				
Area Around Room 'Always' Quiet at Night	300+	47%	-	58%
Doctors 'Always' Communicated Well	300+	75%	-	80%
Home Recovery Information Given	300+	82%	-	82%
Hospital Given 9 or 10 on 10 Point Scale	300+	64%	-	67%
Meds 'Always' Explained Before Given	300+	59%	-	60%
Nurses 'Always' Communicated Well	300+	73%	-	76%
Pain 'Always' Well Controlled	300+	65%	-	69%
Room and Bathroom 'Always' Clean	300+	61%	-	71%
Timely Help 'Always' Received	300+	55%	-	64%
Would Definitely Recommend Hospital	300+	71%	-	69%

Lawrence & Memorial Hospital

365 Montauk Ave
New London, CT 06320
Phone: 860-442-0711
Fax: 860-444-3717
E-mail: kanthony@lmhosp.org
URL: www.lmhospital.org
Type: Acute Care Hospitals
Emergency Services: No
Ownership: Voluntary Non-Profit - Private
Beds: 350

Key Personnel:

CEO/President. . . . . Bruce D Cummings
Cardiac Laboratory. . . . . Gerry Mulholland
Operating Room. . . . . Joe Aldred
Pediatric In-Patient Care . . . . Bernard N Giserman, MD
Quality Assurance . . . . Sherry Strammiello
Radiology. . . . . Donna Blakley
Ambulatory Care . . . . Anthony Coppola, MD
Emergency Room . . . . Ronnie Hanrahan, RN

Measure	Cases	This Hosp.	State Avg.	U.S. Avg.
Heart Attack Care				
ACE Inhibitor or ARB for LVSD[1,2]	18	100%	94%	96%
Aspirin at Arrival[2]	133	98%	99%	99%
Aspirin at Discharge[2]	117	99%	99%	98%
Beta Blocker at Discharge[2]	109	100%	98%	98%
Fibrinolytic Medication Timing[2]	0	-	50%	55%
PCI Within 90 Minutes of Arrival[2]	31	84%	87%	90%
Smoking Cessation Advice[2]	39	100%	100%	99%
Chest Pain/Possible Heart Attack Care				
Aspirin at Arrival	26	100%	97%	95%
Median Time to ECG (minutes)	28	8	8	8
Median Time to Transfer (minutes)[1,3]	2	122	73	61
Fibrinolytic Medication Timing	0	-	37%	54%
Heart Failure Care				
ACE Inhibitor or ARB for LVSD[2]	53	91%	93%	94%
Discharge Instructions[2]	194	79%	86%	88%
Evaluation of LVS Function[2]	287	97%	99%	98%
Smoking Cessation Advice[2]	28	100%	99%	98%
Pneumonia Care				
Appropriate Initial Antibiotic[2]	73	81%	93%	92%
Blood Culture Timing[2]	123	95%	96%	96%
Influenza Vaccine[2]	82	93%	91%	91%
Initial Antibiotic Timing[2]	122	94%	96%	95%
Pneumococcal Vaccine[2]	133	93%	93%	93%
Smoking Cessation Advice[2]	52	100%	98%	97%
Surgical Care Improvement Project				
Appropriate VTP Within 24 Hours[2]	156	92%	95%	92%
Appropriate Hair Removal[2]	426	99%	99%	99%
Appropriate Beta Blocker Usage[2]	150	94%	93%	93%
Controlled Postoperative Blood Glucose[2]	0	-	91%	93%
Prophylactic Antibiotic Timing[2]	301	98%	96%	97%
Prophylactic Antibiotic Timing (Outpatient)	211	96%	92%	92%
Prophylactic Antibiotic Selection[2]	302	97%	97%	97%
Prophylactic Antibiotic Select. (Outpatient)	205	96%	92%	94%
Prophylactic Antibiotic Stopped[2]	296	96%	95%	94%
Recommended VTP Ordered[2]	156	94%	96%	94%
Urinary Catheter Removal[2]	85	92%	91%	90%
Children's Asthma Care				
Received Systemic Corticosteroids	-	-	-	100%
Received Home Management Plan	-	-	-	71%
Received Reliever Medication	-	-	-	100%
Use of Medical Imaging				
Combination Abdominal CT Scan	1,370	0.088	0.120	0.191
Combination Chest CT Scan	1,183	0.000	0.026	0.054
Follow-up Mammogram/Ultrasound	3,080	5.6%	9.2%	8.4%
MRI for Low Back Pain	228	32.0%	26.9%	32.7%
Survey of Patients' Hospital Experiences				
Area Around Room 'Always' Quiet at Night	300+	46%	-	58%
Doctors 'Always' Communicated Well	300+	75%	-	80%
Home Recovery Information Given	300+	80%	-	82%
Hospital Given 9 or 10 on 10 Point Scale	300+	60%	-	67%
Meds 'Always' Explained Before Given	300+	56%	-	60%
Nurses 'Always' Communicated Well	300+	75%	-	76%
Pain 'Always' Well Controlled	300+	69%	-	69%
Room and Bathroom 'Always' Clean	300+	65%	-	71%
Timely Help 'Always' Received	300+	58%	-	64%
Would Definitely Recommend Hospital	300+	69%	-	69%

NOTE: Hospital profiles are in alphabetical order by state, then city, then hospital within the city; Rankings exclude hospitals with less than 25 cases except for patient surveys which excludes hospitals with less than 100 cases; (a) 100–299 cases; (1) The number of cases is too small to be sure how well a hospital is performing; (2) The hospital indicated that the data submitted for this measure were based on a sample of cases; (3) Data was collected during a shorter time period (fewer quarters) than the maximum possible time for this measure; (4) Suppressed for one or more quarters by CMS; (5) No data is available from the hospital for this measure; (6) Fewer than 100 patients completed the HCAHPS survey. Use these rates with caution, as the number of surveys may be too low to reliably assess hospital performance; (7) Survey results are based on less than 12 months of data; (8) Survey results are not available for this reporting period; (9) No or very few patients were eligible for the HCAHPS survey. The scores shown, if any, reflect a very small number of surveys; (10) A state average was not calculated because too few hospitals in the state submitted data; (11) There were discrepancies in the data collection process; Please refer to the User's Guide for a full explanation of data.

New Milford Hospital

21 Elm St
New Milford, CT 06776
Phone: 860-355-2611
Fax: 860-210-7422
URL: www.newmilfordhospital.org
Type: Acute Care Hospitals
Emergency Services: No
Ownership: Voluntary Non-Profit - Private
Beds: 85

Key Personnel:
CEO/President. . . . . Richard E Pugh
Chief of Medical Staff. . . . . Thomas Koobatian, MD
Infection Control. . . . . Brenda Warren, RN
Operating Room. . . . . Courtney E Chambers, RN
Pediatric Ambulatory Care . . . . . . Evan Hack, MD
Pediatric In-Patient Care . . . . . . Evan Hack, MD
Quality Assurance . . . . Linda Vryhof
Radiology. . . . . Andrea Q Crowley, MD

Measure	Cases	This Hosp.	State Avg.	U.S. Avg.
Heart Attack Care				
ACE Inhibitor or ARB for LVSD[1]	2	100%	94%	96%
Aspirin at Arrival[1]	11	100%	99%	99%
Aspirin at Discharge[1]	8	100%	99%	98%
Beta Blocker at Discharge[1]	8	88%	98%	98%
Fibrinolytic Medication Timing	0	-	50%	55%
PCI Within 90 Minutes of Arrival	0	-	87%	90%
Smoking Cessation Advice	0	-	100%	99%
Chest Pain/Possible Heart Attack Care				
Aspirin at Arrival	42	98%	97%	95%
Median Time to ECG (minutes)	41	10	8	8
Median Time to Transfer (minutes)[1]	12	84	73	61
Fibrinolytic Medication Timing	0	-	37%	54%
Heart Failure Care				
ACE Inhibitor or ARB for LVSD[1]	21	90%	93%	94%
Discharge Instructions	41	83%	86%	88%
Evaluation of LVS Function	75	99%	99%	98%
Smoking Cessation Advice[1]	9	100%	99%	98%
Pneumonia Care				
Appropriate Initial Antibiotic	44	93%	93%	92%
Blood Culture Timing	53	92%	96%	96%
Influenza Vaccine	35	77%	91%	91%
Initial Antibiotic Timing	57	100%	96%	95%
Pneumococcal Vaccine	57	81%	93%	93%
Smoking Cessation Advice[1]	16	100%	98%	97%
Surgical Care Improvement Project				
Appropriate VTP Within 24 Hours[2]	76	99%	95%	92%
Appropriate Hair Removal[2]	252	100%	99%	99%
Appropriate Beta Blocker Usage[2]	73	100%	93%	93%
Controlled Postoperative Blood Glucose[2]	0	-	91%	93%
Prophylactic Antibiotic Timing[2]	187	97%	96%	97%
Prophylactic Antibiotic Timing (Outpatient)	77	91%	92%	92%
Prophylactic Antibiotic Selection[2]	189	97%	97%	97%
Prophylactic Antibiotic Select. (Outpatient)	70	99%	92%	94%
Prophylactic Antibiotic Stopped[2]	185	96%	95%	94%
Recommended VTP Ordered[2]	76	99%	96%	94%
Urinary Catheter Removal[1,2]	17	76%	91%	90%
Children's Asthma Care				
Received Systemic Corticosteroids	-	-	-	100%
Received Home Management Plan	-	-	-	71%
Received Reliever Medication	-	-	-	100%
Use of Medical Imaging				
Combination Abdominal CT Scan	628	0.057	0.120	0.191
Combination Chest CT Scan	618	0.005	0.026	0.054
Follow-up Mammogram/Ultrasound	709	4.7%	9.2%	8.4%
MRI for Low Back Pain	84	34.5%	26.9%	32.7%
Survey of Patients' Hospital Experiences				
Area Around Room 'Always' Quiet at Night	300+	56%	-	58%
Doctors 'Always' Communicated Well	300+	81%	-	80%
Home Recovery Information Given	300+	82%	-	82%
Hospital Given 9 or 10 on 10 Point Scale	300+	70%	-	67%
Meds 'Always' Explained Before Given	300+	57%	-	60%
Nurses 'Always' Communicated Well	300+	78%	-	76%
Pain 'Always' Well Controlled	300+	71%	-	69%
Room and Bathroom 'Always' Clean	300+	74%	-	71%
Timely Help 'Always' Received	300+	64%	-	64%
Would Definitely Recommend Hospital	300+	75%	-	69%

Norwalk Hospital Association

24 Stevens Street
Norwalk, CT 06856
Phone: 203-852-2000
Fax: 203-855-3987
E-mail: hr@norwalkhealth.org
URL: www.norwalkhosp.org
Type: Acute Care Hospitals
Emergency Services: No
Ownership: Voluntary Non-Profit - Private
Beds: 328

Key Personnel:
CEO/President. . . . . Dan Deborah
Chief of Medical Staff . . . . Michael Macks, MD
Coronary Care . . . . Debbie Bailey
Infection Control. . . . . Erin Fitzgerald
Pediatric Ambulatory Care . . . . . . Vicki Smetak, MD
Pediatric In-Patient Care . . . . . . Vicki Smetak, MD
Quality Assurance . . . . Claire Davis, RN
Radiology. . . . . Alan Richman MD

Measure	Cases	This Hosp.	State Avg.	U.S. Avg.
Heart Attack Care				
ACE Inhibitor or ARB for LVSD[1]	21	100%	94%	96%
Aspirin at Arrival	161	99%	99%	99%
Aspirin at Discharge	94	100%	99%	98%
Beta Blocker at Discharge	98	99%	98%	98%
Fibrinolytic Medication Timing	0	-	50%	55%
PCI Within 90 Minutes of Arrival	33	94%	87%	90%
Smoking Cessation Advice	26	100%	100%	99%
Chest Pain/Possible Heart Attack Care				
Aspirin at Arrival[1]	15	100%	97%	95%
Median Time to ECG (minutes)[1]	16	12	8	8
Median Time to Transfer (minutes)[5]	0	-	73	61
Fibrinolytic Medication Timing[3]	0	-	37%	54%
Heart Failure Care				
ACE Inhibitor or ARB for LVSD[2]	82	96%	93%	94%
Discharge Instructions[2]	220	72%	86%	88%
Evaluation of LVS Function[2]	330	100%	99%	98%
Smoking Cessation Advice[2]	37	97%	99%	98%
Pneumonia Care				
Appropriate Initial Antibiotic[2]	100	98%	93%	92%
Blood Culture Timing[2]	156	100%	96%	96%
Influenza Vaccine[2]	96	85%	91%	91%
Initial Antibiotic Timing[2]	182	96%	96%	95%
Pneumococcal Vaccine[2]	208	88%	93%	93%
Smoking Cessation Advice[2]	49	100%	98%	97%
Surgical Care Improvement Project				
Appropriate VTP Within 24 Hours	341	94%	95%	92%
Appropriate Hair Removal	765	100%	99%	99%
Appropriate Beta Blocker Usage	207	91%	93%	93%
Controlled Postoperative Blood Glucose[1]	2	100%	91%	93%
Prophylactic Antibiotic Timing	448	99%	96%	97%
Prophylactic Antibiotic Timing (Outpatient)	247	96%	92%	92%
Prophylactic Antibiotic Selection	450	98%	97%	97%
Prophylactic Antibiotic Select. (Outpatient)	242	88%	92%	94%
Prophylactic Antibiotic Stopped	412	97%	95%	94%
Recommended VTP Ordered	341	94%	96%	94%
Urinary Catheter Removal	80	70%	91%	90%
Children's Asthma Care				
Received Systemic Corticosteroids	-	-	-	100%
Received Home Management Plan	-	-	-	71%
Received Reliever Medication	-	-	-	100%
Use of Medical Imaging				
Combination Abdominal CT Scan	758	0.066	0.120	0.191
Combination Chest CT Scan	590	0.059	0.026	0.054
Follow-up Mammogram/Ultrasound	294	14.3%	9.2%	8.4%
MRI for Low Back Pain	397	24.7%	26.9%	32.7%
Survey of Patients' Hospital Experiences				
Area Around Room 'Always' Quiet at Night	300+	38%	-	58%
Doctors 'Always' Communicated Well	300+	80%	-	80%
Home Recovery Information Given	300+	79%	-	82%
Hospital Given 9 or 10 on 10 Point Scale	300+	67%	-	67%
Meds 'Always' Explained Before Given	300+	60%	-	60%
Nurses 'Always' Communicated Well	300+	74%	-	76%
Pain 'Always' Well Controlled	300+	72%	-	69%
Room and Bathroom 'Always' Clean	300+	73%	-	71%
Timely Help 'Always' Received	300+	62%	-	64%
Would Definitely Recommend Hospital	300+	75%	-	69%

William W Backus Hospital

326 Washington St
Norwich, CT 06360
Phone: 860-889-8331
Fax: 860-823-6329
E-mail: smawhiney@wwbh.org
URL: www.backushospital.org
Type: Acute Care Hospitals
Emergency Services: No
Ownership: Voluntary Non-Profit - Other
Beds: 20

Key Personnel:
CEO/President. . . . . Thomas P Pipicelli
Chief of Medical Staff . . . . Peter Shea, MD
Pediatric Ambulatory Care . . . . . . Ravi Prakash, MD
Quality Assurance . . . . Joseph Hughes
Radiology. . . . . Herb Lustberg, MD
Emergency Room . . . . Susan Davis, RN

Measure	Cases	This Hosp.	State Avg.	U.S. Avg.
Heart Attack Care				
ACE Inhibitor or ARB for LVSD[1]	9	100%	94%	96%
Aspirin at Arrival	61	97%	99%	99%
Aspirin at Discharge	39	92%	99%	98%
Beta Blocker at Discharge	37	100%	98%	98%
Fibrinolytic Medication Timing[1]	1	100%	50%	55%
PCI Within 90 Minutes of Arrival	0	-	87%	90%
Smoking Cessation Advice[1]	7	100%	100%	99%
Chest Pain/Possible Heart Attack Care				
Aspirin at Arrival	220	99%	97%	95%
Median Time to ECG (minutes)	224	5	8	8
Median Time to Transfer (minutes)	52	86	73	61
Fibrinolytic Medication Timing[1]	5	40%	37%	54%
Heart Failure Care				
ACE Inhibitor or ARB for LVSD	85	96%	93%	94%
Discharge Instructions	226	84%	86%	88%
Evaluation of LVS Function	305	100%	99%	98%
Smoking Cessation Advice	57	100%	99%	98%
Pneumonia Care				
Appropriate Initial Antibiotic[2]	99	92%	93%	92%
Blood Culture Timing[2]	161	92%	96%	96%
Influenza Vaccine[2]	120	81%	91%	91%
Initial Antibiotic Timing[2]	195	97%	96%	95%
Pneumococcal Vaccine[2]	181	87%	93%	93%
Smoking Cessation Advice[2]	83	100%	98%	97%
Surgical Care Improvement Project				
Appropriate VTP Within 24 Hours[2]	219	92%	95%	92%
Appropriate Hair Removal[2]	481	99%	99%	99%
Appropriate Beta Blocker Usage[2]	143	92%	93%	93%
Controlled Postoperative Blood Glucose[2]	0	-	91%	93%
Prophylactic Antibiotic Timing[2]	323	92%	96%	97%
Prophylactic Antibiotic Timing (Outpatient)	291	92%	92%	92%
Prophylactic Antibiotic Selection[2]	320	97%	97%	97%
Prophylactic Antibiotic Select. (Outpatient)	290	93%	92%	94%
Prophylactic Antibiotic Stopped[2]	307	96%	95%	94%
Recommended VTP Ordered[2]	219	96%	96%	94%
Urinary Catheter Removal[2]	87	92%	91%	90%
Children's Asthma Care				
Received Systemic Corticosteroids	-	-	-	100%
Received Home Management Plan	-	-	-	71%
Received Reliever Medication	-	-	-	100%
Use of Medical Imaging				
Combination Abdominal CT Scan	1,563	0.061	0.120	0.191
Combination Chest CT Scan	1,444	0.006	0.026	0.054
Follow-up Mammogram/Ultrasound	2,020	6.2%	9.2%	8.4%
MRI for Low Back Pain	278	25.2%	26.9%	32.7%
Survey of Patients' Hospital Experiences				
Area Around Room 'Always' Quiet at Night	300+	48%	-	58%
Doctors 'Always' Communicated Well	300+	74%	-	80%
Home Recovery Information Given	300+	82%	-	82%
Hospital Given 9 or 10 on 10 Point Scale	300+	67%	-	67%
Meds 'Always' Explained Before Given	300+	55%	-	60%
Nurses 'Always' Communicated Well	300+	74%	-	76%
Pain 'Always' Well Controlled	300+	64%	-	69%
Room and Bathroom 'Always' Clean	300+	74%	-	71%
Timely Help 'Always' Received	300+	60%	-	64%
Would Definitely Recommend Hospital	300+	71%	-	69%

NOTE: Hospital profiles are in alphabetical order by state, then city, then hospital within the city; Rankings exclude hospitals with less than 25 cases except for patient surveys which excludes hospitals with less than 100 cases; (a) 100–299 cases; (1) The number of cases is too small to be sure how well a hospital is performing; (2) The hospital indicated that the data submitted for this measure were based on a sample of cases; (3) Data was collected during a shorter time period (fewer quarters) than the maximum possible time for this measure; (4) Suppressed for one or more quarters by CMS; (5) No data is available from the hospital for this measure; (6) Fewer than 100 patients completed the HCAHPS survey. Use these rates with caution, as the number of surveys may be too low to reliably assess hospital performance; (7) Survey results are based on less than 12 months of data; (8) Survey results are not available for this reporting period; (9) No or very few patients were eligible for the HCAHPS survey. The scores shown, if any, reflect a very small number of surveys; (10) A state average was not calculated because too few hospitals in the state submitted data; (11) There were discrepancies in the data collection process; Please refer to the User's Guide for a full explanation of data.

Day Kimball Hospital

320 Pomfret Street
Putnam, CT 06260
Phone: 860-928-6541
Fax: 860-963-6375
E-mail: ilisee@daykimball.org
URL: www.daykimball.org
Type: Acute Care Hospitals
Emergency Services: Yes
Ownership: Voluntary Non-Profit - Private
Beds: 103

Key Personnel:
CEO/President. . . . . Ann Errichetti, MD
Chief of Medical Staff. . . . . John Day
Infection Control. . . . . Douglas Waite, MD
Quality Assurance . . . . Elaine Noren
Anesthesiology. . . . . Steven Schimmel, MD
Emergency Room . . . . Joel S Bogner
Intensive Care Unit. . . . . John Modica, MD
Patient Relations . . . . Sandra Bucci

Measure	Cases	This Hosp.	State Avg.	U.S. Avg.
Heart Attack Care				
ACE Inhibitor or ARB for LVSD[1]	5	100%	94%	96%
Aspirin at Arrival	33	94%	99%	99%
Aspirin at Discharge[1]	20	90%	99%	98%
Beta Blocker at Discharge[1]	19	89%	98%	98%
Fibrinolytic Medication Timing	0	-	50%	55%
PCI Within 90 Minutes of Arrival	0	-	87%	90%
Smoking Cessation Advice[1]	1	100%	100%	99%
Chest Pain/Possible Heart Attack Care				
Aspirin at Arrival	115	96%	97%	95%
Median Time to ECG (minutes)	120	8	8	8
Median Time to Transfer (minutes)[1]	13	44	73	61
Fibrinolytic Medication Timing	0	-	37%	54%
Heart Failure Care				
ACE Inhibitor or ARB for LVSD	47	96%	93%	94%
Discharge Instructions	78	81%	86%	88%
Evaluation of LVS Function	114	97%	99%	98%
Smoking Cessation Advice[1]	15	87%	99%	98%
Pneumonia Care				
Appropriate Initial Antibiotic	86	97%	93%	92%
Blood Culture Timing	155	96%	96%	96%
Influenza Vaccine	76	79%	91%	91%
Initial Antibiotic Timing	155	96%	96%	95%
Pneumococcal Vaccine	121	88%	93%	93%
Smoking Cessation Advice	35	100%	98%	97%
Surgical Care Improvement Project				
Appropriate VTP Within 24 Hours	99	90%	95%	92%
Appropriate Hair Removal	328	100%	99%	99%
Appropriate Beta Blocker Usage	100	90%	93%	93%
Controlled Postoperative Blood Glucose	0	-	91%	93%
Prophylactic Antibiotic Timing	258	95%	96%	97%
Prophylactic Antibiotic Timing (Outpatient)	110	90%	92%	92%
Prophylactic Antibiotic Selection	256	98%	97%	97%
Prophylactic Antibiotic Select. (Outpatient)	101	94%	92%	94%
Prophylactic Antibiotic Stopped	249	93%	95%	94%
Recommended VTP Ordered	100	93%	96%	94%
Urinary Catheter Removal[1]	11	100%	91%	90%
Children's Asthma Care				
Received Systemic Corticosteroids	-	-	-	100%
Received Home Management Plan	-	-	-	71%
Received Reliever Medication	-	-	-	100%
Use of Medical Imaging				
Combination Abdominal CT Scan	556	0.052	0.120	0.191
Combination Chest CT Scan	513	0.004	0.026	0.054
Follow-up Mammogram/Ultrasound	1,339	5.5%	9.2%	8.4%
MRI for Low Back Pain	84	26.2%	26.9%	32.7%
Survey of Patients' Hospital Experiences				
Area Around Room 'Always' Quiet at Night	300+	52%	-	58%
Doctors 'Always' Communicated Well	300+	82%	-	80%
Home Recovery Information Given	300+	81%	-	82%
Hospital Given 9 or 10 on 10 Point Scale	300+	64%	-	67%
Meds 'Always' Explained Before Given	300+	60%	-	60%
Nurses 'Always' Communicated Well	300+	79%	-	76%
Pain 'Always' Well Controlled	300+	67%	-	69%
Room and Bathroom 'Always' Clean	300+	80%	-	71%
Timely Help 'Always' Received	300+	67%	-	64%
Would Definitely Recommend Hospital	300+	67%	-	69%

Rockville General Hospital

31 Union St
Rockville, CT 06066
Phone: 860-872-5160
Fax: 860-875-5336
E-mail: info@echn.org
URL: www.echn.org
Type: Acute Care Hospitals
Emergency Services: Yes
Ownership: Voluntary Non-Profit - Other
Beds: 102

Key Personnel:
CEO/President. . . . . Peter J Karl
Chief of Medical Staff. . . . . Joel J Reich
Coronary Care . . . . Richard Slutsky
Operating Room. . . . . Judy Montgomery
Quality Assurance . . . . Dennis P McConville
Patient Relations . . . . Deborah A Parker, RN

Measure	Cases	This Hosp.	State Avg.	U.S. Avg.
Heart Attack Care				
ACE Inhibitor or ARB for LVSD[1]	5	100%	94%	96%
Aspirin at Arrival	26	100%	99%	99%
Aspirin at Discharge[1]	17	100%	99%	98%
Beta Blocker at Discharge[1]	21	100%	98%	98%
Fibrinolytic Medication Timing	0	-	50%	55%
PCI Within 90 Minutes of Arrival	0	-	87%	90%
Smoking Cessation Advice	0	-	100%	99%
Chest Pain/Possible Heart Attack Care				
Aspirin at Arrival	40	88%	97%	95%
Median Time to ECG (minutes)	42	5	8	8
Median Time to Transfer (minutes)[1]	15	84	73	61
Fibrinolytic Medication Timing	0	-	37%	54%
Heart Failure Care				
ACE Inhibitor or ARB for LVSD[1]	20	100%	93%	94%
Discharge Instructions	58	88%	86%	88%
Evaluation of LVS Function	93	100%	99%	98%
Smoking Cessation Advice[1]	12	100%	99%	98%
Pneumonia Care				
Appropriate Initial Antibiotic	74	84%	93%	92%
Blood Culture Timing	128	99%	96%	96%
Influenza Vaccine	92	96%	91%	91%
Initial Antibiotic Timing	106	99%	96%	95%
Pneumococcal Vaccine	117	97%	93%	93%
Smoking Cessation Advice	43	100%	98%	97%
Surgical Care Improvement Project				
Appropriate VTP Within 24 Hours	72	89%	95%	92%
Appropriate Hair Removal	210	100%	99%	99%
Appropriate Beta Blocker Usage	57	89%	93%	93%
Controlled Postoperative Blood Glucose	0	-	91%	93%
Prophylactic Antibiotic Timing	144	99%	96%	97%
Prophylactic Antibiotic Timing (Outpatient)	97	96%	92%	92%
Prophylactic Antibiotic Selection	145	100%	97%	97%
Prophylactic Antibiotic Select. (Outpatient)	94	98%	92%	94%
Prophylactic Antibiotic Stopped	137	99%	95%	94%
Recommended VTP Ordered	72	96%	96%	94%
Urinary Catheter Removal	28	79%	91%	90%
Children's Asthma Care				
Received Systemic Corticosteroids	-	-	-	100%
Received Home Management Plan	-	-	-	71%
Received Reliever Medication	-	-	-	100%
Use of Medical Imaging				
Combination Abdominal CT Scan	546	0.081	0.120	0.191
Combination Chest CT Scan	431	0.023	0.026	0.054
Follow-up Mammogram/Ultrasound	415	6.5%	9.2%	8.4%
MRI for Low Back Pain	95	32.6%	26.9%	32.7%
Survey of Patients' Hospital Experiences				
Area Around Room 'Always' Quiet at Night	300+	55%	-	58%
Doctors 'Always' Communicated Well	300+	75%	-	80%
Home Recovery Information Given	300+	81%	-	82%
Hospital Given 9 or 10 on 10 Point Scale	300+	65%	-	67%
Meds 'Always' Explained Before Given	300+	57%	-	60%
Nurses 'Always' Communicated Well	300+	77%	-	76%
Pain 'Always' Well Controlled	300+	70%	-	69%
Room and Bathroom 'Always' Clean	300+	69%	-	71%
Timely Help 'Always' Received	300+	63%	-	64%
Would Definitely Recommend Hospital	300+	69%	-	69%

Sharon Hospital

50 Hospital Hill Road
Sharon, CT 06069
Phone: 860-364-4228
Fax: 860-364-4470
E-mail: info@sharonhospital.com
URL: www.sharonhospital.com
Type: Acute Care Hospitals
Emergency Services: Yes
Ownership: Proprietary
Beds: 25

Key Personnel:
CEO/President. . . . . Kimberly Lumia
Cardiac Laboratory. . . . . Lee S. Marcu
Chief of Medical Staff . . . . Michael D Parker, MD
Infection Control. . . . . Diana Kelly
Operating Room. . . . . Patricia Carson
Pediatric Ambulatory Care . . . . . Susan Jessen
Pediatric In-Patient Care . . . . Virginia L Gray-Carke
Radiology. . . . . Joseph C Antonio

Measure	Cases	This Hosp.	State Avg.	U.S. Avg.
Heart Attack Care				
ACE Inhibitor or ARB for LVSD[1]	1	0%	94%	96%
Aspirin at Arrival[1]	15	100%	99%	99%
Aspirin at Discharge[1]	7	100%	99%	98%
Beta Blocker at Discharge[1]	11	91%	98%	98%
Fibrinolytic Medication Timing	0	-	50%	55%
PCI Within 90 Minutes of Arrival	0	-	87%	90%
Smoking Cessation Advice[1]	1	100%	100%	99%
Chest Pain/Possible Heart Attack Care				
Aspirin at Arrival	40	98%	97%	95%
Median Time to ECG (minutes)	43	8	8	8
Median Time to Transfer (minutes)[1]	13	160	73	61
Fibrinolytic Medication Timing[1]	4	25%	37%	54%
Heart Failure Care				
ACE Inhibitor or ARB for LVSD[1]	8	100%	93%	94%
Discharge Instructions[1]	21	90%	86%	88%
Evaluation of LVS Function	43	95%	99%	98%
Smoking Cessation Advice[1]	2	100%	99%	98%
Pneumonia Care				
Appropriate Initial Antibiotic	45	87%	93%	92%
Blood Culture Timing	77	96%	96%	96%
Influenza Vaccine	39	100%	91%	91%
Initial Antibiotic Timing	79	100%	96%	95%
Pneumococcal Vaccine	68	100%	93%	93%
Smoking Cessation Advice[1]	15	80%	98%	97%
Surgical Care Improvement Project				
Appropriate VTP Within 24 Hours	52	85%	95%	92%
Appropriate Hair Removal	138	100%	99%	99%
Appropriate Beta Blocker Usage	30	100%	93%	93%
Controlled Postoperative Blood Glucose	0	-	91%	93%
Prophylactic Antibiotic Timing	91	98%	96%	97%
Prophylactic Antibiotic Timing (Outpatient)[1,3]	23	96%	92%	92%
Prophylactic Antibiotic Selection	91	95%	97%	97%
Prophylactic Antibiotic Select. (Outpatient)[1,3]	22	100%	92%	94%
Prophylactic Antibiotic Stopped	87	95%	95%	94%
Recommended VTP Ordered	53	87%	96%	94%
Urinary Catheter Removal[1]	22	82%	91%	90%
Children's Asthma Care				
Received Systemic Corticosteroids	-	-	-	100%
Received Home Management Plan	-	-	-	71%
Received Reliever Medication	-	-	-	100%
Use of Medical Imaging				
Combination Abdominal CT Scan	363	0.694	0.120	0.191
Combination Chest CT Scan	290	0.017	0.026	0.054
Follow-up Mammogram/Ultrasound	887	8.5%	9.2%	8.4%
MRI for Low Back Pain	98	32.7%	26.9%	32.7%
Survey of Patients' Hospital Experiences				
Area Around Room 'Always' Quiet at Night	300+	60%	-	58%
Doctors 'Always' Communicated Well	300+	85%	-	80%
Home Recovery Information Given	300+	84%	-	82%
Hospital Given 9 or 10 on 10 Point Scale	300+	74%	-	67%
Meds 'Always' Explained Before Given	300+	61%	-	60%
Nurses 'Always' Communicated Well	300+	78%	-	76%
Pain 'Always' Well Controlled	300+	73%	-	69%
Room and Bathroom 'Always' Clean	300+	72%	-	71%
Timely Help 'Always' Received	300+	63%	-	64%
Would Definitely Recommend Hospital	300+	75%	-	69%

NOTE: Hospital profiles are in alphabetical order by state, then city, then hospital within the city; Rankings exclude hospitals with less than 25 cases except for patient surveys which excludes hospitals with less than 100 cases; (a) 100–299 cases; (1) The number of cases is too small to be sure how well a hospital is performing; (2) The hospital indicated that the data submitted for this measure were based on a sample of cases; (3) Data was collected during a shorter time period (fewer quarters) than the maximum possible time for this measure; (4) Suppressed for one or more quarters by CMS; (5) No data is available from the hospital for this measure; (6) Fewer than 100 patients completed the HCAHPS survey. Use these rates with caution, as the number of surveys may be too low to reliably assess hospital performance; (7) Survey results are based on less than 12 months of data; (8) Survey results are not available for this reporting period; (9) No or very few patients were eligible for the HCAHPS survey. The scores shown, if any, reflect a very small number of surveys; (10) A state average was not calculated because too few hospitals in the state submitted data; (11) There were discrepancies in the data collection process; Please refer to the User's Guide for a full explanation of data.

Johnson Memorial Hospital

201 Chestnut Hill Rd Phone: 860-684-4251
Stafford Springs, CT 06076 Fax: 860-684-8459
URL: www.johnsonhealthnetwork.com
Type: Acute Care Hospitals Emergency Services: Yes
Ownership: Voluntary Non-Profit - Private Beds: 89

Key Personnel:

CEO/President. . . . . Alfred A Lerz
Cardiac Laboratory. . . . . James Lietz
Chief of Medical Staff. . . . . Nicholas Salerno, MD
Operating Room. . . . . Stephanie Kelley, RN
Quality Assurance . . . . Debra Abel
Radiology. . . . . Richard Buck

Measure	Cases	This Hosp.	State Avg.	U.S. Avg.
Heart Attack Care				
ACE Inhibitor or ARB for LVSD[1]	3	67%	94%	96%
Aspirin at Arrival[1]	11	82%	99%	99%
Aspirin at Discharge[1]	5	80%	99%	98%
Beta Blocker at Discharge[1]	6	83%	98%	98%
Fibrinolytic Medication Timing	0	-	50%	55%
PCI Within 90 Minutes of Arrival	0	-	87%	90%
Smoking Cessation Advice	0	-	100%	99%
Chest Pain/Possible Heart Attack Care				
Aspirin at Arrival	65	97%	97%	95%
Median Time to ECG (minutes)	68	12	8	8
Median Time to Transfer (minutes)[1]	2	328	73	61
Fibrinolytic Medication Timing[1]	9	67%	37%	54%
Heart Failure Care				
ACE Inhibitor or ARB for LVSD	26	92%	93%	94%
Discharge Instructions	77	99%	86%	88%
Evaluation of LVS Function	120	97%	99%	98%
Smoking Cessation Advice[1]	6	100%	99%	98%
Pneumonia Care				
Appropriate Initial Antibiotic	74	95%	93%	92%
Blood Culture Timing	142	97%	96%	96%
Influenza Vaccine	77	96%	91%	91%
Initial Antibiotic Timing	108	94%	96%	95%
Pneumococcal Vaccine	125	98%	93%	93%
Smoking Cessation Advice	39	100%	98%	97%
Surgical Care Improvement Project				
Appropriate VTP Within 24 Hours	96	94%	95%	92%
Appropriate Hair Removal	182	97%	99%	99%
Appropriate Beta Blocker Usage	48	96%	93%	93%
Controlled Postoperative Blood Glucose	0	-	91%	93%
Prophylactic Antibiotic Timing	115	98%	96%	97%
Prophylactic Antibiotic Timing (Outpatient)	113	96%	92%	92%
Prophylactic Antibiotic Selection	114	93%	97%	97%
Prophylactic Antibiotic Select. (Outpatient)	110	90%	92%	94%
Prophylactic Antibiotic Stopped	110	93%	95%	94%
Recommended VTP Ordered	96	96%	96%	94%
Urinary Catheter Removal	45	89%	91%	90%
Children's Asthma Care				
Received Systemic Corticosteroids	-	-	-	100%
Received Home Management Plan	-	-	-	71%
Received Reliever Medication	-	-	-	100%
Use of Medical Imaging				
Combination Abdominal CT Scan	372	0.024	0.120	0.191
Combination Chest CT Scan	276	0.000	0.026	0.054
Follow-up Mammogram/Ultrasound	500	6.4%	9.2%	8.4%
MRI for Low Back Pain	58	31.0%	26.9%	32.7%
Survey of Patients' Hospital Experiences				
Area Around Room 'Always' Quiet at Night	300+	57%	-	58%
Doctors 'Always' Communicated Well	300+	76%	-	80%
Home Recovery Information Given	300+	84%	-	82%
Hospital Given 9 or 10 on 10 Point Scale	300+	61%	-	67%
Meds 'Always' Explained Before Given	300+	55%	-	60%
Nurses 'Always' Communicated Well	300+	73%	-	76%
Pain 'Always' Well Controlled	300+	67%	-	69%
Room and Bathroom 'Always' Clean	300+	69%	-	71%
Timely Help 'Always' Received	300+	55%	-	64%
Would Definitely Recommend Hospital	300+	66%	-	69%

Stamford Hospital

Shelburne Rd & West Broad St Phone: 203-276-1000
Stamford, CT 06904 Fax: 203-325-7223
E-mail: cmurphy@stamhealth.org
URL: www.stamhealth.org
Type: Acute Care Hospitals Emergency Services: Yes
Ownership: Voluntary Non-Profit - Private Beds: 305

Key Personnel:

CEO/President. . . . . Brian G Grissler
Chief of Medical Staff. . . . . William Hines
Infection Control. . . . . Diane Baranowsky
Operating Room. . . . . Beth Wolff, RN
Pediatric Ambulatory Care . . . . . Michael N Suchenski, MD
Quality Assurance . . . . Eva Winjarska
Radiology. . . . . James J McSweeney, MD

Measure	Cases	This Hosp.	State Avg.	U.S. Avg.
Heart Attack Care				
ACE Inhibitor or ARB for LVSD	39	92%	94%	96%
Aspirin at Arrival	195	98%	99%	99%
Aspirin at Discharge	180	98%	99%	98%
Beta Blocker at Discharge	179	98%	98%	98%
Fibrinolytic Medication Timing	0	-	50%	55%
PCI Within 90 Minutes of Arrival	27	81%	87%	90%
Smoking Cessation Advice	36	100%	100%	99%
Chest Pain/Possible Heart Attack Care				
Aspirin at Arrival[3]	0	-	97%	95%
Median Time to ECG (minutes)[3]	0	-	8	8
Median Time to Transfer (minutes)[5]	0	-	73	61
Fibrinolytic Medication Timing[5]	0	-	37%	54%
Heart Failure Care				
ACE Inhibitor or ARB for LVSD	149	93%	93%	94%
Discharge Instructions	216	88%	86%	88%
Evaluation of LVS Function	328	98%	99%	98%
Smoking Cessation Advice	33	100%	99%	98%
Pneumonia Care				
Appropriate Initial Antibiotic	136	92%	93%	92%
Blood Culture Timing	208	100%	96%	96%
Influenza Vaccine	133	92%	91%	91%
Initial Antibiotic Timing	196	96%	96%	95%
Pneumococcal Vaccine	195	96%	93%	93%
Smoking Cessation Advice	48	100%	98%	97%
Surgical Care Improvement Project				
Appropriate VTP Within 24 Hours[2]	152	99%	95%	92%
Appropriate Hair Removal[2]	439	100%	99%	99%
Appropriate Beta Blocker Usage[2]	130	95%	93%	93%
Controlled Postoperative Blood Glucose[2]	36	100%	91%	93%
Prophylactic Antibiotic Timing[2]	297	99%	96%	97%
Prophylactic Antibiotic Timing (Outpatient)	428	96%	92%	92%
Prophylactic Antibiotic Selection[2]	302	99%	97%	97%
Prophylactic Antibiotic Select. (Outpatient)	422	96%	92%	94%
Prophylactic Antibiotic Stopped[2]	287	98%	95%	94%
Recommended VTP Ordered[2]	154	97%	96%	94%
Urinary Catheter Removal[2]	61	95%	91%	90%
Children's Asthma Care				
Received Systemic Corticosteroids	-	-	-	100%
Received Home Management Plan	-	-	-	71%
Received Reliever Medication	-	-	-	100%
Use of Medical Imaging				
Combination Abdominal CT Scan	1,708	0.040	0.120	0.191
Combination Chest CT Scan	1,200	0.002	0.026	0.054
Follow-up Mammogram/Ultrasound	2,159	16.5%	9.2%	8.4%
MRI for Low Back Pain	176	31.3%	26.9%	32.7%
Survey of Patients' Hospital Experiences				
Area Around Room 'Always' Quiet at Night	300+	53%	-	58%
Doctors 'Always' Communicated Well	300+	78%	-	80%
Home Recovery Information Given	300+	74%	-	82%
Hospital Given 9 or 10 on 10 Point Scale	300+	65%	-	67%
Meds 'Always' Explained Before Given	300+	58%	-	60%
Nurses 'Always' Communicated Well	300+	75%	-	76%
Pain 'Always' Well Controlled	300+	70%	-	69%
Room and Bathroom 'Always' Clean	300+	63%	-	71%
Timely Help 'Always' Received	300+	56%	-	64%
Would Definitely Recommend Hospital	300+	70%	-	69%

Charlotte Hungerford Hospital

540 Litchfield St Phone: 860-496-6666
Torrington, CT 06790 Fax: 860-482-8627
URL: www.charlottesweb.hungerford.org
Type: Acute Care Hospitals Emergency Services: Yes
Ownership: Voluntary Non-Profit - Private Beds: 109

Key Personnel:

CEO/President. . . . . Daniel McIntyre
Chief of Medical Staff. . . . . Mark Prete, MD
Infection Control. . . . . Joseph O'Geen
Operating Room. . . . . Timothy Gostkowski
Quality Assurance . . . . Donna Feinstein
Radiology. . . . . Herman Coleman, MD
Emergency Room . . . . Peter Bull
Patient Relations . . . . Marty Mancuso

Measure	Cases	This Hosp.	State Avg.	U.S. Avg.
Heart Attack Care				
ACE Inhibitor or ARB for LVSD[1]	3	100%	94%	96%
Aspirin at Arrival	47	100%	99%	99%
Aspirin at Discharge	36	100%	99%	98%
Beta Blocker at Discharge	38	100%	98%	98%
Fibrinolytic Medication Timing	0	-	50%	55%
PCI Within 90 Minutes of Arrival	0	-	87%	90%
Smoking Cessation Advice[1]	3	100%	100%	99%
Chest Pain/Possible Heart Attack Care				
Aspirin at Arrival	118	96%	97%	95%
Median Time to ECG (minutes)	118	12	8	8
Median Time to Transfer (minutes)[1]	10	80	73	61
Fibrinolytic Medication Timing[1]	11	9%	37%	54%
Heart Failure Care				
ACE Inhibitor or ARB for LVSD	32	88%	93%	94%
Discharge Instructions	73	90%	86%	88%
Evaluation of LVS Function	129	98%	99%	98%
Smoking Cessation Advice[1]	9	100%	99%	98%
Pneumonia Care				
Appropriate Initial Antibiotic	68	90%	93%	92%
Blood Culture Timing	101	98%	96%	96%
Influenza Vaccine	117	97%	91%	91%
Initial Antibiotic Timing	123	95%	96%	95%
Pneumococcal Vaccine	169	96%	93%	93%
Smoking Cessation Advice	44	100%	98%	97%
Surgical Care Improvement Project				
Appropriate VTP Within 24 Hours[2]	101	95%	95%	92%
Appropriate Hair Removal[2]	312	100%	99%	99%
Appropriate Beta Blocker Usage[2]	104	93%	93%	93%
Controlled Postoperative Blood Glucose[2]	0	-	91%	93%
Prophylactic Antibiotic Timing[2]	199	91%	96%	97%
Prophylactic Antibiotic Timing (Outpatient)	160	88%	92%	92%
Prophylactic Antibiotic Selection[2]	199	96%	97%	97%
Prophylactic Antibiotic Select. (Outpatient)	151	95%	92%	94%
Prophylactic Antibiotic Stopped[2]	190	94%	95%	94%
Recommended VTP Ordered[2]	101	97%	96%	94%
Urinary Catheter Removal[2]	26	54%	91%	90%
Children's Asthma Care				
Received Systemic Corticosteroids	-	-	-	100%
Received Home Management Plan	-	-	-	71%
Received Reliever Medication	-	-	-	100%
Use of Medical Imaging				
Combination Abdominal CT Scan	663	0.101	0.120	0.191
Combination Chest CT Scan	562	0.075	0.026	0.054
Follow-up Mammogram/Ultrasound	2,202	10.3%	9.2%	8.4%
MRI for Low Back Pain[1]	7	57.1%	26.9%	32.7%
Survey of Patients' Hospital Experiences				
Area Around Room 'Always' Quiet at Night	300+	48%	-	58%
Doctors 'Always' Communicated Well	300+	79%	-	80%
Home Recovery Information Given	300+	84%	-	82%
Hospital Given 9 or 10 on 10 Point Scale	300+	66%	-	67%
Meds 'Always' Explained Before Given	300+	59%	-	60%
Nurses 'Always' Communicated Well	300+	78%	-	76%
Pain 'Always' Well Controlled	300+	71%	-	69%
Room and Bathroom 'Always' Clean	300+	72%	-	71%
Timely Help 'Always' Received	300+	64%	-	64%
Would Definitely Recommend Hospital	300+	62%	-	69%

NOTE: Hospital profiles are in alphabetical order by state, then city, then hospital within the city; Rankings exclude hospitals with less than 25 cases except for patient surveys which excludes hospitals with less than 100 cases; (a) 100–299 cases; (1) The number of cases is too small to be sure how well a hospital is performing; (2) The hospital indicated that the data submitted for this measure were based on a sample of cases; (3) Data was collected during a shorter time period (fewer quarters) than the maximum possible time for this measure; (4) Suppressed for one or more quarters by CMS; (5) No data is available from the hospital for this measure; (6) Fewer than 100 patients completed the HCAHPS survey. Use these rates with caution, as the number of surveys may be too low to reliably assess hospital performance; (7) Survey results are based on less than 12 months of data; (8) Survey results are not available for this reporting period; (9) No or very few patients were eligible for the HCAHPS survey. The scores shown, if any, reflect a very small number of surveys; (10) A state average was not calculated because too few hospitals in the state submitted data; (11) There were discrepancies in the data collection process; Please refer to the User's Guide for a full explanation of data.

Masonic Home and Hospital

22 Masonic Ave
Wallingford, CT 06492
Phone: 203-679-5900
Fax: 203-679-5038
E-mail: info@masonicare.org
URL: www.masonicare.org
Type: Acute Care Hospitals
Emergency Services: No
Ownership: Voluntary Non-Profit - Private
Beds: 548

Key Personnel:
CEO/President.............. Stephen McPherson
Chief of Medical Staff.......... Ronald Schwartz MD
Infection Control............. Irene Morris RN
Quality Assurance .... Tracey Lemay
Radiology................... Jean Desrosiers
Ambulatory Care .... Carol Herbert RN

Measure	Cases	This Hosp.	State Avg.	U.S. Avg.
Heart Attack Care				
ACE Inhibitor or ARB for LVSD[5]	0	-	94%	96%
Aspirin at Arrival[5]	0	-	99%	99%
Aspirin at Discharge[5]	0	-	99%	98%
Beta Blocker at Discharge[5]	0	-	98%	98%
Fibrinolytic Medication Timing[5]	0	-	50%	55%
PCI Within 90 Minutes of Arrival[5]	0	-	87%	90%
Smoking Cessation Advice[5]	0	-	100%	99%
Chest Pain/Possible Heart Attack Care				
Aspirin at Arrival[5]	0	-	97%	95%
Median Time to ECG (minutes)[5]	0	-	8	8
Median Time to Transfer (minutes)[5]	0	-	73	61
Fibrinolytic Medication Timing[5]	0	-	37%	54%
Heart Failure Care				
ACE Inhibitor or ARB for LVSD[1]	6	50%	93%	94%
Discharge Instructions[1]	8	25%	86%	88%
Evaluation of LVS Function	40	80%	99%	98%
Smoking Cessation Advice	0	-	99%	98%
Pneumonia Care				
Appropriate Initial Antibiotic	0	-	93%	92%
Blood Culture Timing	0	-	96%	96%
Influenza Vaccine[1]	22	91%	91%	91%
Initial Antibiotic Timing[1]	3	33%	96%	95%
Pneumococcal Vaccine	48	94%	93%	93%
Smoking Cessation Advice[1]	1	100%	98%	97%
Surgical Care Improvement Project				
Appropriate VTP Within 24 Hours[5]	0	-	95%	92%
Appropriate Hair Removal[5]	0	-	99%	99%
Appropriate Beta Blocker Usage[5]	0	-	93%	93%
Controlled Postoperative Blood Glucose[5]	0	-	91%	93%
Prophylactic Antibiotic Timing[5]	0	-	96%	97%
Prophylactic Antibiotic Timing (Outpatient)[5]	0	-	92%	92%
Prophylactic Antibiotic Selection[5]	0	-	97%	97%
Prophylactic Antibiotic Select. (Outpatient)[5]	0	-	92%	94%
Prophylactic Antibiotic Stopped[5]	0	-	95%	94%
Recommended VTP Ordered[5]	0	-	96%	94%
Urinary Catheter Removal[5]	0	-	91%	90%
Children's Asthma Care				
Received Systemic Corticosteroids	-	-	-	100%
Received Home Management Plan	-	-	-	71%
Received Reliever Medication	-	-	-	100%
Use of Medical Imaging				
Combination Abdominal CT Scan[5]	0	-	0.120	0.191
Combination Chest CT Scan[5]	0	-	0.026	0.054
Follow-up Mammogram/Ultrasound[5]	0	-	9.2%	8.4%
MRI for Low Back Pain[5]	0	-	26.9%	32.7%
Survey of Patients' Hospital Experiences				
Area Around Room 'Always' Quiet at Night	(a)	43%	-	58%
Doctors 'Always' Communicated Well	(a)	60%	-	80%
Home Recovery Information Given	(a)	77%	-	82%
Hospital Given 9 or 10 on 10 Point Scale	(a)	57%	-	67%
Meds 'Always' Explained Before Given	(a)	40%	-	60%
Nurses 'Always' Communicated Well	(a)	64%	-	76%
Pain 'Always' Well Controlled	(a)	65%	-	69%
Room and Bathroom 'Always' Clean	(a)	69%	-	71%
Timely Help 'Always' Received	(a)	42%	-	64%
Would Definitely Recommend Hospital	(a)	65%	-	69%

Saint Marys Hospital

56 Franklin St
Waterbury, CT 06706
Phone: 203-574-6000
Fax: 203-709-7753
Type: Acute Care Hospitals
Emergency Services: Yes
Ownership: Voluntary Non-Profit - Church
Beds: 347

Key Personnel:
CEO/President.............. Bob Ritz
Operating Room............. Pat Clement
Pediatric Ambulatory Care ...... M Alex Geertsmand
Pediatric In-Patient Care .... M Alex Geertsmand
Radiology................... Robert Lehman, MD
Emergency Room .... Dr Fisher

Measure	Cases	This Hosp.	State Avg.	U.S. Avg.
Heart Attack Care				
ACE Inhibitor or ARB for LVSD	31	100%	94%	96%
Aspirin at Arrival	168	100%	99%	99%
Aspirin at Discharge	164	100%	99%	98%
Beta Blocker at Discharge	155	100%	98%	98%
Fibrinolytic Medication Timing	0	-	50%	55%
PCI Within 90 Minutes of Arrival	42	98%	87%	90%
Smoking Cessation Advice	54	96%	100%	99%
Chest Pain/Possible Heart Attack Care				
Aspirin at Arrival[1,3]	1	100%	97%	95%
Median Time to ECG (minutes)[1,3]	1	4	8	8
Median Time to Transfer (minutes)[3]	0	-	73	61
Fibrinolytic Medication Timing[3]	0	-	37%	54%
Heart Failure Care				
ACE Inhibitor or ARB for LVSD	83	100%	93%	94%
Discharge Instructions	204	100%	86%	88%
Evaluation of LVS Function	301	100%	99%	98%
Smoking Cessation Advice	27	100%	99%	98%
Pneumonia Care				
Appropriate Initial Antibiotic[2]	111	90%	93%	92%
Blood Culture Timing[2]	175	95%	96%	96%
Influenza Vaccine[2]	72	97%	91%	91%
Initial Antibiotic Timing[2]	169	87%	96%	95%
Pneumococcal Vaccine[2]	144	83%	93%	93%
Smoking Cessation Advice[2]	39	97%	98%	97%
Surgical Care Improvement Project				
Appropriate VTP Within 24 Hours[2]	173	94%	95%	92%
Appropriate Hair Removal[2]	615	98%	99%	99%
Appropriate Beta Blocker Usage[2]	193	95%	93%	93%
Controlled Postoperative Blood Glucose[2]	101	96%	91%	93%
Prophylactic Antibiotic Timing[2]	437	93%	96%	97%
Prophylactic Antibiotic Timing (Outpatient)	123	77%	92%	92%
Prophylactic Antibiotic Selection[2]	443	96%	97%	97%
Prophylactic Antibiotic Select. (Outpatient)	104	93%	92%	94%
Prophylactic Antibiotic Stopped[2]	431	92%	95%	94%
Recommended VTP Ordered[2]	173	94%	96%	94%
Urinary Catheter Removal[2]	66	80%	91%	90%
Children's Asthma Care				
Received Systemic Corticosteroids	-	-	-	100%
Received Home Management Plan	-	-	-	71%
Received Reliever Medication	-	-	-	100%
Use of Medical Imaging				
Combination Abdominal CT Scan	846	0.061	0.120	0.191
Combination Chest CT Scan	700	0.003	0.026	0.054
Follow-up Mammogram/Ultrasound	489	11.5%	9.2%	8.4%
MRI for Low Back Pain[1]	37	37.8%	26.9%	32.7%
Survey of Patients' Hospital Experiences				
Area Around Room 'Always' Quiet at Night	300+	48%	-	58%
Doctors 'Always' Communicated Well	300+	78%	-	80%
Home Recovery Information Given	300+	85%	-	82%
Hospital Given 9 or 10 on 10 Point Scale	300+	63%	-	67%
Meds 'Always' Explained Before Given	300+	57%	-	60%
Nurses 'Always' Communicated Well	300+	73%	-	76%
Pain 'Always' Well Controlled	300+	67%	-	69%
Room and Bathroom 'Always' Clean	300+	71%	-	71%
Timely Help 'Always' Received	300+	57%	-	64%
Would Definitely Recommend Hospital	300+	69%	-	69%

Waterbury Hospital

64 Robbins St
Waterbury, CT 06721
Phone: 203-573-6000
Fax: 203-573-7325
URL: www.waterburyhospital.org
Type: Acute Care Hospitals
Emergency Services: No
Ownership: Voluntary Non-Profit - Private
Beds: 357

Key Personnel:
CEO/President.............. John H Tobin
Chief of Medical Staff.......... Steve Eisen, MD
Infection Control............. Maria Villaneuava
Operating Room............. Ellen Polokoff
Quality Assurance .... John Porter
Radiology................... John DeLeon, MD
Anesthesiology............... Neil Peterson, MD
Emergency Room .... Kreig Middleman, MD

Measure	Cases	This Hosp.	State Avg.	U.S. Avg.
Heart Attack Care				
ACE Inhibitor or ARB for LVSD	34	91%	94%	96%
Aspirin at Arrival	227	100%	99%	99%
Aspirin at Discharge	219	100%	99%	98%
Beta Blocker at Discharge	215	100%	98%	98%
Fibrinolytic Medication Timing	0	-	50%	55%
PCI Within 90 Minutes of Arrival	38	89%	87%	90%
Smoking Cessation Advice	64	100%	100%	99%
Chest Pain/Possible Heart Attack Care				
Aspirin at Arrival[5]	0	-	97%	95%
Median Time to ECG (minutes)[5]	0	-	8	8
Median Time to Transfer (minutes)[5]	0	-	73	61
Fibrinolytic Medication Timing[5]	0	-	37%	54%
Heart Failure Care				
ACE Inhibitor or ARB for LVSD[2]	93	84%	93%	94%
Discharge Instructions[2]	203	77%	86%	88%
Evaluation of LVS Function[2]	321	98%	99%	98%
Smoking Cessation Advice[2]	48	100%	99%	98%
Pneumonia Care				
Appropriate Initial Antibiotic[2]	88	86%	93%	92%
Blood Culture Timing[2]	199	94%	96%	96%
Influenza Vaccine[2]	117	79%	91%	91%
Initial Antibiotic Timing[2]	198	93%	96%	95%
Pneumococcal Vaccine[2]	195	90%	93%	93%
Smoking Cessation Advice[2]	79	100%	98%	97%
Surgical Care Improvement Project				
Appropriate VTP Within 24 Hours[2]	155	98%	95%	92%
Appropriate Hair Removal[2]	635	100%	99%	99%
Appropriate Beta Blocker Usage[2]	185	90%	93%	93%
Controlled Postoperative Blood Glucose[2]	87	83%	91%	93%
Prophylactic Antibiotic Timing[2]	449	94%	96%	97%
Prophylactic Antibiotic Timing (Outpatient)	140	91%	92%	92%
Prophylactic Antibiotic Selection[2]	450	97%	97%	97%
Prophylactic Antibiotic Select. (Outpatient)	137	94%	92%	94%
Prophylactic Antibiotic Stopped[2]	438	91%	95%	94%
Recommended VTP Ordered[2]	155	99%	96%	94%
Urinary Catheter Removal[2]	66	95%	91%	90%
Children's Asthma Care				
Received Systemic Corticosteroids	-	-	-	100%
Received Home Management Plan	-	-	-	71%
Received Reliever Medication	-	-	-	100%
Use of Medical Imaging				
Combination Abdominal CT Scan	825	0.028	0.120	0.191
Combination Chest CT Scan	634	0.000	0.026	0.054
Follow-up Mammogram/Ultrasound	298	10.4%	9.2%	8.4%
MRI for Low Back Pain[1]	7	42.9%	26.9%	32.7%
Survey of Patients' Hospital Experiences				
Area Around Room 'Always' Quiet at Night	300+	44%	-	58%
Doctors 'Always' Communicated Well	300+	81%	-	80%
Home Recovery Information Given	300+	88%	-	82%
Hospital Given 9 or 10 on 10 Point Scale	300+	64%	-	67%
Meds 'Always' Explained Before Given	300+	58%	-	60%
Nurses 'Always' Communicated Well	300+	77%	-	76%
Pain 'Always' Well Controlled	300+	69%	-	69%
Room and Bathroom 'Always' Clean	300+	61%	-	71%
Timely Help 'Always' Received	300+	59%	-	64%
Would Definitely Recommend Hospital	300+	70%	-	69%

NOTE: Hospital profiles are in alphabetical order by state, then city, then hospital within the city; Rankings exclude hospitals with less than 25 cases except for patient surveys which excludes hospitals with less than 100 cases; (a) 100–299 cases; (1) The number of cases is too small to be sure how well a hospital is performing; (2) The hospital indicated that the data submitted for this measure were based on a sample of cases; (3) Data was collected during a shorter time period (fewer quarters) than the maximum possible time for this measure; (4) Suppressed for one or more quarters by CMS; (5) No data is available from the hospital for this measure; (6) Fewer than 100 patients completed the HCAHPS survey. Use these rates with caution, as the number of surveys may be too low to reliably assess hospital performance; (7) Survey results are based on less than 12 months of data; (8) Survey results are not available for this reporting period; (9) No or very few patients were eligible for the HCAHPS survey. The scores shown, if any, reflect a very small number of surveys; (10) A state average was not calculated because too few hospitals in the state submitted data; (11) There were discrepancies in the data collection process; Please refer to the User's Guide for a full explanation of data.

Hebrew Home and Hospital

1 Abrahms Boulevard
West Hartford, CT 06117
E-mail: info@hebrewhealthcare.org
URL: www.hebrewhealthcare.org
Type: Acute Care Hospitals
Ownership: Voluntary Non-Profit - Private

Phone: 860-523-3800
Fax: 860-523-3949

Emergency Services: No
Beds: 334

Key Personnel:
CEO/President . . . . Bonnie Gauthier
Chief of Medical Staff . . . . Kathy Mon, MD
Infection Control . . . . Barbara Joy, RN
Quality Assurance . . . . Linda McDonnell
Patient Relations . . . . Jennifer Terray

Measure	Cases	This Hosp.	State Avg.	U.S. Avg.
Heart Attack Care				
ACE Inhibitor or ARB for LVSD[5]	0	-	94%	96%
Aspirin at Arrival[5]	0	-	99%	99%
Aspirin at Discharge[5]	0	-	99%	98%
Beta Blocker at Discharge[5]	0	-	98%	98%
Fibrinolytic Medication Timing[5]	0	-	50%	55%
PCI Within 90 Minutes of Arrival[5]	0	-	87%	90%
Smoking Cessation Advice[5]	0	-	100%	99%
Chest Pain/Possible Heart Attack Care				
Aspirin at Arrival[5]	0	-	97%	95%
Median Time to ECG (minutes)[5]	0	-	8	8
Median Time to Transfer (minutes)[5]	0	-	73	61
Fibrinolytic Medication Timing[5]	0	-	37%	54%
Heart Failure Care				
ACE Inhibitor or ARB for LVSD[1,2]	2	50%	93%	94%
Discharge Instructions[1,2]	1	0%	86%	88%
Evaluation of LVS Function[1,2]	17	94%	99%	98%
Smoking Cessation Advice[1,2]	2	0%	99%	98%
Pneumonia Care				
Appropriate Initial Antibiotic[2]	0	-	93%	92%
Blood Culture Timing[2]	0	-	96%	96%
Influenza Vaccine[1,2]	7	86%	91%	91%
Initial Antibiotic Timing[1,2]	8	100%	96%	95%
Pneumococcal Vaccine[1,2]	14	86%	93%	93%
Smoking Cessation Advice[1,2]	3	0%	98%	97%
Surgical Care Improvement Project				
Appropriate VTP Within 24 Hours[5]	0	-	95%	92%
Appropriate Hair Removal[5]	0	-	99%	99%
Appropriate Beta Blocker Usage[5]	0	-	93%	93%
Controlled Postoperative Blood Glucose[5]	0	-	91%	93%
Prophylactic Antibiotic Timing[5]	0	-	96%	97%
Prophylactic Antibiotic Timing (Outpatient)[5]	0	-	92%	92%
Prophylactic Antibiotic Selection[5]	0	-	97%	97%
Prophylactic Antibiotic Select. (Outpatient)[5]	0	-	92%	94%
Prophylactic Antibiotic Stopped[5]	0	-	95%	94%
Recommended VTP Ordered[5]	0	-	96%	94%
Urinary Catheter Removal[5]	0	-	91%	90%
Children's Asthma Care				
Received Systemic Corticosteroids	-	-	-	100%
Received Home Management Plan	-	-	-	71%
Received Reliever Medication	-	-	-	100%
Use of Medical Imaging				
Combination Abdominal CT Scan[5]	0	-	0.120	0.191
Combination Chest CT Scan[5]	0	-	0.026	0.054
Follow-up Mammogram/Ultrasound[5]	0	-	9.2%	8.4%
MRI for Low Back Pain[5]	0	-	26.9%	32.7%
Survey of Patients' Hospital Experiences				
Area Around Room 'Always' Quiet at Night[6]	<100	54%	-	58%
Doctors 'Always' Communicated Well[6]	<100	72%	-	80%
Home Recovery Information Given[6]	<100	81%	-	82%
Hospital Given 9 or 10 on 10 Point Scale[6]	<100	71%	-	67%
Meds 'Always' Explained Before Given[6]	<100	29%	-	60%
Nurses 'Always' Communicated Well[6]	<100	68%	-	76%
Pain 'Always' Well Controlled[6]	<100	55%	-	69%
Room and Bathroom 'Always' Clean[6]	<100	79%	-	71%
Timely Help 'Always' Received[6]	<100	51%	-	64%
Would Definitely Recommend Hospital[6]	<100	65%	-	69%

West Haven VA Medical Center

950 Campbell Avenue
West Haven, CT 06516
URL: www.visn1.med.va.gov/vact
Type: Acute Care-Veterans Administration
Ownership: Government - Federal

Phone: 203-932-5711
Fax: 203-937-3868

Emergency Services: No
Beds: 191

Key Personnel:
CEO/President . . . . Roger L Johnson
Chief of Medical Staff . . . . Michael H Ebert, MD
Operating Room . . . . Cindy Christensen
Quality Assurance . . . . Catherine Grabowski

Measure	Cases	This Hosp.	State Avg.	U.S. Avg.
Heart Attack Care				
ACE Inhibitor or ARB for LVSD[5]	0	-	94%	96%
Aspirin at Arrival[5]	0	-	99%	99%
Aspirin at Discharge[5]	0	-	99%	98%
Beta Blocker at Discharge[5]	0	-	98%	98%
Fibrinolytic Medication Timing[5]	0	-	50%	55%
PCI Within 90 Minutes of Arrival[5]	0	-	87%	90%
Smoking Cessation Advice[5]	0	-	100%	99%
Chest Pain/Possible Heart Attack Care				
Aspirin at Arrival	-	-	97%	95%
Median Time to ECG (minutes)	-	-	8	8
Median Time to Transfer (minutes)	-	-	73	61
Fibrinolytic Medication Timing	-	-	37%	54%
Heart Failure Care				
ACE Inhibitor or ARB for LVSD	43	100%	93%	94%
Discharge Instructions	161	100%	86%	88%
Evaluation of LVS Function	184	99%	99%	98%
Smoking Cessation Advice	25	100%	99%	98%
Pneumonia Care				
Appropriate Initial Antibiotic	46	93%	93%	92%
Blood Culture Timing	90	98%	96%	96%
Influenza Vaccine	65	95%	91%	91%
Initial Antibiotic Timing	74	77%	96%	95%
Pneumococcal Vaccine	97	99%	93%	93%
Smoking Cessation Advice	33	100%	98%	97%
Surgical Care Improvement Project				
Appropriate VTP Within 24 Hours[2]	142	100%	95%	92%
Appropriate Hair Removal[2]	288	100%	99%	99%
Appropriate Beta Blocker Usage[2]	165	100%	93%	93%
Controlled Postoperative Blood Glucose[2]	60	98%	91%	93%
Prophylactic Antibiotic Timing	189	98%	96%	97%
Prophylactic Antibiotic Timing (Outpatient)	-	-	92%	92%
Prophylactic Antibiotic Selection	203	99%	97%	97%
Prophylactic Antibiotic Select. (Outpatient)	-	-	92%	94%
Prophylactic Antibiotic Stopped	178	92%	95%	94%
Recommended VTP Ordered[2]	142	100%	96%	94%
Urinary Catheter Removal[2]	118	100%	91%	90%
Children's Asthma Care				
Received Systemic Corticosteroids	-	-	-	100%
Received Home Management Plan	-	-	-	71%
Received Reliever Medication	-	-	-	100%
Use of Medical Imaging				
Combination Abdominal CT Scan	-	-	0.120	0.191
Combination Chest CT Scan	-	-	0.026	0.054
Follow-up Mammogram/Ultrasound	-	-	9.2%	8.4%
MRI for Low Back Pain	-	-	26.9%	32.7%
Survey of Patients' Hospital Experiences				
Area Around Room 'Always' Quiet at Night	-	-	-	58%
Doctors 'Always' Communicated Well	-	-	-	80%
Home Recovery Information Given	-	-	-	82%
Hospital Given 9 or 10 on 10 Point Scale	-	-	-	67%
Meds 'Always' Explained Before Given	-	-	-	60%
Nurses 'Always' Communicated Well	-	-	-	76%
Pain 'Always' Well Controlled	-	-	-	69%
Room and Bathroom 'Always' Clean	-	-	-	71%
Timely Help 'Always' Received	-	-	-	64%
Would Definitely Recommend Hospital	-	-	-	69%

Windham Hospital

112 Mansfield Ave
Willimantic, CT 06226
E-mail: info@windhamhospital.org
URL: www.wcmh.org
Type: Acute Care Hospitals
Ownership: Voluntary Non-Profit - Private

Phone: 860-456-9116
Fax: 860-456-6838

Emergency Services: Yes
Beds: 130

Key Personnel:
CEO/President . . . . Duane Carlberg
Chief of Medical Staff . . . . Michael Shore, MD
Operating Room . . . . Francis Siracusa
Pediatric Ambulatory Care . . . . . Thomas Gorin
Pediatric In-Patient Care . . . . . . Thomas Gorin
Quality Assurance . . . . Annette Hansell
Radiology . . . . Bruce Arose, MD

Measure	Cases	This Hosp.	State Avg.	U.S. Avg.
Heart Attack Care				
ACE Inhibitor or ARB for LVSD[1]	2	0%	94%	96%
Aspirin at Arrival	27	96%	99%	99%
Aspirin at Discharge[1]	19	89%	99%	98%
Beta Blocker at Discharge[1]	20	95%	98%	98%
Fibrinolytic Medication Timing[1]	1	0%	50%	55%
PCI Within 90 Minutes of Arrival	0	-	87%	90%
Smoking Cessation Advice[1]	3	100%	100%	99%
Chest Pain/Possible Heart Attack Care				
Aspirin at Arrival	46	100%	97%	95%
Median Time to ECG (minutes)	48	10	8	8
Median Time to Transfer (minutes)[1]	8	54	73	61
Fibrinolytic Medication Timing[1]	5	40%	37%	54%
Heart Failure Care				
ACE Inhibitor or ARB for LVSD	43	79%	93%	94%
Discharge Instructions	91	80%	86%	88%
Evaluation of LVS Function	138	100%	99%	98%
Smoking Cessation Advice[1]	10	100%	99%	98%
Pneumonia Care				
Appropriate Initial Antibiotic	80	95%	93%	92%
Blood Culture Timing	131	98%	96%	96%
Influenza Vaccine	68	87%	91%	91%
Initial Antibiotic Timing	126	100%	96%	95%
Pneumococcal Vaccine	97	88%	93%	93%
Smoking Cessation Advice	41	100%	98%	97%
Surgical Care Improvement Project				
Appropriate VTP Within 24 Hours	88	100%	95%	92%
Appropriate Hair Removal	155	99%	99%	99%
Appropriate Beta Blocker Usage	49	86%	93%	93%
Controlled Postoperative Blood Glucose	0	-	91%	93%
Prophylactic Antibiotic Timing	90	99%	96%	97%
Prophylactic Antibiotic Timing (Outpatient)	63	90%	92%	92%
Prophylactic Antibiotic Selection	90	97%	97%	97%
Prophylactic Antibiotic Select. (Outpatient)	58	78%	92%	94%
Prophylactic Antibiotic Stopped	85	99%	95%	94%
Recommended VTP Ordered	88	100%	96%	94%
Urinary Catheter Removal	39	85%	91%	90%
Children's Asthma Care				
Received Systemic Corticosteroids	-	-	-	100%
Received Home Management Plan	-	-	-	71%
Received Reliever Medication	-	-	-	100%
Use of Medical Imaging				
Combination Abdominal CT Scan	554	0.079	0.120	0.191
Combination Chest CT Scan	434	0.021	0.026	0.054
Follow-up Mammogram/Ultrasound	1,222	9.6%	9.2%	8.4%
MRI for Low Back Pain	127	33.1%	26.9%	32.7%
Survey of Patients' Hospital Experiences				
Area Around Room 'Always' Quiet at Night	300+	43%	-	58%
Doctors 'Always' Communicated Well	300+	79%	-	80%
Home Recovery Information Given	300+	81%	-	82%
Hospital Given 9 or 10 on 10 Point Scale	300+	66%	-	67%
Meds 'Always' Explained Before Given	300+	64%	-	60%
Nurses 'Always' Communicated Well	300+	77%	-	76%
Pain 'Always' Well Controlled	300+	68%	-	69%
Room and Bathroom 'Always' Clean	300+	72%	-	71%
Timely Help 'Always' Received	300+	64%	-	64%
Would Definitely Recommend Hospital	300+	69%	-	69%

Heart Attack Care

1. ACE Inhibitor or ARB for LVSD

Hospital Name	City	Rate	Cases
Beebe Medical Center	Lewes	97%	39
Bayhealth - Kent General Hospital	Dover	94%	49
Christiana Care Health Services	Newark	94%	114
Saint Francis Hospital	Wilmington	94%	33

2. Aspirin at Arrival

Hospital Name	City	Rate	Cases
Beebe Medical Center	Lewes	100%	264
Nanticoke Memorial Hospital	Seaford	100%	97
Bayhealth - Kent General Hospital	Dover	99%	329
Christiana Care Health Services	Newark	99%	484
Saint Francis Hospital	Wilmington	97%	116

3. Aspirin at Discharge

Hospital Name	City	Rate	Cases
Bayhealth - Kent General Hospital	Dover	100%	341
Beebe Medical Center	Lewes	100%	261
Christiana Care Health Services	Newark	99%	632
Nanticoke Memorial Hospital	Seaford	99%	81
Saint Francis Hospital	Wilmington	99%	109

4. Beta Blocker at Discharge

Hospital Name	City	Rate	Cases
Bayhealth - Kent General Hospital	Dover	99%	335
Christiana Care Health Services	Newark	99%	609
Nanticoke Memorial Hospital	Seaford	99%	83
Saint Francis Hospital	Wilmington	99%	102
Beebe Medical Center	Lewes	97%	258

6. PCI Within 90 Minutes of Arrival

Hospital Name	City	Rate	Cases
Beebe Medical Center	Lewes	92%	40
Bayhealth - Kent General Hospital	Dover	91%	53
Christiana Care Health Services	Newark	89%	140

7. Smoking Cessation Advice

Hospital Name	City	Rate	Cases
Beebe Medical Center	Lewes	100%	85
Christiana Care Health Services	Newark	100%	220
Nanticoke Memorial Hospital	Seaford	100%	27
Saint Francis Hospital	Wilmington	100%	49
Bayhealth - Kent General Hospital	Dover	99%	139

Chest Pain/Possible Heart Attack Care

8. Aspirin at Arrival

Hospital Name	City	Rate	Cases
Bayhealth - Kent General Hospital	Dover	100%	31

9. Median Time to ECG (minutes)

Hospital Name	City	Min.	Cases
Bayhealth - Kent General Hospital	Dover	6	32

Heart Failure Care

12. ACE Inhibitor or ARB for LVSD

Hospital Name	City	Rate	Cases
Nanticoke Memorial Hospital	Seaford	100%	37
Bayhealth - Kent General Hospital	Dover	99%	171
Saint Francis Hospital	Wilmington	97%	102
Beebe Medical Center	Lewes	95%	104
Christiana Care Health Services[2]	Newark	89%	284

13. Discharge Instructions

Hospital Name	City	Rate	Cases
Nanticoke Memorial Hospital	Seaford	98%	166
Beebe Medical Center	Lewes	97%	276
Bayhealth - Kent General Hospital	Dover	95%	416
Saint Francis Hospital	Wilmington	94%	205
Wilmington VA Medical Center	Wilmington	90%	49
Christiana Care Health Services[2]	Newark	86%	616

14. Evaluation of LVS Function

Hospital Name	City	Rate	Cases
Bayhealth - Kent General Hospital	Dover	100%	506
Wilmington VA Medical Center	Wilmington	100%	52
Christiana Care Health Services[2]	Newark	99%	802
Nanticoke Memorial Hospital	Seaford	99%	202
Beebe Medical Center	Lewes	98%	353
Saint Francis Hospital	Wilmington	96%	234

15. Smoking Cessation Advice

Hospital Name	City	Rate	Cases
Bayhealth - Kent General Hospital	Dover	100%	123
Christiana Care Health Services[2]	Newark	100%	121
Nanticoke Memorial Hospital	Seaford	100%	39
Saint Francis Hospital	Wilmington	100%	54
Beebe Medical Center	Lewes	98%	59

Pneumonia Care

16. Appropriate Initial Antibiotic

Hospital Name	City	Rate	Cases
Nanticoke Memorial Hospital	Seaford	97%	103
Beebe Medical Center	Lewes	95%	190
Saint Francis Hospital	Wilmington	92%	85
Bayhealth - Kent General Hospital	Dover	90%	303
Christiana Care Health Services[2]	Newark	85%	310

17. Blood Culture Timing

Hospital Name	City	Rate	Cases
Nanticoke Memorial Hospital	Seaford	100%	158
Beebe Medical Center	Lewes	99%	290
Wilmington VA Medical Center	Wilmington	97%	34
Bayhealth - Kent General Hospital	Dover	95%	488
Saint Francis Hospital	Wilmington	93%	122
Christiana Care Health Services[2]	Newark	87%	450

18. Influenza Vaccine

Hospital Name	City	Rate	Cases
Beebe Medical Center	Lewes	98%	165
Bayhealth - Kent General Hospital	Dover	93%	357
Saint Francis Hospital	Wilmington	92%	52
Nanticoke Memorial Hospital	Seaford	89%	136
Christiana Care Health Services[2]	Newark	73%	284

19. Initial Antibiotic Timing

Hospital Name	City	Rate	Cases
Nanticoke Memorial Hospital	Seaford	98%	168
Beebe Medical Center	Lewes	97%	273
Saint Francis Hospital	Wilmington	96%	112
Bayhealth - Kent General Hospital	Dover	93%	497
Christiana Care Health Services[2]	Newark	92%	492
Wilmington VA Medical Center	Wilmington	83%	36

20. Pneumococcal Vaccine

Hospital Name	City	Rate	Cases
Nanticoke Memorial Hospital	Seaford	98%	170
Beebe Medical Center	Lewes	97%	260
Bayhealth - Kent General Hospital	Dover	95%	449
Saint Francis Hospital	Wilmington	90%	68
Christiana Care Health Services[2]	Newark	80%	411

21. Smoking Cessation Advice

Hospital Name	City	Rate	Cases
Christiana Care Health Services[2]	Newark	100%	171
Nanticoke Memorial Hospital	Seaford	100%	94
Saint Francis Hospital	Wilmington	100%	48
Bayhealth - Kent General Hospital	Dover	99%	261
Beebe Medical Center	Lewes	99%	99

Surgical Care Improvement Project

22. Appropriate VTP Within 24 Hours

Hospital Name	City	Rate	Cases
Beebe Medical Center[2]	Lewes	96%	264
Christiana Care Health Services[2]	Newark	95%	278
Saint Francis Hospital	Wilmington	94%	125
Wilmington VA Medical Center[2]	Wilmington	93%	46
Nanticoke Memorial Hospital[2]	Seaford	91%	86
Bayhealth - Kent General Hospital[2]	Dover	88%	329

23. Appropriate Hair Removal

Hospital Name	City	Rate	Cases
Bayhealth - Kent General Hospital[2]	Dover	100%	1203
Beebe Medical Center[2]	Lewes	100%	1279
Christiana Care Health Services[2]	Newark	100%	1096
Nanticoke Memorial Hospital[2]	Seaford	100%	170
Saint Francis Hospital	Wilmington	100%	551
Wilmington VA Medical Center[2]	Wilmington	100%	59

24. Appropriate Beta Blocker Usage

Hospital Name	City	Rate	Cases
Nanticoke Memorial Hospital[2]	Seaford	100%	50
Beebe Medical Center[2]	Lewes	99%	462
Christiana Care Health Services[2]	Newark	97%	321
Saint Francis Hospital	Wilmington	94%	136
Bayhealth - Kent General Hospital[2]	Dover	88%	414

25. Controlled Postoperative Blood Glucose

Hospital Name	City	Rate	Cases
Bayhealth - Kent General Hospital[2]	Dover	99%	158
Beebe Medical Center[2]	Lewes	96%	138
Christiana Care Health Services[2]	Newark	91%	195
Saint Francis Hospital	Wilmington	85%	82

26. Prophylactic Antibiotic Timing

Hospital Name	City	Rate	Cases
Beebe Medical Center[2]	Lewes	98%	982
Christiana Care Health Services[2]	Newark	97%	716
Nanticoke Memorial Hospital[2]	Seaford	97%	69
Bayhealth - Kent General Hospital[2]	Dover	96%	886
Saint Francis Hospital	Wilmington	93%	333

27. Prophylactic Antibiotic Timing (Outpatient)

Hospital Name	City	Rate	Cases
Beebe Medical Center	Lewes	95%	294
Saint Francis Hospital	Wilmington	95%	310
Nanticoke Memorial Hospital	Seaford	93%	103
Christiana Care Health Services	Newark	89%	903
Bayhealth - Kent General Hospital	Dover	83%	211

28. Prophylactic Antibiotic Selection

Hospital Name	City	Rate	Cases
Christiana Care Health Services[2]	Newark	100%	725
Beebe Medical Center[2]	Lewes	99%	988
Bayhealth - Kent General Hospital[2]	Dover	98%	893
Saint Francis Hospital	Wilmington	98%	336
Nanticoke Memorial Hospital[2]	Seaford	97%	70

29. Prophylactic Antibiotic Selection (Outpatient)

Hospital Name	City	Rate	Cases
Beebe Medical Center	Lewes	97%	288
Saint Francis Hospital	Wilmington	94%	304
Bayhealth - Kent General Hospital	Dover	84%	200
Christiana Care Health Services	Newark	83%	872
Nanticoke Memorial Hospital	Seaford	80%	98

30. Prophylactic Antibiotic Stopped

Hospital Name	City	Rate	Cases
Beebe Medical Center[2]	Lewes	100%	981
Christiana Care Health Services[2]	Newark	98%	682
Bayhealth - Kent General Hospital[2]	Dover	95%	808
Saint Francis Hospital	Wilmington	94%	301
Nanticoke Memorial Hospital[2]	Seaford	90%	62

31. Recommended VTP Ordered

Hospital Name	City	Rate	Cases
Christiana Care Health Services[2]	Newark	98%	278
Beebe Medical Center[2]	Lewes	96%	264
Saint Francis Hospital	Wilmington	96%	125
Bayhealth - Kent General Hospital[2]	Dover	95%	329
Nanticoke Memorial Hospital[2]	Seaford	95%	86
Wilmington VA Medical Center[2]	Wilmington	93%	46

32. Urinary Catheter Removal

Hospital Name	City	Rate	Cases
Beebe Medical Center[2]	Lewes	98%	471
Christiana Care Health Services[2]	Newark	94%	249
Bayhealth - Kent General Hospital[2]	Dover	93%	220
Saint Francis Hospital	Wilmington	90%	48

Use of Medical Imaging

36. Combination Abdominal CT Scan

Hospital Name	City	Ratio	Cases
Saint Francis Hospital	Wilmington	0.022	410
Christiana Care Health Services	Newark	0.029	2682
Beebe Medical Center	Lewes	0.076	2079
Nanticoke Memorial Hospital	Seaford	0.268	694
Bayhealth - Kent General Hospital	Dover	0.688	2515

37. Combination Chest CT Scan

Hospital Name	City	Ratio	Cases
Christiana Care Health Services	Newark	0.000	2929
Saint Francis Hospital	Wilmington	0.003	295
Nanticoke Memorial Hospital	Seaford	0.021	521
Beebe Medical Center	Lewes	0.040	1296
Bayhealth - Kent General Hospital	Dover	0.113	1602

NOTE: Hospital profiles are in alphabetical order by state, then city, then hospital within the city; Rankings exclude hospitals with less than 25 cases except for patient surveys which excludes hospitals with less than 100 cases; (a) 100–299 cases; (1) The number of cases is too small to be sure how well a hospital is performing; (2) The hospital indicated that the data submitted for this measure were based on a sample of cases; (3) Data was collected during a shorter time period (fewer quarters) than the maximum possible time for this measure; (4) Suppressed for one or more quarters by CMS; (5) No data is available from the hospital for this measure; (6) Fewer than 100 patients completed the HCAHPS survey. Use these rates with caution, as the number of surveys may be too low to reliably assess hospital performance; (7) Survey results are based on less than 12 months of data; (8) Survey results are not available for this reporting period; (9) No or very few patients were eligible for the HCAHPS survey. The scores shown, if any, reflect a very small number of surveys; (10) A state average was not calculated because too few hospitals in the state submitted data; (11) There were discrepancies in the data collection process; Please refer to the User's Guide for a full explanation of data.

38. Follow-up Mammogram/Ultrasound

Hospital Name	City	Rate	Cases
Saint Francis Hospital	Wilmington	3.5%	864
Beebe Medical Center	Lewes	5.7%	3147
Nanticoke Memorial Hospital	Seaford	6.9%	1178
Christiana Care Health Services	Newark	7.8%	2424
Bayhealth - Kent General Hospital	Dover	9.4%	3440

39. MRI for Low Back Pain

Hospital Name	City	Rate	Cases
Saint Francis Hospital[1]	Wilmington	21.6%	37
Nanticoke Memorial Hospital	Seaford	21.7%	92
Beebe Medical Center	Lewes	23.5%	293
Bayhealth - Kent General Hospital	Dover	23.7%	257
Christiana Care Health Services	Newark	32.5%	252

Survey of Patients' Hospital Experiences

40. Area Around Room 'Always' Quiet at Night

Hospital Name	City	Rate	Cases
Saint Francis Hospital	Wilmington	57%	300+
Bayhealth - Kent General Hospital	Dover	54%	300+
Christiana Care Health Services	Newark	49%	300+
Beebe Medical Center	Lewes	47%	300+
Nanticoke Memorial Hospital	Seaford	44%	300+

41. Doctors 'Always' Communicated Well

Hospital Name	City	Rate	Cases
Nanticoke Memorial Hospital	Seaford	81%	300+
Bayhealth - Kent General Hospital	Dover	80%	300+
Beebe Medical Center	Lewes	79%	300+
Christiana Care Health Services	Newark	78%	300+
Saint Francis Hospital	Wilmington	78%	300+

42. Home Recovery Information Given

Hospital Name	City	Rate	Cases
Bayhealth - Kent General Hospital	Dover	84%	300+
Nanticoke Memorial Hospital	Seaford	84%	300+
Beebe Medical Center	Lewes	83%	300+
Christiana Care Health Services	Newark	79%	300+
Saint Francis Hospital	Wilmington	74%	300+

43. Hospital Given 9 or 10 on 10 Point Scale

Hospital Name	City	Rate	Cases
Beebe Medical Center	Lewes	70%	300+
Christiana Care Health Services	Newark	67%	300+
Bayhealth - Kent General Hospital	Dover	65%	300+
Nanticoke Memorial Hospital	Seaford	61%	300+
Saint Francis Hospital	Wilmington	60%	300+

44. Meds 'Always' Explained Before Given

Hospital Name	City	Rate	Cases
Beebe Medical Center	Lewes	63%	300+
Nanticoke Memorial Hospital	Seaford	62%	300+
Christiana Care Health Services	Newark	61%	300+
Bayhealth - Kent General Hospital	Dover	60%	300+
Saint Francis Hospital	Wilmington	54%	300+

45. Nurses 'Always' Communicated Well

Hospital Name	City	Rate	Cases
Beebe Medical Center	Lewes	79%	300+
Bayhealth - Kent General Hospital	Dover	76%	300+
Christiana Care Health Services	Newark	76%	300+
Nanticoke Memorial Hospital	Seaford	76%	300+
Saint Francis Hospital	Wilmington	71%	300+

46. Pain 'Always' Well Controlled

Hospital Name	City	Rate	Cases
Beebe Medical Center	Lewes	72%	300+
Christiana Care Health Services	Newark	70%	300+
Bayhealth - Kent General Hospital	Dover	69%	300+
Nanticoke Memorial Hospital	Seaford	68%	300+
Saint Francis Hospital	Wilmington	63%	300+

47. Room and Bathroom 'Always' Clean

Hospital Name	City	Rate	Cases
Nanticoke Memorial Hospital	Seaford	70%	300+
Christiana Care Health Services	Newark	69%	300+
Beebe Medical Center	Lewes	68%	300+
Bayhealth - Kent General Hospital	Dover	65%	300+
Saint Francis Hospital	Wilmington	59%	300+

48. Timely Help 'Always' Received

Hospital Name	City	Rate	Cases
Beebe Medical Center	Lewes	68%	300+
Christiana Care Health Services	Newark	66%	300+
Bayhealth - Kent General Hospital	Dover	59%	300+
Nanticoke Memorial Hospital	Seaford	59%	300+
Saint Francis Hospital	Wilmington	59%	300+

49. Would Definitely Recommend Hospital

Hospital Name	City	Rate	Cases
Christiana Care Health Services	Newark	76%	300+
Beebe Medical Center	Lewes	70%	300+
Bayhealth - Kent General Hospital	Dover	66%	300+
Nanticoke Memorial Hospital	Seaford	62%	300+
Saint Francis Hospital	Wilmington	60%	300+

NOTE: Hospital profiles are in alphabetical order by state, then city, then hospital within the city; Rankings exclude hospitals with less than 25 cases except for patient surveys which excludes hospitals with less than 100 cases; (a) 100–299 cases; (1) The number of cases is too small to be sure how well a hospital is performing; (2) The hospital indicated that the data submitted for this measure were based on a sample of cases; (3) Data was collected during a shorter time period (fewer quarters) than the maximum possible time for this measure; (4) Suppressed for one or more quarters by CMS; (5) No data is available from the hospital for this measure; (6) Fewer than 100 patients completed the HCAHPS survey. Use these rates with caution, as the number of surveys may be too low to reliably assess hospital performance; (7) Survey results are based on less than 12 months of data; (8) Survey results are not available for this reporting period; (9) No or very few patients were eligible for the HCAHPS survey. The scores shown, if any, reflect a very small number of surveys; (10) A state average was not calculated because too few hospitals in the state submitted data; (11) There were discrepancies in the data collection process; Please refer to the User's Guide for a full explanation of data.

Bayhealth - Kent General Hospital

640 S State Street Phone: 302-744-7001
Dover, DE 19901 Fax: 302-735-3227
URL: www.bayhealth.org/about/kent.asp
Type: Acute Care Hospitals Emergency Services: Yes
Ownership: Voluntary Non-Profit - Other Beds: 231

Key Personnel:
CEO/President. . . . . Dennis E Klima
Chief of Medical Staff. . . . . William Rosenfeld
Operating Room. . . . . Chris Price
Quality Assurance . . . . Joann Davis
Ambulatory Care . . . . Al Pilong
Anesthesiology. . . . . Brian McCarthy
Emergency Room . . . . Craig Hochstein, MD
Patient Relations . . . . Cathy Marketto

Measure	Cases	This Hosp.	State Avg.	U.S. Avg.
Heart Attack Care				
ACE Inhibitor or ARB for LVSD	49	94%	95%	96%
Aspirin at Arrival	329	99%	99%	99%
Aspirin at Discharge	341	100%	99%	98%
Beta Blocker at Discharge	335	99%	98%	98%
Fibrinolytic Medication Timing	0	-	67%	55%
PCI Within 90 Minutes of Arrival	53	91%	90%	90%
Smoking Cessation Advice	139	99%	100%	99%
Chest Pain/Possible Heart Attack Care				
Aspirin at Arrival	31	100%	100%	95%
Median Time to ECG (minutes)	32	6	6	8
Median Time to Transfer (minutes)[1,3]	5	72	72	61
Fibrinolytic Medication Timing[3]	0	-	0%	54%
Heart Failure Care				
ACE Inhibitor or ARB for LVSD	171	99%	94%	94%
Discharge Instructions	416	95%	92%	88%
Evaluation of LVS Function	506	100%	99%	98%
Smoking Cessation Advice	123	100%	100%	98%
Pneumonia Care				
Appropriate Initial Antibiotic	303	90%	90%	92%
Blood Culture Timing	488	95%	94%	96%
Influenza Vaccine	357	93%	87%	91%
Initial Antibiotic Timing	497	93%	94%	95%
Pneumococcal Vaccine	449	95%	91%	93%
Smoking Cessation Advice	261	99%	100%	97%
Surgical Care Improvement Project				
Appropriate VTP Within 24 Hours[2]	329	88%	93%	92%
Appropriate Hair Removal[2]	1,203	100%	100%	99%
Appropriate Beta Blocker Usage[2]	414	88%	95%	93%
Controlled Postoperative Blood Glucose[2]	158	99%	94%	93%
Prophylactic Antibiotic Timing[2]	886	96%	97%	97%
Prophylactic Antibiotic Timing (Outpatient)	211	83%	90%	92%
Prophylactic Antibiotic Selection[2]	893	98%	99%	97%
Prophylactic Antibiotic Select. (Outpatient)	200	84%	87%	94%
Prophylactic Antibiotic Stopped[2]	808	95%	97%	94%
Recommended VTP Ordered[2]	329	95%	96%	94%
Urinary Catheter Removal[2]	220	93%	95%	90%
Children's Asthma Care				
Received Systemic Corticosteroids	-	-	-	100%
Received Home Management Plan	-	-	-	71%
Received Reliever Medication	-	-	-	100%
Use of Medical Imaging				
Combination Abdominal CT Scan	2,515	0.688	0.258	0.191
Combination Chest CT Scan	1,602	0.113	0.037	0.054
Follow-up Mammogram/Ultrasound	3,440	9.4%	7.3%	8.4%
MRI for Low Back Pain	257	23.7%	25.8%	32.7%
Survey of Patients' Hospital Experiences				
Area Around Room 'Always' Quiet at Night	300+	54%	-	58%
Doctors 'Always' Communicated Well	300+	80%	-	80%
Home Recovery Information Given	300+	84%	-	82%
Hospital Given 9 or 10 on 10 Point Scale	300+	65%	-	67%
Meds 'Always' Explained Before Given	300+	60%	-	60%
Nurses 'Always' Communicated Well	300+	76%	-	76%
Pain 'Always' Well Controlled	300+	69%	-	69%
Room and Bathroom 'Always' Clean	300+	65%	-	71%
Timely Help 'Always' Received	300+	59%	-	64%
Would Definitely Recommend Hospital	300+	66%	-	69%

Beebe Medical Center

424 Savannah Rd Phone: 302-645-3300
Lewes, DE 19958 Fax: 302-645-3585
E-mail: khalen@bbmc.org
URL: www.beebemed.org
Type: Acute Care Hospitals Emergency Services: Yes
Ownership: Proprietary Beds: 138

Key Personnel:
CEO/President. . . . . Jeff Fried
Chief of Medical Staff. . . . . Andrejs Strauss, MD
Operating Room. . . . . Perry Jeffrey
Pediatric Ambulatory Care . . . . . . Sautosh Reddy, MD
Pediatric In-Patient Care . . . . Sautosh Reddy, MD
Quality Assurance . . . . Barbara Reick
Radiology. . . . . Frances Esposito, MD
Patient Relations . . . . Ellen Tolbert

Measure	Cases	This Hosp.	State Avg.	U.S. Avg.
Heart Attack Care				
ACE Inhibitor or ARB for LVSD	39	97%	95%	96%
Aspirin at Arrival	264	100%	99%	99%
Aspirin at Discharge	261	100%	99%	98%
Beta Blocker at Discharge	258	97%	98%	98%
Fibrinolytic Medication Timing	0	-	67%	55%
PCI Within 90 Minutes of Arrival	40	92%	90%	90%
Smoking Cessation Advice	85	100%	100%	99%
Chest Pain/Possible Heart Attack Care				
Aspirin at Arrival[1]	4	100%	100%	95%
Median Time to ECG (minutes)[1]	5	2	6	8
Median Time to Transfer (minutes)[5]	0	-	72	61
Fibrinolytic Medication Timing[5]	0	-	0%	54%
Heart Failure Care				
ACE Inhibitor or ARB for LVSD	104	95%	94%	94%
Discharge Instructions	276	97%	92%	88%
Evaluation of LVS Function	353	98%	99%	98%
Smoking Cessation Advice	59	98%	100%	98%
Pneumonia Care				
Appropriate Initial Antibiotic	190	95%	90%	92%
Blood Culture Timing	290	99%	94%	96%
Influenza Vaccine	165	98%	87%	91%
Initial Antibiotic Timing	273	97%	94%	95%
Pneumococcal Vaccine	260	97%	91%	93%
Smoking Cessation Advice	99	99%	100%	97%
Surgical Care Improvement Project				
Appropriate VTP Within 24 Hours[2]	264	96%	93%	92%
Appropriate Hair Removal[2]	1,279	100%	100%	99%
Appropriate Beta Blocker Usage[2]	462	99%	95%	93%
Controlled Postoperative Blood Glucose[2]	138	96%	94%	93%
Prophylactic Antibiotic Timing[2]	982	98%	97%	97%
Prophylactic Antibiotic Timing (Outpatient)	294	95%	90%	92%
Prophylactic Antibiotic Selection[2]	988	99%	99%	97%
Prophylactic Antibiotic Select. (Outpatient)	288	97%	87%	94%
Prophylactic Antibiotic Stopped[2]	981	100%	97%	94%
Recommended VTP Ordered[2]	264	96%	96%	94%
Urinary Catheter Removal[2]	471	98%	95%	90%
Children's Asthma Care				
Received Systemic Corticosteroids	-	-	-	100%
Received Home Management Plan	-	-	-	71%
Received Reliever Medication	-	-	-	100%
Use of Medical Imaging				
Combination Abdominal CT Scan	2,079	0.076	0.258	0.191
Combination Chest CT Scan	1,296	0.040	0.037	0.054
Follow-up Mammogram/Ultrasound	3,147	5.7%	7.3%	8.4%
MRI for Low Back Pain	293	23.5%	25.8%	32.7%
Survey of Patients' Hospital Experiences				
Area Around Room 'Always' Quiet at Night	300+	47%	-	58%
Doctors 'Always' Communicated Well	300+	79%	-	80%
Home Recovery Information Given	300+	83%	-	82%
Hospital Given 9 or 10 on 10 Point Scale	300+	70%	-	67%
Meds 'Always' Explained Before Given	300+	63%	-	60%
Nurses 'Always' Communicated Well	300+	79%	-	76%
Pain 'Always' Well Controlled	300+	72%	-	69%
Room and Bathroom 'Always' Clean	300+	68%	-	71%
Timely Help 'Always' Received	300+	68%	-	64%
Would Definitely Recommend Hospital	300+	70%	-	69%

Christiana Care Health Services

4755 Ogletown-Stanton Road Phone: 302-733-1000
Newark, DE 19718 Fax: 302-428-5790
URL: www.christianacare.org
Type: Acute Care Hospitals Emergency Services: Yes
Ownership: Voluntary Non-Profit - Private Beds: 250

Key Personnel:
CEO/President. . . . . Robert J Laskowksi

Measure	Cases	This Hosp.	State Avg.	U.S. Avg.
Heart Attack Care				
ACE Inhibitor or ARB for LVSD	114	94%	95%	96%
Aspirin at Arrival	484	99%	99%	99%
Aspirin at Discharge	632	99%	99%	98%
Beta Blocker at Discharge	609	99%	98%	98%
Fibrinolytic Medication Timing[1]	1	0%	67%	55%
PCI Within 90 Minutes of Arrival	140	89%	90%	90%
Smoking Cessation Advice	220	100%	100%	99%
Chest Pain/Possible Heart Attack Care				
Aspirin at Arrival[5]	0	-	100%	95%
Median Time to ECG (minutes)[5]	0	-	6	8
Median Time to Transfer (minutes)[5]	0	-	72	61
Fibrinolytic Medication Timing[5]	0	-	0%	54%
Heart Failure Care				
ACE Inhibitor or ARB for LVSD[2]	284	89%	94%	94%
Discharge Instructions[2]	616	86%	92%	88%
Evaluation of LVS Function[2]	802	99%	99%	98%
Smoking Cessation Advice[2]	121	100%	100%	98%
Pneumonia Care				
Appropriate Initial Antibiotic[2]	310	85%	90%	92%
Blood Culture Timing[2]	450	87%	94%	96%
Influenza Vaccine[2]	284	73%	87%	91%
Initial Antibiotic Timing[2]	492	92%	94%	95%
Pneumococcal Vaccine[2]	411	80%	91%	93%
Smoking Cessation Advice[2]	171	100%	100%	97%
Surgical Care Improvement Project				
Appropriate VTP Within 24 Hours[2]	278	95%	93%	92%
Appropriate Hair Removal[2]	1,096	100%	100%	99%
Appropriate Beta Blocker Usage[2]	321	97%	95%	93%
Controlled Postoperative Blood Glucose[2]	195	91%	94%	93%
Prophylactic Antibiotic Timing[2]	716	97%	97%	97%
Prophylactic Antibiotic Timing (Outpatient)	903	89%	90%	92%
Prophylactic Antibiotic Selection[2]	725	100%	99%	97%
Prophylactic Antibiotic Select. (Outpatient)	872	83%	87%	94%
Prophylactic Antibiotic Stopped[2]	682	98%	97%	94%
Recommended VTP Ordered[2]	278	98%	96%	94%
Urinary Catheter Removal[2]	249	94%	95%	90%
Children's Asthma Care				
Received Systemic Corticosteroids	-	-	-	100%
Received Home Management Plan	-	-	-	71%
Received Reliever Medication	-	-	-	100%
Use of Medical Imaging				
Combination Abdominal CT Scan	2,682	0.029	0.258	0.191
Combination Chest CT Scan	2,929	0.000	0.037	0.054
Follow-up Mammogram/Ultrasound	2,424	7.8%	7.3%	8.4%
MRI for Low Back Pain	252	32.5%	25.8%	32.7%
Survey of Patients' Hospital Experiences				
Area Around Room 'Always' Quiet at Night	300+	49%	-	58%
Doctors 'Always' Communicated Well	300+	78%	-	80%
Home Recovery Information Given	300+	79%	-	82%
Hospital Given 9 or 10 on 10 Point Scale	300+	67%	-	67%
Meds 'Always' Explained Before Given	300+	61%	-	60%
Nurses 'Always' Communicated Well	300+	76%	-	76%
Pain 'Always' Well Controlled	300+	70%	-	69%
Room and Bathroom 'Always' Clean	300+	69%	-	71%
Timely Help 'Always' Received	300+	66%	-	64%
Would Definitely Recommend Hospital	300+	76%	-	69%

NOTE: Hospital profiles are in alphabetical order by state, then city, then hospital within the city; Rankings exclude hospitals with less than 25 cases except for patient surveys which excludes hospitals with less than 100 cases; (a) 100–299 cases; (1) The number of cases is too small to be sure how well a hospital is performing; (2) The hospital indicated that the data submitted for this measure were based on a sample of cases; (3) Data was collected during a shorter time period (fewer quarters) than the maximum possible time for this measure; (4) Suppressed for one or more quarters by CMS; (5) No data is available from the hospital for this measure; (6) Fewer than 100 patients completed the HCAHPS survey. Use these rates with caution, as the number of surveys may be too low to reliably assess hospital performance; (7) Survey results are based on less than 12 months of data; (8) Survey results are not available for this reporting period; (9) No or very few patients were eligible for the HCAHPS survey. The scores shown, if any, reflect a very small number of surveys; (10) A state average was not calculated because too few hospitals in the state submitted data; (11) There were discrepancies in the data collection process; Please refer to the User's Guide for a full explanation of data.

Nanticoke Memorial Hospital

801 Middleford Rd
Seaford, DE 19973
Phone: 302-629-6611
Fax: 302-629-4758
E-mail: nhshr@ce.net
URL: www.nanticoke.org
Type: Acute Care Hospitals
Emergency Services: No
Ownership: Voluntary Non-Profit - Private
Beds: 140

Key Personnel:
CEO/President. . . . . Daniel J Werner
Operating Room. . . . . Stephen D Carey
Pediatric Ambulatory Care . . . . . . Patrick Jarvie, MD
Pediatric In-Patient Care . . . . Patrick Jarvie, MD
Quality Assurance . . . . Barbara Young
Radiology. . . . . Warren Cohen, MD
Emergency Room . . . . Yvonne O'Brien

Measure	Cases	This Hosp.	State Avg.	U.S. Avg.
Heart Attack Care				
ACE Inhibitor or ARB for LVSD[1]	11	100%	95%	96%
Aspirin at Arrival	97	100%	99%	99%
Aspirin at Discharge	81	99%	99%	98%
Beta Blocker at Discharge	83	99%	98%	98%
Fibrinolytic Medication Timing[1]	2	100%	67%	55%
PCI Within 90 Minutes of Arrival[1]	19	100%	90%	90%
Smoking Cessation Advice	27	100%	100%	99%
Chest Pain/Possible Heart Attack Care				
Aspirin at Arrival[1]	15	100%	100%	95%
Median Time to ECG (minutes)[1]	15	7	6	8
Median Time to Transfer (minutes)[5]	0	-	72	61
Fibrinolytic Medication Timing[3]	0	-	0%	54%
Heart Failure Care				
ACE Inhibitor or ARB for LVSD	37	100%	94%	94%
Discharge Instructions	166	98%	92%	88%
Evaluation of LVS Function	202	99%	99%	98%
Smoking Cessation Advice	39	100%	100%	98%
Pneumonia Care				
Appropriate Initial Antibiotic	103	97%	90%	92%
Blood Culture Timing	158	100%	94%	96%
Influenza Vaccine	136	89%	87%	91%
Initial Antibiotic Timing	168	98%	94%	95%
Pneumococcal Vaccine	170	98%	91%	93%
Smoking Cessation Advice	94	100%	100%	97%
Surgical Care Improvement Project				
Appropriate VTP Within 24 Hours[2]	86	91%	93%	92%
Appropriate Hair Removal[2]	170	100%	100%	99%
Appropriate Beta Blocker Usage[2]	50	100%	95%	93%
Controlled Postoperative Blood Glucose[2]	0	-	94%	93%
Prophylactic Antibiotic Timing[2]	69	97%	97%	97%
Prophylactic Antibiotic Timing (Outpatient)	103	93%	90%	92%
Prophylactic Antibiotic Selection[2]	70	97%	99%	97%
Prophylactic Antibiotic Select. (Outpatient)	98	80%	87%	94%
Prophylactic Antibiotic Stopped[2]	62	90%	97%	94%
Recommended VTP Ordered[2]	86	95%	96%	94%
Urinary Catheter Removal[1,2]	18	89%	95%	90%
Children's Asthma Care				
Received Systemic Corticosteroids	-	-	-	100%
Received Home Management Plan	-	-	-	71%
Received Reliever Medication	-	-	-	100%
Use of Medical Imaging				
Combination Abdominal CT Scan	694	0.268	0.258	0.191
Combination Chest CT Scan	521	0.021	0.037	0.054
Follow-up Mammogram/Ultrasound	1,178	6.9%	7.3%	8.4%
MRI for Low Back Pain	92	21.7%	25.8%	32.7%
Survey of Patients' Hospital Experiences				
Area Around Room 'Always' Quiet at Night	300+	44%	-	58%
Doctors 'Always' Communicated Well	300+	81%	-	80%
Home Recovery Information Given	300+	84%	-	82%
Hospital Given 9 or 10 on 10 Point Scale	300+	61%	-	67%
Meds 'Always' Explained Before Given	300+	62%	-	60%
Nurses 'Always' Communicated Well	300+	76%	-	76%
Pain 'Always' Well Controlled	300+	68%	-	69%
Room and Bathroom 'Always' Clean	300+	70%	-	71%
Timely Help 'Always' Received	300+	59%	-	64%
Would Definitely Recommend Hospital	300+	62%	-	69%

Saint Francis Hospital

7th and Clayton Sts
Wilmington, DE 19805
Phone: 302-421-4100
URL: www.stfrancishealthcare.org
Type: Acute Care Hospitals
Emergency Services: Yes
Ownership: Voluntary Non-Profit - Private
Beds: 330

Key Personnel:
CEO/President. . . . . Clarence Laliberty

Measure	Cases	This Hosp.	State Avg.	U.S. Avg.
Heart Attack Care				
ACE Inhibitor or ARB for LVSD	33	94%	95%	96%
Aspirin at Arrival	116	97%	99%	99%
Aspirin at Discharge	109	99%	99%	98%
Beta Blocker at Discharge	102	99%	98%	98%
Fibrinolytic Medication Timing	0	-	67%	55%
PCI Within 90 Minutes of Arrival[1]	11	73%	90%	90%
Smoking Cessation Advice	49	100%	100%	99%
Chest Pain/Possible Heart Attack Care				
Aspirin at Arrival[5]	0	-	100%	95%
Median Time to ECG (minutes)[5]	0	-	6	8
Median Time to Transfer (minutes)[5]	0	-	72	61
Fibrinolytic Medication Timing[5]	0	-	0%	54%
Heart Failure Care				
ACE Inhibitor or ARB for LVSD	102	97%	94%	94%
Discharge Instructions	205	94%	92%	88%
Evaluation of LVS Function	234	96%	99%	98%
Smoking Cessation Advice	54	100%	100%	98%
Pneumonia Care				
Appropriate Initial Antibiotic	85	92%	90%	92%
Blood Culture Timing	122	93%	94%	96%
Influenza Vaccine	52	92%	87%	91%
Initial Antibiotic Timing	112	96%	94%	95%
Pneumococcal Vaccine	68	90%	91%	93%
Smoking Cessation Advice	48	100%	100%	97%
Surgical Care Improvement Project				
Appropriate VTP Within 24 Hours	125	94%	93%	92%
Appropriate Hair Removal	551	100%	100%	99%
Appropriate Beta Blocker Usage	136	94%	95%	93%
Controlled Postoperative Blood Glucose	82	85%	94%	93%
Prophylactic Antibiotic Timing	333	93%	97%	97%
Prophylactic Antibiotic Timing (Outpatient)	310	95%	90%	92%
Prophylactic Antibiotic Selection	336	98%	99%	97%
Prophylactic Antibiotic Select. (Outpatient)	304	94%	87%	94%
Prophylactic Antibiotic Stopped	301	94%	97%	94%
Recommended VTP Ordered	125	96%	96%	94%
Urinary Catheter Removal	48	90%	95%	90%
Children's Asthma Care				
Received Systemic Corticosteroids	-	-	-	100%
Received Home Management Plan	-	-	-	71%
Received Reliever Medication	-	-	-	100%
Use of Medical Imaging				
Combination Abdominal CT Scan	410	0.022	0.258	0.191
Combination Chest CT Scan	295	0.003	0.037	0.054
Follow-up Mammogram/Ultrasound	864	3.5%	7.3%	8.4%
MRI for Low Back Pain[1]	37	21.6%	25.8%	32.7%
Survey of Patients' Hospital Experiences				
Area Around Room 'Always' Quiet at Night	300+	57%	-	58%
Doctors 'Always' Communicated Well	300+	78%	-	80%
Home Recovery Information Given	300+	74%	-	82%
Hospital Given 9 or 10 on 10 Point Scale	300+	60%	-	67%
Meds 'Always' Explained Before Given	300+	54%	-	60%
Nurses 'Always' Communicated Well	300+	71%	-	76%
Pain 'Always' Well Controlled	300+	63%	-	69%
Room and Bathroom 'Always' Clean	300+	59%	-	71%
Timely Help 'Always' Received	300+	59%	-	64%
Would Definitely Recommend Hospital	300+	60%	-	69%

Wilmington VA Medical Center

1601 Kirkwood Highway
Wilmington, DE 19805
Phone: 302-994-2511
Fax: 302-633-5591
URL: www.va.gov/wilmington
Type: Acute Care-Veterans Administration
Emergency Services: No
Ownership: Government - Federal
Beds: 120

Key Personnel:
CEO/President. . . . . Charles M Dorman
Cardiac Laboratory. . . . . Gaddum Reddy, MD
Chief of Medical Staff . . . . Dennis R Witmer, MD
Infection Control. . . . . Ted Martynowicz, DO
Operating Room. . . . . Jeanne Long
Quality Assurance . . . . Melinda Haebel

Measure	Cases	This Hosp.	State Avg.	U.S. Avg.
Heart Attack Care				
ACE Inhibitor or ARB for LVSD[5]	0	-	95%	96%
Aspirin at Arrival[5]	0	-	99%	99%
Aspirin at Discharge[5]	0	-	99%	98%
Beta Blocker at Discharge[5]	0	-	98%	98%
Fibrinolytic Medication Timing[5]	0	-	67%	55%
PCI Within 90 Minutes of Arrival[5]	0	-	90%	90%
Smoking Cessation Advice[5]	0	-	100%	99%
Chest Pain/Possible Heart Attack Care				
Aspirin at Arrival	-	-	100%	95%
Median Time to ECG (minutes)	-	-	6	8
Median Time to Transfer (minutes)	-	-	72	61
Fibrinolytic Medication Timing	-	-	0%	54%
Heart Failure Care				
ACE Inhibitor or ARB for LVSD[1]	21	100%	94%	94%
Discharge Instructions	49	90%	92%	88%
Evaluation of LVS Function	52	100%	99%	98%
Smoking Cessation Advice[1]	9	89%	100%	98%
Pneumonia Care				
Appropriate Initial Antibiotic[1]	21	81%	90%	92%
Blood Culture Timing	34	97%	94%	96%
Influenza Vaccine[1]	21	100%	87%	91%
Initial Antibiotic Timing	36	83%	94%	95%
Pneumococcal Vaccine[1]	19	100%	91%	93%
Smoking Cessation Advice[1]	16	88%	100%	97%
Surgical Care Improvement Project				
Appropriate VTP Within 24 Hours[2]	46	93%	93%	92%
Appropriate Hair Removal[2]	59	100%	100%	99%
Appropriate Beta Blocker Usage[1,2]	23	100%	95%	93%
Controlled Postoperative Blood Glucose[2,5]	0	-	94%	93%
Prophylactic Antibiotic Timing[1]	20	95%	97%	97%
Prophylactic Antibiotic Timing (Outpatient)	-	-	90%	92%
Prophylactic Antibiotic Selection[1]	20	95%	99%	97%
Prophylactic Antibiotic Select. (Outpatient)	-	-	87%	94%
Prophylactic Antibiotic Stopped[1]	20	100%	97%	94%
Recommended VTP Ordered[2]	46	93%	96%	94%
Urinary Catheter Removal[1,2]	20	100%	95%	90%
Children's Asthma Care				
Received Systemic Corticosteroids	-	-	-	100%
Received Home Management Plan	-	-	-	71%
Received Reliever Medication	-	-	-	100%
Use of Medical Imaging				
Combination Abdominal CT Scan	-	-	0.258	0.191
Combination Chest CT Scan	-	-	0.037	0.054
Follow-up Mammogram/Ultrasound	-	-	7.3%	8.4%
MRI for Low Back Pain	-	-	25.8%	32.7%
Survey of Patients' Hospital Experiences				
Area Around Room 'Always' Quiet at Night	-	-	-	58%
Doctors 'Always' Communicated Well	-	-	-	80%
Home Recovery Information Given	-	-	-	82%
Hospital Given 9 or 10 on 10 Point Scale	-	-	-	67%
Meds 'Always' Explained Before Given	-	-	-	60%
Nurses 'Always' Communicated Well	-	-	-	76%
Pain 'Always' Well Controlled	-	-	-	69%
Room and Bathroom 'Always' Clean	-	-	-	71%
Timely Help 'Always' Received	-	-	-	64%
Would Definitely Recommend Hospital	-	-	-	69%

NOTE: Hospital profiles are in alphabetical order by state, then city, then hospital within the city; Rankings exclude hospitals with less than 25 cases except for patient surveys which excludes hospitals with less than 100 cases; (a) 100–299 cases; (1) The number of cases is too small to be sure how well a hospital is performing; (2) The hospital indicated that the data submitted for this measure were based on a sample of cases; (3) Data was collected during a shorter time period (fewer quarters) than the maximum possible time for this measure; (4) Suppressed for one or more quarters by CMS; (5) No data is available from the hospital for this measure; (6) Fewer than 100 patients completed the HCAHPS survey. Use these rates with caution, as the number of surveys may be too low to reliably assess hospital performance; (7) Survey results are based on less than 12 months of data; (8) Survey results are not available for this reporting period; (9) No or very few patients were eligible for the HCAHPS survey. The scores shown, if any, reflect a very small number of surveys; (10) A state average was not calculated because too few hospitals in the state submitted data; (11) There were discrepancies in the data collection process; Please refer to the User's Guide for a full explanation of data.

Heart Attack Care

1. ACE Inhibitor or ARB for LVSD

Hospital Name	City	Rate	Cases
Washington Hospital Center[2]	Washington	97%	78
George Washington Univ Hospital	Washington	91%	33

2. Aspirin at Arrival

Hospital Name	City	Rate	Cases
Washington DC VA Medical Center	Washington	100%	25
George Washington Univ Hospital	Washington	99%	191
Washington Hospital Center[2]	Washington	98%	63
Sibley Memorial Hospital	Washington	97%	32
Providence Hospital	Washington	95%	60
Howard University Hospital	Washington	91%	45

3. Aspirin at Discharge

Hospital Name	City	Rate	Cases
Howard University Hospital	Washington	100%	45
Washington DC VA Medical Center	Washington	100%	31
Washington Hospital Center[2]	Washington	99%	282
George Washington Univ Hospital	Washington	98%	259
Providence Hospital	Washington	89%	45

4. Beta Blocker at Discharge

Hospital Name	City	Rate	Cases
Washington DC VA Medical Center	Washington	100%	29
Washington Hospital Center[2]	Washington	99%	269
George Washington Univ Hospital	Washington	97%	232
Howard University Hospital	Washington	96%	45
Providence Hospital	Washington	81%	43

6. PCI Within 90 Minutes of Arrival

Hospital Name	City	Rate	Cases
George Washington Univ Hospital	Washington	88%	34

7. Smoking Cessation Advice

Hospital Name	City	Rate	Cases
George Washington Univ Hospital	Washington	100%	73
Howard University Hospital	Washington	100%	26
Washington Hospital Center[2]	Washington	100%	79

Chest Pain/Possible Heart Attack Care

8. Aspirin at Arrival

Hospital Name	City	Rate	Cases
Sibley Memorial Hospital	Washington	98%	47
Georgetown University Hospital	Washington	96%	50

9. Median Time to ECG (minutes)

Hospital Name	City	Min.	Cases
Sibley Memorial Hospital	Washington	10	49
Georgetown University Hospital	Washington	14	53

Heart Failure Care

12. ACE Inhibitor or ARB for LVSD

Hospital Name	City	Rate	Cases
Georgetown University Hospital	Washington	100%	37
Howard University Hospital[2]	Washington	97%	154
Sibley Memorial Hospital	Washington	97%	35
Washington Hospital Center[2]	Washington	97%	193
George Washington Univ Hospital	Washington	95%	167
Washington DC VA Medical Center	Washington	94%	160
Providence Hospital	Washington	83%	255
United Medical Center	Washington	81%	122

13. Discharge Instructions

Hospital Name	City	Rate	Cases
George Washington Univ Hospital	Washington	100%	331
Howard University Hospital[2]	Washington	99%	268
Washington DC VA Medical Center	Washington	96%	224
Washington Hospital Center[2]	Washington	93%	355
Georgetown University Hospital	Washington	89%	73
Sibley Memorial Hospital	Washington	83%	102
United Medical Center	Washington	60%	235
Providence Hospital	Washington	24%	504

14. Evaluation of LVS Function

Hospital Name	City	Rate	Cases
Georgetown University Hospital	Washington	99%	90
Sibley Memorial Hospital	Washington	99%	124
Washington DC VA Medical Center	Washington	99%	234
George Washington Univ Hospital	Washington	98%	372

Howard University Hospital[2]	Washington	98%	286
Washington Hospital Center[2]	Washington	98%	393
Providence Hospital	Washington	92%	588
United Medical Center	Washington	91%	270

15. Smoking Cessation Advice

Hospital Name	City	Rate	Cases
George Washington Univ Hospital	Washington	100%	67
Howard University Hospital[2]	Washington	100%	94
Washington DC VA Medical Center	Washington	100%	74
Washington Hospital Center[2]	Washington	100%	72
United Medical Center	Washington	97%	116
Providence Hospital	Washington	95%	101

Pneumonia Care

16. Appropriate Initial Antibiotic

Hospital Name	City	Rate	Cases
United Medical Center	Washington	98%	87
Washington Hospital Center[2]	Washington	98%	58
Washington DC VA Medical Center	Washington	97%	33
Georgetown University Hospital[2]	Washington	95%	38
Howard University Hospital[2]	Washington	92%	64
Sibley Memorial Hospital[2]	Washington	92%	87
Providence Hospital	Washington	85%	120
George Washington Univ Hospital	Washington	71%	55

17. Blood Culture Timing

Hospital Name	City	Rate	Cases
Sibley Memorial Hospital[2]	Washington	98%	135
Washington DC VA Medical Center	Washington	97%	60
George Washington Univ Hospital	Washington	94%	47
Howard University Hospital[2]	Washington	92%	90
Georgetown University Hospital[2]	Washington	87%	60
Washington Hospital Center[2]	Washington	86%	56
Providence Hospital	Washington	82%	170
United Medical Center	Washington	79%	115

18. Influenza Vaccine

Hospital Name	City	Rate	Cases
George Washington Univ Hospital	Washington	95%	43
Washington Hospital Center[2]	Washington	93%	75
Sibley Memorial Hospital[2]	Washington	92%	74
Washington DC VA Medical Center	Washington	90%	50
Howard University Hospital[2]	Washington	89%	57
Georgetown University Hospital[2]	Washington	85%	66
Providence Hospital	Washington	40%	149
United Medical Center	Washington	33%	79

19. Initial Antibiotic Timing

Hospital Name	City	Rate	Cases
Sibley Memorial Hospital[2]	Washington	98%	105
Washington Hospital Center[2]	Washington	98%	111
George Washington Univ Hospital	Washington	97%	69
Georgetown University Hospital[2]	Washington	96%	75
Washington DC VA Medical Center	Washington	88%	57
Providence Hospital	Washington	80%	188
Howard University Hospital[2]	Washington	75%	113
United Medical Center	Washington	67%	153

20. Pneumococcal Vaccine

Hospital Name	City	Rate	Cases
Washington DC VA Medical Center	Washington	96%	49
Washington Hospital Center[2]	Washington	94%	87
Georgetown University Hospital[2]	Washington	93%	60
Sibley Memorial Hospital[2]	Washington	90%	120
George Washington Univ Hospital	Washington	88%	51
Howard University Hospital[2]	Washington	73%	45
Providence Hospital	Washington	50%	158
United Medical Center	Washington	27%	73

21. Smoking Cessation Advice

Hospital Name	City	Rate	Cases
Georgetown University Hospital[2]	Washington	100%	27
Washington Hospital Center[2]	Washington	100%	52
Howard University Hospital[2]	Washington	99%	84
George Washington Univ Hospital	Washington	97%	32
Providence Hospital	Washington	96%	85
United Medical Center	Washington	86%	105

Surgical Care Improvement Project

22. Appropriate VTP Within 24 Hours

Hospital Name	City	Rate	Cases
Georgetown University Hospital[2]	Washington	99%	231
Washington Hospital Center[2]	Washington	99%	299

George Washington Univ Hospital[2]	Washington	98%	215
Sibley Memorial Hospital[2]	Washington	96%	269
Washington DC VA Medical Center[2]	Washington	93%	96
Providence Hospital[2]	Washington	89%	175
Howard University Hospital[2]	Washington	88%	165
United Medical Center	Washington	83%	65

23. Appropriate Hair Removal

Hospital Name	City	Rate	Cases
Georgetown University Hospital[2]	Washington	100%	415
Providence Hospital[2]	Washington	100%	364
Sibley Memorial Hospital[2]	Washington	100%	635
Washington DC VA Medical Center[2]	Washington	100%	227
Washington Hospital Center[2]	Washington	100%	808
United Medical Center	Washington	99%	110
George Washington Univ Hospital[2]	Washington	98%	714
Howard University Hospital[2]	Washington	95%	248

24. Appropriate Beta Blocker Usage

Hospital Name	City	Rate	Cases
Washington DC VA Medical Center[2]	Washington	100%	99
Washington Hospital Center[2]	Washington	98%	306
Georgetown University Hospital[2]	Washington	95%	113
George Washington Univ Hospital[2]	Washington	93%	191
Sibley Memorial Hospital[2]	Washington	93%	135
Howard University Hospital[2]	Washington	82%	45
Providence Hospital[2]	Washington	82%	67

25. Controlled Postoperative Blood Glucose

Hospital Name	City	Rate	Cases
Washington Hospital Center[2]	Washington	98%	209
George Washington Univ Hospital[2]	Washington	96%	160
Washington DC VA Medical Center[2]	Washington	92%	106

26. Prophylactic Antibiotic Timing

Hospital Name	City	Rate	Cases
Washington DC VA Medical Center	Washington	100%	144
George Washington Univ Hospital[2]	Washington	97%	536
Washington Hospital Center[2]	Washington	97%	564
Georgetown University Hospital[2]	Washington	96%	273
Sibley Memorial Hospital[2]	Washington	96%	466
United Medical Center	Washington	93%	27
Providence Hospital[2]	Washington	92%	249
Howard University Hospital[2]	Washington	77%	165

27. Prophylactic Antibiotic Timing (Outpatient)

Hospital Name	City	Rate	Cases
George Washington Univ Hospital	Washington	97%	410
Washington Hospital Center	Washington	95%	526
Georgetown University Hospital	Washington	94%	356
Sibley Memorial Hospital	Washington	91%	265
Providence Hospital	Washington	73%	281
United Medical Center[3]	Washington	40%	25
Howard University Hospital	Washington	23%	147

28. Prophylactic Antibiotic Selection

Hospital Name	City	Rate	Cases
Washington DC VA Medical Center	Washington	99%	145
Washington Hospital Center[2]	Washington	98%	580
Georgetown University Hospital[2]	Washington	97%	279
Sibley Memorial Hospital[2]	Washington	96%	468
United Medical Center	Washington	96%	27
George Washington Univ Hospital[2]	Washington	95%	543
Howard University Hospital[2]	Washington	94%	166
Providence Hospital[2]	Washington	83%	250

29. Prophylactic Antibiotic Selection (Outpatient)

Hospital Name	City	Rate	Cases
Georgetown University Hospital	Washington	96%	352
Washington Hospital Center	Washington	96%	523
George Washington Univ Hospital	Washington	93%	404
Sibley Memorial Hospital	Washington	88%	264
Providence Hospital	Washington	85%	231
Howard University Hospital	Washington	73%	52

30. Prophylactic Antibiotic Stopped

Hospital Name	City	Rate	Cases
Washington DC VA Medical Center	Washington	96%	140
Washington Hospital Center[2]	Washington	96%	553
Georgetown University Hospital[2]	Washington	95%	257
Sibley Memorial Hospital[2]	Washington	94%	454
George Washington Univ Hospital[2]	Washington	92%	450
Howard University Hospital[2]	Washington	84%	160
Providence Hospital[2]	Washington	80%	237
United Medical Center	Washington	68%	25

NOTE: Hospital profiles are in alphabetical order by state, then city, then hospital within the city; Rankings exclude hospitals with less than 25 cases except for patient surveys which excludes hospitals with less than 100 cases; (a) 100–299 cases; (1) The number of cases is too small to be sure how well a hospital is performing; (2) The hospital indicated that the data submitted for this measure were based on a sample of cases; (3) Data was collected during a shorter time period (fewer quarters) than the maximum possible time for this measure; (4) Suppressed for one or more quarters by CMS; (5) No data is available from the hospital for this measure; (6) Fewer than 100 patients completed the HCAHPS survey. Use these rates with caution, as the number of surveys may be too low to reliably assess hospital performance; (7) Survey results are based on less than 12 months of data; (8) Survey results are not available for this reporting period; (9) No or very few patients were eligible for the HCAHPS survey. The scores shown, if any, reflect a very small number of surveys; (10) A state average was not calculated because too few hospitals in the state submitted data; (11) There were discrepancies in the data collection process; Please refer to the User's Guide for a full explanation of data.

31. Recommended VTP Ordered

Hospital Name	City	Rate	Cases
George Washington Univ Hospital[2]	Washington	99%	215
Georgetown University Hospital[2]	Washington	99%	232
Washington Hospital Center[2]	Washington	99%	299
Sibley Memorial Hospital[2]	Washington	97%	269
Washington DC VA Medical Center[2]	Washington	92%	97
Providence Hospital[2]	Washington	91%	175
Howard University Hospital[2]	Washington	88%	165
United Medical Center	Washington	85%	66

32. Urinary Catheter Removal

Hospital Name	City	Rate	Cases
Washington DC VA Medical Center[2]	Washington	99%	87
Sibley Memorial Hospital[2]	Washington	94%	146
Georgetown University Hospital[2]	Washington	92%	119
Washington Hospital Center[2]	Washington	92%	220
Howard University Hospital[2]	Washington	88%	64
George Washington Univ Hospital[2]	Washington	82%	205
Providence Hospital[2]	Washington	78%	93

Children's Asthma Care

33. Received Systemic Corticosteroids

Hospital Name	City	Rate	Cases
Children's Hospital NMC[2]	Washington	100%	419
Georgetown University Hospital[2]	Washington	97%	39
Howard University Hospital[2]	Washington	97%	34

34. Received Home Management Plan of Care

Hospital Name	City	Rate	Cases
Children's Hospital NMC[2]	Washington	71%	417
Georgetown University Hospital[2]	Washington	53%	40
Howard University Hospital[2]	Washington	0%	34

35. Received Reliever Medication

Hospital Name	City	Rate	Cases
Children's Hospital NMC[2]	Washington	100%	420
Georgetown University Hospital[2]	Washington	100%	40
Howard University Hospital[2]	Washington	100%	34

Use of Medical Imaging

36. Combination Abdominal CT Scan

Hospital Name	City	Ratio	Cases
Washington Hospital Center	Washington	0.009	1843
United Medical Center	Washington	0.016	123
Sibley Memorial Hospital	Washington	0.039	1095
Howard University Hospital	Washington	0.061	244
Georgetown University Hospital	Washington	0.081	1367
George Washington Univ Hospital	Washington	0.179	697
Providence Hospital	Washington	0.574	810

37. Combination Chest CT Scan

Hospital Name	City	Ratio	Cases
Washington Hospital Center	Washington	0.002	1377
Sibley Memorial Hospital	Washington	0.003	966
United Medical Center	Washington	0.011	90
Georgetown University Hospital	Washington	0.012	1455
Howard University Hospital	Washington	0.027	187
George Washington Univ Hospital	Washington	0.058	635
Providence Hospital	Washington	0.484	409

38. Follow-up Mammogram/Ultrasound

Hospital Name	City	Rate	Cases
Washington Hospital Center	Washington	4.0%	1845
George Washington Univ Hospital	Washington	5.4%	575
Providence Hospital	Washington	5.7%	1909
United Medical Center	Washington	5.7%	348
Sibley Memorial Hospital	Washington	8.6%	2076
Howard University Hospital	Washington	9.2%	541
Georgetown University Hospital	Washington	10.4%	867

39. MRI for Low Back Pain

Hospital Name	City	Rate	Cases
George Washington Univ Hospital	Washington	26.7%	101
Georgetown University Hospital	Washington	30.3%	109
Sibley Memorial Hospital	Washington	30.8%	263
Washington Hospital Center	Washington	31.0%	245
Providence Hospital	Washington	36.5%	115
Howard University Hospital	Washington	50.0%	38

Survey of Patients' Hospital Experiences

40. Area Around Room 'Always' Quiet at Night

Hospital Name	City	Rate	Cases
Howard University Hospital	Washington	68%	300+
Providence Hospital	Washington	62%	300+
George Washington Univ Hospital	Washington	59%	300+
Georgetown University Hospital	Washington	55%	300+
United Medical Center	Washington	55%	300+
Washington Hospital Center	Washington	53%	300+
Sibley Memorial Hospital	Washington	48%	300+

41. Doctors 'Always' Communicated Well

Hospital Name	City	Rate	Cases
Washington Hospital Center	Washington	79%	300+
Georgetown University Hospital	Washington	77%	300+
Howard University Hospital	Washington	77%	300+
Providence Hospital	Washington	77%	300+
Sibley Memorial Hospital	Washington	77%	300+
George Washington Univ Hospital	Washington	76%	300+
United Medical Center	Washington	68%	300+

42. Home Recovery Information Given

Hospital Name	City	Rate	Cases
Georgetown University Hospital	Washington	87%	300+
Washington Hospital Center	Washington	83%	300+
George Washington Univ Hospital	Washington	80%	300+
Sibley Memorial Hospital	Washington	75%	300+
Howard University Hospital	Washington	74%	300+
Providence Hospital	Washington	74%	300+
United Medical Center	Washington	64%	300+

43. Hospital Given 9 or 10 on 10 Point Scale

Hospital Name	City	Rate	Cases
Georgetown University Hospital	Washington	68%	300+
George Washington Univ Hospital	Washington	62%	300+
Sibley Memorial Hospital	Washington	62%	300+
Providence Hospital	Washington	61%	300+
Washington Hospital Center	Washington	61%	300+
Howard University Hospital	Washington	57%	300+
United Medical Center	Washington	41%	300+

44. Meds 'Always' Explained Before Given

Hospital Name	City	Rate	Cases
Georgetown University Hospital	Washington	61%	300+
Howard University Hospital	Washington	55%	300+
George Washington Univ Hospital	Washington	54%	300+
Providence Hospital	Washington	54%	300+
Sibley Memorial Hospital	Washington	54%	300+
Washington Hospital Center	Washington	53%	300+
United Medical Center	Washington	51%	300+

45. Nurses 'Always' Communicated Well

Hospital Name	City	Rate	Cases
Georgetown University Hospital	Washington	75%	300+
Providence Hospital	Washington	70%	300+
Sibley Memorial Hospital	Washington	69%	300+
Howard University Hospital	Washington	68%	300+
Washington Hospital Center	Washington	67%	300+
George Washington Univ Hospital	Washington	66%	300+
United Medical Center	Washington	61%	300+

46. Pain 'Always' Well Controlled

Hospital Name	City	Rate	Cases
Sibley Memorial Hospital	Washington	69%	300+
Georgetown University Hospital	Washington	67%	300+
Providence Hospital	Washington	64%	300+
Washington Hospital Center	Washington	64%	300+
Howard University Hospital	Washington	63%	300+
George Washington Univ Hospital	Washington	59%	300+
United Medical Center	Washington	58%	300+

47. Room and Bathroom 'Always' Clean

Hospital Name	City	Rate	Cases
Providence Hospital	Washington	67%	300+
Sibley Memorial Hospital	Washington	67%	300+
Howard University Hospital	Washington	64%	300+
Georgetown University Hospital	Washington	63%	300+
United Medical Center	Washington	63%	300+
Washington Hospital Center	Washington	61%	300+
George Washington Univ Hospital	Washington	60%	300+

48. Timely Help 'Always' Received

Hospital Name	City	Rate	Cases
Georgetown University Hospital	Washington	55%	300+

Howard University Hospital	Washington	55%	300+
Providence Hospital	Washington	54%	300+
Sibley Memorial Hospital	Washington	52%	300+
George Washington Univ Hospital	Washington	48%	300+
Washington Hospital Center	Washington	47%	300+
United Medical Center	Washington	45%	300+

49. Would Definitely Recommend Hospital

Hospital Name	City	Rate	Cases
Georgetown University Hospital	Washington	75%	300+
Sibley Memorial Hospital	Washington	72%	300+
George Washington Univ Hospital	Washington	67%	300+
Washington Hospital Center	Washington	66%	300+
Providence Hospital	Washington	63%	300+
Howard University Hospital	Washington	57%	300+
United Medical Center	Washington	36%	300+

NOTE: Hospital profiles are in alphabetical order by state, then city, then hospital within the city; Rankings exclude hospitals with less than 25 cases except for patient surveys which excludes hospitals with less than 100 cases; (a) 100–299 cases; (1) The number of cases is too small to be sure how well a hospital is performing; (2) The hospital indicated that the data submitted for this measure were based on a sample of cases; (3) Data was collected during a shorter time period (fewer quarters) than the maximum possible time for this measure; (4) Suppressed for one or more quarters by CMS; (5) No data is available from the hospital for this measure; (6) Fewer than 100 patients completed the HCAHPS survey. Use these rates with caution, as the number of surveys may be too low to reliably assess hospital performance; (7) Survey results are based on less than 12 months of data; (8) Survey results are not available for this reporting period; (9) No or very few patients were eligible for the HCAHPS survey. The scores shown, if any, reflect a very small number of surveys; (10) A state average was not calculated because too few hospitals in the state submitted data; (11) There were discrepancies in the data collection process; Please refer to the User's Guide for a full explanation of data.

Children's Hospital NMC

111 Michigan Ave, NW Phone: 202-884-5000
Washington, DC 20010 Fax: 202-884-5987
URL: www.dcchildrens.com
Type: Childrens Emergency Services: Yes
Ownership: Voluntary Non-Profit - Private Beds: 279

Key Personnel:
CEO/President. . . . . Edwin K Zechman
Cardiac Laboratory. . . . . Gerard Robert Martin, MD
Chief of Medical Staff. . . . . Peter Holbrook, MD
Operating Room. . . . . Kurt D Newman, MD
Pediatric In-Patient Care . . . . . . Peter Scheidt, MD
Radiology. . . . . David Kushner, MD
Emergency Room . . . . Dr. James Chamberland
Patient Relations . . . . Nellie Robinson, RN/MS

Measure	Cases	This Hosp.	State Avg.	U.S. Avg.
Heart Attack Care				
ACE Inhibitor or ARB for LVSD	-	-	94%	96%
Aspirin at Arrival	-	-	97%	99%
Aspirin at Discharge	-	-	98%	98%
Beta Blocker at Discharge	-	-	96%	98%
Fibrinolytic Medication Timing	-	-	-	55%
PCI Within 90 Minutes of Arrival	-	-	80%	90%
Smoking Cessation Advice	-	-	99%	99%
Chest Pain/Possible Heart Attack Care				
Aspirin at Arrival	-	-	94%	95%
Median Time to ECG (minutes)	-	-	14	8
Median Time to Transfer (minutes)	-	-	104	61
Fibrinolytic Medication Timing	-	-	0%	54%
Heart Failure Care				
ACE Inhibitor or ARB for LVSD	-	-	91%	94%
Discharge Instructions	-	-	72%	88%
Evaluation of LVS Function	-	-	96%	98%
Smoking Cessation Advice	-	-	98%	98%
Pneumonia Care				
Appropriate Initial Antibiotic	-	-	90%	92%
Blood Culture Timing	-	-	88%	96%
Influenza Vaccine	-	-	69%	91%
Initial Antibiotic Timing	-	-	85%	95%
Pneumococcal Vaccine	-	-	71%	93%
Smoking Cessation Advice	-	-	95%	97%
Surgical Care Improvement Project				
Appropriate VTP Within 24 Hours	-	-	95%	92%
Appropriate Hair Removal	-	-	99%	99%
Appropriate Beta Blocker Usage	-	-	92%	93%
Controlled Postoperative Blood Glucose	-	-	96%	93%
Prophylactic Antibiotic Timing	-	-	95%	97%
Prophylactic Antibiotic Timing (Outpatient)	-	-	86%	92%
Prophylactic Antibiotic Selection	-	-	95%	97%
Prophylactic Antibiotic Select. (Outpatient)	-	-	92%	94%
Prophylactic Antibiotic Stopped	-	-	92%	94%
Recommended VTP Ordered	-	-	96%	94%
Urinary Catheter Removal	-	-	88%	90%
Children's Asthma Care				
Received Systemic Corticosteroids[2]	419	100%	-	100%
Received Home Management Plan[2]	417	71%	-	71%
Received Reliever Medication[2]	420	100%	-	100%
Use of Medical Imaging				
Combination Abdominal CT Scan	-	-	0.126	0.191
Combination Chest CT Scan	-	-	0.052	0.054
Follow-up Mammogram/Ultrasound	-	-	6.8%	8.4%
MRI for Low Back Pain	-	-	31.9%	32.7%
Survey of Patients' Hospital Experiences				
Area Around Room 'Always' Quiet at Night	-	-	-	58%
Doctors 'Always' Communicated Well	-	-	-	80%
Home Recovery Information Given	-	-	-	82%
Hospital Given 9 or 10 on 10 Point Scale	-	-	-	67%
Meds 'Always' Explained Before Given	-	-	-	60%
Nurses 'Always' Communicated Well	-	-	-	76%
Pain 'Always' Well Controlled	-	-	-	69%
Room and Bathroom 'Always' Clean	-	-	-	71%
Timely Help 'Always' Received	-	-	-	64%
Would Definitely Recommend Hospital	-	-	-	69%

George Washington Univ Hospital

900 23rd St NW Phone: 202-716-4605
Washington, DC 20037 Fax: 202-715-5206
URL: www.gwhospital.com
Type: Acute Care Hospitals Emergency Services: Yes
Ownership: Voluntary Non-Profit - Other Beds: 371

Key Personnel:
CEO/President. . . . . Richard Becker
Chief of Medical Staff. . . . . Richard Becker
Infection Control. . . . . Rita Smith, RN
Operating Room. . . . . Elizabeth White, RN
Quality Assurance . . . . Melanie Sage
Radiology. . . . . Mark Lerner

Measure	Cases	This Hosp.	State Avg.	U.S. Avg.
Heart Attack Care				
ACE Inhibitor or ARB for LVSD	33	91%	94%	96%
Aspirin at Arrival	191	99%	97%	99%
Aspirin at Discharge	259	98%	98%	98%
Beta Blocker at Discharge	232	97%	96%	98%
Fibrinolytic Medication Timing	0	-	-	55%
PCI Within 90 Minutes of Arrival	34	88%	80%	90%
Smoking Cessation Advice	73	100%	99%	99%
Chest Pain/Possible Heart Attack Care				
Aspirin at Arrival[1,3]	2	50%	94%	95%
Median Time to ECG (minutes)[1,3]	2	228	14	8
Median Time to Transfer (minutes)[5]	0	-	104	61
Fibrinolytic Medication Timing[5]	0	-	0%	54%
Heart Failure Care				
ACE Inhibitor or ARB for LVSD	167	95%	91%	94%
Discharge Instructions	331	100%	72%	88%
Evaluation of LVS Function	372	98%	96%	98%
Smoking Cessation Advice	67	100%	98%	98%
Pneumonia Care				
Appropriate Initial Antibiotic	55	71%	90%	92%
Blood Culture Timing	47	94%	88%	96%
Influenza Vaccine	43	95%	69%	91%
Initial Antibiotic Timing	69	97%	85%	95%
Pneumococcal Vaccine	51	88%	71%	93%
Smoking Cessation Advice	32	97%	95%	97%
Surgical Care Improvement Project				
Appropriate VTP Within 24 Hours[2]	215	98%	95%	92%
Appropriate Hair Removal[2]	714	98%	99%	99%
Appropriate Beta Blocker Usage[2]	191	93%	92%	93%
Controlled Postoperative Blood Glucose[2]	160	96%	96%	93%
Prophylactic Antibiotic Timing[2]	536	97%	95%	97%
Prophylactic Antibiotic Timing (Outpatient)	410	97%	86%	92%
Prophylactic Antibiotic Selection[2]	543	95%	95%	97%
Prophylactic Antibiotic Select. (Outpatient)	404	93%	92%	94%
Prophylactic Antibiotic Stopped[2]	450	92%	92%	94%
Recommended VTP Ordered[2]	215	99%	96%	94%
Urinary Catheter Removal[2]	205	82%	88%	90%
Children's Asthma Care				
Received Systemic Corticosteroids	-	-	-	100%
Received Home Management Plan	-	-	-	71%
Received Reliever Medication	-	-	-	100%
Use of Medical Imaging				
Combination Abdominal CT Scan	697	0.179	0.126	0.191
Combination Chest CT Scan	635	0.058	0.052	0.054
Follow-up Mammogram/Ultrasound	575	5.4%	6.8%	8.4%
MRI for Low Back Pain	101	26.7%	31.9%	32.7%
Survey of Patients' Hospital Experiences				
Area Around Room 'Always' Quiet at Night	300+	59%	-	58%
Doctors 'Always' Communicated Well	300+	76%	-	80%
Home Recovery Information Given	300+	80%	-	82%
Hospital Given 9 or 10 on 10 Point Scale	300+	62%	-	67%
Meds 'Always' Explained Before Given	300+	54%	-	60%
Nurses 'Always' Communicated Well	300+	66%	-	76%
Pain 'Always' Well Controlled	300+	59%	-	69%
Room and Bathroom 'Always' Clean	300+	60%	-	71%
Timely Help 'Always' Received	300+	48%	-	64%
Would Definitely Recommend Hospital	300+	67%	-	69%

Georgetown University Hospital

3800 Reservoir Rd Phone: 202-784-3000
Washington, DC 20007 Fax: 202-444-2875
URL: www.georgetownuniversityhospital.org
Type: Acute Care Hospitals Emergency Services: Yes
Ownership: Govt - Hospital Dist/Auth Beds: 381

Key Personnel:
CEO/President. . . . . Joyce Johnson

Measure	Cases	This Hosp.	State Avg.	U.S. Avg.
Heart Attack Care				
ACE Inhibitor or ARB for LVSD[1,3]	1	100%	94%	96%
Aspirin at Arrival[1,3]	5	100%	97%	99%
Aspirin at Discharge[1,3]	3	100%	98%	98%
Beta Blocker at Discharge[1,3]	3	100%	96%	98%
Fibrinolytic Medication Timing[3]	0	-	-	55%
PCI Within 90 Minutes of Arrival[3]	0	-	80%	90%
Smoking Cessation Advice[1,3]	1	100%	99%	99%
Chest Pain/Possible Heart Attack Care				
Aspirin at Arrival	50	96%	94%	95%
Median Time to ECG (minutes)	53	14	14	8
Median Time to Transfer (minutes)[1,3]	6	84	104	61
Fibrinolytic Medication Timing	0	-	0%	54%
Heart Failure Care				
ACE Inhibitor or ARB for LVSD	37	100%	91%	94%
Discharge Instructions	73	89%	72%	88%
Evaluation of LVS Function	90	99%	96%	98%
Smoking Cessation Advice[1]	22	100%	98%	98%
Pneumonia Care				
Appropriate Initial Antibiotic[2]	38	95%	90%	92%
Blood Culture Timing[2]	60	87%	88%	96%
Influenza Vaccine[2]	66	85%	69%	91%
Initial Antibiotic Timing[2]	75	96%	85%	95%
Pneumococcal Vaccine[2]	60	93%	71%	93%
Smoking Cessation Advice[2]	27	100%	95%	97%
Surgical Care Improvement Project				
Appropriate VTP Within 24 Hours[2]	231	99%	95%	92%
Appropriate Hair Removal[2]	415	100%	99%	99%
Appropriate Beta Blocker Usage[2]	113	95%	92%	93%
Controlled Postoperative Blood Glucose[2]	0	-	96%	93%
Prophylactic Antibiotic Timing[2]	273	96%	95%	97%
Prophylactic Antibiotic Timing (Outpatient)	356	94%	86%	92%
Prophylactic Antibiotic Selection[2]	279	97%	95%	97%
Prophylactic Antibiotic Select. (Outpatient)	352	96%	92%	94%
Prophylactic Antibiotic Stopped[2]	257	95%	92%	94%
Recommended VTP Ordered[2]	232	99%	96%	94%
Urinary Catheter Removal[2]	119	92%	88%	90%
Children's Asthma Care				
Received Systemic Corticosteroids[2]	39	97%	-	100%
Received Home Management Plan[2]	40	53%	-	71%
Received Reliever Medication[2]	40	100%	-	100%
Use of Medical Imaging				
Combination Abdominal CT Scan	1,367	0.081	0.126	0.191
Combination Chest CT Scan	1,455	0.012	0.052	0.054
Follow-up Mammogram/Ultrasound	867	10.4%	6.8%	8.4%
MRI for Low Back Pain	109	30.3%	31.9%	32.7%
Survey of Patients' Hospital Experiences				
Area Around Room 'Always' Quiet at Night	300+	55%	-	58%
Doctors 'Always' Communicated Well	300+	77%	-	80%
Home Recovery Information Given	300+	87%	-	82%
Hospital Given 9 or 10 on 10 Point Scale	300+	68%	-	67%
Meds 'Always' Explained Before Given	300+	61%	-	60%
Nurses 'Always' Communicated Well	300+	75%	-	76%
Pain 'Always' Well Controlled	300+	67%	-	69%
Room and Bathroom 'Always' Clean	300+	63%	-	71%
Timely Help 'Always' Received	300+	55%	-	64%
Would Definitely Recommend Hospital	300+	75%	-	69%

NOTE: Hospital profiles are in alphabetical order by state, then city, then hospital within the city; Rankings exclude hospitals with less than 25 cases except for patient surveys which excludes hospitals with less than 100 cases; (a) 100–299 cases; (1) The number of cases is too small to be sure how well a hospital is performing; (2) The hospital indicated that the data submitted for this measure were based on a sample of cases; (3) Data was collected during a shorter time period (fewer quarters) than the maximum possible time for this measure; (4) Suppressed for one or more quarters by CMS; (5) No data is available from the hospital for this measure; (6) Fewer than 100 patients completed the HCAHPS survey. Use these rates with caution, as the number of surveys may be too low to reliably assess hospital performance; (7) Survey results are based on less than 12 months of data; (8) Survey results are not available for this reporting period; (9) No or very few patients were eligible for the HCAHPS survey. The scores shown, if any, reflect a very small number of surveys; (10) A state average was not calculated because too few hospitals in the state submitted data; (11) There were discrepancies in the data collection process; Please refer to the User's Guide for a full explanation of data.

Howard University Hospital

2041 Georgia Ave NW Phone: 202-745-6100
Washington, DC 20060 Fax: 202-745-3731
URL: www.huhosp.org
Type: Acute Care Hospitals Emergency Services: Yes
Ownership: Voluntary Non-Profit - Other Beds: 482

Key Personnel:
CEO/President. . . . . H Patrick Swygert
Cardiac Laboratory. . . . . Deborah Williams, MD
Chief of Medical Staff . . . . Alvin Thomas, MD
Infection Control. . . . . John I McNeil, MD
Operating Room. . . . . Clive O Callender, MD FACS
Pediatric In-Patient Care . . . . . . Renee Jenkins, MD
Quality Assurance . . . . Norma Bent
Radiology. . . . . Roma V Gumbs, MD

Measure	Cases	This Hosp.	State Avg.	U.S. Avg.
Heart Attack Care				
ACE Inhibitor or ARB for LVSD[1]	9	100%	94%	96%
Aspirin at Arrival	45	91%	97%	99%
Aspirin at Discharge	45	100%	98%	98%
Beta Blocker at Discharge	45	96%	96%	98%
Fibrinolytic Medication Timing	0	-	-	55%
PCI Within 90 Minutes of Arrival[1]	4	0%	80%	90%
Smoking Cessation Advice	26	100%	99%	99%
Chest Pain/Possible Heart Attack Care				
Aspirin at Arrival[1,3]	6	83%	94%	95%
Median Time to ECG (minutes)[1,3]	9	26	14	8
Median Time to Transfer (minutes)[5]	0	-	104	61
Fibrinolytic Medication Timing[5]	0	-	0%	54%
Heart Failure Care				
ACE Inhibitor or ARB for LVSD[2]	154	97%	91%	94%
Discharge Instructions[2]	268	99%	72%	88%
Evaluation of LVS Function[2]	286	98%	96%	98%
Smoking Cessation Advice[2]	94	100%	98%	98%
Pneumonia Care				
Appropriate Initial Antibiotic[2]	64	92%	90%	92%
Blood Culture Timing[2]	90	92%	88%	96%
Influenza Vaccine[2]	57	89%	69%	91%
Initial Antibiotic Timing[2]	113	75%	85%	95%
Pneumococcal Vaccine[2]	45	73%	71%	93%
Smoking Cessation Advice[2]	84	99%	95%	97%
Surgical Care Improvement Project				
Appropriate VTP Within 24 Hours[2]	165	88%	95%	92%
Appropriate Hair Removal[2]	248	95%	99%	99%
Appropriate Beta Blocker Usage[2]	45	82%	92%	93%
Controlled Postoperative Blood Glucose[1,2]	8	62%	96%	93%
Prophylactic Antibiotic Timing[2]	165	77%	95%	97%
Prophylactic Antibiotic Timing (Outpatient)	147	23%	86%	92%
Prophylactic Antibiotic Selection[2]	166	94%	95%	97%
Prophylactic Antibiotic Select. (Outpatient)	52	73%	92%	94%
Prophylactic Antibiotic Stopped[2]	160	84%	92%	94%
Recommended VTP Ordered[2]	165	88%	96%	94%
Urinary Catheter Removal[2]	64	88%	88%	90%
Children's Asthma Care				
Received Systemic Corticosteroids[2]	34	97%	-	100%
Received Home Management Plan[2]	34	0%	-	71%
Received Reliever Medication[2]	34	100%	-	100%
Use of Medical Imaging				
Combination Abdominal CT Scan	244	0.061	0.126	0.191
Combination Chest CT Scan	187	0.027	0.052	0.054
Follow-up Mammogram/Ultrasound	541	9.2%	6.8%	8.4%
MRI for Low Back Pain	38	50.0%	31.9%	32.7%
Survey of Patients' Hospital Experiences				
Area Around Room 'Always' Quiet at Night	300+	68%	-	58%
Doctors 'Always' Communicated Well	300+	77%	-	80%
Home Recovery Information Given	300+	74%	-	82%
Hospital Given 9 or 10 on 10 Point Scale	300+	57%	-	67%
Meds 'Always' Explained Before Given	300+	55%	-	60%
Nurses 'Always' Communicated Well	300+	68%	-	76%
Pain 'Always' Well Controlled	300+	63%	-	69%
Room and Bathroom 'Always' Clean	300+	64%	-	71%
Timely Help 'Always' Received	300+	55%	-	64%
Would Definitely Recommend Hospital	300+	57%	-	69%

Providence Hospital

1150 Varnum St NE Phone: 202-269-7000
Washington, DC 20017 Fax: 202-269-7160
URL: www.provhosp.org
Type: Acute Care Hospitals Emergency Services: Yes
Ownership: Voluntary Non-Profit - Private Beds: 240

Key Personnel:
CEO/President. . . . . Sister Carol Keehan
Chief of Medical Staff. . . . . Robert Simmons
Infection Control. . . . . John Morrissey, MD
Operating Room. . . . . Willie C Blair
Pediatric In-Patient Care . . . . . . Jolan Rhodes, MD
Quality Assurance . . . . Deborah Gill
Radiology. . . . . Joel Bruce Bowers, RN
Intensive Care Unit. . . . . Byron Atkinson, RN

Measure	Cases	This Hosp.	State Avg.	U.S. Avg.
Heart Attack Care				
ACE Inhibitor or ARB for LVSD[1]	17	82%	94%	96%
Aspirin at Arrival	60	95%	97%	99%
Aspirin at Discharge	45	89%	98%	98%
Beta Blocker at Discharge	43	81%	96%	98%
Fibrinolytic Medication Timing	0	-	-	55%
PCI Within 90 Minutes of Arrival[1]	1	0%	80%	90%
Smoking Cessation Advice[1]	14	93%	99%	99%
Chest Pain/Possible Heart Attack Care				
Aspirin at Arrival[1]	12	75%	94%	95%
Median Time to ECG (minutes)[1]	12	33	14	8
Median Time to Transfer (minutes)[1,3]	1	1131	104	61
Fibrinolytic Medication Timing[3]	0	-	0%	54%
Heart Failure Care				
ACE Inhibitor or ARB for LVSD	255	83%	91%	94%
Discharge Instructions	504	24%	72%	88%
Evaluation of LVS Function	588	92%	96%	98%
Smoking Cessation Advice	101	95%	98%	98%
Pneumonia Care				
Appropriate Initial Antibiotic	120	85%	90%	92%
Blood Culture Timing	170	82%	88%	96%
Influenza Vaccine	149	40%	69%	91%
Initial Antibiotic Timing	188	80%	85%	95%
Pneumococcal Vaccine	158	50%	71%	93%
Smoking Cessation Advice	85	96%	95%	97%
Surgical Care Improvement Project				
Appropriate VTP Within 24 Hours[2]	175	89%	95%	92%
Appropriate Hair Removal[2]	364	100%	99%	99%
Appropriate Beta Blocker Usage[2]	67	82%	92%	93%
Controlled Postoperative Blood Glucose[2]	0	-	96%	93%
Prophylactic Antibiotic Timing[2]	249	92%	95%	97%
Prophylactic Antibiotic Timing (Outpatient)	281	73%	86%	92%
Prophylactic Antibiotic Selection[2]	250	83%	95%	97%
Prophylactic Antibiotic Select. (Outpatient)	231	85%	92%	94%
Prophylactic Antibiotic Stopped[2]	237	80%	92%	94%
Recommended VTP Ordered[2]	175	91%	96%	94%
Urinary Catheter Removal[2]	93	78%	88%	90%
Children's Asthma Care				
Received Systemic Corticosteroids	-	-	-	100%
Received Home Management Plan	-	-	-	71%
Received Reliever Medication	-	-	-	100%
Use of Medical Imaging				
Combination Abdominal CT Scan	810	0.574	0.126	0.191
Combination Chest CT Scan	409	0.484	0.052	0.054
Follow-up Mammogram/Ultrasound	1,909	5.7%	6.8%	8.4%
MRI for Low Back Pain	115	36.5%	31.9%	32.7%
Survey of Patients' Hospital Experiences				
Area Around Room 'Always' Quiet at Night	300+	62%	-	58%
Doctors 'Always' Communicated Well	300+	77%	-	80%
Home Recovery Information Given	300+	74%	-	82%
Hospital Given 9 or 10 on 10 Point Scale	300+	61%	-	67%
Meds 'Always' Explained Before Given	300+	54%	-	60%
Nurses 'Always' Communicated Well	300+	70%	-	76%
Pain 'Always' Well Controlled	300+	64%	-	69%
Room and Bathroom 'Always' Clean	300+	67%	-	71%
Timely Help 'Always' Received	300+	54%	-	64%
Would Definitely Recommend Hospital	300+	63%	-	69%

Sibley Memorial Hospital

5255 Loughboro Rd NW Phone: 202-537-4680
Washington, DC 20016 Fax: 202-364-8405
URL: www.sibley.org
Type: Acute Care Hospitals Emergency Services: Yes
Ownership: Voluntary Non-Profit - Other Beds: 328

Key Personnel:
CEO/President. . . . . Robert L Sloan
Operating Room. . . . . Cindy Lee, RN
Patient Relations . . . . Joan Vincent, RN

Measure	Cases	This Hosp.	State Avg.	U.S. Avg.
Heart Attack Care				
ACE Inhibitor or ARB for LVSD[1]	4	100%	94%	96%
Aspirin at Arrival	32	97%	97%	99%
Aspirin at Discharge[1]	19	100%	98%	98%
Beta Blocker at Discharge[1]	18	100%	96%	98%
Fibrinolytic Medication Timing	0	-	-	55%
PCI Within 90 Minutes of Arrival	0	-	80%	90%
Smoking Cessation Advice[1]	2	100%	99%	99%
Chest Pain/Possible Heart Attack Care				
Aspirin at Arrival	47	98%	94%	95%
Median Time to ECG (minutes)	49	10	14	8
Median Time to Transfer (minutes)[1]	13	101	104	61
Fibrinolytic Medication Timing	0	-	0%	54%
Heart Failure Care				
ACE Inhibitor or ARB for LVSD	35	97%	91%	94%
Discharge Instructions	102	83%	72%	88%
Evaluation of LVS Function	124	99%	96%	98%
Smoking Cessation Advice[1]	6	100%	98%	98%
Pneumonia Care				
Appropriate Initial Antibiotic[2]	87	92%	90%	92%
Blood Culture Timing[2]	135	98%	88%	96%
Influenza Vaccine[2]	74	92%	69%	91%
Initial Antibiotic Timing[2]	105	98%	85%	95%
Pneumococcal Vaccine[2]	120	90%	71%	93%
Smoking Cessation Advice[1,2]	22	100%	95%	97%
Surgical Care Improvement Project				
Appropriate VTP Within 24 Hours[2]	269	96%	95%	92%
Appropriate Hair Removal[2]	635	100%	99%	99%
Appropriate Beta Blocker Usage[2]	135	93%	92%	93%
Controlled Postoperative Blood Glucose[2]	0	-	96%	93%
Prophylactic Antibiotic Timing[2]	466	96%	95%	97%
Prophylactic Antibiotic Timing (Outpatient)	265	91%	86%	92%
Prophylactic Antibiotic Selection[2]	468	96%	95%	97%
Prophylactic Antibiotic Select. (Outpatient)	264	88%	92%	94%
Prophylactic Antibiotic Stopped[2]	454	94%	92%	94%
Recommended VTP Ordered[2]	269	97%	96%	94%
Urinary Catheter Removal[2]	146	94%	88%	90%
Children's Asthma Care				
Received Systemic Corticosteroids	-	-	-	100%
Received Home Management Plan	-	-	-	71%
Received Reliever Medication	-	-	-	100%
Use of Medical Imaging				
Combination Abdominal CT Scan	1,095	0.039	0.126	0.191
Combination Chest CT Scan	966	0.003	0.052	0.054
Follow-up Mammogram/Ultrasound	2,076	8.6%	6.8%	8.4%
MRI for Low Back Pain	263	30.8%	31.9%	32.7%
Survey of Patients' Hospital Experiences				
Area Around Room 'Always' Quiet at Night	300+	48%	-	58%
Doctors 'Always' Communicated Well	300+	77%	-	80%
Home Recovery Information Given	300+	75%	-	82%
Hospital Given 9 or 10 on 10 Point Scale	300+	62%	-	67%
Meds 'Always' Explained Before Given	300+	54%	-	60%
Nurses 'Always' Communicated Well	300+	69%	-	76%
Pain 'Always' Well Controlled	300+	69%	-	69%
Room and Bathroom 'Always' Clean	300+	67%	-	71%
Timely Help 'Always' Received	300+	52%	-	64%
Would Definitely Recommend Hospital	300+	72%	-	69%

NOTE: Hospital profiles are in alphabetical order by state, then city, then hospital within the city; Rankings exclude hospitals with less than 25 cases except for patient surveys which excludes hospitals with less than 100 cases; (a) 100–299 cases; (1) The number of cases is too small to be sure how well a hospital is performing; (2) The hospital indicated that the data submitted for this measure were based on a sample of cases; (3) Data was collected during a shorter time period (fewer quarters) than the maximum possible time for this measure; (4) Suppressed for one or more quarters by CMS; (5) No data is available from the hospital for this measure; (6) Fewer than 100 patients completed the HCAHPS survey. Use these rates with caution, as the number of surveys may be too low to reliably assess hospital performance; (7) Survey results are based on less than 12 months of data; (8) Survey results are not available for this reporting period; (9) No or very few patients were eligible for the HCAHPS survey. The scores shown, if any, reflect a very small number of surveys; (10) A state average was not calculated because too few hospitals in the state submitted data; (11) There were discrepancies in the data collection process; Please refer to the User's Guide for a full explanation of data.

United Medical Center

1310 Southern Avenue SE Phone: 202-574-6611
Washington, DC 20032 Fax: 202-574-6110
URL: www.greatersoutheastorg.verizonsupersite.com/home
Type: Acute Care Hospitals Emergency Services: Yes
Ownership: Proprietary Beds: 450

Key Personnel:
CEO/President. . . . . Cyril Allen
Chief of Medical Staff. . . . . Edger Potter
Operating Room. . . . . Ester Espartero, RN
Pediatric Ambulatory Care . . . . . . Gail Crossman, RN
Pediatric In-Patient Care . . . . Gail Crossman, RN
Quality Assurance . . . . Paula Johnson
Radiology. . . . . Alfred Goldson, MD

Measure	Cases	This Hosp.	State Avg.	U.S. Avg.
Heart Attack Care				
ACE Inhibitor or ARB for LVSD[1]	1	0%	94%	96%
Aspirin at Arrival[1]	7	57%	97%	99%
Aspirin at Discharge[1]	4	75%	98%	98%
Beta Blocker at Discharge[1]	4	50%	96%	98%
Fibrinolytic Medication Timing	0	-	-	55%
PCI Within 90 Minutes of Arrival	0	-	80%	90%
Smoking Cessation Advice[1]	1	0%	99%	99%
Chest Pain/Possible Heart Attack Care				
Aspirin at Arrival[1,3]	9	100%	94%	95%
Median Time to ECG (minutes)[1,3]	10	19	14	8
Median Time to Transfer (minutes)[5]	0	-	104	61
Fibrinolytic Medication Timing[3]	0	-	0%	54%
Heart Failure Care				
ACE Inhibitor or ARB for LVSD	122	81%	91%	94%
Discharge Instructions	235	60%	72%	88%
Evaluation of LVS Function	270	91%	96%	98%
Smoking Cessation Advice	116	97%	98%	98%
Pneumonia Care				
Appropriate Initial Antibiotic	87	98%	90%	92%
Blood Culture Timing	115	79%	88%	96%
Influenza Vaccine	79	33%	69%	91%
Initial Antibiotic Timing	153	67%	85%	95%
Pneumococcal Vaccine	73	27%	71%	93%
Smoking Cessation Advice	105	86%	95%	97%
Surgical Care Improvement Project				
Appropriate VTP Within 24 Hours	65	83%	95%	92%
Appropriate Hair Removal	110	99%	99%	99%
Appropriate Beta Blocker Usage[1]	24	50%	92%	93%
Controlled Postoperative Blood Glucose	0	-	96%	93%
Prophylactic Antibiotic Timing	27	93%	95%	97%
Prophylactic Antibiotic Timing (Outpatient)[3]	25	40%	86%	92%
Prophylactic Antibiotic Selection	27	96%	95%	97%
Prophylactic Antibiotic Select. (Outpatient)[1,3]	20	80%	92%	94%
Prophylactic Antibiotic Stopped	25	68%	92%	94%
Recommended VTP Ordered	66	85%	96%	94%
Urinary Catheter Removal[1]	20	75%	88%	90%
Children's Asthma Care				
Received Systemic Corticosteroids	-	-	-	100%
Received Home Management Plan	-	-	-	71%
Received Reliever Medication	-	-	-	100%
Use of Medical Imaging				
Combination Abdominal CT Scan	123	0.016	0.126	0.191
Combination Chest CT Scan	90	0.011	0.052	0.054
Follow-up Mammogram/Ultrasound	348	5.7%	6.8%	8.4%
MRI for Low Back Pain[5]	0	-	31.9%	32.7%
Survey of Patients' Hospital Experiences				
Area Around Room 'Always' Quiet at Night	300+	55%	-	58%
Doctors 'Always' Communicated Well	300+	68%	-	80%
Home Recovery Information Given	300+	64%	-	82%
Hospital Given 9 or 10 on 10 Point Scale	300+	41%	-	67%
Meds 'Always' Explained Before Given	300+	51%	-	60%
Nurses 'Always' Communicated Well	300+	61%	-	76%
Pain 'Always' Well Controlled	300+	58%	-	69%
Room and Bathroom 'Always' Clean	300+	63%	-	71%
Timely Help 'Always' Received	300+	45%	-	64%
Would Definitely Recommend Hospital	300+	36%	-	69%

Washington DC VA Medical Center

50 Irving Street, N.W. Phone: 202-745-8000
Washington, DC 20422 Fax: 202-745-8530
URL: www.washington.va.gov
Type: Acute Care-Veterans Administration Emergency Services: No
Ownership: Government - Federal Beds: 291

Key Personnel:
CEO/President. . . . . Sanford M Garfunkel
Chief of Medical Staff. . . . . David Nashel, MD
Infection Control. . . . . Fred Gordin
Operating Room. . . . . Charles Shuner
Quality Assurance . . . . Cathy Delligatti
Radiology. . . . . Klemens Barth
Patient Relations . . . . Terry Koss

Measure	Cases	This Hosp.	State Avg.	U.S. Avg.
Heart Attack Care				
ACE Inhibitor or ARB for LVSD[1]	6	100%	94%	96%
Aspirin at Arrival	25	100%	97%	99%
Aspirin at Discharge	31	100%	98%	98%
Beta Blocker at Discharge	29	100%	96%	98%
Fibrinolytic Medication Timing[5]	0	-	-	55%
PCI Within 90 Minutes of Arrival[1]	5	80%	80%	90%
Smoking Cessation Advice[1]	12	100%	99%	99%
Chest Pain/Possible Heart Attack Care				
Aspirin at Arrival	-	-	94%	95%
Median Time to ECG (minutes)	-	-	14	8
Median Time to Transfer (minutes)	-	-	104	61
Fibrinolytic Medication Timing	-	-	0%	54%
Heart Failure Care				
ACE Inhibitor or ARB for LVSD	160	94%	91%	94%
Discharge Instructions	224	96%	72%	88%
Evaluation of LVS Function	234	99%	96%	98%
Smoking Cessation Advice	74	100%	98%	98%
Pneumonia Care				
Appropriate Initial Antibiotic	33	97%	90%	92%
Blood Culture Timing	60	97%	88%	96%
Influenza Vaccine	50	90%	69%	91%
Initial Antibiotic Timing	57	88%	85%	95%
Pneumococcal Vaccine	49	96%	71%	93%
Smoking Cessation Advice[1]	17	100%	95%	97%
Surgical Care Improvement Project				
Appropriate VTP Within 24 Hours[2]	96	93%	95%	92%
Appropriate Hair Removal[2]	227	100%	99%	99%
Appropriate Beta Blocker Usage[2]	99	100%	92%	93%
Controlled Postoperative Blood Glucose[2]	106	92%	96%	93%
Prophylactic Antibiotic Timing	144	100%	95%	97%
Prophylactic Antibiotic Timing (Outpatient)	-	-	86%	92%
Prophylactic Antibiotic Selection	145	99%	95%	97%
Prophylactic Antibiotic Select. (Outpatient)	-	-	92%	94%
Prophylactic Antibiotic Stopped	140	96%	92%	94%
Recommended VTP Ordered[2]	97	92%	96%	94%
Urinary Catheter Removal[2]	87	99%	88%	90%
Children's Asthma Care				
Received Systemic Corticosteroids	-	-	-	100%
Received Home Management Plan	-	-	-	71%
Received Reliever Medication	-	-	-	100%
Use of Medical Imaging				
Combination Abdominal CT Scan	-	-	0.126	0.191
Combination Chest CT Scan	-	-	0.052	0.054
Follow-up Mammogram/Ultrasound	-	-	6.8%	8.4%
MRI for Low Back Pain	-	-	31.9%	32.7%
Survey of Patients' Hospital Experiences				
Area Around Room 'Always' Quiet at Night	-	-	-	58%
Doctors 'Always' Communicated Well	-	-	-	80%
Home Recovery Information Given	-	-	-	82%
Hospital Given 9 or 10 on 10 Point Scale	-	-	-	67%
Meds 'Always' Explained Before Given	-	-	-	60%
Nurses 'Always' Communicated Well	-	-	-	76%
Pain 'Always' Well Controlled	-	-	-	69%
Room and Bathroom 'Always' Clean	-	-	-	71%
Timely Help 'Always' Received	-	-	-	64%
Would Definitely Recommend Hospital	-	-	-	69%

Washington Hospital Center

110 Irving St NW Phone: 202-877-7000
Washington, DC 20010 Fax: 202-877-3299
URL: www.whcenter.org
Type: Acute Care Hospitals Emergency Services: Yes
Ownership: Voluntary Non-Profit - Other Beds: 926

Key Personnel:
CEO/President. . . . . Harrison J. Rider, III
Cardiac Laboratory. . . . . Maureen Clancy
Chief of Medical Staff. . . . . Janis M Orlowski MD
Coronary Care . . . . Julio Panza MD
Infection Control. . . . . Nancy Donegan
Operating Room. . . . . John J. Ricotta, MD, FACS
Pediatric Ambulatory Care . . . . . . Zacharia Cherian MD
Radiology. . . . . James Jelinek, MD

Measure	Cases	This Hosp.	State Avg.	U.S. Avg.
Heart Attack Care				
ACE Inhibitor or ARB for LVSD[2]	78	97%	94%	96%
Aspirin at Arrival[2]	63	98%	97%	99%
Aspirin at Discharge[2]	282	99%	98%	98%
Beta Blocker at Discharge[2]	269	99%	96%	98%
Fibrinolytic Medication Timing[2]	0	-	-	55%
PCI Within 90 Minutes of Arrival[1,2]	5	100%	80%	90%
Smoking Cessation Advice[2]	79	100%	99%	99%
Chest Pain/Possible Heart Attack Care				
Aspirin at Arrival[1,3]	1	100%	94%	95%
Median Time to ECG (minutes)[1,3]	1	4	14	8
Median Time to Transfer (minutes)[5]	0	-	104	61
Fibrinolytic Medication Timing[3]	0	-	0%	54%
Heart Failure Care				
ACE Inhibitor or ARB for LVSD[2]	193	97%	91%	94%
Discharge Instructions[2]	355	93%	72%	88%
Evaluation of LVS Function[2]	393	98%	96%	98%
Smoking Cessation Advice[2]	72	100%	98%	98%
Pneumonia Care				
Appropriate Initial Antibiotic[2]	58	98%	90%	92%
Blood Culture Timing[2]	56	86%	88%	96%
Influenza Vaccine[2]	75	93%	69%	91%
Initial Antibiotic Timing[2]	111	98%	85%	95%
Pneumococcal Vaccine[2]	87	94%	71%	93%
Smoking Cessation Advice[2]	52	100%	95%	97%
Surgical Care Improvement Project				
Appropriate VTP Within 24 Hours[2]	299	99%	95%	92%
Appropriate Hair Removal[2]	808	100%	99%	99%
Appropriate Beta Blocker Usage[2]	306	98%	92%	93%
Controlled Postoperative Blood Glucose[2]	209	98%	96%	93%
Prophylactic Antibiotic Timing[2]	564	97%	95%	97%
Prophylactic Antibiotic Timing (Outpatient)	526	95%	86%	92%
Prophylactic Antibiotic Selection[2]	580	98%	95%	97%
Prophylactic Antibiotic Select. (Outpatient)	523	96%	92%	94%
Prophylactic Antibiotic Stopped[2]	553	96%	92%	94%
Recommended VTP Ordered[2]	299	99%	96%	94%
Urinary Catheter Removal[2]	220	92%	88%	90%
Children's Asthma Care				
Received Systemic Corticosteroids	-	-	-	100%
Received Home Management Plan	-	-	-	71%
Received Reliever Medication	-	-	-	100%
Use of Medical Imaging				
Combination Abdominal CT Scan	1,843	0.009	0.126	0.191
Combination Chest CT Scan	1,377	0.002	0.052	0.054
Follow-up Mammogram/Ultrasound	1,845	4.0%	6.8%	8.4%
MRI for Low Back Pain	245	31.0%	31.9%	32.7%
Survey of Patients' Hospital Experiences				
Area Around Room 'Always' Quiet at Night	300+	53%	-	58%
Doctors 'Always' Communicated Well	300+	79%	-	80%
Home Recovery Information Given	300+	83%	-	82%
Hospital Given 9 or 10 on 10 Point Scale	300+	61%	-	67%
Meds 'Always' Explained Before Given	300+	53%	-	60%
Nurses 'Always' Communicated Well	300+	67%	-	76%
Pain 'Always' Well Controlled	300+	64%	-	69%
Room and Bathroom 'Always' Clean	300+	61%	-	71%
Timely Help 'Always' Received	300+	47%	-	64%
Would Definitely Recommend Hospital	300+	66%	-	69%

NOTE: Hospital profiles are in alphabetical order by state, then city, then hospital within the city; Rankings exclude hospitals with less than 25 cases except for patient surveys which excludes hospitals with less than 100 cases; (a) 100–299 cases; (1) The number of cases is too small to be sure how well a hospital is performing; (2) The hospital indicated that the data submitted for this measure were based on a sample of cases; (3) Data was collected during a shorter time period (fewer quarters) than the maximum possible time for this measure; (4) Suppressed for one or more quarters by CMS; (5) No data is available from the hospital for this measure; (6) Fewer than 100 patients completed the HCAHPS survey. Use these rates with caution, as the number of surveys may be too low to reliably assess hospital performance; (7) Survey results are based on less than 12 months of data; (8) Survey results are not available for this reporting period; (9) No or very few patients were eligible for the HCAHPS survey. The scores shown, if any, reflect a very small number of surveys; (10) A state average was not calculated because too few hospitals in the state submitted data; (11) There were discrepancies in the data collection process; Please refer to the User's Guide for a full explanation of data.

Heart Attack Care

1. ACE Inhibitor or ARB for LVSD

Hospital Name	City	Rate	Cases
Central Baptist Hospital	Lexington	100%	95
Saint Elizabeth Medical Center North[2]	Covington	100%	47
Saint Joseph Hospital London	London	100%	40
Western Baptist Hospital	Paducah	100%	62
Hardin Memorial Hospital	Elizabethtown	98%	47
Lourdes Hospital	Paducah	98%	52
King's Daughters' Medical Center[2]	Ashland	97%	103
Lake Cumberland Regional Hospital	Somerset	97%	30
Pikeville Medical Center	Pikeville	97%	33
Saint Joseph East[2]	Lexington	97%	39
Baptist Hospital East	Louisville	96%	80
Jewish Hospital & St Mary's Healthcare	Louisville	96%	165
Norton Hospitals	Louisville	96%	140
University of Kentucky Hospital[2]	Lexington	96%	71
Regional Medical Center of Hopkins County	Madisonville	94%	65
Saint Joseph Hospital[2]	Lexington	92%	83
Owensboro Medical Health System	Owensboro	87%	82
The Medical Center at Bowling Green	Bowling Green	82%	55
Hazard Arh Regional Medical Center[2]	Hazard	81%	52
T J Samson Community Hospital	Glasgow	74%	27

2. Aspirin at Arrival

Hospital Name	City	Rate	Cases
Baptist Hospital East	Louisville	100%	443
Baptist Regional Medical Center	Corbin	100%	53
Frankfort Regional Medical Center	Frankfort	100%	30
Greenview Regional Hospital	Bowling Green	100%	29
Jewish Hospital & St Mary's Healthcare	Louisville	100%	402
Jewish Hospital - Shelbyville	Shelbyville	100%	29
Lourdes Hospital	Paducah	100%	129
Meadowview Regional Medical Center	Maysville	100%	82
Saint Claire Regional Medical Center	Morehead	100%	84
Saint Elizabeth Florence	Florence	100%	104
Saint Elizabeth Ft Thomas	Fort Thomas	100%	129
Saint Elizabeth Medical Center North[2]	Covington	100%	211
Central Baptist Hospital	Lexington	99%	146
Lake Cumberland Regional Hospital	Somerset	99%	178
Owensboro Medical Health System	Owensboro	99%	282
Pikeville Medical Center	Pikeville	99%	163
Regional Medical Center of Hopkins County	Madisonville	99%	180
Saint Joseph Hospital London	London	99%	171
University of Kentucky Hospital[2]	Lexington	99%	127
Ephraim Mcdowell Regional Medical Center	Danville	98%	102
Hardin Memorial Hospital	Elizabethtown	98%	293
King's Daughters' Medical Center[2]	Ashland	98%	452
Lexington-Leestown VA Medical Center	Lexington	98%	128
Norton Hospitals	Louisville	98%	458
Saint Joseph Hospital[2]	Lexington	98%	172
Western Baptist Hospital	Paducah	98%	237
Baptist Hospital Northeast	La Grange	97%	33
Highlands Regional Medical Center	Prestonsburg	97%	30
Saint Joseph East[2]	Lexington	97%	75
University of Louisville Hospital	Louisville	97%	107
Louisville VA Medical Center	Louisville	96%	80
The Medical Center at Bowling Green	Bowling Green	96%	218
Our Lady of Bellefonte Hospital	Ashland	96%	54
Hazard Arh Regional Medical Center[2]	Hazard	93%	111
T J Samson Community Hospital	Glasgow	93%	165

3. Aspirin at Discharge

Hospital Name	City	Rate	Cases
Central Baptist Hospital	Lexington	100%	671
King's Daughters' Medical Center[2]	Ashland	100%	732
Louisville VA Medical Center	Louisville	100%	65
Lourdes Hospital	Paducah	100%	178
Meadowview Regional Medical Center	Maysville	100%	78
Norton Hospitals	Louisville	100%	724
Pikeville Medical Center	Pikeville	100%	224
Saint Elizabeth Florence	Florence	100%	64
Saint Elizabeth Ft Thomas	Fort Thomas	100%	66
Saint Elizabeth Medical Center North[2]	Covington	100%	303
Saint Joseph Hospital London	London	100%	296
Western Baptist Hospital	Paducah	100%	395
Baptist Hospital East	Louisville	99%	474
Ephraim Mcdowell Regional Medical Center	Danville	99%	79
Jewish Hospital & St Mary's Healthcare	Louisville	99%	965
Lexington-Leestown VA Medical Center	Lexington	99%	121
Owensboro Medical Health System	Owensboro	99%	292
Saint Joseph East[2]	Lexington	99%	203
Saint Joseph Hospital[2]	Lexington	99%	437
University of Kentucky Hospital[2]	Lexington	99%	280
Hardin Memorial Hospital	Elizabethtown	98%	291
Lake Cumberland Regional Hospital	Somerset	98%	193
The Medical Center at Bowling Green	Bowling Green	97%	297
Our Lady of Bellefonte Hospital	Ashland	97%	29
Regional Medical Center of Hopkins County	Madisonville	97%	218
Saint Claire Regional Medical Center	Morehead	96%	72
University of Louisville Hospital	Louisville	95%	107
T J Samson Community Hospital	Glasgow	94%	148
Hazard Arh Regional Medical Center[2]	Hazard	92%	167

4. Beta Blocker at Discharge

Hospital Name	City	Rate	Cases
Baptist Hospital East	Louisville	100%	448
Central Baptist Hospital	Lexington	100%	625
Hardin Memorial Hospital	Elizabethtown	100%	294
Louisville VA Medical Center	Louisville	100%	61
Meadowview Regional Medical Center	Maysville	100%	71
Norton Hospitals	Louisville	100%	705
Our Lady of Bellefonte Hospital	Ashland	100%	30
Saint Elizabeth Florence	Florence	100%	59
Saint Elizabeth Ft Thomas	Fort Thomas	100%	67
Saint Elizabeth Medical Center North[2]	Covington	100%	283
Western Baptist Hospital	Paducah	100%	374
King's Daughters' Medical Center[2]	Ashland	99%	712
Lake Cumberland Regional Hospital	Somerset	99%	177
Lexington-Leestown VA Medical Center	Lexington	99%	113
Lourdes Hospital	Paducah	99%	173
Saint Claire Regional Medical Center	Morehead	99%	73
Saint Joseph Hospital London	London	99%	275
Owensboro Medical Health System	Owensboro	98%	283
Pikeville Medical Center	Pikeville	98%	216
Saint Joseph Hospital[2]	Lexington	98%	414
University of Kentucky Hospital[2]	Lexington	98%	269
Jewish Hospital & St Mary's Healthcare	Louisville	97%	921
Regional Medical Center of Hopkins County	Madisonville	97%	202
Saint Joseph East[2]	Lexington	97%	184
University of Louisville Hospital	Louisville	97%	97
Ephraim Mcdowell Regional Medical Center	Danville	96%	78
T J Samson Community Hospital	Glasgow	96%	154
The Medical Center at Bowling Green	Bowling Green	95%	281
Hazard Arh Regional Medical Center[2]	Hazard	89%	170

5. Fibrinolytic Medication Timing

Hospital Name	City	Rate	Cases
Hardin Memorial Hospital	Elizabethtown	67%	36

6. PCI Within 90 Minutes of Arrival

Hospital Name	City	Rate	Cases
Central Baptist Hospital	Lexington	100%	47
Saint Joseph Hospital London	London	98%	42
Regional Medical Center of Hopkins County	Madisonville	97%	32
Saint Elizabeth Medical Center North[2]	Covington	95%	42
King's Daughters' Medical Center[2]	Ashland	92%	84
Baptist Hospital East	Louisville	89%	89
Lake Cumberland Regional Hospital	Somerset	86%	49
The Medical Center at Bowling Green	Bowling Green	86%	49
Western Baptist Hospital	Paducah	86%	36
Owensboro Medical Health System	Owensboro	85%	34
Norton Hospitals	Louisville	84%	70
Pikeville Medical Center	Pikeville	80%	25

7. Smoking Cessation Advice

Hospital Name	City	Rate	Cases
Baptist Hospital East	Louisville	100%	142
Central Baptist Hospital	Lexington	100%	269
Hardin Memorial Hospital	Elizabethtown	100%	116
Jewish Hospital & St Mary's Healthcare	Louisville	100%	411
King's Daughters' Medical Center[2]	Ashland	100%	351
Lake Cumberland Regional Hospital	Somerset	100%	93
Lexington-Leestown VA Medical Center	Lexington	100%	42
Lourdes Hospital	Paducah	100%	84
Meadowview Regional Medical Center	Maysville	100%	37
Norton Hospitals	Louisville	100%	319
Owensboro Medical Health System	Owensboro	100%	137
Pikeville Medical Center	Pikeville	100%	115
Saint Elizabeth Medical Center North[2]	Covington	100%	117
Saint Joseph East[2]	Lexington	100%	100
Saint Joseph Hospital[2]	Lexington	100%	205
Saint Joseph Hospital London	London	100%	165
T J Samson Community Hospital	Glasgow	100%	63
Western Baptist Hospital	Paducah	100%	170
The Medical Center at Bowling Green	Bowling Green	99%	149
Regional Medical Center of Hopkins County	Madisonville	99%	107
University of Kentucky Hospital[2]	Lexington	99%	135
University of Louisville Hospital	Louisville	99%	73
Hazard Arh Regional Medical Center[2]	Hazard	98%	86
Saint Claire Regional Medical Center	Morehead	97%	36
Louisville VA Medical Center	Louisville	96%	25

Chest Pain/Possible Heart Attack Care

8. Aspirin at Arrival

Hospital Name	City	Rate	Cases
Baptist Hospital Northeast	La Grange	100%	29
Frankfort Regional Medical Center	Frankfort	100%	151
Meadowview Regional Medical Center	Maysville	100%	46
Monroe County Medical Center	Tompkinsville	100%	79
Parkway Regional Hospital	Fulton	100%	40
Saint Elizabeth Ft Thomas	Fort Thomas	100%	37
Three Rivers Medical Center	Louisa	100%	142
Georgetown Community Hospital	Georgetown	99%	82
Harrison Memorial Hospital	Cynthiana	99%	101
Saint Claire Regional Medical Center	Morehead	99%	85
Whitesburg ARH Hospital	Whitesburg	99%	124
Baptist Regional Medical Center	Corbin	98%	144
Bourbon Community Hospital	Paris	98%	84
Harlan Appalachian Reg Healthcare Hosp	Harlan	98%	98
Murray-Calloway County Hospital	Murray	98%	125
Our Lady of Bellefonte Hospital	Ashland	98%	65
Paul B Hall Regional Medical Center	Paintsville	98%	125
Saint Joseph Hospital London	London	98%	80
Spring View Hospital	Lebanon	98%	121
Williamson ARH Hospital	S Williamson	98%	45
Jewish Hospital & St Mary's Healthcare	Louisville	97%	385
Saint Elizabeth Florence	Florence	97%	37
Saint Joseph Mount Sterling	Mount Sterling	97%	218
Ephraim Mcdowell Regional Medical Center	Danville	96%	101
Jennie Stuart Medical Center	Hopkinsville	96%	214
Jewish Hospital - Shelbyville	Shelbyville	96%	100
Logan Memorial Hospital	Russellville	96%	128
Saint Joseph Hospital	Lexington	96%	28
Flaget Memorial Hospital	Bardstown	95%	225
Middlesboro Appalachian Reg Hlthcre Hosp	Middlesboro	95%	126
Muhlenberg Community Hospital	Greenville	95%	179
Pattie A Clay Regional Medical Center	Richmond	95%	141
Twin Lakes Regional Medical Center	Leitchfield	95%	101
Kentucky River Medical Center	Jackson	94%	78
Methodist Hospital	Henderson	94%	101
Rockcastle Reg Hosp & Respiratory Care Ctr	Mount Vernon	94%	85
Taylor Regional Hospital	Campbellsville	94%	143
Norton Hospitals[3]	Louisville	92%	36
Crittenden Health System	Marion	91%	33
Westlake Regional Hospital	Columbia	90%	105
Clark Regional Medical Center	Winchester	89%	331
Clinton County Hospital	Albany	89%	28
Pineville Community Hospital	Pineville	89%	46
Fleming County Hospital	Flemingsburg	88%	51
Highlands Regional Medical Center	Prestonsburg	88%	258
Methodist Hospital Union County	Morganfield	88%	73
Russell County Hospital	Russell Springs	87%	38
Hazard Arh Regional Medical Center	Hazard	84%	25

9. Median Time to ECG (minutes)

Hospital Name	City	Min.	Cases
Saint Claire Regional Medical Center	Morehead	1	95
Ephraim Mcdowell Regional Medical Center	Danville	2	104
Meadowview Regional Medical Center	Maysville	2	45
Paul B Hall Regional Medical Center	Paintsville	2	133
T J Samson Community Hospital	Glasgow	2	25
Crittenden Health System	Marion	3	35
Bourbon Community Hospital	Paris	4	87
Jewish Hospital & St Mary's Healthcare	Louisville	4	393
Jewish Hospital - Shelbyville	Shelbyville	4	104
Methodist Hospital	Henderson	4	104
Parkway Regional Hospital	Fulton	4	43
Pattie A Clay Regional Medical Center	Richmond	4	142
Baptist Hospital Northeast	La Grange	5	31
Clinton County Hospital	Albany	5	34
Frankfort Regional Medical Center	Frankfort	5	156
Logan Memorial Hospital	Russellville	5	135
Norton Hospitals[3]	Louisville	5	36
Three Rivers Medical Center	Louisa	5	144
Monroe County Medical Center	Tompkinsville	6	83
Saint Joseph Mount Sterling	Mount Sterling	6	221
Baptist Regional Medical Center	Corbin	7	150
Clark Regional Medical Center	Winchester	7	346
Georgetown Community Hospital	Georgetown	7	84
Middlesboro Appalachian Reg Hlthcre Hosp	Middlesboro	7	130
Saint Joseph Hospital	Lexington	7	31
Spring View Hospital	Lebanon	7	124
Highlands Regional Medical Center	Prestonsburg	8	268
Jennie Stuart Medical Center	Hopkinsville	8	231
Kentucky River Medical Center	Jackson	8	82
Methodist Hospital Union County	Morganfield	8	80
Muhlenberg Community Hospital	Greenville	8	190
Saint Joseph Hospital London	London	8	94
Twin Lakes Regional Medical Center	Leitchfield	8	110
Harrison Memorial Hospital	Cynthiana	9	101
Murray-Calloway County Hospital	Murray	9	124

NOTE: Hospital profiles are in alphabetical order by state, then city, then hospital within the city; Rankings exclude hospitals with less than 25 cases except for patient surveys which excludes hospitals with less than 100 cases; (a) 100–299 cases; (1) The number of cases is too small to be sure how well a hospital is performing; (2) The hospital indicated that the data submitted for this measure were based on a sample of cases; (3) Data was collected during a shorter time period (fewer quarters) than the maximum possible time for this measure; (4) Suppressed for one or more quarters by CMS; (5) No data is available from the hospital for this measure; (6) Fewer than 100 patients completed the HCAHPS survey. Use these rates with caution, as the number of surveys may be too low to reliably assess hospital performance; (7) Survey results are based on less than 12 months of data; (8) Survey results are not available for this reporting period; (9) No or very few patients were eligible for the HCAHPS survey. The scores shown, if any, reflect a very small number of surveys; (10) A state average was not calculated because too few hospitals in the state submitted data; (11) There were discrepancies in the data collection process; Please refer to the User's Guide for a full explanation of data.

Saint Elizabeth Medical Center North	Covington	10	26
Westlake Regional Hospital	Columbia	10	110
Williamson ARH Hospital	S Williamson	10	43
Saint Elizabeth Florence	Florence	11	38
Saint Elizabeth Ft Thomas	Fort Thomas	11	40
Taylor Regional Hospital	Campbellsville	11	147
Flaget Memorial Hospital	Bardstown	12	228
Rockcastle Reg Hosp & Respiratory Care Ctr	Mount Vernon	12	87
Fleming County Hospital	Flemingsburg	13	51
Pineville Community Hospital	Pineville	13	49
Russell County Hospital	Russell Springs	14	40
Harlan Appalachian Reg Healthcare Hosp	Harlan	15	108
Whitesburg ARH Hospital	Whitesburg	17	116
Our Lady of Bellefonte Hospital	Ashland	20	65

10. Median Time to Transfer (minutes)

Hospital Name	City	Min.	Cases
Jewish Hospital & St Mary's Healthcare	Louisville	63	38
Pattie A Clay Regional Medical Center	Richmond	69	35

Heart Failure Care

12. ACE Inhibitor or ARB for LVSD

Hospital Name	City	Rate	Cases
Baptist Regional Medical Center	Corbin	100%	41
Frankfort Regional Medical Center	Frankfort	100%	33
Harlan Appalachian Reg Healthcare Hosp	Harlan	100%	33
Louisville VA Medical Center	Louisville	100%	95
Our Lady of Bellefonte Hospital	Ashland	100%	37
Saint Elizabeth Florence	Florence	100%	68
Saint Elizabeth Ft Thomas	Fort Thomas	100%	44
Saint Elizabeth Medical Center North[2]	Covington	100%	90
Saint Joseph Hospital London	London	100%	90
Western Baptist Hospital	Paducah	100%	171
Central Baptist Hospital	Lexington	99%	137
King's Daughters' Medical Center[2]	Ashland	98%	209
Jackson Purchase Medical Center	Mayfield	97%	29
Three Rivers Medical Center	Louisa	97%	35
University of Kentucky Hospital[2]	Lexington	97%	159
Paul B Hall Regional Medical Center	Paintsville	96%	25
Saint Claire Regional Medical Center	Morehead	96%	49
Whitesburg ARH Hospital	Whitesburg	96%	28
Ephraim Mcdowell Regional Medical Center	Danville	95%	61
Norton Hospitals	Louisville	95%	386
Saint Joseph Hospital[2]	Lexington	95%	112
University of Louisville Hospital	Louisville	95%	111
Jennie Stuart Medical Center	Hopkinsville	94%	81
Middlesboro Appalachian Reg Hlthcre Hosp	Middlesboro	94%	36
Lexington-Leestown VA Medical Center	Lexington	93%	82
Hardin Memorial Hospital	Elizabethtown	92%	144
Lourdes Hospital	Paducah	92%	132
Pattie A Clay Regional Medical Center	Richmond	92%	25
Lake Cumberland Regional Hospital	Somerset	90%	84
Pikeville Medical Center	Pikeville	90%	105
Methodist Hospital	Henderson	89%	53
Regional Medical Center of Hopkins County	Madisonville	89%	134
Saint Joseph East	Lexington	89%	45
Baptist Hospital East	Louisville	88%	255
Owensboro Medical Health System	Owensboro	88%	219
Westlake Regional Hospital	Columbia	88%	42
Jewish Hospital & St Mary's Healthcare	Louisville	86%	438
Highlands Regional Medical Center	Prestonsburg	85%	60
Hazard Arh Regional Medical Center[2]	Hazard	83%	63
The Medical Center at Bowling Green	Bowling Green	77%	183
Pineville Community Hospital	Pineville	77%	56
T J Samson Community Hospital	Glasgow	77%	57
Clinton County Hospital	Albany	62%	37

13. Discharge Instructions

Hospital Name	City	Rate	Cases
Crittenden Health System	Marion	100%	37
Greenview Regional Hospital	Bowling Green	100%	67
Jackson Purchase Medical Center	Mayfield	100%	77
McDowell Arh Hospital	McDowell	100%	51
Meadowview Regional Medical Center	Maysville	100%	55
Memorial Hospital	Manchester	100%	88
Morgan County Arh Hospital	West Liberty	100%	28
Saint Joseph Martin	Martin	100%	49
Spring View Hospital	Lebanon	100%	53
Baptist Regional Medical Center	Corbin	99%	136
Harlan Appalachian Reg Healthcare Hosp	Harlan	99%	153
Lexington-Leestown VA Medical Center	Lexington	99%	255
Louisville VA Medical Center	Louisville	99%	193
Three Rivers Medical Center	Louisa	99%	89
Ephraim Mcdowell Regional Medical Center	Danville	98%	187
Frankfort Regional Medical Center	Frankfort	98%	121
Pattie A Clay Regional Medical Center	Richmond	98%	47
Pikeville Medical Center	Pikeville	98%	279
Highlands Regional Medical Center	Prestonsburg	97%	162
Ephraim Mcdowell Fort Logan Hospital	Stanford	96%	27
Middlesboro Appalachian Reg Hlthcre Hosp	Middlesboro	96%	92
Saint Elizabeth Medical Center North[2]	Covington	96%	273
Western Baptist Hospital	Paducah	95%	390
Bourbon Community Hospital	Paris	94%	34
Breckinridge Memorial Hospital[3]	Hardinsburg	94%	31
Williamson ARH Hospital	S Williamson	94%	110
Saint Joseph Hospital London	London	93%	266
Westlake Regional Hospital	Columbia	93%	170
Baptist Hospital Northeast	La Grange	92%	79
Central Baptist Hospital	Lexington	92%	297
Saint Elizabeth Ft Thomas	Fort Thomas	92%	173
Whitesburg ARH Hospital	Whitesburg	92%	177
King's Daughters' Medical Center[2]	Ashland	91%	783
Owensboro Medical Health System	Owensboro	91%	462
Our Lady of Bellefonte Hospital	Ashland	90%	220
Paul B Hall Regional Medical Center	Paintsville	90%	80
Saint Joseph Mount Sterling	Mount Sterling	90%	30
Lourdes Hospital	Paducah	88%	209
Rockcastle Reg Hosp & Respiratory Care Ctr	Mount Vernon	88%	32
Saint Claire Regional Medical Center	Morehead	88%	104
Saint Elizabeth Florence	Florence	88%	149
Saint Elizabeth Grant	Williamstown	88%	33
Ohio County Hospital	Hartford	86%	28
Muhlenberg Community Hospital	Greenville	85%	39
Flaget Memorial Hospital	Bardstown	84%	43
Lake Cumberland Regional Hospital	Somerset	84%	202
Logan Memorial Hospital	Russellville	84%	80
Methodist Hospital	Henderson	84%	165
Twin Lakes Regional Medical Center[2]	Leitchfield	84%	38
Hardin Memorial Hospital	Elizabethtown	83%	379
Mary Breckinridge Hospital	Hyden	83%	42
Georgetown Community Hospital	Georgetown	82%	34
Harrison Memorial Hospital	Cynthiana	82%	34
Kentucky River Medical Center	Jackson	82%	78
Saint Joseph East	Lexington	82%	101
Saint Joseph Hospital[2]	Lexington	82%	268
Jewish Hospital - Shelbyville	Shelbyville	80%	70
Saint Joseph Berea	Berea	80%	30
Fleming County Hospital[2]	Flemingsburg	78%	78
Regional Medical Center of Hopkins County	Madisonville	78%	191
Baptist Hospital East	Louisville	76%	654
Clark Regional Medical Center	Winchester	76%	45
Clinton County Hospital	Albany	75%	67
Taylor Regional Hospital[2]	Campbellsville	75%	53
University of Louisville Hospital	Louisville	75%	186
University of Kentucky Hospital[2]	Lexington	74%	314
Jennie Stuart Medical Center	Hopkinsville	73%	141
Norton Hospitals	Louisville	73%	1003
T J Samson Community Hospital	Glasgow	69%	154
The Medical Center at Franklin	Franklin	68%	31
Hazard Arh Regional Medical Center[2]	Hazard	67%	276
Monroe County Medical Center	Tompkinsville	67%	86
Jewish Hospital & St Mary's Healthcare	Louisville	66%	1079
Murray-Calloway County Hospital	Murray	65%	101
The Medical Center at Bowling Green	Bowling Green	64%	490
Knox County Hospital	Barbourville	58%	43
Pineville Community Hospital	Pineville	53%	214
Marshall County Hospital	Benton	44%	25
Caverna Memorial Hospital	Horse Cave	42%	26
Cumberland County Hospital	Burkesville	37%	38
Livingston Hospital and Healthcare	Salem	0%	45

14. Evaluation of LVS Function

Hospital Name	City	Rate	Cases
Baptist Hospital East	Louisville	100%	913
Baptist Hospital Northeast	La Grange	100%	107
Baptist Regional Medical Center	Corbin	100%	179
Ephraim Mcdowell Fort Logan Hospital	Stanford	100%	36
Ephraim Mcdowell Regional Medical Center	Danville	100%	228
Frankfort Regional Medical Center	Frankfort	100%	137
Georgetown Community Hospital	Georgetown	100%	42
Greenview Regional Hospital	Bowling Green	100%	96
Harlan Appalachian Reg Healthcare Hosp	Harlan	100%	187
Harrison Memorial Hospital	Cynthiana	100%	49
Kentucky River Medical Center	Jackson	100%	99
King's Daughters' Medical Center[2]	Ashland	100%	901
Lexington-Leestown VA Medical Center	Lexington	100%	270
Louisville VA Medical Center	Louisville	100%	213
Lourdes Hospital	Paducah	100%	272
McDowell Arh Hospital	McDowell	100%	52
Meadowview Regional Medical Center	Maysville	100%	67
Memorial Hospital	Manchester	100%	102
Owensboro Medical Health System	Owensboro	100%	553
Parkway Regional Hospital	Fulton	100%	27
Rockcastle Reg Hosp & Respiratory Care Ctr	Mount Vernon	100%	41
Saint Elizabeth Florence	Florence	100%	200
Saint Elizabeth Ft Thomas	Fort Thomas	100%	234
Saint Elizabeth Grant	Williamstown	100%	34
Saint Elizabeth Medical Center North[2]	Covington	100%	320
Saint Joseph Hospital London	London	100%	295
Spring View Hospital	Lebanon	100%	75
Three Rivers Medical Center	Louisa	100%	98
Western Baptist Hospital	Paducah	100%	462
Central Baptist Hospital	Lexington	99%	331
Hardin Memorial Hospital	Elizabethtown	99%	487
Jewish Hospital & St Mary's Healthcare	Louisville	99%	1301
Jewish Hospital - Shelbyville	Shelbyville	99%	102
Lake Cumberland Regional Hospital	Somerset	99%	235
Middlesboro Appalachian Reg Hlthcre Hosp	Middlesboro	99%	129
Norton Hospitals	Louisville	99%	1290
Paul B Hall Regional Medical Center	Paintsville	99%	105
Pikeville Medical Center	Pikeville	99%	308
Saint Joseph Hospital[2]	Lexington	99%	300
T J Samson Community Hospital	Glasgow	99%	184
Bourbon Community Hospital	Paris	98%	46
Flaget Memorial Hospital	Bardstown	98%	52
Hazard Arh Regional Medical Center[2]	Hazard	98%	306
Jackson Purchase Medical Center	Mayfield	98%	103
Methodist Hospital	Henderson	98%	210
Our Lady of Bellefonte Hospital	Ashland	98%	250
Regional Medical Center of Hopkins County	Madisonville	98%	238
Saint Joseph East	Lexington	98%	108
Saint Joseph Martin	Martin	98%	52
University of Louisville Hospital	Louisville	98%	200
Williamson ARH Hospital	S Williamson	98%	123
Highlands Regional Medical Center	Prestonsburg	97%	201
Logan Memorial Hospital	Russellville	97%	97
Pattie A Clay Regional Medical Center	Richmond	97%	66
Saint Claire Regional Medical Center	Morehead	97%	129
Saint Joseph Berea	Berea	97%	38
University of Kentucky Hospital[2]	Lexington	97%	356
The Medical Center at Bowling Green	Bowling Green	95%	593
Whitesburg ARH Hospital	Whitesburg	95%	201
Clark Regional Medical Center	Winchester	94%	51
Mary Breckinridge Hospital	Hyden	92%	52
Saint Joseph Mount Sterling	Mount Sterling	92%	38
Taylor Regional Hospital[2]	Campbellsville	92%	64
Westlake Regional Hospital	Columbia	92%	221
Morgan County Arh Hospital	West Liberty	91%	32
Murray-Calloway County Hospital	Murray	91%	116
Twin Lakes Regional Medical Center[2]	Leitchfield	91%	44
Pineville Community Hospital	Pineville	90%	241
Crittenden Health System	Marion	89%	61
Ohio County Hospital	Hartford	85%	34
Jennie Stuart Medical Center	Hopkinsville	84%	181
Muhlenberg Community Hospital	Greenville	84%	62
Carroll County Hospital	Carrollton	81%	27
Fleming County Hospital[2]	Flemingsburg	81%	98
Monroe County Medical Center	Tompkinsville	79%	112
Methodist Hospital Union County	Morganfield	78%	27
Clinton County Hospital	Albany	76%	72
The James B Haggin Memorial Hospital	Harrodsburg	75%	40
The Medical Center at Scottsville	Scottsville	75%	32
Russell County Hospital	Russell Springs	74%	31
Knox County Hospital	Barbourville	73%	49
Caverna Memorial Hospital	Horse Cave	55%	38
The Medical Center at Franklin	Franklin	55%	47
Marshall County Hospital	Benton	54%	41
Breckinridge Memorial Hospital[3]	Hardinsburg	44%	41
Livingston Hospital and Healthcare	Salem	39%	56
Cumberland County Hospital	Burkesville	32%	53

15. Smoking Cessation Advice

Hospital Name	City	Rate	Cases
Baptist Hospital East	Louisville	100%	112
Baptist Regional Medical Center	Corbin	100%	30
Central Baptist Hospital	Lexington	100%	56
Harlan Appalachian Reg Healthcare Hosp	Harlan	100%	33
Hazard Arh Regional Medical Center[2]	Hazard	100%	53
Highlands Regional Medical Center	Prestonsburg	100%	33
Jackson Purchase Medical Center	Mayfield	100%	27
King's Daughters' Medical Center[2]	Ashland	100%	185
Lake Cumberland Regional Hospital	Somerset	100%	59
Lexington-Leestown VA Medical Center	Lexington	100%	50
Logan Memorial Hospital	Russellville	100%	29
Lourdes Hospital	Paducah	100%	45
The Medical Center at Bowling Green	Bowling Green	100%	138
Methodist Hospital	Henderson	100%	39
Norton Hospitals	Louisville	100%	311
Our Lady of Bellefonte Hospital	Ashland	100%	46
Owensboro Medical Health System	Owensboro	100%	92
Paul B Hall Regional Medical Center	Paintsville	100%	25
Pikeville Medical Center	Pikeville	100%	62
Regional Medical Center of Hopkins County	Madisonville	100%	64
Saint Elizabeth Florence	Florence	100%	42
Saint Elizabeth Ft Thomas	Fort Thomas	100%	35
Saint Elizabeth Medical Center North[2]	Covington	100%	67
Saint Joseph East	Lexington	100%	30
Saint Joseph Hospital[2]	Lexington	100%	62

NOTE: Hospital profiles are in alphabetical order by state, then city, then hospital within the city; Rankings exclude hospitals with less than 25 cases except for patient surveys which excludes hospitals with less than 100 cases; (a) 100–299 cases; (1) The number of cases is too small to be sure how well a hospital is performing; (2) The hospital indicated that the data submitted for this measure were based on a sample of cases; (3) Data was collected during a shorter time period (fewer quarters) than the maximum possible time for this measure; (4) Suppressed for one or more quarters by CMS; (5) No data is available from the hospital for this measure; (6) Fewer than 100 patients completed the HCAHPS survey. Use these rates with caution, as the number of surveys may be too low to reliably assess hospital performance; (7) Survey results are based on less than 12 months of data; (8) Survey results are not available for this reporting period; (9) No or very few patients were eligible for the HCAHPS survey. The scores shown, if any, reflect a very small number of surveys; (10) A state average was not calculated because too few hospitals in the state submitted data; (11) There were discrepancies in the data collection process; Please refer to the User's Guide for a full explanation of data.

Saint Joseph Hospital London	London	100%	79
T J Samson Community Hospital	Glasgow	100%	40
Three Rivers Medical Center	Louisa	100%	25
University of Louisville Hospital	Louisville	100%	115
Western Baptist Hospital	Paducah	100%	112
Whitesburg ARH Hospital	Whitesburg	100%	41
Williamson ARH Hospital	S Williamson	100%	31
Hardin Memorial Hospital	Elizabethtown	99%	123
Jewish Hospital & St Mary's Healthcare	Louisville	99%	312
Ephraim Mcdowell Regional Medical Center	Danville	98%	44
Louisville VA Medical Center	Louisville	98%	57
Saint Claire Regional Medical Center	Morehead	97%	30
University of Kentucky Hospital[2]	Lexington	97%	115
Jennie Stuart Medical Center	Hopkinsville	91%	55
Westlake Regional Hospital	Columbia	87%	38
Pineville Community Hospital	Pineville	86%	51
Monroe County Medical Center	Tompkinsville	77%	35

Pneumonia Care

16. Appropriate Initial Antibiotic

Hospital Name	City	Rate	Cases
Ephraim Mcdowell Fort Logan Hospital	Stanford	100%	48
Saint Elizabeth Grant	Williamstown	100%	32
Greenview Regional Hospital	Bowling Green	99%	76
Logan Memorial Hospital	Russellville	99%	145
Meadowview Regional Medical Center	Maysville	99%	85
Three Rivers Medical Center	Louisa	99%	94
Paul B Hall Regional Medical Center	Paintsville	98%	122
Frankfort Regional Medical Center	Frankfort	97%	68
Lourdes Hospital	Paducah	97%	148
Bluegrass Community Hospital	Versailles	96%	26
Flaget Memorial Hospital	Bardstown	96%	85
Georgetown Community Hospital	Georgetown	96%	45
Lexington-Leestown VA Medical Center	Lexington	96%	94
Saint Joseph East[2]	Lexington	96%	68
Baptist Regional Medical Center	Corbin	95%	214
Central Baptist Hospital	Lexington	95%	150
Louisville VA Medical Center	Louisville	95%	87
Middlesboro Appalachian Reg Hlthcre Hosp	Middlesboro	95%	130
Pattie A Clay Regional Medical Center	Richmond	95%	114
Spring View Hospital	Lebanon	95%	41
T J Samson Community Hospital[2]	Glasgow	95%	101
Harrison Memorial Hospital	Cynthiana	94%	115
Kentucky River Medical Center	Jackson	94%	64
King's Daughters' Medical Center[2]	Ashland	94%	358
The Medical Center at Franklin	Franklin	94%	70
Saint Elizabeth Ft Thomas	Fort Thomas	94%	157
Saint Joseph Mount Sterling	Mount Sterling	94%	83
Western Baptist Hospital	Paducah	94%	206
Jewish Hospital & St Mary's Healthcare	Louisville	93%	442
Lake Cumberland Regional Hospital	Somerset	93%	236
Norton Hospitals	Louisville	93%	538
Parkway Regional Hospital	Fulton	93%	45
Saint Joseph Hospital[2]	Lexington	93%	95
Westlake Regional Hospital	Columbia	93%	91
Whitesburg ARH Hospital	Whitesburg	93%	150
Hardin Memorial Hospital[2]	Elizabethtown	92%	98
Harlan Appalachian Reg Healthcare Hosp	Harlan	92%	149
Marcum and Wallace Memorial Hospital	Irvine	92%	38
Saint Claire Regional Medical Center	Morehead	92%	106
Owensboro Medical Health System	Owensboro	91%	128
Regional Medical Center of Hopkins County	Madisonville	91%	105
Saint Elizabeth Medical Center North[2]	Covington	91%	68
Trigg County Hospital[2]	Cadiz	91%	32
Twin Lakes Regional Medical Center[2]	Leitchfield	91%	99
Jennie Stuart Medical Center	Hopkinsville	90%	170
Muhlenberg Community Hospital	Greenville	90%	116
Our Lady of Bellefonte Hospital	Ashland	90%	170
Pikeville Medical Center	Pikeville	90%	190
Saint Joseph Hospital London	London	90%	121
Jackson Purchase Medical Center	Mayfield	89%	97
The James B Haggin Memorial Hospital	Harrodsburg	89%	36
Jewish Hospital - Shelbyville	Shelbyville	89%	81
Memorial Hospital	Manchester	89%	173
Morgan County Arh Hospital	West Liberty	89%	72
Rockcastle Reg Hosp & Respiratory Care Ctr[2]	Mount Vernon	89%	35
Bourbon Community Hospital	Paris	88%	33
Ephraim Mcdowell Regional Medical Center[2]	Danville	88%	138
Mary Breckinridge Hospital	Hyden	88%	52
Methodist Hospital Union County	Morganfield	88%	32
Saint Elizabeth Florence	Florence	88%	85
University of Louisville Hospital	Louisville	88%	67
Williamson ARH Hospital	S Williamson	88%	95
Baptist Hospital East	Louisville	87%	385
Saint Joseph Berea	Berea	87%	39
The Medical Center at Bowling Green	Bowling Green	86%	217
Monroe County Medical Center	Tompkinsville	86%	59
Wayne County Hospital	Monticello	86%	37
Ohio County Hospital	Hartford	85%	33
Russell County Hospital	Russell Springs	85%	68
Saint Joseph Martin	Martin	85%	60
Highlands Regional Medical Center	Prestonsburg	84%	144
Casey County Hospital	Liberty	83%	59
Clark Regional Medical Center	Winchester	83%	154
Hazard Arh Regional Medical Center[2]	Hazard	83%	75
Baptist Hospital Northeast	La Grange	82%	84
Fleming County Hospital[2]	Flemingsburg	81%	117
Taylor Regional Hospital	Campbellsville	81%	98
The Medical Center at Scottsville	Scottsville	80%	30
Caldwell Medical Center	Princeton	79%	28
Pineville Community Hospital	Pineville	79%	97
Methodist Hospital	Henderson	77%	150
Clinton County Hospital	Albany	76%	78
University of Kentucky Hospital[2]	Lexington	74%	58
Murray-Calloway County Hospital	Murray	71%	114
Knox County Hospital	Barbourville	70%	63
Breckinridge Memorial Hospital	Hardinsburg	69%	26
Livingston Hospital and Healthcare	Salem	68%	25
McDowell Arh Hospital	McDowell	66%	85
Crittenden Health System	Marion	60%	45
Nicholas County Hospital	Carlisle	59%	29

17. Blood Culture Timing

Hospital Name	City	Rate	Cases
Bluegrass Community Hospital	Versailles	100%	30
Frankfort Regional Medical Center	Frankfort	100%	121
Hazard Arh Regional Medical Center[2]	Hazard	100%	32
Meadowview Regional Medical Center	Maysville	100%	103
Muhlenberg Community Hospital	Greenville	100%	51
Parkway Regional Hospital	Fulton	100%	47
Rockcastle Reg Hosp & Respiratory Care Ctr[2]	Mount Vernon	100%	35
Saint Elizabeth Medical Center North[2]	Covington	100%	62
Saint Joseph Berea	Berea	100%	33
Three Rivers Medical Center	Louisa	100%	84
Methodist Hospital	Henderson	99%	154
Middlesboro Appalachian Reg Hlthcre Hosp	Middlesboro	99%	162
Paul B Hall Regional Medical Center	Paintsville	99%	195
Regional Medical Center of Hopkins County	Madisonville	99%	187
Saint Joseph Hospital[2]	Lexington	99%	145
Western Baptist Hospital	Paducah	99%	250
Baptist Hospital Northeast	La Grange	98%	108
Carroll County Hospital	Carrollton	98%	41
Central Baptist Hospital	Lexington	98%	219
Ephraim Mcdowell Fort Logan Hospital	Stanford	98%	66
Greenview Regional Hospital	Bowling Green	98%	100
Jackson Purchase Medical Center	Mayfield	98%	128
Lexington-Leestown VA Medical Center	Lexington	98%	179
Louisville VA Medical Center	Louisville	98%	151
Saint Joseph Hospital London	London	98%	178
T J Samson Community Hospital[2]	Glasgow	98%	60
Ephraim Mcdowell Regional Medical Center[2]	Danville	97%	180
Logan Memorial Hospital	Russellville	97%	99
Lourdes Hospital	Paducah	97%	183
Mary Breckinridge Hospital	Hyden	97%	69
The Medical Center at Franklin	Franklin	97%	31
Norton Hospitals	Louisville	97%	935
Our Lady of Bellefonte Hospital	Ashland	97%	223
Saint Elizabeth Ft Thomas	Fort Thomas	97%	116
Saint Joseph Martin	Martin	97%	66
Spring View Hospital	Lebanon	97%	67
Taylor Regional Hospital	Campbellsville	97%	103
Baptist Regional Medical Center	Corbin	96%	225
Georgetown Community Hospital	Georgetown	96%	75
Jewish Hospital & St Mary's Healthcare	Louisville	96%	735
Kentucky River Medical Center	Jackson	96%	72
King's Daughters' Medical Center[2]	Ashland	96%	318
Lake Cumberland Regional Hospital	Somerset	96%	196
Murray-Calloway County Hospital	Murray	96%	105
Owensboro Medical Health System	Owensboro	96%	253
Saint Elizabeth Florence	Florence	96%	112
Harlan Appalachian Reg Healthcare Hosp	Harlan	95%	164
Harrison Memorial Hospital	Cynthiana	95%	123
Marcum and Wallace Memorial Hospital	Irvine	95%	42
The Medical Center at Bowling Green	Bowling Green	95%	258
Pikeville Medical Center	Pikeville	95%	252
Saint Joseph Mount Sterling	Mount Sterling	95%	103
Baptist Hospital East	Louisville	94%	620
Crittenden Health System	Marion	94%	31
Knox County Hospital	Barbourville	94%	54
Memorial Hospital	Manchester	94%	152
Ohio County Hospital	Hartford	94%	32
Twin Lakes Regional Medical Center[2]	Leitchfield	94%	110
Wayne County Hospital	Monticello	94%	36
Highlands Regional Medical Center	Prestonsburg	93%	153
Clark Regional Medical Center	Winchester	92%	155
Flaget Memorial Hospital	Bardstown	92%	106
Jennie Stuart Medical Center	Hopkinsville	92%	179
Morgan County Arh Hospital	West Liberty	92%	61
Saint Claire Regional Medical Center	Morehead	92%	216
Saint Joseph East[2]	Lexington	92%	79
Whitesburg ARH Hospital	Whitesburg	92%	108
Bourbon Community Hospital	Paris	91%	53
Fleming County Hospital[2]	Flemingsburg	91%	101
Jewish Hospital - Shelbyville	Shelbyville	90%	92
University of Kentucky Hospital[2]	Lexington	88%	119
Pattie A Clay Regional Medical Center	Richmond	87%	127
Pineville Community Hospital	Pineville	86%	79
Hardin Memorial Hospital[2]	Elizabethtown	83%	103
McDowell Arh Hospital	McDowell	83%	65
University of Louisville Hospital	Louisville	83%	103
The James B Haggin Memorial Hospital	Harrodsburg	80%	50
Russell County Hospital	Russell Springs	77%	65
Williamson ARH Hospital	S Williamson	75%	65
Monroe County Medical Center	Tompkinsville	70%	54

18. Influenza Vaccine

Hospital Name	City	Rate	Cases
Baptist Regional Medical Center	Corbin	100%	188
Frankfort Regional Medical Center	Frankfort	100%	82
Greenview Regional Hospital	Bowling Green	100%	67
Harlan Appalachian Reg Healthcare Hosp	Harlan	100%	104
Knox County Hospital	Barbourville	100%	48
Lourdes Hospital	Paducah	100%	169
Morgan County Arh Hospital	West Liberty	100%	45
Owensboro Medical Health System	Owensboro	100%	191
Parkway Regional Hospital	Fulton	100%	28
Pattie A Clay Regional Medical Center	Richmond	100%	94
Three Rivers Medical Center	Louisa	100%	73
Williamson ARH Hospital	S Williamson	100%	65
Baptist Hospital Northeast	La Grange	99%	80
Central Baptist Hospital	Lexington	99%	170
Our Lady of Bellefonte Hospital	Ashland	99%	217
Ephraim Mcdowell Fort Logan Hospital	Stanford	98%	59
Paul B Hall Regional Medical Center	Paintsville	98%	128
Saint Elizabeth Medical Center North[2]	Covington	98%	90
Saint Joseph Berea	Berea	98%	42
Saint Joseph Hospital London	London	98%	85
T J Samson Community Hospital[2]	Glasgow	98%	95
Ephraim Mcdowell Regional Medical Center	Danville	97%	220
Lake Cumberland Regional Hospital	Somerset	97%	235
Memorial Hospital	Manchester	97%	115
Saint Elizabeth Florence	Florence	97%	118
Saint Joseph Hospital[2]	Lexington	97%	164
Western Baptist Hospital	Paducah	97%	241
Baptist Hospital East	Louisville	96%	492
Clinton County Hospital	Albany	96%	48
Georgetown Community Hospital	Georgetown	96%	49
Middlesboro Appalachian Reg Hlthcre Hosp	Middlesboro	96%	98
Saint Claire Regional Medical Center	Morehead	96%	113
Saint Joseph East[2]	Lexington	96%	72
Saint Joseph Martin	Martin	96%	25
Clark Regional Medical Center	Winchester	95%	86
Highlands Regional Medical Center	Prestonsburg	95%	132
Jewish Hospital - Shelbyville	Shelbyville	95%	73
Kentucky River Medical Center	Jackson	95%	58
King's Daughters' Medical Center[2]	Ashland	95%	421
Logan Memorial Hospital	Russellville	95%	131
Louisville VA Medical Center	Louisville	95%	101
Norton Hospitals	Louisville	95%	671
Rockcastle Reg Hosp & Respiratory Care Ctr	Mount Vernon	95%	42
Saint Elizabeth Ft Thomas	Fort Thomas	95%	133
Spring View Hospital	Lebanon	95%	38
Flaget Memorial Hospital	Bardstown	94%	66
Meadowview Regional Medical Center	Maysville	94%	79
Carroll County Hospital	Carrollton	93%	29
The Medical Center at Bowling Green	Bowling Green	93%	316
Pikeville Medical Center	Pikeville	93%	235
Twin Lakes Regional Medical Center[2]	Leitchfield	93%	83
Fleming County Hospital	Flemingsburg	92%	66
Hardin Memorial Hospital[2]	Elizabethtown	92%	91
Jennie Stuart Medical Center	Hopkinsville	92%	143
Lexington-Leestown VA Medical Center	Lexington	92%	103
Marcum and Wallace Memorial Hospital	Irvine	92%	40
Regional Medical Center of Hopkins County	Madisonville	91%	168
Saint Joseph Mount Sterling	Mount Sterling	91%	54
Harrison Memorial Hospital	Cynthiana	90%	69
Jackson Purchase Medical Center	Mayfield	90%	142
Methodist Hospital Union County	Morganfield	90%	29
Crittenden Health System	Marion	89%	53
Mary Breckinridge Hospital	Hyden	88%	51
Muhlenberg Community Hospital	Greenville	88%	93
Bourbon Community Hospital	Paris	87%	38
Cumberland County Hospital	Burkesville	87%	31
Jewish Hospital & St Mary's Healthcare	Louisville	87%	617
The James B Haggin Memorial Hospital	Harrodsburg	85%	53
McDowell Arh Hospital	McDowell	85%	39
The Medical Center at Franklin	Franklin	85%	62
Methodist Hospital	Henderson	85%	143
University of Kentucky Hospital[2]	Lexington	85%	109

NOTE: Hospital profiles are in alphabetical order by state, then city, then hospital within the city; Rankings exclude hospitals with less than 25 cases except for patient surveys which excludes hospitals with less than 100 cases; (a) 100–299 cases; (1) The number of cases is too small to be sure how well a hospital is performing; (2) The hospital indicated that the data submitted for this measure were based on a sample of cases; (3) Data was collected during a shorter time period (fewer quarters) than the maximum possible time for this measure; (4) Suppressed for one or more quarters by CMS; (5) No data is available from the hospital for this measure; (6) Fewer than 100 patients completed the HCAHPS survey. Use these rates with caution, as the number of surveys may be too low to reliably assess hospital performance; (7) Survey results are based on less than 12 months of data; (8) Survey results are not available for this reporting period; (9) No or very few patients were eligible for the HCAHPS survey. The scores shown, if any, reflect a very small number of surveys; (10) A state average was not calculated because too few hospitals in the state submitted data; (11) There were discrepancies in the data collection process; Please refer to the User's Guide for a full explanation of data.

Pineville Community Hospital	Pineville	83%	94
Whitesburg ARH Hospital	Whitesburg	79%	105
Monroe County Medical Center	Tompkinsville	77%	64
Wayne County Hospital	Monticello	76%	33
Westlake Regional Hospital	Columbia	71%	68
Russell County Hospital	Russell Springs	70%	47
University of Louisville Hospital	Louisville	69%	75
Hazard Arh Regional Medical Center[2]	Hazard	68%	82
Taylor Regional Hospital	Campbellsville	68%	107
Casey County Hospital	Liberty	66%	61
Ohio County Hospital	Hartford	62%	34
Murray-Calloway County Hospital	Murray	55%	118

19. Initial Antibiotic Timing

Hospital Name	City	Rate	Cases
Bluegrass Community Hospital	Versailles	100%	37
Bourbon Community Hospital	Paris	100%	51
Flaget Memorial Hospital	Bardstown	100%	100
Georgetown Community Hospital	Georgetown	100%	75
Kentucky River Medical Center	Jackson	100%	116
Meadowview Regional Medical Center	Maysville	100%	104
Parkway Regional Hospital	Fulton	100%	63
Saint Elizabeth Grant	Williamstown	100%	37
Saint Joseph Berea	Berea	100%	56
Saint Joseph Martin	Martin	100%	70
Three Rivers Medical Center	Louisa	100%	122
Wayne County Hospital	Monticello	100%	48
Harrison Memorial Hospital	Cynthiana	99%	136
Logan Memorial Hospital	Russellville	99%	170
Mary Breckinridge Hospital	Hyden	99%	71
Muhlenberg Community Hospital	Greenville	99%	144
Pattie A Clay Regional Medical Center	Richmond	99%	140
Paul B Hall Regional Medical Center	Paintsville	99%	212
Saint Elizabeth Medical Center North[2]	Covington	99%	122
Saint Joseph Mount Sterling	Mount Sterling	99%	89
Western Baptist Hospital	Paducah	99%	270
Baptist Hospital Northeast	La Grange	98%	113
Baptist Regional Medical Center	Corbin	98%	253
Central Baptist Hospital	Lexington	98%	216
Ephraim Mcdowell Fort Logan Hospital	Stanford	98%	93
Frankfort Regional Medical Center	Frankfort	98%	121
Jackson Purchase Medical Center	Mayfield	98%	161
Lake Cumberland Regional Hospital	Somerset	98%	339
Saint Elizabeth Ft Thomas	Fort Thomas	98%	161
Saint Joseph Hospital London	London	98%	152
Twin Lakes Regional Medical Center[2]	Leitchfield	98%	114
Westlake Regional Hospital	Columbia	98%	121
Whitesburg ARH Hospital	Whitesburg	98%	181
Greenview Regional Hospital	Bowling Green	97%	117
Harlan Appalachian Reg Healthcare Hosp	Harlan	97%	232
Middlesboro Appalachian Reg Hlthcre Hosp	Middlesboro	97%	170
Morgan County Arh Hospital	West Liberty	97%	78
Ohio County Hospital	Hartford	97%	38
Rockcastle Reg Hosp & Respiratory Care Ctr[2]	Mount Vernon	97%	64
Saint Claire Regional Medical Center	Morehead	97%	196
Spring View Hospital	Lebanon	97%	73
T J Samson Community Hospital[2]	Glasgow	97%	154
Trigg County Hospital[2]	Cadiz	97%	36
Baptist Hospital East	Louisville	96%	628
Casey County Hospital	Liberty	96%	91
Clark Regional Medical Center	Winchester	96%	182
Ephraim Mcdowell Regional Medical Center[2]	Danville	96%	285
Jewish Hospital - Shelbyville	Shelbyville	96%	116
King's Daughters' Medical Center[2]	Ashland	96%	493
Lourdes Hospital	Paducah	96%	205
Marcum and Wallace Memorial Hospital	Irvine	96%	51
New Horizons Medical Center	Owenton	96%	28
Our Lady of Bellefonte Hospital	Ashland	96%	275
Saint Joseph Hospital[2]	Lexington	96%	153
Crittenden Health System	Marion	95%	59
Highlands Regional Medical Center	Prestonsburg	95%	240
The James B Haggin Memorial Hospital	Harrodsburg	95%	44
Methodist Hospital	Henderson	95%	231
Norton Hospitals	Louisville	95%	892
Pikeville Medical Center	Pikeville	95%	316
Fleming County Hospital[2]	Flemingsburg	94%	94
Jewish Hospital & St Mary's Healthcare	Louisville	94%	712
Knox County Hospital	Barbourville	94%	78
Louisville VA Medical Center	Louisville	94%	147
The Medical Center at Franklin	Franklin	94%	88
Monroe County Medical Center	Tompkinsville	94%	96
Nicholas County Hospital	Carlisle	94%	36
Russell County Hospital	Russell Springs	94%	89
Williamson ARH Hospital	S Williamson	94%	108
Carroll County Hospital	Carrollton	93%	56
Clinton County Hospital	Albany	93%	57
Hardin Memorial Hospital[2]	Elizabethtown	93%	136
Lexington-Leestown VA Medical Center	Lexington	93%	162
The Medical Center at Bowling Green	Bowling Green	93%	338
Memorial Hospital	Manchester	93%	194
Owensboro Medical Health System	Owensboro	93%	364
Saint Elizabeth Florence	Florence	93%	134
Jane Todd Crawford Hospital	Greensburg	92%	25
Jennie Stuart Medical Center	Hopkinsville	92%	238
Livingston Hospital and Healthcare	Salem	92%	26
Murray-Calloway County Hospital	Murray	92%	161
Regional Medical Center of Hopkins County	Madisonville	92%	271
Caldwell Medical Center	Princeton	91%	34
The Medical Center at Scottsville	Scottsville	91%	35
Methodist Hospital Union County	Morganfield	89%	37
Saint Joseph East[2]	Lexington	89%	83
Hazard Arh Regional Medical Center[2]	Hazard	88%	116
Pineville Community Hospital	Pineville	88%	125
Taylor Regional Hospital	Campbellsville	87%	128
University of Kentucky Hospital[2]	Lexington	84%	123
McDowell Arh Hospital	McDowell	83%	106
Breckinridge Memorial Hospital	Hardinsburg	82%	38
University of Louisville Hospital	Louisville	82%	121
Cumberland County Hospital	Burkesville	76%	45

20. Pneumococcal Vaccine

Hospital Name	City	Rate	Cases
Baptist Regional Medical Center	Corbin	100%	256
Ephraim Mcdowell Fort Logan Hospital	Stanford	100%	83
Frankfort Regional Medical Center	Frankfort	100%	114
Greenview Regional Hospital	Bowling Green	100%	86
Harlan Appalachian Reg Healthcare Hosp	Harlan	100%	125
Kentucky River Medical Center	Jackson	100%	79
Lake Cumberland Regional Hospital	Somerset	100%	285
Lourdes Hospital	Paducah	100%	194
Meadowview Regional Medical Center	Maysville	100%	99
Morgan County Arh Hospital	West Liberty	100%	62
Parkway Regional Hospital	Fulton	100%	53
Rockcastle Reg Hosp & Respiratory Care Ctr[2]	Mount Vernon	100%	66
Saint Elizabeth Grant	Williamstown	100%	28
Saint Joseph Berea	Berea	100%	46
Three Rivers Medical Center	Louisa	100%	72
Baptist Hospital Northeast	La Grange	99%	106
Central Baptist Hospital	Lexington	99%	248
Our Lady of Bellefonte Hospital	Ashland	99%	256
Paul B Hall Regional Medical Center	Paintsville	99%	174
Saint Elizabeth Medical Center North[2]	Covington	99%	115
Saint Joseph Hospital[2]	Lexington	99%	220
T J Samson Community Hospital[2]	Glasgow	99%	153
Western Baptist Hospital	Paducah	99%	267
Williamson ARH Hospital	S Williamson	99%	82
Lexington-Leestown VA Medical Center	Lexington	98%	151
Louisville VA Medical Center	Louisville	98%	117
Pattie A Clay Regional Medical Center	Richmond	98%	120
Saint Joseph Hospital London	London	98%	148
Clark Regional Medical Center	Winchester	97%	116
Ephraim Mcdowell Regional Medical Center[2]	Danville	97%	273
Knox County Hospital	Barbourville	97%	60
Logan Memorial Hospital	Russellville	97%	151
Middlesboro Appalachian Reg Hlthcre Hosp	Middlesboro	97%	110
Owensboro Medical Health System	Owensboro	97%	312
Pikeville Medical Center	Pikeville	97%	308
Regional Medical Center of Hopkins County	Madisonville	97%	220
Saint Elizabeth Ft Thomas	Fort Thomas	97%	174
Harrison Memorial Hospital	Cynthiana	96%	121
Mary Breckinridge Hospital	Hyden	96%	55
The Medical Center at Bowling Green	Bowling Green	96%	380
The Medical Center at Scottsville	Scottsville	96%	28
Memorial Hospital	Manchester	96%	113
Norton Hospitals	Louisville	96%	779
Saint Elizabeth Florence	Florence	96%	164
Saint Joseph East[2]	Lexington	96%	89
Spring View Hospital	Lebanon	96%	55
Baptist Hospital East	Louisville	95%	689
Flaget Memorial Hospital	Bardstown	95%	83
Georgetown Community Hospital	Georgetown	95%	59
King's Daughters' Medical Center[2]	Ashland	95%	536
Carroll County Hospital	Carrollton	94%	35
Hardin Memorial Hospital[2]	Elizabethtown	94%	133
Jackson Purchase Medical Center	Mayfield	94%	212
Saint Joseph Martin	Martin	94%	33
McDowell Arh Hospital	McDowell	93%	45
Jewish Hospital & St Mary's Healthcare	Louisville	92%	724
Jewish Hospital - Shelbyville	Shelbyville	92%	88
Trigg County Hospital[2]	Cadiz	92%	26
Twin Lakes Regional Medical Center[2]	Leitchfield	92%	115
Clinton County Hospital	Albany	91%	58
Methodist Hospital	Henderson	91%	191
Saint Claire Regional Medical Center	Morehead	91%	183
Wayne County Hospital	Monticello	91%	55
Marcum and Wallace Memorial Hospital	Irvine	90%	59
Bourbon Community Hospital	Paris	89%	46
Highlands Regional Medical Center	Prestonsburg	89%	173
Jennie Stuart Medical Center	Hopkinsville	89%	186
The Medical Center at Franklin	Franklin	89%	80
Methodist Hospital Union County	Morganfield	89%	37
Muhlenberg Community Hospital	Greenville	88%	110
Pineville Community Hospital	Pineville	88%	107
Saint Joseph Mount Sterling	Mount Sterling	87%	83
Fleming County Hospital[2]	Flemingsburg	86%	98
Whitesburg ARH Hospital	Whitesburg	86%	113
University of Kentucky Hospital[2]	Lexington	85%	104
The James B Haggin Memorial Hospital	Harrodsburg	82%	71
Monroe County Medical Center	Tompkinsville	81%	86
Cumberland County Hospital	Burkesville	80%	40
University of Louisville Hospital	Louisville	79%	52
Hazard Arh Regional Medical Center[2]	Hazard	78%	88
Westlake Regional Hospital	Columbia	78%	96
Casey County Hospital	Liberty	77%	78
Taylor Regional Hospital	Campbellsville	76%	134
Russell County Hospital	Russell Springs	75%	61
Breckinridge Memorial Hospital	Hardinsburg	73%	30
Crittenden Health System	Marion	72%	69
Caverna Memorial Hospital	Horse Cave	70%	27
Ohio County Hospital	Hartford	69%	39
Murray-Calloway County Hospital	Murray	68%	139
New Horizons Medical Center	Owenton	62%	26

21. Smoking Cessation Advice

Hospital Name	City	Rate	Cases
Baptist Regional Medical Center	Corbin	100%	151
Central Baptist Hospital	Lexington	100%	130
Clinton County Hospital	Albany	100%	39
Crittenden Health System	Marion	100%	33
Ephraim Mcdowell Fort Logan Hospital	Stanford	100%	47
Ephraim Mcdowell Regional Medical Center[2]	Danville	100%	156
Flaget Memorial Hospital	Bardstown	100%	54
Georgetown Community Hospital	Georgetown	100%	34
Greenview Regional Hospital	Bowling Green	100%	68
Harlan Appalachian Reg Healthcare Hosp	Harlan	100%	98
Harrison Memorial Hospital	Cynthiana	100%	53
Highlands Regional Medical Center	Prestonsburg	100%	98
Jackson Purchase Medical Center	Mayfield	100%	93
Jewish Hospital & St Mary's Healthcare	Louisville	100%	475
Jewish Hospital - Shelbyville	Shelbyville	100%	55
Kentucky River Medical Center	Jackson	100%	65
Lexington-Leestown VA Medical Center	Lexington	100%	43
Logan Memorial Hospital	Russellville	100%	82
Louisville VA Medical Center	Louisville	100%	81
Lourdes Hospital	Paducah	100%	94
McDowell Arh Hospital	McDowell	100%	39
Meadowview Regional Medical Center	Maysville	100%	37
The Medical Center at Bowling Green	Bowling Green	100%	199
The Medical Center at Franklin	Franklin	100%	35
Memorial Hospital	Manchester	100%	123
Middlesboro Appalachian Reg Hlthcre Hosp	Middlesboro	100%	75
Norton Hospitals	Louisville	100%	475
Our Lady of Bellefonte Hospital	Ashland	100%	161
Parkway Regional Hospital	Fulton	100%	26
Pattie A Clay Regional Medical Center	Richmond	100%	57
Paul B Hall Regional Medical Center	Paintsville	100%	143
Pikeville Medical Center	Pikeville	100%	195
Rockcastle Reg Hosp & Respiratory Care Ctr[2]	Mount Vernon	100%	34
Saint Elizabeth Florence	Florence	100%	76
Saint Elizabeth Ft Thomas	Fort Thomas	100%	82
Saint Elizabeth Medical Center North[2]	Covington	100%	81
Saint Joseph Berea	Berea	100%	38
Saint Joseph East[2]	Lexington	100%	69
Saint Joseph Hospital[2]	Lexington	100%	105
Saint Joseph Hospital London	London	100%	114
Saint Joseph Martin	Martin	100%	37
T J Samson Community Hospital[2]	Glasgow	100%	95
Three Rivers Medical Center	Louisa	100%	71
Twin Lakes Regional Medical Center[2]	Leitchfield	100%	57
Western Baptist Hospital	Paducah	100%	162
Whitesburg ARH Hospital	Whitesburg	100%	89
Williamson ARH Hospital	S Williamson	100%	55
Baptist Hospital East	Louisville	99%	195
Hazard Arh Regional Medical Center[2]	Hazard	99%	70
King's Daughters' Medical Center[2]	Ashland	99%	368
Lake Cumberland Regional Hospital	Somerset	99%	166
Owensboro Medical Health System	Owensboro	99%	180
Regional Medical Center of Hopkins County	Madisonville	99%	158
University of Louisville Hospital	Louisville	99%	109
Baptist Hospital Northeast	La Grange	98%	44
Clark Regional Medical Center	Winchester	98%	91
Frankfort Regional Medical Center	Frankfort	98%	54
Mary Breckinridge Hospital	Hyden	97%	29
Saint Claire Regional Medical Center	Morehead	97%	108
University of Kentucky Hospital[2]	Lexington	97%	119
Casey County Hospital	Liberty	96%	25
Saint Joseph Mount Sterling	Mount Sterling	96%	46
Jennie Stuart Medical Center	Hopkinsville	95%	101
Hardin Memorial Hospital[2]	Elizabethtown	94%	69
Murray-Calloway County Hospital	Murray	94%	67

NOTE: Hospital profiles are in alphabetical order by state, then city, then hospital within the city; Rankings exclude hospitals with less than 25 cases except for patient surveys which excludes hospitals with less than 100 cases; (a) 100–299 cases; (1) The number of cases is too small to be sure how well a hospital is performing; (2) The hospital indicated that the data submitted for this measure were based on a sample of cases; (3) Data was collected during a shorter time period (fewer quarters) than the maximum possible time for this measure; (4) Suppressed for one or more quarters by CMS; (5) No data is available from the hospital for this measure; (6) Fewer than 100 patients completed the HCAHPS survey. Use these rates with caution, as the number of surveys may be too low to reliably assess hospital performance; (7) Survey results are based on less than 12 months of data; (8) Survey results are not available for this reporting period; (9) No or very few patients were eligible for the HCAHPS survey. The scores shown, if any, reflect a very small number of surveys; (10) A state average was not calculated because too few hospitals in the state submitted data; (11) There were discrepancies in the data collection process; Please refer to the User's Guide for a full explanation of data.

Carroll County Hospital	Carrollton	93%	30
Muhlenberg Community Hospital	Greenville	93%	75
Methodist Hospital	Henderson	92%	105
Knox County Hospital	Barbourville	89%	37
Westlake Regional Hospital	Columbia	89%	63
Russell County Hospital	Russell Springs	85%	41
Fleming County Hospital[2]	Flemingsburg	84%	58
Taylor Regional Hospital	Campbellsville	84%	67
Monroe County Medical Center	Tompkinsville	83%	46
Pineville Community Hospital	Pineville	77%	62
Cumberland County Hospital	Burkesville	68%	34
The James B Haggin Memorial Hospital	Harrodsburg	61%	41

Surgical Care Improvement Project

22. Appropriate VTP Within 24 Hours

Hospital Name	City	Rate	Cases
Harlan Appalachian Reg Healthcare Hosp	Harlan	100%	25
Highlands Regional Medical Center	Prestonsburg	100%	41
Meadowview Regional Medical Center	Maysville	100%	34
Muhlenberg Community Hospital	Greenville	100%	55
Paul B Hall Regional Medical Center	Paintsville	100%	27
Saint Joseph Mount Sterling	Mount Sterling	100%	51
Jackson Purchase Medical Center	Mayfield	99%	185
Saint Joseph Hospital London[2]	London	99%	98
Ephraim Mcdowell Regional Medical Center	Danville	98%	189
Spring View Hospital	Lebanon	98%	80
Baptist Regional Medical Center	Corbin	97%	130
Harrison Memorial Hospital	Cynthiana	97%	38
Saint Elizabeth Ft Thomas[2]	Fort Thomas	97%	123
Williamson ARH Hospital[2]	S Williamson	97%	33
Greenview Regional Hospital	Bowling Green	96%	156
Jennie Stuart Medical Center	Hopkinsville	96%	126
Saint Claire Regional Medical Center[2]	Morehead	96%	92
Central Baptist Hospital	Lexington	95%	587
Flaget Memorial Hospital	Bardstown	95%	74
Lake Cumberland Regional Hospital	Somerset	95%	275
Methodist Hospital[2]	Henderson	95%	75
Saint Elizabeth Medical Center North[2]	Covington	95%	166
Baptist Hospital Northeast	La Grange	94%	98
Frankfort Regional Medical Center	Frankfort	94%	144
Pineville Community Hospital[2]	Pineville	94%	33
Saint Joseph Hospital[2]	Lexington	94%	418
Lourdes Hospital[2]	Paducah	93%	401
Owensboro Medical Health System[2]	Owensboro	92%	266
Pattie A Clay Regional Medical Center	Richmond	92%	89
Saint Joseph Berea	Berea	92%	26
Twin Lakes Regional Medical Center[2]	Leitchfield	92%	80
Western Baptist Hospital	Paducah	92%	473
King's Daughters' Medical Center[2]	Ashland	91%	171
Saint Joseph East[2]	Lexington	91%	176
University of Kentucky Hospital[2]	Lexington	91%	287
Baptist Hospital East	Louisville	90%	1105
Saint Elizabeth Florence[2]	Florence	90%	102
Hazard Arh Regional Medical Center[2]	Hazard	89%	128
Middlesboro Appalachian Reg Hlthcre Hosp	Middlesboro	89%	28
Norton Hospitals[2]	Louisville	89%	969
Pikeville Medical Center[2]	Pikeville	89%	274
Taylor Regional Hospital	Campbellsville	89%	97
Jewish Hospital & St Mary's Healthcare[2]	Louisville	88%	352
Regional Medical Center of Hopkins County[2]	Madisonville	88%	253
Hardin Memorial Hospital[2]	Elizabethtown	87%	191
Our Lady of Bellefonte Hospital	Ashland	85%	148
Clark Regional Medical Center[2]	Winchester	84%	50
The Medical Center at Bowling Green	Bowling Green	84%	402
University of Louisville Hospital[2]	Louisville	84%	160
Jewish Hospital - Shelbyville	Shelbyville	83%	66
Georgetown Community Hospital	Georgetown	81%	43
Murray-Calloway County Hospital	Murray	81%	109
T J Samson Community Hospital[2]	Glasgow	79%	128

23. Appropriate Hair Removal

Hospital Name	City	Rate	Cases
Baptist Hospital Northeast	La Grange	100%	210
Baptist Regional Medical Center	Corbin	100%	316
Bluegrass Community Hospital	Versailles	100%	40
Central Baptist Hospital	Lexington	100%	2109
Clark Regional Medical Center[2]	Winchester	100%	189
Ephraim Mcdowell Fort Logan Hospital	Stanford	100%	30
Ephraim Mcdowell Regional Medical Center	Danville	100%	514
Flaget Memorial Hospital	Bardstown	100%	301
Frankfort Regional Medical Center	Frankfort	100%	253
Georgetown Community Hospital	Georgetown	100%	88
Greenview Regional Hospital	Bowling Green	100%	450
Hardin Memorial Hospital[2]	Elizabethtown	100%	556
Harlan Appalachian Reg Healthcare Hosp	Harlan	100%	65
Hazard Arh Regional Medical Center[2]	Hazard	100%	354
Highlands Regional Medical Center	Prestonsburg	100%	85
Jackson Purchase Medical Center	Mayfield	100%	318
Jewish Hospital - Shelbyville	Shelbyville	100%	138
King's Daughters' Medical Center[2]	Ashland	100%	732
Lake Cumberland Regional Hospital	Somerset	100%	722
Lourdes Hospital[2]	Paducah	100%	955
Meadowview Regional Medical Center	Maysville	100%	74
The Medical Center at Bowling Green	Bowling Green	100%	1480
Middlesboro Appalachian Reg Hlthcre Hosp	Middlesboro	100%	51
Muhlenberg Community Hospital	Greenville	100%	120
Norton Hospitals[2]	Louisville	100%	3536
Our Lady of Bellefonte Hospital	Ashland	100%	544
Parkway Regional Hospital[2]	Fulton	100%	26
Pattie A Clay Regional Medical Center	Richmond	100%	490
Paul B Hall Regional Medical Center	Paintsville	100%	33
Pikeville Medical Center[2]	Pikeville	100%	856
Pineville Community Hospital[2]	Pineville	100%	74
Regional Medical Center of Hopkins County[2]	Madisonville	100%	789
Saint Elizabeth Florence[2]	Florence	100%	252
Saint Elizabeth Ft Thomas[2]	Fort Thomas	100%	215
Saint Elizabeth Medical Center North[2]	Covington	100%	712
Saint Joseph Berea	Berea	100%	41
Saint Joseph East[2]	Lexington	100%	548
Saint Joseph Hospital[2]	Lexington	100%	1230
Saint Joseph Hospital London[2]	London	100%	401
Saint Joseph Mount Sterling	Mount Sterling	100%	219
Spring View Hospital	Lebanon	100%	238
Twin Lakes Regional Medical Center[2]	Leitchfield	100%	189
Western Baptist Hospital	Paducah	100%	1128
Whitesburg ARH Hospital	Whitesburg	100%	63
Williamson ARH Hospital[2]	S Williamson	100%	70
Harrison Memorial Hospital	Cynthiana	99%	77
Jewish Hospital & St Mary's Healthcare[2]	Louisville	99%	1108
Murray-Calloway County Hospital	Murray	99%	268
Owensboro Medical Health System[2]	Owensboro	99%	1045
Saint Claire Regional Medical Center[2]	Morehead	99%	196
Three Rivers Medical Center[2]	Louisa	99%	81
University of Kentucky Hospital[2]	Lexington	99%	761
Baptist Hospital East	Louisville	98%	4190
University of Louisville Hospital[2]	Louisville	96%	421
Taylor Regional Hospital	Campbellsville	94%	223
Jennie Stuart Medical Center	Hopkinsville	93%	421
Methodist Hospital[2]	Henderson	93%	218
T J Samson Community Hospital[2]	Glasgow	89%	292

24. Appropriate Beta Blocker Usage

Hospital Name	City	Rate	Cases
Our Lady of Bellefonte Hospital	Ashland	100%	144
Pattie A Clay Regional Medical Center	Richmond	100%	82
Saint Elizabeth Ft Thomas[2]	Fort Thomas	100%	42
Baptist Regional Medical Center	Corbin	99%	106
Frankfort Regional Medical Center	Frankfort	99%	75
Jackson Purchase Medical Center	Mayfield	99%	95
Owensboro Medical Health System[2]	Owensboro	99%	394
Ephraim Mcdowell Regional Medical Center	Danville	98%	146
Greenview Regional Hospital	Bowling Green	98%	160
Saint Joseph Hospital London[2]	London	98%	176
Spring View Hospital	Lebanon	98%	51
Central Baptist Hospital	Lexington	97%	709
Jewish Hospital - Shelbyville	Shelbyville	97%	35
King's Daughters' Medical Center[2]	Ashland	97%	264
Lake Cumberland Regional Hospital	Somerset	97%	229
Saint Elizabeth Medical Center North[2]	Covington	97%	226
Saint Joseph Mount Sterling	Mount Sterling	96%	80
Baptist Hospital Northeast	La Grange	95%	57
Lourdes Hospital[2]	Paducah	95%	347
Regional Medical Center of Hopkins County[2]	Madisonville	95%	256
Saint Elizabeth Florence[2]	Florence	95%	41
Saint Joseph East[2]	Lexington	95%	157
Hazard Arh Regional Medical Center[2]	Hazard	94%	152
Jewish Hospital & St Mary's Healthcare[2]	Louisville	94%	409
Saint Joseph Hospital[2]	Lexington	94%	496
Methodist Hospital[2]	Henderson	93%	56
Murray-Calloway County Hospital	Murray	93%	69
Norton Hospitals[2]	Louisville	93%	1186
T J Samson Community Hospital[2]	Glasgow	93%	107
Twin Lakes Regional Medical Center[2]	Leitchfield	93%	46
Baptist Hospital East	Louisville	92%	1285
Pikeville Medical Center[2]	Pikeville	92%	334
Saint Claire Regional Medical Center[2]	Morehead	92%	78
Hardin Memorial Hospital[2]	Elizabethtown	90%	186
Flaget Memorial Hospital	Bardstown	87%	98
Jennie Stuart Medical Center	Hopkinsville	85%	85
University of Kentucky Hospital[2]	Lexington	85%	248
Western Baptist Hospital	Paducah	84%	372
Taylor Regional Hospital	Campbellsville	80%	45
The Medical Center at Bowling Green	Bowling Green	79%	461
Clark Regional Medical Center[2]	Winchester	76%	45
University of Louisville Hospital[2]	Louisville	64%	107

25. Controlled Postoperative Blood Glucose

Hospital Name	City	Rate	Cases
King's Daughters' Medical Center[2]	Ashland	100%	124
Hazard Arh Regional Medical Center[2]	Hazard	98%	84
University of Louisville Hospital[2]	Louisville	98%	58
Central Baptist Hospital	Lexington	97%	379
Saint Joseph Hospital London[2]	London	97%	124
Lake Cumberland Regional Hospital	Somerset	96%	83
Norton Hospitals[2]	Louisville	96%	516
Owensboro Medical Health System[2]	Owensboro	96%	219
Hardin Memorial Hospital[2]	Elizabethtown	95%	76
Lourdes Hospital[2]	Paducah	95%	164
Saint Joseph Hospital[2]	Lexington	95%	439
Baptist Hospital East	Louisville	93%	266
The Medical Center at Bowling Green	Bowling Green	92%	245
Saint Elizabeth Medical Center North[2]	Covington	92%	156
Jewish Hospital & St Mary's Healthcare[2]	Louisville	90%	181
University of Kentucky Hospital[2]	Lexington	90%	100
Western Baptist Hospital	Paducah	90%	244
Regional Medical Center of Hopkins County[2]	Madisonville	89%	123
Pikeville Medical Center[2]	Pikeville	85%	124

26. Prophylactic Antibiotic Timing

Hospital Name	City	Rate	Cases
Bluegrass Community Hospital	Versailles	100%	30
Central Baptist Hospital	Lexington	100%	1292
Greenview Regional Hospital	Bowling Green	100%	355
Jackson Purchase Medical Center	Mayfield	100%	253
Meadowview Regional Medical Center	Maysville	100%	53
Middlesboro Appalachian Reg Hlthcre Hosp	Middlesboro	100%	25
Saint Elizabeth Ft Thomas[2]	Fort Thomas	100%	92
Saint Joseph Berea	Berea	100%	27
Three Rivers Medical Center[2]	Louisa	100%	71
Williamson ARH Hospital[2]	S Williamson	100%	42
Ephraim Mcdowell Regional Medical Center	Danville	99%	337
Hazard Arh Regional Medical Center[2]	Hazard	99%	210
Saint Elizabeth Medical Center North[2]	Covington	99%	487
Saint Joseph East[2]	Lexington	99%	398
Saint Joseph Hospital London[2]	London	99%	272
Spring View Hospital	Lebanon	99%	187
Baptist Hospital East	Louisville	98%	2912
Baptist Regional Medical Center	Corbin	98%	222
Frankfort Regional Medical Center	Frankfort	98%	132
Georgetown Community Hospital	Georgetown	98%	42
Lake Cumberland Regional Hospital	Somerset	98%	363
Lourdes Hospital[2]	Paducah	98%	761
Our Lady of Bellefonte Hospital	Ashland	98%	380
Owensboro Medical Health System[2]	Owensboro	98%	791
Pattie A Clay Regional Medical Center	Richmond	98%	372
Saint Elizabeth Florence[2]	Florence	98%	119
Saint Joseph Hospital[2]	Lexington	98%	685
Saint Joseph Mount Sterling	Mount Sterling	98%	185
Twin Lakes Regional Medical Center[2]	Leitchfield	98%	117
Baptist Hospital Northeast	La Grange	97%	146
Ephraim Mcdowell Fort Logan Hospital	Stanford	97%	32
Flaget Memorial Hospital	Bardstown	97%	223
Hardin Memorial Hospital[2]	Elizabethtown	97%	387
Harlan Appalachian Reg Healthcare Hosp	Harlan	97%	39
Highlands Regional Medical Center	Prestonsburg	97%	31
King's Daughters' Medical Center[2]	Ashland	97%	516
Methodist Hospital[2]	Henderson	97%	138
Muhlenberg Community Hospital	Greenville	97%	67
Regional Medical Center of Hopkins County[2]	Madisonville	97%	550
Jewish Hospital & St Mary's Healthcare[2]	Louisville	96%	705
The Medical Center at Bowling Green	Bowling Green	96%	979
Norton Hospitals[2]	Louisville	96%	2460
Whitesburg ARH Hospital	Whitesburg	96%	46
Pikeville Medical Center[2]	Pikeville	95%	623
Taylor Regional Hospital	Campbellsville	95%	135
Western Baptist Hospital	Paducah	95%	713
Clark Regional Medical Center[2]	Winchester	94%	158
University of Kentucky Hospital[2]	Lexington	94%	487
University of Louisville Hospital[2]	Louisville	94%	271
Jennie Stuart Medical Center	Hopkinsville	93%	315
Murray-Calloway County Hospital	Murray	93%	167
Pineville Community Hospital[2]	Pineville	93%	56
Harrison Memorial Hospital	Cynthiana	92%	40
Jewish Hospital - Shelbyville	Shelbyville	92%	65
Saint Claire Regional Medical Center[2]	Morehead	88%	118
T J Samson Community Hospital[2]	Glasgow	83%	260

27. Prophylactic Antibiotic Timing (Outpatient)

Hospital Name	City	Rate	Cases
Kentucky River Medical Center	Jackson	100%	75
Central Baptist Hospital	Lexington	99%	1921
Georgetown Community Hospital	Georgetown	99%	185
Jackson Purchase Medical Center	Mayfield	99%	92
Lake Cumberland Regional Hospital	Somerset	99%	468
Baptist Regional Medical Center	Corbin	98%	215
Saint Joseph East	Lexington	98%	307
Meadowview Regional Medical Center	Maysville	97%	135
Pattie A Clay Regional Medical Center	Richmond	97%	116
Saint Elizabeth Medical Center North	Covington	97%	593

NOTE: Hospital profiles are in alphabetical order by state, then city, then hospital within the city; Rankings exclude hospitals with less than 25 cases except for patient surveys which excludes hospitals with less than 100 cases; (a) 100–299 cases; (1) The number of cases is too small to be sure how well a hospital is performing; (2) The hospital indicated that the data submitted for this measure were based on a sample of cases; (3) Data was collected during a shorter time period (fewer quarters) than the maximum possible time for this measure; (4) Suppressed for one or more quarters by CMS; (5) No data is available from the hospital for this measure; (6) Fewer than 100 patients completed the HCAHPS survey. Use these rates with caution, as the number of surveys may be too low to reliably assess hospital performance; (7) Survey results are based on less than 12 months of data; (8) Survey results are not available for this reporting period; (9) No or very few patients were eligible for the HCAHPS survey. The scores shown, if any, reflect a very small number of surveys; (10) A state average was not calculated because too few hospitals in the state submitted data; (11) There were discrepancies in the data collection process; Please refer to the User's Guide for a full explanation of data.

Baptist Hospital East	Louisville	96%	1548
Greenview Regional Hospital	Bowling Green	96%	168
Hardin Memorial Hospital	Elizabethtown	96%	514
Saint Joseph Hospital London	London	96%	291
Whitesburg ARH Hospital	Whitesburg	96%	121
Frankfort Regional Medical Center	Frankfort	95%	241
Harrison Memorial Hospital	Cynthiana	95%	38
Jewish Hospital & St Mary's Healthcare	Louisville	95%	1033
Lourdes Hospital	Paducah	95%	276
Our Lady of Bellefonte Hospital	Ashland	95%	203
Flaget Memorial Hospital	Bardstown	94%	95
Harlan Appalachian Reg Healthcare Hosp	Harlan	94%	49
Highlands Regional Medical Center	Prestonsburg	94%	141
Methodist Hospital	Henderson	94%	225
Western Baptist Hospital	Paducah	94%	628
Middlesboro Appalachian Reg Hlthcre Hosp	Middlesboro	93%	43
Owensboro Medical Health System	Owensboro	92%	890
Regional Medical Center of Hopkins County	Madisonville	91%	140
Saint Claire Regional Medical Center	Morehead	91%	80
Saint Joseph Mount Sterling	Mount Sterling	91%	35
Norton Hospitals	Louisville	90%	1238
Twin Lakes Regional Medical Center	Leitchfield	90%	41
Saint Elizabeth Florence	Florence	88%	25
Jennie Stuart Medical Center	Hopkinsville	87%	166
Taylor Regional Hospital	Campbellsville	87%	77
University of Kentucky Hospital	Lexington	87%	796
Baptist Hospital Northeast	La Grange	86%	50
Saint Joseph Hospital	Lexington	83%	878
Jewish Hospital - Shelbyville	Shelbyville	82%	33
The Medical Center at Bowling Green	Bowling Green	82%	540
Murray-Calloway County Hospital	Murray	82%	187
King's Daughters' Medical Center	Ashland	81%	343
Williamson ARH Hospital	S Williamson	81%	26
University of Louisville Hospital	Louisville	79%	277
Ephraim Mcdowell Regional Medical Center	Danville	78%	267
Clark Regional Medical Center	Winchester	76%	46
T J Samson Community Hospital	Glasgow	75%	173
Pikeville Medical Center	Pikeville	74%	144
Hazard Arh Regional Medical Center	Hazard	71%	127

28. Prophylactic Antibiotic Selection

Hospital Name	City	Rate	Cases
Bluegrass Community Hospital	Versailles	100%	30
Ephraim Mcdowell Regional Medical Center	Danville	100%	337
Georgetown Community Hospital	Georgetown	100%	41
Harlan Appalachian Reg Healthcare Hosp	Harlan	100%	39
Jackson Purchase Medical Center	Mayfield	100%	254
Meadowview Regional Medical Center	Maysville	100%	53
Saint Joseph Berea	Berea	100%	27
Saint Joseph Mount Sterling	Mount Sterling	100%	185
Spring View Hospital	Lebanon	100%	189
Three Rivers Medical Center[2]	Louisa	100%	73
Williamson ARH Hospital[2]	S Williamson	100%	42
Baptist Hospital Northeast	La Grange	99%	146
Baptist Regional Medical Center	Corbin	99%	223
Central Baptist Hospital	Lexington	99%	1313
Flaget Memorial Hospital	Bardstown	99%	223
Frankfort Regional Medical Center	Frankfort	99%	134
Greenview Regional Hospital	Bowling Green	99%	356
King's Daughters' Medical Center[2]	Ashland	99%	522
Lourdes Hospital[2]	Paducah	99%	773
Methodist Hospital[2]	Henderson	99%	139
Our Lady of Bellefonte Hospital	Ashland	99%	379
Owensboro Medical Health System[2]	Owensboro	99%	799
Pikeville Medical Center[2]	Pikeville	99%	627
Saint Elizabeth Florence[2]	Florence	99%	120
Saint Joseph Hospital London[2]	London	99%	279
Norton Hospitals[2]	Louisville	98%	2490
Pattie A Clay Regional Medical Center	Richmond	98%	370
Regional Medical Center of Hopkins County[2]	Madisonville	98%	557
Saint Elizabeth Ft Thomas[2]	Fort Thomas	98%	92
Saint Elizabeth Medical Center North[2]	Covington	98%	493
Saint Joseph Hospital[2]	Lexington	98%	706
Twin Lakes Regional Medical Center[2]	Leitchfield	98%	119
Western Baptist Hospital	Paducah	98%	724
Baptist Hospital East	Louisville	97%	2935
Clark Regional Medical Center[2]	Winchester	97%	158
Ephraim Mcdowell Fort Logan Hospital	Stanford	97%	32
Highlands Regional Medical Center	Prestonsburg	97%	31
Jennie Stuart Medical Center	Hopkinsville	97%	318
Jewish Hospital & St Mary's Healthcare[2]	Louisville	97%	710
Lake Cumberland Regional Hospital	Somerset	97%	371
The Medical Center at Bowling Green	Bowling Green	97%	987
Saint Claire Regional Medical Center[2]	Morehead	97%	119
Saint Joseph East[2]	Lexington	97%	400
Middlesboro Appalachian Reg Hlthcre Hosp	Middlesboro	96%	26
Taylor Regional Hospital	Campbellsville	96%	134
Muhlenberg Community Hospital	Greenville	95%	66
University of Kentucky Hospital[2]	Lexington	95%	486
University of Louisville Hospital[2]	Louisville	95%	279
Hardin Memorial Hospital[2]	Elizabethtown	94%	393
Harrison Memorial Hospital	Cynthiana	93%	41
Pineville Community Hospital[2]	Pineville	93%	56
T J Samson Community Hospital[2]	Glasgow	92%	261
Jewish Hospital - Shelbyville	Shelbyville	91%	68
Murray-Calloway County Hospital	Murray	91%	169
Whitesburg ARH Hospital	Whitesburg	91%	47
Hazard Arh Regional Medical Center[2]	Hazard	89%	212

29. Prophylactic Antibiotic Selection (Outpatient)

Hospital Name	City	Rate	Cases
Jackson Purchase Medical Center	Mayfield	100%	91
Middlesboro Appalachian Reg Hlthcre Hosp	Middlesboro	100%	40
Saint Joseph Mount Sterling	Mount Sterling	100%	34
Twin Lakes Regional Medical Center	Leitchfield	100%	37
Williamson ARH Hospital	S Williamson	100%	27
Central Baptist Hospital	Lexington	99%	1907
Georgetown Community Hospital	Georgetown	99%	185
Kentucky River Medical Center	Jackson	99%	75
Pattie A Clay Regional Medical Center	Richmond	99%	117
Baptist Hospital Northeast	La Grange	98%	45
Baptist Regional Medical Center	Corbin	98%	210
Greenview Regional Hospital	Bowling Green	98%	166
Saint Joseph Hospital London	London	98%	283
Frankfort Regional Medical Center	Frankfort	97%	234
Jewish Hospital & St Mary's Healthcare	Louisville	97%	1011
Our Lady of Bellefonte Hospital	Ashland	97%	197
Taylor Regional Hospital	Campbellsville	97%	73
Lake Cumberland Regional Hospital	Somerset	96%	468
Saint Elizabeth Medical Center North	Covington	96%	592
Saint Joseph East	Lexington	96%	303
Baptist Hospital East	Louisville	95%	1554
Clark Regional Medical Center	Winchester	95%	41
Meadowview Regional Medical Center	Maysville	95%	132
Harlan Appalachian Reg Healthcare Hosp	Harlan	94%	54
Pikeville Medical Center	Pikeville	94%	108
Hazard Arh Regional Medical Center	Hazard	93%	126
Highlands Regional Medical Center	Prestonsburg	93%	134
Jewish Hospital - Shelbyville	Shelbyville	93%	27
Lourdes Hospital	Paducah	93%	272
University of Kentucky Hospital	Lexington	93%	727
Whitesburg ARH Hospital	Whitesburg	93%	118
Ephraim Mcdowell Regional Medical Center	Danville	92%	231
Jennie Stuart Medical Center	Hopkinsville	92%	165
The Medical Center at Bowling Green	Bowling Green	92%	483
Saint Joseph Hospital	Lexington	92%	868
Hardin Memorial Hospital	Elizabethtown	91%	502
Methodist Hospital	Henderson	91%	220
Regional Medical Center of Hopkins County	Madisonville	91%	138
Saint Claire Regional Medical Center	Morehead	91%	117
Murray-Calloway County Hospital	Murray	90%	168
University of Louisville Hospital	Louisville	90%	238
T J Samson Community Hospital	Glasgow	89%	142
Western Baptist Hospital	Paducah	89%	619
Flaget Memorial Hospital	Bardstown	87%	91
King's Daughters' Medical Center	Ashland	87%	319
Norton Hospitals	Louisville	87%	1190
Harrison Memorial Hospital	Cynthiana	86%	37
Owensboro Medical Health System	Owensboro	86%	901
Saint Elizabeth Florence	Florence	72%	25

30. Prophylactic Antibiotic Stopped

Hospital Name	City	Rate	Cases
Ephraim Mcdowell Fort Logan Hospital	Stanford	100%	31
Harlan Appalachian Reg Healthcare Hosp	Harlan	100%	38
Meadowview Regional Medical Center	Maysville	100%	53
Spring View Hospital	Lebanon	100%	185
Ephraim Mcdowell Regional Medical Center	Danville	99%	321
Our Lady of Bellefonte Hospital	Ashland	99%	341
Owensboro Medical Health System[2]	Owensboro	99%	771
Three Rivers Medical Center[2]	Louisa	99%	68
Baptist Regional Medical Center	Corbin	98%	210
Central Baptist Hospital	Lexington	98%	1234
Greenview Regional Hospital	Bowling Green	98%	342
Jackson Purchase Medical Center	Mayfield	98%	235
Jewish Hospital - Shelbyville	Shelbyville	98%	64
Saint Elizabeth Medical Center North[2]	Covington	98%	460
Saint Joseph Hospital London[2]	London	98%	221
Baptist Hospital Northeast	La Grange	97%	141
Flaget Memorial Hospital	Bardstown	97%	220
Highlands Regional Medical Center	Prestonsburg	97%	30
King's Daughters' Medical Center[2]	Ashland	97%	505
Saint Elizabeth Ft Thomas[2]	Fort Thomas	97%	79
Baptist Hospital East	Louisville	96%	2791
The Medical Center at Bowling Green	Bowling Green	96%	957
Saint Joseph Berea	Berea	96%	26
Saint Joseph East[2]	Lexington	96%	390
Saint Joseph Hospital[2]	Lexington	96%	638
Twin Lakes Regional Medical Center[2]	Leitchfield	96%	114
Hazard Arh Regional Medical Center[2]	Hazard	95%	196
Pattie A Clay Regional Medical Center	Richmond	95%	363
Regional Medical Center of Hopkins County[2]	Madisonville	95%	518
Saint Joseph Mount Sterling	Mount Sterling	95%	183
Frankfort Regional Medical Center	Frankfort	94%	127
Saint Elizabeth Florence[2]	Florence	94%	112
Bluegrass Community Hospital	Versailles	93%	29
Jewish Hospital & St Mary's Healthcare[2]	Louisville	93%	650
Lake Cumberland Regional Hospital	Somerset	93%	342
Lourdes Hospital[2]	Paducah	93%	710
Harrison Memorial Hospital	Cynthiana	92%	39
Middlesboro Appalachian Reg Hlthcre Hosp	Middlesboro	92%	25
Williamson ARH Hospital[2]	S Williamson	92%	39
Muhlenberg Community Hospital	Greenville	91%	64
Pikeville Medical Center[2]	Pikeville	91%	597
University of Kentucky Hospital[2]	Lexington	91%	465
Whitesburg ARH Hospital	Whitesburg	91%	44
Methodist Hospital[2]	Henderson	90%	135
Saint Claire Regional Medical Center[2]	Morehead	90%	116
University of Louisville Hospital[2]	Louisville	90%	246
Norton Hospitals[2]	Louisville	89%	2227
Taylor Regional Hospital	Campbellsville	89%	133
Western Baptist Hospital	Paducah	89%	665
Clark Regional Medical Center[2]	Winchester	88%	153
Jennie Stuart Medical Center	Hopkinsville	87%	307
Georgetown Community Hospital	Georgetown	85%	39
Murray-Calloway County Hospital	Murray	83%	163
T J Samson Community Hospital[2]	Glasgow	80%	260
Hardin Memorial Hospital[2]	Elizabethtown	77%	374
Pineville Community Hospital[2]	Pineville	74%	54

31. Recommended VTP Ordered

Hospital Name	City	Rate	Cases
Harlan Appalachian Reg Healthcare Hosp	Harlan	100%	25
Harrison Memorial Hospital	Cynthiana	100%	38
Highlands Regional Medical Center	Prestonsburg	100%	41
Meadowview Regional Medical Center	Maysville	100%	34
Muhlenberg Community Hospital	Greenville	100%	55
Paul B Hall Regional Medical Center	Paintsville	100%	27
Saint Joseph Berea	Berea	100%	26
Saint Joseph Mount Sterling	Mount Sterling	100%	51
Ephraim Mcdowell Regional Medical Center	Danville	99%	189
Greenview Regional Hospital	Bowling Green	99%	156
Jackson Purchase Medical Center	Mayfield	99%	186
Saint Joseph Hospital London[2]	London	99%	99
Frankfort Regional Medical Center	Frankfort	98%	144
Lourdes Hospital[2]	Paducah	98%	404
Saint Claire Regional Medical Center[2]	Morehead	98%	92
Saint Elizabeth Ft Thomas[2]	Fort Thomas	98%	123
Baptist Regional Medical Center	Corbin	97%	130
Flaget Memorial Hospital	Bardstown	97%	74
Lake Cumberland Regional Hospital	Somerset	97%	275
Saint Elizabeth Medical Center North[2]	Covington	97%	166
Saint Joseph Hospital[2]	Lexington	97%	418
Williamson ARH Hospital[2]	S Williamson	97%	33
Central Baptist Hospital	Lexington	96%	590
Methodist Hospital[2]	Henderson	96%	76
Spring View Hospital	Lebanon	96%	81
Baptist Hospital East	Louisville	95%	1106
Baptist Hospital Northeast	La Grange	95%	98
King's Daughters' Medical Center[2]	Ashland	95%	172
Twin Lakes Regional Medical Center[2]	Leitchfield	95%	80
Western Baptist Hospital	Paducah	95%	484
Owensboro Medical Health System[2]	Owensboro	94%	270
Pikeville Medical Center[2]	Pikeville	94%	276
Pineville Community Hospital[2]	Pineville	94%	33
Saint Joseph East[2]	Lexington	94%	177
Middlesboro Appalachian Reg Hlthcre Hosp	Middlesboro	93%	28
Norton Hospitals[2]	Louisville	93%	977
Clark Regional Medical Center[2]	Winchester	92%	50
Hazard Arh Regional Medical Center[2]	Hazard	92%	128
Jewish Hospital & St Mary's Healthcare[2]	Louisville	92%	354
Pattie A Clay Regional Medical Center	Richmond	92%	89
Saint Elizabeth Florence[2]	Florence	92%	103
University of Kentucky Hospital[2]	Lexington	92%	291
Jennie Stuart Medical Center	Hopkinsville	90%	134
Regional Medical Center of Hopkins County[2]	Madisonville	90%	255
Taylor Regional Hospital	Campbellsville	90%	98
Our Lady of Bellefonte Hospital	Ashland	89%	148
Hardin Memorial Hospital[2]	Elizabethtown	86%	194
University of Louisville Hospital[2]	Louisville	86%	160
The Medical Center at Bowling Green	Bowling Green	85%	405
Georgetown Community Hospital	Georgetown	84%	43
Jewish Hospital - Shelbyville	Shelbyville	82%	67
Murray-Calloway County Hospital	Murray	82%	109
T J Samson Community Hospital[2]	Glasgow	78%	129

32. Urinary Catheter Removal

Hospital Name	City	Rate	Cases
Baptist Regional Medical Center	Corbin	100%	55
Ephraim Mcdowell Regional Medical Center	Danville	100%	102

NOTE: Hospital profiles are in alphabetical order by state, then city, then hospital within the city; Rankings exclude hospitals with less than 25 cases except for patient surveys which excludes hospitals with less than 100 cases; (a) 100–299 cases; (1) The number of cases is too small to be sure how well a hospital is performing; (2) The hospital indicated that the data submitted for this measure were based on a sample of cases; (3) Data was collected during a shorter time period (fewer quarters) than the maximum possible time for this measure; (4) Suppressed for one or more quarters by CMS; (5) No data is available from the hospital for this measure; (6) Fewer than 100 patients completed the HCAHPS survey. Use these rates with caution, as the number of surveys may be too low to reliably assess hospital performance; (7) Survey results are based on less than 12 months of data; (8) Survey results are not available for this reporting period; (9) No or very few patients were eligible for the HCAHPS survey. The scores shown, if any, reflect a very small number of surveys; (10) A state average was not calculated because too few hospitals in the state submitted data; (11) There were discrepancies in the data collection process; Please refer to the User's Guide for a full explanation of data.

Saint Joseph Mount Sterling	Mount Sterling	100%	86
Twin Lakes Regional Medical Center[2]	Leitchfield	100%	42
Frankfort Regional Medical Center	Frankfort	98%	51
Greenview Regional Hospital	Bowling Green	98%	180
Flaget Memorial Hospital	Bardstown	97%	90
Jackson Purchase Medical Center	Mayfield	97%	105
Owensboro Medical Health System[2]	Owensboro	95%	195
Regional Medical Center of Hopkins County[2]	Madisonville	95%	172
The Medical Center at Bowling Green	Bowling Green	94%	377
Murray-Calloway County Hospital	Murray	94%	52
Pattie A Clay Regional Medical Center	Richmond	94%	54
Our Lady of Bellefonte Hospital	Ashland	93%	158
Saint Joseph Hospital London	London	93%	59
Norton Hospitals[2]	Louisville	92%	853
Baptist Hospital East	Louisville	91%	479
Lourdes Hospital[2]	Paducah	90%	173
Central Baptist Hospital	Lexington	88%	433
Hazard Arh Regional Medical Center	Hazard	88%	66
Pikeville Medical Center[2]	Pikeville	88%	257
Hardin Memorial Hospital[2]	Elizabethtown	87%	142
Jewish Hospital & St Mary's Healthcare[2]	Louisville	87%	218
King's Daughters' Medical Center[2]	Ashland	87%	189
Saint Joseph East[2]	Lexington	86%	91
Lake Cumberland Regional Hospital	Somerset	85%	131
Methodist Hospital[2]	Henderson	85%	52
University of Kentucky Hospital[2]	Lexington	85%	143
Clark Regional Medical Center[2]	Winchester	84%	43
Saint Elizabeth Medical Center North[2]	Covington	84%	88
Western Baptist Hospital	Paducah	83%	279
T J Samson Community Hospital[2]	Glasgow	80%	81
Saint Joseph Hospital[2]	Lexington	79%	247
Spring View Hospital	Lebanon	78%	46
University of Louisville Hospital[2]	Louisville	76%	71
Jennie Stuart Medical Center	Hopkinsville	75%	101
Saint Claire Regional Medical Center[2]	Morehead	71%	42

Children's Asthma Care

33. Received Systemic Corticosteroids

Hospital Name	City	Rate	Cases
Norton Hospitals	Louisville	100%	795
Paul B Hall Regional Medical Center	Paintsville	99%	85
University of Kentucky Hospital[2]	Lexington	97%	127

34. Received Home Management Plan of Care

Hospital Name	City	Rate	Cases
Paul B Hall Regional Medical Center	Paintsville	99%	86
Norton Hospitals	Louisville	89%	792
University of Kentucky Hospital[2]	Lexington	61%	127

35. Received Reliever Medication

Hospital Name	City	Rate	Cases
Norton Hospitals	Louisville	100%	795
Paul B Hall Regional Medical Center	Paintsville	100%	88
University of Kentucky Hospital[2]	Lexington	100%	127

Use of Medical Imaging

36. Combination Abdominal CT Scan

Hospital Name	City	Ratio	Cases
Rockcastle Reg Hosp & Respiratory Care Ctr	Mount Vernon	0.000	254
Hazard Arh Regional Medical Center	Hazard	0.006	542
McDowell Arh Hospital	McDowell	0.006	180
Williamson ARH Hospital	S Williamson	0.006	179
Saint Joseph East	Lexington	0.012	257
Pattie A Clay Regional Medical Center	Richmond	0.015	588
Saint Joseph Hospital	Lexington	0.016	565
University of Kentucky Hospital	Lexington	0.020	1583
Morgan County Arh Hospital	West Liberty	0.022	185
Frankfort Regional Medical Center	Frankfort	0.024	533
Saint Elizabeth Ft Thomas	Fort Thomas	0.025	523
Whitesburg ARH Hospital	Whitesburg	0.030	265
Jennie Stuart Medical Center	Hopkinsville	0.032	587
Twin Lakes Regional Medical Center	Leitchfield	0.034	296
Central Baptist Hospital	Lexington	0.035	1358
Pikeville Medical Center	Pikeville	0.040	1272
Crittenden Health System	Marion	0.043	93
Three Rivers Medical Center	Louisa	0.046	241
Flaget Memorial Hospital	Bardstown	0.047	407
King's Daughters' Medical Center	Ashland	0.050	2364
Saint Joseph Hospital London	London	0.052	698
Saint Elizabeth Florence	Florence	0.056	413
Saint Joseph Mount Sterling	Mount Sterling	0.057	477
Georgetown Community Hospital	Georgetown	0.058	345
Saint Elizabeth Medical Center North	Covington	0.061	2226
Saint Elizabeth Grant	Williamstown	0.062	369
Baptist Regional Medical Center	Corbin	0.063	667
Harrison Memorial Hospital	Cynthiana	0.063	272
University of Louisville Hospital	Louisville	0.063	702
The Medical Center at Bowling Green	Bowling Green	0.064	897
Logan Memorial Hospital	Russellville	0.069	218
Baptist Hospital East	Louisville	0.072	2433
Jewish Hospital - Shelbyville	Shelbyville	0.072	349
Regional Medical Center of Hopkins County	Madisonville	0.078	637
Our Lady of Bellefonte Hospital	Ashland	0.083	929
Jewish Hospital & St Mary's Healthcare	Louisville	0.091	3041
Hardin Memorial Hospital	Elizabethtown	0.092	1344
Baptist Hospital Northeast	La Grange	0.101	288
Ephraim Mcdowell Regional Medical Center	Danville	0.107	797
Bourbon Community Hospital	Paris	0.110	264
Western Baptist Hospital	Paducah	0.113	1835
Methodist Hospital Union County	Morganfield	0.134	142
Memorial Hospital	Manchester	0.135	282
Lake Cumberland Regional Hospital	Somerset	0.150	1074
Kentucky River Medical Center	Jackson	0.157	166
Clinton County Hospital	Albany	0.171	152
Methodist Hospital	Henderson	0.177	492
Murray-Calloway County Hospital	Murray	0.182	533
Norton Hospitals	Louisville	0.184	3316
Paul B Hall Regional Medical Center	Paintsville	0.216	328
Spring View Hospital	Lebanon	0.241	224
T J Samson Community Hospital	Glasgow	0.256	841
Pineville Community Hospital	Pineville	0.294	265
Lourdes Hospital	Paducah	0.312	650
Jackson Purchase Medical Center	Mayfield	0.343	335
Highlands Regional Medical Center	Prestonsburg	0.372	1015
Taylor Regional Hospital	Campbellsville	0.414	694
Muhlenberg Community Hospital	Greenville	0.419	191
Harlan Appalachian Reg Healthcare Hosp	Harlan	0.424	420
Owensboro Medical Health System	Owensboro	0.433	1695
Greenview Regional Hospital	Bowling Green	0.436	514
Monroe County Medical Center	Tompkinsville	0.459	196
Westlake Regional Hospital	Columbia	0.462	195
Middlesboro Appalachian Reg Hlthcre Hosp	Middlesboro	0.467	377
Clark Regional Medical Center	Winchester	0.515	443
Parkway Regional Hospital	Fulton	0.577	104
Fleming County Hospital	Flemingsburg	0.581	191
Saint Claire Regional Medical Center	Morehead	0.616	700
Meadowview Regional Medical Center	Maysville	0.649	288
Russell County Hospital	Russell Springs	0.710	248

37. Combination Chest CT Scan

Hospital Name	City	Ratio	Cases
Ephraim Mcdowell Regional Medical Center	Danville	0.000	403
Flaget Memorial Hospital	Bardstown	0.000	290
Frankfort Regional Medical Center	Frankfort	0.000	311
Jackson Purchase Medical Center	Mayfield	0.000	289
Meadowview Regional Medical Center	Maysville	0.000	239
Saint Elizabeth Florence	Florence	0.000	185
Saint Elizabeth Ft Thomas	Fort Thomas	0.000	342
Saint Elizabeth Grant	Williamstown	0.000	144
Saint Joseph East[1]	Lexington	0.000	33
Twin Lakes Regional Medical Center	Leitchfield	0.000	278
Baptist Hospital East	Louisville	0.001	1748
Hardin Memorial Hospital	Elizabethtown	0.001	960
Highlands Regional Medical Center	Prestonsburg	0.002	502
Jewish Hospital & St Mary's Healthcare	Louisville	0.002	3085
Saint Elizabeth Medical Center North	Covington	0.002	1311
Jennie Stuart Medical Center	Hopkinsville	0.003	308
Baptist Hospital Northeast	La Grange	0.005	222
Regional Medical Center of Hopkins County	Madisonville	0.005	367
University of Kentucky Hospital	Lexington	0.005	1979
Harrison Memorial Hospital	Cynthiana	0.006	167
Taylor Regional Hospital	Campbellsville	0.006	537
University of Louisville Hospital	Louisville	0.006	844
Jewish Hospital - Shelbyville	Shelbyville	0.007	290
Bourbon Community Hospital	Paris	0.008	121
Saint Joseph Hospital	Lexington	0.009	115
Saint Joseph Mount Sterling	Mount Sterling	0.009	330
Murray-Calloway County Hospital	Murray	0.011	274
Saint Joseph Hospital London	London	0.011	380
Williamson ARH Hospital	S Williamson	0.011	92
Fleming County Hospital	Flemingsburg	0.012	167
King's Daughters' Medical Center	Ashland	0.013	2154
Logan Memorial Hospital	Russellville	0.013	160
Russell County Hospital	Russell Springs	0.013	151
Central Baptist Hospital	Lexington	0.014	1233
Crittenden Health System	Marion	0.016	63
Hazard Arh Regional Medical Center	Hazard	0.017	233
Methodist Hospital	Henderson	0.018	331
Baptist Regional Medical Center	Corbin	0.019	480
Owensboro Medical Health System	Owensboro	0.020	1282
Pattie A Clay Regional Medical Center	Richmond	0.020	345
Whitesburg ARH Hospital	Whitesburg	0.020	101
Georgetown Community Hospital	Georgetown	0.024	167
Morgan County Arh Hospital	West Liberty	0.026	77
Lourdes Hospital	Paducah	0.036	496
McDowell Arh Hospital	McDowell	0.037	81
Pikeville Medical Center	Pikeville	0.038	797
Saint Claire Regional Medical Center	Morehead	0.039	463
Parkway Regional Hospital	Fulton	0.044	45
Middlesboro Appalachian Reg Hlthcre Hosp	Middlesboro	0.045	222
Western Baptist Hospital	Paducah	0.058	1178
Three Rivers Medical Center	Louisa	0.061	132
Lake Cumberland Regional Hospital	Somerset	0.069	765
Muhlenberg Community Hospital	Greenville	0.075	67
Our Lady of Bellefonte Hospital	Ashland	0.080	522
Greenview Regional Hospital	Bowling Green	0.086	186
Rockcastle Reg Hosp & Respiratory Care Ctr	Mount Vernon	0.127	173
Kentucky River Medical Center	Jackson	0.139	115
Memorial Hospital	Manchester	0.145	138
The Medical Center at Bowling Green	Bowling Green	0.175	417
T J Samson Community Hospital	Glasgow	0.175	605
Methodist Hospital Union County	Morganfield	0.185	81
Spring View Hospital	Lebanon	0.198	131
Westlake Regional Hospital	Columbia	0.225	102
Norton Hospitals	Louisville	0.233	2506
Harlan Appalachian Reg Healthcare Hosp	Harlan	0.235	196
Paul B Hall Regional Medical Center	Paintsville	0.248	218
Clinton County Hospital	Albany	0.298	94
Pineville Community Hospital	Pineville	0.322	90
Monroe County Medical Center	Tompkinsville	0.338	145
Clark Regional Medical Center	Winchester	0.429	282

38. Follow-up Mammogram/Ultrasound

Hospital Name	City	Rate	Cases
Highlands Regional Medical Center	Prestonsburg	1.6%	962
Frankfort Regional Medical Center	Frankfort	1.9%	775
Spring View Hospital	Lebanon	2.1%	419
Saint Joseph East	Lexington	3.1%	739
Clark Regional Medical Center	Winchester	3.3%	480
University of Kentucky Hospital	Lexington	3.4%	357
Pattie A Clay Regional Medical Center	Richmond	3.5%	739
Methodist Hospital	Henderson	3.8%	785
Clinton County Hospital	Albany	4.0%	175
Parkway Regional Hospital	Fulton	4.1%	196
Murray-Calloway County Hospital	Murray	4.6%	1007
Russell County Hospital	Russell Springs	4.6%	326
Jewish Hospital & St Mary's Healthcare	Louisville	4.7%	3462
Morgan County Arh Hospital	West Liberty	4.7%	86
Saint Joseph Hospital	Lexington	4.9%	759
Baptist Hospital Northeast	La Grange	5.0%	555
Ephraim Mcdowell Regional Medical Center	Danville	5.0%	1364
The Medical Center at Bowling Green	Bowling Green	5.1%	803
Methodist Hospital Union County	Morganfield	5.4%	279
Memorial Hospital	Manchester	5.5%	256
Jennie Stuart Medical Center	Hopkinsville	5.6%	1059
Jewish Hospital - Shelbyville	Shelbyville	5.6%	663
Monroe County Medical Center	Tompkinsville	5.7%	106
Muhlenberg Community Hospital	Greenville	5.8%	172
Georgetown Community Hospital	Georgetown	5.9%	354
Owensboro Medical Health System	Owensboro	5.9%	2576
Rockcastle Reg Hosp & Respiratory Care Ctr	Mount Vernon	5.9%	256
Hazard Arh Regional Medical Center	Hazard	6.1%	360
Lake Cumberland Regional Hospital	Somerset	6.1%	1498
Saint Joseph Hospital London	London	6.3%	525
Pineville Community Hospital	Pineville	6.6%	318
Saint Elizabeth Grant	Williamstown	6.8%	235
Twin Lakes Regional Medical Center	Leitchfield	6.8%	428
Baptist Regional Medical Center	Corbin	7.2%	945
Middlesboro Appalachian Reg Hlthcre Hosp	Middlesboro	7.2%	390
Saint Elizabeth Medical Center North	Covington	7.2%	3448
Crittenden Health System	Marion	7.4%	135
Jackson Purchase Medical Center	Mayfield	7.4%	610
King's Daughters' Medical Center	Ashland	7.6%	2425
Saint Elizabeth Florence	Florence	7.6%	514
Whitesburg ARH Hospital	Whitesburg	7.7%	260
University of Louisville Hospital	Louisville	7.8%	1378
Pikeville Medical Center	Pikeville	7.9%	1225
Saint Claire Regional Medical Center	Morehead	7.9%	756
Saint Elizabeth Ft Thomas	Fort Thomas	7.9%	611
T J Samson Community Hospital	Glasgow	8.0%	1292
Bourbon Community Hospital	Paris	8.1%	371
Our Lady of Bellefonte Hospital	Ashland	8.4%	1149
Kentucky River Medical Center	Jackson	8.6%	174
Flaget Memorial Hospital	Bardstown	8.8%	464
Harlan Appalachian Reg Healthcare Hosp	Harlan	8.9%	359
Baptist Hospital East	Louisville	9.1%	2907
Williamson ARH Hospital	S Williamson	9.3%	216
Lourdes Hospital	Paducah	9.6%	353
Norton Hospitals	Louisville	9.6%	4166
Meadowview Regional Medical Center	Maysville	9.9%	436
Greenview Regional Hospital	Bowling Green	10.8%	287
Saint Joseph Mount Sterling	Mount Sterling	11.5%	304
Western Baptist Hospital	Paducah	11.6%	982
Westlake Regional Hospital	Columbia	11.6%	190
Harrison Memorial Hospital	Cynthiana	11.9%	329
McDowell Arh Hospital	McDowell	12.4%	137

NOTE: Hospital profiles are in alphabetical order by state, then city, then hospital within the city; Rankings exclude hospitals with less than 25 cases except for patient surveys which excludes hospitals with less than 100 cases; (a) 100–299 cases; (1) The number of cases is too small to be sure how well a hospital is performing; (2) The hospital indicated that the data submitted for this measure were based on a sample of cases; (3) Data was collected during a shorter time period (fewer quarters) than the maximum possible time for this measure; (4) Suppressed for one or more quarters by CMS; (5) No data is available from the hospital for this measure; (6) Fewer than 100 patients completed the HCAHPS survey. Use these rates with caution, as the number of surveys may be too low to reliably assess hospital performance; (7) Survey results are based on less than 12 months of data; (8) Survey results are not available for this reporting period; (9) No or very few patients were eligible for the HCAHPS survey. The scores shown, if any, reflect a very small number of surveys; (10) A state average was not calculated because too few hospitals in the state submitted data; (11) There were discrepancies in the data collection process; Please refer to the User's Guide for a full explanation of data.

Logan Memorial Hospital	Russellville	13.1%	480
Fleming County Hospital	Flemingsburg	13.5%	237
Hardin Memorial Hospital	Elizabethtown	14.6%	1804
Taylor Regional Hospital	Campbellsville	17.0%	911
Paul B Hall Regional Medical Center	Paintsville	18.1%	127
Three Rivers Medical Center	Louisa	18.1%	149
Central Baptist Hospital	Lexington	19.0%	2541

39. MRI for Low Back Pain

Hospital Name	City	Rate	Cases
Baptist Hospital Northeast	La Grange	23.9%	88
Taylor Regional Hospital	Campbellsville	23.9%	159
Saint Elizabeth Florence[1]	Florence	25.8%	31
Whitesburg ARH Hospital	Whitesburg	26.0%	73
Greenview Regional Hospital	Bowling Green	27.4%	73
King's Daughters' Medical Center	Ashland	28.0%	632
Crittenden Health System[1]	Marion	28.9%	45
University of Kentucky Hospital	Lexington	28.9%	197
Norton Hospitals	Louisville	29.1%	873
Monroe County Medical Center	Tompkinsville	29.3%	58
Rockcastle Reg Hosp & Respiratory Care Ctr	Mount Vernon	30.1%	93
Jewish Hospital - Shelbyville	Shelbyville	30.4%	69
Saint Elizabeth Ft Thomas[1]	Fort Thomas	30.4%	46
Hardin Memorial Hospital	Elizabethtown	31.0%	187
Pattie A Clay Regional Medical Center	Richmond	31.5%	149
Memorial Hospital	Manchester	32.1%	81
Central Baptist Hospital	Lexington	32.5%	157
Frankfort Regional Medical Center[1]	Frankfort	32.6%	43
Jennie Stuart Medical Center	Hopkinsville	32.6%	132
Owensboro Medical Health System	Owensboro	33.2%	416
Saint Joseph Hospital	Lexington	33.7%	98
Western Baptist Hospital	Paducah	33.8%	275
Baptist Hospital East	Louisville	33.9%	584
Ephraim Mcdowell Regional Medical Center	Danville	34.2%	316
The Medical Center at Bowling Green	Bowling Green	34.7%	150
Paul B Hall Regional Medical Center	Paintsville	35.1%	57
Saint Joseph Hospital London	London	35.2%	128
Highlands Regional Medical Center	Prestonsburg	35.3%	156
Pikeville Medical Center	Pikeville	36.0%	397
Twin Lakes Regional Medical Center	Leitchfield	36.0%	86
Lourdes Hospital	Paducah	36.4%	154
Saint Elizabeth Medical Center North	Covington	36.6%	145
Jewish Hospital & St Mary's Healthcare	Louisville	36.9%	718
Middlesboro Appalachian Reg Hlthcre Hosp	Middlesboro	37.5%	136
Saint Joseph East[1]	Lexington	37.5%	32
Logan Memorial Hospital[1]	Russellville	38.5%	26
T J Samson Community Hospital	Glasgow	38.5%	130
Murray-Calloway County Hospital	Murray	39.0%	118
Regional Medical Center of Hopkins County	Madisonville	39.2%	130
Clark Regional Medical Center	Winchester	39.7%	73
Bourbon Community Hospital	Paris	40.0%	40
Our Lady of Bellefonte Hospital	Ashland	40.3%	268
Lake Cumberland Regional Hospital	Somerset	41.5%	258
Jackson Purchase Medical Center	Mayfield	42.2%	64
Harlan Appalachian Reg Healthcare Hosp	Harlan	42.3%	104
Methodist Hospital	Henderson	42.6%	122
Flaget Memorial Hospital	Bardstown	42.7%	117
Saint Claire Regional Medical Center	Morehead	43.4%	143
Three Rivers Medical Center	Louisa	43.9%	57
Hazard Arh Regional Medical Center[1]	Hazard	44.0%	25
Morgan County Arh Hospital[1]	West Liberty	44.1%	34
Saint Elizabeth Grant	Williamstown	44.4%	90
Georgetown Community Hospital	Georgetown	44.8%	58
Spring View Hospital	Lebanon	46.3%	54
Fleming County Hospital[1]	Flemingsburg	46.7%	30
Kentucky River Medical Center	Jackson	48.4%	64
Baptist Regional Medical Center	Corbin	50.0%	208
University of Louisville Hospital	Louisville	50.9%	57
Williamson ARH Hospital	S Williamson	50.9%	57
Muhlenberg Community Hospital	Greenville	51.8%	83
McDowell Arh Hospital[1]	McDowell	72.7%	33

Survey of Patients' Hospital Experiences

40. Area Around Room 'Always' Quiet at Night

Hospital Name	City	Rate	Cases
Westlake Regional Hospital	Columbia	87%	300+
Clinton County Hospital	Albany	79%	300+
McDowell Arh Hospital	McDowell	76%	(a)
Morgan County Arh Hospital	West Liberty	76%	(a)
Marcum and Wallace Memorial Hospital	Irvine	74%	(a)
Our Lady of Bellefonte Hospital	Ashland	73%	300+
Parkway Regional Hospital	Fulton	73%	(a)
Methodist Hospital Union County	Morganfield	69%	(a)
Middlesboro Appalachian Reg Hlthcre Hosp	Middlesboro	69%	300+
T J Samson Community Hospital	Glasgow	68%	300+
Bourbon Community Hospital	Paris	67%	(a)
Saint Elizabeth Grant	Williamstown	67%	(a)
Saint Joseph Berea	Berea	67%	300+
Jackson Purchase Medical Center	Mayfield	66%	300+
Greenview Regional Hospital	Bowling Green	65%	300+
Spring View Hospital	Lebanon	65%	300+
Western Baptist Hospital	Paducah	65%	300+
Fleming County Hospital	Flemingsburg	64%	(a)
Frankfort Regional Medical Center	Frankfort	64%	300+
Logan Memorial Hospital	Russellville	64%	300+
Williamson ARH Hospital	S Williamson	64%	300+
Harlan Appalachian Reg Healthcare Hosp	Harlan	63%	300+
King's Daughters' Medical Center	Ashland	63%	300+
Meadowview Regional Medical Center	Maysville	63%	300+
Georgetown Community Hospital	Georgetown	62%	300+
Hazard Arh Regional Medical Center	Hazard	62%	300+
Monroe County Medical Center	Tompkinsville	62%	300+
Saint Joseph Hospital	Lexington	62%	300+
Three Rivers Medical Center	Louisa	62%	300+
Whitesburg ARH Hospital	Whitesburg	62%	300+
Ephraim Mcdowell Fort Logan Hospital	Stanford	61%	(a)
Kentucky River Medical Center	Jackson	61%	300+
Lake Cumberland Regional Hospital	Somerset	61%	300+
Muhlenberg Community Hospital	Greenville	61%	300+
Pikeville Medical Center	Pikeville	61%	300+
Saint Joseph Martin	Martin	61%	300+
Saint Joseph Mount Sterling	Mount Sterling	61%	(a)
The Medical Center at Bowling Green	Bowling Green	60%	300+
Ohio County Hospital	Hartford	60%	(a)
Paul B Hall Regional Medical Center	Paintsville	60%	300+
Saint Elizabeth Medical Center North	Covington	60%	300+
Saint Joseph East	Lexington	60%	300+
Flaget Memorial Hospital	Bardstown	59%	300+
Rockcastle Reg Hosp & Respiratory Care Ctr	Mount Vernon	59%	(a)
Baptist Hospital East	Louisville	58%	300+
Clark Regional Medical Center	Winchester	58%	300+
Methodist Hospital	Henderson	58%	300+
Norton Hospitals	Louisville	58%	300+
Regional Medical Center of Hopkins County	Madisonville	58%	300+
Taylor Regional Hospital	Campbellsville	58%	300+
Crittenden Health System	Marion	57%	(a)
Jennie Stuart Medical Center	Hopkinsville	57%	300+
Pineville Community Hospital	Pineville	57%	300+
Saint Elizabeth Florence	Florence	57%	300+
Owensboro Medical Health System	Owensboro	56%	300+
Pattie A Clay Regional Medical Center	Richmond	56%	300+
Harrison Memorial Hospital	Cynthiana	55%	300+
Highlands Regional Medical Center	Prestonsburg	55%	300+
Murray-Calloway County Hospital	Murray	55%	300+
Ephraim Mcdowell Regional Medical Center	Danville	54%	300+
Lourdes Hospital	Paducah	54%	300+
Central Baptist Hospital	Lexington	53%	300+
Jewish Hospital & St Mary's Healthcare	Louisville	53%	300+
Twin Lakes Regional Medical Center	Leitchfield	53%	300+
Saint Elizabeth Ft Thomas	Fort Thomas	52%	300+
Saint Joseph Hospital London	London	52%	300+
University of Kentucky Hospital	Lexington	52%	300+
Saint Claire Regional Medical Center	Morehead	49%	300+
Baptist Hospital Northeast	La Grange	48%	300+
Baptist Regional Medical Center	Corbin	48%	300+
University of Louisville Hospital	Louisville	48%	300+
Jewish Hospital - Shelbyville	Shelbyville	47%	300+
Memorial Hospital	Manchester	45%	(a)
Hardin Memorial Hospital	Elizabethtown	44%	300+

41. Doctors 'Always' Communicated Well

Hospital Name	City	Rate	Cases
Westlake Regional Hospital	Columbia	100%	300+
Clinton County Hospital	Albany	92%	300+
Methodist Hospital Union County	Morganfield	92%	(a)
Morgan County Arh Hospital	West Liberty	92%	(a)
Clark Regional Medical Center	Winchester	90%	300+
Muhlenberg Community Hospital	Greenville	89%	300+
Rockcastle Reg Hosp & Respiratory Care Ctr	Mount Vernon	89%	(a)
Harrison Memorial Hospital	Cynthiana	88%	300+
McDowell Arh Hospital	McDowell	88%	(a)
Middlesboro Appalachian Reg Hlthcre Hosp	Middlesboro	88%	300+
Parkway Regional Hospital	Fulton	88%	(a)
Three Rivers Medical Center	Louisa	88%	300+
Crittenden Health System	Marion	87%	(a)
Georgetown Community Hospital	Georgetown	87%	300+
Marcum and Wallace Memorial Hospital	Irvine	87%	(a)
Pikeville Medical Center	Pikeville	87%	300+
Whitesburg ARH Hospital	Whitesburg	87%	300+
Our Lady of Bellefonte Hospital	Ashland	86%	300+
Pineville Community Hospital	Pineville	86%	300+
Saint Joseph Berea	Berea	86%	300+
Saint Joseph Martin	Martin	86%	300+
Bourbon Community Hospital	Paris	85%	(a)
Monroe County Medical Center	Tompkinsville	85%	300+
Saint Claire Regional Medical Center	Morehead	85%	300+
Baptist Regional Medical Center	Corbin	84%	300+
Frankfort Regional Medical Center	Frankfort	84%	300+
Greenview Regional Hospital	Bowling Green	84%	300+
Jackson Purchase Medical Center	Mayfield	84%	300+
Lake Cumberland Regional Hospital	Somerset	84%	300+
Logan Memorial Hospital	Russellville	84%	300+
Methodist Hospital	Henderson	84%	300+
Saint Elizabeth Grant	Williamstown	84%	(a)
T J Samson Community Hospital	Glasgow	84%	300+
Taylor Regional Hospital	Campbellsville	84%	300+
Williamson ARH Hospital	S Williamson	84%	300+
Hardin Memorial Hospital	Elizabethtown	83%	300+
Hazard Arh Regional Medical Center	Hazard	83%	300+
Highlands Regional Medical Center	Prestonsburg	83%	300+
Murray-Calloway County Hospital	Murray	83%	300+
Ohio County Hospital	Hartford	83%	(a)
Regional Medical Center of Hopkins County	Madisonville	83%	300+
Flaget Memorial Hospital	Bardstown	82%	300+
King's Daughters' Medical Center	Ashland	82%	300+
Meadowview Regional Medical Center	Maysville	82%	300+
Owensboro Medical Health System	Owensboro	82%	300+
Saint Joseph Mount Sterling	Mount Sterling	82%	(a)
Central Baptist Hospital	Lexington	81%	300+
Lourdes Hospital	Paducah	81%	300+
The Medical Center at Bowling Green	Bowling Green	81%	300+
Saint Joseph East	Lexington	81%	300+
Saint Joseph Hospital	Lexington	81%	300+
Spring View Hospital	Lebanon	81%	300+
Baptist Hospital East	Louisville	80%	300+
Kentucky River Medical Center	Jackson	80%	300+
Harlan Appalachian Reg Healthcare Hosp	Harlan	79%	300+
Paul B Hall Regional Medical Center	Paintsville	79%	300+
Saint Elizabeth Medical Center North	Covington	79%	300+
Saint Joseph Hospital London	London	79%	300+
Western Baptist Hospital	Paducah	79%	300+
Fleming County Hospital	Flemingsburg	78%	(a)
Norton Hospitals	Louisville	78%	300+
Pattie A Clay Regional Medical Center	Richmond	78%	300+
Baptist Hospital Northeast	La Grange	77%	300+
Ephraim Mcdowell Fort Logan Hospital	Stanford	77%	(a)
Ephraim Mcdowell Regional Medical Center	Danville	77%	300+
Jewish Hospital - Shelbyville	Shelbyville	77%	300+
Twin Lakes Regional Medical Center	Leitchfield	77%	300+
Saint Elizabeth Ft Thomas	Fort Thomas	76%	300+
University of Kentucky Hospital	Lexington	76%	300+
Jennie Stuart Medical Center	Hopkinsville	75%	300+
Memorial Hospital	Manchester	75%	(a)
Saint Elizabeth Florence	Florence	75%	300+
Jewish Hospital & St Mary's Healthcare	Louisville	73%	300+
University of Louisville Hospital	Louisville	73%	300+

42. Home Recovery Information Given

Hospital Name	City	Rate	Cases
Westlake Regional Hospital	Columbia	99%	300+
Morgan County Arh Hospital	West Liberty	91%	(a)
Baptist Hospital East	Louisville	88%	300+
Clark Regional Medical Center	Winchester	88%	300+
McDowell Arh Hospital	McDowell	88%	(a)
Saint Elizabeth Grant	Williamstown	88%	(a)
Bourbon Community Hospital	Paris	87%	(a)
Frankfort Regional Medical Center	Frankfort	87%	300+
Flaget Memorial Hospital	Bardstown	86%	300+
Georgetown Community Hospital	Georgetown	86%	300+
Pikeville Medical Center	Pikeville	86%	300+
Saint Elizabeth Medical Center North	Covington	86%	300+
University of Kentucky Hospital	Lexington	86%	300+
Western Baptist Hospital	Paducah	86%	300+
Greenview Regional Hospital	Bowling Green	85%	300+
The Medical Center at Bowling Green	Bowling Green	85%	300+
Muhlenberg Community Hospital	Greenville	85%	300+
Owensboro Medical Health System	Owensboro	85%	300+
Saint Elizabeth Ft Thomas	Fort Thomas	85%	300+
Saint Joseph East	Lexington	85%	300+
Baptist Hospital Northeast	La Grange	84%	300+
Ephraim Mcdowell Fort Logan Hospital	Stanford	84%	(a)
Middlesboro Appalachian Reg Hlthcre Hosp	Middlesboro	84%	300+
Regional Medical Center of Hopkins County	Madisonville	84%	300+
Saint Joseph Berea	Berea	84%	300+
Saint Joseph Mount Sterling	Mount Sterling	84%	(a)
T J Samson Community Hospital	Glasgow	84%	300+
Whitesburg ARH Hospital	Whitesburg	84%	300+
Harrison Memorial Hospital	Cynthiana	83%	300+
Jackson Purchase Medical Center	Mayfield	83%	300+
Memorial Hospital	Manchester	83%	(a)
Norton Hospitals	Louisville	83%	300+
Ohio County Hospital	Hartford	83%	(a)
Our Lady of Bellefonte Hospital	Ashland	83%	300+
Parkway Regional Hospital	Fulton	83%	(a)
Saint Claire Regional Medical Center	Morehead	83%	300+
Saint Elizabeth Florence	Florence	83%	300+
Saint Joseph Hospital	Lexington	83%	300+
Williamson ARH Hospital	S Williamson	83%	300+
Baptist Regional Medical Center	Corbin	82%	300+

NOTE: Hospital profiles are in alphabetical order by state, then city, then hospital within the city; Rankings exclude hospitals with less than 25 cases except for patient surveys which excludes hospitals with less than 100 cases; (a) 100–299 cases; (1) The number of cases is too small to be sure how well a hospital is performing; (2) The hospital indicated that the data submitted for this measure were based on a sample of cases; (3) Data was collected during a shorter time period (fewer quarters) than the maximum possible time for this measure; (4) Suppressed for one or more quarters by CMS; (5) No data is available from the hospital for this measure; (6) Fewer than 100 patients completed the HCAHPS survey. Use these rates with caution, as the number of surveys may be too low to reliably assess hospital performance; (7) Survey results are based on less than 12 months of data; (8) Survey results are not available for this reporting period; (9) No or very few patients were eligible for the HCAHPS survey. The scores shown, if any, reflect a very small number of surveys; (10) A state average was not calculated because too few hospitals in the state submitted data; (11) There were discrepancies in the data collection process; Please refer to the User's Guide for a full explanation of data.

Fleming County Hospital	Flemingsburg	82%	(a)
King's Daughters' Medical Center	Ashland	82%	300+
Lake Cumberland Regional Hospital	Somerset	82%	300+
Meadowview Regional Medical Center	Maysville	82%	300+
Pattie A Clay Regional Medical Center	Richmond	82%	300+
Central Baptist Hospital	Lexington	81%	300+
Marcum and Wallace Memorial Hospital	Irvine	81%	(a)
Murray-Calloway County Hospital	Murray	81%	300+
Saint Joseph Hospital London	London	81%	300+
Three Rivers Medical Center	Louisa	81%	300+
University of Louisville Hospital	Louisville	81%	300+
Harlan Appalachian Reg Healthcare Hosp	Harlan	80%	300+
Jennie Stuart Medical Center	Hopkinsville	80%	300+
Logan Memorial Hospital	Russellville	80%	300+
Saint Joseph Martin	Martin	80%	300+
Hardin Memorial Hospital	Elizabethtown	79%	300+
Kentucky River Medical Center	Jackson	79%	300+
Lourdes Hospital	Paducah	79%	300+
Methodist Hospital	Henderson	79%	300+
Spring View Hospital	Lebanon	79%	300+
Taylor Regional Hospital	Campbellsville	79%	300+
Ephraim Mcdowell Regional Medical Center	Danville	78%	300+
Hazard Arh Regional Medical Center	Hazard	78%	300+
Methodist Hospital Union County	Morganfield	78%	(a)
Paul B Hall Regional Medical Center	Paintsville	78%	300+
Jewish Hospital & St Mary's Healthcare	Louisville	77%	300+
Pineville Community Hospital	Pineville	77%	300+
Rockcastle Reg Hosp & Respiratory Care Ctr	Mount Vernon	77%	(a)
Twin Lakes Regional Medical Center	Leitchfield	77%	300+
Clinton County Hospital	Albany	76%	300+
Jewish Hospital - Shelbyville	Shelbyville	73%	300+
Monroe County Medical Center	Tompkinsville	73%	300+
Highlands Regional Medical Center	Prestonsburg	70%	300+
Crittenden Health System	Marion	69%	(a)

43. Hospital Given 9 or 10 on 10 Point Scale

Hospital Name	City	Rate	Cases
Clinton County Hospital	Albany	81%	300+
Saint Elizabeth Grant	Williamstown	80%	(a)
Westlake Regional Hospital	Columbia	80%	300+
Morgan County Arh Hospital	West Liberty	79%	(a)
Marcum and Wallace Memorial Hospital	Irvine	78%	(a)
Our Lady of Bellefonte Hospital	Ashland	78%	300+
King's Daughters' Medical Center	Ashland	77%	300+
Fleming County Hospital	Flemingsburg	76%	(a)
Methodist Hospital Union County	Morganfield	76%	(a)
Pikeville Medical Center	Pikeville	76%	300+
Saint Joseph Berea	Berea	76%	300+
Saint Joseph Martin	Martin	76%	300+
Baptist Hospital East	Louisville	75%	300+
McDowell Arh Hospital	McDowell	75%	(a)
Rockcastle Reg Hosp & Respiratory Care Ctr	Mount Vernon	75%	(a)
Central Baptist Hospital	Lexington	74%	300+
Clark Regional Medical Center	Winchester	74%	300+
Flaget Memorial Hospital	Bardstown	74%	300+
Parkway Regional Hospital	Fulton	74%	(a)
Saint Elizabeth Medical Center North	Covington	74%	300+
Williamson ARH Hospital	S Williamson	74%	300+
Greenview Regional Hospital	Bowling Green	73%	300+
Western Baptist Hospital	Paducah	72%	300+
Whitesburg ARH Hospital	Whitesburg	72%	300+
Bourbon Community Hospital	Paris	71%	(a)
Ephraim Mcdowell Fort Logan Hospital	Stanford	71%	(a)
Harrison Memorial Hospital	Cynthiana	71%	300+
Owensboro Medical Health System	Owensboro	71%	300+
Saint Joseph Hospital	Lexington	71%	300+
Georgetown Community Hospital	Georgetown	70%	300+
Jackson Purchase Medical Center	Mayfield	70%	300+
Middlesboro Appalachian Reg Hlthcre Hosp	Middlesboro	70%	300+
Regional Medical Center of Hopkins County	Madisonville	70%	300+
Saint Joseph East	Lexington	70%	300+
Saint Joseph Hospital London	London	70%	300+
T J Samson Community Hospital	Glasgow	70%	300+
Frankfort Regional Medical Center	Frankfort	69%	300+
The Medical Center at Bowling Green	Bowling Green	69%	300+
Norton Hospitals	Louisville	69%	300+
Hazard Arh Regional Medical Center	Hazard	67%	300+
Taylor Regional Hospital	Campbellsville	67%	300+
Three Rivers Medical Center	Louisa	67%	300+
Harlan Appalachian Reg Healthcare Hosp	Harlan	66%	300+
Logan Memorial Hospital	Russellville	66%	300+
Lourdes Hospital	Paducah	66%	300+
Saint Joseph Mount Sterling	Mount Sterling	66%	(a)
Lake Cumberland Regional Hospital	Somerset	65%	300+
Monroe County Medical Center	Tompkinsville	65%	300+
Baptist Hospital Northeast	La Grange	64%	300+
Baptist Regional Medical Center	Corbin	64%	300+
Hardin Memorial Hospital	Elizabethtown	64%	300+
Meadowview Regional Medical Center	Maysville	64%	300+
Muhlenberg Community Hospital	Greenville	64%	300+
Kentucky River Medical Center	Jackson	63%	300+
University of Louisville Hospital	Louisville	63%	300+
Pineville Community Hospital	Pineville	62%	300+
Saint Claire Regional Medical Center	Morehead	62%	300+
Methodist Hospital	Henderson	61%	300+
Saint Elizabeth Florence	Florence	61%	300+
Spring View Hospital	Lebanon	61%	300+
University of Kentucky Hospital	Lexington	61%	300+
Jewish Hospital & St Mary's Healthcare	Louisville	60%	300+
Jewish Hospital - Shelbyville	Shelbyville	60%	300+
Murray-Calloway County Hospital	Murray	60%	300+
Ephraim Mcdowell Regional Medical Center	Danville	59%	300+
Ohio County Hospital	Hartford	59%	(a)
Pattie A Clay Regional Medical Center	Richmond	59%	300+
Saint Elizabeth Ft Thomas	Fort Thomas	59%	300+
Crittenden Health System	Marion	58%	(a)
Highlands Regional Medical Center	Prestonsburg	58%	300+
Paul B Hall Regional Medical Center	Paintsville	58%	300+
Twin Lakes Regional Medical Center	Leitchfield	57%	300+
Jennie Stuart Medical Center	Hopkinsville	54%	300+
Memorial Hospital	Manchester	54%	(a)

44. Meds 'Always' Explained Before Given

Hospital Name	City	Rate	Cases
Westlake Regional Hospital	Columbia	87%	300+
Morgan County Arh Hospital	West Liberty	79%	(a)
Clark Regional Medical Center	Winchester	74%	300+
Marcum and Wallace Memorial Hospital	Irvine	74%	(a)
Saint Joseph Martin	Martin	72%	300+
Three Rivers Medical Center	Louisa	69%	300+
McDowell Arh Hospital	McDowell	68%	(a)
Flaget Memorial Hospital	Bardstown	67%	300+
Muhlenberg Community Hospital	Greenville	67%	300+
Our Lady of Bellefonte Hospital	Ashland	67%	300+
Greenview Regional Hospital	Bowling Green	66%	300+
Regional Medical Center of Hopkins County	Madisonville	66%	300+
Saint Elizabeth Grant	Williamstown	66%	(a)
Saint Joseph Mount Sterling	Mount Sterling	66%	(a)
T J Samson Community Hospital	Glasgow	66%	300+
Williamson ARH Hospital	S Williamson	66%	300+
Ephraim Mcdowell Fort Logan Hospital	Stanford	65%	(a)
Frankfort Regional Medical Center	Frankfort	65%	300+
Harrison Memorial Hospital	Cynthiana	65%	300+
King's Daughters' Medical Center	Ashland	65%	300+
Pikeville Medical Center	Pikeville	65%	300+
Central Baptist Hospital	Lexington	64%	300+
Crittenden Health System	Marion	64%	(a)
Fleming County Hospital	Flemingsburg	64%	(a)
Parkway Regional Hospital	Fulton	64%	(a)
Saint Claire Regional Medical Center	Morehead	64%	300+
Saint Joseph Berea	Berea	64%	300+
Whitesburg ARH Hospital	Whitesburg	64%	300+
Georgetown Community Hospital	Georgetown	63%	300+
Hardin Memorial Hospital	Elizabethtown	63%	300+
Rockcastle Reg Hosp & Respiratory Care Ctr	Mount Vernon	63%	(a)
Saint Elizabeth Medical Center North	Covington	63%	300+
Bourbon Community Hospital	Paris	62%	(a)
Clinton County Hospital	Albany	62%	300+
Jackson Purchase Medical Center	Mayfield	62%	300+
Methodist Hospital Union County	Morganfield	62%	(a)
Saint Joseph Hospital London	London	62%	300+
Harlan Appalachian Reg Healthcare Hosp	Harlan	61%	300+
Lake Cumberland Regional Hospital	Somerset	61%	300+
Middlesboro Appalachian Reg Hlthcre Hosp	Middlesboro	61%	300+
Norton Hospitals	Louisville	61%	300+
Saint Elizabeth Ft Thomas	Fort Thomas	61%	300+
The Medical Center at Bowling Green	Bowling Green	60%	300+
Saint Joseph Hospital	Lexington	60%	300+
Hazard Arh Regional Medical Center	Hazard	59%	300+
Saint Elizabeth Florence	Florence	59%	300+
Taylor Regional Hospital	Campbellsville	59%	300+
Western Baptist Hospital	Paducah	59%	300+
Baptist Regional Medical Center	Corbin	58%	300+
Kentucky River Medical Center	Jackson	58%	300+
Logan Memorial Hospital	Russellville	58%	300+
Methodist Hospital	Henderson	58%	300+
Saint Joseph East	Lexington	58%	300+
Twin Lakes Regional Medical Center	Leitchfield	58%	300+
University of Kentucky Hospital	Lexington	58%	300+
Baptist Hospital East	Louisville	57%	300+
Meadowview Regional Medical Center	Maysville	57%	300+
Monroe County Medical Center	Tompkinsville	57%	300+
Paul B Hall Regional Medical Center	Paintsville	57%	300+
University of Louisville Hospital	Louisville	57%	300+
Highlands Regional Medical Center	Prestonsburg	56%	300+
Murray-Calloway County Hospital	Murray	56%	300+
Owensboro Medical Health System	Owensboro	56%	300+
Pineville Community Hospital	Pineville	56%	300+
Pattie A Clay Regional Medical Center	Richmond	55%	300+
Jennie Stuart Medical Center	Hopkinsville	54%	300+
Jewish Hospital & St Mary's Healthcare	Louisville	54%	300+
Lourdes Hospital	Paducah	54%	300+
Spring View Hospital	Lebanon	54%	300+
Baptist Hospital Northeast	La Grange	53%	300+
Jewish Hospital - Shelbyville	Shelbyville	53%	300+
Ephraim Mcdowell Regional Medical Center	Danville	52%	300+
Memorial Hospital	Manchester	52%	(a)
Ohio County Hospital	Hartford	48%	(a)

45. Nurses 'Always' Communicated Well

Hospital Name	City	Rate	Cases
Westlake Regional Hospital	Columbia	99%	300+
Marcum and Wallace Memorial Hospital	Irvine	91%	(a)
Methodist Hospital Union County	Morganfield	87%	(a)
Saint Joseph Martin	Martin	86%	300+
Clark Regional Medical Center	Winchester	85%	300+
Our Lady of Bellefonte Hospital	Ashland	84%	300+
Clinton County Hospital	Albany	83%	300+
King's Daughters' Medical Center	Ashland	83%	300+
McDowell Arh Hospital	McDowell	83%	(a)
Saint Elizabeth Grant	Williamstown	83%	(a)
Parkway Regional Hospital	Fulton	82%	(a)
Rockcastle Reg Hosp & Respiratory Care Ctr	Mount Vernon	82%	(a)
Saint Joseph Berea	Berea	82%	300+
Whitesburg ARH Hospital	Whitesburg	82%	300+
Bourbon Community Hospital	Paris	81%	(a)
Morgan County Arh Hospital	West Liberty	81%	(a)
Muhlenberg Community Hospital	Greenville	81%	300+
Pikeville Medical Center	Pikeville	81%	300+
T J Samson Community Hospital	Glasgow	81%	300+
Central Baptist Hospital	Lexington	80%	300+
Harrison Memorial Hospital	Cynthiana	80%	300+
Middlesboro Appalachian Reg Hlthcre Hosp	Middlesboro	80%	300+
Regional Medical Center of Hopkins County	Madisonville	80%	300+
Saint Claire Regional Medical Center	Morehead	80%	300+
Saint Joseph Hospital London	London	80%	300+
Three Rivers Medical Center	Louisa	80%	300+
Baptist Hospital East	Louisville	79%	300+
Crittenden Health System	Marion	79%	(a)
Fleming County Hospital	Flemingsburg	79%	(a)
Greenview Regional Hospital	Bowling Green	79%	300+
Ohio County Hospital	Hartford	79%	(a)
Western Baptist Hospital	Paducah	79%	300+
Williamson ARH Hospital	S Williamson	79%	300+
Ephraim Mcdowell Fort Logan Hospital	Stanford	78%	(a)
Flaget Memorial Hospital	Bardstown	78%	300+
Frankfort Regional Medical Center	Frankfort	78%	300+
Logan Memorial Hospital	Russellville	78%	300+
Owensboro Medical Health System	Owensboro	78%	300+
Saint Elizabeth Medical Center North	Covington	78%	300+
Saint Joseph Hospital	Lexington	78%	300+
Saint Joseph Mount Sterling	Mount Sterling	78%	(a)
Baptist Regional Medical Center	Corbin	77%	300+
Georgetown Community Hospital	Georgetown	77%	300+
Hardin Memorial Hospital	Elizabethtown	77%	300+
Harlan Appalachian Reg Healthcare Hosp	Harlan	77%	300+
Hazard Arh Regional Medical Center	Hazard	77%	300+
Meadowview Regional Medical Center	Maysville	77%	300+
The Medical Center at Bowling Green	Bowling Green	77%	300+
Methodist Hospital	Henderson	77%	300+
Monroe County Medical Center	Tompkinsville	77%	300+
Norton Hospitals	Louisville	77%	300+
Taylor Regional Hospital	Campbellsville	77%	300+
Baptist Hospital Northeast	La Grange	76%	300+
Jackson Purchase Medical Center	Mayfield	76%	300+
Kentucky River Medical Center	Jackson	76%	300+
Lake Cumberland Regional Hospital	Somerset	76%	300+
Pineville Community Hospital	Pineville	76%	300+
Highlands Regional Medical Center	Prestonsburg	75%	300+
Saint Elizabeth Ft Thomas	Fort Thomas	75%	300+
Saint Joseph East	Lexington	75%	300+
Spring View Hospital	Lebanon	75%	300+
Lourdes Hospital	Paducah	74%	300+
Murray-Calloway County Hospital	Murray	74%	300+
Saint Elizabeth Florence	Florence	74%	300+
Twin Lakes Regional Medical Center	Leitchfield	74%	300+
University of Kentucky Hospital	Lexington	74%	300+
Jewish Hospital - Shelbyville	Shelbyville	72%	300+
Memorial Hospital	Manchester	72%	(a)
Ephraim Mcdowell Regional Medical Center	Danville	71%	300+
Pattie A Clay Regional Medical Center	Richmond	71%	300+
Paul B Hall Regional Medical Center	Paintsville	71%	300+
University of Louisville Hospital	Louisville	71%	300+
Jewish Hospital & St Mary's Healthcare	Louisville	70%	300+
Jennie Stuart Medical Center	Hopkinsville	67%	300+

46. Pain 'Always' Well Controlled

Hospital Name	City	Rate	Cases
Westlake Regional Hospital	Columbia	99%	300+
Clark Regional Medical Center	Winchester	78%	300+

NOTE: Hospital profiles are in alphabetical order by state, then city, then hospital within the city; Rankings exclude hospitals with less than 25 cases except for patient surveys which excludes hospitals with less than 100 cases; (a) 100–299 cases; (1) The number of cases is too small to be sure how well a hospital is performing; (2) The hospital indicated that the data submitted for this measure were based on a sample of cases; (3) Data was collected during a shorter time period (fewer quarters) than the maximum possible time for this measure; (4) Suppressed for one or more quarters by CMS; (5) No data is available from the hospital for this measure; (6) Fewer than 100 patients completed the HCAHPS survey. Use these rates with caution, as the number of surveys may be too low to reliably assess hospital performance; (7) Survey results are based on less than 12 months of data; (8) Survey results are not available for this reporting period; (9) No or very few patients were eligible for the HCAHPS survey. The scores shown, if any, reflect a very small number of surveys; (10) A state average was not calculated because too few hospitals in the state submitted data; (11) There were discrepancies in the data collection process; Please refer to the User's Guide for a full explanation of data.

Marcum and Wallace Memorial Hospital	Irvine	78%	(a)
Muhlenberg Community Hospital	Greenville	77%	300+
Parkway Regional Hospital	Fulton	77%	(a)
Pikeville Medical Center	Pikeville	77%	300+
Bourbon Community Hospital	Paris	76%	(a)
Morgan County Arh Hospital	West Liberty	76%	(a)
Our Lady of Bellefonte Hospital	Ashland	76%	300+
Methodist Hospital Union County	Morganfield	75%	(a)
Saint Elizabeth Grant	Williamstown	75%	(a)
Flaget Memorial Hospital	Bardstown	74%	300+
King's Daughters' Medical Center	Ashland	74%	300+
Logan Memorial Hospital	Russellville	74%	300+
McDowell Arh Hospital	McDowell	74%	(a)
Ohio County Hospital	Hartford	74%	(a)
Williamson ARH Hospital	S Williamson	74%	300+
Frankfort Regional Medical Center	Frankfort	73%	300+
Lake Cumberland Regional Hospital	Somerset	73%	300+
Regional Medical Center of Hopkins County	Madisonville	73%	300+
Saint Joseph Hospital London	London	73%	300+
Saint Joseph Martin	Martin	73%	300+
T J Samson Community Hospital	Glasgow	73%	300+
Central Baptist Hospital	Lexington	72%	300+
Meadowview Regional Medical Center	Maysville	72%	300+
Rockcastle Reg Hosp & Respiratory Care Ctr	Mount Vernon	72%	(a)
Saint Joseph Berea	Berea	72%	300+
Saint Joseph Mount Sterling	Mount Sterling	72%	(a)
Three Rivers Medical Center	Louisa	72%	300+
Baptist Hospital East	Louisville	71%	300+
Clinton County Hospital	Albany	71%	300+
Georgetown Community Hospital	Georgetown	71%	300+
Greenview Regional Hospital	Bowling Green	71%	300+
Harrison Memorial Hospital	Cynthiana	71%	300+
Methodist Hospital	Henderson	71%	300+
Owensboro Medical Health System	Owensboro	71%	300+
Saint Claire Regional Medical Center	Morehead	71%	300+
Saint Joseph Hospital	Lexington	71%	300+
Whitesburg ARH Hospital	Whitesburg	71%	300+
Fleming County Hospital	Flemingsburg	70%	(a)
Hazard Arh Regional Medical Center	Hazard	70%	300+
The Medical Center at Bowling Green	Bowling Green	70%	300+
Middlesboro Appalachian Reg Hlthcre Hosp	Middlesboro	70%	300+
Monroe County Medical Center	Tompkinsville	70%	300+
Norton Hospitals	Louisville	70%	300+
Saint Elizabeth Medical Center North	Covington	70%	300+
Saint Joseph East	Lexington	70%	300+
Saint Elizabeth Ft Thomas	Fort Thomas	69%	300+
Spring View Hospital	Lebanon	69%	300+
Taylor Regional Hospital	Campbellsville	69%	300+
Crittenden Health System	Marion	68%	(a)
Harlan Appalachian Reg Healthcare Hosp	Harlan	68%	300+
Jackson Purchase Medical Center	Mayfield	68%	300+
Kentucky River Medical Center	Jackson	68%	300+
Saint Elizabeth Florence	Florence	68%	300+
Western Baptist Hospital	Paducah	68%	300+
Baptist Regional Medical Center	Corbin	67%	300+
Hardin Memorial Hospital	Elizabethtown	67%	300+
Twin Lakes Regional Medical Center	Leitchfield	67%	300+
Pattie A Clay Regional Medical Center	Richmond	66%	300+
Pineville Community Hospital	Pineville	66%	300+
Baptist Hospital Northeast	La Grange	65%	300+
Ephraim Mcdowell Fort Logan Hospital	Stanford	65%	(a)
Lourdes Hospital	Paducah	65%	300+
Murray-Calloway County Hospital	Murray	65%	300+
University of Kentucky Hospital	Lexington	65%	300+
Ephraim Mcdowell Regional Medical Center	Danville	64%	300+
Jewish Hospital - Shelbyville	Shelbyville	64%	300+
Highlands Regional Medical Center	Prestonsburg	63%	300+
Jennie Stuart Medical Center	Hopkinsville	63%	300+
Memorial Hospital	Manchester	63%	(a)
University of Louisville Hospital	Louisville	63%	300+
Paul B Hall Regional Medical Center	Paintsville	62%	300+
Jewish Hospital & St Mary's Healthcare	Louisville	61%	300+

47. Room and Bathroom 'Always' Clean

Hospital Name	City	Rate	Cases
Westlake Regional Hospital	Columbia	96%	300+
Marcum and Wallace Memorial Hospital	Irvine	93%	(a)
Clinton County Hospital	Albany	89%	300+
Fleming County Hospital	Flemingsburg	87%	(a)
Morgan County Arh Hospital	West Liberty	86%	(a)
T J Samson Community Hospital	Glasgow	86%	300+
McDowell Arh Hospital	McDowell	85%	(a)
Clark Regional Medical Center	Winchester	84%	300+
Methodist Hospital Union County	Morganfield	84%	(a)
Monroe County Medical Center	Tompkinsville	82%	300+
Saint Joseph Martin	Martin	82%	300+
Rockcastle Reg Hosp & Respiratory Care Ctr	Mount Vernon	81%	(a)
Crittenden Health System	Marion	79%	(a)
Ohio County Hospital	Hartford	79%	(a)
Harrison Memorial Hospital	Cynthiana	78%	300+
Our Lady of Bellefonte Hospital	Ashland	78%	300+
Parkway Regional Hospital	Fulton	78%	(a)
Pineville Community Hospital	Pineville	78%	300+
Saint Elizabeth Grant	Williamstown	78%	(a)
Ephraim Mcdowell Fort Logan Hospital	Stanford	77%	(a)
Flaget Memorial Hospital	Bardstown	75%	300+
Muhlenberg Community Hospital	Greenville	75%	300+
Whitesburg ARH Hospital	Whitesburg	75%	300+
Greenview Regional Hospital	Bowling Green	74%	300+
King's Daughters' Medical Center	Ashland	74%	300+
Meadowview Regional Medical Center	Maysville	74%	300+
Middlesboro Appalachian Reg Hlthcre Hosp	Middlesboro	74%	300+
Three Rivers Medical Center	Louisa	74%	300+
Hazard Arh Regional Medical Center	Hazard	73%	300+
Methodist Hospital	Henderson	73%	300+
Saint Joseph Berea	Berea	73%	300+
Saint Joseph Mount Sterling	Mount Sterling	73%	(a)
Taylor Regional Hospital	Campbellsville	73%	300+
Western Baptist Hospital	Paducah	73%	300+
Bourbon Community Hospital	Paris	72%	(a)
Harlan Appalachian Reg Healthcare Hosp	Harlan	72%	300+
Pikeville Medical Center	Pikeville	72%	300+
Saint Joseph Hospital London	London	72%	300+
Williamson ARH Hospital	S Williamson	72%	300+
Lake Cumberland Regional Hospital	Somerset	71%	300+
Owensboro Medical Health System	Owensboro	71%	300+
Saint Claire Regional Medical Center	Morehead	71%	300+
Saint Elizabeth Ft Thomas	Fort Thomas	71%	300+
Frankfort Regional Medical Center	Frankfort	70%	300+
Norton Hospitals	Louisville	70%	300+
Saint Elizabeth Medical Center North	Covington	70%	300+
Hardin Memorial Hospital	Elizabethtown	69%	300+
Highlands Regional Medical Center	Prestonsburg	69%	300+
Jackson Purchase Medical Center	Mayfield	69%	300+
Kentucky River Medical Center	Jackson	69%	300+
The Medical Center at Bowling Green	Bowling Green	69%	300+
Pattie A Clay Regional Medical Center	Richmond	69%	300+
Regional Medical Center of Hopkins County	Madisonville	69%	300+
Paul B Hall Regional Medical Center	Paintsville	68%	300+
Ephraim Mcdowell Regional Medical Center	Danville	67%	300+
Jewish Hospital - Shelbyville	Shelbyville	67%	300+
Murray-Calloway County Hospital	Murray	67%	300+
Saint Elizabeth Florence	Florence	67%	300+
Twin Lakes Regional Medical Center	Leitchfield	67%	300+
Baptist Hospital East	Louisville	66%	300+
Baptist Regional Medical Center	Corbin	66%	300+
Jennie Stuart Medical Center	Hopkinsville	66%	300+
Memorial Hospital	Manchester	66%	(a)
Saint Joseph Hospital	Lexington	66%	300+
Spring View Hospital	Lebanon	66%	300+
Logan Memorial Hospital	Russellville	65%	300+
Georgetown Community Hospital	Georgetown	64%	300+
Saint Joseph East	Lexington	64%	300+
Baptist Hospital Northeast	La Grange	62%	300+
Central Baptist Hospital	Lexington	62%	300+
Lourdes Hospital	Paducah	61%	300+
University of Louisville Hospital	Louisville	61%	300+
University of Kentucky Hospital	Lexington	60%	300+
Jewish Hospital & St Mary's Healthcare	Louisville	57%	300+

48. Timely Help 'Always' Received

Hospital Name	City	Rate	Cases
Westlake Regional Hospital	Columbia	97%	300+
Saint Elizabeth Grant	Williamstown	83%	(a)
Marcum and Wallace Memorial Hospital	Irvine	82%	(a)
Morgan County Arh Hospital	West Liberty	81%	(a)
McDowell Arh Hospital	McDowell	80%	(a)
Saint Joseph Martin	Martin	79%	300+
Methodist Hospital Union County	Morganfield	77%	(a)
Clark Regional Medical Center	Winchester	76%	300+
Parkway Regional Hospital	Fulton	74%	(a)
T J Samson Community Hospital	Glasgow	74%	300+
Whitesburg ARH Hospital	Whitesburg	74%	300+
Flaget Memorial Hospital	Bardstown	72%	300+
Saint Joseph Hospital London	London	72%	300+
Bourbon Community Hospital	Paris	71%	(a)
Harlan Appalachian Reg Healthcare Hosp	Harlan	70%	300+
Middlesboro Appalachian Reg Hlthcre Hosp	Middlesboro	70%	300+
Our Lady of Bellefonte Hospital	Ashland	70%	300+
Saint Joseph Berea	Berea	70%	300+
Clinton County Hospital	Albany	69%	300+
Ephraim Mcdowell Fort Logan Hospital	Stanford	69%	(a)
Logan Memorial Hospital	Russellville	69%	300+
Ohio County Hospital	Hartford	69%	(a)
King's Daughters' Medical Center	Ashland	68%	300+
Muhlenberg Community Hospital	Greenville	68%	300+
Pikeville Medical Center	Pikeville	68%	300+
Three Rivers Medical Center	Louisa	68%	300+
Williamson ARH Hospital	S Williamson	68%	300+
Baptist Regional Medical Center	Corbin	67%	300+
Crittenden Health System	Marion	66%	(a)
Saint Joseph Mount Sterling	Mount Sterling	66%	(a)
Taylor Regional Hospital	Campbellsville	66%	300+
Central Baptist Hospital	Lexington	65%	300+
Frankfort Regional Medical Center	Frankfort	65%	300+
The Medical Center at Bowling Green	Bowling Green	65%	300+
Rockcastle Reg Hosp & Respiratory Care Ctr	Mount Vernon	65%	(a)
Saint Elizabeth Medical Center North	Covington	65%	300+
Baptist Hospital East	Louisville	64%	300+
Fleming County Hospital	Flemingsburg	64%	(a)
Georgetown Community Hospital	Georgetown	64%	300+
Hazard Arh Regional Medical Center	Hazard	64%	300+
Highlands Regional Medical Center	Prestonsburg	64%	300+
Lake Cumberland Regional Hospital	Somerset	64%	300+
Norton Hospitals	Louisville	64%	300+
Owensboro Medical Health System	Owensboro	64%	300+
Saint Claire Regional Medical Center	Morehead	64%	300+
Twin Lakes Regional Medical Center	Leitchfield	64%	300+
Harrison Memorial Hospital	Cynthiana	63%	300+
Saint Joseph Hospital	Lexington	63%	300+
Greenview Regional Hospital	Bowling Green	62%	300+
Kentucky River Medical Center	Jackson	62%	300+
Western Baptist Hospital	Paducah	62%	300+
Meadowview Regional Medical Center	Maysville	61%	300+
Methodist Hospital	Henderson	61%	300+
Murray-Calloway County Hospital	Murray	61%	300+
Pattie A Clay Regional Medical Center	Richmond	61%	300+
Saint Joseph East	Lexington	61%	300+
Spring View Hospital	Lebanon	61%	300+
University of Kentucky Hospital	Lexington	61%	300+
Jackson Purchase Medical Center	Mayfield	60%	300+
Lourdes Hospital	Paducah	60%	300+
Saint Elizabeth Ft Thomas	Fort Thomas	60%	300+
Pineville Community Hospital	Pineville	59%	300+
Regional Medical Center of Hopkins County	Madisonville	59%	300+
Saint Elizabeth Florence	Florence	59%	300+
Hardin Memorial Hospital	Elizabethtown	58%	300+
Jewish Hospital - Shelbyville	Shelbyville	58%	300+
Paul B Hall Regional Medical Center	Paintsville	57%	300+
Baptist Hospital Northeast	La Grange	56%	300+
Jennie Stuart Medical Center	Hopkinsville	56%	300+
Memorial Hospital	Manchester	56%	(a)
Monroe County Medical Center	Tompkinsville	56%	300+
Ephraim Mcdowell Regional Medical Center	Danville	55%	300+
Jewish Hospital & St Mary's Healthcare	Louisville	52%	300+
University of Louisville Hospital	Louisville	52%	300+

49. Would Definitely Recommend Hospital

Hospital Name	City	Rate	Cases
Westlake Regional Hospital	Columbia	98%	300+
Clinton County Hospital	Albany	85%	300+
Central Baptist Hospital	Lexington	82%	300+
King's Daughters' Medical Center	Ashland	82%	300+
Morgan County Arh Hospital	West Liberty	82%	(a)
Baptist Hospital East	Louisville	81%	300+
Our Lady of Bellefonte Hospital	Ashland	79%	300+
Saint Elizabeth Medical Center North	Covington	79%	300+
Saint Joseph Berea	Berea	79%	300+
Saint Joseph Martin	Martin	79%	300+
Western Baptist Hospital	Paducah	79%	300+
Methodist Hospital Union County	Morganfield	78%	(a)
Pikeville Medical Center	Pikeville	78%	300+
Saint Joseph Hospital	Lexington	77%	300+
Greenview Regional Hospital	Bowling Green	76%	300+
Marcum and Wallace Memorial Hospital	Irvine	76%	(a)
McDowell Arh Hospital	McDowell	76%	(a)
Clark Regional Medical Center	Winchester	75%	300+
Fleming County Hospital	Flemingsburg	75%	(a)
Bourbon Community Hospital	Paris	74%	(a)
The Medical Center at Bowling Green	Bowling Green	74%	300+
Saint Elizabeth Grant	Williamstown	74%	(a)
Saint Joseph East	Lexington	74%	300+
Flaget Memorial Hospital	Bardstown	73%	300+
Rockcastle Reg Hosp & Respiratory Care Ctr	Mount Vernon	73%	(a)
Saint Joseph Hospital London	London	73%	300+
Williamson ARH Hospital	S Williamson	73%	300+
Ephraim Mcdowell Fort Logan Hospital	Stanford	72%	(a)
Norton Hospitals	Louisville	72%	300+
Georgetown Community Hospital	Georgetown	71%	300+
Owensboro Medical Health System	Owensboro	71%	300+
Regional Medical Center of Hopkins County	Madisonville	71%	300+
Whitesburg ARH Hospital	Whitesburg	71%	300+
Lourdes Hospital	Paducah	70%	300+
T J Samson Community Hospital	Glasgow	70%	300+
Jackson Purchase Medical Center	Mayfield	68%	300+
Pineville Community Hospital	Pineville	68%	300+
Baptist Hospital Northeast	La Grange	67%	300+
Harrison Memorial Hospital	Cynthiana	67%	300+
Parkway Regional Hospital	Fulton	67%	(a)
University of Kentucky Hospital	Lexington	67%	300+

NOTE: Hospital profiles are in alphabetical order by state, then city, then hospital within the city; Rankings exclude hospitals with less than 25 cases except for patient surveys which excludes hospitals with less than 100 cases; (a) 100–299 cases; (1) The number of cases is too small to be sure how well a hospital is performing; (2) The hospital indicated that the data submitted for this measure were based on a sample of cases; (3) Data was collected during a shorter time period (fewer quarters) than the maximum possible time for this measure; (4) Suppressed for one or more quarters by CMS; (5) No data is available from the hospital for this measure; (6) Fewer than 100 patients completed the HCAHPS survey. Use these rates with caution, as the number of surveys may be too low to reliably assess hospital performance; (7) Survey results are based on less than 12 months of data; (8) Survey results are not available for this reporting period; (9) No or very few patients were eligible for the HCAHPS survey. The scores shown, if any, reflect a very small number of surveys; (10) A state average was not calculated because too few hospitals in the state submitted data; (11) There were discrepancies in the data collection process; Please refer to the User's Guide for a full explanation of data.

Ohio County Hospital	Hartford	66%	(a)
Saint Claire Regional Medical Center	Morehead	66%	300+
Saint Joseph Mount Sterling	Mount Sterling	66%	(a)
Taylor Regional Hospital	Campbellsville	66%	300+
Hardin Memorial Hospital	Elizabethtown	65%	300+
Lake Cumberland Regional Hospital	Somerset	65%	300+
Meadowview Regional Medical Center	Maysville	65%	300+
Middlesboro Appalachian Reg Hlthcre Hosp	Middlesboro	65%	300+
Three Rivers Medical Center	Louisa	65%	300+
University of Louisville Hospital	Louisville	65%	300+
Baptist Regional Medical Center	Corbin	64%	300+
Frankfort Regional Medical Center	Frankfort	64%	300+
Crittenden Health System	Marion	63%	(a)
Hazard Arh Regional Medical Center	Hazard	63%	300+
Jewish Hospital & St Mary's Healthcare	Louisville	63%	300+
Muhlenberg Community Hospital	Greenville	63%	300+
Saint Elizabeth Florence	Florence	63%	300+
Saint Elizabeth Ft Thomas	Fort Thomas	63%	300+
Ephraim Mcdowell Regional Medical Center	Danville	62%	300+
Harlan Appalachian Reg Healthcare Hosp	Harlan	62%	300+
Logan Memorial Hospital	Russellville	61%	300+
Monroe County Medical Center	Tompkinsville	61%	300+
Pattie A Clay Regional Medical Center	Richmond	61%	300+
Methodist Hospital	Henderson	60%	300+
Murray-Calloway County Hospital	Murray	60%	300+
Spring View Hospital	Lebanon	60%	300+
Highlands Regional Medical Center	Prestonsburg	59%	300+
Kentucky River Medical Center	Jackson	59%	300+
Twin Lakes Regional Medical Center	Leitchfield	59%	300+
Paul B Hall Regional Medical Center	Paintsville	58%	300+
Jewish Hospital - Shelbyville	Shelbyville	57%	300+
Jennie Stuart Medical Center	Hopkinsville	50%	300+
Memorial Hospital	Manchester	49%	(a)

Clinton County Hospital

723 Burkesville Road
Albany, KY 42602
Phone: 606-387-6421
Fax: 606-387-8550
E-mail: info@clintoncountyhospital.com
URL: www.clintoncountyhospital.com
Type: Acute Care Hospitals
Emergency Services: No
Ownership: Proprietary
Beds: 42

Key Personnel:
CEO/President . . . . Randel A Flowers, PhD
Chief of Medical Staff . . . . Vicki Latham
Infection Control . . . . Linda Steele
Operating Room . . . . Tracy Cross
Quality Assurance . . . . Pat Sewell
Radiology . . . . Jai Singh
Emergency Room . . . . Tamara Collins
Intensive Care Unit . . . . Janice Beard

Measure	Cases	This Hosp.	State Avg.	U.S. Avg.
Heart Attack Care				
ACE Inhibitor or ARB for LVSD[3]	0	-	94%	96%
Aspirin at Arrival[1,3]	5	100%	98%	99%
Aspirin at Discharge[1,3]	3	67%	99%	98%
Beta Blocker at Discharge[1,3]	3	67%	98%	98%
Fibrinolytic Medication Timing[3]	0	-	60%	55%
PCI Within 90 Minutes of Arrival[3]	0	-	88%	90%
Smoking Cessation Advice[3]	0	-	100%	99%
Chest Pain/Possible Heart Attack Care				
Aspirin at Arrival	28	89%	95%	95%
Median Time to ECG (minutes)	34	5	7	8
Median Time to Transfer (minutes)[1,3]	2	125	65	61
Fibrinolytic Medication Timing[1]	3	67%	62%	54%
Heart Failure Care				
ACE Inhibitor or ARB for LVSD	37	62%	91%	94%
Discharge Instructions	67	75%	82%	88%
Evaluation of LVS Function	72	76%	96%	98%
Smoking Cessation Advice[1]	15	100%	98%	98%
Pneumonia Care				
Appropriate Initial Antibiotic	78	76%	90%	92%
Blood Culture Timing[1]	19	74%	95%	96%
Influenza Vaccine	48	96%	92%	91%
Initial Antibiotic Timing	57	93%	95%	95%
Pneumococcal Vaccine	58	91%	94%	93%
Smoking Cessation Advice	39	100%	98%	97%
Surgical Care Improvement Project				
Appropriate VTP Within 24 Hours[1,3]	1	100%	91%	92%
Appropriate Hair Removal[1,3]	14	93%	99%	99%
Appropriate Beta Blocker Usage[1,3]	2	0%	93%	93%
Controlled Postoperative Blood Glucose[3]	0	-	94%	93%
Prophylactic Antibiotic Timing[1,3]	8	75%	97%	97%
Prophylactic Antibiotic Timing (Outpatient)[1,3]	2	0%	92%	92%
Prophylactic Antibiotic Selection[1,3]	7	100%	98%	97%
Prophylactic Antibiotic Select. (Outpatient)[3]	0	-	93%	94%
Prophylactic Antibiotic Stopped[1,3]	7	100%	94%	94%
Recommended VTP Ordered[1,3]	1	100%	94%	94%
Urinary Catheter Removal[3]	0	-	89%	90%
Children's Asthma Care				
Received Systemic Corticosteroids	-	-	-	100%
Received Home Management Plan	-	-	-	71%
Received Reliever Medication	-	-	-	100%
Use of Medical Imaging				
Combination Abdominal CT Scan	152	0.171	0.160	0.191
Combination Chest CT Scan	94	0.298	0.054	0.054
Follow-up Mammogram/Ultrasound	175	4.0%	7.9%	8.4%
MRI for Low Back Pain[5]	0	-	35.6%	32.7%
Survey of Patients' Hospital Experiences				
Area Around Room 'Always' Quiet at Night	300+	79%	-	58%
Doctors 'Always' Communicated Well	300+	92%	-	80%
Home Recovery Information Given	300+	76%	-	82%
Hospital Given 9 or 10 on 10 Point Scale	300+	81%	-	67%
Meds 'Always' Explained Before Given	300+	62%	-	60%
Nurses 'Always' Communicated Well	300+	83%	-	76%
Pain 'Always' Well Controlled	300+	71%	-	69%
Room and Bathroom 'Always' Clean	300+	89%	-	71%
Timely Help 'Always' Received	300+	69%	-	64%
Would Definitely Recommend Hospital	300+	85%	-	69%

King's Daughters' Medical Center

2201 Lexington Avenue
Ashland, KY 41101
Phone: 606-327-4000
Fax: 606-327-4805
URL: www.kdmc.com
Type: Acute Care Hospitals
Emergency Services: Yes
Ownership: Proprietary
Beds: 341

Key Personnel:
CEO/President . . . . Fred L Jackson
Chief of Medical Staff . . . . Philip W Fioret
Infection Control . . . . Lea Acord
Pediatric Ambulatory Care . . . . . . John Roger Potter, MD
Pediatric In-Patient Care . . . . John Roger Potter, MD
Quality Assurance . . . . Sheryl Mahaney
Radiology . . . . Chun Kim, MD

Measure	Cases	This Hosp.	State Avg.	U.S. Avg.
Heart Attack Care				
ACE Inhibitor or ARB for LVSD[2]	103	97%	94%	96%
Aspirin at Arrival[2]	452	98%	98%	99%
Aspirin at Discharge[2]	732	100%	99%	98%
Beta Blocker at Discharge[2]	712	99%	98%	98%
Fibrinolytic Medication Timing[2]	0	-	60%	55%
PCI Within 90 Minutes of Arrival[2]	84	92%	88%	90%
Smoking Cessation Advice[2]	351	100%	100%	99%
Chest Pain/Possible Heart Attack Care				
Aspirin at Arrival[5]	0	-	95%	95%
Median Time to ECG (minutes)[5]	0	-	7	8
Median Time to Transfer (minutes)[5]	0	-	65	61
Fibrinolytic Medication Timing[5]	0	-	62%	54%
Heart Failure Care				
ACE Inhibitor or ARB for LVSD[2]	209	98%	91%	94%
Discharge Instructions[2]	783	91%	82%	88%
Evaluation of LVS Function[2]	901	100%	96%	98%
Smoking Cessation Advice[2]	185	100%	98%	98%
Pneumonia Care				
Appropriate Initial Antibiotic[2]	358	94%	90%	92%
Blood Culture Timing[2]	318	96%	95%	96%
Influenza Vaccine[2]	421	95%	92%	91%
Initial Antibiotic Timing[2]	493	96%	95%	95%
Pneumococcal Vaccine[2]	536	95%	94%	93%
Smoking Cessation Advice[2]	368	99%	98%	97%
Surgical Care Improvement Project				
Appropriate VTP Within 24 Hours[2]	171	91%	91%	92%
Appropriate Hair Removal[2]	732	100%	99%	99%
Appropriate Beta Blocker Usage[2]	264	97%	93%	93%
Controlled Postoperative Blood Glucose[2]	124	100%	94%	93%
Prophylactic Antibiotic Timing[2]	516	97%	97%	97%
Prophylactic Antibiotic Timing (Outpatient)	343	81%	92%	92%
Prophylactic Antibiotic Selection[2]	522	99%	98%	97%
Prophylactic Antibiotic Select. (Outpatient)	319	87%	93%	94%
Prophylactic Antibiotic Stopped[2]	505	97%	94%	94%
Recommended VTP Ordered[2]	172	95%	94%	94%
Urinary Catheter Removal[2]	189	87%	89%	90%
Children's Asthma Care				
Received Systemic Corticosteroids	-	-	-	100%
Received Home Management Plan	-	-	-	71%
Received Reliever Medication	-	-	-	100%
Use of Medical Imaging				
Combination Abdominal CT Scan	2,364	0.050	0.160	0.191
Combination Chest CT Scan	2,154	0.013	0.054	0.054
Follow-up Mammogram/Ultrasound	2,425	7.6%	7.9%	8.4%
MRI for Low Back Pain	632	28.0%	35.6%	32.7%
Survey of Patients' Hospital Experiences				
Area Around Room 'Always' Quiet at Night	300+	63%	-	58%
Doctors 'Always' Communicated Well	300+	82%	-	80%
Home Recovery Information Given	300+	82%	-	82%
Hospital Given 9 or 10 on 10 Point Scale	300+	77%	-	67%
Meds 'Always' Explained Before Given	300+	65%	-	60%
Nurses 'Always' Communicated Well	300+	83%	-	76%
Pain 'Always' Well Controlled	300+	74%	-	69%
Room and Bathroom 'Always' Clean	300+	74%	-	71%
Timely Help 'Always' Received	300+	68%	-	64%
Would Definitely Recommend Hospital	300+	82%	-	69%

Our Lady of Bellefonte Hospital

1000 Saint Christopher Drive
Ashland, KY 41101
Phone: 606-833-3600
Fax: 606-833-3593
URL: www.olbh.com
Type: Acute Care Hospitals
Emergency Services: Yes
Ownership: Voluntary Non-Profit - Church
Beds: 214

Key Personnel:
CEO/President . . . . Mark Gordon
Chief of Medical Staff . . . . Eugene DeGiorgio, MD

Measure	Cases	This Hosp.	State Avg.	U.S. Avg.
Heart Attack Care				
ACE Inhibitor or ARB for LVSD[1]	4	100%	94%	96%
Aspirin at Arrival	54	96%	98%	99%
Aspirin at Discharge	29	97%	99%	98%
Beta Blocker at Discharge	30	100%	98%	98%
Fibrinolytic Medication Timing	0	-	60%	55%
PCI Within 90 Minutes of Arrival	0	-	88%	90%
Smoking Cessation Advice[1]	9	100%	100%	99%
Chest Pain/Possible Heart Attack Care				
Aspirin at Arrival	65	98%	95%	95%
Median Time to ECG (minutes)	65	20	7	8
Median Time to Transfer (minutes)[3]	0	-	65	61
Fibrinolytic Medication Timing[1]	1	0%	62%	54%
Heart Failure Care				
ACE Inhibitor or ARB for LVSD	37	100%	91%	94%
Discharge Instructions	220	90%	82%	88%
Evaluation of LVS Function	250	98%	96%	98%
Smoking Cessation Advice	46	100%	98%	98%
Pneumonia Care				
Appropriate Initial Antibiotic	170	90%	90%	92%
Blood Culture Timing	223	97%	95%	96%
Influenza Vaccine	217	99%	92%	91%
Initial Antibiotic Timing	275	96%	95%	95%
Pneumococcal Vaccine	256	99%	94%	93%
Smoking Cessation Advice	161	100%	98%	97%
Surgical Care Improvement Project				
Appropriate VTP Within 24 Hours	148	85%	91%	92%
Appropriate Hair Removal	544	100%	99%	99%
Appropriate Beta Blocker Usage	144	100%	93%	93%
Controlled Postoperative Blood Glucose	0	-	94%	93%
Prophylactic Antibiotic Timing	380	98%	97%	97%
Prophylactic Antibiotic Timing (Outpatient)	203	95%	92%	92%
Prophylactic Antibiotic Selection	379	99%	98%	97%
Prophylactic Antibiotic Select. (Outpatient)	197	97%	93%	94%
Prophylactic Antibiotic Stopped	341	99%	94%	94%
Recommended VTP Ordered	148	89%	94%	94%
Urinary Catheter Removal	158	93%	89%	90%
Children's Asthma Care				
Received Systemic Corticosteroids	-	-	-	100%
Received Home Management Plan	-	-	-	71%
Received Reliever Medication	-	-	-	100%
Use of Medical Imaging				
Combination Abdominal CT Scan	929	0.083	0.160	0.191
Combination Chest CT Scan	522	0.080	0.054	0.054
Follow-up Mammogram/Ultrasound	1,149	8.4%	7.9%	8.4%
MRI for Low Back Pain	268	40.3%	35.6%	32.7%
Survey of Patients' Hospital Experiences				
Area Around Room 'Always' Quiet at Night	300+	73%	-	58%
Doctors 'Always' Communicated Well	300+	86%	-	80%
Home Recovery Information Given	300+	83%	-	82%
Hospital Given 9 or 10 on 10 Point Scale	300+	78%	-	67%
Meds 'Always' Explained Before Given	300+	67%	-	60%
Nurses 'Always' Communicated Well	300+	84%	-	76%
Pain 'Always' Well Controlled	300+	76%	-	69%
Room and Bathroom 'Always' Clean	300+	78%	-	71%
Timely Help 'Always' Received	300+	70%	-	64%
Would Definitely Recommend Hospital	300+	79%	-	69%

NOTE: Hospital profiles are in alphabetical order by state, then city, then hospital within the city; Rankings exclude hospitals with less than 25 cases except for patient surveys which excludes hospitals with less than 100 cases; (a) 100–299 cases; (1) The number of cases is too small to be sure how well a hospital is performing; (2) The hospital indicated that the data submitted for this measure were based on a sample of cases; (3) Data was collected during a shorter time period (fewer quarters) than the maximum possible time for this measure; (4) Suppressed for one or more quarters by CMS; (5) No data is available from the hospital for this measure; (6) Fewer than 100 patients completed the HCAHPS survey. Use these rates with caution, as the number of surveys may be too low to reliably assess hospital performance; (7) Survey results are based on less than 12 months of data; (8) Survey results are not available for this reporting period; (9) No or very few patients were eligible for the HCAHPS survey. The scores shown, if any, reflect a very small number of surveys; (10) A state average was not calculated because too few hospitals in the state submitted data; (11) There were discrepancies in the data collection process; Please refer to the User's Guide for a full explanation of data.

Knox County Hospital

80 Hospital Drive
Barbourville, KY 40906
E-mail: webmaster@knoxcohospital.com
URL: www.knoxcohospital.com
Type: Critical Access Hospitals
Ownership: Proprietary

Phone: 606-546-4175
Fax: 606-545-5511

Emergency Services: Yes
Beds: 58

Key Personnel:
CEO/President . . . . Rebecca Lewis
Quality Assurance . . . . Rita Hammons
Radiology . . . . Mike Standifer

Measure	Cases	This Hosp.	State Avg.	U.S. Avg.
Heart Attack Care				
ACE Inhibitor or ARB for LVSD	0	-	94%	96%
Aspirin at Arrival[1]	11	100%	98%	99%
Aspirin at Discharge[1]	6	100%	99%	98%
Beta Blocker at Discharge[1]	8	88%	98%	98%
Fibrinolytic Medication Timing	0	-	60%	55%
PCI Within 90 Minutes of Arrival	0	-	88%	90%
Smoking Cessation Advice[1]	2	50%	100%	99%
Chest Pain/Possible Heart Attack Care				
Aspirin at Arrival	-	-	95%	95%
Median Time to ECG (minutes)	-	-	7	8
Median Time to Transfer (minutes)	-	-	65	61
Fibrinolytic Medication Timing	-	-	62%	54%
Heart Failure Care				
ACE Inhibitor or ARB for LVSD[1]	12	75%	91%	94%
Discharge Instructions	43	58%	82%	88%
Evaluation of LVS Function	49	73%	96%	98%
Smoking Cessation Advice[1]	10	100%	98%	98%
Pneumonia Care				
Appropriate Initial Antibiotic	63	70%	90%	92%
Blood Culture Timing	54	94%	95%	96%
Influenza Vaccine	48	100%	92%	91%
Initial Antibiotic Timing	78	94%	95%	95%
Pneumococcal Vaccine	60	97%	94%	93%
Smoking Cessation Advice	37	89%	98%	97%
Surgical Care Improvement Project				
Appropriate VTP Within 24 Hours[1,3]	3	67%	91%	92%
Appropriate Hair Removal[1,3]	5	60%	99%	99%
Appropriate Beta Blocker Usage[1,3]	1	0%	93%	93%
Controlled Postoperative Blood Glucose[3]	0	-	94%	93%
Prophylactic Antibiotic Timing[1,3]	2	50%	97%	97%
Prophylactic Antibiotic Timing (Outpatient)	-	-	92%	92%
Prophylactic Antibiotic Selection[1,3]	2	50%	98%	97%
Prophylactic Antibiotic Select. (Outpatient)	-	-	93%	94%
Prophylactic Antibiotic Stopped[1,3]	2	50%	94%	94%
Recommended VTP Ordered[1,3]	3	67%	94%	94%
Urinary Catheter Removal[1,3]	1	100%	89%	90%
Children's Asthma Care				
Received Systemic Corticosteroids	-	-	-	100%
Received Home Management Plan	-	-	-	71%
Received Reliever Medication	-	-	-	100%
Use of Medical Imaging				
Combination Abdominal CT Scan	-	-	0.160	0.191
Combination Chest CT Scan	-	-	0.054	0.054
Follow-up Mammogram/Ultrasound	-	-	7.9%	8.4%
MRI for Low Back Pain	-	-	35.6%	32.7%
Survey of Patients' Hospital Experiences				
Area Around Room 'Always' Quiet at Night[8]	-	-	-	58%
Doctors 'Always' Communicated Well[8]	-	-	-	80%
Home Recovery Information Given[8]	-	-	-	82%
Hospital Given 9 or 10 on 10 Point Scale[8]	-	-	-	67%
Meds 'Always' Explained Before Given[8]	-	-	-	60%
Nurses 'Always' Communicated Well[8]	-	-	-	76%
Pain 'Always' Well Controlled[8]	-	-	-	69%
Room and Bathroom 'Always' Clean[8]	-	-	-	71%
Timely Help 'Always' Received[8]	-	-	-	64%
Would Definitely Recommend Hospital[8]	-	-	-	69%

Flaget Memorial Hospital

4305 New Shepherdsville Road
Bardstown, KY 40004
URL: www.flaget.com
Type: Acute Care Hospitals
Ownership: Voluntary Non-Profit - Private

Phone: 502-350-5000
Fax: 502-350-5036

Emergency Services: Yes
Beds: 52

Key Personnel:
CEO/President . . . . Bruce Klotkarh
Chief of Medical Staff . . . . Mark Abraham, MD
Quality Assurance . . . . Cheri Davidson
Emergency Room . . . . Clara Powell, RN

Measure	Cases	This Hosp.	State Avg.	U.S. Avg.
Heart Attack Care				
ACE Inhibitor or ARB for LVSD	0	-	94%	96%
Aspirin at Arrival[1]	19	95%	98%	99%
Aspirin at Discharge[1]	12	83%	99%	98%
Beta Blocker at Discharge[1]	11	100%	98%	98%
Fibrinolytic Medication Timing	0	-	60%	55%
PCI Within 90 Minutes of Arrival	0	-	88%	90%
Smoking Cessation Advice[1]	1	100%	100%	99%
Chest Pain/Possible Heart Attack Care				
Aspirin at Arrival	225	95%	95%	95%
Median Time to ECG (minutes)	228	12	7	8
Median Time to Transfer (minutes)[1,3]	1	132	65	61
Fibrinolytic Medication Timing[1]	13	77%	62%	54%
Heart Failure Care				
ACE Inhibitor or ARB for LVSD[1]	16	81%	91%	94%
Discharge Instructions	43	84%	82%	88%
Evaluation of LVS Function	52	98%	96%	98%
Smoking Cessation Advice[1]	13	100%	98%	98%
Pneumonia Care				
Appropriate Initial Antibiotic	85	96%	90%	92%
Blood Culture Timing	106	92%	95%	96%
Influenza Vaccine	66	94%	92%	91%
Initial Antibiotic Timing	100	95%	95%	95%
Pneumococcal Vaccine	83	95%	94%	93%
Smoking Cessation Advice	54	100%	98%	97%
Surgical Care Improvement Project				
Appropriate VTP Within 24 Hours	74	95%	91%	92%
Appropriate Hair Removal	301	100%	99%	99%
Appropriate Beta Blocker Usage	98	87%	93%	93%
Controlled Postoperative Blood Glucose	0	-	94%	93%
Prophylactic Antibiotic Timing	223	97%	97%	97%
Prophylactic Antibiotic Timing (Outpatient)	95	94%	92%	92%
Prophylactic Antibiotic Selection	223	99%	98%	97%
Prophylactic Antibiotic Select. (Outpatient)	91	87%	93%	94%
Prophylactic Antibiotic Stopped	220	97%	94%	94%
Recommended VTP Ordered	74	97%	94%	94%
Urinary Catheter Removal	90	97%	89%	90%
Children's Asthma Care				
Received Systemic Corticosteroids	-	-	-	100%
Received Home Management Plan	-	-	-	71%
Received Reliever Medication	-	-	-	100%
Use of Medical Imaging				
Combination Abdominal CT Scan	407	0.047	0.160	0.191
Combination Chest CT Scan	290	0.000	0.054	0.054
Follow-up Mammogram/Ultrasound	464	8.8%	7.9%	8.4%
MRI for Low Back Pain	117	42.7%	35.6%	32.7%
Survey of Patients' Hospital Experiences				
Area Around Room 'Always' Quiet at Night	300+	59%	-	58%
Doctors 'Always' Communicated Well	300+	82%	-	80%
Home Recovery Information Given	300+	86%	-	82%
Hospital Given 9 or 10 on 10 Point Scale	300+	74%	-	67%
Meds 'Always' Explained Before Given	300+	67%	-	60%
Nurses 'Always' Communicated Well	300+	78%	-	76%
Pain 'Always' Well Controlled	300+	74%	-	69%
Room and Bathroom 'Always' Clean	300+	75%	-	71%
Timely Help 'Always' Received	300+	72%	-	64%
Would Definitely Recommend Hospital	300+	73%	-	69%

Marshall County Hospital

615 Old Symsonia Road
Benton, KY 42025
Type: Critical Access Hospitals
Ownership: Govt - Hospital Dist/Auth

Phone: 270-527-4800
Fax: 270-527-4853

Emergency Services: Yes
Beds: 80

Key Personnel:
CEO/President . . . . Kathy Long
Chief of Medical Staff . . . . Glen Van Loon, MD
Coronary Care . . . . Lisa Bowlin
Infection Control . . . . Mary Jo Myers
Operating Room . . . . Robert Beale
Quality Assurance . . . . Lisa Bowlin
Emergency Room . . . . Sharon Sirls
Intensive Care Unit . . . . Lisa Bowlin

Measure	Cases	This Hosp.	State Avg.	U.S. Avg.
Heart Attack Care				
ACE Inhibitor or ARB for LVSD[3]	0	-	94%	96%
Aspirin at Arrival[1,3]	5	60%	98%	99%
Aspirin at Discharge[1,3]	2	50%	99%	98%
Beta Blocker at Discharge[1,3]	3	33%	98%	98%
Fibrinolytic Medication Timing[5]	0	-	60%	55%
PCI Within 90 Minutes of Arrival[5]	0	-	88%	90%
Smoking Cessation Advice[3]	0	-	100%	99%
Chest Pain/Possible Heart Attack Care				
Aspirin at Arrival	-	-	95%	95%
Median Time to ECG (minutes)	-	-	7	8
Median Time to Transfer (minutes)	-	-	65	61
Fibrinolytic Medication Timing	-	-	62%	54%
Heart Failure Care				
ACE Inhibitor or ARB for LVSD[1]	3	33%	91%	94%
Discharge Instructions	25	44%	82%	88%
Evaluation of LVS Function	41	54%	96%	98%
Smoking Cessation Advice[1]	7	57%	98%	98%
Pneumonia Care				
Appropriate Initial Antibiotic[1,2,3]	19	74%	90%	92%
Blood Culture Timing[1,2]	20	70%	95%	96%
Influenza Vaccine[1,2]	15	60%	92%	91%
Initial Antibiotic Timing[1,2]	22	82%	95%	95%
Pneumococcal Vaccine[1,2]	22	55%	94%	93%
Smoking Cessation Advice[1,2]	9	44%	98%	97%
Surgical Care Improvement Project				
Appropriate VTP Within 24 Hours[5]	0	-	91%	92%
Appropriate Hair Removal[5]	0	-	99%	99%
Appropriate Beta Blocker Usage[5]	0	-	93%	93%
Controlled Postoperative Blood Glucose[5]	0	-	94%	93%
Prophylactic Antibiotic Timing[5]	0	-	97%	97%
Prophylactic Antibiotic Timing (Outpatient)	-	-	92%	92%
Prophylactic Antibiotic Selection[5]	0	-	98%	97%
Prophylactic Antibiotic Select. (Outpatient)	-	-	93%	94%
Prophylactic Antibiotic Stopped[5]	0	-	94%	94%
Recommended VTP Ordered[5]	0	-	94%	94%
Urinary Catheter Removal[5]	0	-	89%	90%
Children's Asthma Care				
Received Systemic Corticosteroids	-	-	-	100%
Received Home Management Plan	-	-	-	71%
Received Reliever Medication	-	-	-	100%
Use of Medical Imaging				
Combination Abdominal CT Scan	-	-	0.160	0.191
Combination Chest CT Scan	-	-	0.054	0.054
Follow-up Mammogram/Ultrasound	-	-	7.9%	8.4%
MRI for Low Back Pain	-	-	35.6%	32.7%
Survey of Patients' Hospital Experiences				
Area Around Room 'Always' Quiet at Night[8]	-	-	-	58%
Doctors 'Always' Communicated Well[8]	-	-	-	80%
Home Recovery Information Given[8]	-	-	-	82%
Hospital Given 9 or 10 on 10 Point Scale[8]	-	-	-	67%
Meds 'Always' Explained Before Given[8]	-	-	-	60%
Nurses 'Always' Communicated Well[8]	-	-	-	76%
Pain 'Always' Well Controlled[8]	-	-	-	69%
Room and Bathroom 'Always' Clean[8]	-	-	-	71%
Timely Help 'Always' Received[8]	-	-	-	64%
Would Definitely Recommend Hospital[8]	-	-	-	69%

NOTE: Hospital profiles are in alphabetical order by state, then city, then hospital within the city; Rankings exclude hospitals with less than 25 cases except for patient surveys which excludes hospitals with less than 100 cases; (a) 100–299 cases; (1) The number of cases is too small to be sure how well a hospital is performing; (2) The hospital indicated that the data submitted for this measure was based on a sample of cases; (3) Data was collected during a shorter time period (fewer quarters) than the maximum possible time for this measure; (4) Suppressed for one or more quarters by CMS; (5) No data is available from the hospital for this measure; (6) Fewer than 100 patients completed the HCAHPS survey. Use these rates with caution, as the number of surveys may be too low to reliably assess hospital performance; (7) Survey results are based on less than 12 months of data; (8) Survey results are not available for this reporting period; (9) No or very few patients were eligible for the HCAHPS survey. The scores shown, if any, reflect a very small number of surveys; (10) A state average was not calculated because too few hospitals in the state submitted data; (11) There were discrepancies in the data collection process; Please refer to the User's Guide for a full explanation of data.

Saint Joseph Berea

305 Estill Street
Berea, KY 40403
Phone: 859-986-6500
Fax: 859-986-6768
E-mail: info@bereahospital.org
URL: www.bereahospital.org
Type: Critical Access Hospitals
Emergency Services: Yes
Ownership: Voluntary Non-Profit - Private
Beds: 48

Key Personnel:
CEO/President. . . . . Greg Gerard
Chief of Medical Staff . . . . Saves Desai MD
Infection Control. . . . . Helen Rice
Operating Room. . . . . Kent Kessler
Quality Assurance . . . . Darlene Matekovich
Emergency Room . . . . John Mullins MD
Intensive Care Unit. . . . . Mary Kemper
Patient Relations . . . . Katie Heckman

Measure	Cases	This Hosp.	State Avg.	U.S. Avg.
Heart Attack Care				
ACE Inhibitor or ARB for LVSD[1]	2	100%	94%	96%
Aspirin at Arrival[1]	6	100%	98%	99%
Aspirin at Discharge[1]	3	100%	99%	98%
Beta Blocker at Discharge[1]	5	100%	98%	98%
Fibrinolytic Medication Timing	0	-	60%	55%
PCI Within 90 Minutes of Arrival	0	-	88%	90%
Smoking Cessation Advice[1]	3	100%	100%	99%
Chest Pain/Possible Heart Attack Care				
Aspirin at Arrival	-	-	95%	95%
Median Time to ECG (minutes)	-	-	7	8
Median Time to Transfer (minutes)	-	-	65	61
Fibrinolytic Medication Timing	-	-	62%	54%
Heart Failure Care				
ACE Inhibitor or ARB for LVSD[1]	14	100%	91%	94%
Discharge Instructions	30	80%	82%	88%
Evaluation of LVS Function	38	97%	96%	98%
Smoking Cessation Advice[1]	11	100%	98%	98%
Pneumonia Care				
Appropriate Initial Antibiotic	39	87%	90%	92%
Blood Culture Timing	33	100%	95%	96%
Influenza Vaccine	42	98%	92%	91%
Initial Antibiotic Timing	56	100%	95%	95%
Pneumococcal Vaccine	46	100%	94%	93%
Smoking Cessation Advice	38	100%	98%	97%
Surgical Care Improvement Project				
Appropriate VTP Within 24 Hours	26	92%	91%	92%
Appropriate Hair Removal	41	100%	99%	99%
Appropriate Beta Blocker Usage[1]	10	100%	93%	93%
Controlled Postoperative Blood Glucose	0	-	94%	93%
Prophylactic Antibiotic Timing	27	100%	97%	97%
Prophylactic Antibiotic Timing (Outpatient)	-	-	92%	92%
Prophylactic Antibiotic Selection	27	100%	98%	97%
Prophylactic Antibiotic Select. (Outpatient)	-	-	93%	94%
Prophylactic Antibiotic Stopped	26	96%	94%	94%
Recommended VTP Ordered	26	100%	94%	94%
Urinary Catheter Removal[1]	5	100%	89%	90%
Children's Asthma Care				
Received Systemic Corticosteroids	-	-	-	100%
Received Home Management Plan	-	-	-	71%
Received Reliever Medication	-	-	-	100%
Use of Medical Imaging				
Combination Abdominal CT Scan	-	-	0.160	0.191
Combination Chest CT Scan	-	-	0.054	0.054
Follow-up Mammogram/Ultrasound	-	-	7.9%	8.4%
MRI for Low Back Pain	-	-	35.6%	32.7%
Survey of Patients' Hospital Experiences				
Area Around Room 'Always' Quiet at Night	300+	67%	-	58%
Doctors 'Always' Communicated Well	300+	86%	-	80%
Home Recovery Information Given	300+	84%	-	82%
Hospital Given 9 or 10 on 10 Point Scale	300+	76%	-	67%
Meds 'Always' Explained Before Given	300+	64%	-	60%
Nurses 'Always' Communicated Well	300+	82%	-	76%
Pain 'Always' Well Controlled	300+	72%	-	69%
Room and Bathroom 'Always' Clean	300+	73%	-	71%
Timely Help 'Always' Received	300+	70%	-	64%
Would Definitely Recommend Hospital	300+	79%	-	69%

Greenview Regional Hospital

1801 Ashley Circle
Bowling Green, KY 42104
Phone: 270-793-1000
URL: greenviewhospital.com
Type: Acute Care Hospitals
Emergency Services: Yes
Ownership: Proprietary
Beds: 211

Key Personnel:
CEO . . . . Mark Marsh

Measure	Cases	This Hosp.	State Avg.	U.S. Avg.
Heart Attack Care				
ACE Inhibitor or ARB for LVSD	0	-	94%	96%
Aspirin at Arrival	29	100%	98%	99%
Aspirin at Discharge[1]	20	100%	99%	98%
Beta Blocker at Discharge[1]	22	95%	98%	98%
Fibrinolytic Medication Timing	0	-	60%	55%
PCI Within 90 Minutes of Arrival[1]	1	100%	88%	90%
Smoking Cessation Advice[1]	9	100%	100%	99%
Chest Pain/Possible Heart Attack Care				
Aspirin at Arrival[1]	13	100%	95%	95%
Median Time to ECG (minutes)[1]	13	5	7	8
Median Time to Transfer (minutes)[1,3]	3	65	65	61
Fibrinolytic Medication Timing	0	-	62%	54%
Heart Failure Care				
ACE Inhibitor or ARB for LVSD[1]	20	100%	91%	94%
Discharge Instructions	67	100%	82%	88%
Evaluation of LVS Function	96	100%	96%	98%
Smoking Cessation Advice[1]	11	100%	98%	98%
Pneumonia Care				
Appropriate Initial Antibiotic	76	99%	90%	92%
Blood Culture Timing	100	98%	95%	96%
Influenza Vaccine	67	100%	92%	91%
Initial Antibiotic Timing	117	97%	95%	95%
Pneumococcal Vaccine	86	100%	94%	93%
Smoking Cessation Advice	68	100%	98%	97%
Surgical Care Improvement Project				
Appropriate VTP Within 24 Hours	156	96%	91%	92%
Appropriate Hair Removal	450	100%	99%	99%
Appropriate Beta Blocker Usage	160	98%	93%	93%
Controlled Postoperative Blood Glucose	0	-	94%	93%
Prophylactic Antibiotic Timing	355	100%	97%	97%
Prophylactic Antibiotic Timing (Outpatient)	168	96%	92%	92%
Prophylactic Antibiotic Selection	356	99%	98%	97%
Prophylactic Antibiotic Select. (Outpatient)	166	98%	93%	94%
Prophylactic Antibiotic Stopped	342	98%	94%	94%
Recommended VTP Ordered	156	99%	94%	94%
Urinary Catheter Removal	180	98%	89%	90%
Children's Asthma Care				
Received Systemic Corticosteroids	-	-	-	100%
Received Home Management Plan	-	-	-	71%
Received Reliever Medication	-	-	-	100%
Use of Medical Imaging				
Combination Abdominal CT Scan	514	0.436	0.160	0.191
Combination Chest CT Scan	186	0.086	0.054	0.054
Follow-up Mammogram/Ultrasound	287	10.8%	7.9%	8.4%
MRI for Low Back Pain	73	27.4%	35.6%	32.7%
Survey of Patients' Hospital Experiences				
Area Around Room 'Always' Quiet at Night	300+	65%	-	58%
Doctors 'Always' Communicated Well	300+	84%	-	80%
Home Recovery Information Given	300+	85%	-	82%
Hospital Given 9 or 10 on 10 Point Scale	300+	73%	-	67%
Meds 'Always' Explained Before Given	300+	66%	-	60%
Nurses 'Always' Communicated Well	300+	79%	-	76%
Pain 'Always' Well Controlled	300+	71%	-	69%
Room and Bathroom 'Always' Clean	300+	74%	-	71%
Timely Help 'Always' Received	300+	62%	-	64%
Would Definitely Recommend Hospital	300+	76%	-	69%

The Medical Center at Bowling Green

250 Park Street
Bowling Green, KY 42101
Phone: 270-745-1000
Fax: 270-745-1253
E-mail: SKWebb@mcbg.org
URL: www.mcbg.org
Type: Acute Care Hospitals
Emergency Services: Yes
Ownership: Voluntary Non-Profit - Private
Beds: 330

Key Personnel:
CEO/President. . . . . Connie Smith, MD
Pediatric Ambulatory Care . . . . . . Zahid Fraser, MD
Pediatric In-Patient Care . . . . Zahid Fraser, MD
Quality Assurance . . . . Gerri Glenn
Radiology. . . . . Ken Bartholomew, MD
Hemotology Center . . . . Sandy Durrance, RN
Intensive Care Unit. . . . . Barbara Wolfe, RN

Measure	Cases	This Hosp.	State Avg.	U.S. Avg.
Heart Attack Care				
ACE Inhibitor or ARB for LVSD	55	82%	94%	96%
Aspirin at Arrival	218	96%	98%	99%
Aspirin at Discharge	297	97%	99%	98%
Beta Blocker at Discharge	281	95%	98%	98%
Fibrinolytic Medication Timing	0	-	60%	55%
PCI Within 90 Minutes of Arrival	49	86%	88%	90%
Smoking Cessation Advice	149	99%	100%	99%
Chest Pain/Possible Heart Attack Care				
Aspirin at Arrival[1]	19	79%	95%	95%
Median Time to ECG (minutes)[1]	20	10	7	8
Median Time to Transfer (minutes)[5]	0	-	65	61
Fibrinolytic Medication Timing[5]	0	-	62%	54%
Heart Failure Care				
ACE Inhibitor or ARB for LVSD	183	77%	91%	94%
Discharge Instructions	490	64%	82%	88%
Evaluation of LVS Function	593	95%	96%	98%
Smoking Cessation Advice	138	100%	98%	98%
Pneumonia Care				
Appropriate Initial Antibiotic	217	86%	90%	92%
Blood Culture Timing	258	95%	95%	96%
Influenza Vaccine	316	93%	92%	91%
Initial Antibiotic Timing	338	93%	95%	95%
Pneumococcal Vaccine	380	96%	94%	93%
Smoking Cessation Advice	199	100%	98%	97%
Surgical Care Improvement Project				
Appropriate VTP Within 24 Hours	402	84%	91%	92%
Appropriate Hair Removal	1,480	100%	99%	99%
Appropriate Beta Blocker Usage	461	79%	93%	93%
Controlled Postoperative Blood Glucose	245	92%	94%	93%
Prophylactic Antibiotic Timing	979	96%	97%	97%
Prophylactic Antibiotic Timing (Outpatient)	540	82%	92%	92%
Prophylactic Antibiotic Selection	987	97%	98%	97%
Prophylactic Antibiotic Select. (Outpatient)	483	92%	93%	94%
Prophylactic Antibiotic Stopped	957	96%	94%	94%
Recommended VTP Ordered	405	85%	94%	94%
Urinary Catheter Removal	377	94%	89%	90%
Children's Asthma Care				
Received Systemic Corticosteroids	-	-	-	100%
Received Home Management Plan	-	-	-	71%
Received Reliever Medication	-	-	-	100%
Use of Medical Imaging				
Combination Abdominal CT Scan	897	0.064	0.160	0.191
Combination Chest CT Scan	417	0.175	0.054	0.054
Follow-up Mammogram/Ultrasound	803	5.1%	7.9%	8.4%
MRI for Low Back Pain	150	34.7%	35.6%	32.7%
Survey of Patients' Hospital Experiences				
Area Around Room 'Always' Quiet at Night	300+	60%	-	58%
Doctors 'Always' Communicated Well	300+	81%	-	80%
Home Recovery Information Given	300+	85%	-	82%
Hospital Given 9 or 10 on 10 Point Scale	300+	69%	-	67%
Meds 'Always' Explained Before Given	300+	60%	-	60%
Nurses 'Always' Communicated Well	300+	77%	-	76%
Pain 'Always' Well Controlled	300+	70%	-	69%
Room and Bathroom 'Always' Clean	300+	69%	-	71%
Timely Help 'Always' Received	300+	65%	-	64%
Would Definitely Recommend Hospital	300+	74%	-	69%

NOTE: Hospital profiles are in alphabetical order by state, then city, then hospital within the city; Rankings exclude hospitals with less than 25 cases except for patient surveys which excludes hospitals with less than 100 cases; (a) 100–299 cases; (1) The number of cases is too small to be sure how well a hospital is performing; (2) The hospital indicated that the data submitted for this measure were based on a sample of cases; (3) Data was collected during a shorter time period (fewer quarters) than the maximum possible time for this measure; (4) Suppressed for one or more quarters by CMS; (5) No data is available from the hospital for this measure; (6) Fewer than 100 patients completed the HCAHPS survey. Use these rates with caution, as the number of surveys may be too low to reliably assess hospital performance; (7) Survey results are based on less than 12 months of data; (8) Survey results are not available for this reporting period; (9) No or very few patients were eligible for the HCAHPS survey. The scores shown, if any, reflect a very small number of surveys; (10) A state average was not calculated because too few hospitals in the state submitted data; (11) There were discrepancies in the data collection process; Please refer to the User's Guide for a full explanation of data.

Cumberland County Hospital

299 Glasgow Road
Burkesville, KY 42717
Phone: 270-864-2511
Fax: 270-864-1307
E-mail: administration@cchospital.org
URL: www.cumberlandhospital.org
Type: Critical Access Hospitals
Emergency Services: Yes
Ownership: Voluntary Non-Profit - Other
Beds: 31

Key Personnel:
CEO/President. . . . . Edward J Sanford

Measure	Cases	This Hosp.	State Avg.	U.S. Avg.
Heart Attack Care				
ACE Inhibitor or ARB for LVSD[1]	1	100%	94%	96%
Aspirin at Arrival[1]	5	100%	98%	99%
Aspirin at Discharge[1]	3	100%	99%	98%
Beta Blocker at Discharge[1]	3	67%	98%	98%
Fibrinolytic Medication Timing	0	-	60%	55%
PCI Within 90 Minutes of Arrival	0	-	88%	90%
Smoking Cessation Advice	0	-	100%	99%
Chest Pain/Possible Heart Attack Care				
Aspirin at Arrival	-	-	95%	95%
Median Time to ECG (minutes)	-	-	7	8
Median Time to Transfer (minutes)	-	-	65	61
Fibrinolytic Medication Timing	-	-	62%	54%
Heart Failure Care				
ACE Inhibitor or ARB for LVSD[1]	2	50%	91%	94%
Discharge Instructions	38	37%	82%	88%
Evaluation of LVS Function	53	32%	96%	98%
Smoking Cessation Advice[1]	11	45%	98%	98%
Pneumonia Care				
Appropriate Initial Antibiotic[1]	14	71%	90%	92%
Blood Culture Timing[1]	6	100%	95%	96%
Influenza Vaccine	31	87%	92%	91%
Initial Antibiotic Timing	45	76%	95%	95%
Pneumococcal Vaccine	40	80%	94%	93%
Smoking Cessation Advice	34	68%	98%	97%
Surgical Care Improvement Project				
Appropriate VTP Within 24 Hours[5]	0	-	91%	92%
Appropriate Hair Removal[5]	0	-	99%	99%
Appropriate Beta Blocker Usage[5]	0	-	93%	93%
Controlled Postoperative Blood Glucose[5]	0	-	94%	93%
Prophylactic Antibiotic Timing[5]	0	-	97%	97%
Prophylactic Antibiotic Timing (Outpatient)	-	-	92%	92%
Prophylactic Antibiotic Selection[5]	0	-	98%	97%
Prophylactic Antibiotic Select. (Outpatient)	-	-	93%	94%
Prophylactic Antibiotic Stopped[5]	0	-	94%	94%
Recommended VTP Ordered[5]	0	-	94%	94%
Urinary Catheter Removal[5]	0	-	89%	90%
Children's Asthma Care				
Received Systemic Corticosteroids	-	-	-	100%
Received Home Management Plan	-	-	-	71%
Received Reliever Medication	-	-	-	100%
Use of Medical Imaging				
Combination Abdominal CT Scan	-	-	0.160	0.191
Combination Chest CT Scan	-	-	0.054	0.054
Follow-up Mammogram/Ultrasound	-	-	7.9%	8.4%
MRI for Low Back Pain	-	-	35.6%	32.7%
Survey of Patients' Hospital Experiences				
Area Around Room 'Always' Quiet at Night[8]	-	-	-	58%
Doctors 'Always' Communicated Well[8]	-	-	-	80%
Home Recovery Information Given[8]	-	-	-	82%
Hospital Given 9 or 10 on 10 Point Scale[8]	-	-	-	67%
Meds 'Always' Explained Before Given[8]	-	-	-	60%
Nurses 'Always' Communicated Well[8]	-	-	-	76%
Pain 'Always' Well Controlled[8]	-	-	-	69%
Room and Bathroom 'Always' Clean[8]	-	-	-	71%
Timely Help 'Always' Received[8]	-	-	-	64%
Would Definitely Recommend Hospital[8]	-	-	-	69%

Trigg County Hospital

254 Main Street
Cadiz, KY 42211
Phone: 270-522-3215
Fax: 270-522-6974
URL: www.trigghospital.org
Type: Critical Access Hospitals
Emergency Services: Yes
Ownership: Government - Local
Beds: 25

Key Personnel:
CEO/President. . . . . Alisa Coleman
Cardiac Laboratory. . . . . George Howe
Chief of Medical Staff . . . . Stuart Harris, MD
Infection Control. . . . . Susanna May
Operating Room. . . . . Susanna May
Radiology. . . . . Jill Cunningham
Emergency Room . . . . Frieda Wood
Patient Relations . . . . Nicole Reamer

Measure	Cases	This Hosp.	State Avg.	U.S. Avg.
Heart Attack Care				
ACE Inhibitor or ARB for LVSD[5]	0	-	94%	96%
Aspirin at Arrival[5]	0	-	98%	99%
Aspirin at Discharge[5]	0	-	99%	98%
Beta Blocker at Discharge[5]	0	-	98%	98%
Fibrinolytic Medication Timing[5]	0	-	60%	55%
PCI Within 90 Minutes of Arrival[5]	0	-	88%	90%
Smoking Cessation Advice[5]	0	-	100%	99%
Chest Pain/Possible Heart Attack Care				
Aspirin at Arrival	-	-	95%	95%
Median Time to ECG (minutes)	-	-	7	8
Median Time to Transfer (minutes)	-	-	65	61
Fibrinolytic Medication Timing	-	-	62%	54%
Heart Failure Care				
ACE Inhibitor or ARB for LVSD[1]	2	50%	91%	94%
Discharge Instructions[1]	13	100%	82%	88%
Evaluation of LVS Function[1]	24	29%	96%	98%
Smoking Cessation Advice[1]	5	100%	98%	98%
Pneumonia Care				
Appropriate Initial Antibiotic[2]	32	91%	90%	92%
Blood Culture Timing[1,2]	11	82%	95%	96%
Influenza Vaccine[1,2]	15	93%	92%	91%
Initial Antibiotic Timing[2]	36	97%	95%	95%
Pneumococcal Vaccine[2]	26	92%	94%	93%
Smoking Cessation Advice[1,2]	10	100%	98%	97%
Surgical Care Improvement Project				
Appropriate VTP Within 24 Hours[5]	0	-	91%	92%
Appropriate Hair Removal[5]	0	-	99%	99%
Appropriate Beta Blocker Usage[5]	0	-	93%	93%
Controlled Postoperative Blood Glucose[5]	0	-	94%	93%
Prophylactic Antibiotic Timing[5]	0	-	97%	97%
Prophylactic Antibiotic Timing (Outpatient)	-	-	92%	92%
Prophylactic Antibiotic Selection[5]	0	-	98%	97%
Prophylactic Antibiotic Select. (Outpatient)	-	-	93%	94%
Prophylactic Antibiotic Stopped[5]	0	-	94%	94%
Recommended VTP Ordered[5]	0	-	94%	94%
Urinary Catheter Removal[5]	0	-	89%	90%
Children's Asthma Care				
Received Systemic Corticosteroids	-	-	-	100%
Received Home Management Plan	-	-	-	71%
Received Reliever Medication	-	-	-	100%
Use of Medical Imaging				
Combination Abdominal CT Scan	-	-	0.160	0.191
Combination Chest CT Scan	-	-	0.054	0.054
Follow-up Mammogram/Ultrasound	-	-	7.9%	8.4%
MRI for Low Back Pain	-	-	35.6%	32.7%
Survey of Patients' Hospital Experiences				
Area Around Room 'Always' Quiet at Night[6]	<100	60%	-	58%
Doctors 'Always' Communicated Well[6]	<100	81%	-	80%
Home Recovery Information Given[6]	<100	67%	-	82%
Hospital Given 9 or 10 on 10 Point Scale[6]	<100	60%	-	67%
Meds 'Always' Explained Before Given[6]	<100	66%	-	60%
Nurses 'Always' Communicated Well[6]	<100	80%	-	76%
Pain 'Always' Well Controlled[6]	<100	68%	-	69%
Room and Bathroom 'Always' Clean[6]	<100	75%	-	71%
Timely Help 'Always' Received[6]	<100	67%	-	64%
Would Definitely Recommend Hospital	<100	64%	-	69%

Taylor Regional Hospital

1700 Old Lebanon Road
Campbellsville, KY 42718
Phone: 270-465-3561
Fax: 270-789-5875
URL: www.tchosp.org
Type: Acute Care Hospitals
Emergency Services: Yes
Ownership: Govt - Hospital Dist/Auth
Beds: 90

Key Personnel:
CEO/President. . . . . Jane Wheatley
Chief of Medical Staff . . . . Gary Frazier
Radiology. . . . . Curtis Manning

Measure	Cases	This Hosp.	State Avg.	U.S. Avg.
Heart Attack Care				
ACE Inhibitor or ARB for LVSD[1]	3	67%	94%	96%
Aspirin at Arrival[1]	21	86%	98%	99%
Aspirin at Discharge[1]	8	88%	99%	98%
Beta Blocker at Discharge[1]	11	64%	98%	98%
Fibrinolytic Medication Timing	0	-	60%	55%
PCI Within 90 Minutes of Arrival	0	-	88%	90%
Smoking Cessation Advice[1]	4	100%	100%	99%
Chest Pain/Possible Heart Attack Care				
Aspirin at Arrival	143	94%	95%	95%
Median Time to ECG (minutes)	147	11	7	8
Median Time to Transfer (minutes)[1,3]	3	105	65	61
Fibrinolytic Medication Timing[1]	21	62%	62%	54%
Heart Failure Care				
ACE Inhibitor or ARB for LVSD[1,2]	16	88%	91%	94%
Discharge Instructions[2]	53	75%	82%	88%
Evaluation of LVS Function[2]	64	92%	96%	98%
Smoking Cessation Advice[1,2]	15	100%	98%	98%
Pneumonia Care				
Appropriate Initial Antibiotic	98	81%	90%	92%
Blood Culture Timing	103	97%	95%	96%
Influenza Vaccine	107	68%	92%	91%
Initial Antibiotic Timing	128	87%	95%	95%
Pneumococcal Vaccine	134	76%	94%	93%
Smoking Cessation Advice	67	84%	98%	97%
Surgical Care Improvement Project				
Appropriate VTP Within 24 Hours	97	89%	91%	92%
Appropriate Hair Removal	223	94%	99%	99%
Appropriate Beta Blocker Usage	45	80%	93%	93%
Controlled Postoperative Blood Glucose	0	-	94%	93%
Prophylactic Antibiotic Timing	135	95%	97%	97%
Prophylactic Antibiotic Timing (Outpatient)	77	87%	92%	92%
Prophylactic Antibiotic Selection	134	96%	98%	97%
Prophylactic Antibiotic Select. (Outpatient)	73	97%	93%	94%
Prophylactic Antibiotic Stopped	133	89%	94%	94%
Recommended VTP Ordered	98	90%	94%	94%
Urinary Catheter Removal[1]	16	75%	89%	90%
Children's Asthma Care				
Received Systemic Corticosteroids	-	-	-	100%
Received Home Management Plan	-	-	-	71%
Received Reliever Medication	-	-	-	100%
Use of Medical Imaging				
Combination Abdominal CT Scan	694	0.414	0.160	0.191
Combination Chest CT Scan	537	0.006	0.054	0.054
Follow-up Mammogram/Ultrasound	911	17.0%	7.9%	8.4%
MRI for Low Back Pain	159	23.9%	35.6%	32.7%
Survey of Patients' Hospital Experiences				
Area Around Room 'Always' Quiet at Night	300+	58%	-	58%
Doctors 'Always' Communicated Well	300+	84%	-	80%
Home Recovery Information Given	300+	79%	-	82%
Hospital Given 9 or 10 on 10 Point Scale	300+	67%	-	67%
Meds 'Always' Explained Before Given	300+	59%	-	60%
Nurses 'Always' Communicated Well	300+	77%	-	76%
Pain 'Always' Well Controlled	300+	69%	-	69%
Room and Bathroom 'Always' Clean	300+	73%	-	71%
Timely Help 'Always' Received	300+	66%	-	64%
Would Definitely Recommend Hospital	300+	66%	-	69%

NOTE: Hospital profiles are in alphabetical order by state, then city, then hospital within the city; Rankings exclude hospitals with less than 25 cases except for patient surveys which excludes hospitals with less than 100 cases; (a) 100–299 cases; (1) The number of cases is too small to be sure how well a hospital is performing; (2) The hospital indicated that the data submitted for this measure were based on a sample of cases; (3) Data was collected during a shorter time period (fewer quarters) than the maximum possible time for this measure; (4) Suppressed for one or more quarters by CMS; (5) No data is available from the hospital for this measure; (6) Fewer than 100 patients completed the HCAHPS survey. Use these rates with caution, as the number of surveys may be too low to reliably assess hospital performance; (7) Survey results are based on less than 12 months of data; (8) Survey results are not available for this reporting period; (9) No or very few patients were eligible for the HCAHPS survey. The scores shown, if any, reflect a very small number of surveys; (10) A state average was not calculated because too few hospitals in the state submitted data; (11) There were discrepancies in the data collection process; Please refer to the User's Guide for a full explanation of data.

Nicholas County Hospital

2323 Concrete Road
Carlisle, KY 40311
Phone: 859-289-7181
Fax: 859-289-7510
URL: www.johnsonmathers.org
Type: Critical Access Hospitals
Emergency Services: Yes
Ownership: Voluntary Non-Profit - Other
Beds: 18

Key Personnel:
CEO/President. . . . . Doris Ecton
Chief of Medical Staff . . . . Stephen Besson, MD
Infection Control . . . . Mendy Courtney, RN
Radiology. . . . . Otis Davis
Emergency Room . . . . Carolyn Pope, RN

Measure	Cases	This Hosp.	State Avg.	U.S. Avg.
Heart Attack Care				
ACE Inhibitor or ARB for LVSD[5]	0	-	94%	96%
Aspirin at Arrival[5]	0	-	98%	99%
Aspirin at Discharge[5]	0	-	99%	98%
Beta Blocker at Discharge[5]	0	-	98%	98%
Fibrinolytic Medication Timing[5]	0	-	60%	55%
PCI Within 90 Minutes of Arrival[5]	0	-	88%	90%
Smoking Cessation Advice[5]	0	-	100%	99%
Chest Pain/Possible Heart Attack Care				
Aspirin at Arrival	-	-	95%	95%
Median Time to ECG (minutes)	-	-	7	8
Median Time to Transfer (minutes)	-	-	65	61
Fibrinolytic Medication Timing	-	-	62%	54%
Heart Failure Care				
ACE Inhibitor or ARB for LVSD[1]	2	0%	91%	94%
Discharge Instructions[1]	5	40%	82%	88%
Evaluation of LVS Function[1]	7	100%	96%	98%
Smoking Cessation Advice[1]	1	100%	98%	98%
Pneumonia Care				
Appropriate Initial Antibiotic	29	59%	90%	92%
Blood Culture Timing[1]	24	71%	95%	96%
Influenza Vaccine[1]	23	87%	92%	91%
Initial Antibiotic Timing	36	94%	95%	95%
Pneumococcal Vaccine[1]	19	68%	94%	93%
Smoking Cessation Advice[1]	21	100%	98%	97%
Surgical Care Improvement Project				
Appropriate VTP Within 24 Hours[5]	0	-	91%	92%
Appropriate Hair Removal[5]	0	-	99%	99%
Appropriate Beta Blocker Usage[5]	0	-	93%	93%
Controlled Postoperative Blood Glucose[5]	0	-	94%	93%
Prophylactic Antibiotic Timing[5]	0	-	97%	97%
Prophylactic Antibiotic Timing (Outpatient)	-	-	92%	92%
Prophylactic Antibiotic Selection[5]	0	-	98%	97%
Prophylactic Antibiotic Select. (Outpatient)	-	-	93%	94%
Prophylactic Antibiotic Stopped[5]	0	-	94%	94%
Recommended VTP Ordered[5]	0	-	94%	94%
Urinary Catheter Removal[5]	0	-	89%	90%
Children's Asthma Care				
Received Systemic Corticosteroids	-	-	-	100%
Received Home Management Plan	-	-	-	71%
Received Reliever Medication	-	-	-	100%
Use of Medical Imaging				
Combination Abdominal CT Scan	-	-	0.160	0.191
Combination Chest CT Scan	-	-	0.054	0.054
Follow-up Mammogram/Ultrasound	-	-	7.9%	8.4%
MRI for Low Back Pain	-	-	35.6%	32.7%
Survey of Patients' Hospital Experiences				
Area Around Room 'Always' Quiet at Night[8]	-	-	-	58%
Doctors 'Always' Communicated Well[8]	-	-	-	80%
Home Recovery Information Given[8]	-	-	-	82%
Hospital Given 9 or 10 on 10 Point Scale[8]	-	-	-	67%
Meds 'Always' Explained Before Given[8]	-	-	-	60%
Nurses 'Always' Communicated Well[8]	-	-	-	76%
Pain 'Always' Well Controlled[8]	-	-	-	69%
Room and Bathroom 'Always' Clean[8]	-	-	-	71%
Timely Help 'Always' Received[8]	-	-	-	64%
Would Definitely Recommend Hospital[8]	-	-	-	69%

Carroll County Hospital

309 Eleventh Street
Carrollton, KY 41008
Phone: 502-732-4321
Fax: 502-732-3292
E-mail: mabel.burkhardt@nortonhealthcare.org
Type: Critical Access Hospitals
Emergency Services: Yes
Ownership: Government - Local
Beds: 49

Key Personnel:
CEO/President. . . . . Kim Dees
Chief of Medical Staff . . . . Hari Nagaraj
Operating Room. . . . . Trudy Gould
Emergency Room . . . . Allen Young
Intensive Care Unit. . . . . Rhonda Clark

Measure	Cases	This Hosp.	State Avg.	U.S. Avg.
Heart Attack Care				
ACE Inhibitor or ARB for LVSD[3]	0	-	94%	96%
Aspirin at Arrival[1,3]	4	100%	98%	99%
Aspirin at Discharge[1,3]	3	67%	99%	98%
Beta Blocker at Discharge[1,3]	2	50%	98%	98%
Fibrinolytic Medication Timing[3]	0	-	60%	55%
PCI Within 90 Minutes of Arrival[3]	0	-	88%	90%
Smoking Cessation Advice[3]	0	-	100%	99%
Chest Pain/Possible Heart Attack Care				
Aspirin at Arrival	-	-	95%	95%
Median Time to ECG (minutes)	-	-	7	8
Median Time to Transfer (minutes)	-	-	65	61
Fibrinolytic Medication Timing	-	-	62%	54%
Heart Failure Care				
ACE Inhibitor or ARB for LVSD[1]	6	50%	91%	94%
Discharge Instructions[1]	17	100%	82%	88%
Evaluation of LVS Function	27	81%	96%	98%
Smoking Cessation Advice[1]	5	80%	98%	98%
Pneumonia Care				
Appropriate Initial Antibiotic[1]	22	82%	90%	92%
Blood Culture Timing	41	98%	95%	96%
Influenza Vaccine	29	93%	92%	91%
Initial Antibiotic Timing	56	93%	95%	95%
Pneumococcal Vaccine	35	94%	94%	93%
Smoking Cessation Advice	30	93%	98%	97%
Surgical Care Improvement Project				
Appropriate VTP Within 24 Hours[5]	0	-	91%	92%
Appropriate Hair Removal[5]	0	-	99%	99%
Appropriate Beta Blocker Usage[5]	0	-	93%	93%
Controlled Postoperative Blood Glucose[5]	0	-	94%	93%
Prophylactic Antibiotic Timing[5]	0	-	97%	97%
Prophylactic Antibiotic Timing (Outpatient)	-	-	92%	92%
Prophylactic Antibiotic Selection[5]	0	-	98%	97%
Prophylactic Antibiotic Select. (Outpatient)	-	-	93%	94%
Prophylactic Antibiotic Stopped[5]	0	-	94%	94%
Recommended VTP Ordered[5]	0	-	94%	94%
Urinary Catheter Removal[5]	0	-	89%	90%
Children's Asthma Care				
Received Systemic Corticosteroids	-	-	-	100%
Received Home Management Plan	-	-	-	71%
Received Reliever Medication	-	-	-	100%
Use of Medical Imaging				
Combination Abdominal CT Scan	-	-	0.160	0.191
Combination Chest CT Scan	-	-	0.054	0.054
Follow-up Mammogram/Ultrasound	-	-	7.9%	8.4%
MRI for Low Back Pain	-	-	35.6%	32.7%
Survey of Patients' Hospital Experiences				
Area Around Room 'Always' Quiet at Night[8]	-	-	-	58%
Doctors 'Always' Communicated Well[8]	-	-	-	80%
Home Recovery Information Given[8]	-	-	-	82%
Hospital Given 9 or 10 on 10 Point Scale[8]	-	-	-	67%
Meds 'Always' Explained Before Given[8]	-	-	-	60%
Nurses 'Always' Communicated Well[8]	-	-	-	76%
Pain 'Always' Well Controlled[8]	-	-	-	69%
Room and Bathroom 'Always' Clean[8]	-	-	-	71%
Timely Help 'Always' Received[8]	-	-	-	64%
Would Definitely Recommend Hospital[8]	-	-	-	69%

Westlake Regional Hospital

901 Westlake Drive
Columbia, KY 42728
Phone: 270-384-4753
Fax: 270-384-3742
URL: www.westlake-healthcare.org
Type: Acute Care Hospitals
Emergency Services: Yes
Ownership: Govt - Hospital Dist/Auth
Beds: 80

Key Personnel:
Chief of Medical Staff . . . . Gary Partin, MD
Infection Control. . . . . Sharon Watson
Operating Room. . . . . Kathy Hadley
Quality Assurance . . . . Jim Hagan
Anesthesiology. . . . . Tom Wimmer
Emergency Room . . . . Celia Downey
Intensive Care Unit. . . . . Celia Downey

Measure	Cases	This Hosp.	State Avg.	U.S. Avg.
Heart Attack Care				
ACE Inhibitor or ARB for LVSD	0	-	94%	96%
Aspirin at Arrival[1]	5	100%	98%	99%
Aspirin at Discharge[1]	4	100%	99%	98%
Beta Blocker at Discharge[1]	4	100%	98%	98%
Fibrinolytic Medication Timing	0	-	60%	55%
PCI Within 90 Minutes of Arrival	0	-	88%	90%
Smoking Cessation Advice[1]	1	100%	100%	99%
Chest Pain/Possible Heart Attack Care				
Aspirin at Arrival	105	90%	95%	95%
Median Time to ECG (minutes)	110	10	7	8
Median Time to Transfer (minutes)[1,3]	2	128	65	61
Fibrinolytic Medication Timing[1]	6	67%	62%	54%
Heart Failure Care				
ACE Inhibitor or ARB for LVSD	42	88%	91%	94%
Discharge Instructions	170	93%	82%	88%
Evaluation of LVS Function	221	92%	96%	98%
Smoking Cessation Advice	38	87%	98%	98%
Pneumonia Care				
Appropriate Initial Antibiotic	91	93%	90%	92%
Blood Culture Timing	0	-	95%	96%
Influenza Vaccine	68	71%	92%	91%
Initial Antibiotic Timing	121	98%	95%	95%
Pneumococcal Vaccine	96	78%	94%	93%
Smoking Cessation Advice	63	89%	98%	97%
Surgical Care Improvement Project				
Appropriate VTP Within 24 Hours[5]	0	-	91%	92%
Appropriate Hair Removal[5]	0	-	99%	99%
Appropriate Beta Blocker Usage[5]	0	-	93%	93%
Controlled Postoperative Blood Glucose[5]	0	-	94%	93%
Prophylactic Antibiotic Timing[5]	0	-	97%	97%
Prophylactic Antibiotic Timing (Outpatient)[1,3]	12	83%	92%	92%
Prophylactic Antibiotic Selection[5]	0	-	98%	97%
Prophylactic Antibiotic Select. (Outpatient)[1,3]	10	80%	93%	94%
Prophylactic Antibiotic Stopped[5]	0	-	94%	94%
Recommended VTP Ordered[5]	0	-	94%	94%
Urinary Catheter Removal[5]	0	-	89%	90%
Children's Asthma Care				
Received Systemic Corticosteroids	-	-	-	100%
Received Home Management Plan	-	-	-	71%
Received Reliever Medication	-	-	-	100%
Use of Medical Imaging				
Combination Abdominal CT Scan	195	0.462	0.160	0.191
Combination Chest CT Scan	102	0.225	0.054	0.054
Follow-up Mammogram/Ultrasound	190	11.6%	7.9%	8.4%
MRI for Low Back Pain[5]	0	-	35.6%	32.7%
Survey of Patients' Hospital Experiences				
Area Around Room 'Always' Quiet at Night	300+	87%	-	58%
Doctors 'Always' Communicated Well	300+	100%	-	80%
Home Recovery Information Given	300+	99%	-	82%
Hospital Given 9 or 10 on 10 Point Scale	300+	80%	-	67%
Meds 'Always' Explained Before Given	300+	87%	-	60%
Nurses 'Always' Communicated Well	300+	99%	-	76%
Pain 'Always' Well Controlled	300+	99%	-	69%
Room and Bathroom 'Always' Clean	300+	96%	-	71%
Timely Help 'Always' Received	300+	97%	-	64%
Would Definitely Recommend Hospital	300+	98%	-	69%

NOTE: Hospital profiles are in alphabetical order by state, then city, then hospital within the city; Rankings exclude hospitals with less than 25 cases except for patient surveys which excludes hospitals with less than 100 cases; (a) 100–299 cases; (1) The number of cases is too small to be sure how well a hospital is performing; (2) The hospital indicated that the data submitted for this measure were based on a sample of cases; (3) Data was collected during a shorter time period (fewer quarters) than the maximum possible time for this measure; (4) Suppressed for one or more quarters by CMS; (5) No data is available from the hospital for this measure; (6) Fewer than 100 patients completed the HCAHPS survey. Use these rates with caution, as the number of surveys may be too low to reliably assess hospital performance; (7) Survey results are based on less than 12 months of data; (8) Survey results are not available for this reporting period; (9) No or very few patients were eligible for the HCAHPS survey. The scores shown, if any, reflect a very small number of surveys; (10) A state average was not calculated because too few hospitals in the state submitted data; (11) There were discrepancies in the data collection process; Please refer to the User's Guide for a full explanation of data.

Baptist Regional Medical Center

One Trillium Way Phone: 606-528-1212
Corbin, KY 40701 Fax: 606-528-9996
URL: www.baptistregional.com
Type: Acute Care Hospitals Emergency Services: Yes
Ownership: Voluntary Non-Profit - Private Beds: 240

Key Personnel:
CEO/President.............. John Henson
Chief of Medical Staff......... Ross Halbleib
Infection Control............. Elizabeth Bryant
Operating Room............. George Liu
Quality Assurance .... Theresa Sidebottom
Radiology................... William Daniel II
Intensive Care Unit........... Donna Carroll

Measure	Cases	This Hosp.	State Avg.	U.S. Avg.
Heart Attack Care				
ACE Inhibitor or ARB for LVSD[1]	4	100%	94%	96%
Aspirin at Arrival	53	100%	98%	99%
Aspirin at Discharge[1]	20	100%	99%	98%
Beta Blocker at Discharge[1]	22	100%	98%	98%
Fibrinolytic Medication Timing	0	-	60%	55%
PCI Within 90 Minutes of Arrival	0	-	88%	90%
Smoking Cessation Advice[1]	5	100%	100%	99%
Chest Pain/Possible Heart Attack Care				
Aspirin at Arrival	144	98%	95%	95%
Median Time to ECG (minutes)	150	7	7	8
Median Time to Transfer (minutes)[1,3]	10	58	65	61
Fibrinolytic Medication Timing[1]	2	0%	62%	54%
Heart Failure Care				
ACE Inhibitor or ARB for LVSD	41	100%	91%	94%
Discharge Instructions	136	99%	82%	88%
Evaluation of LVS Function	179	100%	96%	98%
Smoking Cessation Advice	30	100%	98%	98%
Pneumonia Care				
Appropriate Initial Antibiotic	214	95%	90%	92%
Blood Culture Timing	225	96%	95%	96%
Influenza Vaccine	188	100%	92%	91%
Initial Antibiotic Timing	253	98%	95%	95%
Pneumococcal Vaccine	256	100%	94%	93%
Smoking Cessation Advice	151	100%	98%	97%
Surgical Care Improvement Project				
Appropriate VTP Within 24 Hours	130	97%	91%	92%
Appropriate Hair Removal	316	100%	99%	99%
Appropriate Beta Blocker Usage	106	99%	93%	93%
Controlled Postoperative Blood Glucose	0	-	94%	93%
Prophylactic Antibiotic Timing	222	98%	97%	97%
Prophylactic Antibiotic Timing (Outpatient)	215	98%	92%	92%
Prophylactic Antibiotic Selection	223	99%	98%	97%
Prophylactic Antibiotic Select. (Outpatient)	210	98%	93%	94%
Prophylactic Antibiotic Stopped	210	98%	94%	94%
Recommended VTP Ordered	130	97%	94%	94%
Urinary Catheter Removal	55	100%	89%	90%
Children's Asthma Care				
Received Systemic Corticosteroids	-	-	-	100%
Received Home Management Plan	-	-	-	71%
Received Reliever Medication	-	-	-	100%
Use of Medical Imaging				
Combination Abdominal CT Scan	667	0.063	0.160	0.191
Combination Chest CT Scan	480	0.019	0.054	0.054
Follow-up Mammogram/Ultrasound	945	7.2%	7.9%	8.4%
MRI for Low Back Pain	208	50.0%	35.6%	32.7%
Survey of Patients' Hospital Experiences				
Area Around Room 'Always' Quiet at Night	300+	48%	-	58%
Doctors 'Always' Communicated Well	300+	84%	-	80%
Home Recovery Information Given	300+	82%	-	82%
Hospital Given 9 or 10 on 10 Point Scale	300+	64%	-	67%
Meds 'Always' Explained Before Given	300+	58%	-	60%
Nurses 'Always' Communicated Well	300+	77%	-	76%
Pain 'Always' Well Controlled	300+	67%	-	69%
Room and Bathroom 'Always' Clean	300+	66%	-	71%
Timely Help 'Always' Received	300+	67%	-	64%
Would Definitely Recommend Hospital	300+	64%	-	69%

Saint Elizabeth Medical Center North

401 East 20th Street Phone: 859-292-2000
Covington, KY 41014 Fax: 859-301-5178
E-mail: contact@stelizabeth.com
URL: www.stelizabeth.com
Type: Acute Care Hospitals Emergency Services: Yes
Ownership: Voluntary Non-Profit - Church Beds: 684

Key Personnel:
CEO/President............... Joseph W Gross
Chief of Medical Staff.......... Phillip B Schworer, MD
Infection Control.............. Patty Burns
Operating Room.............. Sue Sansone, RN
Pediatric In-Patient Care .... Mary Garamy, RN
Quality Assurance .... Lisa Frey
Radiology................... Lloyd Gill

Measure	Cases	This Hosp.	State Avg.	U.S. Avg.
Heart Attack Care				
ACE Inhibitor or ARB for LVSD[2]	47	100%	94%	96%
Aspirin at Arrival[2]	211	100%	98%	99%
Aspirin at Discharge[2]	303	100%	99%	98%
Beta Blocker at Discharge[2]	283	100%	98%	98%
Fibrinolytic Medication Timing[2]	0	-	60%	55%
PCI Within 90 Minutes of Arrival[2]	42	95%	88%	90%
Smoking Cessation Advice[2]	117	100%	100%	99%
Chest Pain/Possible Heart Attack Care				
Aspirin at Arrival[1]	24	92%	95%	95%
Median Time to ECG (minutes)	26	10	7	8
Median Time to Transfer (minutes)[5]	0	-	65	61
Fibrinolytic Medication Timing[5]	0	-	62%	54%
Heart Failure Care				
ACE Inhibitor or ARB for LVSD[2]	90	100%	91%	94%
Discharge Instructions[2]	273	96%	82%	88%
Evaluation of LVS Function[2]	320	100%	96%	98%
Smoking Cessation Advice[2]	67	100%	98%	98%
Pneumonia Care				
Appropriate Initial Antibiotic[2]	68	91%	90%	92%
Blood Culture Timing[2]	62	100%	95%	96%
Influenza Vaccine[2]	90	98%	92%	91%
Initial Antibiotic Timing[2]	122	99%	95%	95%
Pneumococcal Vaccine[2]	115	99%	94%	93%
Smoking Cessation Advice[2]	81	100%	98%	97%
Surgical Care Improvement Project				
Appropriate VTP Within 24 Hours[2]	166	95%	91%	92%
Appropriate Hair Removal[2]	712	100%	99%	99%
Appropriate Beta Blocker Usage[2]	226	97%	93%	93%
Controlled Postoperative Blood Glucose[2]	156	92%	94%	93%
Prophylactic Antibiotic Timing[2]	487	99%	97%	97%
Prophylactic Antibiotic Timing (Outpatient)	593	97%	92%	92%
Prophylactic Antibiotic Selection[2]	493	98%	98%	97%
Prophylactic Antibiotic Select. (Outpatient)	592	96%	93%	94%
Prophylactic Antibiotic Stopped[2]	460	98%	94%	94%
Recommended VTP Ordered[2]	166	97%	94%	94%
Urinary Catheter Removal[2]	88	84%	89%	90%
Children's Asthma Care				
Received Systemic Corticosteroids	-	-	-	100%
Received Home Management Plan	-	-	-	71%
Received Reliever Medication	-	-	-	100%
Use of Medical Imaging				
Combination Abdominal CT Scan	2,226	0.061	0.160	0.191
Combination Chest CT Scan	1,311	0.002	0.054	0.054
Follow-up Mammogram/Ultrasound	3,448	7.2%	7.9%	8.4%
MRI for Low Back Pain	145	36.6%	35.6%	32.7%
Survey of Patients' Hospital Experiences				
Area Around Room 'Always' Quiet at Night	300+	60%	-	58%
Doctors 'Always' Communicated Well	300+	79%	-	80%
Home Recovery Information Given	300+	86%	-	82%
Hospital Given 9 or 10 on 10 Point Scale	300+	74%	-	67%
Meds 'Always' Explained Before Given	300+	63%	-	60%
Nurses 'Always' Communicated Well	300+	78%	-	76%
Pain 'Always' Well Controlled	300+	70%	-	69%
Room and Bathroom 'Always' Clean	300+	70%	-	71%
Timely Help 'Always' Received	300+	65%	-	64%
Would Definitely Recommend Hospital	300+	79%	-	69%

Harrison Memorial Hospital

1210 Ky Hwy 36 E Phone: 859-234-2300
Cynthiana, KY 41031 Fax: 859-235-3699
URL: www.harrisonmemhosp.com
Type: Acute Care Hospitals Emergency Services: Yes
Ownership: Voluntary Non-Profit - Other Beds: 99

Key Personnel:
Chief of Medical Staff.......... David French
Radiology.................... Douglas C Crutcher
Emergency Room .... M Gainey

Measure	Cases	This Hosp.	State Avg.	U.S. Avg.
Heart Attack Care				
ACE Inhibitor or ARB for LVSD	0	-	94%	96%
Aspirin at Arrival[1]	3	100%	98%	99%
Aspirin at Discharge[1]	2	100%	99%	98%
Beta Blocker at Discharge[1]	2	100%	98%	98%
Fibrinolytic Medication Timing	0	-	60%	55%
PCI Within 90 Minutes of Arrival	0	-	88%	90%
Smoking Cessation Advice	0	-	100%	99%
Chest Pain/Possible Heart Attack Care				
Aspirin at Arrival	101	99%	95%	95%
Median Time to ECG (minutes)	101	9	7	8
Median Time to Transfer (minutes)[1,3]	2	109	65	61
Fibrinolytic Medication Timing[1]	10	60%	62%	54%
Heart Failure Care				
ACE Inhibitor or ARB for LVSD[1]	13	85%	91%	94%
Discharge Instructions	34	82%	82%	88%
Evaluation of LVS Function	49	100%	96%	98%
Smoking Cessation Advice[1]	10	100%	98%	98%
Pneumonia Care				
Appropriate Initial Antibiotic	115	94%	90%	92%
Blood Culture Timing	123	95%	95%	96%
Influenza Vaccine	69	90%	92%	91%
Initial Antibiotic Timing	136	99%	95%	95%
Pneumococcal Vaccine	121	96%	94%	93%
Smoking Cessation Advice	53	100%	98%	97%
Surgical Care Improvement Project				
Appropriate VTP Within 24 Hours	38	97%	91%	92%
Appropriate Hair Removal	77	99%	99%	99%
Appropriate Beta Blocker Usage[1]	20	95%	93%	93%
Controlled Postoperative Blood Glucose	0	-	94%	93%
Prophylactic Antibiotic Timing	40	92%	97%	97%
Prophylactic Antibiotic Timing (Outpatient)	38	95%	92%	92%
Prophylactic Antibiotic Selection	41	93%	98%	97%
Prophylactic Antibiotic Select. (Outpatient)	37	86%	93%	94%
Prophylactic Antibiotic Stopped	39	92%	94%	94%
Recommended VTP Ordered	38	100%	94%	94%
Urinary Catheter Removal[1]	9	100%	89%	90%
Children's Asthma Care				
Received Systemic Corticosteroids	-	-	-	100%
Received Home Management Plan	-	-	-	71%
Received Reliever Medication	-	-	-	100%
Use of Medical Imaging				
Combination Abdominal CT Scan	272	0.063	0.160	0.191
Combination Chest CT Scan	167	0.006	0.054	0.054
Follow-up Mammogram/Ultrasound	329	11.9%	7.9%	8.4%
MRI for Low Back Pain[5]	0	-	35.6%	32.7%
Survey of Patients' Hospital Experiences				
Area Around Room 'Always' Quiet at Night	300+	55%	-	58%
Doctors 'Always' Communicated Well	300+	88%	-	80%
Home Recovery Information Given	300+	83%	-	82%
Hospital Given 9 or 10 on 10 Point Scale	300+	71%	-	67%
Meds 'Always' Explained Before Given	300+	65%	-	60%
Nurses 'Always' Communicated Well	300+	80%	-	76%
Pain 'Always' Well Controlled	300+	71%	-	69%
Room and Bathroom 'Always' Clean	300+	78%	-	71%
Timely Help 'Always' Received	300+	63%	-	64%
Would Definitely Recommend Hospital	300+	67%	-	69%

NOTE: Hospital profiles are in alphabetical order by state, then city, then hospital within the city; Rankings exclude hospitals with less than 25 cases except for patient surveys which excludes hospitals with less than 100 cases; (a) 100–299 cases; (1) The number of cases is too small to be sure how well a hospital is performing; (2) The hospital indicated that the data submitted for this measure were based on a sample of cases; (3) Data was collected during a shorter time period (fewer quarters) than the maximum possible time for this measure; (4) Suppressed for one or more quarters by CMS; (5) No data is available from the hospital for this measure; (6) Fewer than 100 patients completed the HCAHPS survey. Use these rates with caution, as the number of surveys may be too low to reliably assess hospital performance; (7) Survey results are based on less than 12 months of data; (8) Survey results are not available for this reporting period; (9) No or very few patients were eligible for the HCAHPS survey. The scores shown, if any, reflect a very small number of surveys; (10) A state average was not calculated because too few hospitals in the state submitted data; (11) There were discrepancies in the data collection process; Please refer to the User's Guide for a full explanation of data.

Ephraim Mcdowell Regional Medical Center

217 South Third Street
Danville, KY 40422
E-mail: marketing@emhealth.org
URL: www.emrmc.com
Type: Acute Care Hospitals
Ownership: Voluntary Non-Profit - Other
Phone: 859-239-2409
Fax: 859-239-6960
Emergency Services: Yes
Beds: 177

Key Personnel:
CEO/President . . . . Clark Taylor
Chief of Medical Staff . . . . William P Baas
Coronary Care . . . . Beth Carter
Infection Control . . . . Ginger Elliot
Operating Room . . . . Paul DeLuca
Pediatric Ambulatory Care . . . . . . Russel Goodwin, MD
Quality Assurance . . . . Nancy Brooks
Radiology . . . . Shawn D Grant, MD

Measure	Cases	This Hosp.	State Avg.	U.S. Avg.
Heart Attack Care				
ACE Inhibitor or ARB for LVSD[1]	12	100%	94%	96%
Aspirin at Arrival	102	98%	98%	99%
Aspirin at Discharge	79	99%	99%	98%
Beta Blocker at Discharge	78	96%	98%	98%
Fibrinolytic Medication Timing	0	-	60%	55%
PCI Within 90 Minutes of Arrival[1]	9	78%	88%	90%
Smoking Cessation Advice[1]	22	100%	100%	99%
Chest Pain/Possible Heart Attack Care				
Aspirin at Arrival	101	96%	95%	95%
Median Time to ECG (minutes)	104	2	7	8
Median Time to Transfer (minutes)[1,3]	15	65	65	61
Fibrinolytic Medication Timing	0	-	62%	54%
Heart Failure Care				
ACE Inhibitor or ARB for LVSD	61	95%	91%	94%
Discharge Instructions	187	98%	82%	88%
Evaluation of LVS Function	228	100%	96%	98%
Smoking Cessation Advice	44	98%	98%	98%
Pneumonia Care				
Appropriate Initial Antibiotic[2]	138	88%	90%	92%
Blood Culture Timing[2]	180	97%	95%	96%
Influenza Vaccine	220	97%	92%	91%
Initial Antibiotic Timing[2]	285	96%	95%	95%
Pneumococcal Vaccine[2]	273	97%	94%	93%
Smoking Cessation Advice[2]	156	100%	98%	97%
Surgical Care Improvement Project				
Appropriate VTP Within 24 Hours	189	98%	91%	92%
Appropriate Hair Removal	514	100%	99%	99%
Appropriate Beta Blocker Usage	146	98%	93%	93%
Controlled Postoperative Blood Glucose	0	-	94%	93%
Prophylactic Antibiotic Timing	337	99%	97%	97%
Prophylactic Antibiotic Timing (Outpatient)	267	78%	92%	92%
Prophylactic Antibiotic Selection	337	100%	98%	97%
Prophylactic Antibiotic Select. (Outpatient)	231	92%	93%	94%
Prophylactic Antibiotic Stopped	321	99%	94%	94%
Recommended VTP Ordered	189	99%	94%	94%
Urinary Catheter Removal	102	100%	89%	90%
Children's Asthma Care				
Received Systemic Corticosteroids	-	-	-	100%
Received Home Management Plan	-	-	-	71%
Received Reliever Medication	-	-	-	100%
Use of Medical Imaging				
Combination Abdominal CT Scan	797	0.107	0.160	0.191
Combination Chest CT Scan	403	0.000	0.054	0.054
Follow-up Mammogram/Ultrasound	1,364	5.0%	7.9%	8.4%
MRI for Low Back Pain	316	34.2%	35.6%	32.7%
Survey of Patients' Hospital Experiences				
Area Around Room 'Always' Quiet at Night	300+	54%	-	58%
Doctors 'Always' Communicated Well	300+	77%	-	80%
Home Recovery Information Given	300+	78%	-	82%
Hospital Given 9 or 10 on 10 Point Scale	300+	59%	-	67%
Meds 'Always' Explained Before Given	300+	52%	-	60%
Nurses 'Always' Communicated Well	300+	71%	-	76%
Pain 'Always' Well Controlled	300+	64%	-	69%
Room and Bathroom 'Always' Clean	300+	67%	-	71%
Timely Help 'Always' Received	300+	55%	-	64%
Would Definitely Recommend Hospital	300+	62%	-	69%

Hardin Memorial Hospital

913 North Dixie Avenue
Elizabethtown, KY 42701
URL: www.hmh.net
Type: Acute Care Hospitals
Ownership: Government - Local
Phone: 270-737-1212
Fax: 270-706-5125
Emergency Services: Yes
Beds: 300

Key Personnel:
CEO/President . . . . David Gray
Chief of Medical Staff . . . . Cora Veza
Infection Control . . . . Jo Ellen Mackey
Operating Room . . . . Denise Adams
Pediatric Ambulatory Care . . . . . . Robert Padgett, MD
Pediatric In-Patient Care . . . . . . Robert Padgett, MD
Quality Assurance . . . . Vivian Bishoff
Radiology . . . . Michael Oliff, MD

Measure	Cases	This Hosp.	State Avg.	U.S. Avg.
Heart Attack Care				
ACE Inhibitor or ARB for LVSD	47	98%	94%	96%
Aspirin at Arrival	293	98%	98%	99%
Aspirin at Discharge	291	98%	99%	98%
Beta Blocker at Discharge	294	100%	98%	98%
Fibrinolytic Medication Timing	36	67%	60%	55%
PCI Within 90 Minutes of Arrival[1]	8	12%	88%	90%
Smoking Cessation Advice	116	100%	100%	99%
Chest Pain/Possible Heart Attack Care				
Aspirin at Arrival[1]	12	92%	95%	95%
Median Time to ECG (minutes)[1]	12	14	7	8
Median Time to Transfer (minutes)[5]	0	-	65	61
Fibrinolytic Medication Timing[3]	0	-	62%	54%
Heart Failure Care				
ACE Inhibitor or ARB for LVSD	144	92%	91%	94%
Discharge Instructions	379	83%	82%	88%
Evaluation of LVS Function	487	99%	96%	98%
Smoking Cessation Advice	123	99%	98%	98%
Pneumonia Care				
Appropriate Initial Antibiotic[2]	98	92%	90%	92%
Blood Culture Timing[2]	103	83%	95%	96%
Influenza Vaccine[2]	91	92%	92%	91%
Initial Antibiotic Timing[2]	136	93%	95%	95%
Pneumococcal Vaccine[2]	133	94%	94%	93%
Smoking Cessation Advice[2]	69	94%	98%	97%
Surgical Care Improvement Project				
Appropriate VTP Within 24 Hours[2]	191	87%	91%	92%
Appropriate Hair Removal[2]	556	100%	99%	99%
Appropriate Beta Blocker Usage[2]	186	90%	93%	93%
Controlled Postoperative Blood Glucose[2]	76	95%	94%	93%
Prophylactic Antibiotic Timing[2]	387	97%	97%	97%
Prophylactic Antibiotic Timing (Outpatient)	514	96%	92%	92%
Prophylactic Antibiotic Selection[2]	393	94%	98%	97%
Prophylactic Antibiotic Select. (Outpatient)	502	91%	93%	94%
Prophylactic Antibiotic Stopped[2]	374	77%	94%	94%
Recommended VTP Ordered[2]	194	86%	94%	94%
Urinary Catheter Removal[2]	142	87%	89%	90%
Children's Asthma Care				
Received Systemic Corticosteroids	-	-	-	100%
Received Home Management Plan	-	-	-	71%
Received Reliever Medication	-	-	-	100%
Use of Medical Imaging				
Combination Abdominal CT Scan	1,344	0.092	0.160	0.191
Combination Chest CT Scan	960	0.001	0.054	0.054
Follow-up Mammogram/Ultrasound	1,804	14.6%	7.9%	8.4%
MRI for Low Back Pain	187	31.0%	35.6%	32.7%
Survey of Patients' Hospital Experiences				
Area Around Room 'Always' Quiet at Night	300+	44%	-	58%
Doctors 'Always' Communicated Well	300+	83%	-	80%
Home Recovery Information Given	300+	79%	-	82%
Hospital Given 9 or 10 on 10 Point Scale	300+	64%	-	67%
Meds 'Always' Explained Before Given	300+	63%	-	60%
Nurses 'Always' Communicated Well	300+	77%	-	76%
Pain 'Always' Well Controlled	300+	67%	-	69%
Room and Bathroom 'Always' Clean	300+	69%	-	71%
Timely Help 'Always' Received	300+	58%	-	64%
Would Definitely Recommend Hospital	300+	65%	-	69%

Fleming County Hospital

55 Foundation Drive
Flemingsburg, KY 41041
URL: www.flemingcountyhospital.org
Type: Acute Care Hospitals
Ownership: Voluntary Non-Profit - Other
Phone: 606-849-2351
Fax: 606-849-5005
Emergency Services: Yes
Beds: 52

Key Personnel:
CEO/President . . . . Mark Armstrong
Chief of Medical Staff . . . . Samuel W Gehring, MD
Infection Control . . . . Jeanne Conley, RN
Operating Room . . . . Theresa Huber, RN
Quality Assurance . . . . Marsha Gorman
Radiology . . . . Richard S Hartman, RT
Emergency Room . . . . Roland Benton
Intensive Care Unit . . . . Helen McKay, RN

Measure	Cases	This Hosp.	State Avg.	U.S. Avg.
Heart Attack Care				
ACE Inhibitor or ARB for LVSD[2,3]	0	-	94%	96%
Aspirin at Arrival[3,1,2]	3	67%	98%	99%
Aspirin at Discharge[1,2,3]	1	0%	99%	98%
Beta Blocker at Discharge[1,2,3]	1	100%	98%	98%
Fibrinolytic Medication Timing[2,3]	0	-	60%	55%
PCI Within 90 Minutes of Arrival[2,3]	0	-	88%	90%
Smoking Cessation Advice[2,3]	0	-	100%	99%
Chest Pain/Possible Heart Attack Care				
Aspirin at Arrival	51	88%	95%	95%
Median Time to ECG (minutes)	51	13	7	8
Median Time to Transfer (minutes)[1,3]	3	266	65	61
Fibrinolytic Medication Timing[1]	12	67%	62%	54%
Heart Failure Care				
ACE Inhibitor or ARB for LVSD[1,2]	18	61%	91%	94%
Discharge Instructions[2]	78	78%	82%	88%
Evaluation of LVS Function[2]	98	81%	96%	98%
Smoking Cessation Advice[1,2]	12	100%	98%	98%
Pneumonia Care				
Appropriate Initial Antibiotic[2]	117	81%	90%	92%
Blood Culture Timing[2]	101	91%	95%	96%
Influenza Vaccine	66	92%	92%	91%
Initial Antibiotic Timing[2]	94	94%	95%	95%
Pneumococcal Vaccine[2]	98	86%	94%	93%
Smoking Cessation Advice[2]	58	84%	98%	97%
Surgical Care Improvement Project				
Appropriate VTP Within 24 Hours[1,2]	9	89%	91%	92%
Appropriate Hair Removal[1,2]	14	100%	99%	99%
Appropriate Beta Blocker Usage[1,2]	6	33%	93%	93%
Controlled Postoperative Blood Glucose[2]	0	-	94%	93%
Prophylactic Antibiotic Timing[1,2]	10	70%	97%	97%
Prophylactic Antibiotic Timing (Outpatient)[1]	21	81%	92%	92%
Prophylactic Antibiotic Selection[1,2]	10	100%	98%	97%
Prophylactic Antibiotic Select. (Outpatient)[1]	21	90%	93%	94%
Prophylactic Antibiotic Stopped[1,2]	10	80%	94%	94%
Recommended VTP Ordered[1,2]	9	89%	94%	94%
Urinary Catheter Removal[1]	7	100%	89%	90%
Children's Asthma Care				
Received Systemic Corticosteroids	-	-	-	100%
Received Home Management Plan	-	-	-	71%
Received Reliever Medication	-	-	-	100%
Use of Medical Imaging				
Combination Abdominal CT Scan	191	0.581	0.160	0.191
Combination Chest CT Scan	167	0.012	0.054	0.054
Follow-up Mammogram/Ultrasound	237	13.5%	7.9%	8.4%
MRI for Low Back Pain[1]	30	46.7%	35.6%	32.7%
Survey of Patients' Hospital Experiences				
Area Around Room 'Always' Quiet at Night	(a)	64%	-	58%
Doctors 'Always' Communicated Well	(a)	78%	-	80%
Home Recovery Information Given	(a)	82%	-	82%
Hospital Given 9 or 10 on 10 Point Scale	(a)	76%	-	67%
Meds 'Always' Explained Before Given	(a)	64%	-	60%
Nurses 'Always' Communicated Well	(a)	79%	-	76%
Pain 'Always' Well Controlled	(a)	70%	-	69%
Room and Bathroom 'Always' Clean	(a)	87%	-	71%
Timely Help 'Always' Received	(a)	64%	-	64%
Would Definitely Recommend Hospital	(a)	75%	-	69%

NOTE: Hospital profiles are in alphabetical order by state, then city, then hospital within the city; Rankings exclude hospitals with less than 25 cases except for patient surveys which excludes hospitals with less than 100 cases; (a) 100–299 cases; (1) The number of cases is too small to be sure how well a hospital is performing; (2) The hospital indicated that the data submitted for this measure were based on a sample of cases; (3) Data was collected during a shorter time period (fewer quarters) than the maximum possible time for this measure; (4) Suppressed for one or more quarters by CMS; (5) No data is available from the hospital for this measure; (6) Fewer than 100 patients completed the HCAHPS survey. Use these rates with caution, as the number of surveys may be too low to reliably assess hospital performance; (7) Survey results are based on less than 12 months of data; (8) Survey results are not available for this reporting period; (9) No or very few patients were eligible for the HCAHPS survey. The scores shown, if any, reflect a very small number of surveys; (10) A state average was not calculated because too few hospitals in the state submitted data; (11) There were discrepancies in the data collection process; Please refer to the User's Guide for a full explanation of data.

Saint Elizabeth Florence

4900 Houston Road
Florence, KY 41042
Phone: 859-962-5200
Fax: 859-212-5221
URL: www.stlukehospitals.com
Type: Acute Care Hospitals
Emergency Services: Yes
Ownership: Voluntary Non-Profit - Private
Beds: 177

Key Personnel:
CEO/President. . . . . Daniel M Vinson
Operating Room. . . . . Beth Ackerson
Pediatric Ambulatory Care . . . . . Ted Pappas, MD
Pediatric In-Patient Care . . . . . . Ted Pappas, MD
Quality Assurance . . . . Ron Reeser
Radiology. . . . . Carol Milburn, MD

Measure	Cases	This Hosp.	State Avg.	U.S. Avg.
Heart Attack Care				
ACE Inhibitor or ARB for LVSD[1]	15	100%	94%	96%
Aspirin at Arrival	104	100%	98%	99%
Aspirin at Discharge	64	100%	99%	98%
Beta Blocker at Discharge	59	100%	98%	98%
Fibrinolytic Medication Timing	0	-	60%	55%
PCI Within 90 Minutes of Arrival	0	-	88%	90%
Smoking Cessation Advice[1]	22	100%	100%	99%
Chest Pain/Possible Heart Attack Care				
Aspirin at Arrival	37	97%	95%	95%
Median Time to ECG (minutes)	38	11	7	8
Median Time to Transfer (minutes)[1]	23	55	65	61
Fibrinolytic Medication Timing	0	-	62%	54%
Heart Failure Care				
ACE Inhibitor or ARB for LVSD	68	100%	91%	94%
Discharge Instructions	149	88%	82%	88%
Evaluation of LVS Function	200	100%	96%	98%
Smoking Cessation Advice	42	100%	98%	98%
Pneumonia Care				
Appropriate Initial Antibiotic	85	88%	90%	92%
Blood Culture Timing	112	96%	95%	96%
Influenza Vaccine	118	97%	92%	91%
Initial Antibiotic Timing	134	93%	95%	95%
Pneumococcal Vaccine	164	96%	94%	93%
Smoking Cessation Advice	76	100%	98%	97%
Surgical Care Improvement Project				
Appropriate VTP Within 24 Hours[2]	102	90%	91%	92%
Appropriate Hair Removal[2]	252	100%	99%	99%
Appropriate Beta Blocker Usage[2]	41	95%	93%	93%
Controlled Postoperative Blood Glucose[2]	0	-	94%	93%
Prophylactic Antibiotic Timing[2]	119	98%	97%	97%
Prophylactic Antibiotic Timing (Outpatient)	25	88%	92%	92%
Prophylactic Antibiotic Selection[2]	120	99%	98%	97%
Prophylactic Antibiotic Select. (Outpatient)	25	72%	93%	94%
Prophylactic Antibiotic Stopped[2]	112	94%	94%	94%
Recommended VTP Ordered[2]	103	92%	94%	94%
Urinary Catheter Removal[1,2]	18	56%	89%	90%
Children's Asthma Care				
Received Systemic Corticosteroids	-	-	-	100%
Received Home Management Plan	-	-	-	71%
Received Reliever Medication	-	-	-	100%
Use of Medical Imaging				
Combination Abdominal CT Scan	413	0.056	0.160	0.191
Combination Chest CT Scan	185	0.000	0.054	0.054
Follow-up Mammogram/Ultrasound	514	7.6%	7.9%	8.4%
MRI for Low Back Pain[1]	31	25.8%	35.6%	32.7%
Survey of Patients' Hospital Experiences				
Area Around Room 'Always' Quiet at Night	300+	57%	-	58%
Doctors 'Always' Communicated Well	300+	75%	-	80%
Home Recovery Information Given	300+	83%	-	82%
Hospital Given 9 or 10 on 10 Point Scale	300+	61%	-	67%
Meds 'Always' Explained Before Given	300+	59%	-	60%
Nurses 'Always' Communicated Well	300+	74%	-	76%
Pain 'Always' Well Controlled	300+	68%	-	69%
Room and Bathroom 'Always' Clean	300+	67%	-	71%
Timely Help 'Always' Received	300+	59%	-	64%
Would Definitely Recommend Hospital	300+	63%	-	69%

Saint Elizabeth Ft Thomas

85 North Grand Avenue
Fort Thomas, KY 41075
Phone: 859-572-3100
Fax: 859-572-3895
E-mail: lmw@chhs-nkey.org
URL: www.cardinalhill.org
Type: Acute Care Hospitals
Emergency Services: Yes
Ownership: Voluntary Non-Profit - Private
Beds: 33

Key Personnel:
CEO/President. . . . . Kerry Gillihan
Chief of Medical Staff . . . . Patrica Miles

Measure	Cases	This Hosp.	State Avg.	U.S. Avg.
Heart Attack Care				
ACE Inhibitor or ARB for LVSD[1]	12	100%	94%	96%
Aspirin at Arrival	129	100%	98%	99%
Aspirin at Discharge	66	100%	99%	98%
Beta Blocker at Discharge	67	100%	98%	98%
Fibrinolytic Medication Timing	0	-	60%	55%
PCI Within 90 Minutes of Arrival	0	-	88%	90%
Smoking Cessation Advice[1]	22	100%	100%	99%
Chest Pain/Possible Heart Attack Care				
Aspirin at Arrival	37	100%	95%	95%
Median Time to ECG (minutes)	40	11	7	8
Median Time to Transfer (minutes)[1]	14	48	65	61
Fibrinolytic Medication Timing	0	-	62%	54%
Heart Failure Care				
ACE Inhibitor or ARB for LVSD	44	100%	91%	94%
Discharge Instructions	173	92%	82%	88%
Evaluation of LVS Function	234	100%	96%	98%
Smoking Cessation Advice	35	100%	98%	98%
Pneumonia Care				
Appropriate Initial Antibiotic	157	94%	90%	92%
Blood Culture Timing	116	97%	95%	96%
Influenza Vaccine	133	95%	92%	91%
Initial Antibiotic Timing	161	98%	95%	95%
Pneumococcal Vaccine	174	97%	94%	93%
Smoking Cessation Advice	82	100%	98%	97%
Surgical Care Improvement Project				
Appropriate VTP Within 24 Hours[2]	123	97%	91%	92%
Appropriate Hair Removal[2]	215	100%	99%	99%
Appropriate Beta Blocker Usage[2]	42	100%	93%	93%
Controlled Postoperative Blood Glucose[2]	0	-	94%	93%
Prophylactic Antibiotic Timing[2]	92	100%	97%	97%
Prophylactic Antibiotic Timing (Outpatient)[1]	19	63%	92%	92%
Prophylactic Antibiotic Selection[2]	92	98%	98%	97%
Prophylactic Antibiotic Select. (Outpatient)[1]	16	81%	93%	94%
Prophylactic Antibiotic Stopped[2]	79	97%	94%	94%
Recommended VTP Ordered[2]	123	98%	94%	94%
Urinary Catheter Removal[1,2]	24	75%	89%	90%
Children's Asthma Care				
Received Systemic Corticosteroids	-	-	-	100%
Received Home Management Plan	-	-	-	71%
Received Reliever Medication	-	-	-	100%
Use of Medical Imaging				
Combination Abdominal CT Scan	523	0.025	0.160	0.191
Combination Chest CT Scan	342	0.000	0.054	0.054
Follow-up Mammogram/Ultrasound	611	7.9%	7.9%	8.4%
MRI for Low Back Pain[1]	46	30.4%	35.6%	32.7%
Survey of Patients' Hospital Experiences				
Area Around Room 'Always' Quiet at Night	300+	52%	-	58%
Doctors 'Always' Communicated Well	300+	76%	-	80%
Home Recovery Information Given	300+	85%	-	82%
Hospital Given 9 or 10 on 10 Point Scale	300+	59%	-	67%
Meds 'Always' Explained Before Given	300+	61%	-	60%
Nurses 'Always' Communicated Well	300+	75%	-	76%
Pain 'Always' Well Controlled	300+	69%	-	69%
Room and Bathroom 'Always' Clean	300+	71%	-	71%
Timely Help 'Always' Received	300+	60%	-	64%
Would Definitely Recommend Hospital	300+	63%	-	69%

Frankfort Regional Medical Center

299 Kings Daughters Drive
Frankfort, KY 40601
Phone: 502-875-5240
Fax: 502-226-7936
URL: www.frankfortregional.com
Type: Acute Care Hospitals
Emergency Services: Yes
Ownership: Proprietary
Beds: 173

Key Personnel:
CEO/President. . . . . Michael Mayo
Cardiac Laboratory. . . . . Dave Sebastian
Chief of Medical Staff . . . . Allen Haddix, MD
Infection Control. . . . . Emily Mills
Operating Room. . . . . Becky Jernigan
Quality Assurance . . . . Pam Melton
Emergency Room . . . . Timothy K Anderson
Patient Relations . . . . Karen Muzzillo

Measure	Cases	This Hosp.	State Avg.	U.S. Avg.
Heart Attack Care				
ACE Inhibitor or ARB for LVSD[1]	5	100%	94%	96%
Aspirin at Arrival	30	100%	98%	99%
Aspirin at Discharge[1]	16	100%	99%	98%
Beta Blocker at Discharge[1]	16	100%	98%	98%
Fibrinolytic Medication Timing	0	-	60%	55%
PCI Within 90 Minutes of Arrival	0	-	88%	90%
Smoking Cessation Advice[1]	4	100%	100%	99%
Chest Pain/Possible Heart Attack Care				
Aspirin at Arrival	151	100%	95%	95%
Median Time to ECG (minutes)	156	5	7	8
Median Time to Transfer (minutes)[1]	22	51	65	61
Fibrinolytic Medication Timing[1]	2	50%	62%	54%
Heart Failure Care				
ACE Inhibitor or ARB for LVSD	33	100%	91%	94%
Discharge Instructions	121	98%	82%	88%
Evaluation of LVS Function	137	100%	96%	98%
Smoking Cessation Advice[1]	23	100%	98%	98%
Pneumonia Care				
Appropriate Initial Antibiotic	68	97%	90%	92%
Blood Culture Timing	121	100%	95%	96%
Influenza Vaccine	82	100%	92%	91%
Initial Antibiotic Timing	121	98%	95%	95%
Pneumococcal Vaccine	114	100%	94%	93%
Smoking Cessation Advice	54	98%	98%	97%
Surgical Care Improvement Project				
Appropriate VTP Within 24 Hours	144	94%	91%	92%
Appropriate Hair Removal	253	100%	99%	99%
Appropriate Beta Blocker Usage	75	99%	93%	93%
Controlled Postoperative Blood Glucose	0	-	94%	93%
Prophylactic Antibiotic Timing	132	98%	97%	97%
Prophylactic Antibiotic Timing (Outpatient)	241	95%	92%	92%
Prophylactic Antibiotic Selection	134	99%	98%	97%
Prophylactic Antibiotic Select. (Outpatient)	234	97%	93%	94%
Prophylactic Antibiotic Stopped	127	94%	94%	94%
Recommended VTP Ordered	144	98%	94%	94%
Urinary Catheter Removal	51	98%	89%	90%
Children's Asthma Care				
Received Systemic Corticosteroids	-	-	-	100%
Received Home Management Plan	-	-	-	71%
Received Reliever Medication	-	-	-	100%
Use of Medical Imaging				
Combination Abdominal CT Scan	533	0.024	0.160	0.191
Combination Chest CT Scan	311	0.000	0.054	0.054
Follow-up Mammogram/Ultrasound	775	1.9%	7.9%	8.4%
MRI for Low Back Pain[1]	43	32.6%	35.6%	32.7%
Survey of Patients' Hospital Experiences				
Area Around Room 'Always' Quiet at Night	300+	64%	-	58%
Doctors 'Always' Communicated Well	300+	84%	-	80%
Home Recovery Information Given	300+	87%	-	82%
Hospital Given 9 or 10 on 10 Point Scale	300+	69%	-	67%
Meds 'Always' Explained Before Given	300+	65%	-	60%
Nurses 'Always' Communicated Well	300+	78%	-	76%
Pain 'Always' Well Controlled	300+	73%	-	69%
Room and Bathroom 'Always' Clean	300+	70%	-	71%
Timely Help 'Always' Received	300+	65%	-	64%
Would Definitely Recommend Hospital	300+	64%	-	69%

NOTE: Hospital profiles are in alphabetical order by state, then city, then hospital within the city; Rankings exclude hospitals with less than 25 cases except for patient surveys which excludes hospitals with less than 100 cases; (a) 100–299 cases; (1) The number of cases is too small to be sure how well a hospital is performing; (2) The hospital indicated that the data submitted for this measure were based on a sample of cases; (3) Data was collected during a shorter time period (fewer quarters) than the maximum possible time for this measure; (4) Suppressed for one or more quarters by CMS; (5) No data is available from the hospital for this measure; (6) Fewer than 100 patients completed the HCAHPS survey. Use these rates with caution, as the number of surveys may be too low to reliably assess hospital performance; (7) Survey results are based on less than 12 months of data; (8) Survey results are not available for this reporting period; (9) No or very few patients were eligible for the HCAHPS survey. The scores shown, if any, reflect a very small number of surveys; (10) A state average was not calculated because too few hospitals in the state submitted data; (11) There were discrepancies in the data collection process; Please refer to the User's Guide for a full explanation of data.

The Medical Center at Franklin

1100 Brookhaven Road
Franklin, KY 42135
URL: www.mcfrk.org
Type: Critical Access Hospitals
Ownership: Voluntary Non-Profit - Private
Key Personnel:
CEO/President . . . . John C. Desmarais

Phone: 270-598-4800

Emergency Services: Yes
Beds: 25

Measure	Cases	This Hosp.	State Avg.	U.S. Avg.
Heart Attack Care				
ACE Inhibitor or ARB for LVSD[1,3]	1	0%	94%	96%
Aspirin at Arrival[1,3]	2	50%	98%	99%
Aspirin at Discharge[1,3]	1	100%	99%	98%
Beta Blocker at Discharge[1,3]	2	100%	98%	98%
Fibrinolytic Medication Timing[3]	0	-	60%	55%
PCI Within 90 Minutes of Arrival[5]	0	-	88%	90%
Smoking Cessation Advice[1,3]	1	100%	100%	99%
Chest Pain/Possible Heart Attack Care				
Aspirin at Arrival	-	-	95%	95%
Median Time to ECG (minutes)	-	-	7	8
Median Time to Transfer (minutes)	-	-	65	61
Fibrinolytic Medication Timing	-	-	62%	54%
Heart Failure Care				
ACE Inhibitor or ARB for LVSD[1]	9	78%	91%	94%
Discharge Instructions	31	68%	82%	88%
Evaluation of LVS Function	47	55%	96%	98%
Smoking Cessation Advice[1]	3	100%	98%	98%
Pneumonia Care				
Appropriate Initial Antibiotic	70	94%	90%	92%
Blood Culture Timing	31	97%	95%	96%
Influenza Vaccine	62	85%	92%	91%
Initial Antibiotic Timing	88	94%	95%	95%
Pneumococcal Vaccine	80	89%	94%	93%
Smoking Cessation Advice	35	100%	98%	97%
Surgical Care Improvement Project				
Appropriate VTP Within 24 Hours[5]	0	-	91%	92%
Appropriate Hair Removal[5]	0	-	99%	99%
Appropriate Beta Blocker Usage[5]	0	-	93%	93%
Controlled Postoperative Blood Glucose[5]	0	-	94%	93%
Prophylactic Antibiotic Timing[5]	0	-	97%	97%
Prophylactic Antibiotic Timing (Outpatient)	-	-	92%	92%
Prophylactic Antibiotic Selection[5]	0	-	98%	97%
Prophylactic Antibiotic Select. (Outpatient)	-	-	93%	94%
Prophylactic Antibiotic Stopped[5]	0	-	94%	94%
Recommended VTP Ordered[5]	0	-	94%	94%
Urinary Catheter Removal	0	-	89%	90%
Children's Asthma Care				
Received Systemic Corticosteroids	-	-	-	100%
Received Home Management Plan	-	-	-	71%
Received Reliever Medication	-	-	-	100%
Use of Medical Imaging				
Combination Abdominal CT Scan	-	-	0.160	0.191
Combination Chest CT Scan	-	-	0.054	0.054
Follow-up Mammogram/Ultrasound	-	-	7.9%	8.4%
MRI for Low Back Pain	-	-	35.6%	32.7%
Survey of Patients' Hospital Experiences				
Area Around Room 'Always' Quiet at Night[8]	-	-	-	58%
Doctors 'Always' Communicated Well[8]	-	-	-	80%
Home Recovery Information Given[8]	-	-	-	82%
Hospital Given 9 or 10 on 10 Point Scale[8]	-	-	-	67%
Meds 'Always' Explained Before Given[8]	-	-	-	60%
Nurses 'Always' Communicated Well[8]	-	-	-	76%
Pain 'Always' Well Controlled[8]	-	-	-	69%
Room and Bathroom 'Always' Clean[8]	-	-	-	71%
Timely Help 'Always' Received[8]	-	-	-	64%
Would Definitely Recommend Hospital[8]	-	-	-	69%

Parkway Regional Hospital

2000 Holiday Lane
Fulton, KY 42041
Type: Acute Care Hospitals
Ownership: Proprietary
Key Personnel:
CEO/President . . . . Michael Patterson

Phone: 270-472-2522
Fax: 270-472-2438
Emergency Services: Yes
Beds: 70

Measure	Cases	This Hosp.	State Avg.	U.S. Avg.
Heart Attack Care				
ACE Inhibitor or ARB for LVSD	0	-	94%	96%
Aspirin at Arrival[1]	2	100%	98%	99%
Aspirin at Discharge[1]	1	100%	99%	98%
Beta Blocker at Discharge[1]	1	100%	98%	98%
Fibrinolytic Medication Timing	0	-	60%	55%
PCI Within 90 Minutes of Arrival	0	-	88%	90%
Smoking Cessation Advice	0	-	100%	99%
Chest Pain/Possible Heart Attack Care				
Aspirin at Arrival	40	100%	95%	95%
Median Time to ECG (minutes)	43	4	7	8
Median Time to Transfer (minutes)[3]	0	-	65	61
Fibrinolytic Medication Timing[1]	3	67%	62%	54%
Heart Failure Care				
ACE Inhibitor or ARB for LVSD[1]	10	100%	91%	94%
Discharge Instructions[1]	19	100%	82%	88%
Evaluation of LVS Function[1]	27	100%	96%	98%
Smoking Cessation Advice[1]	4	100%	98%	98%
Pneumonia Care				
Appropriate Initial Antibiotic	45	93%	90%	92%
Blood Culture Timing	47	100%	95%	96%
Influenza Vaccine	28	100%	92%	91%
Initial Antibiotic Timing	63	100%	95%	95%
Pneumococcal Vaccine	53	100%	94%	93%
Smoking Cessation Advice	26	100%	98%	97%
Surgical Care Improvement Project				
Appropriate VTP Within 24 Hours[1,2]	7	86%	91%	92%
Appropriate Hair Removal[2]	26	100%	99%	99%
Appropriate Beta Blocker Usage[1,2]	4	100%	93%	93%
Controlled Postoperative Blood Glucose[2]	0	-	94%	93%
Prophylactic Antibiotic Timing[1,2]	14	100%	97%	97%
Prophylactic Antibiotic Timing (Outpatient)[1,3]	1	100%	92%	92%
Prophylactic Antibiotic Selection[1,2]	14	100%	98%	97%
Prophylactic Antibiotic Select. (Outpatient)[1,3]	1	0%	93%	94%
Prophylactic Antibiotic Stopped[1,2]	14	100%	94%	94%
Recommended VTP Ordered[1,2]	7	86%	94%	94%
Urinary Catheter Removal	0	-	89%	90%
Children's Asthma Care				
Received Systemic Corticosteroids	-	-	-	100%
Received Home Management Plan	-	-	-	71%
Received Reliever Medication	-	-	-	100%
Use of Medical Imaging				
Combination Abdominal CT Scan	104	0.577	0.160	0.191
Combination Chest CT Scan	45	0.044	0.054	0.054
Follow-up Mammogram/Ultrasound	196	4.1%	7.9%	8.4%
MRI for Low Back Pain[1]	17	47.1%	35.6%	32.7%
Survey of Patients' Hospital Experiences				
Area Around Room 'Always' Quiet at Night	(a)	73%	-	58%
Doctors 'Always' Communicated Well	(a)	88%	-	80%
Home Recovery Information Given	(a)	83%	-	82%
Hospital Given 9 or 10 on 10 Point Scale	(a)	74%	-	67%
Meds 'Always' Explained Before Given	(a)	64%	-	60%
Nurses 'Always' Communicated Well	(a)	82%	-	76%
Pain 'Always' Well Controlled	(a)	77%	-	69%
Room and Bathroom 'Always' Clean	(a)	78%	-	71%
Timely Help 'Always' Received	(a)	74%	-	64%
Would Definitely Recommend Hospital	(a)	67%	-	69%

Georgetown Community Hospital

1140 Lexington Road
Georgetown, KY 40324
URL: www.georgetowncommunityhospital.com
Type: Acute Care Hospitals
Ownership: Proprietary
Key Personnel:
CEO/President . . . . Michael Clark
Chief of Medical Staff . . . . Kelly Burguss
Emergency Room . . . . Philip Wagner

Phone: 502-868-1100
Fax: 502-868-5607

Emergency Services: Yes
Beds: 75

Measure	Cases	This Hosp.	State Avg.	U.S. Avg.
Heart Attack Care				
ACE Inhibitor or ARB for LVSD[1,3]	2	100%	94%	96%
Aspirin at Arrival[1,3]	5	100%	98%	99%
Aspirin at Discharge[1,3]	3	100%	99%	98%
Beta Blocker at Discharge[1,3]	3	100%	98%	98%
Fibrinolytic Medication Timing[3]	0	-	60%	55%
PCI Within 90 Minutes of Arrival[3]	0	-	88%	90%
Smoking Cessation Advice[3]	0	-	100%	99%
Chest Pain/Possible Heart Attack Care				
Aspirin at Arrival	82	99%	95%	95%
Median Time to ECG (minutes)	84	7	7	8
Median Time to Transfer (minutes)[1,3]	6	82	65	61
Fibrinolytic Medication Timing[1]	2	50%	62%	54%
Heart Failure Care				
ACE Inhibitor or ARB for LVSD[1]	13	92%	91%	94%
Discharge Instructions	34	82%	82%	88%
Evaluation of LVS Function	42	100%	96%	98%
Smoking Cessation Advice[1]	7	100%	98%	98%
Pneumonia Care				
Appropriate Initial Antibiotic	45	96%	90%	92%
Blood Culture Timing	75	96%	95%	96%
Influenza Vaccine	49	96%	92%	91%
Initial Antibiotic Timing	75	100%	95%	95%
Pneumococcal Vaccine	59	95%	94%	93%
Smoking Cessation Advice	34	100%	98%	97%
Surgical Care Improvement Project				
Appropriate VTP Within 24 Hours	43	81%	91%	92%
Appropriate Hair Removal	88	100%	99%	99%
Appropriate Beta Blocker Usage[1]	24	96%	93%	93%
Controlled Postoperative Blood Glucose	0	-	94%	93%
Prophylactic Antibiotic Timing	42	98%	97%	97%
Prophylactic Antibiotic Timing (Outpatient)	185	99%	92%	92%
Prophylactic Antibiotic Selection	41	100%	98%	97%
Prophylactic Antibiotic Select. (Outpatient)	185	99%	93%	94%
Prophylactic Antibiotic Stopped	39	85%	94%	94%
Recommended VTP Ordered	43	84%	94%	94%
Urinary Catheter Removal[1]	13	69%	89%	90%
Children's Asthma Care				
Received Systemic Corticosteroids	-	-	-	100%
Received Home Management Plan	-	-	-	71%
Received Reliever Medication	-	-	-	100%
Use of Medical Imaging				
Combination Abdominal CT Scan	345	0.058	0.160	0.191
Combination Chest CT Scan	167	0.024	0.054	0.054
Follow-up Mammogram/Ultrasound	354	5.9%	7.9%	8.4%
MRI for Low Back Pain	58	44.8%	35.6%	32.7%
Survey of Patients' Hospital Experiences				
Area Around Room 'Always' Quiet at Night	300+	62%	-	58%
Doctors 'Always' Communicated Well	300+	87%	-	80%
Home Recovery Information Given	300+	86%	-	82%
Hospital Given 9 or 10 on 10 Point Scale	300+	70%	-	67%
Meds 'Always' Explained Before Given	300+	63%	-	60%
Nurses 'Always' Communicated Well	300+	77%	-	76%
Pain 'Always' Well Controlled	300+	71%	-	69%
Room and Bathroom 'Always' Clean	300+	64%	-	71%
Timely Help 'Always' Received	300+	64%	-	64%
Would Definitely Recommend Hospital	300+	71%	-	69%

NOTE: Hospital profiles are in alphabetical order by state, then city, then hospital within the city; Rankings exclude hospitals with less than 25 cases except for patient surveys which excludes hospitals with less than 100 cases; (a) 100–299 cases; (1) The number of cases is too small to be sure how well a hospital is performing; (2) The hospital indicated that the data submitted for this measure were based on a sample of cases; (3) Data was collected during a shorter time period (fewer quarters) than the maximum possible time for this measure; (4) Suppressed for one or more quarters by CMS; (5) No data is available from the hospital for this measure; (6) Fewer than 100 patients completed the HCAHPS survey. Use these rates with caution, as the number of surveys may be too low to reliably assess hospital performance; (7) Survey results are based on less than 12 months of data; (8) Survey results are not available for this reporting period; (9) No or very few patients were eligible for the HCAHPS survey. The scores shown, if any, reflect a very small number of surveys; (10) A state average was not calculated because too few hospitals in the state submitted data; (11) There were discrepancies in the data collection process; Please refer to the User's Guide for a full explanation of data.

T J Samson Community Hospital

1301 North Race Street
Glasgow, KY 42141
Phone: 270-651-4159
Fax: 270-651-4848
E-mail: Tjsamson@tjsamson.org
URL: www.tjsamson.org
Type: Acute Care Hospitals
Emergency Services: Yes
Ownership: Voluntary Non-Profit - Other
Beds: 196

Key Personnel:
CEO/President.............. Bill Kindred
Chief of Medical Staff.......... Jeffery Sabolovic, MD
Coronary Care.............. Barbara Buss, RN
Infection Control.......... Millie Delk
Pediatric Ambulatory Care...... Melissa Dennison, MD
Pediatric In-Patient Care....... Melissa Dennison, MD
Quality Assurance........... Melanie Watson
Radiology................ Michael Shadowe

Measure	Cases	This Hosp.	State Avg.	U.S. Avg.
Heart Attack Care				
ACE Inhibitor or ARB for LVSD	27	74%	94%	96%
Aspirin at Arrival	165	93%	98%	99%
Aspirin at Discharge	148	94%	99%	98%
Beta Blocker at Discharge	154	96%	98%	98%
Fibrinolytic Medication Timing[1]	6	33%	60%	55%
PCI Within 90 Minutes of Arrival[1]	21	86%	88%	90%
Smoking Cessation Advice	63	100%	100%	99%
Chest Pain/Possible Heart Attack Care				
Aspirin at Arrival[1]	24	88%	95%	95%
Median Time to ECG (minutes)	25	2	7	8
Median Time to Transfer (minutes)[1,3]	1	42	65	61
Fibrinolytic Medication Timing[1]	4	75%	62%	54%
Heart Failure Care				
ACE Inhibitor or ARB for LVSD	57	77%	91%	94%
Discharge Instructions	154	69%	82%	88%
Evaluation of LVS Function	184	99%	96%	98%
Smoking Cessation Advice	40	100%	98%	98%
Pneumonia Care				
Appropriate Initial Antibiotic[2]	101	95%	90%	92%
Blood Culture Timing[2]	60	98%	95%	96%
Influenza Vaccine[2]	95	98%	92%	91%
Initial Antibiotic Timing[2]	154	97%	95%	95%
Pneumococcal Vaccine[2]	153	99%	94%	93%
Smoking Cessation Advice[2]	95	100%	98%	97%
Surgical Care Improvement Project				
Appropriate VTP Within 24 Hours[2]	128	79%	91%	92%
Appropriate Hair Removal[2]	292	89%	99%	99%
Appropriate Beta Blocker Usage[2]	107	93%	93%	93%
Controlled Postoperative Blood Glucose[2]	0	-	94%	93%
Prophylactic Antibiotic Timing[2]	260	83%	97%	97%
Prophylactic Antibiotic Timing (Outpatient)	173	75%	92%	92%
Prophylactic Antibiotic Selection[2]	261	92%	98%	97%
Prophylactic Antibiotic Select. (Outpatient)	142	89%	93%	94%
Prophylactic Antibiotic Stopped[2]	260	80%	94%	94%
Recommended VTP Ordered[2]	129	78%	94%	94%
Urinary Catheter Removal[2]	81	80%	89%	90%
Children's Asthma Care				
Received Systemic Corticosteroids	-	-	-	100%
Received Home Management Plan	-	-	-	71%
Received Reliever Medication	-	-	-	100%
Use of Medical Imaging				
Combination Abdominal CT Scan	841	0.256	0.160	0.191
Combination Chest CT Scan	605	0.175	0.054	0.054
Follow-up Mammogram/Ultrasound	1,292	8.0%	7.9%	8.4%
MRI for Low Back Pain	130	38.5%	35.6%	32.7%
Survey of Patients' Hospital Experiences				
Area Around Room 'Always' Quiet at Night	300+	68%	-	58%
Doctors 'Always' Communicated Well	300+	84%	-	80%
Home Recovery Information Given	300+	84%	-	82%
Hospital Given 9 or 10 on 10 Point Scale	300+	70%	-	67%
Meds 'Always' Explained Before Given	300+	66%	-	60%
Nurses 'Always' Communicated Well	300+	81%	-	76%
Pain 'Always' Well Controlled	300+	73%	-	69%
Room and Bathroom 'Always' Clean	300+	86%	-	71%
Timely Help 'Always' Received	300+	74%	-	64%
Would Definitely Recommend Hospital	300+	70%	-	69%

Jane Todd Crawford Hospital

202-206 Milby Street
Greensburg, KY 42743
Phone: 270-932-4211
Fax: 270-932-3504
E-mail: jtodd@kih.net
Type: Critical Access Hospitals
Emergency Services: Yes
Ownership: Voluntary Non-Profit - Private
Beds: 64

Key Personnel:
CEO/President.............. Rex A Tungate

Measure	Cases	This Hosp.	State Avg.	U.S. Avg.
Heart Attack Care				
ACE Inhibitor or ARB for LVSD[3]	0	-	94%	96%
Aspirin at Arrival[1,3]	2	100%	98%	99%
Aspirin at Discharge[1,3]	2	50%	99%	98%
Beta Blocker at Discharge[1,3]	1	100%	98%	98%
Fibrinolytic Medication Timing[3]	0	-	60%	55%
PCI Within 90 Minutes of Arrival[3]	0	-	88%	90%
Smoking Cessation Advice[1,3]	1	100%	100%	99%
Chest Pain/Possible Heart Attack Care				
Aspirin at Arrival	-	-	95%	95%
Median Time to ECG (minutes)	-	-	7	8
Median Time to Transfer (minutes)	-	-	65	61
Fibrinolytic Medication Timing	-	-	62%	54%
Heart Failure Care				
ACE Inhibitor or ARB for LVSD[1,3]	1	100%	91%	94%
Discharge Instructions[1,3]	5	80%	82%	88%
Evaluation of LVS Function[1,3]	6	17%	96%	98%
Smoking Cessation Advice[1,3]	3	33%	98%	98%
Pneumonia Care				
Appropriate Initial Antibiotic[1]	22	82%	90%	92%
Blood Culture Timing	0	-	95%	96%
Influenza Vaccine[1]	19	42%	92%	91%
Initial Antibiotic Timing	25	92%	95%	95%
Pneumococcal Vaccine[1]	24	62%	94%	93%
Smoking Cessation Advice[1]	16	94%	98%	97%
Surgical Care Improvement Project				
Appropriate VTP Within 24 Hours[5]	0	-	91%	92%
Appropriate Hair Removal[5]	0	-	99%	99%
Appropriate Beta Blocker Usage[5]	0	-	93%	93%
Controlled Postoperative Blood Glucose[5]	0	-	94%	93%
Prophylactic Antibiotic Timing[5]	0	-	97%	97%
Prophylactic Antibiotic Timing (Outpatient)	-	-	92%	92%
Prophylactic Antibiotic Selection[5]	0	-	98%	97%
Prophylactic Antibiotic Select. (Outpatient)	-	-	93%	94%
Prophylactic Antibiotic Stopped[5]	0	-	94%	94%
Recommended VTP Ordered[5]	0	-	94%	94%
Urinary Catheter Removal[5]	0	-	89%	90%
Children's Asthma Care				
Received Systemic Corticosteroids	-	-	-	100%
Received Home Management Plan	-	-	-	71%
Received Reliever Medication	-	-	-	100%
Use of Medical Imaging				
Combination Abdominal CT Scan	-	-	0.160	0.191
Combination Chest CT Scan	-	-	0.054	0.054
Follow-up Mammogram/Ultrasound	-	-	7.9%	8.4%
MRI for Low Back Pain	-	-	35.6%	32.7%
Survey of Patients' Hospital Experiences				
Area Around Room 'Always' Quiet at Night[8]	-	-	-	58%
Doctors 'Always' Communicated Well[8]	-	-	-	80%
Home Recovery Information Given[8]	-	-	-	82%
Hospital Given 9 or 10 on 10 Point Scale[8]	-	-	-	67%
Meds 'Always' Explained Before Given[8]	-	-	-	60%
Nurses 'Always' Communicated Well[8]	-	-	-	76%
Pain 'Always' Well Controlled[8]	-	-	-	69%
Room and Bathroom 'Always' Clean[8]	-	-	-	71%
Timely Help 'Always' Received[8]	-	-	-	64%
Would Definitely Recommend Hospital[8]	-	-	-	69%

Muhlenberg Community Hospital

440 Hopkinsville Street
Greenville, KY 42345
Phone: 270-338-8000
Fax: 270-338-8278
URL: www.mchky.org
Type: Acute Care Hospitals
Emergency Services: Yes
Ownership: Voluntary Non-Profit - Other
Beds: 135

Key Personnel:
CEO/President.............. Lloyd K Ford, JR
Chief of Medical Staff.......... Brad Sparks, MD
Coronary Care.............. Kim Vender
Infection Control.......... Beckie Penrod
Operating Room............. Fara Stewart
Pediatric Ambulatory Care...... Karla Davis
Pediatric In-Patient Care....... Karla Davis
Quality Assurance........... Michele Vincent

Measure	Cases	This Hosp.	State Avg.	U.S. Avg.
Heart Attack Care				
ACE Inhibitor or ARB for LVSD	0	-	94%	96%
Aspirin at Arrival[1]	5	80%	98%	99%
Aspirin at Discharge[1]	2	100%	99%	98%
Beta Blocker at Discharge[1]	1	100%	98%	98%
Fibrinolytic Medication Timing	0	-	60%	55%
PCI Within 90 Minutes of Arrival	0	-	88%	90%
Smoking Cessation Advice[1]	2	100%	100%	99%
Chest Pain/Possible Heart Attack Care				
Aspirin at Arrival	179	95%	95%	95%
Median Time to ECG (minutes)	190	8	7	8
Median Time to Transfer (minutes)[1]	18	66	65	61
Fibrinolytic Medication Timing[1]	3	33%	62%	54%
Heart Failure Care				
ACE Inhibitor or ARB for LVSD[1]	19	100%	91%	94%
Discharge Instructions	39	85%	82%	88%
Evaluation of LVS Function	62	84%	96%	98%
Smoking Cessation Advice[1]	12	92%	98%	98%
Pneumonia Care				
Appropriate Initial Antibiotic	116	90%	90%	92%
Blood Culture Timing	51	100%	95%	96%
Influenza Vaccine	93	88%	92%	91%
Initial Antibiotic Timing	144	99%	95%	95%
Pneumococcal Vaccine	110	88%	94%	93%
Smoking Cessation Advice	75	93%	98%	97%
Surgical Care Improvement Project				
Appropriate VTP Within 24 Hours	55	100%	91%	92%
Appropriate Hair Removal	120	100%	99%	99%
Appropriate Beta Blocker Usage[1]	23	87%	93%	93%
Controlled Postoperative Blood Glucose	0	-	94%	93%
Prophylactic Antibiotic Timing	67	97%	97%	97%
Prophylactic Antibiotic Timing (Outpatient)[1]	6	17%	92%	92%
Prophylactic Antibiotic Selection	66	95%	98%	97%
Prophylactic Antibiotic Select. (Outpatient)[1]	1	100%	93%	94%
Prophylactic Antibiotic Stopped	64	91%	94%	94%
Recommended VTP Ordered	55	100%	94%	94%
Urinary Catheter Removal[1]	11	91%	89%	90%
Children's Asthma Care				
Received Systemic Corticosteroids	-	-	-	100%
Received Home Management Plan	-	-	-	71%
Received Reliever Medication	-	-	-	100%
Use of Medical Imaging				
Combination Abdominal CT Scan	191	0.419	0.160	0.191
Combination Chest CT Scan	67	0.075	0.054	0.054
Follow-up Mammogram/Ultrasound	172	5.8%	7.9%	8.4%
MRI for Low Back Pain	83	51.8%	35.6%	32.7%
Survey of Patients' Hospital Experiences				
Area Around Room 'Always' Quiet at Night	300+	61%	-	58%
Doctors 'Always' Communicated Well	300+	89%	-	80%
Home Recovery Information Given	300+	85%	-	82%
Hospital Given 9 or 10 on 10 Point Scale	300+	64%	-	67%
Meds 'Always' Explained Before Given	300+	67%	-	60%
Nurses 'Always' Communicated Well	300+	81%	-	76%
Pain 'Always' Well Controlled	300+	77%	-	69%
Room and Bathroom 'Always' Clean	300+	75%	-	71%
Timely Help 'Always' Received	300+	68%	-	64%
Would Definitely Recommend Hospital	300+	63%	-	69%

NOTE: Hospital profiles are in alphabetical order by state, then city, then hospital within the city; Rankings exclude hospitals with less than 25 cases except for patient surveys which excludes hospitals with less than 100 cases; (a) 100–299 cases; (1) The number of cases is too small to be sure how well a hospital is performing; (2) The hospital indicated that the data submitted for this measure were based on a sample of cases; (3) Data was collected during a shorter time period (fewer quarters) than the maximum possible time for this measure; (4) Suppressed for one or more quarters by CMS; (5) No data is available from the hospital for this measure; (6) Fewer than 100 patients completed the HCAHPS survey. Use these rates with caution, as the number of surveys may be too low to reliably assess hospital performance; (7) Survey results are based on less than 12 months of data; (8) Survey results are not available for this reporting period; (9) No or very few patients were eligible for the HCAHPS survey. The scores shown, if any, reflect a very small number of surveys; (10) A state average was not calculated because too few hospitals in the state submitted data; (11) There were discrepancies in the data collection process; Please refer to the User's Guide for a full explanation of data.

Breckinridge Memorial Hospital

1011 Old Highway 60 Phone: 270-756-7000
Hardinsburg, KY 40143 Fax: 270-756-6510
E-mail: info@breckhealth.org
URL: www.breckhealth.org
Type: Critical Access Hospitals Emergency Services: Yes
Ownership: Voluntary Non-Profit - Private Beds: 45

Key Personnel:
CEO/President.............. Michael Cooper
Chief of Medical Staff.......... Robert Chambliss, MD
Operating Room............. Amy Mingus
Quality Assurance .... Ricky Moore
Emergency Room .... Patty White

Measure	Cases	This Hosp.	State Avg.	U.S. Avg.
Heart Attack Care				
ACE Inhibitor or ARB for LVSD[5]	0	-	94%	96%
Aspirin at Arrival[5]	0	-	98%	99%
Aspirin at Discharge[5]	0	-	99%	98%
Beta Blocker at Discharge[5]	0	-	98%	98%
Fibrinolytic Medication Timing[5]	0	-	60%	55%
PCI Within 90 Minutes of Arrival[5]	0	-	88%	90%
Smoking Cessation Advice[5]	0	-	100%	99%
Chest Pain/Possible Heart Attack Care				
Aspirin at Arrival	-	-	95%	95%
Median Time to ECG (minutes)	-	-	7	8
Median Time to Transfer (minutes)	-	-	65	61
Fibrinolytic Medication Timing	-	-	62%	54%
Heart Failure Care				
ACE Inhibitor or ARB for LVSD[1,3]	2	100%	91%	94%
Discharge Instructions[3]	31	94%	82%	88%
Evaluation of LVS Function[3]	41	44%	96%	98%
Smoking Cessation Advice[1,3]	7	71%	98%	98%
Pneumonia Care				
Appropriate Initial Antibiotic	26	69%	90%	92%
Blood Culture Timing[1]	11	64%	95%	96%
Influenza Vaccine[1]	21	57%	92%	91%
Initial Antibiotic Timing	38	82%	95%	95%
Pneumococcal Vaccine	30	73%	94%	93%
Smoking Cessation Advice[1]	19	89%	98%	97%
Surgical Care Improvement Project				
Appropriate VTP Within 24 Hours[5]	0	-	91%	92%
Appropriate Hair Removal[5]	0	-	99%	99%
Appropriate Beta Blocker Usage[5]	0	-	93%	93%
Controlled Postoperative Blood Glucose[5]	0	-	94%	93%
Prophylactic Antibiotic Timing[5]	0	-	97%	97%
Prophylactic Antibiotic Timing (Outpatient)	-	-	92%	92%
Prophylactic Antibiotic Selection[5]	0	-	98%	97%
Prophylactic Antibiotic Select. (Outpatient)	-	-	93%	94%
Prophylactic Antibiotic Stopped[5]	0	-	94%	94%
Recommended VTP Ordered[5]	0	-	94%	94%
Urinary Catheter Removal[5]	0	-	89%	90%
Children's Asthma Care				
Received Systemic Corticosteroids	-	-	-	100%
Received Home Management Plan	-	-	-	71%
Received Reliever Medication	-	-	-	100%
Use of Medical Imaging				
Combination Abdominal CT Scan	-	-	0.160	0.191
Combination Chest CT Scan	-	-	0.054	0.054
Follow-up Mammogram/Ultrasound	-	-	7.9%	8.4%
MRI for Low Back Pain	-	-	35.6%	32.7%
Survey of Patients' Hospital Experiences				
Area Around Room 'Always' Quiet at Night[8]	-	-	-	58%
Doctors 'Always' Communicated Well[8]	-	-	-	80%
Home Recovery Information Given[8]	-	-	-	82%
Hospital Given 9 or 10 on 10 Point Scale[8]	-	-	-	67%
Meds 'Always' Explained Before Given[8]	-	-	-	60%
Nurses 'Always' Communicated Well[8]	-	-	-	76%
Pain 'Always' Well Controlled[8]	-	-	-	69%
Room and Bathroom 'Always' Clean[8]	-	-	-	71%
Timely Help 'Always' Received[8]	-	-	-	64%
Would Definitely Recommend Hospital[8]	-	-	-	69%

Harlan Appalachian Regional Healthcare Hospital

81 Ball Park Road Phone: 606-573-8100
Harlan, KY 40831 Fax: 606-573-8200
URL: www.arh.org
Type: Acute Care Hospitals Emergency Services: Yes
Ownership: Voluntary Non-Profit - Other Beds: 150

Key Personnel:
CEO/President.............. Jerry W Haynes
Cardiac Laboratory............ Johnnie Bargo
Chief of Medical Staff.......... Anna Algridge
Quality Assurance .... Russ Barker
Radiology.................. Gregory Y Tiu
Emergency Room .... Donna Middleton, RN

Measure	Cases	This Hosp.	State Avg.	U.S. Avg.
Heart Attack Care				
ACE Inhibitor or ARB for LVSD	0	-	94%	96%
Aspirin at Arrival[1]	7	71%	98%	99%
Aspirin at Discharge[1]	1	100%	99%	98%
Beta Blocker at Discharge[1]	1	100%	98%	98%
Fibrinolytic Medication Timing	0	-	60%	55%
PCI Within 90 Minutes of Arrival	0	-	88%	90%
Smoking Cessation Advice	0	-	100%	99%
Chest Pain/Possible Heart Attack Care				
Aspirin at Arrival	98	98%	95%	95%
Median Time to ECG (minutes)	108	15	7	8
Median Time to Transfer (minutes)[1,3]	1	83	65	61
Fibrinolytic Medication Timing[1]	6	83%	62%	54%
Heart Failure Care				
ACE Inhibitor or ARB for LVSD	33	100%	91%	94%
Discharge Instructions	153	99%	82%	88%
Evaluation of LVS Function	187	100%	96%	98%
Smoking Cessation Advice	33	100%	98%	98%
Pneumonia Care				
Appropriate Initial Antibiotic	149	92%	90%	92%
Blood Culture Timing	164	95%	95%	96%
Influenza Vaccine	104	100%	92%	91%
Initial Antibiotic Timing	232	97%	95%	95%
Pneumococcal Vaccine	125	100%	94%	93%
Smoking Cessation Advice	98	100%	98%	97%
Surgical Care Improvement Project				
Appropriate VTP Within 24 Hours	25	100%	91%	92%
Appropriate Hair Removal	65	100%	99%	99%
Appropriate Beta Blocker Usage[1]	11	100%	93%	93%
Controlled Postoperative Blood Glucose	0	-	94%	93%
Prophylactic Antibiotic Timing	39	97%	97%	97%
Prophylactic Antibiotic Timing (Outpatient)	49	94%	92%	92%
Prophylactic Antibiotic Selection	39	100%	98%	97%
Prophylactic Antibiotic Select. (Outpatient)	54	94%	93%	94%
Prophylactic Antibiotic Stopped	38	100%	94%	94%
Recommended VTP Ordered	25	100%	94%	94%
Urinary Catheter Removal[1]	4	100%	89%	90%
Children's Asthma Care				
Received Systemic Corticosteroids	-	-	-	100%
Received Home Management Plan	-	-	-	71%
Received Reliever Medication	-	-	-	100%
Use of Medical Imaging				
Combination Abdominal CT Scan	420	0.424	0.160	0.191
Combination Chest CT Scan	196	0.235	0.054	0.054
Follow-up Mammogram/Ultrasound	359	8.9%	7.9%	8.4%
MRI for Low Back Pain	104	42.3%	35.6%	32.7%
Survey of Patients' Hospital Experiences				
Area Around Room 'Always' Quiet at Night	300+	63%	-	58%
Doctors 'Always' Communicated Well	300+	79%	-	80%
Home Recovery Information Given	300+	80%	-	82%
Hospital Given 9 or 10 on 10 Point Scale	300+	66%	-	67%
Meds 'Always' Explained Before Given	300+	61%	-	60%
Nurses 'Always' Communicated Well	300+	77%	-	76%
Pain 'Always' Well Controlled	300+	68%	-	69%
Room and Bathroom 'Always' Clean	300+	72%	-	71%
Timely Help 'Always' Received	300+	70%	-	64%
Would Definitely Recommend Hospital	300+	62%	-	69%

The James B Haggin Memorial Hospital

464 Linden Avenue Phone: 859-734-5441
Harrodsburg, KY 40330 Fax: 859-734-5563
Type: Critical Access Hospitals Emergency Services: Yes
Ownership: Voluntary Non-Profit - Other Beds: 59

Key Personnel:
CEO/President.............. Earl Motzer
Radiology.................. Pervez Siddiqui

Measure	Cases	This Hosp.	State Avg.	U.S. Avg.
Heart Attack Care				
ACE Inhibitor or ARB for LVSD[5]	0	-	94%	96%
Aspirin at Arrival[5]	0	-	98%	99%
Aspirin at Discharge[5]	0	-	99%	98%
Beta Blocker at Discharge[5]	0	-	98%	98%
Fibrinolytic Medication Timing[5]	0	-	60%	55%
PCI Within 90 Minutes of Arrival[5]	0	-	88%	90%
Smoking Cessation Advice[5]	0	-	100%	99%
Chest Pain/Possible Heart Attack Care				
Aspirin at Arrival	-	-	95%	95%
Median Time to ECG (minutes)	-	-	7	8
Median Time to Transfer (minutes)	-	-	65	61
Fibrinolytic Medication Timing	-	-	62%	54%
Heart Failure Care				
ACE Inhibitor or ARB for LVSD[1]	12	83%	91%	94%
Discharge Instructions[1]	24	79%	82%	88%
Evaluation of LVS Function	40	75%	96%	98%
Smoking Cessation Advice[1]	11	73%	98%	98%
Pneumonia Care				
Appropriate Initial Antibiotic	36	89%	90%	92%
Blood Culture Timing	50	80%	95%	96%
Influenza Vaccine	53	85%	92%	91%
Initial Antibiotic Timing	44	95%	95%	95%
Pneumococcal Vaccine	71	82%	94%	93%
Smoking Cessation Advice	41	61%	98%	97%
Surgical Care Improvement Project				
Appropriate VTP Within 24 Hours[5]	0	-	91%	92%
Appropriate Hair Removal[5]	0	-	99%	99%
Appropriate Beta Blocker Usage[5]	0	-	93%	93%
Controlled Postoperative Blood Glucose[5]	0	-	94%	93%
Prophylactic Antibiotic Timing[5]	0	-	97%	97%
Prophylactic Antibiotic Timing (Outpatient)	-	-	92%	92%
Prophylactic Antibiotic Selection[5]	0	-	98%	97%
Prophylactic Antibiotic Select. (Outpatient)	-	-	93%	94%
Prophylactic Antibiotic Stopped[5]	0	-	94%	94%
Recommended VTP Ordered[5]	0	-	94%	94%
Urinary Catheter Removal[5]	0	-	89%	90%
Children's Asthma Care				
Received Systemic Corticosteroids	-	-	-	100%
Received Home Management Plan	-	-	-	71%
Received Reliever Medication	-	-	-	100%
Use of Medical Imaging				
Combination Abdominal CT Scan	-	-	0.160	0.191
Combination Chest CT Scan	-	-	0.054	0.054
Follow-up Mammogram/Ultrasound	-	-	7.9%	8.4%
MRI for Low Back Pain	-	-	35.6%	32.7%
Survey of Patients' Hospital Experiences				
Area Around Room 'Always' Quiet at Night[8]	-	-	-	58%
Doctors 'Always' Communicated Well[8]	-	-	-	80%
Home Recovery Information Given[8]	-	-	-	82%
Hospital Given 9 or 10 on 10 Point Scale[8]	-	-	-	67%
Meds 'Always' Explained Before Given[8]	-	-	-	60%
Nurses 'Always' Communicated Well[8]	-	-	-	76%
Pain 'Always' Well Controlled[8]	-	-	-	69%
Room and Bathroom 'Always' Clean[8]	-	-	-	71%
Timely Help 'Always' Received[8]	-	-	-	64%
Would Definitely Recommend Hospital[8]	-	-	-	69%

NOTE: Hospital profiles are in alphabetical order by state, then city, then hospital within the city; Rankings exclude hospitals with less than 25 cases except for patient surveys which excludes hospitals with less than 100 cases; (a) 100–299 cases; (1) The number of cases is too small to be sure how well a hospital is performing; (2) The hospital indicated that the data submitted for this measure were based on a sample of cases; (3) Data was collected during a shorter time period (fewer quarters) than the maximum possible time for this measure; (4) Suppressed for one or more quarters by CMS; (5) No data is available from the hospital for this measure; (6) Fewer than 100 patients completed the HCAHPS survey. Use these rates with caution, as the number of surveys may be too low to reliably assess hospital performance; (7) Survey results are based on less than 12 months of data; (8) Survey results are not available for this reporting period; (9) No or very few patients were eligible for the HCAHPS survey. The scores shown, if any, reflect a very small number of surveys; (10) A state average was not calculated because too few hospitals in the state submitted data; (11) There were discrepancies in the data collection process; Please refer to the User's Guide for a full explanation of data.

Ohio County Hospital

1211 Old Main Street
Hartford, KY 42347
Phone: 270-298-7411
Fax: 270-298-3758
URL: www.ohiocountyhospital.com
Type: Critical Access Hospitals
Emergency Services: Yes
Ownership: Proprietary
Beds: 68

Key Personnel:

CEO/President. . . . . Blaine Pieper
Chief of Medical Staff. . . . . Leticia Tuker
Radiology. . . . . Bruce Bu
Patient Relations . . . . Brenda Newcom, RN

Measure	Cases	This Hosp.	State Avg.	U.S. Avg.
Heart Attack Care				
ACE Inhibitor or ARB for LVSD[3]	0	-	94%	96%
Aspirin at Arrival[3]	0	-	98%	99%
Aspirin at Discharge[3]	0	-	99%	98%
Beta Blocker at Discharge[3]	0	-	98%	98%
Fibrinolytic Medication Timing[3]	0	-	60%	55%
PCI Within 90 Minutes of Arrival[3]	0	-	88%	90%
Smoking Cessation Advice[3]	0	-	100%	99%
Chest Pain/Possible Heart Attack Care				
Aspirin at Arrival	-	-	95%	95%
Median Time to ECG (minutes)	-	-	7	8
Median Time to Transfer (minutes)	-	-	65	61
Fibrinolytic Medication Timing	-	-	62%	54%
Heart Failure Care				
ACE Inhibitor or ARB for LVSD[1]	7	86%	91%	94%
Discharge Instructions	28	86%	82%	88%
Evaluation of LVS Function	34	85%	96%	98%
Smoking Cessation Advice[1]	5	100%	98%	98%
Pneumonia Care				
Appropriate Initial Antibiotic	33	85%	90%	92%
Blood Culture Timing	32	94%	95%	96%
Influenza Vaccine	34	62%	92%	91%
Initial Antibiotic Timing	38	97%	95%	95%
Pneumococcal Vaccine	39	69%	94%	93%
Smoking Cessation Advice[1]	18	89%	98%	97%
Surgical Care Improvement Project				
Appropriate VTP Within 24 Hours[1]	11	91%	91%	92%
Appropriate Hair Removal[1]	24	100%	99%	99%
Appropriate Beta Blocker Usage[5]	0	-	93%	93%
Controlled Postoperative Blood Glucose	0	-	94%	93%
Prophylactic Antibiotic Timing[1]	20	90%	97%	97%
Prophylactic Antibiotic Timing (Outpatient)	-	-	92%	92%
Prophylactic Antibiotic Selection[1]	20	50%	98%	97%
Prophylactic Antibiotic Select. (Outpatient)	-	-	93%	94%
Prophylactic Antibiotic Stopped[1]	19	89%	94%	94%
Recommended VTP Ordered[1]	11	91%	94%	94%
Urinary Catheter Removal[1]	2	100%	89%	90%
Children's Asthma Care				
Received Systemic Corticosteroids	-	-	-	100%
Received Home Management Plan	-	-	-	71%
Received Reliever Medication	-	-	-	100%
Use of Medical Imaging				
Combination Abdominal CT Scan	-	-	0.160	0.191
Combination Chest CT Scan	-	-	0.054	0.054
Follow-up Mammogram/Ultrasound	-	-	7.9%	8.4%
MRI for Low Back Pain	-	-	35.6%	32.7%
Survey of Patients' Hospital Experiences				
Area Around Room 'Always' Quiet at Night	(a)	60%	-	58%
Doctors 'Always' Communicated Well	(a)	83%	-	80%
Home Recovery Information Given	(a)	83%	-	82%
Hospital Given 9 or 10 on 10 Point Scale	(a)	59%	-	67%
Meds 'Always' Explained Before Given	(a)	48%	-	60%
Nurses 'Always' Communicated Well	(a)	79%	-	76%
Pain 'Always' Well Controlled	(a)	74%	-	69%
Room and Bathroom 'Always' Clean	(a)	79%	-	71%
Timely Help 'Always' Received	(a)	69%	-	64%
Would Definitely Recommend Hospital	(a)	66%	-	69%

Hazard Arh Regional Medical Center

100 Medical Center Drive
Hazard, KY 41701
Phone: 606-439-6600
Fax: 606-439-6682
E-mail: afugate@arh.org
URL: www.arh.org/hazard
Type: Acute Care Hospitals
Emergency Services: Yes
Ownership: Voluntary Non-Profit - Other
Beds: 308

Key Personnel:

CEO/President. . . . . Dennis Chaney
Chief of Medical Staff. . . . . James A Chaney, MD
Infection Control. . . . . Tonda Young
Radiology. . . . . Doug Morgan, RT
Emergency Room . . . . Lisa Hall
Intensive Care Unit. . . . . Wanda Combs, RN

Measure	Cases	This Hosp.	State Avg.	U.S. Avg.
Heart Attack Care				
ACE Inhibitor or ARB for LVSD[2]	52	81%	94%	96%
Aspirin at Arrival[2]	111	93%	98%	99%
Aspirin at Discharge[2]	167	92%	99%	98%
Beta Blocker at Discharge[2]	170	89%	98%	98%
Fibrinolytic Medication Timing[2]	0	-	60%	55%
PCI Within 90 Minutes of Arrival[1,2]	15	60%	88%	90%
Smoking Cessation Advice[2]	86	98%	100%	99%
Chest Pain/Possible Heart Attack Care				
Aspirin at Arrival	25	84%	95%	95%
Median Time to ECG (minutes)[1]	24	9	7	8
Median Time to Transfer (minutes)[5]	0	-	65	61
Fibrinolytic Medication Timing[3]	0	-	62%	54%
Heart Failure Care				
ACE Inhibitor or ARB for LVSD[2]	63	83%	91%	94%
Discharge Instructions[2]	276	67%	82%	88%
Evaluation of LVS Function[2]	306	98%	96%	98%
Smoking Cessation Advice[2]	53	100%	98%	98%
Pneumonia Care				
Appropriate Initial Antibiotic[2]	75	83%	90%	92%
Blood Culture Timing[2]	32	100%	95%	96%
Influenza Vaccine[2]	82	68%	92%	91%
Initial Antibiotic Timing[2]	116	88%	95%	95%
Pneumococcal Vaccine[2]	88	78%	94%	93%
Smoking Cessation Advice[2]	70	99%	98%	97%
Surgical Care Improvement Project				
Appropriate VTP Within 24 Hours[2]	128	89%	91%	92%
Appropriate Hair Removal[2]	354	100%	99%	99%
Appropriate Beta Blocker Usage[2]	152	94%	93%	93%
Controlled Postoperative Blood Glucose[2]	84	98%	94%	93%
Prophylactic Antibiotic Timing[2]	210	99%	97%	97%
Prophylactic Antibiotic Timing (Outpatient)	127	71%	92%	92%
Prophylactic Antibiotic Selection[2]	212	89%	98%	97%
Prophylactic Antibiotic Select. (Outpatient)	126	93%	93%	94%
Prophylactic Antibiotic Stopped[2]	196	95%	94%	94%
Recommended VTP Ordered[2]	128	92%	94%	94%
Urinary Catheter Removal	66	88%	89%	90%
Children's Asthma Care				
Received Systemic Corticosteroids	-	-	-	100%
Received Home Management Plan	-	-	-	71%
Received Reliever Medication	-	-	-	100%
Use of Medical Imaging				
Combination Abdominal CT Scan	542	0.006	0.160	0.191
Combination Chest CT Scan	233	0.017	0.054	0.054
Follow-up Mammogram/Ultrasound	360	6.1%	7.9%	8.4%
MRI for Low Back Pain[1]	25	44.0%	35.6%	32.7%
Survey of Patients' Hospital Experiences				
Area Around Room 'Always' Quiet at Night	300+	62%	-	58%
Doctors 'Always' Communicated Well	300+	83%	-	80%
Home Recovery Information Given	300+	78%	-	82%
Hospital Given 9 or 10 on 10 Point Scale	300+	67%	-	67%
Meds 'Always' Explained Before Given	300+	59%	-	60%
Nurses 'Always' Communicated Well	300+	77%	-	76%
Pain 'Always' Well Controlled	300+	70%	-	69%
Room and Bathroom 'Always' Clean	300+	73%	-	71%
Timely Help 'Always' Received	300+	64%	-	64%
Would Definitely Recommend Hospital	300+	63%	-	69%

Methodist Hospital

1305 N Elm St
Henderson, KY 42420
Phone: 270-827-7700
Fax: 270-827-7129
E-mail: info@methodisthospital.net
URL: www.methodisthospital.net
Type: Acute Care Hospitals
Emergency Services: Yes
Ownership: Voluntary Non-Profit - Church
Beds: 197

Key Personnel:

Cardiac Laboratory. . . . . Sandy Shuler
Chief of Medical Staff. . . . . Mohit K Sheth, MD
Coronary Care . . . . Brenda Dossett
Pediatric In-Patient Care . . . . Rita Barron
Radiology. . . . . Anthony Perkins
Emergency Room . . . . Salim Akrabawi, RN
Intensive Care Unit. . . . . Beverly Skaggs
Patient Relations . . . . Bill Schwartz

Measure	Cases	This Hosp.	State Avg.	U.S. Avg.
Heart Attack Care				
ACE Inhibitor or ARB for LVSD[1]	9	100%	94%	96%
Aspirin at Arrival[1]	23	91%	98%	99%
Aspirin at Discharge[1]	17	76%	99%	98%
Beta Blocker at Discharge[1]	19	84%	98%	98%
Fibrinolytic Medication Timing[1]	1	0%	60%	55%
PCI Within 90 Minutes of Arrival	0	-	88%	90%
Smoking Cessation Advice[1]	6	67%	100%	99%
Chest Pain/Possible Heart Attack Care				
Aspirin at Arrival	101	94%	95%	95%
Median Time to ECG (minutes)	104	4	7	8
Median Time to Transfer (minutes)[1,3]	8	66	65	61
Fibrinolytic Medication Timing	0	-	62%	54%
Heart Failure Care				
ACE Inhibitor or ARB for LVSD	53	89%	91%	94%
Discharge Instructions	165	84%	82%	88%
Evaluation of LVS Function	210	98%	96%	98%
Smoking Cessation Advice	39	100%	98%	98%
Pneumonia Care				
Appropriate Initial Antibiotic	150	77%	90%	92%
Blood Culture Timing	154	99%	95%	96%
Influenza Vaccine	143	85%	92%	91%
Initial Antibiotic Timing	231	95%	95%	95%
Pneumococcal Vaccine	191	91%	94%	93%
Smoking Cessation Advice	105	92%	98%	97%
Surgical Care Improvement Project				
Appropriate VTP Within 24 Hours[2]	75	95%	91%	92%
Appropriate Hair Removal[2]	218	93%	99%	99%
Appropriate Beta Blocker Usage[2]	56	93%	93%	93%
Controlled Postoperative Blood Glucose[2]	0	-	94%	93%
Prophylactic Antibiotic Timing[2]	138	97%	97%	97%
Prophylactic Antibiotic Timing (Outpatient)	225	94%	92%	92%
Prophylactic Antibiotic Selection[2]	139	99%	98%	97%
Prophylactic Antibiotic Select. (Outpatient)	220	91%	93%	94%
Prophylactic Antibiotic Stopped[2]	135	90%	94%	94%
Recommended VTP Ordered[2]	76	96%	94%	94%
Urinary Catheter Removal[2]	52	85%	89%	90%
Children's Asthma Care				
Received Systemic Corticosteroids	-	-	-	100%
Received Home Management Plan	-	-	-	71%
Received Reliever Medication	-	-	-	100%
Use of Medical Imaging				
Combination Abdominal CT Scan	492	0.177	0.160	0.191
Combination Chest CT Scan	331	0.018	0.054	0.054
Follow-up Mammogram/Ultrasound	785	3.8%	7.9%	8.4%
MRI for Low Back Pain	122	42.6%	35.6%	32.7%
Survey of Patients' Hospital Experiences				
Area Around Room 'Always' Quiet at Night	300+	58%	-	58%
Doctors 'Always' Communicated Well	300+	84%	-	80%
Home Recovery Information Given	300+	79%	-	82%
Hospital Given 9 or 10 on 10 Point Scale	300+	61%	-	67%
Meds 'Always' Explained Before Given	300+	58%	-	60%
Nurses 'Always' Communicated Well	300+	77%	-	76%
Pain 'Always' Well Controlled	300+	71%	-	69%
Room and Bathroom 'Always' Clean	300+	73%	-	71%
Timely Help 'Always' Received	300+	61%	-	64%
Would Definitely Recommend Hospital	300+	60%	-	69%

NOTE: Hospital profiles are in alphabetical order by state, then city, then hospital within the city; Rankings exclude hospitals with less than 25 cases except for patient surveys which excludes hospitals with less than 100 cases; (a) 100–299 cases; (1) The number of cases is too small to be sure how well a hospital is performing; (2) The hospital indicated that the data submitted for this measure were based on a sample of cases; (3) Data was collected during a shorter time period (fewer quarters) than the maximum possible time for this measure; (4) Suppressed for one or more quarters by CMS; (5) No data is available from the hospital for this measure; (6) Fewer than 100 patients completed the HCAHPS survey. Use these rates with caution, as the number of surveys may be too low to reliably assess hospital performance; (7) Survey results are based on less than 12 months of data; (8) Survey results are not available for this reporting period; (9) No or very few patients were eligible for the HCAHPS survey. The scores shown, if any, reflect a very small number of surveys; (10) A state average was not calculated because too few hospitals in the state submitted data; (11) There were discrepancies in the data collection process; Please refer to the User's Guide for a full explanation of data.

Jennie Stuart Medical Center

320 West 18th Street
Hopkinsville, KY 42240
URL: www.jsmc.org
Type: Acute Care Hospitals
Ownership: Voluntary Non-Profit - Private

Phone: 270-887-0100
Fax: 270-887-0254

Emergency Services: No
Beds: 194

Key Personnel:
CEO/President . . . . Terry Peeples
Chief of Medical Staff . . . . Travis Calhoun
Infection Control . . . . Betty Jones
Operating Room . . . . J Giannini
Pediatric Ambulatory Care . . . . . . Ronald Howard
Pediatric In-Patient Care . . . . Ronald Howard
Quality Assurance . . . . Eric Lee
Radiology . . . . Michael Clark

Measure	Cases	This Hosp.	State Avg.	U.S. Avg.
Heart Attack Care				
ACE Inhibitor or ARB for LVSD[1]	4	100%	94%	96%
Aspirin at Arrival[1]	20	90%	98%	99%
Aspirin at Discharge[1]	15	87%	99%	98%
Beta Blocker at Discharge[1]	15	100%	98%	98%
Fibrinolytic Medication Timing	0	-	60%	55%
PCI Within 90 Minutes of Arrival	0	-	88%	90%
Smoking Cessation Advice[1]	5	100%	100%	99%
Chest Pain/Possible Heart Attack Care				
Aspirin at Arrival	214	96%	95%	95%
Median Time to ECG (minutes)	231	8	7	8
Median Time to Transfer (minutes)[1]	14	164	65	61
Fibrinolytic Medication Timing[1]	19	37%	62%	54%
Heart Failure Care				
ACE Inhibitor or ARB for LVSD	81	94%	91%	94%
Discharge Instructions	141	73%	82%	88%
Evaluation of LVS Function	181	84%	96%	98%
Smoking Cessation Advice	55	91%	98%	98%
Pneumonia Care				
Appropriate Initial Antibiotic	170	90%	90%	92%
Blood Culture Timing	179	92%	95%	96%
Influenza Vaccine	143	92%	92%	91%
Initial Antibiotic Timing	238	92%	95%	95%
Pneumococcal Vaccine	186	89%	94%	93%
Smoking Cessation Advice	101	95%	98%	97%
Surgical Care Improvement Project				
Appropriate VTP Within 24 Hours	126	96%	91%	92%
Appropriate Hair Removal	421	93%	99%	99%
Appropriate Beta Blocker Usage	85	85%	93%	93%
Controlled Postoperative Blood Glucose	0	-	94%	93%
Prophylactic Antibiotic Timing	315	93%	97%	97%
Prophylactic Antibiotic Timing (Outpatient)	166	87%	92%	92%
Prophylactic Antibiotic Selection	318	97%	98%	97%
Prophylactic Antibiotic Select. (Outpatient)	165	92%	93%	94%
Prophylactic Antibiotic Stopped	307	87%	94%	94%
Recommended VTP Ordered	134	90%	94%	94%
Urinary Catheter Removal	101	75%	89%	90%
Children's Asthma Care				
Received Systemic Corticosteroids	-	-	-	100%
Received Home Management Plan	-	-	-	71%
Received Reliever Medication	-	-	-	100%
Use of Medical Imaging				
Combination Abdominal CT Scan	587	0.032	0.160	0.191
Combination Chest CT Scan	308	0.003	0.054	0.054
Follow-up Mammogram/Ultrasound	1,059	5.6%	7.9%	8.4%
MRI for Low Back Pain	132	32.6%	35.6%	32.7%
Survey of Patients' Hospital Experiences				
Area Around Room 'Always' Quiet at Night	300+	57%	-	58%
Doctors 'Always' Communicated Well	300+	75%	-	80%
Home Recovery Information Given	300+	80%	-	82%
Hospital Given 9 or 10 on 10 Point Scale	300+	54%	-	67%
Meds 'Always' Explained Before Given	300+	54%	-	60%
Nurses 'Always' Communicated Well	300+	67%	-	76%
Pain 'Always' Well Controlled	300+	63%	-	69%
Room and Bathroom 'Always' Clean	300+	66%	-	71%
Timely Help 'Always' Received	300+	56%	-	64%
Would Definitely Recommend Hospital	300+	50%	-	69%

Caverna Memorial Hospital

1501 South Dixie Street
Horse Cave, KY 42749
URL: www.cavernahospital.com
Type: Critical Access Hospitals
Ownership: Voluntary Non-Profit - Private

Phone: 270-786-2191
Fax: 270-786-1557

Emergency Services: Yes
Beds: 25

Key Personnel:
CEO/President . . . . Alan Alexander
Chief of Medical Staff . . . . David N Catlett
Radiology . . . . Jannice Aaron

Measure	Cases	This Hosp.	State Avg.	U.S. Avg.
Heart Attack Care				
ACE Inhibitor or ARB for LVSD[3]	0	-	94%	96%
Aspirin at Arrival[1,3]	4	75%	98%	99%
Aspirin at Discharge[1,3]	2	50%	99%	98%
Beta Blocker at Discharge[1,3]	2	50%	98%	98%
Fibrinolytic Medication Timing[3]	0	-	60%	55%
PCI Within 90 Minutes of Arrival[3]	0	-	88%	90%
Smoking Cessation Advice[1,3]	1	0%	100%	99%
Chest Pain/Possible Heart Attack Care				
Aspirin at Arrival	-	-	95%	95%
Median Time to ECG (minutes)	-	-	7	8
Median Time to Transfer (minutes)	-	-	65	61
Fibrinolytic Medication Timing	-	-	62%	54%
Heart Failure Care				
ACE Inhibitor or ARB for LVSD[1]	4	75%	91%	94%
Discharge Instructions	26	42%	82%	88%
Evaluation of LVS Function	38	55%	96%	98%
Smoking Cessation Advice[1]	8	75%	98%	98%
Pneumonia Care				
Appropriate Initial Antibiotic[1]	14	100%	90%	92%
Blood Culture Timing[1]	17	100%	95%	96%
Influenza Vaccine[1]	19	79%	92%	91%
Initial Antibiotic Timing[1]	1	0%	95%	95%
Pneumococcal Vaccine	27	70%	94%	93%
Smoking Cessation Advice[1]	7	86%	98%	97%
Surgical Care Improvement Project				
Appropriate VTP Within 24 Hours[5]	0	-	91%	92%
Appropriate Hair Removal[5]	0	-	99%	99%
Appropriate Beta Blocker Usage[5]	0	-	93%	93%
Controlled Postoperative Blood Glucose[5]	0	-	94%	93%
Prophylactic Antibiotic Timing[5]	0	-	97%	97%
Prophylactic Antibiotic Timing (Outpatient)	-	-	92%	92%
Prophylactic Antibiotic Selection[5]	0	-	98%	97%
Prophylactic Antibiotic Select. (Outpatient)	-	-	93%	94%
Prophylactic Antibiotic Stopped[5]	0	-	94%	94%
Recommended VTP Ordered[5]	0	-	94%	94%
Urinary Catheter Removal[5]	0	-	89%	90%
Children's Asthma Care				
Received Systemic Corticosteroids	-	-	-	100%
Received Home Management Plan	-	-	-	71%
Received Reliever Medication	-	-	-	100%
Use of Medical Imaging				
Combination Abdominal CT Scan	-	-	0.160	0.191
Combination Chest CT Scan	-	-	0.054	0.054
Follow-up Mammogram/Ultrasound	-	-	7.9%	8.4%
MRI for Low Back Pain	-	-	35.6%	32.7%
Survey of Patients' Hospital Experiences				
Area Around Room 'Always' Quiet at Night[8]	-	-	-	58%
Doctors 'Always' Communicated Well[8]	-	-	-	80%
Home Recovery Information Given[8]	-	-	-	82%
Hospital Given 9 or 10 on 10 Point Scale[8]	-	-	-	67%
Meds 'Always' Explained Before Given[8]	-	-	-	60%
Nurses 'Always' Communicated Well[8]	-	-	-	76%
Pain 'Always' Well Controlled[8]	-	-	-	69%
Room and Bathroom 'Always' Clean[8]	-	-	-	71%
Timely Help 'Always' Received[8]	-	-	-	64%
Would Definitely Recommend Hospital[8]	-	-	-	69%

Mary Breckinridge Hospital

130 Kate Ireland Drive
Hyden, KY 41749
Type: Critical Access Hospitals
Ownership: Voluntary Non-Profit - Private

Phone: 606-672-2901
Fax: 606-672-3626
Emergency Services: Yes
Beds: 40

Key Personnel:
CEO/President . . . . William Hall
Chief of Medical Staff . . . . Roy Varghese, MD
Infection Control . . . . Mona Howard
Operating Room . . . . Linda Craft
Quality Assurance . . . . Betty Helen Couch
Emergency Room . . . . Edith Hensley

Measure	Cases	This Hosp.	State Avg.	U.S. Avg.
Heart Attack Care				
ACE Inhibitor or ARB for LVSD[3]	0	-	94%	96%
Aspirin at Arrival[1,3]	1	100%	98%	99%
Aspirin at Discharge[1,3]	1	100%	99%	98%
Beta Blocker at Discharge[1,3]	1	0%	98%	98%
Fibrinolytic Medication Timing[3]	0	-	60%	55%
PCI Within 90 Minutes of Arrival[3]	0	-	88%	90%
Smoking Cessation Advice[3]	0	-	100%	99%
Chest Pain/Possible Heart Attack Care				
Aspirin at Arrival	-	-	95%	95%
Median Time to ECG (minutes)	-	-	7	8
Median Time to Transfer (minutes)	-	-	65	61
Fibrinolytic Medication Timing	-	-	62%	54%
Heart Failure Care				
ACE Inhibitor or ARB for LVSD[1]	8	100%	91%	94%
Discharge Instructions	42	83%	82%	88%
Evaluation of LVS Function	52	92%	96%	98%
Smoking Cessation Advice[1]	7	100%	98%	98%
Pneumonia Care				
Appropriate Initial Antibiotic	52	88%	90%	92%
Blood Culture Timing	69	97%	95%	96%
Influenza Vaccine	51	88%	92%	91%
Initial Antibiotic Timing	71	99%	95%	95%
Pneumococcal Vaccine	55	96%	94%	93%
Smoking Cessation Advice	29	97%	98%	97%
Surgical Care Improvement Project				
Appropriate VTP Within 24 Hours[5]	0	-	91%	92%
Appropriate Hair Removal[5]	0	-	99%	99%
Appropriate Beta Blocker Usage[5]	0	-	93%	93%
Controlled Postoperative Blood Glucose[5]	0	-	94%	93%
Prophylactic Antibiotic Timing[5]	0	-	97%	97%
Prophylactic Antibiotic Timing (Outpatient)	-	-	92%	92%
Prophylactic Antibiotic Selection[5]	0	-	98%	97%
Prophylactic Antibiotic Select. (Outpatient)	-	-	93%	94%
Prophylactic Antibiotic Stopped[5]	0	-	94%	94%
Recommended VTP Ordered[5]	0	-	94%	94%
Urinary Catheter Removal[5]	0	-	89%	90%
Children's Asthma Care				
Received Systemic Corticosteroids	-	-	-	100%
Received Home Management Plan	-	-	-	71%
Received Reliever Medication	-	-	-	100%
Use of Medical Imaging				
Combination Abdominal CT Scan	-	-	0.160	0.191
Combination Chest CT Scan	-	-	0.054	0.054
Follow-up Mammogram/Ultrasound	-	-	7.9%	8.4%
MRI for Low Back Pain	-	-	35.6%	32.7%
Survey of Patients' Hospital Experiences				
Area Around Room 'Always' Quiet at Night[8]	-	-	-	58%
Doctors 'Always' Communicated Well[8]	-	-	-	80%
Home Recovery Information Given[8]	-	-	-	82%
Hospital Given 9 or 10 on 10 Point Scale[8]	-	-	-	67%
Meds 'Always' Explained Before Given[8]	-	-	-	60%
Nurses 'Always' Communicated Well[8]	-	-	-	76%
Pain 'Always' Well Controlled[8]	-	-	-	69%
Room and Bathroom 'Always' Clean[8]	-	-	-	71%
Timely Help 'Always' Received[8]	-	-	-	64%
Would Definitely Recommend Hospital[8]	-	-	-	69%

NOTE: Hospital profiles are in alphabetical order by state, then city, then hospital within the city; Rankings exclude hospitals with less than 25 cases except for patient surveys which excludes hospitals with less than 100 cases; (a) 100–299 cases; (1) The number of cases is too small to be sure how well a hospital is performing; (2) The hospital indicated that the data submitted for this measure were based on a sample of cases; (3) Data was collected during a shorter time period (fewer quarters) than the maximum possible time for this measure; (4) Suppressed for one or more quarters by CMS; (5) No data is available from the hospital for this measure; (6) Fewer than 100 patients completed the HCAHPS survey. Use these rates with caution, as the number of surveys may be too low to reliably assess hospital performance; (7) Survey results are based on less than 12 months of data; (8) Survey results are not available for this reporting period; (9) No or very few patients were eligible for the HCAHPS survey. The scores shown, if any, reflect a very small number of surveys; (10) A state average was not calculated because too few hospitals in the state submitted data; (11) There were discrepancies in the data collection process; Please refer to the User's Guide for a full explanation of data.

Marcum and Wallace Memorial Hospital

60 Mercy Court
Irvine, KY 40336
Type: Critical Access Hospitals
Ownership: Voluntary Non-Profit - Church

Phone: 606-723-2115
Fax: 606-723-6549
Emergency Services: Yes
Beds: 26

Key Personnel:
CEO/President . . . . Susan Ftarling
Quality Assurance . . . . Susan Ftarling
Emergency Room . . . . Jenith Smith

Measure	Cases	This Hosp.	State Avg.	U.S. Avg.
Heart Attack Care				
ACE Inhibitor or ARB for LVSD[5]	0	-	94%	96%
Aspirin at Arrival[5]	0	-	98%	99%
Aspirin at Discharge[5]	0	-	99%	98%
Beta Blocker at Discharge[5]	0	-	98%	98%
Fibrinolytic Medication Timing[5]	0	-	60%	55%
PCI Within 90 Minutes of Arrival[5]	0	-	88%	90%
Smoking Cessation Advice[5]	0	-	100%	99%
Chest Pain/Possible Heart Attack Care				
Aspirin at Arrival	-	-	95%	95%
Median Time to ECG (minutes)	-	-	7	8
Median Time to Transfer (minutes)	-	-	65	61
Fibrinolytic Medication Timing	-	-	62%	54%
Heart Failure Care				
ACE Inhibitor or ARB for LVSD[1]	2	100%	91%	94%
Discharge Instructions[1]	10	80%	82%	88%
Evaluation of LVS Function[1]	10	70%	96%	98%
Smoking Cessation Advice[1]	0	-	98%	98%
Pneumonia Care				
Appropriate Initial Antibiotic	38	92%	90%	92%
Blood Culture Timing	42	95%	95%	96%
Influenza Vaccine	40	92%	92%	91%
Initial Antibiotic Timing	51	96%	95%	95%
Pneumococcal Vaccine	59	90%	94%	93%
Smoking Cessation Advice[1]	21	95%	98%	97%
Surgical Care Improvement Project				
Appropriate VTP Within 24 Hours[5]	0	-	91%	92%
Appropriate Hair Removal[5]	0	-	99%	99%
Appropriate Beta Blocker Usage[5]	0	-	93%	93%
Controlled Postoperative Blood Glucose[5]	0	-	94%	93%
Prophylactic Antibiotic Timing[5]	0	-	97%	97%
Prophylactic Antibiotic Timing (Outpatient)	-	-	92%	92%
Prophylactic Antibiotic Selection[5]	0	-	98%	97%
Prophylactic Antibiotic Select. (Outpatient)	-	-	93%	94%
Prophylactic Antibiotic Stopped[5]	0	-	94%	94%
Recommended VTP Ordered[5]	0	-	94%	94%
Urinary Catheter Removal[5]	0	-	89%	90%
Children's Asthma Care				
Received Systemic Corticosteroids	-	-	-	100%
Received Home Management Plan	-	-	-	71%
Received Reliever Medication	-	-	-	100%
Use of Medical Imaging				
Combination Abdominal CT Scan	-	-	0.160	0.191
Combination Chest CT Scan	-	-	0.054	0.054
Follow-up Mammogram/Ultrasound	-	-	7.9%	8.4%
MRI for Low Back Pain	-	-	35.6%	32.7%
Survey of Patients' Hospital Experiences				
Area Around Room 'Always' Quiet at Night	(a)	74%	-	58%
Doctors 'Always' Communicated Well	(a)	87%	-	80%
Home Recovery Information Given	(a)	81%	-	82%
Hospital Given 9 or 10 on 10 Point Scale	(a)	78%	-	67%
Meds 'Always' Explained Before Given	(a)	74%	-	60%
Nurses 'Always' Communicated Well	(a)	91%	-	76%
Pain 'Always' Well Controlled	(a)	78%	-	69%
Room and Bathroom 'Always' Clean	(a)	93%	-	71%
Timely Help 'Always' Received	(a)	82%	-	64%
Would Definitely Recommend Hospital	(a)	76%	-	69%

Kentucky River Medical Center

540 Jett Drive
Jackson, KY 41339
URL: www.kentuckyrivermc.com
Type: Acute Care Hospitals
Ownership: Proprietary

Phone: 606-666-6000
Fax: 606-666-6107

Emergency Services: Yes
Beds: 55

Key Personnel:
Quality Assurance . . . . Carolyn S Lipp

Measure	Cases	This Hosp.	State Avg.	U.S. Avg.
Heart Attack Care				
ACE Inhibitor or ARB for LVSD[1]	3	100%	94%	96%
Aspirin at Arrival[1]	24	100%	98%	99%
Aspirin at Discharge[1]	13	100%	98%	98%
Beta Blocker at Discharge[1]	9	89%	98%	98%
Fibrinolytic Medication Timing[1]	0	-	60%	55%
PCI Within 90 Minutes of Arrival[1]	0	-	88%	90%
Smoking Cessation Advice[1]	6	100%	100%	99%
Chest Pain/Possible Heart Attack Care				
Aspirin at Arrival	78	94%	95%	95%
Median Time to ECG (minutes)	82	8	7	8
Median Time to Transfer (minutes)[1,3]	4	72	65	61
Fibrinolytic Medication Timing[1]	9	78%	62%	54%
Heart Failure Care				
ACE Inhibitor or ARB for LVSD[1]	22	95%	91%	94%
Discharge Instructions	78	82%	82%	88%
Evaluation of LVS Function	99	100%	96%	98%
Smoking Cessation Advice[1]	24	100%	98%	98%
Pneumonia Care				
Appropriate Initial Antibiotic	64	94%	90%	92%
Blood Culture Timing	72	96%	95%	96%
Influenza Vaccine	58	95%	92%	91%
Initial Antibiotic Timing	116	100%	95%	95%
Pneumococcal Vaccine	79	100%	94%	93%
Smoking Cessation Advice	65	100%	98%	97%
Surgical Care Improvement Project				
Appropriate VTP Within 24 Hours[1,2]	12	100%	91%	92%
Appropriate Hair Removal[1,2]	21	100%	99%	99%
Appropriate Beta Blocker Usage[1,2]	6	83%	93%	93%
Controlled Postoperative Blood Glucose[2]	0	-	94%	93%
Prophylactic Antibiotic Timing[1,2]	9	100%	97%	97%
Prophylactic Antibiotic Timing (Outpatient)	75	100%	92%	92%
Prophylactic Antibiotic Selection[1,2]	10	90%	98%	97%
Prophylactic Antibiotic Select. (Outpatient)	75	99%	93%	94%
Prophylactic Antibiotic Stopped[1,2]	9	67%	94%	94%
Recommended VTP Ordered[1,2]	12	100%	94%	94%
Urinary Catheter Removal[1]	3	100%	89%	90%
Children's Asthma Care				
Received Systemic Corticosteroids	-	-	-	100%
Received Home Management Plan	-	-	-	71%
Received Reliever Medication	-	-	-	100%
Use of Medical Imaging				
Combination Abdominal CT Scan	166	0.157	0.160	0.191
Combination Chest CT Scan	115	0.139	0.054	0.054
Follow-up Mammogram/Ultrasound	174	8.6%	7.9%	8.4%
MRI for Low Back Pain	64	48.4%	35.6%	32.7%
Survey of Patients' Hospital Experiences				
Area Around Room 'Always' Quiet at Night	300+	61%	-	58%
Doctors 'Always' Communicated Well	300+	80%	-	80%
Home Recovery Information Given	300+	79%	-	82%
Hospital Given 9 or 10 on 10 Point Scale	300+	63%	-	67%
Meds 'Always' Explained Before Given	300+	58%	-	60%
Nurses 'Always' Communicated Well	300+	76%	-	76%
Pain 'Always' Well Controlled	300+	68%	-	69%
Room and Bathroom 'Always' Clean	300+	69%	-	71%
Timely Help 'Always' Received	300+	62%	-	64%
Would Definitely Recommend Hospital	300+	59%	-	69%

Baptist Hospital Northeast

1025 New Moody Lane
La Grange, KY 40031
URL: www.baptistnortheast.com
Type: Acute Care Hospitals
Ownership: Voluntary Non-Profit - Private

Phone: 502-222-5388
Fax: 502-222-3411

Emergency Services: Yes
Beds: 120

Key Personnel:
Cardiac Laboratory . . . . Maureen Holmes
Chief of Medical Staff . . . . Richardzabeth Waggen, MD
Coronary Care . . . . Lynn Rigon
Infection Control . . . . Marilyn Czape
Operating Room . . . . Barbara Ritchie
Quality Assurance . . . . Toby Bilbro
Radiology . . . . Rommi Wadlington

Measure	Cases	This Hosp.	State Avg.	U.S. Avg.
Heart Attack Care				
ACE Inhibitor or ARB for LVSD[1]	3	100%	94%	96%
Aspirin at Arrival	33	97%	98%	99%
Aspirin at Discharge[1]	11	100%	99%	98%
Beta Blocker at Discharge[1]	10	100%	98%	98%
Fibrinolytic Medication Timing[1]	1	0%	60%	55%
PCI Within 90 Minutes of Arrival	0	-	88%	90%
Smoking Cessation Advice[1]	1	100%	100%	99%
Chest Pain/Possible Heart Attack Care				
Aspirin at Arrival	29	100%	95%	95%
Median Time to ECG (minutes)	31	5	7	8
Median Time to Transfer (minutes)[1,3]	5	48	65	61
Fibrinolytic Medication Timing[1]	3	100%	62%	54%
Heart Failure Care				
ACE Inhibitor or ARB for LVSD[1]	15	80%	91%	94%
Discharge Instructions	79	92%	82%	88%
Evaluation of LVS Function	107	100%	96%	98%
Smoking Cessation Advice[1]	14	93%	98%	98%
Pneumonia Care				
Appropriate Initial Antibiotic	84	82%	90%	92%
Blood Culture Timing	108	98%	95%	96%
Influenza Vaccine	80	99%	92%	91%
Initial Antibiotic Timing	113	98%	95%	95%
Pneumococcal Vaccine	106	99%	94%	93%
Smoking Cessation Advice	44	98%	98%	97%
Surgical Care Improvement Project				
Appropriate VTP Within 24 Hours	98	94%	91%	92%
Appropriate Hair Removal	210	100%	99%	99%
Appropriate Beta Blocker Usage	57	95%	93%	93%
Controlled Postoperative Blood Glucose	0	-	94%	93%
Prophylactic Antibiotic Timing	146	97%	97%	97%
Prophylactic Antibiotic Timing (Outpatient)	50	86%	92%	92%
Prophylactic Antibiotic Selection	146	99%	98%	97%
Prophylactic Antibiotic Select. (Outpatient)	45	98%	93%	94%
Prophylactic Antibiotic Stopped	141	97%	94%	94%
Recommended VTP Ordered	98	95%	94%	94%
Urinary Catheter Removal[1]	15	60%	89%	90%
Children's Asthma Care				
Received Systemic Corticosteroids	-	-	-	100%
Received Home Management Plan	-	-	-	71%
Received Reliever Medication	-	-	-	100%
Use of Medical Imaging				
Combination Abdominal CT Scan	288	0.101	0.160	0.191
Combination Chest CT Scan	222	0.005	0.054	0.054
Follow-up Mammogram/Ultrasound	555	5.0%	7.9%	8.4%
MRI for Low Back Pain	88	23.9%	35.6%	32.7%
Survey of Patients' Hospital Experiences				
Area Around Room 'Always' Quiet at Night	300+	48%	-	58%
Doctors 'Always' Communicated Well	300+	77%	-	80%
Home Recovery Information Given	300+	84%	-	82%
Hospital Given 9 or 10 on 10 Point Scale	300+	64%	-	67%
Meds 'Always' Explained Before Given	300+	53%	-	60%
Nurses 'Always' Communicated Well	300+	76%	-	76%
Pain 'Always' Well Controlled	300+	65%	-	69%
Room and Bathroom 'Always' Clean	300+	62%	-	71%
Timely Help 'Always' Received	300+	56%	-	64%
Would Definitely Recommend Hospital	300+	67%	-	69%

NOTE: Hospital profiles are in alphabetical order by state, then city, then hospital within the city; Rankings exclude hospitals with less than 25 cases except for patient surveys which excludes hospitals with less than 100 cases; (a) 100–299 cases; (1) The number of cases is too small to be sure how well a hospital is performing; (2) The hospital indicated that the data submitted for this measure was based on a sample of cases; (3) Data was collected during a shorter time period (fewer quarters) than the maximum possible time for this measure; (4) Suppressed for one or more quarters by CMS; (5) No data is available from the hospital for this measure; (6) Fewer than 100 patients completed the HCAHPS survey. Use these rates with caution, as the number of surveys may be too low to reliably assess hospital performance; (7) Survey results are based on less than 12 months of data; (8) Survey results are not available for this reporting period; (9) No or very few patients were eligible for the HCAHPS survey; (10) A state average was not calculated because too few hospitals in the state submitted data; (11) There were discrepancies in the data collection process; Please refer to the User's Guide for a full explanation of data.

Spring View Hospital

320 Loretto Road
Lebanon, KY 40033
Type: Acute Care Hospitals
Ownership: Proprietary

Phone: 270-692-5145
Fax: 270-692-5155
Emergency Services: No
Beds: 113

Measure	Cases	This Hosp.	State Avg.	U.S. Avg.
Heart Attack Care				
ACE Inhibitor or ARB for LVSD[1,3]	2	100%	94%	96%
Aspirin at Arrival[1,3]	7	100%	98%	99%
Aspirin at Discharge[1,3]	6	100%	99%	98%
Beta Blocker at Discharge[1,3]	6	100%	98%	98%
Fibrinolytic Medication Timing[3]	0	-	60%	55%
PCI Within 90 Minutes of Arrival[3]	0	-	88%	90%
Smoking Cessation Advice[3]	0	-	100%	99%
Chest Pain/Possible Heart Attack Care				
Aspirin at Arrival	121	98%	95%	95%
Median Time to ECG (minutes)	124	7	7	8
Median Time to Transfer (minutes)[5]	0	-	65	61
Fibrinolytic Medication Timing[1]	4	100%	62%	54%
Heart Failure Care				
ACE Inhibitor or ARB for LVSD[1]	18	94%	91%	94%
Discharge Instructions	53	100%	82%	88%
Evaluation of LVS Function	75	100%	96%	98%
Smoking Cessation Advice[1]	11	100%	98%	98%
Pneumonia Care				
Appropriate Initial Antibiotic	41	95%	90%	92%
Blood Culture Timing	67	97%	95%	96%
Influenza Vaccine	38	95%	92%	91%
Initial Antibiotic Timing	73	97%	95%	95%
Pneumococcal Vaccine	55	96%	94%	93%
Smoking Cessation Advice[1]	13	100%	98%	97%
Surgical Care Improvement Project				
Appropriate VTP Within 24 Hours	80	98%	91%	92%
Appropriate Hair Removal	238	100%	99%	99%
Appropriate Beta Blocker Usage	51	98%	93%	93%
Controlled Postoperative Blood Glucose	0	-	94%	93%
Prophylactic Antibiotic Timing	187	99%	97%	97%
Prophylactic Antibiotic Timing (Outpatient)[1]	24	100%	92%	92%
Prophylactic Antibiotic Selection	189	100%	98%	97%
Prophylactic Antibiotic Select. (Outpatient)[1]	24	100%	93%	94%
Prophylactic Antibiotic Stopped	185	100%	94%	94%
Recommended VTP Ordered	81	96%	94%	94%
Urinary Catheter Removal	46	78%	89%	90%
Children's Asthma Care				
Received Systemic Corticosteroids	-	-	-	100%
Received Home Management Plan	-	-	-	71%
Received Reliever Medication	-	-	-	100%
Use of Medical Imaging				
Combination Abdominal CT Scan	224	0.241	0.160	0.191
Combination Chest CT Scan	131	0.198	0.054	0.054
Follow-up Mammogram/Ultrasound	419	2.1%	7.9%	8.4%
MRI for Low Back Pain	54	46.3%	35.6%	32.7%
Survey of Patients' Hospital Experiences				
Area Around Room 'Always' Quiet at Night	300+	65%	-	58%
Doctors 'Always' Communicated Well	300+	81%	-	80%
Home Recovery Information Given	300+	79%	-	82%
Hospital Given 9 or 10 on 10 Point Scale	300+	61%	-	67%
Meds 'Always' Explained Before Given	300+	54%	-	60%
Nurses 'Always' Communicated Well	300+	75%	-	76%
Pain 'Always' Well Controlled	300+	69%	-	69%
Room and Bathroom 'Always' Clean	300+	66%	-	71%
Timely Help 'Always' Received	300+	61%	-	64%
Would Definitely Recommend Hospital	300+	60%	-	69%

Twin Lakes Regional Medical Center

910 Wallace Avenue
Leitchfield, KY 42754
URL: www.tlrmc.com
Type: Acute Care Hospitals
Ownership: Voluntary Non-Profit - Other

Phone: 270-259-9400
Fax: 270-259-9524

Emergency Services: Yes
Beds: 75

Key Personnel:
CEO/President . . . . Stephen L Meredith
Radiology. . . . . Kenneth Dennison

Measure	Cases	This Hosp.	State Avg.	U.S. Avg.
Heart Attack Care				
ACE Inhibitor or ARB for LVSD[3]	0	-	94%	96%
Aspirin at Arrival[1,3]	3	67%	98%	99%
Aspirin at Discharge[1,3]	2	100%	99%	98%
Beta Blocker at Discharge[1,3]	2	100%	98%	98%
Fibrinolytic Medication Timing[3]	0	-	60%	55%
PCI Within 90 Minutes of Arrival[3]	0	-	88%	90%
Smoking Cessation Advice[3]	0	-	100%	99%
Chest Pain/Possible Heart Attack Care				
Aspirin at Arrival	101	95%	95%	95%
Median Time to ECG (minutes)	110	8	7	8
Median Time to Transfer (minutes)[1,3]	2	130	65	61
Fibrinolytic Medication Timing[1]	13	92%	62%	54%
Heart Failure Care				
ACE Inhibitor or ARB for LVSD[1,2]	11	100%	91%	94%
Discharge Instructions[2]	38	84%	82%	88%
Evaluation of LVS Function[2]	44	91%	96%	98%
Smoking Cessation Advice[1,2]	14	100%	98%	98%
Pneumonia Care				
Appropriate Initial Antibiotic[2]	99	91%	90%	92%
Blood Culture Timing[2]	110	94%	95%	96%
Influenza Vaccine[2]	83	93%	92%	91%
Initial Antibiotic Timing[2]	114	98%	95%	95%
Pneumococcal Vaccine[2]	115	92%	94%	93%
Smoking Cessation Advice[2]	57	100%	98%	97%
Surgical Care Improvement Project				
Appropriate VTP Within 24 Hours[2]	80	92%	91%	92%
Appropriate Hair Removal[2]	189	100%	99%	99%
Appropriate Beta Blocker Usage[2]	46	93%	93%	93%
Controlled Postoperative Blood Glucose[2]	0	-	94%	93%
Prophylactic Antibiotic Timing[2]	117	98%	97%	97%
Prophylactic Antibiotic Timing (Outpatient)	41	90%	92%	92%
Prophylactic Antibiotic Selection[2]	119	98%	98%	97%
Prophylactic Antibiotic Select. (Outpatient)	37	100%	93%	94%
Prophylactic Antibiotic Stopped[2]	114	96%	94%	94%
Recommended VTP Ordered[2]	80	95%	94%	94%
Urinary Catheter Removal[2]	42	100%	89%	90%
Children's Asthma Care				
Received Systemic Corticosteroids	-	-	-	100%
Received Home Management Plan	-	-	-	71%
Received Reliever Medication	-	-	-	100%
Use of Medical Imaging				
Combination Abdominal CT Scan	296	0.034	0.160	0.191
Combination Chest CT Scan	278	0.000	0.054	0.054
Follow-up Mammogram/Ultrasound	428	6.8%	7.9%	8.4%
MRI for Low Back Pain	86	36.0%	35.6%	32.7%
Survey of Patients' Hospital Experiences				
Area Around Room 'Always' Quiet at Night	300+	53%	-	58%
Doctors 'Always' Communicated Well	300+	77%	-	80%
Home Recovery Information Given	300+	77%	-	82%
Hospital Given 9 or 10 on 10 Point Scale	300+	57%	-	67%
Meds 'Always' Explained Before Given	300+	58%	-	60%
Nurses 'Always' Communicated Well	300+	74%	-	76%
Pain 'Always' Well Controlled	300+	67%	-	69%
Room and Bathroom 'Always' Clean	300+	67%	-	71%
Timely Help 'Always' Received	300+	64%	-	64%
Would Definitely Recommend Hospital	300+	59%	-	69%

Central Baptist Hospital

1740 Nicholasville Road
Lexington, KY 40503
URL: www.centralbap.com
Type: Acute Care Hospitals
Ownership: Govt - Hospital Dist/Auth

Phone: 859-260-6100
Fax: 859-260-6117

Emergency Services: Yes
Beds: 383

Key Personnel:
CEO/President . . . . William G Sisson
Chief of Medical Staff . . . . Jon Voss, MD
Coronary Care . . . . Norma Lake
Infection Control . . . . Dee Anderson, RN
Operating Room . . . . Kathleen Blair
Pediatric In-Patient Care . . . . Carole Bales
Quality Assurance . . . . Lynn Kolokowski
Radiology. . . . . Bill Broaddis

Measure	Cases	This Hosp.	State Avg.	U.S. Avg.
Heart Attack Care				
ACE Inhibitor or ARB for LVSD	95	100%	94%	96%
Aspirin at Arrival	146	99%	98%	99%
Aspirin at Discharge	671	100%	99%	98%
Beta Blocker at Discharge	625	100%	98%	98%
Fibrinolytic Medication Timing	0	-	60%	55%
PCI Within 90 Minutes of Arrival	47	100%	88%	90%
Smoking Cessation Advice	269	100%	100%	99%
Chest Pain/Possible Heart Attack Care				
Aspirin at Arrival[1,3]	2	100%	95%	95%
Median Time to ECG (minutes)[1,3]	2	2	7	8
Median Time to Transfer (minutes)[5]	0	-	65	61
Fibrinolytic Medication Timing[3]	0	-	62%	54%
Heart Failure Care				
ACE Inhibitor or ARB for LVSD	137	99%	91%	94%
Discharge Instructions	297	92%	82%	88%
Evaluation of LVS Function	331	99%	96%	98%
Smoking Cessation Advice	56	100%	98%	98%
Pneumonia Care				
Appropriate Initial Antibiotic	150	95%	90%	92%
Blood Culture Timing	219	98%	95%	96%
Influenza Vaccine	170	99%	92%	91%
Initial Antibiotic Timing	216	98%	95%	95%
Pneumococcal Vaccine	248	99%	94%	93%
Smoking Cessation Advice	130	100%	98%	97%
Surgical Care Improvement Project				
Appropriate VTP Within 24 Hours	587	95%	91%	92%
Appropriate Hair Removal	2,109	100%	99%	99%
Appropriate Beta Blocker Usage	709	97%	93%	93%
Controlled Postoperative Blood Glucose	379	97%	94%	93%
Prophylactic Antibiotic Timing	1,292	100%	97%	97%
Prophylactic Antibiotic Timing (Outpatient)	1,921	99%	92%	92%
Prophylactic Antibiotic Selection	1,313	99%	98%	97%
Prophylactic Antibiotic Select. (Outpatient)	1,907	99%	93%	94%
Prophylactic Antibiotic Stopped	1,234	98%	94%	94%
Recommended VTP Ordered	590	96%	94%	94%
Urinary Catheter Removal	433	88%	89%	90%
Children's Asthma Care				
Received Systemic Corticosteroids	-	-	-	100%
Received Home Management Plan	-	-	-	71%
Received Reliever Medication	-	-	-	100%
Use of Medical Imaging				
Combination Abdominal CT Scan	1,358	0.035	0.160	0.191
Combination Chest CT Scan	1,233	0.014	0.054	0.054
Follow-up Mammogram/Ultrasound	2,541	19.0%	7.9%	8.4%
MRI for Low Back Pain	157	32.5%	35.6%	32.7%
Survey of Patients' Hospital Experiences				
Area Around Room 'Always' Quiet at Night	300+	53%	-	58%
Doctors 'Always' Communicated Well	300+	81%	-	80%
Home Recovery Information Given	300+	81%	-	82%
Hospital Given 9 or 10 on 10 Point Scale	300+	74%	-	67%
Meds 'Always' Explained Before Given	300+	64%	-	60%
Nurses 'Always' Communicated Well	300+	80%	-	76%
Pain 'Always' Well Controlled	300+	72%	-	69%
Room and Bathroom 'Always' Clean	300+	62%	-	71%
Timely Help 'Always' Received	300+	65%	-	64%
Would Definitely Recommend Hospital	300+	82%	-	69%

NOTE: Hospital profiles are in alphabetical order by state, then city, then hospital within the city; Rankings exclude hospitals with less than 25 cases except for patient surveys which excludes hospitals with less than 100 cases; (a) 100–299 cases; (1) The number of cases is too small to be sure how well a hospital is performing; (2) The hospital indicated that the data submitted for this measure were based on a sample of cases; (3) Data was collected during a shorter time period (fewer quarters) than the maximum possible time for this measure; (4) Suppressed for one or more quarters by CMS; (5) No data is available from the hospital for this measure; (6) Fewer than 100 patients completed the HCAHPS survey. Use these rates with caution, as the number of surveys may be too low to reliably assess hospital performance; (7) Survey results are based on less than 12 months of data; (8) Survey results are not available for this reporting period; (9) No or very few patients were eligible for the HCAHPS survey. The scores shown, if any, reflect a very small number of surveys; (10) A state average was not calculated because too few hospitals in the state submitted data; (11) There were discrepancies in the data collection process; Please refer to the User's Guide for a full explanation of data.

Lexington-Leestown VA Medical Center

2250 Leestown Rd
Lexington, KY 40511
Phone: 859-233-4511
Fax: 859-281-4911
URL: www.lexington.va.gov
Type: Acute Care-Veterans Administration
Emergency Services: No
Ownership: Government - Federal
Beds: 99

Key Personnel:
Chief of Medical Staff . . . . Walter Divers, MD
Operating Room. . . . . Dr. Schwarrcz
Quality Assurance . . . . Linda Cranfill
Ambulatory Care . . . . Dr. James Flueck
Anesthesiology. . . . . Dr. Daniel Reese
Patient Relations . . . . Melinda Washburn, RN, MSN

Measure	Cases	This Hosp.	State Avg.	U.S. Avg.
Heart Attack Care				
ACE Inhibitor or ARB for LVSD[1]	17	100%	94%	96%
Aspirin at Arrival	128	98%	98%	99%
Aspirin at Discharge	121	99%	99%	98%
Beta Blocker at Discharge	113	99%	98%	98%
Fibrinolytic Medication Timing[5]	0	-	60%	55%
PCI Within 90 Minutes of Arrival[1]	12	42%	88%	90%
Smoking Cessation Advice	42	100%	100%	99%
Chest Pain/Possible Heart Attack Care				
Aspirin at Arrival	-	-	95%	95%
Median Time to ECG (minutes)	-	-	7	8
Median Time to Transfer (minutes)	-	-	65	61
Fibrinolytic Medication Timing	-	-	62%	54%
Heart Failure Care				
ACE Inhibitor or ARB for LVSD	82	93%	91%	94%
Discharge Instructions	255	99%	82%	88%
Evaluation of LVS Function	270	100%	96%	98%
Smoking Cessation Advice	50	100%	98%	98%
Pneumonia Care				
Appropriate Initial Antibiotic	94	96%	90%	92%
Blood Culture Timing	179	98%	95%	96%
Influenza Vaccine	103	92%	92%	91%
Initial Antibiotic Timing	162	93%	95%	95%
Pneumococcal Vaccine	151	98%	94%	93%
Smoking Cessation Advice	43	100%	98%	97%
Surgical Care Improvement Project				
Appropriate VTP Within 24 Hours[2,5]	0	-	91%	92%
Appropriate Hair Removal[2,5]	0	-	99%	99%
Appropriate Beta Blocker Usage[2,5]	0	-	93%	93%
Controlled Postoperative Blood Glucose[2,5]	0	-	94%	93%
Prophylactic Antibiotic Timing[5]	0	-	97%	97%
Prophylactic Antibiotic Timing (Outpatient)	-	-	92%	92%
Prophylactic Antibiotic Selection[5]	0	-	98%	97%
Prophylactic Antibiotic Select. (Outpatient)	-	-	93%	94%
Prophylactic Antibiotic Stopped[5]	0	-	94%	94%
Recommended VTP Ordered[2,5]	0	-	94%	94%
Urinary Catheter Removal[2,5]	0	-	89%	90%
Children's Asthma Care				
Received Systemic Corticosteroids	-	-	-	100%
Received Home Management Plan	-	-	-	71%
Received Reliever Medication	-	-	-	100%
Use of Medical Imaging				
Combination Abdominal CT Scan	-	-	0.160	0.191
Combination Chest CT Scan	-	-	0.054	0.054
Follow-up Mammogram/Ultrasound	-	-	7.9%	8.4%
MRI for Low Back Pain	-	-	35.6%	32.7%
Survey of Patients' Hospital Experiences				
Area Around Room 'Always' Quiet at Night	-	-	-	58%
Doctors 'Always' Communicated Well	-	-	-	80%
Home Recovery Information Given	-	-	-	82%
Hospital Given 9 or 10 on 10 Point Scale	-	-	-	67%
Meds 'Always' Explained Before Given	-	-	-	60%
Nurses 'Always' Communicated Well	-	-	-	76%
Pain 'Always' Well Controlled	-	-	-	69%
Room and Bathroom 'Always' Clean	-	-	-	71%
Timely Help 'Always' Received	-	-	-	64%
Would Definitely Recommend Hospital	-	-	-	69%

Saint Joseph East

150 North Eagle Creek Drive
Lexington, KY 40509
Phone: 859-967-5000
Fax: 859-967-5766
URL: www.sjhlex.org
Type: Acute Care Hospitals
Emergency Services: Yes
Ownership: Voluntary Non-Profit - Church
Beds: 174

Key Personnel:
CEO/President. . . . . Gene Woods

Measure	Cases	This Hosp.	State Avg.	U.S. Avg.
Heart Attack Care				
ACE Inhibitor or ARB for LVSD[2]	39	97%	94%	96%
Aspirin at Arrival[2]	75	97%	98%	99%
Aspirin at Discharge[2]	203	99%	99%	98%
Beta Blocker at Discharge[2]	184	97%	98%	98%
Fibrinolytic Medication Timing[2]	0	-	60%	55%
PCI Within 90 Minutes of Arrival[1,2]	18	100%	88%	90%
Smoking Cessation Advice[2]	100	100%	100%	99%
Chest Pain/Possible Heart Attack Care				
Aspirin at Arrival[1]	18	100%	95%	95%
Median Time to ECG (minutes)[1]	18	15	7	8
Median Time to Transfer (minutes)[5]	0	-	65	61
Fibrinolytic Medication Timing[3]	0	-	62%	54%
Heart Failure Care				
ACE Inhibitor or ARB for LVSD	45	89%	91%	94%
Discharge Instructions	101	82%	82%	88%
Evaluation of LVS Function	108	98%	96%	98%
Smoking Cessation Advice	30	100%	98%	98%
Pneumonia Care				
Appropriate Initial Antibiotic[2]	68	96%	90%	92%
Blood Culture Timing[2]	79	92%	95%	96%
Influenza Vaccine[2]	72	96%	92%	91%
Initial Antibiotic Timing[2]	83	89%	95%	95%
Pneumococcal Vaccine[2]	89	96%	94%	93%
Smoking Cessation Advice[2]	69	100%	98%	97%
Surgical Care Improvement Project				
Appropriate VTP Within 24 Hours[2]	176	91%	91%	92%
Appropriate Hair Removal[2]	548	100%	99%	99%
Appropriate Beta Blocker Usage[2]	157	95%	93%	93%
Controlled Postoperative Blood Glucose[2]	0	-	94%	93%
Prophylactic Antibiotic Timing[2]	398	99%	97%	97%
Prophylactic Antibiotic Timing (Outpatient)	307	98%	92%	92%
Prophylactic Antibiotic Selection[2]	400	97%	98%	97%
Prophylactic Antibiotic Select. (Outpatient)	303	96%	93%	94%
Prophylactic Antibiotic Stopped[2]	390	96%	94%	94%
Recommended VTP Ordered[2]	177	94%	94%	94%
Urinary Catheter Removal[2]	91	86%	89%	90%
Children's Asthma Care				
Received Systemic Corticosteroids	-	-	-	100%
Received Home Management Plan	-	-	-	71%
Received Reliever Medication	-	-	-	100%
Use of Medical Imaging				
Combination Abdominal CT Scan	257	0.012	0.160	0.191
Combination Chest CT Scan[1]	33	0.000	0.054	0.054
Follow-up Mammogram/Ultrasound	739	3.1%	7.9%	8.4%
MRI for Low Back Pain[1]	32	37.5%	35.6%	32.7%
Survey of Patients' Hospital Experiences				
Area Around Room 'Always' Quiet at Night	300+	60%	-	58%
Doctors 'Always' Communicated Well	300+	81%	-	80%
Home Recovery Information Given	300+	85%	-	82%
Hospital Given 9 or 10 on 10 Point Scale	300+	70%	-	67%
Meds 'Always' Explained Before Given	300+	58%	-	60%
Nurses 'Always' Communicated Well	300+	75%	-	76%
Pain 'Always' Well Controlled	300+	70%	-	69%
Room and Bathroom 'Always' Clean	300+	64%	-	71%
Timely Help 'Always' Received	300+	61%	-	64%
Would Definitely Recommend Hospital	300+	74%	-	69%

Saint Joseph Hospital

One Saint Joseph Drive
Lexington, KY 40504
Phone: 859-313-1714
Fax: 859-260-6117
URL: www.sjhlex.org
Type: Acute Care Hospitals
Emergency Services: Yes
Ownership: Voluntary Non-Profit - Church
Beds: 468

Key Personnel:
Chief of Medical Staff . . . . Dennis B Kelly, MD
Operating Room. . . . . Judy Behnhardy
Pediatric Ambulatory Care . . . . . . Walter Yates, MD
Pediatric In-Patient Care . . . . Walter Yates, MD
Quality Assurance . . . . Cherri Tichenor
Radiology. . . . . Chris Riley, MD
Anesthesiology. . . . . Wayne Graff, MD
Emergency Room . . . . Barry Parsley, MD

Measure	Cases	This Hosp.	State Avg.	U.S. Avg.
Heart Attack Care				
ACE Inhibitor or ARB for LVSD[2]	83	92%	94%	96%
Aspirin at Arrival[2]	172	98%	98%	99%
Aspirin at Discharge[2]	437	99%	99%	98%
Beta Blocker at Discharge[2]	414	98%	98%	98%
Fibrinolytic Medication Timing[2]	0	-	60%	55%
PCI Within 90 Minutes of Arrival[1,2]	22	86%	88%	90%
Smoking Cessation Advice[2]	205	100%	100%	99%
Chest Pain/Possible Heart Attack Care				
Aspirin at Arrival	28	96%	95%	95%
Median Time to ECG (minutes)	31	7	7	8
Median Time to Transfer (minutes)[5]	0	-	65	61
Fibrinolytic Medication Timing[5]	0	-	62%	54%
Heart Failure Care				
ACE Inhibitor or ARB for LVSD[2]	112	95%	91%	94%
Discharge Instructions[2]	268	82%	82%	88%
Evaluation of LVS Function[2]	300	99%	96%	98%
Smoking Cessation Advice[2]	62	100%	98%	98%
Pneumonia Care				
Appropriate Initial Antibiotic[2]	95	93%	90%	92%
Blood Culture Timing[2]	145	99%	95%	96%
Influenza Vaccine[2]	164	97%	92%	91%
Initial Antibiotic Timing[2]	153	96%	95%	95%
Pneumococcal Vaccine[2]	220	99%	94%	93%
Smoking Cessation Advice[2]	105	100%	98%	97%
Surgical Care Improvement Project				
Appropriate VTP Within 24 Hours[2]	418	94%	91%	92%
Appropriate Hair Removal[2]	1,230	100%	99%	99%
Appropriate Beta Blocker Usage[2]	496	94%	93%	93%
Controlled Postoperative Blood Glucose[2]	439	95%	94%	93%
Prophylactic Antibiotic Timing[2]	685	98%	97%	97%
Prophylactic Antibiotic Timing (Outpatient)	878	83%	92%	92%
Prophylactic Antibiotic Selection[2]	706	98%	98%	97%
Prophylactic Antibiotic Select. (Outpatient)	868	92%	93%	94%
Prophylactic Antibiotic Stopped[2]	638	96%	94%	94%
Recommended VTP Ordered[2]	418	97%	94%	94%
Urinary Catheter Removal[2]	247	79%	89%	90%
Children's Asthma Care				
Received Systemic Corticosteroids	-	-	-	100%
Received Home Management Plan	-	-	-	71%
Received Reliever Medication	-	-	-	100%
Use of Medical Imaging				
Combination Abdominal CT Scan	565	0.016	0.160	0.191
Combination Chest CT Scan	115	0.009	0.054	0.054
Follow-up Mammogram/Ultrasound	759	4.9%	7.9%	8.4%
MRI for Low Back Pain	98	33.7%	35.6%	32.7%
Survey of Patients' Hospital Experiences				
Area Around Room 'Always' Quiet at Night	300+	62%	-	58%
Doctors 'Always' Communicated Well	300+	81%	-	80%
Home Recovery Information Given	300+	83%	-	82%
Hospital Given 9 or 10 on 10 Point Scale	300+	71%	-	67%
Meds 'Always' Explained Before Given	300+	60%	-	60%
Nurses 'Always' Communicated Well	300+	78%	-	76%
Pain 'Always' Well Controlled	300+	71%	-	69%
Room and Bathroom 'Always' Clean	300+	66%	-	71%
Timely Help 'Always' Received	300+	63%	-	64%
Would Definitely Recommend Hospital	300+	77%	-	69%

NOTE: Hospital profiles are in alphabetical order by state, then city, then hospital within the city; Rankings exclude hospitals with less than 25 cases except for patient surveys which excludes hospitals with less than 100 cases; (a) 100–299 cases; (1) The number of cases is too small to be sure how well a hospital is performing; (2) The hospital indicated that the data submitted for this measure were based on a sample of cases; (3) Data was collected during a shorter time period (fewer quarters) than the maximum possible time for this measure; (4) Suppressed for one or more quarters by CMS; (5) No data is available from the hospital for this measure; (6) Fewer than 100 patients completed the HCAHPS survey. Use these rates with caution, as the number of surveys may be too low to reliably assess hospital performance; (7) Survey results are based on less than 12 months of data; (8) Survey results are not available for this reporting period; (9) No or very few patients were eligible for the HCAHPS survey. The scores shown, if any, reflect a very small number of surveys; (10) A state average was not calculated because too few hospitals in the state submitted data; (11) There were discrepancies in the data collection process; Please refer to the User's Guide for a full explanation of data.

University of Kentucky Hospital

800 Rose Street
Lexington, KY 40536
URL: www.uhealthcare.uky.edu
Type: Acute Care Hospitals
Ownership: Government - State

Phone: 859-323-5470
Fax: 859-323-2044

Emergency Services: Yes
Beds: 473

Key Personnel:
Chief of Medical Staff . . . . Courtney Higdon
Coronary Care . . . . Ann Wiard, RN
Infection Control . . . . Martin Evans, MD
Operating Room. . . . . Patricia Seabolt, RN
Pediatric In-Patient Care . . . . . . Sherry Holmes, RN
Quality Assurance . . . . Jennifer Blakeley
Radiology. . . . . Todd Hickey

Measure	Cases	This Hosp.	State Avg.	U.S. Avg.
Heart Attack Care				
ACE Inhibitor or ARB for LVSD[2]	71	96%	94%	96%
Aspirin at Arrival[2]	127	99%	98%	99%
Aspirin at Discharge[2]	280	99%	99%	98%
Beta Blocker at Discharge[2]	269	98%	98%	98%
Fibrinolytic Medication Timing[2]	0	-	60%	55%
PCI Within 90 Minutes of Arrival[1,2]	23	83%	88%	90%
Smoking Cessation Advice[2]	135	99%	100%	99%
Chest Pain/Possible Heart Attack Care				
Aspirin at Arrival[5]	0	-	95%	95%
Median Time to ECG (minutes)[5]	0	-	7	8
Median Time to Transfer (minutes)[5]	0	-	65	61
Fibrinolytic Medication Timing[5]	0	-	62%	54%
Heart Failure Care				
ACE Inhibitor or ARB for LVSD[2]	159	97%	91%	94%
Discharge Instructions[2]	314	74%	82%	88%
Evaluation of LVS Function[2]	356	97%	96%	98%
Smoking Cessation Advice[2]	115	97%	98%	98%
Pneumonia Care				
Appropriate Initial Antibiotic[2]	58	74%	90%	92%
Blood Culture Timing[2]	119	88%	95%	96%
Influenza Vaccine[2]	109	85%	92%	91%
Initial Antibiotic Timing[2]	123	84%	95%	95%
Pneumococcal Vaccine[2]	104	85%	94%	93%
Smoking Cessation Advice[2]	119	97%	98%	97%
Surgical Care Improvement Project				
Appropriate VTP Within 24 Hours[2]	287	91%	91%	92%
Appropriate Hair Removal[2]	761	99%	99%	99%
Appropriate Beta Blocker Usage[2]	248	85%	93%	93%
Controlled Postoperative Blood Glucose[2]	100	90%	94%	93%
Prophylactic Antibiotic Timing[2]	487	94%	97%	97%
Prophylactic Antibiotic Timing (Outpatient)	796	87%	92%	92%
Prophylactic Antibiotic Selection[2]	486	95%	98%	97%
Prophylactic Antibiotic Select. (Outpatient)	727	93%	93%	94%
Prophylactic Antibiotic Stopped[2]	465	91%	94%	94%
Recommended VTP Ordered[2]	291	92%	94%	94%
Urinary Catheter Removal[2]	143	85%	89%	90%
Children's Asthma Care				
Received Systemic Corticosteroids[2]	127	97%	-	100%
Received Home Management Plan[2]	127	61%	-	71%
Received Reliever Medication[2]	127	100%	-	100%
Use of Medical Imaging				
Combination Abdominal CT Scan	1,583	0.020	0.160	0.191
Combination Chest CT Scan	1,979	0.005	0.054	0.054
Follow-up Mammogram/Ultrasound	357	3.4%	7.9%	8.4%
MRI for Low Back Pain	197	28.9%	35.6%	32.7%
Survey of Patients' Hospital Experiences				
Area Around Room 'Always' Quiet at Night	300+	52%	-	58%
Doctors 'Always' Communicated Well	300+	76%	-	80%
Home Recovery Information Given	300+	86%	-	82%
Hospital Given 9 or 10 on 10 Point Scale	300+	61%	-	67%
Meds 'Always' Explained Before Given	300+	58%	-	60%
Nurses 'Always' Communicated Well	300+	74%	-	76%
Pain 'Always' Well Controlled	300+	65%	-	69%
Room and Bathroom 'Always' Clean	300+	60%	-	71%
Timely Help 'Always' Received	300+	61%	-	64%
Would Definitely Recommend Hospital	300+	67%	-	69%

Casey County Hospital

187 Wolford Avenue
Liberty, KY 42539
Type: Critical Access Hospitals
Ownership: Govt - Hospital Dist/Auth

Phone: 606-787-6275
Fax: 606-787-9717
Emergency Services: Yes
Beds: 24

Key Personnel:
CEO/President. . . . . Rusty Tungate
Emergency Room . . . . Linda Mackey

Measure	Cases	This Hosp.	State Avg.	U.S. Avg.
Heart Attack Care				
ACE Inhibitor or ARB for LVSD[3]	0	-	94%	96%
Aspirin at Arrival[3]	0	-	98%	99%
Aspirin at Discharge[3]	0	-	99%	98%
Beta Blocker at Discharge[1,3]	1	100%	98%	98%
Fibrinolytic Medication Timing[3]	0	-	60%	55%
PCI Within 90 Minutes of Arrival[3]	0	-	88%	90%
Smoking Cessation Advice[3]	0	-	100%	99%
Chest Pain/Possible Heart Attack Care				
Aspirin at Arrival	-	-	95%	95%
Median Time to ECG (minutes)	-	-	7	8
Median Time to Transfer (minutes)	-	-	65	61
Fibrinolytic Medication Timing	-	-	62%	54%
Heart Failure Care				
ACE Inhibitor or ARB for LVSD[1]	1	0%	91%	94%
Discharge Instructions[1]	10	70%	82%	88%
Evaluation of LVS Function[1]	16	50%	96%	98%
Smoking Cessation Advice[1]	4	75%	98%	98%
Pneumonia Care				
Appropriate Initial Antibiotic	59	83%	90%	92%
Blood Culture Timing[1]	1	100%	95%	96%
Influenza Vaccine	61	66%	92%	91%
Initial Antibiotic Timing	91	96%	95%	95%
Pneumococcal Vaccine	78	77%	94%	93%
Smoking Cessation Advice	25	96%	98%	97%
Surgical Care Improvement Project				
Appropriate VTP Within 24 Hours[5]	0	-	91%	92%
Appropriate Hair Removal[5]	0	-	99%	99%
Appropriate Beta Blocker Usage[5]	0	-	93%	93%
Controlled Postoperative Blood Glucose[5]	0	-	94%	93%
Prophylactic Antibiotic Timing[5]	0	-	97%	97%
Prophylactic Antibiotic Timing (Outpatient)	-	-	92%	92%
Prophylactic Antibiotic Selection[5]	0	-	98%	97%
Prophylactic Antibiotic Select. (Outpatient)	-	-	93%	94%
Prophylactic Antibiotic Stopped[5]	0	-	94%	94%
Recommended VTP Ordered[5]	0	-	94%	94%
Urinary Catheter Removal[5]	0	-	89%	90%
Children's Asthma Care				
Received Systemic Corticosteroids	-	-	-	100%
Received Home Management Plan	-	-	-	71%
Received Reliever Medication	-	-	-	100%
Use of Medical Imaging				
Combination Abdominal CT Scan	-	-	0.160	0.191
Combination Chest CT Scan	-	-	0.054	0.054
Follow-up Mammogram/Ultrasound	-	-	7.9%	8.4%
MRI for Low Back Pain	-	-	35.6%	32.7%
Survey of Patients' Hospital Experiences				
Area Around Room 'Always' Quiet at Night[8]	-	-	-	58%
Doctors 'Always' Communicated Well[8]	-	-	-	80%
Home Recovery Information Given[8]	-	-	-	82%
Hospital Given 9 or 10 on 10 Point Scale[8]	-	-	-	67%
Meds 'Always' Explained Before Given[8]	-	-	-	60%
Nurses 'Always' Communicated Well[8]	-	-	-	76%
Pain 'Always' Well Controlled[8]	-	-	-	69%
Room and Bathroom 'Always' Clean[8]	-	-	-	71%
Timely Help 'Always' Received[8]	-	-	-	64%
Would Definitely Recommend Hospital[8]	-	-	-	69%

Saint Joseph Hospital London

1001 Saint Joseph Lane
London, KY 40741
URL: www.sjhlex.org
Type: Acute Care Hospitals
Ownership: Voluntary Non-Profit - Private

Phone: 606-330-6000

Emergency Services: Yes

Measure	Cases	This Hosp.	State Avg.	U.S. Avg.
Heart Attack Care				
ACE Inhibitor or ARB for LVSD	40	100%	94%	96%
Aspirin at Arrival	171	99%	98%	99%
Aspirin at Discharge	296	100%	99%	98%
Beta Blocker at Discharge	275	99%	98%	98%
Fibrinolytic Medication Timing	0	-	60%	55%
PCI Within 90 Minutes of Arrival	42	98%	88%	90%
Smoking Cessation Advice	165	100%	100%	99%
Chest Pain/Possible Heart Attack Care				
Aspirin at Arrival	80	98%	95%	95%
Median Time to ECG (minutes)	94	8	7	8
Median Time to Transfer (minutes)[5]	0	-	65	61
Fibrinolytic Medication Timing[3]	0	-	62%	54%
Heart Failure Care				
ACE Inhibitor or ARB for LVSD	90	100%	91%	94%
Discharge Instructions	266	93%	82%	88%
Evaluation of LVS Function	295	100%	96%	98%
Smoking Cessation Advice	79	100%	98%	98%
Pneumonia Care				
Appropriate Initial Antibiotic	121	90%	90%	92%
Blood Culture Timing	178	98%	95%	96%
Influenza Vaccine	85	98%	92%	91%
Initial Antibiotic Timing	152	98%	95%	95%
Pneumococcal Vaccine	148	98%	94%	93%
Smoking Cessation Advice	114	100%	98%	97%
Surgical Care Improvement Project				
Appropriate VTP Within 24 Hours[2]	98	99%	91%	92%
Appropriate Hair Removal[2]	401	100%	99%	99%
Appropriate Beta Blocker Usage[2]	176	98%	93%	93%
Controlled Postoperative Blood Glucose[2]	124	97%	94%	93%
Prophylactic Antibiotic Timing[2]	272	99%	97%	97%
Prophylactic Antibiotic Timing (Outpatient)	291	96%	92%	92%
Prophylactic Antibiotic Selection[2]	279	99%	98%	97%
Prophylactic Antibiotic Select. (Outpatient)	283	98%	93%	94%
Prophylactic Antibiotic Stopped[2]	221	98%	94%	94%
Recommended VTP Ordered[2]	99	99%	94%	94%
Urinary Catheter Removal	59	93%	89%	90%
Children's Asthma Care				
Received Systemic Corticosteroids	-	-	-	100%
Received Home Management Plan	-	-	-	71%
Received Reliever Medication	-	-	-	100%
Use of Medical Imaging				
Combination Abdominal CT Scan	698	0.052	0.160	0.191
Combination Chest CT Scan	380	0.011	0.054	0.054
Follow-up Mammogram/Ultrasound	525	6.3%	7.9%	8.4%
MRI for Low Back Pain	128	35.2%	35.6%	32.7%
Survey of Patients' Hospital Experiences				
Area Around Room 'Always' Quiet at Night	300+	52%	-	58%
Doctors 'Always' Communicated Well	300+	79%	-	80%
Home Recovery Information Given	300+	81%	-	82%
Hospital Given 9 or 10 on 10 Point Scale	300+	70%	-	67%
Meds 'Always' Explained Before Given	300+	62%	-	60%
Nurses 'Always' Communicated Well	300+	80%	-	76%
Pain 'Always' Well Controlled	300+	73%	-	69%
Room and Bathroom 'Always' Clean	300+	72%	-	71%
Timely Help 'Always' Received	300+	72%	-	64%
Would Definitely Recommend Hospital	300+	73%	-	69%

NOTE: Hospital profiles are in alphabetical order by state, then city, then hospital within the city; Rankings exclude hospitals with less than 25 cases except for patient surveys which excludes hospitals with less than 100 cases; (a) 100–299 cases; (1) The number of cases is too small to be sure how well a hospital is performing; (2) The hospital indicated that the data submitted for this measure were based on a sample of cases; (3) Data was collected during a shorter time period (fewer quarters) than the maximum possible time for this measure; (4) Suppressed for one or more quarters by CMS; (5) No data is available from the hospital for this measure; (6) Fewer than 100 patients completed the HCAHPS survey. Use these rates with caution, as the number of surveys may be too low to reliably assess hospital performance; (7) Survey results are based on less than 12 months of data; (8) Survey results are not available for this reporting period; (9) No or very few patients were eligible for the HCAHPS survey. The scores shown, if any, reflect a very small number of surveys; (10) A state average was not calculated because too few hospitals in the state submitted data; (11) There were discrepancies in the data collection process; Please refer to the User's Guide for a full explanation of data.

Three Rivers Medical Center

Highway 644
Louisa, KY 41230
Phone: 606-638-9451
Fax: 606-638-9494
URL: www.threeriversmedicalcenter.com
Type: Acute Care Hospitals
Emergency Services: Yes
Ownership: Proprietary
Beds: 90

Key Personnel:
CEO/President. . . . . Greg Kiser
Cardiac Laboratory. . . . . Joe Bevans
Chief of Medical Staff . . . . Lee Balaklaw
Operating Room. . . . . Barbara Robinson, MD
Quality Assurance . . . . Betty Slone
Radiology. . . . . Paul V Akers
Emergency Room . . . . Dian Ratcliff

Measure	Cases	This Hosp.	State Avg.	U.S. Avg.
Heart Attack Care				
ACE Inhibitor or ARB for LVSD	0	-	94%	96%
Aspirin at Arrival[1]	6	100%	98%	99%
Aspirin at Discharge[1]	2	100%	99%	98%
Beta Blocker at Discharge[1]	2	100%	98%	98%
Fibrinolytic Medication Timing	0	-	60%	55%
PCI Within 90 Minutes of Arrival	0	-	88%	90%
Smoking Cessation Advice	0	-	100%	99%
Chest Pain/Possible Heart Attack Care				
Aspirin at Arrival	142	100%	95%	95%
Median Time to ECG (minutes)	144	5	7	8
Median Time to Transfer (minutes)[1,3]	6	50	65	61
Fibrinolytic Medication Timing[1]	1	100%	62%	54%
Heart Failure Care				
ACE Inhibitor or ARB for LVSD	35	97%	91%	94%
Discharge Instructions	89	99%	82%	88%
Evaluation of LVS Function	98	100%	96%	98%
Smoking Cessation Advice	25	100%	98%	98%
Pneumonia Care				
Appropriate Initial Antibiotic	94	99%	90%	92%
Blood Culture Timing	84	100%	95%	96%
Influenza Vaccine	73	100%	92%	91%
Initial Antibiotic Timing	122	100%	95%	95%
Pneumococcal Vaccine	72	100%	94%	93%
Smoking Cessation Advice	71	100%	98%	97%
Surgical Care Improvement Project				
Appropriate VTP Within 24 Hours[1,2]	17	100%	91%	92%
Appropriate Hair Removal[2]	81	99%	99%	99%
Appropriate Beta Blocker Usage[1,2]	12	100%	93%	93%
Controlled Postoperative Blood Glucose[2]	0	-	94%	93%
Prophylactic Antibiotic Timing[2]	71	100%	97%	97%
Prophylactic Antibiotic Timing (Outpatient)[1]	15	93%	92%	92%
Prophylactic Antibiotic Selection[2]	73	100%	98%	97%
Prophylactic Antibiotic Select. (Outpatient)[1]	15	87%	93%	94%
Prophylactic Antibiotic Stopped[2]	68	99%	94%	94%
Recommended VTP Ordered[1,2]	17	100%	94%	94%
Urinary Catheter Removal	0	-	89%	90%
Children's Asthma Care				
Received Systemic Corticosteroids	-	-	-	100%
Received Home Management Plan	-	-	-	71%
Received Reliever Medication	-	-	-	100%
Use of Medical Imaging				
Combination Abdominal CT Scan	241	0.046	0.160	0.191
Combination Chest CT Scan	132	0.061	0.054	0.054
Follow-up Mammogram/Ultrasound	149	18.1%	7.9%	8.4%
MRI for Low Back Pain	57	43.9%	35.6%	32.7%
Survey of Patients' Hospital Experiences				
Area Around Room 'Always' Quiet at Night	300+	62%	-	58%
Doctors 'Always' Communicated Well	300+	88%	-	80%
Home Recovery Information Given	300+	81%	-	82%
Hospital Given 9 or 10 on 10 Point Scale	300+	67%	-	67%
Meds 'Always' Explained Before Given	300+	69%	-	60%
Nurses 'Always' Communicated Well	300+	80%	-	76%
Pain 'Always' Well Controlled	300+	72%	-	69%
Room and Bathroom 'Always' Clean	300+	74%	-	71%
Timely Help 'Always' Received	300+	68%	-	64%
Would Definitely Recommend Hospital	300+	65%	-	69%

Baptist Hospital East

4000 Kresge Way
Louisville, KY 40207
Phone: 502-897-8100
Fax: 502-897-8020
E-mail: bheinfocenter@bhsi.com
URL: www.baptisteast.com
Type: Acute Care Hospitals
Emergency Services: Yes
Ownership: Voluntary Non-Profit - Private
Beds: 519

Key Personnel:
CEO/President. . . . . David Gray
Infection Control . . . . Connie Baker
Radiology. . . . . Robert Elliott MD
Hemotology Center . . . . Denise Carroll
Intensive Care Unit. . . . . Paul Battes

Measure	Cases	This Hosp.	State Avg.	U.S. Avg.
Heart Attack Care				
ACE Inhibitor or ARB for LVSD	80	96%	94%	96%
Aspirin at Arrival	443	100%	98%	99%
Aspirin at Discharge	474	99%	99%	98%
Beta Blocker at Discharge	448	100%	98%	98%
Fibrinolytic Medication Timing	0	-	60%	55%
PCI Within 90 Minutes of Arrival	89	89%	88%	90%
Smoking Cessation Advice	142	100%	100%	99%
Chest Pain/Possible Heart Attack Care				
Aspirin at Arrival[1]	5	80%	95%	95%
Median Time to ECG (minutes)[1]	5	0	7	8
Median Time to Transfer (minutes)[5]	0	-	65	61
Fibrinolytic Medication Timing[5]	0	-	62%	54%
Heart Failure Care				
ACE Inhibitor or ARB for LVSD	255	88%	91%	94%
Discharge Instructions	654	76%	82%	88%
Evaluation of LVS Function	913	100%	96%	98%
Smoking Cessation Advice	112	100%	98%	98%
Pneumonia Care				
Appropriate Initial Antibiotic	385	87%	90%	92%
Blood Culture Timing	620	94%	95%	96%
Influenza Vaccine	492	96%	92%	91%
Initial Antibiotic Timing	628	96%	95%	95%
Pneumococcal Vaccine	689	95%	94%	93%
Smoking Cessation Advice	195	99%	98%	97%
Surgical Care Improvement Project				
Appropriate VTP Within 24 Hours	1,105	90%	91%	92%
Appropriate Hair Removal	4,190	98%	99%	99%
Appropriate Beta Blocker Usage	1,285	92%	93%	93%
Controlled Postoperative Blood Glucose	266	93%	94%	93%
Prophylactic Antibiotic Timing	2,912	98%	97%	97%
Prophylactic Antibiotic Timing (Outpatient)	1,548	96%	92%	92%
Prophylactic Antibiotic Selection	2,935	97%	98%	97%
Prophylactic Antibiotic Select. (Outpatient)	1,554	95%	93%	94%
Prophylactic Antibiotic Stopped	2,791	96%	94%	94%
Recommended VTP Ordered	1,106	95%	94%	94%
Urinary Catheter Removal	479	91%	89%	90%
Children's Asthma Care				
Received Systemic Corticosteroids	-	-	-	100%
Received Home Management Plan	-	-	-	71%
Received Reliever Medication	-	-	-	100%
Use of Medical Imaging				
Combination Abdominal CT Scan	2,433	0.072	0.160	0.191
Combination Chest CT Scan	1,748	0.001	0.054	0.054
Follow-up Mammogram/Ultrasound	2,907	9.1%	7.9%	8.4%
MRI for Low Back Pain	584	33.9%	35.6%	32.7%
Survey of Patients' Hospital Experiences				
Area Around Room 'Always' Quiet at Night	300+	58%	-	58%
Doctors 'Always' Communicated Well	300+	80%	-	80%
Home Recovery Information Given	300+	88%	-	82%
Hospital Given 9 or 10 on 10 Point Scale	300+	75%	-	67%
Meds 'Always' Explained Before Given	300+	57%	-	60%
Nurses 'Always' Communicated Well	300+	79%	-	76%
Pain 'Always' Well Controlled	300+	71%	-	69%
Room and Bathroom 'Always' Clean	300+	66%	-	71%
Timely Help 'Always' Received	300+	64%	-	64%
Would Definitely Recommend Hospital	300+	81%	-	69%

Jewish Hospital & St Mary's Healthcare

200 Abraham Flexner Way
Louisville, KY 40202
Phone: 502-587-4011
URL: www.jhhs.org
Type: Acute Care Hospitals
Emergency Services: Yes
Ownership: Voluntary Non-Profit - Private

Key Personnel:
CEO/President. . . . . Robert L Shircliff
Chief of Medical Staff . . . . Lynn T Simon, MDMBACHE
Operating Room. . . . . Lisa Jackson
Ambulatory Care . . . . Luis R Scheker, MD
Anesthesiology. . . . . Atul Barry, MD
Emergency Room . . . . Tom Neal

Measure	Cases	This Hosp.	State Avg.	U.S. Avg.
Heart Attack Care				
ACE Inhibitor or ARB for LVSD	165	96%	94%	96%
Aspirin at Arrival	402	100%	98%	99%
Aspirin at Discharge	965	99%	99%	98%
Beta Blocker at Discharge	921	97%	98%	98%
Fibrinolytic Medication Timing	0	-	60%	55%
PCI Within 90 Minutes of Arrival[1]	22	73%	88%	90%
Smoking Cessation Advice	411	100%	100%	99%
Chest Pain/Possible Heart Attack Care				
Aspirin at Arrival	385	97%	95%	95%
Median Time to ECG (minutes)	393	4	7	8
Median Time to Transfer (minutes)	38	63	65	61
Fibrinolytic Medication Timing[1]	2	0%	62%	54%
Heart Failure Care				
ACE Inhibitor or ARB for LVSD	438	86%	91%	94%
Discharge Instructions	1,079	66%	82%	88%
Evaluation of LVS Function	1,301	99%	96%	98%
Smoking Cessation Advice	312	99%	98%	98%
Pneumonia Care				
Appropriate Initial Antibiotic	442	93%	90%	92%
Blood Culture Timing	735	96%	95%	96%
Influenza Vaccine	617	87%	92%	91%
Initial Antibiotic Timing	712	94%	95%	95%
Pneumococcal Vaccine	724	92%	94%	93%
Smoking Cessation Advice	475	100%	98%	97%
Surgical Care Improvement Project				
Appropriate VTP Within 24 Hours[2]	352	88%	91%	92%
Appropriate Hair Removal[2]	1,108	99%	99%	99%
Appropriate Beta Blocker Usage[2]	409	94%	93%	93%
Controlled Postoperative Blood Glucose[2]	181	90%	94%	93%
Prophylactic Antibiotic Timing[2]	705	96%	97%	97%
Prophylactic Antibiotic Timing (Outpatient)	1,033	95%	92%	92%
Prophylactic Antibiotic Selection[2]	710	97%	98%	97%
Prophylactic Antibiotic Select. (Outpatient)	1,011	97%	93%	94%
Prophylactic Antibiotic Stopped[2]	650	93%	94%	94%
Recommended VTP Ordered[2]	354	92%	94%	94%
Urinary Catheter Removal[2]	218	87%	89%	90%
Children's Asthma Care				
Received Systemic Corticosteroids	-	-	-	100%
Received Home Management Plan	-	-	-	71%
Received Reliever Medication	-	-	-	100%
Use of Medical Imaging				
Combination Abdominal CT Scan	3,041	0.091	0.160	0.191
Combination Chest CT Scan	3,085	0.002	0.054	0.054
Follow-up Mammogram/Ultrasound	3,462	4.7%	7.9%	8.4%
MRI for Low Back Pain	718	36.9%	35.6%	32.7%
Survey of Patients' Hospital Experiences				
Area Around Room 'Always' Quiet at Night	300+	53%	-	58%
Doctors 'Always' Communicated Well	300+	73%	-	80%
Home Recovery Information Given	300+	77%	-	82%
Hospital Given 9 or 10 on 10 Point Scale	300+	60%	-	67%
Meds 'Always' Explained Before Given	300+	54%	-	60%
Nurses 'Always' Communicated Well	300+	70%	-	76%
Pain 'Always' Well Controlled	300+	61%	-	69%
Room and Bathroom 'Always' Clean	300+	57%	-	71%
Timely Help 'Always' Received	300+	52%	-	64%
Would Definitely Recommend Hospital	300+	63%	-	69%

NOTE: Hospital profiles are in alphabetical order by state, then city, then hospital within the city; Rankings exclude hospitals with less than 25 cases except for patient surveys which excludes hospitals with less than 100 cases; (a) 100–299 cases; (1) The number of cases is too small to be sure how well a hospital is performing; (2) The hospital indicated that the data submitted for this measure were based on a sample of cases; (3) Data was collected during a shorter time period (fewer quarters) than the maximum possible time for this measure; (4) Suppressed for one or more quarters by CMS; (5) No data is available from the hospital for this measure; (6) Fewer than 100 patients completed the HCAHPS survey. Use these rates with caution, as the number of surveys may be too low to reliably assess hospital performance; (7) Survey results are based on less than 12 months of data; (8) Survey results are not available for this reporting period; (9) No or very few patients were eligible for the HCAHPS survey. The scores shown, if any, reflect a very small number of surveys; (10) A state average was not calculated because too few hospitals in the state submitted data; (11) There were discrepancies in the data collection process; Please refer to the User's Guide for a full explanation of data.

Louisville VA Medical Center

800 Zorn Avenue Phone: 502-287-4000
Louisville, KY 40206 Fax: 502-287-6225
E-mail: sander.larry-j@lousville.va.gov
URL: www.va.gov/603louisville
Type: Acute Care-Veterans Administration Emergency Services: No
Ownership: Government - Federal Beds: 168

Key Personnel:
Chief of Medical Staff . . . . Marylee Rothschild, MD
Infection Control . . . . Alberta Mozee, RN
Quality Assurance . . . . Verena Wheatley
Emergency Room . . . . Ruby Leverson
Patient Relations . . . . Kathleen Rajoevich, RN

Measure	Cases	This Hosp.	State Avg.	U.S. Avg.
Heart Attack Care				
ACE Inhibitor or ARB for LVSD[1]	10	100%	94%	96%
Aspirin at Arrival	80	96%	98%	99%
Aspirin at Discharge	65	100%	99%	98%
Beta Blocker at Discharge	61	100%	98%	98%
Fibrinolytic Medication Timing[5]	0	-	60%	55%
PCI Within 90 Minutes of Arrival[1]	5	60%	88%	90%
Smoking Cessation Advice	25	96%	100%	99%
Chest Pain/Possible Heart Attack Care				
Aspirin at Arrival	-	-	95%	95%
Median Time to ECG (minutes)	-	-	7	8
Median Time to Transfer (minutes)	-	-	65	61
Fibrinolytic Medication Timing	-	-	62%	54%
Heart Failure Care				
ACE Inhibitor or ARB for LVSD	95	100%	91%	94%
Discharge Instructions	193	99%	82%	88%
Evaluation of LVS Function	213	100%	96%	98%
Smoking Cessation Advice	57	98%	98%	98%
Pneumonia Care				
Appropriate Initial Antibiotic	87	95%	90%	92%
Blood Culture Timing	151	98%	95%	96%
Influenza Vaccine	101	95%	92%	91%
Initial Antibiotic Timing	147	94%	95%	95%
Pneumococcal Vaccine	117	98%	94%	93%
Smoking Cessation Advice	81	100%	98%	97%
Surgical Care Improvement Project				
Appropriate VTP Within 24 Hours[2,5]	0	-	91%	92%
Appropriate Hair Removal[2,5]	0	-	99%	99%
Appropriate Beta Blocker Usage[2,5]	0	-	93%	93%
Controlled Postoperative Blood Glucose[2,5]	0	-	94%	93%
Prophylactic Antibiotic Timing[5]	0	-	97%	97%
Prophylactic Antibiotic Timing (Outpatient)	-	-	92%	92%
Prophylactic Antibiotic Selection[5]	0	-	98%	97%
Prophylactic Antibiotic Select. (Outpatient)	-	-	93%	94%
Prophylactic Antibiotic Stopped[5]	0	-	94%	94%
Recommended VTP Ordered[2,5]	0	-	94%	94%
Urinary Catheter Removal[2,5]	0	-	89%	90%
Children's Asthma Care				
Received Systemic Corticosteroids	-	-	-	100%
Received Home Management Plan	-	-	-	71%
Received Reliever Medication	-	-	-	100%
Use of Medical Imaging				
Combination Abdominal CT Scan	-	-	0.160	0.191
Combination Chest CT Scan	-	-	0.054	0.054
Follow-up Mammogram/Ultrasound	-	-	7.9%	8.4%
MRI for Low Back Pain	-	-	35.6%	32.7%
Survey of Patients' Hospital Experiences				
Area Around Room 'Always' Quiet at Night	-	-	-	58%
Doctors 'Always' Communicated Well	-	-	-	80%
Home Recovery Information Given	-	-	-	82%
Hospital Given 9 or 10 on 10 Point Scale	-	-	-	67%
Meds 'Always' Explained Before Given	-	-	-	60%
Nurses 'Always' Communicated Well	-	-	-	76%
Pain 'Always' Well Controlled	-	-	-	69%
Room and Bathroom 'Always' Clean	-	-	-	71%
Timely Help 'Always' Received	-	-	-	64%
Would Definitely Recommend Hospital	-	-	-	69%

Norton Hospitals

200 East Chestnut Street Phone: 502-629-6560
Louisville, KY 40202
URL: www.nortonhealthcare.com
Type: Acute Care Hospitals Emergency Services: Yes
Ownership: Voluntary Non-Profit - Private

Key Personnel:
CEO/President. . . . . Kevin S. Wardell

Measure	Cases	This Hosp.	State Avg.	U.S. Avg.
Heart Attack Care				
ACE Inhibitor or ARB for LVSD	140	96%	94%	96%
Aspirin at Arrival	458	98%	98%	99%
Aspirin at Discharge	724	100%	99%	98%
Beta Blocker at Discharge	705	100%	98%	98%
Fibrinolytic Medication Timing	0	-	60%	55%
PCI Within 90 Minutes of Arrival	70	84%	88%	90%
Smoking Cessation Advice	319	100%	100%	99%
Chest Pain/Possible Heart Attack Care				
Aspirin at Arrival[3]	36	92%	95%	95%
Median Time to ECG (minutes)[3]	36	5	7	8
Median Time to Transfer (minutes)[3,1]	8	56	65	61
Fibrinolytic Medication Timing[3]	0	-	62%	54%
Heart Failure Care				
ACE Inhibitor or ARB for LVSD	386	95%	91%	94%
Discharge Instructions	1,003	73%	82%	88%
Evaluation of LVS Function	1,290	99%	96%	98%
Smoking Cessation Advice	311	100%	98%	98%
Pneumonia Care				
Appropriate Initial Antibiotic	538	93%	90%	92%
Blood Culture Timing	935	97%	95%	96%
Influenza Vaccine	671	95%	92%	91%
Initial Antibiotic Timing	892	95%	95%	95%
Pneumococcal Vaccine	779	96%	94%	93%
Smoking Cessation Advice	475	100%	98%	97%
Surgical Care Improvement Project				
Appropriate VTP Within 24 Hours[2]	969	89%	91%	92%
Appropriate Hair Removal[2]	3,536	100%	99%	99%
Appropriate Beta Blocker Usage[2]	1,186	93%	93%	93%
Controlled Postoperative Blood Glucose[2]	516	96%	94%	93%
Prophylactic Antibiotic Timing[2]	2,460	96%	97%	97%
Prophylactic Antibiotic Timing (Outpatient)	1,238	90%	92%	92%
Prophylactic Antibiotic Selection[2]	2,490	98%	98%	97%
Prophylactic Antibiotic Select. (Outpatient)	1,190	87%	93%	94%
Prophylactic Antibiotic Stopped[2]	2,227	89%	94%	94%
Recommended VTP Ordered[2]	977	93%	94%	94%
Urinary Catheter Removal[2]	853	92%	89%	90%
Children's Asthma Care				
Received Systemic Corticosteroids	795	100%	-	100%
Received Home Management Plan	792	89%	-	71%
Received Reliever Medication	795	100%	-	100%
Use of Medical Imaging				
Combination Abdominal CT Scan	3,316	0.184	0.160	0.191
Combination Chest CT Scan	2,506	0.233	0.054	0.054
Follow-up Mammogram/Ultrasound	4,166	9.6%	7.9%	8.4%
MRI for Low Back Pain	873	29.1%	35.6%	32.7%
Survey of Patients' Hospital Experiences				
Area Around Room 'Always' Quiet at Night	300+	58%	-	58%
Doctors 'Always' Communicated Well	300+	78%	-	80%
Home Recovery Information Given	300+	83%	-	82%
Hospital Given 9 or 10 on 10 Point Scale	300+	69%	-	67%
Meds 'Always' Explained Before Given	300+	61%	-	60%
Nurses 'Always' Communicated Well	300+	77%	-	76%
Pain 'Always' Well Controlled	300+	70%	-	69%
Room and Bathroom 'Always' Clean	300+	70%	-	71%
Timely Help 'Always' Received	300+	64%	-	64%
Would Definitely Recommend Hospital	300+	72%	-	69%

University of Louisville Hospital

530 South Jackson Street Phone: 502-562-3000
Louisville, KY 40202 Fax: 502-562-3593
URL: www.uoflhealthcare.org
Type: Acute Care Hospitals Emergency Services: No
Ownership: Voluntary Non-Profit - Private Beds: 404

Key Personnel:
CEO/President. . . . . James H Taylor
Operating Room. . . . . Patty Melvin
Anesthesiology. . . . . Anupama Wadhwa

Measure	Cases	This Hosp.	State Avg.	U.S. Avg.
Heart Attack Care				
ACE Inhibitor or ARB for LVSD[1]	16	94%	94%	96%
Aspirin at Arrival	107	97%	98%	99%
Aspirin at Discharge	107	95%	99%	98%
Beta Blocker at Discharge	97	97%	98%	98%
Fibrinolytic Medication Timing	0	-	60%	55%
PCI Within 90 Minutes of Arrival[1]	22	91%	88%	90%
Smoking Cessation Advice	73	99%	100%	99%
Chest Pain/Possible Heart Attack Care				
Aspirin at Arrival[5]	0	-	95%	95%
Median Time to ECG (minutes)[5]	0	-	7	8
Median Time to Transfer (minutes)[5]	0	-	65	61
Fibrinolytic Medication Timing[5]	0	-	62%	54%
Heart Failure Care				
ACE Inhibitor or ARB for LVSD	111	95%	91%	94%
Discharge Instructions	186	75%	82%	88%
Evaluation of LVS Function	200	98%	96%	98%
Smoking Cessation Advice	115	100%	98%	98%
Pneumonia Care				
Appropriate Initial Antibiotic	67	88%	90%	92%
Blood Culture Timing	103	83%	95%	96%
Influenza Vaccine	75	69%	92%	91%
Initial Antibiotic Timing	121	82%	95%	95%
Pneumococcal Vaccine	52	79%	94%	93%
Smoking Cessation Advice	109	99%	98%	97%
Surgical Care Improvement Project				
Appropriate VTP Within 24 Hours[2]	160	84%	91%	92%
Appropriate Hair Removal[2]	421	96%	99%	99%
Appropriate Beta Blocker Usage[2]	107	64%	93%	93%
Controlled Postoperative Blood Glucose[2]	58	98%	94%	93%
Prophylactic Antibiotic Timing[2]	271	94%	97%	97%
Prophylactic Antibiotic Timing (Outpatient)	277	79%	92%	92%
Prophylactic Antibiotic Selection[2]	279	95%	98%	97%
Prophylactic Antibiotic Select. (Outpatient)	238	90%	93%	94%
Prophylactic Antibiotic Stopped[2]	246	90%	94%	94%
Recommended VTP Ordered[2]	160	86%	94%	94%
Urinary Catheter Removal[2]	71	76%	89%	90%
Children's Asthma Care				
Received Systemic Corticosteroids	-	-	-	100%
Received Home Management Plan	-	-	-	71%
Received Reliever Medication	-	-	-	100%
Use of Medical Imaging				
Combination Abdominal CT Scan	702	0.063	0.160	0.191
Combination Chest CT Scan	844	0.006	0.054	0.054
Follow-up Mammogram/Ultrasound	1,378	7.8%	7.9%	8.4%
MRI for Low Back Pain	57	50.9%	35.6%	32.7%
Survey of Patients' Hospital Experiences				
Area Around Room 'Always' Quiet at Night	300+	48%	-	58%
Doctors 'Always' Communicated Well	300+	73%	-	80%
Home Recovery Information Given	300+	81%	-	82%
Hospital Given 9 or 10 on 10 Point Scale	300+	63%	-	67%
Meds 'Always' Explained Before Given	300+	57%	-	60%
Nurses 'Always' Communicated Well	300+	71%	-	76%
Pain 'Always' Well Controlled	300+	63%	-	69%
Room and Bathroom 'Always' Clean	300+	61%	-	71%
Timely Help 'Always' Received	300+	52%	-	64%
Would Definitely Recommend Hospital	300+	65%	-	69%

NOTE: Hospital profiles are in alphabetical order by state, then city, then hospital within the city; Rankings exclude hospitals with less than 25 cases except for patient surveys which excludes hospitals with less than 100 cases; (a) 100–299 cases; (1) The number of cases is too small to be sure how well a hospital is performing; (2) The hospital indicated that the data submitted for this measure were based on a sample of cases; (3) Data was collected during a shorter time period (fewer quarters) than the maximum possible time for this measure; (4) Suppressed for one or more quarters by CMS; (5) No data is available from the hospital for this measure; (6) Fewer than 100 patients completed the HCAHPS survey. Use these rates with caution, as the number of surveys may be too low to reliably assess hospital performance; (7) Survey results are based on less than 12 months of data; (8) Survey results are not available for this reporting period; (9) No or very few patients were eligible for the HCAHPS survey. The scores shown, if any, reflect a very small number of surveys; (10) A state average was not calculated because too few hospitals in the state submitted data; (11) There were discrepancies in the data collection process; Please refer to the User's Guide for a full explanation of data.

Regional Medical Center of Hopkins County

900 Hospital Drive
Madisonville, KY 42431
Phone: 270-825-5100
Fax: 270-825-6650
E-mail: info@trover.org
URL: www.troverfoundation.org
Type: Acute Care Hospitals
Emergency Services: Yes
Ownership: Voluntary Non-Profit - Private
Beds: 410

Key Personnel:
CEO/President. . . . . Bobby Dampier
Radiology. . . . . Kavita Erickson

Measure	Cases	This Hosp.	State Avg.	U.S. Avg.
Heart Attack Care				
ACE Inhibitor or ARB for LVSD	65	94%	94%	96%
Aspirin at Arrival	180	99%	98%	99%
Aspirin at Discharge	218	97%	99%	98%
Beta Blocker at Discharge	202	97%	98%	98%
Fibrinolytic Medication Timing	0	-	60%	55%
PCI Within 90 Minutes of Arrival	32	97%	88%	90%
Smoking Cessation Advice	107	99%	100%	99%
Chest Pain/Possible Heart Attack Care				
Aspirin at Arrival[1]	6	83%	95%	95%
Median Time to ECG (minutes)[1]	7	3	7	8
Median Time to Transfer (minutes)[5]	0	-	65	61
Fibrinolytic Medication Timing[3]	0	-	62%	54%
Heart Failure Care				
ACE Inhibitor or ARB for LVSD	134	89%	91%	94%
Discharge Instructions	191	78%	82%	88%
Evaluation of LVS Function	238	98%	96%	98%
Smoking Cessation Advice	64	100%	98%	98%
Pneumonia Care				
Appropriate Initial Antibiotic	105	91%	90%	92%
Blood Culture Timing	187	99%	95%	96%
Influenza Vaccine	168	91%	92%	91%
Initial Antibiotic Timing	271	92%	95%	95%
Pneumococcal Vaccine	220	97%	94%	93%
Smoking Cessation Advice	158	99%	98%	97%
Surgical Care Improvement Project				
Appropriate VTP Within 24 Hours[2]	253	88%	91%	92%
Appropriate Hair Removal[2]	789	100%	99%	99%
Appropriate Beta Blocker Usage[2]	256	95%	93%	93%
Controlled Postoperative Blood Glucose[2]	123	89%	94%	93%
Prophylactic Antibiotic Timing[2]	550	97%	97%	97%
Prophylactic Antibiotic Timing (Outpatient)	140	91%	92%	92%
Prophylactic Antibiotic Selection[2]	557	98%	98%	97%
Prophylactic Antibiotic Select. (Outpatient)	138	91%	93%	94%
Prophylactic Antibiotic Stopped[2]	518	95%	94%	94%
Recommended VTP Ordered[2]	255	90%	94%	94%
Urinary Catheter Removal[2]	172	95%	89%	90%
Children's Asthma Care				
Received Systemic Corticosteroids	-	-	-	100%
Received Home Management Plan	-	-	-	71%
Received Reliever Medication	-	-	-	100%
Use of Medical Imaging				
Combination Abdominal CT Scan	637	0.078	0.160	0.191
Combination Chest CT Scan	367	0.005	0.054	0.054
Follow-up Mammogram/Ultrasound[5]	0	-	7.9%	8.4%
MRI for Low Back Pain	130	39.2%	35.6%	32.7%
Survey of Patients' Hospital Experiences				
Area Around Room 'Always' Quiet at Night	300+	58%	-	58%
Doctors 'Always' Communicated Well	300+	83%	-	80%
Home Recovery Information Given	300+	84%	-	82%
Hospital Given 9 or 10 on 10 Point Scale	300+	70%	-	67%
Meds 'Always' Explained Before Given	300+	66%	-	60%
Nurses 'Always' Communicated Well	300+	80%	-	76%
Pain 'Always' Well Controlled	300+	73%	-	69%
Room and Bathroom 'Always' Clean	300+	69%	-	71%
Timely Help 'Always' Received	300+	59%	-	64%
Would Definitely Recommend Hospital	300+	71%	-	69%

Memorial Hospital

210 Marie Langdon Drive
Manchester, KY 40962
Phone: 606-598-5104
Fax: 606-598-7008
E-mail: rosann.may@ahss.org
URL: www.manchestermemorial.com
Type: Acute Care Hospitals
Emergency Services: Yes
Ownership: Voluntary Non-Profit - Church
Beds: 63

Key Personnel:
CEO/President. . . . . Dennis Meyers
Chief of Medical Staff . . . . Kishore Javhav
Quality Assurance . . . . Melissa Culver
Emergency Room . . . . Kathy Campbell

Measure	Cases	This Hosp.	State Avg.	U.S. Avg.
Heart Attack Care				
ACE Inhibitor or ARB for LVSD[1]	2	100%	94%	96%
Aspirin at Arrival[1]	13	100%	98%	99%
Aspirin at Discharge[1]	6	100%	99%	98%
Beta Blocker at Discharge[1]	4	100%	98%	98%
Fibrinolytic Medication Timing	0	-	60%	55%
PCI Within 90 Minutes of Arrival	0	-	88%	90%
Smoking Cessation Advice[1]	2	100%	100%	99%
Chest Pain/Possible Heart Attack Care				
Aspirin at Arrival[1]	11	91%	95%	95%
Median Time to ECG (minutes)[1]	11	12	7	8
Median Time to Transfer (minutes)[5]	0	-	65	61
Fibrinolytic Medication Timing[5]	0	-	62%	54%
Heart Failure Care				
ACE Inhibitor or ARB for LVSD[1]	17	94%	91%	94%
Discharge Instructions	88	100%	82%	88%
Evaluation of LVS Function	102	100%	96%	98%
Smoking Cessation Advice[1]	20	100%	98%	98%
Pneumonia Care				
Appropriate Initial Antibiotic	173	89%	90%	92%
Blood Culture Timing	152	94%	95%	96%
Influenza Vaccine	115	97%	92%	91%
Initial Antibiotic Timing	194	93%	95%	95%
Pneumococcal Vaccine	113	96%	94%	93%
Smoking Cessation Advice	123	100%	98%	97%
Surgical Care Improvement Project				
Appropriate VTP Within 24 Hours[1]	19	63%	91%	92%
Appropriate Hair Removal[1]	24	100%	99%	99%
Appropriate Beta Blocker Usage[1]	5	100%	93%	93%
Controlled Postoperative Blood Glucose	0	-	94%	93%
Prophylactic Antibiotic Timing[1]	3	100%	97%	97%
Prophylactic Antibiotic Timing (Outpatient)[1]	24	79%	92%	92%
Prophylactic Antibiotic Selection[1]	3	100%	98%	97%
Prophylactic Antibiotic Select. (Outpatient)[1]	19	79%	93%	94%
Prophylactic Antibiotic Stopped[1]	3	67%	94%	94%
Recommended VTP Ordered[1]	19	68%	94%	94%
Urinary Catheter Removal[1]	3	67%	89%	90%
Children's Asthma Care				
Received Systemic Corticosteroids	-	-	-	100%
Received Home Management Plan	-	-	-	71%
Received Reliever Medication	-	-	-	100%
Use of Medical Imaging				
Combination Abdominal CT Scan	282	0.135	0.160	0.191
Combination Chest CT Scan	138	0.145	0.054	0.054
Follow-up Mammogram/Ultrasound	256	5.5%	7.9%	8.4%
MRI for Low Back Pain	81	32.1%	35.6%	32.7%
Survey of Patients' Hospital Experiences				
Area Around Room 'Always' Quiet at Night	(a)	45%	-	58%
Doctors 'Always' Communicated Well	(a)	75%	-	80%
Home Recovery Information Given	(a)	83%	-	82%
Hospital Given 9 or 10 on 10 Point Scale	(a)	54%	-	67%
Meds 'Always' Explained Before Given	(a)	52%	-	60%
Nurses 'Always' Communicated Well	(a)	72%	-	76%
Pain 'Always' Well Controlled	(a)	63%	-	69%
Room and Bathroom 'Always' Clean	(a)	66%	-	71%
Timely Help 'Always' Received	(a)	56%	-	64%
Would Definitely Recommend Hospital	(a)	49%	-	69%

Crittenden Health System

520 West Gum Street
Marion, KY 42064
Phone: 270-965-5281
Fax: 270-965-1061
URL: www.crittenden-health.org
Type: Acute Care Hospitals
Emergency Services: Yes
Ownership: Proprietary
Beds: 50

Key Personnel:
CEO/President. . . . . Jim Cristenson
Radiology. . . . . Carl Watkins

Measure	Cases	This Hosp.	State Avg.	U.S. Avg.
Heart Attack Care				
ACE Inhibitor or ARB for LVSD	0	-	94%	96%
Aspirin at Arrival[1]	11	91%	98%	99%
Aspirin at Discharge[1]	6	67%	99%	98%
Beta Blocker at Discharge[1]	7	86%	98%	98%
Fibrinolytic Medication Timing	0	-	60%	55%
PCI Within 90 Minutes of Arrival	0	-	88%	90%
Smoking Cessation Advice[1]	3	100%	100%	99%
Chest Pain/Possible Heart Attack Care				
Aspirin at Arrival	33	91%	95%	95%
Median Time to ECG (minutes)	35	3	7	8
Median Time to Transfer (minutes)[1,3]	2	88	65	61
Fibrinolytic Medication Timing[1]	5	80%	62%	54%
Heart Failure Care				
ACE Inhibitor or ARB for LVSD[1]	11	82%	91%	94%
Discharge Instructions	37	100%	82%	88%
Evaluation of LVS Function	61	89%	96%	98%
Smoking Cessation Advice[1]	11	100%	98%	98%
Pneumonia Care				
Appropriate Initial Antibiotic	45	60%	90%	92%
Blood Culture Timing	31	94%	95%	96%
Influenza Vaccine	53	89%	92%	91%
Initial Antibiotic Timing	59	95%	95%	95%
Pneumococcal Vaccine	69	72%	94%	93%
Smoking Cessation Advice	33	100%	98%	97%
Surgical Care Improvement Project				
Appropriate VTP Within 24 Hours[1,3]	2	50%	91%	92%
Appropriate Hair Removal[1,3]	5	60%	99%	99%
Appropriate Beta Blocker Usage[1,3]	1	0%	93%	93%
Controlled Postoperative Blood Glucose[3]	0	-	94%	93%
Prophylactic Antibiotic Timing[1,3]	4	50%	97%	97%
Prophylactic Antibiotic Timing (Outpatient)[1,3]	5	0%	92%	92%
Prophylactic Antibiotic Selection[1,3]	4	0%	98%	97%
Prophylactic Antibiotic Select. (Outpatient)[3]	0	-	93%	94%
Prophylactic Antibiotic Stopped[1,3]	4	25%	94%	94%
Recommended VTP Ordered[1,3]	2	50%	94%	94%
Urinary Catheter Removal[1,3]	1	0%	89%	90%
Children's Asthma Care				
Received Systemic Corticosteroids	-	-	-	100%
Received Home Management Plan	-	-	-	71%
Received Reliever Medication	-	-	-	100%
Use of Medical Imaging				
Combination Abdominal CT Scan	93	0.043	0.160	0.191
Combination Chest CT Scan	63	0.016	0.054	0.054
Follow-up Mammogram/Ultrasound	135	7.4%	7.9%	8.4%
MRI for Low Back Pain[1]	45	28.9%	35.6%	32.7%
Survey of Patients' Hospital Experiences				
Area Around Room 'Always' Quiet at Night	(a)	57%	-	58%
Doctors 'Always' Communicated Well	(a)	87%	-	80%
Home Recovery Information Given	(a)	69%	-	82%
Hospital Given 9 or 10 on 10 Point Scale	(a)	58%	-	67%
Meds 'Always' Explained Before Given	(a)	64%	-	60%
Nurses 'Always' Communicated Well	(a)	79%	-	76%
Pain 'Always' Well Controlled	(a)	68%	-	69%
Room and Bathroom 'Always' Clean	(a)	79%	-	71%
Timely Help 'Always' Received	(a)	66%	-	64%
Would Definitely Recommend Hospital	(a)	63%	-	69%

NOTE: Hospital profiles are in alphabetical order by state, then city, then hospital within the city; Rankings exclude hospitals with less than 25 cases except for patient surveys which excludes hospitals with less than 100 cases; (a) 100–299 cases; (1) The number of cases is too small to be sure how well a hospital is performing; (2) The hospital indicated that the data submitted for this measure were based on a sample of cases; (3) Data was collected during a shorter time period (fewer quarters) than the maximum possible time for this measure; (4) Suppressed for one or more quarters by CMS; (5) No data is available from the hospital for this measure; (6) Fewer than 100 patients completed the HCAHPS survey. Use these rates with caution, as the number of surveys may be too low to reliably assess hospital performance; (7) Survey results are based on less than 12 months of data; (8) Survey results are not available for this reporting period; (9) No or very few patients were eligible for the HCAHPS survey. The scores shown, if any, reflect a very small number of surveys; (10) A state average was not calculated because too few hospitals in the state submitted data; (11) There were discrepancies in the data collection process; Please refer to the User's Guide for a full explanation of data.

Saint Joseph Martin

11203 Main Street
Martin, KY 41649
Phone: 606-285-5181
URL: www.catholichealth.net
Type: Critical Access Hospitals
Emergency Services: Yes
Ownership: Voluntary Non-Profit - Private
Beds: 25

Key Personnel:

CEO/President . . . . Kathy Stumbo
Infection Control . . . . Mary Martin, RN/CIC
Operating Room . . . . Danita Hampton, RN BSN
Pediatric In-Patient Care . . . . Mary Little, RN BSN
Quality Assurance . . . . Olive Martin, MT
Anesthesiology . . . . William Montgomery, CRNA
Emergency Room . . . . Ronald Ross, RN BSN

Measure	Cases	This Hosp.	State Avg.	U.S. Avg.
Heart Attack Care				
ACE Inhibitor or ARB for LVSD[5]	0	-	94%	96%
Aspirin at Arrival[5]	0	-	98%	99%
Aspirin at Discharge[5]	0	-	99%	98%
Beta Blocker at Discharge[5]	0	-	98%	98%
Fibrinolytic Medication Timing[5]	0	-	60%	55%
PCI Within 90 Minutes of Arrival[5]	0	-	88%	90%
Smoking Cessation Advice[5]	0	-	100%	99%
Chest Pain/Possible Heart Attack Care				
Aspirin at Arrival	-	-	95%	95%
Median Time to ECG (minutes)	-	-	7	8
Median Time to Transfer (minutes)	-	-	65	61
Fibrinolytic Medication Timing	-	-	62%	54%
Heart Failure Care				
ACE Inhibitor or ARB for LVSD[1]	16	81%	91%	94%
Discharge Instructions	49	100%	82%	88%
Evaluation of LVS Function	52	98%	96%	98%
Smoking Cessation Advice[1]	7	100%	98%	98%
Pneumonia Care				
Appropriate Initial Antibiotic	60	85%	90%	92%
Blood Culture Timing	66	97%	95%	96%
Influenza Vaccine	25	96%	92%	91%
Initial Antibiotic Timing	70	100%	95%	95%
Pneumococcal Vaccine	33	94%	94%	93%
Smoking Cessation Advice	37	100%	98%	97%
Surgical Care Improvement Project				
Appropriate VTP Within 24 Hours[5]	0	-	91%	92%
Appropriate Hair Removal[5]	0	-	99%	99%
Appropriate Beta Blocker Usage[5]	0	-	93%	93%
Controlled Postoperative Blood Glucose[5]	0	-	94%	93%
Prophylactic Antibiotic Timing[5]	0	-	97%	97%
Prophylactic Antibiotic Timing (Outpatient)	-	-	92%	92%
Prophylactic Antibiotic Selection[5]	0	-	98%	97%
Prophylactic Antibiotic Select. (Outpatient)	-	-	93%	94%
Prophylactic Antibiotic Stopped[5]	0	-	94%	94%
Recommended VTP Ordered[5]	0	-	94%	94%
Urinary Catheter Removal[5]	0	-	89%	90%
Children's Asthma Care				
Received Systemic Corticosteroids	-	-	-	100%
Received Home Management Plan	-	-	-	71%
Received Reliever Medication	-	-	-	100%
Use of Medical Imaging				
Combination Abdominal CT Scan	-	-	0.160	0.191
Combination Chest CT Scan	-	-	0.054	0.054
Follow-up Mammogram/Ultrasound	-	-	7.9%	8.4%
MRI for Low Back Pain	-	-	35.6%	32.7%
Survey of Patients' Hospital Experiences				
Area Around Room 'Always' Quiet at Night	300+	61%	-	58%
Doctors 'Always' Communicated Well	300+	86%	-	80%
Home Recovery Information Given	300+	80%	-	82%
Hospital Given 9 or 10 on 10 Point Scale	300+	76%	-	67%
Meds 'Always' Explained Before Given	300+	72%	-	60%
Nurses 'Always' Communicated Well	300+	86%	-	76%
Pain 'Always' Well Controlled	300+	73%	-	69%
Room and Bathroom 'Always' Clean	300+	82%	-	71%
Timely Help 'Always' Received	300+	79%	-	64%
Would Definitely Recommend Hospital	300+	79%	-	69%

Jackson Purchase Medical Center

1099 Medical Center Circle
Mayfield, KY 42066
Phone: 270-251-4500
Fax: 270-251-4507
URL: www.jacksonpurchase.com
Type: Acute Care Hospitals
Emergency Services: Yes
Ownership: Govt - Hospital Dist/Auth
Beds: 107

Key Personnel:

CEO/President . . . . Mary Jo Lewis
Chief of Medical Staff . . . . David Zetter, MD
Infection Control . . . . Ronnica Adams, RD, LD
Operating Room . . . . Edward McWhirt, RN, BSN
Quality Assurance . . . . Denise Hawks
Radiology . . . . John J Beasley, RT(R)
Emergency Room . . . . Della Thurston, RN
Intensive Care Unit . . . . Julia Grove

Measure	Cases	This Hosp.	State Avg.	U.S. Avg.
Heart Attack Care				
ACE Inhibitor or ARB for LVSD[1]	3	100%	94%	96%
Aspirin at Arrival[1]	20	95%	98%	99%
Aspirin at Discharge[1]	13	100%	99%	98%
Beta Blocker at Discharge[1]	13	100%	98%	98%
Fibrinolytic Medication Timing	0	-	60%	55%
PCI Within 90 Minutes of Arrival	0	-	88%	90%
Smoking Cessation Advice[1]	4	100%	100%	99%
Chest Pain/Possible Heart Attack Care				
Aspirin at Arrival[1]	10	90%	95%	95%
Median Time to ECG (minutes)[1]	12	4	7	8
Median Time to Transfer (minutes)[1,3]	1	185	65	61
Fibrinolytic Medication Timing[3]	0	-	62%	54%
Heart Failure Care				
ACE Inhibitor or ARB for LVSD	29	97%	91%	94%
Discharge Instructions	77	100%	82%	88%
Evaluation of LVS Function	103	98%	96%	98%
Smoking Cessation Advice	27	100%	98%	98%
Pneumonia Care				
Appropriate Initial Antibiotic	97	89%	90%	92%
Blood Culture Timing	128	98%	95%	96%
Influenza Vaccine	142	90%	92%	91%
Initial Antibiotic Timing	161	98%	95%	95%
Pneumococcal Vaccine	212	94%	94%	93%
Smoking Cessation Advice	93	100%	98%	97%
Surgical Care Improvement Project				
Appropriate VTP Within 24 Hours	185	99%	91%	92%
Appropriate Hair Removal	318	100%	99%	99%
Appropriate Beta Blocker Usage	95	99%	93%	93%
Controlled Postoperative Blood Glucose	0	-	94%	93%
Prophylactic Antibiotic Timing	253	100%	97%	97%
Prophylactic Antibiotic Timing (Outpatient)	92	99%	92%	92%
Prophylactic Antibiotic Selection	254	100%	98%	97%
Prophylactic Antibiotic Select. (Outpatient)	91	100%	93%	94%
Prophylactic Antibiotic Stopped	235	98%	94%	94%
Recommended VTP Ordered	186	99%	94%	94%
Urinary Catheter Removal	105	97%	89%	90%
Children's Asthma Care				
Received Systemic Corticosteroids	-	-	-	100%
Received Home Management Plan	-	-	-	71%
Received Reliever Medication	-	-	-	100%
Use of Medical Imaging				
Combination Abdominal CT Scan	335	0.343	0.160	0.191
Combination Chest CT Scan	289	0.000	0.054	0.054
Follow-up Mammogram/Ultrasound	610	7.4%	7.9%	8.4%
MRI for Low Back Pain	64	42.2%	35.6%	32.7%
Survey of Patients' Hospital Experiences				
Area Around Room 'Always' Quiet at Night	300+	66%	-	58%
Doctors 'Always' Communicated Well	300+	84%	-	80%
Home Recovery Information Given	300+	83%	-	82%
Hospital Given 9 or 10 on 10 Point Scale	300+	70%	-	67%
Meds 'Always' Explained Before Given	300+	62%	-	60%
Nurses 'Always' Communicated Well	300+	76%	-	76%
Pain 'Always' Well Controlled	300+	68%	-	69%
Room and Bathroom 'Always' Clean	300+	69%	-	71%
Timely Help 'Always' Received	300+	60%	-	64%
Would Definitely Recommend Hospital	300+	68%	-	69%

Meadowview Regional Medical Center

989 Medical Park Drive
Maysville, KY 41056
Phone: 606-759-5311
Fax: 606-759-5616
URL: www.meadowviewregional.com
Type: Acute Care Hospitals
Emergency Services: Yes
Ownership: Proprietary
Beds: 101

Key Personnel:

CEO/President . . . . Curtis Courtney
Chief of Medical Staff . . . . Rick Hartman
Infection Control . . . . Clare Vetter
Quality Assurance . . . . Pam Brant, RN
Radiology . . . . Richard Hartman
Emergency Room . . . . June Fultz
Intensive Care Unit . . . . June Fultz

Measure	Cases	This Hosp.	State Avg.	U.S. Avg.
Heart Attack Care				
ACE Inhibitor or ARB for LVSD[1]	10	100%	94%	96%
Aspirin at Arrival	82	100%	98%	99%
Aspirin at Discharge	78	100%	99%	98%
Beta Blocker at Discharge	71	100%	98%	98%
Fibrinolytic Medication Timing	0	-	60%	55%
PCI Within 90 Minutes of Arrival[1]	17	94%	88%	90%
Smoking Cessation Advice	37	100%	100%	99%
Chest Pain/Possible Heart Attack Care				
Aspirin at Arrival	46	100%	95%	95%
Median Time to ECG (minutes)	45	2	7	8
Median Time to Transfer (minutes)[1,3]	2	116	65	61
Fibrinolytic Medication Timing[3]	0	-	62%	54%
Heart Failure Care				
ACE Inhibitor or ARB for LVSD[1]	22	100%	91%	94%
Discharge Instructions	55	100%	82%	88%
Evaluation of LVS Function	67	100%	96%	98%
Smoking Cessation Advice[1]	11	100%	98%	98%
Pneumonia Care				
Appropriate Initial Antibiotic	85	99%	90%	92%
Blood Culture Timing	103	100%	95%	96%
Influenza Vaccine	79	94%	92%	91%
Initial Antibiotic Timing	104	100%	95%	95%
Pneumococcal Vaccine	99	100%	94%	93%
Smoking Cessation Advice	37	100%	98%	97%
Surgical Care Improvement Project				
Appropriate VTP Within 24 Hours	34	100%	91%	92%
Appropriate Hair Removal	74	100%	99%	99%
Appropriate Beta Blocker Usage[1]	19	100%	93%	93%
Controlled Postoperative Blood Glucose	0	-	94%	93%
Prophylactic Antibiotic Timing	53	100%	97%	97%
Prophylactic Antibiotic Timing (Outpatient)	135	97%	92%	92%
Prophylactic Antibiotic Selection	53	100%	98%	97%
Prophylactic Antibiotic Select. (Outpatient)	132	95%	93%	94%
Prophylactic Antibiotic Stopped	53	100%	94%	94%
Recommended VTP Ordered	34	100%	94%	94%
Urinary Catheter Removal[1]	20	100%	89%	90%
Children's Asthma Care				
Received Systemic Corticosteroids	-	-	-	100%
Received Home Management Plan	-	-	-	71%
Received Reliever Medication	-	-	-	100%
Use of Medical Imaging				
Combination Abdominal CT Scan	288	0.649	0.160	0.191
Combination Chest CT Scan	239	0.000	0.054	0.054
Follow-up Mammogram/Ultrasound	436	9.9%	7.9%	8.4%
MRI for Low Back Pain[1]	6	66.7%	35.6%	32.7%
Survey of Patients' Hospital Experiences				
Area Around Room 'Always' Quiet at Night	300+	63%	-	58%
Doctors 'Always' Communicated Well	300+	82%	-	80%
Home Recovery Information Given	300+	82%	-	82%
Hospital Given 9 or 10 on 10 Point Scale	300+	64%	-	67%
Meds 'Always' Explained Before Given	300+	57%	-	60%
Nurses 'Always' Communicated Well	300+	77%	-	76%
Pain 'Always' Well Controlled	300+	72%	-	69%
Room and Bathroom 'Always' Clean	300+	74%	-	71%
Timely Help 'Always' Received	300+	61%	-	64%
Would Definitely Recommend Hospital	300+	65%	-	69%

NOTE: Hospital profiles are in alphabetical order by state, then city, then hospital within the city; Rankings exclude hospitals with less than 25 cases except for patient surveys which excludes hospitals with less than 100 cases; (a) 100–299 cases; (1) The number of cases is too small to be sure how well a hospital is performing; (2) The hospital indicated that the data submitted for this measure were based on a sample of cases; (3) Data was collected during a shorter time period (fewer quarters) than the maximum possible time for this measure; (4) Suppressed for one or more quarters by CMS; (5) No data is available from the hospital for this measure; (6) Fewer than 100 patients completed the HCAHPS survey. Use these rates with caution, as the number of surveys may be too low to reliably assess hospital performance; (7) Survey results are based on less than 12 months of data; (8) Survey results are not available for this reporting period; (9) No or very few patients were eligible for the HCAHPS survey. The scores shown, if any, reflect a very small number of surveys; (10) A state average was not calculated because too few hospitals in the state submitted data; (11) There were discrepancies in the data collection process; Please refer to the User's Guide for a full explanation of data.

McDowell Arh Hospital

9879 Kentucky Route 122
McDowell, KY 41647
E-mail: mcdowellarh@arh.org
URL: www.arh.org/mcdowell
Type: Critical Access Hospitals
Ownership: Voluntary Non-Profit - Private

Phone: 606-377-3400
Fax: 606-377-3433

Emergency Services: Yes
Beds: 25

Key Personnel:
CEO/President . . . . R Barker
Chief of Medical Staff . . . . Donna Johnson
Operating Room . . . . Josephine Akers
Pediatric In-Patient Care . . . . Vivian Ong, MD
Quality Assurance . . . . Jeff Frazier
Radiology . . . . Dhirenkumar I Desai, MD
Anesthesiology . . . . Kerry Slona, CRNA
Emergency Room . . . . Francisco G Rivera, MD

Measure	Cases	This Hosp.	State Avg.	U.S. Avg.
Heart Attack Care				
ACE Inhibitor or ARB for LVSD[3]	0	-	94%	96%
Aspirin at Arrival[3]	0	-	98%	99%
Aspirin at Discharge[3]	0	-	99%	98%
Beta Blocker at Discharge[3]	0	-	98%	98%
Fibrinolytic Medication Timing[3]	0	-	60%	55%
PCI Within 90 Minutes of Arrival[3]	0	-	88%	90%
Smoking Cessation Advice[3]	0	-	100%	99%
Chest Pain/Possible Heart Attack Care				
Aspirin at Arrival[5]	0	-	95%	95%
Median Time to ECG (minutes)[5]	0	-	7	8
Median Time to Transfer (minutes)[5]	0	-	65	61
Fibrinolytic Medication Timing[5]	0	-	62%	54%
Heart Failure Care				
ACE Inhibitor or ARB for LVSD[1]	16	94%	91%	94%
Discharge Instructions	51	100%	82%	88%
Evaluation of LVS Function	52	100%	96%	98%
Smoking Cessation Advice[1]	15	100%	98%	98%
Pneumonia Care				
Appropriate Initial Antibiotic	85	66%	90%	92%
Blood Culture Timing	65	83%	95%	96%
Influenza Vaccine	39	85%	92%	91%
Initial Antibiotic Timing	106	83%	95%	95%
Pneumococcal Vaccine	45	93%	94%	93%
Smoking Cessation Advice	39	100%	98%	97%
Surgical Care Improvement Project				
Appropriate VTP Within 24 Hours[5]	0	-	91%	92%
Appropriate Hair Removal[5]	0	-	99%	99%
Appropriate Beta Blocker Usage[5]	0	-	93%	93%
Controlled Postoperative Blood Glucose[5]	0	-	94%	93%
Prophylactic Antibiotic Timing[5]	0	-	97%	97%
Prophylactic Antibiotic Timing (Outpatient)[5]	0	-	92%	92%
Prophylactic Antibiotic Selection[5]	0	-	98%	97%
Prophylactic Antibiotic Select. (Outpatient)[5]	0	-	93%	94%
Prophylactic Antibiotic Stopped[5]	0	-	94%	94%
Recommended VTP Ordered[5]	0	-	94%	94%
Urinary Catheter Removal[5]	0	-	89%	90%
Children's Asthma Care				
Received Systemic Corticosteroids	-	-	-	100%
Received Home Management Plan	-	-	-	71%
Received Reliever Medication	-	-	-	100%
Use of Medical Imaging				
Combination Abdominal CT Scan	180	0.006	0.160	0.191
Combination Chest CT Scan	81	0.037	0.054	0.054
Follow-up Mammogram/Ultrasound	137	12.4%	7.9%	8.4%
MRI for Low Back Pain[1]	33	72.7%	35.6%	32.7%
Survey of Patients' Hospital Experiences				
Area Around Room 'Always' Quiet at Night	(a)	76%	-	58%
Doctors 'Always' Communicated Well	(a)	88%	-	80%
Home Recovery Information Given	(a)	88%	-	82%
Hospital Given 9 or 10 on 10 Point Scale	(a)	75%	-	67%
Meds 'Always' Explained Before Given	(a)	68%	-	60%
Nurses 'Always' Communicated Well	(a)	83%	-	76%
Pain 'Always' Well Controlled	(a)	74%	-	69%
Room and Bathroom 'Always' Clean	(a)	85%	-	71%
Timely Help 'Always' Received	(a)	80%	-	64%
Would Definitely Recommend Hospital	(a)	76%	-	69%

Middlesboro Appalachian Regional Healthcare Hospital

3600 West Cumberland Avenue
Middlesboro, KY 40965
URL: www.arh.org/middlesboro
Type: Acute Care Hospitals
Ownership: Voluntary Non-Profit - Private

Phone: 606-242-1101
Fax: 606-248-3903

Emergency Services: Yes
Beds: 96

Key Personnel:
CEO/President . . . . Jerry W Haynes
Chief of Medical Staff . . . . Vicente Kaw, MD
Infection Control . . . . Shirley Lovell
Operating Room . . . . Charles Crumley, RN
Pediatric Ambulatory Care . . . . . Houshang Khorram, MD
Pediatric In-Patient Care . . . . . . Houshang Khorram, MD
Quality Assurance . . . . Lisa Dooley
Radiology . . . . Ashok R Patel, MD

Measure	Cases	This Hosp.	State Avg.	U.S. Avg.
Heart Attack Care				
ACE Inhibitor or ARB for LVSD[1]	5	80%	94%	96%
Aspirin at Arrival[1]	6	100%	98%	99%
Aspirin at Discharge[1]	5	100%	99%	98%
Beta Blocker at Discharge[1]	7	100%	98%	98%
Fibrinolytic Medication Timing	0	-	60%	55%
PCI Within 90 Minutes of Arrival	0	-	88%	90%
Smoking Cessation Advice	0	-	100%	99%
Chest Pain/Possible Heart Attack Care				
Aspirin at Arrival	126	95%	95%	95%
Median Time to ECG (minutes)	130	7	7	8
Median Time to Transfer (minutes)[1]	9	60	65	61
Fibrinolytic Medication Timing	0	-	62%	54%
Heart Failure Care				
ACE Inhibitor or ARB for LVSD	36	94%	91%	94%
Discharge Instructions	92	96%	82%	88%
Evaluation of LVS Function	129	99%	96%	98%
Smoking Cessation Advice[1]	18	100%	98%	98%
Pneumonia Care				
Appropriate Initial Antibiotic	130	95%	90%	92%
Blood Culture Timing	162	99%	95%	96%
Influenza Vaccine	98	96%	92%	91%
Initial Antibiotic Timing	170	97%	95%	95%
Pneumococcal Vaccine	110	97%	94%	93%
Smoking Cessation Advice	75	100%	98%	97%
Surgical Care Improvement Project				
Appropriate VTP Within 24 Hours	28	89%	91%	92%
Appropriate Hair Removal	51	100%	99%	99%
Appropriate Beta Blocker Usage[1]	10	90%	93%	93%
Controlled Postoperative Blood Glucose	0	-	94%	93%
Prophylactic Antibiotic Timing	25	100%	97%	97%
Prophylactic Antibiotic Timing (Outpatient)	43	93%	92%	92%
Prophylactic Antibiotic Selection	26	96%	98%	97%
Prophylactic Antibiotic Select. (Outpatient)	40	100%	93%	94%
Prophylactic Antibiotic Stopped	25	92%	94%	94%
Recommended VTP Ordered	28	93%	94%	94%
Urinary Catheter Removal[1]	4	75%	89%	90%
Children's Asthma Care				
Received Systemic Corticosteroids	-	-	-	100%
Received Home Management Plan	-	-	-	71%
Received Reliever Medication	-	-	-	100%
Use of Medical Imaging				
Combination Abdominal CT Scan	377	0.467	0.160	0.191
Combination Chest CT Scan	222	0.045	0.054	0.054
Follow-up Mammogram/Ultrasound	390	7.2%	7.9%	8.4%
MRI for Low Back Pain	136	37.5%	35.6%	32.7%
Survey of Patients' Hospital Experiences				
Area Around Room 'Always' Quiet at Night	300+	69%	-	58%
Doctors 'Always' Communicated Well	300+	88%	-	80%
Home Recovery Information Given	300+	84%	-	82%
Hospital Given 9 or 10 on 10 Point Scale	300+	70%	-	67%
Meds 'Always' Explained Before Given	300+	61%	-	60%
Nurses 'Always' Communicated Well	300+	80%	-	76%
Pain 'Always' Well Controlled	300+	70%	-	69%
Room and Bathroom 'Always' Clean	300+	74%	-	71%
Timely Help 'Always' Received	300+	70%	-	64%
Would Definitely Recommend Hospital	300+	65%	-	69%

Wayne County Hospital

166 Hospital Street
Monticello, KY 42633
E-mail: wchospital@kih.net
Type: Critical Access Hospitals
Ownership: Voluntary Non-Profit - Other

Phone: 606-348-9343
Fax: 606-348-5796

Emergency Services: Yes
Beds: 30

Key Personnel:
CEO/President . . . . Pat Brinson
Chief of Medical Staff . . . . Walter Koscrenski
Emergency Room . . . . Patricia Brenson

Measure	Cases	This Hosp.	State Avg.	U.S. Avg.
Heart Attack Care				
ACE Inhibitor or ARB for LVSD[3]	0	-	94%	96%
Aspirin at Arrival[1,3]	1	100%	98%	99%
Aspirin at Discharge[3]	0	-	99%	98%
Beta Blocker at Discharge[3]	0	-	98%	98%
Fibrinolytic Medication Timing[3]	0	-	60%	55%
PCI Within 90 Minutes of Arrival[3]	0	-	88%	90%
Smoking Cessation Advice[3]	0	-	100%	99%
Chest Pain/Possible Heart Attack Care				
Aspirin at Arrival	-	-	95%	95%
Median Time to ECG (minutes)	-	-	7	8
Median Time to Transfer (minutes)	-	-	65	61
Fibrinolytic Medication Timing	-	-	62%	54%
Heart Failure Care				
ACE Inhibitor or ARB for LVSD[1]	6	67%	91%	94%
Discharge Instructions	15	73%	82%	88%
Evaluation of LVS Function[1]	19	68%	96%	98%
Smoking Cessation Advice[1]	2	100%	98%	98%
Pneumonia Care				
Appropriate Initial Antibiotic	37	86%	90%	92%
Blood Culture Timing	36	94%	95%	96%
Influenza Vaccine	33	76%	92%	91%
Initial Antibiotic Timing	48	100%	95%	95%
Pneumococcal Vaccine	55	91%	94%	93%
Smoking Cessation Advice[1]	16	81%	98%	97%
Surgical Care Improvement Project				
Appropriate VTP Within 24 Hours[5]	0	-	91%	92%
Appropriate Hair Removal[5]	0	-	99%	99%
Appropriate Beta Blocker Usage[5]	0	-	93%	93%
Controlled Postoperative Blood Glucose[5]	0	-	94%	93%
Prophylactic Antibiotic Timing[5]	0	-	97%	97%
Prophylactic Antibiotic Timing (Outpatient)	-	-	92%	92%
Prophylactic Antibiotic Selection[5]	0	-	98%	97%
Prophylactic Antibiotic Select. (Outpatient)	-	-	93%	94%
Prophylactic Antibiotic Stopped[5]	0	-	94%	94%
Recommended VTP Ordered[5]	0	-	94%	94%
Urinary Catheter Removal[5]	0	-	89%	90
Children's Asthma Care				
Received Systemic Corticosteroids	-	-	-	100%
Received Home Management Plan	-	-	-	71%
Received Reliever Medication	-	-	-	100%
Use of Medical Imaging				
Combination Abdominal CT Scan	-	-	0.160	0.191
Combination Chest CT Scan	-	-	0.054	0.054
Follow-up Mammogram/Ultrasound	-	-	7.9%	8.4%
MRI for Low Back Pain	-	-	35.6%	32.7%
Survey of Patients' Hospital Experiences				
Area Around Room 'Always' Quiet at Night[8]	-	-	-	58%
Doctors 'Always' Communicated Well[8]	-	-	-	80%
Home Recovery Information Given[8]	-	-	-	82%
Hospital Given 9 or 10 on 10 Point Scale[8]	-	-	-	67%
Meds 'Always' Explained Before Given[8]	-	-	-	60%
Nurses 'Always' Communicated Well[8]	-	-	-	76%
Pain 'Always' Well Controlled[8]	-	-	-	69%
Room and Bathroom 'Always' Clean[8]	-	-	-	71%
Timely Help 'Always' Received[8]	-	-	-	64%
Would Definitely Recommend Hospital[8]	-	-	-	69%

NOTE: Hospital profiles are in alphabetical order by state, then city, then hospital within the city; Rankings exclude hospitals with less than 25 cases except for patient surveys which excludes hospitals with less than 100 cases; (a) 100–299 cases; (1) The number of cases is too small to be sure how well a hospital is performing; (2) The hospital indicated that the data submitted for this measure were based on a sample of cases; (3) Data was collected during a shorter time period (fewer quarters) than the maximum possible time for this measure; (4) Suppressed for one or more quarters by CMS; (5) No data is available from the hospital for this measure; (6) Fewer than 100 patients completed the HCAHPS survey. Use these rates with caution, as the number of surveys may be too low to reliably assess hospital performance; (7) Survey results are based on less than 12 months of data; (8) Survey results are not available for this reporting period; (9) No or very few patients were eligible for the HCAHPS survey. The scores shown, if any, reflect a very small number of surveys; (10) A state average was not calculated because too few hospitals in the state submitted data; (11) There were discrepancies in the data collection process; Please refer to the User's Guide for a full explanation of data.

Saint Claire Regional Medical Center

222 Medical Circle — Phone: 606-783-6500
Morehead, KY 40351 — Fax: 606-783-6503
E-mail: mjneff@st-claire.org
URL: www.st-claire.org
Type: Acute Care Hospitals — Emergency Services: Yes
Ownership: Voluntary Non-Profit - Church — Beds: 159

Key Personnel:
CEO/President.............. Mark J Neff
Cardiac Laboratory........... Charlotte Lewis
Chief of Medical Staff.......... Will Mehlan, MD
Infection Control............. Charlette Kinney
Operating Room.............. Lisa Amburgery
Pediatric In-Patient Care .... Nancy Maggard
Quality Assurance .... Linda Fultz
Radiology.................. Charles Butler

Measure	Cases	This Hosp.	State Avg.	U.S. Avg.
Heart Attack Care				
ACE Inhibitor or ARB for LVSD[1]	14	79%	94%	96%
Aspirin at Arrival	84	100%	98%	99%
Aspirin at Discharge	72	96%	99%	98%
Beta Blocker at Discharge	73	99%	98%	98%
Fibrinolytic Medication Timing	0	-	60%	55%
PCI Within 90 Minutes of Arrival[1]	10	100%	88%	90%
Smoking Cessation Advice	36	97%	100%	99%
Chest Pain/Possible Heart Attack Care				
Aspirin at Arrival	85	99%	95%	95%
Median Time to ECG (minutes)	95	1	7	8
Median Time to Transfer (minutes)[1]	4	54	65	61
Fibrinolytic Medication Timing[1]	3	33%	62%	54%
Heart Failure Care				
ACE Inhibitor or ARB for LVSD	49	96%	91%	94%
Discharge Instructions	104	88%	82%	88%
Evaluation of LVS Function	129	97%	96%	98%
Smoking Cessation Advice	30	97%	98%	98%
Pneumonia Care				
Appropriate Initial Antibiotic	106	92%	90%	92%
Blood Culture Timing	216	92%	95%	96%
Influenza Vaccine	113	96%	92%	91%
Initial Antibiotic Timing	196	97%	95%	95%
Pneumococcal Vaccine	183	91%	94%	93%
Smoking Cessation Advice	108	97%	98%	97%
Surgical Care Improvement Project				
Appropriate VTP Within 24 Hours[2]	92	96%	91%	92%
Appropriate Hair Removal[2]	196	99%	99%	99%
Appropriate Beta Blocker Usage[2]	78	92%	93%	93%
Controlled Postoperative Blood Glucose[2]	0	-	94%	93%
Prophylactic Antibiotic Timing[2]	118	88%	97%	97%
Prophylactic Antibiotic Timing (Outpatient)	80	91%	92%	92%
Prophylactic Antibiotic Selection[2]	119	97%	98%	97%
Prophylactic Antibiotic Select. (Outpatient)	117	91%	93%	94%
Prophylactic Antibiotic Stopped[2]	116	90%	94%	94%
Recommended VTP Ordered[2]	92	98%	94%	94%
Urinary Catheter Removal[2]	42	71%	89%	90%
Children's Asthma Care				
Received Systemic Corticosteroids[1]	4	100%	-	100%
Received Home Management Plan[1]	5	80%	-	71%
Received Reliever Medication[1]	5	100%	-	100%
Use of Medical Imaging				
Combination Abdominal CT Scan	700	0.616	0.160	0.191
Combination Chest CT Scan	463	0.039	0.054	0.054
Follow-up Mammogram/Ultrasound	756	7.9%	7.9%	8.4%
MRI for Low Back Pain	143	43.4%	35.6%	32.7%
Survey of Patients' Hospital Experiences				
Area Around Room 'Always' Quiet at Night	300+	49%	-	58%
Doctors 'Always' Communicated Well	300+	85%	-	80%
Home Recovery Information Given	300+	83%	-	82%
Hospital Given 9 or 10 on 10 Point Scale	300+	62%	-	67%
Meds 'Always' Explained Before Given	300+	64%	-	60%
Nurses 'Always' Communicated Well	300+	80%	-	76%
Pain 'Always' Well Controlled	300+	71%	-	69%
Room and Bathroom 'Always' Clean	300+	71%	-	71%
Timely Help 'Always' Received	300+	64%	-	64%
Would Definitely Recommend Hospital	300+	66%	-	69%

Methodist Hospital Union County

4604 Us Highway 60 West — Phone: 270-389-3030
Morganfield, KY 42437 — Fax: 270-389-5059
E-mail: pdonahue@methodisthospital.net
URL: www.methodisthospitaluc.net
Type: Critical Access Hospitals — Emergency Services: Yes
Ownership: Voluntary Non-Profit - Church — Beds: 25

Key Personnel:
Chief of Medical Staff.......... William Guyette, MD
Coronary Care............... Peggy Creighton, RN
Infection Control............. Marie White, RN
Operating Room.............. Vinod Joni, MD
Pediatric In-Patient Care .... Peggy Creighton, RN
Quality Assurance .... Marie Whits, RN
Radiology.................. William Guyette, MD
Emergency Room .... William Clapp, MD

Measure	Cases	This Hosp.	State Avg.	U.S. Avg.
Heart Attack Care				
ACE Inhibitor or ARB for LVSD[1,3]	1	100%	94%	96%
Aspirin at Arrival[1,3]	1	100%	98%	99%
Aspirin at Discharge[1,3]	1	100%	99%	98%
Beta Blocker at Discharge[1,3]	1	100%	98%	98%
Fibrinolytic Medication Timing[3]	0	-	60%	55%
PCI Within 90 Minutes of Arrival[3]	0	-	88%	90%
Smoking Cessation Advice[3]	0	-	100%	99%
Chest Pain/Possible Heart Attack Care				
Aspirin at Arrival	73	88%	95%	95%
Median Time to ECG (minutes)	80	8	7	8
Median Time to Transfer (minutes)[5]	0	-	65	61
Fibrinolytic Medication Timing[3]	0	-	62%	54%
Heart Failure Care				
ACE Inhibitor or ARB for LVSD[1]	10	80%	91%	94%
Discharge Instructions[1]	24	100%	82%	88%
Evaluation of LVS Function	27	78%	96%	98%
Smoking Cessation Advice[1]	4	100%	98%	98%
Pneumonia Care				
Appropriate Initial Antibiotic	32	88%	90%	92%
Blood Culture Timing[1]	23	78%	95%	96%
Influenza Vaccine	29	90%	92%	91%
Initial Antibiotic Timing	37	89%	95%	95%
Pneumococcal Vaccine	37	89%	94%	93%
Smoking Cessation Advice[1]	14	100%	98%	97%
Surgical Care Improvement Project				
Appropriate VTP Within 24 Hours[5]	0	-	91%	92%
Appropriate Hair Removal[5]	0	-	99%	99%
Appropriate Beta Blocker Usage[5]	0	-	93%	93%
Controlled Postoperative Blood Glucose[5]	0	-	94%	93%
Prophylactic Antibiotic Timing[5]	0	-	97%	97%
Prophylactic Antibiotic Timing (Outpatient)[5]	0	-	92%	92%
Prophylactic Antibiotic Selection[5]	0	-	98%	97%
Prophylactic Antibiotic Select. (Outpatient)[5]	0	-	93%	94%
Prophylactic Antibiotic Stopped[5]	0	-	94%	94%
Recommended VTP Ordered[5]	0	-	94%	94%
Urinary Catheter Removal[5]	0	-	89%	90%
Children's Asthma Care				
Received Systemic Corticosteroids	-	-	-	100%
Received Home Management Plan	-	-	-	71%
Received Reliever Medication	-	-	-	100%
Use of Medical Imaging				
Combination Abdominal CT Scan	142	0.134	0.160	0.191
Combination Chest CT Scan	81	0.185	0.054	0.054
Follow-up Mammogram/Ultrasound	279	5.4%	7.9%	8.4%
MRI for Low Back Pain[5]	0	-	35.6%	32.7%
Survey of Patients' Hospital Experiences				
Area Around Room 'Always' Quiet at Night	(a)	69%	-	58%
Doctors 'Always' Communicated Well	(a)	92%	-	80%
Home Recovery Information Given	(a)	78%	-	82%
Hospital Given 9 or 10 on 10 Point Scale	(a)	76%	-	67%
Meds 'Always' Explained Before Given	(a)	62%	-	60%
Nurses 'Always' Communicated Well	(a)	87%	-	76%
Pain 'Always' Well Controlled	(a)	75%	-	69%
Room and Bathroom 'Always' Clean	(a)	84%	-	71%
Timely Help 'Always' Received	(a)	77%	-	64%
Would Definitely Recommend Hospital	(a)	78%	-	69%

Saint Joseph Mount Sterling

50 Sterling Avenue — Phone: 859-498-1220
Mount Sterling, KY 40353 — Fax: 859-498-5155
URL: www.marychiles.org
Type: Acute Care Hospitals — Emergency Services: Yes
Ownership: Voluntary Non-Profit - Church — Beds: 63

Key Personnel:
CEO/President.............. Patrick A Romano, JR
Chief of Medical Staff.......... John Merryman, MD
Infection Control............. Lisa Ray, RN
Operating Room.............. Sheila Barnes, RN
Pediatric In-Patient Care .... Rick Hall, MD
Radiology.................. Tim Damron
Patient Relations .... Tammye Hood, RN

Measure	Cases	This Hosp.	State Avg.	U.S. Avg.
Heart Attack Care				
ACE Inhibitor or ARB for LVSD[1]	1	0%	94%	96%
Aspirin at Arrival[1]	5	100%	98%	99%
Aspirin at Discharge[1]	3	100%	99%	98%
Beta Blocker at Discharge[1]	3	100%	98%	98%
Fibrinolytic Medication Timing	0	-	60%	55%
PCI Within 90 Minutes of Arrival	0	-	88%	90%
Smoking Cessation Advice	0	-	100%	99%
Chest Pain/Possible Heart Attack Care				
Aspirin at Arrival	218	97%	95%	95%
Median Time to ECG (minutes)	221	6	7	8
Median Time to Transfer (minutes)[1,3]	1	52	65	61
Fibrinolytic Medication Timing[1]	15	53%	62%	54%
Heart Failure Care				
ACE Inhibitor or ARB for LVSD[1]	7	100%	91%	94%
Discharge Instructions	30	90%	82%	88%
Evaluation of LVS Function	38	92%	96%	98%
Smoking Cessation Advice[1]	12	100%	98%	98%
Pneumonia Care				
Appropriate Initial Antibiotic	83	94%	90%	92%
Blood Culture Timing	103	95%	95%	96%
Influenza Vaccine	54	91%	92%	91%
Initial Antibiotic Timing	89	99%	95%	95%
Pneumococcal Vaccine	83	87%	94%	93%
Smoking Cessation Advice	46	96%	98%	97%
Surgical Care Improvement Project				
Appropriate VTP Within 24 Hours	51	100%	91%	92%
Appropriate Hair Removal	219	100%	99%	99%
Appropriate Beta Blocker Usage	80	96%	93%	93%
Controlled Postoperative Blood Glucose	0	-	94%	93%
Prophylactic Antibiotic Timing	185	98%	97%	97%
Prophylactic Antibiotic Timing (Outpatient)	35	91%	92%	92%
Prophylactic Antibiotic Selection	185	100%	98%	97%
Prophylactic Antibiotic Select. (Outpatient)	34	100%	93%	94%
Prophylactic Antibiotic Stopped	183	95%	94%	94%
Recommended VTP Ordered	51	100%	94%	94%
Urinary Catheter Removal	86	100%	89%	90%
Children's Asthma Care				
Received Systemic Corticosteroids	-	-	-	100%
Received Home Management Plan	-	-	-	71%
Received Reliever Medication	-	-	-	100%
Use of Medical Imaging				
Combination Abdominal CT Scan	477	0.057	0.160	0.191
Combination Chest CT Scan	330	0.009	0.054	0.054
Follow-up Mammogram/Ultrasound	304	11.5%	7.9%	8.4%
MRI for Low Back Pain[5]	0	-	35.6%	32.7%
Survey of Patients' Hospital Experiences				
Area Around Room 'Always' Quiet at Night	(a)	61%	-	58%
Doctors 'Always' Communicated Well	(a)	82%	-	80%
Home Recovery Information Given	(a)	84%	-	82%
Hospital Given 9 or 10 on 10 Point Scale	(a)	66%	-	67%
Meds 'Always' Explained Before Given	(a)	66%	-	60%
Nurses 'Always' Communicated Well	(a)	78%	-	76%
Pain 'Always' Well Controlled	(a)	72%	-	69%
Room and Bathroom 'Always' Clean	(a)	73%	-	71%
Timely Help 'Always' Received	(a)	66%	-	64%
Would Definitely Recommend Hospital	(a)	66%	-	69%

NOTE: Hospital profiles are in alphabetical order by state, then city, then hospital within the city; Rankings exclude hospitals with less than 25 cases except for patient surveys which excludes hospitals with less than 100 cases; (a) 100–299 cases; (1) The number of cases is too small to be sure how well a hospital is performing; (2) The hospital indicated that the data submitted for this measure were based on a sample of cases; (3) Data was collected during a shorter time period (fewer quarters) than the maximum possible time for this measure; (4) Suppressed for one or more quarters by CMS; (5) No data is available from the hospital for this measure; (6) Fewer than 100 patients completed the HCAHPS survey. Use these rates with caution, as the number of surveys may be too low to reliably assess hospital performance; (7) Survey results are based on less than 12 months of data; (8) Survey results are not available for this reporting period; (9) No or very few patients were eligible for the HCAHPS survey. The scores shown, if any, reflect a very small number of surveys; (10) A state average was not calculated because too few hospitals in the state submitted data; (11) There were discrepancies in the data collection process; Please refer to the User's Guide for a full explanation of data.

Rockcastle Regional Hospital & Respiratory Care Center

145 Newcomb Avenue
Mount Vernon, KY 40456
Phone: 606-256-2195
Fax: 606-256-3232
URL: www.rockcastlehospital.com
Type: Acute Care Hospitals
Emergency Services: No
Ownership: Voluntary Non-Profit - Private
Beds: 86

Key Personnel:

CEO/President. . . . . Stephen A Estes
Chief of Medical Staff . . . . Jon Arvin
Infection Control. . . . . Traci Bullens
Operating Room. . . . . Christian Knecht
Quality Assurance . . . . Stephen Estes
Radiology. . . . . Eduard Gomez
Anesthesiology. . . . . Tiffany Patrick
Emergency Room . . . . William P McElwain, MD

Measure	Cases	This Hosp.	State Avg.	U.S. Avg.
Heart Attack Care				
ACE Inhibitor or ARB for LVSD[1]	1	100%	94%	96%
Aspirin at Arrival[1]	4	100%	98%	99%
Aspirin at Discharge[1]	3	100%	99%	98%
Beta Blocker at Discharge[1]	3	100%	98%	98%
Fibrinolytic Medication Timing	0	-	60%	55%
PCI Within 90 Minutes of Arrival	0	-	88%	90%
Smoking Cessation Advice	0	-	100%	99%
Chest Pain/Possible Heart Attack Care				
Aspirin at Arrival	85	94%	95%	95%
Median Time to ECG (minutes)	87	12	7	8
Median Time to Transfer (minutes)[1]	10	72	65	61
Fibrinolytic Medication Timing[1]	1	0%	62%	54%
Heart Failure Care				
ACE Inhibitor or ARB for LVSD[1]	12	92%	91%	94%
Discharge Instructions	32	88%	82%	88%
Evaluation of LVS Function	41	100%	96%	98%
Smoking Cessation Advice[1]	6	100%	98%	98%
Pneumonia Care				
Appropriate Initial Antibiotic[2]	35	89%	90%	92%
Blood Culture Timing[2]	35	100%	95%	96%
Influenza Vaccine	42	95%	92%	91%
Initial Antibiotic Timing[2]	64	97%	95%	95%
Pneumococcal Vaccine[2]	66	100%	94%	93%
Smoking Cessation Advice[2]	34	100%	98%	97%
Surgical Care Improvement Project				
Appropriate VTP Within 24 Hours[1,3]	1	100%	91%	92%
Appropriate Hair Removal[1,3]	1	100%	99%	99%
Appropriate Beta Blocker Usage[3]	0	-	93%	93%
Controlled Postoperative Blood Glucose[3]	0	-	94%	93%
Prophylactic Antibiotic Timing[1,3]	1	0%	97%	97%
Prophylactic Antibiotic Timing (Outpatient)[1,3]	2	50%	92%	92%
Prophylactic Antibiotic Selection[1,3]	1	100%	98%	97%
Prophylactic Antibiotic Select. (Outpatient)[1,3]	1	100%	93%	94%
Prophylactic Antibiotic Stopped[1,3]	1	100%	94%	94%
Recommended VTP Ordered[1,3]	1	100%	94%	94%
Urinary Catheter Removal[1,3]	1	100%	89%	90%
Children's Asthma Care				
Received Systemic Corticosteroids	-	-	-	100%
Received Home Management Plan	-	-	-	71%
Received Reliever Medication	-	-	-	100%
Use of Medical Imaging				
Combination Abdominal CT Scan	254	0.000	0.160	0.191
Combination Chest CT Scan	173	0.127	0.054	0.054
Follow-up Mammogram/Ultrasound	256	5.9%	7.9%	8.4%
MRI for Low Back Pain	93	30.1%	35.6%	32.7%
Survey of Patients' Hospital Experiences				
Area Around Room 'Always' Quiet at Night	(a)	59%	-	58%
Doctors 'Always' Communicated Well	(a)	89%	-	80%
Home Recovery Information Given	(a)	77%	-	82%
Hospital Given 9 or 10 on 10 Point Scale	(a)	75%	-	67%
Meds 'Always' Explained Before Given	(a)	63%	-	60%
Nurses 'Always' Communicated Well	(a)	82%	-	76%
Pain 'Always' Well Controlled	(a)	72%	-	69%
Room and Bathroom 'Always' Clean	(a)	81%	-	71%
Timely Help 'Always' Received	(a)	65%	-	64%
Would Definitely Recommend Hospital	(a)	73%	-	69%

Murray-Calloway County Hospital

803 Poplar Street
Murray, KY 42071
Phone: 270-762-1100
Fax: 270-767-3600
E-mail: info@murrayhospital.org
URL: www.murrayhospital.org
Type: Acute Care Hospitals
Emergency Services: No
Ownership: Voluntary Non-Profit - Other
Beds: 366

Key Personnel:

CEO/President. . . . . John O'Shaughnessy
Chief of Medical Staff . . . . Dr Richard Crouch, MD
Infection Control. . . . . Lisa Ray, RN
Operating Room. . . . . Mary Hension, RN
Radiology. . . . . Felipe Patino
Emergency Room . . . . Jerry Edwards, MD
Intensive Care Unit. . . . . Jeanne Mathis, RN
Patient Relations . . . . Allen Peters

Measure	Cases	This Hosp.	State Avg.	U.S. Avg.
Heart Attack Care				
ACE Inhibitor or ARB for LVSD[1]	3	67%	94%	96%
Aspirin at Arrival[1]	18	83%	98%	99%
Aspirin at Discharge[1]	11	100%	99%	98%
Beta Blocker at Discharge[1]	12	92%	98%	98%
Fibrinolytic Medication Timing	0	-	60%	55%
PCI Within 90 Minutes of Arrival	0	-	88%	90%
Smoking Cessation Advice[1]	2	50%	100%	99%
Chest Pain/Possible Heart Attack Care				
Aspirin at Arrival	125	98%	95%	95%
Median Time to ECG (minutes)	124	9	7	8
Median Time to Transfer (minutes)[1]	5	55	65	61
Fibrinolytic Medication Timing[1]	5	20%	62%	54%
Heart Failure Care				
ACE Inhibitor or ARB for LVSD[1]	21	67%	91%	94%
Discharge Instructions	101	65%	82%	88%
Evaluation of LVS Function	116	91%	96%	98%
Smoking Cessation Advice[1]	13	92%	98%	98%
Pneumonia Care				
Appropriate Initial Antibiotic	114	71%	90%	92%
Blood Culture Timing	105	96%	95%	96%
Influenza Vaccine	118	55%	92%	91%
Initial Antibiotic Timing	161	92%	95%	95%
Pneumococcal Vaccine	139	68%	94%	93%
Smoking Cessation Advice	67	94%	98%	97%
Surgical Care Improvement Project				
Appropriate VTP Within 24 Hours	109	81%	91%	92%
Appropriate Hair Removal	268	99%	99%	99%
Appropriate Beta Blocker Usage	69	93%	93%	93%
Controlled Postoperative Blood Glucose	0	-	94%	93%
Prophylactic Antibiotic Timing	167	93%	97%	97%
Prophylactic Antibiotic Timing (Outpatient)	187	82%	92%	92%
Prophylactic Antibiotic Selection	169	91%	98%	97%
Prophylactic Antibiotic Select. (Outpatient)	168	90%	93%	94%
Prophylactic Antibiotic Stopped	163	83%	94%	94%
Recommended VTP Ordered	109	82%	94%	94%
Urinary Catheter Removal	52	94%	89%	90%
Children's Asthma Care				
Received Systemic Corticosteroids	-	-	-	100%
Received Home Management Plan	-	-	-	71%
Received Reliever Medication	-	-	-	100%
Use of Medical Imaging				
Combination Abdominal CT Scan	533	0.182	0.160	0.191
Combination Chest CT Scan	274	0.011	0.054	0.054
Follow-up Mammogram/Ultrasound	1,007	4.6%	7.9%	8.4%
MRI for Low Back Pain	118	39.0%	35.6%	32.7%
Survey of Patients' Hospital Experiences				
Area Around Room 'Always' Quiet at Night	300+	55%	-	58%
Doctors 'Always' Communicated Well	300+	83%	-	80%
Home Recovery Information Given	300+	81%	-	82%
Hospital Given 9 or 10 on 10 Point Scale	300+	60%	-	67%
Meds 'Always' Explained Before Given	300+	56%	-	60%
Nurses 'Always' Communicated Well	300+	74%	-	76%
Pain 'Always' Well Controlled	300+	65%	-	69%
Room and Bathroom 'Always' Clean	300+	67%	-	71%
Timely Help 'Always' Received	300+	61%	-	64%
Would Definitely Recommend Hospital	300+	60%	-	69%

Owensboro Medical Health System

811 East Parrish Avenue
Owensboro, KY 42303
Phone: 502-688-2000
Fax: 270-685-7195
URL: www.omhs.org
Type: Acute Care Hospitals
Emergency Services: Yes
Ownership: Voluntary Non-Profit - Private
Beds: 447

Key Personnel:

CEO/President. . . . . Jeff Barber
Cardiac Laboratory. . . . . Liz Belt
Chief of Medical Staff . . . . Wathen Medley MD
Operating Room. . . . . Marti Gaw
Quality Assurance . . . . Pam Cox
Radiology. . . . . Donna Ross
Emergency Room . . . . Debbie Eoch
Intensive Care Unit. . . . . Lisa Burnett

Measure	Cases	This Hosp.	State Avg.	U.S. Avg.
Heart Attack Care				
ACE Inhibitor or ARB for LVSD	82	87%	94%	96%
Aspirin at Arrival	282	99%	98%	99%
Aspirin at Discharge	292	99%	99%	98%
Beta Blocker at Discharge	283	98%	98%	98%
Fibrinolytic Medication Timing	0	-	60%	55%
PCI Within 90 Minutes of Arrival	34	85%	88%	90%
Smoking Cessation Advice	137	100%	100%	99%
Chest Pain/Possible Heart Attack Care				
Aspirin at Arrival[1,3]	1	100%	95%	95%
Median Time to ECG (minutes)[1,3]	1	0	7	8
Median Time to Transfer (minutes)[5]	0	-	65	61
Fibrinolytic Medication Timing[5]	0	-	62%	54%
Heart Failure Care				
ACE Inhibitor or ARB for LVSD	219	88%	91%	94%
Discharge Instructions	462	91%	82%	88%
Evaluation of LVS Function	553	100%	96%	98%
Smoking Cessation Advice	92	100%	98%	98%
Pneumonia Care				
Appropriate Initial Antibiotic	128	91%	90%	92%
Blood Culture Timing	253	96%	95%	96%
Influenza Vaccine	191	100%	92%	91%
Initial Antibiotic Timing	364	93%	95%	95%
Pneumococcal Vaccine	312	97%	94%	93%
Smoking Cessation Advice	180	99%	98%	97%
Surgical Care Improvement Project				
Appropriate VTP Within 24 Hours[2]	266	92%	91%	92%
Appropriate Hair Removal[2]	1,045	99%	99%	99%
Appropriate Beta Blocker Usage[2]	394	99%	93%	93%
Controlled Postoperative Blood Glucose[2]	219	96%	94%	93%
Prophylactic Antibiotic Timing[2]	791	98%	97%	97%
Prophylactic Antibiotic Timing (Outpatient)	890	92%	92%	92%
Prophylactic Antibiotic Selection[2]	799	99%	98%	97%
Prophylactic Antibiotic Select. (Outpatient)	901	86%	93%	94%
Prophylactic Antibiotic Stopped[2]	771	99%	94%	94%
Recommended VTP Ordered[2]	270	94%	94%	94%
Urinary Catheter Removal[2]	195	95%	89%	90%
Children's Asthma Care				
Received Systemic Corticosteroids	-	-	-	100%
Received Home Management Plan	-	-	-	71%
Received Reliever Medication	-	-	-	100%
Use of Medical Imaging				
Combination Abdominal CT Scan	1,695	0.433	0.160	0.191
Combination Chest CT Scan	1,282	0.020	0.054	0.054
Follow-up Mammogram/Ultrasound	2,576	5.9%	7.9%	8.4%
MRI for Low Back Pain	416	33.2%	35.6%	32.7%
Survey of Patients' Hospital Experiences				
Area Around Room 'Always' Quiet at Night	300+	56%	-	58%
Doctors 'Always' Communicated Well	300+	82%	-	80%
Home Recovery Information Given	300+	85%	-	82%
Hospital Given 9 or 10 on 10 Point Scale	300+	71%	-	67%
Meds 'Always' Explained Before Given	300+	56%	-	60%
Nurses 'Always' Communicated Well	300+	78%	-	76%
Pain 'Always' Well Controlled	300+	71%	-	69%
Room and Bathroom 'Always' Clean	300+	71%	-	71%
Timely Help 'Always' Received	300+	64%	-	64%
Would Definitely Recommend Hospital	300+	71%	-	69%

NOTE: Hospital profiles are in alphabetical order by state, then city, then hospital within the city; Rankings exclude hospitals with less than 25 cases except for patient surveys which excludes hospitals with less than 100 cases; (a) 100–299 cases; (1) The number of cases is too small to be sure how well a hospital is performing; (2) The hospital indicated that the data submitted for this measure were based on a sample of cases; (3) Data was collected during a shorter time period (fewer quarters) than the maximum possible time for this measure; (4) Suppressed for one or more quarters by CMS; (5) No data is available from the hospital for this measure; (6) Fewer than 100 patients completed the HCAHPS survey. Use these rates with caution, as the number of surveys may be too low to reliably assess hospital performance; (7) Survey results are based on less than 12 months of data; (8) Survey results are not available for this reporting period; (9) No or very few patients were eligible for the HCAHPS survey. The scores shown, if any, reflect a very small number of surveys; (10) A state average was not calculated because too few hospitals in the state submitted data; (11) There were discrepancies in the data collection process; Please refer to the User's Guide for a full explanation of data.

New Horizons Medical Center

330 Roland Avenue — Phone: 502-484-4656
Owenton, KY 40359
URL: www.newhorizonsmedicalcenter.org
Type: Critical Access Hospitals — Emergency Services: Yes
Ownership: Proprietary

Key Personnel:
CEO/President. . . . . Bernard T Poe

Measure	Cases	This Hosp.	State Avg.	U.S. Avg.
Heart Attack Care				
ACE Inhibitor or ARB for LVSD[5]	0	-	94%	96%
Aspirin at Arrival[5]	0	-	98%	99%
Aspirin at Discharge[5]	0	-	99%	98%
Beta Blocker at Discharge[5]	0	-	98%	98%
Fibrinolytic Medication Timing[5]	0	-	60%	55%
PCI Within 90 Minutes of Arrival[5]	0	-	88%	90%
Smoking Cessation Advice[5]	0	-	100%	99%
Chest Pain/Possible Heart Attack Care				
Aspirin at Arrival	-	-	95%	95%
Median Time to ECG (minutes)	-	-	7	8
Median Time to Transfer (minutes)	-	-	65	61
Fibrinolytic Medication Timing	-	-	62%	54%
Heart Failure Care				
ACE Inhibitor or ARB for LVSD[1]	6	100%	91%	94%
Discharge Instructions[1]	13	54%	82%	88%
Evaluation of LVS Function[1]	18	83%	96%	98%
Smoking Cessation Advice[1]	4	75%	98%	98%
Pneumonia Care				
Appropriate Initial Antibiotic[1]	15	87%	90%	92%
Blood Culture Timing[1]	14	93%	95%	96%
Influenza Vaccine[1]	15	80%	92%	91%
Initial Antibiotic Timing	28	96%	95%	95%
Pneumococcal Vaccine	26	62%	94%	93%
Smoking Cessation Advice[1]	7	71%	98%	97%
Surgical Care Improvement Project				
Appropriate VTP Within 24 Hours[5]	0	-	91%	92%
Appropriate Hair Removal[5]	0	-	99%	99%
Appropriate Beta Blocker Usage[5]	0	-	93%	93%
Controlled Postoperative Blood Glucose[5]	0	-	94%	93%
Prophylactic Antibiotic Timing[5]	0	-	97%	97%
Prophylactic Antibiotic Timing (Outpatient)	-	-	92%	92%
Prophylactic Antibiotic Selection[5]	0	-	98%	97%
Prophylactic Antibiotic Select. (Outpatient)	-	-	93%	94%
Prophylactic Antibiotic Stopped[5]	0	-	94%	94%
Recommended VTP Ordered[5]	0	-	94%	94%
Urinary Catheter Removal[5]	0	-	89%	90%
Children's Asthma Care				
Received Systemic Corticosteroids	-	-	-	100%
Received Home Management Plan	-	-	-	71%
Received Reliever Medication	-	-	-	100%
Use of Medical Imaging				
Combination Abdominal CT Scan	-	-	0.160	0.191
Combination Chest CT Scan	-	-	0.054	0.054
Follow-up Mammogram/Ultrasound	-	-	7.9%	8.4%
MRI for Low Back Pain	-	-	35.6%	32.7%
Survey of Patients' Hospital Experiences				
Area Around Room 'Always' Quiet at Night[8]	-	-	-	58%
Doctors 'Always' Communicated Well[8]	-	-	-	80%
Home Recovery Information Given[8]	-	-	-	82%
Hospital Given 9 or 10 on 10 Point Scale[8]	-	-	-	67%
Meds 'Always' Explained Before Given[8]	-	-	-	60%
Nurses 'Always' Communicated Well[8]	-	-	-	76%
Pain 'Always' Well Controlled[8]	-	-	-	69%
Room and Bathroom 'Always' Clean[8]	-	-	-	71%
Timely Help 'Always' Received[8]	-	-	-	64%
Would Definitely Recommend Hospital[8]	-	-	-	69%

Lourdes Hospital

1530 Lone Oak Road — Phone: 270-444-2444
Paducah, KY 42001 — Fax: 270-444-2980
URL: www.ehealthconnection.com
Type: Acute Care Hospitals — Emergency Services: Yes
Ownership: Voluntary Non-Profit - Church — Beds: 389

Key Personnel:
CEO/President. . . . . Steven Grinnell
Chief of Medical Staff . . . . Daniel Howard
Operating Room. . . . . Jason David Banister
Quality Assurance . . . . Jan Kincer
Radiology. . . . . William E Adams, MD
Anesthesiology. . . . . Blane Graw, MD
Emergency Room . . . . Philip E Anderson

Measure	Cases	This Hosp.	State Avg.	U.S. Avg.
Heart Attack Care				
ACE Inhibitor or ARB for LVSD	52	98%	94%	96%
Aspirin at Arrival	129	100%	98%	99%
Aspirin at Discharge	178	100%	99%	98%
Beta Blocker at Discharge	173	99%	98%	98%
Fibrinolytic Medication Timing	0	-	60%	55%
PCI Within 90 Minutes of Arrival[1]	20	90%	88%	90%
Smoking Cessation Advice	84	100%	100%	99%
Chest Pain/Possible Heart Attack Care				
Aspirin at Arrival[1,3]	2	100%	95%	95%
Median Time to ECG (minutes)[1,3]	2	13	7	8
Median Time to Transfer (minutes)[5]	0	-	65	61
Fibrinolytic Medication Timing[5]	0	-	62%	54%
Heart Failure Care				
ACE Inhibitor or ARB for LVSD	132	92%	91%	94%
Discharge Instructions	209	88%	82%	88%
Evaluation of LVS Function	272	100%	96%	98%
Smoking Cessation Advice	45	100%	98%	98%
Pneumonia Care				
Appropriate Initial Antibiotic	148	97%	90%	92%
Blood Culture Timing	183	97%	95%	96%
Influenza Vaccine	169	100%	92%	91%
Initial Antibiotic Timing	205	96%	95%	95%
Pneumococcal Vaccine	194	100%	94%	93%
Smoking Cessation Advice	94	100%	98%	97%
Surgical Care Improvement Project				
Appropriate VTP Within 24 Hours[2]	401	93%	91%	92%
Appropriate Hair Removal[2]	955	100%	99%	99%
Appropriate Beta Blocker Usage[2]	347	95%	93%	93%
Controlled Postoperative Blood Glucose[2]	164	95%	94%	93%
Prophylactic Antibiotic Timing[2]	761	98%	97%	97%
Prophylactic Antibiotic Timing (Outpatient)	276	95%	92%	92%
Prophylactic Antibiotic Selection[2]	773	99%	98%	97%
Prophylactic Antibiotic Select. (Outpatient)	272	93%	93%	94%
Prophylactic Antibiotic Stopped[2]	710	93%	94%	94%
Recommended VTP Ordered[2]	404	98%	94%	94%
Urinary Catheter Removal[2]	173	90%	89%	90%
Children's Asthma Care				
Received Systemic Corticosteroids	-	-	-	100%
Received Home Management Plan	-	-	-	71%
Received Reliever Medication	-	-	-	100%
Use of Medical Imaging				
Combination Abdominal CT Scan	650	0.312	0.160	0.191
Combination Chest CT Scan	496	0.036	0.054	0.054
Follow-up Mammogram/Ultrasound	353	9.6%	7.9%	8.4%
MRI for Low Back Pain	154	36.4%	35.6%	32.7%
Survey of Patients' Hospital Experiences				
Area Around Room 'Always' Quiet at Night	300+	54%	-	58%
Doctors 'Always' Communicated Well	300+	81%	-	80%
Home Recovery Information Given	300+	79%	-	82%
Hospital Given 9 or 10 on 10 Point Scale	300+	66%	-	67%
Meds 'Always' Explained Before Given	300+	54%	-	60%
Nurses 'Always' Communicated Well	300+	74%	-	76%
Pain 'Always' Well Controlled	300+	65%	-	69%
Room and Bathroom 'Always' Clean	300+	61%	-	71%
Timely Help 'Always' Received	300+	60%	-	64%
Would Definitely Recommend Hospital	300+	70%	-	69%

Western Baptist Hospital

2501 Kentucky Avenue — Phone: 270-575-2300
Paducah, KY 42003 — Fax: 270-575-2217
URL: www.westernbaptist.com
Type: Acute Care Hospitals — Emergency Services: Yes
Ownership: Voluntary Non-Profit - Church — Beds: 349

Key Personnel:
CEO/President. . . . . Scott Ware
Chief of Medical Staff . . . . Eric Shields, MD
Infection Control. . . . . Chris Nutty
Operating Room. . . . . Ted Henderson
Pediatric Ambulatory Care . . . . . . Glenda Channey, MD
Pediatric In-Patient Care . . . . Glenda Channey, MD
Quality Assurance . . . . Meri Curtis
Radiology. . . . . Bob Seely

Measure	Cases	This Hosp.	State Avg.	U.S. Avg.
Heart Attack Care				
ACE Inhibitor or ARB for LVSD	62	100%	94%	96%
Aspirin at Arrival	237	98%	98%	99%
Aspirin at Discharge	395	100%	99%	98%
Beta Blocker at Discharge	374	100%	98%	98%
Fibrinolytic Medication Timing	0	-	60%	55%
PCI Within 90 Minutes of Arrival	36	86%	88%	90%
Smoking Cessation Advice	170	100%	100%	99%
Chest Pain/Possible Heart Attack Care				
Aspirin at Arrival[1,3]	1	100%	95%	95%
Median Time to ECG (minutes)[1,3]	1	0	7	8
Median Time to Transfer (minutes)[5]	0	-	65	61
Fibrinolytic Medication Timing[5]	0	-	62%	54%
Heart Failure Care				
ACE Inhibitor or ARB for LVSD	171	100%	91%	94%
Discharge Instructions	390	95%	82%	88%
Evaluation of LVS Function	462	100%	96%	98%
Smoking Cessation Advice	112	100%	98%	98%
Pneumonia Care				
Appropriate Initial Antibiotic	206	94%	90%	92%
Blood Culture Timing	250	99%	95%	96%
Influenza Vaccine	241	97%	92%	91%
Initial Antibiotic Timing	270	99%	95%	95%
Pneumococcal Vaccine	267	99%	94%	93%
Smoking Cessation Advice	162	100%	98%	97%
Surgical Care Improvement Project				
Appropriate VTP Within 24 Hours	473	92%	91%	92%
Appropriate Hair Removal	1,128	100%	99%	99%
Appropriate Beta Blocker Usage	372	84%	93%	93%
Controlled Postoperative Blood Glucose	244	90%	94%	93%
Prophylactic Antibiotic Timing	713	95%	97%	97%
Prophylactic Antibiotic Timing (Outpatient)	628	94%	92%	92%
Prophylactic Antibiotic Selection	724	98%	98%	97%
Prophylactic Antibiotic Select. (Outpatient)	619	89%	93%	94%
Prophylactic Antibiotic Stopped	665	89%	94%	94%
Recommended VTP Ordered	484	95%	94%	94%
Urinary Catheter Removal	279	83%	89%	90%
Children's Asthma Care				
Received Systemic Corticosteroids	-	-	-	100%
Received Home Management Plan	-	-	-	71%
Received Reliever Medication	-	-	-	100%
Use of Medical Imaging				
Combination Abdominal CT Scan	1,835	0.113	0.160	0.191
Combination Chest CT Scan	1,178	0.058	0.054	0.054
Follow-up Mammogram/Ultrasound	982	11.6%	7.9%	8.4%
MRI for Low Back Pain	275	33.8%	35.6%	32.7%
Survey of Patients' Hospital Experiences				
Area Around Room 'Always' Quiet at Night	300+	65%	-	58%
Doctors 'Always' Communicated Well	300+	79%	-	80%
Home Recovery Information Given	300+	86%	-	82%
Hospital Given 9 or 10 on 10 Point Scale	300+	72%	-	67%
Meds 'Always' Explained Before Given	300+	59%	-	60%
Nurses 'Always' Communicated Well	300+	79%	-	76%
Pain 'Always' Well Controlled	300+	68%	-	69%
Room and Bathroom 'Always' Clean	300+	73%	-	71%
Timely Help 'Always' Received	300+	62%	-	64%
Would Definitely Recommend Hospital	300+	79%	-	69%

NOTE: Hospital profiles are in alphabetical order by state, then city, then hospital within the city; Rankings exclude hospitals with less than 25 cases except for patient surveys which excludes hospitals with less than 100 cases; (a) 100–299 cases; (1) The number of cases is too small to be sure how well a hospital is performing; (2) The hospital indicated that the data submitted for this measure were based on a sample of cases; (3) Data was collected during a shorter time period (fewer quarters) than the maximum possible time for this measure; (4) Suppressed for one or more quarters by CMS; (5) No data is available from the hospital for this measure; (6) Fewer than 100 patients completed the HCAHPS survey. Use these rates with caution, as the number of surveys may be too low to reliably assess hospital performance; (7) Survey results are based on less than 12 months of data; (8) Survey results are not available for this reporting period; (9) No or very few patients were eligible for the HCAHPS survey. The scores shown, if any, reflect a very small number of surveys; (10) A state average was not calculated because too few hospitals in the state submitted data; (11) There were discrepancies in the data collection process; Please refer to the User's Guide for a full explanation of data.

Paul B Hall Regional Medical Center

625 James S Trimble Blvd
Paintsville, KY 41240
URL: www.pbhrmc.com
Type: Acute Care Hospitals
Ownership: Proprietary

Phone: 606-789-3511
Fax: 606-789-6486
Emergency Services: Yes
Beds: 72

Key Personnel:
CEO/President.............. Deborah L Trimble
Operating Room.............. JoAnn Allen
Radiology.............. Jon E Anderson
Emergency Room .... Willard C Arnold
Intensive Care Unit.............. Patricia Foley

Measure	Cases	This Hosp.	State Avg.	U.S. Avg.
Heart Attack Care				
ACE Inhibitor or ARB for LVSD[1]	1	100%	94%	96%
Aspirin at Arrival[1]	5	100%	98%	99%
Aspirin at Discharge[1]	3	100%	99%	98%
Beta Blocker at Discharge[1]	3	100%	98%	98%
Fibrinolytic Medication Timing	0	-	60%	55%
PCI Within 90 Minutes of Arrival	0	-	88%	90%
Smoking Cessation Advice[1]	1	100%	100%	99%
Chest Pain/Possible Heart Attack Care				
Aspirin at Arrival	125	98%	95%	95%
Median Time to ECG (minutes)	133	2	7	8
Median Time to Transfer (minutes)[1,3]	1	165	65	61
Fibrinolytic Medication Timing[1]	5	80%	62%	54%
Heart Failure Care				
ACE Inhibitor or ARB for LVSD	25	96%	91%	94%
Discharge Instructions	80	90%	82%	88%
Evaluation of LVS Function	105	99%	96%	98%
Smoking Cessation Advice	25	100%	98%	98%
Pneumonia Care				
Appropriate Initial Antibiotic	122	98%	90%	92%
Blood Culture Timing	195	99%	95%	96%
Influenza Vaccine	128	98%	92%	91%
Initial Antibiotic Timing	212	99%	95%	95%
Pneumococcal Vaccine	174	99%	94%	93%
Smoking Cessation Advice	143	100%	98%	97%
Surgical Care Improvement Project				
Appropriate VTP Within 24 Hours	27	100%	91%	92%
Appropriate Hair Removal	33	100%	99%	99%
Appropriate Beta Blocker Usage[1]	6	100%	93%	93%
Controlled Postoperative Blood Glucose	0	-	94%	93%
Prophylactic Antibiotic Timing[1]	11	100%	97%	97%
Prophylactic Antibiotic Timing (Outpatient)[1,3]	2	50%	92%	92%
Prophylactic Antibiotic Selection[1]	11	100%	98%	97%
Prophylactic Antibiotic Select. (Outpatient)[1,3]	1	100%	93%	94%
Prophylactic Antibiotic Stopped[1]	3	67%	94%	94%
Recommended VTP Ordered	27	100%	94%	94%
Urinary Catheter Removal	0	-	89%	90%
Children's Asthma Care				
Received Systemic Corticosteroids	85	99%	-	100%
Received Home Management Plan	86	99%	-	71%
Received Reliever Medication	88	100%	-	100%
Use of Medical Imaging				
Combination Abdominal CT Scan	328	0.216	0.160	0.191
Combination Chest CT Scan	218	0.248	0.054	0.054
Follow-up Mammogram/Ultrasound	127	18.1%	7.9%	8.4%
MRI for Low Back Pain	57	35.1%	35.6%	32.7%
Survey of Patients' Hospital Experiences				
Area Around Room 'Always' Quiet at Night	300+	60%	-	58%
Doctors 'Always' Communicated Well	300+	79%	-	80%
Home Recovery Information Given	300+	78%	-	82%
Hospital Given 9 or 10 on 10 Point Scale	300+	58%	-	67%
Meds 'Always' Explained Before Given	300+	57%	-	60%
Nurses 'Always' Communicated Well	300+	71%	-	76%
Pain 'Always' Well Controlled	300+	62%	-	69%
Room and Bathroom 'Always' Clean	300+	68%	-	71%
Timely Help 'Always' Received	300+	57%	-	64%
Would Definitely Recommend Hospital	300+	58%	-	69%

Bourbon Community Hospital

9 Linville Drive
Paris, KY 40361
URL: www.bourbonhospital.com
Type: Acute Care Hospitals
Ownership: Proprietary

Phone: 859-987-3600
Fax: 859-987-1003
Emergency Services: No
Beds: 58

Key Personnel:
CEO/President.............. Kerry Wehmeyer
Chief of Medical Staff.............. Charles Allran
Infection Control.............. Marsha Haney, RN
Operating Room.............. C Schulstad, RN
Quality Assurance .... Jennie Rockidge, RN
Radiology.............. Jerry Anderson
Emergency Room .... Robert Biddle, MD
Intensive Care Unit.............. Donna Davis, RN

Measure	Cases	This Hosp.	State Avg.	U.S. Avg.
Heart Attack Care				
ACE Inhibitor or ARB for LVSD[3]	0	-	94%	96%
Aspirin at Arrival[1,3]	4	75%	98%	99%
Aspirin at Discharge[1,3]	2	100%	99%	98%
Beta Blocker at Discharge[1,3]	1	100%	98%	98%
Fibrinolytic Medication Timing[3]	0	-	60%	55%
PCI Within 90 Minutes of Arrival[3]	0	-	88%	90%
Smoking Cessation Advice[3]	0	-	100%	99%
Chest Pain/Possible Heart Attack Care				
Aspirin at Arrival	84	98%	95%	95%
Median Time to ECG (minutes)	87	4	7	8
Median Time to Transfer (minutes)[1,3]	4	119	65	61
Fibrinolytic Medication Timing[1]	1	100%	62%	54%
Heart Failure Care				
ACE Inhibitor or ARB for LVSD[1]	7	71%	91%	94%
Discharge Instructions	34	94%	82%	88%
Evaluation of LVS Function	46	98%	96%	98%
Smoking Cessation Advice[1]	14	100%	98%	98%
Pneumonia Care				
Appropriate Initial Antibiotic	33	88%	90%	92%
Blood Culture Timing	53	91%	95%	96%
Influenza Vaccine	38	87%	92%	91%
Initial Antibiotic Timing	51	100%	95%	95%
Pneumococcal Vaccine	46	89%	94%	93%
Smoking Cessation Advice[1]	18	100%	98%	97%
Surgical Care Improvement Project				
Appropriate VTP Within 24 Hours[1]	9	78%	91%	92%
Appropriate Hair Removal[1]	13	100%	99%	99%
Appropriate Beta Blocker Usage[1]	5	80%	93%	93%
Controlled Postoperative Blood Glucose	0	-	94%	93%
Prophylactic Antibiotic Timing[1]	6	100%	97%	97%
Prophylactic Antibiotic Timing (Outpatient)[1,3]	5	80%	92%	92%
Prophylactic Antibiotic Selection[1]	6	83%	98%	97%
Prophylactic Antibiotic Select. (Outpatient)[1,3]	4	100%	93%	94%
Prophylactic Antibiotic Stopped[1]	6	100%	94%	94%
Recommended VTP Ordered[1]	9	89%	94%	94%
Urinary Catheter Removal	0	-	89%	90%
Children's Asthma Care				
Received Systemic Corticosteroids	-	-	-	100%
Received Home Management Plan	-	-	-	71%
Received Reliever Medication	-	-	-	100%
Use of Medical Imaging				
Combination Abdominal CT Scan	264	0.110	0.160	0.191
Combination Chest CT Scan	121	0.008	0.054	0.054
Follow-up Mammogram/Ultrasound	371	8.1%	7.9%	8.4%
MRI for Low Back Pain	40	40.0%	35.6%	32.7%
Survey of Patients' Hospital Experiences				
Area Around Room 'Always' Quiet at Night	(a)	67%	-	58%
Doctors 'Always' Communicated Well	(a)	85%	-	80%
Home Recovery Information Given	(a)	87%	-	82%
Hospital Given 9 or 10 on 10 Point Scale	(a)	71%	-	67%
Meds 'Always' Explained Before Given	(a)	62%	-	60%
Nurses 'Always' Communicated Well	(a)	81%	-	76%
Pain 'Always' Well Controlled	(a)	76%	-	69%
Room and Bathroom 'Always' Clean	(a)	72%	-	71%
Timely Help 'Always' Received	(a)	71%	-	64%
Would Definitely Recommend Hospital	(a)	74%	-	69%

Pikeville Medical Center

911 Bypass Road
Pikeville, KY 41501
URL: www.pikevillehospital.org
Type: Acute Care Hospitals
Ownership: Voluntary Non-Profit - Private

Phone: 606-437-3500
Fax: 606-437-4996
Emergency Services: Yes
Beds: 221

Key Personnel:
CEO/President.............. Walter E May
Chief of Medical Staff.............. William M Johnson
Operating Room.............. Ernestine Mullins
Pediatric Ambulatory Care .... Willena Moore
Pediatric In-Patient Care .... Sheila Belcher
Quality Assurance .... Mary Combs
Radiology.............. Dennis H Halbert
Patient Relations .... Patty Thompson

Measure	Cases	This Hosp.	State Avg.	U.S. Avg.
Heart Attack Care				
ACE Inhibitor or ARB for LVSD	33	97%	94%	96%
Aspirin at Arrival	163	99%	98%	99%
Aspirin at Discharge	224	100%	99%	98%
Beta Blocker at Discharge	216	98%	98%	98%
Fibrinolytic Medication Timing	0	-	60%	55%
PCI Within 90 Minutes of Arrival	25	80%	88%	90%
Smoking Cessation Advice	115	100%	100%	99%
Chest Pain/Possible Heart Attack Care				
Aspirin at Arrival[5]	0	-	95%	95%
Median Time to ECG (minutes)[5]	0	-	7	8
Median Time to Transfer (minutes)[5]	0	-	65	61
Fibrinolytic Medication Timing[5]	0	-	62%	54%
Heart Failure Care				
ACE Inhibitor or ARB for LVSD	105	90%	91%	94%
Discharge Instructions	279	98%	82%	88%
Evaluation of LVS Function	308	99%	96%	98%
Smoking Cessation Advice	62	100%	98%	98%
Pneumonia Care				
Appropriate Initial Antibiotic	190	90%	90%	92%
Blood Culture Timing	252	95%	95%	96%
Influenza Vaccine	235	93%	92%	91%
Initial Antibiotic Timing	316	95%	95%	95%
Pneumococcal Vaccine	308	97%	94%	93%
Smoking Cessation Advice	195	100%	98%	97%
Surgical Care Improvement Project				
Appropriate VTP Within 24 Hours[2]	274	89%	91%	92%
Appropriate Hair Removal[2]	856	100%	99%	99%
Appropriate Beta Blocker Usage[2]	334	92%	93%	93%
Controlled Postoperative Blood Glucose[2]	124	85%	94%	93%
Prophylactic Antibiotic Timing[2]	623	95%	97%	97%
Prophylactic Antibiotic Timing (Outpatient)	144	74%	92%	92%
Prophylactic Antibiotic Selection[2]	627	99%	98%	97%
Prophylactic Antibiotic Select. (Outpatient)	108	94%	93%	94%
Prophylactic Antibiotic Stopped[2]	597	91%	94%	94%
Recommended VTP Ordered[2]	276	94%	94%	94%
Urinary Catheter Removal[2]	257	88%	89%	90%
Children's Asthma Care				
Received Systemic Corticosteroids	-	-	-	100%
Received Home Management Plan	-	-	-	71%
Received Reliever Medication	-	-	-	100%
Use of Medical Imaging				
Combination Abdominal CT Scan	1,272	0.040	0.160	0.191
Combination Chest CT Scan	797	0.038	0.054	0.054
Follow-up Mammogram/Ultrasound	1,225	7.9%	7.9%	8.4%
MRI for Low Back Pain	397	36.0%	35.6%	32.7%
Survey of Patients' Hospital Experiences				
Area Around Room 'Always' Quiet at Night	300+	61%	-	58%
Doctors 'Always' Communicated Well	300+	87%	-	80%
Home Recovery Information Given	300+	86%	-	82%
Hospital Given 9 or 10 on 10 Point Scale	300+	76%	-	67%
Meds 'Always' Explained Before Given	300+	65%	-	60%
Nurses 'Always' Communicated Well	300+	81%	-	76%
Pain 'Always' Well Controlled	300+	77%	-	69%
Room and Bathroom 'Always' Clean	300+	72%	-	71%
Timely Help 'Always' Received	300+	68%	-	64%
Would Definitely Recommend Hospital	300+	78%	-	69%

NOTE: Hospital profiles are in alphabetical order by state, then city, then hospital within the city; Rankings exclude hospitals with less than 25 cases except for patient surveys which excludes hospitals with less than 100 cases; (a) 100–299 cases; (1) The number of cases is too small to be sure how well a hospital is performing; (2) The hospital indicated that the data submitted for this measure were based on a sample of cases; (3) Data was collected during a shorter time period (fewer quarters) than the maximum possible time for this measure; (4) Suppressed for one or more quarters by CMS; (5) No data is available from the hospital for this measure; (6) Fewer than 100 patients completed the HCAHPS survey. Use these rates with caution, as the number of surveys may be too low to reliably assess hospital performance; (7) Survey results are based on less than 12 months of data; (8) Survey results are not available for this reporting period; (9) No or very few patients were eligible for the HCAHPS survey. The scores shown, if any, reflect a very small number of surveys; (10) A state average was not calculated because too few hospitals in the state submitted data; (11) There were discrepancies in the data collection process; Please refer to the User's Guide for a full explanation of data.

Pineville Community Hospital

850 Riverview Avenue
Pineville, KY 40977
Phone: 606-337-3051
Fax: 606-337-4284
Type: Acute Care Hospitals
Emergency Services: Yes
Ownership: Voluntary Non-Profit - Other
Beds: 150

Key Personnel:
Operating Room. . . . . Scott Emerick
Quality Assurance . . . . Brooke Jones
Anesthesiology. . . . . Shannon Cheech, CRNA
Emergency Room . . . . Nora Ciford

Measure	Cases	This Hosp.	State Avg.	U.S. Avg.
Heart Attack Care				
ACE Inhibitor or ARB for LVSD[1]	1	0%	94%	96%
Aspirin at Arrival[1]	8	75%	98%	99%
Aspirin at Discharge[1]	4	75%	99%	98%
Beta Blocker at Discharge[1]	4	50%	98%	98%
Fibrinolytic Medication Timing	0	-	60%	55%
PCI Within 90 Minutes of Arrival	0	-	88%	90%
Smoking Cessation Advice[1]	2	0%	100%	99%
Chest Pain/Possible Heart Attack Care				
Aspirin at Arrival	46	89%	95%	95%
Median Time to ECG (minutes)	49	13	7	8
Median Time to Transfer (minutes)[1]	6	102	65	61
Fibrinolytic Medication Timing[1]	3	0%	62%	54%
Heart Failure Care				
ACE Inhibitor or ARB for LVSD	56	77%	91%	94%
Discharge Instructions	214	53%	82%	88%
Evaluation of LVS Function	241	90%	96%	98%
Smoking Cessation Advice	51	86%	98%	98%
Pneumonia Care				
Appropriate Initial Antibiotic	97	79%	90%	92%
Blood Culture Timing	79	86%	95%	96%
Influenza Vaccine	94	83%	92%	91%
Initial Antibiotic Timing	125	88%	95%	95%
Pneumococcal Vaccine	107	88%	94%	93%
Smoking Cessation Advice	62	77%	98%	97%
Surgical Care Improvement Project				
Appropriate VTP Within 24 Hours[2]	33	94%	91%	92%
Appropriate Hair Removal[2]	74	100%	99%	99%
Appropriate Beta Blocker Usage[1,2]	11	73%	93%	93%
Controlled Postoperative Blood Glucose[2]	0	-	94%	93%
Prophylactic Antibiotic Timing[2]	56	93%	97%	97%
Prophylactic Antibiotic Timing (Outpatient)[5]	0	-	92%	92%
Prophylactic Antibiotic Selection[2]	56	93%	98%	97%
Prophylactic Antibiotic Select. (Outpatient)[5]	0	-	93%	94%
Prophylactic Antibiotic Stopped[2]	54	74%	94%	94%
Recommended VTP Ordered[2]	33	94%	94%	94%
Urinary Catheter Removal[1,2]	3	33%	89%	90%
Children's Asthma Care				
Received Systemic Corticosteroids	-	-	-	100%
Received Home Management Plan	-	-	-	71%
Received Reliever Medication	-	-	-	100%
Use of Medical Imaging				
Combination Abdominal CT Scan	265	0.294	0.160	0.191
Combination Chest CT Scan	90	0.322	0.054	0.054
Follow-up Mammogram/Ultrasound	318	6.6%	7.9%	8.4%
MRI for Low Back Pain[5]	0	-	35.6%	32.7%
Survey of Patients' Hospital Experiences				
Area Around Room 'Always' Quiet at Night	300+	57%	-	58%
Doctors 'Always' Communicated Well	300+	86%	-	80%
Home Recovery Information Given	300+	77%	-	82%
Hospital Given 9 or 10 on 10 Point Scale	300+	62%	-	67%
Meds 'Always' Explained Before Given	300+	56%	-	60%
Nurses 'Always' Communicated Well	300+	76%	-	76%
Pain 'Always' Well Controlled	300+	66%	-	69%
Room and Bathroom 'Always' Clean	300+	78%	-	71%
Timely Help 'Always' Received	300+	59%	-	64%
Would Definitely Recommend Hospital	300+	68%	-	69%

Highlands Regional Medical Center

5000 Kentucky Rte 321
Prestonsburg, KY 41653
Phone: 606-886-8511
Fax: 606-886-7534
E-mail: info@hrmc.org
URL: www.hrmc.org
Type: Acute Care Hospitals
Emergency Services: Yes
Ownership: Voluntary Non-Profit - Other
Beds: 184

Key Personnel:
Chief of Medical Staff. . . . . Sujatha Reddy
Infection Control. . . . . Norcie Jervis
Operating Room. . . . . Faruque Ahmed
Quality Assurance . . . . Eunice Hull
Anesthesiology. . . . . Jonathan Korshin
Emergency Room . . . . Dena Patton
Intensive Care Unit. . . . . Sharon Dingus

Measure	Cases	This Hosp.	State Avg.	U.S. Avg.
Heart Attack Care				
ACE Inhibitor or ARB for LVSD[1]	4	100%	94%	96%
Aspirin at Arrival	30	97%	98%	99%
Aspirin at Discharge[1]	20	100%	99%	98%
Beta Blocker at Discharge[1]	20	95%	98%	98%
Fibrinolytic Medication Timing	0	-	60%	55%
PCI Within 90 Minutes of Arrival	0	-	88%	90%
Smoking Cessation Advice[1]	5	100%	100%	99%
Chest Pain/Possible Heart Attack Care				
Aspirin at Arrival	258	88%	95%	95%
Median Time to ECG (minutes)	268	8	7	8
Median Time to Transfer (minutes)[1,3]	11	183	65	61
Fibrinolytic Medication Timing[1]	4	50%	62%	54%
Heart Failure Care				
ACE Inhibitor or ARB for LVSD	60	85%	91%	94%
Discharge Instructions	162	97%	82%	88%
Evaluation of LVS Function	201	97%	96%	98%
Smoking Cessation Advice	33	100%	98%	98%
Pneumonia Care				
Appropriate Initial Antibiotic	144	84%	90%	92%
Blood Culture Timing	153	93%	95%	96%
Influenza Vaccine	132	95%	92%	91%
Initial Antibiotic Timing	240	95%	95%	95%
Pneumococcal Vaccine	173	89%	94%	93%
Smoking Cessation Advice	98	100%	98%	97%
Surgical Care Improvement Project				
Appropriate VTP Within 24 Hours	41	100%	91%	92%
Appropriate Hair Removal	85	100%	99%	99%
Appropriate Beta Blocker Usage[1]	16	100%	93%	93%
Controlled Postoperative Blood Glucose	0	-	94%	93%
Prophylactic Antibiotic Timing	31	97%	97%	97%
Prophylactic Antibiotic Timing (Outpatient)	141	94%	92%	92%
Prophylactic Antibiotic Selection	31	97%	98%	97%
Prophylactic Antibiotic Select. (Outpatient)	134	93%	93%	94%
Prophylactic Antibiotic Stopped	30	97%	94%	94%
Recommended VTP Ordered	41	100%	94%	94%
Urinary Catheter Removal[1]	16	88%	89%	90%
Children's Asthma Care				
Received Systemic Corticosteroids	-	-	-	100%
Received Home Management Plan	-	-	-	71%
Received Reliever Medication	-	-	-	100%
Use of Medical Imaging				
Combination Abdominal CT Scan	1,015	0.372	0.160	0.191
Combination Chest CT Scan	502	0.002	0.054	0.054
Follow-up Mammogram/Ultrasound	962	1.6%	7.9%	8.4%
MRI for Low Back Pain	156	35.3%	35.6%	32.7%
Survey of Patients' Hospital Experiences				
Area Around Room 'Always' Quiet at Night	300+	55%	-	58%
Doctors 'Always' Communicated Well	300+	83%	-	80%
Home Recovery Information Given	300+	70%	-	82%
Hospital Given 9 or 10 on 10 Point Scale	300+	58%	-	67%
Meds 'Always' Explained Before Given	300+	56%	-	60%
Nurses 'Always' Communicated Well	300+	75%	-	76%
Pain 'Always' Well Controlled	300+	63%	-	69%
Room and Bathroom 'Always' Clean	300+	69%	-	71%
Timely Help 'Always' Received	300+	64%	-	64%
Would Definitely Recommend Hospital	300+	59%	-	69%

Caldwell Medical Center

100 Medical Center Drive
Princeton, KY 42445
Phone: 270-365-0300
Fax: 270-365-6694
E-mail: info@CaldwellHosp.org
URL: www.caldwellhosp.org
Type: Critical Access Hospitals
Emergency Services: Yes
Ownership: Govt - Hospital Dist/Auth
Beds: 25

Key Personnel:
CEO/President. . . . . Charles Zorell Jr., CEO
Infection Control. . . . . Tonya Magowan
Operating Room. . . . . Tammy Mcconnel
Radiology. . . . . Sandy Stephans

Measure	Cases	This Hosp.	State Avg.	U.S. Avg.
Heart Attack Care				
ACE Inhibitor or ARB for LVSD[5]	0	-	94%	96%
Aspirin at Arrival[5]	0	-	98%	99%
Aspirin at Discharge[5]	0	-	99%	98%
Beta Blocker at Discharge[5]	0	-	98%	98%
Fibrinolytic Medication Timing[5]	0	-	60%	55%
PCI Within 90 Minutes of Arrival[5]	0	-	88%	90%
Smoking Cessation Advice[5]	0	-	100%	99%
Chest Pain/Possible Heart Attack Care				
Aspirin at Arrival	-	-	95%	95%
Median Time to ECG (minutes)	-	-	7	8
Median Time to Transfer (minutes)	-	-	65	61
Fibrinolytic Medication Timing	-	-	62%	54%
Heart Failure Care				
ACE Inhibitor or ARB for LVSD[1]	6	83%	91%	94%
Discharge Instructions[1]	15	100%	82%	88%
Evaluation of LVS Function[1]	21	86%	96%	98%
Smoking Cessation Advice[1]	3	100%	98%	98%
Pneumonia Care				
Appropriate Initial Antibiotic	28	79%	90%	92%
Blood Culture Timing[1]	23	87%	95%	96%
Influenza Vaccine[1]	14	86%	92%	91%
Initial Antibiotic Timing	34	91%	95%	95%
Pneumococcal Vaccine[1]	23	83%	94%	93%
Smoking Cessation Advice[1]	4	100%	98%	97%
Surgical Care Improvement Project				
Appropriate VTP Within 24 Hours[5]	0	-	91%	92%
Appropriate Hair Removal[5]	0	-	99%	99%
Appropriate Beta Blocker Usage[5]	0	-	93%	93%
Controlled Postoperative Blood Glucose[5]	0	-	94%	93%
Prophylactic Antibiotic Timing[5]	0	-	97%	97%
Prophylactic Antibiotic Timing (Outpatient)	-	-	92%	92%
Prophylactic Antibiotic Selection[5]	0	-	98%	97%
Prophylactic Antibiotic Select. (Outpatient)	-	-	93%	94%
Prophylactic Antibiotic Stopped[5]	0	-	94%	94%
Recommended VTP Ordered[5]	0	-	94%	94%
Urinary Catheter Removal[5]	0	-	89%	90%
Children's Asthma Care				
Received Systemic Corticosteroids	-	-	-	100%
Received Home Management Plan	-	-	-	71%
Received Reliever Medication	-	-	-	100%
Use of Medical Imaging				
Combination Abdominal CT Scan	-	-	0.160	0.191
Combination Chest CT Scan	-	-	0.054	0.054
Follow-up Mammogram/Ultrasound	-	-	7.9%	8.4%
MRI for Low Back Pain	-	-	35.6%	32.7%
Survey of Patients' Hospital Experiences				
Area Around Room 'Always' Quiet at Night[8]	-	-	-	58%
Doctors 'Always' Communicated Well[8]	-	-	-	80%
Home Recovery Information Given[8]	-	-	-	82%
Hospital Given 9 or 10 on 10 Point Scale[8]	-	-	-	67%
Meds 'Always' Explained Before Given[8]	-	-	-	60%
Nurses 'Always' Communicated Well[8]	-	-	-	76%
Pain 'Always' Well Controlled[8]	-	-	-	69%
Room and Bathroom 'Always' Clean[8]	-	-	-	71%
Timely Help 'Always' Received[8]	-	-	-	64%
Would Definitely Recommend Hospital[8]	-	-	-	69%

NOTE: Hospital profiles are in alphabetical order by state, then city, then hospital within the city; Rankings exclude hospitals with less than 25 cases except for patient surveys which excludes hospitals with less than 100 cases; (a) 100–299 cases; (1) The number of cases is too small to be sure how well a hospital is performing; (2) The hospital indicated that the data submitted for this measure were based on a sample of cases; (3) Data was collected during a shorter time period (fewer quarters) than the maximum possible time for this measure; (4) Suppressed for one or more quarters by CMS; (5) No data is available from the hospital for this measure; (6) Fewer than 100 patients completed the HCAHPS survey. Use these rates with caution, as the number of surveys may be too low to reliably assess hospital performance; (7) Survey results are based on less than 12 months of data; (8) Survey results are not available for this reporting period; (9) No or very few patients were eligible for the HCAHPS survey. The scores shown, if any, reflect a very small number of surveys; (10) A state average was not calculated because too few hospitals in the state submitted data; (11) There were discrepancies in the data collection process; Please refer to the User's Guide for a full explanation of data.

Pattie A Clay Regional Medical Center

801 Eastern Bypass
Richmond, KY 40475
Phone: 859-623-3131
Fax: 859-625-3535
URL: www.pattieaclay.org
Type: Acute Care Hospitals
Emergency Services: Yes
Ownership: Voluntary Non-Profit - Private
Beds: 105

Key Personnel:
CEO/President. . . . . Robert J Hudson
Cardiac Laboratory. . . . . Shelia Powell, RN
Chief of Medical Staff. . . . . Patricia Barnwell
Operating Room. . . . . S Fritz, RN
Quality Assurance . . . . Janie Rosanbalm, RN
Emergency Room . . . . Pat Cornelison, RN

Measure	Cases	This Hosp.	State Avg.	U.S. Avg.
Heart Attack Care				
ACE Inhibitor or ARB for LVSD[1]	7	100%	94%	96%
Aspirin at Arrival[1]	22	95%	98%	99%
Aspirin at Discharge[1]	13	100%	99%	98%
Beta Blocker at Discharge[1]	16	100%	98%	98%
Fibrinolytic Medication Timing	0	-	60%	55%
PCI Within 90 Minutes of Arrival	0	-	88%	90%
Smoking Cessation Advice[1]	4	100%	100%	99%
Chest Pain/Possible Heart Attack Care				
Aspirin at Arrival	141	95%	95%	95%
Median Time to ECG (minutes)	142	4	7	8
Median Time to Transfer (minutes)	35	69	65	61
Fibrinolytic Medication Timing[1]	4	0%	62%	54%
Heart Failure Care				
ACE Inhibitor or ARB for LVSD	25	92%	91%	94%
Discharge Instructions	47	98%	82%	88%
Evaluation of LVS Function	66	97%	96%	98%
Smoking Cessation Advice[1]	9	100%	98%	98%
Pneumonia Care				
Appropriate Initial Antibiotic	114	95%	90%	92%
Blood Culture Timing	127	87%	95%	96%
Influenza Vaccine	94	100%	92%	91%
Initial Antibiotic Timing	140	99%	95%	95%
Pneumococcal Vaccine	120	98%	94%	93%
Smoking Cessation Advice	57	100%	98%	97%
Surgical Care Improvement Project				
Appropriate VTP Within 24 Hours	89	92%	91%	92%
Appropriate Hair Removal	490	100%	99%	99%
Appropriate Beta Blocker Usage	82	100%	93%	93%
Controlled Postoperative Blood Glucose	0	-	94%	93%
Prophylactic Antibiotic Timing	372	98%	97%	97%
Prophylactic Antibiotic Timing (Outpatient)	116	97%	92%	92%
Prophylactic Antibiotic Selection	370	98%	98%	97%
Prophylactic Antibiotic Select. (Outpatient)	117	99%	93%	94%
Prophylactic Antibiotic Stopped	363	95%	94%	94%
Recommended VTP Ordered	89	92%	94%	94%
Urinary Catheter Removal	54	94%	89%	90%
Children's Asthma Care				
Received Systemic Corticosteroids	-	-	-	100%
Received Home Management Plan	-	-	-	71%
Received Reliever Medication	-	-	-	100%
Use of Medical Imaging				
Combination Abdominal CT Scan	588	0.015	0.160	0.191
Combination Chest CT Scan	345	0.020	0.054	0.054
Follow-up Mammogram/Ultrasound	739	3.5%	7.9%	8.4%
MRI for Low Back Pain	149	31.5%	35.6%	32.7%
Survey of Patients' Hospital Experiences				
Area Around Room 'Always' Quiet at Night	300+	56%	-	58%
Doctors 'Always' Communicated Well	300+	78%	-	80%
Home Recovery Information Given	300+	82%	-	82%
Hospital Given 9 or 10 on 10 Point Scale	300+	59%	-	67%
Meds 'Always' Explained Before Given	300+	55%	-	60%
Nurses 'Always' Communicated Well	300+	71%	-	76%
Pain 'Always' Well Controlled	300+	66%	-	69%
Room and Bathroom 'Always' Clean	300+	69%	-	71%
Timely Help 'Always' Received	300+	61%	-	64%
Would Definitely Recommend Hospital	300+	61%	-	69%

Russell County Hospital

153 Dowell Road
Russell Springs, KY 42642
Phone: 270-866-4141
Fax: 270-866-2136
URL: www.russellcohospital.org
Type: Critical Access Hospitals
Emergency Services: Yes
Ownership: Govt - Hospital Dist/Auth
Beds: 45

Key Personnel:
CEO/President. . . . . Gary Delsorge
Operating Room. . . . . Vijay Jain, MD
Radiology. . . . . Jerry Westerfield, MD
Emergency Room . . . . Paula Roy, MD

Measure	Cases	This Hosp.	State Avg.	U.S. Avg.
Heart Attack Care				
ACE Inhibitor or ARB for LVSD[1]	1	100%	94%	96%
Aspirin at Arrival[1]	8	62%	98%	99%
Aspirin at Discharge[1]	8	62%	99%	98%
Beta Blocker at Discharge[1]	8	62%	98%	98%
Fibrinolytic Medication Timing	0	-	60%	55%
PCI Within 90 Minutes of Arrival	0	-	88%	90%
Smoking Cessation Advice	0	-	100%	99%
Chest Pain/Possible Heart Attack Care				
Aspirin at Arrival	38	87%	95%	95%
Median Time to ECG (minutes)	40	14	7	8
Median Time to Transfer (minutes)[1,3]	3	140	65	61
Fibrinolytic Medication Timing[1,3]	1	0%	62%	54%
Heart Failure Care				
ACE Inhibitor or ARB for LVSD[1]	5	60%	91%	94%
Discharge Instructions[1]	24	92%	82%	88%
Evaluation of LVS Function	31	74%	96%	98%
Smoking Cessation Advice[1]	8	100%	98%	98%
Pneumonia Care				
Appropriate Initial Antibiotic	68	85%	90%	92%
Blood Culture Timing	65	77%	95%	96%
Influenza Vaccine	47	70%	92%	91%
Initial Antibiotic Timing	89	94%	95%	95%
Pneumococcal Vaccine	61	75%	94%	93%
Smoking Cessation Advice	41	85%	98%	97%
Surgical Care Improvement Project				
Appropriate VTP Within 24 Hours[5]	0	-	91%	92%
Appropriate Hair Removal[5]	0	-	99%	99%
Appropriate Beta Blocker Usage[5]	0	-	93%	93%
Controlled Postoperative Blood Glucose[5]	0	-	94%	93%
Prophylactic Antibiotic Timing[5]	0	-	97%	97%
Prophylactic Antibiotic Timing (Outpatient)[5]	0	-	92%	92%
Prophylactic Antibiotic Selection[5]	0	-	98%	97%
Prophylactic Antibiotic Select. (Outpatient)[5]	0	-	93%	94%
Prophylactic Antibiotic Stopped[5]	0	-	94%	94%
Recommended VTP Ordered[5]	0	-	94%	94%
Urinary Catheter Removal[5]	0	-	89%	90%
Children's Asthma Care				
Received Systemic Corticosteroids	-	-	-	100%
Received Home Management Plan	-	-	-	71%
Received Reliever Medication	-	-	-	100%
Use of Medical Imaging				
Combination Abdominal CT Scan	248	0.710	0.160	0.191
Combination Chest CT Scan	151	0.013	0.054	0.054
Follow-up Mammogram/Ultrasound	326	4.6%	7.9%	8.4%
MRI for Low Back Pain[5]	0	-	35.6%	32.7%
Survey of Patients' Hospital Experiences				
Area Around Room 'Always' Quiet at Night[8]	-	-	-	58%
Doctors 'Always' Communicated Well[8]	-	-	-	80%
Home Recovery Information Given[8]	-	-	-	82%
Hospital Given 9 or 10 on 10 Point Scale[8]	-	-	-	67%
Meds 'Always' Explained Before Given[8]	-	-	-	60%
Nurses 'Always' Communicated Well[8]	-	-	-	76%
Pain 'Always' Well Controlled[8]	-	-	-	69%
Room and Bathroom 'Always' Clean[8]	-	-	-	71%
Timely Help 'Always' Received[8]	-	-	-	64%
Would Definitely Recommend Hospital[8]	-	-	-	69%

Logan Memorial Hospital

1625 Nashville Street
Russellville, KY 42276
Phone: 270-726-4011
Fax: 270-726-7465
URL: www.loganmemorial.com
Type: Acute Care Hospitals
Emergency Services: Yes
Ownership: Proprietary
Beds: 100

Key Personnel:
CEO/President. . . . . William Haugh
Cardiac Laboratory. . . . . Shirley Blick
Chief of Medical Staff. . . . . Muhammad Ahmad, MD
Infection Control. . . . . Joyce Noe
Operating Room. . . . . Adam Ellis
Quality Assurance . . . . June Massingille
Radiology. . . . . Todd Talmadge

Measure	Cases	This Hosp.	State Avg.	U.S. Avg.
Heart Attack Care				
ACE Inhibitor or ARB for LVSD	0	-	94%	96%
Aspirin at Arrival[1]	4	75%	98%	99%
Aspirin at Discharge[1]	2	100%	99%	98%
Beta Blocker at Discharge[1]	2	100%	98%	98%
Fibrinolytic Medication Timing	0	-	60%	55%
PCI Within 90 Minutes of Arrival	0	-	88%	90%
Smoking Cessation Advice[1]	1	100%	100%	99%
Chest Pain/Possible Heart Attack Care				
Aspirin at Arrival	128	96%	95%	95%
Median Time to ECG (minutes)	135	5	7	8
Median Time to Transfer (minutes)[1,3]	2	92	65	61
Fibrinolytic Medication Timing[1]	10	90%	62%	54%
Heart Failure Care				
ACE Inhibitor or ARB for LVSD[1]	22	86%	91%	94%
Discharge Instructions	80	84%	82%	88%
Evaluation of LVS Function	97	97%	96%	98%
Smoking Cessation Advice	29	100%	98%	98%
Pneumonia Care				
Appropriate Initial Antibiotic	145	99%	90%	92%
Blood Culture Timing	99	97%	95%	96%
Influenza Vaccine	131	95%	92%	91%
Initial Antibiotic Timing	170	99%	95%	95%
Pneumococcal Vaccine	151	97%	94%	93%
Smoking Cessation Advice	82	100%	98%	97%
Surgical Care Improvement Project				
Appropriate VTP Within 24 Hours[1]	16	94%	91%	92%
Appropriate Hair Removal[1]	23	100%	99%	99%
Appropriate Beta Blocker Usage[1]	9	78%	93%	93%
Controlled Postoperative Blood Glucose	0	-	94%	93%
Prophylactic Antibiotic Timing[1]	12	92%	97%	97%
Prophylactic Antibiotic Timing (Outpatient)[1]	18	94%	92%	92%
Prophylactic Antibiotic Selection[1]	12	100%	98%	97%
Prophylactic Antibiotic Select. (Outpatient)[1]	18	89%	93%	94%
Prophylactic Antibiotic Stopped[1]	11	100%	94%	94%
Recommended VTP Ordered[1]	16	94%	94%	94%
Urinary Catheter Removal[1]	4	100%	89%	90%
Children's Asthma Care				
Received Systemic Corticosteroids[1]	5	100%	-	100%
Received Home Management Plan[1]	6	83%	-	71%
Received Reliever Medication[1]	6	100%	-	100%
Use of Medical Imaging				
Combination Abdominal CT Scan	218	0.069	0.160	0.191
Combination Chest CT Scan	160	0.013	0.054	0.054
Follow-up Mammogram/Ultrasound	480	13.1%	7.9%	8.4%
MRI for Low Back Pain[1]	26	38.5%	35.6%	32.7%
Survey of Patients' Hospital Experiences				
Area Around Room 'Always' Quiet at Night	300+	64%	-	58%
Doctors 'Always' Communicated Well	300+	84%	-	80%
Home Recovery Information Given	300+	80%	-	82%
Hospital Given 9 or 10 on 10 Point Scale	300+	66%	-	67%
Meds 'Always' Explained Before Given	300+	58%	-	60%
Nurses 'Always' Communicated Well	300+	78%	-	76%
Pain 'Always' Well Controlled	300+	74%	-	69%
Room and Bathroom 'Always' Clean	300+	65%	-	71%
Timely Help 'Always' Received	300+	69%	-	64%
Would Definitely Recommend Hospital	300+	61%	-	69%

NOTE: Hospital profiles are in alphabetical order by state, then city, then hospital within the city; Rankings exclude hospitals with less than 25 cases except for patient surveys which excludes hospitals with less than 100 cases; (a) 100–299 cases; (1) The number of cases is too small to be sure how well a hospital is performing; (2) The hospital indicated that the data submitted for this measure were based on a sample of cases; (3) Data was collected during a shorter time period (fewer quarters) than the maximum possible time for this measure; (4) Suppressed for one or more quarters by CMS; (5) No data is available from the hospital for this measure; (6) Fewer than 100 patients completed the HCAHPS survey. Use these rates with caution, as the number of surveys may be too low to reliably assess hospital performance; (7) Survey results are based on less than 12 months of data; (8) Survey results are not available for this reporting period; (9) No or very few patients were eligible for the HCAHPS survey. The scores shown, if any, reflect a very small number of surveys; (10) A state average was not calculated because too few hospitals in the state submitted data; (11) There were discrepancies in the data collection process; Please refer to the User's Guide for a full explanation of data.

Livingston Hospital and Healthcare

131 Hospital Drive
Salem, KY 42078
URL: www.lhhs.org
Type: Critical Access Hospitals
Ownership: Proprietary

Phone: 270-988-2299
Fax: 270-988-3900

Emergency Services: Yes
Beds: 25

Key Personnel:
CEO/President . . . . Mike Budnick
Quality Assurance . . . . Pat Fletcher
Radiology . . . . William Guyette

Measure	Cases	This Hosp.	State Avg.	U.S. Avg.
Heart Attack Care				
ACE Inhibitor or ARB for LVSD[3]	0	-	94%	96%
Aspirin at Arrival[1,3]	6	33%	98%	99%
Aspirin at Discharge[1,3]	6	83%	99%	98%
Beta Blocker at Discharge[1,3]	6	83%	98%	98%
Fibrinolytic Medication Timing[5]	0	-	60%	55%
PCI Within 90 Minutes of Arrival[5]	0	-	88%	90%
Smoking Cessation Advice[1,3]	1	0%	100%	99%
Chest Pain/Possible Heart Attack Care				
Aspirin at Arrival	-		95%	95%
Median Time to ECG (minutes)	-		7	8
Median Time to Transfer (minutes)	-	-	65	61
Fibrinolytic Medication Timing	-		62%	54%
Heart Failure Care				
ACE Inhibitor or ARB for LVSD[1]	4	50%	91%	94%
Discharge Instructions	45	0%	82%	88%
Evaluation of LVS Function	56	39%	96%	98%
Smoking Cessation Advice[1]	10	100%	98%	98%
Pneumonia Care				
Appropriate Initial Antibiotic	25	68%	90%	92%
Blood Culture Timing[1]	3	67%	95%	96%
Influenza Vaccine[1]	15	13%	92%	91%
Initial Antibiotic Timing	26	92%	95%	95%
Pneumococcal Vaccine[1]	21	29%	94%	93%
Smoking Cessation Advice[1]	14	86%	98%	97%
Surgical Care Improvement Project				
Appropriate VTP Within 24 Hours[5]	0	-	91%	92%
Appropriate Hair Removal[5]	0	-	99%	99%
Appropriate Beta Blocker Usage[5]	0	-	93%	93%
Controlled Postoperative Blood Glucose[5]	0	-	94%	93%
Prophylactic Antibiotic Timing[5]	0	-	97%	97%
Prophylactic Antibiotic Timing (Outpatient)	-		92%	92%
Prophylactic Antibiotic Selection[5]	0	-	98%	97%
Prophylactic Antibiotic Select. (Outpatient)	-		93%	94%
Prophylactic Antibiotic Stopped[5]	0	-	94%	94%
Recommended VTP Ordered[5]	0	-	94%	94%
Urinary Catheter Removal[5]	0	-	89%	90%
Children's Asthma Care				
Received Systemic Corticosteroids	-	-	-	100%
Received Home Management Plan	-	-	-	71%
Received Reliever Medication	-	-	-	100%
Use of Medical Imaging				
Combination Abdominal CT Scan	-		0.160	0.191
Combination Chest CT Scan	-		0.054	0.054
Follow-up Mammogram/Ultrasound	-		7.9%	8.4%
MRI for Low Back Pain	-		35.6%	32.7%
Survey of Patients' Hospital Experiences				
Area Around Room 'Always' Quiet at Night[8]	-	-	-	58%
Doctors 'Always' Communicated Well[8]	-	-	-	80%
Home Recovery Information Given[8]	-	-	-	82%
Hospital Given 9 or 10 on 10 Point Scale[8]	-	-	-	67%
Meds 'Always' Explained Before Given[8]	-	-	-	60%
Nurses 'Always' Communicated Well[8]	-	-	-	76%
Pain 'Always' Well Controlled[8]	-	-	-	69%
Room and Bathroom 'Always' Clean[8]	-	-	-	71%
Timely Help 'Always' Received[8]	-	-	-	64%
Would Definitely Recommend Hospital[8]	-	-	-	69%

The Medical Center at Scottsville

456 Burnley Road
Scottsville, KY 42164
Type: Critical Access Hospitals
Ownership: Voluntary Non-Profit - Private

Phone: 270-622-2800
Fax: 270-622-2208
Emergency Services: Yes
Beds: 157

Measure	Cases	This Hosp.	State Avg.	U.S. Avg.
Heart Attack Care				
ACE Inhibitor or ARB for LVSD[5]	0	-	94%	96%
Aspirin at Arrival[5]	0	-	98%	99%
Aspirin at Discharge[5]	0	-	99%	98%
Beta Blocker at Discharge[5]	0	-	98%	98%
Fibrinolytic Medication Timing[5]	0	-	60%	55%
PCI Within 90 Minutes of Arrival[5]	0	-	88%	90%
Smoking Cessation Advice[5]	0	-	100%	99%
Chest Pain/Possible Heart Attack Care				
Aspirin at Arrival	-		95%	95%
Median Time to ECG (minutes)	-		7	8
Median Time to Transfer (minutes)	-		65	61
Fibrinolytic Medication Timing	-		62%	54%
Heart Failure Care				
ACE Inhibitor or ARB for LVSD[1]	4	75%	91%	94%
Discharge Instructions[1]	20	30%	82%	88%
Evaluation of LVS Function	32	75%	96%	98%
Smoking Cessation Advice[1]	6	100%	98%	98%
Pneumonia Care				
Appropriate Initial Antibiotic	30	80%	90%	92%
Blood Culture Timing[1]	8	100%	95%	96%
Influenza Vaccine[1]	19	84%	92%	91%
Initial Antibiotic Timing	35	91%	95%	95%
Pneumococcal Vaccine	28	96%	94%	93%
Smoking Cessation Advice[1]	9	100%	98%	97%
Surgical Care Improvement Project				
Appropriate VTP Within 24 Hours[5]	0	-	91%	92%
Appropriate Hair Removal[5]	0	-	99%	99%
Appropriate Beta Blocker Usage[5]	0	-	93%	93%
Controlled Postoperative Blood Glucose[5]	0	-	94%	93%
Prophylactic Antibiotic Timing[5]	0	-	97%	97%
Prophylactic Antibiotic Timing (Outpatient)	-		92%	92%
Prophylactic Antibiotic Selection[5]	0	-	98%	97%
Prophylactic Antibiotic Select. (Outpatient)	-		93%	94%
Prophylactic Antibiotic Stopped[5]	0	-	94%	94%
Recommended VTP Ordered[5]	0	-	94%	94%
Urinary Catheter Removal[5]	0	-	89%	90%
Children's Asthma Care				
Received Systemic Corticosteroids	-	-	-	100%
Received Home Management Plan	-	-	-	71%
Received Reliever Medication	-	-	-	100%
Use of Medical Imaging				
Combination Abdominal CT Scan	-		0.160	0.191
Combination Chest CT Scan	-		0.054	0.054
Follow-up Mammogram/Ultrasound	-		7.9%	8.4%
MRI for Low Back Pain	-		35.6%	32.7%
Survey of Patients' Hospital Experiences				
Area Around Room 'Always' Quiet at Night[8]	-	-	-	58%
Doctors 'Always' Communicated Well[8]	-	-	-	80%
Home Recovery Information Given[8]	-	-	-	82%
Hospital Given 9 or 10 on 10 Point Scale[8]	-	-	-	67%
Meds 'Always' Explained Before Given[8]	-	-	-	60%
Nurses 'Always' Communicated Well[8]	-	-	-	76%
Pain 'Always' Well Controlled[8]	-	-	-	69%
Room and Bathroom 'Always' Clean[8]	-	-	-	71%
Timely Help 'Always' Received[8]	-	-	-	64%
Would Definitely Recommend Hospital[8]	-	-	-	69%

Jewish Hospital - Shelbyville

727 Hospital Drive
Shelbyville, KY 40065
Type: Acute Care Hospitals
Ownership: Voluntary Non-Profit - Private

Phone: 502-647-4300

Emergency Services: Yes

Measure	Cases	This Hosp.	State Avg.	U.S. Avg.
Heart Attack Care				
ACE Inhibitor or ARB for LVSD[1]	1	100%	94%	96%
Aspirin at Arrival	29	100%	98%	99%
Aspirin at Discharge[1]	12	100%	99%	98%
Beta Blocker at Discharge[1]	11	91%	98%	98%
Fibrinolytic Medication Timing	0	-	60%	55%
PCI Within 90 Minutes of Arrival	0	-	88%	90%
Smoking Cessation Advice	0	-	100%	99%
Chest Pain/Possible Heart Attack Care				
Aspirin at Arrival	100	96%	95%	95%
Median Time to ECG (minutes)	104	4	7	8
Median Time to Transfer (minutes)[1,3]	1	125	65	61
Fibrinolytic Medication Timing[1]	13	54%	62%	54%
Heart Failure Care				
ACE Inhibitor or ARB for LVSD[1]	16	75%	91%	94%
Discharge Instructions	70	80%	82%	88%
Evaluation of LVS Function	102	99%	96%	98%
Smoking Cessation Advice[1]	24	100%	98%	98%
Pneumonia Care				
Appropriate Initial Antibiotic	81	89%	90%	92%
Blood Culture Timing	92	90%	95%	96%
Influenza Vaccine	73	95%	92%	91%
Initial Antibiotic Timing	116	96%	95%	95%
Pneumococcal Vaccine	88	92%	94%	93%
Smoking Cessation Advice	55	100%	98%	97%
Surgical Care Improvement Project				
Appropriate VTP Within 24 Hours	66	83%	91%	92%
Appropriate Hair Removal	138	100%	99%	99%
Appropriate Beta Blocker Usage	35	97%	93%	93%
Controlled Postoperative Blood Glucose	0	-	94%	93%
Prophylactic Antibiotic Timing	65	92%	97%	97%
Prophylactic Antibiotic Timing (Outpatient)	33	82%	92%	92%
Prophylactic Antibiotic Selection	68	91%	98%	97%
Prophylactic Antibiotic Select. (Outpatient)	27	93%	93%	94%
Prophylactic Antibiotic Stopped	64	98%	94%	94%
Recommended VTP Ordered	67	82%	94%	94%
Urinary Catheter Removal[1]	24	83%	89%	90%
Children's Asthma Care				
Received Systemic Corticosteroids	-	-	-	100%
Received Home Management Plan	-	-	-	71%
Received Reliever Medication	-	-	-	100%
Use of Medical Imaging				
Combination Abdominal CT Scan	349	0.072	0.160	0.191
Combination Chest CT Scan	290	0.007	0.054	0.054
Follow-up Mammogram/Ultrasound	663	5.6%	7.9%	8.4%
MRI for Low Back Pain	69	30.4%	35.6%	32.7%
Survey of Patients' Hospital Experiences				
Area Around Room 'Always' Quiet at Night	300+	47%	-	58%
Doctors 'Always' Communicated Well	300+	77%	-	80%
Home Recovery Information Given	300+	73%	-	82%
Hospital Given 9 or 10 on 10 Point Scale	300+	60%	-	67%
Meds 'Always' Explained Before Given	300+	53%	-	60%
Nurses 'Always' Communicated Well	300+	72%	-	76%
Pain 'Always' Well Controlled	300+	64%	-	69%
Room and Bathroom 'Always' Clean	300+	67%	-	71%
Timely Help 'Always' Received	300+	58%	-	64%
Would Definitely Recommend Hospital	300+	57%	-	69%

Lake Cumberland Regional Hospital

305 Langdon Street, Somerset, KY 42503
Phone: 606-679-7441
Fax: 606-678-9919
Type: Acute Care Hospitals
Emergency Services: Yes
Ownership: Proprietary
Beds: 234

Key Personnel:
CEO/President. . . . . Jeff Seraphine
Chief of Medical Staff . . . . Michael Citalo
Infection Control. . . . . Judy Kaen RN
Operating Room. . . . . Lindae Cook
Quality Assurance . . . . Pat Brinson
Radiology. . . . . William M Baker
Emergency Room . . . . Mel Medroso MD
Intensive Care Unit. . . . . Dottie Campbell RN

Measure	Cases	This Hosp.	State Avg.	U.S. Avg.
Heart Attack Care				
ACE Inhibitor or ARB for LVSD	30	97%	94%	96%
Aspirin at Arrival	178	99%	98%	99%
Aspirin at Discharge	193	98%	99%	98%
Beta Blocker at Discharge	177	99%	98%	98%
Fibrinolytic Medication Timing	0	-	60%	55%
PCI Within 90 Minutes of Arrival	49	86%	88%	90%
Smoking Cessation Advice	93	100%	100%	99%
Chest Pain/Possible Heart Attack Care				
Aspirin at Arrival[1]	23	87%	95%	95%
Median Time to ECG (minutes)[1]	23	6	7	8
Median Time to Transfer (minutes)[5]	0	-	65	61
Fibrinolytic Medication Timing[5]	0	-	62%	54%
Heart Failure Care				
ACE Inhibitor or ARB for LVSD	84	90%	91%	94%
Discharge Instructions	202	84%	82%	88%
Evaluation of LVS Function	235	99%	96%	98%
Smoking Cessation Advice	59	100%	98%	98%
Pneumonia Care				
Appropriate Initial Antibiotic	236	93%	90%	92%
Blood Culture Timing	196	96%	95%	96%
Influenza Vaccine	235	97%	92%	91%
Initial Antibiotic Timing	339	98%	95%	95%
Pneumococcal Vaccine	285	100%	94%	93%
Smoking Cessation Advice	166	99%	98%	97%
Surgical Care Improvement Project				
Appropriate VTP Within 24 Hours	275	95%	91%	92%
Appropriate Hair Removal	722	100%	99%	99%
Appropriate Beta Blocker Usage	229	97%	93%	93%
Controlled Postoperative Blood Glucose	83	96%	94%	93%
Prophylactic Antibiotic Timing	363	98%	97%	97%
Prophylactic Antibiotic Timing (Outpatient)	468	99%	92%	92%
Prophylactic Antibiotic Selection	371	97%	98%	97%
Prophylactic Antibiotic Select. (Outpatient)	468	96%	93%	94%
Prophylactic Antibiotic Stopped	342	93%	94%	94%
Recommended VTP Ordered	275	97%	94%	94%
Urinary Catheter Removal	131	85%	89%	90%
Children's Asthma Care				
Received Systemic Corticosteroids	-	-	-	100%
Received Home Management Plan	-	-	-	71%
Received Reliever Medication	-	-	-	100%
Use of Medical Imaging				
Combination Abdominal CT Scan	1,074	0.150	0.160	0.191
Combination Chest CT Scan	765	0.069	0.054	0.054
Follow-up Mammogram/Ultrasound	1,498	6.1%	7.9%	8.4%
MRI for Low Back Pain	258	41.5%	35.6%	32.7%
Survey of Patients' Hospital Experiences				
Area Around Room 'Always' Quiet at Night	300+	61%	-	58%
Doctors 'Always' Communicated Well	300+	84%	-	80%
Home Recovery Information Given	300+	82%	-	82%
Hospital Given 9 or 10 on 10 Point Scale	300+	65%	-	67%
Meds 'Always' Explained Before Given	300+	61%	-	60%
Nurses 'Always' Communicated Well	300+	76%	-	76%
Pain 'Always' Well Controlled	300+	73%	-	69%
Room and Bathroom 'Always' Clean	300+	71%	-	71%
Timely Help 'Always' Received	300+	64%	-	64%
Would Definitely Recommend Hospital	300+	65%	-	69%

Williamson ARH Hospital

260 Hospital Drive, South Williamson, KY 41503
Phone: 606-237-1700
Fax: 606-237-1701
URL: www.arh.org
Type: Acute Care Hospitals
Emergency Services: Yes
Ownership: Proprietary
Beds: 113

Key Personnel:
CEO/President. . . . . Wes Dangerfield
Chief of Medical Staff . . . . Mansoor Mahmood, MD
Coronary Care . . . . Elizabeth Smith, RN
Infection Control. . . . . Sheila Hall, RN
Pediatric Ambulatory Care . . . . . . Charles Johnson, MD
Pediatric In-Patient Care . . . . Charles Johnson, MD
Quality Assurance . . . . Karen Reed
Radiology. . . . . Jagadishwar Dev, MD

Measure	Cases	This Hosp.	State Avg.	U.S. Avg.
Heart Attack Care				
ACE Inhibitor or ARB for LVSD	0	-	94%	96%
Aspirin at Arrival[1]	10	90%	98%	99%
Aspirin at Discharge[1]	4	100%	99%	98%
Beta Blocker at Discharge[1]	6	100%	98%	98%
Fibrinolytic Medication Timing	0	-	60%	55%
PCI Within 90 Minutes of Arrival	0	-	88%	90%
Smoking Cessation Advice[1]	2	100%	100%	99%
Chest Pain/Possible Heart Attack Care				
Aspirin at Arrival	45	98%	95%	95%
Median Time to ECG (minutes)	43	10	7	8
Median Time to Transfer (minutes)[5]	0	-	65	61
Fibrinolytic Medication Timing[1]	1	100%	62%	54%
Heart Failure Care				
ACE Inhibitor or ARB for LVSD[1]	17	100%	91%	94%
Discharge Instructions	110	94%	82%	88%
Evaluation of LVS Function	123	98%	96%	98%
Smoking Cessation Advice	31	100%	98%	98%
Pneumonia Care				
Appropriate Initial Antibiotic	95	88%	90%	92%
Blood Culture Timing	65	75%	95%	96%
Influenza Vaccine	65	100%	92%	91%
Initial Antibiotic Timing	108	94%	95%	95%
Pneumococcal Vaccine	82	99%	94%	93%
Smoking Cessation Advice	55	100%	98%	97%
Surgical Care Improvement Project				
Appropriate VTP Within 24 Hours[2]	33	97%	91%	92%
Appropriate Hair Removal[2]	70	100%	99%	99%
Appropriate Beta Blocker Usage[1,2]	22	95%	93%	93%
Controlled Postoperative Blood Glucose[2]	0	-	94%	93%
Prophylactic Antibiotic Timing[2]	42	100%	97%	97%
Prophylactic Antibiotic Timing (Outpatient)	26	81%	92%	92%
Prophylactic Antibiotic Selection[2]	42	100%	98%	97%
Prophylactic Antibiotic Select. (Outpatient)	27	100%	93%	94%
Prophylactic Antibiotic Stopped[2]	39	92%	94%	94%
Recommended VTP Ordered[2]	33	97%	94%	94%
Urinary Catheter Removal[1]	10	80%	89%	90%
Children's Asthma Care				
Received Systemic Corticosteroids	-	-	-	100%
Received Home Management Plan	-	-	-	71%
Received Reliever Medication	-	-	-	100%
Use of Medical Imaging				
Combination Abdominal CT Scan	179	0.006	0.160	0.191
Combination Chest CT Scan	92	0.011	0.054	0.054
Follow-up Mammogram/Ultrasound	216	9.3%	7.9%	8.4%
MRI for Low Back Pain	57	50.9%	35.6%	32.7%
Survey of Patients' Hospital Experiences				
Area Around Room 'Always' Quiet at Night	300+	64%	-	58%
Doctors 'Always' Communicated Well	300+	84%	-	80%
Home Recovery Information Given	300+	83%	-	82%
Hospital Given 9 or 10 on 10 Point Scale	300+	74%	-	67%
Meds 'Always' Explained Before Given	300+	66%	-	60%
Nurses 'Always' Communicated Well	300+	79%	-	76%
Pain 'Always' Well Controlled	300+	74%	-	69%
Room and Bathroom 'Always' Clean	300+	72%	-	71%
Timely Help 'Always' Received	300+	68%	-	64%
Would Definitely Recommend Hospital	300+	73%	-	69%

Ephraim Mcdowell Fort Logan Hospital

110 Metker Trail, Stanford, KY 40484
Phone: 606-365-4600
Fax: 606-365-7900
E-mail: flh@searnet.com
URL: www.emhealth.org
Type: Critical Access Hospitals
Emergency Services: Yes
Ownership: Voluntary Non-Profit - Private
Beds: 25

Key Personnel:
CEO/President. . . . . Vicki A Darnell
Chief of Medical Staff . . . . Narea James, MD
Infection Control. . . . . Mary Lou Lynn, RN
Radiology. . . . . Shawn D Grant
Anesthesiology. . . . . Balazs Makaj, MD
Emergency Room . . . . Paula Ledford, DON

Measure	Cases	This Hosp.	State Avg.	U.S. Avg.
Heart Attack Care				
ACE Inhibitor or ARB for LVSD	0	-	94%	96%
Aspirin at Arrival[1]	7	86%	98%	99%
Aspirin at Discharge[1]	2	100%	99%	98%
Beta Blocker at Discharge[1]	2	100%	98%	98%
Fibrinolytic Medication Timing	0	-	60%	55%
PCI Within 90 Minutes of Arrival	0	-	88%	90%
Smoking Cessation Advice[1]	1	100%	100%	99%
Chest Pain/Possible Heart Attack Care				
Aspirin at Arrival	-	-	95%	95%
Median Time to ECG (minutes)	-	-	7	8
Median Time to Transfer (minutes)	-	-	65	61
Fibrinolytic Medication Timing	-	-	62%	54%
Heart Failure Care				
ACE Inhibitor or ARB for LVSD[1]	9	89%	91%	94%
Discharge Instructions	27	96%	82%	88%
Evaluation of LVS Function	36	100%	96%	98%
Smoking Cessation Advice[1]	7	100%	98%	98%
Pneumonia Care				
Appropriate Initial Antibiotic	48	100%	90%	92%
Blood Culture Timing	66	98%	95%	96%
Influenza Vaccine	59	98%	92%	91%
Initial Antibiotic Timing	93	98%	95%	95%
Pneumococcal Vaccine	83	100%	94%	93%
Smoking Cessation Advice	47	100%	98%	97%
Surgical Care Improvement Project				
Appropriate VTP Within 24 Hours[1]	1	100%	91%	92%
Appropriate Hair Removal	30	100%	99%	99%
Appropriate Beta Blocker Usage[1]	4	75%	93%	93%
Controlled Postoperative Blood Glucose[5]	0	-	94%	93%
Prophylactic Antibiotic Timing	32	97%	97%	97%
Prophylactic Antibiotic Timing (Outpatient)	-	-	92%	92%
Prophylactic Antibiotic Selection	32	97%	98%	97%
Prophylactic Antibiotic Select. (Outpatient)	-	-	93%	94%
Prophylactic Antibiotic Stopped	31	100%	94%	94%
Recommended VTP Ordered[1]	1	100%	94%	94%
Urinary Catheter Removal	0	-	89%	90%
Children's Asthma Care				
Received Systemic Corticosteroids	-	-	-	100%
Received Home Management Plan	-	-	-	71%
Received Reliever Medication	-	-	-	100%
Use of Medical Imaging				
Combination Abdominal CT Scan	-	-	0.160	0.191
Combination Chest CT Scan	-	-	0.054	0.054
Follow-up Mammogram/Ultrasound	-	-	7.9%	8.4%
MRI for Low Back Pain	-	-	35.6%	32.7%
Survey of Patients' Hospital Experiences				
Area Around Room 'Always' Quiet at Night	(a)	61%	-	58%
Doctors 'Always' Communicated Well	(a)	77%	-	80%
Home Recovery Information Given	(a)	84%	-	82%
Hospital Given 9 or 10 on 10 Point Scale	(a)	71%	-	67%
Meds 'Always' Explained Before Given	(a)	65%	-	60%
Nurses 'Always' Communicated Well	(a)	78%	-	76%
Pain 'Always' Well Controlled	(a)	65%	-	69%
Room and Bathroom 'Always' Clean	(a)	77%	-	71%
Timely Help 'Always' Received	(a)	69%	-	64%
Would Definitely Recommend Hospital	(a)	72%	-	69%

NOTE: Hospital profiles are in alphabetical order by state, then city, then hospital within the city; Rankings exclude hospitals with less than 25 cases except for patient surveys which excludes hospitals with less than 100 cases; (a) 100–299 cases; (1) The number of cases is too small to be sure how well a hospital is performing; (2) The hospital indicated that the data submitted for this measure were based on a sample of cases; (3) Data was collected during a shorter time period (fewer quarters) than the maximum possible time for this measure; (4) Suppressed for one or more quarters by CMS; (5) No data is available from the hospital for this measure; (6) Fewer than 100 patients completed the HCAHPS survey. Use these rates with caution, as the number of surveys may be too low to reliably assess hospital performance; (7) Survey results are based on less than 12 months of data; (8) Survey results are not available for this reporting period; (9) No or very few patients were eligible for the HCAHPS survey. The scores shown, if any, reflect a very small number of surveys; (10) A state average was not calculated because too few hospitals in the state submitted data; (11) There were discrepancies in the data collection process; Please refer to the User's Guide for a full explanation of data.

Monroe County Medical Center

529 Capp Harlan Road
Tompkinsville, KY 42167
URL: www.mcmccares.com
Type: Acute Care Hospitals
Ownership: Voluntary Non-Profit - Private

Phone: 270-487-9231
Fax: 270-487-5784

Emergency Services: Yes
Beds: 49

Key Personnel:
CEO/President . . . . Vicky McFall
Chief of Medical Staff . . . . Anthony C Carter
Infection Control . . . . Lisa Davis RN
Quality Assurance . . . . Dana Hammer
Radiology . . . . Joseph J Brennan
Emergency Room . . . . Moujahed Achtar

Measure	Cases	This Hosp.	State Avg.	U.S. Avg.
Heart Attack Care				
ACE Inhibitor or ARB for LVSD[1]	3	67%	94%	96%
Aspirin at Arrival[1]	9	78%	98%	99%
Aspirin at Discharge[1]	4	75%	99%	98%
Beta Blocker at Discharge[1]	5	60%	98%	98%
Fibrinolytic Medication Timing	0	-	60%	55%
PCI Within 90 Minutes of Arrival	0	-	88%	90%
Smoking Cessation Advice[1]	2	100%	100%	99%
Chest Pain/Possible Heart Attack Care				
Aspirin at Arrival	79	100%	95%	95%
Median Time to ECG (minutes)	83	6	7	8
Median Time to Transfer (minutes)[1,3]	1	182	65	61
Fibrinolytic Medication Timing[1]	5	80%	62%	54%
Heart Failure Care				
ACE Inhibitor or ARB for LVSD[1]	21	71%	91%	94%
Discharge Instructions	86	67%	82%	88%
Evaluation of LVS Function	112	79%	96%	98%
Smoking Cessation Advice	35	77%	98%	98%
Pneumonia Care				
Appropriate Initial Antibiotic	59	86%	90%	92%
Blood Culture Timing	54	70%	95%	96%
Influenza Vaccine	64	77%	92%	91%
Initial Antibiotic Timing	96	94%	95%	95%
Pneumococcal Vaccine	86	81%	94%	93%
Smoking Cessation Advice	46	83%	98%	97%
Surgical Care Improvement Project				
Appropriate VTP Within 24 Hours[5]	0	-	91%	92%
Appropriate Hair Removal[5]	0	-	99%	99%
Appropriate Beta Blocker Usage[5]	0	-	93%	93%
Controlled Postoperative Blood Glucose[5]	0	-	94%	93%
Prophylactic Antibiotic Timing[5]	0	-	97%	97%
Prophylactic Antibiotic Timing (Outpatient)[5]	0	-	92%	92%
Prophylactic Antibiotic Selection[5]	0	-	98%	97%
Prophylactic Antibiotic Select. (Outpatient)[5]	0	-	93%	94%
Prophylactic Antibiotic Stopped[5]	0	-	94%	94%
Recommended VTP Ordered[5]	0	-	94%	94%
Urinary Catheter Removal[5]	0	-	89%	90%
Children's Asthma Care				
Received Systemic Corticosteroids	-	-	-	100%
Received Home Management Plan	-	-	-	71%
Received Reliever Medication	-	-	-	100%
Use of Medical Imaging				
Combination Abdominal CT Scan	196	0.459	0.160	0.191
Combination Chest CT Scan	145	0.338	0.054	0.054
Follow-up Mammogram/Ultrasound	106	5.7%	7.9%	8.4%
MRI for Low Back Pain	58	29.3%	35.6%	32.7%
Survey of Patients' Hospital Experiences				
Area Around Room 'Always' Quiet at Night	300+	62%	-	58%
Doctors 'Always' Communicated Well	300+	85%	-	80%
Home Recovery Information Given	300+	73%	-	82%
Hospital Given 9 or 10 on 10 Point Scale	300+	65%	-	67%
Meds 'Always' Explained Before Given	300+	57%	-	60%
Nurses 'Always' Communicated Well	300+	77%	-	76%
Pain 'Always' Well Controlled	300+	70%	-	69%
Room and Bathroom 'Always' Clean	300+	82%	-	71%
Timely Help 'Always' Received	300+	56%	-	64%
Would Definitely Recommend Hospital	300+	61%	-	69%

Bluegrass Community Hospital

360 Amsden Avenue
Versailles, KY 40383
Type: Critical Access Hospitals
Ownership: Proprietary

Phone: 859-879-2300
Fax: 859-873-1016
Emergency Services: Yes
Beds: 73

Key Personnel:
CEO/President . . . . Nancy Littrell
Chief of Medical Staff . . . . W Foley
Infection Control . . . . Tina Cairell
Operating Room . . . . Sherri Taylor, RN
Pediatric Ambulatory Care . . . . . C Rener
Pediatric In-Patient Care . . . . . . C Rener
Quality Assurance . . . . Barbara Kauppi
Intensive Care Unit . . . . Dale Goodin, MD

Measure	Cases	This Hosp.	State Avg.	U.S. Avg.
Heart Attack Care				
ACE Inhibitor or ARB for LVSD[5]	0	-	94%	96%
Aspirin at Arrival[5]	0	-	98%	99%
Aspirin at Discharge[5]	0	-	99%	98%
Beta Blocker at Discharge[5]	0	-	98%	98%
Fibrinolytic Medication Timing[5]	0	-	60%	55%
PCI Within 90 Minutes of Arrival[5]	0	-	88%	90%
Smoking Cessation Advice[5]	0	-	100%	99%
Chest Pain/Possible Heart Attack Care				
Aspirin at Arrival	-	-	95%	95%
Median Time to ECG (minutes)	-	-	7	8
Median Time to Transfer (minutes)	-	-	65	61
Fibrinolytic Medication Timing	-	-	62%	54%
Heart Failure Care				
ACE Inhibitor or ARB for LVSD[1]	3	100%	91%	94%
Discharge Instructions[1]	11	100%	82%	88%
Evaluation of LVS Function[1]	13	100%	96%	98%
Smoking Cessation Advice[1]	3	100%	98%	98%
Pneumonia Care				
Appropriate Initial Antibiotic	26	96%	90%	92%
Blood Culture Timing	30	100%	95%	96%
Influenza Vaccine[1]	24	100%	92%	91%
Initial Antibiotic Timing	37	100%	95%	95%
Pneumococcal Vaccine[1]	24	100%	94%	93%
Smoking Cessation Advice[1]	18	100%	98%	97%
Surgical Care Improvement Project				
Appropriate VTP Within 24 Hours[1]	12	92%	91%	92%
Appropriate Hair Removal	40	100%	99%	99%
Appropriate Beta Blocker Usage[1,3]	8	100%	93%	93%
Controlled Postoperative Blood Glucose	0	-	94%	93%
Prophylactic Antibiotic Timing	30	100%	97%	97%
Prophylactic Antibiotic Timing (Outpatient)	-	-	92%	92%
Prophylactic Antibiotic Selection	30	100%	98%	97%
Prophylactic Antibiotic Select. (Outpatient)	-	-	93%	94%
Prophylactic Antibiotic Stopped	29	93%	94%	94%
Recommended VTP Ordered[1]	12	92%	94%	94%
Urinary Catheter Removal[1]	10	100%	89%	90%
Children's Asthma Care				
Received Systemic Corticosteroids	-	-	-	100%
Received Home Management Plan	-	-	-	71%
Received Reliever Medication	-	-	-	100%
Use of Medical Imaging				
Combination Abdominal CT Scan	-	-	0.160	0.191
Combination Chest CT Scan	-	-	0.054	0.054
Follow-up Mammogram/Ultrasound	-	-	7.9%	8.4%
MRI for Low Back Pain	-	-	35.6%	32.7%
Survey of Patients' Hospital Experiences				
Area Around Room 'Always' Quiet at Night[6]	<100	65%	-	58%
Doctors 'Always' Communicated Well[6]	<100	82%	-	80%
Home Recovery Information Given[6]	<100	83%	-	82%
Hospital Given 9 or 10 on 10 Point Scale[6]	<100	81%	-	67%
Meds 'Always' Explained Before Given[6]	<100	51%	-	60%
Nurses 'Always' Communicated Well[6]	<100	78%	-	76%
Pain 'Always' Well Controlled[6]	<100	66%	-	69%
Room and Bathroom 'Always' Clean[6]	<100	77%	-	71%
Timely Help 'Always' Received[6]	<100	69%	-	64%
Would Definitely Recommend Hospital	<100	66%	-	69%

Morgan County Arh Hospital

476 Liberty Road
West Liberty, KY 41472
URL: www.arh.org/morgan
Type: Critical Access Hospitals
Ownership: Voluntary Non-Profit - Private

Phone: 606-743-3186
Fax: 606-743-9604

Emergency Services: Yes
Beds: 50

Key Personnel:
CEO/President . . . . Timothy A Hatfield
Chief of Medical Staff . . . . Diana V Soarici, MD
Infection Control . . . . Patricia Lewis, RN
Quality Assurance . . . . Dolores Luke
Emergency Room . . . . Gail Perry, RN

Measure	Cases	This Hosp.	State Avg.	U.S. Avg.
Heart Attack Care				
ACE Inhibitor or ARB for LVSD[3]	0	-	94%	96%
Aspirin at Arrival[3]	0	-	98%	99%
Aspirin at Discharge[3]	0	-	99%	98%
Beta Blocker at Discharge[3]	0	-	98%	98%
Fibrinolytic Medication Timing[3]	0	-	60%	55%
PCI Within 90 Minutes of Arrival[3]	0	-	88%	90%
Smoking Cessation Advice[3]	0	-	100%	99%
Chest Pain/Possible Heart Attack Care				
Aspirin at Arrival[5]	0	-	95%	95%
Median Time to ECG (minutes)[5]	0	-	7	8
Median Time to Transfer (minutes)[5]	0	-	65	61
Fibrinolytic Medication Timing[5]	0	-	62%	54%
Heart Failure Care				
ACE Inhibitor or ARB for LVSD[1]	6	67%	91%	94%
Discharge Instructions	28	100%	82%	88%
Evaluation of LVS Function	32	91%	96%	98%
Smoking Cessation Advice[1]	6	100%	98%	98%
Pneumonia Care				
Appropriate Initial Antibiotic	72	89%	90%	92%
Blood Culture Timing	61	92%	95%	96%
Influenza Vaccine	45	100%	92%	91%
Initial Antibiotic Timing	78	97%	95%	95%
Pneumococcal Vaccine	62	100%	94%	93%
Smoking Cessation Advice[1]	21	100%	98%	97%
Surgical Care Improvement Project				
Appropriate VTP Within 24 Hours[5]	0	-	91%	92%
Appropriate Hair Removal[5]	0	-	99%	99%
Appropriate Beta Blocker Usage[5]	0	-	93%	93%
Controlled Postoperative Blood Glucose[5]	0	-	94%	93%
Prophylactic Antibiotic Timing[5]	0	-	97%	97%
Prophylactic Antibiotic Timing (Outpatient)[5]	0	-	92%	92%
Prophylactic Antibiotic Selection[5]	0	-	98%	97%
Prophylactic Antibiotic Select. (Outpatient)[5]	0	-	93%	94%
Prophylactic Antibiotic Stopped[5]	0	-	94%	94%
Recommended VTP Ordered[5]	0	-	94%	94%
Urinary Catheter Removal[5]	0	-	89%	90%
Children's Asthma Care				
Received Systemic Corticosteroids	-	-	-	100%
Received Home Management Plan	-	-	-	71%
Received Reliever Medication	-	-	-	100%
Use of Medical Imaging				
Combination Abdominal CT Scan	185	0.022	0.160	0.191
Combination Chest CT Scan	77	0.026	0.054	0.054
Follow-up Mammogram/Ultrasound	86	4.7%	7.9%	8.4%
MRI for Low Back Pain[1]	34	44.1%	35.6%	32.7%
Survey of Patients' Hospital Experiences				
Area Around Room 'Always' Quiet at Night	(a)	76%	-	58%
Doctors 'Always' Communicated Well	(a)	92%	-	80%
Home Recovery Information Given	(a)	91%	-	82%
Hospital Given 9 or 10 on 10 Point Scale	(a)	79%	-	67%
Meds 'Always' Explained Before Given	(a)	79%	-	60%
Nurses 'Always' Communicated Well	(a)	81%	-	76%
Pain 'Always' Well Controlled	(a)	76%	-	69%
Room and Bathroom 'Always' Clean	(a)	86%	-	71%
Timely Help 'Always' Received	(a)	81%	-	64%
Would Definitely Recommend Hospital	(a)	82%	-	69%

NOTE: Hospital profiles are in alphabetical order by state, then city, then hospital within the city; Rankings exclude hospitals with less than 25 cases except for patient surveys which excludes hospitals with less than 100 cases; (a) 100–299 cases; (1) The number of cases is too small to be sure how well a hospital is performing; (2) The hospital indicated that the data submitted for this measure were based on a sample of cases; (3) Data was collected during a shorter time period (fewer quarters) than the maximum possible time for this measure; (4) Suppressed for one or more quarters by CMS; (5) No data is available from the hospital for this measure; (6) Fewer than 100 patients completed the HCAHPS survey. Use these rates with caution, as the number of surveys may be too low to reliably assess hospital performance; (7) Survey results are based on less than 12 months of data; (8) Survey results are not available for this reporting period; (9) No or very few patients were eligible for the HCAHPS survey. The scores shown, if any, reflect a very small number of surveys; (10) A state average was not calculated because too few hospitals in the state submitted data; (11) There were discrepancies in the data collection process; Please refer to the User's Guide for a full explanation of data.

Whitesburg ARH Hospital

240 Hospital Road
Whitesburg, KY 41858
URL: www.arh.org/whitesburg
Type: Acute Care Hospitals
Ownership: Voluntary Non-Profit - Other

Phone: 606-633-3500
Fax: 606-633-3652

Emergency Services: Yes
Beds: 82

Key Personnel:

CEO/President	Jerry W Haynes
Chief of Medical Staff	PS Chandra Shekar, MD
Coronary Care	Teresa Hogg
Infection Control	Glenda Helton
Operating Room	Charles Crumley
Quality Assurance	Gail McConnell
Radiology	John J Beasley
Patient Relations	Heather Burton

Measure	Cases	This Hosp.	State Avg.	U.S. Avg.
Heart Attack Care				
ACE Inhibitor or ARB for LVSD[1]	1	100%	94%	96%
Aspirin at Arrival[1]	7	100%	98%	99%
Aspirin at Discharge[1]	4	100%	99%	98%
Beta Blocker at Discharge[1]	3	100%	98%	98%
Fibrinolytic Medication Timing[1]	1	100%	60%	55%
PCI Within 90 Minutes of Arrival	0	-	88%	90%
Smoking Cessation Advice[1]	2	100%	100%	99%
Chest Pain/Possible Heart Attack Care				
Aspirin at Arrival	124	99%	95%	95%
Median Time to ECG (minutes)	116	17	7	8
Median Time to Transfer (minutes)[5]	0	-	65	61
Fibrinolytic Medication Timing[1]	3	100%	62%	54%
Heart Failure Care				
ACE Inhibitor or ARB for LVSD	28	96%	91%	94%
Discharge Instructions	177	92%	82%	88%
Evaluation of LVS Function	201	95%	96%	98%
Smoking Cessation Advice	41	100%	98%	98%
Pneumonia Care				
Appropriate Initial Antibiotic	150	93%	90%	92%
Blood Culture Timing	108	92%	95%	96%
Influenza Vaccine	105	79%	92%	91%
Initial Antibiotic Timing	181	98%	95%	95%
Pneumococcal Vaccine	113	86%	94%	93%
Smoking Cessation Advice	89	100%	98%	97%
Surgical Care Improvement Project				
Appropriate VTP Within 24 Hours[1]	20	100%	91%	92%
Appropriate Hair Removal	63	100%	99%	99%
Appropriate Beta Blocker Usage[1]	12	92%	93%	93%
Controlled Postoperative Blood Glucose	0	-	94%	93%
Prophylactic Antibiotic Timing	46	96%	97%	97%
Prophylactic Antibiotic Timing (Outpatient)	121	96%	92%	92%
Prophylactic Antibiotic Selection	47	91%	98%	97%
Prophylactic Antibiotic Select. (Outpatient)	118	93%	93%	94%
Prophylactic Antibiotic Stopped	44	91%	94%	94%
Recommended VTP Ordered[1]	20	100%	94%	94%
Urinary Catheter Removal[1]	2	100%	89%	90%
Children's Asthma Care				
Received Systemic Corticosteroids	-	-	-	100%
Received Home Management Plan	-	-	-	71%
Received Reliever Medication	-	-	-	100%
Use of Medical Imaging				
Combination Abdominal CT Scan	265	0.030	0.160	0.191
Combination Chest CT Scan	101	0.020	0.054	0.054
Follow-up Mammogram/Ultrasound	260	7.7%	7.9%	8.4%
MRI for Low Back Pain	73	26.0%	35.6%	32.7%
Survey of Patients' Hospital Experiences				
Area Around Room 'Always' Quiet at Night	300+	62%	-	58%
Doctors 'Always' Communicated Well	300+	87%	-	80%
Home Recovery Information Given	300+	84%	-	82%
Hospital Given 9 or 10 on 10 Point Scale	300+	72%	-	67%
Meds 'Always' Explained Before Given	300+	64%	-	60%
Nurses 'Always' Communicated Well	300+	82%	-	76%
Pain 'Always' Well Controlled	300+	71%	-	69%
Room and Bathroom 'Always' Clean	300+	75%	-	71%
Timely Help 'Always' Received	300+	74%	-	64%
Would Definitely Recommend Hospital	300+	71%	-	69%

Saint Elizabeth Grant

238 Barnes Road
Williamstown, KY 41097
URL: www.stelizabeth.com
Type: Critical Access Hospitals
Ownership: Voluntary Non-Profit - Church

Phone: 859-824-8240
Fax: 859-824-8118

Emergency Services: Yes
Beds: 30

Key Personnel:

CEO/President	Joseph Gross
Chief of Medical Staff	LeRoy Kendall, MD

Measure	Cases	This Hosp.	State Avg.	U.S. Avg.
Heart Attack Care				
ACE Inhibitor or ARB for LVSD[3]	0	-	94%	96%
Aspirin at Arrival[1,3]	1	100%	98%	99%
Aspirin at Discharge[3]	0	-	99%	98%
Beta Blocker at Discharge[3]	0	-	98%	98%
Fibrinolytic Medication Timing[3]	0	-	60%	55%
PCI Within 90 Minutes of Arrival[3]	0	-	88%	90%
Smoking Cessation Advice[3]	0	-	100%	99%
Chest Pain/Possible Heart Attack Care				
Aspirin at Arrival[5]	0	-	95%	95%
Median Time to ECG (minutes)[5]	0	-	7	8
Median Time to Transfer (minutes)[5]	0	-	65	61
Fibrinolytic Medication Timing[5]	0	-	62%	54%
Heart Failure Care				
ACE Inhibitor or ARB for LVSD[1]	4	100%	91%	94%
Discharge Instructions	33	88%	82%	88%
Evaluation of LVS Function	34	100%	96%	98%
Smoking Cessation Advice[1]	8	100%	98%	98%
Pneumonia Care				
Appropriate Initial Antibiotic	32	100%	90%	92%
Blood Culture Timing[1]	12	100%	95%	96%
Influenza Vaccine[1]	18	100%	92%	91%
Initial Antibiotic Timing	37	100%	95%	95%
Pneumococcal Vaccine	28	100%	94%	93%
Smoking Cessation Advice[1]	12	100%	98%	97%
Surgical Care Improvement Project				
Appropriate VTP Within 24 Hours[5]	0	-	91%	92%
Appropriate Hair Removal[5]	0	-	99%	99%
Appropriate Beta Blocker Usage[5]	0	-	93%	93%
Controlled Postoperative Blood Glucose[5]	0	-	94%	93%
Prophylactic Antibiotic Timing[5]	0	-	97%	97%
Prophylactic Antibiotic Timing (Outpatient)[5]	0	-	92%	92%
Prophylactic Antibiotic Selection[5]	0	-	98%	97%
Prophylactic Antibiotic Select. (Outpatient)[5]	0	-	93%	94%
Prophylactic Antibiotic Stopped[5]	0	-	94%	94%
Recommended VTP Ordered[5]	0	-	94%	94%
Urinary Catheter Removal[5]	0	-	89%	90%
Children's Asthma Care				
Received Systemic Corticosteroids	-	-	-	100%
Received Home Management Plan	-	-	-	71%
Received Reliever Medication	-	-	-	100%
Use of Medical Imaging				
Combination Abdominal CT Scan	369	0.062	0.160	0.191
Combination Chest CT Scan	144	0.000	0.054	0.054
Follow-up Mammogram/Ultrasound	235	6.8%	7.9%	8.4%
MRI for Low Back Pain	90	44.4%	35.6%	32.7%
Survey of Patients' Hospital Experiences				
Area Around Room 'Always' Quiet at Night	(a)	67%	-	58%
Doctors 'Always' Communicated Well	(a)	84%	-	80%
Home Recovery Information Given	(a)	88%	-	82%
Hospital Given 9 or 10 on 10 Point Scale	(a)	80%	-	67%
Meds 'Always' Explained Before Given	(a)	66%	-	60%
Nurses 'Always' Communicated Well	(a)	83%	-	76%
Pain 'Always' Well Controlled	(a)	75%	-	69%
Room and Bathroom 'Always' Clean	(a)	78%	-	71%
Timely Help 'Always' Received	(a)	83%	-	64%
Would Definitely Recommend Hospital	(a)	74%	-	69%

Clark Regional Medical Center

1107 West Lexington Avenue
Winchester, KY 40391
URL: www.clarkregional.org
Type: Acute Care Hospitals
Ownership: Voluntary Non-Profit - Private

Phone: 859-745-3500
Fax: 859-744-6408

Emergency Services: Yes
Beds: 100

Key Personnel:

CEO/President	Robert Fraraccio
Chief of Medical Staff	Richard Chamberlin, MD
Radiology	William Cooper

Measure	Cases	This Hosp.	State Avg.	U.S. Avg.
Heart Attack Care				
ACE Inhibitor or ARB for LVSD[1]	4	50%	94%	96%
Aspirin at Arrival[1]	11	91%	98%	99%
Aspirin at Discharge[1]	7	100%	99%	98%
Beta Blocker at Discharge[1]	7	100%	98%	98%
Fibrinolytic Medication Timing	0	-	60%	55%
PCI Within 90 Minutes of Arrival	0	-	88%	90%
Smoking Cessation Advice[1]	2	100%	100%	99%
Chest Pain/Possible Heart Attack Care				
Aspirin at Arrival	331	89%	95%	95%
Median Time to ECG (minutes)	346	7	7	8
Median Time to Transfer (minutes)[1,3]	4	76	65	61
Fibrinolytic Medication Timing[1]	1	0%	62%	54%
Heart Failure Care				
ACE Inhibitor or ARB for LVSD[1]	19	58%	91%	94%
Discharge Instructions	45	76%	82%	88%
Evaluation of LVS Function	51	94%	96%	98%
Smoking Cessation Advice[1]	11	100%	98%	98%
Pneumonia Care				
Appropriate Initial Antibiotic	154	83%	90%	92%
Blood Culture Timing	155	92%	95%	96%
Influenza Vaccine	86	95%	92%	91%
Initial Antibiotic Timing	182	96%	95%	95%
Pneumococcal Vaccine	116	97%	94%	93%
Smoking Cessation Advice	91	98%	98%	97%
Surgical Care Improvement Project				
Appropriate VTP Within 24 Hours[2]	50	84%	91%	92%
Appropriate Hair Removal[2]	189	100%	99%	99%
Appropriate Beta Blocker Usage[2]	45	76%	93%	93%
Controlled Postoperative Blood Glucose[2]	0	-	94%	93%
Prophylactic Antibiotic Timing[2]	158	94%	97%	97%
Prophylactic Antibiotic Timing (Outpatient)	46	76%	92%	92%
Prophylactic Antibiotic Selection[2]	158	97%	98%	97%
Prophylactic Antibiotic Select. (Outpatient)	41	95%	93%	94%
Prophylactic Antibiotic Stopped[2]	153	88%	94%	94%
Recommended VTP Ordered[2]	50	92%	94%	94%
Urinary Catheter Removal[2]	43	84%	89%	90%
Children's Asthma Care				
Received Systemic Corticosteroids	-	-	-	100%
Received Home Management Plan	-	-	-	71%
Received Reliever Medication	-	-	-	100%
Use of Medical Imaging				
Combination Abdominal CT Scan	443	0.515	0.160	0.191
Combination Chest CT Scan	282	0.429	0.054	0.054
Follow-up Mammogram/Ultrasound	480	3.3%	7.9%	8.4%
MRI for Low Back Pain	73	39.7%	35.6%	32.7%
Survey of Patients' Hospital Experiences				
Area Around Room 'Always' Quiet at Night	300+	58%	-	58%
Doctors 'Always' Communicated Well	300+	90%	-	80%
Home Recovery Information Given	300+	88%	-	82%
Hospital Given 9 or 10 on 10 Point Scale	300+	74%	-	67%
Meds 'Always' Explained Before Given	300+	74%	-	60%
Nurses 'Always' Communicated Well	300+	85%	-	76%
Pain 'Always' Well Controlled	300+	78%	-	69%
Room and Bathroom 'Always' Clean	300+	84%	-	71%
Timely Help 'Always' Received	300+	76%	-	64%
Would Definitely Recommend Hospital	300+	75%	-	69%

Heart Attack Care

1. ACE Inhibitor or ARB for LVSD

Hospital Name	City	Rate	Cases
Eastern Maine Medical Center	Bangor	99%	110
Maine Medical Center	Portland	99%	100
Central Maine Medical Center[2]	Lewiston	97%	31

2. Aspirin at Arrival

Hospital Name	City	Rate	Cases
Cary Medical Center	Caribou	100%	28
Eastern Maine Medical Center	Bangor	100%	247
Maine Coast Memorial Hospital	Ellsworth	100%	47
Mercy Hospital	Portland	100%	55
Mid Coast Hospital	Brunswick	100%	49
Penobscot Bay Medical Center	Rockport	100%	38
Saint Joseph Hospital	Bangor	100%	78
York Hospital	York	100%	71
Central Maine Medical Center[2]	Lewiston	99%	176
Maine General Medical Center	Augusta	99%	166
Maine Medical Center	Portland	99%	372
Southern Maine Medical Center	Biddeford	99%	99
Saint Marys Regional Medical Center	Lewiston	98%	51
Aroostook Medical Center	Presque Isle	96%	49
Henrietta D Goodall Hospital	Sanford	94%	36

3. Aspirin at Discharge

Hospital Name	City	Rate	Cases
Central Maine Medical Center[2]	Lewiston	100%	289
Maine Medical Center	Portland	100%	988
Mercy Hospital	Portland	100%	32
Mid Coast Hospital	Brunswick	100%	31
Penobscot Bay Medical Center	Rockport	100%	25
Saint Marys Regional Medical Center	Lewiston	100%	37
Eastern Maine Medical Center	Bangor	99%	921
Southern Maine Medical Center	Biddeford	99%	67
Maine General Medical Center	Augusta	98%	89
Saint Joseph Hospital	Bangor	98%	51
York Hospital	York	98%	60
Aroostook Medical Center	Presque Isle	97%	36
Maine Coast Memorial Hospital	Ellsworth	96%	27

4. Beta Blocker at Discharge

Hospital Name	City	Rate	Cases
Eastern Maine Medical Center	Bangor	100%	880
Henrietta D Goodall Hospital	Sanford	100%	26
Maine General Medical Center	Augusta	100%	100
Mid Coast Hospital	Brunswick	100%	31
Saint Joseph Hospital	Bangor	100%	50
Southern Maine Medical Center	Biddeford	100%	70
York Hospital	York	100%	59
Maine Medical Center	Portland	99%	979
Central Maine Medical Center[2]	Lewiston	97%	278
Mercy Hospital	Portland	97%	31
Aroostook Medical Center	Presque Isle	95%	37
Saint Marys Regional Medical Center	Lewiston	94%	35

6. PCI Within 90 Minutes of Arrival

Hospital Name	City	Rate	Cases
Eastern Maine Medical Center	Bangor	95%	38
Maine Medical Center	Portland	92%	76

7. Smoking Cessation Advice

Hospital Name	City	Rate	Cases
Central Maine Medical Center[2]	Lewiston	100%	109
Eastern Maine Medical Center	Bangor	100%	310
Maine Medical Center	Portland	99%	286

Chest Pain/Possible Heart Attack Care

8. Aspirin at Arrival

Hospital Name	City	Rate	Cases
Down East Community Hospital	Machias	100%	81
Inland Hospital	Waterville	100%	74
Penobscot Bay Medical Center	Rockport	100%	49
Saint Andrews Hospital[3]	Boothbay Hrbr	100%	49
Southern Maine Medical Center	Biddeford	100%	73
Maine General Medical Center	Augusta	99%	113
Aroostook Medical Center	Presque Isle	98%	50
Mid Coast Hospital	Brunswick	98%	60
Stephens Memorial Hospital	Norway	98%	58
Henrietta D Goodall Hospital	Sanford	96%	50
Maine Coast Memorial Hospital	Ellsworth	96%	47
Miles Memorial Hospital	Damariscotta	96%	77
Redington Fairview General Hospital[3]	Skowhegan	93%	29
Franklin Memorial Hospital	Farmington	92%	39

9. Median Time to ECG (minutes)

Hospital Name	City	Min.	Cases
Aroostook Medical Center	Presque Isle	3	50
Henrietta D Goodall Hospital	Sanford	3	50
Mid Coast Hospital	Brunswick	4	61
Inland Hospital	Waterville	5	77
Maine General Medical Center	Augusta	5	118
Redington Fairview General Hospital[3]	Skowhegan	5	33
Miles Memorial Hospital	Damariscotta	6	78
Penobscot Bay Medical Center	Rockport	6	51
Saint Andrews Hospital[3]	Boothbay Hrbr	7	49
Franklin Memorial Hospital	Farmington	8	39
Stephens Memorial Hospital	Norway	8	58
Down East Community Hospital	Machias	10	85
Maine Coast Memorial Hospital	Ellsworth	10	47
Southern Maine Medical Center	Biddeford	11	73

10. Median Time to Transfer (minutes)

Hospital Name	City	Min.	Cases
Southern Maine Medical Center	Biddeford	26	32

11. Fibrinolytic Medication Timing

Hospital Name	City	Rate	Cases
Maine General Medical Center	Augusta	88%	43

Heart Failure Care

12. ACE Inhibitor or ARB for LVSD

Hospital Name	City	Rate	Cases
Eastern Maine Medical Center	Bangor	100%	118
Mid Coast Hospital	Brunswick	100%	42
Saint Joseph Hospital	Bangor	100%	35
Central Maine Medical Center	Lewiston	99%	79
Southern Maine Medical Center[2]	Biddeford	98%	40
Maine General Medical Center	Augusta	96%	68
Maine Medical Center	Portland	96%	160

13. Discharge Instructions

Hospital Name	City	Rate	Cases
Down East Community Hospital	Machias	100%	29
Houlton Regional Hospital	Houlton	100%	26
Mid Coast Hospital	Brunswick	100%	75
Sebasticook Valley Hospital	Pittsfield	100%	38
Central Maine Medical Center	Lewiston	99%	194
Franklin Memorial Hospital	Farmington	99%	67
Mercy Hospital	Portland	99%	98
Cary Medical Center	Caribou	98%	52
Saint Joseph Hospital	Bangor	98%	109
Penobscot Bay Medical Center	Rockport	96%	80
York Hospital	York	96%	93
Saint Marys Regional Medical Center	Lewiston	93%	68
Maine General Medical Center	Augusta	92%	167
Miles Memorial Hospital	Damariscotta	91%	54
Bridgton Hospital	Bridgton	90%	30
Eastern Maine Medical Center	Bangor	90%	301
Southern Maine Medical Center[2]	Biddeford	90%	141
Togus VA Medical Center	Augusta	88%	64
Parkview Adventist Medical Center	Brunswick	87%	38
Henrietta D Goodall Hospital	Sanford	86%	65
Maine Medical Center	Portland	86%	477
Redington Fairview General Hospital	Skowhegan	84%	38
Inland Hospital	Waterville	83%	29
Aroostook Medical Center	Presque Isle	81%	58
Millinocket Regional Hospital	Millinocket	81%	27
Maine Coast Memorial Hospital	Ellsworth	79%	43

14. Evaluation of LVS Function

Hospital Name	City	Rate	Cases
Cary Medical Center	Caribou	100%	69
Central Maine Medical Center	Lewiston	100%	258
Down East Community Hospital	Machias	100%	39
Eastern Maine Medical Center	Bangor	100%	375
Inland Hospital	Waterville	100%	56
Maine Coast Memorial Hospital	Ellsworth	100%	63
Maine General Medical Center	Augusta	100%	215
Mercy Hospital	Portland	100%	166
Mid Coast Hospital	Brunswick	100%	95
Miles Memorial Hospital	Damariscotta	100%	68
Northern Maine Medical Center	Fort Kent	100%	32
Saint Joseph Hospital	Bangor	100%	144
Southern Maine Medical Center[2]	Biddeford	100%	207
Togus VA Medical Center	Augusta	100%	78
Aroostook Medical Center	Presque Isle	99%	67
Henrietta D Goodall Hospital	Sanford	99%	90
Maine Medical Center	Portland	99%	619
Penobscot Bay Medical Center	Rockport	99%	116
Saint Marys Regional Medical Center	Lewiston	99%	133
Houlton Regional Hospital	Houlton	98%	50
Redington Fairview General Hospital	Skowhegan	98%	52
York Hospital	York	98%	122
Millinocket Regional Hospital	Millinocket	97%	35
Mount Desert Island Hospital	Bar Harbor	97%	29
Rumford Hospital	Rumford	97%	35
Franklin Memorial Hospital	Farmington	95%	91
Bridgton Hospital	Bridgton	94%	31
Sebasticook Valley Hospital	Pittsfield	93%	44
Waldo County General Hospital	Belfast	93%	30
Parkview Adventist Medical Center	Brunswick	92%	48
Stephens Memorial Hospital	Norway	86%	35

15. Smoking Cessation Advice

Hospital Name	City	Rate	Cases
Central Maine Medical Center	Lewiston	100%	42
Maine General Medical Center	Augusta	100%	28
Eastern Maine Medical Center	Bangor	99%	73
Maine Medical Center	Portland	93%	67
Mercy Hospital	Portland	93%	30

Pneumonia Care

16. Appropriate Initial Antibiotic

Hospital Name	City	Rate	Cases
Penobscot Valley Hospital	Lincoln	100%	27
Redington Fairview General Hospital	Skowhegan	100%	72
Mid Coast Hospital[2]	Brunswick	99%	83
Saint Joseph Hospital	Bangor	99%	121
Cary Medical Center	Caribou	97%	32
Central Maine Medical Center[2]	Lewiston	97%	69
Franklin Memorial Hospital	Farmington	97%	30
Maine General Medical Center	Augusta	97%	154
York Hospital	York	97%	65
Calais Regional Hospital	Calais	96%	45
Henrietta D Goodall Hospital	Sanford	96%	71
Southern Maine Medical Center[2]	Biddeford	96%	80
Waldo County General Hospital	Belfast	96%	56
Houlton Regional Hospital	Houlton	95%	62
Maine Coast Memorial Hospital	Ellsworth	95%	44
Miles Memorial Hospital	Damariscotta	94%	49
Penobscot Bay Medical Center	Rockport	94%	64
Maine Medical Center	Portland	93%	111
Saint Marys Regional Medical Center	Lewiston	93%	58
Sebasticook Valley Hospital	Pittsfield	93%	41
Northern Maine Medical Center	Fort Kent	92%	38
Togus VA Medical Center	Augusta	92%	36
Bridgton Hospital	Bridgton	91%	46
Eastern Maine Medical Center	Bangor	91%	108
Mayo Regional Hospital	Dover Foxcroft	91%	35
Stephens Memorial Hospital[2]	Norway	91%	45
Aroostook Medical Center	Presque Isle	89%	44
Inland Hospital	Waterville	89%	27
Mercy Hospital	Portland	88%	115
Parkview Adventist Medical Center	Brunswick	82%	39
Down East Community Hospital	Machias	81%	26

17. Blood Culture Timing

Hospital Name	City	Rate	Cases
Cary Medical Center	Caribou	100%	39
Henrietta D Goodall Hospital	Sanford	100%	103
Houlton Regional Hospital	Houlton	100%	78
Inland Hospital	Waterville	100%	52
Millinocket Regional Hospital	Millinocket	100%	30
Mount Desert Island Hospital	Bar Harbor	100%	31
Penobscot Valley Hospital	Lincoln	100%	36
Waldo County General Hospital	Belfast	100%	34
Miles Memorial Hospital	Damariscotta	99%	75
Eastern Maine Medical Center	Bangor	98%	220
Northern Maine Medical Center	Fort Kent	98%	45
Redington Fairview General Hospital	Skowhegan	98%	105
Sebasticook Valley Hospital	Pittsfield	98%	47
Bridgton Hospital	Bridgton	97%	58
Maine General Medical Center	Augusta	97%	235
Penobscot Bay Medical Center	Rockport	97%	92
Stephens Memorial Hospital[2]	Norway	97%	71
York Hospital	York	97%	67
Saint Joseph Hospital	Bangor	96%	162
Aroostook Medical Center	Presque Isle	95%	83
Saint Marys Regional Medical Center	Lewiston	95%	44
Blue Hill Memorial Hospital	Blue Hill	94%	31
Down East Community Hospital	Machias	94%	47
Franklin Memorial Hospital	Farmington	94%	71
Mayo Regional Hospital	Dover Foxcroft	93%	46
Mercy Hospital	Portland	92%	149
Central Maine Medical Center[2]	Lewiston	91%	139
Parkview Adventist Medical Center	Brunswick	91%	46
Maine Medical Center	Portland	89%	338
Mid Coast Hospital[2]	Brunswick	89%	66

NOTE: Hospital profiles are in alphabetical order by state, then city, then hospital within the city; Rankings exclude hospitals with less than 25 cases except for patient surveys which excludes hospitals with less than 100 cases; (a) 100–299 cases; (1) The number of cases is too small to be sure how well a hospital is performing; (2) The hospital indicated that the data submitted for this measure were based on a sample of cases; (3) Data was collected during a shorter time period (fewer quarters) than the maximum possible time for this measure; (4) Suppressed for one or more quarters by CMS; (5) No data is available from the hospital for this measure; (6) Fewer than 100 patients completed the HCAHPS survey. Use these rates with caution, as the number of surveys may be too low to reliably assess hospital performance; (7) Survey results are based on less than 12 months of data; (8) Survey results are not available for this reporting period; (9) No or very few patients were eligible for the HCAHPS survey. The scores shown, if any, reflect a very small number of surveys; (10) A state average was not calculated because too few hospitals in the state submitted data; (11) There were discrepancies in the data collection process; Please refer to the User's Guide for a full explanation of data.

Southern Maine Medical Center[2]	Biddeford	89%	81
Togus VA Medical Center	Augusta	88%	41
Maine Coast Memorial Hospital	Ellsworth	87%	55
Rumford Hospital	Rumford	86%	44

18. Influenza Vaccine

Hospital Name	City	Rate	Cases
Aroostook Medical Center	Presque Isle	100%	33
Calais Regional Hospital	Calais	100%	26
Franklin Memorial Hospital	Farmington	100%	46
Henrietta D Goodall Hospital	Sanford	100%	82
Mayo Regional Hospital	Dover Foxcroft	100%	29
Mid Coast Hospital[2]	Brunswick	100%	78
Miles Memorial Hospital	Damariscotta	100%	43
Redington Fairview General Hospital	Skowhegan	100%	92
Rumford Hospital	Rumford	100%	28
Saint Joseph Hospital	Bangor	100%	116
Waldo County General Hospital	Belfast	100%	46
York Hospital	York	100%	66
Maine General Medical Center	Augusta	99%	167
Eastern Maine Medical Center	Bangor	98%	191
Houlton Regional Hospital	Houlton	98%	51
Penobscot Bay Medical Center	Rockport	98%	65
Southern Maine Medical Center[2]	Biddeford	98%	91
Stephens Memorial Hospital	Norway	98%	49
Inland Hospital	Waterville	97%	32
Maine Medical Center	Portland	97%	207
Parkview Adventist Medical Center	Brunswick	97%	33
Mercy Hospital	Portland	95%	103
Togus VA Medical Center	Augusta	95%	43
Bridgton Hospital	Bridgton	94%	36
Northern Maine Medical Center	Fort Kent	94%	34
Central Maine Medical Center[2]	Lewiston	91%	90
Saint Marys Regional Medical Center	Lewiston	82%	62
Maine Coast Memorial Hospital	Ellsworth	59%	51

19. Initial Antibiotic Timing

Hospital Name	City	Rate	Cases
Calais Regional Hospital	Calais	100%	53
Cary Medical Center	Caribou	100%	41
Central Maine Medical Center[2]	Lewiston	100%	137
Inland Hospital	Waterville	100%	43
Mount Desert Island Hospital	Bar Harbor	100%	27
Penobscot Valley Hospital	Lincoln	100%	38
Rumford Hospital	Rumford	100%	42
Sebasticook Valley Hospital	Pittsfield	100%	43
Waldo County General Hospital	Belfast	100%	76
Henrietta D Goodall Hospital	Sanford	99%	105
Mid Coast Hospital[2]	Brunswick	99%	104
Miles Memorial Hospital	Damariscotta	99%	73
Redington Fairview General Hospital	Skowhegan	99%	124
Southern Maine Medical Center[2]	Biddeford	99%	125
York Hospital	York	99%	95
Eastern Maine Medical Center	Bangor	98%	201
Northern Maine Medical Center	Fort Kent	98%	58
Parkview Adventist Medical Center	Brunswick	98%	53
Penobscot Bay Medical Center	Rockport	98%	88
Stephens Memorial Hospital[2]	Norway	98%	94
Houlton Regional Hospital	Houlton	97%	74
Maine Coast Memorial Hospital	Ellsworth	97%	74
Maine Medical Center	Portland	97%	303
Mercy Hospital	Portland	97%	155
Saint Joseph Hospital	Bangor	97%	184
Aroostook Medical Center	Presque Isle	96%	72
Maine General Medical Center	Augusta	96%	248
Millinocket Regional Hospital	Millinocket	96%	27
Bridgton Hospital	Bridgton	95%	59
Mayo Regional Hospital	Dover Foxcroft	95%	55
Saint Marys Regional Medical Center	Lewiston	95%	79
Franklin Memorial Hospital	Farmington	94%	88
Togus VA Medical Center	Augusta	93%	43
Down East Community Hospital	Machias	90%	42

20. Pneumococcal Vaccine

Hospital Name	City	Rate	Cases
Calais Regional Hospital	Calais	100%	43
Cary Medical Center	Caribou	100%	39
Henrietta D Goodall Hospital	Sanford	100%	106
Inland Hospital	Waterville	100%	51
Mayo Regional Hospital	Dover Foxcroft	100%	48
Millinocket Regional Hospital	Millinocket	100%	28
Mount Desert Island Hospital	Bar Harbor	100%	30
Penobscot Valley Hospital	Lincoln	100%	35
Redington Fairview General Hospital	Skowhegan	100%	117
Houlton Regional Hospital	Houlton	99%	77
Maine Coast Memorial Hospital	Ellsworth	99%	94
Maine General Medical Center	Augusta	99%	216
Mid Coast Hospital[2]	Brunswick	99%	120
Southern Maine Medical Center[2]	Biddeford	99%	121
Waldo County General Hospital	Belfast	99%	79
Eastern Maine Medical Center	Bangor	98%	212
Miles Memorial Hospital	Damariscotta	98%	65
Saint Joseph Hospital	Bangor	98%	177
Stephens Memorial Hospital[2]	Norway	98%	85
Mercy Hospital	Portland	97%	144
Penobscot Bay Medical Center	Rockport	97%	90
Aroostook Medical Center	Presque Isle	96%	74
Franklin Memorial Hospital	Farmington	96%	68
Maine Medical Center	Portland	96%	302
Northern Maine Medical Center	Fort Kent	96%	49
Parkview Adventist Medical Center	Brunswick	96%	48
Togus VA Medical Center	Augusta	96%	49
Central Maine Medical Center[2]	Lewiston	95%	120
Saint Marys Regional Medical Center	Lewiston	95%	82
York Hospital	York	95%	95
Down East Community Hospital	Machias	93%	43
Rumford Hospital	Rumford	93%	42
Bridgton Hospital	Bridgton	92%	53
Sebasticook Valley Hospital	Pittsfield	92%	40
Blue Hill Memorial Hospital	Blue Hill	85%	27

21. Smoking Cessation Advice

Hospital Name	City	Rate	Cases
Central Maine Medical Center[2]	Lewiston	100%	60
Eastern Maine Medical Center	Bangor	100%	144
Henrietta D Goodall Hospital	Sanford	100%	37
Maine Coast Memorial Hospital	Ellsworth	100%	42
Maine Medical Center	Portland	100%	91
Mercy Hospital	Portland	100%	50
Mid Coast Hospital[2]	Brunswick	100%	25
Penobscot Bay Medical Center	Rockport	100%	37
Saint Joseph Hospital	Bangor	100%	66
Saint Marys Regional Medical Center	Lewiston	100%	31
Maine General Medical Center	Augusta	98%	84
Redington Fairview General Hospital	Skowhegan	97%	29
Southern Maine Medical Center[2]	Biddeford	97%	38
Aroostook Medical Center	Presque Isle	96%	28
Togus VA Medical Center	Augusta	96%	28
York Hospital	York	96%	25

Surgical Care Improvement Project

22. Appropriate VTP Within 24 Hours

Hospital Name	City	Rate	Cases
Henrietta D Goodall Hospital	Sanford	100%	55
Inland Hospital	Waterville	100%	70
Redington Fairview General Hospital	Skowhegan	100%	48
Aroostook Medical Center	Presque Isle	99%	127
Maine Coast Memorial Hospital[2]	Ellsworth	99%	177
Maine Medical Center[2]	Portland	99%	208
Eastern Maine Medical Center[2]	Bangor	98%	403
Parkview Adventist Medical Center	Brunswick	98%	44
Saint Joseph Hospital[2]	Bangor	98%	199
York Hospital	York	98%	117
Miles Memorial Hospital	Damariscotta	97%	64
Cary Medical Center	Caribou	96%	47
Maine General Medical Center[2]	Augusta	96%	222
Mid Coast Hospital	Brunswick	96%	90
Sebasticook Valley Hospital	Pittsfield	96%	28
Central Maine Medical Center[2]	Lewiston	95%	171
Saint Marys Regional Medical Center[2]	Lewiston	94%	136
Southern Maine Medical Center[2]	Biddeford	94%	101
Togus VA Medical Center[2]	Augusta	94%	86
Penobscot Bay Medical Center	Rockport	92%	74
Stephens Memorial Hospital	Norway	92%	50
Mayo Regional Hospital[2]	Dover Foxcroft	90%	42
Mercy Hospital[2]	Portland	90%	126
Franklin Memorial Hospital	Farmington	88%	73
Waldo County General Hospital	Belfast	88%	51

23. Appropriate Hair Removal

Hospital Name	City	Rate	Cases
Aroostook Medical Center	Presque Isle	100%	182
Blue Hill Memorial Hospital	Blue Hill	100%	51
Bridgton Hospital	Bridgton	100%	27
Calais Regional Hospital	Calais	100%	51
Cary Medical Center	Caribou	100%	107
Central Maine Medical Center[2]	Lewiston	100%	655
Eastern Maine Medical Center[2]	Bangor	100%	1492
Franklin Memorial Hospital	Farmington	100%	222
Henrietta D Goodall Hospital	Sanford	100%	151
Houlton Regional Hospital	Houlton	100%	30
Inland Hospital	Waterville	100%	125
Maine Coast Memorial Hospital[2]	Ellsworth	100%	240
Maine General Medical Center[2]	Augusta	100%	751
Mayo Regional Hospital[2]	Dover Foxcroft	100%	148
Mercy Hospital[2]	Portland	100%	447
Mid Coast Hospital	Brunswick	100%	227
Miles Memorial Hospital	Damariscotta	100%	146
Mount Desert Island Hospital[2]	Bar Harbor	100%	56
Northern Maine Medical Center	Fort Kent	100%	39
Parkview Adventist Medical Center	Brunswick	100%	68
Penobscot Bay Medical Center	Rockport	100%	270
Redington Fairview General Hospital	Skowhegan	100%	70
Saint Joseph Hospital[2]	Bangor	100%	507
Saint Marys Regional Medical Center[2]	Lewiston	100%	532
Sebasticook Valley Hospital	Pittsfield	100%	43
Southern Maine Medical Center[2]	Biddeford	100%	304
Stephens Memorial Hospital	Norway	100%	172
Togus VA Medical Center[2]	Augusta	100%	155
York Hospital	York	100%	275
Waldo County General Hospital	Belfast	99%	154
Millinocket Regional Hospital	Millinocket	98%	44
Maine Medical Center[2]	Portland	97%	818

24. Appropriate Beta Blocker Usage

Hospital Name	City	Rate	Cases
Aroostook Medical Center	Presque Isle	100%	58
Henrietta D Goodall Hospital	Sanford	100%	41
Mercy Hospital[2]	Portland	100%	113
Mid Coast Hospital	Brunswick	100%	45
Eastern Maine Medical Center[2]	Bangor	99%	592
York Hospital	York	99%	85
Saint Joseph Hospital[2]	Bangor	97%	134
Saint Marys Regional Medical Center[2]	Lewiston	97%	162
Maine Medical Center[2]	Portland	96%	316
Penobscot Bay Medical Center	Rockport	96%	76
Stephens Memorial Hospital	Norway	96%	45
Waldo County General Hospital	Belfast	96%	49
Togus VA Medical Center[2]	Augusta	95%	55
Cary Medical Center	Caribou	94%	36
Franklin Memorial Hospital	Farmington	94%	66
Mayo Regional Hospital[2]	Dover Foxcroft	94%	47
Maine General Medical Center[2]	Augusta	91%	222
Southern Maine Medical Center[2]	Biddeford	90%	102
Maine Coast Memorial Hospital[2]	Ellsworth	89%	73
Central Maine Medical Center[2]	Lewiston	88%	199
Miles Memorial Hospital	Damariscotta	88%	41

25. Controlled Postoperative Blood Glucose

Hospital Name	City	Rate	Cases
Eastern Maine Medical Center[2]	Bangor	97%	386
Maine Medical Center[2]	Portland	96%	174
Central Maine Medical Center[2]	Lewiston	95%	121

26. Prophylactic Antibiotic Timing

Hospital Name	City	Rate	Cases
Henrietta D Goodall Hospital	Sanford	100%	127
Millinocket Regional Hospital	Millinocket	100%	42
Redington Fairview General Hospital	Skowhegan	100%	45
Saint Joseph Hospital[2]	Bangor	100%	380
Sebasticook Valley Hospital	Pittsfield	100%	35
Cary Medical Center	Caribou	99%	67
Eastern Maine Medical Center[2]	Bangor	99%	1031
Maine Medical Center[2]	Portland	99%	606
Mayo Regional Hospital[2]	Dover Foxcroft	99%	134
Mid Coast Hospital	Brunswick	99%	175
Saint Marys Regional Medical Center[2]	Lewiston	99%	403
Aroostook Medical Center	Presque Isle	98%	135
Franklin Memorial Hospital	Farmington	98%	167
Inland Hospital	Waterville	98%	87
Maine General Medical Center[2]	Augusta	98%	598
Penobscot Bay Medical Center	Rockport	98%	210
Stephens Memorial Hospital	Norway	98%	118
York Hospital	York	98%	164
Calais Regional Hospital	Calais	97%	39
Mercy Hospital[2]	Portland	97%	318
Southern Maine Medical Center[2]	Biddeford	97%	194
Waldo County General Hospital	Belfast	97%	112
Central Maine Medical Center[2]	Lewiston	96%	477
Maine Coast Memorial Hospital[2]	Ellsworth	96%	159
Mount Desert Island Hospital[2]	Bar Harbor	95%	41
Togus VA Medical Center	Augusta	95%	105
Miles Memorial Hospital	Damariscotta	94%	127
Northern Maine Medical Center	Fort Kent	94%	33
Parkview Adventist Medical Center	Brunswick	93%	43
Houlton Regional Hospital	Houlton	92%	26

27. Prophylactic Antibiotic Timing (Outpatient)

Hospital Name	City	Rate	Cases
Mid Coast Hospital	Brunswick	99%	151
Inland Hospital	Waterville	98%	166
Saint Joseph Hospital	Bangor	98%	328
Maine General Medical Center	Augusta	97%	398
Central Maine Medical Center	Lewiston	96%	502
Stephens Memorial Hospital	Norway	96%	93
York Hospital	York	96%	98

NOTE: Hospital profiles are in alphabetical order by state, then city, then hospital within the city; Rankings exclude hospitals with less than 25 cases except for patient surveys which excludes hospitals with less than 100 cases; (a) 100–299 cases; (1) The number of cases is too small to be sure how well a hospital is performing; (2) The hospital indicated that the data submitted for this measure were based on a sample of cases; (3) Data was collected during a shorter time period (fewer quarters) than the maximum possible time for this measure; (4) Suppressed for one or more quarters by CMS; (5) No data is available from the hospital for this measure; (6) Fewer than 100 patients completed the HCAHPS survey. Use these rates with caution, as the number of surveys may be too low to reliably assess hospital performance; (7) Survey results are based on less than 12 months of data; (8) Survey results are not available for this reporting period; (9) No or very few patients were eligible for the HCAHPS survey. The scores shown, if any, reflect a very small number of surveys; (10) A state average was not calculated because too few hospitals in the state submitted data; (11) There were discrepancies in the data collection process; Please refer to the User's Guide for a full explanation of data.

Eastern Maine Medical Center	Bangor	95%	820
Down East Community Hospital	Machias	94%	49
Henrietta D Goodall Hospital	Sanford	93%	45
Maine Medical Center	Portland	93%	883
Miles Memorial Hospital	Damariscotta	93%	30
Southern Maine Medical Center	Biddeford	93%	61
Aroostook Medical Center	Presque Isle	92%	78
Franklin Memorial Hospital	Farmington	92%	50
Saint Marys Regional Medical Center	Lewiston	92%	140
Mercy Hospital	Portland	86%	629
Penobscot Bay Medical Center	Rockport	86%	59
Maine Coast Memorial Hospital	Ellsworth	85%	34
Northern Maine Medical Center	Fort Kent	76%	29
Cary Medical Center	Caribou	54%	28
Parkview Adventist Medical Center	Brunswick	48%	33

28. Prophylactic Antibiotic Selection

Hospital Name	City	Rate	Cases
Houlton Regional Hospital	Houlton	100%	26
Maine Coast Memorial Hospital[2]	Ellsworth	100%	159
Millinocket Regional Hospital	Millinocket	100%	43
Mount Desert Island Hospital[2]	Bar Harbor	100%	42
Northern Maine Medical Center	Fort Kent	100%	33
Redington Fairview General Hospital	Skowhegan	100%	45
Saint Marys Regional Medical Center[2]	Lewiston	100%	405
Sebasticook Valley Hospital	Pittsfield	100%	35
Aroostook Medical Center	Presque Isle	99%	135
Eastern Maine Medical Center[2]	Bangor	99%	1058
Henrietta D Goodall Hospital	Sanford	99%	127
Maine General Medical Center[2]	Augusta	99%	600
Maine Medical Center[2]	Portland	99%	615
Mayo Regional Hospital[2]	Dover Foxcroft	99%	134
Mid Coast Hospital	Brunswick	99%	175
Miles Memorial Hospital	Damariscotta	99%	127
Saint Joseph Hospital[2]	Bangor	99%	381
Central Maine Medical Center[2]	Lewiston	98%	485
Franklin Memorial Hospital	Farmington	98%	167
Inland Hospital	Waterville	98%	87
Mercy Hospital[2]	Portland	98%	316
Penobscot Bay Medical Center	Rockport	98%	211
Waldo County General Hospital	Belfast	98%	112
York Hospital	York	98%	165
Calais Regional Hospital	Calais	97%	39
Cary Medical Center	Caribou	97%	67
Southern Maine Medical Center[2]	Biddeford	97%	194
Stephens Memorial Hospital	Norway	97%	118
Togus VA Medical Center	Augusta	95%	104
Parkview Adventist Medical Center	Brunswick	91%	43

29. Prophylactic Antibiotic Selection (Outpatient)

Hospital Name	City	Rate	Cases
Maine General Medical Center	Augusta	99%	393
Saint Joseph Hospital	Bangor	99%	325
York Hospital	York	99%	97
Maine Medical Center	Portland	98%	858
Miles Memorial Hospital	Damariscotta	97%	36
Northern Maine Medical Center	Fort Kent	97%	34
Aroostook Medical Center	Presque Isle	96%	73
Mid Coast Hospital	Brunswick	96%	167
Penobscot Bay Medical Center	Rockport	96%	84
Eastern Maine Medical Center	Bangor	95%	960
Henrietta D Goodall Hospital	Sanford	95%	42
Inland Hospital	Waterville	95%	165
Central Maine Medical Center	Lewiston	94%	600
Maine Coast Memorial Hospital	Ellsworth	94%	79
Stephens Memorial Hospital	Norway	94%	90
Down East Community Hospital	Machias	92%	49
Franklin Memorial Hospital	Farmington	92%	59
Saint Marys Regional Medical Center	Lewiston	91%	137
Southern Maine Medical Center	Biddeford	91%	58
Cary Medical Center	Caribou	90%	70
Mercy Hospital	Portland	90%	587

30. Prophylactic Antibiotic Stopped

Hospital Name	City	Rate	Cases
Mayo Regional Hospital[2]	Dover Foxcroft	100%	134
Mount Desert Island Hospital[2]	Bar Harbor	100%	41
Saint Joseph Hospital[2]	Bangor	100%	376
Sebasticook Valley Hospital	Pittsfield	100%	35
Southern Maine Medical Center[2]	Biddeford	100%	190
Mid Coast Hospital	Brunswick	99%	168
Aroostook Medical Center	Presque Isle	98%	129
Eastern Maine Medical Center[2]	Bangor	98%	974
Maine Medical Center[2]	Portland	98%	599
Mercy Hospital[2]	Portland	98%	312
Millinocket Regional Hospital	Millinocket	98%	40
Redington Fairview General Hospital	Skowhegan	98%	43
Calais Regional Hospital	Calais	97%	38
Cary Medical Center	Caribou	97%	65
Henrietta D Goodall Hospital	Sanford	97%	123
Miles Memorial Hospital	Damariscotta	97%	121
Saint Marys Regional Medical Center[2]	Lewiston	97%	394
Stephens Memorial Hospital	Norway	97%	118
York Hospital	York	97%	163
Maine General Medical Center[2]	Augusta	96%	586
Penobscot Bay Medical Center	Rockport	96%	208
Waldo County General Hospital	Belfast	96%	105
Central Maine Medical Center[2]	Lewiston	95%	452
Franklin Memorial Hospital	Farmington	95%	165
Parkview Adventist Medical Center	Brunswick	95%	42
Maine Coast Memorial Hospital[2]	Ellsworth	94%	151
Togus VA Medical Center	Augusta	94%	103
Inland Hospital	Waterville	92%	86
Northern Maine Medical Center	Fort Kent	82%	33

31. Recommended VTP Ordered

Hospital Name	City	Rate	Cases
Henrietta D Goodall Hospital	Sanford	100%	55
Inland Hospital	Waterville	100%	70
Maine Medical Center[2]	Portland	100%	208
Redington Fairview General Hospital	Skowhegan	100%	48
Sebasticook Valley Hospital	Pittsfield	100%	28
Aroostook Medical Center	Presque Isle	99%	127
Eastern Maine Medical Center[2]	Bangor	99%	403
Maine Coast Memorial Hospital[2]	Ellsworth	99%	177
Saint Joseph Hospital[2]	Bangor	99%	199
Cary Medical Center	Caribou	98%	47
Mid Coast Hospital	Brunswick	98%	90
Parkview Adventist Medical Center	Brunswick	98%	44
York Hospital	York	98%	117
Miles Memorial Hospital	Damariscotta	97%	64
Central Maine Medical Center[2]	Lewiston	96%	172
Maine General Medical Center[2]	Augusta	96%	222
Saint Marys Regional Medical Center[2]	Lewiston	96%	136
Stephens Memorial Hospital	Norway	96%	50
Penobscot Bay Medical Center	Rockport	95%	74
Southern Maine Medical Center[2]	Biddeford	94%	102
Togus VA Medical Center[2]	Augusta	94%	87
Franklin Memorial Hospital	Farmington	92%	73
Mercy Hospital[2]	Portland	92%	127
Mayo Regional Hospital[2]	Dover Foxcroft	90%	42
Waldo County General Hospital	Belfast	88%	51

32. Urinary Catheter Removal

Hospital Name	City	Rate	Cases
Henrietta D Goodall Hospital	Sanford	100%	52
Mayo Regional Hospital[2]	Dover Foxcroft	100%	45
Miles Memorial Hospital	Damariscotta	97%	38
Aroostook Medical Center	Presque Isle	96%	50
Southern Maine Medical Center[2]	Biddeford	96%	57
York Hospital	York	96%	50
Maine General Medical Center[2]	Augusta	94%	227
Maine Medical Center[2]	Portland	94%	164
Eastern Maine Medical Center[2]	Bangor	93%	409
Franklin Memorial Hospital	Farmington	93%	45
Stephens Memorial Hospital	Norway	93%	56
Waldo County General Hospital	Belfast	93%	43
Mercy Hospital[2]	Portland	92%	131
Maine Coast Memorial Hospital	Ellsworth	86%	73
Saint Joseph Hospital[2]	Bangor	86%	28
Central Maine Medical Center[2]	Lewiston	84%	92
Inland Hospital	Waterville	81%	47
Togus VA Medical Center[2]	Augusta	79%	28
Saint Marys Regional Medical Center[2]	Lewiston	78%	58

Use of Medical Imaging

36. Combination Abdominal CT Scan

Hospital Name	City	Ratio	Cases
Inland Hospital	Waterville	0.023	308
Eastern Maine Medical Center	Bangor	0.029	1584
Southern Maine Medical Center	Biddeford	0.037	756
Maine General Medical Center	Augusta	0.043	1618
Saint Andrews Hospital	Boothbay Hrbr	0.047	85
Mercy Hospital	Portland	0.049	594
Miles Memorial Hospital	Damariscotta	0.052	289
Saint Joseph Hospital	Bangor	0.058	567
Saint Marys Regional Medical Center	Lewiston	0.071	722
Parkview Adventist Medical Center	Brunswick	0.078	230
Maine Coast Memorial Hospital	Ellsworth	0.080	386
Penobscot Bay Medical Center	Rockport	0.080	552
Central Maine Medical Center	Lewiston	0.084	1073
Henrietta D Goodall Hospital	Sanford	0.096	457
Maine Medical Center	Portland	0.102	1961
Redington Fairview General Hospital	Skowhegan	0.123	481
York Hospital	York	0.131	657
Franklin Memorial Hospital	Farmington	0.148	438
Mid Coast Hospital	Brunswick	0.161	639
Down East Community Hospital	Machias	0.233	283
Mount Desert Island Hospital	Bar Harbor	0.259	259
Northern Maine Medical Center	Fort Kent	0.345	203
Calais Regional Hospital	Calais	0.391	230
Aroostook Medical Center	Presque Isle	0.475	577
Cary Medical Center	Caribou	0.558	403
Stephens Memorial Hospital	Norway	0.609	330

37. Combination Chest CT Scan

Hospital Name	City	Ratio	Cases
Inland Hospital	Waterville	0.000	125
Maine Coast Memorial Hospital	Ellsworth	0.000	266
Saint Joseph Hospital	Bangor	0.000	401
Southern Maine Medical Center	Biddeford	0.000	470
Central Maine Medical Center	Lewiston	0.001	873
Eastern Maine Medical Center	Bangor	0.002	1475
Mid Coast Hospital	Brunswick	0.002	499
Penobscot Bay Medical Center	Rockport	0.002	480
Maine Medical Center	Portland	0.004	2037
Maine General Medical Center	Augusta	0.006	1388
Mercy Hospital	Portland	0.008	597
Saint Marys Regional Medical Center	Lewiston	0.008	633
York Hospital	York	0.008	502
Franklin Memorial Hospital	Farmington	0.009	322
Miles Memorial Hospital	Damariscotta	0.010	203
Stephens Memorial Hospital	Norway	0.013	380
Northern Maine Medical Center	Fort Kent	0.023	215
Parkview Adventist Medical Center	Brunswick	0.025	120
Henrietta D Goodall Hospital	Sanford	0.027	369
Saint Andrews Hospital	Boothbay Hrbr	0.038	53
Redington Fairview General Hospital	Skowhegan	0.066	196
Mount Desert Island Hospital	Bar Harbor	0.147	109
Down East Community Hospital	Machias	0.176	255
Aroostook Medical Center	Presque Isle	0.290	486
Cary Medical Center	Caribou	0.400	443
Calais Regional Hospital	Calais	0.461	152

38. Follow-up Mammogram/Ultrasound

Hospital Name	City	Rate	Cases
Maine Coast Memorial Hospital	Ellsworth	3.0%	946
Calais Regional Hospital	Calais	4.5%	397
Central Maine Medical Center	Lewiston	4.8%	1410
Mount Desert Island Hospital	Bar Harbor	4.9%	367
Saint Joseph Hospital	Bangor	4.9%	2577
Eastern Maine Medical Center	Bangor	5.4%	1435
Miles Memorial Hospital	Damariscotta	5.4%	706
Mercy Hospital	Portland	5.7%	2053
Maine General Medical Center	Augusta	6.5%	3702
Southern Maine Medical Center	Biddeford	7.2%	1344
Franklin Memorial Hospital	Farmington	7.5%	1189
Northern Maine Medical Center	Fort Kent	7.9%	692
Mid Coast Hospital	Brunswick	8.0%	1088
Inland Hospital	Waterville	8.1%	419
Stephens Memorial Hospital	Norway	8.5%	1139
Henrietta D Goodall Hospital	Sanford	8.7%	967
Redington Fairview General Hospital	Skowhegan	8.7%	932
Saint Marys Regional Medical Center	Lewiston	9.3%	1273
Aroostook Medical Center	Presque Isle	10.1%	999
Parkview Adventist Medical Center	Brunswick	10.7%	718
York Hospital	York	10.7%	1207
Maine Medical Center	Portland	11.0%	2473
Down East Community Hospital	Machias	11.9%	571
Saint Andrews Hospital	Boothbay Hrbr	13.7%	190
Cary Medical Center	Caribou	14.2%	773

39. MRI for Low Back Pain

Hospital Name	City	Rate	Cases
York Hospital	York	26.2%	141
Mid Coast Hospital	Brunswick	29.3%	147
Saint Marys Regional Medical Center	Lewiston	29.8%	208
Saint Joseph Hospital	Bangor	32.8%	262
Maine Medical Center	Portland	33.6%	149
Maine Coast Memorial Hospital	Ellsworth	34.8%	141
Mercy Hospital	Portland	35.5%	211
Eastern Maine Medical Center	Bangor	36.9%	293
Henrietta D Goodall Hospital	Sanford	37.1%	105
Southern Maine Medical Center	Biddeford	37.1%	175
Franklin Memorial Hospital	Farmington	43.7%	135
Parkview Adventist Medical Center	Brunswick	44.1%	59
Cary Medical Center	Caribou	44.3%	70
Stephens Memorial Hospital	Norway	49.4%	79
Northern Maine Medical Center	Fort Kent	56.8%	74

Survey of Patients' Hospital Experiences

40. Area Around Room 'Always' Quiet at Night

Hospital Name	City	Rate	Cases
Calais Regional Hospital	Calais	71%	(a)

NOTE: Hospital profiles are in alphabetical order by state, then city, then hospital within the city; Rankings exclude hospitals with less than 25 cases except for patient surveys which excludes hospitals with less than 100 cases; (a) 100–299 cases; (1) The number of cases is too small to be sure how well a hospital is performing; (2) The hospital indicated that the data submitted for this measure were based on a sample of cases; (3) Data was collected during a shorter time period (fewer quarters) than the maximum possible time for this measure; (4) Suppressed for one or more quarters by CMS; (5) No data is available from the hospital for this measure; (6) Fewer than 100 patients completed the HCAHPS survey. Use these rates with caution, as the number of surveys may be too low to reliably assess hospital performance; (7) Survey results are based on less than 12 months of data; (8) Survey results are not available for this reporting period; (9) No or very few patients were eligible for the HCAHPS survey. The scores shown, if any, reflect a very small number of surveys; (10) A state average was not calculated because too few hospitals in the state submitted data; (11) There were discrepancies in the data collection process; Please refer to the User's Guide for a full explanation of data.

Inland Hospital	Waterville	69%	(a)
Rumford Hospital	Rumford	69%	(a)
Millinocket Regional Hospital	Millinocket	66%	(a)
Down East Community Hospital	Machias	65%	(a)
Mount Desert Island Hospital	Bar Harbor	63%	(a)
Mercy Hospital	Portland	62%	300+
Penobscot Valley Hospital	Lincoln	62%	(a)
Waldo County General Hospital	Belfast	62%	(a)
Bridgton Hospital	Bridgton	61%	300+
Cary Medical Center	Caribou	60%	300+
Redington Fairview General Hospital	Skowhegan	60%	300+
Henrietta D Goodall Hospital	Sanford	59%	300+
Saint Joseph Hospital	Bangor	59%	300+
Houlton Regional Hospital	Houlton	58%	300+
Saint Marys Regional Medical Center	Lewiston	58%	300+
York Hospital	York	58%	300+
Blue Hill Memorial Hospital	Blue Hill	57%	(a)
Mayo Regional Hospital	Dover Foxcroft	57%	(a)
Northern Maine Medical Center	Fort Kent	57%	(a)
Stephens Memorial Hospital	Norway	56%	300+
Maine Coast Memorial Hospital	Ellsworth	55%	300+
Parkview Adventist Medical Center	Brunswick	55%	300+
Franklin Memorial Hospital	Farmington	53%	300+
Miles Memorial Hospital	Damariscotta	53%	300+
Penobscot Bay Medical Center	Rockport	53%	300+
Mid Coast Hospital	Brunswick	52%	300+
Central Maine Medical Center	Lewiston	50%	300+
Maine Medical Center	Portland	49%	300+
Southern Maine Medical Center	Biddeford	48%	300+
Aroostook Medical Center	Presque Isle	46%	300+
Sebasticook Valley Hospital	Pittsfield	46%	(a)
Maine General Medical Center	Augusta	45%	300+
Eastern Maine Medical Center	Bangor	44%	300+

41. Doctors 'Always' Communicated Well

Hospital Name	City	Rate	Cases
Mount Desert Island Hospital	Bar Harbor	90%	(a)
Cary Medical Center	Caribou	87%	300+
Mayo Regional Hospital	Dover Foxcroft	87%	(a)
Millinocket Regional Hospital	Millinocket	87%	(a)
York Hospital	York	87%	300+
Bridgton Hospital	Bridgton	86%	300+
Down East Community Hospital	Machias	86%	(a)
Maine Coast Memorial Hospital	Ellsworth	86%	300+
Redington Fairview General Hospital	Skowhegan	85%	300+
Houlton Regional Hospital	Houlton	84%	300+
Miles Memorial Hospital	Damariscotta	84%	300+
Parkview Adventist Medical Center	Brunswick	84%	300+
Penobscot Valley Hospital	Lincoln	84%	(a)
Stephens Memorial Hospital	Norway	84%	300+
Waldo County General Hospital	Belfast	83%	(a)
Saint Joseph Hospital	Bangor	82%	300+
Calais Regional Hospital	Calais	81%	(a)
Northern Maine Medical Center	Fort Kent	81%	(a)
Southern Maine Medical Center	Biddeford	81%	300+
Franklin Memorial Hospital	Farmington	80%	300+
Penobscot Bay Medical Center	Rockport	80%	300+
Saint Marys Regional Medical Center	Lewiston	80%	300+
Blue Hill Memorial Hospital	Blue Hill	79%	(a)
Henrietta D Goodall Hospital	Sanford	79%	300+
Inland Hospital	Waterville	79%	(a)
Maine General Medical Center	Augusta	79%	300+
Mercy Hospital	Portland	78%	300+
Mid Coast Hospital	Brunswick	78%	300+
Central Maine Medical Center	Lewiston	77%	300+
Eastern Maine Medical Center	Bangor	77%	300+
Maine Medical Center	Portland	77%	300+
Sebasticook Valley Hospital	Pittsfield	76%	(a)
Aroostook Medical Center	Presque Isle	74%	300+
Rumford Hospital	Rumford	72%	(a)

42. Home Recovery Information Given

Hospital Name	City	Rate	Cases
Redington Fairview General Hospital	Skowhegan	91%	300+
Bridgton Hospital	Bridgton	90%	300+
Mount Desert Island Hospital	Bar Harbor	90%	(a)
Stephens Memorial Hospital	Norway	90%	300+
Saint Joseph Hospital	Bangor	89%	300+
Waldo County General Hospital	Belfast	89%	(a)
Cary Medical Center	Caribou	88%	300+
Henrietta D Goodall Hospital	Sanford	88%	300+
Maine Coast Memorial Hospital	Ellsworth	88%	300+
Maine General Medical Center	Augusta	88%	300+
Mayo Regional Hospital	Dover Foxcroft	88%	(a)
Penobscot Bay Medical Center	Rockport	88%	300+
Penobscot Valley Hospital	Lincoln	88%	(a)
Rumford Hospital	Rumford	88%	(a)
Sebasticook Valley Hospital	Pittsfield	88%	(a)
Millinocket Regional Hospital	Millinocket	87%	(a)
Parkview Adventist Medical Center	Brunswick	87%	300+
Saint Marys Regional Medical Center	Lewiston	87%	300+
York Hospital	York	87%	300+
Franklin Memorial Hospital	Farmington	86%	300+
Houlton Regional Hospital	Houlton	86%	300+
Mercy Hospital	Portland	86%	300+
Southern Maine Medical Center	Biddeford	86%	300+
Central Maine Medical Center	Lewiston	85%	300+
Eastern Maine Medical Center	Bangor	85%	300+
Inland Hospital	Waterville	85%	(a)
Mid Coast Hospital	Brunswick	85%	300+
Maine Medical Center	Portland	84%	300+
Down East Community Hospital	Machias	83%	(a)
Miles Memorial Hospital	Damariscotta	83%	300+
Calais Regional Hospital	Calais	82%	(a)
Northern Maine Medical Center	Fort Kent	81%	(a)
Blue Hill Memorial Hospital	Blue Hill	80%	(a)
Aroostook Medical Center	Presque Isle	76%	300+

43. Hospital Given 9 or 10 on 10 Point Scale

Hospital Name	City	Rate	Cases
Mount Desert Island Hospital	Bar Harbor	84%	(a)
York Hospital	York	84%	300+
Parkview Adventist Medical Center	Brunswick	83%	300+
Saint Joseph Hospital	Bangor	80%	300+
Millinocket Regional Hospital	Millinocket	79%	(a)
Waldo County General Hospital	Belfast	79%	(a)
Maine Coast Memorial Hospital	Ellsworth	78%	300+
Bridgton Hospital	Bridgton	76%	300+
Houlton Regional Hospital	Houlton	74%	300+
Mercy Hospital	Portland	74%	300+
Stephens Memorial Hospital	Norway	74%	300+
Mayo Regional Hospital	Dover Foxcroft	73%	(a)
Redington Fairview General Hospital	Skowhegan	73%	300+
Miles Memorial Hospital	Damariscotta	72%	300+
Down East Community Hospital	Machias	71%	(a)
Saint Marys Regional Medical Center	Lewiston	71%	300+
Inland Hospital	Waterville	70%	(a)
Maine Medical Center	Portland	70%	300+
Mid Coast Hospital	Brunswick	70%	300+
Rumford Hospital	Rumford	70%	(a)
Cary Medical Center	Caribou	69%	300+
Eastern Maine Medical Center	Bangor	69%	300+
Franklin Memorial Hospital	Farmington	68%	300+
Penobscot Valley Hospital	Lincoln	68%	(a)
Central Maine Medical Center	Lewiston	67%	300+
Sebasticook Valley Hospital	Pittsfield	67%	(a)
Calais Regional Hospital	Calais	66%	(a)
Penobscot Bay Medical Center	Rockport	66%	300+
Southern Maine Medical Center	Biddeford	66%	300+
Blue Hill Memorial Hospital	Blue Hill	64%	(a)
Maine General Medical Center	Augusta	63%	300+
Aroostook Medical Center	Presque Isle	61%	300+
Northern Maine Medical Center	Fort Kent	60%	(a)
Henrietta D Goodall Hospital	Sanford	57%	300+

44. Meds 'Always' Explained Before Given

Hospital Name	City	Rate	Cases
Millinocket Regional Hospital	Millinocket	74%	(a)
Maine Coast Memorial Hospital	Ellsworth	73%	300+
Mount Desert Island Hospital	Bar Harbor	72%	(a)
Redington Fairview General Hospital	Skowhegan	70%	300+
Bridgton Hospital	Bridgton	69%	300+
Penobscot Valley Hospital	Lincoln	69%	(a)
Calais Regional Hospital	Calais	68%	(a)
Down East Community Hospital	Machias	68%	(a)
Waldo County General Hospital	Belfast	68%	(a)
Northern Maine Medical Center	Fort Kent	67%	(a)
York Hospital	York	67%	300+
Maine General Medical Center	Augusta	66%	300+
Miles Memorial Hospital	Damariscotta	66%	300+
Mayo Regional Hospital	Dover Foxcroft	65%	(a)
Parkview Adventist Medical Center	Brunswick	65%	300+
Sebasticook Valley Hospital	Pittsfield	65%	(a)
Blue Hill Memorial Hospital	Blue Hill	64%	(a)
Mercy Hospital	Portland	64%	300+
Stephens Memorial Hospital	Norway	64%	300+
Houlton Regional Hospital	Houlton	63%	300+
Saint Joseph Hospital	Bangor	63%	300+
Franklin Memorial Hospital	Farmington	62%	300+
Penobscot Bay Medical Center	Rockport	62%	300+
Southern Maine Medical Center	Biddeford	62%	300+
Cary Medical Center	Caribou	61%	300+
Henrietta D Goodall Hospital	Sanford	61%	300+
Saint Marys Regional Medical Center	Lewiston	61%	300+
Inland Hospital	Waterville	60%	(a)
Maine Medical Center	Portland	60%	300+
Mid Coast Hospital	Brunswick	60%	300+
Central Maine Medical Center	Lewiston	59%	300+
Eastern Maine Medical Center	Bangor	59%	300+
Aroostook Medical Center	Presque Isle	53%	300+
Rumford Hospital	Rumford	53%	(a)

45. Nurses 'Always' Communicated Well

Hospital Name	City	Rate	Cases
Millinocket Regional Hospital	Millinocket	87%	(a)
Mount Desert Island Hospital	Bar Harbor	86%	(a)
Down East Community Hospital	Machias	85%	(a)
Maine Coast Memorial Hospital	Ellsworth	85%	300+
Waldo County General Hospital	Belfast	84%	(a)
York Hospital	York	84%	300+
Houlton Regional Hospital	Houlton	83%	300+
Inland Hospital	Waterville	83%	(a)
Redington Fairview General Hospital	Skowhegan	83%	300+
Cary Medical Center	Caribou	81%	300+
Saint Joseph Hospital	Bangor	81%	300+
Calais Regional Hospital	Calais	80%	(a)
Parkview Adventist Medical Center	Brunswick	80%	300+
Penobscot Valley Hospital	Lincoln	80%	(a)
Bridgton Hospital	Bridgton	79%	300+
Franklin Memorial Hospital	Farmington	79%	300+
Mayo Regional Hospital	Dover Foxcroft	79%	(a)
Miles Memorial Hospital	Damariscotta	79%	300+
Northern Maine Medical Center	Fort Kent	79%	(a)
Saint Marys Regional Medical Center	Lewiston	79%	300+
Maine General Medical Center	Augusta	78%	300+
Southern Maine Medical Center	Biddeford	78%	300+
Eastern Maine Medical Center	Bangor	77%	300+
Mercy Hospital	Portland	77%	300+
Sebasticook Valley Hospital	Pittsfield	77%	(a)
Stephens Memorial Hospital	Norway	77%	300+
Penobscot Bay Medical Center	Rockport	76%	300+
Aroostook Medical Center	Presque Isle	75%	300+
Blue Hill Memorial Hospital	Blue Hill	75%	(a)
Central Maine Medical Center	Lewiston	75%	300+
Maine Medical Center	Portland	75%	300+
Mid Coast Hospital	Brunswick	75%	300+
Rumford Hospital	Rumford	75%	(a)
Henrietta D Goodall Hospital	Sanford	73%	300+

46. Pain 'Always' Well Controlled

Hospital Name	City	Rate	Cases
Down East Community Hospital	Machias	82%	(a)
Waldo County General Hospital	Belfast	81%	(a)
Maine Coast Memorial Hospital	Ellsworth	80%	300+
Penobscot Valley Hospital	Lincoln	79%	(a)
Calais Regional Hospital	Calais	78%	(a)
Millinocket Regional Hospital	Millinocket	76%	(a)
Mount Desert Island Hospital	Bar Harbor	76%	(a)
Bridgton Hospital	Bridgton	75%	300+
York Hospital	York	75%	300+
Mayo Regional Hospital	Dover Foxcroft	73%	(a)
Miles Memorial Hospital	Damariscotta	73%	300+
Redington Fairview General Hospital	Skowhegan	73%	300+
Saint Joseph Hospital	Bangor	73%	300+
Cary Medical Center	Caribou	72%	300+
Inland Hospital	Waterville	72%	(a)
Parkview Adventist Medical Center	Brunswick	72%	300+
Houlton Regional Hospital	Houlton	71%	300+
Maine General Medical Center	Augusta	71%	300+
Stephens Memorial Hospital	Norway	71%	300+
Franklin Memorial Hospital	Farmington	70%	300+
Maine Medical Center	Portland	70%	300+
Mid Coast Hospital	Brunswick	70%	300+
Penobscot Bay Medical Center	Rockport	70%	300+
Southern Maine Medical Center	Biddeford	70%	300+
Eastern Maine Medical Center	Bangor	69%	300+
Northern Maine Medical Center	Fort Kent	69%	(a)
Central Maine Medical Center	Lewiston	68%	300+
Rumford Hospital	Rumford	68%	(a)
Saint Marys Regional Medical Center	Lewiston	68%	300+
Henrietta D Goodall Hospital	Sanford	67%	300+
Mercy Hospital	Portland	66%	300+
Blue Hill Memorial Hospital	Blue Hill	65%	(a)
Aroostook Medical Center	Presque Isle	63%	300+
Sebasticook Valley Hospital	Pittsfield	59%	(a)

47. Room and Bathroom 'Always' Clean

Hospital Name	City	Rate	Cases
Millinocket Regional Hospital	Millinocket	91%	(a)
Down East Community Hospital	Machias	86%	(a)
Maine Coast Memorial Hospital	Ellsworth	86%	300+
Mount Desert Island Hospital	Bar Harbor	86%	(a)
Parkview Adventist Medical Center	Brunswick	86%	300+
Rumford Hospital	Rumford	85%	(a)
Waldo County General Hospital	Belfast	85%	(a)
Sebasticook Valley Hospital	Pittsfield	84%	(a)
Redington Fairview General Hospital	Skowhegan	83%	300+
Mayo Regional Hospital	Dover Foxcroft	82%	(a)
Penobscot Valley Hospital	Lincoln	82%	(a)

NOTE: Hospital profiles are in alphabetical order by state, then city, then hospital within the city; Rankings exclude hospitals with less than 25 cases except for patient surveys which excludes hospitals with less than 100 cases; (a) 100–299 cases; (1) The number of cases is too small to be sure how well a hospital is performing; (2) The hospital indicated that the data submitted for this measure were based on a sample of cases; (3) Data was collected during a shorter time period (fewer quarters) than the maximum possible time for this measure; (4) Suppressed for one or more quarters by CMS; (5) No data is available from the hospital for this measure; (6) Fewer than 100 patients completed the HCAHPS survey. Use these rates with caution, as the number of surveys may be too low to reliably assess hospital performance; (7) Survey results are based on less than 12 months of data; (8) Survey results are not available for this reporting period; (9) No or very few patients were eligible for the HCAHPS survey. The scores shown, if any, reflect a very small number of surveys; (10) A state average was not calculated because too few hospitals in the state submitted data; (11) There were discrepancies in the data collection process; Please refer to the User's Guide for a full explanation of data.

Hospital Name	City	Rate	Cases
Franklin Memorial Hospital	Farmington	81%	300+
Northern Maine Medical Center	Fort Kent	80%	(a)
Aroostook Medical Center	Presque Isle	79%	300+
Bridgton Hospital	Bridgton	79%	300+
Calais Regional Hospital	Calais	79%	(a)
Houlton Regional Hospital	Houlton	79%	300+
Saint Joseph Hospital	Bangor	79%	300+
Blue Hill Memorial Hospital	Blue Hill	78%	(a)
Saint Marys Regional Medical Center	Lewiston	78%	300+
Inland Hospital	Waterville	77%	(a)
Maine General Medical Center	Augusta	77%	300+
Stephens Memorial Hospital	Norway	77%	300+
York Hospital	York	77%	300+
Miles Memorial Hospital	Damariscotta	76%	300+
Henrietta D Goodall Hospital	Sanford	75%	300+
Mid Coast Hospital	Brunswick	74%	300+
Cary Medical Center	Caribou	73%	300+
Eastern Maine Medical Center	Bangor	73%	300+
Penobscot Bay Medical Center	Rockport	73%	300+
Southern Maine Medical Center	Biddeford	73%	300+
Mercy Hospital	Portland	71%	300+
Central Maine Medical Center	Lewiston	69%	300+
Maine Medical Center	Portland	69%	300+

Hospital Name	City	Rate	Cases
Sebasticook Valley Hospital	Pittsfield	68%	(a)
Northern Maine Medical Center	Fort Kent	67%	(a)
Penobscot Valley Hospital	Lincoln	67%	(a)
Calais Regional Hospital	Calais	66%	(a)
Blue Hill Memorial Hospital	Blue Hill	63%	(a)
Henrietta D Goodall Hospital	Sanford	60%	300+
Aroostook Medical Center	Presque Isle	56%	300+

48. Timely Help 'Always' Received

Hospital Name	City	Rate	Cases
Millinocket Regional Hospital	Millinocket	85%	(a)
Mount Desert Island Hospital	Bar Harbor	82%	(a)
Houlton Regional Hospital	Houlton	80%	300+
Waldo County General Hospital	Belfast	79%	(a)
Calais Regional Hospital	Calais	78%	(a)
Down East Community Hospital	Machias	77%	(a)
Maine Coast Memorial Hospital	Ellsworth	77%	300+
Mayo Regional Hospital	Dover Foxcroft	75%	(a)
Bridgton Hospital	Bridgton	74%	300+
Cary Medical Center	Caribou	72%	300+
Inland Hospital	Waterville	72%	(a)
Parkview Adventist Medical Center	Brunswick	72%	300+
York Hospital	York	72%	300+
Redington Fairview General Hospital	Skowhegan	71%	300+
Rumford Hospital	Rumford	71%	(a)
Blue Hill Memorial Hospital	Blue Hill	70%	(a)
Miles Memorial Hospital	Damariscotta	70%	300+
Northern Maine Medical Center	Fort Kent	70%	(a)
Penobscot Valley Hospital	Lincoln	69%	(a)
Penobscot Bay Medical Center	Rockport	67%	300+
Aroostook Medical Center	Presque Isle	66%	300+
Saint Joseph Hospital	Bangor	65%	300+
Central Maine Medical Center	Lewiston	64%	300+
Franklin Memorial Hospital	Farmington	64%	300+
Henrietta D Goodall Hospital	Sanford	64%	300+
Maine General Medical Center	Augusta	64%	300+
Stephens Memorial Hospital	Norway	63%	300+
Eastern Maine Medical Center	Bangor	62%	300+
Maine Medical Center	Portland	62%	300+
Sebasticook Valley Hospital	Pittsfield	62%	(a)
Southern Maine Medical Center	Biddeford	62%	300+
Saint Marys Regional Medical Center	Lewiston	61%	300+
Mercy Hospital	Portland	60%	300+
Mid Coast Hospital	Brunswick	60%	300+

49. Would Definitely Recommend Hospital

Hospital Name	City	Rate	Cases
York Hospital	York	90%	300+
Mount Desert Island Hospital	Bar Harbor	87%	(a)
Parkview Adventist Medical Center	Brunswick	87%	300+
Saint Joseph Hospital	Bangor	83%	300+
Maine Coast Memorial Hospital	Ellsworth	82%	300+
Millinocket Regional Hospital	Millinocket	81%	(a)
Mercy Hospital	Portland	79%	300+
Miles Memorial Hospital	Damariscotta	79%	300+
Saint Marys Regional Medical Center	Lewiston	79%	300+
Inland Hospital	Waterville	78%	(a)
Mid Coast Hospital	Brunswick	78%	300+
Waldo County General Hospital	Belfast	78%	(a)
Central Maine Medical Center	Lewiston	77%	300+
Maine Medical Center	Portland	77%	300+
Redington Fairview General Hospital	Skowhegan	77%	300+
Eastern Maine Medical Center	Bangor	76%	300+
Southern Maine Medical Center	Biddeford	76%	300+
Stephens Memorial Hospital	Norway	76%	300+
Bridgton Hospital	Bridgton	75%	300+
Mayo Regional Hospital	Dover Foxcroft	75%	(a)
Houlton Regional Hospital	Houlton	73%	300+
Cary Medical Center	Caribou	72%	300+
Maine General Medical Center	Augusta	70%	300+
Down East Community Hospital	Machias	69%	(a)
Penobscot Bay Medical Center	Rockport	69%	300+
Rumford Hospital	Rumford	69%	(a)
Franklin Memorial Hospital	Farmington	68%	300+

NOTE: Hospital profiles are in alphabetical order by state, then city, then hospital within the city; Rankings exclude hospitals with less than 25 cases except for patient surveys which excludes hospitals with less than 100 cases; (a) 100–299 cases; (1) The number of cases is too small to be sure how well a hospital is performing; (2) The hospital indicated that the data submitted for this measure were based on a sample of cases; (3) Data was collected during a shorter time period (fewer quarters) than the maximum possible time for this measure; (4) Suppressed for one or more quarters by CMS; (5) No data is available from the hospital for this measure; (6) Fewer than 100 patients completed the HCAHPS survey. Use these rates with caution, as the number of surveys may be too low to reliably assess hospital performance; (7) Survey results are based on less than 12 months of data; (8) Survey results are not available for this reporting period; (9) No or very few patients were eligible for the HCAHPS survey. The scores shown, if any, reflect a very small number of surveys; (10) A state average was not calculated because too few hospitals in the state submitted data; (11) There were discrepancies in the data collection process; Please refer to the User's Guide for a full explanation of data.

Maine General Medical Center

6 E Chestnut St
Augusta, ME 04330
Phone: 207-872-1000
Fax: 207-872-4665
URL: www.mainegeneral.org
Type: Acute Care Hospitals
Emergency Services: Yes
Ownership: Voluntary Non-Profit - Other
Beds: 246

Key Personnel:
CEO/President. . . . . Scott B Bullock
Chief of Medical Staff. . . . . Thomas J Keating
Radiology. . . . . Paul D Gagliardi

Measure	Cases	This Hosp.	State Avg.	U.S. Avg.
Heart Attack Care				
ACE Inhibitor or ARB for LVSD[1]	17	94%	98%	96%
Aspirin at Arrival	166	99%	99%	99%
Aspirin at Discharge	89	98%	99%	98%
Beta Blocker at Discharge	100	100%	99%	98%
Fibrinolytic Medication Timing	0	-	43%	55%
PCI Within 90 Minutes of Arrival	0	-	94%	90%
Smoking Cessation Advice[1]	10	100%	100%	99%
Chest Pain/Possible Heart Attack Care				
Aspirin at Arrival	113	99%	98%	95%
Median Time to ECG (minutes)	118	5	7	8
Median Time to Transfer (minutes)[1]	3	165	46	61
Fibrinolytic Medication Timing	43	88%	75%	54%
Heart Failure Care				
ACE Inhibitor or ARB for LVSD	68	96%	97%	94%
Discharge Instructions	167	92%	91%	88%
Evaluation of LVS Function	215	100%	99%	98%
Smoking Cessation Advice	28	100%	97%	98%
Pneumonia Care				
Appropriate Initial Antibiotic	154	97%	94%	92%
Blood Culture Timing	235	97%	95%	96%
Influenza Vaccine	167	99%	97%	91%
Initial Antibiotic Timing	248	96%	98%	95%
Pneumococcal Vaccine	216	99%	97%	93%
Smoking Cessation Advice	84	98%	99%	97%
Surgical Care Improvement Project				
Appropriate VTP Within 24 Hours[2]	222	96%	96%	92%
Appropriate Hair Removal[2]	751	100%	100%	99%
Appropriate Beta Blocker Usage[2]	222	91%	95%	93%
Controlled Postoperative Blood Glucose[2]	0	-	97%	93%
Prophylactic Antibiotic Timing[2]	598	98%	98%	97%
Prophylactic Antibiotic Timing (Outpatient)	398	97%	93%	92%
Prophylactic Antibiotic Selection[2]	600	99%	99%	97%
Prophylactic Antibiotic Select. (Outpatient)	393	99%	95%	94%
Prophylactic Antibiotic Stopped[2]	586	96%	97%	94%
Recommended VTP Ordered[2]	222	96%	97%	94%
Urinary Catheter Removal[2]	227	94%	92%	90%
Children's Asthma Care				
Received Systemic Corticosteroids	-	-	-	100%
Received Home Management Plan	-	-	-	71%
Received Reliever Medication	-	-	-	100%
Use of Medical Imaging				
Combination Abdominal CT Scan	1,618	0.043	0.133	0.191
Combination Chest CT Scan	1,388	0.006	0.045	0.054
Follow-up Mammogram/Ultrasound	3,702	6.5%	7.6%	8.4%
MRI for Low Back Pain[1]	4	50.0%	36.7%	32.7%
Survey of Patients' Hospital Experiences				
Area Around Room 'Always' Quiet at Night	300+	45%	-	58%
Doctors 'Always' Communicated Well	300+	79%	-	80%
Home Recovery Information Given	300+	88%	-	82%
Hospital Given 9 or 10 on 10 Point Scale	300+	63%	-	67%
Meds 'Always' Explained Before Given	300+	66%	-	60%
Nurses 'Always' Communicated Well	300+	78%	-	76%
Pain 'Always' Well Controlled	300+	71%	-	69%
Room and Bathroom 'Always' Clean	300+	77%	-	71%
Timely Help 'Always' Received	300+	64%	-	64%
Would Definitely Recommend Hospital	300+	70%	-	69%

Togus VA Medical Center

1 VA Center
Augusta, ME 04330
Phone: 207-623-8411
URL: www.maine.va.gov
Type: Acute Care-Veterans Administration
Emergency Services: No
Ownership: Government - Federal
Beds: 67

Measure	Cases	This Hosp.	State Avg.	U.S. Avg.
Heart Attack Care				
ACE Inhibitor or ARB for LVSD[5]	0	-	98%	96%
Aspirin at Arrival[5]	0	-	99%	99%
Aspirin at Discharge[5]	0	-	99%	98%
Beta Blocker at Discharge[5]	0	-	99%	98%
Fibrinolytic Medication Timing[5]	0	-	43%	55%
PCI Within 90 Minutes of Arrival[5]	0	-	94%	90%
Smoking Cessation Advice[5]	0	-	100%	99%
Chest Pain/Possible Heart Attack Care				
Aspirin at Arrival	-	-	98%	95%
Median Time to ECG (minutes)	-	-	7	8
Median Time to Transfer (minutes)	-	-	46	61
Fibrinolytic Medication Timing	-	-	75%	54%
Heart Failure Care				
ACE Inhibitor or ARB for LVSD[1]	20	85%	97%	94%
Discharge Instructions	64	88%	91%	88%
Evaluation of LVS Function	78	100%	99%	98%
Smoking Cessation Advice[1]	17	82%	97%	98%
Pneumonia Care				
Appropriate Initial Antibiotic	36	92%	94%	92%
Blood Culture Timing	41	88%	95%	96%
Influenza Vaccine	43	95%	97%	91%
Initial Antibiotic Timing	43	93%	98%	95%
Pneumococcal Vaccine	49	96%	97%	93%
Smoking Cessation Advice	28	96%	99%	97%
Surgical Care Improvement Project				
Appropriate VTP Within 24 Hours[2]	86	94%	96%	92%
Appropriate Hair Removal[2]	155	100%	100%	99%
Appropriate Beta Blocker Usage[2]	55	95%	95%	93%
Controlled Postoperative Blood Glucose[2,5]	0	-	97%	93%
Prophylactic Antibiotic Timing	105	95%	98%	97%
Prophylactic Antibiotic Timing (Outpatient)	-	-	93%	92%
Prophylactic Antibiotic Selection	104	95%	99%	97%
Prophylactic Antibiotic Select. (Outpatient)	-	-	95%	94%
Prophylactic Antibiotic Stopped	103	94%	97%	94%
Recommended VTP Ordered[2]	87	94%	97%	94%
Urinary Catheter Removal[2]	28	79%	92%	90%
Children's Asthma Care				
Received Systemic Corticosteroids	-	-	-	100%
Received Home Management Plan	-	-	-	71%
Received Reliever Medication	-	-	-	100%
Use of Medical Imaging				
Combination Abdominal CT Scan	-	-	0.133	0.191
Combination Chest CT Scan	-	-	0.045	0.054
Follow-up Mammogram/Ultrasound	-	-	7.6%	8.4%
MRI for Low Back Pain	-	-	36.7%	32.7%
Survey of Patients' Hospital Experiences				
Area Around Room 'Always' Quiet at Night	-	-	-	58%
Doctors 'Always' Communicated Well	-	-	-	80%
Home Recovery Information Given	-	-	-	82%
Hospital Given 9 or 10 on 10 Point Scale	-	-	-	67%
Meds 'Always' Explained Before Given	-	-	-	60%
Nurses 'Always' Communicated Well	-	-	-	76%
Pain 'Always' Well Controlled	-	-	-	69%
Room and Bathroom 'Always' Clean	-	-	-	71%
Timely Help 'Always' Received	-	-	-	64%
Would Definitely Recommend Hospital	-	-	-	69%

Eastern Maine Medical Center

489 State St
Bangor, ME 04401
Phone: 207-973-7000
Fax: 207-973-7865
URL: www.emh.org
Type: Acute Care Hospitals
Emergency Services: Yes
Ownership: Voluntary Non-Profit - Private
Beds: 441

Key Personnel:
CEO/President. . . . . Deborah Carey Johnson, RN
Chief of Medical Staff. . . . . James A Raczek, MD

Measure	Cases	This Hosp.	State Avg.	U.S. Avg.
Heart Attack Care				
ACE Inhibitor or ARB for LVSD	110	99%	98%	96%
Aspirin at Arrival	247	100%	99%	99%
Aspirin at Discharge	921	99%	99%	98%
Beta Blocker at Discharge	880	100%	99%	98%
Fibrinolytic Medication Timing	0	-	43%	55%
PCI Within 90 Minutes of Arrival	38	95%	94%	90%
Smoking Cessation Advice	310	100%	100%	99%
Chest Pain/Possible Heart Attack Care				
Aspirin at Arrival[1]	6	100%	98%	95%
Median Time to ECG (minutes)[1]	6	16	7	8
Median Time to Transfer (minutes)[5]	0	-	46	61
Fibrinolytic Medication Timing[5]	0	-	75%	54%
Heart Failure Care				
ACE Inhibitor or ARB for LVSD	118	100%	97%	94%
Discharge Instructions	301	90%	91%	88%
Evaluation of LVS Function	375	100%	99%	98%
Smoking Cessation Advice	73	99%	97%	98%
Pneumonia Care				
Appropriate Initial Antibiotic	108	91%	94%	92%
Blood Culture Timing	220	98%	95%	96%
Influenza Vaccine	191	98%	97%	91%
Initial Antibiotic Timing	201	98%	98%	95%
Pneumococcal Vaccine	212	98%	97%	93%
Smoking Cessation Advice	144	100%	99%	97%
Surgical Care Improvement Project				
Appropriate VTP Within 24 Hours[2]	403	98%	96%	92%
Appropriate Hair Removal[2]	1,492	100%	100%	99%
Appropriate Beta Blocker Usage[2]	592	99%	95%	93%
Controlled Postoperative Blood Glucose[2]	386	97%	97%	93%
Prophylactic Antibiotic Timing[2]	1,031	99%	98%	97%
Prophylactic Antibiotic Timing (Outpatient)	820	95%	93%	92%
Prophylactic Antibiotic Selection[2]	1,058	99%	99%	97%
Prophylactic Antibiotic Select. (Outpatient)	960	95%	95%	94%
Prophylactic Antibiotic Stopped[2]	974	98%	97%	94%
Recommended VTP Ordered[2]	403	99%	97%	94%
Urinary Catheter Removal[2]	409	93%	92%	90%
Children's Asthma Care				
Received Systemic Corticosteroids	-	-	-	100%
Received Home Management Plan	-	-	-	71%
Received Reliever Medication	-	-	-	100%
Use of Medical Imaging				
Combination Abdominal CT Scan	1,584	0.029	0.133	0.191
Combination Chest CT Scan	1,475	0.002	0.045	0.054
Follow-up Mammogram/Ultrasound	1,435	5.4%	7.6%	8.4%
MRI for Low Back Pain	293	36.9%	36.7%	32.7%
Survey of Patients' Hospital Experiences				
Area Around Room 'Always' Quiet at Night	300+	44%	-	58%
Doctors 'Always' Communicated Well	300+	77%	-	80%
Home Recovery Information Given	300+	85%	-	82%
Hospital Given 9 or 10 on 10 Point Scale	300+	69%	-	67%
Meds 'Always' Explained Before Given	300+	59%	-	60%
Nurses 'Always' Communicated Well	300+	77%	-	76%
Pain 'Always' Well Controlled	300+	69%	-	69%
Room and Bathroom 'Always' Clean	300+	73%	-	71%
Timely Help 'Always' Received	300+	62%	-	64%
Would Definitely Recommend Hospital	300+	76%	-	69%

NOTE: Hospital profiles are in alphabetical order by state, then city, then hospital within the city; Rankings exclude hospitals with less than 25 cases except for patient surveys which excludes hospitals with less than 100 cases; (a) 100–299 cases; (1) The number of cases is too small to be sure how well a hospital is performing; (2) The hospital indicated that the data submitted for this measure were based on a sample of cases; (3) Data was collected during a shorter time period (fewer quarters) than the maximum possible time for this measure; (4) Suppressed for one or more quarters by CMS; (5) No data is available from the hospital for this measure; (6) Fewer than 100 patients completed the HCAHPS survey. Use these rates with caution, as the number of surveys may be too low to reliably assess hospital performance; (7) Survey results are based on less than 12 months of data; (8) Survey results are not available for this reporting period; (9) No or very few patients were eligible for the HCAHPS survey. The scores shown, if any, reflect a very small number of surveys; (10) A state average was not calculated because too few hospitals in the state submitted data; (11) There were discrepancies in the data collection process; Please refer to the User's Guide for a full explanation of data.

Saint Joseph Hospital

360 Broadway
Bangor, ME 04401
Phone: 207-262-1000
Fax: 207-262-1922
URL: www.stjoeshealing.com
Type: Acute Care Hospitals
Emergency Services: No
Ownership: Voluntary Non-Profit - Church
Beds: 100

Key Personnel:

CEO/President. . . . . Sister Mary Norberta, CSSF
Chief of Medical Staff. . . . . David Renedo, MD
Radiology. . . . . David Ahola
Patient Relations . . . . Dianne Swandal, BSN

Measure	Cases	This Hosp.	State Avg.	U.S. Avg.
Heart Attack Care				
ACE Inhibitor or ARB for LVSD[1]	8	100%	98%	96%
Aspirin at Arrival	78	100%	99%	99%
Aspirin at Discharge	51	98%	99%	98%
Beta Blocker at Discharge	50	100%	99%	98%
Fibrinolytic Medication Timing	0	-	43%	55%
PCI Within 90 Minutes of Arrival	0	-	94%	90%
Smoking Cessation Advice[1]	8	100%	100%	99%
Chest Pain/Possible Heart Attack Care				
Aspirin at Arrival[1]	23	100%	98%	95%
Median Time to ECG (minutes)[1]	24	20	7	8
Median Time to Transfer (minutes)[1]	9	55	46	61
Fibrinolytic Medication Timing	0	-	75%	54%
Heart Failure Care				
ACE Inhibitor or ARB for LVSD	35	100%	97%	94%
Discharge Instructions	109	98%	91%	88%
Evaluation of LVS Function	144	100%	99%	98%
Smoking Cessation Advice[1]	22	100%	97%	98%
Pneumonia Care				
Appropriate Initial Antibiotic	121	99%	94%	92%
Blood Culture Timing	162	96%	95%	96%
Influenza Vaccine	116	100%	97%	91%
Initial Antibiotic Timing	184	97%	98%	95%
Pneumococcal Vaccine	177	98%	97%	93%
Smoking Cessation Advice	66	100%	99%	97%
Surgical Care Improvement Project				
Appropriate VTP Within 24 Hours[2]	199	98%	96%	92%
Appropriate Hair Removal[2]	507	100%	100%	99%
Appropriate Beta Blocker Usage[2]	134	97%	95%	93%
Controlled Postoperative Blood Glucose[2]	0	-	97%	93%
Prophylactic Antibiotic Timing[2]	380	100%	98%	97%
Prophylactic Antibiotic Timing (Outpatient)	328	98%	93%	92%
Prophylactic Antibiotic Selection[2]	381	99%	99%	97%
Prophylactic Antibiotic Select. (Outpatient)	325	99%	95%	94%
Prophylactic Antibiotic Stopped[2]	376	100%	97%	94%
Recommended VTP Ordered[2]	199	99%	97%	94%
Urinary Catheter Removal[2]	28	86%	92%	90%
Children's Asthma Care				
Received Systemic Corticosteroids	-	-	-	100%
Received Home Management Plan	-	-	-	71%
Received Reliever Medication	-	-	-	100%
Use of Medical Imaging				
Combination Abdominal CT Scan	567	0.058	0.133	0.191
Combination Chest CT Scan	401	0.000	0.045	0.054
Follow-up Mammogram/Ultrasound	2,577	4.9%	7.6%	8.4%
MRI for Low Back Pain	262	32.8%	36.7%	32.7%
Survey of Patients' Hospital Experiences				
Area Around Room 'Always' Quiet at Night	300+	59%	-	58%
Doctors 'Always' Communicated Well	300+	82%	-	80%
Home Recovery Information Given	300+	89%	-	82%
Hospital Given 9 or 10 on 10 Point Scale	300+	80%	-	67%
Meds 'Always' Explained Before Given	300+	63%	-	60%
Nurses 'Always' Communicated Well	300+	81%	-	76%
Pain 'Always' Well Controlled	300+	73%	-	69%
Room and Bathroom 'Always' Clean	300+	79%	-	71%
Timely Help 'Always' Received	300+	65%	-	64%
Would Definitely Recommend Hospital	300+	83%	-	69%

Mount Desert Island Hospital

10 Wayman Lane
Bar Harbor, ME 04609
Phone: 207-288-5081
Fax: 207-288-5874
E-mail: crdev@mdihospital.org
URL: www.mdihospital.com
Type: Critical Access Hospitals
Emergency Services: Yes
Ownership: Voluntary Non-Profit - Private
Beds: 49

Key Personnel:

CEO/President. . . . . Arthur J Blank
Chief of Medical Staff . . . . John M Benson, MD
Quality Assurance . . . . Jean Wolf
Emergency Room . . . . Michael Lewin, MD

Measure	Cases	This Hosp.	State Avg.	U.S. Avg.
Heart Attack Care				
ACE Inhibitor or ARB for LVSD[1]	1	100%	98%	96%
Aspirin at Arrival[1]	12	100%	99%	99%
Aspirin at Discharge[1]	6	100%	99%	98%
Beta Blocker at Discharge[1]	5	80%	99%	98%
Fibrinolytic Medication Timing	0	-	43%	55%
PCI Within 90 Minutes of Arrival	0	-	94%	90%
Smoking Cessation Advice[1]	1	100%	100%	99%
Chest Pain/Possible Heart Attack Care				
Aspirin at Arrival[5]	0	-	98%	95%
Median Time to ECG (minutes)[5]	0	-	7	8
Median Time to Transfer (minutes)[5]	0	-	46	61
Fibrinolytic Medication Timing[5]	0	-	75%	54%
Heart Failure Care				
ACE Inhibitor or ARB for LVSD[1]	8	88%	97%	94%
Discharge Instructions[1]	14	100%	91%	88%
Evaluation of LVS Function	29	97%	99%	98%
Smoking Cessation Advice[1]	1	100%	97%	98%
Pneumonia Care				
Appropriate Initial Antibiotic[1]	17	88%	94%	92%
Blood Culture Timing	31	100%	95%	96%
Influenza Vaccine[1]	14	100%	97%	91%
Initial Antibiotic Timing	27	100%	98%	95%
Pneumococcal Vaccine	30	100%	97%	93%
Smoking Cessation Advice[1]	1	100%	99%	97%
Surgical Care Improvement Project				
Appropriate VTP Within 24 Hours[1,2]	22	95%	96%	92%
Appropriate Hair Removal[2]	56	100%	100%	99%
Appropriate Beta Blocker Usage[1,2]	7	86%	95%	93%
Controlled Postoperative Blood Glucose[2]	0	-	97%	93%
Prophylactic Antibiotic Timing[2]	41	95%	98%	97%
Prophylactic Antibiotic Timing (Outpatient)[5]	0	-	93%	92%
Prophylactic Antibiotic Selection[2]	42	100%	99%	97%
Prophylactic Antibiotic Select. (Outpatient)[5]	0	-	95%	94%
Prophylactic Antibiotic Stopped[2]	41	100%	97%	94%
Recommended VTP Ordered[1,2]	23	91%	97%	94%
Urinary Catheter Removal[1,2]	20	95%	92%	90%
Children's Asthma Care				
Received Systemic Corticosteroids	-	-	-	100%
Received Home Management Plan	-	-	-	71%
Received Reliever Medication	-	-	-	100%
Use of Medical Imaging				
Combination Abdominal CT Scan	259	0.259	0.133	0.191
Combination Chest CT Scan	109	0.147	0.045	0.054
Follow-up Mammogram/Ultrasound	367	4.9%	7.6%	8.4%
MRI for Low Back Pain[5]	0	-	36.7%	32.7%
Survey of Patients' Hospital Experiences				
Area Around Room 'Always' Quiet at Night	(a)	63%	-	58%
Doctors 'Always' Communicated Well	(a)	90%	-	80%
Home Recovery Information Given	(a)	90%	-	82%
Hospital Given 9 or 10 on 10 Point Scale	(a)	84%	-	67%
Meds 'Always' Explained Before Given	(a)	72%	-	60%
Nurses 'Always' Communicated Well	(a)	86%	-	76%
Pain 'Always' Well Controlled	(a)	76%	-	69%
Room and Bathroom 'Always' Clean	(a)	86%	-	71%
Timely Help 'Always' Received	(a)	82%	-	64%
Would Definitely Recommend Hospital	(a)	87%	-	69%

Waldo County General Hospital

118 Northport Ave
Belfast, ME 04915
Phone: 207-338-2500
Fax: 207-338-9382
E-mail: inquires@wchi.com
URL: www.wchi.com
Type: Critical Access Hospitals
Emergency Services: Yes
Ownership: Voluntary Non-Profit - Private
Beds: 25

Key Personnel:

CEO/President. . . . . Mark Biscone
Radiology. . . . . John P Gay
Emergency Room . . . . Camille C Canova

Measure	Cases	This Hosp.	State Avg.	U.S. Avg.
Heart Attack Care				
ACE Inhibitor or ARB for LVSD[1]	6	100%	98%	96%
Aspirin at Arrival[1]	19	95%	99%	99%
Aspirin at Discharge[1]	15	100%	99%	98%
Beta Blocker at Discharge[1]	15	100%	99%	98%
Fibrinolytic Medication Timing	0	-	43%	55%
PCI Within 90 Minutes of Arrival[5]	0	-	94%	90%
Smoking Cessation Advice[1]	2	100%	100%	99%
Chest Pain/Possible Heart Attack Care				
Aspirin at Arrival	-	-	98%	95%
Median Time to ECG (minutes)	-	-	7	8
Median Time to Transfer (minutes)	-	-	46	61
Fibrinolytic Medication Timing	-	-	75%	54%
Heart Failure Care				
ACE Inhibitor or ARB for LVSD[1]	4	100%	97%	94%
Discharge Instructions[1]	22	86%	91%	88%
Evaluation of LVS Function	30	93%	99%	98%
Smoking Cessation Advice[1]	6	100%	97%	98%
Pneumonia Care				
Appropriate Initial Antibiotic	56	96%	94%	92%
Blood Culture Timing	34	100%	95%	96%
Influenza Vaccine	46	100%	97%	91%
Initial Antibiotic Timing	76	100%	98%	95%
Pneumococcal Vaccine	79	99%	97%	93%
Smoking Cessation Advice[1]	18	100%	99%	97%
Surgical Care Improvement Project				
Appropriate VTP Within 24 Hours	51	88%	96%	92%
Appropriate Hair Removal	154	99%	100%	99%
Appropriate Beta Blocker Usage	49	96%	95%	93%
Controlled Postoperative Blood Glucose	0	-	97%	93%
Prophylactic Antibiotic Timing	112	97%	98%	97%
Prophylactic Antibiotic Timing (Outpatient)	-	-	93%	92%
Prophylactic Antibiotic Selection	112	98%	99%	97%
Prophylactic Antibiotic Select. (Outpatient)	-	-	95%	94%
Prophylactic Antibiotic Stopped	105	96%	97%	94%
Recommended VTP Ordered	51	88%	97%	94%
Urinary Catheter Removal	43	93%	92%	90%
Children's Asthma Care				
Received Systemic Corticosteroids	-	-	-	100%
Received Home Management Plan	-	-	-	71%
Received Reliever Medication	-	-	-	100%
Use of Medical Imaging				
Combination Abdominal CT Scan	-	-	0.133	0.191
Combination Chest CT Scan	-	-	0.045	0.054
Follow-up Mammogram/Ultrasound	-	-	7.6%	8.4%
MRI for Low Back Pain	-	-	36.7%	32.7%
Survey of Patients' Hospital Experiences				
Area Around Room 'Always' Quiet at Night	(a)	62%	-	58%
Doctors 'Always' Communicated Well	(a)	83%	-	80%
Home Recovery Information Given	(a)	89%	-	82%
Hospital Given 9 or 10 on 10 Point Scale	(a)	79%	-	67%
Meds 'Always' Explained Before Given	(a)	68%	-	60%
Nurses 'Always' Communicated Well	(a)	84%	-	76%
Pain 'Always' Well Controlled	(a)	81%	-	69%
Room and Bathroom 'Always' Clean	(a)	85%	-	71%
Timely Help 'Always' Received	(a)	79%	-	64%
Would Definitely Recommend Hospital	(a)	78%	-	69%

NOTE: Hospital profiles are in alphabetical order by state, then city, then hospital within the city; Rankings exclude hospitals with less than 25 cases except for patient surveys which excludes hospitals with less than 100 cases; (a) 100–299 cases; (1) The number of cases is too small to be sure how well a hospital is performing; (2) The hospital indicated that the data submitted for this measure were based on a sample of cases; (3) Data was collected during a shorter time period (fewer quarters) than the maximum possible time for this measure; (4) Suppressed for one or more quarters by CMS; (5) No data is available from the hospital for this measure; (6) Fewer than 100 patients completed the HCAHPS survey. Use these rates with caution, as the number of surveys may be too low to reliably assess hospital performance; (7) Survey results are based on less than 12 months of data; (8) Survey results are not available for this reporting period; (9) No or very few patients were eligible for the HCAHPS survey. The scores shown, if any, reflect a very small number of surveys; (10) A state average was not calculated because too few hospitals in the state submitted data; (11) There were discrepancies in the data collection process; Please refer to the User's Guide for a full explanation of data.

Southern Maine Medical Center

1 Medical Center Drive — Phone: 207-283-7000
Biddeford, ME 04005 — Fax: 207-283-7020
E-mail: info@smmc.org
URL: www.smmc.org
Type: Acute Care Hospitals — Emergency Services: Yes
Ownership: Voluntary Non-Profit - Private — Beds: 150

Key Personnel:
CEO/President. . . . . Edward J McGeachey
Chief of Medical Staff . . . . Robert Fernandez, MD
Coronary Care . . . . Kathy Viger, RN
Operating Room. . . . . Toni Clark, RN
Quality Assurance . . . . Melissa McClay
Radiology. . . . . Stephen M Madigan
Emergency Room . . . . Gina Quinn-Skillings, MD

Measure	Cases	This Hosp.	State Avg.	U.S. Avg.
Heart Attack Care				
ACE Inhibitor or ARB for LVSD[1]	12	100%	98%	96%
Aspirin at Arrival	99	99%	99%	99%
Aspirin at Discharge	67	99%	99%	98%
Beta Blocker at Discharge	70	100%	99%	98%
Fibrinolytic Medication Timing	0	-	43%	55%
PCI Within 90 Minutes of Arrival	0	-	94%	90%
Smoking Cessation Advice[1]	10	100%	100%	99%
Chest Pain/Possible Heart Attack Care				
Aspirin at Arrival	73	100%	98%	95%
Median Time to ECG (minutes)	73	11	7	8
Median Time to Transfer (minutes)	32	26	46	61
Fibrinolytic Medication Timing[1]	1	100%	75%	54%
Heart Failure Care				
ACE Inhibitor or ARB for LVSD[2]	40	98%	97%	94%
Discharge Instructions[2]	141	90%	91%	88%
Evaluation of LVS Function[2]	207	100%	99%	98%
Smoking Cessation Advice[1,2]	16	100%	97%	98%
Pneumonia Care				
Appropriate Initial Antibiotic[2]	80	96%	94%	92%
Blood Culture Timing[2]	81	89%	95%	96%
Influenza Vaccine[2]	91	98%	97%	91%
Initial Antibiotic Timing[2]	125	99%	98%	95%
Pneumococcal Vaccine[2]	121	99%	97%	93%
Smoking Cessation Advice[2]	38	97%	99%	97%
Surgical Care Improvement Project				
Appropriate VTP Within 24 Hours[2]	101	94%	96%	92%
Appropriate Hair Removal[2]	304	100%	100%	99%
Appropriate Beta Blocker Usage[2]	102	90%	95%	93%
Controlled Postoperative Blood Glucose[2]	0	-	97%	93%
Prophylactic Antibiotic Timing[2]	194	97%	98%	97%
Prophylactic Antibiotic Timing (Outpatient)	61	93%	93%	92%
Prophylactic Antibiotic Selection[2]	194	97%	99%	97%
Prophylactic Antibiotic Select. (Outpatient)	58	91%	95%	94%
Prophylactic Antibiotic Stopped[2]	190	100%	97%	94%
Recommended VTP Ordered[2]	102	94%	97%	94%
Urinary Catheter Removal[2]	57	96%	92%	90%
Children's Asthma Care				
Received Systemic Corticosteroids	-	-	-	100%
Received Home Management Plan	-	-	-	71%
Received Reliever Medication	-	-	-	100%
Use of Medical Imaging				
Combination Abdominal CT Scan	756	0.037	0.133	0.191
Combination Chest CT Scan	470	0.000	0.045	0.054
Follow-up Mammogram/Ultrasound	1,344	7.2%	7.6%	8.4%
MRI for Low Back Pain	175	37.1%	36.7%	32.7%
Survey of Patients' Hospital Experiences				
Area Around Room 'Always' Quiet at Night	300+	48%	-	58%
Doctors 'Always' Communicated Well	300+	81%	-	80%
Home Recovery Information Given	300+	86%	-	82%
Hospital Given 9 or 10 on 10 Point Scale	300+	66%	-	67%
Meds 'Always' Explained Before Given	300+	62%	-	60%
Nurses 'Always' Communicated Well	300+	78%	-	76%
Pain 'Always' Well Controlled	300+	70%	-	69%
Room and Bathroom 'Always' Clean	300+	73%	-	71%
Timely Help 'Always' Received	300+	62%	-	64%
Would Definitely Recommend Hospital	300+	76%	-	69%

Blue Hill Memorial Hospital

57 Water Street — Phone: 207-374-2836
Blue Hill, ME 04614 — Fax: 207-374-5368
URL: bhmh.org/default.html
Type: Critical Access Hospitals — Emergency Services: Yes
Ownership: Government - Local — Beds: 25

Key Personnel:
CEO/President. . . . . Erik N Steele
Chief of Medical Staff . . . . Robert Baroody
Radiology. . . . . Richard Seger

Measure	Cases	This Hosp.	State Avg.	U.S. Avg.
Heart Attack Care				
ACE Inhibitor or ARB for LVSD[1]	3	100%	98%	96%
Aspirin at Arrival[1]	10	100%	99%	99%
Aspirin at Discharge[1]	8	88%	99%	98%
Beta Blocker at Discharge[1]	8	100%	99%	98%
Fibrinolytic Medication Timing	0	-	43%	55%
PCI Within 90 Minutes of Arrival[5]	0	-	94%	90%
Smoking Cessation Advice[1]	1	100%	100%	99%
Chest Pain/Possible Heart Attack Care				
Aspirin at Arrival	-	-	98%	95%
Median Time to ECG (minutes)	-	-	7	8
Median Time to Transfer (minutes)	-	-	46	61
Fibrinolytic Medication Timing	-	-	75%	54%
Heart Failure Care				
ACE Inhibitor or ARB for LVSD[1]	5	100%	97%	94%
Discharge Instructions[1]	16	100%	91%	88%
Evaluation of LVS Function[1]	18	94%	99%	98%
Smoking Cessation Advice[1]	2	100%	97%	98%
Pneumonia Care				
Appropriate Initial Antibiotic[1]	24	92%	94%	92%
Blood Culture Timing	31	94%	95%	96%
Influenza Vaccine[1]	18	89%	97%	91%
Initial Antibiotic Timing[1]	23	100%	98%	95%
Pneumococcal Vaccine	27	85%	97%	93%
Smoking Cessation Advice[1]	6	100%	99%	97%
Surgical Care Improvement Project				
Appropriate VTP Within 24 Hours[1]	15	93%	96%	92%
Appropriate Hair Removal	51	100%	100%	99%
Appropriate Beta Blocker Usage[1]	10	90%	95%	93%
Controlled Postoperative Blood Glucose	0	-	97%	93%
Prophylactic Antibiotic Timing[1]	20	95%	98%	97%
Prophylactic Antibiotic Timing (Outpatient)	-	-	93%	92%
Prophylactic Antibiotic Selection[1]	21	95%	99%	97%
Prophylactic Antibiotic Select. (Outpatient)	-	-	95%	94%
Prophylactic Antibiotic Stopped[1]	20	95%	97%	94%
Recommended VTP Ordered[1]	15	93%	97%	94%
Urinary Catheter Removal[1]	1	100%	92%	90%
Children's Asthma Care				
Received Systemic Corticosteroids	-	-	-	100%
Received Home Management Plan	-	-	-	71%
Received Reliever Medication	-	-	-	100%
Use of Medical Imaging				
Combination Abdominal CT Scan	-	-	0.133	0.191
Combination Chest CT Scan	-	-	0.045	0.054
Follow-up Mammogram/Ultrasound	-	-	7.6%	8.4%
MRI for Low Back Pain	-	-	36.7%	32.7%
Survey of Patients' Hospital Experiences				
Area Around Room 'Always' Quiet at Night	(a)	57%	-	58%
Doctors 'Always' Communicated Well	(a)	79%	-	80%
Home Recovery Information Given	(a)	80%	-	82%
Hospital Given 9 or 10 on 10 Point Scale	(a)	64%	-	67%
Meds 'Always' Explained Before Given	(a)	64%	-	60%
Nurses 'Always' Communicated Well	(a)	75%	-	76%
Pain 'Always' Well Controlled	(a)	65%	-	69%
Room and Bathroom 'Always' Clean	(a)	78%	-	71%
Timely Help 'Always' Received	(a)	70%	-	64%
Would Definitely Recommend Hospital	(a)	63%	-	69%

Saint Andrews Hospital

2st Andrews Lane — Phone: 207-633-2121
Boothbay Hrbr, ME 04538 — Fax: 207-633-5173
E-mail: mpinkham@standrewshealthcare.org
URL: www.standrewshealthcare.org
Type: Critical Access Hospitals — Emergency Services: Yes
Ownership: Voluntary Non-Profit - Private — Beds: 15

Key Personnel:
CEO/President. . . . . James W Donovan
Chief of Medical Staff . . . . Jana Kazalski, DO
Infection Control. . . . . Joan Taylor
Quality Assurance . . . . Charles White
Radiology. . . . . Bernadette V Jakomin, MD
Emergency Room . . . . Matthew Sleeth, MD

Measure	Cases	This Hosp.	State Avg.	U.S. Avg.
Heart Attack Care				
ACE Inhibitor or ARB for LVSD[3]	0	-	98%	96%
Aspirin at Arrival[1,3]	1	100%	99%	99%
Aspirin at Discharge[3]	0	-	99%	98%
Beta Blocker at Discharge[1,3]	1	100%	99%	98%
Fibrinolytic Medication Timing[3]	0	-	43%	55%
PCI Within 90 Minutes of Arrival[3]	0	-	94%	90%
Smoking Cessation Advice[3]	0	-	100%	99%
Chest Pain/Possible Heart Attack Care				
Aspirin at Arrival[3]	49	100%	98%	95%
Median Time to ECG (minutes)[3]	49	7	7	8
Median Time to Transfer (minutes)[5]	0	-	46	61
Fibrinolytic Medication Timing[1,3]	3	67%	75%	54%
Heart Failure Care				
ACE Inhibitor or ARB for LVSD[1,3]	2	100%	97%	94%
Discharge Instructions[1,3]	4	75%	91%	88%
Evaluation of LVS Function[1,3]	9	89%	99%	98%
Smoking Cessation Advice[1,3]	1	100%	97%	98%
Pneumonia Care				
Appropriate Initial Antibiotic[1,3]	5	100%	94%	92%
Blood Culture Timing[1,3]	4	100%	95%	96%
Influenza Vaccine[1]	7	100%	97%	91%
Initial Antibiotic Timing[1,3]	9	100%	98%	95%
Pneumococcal Vaccine[1,3]	10	90%	97%	93%
Smoking Cessation Advice[1,3]	1	100%	99%	97%
Surgical Care Improvement Project				
Appropriate VTP Within 24 Hours[5]	0	-	96%	92%
Appropriate Hair Removal[5]	0	-	100%	99%
Appropriate Beta Blocker Usage[5]	0	-	95%	93%
Controlled Postoperative Blood Glucose[5]	0	-	97%	93%
Prophylactic Antibiotic Timing[5]	0	-	98%	97%
Prophylactic Antibiotic Timing (Outpatient)[5]	0	-	93%	92%
Prophylactic Antibiotic Selection[5]	0	-	99%	97%
Prophylactic Antibiotic Select. (Outpatient)[5]	0	-	95%	94%
Prophylactic Antibiotic Stopped[5]	0	-	97%	94%
Recommended VTP Ordered[5]	0	-	97%	94%
Urinary Catheter Removal[5]	0	-	92%	90%
Children's Asthma Care				
Received Systemic Corticosteroids	-	-	-	100%
Received Home Management Plan	-	-	-	71%
Received Reliever Medication	-	-	-	100%
Use of Medical Imaging				
Combination Abdominal CT Scan	85	0.047	0.133	0.191
Combination Chest CT Scan	53	0.038	0.045	0.054
Follow-up Mammogram/Ultrasound	190	13.7%	7.6%	8.4%
MRI for Low Back Pain[5]	0	-	36.7%	32.7%
Survey of Patients' Hospital Experiences				
Area Around Room 'Always' Quiet at Night[6]	<100	47%	-	58%
Doctors 'Always' Communicated Well[6]	<100	87%	-	80%
Home Recovery Information Given[6]	<100	91%	-	82%
Hospital Given 9 or 10 on 10 Point Scale[6]	<100	69%	-	67%
Meds 'Always' Explained Before Given[6]	<100	73%	-	60%
Nurses 'Always' Communicated Well[6]	<100	75%	-	76%
Pain 'Always' Well Controlled[6]	<100	65%	-	69%
Room and Bathroom 'Always' Clean[6]	<100	66%	-	71%
Timely Help 'Always' Received[6]	<100	61%	-	64%
Would Definitely Recommend Hospital	<100	78%	-	69%

NOTE: Hospital profiles are in alphabetical order by state, then city, then hospital within the city; Rankings exclude hospitals with less than 25 cases except for patient surveys which excludes hospitals with less than 100 cases; (a) 100–299 cases; (1) The number of cases is too small to be sure how well a hospital is performing; (2) The hospital indicated that the data submitted for this measure were based on a sample of cases; (3) Data was collected during a shorter time period (fewer quarters) than the maximum possible time for this measure; (4) Suppressed for one or more quarters by CMS; (5) No data is available from the hospital for this measure; (6) Fewer than 100 patients completed the HCAHPS survey. Use these rates with caution, as the number of surveys may be too low to reliably assess hospital performance; (7) Survey results are based on less than 12 months of data; (8) Survey results are not available for this reporting period; (9) No or very few patients were eligible for the HCAHPS survey. The scores shown, if any, reflect a very small number of surveys; (10) A state average was not calculated because too few hospitals in the state submitted data; (11) There were discrepancies in the data collection process; Please refer to the User's Guide for a full explanation of data.

Bridgton Hospital

10 Hospital Drive
Bridgton, ME 04009
E-mail: dubay@bh.com
URL: www.bridgtonhospital.com
Type: Critical Access Hospitals
Ownership: Voluntary Non-Profit - Private
Phone: 207-647-6000
Fax: 207-647-4209
Emergency Services: Yes
Beds: 40

Key Personnel:
Chief of Medical Staff.......... Henry Roy, III, MD
Infection Control.............. Marcia Elliott, RN
Operating Room.............. Genise Knowlton, RN
Pediatric Ambulatory Care...... Wenda L Saunders, MD
Pediatric In-Patient Care....... Wenda L Saunders, MD
Quality Assurance............ Kathy Wohlenberg

Measure	Cases	This Hosp.	State Avg.	U.S. Avg.
Heart Attack Care				
ACE Inhibitor or ARB for LVSD[5]	0	-	98%	96%
Aspirin at Arrival[5]	0	-	99%	99%
Aspirin at Discharge[5]	0	-	99%	98%
Beta Blocker at Discharge[5]	0	-	99%	98%
Fibrinolytic Medication Timing[5]	0	-	43%	55%
PCI Within 90 Minutes of Arrival[5]	0	-	94%	90%
Smoking Cessation Advice[5]	0	-	100%	99%
Chest Pain/Possible Heart Attack Care				
Aspirin at Arrival	-	-	98%	95%
Median Time to ECG (minutes)	-	-	7	8
Median Time to Transfer (minutes)	-	-	46	61
Fibrinolytic Medication Timing	-	-	75%	54%
Heart Failure Care				
ACE Inhibitor or ARB for LVSD[1]	2	100%	97%	94%
Discharge Instructions	30	90%	91%	88%
Evaluation of LVS Function	31	94%	99%	98%
Smoking Cessation Advice[1]	5	100%	97%	98%
Pneumonia Care				
Appropriate Initial Antibiotic	46	91%	94%	92%
Blood Culture Timing	58	97%	95%	96%
Influenza Vaccine	36	94%	97%	91%
Initial Antibiotic Timing	59	95%	98%	95%
Pneumococcal Vaccine	53	92%	97%	93%
Smoking Cessation Advice[1]	16	100%	99%	97%
Surgical Care Improvement Project				
Appropriate VTP Within 24 Hours[1]	10	90%	96%	92%
Appropriate Hair Removal	27	100%	100%	99%
Appropriate Beta Blocker Usage[5]	0	-	95%	93%
Controlled Postoperative Blood Glucose	0	-	97%	93%
Prophylactic Antibiotic Timing[1]	20	95%	98%	97%
Prophylactic Antibiotic Timing (Outpatient)	-	-	93%	92%
Prophylactic Antibiotic Selection[1]	21	100%	99%	97%
Prophylactic Antibiotic Select. (Outpatient)	-	-	95%	94%
Prophylactic Antibiotic Stopped[1]	20	90%	97%	94%
Recommended VTP Ordered[1]	10	100%	97%	94%
Urinary Catheter Removal[1]	1	100%	92%	90%
Children's Asthma Care				
Received Systemic Corticosteroids	-	-	-	100%
Received Home Management Plan	-	-	-	71%
Received Reliever Medication	-	-	-	100%
Use of Medical Imaging				
Combination Abdominal CT Scan	-	-	0.133	0.191
Combination Chest CT Scan	-	-	0.045	0.054
Follow-up Mammogram/Ultrasound	-	-	7.6%	8.4%
MRI for Low Back Pain	-	-	36.7%	32.7%
Survey of Patients' Hospital Experiences				
Area Around Room 'Always' Quiet at Night	300+	61%	-	58%
Doctors 'Always' Communicated Well	300+	86%	-	80%
Home Recovery Information Given	300+	90%	-	82%
Hospital Given 9 or 10 on 10 Point Scale	300+	76%	-	67%
Meds 'Always' Explained Before Given	300+	69%	-	60%
Nurses 'Always' Communicated Well	300+	79%	-	76%
Pain 'Always' Well Controlled	300+	75%	-	69%
Room and Bathroom 'Always' Clean	300+	79%	-	71%
Timely Help 'Always' Received	300+	74%	-	64%
Would Definitely Recommend Hospital	300+	75%	-	69%

Mid Coast Hospital

123 Medical Center Drive
Brunswick, ME 04011
URL: www.midcoasthealth.com
Type: Acute Care Hospitals
Ownership: Voluntary Non-Profit - Private
Phone: 207-729-0181
Fax: 207-373-6744
Emergency Services: Yes
Beds: 104

Key Personnel:
CEO/President.............. Herbert Paris
Chief of Medical Staff.......... Scott Mills, MD
Infection Control.............. Lorna MacKinnon, RN
Quality Assurance............ George Hunter
Radiology.................. John J Chomyn
Emergency Room............ Marlene Cormier
Intensive Care Unit........... Brian Viele

Measure	Cases	This Hosp.	State Avg.	U.S. Avg.
Heart Attack Care				
ACE Inhibitor or ARB for LVSD[1]	11	100%	98%	96%
Aspirin at Arrival	49	100%	99%	99%
Aspirin at Discharge	31	100%	99%	98%
Beta Blocker at Discharge	31	100%	99%	98%
Fibrinolytic Medication Timing	0	-	43%	55%
PCI Within 90 Minutes of Arrival	0	-	94%	90%
Smoking Cessation Advice[1]	5	100%	100%	99%
Chest Pain/Possible Heart Attack Care				
Aspirin at Arrival	60	98%	98%	95%
Median Time to ECG (minutes)	61	4	7	8
Median Time to Transfer (minutes)	0	-	46	61
Fibrinolytic Medication Timing[1]	20	80%	75%	54%
Heart Failure Care				
ACE Inhibitor or ARB for LVSD	42	100%	97%	94%
Discharge Instructions	75	100%	91%	88%
Evaluation of LVS Function	95	100%	99%	98%
Smoking Cessation Advice[1]	15	100%	97%	98%
Pneumonia Care				
Appropriate Initial Antibiotic[2]	83	99%	94%	92%
Blood Culture Timing[2]	66	89%	95%	96%
Influenza Vaccine[2]	78	100%	97%	91%
Initial Antibiotic Timing[2]	104	99%	98%	95%
Pneumococcal Vaccine[2]	120	99%	97%	93%
Smoking Cessation Advice[2]	25	100%	99%	97%
Surgical Care Improvement Project				
Appropriate VTP Within 24 Hours	90	96%	96%	92%
Appropriate Hair Removal	227	100%	100%	99%
Appropriate Beta Blocker Usage	45	100%	95%	93%
Controlled Postoperative Blood Glucose	0	-	97%	93%
Prophylactic Antibiotic Timing	175	99%	98%	97%
Prophylactic Antibiotic Timing (Outpatient)	151	99%	93%	92%
Prophylactic Antibiotic Selection	175	99%	99%	97%
Prophylactic Antibiotic Select. (Outpatient)	167	96%	95%	94%
Prophylactic Antibiotic Stopped	168	99%	97%	94%
Recommended VTP Ordered	90	98%	97%	94%
Urinary Catheter Removal[1]	13	92%	92%	90%
Children's Asthma Care				
Received Systemic Corticosteroids	-	-	-	100%
Received Home Management Plan	-	-	-	71%
Received Reliever Medication	-	-	-	100%
Use of Medical Imaging				
Combination Abdominal CT Scan	639	0.161	0.133	0.191
Combination Chest CT Scan	499	0.002	0.045	0.054
Follow-up Mammogram/Ultrasound	1,088	8.0%	7.6%	8.4%
MRI for Low Back Pain	147	29.3%	36.7%	32.7%
Survey of Patients' Hospital Experiences				
Area Around Room 'Always' Quiet at Night	300+	52%	-	58%
Doctors 'Always' Communicated Well	300+	78%	-	80%
Home Recovery Information Given	300+	85%	-	82%
Hospital Given 9 or 10 on 10 Point Scale	300+	70%	-	67%
Meds 'Always' Explained Before Given	300+	60%	-	60%
Nurses 'Always' Communicated Well	300+	75%	-	76%
Pain 'Always' Well Controlled	300+	70%	-	69%
Room and Bathroom 'Always' Clean	300+	74%	-	71%
Timely Help 'Always' Received	300+	60%	-	64%
Would Definitely Recommend Hospital	300+	78%	-	69%

Parkview Adventist Medical Center

329 Main St
Brunswick, ME 04011
URL: www.parkviewamc.org
Type: Acute Care Hospitals
Ownership: Voluntary Non-Profit - Church
Phone: 207-373-2000
Fax: 207-373-2161
Emergency Services: No
Beds: 55

Key Personnel:
CEO/President.............. Ted Lewis
Pediatric Ambulatory Care...... Larry Losey, MD
Pediatric In-Patient Care....... Larry Losey, MD
Radiology.................. K. Fleming
Hemotology Center........... Trudi Chase

Measure	Cases	This Hosp.	State Avg.	U.S. Avg.
Heart Attack Care				
ACE Inhibitor or ARB for LVSD[1]	7	86%	98%	96%
Aspirin at Arrival[1]	9	78%	99%	99%
Aspirin at Discharge[1]	6	83%	99%	98%
Beta Blocker at Discharge[1]	7	100%	99%	98%
Fibrinolytic Medication Timing	0	-	43%	55%
PCI Within 90 Minutes of Arrival	0	-	94%	90%
Smoking Cessation Advice[1]	1	100%	100%	99%
Chest Pain/Possible Heart Attack Care				
Aspirin at Arrival[1]	22	100%	98%	95%
Median Time to ECG (minutes)[1]	22	12	7	8
Median Time to Transfer (minutes)[1,3]	4	55	46	61
Fibrinolytic Medication Timing[1,3]	1	100%	75%	54%
Heart Failure Care				
ACE Inhibitor or ARB for LVSD[1]	16	94%	97%	94%
Discharge Instructions	38	87%	91%	88%
Evaluation of LVS Function	48	92%	99%	98%
Smoking Cessation Advice[1]	3	100%	97%	98%
Pneumonia Care				
Appropriate Initial Antibiotic	39	82%	94%	92%
Blood Culture Timing	46	91%	95%	96%
Influenza Vaccine	33	97%	97%	91%
Initial Antibiotic Timing	53	98%	98%	95%
Pneumococcal Vaccine	48	96%	97%	93%
Smoking Cessation Advice[1]	10	100%	99%	97%
Surgical Care Improvement Project				
Appropriate VTP Within 24 Hours	44	98%	96%	92%
Appropriate Hair Removal	68	100%	100%	99%
Appropriate Beta Blocker Usage[1]	21	100%	95%	93%
Controlled Postoperative Blood Glucose	0	-	97%	93%
Prophylactic Antibiotic Timing	43	93%	98%	97%
Prophylactic Antibiotic Timing (Outpatient)	33	48%	93%	92%
Prophylactic Antibiotic Selection	43	91%	99%	97%
Prophylactic Antibiotic Select. (Outpatient)[1]	16	94%	95%	94%
Prophylactic Antibiotic Stopped	42	95%	97%	94%
Recommended VTP Ordered	44	98%	97%	94%
Urinary Catheter Removal[1]	5	60%	92%	90%
Children's Asthma Care				
Received Systemic Corticosteroids	-	-	-	100%
Received Home Management Plan	-	-	-	71%
Received Reliever Medication	-	-	-	100%
Use of Medical Imaging				
Combination Abdominal CT Scan	230	0.078	0.133	0.191
Combination Chest CT Scan	120	0.025	0.045	0.054
Follow-up Mammogram/Ultrasound	718	10.7%	7.6%	8.4%
MRI for Low Back Pain	59	44.1%	36.7%	32.7%
Survey of Patients' Hospital Experiences				
Area Around Room 'Always' Quiet at Night	300+	55%	-	58%
Doctors 'Always' Communicated Well	300+	84%	-	80%
Home Recovery Information Given	300+	87%	-	82%
Hospital Given 9 or 10 on 10 Point Scale	300+	83%	-	67%
Meds 'Always' Explained Before Given	300+	65%	-	60%
Nurses 'Always' Communicated Well	300+	80%	-	76%
Pain 'Always' Well Controlled	300+	72%	-	69%
Room and Bathroom 'Always' Clean	300+	86%	-	71%
Timely Help 'Always' Received	300+	72%	-	64%
Would Definitely Recommend Hospital	300+	87%	-	69%

NOTE: Hospital profiles are in alphabetical order by state, then city, then hospital within the city; Rankings exclude hospitals with less than 25 cases except for patient surveys which excludes hospitals with less than 100 cases; (a) 100–299 cases; (1) The number of cases is too small to be sure how well a hospital is performing; (2) The hospital indicated that the data submitted for this measure were based on a sample of cases; (3) Data was collected during a shorter time period (fewer quarters) than the maximum possible time for this measure; (4) Suppressed for one or more quarters by CMS; (5) No data is available from the hospital for this measure; (6) Fewer than 100 patients completed the HCAHPS survey. Use these rates with caution, as the number of surveys may be too low to reliably assess hospital performance; (7) Survey results are based on less than 12 months of data; (8) Survey results are not available for this reporting period; (9) No or very few patients were eligible for the HCAHPS survey. The scores shown, if any, reflect a very small number of surveys; (10) A state average was not calculated because too few hospitals in the state submitted data; (11) There were discrepancies in the data collection process; Please refer to the User's Guide for a full explanation of data.

Calais Regional Hospital

24 Hospital Lane
Calais, ME 04619
URL: www.calaishospital.com
Type: Critical Access Hospitals
Ownership: Voluntary Non-Profit - Private

Phone: 207-454-7521
Fax: 207-454-3616

Emergency Services: Yes
Beds: 49

Key Personnel:
CEO/President . . . . Ray H Davis, Jr
Chief of Medical Staff . . . . Peter S Wilkinson, DO
Infection Control . . . . Stacey Doten
Operating Room . . . . Robert Chagrasulis, RN
Quality Assurance . . . . Stacey Doten
Radiology . . . . Edward Barrera, MD
Emergency Room . . . . Cressey Brazier, MD
Intensive Care Unit . . . . Barbara Wheaton, RN

Measure	Cases	This Hosp.	State Avg.	U.S. Avg.
Heart Attack Care				
ACE Inhibitor or ARB for LVSD[1]	4	100%	98%	96%
Aspirin at Arrival[1]	15	100%	99%	99%
Aspirin at Discharge[1]	11	100%	99%	98%
Beta Blocker at Discharge[1]	10	90%	99%	98%
Fibrinolytic Medication Timing	0	-	43%	55%
PCI Within 90 Minutes of Arrival	0	-	94%	90%
Smoking Cessation Advice[1]	1	100%	100%	99%
Chest Pain/Possible Heart Attack Care				
Aspirin at Arrival[5]	0	-	98%	95%
Median Time to ECG (minutes)[5]	0	-	7	8
Median Time to Transfer (minutes)[5]	0	-	46	61
Fibrinolytic Medication Timing[5]	0	-	75%	54%
Heart Failure Care				
ACE Inhibitor or ARB for LVSD[1]	2	100%	97%	94%
Discharge Instructions[1]	16	94%	91%	88%
Evaluation of LVS Function[1]	22	100%	99%	98%
Smoking Cessation Advice[1]	4	75%	97%	98%
Pneumonia Care				
Appropriate Initial Antibiotic	45	96%	94%	92%
Blood Culture Timing[5]	0	-	95%	96%
Influenza Vaccine	26	100%	97%	91%
Initial Antibiotic Timing	53	100%	98%	95%
Pneumococcal Vaccine	43	100%	97%	93%
Smoking Cessation Advice[1]	15	93%	99%	97%
Surgical Care Improvement Project				
Appropriate VTP Within 24 Hours[1]	19	100%	96%	92%
Appropriate Hair Removal	51	100%	100%	99%
Appropriate Beta Blocker Usage[1]	13	100%	95%	93%
Controlled Postoperative Blood Glucose	0	-	97%	93%
Prophylactic Antibiotic Timing	39	97%	98%	97%
Prophylactic Antibiotic Timing (Outpatient)[5]	0	-	93%	92%
Prophylactic Antibiotic Selection	39	97%	99%	97%
Prophylactic Antibiotic Select. (Outpatient)[5]	0	-	95%	94%
Prophylactic Antibiotic Stopped	38	97%	97%	94%
Recommended VTP Ordered[1]	19	100%	97%	94%
Urinary Catheter Removal[1]	19	100%	92%	90%
Children's Asthma Care				
Received Systemic Corticosteroids	-	-	-	100%
Received Home Management Plan	-	-	-	71%
Received Reliever Medication	-	-	-	100%
Use of Medical Imaging				
Combination Abdominal CT Scan	230	0.391	0.133	0.191
Combination Chest CT Scan	152	0.461	0.045	0.054
Follow-up Mammogram/Ultrasound	397	4.5%	7.6%	8.4%
MRI for Low Back Pain	23	52.2%	36.7%	32.7%
Survey of Patients' Hospital Experiences				
Area Around Room 'Always' Quiet at Night	(a)	71%	-	58%
Doctors 'Always' Communicated Well	(a)	81%	-	80%
Home Recovery Information Given	(a)	82%	-	82%
Hospital Given 9 or 10 on 10 Point Scale	(a)	66%	-	67%
Meds 'Always' Explained Before Given	(a)	68%	-	60%
Nurses 'Always' Communicated Well	(a)	80%	-	76%
Pain 'Always' Well Controlled	(a)	78%	-	69%
Room and Bathroom 'Always' Clean	(a)	79%	-	71%
Timely Help 'Always' Received	(a)	78%	-	64%
Would Definitely Recommend Hospital	(a)	66%	-	69%

Cary Medical Center

163 Van Buren Rd, Suite 1
Caribou, ME 04736
E-mail: mfreeman@cary.carymed.org
URL: www.carymedicalcenter.org
Type: Acute Care Hospitals
Ownership: Government - Local

Phone: 207-498-3111
Fax: 207-496-2631

Emergency Services: Yes
Beds: 65

Key Personnel:
CEO/President . . . . Kris Doody, RN
Cardiac Laboratory . . . . Gus Cains
Chief of Medical Staff . . . . Krista Burchill
Quality Assurance . . . . Darlene Higgins
Radiology . . . . John Stewart
Emergency Room . . . . Daniel Harrigan, MD
Intensive Care Unit . . . . Jackie Deboe

Measure	Cases	This Hosp.	State Avg.	U.S. Avg.
Heart Attack Care				
ACE Inhibitor or ARB for LVSD[1]	2	100%	98%	96%
Aspirin at Arrival	28	100%	99%	99%
Aspirin at Discharge[1]	18	100%	99%	98%
Beta Blocker at Discharge[1]	19	100%	99%	98%
Fibrinolytic Medication Timing	0	-	43%	55%
PCI Within 90 Minutes of Arrival	0	-	94%	90%
Smoking Cessation Advice[1]	1	100%	100%	99%
Chest Pain/Possible Heart Attack Care				
Aspirin at Arrival[1]	8	100%	98%	95%
Median Time to ECG (minutes)[1]	9	0	7	8
Median Time to Transfer (minutes)[3]	0	-	46	61
Fibrinolytic Medication Timing[1]	4	50%	75%	54%
Heart Failure Care				
ACE Inhibitor or ARB for LVSD[1]	9	100%	97%	94%
Discharge Instructions	52	98%	91%	88%
Evaluation of LVS Function	69	100%	99%	98%
Smoking Cessation Advice[1]	4	100%	97%	98%
Pneumonia Care				
Appropriate Initial Antibiotic	32	97%	94%	92%
Blood Culture Timing	39	100%	95%	96%
Influenza Vaccine[1]	22	100%	97%	91%
Initial Antibiotic Timing	41	100%	98%	95%
Pneumococcal Vaccine	39	100%	97%	93%
Smoking Cessation Advice[1]	9	89%	99%	97%
Surgical Care Improvement Project				
Appropriate VTP Within 24 Hours	47	96%	96%	92%
Appropriate Hair Removal	107	100%	100%	99%
Appropriate Beta Blocker Usage	36	94%	95%	93%
Controlled Postoperative Blood Glucose	0	-	97%	93%
Prophylactic Antibiotic Timing	67	99%	98%	97%
Prophylactic Antibiotic Timing (Outpatient)	28	54%	93%	92%
Prophylactic Antibiotic Selection	67	97%	99%	97%
Prophylactic Antibiotic Select. (Outpatient)	70	90%	95%	94%
Prophylactic Antibiotic Stopped	65	97%	97%	94%
Recommended VTP Ordered	47	98%	97%	94%
Urinary Catheter Removal[1]	18	94%	92%	90%
Children's Asthma Care				
Received Systemic Corticosteroids	-	-	-	100%
Received Home Management Plan	-	-	-	71%
Received Reliever Medication	-	-	-	100%
Use of Medical Imaging				
Combination Abdominal CT Scan	403	0.558	0.133	0.191
Combination Chest CT Scan	443	0.400	0.045	0.054
Follow-up Mammogram/Ultrasound	773	14.2%	7.6%	8.4%
MRI for Low Back Pain	70	44.3%	36.7%	32.7%
Survey of Patients' Hospital Experiences				
Area Around Room 'Always' Quiet at Night	300+	60%	-	58%
Doctors 'Always' Communicated Well	300+	87%	-	80%
Home Recovery Information Given	300+	88%	-	82%
Hospital Given 9 or 10 on 10 Point Scale	300+	69%	-	67%
Meds 'Always' Explained Before Given	300+	61%	-	60%
Nurses 'Always' Communicated Well	300+	81%	-	76%
Pain 'Always' Well Controlled	300+	72%	-	69%
Room and Bathroom 'Always' Clean	300+	73%	-	71%
Timely Help 'Always' Received	300+	72%	-	64%
Would Definitely Recommend Hospital	300+	72%	-	69%

Miles Memorial Hospital

35 Miles Street
Damariscotta, ME 04543
E-mail: info@mileshealthcare.org
URL: www.mileshealthcare.org
Type: Acute Care Hospitals
Ownership: Voluntary Non-Profit - Private

Phone: 207-563-1234
Fax: 207-563-4710

Emergency Services: No
Beds: 35

Key Personnel:
CEO/President . . . . Judith C Tarr
Chief of Medical Staff . . . . Timothy Goltz
Anesthesiology . . . . Russ Maek, MD
Emergency Room . . . . Janet Fowle
Patient Relations . . . . Vicky Bell

Measure	Cases	This Hosp.	State Avg.	U.S. Avg.
Heart Attack Care				
ACE Inhibitor or ARB for LVSD[1]	0	-	98%	96%
Aspirin at Arrival[1]	5	100%	99%	99%
Aspirin at Discharge[1]	2	100%	99%	98%
Beta Blocker at Discharge[1]	2	100%	99%	98%
Fibrinolytic Medication Timing	0	-	43%	55%
PCI Within 90 Minutes of Arrival	0	-	94%	90%
Smoking Cessation Advice	0	-	100%	99%
Chest Pain/Possible Heart Attack Care				
Aspirin at Arrival	77	96%	98%	95%
Median Time to ECG (minutes)	78	6	7	8
Median Time to Transfer (minutes)[1,3]	1	193	46	61
Fibrinolytic Medication Timing[1]	6	100%	75%	54%
Heart Failure Care				
ACE Inhibitor or ARB for LVSD[1]	18	89%	97%	94%
Discharge Instructions	54	91%	91%	88%
Evaluation of LVS Function	68	100%	99%	98%
Smoking Cessation Advice[1]	7	100%	97%	98%
Pneumonia Care				
Appropriate Initial Antibiotic	49	94%	94%	92%
Blood Culture Timing	75	99%	95%	96%
Influenza Vaccine	43	100%	97%	91%
Initial Antibiotic Timing	73	99%	98%	95%
Pneumococcal Vaccine	65	98%	97%	93%
Smoking Cessation Advice[1]	21	100%	99%	97%
Surgical Care Improvement Project				
Appropriate VTP Within 24 Hours	64	97%	96%	92%
Appropriate Hair Removal	146	100%	100%	99%
Appropriate Beta Blocker Usage	41	88%	95%	93%
Controlled Postoperative Blood Glucose	0	-	97%	93%
Prophylactic Antibiotic Timing	127	94%	98%	97%
Prophylactic Antibiotic Timing (Outpatient)	30	93%	93%	92%
Prophylactic Antibiotic Selection	127	99%	99%	97%
Prophylactic Antibiotic Select. (Outpatient)	36	97%	95%	94%
Prophylactic Antibiotic Stopped	121	97%	97%	94%
Recommended VTP Ordered	64	97%	97%	94%
Urinary Catheter Removal	38	97%	92%	90%
Children's Asthma Care				
Received Systemic Corticosteroids	-	-	-	100%
Received Home Management Plan	-	-	-	71%
Received Reliever Medication	-	-	-	100%
Use of Medical Imaging				
Combination Abdominal CT Scan	289	0.052	0.133	0.191
Combination Chest CT Scan	203	0.010	0.045	0.054
Follow-up Mammogram/Ultrasound	706	5.4%	7.6%	8.4%
MRI for Low Back Pain[5]	0	-	36.7%	32.7%
Survey of Patients' Hospital Experiences				
Area Around Room 'Always' Quiet at Night	300+	53%	-	58%
Doctors 'Always' Communicated Well	300+	84%	-	80%
Home Recovery Information Given	300+	83%	-	82%
Hospital Given 9 or 10 on 10 Point Scale	300+	72%	-	67%
Meds 'Always' Explained Before Given	300+	66%	-	60%
Nurses 'Always' Communicated Well	300+	79%	-	76%
Pain 'Always' Well Controlled	300+	73%	-	69%
Room and Bathroom 'Always' Clean	300+	76%	-	71%
Timely Help 'Always' Received	300+	70%	-	64%
Would Definitely Recommend Hospital	300+	79%	-	69%

Mayo Regional Hospital

897 West Main Street
Dover Foxcroft, ME 04426
E-mail: tlizotte@mayohospital.com
URL: www.mayohospital.com
Type: Critical Access Hospitals
Ownership: Govt - Hospital Dist/Auth

Phone: 207-564-4251
Fax: 207-564-4356

Emergency Services: Yes
Beds: 25

Key Personnel:
CEO/President . . . . Ralph Gabarro
Chief of Medical Staff . . . . Thomas Murray, MD
Infection Control . . . . Kristy Pratley, RN
Operating Room . . . . Linda Zimmerman
Quality Assurance . . . . Cheryl Roberts
Radiology . . . . Joan Lovell

Measure	Cases	This Hosp.	State Avg.	U.S. Avg.
Heart Attack Care				
ACE Inhibitor or ARB for LVSD[1]	2	100%	98%	96%
Aspirin at Arrival[1]	19	100%	99%	99%
Aspirin at Discharge[1]	12	100%	99%	98%
Beta Blocker at Discharge[1]	11	100%	99%	98%
Fibrinolytic Medication Timing[1]	1	100%	43%	55%
PCI Within 90 Minutes of Arrival	0	-	94%	90%
Smoking Cessation Advice[1]	1	100%	100%	99%
Chest Pain/Possible Heart Attack Care				
Aspirin at Arrival	-	-	98%	95%
Median Time to ECG (minutes)	-	-	7	8
Median Time to Transfer (minutes)	-	-	46	61
Fibrinolytic Medication Timing	-	-	75%	54%
Heart Failure Care				
ACE Inhibitor or ARB for LVSD[1]	6	100%	97%	94%
Discharge Instructions[1]	16	88%	91%	88%
Evaluation of LVS Function[1]	21	100%	99%	98%
Smoking Cessation Advice[1]	5	100%	97%	98%
Pneumonia Care				
Appropriate Initial Antibiotic	35	91%	94%	92%
Blood Culture Timing	46	93%	95%	96%
Influenza Vaccine	29	100%	97%	91%
Initial Antibiotic Timing	55	95%	98%	95%
Pneumococcal Vaccine	48	100%	97%	93%
Smoking Cessation Advice[1]	13	92%	99%	97%
Surgical Care Improvement Project				
Appropriate VTP Within 24 Hours[2]	42	90%	96%	92%
Appropriate Hair Removal[2]	148	100%	100%	99%
Appropriate Beta Blocker Usage[2]	47	94%	95%	93%
Controlled Postoperative Blood Glucose[2]	0	-	97%	93%
Prophylactic Antibiotic Timing[2]	134	99%	98%	97%
Prophylactic Antibiotic Timing (Outpatient)	-	-	93%	92%
Prophylactic Antibiotic Selection[2]	134	99%	99%	97%
Prophylactic Antibiotic Select. (Outpatient)	-	-	95%	94%
Prophylactic Antibiotic Stopped[2]	134	100%	97%	94%
Recommended VTP Ordered[2]	42	90%	97%	94%
Urinary Catheter Removal[2]	45	100%	92%	90%
Children's Asthma Care				
Received Systemic Corticosteroids	-	-	-	100%
Received Home Management Plan	-	-	-	71%
Received Reliever Medication	-	-	-	100%
Use of Medical Imaging				
Combination Abdominal CT Scan	-	-	0.133	0.191
Combination Chest CT Scan	-	-	0.045	0.054
Follow-up Mammogram/Ultrasound	-	-	7.6%	8.4%
MRI for Low Back Pain	-	-	36.7%	32.7%
Survey of Patients' Hospital Experiences				
Area Around Room 'Always' Quiet at Night	(a)	57%	-	58%
Doctors 'Always' Communicated Well	(a)	87%	-	80%
Home Recovery Information Given	(a)	88%	-	82%
Hospital Given 9 or 10 on 10 Point Scale	(a)	73%	-	67%
Meds 'Always' Explained Before Given	(a)	65%	-	60%
Nurses 'Always' Communicated Well	(a)	79%	-	76%
Pain 'Always' Well Controlled	(a)	73%	-	69%
Room and Bathroom 'Always' Clean	(a)	82%	-	71%
Timely Help 'Always' Received	(a)	75%	-	64%
Would Definitely Recommend Hospital	(a)	75%	-	69%

Maine Coast Memorial Hospital

50 Union St
Ellsworth, ME 04605
E-mail: dbunker@mainehospital.org
URL: www.mainehospital.org
Type: Acute Care Hospitals
Ownership: Voluntary Non-Profit - Other

Phone: 207-667-5311
Fax: 207-664-5305

Emergency Services: No
Beds: 64

Key Personnel:
CEO/President . . . . Douglas Jones
Chief of Medical Staff . . . . Peter Ossanna, MD
Emergency Room . . . . Kenneth Christian, MD

Measure	Cases	This Hosp.	State Avg.	U.S. Avg.
Heart Attack Care				
ACE Inhibitor or ARB for LVSD[1]	2	100%	98%	96%
Aspirin at Arrival	47	100%	99%	99%
Aspirin at Discharge	27	96%	99%	98%
Beta Blocker at Discharge[1]	24	96%	99%	98%
Fibrinolytic Medication Timing[1]	1	100%	43%	55%
PCI Within 90 Minutes of Arrival	0	-	94%	90%
Smoking Cessation Advice[1]	4	100%	100%	99%
Chest Pain/Possible Heart Attack Care				
Aspirin at Arrival	47	96%	98%	95%
Median Time to ECG (minutes)	47	10	7	8
Median Time to Transfer (minutes)[1,3]	1	85	46	61
Fibrinolytic Medication Timing[1]	9	44%	75%	54%
Heart Failure Care				
ACE Inhibitor or ARB for LVSD[1]	19	89%	97%	94%
Discharge Instructions	43	79%	91%	88%
Evaluation of LVS Function	63	100%	99%	98%
Smoking Cessation Advice[1]	3	100%	97%	98%
Pneumonia Care				
Appropriate Initial Antibiotic	44	95%	94%	92%
Blood Culture Timing	55	87%	95%	96%
Influenza Vaccine	51	59%	97%	91%
Initial Antibiotic Timing	74	97%	98%	95%
Pneumococcal Vaccine	94	99%	97%	93%
Smoking Cessation Advice	42	100%	99%	97%
Surgical Care Improvement Project				
Appropriate VTP Within 24 Hours[2]	177	99%	96%	92%
Appropriate Hair Removal[2]	240	100%	100%	99%
Appropriate Beta Blocker Usage[2]	73	89%	95%	93%
Controlled Postoperative Blood Glucose[2]	0	-	97%	93%
Prophylactic Antibiotic Timing[2]	159	96%	98%	97%
Prophylactic Antibiotic Timing (Outpatient)	34	85%	93%	92%
Prophylactic Antibiotic Selection[2]	159	100%	99%	97%
Prophylactic Antibiotic Select. (Outpatient)	79	94%	95%	94%
Prophylactic Antibiotic Stopped[2]	151	94%	97%	94%
Recommended VTP Ordered[2]	177	99%	97%	94%
Urinary Catheter Removal	73	86%	92%	90%
Children's Asthma Care				
Received Systemic Corticosteroids	-	-	-	100%
Received Home Management Plan	-	-	-	71%
Received Reliever Medication	-	-	-	100%
Use of Medical Imaging				
Combination Abdominal CT Scan	386	0.080	0.133	0.191
Combination Chest CT Scan	266	0.000	0.045	0.054
Follow-up Mammogram/Ultrasound	946	3.0%	7.6%	8.4%
MRI for Low Back Pain	141	34.8%	36.7%	32.7%
Survey of Patients' Hospital Experiences				
Area Around Room 'Always' Quiet at Night	300+	55%	-	58%
Doctors 'Always' Communicated Well	300+	86%	-	80%
Home Recovery Information Given	300+	88%	-	82%
Hospital Given 9 or 10 on 10 Point Scale	300+	78%	-	67%
Meds 'Always' Explained Before Given	300+	73%	-	60%
Nurses 'Always' Communicated Well	300+	85%	-	76%
Pain 'Always' Well Controlled	300+	80%	-	69%
Room and Bathroom 'Always' Clean	300+	86%	-	71%
Timely Help 'Always' Received	300+	77%	-	64%
Would Definitely Recommend Hospital	300+	82%	-	69%

Franklin Memorial Hospital

111 Franklin Health Commons
Farmington, ME 04938
E-mail: batt@fchn.org
URL: www.fchn.org
Type: Acute Care Hospitals
Ownership: Voluntary Non-Profit - Private

Phone: 207-778-6031
Fax: 207-779-2548

Emergency Services: Yes
Beds: 70

Key Personnel:
CEO/President . . . . Richard A Batt
Cardiac Laboratory . . . . Joel Chandler
Chief of Medical Staff . . . . Rodrick Prior, MD
Quality Assurance . . . . Mary Drake
Emergency Room . . . . Steven Zanella

Measure	Cases	This Hosp.	State Avg.	U.S. Avg.
Heart Attack Care				
ACE Inhibitor or ARB for LVSD[1]	4	100%	98%	96%
Aspirin at Arrival[1]	18	100%	99%	99%
Aspirin at Discharge[1]	12	100%	99%	98%
Beta Blocker at Discharge[1]	13	100%	99%	98%
Fibrinolytic Medication Timing	0	-	43%	55%
PCI Within 90 Minutes of Arrival	0	-	94%	90%
Smoking Cessation Advice[1]	2	50%	100%	99%
Chest Pain/Possible Heart Attack Care				
Aspirin at Arrival	39	92%	98%	95%
Median Time to ECG (minutes)	39	8	7	8
Median Time to Transfer (minutes)[3]	0	-	46	61
Fibrinolytic Medication Timing[1]	2	50%	75%	54%
Heart Failure Care				
ACE Inhibitor or ARB for LVSD[1]	23	83%	97%	94%
Discharge Instructions	67	99%	91%	88%
Evaluation of LVS Function	91	95%	99%	98%
Smoking Cessation Advice[1]	8	100%	97%	98%
Pneumonia Care				
Appropriate Initial Antibiotic	30	97%	94%	92%
Blood Culture Timing	71	94%	95%	96%
Influenza Vaccine	46	100%	97%	91%
Initial Antibiotic Timing	88	94%	98%	95%
Pneumococcal Vaccine	68	96%	97%	93%
Smoking Cessation Advice[1]	17	100%	99%	97%
Surgical Care Improvement Project				
Appropriate VTP Within 24 Hours	73	88%	96%	92%
Appropriate Hair Removal	222	100%	100%	99%
Appropriate Beta Blocker Usage	66	94%	95%	93%
Controlled Postoperative Blood Glucose	0	-	97%	93%
Prophylactic Antibiotic Timing	167	98%	98%	97%
Prophylactic Antibiotic Timing (Outpatient)	50	92%	93%	92%
Prophylactic Antibiotic Selection	167	98%	99%	97%
Prophylactic Antibiotic Select. (Outpatient)	59	92%	95%	94%
Prophylactic Antibiotic Stopped	165	95%	97%	94%
Recommended VTP Ordered	73	92%	97%	94%
Urinary Catheter Removal	45	93%	92%	90%
Children's Asthma Care				
Received Systemic Corticosteroids	-	-	-	100%
Received Home Management Plan	-	-	-	71%
Received Reliever Medication	-	-	-	100%
Use of Medical Imaging				
Combination Abdominal CT Scan	438	0.148	0.133	0.191
Combination Chest CT Scan	322	0.009	0.045	0.054
Follow-up Mammogram/Ultrasound	1,189	7.5%	7.6%	8.4%
MRI for Low Back Pain	135	43.7%	36.7%	32.7%
Survey of Patients' Hospital Experiences				
Area Around Room 'Always' Quiet at Night	300+	53%	-	58%
Doctors 'Always' Communicated Well	300+	80%	-	80%
Home Recovery Information Given	300+	86%	-	82%
Hospital Given 9 or 10 on 10 Point Scale	300+	68%	-	67%
Meds 'Always' Explained Before Given	300+	62%	-	60%
Nurses 'Always' Communicated Well	300+	79%	-	76%
Pain 'Always' Well Controlled	300+	70%	-	69%
Room and Bathroom 'Always' Clean	300+	81%	-	71%
Timely Help 'Always' Received	300+	64%	-	64%
Would Definitely Recommend Hospital	300+	68%	-	69%

Northern Maine Medical Center

194 E Main St
Fort Kent, ME 04743
E-mail: robin.damboise@nmmc.org
URL: www.nmmc.org
Type: Acute Care Hospitals
Ownership: Voluntary Non-Profit - Private

Phone: 207-834-3195
Fax: 207-834-2202

Emergency Services: Yes
Beds: 52

Key Personnel:

CEO/President	Martin B Bernstein
Cardiac Laboratory	Don Thersault
Chief of Medical Staff	Dr. Guy Raymond
Infection Control	Tina Soucy
Operating Room	Jill Daigle
Quality Assurance	Sue Devoe
Radiology	Michael Puttkammer

Measure	Cases	This Hosp.	State Avg.	U.S. Avg.
Heart Attack Care				
ACE Inhibitor or ARB for LVSD[1]	1	100%	98%	96%
Aspirin at Arrival[1]	9	100%	99%	99%
Aspirin at Discharge[1]	4	100%	99%	98%
Beta Blocker at Discharge[1]	4	100%	99%	98%
Fibrinolytic Medication Timing[1]	1	0%	43%	55%
PCI Within 90 Minutes of Arrival	0	-	94%	90%
Smoking Cessation Advice	0	-	100%	99%
Chest Pain/Possible Heart Attack Care				
Aspirin at Arrival[1]	19	100%	98%	95%
Median Time to ECG (minutes)[1]	18	6	7	8
Median Time to Transfer (minutes)[5]	0	-	46	61
Fibrinolytic Medication Timing[1]	4	100%	75%	54%
Heart Failure Care				
ACE Inhibitor or ARB for LVSD[1]	11	100%	97%	94%
Discharge Instructions[1]	21	90%	91%	88%
Evaluation of LVS Function	32	100%	99%	98%
Smoking Cessation Advice[1]	4	100%	97%	98%
Pneumonia Care				
Appropriate Initial Antibiotic	38	92%	94%	92%
Blood Culture Timing	45	98%	95%	96%
Influenza Vaccine	34	94%	97%	91%
Initial Antibiotic Timing	58	98%	98%	95%
Pneumococcal Vaccine	49	96%	97%	93%
Smoking Cessation Advice[1]	10	90%	99%	97%
Surgical Care Improvement Project				
Appropriate VTP Within 24 Hours[1]	23	87%	96%	92%
Appropriate Hair Removal	39	100%	100%	99%
Appropriate Beta Blocker Usage[1]	9	100%	95%	93%
Controlled Postoperative Blood Glucose	0	-	97%	93%
Prophylactic Antibiotic Timing	33	94%	98%	97%
Prophylactic Antibiotic Timing (Outpatient)	29	76%	93%	92%
Prophylactic Antibiotic Selection	33	100%	99%	97%
Prophylactic Antibiotic Select. (Outpatient)	34	97%	95%	94%
Prophylactic Antibiotic Stopped	33	82%	97%	94%
Recommended VTP Ordered[1]	23	100%	97%	94%
Urinary Catheter Removal[1]	21	100%	92%	90%
Children's Asthma Care				
Received Systemic Corticosteroids	-	-	-	100%
Received Home Management Plan	-	-	-	71%
Received Reliever Medication	-	-	-	100%
Use of Medical Imaging				
Combination Abdominal CT Scan	203	0.345	0.133	0.191
Combination Chest CT Scan	215	0.023	0.045	0.054
Follow-up Mammogram/Ultrasound	692	7.9%	7.6%	8.4%
MRI for Low Back Pain	74	56.8%	36.7%	32.7%
Survey of Patients' Hospital Experiences				
Area Around Room 'Always' Quiet at Night	(a)	57%	-	58%
Doctors 'Always' Communicated Well	(a)	81%	-	80%
Home Recovery Information Given	(a)	81%	-	82%
Hospital Given 9 or 10 on 10 Point Scale	(a)	60%	-	67%
Meds 'Always' Explained Before Given	(a)	67%	-	60%
Nurses 'Always' Communicated Well	(a)	79%	-	76%
Pain 'Always' Well Controlled	(a)	69%	-	69%
Room and Bathroom 'Always' Clean	(a)	80%	-	71%
Timely Help 'Always' Received	(a)	70%	-	64%
Would Definitely Recommend Hospital	(a)	67%	-	69%

Charles A Dean Memorial Hospital

Pritham Avenue
Greenville, ME 04441
URL: cadean.org/default.htm
Type: Critical Access Hospitals
Ownership: Voluntary Non-Profit - Private

Phone: 207-695-5200
Fax: 207-695-2329

Emergency Services: Yes
Beds: 14

Key Personnel:

CEO/President	Geno Murray
Patient Relations	Dan Blue

Measure	Cases	This Hosp.	State Avg.	U.S. Avg.
Heart Attack Care				
ACE Inhibitor or ARB for LVSD[3]	0	-	98%	96%
Aspirin at Arrival[3]	0	-	99%	99%
Aspirin at Discharge[3]	0	-	99%	98%
Beta Blocker at Discharge[3]	0	-	99%	98%
Fibrinolytic Medication Timing[3]	0	-	43%	55%
PCI Within 90 Minutes of Arrival[3]	0	-	94%	90%
Smoking Cessation Advice[3]	0	-	100%	99%
Chest Pain/Possible Heart Attack Care				
Aspirin at Arrival	-	-	98%	95%
Median Time to ECG (minutes)	-	-	7	8
Median Time to Transfer (minutes)	-	-	46	61
Fibrinolytic Medication Timing	-	-	75%	54%
Heart Failure Care				
ACE Inhibitor or ARB for LVSD[3]	0	-	97%	94%
Discharge Instructions[1,3]	2	100%	91%	88%
Evaluation of LVS Function[1,3]	4	100%	99%	98%
Smoking Cessation Advice[3]	0	-	97%	98%
Pneumonia Care				
Appropriate Initial Antibiotic[1]	1	100%	94%	92%
Blood Culture Timing[1]	11	91%	95%	96%
Influenza Vaccine[1]	4	100%	97%	91%
Initial Antibiotic Timing[1]	11	100%	98%	95%
Pneumococcal Vaccine[1]	8	100%	97%	93%
Smoking Cessation Advice[1]	2	100%	99%	97%
Surgical Care Improvement Project				
Appropriate VTP Within 24 Hours[3]	0	-	96%	92%
Appropriate Hair Removal[1,3]	2	100%	100%	99%
Appropriate Beta Blocker Usage[5]	0	-	95%	93%
Controlled Postoperative Blood Glucose[3]	0	-	97%	93%
Prophylactic Antibiotic Timing[1,3]	2	100%	98%	97%
Prophylactic Antibiotic Timing (Outpatient)	-	-	93%	92%
Prophylactic Antibiotic Selection[1,3]	2	50%	99%	97%
Prophylactic Antibiotic Select. (Outpatient)	-	-	95%	94%
Prophylactic Antibiotic Stopped[1,3]	2	100%	97%	94%
Recommended VTP Ordered[3]	0	-	97%	94%
Urinary Catheter Removal[3]	0	-	92%	90%
Children's Asthma Care				
Received Systemic Corticosteroids	-	-	-	100%
Received Home Management Plan	-	-	-	71%
Received Reliever Medication	-	-	-	100%
Use of Medical Imaging				
Combination Abdominal CT Scan	-	-	0.133	0.191
Combination Chest CT Scan	-	-	0.045	0.054
Follow-up Mammogram/Ultrasound	-	-	7.6%	8.4%
MRI for Low Back Pain	-	-	36.7%	32.7%
Survey of Patients' Hospital Experiences				
Area Around Room 'Always' Quiet at Night[6]	<100	63%	-	58%
Doctors 'Always' Communicated Well[6]	<100	92%	-	80%
Home Recovery Information Given[6]	<100	88%	-	82%
Hospital Given 9 or 10 on 10 Point Scale[6]	<100	81%	-	67%
Meds 'Always' Explained Before Given[6]	<100	76%	-	60%
Nurses 'Always' Communicated Well[6]	<100	92%	-	76%
Pain 'Always' Well Controlled[6]	<100	82%	-	69%
Room and Bathroom 'Always' Clean[6]	<100	82%	-	71%
Timely Help 'Always' Received[6]	<100	91%	-	64%
Would Definitely Recommend Hospital	<100	88%	-	69%

Houlton Regional Hospital

20 Hartford Street
Houlton, ME 04730
E-mail: info@houltonregional.org
URL: www.houlton.net/hrh
Type: Critical Access Hospitals
Ownership: Voluntary Non-Profit - Other

Phone: 207-532-2900
Fax: 207-532-4755

Emergency Services: Yes
Beds: 91

Key Personnel:

CEO/President	Thomas J Moakler
Chief of Medical Staff	Philip Mc Farnei, MD

Measure	Cases	This Hosp.	State Avg.	U.S. Avg.
Heart Attack Care				
ACE Inhibitor or ARB for LVSD[1]	1	100%	98%	96%
Aspirin at Arrival[1]	9	89%	99%	99%
Aspirin at Discharge[1]	3	67%	99%	98%
Beta Blocker at Discharge[1]	2	100%	99%	98%
Fibrinolytic Medication Timing[1]	1	0%	43%	55%
PCI Within 90 Minutes of Arrival	0	-	94%	90%
Smoking Cessation Advice	0	-	100%	99%
Chest Pain/Possible Heart Attack Care				
Aspirin at Arrival	-	-	98%	95%
Median Time to ECG (minutes)	-	-	7	8
Median Time to Transfer (minutes)	-	-	46	61
Fibrinolytic Medication Timing	-	-	75%	54%
Heart Failure Care				
ACE Inhibitor or ARB for LVSD[1]	5	100%	97%	94%
Discharge Instructions	26	100%	91%	88%
Evaluation of LVS Function	50	98%	99%	98%
Smoking Cessation Advice[1]	8	100%	97%	98%
Pneumonia Care				
Appropriate Initial Antibiotic	62	95%	94%	92%
Blood Culture Timing	78	100%	95%	96%
Influenza Vaccine	51	98%	97%	91%
Initial Antibiotic Timing	74	97%	98%	95%
Pneumococcal Vaccine	77	99%	97%	93%
Smoking Cessation Advice[1]	21	100%	99%	97%
Surgical Care Improvement Project				
Appropriate VTP Within 24 Hours[1]	12	100%	96%	92%
Appropriate Hair Removal	30	100%	100%	99%
Appropriate Beta Blocker Usage[1]	7	100%	95%	93%
Controlled Postoperative Blood Glucose	0	-	97%	93%
Prophylactic Antibiotic Timing	26	92%	98%	97%
Prophylactic Antibiotic Timing (Outpatient)	-	-	93%	92%
Prophylactic Antibiotic Selection	26	100%	99%	97%
Prophylactic Antibiotic Select. (Outpatient)	-	-	95%	94%
Prophylactic Antibiotic Stopped[1]	23	96%	97%	94%
Recommended VTP Ordered[1]	12	100%	97%	94%
Urinary Catheter Removal[1]	5	80%	92%	90%
Children's Asthma Care				
Received Systemic Corticosteroids	-	-	-	100%
Received Home Management Plan	-	-	-	71%
Received Reliever Medication	-	-	-	100%
Use of Medical Imaging				
Combination Abdominal CT Scan	-	-	0.133	0.191
Combination Chest CT Scan	-	-	0.045	0.054
Follow-up Mammogram/Ultrasound	-	-	7.6%	8.4%
MRI for Low Back Pain	-	-	36.7%	32.7%
Survey of Patients' Hospital Experiences				
Area Around Room 'Always' Quiet at Night	300+	58%	-	58%
Doctors 'Always' Communicated Well	300+	84%	-	80%
Home Recovery Information Given	300+	86%	-	82%
Hospital Given 9 or 10 on 10 Point Scale	300+	74%	-	67%
Meds 'Always' Explained Before Given	300+	63%	-	60%
Nurses 'Always' Communicated Well	300+	83%	-	76%
Pain 'Always' Well Controlled	300+	71%	-	69%
Room and Bathroom 'Always' Clean	300+	79%	-	71%
Timely Help 'Always' Received	300+	80%	-	64%
Would Definitely Recommend Hospital	300+	73%	-	69%

NOTE: Hospital profiles are in alphabetical order by state, then city, then hospital within the city; Rankings exclude hospitals with less than 25 cases except for patient surveys which excludes hospitals with less than 100 cases; (a) 100–299 cases; (1) The number of cases is too small to be sure how well a hospital is performing; (2) The hospital indicated that the data submitted for this measure were based on a sample of cases; (3) Data was collected during a shorter time period (fewer quarters) than the maximum possible time for this measure; (4) Suppressed for one or more quarters by CMS; (5) No data is available from the hospital for this measure; (6) Fewer than 100 patients completed the HCAHPS survey. Use these rates with caution, as the number of surveys may be too low to reliably assess hospital performance; (7) Survey results are based on less than 12 months of data; (8) Survey results are not available for this reporting period; (9) No or very few patients were eligible for the HCAHPS survey. The scores shown, if any, reflect a very small number of surveys; (10) A state average was not calculated because too few hospitals in the state submitted data; (11) There were discrepancies in the data collection process; Please refer to the User's Guide for a full explanation of data.

Central Maine Medical Center

300 Main St
Lewiston, ME 04240
E-mail: cmmc@cmmc.org
URL: www.cmmc.org
Type: Acute Care Hospitals
Ownership: Voluntary Non-Profit - Private

Phone: 207-795-0111
Fax: 207-795-5687

Emergency Services: Yes
Beds: 250

Key Personnel:
CEO/President . . . . Peter Chalke
Cardiac Laboratory . . . . Susan Horton
Chief of Medical Staff . . . . Lanny Oliver
Pediatric Ambulatory Care . . . . . Stephen Jacobs, MD
Pediatric In-Patient Care . . . . . . Stephen Jacobs, MD
Quality Assurance . . . . Sharon King
Radiology . . . . Barry Kutzen, MD
Emergency Room . . . . John Fields, RN

Measure	Cases	This Hosp.	State Avg.	U.S. Avg.
Heart Attack Care				
ACE Inhibitor or ARB for LVSD[2]	31	97%	98%	96%
Aspirin at Arrival[2]	176	99%	99%	99%
Aspirin at Discharge[2]	289	100%	99%	98%
Beta Blocker at Discharge[2]	278	97%	99%	98%
Fibrinolytic Medication Timing[2]	0	-	43%	55%
PCI Within 90 Minutes of Arrival[1,2]	23	100%	94%	90%
Smoking Cessation Advice[2]	109	100%	100%	99%
Chest Pain/Possible Heart Attack Care				
Aspirin at Arrival[1]	4	100%	98%	95%
Median Time to ECG (minutes)[1]	5	3	7	8
Median Time to Transfer (minutes)[5]	0	-	46	61
Fibrinolytic Medication Timing[1,3]	1	0%	75%	54%
Heart Failure Care				
ACE Inhibitor or ARB for LVSD	79	99%	97%	94%
Discharge Instructions	194	99%	91%	88%
Evaluation of LVS Function	258	100%	99%	98%
Smoking Cessation Advice	42	100%	97%	98%
Pneumonia Care				
Appropriate Initial Antibiotic[2]	69	97%	94%	92%
Blood Culture Timing[2]	139	91%	95%	96%
Influenza Vaccine[2]	90	91%	97%	91%
Initial Antibiotic Timing[2]	137	100%	98%	95%
Pneumococcal Vaccine[2]	120	95%	97%	93%
Smoking Cessation Advice[2]	60	100%	99%	97%
Surgical Care Improvement Project				
Appropriate VTP Within 24 Hours[2]	171	95%	96%	92%
Appropriate Hair Removal[2]	655	100%	100%	99%
Appropriate Beta Blocker Usage[2]	199	88%	95%	93%
Controlled Postoperative Blood Glucose[2]	121	95%	97%	93%
Prophylactic Antibiotic Timing[2]	477	96%	98%	97%
Prophylactic Antibiotic Timing (Outpatient)	502	96%	93%	92%
Prophylactic Antibiotic Selection[2]	485	98%	99%	97%
Prophylactic Antibiotic Select. (Outpatient)	600	94%	95%	94%
Prophylactic Antibiotic Stopped[2]	452	95%	97%	94%
Recommended VTP Ordered[2]	172	96%	97%	94%
Urinary Catheter Removal[2]	92	84%	92%	90%
Children's Asthma Care				
Received Systemic Corticosteroids	-	-	-	100%
Received Home Management Plan	-	-	-	71%
Received Reliever Medication	-	-	-	100%
Use of Medical Imaging				
Combination Abdominal CT Scan	1,073	0.084	0.133	0.191
Combination Chest CT Scan	873	0.001	0.045	0.054
Follow-up Mammogram/Ultrasound	1,410	4.8%	7.6%	8.4%
MRI for Low Back Pain[5]	0	-	36.7%	32.7%
Survey of Patients' Hospital Experiences				
Area Around Room 'Always' Quiet at Night	300+	50%	-	58%
Doctors 'Always' Communicated Well	300+	77%	-	80%
Home Recovery Information Given	300+	85%	-	82%
Hospital Given 9 or 10 on 10 Point Scale	300+	67%	-	67%
Meds 'Always' Explained Before Given	300+	59%	-	60%
Nurses 'Always' Communicated Well	300+	75%	-	76%
Pain 'Always' Well Controlled	300+	68%	-	69%
Room and Bathroom 'Always' Clean	300+	69%	-	71%
Timely Help 'Always' Received	300+	64%	-	64%
Would Definitely Recommend Hospital	300+	77%	-	69%

Saint Marys Regional Medical Center

Campus Avenue
Lewiston, ME 04240
URL: www.stmarysmaine.com
Type: Acute Care Hospitals
Ownership: Voluntary Non-Profit - Private

Phone: 207-777-8100
Fax: 207-777-8800

Emergency Services: Yes
Beds: 233

Key Personnel:
CEO/President . . . . James Cassidy
Chief of Medical Staff . . . . Peter Beeckel
Infection Control . . . . Diane Theriault, RN
Operating Room . . . . Justin Clark
Pediatric Ambulatory Care . . . . . Linda Glass, MD
Pediatric In-Patient Care . . . . . . Linda Glass, MD
Quality Assurance . . . . Kathleen Bremer
Radiology . . . . Cindy Brousseau

Measure	Cases	This Hosp.	State Avg.	U.S. Avg.
Heart Attack Care				
ACE Inhibitor or ARB for LVSD[1]	4	100%	98%	96%
Aspirin at Arrival	51	98%	99%	99%
Aspirin at Discharge	37	100%	99%	98%
Beta Blocker at Discharge	35	94%	99%	98%
Fibrinolytic Medication Timing	0	-	43%	55%
PCI Within 90 Minutes of Arrival	0	-	94%	90%
Smoking Cessation Advice[1]	7	100%	100%	99%
Chest Pain/Possible Heart Attack Care				
Aspirin at Arrival[1]	21	95%	98%	95%
Median Time to ECG (minutes)[1]	22	8	7	8
Median Time to Transfer (minutes)[1]	7	56	46	61
Fibrinolytic Medication Timing[1]	1	0%	75%	54%
Heart Failure Care				
ACE Inhibitor or ARB for LVSD[1]	21	90%	97%	94%
Discharge Instructions	68	93%	91%	88%
Evaluation of LVS Function	133	99%	99%	98%
Smoking Cessation Advice[1]	14	100%	97%	98%
Pneumonia Care				
Appropriate Initial Antibiotic	58	93%	94%	92%
Blood Culture Timing	44	95%	95%	96%
Influenza Vaccine	62	82%	97%	91%
Initial Antibiotic Timing	79	95%	98%	95%
Pneumococcal Vaccine	82	95%	97%	93%
Smoking Cessation Advice	31	100%	99%	97%
Surgical Care Improvement Project				
Appropriate VTP Within 24 Hours[2]	136	94%	96%	92%
Appropriate Hair Removal[2]	532	100%	100%	99%
Appropriate Beta Blocker Usage[2]	162	97%	95%	93%
Controlled Postoperative Blood Glucose[2]	0	-	97%	93%
Prophylactic Antibiotic Timing[2]	403	99%	98%	97%
Prophylactic Antibiotic Timing (Outpatient)	140	92%	93%	92%
Prophylactic Antibiotic Selection[2]	405	100%	99%	97%
Prophylactic Antibiotic Select. (Outpatient)	137	91%	95%	94%
Prophylactic Antibiotic Stopped[2]	394	97%	97%	94%
Recommended VTP Ordered[2]	136	96%	97%	94%
Urinary Catheter Removal[2]	58	78%	92%	90%
Children's Asthma Care				
Received Systemic Corticosteroids	-	-	-	100%
Received Home Management Plan	-	-	-	71%
Received Reliever Medication	-	-	-	100%
Use of Medical Imaging				
Combination Abdominal CT Scan	722	0.071	0.133	0.191
Combination Chest CT Scan	633	0.008	0.045	0.054
Follow-up Mammogram/Ultrasound	1,273	9.3%	7.6%	8.4%
MRI for Low Back Pain	208	29.8%	36.7%	32.7%
Survey of Patients' Hospital Experiences				
Area Around Room 'Always' Quiet at Night	300+	58%	-	58%
Doctors 'Always' Communicated Well	300+	80%	-	80%
Home Recovery Information Given	300+	87%	-	82%
Hospital Given 9 or 10 on 10 Point Scale	300+	71%	-	67%
Meds 'Always' Explained Before Given	300+	61%	-	60%
Nurses 'Always' Communicated Well	300+	79%	-	76%
Pain 'Always' Well Controlled	300+	68%	-	69%
Room and Bathroom 'Always' Clean	300+	78%	-	71%
Timely Help 'Always' Received	300+	61%	-	64%
Would Definitely Recommend Hospital	300+	79%	-	69%

Penobscot Valley Hospital

7 Transalpine Road
Lincoln, ME 04457
E-mail: info@pvhhealthcare.org
URL: www.pvhhealthcare.org
Type: Critical Access Hospitals
Ownership: Voluntary Non-Profit - Private

Phone: 207-794-3321
Fax: 207-794-6490

Emergency Services: Yes
Beds: 25

Key Personnel:
CEO/President . . . . Ronald Victory
Quality Assurance . . . . Penelope Kneeland
Emergency Room . . . . David Ettinger

Measure	Cases	This Hosp.	State Avg.	U.S. Avg.
Heart Attack Care				
ACE Inhibitor or ARB for LVSD	0	-	98%	96%
Aspirin at Arrival[1]	6	100%	99%	99%
Aspirin at Discharge[1]	2	100%	99%	98%
Beta Blocker at Discharge[1]	2	100%	99%	98%
Fibrinolytic Medication Timing	0	-	43%	55%
PCI Within 90 Minutes of Arrival	0	-	94%	90%
Smoking Cessation Advice	0	-	100%	99%
Chest Pain/Possible Heart Attack Care				
Aspirin at Arrival	-	-	98%	95%
Median Time to ECG (minutes)	-	-	7	8
Median Time to Transfer (minutes)	-	-	46	61
Fibrinolytic Medication Timing	-	-	75%	54%
Heart Failure Care				
ACE Inhibitor or ARB for LVSD[1]	4	100%	97%	94%
Discharge Instructions[1]	9	78%	91%	88%
Evaluation of LVS Function[1]	12	100%	99%	98%
Smoking Cessation Advice	0	-	97%	98%
Pneumonia Care				
Appropriate Initial Antibiotic	27	100%	94%	92%
Blood Culture Timing	36	100%	95%	96%
Influenza Vaccine[1]	17	100%	97%	91%
Initial Antibiotic Timing	38	100%	98%	95%
Pneumococcal Vaccine	35	100%	97%	93%
Smoking Cessation Advice[1]	10	90%	99%	97%
Surgical Care Improvement Project				
Appropriate VTP Within 24 Hours[1]	6	100%	96%	92%
Appropriate Hair Removal[1]	8	100%	100%	99%
Appropriate Beta Blocker Usage[1]	3	100%	95%	93%
Controlled Postoperative Blood Glucose	0	-	97%	93%
Prophylactic Antibiotic Timing[1]	7	100%	98%	97%
Prophylactic Antibiotic Timing (Outpatient)	-	-	93%	92%
Prophylactic Antibiotic Selection[1]	7	100%	99%	97%
Prophylactic Antibiotic Select. (Outpatient)	-	-	95%	94%
Prophylactic Antibiotic Stopped[1]	7	100%	97%	94%
Recommended VTP Ordered[1]	6	100%	97%	94%
Urinary Catheter Removal[1]	1	100%	92%	90%
Children's Asthma Care				
Received Systemic Corticosteroids	-	-	-	100%
Received Home Management Plan	-	-	-	71%
Received Reliever Medication	-	-	-	100%
Use of Medical Imaging				
Combination Abdominal CT Scan	-	-	0.133	0.191
Combination Chest CT Scan	-	-	0.045	0.054
Follow-up Mammogram/Ultrasound	-	-	7.6%	8.4%
MRI for Low Back Pain	-	-	36.7%	32.7%
Survey of Patients' Hospital Experiences				
Area Around Room 'Always' Quiet at Night	(a)	62%	-	58%
Doctors 'Always' Communicated Well	(a)	84%	-	80%
Home Recovery Information Given	(a)	88%	-	82%
Hospital Given 9 or 10 on 10 Point Scale	(a)	68%	-	67%
Meds 'Always' Explained Before Given	(a)	69%	-	60%
Nurses 'Always' Communicated Well	(a)	80%	-	76%
Pain 'Always' Well Controlled	(a)	79%	-	69%
Room and Bathroom 'Always' Clean	(a)	82%	-	71%
Timely Help 'Always' Received	(a)	69%	-	64%
Would Definitely Recommend Hospital	(a)	67%	-	69%

NOTE: Hospital profiles are in alphabetical order by state, then city, then hospital within the city; Rankings exclude hospitals with less than 25 cases except for patient surveys which excludes hospitals with less than 100 cases; (a) 100–299 cases; (1) The number of cases is too small to be sure how well a hospital is performing; (2) The hospital indicated that the data submitted for this measure were based on a sample of cases; (3) Data was collected during a shorter time period (fewer quarters) than the maximum possible time for this measure; (4) Suppressed for one or more quarters by CMS; (5) No data is available from the hospital for this measure; (6) Fewer than 100 patients completed the HCAHPS survey. Use these rates with caution, as the number of surveys may be too low to reliably assess hospital performance; (7) Survey results are based on less than 12 months of data; (8) Survey results are not available for this reporting period; (9) No or very few patients were eligible for the HCAHPS survey. The scores shown, if any, reflect a very small number of surveys; (10) A state average was not calculated because too few hospitals in the state submitted data; (11) There were discrepancies in the data collection process; Please refer to the User's Guide for a full explanation of data.

Down East Community Hospital

11 Hospital Drive
Machias, ME 04654
Phone: 207-255-3356
Fax: 207-255-0427
E-mail: mjgripp@dech.org
URL: www.dech.org
Type: Critical Access Hospitals
Emergency Services: Yes
Ownership: Voluntary Non-Profit - Private
Beds: 36

Key Personnel:
CEO/President. . . . . Wayne T Dodwell
Chief of Medical Staff . . . . David Rioux, DO
Infection Control. . . . . Bart Brizee, RN
Operating Room. . . . . Jane Foshay, RN, CRNFA
Quality Assurance . . . . Sue Jones-Burr
Radiology. . . . . Karen Krigman, MD
Emergency Room . . . . Kristzina Morin, DO
Patient Relations . . . . Vicki Brown

Measure	Cases	This Hosp.	State Avg.	U.S. Avg.
Heart Attack Care				
ACE Inhibitor or ARB for LVSD[1]	1	100%	98%	96%
Aspirin at Arrival[1]	17	94%	99%	99%
Aspirin at Discharge[1]	16	81%	99%	98%
Beta Blocker at Discharge[1]	16	94%	99%	98%
Fibrinolytic Medication Timing	0	-	43%	55%
PCI Within 90 Minutes of Arrival	0	-	94%	90%
Smoking Cessation Advice[1]	1	100%	100%	99%
Chest Pain/Possible Heart Attack Care				
Aspirin at Arrival	81	100%	98%	95%
Median Time to ECG (minutes)	85	10	7	8
Median Time to Transfer (minutes)[3]	0	-	46	61
Fibrinolytic Medication Timing[1]	3	67%	75%	54%
Heart Failure Care				
ACE Inhibitor or ARB for LVSD[1]	9	100%	97%	94%
Discharge Instructions	29	100%	91%	88%
Evaluation of LVS Function	39	100%	99%	98%
Smoking Cessation Advice[1]	6	100%	97%	98%
Pneumonia Care				
Appropriate Initial Antibiotic	26	81%	94%	92%
Blood Culture Timing	47	94%	95%	96%
Influenza Vaccine[1]	18	89%	97%	91%
Initial Antibiotic Timing	42	90%	98%	95%
Pneumococcal Vaccine	43	93%	97%	93%
Smoking Cessation Advice[1]	10	100%	99%	97%
Surgical Care Improvement Project				
Appropriate VTP Within 24 Hours[1]	6	100%	96%	92%
Appropriate Hair Removal[1]	15	100%	100%	99%
Appropriate Beta Blocker Usage[1]	2	100%	95%	93%
Controlled Postoperative Blood Glucose	0	-	97%	93%
Prophylactic Antibiotic Timing[1]	10	100%	98%	97%
Prophylactic Antibiotic Timing (Outpatient)	49	94%	93%	92%
Prophylactic Antibiotic Selection[1]	10	100%	99%	97%
Prophylactic Antibiotic Select. (Outpatient)	49	92%	95%	94%
Prophylactic Antibiotic Stopped[1]	10	100%	97%	94%
Recommended VTP Ordered[1]	6	100%	97%	94%
Urinary Catheter Removal	0	-	92%	90%
Children's Asthma Care				
Received Systemic Corticosteroids	-	-	-	100%
Received Home Management Plan	-	-	-	71%
Received Reliever Medication	-	-	-	100%
Use of Medical Imaging				
Combination Abdominal CT Scan	283	0.233	0.133	0.191
Combination Chest CT Scan	255	0.176	0.045	0.054
Follow-up Mammogram/Ultrasound	571	11.9%	7.6%	8.4%
MRI for Low Back Pain[5]	0	-	36.7%	32.7%
Survey of Patients' Hospital Experiences				
Area Around Room 'Always' Quiet at Night	(a)	65%	-	58%
Doctors 'Always' Communicated Well	(a)	86%	-	80%
Home Recovery Information Given	(a)	83%	-	82%
Hospital Given 9 or 10 on 10 Point Scale	(a)	71%	-	67%
Meds 'Always' Explained Before Given	(a)	68%	-	60%
Nurses 'Always' Communicated Well	(a)	85%	-	76%
Pain 'Always' Well Controlled	(a)	82%	-	69%
Room and Bathroom 'Always' Clean	(a)	86%	-	71%
Timely Help 'Always' Received	(a)	77%	-	64%
Would Definitely Recommend Hospital	(a)	69%	-	69%

Millinocket Regional Hospital

200 Somerset Street
Millinocket, ME 04462
Phone: 207-723-5161
Fax: 207-723-4913
URL: www.mrhme.org
Type: Critical Access Hospitals
Emergency Services: Yes
Ownership: Voluntary Non-Profit - Private
Beds: 42

Key Personnel:
CEO/President. . . . . Marie Vienneau
Chief of Medical Staff . . . . Daniel Herbert, MD
Quality Assurance . . . . Mary Marter, RN
Radiology. . . . . John Connolly
Emergency Room . . . . Stephanie Thompson, RN

Measure	Cases	This Hosp.	State Avg.	U.S. Avg.
Heart Attack Care				
ACE Inhibitor or ARB for LVSD	0	-	98%	96%
Aspirin at Arrival[1]	8	100%	99%	99%
Aspirin at Discharge[1]	7	100%	99%	98%
Beta Blocker at Discharge[1]	7	100%	99%	98%
Fibrinolytic Medication Timing	0	-	43%	55%
PCI Within 90 Minutes of Arrival	0	-	94%	90%
Smoking Cessation Advice	0	-	100%	99%
Chest Pain/Possible Heart Attack Care				
Aspirin at Arrival	-	-	98%	95%
Median Time to ECG (minutes)	-	-	7	8
Median Time to Transfer (minutes)	-	-	46	61
Fibrinolytic Medication Timing	-	-	75%	54%
Heart Failure Care				
ACE Inhibitor or ARB for LVSD[1]	8	100%	97%	94%
Discharge Instructions	27	81%	91%	88%
Evaluation of LVS Function	35	97%	99%	98%
Smoking Cessation Advice[1]	5	100%	97%	98%
Pneumonia Care				
Appropriate Initial Antibiotic[1]	20	95%	94%	92%
Blood Culture Timing	30	100%	95%	96%
Influenza Vaccine[1]	15	100%	97%	91%
Initial Antibiotic Timing	27	96%	98%	95%
Pneumococcal Vaccine	28	100%	97%	93%
Smoking Cessation Advice[1]	5	100%	99%	97%
Surgical Care Improvement Project				
Appropriate VTP Within 24 Hours[1]	23	100%	96%	92%
Appropriate Hair Removal	44	98%	100%	99%
Appropriate Beta Blocker Usage[1]	11	100%	95%	93%
Controlled Postoperative Blood Glucose	0	-	97%	93%
Prophylactic Antibiotic Timing	42	100%	98%	97%
Prophylactic Antibiotic Timing (Outpatient)	-	-	93%	92%
Prophylactic Antibiotic Selection	43	100%	99%	97%
Prophylactic Antibiotic Select. (Outpatient)	-	-	95%	94%
Prophylactic Antibiotic Stopped	40	98%	97%	94%
Recommended VTP Ordered[1]	23	100%	97%	94%
Urinary Catheter Removal[1]	18	94%	92%	90%
Children's Asthma Care				
Received Systemic Corticosteroids	-	-	-	100%
Received Home Management Plan	-	-	-	71%
Received Reliever Medication	-	-	-	100%
Use of Medical Imaging				
Combination Abdominal CT Scan	-	-	0.133	0.191
Combination Chest CT Scan	-	-	0.045	0.054
Follow-up Mammogram/Ultrasound	-	-	7.6%	8.4%
MRI for Low Back Pain	-	-	36.7%	32.7%
Survey of Patients' Hospital Experiences				
Area Around Room 'Always' Quiet at Night	(a)	66%	-	58%
Doctors 'Always' Communicated Well	(a)	87%	-	80%
Home Recovery Information Given	(a)	87%	-	82%
Hospital Given 9 or 10 on 10 Point Scale	(a)	79%	-	67%
Meds 'Always' Explained Before Given	(a)	74%	-	60%
Nurses 'Always' Communicated Well	(a)	87%	-	76%
Pain 'Always' Well Controlled	(a)	76%	-	69%
Room and Bathroom 'Always' Clean	(a)	91%	-	71%
Timely Help 'Always' Received	(a)	85%	-	64%
Would Definitely Recommend Hospital	(a)	81%	-	69%

Stephens Memorial Hospital

181 Main Street
Norway, ME 04268
Phone: 207-743-5933
Fax: 207-743-1566
URL: www.wmhcc.com
Type: Acute Care Hospitals
Emergency Services: Yes
Ownership: Voluntary Non-Profit - Private
Beds: 50

Key Personnel:
CEO/President. . . . . Timothy A Churchill
Chief of Medical Staff . . . . Kate Herlihy
Radiology. . . . . William Portner

Measure	Cases	This Hosp.	State Avg.	U.S. Avg.
Heart Attack Care				
ACE Inhibitor or ARB for LVSD[1]	2	50%	98%	96%
Aspirin at Arrival[1]	12	100%	99%	99%
Aspirin at Discharge[1]	12	100%	99%	98%
Beta Blocker at Discharge[1]	11	91%	99%	98%
Fibrinolytic Medication Timing[1]	1	0%	43%	55%
PCI Within 90 Minutes of Arrival	0	-	94%	90%
Smoking Cessation Advice	0	-	100%	99%
Chest Pain/Possible Heart Attack Care				
Aspirin at Arrival	58	98%	98%	95%
Median Time to ECG (minutes)	58	8	7	8
Median Time to Transfer (minutes)[1,3]	4	35	46	61
Fibrinolytic Medication Timing[1]	7	71%	75%	54%
Heart Failure Care				
ACE Inhibitor or ARB for LVSD[1]	8	100%	97%	94%
Discharge Instructions[1]	23	91%	91%	88%
Evaluation of LVS Function	35	86%	99%	98%
Smoking Cessation Advice[1]	2	100%	97%	98%
Pneumonia Care				
Appropriate Initial Antibiotic[2]	45	91%	94%	92%
Blood Culture Timing[2]	71	97%	95%	96%
Influenza Vaccine	49	98%	97%	91%
Initial Antibiotic Timing[2]	94	98%	98%	95%
Pneumococcal Vaccine[2]	85	98%	97%	93%
Smoking Cessation Advice[1,2]	17	100%	99%	97%
Surgical Care Improvement Project				
Appropriate VTP Within 24 Hours	50	92%	96%	92%
Appropriate Hair Removal	172	100%	100%	99%
Appropriate Beta Blocker Usage	45	96%	95%	93%
Controlled Postoperative Blood Glucose	0	-	97%	93%
Prophylactic Antibiotic Timing	118	98%	98%	97%
Prophylactic Antibiotic Timing (Outpatient)	93	96%	93%	92%
Prophylactic Antibiotic Selection	118	97%	99%	97%
Prophylactic Antibiotic Select. (Outpatient)	90	94%	95%	94%
Prophylactic Antibiotic Stopped	118	97%	97%	94%
Recommended VTP Ordered	50	96%	97%	94%
Urinary Catheter Removal	56	93%	92%	90%
Children's Asthma Care				
Received Systemic Corticosteroids	-	-	-	100%
Received Home Management Plan	-	-	-	71%
Received Reliever Medication	-	-	-	100%
Use of Medical Imaging				
Combination Abdominal CT Scan	330	0.609	0.133	0.191
Combination Chest CT Scan	380	0.013	0.045	0.054
Follow-up Mammogram/Ultrasound	1,139	8.5%	7.6%	8.4%
MRI for Low Back Pain	79	49.4%	36.7%	32.7%
Survey of Patients' Hospital Experiences				
Area Around Room 'Always' Quiet at Night	300+	56%	-	58%
Doctors 'Always' Communicated Well	300+	84%	-	80%
Home Recovery Information Given	300+	90%	-	82%
Hospital Given 9 or 10 on 10 Point Scale	300+	74%	-	67%
Meds 'Always' Explained Before Given	300+	64%	-	60%
Nurses 'Always' Communicated Well	300+	77%	-	76%
Pain 'Always' Well Controlled	300+	71%	-	69%
Room and Bathroom 'Always' Clean	300+	77%	-	71%
Timely Help 'Always' Received	300+	63%	-	64%
Would Definitely Recommend Hospital	300+	76%	-	69%

NOTE: Hospital profiles are in alphabetical order by state, then city, then hospital within the city; Rankings exclude hospitals with less than 25 cases except for patient surveys which excludes hospitals with less than 100 cases; (a) 100–299 cases; (1) The number of cases is too small to be sure how well a hospital is performing; (2) The hospital indicated that the data submitted for this measure were based on a sample of cases; (3) Data was collected during a shorter time period (fewer quarters) than the maximum possible time for this measure; (4) Suppressed for one or more quarters by CMS; (5) No data is available from the hospital for this measure; (6) Fewer than 100 patients completed the HCAHPS survey. Use these rates with caution, as the number of surveys may be too low to reliably assess hospital performance; (7) Survey results are based on less than 12 months of data; (8) Survey results are not available for this reporting period; (9) No or very few patients were eligible for the HCAHPS survey. The scores shown, if any, reflect a very small number of surveys; (10) A state average was not calculated because too few hospitals in the state submitted data; (11) There were discrepancies in the data collection process; Please refer to the User's Guide for a full explanation of data.

Sebasticook Valley Hospital

447 North Main Street
Pittsfield, ME 04967
URL: sebasticookhospital.org
Type: Critical Access Hospitals
Ownership: Voluntary Non-Profit - Private
Phone: 207-487-5141
Fax: 207-487-3204
Emergency Services: Yes
Beds: 25

Key Personnel:
CEO/President. . . . . Jack May
Chief of Medical Staff . . . . Brad Huot, MD
Quality Assurance . . . . Sharon King

Measure	Cases	This Hosp.	State Avg.	U.S. Avg.
Heart Attack Care				
ACE Inhibitor or ARB for LVSD[1]	1	100%	98%	96%
Aspirin at Arrival[1]	7	100%	99%	99%
Aspirin at Discharge[1]	7	100%	99%	98%
Beta Blocker at Discharge[1]	6	100%	99%	98%
Fibrinolytic Medication Timing	0	-	43%	55%
PCI Within 90 Minutes of Arrival	0	-	94%	90%
Smoking Cessation Advice	0	-	100%	99%
Chest Pain/Possible Heart Attack Care				
Aspirin at Arrival	-	-	98%	95%
Median Time to ECG (minutes)	-	-	7	8
Median Time to Transfer (minutes)	-	-	46	61
Fibrinolytic Medication Timing	-	-	75%	54%
Heart Failure Care				
ACE Inhibitor or ARB for LVSD[1]	4	100%	97%	94%
Discharge Instructions	38	100%	91%	88%
Evaluation of LVS Function	44	93%	99%	98%
Smoking Cessation Advice[1]	5	100%	97%	98%
Pneumonia Care				
Appropriate Initial Antibiotic	41	93%	94%	92%
Blood Culture Timing	47	98%	95%	96%
Influenza Vaccine[1]	18	100%	97%	91%
Initial Antibiotic Timing	43	100%	98%	95%
Pneumococcal Vaccine	40	92%	97%	93%
Smoking Cessation Advice[1]	14	100%	99%	97%
Surgical Care Improvement Project				
Appropriate VTP Within 24 Hours	28	96%	96%	92%
Appropriate Hair Removal	43	100%	100%	99%
Appropriate Beta Blocker Usage[5]	0	-	95%	93%
Controlled Postoperative Blood Glucose	0	-	97%	93%
Prophylactic Antibiotic Timing	35	100%	98%	97%
Prophylactic Antibiotic Timing (Outpatient)	-	-	93%	92%
Prophylactic Antibiotic Selection	35	100%	99%	97%
Prophylactic Antibiotic Select. (Outpatient)	-	-	95%	94%
Prophylactic Antibiotic Stopped	35	100%	97%	94%
Recommended VTP Ordered	28	100%	97%	94%
Urinary Catheter Removal[1]	13	92%	92%	90%
Children's Asthma Care				
Received Systemic Corticosteroids	-	-	-	100%
Received Home Management Plan	-	-	-	71%
Received Reliever Medication	-	-	-	100%
Use of Medical Imaging				
Combination Abdominal CT Scan	-	-	0.133	0.191
Combination Chest CT Scan	-	-	0.045	0.054
Follow-up Mammogram/Ultrasound	-	-	7.6%	8.4%
MRI for Low Back Pain	-	-	36.7%	32.7%
Survey of Patients' Hospital Experiences				
Area Around Room 'Always' Quiet at Night	(a)	46%	-	58%
Doctors 'Always' Communicated Well	(a)	76%	-	80%
Home Recovery Information Given	(a)	88%	-	82%
Hospital Given 9 or 10 on 10 Point Scale	(a)	67%	-	67%
Meds 'Always' Explained Before Given	(a)	65%	-	60%
Nurses 'Always' Communicated Well	(a)	77%	-	76%
Pain 'Always' Well Controlled	(a)	59%	-	69%
Room and Bathroom 'Always' Clean	(a)	84%	-	71%
Timely Help 'Always' Received	(a)	62%	-	64%
Would Definitely Recommend Hospital	(a)	68%	-	69%

Maine Medical Center

22 Bramhall St
Portland, ME 04102
URL: www.mmc.org
Type: Acute Care Hospitals
Ownership: Voluntary Non-Profit - Private
Phone: 207-662-0111
Fax: 207-871-6212
Emergency Services: Yes
Beds: 605

Key Personnel:
Operating Room. . . . . Karen Dumond

Measure	Cases	This Hosp.	State Avg.	U.S. Avg.
Heart Attack Care				
ACE Inhibitor or ARB for LVSD	100	99%	98%	96%
Aspirin at Arrival	372	99%	99%	99%
Aspirin at Discharge	988	100%	99%	98%
Beta Blocker at Discharge	979	99%	99%	98%
Fibrinolytic Medication Timing[1]	2	50%	43%	55%
PCI Within 90 Minutes of Arrival	76	92%	94%	90%
Smoking Cessation Advice	286	99%	100%	99%
Chest Pain/Possible Heart Attack Care				
Aspirin at Arrival[3]	0	-	98%	95%
Median Time to ECG (minutes)[3]	0	-	7	8
Median Time to Transfer (minutes)[5]	0	-	46	61
Fibrinolytic Medication Timing[5]	0	-	75%	54%
Heart Failure Care				
ACE Inhibitor or ARB for LVSD	160	96%	97%	94%
Discharge Instructions	477	86%	91%	88%
Evaluation of LVS Function	619	99%	99%	98%
Smoking Cessation Advice	67	93%	97%	98%
Pneumonia Care				
Appropriate Initial Antibiotic	111	93%	94%	92%
Blood Culture Timing	338	89%	95%	96%
Influenza Vaccine	207	97%	97%	91%
Initial Antibiotic Timing	303	97%	98%	95%
Pneumococcal Vaccine	302	96%	97%	93%
Smoking Cessation Advice	91	100%	99%	97%
Surgical Care Improvement Project				
Appropriate VTP Within 24 Hours[2]	208	99%	96%	92%
Appropriate Hair Removal[2]	818	97%	100%	99%
Appropriate Beta Blocker Usage[2]	316	96%	95%	93%
Controlled Postoperative Blood Glucose[2]	174	96%	97%	93%
Prophylactic Antibiotic Timing[2]	606	99%	98%	97%
Prophylactic Antibiotic Timing (Outpatient)	883	93%	93%	92%
Prophylactic Antibiotic Selection[2]	615	99%	99%	97%
Prophylactic Antibiotic Select. (Outpatient)	858	98%	95%	94%
Prophylactic Antibiotic Stopped[2]	599	98%	97%	94%
Recommended VTP Ordered[2]	208	100%	97%	94%
Urinary Catheter Removal[2]	164	94%	92%	90%
Children's Asthma Care				
Received Systemic Corticosteroids	-	-	-	100%
Received Home Management Plan	-	-	-	71%
Received Reliever Medication	-	-	-	100%
Use of Medical Imaging				
Combination Abdominal CT Scan	1,961	0.102	0.133	0.191
Combination Chest CT Scan	2,037	0.004	0.045	0.054
Follow-up Mammogram/Ultrasound	2,473	11.0%	7.6%	8.4%
MRI for Low Back Pain	149	33.6%	36.7%	32.7%
Survey of Patients' Hospital Experiences				
Area Around Room 'Always' Quiet at Night	300+	49%	-	58%
Doctors 'Always' Communicated Well	300+	77%	-	80%
Home Recovery Information Given	300+	84%	-	82%
Hospital Given 9 or 10 on 10 Point Scale	300+	70%	-	67%
Meds 'Always' Explained Before Given	300+	60%	-	60%
Nurses 'Always' Communicated Well	300+	75%	-	76%
Pain 'Always' Well Controlled	300+	70%	-	69%
Room and Bathroom 'Always' Clean	300+	69%	-	71%
Timely Help 'Always' Received	300+	62%	-	64%
Would Definitely Recommend Hospital	300+	77%	-	69%

Mercy Hospital

144 State St
Portland, ME 04101
URL: www.mercyhospital.com
Type: Acute Care Hospitals
Ownership: Voluntary Non-Profit - Church
Phone: 207-879-3000
Fax: 207-879-3666
Emergency Services: Yes

Key Personnel:
CEO/President. . . . . Eileen F Skinner
Chief of Medical Staff . . . . Stephen Sears, MD
Radiology. . . . . Greatorex David
Emergency Room . . . . Rebecca Bloch
Patient Relations . . . . Jill Berry Bowen, RN, CHE

Measure	Cases	This Hosp.	State Avg.	U.S. Avg.
Heart Attack Care				
ACE Inhibitor or ARB for LVSD[1]	4	100%	98%	96%
Aspirin at Arrival	55	100%	99%	99%
Aspirin at Discharge	32	100%	99%	98%
Beta Blocker at Discharge	31	97%	99%	98%
Fibrinolytic Medication Timing	0	-	43%	55%
PCI Within 90 Minutes of Arrival	0	-	94%	90%
Smoking Cessation Advice[1]	7	100%	100%	99%
Chest Pain/Possible Heart Attack Care				
Aspirin at Arrival[1]	23	100%	98%	95%
Median Time to ECG (minutes)[1]	22	17	7	8
Median Time to Transfer (minutes)[1,3]	9	94	46	61
Fibrinolytic Medication Timing	0	-	75%	54%
Heart Failure Care				
ACE Inhibitor or ARB for LVSD[1]	24	96%	97%	94%
Discharge Instructions	98	99%	91%	88%
Evaluation of LVS Function	166	100%	99%	98%
Smoking Cessation Advice	30	93%	97%	98%
Pneumonia Care				
Appropriate Initial Antibiotic	115	88%	94%	92%
Blood Culture Timing	149	92%	95%	96%
Influenza Vaccine	103	95%	97%	91%
Initial Antibiotic Timing	155	97%	98%	95%
Pneumococcal Vaccine	144	97%	97%	93%
Smoking Cessation Advice	50	100%	99%	97%
Surgical Care Improvement Project				
Appropriate VTP Within 24 Hours[2]	126	90%	96%	92%
Appropriate Hair Removal[2]	447	100%	100%	99%
Appropriate Beta Blocker Usage[2]	113	100%	95%	93%
Controlled Postoperative Blood Glucose[2]	0	-	97%	93%
Prophylactic Antibiotic Timing[2]	318	97%	98%	97%
Prophylactic Antibiotic Timing (Outpatient)	629	86%	93%	92%
Prophylactic Antibiotic Selection[2]	316	98%	99%	97%
Prophylactic Antibiotic Select. (Outpatient)	587	90%	95%	94%
Prophylactic Antibiotic Stopped[2]	312	98%	97%	94%
Recommended VTP Ordered[2]	127	92%	97%	94%
Urinary Catheter Removal[2]	131	92%	92%	90%
Children's Asthma Care				
Received Systemic Corticosteroids	-	-	-	100%
Received Home Management Plan	-	-	-	71%
Received Reliever Medication	-	-	-	100%
Use of Medical Imaging				
Combination Abdominal CT Scan	594	0.049	0.133	0.191
Combination Chest CT Scan	597	0.008	0.045	0.054
Follow-up Mammogram/Ultrasound	2,053	5.7%	7.6%	8.4%
MRI for Low Back Pain	211	35.5%	36.7%	32.7%
Survey of Patients' Hospital Experiences				
Area Around Room 'Always' Quiet at Night	300+	62%	-	58%
Doctors 'Always' Communicated Well	300+	78%	-	80%
Home Recovery Information Given	300+	86%	-	82%
Hospital Given 9 or 10 on 10 Point Scale	300+	74%	-	67%
Meds 'Always' Explained Before Given	300+	64%	-	60%
Nurses 'Always' Communicated Well	300+	77%	-	76%
Pain 'Always' Well Controlled	300+	66%	-	69%
Room and Bathroom 'Always' Clean	300+	71%	-	71%
Timely Help 'Always' Received	300+	60%	-	64%
Would Definitely Recommend Hospital	300+	79%	-	69%

NOTE: Hospital profiles are in alphabetical order by state, then city, then hospital within the city; Rankings exclude hospitals with less than 25 cases except for patient surveys which excludes hospitals with less than 100 cases; (a) 100–299 cases; (1) The number of cases is too small to be sure how well a hospital is performing; (2) The hospital indicated that the data submitted for this measure were based on a sample of cases; (3) Data was collected during a shorter time period (fewer quarters) than the maximum possible time for this measure; (4) Suppressed for one or more quarters by CMS; (5) No data is available from the hospital for this measure; (6) Fewer than 100 patients completed the HCAHPS survey. Use these rates with caution, as the number of surveys may be too low to reliably assess hospital performance; (7) Survey results are based on less than 12 months of data; (8) Survey results are not available for this reporting period; (9) No or very few patients were eligible for the HCAHPS survey. The scores shown, if any, reflect a very small number of surveys; (10) A state average was not calculated because too few hospitals in the state submitted data; (11) There were discrepancies in the data collection process; Please refer to the User's Guide for a full explanation of data.

Aroostook Medical Center

140 Academy Street
Presque Isle, ME 04769
URL: www.tamc.org
Phone: 207-768-4000
Fax: 207-768-4226
Type: Acute Care Hospitals
Emergency Services: No
Ownership: Voluntary Non-Profit - Private
Beds: 177

Key Personnel:
CEO/President.............. David A Peterson
Chief of Medical Staff.......... Lawrence Crystal
Quality Assurance .... Stephen A Poitras
Emergency Room .... Sharon Lesbear

Measure	Cases	This Hosp.	State Avg.	U.S. Avg.
Heart Attack Care				
ACE Inhibitor or ARB for LVSD[1]	5	80%	98%	96%
Aspirin at Arrival	49	96%	99%	99%
Aspirin at Discharge	36	97%	99%	98%
Beta Blocker at Discharge	37	95%	99%	98%
Fibrinolytic Medication Timing	0	-	43%	55%
PCI Within 90 Minutes of Arrival	0	-	94%	90%
Smoking Cessation Advice[1]	3	100%	100%	99%
Chest Pain/Possible Heart Attack Care				
Aspirin at Arrival	50	98%	98%	95%
Median Time to ECG (minutes)	50	3	7	8
Median Time to Transfer (minutes)[3]	0	-	46	61
Fibrinolytic Medication Timing[1]	6	67%	75%	54%
Heart Failure Care				
ACE Inhibitor or ARB for LVSD[1]	17	100%	97%	94%
Discharge Instructions	58	81%	91%	88%
Evaluation of LVS Function	67	99%	99%	98%
Smoking Cessation Advice[1]	7	100%	97%	98%
Pneumonia Care				
Appropriate Initial Antibiotic	44	89%	94%	92%
Blood Culture Timing	83	95%	95%	96%
Influenza Vaccine	33	100%	97%	91%
Initial Antibiotic Timing	72	96%	98%	95%
Pneumococcal Vaccine	74	96%	97%	93%
Smoking Cessation Advice	28	96%	99%	97%
Surgical Care Improvement Project				
Appropriate VTP Within 24 Hours	127	99%	96%	92%
Appropriate Hair Removal	182	100%	100%	99%
Appropriate Beta Blocker Usage	58	100%	95%	93%
Controlled Postoperative Blood Glucose	0	-	97%	93%
Prophylactic Antibiotic Timing	135	98%	98%	97%
Prophylactic Antibiotic Timing (Outpatient)	78	92%	93%	92%
Prophylactic Antibiotic Selection	135	99%	99%	97%
Prophylactic Antibiotic Select. (Outpatient)	73	96%	95%	94%
Prophylactic Antibiotic Stopped	129	98%	97%	94%
Recommended VTP Ordered	127	99%	97%	94%
Urinary Catheter Removal	50	96%	92%	90%
Children's Asthma Care				
Received Systemic Corticosteroids	-	-	-	100%
Received Home Management Plan	-	-	-	71%
Received Reliever Medication	-	-	-	100%
Use of Medical Imaging				
Combination Abdominal CT Scan	577	0.475	0.133	0.191
Combination Chest CT Scan	486	0.290	0.045	0.054
Follow-up Mammogram/Ultrasound	999	10.1%	7.6%	8.4%
MRI for Low Back Pain[5]	0	-	36.7%	32.7%
Survey of Patients' Hospital Experiences				
Area Around Room 'Always' Quiet at Night	300+	46%	-	58%
Doctors 'Always' Communicated Well	300+	74%	-	80%
Home Recovery Information Given	300+	76%	-	82%
Hospital Given 9 or 10 on 10 Point Scale	300+	61%	-	67%
Meds 'Always' Explained Before Given	300+	53%	-	60%
Nurses 'Always' Communicated Well	300+	75%	-	76%
Pain 'Always' Well Controlled	300+	63%	-	69%
Room and Bathroom 'Always' Clean	300+	79%	-	71%
Timely Help 'Always' Received	300+	66%	-	64%
Would Definitely Recommend Hospital	300+	56%	-	69%

Penobscot Bay Medical Center

6 Glen Cove Drive
Rockport, ME 04856
URL: www.nehealth.org
Phone: 207-596-8000
Fax: 207-593-6710
Type: Acute Care Hospitals
Emergency Services: No
Ownership: Voluntary Non-Profit - Private
Beds: 106

Key Personnel:
CEO/President.............. Roy Hitthing
Radiology.................. Charles A Crans Jr

Measure	Cases	This Hosp.	State Avg.	U.S. Avg.
Heart Attack Care				
ACE Inhibitor or ARB for LVSD[1]	1	100%	98%	96%
Aspirin at Arrival	38	100%	99%	99%
Aspirin at Discharge	25	100%	99%	98%
Beta Blocker at Discharge[1]	23	100%	99%	98%
Fibrinolytic Medication Timing	0	-	43%	55%
PCI Within 90 Minutes of Arrival	0	-	94%	90%
Smoking Cessation Advice[1]	3	100%	100%	99%
Chest Pain/Possible Heart Attack Care				
Aspirin at Arrival	49	100%	98%	95%
Median Time to ECG (minutes)	51	6	7	8
Median Time to Transfer (minutes)[3]	0	-	46	61
Fibrinolytic Medication Timing[1]	13	69%	75%	54%
Heart Failure Care				
ACE Inhibitor or ARB for LVSD[1]	20	100%	97%	94%
Discharge Instructions	80	96%	91%	88%
Evaluation of LVS Function	116	99%	99%	98%
Smoking Cessation Advice[1]	10	90%	97%	98%
Pneumonia Care				
Appropriate Initial Antibiotic	64	94%	94%	92%
Blood Culture Timing	92	97%	95%	96%
Influenza Vaccine	65	98%	97%	91%
Initial Antibiotic Timing	88	98%	98%	95%
Pneumococcal Vaccine	90	97%	97%	93%
Smoking Cessation Advice	37	100%	99%	97%
Surgical Care Improvement Project				
Appropriate VTP Within 24 Hours	74	92%	96%	92%
Appropriate Hair Removal	270	100%	100%	99%
Appropriate Beta Blocker Usage	76	96%	95%	93%
Controlled Postoperative Blood Glucose	0	-	97%	93%
Prophylactic Antibiotic Timing	210	98%	98%	97%
Prophylactic Antibiotic Timing (Outpatient)	59	86%	93%	92%
Prophylactic Antibiotic Selection	211	98%	99%	97%
Prophylactic Antibiotic Select. (Outpatient)	84	96%	95%	94%
Prophylactic Antibiotic Stopped	208	96%	97%	94%
Recommended VTP Ordered	74	95%	97%	94%
Urinary Catheter Removal[1]	10	80%	92%	90%
Children's Asthma Care				
Received Systemic Corticosteroids	-	-	-	100%
Received Home Management Plan	-	-	-	71%
Received Reliever Medication	-	-	-	100%
Use of Medical Imaging				
Combination Abdominal CT Scan	552	0.080	0.133	0.191
Combination Chest CT Scan	480	0.002	0.045	0.054
Follow-up Mammogram/Ultrasound[5]	0	-	7.6%	8.4%
MRI for Low Back Pain[1]	4	25.0%	36.7%	32.7%
Survey of Patients' Hospital Experiences				
Area Around Room 'Always' Quiet at Night	300+	53%	-	58%
Doctors 'Always' Communicated Well	300+	80%	-	80%
Home Recovery Information Given	300+	88%	-	82%
Hospital Given 9 or 10 on 10 Point Scale	300+	66%	-	67%
Meds 'Always' Explained Before Given	300+	62%	-	60%
Nurses 'Always' Communicated Well	300+	76%	-	76%
Pain 'Always' Well Controlled	300+	70%	-	69%
Room and Bathroom 'Always' Clean	300+	73%	-	71%
Timely Help 'Always' Received	300+	67%	-	64%
Would Definitely Recommend Hospital	300+	69%	-	69%

Rumford Hospital

420 Franklin Street
Rumford, ME 04276
URL: www.rumfordhospital.org
Phone: 207-364-4561
Fax: 207-369-0834
Type: Critical Access Hospitals
Emergency Services: Yes
Ownership: Voluntary Non-Profit - Private
Beds: 49

Key Personnel:
CEO/President.............. John Welsh
Radiology.................. John J Bennett

Measure	Cases	This Hosp.	State Avg.	U.S. Avg.
Heart Attack Care				
ACE Inhibitor or ARB for LVSD[1,3]	1	100%	98%	96%
Aspirin at Arrival[1,3]	2	100%	99%	99%
Aspirin at Discharge[1,3]	4	100%	99%	98%
Beta Blocker at Discharge[1,3]	5	100%	99%	98%
Fibrinolytic Medication Timing[3]	0	-	43%	55%
PCI Within 90 Minutes of Arrival[3]	0	-	94%	90%
Smoking Cessation Advice[3]	0	-	100%	99%
Chest Pain/Possible Heart Attack Care				
Aspirin at Arrival	-	-	98%	95%
Median Time to ECG (minutes)	-	-	7	8
Median Time to Transfer (minutes)	-	-	46	61
Fibrinolytic Medication Timing	-	-	75%	54%
Heart Failure Care				
ACE Inhibitor or ARB for LVSD[1]	6	83%	97%	94%
Discharge Instructions[1]	24	96%	91%	88%
Evaluation of LVS Function	35	97%	99%	98%
Smoking Cessation Advice[1]	1	100%	97%	98%
Pneumonia Care				
Appropriate Initial Antibiotic[1]	23	91%	94%	92%
Blood Culture Timing	44	86%	95%	96%
Influenza Vaccine	28	100%	97%	91%
Initial Antibiotic Timing	42	100%	98%	95%
Pneumococcal Vaccine	42	93%	97%	93%
Smoking Cessation Advice[1]	13	100%	99%	97%
Surgical Care Improvement Project				
Appropriate VTP Within 24 Hours[5]	0	-	96%	92%
Appropriate Hair Removal[5]	0	-	100%	99%
Appropriate Beta Blocker Usage[5]	0	-	95%	93%
Controlled Postoperative Blood Glucose[5]	0	-	97%	93%
Prophylactic Antibiotic Timing[5]	0	-	98%	97%
Prophylactic Antibiotic Timing (Outpatient)	-	-	93%	92%
Prophylactic Antibiotic Selection[5]	0	-	99%	97%
Prophylactic Antibiotic Select. (Outpatient)	-	-	95%	94%
Prophylactic Antibiotic Stopped[5]	0	-	97%	94%
Recommended VTP Ordered[5]	0	-	97%	94%
Urinary Catheter Removal[5]	0	-	92%	90%
Children's Asthma Care				
Received Systemic Corticosteroids	-	-	-	100%
Received Home Management Plan	-	-	-	71%
Received Reliever Medication	-	-	-	100%
Use of Medical Imaging				
Combination Abdominal CT Scan	-	-	0.133	0.191
Combination Chest CT Scan	-	-	0.045	0.054
Follow-up Mammogram/Ultrasound	-	-	7.6%	8.4%
MRI for Low Back Pain	-	-	36.7%	32.7%
Survey of Patients' Hospital Experiences				
Area Around Room 'Always' Quiet at Night	(a)	69%	-	58%
Doctors 'Always' Communicated Well	(a)	72%	-	80%
Home Recovery Information Given	(a)	88%	-	82%
Hospital Given 9 or 10 on 10 Point Scale	(a)	70%	-	67%
Meds 'Always' Explained Before Given	(a)	53%	-	60%
Nurses 'Always' Communicated Well	(a)	75%	-	76%
Pain 'Always' Well Controlled	(a)	68%	-	69%
Room and Bathroom 'Always' Clean	(a)	85%	-	71%
Timely Help 'Always' Received	(a)	71%	-	64%
Would Definitely Recommend Hospital	(a)	69%	-	69%

NOTE: Hospital profiles are in alphabetical order by state, then city, then hospital within the city; Rankings exclude hospitals with less than 25 cases except for patient surveys which excludes hospitals with less than 100 cases; (a) 100–299 cases; (1) The number of cases is too small to be sure how well a hospital is performing; (2) The hospital indicated that the data submitted for this measure were based on a sample of cases; (3) Data was collected during a shorter time period (fewer quarters) than the maximum possible time for this measure; (4) Suppressed for one or more quarters by CMS; (5) No data is available from the hospital for this measure; (6) Fewer than 100 patients completed the HCAHPS survey. Use these rates with caution, as the number of surveys may be too low to reliably assess hospital performance; (7) Survey results are based on less than 12 months of data; (8) Survey results are not available for this reporting period; (9) No or very few patients were eligible for the HCAHPS survey. The scores shown, if any, reflect a very small number of surveys; (10) A state average was not calculated because too few hospitals in the state submitted data; (11) There were discrepancies in the data collection process; Please refer to the User's Guide for a full explanation of data.

Henrietta D Goodall Hospital

25 June St
Sanford, ME 04073
Phone: 207-324-4310
Fax: 207-490-7328
E-mail: mfroning@goodallhospital.org
URL: www.goodallhospital.org
Type: Acute Care Hospitals
Emergency Services: Yes
Ownership: Voluntary Non-Profit - Private
Beds: 137

Key Personnel:
CEO/President. . . . . Darlene Stromstad
Chief of Medical Staff. . . . . Mark A Rautenberg
Operating Room. . . . . Ken Gillis
Quality Assurance . . . . Eliot Sanantagosl
Radiology. . . . . Edward M Cruz
Anesthesiology. . . . . Leonid I Temkin, MD
Emergency Room . . . . John Bartley, MD
Patient Relations . . . . Lorraine D Masure

Measure	Cases	This Hosp.	State Avg.	U.S. Avg.
Heart Attack Care				
ACE Inhibitor or ARB for LVSD[1]	5	100%	98%	96%
Aspirin at Arrival	36	94%	99%	99%
Aspirin at Discharge[1]	21	95%	99%	98%
Beta Blocker at Discharge	26	100%	99%	98%
Fibrinolytic Medication Timing	0	-	43%	55%
PCI Within 90 Minutes of Arrival	0	-	94%	90%
Smoking Cessation Advice[1]	1	100%	100%	99%
Chest Pain/Possible Heart Attack Care				
Aspirin at Arrival	50	96%	98%	95%
Median Time to ECG (minutes)	50	3	7	8
Median Time to Transfer (minutes)[1,3]	2	48	46	61
Fibrinolytic Medication Timing[1]	14	64%	75%	54%
Heart Failure Care				
ACE Inhibitor or ARB for LVSD[1]	9	100%	97%	94%
Discharge Instructions	65	86%	91%	88%
Evaluation of LVS Function	90	99%	99%	98%
Smoking Cessation Advice[1]	13	100%	97%	98%
Pneumonia Care				
Appropriate Initial Antibiotic	71	96%	94%	92%
Blood Culture Timing	103	100%	95%	96%
Influenza Vaccine	82	100%	97%	91%
Initial Antibiotic Timing	105	99%	98%	95%
Pneumococcal Vaccine	106	100%	97%	93%
Smoking Cessation Advice	37	100%	99%	97%
Surgical Care Improvement Project				
Appropriate VTP Within 24 Hours	55	100%	96%	92%
Appropriate Hair Removal	151	100%	100%	99%
Appropriate Beta Blocker Usage	41	100%	95%	93%
Controlled Postoperative Blood Glucose	0	-	97%	93%
Prophylactic Antibiotic Timing	127	100%	98%	97%
Prophylactic Antibiotic Timing (Outpatient)	45	93%	93%	92%
Prophylactic Antibiotic Selection	127	99%	99%	97%
Prophylactic Antibiotic Select. (Outpatient)	42	95%	95%	94%
Prophylactic Antibiotic Stopped	123	97%	97%	94%
Recommended VTP Ordered	55	100%	97%	94%
Urinary Catheter Removal	52	100%	92%	90%
Children's Asthma Care				
Received Systemic Corticosteroids	-	-	-	100%
Received Home Management Plan	-	-	-	71%
Received Reliever Medication	-	-	-	100%
Use of Medical Imaging				
Combination Abdominal CT Scan	457	0.096	0.133	0.191
Combination Chest CT Scan	369	0.027	0.045	0.054
Follow-up Mammogram/Ultrasound	967	8.7%	7.6%	8.4%
MRI for Low Back Pain	105	37.1%	36.7%	32.7%
Survey of Patients' Hospital Experiences				
Area Around Room 'Always' Quiet at Night	300+	59%	-	58%
Doctors 'Always' Communicated Well	300+	79%	-	80%
Home Recovery Information Given	300+	88%	-	82%
Hospital Given 9 or 10 on 10 Point Scale	300+	57%	-	67%
Meds 'Always' Explained Before Given	300+	61%	-	60%
Nurses 'Always' Communicated Well	300+	73%	-	76%
Pain 'Always' Well Controlled	300+	67%	-	69%
Room and Bathroom 'Always' Clean	300+	75%	-	71%
Timely Help 'Always' Received	300+	64%	-	64%
Would Definitely Recommend Hospital	300+	60%	-	69%

Redington Fairview General Hospital

46 Fairview Ave
Skowhegan, ME 04976
Phone: 207-474-5121
Fax: 207-474-5121
E-mail: info@rfgh.net
URL: www.rfgh.net
Type: Critical Access Hospitals
Emergency Services: Yes
Ownership: Voluntary Non-Profit - Other
Beds: 65

Key Personnel:
CEO/President. . . . . Richard Willett
Chief of Medical Staff. . . . . Roger Renfrew, MD
Infection Control. . . . . Peg Shore
Pediatric Ambulatory Care . . . . . . Ruby Rodriguez
Pediatric In-Patient Care . . . . Ruby Rodriguez
Quality Assurance . . . . Alma Fournier, RN
Radiology. . . . . Anthony Van Dyck, MD
Intensive Care Unit. . . . . Sandy Whiting

Measure	Cases	This Hosp.	State Avg.	U.S. Avg.
Heart Attack Care				
ACE Inhibitor or ARB for LVSD[1]	1	100%	98%	96%
Aspirin at Arrival[1]	21	100%	99%	99%
Aspirin at Discharge[1]	11	100%	99%	98%
Beta Blocker at Discharge[1]	11	100%	99%	98%
Fibrinolytic Medication Timing	0	-	43%	55%
PCI Within 90 Minutes of Arrival	0	-	94%	90%
Smoking Cessation Advice[1]	2	100%	100%	99%
Chest Pain/Possible Heart Attack Care				
Aspirin at Arrival[3]	29	93%	98%	95%
Median Time to ECG (minutes)[3]	33	5	7	8
Median Time to Transfer (minutes)[1,3]	2	440	46	61
Fibrinolytic Medication Timing[1,3]	6	67%	75%	54%
Heart Failure Care				
ACE Inhibitor or ARB for LVSD[1]	10	100%	97%	94%
Discharge Instructions	38	84%	91%	88%
Evaluation of LVS Function	52	98%	99%	98%
Smoking Cessation Advice[1]	3	100%	97%	98%
Pneumonia Care				
Appropriate Initial Antibiotic	72	100%	94%	92%
Blood Culture Timing	105	98%	95%	96%
Influenza Vaccine	92	100%	97%	91%
Initial Antibiotic Timing	124	99%	98%	95%
Pneumococcal Vaccine	117	100%	97%	93%
Smoking Cessation Advice	29	97%	99%	97%
Surgical Care Improvement Project				
Appropriate VTP Within 24 Hours	48	100%	96%	92%
Appropriate Hair Removal	70	100%	100%	99%
Appropriate Beta Blocker Usage[5]	0	-	95%	93%
Controlled Postoperative Blood Glucose	0	-	97%	93%
Prophylactic Antibiotic Timing	45	100%	98%	97%
Prophylactic Antibiotic Timing (Outpatient)[1,3]	9	100%	93%	92%
Prophylactic Antibiotic Selection	45	100%	99%	97%
Prophylactic Antibiotic Select. (Outpatient)[1,3]	9	100%	95%	94%
Prophylactic Antibiotic Stopped	43	98%	97%	94%
Recommended VTP Ordered	48	100%	97%	94%
Urinary Catheter Removal[1]	20	90%	92%	90%
Children's Asthma Care				
Received Systemic Corticosteroids	-	-	-	100%
Received Home Management Plan	-	-	-	71%
Received Reliever Medication	-	-	-	100%
Use of Medical Imaging				
Combination Abdominal CT Scan	481	0.123	0.133	0.191
Combination Chest CT Scan	196	0.066	0.045	0.054
Follow-up Mammogram/Ultrasound	932	8.7%	7.6%	8.4%
MRI for Low Back Pain[5]	0	-	36.7%	32.7%
Survey of Patients' Hospital Experiences				
Area Around Room 'Always' Quiet at Night	300+	60%	-	58%
Doctors 'Always' Communicated Well	300+	85%	-	80%
Home Recovery Information Given	300+	91%	-	82%
Hospital Given 9 or 10 on 10 Point Scale	300+	73%	-	67%
Meds 'Always' Explained Before Given	300+	70%	-	60%
Nurses 'Always' Communicated Well	300+	83%	-	76%
Pain 'Always' Well Controlled	300+	73%	-	69%
Room and Bathroom 'Always' Clean	300+	83%	-	71%
Timely Help 'Always' Received	300+	71%	-	64%
Would Definitely Recommend Hospital	300+	77%	-	69%

Inland Hospital

200 Kennedy Memorial Drive
Waterville, ME 04901
Phone: 207-861-3000
URL: www.inlandhospital.org
Type: Acute Care Hospitals
Emergency Services: Yes
Ownership: Voluntary Non-Profit - Private
Beds: 78

Key Personnel:
CEO/President. . . . . John Dalton
Chief of Medical Staff. . . . . Michael Palumbo
Radiology. . . . . Hugh R Caggiano

Measure	Cases	This Hosp.	State Avg.	U.S. Avg.
Heart Attack Care				
ACE Inhibitor or ARB for LVSD	0	-	98%	96%
Aspirin at Arrival[1]	6	100%	99%	99%
Aspirin at Discharge[1]	1	100%	99%	98%
Beta Blocker at Discharge[1]	1	100%	99%	98%
Fibrinolytic Medication Timing	0	-	43%	55%
PCI Within 90 Minutes of Arrival	0	-	94%	90%
Smoking Cessation Advice	0	-	100%	99%
Chest Pain/Possible Heart Attack Care				
Aspirin at Arrival	74	100%	98%	95%
Median Time to ECG (minutes)	77	5	7	8
Median Time to Transfer (minutes)[1,3]	2	135	46	61
Fibrinolytic Medication Timing[1]	3	67%	75%	54%
Heart Failure Care				
ACE Inhibitor or ARB for LVSD[1]	8	75%	97%	94%
Discharge Instructions	29	83%	91%	88%
Evaluation of LVS Function	56	100%	99%	98%
Smoking Cessation Advice[1]	12	92%	97%	98%
Pneumonia Care				
Appropriate Initial Antibiotic	27	89%	94%	92%
Blood Culture Timing	52	100%	95%	96%
Influenza Vaccine	32	97%	97%	91%
Initial Antibiotic Timing	43	100%	98%	95%
Pneumococcal Vaccine	51	100%	97%	93%
Smoking Cessation Advice[1]	14	100%	99%	97%
Surgical Care Improvement Project				
Appropriate VTP Within 24 Hours	70	100%	96%	92%
Appropriate Hair Removal	125	100%	100%	99%
Appropriate Beta Blocker Usage[1]	20	70%	95%	93%
Controlled Postoperative Blood Glucose	0	-	97%	93%
Prophylactic Antibiotic Timing	87	98%	98%	97%
Prophylactic Antibiotic Timing (Outpatient)	166	98%	93%	92%
Prophylactic Antibiotic Selection	87	98%	99%	97%
Prophylactic Antibiotic Select. (Outpatient)	165	95%	95%	94%
Prophylactic Antibiotic Stopped	86	92%	97%	94%
Recommended VTP Ordered	70	100%	97%	94%
Urinary Catheter Removal	47	81%	92%	90%
Children's Asthma Care				
Received Systemic Corticosteroids	-	-	-	100%
Received Home Management Plan	-	-	-	71%
Received Reliever Medication	-	-	-	100%
Use of Medical Imaging				
Combination Abdominal CT Scan	308	0.023	0.133	0.191
Combination Chest CT Scan	125	0.000	0.045	0.054
Follow-up Mammogram/Ultrasound	419	8.1%	7.6%	8.4%
MRI for Low Back Pain[5]	0	-	36.7%	32.7%
Survey of Patients' Hospital Experiences				
Area Around Room 'Always' Quiet at Night	(a)	69%	-	58%
Doctors 'Always' Communicated Well	(a)	79%	-	80%
Home Recovery Information Given	(a)	85%	-	82%
Hospital Given 9 or 10 on 10 Point Scale	(a)	70%	-	67%
Meds 'Always' Explained Before Given	(a)	60%	-	60%
Nurses 'Always' Communicated Well	(a)	83%	-	76%
Pain 'Always' Well Controlled	(a)	72%	-	69%
Room and Bathroom 'Always' Clean	(a)	77%	-	71%
Timely Help 'Always' Received	(a)	72%	-	64%
Would Definitely Recommend Hospital	(a)	78%	-	69%

NOTE: Hospital profiles are in alphabetical order by state, then city, then hospital within the city; Rankings exclude hospitals with less than 25 cases except for patient surveys which excludes hospitals with less than 100 cases; (a) 100–299 cases; (1) The number of cases is too small to be sure how well a hospital is performing; (2) The hospital indicated that the data submitted for this measure were based on a sample of cases; (3) Data was collected during a shorter time period (fewer quarters) than the maximum possible time for this measure; (4) Suppressed for one or more quarters by CMS; (5) No data is available from the hospital for this measure; (6) Fewer than 100 patients completed the HCAHPS survey. Use these rates with caution, as the number of surveys may be too low to reliably assess hospital performance; (7) Survey results are based on less than 12 months of data; (8) Survey results are not available for this reporting period; (9) No or very few patients were eligible for the HCAHPS survey. The scores shown, if any, reflect a very small number of surveys; (10) A state average was not calculated because too few hospitals in the state submitted data; (11) There were discrepancies in the data collection process; Please refer to the User's Guide for a full explanation of data.

York Hospital

15 Hospital Dr
York, ME 03909
E-mail: cr@yorkhospital.com
URL: www.yorkhospital.com
Type: Acute Care Hospitals
Ownership: Voluntary Non-Profit - Private

Phone: 207-363-4321
Fax: 207-363-3858

Emergency Services: No
Beds: 79

Key Personnel:
Coronary Care . . . . Larry Pedrovich
Infection Control . . . . Shirley Peverly
Quality Assurance . . . . Eliot Smith, MD
Radiology. . . . . Edward Michael Cruz
Emergency Room . . . . Elliot Smith, MD

Measure	Cases	This Hosp.	State Avg.	U.S. Avg.
Heart Attack Care				
ACE Inhibitor or ARB for LVSD[1]	9	100%	98%	96%
Aspirin at Arrival	71	100%	99%	99%
Aspirin at Discharge	60	98%	99%	98%
Beta Blocker at Discharge	59	100%	99%	98%
Fibrinolytic Medication Timing	0	-	43%	55%
PCI Within 90 Minutes of Arrival[1]	10	90%	94%	90%
Smoking Cessation Advice[1]	13	100%	100%	99%
Chest Pain/Possible Heart Attack Care				
Aspirin at Arrival[1,3]	6	100%	98%	95%
Median Time to ECG (minutes)[1,3]	6	10	7	8
Median Time to Transfer (minutes)[5]	0	-	46	61
Fibrinolytic Medication Timing[3]	0	-	75%	54%
Heart Failure Care				
ACE Inhibitor or ARB for LVSD[1]	22	95%	97%	94%
Discharge Instructions	93	96%	91%	88%
Evaluation of LVS Function	122	98%	99%	98%
Smoking Cessation Advice[1]	6	100%	97%	98%
Pneumonia Care				
Appropriate Initial Antibiotic	65	97%	94%	92%
Blood Culture Timing	67	97%	95%	96%
Influenza Vaccine	66	100%	97%	91%
Initial Antibiotic Timing	95	99%	98%	95%
Pneumococcal Vaccine	95	95%	97%	93%
Smoking Cessation Advice	25	96%	99%	97%
Surgical Care Improvement Project				
Appropriate VTP Within 24 Hours	117	98%	96%	92%
Appropriate Hair Removal	275	100%	100%	99%
Appropriate Beta Blocker Usage	85	99%	95%	93%
Controlled Postoperative Blood Glucose	0	-	97%	93%
Prophylactic Antibiotic Timing	164	98%	98%	97%
Prophylactic Antibiotic Timing (Outpatient)	98	96%	93%	92%
Prophylactic Antibiotic Selection	165	98%	99%	97%
Prophylactic Antibiotic Select. (Outpatient)	97	99%	95%	94%
Prophylactic Antibiotic Stopped	163	97%	97%	94%
Recommended VTP Ordered	117	98%	97%	94%
Urinary Catheter Removal	50	96%	92%	90%
Children's Asthma Care				
Received Systemic Corticosteroids	-	-	-	100%
Received Home Management Plan	-	-	-	71%
Received Reliever Medication	-	-	-	100%
Use of Medical Imaging				
Combination Abdominal CT Scan	657	0.131	0.133	0.191
Combination Chest CT Scan	502	0.008	0.045	0.054
Follow-up Mammogram/Ultrasound	1,207	10.7%	7.6%	8.4%
MRI for Low Back Pain	141	26.2%	36.7%	32.7%
Survey of Patients' Hospital Experiences				
Area Around Room 'Always' Quiet at Night	300+	58%	-	58%
Doctors 'Always' Communicated Well	300+	87%	-	80%
Home Recovery Information Given	300+	87%	-	82%
Hospital Given 9 or 10 on 10 Point Scale	300+	84%	-	67%
Meds 'Always' Explained Before Given	300+	67%	-	60%
Nurses 'Always' Communicated Well	300+	84%	-	76%
Pain 'Always' Well Controlled	300+	75%	-	69%
Room and Bathroom 'Always' Clean	300+	77%	-	71%
Timely Help 'Always' Received	300+	72%	-	64%
Would Definitely Recommend Hospital	300+	90%	-	69%

NOTE: Hospital profiles are in alphabetical order by state, then city, then hospital within the city; Rankings exclude hospitals with less than 25 cases except for patient surveys which excludes hospitals with less than 100 cases; (a) 100–299 cases; (1) The number of cases is too small to be sure how well a hospital is performing; (2) The hospital indicated that the data submitted for this measure were based on a sample of cases; (3) Data was collected during a shorter time period (fewer quarters) than the maximum possible time for this measure; (4) Suppressed for one or more quarters by CMS; (5) No data is available from the hospital for this measure; (6) Fewer than 100 patients completed the HCAHPS survey. Use these rates with caution, as the number of surveys may be too low to reliably assess hospital performance; (7) Survey results are based on less than 12 months of data; (8) Survey results are not available for this reporting period; (9) No or very few patients were eligible for the HCAHPS survey. The scores shown, if any, reflect a very small number of surveys; (10) A state average was not calculated because too few hospitals in the state submitted data; (11) There were discrepancies in the data collection process; Please refer to the User's Guide for a full explanation of data.

Heart Attack Care

1. ACE Inhibitor or ARB for LVSD

Hospital Name	City	Rate	Cases
The Johns Hopkins Hospital[2]	Baltimore	100%	44
Saint Agnes Hospital	Baltimore	100%	27
Saint Joseph Medical Center[2]	Towson	100%	54
Upper Chesapeake Medical Center	Bel Air	100%	30
Frederick Memorial Hospital	Frederick	96%	27
Johns Hopkins Bayview Medical Center	Baltimore	96%	28
Shady Grove Adventist Hospital	Rockville	96%	27
Washington Adventist Hospital[2]	Takoma Park	96%	71
Peninsula Regional Medical Center	Salisbury	95%	100
Suburban Hospital	Bethesda	95%	44
Union Memorial Hospital	Baltimore	94%	108
University of Maryland Medical Center	Baltimore	92%	77
Prince Georges Hospital Center	Cheverly	87%	30
Sinai Hospital of Baltimore	Baltimore	86%	71
Southern Maryland Hospital Center	Clinton	85%	34
Western Maryland Regional Medical Center	Cumberland	83%	46

2. Aspirin at Arrival

Hospital Name	City	Rate	Cases
Civista Medical Center	La Plata	100%	36
Harbor Hospital	Brooklyn	100%	42
Holy Cross Hospital	Silver Spring	100%	188
Johns Hopkins Bayview Medical Center	Baltimore	100%	172
The Johns Hopkins Hospital[2]	Baltimore	100%	90
Memorial Hospital at Easton	Easton	100%	84
Meritus Medical Center	Hagerstown	100%	156
Montgomery General Hospital	Olney	100%	48
Saint Joseph Medical Center[2]	Towson	100%	172
Shady Grove Adventist Hospital	Rockville	100%	180
Sinai Hospital of Baltimore	Baltimore	100%	210
Union Hospital of Cecil County	Elkton	100%	55
VA Maryland Healthcare System - Baltimore	Baltimore	100%	36
Baltimore Washington Medical Center	Glen Burnie	99%	202
Franklin Square Hospital Center	Baltimore	99%	203
Suburban Hospital	Bethesda	99%	177
University of Maryland Medical Center	Baltimore	99%	83
Upper Chesapeake Medical Center	Bel Air	99%	202
Washington Adventist Hospital[2]	Takoma Park	99%	83
Anne Arundel Medical Center	Annapolis	98%	208
Carroll Hospital Center	Westminster	98%	150
Howard County General Hospital	Columbia	98%	129
Frederick Memorial Hospital	Frederick	97%	164
Harford Memorial Hospital	Havre De Grace	97%	36
Peninsula Regional Medical Center	Salisbury	97%	403
Saint Mary's Hospital	Leonardtown	97%	38
Western Maryland Regional Medical Center	Cumberland	97%	193
Good Samaritan Hospital	Baltimore	96%	103
Laurel Regional Medical Center	Laurel	96%	55
Northwest Hospital Center	Randallstown	96%	93
Southern Maryland Hospital Center	Clinton	96%	159
Union Memorial Hospital	Baltimore	96%	116
Calvert Memorial Hospital	Prince Frederick	95%	43
Saint Agnes Hospital	Baltimore	95%	133
Bon Secours Hospital	Baltimore	93%	29
Prince Georges Hospital Center	Cheverly	91%	171
Doctors' Community Hospital	Lanham	90%	50

3. Aspirin at Discharge

Hospital Name	City	Rate	Cases
Franklin Square Hospital Center	Baltimore	100%	123
Holy Cross Hospital	Silver Spring	100%	110
Howard County General Hospital	Columbia	100%	90
Memorial Hospital at Easton	Easton	100%	47
Meritus Medical Center	Hagerstown	100%	129
Anne Arundel Medical Center	Annapolis	99%	153
Carroll Hospital Center	Westminster	99%	93
The Johns Hopkins Hospital[2]	Baltimore	99%	301
Peninsula Regional Medical Center	Salisbury	99%	540
Saint Agnes Hospital	Baltimore	99%	105
Saint Joseph Medical Center[2]	Towson	99%	323
Shady Grove Adventist Hospital	Rockville	99%	159
Suburban Hospital	Bethesda	99%	241
Union Memorial Hospital	Baltimore	99%	696
Baltimore Washington Medical Center	Glen Burnie	98%	124
Frederick Memorial Hospital	Frederick	98%	134
Johns Hopkins Bayview Medical Center	Baltimore	98%	129
Sinai Hospital of Baltimore	Baltimore	98%	379
Southern Maryland Hospital Center	Clinton	98%	123
University of Maryland Medical Center	Baltimore	98%	471
Washington Adventist Hospital[2]	Takoma Park	98%	292
Western Maryland Regional Medical Center	Cumberland	98%	219
Upper Chesapeake Medical Center	Bel Air	97%	145
Calvert Memorial Hospital	Prince Frederick	96%	27
Good Samaritan Hospital	Baltimore	95%	81
Northwest Hospital Center	Randallstown	95%	56
VA Maryland Healthcare System - Baltimore	Baltimore	93%	29
Prince Georges Hospital Center	Cheverly	86%	170
Laurel Regional Medical Center	Laurel	81%	27

4. Beta Blocker at Discharge

Hospital Name	City	Rate	Cases
Calvert Memorial Hospital	Prince Frederick	100%	27
Good Samaritan Hospital	Baltimore	100%	81
Anne Arundel Medical Center	Annapolis	99%	153
Franklin Square Hospital Center	Baltimore	99%	121
Holy Cross Hospital	Silver Spring	99%	114
Howard County General Hospital	Columbia	99%	90
The Johns Hopkins Hospital[2]	Baltimore	99%	284
Meritus Medical Center	Hagerstown	99%	128
Peninsula Regional Medical Center	Salisbury	99%	536
Saint Agnes Hospital	Baltimore	99%	105
Saint Joseph Medical Center[2]	Towson	99%	321
Shady Grove Adventist Hospital	Rockville	99%	156
Upper Chesapeake Medical Center	Bel Air	99%	145
Johns Hopkins Bayview Medical Center	Baltimore	98%	127
Memorial Hospital at Easton	Easton	98%	46
Suburban Hospital	Bethesda	98%	240
Washington Adventist Hospital[2]	Takoma Park	98%	282
Carroll Hospital Center	Westminster	97%	89
Frederick Memorial Hospital	Frederick	97%	135
Sinai Hospital of Baltimore	Baltimore	97%	372
Southern Maryland Hospital Center	Clinton	97%	118
University of Maryland Medical Center	Baltimore	97%	444
VA Maryland Healthcare System - Baltimore	Baltimore	97%	29
Baltimore Washington Medical Center	Glen Burnie	96%	127
Northwest Hospital Center	Randallstown	96%	57
Union Memorial Hospital	Baltimore	96%	674
Laurel Regional Medical Center	Laurel	93%	29
Western Maryland Regional Medical Center	Cumberland	91%	213
Prince Georges Hospital Center	Cheverly	90%	165

6. PCI Within 90 Minutes of Arrival

Hospital Name	City	Rate	Cases
Frederick Memorial Hospital	Frederick	98%	63
Johns Hopkins Bayview Medical Center	Baltimore	93%	27
Holy Cross Hospital	Silver Spring	89%	38
Meritus Medical Center	Hagerstown	89%	46
Carroll Hospital Center	Westminster	88%	48
Shady Grove Adventist Hospital	Rockville	87%	71
Southern Maryland Hospital Center	Clinton	87%	38
Upper Chesapeake Medical Center	Bel Air	86%	79
Baltimore Washington Medical Center	Glen Burnie	84%	83
Franklin Square Hospital Center	Baltimore	84%	56
Sinai Hospital of Baltimore	Baltimore	82%	51
Anne Arundel Medical Center	Annapolis	80%	70
Peninsula Regional Medical Center	Salisbury	80%	91
Saint Agnes Hospital	Baltimore	80%	50
Howard County General Hospital	Columbia	78%	64
Suburban Hospital	Bethesda	72%	36
Prince Georges Hospital Center	Cheverly	42%	31

7. Smoking Cessation Advice

Hospital Name	City	Rate	Cases
Anne Arundel Medical Center	Annapolis	100%	53
Baltimore Washington Medical Center	Glen Burnie	100%	35
Carroll Hospital Center	Westminster	100%	25
Howard County General Hospital	Columbia	100%	30
Johns Hopkins Bayview Medical Center	Baltimore	100%	55
The Johns Hopkins Hospital[2]	Baltimore	100%	110
Meritus Medical Center	Hagerstown	100%	49
Saint Joseph Medical Center[2]	Towson	100%	87
Sinai Hospital of Baltimore	Baltimore	100%	129
Southern Maryland Hospital Center	Clinton	100%	43
Suburban Hospital	Bethesda	100%	38
Upper Chesapeake Medical Center	Bel Air	100%	54
Washington Adventist Hospital[2]	Takoma Park	100%	81
Peninsula Regional Medical Center	Salisbury	99%	172
University of Maryland Medical Center	Baltimore	99%	166
Western Maryland Regional Medical Center	Cumberland	99%	86
Prince Georges Hospital Center	Cheverly	98%	64
Shady Grove Adventist Hospital	Rockville	98%	59
Frederick Memorial Hospital	Frederick	97%	39
Franklin Square Hospital Center	Baltimore	95%	44
Saint Agnes Hospital	Baltimore	95%	40
Union Memorial Hospital	Baltimore	93%	252

Heart Failure Care

12. ACE Inhibitor or ARB for LVSD

Hospital Name	City	Rate	Cases
Calvert Memorial Hospital[2]	Prince Frederick	100%	67
Shady Grove Adventist Hospital	Rockville	100%	140
Holy Cross Hospital[2]	Silver Spring	99%	134
Meritus Medical Center	Hagerstown	99%	101
Saint Joseph Medical Center[2]	Towson	99%	94
Harford Memorial Hospital	Havre De Grace	98%	58
The Johns Hopkins Hospital[2]	Baltimore	98%	200
Laurel Regional Medical Center	Laurel	98%	50
Northwest Hospital Center	Randallstown	98%	185
Peninsula Regional Medical Center	Salisbury	98%	265
Atlantic General Hospital	Berlin	97%	38
Franklin Square Hospital Center	Baltimore	97%	218
Saint Mary's Hospital	Leonardtown	97%	68
Howard County General Hospital[2]	Columbia	96%	77
Johns Hopkins Bayview Medical Center	Baltimore	96%	234
Montgomery General Hospital	Olney	96%	77
Union Hospital of Cecil County	Elkton	96%	68
Upper Chesapeake Medical Center	Bel Air	96%	78
Mercy Medical Center	Baltimore	95%	153
Washington Adventist Hospital[2]	Takoma Park	95%	182
Baltimore Washington Medical Center	Glen Burnie	94%	196
Memorial Hospital at Easton	Easton	94%	154
Southern Maryland Hospital Center	Clinton	94%	277
University of Maryland Medical Center	Baltimore	94%	251
Frederick Memorial Hospital	Frederick	93%	153
Good Samaritan Hospital	Baltimore	93%	264
Sinai Hospital of Baltimore	Baltimore	93%	249
VA Maryland Healthcare System - Baltimore	Baltimore	93%	117
Western Maryland Regional Medical Center	Cumberland	93%	183
Greater Baltimore Medical Center	Baltimore	92%	62
Union Memorial Hospital	Baltimore	92%	311
Harbor Hospital	Brooklyn	91%	129
Saint Agnes Hospital	Baltimore	91%	285
Civista Medical Center[2]	La Plata	90%	79
Doctors' Community Hospital	Lanham	90%	195
Suburban Hospital[2]	Bethesda	90%	108
Carroll Hospital Center[2]	Westminster	89%	80
Garrett County Memorial Hospital	Oakland	89%	27
Prince Georges Hospital Center[2]	Cheverly	89%	105
Bon Secours Hospital	Baltimore	88%	113
Anne Arundel Medical Center	Annapolis	87%	171
Fort Washington Hospital	Fort Washington	86%	66
Chester River Hospital Center	Chestertown	85%	41
Maryland General Hospital	Baltimore	80%	123

13. Discharge Instructions

Hospital Name	City	Rate	Cases
Atlantic General Hospital	Berlin	99%	100
Maryland General Hospital	Baltimore	99%	242
Suburban Hospital[2]	Bethesda	99%	198
Harford Memorial Hospital	Havre De Grace	98%	183
VA Maryland Healthcare System - Baltimore	Baltimore	98%	252
Greater Baltimore Medical Center	Baltimore	97%	173
Upper Chesapeake Medical Center	Bel Air	97%	301
Calvert Memorial Hospital[2]	Prince Frederick	96%	174
Laurel Regional Medical Center	Laurel	96%	112
Mercy Medical Center	Baltimore	96%	339
Meritus Medical Center	Hagerstown	96%	281
Shady Grove Adventist Hospital	Rockville	96%	284
Bon Secours Hospital	Baltimore	95%	313
Fort Washington Hospital	Fort Washington	95%	150
Civista Medical Center[2]	La Plata	94%	226
Howard County General Hospital[2]	Columbia	94%	217
Saint Joseph Medical Center[2]	Towson	94%	252
Saint Mary's Hospital	Leonardtown	94%	215
Southern Maryland Hospital Center	Clinton	94%	661
Union Hospital of Cecil County	Elkton	93%	161
Union Memorial Hospital	Baltimore	93%	620
Carroll Hospital Center[2]	Westminster	92%	205
Holy Cross Hospital[2]	Silver Spring	89%	316
Montgomery General Hospital	Olney	89%	152
Good Samaritan Hospital	Baltimore	88%	624
The Johns Hopkins Hospital[2]	Baltimore	88%	361
Peninsula Regional Medical Center	Salisbury	88%	727
Prince Georges Hospital Center[2]	Cheverly	85%	276
Baltimore Washington Medical Center	Glen Burnie	84%	608
Northwest Hospital Center	Randallstown	84%	344
Western Maryland Regional Medical Center	Cumberland	84%	361
Memorial Hosp & Med Ctr of Cumberland[3]	Cumberland	82%	34
Anne Arundel Medical Center	Annapolis	79%	418
Doctors' Community Hospital	Lanham	79%	440
Franklin Square Hospital Center	Baltimore	79%	594
Harbor Hospital	Brooklyn	79%	309
University of Maryland Medical Center	Baltimore	78%	391
Johns Hopkins Bayview Medical Center	Baltimore	77%	509
Washington Adventist Hospital[2]	Takoma Park	77%	311
Chester River Hospital Center	Chestertown	76%	97
Frederick Memorial Hospital	Frederick	76%	378
Saint Agnes Hospital	Baltimore	76%	492
Garrett County Memorial Hospital	Oakland	75%	64
Memorial Hospital at Easton	Easton	75%	420
Sinai Hospital of Baltimore	Baltimore	67%	587

NOTE: Hospital profiles are in alphabetical order by state, then city, then hospital within the city; Rankings exclude hospitals with less than 25 cases except for patient surveys which excludes hospitals with less than 100 cases; (a) 100–299 cases; (1) The number of cases is too small to be sure how well a hospital is performing; (2) The hospital indicated that the data submitted for this measure were based on a sample of cases; (3) Data was collected during a shorter time period (fewer quarters) than the maximum possible time for this measure; (4) Suppressed for one or more quarters by CMS; (5) No data is available from the hospital for this measure; (6) Fewer than 100 patients completed the HCAHPS survey. Use these rates with caution, as the number of surveys may be too low to reliably assess hospital performance; (7) Survey results are based on less than 12 months of data; (8) Survey results are not available for this reporting period; (9) No or very few patients were eligible for the HCAHPS survey. The scores shown, if any, reflect a very small number of surveys; (10) A state average was not calculated because too few hospitals in the state submitted data; (11) There were discrepancies in the data collection process; Please refer to the User's Guide for a full explanation of data.

14. Evaluation of LVS Function

Hospital Name	City	Rate	Cases
Calvert Memorial Hospital[2]	Prince Frederick	100%	233
Franklin Square Hospital Center	Baltimore	100%	753
Frederick Memorial Hospital	Frederick	100%	489
Harford Memorial Hospital	Havre De Grace	100%	223
Meritus Medical Center	Hagerstown	100%	344
Saint Joseph Medical Center[2]	Towson	100%	325
Saint Mary's Hospital	Leonardtown	100%	254
Shady Grove Adventist Hospital	Rockville	100%	377
Upper Chesapeake Medical Center	Bel Air	100%	374
VA Maryland Healthcare System - Baltimore	Baltimore	100%	252
Baltimore Washington Medical Center	Glen Burnie	99%	715
Civista Medical Center[2]	La Plata	99%	270
Harbor Hospital	Brooklyn	99%	343
Holy Cross Hospital[2]	Silver Spring	99%	414
Howard County General Hospital[2]	Columbia	99%	281
Johns Hopkins Bayview Medical Center	Baltimore	99%	671
The Johns Hopkins Hospital[2]	Baltimore	99%	404
Mercy Medical Center	Baltimore	99%	369
Montgomery General Hospital	Olney	99%	215
Northwest Hospital Center	Randallstown	99%	470
Western Maryland Regional Medical Center	Cumberland	99%	472
Atlantic General Hospital	Berlin	98%	125
Memorial Hospital at Easton	Easton	98%	516
Southern Maryland Hospital Center	Clinton	98%	752
Suburban Hospital[2]	Bethesda	98%	288
Union Hospital of Cecil County	Elkton	98%	199
University of Maryland Medical Center	Baltimore	98%	429
Anne Arundel Medical Center	Annapolis	97%	535
Garrett County Memorial Hospital	Oakland	97%	89
Good Samaritan Hospital	Baltimore	97%	829
Greater Baltimore Medical Center	Baltimore	97%	261
Sinai Hospital of Baltimore	Baltimore	97%	708
Laurel Regional Medical Center	Laurel	96%	160
Memorial Hosp & Med Ctr of Cumberland[3]	Cumberland	96%	50
Peninsula Regional Medical Center	Salisbury	96%	932
Washington Adventist Hospital[2]	Takoma Park	96%	398
Carroll Hospital Center[2]	Westminster	95%	269
Doctors' Community Hospital	Lanham	95%	495
Saint Agnes Hospital	Baltimore	95%	635
Union Memorial Hospital	Baltimore	95%	739
Fort Washington Hospital	Fort Washington	94%	170
Maryland General Hospital	Baltimore	94%	300
Bon Secours Hospital	Baltimore	92%	376
Chester River Hospital Center	Chestertown	90%	126
Prince Georges Hospital Center[2]	Cheverly	89%	304

15. Smoking Cessation Advice

Hospital Name	City	Rate	Cases
Anne Arundel Medical Center	Annapolis	100%	69
Atlantic General Hospital	Berlin	100%	29
Baltimore Washington Medical Center	Glen Burnie	100%	96
Carroll Hospital Center[2]	Westminster	100%	39
Civista Medical Center[2]	La Plata	100%	42
Doctors' Community Hospital	Lanham	100%	86
Frederick Memorial Hospital	Frederick	100%	45
Harford Memorial Hospital	Havre De Grace	100%	30
Holy Cross Hospital[2]	Silver Spring	100%	43
Memorial Hospital at Easton	Easton	100%	90
Meritus Medical Center	Hagerstown	100%	53
Northwest Hospital Center	Randallstown	100%	58
Saint Joseph Medical Center[2]	Towson	100%	38
Saint Mary's Hospital	Leonardtown	100%	40
Shady Grove Adventist Hospital	Rockville	100%	39
Southern Maryland Hospital Center	Clinton	100%	123
University of Maryland Medical Center	Baltimore	100%	115
Upper Chesapeake Medical Center	Bel Air	100%	46
VA Maryland Healthcare System - Baltimore	Baltimore	100%	57
Washington Adventist Hospital[2]	Takoma Park	100%	50
Johns Hopkins Bayview Medical Center	Baltimore	99%	197
Mercy Medical Center	Baltimore	99%	111
Sinai Hospital of Baltimore	Baltimore	99%	139
Harbor Hospital	Brooklyn	98%	114
Peninsula Regional Medical Center	Salisbury	98%	151
Prince Georges Hospital Center[2]	Cheverly	98%	99
Saint Agnes Hospital	Baltimore	98%	124
Western Maryland Regional Medical Center	Cumberland	98%	51
Bon Secours Hospital	Baltimore	97%	128
Good Samaritan Hospital	Baltimore	97%	123
The Johns Hopkins Hospital[2]	Baltimore	97%	109
Laurel Regional Medical Center	Laurel	96%	28
Maryland General Hospital	Baltimore	96%	139
Union Memorial Hospital	Baltimore	94%	196
Franklin Square Hospital Center	Baltimore	93%	121
Union Hospital of Cecil County	Elkton	89%	45

Pneumonia Care

16. Appropriate Initial Antibiotic

Hospital Name	City	Rate	Cases
Chester River Hospital Center[3]	Chestertown	100%	29
Carroll Hospital Center[2]	Westminster	99%	105
Montgomery General Hospital	Olney	99%	151
Bon Secours Hospital	Baltimore	98%	94
Upper Chesapeake Medical Center	Bel Air	98%	249
Civista Medical Center[2]	La Plata	97%	124
Frederick Memorial Hospital	Frederick	97%	250
Saint Mary's Hospital	Leonardtown	97%	73
Calvert Memorial Hospital[2]	Prince Frederick	96%	116
Mercy Medical Center	Baltimore	96%	110
Northwest Hospital Center	Randallstown	96%	220
VA Maryland Healthcare System - Baltimore	Baltimore	96%	100
Washington Adventist Hospital[2]	Takoma Park	96%	55
Doctors' Community Hospital	Lanham	95%	219
Harford Memorial Hospital	Havre De Grace	95%	132
Howard County General Hospital[2]	Columbia	95%	84
Atlantic General Hospital	Berlin	94%	83
Greater Baltimore Medical Center	Baltimore	94%	156
Holy Cross Hospital[2]	Silver Spring	94%	168
Memorial Hospital at Easton	Easton	94%	216
The Johns Hopkins Hospital[2]	Baltimore	93%	69
Saint Agnes Hospital[2]	Baltimore	93%	72
Shady Grove Adventist Hospital[2]	Rockville	93%	90
Baltimore Washington Medical Center	Glen Burnie	92%	452
Good Samaritan Hospital	Baltimore	92%	181
Saint Joseph Medical Center[2]	Towson	92%	95
Union Hospital of Cecil County	Elkton	92%	116
Franklin Square Hospital Center	Baltimore	91%	306
Peninsula Regional Medical Center[2]	Salisbury	91%	186
Union Memorial Hospital	Baltimore	91%	118
University of Maryland Medical Center	Baltimore	91%	98
Anne Arundel Medical Center	Annapolis	90%	252
Meritus Medical Center	Hagerstown	90%	320
Harbor Hospital	Brooklyn	89%	254
Johns Hopkins Bayview Medical Center	Baltimore	89%	183
Sinai Hospital of Baltimore	Baltimore	89%	158
Southern Maryland Hospital Center[2]	Clinton	89%	123
Laurel Regional Medical Center	Laurel	88%	98
Suburban Hospital[2]	Bethesda	88%	146
Maryland General Hospital	Baltimore	84%	69
Prince Georges Hospital Center[2]	Cheverly	84%	63
Western Maryland Regional Medical Center	Cumberland	84%	183
Memorial Hosp & Med Ctr of Cumberland[3]	Cumberland	81%	31
Garrett County Memorial Hospital	Oakland	74%	27

17. Blood Culture Timing

Hospital Name	City	Rate	Cases
Garrett County Memorial Hospital	Oakland	100%	38
Civista Medical Center[2]	La Plata	99%	203
Upper Chesapeake Medical Center	Bel Air	99%	446
VA Maryland Healthcare System - Baltimore	Baltimore	99%	157
Carroll Hospital Center[2]	Westminster	98%	184
The Johns Hopkins Hospital[2]	Baltimore	98%	65
Union Hospital of Cecil County	Elkton	98%	196
Washington Adventist Hospital[2]	Takoma Park	98%	112
Atlantic General Hospital	Berlin	97%	118
Montgomery General Hospital	Olney	97%	212
Saint Mary's Hospital	Leonardtown	97%	111
Holy Cross Hospital[2]	Silver Spring	96%	175
Saint Joseph Medical Center[2]	Towson	96%	135
Memorial Hospital at Easton	Easton	95%	306
Mercy Medical Center	Baltimore	95%	136
Franklin Square Hospital Center	Baltimore	94%	391
Johns Hopkins Bayview Medical Center	Baltimore	94%	273
Meritus Medical Center	Hagerstown	94%	346
Peninsula Regional Medical Center[2]	Salisbury	94%	264
Shady Grove Adventist Hospital[2]	Rockville	94%	101
Baltimore Washington Medical Center	Glen Burnie	93%	653
Harbor Hospital	Brooklyn	93%	356
Laurel Regional Medical Center	Laurel	93%	175
Northwest Hospital Center	Randallstown	93%	311
Calvert Memorial Hospital[2]	Prince Frederick	92%	168
Harford Memorial Hospital	Havre De Grace	92%	211
Memorial Hosp & Med Ctr of Cumberland[3]	Cumberland	92%	26
Bon Secours Hospital	Baltimore	91%	183
Fort Washington Hospital	Fort Washington	91%	106
Western Maryland Regional Medical Center	Cumberland	91%	180
Frederick Memorial Hospital	Frederick	90%	216
Good Samaritan Hospital	Baltimore	90%	271
Sinai Hospital of Baltimore	Baltimore	90%	296
Chester River Hospital Center[3]	Chestertown	89%	37
Anne Arundel Medical Center	Annapolis	88%	423
Union Memorial Hospital	Baltimore	88%	185
University of Maryland Medical Center	Baltimore	88%	229
Doctors' Community Hospital	Lanham	87%	343
Maryland General Hospital	Baltimore	87%	189
Prince Georges Hospital Center[2]	Cheverly	87%	84
Saint Agnes Hospital[2]	Baltimore	87%	166
Greater Baltimore Medical Center	Baltimore	86%	249
Suburban Hospital[2]	Bethesda	86%	241
Southern Maryland Hospital Center[2]	Clinton	85%	160
Howard County General Hospital[2]	Columbia	84%	110

18. Influenza Vaccine

Hospital Name	City	Rate	Cases
Garrett County Memorial Hospital	Oakland	100%	26
Meritus Medical Center	Hagerstown	100%	218
Union Hospital of Cecil County	Elkton	100%	115
Atlantic General Hospital	Berlin	99%	76
Holy Cross Hospital[2]	Silver Spring	98%	176
Northwest Hospital Center	Randallstown	97%	210
Franklin Square Hospital Center	Baltimore	96%	299
Carroll Hospital Center[2]	Westminster	95%	100
Civista Medical Center[2]	La Plata	95%	99
Fort Washington Hospital	Fort Washington	95%	38
Saint Mary's Hospital	Leonardtown	95%	85
Southern Maryland Hospital Center[2]	Clinton	95%	95
Montgomery General Hospital	Olney	94%	152
Saint Agnes Hospital[2]	Baltimore	94%	79
Union Memorial Hospital	Baltimore	94%	138
Baltimore Washington Medical Center	Glen Burnie	93%	389
Frederick Memorial Hospital	Frederick	93%	236
Harford Memorial Hospital	Havre De Grace	93%	104
Sinai Hospital of Baltimore	Baltimore	93%	190
Upper Chesapeake Medical Center	Bel Air	93%	199
Calvert Memorial Hospital[2]	Prince Frederick	92%	88
Chester River Hospital Center	Chestertown	92%	50
Mercy Medical Center	Baltimore	92%	77
Good Samaritan Hospital	Baltimore	91%	173
Greater Baltimore Medical Center	Baltimore	91%	203
Harbor Hospital	Brooklyn	91%	191
Howard County General Hospital[2]	Columbia	91%	79
University of Maryland Medical Center	Baltimore	91%	150
VA Maryland Healthcare System - Baltimore	Baltimore	91%	81
Peninsula Regional Medical Center[2]	Salisbury	87%	191
Saint Joseph Medical Center[2]	Towson	87%	54
Memorial Hospital at Easton	Easton	86%	162
Anne Arundel Medical Center	Annapolis	83%	271
Western Maryland Regional Medical Center	Cumberland	82%	196
Suburban Hospital[2]	Bethesda	80%	133
Laurel Regional Medical Center	Laurel	79%	110
Shady Grove Adventist Hospital[2]	Rockville	78%	80
The Johns Hopkins Hospital[2]	Baltimore	75%	109
Washington Adventist Hospital[2]	Takoma Park	72%	67
Johns Hopkins Bayview Medical Center	Baltimore	68%	241
Bon Secours Hospital	Baltimore	64%	102
Doctors' Community Hospital	Lanham	64%	177
Maryland General Hospital	Baltimore	58%	125
Prince Georges Hospital Center[2]	Cheverly	47%	73

19. Initial Antibiotic Timing

Hospital Name	City	Rate	Cases
Montgomery General Hospital	Olney	99%	190
Atlantic General Hospital	Berlin	98%	116
Calvert Memorial Hospital[2]	Prince Frederick	98%	172
Carroll Hospital Center[2]	Westminster	98%	171
Garrett County Memorial Hospital	Oakland	98%	43
Mercy Medical Center	Baltimore	98%	170
Saint Mary's Hospital	Leonardtown	98%	125
Franklin Square Hospital Center	Baltimore	97%	474
Harbor Hospital	Brooklyn	97%	341
Howard County General Hospital[2]	Columbia	97%	95
The Johns Hopkins Hospital[2]	Baltimore	97%	142
Memorial Hospital at Easton	Easton	97%	293
Shady Grove Adventist Hospital[2]	Rockville	97%	121
Washington Adventist Hospital[2]	Takoma Park	97%	117
Baltimore Washington Medical Center	Glen Burnie	96%	581
Civista Medical Center[2]	La Plata	96%	204
Frederick Memorial Hospital	Frederick	96%	411
Holy Cross Hospital[2]	Silver Spring	96%	241
Suburban Hospital[2]	Bethesda	96%	209
Union Memorial Hospital	Baltimore	96%	219
Upper Chesapeake Medical Center	Bel Air	96%	387
Chester River Hospital Center[3]	Chestertown	95%	41
Doctors' Community Hospital	Lanham	95%	301
Northwest Hospital Center	Randallstown	95%	410
Peninsula Regional Medical Center[2]	Salisbury	95%	343
Saint Joseph Medical Center[2]	Towson	95%	148
Harford Memorial Hospital	Havre De Grace	94%	183
Sinai Hospital of Baltimore	Baltimore	94%	290
Union Hospital of Cecil County	Elkton	94%	202
Good Samaritan Hospital	Baltimore	93%	302
Saint Agnes Hospital[2]	Baltimore	93%	162
Southern Maryland Hospital Center[2]	Clinton	93%	182
University of Maryland Medical Center	Baltimore	93%	223
Greater Baltimore Medical Center	Baltimore	92%	236

NOTE: Hospital profiles are in alphabetical order by state, then city, then hospital within the city; Rankings exclude hospitals with less than 25 cases except for patient surveys which excludes hospitals with less than 100 cases; (a) 100–299 cases; (1) The number of cases is too small to be sure how well a hospital is performing; (2) The hospital indicated that the data submitted for this measure were based on a sample of cases; (3) Data was collected during a shorter time period (fewer quarters) than the maximum possible time for this measure; (4) Suppressed for one or more quarters by CMS; (5) No data is available from the hospital for this measure; (6) Fewer than 100 patients completed the HCAHPS survey. Use these rates with caution, as the number of surveys may be too low to reliably assess hospital performance; (7) Survey results are based on less than 12 months of data; (8) Survey results are not available for this reporting period; (9) No or very few patients were eligible for the HCAHPS survey. The scores shown, if any, reflect a very small number of surveys; (10) A state average was not calculated because too few hospitals in the state submitted data; (11) There were discrepancies in the data collection process; Please refer to the User's Guide for a full explanation of data.

VA Maryland Healthcare System - Baltimore	Baltimore	92%	159
Anne Arundel Medical Center	Annapolis	91%	371
Fort Washington Hospital	Fort Washington	91%	106
Laurel Regional Medical Center	Laurel	91%	159
Meritus Medical Center	Hagerstown	90%	517
Bon Secours Hospital	Baltimore	89%	167
Johns Hopkins Bayview Medical Center	Baltimore	89%	342
Maryland General Hospital	Baltimore	86%	190
Prince Georges Hospital Center[2]	Cheverly	85%	46
Western Maryland Regional Medical Center	Cumberland	85%	267
Memorial Hosp & Med Ctr of Cumberland[3]	Cumberland	83%	46

20. Pneumococcal Vaccine

Hospital Name	City	Rate	Cases
Garrett County Memorial Hospital	Oakland	100%	33
VA Maryland Healthcare System - Baltimore	Baltimore	100%	103
Holy Cross Hospital[2]	Silver Spring	99%	262
Atlantic General Hospital	Berlin	98%	126
Baltimore Washington Medical Center	Glen Burnie	98%	493
Civista Medical Center[2]	La Plata	98%	160
Meritus Medical Center	Hagerstown	98%	429
Montgomery General Hospital	Olney	98%	211
Northwest Hospital Center	Randallstown	98%	287
Saint Mary's Hospital	Leonardtown	98%	102
Upper Chesapeake Medical Center	Bel Air	98%	278
Franklin Square Hospital Center	Baltimore	97%	399
Calvert Memorial Hospital[2]	Prince Frederick	96%	141
Carroll Hospital Center[2]	Westminster	96%	146
Chester River Hospital Center[3]	Chestertown	96%	54
Fort Washington Hospital	Fort Washington	96%	56
Frederick Memorial Hospital	Frederick	96%	415
Good Samaritan Hospital	Baltimore	96%	183
Harford Memorial Hospital	Havre De Grace	96%	125
Saint Joseph Medical Center[2]	Towson	96%	164
Southern Maryland Hospital Center[2]	Clinton	96%	131
Union Hospital of Cecil County	Elkton	96%	165
Union Memorial Hospital	Baltimore	96%	159
Mercy Medical Center	Baltimore	94%	81
Saint Agnes Hospital[2]	Baltimore	94%	108
Anne Arundel Medical Center	Annapolis	93%	407
Sinai Hospital of Baltimore	Baltimore	93%	251
Greater Baltimore Medical Center	Baltimore	92%	298
University of Maryland Medical Center	Baltimore	92%	131
Harbor Hospital	Brooklyn	91%	215
Howard County General Hospital[2]	Columbia	91%	122
Memorial Hospital at Easton	Easton	91%	260
Western Maryland Regional Medical Center	Cumberland	87%	260
Peninsula Regional Medical Center[2]	Salisbury	86%	354
Doctors' Community Hospital	Lanham	85%	226
Maryland General Hospital	Baltimore	85%	110
Washington Adventist Hospital[2]	Takoma Park	81%	119
Johns Hopkins Bayview Medical Center	Baltimore	77%	304
Laurel Regional Medical Center	Laurel	77%	135
The Johns Hopkins Hospital[2]	Baltimore	76%	71
Shady Grove Adventist Hospital[2]	Rockville	73%	133
Suburban Hospital[2]	Bethesda	73%	224
Bon Secours Hospital	Baltimore	68%	78
Memorial Hosp & Med Ctr of Cumberland[3]	Cumberland	68%	28
Prince Georges Hospital Center[2]	Cheverly	47%	88

21. Smoking Cessation Advice

Hospital Name	City	Rate	Cases
Anne Arundel Medical Center	Annapolis	100%	130
Baltimore Washington Medical Center	Glen Burnie	100%	220
Calvert Memorial Hospital[2]	Prince Frederick	100%	59
Carroll Hospital Center[2]	Westminster	100%	38
Civista Medical Center[2]	La Plata	100%	63
Doctors' Community Hospital	Lanham	100%	82
Fort Washington Hospital	Fort Washington	100%	25
Harford Memorial Hospital	Havre De Grace	100%	82
Holy Cross Hospital[2]	Silver Spring	100%	50
Howard County General Hospital[2]	Columbia	100%	35
The Johns Hopkins Hospital[2]	Baltimore	100%	117
Laurel Regional Medical Center	Laurel	100%	35
Memorial Hospital at Easton	Easton	100%	96
Meritus Medical Center	Hagerstown	100%	211
Northwest Hospital Center	Randallstown	100%	100
Saint Joseph Medical Center[2]	Towson	100%	38
Saint Mary's Hospital	Leonardtown	100%	40
Sinai Hospital of Baltimore	Baltimore	100%	112
Southern Maryland Hospital Center[2]	Clinton	100%	66
Upper Chesapeake Medical Center	Bel Air	100%	113
VA Maryland Healthcare System - Baltimore	Baltimore	100%	70
Frederick Memorial Hospital	Frederick	99%	150
Harbor Hospital	Brooklyn	99%	218
University of Maryland Medical Center	Baltimore	99%	190
Greater Baltimore Medical Center	Baltimore	98%	48
Mercy Medical Center	Baltimore	98%	100
Montgomery General Hospital	Olney	98%	41
Bon Secours Hospital	Baltimore	97%	150

Johns Hopkins Bayview Medical Center	Baltimore	96%	187
Maryland General Hospital	Baltimore	96%	163
Peninsula Regional Medical Center[2]	Salisbury	95%	104
Atlantic General Hospital	Berlin	94%	33
Shady Grove Adventist Hospital[2]	Rockville	94%	36
Good Samaritan Hospital	Baltimore	92%	103
Saint Agnes Hospital[2]	Baltimore	92%	62
Union Hospital of Cecil County	Elkton	92%	143
Union Memorial Hospital	Baltimore	91%	86
Prince Georges Hospital Center[2]	Cheverly	90%	60
Western Maryland Regional Medical Center	Cumberland	90%	87
Franklin Square Hospital Center	Baltimore	89%	199

Surgical Care Improvement Project

22. Appropriate VTP Within 24 Hours

Hospital Name	City	Rate	Cases
Johns Hopkins Bayview Medical Center[2]	Baltimore	99%	259
Saint Agnes Hospital[2]	Baltimore	99%	177
The Johns Hopkins Hospital[2]	Baltimore	98%	238
Upper Chesapeake Medical Center[2]	Bel Air	98%	181
Saint Joseph Medical Center[2]	Towson	97%	102
Union Memorial Hospital[2]	Baltimore	97%	250
Holy Cross Hospital[2]	Silver Spring	96%	234
Mercy Medical Center[2]	Baltimore	96%	248
Meritus Medical Center	Hagerstown	96%	350
University of Maryland Medical Center[2]	Baltimore	96%	669
Saint Mary's Hospital[2]	Leonardtown	95%	66
VA Maryland Healthcare System - Baltimore[2]	Baltimore	95%	113
Garrett County Memorial Hospital	Oakland	94%	70
Good Samaritan Hospital	Baltimore	94%	324
Southern Maryland Hospital Center[2]	Clinton	94%	208
Atlantic General Hospital	Berlin	93%	153
Civista Medical Center[2]	La Plata	93%	153
Franklin Square Hospital Center[2]	Baltimore	93%	335
Harford Memorial Hospital	Havre De Grace	93%	75
Howard County General Hospital[2]	Columbia	93%	144
Montgomery General Hospital	Olney	93%	182
Calvert Memorial Hospital[2]	Prince Frederick	92%	72
Fort Washington Hospital	Fort Washington	92%	75
Suburban Hospital[2]	Bethesda	92%	258
Frederick Memorial Hospital[2]	Frederick	91%	172
Harbor Hospital[2]	Brooklyn	91%	199
Shady Grove Adventist Hospital[2]	Rockville	91%	152
Greater Baltimore Medical Center	Baltimore	89%	336
Northwest Hospital Center	Randallstown	89%	177
Union Hospital of Cecil County	Elkton	89%	142
Washington Adventist Hospital[2]	Takoma Park	89%	123
Sinai Hospital of Baltimore[2]	Baltimore	88%	299
Doctors' Community Hospital[2]	Lanham	87%	233
Anne Arundel Medical Center[2]	Annapolis	86%	290
Carroll Hospital Center[2]	Westminster	86%	145
Bon Secours Hospital	Baltimore	83%	83
Memorial Hosp & Med Ctr of Cumberland[3]	Cumberland	83%	48
Memorial Hospital at Easton	Easton	83%	222
Laurel Regional Medical Center	Laurel	82%	50
Baltimore Washington Medical Center[2]	Glen Burnie	80%	322
Western Maryland Regional Medical Center	Cumberland	79%	214
Maryland General Hospital	Baltimore	78%	102
Peninsula Regional Medical Center[2]	Salisbury	72%	133
Chester River Hospital Center	Chestertown	61%	54
Prince Georges Hospital Center[2]	Cheverly	45%	105

23. Appropriate Hair Removal

Hospital Name	City	Rate	Cases
Anne Arundel Medical Center[2]	Annapolis	100%	1356
Calvert Memorial Hospital[2]	Prince Frederick	100%	326
Carroll Hospital Center[2]	Westminster	100%	506
Civista Medical Center[2]	La Plata	100%	394
Doctors' Community Hospital[2]	Lanham	100%	482
Fort Washington Hospital	Fort Washington	100%	203
Frederick Memorial Hospital[2]	Frederick	100%	730
Garrett County Memorial Hospital	Oakland	100%	202
Good Samaritan Hospital	Baltimore	100%	977
Greater Baltimore Medical Center	Baltimore	100%	1220
Harford Memorial Hospital	Havre De Grace	100%	220
Holy Cross Hospital[2]	Silver Spring	100%	680
Howard County General Hospital[2]	Columbia	100%	440
Johns Hopkins Bayview Medical Center[2]	Baltimore	100%	743
The Johns Hopkins Hospital[2]	Baltimore	100%	877
Laurel Regional Medical Center	Laurel	100%	167
Maryland General Hospital	Baltimore	100%	219
Memorial Hosp & Med Ctr of Cumberland[3]	Cumberland	100%	245
Memorial Hospital at Easton	Easton	100%	881
Meritus Medical Center	Hagerstown	100%	1338
Montgomery General Hospital	Olney	100%	478
Northwest Hospital Center	Randallstown	100%	460
Peninsula Regional Medical Center[2]	Salisbury	100%	566
Saint Mary's Hospital[2]	Leonardtown	100%	369
Shady Grove Adventist Hospital[2]	Rockville	100%	464

Sinai Hospital of Baltimore[2]	Baltimore	100%	985
Southern Maryland Hospital Center[2]	Clinton	100%	682
Suburban Hospital[2]	Bethesda	100%	1268
Union Hospital of Cecil County	Elkton	100%	429
Upper Chesapeake Medical Center[2]	Bel Air	100%	607
VA Maryland Healthcare System - Baltimore[2]	Baltimore	100%	140
Washington Adventist Hospital[2]	Takoma Park	100%	492
Western Maryland Regional Medical Center	Cumberland	100%	768
Atlantic General Hospital	Berlin	99%	304
Baltimore Washington Medical Center[2]	Glen Burnie	99%	958
Bon Secours Hospital	Baltimore	99%	130
Chester River Hospital Center	Chestertown	99%	135
Franklin Square Hospital Center[2]	Baltimore	99%	1077
Harbor Hospital[2]	Brooklyn	99%	820
Mercy Medical Center[2]	Baltimore	99%	1112
Prince Georges Hospital Center[2]	Cheverly	99%	250
Saint Agnes Hospital[2]	Baltimore	99%	686
Saint Joseph Medical Center[2]	Towson	99%	568
Union Memorial Hospital[2]	Baltimore	99%	1727
University of Maryland Medical Center[2]	Baltimore	97%	1727

24. Appropriate Beta Blocker Usage

Hospital Name	City	Rate	Cases
Chester River Hospital Center	Chestertown	100%	39
Harford Memorial Hospital	Havre De Grace	100%	64
Saint Mary's Hospital[2]	Leonardtown	100%	86
Atlantic General Hospital	Berlin	99%	95
Holy Cross Hospital[2]	Silver Spring	99%	146
Saint Agnes Hospital[2]	Baltimore	98%	161
Suburban Hospital[2]	Bethesda	98%	384
VA Maryland Healthcare System - Baltimore[2]	Baltimore	98%	51
Good Samaritan Hospital	Baltimore	97%	276
Johns Hopkins Bayview Medical Center[2]	Baltimore	97%	233
Calvert Memorial Hospital[2,3]	Prince Frederick	96%	54
Union Memorial Hospital[2]	Baltimore	96%	506
Meritus Medical Center	Hagerstown	95%	375
Montgomery General Hospital	Olney	95%	110
Saint Joseph Medical Center[2]	Towson	95%	224
Sinai Hospital of Baltimore[2]	Baltimore	95%	274
Shady Grove Adventist Hospital[2]	Rockville	94%	123
Frederick Memorial Hospital[2]	Frederick	93%	241
Southern Maryland Hospital Center[2]	Clinton	93%	153
The Johns Hopkins Hospital[2]	Baltimore	92%	320
Upper Chesapeake Medical Center[2]	Bel Air	92%	181
Anne Arundel Medical Center[2]	Annapolis	91%	318
Harbor Hospital[2]	Brooklyn	91%	194
Franklin Square Hospital Center[2]	Baltimore	90%	348
Mercy Medical Center[2]	Baltimore	90%	250
Garrett County Memorial Hospital	Oakland	89%	61
Laurel Regional Medical Center	Laurel	89%	37
Memorial Hospital at Easton	Easton	89%	253
Northwest Hospital Center	Randallstown	89%	113
Carroll Hospital Center[2]	Westminster	88%	122
Howard County General Hospital[2]	Columbia	88%	88
Peninsula Regional Medical Center[2]	Salisbury	88%	209
Union Hospital of Cecil County	Elkton	88%	92
Baltimore Washington Medical Center[2]	Glen Burnie	86%	326
Civista Medical Center[2]	La Plata	84%	77
Greater Baltimore Medical Center	Baltimore	83%	334
Western Maryland Regional Medical Center	Cumberland	83%	263
Memorial Hosp & Med Ctr of Cumberland[3]	Cumberland	80%	90
Washington Adventist Hospital[2]	Takoma Park	79%	169
University of Maryland Medical Center[2]	Baltimore	78%	603
Maryland General Hospital	Baltimore	75%	44

25. Controlled Postoperative Blood Glucose

Hospital Name	City	Rate	Cases
Saint Joseph Medical Center[2]	Towson	96%	118
The Johns Hopkins Hospital[2]	Baltimore	94%	330
Suburban Hospital[2]	Bethesda	93%	205
University of Maryland Medical Center[2]	Baltimore	93%	510
Sinai Hospital of Baltimore[2]	Baltimore	91%	233
Peninsula Regional Medical Center[2]	Salisbury	89%	129
Union Memorial Hospital[2]	Baltimore	88%	173
Western Maryland Regional Medical Center	Cumberland	88%	206
Washington Adventist Hospital[2]	Takoma Park	86%	137

26. Prophylactic Antibiotic Timing

Hospital Name	City	Rate	Cases
Howard County General Hospital[2]	Columbia	99%	265
The Johns Hopkins Hospital[2]	Baltimore	99%	567
Saint Mary's Hospital[2]	Leonardtown	99%	302
Southern Maryland Hospital Center[2]	Clinton	99%	476
Franklin Square Hospital Center[2]	Baltimore	98%	797
Frederick Memorial Hospital[2]	Frederick	98%	590
Johns Hopkins Bayview Medical Center[2]	Baltimore	98%	579
Memorial Hospital at Easton	Easton	98%	609
Meritus Medical Center	Hagerstown	98%	916
Union Hospital of Cecil County	Elkton	98%	272

NOTE: Hospital profiles are in alphabetical order by state, then city, then hospital within the city; Rankings exclude hospitals with less than 25 cases except for patient surveys which excludes hospitals with less than 100 cases; (a) 100–299 cases; (1) The number of cases is too small to be sure how well a hospital is performing; (2) The hospital indicated that the data submitted for this measure were based on a sample of cases; (3) Data was collected during a shorter time period (fewer quarters) than the maximum possible time for this measure; (4) Suppressed for one or more quarters by CMS; (5) No data is available from the hospital for this measure; (6) Fewer than 100 patients completed the HCAHPS survey. Use these rates with caution, as the number of surveys may be too low to reliably assess hospital performance; (7) Survey results are based on less than 12 months of data; (8) Survey results are not available for this reporting period; (9) No or very few patients were eligible for the HCAHPS survey. The scores shown, if any, reflect a very small number of surveys; (10) A state average was not calculated because too few hospitals in the state submitted data; (11) There were discrepancies in the data collection process; Please refer to the User's Guide for a full explanation of data.

VA Maryland Healthcare System - Baltimore	Baltimore	98%	66
Atlantic General Hospital	Berlin	97%	197
Doctors' Community Hospital[2]	Lanham	97%	353
Harbor Hospital[2]	Brooklyn	97%	665
Laurel Regional Medical Center	Laurel	97%	112
Mercy Medical Center[2]	Baltimore	97%	910
Montgomery General Hospital	Olney	97%	305
Saint Agnes Hospital[2]	Baltimore	97%	519
Saint Joseph Medical Center[2]	Towson	97%	369
Sinai Hospital of Baltimore[2]	Baltimore	97%	677
Washington Adventist Hospital[2]	Takoma Park	97%	344
Calvert Memorial Hospital[2]	Prince Frederick	96%	258
Civista Medical Center[2]	La Plata	96%	240
Good Samaritan Hospital	Baltimore	96%	635
Holy Cross Hospital[2]	Silver Spring	96%	396
Shady Grove Adventist Hospital[2]	Rockville	96%	325
Union Memorial Hospital[2]	Baltimore	96%	1511
Baltimore Washington Medical Center[2]	Glen Burnie	95%	659
Northwest Hospital Center	Randallstown	95%	280
Peninsula Regional Medical Center[2]	Salisbury	95%	411
Suburban Hospital[2]	Bethesda	95%	1065
University of Maryland Medical Center[2]	Baltimore	95%	823
Upper Chesapeake Medical Center[2]	Bel Air	95%	421
Harford Memorial Hospital	Havre De Grace	94%	146
Maryland General Hospital	Baltimore	94%	120
Carroll Hospital Center[2]	Westminster	93%	334
Garrett County Memorial Hospital	Oakland	93%	155
Fort Washington Hospital	Fort Washington	92%	130
Greater Baltimore Medical Center	Baltimore	91%	703
Memorial Hosp & Med Ctr of Cumberland[3]	Cumberland	91%	190
Prince Georges Hospital Center[2]	Cheverly	91%	135
Western Maryland Regional Medical Center	Cumberland	91%	503
Anne Arundel Medical Center[2]	Annapolis	90%	1050
Chester River Hospital Center	Chestertown	84%	95
Bon Secours Hospital	Baltimore	83%	42

28. Prophylactic Antibiotic Selection

Hospital Name	City	Rate	Cases
Civista Medical Center[2]	La Plata	99%	239
Doctors' Community Hospital[2]	Lanham	99%	356
Frederick Memorial Hospital[2]	Frederick	99%	589
Good Samaritan Hospital	Baltimore	99%	643
Memorial Hosp & Med Ctr of Cumberland[3]	Cumberland	99%	194
Memorial Hospital at Easton	Easton	99%	614
Mercy Medical Center[2]	Baltimore	99%	917
Meritus Medical Center	Hagerstown	99%	917
Union Memorial Hospital[2]	Baltimore	99%	1512
Atlantic General Hospital	Berlin	98%	198
Harford Memorial Hospital	Havre De Grace	98%	152
Howard County General Hospital[2]	Columbia	98%	266
Johns Hopkins Bayview Medical Center[2]	Baltimore	98%	578
The Johns Hopkins Hospital[2]	Baltimore	98%	581
Montgomery General Hospital	Olney	98%	314
Northwest Hospital Center	Randallstown	98%	281
Saint Agnes Hospital[2]	Baltimore	98%	521
Saint Joseph Medical Center[2]	Towson	98%	384
Saint Mary's Hospital[2]	Leonardtown	98%	304
University of Maryland Medical Center[2]	Baltimore	98%	857
VA Maryland Healthcare System - Baltimore	Baltimore	98%	66
Washington Adventist Hospital[2]	Takoma Park	98%	351
Western Maryland Regional Medical Center	Cumberland	98%	512
Baltimore Washington Medical Center[2]	Glen Burnie	97%	668
Calvert Memorial Hospital[2]	Prince Frederick	97%	260
Carroll Hospital Center[2]	Westminster	97%	335
Shady Grove Adventist Hospital[2]	Rockville	97%	323
Sinai Hospital of Baltimore[2]	Baltimore	97%	685
Suburban Hospital[2]	Bethesda	97%	1067
Greater Baltimore Medical Center	Baltimore	96%	712
Holy Cross Hospital[2]	Silver Spring	96%	395
Franklin Square Hospital Center[2]	Baltimore	95%	809
Peninsula Regional Medical Center[2]	Salisbury	95%	419
Southern Maryland Hospital Center[2]	Clinton	95%	481
Union Hospital of Cecil County	Elkton	95%	276
Anne Arundel Medical Center[2]	Annapolis	94%	1046
Harbor Hospital[2]	Brooklyn	94%	669
Laurel Regional Medical Center	Laurel	94%	112
Maryland General Hospital	Baltimore	94%	117
Upper Chesapeake Medical Center[2]	Bel Air	94%	435
Chester River Hospital Center	Chestertown	93%	95
Garrett County Memorial Hospital	Oakland	93%	156
Prince Georges Hospital Center[2]	Cheverly	93%	137
Fort Washington Hospital	Fort Washington	92%	133
Bon Secours Hospital	Baltimore	86%	44

30. Prophylactic Antibiotic Stopped

Hospital Name	City	Rate	Cases
Franklin Square Hospital Center[2]	Baltimore	99%	746
Good Samaritan Hospital	Baltimore	98%	608
Harford Memorial Hospital	Havre De Grace	98%	139
Memorial Hospital at Easton	Easton	98%	601
Holy Cross Hospital[2]	Silver Spring	97%	381
Meritus Medical Center	Hagerstown	97%	867
Northwest Hospital Center	Randallstown	97%	260
Saint Joseph Medical Center[2]	Towson	97%	340
Saint Mary's Hospital[2]	Leonardtown	97%	297
Union Memorial Hospital[2]	Baltimore	97%	1487
VA Maryland Healthcare System - Baltimore	Baltimore	97%	63
Civista Medical Center[2]	La Plata	96%	206
Anne Arundel Medical Center[2]	Annapolis	95%	1006
Calvert Memorial Hospital[2]	Prince Frederick	95%	254
The Johns Hopkins Hospital[2]	Baltimore	95%	541
Mercy Medical Center[2]	Baltimore	95%	884
Peninsula Regional Medical Center[2]	Salisbury	95%	396
Sinai Hospital of Baltimore[2]	Baltimore	95%	626
Southern Maryland Hospital Center[2]	Clinton	95%	460
Atlantic General Hospital	Berlin	94%	188
Carroll Hospital Center[2]	Westminster	94%	328
Johns Hopkins Bayview Medical Center[2]	Baltimore	94%	567
Saint Agnes Hospital[2]	Baltimore	94%	489
Suburban Hospital[2]	Bethesda	94%	1058
Union Hospital of Cecil County	Elkton	94%	261
Upper Chesapeake Medical Center[2]	Bel Air	94%	407
Washington Adventist Hospital[2]	Takoma Park	94%	334
Frederick Memorial Hospital[2]	Frederick	93%	569
University of Maryland Medical Center[2]	Baltimore	93%	780
Fort Washington Hospital	Fort Washington	92%	130
Greater Baltimore Medical Center	Baltimore	92%	683
Harbor Hospital[2]	Brooklyn	92%	653
Montgomery General Hospital	Olney	92%	292
Howard County General Hospital[2]	Columbia	91%	246
Shady Grove Adventist Hospital[2]	Rockville	91%	310
Baltimore Washington Medical Center[2]	Glen Burnie	89%	628
Doctors' Community Hospital[2]	Lanham	89%	339
Laurel Regional Medical Center	Laurel	89%	108
Memorial Hosp & Med Ctr of Cumberland[3]	Cumberland	89%	189
Chester River Hospital Center	Chestertown	88%	91
Garrett County Memorial Hospital	Oakland	88%	151
Western Maryland Regional Medical Center	Cumberland	88%	488
Maryland General Hospital	Baltimore	87%	116
Prince Georges Hospital Center[2]	Cheverly	75%	126
Bon Secours Hospital	Baltimore	65%	40

31. Recommended VTP Ordered

Hospital Name	City	Rate	Cases
Calvert Memorial Hospital[2]	Prince Frederick	99%	72
Johns Hopkins Bayview Medical Center[2]	Baltimore	99%	259
Meritus Medical Center	Hagerstown	99%	350
The Johns Hopkins Hospital[2]	Baltimore	98%	238
Mercy Medical Center[2]	Baltimore	98%	248
Saint Agnes Hospital[2]	Baltimore	98%	178
Saint Joseph Medical Center[2]	Towson	98%	102
Upper Chesapeake Medical Center[2]	Bel Air	98%	181
Franklin Square Hospital Center[2]	Baltimore	97%	335
Howard County General Hospital[2]	Columbia	97%	144
Southern Maryland Hospital Center[2]	Clinton	97%	208
Union Memorial Hospital[2]	Baltimore	97%	250
University of Maryland Medical Center[2]	Baltimore	97%	673
Good Samaritan Hospital	Baltimore	96%	324
Holy Cross Hospital[2]	Silver Spring	96%	234
VA Maryland Healthcare System - Baltimore[2]	Baltimore	96%	113
Saint Mary's Hospital[2]	Leonardtown	95%	66
Carroll Hospital Center[2]	Westminster	94%	145
Civista Medical Center[2]	La Plata	94%	153
Shady Grove Adventist Hospital[2]	Rockville	94%	152
Washington Adventist Hospital[2]	Takoma Park	94%	123
Atlantic General Hospital	Berlin	93%	153
Garrett County Memorial Hospital	Oakland	93%	71
Harbor Hospital[2]	Brooklyn	93%	199
Harford Memorial Hospital	Havre De Grace	93%	75
Montgomery General Hospital	Olney	93%	182
Doctors' Community Hospital[2]	Lanham	92%	233
Fort Washington Hospital	Fort Washington	92%	75
Frederick Memorial Hospital[2]	Frederick	92%	172
Suburban Hospital[2]	Bethesda	91%	261
Union Hospital of Cecil County	Elkton	90%	142
Anne Arundel Medical Center[2]	Annapolis	89%	291
Greater Baltimore Medical Center	Baltimore	89%	336
Memorial Hospital at Easton	Easton	89%	224
Northwest Hospital Center	Randallstown	89%	177
Sinai Hospital of Baltimore[2]	Baltimore	89%	299
Bon Secours Hospital	Baltimore	85%	87
Laurel Regional Medical Center	Laurel	84%	51
Memorial Hosp & Med Ctr of Cumberland[3]	Cumberland	84%	50
Baltimore Washington Medical Center[2]	Glen Burnie	81%	323
Western Maryland Regional Medical Center	Cumberland	80%	216
Maryland General Hospital	Baltimore	76%	106
Peninsula Regional Medical Center[2]	Salisbury	74%	133
Chester River Hospital Center	Chestertown	61%	54
Prince Georges Hospital Center[2]	Cheverly	50%	105

32. Urinary Catheter Removal

Hospital Name	City	Rate	Cases
Holy Cross Hospital[2]	Silver Spring	99%	71
Johns Hopkins Bayview Medical Center[2]	Baltimore	99%	284
Shady Grove Adventist Hospital[2]	Rockville	99%	118
Suburban Hospital[2]	Bethesda	99%	337
Saint Mary's Hospital[2]	Leonardtown	98%	118
Calvert Memorial Hospital[2]	Prince Frederick	97%	64
Harford Memorial Hospital	Havre De Grace	97%	68
Mercy Medical Center[2]	Baltimore	97%	411
Frederick Memorial Hospital[2]	Frederick	95%	288
Saint Agnes Hospital[2]	Baltimore	95%	129
Franklin Square Hospital Center[2]	Baltimore	94%	232
Northwest Hospital Center	Randallstown	94%	34
Good Samaritan Hospital	Baltimore	93%	329
Montgomery General Hospital	Olney	93%	166
Anne Arundel Medical Center[2]	Annapolis	92%	309
Howard County General Hospital[2]	Columbia	92%	80
Sinai Hospital of Baltimore[2]	Baltimore	92%	276
Memorial Hospital at Easton	Easton	91%	217
Southern Maryland Hospital Center[2]	Clinton	91%	69
Union Hospital of Cecil County	Elkton	91%	98
Union Memorial Hospital[2]	Baltimore	91%	116
Upper Chesapeake Medical Center[2]	Bel Air	91%	140
Meritus Medical Center	Hagerstown	90%	173
Washington Adventist Hospital[2]	Takoma Park	90%	125
Peninsula Regional Medical Center[2]	Salisbury	89%	142
Saint Joseph Medical Center[2]	Towson	88%	74
VA Maryland Healthcare System - Baltimore[2]	Baltimore	88%	49
Atlantic General Hospital	Berlin	87%	93
Doctors' Community Hospital[2]	Lanham	87%	122
Harbor Hospital[2]	Brooklyn	86%	141
Civista Medical Center	La Plata	85%	88
Greater Baltimore Medical Center	Baltimore	85%	310
Baltimore Washington Medical Center[2]	Glen Burnie	82%	156
Bon Secours Hospital	Baltimore	80%	25
University of Maryland Medical Center[2]	Baltimore	80%	455
The Johns Hopkins Hospital[2]	Baltimore	75%	190
Carroll Hospital Center[2]	Westminster	74%	43
Chester River Hospital Center	Chestertown	73%	33
Prince Georges Hospital Center[2]	Cheverly	65%	48
Western Maryland Regional Medical Center	Cumberland	63%	76
Maryland General Hospital	Baltimore	62%	39
Garrett County Memorial Hospital	Oakland	36%	64

Children's Asthma Care

33. Received Systemic Corticosteroids

Hospital Name	City	Rate	Cases
Baltimore Washington Medical Center	Glen Burnie	100%	121

34. Received Home Management Plan of Care

Hospital Name	City	Rate	Cases
Baltimore Washington Medical Center	Glen Burnie	84%	116

35. Received Reliever Medication

Hospital Name	City	Rate	Cases
Baltimore Washington Medical Center	Glen Burnie	100%	121

Use of Medical Imaging

36. Combination Abdominal CT Scan

Hospital Name	City	Ratio	Cases
Memorial Hosp & Med Ctr of Cumberland	Cumberland	0.017	476
Holy Cross Hospital	Silver Spring	0.026	538
Western Maryland Regional Medical Center	Cumberland	0.062	1176

37. Combination Chest CT Scan

Hospital Name	City	Ratio	Cases
Memorial Hosp & Med Ctr of Cumberland	Cumberland	0.003	377
Holy Cross Hospital	Silver Spring	0.004	265
Western Maryland Regional Medical Center	Cumberland	0.010	1007

38. Follow-up Mammogram/Ultrasound

Hospital Name	City	Rate	Cases
Western Maryland Regional Medical Center	Cumberland	7.4%	1400
Holy Cross Hospital	Silver Spring	9.9%	111

39. MRI for Low Back Pain

Hospital Name	City	Rate	Cases
Western Maryland Regional Medical Center	Cumberland	36.1%	183
Holy Cross Hospital	Silver Spring	38.6%	44

NOTE: Hospital profiles are in alphabetical order by state, then city, then hospital within the city; Rankings exclude hospitals with less than 25 cases except for patient surveys which excludes hospitals with less than 100 cases; (a) 100–299 cases; (1) The number of cases is too small to be sure how well a hospital is performing; (2) The hospital indicated that the data submitted for this measure were based on a sample of cases; (3) Data was collected during a shorter time period (fewer quarters) than the maximum possible time for this measure; (4) Suppressed for one or more quarters by CMS; (5) No data is available from the hospital for this measure; (6) Fewer than 100 patients completed the HCAHPS survey. Use these rates with caution, as the number of surveys may be too low to reliably assess hospital performance; (7) Survey results are based on less than 12 months of data; (8) Survey results are not available for this reporting period; (9) No or very few patients were eligible for the HCAHPS survey. The scores shown, if any, reflect a very small number of surveys; (10) A state average was not calculated because too few hospitals in the state submitted data; (11) There were discrepancies in the data collection process; Please refer to the User's Guide for a full explanation of data.

Survey of Patients' Hospital Experiences

40. Area Around Room 'Always' Quiet at Night

Hospital Name	City	Rate	Cases
Bon Secours Hospital	Baltimore	63%	300+
Union Memorial Hospital	Baltimore	63%	300+
Good Samaritan Hospital	Baltimore	62%	300+
Anne Arundel Medical Center	Annapolis	61%	300+
Edward Mccready Memorial Hospital	Crisfield	61%	(a)
Maryland General Hospital	Baltimore	61%	300+
Mercy Medical Center	Baltimore	59%	300+
Chester River Hospital Center	Chestertown	58%	300+
Upper Chesapeake Medical Center	Bel Air	58%	300+
Memorial Hospital at Easton	Easton	57%	300+
Saint Mary's Hospital	Leonardtown	57%	300+
Union Hospital of Cecil County	Elkton	57%	300+
Baltimore Washington Medical Center	Glen Burnie	56%	300+
Civista Medical Center	La Plata	56%	300+
Fort Washington Hospital	Fort Washington	56%	300+
Holy Cross Hospital	Silver Spring	56%	300+
The Johns Hopkins Hospital	Baltimore	56%	300+
Saint Joseph Medical Center	Towson	56%	300+
Harbor Hospital	Brooklyn	55%	300+
Harford Memorial Hospital	Havre De Grace	55%	300+
Northwest Hospital Center	Randallstown	55%	300+
Calvert Memorial Hospital	Prince Frederick	54%	300+
Saint Agnes Hospital	Baltimore	54%	300+
Howard County General Hospital	Columbia	53%	300+
University of Maryland Medical Center	Baltimore	53%	300+
Laurel Regional Medical Center	Laurel	52%	300+
Frederick Memorial Hospital	Frederick	51%	300+
Greater Baltimore Medical Center	Baltimore	51%	300+
Shady Grove Adventist Hospital	Rockville	51%	300+
Sinai Hospital of Baltimore	Baltimore	51%	300+
Suburban Hospital	Bethesda	51%	300+
Atlantic General Hospital	Berlin	50%	300+
Garrett County Memorial Hospital	Oakland	50%	300+
Doctors' Community Hospital	Lanham	49%	300+
Prince Georges Hospital Center	Cheverly	49%	300+
Franklin Square Hospital Center	Baltimore	48%	300+
Johns Hopkins Bayview Medical Center	Baltimore	48%	300+
Peninsula Regional Medical Center	Salisbury	48%	300+
Western Maryland Regional Medical Center	Cumberland	48%	300+
Carroll Hospital Center	Westminster	47%	300+
Washington Adventist Hospital	Takoma Park	47%	300+
Montgomery General Hospital	Olney	45%	300+
Southern Maryland Hospital Center	Clinton	43%	300+
Meritus Medical Center	Hagerstown	39%	300+

41. Doctors 'Always' Communicated Well

Hospital Name	City	Rate	Cases
Edward Mccready Memorial Hospital	Crisfield	86%	(a)
Garrett County Memorial Hospital	Oakland	85%	300+
Mercy Medical Center	Baltimore	84%	300+
Greater Baltimore Medical Center	Baltimore	81%	300+
Memorial Hospital at Easton	Easton	81%	300+
Union Hospital of Cecil County	Elkton	81%	300+
Union Memorial Hospital	Baltimore	81%	300+
Anne Arundel Medical Center	Annapolis	80%	300+
Good Samaritan Hospital	Baltimore	80%	300+
Saint Joseph Medical Center	Towson	80%	300+
Saint Mary's Hospital	Leonardtown	80%	300+
Johns Hopkins Bayview Medical Center	Baltimore	79%	300+
The Johns Hopkins Hospital	Baltimore	79%	300+
Suburban Hospital	Bethesda	79%	300+
Calvert Memorial Hospital	Prince Frederick	78%	300+
Chester River Hospital Center	Chestertown	78%	300+
Harbor Hospital	Brooklyn	78%	300+
Harford Memorial Hospital	Havre De Grace	78%	300+
Maryland General Hospital	Baltimore	78%	300+
Saint Agnes Hospital	Baltimore	78%	300+
University of Maryland Medical Center	Baltimore	78%	300+
Atlantic General Hospital	Berlin	77%	300+
Baltimore Washington Medical Center	Glen Burnie	77%	300+
Bon Secours Hospital	Baltimore	77%	300+
Franklin Square Hospital Center	Baltimore	77%	300+
Carroll Hospital Center	Westminster	76%	300+
Fort Washington Hospital	Fort Washington	76%	300+
Frederick Memorial Hospital	Frederick	76%	300+
Washington Adventist Hospital	Takoma Park	76%	300+
Holy Cross Hospital	Silver Spring	75%	300+
Howard County General Hospital	Columbia	75%	300+
Upper Chesapeake Medical Center	Bel Air	75%	300+
Western Maryland Regional Medical Center	Cumberland	75%	300+
Doctors' Community Hospital	Lanham	74%	300+
Peninsula Regional Medical Center	Salisbury	74%	300+
Civista Medical Center	La Plata	73%	300+
Meritus Medical Center	Hagerstown	73%	300+
Montgomery General Hospital	Olney	73%	300+
Shady Grove Adventist Hospital	Rockville	73%	300+
Sinai Hospital of Baltimore	Baltimore	73%	300+
Southern Maryland Hospital Center	Clinton	72%	300+
Northwest Hospital Center	Randallstown	71%	300+
Prince Georges Hospital Center	Cheverly	69%	300+
Laurel Regional Medical Center	Laurel	68%	300+

42. Home Recovery Information Given

Hospital Name	City	Rate	Cases
Edward Mccready Memorial Hospital	Crisfield	87%	(a)
Mercy Medical Center	Baltimore	87%	300+
Anne Arundel Medical Center	Annapolis	86%	300+
Memorial Hospital at Easton	Easton	86%	300+
University of Maryland Medical Center	Baltimore	86%	300+
Garrett County Memorial Hospital	Oakland	85%	300+
Good Samaritan Hospital	Baltimore	85%	300+
The Johns Hopkins Hospital	Baltimore	85%	300+
Atlantic General Hospital	Berlin	84%	300+
Chester River Hospital Center	Chestertown	84%	300+
Johns Hopkins Bayview Medical Center	Baltimore	84%	300+
Meritus Medical Center	Hagerstown	84%	300+
Montgomery General Hospital	Olney	84%	300+
Calvert Memorial Hospital	Prince Frederick	83%	300+
Union Memorial Hospital	Baltimore	83%	300+
Upper Chesapeake Medical Center	Bel Air	83%	300+
Western Maryland Regional Medical Center	Cumberland	83%	300+
Saint Agnes Hospital	Baltimore	82%	300+
Union Hospital of Cecil County	Elkton	82%	300+
Baltimore Washington Medical Center	Glen Burnie	81%	300+
Harford Memorial Hospital	Havre De Grace	81%	300+
Howard County General Hospital	Columbia	81%	300+
Peninsula Regional Medical Center	Salisbury	81%	300+
Saint Mary's Hospital	Leonardtown	81%	300+
Franklin Square Hospital Center	Baltimore	80%	300+
Frederick Memorial Hospital	Frederick	80%	300+
Saint Joseph Medical Center	Towson	80%	300+
Harbor Hospital	Brooklyn	79%	300+
Maryland General Hospital	Baltimore	79%	300+
Suburban Hospital	Bethesda	79%	300+
Carroll Hospital Center	Westminster	78%	300+
Sinai Hospital of Baltimore	Baltimore	78%	300+
Bon Secours Hospital	Baltimore	77%	300+
Doctors' Community Hospital	Lanham	77%	300+
Greater Baltimore Medical Center	Baltimore	77%	300+
Washington Adventist Hospital	Takoma Park	77%	300+
Civista Medical Center	La Plata	76%	300+
Fort Washington Hospital	Fort Washington	75%	300+
Shady Grove Adventist Hospital	Rockville	75%	300+
Holy Cross Hospital	Silver Spring	74%	300+
Prince Georges Hospital Center	Cheverly	73%	300+
Northwest Hospital Center	Randallstown	71%	300+
Southern Maryland Hospital Center	Clinton	71%	300+
Laurel Regional Medical Center	Laurel	70%	300+

43. Hospital Given 9 or 10 on 10 Point Scale

Hospital Name	City	Rate	Cases
The Johns Hopkins Hospital	Baltimore	76%	300+
Anne Arundel Medical Center	Annapolis	74%	300+
Edward Mccready Memorial Hospital	Crisfield	73%	(a)
Mercy Medical Center	Baltimore	72%	300+
Union Memorial Hospital	Baltimore	72%	300+
Good Samaritan Hospital	Baltimore	70%	300+
Memorial Hospital at Easton	Easton	70%	300+
Atlantic General Hospital	Berlin	69%	300+
Garrett County Memorial Hospital	Oakland	68%	300+
Union Hospital of Cecil County	Elkton	68%	300+
Greater Baltimore Medical Center	Baltimore	67%	300+
Saint Joseph Medical Center	Towson	67%	300+
University of Maryland Medical Center	Baltimore	67%	300+
Baltimore Washington Medical Center	Glen Burnie	66%	300+
Carroll Hospital Center	Westminster	66%	300+
Frederick Memorial Hospital	Frederick	66%	300+
Johns Hopkins Bayview Medical Center	Baltimore	66%	300+
Chester River Hospital Center	Chestertown	65%	300+
Harbor Hospital	Brooklyn	65%	300+
Saint Mary's Hospital	Leonardtown	65%	300+
Calvert Memorial Hospital	Prince Frederick	64%	300+
Harford Memorial Hospital	Havre De Grace	64%	300+
Howard County General Hospital	Columbia	64%	300+
Upper Chesapeake Medical Center	Bel Air	64%	300+
Suburban Hospital	Bethesda	62%	300+
Northwest Hospital Center	Randallstown	61%	300+
Saint Agnes Hospital	Baltimore	61%	300+
Peninsula Regional Medical Center	Salisbury	60%	300+
Western Maryland Regional Medical Center	Cumberland	60%	300+
Franklin Square Hospital Center	Baltimore	59%	300+
Doctors' Community Hospital	Lanham	58%	300+
Holy Cross Hospital	Silver Spring	58%	300+
Montgomery General Hospital	Olney	58%	300+
Sinai Hospital of Baltimore	Baltimore	58%	300+
Maryland General Hospital	Baltimore	57%	300+
Civista Medical Center	La Plata	56%	300+
Meritus Medical Center	Hagerstown	55%	300+
Fort Washington Hospital	Fort Washington	53%	300+
Washington Adventist Hospital	Takoma Park	53%	300+
Bon Secours Hospital	Baltimore	52%	300+
Shady Grove Adventist Hospital	Rockville	51%	300+
Laurel Regional Medical Center	Laurel	44%	300+
Prince Georges Hospital Center	Cheverly	44%	300+
Southern Maryland Hospital Center	Clinton	42%	300+

44. Meds 'Always' Explained Before Given

Hospital Name	City	Rate	Cases
Edward Mccready Memorial Hospital	Crisfield	68%	(a)
Saint Mary's Hospital	Leonardtown	64%	300+
Carroll Hospital Center	Westminster	63%	300+
Garrett County Memorial Hospital	Oakland	63%	300+
The Johns Hopkins Hospital	Baltimore	62%	300+
Anne Arundel Medical Center	Annapolis	61%	300+
Chester River Hospital Center	Chestertown	61%	300+
Harford Memorial Hospital	Havre De Grace	61%	300+
Memorial Hospital at Easton	Easton	61%	300+
Mercy Medical Center	Baltimore	61%	300+
University of Maryland Medical Center	Baltimore	61%	300+
Union Hospital of Cecil County	Elkton	60%	300+
Johns Hopkins Bayview Medical Center	Baltimore	59%	300+
Meritus Medical Center	Hagerstown	59%	300+
Union Memorial Hospital	Baltimore	59%	300+
Calvert Memorial Hospital	Prince Frederick	58%	300+
Frederick Memorial Hospital	Frederick	58%	300+
Greater Baltimore Medical Center	Baltimore	58%	300+
Montgomery General Hospital	Olney	58%	300+
Suburban Hospital	Bethesda	58%	300+
Atlantic General Hospital	Berlin	57%	300+
Civista Medical Center	La Plata	57%	300+
Upper Chesapeake Medical Center	Bel Air	57%	300+
Good Samaritan Hospital	Baltimore	56%	300+
Harbor Hospital	Brooklyn	56%	300+
Maryland General Hospital	Baltimore	56%	300+
Saint Agnes Hospital	Baltimore	56%	300+
Sinai Hospital of Baltimore	Baltimore	56%	300+
Northwest Hospital Center	Randallstown	55%	300+
Baltimore Washington Medical Center	Glen Burnie	54%	300+
Howard County General Hospital	Columbia	54%	300+
Saint Joseph Medical Center	Towson	53%	300+
Western Maryland Regional Medical Center	Cumberland	53%	300+
Bon Secours Hospital	Baltimore	52%	300+
Fort Washington Hospital	Fort Washington	52%	300+
Southern Maryland Hospital Center	Clinton	52%	300+
Franklin Square Hospital Center	Baltimore	51%	300+
Laurel Regional Medical Center	Laurel	51%	300+
Doctors' Community Hospital	Lanham	50%	300+
Holy Cross Hospital	Silver Spring	50%	300+
Peninsula Regional Medical Center	Salisbury	50%	300+
Prince Georges Hospital Center	Cheverly	49%	300+
Shady Grove Adventist Hospital	Rockville	48%	300+
Washington Adventist Hospital	Takoma Park	47%	300+

45. Nurses 'Always' Communicated Well

Hospital Name	City	Rate	Cases
Edward Mccready Memorial Hospital	Crisfield	86%	(a)
Garrett County Memorial Hospital	Oakland	80%	300+
Saint Mary's Hospital	Leonardtown	80%	300+
Memorial Hospital at Easton	Easton	79%	300+
Anne Arundel Medical Center	Annapolis	78%	300+
Frederick Memorial Hospital	Frederick	78%	300+
Mercy Medical Center	Baltimore	78%	300+
The Johns Hopkins Hospital	Baltimore	77%	300+
Atlantic General Hospital	Berlin	76%	300+
Carroll Hospital Center	Westminster	76%	300+
Chester River Hospital Center	Chestertown	76%	300+
Good Samaritan Hospital	Baltimore	76%	300+
Harford Memorial Hospital	Havre De Grace	76%	300+
Union Hospital of Cecil County	Elkton	76%	300+
Meritus Medical Center	Hagerstown	75%	300+
Upper Chesapeake Medical Center	Bel Air	75%	300+
Baltimore Washington Medical Center	Glen Burnie	74%	300+
Harbor Hospital	Brooklyn	74%	300+
Johns Hopkins Bayview Medical Center	Baltimore	74%	300+
Saint Joseph Medical Center	Towson	74%	300+
Union Memorial Hospital	Baltimore	74%	300+
University of Maryland Medical Center	Baltimore	74%	300+
Civista Medical Center	La Plata	73%	300+
Greater Baltimore Medical Center	Baltimore	73%	300+
Calvert Memorial Hospital	Prince Frederick	72%	300+
Franklin Square Hospital Center	Baltimore	72%	300+
Howard County General Hospital	Columbia	72%	300+
Maryland General Hospital	Baltimore	72%	300+
Northwest Hospital Center	Randallstown	72%	300+
Saint Agnes Hospital	Baltimore	72%	300+
Western Maryland Regional Medical Center	Cumberland	71%	300+

NOTE: Hospital profiles are in alphabetical order by state, then city, then hospital within the city; Rankings exclude hospitals with less than 25 cases except for patient surveys which excludes hospitals with less than 100 cases; (a) 100–299 cases; (1) The number of cases is too small to be sure how well a hospital is performing; (2) The hospital indicated that the data submitted for this measure were based on a sample of cases; (3) Data was collected during a shorter time period (fewer quarters) than the maximum possible time for this measure; (4) Suppressed for one or more quarters by CMS; (5) No data is available from the hospital for this measure; (6) Fewer than 100 patients completed the HCAHPS survey. Use these rates with caution, as the number of surveys may be too low to reliably assess hospital performance; (7) Survey results are based on less than 12 months of data; (8) Survey results are not available for this reporting period; (9) No or very few patients were eligible for the HCAHPS survey. The scores shown, if any, reflect a very small number of surveys; (10) A state average was not calculated because too few hospitals in the state submitted data; (11) There were discrepancies in the data collection process; Please refer to the User's Guide for a full explanation of data.

Fort Washington Hospital	Fort Washington	70%	300+
Peninsula Regional Medical Center	Salisbury	70%	300+
Sinai Hospital of Baltimore	Baltimore	70%	300+
Montgomery General Hospital	Olney	69%	300+
Suburban Hospital	Bethesda	69%	300+
Bon Secours Hospital	Baltimore	68%	300+
Doctors' Community Hospital	Lanham	67%	300+
Holy Cross Hospital	Silver Spring	67%	300+
Southern Maryland Hospital Center	Clinton	66%	300+
Washington Adventist Hospital	Takoma Park	64%	300+
Laurel Regional Medical Center	Laurel	62%	300+
Shady Grove Adventist Hospital	Rockville	62%	300+
Prince Georges Hospital Center	Cheverly	60%	300+

46. Pain 'Always' Well Controlled

Hospital Name	City	Rate	Cases
Edward Mccready Memorial Hospital	Crisfield	80%	(a)
Mercy Medical Center	Baltimore	73%	300+
Garrett County Memorial Hospital	Oakland	72%	300+
Memorial Hospital at Easton	Easton	72%	300+
Anne Arundel Medical Center	Annapolis	70%	300+
Frederick Memorial Hospital	Frederick	70%	300+
The Johns Hopkins Hospital	Baltimore	70%	300+
Atlantic General Hospital	Berlin	69%	300+
Chester River Hospital Center	Chestertown	69%	300+
Good Samaritan Hospital	Baltimore	69%	300+
Saint Joseph Medical Center	Towson	69%	300+
Carroll Hospital Center	Westminster	68%	300+
Greater Baltimore Medical Center	Baltimore	68%	300+
Harford Memorial Hospital	Havre De Grace	68%	300+
Baltimore Washington Medical Center	Glen Burnie	67%	300+
Saint Agnes Hospital	Baltimore	67%	300+
Saint Mary's Hospital	Leonardtown	67%	300+
Union Hospital of Cecil County	Elkton	67%	300+
Union Memorial Hospital	Baltimore	67%	300+
University of Maryland Medical Center	Baltimore	67%	300+
Upper Chesapeake Medical Center	Bel Air	67%	300+
Calvert Memorial Hospital	Prince Frederick	66%	300+
Howard County General Hospital	Columbia	66%	300+
Meritus Medical Center	Hagerstown	66%	300+
Civista Medical Center	La Plata	65%	300+
Harbor Hospital	Brooklyn	65%	300+
Suburban Hospital	Bethesda	65%	300+
Western Maryland Regional Medical Center	Cumberland	65%	300+
Bon Secours Hospital	Baltimore	64%	300+
Peninsula Regional Medical Center	Salisbury	64%	300+
Southern Maryland Hospital Center	Clinton	64%	300+
Fort Washington Hospital	Fort Washington	63%	300+
Holy Cross Hospital	Silver Spring	63%	300+
Johns Hopkins Bayview Medical Center	Baltimore	63%	300+
Franklin Square Hospital Center	Baltimore	62%	300+
Maryland General Hospital	Baltimore	62%	300+
Northwest Hospital Center	Randallstown	62%	300+
Doctors' Community Hospital	Lanham	61%	300+
Montgomery General Hospital	Olney	60%	300+
Sinai Hospital of Baltimore	Baltimore	59%	300+
Laurel Regional Medical Center	Laurel	58%	300+
Shady Grove Adventist Hospital	Rockville	58%	300+
Washington Adventist Hospital	Takoma Park	58%	300+
Prince Georges Hospital Center	Cheverly	56%	300+

47. Room and Bathroom 'Always' Clean

Hospital Name	City	Rate	Cases
Edward Mccready Memorial Hospital	Crisfield	78%	(a)
Chester River Hospital Center	Chestertown	73%	300+
Good Samaritan Hospital	Baltimore	72%	300+
Saint Mary's Hospital	Leonardtown	72%	300+
Doctors' Community Hospital	Lanham	71%	300+
Garrett County Memorial Hospital	Oakland	71%	300+
Memorial Hospital at Easton	Easton	71%	300+
Frederick Memorial Hospital	Frederick	70%	300+
Howard County General Hospital	Columbia	70%	300+
Western Maryland Regional Medical Center	Cumberland	69%	300+
Meritus Medical Center	Hagerstown	68%	300+
Union Memorial Hospital	Baltimore	68%	300+
Anne Arundel Medical Center	Annapolis	66%	300+
Baltimore Washington Medical Center	Glen Burnie	66%	300+
Harford Memorial Hospital	Havre De Grace	66%	300+
Union Hospital of Cecil County	Elkton	66%	300+
Atlantic General Hospital	Berlin	65%	300+
Bon Secours Hospital	Baltimore	65%	300+
Calvert Memorial Hospital	Prince Frederick	65%	300+
Civista Medical Center	La Plata	65%	300+
The Johns Hopkins Hospital	Baltimore	65%	300+
Carroll Hospital Center	Westminster	64%	300+
Upper Chesapeake Medical Center	Bel Air	64%	300+
Mercy Medical Center	Baltimore	63%	300+
Peninsula Regional Medical Center	Salisbury	63%	300+
Suburban Hospital	Bethesda	63%	300+
Northwest Hospital Center	Randallstown	62%	300+
Fort Washington Hospital	Fort Washington	61%	300+
Maryland General Hospital	Baltimore	60%	300+
Greater Baltimore Medical Center	Baltimore	59%	300+
Holy Cross Hospital	Silver Spring	59%	300+
Johns Hopkins Bayview Medical Center	Baltimore	59%	300+
Prince Georges Hospital Center	Cheverly	59%	300+
Saint Joseph Medical Center	Towson	59%	300+
Sinai Hospital of Baltimore	Baltimore	59%	300+
Harbor Hospital	Brooklyn	58%	300+
University of Maryland Medical Center	Baltimore	58%	300+
Montgomery General Hospital	Olney	57%	300+
Saint Agnes Hospital	Baltimore	56%	300+
Laurel Regional Medical Center	Laurel	55%	300+
Washington Adventist Hospital	Takoma Park	54%	300+
Franklin Square Hospital Center	Baltimore	53%	300+
Shady Grove Adventist Hospital	Rockville	53%	300+
Southern Maryland Hospital Center	Clinton	53%	300+

48. Timely Help 'Always' Received

Hospital Name	City	Rate	Cases
Edward Mccready Memorial Hospital	Crisfield	80%	(a)
Garrett County Memorial Hospital	Oakland	70%	300+
Chester River Hospital Center	Chestertown	68%	300+
Memorial Hospital at Easton	Easton	68%	300+
Anne Arundel Medical Center	Annapolis	65%	300+
Atlantic General Hospital	Berlin	63%	300+
Saint Mary's Hospital	Leonardtown	63%	300+
Carroll Hospital Center	Westminster	61%	300+
Civista Medical Center	La Plata	61%	300+
The Johns Hopkins Hospital	Baltimore	61%	300+
Western Maryland Regional Medical Center	Cumberland	61%	300+
Saint Joseph Medical Center	Towson	60%	300+
Union Memorial Hospital	Baltimore	60%	300+
Baltimore Washington Medical Center	Glen Burnie	59%	300+
Calvert Memorial Hospital	Prince Frederick	59%	300+
University of Maryland Medical Center	Baltimore	59%	300+
Good Samaritan Hospital	Baltimore	58%	300+
Johns Hopkins Bayview Medical Center	Baltimore	58%	300+
Maryland General Hospital	Baltimore	58%	300+
Meritus Medical Center	Hagerstown	58%	300+
Fort Washington Hospital	Fort Washington	57%	300+
Frederick Memorial Hospital	Frederick	57%	300+
Greater Baltimore Medical Center	Baltimore	57%	300+
Harford Memorial Hospital	Havre De Grace	57%	300+
Mercy Medical Center	Baltimore	57%	300+
Union Hospital of Cecil County	Elkton	57%	300+
Howard County General Hospital	Columbia	56%	300+
Upper Chesapeake Medical Center	Bel Air	56%	300+
Northwest Hospital Center	Randallstown	55%	300+
Bon Secours Hospital	Baltimore	54%	300+
Montgomery General Hospital	Olney	54%	300+
Saint Agnes Hospital	Baltimore	54%	300+
Suburban Hospital	Bethesda	54%	300+
Franklin Square Hospital Center	Baltimore	53%	300+
Harbor Hospital	Brooklyn	52%	300+
Holy Cross Hospital	Silver Spring	52%	300+
Southern Maryland Hospital Center	Clinton	52%	300+
Peninsula Regional Medical Center	Salisbury	51%	300+
Sinai Hospital of Baltimore	Baltimore	51%	300+
Doctors' Community Hospital	Lanham	50%	300+
Laurel Regional Medical Center	Laurel	45%	300+
Washington Adventist Hospital	Takoma Park	44%	300+
Prince Georges Hospital Center	Cheverly	39%	300+
Shady Grove Adventist Hospital	Rockville	39%	300+

49. Would Definitely Recommend Hospital

Hospital Name	City	Rate	Cases
The Johns Hopkins Hospital	Baltimore	82%	300+
Anne Arundel Medical Center	Annapolis	81%	300+
Union Memorial Hospital	Baltimore	77%	300+
Good Samaritan Hospital	Baltimore	76%	300+
Greater Baltimore Medical Center	Baltimore	76%	300+
Atlantic General Hospital	Berlin	75%	300+
Edward Mccready Memorial Hospital	Crisfield	74%	(a)
Mercy Medical Center	Baltimore	74%	300+
Saint Joseph Medical Center	Towson	74%	300+
Suburban Hospital	Bethesda	73%	300+
University of Maryland Medical Center	Baltimore	73%	300+
Howard County General Hospital	Columbia	71%	300+
Frederick Memorial Hospital	Frederick	70%	300+
Baltimore Washington Medical Center	Glen Burnie	69%	300+
Garrett County Memorial Hospital	Oakland	69%	300+
Johns Hopkins Bayview Medical Center	Baltimore	69%	300+
Memorial Hospital at Easton	Easton	68%	300+
Carroll Hospital Center	Westminster	66%	300+
Harbor Hospital	Brooklyn	66%	300+
Calvert Memorial Hospital	Prince Frederick	65%	300+
Saint Agnes Hospital	Baltimore	65%	300+
Saint Mary's Hospital	Leonardtown	65%	300+
Union Hospital of Cecil County	Elkton	65%	300+
Upper Chesapeake Medical Center	Bel Air	65%	300+
Harford Memorial Hospital	Havre De Grace	64%	300+
Montgomery General Hospital	Olney	64%	300+
Peninsula Regional Medical Center	Salisbury	64%	300+
Western Maryland Regional Medical Center	Cumberland	64%	300+
Doctors' Community Hospital	Lanham	63%	300+
Holy Cross Hospital	Silver Spring	63%	300+
Sinai Hospital of Baltimore	Baltimore	63%	300+
Chester River Hospital Center	Chestertown	62%	300+
Northwest Hospital Center	Randallstown	62%	300+
Washington Adventist Hospital	Takoma Park	60%	300+
Civista Medical Center	La Plata	59%	300+
Franklin Square Hospital Center	Baltimore	59%	300+
Meritus Medical Center	Hagerstown	58%	300+
Shady Grove Adventist Hospital	Rockville	57%	300+
Fort Washington Hospital	Fort Washington	56%	300+
Maryland General Hospital	Baltimore	56%	300+
Bon Secours Hospital	Baltimore	49%	300+
Laurel Regional Medical Center	Laurel	44%	300+
Southern Maryland Hospital Center	Clinton	42%	300+
Prince Georges Hospital Center	Cheverly	41%	300+

NOTE: Hospital profiles are in alphabetical order by state, then city, then hospital within the city; Rankings exclude hospitals with less than 25 cases except for patient surveys which excludes hospitals with less than 100 cases; (a) 100–299 cases; (1) The number of cases is too small to be sure how well a hospital is performing; (2) The hospital indicated that the data submitted for this measure were based on a sample of cases; (3) Data was collected during a shorter time period (fewer quarters) than the maximum possible time for this measure; (4) Suppressed for one or more quarters by CMS; (5) No data is available from the hospital for this measure; (6) Fewer than 100 patients completed the HCAHPS survey. Use these rates with caution, as the number of surveys may be too low to reliably assess hospital performance; (7) Survey results are based on less than 12 months of data; (8) Survey results are not available for this reporting period; (9) No or very few patients were eligible for the HCAHPS survey. The scores shown, if any, reflect a very small number of surveys; (10) A state average was not calculated because too few hospitals in the state submitted data; (11) There were discrepancies in the data collection process; Please refer to the User's Guide for a full explanation of data.

Anne Arundel Medical Center

2001 Medical Parkway
Annapolis, MD 21401
URL: www.aahs.org
Type: Acute Care Hospitals
Ownership: Voluntary Non-Profit - Private

Phone: 443-481-1307
Fax: 443-481-4707
Emergency Services: Yes
Beds: 316

Key Personnel:
CEO/President. . . . . Martin L Doordan
Chief of Medical Staff. . . . . Joseph A Moser, MD
Infection Control. . . . . Mary Clance, MD
Operating Room. . . . . Sue Patton, RN
Pediatric In-Patient Care . . . . Karen Peddicord, PhD
Quality Assurance . . . . Shirley J Knelly

Measure	Cases	This Hosp.	State Avg.	U.S. Avg.
Heart Attack Care				
ACE Inhibitor or ARB for LVSD[1]	24	100%	94%	96%
Aspirin at Arrival	208	98%	98%	99%
Aspirin at Discharge	153	99%	98%	98%
Beta Blocker at Discharge	153	99%	97%	98%
Fibrinolytic Medication Timing	0	-	42%	55%
PCI Within 90 Minutes of Arrival	70	80%	83%	90%
Smoking Cessation Advice	53	100%	98%	99%
Chest Pain/Possible Heart Attack Care				
Aspirin at Arrival	-	-	0%	95%
Median Time to ECG (minutes)	-	-	0	8
Median Time to Transfer (minutes)	-	-	0	61
Fibrinolytic Medication Timing	-	-	0%	54%
Heart Failure Care				
ACE Inhibitor or ARB for LVSD	171	87%	94%	94%
Discharge Instructions	418	79%	86%	88%
Evaluation of LVS Function	535	97%	97%	98%
Smoking Cessation Advice	69	100%	98%	98%
Pneumonia Care				
Appropriate Initial Antibiotic	252	90%	92%	92%
Blood Culture Timing	423	88%	92%	96%
Influenza Vaccine	271	83%	88%	91%
Initial Antibiotic Timing	371	91%	94%	95%
Pneumococcal Vaccine	407	93%	92%	93%
Smoking Cessation Advice	130	100%	97%	97%
Surgical Care Improvement Project				
Appropriate VTP Within 24 Hours[2]	290	86%	90%	92%
Appropriate Hair Removal[2]	1,356	100%	100%	99%
Appropriate Beta Blocker Usage[2]	318	91%	91%	93%
Controlled Postoperative Blood Glucose[2]	0	-	91%	93%
Prophylactic Antibiotic Timing[2]	1,050	90%	96%	97%
Prophylactic Antibiotic Timing (Outpatient)	-	-	0%	92%
Prophylactic Antibiotic Selection[2]	1,046	94%	97%	97%
Prophylactic Antibiotic Select. (Outpatient)	-	-	0%	94%
Prophylactic Antibiotic Stopped[2]	1,006	95%	94%	94%
Recommended VTP Ordered[2]	291	89%	92%	94%
Urinary Catheter Removal[2]	309	92%	89%	90%
Children's Asthma Care				
Received Systemic Corticosteroids	-	-	-	100%
Received Home Management Plan	-	-	-	71%
Received Reliever Medication	-	-	-	100%
Use of Medical Imaging				
Combination Abdominal CT Scan	-	-	0.064	0.191
Combination Chest CT Scan	-	-	0.013	0.054
Follow-up Mammogram/Ultrasound	-	-	8.6%	8.4%
MRI for Low Back Pain	-	-	31.7%	32.7%
Survey of Patients' Hospital Experiences				
Area Around Room 'Always' Quiet at Night	300+	61%	-	58%
Doctors 'Always' Communicated Well	300+	80%	-	80%
Home Recovery Information Given	300+	86%	-	82%
Hospital Given 9 or 10 on 10 Point Scale	300+	74%	-	67%
Meds 'Always' Explained Before Given	300+	61%	-	60%
Nurses 'Always' Communicated Well	300+	78%	-	76%
Pain 'Always' Well Controlled	300+	70%	-	69%
Room and Bathroom 'Always' Clean	300+	66%	-	71%
Timely Help 'Always' Received	300+	65%	-	64%
Would Definitely Recommend Hospital	300+	81%	-	69%

Bon Secours Hospital

2000 W Baltimore Street
Baltimore, MD 21223
URL: www.bonsecours.org/baltimore
Type: Acute Care Hospitals
Ownership: Voluntary Non-Profit - Private

Phone: 410-362-3000
Fax: 410-442-1082
Emergency Services: Yes
Beds: 208

Key Personnel:
CEO/President. . . . . Dr Samuel L Ross, FACHE
Chief of Medical Staff. . . . . Efem Imoke, MD
Quality Assurance . . . . William Law, MD
Radiology. . . . . Adolfo M Alonso, MD
Ambulatory Care . . . . Reed Winston, MD
Patient Relations . . . . Jean Phaire

Measure	Cases	This Hosp.	State Avg.	U.S. Avg.
Heart Attack Care				
ACE Inhibitor or ARB for LVSD[1]	5	80%	94%	96%
Aspirin at Arrival	29	93%	98%	99%
Aspirin at Discharge[1]	19	95%	98%	98%
Beta Blocker at Discharge[1]	20	95%	97%	98%
Fibrinolytic Medication Timing	0	-	42%	55%
PCI Within 90 Minutes of Arrival	0	-	83%	90%
Smoking Cessation Advice[1]	8	100%	98%	99%
Chest Pain/Possible Heart Attack Care				
Aspirin at Arrival	-	-	0%	95%
Median Time to ECG (minutes)	-	-	0	8
Median Time to Transfer (minutes)	-	-	0	61
Fibrinolytic Medication Timing	-	-	0%	54%
Heart Failure Care				
ACE Inhibitor or ARB for LVSD	113	88%	94%	94%
Discharge Instructions	313	95%	86%	88%
Evaluation of LVS Function	376	92%	97%	98%
Smoking Cessation Advice	128	97%	98%	98%
Pneumonia Care				
Appropriate Initial Antibiotic	94	98%	92%	92%
Blood Culture Timing	183	91%	92%	96%
Influenza Vaccine	102	64%	88%	91%
Initial Antibiotic Timing	167	89%	94%	95%
Pneumococcal Vaccine	78	68%	92%	93%
Smoking Cessation Advice	150	97%	97%	97%
Surgical Care Improvement Project				
Appropriate VTP Within 24 Hours	83	83%	90%	92%
Appropriate Hair Removal	130	99%	100%	99%
Appropriate Beta Blocker Usage[1]	22	82%	91%	93%
Controlled Postoperative Blood Glucose	0	-	91%	93%
Prophylactic Antibiotic Timing	42	83%	96%	97%
Prophylactic Antibiotic Timing (Outpatient)	-	-	0%	92%
Prophylactic Antibiotic Selection	44	86%	97%	97%
Prophylactic Antibiotic Select. (Outpatient)	-	-	0%	94%
Prophylactic Antibiotic Stopped	40	65%	94%	94%
Recommended VTP Ordered	87	85%	92%	94%
Urinary Catheter Removal	25	80%	89%	90%
Children's Asthma Care				
Received Systemic Corticosteroids	-	-	-	100%
Received Home Management Plan	-	-	-	71%
Received Reliever Medication	-	-	-	100%
Use of Medical Imaging				
Combination Abdominal CT Scan	-	-	0.064	0.191
Combination Chest CT Scan	-	-	0.013	0.054
Follow-up Mammogram/Ultrasound	-	-	8.6%	8.4%
MRI for Low Back Pain	-	-	31.7%	32.7%
Survey of Patients' Hospital Experiences				
Area Around Room 'Always' Quiet at Night	300+	63%	-	58%
Doctors 'Always' Communicated Well	300+	77%	-	80%
Home Recovery Information Given	300+	77%	-	82%
Hospital Given 9 or 10 on 10 Point Scale	300+	52%	-	67%
Meds 'Always' Explained Before Given	300+	52%	-	60%
Nurses 'Always' Communicated Well	300+	68%	-	76%
Pain 'Always' Well Controlled	300+	64%	-	69%
Room and Bathroom 'Always' Clean	300+	65%	-	71%
Timely Help 'Always' Received	300+	54%	-	64%
Would Definitely Recommend Hospital	300+	49%	-	69%

Franklin Square Hospital Center

9000 Franklin Square Dr
Baltimore, MD 21237
URL: www.franklinsquare.org
Type: Acute Care Hospitals
Ownership: Voluntary Non-Profit - Private

Phone: 443-777-7850
Fax: 443-777-7904
Emergency Services: Yes
Beds: 380

Key Personnel:
CEO/President. . . . . Carl Schindelar
Chief of Medical Staff. . . . . Anthony Sclama
Operating Room. . . . . Beth Leilich RN
Pediatric Ambulatory Care . . . . . . Scott Krugman MD
Quality Assurance . . . . Jacqueline Spielman
Radiology. . . . . Blair Andrew
Emergency Room . . . . Michael Pipkin MD

Measure	Cases	This Hosp.	State Avg.	U.S. Avg.
Heart Attack Care				
ACE Inhibitor or ARB for LVSD[1]	20	100%	94%	96%
Aspirin at Arrival	203	99%	98%	99%
Aspirin at Discharge	123	100%	98%	98%
Beta Blocker at Discharge	121	99%	97%	98%
Fibrinolytic Medication Timing	0	-	42%	55%
PCI Within 90 Minutes of Arrival	56	84%	83%	90%
Smoking Cessation Advice	44	95%	98%	99%
Chest Pain/Possible Heart Attack Care				
Aspirin at Arrival	-	-	0%	95%
Median Time to ECG (minutes)	-	-	0	8
Median Time to Transfer (minutes)	-	-	0	61
Fibrinolytic Medication Timing	-	-	0%	54%
Heart Failure Care				
ACE Inhibitor or ARB for LVSD	218	97%	94%	94%
Discharge Instructions	594	79%	86%	88%
Evaluation of LVS Function	753	100%	97%	98%
Smoking Cessation Advice	121	93%	98%	98%
Pneumonia Care				
Appropriate Initial Antibiotic	306	91%	92%	92%
Blood Culture Timing	391	94%	92%	96%
Influenza Vaccine	299	96%	88%	91%
Initial Antibiotic Timing	474	97%	94%	95%
Pneumococcal Vaccine	399	97%	92%	93%
Smoking Cessation Advice	199	89%	97%	97%
Surgical Care Improvement Project				
Appropriate VTP Within 24 Hours[2]	335	93%	90%	92%
Appropriate Hair Removal[2]	1,077	99%	100%	99%
Appropriate Beta Blocker Usage[2]	348	90%	91%	93%
Controlled Postoperative Blood Glucose[2]	0	-	91%	93%
Prophylactic Antibiotic Timing[2]	797	98%	96%	97%
Prophylactic Antibiotic Timing (Outpatient)	-	-	0%	92%
Prophylactic Antibiotic Selection[2]	809	95%	97%	97%
Prophylactic Antibiotic Select. (Outpatient)	-	-	0%	94%
Prophylactic Antibiotic Stopped[2]	746	99%	94%	94%
Recommended VTP Ordered[2]	335	97%	92%	94%
Urinary Catheter Removal[2]	232	94%	89%	90%
Children's Asthma Care				
Received Systemic Corticosteroids	-	-	-	100%
Received Home Management Plan	-	-	-	71%
Received Reliever Medication	-	-	-	100%
Use of Medical Imaging				
Combination Abdominal CT Scan	-	-	0.064	0.191
Combination Chest CT Scan	-	-	0.013	0.054
Follow-up Mammogram/Ultrasound	-	-	8.6%	8.4%
MRI for Low Back Pain	-	-	31.7%	32.7%
Survey of Patients' Hospital Experiences				
Area Around Room 'Always' Quiet at Night	300+	48%	-	58%
Doctors 'Always' Communicated Well	300+	77%	-	80%
Home Recovery Information Given	300+	80%	-	82%
Hospital Given 9 or 10 on 10 Point Scale	300+	59%	-	67%
Meds 'Always' Explained Before Given	300+	51%	-	60%
Nurses 'Always' Communicated Well	300+	72%	-	76%
Pain 'Always' Well Controlled	300+	62%	-	69%
Room and Bathroom 'Always' Clean	300+	53%	-	71%
Timely Help 'Always' Received	300+	53%	-	64%
Would Definitely Recommend Hospital	300+	59%	-	69%

NOTE: Hospital profiles are in alphabetical order by state, then city, then hospital within the city; Rankings exclude hospitals with less than 25 cases except for patient surveys which excludes hospitals with less than 100 cases; (a) 100–299 cases; (1) The number of cases is too small to be sure how well a hospital is performing; (2) The hospital indicated that the data submitted for this measure were based on a sample of cases; (3) Data was collected during a shorter time period (fewer quarters) than the maximum possible time for this measure; (4) Suppressed for one or more quarters by CMS; (5) No data is available from the hospital for this measure; (6) Fewer than 100 patients completed the HCAHPS survey. Use these rates with caution, as the number of surveys may be too low to reliably assess hospital performance; (7) Survey results are based on less than 12 months of data; (8) Survey results are not available for this reporting period; (9) No or very few patients were eligible for the HCAHPS survey. The scores shown, if any, reflect a very small number of surveys; (10) A state average was not calculated because too few hospitals in the state submitted data; (11) There were discrepancies in the data collection process; Please refer to the User's Guide for a full explanation of data.

Good Samaritan Hospital

5601 Loch Raven Blvd
Baltimore, MD 21239
Phone: 443-444-3902
Fax: 410-532-5929
URL: www.goodsam-md.org
Type: Acute Care Hospitals
Emergency Services: Yes
Ownership: Voluntary Non-Profit - Other
Beds: 317

Key Personnel:

CEO/President.............. Jeffrey Matton
Cardiac Laboratory.............. Linda Hawes RN
Chief of Medical Staff......... Chandralekha Banerjee MD
Operating Room.............. Jeremy Weiner, MD
Quality Assurance .... Ken Walsch
Radiology.............. Allan Weksberg MD
Anesthesiology.............. Michael Sendak MD
Emergency Room .... Kevin Scruggs MD

Measure	Cases	This Hosp.	State Avg.	U.S. Avg.
Heart Attack Care				
ACE Inhibitor or ARB for LVSD[1]	23	100%	94%	96%
Aspirin at Arrival	103	96%	98%	99%
Aspirin at Discharge	81	95%	98%	98%
Beta Blocker at Discharge	81	100%	97%	98%
Fibrinolytic Medication Timing	0	-	42%	55%
PCI Within 90 Minutes of Arrival	0	-	83%	90%
Smoking Cessation Advice[1]	13	100%	98%	99%
Chest Pain/Possible Heart Attack Care				
Aspirin at Arrival	-	-	0%	95%
Median Time to ECG (minutes)	-	-	0	8
Median Time to Transfer (minutes)	-	-	0	61
Fibrinolytic Medication Timing	-	-	0%	54%
Heart Failure Care				
ACE Inhibitor or ARB for LVSD	264	93%	94%	94%
Discharge Instructions	624	88%	86%	88%
Evaluation of LVS Function	829	97%	97%	98%
Smoking Cessation Advice	123	97%	98%	98%
Pneumonia Care				
Appropriate Initial Antibiotic	181	92%	92%	92%
Blood Culture Timing	271	90%	92%	96%
Influenza Vaccine	173	91%	88%	91%
Initial Antibiotic Timing	302	93%	94%	95%
Pneumococcal Vaccine	183	96%	92%	93%
Smoking Cessation Advice	103	92%	97%	97%
Surgical Care Improvement Project				
Appropriate VTP Within 24 Hours	324	94%	90%	92%
Appropriate Hair Removal	977	100%	100%	99%
Appropriate Beta Blocker Usage	276	97%	91%	93%
Controlled Postoperative Blood Glucose	0	-	91%	93%
Prophylactic Antibiotic Timing	635	96%	96%	97%
Prophylactic Antibiotic Timing (Outpatient)	-	-	0%	92%
Prophylactic Antibiotic Selection	643	99%	97%	97%
Prophylactic Antibiotic Select. (Outpatient)	-	-	0%	94%
Prophylactic Antibiotic Stopped	608	98%	94%	94%
Recommended VTP Ordered	324	96%	92%	94%
Urinary Catheter Removal	329	93%	89%	90%
Children's Asthma Care				
Received Systemic Corticosteroids	-	-	-	100%
Received Home Management Plan	-	-	-	71%
Received Reliever Medication	-	-	-	100%
Use of Medical Imaging				
Combination Abdominal CT Scan	-	-	0.064	0.191
Combination Chest CT Scan	-	-	0.013	0.054
Follow-up Mammogram/Ultrasound	-	-	8.6%	8.4%
MRI for Low Back Pain	-	-	31.7%	32.7%
Survey of Patients' Hospital Experiences				
Area Around Room 'Always' Quiet at Night	300+	62%	-	58%
Doctors 'Always' Communicated Well	300+	80%	-	80%
Home Recovery Information Given	300+	85%	-	82%
Hospital Given 9 or 10 on 10 Point Scale	300+	70%	-	67%
Meds 'Always' Explained Before Given	300+	56%	-	60%
Nurses 'Always' Communicated Well	300+	76%	-	76%
Pain 'Always' Well Controlled	300+	69%	-	69%
Room and Bathroom 'Always' Clean	300+	72%	-	71%
Timely Help 'Always' Received	300+	58%	-	64%
Would Definitely Recommend Hospital	300+	76%	-	69%

Greater Baltimore Medical Center

6701 North Charles Street
Baltimore, MD 21204
Phone: 443-849-2121
Fax: 410-828-3024
URL: www.gbmc.org
Type: Acute Care Hospitals
Emergency Services: Yes
Ownership: Voluntary Non-Profit - Private
Beds: 372

Key Personnel:

CEO/President.............. Lawrence M Merlis
Chief of Medical Staff.......... Rodney Williams, MD, JD
Operating Room.............. Dale Buchbinder, MD
Pediatric Ambulatory Care ...... Timothy F Doran, MD
Quality Assurance .... Paul Masser
Radiology.................. H Alexander Munitz, MD
Emergency Room .... Kim Bushnell, RN
Hemotology Center .... Laurie Mead

Measure	Cases	This Hosp.	State Avg.	U.S. Avg.
Heart Attack Care				
ACE Inhibitor or ARB for LVSD[1]	2	100%	94%	96%
Aspirin at Arrival[1]	15	93%	98%	99%
Aspirin at Discharge[1]	7	100%	98%	98%
Beta Blocker at Discharge[1]	6	100%	97%	98%
Fibrinolytic Medication Timing	0	-	42%	55%
PCI Within 90 Minutes of Arrival	0	-	83%	90%
Smoking Cessation Advice[1]	1	100%	98%	99%
Chest Pain/Possible Heart Attack Care				
Aspirin at Arrival	-	-	0%	95%
Median Time to ECG (minutes)	-	-	0	8
Median Time to Transfer (minutes)	-	-	0	61
Fibrinolytic Medication Timing	-	-	0%	54%
Heart Failure Care				
ACE Inhibitor or ARB for LVSD	62	92%	94%	94%
Discharge Instructions	173	97%	86%	88%
Evaluation of LVS Function	261	97%	97%	98%
Smoking Cessation Advice[1]	19	100%	98%	98%
Pneumonia Care				
Appropriate Initial Antibiotic	156	94%	92%	92%
Blood Culture Timing	249	86%	92%	96%
Influenza Vaccine	203	91%	88%	91%
Initial Antibiotic Timing	236	92%	94%	95%
Pneumococcal Vaccine	298	92%	92%	93%
Smoking Cessation Advice	48	98%	97%	97%
Surgical Care Improvement Project				
Appropriate VTP Within 24 Hours	336	89%	90%	92%
Appropriate Hair Removal	1,220	100%	100%	99%
Appropriate Beta Blocker Usage	334	83%	91%	93%
Controlled Postoperative Blood Glucose	0	-	91%	93%
Prophylactic Antibiotic Timing	703	91%	96%	97%
Prophylactic Antibiotic Timing (Outpatient)	-	-	0%	92%
Prophylactic Antibiotic Selection	712	96%	97%	97%
Prophylactic Antibiotic Select. (Outpatient)	-	-	0%	94%
Prophylactic Antibiotic Stopped	683	92%	94%	94%
Recommended VTP Ordered	336	89%	92%	94%
Urinary Catheter Removal	310	85%	89%	90%
Children's Asthma Care				
Received Systemic Corticosteroids	-	-	-	100%
Received Home Management Plan	-	-	-	71%
Received Reliever Medication	-	-	-	100%
Use of Medical Imaging				
Combination Abdominal CT Scan	-	-	0.064	0.191
Combination Chest CT Scan	-	-	0.013	0.054
Follow-up Mammogram/Ultrasound	-	-	8.6%	8.4%
MRI for Low Back Pain	-	-	31.7%	32.7%
Survey of Patients' Hospital Experiences				
Area Around Room 'Always' Quiet at Night	300+	51%	-	58%
Doctors 'Always' Communicated Well	300+	81%	-	80%
Home Recovery Information Given	300+	77%	-	82%
Hospital Given 9 or 10 on 10 Point Scale	300+	67%	-	67%
Meds 'Always' Explained Before Given	300+	58%	-	60%
Nurses 'Always' Communicated Well	300+	73%	-	76%
Pain 'Always' Well Controlled	300+	68%	-	69%
Room and Bathroom 'Always' Clean	300+	59%	-	71%
Timely Help 'Always' Received	300+	57%	-	64%
Would Definitely Recommend Hospital	300+	76%	-	69%

Johns Hopkins Bayview Medical Center

4940 Eastern Avenue
Baltimore, MD 21224
Phone: 410-550-0123
Fax: 410-550-0184
URL: www.hopkinsbayview.org
Type: Acute Care Hospitals
Emergency Services: Yes
Ownership: Voluntary Non-Profit - Private
Beds: 565

Key Personnel:

CEO/President.............. Richard Bennett, MD
Chief of Medical Staff.......... David Hellmann,, MD
Coronary Care.............. Robert Gibson, MD
Infection Control.............. Jeanne LeClair
Operating Room.............. Thomas Magnuson, MD
Pediatric Ambulatory Care ...... Mike Crocetti, MD
Pediatric In-Patient Care .... Archie Golden, MD
Radiology.................. Mark Bohlman, MD

Measure	Cases	This Hosp.	State Avg.	U.S. Avg.
Heart Attack Care				
ACE Inhibitor or ARB for LVSD	28	96%	94%	96%
Aspirin at Arrival	172	100%	98%	99%
Aspirin at Discharge	129	98%	98%	98%
Beta Blocker at Discharge	127	98%	97%	98%
Fibrinolytic Medication Timing	0	-	42%	55%
PCI Within 90 Minutes of Arrival	27	93%	83%	90%
Smoking Cessation Advice	55	100%	98%	99%
Chest Pain/Possible Heart Attack Care				
Aspirin at Arrival	-	-	0%	95%
Median Time to ECG (minutes)	-	-	0	8
Median Time to Transfer (minutes)	-	-	0	61
Fibrinolytic Medication Timing	-	-	0%	54%
Heart Failure Care				
ACE Inhibitor or ARB for LVSD	234	96%	94%	94%
Discharge Instructions	509	77%	86%	88%
Evaluation of LVS Function	671	99%	97%	98%
Smoking Cessation Advice	197	99%	98%	98%
Pneumonia Care				
Appropriate Initial Antibiotic	183	89%	92%	92%
Blood Culture Timing	273	94%	92%	96%
Influenza Vaccine	241	68%	88%	91%
Initial Antibiotic Timing	342	89%	94%	95%
Pneumococcal Vaccine	304	77%	92%	93%
Smoking Cessation Advice	187	96%	97%	97%
Surgical Care Improvement Project				
Appropriate VTP Within 24 Hours[2]	259	99%	90%	92%
Appropriate Hair Removal[2]	743	100%	100%	99%
Appropriate Beta Blocker Usage[2]	233	97%	91%	93%
Controlled Postoperative Blood Glucose[2]	0	-	91%	93%
Prophylactic Antibiotic Timing[2]	579	98%	96%	97%
Prophylactic Antibiotic Timing (Outpatient)	-	-	0%	92%
Prophylactic Antibiotic Selection[2]	578	98%	97%	97%
Prophylactic Antibiotic Select. (Outpatient)	-	-	0%	94%
Prophylactic Antibiotic Stopped[2]	567	94%	94%	94%
Recommended VTP Ordered[2]	259	99%	92%	94%
Urinary Catheter Removal[2]	284	99%	89%	90%
Children's Asthma Care				
Received Systemic Corticosteroids	-	-	-	100%
Received Home Management Plan	-	-	-	71%
Received Reliever Medication	-	-	-	100%
Use of Medical Imaging				
Combination Abdominal CT Scan	-	-	0.064	0.191
Combination Chest CT Scan	-	-	0.013	0.054
Follow-up Mammogram/Ultrasound	-	-	8.6%	8.4%
MRI for Low Back Pain	-	-	31.7%	32.7%
Survey of Patients' Hospital Experiences				
Area Around Room 'Always' Quiet at Night	300+	48%	-	58%
Doctors 'Always' Communicated Well	300+	79%	-	80%
Home Recovery Information Given	300+	84%	-	82%
Hospital Given 9 or 10 on 10 Point Scale	300+	66%	-	67%
Meds 'Always' Explained Before Given	300+	59%	-	60%
Nurses 'Always' Communicated Well	300+	74%	-	76%
Pain 'Always' Well Controlled	300+	63%	-	69%
Room and Bathroom 'Always' Clean	300+	59%	-	71%
Timely Help 'Always' Received	300+	58%	-	64%
Would Definitely Recommend Hospital	300+	69%	-	69%

NOTE: Hospital profiles are in alphabetical order by state, then city, then hospital within the city; Rankings exclude hospitals with less than 25 cases except for patient surveys which excludes hospitals with less than 100 cases; (a) 100–299 cases; (1) The number of cases is too small to be sure how well a hospital is performing; (2) The hospital indicated that the data submitted for this measure were based on a sample of cases; (3) Data was collected during a shorter time period (fewer quarters) than the maximum possible time for this measure; (4) Suppressed for one or more quarters by CMS; (5) No data is available from the hospital for this measure; (6) Fewer than 100 patients completed the HCAHPS survey. Use these rates with caution, as the number of surveys may be too low to reliably assess hospital performance; (7) Survey results are based on less than 12 months of data; (8) Survey results are not available for this reporting period; (9) No or very few patients were eligible for the HCAHPS survey. The scores shown, if any, reflect a very small number of surveys; (10) A state average was not calculated because too few hospitals in the state submitted data; (11) There were discrepancies in the data collection process; Please refer to the User's Guide for a full explanation of data.

The Johns Hopkins Hospital

600 North Wolfe Street
Baltimore, MD 21287
E-mail: drichma@jhmi.edu
URL: www.jhmi.edu
Phone: 410-955-9540
Fax: 410-955-0890
Type: Acute Care Hospitals
Ownership: Voluntary Non-Profit - Private
Emergency Services: Yes
Beds: 1,036

Key Personnel:
CEO/President. . . . . Ronald R Peterson, MD
Chief of Medical Staff. . . . . Edward Benz, MD
Infection Control. . . . . John Froggatt, III, DP
Pediatric Ambulatory Care . . . . . . George Dover, MD
Pediatric In-Patient Care . . . . . . George Dover, MD
Quality Assurance . . . . Rick Kidwell
Radiology. . . . . George Saba

Measure	Cases	This Hosp.	State Avg.	U.S. Avg.
Heart Attack Care				
ACE Inhibitor or ARB for LVSD[2]	44	100%	94%	96%
Aspirin at Arrival[2]	90	100%	98%	99%
Aspirin at Discharge[2]	301	99%	98%	98%
Beta Blocker at Discharge[2]	284	99%	97%	98%
Fibrinolytic Medication Timing[2]	0	-	42%	55%
PCI Within 90 Minutes of Arrival[1,2]	11	55%	83%	90%
Smoking Cessation Advice[2]	110	100%	98%	99%
Chest Pain/Possible Heart Attack Care				
Aspirin at Arrival	-	-	0%	95%
Median Time to ECG (minutes)	-	-	0	8
Median Time to Transfer (minutes)	-	-	0	61
Fibrinolytic Medication Timing	-	-	0%	54%
Heart Failure Care				
ACE Inhibitor or ARB for LVSD[2]	200	98%	94%	94%
Discharge Instructions[2]	361	88%	86%	88%
Evaluation of LVS Function[2]	404	99%	97%	98%
Smoking Cessation Advice[2]	109	97%	98%	98%
Pneumonia Care				
Appropriate Initial Antibiotic[2]	69	93%	92%	92%
Blood Culture Timing[2]	65	98%	92%	96%
Influenza Vaccine[2]	109	75%	88%	91%
Initial Antibiotic Timing[2]	142	97%	94%	95%
Pneumococcal Vaccine[2]	71	76%	92%	93%
Smoking Cessation Advice[2]	117	100%	97%	97%
Surgical Care Improvement Project				
Appropriate VTP Within 24 Hours[2]	238	98%	90%	92%
Appropriate Hair Removal[2]	877	100%	100%	99%
Appropriate Beta Blocker Usage[2]	320	92%	91%	93%
Controlled Postoperative Blood Glucose[2]	330	94%	91%	93%
Prophylactic Antibiotic Timing[2]	567	99%	96%	97%
Prophylactic Antibiotic Timing (Outpatient)	-	-	0%	92%
Prophylactic Antibiotic Selection[2]	581	98%	97%	97%
Prophylactic Antibiotic Select. (Outpatient)	-	-	0%	94%
Prophylactic Antibiotic Stopped[2]	541	95%	94%	94%
Recommended VTP Ordered[2]	238	98%	92%	94%
Urinary Catheter Removal[2]	190	75%	89%	90%
Children's Asthma Care				
Received Systemic Corticosteroids	-	-	-	100%
Received Home Management Plan	-	-	-	71%
Received Reliever Medication	-	-	-	100%
Use of Medical Imaging				
Combination Abdominal CT Scan	-	-	0.064	0.191
Combination Chest CT Scan	-	-	0.013	0.054
Follow-up Mammogram/Ultrasound	-	-	8.6%	8.4%
MRI for Low Back Pain	-	-	31.7%	32.7%
Survey of Patients' Hospital Experiences				
Area Around Room 'Always' Quiet at Night	300+	56%	-	58%
Doctors 'Always' Communicated Well	300+	79%	-	80%
Home Recovery Information Given	300+	85%	-	82%
Hospital Given 9 or 10 on 10 Point Scale	300+	76%	-	67%
Meds 'Always' Explained Before Given	300+	62%	-	60%
Nurses 'Always' Communicated Well	300+	77%	-	76%
Pain 'Always' Well Controlled	300+	70%	-	69%
Room and Bathroom 'Always' Clean	300+	65%	-	71%
Timely Help 'Always' Received	300+	61%	-	64%
Would Definitely Recommend Hospital	300+	82%	-	69%

Maryland General Hospital

827 Linden Ave
Baltimore, MD 21201
URL: www.marylandgeneral.org
Phone: 410-225-8996
Fax: 410-669-8368
Type: Acute Care Hospitals
Ownership: Voluntary Non-Profit - Other
Emergency Services: Yes
Beds: 238

Key Personnel:
CEO/President. . . . . Sylvia Smith Johnson
Chief of Medical Staff. . . . . William Anthony, MD
Operating Room. . . . . Jeanne Queen, RN
Pediatric In-Patient Care . . . . . . Mario Gonzalez
Ambulatory Care . . . . Brian Krebs
Emergency Room . . . . Rhamin Ligon, MD

Measure	Cases	This Hosp.	State Avg.	U.S. Avg.
Heart Attack Care				
ACE Inhibitor or ARB for LVSD[1]	5	60%	94%	96%
Aspirin at Arrival[1]	24	100%	98%	99%
Aspirin at Discharge[1]	17	88%	98%	98%
Beta Blocker at Discharge[1]	18	83%	97%	98%
Fibrinolytic Medication Timing	0	-	42%	55%
PCI Within 90 Minutes of Arrival	0	-	83%	90%
Smoking Cessation Advice[1]	5	100%	98%	99%
Chest Pain/Possible Heart Attack Care				
Aspirin at Arrival	-	-	0%	95%
Median Time to ECG (minutes)	-	-	0	8
Median Time to Transfer (minutes)	-	-	0	61
Fibrinolytic Medication Timing	-	-	0%	54%
Heart Failure Care				
ACE Inhibitor or ARB for LVSD	123	80%	94%	94%
Discharge Instructions	242	99%	86%	88%
Evaluation of LVS Function	300	94%	97%	98%
Smoking Cessation Advice	139	96%	98%	98%
Pneumonia Care				
Appropriate Initial Antibiotic	69	84%	92%	92%
Blood Culture Timing	189	87%	92%	96%
Influenza Vaccine	125	58%	88%	91%
Initial Antibiotic Timing	190	86%	94%	95%
Pneumococcal Vaccine	110	85%	92%	93%
Smoking Cessation Advice	163	96%	97%	97%
Surgical Care Improvement Project				
Appropriate VTP Within 24 Hours	102	78%	90%	92%
Appropriate Hair Removal	219	100%	100%	99%
Appropriate Beta Blocker Usage	44	75%	91%	93%
Controlled Postoperative Blood Glucose	0	-	91%	93%
Prophylactic Antibiotic Timing	120	94%	96%	97%
Prophylactic Antibiotic Timing (Outpatient)	-	-	0%	92%
Prophylactic Antibiotic Selection	117	94%	97%	97%
Prophylactic Antibiotic Select. (Outpatient)	-	-	0%	94%
Prophylactic Antibiotic Stopped	116	87%	94%	94%
Recommended VTP Ordered	106	76%	92%	94%
Urinary Catheter Removal	39	62%	89%	90%
Children's Asthma Care				
Received Systemic Corticosteroids	-	-	-	100%
Received Home Management Plan	-	-	-	71%
Received Reliever Medication	-	-	-	100%
Use of Medical Imaging				
Combination Abdominal CT Scan	-	-	0.064	0.191
Combination Chest CT Scan	-	-	0.013	0.054
Follow-up Mammogram/Ultrasound	-	-	8.6%	8.4%
MRI for Low Back Pain	-	-	31.7%	32.7%
Survey of Patients' Hospital Experiences				
Area Around Room 'Always' Quiet at Night	300+	61%	-	58%
Doctors 'Always' Communicated Well	300+	78%	-	80%
Home Recovery Information Given	300+	79%	-	82%
Hospital Given 9 or 10 on 10 Point Scale	300+	57%	-	67%
Meds 'Always' Explained Before Given	300+	56%	-	60%
Nurses 'Always' Communicated Well	300+	72%	-	76%
Pain 'Always' Well Controlled	300+	62%	-	69%
Room and Bathroom 'Always' Clean	300+	60%	-	71%
Timely Help 'Always' Received	300+	58%	-	64%
Would Definitely Recommend Hospital	300+	56%	-	69%

Mercy Medical Center

301 St Paul Place
Baltimore, MD 21202
Phone: 410-332-9237
Type: Acute Care Hospitals
Emergency Services: Yes
Ownership: Voluntary Non-Profit - Church

Key Personnel:
CEO/President. . . . . Thomas Mullen

Measure	Cases	This Hosp.	State Avg.	U.S. Avg.
Heart Attack Care				
ACE Inhibitor or ARB for LVSD[1]	3	100%	94%	96%
Aspirin at Arrival[1]	18	100%	98%	99%
Aspirin at Discharge[1]	14	100%	98%	98%
Beta Blocker at Discharge[1]	13	100%	97%	98%
Fibrinolytic Medication Timing	0	-	42%	55%
PCI Within 90 Minutes of Arrival	0	-	83%	90%
Smoking Cessation Advice[1]	5	100%	98%	99%
Chest Pain/Possible Heart Attack Care				
Aspirin at Arrival	-	-	0%	95%
Median Time to ECG (minutes)	-	-	0	8
Median Time to Transfer (minutes)	-	-	0	61
Fibrinolytic Medication Timing	-	-	0%	54%
Heart Failure Care				
ACE Inhibitor or ARB for LVSD	153	95%	94%	94%
Discharge Instructions	339	96%	86%	88%
Evaluation of LVS Function	369	99%	97%	98%
Smoking Cessation Advice	111	99%	98%	98%
Pneumonia Care				
Appropriate Initial Antibiotic	110	96%	92%	92%
Blood Culture Timing	136	95%	92%	96%
Influenza Vaccine	77	92%	88%	91%
Initial Antibiotic Timing	170	98%	94%	95%
Pneumococcal Vaccine	81	94%	92%	93%
Smoking Cessation Advice	100	98%	97%	97%
Surgical Care Improvement Project				
Appropriate VTP Within 24 Hours[2]	248	96%	90%	92%
Appropriate Hair Removal[2]	1,112	99%	100%	99%
Appropriate Beta Blocker Usage[2]	250	90%	91%	93%
Controlled Postoperative Blood Glucose[2]	0	-	91%	93%
Prophylactic Antibiotic Timing[2]	910	97%	96%	97%
Prophylactic Antibiotic Timing (Outpatient)	-	-	0%	92%
Prophylactic Antibiotic Selection[2]	917	99%	97%	97%
Prophylactic Antibiotic Select. (Outpatient)	-	-	0%	94%
Prophylactic Antibiotic Stopped[2]	884	95%	94%	94%
Recommended VTP Ordered[2]	248	98%	92%	94%
Urinary Catheter Removal[2]	411	97%	89%	90%
Children's Asthma Care				
Received Systemic Corticosteroids	-	-	-	100%
Received Home Management Plan	-	-	-	71%
Received Reliever Medication	-	-	-	100%
Use of Medical Imaging				
Combination Abdominal CT Scan	-	-	0.064	0.191
Combination Chest CT Scan	-	-	0.013	0.054
Follow-up Mammogram/Ultrasound	-	-	8.6%	8.4%
MRI for Low Back Pain	-	-	31.7%	32.7%
Survey of Patients' Hospital Experiences				
Area Around Room 'Always' Quiet at Night	300+	59%	-	58%
Doctors 'Always' Communicated Well	300+	84%	-	80%
Home Recovery Information Given	300+	87%	-	82%
Hospital Given 9 or 10 on 10 Point Scale	300+	72%	-	67%
Meds 'Always' Explained Before Given	300+	61%	-	60%
Nurses 'Always' Communicated Well	300+	78%	-	76%
Pain 'Always' Well Controlled	300+	73%	-	69%
Room and Bathroom 'Always' Clean	300+	63%	-	71%
Timely Help 'Always' Received	300+	57%	-	64%
Would Definitely Recommend Hospital	300+	74%	-	69%

NOTE: Hospital profiles are in alphabetical order by state, then city, then hospital within the city; Rankings exclude hospitals with less than 25 cases except for patient surveys which excludes hospitals with less than 100 cases; (a) 100–299 cases; (1) The number of cases is too small to be sure how well a hospital is performing; (2) The hospital indicated that the data submitted for this measure were based on a sample of cases; (3) Data was collected during a shorter time period (fewer quarters) than the maximum possible time for this measure; (4) Suppressed for one or more quarters by CMS; (5) No data is available from the hospital for this measure; (6) Fewer than 100 patients completed the HCAHPS survey. Use these rates with caution, as the number of surveys may be too low to reliably assess hospital performance; (7) Survey results are based on less than 12 months of data; (8) Survey results are not available for this reporting period; (9) No or very few patients were eligible for the HCAHPS survey. The scores shown, if any, reflect a very small number of surveys; (10) A state average was not calculated because too few hospitals in the state submitted data; (11) There were discrepancies in the data collection process; Please refer to the User's Guide for a full explanation of data.

Saint Agnes Hospital

Wilkens & Caton Avenues
Baltimore, MD 21229
E-mail: info@stagnes.org
URL: www.stagnes.org
Phone: 410-368-2101
Fax: 410-368-3536
Type: Acute Care Hospitals
Ownership: Voluntary Non-Profit - Church
Emergency Services: Yes
Beds: 323

Key Personnel:
CEO/President. . . . . Bonnie Phipps
Chief of Medical Staff . . . . Adrian Long, MD
Operating Room. . . . . Dorothy James
Pediatric In-Patient Care . . . . Michael Burke, MD
Quality Assurance . . . . Mike Moriarty, MD
Radiology. . . . . Robert Stroud, MD
Emergency Room . . . . Kevin Scruggs
Patient Relations . . . . Yolanda Copeland

Measure	Cases	This Hosp.	State Avg.	U.S. Avg.
Heart Attack Care				
ACE Inhibitor or ARB for LVSD	27	100%	94%	96%
Aspirin at Arrival	133	95%	98%	99%
Aspirin at Discharge	105	99%	98%	98%
Beta Blocker at Discharge	105	99%	97%	98%
Fibrinolytic Medication Timing[1]	2	0%	42%	55%
PCI Within 90 Minutes of Arrival	50	80%	83%	90%
Smoking Cessation Advice	40	95%	98%	99%
Chest Pain/Possible Heart Attack Care				
Aspirin at Arrival	-	-	0%	95%
Median Time to ECG (minutes)	-	-	0	8
Median Time to Transfer (minutes)	-	-	0	61
Fibrinolytic Medication Timing	-	-	0%	54%
Heart Failure Care				
ACE Inhibitor or ARB for LVSD	285	91%	94%	94%
Discharge Instructions	492	76%	86%	88%
Evaluation of LVS Function	635	95%	97%	98%
Smoking Cessation Advice	124	98%	98%	98%
Pneumonia Care				
Appropriate Initial Antibiotic[2]	72	93%	92%	92%
Blood Culture Timing[2]	166	87%	92%	96%
Influenza Vaccine[2]	79	94%	88%	91%
Initial Antibiotic Timing[2]	162	93%	94%	95%
Pneumococcal Vaccine[2]	108	94%	92%	93%
Smoking Cessation Advice[2]	62	92%	97%	97%
Surgical Care Improvement Project				
Appropriate VTP Within 24 Hours[2]	177	99%	90%	92%
Appropriate Hair Removal[2]	686	99%	100%	99%
Appropriate Beta Blocker Usage[2]	161	98%	91%	93%
Controlled Postoperative Blood Glucose[2]	0	-	91%	93%
Prophylactic Antibiotic Timing[2]	519	97%	96%	97%
Prophylactic Antibiotic Timing (Outpatient)	-	-	0%	92%
Prophylactic Antibiotic Selection[2]	521	98%	97%	97%
Prophylactic Antibiotic Select. (Outpatient)	-	-	0%	94%
Prophylactic Antibiotic Stopped[2]	489	94%	94%	94%
Recommended VTP Ordered[2]	178	98%	92%	94%
Urinary Catheter Removal[2]	129	95%	89%	90%
Children's Asthma Care				
Received Systemic Corticosteroids	-	-	-	100%
Received Home Management Plan	-	-	-	71%
Received Reliever Medication	-	-	-	100%
Use of Medical Imaging				
Combination Abdominal CT Scan	-	-	0.064	0.191
Combination Chest CT Scan	-	-	0.013	0.054
Follow-up Mammogram/Ultrasound	-	-	8.6%	8.4%
MRI for Low Back Pain	-	-	31.7%	32.7%
Survey of Patients' Hospital Experiences				
Area Around Room 'Always' Quiet at Night	300+	54%	-	58%
Doctors 'Always' Communicated Well	300+	78%	-	80%
Home Recovery Information Given	300+	82%	-	82%
Hospital Given 9 or 10 on 10 Point Scale	300+	61%	-	67%
Meds 'Always' Explained Before Given	300+	56%	-	60%
Nurses 'Always' Communicated Well	300+	72%	-	76%
Pain 'Always' Well Controlled	300+	67%	-	69%
Room and Bathroom 'Always' Clean	300+	56%	-	71%
Timely Help 'Always' Received	300+	54%	-	64%
Would Definitely Recommend Hospital	300+	65%	-	69%

Sinai Hospital of Baltimore

2401 West Belvedere Ave
Baltimore, MD 21215
URL: www.sinai-balt.com
Phone: 410-601-5131
Fax: 410-601-9055
Type: Acute Care Hospitals
Ownership: Voluntary Non-Profit - Other
Emergency Services: Yes
Beds: 467

Key Personnel:
CEO/President. . . . . Neil Meltzer
Chief of Medical Staff . . . . Lorrie Liang, MD
Coronary Care . . . . Valerie Allen
Infection Control. . . . . Katleen Arias
Pediatric Ambulatory Care . . . . . . Joseph M Wiley, MD
Pediatric In-Patient Care . . . . Joseph M Wiley, MD
Quality Assurance . . . . Sheila McClahahan
Radiology. . . . . Noah I Lightman, MD

Measure	Cases	This Hosp.	State Avg.	U.S. Avg.
Heart Attack Care				
ACE Inhibitor or ARB for LVSD	71	86%	94%	96%
Aspirin at Arrival	210	100%	98%	99%
Aspirin at Discharge	379	98%	98%	98%
Beta Blocker at Discharge	372	97%	97%	98%
Fibrinolytic Medication Timing	0	-	42%	55%
PCI Within 90 Minutes of Arrival	51	82%	83%	90%
Smoking Cessation Advice	129	100%	98%	99%
Chest Pain/Possible Heart Attack Care				
Aspirin at Arrival	-	-	0%	95%
Median Time to ECG (minutes)	-	-	0	8
Median Time to Transfer (minutes)	-	-	0	61
Fibrinolytic Medication Timing	-	-	0%	54%
Heart Failure Care				
ACE Inhibitor or ARB for LVSD	249	93%	94%	94%
Discharge Instructions	587	67%	86%	88%
Evaluation of LVS Function	708	97%	97%	98%
Smoking Cessation Advice	139	99%	98%	98%
Pneumonia Care				
Appropriate Initial Antibiotic	158	89%	92%	92%
Blood Culture Timing	296	90%	92%	96%
Influenza Vaccine	190	93%	88%	91%
Initial Antibiotic Timing	290	94%	94%	95%
Pneumococcal Vaccine	251	93%	92%	93%
Smoking Cessation Advice	112	100%	97%	97%
Surgical Care Improvement Project				
Appropriate VTP Within 24 Hours[2]	299	88%	90%	92%
Appropriate Hair Removal[2]	985	100%	100%	99%
Appropriate Beta Blocker Usage[2]	274	95%	91%	93%
Controlled Postoperative Blood Glucose[2]	233	91%	91%	93%
Prophylactic Antibiotic Timing[2]	677	97%	96%	97%
Prophylactic Antibiotic Timing (Outpatient)	-	-	0%	92%
Prophylactic Antibiotic Selection[2]	685	97%	97%	97%
Prophylactic Antibiotic Select. (Outpatient)	-	-	0%	94%
Prophylactic Antibiotic Stopped[2]	626	95%	94%	94%
Recommended VTP Ordered[2]	299	89%	92%	94%
Urinary Catheter Removal[2]	276	92%	89%	90%
Children's Asthma Care				
Received Systemic Corticosteroids	-	-	-	100%
Received Home Management Plan	-	-	-	71%
Received Reliever Medication	-	-	-	100%
Use of Medical Imaging				
Combination Abdominal CT Scan	-	-	0.064	0.191
Combination Chest CT Scan	-	-	0.013	0.054
Follow-up Mammogram/Ultrasound	-	-	8.6%	8.4%
MRI for Low Back Pain	-	-	31.7%	32.7%
Survey of Patients' Hospital Experiences				
Area Around Room 'Always' Quiet at Night	300+	51%	-	58%
Doctors 'Always' Communicated Well	300+	73%	-	80%
Home Recovery Information Given	300+	78%	-	82%
Hospital Given 9 or 10 on 10 Point Scale	300+	58%	-	67%
Meds 'Always' Explained Before Given	300+	56%	-	60%
Nurses 'Always' Communicated Well	300+	70%	-	76%
Pain 'Always' Well Controlled	300+	59%	-	69%
Room and Bathroom 'Always' Clean	300+	59%	-	71%
Timely Help 'Always' Received	300+	51%	-	64%
Would Definitely Recommend Hospital	300+	63%	-	69%

Union Memorial Hospital

201 E University Pky
Baltimore, MD 21218
URL: www.unionmemorial.org
Phone: 410-554-2227
Fax: 410-554-2652
Type: Acute Care Hospitals
Ownership: Voluntary Non-Profit - Other
Emergency Services: Yes
Beds: 283

Key Personnel:
CEO/President. . . . . Harrison J Rider III
Chief of Medical Staff . . . . Robert Ferguson, MD
Infection Control. . . . . Barbara Elau
Operating Room. . . . . Kathy Mucei
Pediatric Ambulatory Care . . . . . . Jay Gopal, MD
Quality Assurance . . . . Anne Flood
Radiology. . . . . Carlton Sexton

Measure	Cases	This Hosp.	State Avg.	U.S. Avg.
Heart Attack Care				
ACE Inhibitor or ARB for LVSD	108	94%	94%	96%
Aspirin at Arrival	116	96%	98%	99%
Aspirin at Discharge	696	99%	98%	98%
Beta Blocker at Discharge	674	96%	97%	98%
Fibrinolytic Medication Timing	0	-	42%	55%
PCI Within 90 Minutes of Arrival[1]	18	83%	83%	90%
Smoking Cessation Advice	252	93%	98%	99%
Chest Pain/Possible Heart Attack Care				
Aspirin at Arrival	-	-	0%	95%
Median Time to ECG (minutes)	-	-	0	8
Median Time to Transfer (minutes)	-	-	0	61
Fibrinolytic Medication Timing	-	-	0%	54%
Heart Failure Care				
ACE Inhibitor or ARB for LVSD	311	92%	94%	94%
Discharge Instructions	620	93%	86%	88%
Evaluation of LVS Function	739	95%	97%	98%
Smoking Cessation Advice	196	94%	98%	98%
Pneumonia Care				
Appropriate Initial Antibiotic	118	91%	92%	92%
Blood Culture Timing	185	88%	92%	96%
Influenza Vaccine	138	94%	88%	91%
Initial Antibiotic Timing	219	96%	94%	95%
Pneumococcal Vaccine	159	96%	92%	93%
Smoking Cessation Advice	86	91%	97%	97%
Surgical Care Improvement Project				
Appropriate VTP Within 24 Hours[2]	250	97%	90%	92%
Appropriate Hair Removal[2]	1,727	99%	100%	99%
Appropriate Beta Blocker Usage[2]	506	96%	91%	93%
Controlled Postoperative Blood Glucose[2]	173	88%	91%	93%
Prophylactic Antibiotic Timing[2]	1,511	96%	96%	97%
Prophylactic Antibiotic Timing (Outpatient)	-	-	0%	92%
Prophylactic Antibiotic Selection[2]	1,512	99%	97%	97%
Prophylactic Antibiotic Select. (Outpatient)	-	-	0%	94%
Prophylactic Antibiotic Stopped[2]	1,487	97%	94%	94%
Recommended VTP Ordered[2]	250	97%	92%	94%
Urinary Catheter Removal[2]	116	91%	89%	90%
Children's Asthma Care				
Received Systemic Corticosteroids	-	-	-	100%
Received Home Management Plan	-	-	-	71%
Received Reliever Medication	-	-	-	100%
Use of Medical Imaging				
Combination Abdominal CT Scan	-	-	0.064	0.191
Combination Chest CT Scan	-	-	0.013	0.054
Follow-up Mammogram/Ultrasound	-	-	8.6%	8.4%
MRI for Low Back Pain	-	-	31.7%	32.7%
Survey of Patients' Hospital Experiences				
Area Around Room 'Always' Quiet at Night	300+	63%	-	58%
Doctors 'Always' Communicated Well	300+	81%	-	80%
Home Recovery Information Given	300+	83%	-	82%
Hospital Given 9 or 10 on 10 Point Scale	300+	72%	-	67%
Meds 'Always' Explained Before Given	300+	59%	-	60%
Nurses 'Always' Communicated Well	300+	74%	-	76%
Pain 'Always' Well Controlled	300+	67%	-	69%
Room and Bathroom 'Always' Clean	300+	68%	-	71%
Timely Help 'Always' Received	300+	60%	-	64%
Would Definitely Recommend Hospital	300+	77%	-	69%

NOTE: Hospital profiles are in alphabetical order by state, then city, then hospital within the city; Rankings exclude hospitals with less than 25 cases except for patient surveys which excludes hospitals with less than 100 cases; (a) 100–299 cases; (1) The number of cases is too small to be sure how well a hospital is performing; (2) The hospital indicated that the data submitted for this measure were based on a sample of cases; (3) Data was collected during a shorter time period (fewer quarters) than the maximum possible time for this measure; (4) Suppressed for one or more quarters by CMS; (5) No data is available from the hospital for this measure; (6) Fewer than 100 patients completed the HCAHPS survey. Use these rates with caution, as the number of surveys may be too low to reliably assess hospital performance; (7) Survey results are based on less than 12 months of data; (8) Survey results are not available for this reporting period; (9) No or very few patients were eligible for the HCAHPS survey. The scores shown, if any, reflect a very small number of surveys; (10) A state average was not calculated because too few hospitals in the state submitted data; (11) There were discrepancies in the data collection process; Please refer to the User's Guide for a full explanation of data.

University of Maryland Medical Center

22 S Greene St | Phone: 410-328-0313
Baltimore, MD 21201 | Fax: 410-328-8664
URL: www.umm.edu
Type: Acute Care Hospitals | Emergency Services: Yes
Ownership: Voluntary Non-Profit - Private | Beds: 650

Key Personnel:
CEO/President. . . . . Morton I Rapoport, MD
Chief of Medical Staff. . . . . Frank Calia, MD
Infection Control. . . . . Joan Hebden
Pediatric Ambulatory Care . . . . . . Michael Berman, MD
Pediatric In-Patient Care . . . . Michael Berman, MD
Quality Assurance . . . . Josephine Goode-Johnson
Radiology. . . . . Philip A Templeton, MD
Emergency Room . . . . Robert Barish, MD

Measure	Cases	This Hosp.	State Avg.	U.S. Avg.
Heart Attack Care				
ACE Inhibitor or ARB for LVSD	77	92%	94%	96%
Aspirin at Arrival	83	99%	98%	99%
Aspirin at Discharge	471	98%	98%	98%
Beta Blocker at Discharge	444	97%	97%	98%
Fibrinolytic Medication Timing	0	-	42%	55%
PCI Within 90 Minutes of Arrival[1]	15	60%	83%	90%
Smoking Cessation Advice	166	99%	98%	99%
Chest Pain/Possible Heart Attack Care				
Aspirin at Arrival	-	-	0%	95%
Median Time to ECG (minutes)	-	-	0	8
Median Time to Transfer (minutes)	-	-	0	61
Fibrinolytic Medication Timing	-	-	0%	54%
Heart Failure Care				
ACE Inhibitor or ARB for LVSD	251	94%	94%	94%
Discharge Instructions	391	78%	86%	88%
Evaluation of LVS Function	429	98%	97%	98%
Smoking Cessation Advice	115	100%	98%	98%
Pneumonia Care				
Appropriate Initial Antibiotic	98	91%	92%	92%
Blood Culture Timing	229	88%	92%	96%
Influenza Vaccine	150	91%	88%	91%
Initial Antibiotic Timing	223	93%	94%	95%
Pneumococcal Vaccine	131	92%	92%	93%
Smoking Cessation Advice	190	99%	97%	97%
Surgical Care Improvement Project				
Appropriate VTP Within 24 Hours[2]	669	96%	90%	92%
Appropriate Hair Removal[2]	1,727	97%	100%	99%
Appropriate Beta Blocker Usage[2]	603	78%	91%	93%
Controlled Postoperative Blood Glucose[2]	510	93%	91%	93%
Prophylactic Antibiotic Timing[2]	823	95%	96%	97%
Prophylactic Antibiotic Timing (Outpatient)	-	-	0%	92%
Prophylactic Antibiotic Selection[2]	857	98%	97%	97%
Prophylactic Antibiotic Select. (Outpatient)	-	-	0%	94%
Prophylactic Antibiotic Stopped[2]	780	93%	94%	94%
Recommended VTP Ordered[2]	673	97%	92%	94%
Urinary Catheter Removal[2]	455	80%	89%	90%
Children's Asthma Care				
Received Systemic Corticosteroids	-	-	-	100%
Received Home Management Plan	-	-	-	71%
Received Reliever Medication	-	-	-	100%
Use of Medical Imaging				
Combination Abdominal CT Scan	-	-	0.064	0.191
Combination Chest CT Scan	-	-	0.013	0.054
Follow-up Mammogram/Ultrasound	-	-	8.6%	8.4%
MRI for Low Back Pain	-	-	31.7%	32.7%
Survey of Patients' Hospital Experiences				
Area Around Room 'Always' Quiet at Night	300+	53%	-	58%
Doctors 'Always' Communicated Well	300+	78%	-	80%
Home Recovery Information Given	300+	86%	-	82%
Hospital Given 9 or 10 on 10 Point Scale	300+	67%	-	67%
Meds 'Always' Explained Before Given	300+	61%	-	60%
Nurses 'Always' Communicated Well	300+	74%	-	76%
Pain 'Always' Well Controlled	300+	67%	-	69%
Room and Bathroom 'Always' Clean	300+	58%	-	71%
Timely Help 'Always' Received	300+	59%	-	64%
Would Definitely Recommend Hospital	300+	73%	-	69%

VA Maryland Healthcare System - Baltimore

10 North Greene Street | Phone: 410-605-7016
Baltimore, MD 21201
URL: www.maryland.va.gov
Type: Acute Care-Veterans Administration | Emergency Services: No
Ownership: Government - Federal | Beds: 137

Measure	Cases	This Hosp.	State Avg.	U.S. Avg.
Heart Attack Care				
ACE Inhibitor or ARB for LVSD[1]	3	100%	94%	96%
Aspirin at Arrival	36	100%	98%	99%
Aspirin at Discharge	29	93%	98%	98%
Beta Blocker at Discharge	29	97%	97%	98%
Fibrinolytic Medication Timing[5]	0	-	42%	55%
PCI Within 90 Minutes of Arrival[1]	2	0%	83%	90%
Smoking Cessation Advice[1]	12	100%	98%	99%
Chest Pain/Possible Heart Attack Care				
Aspirin at Arrival	-	-	0%	95%
Median Time to ECG (minutes)	-	-	0	8
Median Time to Transfer (minutes)	-	-	0	61
Fibrinolytic Medication Timing	-	-	0%	54%
Heart Failure Care				
ACE Inhibitor or ARB for LVSD	117	93%	94%	94%
Discharge Instructions	252	98%	86%	88%
Evaluation of LVS Function	252	100%	97%	98%
Smoking Cessation Advice	57	100%	98%	98%
Pneumonia Care				
Appropriate Initial Antibiotic	100	96%	92%	92%
Blood Culture Timing	157	99%	92%	96%
Influenza Vaccine	81	91%	88%	91%
Initial Antibiotic Timing	159	92%	94%	95%
Pneumococcal Vaccine	103	100%	92%	93%
Smoking Cessation Advice	70	100%	97%	97%
Surgical Care Improvement Project				
Appropriate VTP Within 24 Hours[2]	113	95%	90%	92%
Appropriate Hair Removal[2]	140	100%	100%	99%
Appropriate Beta Blocker Usage[2]	51	98%	91%	93%
Controlled Postoperative Blood Glucose[2,5]	0	-	91%	93%
Prophylactic Antibiotic Timing	66	98%	96%	97%
Prophylactic Antibiotic Timing (Outpatient)	-	-	0%	92%
Prophylactic Antibiotic Selection	66	98%	97%	97%
Prophylactic Antibiotic Select. (Outpatient)	-	-	0%	94%
Prophylactic Antibiotic Stopped	63	97%	94%	94%
Recommended VTP Ordered[2]	113	96%	92%	94%
Urinary Catheter Removal[2]	49	88%	89%	90%
Children's Asthma Care				
Received Systemic Corticosteroids	-	-	-	100%
Received Home Management Plan	-	-	-	71%
Received Reliever Medication	-	-	-	100%
Use of Medical Imaging				
Combination Abdominal CT Scan	-	-	0.064	0.191
Combination Chest CT Scan	-	-	0.013	0.054
Follow-up Mammogram/Ultrasound	-	-	8.6%	8.4%
MRI for Low Back Pain	-	-	31.7%	32.7%
Survey of Patients' Hospital Experiences				
Area Around Room 'Always' Quiet at Night	-	-	-	58%
Doctors 'Always' Communicated Well	-	-	-	80%
Home Recovery Information Given	-	-	-	82%
Hospital Given 9 or 10 on 10 Point Scale	-	-	-	67%
Meds 'Always' Explained Before Given	-	-	-	60%
Nurses 'Always' Communicated Well	-	-	-	76%
Pain 'Always' Well Controlled	-	-	-	69%
Room and Bathroom 'Always' Clean	-	-	-	71%
Timely Help 'Always' Received	-	-	-	64%
Would Definitely Recommend Hospital	-	-	-	69%

Upper Chesapeake Medical Center

500 Upper Chesapeake Drive | Phone: 443-643-3303
Bel Air, MD 21014 | Fax: 443-643-4210
URL: www.uchs.org
Type: Acute Care Hospitals | Emergency Services: Yes
Ownership: Voluntary Non-Profit - Other | Beds: 143

Key Personnel:
CEO/President. . . . . Lyle Ernest Sheldon, FACHE
Chief of Medical Staff. . . . . Peggy Vaughan, MD
Operating Room. . . . . Robert Hoofnagle
Pediatric In-Patient Care . . . . Marianne Fridberg, MD
Quality Assurance . . . . Jane Gordon
Radiology. . . . . Richard Mones, MD
Emergency Room . . . . Charlotte Meck
Intensive Care Unit. . . . . Antoinette Spevetz, MD

Measure	Cases	This Hosp.	State Avg.	U.S. Avg.
Heart Attack Care				
ACE Inhibitor or ARB for LVSD	30	100%	94%	96%
Aspirin at Arrival	202	99%	98%	99%
Aspirin at Discharge	145	97%	98%	98%
Beta Blocker at Discharge	145	99%	97%	98%
Fibrinolytic Medication Timing	0	-	42%	55%
PCI Within 90 Minutes of Arrival	79	86%	83%	90%
Smoking Cessation Advice	54	100%	98%	99%
Chest Pain/Possible Heart Attack Care				
Aspirin at Arrival	-	-	0%	95%
Median Time to ECG (minutes)	-	-	0	8
Median Time to Transfer (minutes)	-	-	0	61
Fibrinolytic Medication Timing	-	-	0%	54%
Heart Failure Care				
ACE Inhibitor or ARB for LVSD	78	96%	94%	94%
Discharge Instructions	301	97%	86%	88%
Evaluation of LVS Function	374	100%	97%	98%
Smoking Cessation Advice	46	100%	98%	98%
Pneumonia Care				
Appropriate Initial Antibiotic	249	98%	92%	92%
Blood Culture Timing	446	99%	92%	96%
Influenza Vaccine	199	93%	88%	91%
Initial Antibiotic Timing	387	96%	94%	95%
Pneumococcal Vaccine	278	98%	92%	93%
Smoking Cessation Advice	113	100%	97%	97%
Surgical Care Improvement Project				
Appropriate VTP Within 24 Hours[2]	181	98%	90%	92%
Appropriate Hair Removal[2]	607	100%	100%	99%
Appropriate Beta Blocker Usage[2]	181	92%	91%	93%
Controlled Postoperative Blood Glucose[2]	0	-	91%	93%
Prophylactic Antibiotic Timing[2]	421	95%	96%	97%
Prophylactic Antibiotic Timing (Outpatient)	-	-	0%	92%
Prophylactic Antibiotic Selection[2]	435	94%	97%	97%
Prophylactic Antibiotic Select. (Outpatient)	-	-	0%	94%
Prophylactic Antibiotic Stopped[2]	407	94%	94%	94%
Recommended VTP Ordered[2]	181	98%	92%	94%
Urinary Catheter Removal[2]	140	91%	89%	90%
Children's Asthma Care				
Received Systemic Corticosteroids	-	-	-	100%
Received Home Management Plan	-	-	-	71%
Received Reliever Medication	-	-	-	100%
Use of Medical Imaging				
Combination Abdominal CT Scan	-	-	0.064	0.191
Combination Chest CT Scan	-	-	0.013	0.054
Follow-up Mammogram/Ultrasound	-	-	8.6%	8.4%
MRI for Low Back Pain	-	-	31.7%	32.7%
Survey of Patients' Hospital Experiences				
Area Around Room 'Always' Quiet at Night	300+	58%	-	58%
Doctors 'Always' Communicated Well	300+	75%	-	80%
Home Recovery Information Given	300+	83%	-	82%
Hospital Given 9 or 10 on 10 Point Scale	300+	64%	-	67%
Meds 'Always' Explained Before Given	300+	57%	-	60%
Nurses 'Always' Communicated Well	300+	75%	-	76%
Pain 'Always' Well Controlled	300+	67%	-	69%
Room and Bathroom 'Always' Clean	300+	64%	-	71%
Timely Help 'Always' Received	300+	56%	-	64%
Would Definitely Recommend Hospital	300+	65%	-	69%

NOTE: Hospital profiles are in alphabetical order by state, then city, then hospital within the city; Rankings exclude hospitals with less than 25 cases except for patient surveys which excludes hospitals with less than 100 cases; (a) 100–299 cases; (1) The number of cases is too small to be sure how well a hospital is performing; (2) The hospital indicated that the data submitted for this measure were based on a sample of cases; (3) Data was collected during a shorter time period (fewer quarters) than the maximum possible time for this measure; (4) Suppressed for one or more quarters by CMS; (5) No data is available from the hospital for this measure; (6) Fewer than 100 patients completed the HCAHPS survey. Use these rates with caution, as the number of surveys may be too low to reliably assess hospital performance; (7) Survey results are based on less than 12 months of data; (8) Survey results are not available for this reporting period; (9) No or very few patients were eligible for the HCAHPS survey. The scores shown, if any, reflect a very small number of surveys; (10) A state average was not calculated because too few hospitals in the state submitted data; (11) There were discrepancies in the data collection process; Please refer to the User's Guide for a full explanation of data.

Atlantic General Hospital

9733 Healthway Drive
Berlin, MD 21811
Phone: 410-641-9601
Fax: 410-641-9670
E-mail: agh@atlanticgeneral.org
URL: www.atlanticgeneral.org
Type: Acute Care Hospitals
Emergency Services: Yes
Ownership: Voluntary Non-Profit - Private
Beds: 62

Key Personnel:
CEO/President. . . . . Michael Franklin, CHE
Chief of Medical Staff. . . . . Edwin Castaneda
Coronary Care . . . . Scott Rose
Infection Control. . . . . Michaelann Frate, RN
Operating Room. . . . . Shirley Spirk
Quality Assurance . . . . Charles Gizora
Radiology. . . . . Simmi Chawla

Measure	Cases	This Hosp.	State Avg.	U.S. Avg.
Heart Attack Care				
ACE Inhibitor or ARB for LVSD	0	-	94%	96%
Aspirin at Arrival[1]	7	100%	98%	99%
Aspirin at Discharge[1]	4	100%	98%	98%
Beta Blocker at Discharge[1]	5	100%	97%	98%
Fibrinolytic Medication Timing[5]	0	-	42%	55%
PCI Within 90 Minutes of Arrival[5]	0	-	83%	90%
Smoking Cessation Advice	0	-	98%	99%
Chest Pain/Possible Heart Attack Care				
Aspirin at Arrival	-	-	0%	95%
Median Time to ECG (minutes)	-	-	0	8
Median Time to Transfer (minutes)	-	-	0	61
Fibrinolytic Medication Timing	-	-	0%	54%
Heart Failure Care				
ACE Inhibitor or ARB for LVSD	38	97%	94%	94%
Discharge Instructions	100	99%	86%	88%
Evaluation of LVS Function	125	98%	97%	98%
Smoking Cessation Advice	29	100%	98%	98%
Pneumonia Care				
Appropriate Initial Antibiotic	83	94%	92%	92%
Blood Culture Timing	118	97%	92%	96%
Influenza Vaccine	76	99%	88%	91%
Initial Antibiotic Timing	116	98%	94%	95%
Pneumococcal Vaccine	126	98%	92%	93%
Smoking Cessation Advice	33	94%	97%	97%
Surgical Care Improvement Project				
Appropriate VTP Within 24 Hours	153	93%	90%	92%
Appropriate Hair Removal	304	99%	100%	99%
Appropriate Beta Blocker Usage	95	99%	91%	93%
Controlled Postoperative Blood Glucose	0	-	91%	93%
Prophylactic Antibiotic Timing	197	97%	96%	97%
Prophylactic Antibiotic Timing (Outpatient)	-	-	0%	92%
Prophylactic Antibiotic Selection	198	98%	97%	97%
Prophylactic Antibiotic Select. (Outpatient)	-	-	0%	94%
Prophylactic Antibiotic Stopped	188	94%	94%	94%
Recommended VTP Ordered	153	93%	92%	94%
Urinary Catheter Removal	93	87%	89%	90%
Children's Asthma Care				
Received Systemic Corticosteroids	-	-	-	100%
Received Home Management Plan	-	-	-	71%
Received Reliever Medication	-	-	-	100%
Use of Medical Imaging				
Combination Abdominal CT Scan	-	-	0.064	0.191
Combination Chest CT Scan	-	-	0.013	0.054
Follow-up Mammogram/Ultrasound	-	-	8.6%	8.4%
MRI for Low Back Pain	-	-	31.7%	32.7%
Survey of Patients' Hospital Experiences				
Area Around Room 'Always' Quiet at Night	300+	50%	-	58%
Doctors 'Always' Communicated Well	300+	77%	-	80%
Home Recovery Information Given	300+	84%	-	82%
Hospital Given 9 or 10 on 10 Point Scale	300+	69%	-	67%
Meds 'Always' Explained Before Given	300+	57%	-	60%
Nurses 'Always' Communicated Well	300+	76%	-	76%
Pain 'Always' Well Controlled	300+	69%	-	69%
Room and Bathroom 'Always' Clean	300+	65%	-	71%
Timely Help 'Always' Received	300+	63%	-	64%
Would Definitely Recommend Hospital	300+	75%	-	69%

Suburban Hospital

8600 Old Georgetown Rd
Bethesda, MD 20814
Phone: 301-896-2576
Fax: 301-897-1339
URL: www.suburbanhospital.org
Type: Acute Care Hospitals
Emergency Services: Yes
Ownership: Voluntary Non-Profit - Private
Beds: 366

Key Personnel:
CEO/President. . . . . Brian Gragnolati
Chief of Medical Staff . . . . Dr Eugene Passamani
Infection Control. . . . . Fred Gill, MD
Quality Assurance . . . . Mary Monen
Radiology. . . . . Stephan Cisternino, MD
Anesthesiology. . . . . Steven Hopper, MD
Emergency Room . . . . Robert J Rothstein, MD
Patient Relations . . . . Jacky Schultz

Measure	Cases	This Hosp.	State Avg.	U.S. Avg.
Heart Attack Care				
ACE Inhibitor or ARB for LVSD	44	95%	94%	96%
Aspirin at Arrival	177	99%	98%	99%
Aspirin at Discharge	241	99%	98%	98%
Beta Blocker at Discharge	240	98%	97%	98%
Fibrinolytic Medication Timing	0	-	42%	55%
PCI Within 90 Minutes of Arrival	36	72%	83%	90%
Smoking Cessation Advice	38	100%	98%	99%
Chest Pain/Possible Heart Attack Care				
Aspirin at Arrival	-	-	0%	95%
Median Time to ECG (minutes)	-	-	0	8
Median Time to Transfer (minutes)	-	-	0	61
Fibrinolytic Medication Timing	-	-	0%	54%
Heart Failure Care				
ACE Inhibitor or ARB for LVSD[2]	108	90%	94%	94%
Discharge Instructions[2]	198	99%	86%	88%
Evaluation of LVS Function[2]	288	98%	97%	98%
Smoking Cessation Advice[1,2]	7	100%	98%	98%
Pneumonia Care				
Appropriate Initial Antibiotic[2]	146	88%	92%	92%
Blood Culture Timing[2]	241	86%	92%	96%
Influenza Vaccine[2]	133	80%	88%	91%
Initial Antibiotic Timing[2]	209	96%	94%	95%
Pneumococcal Vaccine[2]	224	73%	92%	93%
Smoking Cessation Advice[1,2]	21	100%	97%	97%
Surgical Care Improvement Project				
Appropriate VTP Within 24 Hours[2]	258	92%	90%	92%
Appropriate Hair Removal[2]	1,268	100%	100%	99%
Appropriate Beta Blocker Usage[2]	384	98%	91%	93%
Controlled Postoperative Blood Glucose[2]	205	93%	91%	93%
Prophylactic Antibiotic Timing[2]	1,065	95%	96%	97%
Prophylactic Antibiotic Timing (Outpatient)	-	-	0%	92%
Prophylactic Antibiotic Selection[2]	1,067	97%	97%	97%
Prophylactic Antibiotic Select. (Outpatient)	-	-	0%	94%
Prophylactic Antibiotic Stopped[2]	1,058	94%	94%	94%
Recommended VTP Ordered[2]	261	91%	92%	94%
Urinary Catheter Removal[2]	337	99%	89%	90%
Children's Asthma Care				
Received Systemic Corticosteroids	-	-	-	100%
Received Home Management Plan	-	-	-	71%
Received Reliever Medication	-	-	-	100%
Use of Medical Imaging				
Combination Abdominal CT Scan	-	-	0.064	0.191
Combination Chest CT Scan	-	-	0.013	0.054
Follow-up Mammogram/Ultrasound	-	-	8.6%	8.4%
MRI for Low Back Pain	-	-	31.7%	32.7%
Survey of Patients' Hospital Experiences				
Area Around Room 'Always' Quiet at Night	300+	51%	-	58%
Doctors 'Always' Communicated Well	300+	79%	-	80%
Home Recovery Information Given	300+	79%	-	82%
Hospital Given 9 or 10 on 10 Point Scale	300+	62%	-	67%
Meds 'Always' Explained Before Given	300+	58%	-	60%
Nurses 'Always' Communicated Well	300+	69%	-	76%
Pain 'Always' Well Controlled	300+	65%	-	69%
Room and Bathroom 'Always' Clean	300+	63%	-	71%
Timely Help 'Always' Received	300+	54%	-	64%
Would Definitely Recommend Hospital	300+	73%	-	69%

Harbor Hospital

3001 S Hanover Street
Brooklyn, MD 21225
Phone: 410-350-3201
Fax: 410-350-2052
URL: www.harborhospital.org
Type: Acute Care Hospitals
Emergency Services: Yes
Ownership: Voluntary Non-Profit - Private
Beds: 182

Key Personnel:
CEO/President. . . . . David Pitman
Operating Room. . . . . Ashok Agrawal, RN
Pediatric In-Patient Care . . . . Shahid Aziz, MD
Quality Assurance . . . . Christine Swearingen
Radiology. . . . . Mohsen Gharib
Ambulatory Care . . . . Joel N Bryan
Anesthesiology. . . . . Allan Birenberg, MD
Emergency Room . . . . Tammy Kile, MD

Measure	Cases	This Hosp.	State Avg.	U.S. Avg.
Heart Attack Care				
ACE Inhibitor or ARB for LVSD[1]	4	100%	94%	96%
Aspirin at Arrival	42	100%	98%	99%
Aspirin at Discharge[1]	13	100%	98%	98%
Beta Blocker at Discharge[1]	14	100%	97%	98%
Fibrinolytic Medication Timing	0	-	42%	55%
PCI Within 90 Minutes of Arrival	0	-	83%	90%
Smoking Cessation Advice[1]	3	100%	98%	99%
Chest Pain/Possible Heart Attack Care				
Aspirin at Arrival	-	-	0%	95%
Median Time to ECG (minutes)	-	-	0	8
Median Time to Transfer (minutes)	-	-	0	61
Fibrinolytic Medication Timing	-	-	0%	54%
Heart Failure Care				
ACE Inhibitor or ARB for LVSD	129	91%	94%	94%
Discharge Instructions	309	79%	86%	88%
Evaluation of LVS Function	343	99%	97%	98%
Smoking Cessation Advice	114	98%	98%	98%
Pneumonia Care				
Appropriate Initial Antibiotic	254	89%	92%	92%
Blood Culture Timing	356	93%	92%	96%
Influenza Vaccine	191	91%	88%	91%
Initial Antibiotic Timing	341	97%	94%	95%
Pneumococcal Vaccine	215	91%	92%	93%
Smoking Cessation Advice	218	99%	97%	97%
Surgical Care Improvement Project				
Appropriate VTP Within 24 Hours[2]	199	91%	90%	92%
Appropriate Hair Removal[2]	820	99%	100%	99%
Appropriate Beta Blocker Usage[2]	194	91%	91%	93%
Controlled Postoperative Blood Glucose[2]	0	-	91%	93%
Prophylactic Antibiotic Timing[2]	665	97%	96%	97%
Prophylactic Antibiotic Timing (Outpatient)	-	-	0%	92%
Prophylactic Antibiotic Selection[2]	669	94%	97%	97%
Prophylactic Antibiotic Select. (Outpatient)	-	-	0%	94%
Prophylactic Antibiotic Stopped[2]	653	92%	94%	94%
Recommended VTP Ordered[2]	199	93%	92%	94%
Urinary Catheter Removal[2]	141	86%	89%	90%
Children's Asthma Care				
Received Systemic Corticosteroids	-	-	-	100%
Received Home Management Plan	-	-	-	71%
Received Reliever Medication	-	-	-	100%
Use of Medical Imaging				
Combination Abdominal CT Scan	-	-	0.064	0.191
Combination Chest CT Scan	-	-	0.013	0.054
Follow-up Mammogram/Ultrasound	-	-	8.6%	8.4%
MRI for Low Back Pain	-	-	31.7%	32.7%
Survey of Patients' Hospital Experiences				
Area Around Room 'Always' Quiet at Night	300+	55%	-	58%
Doctors 'Always' Communicated Well	300+	78%	-	80%
Home Recovery Information Given	300+	79%	-	82%
Hospital Given 9 or 10 on 10 Point Scale	300+	65%	-	67%
Meds 'Always' Explained Before Given	300+	56%	-	60%
Nurses 'Always' Communicated Well	300+	74%	-	76%
Pain 'Always' Well Controlled	300+	65%	-	69%
Room and Bathroom 'Always' Clean	300+	58%	-	71%
Timely Help 'Always' Received	300+	52%	-	64%
Would Definitely Recommend Hospital	300+	66%	-	69%

NOTE: Hospital profiles are in alphabetical order by state, then city, then hospital within the city; Rankings exclude hospitals with less than 25 cases except for patient surveys which excludes hospitals with less than 100 cases; (a) 100–299 cases; (1) The number of cases is too small to be sure how well a hospital is performing; (2) The hospital indicated that the data submitted for this measure were based on a sample of cases; (3) Data was collected during a shorter time period (fewer quarters) than the maximum possible time for this measure; (4) Suppressed for one or more quarters by CMS; (5) No data is available from the hospital for this measure; (6) Fewer than 100 patients completed the HCAHPS survey. Use these rates with caution, as the number of surveys may be too low to reliably assess hospital performance; (7) Survey results are based on less than 12 months of data; (8) Survey results are not available for this reporting period; (9) No or very few patients were eligible for the HCAHPS survey. The scores shown, if any, reflect a very small number of surveys; (10) A state average was not calculated because too few hospitals in the state submitted data; (11) There were discrepancies in the data collection process; Please refer to the User's Guide for a full explanation of data.

Chester River Hospital Center

100 Brown St | Phone: 410-778-7668
Chestertown, MD 21620
Type: Acute Care Hospitals | Emergency Services: Yes
Ownership: Voluntary Non-Profit - Private

Key Personnel:
CEO/President. . . . . William R Kirk Jr

Measure	Cases	This Hosp.	State Avg.	U.S. Avg.
Heart Attack Care				
ACE Inhibitor or ARB for LVSD[1,3]	3	67%	94%	96%
Aspirin at Arrival[1,3]	12	83%	98%	99%
Aspirin at Discharge[1,3]	8	88%	98%	98%
Beta Blocker at Discharge[1,3]	9	89%	97%	98%
Fibrinolytic Medication Timing[3]	0	-	42%	55%
PCI Within 90 Minutes of Arrival[3]	0	-	83%	90%
Smoking Cessation Advice[1,3]	1	100%	98%	99%
Chest Pain/Possible Heart Attack Care				
Aspirin at Arrival	-	-	0%	95%
Median Time to ECG (minutes)	-	-	0	8
Median Time to Transfer (minutes)	-	-	0	61
Fibrinolytic Medication Timing	-	-	0%	54%
Heart Failure Care				
ACE Inhibitor or ARB for LVSD	41	85%	94%	94%
Discharge Instructions	97	76%	86%	88%
Evaluation of LVS Function	126	90%	97%	98%
Smoking Cessation Advice[1]	20	95%	98%	98%
Pneumonia Care				
Appropriate Initial Antibiotic[3]	29	100%	92%	92%
Blood Culture Timing[3]	37	89%	92%	96%
Influenza Vaccine	50	92%	88%	91%
Initial Antibiotic Timing[3]	41	95%	94%	95%
Pneumococcal Vaccine[3]	54	96%	92%	93%
Smoking Cessation Advice[1,3]	14	93%	97%	97%
Surgical Care Improvement Project				
Appropriate VTP Within 24 Hours	54	61%	90%	92%
Appropriate Hair Removal	135	99%	100%	99%
Appropriate Beta Blocker Usage	39	100%	91%	93%
Controlled Postoperative Blood Glucose	0	-	91%	93%
Prophylactic Antibiotic Timing	95	84%	96%	97%
Prophylactic Antibiotic Timing (Outpatient)	-	-	0%	92%
Prophylactic Antibiotic Selection	95	93%	97%	97%
Prophylactic Antibiotic Select. (Outpatient)	-	-	0%	94%
Prophylactic Antibiotic Stopped	91	88%	94%	94%
Recommended VTP Ordered	54	61%	92%	94%
Urinary Catheter Removal	33	73%	89%	90%
Children's Asthma Care				
Received Systemic Corticosteroids	-	-	-	100%
Received Home Management Plan	-	-	-	71%
Received Reliever Medication	-	-	-	100%
Use of Medical Imaging				
Combination Abdominal CT Scan	-	-	0.064	0.191
Combination Chest CT Scan	-	-	0.013	0.054
Follow-up Mammogram/Ultrasound	-	-	8.6%	8.4%
MRI for Low Back Pain	-	-	31.7%	32.7%
Survey of Patients' Hospital Experiences				
Area Around Room 'Always' Quiet at Night	300+	58%	-	58%
Doctors 'Always' Communicated Well	300+	78%	-	80%
Home Recovery Information Given	300+	84%	-	82%
Hospital Given 9 or 10 on 10 Point Scale	300+	65%	-	67%
Meds 'Always' Explained Before Given	300+	61%	-	60%
Nurses 'Always' Communicated Well	300+	76%	-	76%
Pain 'Always' Well Controlled	300+	69%	-	69%
Room and Bathroom 'Always' Clean	300+	73%	-	71%
Timely Help 'Always' Received	300+	68%	-	64%
Would Definitely Recommend Hospital	300+	62%	-	69%

Prince Georges Hospital Center

3001 Hospital Drive | Phone: 301-618-2000
Cheverly, MD 20785 | Fax: 301-618-2547
URL: www.princegeorgeshospital.org
Type: Acute Care Hospitals | Emergency Services: Yes
Ownership: Voluntary Non-Profit - Private | Beds: 290

Key Personnel:
CEO/President. . . . . G.T, Dunlop Ecker
Chief of Medical Staff . . . . Shirley Morgan
Infection Control. . . . . Jackie Cohran
Pediatric Ambulatory Care . . . . . . Frederick Corder, MD
Pediatric In-Patient Care . . . . Frederick Corder, MD
Quality Assurance . . . . Brigid Krizek
Radiology. . . . . David Blanton, MD

Measure	Cases	This Hosp.	State Avg.	U.S. Avg.
Heart Attack Care				
ACE Inhibitor or ARB for LVSD	30	87%	94%	96%
Aspirin at Arrival	171	91%	98%	99%
Aspirin at Discharge	170	86%	98%	98%
Beta Blocker at Discharge	165	90%	97%	98%
Fibrinolytic Medication Timing	0	-	42%	55%
PCI Within 90 Minutes of Arrival	31	42%	83%	90%
Smoking Cessation Advice	64	98%	98%	99%
Chest Pain/Possible Heart Attack Care				
Aspirin at Arrival	-	-	0%	95%
Median Time to ECG (minutes)	-	-	0	8
Median Time to Transfer (minutes)	-	-	0	61
Fibrinolytic Medication Timing	-	-	0%	54%
Heart Failure Care				
ACE Inhibitor or ARB for LVSD[2]	105	89%	94%	94%
Discharge Instructions[2]	276	85%	86%	88%
Evaluation of LVS Function[2]	304	89%	97%	98%
Smoking Cessation Advice[2]	99	98%	98%	98%
Pneumonia Care				
Appropriate Initial Antibiotic[2]	63	84%	92%	92%
Blood Culture Timing[2]	84	87%	92%	96%
Influenza Vaccine[2]	73	47%	88%	91%
Initial Antibiotic Timing[2]	46	85%	94%	95%
Pneumococcal Vaccine[2]	88	47%	92%	93%
Smoking Cessation Advice[2]	60	90%	97%	97%
Surgical Care Improvement Project				
Appropriate VTP Within 24 Hours[2]	105	45%	90%	92%
Appropriate Hair Removal[2]	250	99%	100%	99%
Appropriate Beta Blocker Usage[5]	0	-	91%	93%
Controlled Postoperative Blood Glucose[1,2]	14	86%	91%	93%
Prophylactic Antibiotic Timing[2]	135	91%	96%	97%
Prophylactic Antibiotic Timing (Outpatient)	-	-	0%	92%
Prophylactic Antibiotic Selection[2]	137	93%	97%	97%
Prophylactic Antibiotic Select. (Outpatient)	-	-	0%	94%
Prophylactic Antibiotic Stopped[2]	126	75%	94%	94%
Recommended VTP Ordered[2]	105	50%	92%	94%
Urinary Catheter Removal[2]	48	65%	89%	90%
Children's Asthma Care				
Received Systemic Corticosteroids[1]	7	100%	-	100%
Received Home Management Plan[1]	7	0%	-	71%
Received Reliever Medication[1]	7	100%	-	100%
Use of Medical Imaging				
Combination Abdominal CT Scan	-	-	0.064	0.191
Combination Chest CT Scan	-	-	0.013	0.054
Follow-up Mammogram/Ultrasound	-	-	8.6%	8.4%
MRI for Low Back Pain	-	-	31.7%	32.7%
Survey of Patients' Hospital Experiences				
Area Around Room 'Always' Quiet at Night	300+	49%	-	58%
Doctors 'Always' Communicated Well	300+	69%	-	80%
Home Recovery Information Given	300+	73%	-	82%
Hospital Given 9 or 10 on 10 Point Scale	300+	44%	-	67%
Meds 'Always' Explained Before Given	300+	49%	-	60%
Nurses 'Always' Communicated Well	300+	60%	-	76%
Pain 'Always' Well Controlled	300+	56%	-	69%
Room and Bathroom 'Always' Clean	300+	59%	-	71%
Timely Help 'Always' Received	300+	39%	-	64%
Would Definitely Recommend Hospital	300+	41%	-	69%

Southern Maryland Hospital Center

7503 Surratts Rd | Phone: 301-877-4530
Clinton, MD 20735 | Fax: 301-877-9687
URL: www.smhchealth.org
Type: Acute Care Hospitals | Emergency Services: Yes
Ownership: Proprietary | Beds: 358

Key Personnel:
CEO/President. . . . . Michael J Chiatamonte
Radiology. . . . . Daniel Njinimbot
Intensive Care Unit. . . . . Sandy McClean RN

Measure	Cases	This Hosp.	State Avg.	U.S. Avg.
Heart Attack Care				
ACE Inhibitor or ARB for LVSD	34	85%	94%	96%
Aspirin at Arrival	159	96%	98%	99%
Aspirin at Discharge	123	98%	98%	98%
Beta Blocker at Discharge	118	97%	97%	98%
Fibrinolytic Medication Timing[1]	2	100%	42%	55%
PCI Within 90 Minutes of Arrival	38	87%	83%	90%
Smoking Cessation Advice	43	100%	98%	99%
Chest Pain/Possible Heart Attack Care				
Aspirin at Arrival	-	-	0%	95%
Median Time to ECG (minutes)	-	-	0	8
Median Time to Transfer (minutes)	-	-	0	61
Fibrinolytic Medication Timing	-	-	0%	54%
Heart Failure Care				
ACE Inhibitor or ARB for LVSD	277	94%	94%	94%
Discharge Instructions	661	94%	86%	88%
Evaluation of LVS Function	752	98%	97%	98%
Smoking Cessation Advice	123	100%	98%	98%
Pneumonia Care				
Appropriate Initial Antibiotic[2]	123	89%	92%	92%
Blood Culture Timing[2]	160	85%	92%	96%
Influenza Vaccine[2]	95	95%	88%	91%
Initial Antibiotic Timing[2]	182	93%	94%	95%
Pneumococcal Vaccine[2]	131	96%	92%	93%
Smoking Cessation Advice[2]	66	100%	97%	97%
Surgical Care Improvement Project				
Appropriate VTP Within 24 Hours[2]	208	94%	90%	92%
Appropriate Hair Removal[2]	682	100%	100%	99%
Appropriate Beta Blocker Usage[2]	153	93%	91%	93%
Controlled Postoperative Blood Glucose[2]	0	-	91%	93%
Prophylactic Antibiotic Timing[2]	476	99%	96%	97%
Prophylactic Antibiotic Timing (Outpatient)	-	-	0%	92%
Prophylactic Antibiotic Selection[2]	481	95%	97%	97%
Prophylactic Antibiotic Select. (Outpatient)	-	-	0%	94%
Prophylactic Antibiotic Stopped[2]	460	95%	94%	94%
Recommended VTP Ordered[2]	208	97%	92%	94%
Urinary Catheter Removal[2]	69	91%	89%	90%
Children's Asthma Care				
Received Systemic Corticosteroids	-	-	-	100%
Received Home Management Plan	-	-	-	71%
Received Reliever Medication	-	-	-	100%
Use of Medical Imaging				
Combination Abdominal CT Scan	-	-	0.064	0.191
Combination Chest CT Scan	-	-	0.013	0.054
Follow-up Mammogram/Ultrasound	-	-	8.6%	8.4%
MRI for Low Back Pain	-	-	31.7%	32.7%
Survey of Patients' Hospital Experiences				
Area Around Room 'Always' Quiet at Night	300+	43%	-	58%
Doctors 'Always' Communicated Well	300+	72%	-	80%
Home Recovery Information Given	300+	71%	-	82%
Hospital Given 9 or 10 on 10 Point Scale	300+	42%	-	67%
Meds 'Always' Explained Before Given	300+	52%	-	60%
Nurses 'Always' Communicated Well	300+	66%	-	76%
Pain 'Always' Well Controlled	300+	64%	-	69%
Room and Bathroom 'Always' Clean	300+	53%	-	71%
Timely Help 'Always' Received	300+	52%	-	64%
Would Definitely Recommend Hospital	300+	42%	-	69%

NOTE: Hospital profiles are in alphabetical order by state, then city, then hospital within the city; Rankings exclude hospitals with less than 25 cases except for patient surveys which excludes hospitals with less than 100 cases; (a) 100–299 cases; (1) The number of cases is too small to be sure how well a hospital is performing; (2) The hospital indicated that the data submitted for this measure were based on a sample of cases; (3) Data was collected during a shorter time period (fewer quarters) than the maximum possible time for this measure; (4) Suppressed for one or more quarters by CMS; (5) No data is available from the hospital for this measure; (6) Fewer than 100 patients completed the HCAHPS survey. Use these rates with caution, as the number of surveys may be too low to reliably assess hospital performance; (7) Survey results are based on less than 12 months of data; (8) Survey results are not available for this reporting period; (9) No or very few patients were eligible for the HCAHPS survey. The scores shown, if any, reflect a very small number of surveys; (10) A state average was not calculated because too few hospitals in the state submitted data; (11) There were discrepancies in the data collection process; Please refer to the User's Guide for a full explanation of data.

Howard County General Hospital

5755 Cedar Lane
Columbia, MD 21044
URL: www.hcgh.org
Type: Acute Care Hospitals
Ownership: Voluntary Non-Profit - Private

Phone: 410-740-7710
Fax: 410-740-7610

Emergency Services: Yes
Beds: 208

Key Personnel:
Chief of Medical Staff . . . . Jonathan Fish, MD
Operating Room. . . . . Francine Black
Quality Assurance . . . . Judy Brown
Radiology. . . . . John Dunn

Measure	Cases	This Hosp.	State Avg.	U.S. Avg.
Heart Attack Care				
ACE Inhibitor or ARB for LVSD[1]	10	100%	94%	96%
Aspirin at Arrival	129	98%	98%	99%
Aspirin at Discharge	90	100%	98%	98%
Beta Blocker at Discharge	90	99%	97%	98%
Fibrinolytic Medication Timing	0	-	42%	55%
PCI Within 90 Minutes of Arrival	64	78%	83%	90%
Smoking Cessation Advice	30	100%	98%	99%
Chest Pain/Possible Heart Attack Care				
Aspirin at Arrival	-	-	0%	95%
Median Time to ECG (minutes)	-	-	0	8
Median Time to Transfer (minutes)	-	-	0	61
Fibrinolytic Medication Timing	-	-	0%	54%
Heart Failure Care				
ACE Inhibitor or ARB for LVSD[2]	77	96%	94%	94%
Discharge Instructions[2]	217	94%	86%	88%
Evaluation of LVS Function[2]	281	99%	97%	98%
Smoking Cessation Advice[1,2]	21	100%	98%	98%
Pneumonia Care				
Appropriate Initial Antibiotic[2]	84	95%	92%	92%
Blood Culture Timing[2]	110	84%	92%	96%
Influenza Vaccine[2]	79	91%	88%	91%
Initial Antibiotic Timing[2]	95	97%	94%	95%
Pneumococcal Vaccine[2]	122	91%	92%	93%
Smoking Cessation Advice[2]	35	100%	97%	97%
Surgical Care Improvement Project				
Appropriate VTP Within 24 Hours[2]	144	93%	90%	92%
Appropriate Hair Removal[2]	440	100%	100%	99%
Appropriate Beta Blocker Usage[2]	88	88%	91%	93%
Controlled Postoperative Blood Glucose[2]	0	-	91%	93%
Prophylactic Antibiotic Timing[2]	265	99%	96%	97%
Prophylactic Antibiotic Timing (Outpatient)	-	-	0%	92%
Prophylactic Antibiotic Selection[2]	266	98%	97%	97%
Prophylactic Antibiotic Select. (Outpatient)	-	-	0%	94%
Prophylactic Antibiotic Stopped[2]	246	91%	94%	94%
Recommended VTP Ordered[2]	144	97%	92%	94%
Urinary Catheter Removal[2]	80	92%	89%	90%
Children's Asthma Care				
Received Systemic Corticosteroids	-	-	-	100%
Received Home Management Plan	-	-	-	71%
Received Reliever Medication	-	-	-	100%
Use of Medical Imaging				
Combination Abdominal CT Scan	-	-	0.064	0.191
Combination Chest CT Scan	-	-	0.013	0.054
Follow-up Mammogram/Ultrasound	-	-	8.6%	8.4%
MRI for Low Back Pain	-	-	31.7%	32.7%
Survey of Patients' Hospital Experiences				
Area Around Room 'Always' Quiet at Night	300+	53%	-	58%
Doctors 'Always' Communicated Well	300+	75%	-	80%
Home Recovery Information Given	300+	81%	-	82%
Hospital Given 9 or 10 on 10 Point Scale	300+	64%	-	67%
Meds 'Always' Explained Before Given	300+	54%	-	60%
Nurses 'Always' Communicated Well	300+	72%	-	76%
Pain 'Always' Well Controlled	300+	66%	-	69%
Room and Bathroom 'Always' Clean	300+	70%	-	71%
Timely Help 'Always' Received	300+	56%	-	64%
Would Definitely Recommend Hospital	300+	71%	-	69%

Edward Mccready Memorial Hospital

201 Hall Highway
Crisfield, MD 21817
E-mail: mccreadyhospital@aol.com
Type: Acute Care Hospitals
Ownership: Voluntary Non-Profit - Private

Phone: 410-968-3011
Fax: 410-968-3005

Emergency Services: Yes
Beds: 104

Key Personnel:
CEO/President. . . . . Charles F Pinkernan
Chief of Medical Staff . . . . Michael Atkins
Radiology. . . . . t Mary Lynne Everett

Measure	Cases	This Hosp.	State Avg.	U.S. Avg.
Heart Attack Care				
ACE Inhibitor or ARB for LVSD[3]	0	-	94%	96%
Aspirin at Arrival[1,3]	2	100%	98%	99%
Aspirin at Discharge[1,3]	2	100%	98%	98%
Beta Blocker at Discharge[1,3]	2	100%	97%	98%
Fibrinolytic Medication Timing[3]	0	-	42%	55%
PCI Within 90 Minutes of Arrival[3]	0	-	83%	90%
Smoking Cessation Advice[3]	0	-	98%	99%
Chest Pain/Possible Heart Attack Care				
Aspirin at Arrival	-	-	0%	95%
Median Time to ECG (minutes)	-	-	0	8
Median Time to Transfer (minutes)	-	-	0	61
Fibrinolytic Medication Timing	-	-	0%	54%
Heart Failure Care				
ACE Inhibitor or ARB for LVSD[1,3]	9	100%	94%	94%
Discharge Instructions[1,3]	14	79%	86%	88%
Evaluation of LVS Function[1,3]	20	100%	97%	98%
Smoking Cessation Advice[1,3]	5	100%	98%	98%
Pneumonia Care				
Appropriate Initial Antibiotic[1,3]	14	79%	92%	92%
Blood Culture Timing[1,3]	16	100%	92%	96%
Influenza Vaccine[1]	15	100%	88%	91%
Initial Antibiotic Timing[1,3]	21	100%	94%	95%
Pneumococcal Vaccine[1,3]	17	94%	92%	93%
Smoking Cessation Advice[1,3]	3	100%	97%	97%
Surgical Care Improvement Project				
Appropriate VTP Within 24 Hours[1,3]	4	100%	90%	92%
Appropriate Hair Removal[1,3]	4	100%	100%	99%
Appropriate Beta Blocker Usage[1,3]	2	100%	91%	93%
Controlled Postoperative Blood Glucose[3]	0	-	91%	93%
Prophylactic Antibiotic Timing[1,3]	2	100%	96%	97%
Prophylactic Antibiotic Timing (Outpatient)	-	-	0%	92%
Prophylactic Antibiotic Selection[1,3]	2	100%	97%	97%
Prophylactic Antibiotic Select. (Outpatient)	-	-	0%	94%
Prophylactic Antibiotic Stopped[1,3]	2	100%	94%	94%
Recommended VTP Ordered[1,3]	4	100%	92%	94%
Urinary Catheter Removal[1,3]	2	100%	89%	90%
Children's Asthma Care				
Received Systemic Corticosteroids	-	-	-	100%
Received Home Management Plan	-	-	-	71%
Received Reliever Medication	-	-	-	100%
Use of Medical Imaging				
Combination Abdominal CT Scan	-	-	0.064	0.191
Combination Chest CT Scan	-	-	0.013	0.054
Follow-up Mammogram/Ultrasound	-	-	8.6%	8.4%
MRI for Low Back Pain	-	-	31.7%	32.7%
Survey of Patients' Hospital Experiences				
Area Around Room 'Always' Quiet at Night	(a)	61%	-	58%
Doctors 'Always' Communicated Well	(a)	86%	-	80%
Home Recovery Information Given	(a)	87%	-	82%
Hospital Given 9 or 10 on 10 Point Scale	(a)	73%	-	67%
Meds 'Always' Explained Before Given	(a)	68%	-	60%
Nurses 'Always' Communicated Well	(a)	86%	-	76%
Pain 'Always' Well Controlled	(a)	80%	-	69%
Room and Bathroom 'Always' Clean	(a)	78%	-	71%
Timely Help 'Always' Received	(a)	80%	-	64%
Would Definitely Recommend Hospital	(a)	74%	-	69%

Memorial Hospital & Medical Center of Cumberland

600 Memorial Ave
Cumberland, MD 21502
E-mail: cruffo@wmhs.com
Type: Acute Care Hospitals
Ownership: Voluntary Non-Profit - Private

Phone: 301-723-4000
Fax: 301-723-4045

Emergency Services: Yes
Beds: 222

Key Personnel:
CEO/President. . . . . Barry Ronan
Chief of Medical Staff . . . . Dr. James Rower
Coronary Care . . . . Pat Foley
Operating Room. . . . . Shelley Miller
Pediatric Ambulatory Care . . . . . . Debbie Jenkins
Pediatric In-Patient Care . . . . Debbie Jenkins
Quality Assurance . . . . Mary Ann Bloom
Radiology. . . . . Steve Black

Measure	Cases	This Hosp.	State Avg.	U.S. Avg.
Heart Attack Care				
ACE Inhibitor or ARB for LVSD[1,3]	1	100%	94%	96%
Aspirin at Arrival[1,3]	12	92%	98%	99%
Aspirin at Discharge[1,3]	8	100%	98%	98%
Beta Blocker at Discharge[1,3]	9	100%	97%	98%
Fibrinolytic Medication Timing[3]	0	-	42%	55%
PCI Within 90 Minutes of Arrival[3]	0	-	83%	90%
Smoking Cessation Advice[3]	0	-	98%	99%
Chest Pain/Possible Heart Attack Care				
Aspirin at Arrival[5]	0	-	0%	95%
Median Time to ECG (minutes)[5]	0	-	0	8
Median Time to Transfer (minutes)[5]	0	-	0	61
Fibrinolytic Medication Timing[5]	0	-	0%	54%
Heart Failure Care				
ACE Inhibitor or ARB for LVSD[1,3]	18	83%	94%	94%
Discharge Instructions[3]	34	82%	86%	88%
Evaluation of LVS Function[3]	50	96%	97%	98%
Smoking Cessation Advice[1,3]	7	100%	98%	98%
Pneumonia Care				
Appropriate Initial Antibiotic[3]	31	81%	92%	92%
Blood Culture Timing[3]	26	92%	92%	96%
Influenza Vaccine[1,3]	21	76%	88%	91%
Initial Antibiotic Timing[3]	46	83%	94%	95%
Pneumococcal Vaccine[3]	28	68%	92%	93%
Smoking Cessation Advice[1,3]	21	90%	97%	97%
Surgical Care Improvement Project				
Appropriate VTP Within 24 Hours[3]	48	83%	90%	92%
Appropriate Hair Removal[3]	245	100%	100%	99%
Appropriate Beta Blocker Usage[3]	90	80%	91%	93%
Controlled Postoperative Blood Glucose[3]	0	-	91%	93%
Prophylactic Antibiotic Timing[3]	190	91%	96%	97%
Prophylactic Antibiotic Timing (Outpatient)[5]	0	-	0%	92%
Prophylactic Antibiotic Selection[3]	194	99%	97%	97%
Prophylactic Antibiotic Select. (Outpatient)[5]	0	-	0%	94%
Prophylactic Antibiotic Stopped[3]	189	89%	94%	94%
Recommended VTP Ordered[3]	50	84%	92%	94%
Urinary Catheter Removal	0	-	89%	90%
Children's Asthma Care				
Received Systemic Corticosteroids	-	-	-	100%
Received Home Management Plan	-	-	-	71%
Received Reliever Medication	-	-	-	100%
Use of Medical Imaging				
Combination Abdominal CT Scan	476	0.017	0.064	0.191
Combination Chest CT Scan	377	0.003	0.013	0.054
Follow-up Mammogram/Ultrasound[5]	0	-	8.6%	8.4%
MRI for Low Back Pain[1]	1	0.0%	31.7%	32.7%
Survey of Patients' Hospital Experiences				
Area Around Room 'Always' Quiet at Night[8]	-	-	-	58%
Doctors 'Always' Communicated Well[8]	-	-	-	80%
Home Recovery Information Given[8]	-	-	-	82%
Hospital Given 9 or 10 on 10 Point Scale[8]	-	-	-	67%
Meds 'Always' Explained Before Given[8]	-	-	-	60%
Nurses 'Always' Communicated Well[8]	-	-	-	76%
Pain 'Always' Well Controlled[8]	-	-	-	69%
Room and Bathroom 'Always' Clean[8]	-	-	-	71%
Timely Help 'Always' Received[8]	-	-	-	64%
Would Definitely Recommend Hospital[8]	-	-	-	69%

NOTE: Hospital profiles are in alphabetical order by state, then city, then hospital within the city; Rankings exclude hospitals with less than 25 cases except for patient surveys which excludes hospitals with less than 100 cases; (a) 100–299 cases; (1) The number of cases is too small to be sure how well a hospital is performing; (2) The hospital indicated that the data submitted for this measure were based on a shorter time period (fewer quarters) than the maximum possible time for this measure; (4) Suppressed for one or more quarters by CMS; (5) No data is available from the hospital for this measure; (6) Fewer than 100 patients completed the HCAHPS survey. Use these rates with caution, as the number of surveys may be too low to reliably assess hospital performance; (7) Survey results are based on less than 12 months of data; (8) Survey results are not available for this reporting period; (9) No or very few patients were eligible for the HCAHPS survey. The scores shown, if any, reflect a very small number of surveys; (10) A state average was not calculated because too few hospitals in the state submitted data; (11) There were discrepancies in the data collection process; Please refer to the User's Guide for a full explanation of data.

Western Maryland Regional Medical Center

12500 Willowbrook Road   Phone: 240-964-8001
Cumberland, MD 21502
URL: www.wmhs.com
Type: Acute Care Hospitals   Emergency Services: Yes
Ownership: Voluntary Non-Profit - Private   Beds: 275

Measure	Cases	This Hosp.	State Avg.	U.S. Avg.
Heart Attack Care				
ACE Inhibitor or ARB for LVSD	46	83%	94%	96%
Aspirin at Arrival	193	97%	98%	99%
Aspirin at Discharge	219	98%	98%	98%
Beta Blocker at Discharge	213	91%	97%	98%
Fibrinolytic Medication Timing	0	-	42%	55%
PCI Within 90 Minutes of Arrival[1]	7	86%	83%	90%
Smoking Cessation Advice	86	99%	98%	99%
Chest Pain/Possible Heart Attack Care				
Aspirin at Arrival[5]	0	-	0%	95%
Median Time to ECG (minutes)[5]	0	-	0	8
Median Time to Transfer (minutes)[5]	0	-	0	61
Fibrinolytic Medication Timing[5]	0	-	0%	54%
Heart Failure Care				
ACE Inhibitor or ARB for LVSD	183	93%	94%	94%
Discharge Instructions	361	84%	86%	88%
Evaluation of LVS Function	472	99%	97%	98%
Smoking Cessation Advice	51	98%	98%	98%
Pneumonia Care				
Appropriate Initial Antibiotic	183	84%	92%	92%
Blood Culture Timing	180	91%	92%	96%
Influenza Vaccine	196	82%	88%	91%
Initial Antibiotic Timing	267	85%	94%	95%
Pneumococcal Vaccine	260	87%	92%	93%
Smoking Cessation Advice	87	90%	97%	97%
Surgical Care Improvement Project				
Appropriate VTP Within 24 Hours	214	79%	90%	92%
Appropriate Hair Removal	768	100%	100%	99%
Appropriate Beta Blocker Usage	263	83%	91%	93%
Controlled Postoperative Blood Glucose	206	88%	91%	93%
Prophylactic Antibiotic Timing	503	91%	96%	97%
Prophylactic Antibiotic Timing (Outpatient)[5]	0	-	0%	92%
Prophylactic Antibiotic Selection	512	98%	97%	97%
Prophylactic Antibiotic Select. (Outpatient)[5]	0	-	0%	94%
Prophylactic Antibiotic Stopped	488	88%	94%	94%
Recommended VTP Ordered	216	80%	92%	94%
Urinary Catheter Removal	76	63%	89%	90%
Children's Asthma Care				
Received Systemic Corticosteroids	-	-	-	100%
Received Home Management Plan	-	-	-	71%
Received Reliever Medication	-	-	-	100%
Use of Medical Imaging				
Combination Abdominal CT Scan	1,176	0.062	0.064	0.191
Combination Chest CT Scan	1,007	0.010	0.013	0.054
Follow-up Mammogram/Ultrasound	1,400	7.4%	8.6%	8.4%
MRI for Low Back Pain	183	36.1%	31.7%	32.7%
Survey of Patients' Hospital Experiences				
Area Around Room 'Always' Quiet at Night	300+	48%	-	58%
Doctors 'Always' Communicated Well	300+	75%	-	80%
Home Recovery Information Given	300+	83%	-	82%
Hospital Given 9 or 10 on 10 Point Scale	300+	60%	-	67%
Meds 'Always' Explained Before Given	300+	53%	-	60%
Nurses 'Always' Communicated Well	300+	71%	-	76%
Pain 'Always' Well Controlled	300+	65%	-	69%
Room and Bathroom 'Always' Clean	300+	69%	-	71%
Timely Help 'Always' Received	300+	61%	-	64%
Would Definitely Recommend Hospital	300+	64%	-	69%

Memorial Hospital at Easton

219 S Washington St   Phone: 410-822-1000
Easton, MD 21601   Fax: 410-740-8603
URL: www.shorehealth.org
Type: Acute Care Hospitals   Emergency Services: Yes
Ownership: Voluntary Non-Profit - Private   Beds: 250
Key Personnel:
CEO/President . . . . Joseph Ross
Chief of Medical Staff . . . . John Condit, MD
Pediatric Ambulatory Care . . . . . . Brian Corden
Pediatric In-Patient Care . . . . Brian Corden
Quality Assurance . . . . Jeanne Lusby
Radiology . . . . Stephen Brigham

Measure	Cases	This Hosp.	State Avg.	U.S. Avg.
Heart Attack Care				
ACE Inhibitor or ARB for LVSD[1]	11	91%	94%	96%
Aspirin at Arrival	84	100%	98%	99%
Aspirin at Discharge	47	100%	98%	98%
Beta Blocker at Discharge	46	98%	97%	98%
Fibrinolytic Medication Timing[1]	12	42%	42%	55%
PCI Within 90 Minutes of Arrival[5]	0	-	83%	90%
Smoking Cessation Advice[1]	13	100%	98%	99%
Chest Pain/Possible Heart Attack Care				
Aspirin at Arrival	-	-	0%	95%
Median Time to ECG (minutes)	-	-	0	8
Median Time to Transfer (minutes)	-	-	0	61
Fibrinolytic Medication Timing	-	-	0%	54%
Heart Failure Care				
ACE Inhibitor or ARB for LVSD	154	94%	94%	94%
Discharge Instructions	420	75%	86%	88%
Evaluation of LVS Function	516	98%	97%	98%
Smoking Cessation Advice	90	100%	98%	98%
Pneumonia Care				
Appropriate Initial Antibiotic	216	94%	92%	92%
Blood Culture Timing	306	95%	92%	96%
Influenza Vaccine	162	86%	88%	91%
Initial Antibiotic Timing	293	97%	94%	95%
Pneumococcal Vaccine	260	91%	92%	93%
Smoking Cessation Advice	96	100%	97%	97%
Surgical Care Improvement Project				
Appropriate VTP Within 24 Hours	222	83%	90%	92%
Appropriate Hair Removal	881	100%	100%	99%
Appropriate Beta Blocker Usage	253	89%	91%	93%
Controlled Postoperative Blood Glucose	0	-	91%	93%
Prophylactic Antibiotic Timing	609	98%	96%	97%
Prophylactic Antibiotic Timing (Outpatient)	-	-	0%	92%
Prophylactic Antibiotic Selection	614	99%	97%	97%
Prophylactic Antibiotic Select. (Outpatient)	-	-	0%	94%
Prophylactic Antibiotic Stopped	601	98%	94%	94%
Recommended VTP Ordered	224	89%	92%	94%
Urinary Catheter Removal	217	91%	89%	90%
Children's Asthma Care				
Received Systemic Corticosteroids	-	-	-	100%
Received Home Management Plan	-	-	-	71%
Received Reliever Medication	-	-	-	100%
Use of Medical Imaging				
Combination Abdominal CT Scan	-	-	0.064	0.191
Combination Chest CT Scan	-	-	0.013	0.054
Follow-up Mammogram/Ultrasound	-	-	8.6%	8.4%
MRI for Low Back Pain	-	-	31.7%	32.7%
Survey of Patients' Hospital Experiences				
Area Around Room 'Always' Quiet at Night	300+	57%	-	58%
Doctors 'Always' Communicated Well	300+	81%	-	80%
Home Recovery Information Given	300+	86%	-	82%
Hospital Given 9 or 10 on 10 Point Scale	300+	70%	-	67%
Meds 'Always' Explained Before Given	300+	61%	-	60%
Nurses 'Always' Communicated Well	300+	79%	-	76%
Pain 'Always' Well Controlled	300+	72%	-	69%
Room and Bathroom 'Always' Clean	300+	71%	-	71%
Timely Help 'Always' Received	300+	68%	-	64%
Would Definitely Recommend Hospital	300+	68%	-	69%

Union Hospital of Cecil County

106 Bow Street   Phone: 410-392-7009
Elkton, MD 21921   Fax: 410-392-9486
URL: www.uhcc.com
Type: Acute Care Hospitals   Emergency Services: Yes
Ownership: Voluntary Non-Profit - Private   Beds: 116
Key Personnel:
CEO/President . . . . Kenneth S Lewis, MD
Chief of Medical Staff . . . . Paticia Clark
Infection Control . . . . Helen Paxton
Quality Assurance . . . . Michelle Adams
Radiology . . . . Constance Gerassimak
Emergency Room . . . . Jeffrey Tiongson, MD

Measure	Cases	This Hosp.	State Avg.	U.S. Avg.
Heart Attack Care				
ACE Inhibitor or ARB for LVSD[1]	5	100%	94%	96%
Aspirin at Arrival	55	100%	98%	99%
Aspirin at Discharge[1]	14	100%	98%	98%
Beta Blocker at Discharge[1]	16	94%	97%	98%
Fibrinolytic Medication Timing	0	-	42%	55%
PCI Within 90 Minutes of Arrival	0	-	83%	90%
Smoking Cessation Advice[1]	3	100%	98%	99%
Chest Pain/Possible Heart Attack Care				
Aspirin at Arrival	-	-	0%	95%
Median Time to ECG (minutes)	-	-	0	8
Median Time to Transfer (minutes)	-	-	0	61
Fibrinolytic Medication Timing	-	-	0%	54%
Heart Failure Care				
ACE Inhibitor or ARB for LVSD	68	96%	94%	94%
Discharge Instructions	161	93%	86%	88%
Evaluation of LVS Function	199	98%	97%	98%
Smoking Cessation Advice	45	89%	98%	98%
Pneumonia Care				
Appropriate Initial Antibiotic	116	92%	92%	92%
Blood Culture Timing	196	98%	92%	96%
Influenza Vaccine	115	100%	88%	91%
Initial Antibiotic Timing	202	94%	94%	95%
Pneumococcal Vaccine	165	96%	92%	93%
Smoking Cessation Advice	143	92%	97%	97%
Surgical Care Improvement Project				
Appropriate VTP Within 24 Hours	142	89%	90%	92%
Appropriate Hair Removal	429	100%	100%	99%
Appropriate Beta Blocker Usage	92	88%	91%	93%
Controlled Postoperative Blood Glucose	0	-	91%	93%
Prophylactic Antibiotic Timing	272	98%	96%	97%
Prophylactic Antibiotic Timing (Outpatient)	-	-	0%	92%
Prophylactic Antibiotic Selection	276	95%	97%	97%
Prophylactic Antibiotic Select. (Outpatient)	-	-	0%	94%
Prophylactic Antibiotic Stopped	261	94%	94%	94%
Recommended VTP Ordered	142	90%	92%	94%
Urinary Catheter Removal	98	91%	89%	90%
Children's Asthma Care				
Received Systemic Corticosteroids	-	-	-	100%
Received Home Management Plan	-	-	-	71%
Received Reliever Medication	-	-	-	100%
Use of Medical Imaging				
Combination Abdominal CT Scan	-	-	0.064	0.191
Combination Chest CT Scan	-	-	0.013	0.054
Follow-up Mammogram/Ultrasound	-	-	8.6%	8.4%
MRI for Low Back Pain	-	-	31.7%	32.7%
Survey of Patients' Hospital Experiences				
Area Around Room 'Always' Quiet at Night	300+	57%	-	58%
Doctors 'Always' Communicated Well	300+	81%	-	80%
Home Recovery Information Given	300+	82%	-	82%
Hospital Given 9 or 10 on 10 Point Scale	300+	68%	-	67%
Meds 'Always' Explained Before Given	300+	60%	-	60%
Nurses 'Always' Communicated Well	300+	76%	-	76%
Pain 'Always' Well Controlled	300+	67%	-	69%
Room and Bathroom 'Always' Clean	300+	66%	-	71%
Timely Help 'Always' Received	300+	57%	-	64%
Would Definitely Recommend Hospital	300+	65%	-	69%

NOTE: Hospital profiles are in alphabetical order by state, then city, then hospital within the city; Rankings exclude hospitals with less than 25 cases except for patient surveys which excludes hospitals with less than 100 cases; (a) 100–299 cases; (1) The number of cases is too small to be sure how well a hospital is performing; (2) The hospital indicated that the data submitted for this measure were based on a sample of cases; (3) Data was collected during a shorter time period (fewer quarters) than the maximum possible time for this measure; (4) Suppressed for one or more quarters by CMS; (5) No data is available from the hospital for this measure; (6) Fewer than 100 patients completed the HCAHPS survey. Use these rates with caution, as the number of surveys may be too low to reliably assess hospital performance; (7) Survey results are based on less than 12 months of data; (8) Survey results are not available for this reporting period; (9) No or very few patients were eligible for the HCAHPS survey. The scores shown, if any, reflect a very small number of surveys; (10) A state average was not calculated because too few hospitals in the state submitted data; (11) There were discrepancies in the data collection process; Please refer to the User's Guide for a full explanation of data.

Fort Washington Hospital

11711 Livingston Road
Fort Washington, MD 20744
URL: www.fortwashington.org
Type: Acute Care Hospitals
Ownership: Voluntary Non-Profit - Other

Phone: 301-292-7000
Fax: 301-203-2216

Emergency Services: Yes
Beds: 43

Key Personnel:
CEO/President . . . . Verna Meacham, CEO
Chief of Medical Staff . . . . Samir Azer, MD
Infection Control . . . . Carmen Resusseccion, RN
Operating Room . . . . Socorro Obedoza
Anesthesiology . . . . Christopher Smith, MD
Emergency Room . . . . Patrick Daly, MD
Intensive Care Unit . . . . Amir Mirza-Alikhani, MD

Measure	Cases	This Hosp.	State Avg.	U.S. Avg.
Heart Attack Care				
ACE Inhibitor or ARB for LVSD	0	-	94%	96%
Aspirin at Arrival[1]	4	100%	98%	99%
Aspirin at Discharge[1]	2	50%	98%	98%
Beta Blocker at Discharge[1]	3	33%	97%	98%
Fibrinolytic Medication Timing	0	-	42%	55%
PCI Within 90 Minutes of Arrival[5]	0	-	83%	90%
Smoking Cessation Advice	0	-	98%	99%
Chest Pain/Possible Heart Attack Care				
Aspirin at Arrival	-	-	0%	95%
Median Time to ECG (minutes)	-	-	0	8
Median Time to Transfer (minutes)	-	-	0	61
Fibrinolytic Medication Timing	-	-	0%	54%
Heart Failure Care				
ACE Inhibitor or ARB for LVSD	66	86%	94%	94%
Discharge Instructions	150	95%	86%	88%
Evaluation of LVS Function	170	94%	97%	98%
Smoking Cessation Advice[1]	21	100%	98%	98%
Pneumonia Care				
Appropriate Initial Antibiotic[1]	18	61%	92%	92%
Blood Culture Timing	106	91%	92%	96%
Influenza Vaccine	38	95%	88%	91%
Initial Antibiotic Timing	106	91%	94%	95%
Pneumococcal Vaccine	56	96%	92%	93%
Smoking Cessation Advice	25	100%	97%	97%
Surgical Care Improvement Project				
Appropriate VTP Within 24 Hours	75	92%	90%	92%
Appropriate Hair Removal	203	100%	100%	99%
Appropriate Beta Blocker Usage[1,3]	20	85%	91%	93%
Controlled Postoperative Blood Glucose[3]	0	-	91%	93%
Prophylactic Antibiotic Timing	130	92%	96%	97%
Prophylactic Antibiotic Timing (Outpatient)	-	-	0%	92%
Prophylactic Antibiotic Selection	133	92%	97%	97%
Prophylactic Antibiotic Select. (Outpatient)	-	-	0%	94%
Prophylactic Antibiotic Stopped	130	92%	94%	94%
Recommended VTP Ordered	75	92%	92%	94%
Urinary Catheter Removal[1]	17	65%	89%	90%
Children's Asthma Care				
Received Systemic Corticosteroids	-	-	-	100%
Received Home Management Plan	-	-	-	71%
Received Reliever Medication	-	-	-	100%
Use of Medical Imaging				
Combination Abdominal CT Scan	-	-	0.064	0.191
Combination Chest CT Scan	-	-	0.013	0.054
Follow-up Mammogram/Ultrasound	-	-	8.6%	8.4%
MRI for Low Back Pain	-	-	31.7%	32.7%
Survey of Patients' Hospital Experiences				
Area Around Room 'Always' Quiet at Night	300+	56%	-	58%
Doctors 'Always' Communicated Well	300+	76%	-	80%
Home Recovery Information Given	300+	75%	-	82%
Hospital Given 9 or 10 on 10 Point Scale	300+	53%	-	67%
Meds 'Always' Explained Before Given	300+	52%	-	60%
Nurses 'Always' Communicated Well	300+	70%	-	76%
Pain 'Always' Well Controlled	300+	63%	-	69%
Room and Bathroom 'Always' Clean	300+	61%	-	71%
Timely Help 'Always' Received	300+	57%	-	64%
Would Definitely Recommend Hospital	300+	56%	-	69%

Frederick Memorial Hospital

400 West Seventh St
Frederick, MD 21701
URL: www.fmh.org
Type: Acute Care Hospitals
Ownership: Voluntary Non-Profit - Private

Phone: 240-566-3300
Fax: 301-698-3292

Emergency Services: Yes
Beds: 253

Key Personnel:
CEO/President . . . . Thomas A Kleinhanzl
Cardiac Laboratory . . . . Michael Levangie
Chief of Medical Staff . . . . Gene Ashe
Operating Room . . . . Katherine Smith, RN
Pediatric In-Patient Care . . . . James Lee
Quality Assurance . . . . Craig Rosendale
Radiology . . . . Tom Bonnor
Emergency Room . . . . Laila Beaulieu

Measure	Cases	This Hosp.	State Avg.	U.S. Avg.
Heart Attack Care				
ACE Inhibitor or ARB for LVSD	27	96%	94%	96%
Aspirin at Arrival	164	97%	98%	99%
Aspirin at Discharge	134	98%	98%	98%
Beta Blocker at Discharge	135	97%	97%	98%
Fibrinolytic Medication Timing	0	-	42%	55%
PCI Within 90 Minutes of Arrival	63	98%	83%	90%
Smoking Cessation Advice	39	97%	98%	99%
Chest Pain/Possible Heart Attack Care				
Aspirin at Arrival	-	-	0%	95%
Median Time to ECG (minutes)	-	-	0	8
Median Time to Transfer (minutes)	-	-	0	61
Fibrinolytic Medication Timing	-	-	0%	54%
Heart Failure Care				
ACE Inhibitor or ARB for LVSD	153	93%	94%	94%
Discharge Instructions	378	76%	86%	88%
Evaluation of LVS Function	489	100%	97%	98%
Smoking Cessation Advice	45	100%	98%	98%
Pneumonia Care				
Appropriate Initial Antibiotic	250	97%	92%	92%
Blood Culture Timing	216	90%	92%	96%
Influenza Vaccine	236	93%	88%	91%
Initial Antibiotic Timing	411	96%	94%	95%
Pneumococcal Vaccine	415	96%	92%	93%
Smoking Cessation Advice	150	99%	97%	97%
Surgical Care Improvement Project				
Appropriate VTP Within 24 Hours[2]	172	91%	90%	92%
Appropriate Hair Removal[2]	730	100%	100%	99%
Appropriate Beta Blocker Usage[2]	241	93%	91%	93%
Controlled Postoperative Blood Glucose[2]	0	-	91%	93%
Prophylactic Antibiotic Timing[2]	590	98%	96%	97%
Prophylactic Antibiotic Timing (Outpatient)	-	-	0%	92%
Prophylactic Antibiotic Selection[2]	589	99%	97%	97%
Prophylactic Antibiotic Select. (Outpatient)	-	-	0%	94%
Prophylactic Antibiotic Stopped[2]	569	93%	94%	94%
Recommended VTP Ordered[2]	172	92%	92%	94%
Urinary Catheter Removal[2]	288	95%	89%	90%
Children's Asthma Care				
Received Systemic Corticosteroids	-	-	-	100%
Received Home Management Plan	-	-	-	71%
Received Reliever Medication	-	-	-	100%
Use of Medical Imaging				
Combination Abdominal CT Scan	-	-	0.064	0.191
Combination Chest CT Scan	-	-	0.013	0.054
Follow-up Mammogram/Ultrasound	-	-	8.6%	8.4%
MRI for Low Back Pain	-	-	31.7%	32.7%
Survey of Patients' Hospital Experiences				
Area Around Room 'Always' Quiet at Night	300+	51%	-	58%
Doctors 'Always' Communicated Well	300+	76%	-	80%
Home Recovery Information Given	300+	80%	-	82%
Hospital Given 9 or 10 on 10 Point Scale	300+	66%	-	67%
Meds 'Always' Explained Before Given	300+	58%	-	60%
Nurses 'Always' Communicated Well	300+	78%	-	76%
Pain 'Always' Well Controlled	300+	70%	-	69%
Room and Bathroom 'Always' Clean	300+	70%	-	71%
Timely Help 'Always' Received	300+	57%	-	64%
Would Definitely Recommend Hospital	300+	70%	-	69%

Baltimore Washington Medical Center

301 Hospital Dr
Glen Burnie, MD 21061
URL: www.bwmc.umms.org
Type: Acute Care Hospitals
Ownership: Voluntary Non-Profit - Other

Phone: 410-787-4400
Fax: 410-595-1958

Emergency Services: Yes
Beds: 286

Key Personnel:
CEO/President . . . . James R Walker
Chief of Medical Staff . . . . Dr Larry Linder
Infection Control . . . . Donna Lemmert
Operating Room . . . . Joyce Myers, RN
Pediatric Ambulatory Care . . . . . . Eric Sundel, MD
Quality Assurance . . . . Lynda Dabrowski
Radiology . . . . James Cary
Emergency Room . . . . Carol Ann Sperry, RN

Measure	Cases	This Hosp.	State Avg.	U.S. Avg.
Heart Attack Care				
ACE Inhibitor or ARB for LVSD[1]	11	91%	94%	96%
Aspirin at Arrival	202	99%	98%	99%
Aspirin at Discharge	124	98%	98%	98%
Beta Blocker at Discharge	127	96%	97%	98%
Fibrinolytic Medication Timing	0	-	42%	55%
PCI Within 90 Minutes of Arrival	83	84%	83%	90%
Smoking Cessation Advice	35	100%	98%	99%
Chest Pain/Possible Heart Attack Care				
Aspirin at Arrival	-	-	0%	95%
Median Time to ECG (minutes)	-	-	0	8
Median Time to Transfer (minutes)	-	-	0	61
Fibrinolytic Medication Timing	-	-	0%	54%
Heart Failure Care				
ACE Inhibitor or ARB for LVSD	196	94%	94%	94%
Discharge Instructions	608	84%	86%	88%
Evaluation of LVS Function	715	99%	97%	98%
Smoking Cessation Advice	96	100%	98%	98%
Pneumonia Care				
Appropriate Initial Antibiotic	452	92%	92%	92%
Blood Culture Timing	653	93%	92%	96%
Influenza Vaccine	389	93%	88%	91%
Initial Antibiotic Timing	581	96%	94%	95%
Pneumococcal Vaccine	493	98%	92%	93%
Smoking Cessation Advice	220	100%	97%	97%
Surgical Care Improvement Project				
Appropriate VTP Within 24 Hours[2]	322	80%	90%	92%
Appropriate Hair Removal[2]	958	99%	100%	99%
Appropriate Beta Blocker Usage[2]	326	86%	91%	93%
Controlled Postoperative Blood Glucose[5]	0	-	91%	93%
Prophylactic Antibiotic Timing[2]	659	95%	96%	97%
Prophylactic Antibiotic Timing (Outpatient)	-	-	0%	92%
Prophylactic Antibiotic Selection[2]	668	97%	97%	97%
Prophylactic Antibiotic Select. (Outpatient)	-	-	0%	94%
Prophylactic Antibiotic Stopped[2]	628	89%	94%	94%
Recommended VTP Ordered[2]	323	81%	92%	94%
Urinary Catheter Removal[2]	156	82%	89%	90%
Children's Asthma Care				
Received Systemic Corticosteroids	121	100%	-	100%
Received Home Management Plan	116	84%	-	71%
Received Reliever Medication	121	100%	-	100%
Use of Medical Imaging				
Combination Abdominal CT Scan	-	-	0.064	0.191
Combination Chest CT Scan	-	-	0.013	0.054
Follow-up Mammogram/Ultrasound	-	-	8.6%	8.4%
MRI for Low Back Pain	-	-	31.7%	32.7%
Survey of Patients' Hospital Experiences				
Area Around Room 'Always' Quiet at Night	300+	56%	-	58%
Doctors 'Always' Communicated Well	300+	77%	-	80%
Home Recovery Information Given	300+	81%	-	82%
Hospital Given 9 or 10 on 10 Point Scale	300+	66%	-	67%
Meds 'Always' Explained Before Given	300+	54%	-	60%
Nurses 'Always' Communicated Well	300+	74%	-	76%
Pain 'Always' Well Controlled	300+	67%	-	69%
Room and Bathroom 'Always' Clean	300+	66%	-	71%
Timely Help 'Always' Received	300+	59%	-	64%
Would Definitely Recommend Hospital	300+	69%	-	69%

NOTE: Hospital profiles are in alphabetical order by state, then city, then hospital within the city; Rankings exclude hospitals with less than 25 cases except for patient surveys which excludes hospitals with less than 100 cases; (a) 100–299 cases; (1) The number of cases is too small to be sure how well a hospital is performing; (2) The hospital indicated that the data submitted for this measure were based on a sample of cases; (3) Data was collected during a shorter time period (fewer quarters) than the maximum possible time for this measure; (4) Suppressed for one or more quarters by CMS; (5) No data is available from the hospital for this measure; (6) Fewer than 100 patients completed the HCAHPS survey. Use these rates with caution, as the number of surveys may be too low to reliably assess hospital performance; (7) Survey results are based on less than 12 months of data; (8) Survey results are not available for this reporting period; (9) No or very few patients were eligible for the HCAHPS survey. The scores shown, if any, reflect a very small number of surveys; (10) A state average was not calculated because too few hospitals in the state submitted data; (11) There were discrepancies in the data collection process; Please refer to the User's Guide for a full explanation of data.

Meritus Medical Center

11116 Medical Campus Road   Phone: 240-313-9500
Hagerstown, MD 21742
URL: www.meritushealth.com
Type: Acute Care Hospitals   Emergency Services: Yes
Ownership: Voluntary Non-Profit - Private   Beds: 341
Key Personnel:
President/CEO . . . . Joseph P Ross

Measure	Cases	This Hosp.	State Avg.	U.S. Avg.
Heart Attack Care				
ACE Inhibitor or ARB for LVSD[1]	20	100%	94%	96%
Aspirin at Arrival	156	100%	98%	99%
Aspirin at Discharge	129	100%	98%	98%
Beta Blocker at Discharge	128	99%	97%	98%
Fibrinolytic Medication Timing	0	-	42%	55%
PCI Within 90 Minutes of Arrival	46	89%	83%	90%
Smoking Cessation Advice	49	100%	98%	99%
Chest Pain/Possible Heart Attack Care				
Aspirin at Arrival	-	-	0%	95%
Median Time to ECG (minutes)	-	-	0	8
Median Time to Transfer (minutes)	-	-	0	61
Fibrinolytic Medication Timing	-	-	0%	54%
Heart Failure Care				
ACE Inhibitor or ARB for LVSD	101	99%	94%	94%
Discharge Instructions	281	96%	86%	88%
Evaluation of LVS Function	344	100%	97%	98%
Smoking Cessation Advice	53	100%	98%	98%
Pneumonia Care				
Appropriate Initial Antibiotic	320	90%	92%	92%
Blood Culture Timing	346	94%	92%	96%
Influenza Vaccine	218	100%	88%	91%
Initial Antibiotic Timing	517	90%	94%	95%
Pneumococcal Vaccine	429	98%	92%	93%
Smoking Cessation Advice	211	100%	97%	97%
Surgical Care Improvement Project				
Appropriate VTP Within 24 Hours	350	96%	90%	92%
Appropriate Hair Removal	1,338	100%	100%	99%
Appropriate Beta Blocker Usage	375	95%	91%	93%
Controlled Postoperative Blood Glucose	0	-	91%	93%
Prophylactic Antibiotic Timing	916	98%	96%	97%
Prophylactic Antibiotic Timing (Outpatient)	-	-	0%	92%
Prophylactic Antibiotic Selection	917	99%	97%	97%
Prophylactic Antibiotic Select. (Outpatient)	-	-	0%	94%
Prophylactic Antibiotic Stopped	867	97%	94%	94%
Recommended VTP Ordered	350	99%	92%	94%
Urinary Catheter Removal	173	90%	89%	90%
Children's Asthma Care				
Received Systemic Corticosteroids	-	-	-	100%
Received Home Management Plan	-	-	-	71%
Received Reliever Medication	-	-	-	100%
Use of Medical Imaging				
Combination Abdominal CT Scan	-	-	0.064	0.191
Combination Chest CT Scan	-	-	0.013	0.054
Follow-up Mammogram/Ultrasound	-	-	8.6%	8.4%
MRI for Low Back Pain	-	-	31.7%	32.7%
Survey of Patients' Hospital Experiences				
Area Around Room 'Always' Quiet at Night	300+	39%	-	58%
Doctors 'Always' Communicated Well	300+	73%	-	80%
Home Recovery Information Given	300+	84%	-	82%
Hospital Given 9 or 10 on 10 Point Scale	300+	55%	-	67%
Meds 'Always' Explained Before Given	300+	59%	-	60%
Nurses 'Always' Communicated Well	300+	75%	-	76%
Pain 'Always' Well Controlled	300+	66%	-	69%
Room and Bathroom 'Always' Clean	300+	68%	-	71%
Timely Help 'Always' Received	300+	58%	-	64%
Would Definitely Recommend Hospital	300+	58%	-	69%

Harford Memorial Hospital

501 S Union Ave   Phone: 443-643-3303
Havre De Grace, MD 21078   Fax: 443-643-3404
URL: www.uchs.org
Type: Acute Care Hospitals   Emergency Services: Yes
Ownership: Voluntary Non-Profit - Private   Beds: 102
Key Personnel:
CEO/President . . . . Lyle Ernest Sheldon
Chief of Medical Staff . . . . Peggy Vaughan

Measure	Cases	This Hosp.	State Avg.	U.S. Avg.
Heart Attack Care				
ACE Inhibitor or ARB for LVSD[1]	4	100%	94%	96%
Aspirin at Arrival	36	97%	98%	99%
Aspirin at Discharge[1]	19	95%	98%	98%
Beta Blocker at Discharge[1]	21	95%	97%	98%
Fibrinolytic Medication Timing	0	-	42%	55%
PCI Within 90 Minutes of Arrival[5]	0	-	83%	90%
Smoking Cessation Advice[1]	3	100%	98%	99%
Chest Pain/Possible Heart Attack Care				
Aspirin at Arrival	-	-	0%	95%
Median Time to ECG (minutes)	-	-	0	8
Median Time to Transfer (minutes)	-	-	0	61
Fibrinolytic Medication Timing	-	-	0%	54%
Heart Failure Care				
ACE Inhibitor or ARB for LVSD	58	98%	94%	94%
Discharge Instructions	183	98%	86%	88%
Evaluation of LVS Function	223	100%	97%	98%
Smoking Cessation Advice	30	100%	98%	98%
Pneumonia Care				
Appropriate Initial Antibiotic	132	95%	92%	92%
Blood Culture Timing	211	92%	92%	96%
Influenza Vaccine	104	93%	88%	91%
Initial Antibiotic Timing	183	94%	94%	95%
Pneumococcal Vaccine	125	96%	92%	93%
Smoking Cessation Advice	82	100%	97%	97%
Surgical Care Improvement Project				
Appropriate VTP Within 24 Hours	75	93%	90%	92%
Appropriate Hair Removal	220	100%	100%	99%
Appropriate Beta Blocker Usage	64	100%	91%	93%
Controlled Postoperative Blood Glucose	0	-	91%	93%
Prophylactic Antibiotic Timing	146	94%	96%	97%
Prophylactic Antibiotic Timing (Outpatient)	-	-	0%	92%
Prophylactic Antibiotic Selection	152	98%	97%	97%
Prophylactic Antibiotic Select. (Outpatient)	-	-	0%	94%
Prophylactic Antibiotic Stopped	139	98%	94%	94%
Recommended VTP Ordered	75	93%	92%	94%
Urinary Catheter Removal	68	97%	89%	90%
Children's Asthma Care				
Received Systemic Corticosteroids	-	-	-	100%
Received Home Management Plan	-	-	-	71%
Received Reliever Medication	-	-	-	100%
Use of Medical Imaging				
Combination Abdominal CT Scan	-	-	0.064	0.191
Combination Chest CT Scan	-	-	0.013	0.054
Follow-up Mammogram/Ultrasound	-	-	8.6%	8.4%
MRI for Low Back Pain	-	-	31.7%	32.7%
Survey of Patients' Hospital Experiences				
Area Around Room 'Always' Quiet at Night	300+	55%	-	58%
Doctors 'Always' Communicated Well	300+	78%	-	80%
Home Recovery Information Given	300+	81%	-	82%
Hospital Given 9 or 10 on 10 Point Scale	300+	64%	-	67%
Meds 'Always' Explained Before Given	300+	61%	-	60%
Nurses 'Always' Communicated Well	300+	76%	-	76%
Pain 'Always' Well Controlled	300+	68%	-	69%
Room and Bathroom 'Always' Clean	300+	66%	-	71%
Timely Help 'Always' Received	300+	57%	-	64%
Would Definitely Recommend Hospital	300+	64%	-	69%

Civista Medical Center

5 Garrett Avenue   Phone: 301-609-4265
La Plata, MD 20646   Fax: 301-609-4191
E-mail: civistatoday@civista.org
URL: www.civista.org
Type: Acute Care Hospitals   Emergency Services: Yes
Ownership: Voluntary Non-Profit - Other   Beds: 116
Key Personnel:
CEO/President . . . . Christine Stefanides
Chief of Medical Staff . . . . Seetaramayya Nagula, MD
Infection Control . . . . James Dunn
Quality Assurance . . . . Florence Moran
Radiology . . . . Edward Druy
Emergency Room . . . . Stephen M Smith
Intensive Care Unit . . . . Dana Smith

Measure	Cases	This Hosp.	State Avg.	U.S. Avg.
Heart Attack Care				
ACE Inhibitor or ARB for LVSD[1]	6	100%	94%	96%
Aspirin at Arrival	36	100%	98%	99%
Aspirin at Discharge[1]	14	100%	98%	98%
Beta Blocker at Discharge[1]	18	89%	97%	98%
Fibrinolytic Medication Timing	0	-	42%	55%
PCI Within 90 Minutes of Arrival[5]	0	-	83%	90%
Smoking Cessation Advice[1]	6	100%	98%	99%
Chest Pain/Possible Heart Attack Care				
Aspirin at Arrival	-	-	0%	95%
Median Time to ECG (minutes)	-	-	0	8
Median Time to Transfer (minutes)	-	-	0	61
Fibrinolytic Medication Timing	-	-	0%	54%
Heart Failure Care				
ACE Inhibitor or ARB for LVSD[2]	79	90%	94%	94%
Discharge Instructions[2]	226	94%	86%	88%
Evaluation of LVS Function[2]	270	99%	97%	98%
Smoking Cessation Advice[2]	42	100%	98%	98%
Pneumonia Care				
Appropriate Initial Antibiotic[2]	124	97%	92%	92%
Blood Culture Timing[2]	203	99%	92%	96%
Influenza Vaccine[2]	99	95%	88%	91%
Initial Antibiotic Timing[2]	204	96%	94%	95%
Pneumococcal Vaccine[2]	160	98%	92%	93%
Smoking Cessation Advice[2]	63	100%	97%	97%
Surgical Care Improvement Project				
Appropriate VTP Within 24 Hours[2]	153	93%	90%	92%
Appropriate Hair Removal[2]	394	100%	100%	99%
Appropriate Beta Blocker Usage[2]	77	84%	91%	93%
Controlled Postoperative Blood Glucose[2]	0	-	91%	93%
Prophylactic Antibiotic Timing[2]	240	96%	96%	97%
Prophylactic Antibiotic Timing (Outpatient)	-	-	0%	92%
Prophylactic Antibiotic Selection[2]	239	99%	97%	97%
Prophylactic Antibiotic Select. (Outpatient)	-	-	0%	94%
Prophylactic Antibiotic Stopped[2]	206	96%	94%	94%
Recommended VTP Ordered[2]	153	94%	92%	94%
Urinary Catheter Removal	88	85%	89%	90%
Children's Asthma Care				
Received Systemic Corticosteroids	-	-	-	100%
Received Home Management Plan	-	-	-	71%
Received Reliever Medication	-	-	-	100%
Use of Medical Imaging				
Combination Abdominal CT Scan	-	-	0.064	0.191
Combination Chest CT Scan	-	-	0.013	0.054
Follow-up Mammogram/Ultrasound	-	-	8.6%	8.4%
MRI for Low Back Pain	-	-	31.7%	32.7%
Survey of Patients' Hospital Experiences				
Area Around Room 'Always' Quiet at Night	300+	56%	-	58%
Doctors 'Always' Communicated Well	300+	73%	-	80%
Home Recovery Information Given	300+	76%	-	82%
Hospital Given 9 or 10 on 10 Point Scale	300+	56%	-	67%
Meds 'Always' Explained Before Given	300+	57%	-	60%
Nurses 'Always' Communicated Well	300+	73%	-	76%
Pain 'Always' Well Controlled	300+	65%	-	69%
Room and Bathroom 'Always' Clean	300+	65%	-	71%
Timely Help 'Always' Received	300+	61%	-	64%
Would Definitely Recommend Hospital	300+	59%	-	69%

NOTE: Hospital profiles are in alphabetical order by state, then city, then hospital within the city; Rankings exclude hospitals with less than 25 cases except for patient surveys which excludes hospitals with less than 100 cases; (a) 100–299 cases; (1) The number of cases is too small to be sure how well a hospital is performing; (2) The hospital indicated that the data submitted for this measure were based on a sample of cases; (3) Data was collected during a shorter time period (fewer quarters) than the maximum possible time for this measure; (4) Suppressed for one or more quarters by CMS; (5) No data is available from the hospital for this measure; (6) Fewer than 100 patients completed the HCAHPS survey. Use these rates with caution, as the number of surveys may be too low to reliably assess hospital performance; (7) Survey results are based on less than 12 months of data; (8) Survey results are not available for this reporting period; (9) No or very few patients were eligible for the HCAHPS survey. The scores shown, if any, reflect a very small number of surveys; (10) A state average was not calculated because too few hospitals in the state submitted data; (11) There were discrepancies in the data collection process; Please refer to the User's Guide for a full explanation of data.

Doctors' Community Hospital

8118 Good Luck Road
Lanham, MD 20706
URL: www.DCHweb.org
Type: Acute Care Hospitals
Ownership: Proprietary
Phone: 301-552-8085
Fax: 301-552-7937
Emergency Services: Yes
Beds: 250

Key Personnel:

CEO/President. . . . . Philip Down
Cardiac Laboratory. . . . . Cecily Ludka
Quality Assurance . . . . Peg Kostopoulos
Radiology. . . . . Louis Kirschner, MD
Emergency Room . . . . Nancy Haupt, RN

Measure	Cases	This Hosp.	State Avg.	U.S. Avg.
Heart Attack Care				
ACE Inhibitor or ARB for LVSD[1]	8	100%	94%	96%
Aspirin at Arrival	50	90%	98%	99%
Aspirin at Discharge[1]	20	85%	98%	98%
Beta Blocker at Discharge[1]	22	86%	97%	98%
Fibrinolytic Medication Timing	0	-	42%	55%
PCI Within 90 Minutes of Arrival	0	-	83%	90%
Smoking Cessation Advice[1]	1	100%	98%	99%
Chest Pain/Possible Heart Attack Care				
Aspirin at Arrival	-	-	0%	95%
Median Time to ECG (minutes)	-	-	0	8
Median Time to Transfer (minutes)	-	-	0	61
Fibrinolytic Medication Timing	-	-	0%	54%
Heart Failure Care				
ACE Inhibitor or ARB for LVSD	195	90%	94%	94%
Discharge Instructions	440	79%	86%	88%
Evaluation of LVS Function	495	95%	97%	98%
Smoking Cessation Advice	86	100%	98%	98%
Pneumonia Care				
Appropriate Initial Antibiotic	219	95%	92%	92%
Blood Culture Timing	343	87%	92%	96%
Influenza Vaccine	177	64%	88%	91%
Initial Antibiotic Timing	301	95%	94%	95%
Pneumococcal Vaccine	226	85%	92%	93%
Smoking Cessation Advice	82	100%	97%	97%
Surgical Care Improvement Project				
Appropriate VTP Within 24 Hours[2]	233	87%	90%	92%
Appropriate Hair Removal[2]	482	100%	100%	99%
Appropriate Beta Blocker Usage[5]	0	-	91%	93%
Controlled Postoperative Blood Glucose[2]	0	-	91%	93%
Prophylactic Antibiotic Timing[2]	353	97%	96%	97%
Prophylactic Antibiotic Timing (Outpatient)	-	-	0%	92%
Prophylactic Antibiotic Selection[2]	356	99%	97%	97%
Prophylactic Antibiotic Select. (Outpatient)	-	-	0%	94%
Prophylactic Antibiotic Stopped[2]	339	89%	94%	94%
Recommended VTP Ordered[2]	233	92%	92%	94%
Urinary Catheter Removal[2]	122	87%	89%	90%
Children's Asthma Care				
Received Systemic Corticosteroids	-	-	-	100%
Received Home Management Plan	-	-	-	71%
Received Reliever Medication	-	-	-	100%
Use of Medical Imaging				
Combination Abdominal CT Scan	-	-	0.064	0.191
Combination Chest CT Scan	-	-	0.013	0.054
Follow-up Mammogram/Ultrasound	-	-	8.6%	8.4%
MRI for Low Back Pain	-	-	31.7%	32.7%
Survey of Patients' Hospital Experiences				
Area Around Room 'Always' Quiet at Night	300+	49%	-	58%
Doctors 'Always' Communicated Well	300+	74%	-	80%
Home Recovery Information Given	300+	77%	-	82%
Hospital Given 9 or 10 on 10 Point Scale	300+	58%	-	67%
Meds 'Always' Explained Before Given	300+	50%	-	60%
Nurses 'Always' Communicated Well	300+	67%	-	76%
Pain 'Always' Well Controlled	300+	61%	-	69%
Room and Bathroom 'Always' Clean	300+	71%	-	71%
Timely Help 'Always' Received	300+	50%	-	64%
Would Definitely Recommend Hospital	300+	63%	-	69%

Laurel Regional Medical Center

7300 Van Dusen Road
Laurel, MD 20707
URL: www.laurelregionalhospital.org
Type: Acute Care Hospitals
Ownership: Voluntary Non-Profit - Private
Phone: 301-497-7953
Fax: 301-497-7953
Emergency Services: Yes
Beds: 146

Key Personnel:

CEO/President. . . . . Douglas Shepherd
Chief of Medical Staff. . . . . Neil Meade
Infection Control. . . . . Barbara Thieman
Radiology. . . . . Meghal Antani
Anesthesiology. . . . . Jon Newsome, MD
Emergency Room . . . . Gerald Apollon
Patient Relations . . . . Suzy Novotny

Measure	Cases	This Hosp.	State Avg.	U.S. Avg.
Heart Attack Care				
ACE Inhibitor or ARB for LVSD[1]	4	100%	94%	96%
Aspirin at Arrival	55	96%	98%	99%
Aspirin at Discharge	27	81%	98%	98%
Beta Blocker at Discharge	29	93%	97%	98%
Fibrinolytic Medication Timing[1]	1	0%	42%	55%
PCI Within 90 Minutes of Arrival	0	-	83%	90%
Smoking Cessation Advice[1]	2	100%	98%	99%
Chest Pain/Possible Heart Attack Care				
Aspirin at Arrival	-	-	0%	95%
Median Time to ECG (minutes)	-	-	0	8
Median Time to Transfer (minutes)	-	-	0	61
Fibrinolytic Medication Timing	-	-	0%	54%
Heart Failure Care				
ACE Inhibitor or ARB for LVSD	50	98%	94%	94%
Discharge Instructions	112	96%	86%	88%
Evaluation of LVS Function	160	96%	97%	98%
Smoking Cessation Advice	28	96%	98%	98%
Pneumonia Care				
Appropriate Initial Antibiotic	98	88%	92%	92%
Blood Culture Timing	175	93%	92%	96%
Influenza Vaccine	110	79%	88%	91%
Initial Antibiotic Timing	159	91%	94%	95%
Pneumococcal Vaccine	135	77%	92%	93%
Smoking Cessation Advice	35	100%	97%	97%
Surgical Care Improvement Project				
Appropriate VTP Within 24 Hours	50	82%	90%	92%
Appropriate Hair Removal	167	100%	100%	99%
Appropriate Beta Blocker Usage	37	89%	91%	93%
Controlled Postoperative Blood Glucose	0	-	91%	93%
Prophylactic Antibiotic Timing	112	97%	96%	97%
Prophylactic Antibiotic Timing (Outpatient)	-	-	0%	92%
Prophylactic Antibiotic Selection	112	94%	97%	97%
Prophylactic Antibiotic Select. (Outpatient)	-	-	0%	94%
Prophylactic Antibiotic Stopped	108	89%	94%	94%
Recommended VTP Ordered	51	84%	92%	94%
Urinary Catheter Removal[1]	23	87%	89%	90%
Children's Asthma Care				
Received Systemic Corticosteroids	-	-	-	100%
Received Home Management Plan	-	-	-	71%
Received Reliever Medication	-	-	-	100%
Use of Medical Imaging				
Combination Abdominal CT Scan	-	-	0.064	0.191
Combination Chest CT Scan	-	-	0.013	0.054
Follow-up Mammogram/Ultrasound	-	-	8.6%	8.4%
MRI for Low Back Pain	-	-	31.7%	32.7%
Survey of Patients' Hospital Experiences				
Area Around Room 'Always' Quiet at Night	300+	52%	-	58%
Doctors 'Always' Communicated Well	300+	68%	-	80%
Home Recovery Information Given	300+	70%	-	82%
Hospital Given 9 or 10 on 10 Point Scale	300+	44%	-	67%
Meds 'Always' Explained Before Given	300+	51%	-	60%
Nurses 'Always' Communicated Well	300+	62%	-	76%
Pain 'Always' Well Controlled	300+	58%	-	69%
Room and Bathroom 'Always' Clean	300+	55%	-	71%
Timely Help 'Always' Received	300+	45%	-	64%
Would Definitely Recommend Hospital	300+	44%	-	69%

Saint Mary's Hospital

PO Box 527
Leonardtown, MD 20650
URL: www.smhwecare.com
Type: Acute Care Hospitals
Ownership: Voluntary Non-Profit - Private
Phone: 301-475-6001
Fax: 301-475-5388
Emergency Services: Yes
Beds: 110

Key Personnel:

CEO/President. . . . . Christine Wray
Chief of Medical Staff . . . . Cindy Daly, MD
Radiology. . . . . Bolivia Davis
Emergency Room . . . . Eveline Ane

Measure	Cases	This Hosp.	State Avg.	U.S. Avg.
Heart Attack Care				
ACE Inhibitor or ARB for LVSD[1]	3	100%	94%	96%
Aspirin at Arrival	38	97%	98%	99%
Aspirin at Discharge[1]	16	100%	98%	98%
Beta Blocker at Discharge[1]	15	100%	97%	98%
Fibrinolytic Medication Timing	0	-	42%	55%
PCI Within 90 Minutes of Arrival	0	-	83%	90%
Smoking Cessation Advice[1]	1	100%	98%	99%
Chest Pain/Possible Heart Attack Care				
Aspirin at Arrival	-	-	0%	95%
Median Time to ECG (minutes)	-	-	0	8
Median Time to Transfer (minutes)	-	-	0	61
Fibrinolytic Medication Timing	-	-	0%	54%
Heart Failure Care				
ACE Inhibitor or ARB for LVSD	68	97%	94%	94%
Discharge Instructions	215	94%	86%	88%
Evaluation of LVS Function	254	100%	97%	98%
Smoking Cessation Advice	40	100%	98%	98%
Pneumonia Care				
Appropriate Initial Antibiotic	73	97%	92%	92%
Blood Culture Timing	111	97%	92%	96%
Influenza Vaccine	85	95%	88%	91%
Initial Antibiotic Timing	125	98%	94%	95%
Pneumococcal Vaccine	102	98%	92%	93%
Smoking Cessation Advice	40	100%	97%	97%
Surgical Care Improvement Project				
Appropriate VTP Within 24 Hours[2]	66	95%	90%	92%
Appropriate Hair Removal[2]	369	100%	100%	99%
Appropriate Beta Blocker Usage[2]	86	100%	91%	93%
Controlled Postoperative Blood Glucose[2]	0	-	91%	93%
Prophylactic Antibiotic Timing[2]	302	99%	96%	97%
Prophylactic Antibiotic Timing (Outpatient)	-	-	0%	92%
Prophylactic Antibiotic Selection[2]	304	98%	97%	97%
Prophylactic Antibiotic Select. (Outpatient)	-	-	0%	94%
Prophylactic Antibiotic Stopped[2]	297	97%	94%	94%
Recommended VTP Ordered[2]	66	95%	92%	94%
Urinary Catheter Removal[2]	118	98%	89%	90%
Children's Asthma Care				
Received Systemic Corticosteroids	-	-	-	100%
Received Home Management Plan	-	-	-	71%
Received Reliever Medication	-	-	-	100%
Use of Medical Imaging				
Combination Abdominal CT Scan	-	-	0.064	0.191
Combination Chest CT Scan	-	-	0.013	0.054
Follow-up Mammogram/Ultrasound	-	-	8.6%	8.4%
MRI for Low Back Pain	-	-	31.7%	32.7%
Survey of Patients' Hospital Experiences				
Area Around Room 'Always' Quiet at Night	300+	57%	-	58%
Doctors 'Always' Communicated Well	300+	80%	-	80%
Home Recovery Information Given	300+	81%	-	82%
Hospital Given 9 or 10 on 10 Point Scale	300+	65%	-	67%
Meds 'Always' Explained Before Given	300+	64%	-	60%
Nurses 'Always' Communicated Well	300+	80%	-	76%
Pain 'Always' Well Controlled	300+	67%	-	69%
Room and Bathroom 'Always' Clean	300+	72%	-	71%
Timely Help 'Always' Received	300+	63%	-	64%
Would Definitely Recommend Hospital	300+	65%	-	69%

NOTE: Hospital profiles are in alphabetical order by state, then city, then hospital within the city; Rankings exclude hospitals with less than 25 cases except for patient surveys which excludes hospitals with less than 100 cases; (a) 100–299 cases; (1) The number of cases is too small to be sure how well a hospital is performing; (2) The hospital indicated that the data submitted for this measure were based on a sample of cases; (3) Data was collected during a shorter time period (fewer quarters) than the maximum possible time for this measure; (4) Suppressed for one or more quarters by CMS; (5) No data is available from the hospital for this measure; (6) Fewer than 100 patients completed the HCAHPS survey. Use these rates with caution, as the number of surveys may be too low to reliably assess hospital performance; (7) Survey results are based on less than 12 months of data; (8) Survey results are not available for this reporting period; (9) No or very few patients were eligible for the HCAHPS survey. The scores shown, if any, reflect a very small number of surveys; (10) A state average was not calculated because too few hospitals in the state submitted data; (11) There were discrepancies in the data collection process; Please refer to the User's Guide for a full explanation of data.

Garrett County Memorial Hospital

251 N Fourth St   Phone: 301-533-4173
Oakland, MD 21550   Fax: 301-533-4328
URL: www.gcmh.com
Type: Acute Care Hospitals   Emergency Services: Yes
Ownership: Voluntary Non-Profit - Other   Beds: 76

Key Personnel:
CEO/President . . . . Donald P Battista
Chief of Medical Staff . . . . Richard Perry, MD
Coronary Care . . . . Dale Hair, RN
Infection Control . . . . Linda Danjou, RN
Operating Room . . . . Elaine Geroski, RN
Radiology . . . . James K Benjamin

Measure	Cases	This Hosp.	State Avg.	U.S. Avg.
Heart Attack Care				
ACE Inhibitor or ARB for LVSD[1]	1	100%	94%	96%
Aspirin at Arrival[1]	13	92%	98%	99%
Aspirin at Discharge[1]	7	86%	98%	98%
Beta Blocker at Discharge[1]	8	88%	97%	98%
Fibrinolytic Medication Timing	0	-	42%	55%
PCI Within 90 Minutes of Arrival	0	-	83%	90%
Smoking Cessation Advice[1]	3	100%	98%	99%
Chest Pain/Possible Heart Attack Care				
Aspirin at Arrival	-	-	0%	95%
Median Time to ECG (minutes)	-	-	0	8
Median Time to Transfer (minutes)	-	-	0	61
Fibrinolytic Medication Timing	-	-	0%	54%
Heart Failure Care				
ACE Inhibitor or ARB for LVSD	27	89%	94%	94%
Discharge Instructions	64	75%	86%	88%
Evaluation of LVS Function	89	97%	97%	98%
Smoking Cessation Advice[1]	9	100%	98%	98%
Pneumonia Care				
Appropriate Initial Antibiotic	27	74%	92%	92%
Blood Culture Timing	38	100%	92%	96%
Influenza Vaccine	26	100%	88%	91%
Initial Antibiotic Timing	43	98%	94%	95%
Pneumococcal Vaccine	33	100%	92%	93%
Smoking Cessation Advice[1]	11	91%	97%	97%
Surgical Care Improvement Project				
Appropriate VTP Within 24 Hours	70	94%	90%	92%
Appropriate Hair Removal	202	100%	100%	99%
Appropriate Beta Blocker Usage	61	89%	91%	93%
Controlled Postoperative Blood Glucose	0	-	91%	93%
Prophylactic Antibiotic Timing	155	93%	96%	97%
Prophylactic Antibiotic Timing (Outpatient)	-	-	0%	92%
Prophylactic Antibiotic Selection	156	93%	97%	97%
Prophylactic Antibiotic Select. (Outpatient)	-	-	0%	94%
Prophylactic Antibiotic Stopped	151	88%	94%	94%
Recommended VTP Ordered	71	93%	92%	94%
Urinary Catheter Removal	64	36%	89%	90%
Children's Asthma Care				
Received Systemic Corticosteroids	-	-	-	100%
Received Home Management Plan	-	-	-	71%
Received Reliever Medication	-	-	-	100%
Use of Medical Imaging				
Combination Abdominal CT Scan	-	-	0.064	0.191
Combination Chest CT Scan	-	-	0.013	0.054
Follow-up Mammogram/Ultrasound	-	-	8.6%	8.4%
MRI for Low Back Pain	-	-	31.7%	32.7%
Survey of Patients' Hospital Experiences				
Area Around Room 'Always' Quiet at Night	300+	50%	-	58%
Doctors 'Always' Communicated Well	300+	85%	-	80%
Home Recovery Information Given	300+	85%	-	82%
Hospital Given 9 or 10 on 10 Point Scale	300+	68%	-	67%
Meds 'Always' Explained Before Given	300+	63%	-	60%
Nurses 'Always' Communicated Well	300+	80%	-	76%
Pain 'Always' Well Controlled	300+	72%	-	69%
Room and Bathroom 'Always' Clean	300+	71%	-	71%
Timely Help 'Always' Received	300+	70%	-	64%
Would Definitely Recommend Hospital	300+	69%	-	69%

Montgomery General Hospital

18101 Prince Philip Drive   Phone: 301-774-8771
Olney, MD 20832   Fax: 301-774-7389
URL: www.montgomerygeneral.com
Type: Acute Care Hospitals   Emergency Services: Yes
Ownership: Voluntary Non-Profit - Private   Beds: 244

Key Personnel:
CEO/President . . . . Peter W Monge
Chief of Medical Staff . . . . Roger F Leonard, MD
Operating Room . . . . Rene Gelber
Pediatric Ambulatory Care . . . . . Sheila Ideerda, MD
Pediatric In-Patient Care . . . . Sheila Ideerda, MD
Quality Assurance . . . . Nancy Barlow
Emergency Room . . . . Andy Divine

Measure	Cases	This Hosp.	State Avg.	U.S. Avg.
Heart Attack Care				
ACE Inhibitor or ARB for LVSD[1]	7	100%	94%	96%
Aspirin at Arrival	48	100%	98%	99%
Aspirin at Discharge[1]	22	100%	98%	98%
Beta Blocker at Discharge[1]	23	100%	97%	98%
Fibrinolytic Medication Timing[1]	5	40%	42%	55%
PCI Within 90 Minutes of Arrival	0	-	83%	90%
Smoking Cessation Advice[1]	1	100%	98%	99%
Chest Pain/Possible Heart Attack Care				
Aspirin at Arrival	-	-	0%	95%
Median Time to ECG (minutes)	-	-	0	8
Median Time to Transfer (minutes)	-	-	0	61
Fibrinolytic Medication Timing	-	-	0%	54%
Heart Failure Care				
ACE Inhibitor or ARB for LVSD	77	96%	94%	94%
Discharge Instructions	152	89%	86%	88%
Evaluation of LVS Function	215	99%	97%	98%
Smoking Cessation Advice[1]	16	100%	98%	98%
Pneumonia Care				
Appropriate Initial Antibiotic	151	99%	92%	92%
Blood Culture Timing	212	97%	92%	96%
Influenza Vaccine	152	94%	88%	91%
Initial Antibiotic Timing	190	99%	94%	95%
Pneumococcal Vaccine	211	98%	92%	93%
Smoking Cessation Advice	41	98%	97%	97%
Surgical Care Improvement Project				
Appropriate VTP Within 24 Hours	182	93%	90%	92%
Appropriate Hair Removal	478	100%	100%	99%
Appropriate Beta Blocker Usage	110	95%	91%	93%
Controlled Postoperative Blood Glucose	0	-	91%	93%
Prophylactic Antibiotic Timing	305	97%	96%	97%
Prophylactic Antibiotic Timing (Outpatient)	-	-	0%	92%
Prophylactic Antibiotic Selection	314	98%	97%	97%
Prophylactic Antibiotic Select. (Outpatient)	-	-	0%	94%
Prophylactic Antibiotic Stopped	292	92%	94%	94%
Recommended VTP Ordered	182	93%	92%	94%
Urinary Catheter Removal	166	93%	89%	90%
Children's Asthma Care				
Received Systemic Corticosteroids	-	-	-	100%
Received Home Management Plan	-	-	-	71%
Received Reliever Medication	-	-	-	100%
Use of Medical Imaging				
Combination Abdominal CT Scan	-	-	0.064	0.191
Combination Chest CT Scan	-	-	0.013	0.054
Follow-up Mammogram/Ultrasound	-	-	8.6%	8.4%
MRI for Low Back Pain	-	-	31.7%	32.7%
Survey of Patients' Hospital Experiences				
Area Around Room 'Always' Quiet at Night	300+	45%	-	58%
Doctors 'Always' Communicated Well	300+	73%	-	80%
Home Recovery Information Given	300+	84%	-	82%
Hospital Given 9 or 10 on 10 Point Scale	300+	58%	-	67%
Meds 'Always' Explained Before Given	300+	58%	-	60%
Nurses 'Always' Communicated Well	300+	69%	-	76%
Pain 'Always' Well Controlled	300+	60%	-	69%
Room and Bathroom 'Always' Clean	300+	57%	-	71%
Timely Help 'Always' Received	300+	54%	-	64%
Would Definitely Recommend Hospital	300+	64%	-	69%

Calvert Memorial Hospital

100 Hospital Road   Phone: 410-535-8239
Prince Frederick, MD 20678   Fax: 410-535-4125
URL: www.calverthospital.com
Type: Acute Care Hospitals   Emergency Services: Yes
Ownership: Voluntary Non-Profit - Other   Beds: 88

Key Personnel:
CEO/President . . . . James J Xinis
Chief of Medical Staff . . . . Robert Schlager, MD
Infection Control . . . . Judith Sturgis
Operating Room . . . . Gretchen West
Quality Assurance . . . . Susan Dohony
Radiology . . . . Guillermo Zambrano
Intensive Care Unit . . . . Annie Lockhart
Patient Relations . . . . Mattie Lowery

Measure	Cases	This Hosp.	State Avg.	U.S. Avg.
Heart Attack Care				
ACE Inhibitor or ARB for LVSD[1]	4	100%	94%	96%
Aspirin at Arrival	43	95%	98%	99%
Aspirin at Discharge	27	96%	98%	98%
Beta Blocker at Discharge	27	100%	97%	98%
Fibrinolytic Medication Timing	0	-	42%	55%
PCI Within 90 Minutes of Arrival[5]	0	-	83%	90%
Smoking Cessation Advice[1]	2	100%	98%	99%
Chest Pain/Possible Heart Attack Care				
Aspirin at Arrival	-	-	0%	95%
Median Time to ECG (minutes)	-	-	0	8
Median Time to Transfer (minutes)	-	-	0	61
Fibrinolytic Medication Timing	-	-	0%	54%
Heart Failure Care				
ACE Inhibitor or ARB for LVSD[2]	67	100%	94%	94%
Discharge Instructions[2]	174	96%	86%	88%
Evaluation of LVS Function[2]	233	100%	97%	98%
Smoking Cessation Advice[1,2]	21	100%	98%	98%
Pneumonia Care				
Appropriate Initial Antibiotic[2]	116	96%	92%	92%
Blood Culture Timing[2]	168	92%	92%	96%
Influenza Vaccine[2]	88	92%	88%	91%
Initial Antibiotic Timing[2]	172	98%	94%	95%
Pneumococcal Vaccine[2]	141	96%	92%	93%
Smoking Cessation Advice[2]	59	100%	97%	97%
Surgical Care Improvement Project				
Appropriate VTP Within 24 Hours[2]	72	92%	90%	92%
Appropriate Hair Removal[2]	326	100%	100%	99%
Appropriate Beta Blocker Usage[2,3]	54	96%	91%	93%
Controlled Postoperative Blood Glucose[2]	0	-	91%	93%
Prophylactic Antibiotic Timing[2]	258	96%	96%	97%
Prophylactic Antibiotic Timing (Outpatient)	-	-	0%	92%
Prophylactic Antibiotic Selection[2]	260	97%	97%	97%
Prophylactic Antibiotic Select. (Outpatient)	-	-	0%	94%
Prophylactic Antibiotic Stopped[2]	254	95%	94%	94%
Recommended VTP Ordered[2]	72	99%	92%	94%
Urinary Catheter Removal[2]	64	97%	89%	90%
Children's Asthma Care				
Received Systemic Corticosteroids	-	-	-	100%
Received Home Management Plan	-	-	-	71%
Received Reliever Medication	-	-	-	100%
Use of Medical Imaging				
Combination Abdominal CT Scan	-	-	0.064	0.191
Combination Chest CT Scan	-	-	0.013	0.054
Follow-up Mammogram/Ultrasound	-	-	8.6%	8.4%
MRI for Low Back Pain	-	-	31.7%	32.7%
Survey of Patients' Hospital Experiences				
Area Around Room 'Always' Quiet at Night	300+	54%	-	58%
Doctors 'Always' Communicated Well	300+	78%	-	80%
Home Recovery Information Given	300+	83%	-	82%
Hospital Given 9 or 10 on 10 Point Scale	300+	64%	-	67%
Meds 'Always' Explained Before Given	300+	58%	-	60%
Nurses 'Always' Communicated Well	300+	72%	-	76%
Pain 'Always' Well Controlled	300+	66%	-	69%
Room and Bathroom 'Always' Clean	300+	65%	-	71%
Timely Help 'Always' Received	300+	59%	-	64%
Would Definitely Recommend Hospital	300+	65%	-	69%

NOTE: Hospital profiles are in alphabetical order by state, then city, then hospital within the city; Rankings exclude hospitals with less than 25 cases except for patient surveys which excludes hospitals with less than 100 cases; (a) 100–299 cases; (1) The number of cases is too small to be sure how well a hospital is performing; (2) The hospital indicated that the data submitted for this measure were based on a sample of cases; (3) Data was collected during a shorter time period (fewer quarters) than the maximum possible time for this measure; (4) Suppressed for one or more quarters by CMS; (5) No data is available from the hospital for this measure; (6) Fewer than 100 patients completed the HCAHPS survey. Use these rates with caution, as the number of surveys may be too low to reliably assess hospital performance; (7) Survey results are based on less than 12 months of data; (8) Survey results are not available for this reporting period; (9) No or very few patients were eligible for the HCAHPS survey. The scores shown, if any, reflect a very small number of surveys; (10) A state average was not calculated because too few hospitals in the state submitted data; (11) There were discrepancies in the data collection process; Please refer to the User's Guide for a full explanation of data.

Northwest Hospital Center

5401 Old Court Rd
Randallstown, MD 21133
URL: www.lifebridgehealth.org
Type: Acute Care Hospitals
Ownership: Voluntary Non-Profit - Other

Phone: 410-521-5995
Fax: 410-521-7269

Emergency Services: Yes
Beds: 240

Key Personnel:
CEO/President . . . . Dave Krajewski
Quality Assurance . . . . Candy Hamner
Radiology . . . . George Allen
Anesthesiology . . . . Charles Leve, MD
Emergency Room . . . . Deborah Macy
Intensive Care Unit . . . . Christopher Lee, RN
Patient Relations . . . . Sue Jalbert

Measure	Cases	This Hosp.	State Avg.	U.S. Avg.
Heart Attack Care				
ACE Inhibitor or ARB for LVSD[1]	12	75%	94%	96%
Aspirin at Arrival	93	96%	98%	99%
Aspirin at Discharge	56	95%	98%	98%
Beta Blocker at Discharge	57	96%	97%	98%
Fibrinolytic Medication Timing	0	-	42%	55%
PCI Within 90 Minutes of Arrival[5]	0	-	83%	90%
Smoking Cessation Advice[1]	1	100%	98%	99%
Chest Pain/Possible Heart Attack Care				
Aspirin at Arrival	-	-	0%	95%
Median Time to ECG (minutes)	-	-	0	8
Median Time to Transfer (minutes)	-	-	0	61
Fibrinolytic Medication Timing	-	-	0%	54%
Heart Failure Care				
ACE Inhibitor or ARB for LVSD	185	98%	94%	94%
Discharge Instructions	344	84%	86%	88%
Evaluation of LVS Function	470	99%	97%	98%
Smoking Cessation Advice	58	100%	98%	98%
Pneumonia Care				
Appropriate Initial Antibiotic	220	96%	92%	92%
Blood Culture Timing	311	93%	92%	96%
Influenza Vaccine	210	97%	88%	91%
Initial Antibiotic Timing	410	95%	94%	95%
Pneumococcal Vaccine	287	98%	92%	93%
Smoking Cessation Advice	100	100%	97%	97%
Surgical Care Improvement Project				
Appropriate VTP Within 24 Hours	177	89%	90%	92%
Appropriate Hair Removal	460	100%	100%	99%
Appropriate Beta Blocker Usage	113	89%	91%	93%
Controlled Postoperative Blood Glucose[1]	1	100%	91%	93%
Prophylactic Antibiotic Timing	280	95%	96%	97%
Prophylactic Antibiotic Timing (Outpatient)	-	-	0%	92%
Prophylactic Antibiotic Selection	281	98%	97%	97%
Prophylactic Antibiotic Select. (Outpatient)	-	-	0%	94%
Prophylactic Antibiotic Stopped	260	97%	94%	94%
Recommended VTP Ordered	177	89%	92%	94%
Urinary Catheter Removal	34	94%	89%	90%
Children's Asthma Care				
Received Systemic Corticosteroids	-	-	-	100%
Received Home Management Plan	-	-	-	71%
Received Reliever Medication	-	-	-	100%
Use of Medical Imaging				
Combination Abdominal CT Scan	-	-	0.064	0.191
Combination Chest CT Scan	-	-	0.013	0.054
Follow-up Mammogram/Ultrasound	-	-	8.6%	8.4%
MRI for Low Back Pain	-	-	31.7%	32.7%
Survey of Patients' Hospital Experiences				
Area Around Room 'Always' Quiet at Night	300+	55%	-	58%
Doctors 'Always' Communicated Well	300+	71%	-	80%
Home Recovery Information Given	300+	71%	-	82%
Hospital Given 9 or 10 on 10 Point Scale	300+	61%	-	67%
Meds 'Always' Explained Before Given	300+	55%	-	60%
Nurses 'Always' Communicated Well	300+	72%	-	76%
Pain 'Always' Well Controlled	300+	62%	-	69%
Room and Bathroom 'Always' Clean	300+	62%	-	71%
Timely Help 'Always' Received	300+	55%	-	64%
Would Definitely Recommend Hospital	300+	62%	-	69%

Shady Grove Adventist Hospital

9901 Medical Center Dr
Rockville, MD 20850
URL: www.adventisthealthcare.com/SGAH
Type: Acute Care Hospitals
Ownership: Voluntary Non-Profit - Church

Phone: 240-826-6472
Fax: 301-315-3043

Emergency Services: Yes
Beds: 268

Key Personnel:
CEO/President . . . . Deborah A Yancer
Chief of Medical Staff . . . . Robert Eisdorfer, MD

Measure	Cases	This Hosp.	State Avg.	U.S. Avg.
Heart Attack Care				
ACE Inhibitor or ARB for LVSD	27	96%	94%	96%
Aspirin at Arrival	180	100%	98%	99%
Aspirin at Discharge	159	99%	98%	98%
Beta Blocker at Discharge	156	99%	97%	98%
Fibrinolytic Medication Timing	0	-	42%	55%
PCI Within 90 Minutes of Arrival	71	87%	83%	90%
Smoking Cessation Advice	59	98%	98%	99%
Chest Pain/Possible Heart Attack Care				
Aspirin at Arrival	-	-	0%	95%
Median Time to ECG (minutes)	-	-	0	8
Median Time to Transfer (minutes)	-	-	0	61
Fibrinolytic Medication Timing	-	-	0%	54%
Heart Failure Care				
ACE Inhibitor or ARB for LVSD	140	100%	94%	94%
Discharge Instructions	284	96%	86%	88%
Evaluation of LVS Function	377	100%	97%	98%
Smoking Cessation Advice	39	100%	98%	98%
Pneumonia Care				
Appropriate Initial Antibiotic[2]	90	93%	92%	92%
Blood Culture Timing[2]	101	94%	92%	96%
Influenza Vaccine[2]	80	78%	88%	91%
Initial Antibiotic Timing[2]	121	97%	94%	95%
Pneumococcal Vaccine[2]	133	73%	92%	93%
Smoking Cessation Advice[2]	36	94%	97%	97%
Surgical Care Improvement Project				
Appropriate VTP Within 24 Hours[2]	152	91%	90%	92%
Appropriate Hair Removal[2]	464	100%	100%	99%
Appropriate Beta Blocker Usage[2]	123	94%	91%	93%
Controlled Postoperative Blood Glucose[2]	0	-	91%	93%
Prophylactic Antibiotic Timing[2]	325	96%	96%	97%
Prophylactic Antibiotic Timing (Outpatient)	-	-	0%	92%
Prophylactic Antibiotic Selection[2]	323	97%	97%	97%
Prophylactic Antibiotic Select. (Outpatient)	-	-	0%	94%
Prophylactic Antibiotic Stopped[2]	310	91%	94%	94%
Recommended VTP Ordered[2]	152	94%	92%	94%
Urinary Catheter Removal[2]	118	99%	89%	90%
Children's Asthma Care				
Received Systemic Corticosteroids	-	-	-	100%
Received Home Management Plan	-	-	-	71%
Received Reliever Medication	-	-	-	100%
Use of Medical Imaging				
Combination Abdominal CT Scan	-	-	0.064	0.191
Combination Chest CT Scan	-	-	0.013	0.054
Follow-up Mammogram/Ultrasound	-	-	8.6%	8.4%
MRI for Low Back Pain	-	-	31.7%	32.7%
Survey of Patients' Hospital Experiences				
Area Around Room 'Always' Quiet at Night	300+	51%	-	58%
Doctors 'Always' Communicated Well	300+	73%	-	80%
Home Recovery Information Given	300+	75%	-	82%
Hospital Given 9 or 10 on 10 Point Scale	300+	51%	-	67%
Meds 'Always' Explained Before Given	300+	48%	-	60%
Nurses 'Always' Communicated Well	300+	62%	-	76%
Pain 'Always' Well Controlled	300+	58%	-	69%
Room and Bathroom 'Always' Clean	300+	53%	-	71%
Timely Help 'Always' Received	300+	39%	-	64%
Would Definitely Recommend Hospital	300+	57%	-	69%

Peninsula Regional Medical Center

100 E Carroll Ave
Salisbury, MD 21801
URL: www.peninsula.org
Type: Acute Care Hospitals
Ownership: Voluntary Non-Profit - Private

Phone: 410-543-7116
Fax: 410-543-7179

Emergency Services: Yes
Beds: 362

Key Personnel:
CEO/President . . . . Peggy Naleppa
Chief of Medical Staff . . . . Thomas P Lawrence, MD
Coronary Care . . . . Mary Beth D'Amico
Infection Control . . . . Karen Mihalik RN
Pediatric Ambulatory Care . . . . . . Andras Kovacs, MD
Quality Assurance . . . . Susan McDonald
Radiology . . . . Mary Lou Melhorn

Measure	Cases	This Hosp.	State Avg.	U.S. Avg.
Heart Attack Care				
ACE Inhibitor or ARB for LVSD	100	95%	94%	96%
Aspirin at Arrival	403	97%	98%	99%
Aspirin at Discharge	540	99%	98%	98%
Beta Blocker at Discharge	536	99%	97%	98%
Fibrinolytic Medication Timing	0	-	42%	55%
PCI Within 90 Minutes of Arrival	91	80%	83%	90%
Smoking Cessation Advice	172	99%	98%	99%
Chest Pain/Possible Heart Attack Care				
Aspirin at Arrival	-	-	0%	95%
Median Time to ECG (minutes)	-	-	0	8
Median Time to Transfer (minutes)	-	-	0	61
Fibrinolytic Medication Timing	-	-	0%	54%
Heart Failure Care				
ACE Inhibitor or ARB for LVSD	265	98%	94%	94%
Discharge Instructions	727	88%	86%	88%
Evaluation of LVS Function	932	96%	97%	98%
Smoking Cessation Advice	151	98%	98%	98%
Pneumonia Care				
Appropriate Initial Antibiotic[2]	186	91%	92%	92%
Blood Culture Timing[2]	264	94%	92%	96%
Influenza Vaccine[2]	191	87%	88%	91%
Initial Antibiotic Timing[2]	343	95%	94%	95%
Pneumococcal Vaccine[2]	354	86%	92%	93%
Smoking Cessation Advice[2]	104	95%	97%	97%
Surgical Care Improvement Project				
Appropriate VTP Within 24 Hours[2]	133	72%	90%	92%
Appropriate Hair Removal[2]	566	100%	100%	99%
Appropriate Beta Blocker Usage[2]	209	88%	91%	93%
Controlled Postoperative Blood Glucose[2]	129	89%	91%	93%
Prophylactic Antibiotic Timing[2]	411	95%	96%	97%
Prophylactic Antibiotic Timing (Outpatient)	-	-	0%	92%
Prophylactic Antibiotic Selection[2]	419	97%	97%	97%
Prophylactic Antibiotic Select. (Outpatient)	-	-	0%	94%
Prophylactic Antibiotic Stopped[2]	396	95%	94%	94%
Recommended VTP Ordered[2]	133	74%	92%	94%
Urinary Catheter Removal[2]	142	89%	89%	90%
Children's Asthma Care				
Received Systemic Corticosteroids	-	-	-	100%
Received Home Management Plan	-	-	-	71%
Received Reliever Medication	-	-	-	100%
Use of Medical Imaging				
Combination Abdominal CT Scan	-	-	0.064	0.191
Combination Chest CT Scan	-	-	0.013	0.054
Follow-up Mammogram/Ultrasound	-	-	8.6%	8.4%
MRI for Low Back Pain	-	-	31.7%	32.7%
Survey of Patients' Hospital Experiences				
Area Around Room 'Always' Quiet at Night	300+	48%	-	58%
Doctors 'Always' Communicated Well	300+	74%	-	80%
Home Recovery Information Given	300+	81%	-	82%
Hospital Given 9 or 10 on 10 Point Scale	300+	60%	-	67%
Meds 'Always' Explained Before Given	300+	50%	-	60%
Nurses 'Always' Communicated Well	300+	70%	-	76%
Pain 'Always' Well Controlled	300+	64%	-	69%
Room and Bathroom 'Always' Clean	300+	63%	-	71%
Timely Help 'Always' Received	300+	51%	-	64%
Would Definitely Recommend Hospital	300+	64%	-	69%

Holy Cross Hospital

1500 Forest Glen Road   Phone: 301-754-7010
Silver Spring, MD 20910   Fax: 301-754-7031
URL: www.holycrosshealth.org
Type: Acute Care Hospitals   Emergency Services: Yes
Ownership: Voluntary Non-Profit - Church   Beds: 425

Key Personnel:
CEO/President.............. Joseph Swedish
Chief of Medical Staff.......... Blair Eig, MD
Infection Control.............. Mary Mohla
Pediatric In-Patient Care .... Jane Chase
Quality Assurance .... Carolyn Simonsen
Radiology................... Robert Zimmermann, MD
Emergency Room .... Laurence Oufiero, MD
Intensive Care Unit............ Crystal Beckford, RN

Measure	Cases	This Hosp.	State Avg.	U.S. Avg.
Heart Attack Care				
ACE Inhibitor or ARB for LVSD[1]	21	95%	94%	96%
Aspirin at Arrival	188	100%	98%	99%
Aspirin at Discharge	110	100%	98%	98%
Beta Blocker at Discharge	114	99%	97%	98%
Fibrinolytic Medication Timing	0	-	42%	55%
PCI Within 90 Minutes of Arrival	38	89%	83%	90%
Smoking Cessation Advice[1]	15	100%	98%	99%
Chest Pain/Possible Heart Attack Care				
Aspirin at Arrival[5]	0	-	0%	95%
Median Time to ECG (minutes)[5]	0	-	0	8
Median Time to Transfer (minutes)[5]	0	-	0	61
Fibrinolytic Medication Timing[5]	0	-	0%	54%
Heart Failure Care				
ACE Inhibitor or ARB for LVSD[2]	134	99%	94%	94%
Discharge Instructions[2]	316	89%	86%	88%
Evaluation of LVS Function[2]	414	99%	97%	98%
Smoking Cessation Advice[2]	43	100%	98%	98%
Pneumonia Care				
Appropriate Initial Antibiotic[2]	168	94%	92%	92%
Blood Culture Timing[2]	175	96%	92%	96%
Influenza Vaccine[2]	176	98%	88%	91%
Initial Antibiotic Timing[2]	241	96%	94%	95%
Pneumococcal Vaccine[2]	262	99%	92%	93%
Smoking Cessation Advice[2]	50	100%	97%	97%
Surgical Care Improvement Project				
Appropriate VTP Within 24 Hours[2]	234	96%	90%	92%
Appropriate Hair Removal[2]	680	100%	100%	99%
Appropriate Beta Blocker Usage[2]	146	99%	91%	93%
Controlled Postoperative Blood Glucose[2]	0	-	91%	93%
Prophylactic Antibiotic Timing[2]	396	96%	96%	97%
Prophylactic Antibiotic Timing (Outpatient)[5]	0	-	0%	92%
Prophylactic Antibiotic Selection[2]	395	96%	97%	97%
Prophylactic Antibiotic Select. (Outpatient)[5]	0	-	0%	94%
Prophylactic Antibiotic Stopped[2]	381	97%	94%	94%
Recommended VTP Ordered[2]	234	96%	92%	94%
Urinary Catheter Removal[2]	71	99%	89%	90%
Children's Asthma Care				
Received Systemic Corticosteroids	-	-	-	100%
Received Home Management Plan	-	-	-	71%
Received Reliever Medication	-	-	-	100%
Use of Medical Imaging				
Combination Abdominal CT Scan	538	0.026	0.064	0.191
Combination Chest CT Scan	265	0.004	0.013	0.054
Follow-up Mammogram/Ultrasound	111	9.9%	8.6%	8.4%
MRI for Low Back Pain	44	38.6%	31.7%	32.7%
Survey of Patients' Hospital Experiences				
Area Around Room 'Always' Quiet at Night	300+	56%	-	58%
Doctors 'Always' Communicated Well	300+	75%	-	80%
Home Recovery Information Given	300+	74%	-	82%
Hospital Given 9 or 10 on 10 Point Scale	300+	58%	-	67%
Meds 'Always' Explained Before Given	300+	50%	-	60%
Nurses 'Always' Communicated Well	300+	67%	-	76%
Pain 'Always' Well Controlled	300+	63%	-	69%
Room and Bathroom 'Always' Clean	300+	59%	-	71%
Timely Help 'Always' Received	300+	52%	-	64%
Would Definitely Recommend Hospital	300+	63%	-	69%

Washington Adventist Hospital

7600 Carroll Ave   Phone: 301-891-5651
Takoma Park, MD 20912
URL: www.adventisthealthcare.com/WAH
Type: Acute Care Hospitals   Emergency Services: No
Ownership: Voluntary Non-Profit - Church   Beds: 292

Key Personnel:
CEO/President.............. Jere Stocks
Chief of Medical Staff.......... Stephen Michaels MD

Measure	Cases	This Hosp.	State Avg.	U.S. Avg.
Heart Attack Care				
ACE Inhibitor or ARB for LVSD[2]	71	96%	94%	96%
Aspirin at Arrival[2]	83	99%	98%	99%
Aspirin at Discharge[2]	292	98%	98%	98%
Beta Blocker at Discharge[2]	282	98%	97%	98%
Fibrinolytic Medication Timing[1,2]	1	0%	42%	55%
PCI Within 90 Minutes of Arrival[1,2]	20	95%	83%	90%
Smoking Cessation Advice[2]	81	100%	98%	99%
Chest Pain/Possible Heart Attack Care				
Aspirin at Arrival	-	-	0%	95%
Median Time to ECG (minutes)	-	-	0	8
Median Time to Transfer (minutes)	-	-	0	61
Fibrinolytic Medication Timing	-	-	0%	54%
Heart Failure Care				
ACE Inhibitor or ARB for LVSD[2]	182	95%	94%	94%
Discharge Instructions[2]	311	77%	86%	88%
Evaluation of LVS Function[2]	398	96%	97%	98%
Smoking Cessation Advice[2]	50	100%	98%	98%
Pneumonia Care				
Appropriate Initial Antibiotic[2]	55	96%	92%	92%
Blood Culture Timing[2]	112	98%	92%	96%
Influenza Vaccine[2]	67	72%	88%	91%
Initial Antibiotic Timing[2]	117	97%	94%	95%
Pneumococcal Vaccine[2]	119	81%	92%	93%
Smoking Cessation Advice[1,2]	18	100%	97%	97%
Surgical Care Improvement Project				
Appropriate VTP Within 24 Hours[2]	123	89%	90%	92%
Appropriate Hair Removal[2]	492	100%	100%	99%
Appropriate Beta Blocker Usage[2]	169	79%	91%	93%
Controlled Postoperative Blood Glucose[2]	137	86%	91%	93%
Prophylactic Antibiotic Timing[2]	344	97%	96%	97%
Prophylactic Antibiotic Timing (Outpatient)	-	-	0%	92%
Prophylactic Antibiotic Selection[2]	351	98%	97%	97%
Prophylactic Antibiotic Select. (Outpatient)	-	-	0%	94%
Prophylactic Antibiotic Stopped[2]	334	94%	94%	94%
Recommended VTP Ordered[2]	123	94%	92%	94%
Urinary Catheter Removal[2]	125	90%	89%	90%
Children's Asthma Care				
Received Systemic Corticosteroids	-	-	-	100%
Received Home Management Plan	-	-	-	71%
Received Reliever Medication	-	-	-	100%
Use of Medical Imaging				
Combination Abdominal CT Scan	-	-	0.064	0.191
Combination Chest CT Scan	-	-	0.013	0.054
Follow-up Mammogram/Ultrasound	-	-	8.6%	8.4%
MRI for Low Back Pain	-	-	31.7%	32.7%
Survey of Patients' Hospital Experiences				
Area Around Room 'Always' Quiet at Night	300+	47%	-	58%
Doctors 'Always' Communicated Well	300+	76%	-	80%
Home Recovery Information Given	300+	77%	-	82%
Hospital Given 9 or 10 on 10 Point Scale	300+	53%	-	67%
Meds 'Always' Explained Before Given	300+	47%	-	60%
Nurses 'Always' Communicated Well	300+	64%	-	76%
Pain 'Always' Well Controlled	300+	58%	-	69%
Room and Bathroom 'Always' Clean	300+	54%	-	71%
Timely Help 'Always' Received	300+	44%	-	64%
Would Definitely Recommend Hospital	300+	60%	-	69%

Saint Joseph Medical Center

7601 Osler Drive   Phone: 410-337-1200
Towson, MD 21204
URL: www.sjmcmd.org
Type: Acute Care Hospitals   Emergency Services: Yes
Ownership: Voluntary Non-Profit - Church   Beds: 364

Key Personnel:
CEO/President.............. Jeffrey K Norman

Measure	Cases	This Hosp.	State Avg.	U.S. Avg.
Heart Attack Care				
ACE Inhibitor or ARB for LVSD[2]	54	100%	94%	96%
Aspirin at Arrival[2]	172	100%	98%	99%
Aspirin at Discharge[2]	323	99%	98%	98%
Beta Blocker at Discharge[2]	321	99%	97%	98%
Fibrinolytic Medication Timing[2]	0	-	42%	55%
PCI Within 90 Minutes of Arrival[1,2]	20	75%	83%	90%
Smoking Cessation Advice[2]	87	100%	98%	99%
Chest Pain/Possible Heart Attack Care				
Aspirin at Arrival	-	-	0%	95%
Median Time to ECG (minutes)	-	-	0	8
Median Time to Transfer (minutes)	-	-	0	61
Fibrinolytic Medication Timing	-	-	0%	54%
Heart Failure Care				
ACE Inhibitor or ARB for LVSD[2]	94	99%	94%	94%
Discharge Instructions[2]	252	94%	86%	88%
Evaluation of LVS Function[2]	325	100%	97%	98%
Smoking Cessation Advice[2]	38	100%	98%	98%
Pneumonia Care				
Appropriate Initial Antibiotic[2]	95	92%	92%	92%
Blood Culture Timing[2]	135	96%	92%	96%
Influenza Vaccine[2]	54	87%	88%	91%
Initial Antibiotic Timing[2]	148	95%	94%	95%
Pneumococcal Vaccine[2]	164	96%	92%	93%
Smoking Cessation Advice[2]	38	100%	97%	97%
Surgical Care Improvement Project				
Appropriate VTP Within 24 Hours[2]	102	97%	90%	92%
Appropriate Hair Removal[2]	568	99%	100%	99%
Appropriate Beta Blocker Usage[2]	224	95%	91%	93%
Controlled Postoperative Blood Glucose[2]	118	96%	91%	93%
Prophylactic Antibiotic Timing[2]	369	97%	96%	97%
Prophylactic Antibiotic Timing (Outpatient)	-	-	0%	92%
Prophylactic Antibiotic Selection[2]	384	98%	97%	97%
Prophylactic Antibiotic Select. (Outpatient)	-	-	0%	94%
Prophylactic Antibiotic Stopped[2]	340	97%	94%	94%
Recommended VTP Ordered[2]	102	98%	92%	94%
Urinary Catheter Removal[2]	74	88%	89%	90%
Children's Asthma Care				
Received Systemic Corticosteroids	-	-	-	100%
Received Home Management Plan	-	-	-	71%
Received Reliever Medication	-	-	-	100%
Use of Medical Imaging				
Combination Abdominal CT Scan	-	-	0.064	0.191
Combination Chest CT Scan	-	-	0.013	0.054
Follow-up Mammogram/Ultrasound	-	-	8.6%	8.4%
MRI for Low Back Pain	-	-	31.7%	32.7%
Survey of Patients' Hospital Experiences				
Area Around Room 'Always' Quiet at Night	300+	56%	-	58%
Doctors 'Always' Communicated Well	300+	80%	-	80%
Home Recovery Information Given	300+	80%	-	82%
Hospital Given 9 or 10 on 10 Point Scale	300+	67%	-	67%
Meds 'Always' Explained Before Given	300+	53%	-	60%
Nurses 'Always' Communicated Well	300+	74%	-	76%
Pain 'Always' Well Controlled	300+	69%	-	69%
Room and Bathroom 'Always' Clean	300+	59%	-	71%
Timely Help 'Always' Received	300+	60%	-	64%
Would Definitely Recommend Hospital	300+	74%	-	69%

NOTE: Hospital profiles are in alphabetical order by state, then city, then hospital within the city; Rankings exclude hospitals with less than 25 cases except for patient surveys which excludes hospitals with less than 100 cases; (a) 100–299 cases; (1) The number of cases is too small to be sure how well a hospital is performing; (2) The hospital indicated that the data submitted for this measure were based on a sample of cases; (3) Data was collected during a shorter time period (fewer quarters) than the maximum possible time for this measure; (4) Suppressed for one or more quarters by CMS; (5) No data is available from the hospital for this measure; (6) Fewer than 100 patients completed the HCAHPS survey. Use these rates with caution, as the number of surveys may be too low to reliably assess hospital performance; (7) Survey results are based on less than 12 months of data; (8) Survey results are not available for this reporting period; (9) No or very few patients were eligible for the HCAHPS survey. The scores shown, if any, reflect a very small number of surveys; (10) A state average was not calculated because too few hospitals in the state submitted data; (11) There were discrepancies in the data collection process; Please refer to the User's Guide for a full explanation of data.

Carroll Hospital Center

200 Memorial Ave
Westminster, MD 21157
E-mail: info@CarrollHospitalCenter.org
URL: www.carrollhospitalcenter.org
Type: Acute Care Hospitals
Ownership: Voluntary Non-Profit - Private

Phone: 410-871-6900
Fax: 410-871-6325

Emergency Services: Yes
Beds: 200

Key Personnel:
CEO/President . . . . John M Sernulka, CEO
Operating Room . . . . Kate Painter
Pediatric In-Patient Care . . . . Linda Grogan
Quality Assurance . . . . Mary Ann Kowalczyk
Radiology . . . . Sandy D'Arrigo
Patient Relations . . . . Leslie Simmons

Measure	Cases	This Hosp.	State Avg.	U.S. Avg.
Heart Attack Care				
ACE Inhibitor or ARB for LVSD[1]	20	100%	94%	96%
Aspirin at Arrival	150	98%	98%	99%
Aspirin at Discharge	93	99%	98%	98%
Beta Blocker at Discharge	89	97%	97%	98%
Fibrinolytic Medication Timing[1]	1	100%	42%	55%
PCI Within 90 Minutes of Arrival	48	88%	83%	90%
Smoking Cessation Advice	25	100%	98%	99%
Chest Pain/Possible Heart Attack Care				
Aspirin at Arrival	-	-	0%	95%
Median Time to ECG (minutes)	-	-	0	8
Median Time to Transfer (minutes)	-	-	0	61
Fibrinolytic Medication Timing	-	-	0%	54%
Heart Failure Care				
ACE Inhibitor or ARB for LVSD[2]	80	89%	94%	94%
Discharge Instructions[2]	205	92%	86%	88%
Evaluation of LVS Function[2]	269	95%	97%	98%
Smoking Cessation Advice[2]	39	100%	98%	98%
Pneumonia Care				
Appropriate Initial Antibiotic[2]	105	99%	92%	92%
Blood Culture Timing[2]	184	98%	92%	96%
Influenza Vaccine[2]	100	95%	88%	91%
Initial Antibiotic Timing[2]	171	98%	94%	95%
Pneumococcal Vaccine[2]	146	96%	92%	93%
Smoking Cessation Advice[2]	38	100%	97%	97%
Surgical Care Improvement Project				
Appropriate VTP Within 24 Hours[2]	145	86%	90%	92%
Appropriate Hair Removal[2]	506	100%	100%	99%
Appropriate Beta Blocker Usage[2]	122	88%	91%	93%
Controlled Postoperative Blood Glucose[2]	0	-	91%	93%
Prophylactic Antibiotic Timing[2]	334	93%	96%	97%
Prophylactic Antibiotic Timing (Outpatient)	-	-	0%	92%
Prophylactic Antibiotic Selection[2]	335	97%	97%	97%
Prophylactic Antibiotic Select. (Outpatient)	-	-	0%	94%
Prophylactic Antibiotic Stopped[2]	328	94%	94%	94%
Recommended VTP Ordered[2]	145	94%	92%	94%
Urinary Catheter Removal[2]	43	74%	89%	90%
Children's Asthma Care				
Received Systemic Corticosteroids	-	-	-	100%
Received Home Management Plan	-	-	-	71%
Received Reliever Medication	-	-	-	100%
Use of Medical Imaging				
Combination Abdominal CT Scan	-	-	0.064	0.191
Combination Chest CT Scan	-	-	0.013	0.054
Follow-up Mammogram/Ultrasound	-	-	8.6%	8.4%
MRI for Low Back Pain	-	-	31.7%	32.7%
Survey of Patients' Hospital Experiences				
Area Around Room 'Always' Quiet at Night	300+	47%	-	58%
Doctors 'Always' Communicated Well	300+	76%	-	80%
Home Recovery Information Given	300+	78%	-	82%
Hospital Given 9 or 10 on 10 Point Scale	300+	66%	-	67%
Meds 'Always' Explained Before Given	300+	63%	-	60%
Nurses 'Always' Communicated Well	300+	76%	-	76%
Pain 'Always' Well Controlled	300+	68%	-	69%
Room and Bathroom 'Always' Clean	300+	64%	-	71%
Timely Help 'Always' Received	300+	61%	-	64%
Would Definitely Recommend Hospital	300+	66%	-	69%

NOTE: Hospital profiles are in alphabetical order by state, then city, then hospital within the city; Rankings exclude hospitals with less than 25 cases except for patient surveys which excludes hospitals with less than 100 cases; (a) 100–299 cases; (1) The number of cases is too small to be sure how well a hospital is performing; (2) The hospital indicated that the data submitted for this measure were based on a sample of cases; (3) Data was collected during a shorter time period (fewer quarters) than the maximum possible time for this measure; (4) Suppressed for one or more quarters by CMS; (5) No data is available from the hospital for this measure; (6) Fewer than 100 patients completed the HCAHPS survey. Use these rates with caution, as the number of surveys may be too low to reliably assess hospital performance; (7) Survey results are based on less than 12 months of data; (8) Survey results are not available for this reporting period; (9) No or very few patients were eligible for the HCAHPS survey. The scores shown, if any, reflect a very small number of surveys; (10) A state average was not calculated because too few hospitals in the state submitted data; (11) There were discrepancies in the data collection process; Please refer to the User's Guide for a full explanation of data.

Heart Attack Care

1. ACE Inhibitor or ARB for LVSD

Hospital Name	City	Rate	Cases
Metrowest Medical Center	Framingham	100%	30
Mount Auburn Hospital	Cambridge	100%	38
North Shore Medical Center	Salem	100%	46
Tufts Medical Center	Boston	100%	90
Massachusetts General Hospital[2]	Boston	99%	79
UMass Memorial Medical Center[2]	Worcester	98%	151
Saint Vincent Hospital	Worcester	97%	73
Lahey Clinic Hospital	Burlington	96%	139
Baystate Medical Center	Springfield	93%	193
Beverly Hospital Corporation	Beverly	93%	27
Boston Medical Center Corporation	Boston	93%	67
Beth Israel Deaconess Medical Center	Boston	92%	88
Brigham and Women's Hospital	Boston	92%	98
South Shore Hospital	S Weymouth	89%	38
Good Samaritan Medical Center	Brockton	85%	27
Southcoast Hospital Group	Fall River	84%	148
Saint Elizabeth's Medical Center	Brighton	83%	71
Cape Cod Hospital[2]	Hyannis	82%	38

2. Aspirin at Arrival

Hospital Name	City	Rate	Cases
Baystate Medical Center	Springfield	100%	500
Berkshire Medical Center	Pittsfield	100%	88
Beth Israel Deaconess Medical Center	Boston	100%	170
Beverly Hospital Corporation	Beverly	100%	188
Boston Medical Center Corporation	Boston	100%	159
Brigham and Women's Hospital	Boston	100%	270
The Cooley Dickinson Hospital	Northampton	100%	47
Falmouth Hospital	Falmouth	100%	94
Good Samaritan Medical Center	Brockton	100%	173
Hallmark Health System	Melrose	100%	112
Healthalliance Hospitals	Leominster	100%	96
Heywood Hospital[2]	Gardner	100%	49
Jordan Hospital	Plymouth	100%	82
Lahey Clinic Hospital	Burlington	100%	298
Lowell General Hospital	Lowell	100%	137
Marlborough Hospital	Marlborough	100%	36
Massachusetts General Hospital[2]	Boston	100%	273
Metrowest Medical Center	Framingham	100%	121
Milford Regional Medical Center	Milford	100%	72
Newton-Wellesley Hospital	Newton	100%	59
Noble Hospital	Westfield	100%	26
North Adams Regional Hospital	North Adams	100%	37
North Shore Medical Center	Salem	100%	298
Norwood Hospital	Norwood	100%	142
Quincy Medical Center	Quincy	100%	70
Saint Anne's Hospital	Fall River	100%	54
Saint Vincent Hospital	Worcester	100%	368
Signature Healthcare Brockton Hospital	Brockton	100%	188
South Shore Hospital	S Weymouth	100%	281
Tufts Medical Center	Boston	100%	73
Cape Cod Hospital[2]	Hyannis	99%	256
Lawrence General Hospital	Lawrence	99%	102
Mount Auburn Hospital	Cambridge	99%	191
Saint Elizabeth's Medical Center	Brighton	99%	107
Saints Medical Center	Lowell	99%	137
UMass Memorial Medical Center[2]	Worcester	99%	353
Mercy Medical Center	Springfield	98%	87
Milton Hospital	Milton	98%	60
Morton Hospital & Medical Center	Taunton	98%	52
Southcoast Hospital Group	Fall River	98%	640
Winchester Hospital[2]	Winchester	98%	94
Baystate Franklin Medical Center	Greenfield	97%	29
Cambridge Health Alliance	Cambridge	97%	70
Emerson Hospital	West Concord	97%	60
Holy Family Hospital	Methuen	97%	79
Sturdy Memorial Hospital	Attleboro	97%	30
Anna Jaques Hospital	Newburyport	96%	54
Harrington Memorial Hospital	Southbridge	96%	27
Holyoke Medical Center	Holyoke	95%	110
Merrimack Valley Hospital	Haverhill	95%	41

3. Aspirin at Discharge

Hospital Name	City	Rate	Cases
Baystate Medical Center	Springfield	100%	1055
Berkshire Medical Center	Pittsfield	100%	58
Beth Israel Deaconess Medical Center	Boston	100%	529
Beverly Hospital Corporation	Beverly	100%	123
Boston Medical Center Corporation	Boston	100%	456
Brigham and Women's Hospital	Boston	100%	598
Cambridge Health Alliance	Cambridge	100%	52
Emerson Hospital	West Concord	100%	33
Falmouth Hospital	Falmouth	100%	68
Good Samaritan Medical Center	Brockton	100%	127
Hallmark Health System	Melrose	100%	79
Holy Family Hospital	Methuen	100%	50
Lahey Clinic Hospital	Burlington	100%	703
Lowell General Hospital	Lowell	100%	115
Massachusetts General Hospital[2]	Boston	100%	758
Metrowest Medical Center	Framingham	100%	107
Milton Hospital	Milton	100%	42
Mount Auburn Hospital	Cambridge	100%	228
Newton-Wellesley Hospital	Newton	100%	38
North Adams Regional Hospital	North Adams	100%	27
North Shore Medical Center	Salem	100%	301
Quincy Medical Center	Quincy	100%	51
Saint Vincent Hospital	Worcester	100%	446
Tufts Medical Center	Boston	100%	398
UMass Memorial Medical Center[2]	Worcester	100%	825
Winchester Hospital[2]	Winchester	100%	67
Cape Cod Hospital[2]	Hyannis	99%	289
Healthalliance Hospitals	Leominster	99%	69
Lawrence General Hospital	Lawrence	99%	74
Saints Medical Center	Lowell	99%	110
Signature Healthcare Brockton Hospital	Brockton	99%	145
South Shore Hospital	S Weymouth	99%	240
Southcoast Hospital Group	Fall River	99%	687
Mercy Medical Center	Springfield	98%	55
Norwood Hospital	Norwood	98%	101
The Cooley Dickinson Hospital	Northampton	97%	39
Merrimack Valley Hospital	Haverhill	97%	31
Morton Hospital & Medical Center	Taunton	97%	34
Saint Anne's Hospital	Fall River	97%	31
Milford Regional Medical Center	Milford	96%	56
Saint Elizabeth's Medical Center	Brighton	96%	326
Holyoke Medical Center	Holyoke	94%	69
Jordan Hospital	Plymouth	94%	48
Heywood Hospital[2]	Gardner	89%	28

4. Beta Blocker at Discharge

Hospital Name	City	Rate	Cases
Anna Jaques Hospital	Newburyport	100%	26
Berkshire Medical Center	Pittsfield	100%	64
Beth Israel Deaconess Medical Center	Boston	100%	503
Beverly Hospital Corporation	Beverly	100%	127
Boston Medical Center Corporation	Boston	100%	430
Good Samaritan Medical Center	Brockton	100%	120
Jordan Hospital	Plymouth	100%	56
Lawrence General Hospital	Lawrence	100%	75
Lowell General Hospital	Lowell	100%	121
Merrimack Valley Hospital	Haverhill	100%	29
Metrowest Medical Center	Framingham	100%	104
Morton Hospital & Medical Center	Taunton	100%	35
Mount Auburn Hospital	Cambridge	100%	225
Newton-Wellesley Hospital	Newton	100%	41
North Adams Regional Hospital	North Adams	100%	26
North Shore Medical Center	Salem	100%	304
Norwood Hospital	Norwood	100%	96
Saint Anne's Hospital	Fall River	100%	30
Signature Healthcare Brockton Hospital	Brockton	100%	144
South Shore Hospital	S Weymouth	100%	233
UMass Memorial Medical Center[2]	Worcester	100%	793
Baystate Medical Center	Springfield	99%	1015
Healthalliance Hospitals	Leominster	99%	74
Lahey Clinic Hospital	Burlington	99%	687
Massachusetts General Hospital[2]	Boston	99%	727
Saint Vincent Hospital	Worcester	99%	434
Tufts Medical Center	Boston	99%	376
Winchester Hospital[2]	Winchester	99%	74
Brigham and Women's Hospital	Boston	98%	575
Cambridge Health Alliance	Cambridge	98%	50
Cape Cod Hospital[2]	Hyannis	98%	276
Falmouth Hospital	Falmouth	98%	61
Mercy Medical Center	Springfield	98%	60
Milford Regional Medical Center	Milford	98%	53
Quincy Medical Center	Quincy	98%	50
Southcoast Hospital Group	Fall River	98%	706
The Cooley Dickinson Hospital	Northampton	97%	34
Emerson Hospital	West Concord	97%	33
Hallmark Health System	Melrose	97%	79
Heywood Hospital[2]	Gardner	97%	35
Saints Medical Center	Lowell	97%	105
Holyoke Medical Center	Holyoke	96%	71
Saint Elizabeth's Medical Center	Brighton	96%	307
Holy Family Hospital	Methuen	95%	57
Milton Hospital	Milton	95%	41

6. PCI Within 90 Minutes of Arrival

Hospital Name	City	Rate	Cases
Beth Israel Deaconess Medical Center	Boston	100%	27
Cape Cod Hospital[2]	Hyannis	100%	37
Norwood Hospital	Norwood	100%	40
Lowell General Hospital	Lowell	98%	43
North Shore Medical Center	Salem	98%	91
Saint Vincent Hospital	Worcester	98%	44
Signature Healthcare Brockton Hospital	Brockton	98%	44
Baystate Medical Center	Springfield	96%	138
Boston Medical Center Corporation	Boston	96%	28
UMass Memorial Medical Center[2]	Worcester	96%	81
Massachusetts General Hospital[2]	Boston	95%	57
Metrowest Medical Center	Framingham	95%	42
South Shore Hospital	S Weymouth	94%	89
Lahey Clinic Hospital	Burlington	93%	69
Lawrence General Hospital	Lawrence	92%	36
Mount Auburn Hospital	Cambridge	92%	36
Holy Family Hospital	Methuen	88%	26
Brigham and Women's Hospital	Boston	86%	42
Saints Medical Center	Lowell	84%	32
Southcoast Hospital Group	Fall River	84%	58
Good Samaritan Medical Center	Brockton	83%	63

7. Smoking Cessation Advice

Hospital Name	City	Rate	Cases
Baystate Medical Center	Springfield	100%	311
Beth Israel Deaconess Medical Center	Boston	100%	107
Boston Medical Center Corporation	Boston	100%	161
Good Samaritan Medical Center	Brockton	100%	34
Lowell General Hospital	Lowell	100%	27
Massachusetts General Hospital[2]	Boston	100%	197
Metrowest Medical Center	Framingham	100%	25
Mount Auburn Hospital	Cambridge	100%	39
North Shore Medical Center	Salem	100%	106
Saint Vincent Hospital	Worcester	100%	127
Saints Medical Center	Lowell	100%	39
Signature Healthcare Brockton Hospital	Brockton	100%	54
UMass Memorial Medical Center[2]	Worcester	100%	261
Lahey Clinic Hospital	Burlington	99%	156
Saint Elizabeth's Medical Center	Brighton	99%	96
South Shore Hospital	S Weymouth	99%	70
Tufts Medical Center	Boston	99%	103
Brigham and Women's Hospital	Boston	98%	139
Cape Cod Hospital[2]	Hyannis	92%	65
Southcoast Hospital Group	Fall River	92%	195

Chest Pain/Possible Heart Attack Care

8. Aspirin at Arrival

Hospital Name	City	Rate	Cases
Berkshire Medical Center	Pittsfield	100%	109
Good Samaritan Medical Center	Brockton	100%	61
Hallmark Health System	Melrose	100%	104
Marlborough Hospital	Marlborough	100%	79
Norwood Hospital	Norwood	100%	54
Quincy Medical Center	Quincy	100%	59
Beverly Hospital Corporation	Beverly	99%	144
Emerson Hospital	West Concord	99%	70
Milton Hospital	Milton	99%	73
Morton Hospital & Medical Center	Taunton	99%	89
Anna Jaques Hospital	Newburyport	98%	57
Baystate Franklin Medical Center	Greenfield	98%	45
The Cooley Dickinson Hospital	Northampton	98%	83
Heywood Hospital	Gardner	98%	160
Jordan Hospital	Plymouth	98%	165
Merrimack Valley Hospital	Haverhill	98%	46
Metrowest Medical Center	Framingham	98%	55
Nashoba Valley Medical Center	Ayer	98%	96
Noble Hospital	Westfield	98%	40
Healthalliance Hospitals	Leominster	97%	159
Faulkner Hospital	Boston	96%	49
North Adams Regional Hospital	North Adams	96%	48
Sturdy Memorial Hospital	Attleboro	96%	141
Baystate Mary Lane Hospital	Ware	95%	43
Falmouth Hospital	Falmouth	95%	38
Milford Regional Medical Center	Milford	95%	88
Newton-Wellesley Hospital	Newton	95%	56
Beth Israel Deaconess Hospital - Needham	Needham	94%	85
Cambridge Health Alliance	Cambridge	94%	86
Holyoke Medical Center	Holyoke	94%	49
Southcoast Hospital Group	Fall River	94%	128
Lawrence General Hospital	Lawrence	93%	60
Mercy Medical Center	Springfield	93%	46
Winchester Hospital	Winchester	93%	122
Saint Anne's Hospital	Fall River	92%	25
Holy Family Hospital	Methuen	91%	64
South Shore Hospital	S Weymouth	90%	51
Harrington Memorial Hospital	Southbridge	88%	146
Nantucket Cottage Hospital[3]	Nantucket	88%	25
Wing Memorial Hospital and Medical Center	Palmer	85%	41

9. Median Time to ECG (minutes)

Hospital Name	City	Min.	Cases
Newton-Wellesley Hospital	Newton	0	58
Metrowest Medical Center	Framingham	2	56
Good Samaritan Medical Center	Brockton	3	69

NOTE: Hospital profiles are in alphabetical order by state, then city, then hospital within the city; Rankings exclude hospitals with less than 25 cases except for patient surveys which excludes hospitals with less than 100 cases; (a) 100–299 cases; (1) The number of cases is too small to be sure how well a hospital is performing; (2) The hospital indicated that the data submitted for this measure were based on a sample of cases; (3) Data was collected during a shorter time period (fewer quarters) than the maximum possible time for this measure; (4) Suppressed for one or more quarters by CMS; (5) No data is available from the hospital for this measure; (6) Fewer than 100 patients completed the HCAHPS survey. Use these rates with caution, as the number of surveys may be too low to reliably assess hospital performance; (7) Survey results are based on less than 12 months of data; (8) Survey results are not available for this reporting period; (9) No or very few patients were eligible for the HCAHPS survey. The scores shown, if any, reflect a very small number of surveys; (10) A state average was not calculated because too few hospitals in the state submitted data; (11) There were discrepancies in the data collection process; Please refer to the User's Guide for a full explanation of data.

Beth Israel Deaconess Hospital - Needham	Needham	4	89
Nantucket Cottage Hospital[3]	Nantucket	4	26
Cambridge Health Alliance	Cambridge	5	90
Marlborough Hospital	Marlborough	5	81
Noble Hospital	Westfield	6	41
North Adams Regional Hospital	North Adams	6	52
Southcoast Hospital Group	Fall River	6	133
Anna Jaques Hospital	Newburyport	7	56
Baystate Franklin Medical Center	Greenfield	7	48
Emerson Hospital	West Concord	7	71
Healthalliance Hospitals	Leominster	7	159
Mercy Medical Center	Springfield	7	49
Merrimack Valley Hospital	Haverhill	7	49
Berkshire Medical Center	Pittsfield	8	109
The Cooley Dickinson Hospital	Northampton	8	82
Falmouth Hospital	Falmouth	8	39
Holy Family Hospital	Methuen	8	69
Milton Hospital	Milton	8	76
Norwood Hospital	Norwood	8	57
South Shore Hospital	S Weymouth	9	54
Beverly Hospital Corporation	Beverly	10	149
Sturdy Memorial Hospital	Attleboro	10	144
Nashoba Valley Medical Center	Ayer	11	100
Saint Anne's Hospital	Fall River	11	27
Winchester Hospital	Winchester	11	127
Hallmark Health System	Melrose	12	116
Wing Memorial Hospital and Medical Center	Palmer	12	46
Holyoke Medical Center	Holyoke	13	50
Lawrence General Hospital	Lawrence	13	61
Faulkner Hospital	Boston	15	51
Milford Regional Medical Center	Milford	15	91
Morton Hospital & Medical Center	Taunton	16	95
Baystate Mary Lane Hospital	Ware	17	45
Quincy Medical Center	Quincy	17	63
Harrington Memorial Hospital	Southbridge	18	152
Heywood Hospital	Gardner	18	173
Jordan Hospital	Plymouth	22	174

10. Median Time to Transfer (minutes)

Hospital Name	City	Min.	Cases
The Cooley Dickinson Hospital	Northampton	55	33
Beverly Hospital Corporation	Beverly	56	44
Healthalliance Hospitals	Leominster	57	29
Southcoast Hospital Group	Fall River	69	45
Milford Regional Medical Center	Milford	76	31

11. Fibrinolytic Medication Timing

Hospital Name	City	Rate	Cases
Berkshire Medical Center	Pittsfield	81%	31

Heart Failure Care

12. ACE Inhibitor or ARB for LVSD

Hospital Name	City	Rate	Cases
Berkshire Medical Center	Pittsfield	100%	55
Falmouth Hospital	Falmouth	100%	46
Faulkner Hospital[2]	Boston	100%	38
Mount Auburn Hospital	Cambridge	100%	82
Noble Hospital	Westfield	100%	30
Sturdy Memorial Hospital	Attleboro	100%	54
Carney Hospital	Boston	99%	73
Signature Healthcare Brockton Hospital	Brockton	99%	96
Tufts Medical Center	Boston	99%	193
Cambridge Health Alliance	Cambridge	98%	48
The Cooley Dickinson Hospital	Northampton	98%	53
Emerson Hospital	West Concord	98%	45
Jordan Hospital	Plymouth	98%	56
Milford Regional Medical Center	Milford	98%	59
North Shore Medical Center	Salem	98%	108
Quincy Medical Center	Quincy	98%	61
Saint Vincent Hospital	Worcester	98%	138
Beverly Hospital Corporation	Beverly	97%	94
Mercy Medical Center	Springfield	97%	79
Norwood Hospital	Norwood	97%	58
Baystate Medical Center	Springfield	96%	311
Hallmark Health System[2]	Melrose	96%	70
Holy Family Hospital	Methuen	96%	56
Marlborough Hospital	Marlborough	96%	28
Massachusetts General Hospital[2]	Boston	96%	72
Metrowest Medical Center	Framingham	96%	154
Newton-Wellesley Hospital[2]	Newton	96%	54
Winchester Hospital[2]	Winchester	96%	51
Boston Medical Center Corporation	Boston	95%	325
Brigham and Women's Hospital[2]	Boston	95%	96
Good Samaritan Medical Center	Brockton	95%	87
Healthalliance Hospitals	Leominster	95%	41
Milton Hospital	Milton	95%	38
Lowell General Hospital[2]	Lowell	93%	59
Morton Hospital & Medical Center	Taunton	93%	73
UMass Memorial Medical Center[2]	Worcester	93%	247
Merrimack Valley Hospital	Haverhill	92%	36
Beth Israel Deaconess Medical Center[2]	Boston	91%	138
Harrington Memorial Hospital	Southbridge	89%	36
Southcoast Hospital Group	Fall River	89%	362
Anna Jaques Hospital	Newburyport	88%	51
Heywood Hospital[2]	Gardner	88%	25
Lahey Clinic Hospital[2]	Burlington	88%	66
VA Boston Healthcare System - Jamaica Plain	Jamaica Plain	88%	97
Holyoke Medical Center	Holyoke	87%	53
Saints Medical Center	Lowell	86%	64
Saint Elizabeth's Medical Center	Brighton	84%	101
South Shore Hospital	S Weymouth	84%	176
Cape Cod Hospital[2]	Hyannis	79%	87
Lawrence General Hospital	Lawrence	79%	119

13. Discharge Instructions

Hospital Name	City	Rate	Cases
Baystate Mary Lane Hospital	Ware	100%	37
Berkshire Medical Center	Pittsfield	100%	201
Clinton Hospital Association	Clinton	100%	31
Faulkner Hospital[2]	Boston	100%	151
Mount Auburn Hospital	Cambridge	100%	264
New England Baptist Hospital	Boston	100%	29
VA Boston Healthcare System - Jamaica Plain	Jamaica Plain	100%	236
Boston Medical Center Corporation	Boston	99%	697
Brigham and Women's Hospital[2]	Boston	99%	244
Milton Hospital	Milton	99%	133
Hallmark Health System[2]	Melrose	98%	211
Merrimack Valley Hospital	Haverhill	98%	122
Sturdy Memorial Hospital	Attleboro	98%	140
Baystate Medical Center	Springfield	97%	750
Metrowest Medical Center	Framingham	97%	320
Saint Vincent Hospital	Worcester	97%	396
Signature Healthcare Brockton Hospital	Brockton	97%	206
Tufts Medical Center	Boston	97%	348
Quincy Medical Center	Quincy	96%	164
Wing Memorial Hospital and Medical Center[2]	Palmer	96%	103
Baystate Franklin Medical Center	Greenfield	95%	99
Beth Israel Deaconess Medical Center[2]	Boston	95%	433
Newton-Wellesley Hospital[2]	Newton	95%	193
North Adams Regional Hospital	North Adams	95%	75
North Shore Medical Center	Salem	95%	425
Athol Memorial Hospital	Athol	94%	31
The Cooley Dickinson Hospital	Northampton	94%	122
Anna Jaques Hospital	Newburyport	93%	138
Cambridge Health Alliance	Cambridge	93%	191
Lahey Clinic Hospital[2]	Burlington	93%	217
Noble Hospital	Westfield	93%	82
Saint Elizabeth's Medical Center	Brighton	93%	303
Fairview Hospital	Great Barrington	91%	44
Massachusetts General Hospital[2]	Boston	91%	217
Milford Regional Medical Center	Milford	91%	178
Morton Hospital & Medical Center	Taunton	91%	166
UMass Memorial Medical Center[2]	Worcester	91%	553
Falmouth Hospital	Falmouth	90%	177
Norwood Hospital	Norwood	90%	164
Winchester Hospital[2]	Winchester	90%	175
Beverly Hospital Corporation	Beverly	89%	251
Carney Hospital	Boston	88%	144
Nashoba Valley Medical Center	Ayer	88%	64
Saints Medical Center	Lowell	88%	217
Healthalliance Hospitals	Leominster	87%	205
Holy Family Hospital	Methuen	86%	160
Holyoke Medical Center	Holyoke	85%	123
Good Samaritan Medical Center	Brockton	83%	243
Marlborough Hospital	Marlborough	83%	75
Jordan Hospital	Plymouth	82%	194
Beth Israel Deaconess Hospital - Needham	Needham	81%	72
Emerson Hospital	West Concord	78%	127
Saint Anne's Hospital	Fall River	78%	144
Mercy Medical Center	Springfield	77%	249
Heywood Hospital[2]	Gardner	76%	86
Lowell General Hospital[2]	Lowell	76%	249
Cape Cod Hospital[2]	Hyannis	73%	192
Lawrence General Hospital	Lawrence	70%	282
Southcoast Hospital Group	Fall River	66%	872
South Shore Hospital	S Weymouth	64%	540
Harrington Memorial Hospital	Southbridge	61%	90

14. Evaluation of LVS Function

Hospital Name	City	Rate	Cases
Baystate Mary Lane Hospital	Ware	100%	50
Berkshire Medical Center	Pittsfield	100%	284
Beth Israel Deaconess Medical Center[2]	Boston	100%	431
Beverly Hospital Corporation	Beverly	100%	396
Boston Medical Center Corporation	Boston	100%	831
Cambridge Health Alliance	Cambridge	100%	276
Cape Cod Hospital[2]	Hyannis	100%	295
Fairview Hospital	Great Barrington	100%	56
Falmouth Hospital	Falmouth	100%	261
Faulkner Hospital[2]	Boston	100%	211
Good Samaritan Medical Center	Brockton	100%	387
Holy Family Hospital	Methuen	100%	242
Holyoke Medical Center	Holyoke	100%	191
Marlborough Hospital	Marlborough	100%	130
Morton Hospital & Medical Center	Taunton	100%	245
Mount Auburn Hospital	Cambridge	100%	347
New England Baptist Hospital	Boston	100%	38
Newton-Wellesley Hospital[2]	Newton	100%	264
North Adams Regional Hospital	North Adams	100%	101
North Shore Medical Center	Salem	100%	596
Saint Anne's Hospital	Fall River	100%	185
Saint Vincent Hospital	Worcester	100%	592
Signature Healthcare Brockton Hospital	Brockton	100%	290
Tufts Medical Center	Boston	100%	417
UMass Memorial Medical Center[2]	Worcester	100%	799
VA Boston Healthcare System - Jamaica Plain	Jamaica Plain	100%	289
Wing Memorial Hospital and Medical Center[2]	Palmer	100%	143
Brigham and Women's Hospital[2]	Boston	99%	281
Carney Hospital	Boston	99%	195
The Cooley Dickinson Hospital	Northampton	99%	163
Emerson Hospital	West Concord	99%	193
Hallmark Health System[2]	Melrose	99%	298
Healthalliance Hospitals	Leominster	99%	271
Lahey Clinic Hospital[2]	Burlington	99%	278
Massachusetts General Hospital[2]	Boston	99%	270
Mercy Medical Center	Springfield	99%	321
Merrimack Valley Hospital	Haverhill	99%	193
Metrowest Medical Center	Framingham	99%	459
Milford Regional Medical Center	Milford	99%	276
Norwood Hospital	Norwood	99%	271
Quincy Medical Center	Quincy	99%	246
Saints Medical Center	Lowell	99%	321
South Shore Hospital	S Weymouth	99%	858
Winchester Hospital[2]	Winchester	99%	262
Baystate Medical Center	Springfield	98%	967
Beth Israel Deaconess Hospital - Needham	Needham	98%	128
Clinton Hospital Association	Clinton	98%	44
Saint Elizabeth's Medical Center	Brighton	98%	404
Baystate Franklin Medical Center	Greenfield	97%	143
Harrington Memorial Hospital	Southbridge	97%	128
Jordan Hospital	Plymouth	97%	268
Lowell General Hospital[2]	Lowell	97%	329
Milton Hospital	Milton	97%	175
Anna Jaques Hospital	Newburyport	96%	204
Nashoba Valley Medical Center	Ayer	96%	95
Southcoast Hospital Group	Fall River	95%	1287
Sturdy Memorial Hospital	Attleboro	95%	202
Heywood Hospital[2]	Gardner	93%	116
Lawrence General Hospital	Lawrence	92%	408
Noble Hospital	Westfield	91%	104
Athol Memorial Hospital	Athol	88%	48
Martha's Vineyard Hospital[2]	Oak Bluffs	84%	32

15. Smoking Cessation Advice

Hospital Name	City	Rate	Cases
Berkshire Medical Center	Pittsfield	100%	29
Beth Israel Deaconess Medical Center[2]	Boston	100%	61
Beverly Hospital Corporation	Beverly	100%	34
Boston Medical Center Corporation	Boston	100%	216
Carney Hospital	Boston	100%	32
Hallmark Health System[2]	Melrose	100%	33
Healthalliance Hospitals	Leominster	100%	28
Lawrence General Hospital	Lawrence	100%	41
Massachusetts General Hospital[2]	Boston	100%	41
Merrimack Valley Hospital	Haverhill	100%	26
Morton Hospital & Medical Center	Taunton	100%	26
Mount Auburn Hospital	Cambridge	100%	30
North Shore Medical Center	Salem	100%	54
Norwood Hospital	Norwood	100%	25
Quincy Medical Center	Quincy	100%	30
Saint Anne's Hospital	Fall River	100%	25
Saint Vincent Hospital	Worcester	100%	53
Saints Medical Center	Lowell	100%	40
Signature Healthcare Brockton Hospital	Brockton	100%	60
Sturdy Memorial Hospital	Attleboro	100%	30
Tufts Medical Center	Boston	100%	59
UMass Memorial Medical Center[2]	Worcester	100%	103
VA Boston Healthcare System - Jamaica Plain	Jamaica Plain	100%	27
Brigham and Women's Hospital[2]	Boston	98%	43
Mercy Medical Center	Springfield	98%	61
Metrowest Medical Center	Framingham	98%	41
Saint Elizabeth's Medical Center	Brighton	98%	57
Baystate Medical Center	Springfield	97%	166
Good Samaritan Medical Center	Brockton	96%	48
South Shore Hospital	S Weymouth	96%	82
Holyoke Medical Center	Holyoke	92%	26
Cambridge Health Alliance	Cambridge	89%	45
Cape Cod Hospital[2]	Hyannis	84%	31

NOTE: Hospital profiles are in alphabetical order by state, then city, then hospital within the city; Rankings exclude hospitals with less than 25 cases except for patient surveys which excludes hospitals with less than 100 cases; (a) 100–299 cases; (1) The number of cases is too small to be sure how well a hospital is performing; (2) The hospital indicated that the data submitted for this measure were based on a sample of cases; (3) Data was collected during a shorter time period (fewer quarters) than the maximum possible time for this measure; (4) Suppressed for one or more quarters by CMS; (5) No data is available from the hospital for this measure; (6) Fewer than 100 patients completed the HCAHPS survey. Use these rates with caution, as the number of surveys may be too low to reliably assess hospital performance; (7) Survey results are based on less than 12 months of data; (8) Survey results are not available for this reporting period; (9) No or very few patients were eligible for the HCAHPS survey. The scores shown, if any, reflect a very small number of surveys; (10) A state average was not calculated because too few hospitals in the state submitted data; (11) There were discrepancies in the data collection process; Please refer to the User's Guide for a full explanation of data.

Lowell General Hospital[2]	Lowell	83%	30
Southcoast Hospital Group	Fall River	81%	139

Pneumonia Care

16. Appropriate Initial Antibiotic

Hospital Name	City	Rate	Cases
Clinton Hospital Association	Clinton	100%	31
Fairview Hospital	Great Barrington	100%	38
Berkshire Medical Center	Pittsfield	99%	148
Falmouth Hospital	Falmouth	99%	106
Mount Auburn Hospital	Cambridge	99%	175
Newton-Wellesley Hospital[2]	Newton	99%	72
Good Samaritan Medical Center	Brockton	98%	233
North Adams Regional Hospital	North Adams	98%	65
Signature Healthcare Brockton Hospital	Brockton	98%	114
Beverly Hospital Corporation	Beverly	97%	229
Lowell General Hospital[2]	Lowell	97%	146
Mercy Medical Center	Springfield	97%	146
North Shore Medical Center	Salem	97%	334
South Shore Hospital	S Weymouth	97%	251
VA Boston Healthcare System - Jamaica Plain	Jamaica Plain	97%	87
Cambridge Health Alliance	Cambridge	96%	156
The Cooley Dickinson Hospital	Northampton	96%	124
Marlborough Hospital	Marlborough	96%	81
Metrowest Medical Center	Framingham	96%	231
Quincy Medical Center	Quincy	96%	138
Anna Jaques Hospital	Newburyport	95%	124
Baystate Franklin Medical Center	Greenfield	95%	78
Beth Israel Deaconess Hospital - Needham	Needham	95%	61
Lahey Clinic Hospital[2]	Burlington	95%	55
Milford Regional Medical Center	Milford	95%	170
Nashoba Valley Medical Center	Ayer	95%	76
Norwood Hospital	Norwood	95%	133
Saint Vincent Hospital	Worcester	95%	236
Saints Medical Center	Lowell	95%	129
Tufts Medical Center	Boston	95%	96
Emerson Hospital	West Concord	94%	87
Jordan Hospital	Plymouth	94%	203
Massachusetts General Hospital[2]	Boston	94%	63
Morton Hospital & Medical Center	Taunton	94%	125
Beth Israel Deaconess Medical Center[2]	Boston	93%	113
Boston Medical Center Corporation	Boston	93%	144
Sturdy Memorial Hospital	Attleboro	93%	196
Baystate Mary Lane Hospital	Ware	92%	37
Cape Cod Hospital	Hyannis	92%	214
Hallmark Health System[2]	Melrose	92%	117
Holy Family Hospital	Methuen	92%	111
Wing Memorial Hospital and Medical Center	Palmer	92%	64
Baystate Medical Center	Springfield	91%	268
Milton Hospital	Milton	91%	89
Saint Anne's Hospital	Fall River	91%	128
UMass Memorial Medical Center[2]	Worcester	91%	174
Winchester Hospital	Winchester	91%	208
Faulkner Hospital[2]	Boston	90%	86
Healthalliance Hospitals	Leominster	90%	143
Merrimack Valley Hospital	Haverhill	90%	105
Saint Elizabeth's Medical Center	Brighton	90%	106
Carney Hospital	Boston	89%	62
Heywood Hospital	Gardner	89%	95
Noble Hospital	Westfield	88%	85
Holyoke Medical Center	Holyoke	87%	108
Lawrence General Hospital	Lawrence	86%	127
Harrington Memorial Hospital	Southbridge	85%	107
Southcoast Hospital Group	Fall River	85%	684

17. Blood Culture Timing

Hospital Name	City	Rate	Cases
Anna Jaques Hospital	Newburyport	99%	136
Berkshire Medical Center	Pittsfield	99%	283
Falmouth Hospital	Falmouth	99%	197
Lahey Clinic Hospital[2]	Burlington	99%	81
Newton-Wellesley Hospital[2]	Newton	99%	139
Signature Healthcare Brockton Hospital	Brockton	99%	83
Sturdy Memorial Hospital	Attleboro	99%	280
Wing Memorial Hospital and Medical Center	Palmer	99%	119
Baystate Mary Lane Hospital	Ware	98%	47
Brigham and Women's Hospital[2]	Boston	98%	65
Fairview Hospital	Great Barrington	98%	63
Metrowest Medical Center	Framingham	98%	209
Saint Vincent Hospital	Worcester	98%	348
Beverly Hospital Corporation	Beverly	97%	373
Emerson Hospital	West Concord	97%	171
Faulkner Hospital[2]	Boston	97%	143
Good Samaritan Medical Center	Brockton	97%	233
Healthalliance Hospitals	Leominster	97%	275
Mount Auburn Hospital	Cambridge	97%	280
North Adams Regional Hospital	North Adams	97%	124
Norwood Hospital	Norwood	97%	146
Tufts Medical Center	Boston	97%	167
Baystate Franklin Medical Center	Greenfield	96%	137
Beth Israel Deaconess Medical Center[2]	Boston	96%	248
Boston Medical Center Corporation	Boston	96%	136
The Cooley Dickinson Hospital	Northampton	96%	194
Heywood Hospital	Gardner	96%	111
Holy Family Hospital	Methuen	96%	98
Jordan Hospital	Plymouth	96%	277
Mercy Medical Center	Springfield	96%	213
Milford Regional Medical Center	Milford	96%	283
Saint Anne's Hospital	Fall River	96%	103
VA Boston Healthcare System - Jamaica Plain	Jamaica Plain	96%	112
Beth Israel Deaconess Hospital - Needham	Needham	95%	84
Cambridge Health Alliance	Cambridge	95%	278
Morton Hospital & Medical Center	Taunton	95%	177
Hallmark Health System[2]	Melrose	94%	187
Lawrence General Hospital	Lawrence	94%	160
Marlborough Hospital	Marlborough	94%	157
Massachusetts General Hospital[2]	Boston	94%	82
Merrimack Valley Hospital	Haverhill	94%	168
North Shore Medical Center	Salem	94%	526
Saint Elizabeth's Medical Center	Brighton	94%	128
Saints Medical Center	Lowell	94%	189
Athol Memorial Hospital	Athol	93%	45
Carney Hospital	Boston	93%	69
Nashoba Valley Medical Center	Ayer	93%	107
Lowell General Hospital[2]	Lowell	92%	143
UMass Memorial Medical Center[2]	Worcester	92%	310
Winchester Hospital	Winchester	92%	240
Cape Cod Hospital	Hyannis	91%	251
Holyoke Medical Center	Holyoke	91%	201
Noble Hospital	Westfield	91%	131
Quincy Medical Center	Quincy	90%	163
South Shore Hospital	S Weymouth	90%	263
Southcoast Hospital Group	Fall River	90%	853
Harrington Memorial Hospital	Southbridge	89%	113
Milton Hospital	Milton	88%	89
Baystate Medical Center	Springfield	84%	410
Clinton Hospital Association	Clinton	83%	36

18. Influenza Vaccine

Hospital Name	City	Rate	Cases
Fairview Hospital	Great Barrington	100%	42
Marlborough Hospital	Marlborough	100%	99
New England Baptist Hospital	Boston	100%	26
Noble Hospital	Westfield	100%	91
Healthalliance Hospitals	Leominster	99%	148
Nashoba Valley Medical Center	Ayer	99%	73
Newton-Wellesley Hospital[2]	Newton	99%	85
VA Boston Healthcare System - Jamaica Plain	Jamaica Plain	99%	135
Anna Jaques Hospital	Newburyport	98%	112
Faulkner Hospital[2]	Boston	98%	91
Holyoke Medical Center	Holyoke	98%	121
Saint Vincent Hospital	Worcester	98%	317
South Shore Hospital	S Weymouth	98%	283
North Adams Regional Hospital	North Adams	97%	64
Wing Memorial Hospital and Medical Center	Palmer	97%	100
Good Samaritan Medical Center	Brockton	96%	255
Holy Family Hospital	Methuen	96%	107
Mercy Medical Center	Springfield	96%	140
Milton Hospital	Milton	96%	76
Berkshire Medical Center	Pittsfield	95%	195
Beth Israel Deaconess Hospital - Needham	Needham	95%	64
Cambridge Health Alliance	Cambridge	95%	159
Cape Cod Hospital	Hyannis	95%	173
The Cooley Dickinson Hospital	Northampton	95%	131
Emerson Hospital	West Concord	95%	113
Heywood Hospital	Gardner	95%	76
Massachusetts General Hospital[2]	Boston	95%	61
Metrowest Medical Center	Framingham	95%	204
North Shore Medical Center	Salem	95%	352
Falmouth Hospital	Falmouth	94%	124
Lowell General Hospital[2]	Lowell	94%	78
Tufts Medical Center	Boston	94%	174
Baystate Franklin Medical Center	Greenfield	93%	76
Merrimack Valley Hospital	Haverhill	93%	87
Mount Auburn Hospital	Cambridge	93%	193
Brigham and Women's Hospital[2]	Boston	92%	73
Carney Hospital	Boston	92%	61
Jordan Hospital	Plymouth	92%	220
Saint Anne's Hospital	Fall River	92%	156
Athol Memorial Hospital	Athol	91%	34
Beth Israel Deaconess Medical Center[2]	Boston	91%	75
Hallmark Health System[2]	Melrose	91%	133
Signature Healthcare Brockton Hospital	Brockton	91%	105
Southcoast Hospital Group	Fall River	91%	621
Lahey Clinic Hospital[2]	Burlington	90%	78
Milford Regional Medical Center	Milford	90%	174
Sturdy Memorial Hospital	Attleboro	90%	200
Beverly Hospital Corporation	Beverly	89%	211
Norwood Hospital	Norwood	89%	113
Quincy Medical Center	Quincy	88%	104
Baystate Medical Center	Springfield	86%	301
Saints Medical Center	Lowell	84%	149
Saint Elizabeth's Medical Center	Brighton	83%	129
Harrington Memorial Hospital	Southbridge	82%	84
Boston Medical Center Corporation	Boston	80%	230
UMass Memorial Medical Center[2]	Worcester	79%	289
Winchester Hospital	Winchester	79%	204
Lawrence General Hospital	Lawrence	78%	125

19. Initial Antibiotic Timing

Hospital Name	City	Rate	Cases
Fairview Hospital	Great Barrington	100%	59
Martha's Vineyard Hospital[2]	Oak Bluffs	100%	38
Mount Auburn Hospital	Cambridge	100%	254
Newton-Wellesley Hospital[2]	Newton	100%	116
Beverly Hospital Corporation	Beverly	99%	362
Brigham and Women's Hosptial[2]	Boston	99%	68
Mercy Medical Center	Springfield	99%	211
Merrimack Valley Hospital	Haverhill	99%	152
Saint Anne's Hospital	Fall River	99%	224
Signature Healthcare Brockton Hospital	Brockton	99%	176
Athol Memorial Hospital	Athol	98%	45
Berkshire Medical Center	Pittsfield	98%	250
Cambridge Health Alliance	Cambridge	98%	248
Cape Cod Hospital	Hyannis	98%	284
Falmouth Hospital	Falmouth	98%	181
Massachusetts General Hospital[2]	Boston	98%	101
Metrowest Medical Center	Framingham	98%	327
Milford Regional Medical Center	Milford	98%	253
North Adams Regional Hospital	North Adams	98%	116
Norwood Hospital	Norwood	98%	189
Anna Jaques Hospital	Newburyport	97%	181
Beth Israel Deaconess Hospital - Needham	Needham	97%	78
Beth Israel Deaconess Medical Center[2]	Boston	97%	210
Carney Hospital	Boston	97%	86
Clinton Hospital Association	Clinton	97%	39
Emerson Hospital	West Concord	97%	172
Faulkner Hospital[2]	Boston	97%	148
Hallmark Health System[2]	Melrose	97%	188
Harrington Memorial Hospital	Southbridge	97%	130
Healthalliance Hospitals	Leominster	97%	241
Heywood Hospital	Gardner	97%	134
Jordan Hospital	Plymouth	97%	372
Marlborough Hospital	Marlborough	97%	148
Morton Hospital & Medical Center	Taunton	97%	197
Nashoba Valley Medical Center	Ayer	97%	92
Wing Memorial Hospital and Medical Center	Palmer	97%	117
Boston Medical Center Corporation	Boston	96%	230
The Cooley Dickinson Hospital	Northampton	96%	196
Holy Family Hospital	Methuen	96%	155
Lowell General Hospital[2]	Lowell	96%	187
Milton Hospital	Milton	96%	139
Noble Hospital	Westfield	96%	126
Quincy Medical Center	Quincy	96%	176
Saint Elizabeth's Medical Center	Brighton	96%	169
Saint Vincent Hospital	Worcester	96%	436
Saints Medical Center	Lowell	96%	230
South Shore Hospital	S Weymouth	96%	492
Sturdy Memorial Hospital	Attleboro	96%	321
Winchester Hospital	Winchester	96%	276
Baystate Mary Lane Hospital	Ware	95%	38
Tufts Medical Center	Boston	95%	193
Baystate Franklin Medical Center	Greenfield	94%	133
Good Samaritan Medical Center	Brockton	94%	375
North Shore Medical Center	Salem	94%	493
VA Boston Healthcare System - Jamaica Plain	Jamaica Plain	94%	124
Holyoke Medical Center	Holyoke	93%	188
Lawrence General Hospital	Lawrence	93%	220
UMass Memorial Medical Center[2]	Worcester	93%	329
Baystate Medical Center	Springfield	91%	503
Southcoast Hospital Group	Fall River	89%	1053
Lahey Clinic Hospital[2]	Burlington	87%	95

20. Pneumococcal Vaccine

Hospital Name	City	Rate	Cases
New England Baptist Hospital	Boston	100%	28
Noble Hospital	Westfield	100%	119
Faulkner Hospital[2]	Boston	99%	142
Holyoke Medical Center	Holyoke	99%	159
Newton-Wellesley Hospital[2]	Newton	99%	148
North Adams Regional Hospital	North Adams	99%	113
VA Boston Healthcare System - Jamaica Plain	Jamaica Plain	99%	143
Anna Jaques Hospital	Newburyport	98%	171
Athol Memorial Hospital	Athol	98%	43
Berkshire Medical Center	Pittsfield	98%	282
Brigham and Women's Hosptial[2]	Boston	98%	86
Fairview Hospital	Great Barrington	98%	65
Healthalliance Hospitals	Leominster	98%	206
Marlborough Hospital	Marlborough	98%	148

NOTE: Hospital profiles are in alphabetical order by state, then city, then hospital within the city; Rankings exclude hospitals with less than 25 cases except for patient surveys which excludes hospitals with less than 100 cases; (a) 100–299 cases; (1) The number of cases is too small to be sure how well a hospital is performing; (2) The hospital indicated that the data submitted for this measure were based on a sample of cases; (3) Data was collected during a shorter time period (fewer quarters) than the maximum possible time for this measure; (4) Suppressed for one or more quarters by CMS; (5) No data is available from the hospital for this measure; (6) Fewer than 100 patients completed the HCAHPS survey. Use these rates with caution, as the number of surveys may be too low to reliably assess hospital performance; (7) Survey results are based on less than 12 months of data; (8) Survey results are not available for this reporting period; (9) No or very few patients were eligible for the HCAHPS survey. The scores shown, if any, reflect a very small number of surveys; (10) A state average was not calculated because too few hospitals in the state submitted data; (11) There were discrepancies in the data collection process; Please refer to the User's Guide for a full explanation of data.

Nashoba Valley Medical Center	Ayer	98%	102
Saint Vincent Hospital	Worcester	98%	451
South Shore Hospital	S Weymouth	98%	481
Wing Memorial Hospital and Medical Center	Palmer	98%	124
Baystate Mary Lane Hospital	Ware	97%	34
Cambridge Health Alliance	Cambridge	97%	206
Carney Hospital	Boston	97%	88
Falmouth Hospital	Falmouth	97%	177
Morton Hospital & Medical Center	Taunton	97%	146
Mount Auburn Hospital	Cambridge	97%	254
Saint Anne's Hospital	Fall River	96%	226
The Cooley Dickinson Hospital	Northampton	95%	168
Emerson Hospital	West Concord	95%	188
Hallmark Health System[2]	Melrose	95%	204
Lawrence General Hospital	Lawrence	95%	205
Metrowest Medical Center	Framingham	95%	303
Milton Hospital	Milton	95%	130
Signature Healthcare Brockton Hospital	Brockton	95%	178
Baystate Franklin Medical Center	Greenfield	94%	133
Heywood Hospital	Gardner	94%	125
Mercy Medical Center	Springfield	94%	190
Cape Cod Hospital	Hyannis	93%	301
Jordan Hospital	Plymouth	93%	301
Milford Regional Medical Center	Milford	93%	246
Southcoast Hospital Group	Fall River	93%	921
Sturdy Memorial Hospital	Attleboro	93%	261
Tufts Medical Center	Boston	93%	218
Beverly Hospital Corporation	Beverly	92%	322
Holy Family Hospital	Methuen	92%	154
Good Samaritan Medical Center	Brockton	91%	348
Massachusetts General Hospital[2]	Boston	91%	161
Merrimack Valley Hospital	Haverhill	91%	140
Norwood Hospital	Norwood	91%	154
Saints Medical Center	Lowell	91%	203
Lahey Clinic Hospital[2]	Burlington	90%	133
North Shore Medical Center	Salem	90%	502
Quincy Medical Center	Quincy	90%	155
Saint Elizabeth's Medical Center	Brighton	90%	184
Baystate Medical Center	Springfield	89%	386
UMass Memorial Medical Center[2]	Worcester	89%	413
Winchester Hospital	Winchester	88%	301
Beth Israel Deaconess Hospital - Needham	Needham	87%	100
Lowell General Hospital[2]	Lowell	87%	157
Harrington Memorial Hospital	Southbridge	86%	138
Boston Medical Center Corporation	Boston	85%	231
Beth Israel Deaconess Medical Center[2]	Boston	84%	245
Clinton Hospital Association	Clinton	82%	50
Martha's Vineyard Hospital[2]	Oak Bluffs	42%	40

21. Smoking Cessation Advice

Hospital Name	City	Rate	Cases
Anna Jaques Hospital	Newburyport	100%	55
Baystate Franklin Medical Center	Greenfield	100%	29
Berkshire Medical Center	Pittsfield	100%	69
Beth Israel Deaconess Medical Center[2]	Boston	100%	75
Beverly Hospital Corporation	Beverly	100%	88
Carney Hospital	Boston	100%	42
Falmouth Hospital	Falmouth	100%	40
Faulkner Hospital[2]	Boston	100%	25
Marlborough Hospital	Marlborough	100%	41
Massachusetts General Hospital[2]	Boston	100%	39
Merrimack Valley Hospital	Haverhill	100%	47
Morton Hospital & Medical Center	Taunton	100%	39
Mount Auburn Hospital	Cambridge	100%	60
Noble Hospital	Westfield	100%	26
Norwood Hospital	Norwood	100%	57
Quincy Medical Center	Quincy	100%	72
Saint Anne's Hospital	Fall River	100%	81
Saints Medical Center	Lowell	100%	87
Signature Healthcare Brockton Hospital	Brockton	100%	95
UMass Memorial Medical Center[2]	Worcester	100%	144
VA Boston Healthcare System - Jamaica Plain	Jamaica Plain	100%	45
Winchester Hospital	Winchester	100%	69
Metrowest Medical Center	Framingham	99%	83
South Shore Hospital	S Weymouth	99%	101
Hallmark Health System[2]	Melrose	98%	45
Jordan Hospital	Plymouth	98%	94
North Shore Medical Center	Salem	98%	150
Saint Vincent Hospital	Worcester	98%	142
Sturdy Memorial Hospital	Attleboro	98%	100
Wing Memorial Hospital and Medical Center	Palmer	98%	48
Boston Medical Center Corporation	Boston	97%	260
Mercy Medical Center	Springfield	97%	75
North Adams Regional Hospital	North Adams	97%	37
Brigham and Women's Hospital[2]	Boston	96%	25
Good Samaritan Medical Center	Brockton	96%	109
Milton Hospital	Milton	96%	28
Baystate Medical Center	Springfield	95%	158
Healthalliance Hospitals	Leominster	95%	75
Tufts Medical Center	Boston	95%	102
The Cooley Dickinson Hospital	Northampton	94%	66
Holy Family Hospital	Methuen	94%	63
Cambridge Health Alliance	Cambridge	93%	117
Lowell General Hospital[2]	Lowell	93%	60
Cape Cod Hospital	Hyannis	92%	80
Heywood Hospital	Gardner	90%	58
Saint Elizabeth's Medical Center	Brighton	89%	47
Southcoast Hospital Group	Fall River	88%	317
Lawrence General Hospital	Lawrence	85%	61
Milford Regional Medical Center	Milford	85%	61
Harrington Memorial Hospital	Southbridge	83%	42
Holyoke Medical Center	Holyoke	83%	66
Lahey Clinic Hospital[2]	Burlington	77%	26

Surgical Care Improvement Project

22. Appropriate VTP Within 24 Hours

Hospital Name	City	Rate	Cases
Beth Israel Deaconess Hospital - Needham	Needham	100%	60
Boston Medical Center Corporation[2]	Boston	100%	551
Lahey Clinic Hospital[2]	Burlington	100%	231
Noble Hospital	Westfield	100%	40
Norwood Hospital[2]	Norwood	100%	256
Saint Vincent Hospital	Worcester	100%	445
VA Boston Healthcare System - Jamaica Plain[2]	Jamaica Plain	100%	239
Wing Memorial Hospital and Medical Center	Palmer	100%	25
Baystate Medical Center[2]	Springfield	99%	320
Beth Israel Deaconess Medical Center[2]	Boston	99%	417
Cape Cod Hospital[2]	Hyannis	99%	360
Faulkner Hospital[2]	Boston	99%	84
Good Samaritan Medical Center[2]	Brockton	99%	247
Jordan Hospital	Plymouth	99%	159
North Adams Regional Hospital	North Adams	99%	74
Signature Healthcare Brockton Hospital	Brockton	99%	186
Berkshire Medical Center[2]	Pittsfield	98%	335
Beverly Hospital Corporation[2]	Beverly	98%	448
Brigham and Women's Hospital[2]	Boston	98%	252
Carney Hospital[2]	Boston	98%	142
Mercy Medical Center	Springfield	98%	482
Mount Auburn Hospital	Cambridge	98%	432
Quincy Medical Center	Quincy	98%	210
South Shore Hospital	S Weymouth	98%	479
UMass Memorial Medical Center[2]	Worcester	98%	169
Cambridge Health Alliance[2]	Cambridge	97%	172
Fairview Hospital	Great Barrington	97%	33
New England Baptist Hospital[2]	Boston	97%	1849
North Shore Medical Center[2]	Salem	97%	157
Saint Anne's Hospital[2]	Fall River	97%	112
Saint Elizabeth's Medical Center[2]	Brighton	97%	190
Baystate Franklin Medical Center[2]	Greenfield	96%	141
Marlborough Hospital	Marlborough	96%	93
Massachusetts General Hospital[2]	Boston	96%	267
Tufts Medical Center[2]	Boston	96%	245
Anna Jaques Hospital	Newburyport	95%	204
Falmouth Hospital[2]	Falmouth	95%	202
Healthalliance Hospitals	Leominster	95%	186
Milton Hospital	Milton	95%	199
Winchester Hospital	Winchester	95%	333
Merrimack Valley Hospital	Haverhill	94%	82
Metrowest Medical Center[2]	Framingham	94%	259
Milford Regional Medical Center	Milford	94%	118
Sturdy Memorial Hospital	Attleboro	94%	337
Lowell General Hospital[2]	Lowell	92%	172
Morton Hospital & Medical Center	Taunton	92%	181
Nashoba Valley Medical Center	Ayer	92%	71
Emerson Hospital	West Concord	91%	217
Newton-Wellesley Hospital[2]	Newton	91%	92
Hallmark Health System[2]	Melrose	90%	193
The Cooley Dickinson Hospital[2]	Northampton	89%	145
Saints Medical Center	Lowell	89%	148
Southcoast Hospital Group	Fall River	87%	1022
Holy Family Hospital[2]	Methuen	86%	123
Harrington Memorial Hospital	Southbridge	85%	66
Heywood Hospital	Gardner	85%	96
Holyoke Medical Center	Holyoke	85%	114
Lawrence General Hospital	Lawrence	79%	145

23. Appropriate Hair Removal

Hospital Name	City	Rate	Cases
Anna Jaques Hospital	Newburyport	100%	346
Baystate Franklin Medical Center[2]	Greenfield	100%	205
Baystate Mary Lane Hospital	Ware	100%	45
Baystate Medical Center[2]	Springfield	100%	1670
Berkshire Medical Center[2]	Pittsfield	100%	721
Beverly Hospital Corporation[2]	Beverly	100%	1136
Boston Medical Center Corporation[2]	Boston	100%	1127
Brigham and Women's Hospital[2]	Boston	100%	691
Cambridge Health Alliance[2]	Cambridge	100%	289
Cape Cod Hospital[2]	Hyannis	100%	1174
Carney Hospital[2]	Boston	100%	208
The Cooley Dickinson Hospital[2]	Northampton	100%	456
Emerson Hospital	West Concord	100%	529
Fairview Hospital	Great Barrington	100%	80
Falmouth Hospital[2]	Falmouth	100%	644
Good Samaritan Medical Center[2]	Brockton	100%	706
Hallmark Health System[2]	Melrose	100%	389
Healthalliance Hospitals	Leominster	100%	404
Holy Family Hospital[2]	Methuen	100%	529
Holyoke Medical Center	Holyoke	100%	234
Jordan Hospital	Plymouth	100%	579
Lahey Clinic Hospital[2]	Burlington	100%	641
Lowell General Hospital[2]	Lowell	100%	606
Mercy Medical Center	Springfield	100%	977
Merrimack Valley Hospital	Haverhill	100%	191
Metrowest Medical Center[2]	Framingham	100%	626
Milton Hospital	Milton	100%	313
Morton Hospital & Medical Center	Taunton	100%	437
Mount Auburn Hospital	Cambridge	100%	1018
Nashoba Valley Medical Center	Ayer	100%	101
New England Baptist Hospital[2]	Boston	100%	4252
Noble Hospital	Westfield	100%	73
North Adams Regional Hospital	North Adams	100%	214
North Shore Medical Center[2]	Salem	100%	525
Norwood Hospital[2]	Norwood	100%	378
Saint Anne's Hospital[2]	Fall River	100%	193
Saint Elizabeth's Medical Center[2]	Brighton	100%	631
Saint Vincent Hospital	Worcester	100%	1593
Saints Medical Center	Lowell	100%	435
Signature Healthcare Brockton Hospital	Brockton	100%	447
Southcoast Hospital Group	Fall River	100%	2258
UMass Memorial Medical Center[2]	Worcester	100%	607
VA Boston Healthcare System - Jamaica Plain[2]	Jamaica Plain	100%	510
Winchester Hospital	Winchester	100%	903
Wing Memorial Hospital and Medical Center	Palmer	100%	46
Beth Israel Deaconess Hospital - Needham	Needham	99%	127
Beth Israel Deaconess Medical Center[2]	Boston	99%	1243
Harrington Memorial Hospital	Southbridge	99%	139
Milford Regional Medical Center	Milford	99%	388
Newton-Wellesley Hospital[2]	Newton	99%	326
Quincy Medical Center	Quincy	99%	395
Sturdy Memorial Hospital	Attleboro	99%	609
Faulkner Hospital[2]	Boston	98%	242
Heywood Hospital	Gardner	98%	282
Marlborough Hospital	Marlborough	98%	208
Tufts Medical Center[2]	Boston	98%	923
South Shore Hospital	S Weymouth	97%	1123
Massachusetts General Hospital[2]	Boston	96%	752
Lawrence General Hospital	Lawrence	95%	301

24. Appropriate Beta Blocker Usage

Hospital Name	City	Rate	Cases
Berkshire Medical Center[2]	Pittsfield	100%	236
Beth Israel Deaconess Medical Center[2]	Boston	100%	482
Falmouth Hospital[2]	Falmouth	100%	143
Faulkner Hospital[2]	Boston	100%	49
Harrington Memorial Hospital	Southbridge	100%	35
Lahey Clinic Hospital[2]	Burlington	100%	262
Merrimack Valley Hospital	Haverhill	100%	62
Nashoba Valley Medical Center	Ayer	100%	40
Saint Vincent Hospital	Worcester	100%	585
VA Boston Healthcare System - Jamaica Plain[2]	Jamaica Plain	100%	272
New England Baptist Hospital[2]	Boston	99%	1125
Signature Healthcare Brockton Hospital	Brockton	99%	144
Carney Hospital[2]	Boston	98%	62
The Cooley Dickinson Hospital[2]	Northampton	98%	109
Good Samaritan Medical Center[2]	Brockton	98%	215
Metrowest Medical Center[2]	Framingham	98%	220
Milford Regional Medical Center	Milford	98%	128
Winchester Hospital	Winchester	98%	322
Baystate Medical Center[2]	Springfield	97%	580
Beverly Hospital Corporation[2]	Beverly	97%	339
Holy Family Hospital[2]	Methuen	97%	182
North Shore Medical Center[2]	Salem	97%	222
Saint Anne's Hospital[2]	Fall River	97%	74
Saint Elizabeth's Medical Center[2]	Brighton	97%	228
UMass Memorial Medical Center[2]	Worcester	97%	237
Cambridge Health Alliance[2]	Cambridge	96%	70
Fairview Hospital	Great Barrington	96%	27
Norwood Hospital[2]	Norwood	96%	157
Southcoast Hospital Group	Fall River	96%	670
Sturdy Memorial Hospital	Attleboro	96%	183
Cape Cod Hospital[2]	Hyannis	95%	404
Newton-Wellesley Hospital[2]	Newton	95%	74
North Adams Regional Hospital	North Adams	95%	55
Baystate Franklin Medical Center[2]	Greenfield	94%	64
Healthalliance Hospitals	Leominster	94%	124
Lowell General Hospital[2]	Lowell	94%	201
Massachusetts General Hospital[2]	Boston	94%	279
Saints Medical Center	Lowell	94%	133
Anna Jaques Hospital	Newburyport	93%	115

NOTE: Hospital profiles are in alphabetical order by state, then city, then hospital within the city; Rankings exclude hospitals with less than 25 cases except for patient surveys which excludes hospitals with less than 100 cases; (a) 100–299 cases; (1) The number of cases is too small to be sure how well a hospital is performing; (2) The hospital indicated that the data submitted for this measure were based on a sample of cases; (3) Data was collected during a shorter time period (fewer quarters) than the maximum possible time for this measure; (4) Suppressed for one or more quarters by CMS; (5) No data is available from the hospital for this measure; (6) Fewer than 100 patients completed the HCAHPS survey. Use these rates with caution, as the number of surveys may be too low to reliably assess hospital performance; (7) Survey results are based on less than 12 months of data; (8) Survey results are not available for this reporting period; (9) No or very few patients were eligible for the HCAHPS survey. The scores shown, if any, reflect a very small number of surveys; (10) A state average was not calculated because too few hospitals in the state submitted data; (11) There were discrepancies in the data collection process; Please refer to the User's Guide for a full explanation of data.

Beth Israel Deaconess Hospital - Needham	Needham	93%	43
Brigham and Women's Hospital[2]	Boston	93%	256
Lawrence General Hospital	Lawrence	93%	86
Mercy Medical Center	Springfield	93%	256
Boston Medical Center Corporation[2]	Boston	92%	462
Hallmark Health System[2]	Melrose	92%	133
Heywood Hospital	Gardner	92%	87
Marlborough Hospital	Marlborough	92%	64
Mount Auburn Hospital	Cambridge	92%	358
Emerson Hospital	West Concord	91%	139
Holyoke Medical Center	Holyoke	91%	69
Jordan Hospital	Plymouth	91%	174
Quincy Medical Center	Quincy	91%	119
Milton Hospital	Milton	89%	106
Morton Hospital & Medical Center	Taunton	89%	151
South Shore Hospital	S Weymouth	89%	371
Tufts Medical Center[2]	Boston	89%	414

25. Controlled Postoperative Blood Glucose

Hospital Name	City	Rate	Cases
North Shore Medical Center[2]	Salem	100%	114
UMass Memorial Medical Center[2]	Worcester	99%	121
Saint Elizabeth's Medical Center[2]	Brighton	98%	178
Baystate Medical Center[2]	Springfield	97%	341
Brigham and Women's Hospital[2]	Boston	97%	147
Boston Medical Center Corporation[2]	Boston	96%	247
Beth Israel Deaconess Medical Center[2]	Boston	95%	242
Southcoast Hospital Group	Fall River	95%	283
Mount Auburn Hospital	Cambridge	94%	181
Cape Cod Hospital[2]	Hyannis	93%	184
Massachusetts General Hospital[2]	Boston	93%	129
Saint Vincent Hospital	Worcester	93%	165
Tufts Medical Center[2]	Boston	92%	336
Lahey Clinic Hospital[2]	Burlington	88%	126
VA Boston Healthcare System - Jamaica Plain[2]	Jamaica Plain	86%	151

26. Prophylactic Antibiotic Timing

Hospital Name	City	Rate	Cases
Fairview Hospital	Great Barrington	100%	55
Milford Regional Medical Center	Milford	100%	231
North Adams Regional Hospital	North Adams	100%	146
Signature Healthcare Brockton Hospital	Brockton	100%	261
VA Boston Healthcare System - Jamaica Plain	Jamaica Plain	100%	397
Wing Memorial Hospital and Medical Center	Palmer	100%	28
Anna Jaques Hospital	Newburyport	99%	220
Baystate Medical Center[2]	Springfield	99%	1436
Beth Israel Deaconess Medical Center[2]	Boston	99%	632
Beverly Hospital Corporation[2]	Beverly	99%	838
Brigham and Women's Hospital[2]	Boston	99%	427
Cape Cod Hospital[2]	Hyannis	99%	969
Falmouth Hospital[2]	Falmouth	99%	506
Faulkner Hospital[2]	Boston	99%	134
Heywood Hospital	Gardner	99%	232
Lahey Clinic Hospital[2]	Burlington	99%	396
Saint Elizabeth's Medical Center[2]	Brighton	99%	491
Baystate Franklin Medical Center[2]	Greenfield	98%	119
Berkshire Medical Center[2]	Pittsfield	98%	441
Boston Medical Center Corporation[2]	Boston	98%	884
Carney Hospital[2]	Boston	98%	127
The Cooley Dickinson Hospital[2]	Northampton	98%	292
Good Samaritan Medical Center[2]	Brockton	98%	559
Hallmark Health System[2]	Melrose	98%	249
Holy Family Hospital[2]	Methuen	98%	411
Lawrence General Hospital	Lawrence	98%	137
Massachusetts General Hospital[2]	Boston	98%	440
Morton Hospital & Medical Center	Taunton	98%	298
Mount Auburn Hospital	Cambridge	98%	727
North Shore Medical Center[2]	Salem	98%	388
Saint Anne's Hospital[2]	Fall River	98%	120
Saints Medical Center	Lowell	98%	297
South Shore Hospital	S Weymouth	98%	725
Tufts Medical Center[2]	Boston	98%	714
Healthalliance Hospitals	Leominster	97%	283
Lowell General Hospital[2]	Lowell	97%	428
Nashoba Valley Medical Center	Ayer	97%	65
New England Baptist Hospital[2]	Boston	97%	3872
Newton-Wellesley Hospital[2]	Newton	97%	217
Southcoast Hospital Group	Fall River	97%	1488
UMass Memorial Medical Center[2]	Worcester	97%	398
Holyoke Medical Center	Holyoke	96%	147
Jordan Hospital	Plymouth	96%	428
Merrimack Valley Hospital	Haverhill	96%	124
Milton Hospital	Milton	96%	210
Noble Hospital	Westfield	96%	49
Saint Vincent Hospital	Worcester	96%	954
Cambridge Health Alliance[2]	Cambridge	95%	185
Marlborough Hospital	Marlborough	95%	155
Mercy Medical Center	Springfield	95%	532
Norwood Hospital[2]	Norwood	95%	205
Winchester Hospital	Winchester	95%	602
Baystate Mary Lane Hospital	Ware	94%	35
Beth Israel Deaconess Hospital - Needham	Needham	94%	84
Metrowest Medical Center[2]	Framingham	94%	371
Sturdy Memorial Hospital	Attleboro	93%	374
Emerson Hospital	West Concord	92%	361
Harrington Memorial Hospital	Southbridge	88%	83
Quincy Medical Center	Quincy	81%	97

27. Prophylactic Antibiotic Timing (Outpatient)

Hospital Name	City	Rate	Cases
Falmouth Hospital	Falmouth	100%	80
The Cooley Dickinson Hospital	Northampton	99%	149
Milton Hospital	Milton	99%	77
Morton Hospital & Medical Center	Taunton	99%	92
North Shore Medical Center	Salem	99%	505
UMass Memorial Medical Center	Worcester	99%	451
Baystate Franklin Medical Center	Greenfield	98%	85
Berkshire Medical Center	Pittsfield	98%	279
Mount Auburn Hospital	Cambridge	98%	406
Beverly Hospital Corporation	Beverly	97%	280
Faulkner Hospital	Boston	97%	224
Beth Israel Deaconess Hospital - Needham	Needham	96%	70
Cape Cod Hospital	Hyannis	96%	470
Holyoke Medical Center	Holyoke	96%	84
Mercy Medical Center	Springfield	96%	658
New England Baptist Hospital	Boston	96%	549
Newton-Wellesley Hospital	Newton	96%	254
North Adams Regional Hospital	North Adams	96%	56
Saint Vincent Hospital	Worcester	96%	781
Saints Medical Center	Lowell	96%	165
Jordan Hospital	Plymouth	95%	77
Milford Regional Medical Center	Milford	95%	168
Emerson Hospital	West Concord	94%	278
Hallmark Health System	Melrose	94%	117
Marlborough Hospital	Marlborough	94%	52
Saint Elizabeth's Medical Center	Brighton	94%	138
South Shore Hospital	S Weymouth	94%	356
Anna Jaques Hospital	Newburyport	93%	133
Lowell General Hospital	Lowell	93%	290
Baystate Medical Center	Springfield	92%	669
Good Samaritan Medical Center	Brockton	92%	219
Signature Healthcare Brockton Hospital	Brockton	92%	87
Sturdy Memorial Hospital	Attleboro	92%	160
Tufts Medical Center	Boston	92%	237
Brigham and Women's Hosptial	Boston	91%	364
Southcoast Hospital Group	Fall River	91%	834
Cambridge Health Alliance	Cambridge	90%	71
Saint Anne's Hospital	Fall River	90%	49
Boston Medical Center Corporation	Boston	89%	298
Nashoba Valley Medical Center	Ayer	89%	47
Norwood Hospital	Norwood	89%	127
Healthalliance Hospitals	Leominster	88%	86
Winchester Hospital	Winchester	88%	241
Holy Family Hospital	Methuen	87%	112
Merrimack Valley Hospital	Haverhill	87%	31
Lahey Clinic Hospital	Burlington	86%	370
Beth Israel Deaconess Medical Center	Boston	85%	480
Harrington Memorial Hospital	Southbridge	85%	125
Quincy Medical Center	Quincy	85%	75
Metrowest Medical Center	Framingham	84%	325
Massachusetts General Hospital	Boston	74%	479
Lawrence General Hospital	Lawrence	71%	85
Carney Hospital	Boston	65%	34
Heywood Hospital	Gardner	48%	81

28. Prophylactic Antibiotic Selection

Hospital Name	City	Rate	Cases
Baystate Medical Center[2]	Springfield	100%	1446
Fairview Hospital	Great Barrington	100%	56
Healthalliance Hospitals	Leominster	100%	283
Holyoke Medical Center	Holyoke	100%	146
Lahey Clinic Hospital[2]	Burlington	100%	398
Milton Hospital	Milton	100%	208
Nashoba Valley Medical Center	Ayer	100%	65
New England Baptist Hospital[2]	Boston	100%	3874
Wing Memorial Hospital and Medical Center	Palmer	100%	28
Baystate Franklin Medical Center[2]	Greenfield	99%	119
Beth Israel Deaconess Hospital - Needham	Needham	99%	85
Beverly Hospital Corporation[2]	Beverly	99%	841
Boston Medical Center Corporation[2]	Boston	99%	895
Emerson Hospital	West Concord	99%	361
Marlborough Hospital	Marlborough	99%	155
Saint Elizabeth's Medical Center[2]	Brighton	99%	492
Saints Medical Center	Lowell	99%	297
Tufts Medical Center[2]	Boston	99%	727
Berkshire Medical Center[2]	Pittsfield	98%	441
Beth Israel Deaconess Medical Center[2]	Boston	98%	707
Brigham and Women's Hospital[2]	Boston	98%	435
Cape Cod Hospital[2]	Hyannis	98%	979
The Cooley Dickinson Hospital[2]	Northampton	98%	293
Falmouth Hospital[2]	Falmouth	98%	509
Faulkner Hospital[2]	Boston	98%	137
Good Samaritan Medical Center[2]	Brockton	98%	560
Heywood Hospital	Gardner	98%	232
Jordan Hospital	Plymouth	98%	429
Lowell General Hospital[2]	Lowell	98%	429
Merrimack Valley Hospital	Haverhill	98%	124
Metrowest Medical Center[2]	Framingham	98%	371
Newton-Wellesley Hospital[2]	Newton	98%	217
North Shore Medical Center[2]	Salem	98%	399
Norwood Hospital[2]	Norwood	98%	207
Saint Anne's Hospital[2]	Fall River	98%	120
Saint Vincent Hospital	Worcester	98%	959
Signature Healthcare Brockton Hospital	Brockton	98%	264
South Shore Hospital	S Weymouth	98%	725
VA Boston Healthcare System - Jamaica Plain	Jamaica Plain	98%	402
Anna Jaques Hospital	Newburyport	97%	222
Baystate Mary Lane Hospital	Ware	97%	34
Cambridge Health Alliance[2]	Cambridge	97%	189
Holy Family Hospital[2]	Methuen	97%	413
Mercy Medical Center	Springfield	97%	537
Morton Hospital & Medical Center	Taunton	97%	301
Mount Auburn Hospital	Cambridge	97%	732
Sturdy Memorial Hospital	Attleboro	97%	376
UMass Memorial Medical Center[2]	Worcester	97%	409
Winchester Hospital	Winchester	97%	604
Massachusetts General Hospital[2]	Boston	96%	446
Noble Hospital	Westfield	96%	49
North Adams Regional Hospital	North Adams	96%	146
Southcoast Hospital Group	Fall River	96%	1507
Hallmark Health System[2]	Melrose	95%	250
Harrington Memorial Hospital	Southbridge	95%	83
Milford Regional Medical Center	Milford	95%	231
Quincy Medical Center	Quincy	95%	95
Carney Hospital[2]	Boston	94%	126
Lawrence General Hospital	Lawrence	88%	146

29. Prophylactic Antibiotic Selection (Outpatient)

Hospital Name	City	Rate	Cases
The Cooley Dickinson Hospital	Northampton	100%	148
New England Baptist Hospital	Boston	100%	547
North Adams Regional Hospital	North Adams	100%	55
Cambridge Health Alliance	Cambridge	99%	71
North Shore Medical Center	Salem	99%	501
Baystate Medical Center	Springfield	98%	645
Berkshire Medical Center	Pittsfield	98%	276
Holyoke Medical Center	Holyoke	98%	82
Lowell General Hospital	Lowell	98%	283
Mercy Medical Center	Springfield	98%	654
Newton-Wellesley Hospital	Newton	98%	251
Jordan Hospital	Plymouth	97%	76
Mount Auburn Hospital	Cambridge	97%	405
Beverly Hospital Corporation	Beverly	96%	278
Emerson Hospital	West Concord	96%	272
Falmouth Hospital	Falmouth	96%	80
Faulkner Hospital	Boston	96%	224
Lahey Clinic Hospital	Burlington	96%	596
Nashoba Valley Medical Center	Ayer	96%	46
Tufts Medical Center	Boston	96%	381
UMass Memorial Medical Center	Worcester	96%	449
Cape Cod Hospital	Hyannis	95%	465
Good Samaritan Medical Center	Brockton	95%	202
Saint Vincent Hospital	Worcester	95%	780
Beth Israel Deaconess Hospital - Needham	Needham	94%	70
Hallmark Health System	Melrose	94%	113
Heywood Hospital	Gardner	94%	66
Saint Anne's Hospital	Fall River	94%	49
Southcoast Hospital Group	Fall River	94%	799
Winchester Hospital	Winchester	94%	231
Baystate Franklin Medical Center	Greenfield	93%	84
Boston Medical Center Corporation	Boston	93%	297
Brigham and Women's Hospital	Boston	93%	352
Holy Family Hospital	Methuen	93%	100
Lawrence General Hospital	Lawrence	93%	81
Metrowest Medical Center	Framingham	93%	290
South Shore Hospital	S Weymouth	93%	345
Marlborough Hospital	Marlborough	92%	49
Morton Hospital & Medical Center	Taunton	92%	93
Saint Elizabeth's Medical Center	Brighton	92%	133
Saints Medical Center	Lowell	92%	163
Sturdy Memorial Hospital	Attleboro	92%	154
Anna Jaques Hospital	Newburyport	91%	131
Healthalliance Hospitals	Leominster	91%	89
Signature Healthcare Brockton Hospital	Brockton	91%	82
Massachusetts General Hospital	Boston	90%	477
Beth Israel Deaconess Medical Center	Boston	89%	448
Norwood Hospital	Norwood	89%	123
Carney Hospital	Boston	88%	26
Milford Regional Medical Center	Milford	88%	161
Milton Hospital	Milton	88%	77

NOTE: Hospital profiles are in alphabetical order by state, then city, then hospital within the city; Rankings exclude hospitals with less than 25 cases except for patient surveys which excludes hospitals with less than 100 cases; (a) 100–299 cases; (1) The number of cases is too small to be sure how well a hospital is performing; (2) The hospital indicated that the data submitted for this measure were based on a sample of cases; (3) Data was collected during a shorter time period (fewer quarters) than the maximum possible time for this measure; (4) Suppressed for one or more quarters by CMS; (5) No data is available from the hospital for this measure; (6) Fewer than 100 patients completed the HCAHPS survey. Use these rates with caution, as the number of surveys may be too low to reliably assess hospital performance; (7) Survey results are based on less than 12 months of data; (8) Survey results are not available for this reporting period; (9) No or very few patients were eligible for the HCAHPS survey. The scores shown, if any, reflect a very small number of surveys; (10) A state average was not calculated because too few hospitals in the state submitted data; (11) There were discrepancies in the data collection process; Please refer to the User's Guide for a full explanation of data.

Harrington Memorial Hospital	Southbridge	87%	122
Quincy Medical Center	Quincy	81%	67
Merrimack Valley Hospital	Haverhill	79%	28

30. Prophylactic Antibiotic Stopped

Hospital Name	City	Rate	Cases
The Cooley Dickinson Hospital[2]	Northampton	100%	284
Fairview Hospital	Great Barrington	100%	55
Noble Hospital	Westfield	100%	46
VA Boston Healthcare System - Jamaica Plain	Jamaica Plain	100%	397
Wing Memorial Hospital and Medical Center	Palmer	100%	26
Baystate Medical Center[2]	Springfield	99%	1380
Beth Israel Deaconess Hospital - Needham	Needham	99%	81
Beverly Hospital Corporation[2]	Beverly	99%	803
Falmouth Hospital[2]	Falmouth	99%	490
Heywood Hospital	Gardner	99%	226
Jordan Hospital	Plymouth	99%	420
Mount Auburn Hospital	Cambridge	99%	712
North Adams Regional Hospital	North Adams	99%	141
Berkshire Medical Center[2]	Pittsfield	98%	432
Beth Israel Deaconess Medical Center[2]	Boston	98%	614
Cambridge Health Alliance[2]	Cambridge	98%	180
Emerson Hospital	West Concord	98%	345
Faulkner Hospital[2]	Boston	98%	131
Merrimack Valley Hospital	Haverhill	98%	122
Saints Medical Center	Lowell	98%	292
Signature Healthcare Brockton Hospital	Brockton	98%	248
Baystate Mary Lane Hospital	Ware	97%	34
Cape Cod Hospital[2]	Hyannis	97%	943
Healthalliance Hospitals	Leominster	97%	272
Metrowest Medical Center[2]	Framingham	97%	359
North Shore Medical Center[2]	Salem	97%	365
Saint Vincent Hospital	Worcester	97%	828
Southcoast Hospital Group	Fall River	97%	1443
Winchester Hospital	Winchester	97%	592
Hallmark Health System[2]	Melrose	96%	240
Holy Family Hospital[2]	Methuen	96%	402
Mercy Medical Center	Springfield	96%	497
Morton Hospital & Medical Center	Taunton	96%	290
New England Baptist Hospital[2]	Boston	96%	3864
Newton-Wellesley Hospital[2]	Newton	96%	213
South Shore Hospital	S Weymouth	96%	712
Anna Jaques Hospital	Newburyport	95%	213
Holyoke Medical Center	Holyoke	95%	138
Lahey Clinic Hospital[2]	Burlington	95%	376
Marlborough Hospital	Marlborough	95%	152
Milford Regional Medical Center	Milford	95%	227
Norwood Hospital[2]	Norwood	95%	191
Saint Anne's Hospital[2]	Fall River	95%	110
Saint Elizabeth's Medical Center[2]	Brighton	95%	480
UMass Memorial Medical Center[2]	Worcester	95%	377
Baystate Franklin Medical Center[2]	Greenfield	94%	115
Brigham and Women's Hospital[2]	Boston	94%	415
Good Samaritan Medical Center[2]	Brockton	94%	534
Harrington Memorial Hospital	Southbridge	94%	78
Massachusetts General Hospital[2]	Boston	94%	377
Milton Hospital	Milton	94%	200
Sturdy Memorial Hospital	Attleboro	94%	368
Lowell General Hospital[2]	Lowell	93%	404
Tufts Medical Center[2]	Boston	93%	690
Nashoba Valley Medical Center	Ayer	92%	63
Carney Hospital[2]	Boston	90%	116
Lawrence General Hospital	Lawrence	90%	131
Quincy Medical Center	Quincy	89%	87
Boston Medical Center Corporation[2]	Boston	87%	865

31. Recommended VTP Ordered

Hospital Name	City	Rate	Cases
Baystate Medical Center[2]	Springfield	100%	320
Beth Israel Deaconess Hospital - Needham	Needham	100%	60
Boston Medical Center Corporation[2]	Boston	100%	551
Lahey Clinic Hospital[2]	Burlington	100%	231
Massachusetts General Hospital[2]	Boston	100%	268
Noble Hospital	Westfield	100%	40
North Adams Regional Hospital	North Adams	100%	74
Norwood Hospital[2]	Norwood	100%	256
Quincy Medical Center	Quincy	100%	210
Saint Vincent Hospital	Worcester	100%	445
VA Boston Healthcare System - Jamaica Plain[2]	Jamaica Plain	100%	239
Wing Memorial Hospital and Medical Center	Palmer	100%	25
Baystate Franklin Medical Center[2]	Greenfield	99%	141
Beth Israel Deaconess Medical Center[2]	Boston	99%	417
Cape Cod Hospital[2]	Hyannis	99%	360
Faulkner Hospital[2]	Boston	99%	84
Good Samaritan Medical Center[2]	Brockton	99%	247
Jordan Hospital	Plymouth	99%	160
Mercy Medical Center	Springfield	99%	482
Mount Auburn Hospital	Cambridge	99%	432
Saint Anne's Hospital[2]	Fall River	99%	112
Signature Healthcare Brockton Hospital	Brockton	99%	186
UMass Memorial Medical Center[2]	Worcester	99%	169
Berkshire Medical Center[2]	Pittsfield	98%	335
Beverly Hospital Corporation[2]	Beverly	98%	448
Brigham and Women's Hosptial[2]	Boston	98%	254
Cambridge Health Alliance[2]	Cambridge	98%	173
Carney Hospital[2]	Boston	98%	142
North Shore Medical Center[2]	Salem	98%	159
Saint Elizabeth's Medical Center[2]	Brighton	98%	190
South Shore Hospital	S Weymouth	98%	481
Tufts Medical Center[2]	Boston	98%	245
Fairview Hospital	Great Barrington	97%	33
Healthalliance Hospitals	Leominster	97%	186
Nashoba Valley Medical Center	Ayer	97%	71
New England Baptist Hospital[2]	Boston	97%	1855
Emerson Hospital	West Concord	96%	217
Marlborough Hospital	Marlborough	96%	93
Milton Hospital	Milton	96%	199
Sturdy Memorial Hospital	Attleboro	96%	337
Anna Jaques Hospital	Newburyport	95%	204
Falmouth Hospital[2]	Falmouth	95%	202
Milford Regional Medical Center	Milford	95%	118
Winchester Hospital	Winchester	95%	333
Merrimack Valley Hospital	Haverhill	94%	82
Metrowest Medical Center[2]	Framingham	94%	259
Morton Hospital & Medical Center	Taunton	94%	182
Lowell General Hospital[2]	Lowell	93%	172
The Cooley Dickinson Hospital[2]	Northampton	92%	147
Newton-Wellesley Hospital[2]	Newton	92%	92
Hallmark Health System[2]	Melrose	91%	194
Saints Medical Center	Lowell	91%	148
Southcoast Hospital Group	Fall River	91%	1025
Heywood Hospital	Gardner	90%	96
Holyoke Medical Center	Holyoke	88%	114
Holy Family Hospital[2]	Methuen	87%	123
Harrington Memorial Hospital	Southbridge	85%	66
Lawrence General Hospital	Lawrence	83%	145

32. Urinary Catheter Removal

Hospital Name	City	Rate	Cases
Baystate Medical Center[2]	Springfield	100%	687
Milford Regional Medical Center	Milford	100%	101
VA Boston Healthcare System - Jamaica Plain[2]	Jamaica Plain	100%	185
Saint Vincent Hospital	Worcester	99%	411
Boston Medical Center Corporation[2]	Boston	98%	266
Falmouth Hospital[2]	Falmouth	98%	225
Lowell General Hospital[2]	Lowell	98%	107
Beth Israel Deaconess Hospital - Needham	Needham	97%	33
Cambridge Health Alliance[2]	Cambridge	97%	87
Harrington Memorial Hospital	Southbridge	97%	36
Faulkner Hospital[2]	Boston	96%	45
Healthalliance Hospitals	Leominster	96%	98
Beverly Hospital Corporation	Beverly	95%	344
Cape Cod Hospital[2]	Hyannis	94%	321
The Cooley Dickinson Hospital[2]	Northampton	94%	162
Tufts Medical Center[2]	Boston	94%	197
Berkshire Medical Center[2]	Pittsfield	93%	166
Metrowest Medical Center[2]	Framingham	92%	156
Morton Hospital & Medical Center	Taunton	92%	93
New England Baptist Hospital[2]	Boston	92%	1771
Beth Israel Deaconess Medical Center[2]	Boston	91%	264
Jordan Hospital	Plymouth	91%	77
Winchester Hospital	Winchester	91%	239
Hallmark Health System[2]	Melrose	89%	98
Newton-Wellesley Hospital[2]	Newton	89%	54
Emerson Hospital	West Concord	88%	176
Massachusetts General Hospital[2]	Boston	88%	179
Merrimack Valley Hospital	Haverhill	88%	41
Brigham and Women's Hosptial[2]	Boston	87%	167
Milton Hospital	Milton	87%	92
Signature Healthcare Brockton Hospital	Brockton	87%	52
Mercy Medical Center	Springfield	86%	216
Saint Elizabeth's Medical Center[2]	Brighton	86%	157
Holy Family Hospital[2]	Methuen	84%	167
Saint Anne's Hospital	Fall River	84%	51
Carney Hospital[2]	Boston	83%	30
Heywood Hospital	Gardner	82%	94
Marlborough Hospital	Marlborough	81%	68
Sturdy Memorial Hospital	Attleboro	81%	174
Lahey Clinic Hospital[2]	Burlington	80%	95
UMass Memorial Medical Center[2]	Worcester	79%	104
Anna Jaques Hospital	Newburyport	78%	41
North Shore Medical Center[2]	Salem	78%	122
Saints Medical Center	Lowell	78%	58
Good Samaritan Medical Center[2]	Brockton	76%	34
Holyoke Medical Center	Holyoke	76%	46
Nashoba Valley Medical Center	Ayer	76%	29
South Shore Hospital	S Weymouth	75%	159
Mount Auburn Hospital	Cambridge	73%	311
Southcoast Hospital Group	Fall River	73%	501
Baystate Franklin Medical Center	Greenfield	69%	32
Norwood Hospital[2]	Norwood	66%	89
Lawrence General Hospital	Lawrence	58%	50
Quincy Medical Center	Quincy	54%	46

Children's Asthma Care

33. Received Systemic Corticosteroids

Hospital Name	City	Rate	Cases
Baystate Medical Center	Springfield	100%	129
Children's Hospital Boston[2]	Boston	100%	364

34. Received Home Management Plan of Care

Hospital Name	City	Rate	Cases
Baystate Medical Center	Springfield	75%	129
Children's Hospital Boston[2]	Boston	67%	364

35. Received Reliever Medication

Hospital Name	City	Rate	Cases
Children's Hospital Boston[2]	Boston	100%	364
Baystate Medical Center	Springfield	99%	129

Use of Medical Imaging

36. Combination Abdominal CT Scan

Hospital Name	City	Ratio	Cases
Noble Hospital	Westfield	0.018	439
Heywood Hospital	Gardner	0.020	301
Clinton Hospital Association	Clinton	0.024	126
Baystate Mary Lane Hospital	Ware	0.035	230
Saint Vincent Hospital	Worcester	0.035	606
Morton Hospital & Medical Center	Taunton	0.036	831
New England Baptist Hospital	Boston	0.040	329
Anna Jaques Hospital	Newburyport	0.041	636
Baystate Medical Center	Springfield	0.042	1645
Healthalliance Hospitals	Leominster	0.042	601
Lowell General Hospital	Lowell	0.048	1021
Marlborough Hospital	Marlborough	0.050	361
Holyoke Medical Center	Holyoke	0.053	865
The Cooley Dickinson Hospital	Northampton	0.055	740
Emerson Hospital	West Concord	0.055	686
Nantucket Cottage Hospital	Nantucket	0.055	110
Wing Memorial Hospital and Medical Center	Palmer	0.056	444
Signature Healthcare Brockton Hospital	Brockton	0.057	714
Beverly Hospital Corporation	Beverly	0.060	1246
Massachusetts General Hospital	Boston	0.062	3641
Merrimack Valley Hospital	Haverhill	0.064	498
Boston Medical Center Corporation	Boston	0.065	1366
Good Samaritan Medical Center	Brockton	0.065	1131
Quincy Medical Center	Quincy	0.067	751
Faulkner Hospital	Boston	0.070	812
Winchester Hospital	Winchester	0.070	1193
Lawrence General Hospital	Lawrence	0.072	782
Saint Anne's Hospital	Fall River	0.072	666
Southcoast Hospital Group	Fall River	0.075	2982
Norwood Hospital	Norwood	0.078	605
Sturdy Memorial Hospital	Attleboro	0.078	838
Falmouth Hospital	Falmouth	0.079	1145
Brigham and Women's Hosptial	Boston	0.083	2296
Mercy Medical Center	Springfield	0.087	1387
Metrowest Medical Center	Framingham	0.087	1060
Milford Regional Medical Center	Milford	0.089	879
Berkshire Medical Center	Pittsfield	0.090	1989
North Shore Medical Center	Salem	0.091	2380
Newton-Wellesley Hospital	Newton	0.097	1181
Cape Cod Hospital	Hyannis	0.098	2516
South Shore Hospital	S Weymouth	0.105	1304
Hallmark Health System	Melrose	0.110	1549
Mount Auburn Hospital	Cambridge	0.127	938
Baystate Franklin Medical Center	Greenfield	0.132	705
UMass Memorial Medical Center	Worcester	0.135	2202
Carney Hospital	Boston	0.139	482
North Adams Regional Hospital	North Adams	0.149	609
Jordan Hospital	Plymouth	0.159	1338
Nashoba Valley Medical Center	Ayer	0.160	338
Milton Hospital	Milton	0.167	408
Saint Elizabeth's Medical Center	Brighton	0.169	709
Saints Medical Center	Lowell	0.191	770
Cambridge Health Alliance	Cambridge	0.196	657
Lahey Clinic Hospital	Burlington	0.208	2824
Beth Israel Deaconess Hospital - Needham	Needham	0.234	291
Harrington Memorial Hospital	Southbridge	0.235	323
Tufts Medical Center	Boston	0.242	829
Beth Israel Deaconess Medical Center	Boston	0.247	2159
Holy Family Hospital	Methuen	0.410	882

37. Combination Chest CT Scan

Hospital Name	City	Ratio	Cases
Baystate Mary Lane Hospital	Ware	0.000	149

NOTE: Hospital profiles are in alphabetical order by state, then city, then hospital within the city; Rankings exclude hospitals with less than 25 cases except for patient surveys which excludes hospitals with less than 100 cases; (a) 100–299 cases; (1) The number of cases is too small to be sure how well a hospital is performing; (2) The hospital indicated that the data submitted for this measure were based on a sample of cases; (3) Data was collected during a shorter time period (fewer quarters) than the maximum possible time for this measure; (4) Suppressed for one or more quarters by CMS; (5) No data is available from the hospital for this measure; (6) Fewer than 100 patients completed the HCAHPS survey. Use these rates with caution, as the number of surveys may be too low to reliably assess hospital performance; (7) Survey results are based on less than 12 months of data; (8) Survey results are not available for this reporting period; (9) No or very few patients were eligible for the HCAHPS survey. The scores shown, if any, reflect a very small number of surveys; (10) A state average was not calculated because too few hospitals in the state submitted data; (11) There were discrepancies in the data collection process; Please refer to the User's Guide for a full explanation of data.

Clinton Hospital Association	Clinton	0.000	63
The Cooley Dickinson Hospital	Northampton	0.000	535
Heywood Hospital	Gardner	0.000	292
Holyoke Medical Center	Holyoke	0.000	315
Marlborough Hospital	Marlborough	0.000	178
Massachusetts Eye and Ear Infirmary	Boston	0.000	279
Milton Hospital	Milton	0.000	243
Mount Auburn Hospital	Cambridge	0.000	627
Nantucket Cottage Hospital	Nantucket	0.000	73
Noble Hospital	Westfield	0.000	234
Saint Vincent Hospital	Worcester	0.000	431
Winchester Hospital	Winchester	0.000	1052
Baystate Medical Center	Springfield	0.001	1406
Beverly Hospital Corporation	Beverly	0.001	998
Brigham and Women's Hosptial	Boston	0.001	3685
Good Samaritan Medical Center	Brockton	0.001	1024
Lahey Clinic Hospital	Burlington	0.001	2722
Lowell General Hospital	Lowell	0.001	683
Massachusetts General Hospital	Boston	0.001	4973
Milford Regional Medical Center	Milford	0.001	693
North Shore Medical Center	Salem	0.001	2048
Baystate Franklin Medical Center	Greenfield	0.002	419
Beth Israel Deaconess Medical Center	Boston	0.002	2491
Emerson Hospital	West Concord	0.002	614
Faulkner Hospital	Boston	0.002	950
Norwood Hospital	Norwood	0.002	444
Saints Medical Center	Lowell	0.002	507
Wing Memorial Hospital and Medical Center	Palmer	0.002	442
Cambridge Health Alliance	Cambridge	0.003	348
Morton Hospital & Medical Center	Taunton	0.003	642
Newton-Wellesley Hospital	Newton	0.003	1135
Saint Anne's Hospital	Fall River	0.003	587
Healthalliance Hospitals	Leominster	0.004	520
Saint Elizabeth's Medical Center	Brighton	0.005	745
Southcoast Hospital Group	Fall River	0.005	2408
Tufts Medical Center	Boston	0.005	971
Metrowest Medical Center	Framingham	0.006	1024
UMass Memorial Medical Center	Worcester	0.006	1687
Anna Jaques Hospital	Newburyport	0.009	585
North Adams Regional Hospital	North Adams	0.009	555
Mercy Medical Center	Springfield	0.011	760
Nashoba Valley Medical Center	Ayer	0.011	186
Carney Hospital	Boston	0.012	346
Jordan Hospital	Plymouth	0.012	893
Merrimack Valley Hospital	Haverhill	0.016	372
Quincy Medical Center	Quincy	0.016	435
Cape Cod Hospital	Hyannis	0.018	2213
New England Baptist Hospital	Boston	0.021	284
Boston Medical Center Corporation	Boston	0.023	1070
Hallmark Health System	Melrose	0.025	1219
Falmouth Hospital	Falmouth	0.027	1065
Signature Healthcare Brockton Hospital	Brockton	0.030	535
Holy Family Hospital	Methuen	0.031	551
Lawrence General Hospital	Lawrence	0.032	467
Harrington Memorial Hospital	Southbridge	0.037	294
South Shore Hospital	S Weymouth	0.042	945
Berkshire Medical Center	Pittsfield	0.059	1860
Sturdy Memorial Hospital	Attleboro	0.105	466
Beth Israel Deaconess Hospital - Needham	Needham	0.158	203

38. Follow-up Mammogram/Ultrasound

Hospital Name	City	Rate	Cases
Tufts Medical Center	Boston	1.1%	1042
Clinton Hospital Association	Clinton	2.9%	342
Marlborough Hospital	Marlborough	3.3%	694
Nantucket Cottage Hospital	Nantucket	3.7%	134
North Adams Regional Hospital	North Adams	4.5%	1369
Quincy Medical Center	Quincy	4.7%	975
Milton Hospital	Milton	5.2%	878
Wing Memorial Hospital and Medical Center	Palmer	5.2%	639
Baystate Mary Lane Hospital	Ware	5.4%	298
Massachusetts General Hospital	Boston	5.6%	6012
Berkshire Medical Center	Pittsfield	5.7%	2984
Beth Israel Deaconess Medical Center	Boston	5.8%	1884
Boston Medical Center Corporation	Boston	6.0%	2567
Morton Hospital & Medical Center	Taunton	6.3%	1926
The Cooley Dickinson Hospital	Northampton	6.4%	1628
Holy Family Hospital	Methuen	6.4%	929
Holyoke Medical Center	Holyoke	6.5%	1546
UMass Memorial Medical Center	Worcester	6.8%	2418
Heywood Hospital	Gardner	6.9%	596
Mount Auburn Hospital	Cambridge	6.9%	1618
Milford Regional Medical Center	Milford	7.1%	1520
Baystate Medical Center	Springfield	7.2%	1662
Healthalliance Hospitals	Leominster	7.2%	1107
Saint Vincent Hospital	Worcester	7.2%	377
Falmouth Hospital	Falmouth	7.9%	2764
Beverly Hospital Corporation	Beverly	8.1%	3148
Baystate Franklin Medical Center	Greenfield	8.2%	575
Lowell General Hospital	Lowell	8.2%	1083
Saint Anne's Hospital	Fall River	8.2%	1299
Sturdy Memorial Hospital	Attleboro	8.3%	1840
Cambridge Health Alliance	Cambridge	8.4%	1396
North Shore Medical Center	Salem	8.5%	5237
Saint Elizabeth's Medical Center	Brighton	9.3%	1072
Anna Jaques Hospital	Newburyport	9.4%	1792
Saints Medical Center	Lowell	9.4%	1155
Winchester Hospital	Winchester	9.4%	2478
Brigham and Women's Hosptial	Boston	9.5%	3398
Good Samaritan Medical Center	Brockton	9.5%	1342
South Shore Hospital	S Weymouth	9.7%	1772
Jordan Hospital	Plymouth	9.8%	1832
Signature Healthcare Brockton Hospital	Brockton	9.8%	860
Southcoast Hospital Group	Fall River	10.0%	6895
Beth Israel Deaconess Hospital - Needham	Needham	10.4%	473
Harrington Memorial Hospital	Southbridge	10.4%	628
Hallmark Health System	Melrose	10.7%	3532
Lahey Clinic Hospital	Burlington	10.8%	3572
Noble Hospital	Westfield	10.9%	832
Newton-Wellesley Hospital	Newton	11.0%	2613
Lawrence General Hospital	Lawrence	11.4%	729
Merrimack Valley Hospital	Haverhill	11.5%	1126
Mercy Medical Center	Springfield	12.5%	1941
Faulkner Hospital	Boston	13.3%	5107
Emerson Hospital	West Concord	14.5%	1698
Cape Cod Hospital	Hyannis	16.8%	3645
Metrowest Medical Center	Framingham	17.8%	2148
Nashoba Valley Medical Center	Ayer	18.5%	351
Norwood Hospital	Norwood	18.8%	704
Carney Hospital	Boston	26.8%	895

39. MRI for Low Back Pain

Hospital Name	City	Rate	Cases
Saint Vincent Hospital	Worcester	17.6%	74
The Cooley Dickinson Hospital	Northampton	22.2%	234
Beverly Hospital Corporation	Beverly	22.6%	221
Tufts Medical Center	Boston	23.6%	144
Nantucket Cottage Hospital[1]	Nantucket	25.8%	31
Beth Israel Deaconess Medical Center	Boston	25.9%	282
Sturdy Memorial Hospital	Attleboro	26.6%	263
Massachusetts General Hospital	Boston	27.1%	439
Baystate Medical Center	Springfield	27.3%	121
Beth Israel Deaconess Hospital - Needham	Needham	27.8%	79
Norwood Hospital[1]	Norwood	28.0%	25
New England Baptist Hospital	Boston	28.1%	484
Boston Medical Center Corporation	Boston	28.2%	248
Cambridge Health Alliance	Cambridge	28.6%	119
Newton-Wellesley Hospital	Newton	28.9%	159
Faulkner Hospital	Boston	29.0%	69
Jordan Hospital	Plymouth	29.0%	255
Lowell General Hospital	Lowell	29.2%	154
Berkshire Medical Center	Pittsfield	29.3%	399
Nashoba Valley Medical Center	Ayer	29.3%	58
Falmouth Hospital	Falmouth	29.4%	289
Morton Hospital & Medical Center	Taunton	29.6%	152
Saint Anne's Hospital	Fall River	29.8%	104
Southcoast Hospital Group	Fall River	29.9%	298
Brigham and Women's Hosptial	Boston	30.2%	394
Milton Hospital	Milton	30.2%	149
South Shore Hospital	S Weymouth	30.2%	139
Hallmark Health System	Melrose	30.3%	400
Winchester Hospital	Winchester	30.3%	228
Lahey Clinic Hospital	Burlington	30.8%	454
Cape Cod Hospital	Hyannis	31.3%	587
North Shore Medical Center	Salem	31.5%	375
Emerson Hospital	West Concord	32.2%	205
Milford Regional Medical Center	Milford	32.4%	207
Mount Auburn Hospital	Cambridge	32.4%	290
Noble Hospital	Westfield	33.3%	78
Heywood Hospital	Gardner	36.0%	136
Holyoke Medical Center	Holyoke	36.0%	222
Merrimack Valley Hospital	Haverhill	36.1%	119
North Adams Regional Hospital	North Adams	36.1%	133
Good Samaritan Medical Center	Brockton	36.6%	112
Harrington Memorial Hospital	Southbridge	38.1%	63
Signature Healthcare Brockton Hospital	Brockton	38.5%	104
Saint Elizabeth's Medical Center	Brighton	39.1%	174
Carney Hospital	Boston	44.6%	101

Survey of Patients' Hospital Experiences

40. Area Around Room 'Always' Quiet at Night

Hospital Name	City	Rate	Cases
Baystate Mary Lane Hospital	Ware	64%	(a)
Clinton Hospital Association	Clinton	63%	(a)
Nashoba Valley Medical Center	Ayer	62%	300+
Fairview Hospital	Great Barrington	61%	300+
Carney Hospital	Boston	59%	300+
Wing Memorial Hospital and Medical Center	Palmer	58%	300+
Saints Medical Center	Lowell	57%	300+
North Adams Regional Hospital	North Adams	56%	300+
Martha's Vineyard Hospital	Oak Bluffs	55%	(a)
Newton-Wellesley Hospital	Newton	55%	300+
Tufts Medical Center	Boston	55%	300+
The Cooley Dickinson Hospital	Northampton	54%	300+
Faulkner Hospital	Boston	54%	300+
Metrowest Medical Center	Framingham	54%	300+
Brigham and Women's Hosptial	Boston	53%	300+
Cambridge Health Alliance	Cambridge	53%	300+
Heywood Hospital	Gardner	53%	300+
Holyoke Medical Center	Holyoke	53%	300+
North Shore Medical Center	Salem	53%	300+
Lowell General Hospital	Lowell	52%	300+
Milton Hospital	Milton	52%	300+
Noble Hospital	Westfield	52%	300+
Saint Anne's Hospital	Fall River	52%	300+
Saint Elizabeth's Medical Center	Brighton	52%	300+
South Shore Hospital	S Weymouth	52%	300+
Cape Cod Hospital	Hyannis	51%	300+
Hallmark Health System[11]	Melrose	51%	300+
Milford Regional Medical Center	Milford	51%	300+
Southcoast Hospital Group	Fall River	51%	300+
Anna Jaques Hospital	Newburyport	50%	300+
Beth Israel Deaconess Hospital - Needham	Needham	50%	300+
Beth Israel Deaconess Medical Center	Boston	50%	300+
Emerson Hospital	West Concord	50%	300+
Harrington Memorial Hospital	Southbridge	50%	300+
Healthalliance Hospitals	Leominster	50%	300+
Holy Family Hospital	Methuen	50%	300+
Lawrence General Hospital	Lawrence	50%	300+
Massachusetts General Hospital	Boston	50%	300+
Mount Auburn Hospital	Cambridge	50%	300+
New England Baptist Hospital	Boston	50%	300+
Baystate Franklin Medical Center	Greenfield	49%	300+
Boston Medical Center Corporation	Boston	49%	300+
Morton Hospital & Medical Center	Taunton	49%	300+
Winchester Hospital	Winchester	49%	300+
Beverly Hospital Corporation	Beverly	48%	300+
Falmouth Hospital	Falmouth	47%	300+
Good Samaritan Medical Center	Brockton	47%	300+
Sturdy Memorial Hospital	Attleboro	47%	300+
Merrimack Valley Hospital	Haverhill	46%	300+
Jordan Hospital	Plymouth	45%	300+
UMass Memorial Medical Center	Worcester	45%	300+
Lahey Clinic Hospital	Burlington	44%	300+
Massachusetts Eye and Ear Infirmary	Boston	44%	300+
Quincy Medical Center	Quincy	44%	300+
Saint Vincent Hospital	Worcester	44%	300+
Berkshire Medical Center	Pittsfield	43%	300+
Baystate Medical Center	Springfield	42%	300+
Norwood Hospital	Norwood	41%	300+
Signature Healthcare Brockton Hospital	Brockton	41%	300+
Marlborough Hospital	Marlborough	40%	300+
Mercy Medical Center	Springfield	37%	300+

41. Doctors 'Always' Communicated Well

Hospital Name	City	Rate	Cases
Fairview Hospital	Great Barrington	84%	300+
Faulkner Hospital	Boston	84%	300+
Martha's Vineyard Hospital	Oak Bluffs	84%	(a)
Carney Hospital	Boston	83%	300+
Milford Regional Medical Center	Milford	83%	300+
Wing Memorial Hospital and Medical Center	Palmer	83%	300+
Emerson Hospital	West Concord	82%	300+
New England Baptist Hospital	Boston	82%	300+
Newton-Wellesley Hospital	Newton	82%	300+
Cape Cod Hospital	Hyannis	81%	300+
Hallmark Health System[11]	Melrose	81%	300+
Massachusetts Eye and Ear Infirmary	Boston	81%	300+
North Adams Regional Hospital	North Adams	81%	300+
Saint Elizabeth's Medical Center	Brighton	81%	300+
Saints Medical Center	Lowell	81%	300+
Winchester Hospital	Winchester	81%	300+
Anna Jaques Hospital	Newburyport	80%	300+
Baystate Mary Lane Hospital	Ware	80%	(a)
Baystate Medical Center	Springfield	80%	300+
Boston Medical Center Corporation	Boston	80%	300+
Clinton Hospital Association	Clinton	80%	(a)
Heywood Hospital	Gardner	80%	300+
Metrowest Medical Center	Framingham	80%	300+
Milton Hospital	Milton	80%	300+
Mount Auburn Hospital	Cambridge	80%	300+
Noble Hospital	Westfield	80%	300+
Norwood Hospital	Norwood	80%	300+
Tufts Medical Center	Boston	80%	300+
Beth Israel Deaconess Hospital - Needham	Needham	79%	300+
Brigham and Women's Hosptial	Boston	79%	300+
Healthalliance Hospitals	Leominster	79%	300+
Holy Family Hospital	Methuen	79%	300+
Nashoba Valley Medical Center	Ayer	79%	300+

NOTE: Hospital profiles are in alphabetical order by state, then city, then hospital within the city; Rankings exclude hospitals with less than 25 cases except for patient surveys which excludes hospitals with less than 100 cases; (a) 100–299 cases; (1) The number of cases is too small to be sure how well a hospital is performing; (2) The hospital indicated that the data submitted for this measure were based on a sample of cases; (3) Data was collected during a shorter time period (fewer quarters) than the maximum possible time for this measure; (4) Suppressed for one or more quarters by CMS; (5) No data is available from the hospital for this measure; (6) Fewer than 100 patients completed the HCAHPS survey. Use these rates with caution, as the number of surveys may be too low to reliably assess hospital performance; (7) Survey results are based on less than 12 months of data; (8) Survey results are not available for this reporting period; (9) No or very few patients were eligible for the HCAHPS survey. The scores shown, if any, reflect a very small number of surveys; (10) A state average was not calculated because too few hospitals in the state submitted data; (11) There were discrepancies in the data collection process; Please refer to the User's Guide for a full explanation of data.

South Shore Hospital	S Weymouth	79%	300+
Southcoast Hospital Group	Fall River	79%	300+
Beth Israel Deaconess Medical Center	Boston	78%	300+
Beverly Hospital Corporation	Beverly	78%	300+
Cambridge Health Alliance	Cambridge	78%	300+
The Cooley Dickinson Hospital	Northampton	78%	300+
Good Samaritan Medical Center	Brockton	78%	300+
Harrington Memorial Hospital	Southbridge	78%	300+
Jordan Hospital	Plymouth	78%	300+
Lawrence General Hospital	Lawrence	78%	300+
Lowell General Hospital	Lowell	78%	300+
Massachusetts General Hospital	Boston	78%	300+
Merrimack Valley Hospital	Haverhill	78%	300+
Morton Hospital & Medical Center	Taunton	78%	300+
Saint Anne's Hospital	Fall River	78%	300+
Saint Vincent Hospital	Worcester	78%	300+
Sturdy Memorial Hospital	Attleboro	78%	300+
Falmouth Hospital	Falmouth	77%	300+
Lahey Clinic Hospital	Burlington	77%	300+
Marlborough Hospital	Marlborough	77%	300+
Mercy Medical Center	Springfield	77%	300+
Baystate Franklin Medical Center	Greenfield	76%	300+
Berkshire Medical Center	Pittsfield	76%	300+
North Shore Medical Center	Salem	76%	300+
Signature Healthcare Brockton Hospital	Brockton	76%	300+
Holyoke Medical Center	Holyoke	75%	300+
UMass Memorial Medical Center	Worcester	74%	300+
Quincy Medical Center	Quincy	73%	300+

42. Home Recovery Information Given

Hospital Name	City	Rate	Cases
New England Baptist Hospital	Boston	93%	300+
Berkshire Medical Center	Pittsfield	91%	300+
Noble Hospital	Westfield	90%	300+
Faulkner Hospital	Boston	89%	300+
North Adams Regional Hospital	North Adams	89%	300+
Wing Memorial Hospital and Medical Center	Palmer	89%	300+
Baystate Mary Lane Hospital	Ware	88%	(a)
Brigham and Women's Hosptial	Boston	88%	300+
Fairview Hospital	Great Barrington	88%	300+
Healthalliance Hospitals	Leominster	88%	300+
Milford Regional Medical Center	Milford	88%	300+
South Shore Hospital	S Weymouth	88%	300+
UMass Memorial Medical Center	Worcester	88%	300+
Anna Jaques Hospital	Newburyport	87%	300+
Beth Israel Deaconess Medical Center	Boston	87%	300+
Boston Medical Center Corporation	Boston	87%	300+
Carney Hospital	Boston	87%	300+
Clinton Hospital Association	Clinton	87%	(a)
Holyoke Medical Center	Holyoke	87%	300+
Martha's Vineyard Hospital	Oak Bluffs	87%	(a)
Massachusetts General Hospital	Boston	87%	300+
Merrimack Valley Hospital	Haverhill	87%	300+
Nashoba Valley Medical Center	Ayer	87%	300+
Newton-Wellesley Hospital	Newton	87%	300+
Saints Medical Center	Lowell	87%	300+
Cambridge Health Alliance	Cambridge	86%	300+
The Cooley Dickinson Hospital	Northampton	86%	300+
Emerson Hospital	West Concord	86%	300+
Heywood Hospital	Gardner	86%	300+
Mercy Medical Center	Springfield	86%	300+
Saint Anne's Hospital	Fall River	86%	300+
Southcoast Hospital Group	Fall River	86%	300+
Sturdy Memorial Hospital	Attleboro	86%	300+
Baystate Franklin Medical Center	Greenfield	85%	300+
Baystate Medical Center	Springfield	85%	300+
Beverly Hospital Corporation	Beverly	85%	300+
Falmouth Hospital	Falmouth	85%	300+
Lahey Clinic Hospital	Burlington	85%	300+
Marlborough Hospital	Marlborough	85%	300+
Massachusetts Eye and Ear Infirmary	Boston	85%	300+
Mount Auburn Hospital	Cambridge	85%	300+
North Shore Medical Center	Salem	85%	300+
Quincy Medical Center	Quincy	85%	300+
Signature Healthcare Brockton Hospital	Brockton	85%	300+
Tufts Medical Center	Boston	85%	300+
Cape Cod Hospital	Hyannis	84%	300+
Good Samaritan Medical Center	Brockton	84%	300+
Hallmark Health System[11]	Melrose	84%	300+
Saint Vincent Hospital	Worcester	84%	300+
Winchester Hospital	Winchester	84%	300+
Beth Israel Deaconess Hospital - Needham	Needham	83%	300+
Harrington Memorial Hospital	Southbridge	83%	300+
Holy Family Hospital	Methuen	83%	300+
Morton Hospital & Medical Center	Taunton	83%	300+
Norwood Hospital	Norwood	83%	300+
Saint Elizabeth's Medical Center	Brighton	83%	300+
Metrowest Medical Center	Framingham	82%	300+
Lawrence General Hospital	Lawrence	81%	300+
Lowell General Hospital	Lowell	81%	300+
Milton Hospital	Milton	81%	300+
Jordan Hospital	Plymouth	80%	300+

43. Hospital Given 9 or 10 on 10 Point Scale

Hospital Name	City	Rate	Cases
Fairview Hospital	Great Barrington	85%	300+
New England Baptist Hospital	Boston	84%	300+
Brigham and Women's Hosptial	Boston	79%	300+
Faulkner Hospital	Boston	78%	300+
Massachusetts General Hospital	Boston	78%	300+
Milford Regional Medical Center	Milford	77%	300+
Cape Cod Hospital	Hyannis	76%	300+
Clinton Hospital Association	Clinton	75%	(a)
Winchester Hospital	Winchester	75%	300+
Emerson Hospital	West Concord	74%	300+
Baystate Mary Lane Hospital	Ware	73%	(a)
Beth Israel Deaconess Medical Center	Boston	73%	300+
Beth Israel Deaconess Hospital - Needham	Needham	72%	300+
Newton-Wellesley Hospital	Newton	72%	300+
Mount Auburn Hospital	Cambridge	71%	300+
Wing Memorial Hospital and Medical Center	Palmer	71%	300+
Saint Vincent Hospital	Worcester	70%	300+
Tufts Medical Center	Boston	70%	300+
South Shore Hospital	S Weymouth	69%	300+
Beverly Hospital Corporation	Beverly	68%	300+
The Cooley Dickinson Hospital	Northampton	68%	300+
Falmouth Hospital	Falmouth	68%	300+
Lahey Clinic Hospital	Burlington	68%	300+
Saint Elizabeth's Medical Center	Brighton	68%	300+
Saints Medical Center	Lowell	68%	300+
Boston Medical Center Corporation	Boston	67%	300+
Harrington Memorial Hospital	Southbridge	67%	300+
Massachusetts Eye and Ear Infirmary	Boston	67%	300+
Nashoba Valley Medical Center	Ayer	67%	300+
Noble Hospital	Westfield	67%	300+
Sturdy Memorial Hospital	Attleboro	67%	300+
Berkshire Medical Center	Pittsfield	66%	300+
Heywood Hospital	Gardner	66%	300+
Metrowest Medical Center	Framingham	66%	300+
Milton Hospital	Milton	66%	300+
North Shore Medical Center	Salem	66%	300+
Saint Anne's Hospital	Fall River	66%	300+
UMass Memorial Medical Center	Worcester	66%	300+
Baystate Medical Center	Springfield	65%	300+
Carney Hospital	Boston	65%	300+
Hallmark Health System[11]	Melrose	65%	300+
Jordan Hospital	Plymouth	65%	300+
Lowell General Hospital	Lowell	65%	300+
North Adams Regional Hospital	North Adams	65%	300+
Baystate Franklin Medical Center	Greenfield	64%	300+
Merrimack Valley Hospital	Haverhill	64%	300+
Holy Family Hospital	Methuen	63%	300+
Norwood Hospital	Norwood	63%	300+
Anna Jaques Hospital	Newburyport	62%	300+
Good Samaritan Medical Center	Brockton	62%	300+
Southcoast Hospital Group	Fall River	62%	300+
Martha's Vineyard Hospital	Oak Bluffs	61%	(a)
Mercy Medical Center	Springfield	61%	300+
Healthalliance Hospitals	Leominster	60%	300+
Holyoke Medical Center	Holyoke	60%	300+
Marlborough Hospital	Marlborough	60%	300+
Signature Healthcare Brockton Hospital	Brockton	60%	300+
Cambridge Health Alliance	Cambridge	59%	300+
Quincy Medical Center	Quincy	59%	300+
Lawrence General Hospital	Lawrence	57%	300+
Morton Hospital & Medical Center	Taunton	57%	300+

44. Meds 'Always' Explained Before Given

Hospital Name	City	Rate	Cases
Fairview Hospital	Great Barrington	76%	300+
Clinton Hospital Association	Clinton	72%	(a)
Carney Hospital	Boston	66%	300+
Emerson Hospital	West Concord	66%	300+
Milford Regional Medical Center	Milford	65%	300+
Saint Elizabeth's Medical Center	Brighton	65%	300+
South Shore Hospital	S Weymouth	65%	300+
Winchester Hospital	Winchester	65%	300+
Beth Israel Deaconess Hospital - Needham	Needham	64%	300+
Heywood Hospital	Gardner	64%	300+
Martha's Vineyard Hospital	Oak Bluffs	64%	(a)
Mount Auburn Hospital	Cambridge	64%	300+
New England Baptist Hospital	Boston	64%	300+
North Adams Regional Hospital	North Adams	64%	300+
Baystate Mary Lane Hospital	Ware	63%	(a)
Baystate Medical Center	Springfield	63%	300+
Beth Israel Deaconess Medical Center	Boston	63%	300+
Cape Cod Hospital	Hyannis	63%	300+
Faulkner Hospital	Boston	63%	300+
Holy Family Hospital	Methuen	63%	300+
Lawrence General Hospital	Lawrence	63%	300+
Marlborough Hospital	Marlborough	63%	300+
Massachusetts General Hospital	Boston	63%	300+
Newton-Wellesley Hospital	Newton	63%	300+
Noble Hospital	Westfield	63%	300+
Anna Jaques Hospital	Newburyport	62%	300+
Cambridge Health Alliance	Cambridge	62%	300+
Healthalliance Hospitals	Leominster	62%	300+
Metrowest Medical Center	Framingham	62%	300+
Norwood Hospital	Norwood	62%	300+
Wing Memorial Hospital and Medical Center	Palmer	62%	300+
Boston Medical Center Corporation	Boston	61%	300+
Brigham and Women's Hosptial	Boston	61%	300+
Hallmark Health System[11]	Melrose	61%	300+
Harrington Memorial Hospital	Southbridge	61%	300+
Lahey Clinic Hospital	Burlington	61%	300+
Saint Anne's Hospital	Fall River	61%	300+
Saints Medical Center	Lowell	61%	300+
Tufts Medical Center	Boston	61%	300+
Baystate Franklin Medical Center	Greenfield	60%	300+
Beverly Hospital Corporation	Beverly	60%	300+
Good Samaritan Medical Center	Brockton	60%	300+
Jordan Hospital	Plymouth	60%	300+
Lowell General Hospital	Lowell	60%	300+
Milton Hospital	Milton	60%	300+
Morton Hospital & Medical Center	Taunton	60%	300+
North Shore Medical Center	Salem	60%	300+
Sturdy Memorial Hospital	Attleboro	60%	300+
The Cooley Dickinson Hospital	Northampton	59%	300+
Holyoke Medical Center	Holyoke	59%	300+
Merrimack Valley Hospital	Haverhill	59%	300+
Nashoba Valley Medical Center	Ayer	59%	300+
Quincy Medical Center	Quincy	59%	300+
Saint Vincent Hospital	Worcester	59%	300+
Southcoast Hospital Group	Fall River	59%	300+
UMass Memorial Medical Center	Worcester	59%	300+
Berkshire Medical Center	Pittsfield	58%	300+
Falmouth Hospital	Falmouth	58%	300+
Massachusetts Eye and Ear Infirmary	Boston	58%	300+
Signature Healthcare Brockton Hospital	Brockton	58%	300+
Mercy Medical Center	Springfield	57%	300+

45. Nurses 'Always' Communicated Well

Hospital Name	City	Rate	Cases
Fairview Hospital	Great Barrington	87%	300+
Clinton Hospital Association	Clinton	85%	(a)
New England Baptist Hospital	Boston	84%	300+
Faulkner Hospital	Boston	83%	300+
Milford Regional Medical Center	Milford	82%	300+
Baystate Mary Lane Hospital	Ware	81%	(a)
Emerson Hospital	West Concord	81%	300+
Berkshire Medical Center	Pittsfield	80%	300+
Cape Cod Hospital	Hyannis	80%	300+
Carney Hospital	Boston	80%	300+
Hallmark Health System[11]	Melrose	80%	300+
Mount Auburn Hospital	Cambridge	80%	300+
Winchester Hospital	Winchester	80%	300+
Anna Jaques Hospital	Newburyport	79%	300+
Brigham and Women's Hosptial	Boston	79%	300+
Lowell General Hospital	Lowell	79%	300+
Metrowest Medical Center	Framingham	79%	300+
Noble Hospital	Westfield	79%	300+
North Adams Regional Hospital	North Adams	79%	300+
Norwood Hospital	Norwood	79%	300+
Saint Anne's Hospital	Fall River	79%	300+
Tufts Medical Center	Boston	79%	300+
Wing Memorial Hospital and Medical Center	Palmer	79%	300+
Beth Israel Deaconess Hospital - Needham	Needham	78%	300+
Beverly Hospital Corporation	Beverly	78%	300+
Good Samaritan Medical Center	Brockton	78%	300+
Healthalliance Hospitals	Leominster	78%	300+
Massachusetts General Hospital	Boston	78%	300+
Nashoba Valley Medical Center	Ayer	78%	300+
Newton-Wellesley Hospital	Newton	78%	300+
Saints Medical Center	Lowell	78%	300+
South Shore Hospital	S Weymouth	78%	300+
Baystate Franklin Medical Center	Greenfield	77%	300+
Baystate Medical Center	Springfield	77%	300+
Beth Israel Deaconess Medical Center	Boston	77%	300+
Falmouth Hospital	Falmouth	77%	300+
Heywood Hospital	Gardner	77%	300+
Holy Family Hospital	Methuen	77%	300+
Martha's Vineyard Hospital	Oak Bluffs	77%	(a)
Saint Elizabeth's Medical Center	Brighton	77%	300+
Signature Healthcare Brockton Hospital	Brockton	76%	300+
Sturdy Memorial Hospital	Attleboro	76%	300+
The Cooley Dickinson Hospital	Northampton	75%	300+
Harrington Memorial Hospital	Southbridge	75%	300+
Lawrence General Hospital	Lawrence	75%	300+
Marlborough Hospital	Marlborough	75%	300+
Milton Hospital	Milton	75%	300+

NOTE: Hospital profiles are in alphabetical order by state, then city, then hospital within the city; Rankings exclude hospitals with less than 25 cases except for patient surveys which excludes hospitals with less than 100 cases; (a) 100–299 cases; (1) The number of cases is too small to be sure how well a hospital is performing; (2) The hospital indicated that the data submitted for this measure were based on a sample of cases; (3) Data was collected during a shorter time period (fewer quarters) than the maximum possible time for this measure; (4) Suppressed for one or more quarters by CMS; (5) No data is available from the hospital for this measure; (6) Fewer than 100 patients completed the HCAHPS survey. Use these rates with caution, as the number of surveys may be too low to reliably assess hospital performance; (7) Survey results are based on less than 12 months of data; (8) Survey results are not available for this reporting period; (9) No or very few patients were eligible for the HCAHPS survey. The scores shown, if any, reflect a very small number of surveys; (10) A state average was not calculated because too few hospitals in the state submitted data; (11) There were discrepancies in the data collection process; Please refer to the User's Guide for a full explanation of data.

Morton Hospital & Medical Center	Taunton	75%	300+
North Shore Medical Center	Salem	75%	300+
Southcoast Hospital Group	Fall River	75%	300+
Boston Medical Center Corporation	Boston	74%	300+
Merrimack Valley Hospital	Haverhill	74%	300+
Quincy Medical Center	Quincy	74%	300+
Holyoke Medical Center	Holyoke	73%	300+
Jordan Hospital	Plymouth	73%	300+
Saint Vincent Hospital	Worcester	73%	300+
Cambridge Health Alliance	Cambridge	72%	300+
Lahey Clinic Hospital	Burlington	72%	300+
Mercy Medical Center	Springfield	72%	300+
UMass Memorial Medical Center	Worcester	72%	300+
Massachusetts Eye and Ear Infirmary	Boston	71%	300+

46. Pain 'Always' Well Controlled

Hospital Name	City	Rate	Cases
Clinton Hospital Association	Clinton	80%	(a)
Fairview Hospital	Great Barrington	79%	300+
Faulkner Hospital	Boston	76%	300+
Nashoba Valley Medical Center	Ayer	76%	300+
Noble Hospital	Westfield	76%	300+
Emerson Hospital	West Concord	75%	300+
Hallmark Health System[11]	Melrose	75%	300+
Heywood Hospital	Gardner	75%	300+
Martha's Vineyard Hospital	Oak Bluffs	75%	(a)
Milford Regional Medical Center	Milford	75%	300+
Anna Jaques Hospital	Newburyport	74%	300+
Beverly Hospital Corporation	Beverly	74%	300+
Norwood Hospital	Norwood	74%	300+
Jordan Hospital	Plymouth	73%	300+
Marlborough Hospital	Marlborough	73%	300+
Mount Auburn Hospital	Cambridge	73%	300+
North Adams Regional Hospital	North Adams	73%	300+
Saints Medical Center	Lowell	73%	300+
Wing Memorial Hospital and Medical Center	Palmer	73%	300+
Baystate Mary Lane Hospital	Ware	72%	(a)
Berkshire Medical Center	Pittsfield	72%	300+
Cape Cod Hospital	Hyannis	72%	300+
Holy Family Hospital	Methuen	72%	300+
Lawrence General Hospital	Lawrence	72%	300+
Massachusetts Eye and Ear Infirmary	Boston	72%	300+
Metrowest Medical Center	Framingham	72%	300+
Quincy Medical Center	Quincy	72%	300+
Saint Vincent Hospital	Worcester	72%	300+
Brigham and Women's Hospital	Boston	71%	300+
Carney Hospital	Boston	71%	300+
Harrington Memorial Hospital	Southbridge	71%	300+
Healthalliance Hospitals	Leominster	71%	300+
New England Baptist Hospital	Boston	71%	300+
Newton-Wellesley Hospital	Newton	71%	300+
Saint Elizabeth's Medical Center	Brighton	71%	300+
Winchester Hospital	Winchester	71%	300+
Falmouth Hospital	Falmouth	70%	300+
Massachusetts General Hospital	Boston	70%	300+
Merrimack Valley Hospital	Haverhill	70%	300+
Morton Hospital & Medical Center	Taunton	70%	300+
North Shore Medical Center	Salem	70%	300+
South Shore Hospital	S Weymouth	70%	300+
Sturdy Memorial Hospital	Attleboro	70%	300+
Baystate Medical Center	Springfield	69%	300+
Beth Israel Deaconess Hospital - Needham	Needham	69%	300+
Lowell General Hospital	Lowell	69%	300+
Saint Anne's Hospital	Fall River	69%	300+
Beth Israel Deaconess Medical Center	Boston	68%	300+
Good Samaritan Medical Center	Brockton	68%	300+
Baystate Franklin Medical Center	Greenfield	67%	300+
Cambridge Health Alliance	Cambridge	67%	300+
The Cooley Dickinson Hospital	Northampton	67%	300+
Holyoke Medical Center	Holyoke	67%	300+
Milton Hospital	Milton	67%	300+
Signature Healthcare Brockton Hospital	Brockton	67%	300+
Southcoast Hospital Group	Fall River	67%	300+
Tufts Medical Center	Boston	67%	300+
Boston Medical Center Corporation	Boston	66%	300+
UMass Memorial Medical Center	Worcester	65%	300+
Mercy Medical Center	Springfield	64%	300+
Lahey Clinic Hospital	Burlington	63%	300+

47. Room and Bathroom 'Always' Clean

Hospital Name	City	Rate	Cases
Fairview Hospital	Great Barrington	86%	300+
Beth Israel Deaconess Hospital - Needham	Needham	80%	300+
Clinton Hospital Association	Clinton	79%	(a)
Harrington Memorial Hospital	Southbridge	79%	300+
Milford Regional Medical Center	Milford	79%	300+
Cape Cod Hospital	Hyannis	78%	300+
New England Baptist Hospital	Boston	78%	300+
Noble Hospital	Westfield	78%	300+
Sturdy Memorial Hospital	Attleboro	78%	300+
Nashoba Valley Medical Center	Ayer	77%	300+
North Adams Regional Hospital	North Adams	77%	300+
Baystate Mary Lane Hospital	Ware	76%	(a)
Berkshire Medical Center	Pittsfield	76%	300+
Carney Hospital	Boston	76%	300+
The Cooley Dickinson Hospital	Northampton	76%	300+
Newton-Wellesley Hospital	Newton	76%	300+
Saints Medical Center	Lowell	76%	300+
Holyoke Medical Center	Holyoke	75%	300+
Norwood Hospital	Norwood	75%	300+
Saint Anne's Hospital	Fall River	75%	300+
Wing Memorial Hospital and Medical Center	Palmer	75%	300+
Falmouth Hospital	Falmouth	73%	300+
Faulkner Hospital	Boston	73%	300+
Saint Elizabeth's Medical Center	Brighton	73%	300+
South Shore Hospital	S Weymouth	73%	300+
Southcoast Hospital Group	Fall River	73%	300+
Winchester Hospital	Winchester	73%	300+
Healthalliance Hospitals	Leominster	72%	300+
Martha's Vineyard Hospital	Oak Bluffs	72%	(a)
Metrowest Medical Center	Framingham	72%	300+
Milton Hospital	Milton	72%	300+
Morton Hospital & Medical Center	Taunton	72%	300+
Mount Auburn Hospital	Cambridge	72%	300+
Massachusetts General Hospital	Boston	71%	300+
Beth Israel Deaconess Medical Center	Boston	70%	300+
Beverly Hospital Corporation	Beverly	70%	300+
Brigham and Women's Hospital	Boston	70%	300+
Heywood Hospital	Gardner	70%	300+
Marlborough Hospital	Marlborough	70%	300+
Quincy Medical Center	Quincy	70%	300+
North Shore Medical Center	Salem	69%	300+
Saint Vincent Hospital	Worcester	69%	300+
Signature Healthcare Brockton Hospital	Brockton	69%	300+
Boston Medical Center Corporation	Boston	68%	300+
Emerson Hospital	West Concord	68%	300+
Lowell General Hospital	Lowell	68%	300+
Tufts Medical Center	Boston	68%	300+
Anna Jaques Hospital	Newburyport	67%	300+
Cambridge Health Alliance	Cambridge	67%	300+
Good Samaritan Medical Center	Brockton	67%	300+
Hallmark Health System[11]	Melrose	67%	300+
Holy Family Hospital	Methuen	67%	300+
Lawrence General Hospital	Lawrence	67%	300+
Mercy Medical Center	Springfield	67%	300+
Baystate Franklin Medical Center	Greenfield	66%	300+
Baystate Medical Center	Springfield	66%	300+
Merrimack Valley Hospital	Haverhill	66%	300+
Lahey Clinic Hospital	Burlington	65%	300+
Jordan Hospital	Plymouth	64%	300+
Massachusetts Eye and Ear Infirmary	Boston	61%	300+
UMass Memorial Medical Center	Worcester	60%	300+

48. Timely Help 'Always' Received

Hospital Name	City	Rate	Cases
Fairview Hospital	Great Barrington	84%	300+
Clinton Hospital Association	Clinton	76%	(a)
Baystate Mary Lane Hospital	Ware	73%	(a)
Faulkner Hospital	Boston	71%	300+
Noble Hospital	Westfield	71%	300+
New England Baptist Hospital	Boston	70%	300+
Anna Jaques Hospital	Newburyport	68%	300+
Carney Hospital	Boston	68%	300+
Mount Auburn Hospital	Cambridge	68%	300+
Hallmark Health System[11]	Melrose	67%	300+
Harrington Memorial Hospital	Southbridge	67%	300+
Milford Regional Medical Center	Milford	67%	300+
Winchester Hospital	Winchester	67%	300+
Beth Israel Deaconess Hospital - Needham	Needham	66%	300+
Metrowest Medical Center	Framingham	66%	300+
Wing Memorial Hospital and Medical Center	Palmer	66%	300+
Brigham and Women's Hospital	Boston	65%	300+
North Adams Regional Hospital	North Adams	65%	300+
Norwood Hospital	Norwood	65%	300+
Saints Medical Center	Lowell	65%	300+
South Shore Hospital	S Weymouth	65%	300+
Baystate Franklin Medical Center	Greenfield	64%	300+
Berkshire Medical Center	Pittsfield	64%	300+
Cape Cod Hospital	Hyannis	64%	300+
Emerson Hospital	West Concord	64%	300+
Heywood Hospital	Gardner	64%	300+
Beverly Hospital Corporation	Beverly	63%	300+
The Cooley Dickinson Hospital	Northampton	63%	300+
Holy Family Hospital	Methuen	63%	300+
Jordan Hospital	Plymouth	63%	300+
Newton-Wellesley Hospital	Newton	63%	300+
North Shore Medical Center	Salem	63%	300+
Saint Anne's Hospital	Fall River	63%	300+
Saint Elizabeth's Medical Center	Brighton	63%	300+
Signature Healthcare Brockton Hospital	Brockton	63%	300+
Healthalliance Hospitals	Leominster	62%	300+
Massachusetts General Hospital	Boston	62%	300+
Merrimack Valley Hospital	Haverhill	62%	300+
Morton Hospital & Medical Center	Taunton	62%	300+
Falmouth Hospital	Falmouth	61%	300+
Lowell General Hospital	Lowell	61%	300+
Martha's Vineyard Hospital	Oak Bluffs	61%	(a)
Sturdy Memorial Hospital	Attleboro	61%	300+
Lawrence General Hospital	Lawrence	60%	300+
Milton Hospital	Milton	60%	300+
Tufts Medical Center	Boston	60%	300+
Marlborough Hospital	Marlborough	59%	300+
Massachusetts Eye and Ear Infirmary	Boston	59%	300+
Nashoba Valley Medical Center	Ayer	59%	300+
Quincy Medical Center	Quincy	59%	300+
Saint Vincent Hospital	Worcester	59%	300+
Beth Israel Deaconess Medical Center	Boston	58%	300+
Southcoast Hospital Group	Fall River	58%	300+
Baystate Medical Center	Springfield	57%	300+
Boston Medical Center Corporation	Boston	57%	300+
Cambridge Health Alliance	Cambridge	57%	300+
Mercy Medical Center	Springfield	57%	300+
Good Samaritan Medical Center	Brockton	56%	300+
Lahey Clinic Hospital	Burlington	56%	300+
Holyoke Medical Center	Holyoke	55%	300+
UMass Memorial Medical Center	Worcester	55%	300+

49. Would Definitely Recommend Hospital

Hospital Name	City	Rate	Cases
New England Baptist Hospital	Boston	91%	300+
Fairview Hospital	Great Barrington	88%	300+
Massachusetts General Hospital	Boston	88%	300+
Brigham and Women's Hospital	Boston	87%	300+
Cape Cod Hospital	Hyannis	81%	300+
Milford Regional Medical Center	Milford	81%	300+
Newton-Wellesley Hospital	Newton	81%	300+
Winchester Hospital	Winchester	81%	300+
Beth Israel Deaconess Medical Center	Boston	80%	300+
Clinton Hospital Association	Clinton	80%	(a)
Emerson Hospital	West Concord	80%	300+
Faulkner Hospital	Boston	79%	300+
Beth Israel Deaconess Hospital - Needham	Needham	78%	300+
Massachusetts Eye and Ear Infirmary	Boston	78%	300+
Mount Auburn Hospital	Cambridge	77%	300+
Tufts Medical Center	Boston	77%	300+
Wing Memorial Hospital and Medical Center	Palmer	77%	300+
Saint Vincent Hospital	Worcester	76%	300+
Baystate Mary Lane Hospital	Ware	75%	(a)
Baystate Medical Center	Springfield	75%	300+
UMass Memorial Medical Center	Worcester	75%	300+
Beverly Hospital Corporation	Beverly	74%	300+
Falmouth Hospital	Falmouth	74%	300+
Lahey Clinic Hospital	Burlington	74%	300+
Lowell General Hospital	Lowell	74%	300+
North Shore Medical Center	Salem	74%	300+
South Shore Hospital	S Weymouth	74%	300+
Heywood Hospital	Gardner	73%	300+
Saint Elizabeth's Medical Center	Brighton	73%	300+
Boston Medical Center Corporation	Boston	72%	300+
The Cooley Dickinson Hospital	Northampton	72%	300+
Martha's Vineyard Hospital	Oak Bluffs	72%	(a)
Metrowest Medical Center	Framingham	72%	300+
Milton Hospital	Milton	72%	300+
Nashoba Valley Medical Center	Ayer	72%	300+
Saint Anne's Hospital	Fall River	72%	300+
Saints Medical Center	Lowell	72%	300+
Sturdy Memorial Hospital	Attleboro	72%	300+
Harrington Memorial Hospital	Southbridge	71%	300+
Anna Jaques Hospital	Newburyport	70%	300+
Baystate Franklin Medical Center	Greenfield	70%	300+
Hallmark Health System[11]	Melrose	70%	300+
Jordan Hospital	Plymouth	70%	300+
North Adams Regional Hospital	North Adams	70%	300+
Berkshire Medical Center	Pittsfield	69%	300+
Holy Family Hospital	Methuen	69%	300+
Mercy Medical Center	Springfield	69%	300+
Noble Hospital	Westfield	69%	300+
Holyoke Medical Center	Holyoke	68%	300+
Lawrence General Hospital	Lawrence	68%	300+
Southcoast Hospital Group	Fall River	68%	300+
Good Samaritan Medical Center	Brockton	66%	300+
Marlborough Hospital	Marlborough	66%	300+
Carney Hospital	Boston	65%	300+
Healthalliance Hospitals	Leominster	65%	300+
Signature Healthcare Brockton Hospital	Brockton	65%	300+
Cambridge Health Alliance	Cambridge	64%	300+
Norwood Hospital	Norwood	64%	300+
Merrimack Valley Hospital	Haverhill	63%	300+
Quincy Medical Center	Quincy	61%	300+
Morton Hospital & Medical Center	Taunton	57%	300+

NOTE: Hospital profiles are in alphabetical order by state, then city, then hospital within the city; Rankings exclude hospitals with less than 25 cases except for patient surveys which excludes hospitals with less than 100 cases; (a) 100–299 cases; (1) The number of cases is too small to be sure how well a hospital is performing; (2) The hospital indicated that the data submitted for this measure were based on a sample of cases; (3) Data was collected during a shorter time period (fewer quarters) than the maximum possible time for this measure; (4) Suppressed for one or more quarters by CMS; (5) No data is available from the hospital for this measure; (6) Fewer than 100 patients completed the HCAHPS survey. Use these rates with caution, as the number of surveys may be too low to reliably assess hospital performance; (7) Survey results are based on less than 12 months of data; (8) Survey results are not available for this reporting period; (9) No or very few patients were eligible for the HCAHPS survey. The scores shown, if any, reflect a very small number of surveys; (10) A state average was not calculated because too few hospitals in the state submitted data; (11) There were discrepancies in the data collection process; Please refer to the User's Guide for a full explanation of data.

Athol Memorial Hospital

2033 Main Street
Athol, MA 01331
URL: www.atholhospital.org
Type: Critical Access Hospitals
Ownership: Voluntary Non-Profit - Private

Phone: 978-249-3511
Fax: 978-249-2651

Emergency Services: Yes
Beds: 33

Key Personnel:
CEO/President . . . . Steven Penka
Chief of Medical Staff . . . . Mohsen Noreldin, MD
Radiology . . . . Paul Sabel
Emergency Room . . . . John Skrzypczak, MD

Measure	Cases	This Hosp.	State Avg.	U.S. Avg.
Heart Attack Care				
ACE Inhibitor or ARB for LVSD[3]	0	-	94%	96%
Aspirin at Arrival[1,3]	5	80%	99%	99%
Aspirin at Discharge[1,3]	5	100%	99%	98%
Beta Blocker at Discharge[1,3]	6	100%	99%	98%
Fibrinolytic Medication Timing[3]	0	-	50%	55%
PCI Within 90 Minutes of Arrival[3]	0	-	93%	90%
Smoking Cessation Advice[3]	0	-	99%	99%
Chest Pain/Possible Heart Attack Care				
Aspirin at Arrival	-	-	96%	95%
Median Time to ECG (minutes)	-	-	10	8
Median Time to Transfer (minutes)	-	-	65	61
Fibrinolytic Medication Timing	-	-	78%	54%
Heart Failure Care				
ACE Inhibitor or ARB for LVSD[1]	9	100%	94%	94%
Discharge Instructions	31	94%	89%	88%
Evaluation of LVS Function	48	88%	98%	98%
Smoking Cessation Advice[1]	2	100%	97%	98%
Pneumonia Care				
Appropriate Initial Antibiotic[1]	24	79%	93%	92%
Blood Culture Timing	45	93%	95%	96%
Influenza Vaccine	34	91%	92%	91%
Initial Antibiotic Timing	45	98%	96%	95%
Pneumococcal Vaccine	43	98%	93%	93%
Smoking Cessation Advice[1]	9	100%	96%	97%
Surgical Care Improvement Project				
Appropriate VTP Within 24 Hours[1]	11	100%	96%	92%
Appropriate Hair Removal[1]	19	100%	100%	99%
Appropriate Beta Blocker Usage[1]	6	67%	96%	93%
Controlled Postoperative Blood Glucose	0	-	95%	93%
Prophylactic Antibiotic Timing[1]	15	100%	97%	97%
Prophylactic Antibiotic Timing (Outpatient)	-	-	92%	92%
Prophylactic Antibiotic Selection[1]	15	93%	98%	97%
Prophylactic Antibiotic Select. (Outpatient)	-	-	95%	94%
Prophylactic Antibiotic Stopped[1]	15	93%	96%	94%
Recommended VTP Ordered[1]	12	92%	97%	94%
Urinary Catheter Removal[1]	8	100%	89%	90%
Children's Asthma Care				
Received Systemic Corticosteroids	-	-	-	100%
Received Home Management Plan	-	-	-	71%
Received Reliever Medication	-	-	-	100%
Use of Medical Imaging				
Combination Abdominal CT Scan	-	-	0.109	0.191
Combination Chest CT Scan	-	-	0.010	0.054
Follow-up Mammogram/Ultrasound	-	-	9.2%	8.4%
MRI for Low Back Pain	-	-	30.1%	32.7%
Survey of Patients' Hospital Experiences				
Area Around Room 'Always' Quiet at Night[8]	-	-	-	58%
Doctors 'Always' Communicated Well[8]	-	-	-	80%
Home Recovery Information Given[8]	-	-	-	82%
Hospital Given 9 or 10 on 10 Point Scale[8]	-	-	-	67%
Meds 'Always' Explained Before Given[8]	-	-	-	60%
Nurses 'Always' Communicated Well[8]	-	-	-	76%
Pain 'Always' Well Controlled[8]	-	-	-	69%
Room and Bathroom 'Always' Clean[8]	-	-	-	71%
Timely Help 'Always' Received[8]	-	-	-	64%
Would Definitely Recommend Hospital[8]	-	-	-	69%

Sturdy Memorial Hospital

211 Park Street
Attleboro, MA 02703
Type: Acute Care Hospitals
Ownership: Voluntary Non-Profit - Other

Phone: 508-222-5200
Fax: 508-236-7909
Emergency Services: Yes
Beds: 138

Key Personnel:
CEO/President . . . . Linda J Shyavitz
Chief of Medical Staff . . . . Daniel Pietro
Pediatric Ambulatory Care . . . . . Heather Collupy
Pediatric In-Patient Care . . . . . . Heather Collupy
Quality Assurance . . . . Sharon Simmoneau
Radiology . . . . Jay Daly, MD
Emergency Room . . . . Bruce Auerbach

Measure	Cases	This Hosp.	State Avg.	U.S. Avg.
Heart Attack Care				
ACE Inhibitor or ARB for LVSD[1]	6	100%	94%	96%
Aspirin at Arrival	30	97%	99%	99%
Aspirin at Discharge[1]	20	100%	99%	98%
Beta Blocker at Discharge[1]	20	100%	99%	98%
Fibrinolytic Medication Timing	0	-	50%	55%
PCI Within 90 Minutes of Arrival	0	-	93%	90%
Smoking Cessation Advice[1]	3	100%	99%	99%
Chest Pain/Possible Heart Attack Care				
Aspirin at Arrival	141	96%	96%	95%
Median Time to ECG (minutes)	144	10	10	8
Median Time to Transfer (minutes)[1]	23	45	65	61
Fibrinolytic Medication Timing	0	-	78%	54%
Heart Failure Care				
ACE Inhibitor or ARB for LVSD	54	100%	94%	94%
Discharge Instructions	140	98%	89%	88%
Evaluation of LVS Function	202	95%	98%	98%
Smoking Cessation Advice	30	100%	97%	98%
Pneumonia Care				
Appropriate Initial Antibiotic	196	93%	93%	92%
Blood Culture Timing	280	99%	95%	96%
Influenza Vaccine	200	90%	92%	91%
Initial Antibiotic Timing	321	96%	96%	95%
Pneumococcal Vaccine	261	93%	93%	93%
Smoking Cessation Advice	100	98%	96%	97%
Surgical Care Improvement Project				
Appropriate VTP Within 24 Hours	337	94%	96%	92%
Appropriate Hair Removal	609	99%	100%	99%
Appropriate Beta Blocker Usage	183	96%	96%	93%
Controlled Postoperative Blood Glucose	0	-	95%	93%
Prophylactic Antibiotic Timing	374	93%	97%	97%
Prophylactic Antibiotic Timing (Outpatient)	160	92%	92%	92%
Prophylactic Antibiotic Selection	376	97%	98%	97%
Prophylactic Antibiotic Select. (Outpatient)	154	92%	95%	94%
Prophylactic Antibiotic Stopped	368	94%	96%	94%
Recommended VTP Ordered	337	96%	97%	94%
Urinary Catheter Removal	174	81%	89%	90%
Children's Asthma Care				
Received Systemic Corticosteroids	-	-	-	100%
Received Home Management Plan	-	-	-	71%
Received Reliever Medication	-	-	-	100%
Use of Medical Imaging				
Combination Abdominal CT Scan	838	0.078	0.109	0.191
Combination Chest CT Scan	466	0.105	0.010	0.054
Follow-up Mammogram/Ultrasound	1,840	8.3%	9.2%	8.4%
MRI for Low Back Pain	263	26.6%	30.1%	32.7%
Survey of Patients' Hospital Experiences				
Area Around Room 'Always' Quiet at Night	300+	47%	-	58%
Doctors 'Always' Communicated Well	300+	78%	-	80%
Home Recovery Information Given	300+	86%	-	82%
Hospital Given 9 or 10 on 10 Point Scale	300+	67%	-	67%
Meds 'Always' Explained Before Given	300+	60%	-	60%
Nurses 'Always' Communicated Well	300+	76%	-	76%
Pain 'Always' Well Controlled	300+	70%	-	69%
Room and Bathroom 'Always' Clean	300+	78%	-	71%
Timely Help 'Always' Received	300+	61%	-	64%
Would Definitely Recommend Hospital	300+	72%	-	69%

Nashoba Valley Medical Center

200 Groton Road
Ayer, MA 01432
URL: www.nashobamed.com
Type: Acute Care Hospitals
Ownership: Voluntary Non-Profit - Private

Phone: 978-784-9000
Fax: 978-784-9690

Emergency Services: Yes
Beds: 49

Key Personnel:
CEO/President . . . . Steve Roach
Chief of Medical Staff . . . . Michelle Gordon
Radiology . . . . Jerome M Auerbach

Measure	Cases	This Hosp.	State Avg.	U.S. Avg.
Heart Attack Care				
ACE Inhibitor or ARB for LVSD[1]	4	100%	94%	96%
Aspirin at Arrival[1]	18	100%	99%	99%
Aspirin at Discharge[1]	12	100%	99%	98%
Beta Blocker at Discharge[1]	14	100%	99%	98%
Fibrinolytic Medication Timing	0	-	50%	55%
PCI Within 90 Minutes of Arrival	0	-	93%	90%
Smoking Cessation Advice[1]	1	100%	99%	99%
Chest Pain/Possible Heart Attack Care				
Aspirin at Arrival	96	98%	96%	95%
Median Time to ECG (minutes)	100	11	10	8
Median Time to Transfer (minutes)[1,3]	9	45	65	61
Fibrinolytic Medication Timing	0	-	78%	54%
Heart Failure Care				
ACE Inhibitor or ARB for LVSD[1]	22	100%	94%	94%
Discharge Instructions	64	88%	89%	88%
Evaluation of LVS Function	95	96%	98%	98%
Smoking Cessation Advice[1]	7	71%	97%	98%
Pneumonia Care				
Appropriate Initial Antibiotic	76	95%	93%	92%
Blood Culture Timing	107	93%	95%	96%
Influenza Vaccine	73	99%	92%	91%
Initial Antibiotic Timing	92	97%	96%	95%
Pneumococcal Vaccine	102	98%	93%	93%
Smoking Cessation Advice[1]	24	92%	96%	97%
Surgical Care Improvement Project				
Appropriate VTP Within 24 Hours	71	92%	96%	92%
Appropriate Hair Removal	101	100%	100%	99%
Appropriate Beta Blocker Usage	40	100%	96%	93%
Controlled Postoperative Blood Glucose	0	-	95%	93%
Prophylactic Antibiotic Timing	65	97%	97%	97%
Prophylactic Antibiotic Timing (Outpatient)	47	89%	92%	92%
Prophylactic Antibiotic Selection	65	100%	98%	97%
Prophylactic Antibiotic Select. (Outpatient)	46	96%	95%	94%
Prophylactic Antibiotic Stopped	63	92%	96%	94%
Recommended VTP Ordered	71	97%	97%	94%
Urinary Catheter Removal	29	76%	89%	90%
Children's Asthma Care				
Received Systemic Corticosteroids	-	-	-	100%
Received Home Management Plan	-	-	-	71%
Received Reliever Medication	-	-	-	100%
Use of Medical Imaging				
Combination Abdominal CT Scan	338	0.160	0.109	0.191
Combination Chest CT Scan	186	0.011	0.010	0.054
Follow-up Mammogram/Ultrasound	351	18.5%	9.2%	8.4%
MRI for Low Back Pain	58	29.3%	30.1%	32.7%
Survey of Patients' Hospital Experiences				
Area Around Room 'Always' Quiet at Night	300+	62%	-	58%
Doctors 'Always' Communicated Well	300+	79%	-	80%
Home Recovery Information Given	300+	87%	-	82%
Hospital Given 9 or 10 on 10 Point Scale	300+	67%	-	67%
Meds 'Always' Explained Before Given	300+	59%	-	60%
Nurses 'Always' Communicated Well	300+	78%	-	76%
Pain 'Always' Well Controlled	300+	76%	-	69%
Room and Bathroom 'Always' Clean	300+	77%	-	71%
Timely Help 'Always' Received	300+	59%	-	64%
Would Definitely Recommend Hospital	300+	72%	-	69%

NOTE: Hospital profiles are in alphabetical order by state, then city, then hospital within the city; Rankings exclude hospitals with less than 25 cases except for patient surveys which excludes hospitals with less than 100 cases; (a) 100–299 cases; (1) The number of cases is too small to be sure how well a hospital is performing; (2) The hospital indicated that the data submitted for this measure were based on a sample of cases; (3) Data was collected during a shorter time period (fewer quarters) than the maximum possible time for this measure; (4) Suppressed for one or more quarters by CMS; (5) No data is available from the hospital for this measure; (6) Fewer than 100 patients completed the HCAHPS survey. Use these rates with caution, as the number of surveys may be too low to reliably assess hospital performance; (7) Survey results are based on less than 12 months of data; (8) Survey results are not available for this reporting period; (9) No or very few patients were eligible for the HCAHPS survey. The scores shown, if any, reflect a very small number of surveys; (10) A state average was not calculated because too few hospitals in the state submitted data; (11) There were discrepancies in the data collection process; Please refer to the User's Guide for a full explanation of data.

Bedford VA Medical Center

200 Springs Road Phone: 781-275-7500
Bedford, MA 01730 Fax: 781-687-2101
URL: www.visn1.med.va.gov/bedford
Type: Acute Care-Veterans Administration Emergency Services: No
Ownership: Government - Federal Beds: 502

Key Personnel:
CEO/President. . . . . Tammy A Follensbee
Chief of Medical Staff. . . . . Gregory Binus, MD
Infection Control. . . . . Gloria Jarnis
Quality Assurance . . . . Michael Carey
Radiology. . . . . Pat Sacco
Ambulatory Care . . . . James Schlosser, MD
Patient Relations . . . . Karen Kubik

Measure	Cases	This Hosp.	State Avg.	U.S. Avg.
Heart Attack Care				
ACE Inhibitor or ARB for LVSD[5]	0	-	94%	96%
Aspirin at Arrival[5]	0	-	99%	99%
Aspirin at Discharge[5]	0	-	99%	98%
Beta Blocker at Discharge[5]	0	-	99%	98%
Fibrinolytic Medication Timing[5]	0	-	50%	55%
PCI Within 90 Minutes of Arrival[5]	0	-	93%	90%
Smoking Cessation Advice[5]	0	-	99%	99%
Chest Pain/Possible Heart Attack Care				
Aspirin at Arrival	-	-	96%	95%
Median Time to ECG (minutes)	-	-	10	8
Median Time to Transfer (minutes)	-	-	65	61
Fibrinolytic Medication Timing	-	-	78%	54%
Heart Failure Care				
ACE Inhibitor or ARB for LVSD[5]	0	-	94%	94%
Discharge Instructions[5]	0	-	89%	88%
Evaluation of LVS Function[5]	0	-	98%	98%
Smoking Cessation Advice[5]	0	-	97%	98%
Pneumonia Care				
Appropriate Initial Antibiotic[5]	0	-	93%	92%
Blood Culture Timing[5]	0	-	95%	96%
Influenza Vaccine[5]	0	-	92%	91%
Initial Antibiotic Timing[5]	0	-	96%	95%
Pneumococcal Vaccine[5]	0	-	93%	93%
Smoking Cessation Advice[5]	0	-	96%	97%
Surgical Care Improvement Project				
Appropriate VTP Within 24 Hours[2,5]	0	-	96%	92%
Appropriate Hair Removal[2,5]	0	-	100%	99%
Appropriate Beta Blocker Usage[2,5]	0	-	96%	93%
Controlled Postoperative Blood Glucose[2,5]	0	-	95%	93%
Prophylactic Antibiotic Timing[5]	0	-	97%	97%
Prophylactic Antibiotic Timing (Outpatient)	-	-	92%	92%
Prophylactic Antibiotic Selection[5]	0	-	98%	97%
Prophylactic Antibiotic Select. (Outpatient)	-	-	95%	94%
Prophylactic Antibiotic Stopped[5]	0	-	96%	94%
Recommended VTP Ordered[2,5]	0	-	97%	94%
Urinary Catheter Removal[2,5]	0	-	89%	90%
Children's Asthma Care				
Received Systemic Corticosteroids	-	-	-	100%
Received Home Management Plan	-	-	-	71%
Received Reliever Medication	-	-	-	100%
Use of Medical Imaging				
Combination Abdominal CT Scan	-	-	0.109	0.191
Combination Chest CT Scan	-	-	0.010	0.054
Follow-up Mammogram/Ultrasound	-	-	9.2%	8.4%
MRI for Low Back Pain	-	-	30.1%	32.7%
Survey of Patients' Hospital Experiences				
Area Around Room 'Always' Quiet at Night	-	-	-	58%
Doctors 'Always' Communicated Well	-	-	-	80%
Home Recovery Information Given	-	-	-	82%
Hospital Given 9 or 10 on 10 Point Scale	-	-	-	67%
Meds 'Always' Explained Before Given	-	-	-	60%
Nurses 'Always' Communicated Well	-	-	-	76%
Pain 'Always' Well Controlled	-	-	-	69%
Room and Bathroom 'Always' Clean	-	-	-	71%
Timely Help 'Always' Received	-	-	-	64%
Would Definitely Recommend Hospital	-	-	-	69%

Beverly Hospital Corporation

85 Herrick Street Phone: 978-922-3000
Beverly, MA 01915 Fax: 978-921-7025
URL: www.beverlyhospital.org
Type: Acute Care Hospitals Emergency Services: Yes
Ownership: Voluntary Non-Profit - Private Beds: 227

Key Personnel:
CEO/President. . . . . Stephen R Laverty
Chief of Medical Staff. . . . . Augustine O'Keeffe, MD
Radiology. . . . . Stephen A Barrand

Measure	Cases	This Hosp.	State Avg.	U.S. Avg.
Heart Attack Care				
ACE Inhibitor or ARB for LVSD	27	93%	94%	96%
Aspirin at Arrival	188	100%	99%	99%
Aspirin at Discharge	123	100%	99%	98%
Beta Blocker at Discharge	127	100%	99%	98%
Fibrinolytic Medication Timing	0	-	50%	55%
PCI Within 90 Minutes of Arrival	0	-	93%	90%
Smoking Cessation Advice[1]	14	100%	99%	99%
Chest Pain/Possible Heart Attack Care				
Aspirin at Arrival	144	99%	96%	95%
Median Time to ECG (minutes)	149	10	10	8
Median Time to Transfer (minutes)	44	56	65	61
Fibrinolytic Medication Timing	0	-	78%	54%
Heart Failure Care				
ACE Inhibitor or ARB for LVSD	94	97%	94%	94%
Discharge Instructions	251	89%	89%	88%
Evaluation of LVS Function	396	100%	98%	98%
Smoking Cessation Advice	34	100%	97%	98%
Pneumonia Care				
Appropriate Initial Antibiotic	229	97%	93%	92%
Blood Culture Timing	373	97%	95%	96%
Influenza Vaccine	211	89%	92%	91%
Initial Antibiotic Timing	362	99%	96%	95%
Pneumococcal Vaccine	322	92%	93%	93%
Smoking Cessation Advice	88	100%	96%	97%
Surgical Care Improvement Project				
Appropriate VTP Within 24 Hours[2]	448	98%	96%	92%
Appropriate Hair Removal[2]	1,136	100%	100%	99%
Appropriate Beta Blocker Usage[2]	339	97%	96%	93%
Controlled Postoperative Blood Glucose[2]	0	-	95%	93%
Prophylactic Antibiotic Timing[2]	838	99%	97%	97%
Prophylactic Antibiotic Timing (Outpatient)	280	97%	92%	92%
Prophylactic Antibiotic Selection[2]	841	99%	98%	97%
Prophylactic Antibiotic Select. (Outpatient)	278	96%	95%	94%
Prophylactic Antibiotic Stopped[2]	803	99%	96%	94%
Recommended VTP Ordered[2]	448	98%	97%	94%
Urinary Catheter Removal	344	95%	89%	90%
Children's Asthma Care				
Received Systemic Corticosteroids	-	-	-	100%
Received Home Management Plan	-	-	-	71%
Received Reliever Medication	-	-	-	100%
Use of Medical Imaging				
Combination Abdominal CT Scan	1,246	0.060	0.109	0.191
Combination Chest CT Scan	998	0.001	0.010	0.054
Follow-up Mammogram/Ultrasound	3,148	8.1%	9.2%	8.4%
MRI for Low Back Pain	221	22.6%	30.1%	32.7%
Survey of Patients' Hospital Experiences				
Area Around Room 'Always' Quiet at Night	300+	48%	-	58%
Doctors 'Always' Communicated Well	300+	78%	-	80%
Home Recovery Information Given	300+	85%	-	82%
Hospital Given 9 or 10 on 10 Point Scale	300+	68%	-	67%
Meds 'Always' Explained Before Given	300+	60%	-	60%
Nurses 'Always' Communicated Well	300+	78%	-	76%
Pain 'Always' Well Controlled	300+	74%	-	69%
Room and Bathroom 'Always' Clean	300+	70%	-	71%
Timely Help 'Always' Received	300+	63%	-	64%
Would Definitely Recommend Hospital	300+	74%	-	69%

Beth Israel Deaconess Medical Center

330 Brookline Avenue Phone: 617-667-7000
Boston, MA 02215 Fax: 617-667-8155
URL: www.bidmc.harvard.edu
Type: Acute Care Hospitals Emergency Services: Yes
Ownership: Voluntary Non-Profit - Private Beds: 591

Key Personnel:
CEO/President. . . . . Paul F Levy
Chief of Medical Staff. . . . . Robert Moellering, MD
Infection Control. . . . . AW Karchmer, MD
Quality Assurance . . . . Beverly Waite, RN
Radiology. . . . . Melvin Clouse, MD
Emergency Room . . . . Richard Wolfe
Hemotology Center . . . . Jerome Groopman, MD
Intensive Care Unit. . . . . Ronald Silvestri, MD

Measure	Cases	This Hosp.	State Avg.	U.S. Avg.
Heart Attack Care				
ACE Inhibitor or ARB for LVSD	88	92%	94%	96%
Aspirin at Arrival	170	100%	99%	99%
Aspirin at Discharge	529	100%	99%	98%
Beta Blocker at Discharge	503	100%	99%	98%
Fibrinolytic Medication Timing	0	-	50%	55%
PCI Within 90 Minutes of Arrival	27	100%	93%	90%
Smoking Cessation Advice	107	100%	99%	99%
Chest Pain/Possible Heart Attack Care				
Aspirin at Arrival[5]	0	-	96%	95%
Median Time to ECG (minutes)[5]	0	-	10	8
Median Time to Transfer (minutes)[5]	0	-	65	61
Fibrinolytic Medication Timing[5]	0	-	78%	54%
Heart Failure Care				
ACE Inhibitor or ARB for LVSD[2]	138	91%	94%	94%
Discharge Instructions[2]	433	95%	89%	88%
Evaluation of LVS Function[2]	431	100%	98%	98%
Smoking Cessation Advice[2]	61	100%	97%	98%
Pneumonia Care				
Appropriate Initial Antibiotic[2]	113	93%	93%	92%
Blood Culture Timing[2]	248	96%	95%	96%
Influenza Vaccine[2]	75	91%	92%	91%
Initial Antibiotic Timing[2]	210	97%	96%	95%
Pneumococcal Vaccine[2]	245	84%	93%	93%
Smoking Cessation Advice[2]	75	100%	96%	97%
Surgical Care Improvement Project				
Appropriate VTP Within 24 Hours[2]	417	99%	96%	92%
Appropriate Hair Removal[2]	1,243	99%	100%	99%
Appropriate Beta Blocker Usage[2]	482	100%	96%	93%
Controlled Postoperative Blood Glucose[2]	242	95%	95%	93%
Prophylactic Antibiotic Timing[2]	632	99%	97%	97%
Prophylactic Antibiotic Timing (Outpatient)	480	85%	92%	92%
Prophylactic Antibiotic Selection[2]	707	98%	98%	97%
Prophylactic Antibiotic Select. (Outpatient)	448	89%	95%	94%
Prophylactic Antibiotic Stopped[2]	614	98%	96%	94%
Recommended VTP Ordered[2]	417	99%	97%	94%
Urinary Catheter Removal[2]	264	91%	89%	90%
Children's Asthma Care				
Received Systemic Corticosteroids	-	-	-	100%
Received Home Management Plan	-	-	-	71%
Received Reliever Medication	-	-	-	100%
Use of Medical Imaging				
Combination Abdominal CT Scan	2,159	0.247	0.109	0.191
Combination Chest CT Scan	2,491	0.002	0.010	0.054
Follow-up Mammogram/Ultrasound	1,884	5.8%	9.2%	8.4%
MRI for Low Back Pain	282	25.9%	30.1%	32.7%
Survey of Patients' Hospital Experiences				
Area Around Room 'Always' Quiet at Night	300+	50%	-	58%
Doctors 'Always' Communicated Well	300+	78%	-	80%
Home Recovery Information Given	300+	87%	-	82%
Hospital Given 9 or 10 on 10 Point Scale	300+	73%	-	67%
Meds 'Always' Explained Before Given	300+	63%	-	60%
Nurses 'Always' Communicated Well	300+	77%	-	76%
Pain 'Always' Well Controlled	300+	68%	-	69%
Room and Bathroom 'Always' Clean	300+	70%	-	71%
Timely Help 'Always' Received	300+	58%	-	64%
Would Definitely Recommend Hospital	300+	80%	-	69%

NOTE: Hospital profiles are in alphabetical order by state, then city, then hospital within the city; Rankings exclude hospitals with less than 25 cases except for patient surveys which excludes hospitals with less than 100 cases; (a) 100–299 cases; (1) The number of cases is too small to be sure how well a hospital is performing; (2) The hospital indicated that the data submitted for this measure were based on a sample of cases; (3) Data was collected during a shorter time period (fewer quarters) than the maximum possible time for this measure; (4) Suppressed for one or more quarters by CMS; (5) No data is available from the hospital for this measure; (6) Fewer than 100 patients completed the HCAHPS survey. Use these rates with caution, as the number of surveys may be too low to reliably assess hospital performance; (7) Survey results are based on less than 12 months of data; (8) Survey results are not available for this reporting period; (9) No or very few patients were eligible for the HCAHPS survey. The scores shown, if any, reflect a very small number of surveys; (10) A state average was not calculated because too few hospitals in the state submitted data; (11) There were discrepancies in the data collection process; Please refer to the User's Guide for a full explanation of data.

Boston Medical Center Corporation

1 Boston Medical Center Place
Boston, MA 02118
URL: www.bmc.org
Type: Acute Care Hospitals
Ownership: Voluntary Non-Profit - Private

Phone: 617-638-8000
Fax: 617-638-8538

Emergency Services: Yes
Beds: 581

Key Personnel:
CEO/President . . . . Elaine Ullian
Cardiac Laboratory . . . . Alice Jacobs, MD
Coronary Care . . . . Peter Burke, MD
Operating Room . . . . Keith Lewis, MD
Pediatric Ambulatory Care . . . . Doug Hoffman, MD
Pediatric In-Patient Care . . . . Chi-Cheng Huang, MD
Quality Assurance . . . . Denise Mehegan
Radiology . . . . Alexander Norbash, MD

Measure	Cases	This Hosp.	State Avg.	U.S. Avg.
Heart Attack Care				
ACE Inhibitor or ARB for LVSD	67	93%	94%	96%
Aspirin at Arrival	159	100%	99%	99%
Aspirin at Discharge	456	100%	99%	98%
Beta Blocker at Discharge	430	100%	99%	98%
Fibrinolytic Medication Timing	0	-	50%	55%
PCI Within 90 Minutes of Arrival	28	96%	93%	90%
Smoking Cessation Advice	161	100%	99%	99%
Chest Pain/Possible Heart Attack Care				
Aspirin at Arrival[1,3]	6	100%	96%	95%
Median Time to ECG (minutes)[1,3]	6	18	10	8
Median Time to Transfer (minutes)[5]	0	-	65	61
Fibrinolytic Medication Timing[5]	0	-	78%	54%
Heart Failure Care				
ACE Inhibitor or ARB for LVSD	325	95%	94%	94%
Discharge Instructions	697	99%	89%	88%
Evaluation of LVS Function	831	100%	98%	98%
Smoking Cessation Advice	216	100%	97%	98%
Pneumonia Care				
Appropriate Initial Antibiotic	144	93%	93%	92%
Blood Culture Timing	136	96%	95%	96%
Influenza Vaccine	230	80%	92%	91%
Initial Antibiotic Timing	230	96%	96%	95%
Pneumococcal Vaccine	231	85%	93%	93%
Smoking Cessation Advice	260	97%	96%	97%
Surgical Care Improvement Project				
Appropriate VTP Within 24 Hours[2]	551	100%	96%	92%
Appropriate Hair Removal[2]	1,127	100%	100%	99%
Appropriate Beta Blocker Usage[2]	462	92%	96%	93%
Controlled Postoperative Blood Glucose[2]	247	96%	95%	93%
Prophylactic Antibiotic Timing[2]	884	98%	97%	97%
Prophylactic Antibiotic Timing (Outpatient)	298	89%	92%	92%
Prophylactic Antibiotic Selection[2]	895	99%	98%	97%
Prophylactic Antibiotic Select. (Outpatient)	297	93%	95%	94%
Prophylactic Antibiotic Stopped[2]	865	87%	96%	94%
Recommended VTP Ordered[2]	551	100%	97%	94%
Urinary Catheter Removal[2]	266	98%	89%	90%
Children's Asthma Care				
Received Systemic Corticosteroids	-	-	-	100%
Received Home Management Plan	-	-	-	71%
Received Reliever Medication	-	-	-	100%
Use of Medical Imaging				
Combination Abdominal CT Scan	1,366	0.065	0.109	0.191
Combination Chest CT Scan	1,070	0.023	0.010	0.054
Follow-up Mammogram/Ultrasound	2,567	6.0%	9.2%	8.4%
MRI for Low Back Pain	248	28.2%	30.1%	32.7%
Survey of Patients' Hospital Experiences				
Area Around Room 'Always' Quiet at Night	300+	49%	-	58%
Doctors 'Always' Communicated Well	300+	80%	-	80%
Home Recovery Information Given	300+	87%	-	82%
Hospital Given 9 or 10 on 10 Point Scale	300+	67%	-	67%
Meds 'Always' Explained Before Given	300+	61%	-	60%
Nurses 'Always' Communicated Well	300+	74%	-	76%
Pain 'Always' Well Controlled	300+	66%	-	69%
Room and Bathroom 'Always' Clean	300+	68%	-	71%
Timely Help 'Always' Received	300+	57%	-	64%
Would Definitely Recommend Hospital	300+	72%	-	69%

Brigham and Women's Hosptial

75 Francis Street
Boston, MA 02115
URL: www.brighamandwomens.org
Type: Acute Care Hospitals
Ownership: Voluntary Non-Profit - Private

Phone: 617-732-5500
Fax: 617-582-6130

Emergency Services: Yes
Beds: 725

Key Personnel:
CEO/President . . . . Gary Gottlieb, MD, MBA
Chief of Medical Staff . . . . Anthony Whittemore
Radiology . . . . Piran Aliabadi
Anesthesiology . . . . Charles Vacante, MD
Emergency Room . . . . Ron Walls, MD

Measure	Cases	This Hosp.	State Avg.	U.S. Avg.
Heart Attack Care				
ACE Inhibitor or ARB for LVSD	98	92%	94%	96%
Aspirin at Arrival	270	100%	99%	99%
Aspirin at Discharge	598	100%	99%	98%
Beta Blocker at Discharge	575	98%	99%	98%
Fibrinolytic Medication Timing	0	-	50%	55%
PCI Within 90 Minutes of Arrival	42	86%	93%	90%
Smoking Cessation Advice	139	98%	99%	99%
Chest Pain/Possible Heart Attack Care				
Aspirin at Arrival[5]	0	-	96%	95%
Median Time to ECG (minutes)[5]	0	-	10	8
Median Time to Transfer (minutes)[5]	0	-	65	61
Fibrinolytic Medication Timing[5]	0	-	78%	54%
Heart Failure Care				
ACE Inhibitor or ARB for LVSD[2]	96	95%	94%	94%
Discharge Instructions[2]	244	99%	89%	88%
Evaluation of LVS Function[2]	281	99%	98%	98%
Smoking Cessation Advice[2]	43	98%	97%	98%
Pneumonia Care				
Appropriate Initial Antibiotic[1,2]	23	100%	93%	92%
Blood Culture Timing[2]	65	98%	95%	96%
Influenza Vaccine[2]	73	92%	92%	91%
Initial Antibiotic Timing[2]	68	99%	96%	95%
Pneumococcal Vaccine[2]	86	98%	93%	93%
Smoking Cessation Advice[2]	25	96%	96%	97%
Surgical Care Improvement Project				
Appropriate VTP Within 24 Hours[2]	252	98%	96%	92%
Appropriate Hair Removal[2]	691	100%	100%	99%
Appropriate Beta Blocker Usage[2]	256	93%	96%	93%
Controlled Postoperative Blood Glucose[2]	147	97%	95%	93%
Prophylactic Antibiotic Timing[2]	427	99%	97%	97%
Prophylactic Antibiotic Timing (Outpatient)	364	91%	92%	92%
Prophylactic Antibiotic Selection[2]	435	98%	98%	97%
Prophylactic Antibiotic Select. (Outpatient)	352	93%	95%	94%
Prophylactic Antibiotic Stopped[2]	415	94%	96%	94%
Recommended VTP Ordered[2]	254	98%	97%	94%
Urinary Catheter Removal[2]	167	87%	89%	90%
Children's Asthma Care				
Received Systemic Corticosteroids	-	-	-	100%
Received Home Management Plan	-	-	-	71%
Received Reliever Medication	-	-	-	100%
Use of Medical Imaging				
Combination Abdominal CT Scan	2,296	0.083	0.109	0.191
Combination Chest CT Scan	3,685	0.001	0.010	0.054
Follow-up Mammogram/Ultrasound	3,398	9.5%	9.2%	8.4%
MRI for Low Back Pain	394	30.2%	30.1%	32.7%
Survey of Patients' Hospital Experiences				
Area Around Room 'Always' Quiet at Night	300+	53%	-	58%
Doctors 'Always' Communicated Well	300+	79%	-	80%
Home Recovery Information Given	300+	88%	-	82%
Hospital Given 9 or 10 on 10 Point Scale	300+	79%	-	67%
Meds 'Always' Explained Before Given	300+	61%	-	60%
Nurses 'Always' Communicated Well	300+	79%	-	76%
Pain 'Always' Well Controlled	300+	71%	-	69%
Room and Bathroom 'Always' Clean	300+	70%	-	71%
Timely Help 'Always' Received	300+	65%	-	64%
Would Definitely Recommend Hospital	300+	87%	-	69%

Carney Hospital

2100 Dorchester Avenue
Boston, MA 02124
E-mail: chmail@cchcs.org
URL: www.caritascarney.org
Type: Acute Care Hospitals
Ownership: Proprietary

Phone: 617-506-2000

Emergency Services: Yes
Beds: 228

Key Personnel:
CEO/President . . . . Daniel H O'Leary
Cardiac Laboratory . . . . Francis Hubbard, MD
Chief of Medical Staff . . . . Gregory McSweeney
Infection Control . . . . Philip Carling, MD
Operating Room . . . . Cadet, Nissage, RN
Pediatric Ambulatory Care . . . . . . Claudia Lavin, MD
Quality Assurance . . . . Carol Torosian
Radiology . . . . Alexander L Feinstein, MD

Measure	Cases	This Hosp.	State Avg.	U.S. Avg.
Heart Attack Care				
ACE Inhibitor or ARB for LVSD[1]	5	100%	94%	96%
Aspirin at Arrival[1]	13	100%	99%	99%
Aspirin at Discharge[1]	9	100%	99%	98%
Beta Blocker at Discharge[1]	7	100%	99%	98%
Fibrinolytic Medication Timing	0	-	50%	55%
PCI Within 90 Minutes of Arrival	0	-	93%	90%
Smoking Cessation Advice	0	-	99%	99%
Chest Pain/Possible Heart Attack Care				
Aspirin at Arrival[1]	22	91%	96%	95%
Median Time to ECG (minutes)[1]	24	13	10	8
Median Time to Transfer (minutes)[1,3]	7	65	65	61
Fibrinolytic Medication Timing[3]	0	-	78%	54%
Heart Failure Care				
ACE Inhibitor or ARB for LVSD	73	99%	94%	94%
Discharge Instructions	144	88%	89%	88%
Evaluation of LVS Function	195	99%	98%	98%
Smoking Cessation Advice	32	100%	97%	98%
Pneumonia Care				
Appropriate Initial Antibiotic	62	89%	93%	92%
Blood Culture Timing	69	93%	95%	96%
Influenza Vaccine	61	92%	92%	91%
Initial Antibiotic Timing	86	97%	96%	95%
Pneumococcal Vaccine	88	97%	93%	93%
Smoking Cessation Advice	42	100%	96%	97%
Surgical Care Improvement Project				
Appropriate VTP Within 24 Hours[2]	142	98%	96%	92%
Appropriate Hair Removal[2]	208	100%	100%	99%
Appropriate Beta Blocker Usage[2]	62	98%	96%	93%
Controlled Postoperative Blood Glucose[2]	0	-	95%	93%
Prophylactic Antibiotic Timing[2]	127	98%	97%	97%
Prophylactic Antibiotic Timing (Outpatient)	34	65%	92%	92%
Prophylactic Antibiotic Selection[2]	126	94%	98%	97%
Prophylactic Antibiotic Select. (Outpatient)	26	88%	95%	94%
Prophylactic Antibiotic Stopped[2]	116	90%	96%	94%
Recommended VTP Ordered[2]	142	98%	97%	94%
Urinary Catheter Removal[2]	30	83%	89%	90%
Children's Asthma Care				
Received Systemic Corticosteroids	-	-	-	100%
Received Home Management Plan	-	-	-	71%
Received Reliever Medication	-	-	-	100%
Use of Medical Imaging				
Combination Abdominal CT Scan	482	0.139	0.109	0.191
Combination Chest CT Scan	346	0.012	0.010	0.054
Follow-up Mammogram/Ultrasound	895	26.8%	9.2%	8.4%
MRI for Low Back Pain	101	44.6%	30.1%	32.7%
Survey of Patients' Hospital Experiences				
Area Around Room 'Always' Quiet at Night	300+	59%	-	58%
Doctors 'Always' Communicated Well	300+	83%	-	80%
Home Recovery Information Given	300+	87%	-	82%
Hospital Given 9 or 10 on 10 Point Scale	300+	65%	-	67%
Meds 'Always' Explained Before Given	300+	66%	-	60%
Nurses 'Always' Communicated Well	300+	80%	-	76%
Pain 'Always' Well Controlled	300+	71%	-	69%
Room and Bathroom 'Always' Clean	300+	76%	-	71%
Timely Help 'Always' Received	300+	68%	-	64%
Would Definitely Recommend Hospital	300+	65%	-	69%

NOTE: Hospital profiles are in alphabetical order by state, then city, then hospital within the city; Rankings exclude hospitals with less than 25 cases except for patient surveys which excludes hospitals with less than 100 cases; (a) 100–299 cases; (1) The number of cases is too small to be sure how well a hospital is performing; (2) The hospital indicated that the data submitted for this measure were based on a sample of cases; (3) Data was collected during a shorter time period (fewer quarters) than the maximum possible time for this measure; (4) Suppressed for one or more quarters by CMS; (5) No data is available from the hospital for this measure; (6) Fewer than 100 patients completed the HCAHPS survey. Use these rates with caution, as the number of surveys may be too low to reliably assess hospital performance; (7) Survey results are based on less than 12 months of data; (8) Survey results are not available for this reporting period; (9) No or very few patients were eligible for the HCAHPS survey. The scores shown, if any, reflect a very small number of surveys; (10) A state average was not calculated because too few hospitals in the state submitted data; (11) There were discrepancies in the data collection process; Please refer to the User's Guide for a full explanation of data.

Children's Hospital Boston

300 Longwood Avenue
Boston, MA 02115
Phone: 617-735-6000
URL: www.childrenshospital.org
Type: Childrens
Emergency Services: Yes
Ownership: Voluntary Non-Profit - Private
Beds: 396

Key Personnel:
CEO . . . . Dr James Mandell
President . . . . Sandra Fenwick
Cardiology . . . . James Lock, PhD
Radiology . . . . Richard L Robertson

Measure	Cases	This Hosp.	State Avg.	U.S. Avg.
Heart Attack Care				
ACE Inhibitor or ARB for LVSD	-	-	94%	96%
Aspirin at Arrival	-	-	99%	99%
Aspirin at Discharge	-	-	99%	98%
Beta Blocker at Discharge	-	-	99%	98%
Fibrinolytic Medication Timing	-	-	50%	55%
PCI Within 90 Minutes of Arrival	-	-	93%	90%
Smoking Cessation Advice	-	-	99%	99%
Chest Pain/Possible Heart Attack Care				
Aspirin at Arrival	-	-	96%	95%
Median Time to ECG (minutes)	-	-	10	8
Median Time to Transfer (minutes)	-	-	65	61
Fibrinolytic Medication Timing	-	-	78%	54%
Heart Failure Care				
ACE Inhibitor or ARB for LVSD	-	-	94%	94%
Discharge Instructions	-	-	89%	88%
Evaluation of LVS Function	-	-	98%	98%
Smoking Cessation Advice	-	-	97%	98%
Pneumonia Care				
Appropriate Initial Antibiotic	-	-	93%	92%
Blood Culture Timing	-	-	95%	96%
Influenza Vaccine	-	-	92%	91%
Initial Antibiotic Timing	-	-	96%	95%
Pneumococcal Vaccine	-	-	93%	93%
Smoking Cessation Advice	-	-	96%	97%
Surgical Care Improvement Project				
Appropriate VTP Within 24 Hours	-	-	96%	92%
Appropriate Hair Removal	-	-	100%	99%
Appropriate Beta Blocker Usage	-	-	96%	93%
Controlled Postoperative Blood Glucose	-	-	95%	93%
Prophylactic Antibiotic Timing	-	-	97%	97%
Prophylactic Antibiotic Timing (Outpatient)	-	-	92%	92%
Prophylactic Antibiotic Selection	-	-	98%	97%
Prophylactic Antibiotic Select. (Outpatient)	-	-	95%	94%
Prophylactic Antibiotic Stopped	-	-	96%	94%
Recommended VTP Ordered	-	-	97%	94%
Urinary Catheter Removal	-	-	89%	90%
Children's Asthma Care				
Received Systemic Corticosteroids[2]	364	100%	-	100%
Received Home Management Plan[2]	364	67%	-	71%
Received Reliever Medication[2]	364	100%	-	100%
Use of Medical Imaging				
Combination Abdominal CT Scan	-	-	0.109	0.191
Combination Chest CT Scan	-	-	0.010	0.054
Follow-up Mammogram/Ultrasound	-	-	9.2%	8.4%
MRI for Low Back Pain	-	-	30.1%	32.7%
Survey of Patients' Hospital Experiences				
Area Around Room 'Always' Quiet at Night	-	-	-	58%
Doctors 'Always' Communicated Well	-	-	-	80%
Home Recovery Information Given	-	-	-	82%
Hospital Given 9 or 10 on 10 Point Scale	-	-	-	67%
Meds 'Always' Explained Before Given	-	-	-	60%
Nurses 'Always' Communicated Well	-	-	-	76%
Pain 'Always' Well Controlled	-	-	-	69%
Room and Bathroom 'Always' Clean	-	-	-	71%
Timely Help 'Always' Received	-	-	-	64%
Would Definitely Recommend Hospital	-	-	-	69%

Dana-Farber Cancer Institute

44 Binney Street
Boston, MA 02115
Phone: 617-632-3000
Fax: 617-667-9619
E-mail: dana-farbercontactus@dfci.harvard.edu
URL: www.dana-farber.org
Type: Acute Care Hospitals
Emergency Services: No
Ownership: Voluntary Non-Profit - Private
Beds: 57

Key Personnel:
CEO/President . . . . Edward J Benz Jr, MD
Chief of Medical Staff . . . . Lawrence N Shulman, MD
Pediatric Ambulatory Care . . . . . . Stuart H Orkin, MD
Radiology . . . . Jay R Harris, MD
Hemotology Center . . . . James D Griffin, MD
Patient Relations . . . . Patricia Reid Ponte, RN

Measure	Cases	This Hosp.	State Avg.	U.S. Avg.
Heart Attack Care				
ACE Inhibitor or ARB for LVSD[5]	0	-	94%	96%
Aspirin at Arrival[5]	0	-	99%	99%
Aspirin at Discharge[5]	0	-	99%	98%
Beta Blocker at Discharge[5]	0	-	99%	98%
Fibrinolytic Medication Timing[5]	0	-	50%	55%
PCI Within 90 Minutes of Arrival[5]	0	-	93%	90%
Smoking Cessation Advice[5]	0	-	99%	99%
Chest Pain/Possible Heart Attack Care				
Aspirin at Arrival	-	-	96%	95%
Median Time to ECG (minutes)	-	-	10	8
Median Time to Transfer (minutes)	-	-	65	61
Fibrinolytic Medication Timing	-	-	78%	54%
Heart Failure Care				
ACE Inhibitor or ARB for LVSD[5]	0	-	94%	94%
Discharge Instructions[5]	0	-	89%	88%
Evaluation of LVS Function[5]	0	-	98%	98%
Smoking Cessation Advice[5]	0	-	97%	98%
Pneumonia Care				
Appropriate Initial Antibiotic[1]	2	100%	93%	92%
Blood Culture Timing[1]	14	100%	95%	96%
Influenza Vaccine[1]	15	87%	92%	91%
Initial Antibiotic Timing[1]	7	100%	96%	95%
Pneumococcal Vaccine[1]	14	93%	93%	93%
Smoking Cessation Advice[1]	4	100%	96%	97%
Surgical Care Improvement Project				
Appropriate VTP Within 24 Hours[5]	0	-	96%	92%
Appropriate Hair Removal[5]	0	-	100%	99%
Appropriate Beta Blocker Usage[5]	0	-	96%	93%
Controlled Postoperative Blood Glucose[5]	0	-	95%	93%
Prophylactic Antibiotic Timing[5]	0	-	97%	97%
Prophylactic Antibiotic Timing (Outpatient)	-	-	92%	92%
Prophylactic Antibiotic Selection[5]	0	-	98%	97%
Prophylactic Antibiotic Select. (Outpatient)	-	-	95%	94%
Prophylactic Antibiotic Stopped[5]	0	-	96%	94%
Recommended VTP Ordered[5]	0	-	97%	94%
Urinary Catheter Removal[5]	0	-	89%	90%
Children's Asthma Care				
Received Systemic Corticosteroids	-	-	-	100%
Received Home Management Plan	-	-	-	71%
Received Reliever Medication	-	-	-	100%
Use of Medical Imaging				
Combination Abdominal CT Scan	-	-	0.109	0.191
Combination Chest CT Scan	-	-	0.010	0.054
Follow-up Mammogram/Ultrasound	-	-	9.2%	8.4%
MRI for Low Back Pain	-	-	30.1%	32.7%
Survey of Patients' Hospital Experiences				
Area Around Room 'Always' Quiet at Night[8]	-	-	-	58%
Doctors 'Always' Communicated Well[8]	-	-	-	80%
Home Recovery Information Given[8]	-	-	-	82%
Hospital Given 9 or 10 on 10 Point Scale[8]	-	-	-	67%
Meds 'Always' Explained Before Given[8]	-	-	-	60%
Nurses 'Always' Communicated Well[8]	-	-	-	76%
Pain 'Always' Well Controlled[8]	-	-	-	69%
Room and Bathroom 'Always' Clean[8]	-	-	-	71%
Timely Help 'Always' Received[8]	-	-	-	64%
Would Definitely Recommend Hospital[8]	-	-	-	69%

Faulkner Hospital

1153 Centre Street
Boston, MA 02130
Phone: 617-983-7000
Fax: 617-524-8663
Type: Acute Care Hospitals
Emergency Services: No
Ownership: Govt - Hospital Dist/Auth
Beds: 150

Key Personnel:
CEO/President . . . . David J Trull
Chief of Medical Staff . . . . Geoffrey Sherwood
Radiology . . . . James Mastromatteo
Anesthesiology . . . . James Gessner
Emergency Room . . . . Ashley Yeats
Patient Relations . . . . Rosemarie Shortt

Measure	Cases	This Hosp.	State Avg.	U.S. Avg.
Heart Attack Care				
ACE Inhibitor or ARB for LVSD[1]	1	100%	94%	96%
Aspirin at Arrival[1]	22	100%	99%	99%
Aspirin at Discharge[1]	18	100%	99%	98%
Beta Blocker at Discharge[1]	18	100%	99%	98%
Fibrinolytic Medication Timing	0	-	50%	55%
PCI Within 90 Minutes of Arrival	0	-	93%	90%
Smoking Cessation Advice[1]	2	100%	99%	99%
Chest Pain/Possible Heart Attack Care				
Aspirin at Arrival	49	96%	96%	95%
Median Time to ECG (minutes)	51	15	10	8
Median Time to Transfer (minutes)[1]	11	58	65	61
Fibrinolytic Medication Timing	0	-	78%	54%
Heart Failure Care				
ACE Inhibitor or ARB for LVSD[2]	38	100%	94%	94%
Discharge Instructions[2]	151	100%	89%	88%
Evaluation of LVS Function[2]	211	100%	98%	98%
Smoking Cessation Advice[1,2]	12	100%	97%	98%
Pneumonia Care				
Appropriate Initial Antibiotic[2]	86	90%	93%	92%
Blood Culture Timing[2]	143	97%	95%	96%
Influenza Vaccine[2]	91	98%	92%	91%
Initial Antibiotic Timing[2]	148	97%	96%	95%
Pneumococcal Vaccine[2]	142	99%	93%	93%
Smoking Cessation Advice[2]	25	100%	96%	97%
Surgical Care Improvement Project				
Appropriate VTP Within 24 Hours[2]	84	99%	96%	92%
Appropriate Hair Removal[2]	242	98%	100%	99%
Appropriate Beta Blocker Usage[2]	49	100%	96%	93%
Controlled Postoperative Blood Glucose[2]	0	-	95%	93%
Prophylactic Antibiotic Timing[2]	134	99%	97%	97%
Prophylactic Antibiotic Timing (Outpatient)	224	97%	92%	92%
Prophylactic Antibiotic Selection[2]	137	98%	98%	97%
Prophylactic Antibiotic Select. (Outpatient)	224	96%	95%	94%
Prophylactic Antibiotic Stopped[2]	131	98%	96%	94%
Recommended VTP Ordered[2]	84	99%	97%	94%
Urinary Catheter Removal[2]	45	96%	89%	90%
Children's Asthma Care				
Received Systemic Corticosteroids	-	-	-	100%
Received Home Management Plan	-	-	-	71%
Received Reliever Medication	-	-	-	100%
Use of Medical Imaging				
Combination Abdominal CT Scan	812	0.070	0.109	0.191
Combination Chest CT Scan	950	0.002	0.010	0.054
Follow-up Mammogram/Ultrasound	5,107	13.3%	9.2%	8.4%
MRI for Low Back Pain	69	29.0%	30.1%	32.7%
Survey of Patients' Hospital Experiences				
Area Around Room 'Always' Quiet at Night	300+	54%	-	58%
Doctors 'Always' Communicated Well	300+	84%	-	80%
Home Recovery Information Given	300+	89%	-	82%
Hospital Given 9 or 10 on 10 Point Scale	300+	78%	-	67%
Meds 'Always' Explained Before Given	300+	63%	-	60%
Nurses 'Always' Communicated Well	300+	83%	-	76%
Pain 'Always' Well Controlled	300+	76%	-	69%
Room and Bathroom 'Always' Clean	300+	73%	-	71%
Timely Help 'Always' Received	300+	71%	-	64%
Would Definitely Recommend Hospital	300+	79%	-	69%

NOTE: Hospital profiles are in alphabetical order by state, then city, then hospital within the city; Rankings exclude hospitals with less than 25 cases except for patient surveys which excludes hospitals with less than 100 cases; (a) 100–299 cases; (1) The number of cases is too small to be sure how well a hospital is performing; (2) The hospital indicated that the data submitted for this measure were based on a sample of cases; (3) Data was collected during a shorter time period (fewer quarters) than the maximum possible time for this measure; (4) Suppressed for one or more quarters by CMS; (5) No data is available from the hospital for this measure; (6) Fewer than 100 patients completed the HCAHPS survey. Use these rates with caution, as the number of surveys may be too low to reliably assess hospital performance; (7) Survey results are based on less than 12 months of data; (8) Survey results are not available for this reporting period; (9) No or very few patients were eligible for the HCAHPS survey. The scores shown, if any, reflect a very small number of surveys; (10) A state average was not calculated because too few hospitals in the state submitted data; (11) There were discrepancies in the data collection process; Please refer to the User's Guide for a full explanation of data.

Massachusetts Eye and Ear Infirmary

243 Charles Street
Boston, MA 02114
URL: www.meei.harvard.edu
Type: Acute Care Hospitals
Ownership: Voluntary Non-Profit - Private

Phone: 617-523-7900
Fax: 617-573-3444

Emergency Services: Yes
Beds: 42

Key Personnel:
CEO/President . . . . John Fernandez
Chief of Medical Staff . . . . Robert Kiskaddon, MD
Radiology. . . . . Paul Caruso
Anesthesiology. . . . . Salvatore Zasta, MD
Emergency Room . . . . Matthew Gardiner, MD
Patient Relations . . . . Carol Covell, RN

Measure	Cases	This Hosp.	State Avg.	U.S. Avg.
Heart Attack Care				
ACE Inhibitor or ARB for LVSD[5]	0	-	94%	96%
Aspirin at Arrival[5]	0	-	99%	99%
Aspirin at Discharge[5]	0	-	99%	98%
Beta Blocker at Discharge[5]	0	-	99%	98%
Fibrinolytic Medication Timing[5]	0	-	50%	55%
PCI Within 90 Minutes of Arrival[5]	0	-	93%	90%
Smoking Cessation Advice[5]	0	-	99%	99%
Chest Pain/Possible Heart Attack Care				
Aspirin at Arrival[1,3]	3	33%	96%	95%
Median Time to ECG (minutes)[3]	0	-	10	8
Median Time to Transfer (minutes)[5]	0	-	65	61
Fibrinolytic Medication Timing[5]	0	-	78%	54%
Heart Failure Care				
ACE Inhibitor or ARB for LVSD[5]	0	-	94%	94%
Discharge Instructions[5]	0	-	89%	88%
Evaluation of LVS Function[5]	0	-	98%	98%
Smoking Cessation Advice[5]	0	-	97%	98%
Pneumonia Care				
Appropriate Initial Antibiotic[5]	0	-	93%	92%
Blood Culture Timing[5]	0	-	95%	96%
Influenza Vaccine[5]	0	-	92%	91%
Initial Antibiotic Timing[5]	0	-	96%	95%
Pneumococcal Vaccine[5]	0	-	93%	93%
Smoking Cessation Advice[5]	0	-	96%	97%
Surgical Care Improvement Project				
Appropriate VTP Within 24 Hours[1,3]	2	100%	96%	92%
Appropriate Hair Removal[1,3]	7	100%	100%	99%
Appropriate Beta Blocker Usage[3]	0	-	96%	93%
Controlled Postoperative Blood Glucose[3]	0	-	95%	93%
Prophylactic Antibiotic Timing[3]	0	-	97%	97%
Prophylactic Antibiotic Timing (Outpatient)[1]	12	42%	92%	92%
Prophylactic Antibiotic Selection[3]	0	-	98%	97%
Prophylactic Antibiotic Select. (Outpatient)[1]	11	36%	95%	94%
Prophylactic Antibiotic Stopped[3]	0	-	96%	94%
Recommended VTP Ordered[1,3]	2	100%	97%	94%
Urinary Catheter Removal[1,3]	3	100%	89%	90%
Children's Asthma Care				
Received Systemic Corticosteroids	-	-	-	100%
Received Home Management Plan	-	-	-	71%
Received Reliever Medication	-	-	-	100%
Use of Medical Imaging				
Combination Abdominal CT Scan[1]	4	0.000	0.109	0.191
Combination Chest CT Scan	279	0.000	0.010	0.054
Follow-up Mammogram/Ultrasound[5]	0	-	9.2%	8.4%
MRI for Low Back Pain[5]	0	-	30.1%	32.7%
Survey of Patients' Hospital Experiences				
Area Around Room 'Always' Quiet at Night	300+	44%	-	58%
Doctors 'Always' Communicated Well	300+	81%	-	80%
Home Recovery Information Given	300+	85%	-	82%
Hospital Given 9 or 10 on 10 Point Scale	300+	67%	-	67%
Meds 'Always' Explained Before Given	300+	58%	-	60%
Nurses 'Always' Communicated Well	300+	71%	-	76%
Pain 'Always' Well Controlled	300+	72%	-	69%
Room and Bathroom 'Always' Clean	300+	61%	-	71%
Timely Help 'Always' Received	300+	59%	-	64%
Would Definitely Recommend Hospital	300+	78%	-	69%

Massachusetts General Hospital

55 Fruit Street
Boston, MA 02114
URL: www.massgeneral.org
Type: Acute Care Hospitals
Ownership: Voluntary Non-Profit - Private

Phone: 617-726-2000
Fax: 617-724-7632

Emergency Services: Yes
Beds: 868

Key Personnel:
Pediatric In-Patient Care . . . . Joseph Vacanti, MD
Radiology. . . . . James H Thrall, MD
Anesthesiology. . . . . Jeanine Wiener Kronish MD
Hemotology Center . . . . Zareh N. Demirjian

Measure	Cases	This Hosp.	State Avg.	U.S. Avg.
Heart Attack Care				
ACE Inhibitor or ARB for LVSD[2]	79	99%	94%	96%
Aspirin at Arrival[2]	273	100%	99%	99%
Aspirin at Discharge[2]	758	100%	99%	98%
Beta Blocker at Discharge[2]	727	99%	99%	98%
Fibrinolytic Medication Timing[2]	0	-	50%	55%
PCI Within 90 Minutes of Arrival[2]	57	95%	93%	90%
Smoking Cessation Advice[2]	197	100%	99%	99%
Chest Pain/Possible Heart Attack Care				
Aspirin at Arrival[1]	12	100%	96%	95%
Median Time to ECG (minutes)[1]	13	9	10	8
Median Time to Transfer (minutes)[5]	0	-	65	61
Fibrinolytic Medication Timing[5]	0	-	78%	54%
Heart Failure Care				
ACE Inhibitor or ARB for LVSD[2]	72	96%	94%	94%
Discharge Instructions[2]	217	91%	89%	88%
Evaluation of LVS Function[2]	270	99%	98%	98%
Smoking Cessation Advice[2]	41	100%	97%	98%
Pneumonia Care				
Appropriate Initial Antibiotic[2]	63	94%	93%	92%
Blood Culture Timing[2]	82	94%	95%	96%
Influenza Vaccine[2]	61	95%	92%	91%
Initial Antibiotic Timing[2]	101	98%	96%	95%
Pneumococcal Vaccine[2]	161	91%	93%	93%
Smoking Cessation Advice[2]	39	100%	96%	97%
Surgical Care Improvement Project				
Appropriate VTP Within 24 Hours[2]	267	96%	96%	92%
Appropriate Hair Removal[2]	752	96%	100%	99%
Appropriate Beta Blocker Usage[2]	279	94%	96%	93%
Controlled Postoperative Blood Glucose[2]	129	93%	95%	93%
Prophylactic Antibiotic Timing[2]	440	98%	97%	97%
Prophylactic Antibiotic Timing (Outpatient)[2]	479	74%	92%	92%
Prophylactic Antibiotic Selection[2]	446	96%	98%	97%
Prophylactic Antibiotic Select. (Outpatient)[2]	477	90%	95%	94%
Prophylactic Antibiotic Stopped[2]	377	94%	96%	94%
Recommended VTP Ordered[2]	268	100%	97%	94%
Urinary Catheter Removal[2]	179	88%	89%	90%
Children's Asthma Care				
Received Systemic Corticosteroids	-	-	-	100%
Received Home Management Plan	-	-	-	71%
Received Reliever Medication	-	-	-	100%
Use of Medical Imaging				
Combination Abdominal CT Scan	3,641	0.062	0.109	0.191
Combination Chest CT Scan	4,973	0.001	0.010	0.054
Follow-up Mammogram/Ultrasound	6,012	5.6%	9.2%	8.4%
MRI for Low Back Pain	439	27.1%	30.1%	32.7%
Survey of Patients' Hospital Experiences				
Area Around Room 'Always' Quiet at Night	300+	50%	-	58%
Doctors 'Always' Communicated Well	300+	78%	-	80%
Home Recovery Information Given	300+	87%	-	82%
Hospital Given 9 or 10 on 10 Point Scale	300+	78%	-	67%
Meds 'Always' Explained Before Given	300+	63%	-	60%
Nurses 'Always' Communicated Well	300+	78%	-	76%
Pain 'Always' Well Controlled	300+	70%	-	69%
Room and Bathroom 'Always' Clean	300+	71%	-	71%
Timely Help 'Always' Received	300+	62%	-	64%
Would Definitely Recommend Hospital	300+	88%	-	69%

New England Baptist Hospital

125 Parker Hill Avenue
Boston, MA 02120
E-mail: nebhweb@caregroup.harvard.edu
URL: www.nebh.caregroup.org
Type: Acute Care Hospitals
Ownership: Voluntary Non-Profit - Private

Phone: 617-754-5800
Fax: 617-754-5800

Emergency Services: No
Beds: 141

Key Personnel:
CEO/President . . . . Helen R Strieder
Chief of Medical Staff . . . . James F Green
Operating Room . . . . Pauline Robitaille, RN
Pediatric In-Patient Care . . . . Marylou Buyse
Quality Assurance . . . . Marcella Malay
Radiology. . . . . James R Hill, MD
Anesthesiology. . . . . Rueben Azocar
Hemotology Center . . . . Elie Choufani

Measure	Cases	This Hosp.	State Avg.	U.S. Avg.
Heart Attack Care				
ACE Inhibitor or ARB for LVSD[3]	0	-	94%	96%
Aspirin at Arrival[1,3]	3	100%	99%	99%
Aspirin at Discharge[1,3]	1	0%	99%	98%
Beta Blocker at Discharge[3,1]	1	100%	99%	98%
Fibrinolytic Medication Timing[3]	0	-	50%	55%
PCI Within 90 Minutes of Arrival[3]	0	-	93%	90%
Smoking Cessation Advice[3]	0	-	99%	99%
Chest Pain/Possible Heart Attack Care				
Aspirin at Arrival[5]	0	-	96%	95%
Median Time to ECG (minutes)[5]	0	-	10	8
Median Time to Transfer (minutes)[5]	0	-	65	61
Fibrinolytic Medication Timing[5]	0	-	78%	54%
Heart Failure Care				
ACE Inhibitor or ARB for LVSD[1]	8	100%	94%	94%
Discharge Instructions	29	100%	89%	88%
Evaluation of LVS Function	38	100%	98%	98%
Smoking Cessation Advice[1]	3	100%	97%	98%
Pneumonia Care				
Appropriate Initial Antibiotic[1]	17	100%	93%	92%
Blood Culture Timing	0	-	95%	96%
Influenza Vaccine	26	100%	92%	91%
Initial Antibiotic Timing[1]	18	100%	96%	95%
Pneumococcal Vaccine	28	100%	93%	93%
Smoking Cessation Advice[1]	3	100%	96%	97%
Surgical Care Improvement Project				
Appropriate VTP Within 24 Hours[2]	1,849	97%	96%	92%
Appropriate Hair Removal[2]	4,252	100%	100%	99%
Appropriate Beta Blocker Usage[2]	1,125	99%	96%	93%
Controlled Postoperative Blood Glucose[2]	0	-	95%	93%
Prophylactic Antibiotic Timing[2]	3,872	97%	97%	97%
Prophylactic Antibiotic Timing (Outpatient)	549	96%	92%	92%
Prophylactic Antibiotic Selection[2]	3,874	100%	98%	97%
Prophylactic Antibiotic Select. (Outpatient)	547	100%	95%	94%
Prophylactic Antibiotic Stopped[2]	3,864	96%	96%	94%
Recommended VTP Ordered[2]	1,855	97%	97%	94%
Urinary Catheter Removal[2]	1,771	92%	89%	90%
Children's Asthma Care				
Received Systemic Corticosteroids	-	-	-	100%
Received Home Management Plan	-	-	-	71%
Received Reliever Medication	-	-	-	100%
Use of Medical Imaging				
Combination Abdominal CT Scan	329	0.040	0.109	0.191
Combination Chest CT Scan	284	0.021	0.010	0.054
Follow-up Mammogram/Ultrasound[5]	0	-	9.2%	8.4%
MRI for Low Back Pain	484	28.1%	30.1%	32.7%
Survey of Patients' Hospital Experiences				
Area Around Room 'Always' Quiet at Night	300+	50%	-	58%
Doctors 'Always' Communicated Well	300+	82%	-	80%
Home Recovery Information Given	300+	93%	-	82%
Hospital Given 9 or 10 on 10 Point Scale	300+	84%	-	67%
Meds 'Always' Explained Before Given	300+	64%	-	60%
Nurses 'Always' Communicated Well	300+	84%	-	76%
Pain 'Always' Well Controlled	300+	71%	-	69%
Room and Bathroom 'Always' Clean	300+	78%	-	71%
Timely Help 'Always' Received	300+	70%	-	64%
Would Definitely Recommend Hospital	300+	91%	-	69%

Tufts Medical Center

800 Washington Street Phone: 617-636-5000
Boston, MA 02111 Fax: 617-636-4658
URL: www.tuftsmedicalcenter.org
Type: Acute Care Hospitals Emergency Services: Yes
Ownership: Voluntary Non-Profit - Private Beds: 515
Key Personnel:
CEO/President.............. Ellen Zane
Chief of Medical Staff.......... David Fairchild
Infection Control............. David Syndeman MD
Pediatric Ambulatory Care...... John Schreiber
Quality Assurance............ Susan Fletcher
Radiology.................. Kent Yusel MD
Emergency Room............ Brien Barnewolt MD
Intensive Care Unit........... Chris Veary RN

Measure	Cases	This Hosp.	State Avg.	U.S. Avg.
Heart Attack Care				
ACE Inhibitor or ARB for LVSD	90	100%	94%	96%
Aspirin at Arrival	73	100%	99%	99%
Aspirin at Discharge	398	100%	99%	98%
Beta Blocker at Discharge	376	99%	99%	98%
Fibrinolytic Medication Timing	0	-	50%	55%
PCI Within 90 Minutes of Arrival[1]	8	100%	93%	90%
Smoking Cessation Advice	103	99%	99%	99%
Chest Pain/Possible Heart Attack Care				
Aspirin at Arrival[1,3]	2	100%	96%	95%
Median Time to ECG (minutes)[1,3]	2	16	10	8
Median Time to Transfer (minutes)[5]	0	-	65	61
Fibrinolytic Medication Timing[5]	0	-	78%	54%
Heart Failure Care				
ACE Inhibitor or ARB for LVSD	193	99%	94%	94%
Discharge Instructions	348	97%	89%	88%
Evaluation of LVS Function	417	100%	98%	98%
Smoking Cessation Advice	59	100%	97%	98%
Pneumonia Care				
Appropriate Initial Antibiotic	96	95%	93%	92%
Blood Culture Timing	167	97%	95%	96%
Influenza Vaccine	174	94%	92%	91%
Initial Antibiotic Timing	193	95%	96%	95%
Pneumococcal Vaccine	218	93%	93%	93%
Smoking Cessation Advice	102	95%	96%	97%
Surgical Care Improvement Project				
Appropriate VTP Within 24 Hours[2]	245	96%	96%	92%
Appropriate Hair Removal[2]	923	98%	100%	99%
Appropriate Beta Blocker Usage[2]	414	89%	96%	93%
Controlled Postoperative Blood Glucose[2]	336	92%	95%	93%
Prophylactic Antibiotic Timing[2]	714	98%	97%	97%
Prophylactic Antibiotic Timing (Outpatient)	237	92%	92%	92%
Prophylactic Antibiotic Selection[2]	727	99%	98%	97%
Prophylactic Antibiotic Select. (Outpatient)	381	96%	95%	94%
Prophylactic Antibiotic Stopped[2]	690	93%	96%	94%
Recommended VTP Ordered[2]	245	98%	97%	94%
Urinary Catheter Removal[2]	197	94%	89%	90%
Children's Asthma Care				
Received Systemic Corticosteroids	-	-	-	100%
Received Home Management Plan	-	-	-	71%
Received Reliever Medication	-	-	-	100%
Use of Medical Imaging				
Combination Abdominal CT Scan	829	0.242	0.109	0.191
Combination Chest CT Scan	971	0.005	0.010	0.054
Follow-up Mammogram/Ultrasound	1,042	1.1%	9.2%	8.4%
MRI for Low Back Pain	144	23.6%	30.1%	32.7%
Survey of Patients' Hospital Experiences				
Area Around Room 'Always' Quiet at Night	300+	55%	-	58%
Doctors 'Always' Communicated Well	300+	80%	-	80%
Home Recovery Information Given	300+	85%	-	82%
Hospital Given 9 or 10 on 10 Point Scale	300+	70%	-	67%
Meds 'Always' Explained Before Given	300+	61%	-	60%
Nurses 'Always' Communicated Well	300+	79%	-	76%
Pain 'Always' Well Controlled	300+	67%	-	69%
Room and Bathroom 'Always' Clean	300+	68%	-	71%
Timely Help 'Always' Received	300+	60%	-	64%
Would Definitely Recommend Hospital	300+	77%	-	69%

Saint Elizabeth's Medical Center

736 Cambridge Street Phone: 617-789-3000
Brighton, MA 02135 Fax: 617-789-2438
E-mail: semcmail@cchcs.org
URL: www.semc.org
Type: Acute Care Hospitals Emergency Services: Yes
Ownership: Proprietary Beds: 317
Key Personnel:
CEO/President.............. John Holiver
Chief of Medical Staff.......... John O Pastore, MD
Infection Control............. Christine Duffy, RN
Operating Room.............. Carol Hinar
Pediatric Ambulatory Care...... Ronald Pye, MD
Pediatric In-Patient Care....... Ronald Pye, MD
Quality Assurance............ Barbara Lightizer
Radiology.................. R Eugene Langevin, Jr, DM

Measure	Cases	This Hosp.	State Avg.	U.S. Avg.
Heart Attack Care				
ACE Inhibitor or ARB for LVSD	71	83%	94%	96%
Aspirin at Arrival	107	99%	99%	99%
Aspirin at Discharge	326	96%	99%	98%
Beta Blocker at Discharge	307	96%	99%	98%
Fibrinolytic Medication Timing	0	-	50%	55%
PCI Within 90 Minutes of Arrival[1]	16	75%	93%	90%
Smoking Cessation Advice	96	99%	99%	99%
Chest Pain/Possible Heart Attack Care				
Aspirin at Arrival[1,3]	1	100%	96%	95%
Median Time to ECG (minutes)[1,3]	1	21	10	8
Median Time to Transfer (minutes)[5]	0	-	65	61
Fibrinolytic Medication Timing[3]	0	-	78%	54%
Heart Failure Care				
ACE Inhibitor or ARB for LVSD	101	84%	94%	94%
Discharge Instructions	303	93%	89%	88%
Evaluation of LVS Function	404	98%	98%	98%
Smoking Cessation Advice	57	98%	97%	98%
Pneumonia Care				
Appropriate Initial Antibiotic	106	90%	93%	92%
Blood Culture Timing	128	94%	95%	96%
Influenza Vaccine	129	83%	92%	91%
Initial Antibiotic Timing	169	96%	96%	95%
Pneumococcal Vaccine	184	90%	93%	93%
Smoking Cessation Advice	47	89%	96%	97%
Surgical Care Improvement Project				
Appropriate VTP Within 24 Hours[2]	190	97%	96%	92%
Appropriate Hair Removal[2]	631	100%	100%	99%
Appropriate Beta Blocker Usage[2]	228	97%	96%	93%
Controlled Postoperative Blood Glucose[2]	178	98%	95%	93%
Prophylactic Antibiotic Timing[2]	491	99%	97%	97%
Prophylactic Antibiotic Timing (Outpatient)	138	94%	92%	92%
Prophylactic Antibiotic Selection[2]	492	99%	98%	97%
Prophylactic Antibiotic Select. (Outpatient)	133	92%	95%	94%
Prophylactic Antibiotic Stopped[2]	480	95%	96%	94%
Recommended VTP Ordered[2]	190	98%	97%	94%
Urinary Catheter Removal[2]	157	86%	89%	90%
Children's Asthma Care				
Received Systemic Corticosteroids	-	-	-	100%
Received Home Management Plan	-	-	-	71%
Received Reliever Medication	-	-	-	100%
Use of Medical Imaging				
Combination Abdominal CT Scan	709	0.169	0.109	0.191
Combination Chest CT Scan	745	0.005	0.010	0.054
Follow-up Mammogram/Ultrasound	1,072	9.3%	9.2%	8.4%
MRI for Low Back Pain	174	39.1%	30.1%	32.7%
Survey of Patients' Hospital Experiences				
Area Around Room 'Always' Quiet at Night	300+	52%	-	58%
Doctors 'Always' Communicated Well	300+	81%	-	80%
Home Recovery Information Given	300+	83%	-	82%
Hospital Given 9 or 10 on 10 Point Scale	300+	68%	-	67%
Meds 'Always' Explained Before Given	300+	65%	-	60%
Nurses 'Always' Communicated Well	300+	77%	-	76%
Pain 'Always' Well Controlled	300+	71%	-	69%
Room and Bathroom 'Always' Clean	300+	73%	-	71%
Timely Help 'Always' Received	300+	63%	-	64%
Would Definitely Recommend Hospital	300+	73%	-	69%

Good Samaritan Medical Center

235 North Pearl Street Phone: 508-427-3000
Brockton, MA 02301
Type: Acute Care Hospitals Emergency Services: Yes
Ownership: Proprietary
Key Personnel:
CEO/President................ John J Holiver

Measure	Cases	This Hosp.	State Avg.	U.S. Avg.
Heart Attack Care				
ACE Inhibitor or ARB for LVSD	27	85%	94%	96%
Aspirin at Arrival	173	100%	99%	99%
Aspirin at Discharge	127	100%	99%	98%
Beta Blocker at Discharge	120	100%	99%	98%
Fibrinolytic Medication Timing	0	-	50%	55%
PCI Within 90 Minutes of Arrival	63	83%	93%	90%
Smoking Cessation Advice	34	100%	99%	99%
Chest Pain/Possible Heart Attack Care				
Aspirin at Arrival	61	100%	96%	95%
Median Time to ECG (minutes)	69	3	10	8
Median Time to Transfer (minutes)[3]	0	-	65	61
Fibrinolytic Medication Timing[3]	0	-	78%	54%
Heart Failure Care				
ACE Inhibitor or ARB for LVSD	87	95%	94%	94%
Discharge Instructions	243	83%	89%	88%
Evaluation of LVS Function	387	100%	98%	98%
Smoking Cessation Advice	48	96%	97%	98%
Pneumonia Care				
Appropriate Initial Antibiotic	233	98%	93%	92%
Blood Culture Timing	233	97%	95%	96%
Influenza Vaccine	255	96%	92%	91%
Initial Antibiotic Timing	375	94%	96%	95%
Pneumococcal Vaccine	348	91%	93%	93%
Smoking Cessation Advice	109	96%	96%	97%
Surgical Care Improvement Project				
Appropriate VTP Within 24 Hours[2]	247	99%	96%	92%
Appropriate Hair Removal[2]	706	100%	100%	99%
Appropriate Beta Blocker Usage[2]	215	98%	96%	93%
Controlled Postoperative Blood Glucose[2]	0	-	95%	93%
Prophylactic Antibiotic Timing[2]	559	98%	97%	97%
Prophylactic Antibiotic Timing (Outpatient)	219	92%	92%	92%
Prophylactic Antibiotic Selection[2]	560	98%	98%	97%
Prophylactic Antibiotic Select. (Outpatient)	202	95%	95%	94%
Prophylactic Antibiotic Stopped[2]	534	94%	96%	94%
Recommended VTP Ordered[2]	247	99%	97%	94%
Urinary Catheter Removal[2]	34	76%	89%	90%
Children's Asthma Care				
Received Systemic Corticosteroids	-	-	-	100%
Received Home Management Plan	-	-	-	71%
Received Reliever Medication	-	-	-	100%
Use of Medical Imaging				
Combination Abdominal CT Scan	1,131	0.065	0.109	0.191
Combination Chest CT Scan	1,024	0.001	0.010	0.054
Follow-up Mammogram/Ultrasound	1,342	9.5%	9.2%	8.4%
MRI for Low Back Pain	112	36.6%	30.1%	32.7%
Survey of Patients' Hospital Experiences				
Area Around Room 'Always' Quiet at Night	300+	47%	-	58%
Doctors 'Always' Communicated Well	300+	78%	-	80%
Home Recovery Information Given	300+	84%	-	82%
Hospital Given 9 or 10 on 10 Point Scale	300+	62%	-	67%
Meds 'Always' Explained Before Given	300+	60%	-	60%
Nurses 'Always' Communicated Well	300+	78%	-	76%
Pain 'Always' Well Controlled	300+	68%	-	69%
Room and Bathroom 'Always' Clean	300+	67%	-	71%
Timely Help 'Always' Received	300+	56%	-	64%
Would Definitely Recommend Hospital	300+	66%	-	69%

NOTE: Hospital profiles are in alphabetical order by state, then city, then hospital within the city; Rankings exclude hospitals with less than 25 cases except for patient surveys which excludes hospitals with less than 100 cases; (a) 100–299 cases; (1) The number of cases is too small to be sure how well a hospital is performing; (2) The hospital indicated that the data submitted for this measure were based on a sample of cases; (3) Data was collected during a shorter time period (fewer quarters) than the maximum possible time for this measure; (4) Suppressed for one or more quarters by CMS; (5) No data is available from the hospital for this measure; (6) Fewer than 100 patients completed the HCAHPS survey. Use these rates with caution, as the number of surveys may be too low to reliably assess hospital performance; (7) Survey results are based on less than 12 months of data; (8) Survey results are not available for this reporting period; (9) No or very few patients were eligible for the HCAHPS survey. The scores shown, if any, reflect a very small number of surveys; (10) A state average was not calculated because too few hospitals in the state submitted data; (11) There were discrepancies in the data collection process; Please refer to the User's Guide for a full explanation of data.

Signature Healthcare Brockton Hospital

680 Center Street
Brockton, MA 02302
Phone: 508-941-7000
Fax: 508-941-6300
URL: www.brocktonhospital.com
Type: Acute Care Hospitals
Emergency Services: Yes
Ownership: Voluntary Non-Profit - Other
Beds: 268

Key Personnel:
CEO/President. . . . . Dr Goodman
Chief of Medical Staff . . . . Burton J Polanski, MD
Emergency Room . . . . Kate McMenon

Measure	Cases	This Hosp.	State Avg.	U.S. Avg.
Heart Attack Care				
ACE Inhibitor or ARB for LVSD[1]	22	100%	94%	96%
Aspirin at Arrival	188	100%	99%	99%
Aspirin at Discharge	145	99%	99%	98%
Beta Blocker at Discharge	144	100%	99%	98%
Fibrinolytic Medication Timing	0	-	50%	55%
PCI Within 90 Minutes of Arrival	44	98%	93%	90%
Smoking Cessation Advice	54	100%	99%	99%
Chest Pain/Possible Heart Attack Care				
Aspirin at Arrival[1]	18	100%	96%	95%
Median Time to ECG (minutes)[1]	20	6	10	8
Median Time to Transfer (minutes)[5]	0	-	65	61
Fibrinolytic Medication Timing[5]	0	-	78%	54%
Heart Failure Care				
ACE Inhibitor or ARB for LVSD	96	99%	94%	94%
Discharge Instructions	206	97%	89%	88%
Evaluation of LVS Function	290	100%	98%	98%
Smoking Cessation Advice	60	100%	97%	98%
Pneumonia Care				
Appropriate Initial Antibiotic	114	98%	93%	92%
Blood Culture Timing	83	99%	95%	96%
Influenza Vaccine	105	91%	92%	91%
Initial Antibiotic Timing	176	99%	96%	95%
Pneumococcal Vaccine	178	95%	93%	93%
Smoking Cessation Advice	95	100%	96%	97%
Surgical Care Improvement Project				
Appropriate VTP Within 24 Hours	186	99%	96%	92%
Appropriate Hair Removal	447	100%	100%	99%
Appropriate Beta Blocker Usage	144	99%	96%	93%
Controlled Postoperative Blood Glucose	0	-	95%	93%
Prophylactic Antibiotic Timing	261	100%	97%	97%
Prophylactic Antibiotic Timing (Outpatient)	87	92%	92%	92%
Prophylactic Antibiotic Selection	264	98%	98%	97%
Prophylactic Antibiotic Select. (Outpatient)	82	91%	95%	94%
Prophylactic Antibiotic Stopped	248	98%	96%	94%
Recommended VTP Ordered	186	99%	97%	94%
Urinary Catheter Removal	52	87%	89%	90%
Children's Asthma Care				
Received Systemic Corticosteroids	-	-	-	100%
Received Home Management Plan	-	-	-	71%
Received Reliever Medication	-	-	-	100%
Use of Medical Imaging				
Combination Abdominal CT Scan	714	0.057	0.109	0.191
Combination Chest CT Scan	535	0.030	0.010	0.054
Follow-up Mammogram/Ultrasound	860	9.8%	9.2%	8.4%
MRI for Low Back Pain	104	38.5%	30.1%	32.7%
Survey of Patients' Hospital Experiences				
Area Around Room 'Always' Quiet at Night	300+	41%	-	58%
Doctors 'Always' Communicated Well	300+	76%	-	80%
Home Recovery Information Given	300+	85%	-	82%
Hospital Given 9 or 10 on 10 Point Scale	300+	60%	-	67%
Meds 'Always' Explained Before Given	300+	58%	-	60%
Nurses 'Always' Communicated Well	300+	76%	-	76%
Pain 'Always' Well Controlled	300+	67%	-	69%
Room and Bathroom 'Always' Clean	300+	69%	-	71%
Timely Help 'Always' Received	300+	63%	-	64%
Would Definitely Recommend Hospital	300+	65%	-	69%

Lahey Clinic Hospital

41 & 45 Mall Road
Burlington, MA 01803
Phone: 781-744-5100
Fax: 781-744-8920
URL: www.lahey.org
Type: Acute Care Hospitals
Emergency Services: Yes
Ownership: Voluntary Non-Profit - Other
Beds: 317

Key Personnel:
CEO/President. . . . . David M Barret MD
Operating Room. . . . . Roger L Jenkins, MD
Pediatric In-Patient Care . . . . Claire Wilson, MD
Quality Assurance . . . . Joseph M Healy, PhD
Radiology. . . . . Anna Chacko, MD
Anesthesiology. . . . . Micheal Entrup MD
Emergency Room . . . . Jean Brown
Patient Relations . . . . Roger J Cameron

Measure	Cases	This Hosp.	State Avg.	U.S. Avg.
Heart Attack Care				
ACE Inhibitor or ARB for LVSD	139	96%	94%	96%
Aspirin at Arrival	298	100%	99%	99%
Aspirin at Discharge	703	100%	99%	98%
Beta Blocker at Discharge	687	99%	99%	98%
Fibrinolytic Medication Timing[1]	1	100%	50%	55%
PCI Within 90 Minutes of Arrival	69	93%	93%	90%
Smoking Cessation Advice	156	99%	99%	99%
Chest Pain/Possible Heart Attack Care				
Aspirin at Arrival[1,3]	6	83%	96%	95%
Median Time to ECG (minutes)[1,3]	6	9	10	8
Median Time to Transfer (minutes)[5]	0	-	65	61
Fibrinolytic Medication Timing[5]	0	-	78%	54%
Heart Failure Care				
ACE Inhibitor or ARB for LVSD[2]	66	88%	94%	94%
Discharge Instructions[2]	217	93%	89%	88%
Evaluation of LVS Function[2]	278	99%	98%	98%
Smoking Cessation Advice[1,2]	22	100%	97%	98%
Pneumonia Care				
Appropriate Initial Antibiotic[2]	55	95%	93%	92%
Blood Culture Timing[2]	81	99%	95%	96%
Influenza Vaccine[2]	78	90%	92%	91%
Initial Antibiotic Timing[2]	95	87%	96%	95%
Pneumococcal Vaccine[2]	133	90%	93%	93%
Smoking Cessation Advice[2]	26	77%	96%	97%
Surgical Care Improvement Project				
Appropriate VTP Within 24 Hours[2]	231	100%	96%	92%
Appropriate Hair Removal[2]	641	100%	100%	99%
Appropriate Beta Blocker Usage[2]	262	100%	96%	93%
Controlled Postoperative Blood Glucose[2]	126	88%	95%	93%
Prophylactic Antibiotic Timing[2]	396	99%	97%	97%
Prophylactic Antibiotic Timing (Outpatient)	370	86%	92%	92%
Prophylactic Antibiotic Selection[2]	398	100%	98%	97%
Prophylactic Antibiotic Select. (Outpatient)	596	96%	95%	94%
Prophylactic Antibiotic Stopped[2]	376	95%	96%	94%
Recommended VTP Ordered[2]	231	100%	97%	94%
Urinary Catheter Removal[2]	95	80%	89%	90%
Children's Asthma Care				
Received Systemic Corticosteroids	-	-	-	100%
Received Home Management Plan	-	-	-	71%
Received Reliever Medication	-	-	-	100%
Use of Medical Imaging				
Combination Abdominal CT Scan	2,824	0.208	0.109	0.191
Combination Chest CT Scan	2,722	0.001	0.010	0.054
Follow-up Mammogram/Ultrasound	3,572	10.8%	9.2%	8.4%
MRI for Low Back Pain	454	30.8%	30.1%	32.7%
Survey of Patients' Hospital Experiences				
Area Around Room 'Always' Quiet at Night	300+	44%	-	58%
Doctors 'Always' Communicated Well	300+	77%	-	80%
Home Recovery Information Given	300+	85%	-	82%
Hospital Given 9 or 10 on 10 Point Scale	300+	68%	-	67%
Meds 'Always' Explained Before Given	300+	61%	-	60%
Nurses 'Always' Communicated Well	300+	72%	-	76%
Pain 'Always' Well Controlled	300+	63%	-	69%
Room and Bathroom 'Always' Clean	300+	65%	-	71%
Timely Help 'Always' Received	300+	56%	-	64%
Would Definitely Recommend Hospital	300+	74%	-	69%

Cambridge Health Alliance

1493 Cambridge Street
Cambridge, MA 02138
Phone: 617-665-2300
Fax: 617-665-3545
Type: Acute Care Hospitals
Emergency Services: Yes
Ownership: Government - Local
Beds: 270

Key Personnel:
CEO/President. . . . . Chirad Pels
Chief of Medical Staff . . . . David Osler, MD
Emergency Room . . . . Thomas Workman

Measure	Cases	This Hosp.	State Avg.	U.S. Avg.
Heart Attack Care				
ACE Inhibitor or ARB for LVSD[1]	11	100%	94%	96%
Aspirin at Arrival	70	97%	99%	99%
Aspirin at Discharge	52	100%	99%	98%
Beta Blocker at Discharge	50	98%	99%	98%
Fibrinolytic Medication Timing	0	-	50%	55%
PCI Within 90 Minutes of Arrival	0	-	93%	90%
Smoking Cessation Advice[1]	11	100%	99%	99%
Chest Pain/Possible Heart Attack Care				
Aspirin at Arrival	86	94%	96%	95%
Median Time to ECG (minutes)	90	5	10	8
Median Time to Transfer (minutes)[1]	13	56	65	61
Fibrinolytic Medication Timing	0	-	78%	54%
Heart Failure Care				
ACE Inhibitor or ARB for LVSD	48	98%	94%	94%
Discharge Instructions	191	93%	89%	88%
Evaluation of LVS Function	276	100%	98%	98%
Smoking Cessation Advice	45	89%	97%	98%
Pneumonia Care				
Appropriate Initial Antibiotic	156	96%	93%	92%
Blood Culture Timing	278	95%	95%	96%
Influenza Vaccine	159	95%	92%	91%
Initial Antibiotic Timing	248	98%	96%	95%
Pneumococcal Vaccine	206	97%	93%	93%
Smoking Cessation Advice	117	93%	96%	97%
Surgical Care Improvement Project				
Appropriate VTP Within 24 Hours[2]	172	97%	96%	92%
Appropriate Hair Removal[2]	289	100%	100%	99%
Appropriate Beta Blocker Usage[2]	70	96%	96%	93%
Controlled Postoperative Blood Glucose[2]	0	-	95%	93%
Prophylactic Antibiotic Timing[2]	185	95%	97%	97%
Prophylactic Antibiotic Timing (Outpatient)	71	90%	92%	92%
Prophylactic Antibiotic Selection[2]	189	97%	98%	97%
Prophylactic Antibiotic Select. (Outpatient)	71	99%	95%	94%
Prophylactic Antibiotic Stopped[2]	180	98%	96%	94%
Recommended VTP Ordered[2]	173	98%	97%	94%
Urinary Catheter Removal[2]	87	97%	89%	90%
Children's Asthma Care				
Received Systemic Corticosteroids	-	-	-	100%
Received Home Management Plan	-	-	-	71%
Received Reliever Medication	-	-	-	100%
Use of Medical Imaging				
Combination Abdominal CT Scan	657	0.196	0.109	0.191
Combination Chest CT Scan	348	0.003	0.010	0.054
Follow-up Mammogram/Ultrasound	1,396	8.4%	9.2%	8.4%
MRI for Low Back Pain	119	28.6%	30.1%	32.7%
Survey of Patients' Hospital Experiences				
Area Around Room 'Always' Quiet at Night	300+	53%	-	58%
Doctors 'Always' Communicated Well	300+	78%	-	80%
Home Recovery Information Given	300+	86%	-	82%
Hospital Given 9 or 10 on 10 Point Scale	300+	59%	-	67%
Meds 'Always' Explained Before Given	300+	62%	-	60%
Nurses 'Always' Communicated Well	300+	72%	-	76%
Pain 'Always' Well Controlled	300+	67%	-	69%
Room and Bathroom 'Always' Clean	300+	67%	-	71%
Timely Help 'Always' Received	300+	57%	-	64%
Would Definitely Recommend Hospital	300+	64%	-	69%

NOTE: Hospital profiles are in alphabetical order by state, then city, then hospital within the city; Rankings exclude hospitals with less than 25 cases except for patient surveys which excludes hospitals with less than 100 cases; (a) 100–299 cases; (1) The number of cases is too small to be sure how well a hospital is performing; (2) The hospital indicated that the data submitted for this measure were based on a sample of cases; (3) Data was collected during a shorter time period (fewer quarters) than the maximum possible time for this measure; (4) Suppressed for one or more quarters by CMS; (5) No data is available from the hospital for this measure; (6) Fewer than 100 patients completed the HCAHPS survey. Use these rates with caution, as the number of surveys may be too low to reliably assess hospital performance; (7) Survey results are based on less than 12 months of data; (8) Survey results are not available for this reporting period; (9) No or very few patients were eligible for the HCAHPS survey. The scores shown, if any, reflect a very small number of surveys; (10) A state average was not calculated because too few hospitals in the state submitted data; (11) There were discrepancies in the data collection process; Please refer to the User's Guide for a full explanation of data.

Mount Auburn Hospital

330 Mount Auburn Street
Cambridge, MA 02138
Phone: 617-492-3500
Fax: 617-499-5168
Type: Acute Care Hospitals
Emergency Services: Yes
Ownership: Voluntary Non-Profit - Private
Beds: 183

Key Personnel:
CEO/President. . . . . Jeanette Clough
Cardiac Laboratory. . . . . Spanley Forwand, MD
Chief of Medical Staff. . . . . Ryan Sullivan, MD
Operating Room. . . . . Frederick F Bartlett
Pediatric In-Patient Care . . . . David A Link
Quality Assurance . . . . Janet Long
Radiology. . . . . Madeline S Crivello, MD
Emergency Room . . . . Jeanne Donvon

Measure	Cases	This Hosp.	State Avg.	U.S. Avg.
Heart Attack Care				
ACE Inhibitor or ARB for LVSD	38	100%	94%	96%
Aspirin at Arrival	191	99%	99%	99%
Aspirin at Discharge	228	100%	99%	98%
Beta Blocker at Discharge	225	100%	99%	98%
Fibrinolytic Medication Timing	0	-	50%	55%
PCI Within 90 Minutes of Arrival	36	92%	93%	90%
Smoking Cessation Advice	39	100%	99%	99%
Chest Pain/Possible Heart Attack Care				
Aspirin at Arrival[1,3]	2	100%	96%	95%
Median Time to ECG (minutes)[1,3]	2	30	10	8
Median Time to Transfer (minutes)[5]	0	-	65	61
Fibrinolytic Medication Timing[5]	0	-	78%	54%
Heart Failure Care				
ACE Inhibitor or ARB for LVSD	82	100%	94%	94%
Discharge Instructions	264	100%	89%	88%
Evaluation of LVS Function	347	100%	98%	98%
Smoking Cessation Advice	30	100%	97%	98%
Pneumonia Care				
Appropriate Initial Antibiotic	175	99%	93%	92%
Blood Culture Timing	280	97%	95%	96%
Influenza Vaccine	193	93%	92%	91%
Initial Antibiotic Timing	254	100%	96%	95%
Pneumococcal Vaccine	254	97%	93%	93%
Smoking Cessation Advice	60	100%	96%	97%
Surgical Care Improvement Project				
Appropriate VTP Within 24 Hours	432	98%	96%	92%
Appropriate Hair Removal	1,018	100%	100%	99%
Appropriate Beta Blocker Usage	358	92%	96%	93%
Controlled Postoperative Blood Glucose	181	94%	95%	93%
Prophylactic Antibiotic Timing	727	98%	97%	97%
Prophylactic Antibiotic Timing (Outpatient)	406	98%	92%	92%
Prophylactic Antibiotic Selection	732	97%	98%	97%
Prophylactic Antibiotic Select. (Outpatient)	405	97%	95%	94%
Prophylactic Antibiotic Stopped	712	99%	96%	94%
Recommended VTP Ordered	432	99%	97%	94%
Urinary Catheter Removal	311	73%	89%	90%
Children's Asthma Care				
Received Systemic Corticosteroids	-	-	-	100%
Received Home Management Plan	-	-	-	71%
Received Reliever Medication	-	-	-	100%
Use of Medical Imaging				
Combination Abdominal CT Scan	938	0.127	0.109	0.191
Combination Chest CT Scan	627	0.000	0.010	0.054
Follow-up Mammogram/Ultrasound	1,618	6.9%	9.2%	8.4%
MRI for Low Back Pain	290	32.4%	30.1%	32.7%
Survey of Patients' Hospital Experiences				
Area Around Room 'Always' Quiet at Night	300+	50%	-	58%
Doctors 'Always' Communicated Well	300+	80%	-	80%
Home Recovery Information Given	300+	85%	-	82%
Hospital Given 9 or 10 on 10 Point Scale	300+	71%	-	67%
Meds 'Always' Explained Before Given	300+	64%	-	60%
Nurses 'Always' Communicated Well	300+	80%	-	76%
Pain 'Always' Well Controlled	300+	73%	-	69%
Room and Bathroom 'Always' Clean	300+	72%	-	71%
Timely Help 'Always' Received	300+	68%	-	64%
Would Definitely Recommend Hospital	300+	77%	-	69%

Soldiers Home in Massachusetts

91 Crest Avenue
Chelsea, MA 02150
Phone: 617-884-5660
Fax: 617-884-1162
Type: Acute Care Hospitals
Emergency Services: No
Ownership: Government - State
Beds: 188

Key Personnel:
CEO/President. . . . . Michael Resca
Chief of Medical Staff . . . . John Bolzan, MD
Emergency Room . . . . David J Cancian, MD

Measure	Cases	This Hosp.	State Avg.	U.S. Avg.
Heart Attack Care				
ACE Inhibitor or ARB for LVSD	-	-	94%	96%
Aspirin at Arrival	-	-	99%	99%
Aspirin at Discharge	-	-	99%	98%
Beta Blocker at Discharge	-	-	99%	98%
Fibrinolytic Medication Timing	-	-	50%	55%
PCI Within 90 Minutes of Arrival	-	-	93%	90%
Smoking Cessation Advice	-	-	99%	99%
Chest Pain/Possible Heart Attack Care				
Aspirin at Arrival[5]	0	-	96%	95%
Median Time to ECG (minutes)[5]	0	-	10	8
Median Time to Transfer (minutes)[5]	0	-	65	61
Fibrinolytic Medication Timing[5]	0	-	78%	54%
Heart Failure Care				
ACE Inhibitor or ARB for LVSD	-	-	94%	94%
Discharge Instructions	-	-	89%	88%
Evaluation of LVS Function	-	-	98%	98%
Smoking Cessation Advice	-	-	97%	98%
Pneumonia Care				
Appropriate Initial Antibiotic	-	-	93%	92%
Blood Culture Timing	-	-	95%	96%
Influenza Vaccine	-	-	92%	91%
Initial Antibiotic Timing	-	-	96%	95%
Pneumococcal Vaccine	-	-	93%	93%
Smoking Cessation Advice	-	-	96%	97%
Surgical Care Improvement Project				
Appropriate VTP Within 24 Hours	-	-	96%	92%
Appropriate Hair Removal	-	-	100%	99%
Appropriate Beta Blocker Usage	-	-	96%	93%
Controlled Postoperative Blood Glucose	-	-	95%	93%
Prophylactic Antibiotic Timing	-	-	97%	97%
Prophylactic Antibiotic Timing (Outpatient)[5]	0	-	92%	92%
Prophylactic Antibiotic Selection	-	-	98%	97%
Prophylactic Antibiotic Select. (Outpatient)[5]	0	-	95%	94%
Prophylactic Antibiotic Stopped	-	-	96%	94%
Recommended VTP Ordered	-	-	97%	94%
Urinary Catheter Removal	-	-	89%	90%
Children's Asthma Care				
Received Systemic Corticosteroids	-	-	-	100%
Received Home Management Plan	-	-	-	71%
Received Reliever Medication	-	-	-	100%
Use of Medical Imaging				
Combination Abdominal CT Scan[5]	0	-	0.109	0.191
Combination Chest CT Scan[5]	0	-	0.010	0.054
Follow-up Mammogram/Ultrasound[5]	0	-	9.2%	8.4%
MRI for Low Back Pain[5]	0	-	30.1%	32.7%
Survey of Patients' Hospital Experiences				
Area Around Room 'Always' Quiet at Night	-	-	-	58%
Doctors 'Always' Communicated Well	-	-	-	80%
Home Recovery Information Given	-	-	-	82%
Hospital Given 9 or 10 on 10 Point Scale	-	-	-	67%
Meds 'Always' Explained Before Given	-	-	-	60%
Nurses 'Always' Communicated Well	-	-	-	76%
Pain 'Always' Well Controlled	-	-	-	69%
Room and Bathroom 'Always' Clean	-	-	-	71%
Timely Help 'Always' Received	-	-	-	64%
Would Definitely Recommend Hospital	-	-	-	69%

Clinton Hospital Association

201 Highland Street
Clinton, MA 01510
Phone: 978-368-3000
Fax: 978-368-3766
URL: www.umassmemorial.org
Type: Acute Care Hospitals
Emergency Services: Yes
Ownership: Voluntary Non-Profit - Other
Beds: 781

Key Personnel:
CEO/President. . . . . Walter Ettinger, MD
Cardiac Laboratory. . . . . Daniel Fisher, MD, PhD
Chief of Medical Staff . . . . Cheryl Lapriore, MD
Coronary Care . . . . Craig Smith, MD
Infection Control. . . . . Lawrence Madoff, MD
Pediatric In-Patient Care . . . . Marianne Felice, MD
Quality Assurance . . . . Karen Plainte, RN, MBA
Radiology. . . . . JosephA Ferrucci, MD

Measure	Cases	This Hosp.	State Avg.	U.S. Avg.
Heart Attack Care				
ACE Inhibitor or ARB for LVSD[1]	1	100%	94%	96%
Aspirin at Arrival[1]	9	100%	99%	99%
Aspirin at Discharge[1]	8	88%	99%	98%
Beta Blocker at Discharge[1]	7	100%	99%	98%
Fibrinolytic Medication Timing	0	-	50%	55%
PCI Within 90 Minutes of Arrival	0	-	93%	90%
Smoking Cessation Advice[1]	1	100%	99%	99%
Chest Pain/Possible Heart Attack Care				
Aspirin at Arrival[1,3]	13	92%	96%	95%
Median Time to ECG (minutes)[1,3]	13	3	10	8
Median Time to Transfer (minutes)[1,3]	3	60	65	61
Fibrinolytic Medication Timing[1,3]	1	100%	78%	54%
Heart Failure Care				
ACE Inhibitor or ARB for LVSD[1]	5	100%	94%	94%
Discharge Instructions	31	100%	89%	88%
Evaluation of LVS Function	44	98%	98%	98%
Smoking Cessation Advice[1]	6	100%	97%	98%
Pneumonia Care				
Appropriate Initial Antibiotic	31	100%	93%	92%
Blood Culture Timing	36	83%	95%	96%
Influenza Vaccine[1]	24	92%	92%	91%
Initial Antibiotic Timing	39	97%	96%	95%
Pneumococcal Vaccine	50	82%	93%	93%
Smoking Cessation Advice[1]	7	100%	96%	97%
Surgical Care Improvement Project				
Appropriate VTP Within 24 Hours[1,3]	4	75%	96%	92%
Appropriate Hair Removal[1,3]	5	100%	100%	99%
Appropriate Beta Blocker Usage[1,3]	3	100%	96%	93%
Controlled Postoperative Blood Glucose[3]	0	-	95%	93%
Prophylactic Antibiotic Timing[1,3]	1	100%	97%	97%
Prophylactic Antibiotic Timing (Outpatient)[5]	0	-	92%	92%
Prophylactic Antibiotic Selection[1,3]	1	0%	98%	97%
Prophylactic Antibiotic Select. (Outpatient)[5]	0	-	95%	94%
Prophylactic Antibiotic Stopped[1,3]	1	100%	96%	94%
Recommended VTP Ordered[1,3]	4	75%	97%	94%
Urinary Catheter Removal[3]	0	-	89%	90%
Children's Asthma Care				
Received Systemic Corticosteroids	-	-	-	100%
Received Home Management Plan	-	-	-	71%
Received Reliever Medication	-	-	-	100%
Use of Medical Imaging				
Combination Abdominal CT Scan	126	0.024	0.109	0.191
Combination Chest CT Scan	63	0.000	0.010	0.054
Follow-up Mammogram/Ultrasound	342	2.9%	9.2%	8.4%
MRI for Low Back Pain[1]	17	29.4%	30.1%	32.7%
Survey of Patients' Hospital Experiences				
Area Around Room 'Always' Quiet at Night	(a)	63%	-	58%
Doctors 'Always' Communicated Well	(a)	80%	-	80%
Home Recovery Information Given	(a)	87%	-	82%
Hospital Given 9 or 10 on 10 Point Scale	(a)	75%	-	67%
Meds 'Always' Explained Before Given	(a)	72%	-	60%
Nurses 'Always' Communicated Well	(a)	85%	-	76%
Pain 'Always' Well Controlled	(a)	80%	-	69%
Room and Bathroom 'Always' Clean	(a)	79%	-	71%
Timely Help 'Always' Received	(a)	76%	-	64%
Would Definitely Recommend Hospital	(a)	80%	-	69%

NOTE: Hospital profiles are in alphabetical order by state, then city, then hospital within the city; Rankings exclude hospitals with less than 25 cases except for patient surveys which excludes hospitals with less than 100 cases; (a) 100–299 cases; (1) The number of cases is too small to be sure how well a hospital is performing; (2) The hospital indicated that the data submitted for this measure were based on a sample of cases; (3) Data was collected during a shorter time period (fewer quarters) than the maximum possible time for this measure; (4) Suppressed for one or more quarters by CMS; (5) No data is available from the hospital for this measure; (6) Fewer than 100 patients completed the HCAHPS survey. Use these rates with caution, as the number of surveys may be too low to reliably assess hospital performance; (7) Survey results are based on less than 12 months of data; (8) Survey results are not available for this reporting period; (9) No or very few patients were eligible for the HCAHPS survey. The scores shown, if any, reflect a very small number of surveys; (10) A state average was not calculated because too few hospitals in the state submitted data; (11) There were discrepancies in the data collection process; Please refer to the User's Guide for a full explanation of data.

Saint Anne's Hospital

795 Middle Street
Fall River, MA 02721
Phone: 508-674-5600
Fax: 508-675-5647
E-mail: sahmail@cchcs.org
URL: www.saintanneshospital.org
Type: Acute Care Hospitals
Emergency Services: Yes
Ownership: Proprietary
Beds: 165

Key Personnel:
CEO/President. . . . . Michael Metzler
Chief of Medical Staff. . . . . Malcolm W MacDonald
Coronary Care . . . . Kristine Walker, RN
Infection Control. . . . . Diane Gauvin, RN
Pediatric Ambulatory Care . . . . . . Joan Benevides, RN
Pediatric In-Patient Care . . . . . . Nellie Jacob
Quality Assurance . . . . Jane Benevides, RN
Radiology. . . . . Franklin A DePeters

Measure	Cases	This Hosp.	State Avg.	U.S. Avg.
Heart Attack Care				
ACE Inhibitor or ARB for LVSD[1]	6	100%	94%	96%
Aspirin at Arrival	54	100%	99%	99%
Aspirin at Discharge	31	97%	99%	98%
Beta Blocker at Discharge	30	100%	99%	98%
Fibrinolytic Medication Timing	0	-	50%	55%
PCI Within 90 Minutes of Arrival	0	-	93%	90%
Smoking Cessation Advice[1]	6	100%	99%	99%
Chest Pain/Possible Heart Attack Care				
Aspirin at Arrival	25	92%	96%	95%
Median Time to ECG (minutes)	27	11	10	8
Median Time to Transfer (minutes)[1,3]	13	54	65	61
Fibrinolytic Medication Timing	0	-	78%	54%
Heart Failure Care				
ACE Inhibitor or ARB for LVSD[1]	24	100%	94%	94%
Discharge Instructions	144	78%	89%	88%
Evaluation of LVS Function	185	100%	98%	98%
Smoking Cessation Advice	25	100%	97%	98%
Pneumonia Care				
Appropriate Initial Antibiotic	128	91%	93%	92%
Blood Culture Timing	103	96%	95%	96%
Influenza Vaccine	156	92%	92%	91%
Initial Antibiotic Timing	224	99%	96%	95%
Pneumococcal Vaccine	226	96%	93%	93%
Smoking Cessation Advice	81	100%	96%	97%
Surgical Care Improvement Project				
Appropriate VTP Within 24 Hours[2]	112	97%	96%	92%
Appropriate Hair Removal[2]	193	100%	100%	99%
Appropriate Beta Blocker Usage[2]	74	97%	96%	93%
Controlled Postoperative Blood Glucose[2]	0	-	95%	93%
Prophylactic Antibiotic Timing[2]	120	98%	97%	97%
Prophylactic Antibiotic Timing (Outpatient)	49	90%	92%	92%
Prophylactic Antibiotic Selection[2]	120	98%	98%	97%
Prophylactic Antibiotic Select. (Outpatient)	49	94%	95%	94%
Prophylactic Antibiotic Stopped[2]	110	95%	96%	94%
Recommended VTP Ordered[2]	112	99%	97%	94%
Urinary Catheter Removal	51	84%	89%	90%
Children's Asthma Care				
Received Systemic Corticosteroids	-	-	-	100%
Received Home Management Plan	-	-	-	71%
Received Reliever Medication	-	-	-	100%
Use of Medical Imaging				
Combination Abdominal CT Scan	666	0.072	0.109	0.191
Combination Chest CT Scan	587	0.003	0.010	0.054
Follow-up Mammogram/Ultrasound	1,299	8.2%	9.2%	8.4%
MRI for Low Back Pain	104	29.8%	30.1%	32.7%
Survey of Patients' Hospital Experiences				
Area Around Room 'Always' Quiet at Night	300+	52%	-	58%
Doctors 'Always' Communicated Well	300+	78%	-	80%
Home Recovery Information Given	300+	86%	-	82%
Hospital Given 9 or 10 on 10 Point Scale	300+	66%	-	67%
Meds 'Always' Explained Before Given	300+	61%	-	60%
Nurses 'Always' Communicated Well	300+	79%	-	76%
Pain 'Always' Well Controlled	300+	69%	-	69%
Room and Bathroom 'Always' Clean	300+	75%	-	71%
Timely Help 'Always' Received	300+	63%	-	64%
Would Definitely Recommend Hospital	300+	72%	-	69%

Southcoast Hospital Group

363 Highland Avenue
Fall River, MA 02720
Phone: 508-679-3131
Fax: 508-679-7144
URL: www.southcoast.org/charlton
Type: Acute Care Hospitals
Emergency Services: Yes
Ownership: Voluntary Non-Profit - Private
Beds: 362

Key Personnel:
CEO/President. . . . . John B Day
Chief of Medical Staff . . . . Eugene McMahon, MD, MBA

Measure	Cases	This Hosp.	State Avg.	U.S. Avg.
Heart Attack Care				
ACE Inhibitor or ARB for LVSD	148	84%	94%	96%
Aspirin at Arrival	640	98%	99%	99%
Aspirin at Discharge	687	99%	99%	98%
Beta Blocker at Discharge	706	98%	99%	98%
Fibrinolytic Medication Timing	0	-	50%	55%
PCI Within 90 Minutes of Arrival	58	84%	93%	90%
Smoking Cessation Advice	195	92%	99%	99%
Chest Pain/Possible Heart Attack Care				
Aspirin at Arrival	128	94%	96%	95%
Median Time to ECG (minutes)	133	6	10	8
Median Time to Transfer (minutes)	45	69	65	61
Fibrinolytic Medication Timing[1]	1	0%	78%	54%
Heart Failure Care				
ACE Inhibitor or ARB for LVSD	362	89%	94%	94%
Discharge Instructions	872	66%	89%	88%
Evaluation of LVS Function	1,287	95%	98%	98%
Smoking Cessation Advice	139	81%	97%	98%
Pneumonia Care				
Appropriate Initial Antibiotic	684	85%	93%	92%
Blood Culture Timing	853	90%	95%	96%
Influenza Vaccine	621	91%	92%	91%
Initial Antibiotic Timing	1,053	89%	96%	95%
Pneumococcal Vaccine	921	93%	93%	93%
Smoking Cessation Advice	317	88%	96%	97%
Surgical Care Improvement Project				
Appropriate VTP Within 24 Hours	1,022	87%	96%	92%
Appropriate Hair Removal	2,258	100%	100%	99%
Appropriate Beta Blocker Usage	670	96%	96%	93%
Controlled Postoperative Blood Glucose	283	95%	95%	93%
Prophylactic Antibiotic Timing	1,488	97%	97%	97%
Prophylactic Antibiotic Timing (Outpatient)	834	91%	92%	92%
Prophylactic Antibiotic Selection	1,507	96%	98%	97%
Prophylactic Antibiotic Select. (Outpatient)	799	94%	95%	94%
Prophylactic Antibiotic Stopped	1,443	97%	96%	94%
Recommended VTP Ordered	1,025	91%	97%	94%
Urinary Catheter Removal	501	73%	89%	90%
Children's Asthma Care				
Received Systemic Corticosteroids	-	-	-	100%
Received Home Management Plan	-	-	-	71%
Received Reliever Medication	-	-	-	100%
Use of Medical Imaging				
Combination Abdominal CT Scan	2,982	0.075	0.109	0.191
Combination Chest CT Scan	2,408	0.005	0.010	0.054
Follow-up Mammogram/Ultrasound	6,895	10.0%	9.2%	8.4%
MRI for Low Back Pain	298	29.9%	30.1%	32.7%
Survey of Patients' Hospital Experiences				
Area Around Room 'Always' Quiet at Night	300+	51%	-	58%
Doctors 'Always' Communicated Well	300+	79%	-	80%
Home Recovery Information Given	300+	86%	-	82%
Hospital Given 9 or 10 on 10 Point Scale	300+	62%	-	67%
Meds 'Always' Explained Before Given	300+	59%	-	60%
Nurses 'Always' Communicated Well	300+	75%	-	76%
Pain 'Always' Well Controlled	300+	67%	-	69%
Room and Bathroom 'Always' Clean	300+	73%	-	71%
Timely Help 'Always' Received	300+	58%	-	64%
Would Definitely Recommend Hospital	300+	68%	-	69%

Falmouth Hospital

67 & 100 Ter Heun Drive
Falmouth, MA 02540
Phone: 508-548-5300
Fax: 508-457-3857
URL: www.capecodhealth.com
Type: Acute Care Hospitals
Emergency Services: Yes
Ownership: Voluntary Non-Profit - Private
Beds: 95

Key Personnel:
CEO/President. . . . . Susan Wing
Radiology. . . . . Kenneth L Caswell
Emergency Room . . . . Herbert Gray, MD

Measure	Cases	This Hosp.	State Avg.	U.S. Avg.
Heart Attack Care				
ACE Inhibitor or ARB for LVSD[1]	10	100%	94%	96%
Aspirin at Arrival	94	100%	99%	99%
Aspirin at Discharge	68	100%	99%	98%
Beta Blocker at Discharge	61	98%	99%	98%
Fibrinolytic Medication Timing	0	-	50%	55%
PCI Within 90 Minutes of Arrival	0	-	93%	90%
Smoking Cessation Advice[1]	3	100%	99%	99%
Chest Pain/Possible Heart Attack Care				
Aspirin at Arrival	38	95%	96%	95%
Median Time to ECG (minutes)	39	8	10	8
Median Time to Transfer (minutes)	0	-	65	61
Fibrinolytic Medication Timing	0	-	78%	54%
Heart Failure Care				
ACE Inhibitor or ARB for LVSD	46	100%	94%	94%
Discharge Instructions	177	90%	89%	88%
Evaluation of LVS Function	261	100%	98%	98%
Smoking Cessation Advice[1]	19	95%	97%	98%
Pneumonia Care				
Appropriate Initial Antibiotic	106	99%	93%	92%
Blood Culture Timing	197	99%	95%	96%
Influenza Vaccine	124	94%	92%	91%
Initial Antibiotic Timing	181	98%	96%	95%
Pneumococcal Vaccine	177	97%	93%	93%
Smoking Cessation Advice	40	100%	96%	97%
Surgical Care Improvement Project				
Appropriate VTP Within 24 Hours[2]	202	95%	96%	92%
Appropriate Hair Removal[2]	644	100%	100%	99%
Appropriate Beta Blocker Usage[2]	143	100%	96%	93%
Controlled Postoperative Blood Glucose[2]	0	-	95%	93%
Prophylactic Antibiotic Timing[2]	506	99%	97%	97%
Prophylactic Antibiotic Timing (Outpatient)	80	100%	92%	92%
Prophylactic Antibiotic Selection[2]	509	98%	98%	97%
Prophylactic Antibiotic Select. (Outpatient)	80	96%	95%	94%
Prophylactic Antibiotic Stopped[2]	490	99%	96%	94%
Recommended VTP Ordered[2]	202	95%	97%	94%
Urinary Catheter Removal[2]	225	98%	89%	90%
Children's Asthma Care				
Received Systemic Corticosteroids	-	-	-	100%
Received Home Management Plan	-	-	-	71%
Received Reliever Medication	-	-	-	100%
Use of Medical Imaging				
Combination Abdominal CT Scan	1,145	0.079	0.109	0.191
Combination Chest CT Scan	1,065	0.027	0.010	0.054
Follow-up Mammogram/Ultrasound	2,764	7.9%	9.2%	8.4%
MRI for Low Back Pain	289	29.4%	30.1%	32.7%
Survey of Patients' Hospital Experiences				
Area Around Room 'Always' Quiet at Night	300+	47%	-	58%
Doctors 'Always' Communicated Well	300+	77%	-	80%
Home Recovery Information Given	300+	85%	-	82%
Hospital Given 9 or 10 on 10 Point Scale	300+	68%	-	67%
Meds 'Always' Explained Before Given	300+	58%	-	60%
Nurses 'Always' Communicated Well	300+	77%	-	76%
Pain 'Always' Well Controlled	300+	70%	-	69%
Room and Bathroom 'Always' Clean	300+	73%	-	71%
Timely Help 'Always' Received	300+	61%	-	64%
Would Definitely Recommend Hospital	300+	74%	-	69%

NOTE: Hospital profiles are in alphabetical order by state, then city, then hospital within the city; Rankings exclude hospitals with less than 25 cases except for patient surveys which excludes hospitals with less than 100 cases; (a) 100–299 cases; (1) The number of cases is too small to be sure how well a hospital is performing; (2) The hospital indicated that the data submitted for this measure were based on a sample of cases; (3) Data was collected during a shorter time period (fewer quarters) than the maximum possible time for this measure; (4) Suppressed for one or more quarters by CMS; (5) No data is available from the hospital for this measure; (6) Fewer than 100 patients completed the HCAHPS survey. Use these rates with caution, as the number of surveys may be too low to reliably assess hospital performance; (7) Survey results are based on less than 12 months of data; (8) Survey results are not available for this reporting period; (9) No or very few patients were eligible for the HCAHPS survey. The scores shown, if any, reflect a very small number of surveys; (10) A state average was not calculated because too few hospitals in the state submitted data; (11) There were discrepancies in the data collection process; Please refer to the User's Guide for a full explanation of data.

Metrowest Medical Center

115 Lincoln Street
Framingham, MA 01701
E-mail: webmaster@mwmc.com
URL: www.mwmc.com
Type: Acute Care Hospitals
Ownership: Voluntary Non-Profit - Private
Phone: 508-383-1000
Fax: 508-383-1011
Emergency Services: Yes
Beds: 368

Key Personnel:
CEO/President. . . . . Andrei Soran
Cardiac Laboratory. . . . . James Alderman, MD
Emergency Room . . . . Janice Whitney, RN

Measure	Cases	This Hosp.	State Avg.	U.S. Avg.
Heart Attack Care				
ACE Inhibitor or ARB for LVSD	30	100%	94%	96%
Aspirin at Arrival	121	100%	99%	99%
Aspirin at Discharge	107	100%	99%	98%
Beta Blocker at Discharge	104	100%	99%	98%
Fibrinolytic Medication Timing	0	-	50%	55%
PCI Within 90 Minutes of Arrival	42	95%	93%	90%
Smoking Cessation Advice	25	100%	99%	99%
Chest Pain/Possible Heart Attack Care				
Aspirin at Arrival	55	98%	96%	95%
Median Time to ECG (minutes)	56	2	10	8
Median Time to Transfer (minutes)[1,3]	2	84	65	61
Fibrinolytic Medication Timing	0	-	78%	54%
Heart Failure Care				
ACE Inhibitor or ARB for LVSD	154	96%	94%	94%
Discharge Instructions	320	97%	89%	88%
Evaluation of LVS Function	459	99%	98%	98%
Smoking Cessation Advice	41	98%	97%	98%
Pneumonia Care				
Appropriate Initial Antibiotic	231	96%	93%	92%
Blood Culture Timing	209	98%	95%	96%
Influenza Vaccine	204	95%	92%	91%
Initial Antibiotic Timing	327	98%	96%	95%
Pneumococcal Vaccine	303	95%	93%	93%
Smoking Cessation Advice	83	99%	96%	97%
Surgical Care Improvement Project				
Appropriate VTP Within 24 Hours[2]	259	94%	96%	92%
Appropriate Hair Removal[2]	626	100%	100%	99%
Appropriate Beta Blocker Usage[2]	220	98%	96%	93%
Controlled Postoperative Blood Glucose[2]	0	-	95%	93%
Prophylactic Antibiotic Timing[2]	371	94%	97%	97%
Prophylactic Antibiotic Timing (Outpatient)	325	84%	92%	92%
Prophylactic Antibiotic Selection[2]	371	98%	98%	97%
Prophylactic Antibiotic Select. (Outpatient)	290	93%	95%	94%
Prophylactic Antibiotic Stopped[2]	359	97%	96%	94%
Recommended VTP Ordered[2]	259	94%	97%	94%
Urinary Catheter Removal[2]	156	92%	89%	90%
Children's Asthma Care				
Received Systemic Corticosteroids	-	-	-	100%
Received Home Management Plan	-	-	-	71%
Received Reliever Medication	-	-	-	100%
Use of Medical Imaging				
Combination Abdominal CT Scan	1,060	0.087	0.109	0.191
Combination Chest CT Scan	1,024	0.006	0.010	0.054
Follow-up Mammogram/Ultrasound	2,148	17.8%	9.2%	8.4%
MRI for Low Back Pain[5]	0	-	30.1%	32.7%
Survey of Patients' Hospital Experiences				
Area Around Room 'Always' Quiet at Night	300+	54%	-	58%
Doctors 'Always' Communicated Well	300+	80%	-	80%
Home Recovery Information Given	300+	82%	-	82%
Hospital Given 9 or 10 on 10 Point Scale	300+	66%	-	67%
Meds 'Always' Explained Before Given	300+	62%	-	60%
Nurses 'Always' Communicated Well	300+	79%	-	76%
Pain 'Always' Well Controlled	300+	72%	-	69%
Room and Bathroom 'Always' Clean	300+	72%	-	71%
Timely Help 'Always' Received	300+	66%	-	64%
Would Definitely Recommend Hospital	300+	72%	-	69%

Heywood Hospital

242 Green Street
Gardner, MA 01440
Type: Acute Care Hospitals
Ownership: Voluntary Non-Profit - Private
Phone: 978-632-3420
Fax: 978-630-6596
Emergency Services: Yes
Beds: 132

Key Personnel:
CEO/President. . . . . Daniel Moen
Chief of Medical Staff. . . . . Michael Mutchler
Emergency Room . . . . Kunle Fajana, MD

Measure	Cases	This Hosp.	State Avg.	U.S. Avg.
Heart Attack Care				
ACE Inhibitor or ARB for LVSD[1,2]	12	83%	94%	96%
Aspirin at Arrival[2]	49	100%	99%	99%
Aspirin at Discharge[2]	28	89%	99%	98%
Beta Blocker at Discharge[2]	35	97%	99%	98%
Fibrinolytic Medication Timing[2]	0	-	50%	55%
PCI Within 90 Minutes of Arrival[2]	0	-	93%	90%
Smoking Cessation Advice[1,2]	1	100%	99%	99%
Chest Pain/Possible Heart Attack Care				
Aspirin at Arrival	160	98%	96%	95%
Median Time to ECG (minutes)	173	18	10	8
Median Time to Transfer (minutes)[1]	12	95	65	61
Fibrinolytic Medication Timing	0	-	78%	54%
Heart Failure Care				
ACE Inhibitor or ARB for LVSD[2]	25	88%	94%	94%
Discharge Instructions[2]	86	76%	89%	88%
Evaluation of LVS Function[2]	116	93%	98%	98%
Smoking Cessation Advice[2,1]	10	100%	97%	98%
Pneumonia Care				
Appropriate Initial Antibiotic	95	89%	93%	92%
Blood Culture Timing	111	96%	95%	96%
Influenza Vaccine	76	95%	92%	91%
Initial Antibiotic Timing	134	97%	96%	95%
Pneumococcal Vaccine	125	94%	93%	93%
Smoking Cessation Advice	58	90%	96%	97%
Surgical Care Improvement Project				
Appropriate VTP Within 24 Hours	96	85%	96%	92%
Appropriate Hair Removal	282	98%	100%	99%
Appropriate Beta Blocker Usage	87	92%	96%	93%
Controlled Postoperative Blood Glucose	0	-	95%	93%
Prophylactic Antibiotic Timing	232	99%	97%	97%
Prophylactic Antibiotic Timing (Outpatient)	81	48%	92%	92%
Prophylactic Antibiotic Selection	232	98%	98%	97%
Prophylactic Antibiotic Select. (Outpatient)	66	94%	95%	94%
Prophylactic Antibiotic Stopped	226	99%	96%	94%
Recommended VTP Ordered	96	90%	97%	94%
Urinary Catheter Removal	94	82%	89%	90%
Children's Asthma Care				
Received Systemic Corticosteroids	-	-	-	100%
Received Home Management Plan	-	-	-	71%
Received Reliever Medication	-	-	-	100%
Use of Medical Imaging				
Combination Abdominal CT Scan	301	0.020	0.109	0.191
Combination Chest CT Scan	292	0.000	0.010	0.054
Follow-up Mammogram/Ultrasound	596	6.9%	9.2%	8.4%
MRI for Low Back Pain	136	36.0%	30.1%	32.7%
Survey of Patients' Hospital Experiences				
Area Around Room 'Always' Quiet at Night	300+	53%	-	58%
Doctors 'Always' Communicated Well	300+	80%	-	80%
Home Recovery Information Given	300+	86%	-	82%
Hospital Given 9 or 10 on 10 Point Scale	300+	66%	-	67%
Meds 'Always' Explained Before Given	300+	64%	-	60%
Nurses 'Always' Communicated Well	300+	77%	-	76%
Pain 'Always' Well Controlled	300+	75%	-	69%
Room and Bathroom 'Always' Clean	300+	70%	-	71%
Timely Help 'Always' Received	300+	64%	-	64%
Would Definitely Recommend Hospital	300+	73%	-	69%

Fairview Hospital

29 Lewis Avenue
Great Barrington, MA 01230
E-mail: bholcomb@bhsl.org
URL: www.berkshirehealthsystems.com
Type: Critical Access Hospitals
Ownership: Voluntary Non-Profit - Other
Phone: 413-528-0790
Fax: 413-528-0290
Emergency Services: Yes
Beds: 24

Key Personnel:
CEO/President. . . . . Eugene Dellea
Cardiac Laboratory. . . . . Phillip Bhark
Chief of Medical Staff. . . . . Brian Burke
Infection Control. . . . . Geraldine McQuoid
Operating Room. . . . . Donna Wichman
Quality Assurance . . . . Pavani Rangachari
Radiology. . . . . Bob Dillon
Emergency Room . . . . Donna Sena

Measure	Cases	This Hosp.	State Avg.	U.S. Avg.
Heart Attack Care				
ACE Inhibitor or ARB for LVSD[1,3]	2	100%	94%	96%
Aspirin at Arrival[1,3]	8	100%	99%	99%
Aspirin at Discharge[1,3]	7	100%	99%	98%
Beta Blocker at Discharge[1,3]	9	100%	99%	98%
Fibrinolytic Medication Timing[3]	0	-	50%	55%
PCI Within 90 Minutes of Arrival[5]	0	-	93%	90%
Smoking Cessation Advice[3]	0	-	99%	99%
Chest Pain/Possible Heart Attack Care				
Aspirin at Arrival	-	-	96%	95%
Median Time to ECG (minutes)	-	-	10	8
Median Time to Transfer (minutes)	-	-	65	61
Fibrinolytic Medication Timing	-	-	78%	54%
Heart Failure Care				
ACE Inhibitor or ARB for LVSD[1]	17	100%	94%	94%
Discharge Instructions	44	91%	89%	88%
Evaluation of LVS Function	56	100%	98%	98%
Smoking Cessation Advice[1]	6	100%	97%	98%
Pneumonia Care				
Appropriate Initial Antibiotic	38	100%	93%	92%
Blood Culture Timing	63	98%	95%	96%
Influenza Vaccine	42	100%	92%	91%
Initial Antibiotic Timing	59	100%	96%	95%
Pneumococcal Vaccine	65	98%	93%	93%
Smoking Cessation Advice[1]	16	100%	96%	97%
Surgical Care Improvement Project				
Appropriate VTP Within 24 Hours	33	97%	96%	92%
Appropriate Hair Removal	80	100%	100%	99%
Appropriate Beta Blocker Usage	27	96%	96%	93%
Controlled Postoperative Blood Glucose	0	-	95%	93%
Prophylactic Antibiotic Timing	55	100%	97%	97%
Prophylactic Antibiotic Timing (Outpatient)	-	-	92%	92%
Prophylactic Antibiotic Selection	56	100%	98%	97%
Prophylactic Antibiotic Select. (Outpatient)	-	-	95%	94%
Prophylactic Antibiotic Stopped	55	100%	96%	94%
Recommended VTP Ordered	33	97%	97%	94%
Urinary Catheter Removal[1]	7	100%	89%	90%
Children's Asthma Care				
Received Systemic Corticosteroids	-	-	-	100%
Received Home Management Plan	-	-	-	71%
Received Reliever Medication	-	-	-	100%
Use of Medical Imaging				
Combination Abdominal CT Scan	-	-	0.109	0.191
Combination Chest CT Scan	-	-	0.010	0.054
Follow-up Mammogram/Ultrasound	-	-	9.2%	8.4%
MRI for Low Back Pain	-	-	30.1%	32.7%
Survey of Patients' Hospital Experiences				
Area Around Room 'Always' Quiet at Night	300+	61%	-	58%
Doctors 'Always' Communicated Well	300+	84%	-	80%
Home Recovery Information Given	300+	88%	-	82%
Hospital Given 9 or 10 on 10 Point Scale	300+	85%	-	67%
Meds 'Always' Explained Before Given	300+	76%	-	60%
Nurses 'Always' Communicated Well	300+	87%	-	76%
Pain 'Always' Well Controlled	300+	79%	-	69%
Room and Bathroom 'Always' Clean	300+	86%	-	71%
Timely Help 'Always' Received	300+	84%	-	64%
Would Definitely Recommend Hospital	300+	88%	-	69%

NOTE: Hospital profiles are in alphabetical order by state, then city, then hospital within the city; Rankings exclude hospitals with less than 25 cases except for patient surveys which excludes hospitals with less than 100 cases; (a) 100–299 cases; (1) The number of cases is too small to be sure how well a hospital is performing; (2) The hospital indicated that the data submitted for this measure were based on a sample of cases; (3) Data was collected during a shorter time period (fewer quarters) than the maximum possible time for this measure; (4) Suppressed for one or more quarters by CMS; (5) No data is available from the hospital for this measure; (6) Fewer than 100 patients completed the HCAHPS survey. Use these rates with caution, as the number of surveys may be too low to reliably assess hospital performance; (7) Survey results are based on less than 12 months of data; (8) Survey results are not available for this reporting period; (9) No or very few patients were eligible for the HCAHPS survey. The scores shown, if any, reflect a very small number of surveys; (10) A state average was not calculated because too few hospitals in the state submitted data; (11) There were discrepancies in the data collection process; Please refer to the User's Guide for a full explanation of data.

Baystate Franklin Medical Center

164 High Street
Greenfield, MA 01301
URL: www.baystatehealth.com
Type: Acute Care Hospitals
Ownership: Voluntary Non-Profit - Private

Phone: 413-773-0211

Emergency Services: Yes
Beds: 93

Key Personnel:
CEO/President . . . . Chuck Gijanto

Measure	Cases	This Hosp.	State Avg.	U.S. Avg.
Heart Attack Care				
ACE Inhibitor or ARB for LVSD[1]	3	100%	94%	96%
Aspirin at Arrival	29	97%	99%	99%
Aspirin at Discharge[1]	15	93%	99%	98%
Beta Blocker at Discharge[1]	17	100%	99%	98%
Fibrinolytic Medication Timing[1]	2	50%	50%	55%
PCI Within 90 Minutes of Arrival	0	-	93%	90%
Smoking Cessation Advice[1]	1	100%	99%	99%
Chest Pain/Possible Heart Attack Care				
Aspirin at Arrival	45	98%	96%	95%
Median Time to ECG (minutes)	48	7	10	8
Median Time to Transfer (minutes)[1,3]	6	70	65	61
Fibrinolytic Medication Timing[1]	11	73%	78%	54%
Heart Failure Care				
ACE Inhibitor or ARB for LVSD[1]	23	100%	94%	94%
Discharge Instructions	99	95%	89%	88%
Evaluation of LVS Function	143	97%	98%	98%
Smoking Cessation Advice[1]	20	100%	97%	98%
Pneumonia Care				
Appropriate Initial Antibiotic	78	95%	93%	92%
Blood Culture Timing	137	96%	95%	96%
Influenza Vaccine	76	93%	92%	91%
Initial Antibiotic Timing	133	94%	96%	95%
Pneumococcal Vaccine	133	94%	93%	93%
Smoking Cessation Advice	29	100%	96%	97%
Surgical Care Improvement Project				
Appropriate VTP Within 24 Hours[2]	141	96%	96%	92%
Appropriate Hair Removal[2]	205	100%	100%	99%
Appropriate Beta Blocker Usage[2]	64	94%	96%	93%
Controlled Postoperative Blood Glucose[2]	0	-	95%	93%
Prophylactic Antibiotic Timing[2]	119	98%	97%	97%
Prophylactic Antibiotic Timing (Outpatient)	85	98%	92%	92%
Prophylactic Antibiotic Selection[2]	119	99%	98%	97%
Prophylactic Antibiotic Select. (Outpatient)	84	93%	95%	94%
Prophylactic Antibiotic Stopped[2]	115	94%	96%	94%
Recommended VTP Ordered[2]	141	99%	97%	94%
Urinary Catheter Removal	32	69%	89%	90%
Children's Asthma Care				
Received Systemic Corticosteroids	-	-	-	100%
Received Home Management Plan	-	-	-	71%
Received Reliever Medication	-	-	-	100%
Use of Medical Imaging				
Combination Abdominal CT Scan	705	0.132	0.109	0.191
Combination Chest CT Scan	419	0.002	0.010	0.054
Follow-up Mammogram/Ultrasound	575	8.2%	9.2%	8.4%
MRI for Low Back Pain[1]	2	0.0%	30.1%	32.7%
Survey of Patients' Hospital Experiences				
Area Around Room 'Always' Quiet at Night	300+	49%	-	58%
Doctors 'Always' Communicated Well	300+	76%	-	80%
Home Recovery Information Given	300+	85%	-	82%
Hospital Given 9 or 10 on 10 Point Scale	300+	64%	-	67%
Meds 'Always' Explained Before Given	300+	60%	-	60%
Nurses 'Always' Communicated Well	300+	77%	-	76%
Pain 'Always' Well Controlled	300+	67%	-	69%
Room and Bathroom 'Always' Clean	300+	66%	-	71%
Timely Help 'Always' Received	300+	64%	-	64%
Would Definitely Recommend Hospital	300+	70%	-	69%

Merrimack Valley Hospital

140 Lincoln Avenue
Haverhill, MA 01830
E-mail: lester.schindel@merrimackvalleyhospital.com
URL: www.merrimackvalleyhospital.com
Type: Acute Care Hospitals
Ownership: Proprietary

Phone: 978-374-2000
Fax: 978-521-8138

Emergency Services: Yes
Beds: 108

Key Personnel:
CEO/President . . . . Michael Collins
Chief of Medical Staff . . . . George F Kwass, MD
Infection Control . . . . Doris Bobryk-Rana, RN
Operating Room . . . . Cheryl Durkee, RN
Quality Assurance . . . . Gloria Swanbon
Radiology . . . . Lawrence M Casha MD, MD

Measure	Cases	This Hosp.	State Avg.	U.S. Avg.
Heart Attack Care				
ACE Inhibitor or ARB for LVSD[1]	3	67%	94%	96%
Aspirin at Arrival	41	95%	99%	99%
Aspirin at Discharge	31	97%	99%	98%
Beta Blocker at Discharge	29	100%	99%	98%
Fibrinolytic Medication Timing	0	-	50%	55%
PCI Within 90 Minutes of Arrival	0	-	93%	90%
Smoking Cessation Advice[1]	5	100%	99%	99%
Chest Pain/Possible Heart Attack Care				
Aspirin at Arrival	46	98%	96%	95%
Median Time to ECG (minutes)	49	7	10	8
Median Time to Transfer (minutes)[1]	17	51	65	61
Fibrinolytic Medication Timing	0	-	78%	54%
Heart Failure Care				
ACE Inhibitor or ARB for LVSD	36	92%	94%	94%
Discharge Instructions	122	98%	89%	88%
Evaluation of LVS Function	193	98%	98%	98%
Smoking Cessation Advice	26	100%	97%	98%
Pneumonia Care				
Appropriate Initial Antibiotic	105	90%	93%	92%
Blood Culture Timing	168	94%	95%	96%
Influenza Vaccine	87	93%	92%	91%
Initial Antibiotic Timing	152	99%	96%	95%
Pneumococcal Vaccine	140	91%	93%	93%
Smoking Cessation Advice	47	100%	96%	97%
Surgical Care Improvement Project				
Appropriate VTP Within 24 Hours	82	94%	96%	92%
Appropriate Hair Removal	191	100%	100%	99%
Appropriate Beta Blocker Usage	62	100%	96%	93%
Controlled Postoperative Blood Glucose	0	-	95%	93%
Prophylactic Antibiotic Timing	124	96%	97%	97%
Prophylactic Antibiotic Timing (Outpatient)	31	87%	92%	92%
Prophylactic Antibiotic Selection	124	98%	98%	97%
Prophylactic Antibiotic Select. (Outpatient)	28	79%	95%	94%
Prophylactic Antibiotic Stopped	122	98%	96%	94%
Recommended VTP Ordered	82	94%	97%	94%
Urinary Catheter Removal	41	88%	89%	90%
Children's Asthma Care				
Received Systemic Corticosteroids	-	-	-	100%
Received Home Management Plan	-	-	-	71%
Received Reliever Medication	-	-	-	100%
Use of Medical Imaging				
Combination Abdominal CT Scan	498	0.064	0.109	0.191
Combination Chest CT Scan	372	0.016	0.010	0.054
Follow-up Mammogram/Ultrasound	1,126	11.5%	9.2%	8.4%
MRI for Low Back Pain	119	36.1%	30.1%	32.7%
Survey of Patients' Hospital Experiences				
Area Around Room 'Always' Quiet at Night	300+	46%	-	58%
Doctors 'Always' Communicated Well	300+	78%	-	80%
Home Recovery Information Given	300+	87%	-	82%
Hospital Given 9 or 10 on 10 Point Scale	300+	64%	-	67%
Meds 'Always' Explained Before Given	300+	59%	-	60%
Nurses 'Always' Communicated Well	300+	74%	-	76%
Pain 'Always' Well Controlled	300+	70%	-	69%
Room and Bathroom 'Always' Clean	300+	66%	-	71%
Timely Help 'Always' Received	300+	62%	-	64%
Would Definitely Recommend Hospital	300+	63%	-	69%

Holyoke Medical Center

575 Beech Street
Holyoke, MA 01040
URL: www.holyokehealth.com
Type: Acute Care Hospitals
Ownership: Voluntary Non-Profit - Private

Phone: 413-534-2500
Fax: 413-534-2664

Emergency Services: Yes
Beds: 202

Key Personnel:
CEO/President . . . . Hank J Porten
Chief of Medical Staff . . . . M Saleem Bajwa
Operating Room . . . . Brigid Glackin
Quality Assurance . . . . Clark Fenn
Radiology . . . . Won Park
Emergency Room . . . . Joseph Chang

Measure	Cases	This Hosp.	State Avg.	U.S. Avg.
Heart Attack Care				
ACE Inhibitor or ARB for LVSD[1]	14	93%	94%	96%
Aspirin at Arrival	110	95%	99%	99%
Aspirin at Discharge	69	94%	99%	98%
Beta Blocker at Discharge	71	96%	99%	98%
Fibrinolytic Medication Timing	0	-	50%	55%
PCI Within 90 Minutes of Arrival	0	-	93%	90%
Smoking Cessation Advice[1]	6	83%	99%	99%
Chest Pain/Possible Heart Attack Care				
Aspirin at Arrival	49	94%	96%	95%
Median Time to ECG (minutes)	50	13	10	8
Median Time to Transfer (minutes)[1]	21	65	65	61
Fibrinolytic Medication Timing	0	-	78%	54%
Heart Failure Care				
ACE Inhibitor or ARB for LVSD	53	87%	94%	94%
Discharge Instructions	123	85%	89%	88%
Evaluation of LVS Function	191	100%	98%	98%
Smoking Cessation Advice	26	92%	97%	98%
Pneumonia Care				
Appropriate Initial Antibiotic	108	87%	93%	92%
Blood Culture Timing	201	91%	95%	96%
Influenza Vaccine	121	98%	92%	91%
Initial Antibiotic Timing	188	93%	96%	95%
Pneumococcal Vaccine	159	96%	93%	93%
Smoking Cessation Advice	66	83%	96%	97%
Surgical Care Improvement Project				
Appropriate VTP Within 24 Hours	114	85%	96%	92%
Appropriate Hair Removal	234	100%	100%	99%
Appropriate Beta Blocker Usage	69	91%	96%	93%
Controlled Postoperative Blood Glucose	0	-	95%	93%
Prophylactic Antibiotic Timing	147	96%	97%	97%
Prophylactic Antibiotic Timing (Outpatient)	84	96%	92%	92%
Prophylactic Antibiotic Selection	146	100%	98%	97%
Prophylactic Antibiotic Select. (Outpatient)	82	98%	95%	94%
Prophylactic Antibiotic Stopped	138	95%	96%	94%
Recommended VTP Ordered	114	88%	97%	94%
Urinary Catheter Removal	46	76%	89%	90%
Children's Asthma Care				
Received Systemic Corticosteroids	-	-	-	100%
Received Home Management Plan	-	-	-	71%
Received Reliever Medication	-	-	-	100%
Use of Medical Imaging				
Combination Abdominal CT Scan	865	0.053	0.109	0.191
Combination Chest CT Scan	315	0.000	0.010	0.054
Follow-up Mammogram/Ultrasound	1,546	6.5%	9.2%	8.4%
MRI for Low Back Pain	222	36.0%	30.1%	32.7%
Survey of Patients' Hospital Experiences				
Area Around Room 'Always' Quiet at Night	300+	53%	-	58%
Doctors 'Always' Communicated Well	300+	75%	-	80%
Home Recovery Information Given	300+	87%	-	82%
Hospital Given 9 or 10 on 10 Point Scale	300+	60%	-	67%
Meds 'Always' Explained Before Given	300+	59%	-	60%
Nurses 'Always' Communicated Well	300+	73%	-	76%
Pain 'Always' Well Controlled	300+	67%	-	69%
Room and Bathroom 'Always' Clean	300+	75%	-	71%
Timely Help 'Always' Received	300+	55%	-	64%
Would Definitely Recommend Hospital	300+	68%	-	69%

Cape Cod Hospital

88 Lewis Bay Road Phone: 508-771-1800
Hyannis, MA 02601 Fax: 508-790-7964
URL: www.capecodhealth.org
Type: Acute Care Hospitals Emergency Services: Yes
Ownership: Voluntary Non-Profit - Private Beds: 272

Key Personnel:
CEO/President. . . . . Richard Salluzzo
Chief of Medical Staff . . . . James Butterick
Operating Room. . . . . Bonnie Finkle, RN
Pediatric Ambulatory Care . . . . . . Kenneth Colmer, MD
Pediatric In-Patient Care . . . . Kenneth Colmer, MD
Radiology. . . . . Gordan Kanzer, MD
Emergency Room . . . . Dwayne Hendrick

Measure	Cases	This Hosp.	State Avg.	U.S. Avg.
Heart Attack Care				
ACE Inhibitor or ARB for LVSD[2]	38	82%	94%	96%
Aspirin at Arrival[2]	256	99%	99%	99%
Aspirin at Discharge[2]	289	99%	99%	98%
Beta Blocker at Discharge[2]	276	98%	99%	98%
Fibrinolytic Medication Timing[2]	0	-	50%	55%
PCI Within 90 Minutes of Arrival[2]	37	100%	93%	90%
Smoking Cessation Advice[2]	65	92%	99%	99%
Chest Pain/Possible Heart Attack Care				
Aspirin at Arrival[1]	18	94%	96%	95%
Median Time to ECG (minutes)[1]	19	5	10	8
Median Time to Transfer (minutes)[5]	0	-	65	61
Fibrinolytic Medication Timing[5]	0	-	78%	54%
Heart Failure Care				
ACE Inhibitor or ARB for LVSD[2]	87	79%	94%	94%
Discharge Instructions[2]	192	73%	89%	88%
Evaluation of LVS Function[2]	295	100%	98%	98%
Smoking Cessation Advice[2]	31	84%	97%	98%
Pneumonia Care				
Appropriate Initial Antibiotic	214	92%	93%	92%
Blood Culture Timing	251	91%	95%	96%
Influenza Vaccine	173	95%	92%	91%
Initial Antibiotic Timing	284	98%	96%	95%
Pneumococcal Vaccine	301	93%	93%	93%
Smoking Cessation Advice	80	92%	96%	97%
Surgical Care Improvement Project				
Appropriate VTP Within 24 Hours[2]	360	99%	96%	92%
Appropriate Hair Removal[2]	1,174	100%	100%	99%
Appropriate Beta Blocker Usage[2]	404	95%	96%	93%
Controlled Postoperative Blood Glucose[2]	184	93%	95%	93%
Prophylactic Antibiotic Timing[2]	969	99%	97%	97%
Prophylactic Antibiotic Timing (Outpatient)	470	96%	92%	92%
Prophylactic Antibiotic Selection[2]	979	98%	98%	97%
Prophylactic Antibiotic Select. (Outpatient)	465	95%	95%	94%
Prophylactic Antibiotic Stopped[2]	943	97%	96%	94%
Recommended VTP Ordered[2]	360	99%	97%	94%
Urinary Catheter Removal[2]	321	94%	89%	90%
Children's Asthma Care				
Received Systemic Corticosteroids	-	-	-	100%
Received Home Management Plan	-	-	-	71%
Received Reliever Medication	-	-	-	100%
Use of Medical Imaging				
Combination Abdominal CT Scan	2,516	0.098	0.109	0.191
Combination Chest CT Scan	2,213	0.018	0.010	0.054
Follow-up Mammogram/Ultrasound	3,645	16.8%	9.2%	8.4%
MRI for Low Back Pain	587	31.3%	30.1%	32.7%
Survey of Patients' Hospital Experiences				
Area Around Room 'Always' Quiet at Night	300+	51%	-	58%
Doctors 'Always' Communicated Well	300+	81%	-	80%
Home Recovery Information Given	300+	84%	-	82%
Hospital Given 9 or 10 on 10 Point Scale	300+	76%	-	67%
Meds 'Always' Explained Before Given	300+	63%	-	60%
Nurses 'Always' Communicated Well	300+	80%	-	76%
Pain 'Always' Well Controlled	300+	72%	-	69%
Room and Bathroom 'Always' Clean	300+	78%	-	71%
Timely Help 'Always' Received	300+	64%	-	64%
Would Definitely Recommend Hospital	300+	81%	-	69%

VA Boston Healthcare System - Jamaica Plain

150 S. Huntington Avenue Phone: 617-232-9500
Jamaica Plain, MA 02130
URL: www.vaww.visn1.med.va.gov/boston
Type: Acute Care-Veterans Administration Emergency Services: No
Ownership: Government - Federal Beds: 376

Key Personnel:
Chief of Medical Staff . . . . Michael E Charness, MD
Quality Assurance . . . . Lynn Cannavho, RN
Emergency Room . . . . Arthur Robins, MD

Measure	Cases	This Hosp.	State Avg.	U.S. Avg.
Heart Attack Care				
ACE Inhibitor or ARB for LVSD[5]	0	-	94%	96%
Aspirin at Arrival[5]	0	-	99%	99%
Aspirin at Discharge[5]	0	-	99%	98%
Beta Blocker at Discharge[5]	0	-	99%	98%
Fibrinolytic Medication Timing[5]	0	-	50%	55%
PCI Within 90 Minutes of Arrival[5]	0	-	93%	90%
Smoking Cessation Advice[5]	0	-	99%	99%
Chest Pain/Possible Heart Attack Care				
Aspirin at Arrival	-	-	96%	95%
Median Time to ECG (minutes)	-	-	10	8
Median Time to Transfer (minutes)	-	-	65	61
Fibrinolytic Medication Timing	-	-	78%	54%
Heart Failure Care				
ACE Inhibitor or ARB for LVSD	97	88%	94%	94%
Discharge Instructions	236	100%	89%	88%
Evaluation of LVS Function	289	100%	98%	98%
Smoking Cessation Advice	27	100%	97%	98%
Pneumonia Care				
Appropriate Initial Antibiotic	87	97%	93%	92%
Blood Culture Timing	112	96%	95%	96%
Influenza Vaccine	135	99%	92%	91%
Initial Antibiotic Timing	124	94%	96%	95%
Pneumococcal Vaccine	143	99%	93%	93%
Smoking Cessation Advice	45	100%	96%	97%
Surgical Care Improvement Project				
Appropriate VTP Within 24 Hours[2]	239	100%	96%	92%
Appropriate Hair Removal[2]	510	100%	100%	99%
Appropriate Beta Blocker Usage[2]	272	100%	96%	93%
Controlled Postoperative Blood Glucose[2]	151	86%	95%	93%
Prophylactic Antibiotic Timing	397	100%	97%	97%
Prophylactic Antibiotic Timing (Outpatient)	-	-	92%	92%
Prophylactic Antibiotic Selection	402	98%	98%	97%
Prophylactic Antibiotic Select. (Outpatient)	-	-	95%	94%
Prophylactic Antibiotic Stopped	397	100%	96%	94%
Recommended VTP Ordered[2]	239	100%	97%	94%
Urinary Catheter Removal[2]	185	100%	89%	90%
Children's Asthma Care				
Received Systemic Corticosteroids	-	-	-	100%
Received Home Management Plan	-	-	-	71%
Received Reliever Medication	-	-	-	100%
Use of Medical Imaging				
Combination Abdominal CT Scan	-	-	0.109	0.191
Combination Chest CT Scan	-	-	0.010	0.054
Follow-up Mammogram/Ultrasound	-	-	9.2%	8.4%
MRI for Low Back Pain	-	-	30.1%	32.7%
Survey of Patients' Hospital Experiences				
Area Around Room 'Always' Quiet at Night	-	-	-	58%
Doctors 'Always' Communicated Well	-	-	-	80%
Home Recovery Information Given	-	-	-	82%
Hospital Given 9 or 10 on 10 Point Scale	-	-	-	67%
Meds 'Always' Explained Before Given	-	-	-	60%
Nurses 'Always' Communicated Well	-	-	-	76%
Pain 'Always' Well Controlled	-	-	-	69%
Room and Bathroom 'Always' Clean	-	-	-	71%
Timely Help 'Always' Received	-	-	-	64%
Would Definitely Recommend Hospital	-	-	-	69%

Lawrence General Hospital

One General Street Phone: 978-683-4000
Lawrence, MA 01842 Fax: 978-946-8175
URL: www.lawrencegeneral.org
Type: Acute Care Hospitals Emergency Services: Yes
Ownership: Voluntary Non-Profit - Private Beds: 190

Key Personnel:
CEO/President. . . . . Joseph S McManus
Chief of Medical Staff . . . . Brian Callahan
Quality Assurance . . . . Janet Nelson
Emergency Room . . . . Patrick Curran

Measure	Cases	This Hosp.	State Avg.	U.S. Avg.
Heart Attack Care				
ACE Inhibitor or ARB for LVSD[1]	14	93%	94%	96%
Aspirin at Arrival	102	99%	99%	99%
Aspirin at Discharge	74	99%	99%	98%
Beta Blocker at Discharge	75	100%	99%	98%
Fibrinolytic Medication Timing	0	-	50%	55%
PCI Within 90 Minutes of Arrival	36	92%	93%	90%
Smoking Cessation Advice[1]	13	92%	99%	99%
Chest Pain/Possible Heart Attack Care				
Aspirin at Arrival	60	93%	96%	95%
Median Time to ECG (minutes)	61	13	10	8
Median Time to Transfer (minutes)[1,3]	1	71	65	61
Fibrinolytic Medication Timing	0	-	78%	54%
Heart Failure Care				
ACE Inhibitor or ARB for LVSD	119	79%	94%	94%
Discharge Instructions	282	70%	89%	88%
Evaluation of LVS Function	408	92%	98%	98%
Smoking Cessation Advice	41	100%	97%	98%
Pneumonia Care				
Appropriate Initial Antibiotic	127	86%	93%	92%
Blood Culture Timing	160	94%	95%	96%
Influenza Vaccine	125	78%	92%	91%
Initial Antibiotic Timing	220	93%	96%	95%
Pneumococcal Vaccine	205	95%	93%	93%
Smoking Cessation Advice	61	85%	96%	97%
Surgical Care Improvement Project				
Appropriate VTP Within 24 Hours	145	79%	96%	92%
Appropriate Hair Removal	301	95%	100%	99%
Appropriate Beta Blocker Usage	86	93%	96%	93%
Controlled Postoperative Blood Glucose	0	-	95%	93%
Prophylactic Antibiotic Timing	137	98%	97%	97%
Prophylactic Antibiotic Timing (Outpatient)	85	71%	92%	92%
Prophylactic Antibiotic Selection	146	88%	98%	97%
Prophylactic Antibiotic Select. (Outpatient)	81	93%	95%	94%
Prophylactic Antibiotic Stopped	131	90%	96%	94%
Recommended VTP Ordered	145	83%	97%	94%
Urinary Catheter Removal	50	58%	89%	90%
Children's Asthma Care				
Received Systemic Corticosteroids	-	-	-	100%
Received Home Management Plan	-	-	-	71%
Received Reliever Medication	-	-	-	100%
Use of Medical Imaging				
Combination Abdominal CT Scan	782	0.072	0.109	0.191
Combination Chest CT Scan	467	0.032	0.010	0.054
Follow-up Mammogram/Ultrasound	729	11.4%	9.2%	8.4%
MRI for Low Back Pain[5]	0	-	30.1%	32.7%
Survey of Patients' Hospital Experiences				
Area Around Room 'Always' Quiet at Night	300+	50%	-	58%
Doctors 'Always' Communicated Well	300+	78%	-	80%
Home Recovery Information Given	300+	81%	-	82%
Hospital Given 9 or 10 on 10 Point Scale	300+	57%	-	67%
Meds 'Always' Explained Before Given	300+	63%	-	60%
Nurses 'Always' Communicated Well	300+	75%	-	76%
Pain 'Always' Well Controlled	300+	72%	-	69%
Room and Bathroom 'Always' Clean	300+	67%	-	71%
Timely Help 'Always' Received	300+	60%	-	64%
Would Definitely Recommend Hospital	300+	68%	-	69%

NOTE: Hospital profiles are in alphabetical order by state, then city, then hospital within the city; Rankings exclude hospitals with less than 25 cases except for patient surveys which excludes hospitals with less than 100 cases; (a) 100–299 cases; (1) The number of cases is too small to be sure how well a hospital is performing; (2) The hospital indicated that the data submitted for this measure were based on a sample of cases; (3) Data was collected during a shorter time period (fewer quarters) than the maximum possible time for this measure; (4) Suppressed for one or more quarters by CMS; (5) No data is available from the hospital for this measure; (6) Fewer than 100 patients completed the HCAHPS survey. Use these rates with caution, as the number of surveys may be too low to reliably assess hospital performance; (7) Survey results are based on less than 12 months of data; (8) Survey results are not available for this reporting period; (9) No or very few patients were eligible for the HCAHPS survey. The scores shown, if any, reflect a very small number of surveys; (10) A state average was not calculated because too few hospitals in the state submitted data; (11) There were discrepancies in the data collection process; Please refer to the User's Guide for a full explanation of data.

Northampton VA Medical Center

421 N Main St
Leeds, MA 01053
E-mail: lastname.firstname@med.va.gov
URL: www.visn1.med.va.gov/northampton
Type: Acute Care-Veterans Administration
Ownership: Government - Federal

Phone: 413-584-4040
Fax: 413-582-3040

Emergency Services: No
Beds: 167

Key Personnel:
CEO/President . . . . Mary A Dowling
Chief of Medical Staff . . . . George Fuller MD
Infection Control . . . . Don Braman
Quality Assurance . . . . Michael Walsh
Patient Relations . . . . Rosemary Westerman

Measure	Cases	This Hosp.	State Avg.	U.S. Avg.
Heart Attack Care				
ACE Inhibitor or ARB for LVSD[5]	0	-	94%	96%
Aspirin at Arrival[5]	0	-	99%	99%
Aspirin at Discharge[5]	0	-	99%	98%
Beta Blocker at Discharge[5]	0	-	99%	98%
Fibrinolytic Medication Timing[5]	0	-	50%	55%
PCI Within 90 Minutes of Arrival[5]	0	-	93%	90%
Smoking Cessation Advice[5]	0	-	99%	99%
Chest Pain/Possible Heart Attack Care				
Aspirin at Arrival	-		96%	95%
Median Time to ECG (minutes)	-		10	8
Median Time to Transfer (minutes)	-		65	61
Fibrinolytic Medication Timing	-		78%	54%
Heart Failure Care				
ACE Inhibitor or ARB for LVSD[5]	0	-	94%	94%
Discharge Instructions[5]	0	-	89%	88%
Evaluation of LVS Function[5]	0	-	98%	98%
Smoking Cessation Advice[5]	0	-	97%	98%
Pneumonia Care				
Appropriate Initial Antibiotic[5]	0	-	93%	92%
Blood Culture Timing[5]	0	-	95%	96%
Influenza Vaccine[5]	0	-	92%	91%
Initial Antibiotic Timing[5]	0	-	96%	95%
Pneumococcal Vaccine[5]	0	-	93%	93%
Smoking Cessation Advice[5]	0	-	96%	97%
Surgical Care Improvement Project				
Appropriate VTP Within 24 Hours[2,5]	0	-	96%	92%
Appropriate Hair Removal[2,5]	0	-	100%	99%
Appropriate Beta Blocker Usage[2,5]	0	-	96%	93%
Controlled Postoperative Blood Glucose[2,5]	0	-	95%	93%
Prophylactic Antibiotic Timing[5]	0	-	97%	97%
Prophylactic Antibiotic Timing (Outpatient)	-		92%	92%
Prophylactic Antibiotic Selection[5]	0	-	98%	97%
Prophylactic Antibiotic Select. (Outpatient)	-		95%	94%
Prophylactic Antibiotic Stopped[5]	0	-	96%	94%
Recommended VTP Ordered[2,5]	0	-	97%	94%
Urinary Catheter Removal[2,5]	0	-	89%	90%
Children's Asthma Care				
Received Systemic Corticosteroids	-	-		100%
Received Home Management Plan	-	-		71%
Received Reliever Medication	-	-		100%
Use of Medical Imaging				
Combination Abdominal CT Scan	-	-	0.109	0.191
Combination Chest CT Scan	-	-	0.010	0.054
Follow-up Mammogram/Ultrasound	-	-	9.2%	8.4%
MRI for Low Back Pain	-	-	30.1%	32.7%
Survey of Patients' Hospital Experiences				
Area Around Room 'Always' Quiet at Night	-	-		58%
Doctors 'Always' Communicated Well	-	-		80%
Home Recovery Information Given	-	-		82%
Hospital Given 9 or 10 on 10 Point Scale	-	-		67%
Meds 'Always' Explained Before Given	-	-		60%
Nurses 'Always' Communicated Well	-	-		76%
Pain 'Always' Well Controlled	-	-		69%
Room and Bathroom 'Always' Clean	-	-		71%
Timely Help 'Always' Received	-	-		64%
Would Definitely Recommend Hospital	-	-		69%

Healthalliance Hospitals

60 Hospital Road
Leominster, MA 01453
URL: www.healthalliance.com
Type: Acute Care Hospitals
Ownership: Voluntary Non-Profit - Other

Phone: 978-466-2000
Fax: 978-466-2200

Emergency Services: Yes
Beds: 154

Key Personnel:
CEO/President . . . . Patrick Muldoon
Chief of Medical Staff . . . . Val Slayton, MD
Operating Room . . . . Benjamin Grajales
Quality Assurance . . . . Cathy Hawke
Radiology . . . . Daniel P Berman

Measure	Cases	This Hosp.	State Avg.	U.S. Avg.
Heart Attack Care				
ACE Inhibitor or ARB for LVSD[1]	5	100%	94%	96%
Aspirin at Arrival	96	100%	99%	99%
Aspirin at Discharge	69	99%	99%	98%
Beta Blocker at Discharge	74	99%	99%	98%
Fibrinolytic Medication Timing	0	-	50%	55%
PCI Within 90 Minutes of Arrival	0	-	93%	90%
Smoking Cessation Advice[1]	18	100%	99%	99%
Chest Pain/Possible Heart Attack Care				
Aspirin at Arrival	159	97%	96%	95%
Median Time to ECG (minutes)	159	7	10	8
Median Time to Transfer (minutes)	29	57	65	61
Fibrinolytic Medication Timing	0	-	78%	54%
Heart Failure Care				
ACE Inhibitor or ARB for LVSD	41	95%	94%	94%
Discharge Instructions	205	87%	89%	88%
Evaluation of LVS Function	271	99%	98%	98%
Smoking Cessation Advice	28	100%	97%	98%
Pneumonia Care				
Appropriate Initial Antibiotic	143	90%	93%	92%
Blood Culture Timing	275	97%	95%	96%
Influenza Vaccine	148	99%	92%	91%
Initial Antibiotic Timing	241	97%	96%	95%
Pneumococcal Vaccine	206	98%	93%	93%
Smoking Cessation Advice	75	95%	96%	97%
Surgical Care Improvement Project				
Appropriate VTP Within 24 Hours	186	95%	96%	92%
Appropriate Hair Removal	404	100%	100%	99%
Appropriate Beta Blocker Usage	124	94%	96%	93%
Controlled Postoperative Blood Glucose	0	-	95%	93%
Prophylactic Antibiotic Timing	283	97%	97%	97%
Prophylactic Antibiotic Timing (Outpatient)	86	88%	92%	92%
Prophylactic Antibiotic Selection	283	100%	98%	97%
Prophylactic Antibiotic Select. (Outpatient)	89	91%	95%	94%
Prophylactic Antibiotic Stopped	272	97%	96%	94%
Recommended VTP Ordered	186	97%	97%	94%
Urinary Catheter Removal	98	96%	89%	90%
Children's Asthma Care				
Received Systemic Corticosteroids	-	-		100%
Received Home Management Plan	-	-		71%
Received Reliever Medication	-	-		100%
Use of Medical Imaging				
Combination Abdominal CT Scan	601	0.042	0.109	0.191
Combination Chest CT Scan	520	0.004	0.010	0.054
Follow-up Mammogram/Ultrasound	1,107	7.2%	9.2%	8.4%
MRI for Low Back Pain	0	-	30.1%	32.7%
Survey of Patients' Hospital Experiences				
Area Around Room 'Always' Quiet at Night	300+	50%	-	58%
Doctors 'Always' Communicated Well	300+	79%	-	80%
Home Recovery Information Given	300+	88%	-	82%
Hospital Given 9 or 10 on 10 Point Scale	300+	60%	-	67%
Meds 'Always' Explained Before Given	300+	62%	-	60%
Nurses 'Always' Communicated Well	300+	78%	-	76%
Pain 'Always' Well Controlled	300+	71%	-	69%
Room and Bathroom 'Always' Clean	300+	72%	-	71%
Timely Help 'Always' Received	300+	62%	-	64%
Would Definitely Recommend Hospital	300+	65%	-	69%

Lowell General Hospital

295 Varnum Avenue
Lowell, MA 01854
URL: www.lowellgeneral.org
Type: Acute Care Hospitals
Ownership: Voluntary Non-Profit - Private

Phone: 978-937-6000
Fax: 978-452-4169

Emergency Services: Yes
Beds: 208

Key Personnel:
CEO/President . . . . Normand E Deschene
Chief of Medical Staff . . . . Wayne E Pasanen, MD
Coronary Care . . . . Patricia Morse
Infection Control . . . . Karen Kennet
Operating Room . . . . Nicholas Spirito
Pediatric Ambulatory Care . . . . . Michelle Saboliauskas
Quality Assurance . . . . Gina O'Connor
Radiology . . . . Scott D Abel

Measure	Cases	This Hosp.	State Avg.	U.S. Avg.
Heart Attack Care				
ACE Inhibitor or ARB for LVSD[1]	20	100%	94%	96%
Aspirin at Arrival	137	100%	99%	99%
Aspirin at Discharge	115	100%	99%	98%
Beta Blocker at Discharge	121	100%	99%	98%
Fibrinolytic Medication Timing	0	-	50%	55%
PCI Within 90 Minutes of Arrival	43	98%	93%	90%
Smoking Cessation Advice	27	100%	99%	99%
Chest Pain/Possible Heart Attack Care				
Aspirin at Arrival[1]	8	88%	96%	95%
Median Time to ECG (minutes)[1]	8	6	10	8
Median Time to Transfer (minutes)[5]	0	-	65	61
Fibrinolytic Medication Timing[3]	0	-	78%	54%
Heart Failure Care				
ACE Inhibitor or ARB for LVSD[2]	59	93%	94%	94%
Discharge Instructions[2]	249	76%	89%	88%
Evaluation of LVS Function[2]	329	97%	98%	98%
Smoking Cessation Advice[2]	30	83%	97%	98%
Pneumonia Care				
Appropriate Initial Antibiotic[2]	146	97%	93%	92%
Blood Culture Timing[2]	143	92%	95%	96%
Influenza Vaccine[2]	78	94%	92%	91%
Initial Antibiotic Timing[2]	187	96%	96%	95%
Pneumococcal Vaccine[2]	157	87%	93%	93%
Smoking Cessation Advice[2]	60	93%	96%	97%
Surgical Care Improvement Project				
Appropriate VTP Within 24 Hours[2]	172	92%	96%	92%
Appropriate Hair Removal[2]	606	100%	100%	99%
Appropriate Beta Blocker Usage[2]	201	94%	96%	93%
Controlled Postoperative Blood Glucose[2]	0	-	95%	93%
Prophylactic Antibiotic Timing[2]	428	97%	97%	97%
Prophylactic Antibiotic Timing (Outpatient)	290	93%	92%	92%
Prophylactic Antibiotic Selection[2]	429	98%	98%	97%
Prophylactic Antibiotic Select. (Outpatient)	283	98%	95%	94%
Prophylactic Antibiotic Stopped[2]	404	93%	96%	94%
Recommended VTP Ordered[2]	172	93%	97%	94%
Urinary Catheter Removal[2]	107	98%	89%	90%
Children's Asthma Care				
Received Systemic Corticosteroids	-	-		100%
Received Home Management Plan	-	-		71%
Received Reliever Medication	-	-		100%
Use of Medical Imaging				
Combination Abdominal CT Scan	1,021	0.048	0.109	0.191
Combination Chest CT Scan	683	0.001	0.010	0.054
Follow-up Mammogram/Ultrasound	1,083	8.2%	9.2%	8.4%
MRI for Low Back Pain	154	29.2%	30.1%	32.7%
Survey of Patients' Hospital Experiences				
Area Around Room 'Always' Quiet at Night	300+	52%	-	58%
Doctors 'Always' Communicated Well	300+	78%	-	80%
Home Recovery Information Given	300+	81%	-	82%
Hospital Given 9 or 10 on 10 Point Scale	300+	65%	-	67%
Meds 'Always' Explained Before Given	300+	60%	-	60%
Nurses 'Always' Communicated Well	300+	79%	-	76%
Pain 'Always' Well Controlled	300+	69%	-	69%
Room and Bathroom 'Always' Clean	300+	68%	-	71%
Timely Help 'Always' Received	300+	61%	-	64%
Would Definitely Recommend Hospital	300+	74%	-	69%

NOTE: Hospital profiles are in alphabetical order by state, then city, then hospital within the city; Rankings exclude hospitals with less than 25 cases except for patient surveys which excludes hospitals with less than 100 cases; (a) 100–299 cases; (1) The number of cases is too small to be sure how well a hospital is performing; (2) The hospital indicated that the data submitted for this measure were based on a sample of cases; (3) Data was collected during a shorter time period (fewer quarters) than the maximum possible time for this measure; (4) Suppressed for one or more quarters by CMS; (5) No data is available from the hospital for this measure; (6) Fewer than 100 results are not available for this reporting period; (7) Survey results are based on less than 12 months of data; (8) Survey results completed the HCAHPS survey. Use these rates with caution, as the number of surveys may be too low to reliably assess hospital performance; (9) No or very few patients were eligible for the HCAHPS survey. The scores shown, if any, reflect a very small number of surveys; (10) A state average was not calculated because too few hospitals in the state submitted data; (11) There were discrepancies in the data collection process; Please refer to the User's Guide for a full explanation of data.

Saints Medical Center

1 Hospital Drive
Lowell, MA 01852
Phone: 978-458-1411
Fax: 978-458-8369
Type: Acute Care Hospitals
Emergency Services: Yes
Ownership: Voluntary Non-Profit - Church
Beds: 225

Key Personnel:
CEO/President. . . . . Tom Clark
Cardiac Laboratory. . . . . Pammella Waksmonski
Chief of Medical Staff . . . . Peter S Connolly
Operating Room. . . . . Winnie Beaton
Quality Assurance . . . . Marjorie Boldt
Radiology. . . . . Paul S Tower
Emergency Room . . . . Margrett Thibault

Measure	Cases	This Hosp.	State Avg.	U.S. Avg.
Heart Attack Care				
ACE Inhibitor or ARB for LVSD[1]	11	100%	94%	96%
Aspirin at Arrival	137	99%	99%	99%
Aspirin at Discharge	110	99%	99%	98%
Beta Blocker at Discharge	105	97%	99%	98%
Fibrinolytic Medication Timing	0	-	50%	55%
PCI Within 90 Minutes of Arrival	32	84%	93%	90%
Smoking Cessation Advice	39	100%	99%	99%
Chest Pain/Possible Heart Attack Care				
Aspirin at Arrival[1]	17	88%	96%	95%
Median Time to ECG (minutes)[1]	17	6	10	8
Median Time to Transfer (minutes)[5]	0	-	65	61
Fibrinolytic Medication Timing[3]	0	-	78%	54%
Heart Failure Care				
ACE Inhibitor or ARB for LVSD	64	86%	94%	94%
Discharge Instructions	217	88%	89%	88%
Evaluation of LVS Function	321	99%	98%	98%
Smoking Cessation Advice	40	100%	97%	98%
Pneumonia Care				
Appropriate Initial Antibiotic	129	95%	93%	92%
Blood Culture Timing	189	94%	95%	96%
Influenza Vaccine	149	84%	92%	91%
Initial Antibiotic Timing	230	96%	96%	95%
Pneumococcal Vaccine	203	91%	93%	93%
Smoking Cessation Advice	87	100%	96%	97%
Surgical Care Improvement Project				
Appropriate VTP Within 24 Hours	148	89%	96%	92%
Appropriate Hair Removal	435	100%	100%	99%
Appropriate Beta Blocker Usage	133	94%	96%	93%
Controlled Postoperative Blood Glucose	0	-	95%	93%
Prophylactic Antibiotic Timing	297	98%	97%	97%
Prophylactic Antibiotic Timing (Outpatient)	165	96%	92%	92%
Prophylactic Antibiotic Selection	297	99%	98%	97%
Prophylactic Antibiotic Select. (Outpatient)	163	92%	95%	94%
Prophylactic Antibiotic Stopped	292	98%	96%	94%
Recommended VTP Ordered	148	91%	97%	94%
Urinary Catheter Removal	58	78%	89%	90%
Children's Asthma Care				
Received Systemic Corticosteroids	-	-	-	100%
Received Home Management Plan	-	-	-	71%
Received Reliever Medication	-	-	-	100%
Use of Medical Imaging				
Combination Abdominal CT Scan	770	0.191	0.109	0.191
Combination Chest CT Scan	507	0.002	0.010	0.054
Follow-up Mammogram/Ultrasound	1,155	9.4%	9.2%	8.4%
MRI for Low Back Pain[5]	0	-	30.1%	32.7%
Survey of Patients' Hospital Experiences				
Area Around Room 'Always' Quiet at Night	300+	57%	-	58%
Doctors 'Always' Communicated Well	300+	81%	-	80%
Home Recovery Information Given	300+	87%	-	82%
Hospital Given 9 or 10 on 10 Point Scale	300+	68%	-	67%
Meds 'Always' Explained Before Given	300+	61%	-	60%
Nurses 'Always' Communicated Well	300+	78%	-	76%
Pain 'Always' Well Controlled	300+	73%	-	69%
Room and Bathroom 'Always' Clean	300+	76%	-	71%
Timely Help 'Always' Received	300+	65%	-	64%
Would Definitely Recommend Hospital	300+	72%	-	69%

Marlborough Hospital

157 Union Street
Marlborough, MA 01752
Phone: 508-481-5000
Fax: 508-485-9123
E-mail: gorfinkb@ummhc.org
Type: Acute Care Hospitals
Emergency Services: Yes
Ownership: Voluntary Non-Profit - Private
Beds: 104

Key Personnel:
CEO/President. . . . . John Polanowicz
Cardiac Laboratory. . . . . Carlucci Daniel
Chief of Medical Staff . . . . Bhalchandra Parulkar, MD
Operating Room. . . . . Markian Stecyk, MD
Pediatric Ambulatory Care . . . . . . Ricardo Lewitus, MD
Quality Assurance . . . . Sue Scott
Radiology. . . . . Mark Sykes, MD
Emergency Room . . . . Katharyn Kennedy, MD

Measure	Cases	This Hosp.	State Avg.	U.S. Avg.
Heart Attack Care				
ACE Inhibitor or ARB for LVSD[1]	8	100%	94%	96%
Aspirin at Arrival	36	100%	99%	99%
Aspirin at Discharge[1]	24	100%	99%	98%
Beta Blocker at Discharge[1]	23	100%	99%	98%
Fibrinolytic Medication Timing	0	-	50%	55%
PCI Within 90 Minutes of Arrival	0	-	93%	90%
Smoking Cessation Advice[1]	3	100%	99%	99%
Chest Pain/Possible Heart Attack Care				
Aspirin at Arrival	79	100%	96%	95%
Median Time to ECG (minutes)	81	5	10	8
Median Time to Transfer (minutes)[1]	22	36	65	61
Fibrinolytic Medication Timing	0	-	78%	54%
Heart Failure Care				
ACE Inhibitor or ARB for LVSD	28	96%	94%	94%
Discharge Instructions	75	83%	89%	88%
Evaluation of LVS Function	130	100%	98%	98%
Smoking Cessation Advice[1]	11	100%	97%	98%
Pneumonia Care				
Appropriate Initial Antibiotic	81	96%	93%	92%
Blood Culture Timing	157	94%	95%	96%
Influenza Vaccine	99	100%	92%	91%
Initial Antibiotic Timing	148	97%	96%	95%
Pneumococcal Vaccine	148	98%	93%	93%
Smoking Cessation Advice	41	100%	96%	97%
Surgical Care Improvement Project				
Appropriate VTP Within 24 Hours	93	96%	96%	92%
Appropriate Hair Removal	208	98%	100%	99%
Appropriate Beta Blocker Usage	64	92%	96%	93%
Controlled Postoperative Blood Glucose	0	-	95%	93%
Prophylactic Antibiotic Timing	155	95%	97%	97%
Prophylactic Antibiotic Timing (Outpatient)	52	94%	92%	92%
Prophylactic Antibiotic Selection	155	99%	98%	97%
Prophylactic Antibiotic Select. (Outpatient)	49	92%	95%	94%
Prophylactic Antibiotic Stopped	152	95%	96%	94%
Recommended VTP Ordered	93	96%	97%	94%
Urinary Catheter Removal	68	81%	89%	90%
Children's Asthma Care				
Received Systemic Corticosteroids	-	-	-	100%
Received Home Management Plan	-	-	-	71%
Received Reliever Medication	-	-	-	100%
Use of Medical Imaging				
Combination Abdominal CT Scan	361	0.050	0.109	0.191
Combination Chest CT Scan	178	0.000	0.010	0.054
Follow-up Mammogram/Ultrasound	694	3.3%	9.2%	8.4%
MRI for Low Back Pain[5]	0	-	30.1%	32.7%
Survey of Patients' Hospital Experiences				
Area Around Room 'Always' Quiet at Night	300+	40%	-	58%
Doctors 'Always' Communicated Well	300+	77%	-	80%
Home Recovery Information Given	300+	85%	-	82%
Hospital Given 9 or 10 on 10 Point Scale	300+	60%	-	67%
Meds 'Always' Explained Before Given	300+	63%	-	60%
Nurses 'Always' Communicated Well	300+	75%	-	76%
Pain 'Always' Well Controlled	300+	73%	-	69%
Room and Bathroom 'Always' Clean	300+	70%	-	71%
Timely Help 'Always' Received	300+	59%	-	64%
Would Definitely Recommend Hospital	300+	66%	-	69%

Hallmark Health System

585 Lebanon Street
Melrose, MA 02176
Phone: 781-979-3000
Fax: 781-979-3069
URL: www.hallmarkhealth.org
Type: Acute Care Hospitals
Emergency Services: Yes
Ownership: Voluntary Non-Profit - Private
Beds: 234

Key Personnel:
CEO/President. . . . . Michael V Sack
Chief of Medical Staff . . . . Mike Summerer, MD
Pediatric In-Patient Care . . . . Karen Harvey-Wilkes, MD
Radiology. . . . . Eric Henrikson, MD
Anesthesiology. . . . . Fathalla Mashali, MD
Emergency Room . . . . Joseph Pennacchio, MD

Measure	Cases	This Hosp.	State Avg.	U.S. Avg.
Heart Attack Care				
ACE Inhibitor or ARB for LVSD[1]	15	93%	94%	96%
Aspirin at Arrival	112	100%	99%	99%
Aspirin at Discharge	79	100%	99%	98%
Beta Blocker at Discharge	79	97%	99%	98%
Fibrinolytic Medication Timing	0	-	50%	55%
PCI Within 90 Minutes of Arrival[1]	17	76%	93%	90%
Smoking Cessation Advice[1]	21	100%	99%	99%
Chest Pain/Possible Heart Attack Care				
Aspirin at Arrival	104	100%	96%	95%
Median Time to ECG (minutes)	116	12	10	8
Median Time to Transfer (minutes)[1]	10	72	65	61
Fibrinolytic Medication Timing	0	-	78%	54%
Heart Failure Care				
ACE Inhibitor or ARB for LVSD[2]	70	96%	94%	94%
Discharge Instructions[2]	211	98%	89%	88%
Evaluation of LVS Function[2]	298	99%	98%	98%
Smoking Cessation Advice[2]	33	100%	97%	98%
Pneumonia Care				
Appropriate Initial Antibiotic[2]	117	92%	93%	92%
Blood Culture Timing[2]	187	94%	95%	96%
Influenza Vaccine[2]	133	91%	92%	91%
Initial Antibiotic Timing[2]	188	97%	96%	95%
Pneumococcal Vaccine[2]	204	95%	93%	93%
Smoking Cessation Advice[2]	45	98%	96%	97%
Surgical Care Improvement Project				
Appropriate VTP Within 24 Hours[2]	193	90%	96%	92%
Appropriate Hair Removal[2]	389	100%	100%	99%
Appropriate Beta Blocker Usage[2]	133	92%	96%	93%
Controlled Postoperative Blood Glucose[1,2]	1	0%	95%	93%
Prophylactic Antibiotic Timing[2]	249	98%	97%	97%
Prophylactic Antibiotic Timing (Outpatient)	117	94%	92%	92%
Prophylactic Antibiotic Selection[2]	250	95%	98%	97%
Prophylactic Antibiotic Select. (Outpatient)	113	94%	95%	94%
Prophylactic Antibiotic Stopped[2]	240	96%	96%	94%
Recommended VTP Ordered[2]	194	91%	97%	94%
Urinary Catheter Removal[2]	98	89%	89%	90%
Children's Asthma Care				
Received Systemic Corticosteroids	-	-	-	100%
Received Home Management Plan	-	-	-	71%
Received Reliever Medication	-	-	-	100%
Use of Medical Imaging				
Combination Abdominal CT Scan	1,549	0.110	0.109	0.191
Combination Chest CT Scan	1,219	0.025	0.010	0.054
Follow-up Mammogram/Ultrasound	3,532	10.7%	9.2%	8.4%
MRI for Low Back Pain	400	30.3%	30.1%	32.7%
Survey of Patients' Hospital Experiences				
Area Around Room 'Always' Quiet at Night[11]	300+	51%	-	58%
Doctors 'Always' Communicated Well[11]	300+	81%	-	80%
Home Recovery Information Given[11]	300+	84%	-	82%
Hospital Given 9 or 10 on 10 Point Scale[11]	300+	65%	-	67%
Meds 'Always' Explained Before Given[11]	300+	61%	-	60%
Nurses 'Always' Communicated Well[11]	300+	80%	-	76%
Pain 'Always' Well Controlled[11]	300+	75%	-	69%
Room and Bathroom 'Always' Clean[11]	300+	67%	-	71%
Timely Help 'Always' Received[11]	300+	67%	-	64%
Would Definitely Recommend Hospital[11]	300+	70%	-	69%

NOTE: Hospital profiles are in alphabetical order by state, then city, then hospital within the city; Rankings exclude hospitals with less than 25 cases except for patient surveys which excludes hospitals with less than 100 cases; (a) 100–299 cases; (1) The number of cases is too small to be sure how well a hospital is performing; (2) The hospital indicated that the data submitted for this measure were based on a sample of cases; (3) Data was collected during a shorter time period (fewer quarters) than the maximum possible time for this measure; (4) Suppressed for one or more quarters by CMS; (5) No data is available from the hospital for this measure; (6) Fewer than 100 patients completed the HCAHPS survey. Use these rates with caution, as the number of surveys may be too low to reliably assess hospital performance; (7) Survey results are based on less than 12 months of data; (8) Survey results are not available for this reporting period; (9) No or very few patients were eligible for the HCAHPS survey. The scores shown, if any, reflect a very small number of surveys; (10) A state average was not calculated because too few hospitals in the state submitted data; (11) There were discrepancies in the data collection process; Please refer to the User's Guide for a full explanation of data.

Holy Family Hospital

70 East Street
Methuen, MA 01844
Phone: 978-687-0156
Fax: 978-688-7689
E-mail: hfhmail@cchcs.org
URL: www.holyfamilyhosp.org
Type: Acute Care Hospitals
Emergency Services: Yes
Ownership: Proprietary
Beds: 271

Key Personnel:

CEO/President. . . . . Lester P. Schindel
Chief of Medical Staff. . . . . Sally A Hood, MD
Pediatric Ambulatory Care . . . . . . David Avila, DO
Pediatric In-Patient Care . . . . David Avila, DO
Quality Assurance . . . . Carolyn Candiello
Radiology. . . . . Robert C Hannon, MD
Emergency Room . . . . Laurie Crawford, RN

Measure	Cases	This Hosp.	State Avg.	U.S. Avg.
Heart Attack Care				
ACE Inhibitor or ARB for LVSD[1]	10	90%	94%	96%
Aspirin at Arrival	79	97%	99%	99%
Aspirin at Discharge	50	100%	99%	98%
Beta Blocker at Discharge	57	95%	99%	98%
Fibrinolytic Medication Timing	0	-	50%	55%
PCI Within 90 Minutes of Arrival	26	88%	93%	90%
Smoking Cessation Advice[1]	16	100%	99%	99%
Chest Pain/Possible Heart Attack Care				
Aspirin at Arrival	64	91%	96%	95%
Median Time to ECG (minutes)	69	8	10	8
Median Time to Transfer (minutes)[1,3]	2	56	65	61
Fibrinolytic Medication Timing	0	-	78%	54%
Heart Failure Care				
ACE Inhibitor or ARB for LVSD	56	96%	94%	94%
Discharge Instructions	160	86%	89%	88%
Evaluation of LVS Function	242	100%	98%	98%
Smoking Cessation Advice[1]	21	90%	97%	98%
Pneumonia Care				
Appropriate Initial Antibiotic	111	92%	93%	92%
Blood Culture Timing	98	96%	95%	96%
Influenza Vaccine	107	96%	92%	91%
Initial Antibiotic Timing	155	96%	96%	95%
Pneumococcal Vaccine	154	92%	93%	93%
Smoking Cessation Advice	63	94%	96%	97%
Surgical Care Improvement Project				
Appropriate VTP Within 24 Hours[2]	123	86%	96%	92%
Appropriate Hair Removal[2]	529	100%	100%	99%
Appropriate Beta Blocker Usage[2]	182	97%	96%	93%
Controlled Postoperative Blood Glucose[2]	0	-	95%	93%
Prophylactic Antibiotic Timing[2]	411	98%	97%	97%
Prophylactic Antibiotic Timing (Outpatient)	112	87%	92%	92%
Prophylactic Antibiotic Selection[2]	413	97%	98%	97%
Prophylactic Antibiotic Select. (Outpatient)	100	93%	95%	94%
Prophylactic Antibiotic Stopped[2]	402	96%	96%	94%
Recommended VTP Ordered[2]	123	87%	97%	94%
Urinary Catheter Removal[2]	167	84%	89%	90%
Children's Asthma Care				
Received Systemic Corticosteroids	-	-	-	100%
Received Home Management Plan	-	-	-	71%
Received Reliever Medication	-	-	-	100%
Use of Medical Imaging				
Combination Abdominal CT Scan	882	0.410	0.109	0.191
Combination Chest CT Scan	551	0.031	0.010	0.054
Follow-up Mammogram/Ultrasound	929	6.4%	9.2%	8.4%
MRI for Low Back Pain[5]	0	-	30.1%	32.7%
Survey of Patients' Hospital Experiences				
Area Around Room 'Always' Quiet at Night	300+	50%	-	58%
Doctors 'Always' Communicated Well	300+	79%	-	80%
Home Recovery Information Given	300+	83%	-	82%
Hospital Given 9 or 10 on 10 Point Scale	300+	63%	-	67%
Meds 'Always' Explained Before Given	300+	63%	-	60%
Nurses 'Always' Communicated Well	300+	77%	-	76%
Pain 'Always' Well Controlled	300+	72%	-	69%
Room and Bathroom 'Always' Clean	300+	67%	-	71%
Timely Help 'Always' Received	300+	63%	-	64%
Would Definitely Recommend Hospital	300+	69%	-	69%

Milford Regional Medical Center

14 Prospect Street
Milford, MA 01757
Phone: 508-473-1190
Fax: 508-634-9124
URL: www.milfordregional.org
Type: Acute Care Hospitals
Emergency Services: Yes
Ownership: Voluntary Non-Profit - Other
Beds: 121

Key Personnel:

CEO/President. . . . . Francis M Saba
Cardiac Laboratory. . . . . Nancy Tomaso
Chief of Medical Staff . . . . Albert A Crimaldi, MD
Infection Control. . . . . Kim Knox, RN
Operating Room. . . . . Tom Cook, RN
Quality Assurance . . . . Ann Northrop
Emergency Room . . . . Donna Auger
Intensive Care Unit. . . . . Mary Small

Measure	Cases	This Hosp.	State Avg.	U.S. Avg.
Heart Attack Care				
ACE Inhibitor or ARB for LVSD[1]	10	100%	94%	96%
Aspirin at Arrival	72	100%	99%	99%
Aspirin at Discharge	56	96%	99%	98%
Beta Blocker at Discharge	53	98%	99%	98%
Fibrinolytic Medication Timing	0	-	50%	55%
PCI Within 90 Minutes of Arrival	0	-	93%	90%
Smoking Cessation Advice[1]	4	75%	99%	99%
Chest Pain/Possible Heart Attack Care				
Aspirin at Arrival	88	95%	96%	95%
Median Time to ECG (minutes)	91	15	10	8
Median Time to Transfer (minutes)	31	76	65	61
Fibrinolytic Medication Timing	0	-	78%	54%
Heart Failure Care				
ACE Inhibitor or ARB for LVSD	59	98%	94%	94%
Discharge Instructions	178	91%	89%	88%
Evaluation of LVS Function	276	99%	98%	98%
Smoking Cessation Advice[1]	18	83%	97%	98%
Pneumonia Care				
Appropriate Initial Antibiotic	170	95%	93%	92%
Blood Culture Timing	283	96%	95%	96%
Influenza Vaccine	174	90%	92%	91%
Initial Antibiotic Timing	253	98%	96%	95%
Pneumococcal Vaccine	246	93%	93%	93%
Smoking Cessation Advice	61	85%	96%	97%
Surgical Care Improvement Project				
Appropriate VTP Within 24 Hours	118	94%	96%	92%
Appropriate Hair Removal	388	99%	100%	99%
Appropriate Beta Blocker Usage	128	98%	96%	93%
Controlled Postoperative Blood Glucose	0	-	95%	93%
Prophylactic Antibiotic Timing	231	100%	97%	97%
Prophylactic Antibiotic Timing (Outpatient)	168	95%	92%	92%
Prophylactic Antibiotic Selection	231	95%	98%	97%
Prophylactic Antibiotic Select. (Outpatient)	161	88%	95%	94%
Prophylactic Antibiotic Stopped	227	95%	96%	94%
Recommended VTP Ordered	118	95%	97%	94%
Urinary Catheter Removal	101	100%	89%	90%
Children's Asthma Care				
Received Systemic Corticosteroids	-	-	-	100%
Received Home Management Plan	-	-	-	71%
Received Reliever Medication	-	-	-	100%
Use of Medical Imaging				
Combination Abdominal CT Scan	879	0.089	0.109	0.191
Combination Chest CT Scan	693	0.001	0.010	0.054
Follow-up Mammogram/Ultrasound	1,520	7.1%	9.2%	8.4%
MRI for Low Back Pain	207	32.4%	30.1%	32.7%
Survey of Patients' Hospital Experiences				
Area Around Room 'Always' Quiet at Night	300+	51%	-	58%
Doctors 'Always' Communicated Well	300+	83%	-	80%
Home Recovery Information Given	300+	88%	-	82%
Hospital Given 9 or 10 on 10 Point Scale	300+	77%	-	67%
Meds 'Always' Explained Before Given	300+	65%	-	60%
Nurses 'Always' Communicated Well	300+	82%	-	76%
Pain 'Always' Well Controlled	300+	75%	-	69%
Room and Bathroom 'Always' Clean	300+	79%	-	71%
Timely Help 'Always' Received	300+	67%	-	64%
Would Definitely Recommend Hospital	300+	81%	-	69%

Milton Hospital

199 Reedsdale Road
Milton, MA 02186
Phone: 617-696-4600
Fax: 617-696-8323
E-mail: webmaster@miltonhospital.org
URL: www.miltonhosital.org
Type: Acute Care Hospitals
Emergency Services: No
Ownership: Government - Federal
Beds: 113

Key Personnel:

CEO/President. . . . . Joseph V Morrsey
Chief of Medical Staff . . . . Joseph Raduazzo, MD
Radiology. . . . . Patricia Donahue
Emergency Room . . . . Joy Bitner, MD
Intensive Care Unit. . . . . Deebble Sulo
Patient Relations . . . . Cynthia Page

Measure	Cases	This Hosp.	State Avg.	U.S. Avg.
Heart Attack Care				
ACE Inhibitor or ARB for LVSD[1]	7	100%	94%	96%
Aspirin at Arrival	60	98%	99%	99%
Aspirin at Discharge	42	100%	99%	98%
Beta Blocker at Discharge	41	95%	99%	98%
Fibrinolytic Medication Timing	0	-	50%	55%
PCI Within 90 Minutes of Arrival	0	-	93%	90%
Smoking Cessation Advice[1]	3	100%	99%	99%
Chest Pain/Possible Heart Attack Care				
Aspirin at Arrival	73	99%	96%	95%
Median Time to ECG (minutes)	76	8	10	8
Median Time to Transfer (minutes)[1]	17	89	65	61
Fibrinolytic Medication Timing	0	-	78%	54%
Heart Failure Care				
ACE Inhibitor or ARB for LVSD	38	95%	94%	94%
Discharge Instructions	133	99%	89%	88%
Evaluation of LVS Function	175	97%	98%	98%
Smoking Cessation Advice[1]	7	100%	97%	98%
Pneumonia Care				
Appropriate Initial Antibiotic	89	91%	93%	92%
Blood Culture Timing	89	88%	95%	96%
Influenza Vaccine	76	96%	92%	91%
Initial Antibiotic Timing	139	96%	96%	95%
Pneumococcal Vaccine	130	95%	93%	93%
Smoking Cessation Advice	28	96%	96%	97%
Surgical Care Improvement Project				
Appropriate VTP Within 24 Hours	199	95%	96%	92%
Appropriate Hair Removal	313	100%	100%	99%
Appropriate Beta Blocker Usage	106	89%	96%	93%
Controlled Postoperative Blood Glucose	0	-	95%	93%
Prophylactic Antibiotic Timing	210	96%	97%	97%
Prophylactic Antibiotic Timing (Outpatient)	77	99%	92%	92%
Prophylactic Antibiotic Selection	208	100%	98%	97%
Prophylactic Antibiotic Select. (Outpatient)	77	88%	95%	94%
Prophylactic Antibiotic Stopped	200	94%	96%	94%
Recommended VTP Ordered	199	96%	97%	94%
Urinary Catheter Removal	92	87%	89%	90%
Children's Asthma Care				
Received Systemic Corticosteroids	-	-	-	100%
Received Home Management Plan	-	-	-	71%
Received Reliever Medication	-	-	-	100%
Use of Medical Imaging				
Combination Abdominal CT Scan	408	0.167	0.109	0.191
Combination Chest CT Scan	243	0.000	0.010	0.054
Follow-up Mammogram/Ultrasound	878	5.2%	9.2%	8.4%
MRI for Low Back Pain	149	30.2%	30.1%	32.7%
Survey of Patients' Hospital Experiences				
Area Around Room 'Always' Quiet at Night	300+	52%	-	58%
Doctors 'Always' Communicated Well	300+	80%	-	80%
Home Recovery Information Given	300+	81%	-	82%
Hospital Given 9 or 10 on 10 Point Scale	300+	66%	-	67%
Meds 'Always' Explained Before Given	300+	60%	-	60%
Nurses 'Always' Communicated Well	300+	75%	-	76%
Pain 'Always' Well Controlled	300+	67%	-	69%
Room and Bathroom 'Always' Clean	300+	72%	-	71%
Timely Help 'Always' Received	300+	60%	-	64%
Would Definitely Recommend Hospital	300+	72%	-	69%

NOTE: Hospital profiles are in alphabetical order by state, then city, then hospital within the city; Rankings exclude hospitals with less than 25 cases except for patient surveys which excludes hospitals with less than 100 cases; (a) 100–299 cases; (1) The number of cases is too small to be sure how well a hospital is performing; (2) The hospital indicated that the data submitted for this measure were based on a sample of cases; (3) Data was collected during a shorter time period (fewer quarters) than the maximum possible time for this measure; (4) Suppressed for one or more quarters by CMS; (5) No data is available from the hospital for this measure; (6) Fewer than 100 patients completed the HCAHPS survey. Use these rates with caution, as the number of surveys may be too low to reliably assess hospital performance; (7) Survey results are based on less than 12 months of data; (8) Survey results are not available for this reporting period; (9) No or very few patients were eligible for the HCAHPS survey. The scores shown, if any, reflect a very small number of surveys; (10) A state average was not calculated because too few hospitals in the state submitted data; (11) There were discrepancies in the data collection process; Please refer to the User's Guide for a full explanation of data.

Nantucket Cottage Hospital

57 Prospect Street
Nantucket, MA 02554
Phone: 508-228-1200
Fax: 508-825-8249
E-mail: crdcontact@ackhosp.org
URL: www.nantuckehospital.org
Type: Acute Care Hospitals
Emergency Services: Yes
Ownership: Voluntary Non-Profit - Private
Beds: 19

Key Personnel:

CEO/President. . . . . Sylvia Getman
Chief of Medical Staff. . . . . Timothy J Lepore, MD
Infection Control. . . . . Charlene Chadwick, RN
Operating Room. . . . . Kevin Lurie, RN
Quality Assurance . . . . Jan Ellsworth
Radiology. . . . . Oliver Pomeroy
Patient Relations . . . . Jane Bonvini, RN

Measure	Cases	This Hosp.	State Avg.	U.S. Avg.
Heart Attack Care				
ACE Inhibitor or ARB for LVSD[3]	0	-	94%	96%
Aspirin at Arrival[3]	0	-	99%	99%
Aspirin at Discharge[3]	0	-	99%	98%
Beta Blocker at Discharge[3]	0	-	99%	98%
Fibrinolytic Medication Timing[3]	0	-	50%	55%
PCI Within 90 Minutes of Arrival[3]	0	-	93%	90%
Smoking Cessation Advice[3]	0	-	99%	99%
Chest Pain/Possible Heart Attack Care				
Aspirin at Arrival[3]	25	88%	96%	95%
Median Time to ECG (minutes)[3]	26	4	10	8
Median Time to Transfer (minutes)[5]	0	-	65	61
Fibrinolytic Medication Timing[3]	0	-	78%	54%
Heart Failure Care				
ACE Inhibitor or ARB for LVSD[1]	1	0%	94%	94%
Discharge Instructions[1]	9	78%	89%	88%
Evaluation of LVS Function[1]	11	45%	98%	98%
Smoking Cessation Advice	0	-	97%	98%
Pneumonia Care				
Appropriate Initial Antibiotic[1]	5	100%	93%	92%
Blood Culture Timing[1]	5	100%	95%	96%
Influenza Vaccine[1]	2	100%	92%	91%
Initial Antibiotic Timing[1]	2	100%	96%	95%
Pneumococcal Vaccine[1]	5	100%	93%	93%
Smoking Cessation Advice[1]	1	100%	96%	97%
Surgical Care Improvement Project				
Appropriate VTP Within 24 Hours[3]	0	-	96%	92%
Appropriate Hair Removal[1,3]	1	100%	100%	99%
Appropriate Beta Blocker Usage[3]	0	-	96%	93%
Controlled Postoperative Blood Glucose[3]	0	-	95%	93%
Prophylactic Antibiotic Timing[3]	0	-	97%	97%
Prophylactic Antibiotic Timing (Outpatient)[1,3]	1	0%	92%	92%
Prophylactic Antibiotic Selection[3]	0	-	98%	97%
Prophylactic Antibiotic Select. (Outpatient)[1,3]	1	100%	95%	94%
Prophylactic Antibiotic Stopped[3]	0	-	96%	94%
Recommended VTP Ordered[1,3]	1	0%	97%	94%
Urinary Catheter Removal[1,3]	1	0%	89%	90%
Children's Asthma Care				
Received Systemic Corticosteroids	-	-	-	100%
Received Home Management Plan	-	-	-	71%
Received Reliever Medication	-	-	-	100%
Use of Medical Imaging				
Combination Abdominal CT Scan	110	0.055	0.109	0.191
Combination Chest CT Scan	73	0.000	0.010	0.054
Follow-up Mammogram/Ultrasound	134	3.7%	9.2%	8.4%
MRI for Low Back Pain[1]	31	25.8%	30.1%	32.7%
Survey of Patients' Hospital Experiences				
Area Around Room 'Always' Quiet at Night[6]	<100	65%	-	58%
Doctors 'Always' Communicated Well[6]	<100	88%	-	80%
Home Recovery Information Given[6]	<100	74%	-	82%
Hospital Given 9 or 10 on 10 Point Scale[6]	<100	74%	-	67%
Meds 'Always' Explained Before Given[6]	<100	61%	-	60%
Nurses 'Always' Communicated Well[6]	<100	84%	-	76%
Pain 'Always' Well Controlled[6]	<100	78%	-	69%
Room and Bathroom 'Always' Clean[6]	<100	73%	-	71%
Timely Help 'Always' Received[6]	<100	87%	-	64%
Would Definitely Recommend Hospital	<100	82%	-	69%

Beth Israel Deaconess Hospital - Needham

148 Chestnut Street
Needham, MA 02494
Phone: 781-453-3000
Fax: 781-453-5786
URL: www.caregroup.org
Type: Acute Care Hospitals
Emergency Services: Yes
Ownership: Government - Local
Beds: 58

Key Personnel:

CEO/President. . . . . Paul Levy
Cardiac Laboratory. . . . . Joseph P Kannam, MD
Radiology. . . . . Mary Hochman

Measure	Cases	This Hosp.	State Avg.	U.S. Avg.
Heart Attack Care				
ACE Inhibitor or ARB for LVSD[1]	2	100%	94%	96%
Aspirin at Arrival[1]	13	100%	99%	99%
Aspirin at Discharge[1]	8	100%	99%	98%
Beta Blocker at Discharge[1]	9	100%	99%	98%
Fibrinolytic Medication Timing	0	-	50%	55%
PCI Within 90 Minutes of Arrival	0	-	93%	90%
Smoking Cessation Advice	0	-	99%	99%
Chest Pain/Possible Heart Attack Care				
Aspirin at Arrival	85	94%	96%	95%
Median Time to ECG (minutes)	89	4	10	8
Median Time to Transfer (minutes)[1]	14	66	65	61
Fibrinolytic Medication Timing	0	-	78%	54%
Heart Failure Care				
ACE Inhibitor or ARB for LVSD[1]	24	96%	94%	94%
Discharge Instructions	72	81%	89%	88%
Evaluation of LVS Function	128	98%	98%	98%
Smoking Cessation Advice[1]	9	78%	97%	98%
Pneumonia Care				
Appropriate Initial Antibiotic	61	95%	93%	92%
Blood Culture Timing	84	95%	95%	96%
Influenza Vaccine	64	95%	92%	91%
Initial Antibiotic Timing	78	97%	96%	95%
Pneumococcal Vaccine	100	87%	93%	93%
Smoking Cessation Advice[1]	9	89%	96%	97%
Surgical Care Improvement Project				
Appropriate VTP Within 24 Hours	60	100%	96%	92%
Appropriate Hair Removal	127	99%	100%	99%
Appropriate Beta Blocker Usage	43	93%	96%	93%
Controlled Postoperative Blood Glucose	0	-	95%	93%
Prophylactic Antibiotic Timing	84	94%	97%	97%
Prophylactic Antibiotic Timing (Outpatient)	70	96%	92%	92%
Prophylactic Antibiotic Selection	85	99%	98%	97%
Prophylactic Antibiotic Select. (Outpatient)	70	94%	95%	94%
Prophylactic Antibiotic Stopped	81	99%	96%	94%
Recommended VTP Ordered	60	100%	97%	94%
Urinary Catheter Removal	33	97%	89%	90%
Children's Asthma Care				
Received Systemic Corticosteroids	-	-	-	100%
Received Home Management Plan	-	-	-	71%
Received Reliever Medication	-	-	-	100%
Use of Medical Imaging				
Combination Abdominal CT Scan	291	0.234	0.109	0.191
Combination Chest CT Scan	203	0.158	0.010	0.054
Follow-up Mammogram/Ultrasound	473	10.4%	9.2%	8.4%
MRI for Low Back Pain	79	27.8%	30.1%	32.7%
Survey of Patients' Hospital Experiences				
Area Around Room 'Always' Quiet at Night	300+	50%	-	58%
Doctors 'Always' Communicated Well	300+	79%	-	80%
Home Recovery Information Given	300+	83%	-	82%
Hospital Given 9 or 10 on 10 Point Scale	300+	72%	-	67%
Meds 'Always' Explained Before Given	300+	64%	-	60%
Nurses 'Always' Communicated Well	300+	78%	-	76%
Pain 'Always' Well Controlled	300+	69%	-	69%
Room and Bathroom 'Always' Clean	300+	80%	-	71%
Timely Help 'Always' Received	300+	66%	-	64%
Would Definitely Recommend Hospital	300+	78%	-	69%

Anna Jaques Hospital

25 Highland Avenue
Newburyport, MA 01950
Phone: 978-463-1000
Fax: 978-463-1250
URL: www.ajh.org
Type: Acute Care Hospitals
Emergency Services: Yes
Ownership: Voluntary Non-Profit - Private
Beds: 123

Key Personnel:

CEO/President. . . . . Stot W Goodsteed
Cardiac Laboratory. . . . . Jackie Carroll
Chief of Medical Staff . . . . Les Sebba
Quality Assurance . . . . Kathy Lucy, RN
Radiology. . . . . Maximina Boutes, MD
Anesthesiology. . . . . Eduardo D'Agostino, MD
Emergency Room . . . . Joe Hull, MD
Hemotology Center . . . . Paul Spieler, MD

Measure	Cases	This Hosp.	State Avg.	U.S. Avg.
Heart Attack Care				
ACE Inhibitor or ARB for LVSD[1]	7	86%	94%	96%
Aspirin at Arrival	54	96%	99%	99%
Aspirin at Discharge[1]	24	96%	99%	98%
Beta Blocker at Discharge	26	100%	99%	98%
Fibrinolytic Medication Timing	0	-	50%	55%
PCI Within 90 Minutes of Arrival	0	-	93%	90%
Smoking Cessation Advice[1]	3	100%	99%	99%
Chest Pain/Possible Heart Attack Care				
Aspirin at Arrival	57	98%	96%	95%
Median Time to ECG (minutes)	56	7	10	8
Median Time to Transfer (minutes)[1]	24	77	65	61
Fibrinolytic Medication Timing	0	-	78%	54%
Heart Failure Care				
ACE Inhibitor or ARB for LVSD	51	88%	94%	94%
Discharge Instructions	138	93%	89%	88%
Evaluation of LVS Function	204	96%	98%	98%
Smoking Cessation Advice[1]	18	100%	97%	98%
Pneumonia Care				
Appropriate Initial Antibiotic	124	95%	93%	92%
Blood Culture Timing	136	99%	95%	96%
Influenza Vaccine	112	98%	92%	91%
Initial Antibiotic Timing	181	97%	96%	95%
Pneumococcal Vaccine	171	98%	93%	93%
Smoking Cessation Advice	55	100%	96%	97%
Surgical Care Improvement Project				
Appropriate VTP Within 24 Hours	204	95%	96%	92%
Appropriate Hair Removal	346	100%	100%	99%
Appropriate Beta Blocker Usage	115	93%	96%	93%
Controlled Postoperative Blood Glucose	0	-	95%	93%
Prophylactic Antibiotic Timing	220	99%	97%	97%
Prophylactic Antibiotic Timing (Outpatient)	133	93%	92%	92%
Prophylactic Antibiotic Selection	222	97%	98%	97%
Prophylactic Antibiotic Select. (Outpatient)	131	91%	95%	94%
Prophylactic Antibiotic Stopped	213	95%	96%	94%
Recommended VTP Ordered	204	95%	97%	94%
Urinary Catheter Removal	41	78%	89%	90%
Children's Asthma Care				
Received Systemic Corticosteroids	-	-	-	100%
Received Home Management Plan	-	-	-	71%
Received Reliever Medication	-	-	-	100%
Use of Medical Imaging				
Combination Abdominal CT Scan	636	0.041	0.109	0.191
Combination Chest CT Scan	585	0.009	0.010	0.054
Follow-up Mammogram/Ultrasound	1,792	9.4%	9.2%	8.4%
MRI for Low Back Pain[5]	0	-	30.1%	32.7%
Survey of Patients' Hospital Experiences				
Area Around Room 'Always' Quiet at Night	300+	50%	-	58%
Doctors 'Always' Communicated Well	300+	80%	-	80%
Home Recovery Information Given	300+	87%	-	82%
Hospital Given 9 or 10 on 10 Point Scale	300+	62%	-	67%
Meds 'Always' Explained Before Given	300+	62%	-	60%
Nurses 'Always' Communicated Well	300+	79%	-	76%
Pain 'Always' Well Controlled	300+	74%	-	69%
Room and Bathroom 'Always' Clean	300+	67%	-	71%
Timely Help 'Always' Received	300+	68%	-	64%
Would Definitely Recommend Hospital	300+	70%	-	69%

NOTE: Hospital profiles are in alphabetical order by state, then city, then hospital within the city; Rankings exclude hospitals with less than 25 cases except for patient surveys which excludes hospitals with less than 100 cases; (a) 100–299 cases; (1) The number of cases is too small to be sure how well a hospital is performing; (2) The hospital indicated that the data submitted for this measure were based on a sample of cases; (3) Data was collected during a shorter time period (fewer quarters) than the maximum possible time for this measure; (4) Suppressed for one or more quarters by CMS; (5) No data is available from the hospital for this measure; (6) Fewer than 100 patients completed the HCAHPS survey. Use these rates with caution, as the number of surveys may be too low to reliably assess hospital performance; (7) Survey results are based on less than 12 months of data; (8) Survey results are not available for this reporting period; (9) No or very few patients were eligible for the HCAHPS survey. The scores shown, if any, reflect a very small number of surveys; (10) A state average was not calculated because too few hospitals in the state submitted data; (11) There were discrepancies in the data collection process; Please refer to the User's Guide for a full explanation of data.

Newton-Wellesley Hospital

2014 Washington Street
Newton, MA 02462
URL: www.nwh.org
Phone: 617-243-6000
Fax: 617-243-6990
Type: Acute Care Hospitals
Emergency Services: Yes
Ownership: Voluntary Non-Profit - Other
Beds: 290

Key Personnel:

CEO/President. . . . . Michael Jellinek, MD
Chief of Medical Staff. . . . . Laurence Friedman, MD
Infection Control. . . . . Sue MacDonald
Operating Room. . . . . Anna DaSilva, RN
Pediatric Ambulatory Care . . . . . . Joel Bass, MD
Pediatric In-Patient Care . . . . . . Joel Bass, MD
Quality Assurance . . . . Marci Cass
Radiology. . . . . Steven Miller, MD

Measure	Cases	This Hosp.	State Avg.	U.S. Avg.
Heart Attack Care				
ACE Inhibitor or ARB for LVSD[1]	8	100%	94%	96%
Aspirin at Arrival	59	100%	99%	99%
Aspirin at Discharge	38	100%	99%	98%
Beta Blocker at Discharge	41	100%	99%	98%
Fibrinolytic Medication Timing	0	-	50%	55%
PCI Within 90 Minutes of Arrival	0	-	93%	90%
Smoking Cessation Advice[1]	3	100%	99%	99%
Chest Pain/Possible Heart Attack Care				
Aspirin at Arrival	56	95%	96%	95%
Median Time to ECG (minutes)	58	0	10	8
Median Time to Transfer (minutes)[1]	3	65	65	61
Fibrinolytic Medication Timing	0	-	78%	54%
Heart Failure Care				
ACE Inhibitor or ARB for LVSD[2]	54	96%	94%	94%
Discharge Instructions[2]	193	95%	89%	88%
Evaluation of LVS Function[2]	264	100%	98%	98%
Smoking Cessation Advice[1,2]	16	100%	97%	98%
Pneumonia Care				
Appropriate Initial Antibiotic[2]	72	99%	93%	92%
Blood Culture Timing[2]	139	99%	95%	96%
Influenza Vaccine[2]	85	99%	92%	91%
Initial Antibiotic Timing[2]	116	100%	96%	95%
Pneumococcal Vaccine[2]	148	99%	93%	93%
Smoking Cessation Advice[1,2]	23	96%	96%	97%
Surgical Care Improvement Project				
Appropriate VTP Within 24 Hours[2]	92	91%	96%	92%
Appropriate Hair Removal[2]	326	99%	100%	99%
Appropriate Beta Blocker Usage[2]	74	95%	96%	93%
Controlled Postoperative Blood Glucose[2]	0	-	95%	93%
Prophylactic Antibiotic Timing[2]	217	97%	97%	97%
Prophylactic Antibiotic Timing (Outpatient)	254	96%	92%	92%
Prophylactic Antibiotic Selection[2]	217	98%	98%	97%
Prophylactic Antibiotic Select. (Outpatient)	251	98%	95%	94%
Prophylactic Antibiotic Stopped[2]	213	96%	96%	94%
Recommended VTP Ordered[2]	92	92%	97%	94%
Urinary Catheter Removal[2]	54	89%	89%	90%
Children's Asthma Care				
Received Systemic Corticosteroids	-	-	-	100%
Received Home Management Plan	-	-	-	71%
Received Reliever Medication	-	-	-	100%
Use of Medical Imaging				
Combination Abdominal CT Scan	1,181	0.097	0.109	0.191
Combination Chest CT Scan	1,135	0.003	0.010	0.054
Follow-up Mammogram/Ultrasound	2,613	11.0%	9.2%	8.4%
MRI for Low Back Pain	159	28.9%	30.1%	32.7%
Survey of Patients' Hospital Experiences				
Area Around Room 'Always' Quiet at Night	300+	55%	-	58%
Doctors 'Always' Communicated Well	300+	82%	-	80%
Home Recovery Information Given	300+	87%	-	82%
Hospital Given 9 or 10 on 10 Point Scale	300+	72%	-	67%
Meds 'Always' Explained Before Given	300+	63%	-	60%
Nurses 'Always' Communicated Well	300+	78%	-	76%
Pain 'Always' Well Controlled	300+	71%	-	69%
Room and Bathroom 'Always' Clean	300+	76%	-	71%
Timely Help 'Always' Received	300+	63%	-	64%
Would Definitely Recommend Hospital	300+	81%	-	69%

North Adams Regional Hospital

71 Hospital Avenue
North Adams, MA 01247
URL: www.nbhealth.org
Phone: 413-664-5000
Fax: 413-664-5028
Type: Acute Care Hospitals
Emergency Services: Yes
Ownership: Voluntary Non-Profit - Private
Beds: 134

Key Personnel:

CEO/President. . . . . Richard T Palmisano
Chief of Medical Staff . . . . Paul Donovan, MD

Measure	Cases	This Hosp.	State Avg.	U.S. Avg.
Heart Attack Care				
ACE Inhibitor or ARB for LVSD[1]	8	100%	94%	96%
Aspirin at Arrival	37	100%	99%	99%
Aspirin at Discharge	27	100%	99%	98%
Beta Blocker at Discharge	26	100%	99%	98%
Fibrinolytic Medication Timing	0	-	50%	55%
PCI Within 90 Minutes of Arrival	0	-	93%	90%
Smoking Cessation Advice[1]	5	100%	99%	99%
Chest Pain/Possible Heart Attack Care				
Aspirin at Arrival	48	96%	96%	95%
Median Time to ECG (minutes)	52	6	10	8
Median Time to Transfer (minutes)[3]	0	-	65	61
Fibrinolytic Medication Timing[1]	15	80%	78%	54%
Heart Failure Care				
ACE Inhibitor or ARB for LVSD[1]	22	91%	94%	94%
Discharge Instructions	75	95%	89%	88%
Evaluation of LVS Function	101	100%	98%	98%
Smoking Cessation Advice[1]	13	100%	97%	98%
Pneumonia Care				
Appropriate Initial Antibiotic	65	98%	93%	92%
Blood Culture Timing	124	97%	95%	96%
Influenza Vaccine	64	97%	92%	91%
Initial Antibiotic Timing	116	98%	96%	95%
Pneumococcal Vaccine	113	99%	93%	93%
Smoking Cessation Advice	37	97%	96%	97%
Surgical Care Improvement Project				
Appropriate VTP Within 24 Hours	74	99%	96%	92%
Appropriate Hair Removal	214	100%	100%	99%
Appropriate Beta Blocker Usage	55	95%	96%	93%
Controlled Postoperative Blood Glucose	0	-	95%	93%
Prophylactic Antibiotic Timing	146	100%	97%	97%
Prophylactic Antibiotic Timing (Outpatient)	56	96%	92%	92%
Prophylactic Antibiotic Selection	146	96%	98%	97%
Prophylactic Antibiotic Select. (Outpatient)	55	100%	95%	94%
Prophylactic Antibiotic Stopped	141	99%	96%	94%
Recommended VTP Ordered	74	100%	97%	94%
Urinary Catheter Removal[1]	23	91%	89%	90%
Children's Asthma Care				
Received Systemic Corticosteroids	-	-	-	100%
Received Home Management Plan	-	-	-	71%
Received Reliever Medication	-	-	-	100%
Use of Medical Imaging				
Combination Abdominal CT Scan	609	0.149	0.109	0.191
Combination Chest CT Scan	555	0.009	0.010	0.054
Follow-up Mammogram/Ultrasound	1,369	4.5%	9.2%	8.4%
MRI for Low Back Pain	133	36.1%	30.1%	32.7%
Survey of Patients' Hospital Experiences				
Area Around Room 'Always' Quiet at Night	300+	56%	-	58%
Doctors 'Always' Communicated Well	300+	81%	-	80%
Home Recovery Information Given	300+	89%	-	82%
Hospital Given 9 or 10 on 10 Point Scale	300+	65%	-	67%
Meds 'Always' Explained Before Given	300+	64%	-	60%
Nurses 'Always' Communicated Well	300+	79%	-	76%
Pain 'Always' Well Controlled	300+	73%	-	69%
Room and Bathroom 'Always' Clean	300+	77%	-	71%
Timely Help 'Always' Received	300+	65%	-	64%
Would Definitely Recommend Hospital	300+	70%	-	69%

The Cooley Dickinson Hospital

30 Locust Street
Northampton, MA 01060
URL: www.cooley-dickinson.org
Phone: 413-582-2000
Fax: 413-582-2951
Type: Acute Care Hospitals
Emergency Services: Yes
Ownership: Voluntary Non-Profit - Private
Beds: 125

Key Personnel:

CEO/President. . . . . Craig Melin
Chief of Medical Staff . . . . Jay Fleitman, MD
Quality Assurance . . . . Joanne LaBelle
Radiology. . . . . George G Hartnell

Measure	Cases	This Hosp.	State Avg.	U.S. Avg.
Heart Attack Care				
ACE Inhibitor or ARB for LVSD[1]	8	88%	94%	96%
Aspirin at Arrival	47	100%	99%	99%
Aspirin at Discharge	39	97%	99%	98%
Beta Blocker at Discharge	34	97%	99%	98%
Fibrinolytic Medication Timing	0	-	50%	55%
PCI Within 90 Minutes of Arrival	0	-	93%	90%
Smoking Cessation Advice[1]	2	100%	99%	99%
Chest Pain/Possible Heart Attack Care				
Aspirin at Arrival	83	98%	96%	95%
Median Time to ECG (minutes)	82	8	10	8
Median Time to Transfer (minutes)	33	55	65	61
Fibrinolytic Medication Timing	0	-	78%	54%
Heart Failure Care				
ACE Inhibitor or ARB for LVSD	53	98%	94%	94%
Discharge Instructions	122	94%	89%	88%
Evaluation of LVS Function	163	99%	98%	98%
Smoking Cessation Advice[1]	13	100%	97%	98%
Pneumonia Care				
Appropriate Initial Antibiotic	124	96%	93%	92%
Blood Culture Timing	194	96%	95%	96%
Influenza Vaccine	131	95%	92%	91%
Initial Antibiotic Timing	196	96%	96%	95%
Pneumococcal Vaccine	168	95%	93%	93%
Smoking Cessation Advice	66	94%	96%	97%
Surgical Care Improvement Project				
Appropriate VTP Within 24 Hours[2]	145	89%	96%	92%
Appropriate Hair Removal[2]	456	100%	100%	99%
Appropriate Beta Blocker Usage[2]	109	98%	96%	93%
Controlled Postoperative Blood Glucose[2]	0	-	95%	93%
Prophylactic Antibiotic Timing[2]	292	98%	97%	97%
Prophylactic Antibiotic Timing (Outpatient)	149	99%	92%	92%
Prophylactic Antibiotic Selection[2]	293	98%	98%	97%
Prophylactic Antibiotic Select. (Outpatient)	148	100%	95%	94%
Prophylactic Antibiotic Stopped[2]	284	100%	96%	94%
Recommended VTP Ordered[2]	147	92%	97%	94%
Urinary Catheter Removal[2]	162	94%	89%	90%
Children's Asthma Care				
Received Systemic Corticosteroids	-	-	-	100%
Received Home Management Plan	-	-	-	71%
Received Reliever Medication	-	-	-	100%
Use of Medical Imaging				
Combination Abdominal CT Scan	740	0.055	0.109	0.191
Combination Chest CT Scan	535	0.000	0.010	0.054
Follow-up Mammogram/Ultrasound	1,628	6.4%	9.2%	8.4%
MRI for Low Back Pain	234	22.2%	30.1%	32.7%
Survey of Patients' Hospital Experiences				
Area Around Room 'Always' Quiet at Night	300+	54%	-	58%
Doctors 'Always' Communicated Well	300+	78%	-	80%
Home Recovery Information Given	300+	86%	-	82%
Hospital Given 9 or 10 on 10 Point Scale	300+	68%	-	67%
Meds 'Always' Explained Before Given	300+	59%	-	60%
Nurses 'Always' Communicated Well	300+	75%	-	76%
Pain 'Always' Well Controlled	300+	67%	-	69%
Room and Bathroom 'Always' Clean	300+	76%	-	71%
Timely Help 'Always' Received	300+	63%	-	64%
Would Definitely Recommend Hospital	300+	72%	-	69%

NOTE: Hospital profiles are in alphabetical order by state, then city, then hospital within the city; Rankings exclude hospitals with less than 25 cases except for patient surveys which excludes hospitals with less than 100 cases; (a) 100–299 cases; (1) The number of cases is too small to be sure how well a hospital is performing; (2) The hospital indicated that the data submitted for this measure were based on a sample of cases; (3) Data was collected during a shorter time period (fewer quarters) than the maximum possible time for this measure; (4) Suppressed for one or more quarters by CMS; (5) No data is available from the hospital for this measure; (6) Fewer than 100 patients completed the HCAHPS survey. Use these rates with caution, as the number of surveys may be too low to reliably assess hospital performance; (7) Survey results are based on less than 12 months of data; (8) Survey results are not available for this reporting period; (9) No or very few patients were eligible for the HCAHPS survey. The scores shown, if any, reflect a very small number of surveys; (10) A state average was not calculated because too few hospitals in the state submitted data; (11) There were discrepancies in the data collection process; Please refer to the User's Guide for a full explanation of data.

Norwood Hospital

800 Washington Street
Norwood, MA 02062
URL: www.caritasnorwood.org
Type: Acute Care Hospitals
Ownership: Proprietary
Phone: 508-772-1000
Fax: 781-278-6820
Emergency Services: Yes
Beds: 265

Key Personnel:
CEO/President.............. Margaret Hanson
Cardiac Laboratory........... John Kinch, MD
Chief of Medical Staff.......... Michael Ginsburg, MD
Pediatric Ambulatory Care...... Bruce Weinstock, MD
Quality Assurance............ Kathleen Turke
Radiology.................. Kevin Loughlin, MD

Measure	Cases	This Hosp.	State Avg.	U.S. Avg.
Heart Attack Care				
ACE Inhibitor or ARB for LVSD[1]	18	100%	94%	96%
Aspirin at Arrival	142	100%	99%	99%
Aspirin at Discharge	101	98%	99%	98%
Beta Blocker at Discharge	96	100%	99%	98%
Fibrinolytic Medication Timing	0	-	50%	55%
PCI Within 90 Minutes of Arrival	40	100%	93%	90%
Smoking Cessation Advice[1]	23	100%	99%	99%
Chest Pain/Possible Heart Attack Care				
Aspirin at Arrival	54	100%	96%	95%
Median Time to ECG (minutes)	57	8	10	8
Median Time to Transfer (minutes)[1,3]	1	47	65	61
Fibrinolytic Medication Timing	0	-	78%	54%
Heart Failure Care				
ACE Inhibitor or ARB for LVSD	58	97%	94%	94%
Discharge Instructions	164	90%	89%	88%
Evaluation of LVS Function	271	99%	98%	98%
Smoking Cessation Advice	25	100%	97%	98%
Pneumonia Care				
Appropriate Initial Antibiotic	133	95%	93%	92%
Blood Culture Timing	146	97%	95%	96%
Influenza Vaccine	113	89%	92%	91%
Initial Antibiotic Timing	189	98%	96%	95%
Pneumococcal Vaccine	154	91%	93%	93%
Smoking Cessation Advice	57	100%	96%	97%
Surgical Care Improvement Project				
Appropriate VTP Within 24 Hours[2]	256	100%	96%	92%
Appropriate Hair Removal[2]	378	100%	100%	99%
Appropriate Beta Blocker Usage[2]	157	96%	96%	93%
Controlled Postoperative Blood Glucose[2]	0	-	95%	93%
Prophylactic Antibiotic Timing[2]	205	95%	97%	97%
Prophylactic Antibiotic Timing (Outpatient)	127	89%	92%	92%
Prophylactic Antibiotic Selection[2]	207	98%	98%	97%
Prophylactic Antibiotic Select. (Outpatient)	123	89%	95%	94%
Prophylactic Antibiotic Stopped[2]	191	95%	96%	94%
Recommended VTP Ordered[2]	256	100%	97%	94%
Urinary Catheter Removal[2]	89	66%	89%	90%
Children's Asthma Care				
Received Systemic Corticosteroids	-	-	-	100%
Received Home Management Plan	-	-	-	71%
Received Reliever Medication	-	-	-	100%
Use of Medical Imaging				
Combination Abdominal CT Scan	605	0.078	0.109	0.191
Combination Chest CT Scan	444	0.002	0.010	0.054
Follow-up Mammogram/Ultrasound	704	18.8%	9.2%	8.4%
MRI for Low Back Pain[1]	25	28.0%	30.1%	32.7%
Survey of Patients' Hospital Experiences				
Area Around Room 'Always' Quiet at Night	300+	41%	-	58%
Doctors 'Always' Communicated Well	300+	80%	-	80%
Home Recovery Information Given	300+	83%	-	82%
Hospital Given 9 or 10 on 10 Point Scale	300+	63%	-	67%
Meds 'Always' Explained Before Given	300+	62%	-	60%
Nurses 'Always' Communicated Well	300+	79%	-	76%
Pain 'Always' Well Controlled	300+	74%	-	69%
Room and Bathroom 'Always' Clean	300+	75%	-	71%
Timely Help 'Always' Received	300+	65%	-	64%
Would Definitely Recommend Hospital	300+	64%	-	69%

Martha's Vineyard Hospital

One Hospital Road
Oak Bluffs, MA 02557
URL: www.marthasvineyardhospital.com
Type: Critical Access Hospitals
Ownership: Voluntary Non-Profit - Private
Phone: 508-693-0410
Fax: 508-693-5971
Emergency Services: Yes
Beds: 32

Key Personnel:
CEO/President.............. Timothy Walsh
Cardiac Laboratory........... Timothy Gurey, MD
Chief of Medical Staff.......... Michael Goldfein, MD
Operating Room............. Denise Fraser, MD
Pediatric In-Patient Care....... Michael Goldfein, MD
Quality Assurance............ Dedie Wieler
Radiology.................. Stephen Miller, MD
Emergency Room........... Jeffrey Zack, MD

Measure	Cases	This Hosp.	State Avg.	U.S. Avg.
Heart Attack Care				
ACE Inhibitor or ARB for LVSD[5]	0	-	94%	96%
Aspirin at Arrival[5]	0	-	99%	99%
Aspirin at Discharge[5]	0	-	99%	98%
Beta Blocker at Discharge[5]	0	-	99%	98%
Fibrinolytic Medication Timing[5]	0	-	50%	55%
PCI Within 90 Minutes of Arrival[5]	0	-	93%	90%
Smoking Cessation Advice[5]	0	-	99%	99%
Chest Pain/Possible Heart Attack Care				
Aspirin at Arrival	-	-	96%	95%
Median Time to ECG (minutes)	-	-	10	8
Median Time to Transfer (minutes)	-	-	65	61
Fibrinolytic Medication Timing	-	-	78%	54%
Heart Failure Care				
ACE Inhibitor or ARB for LVSD[1,2]	8	88%	94%	94%
Discharge Instructions[1,2]	21	90%	89%	88%
Evaluation of LVS Function[2]	32	84%	98%	98%
Smoking Cessation Advice[1,2]	3	67%	97%	98%
Pneumonia Care				
Appropriate Initial Antibiotic[1,2]	24	88%	93%	92%
Blood Culture Timing[1,2]	23	91%	95%	96%
Influenza Vaccine[1,2]	18	50%	92%	91%
Initial Antibiotic Timing[2]	38	100%	96%	95%
Pneumococcal Vaccine[2]	40	42%	93%	93%
Smoking Cessation Advice[1,2]	3	100%	96%	97%
Surgical Care Improvement Project				
Appropriate VTP Within 24 Hours[5]	0	-	96%	92%
Appropriate Hair Removal[5]	0	-	100%	99%
Appropriate Beta Blocker Usage[5]	0	-	96%	93%
Controlled Postoperative Blood Glucose[5]	0	-	95%	93%
Prophylactic Antibiotic Timing[5]	0	-	97%	97%
Prophylactic Antibiotic Timing (Outpatient)	-	-	92%	92%
Prophylactic Antibiotic Selection[5]	0	-	98%	97%
Prophylactic Antibiotic Select. (Outpatient)	-	-	95%	94%
Prophylactic Antibiotic Stopped[5]	0	-	96%	94%
Recommended VTP Ordered[5]	0	-	97%	94%
Urinary Catheter Removal[5]	0	-	89%	90%
Children's Asthma Care				
Received Systemic Corticosteroids	-	-	-	100%
Received Home Management Plan	-	-	-	71%
Received Reliever Medication	-	-	-	100%
Use of Medical Imaging				
Combination Abdominal CT Scan	-	-	0.109	0.191
Combination Chest CT Scan	-	-	0.010	0.054
Follow-up Mammogram/Ultrasound	-	-	9.2%	8.4%
MRI for Low Back Pain	-	-	30.1%	32.7%
Survey of Patients' Hospital Experiences				
Area Around Room 'Always' Quiet at Night	(a)	55%	-	58%
Doctors 'Always' Communicated Well	(a)	84%	-	80%
Home Recovery Information Given	(a)	87%	-	82%
Hospital Given 9 or 10 on 10 Point Scale	(a)	61%	-	67%
Meds 'Always' Explained Before Given	(a)	64%	-	60%
Nurses 'Always' Communicated Well	(a)	77%	-	76%
Pain 'Always' Well Controlled	(a)	75%	-	69%
Room and Bathroom 'Always' Clean	(a)	72%	-	71%
Timely Help 'Always' Received	(a)	61%	-	64%
Would Definitely Recommend Hospital	(a)	72%	-	69%

Wing Memorial Hospital and Medical Center

40 Wright Street
Palmer, MA 01069
URL: www.winghealth.org
Type: Acute Care Hospitals
Ownership: Voluntary Non-Profit - Other
Phone: 413-283-7651
Fax: 413-284-5117
Emergency Services: Yes
Beds: 74

Key Personnel:
CEO/President.............. Charles Cavagnaro III, MD
Chief of Medical Staff.......... David Maguire, MD
Operating Room............. Sue Keenan, RN
Quality Assurance............ Ronald Krystofik
Radiology.................. Susaney C Londie
Emergency Room............ Lori Striplin, RN
Patient Relations............ Maria Darasz

Measure	Cases	This Hosp.	State Avg.	U.S. Avg.
Heart Attack Care				
ACE Inhibitor or ARB for LVSD[1]	6	83%	94%	96%
Aspirin at Arrival[1]	17	100%	99%	99%
Aspirin at Discharge[1]	11	100%	99%	98%
Beta Blocker at Discharge[1]	11	100%	99%	98%
Fibrinolytic Medication Timing	0	-	50%	55%
PCI Within 90 Minutes of Arrival	0	-	93%	90%
Smoking Cessation Advice[1]	2	100%	99%	99%
Chest Pain/Possible Heart Attack Care				
Aspirin at Arrival	41	85%	96%	95%
Median Time to ECG (minutes)	46	12	10	8
Median Time to Transfer (minutes)[1]	10	48	65	61
Fibrinolytic Medication Timing[1]	1	0%	78%	54%
Heart Failure Care				
ACE Inhibitor or ARB for LVSD[1,2]	21	90%	94%	94%
Discharge Instructions[2]	103	96%	89%	88%
Evaluation of LVS Function[2]	143	100%	98%	98%
Smoking Cessation Advice[1,2]	15	100%	97%	98%
Pneumonia Care				
Appropriate Initial Antibiotic	64	92%	93%	92%
Blood Culture Timing	119	99%	95%	96%
Influenza Vaccine	100	97%	92%	91%
Initial Antibiotic Timing	117	97%	96%	95%
Pneumococcal Vaccine	124	98%	93%	93%
Smoking Cessation Advice	48	98%	96%	97%
Surgical Care Improvement Project				
Appropriate VTP Within 24 Hours	25	100%	96%	92%
Appropriate Hair Removal	46	100%	100%	99%
Appropriate Beta Blocker Usage[1]	20	100%	96%	93%
Controlled Postoperative Blood Glucose	0	-	95%	93%
Prophylactic Antibiotic Timing	28	100%	97%	97%
Prophylactic Antibiotic Timing (Outpatient)[1,3]	23	83%	92%	92%
Prophylactic Antibiotic Selection	28	100%	98%	97%
Prophylactic Antibiotic Select. (Outpatient)[1,3]	19	100%	95%	94%
Prophylactic Antibiotic Stopped	26	100%	96%	94%
Recommended VTP Ordered	25	100%	97%	94%
Urinary Catheter Removal[1]	1	100%	89%	90%
Children's Asthma Care				
Received Systemic Corticosteroids	-	-	-	100%
Received Home Management Plan	-	-	-	71%
Received Reliever Medication	-	-	-	100%
Use of Medical Imaging				
Combination Abdominal CT Scan	444	0.056	0.109	0.191
Combination Chest CT Scan	442	0.002	0.010	0.054
Follow-up Mammogram/Ultrasound	639	5.2%	9.2%	8.4%
MRI for Low Back Pain[5]	0	-	30.1%	32.7%
Survey of Patients' Hospital Experiences				
Area Around Room 'Always' Quiet at Night	300+	58%	-	58%
Doctors 'Always' Communicated Well	300+	83%	-	80%
Home Recovery Information Given	300+	89%	-	82%
Hospital Given 9 or 10 on 10 Point Scale	300+	71%	-	67%
Meds 'Always' Explained Before Given	300+	62%	-	60%
Nurses 'Always' Communicated Well	300+	79%	-	76%
Pain 'Always' Well Controlled	300+	73%	-	69%
Room and Bathroom 'Always' Clean	300+	75%	-	71%
Timely Help 'Always' Received	300+	66%	-	64%
Would Definitely Recommend Hospital	300+	77%	-	69%

NOTE: Hospital profiles are in alphabetical order by state, then city, then hospital within the city; Rankings exclude hospitals with less than 25 cases except for patient surveys which excludes hospitals with less than 100 cases; (a) 100–299 cases; (1) The number of cases is too small to be sure how well a hospital is performing; (2) The hospital indicated that the data submitted for this measure were based on a sample of cases; (3) Data was collected during a shorter time period (fewer quarters) than the maximum possible time for this measure; (4) Suppressed for one or more quarters by CMS; (5) No data is available from the hospital for this measure; (6) Fewer than 100 patients completed the HCAHPS survey. Use these rates with caution, as the number of surveys may be too low to reliably assess hospital performance; (7) Survey results are based on less than 12 months of data; (8) Survey results are not available for this reporting period; (9) No or very few patients were eligible for the HCAHPS survey. The scores shown, if any, reflect a very small number of surveys; (10) A state average was not calculated because too few hospitals in the state submitted data; (11) There were discrepancies in the data collection process; Please refer to the User's Guide for a full explanation of data.

Berkshire Medical Center

725 North Street
Pittsfield, MA 01201
URL: www.berkshirehealthsystems.org
Type: Acute Care Hospitals
Ownership: Voluntary Non-Profit - Other

Phone: 413-447-2000
Fax: 413-447-2091

Emergency Services: Yes
Beds: 302

Key Personnel:
CEO/President . . . . David E Phelps
Chief of Medical Staff . . . . Robert Wespier MD
Operating Room . . . . Diana Vallone RN
Pediatric In-Patient Care . . . . . . Michael Fabrizio MD
Radiology . . . . Anthony Depasquale

Measure	Cases	This Hosp.	State Avg.	U.S. Avg.
Heart Attack Care				
ACE Inhibitor or ARB for LVSD[1]	9	100%	94%	96%
Aspirin at Arrival	88	100%	99%	99%
Aspirin at Discharge	58	100%	99%	98%
Beta Blocker at Discharge	64	100%	99%	98%
Fibrinolytic Medication Timing[1]	1	0%	50%	55%
PCI Within 90 Minutes of Arrival	0	-	93%	90%
Smoking Cessation Advice[1]	7	100%	99%	99%
Chest Pain/Possible Heart Attack Care				
Aspirin at Arrival	109	100%	96%	95%
Median Time to ECG (minutes)	109	8	10	8
Median Time to Transfer (minutes)[1,3]	1	55	65	61
Fibrinolytic Medication Timing	31	81%	78%	54%
Heart Failure Care				
ACE Inhibitor or ARB for LVSD	55	100%	94%	94%
Discharge Instructions	201	100%	89%	88%
Evaluation of LVS Function	284	100%	98%	98%
Smoking Cessation Advice	29	100%	97%	98%
Pneumonia Care				
Appropriate Initial Antibiotic	148	99%	93%	92%
Blood Culture Timing	283	99%	95%	96%
Influenza Vaccine	195	95%	92%	91%
Initial Antibiotic Timing	250	98%	96%	95%
Pneumococcal Vaccine	282	98%	93%	93%
Smoking Cessation Advice	69	100%	96%	97%
Surgical Care Improvement Project				
Appropriate VTP Within 24 Hours[2]	335	98%	96%	92%
Appropriate Hair Removal[2]	721	100%	100%	99%
Appropriate Beta Blocker Usage[2]	236	100%	96%	93%
Controlled Postoperative Blood Glucose[2]	0	-	95%	93%
Prophylactic Antibiotic Timing[2]	441	98%	97%	97%
Prophylactic Antibiotic Timing (Outpatient)	279	98%	92%	92%
Prophylactic Antibiotic Selection[2]	441	98%	98%	97%
Prophylactic Antibiotic Select. (Outpatient)	276	98%	95%	94%
Prophylactic Antibiotic Stopped[2]	432	98%	96%	94%
Recommended VTP Ordered[2]	335	98%	97%	94%
Urinary Catheter Removal[2]	166	93%	89%	90%
Children's Asthma Care				
Received Systemic Corticosteroids	-	-	-	100%
Received Home Management Plan	-	-	-	71%
Received Reliever Medication	-	-	-	100%
Use of Medical Imaging				
Combination Abdominal CT Scan	1,989	0.090	0.109	0.191
Combination Chest CT Scan	1,860	0.059	0.010	0.054
Follow-up Mammogram/Ultrasound	2,984	5.7%	9.2%	8.4%
MRI for Low Back Pain	399	29.3%	30.1%	32.7%
Survey of Patients' Hospital Experiences				
Area Around Room 'Always' Quiet at Night	300+	43%	-	58%
Doctors 'Always' Communicated Well	300+	76%	-	80%
Home Recovery Information Given	300+	91%	-	82%
Hospital Given 9 or 10 on 10 Point Scale	300+	66%	-	67%
Meds 'Always' Explained Before Given	300+	58%	-	60%
Nurses 'Always' Communicated Well	300+	80%	-	76%
Pain 'Always' Well Controlled	300+	72%	-	69%
Room and Bathroom 'Always' Clean	300+	76%	-	71%
Timely Help 'Always' Received	300+	64%	-	64%
Would Definitely Recommend Hospital	300+	69%	-	69%

Jordan Hospital

275 Sandwich Street
Plymouth, MA 02360
URL: www.jordanhospital.org
Type: Acute Care Hospitals
Ownership: Voluntary Non-Profit - Private

Phone: 508-746-2000
Fax: 508-830-1131

Emergency Services: No
Beds: 139

Key Personnel:
CEO/President . . . . Peter J Holden
Chief of Medical Staff . . . . Harvey J Kowaloff, MD, MMM
Radiology . . . . David Betteridge
Emergency Room . . . . Erin Ackland, MD
Patient Relations . . . . Carrol Dillitlane

Measure	Cases	This Hosp.	State Avg.	U.S. Avg.
Heart Attack Care				
ACE Inhibitor or ARB for LVSD[1]	11	100%	94%	96%
Aspirin at Arrival	82	100%	99%	99%
Aspirin at Discharge	48	94%	99%	98%
Beta Blocker at Discharge	56	100%	99%	98%
Fibrinolytic Medication Timing	0	-	50%	55%
PCI Within 90 Minutes of Arrival	0	-	93%	90%
Smoking Cessation Advice[1]	3	67%	99%	99%
Chest Pain/Possible Heart Attack Care				
Aspirin at Arrival	165	98%	96%	95%
Median Time to ECG (minutes)	174	22	10	8
Median Time to Transfer (minutes)	0	-	65	61
Fibrinolytic Medication Timing	0	-	78%	54%
Heart Failure Care				
ACE Inhibitor or ARB for LVSD	56	98%	94%	94%
Discharge Instructions	194	82%	89%	88%
Evaluation of LVS Function	268	97%	98%	98%
Smoking Cessation Advice[1]	20	100%	97%	98%
Pneumonia Care				
Appropriate Initial Antibiotic	203	94%	93%	92%
Blood Culture Timing	277	96%	95%	96%
Influenza Vaccine	220	92%	92%	91%
Initial Antibiotic Timing	372	97%	96%	95%
Pneumococcal Vaccine	301	93%	93%	93%
Smoking Cessation Advice	94	98%	96%	97%
Surgical Care Improvement Project				
Appropriate VTP Within 24 Hours	159	99%	96%	92%
Appropriate Hair Removal	579	100%	100%	99%
Appropriate Beta Blocker Usage	174	91%	96%	93%
Controlled Postoperative Blood Glucose	0	-	95%	93%
Prophylactic Antibiotic Timing	428	96%	97%	97%
Prophylactic Antibiotic Timing (Outpatient)	77	95%	92%	92%
Prophylactic Antibiotic Selection	429	98%	98%	97%
Prophylactic Antibiotic Select. (Outpatient)	76	97%	95%	94%
Prophylactic Antibiotic Stopped	420	99%	96%	94%
Recommended VTP Ordered	160	99%	97%	94%
Urinary Catheter Removal	77	91%	89%	90%
Children's Asthma Care				
Received Systemic Corticosteroids	-	-	-	100%
Received Home Management Plan	-	-	-	71%
Received Reliever Medication	-	-	-	100%
Use of Medical Imaging				
Combination Abdominal CT Scan	1,338	0.159	0.109	0.191
Combination Chest CT Scan	893	0.012	0.010	0.054
Follow-up Mammogram/Ultrasound	1,832	9.8%	9.2%	8.4%
MRI for Low Back Pain	255	29.0%	30.1%	32.7%
Survey of Patients' Hospital Experiences				
Area Around Room 'Always' Quiet at Night	300+	45%	-	58%
Doctors 'Always' Communicated Well	300+	78%	-	80%
Home Recovery Information Given	300+	80%	-	82%
Hospital Given 9 or 10 on 10 Point Scale	300+	65%	-	67%
Meds 'Always' Explained Before Given	300+	60%	-	60%
Nurses 'Always' Communicated Well	300+	73%	-	76%
Pain 'Always' Well Controlled	300+	73%	-	69%
Room and Bathroom 'Always' Clean	300+	64%	-	71%
Timely Help 'Always' Received	300+	63%	-	64%
Would Definitely Recommend Hospital	300+	70%	-	69%

Quincy Medical Center

114 Whitwell Street
Quincy, MA 02169
URL: www.quincymc.org
Type: Acute Care Hospitals
Ownership: Voluntary Non-Profit - Private

Phone: 617-773-6100
Fax: 617-376-4019

Emergency Services: Yes
Beds: 282

Key Personnel:
CEO/President . . . . Gary Gevans
Quality Assurance . . . . Sandi Austin

Measure	Cases	This Hosp.	State Avg.	U.S. Avg.
Heart Attack Care				
ACE Inhibitor or ARB for LVSD[1]	10	100%	94%	96%
Aspirin at Arrival	70	100%	99%	99%
Aspirin at Discharge	51	100%	99%	98%
Beta Blocker at Discharge	50	98%	99%	98%
Fibrinolytic Medication Timing	0	-	50%	55%
PCI Within 90 Minutes of Arrival	0	-	93%	90%
Smoking Cessation Advice[1]	6	83%	99%	99%
Chest Pain/Possible Heart Attack Care				
Aspirin at Arrival	59	100%	96%	95%
Median Time to ECG (minutes)	63	17	10	8
Median Time to Transfer (minutes)[1]	22	91	65	61
Fibrinolytic Medication Timing	0	-	78%	54%
Heart Failure Care				
ACE Inhibitor or ARB for LVSD	61	98%	94%	94%
Discharge Instructions	164	96%	89%	88%
Evaluation of LVS Function	246	99%	98%	98%
Smoking Cessation Advice	30	100%	97%	98%
Pneumonia Care				
Appropriate Initial Antibiotic	138	96%	93%	92%
Blood Culture Timing	163	90%	95%	96%
Influenza Vaccine	104	88%	92%	91%
Initial Antibiotic Timing	176	96%	96%	95%
Pneumococcal Vaccine	155	90%	93%	93%
Smoking Cessation Advice	72	100%	96%	97%
Surgical Care Improvement Project				
Appropriate VTP Within 24 Hours	210	98%	96%	92%
Appropriate Hair Removal	395	99%	100%	99%
Appropriate Beta Blocker Usage	119	91%	96%	93%
Controlled Postoperative Blood Glucose	0	-	95%	93%
Prophylactic Antibiotic Timing	97	81%	97%	97%
Prophylactic Antibiotic Timing (Outpatient)	75	85%	92%	92%
Prophylactic Antibiotic Selection	95	95%	98%	97%
Prophylactic Antibiotic Select. (Outpatient)	67	81%	95%	94%
Prophylactic Antibiotic Stopped	87	89%	96%	94%
Recommended VTP Ordered	210	100%	97%	94%
Urinary Catheter Removal	46	54%	89%	90%
Children's Asthma Care				
Received Systemic Corticosteroids	-	-	-	100%
Received Home Management Plan	-	-	-	71%
Received Reliever Medication	-	-	-	100%
Use of Medical Imaging				
Combination Abdominal CT Scan	751	0.067	0.109	0.191
Combination Chest CT Scan	435	0.016	0.010	0.054
Follow-up Mammogram/Ultrasound	975	4.7%	9.2%	8.4%
MRI for Low Back Pain[5]	0	-	30.1%	32.7%
Survey of Patients' Hospital Experiences				
Area Around Room 'Always' Quiet at Night	300+	44%	-	58%
Doctors 'Always' Communicated Well	300+	73%	-	80%
Home Recovery Information Given	300+	85%	-	82%
Hospital Given 9 or 10 on 10 Point Scale	300+	59%	-	67%
Meds 'Always' Explained Before Given	300+	59%	-	60%
Nurses 'Always' Communicated Well	300+	74%	-	76%
Pain 'Always' Well Controlled	300+	72%	-	69%
Room and Bathroom 'Always' Clean	300+	70%	-	71%
Timely Help 'Always' Received	300+	59%	-	64%
Would Definitely Recommend Hospital	300+	61%	-	69%

NOTE: Hospital profiles are in alphabetical order by state, then city, then hospital within the city; Rankings exclude hospitals with less than 25 cases except for patient surveys which excludes hospitals with less than 100 cases; (a) 100–299 cases; (1) The number of cases is too small to be sure how well a hospital is performing; (2) The hospital indicated that the data submitted for this measure were based on a sample of cases; (3) Data was collected during a shorter time period (fewer quarters) than the maximum possible time for this measure; (4) Suppressed for one or more quarters by CMS; (5) No data is available from the hospital for this measure; (6) Fewer than 100 patients completed the HCAHPS survey. Use these rates with caution, as the number of surveys may be too low to reliably assess hospital performance; (7) Survey results are based on less than 12 months of data; (8) Survey results are not available for this reporting period; (9) No or very few patients were eligible for the HCAHPS survey. The scores shown, if any, reflect a very small number of surveys; (10) A state average was not calculated because too few hospitals in the state submitted data; (11) There were discrepancies in the data collection process; Please refer to the User's Guide for a full explanation of data.

North Shore Medical Center

81 Highland Avenue
Salem, MA 01970
Phone: 978-741-1215
Fax: 978-744-9110
Type: Acute Care Hospitals
Emergency Services: Yes
Ownership: Voluntary Non-Profit - Private
Beds: 260

Key Personnel:
CEO/President. . . . . Robert Rorton
Cardiac Laboratory. . . . . David Roberts
Chief of Medical Staff. . . . . Mitchell Rein
Emergency Room . . . . Vivian Kane

Measure	Cases	This Hosp.	State Avg.	U.S. Avg.
Heart Attack Care				
ACE Inhibitor or ARB for LVSD	46	100%	94%	96%
Aspirin at Arrival	298	100%	99%	99%
Aspirin at Discharge	301	100%	99%	98%
Beta Blocker at Discharge	304	100%	99%	98%
Fibrinolytic Medication Timing	0	-	50%	55%
PCI Within 90 Minutes of Arrival	91	98%	93%	90%
Smoking Cessation Advice	106	100%	99%	99%
Chest Pain/Possible Heart Attack Care				
Aspirin at Arrival[1,3]	3	100%	96%	95%
Median Time to ECG (minutes)[1,3]	3	9	10	8
Median Time to Transfer (minutes)[5]	0	-	65	61
Fibrinolytic Medication Timing[3]	0	-	78%	54%
Heart Failure Care				
ACE Inhibitor or ARB for LVSD	108	98%	94%	94%
Discharge Instructions	425	95%	89%	88%
Evaluation of LVS Function	596	100%	98%	98%
Smoking Cessation Advice	54	100%	97%	98%
Pneumonia Care				
Appropriate Initial Antibiotic	334	97%	93%	92%
Blood Culture Timing	526	94%	95%	96%
Influenza Vaccine	352	95%	92%	91%
Initial Antibiotic Timing	493	94%	96%	95%
Pneumococcal Vaccine	502	90%	93%	93%
Smoking Cessation Advice	150	98%	96%	97%
Surgical Care Improvement Project				
Appropriate VTP Within 24 Hours[2]	157	97%	96%	92%
Appropriate Hair Removal[2]	525	100%	100%	99%
Appropriate Beta Blocker Usage[2]	222	97%	96%	93%
Controlled Postoperative Blood Glucose[2]	114	100%	95%	93%
Prophylactic Antibiotic Timing[2]	388	98%	97%	97%
Prophylactic Antibiotic Timing (Outpatient)	505	99%	92%	92%
Prophylactic Antibiotic Selection[2]	399	98%	98%	97%
Prophylactic Antibiotic Select. (Outpatient)	501	99%	95%	94%
Prophylactic Antibiotic Stopped[2]	365	97%	96%	94%
Recommended VTP Ordered[2]	159	98%	97%	94%
Urinary Catheter Removal[2]	122	78%	89%	90%
Children's Asthma Care				
Received Systemic Corticosteroids	-	-	-	100%
Received Home Management Plan	-	-	-	71%
Received Reliever Medication	-	-	-	100%
Use of Medical Imaging				
Combination Abdominal CT Scan	2,380	0.091	0.109	0.191
Combination Chest CT Scan	2,048	0.001	0.010	0.054
Follow-up Mammogram/Ultrasound	5,237	8.5%	9.2%	8.4%
MRI for Low Back Pain	375	31.5%	30.1%	32.7%
Survey of Patients' Hospital Experiences				
Area Around Room 'Always' Quiet at Night	300+	53%	-	58%
Doctors 'Always' Communicated Well	300+	76%	-	80%
Home Recovery Information Given	300+	85%	-	82%
Hospital Given 9 or 10 on 10 Point Scale	300+	66%	-	67%
Meds 'Always' Explained Before Given	300+	60%	-	60%
Nurses 'Always' Communicated Well	300+	75%	-	76%
Pain 'Always' Well Controlled	300+	70%	-	69%
Room and Bathroom 'Always' Clean	300+	69%	-	71%
Timely Help 'Always' Received	300+	63%	-	64%
Would Definitely Recommend Hospital	300+	74%	-	69%

South Shore Hospital

55 Fogg Road
South Weymouth, MA 02190
Phone: 781-340-8000
Fax: 781-337-3768
URL: www.southshorehospital.org
Type: Acute Care Hospitals
Emergency Services: Yes
Ownership: Voluntary Non-Profit - Private
Beds: 303

Key Personnel:
CEO/President. . . . . Richard Aubut
Chief of Medical Staff. . . . . Brian Battista
Radiology. . . . . Russell Kelley

Measure	Cases	This Hosp.	State Avg.	U.S. Avg.
Heart Attack Care				
ACE Inhibitor or ARB for LVSD	38	89%	94%	96%
Aspirin at Arrival	281	100%	99%	99%
Aspirin at Discharge	240	99%	99%	98%
Beta Blocker at Discharge	233	100%	99%	98%
Fibrinolytic Medication Timing	0	-	50%	55%
PCI Within 90 Minutes of Arrival	89	94%	93%	90%
Smoking Cessation Advice	70	99%	99%	99%
Chest Pain/Possible Heart Attack Care				
Aspirin at Arrival	51	90%	96%	95%
Median Time to ECG (minutes)	54	9	10	8
Median Time to Transfer (minutes)[1,3]	2	188	65	61
Fibrinolytic Medication Timing[3]	0	-	78%	54%
Heart Failure Care				
ACE Inhibitor or ARB for LVSD	176	84%	94%	94%
Discharge Instructions	540	64%	89%	88%
Evaluation of LVS Function	858	99%	98%	98%
Smoking Cessation Advice	82	96%	97%	98%
Pneumonia Care				
Appropriate Initial Antibiotic	251	97%	93%	92%
Blood Culture Timing	263	90%	95%	96%
Influenza Vaccine	283	98%	92%	91%
Initial Antibiotic Timing	492	96%	96%	95%
Pneumococcal Vaccine	481	98%	93%	93%
Smoking Cessation Advice	101	99%	96%	97%
Surgical Care Improvement Project				
Appropriate VTP Within 24 Hours	479	98%	96%	92%
Appropriate Hair Removal	1,123	97%	100%	99%
Appropriate Beta Blocker Usage	371	89%	96%	93%
Controlled Postoperative Blood Glucose	0	-	95%	93%
Prophylactic Antibiotic Timing	725	98%	97%	97%
Prophylactic Antibiotic Timing (Outpatient)	356	94%	92%	92%
Prophylactic Antibiotic Selection	725	98%	98%	97%
Prophylactic Antibiotic Select. (Outpatient)	345	93%	95%	94%
Prophylactic Antibiotic Stopped	712	96%	96%	94%
Recommended VTP Ordered	481	98%	97%	94%
Urinary Catheter Removal	159	75%	89%	90%
Children's Asthma Care				
Received Systemic Corticosteroids	-	-	-	100%
Received Home Management Plan	-	-	-	71%
Received Reliever Medication	-	-	-	100%
Use of Medical Imaging				
Combination Abdominal CT Scan	1,304	0.105	0.109	0.191
Combination Chest CT Scan	945	0.042	0.010	0.054
Follow-up Mammogram/Ultrasound	1,772	9.7%	9.2%	8.4%
MRI for Low Back Pain	139	30.2%	30.1%	32.7%
Survey of Patients' Hospital Experiences				
Area Around Room 'Always' Quiet at Night	300+	52%	-	58%
Doctors 'Always' Communicated Well	300+	79%	-	80%
Home Recovery Information Given	300+	88%	-	82%
Hospital Given 9 or 10 on 10 Point Scale	300+	69%	-	67%
Meds 'Always' Explained Before Given	300+	65%	-	60%
Nurses 'Always' Communicated Well	300+	78%	-	76%
Pain 'Always' Well Controlled	300+	70%	-	69%
Room and Bathroom 'Always' Clean	300+	73%	-	71%
Timely Help 'Always' Received	300+	65%	-	64%
Would Definitely Recommend Hospital	300+	74%	-	69%

Harrington Memorial Hospital

100 South Street
Southbridge, MA 01550
Phone: 508-765-9771
Fax: 508-764-2486
E-mail: hr@harringtonhospital.org
URL: www.harringtonhospital.org
Type: Acute Care Hospitals
Emergency Services: Yes
Ownership: Voluntary Non-Profit - Private
Beds: 113

Key Personnel:
CEO/President. . . . . Ed Moore
Chief of Medical Staff . . . . Vladas Litani, MD
Infection Control. . . . . Judith Zaido
Operating Room. . . . . Laura Fortin
Pediatric In-Patient Care . . . . Ann Beaudry
Quality Assurance . . . . Marlene Mach
Emergency Room . . . . Michael P Gaudet
Intensive Care Unit. . . . . Marsha Woodard

Measure	Cases	This Hosp.	State Avg.	U.S. Avg.
Heart Attack Care				
ACE Inhibitor or ARB for LVSD[1]	3	100%	94%	96%
Aspirin at Arrival	27	96%	99%	99%
Aspirin at Discharge[1]	20	100%	99%	98%
Beta Blocker at Discharge[1]	21	95%	99%	98%
Fibrinolytic Medication Timing	0	-	50%	55%
PCI Within 90 Minutes of Arrival	0	-	93%	90%
Smoking Cessation Advice[1]	3	100%	99%	99%
Chest Pain/Possible Heart Attack Care				
Aspirin at Arrival	146	88%	96%	95%
Median Time to ECG (minutes)	152	18	10	8
Median Time to Transfer (minutes)[1]	17	117	65	61
Fibrinolytic Medication Timing	0	-	78%	54%
Heart Failure Care				
ACE Inhibitor or ARB for LVSD	36	89%	94%	94%
Discharge Instructions	90	61%	89%	88%
Evaluation of LVS Function	128	97%	98%	98%
Smoking Cessation Advice[1]	9	100%	97%	98%
Pneumonia Care				
Appropriate Initial Antibiotic	107	85%	93%	92%
Blood Culture Timing	113	89%	95%	96%
Influenza Vaccine	84	82%	92%	91%
Initial Antibiotic Timing	130	97%	96%	95%
Pneumococcal Vaccine	138	86%	93%	93%
Smoking Cessation Advice	42	83%	96%	97%
Surgical Care Improvement Project				
Appropriate VTP Within 24 Hours	66	85%	96%	92%
Appropriate Hair Removal	139	99%	100%	99%
Appropriate Beta Blocker Usage	35	100%	96%	93%
Controlled Postoperative Blood Glucose	0	-	95%	93%
Prophylactic Antibiotic Timing	83	88%	97%	97%
Prophylactic Antibiotic Timing (Outpatient)	125	85%	92%	92%
Prophylactic Antibiotic Selection	83	95%	98%	97%
Prophylactic Antibiotic Select. (Outpatient)	122	87%	95%	94%
Prophylactic Antibiotic Stopped	78	94%	96%	94%
Recommended VTP Ordered	66	85%	97%	94%
Urinary Catheter Removal	36	97%	89%	90%
Children's Asthma Care				
Received Systemic Corticosteroids	-	-	-	100%
Received Home Management Plan	-	-	-	71%
Received Reliever Medication	-	-	-	100%
Use of Medical Imaging				
Combination Abdominal CT Scan	323	0.235	0.109	0.191
Combination Chest CT Scan	294	0.037	0.010	0.054
Follow-up Mammogram/Ultrasound	628	10.4%	9.2%	8.4%
MRI for Low Back Pain	63	38.1%	30.1%	32.7%
Survey of Patients' Hospital Experiences				
Area Around Room 'Always' Quiet at Night	300+	50%	-	58%
Doctors 'Always' Communicated Well	300+	78%	-	80%
Home Recovery Information Given	300+	83%	-	82%
Hospital Given 9 or 10 on 10 Point Scale	300+	67%	-	67%
Meds 'Always' Explained Before Given	300+	61%	-	60%
Nurses 'Always' Communicated Well	300+	75%	-	76%
Pain 'Always' Well Controlled	300+	71%	-	69%
Room and Bathroom 'Always' Clean	300+	79%	-	71%
Timely Help 'Always' Received	300+	67%	-	64%
Would Definitely Recommend Hospital	300+	71%	-	69%

NOTE: Hospital profiles are in alphabetical order by state, then city, then hospital within the city; Rankings exclude hospitals with less than 25 cases except for patient surveys which excludes hospitals with less than 100 cases; (a) 100–299 cases; (1) The number of cases is too small to be sure how well a hospital is performing; (2) The hospital indicated that the data submitted for this measure were based on a sample of cases; (3) Data was collected during a shorter time period (fewer quarters) than the maximum possible time for this measure; (4) Suppressed for one or more quarters by CMS; (5) No data is available from the hospital for this measure; (6) Fewer than 100 patients completed the HCAHPS survey. Use these rates with caution, as the number of surveys may be too low to reliably assess hospital performance; (7) Survey results are based on less than 12 months of data; (8) Survey results are not available for this reporting period; (9) No or very few patients were eligible for the HCAHPS survey. The scores shown, if any, reflect a very small number of surveys; (10) A state average was not calculated because too few hospitals in the state submitted data; (11) There were discrepancies in the data collection process; Please refer to the User's Guide for a full explanation of data.

Baystate Medical Center

759 Chestnut Street
Springfield, MA 01199
Phone: 413-794-0000
Fax: 413-794-3832
URL: www.baystatehealth.com
Type: Acute Care Hospitals
Emergency Services: Yes
Ownership: Voluntary Non-Profit - Private
Beds: 653

Key Personnel:

CEO/President. . . . . Mark R Tolosky
Chief of Medical Staff . . . . Martin Broder, MD
Operating Room. . . . . Deborah A. Provost
Pediatric Ambulatory Care . . . . . . Edward Reiter, MD
Pediatric In-Patient Care . . . . Edward Reiter, MD
Quality Assurance . . . . Evan M. Benjamin, MD
Radiology. . . . . Eckert Sachsse, MD
Emergency Room . . . . John Santoro, MD

Measure	Cases	This Hosp.	State Avg.	U.S. Avg.
Heart Attack Care				
ACE Inhibitor or ARB for LVSD	193	93%	94%	96%
Aspirin at Arrival	500	100%	99%	99%
Aspirin at Discharge	1,055	100%	99%	98%
Beta Blocker at Discharge	1,015	99%	99%	98%
Fibrinolytic Medication Timing[1]	1	100%	50%	55%
PCI Within 90 Minutes of Arrival	138	96%	93%	90%
Smoking Cessation Advice	311	100%	99%	99%
Chest Pain/Possible Heart Attack Care				
Aspirin at Arrival[1,3]	1	100%	96%	95%
Median Time to ECG (minutes)[1,3]	2	8	10	8
Median Time to Transfer (minutes)[5]	0	-	65	61
Fibrinolytic Medication Timing[5]	0	-	78%	54%
Heart Failure Care				
ACE Inhibitor or ARB for LVSD	311	96%	94%	94%
Discharge Instructions	750	97%	89%	88%
Evaluation of LVS Function	967	98%	98%	98%
Smoking Cessation Advice	166	97%	97%	98%
Pneumonia Care				
Appropriate Initial Antibiotic	268	91%	93%	92%
Blood Culture Timing	410	84%	95%	96%
Influenza Vaccine	301	86%	92%	91%
Initial Antibiotic Timing	503	91%	96%	95%
Pneumococcal Vaccine	386	89%	93%	93%
Smoking Cessation Advice	158	95%	96%	97%
Surgical Care Improvement Project				
Appropriate VTP Within 24 Hours[2]	320	99%	96%	92%
Appropriate Hair Removal[2]	1,670	100%	100%	99%
Appropriate Beta Blocker Usage[2]	580	97%	96%	93%
Controlled Postoperative Blood Glucose[2]	341	97%	95%	93%
Prophylactic Antibiotic Timing[2]	1,436	99%	97%	97%
Prophylactic Antibiotic Timing (Outpatient)	669	92%	92%	92%
Prophylactic Antibiotic Selection[2]	1,446	100%	98%	97%
Prophylactic Antibiotic Select. (Outpatient)	645	98%	95%	94%
Prophylactic Antibiotic Stopped[2]	1,380	99%	96%	94%
Recommended VTP Ordered[2]	320	100%	97%	94%
Urinary Catheter Removal[2]	687	100%	89%	90%
Children's Asthma Care				
Received Systemic Corticosteroids	129	100%	-	100%
Received Home Management Plan	129	75%	-	71%
Received Reliever Medication	129	99%	-	100%
Use of Medical Imaging				
Combination Abdominal CT Scan	1,645	0.042	0.109	0.191
Combination Chest CT Scan	1,406	0.001	0.010	0.054
Follow-up Mammogram/Ultrasound	1,662	7.2%	9.2%	8.4%
MRI for Low Back Pain	121	27.3%	30.1%	32.7%
Survey of Patients' Hospital Experiences				
Area Around Room 'Always' Quiet at Night	300+	42%	-	58%
Doctors 'Always' Communicated Well	300+	80%	-	80%
Home Recovery Information Given	300+	85%	-	82%
Hospital Given 9 or 10 on 10 Point Scale	300+	65%	-	67%
Meds 'Always' Explained Before Given	300+	63%	-	60%
Nurses 'Always' Communicated Well	300+	77%	-	76%
Pain 'Always' Well Controlled	300+	69%	-	69%
Room and Bathroom 'Always' Clean	300+	66%	-	71%
Timely Help 'Always' Received	300+	57%	-	64%
Would Definitely Recommend Hospital	300+	75%	-	69%

Mercy Medical Center

271 Carew Street
Springfield, MA 01104
Phone: 413-748-9000
Fax: 413-748-9609
URL: www.mercycares.com
Type: Acute Care Hospitals
Emergency Services: Yes
Ownership: Voluntary Non-Profit - Private
Beds: 182

Key Personnel:

CEO/President. . . . . Vince J McCorkle
Chief of Medical Staff . . . . P Henri Lamonthe
Radiology. . . . . Gregory Blackman

Measure	Cases	This Hosp.	State Avg.	U.S. Avg.
Heart Attack Care				
ACE Inhibitor or ARB for LVSD[1]	6	83%	94%	96%
Aspirin at Arrival	87	98%	99%	99%
Aspirin at Discharge	55	98%	99%	98%
Beta Blocker at Discharge	60	98%	99%	98%
Fibrinolytic Medication Timing	0	-	50%	55%
PCI Within 90 Minutes of Arrival	0	-	93%	90%
Smoking Cessation Advice[1]	5	100%	99%	99%
Chest Pain/Possible Heart Attack Care				
Aspirin at Arrival	46	93%	96%	95%
Median Time to ECG (minutes)	49	7	10	8
Median Time to Transfer (minutes)[1]	15	71	65	61
Fibrinolytic Medication Timing	0	-	78%	54%
Heart Failure Care				
ACE Inhibitor or ARB for LVSD	79	97%	94%	94%
Discharge Instructions	249	77%	89%	88%
Evaluation of LVS Function	321	99%	98%	98%
Smoking Cessation Advice	61	98%	97%	98%
Pneumonia Care				
Appropriate Initial Antibiotic	146	97%	93%	92%
Blood Culture Timing	213	96%	95%	96%
Influenza Vaccine	140	96%	92%	91%
Initial Antibiotic Timing	211	99%	96%	95%
Pneumococcal Vaccine	190	94%	93%	93%
Smoking Cessation Advice	75	97%	96%	97%
Surgical Care Improvement Project				
Appropriate VTP Within 24 Hours	482	98%	96%	92%
Appropriate Hair Removal	977	100%	100%	99%
Appropriate Beta Blocker Usage	256	93%	96%	93%
Controlled Postoperative Blood Glucose	0	-	95%	93%
Prophylactic Antibiotic Timing	532	95%	97%	97%
Prophylactic Antibiotic Timing (Outpatient)	658	96%	92%	92%
Prophylactic Antibiotic Selection	537	97%	98%	97%
Prophylactic Antibiotic Select. (Outpatient)	654	98%	95%	94%
Prophylactic Antibiotic Stopped	497	96%	96%	94%
Recommended VTP Ordered	482	99%	97%	94%
Urinary Catheter Removal	216	86%	89%	90%
Children's Asthma Care				
Received Systemic Corticosteroids	-	-	-	100%
Received Home Management Plan	-	-	-	71%
Received Reliever Medication	-	-	-	100%
Use of Medical Imaging				
Combination Abdominal CT Scan	1,387	0.087	0.109	0.191
Combination Chest CT Scan	760	0.011	0.010	0.054
Follow-up Mammogram/Ultrasound	1,941	12.5%	9.2%	8.4%
MRI for Low Back Pain[5]	0	-	30.1%	32.7%
Survey of Patients' Hospital Experiences				
Area Around Room 'Always' Quiet at Night	300+	37%	-	58%
Doctors 'Always' Communicated Well	300+	77%	-	80%
Home Recovery Information Given	300+	86%	-	82%
Hospital Given 9 or 10 on 10 Point Scale	300+	61%	-	67%
Meds 'Always' Explained Before Given	300+	57%	-	60%
Nurses 'Always' Communicated Well	300+	72%	-	76%
Pain 'Always' Well Controlled	300+	64%	-	69%
Room and Bathroom 'Always' Clean	300+	67%	-	71%
Timely Help 'Always' Received	300+	57%	-	64%
Would Definitely Recommend Hospital	300+	69%	-	69%

Morton Hospital & Medical Center

88 Washington Street
Taunton, MA 02780
Phone: 508-828-7000
Fax: 508-824-6947
URL: www.mortonhospital.org
Type: Acute Care Hospitals
Emergency Services: Yes
Ownership: Voluntary Non-Profit - Private
Beds: 152

Key Personnel:

CEO/President. . . . . Thomas C Porter
Infection Control. . . . . Marie Lebrun, RN
Quality Assurance . . . . Richard J Slavick
Radiology. . . . . Richard S Jennis
Anesthesiology. . . . . Bijan Naikai, MD
Intensive Care Unit. . . . . Donna Chase, RN

Measure	Cases	This Hosp.	State Avg.	U.S. Avg.
Heart Attack Care				
ACE Inhibitor or ARB for LVSD[1]	8	100%	94%	96%
Aspirin at Arrival	52	98%	99%	99%
Aspirin at Discharge	34	97%	99%	98%
Beta Blocker at Discharge	35	100%	99%	98%
Fibrinolytic Medication Timing	0	-	50%	55%
PCI Within 90 Minutes of Arrival	0	-	93%	90%
Smoking Cessation Advice[1]	1	100%	99%	99%
Chest Pain/Possible Heart Attack Care				
Aspirin at Arrival	89	99%	96%	95%
Median Time to ECG (minutes)	95	16	10	8
Median Time to Transfer (minutes)[1]	17	113	65	61
Fibrinolytic Medication Timing	0	-	78%	54%
Heart Failure Care				
ACE Inhibitor or ARB for LVSD	73	93%	94%	94%
Discharge Instructions	166	91%	89%	88%
Evaluation of LVS Function	245	100%	98%	98%
Smoking Cessation Advice	26	100%	97%	98%
Pneumonia Care				
Appropriate Initial Antibiotic	125	94%	93%	92%
Blood Culture Timing	177	95%	95%	96%
Influenza Vaccine[1]	6	100%	92%	91%
Initial Antibiotic Timing	197	97%	96%	95%
Pneumococcal Vaccine	146	97%	93%	93%
Smoking Cessation Advice	39	100%	96%	97%
Surgical Care Improvement Project				
Appropriate VTP Within 24 Hours	181	92%	96%	92%
Appropriate Hair Removal	437	100%	100%	99%
Appropriate Beta Blocker Usage	151	89%	96%	93%
Controlled Postoperative Blood Glucose	0	-	95%	93%
Prophylactic Antibiotic Timing	298	98%	97%	97%
Prophylactic Antibiotic Timing (Outpatient)	92	99%	92%	92%
Prophylactic Antibiotic Selection	301	97%	98%	97%
Prophylactic Antibiotic Select. (Outpatient)	93	92%	95%	94%
Prophylactic Antibiotic Stopped	290	96%	96%	94%
Recommended VTP Ordered	182	94%	97%	94%
Urinary Catheter Removal	93	92%	89%	90%
Children's Asthma Care				
Received Systemic Corticosteroids	-	-	-	100%
Received Home Management Plan	-	-	-	71%
Received Reliever Medication	-	-	-	100%
Use of Medical Imaging				
Combination Abdominal CT Scan	831	0.036	0.109	0.191
Combination Chest CT Scan	642	0.003	0.010	0.054
Follow-up Mammogram/Ultrasound	1,926	6.3%	9.2%	8.4%
MRI for Low Back Pain	152	29.6%	30.1%	32.7%
Survey of Patients' Hospital Experiences				
Area Around Room 'Always' Quiet at Night	300+	49%	-	58%
Doctors 'Always' Communicated Well	300+	78%	-	80%
Home Recovery Information Given	300+	83%	-	82%
Hospital Given 9 or 10 on 10 Point Scale	300+	57%	-	67%
Meds 'Always' Explained Before Given	300+	60%	-	60%
Nurses 'Always' Communicated Well	300+	75%	-	76%
Pain 'Always' Well Controlled	300+	70%	-	69%
Room and Bathroom 'Always' Clean	300+	72%	-	71%
Timely Help 'Always' Received	300+	62%	-	64%
Would Definitely Recommend Hospital	300+	57%	-	69%

NOTE: Hospital profiles are in alphabetical order by state, then city, then hospital within the city; Rankings exclude hospitals with less than 25 cases except for patient surveys which excludes hospitals with less than 100 cases; (a) 100–299 cases; (1) The number of cases is too small to be sure how well a hospital is performing; (2) The hospital indicated that the data submitted for this measure were based on a sample of cases; (3) Data was collected during a shorter time period (fewer quarters) than the maximum possible time for this measure; (4) Suppressed for one or more quarters by CMS; (5) No data is available from the hospital for this measure; (6) Fewer than 100 patients completed the HCAHPS survey. Use these rates with caution, as the number of surveys may be too low to reliably assess hospital performance; (7) Survey results are based on less than 12 months of data; (8) Survey results are not available for this reporting period; (9) No or very few patients were eligible for the HCAHPS survey. The scores shown, if any, reflect a very small number of surveys; (10) A state average was not calculated because too few hospitals in the state submitted data; (11) There were discrepancies in the data collection process; Please refer to the User's Guide for a full explanation of data.

Baystate Mary Lane Hospital

85 South Street
Ware, MA 01082
URL: www.baystatehealth.com
Type: Acute Care Hospitals
Ownership: Voluntary Non-Profit - Private

Phone: 413-967-6211
Fax: 413-967-2109

Emergency Services: Yes
Beds: 31

Key Personnel:
CEO/President. . . . . Christine F Shirtcliff
Chief of Medical Staff. . . . . Richard Gerstein, MD
Coronary Care . . . . Tina Frazier, RN
Infection Control. . . . . Rosalie Rymarski, RN
Pediatric Ambulatory Care . . . . . Jeannette Tokarz, MD
Pediatric In-Patient Care . . . . . . Jeannette Tokarz, MD
Quality Assurance . . . . Clare Burgess
Radiology. . . . . Eckart Sachsse

Measure	Cases	This Hosp.	State Avg.	U.S. Avg.
Heart Attack Care				
ACE Inhibitor or ARB for LVSD[1]	3	100%	94%	96%
Aspirin at Arrival[1]	13	100%	99%	99%
Aspirin at Discharge[1]	4	100%	99%	98%
Beta Blocker at Discharge[1]	6	100%	99%	98%
Fibrinolytic Medication Timing[1]	1	0%	50%	55%
PCI Within 90 Minutes of Arrival	0	-	93%	90%
Smoking Cessation Advice[1]	1	100%	99%	99%
Chest Pain/Possible Heart Attack Care				
Aspirin at Arrival	43	95%	96%	95%
Median Time to ECG (minutes)	45	17	10	8
Median Time to Transfer (minutes)[1,3]	6	118	65	61
Fibrinolytic Medication Timing[1]	4	100%	78%	54%
Heart Failure Care				
ACE Inhibitor or ARB for LVSD[1]	10	100%	94%	94%
Discharge Instructions	37	100%	89%	88%
Evaluation of LVS Function	50	100%	98%	98%
Smoking Cessation Advice[1]	3	100%	97%	98%
Pneumonia Care				
Appropriate Initial Antibiotic	37	92%	93%	92%
Blood Culture Timing	47	98%	95%	96%
Influenza Vaccine[1]	23	100%	92%	91%
Initial Antibiotic Timing	38	95%	96%	95%
Pneumococcal Vaccine	34	97%	93%	93%
Smoking Cessation Advice[1]	15	100%	96%	97%
Surgical Care Improvement Project				
Appropriate VTP Within 24 Hours[1]	13	100%	96%	92%
Appropriate Hair Removal	45	100%	100%	99%
Appropriate Beta Blocker Usage[1]	10	100%	96%	93%
Controlled Postoperative Blood Glucose	0	-	95%	93%
Prophylactic Antibiotic Timing	35	94%	97%	97%
Prophylactic Antibiotic Timing (Outpatient)[1,3]	1	100%	92%	92%
Prophylactic Antibiotic Selection	34	97%	98%	97%
Prophylactic Antibiotic Select. (Outpatient)[1,3]	1	100%	95%	94%
Prophylactic Antibiotic Stopped	34	97%	96%	94%
Recommended VTP Ordered[1]	13	100%	97%	94%
Urinary Catheter Removal[1]	4	100%	89%	90%
Children's Asthma Care				
Received Systemic Corticosteroids	-	-	-	100%
Received Home Management Plan	-	-	-	71%
Received Reliever Medication	-	-	-	100%
Use of Medical Imaging				
Combination Abdominal CT Scan	230	0.035	0.109	0.191
Combination Chest CT Scan	149	0.000	0.010	0.054
Follow-up Mammogram/Ultrasound	298	5.4%	9.2%	8.4%
MRI for Low Back Pain[5]	0	-	30.1%	32.7%
Survey of Patients' Hospital Experiences				
Area Around Room 'Always' Quiet at Night	(a)	64%	-	58%
Doctors 'Always' Communicated Well	(a)	80%	-	80%
Home Recovery Information Given	(a)	88%	-	82%
Hospital Given 9 or 10 on 10 Point Scale	(a)	73%	-	67%
Meds 'Always' Explained Before Given	(a)	63%	-	60%
Nurses 'Always' Communicated Well	(a)	81%	-	76%
Pain 'Always' Well Controlled	(a)	72%	-	69%
Room and Bathroom 'Always' Clean	(a)	76%	-	71%
Timely Help 'Always' Received	(a)	73%	-	64%
Would Definitely Recommend Hospital	(a)	75%	-	69%

Emerson Hospital

Old Road To 9 Acre Corner
West Concord, MA 01742
Type: Acute Care Hospitals
Ownership: Voluntary Non-Profit - Private

Phone: 978-369-1400
Fax: 978-287-3726
Emergency Services: Yes
Beds: 167

Key Personnel:
CEO/President. . . . . Christine C Schuster
Chief of Medical Staff. . . . . Robert Hopkins
Operating Room. . . . . Diane Kalinowski
Pediatric In-Patient Care . . . . . . Marianne Sutton
Quality Assurance . . . . Regina Vurzynski
Radiology. . . . . Mark A Connaughton, MD
Emergency Room . . . . Alan Woodward

Measure	Cases	This Hosp.	State Avg.	U.S. Avg.
Heart Attack Care				
ACE Inhibitor or ARB for LVSD[1]	6	100%	94%	96%
Aspirin at Arrival	60	97%	99%	99%
Aspirin at Discharge	33	100%	99%	98%
Beta Blocker at Discharge	33	97%	99%	98%
Fibrinolytic Medication Timing	0	-	50%	55%
PCI Within 90 Minutes of Arrival	0	-	93%	90%
Smoking Cessation Advice[1]	5	80%	99%	99%
Chest Pain/Possible Heart Attack Care				
Aspirin at Arrival	70	99%	96%	95%
Median Time to ECG (minutes)	71	7	10	8
Median Time to Transfer (minutes)[1]	22	70	65	61
Fibrinolytic Medication Timing	0	-	78%	54%
Heart Failure Care				
ACE Inhibitor or ARB for LVSD	45	98%	94%	94%
Discharge Instructions	127	78%	89%	88%
Evaluation of LVS Function	193	99%	98%	98%
Smoking Cessation Advice[1]	10	100%	97%	98%
Pneumonia Care				
Appropriate Initial Antibiotic	87	94%	93%	92%
Blood Culture Timing	171	97%	95%	96%
Influenza Vaccine	113	95%	92%	91%
Initial Antibiotic Timing	172	97%	96%	95%
Pneumococcal Vaccine	188	95%	93%	93%
Smoking Cessation Advice[1]	24	96%	96%	97%
Surgical Care Improvement Project				
Appropriate VTP Within 24 Hours	217	91%	96%	92%
Appropriate Hair Removal	529	100%	100%	99%
Appropriate Beta Blocker Usage	139	91%	96%	93%
Controlled Postoperative Blood Glucose	0	-	95%	93%
Prophylactic Antibiotic Timing	361	92%	97%	97%
Prophylactic Antibiotic Timing (Outpatient)	278	94%	92%	92%
Prophylactic Antibiotic Selection	361	99%	98%	97%
Prophylactic Antibiotic Select. (Outpatient)	272	96%	95%	94%
Prophylactic Antibiotic Stopped	345	98%	96%	94%
Recommended VTP Ordered	217	96%	97%	94%
Urinary Catheter Removal	176	88%	89%	90%
Children's Asthma Care				
Received Systemic Corticosteroids	-	-	-	100%
Received Home Management Plan	-	-	-	71%
Received Reliever Medication	-	-	-	100%
Use of Medical Imaging				
Combination Abdominal CT Scan	686	0.055	0.109	0.191
Combination Chest CT Scan	614	0.002	0.010	0.054
Follow-up Mammogram/Ultrasound	1,698	14.5%	9.2%	8.4%
MRI for Low Back Pain	205	32.2%	30.1%	32.7%
Survey of Patients' Hospital Experiences				
Area Around Room 'Always' Quiet at Night	300+	50%	-	58%
Doctors 'Always' Communicated Well	300+	82%	-	80%
Home Recovery Information Given	300+	86%	-	82%
Hospital Given 9 or 10 on 10 Point Scale	300+	74%	-	67%
Meds 'Always' Explained Before Given	300+	66%	-	60%
Nurses 'Always' Communicated Well	300+	81%	-	76%
Pain 'Always' Well Controlled	300+	75%	-	69%
Room and Bathroom 'Always' Clean	300+	68%	-	71%
Timely Help 'Always' Received	300+	64%	-	64%
Would Definitely Recommend Hospital	300+	80%	-	69%

Noble Hospital

115 West Silver Street
Westfield, MA 01085
E-mail: hcote@noblehealth.org
URL: www.noblehospital.org
Type: Acute Care Hospitals
Ownership: Government - Federal

Phone: 413-568-2811
Fax: 413-562-5855

Emergency Services: No
Beds: 97

Key Personnel:
CEO/President. . . . . George Koller
Chief of Medical Staff. . . . . Stanley Strzemeko
Emergency Room . . . . David B Peterson

Measure	Cases	This Hosp.	State Avg.	U.S. Avg.
Heart Attack Care				
ACE Inhibitor or ARB for LVSD[1]	2	100%	94%	96%
Aspirin at Arrival	26	100%	99%	99%
Aspirin at Discharge[1]	20	100%	99%	98%
Beta Blocker at Discharge[1]	22	100%	99%	98%
Fibrinolytic Medication Timing	0	-	50%	55%
PCI Within 90 Minutes of Arrival	0	-	93%	90%
Smoking Cessation Advice[1]	5	100%	99%	99%
Chest Pain/Possible Heart Attack Care				
Aspirin at Arrival	40	98%	96%	95%
Median Time to ECG (minutes)	41	6	10	8
Median Time to Transfer (minutes)[1]	17	34	65	61
Fibrinolytic Medication Timing	0	-	78%	54%
Heart Failure Care				
ACE Inhibitor or ARB for LVSD	30	100%	94%	94%
Discharge Instructions	82	93%	89%	88%
Evaluation of LVS Function	104	91%	98%	98%
Smoking Cessation Advice[1]	8	100%	97%	98%
Pneumonia Care				
Appropriate Initial Antibiotic	85	88%	93%	92%
Blood Culture Timing	131	91%	95%	96%
Influenza Vaccine	91	100%	92%	91%
Initial Antibiotic Timing	126	96%	96%	95%
Pneumococcal Vaccine	119	100%	93%	93%
Smoking Cessation Advice	26	100%	96%	97%
Surgical Care Improvement Project				
Appropriate VTP Within 24 Hours	40	100%	96%	92%
Appropriate Hair Removal	73	100%	100%	99%
Appropriate Beta Blocker Usage[1]	23	100%	96%	93%
Controlled Postoperative Blood Glucose	0	-	95%	93%
Prophylactic Antibiotic Timing	49	96%	97%	97%
Prophylactic Antibiotic Timing (Outpatient)[1]	23	96%	92%	92%
Prophylactic Antibiotic Selection	49	96%	98%	97%
Prophylactic Antibiotic Select. (Outpatient)[1]	23	96%	95%	94%
Prophylactic Antibiotic Stopped	46	100%	96%	94%
Recommended VTP Ordered	40	100%	97%	94%
Urinary Catheter Removal[1]	9	89%	89%	90%
Children's Asthma Care				
Received Systemic Corticosteroids	-	-	-	100%
Received Home Management Plan	-	-	-	71%
Received Reliever Medication	-	-	-	100%
Use of Medical Imaging				
Combination Abdominal CT Scan	439	0.018	0.109	0.191
Combination Chest CT Scan	234	0.000	0.010	0.054
Follow-up Mammogram/Ultrasound	832	10.9%	9.2%	8.4%
MRI for Low Back Pain	78	33.3%	30.1%	32.7%
Survey of Patients' Hospital Experiences				
Area Around Room 'Always' Quiet at Night	300+	52%	-	58%
Doctors 'Always' Communicated Well	300+	80%	-	80%
Home Recovery Information Given	300+	90%	-	82%
Hospital Given 9 or 10 on 10 Point Scale	300+	67%	-	67%
Meds 'Always' Explained Before Given	300+	63%	-	60%
Nurses 'Always' Communicated Well	300+	79%	-	76%
Pain 'Always' Well Controlled	300+	76%	-	69%
Room and Bathroom 'Always' Clean	300+	78%	-	71%
Timely Help 'Always' Received	300+	71%	-	64%
Would Definitely Recommend Hospital	300+	69%	-	69%

NOTE: Hospital profiles are in alphabetical order by state, then city, then hospital within the city; Rankings exclude hospitals with less than 25 cases except for patient surveys which excludes hospitals with less than 100 cases; (a) 100–299 cases; (1) The number of cases is too small to be sure how well a hospital is performing; (2) The hospital indicated that the data submitted for this measure were based on a sample of cases; (3) Data was collected during a shorter time period (fewer quarters) than the maximum possible time for this measure; (4) Suppressed for one or more quarters by CMS; (5) No data is available from the hospital for this measure; (6) Fewer than 100 patients completed the HCAHPS survey. Use these rates with caution, as the number of surveys may be too low to reliably assess hospital performance; (7) Survey results are based on less than 12 months of data; (8) Survey results are not available for this reporting period; (9) No or very few patients were eligible for the HCAHPS survey. The scores shown, if any, reflect a very small number of surveys; (10) A state average was not calculated because too few hospitals in the state submitted data; (11) There were discrepancies in the data collection process; Please refer to the User's Guide for a full explanation of data.

Winchester Hospital

41 Highland Avenue
Winchester, MA 01890
URL: www.winchesterhospital.org
Type: Acute Care Hospitals
Ownership: Voluntary Non-Profit - Other

Phone: 781-729-9000
Fax: 781-756-2923

Emergency Services: Yes
Beds: 200

Key Personnel:
CEO/President . . . . Dale Lodge
Cardiac Laboratory . . . . Joseph Pappalardo
Chief of Medical Staff . . . . Donald J Deraska
Infection Control . . . . Kay Deackoff, RN
Operating Room . . . . Claire O'Brien
Pediatric Ambulatory Care . . . . . . Martha McCarty, MD
Quality Assurance . . . . Celeste Steele

Measure	Cases	This Hosp.	State Avg.	U.S. Avg.
Heart Attack Care				
ACE Inhibitor or ARB for LVSD[1,2]	13	100%	94%	96%
Aspirin at Arrival[2]	94	98%	99%	99%
Aspirin at Discharge[2]	67	100%	99%	98%
Beta Blocker at Discharge[2]	74	99%	99%	98%
Fibrinolytic Medication Timing[2]	0	-	50%	55%
PCI Within 90 Minutes of Arrival[2]	0	-	93%	90%
Smoking Cessation Advice[1,2]	8	100%	99%	99%
Chest Pain/Possible Heart Attack Care				
Aspirin at Arrival	122	93%	96%	95%
Median Time to ECG (minutes)	127	11	10	8
Median Time to Transfer (minutes)[1]	22	66	65	61
Fibrinolytic Medication Timing	0	-	78%	54%
Heart Failure Care				
ACE Inhibitor or ARB for LVSD[2]	51	96%	94%	94%
Discharge Instructions[2]	175	90%	89%	88%
Evaluation of LVS Function[2]	262	99%	98%	98%
Smoking Cessation Advice[1,2]	13	100%	97%	98%
Pneumonia Care				
Appropriate Initial Antibiotic	208	91%	93%	92%
Blood Culture Timing	240	92%	95%	96%
Influenza Vaccine	204	79%	92%	91%
Initial Antibiotic Timing	276	96%	96%	95%
Pneumococcal Vaccine	301	88%	93%	93%
Smoking Cessation Advice	69	100%	96%	97%
Surgical Care Improvement Project				
Appropriate VTP Within 24 Hours	333	95%	96%	92%
Appropriate Hair Removal	903	100%	100%	99%
Appropriate Beta Blocker Usage	322	98%	96%	93%
Controlled Postoperative Blood Glucose	0	-	95%	93%
Prophylactic Antibiotic Timing	602	95%	97%	97%
Prophylactic Antibiotic Timing (Outpatient)	241	88%	92%	92%
Prophylactic Antibiotic Selection	604	97%	98%	97%
Prophylactic Antibiotic Select. (Outpatient)	231	94%	95%	94%
Prophylactic Antibiotic Stopped	592	97%	96%	94%
Recommended VTP Ordered	333	95%	97%	94%
Urinary Catheter Removal	239	91%	89%	90%
Children's Asthma Care				
Received Systemic Corticosteroids	-	-	-	100%
Received Home Management Plan	-	-	-	71%
Received Reliever Medication	-	-	-	100%
Use of Medical Imaging				
Combination Abdominal CT Scan	1,193	0.070	0.109	0.191
Combination Chest CT Scan	1,052	0.000	0.010	0.054
Follow-up Mammogram/Ultrasound	2,478	9.4%	9.2%	8.4%
MRI for Low Back Pain	228	30.3%	30.1%	32.7%
Survey of Patients' Hospital Experiences				
Area Around Room 'Always' Quiet at Night	300+	49%	-	58%
Doctors 'Always' Communicated Well	300+	81%	-	80%
Home Recovery Information Given	300+	84%	-	82%
Hospital Given 9 or 10 on 10 Point Scale	300+	75%	-	67%
Meds 'Always' Explained Before Given	300+	65%	-	60%
Nurses 'Always' Communicated Well	300+	80%	-	76%
Pain 'Always' Well Controlled	300+	71%	-	69%
Room and Bathroom 'Always' Clean	300+	73%	-	71%
Timely Help 'Always' Received	300+	67%	-	64%
Would Definitely Recommend Hospital	300+	81%	-	69%

Adcare Hospital of Worcester

107 Lincoln Street
Worcester, MA 01605
E-mail: info@adcare.com
URL:
Type: Acute Care Hospitals
Ownership: Proprietary

Phone: 508-799-9000
Fax: 508-753-3733

Emergency Services: No
Beds: 114

Key Personnel:
CEO/President . . . . David W Hillis
Chief of Medical Staff . . . . Ronald F Pike, MD
Operating Room . . . . Petrice Muchowski
Quality Assurance . . . . Karole A Mesier

Measure	Cases	This Hosp.	State Avg.	U.S. Avg.
Heart Attack Care				
ACE Inhibitor or ARB for LVSD[5]	0	-	94%	96%
Aspirin at Arrival[5]	0	-	99%	99%
Aspirin at Discharge[5]	0	-	99%	98%
Beta Blocker at Discharge[5]	0	-	99%	98%
Fibrinolytic Medication Timing[5]	0	-	50%	55%
PCI Within 90 Minutes of Arrival[5]	0	-	93%	90%
Smoking Cessation Advice[5]	0	-	99%	99%
Chest Pain/Possible Heart Attack Care				
Aspirin at Arrival[5]	0	-	96%	95%
Median Time to ECG (minutes)[5]	0	-	10	8
Median Time to Transfer (minutes)[5]	0	-	65	61
Fibrinolytic Medication Timing[5]	0	-	78%	54%
Heart Failure Care				
ACE Inhibitor or ARB for LVSD[5]	0	-	94%	94%
Discharge Instructions[5]	0	-	89%	88%
Evaluation of LVS Function[5]	0	-	98%	98%
Smoking Cessation Advice[5]	0	-	97%	98%
Pneumonia Care				
Appropriate Initial Antibiotic[5]	0	-	93%	92%
Blood Culture Timing[5]	0	-	95%	96%
Influenza Vaccine[5]	0	-	92%	91%
Initial Antibiotic Timing[5]	0	-	96%	95%
Pneumococcal Vaccine[5]	0	-	93%	93%
Smoking Cessation Advice[5]	0	-	96%	97%
Surgical Care Improvement Project				
Appropriate VTP Within 24 Hours[5]	0	-	96%	92%
Appropriate Hair Removal[5]	0	-	100%	99%
Appropriate Beta Blocker Usage[5]	0	-	96%	93%
Controlled Postoperative Blood Glucose[5]	0	-	95%	93%
Prophylactic Antibiotic Timing[5]	0	-	97%	97%
Prophylactic Antibiotic Timing (Outpatient)[5]	0	-	92%	92%
Prophylactic Antibiotic Selection[5]	0	-	98%	97%
Prophylactic Antibiotic Select. (Outpatient)[5]	0	-	95%	94%
Prophylactic Antibiotic Stopped[5]	0	-	96%	94%
Recommended VTP Ordered[5]	0	-	97%	94%
Urinary Catheter Removal[5]	0	-	89%	90%
Children's Asthma Care				
Received Systemic Corticosteroids	-	-	-	100%
Received Home Management Plan	-	-	-	71%
Received Reliever Medication	-	-	-	100%
Use of Medical Imaging				
Combination Abdominal CT Scan[5]	0	-	0.109	0.191
Combination Chest CT Scan[5]	0	-	0.010	0.054
Follow-up Mammogram/Ultrasound[5]	0	-	9.2%	8.4%
MRI for Low Back Pain[5]	0	-	30.1%	32.7%
Survey of Patients' Hospital Experiences				
Area Around Room 'Always' Quiet at Night[9]	-	-	-	58%
Doctors 'Always' Communicated Well[9]	-	-	-	80%
Home Recovery Information Given[9]	-	-	-	82%
Hospital Given 9 or 10 on 10 Point Scale[9]	-	-	-	67%
Meds 'Always' Explained Before Given[9]	-	-	-	60%
Nurses 'Always' Communicated Well[9]	-	-	-	76%
Pain 'Always' Well Controlled[9]	-	-	-	69%
Room and Bathroom 'Always' Clean[9]	-	-	-	71%
Timely Help 'Always' Received[9]	-	-	-	64%
Would Definitely Recommend Hospital[9]	-	-	-	69%

Saint Vincent Hospital

123 Summer Street
Worcester, MA 01608
E-mail: dennis.irish@tenethealth.com
URL: www.stvincenthospital.com
Type: Acute Care Hospitals
Ownership: Proprietary

Phone: 508-363-5000
Fax: 508-363-5387

Emergency Services: Yes
Beds: 349

Key Personnel:
CEO/President . . . . John Smithhisler, Jr
Cardiac Laboratory . . . . Gordon Saperia
Chief of Medical Staff . . . . Harvey Kowaloff, MD
Pediatric Ambulatory Care . . . . . . William Horgan, OD
Quality Assurance . . . . Jill Lyons, RN
Radiology . . . . Paul Sabel, MD
Emergency Room . . . . Mary Auffrey, RN

Measure	Cases	This Hosp.	State Avg.	U.S. Avg.
Heart Attack Care				
ACE Inhibitor or ARB for LVSD	73	97%	94%	96%
Aspirin at Arrival	368	100%	99%	99%
Aspirin at Discharge	446	100%	99%	98%
Beta Blocker at Discharge	434	99%	99%	98%
Fibrinolytic Medication Timing	0	-	50%	55%
PCI Within 90 Minutes of Arrival	44	98%	93%	90%
Smoking Cessation Advice	127	100%	99%	99%
Chest Pain/Possible Heart Attack Care				
Aspirin at Arrival[1]	7	100%	96%	95%
Median Time to ECG (minutes)[1]	7	9	10	8
Median Time to Transfer (minutes)[5]	0	-	65	61
Fibrinolytic Medication Timing[5]	0	-	78%	54%
Heart Failure Care				
ACE Inhibitor or ARB for LVSD	138	98%	94%	94%
Discharge Instructions	396	97%	89%	88%
Evaluation of LVS Function	592	100%	98%	98%
Smoking Cessation Advice	53	100%	97%	98%
Pneumonia Care				
Appropriate Initial Antibiotic	236	95%	93%	92%
Blood Culture Timing	348	98%	95%	96%
Influenza Vaccine	317	98%	92%	91%
Initial Antibiotic Timing	436	96%	96%	95%
Pneumococcal Vaccine	451	98%	93%	93%
Smoking Cessation Advice	142	98%	96%	97%
Surgical Care Improvement Project				
Appropriate VTP Within 24 Hours	445	100%	96%	92%
Appropriate Hair Removal	1,593	100%	100%	99%
Appropriate Beta Blocker Usage	585	100%	96%	93%
Controlled Postoperative Blood Glucose	165	93%	95%	93%
Prophylactic Antibiotic Timing	954	96%	97%	97%
Prophylactic Antibiotic Timing (Outpatient)	781	96%	92%	92%
Prophylactic Antibiotic Selection	959	98%	98%	97%
Prophylactic Antibiotic Select. (Outpatient)	780	95%	95%	94%
Prophylactic Antibiotic Stopped	828	97%	96%	94%
Recommended VTP Ordered	445	100%	97%	94%
Urinary Catheter Removal	411	99%	89%	90%
Children's Asthma Care				
Received Systemic Corticosteroids	-	-	-	100%
Received Home Management Plan	-	-	-	71%
Received Reliever Medication	-	-	-	100%
Use of Medical Imaging				
Combination Abdominal CT Scan	606	0.035	0.109	0.191
Combination Chest CT Scan	431	0.000	0.010	0.054
Follow-up Mammogram/Ultrasound	377	7.2%	9.2%	8.4%
MRI for Low Back Pain	74	17.6%	30.1%	32.7%
Survey of Patients' Hospital Experiences				
Area Around Room 'Always' Quiet at Night	300+	44%	-	58%
Doctors 'Always' Communicated Well	300+	78%	-	80%
Home Recovery Information Given	300+	84%	-	82%
Hospital Given 9 or 10 on 10 Point Scale	300+	70%	-	67%
Meds 'Always' Explained Before Given	300+	59%	-	60%
Nurses 'Always' Communicated Well	300+	73%	-	76%
Pain 'Always' Well Controlled	300+	72%	-	69%
Room and Bathroom 'Always' Clean	300+	69%	-	71%
Timely Help 'Always' Received	300+	59%	-	64%
Would Definitely Recommend Hospital	300+	76%	-	69%

UMass Memorial Medical Center

55 Lake Avenue North
Worcester, MA 01655
URL: www.umassmemorial.org
Type: Acute Care Hospitals
Ownership: Voluntary Non-Profit - Private

Phone: 508-334-1000
Fax: 508-856-5225

Emergency Services: Yes
Beds: 771

Key Personnel:

CEO/President................John O'Brien
Cardiac Laboratory...........Robert Phillips, MD
Chief of Medical Staff........Stephen Tosi, MD
Operating Room..............David Ayers, MD
Pediatric Ambulatory Care......Marianne Felice, MD
Pediatric In-Patient Care......Marianne Felice, MD
Radiology...................Krishna Kandarpa, MD

Measure	Cases	This Hosp.	State Avg.	U.S. Avg.
Heart Attack Care				
ACE Inhibitor or ARB for LVSD[2]	151	98%	94%	96%
Aspirin at Arrival[2]	353	99%	99%	99%
Aspirin at Discharge[2]	825	100%	99%	98%
Beta Blocker at Discharge[2]	793	100%	99%	98%
Fibrinolytic Medication Timing[2]	0	-	50%	55%
PCI Within 90 Minutes of Arrival[2]	81	96%	93%	90%
Smoking Cessation Advice[2]	261	100%	99%	99%
Chest Pain/Possible Heart Attack Care				
Aspirin at Arrival[5]	0	-	96%	95%
Median Time to ECG (minutes)[5]	0	-	10	8
Median Time to Transfer (minutes)[5]	0	-	65	61
Fibrinolytic Medication Timing[5]	0	-	78%	54%
Heart Failure Care				
ACE Inhibitor or ARB for LVSD[2]	247	93%	94%	94%
Discharge Instructions[2]	553	91%	89%	88%
Evaluation of LVS Function[2]	799	100%	98%	98%
Smoking Cessation Advice[2]	103	100%	97%	98%
Pneumonia Care				
Appropriate Initial Antibiotic[2]	174	91%	93%	92%
Blood Culture Timing[2]	310	92%	95%	96%
Influenza Vaccine[2]	289	79%	92%	91%
Initial Antibiotic Timing[2]	329	93%	96%	95%
Pneumococcal Vaccine[2]	413	89%	93%	93%
Smoking Cessation Advice[2]	144	100%	96%	97%
Surgical Care Improvement Project				
Appropriate VTP Within 24 Hours[2]	169	98%	96%	92%
Appropriate Hair Removal[2]	607	100%	100%	99%
Appropriate Beta Blocker Usage[2]	237	97%	96%	93%
Controlled Postoperative Blood Glucose[2]	121	99%	95%	93%
Prophylactic Antibiotic Timing[2]	398	97%	97%	97%
Prophylactic Antibiotic Timing (Outpatient)[2]	451	99%	92%	92%
Prophylactic Antibiotic Selection[2]	409	97%	98%	97%
Prophylactic Antibiotic Select. (Outpatient)[2]	449	96%	95%	94%
Prophylactic Antibiotic Stopped[2]	377	95%	96%	94%
Recommended VTP Ordered[2]	169	99%	97%	94%
Urinary Catheter Removal[2]	104	79%	89%	90%
Children's Asthma Care				
Received Systemic Corticosteroids	-	-	-	100%
Received Home Management Plan	-	-	-	71%
Received Reliever Medication	-	-	-	100%
Use of Medical Imaging				
Combination Abdominal CT Scan	2,202	0.135	0.109	0.191
Combination Chest CT Scan	1,687	0.006	0.010	0.054
Follow-up Mammogram/Ultrasound	2,418	6.8%	9.2%	8.4%
MRI for Low Back Pain[5]	0	-	30.1%	32.7%
Survey of Patients' Hospital Experiences				
Area Around Room 'Always' Quiet at Night	300+	45%	-	58%
Doctors 'Always' Communicated Well	300+	74%	-	80%
Home Recovery Information Given	300+	88%	-	82%
Hospital Given 9 or 10 on 10 Point Scale	300+	66%	-	67%
Meds 'Always' Explained Before Given	300+	59%	-	60%
Nurses 'Always' Communicated Well	300+	72%	-	76%
Pain 'Always' Well Controlled	300+	65%	-	69%
Room and Bathroom 'Always' Clean	300+	60%	-	71%
Timely Help 'Always' Received	300+	55%	-	64%
Would Definitely Recommend Hospital	300+	75%	-	69%

NOTE: Hospital profiles are in alphabetical order by state, then city, then hospital within the city; Rankings exclude hospitals with less than 25 cases except for patient surveys which excludes hospitals with less than 100 cases; (a) 100–299 cases; (1) The number of cases is too small to be sure how well a hospital is performing; (2) The hospital indicated that the data submitted for this measure were based on a sample of cases; (3) Data was collected during a shorter time period (fewer quarters) than the maximum possible time for this measure; (4) Suppressed for one or more quarters by CMS; (5) No data is available from the hospital for this measure; (6) Fewer than 100 patients completed the HCAHPS survey. Use these rates with caution, as the number of surveys may be too low to reliably assess hospital performance; (7) Survey results are based on less than 12 months of data; (8) Survey results are not available for this reporting period; (9) No or very few patients were eligible for the HCAHPS survey. The scores shown, if any, reflect a very small number of surveys; (10) A state average was not calculated because too few hospitals in the state submitted data; (11) There were discrepancies in the data collection process; Please refer to the User's Guide for a full explanation of data.

Heart Attack Care

1. ACE Inhibitor or ARB for LVSD

Hospital Name	City	Rate	Cases
Catholic Medical Center	Manchester	100%	76
Concord Hospital	Concord	100%	29
Portsmouth Regional Hospital	Portsmouth	100%	35
Southern Nh Medical Center	Nashua	96%	28
Mary Hitchcock Memorial Hospital[2]	Lebanon	94%	51

2. Aspirin at Arrival

Hospital Name	City	Rate	Cases
Catholic Medical Center	Manchester	100%	213
Cheshire Medical Center	Keene	100%	31
Concord Hospital	Concord	100%	165
Elliot Hospital	Manchester	100%	139
Exeter Hospital	Exeter	100%	118
Mary Hitchcock Memorial Hospital[2]	Lebanon	100%	88
Parkland Medical Center	Derry	100%	85
Portsmouth Regional Hospital	Portsmouth	100%	150
Saint Joseph Hospital[2]	Nashua	100%	65
Southern Nh Medical Center	Nashua	100%	148
Wentworth-Douglass Hospital	Dover	100%	77
Lakes Region General Hospital	Laconia	98%	44

3. Aspirin at Discharge

Hospital Name	City	Rate	Cases
Catholic Medical Center	Manchester	100%	460
Concord Hospital	Concord	100%	228
Elliot Hospital	Manchester	100%	118
Lakes Region General Hospital	Laconia	100%	26
Parkland Medical Center	Derry	100%	73
Portsmouth Regional Hospital	Portsmouth	100%	278
Saint Joseph Hospital[2]	Nashua	100%	46
Exeter Hospital	Exeter	99%	96
Mary Hitchcock Memorial Hospital[2]	Lebanon	99%	510
Southern Nh Medical Center	Nashua	98%	123
Wentworth-Douglass Hospital	Dover	97%	74

4. Beta Blocker at Discharge

Hospital Name	City	Rate	Cases
Catholic Medical Center	Manchester	100%	451
Concord Hospital	Concord	100%	226
Elliot Hospital	Manchester	100%	104
Exeter Hospital	Exeter	100%	88
Parkland Medical Center	Derry	100%	74
Portsmouth Regional Hospital	Portsmouth	100%	267
Saint Joseph Hospital[2]	Nashua	100%	44
Southern Nh Medical Center	Nashua	100%	122
Wentworth-Douglass Hospital	Dover	100%	72
Mary Hitchcock Memorial Hospital[2]	Lebanon	99%	498

6. PCI Within 90 Minutes of Arrival

Hospital Name	City	Rate	Cases
Concord Hospital	Concord	96%	48
Catholic Medical Center	Manchester	95%	43
Exeter Hospital	Exeter	94%	32
Portsmouth Regional Hospital	Portsmouth	93%	28

7. Smoking Cessation Advice

Hospital Name	City	Rate	Cases
Catholic Medical Center	Manchester	100%	148
Concord Hospital	Concord	100%	69
Elliot Hospital	Manchester	100%	37
Exeter Hospital	Exeter	100%	29
Parkland Medical Center	Derry	100%	25
Portsmouth Regional Hospital	Portsmouth	100%	81
Southern Nh Medical Center	Nashua	100%	34
Wentworth-Douglass Hospital	Dover	100%	26
Mary Hitchcock Memorial Hospital[2]	Lebanon	95%	152

Chest Pain/Possible Heart Attack Care

8. Aspirin at Arrival

Hospital Name	City	Rate	Cases
Franklin Regional Hospital	Franklin	100%	31
Saint Joseph Hospital	Nashua	100%	31
Speare Memorial Hospital	Plymouth	100%	40
Cheshire Medical Center	Keene	99%	98
Weeks Medical Center	Lancaster	98%	60
Lakes Region General Hospital	Laconia	97%	135
Upper Connecticut Valley Hospital	Colebrook	97%	38
New London Hospital	New London	95%	37
Monadnock Community Hospital	Peterborough	94%	33
Frisbie Memorial Hospital	Rochester	89%	37

9. Median Time to ECG (minutes)

Hospital Name	City	Min.	Cases
Cheshire Medical Center	Keene	5	99
Frisbie Memorial Hospital	Rochester	5	37
Franklin Regional Hospital	Franklin	7	31
Lakes Region General Hospital	Laconia	7	137
Saint Joseph Hospital	Nashua	8	32
New London Hospital	New London	10	38
Upper Connecticut Valley Hospital	Colebrook	10	38
Monadnock Community Hospital	Peterborough	11	35
Weeks Medical Center	Lancaster	11	65
Speare Memorial Hospital	Plymouth	14	40

10. Median Time to Transfer (minutes)

Hospital Name	City	Min.	Cases
Lakes Region General Hospital	Laconia	36	34

Heart Failure Care

12. ACE Inhibitor or ARB for LVSD

Hospital Name	City	Rate	Cases
Catholic Medical Center[2]	Manchester	100%	102
Parkland Medical Center	Derry	100%	27
Portsmouth Regional Hospital	Portsmouth	100%	29
Saint Joseph Hospital[2]	Nashua	100%	59
Wentworth-Douglass Hospital	Dover	100%	48
Concord Hospital	Concord	99%	86
Elliot Hospital	Manchester	98%	56
Southern Nh Medical Center	Nashua	98%	42
Mary Hitchcock Memorial Hospital	Lebanon	93%	104
Exeter Hospital	Exeter	92%	39

13. Discharge Instructions

Hospital Name	City	Rate	Cases
Exeter Hospital	Exeter	100%	137
Speare Memorial Hospital	Plymouth	100%	30
Southern Nh Medical Center	Nashua	99%	189
Wentworth-Douglass Hospital	Dover	99%	165
Parkland Medical Center	Derry	98%	104
Catholic Medical Center[2]	Manchester	97%	208
The Memorial Hospital	North Conway	97%	30
New London Hospital	New London	97%	32
Concord Hospital	Concord	96%	261
Frisbie Memorial Hospital	Rochester	95%	81
Elliot Hospital	Manchester	91%	135
Cheshire Medical Center	Keene	90%	70
Portsmouth Regional Hospital	Portsmouth	90%	78
Mary Hitchcock Memorial Hospital	Lebanon	84%	239
Saint Joseph Hospital[2]	Nashua	84%	123
Androscoggin Valley Hospital	Berlin	70%	27
Lakes Region General Hospital	Laconia	65%	62

14. Evaluation of LVS Function

Hospital Name	City	Rate	Cases
Catholic Medical Center[2]	Manchester	100%	260
Cheshire Medical Center	Keene	100%	97
Concord Hospital	Concord	100%	343
Exeter Hospital	Exeter	100%	185
Mary Hitchcock Memorial Hospital	Lebanon	100%	281
New London Hospital	New London	100%	38
Parkland Medical Center	Derry	100%	146
Portsmouth Regional Hospital	Portsmouth	100%	109
Saint Joseph Hospital[2]	Nashua	100%	201
Southern Nh Medical Center	Nashua	100%	227
Speare Memorial Hospital	Plymouth	100%	33
Weeks Medical Center	Lancaster	100%	34
Elliot Hospital	Manchester	99%	195
Frisbie Memorial Hospital	Rochester	99%	108
Wentworth-Douglass Hospital	Dover	99%	203
Androscoggin Valley Hospital	Berlin	98%	41
Huggins Hospital	Wolfeboro	98%	41
Lakes Region General Hospital	Laconia	97%	90
Monadnock Community Hospital	Peterborough	97%	29
The Memorial Hospital	North Conway	88%	43
Franklin Regional Hospital	Franklin	87%	30

15. Smoking Cessation Advice

Hospital Name	City	Rate	Cases
Catholic Medical Center[2]	Manchester	100%	40
Concord Hospital	Concord	100%	53
Southern Nh Medical Center	Nashua	100%	37
Mary Hitchcock Memorial Hospital	Lebanon	98%	46

Pneumonia Care

16. Appropriate Initial Antibiotic

Hospital Name	City	Rate	Cases
Catholic Medical Center[2]	Manchester	100%	80
Portsmouth Regional Hospital	Portsmouth	100%	59
Speare Memorial Hospital	Plymouth	100%	27
Valley Regional Hospital	Claremont	100%	26
Weeks Medical Center	Lancaster	100%	28
Southern Nh Medical Center	Nashua	99%	86
Franklin Regional Hospital	Franklin	98%	44
Parkland Medical Center	Derry	98%	58
Wentworth-Douglass Hospital[2]	Dover	98%	99
New London Hospital	New London	97%	29
Monadnock Community Hospital	Peterborough	96%	52
Cheshire Medical Center[2]	Keene	95%	87
Concord Hospital	Concord	95%	196
Exeter Hospital	Exeter	94%	123
Huggins Hospital	Wolfeboro	94%	34
Elliot Hospital[2]	Manchester	93%	88
Frisbie Memorial Hospital	Rochester	92%	97
Lakes Region General Hospital[2]	Laconia	91%	79
The Memorial Hospital[2]	North Conway	89%	27
Saint Joseph Hospital[2]	Nashua	89%	84
Mary Hitchcock Memorial Hospital[2]	Lebanon	88%	74

17. Blood Culture Timing

Hospital Name	City	Rate	Cases
Androscoggin Valley Hospital	Berlin	100%	37
Saint Joseph Hospital[2]	Nashua	100%	114
Speare Memorial Hospital	Plymouth	100%	30
Monadnock Community Hospital	Peterborough	99%	96
Parkland Medical Center	Derry	99%	96
Wentworth-Douglass Hospital[2]	Dover	99%	135
Catholic Medical Center[2]	Manchester	98%	139
Franklin Regional Hospital	Franklin	98%	64
Portsmouth Regional Hospital	Portsmouth	98%	111
Southern Nh Medical Center	Nashua	98%	167
Weeks Medical Center	Lancaster	98%	46
Cheshire Medical Center[2]	Keene	97%	144
Cottage Hospital	Woodsville	97%	30
Lakes Region General Hospital[2]	Laconia	97%	87
New London Hospital	New London	97%	36
Concord Hospital	Concord	96%	285
Exeter Hospital	Exeter	96%	166
Frisbie Memorial Hospital	Rochester	96%	122
Huggins Hospital	Wolfeboro	96%	55
Mary Hitchcock Memorial Hospital[2]	Lebanon	95%	128
The Memorial Hospital[2]	North Conway	93%	29
Valley Regional Hospital	Claremont	92%	36
Elliot Hospital[2]	Manchester	90%	127

18. Influenza Vaccine

Hospital Name	City	Rate	Cases
Portsmouth Regional Hospital	Portsmouth	100%	59
Weeks Medical Center	Lancaster	100%	34
Catholic Medical Center[2]	Manchester	99%	93
Saint Joseph Hospital[2]	Nashua	99%	78
Cheshire Medical Center[2]	Keene	98%	81
Mary Hitchcock Memorial Hospital[2]	Lebanon	98%	147
Parkland Medical Center	Derry	98%	63
Concord Hospital	Concord	97%	186
New London Hospital	New London	97%	31
Southern Nh Medical Center	Nashua	97%	116
Exeter Hospital	Exeter	95%	111
Monadnock Community Hospital	Peterborough	94%	52
Wentworth-Douglass Hospital[2]	Dover	94%	82
Franklin Regional Hospital	Franklin	91%	53
Valley Regional Hospital	Claremont	89%	27
Frisbie Memorial Hospital	Rochester	88%	95
Lakes Region General Hospital[2]	Laconia	87%	78
Elliot Hospital[2]	Manchester	84%	77

19. Initial Antibiotic Timing

Hospital Name	City	Rate	Cases
Androscoggin Valley Hospital	Berlin	100%	36
Cottage Hospital	Woodsville	100%	32
Parkland Medical Center	Derry	100%	76
Portsmouth Regional Hospital	Portsmouth	100%	101
Speare Memorial Hospital	Plymouth	100%	43
Valley Regional Hospital	Claremont	100%	31
Catholic Medical Center[2]	Manchester	99%	125
Elliot Hospital[2]	Manchester	99%	135
Monadnock Community Hospital	Peterborough	99%	84
Frisbie Memorial Hospital	Rochester	98%	100
Huggins Hospital	Wolfeboro	98%	54
Lakes Region General Hospital[2]	Laconia	98%	120
Weeks Medical Center	Lancaster	98%	55
Cheshire Medical Center[2]	Keene	97%	146

NOTE: Hospital profiles are in alphabetical order by state, then city, then hospital within the city; Rankings exclude hospitals with less than 25 cases except for patient surveys which excludes hospitals with less than 100 cases; (a) 100–299 cases; (1) The number of cases is too small to be sure how well a hospital is performing; (2) The hospital indicated that the data submitted for this measure were based on a sample of cases; (3) Data was collected during a shorter time period (fewer quarters) than the maximum possible time for this measure; (4) Suppressed for one or more quarters by CMS; (5) No data is available from the hospital for this measure; (6) Fewer than 100 patients completed the HCAHPS survey. Use these rates with caution, as the number of surveys may be too low to reliably assess hospital performance; (7) Survey results are based on less than 12 months of data; (8) Survey results are not available for this reporting period; (9) No or very few patients were eligible for the HCAHPS survey. The scores shown, if any, reflect a very small number of surveys; (10) A state average was not calculated because too few hospitals in the state submitted data; (11) There were discrepancies in the data collection process; Please refer to the User's Guide for a full explanation of data.

Concord Hospital	Concord	97%	284
The Memorial Hospital[2]	North Conway	97%	29
New London Hospital	New London	97%	33
Southern Nh Medical Center	Nashua	97%	174
Wentworth-Douglass Hospital[2]	Dover	96%	139
Exeter Hospital	Exeter	95%	182
Littleton Regional Hospital	Littleton	94%	33
Franklin Regional Hospital	Franklin	93%	68
Mary Hitchcock Memorial Hospital[2]	Lebanon	92%	133
Saint Joseph Hospital[2]	Nashua	92%	131

20. Pneumococcal Vaccine

Hospital Name	City	Rate	Cases
Catholic Medical Center[2]	Manchester	100%	130
Cottage Hospital	Woodsville	100%	32
Franklin Regional Hospital	Franklin	100%	80
Huggins Hospital	Wolfeboro	100%	44
Portsmouth Regional Hospital	Portsmouth	100%	101
Speare Memorial Hospital	Plymouth	100%	38
Cheshire Medical Center[2]	Keene	99%	123
Elliot Hospital[2]	Manchester	99%	119
Parkland Medical Center	Derry	99%	93
New London Hospital	New London	98%	46
Weeks Medical Center	Lancaster	98%	49
The Memorial Hospital[2]	North Conway	97%	29
Monadnock Community Hospital	Peterborough	97%	71
Saint Joseph Hospital[2]	Nashua	97%	125
Frisbie Memorial Hospital	Rochester	96%	112
Mary Hitchcock Memorial Hospital[2]	Lebanon	96%	159
Androscoggin Valley Hospital	Berlin	95%	44
Concord Hospital	Concord	95%	273
Southern Nh Medical Center	Nashua	95%	144
Exeter Hospital	Exeter	94%	165
Lakes Region General Hospital[2]	Laconia	93%	107
Wentworth-Douglass Hospital[2]	Dover	93%	116
Valley Regional Hospital	Claremont	88%	32
Littleton Regional Hospital	Littleton	64%	36

21. Smoking Cessation Advice

Hospital Name	City	Rate	Cases
Catholic Medical Center[2]	Manchester	100%	50
Exeter Hospital	Exeter	100%	59
Frisbie Memorial Hospital	Rochester	100%	59
Parkland Medical Center	Derry	100%	33
Saint Joseph Hospital[2]	Nashua	100%	27
Southern Nh Medical Center	Nashua	100%	67
Cheshire Medical Center[2]	Keene	98%	50
Concord Hospital	Concord	97%	104
Lakes Region General Hospital[2]	Laconia	97%	36
Wentworth-Douglass Hospital[2]	Dover	97%	38
Elliot Hospital[2]	Manchester	93%	42
Monadnock Community Hospital	Peterborough	92%	26
Mary Hitchcock Memorial Hospital[2]	Lebanon	87%	77

Surgical Care Improvement Project

22. Appropriate VTP Within 24 Hours

Hospital Name	City	Rate	Cases
Elliot Hospital[2]	Manchester	100%	131
Huggins Hospital	Wolfeboro	100%	41
The Memorial Hospital	North Conway	100%	29
Valley Regional Hospital	Claremont	100%	49
Mary Hitchcock Memorial Hospital[2]	Lebanon	99%	269
Saint Joseph Hospital[2]	Nashua	99%	151
Monadnock Community Hospital	Peterborough	97%	36
Portsmouth Regional Hospital[2]	Portsmouth	97%	166
Catholic Medical Center[2]	Manchester	96%	81
Cheshire Medical Center	Keene	95%	110
Exeter Hospital	Exeter	94%	141
Lakes Region General Hospital[2]	Laconia	94%	199
Parkland Medical Center	Derry	94%	70
Southern Nh Medical Center	Nashua	94%	215
Wentworth-Douglass Hospital[2]	Dover	93%	152
Concord Hospital[2]	Concord	92%	122
Frisbie Memorial Hospital	Rochester	92%	80
New London Hospital	New London	91%	35
Alice Peck Day Memorial Hospital[2]	Lebanon	89%	27
Littleton Regional Hospital	Littleton	87%	61

23. Appropriate Hair Removal

Hospital Name	City	Rate	Cases
Androscoggin Valley Hospital	Berlin	100%	44
Catholic Medical Center[2]	Manchester	100%	524
Cheshire Medical Center	Keene	100%	263
Concord Hospital[2]	Concord	100%	464
Cottage Hospital	Woodsville	100%	58
Elliot Hospital[2]	Manchester	100%	377
Exeter Hospital	Exeter	100%	543
Franklin Regional Hospital[2]	Franklin	100%	28
Frisbie Memorial Hospital	Rochester	100%	258
Lakes Region General Hospital[2]	Laconia	100%	448
Littleton Regional Hospital	Littleton	100%	204
Mary Hitchcock Memorial Hospital[2]	Lebanon	100%	871
The Memorial Hospital	North Conway	100%	62
Monadnock Community Hospital	Peterborough	100%	128
New London Hospital	New London	100%	112
Parkland Medical Center	Derry	100%	161
Portsmouth Regional Hospital[2]	Portsmouth	100%	595
Saint Joseph Hospital[2]	Nashua	100%	312
Southern Nh Medical Center	Nashua	100%	589
Speare Memorial Hospital	Plymouth	100%	73
Valley Regional Hospital	Claremont	100%	94
Weeks Medical Center	Lancaster	100%	29
Wentworth-Douglass Hospital[2]	Dover	100%	448
Huggins Hospital	Wolfeboro	99%	91
Alice Peck Day Memorial Hospital[2]	Lebanon	90%	62

24. Appropriate Beta Blocker Usage

Hospital Name	City	Rate	Cases
Frisbie Memorial Hospital	Rochester	100%	92
Huggins Hospital	Wolfeboro	100%	30
New London Hospital	New London	100%	27
Parkland Medical Center	Derry	100%	41
Portsmouth Regional Hospital[2]	Portsmouth	100%	256
Cheshire Medical Center	Keene	99%	69
Concord Hospital[2]	Concord	99%	172
Saint Joseph Hospital[2]	Nashua	98%	82
Southern Nh Medical Center	Nashua	98%	137
Catholic Medical Center[2]	Manchester	94%	226
Lakes Region General Hospital[2]	Laconia	94%	133
Exeter Hospital	Exeter	93%	212
Wentworth-Douglass Hospital[2]	Dover	92%	119
Mary Hitchcock Memorial Hospital[2]	Lebanon	89%	348
Littleton Regional Hospital	Littleton	87%	45
Elliot Hospital[2]	Manchester	86%	86

25. Controlled Postoperative Blood Glucose

Hospital Name	City	Rate	Cases
Catholic Medical Center[2]	Manchester	98%	131
Mary Hitchcock Memorial Hospital[2]	Lebanon	96%	207
Concord Hospital[2]	Concord	95%	106
Portsmouth Regional Hospital[2]	Portsmouth	92%	170

26. Prophylactic Antibiotic Timing

Hospital Name	City	Rate	Cases
Portsmouth Regional Hospital[2]	Portsmouth	100%	373
Southern Nh Medical Center	Nashua	100%	422
Wentworth-Douglass Hospital[2]	Dover	100%	307
Exeter Hospital	Exeter	99%	395
Alice Peck Day Memorial Hospital[2]	Lebanon	98%	48
Catholic Medical Center[2]	Manchester	98%	376
Cheshire Medical Center	Keene	98%	194
Elliot Hospital[2]	Manchester	98%	255
Huggins Hospital	Wolfeboro	98%	56
Parkland Medical Center	Derry	98%	56
Speare Memorial Hospital	Plymouth	98%	60
Valley Regional Hospital	Claremont	98%	82
Frisbie Memorial Hospital	Rochester	97%	174
Mary Hitchcock Memorial Hospital[2]	Lebanon	97%	633
Monadnock Community Hospital	Peterborough	97%	111
Concord Hospital[2]	Concord	96%	360
Lakes Region General Hospital[2]	Laconia	96%	311
Littleton Regional Hospital	Littleton	96%	150
Saint Joseph Hospital[2]	Nashua	96%	218
The Memorial Hospital	North Conway	95%	59
Androscoggin Valley Hospital	Berlin	94%	35
Cottage Hospital	Woodsville	93%	42
Weeks Medical Center	Lancaster	92%	26
New London Hospital	New London	76%	97

27. Prophylactic Antibiotic Timing (Outpatient)

Hospital Name	City	Rate	Cases
Parkland Medical Center	Derry	100%	80
Speare Memorial Hospital	Plymouth	100%	59
Exeter Hospital	Exeter	99%	195
Portsmouth Regional Hospital	Portsmouth	99%	259
Wentworth-Douglass Hospital	Dover	99%	346
Concord Hospital	Concord	98%	406
Monadnock Community Hospital	Peterborough	98%	45
Mary Hitchcock Memorial Hospital	Lebanon	97%	608
Cheshire Medical Center	Keene	96%	110
Elliot Hospital	Manchester	96%	466
Southern Nh Medical Center	Nashua	96%	224
Catholic Medical Center	Manchester	95%	316
Frisbie Memorial Hospital	Rochester	94%	78
Saint Joseph Hospital	Nashua	94%	140
Lakes Region General Hospital	Laconia	93%	182
New London Hospital	New London	75%	83

28. Prophylactic Antibiotic Selection

Hospital Name	City	Rate	Cases
Parkland Medical Center	Derry	100%	55
Portsmouth Regional Hospital[2]	Portsmouth	100%	407
Speare Memorial Hospital	Plymouth	100%	59
Weeks Medical Center	Lancaster	100%	26
Cheshire Medical Center	Keene	99%	194
Elliot Hospital[2]	Manchester	99%	257
Frisbie Memorial Hospital	Rochester	99%	177
Mary Hitchcock Memorial Hospital[2]	Lebanon	99%	647
New London Hospital	New London	99%	98
Saint Joseph Hospital[2]	Nashua	99%	219
Southern Nh Medical Center	Nashua	99%	428
Wentworth-Douglass Hospital[2]	Dover	99%	310
Catholic Medical Center[2]	Manchester	98%	383
Cottage Hospital	Woodsville	98%	42
Exeter Hospital	Exeter	98%	399
Littleton Regional Hospital	Littleton	98%	150
The Memorial Hospital	North Conway	98%	58
Valley Regional Hospital	Claremont	98%	81
Concord Hospital[2]	Concord	97%	369
Lakes Region General Hospital[2]	Laconia	97%	314
Alice Peck Day Memorial Hospital[2]	Lebanon	96%	48
Monadnock Community Hospital	Peterborough	96%	115
Androscoggin Valley Hospital	Berlin	91%	35
Huggins Hospital	Wolfeboro	91%	56

29. Prophylactic Antibiotic Selection (Outpatient)

Hospital Name	City	Rate	Cases
New London Hospital	New London	99%	81
Portsmouth Regional Hospital	Portsmouth	99%	258
Southern Nh Medical Center	Nashua	99%	216
Catholic Medical Center	Manchester	98%	320
Elliot Hospital	Manchester	98%	463
Mary Hitchcock Memorial Hospital	Lebanon	98%	640
Wentworth-Douglass Hospital	Dover	98%	345
Speare Memorial Hospital	Plymouth	97%	59
Cheshire Medical Center	Keene	96%	109
Concord Hospital	Concord	96%	402
Exeter Hospital	Exeter	96%	194
Monadnock Community Hospital	Peterborough	96%	45
Saint Joseph Hospital	Nashua	96%	139
Lakes Region General Hospital	Laconia	95%	175
Parkland Medical Center	Derry	94%	116
Frisbie Memorial Hospital	Rochester	89%	73

30. Prophylactic Antibiotic Stopped

Hospital Name	City	Rate	Cases
Alice Peck Day Memorial Hospital[2]	Lebanon	100%	48
Cheshire Medical Center	Keene	99%	191
Frisbie Memorial Hospital	Rochester	99%	169
New London Hospital	New London	99%	96
Valley Regional Hospital	Claremont	99%	79
Wentworth-Douglass Hospital[2]	Dover	99%	302
Huggins Hospital	Wolfeboro	98%	55
Monadnock Community Hospital	Peterborough	98%	107
Parkland Medical Center	Derry	98%	52
Portsmouth Regional Hospital[2]	Portsmouth	98%	348
Southern Nh Medical Center	Nashua	98%	419
Catholic Medical Center[2]	Manchester	97%	362
Exeter Hospital	Exeter	97%	386
Elliot Hospital[2]	Manchester	96%	244
Mary Hitchcock Memorial Hospital[2]	Lebanon	96%	615
Saint Joseph Hospital[2]	Nashua	96%	211
Weeks Medical Center	Lancaster	96%	25
Concord Hospital[2]	Concord	95%	355
Lakes Region General Hospital[2]	Laconia	95%	301
Littleton Regional Hospital	Littleton	95%	150
Speare Memorial Hospital	Plymouth	95%	57
Cottage Hospital	Woodsville	90%	42
Androscoggin Valley Hospital	Berlin	88%	32
The Memorial Hospital	North Conway	86%	57

31. Recommended VTP Ordered

Hospital Name	City	Rate	Cases
Elliot Hospital[2]	Manchester	100%	131
Huggins Hospital	Wolfeboro	100%	41
The Memorial Hospital	North Conway	100%	29
Monadnock Community Hospital	Peterborough	100%	36
Parkland Medical Center	Derry	100%	70
Valley Regional Hospital	Claremont	100%	49
Mary Hitchcock Memorial Hospital[2]	Lebanon	99%	270
Portsmouth Regional Hospital[2]	Portsmouth	99%	166
Saint Joseph Hospital[2]	Nashua	99%	151
Catholic Medical Center[2]	Manchester	98%	81
Cheshire Medical Center	Keene	97%	110
Exeter Hospital	Exeter	97%	141

NOTE: Hospital profiles are in alphabetical order by state, then city, then hospital within the city; Rankings exclude hospitals with less than 25 cases except for patient surveys which excludes hospitals with less than 100 cases; (a) 100–299 cases; (1) The number of cases is too small to be sure how well a hospital is performing; (2) The hospital indicated that the data submitted for this measure were based on a sample of cases; (3) Data was collected during a shorter time period (fewer quarters) than the maximum possible time for this measure; (4) Suppressed for one or more quarters by CMS; (5) No data is available from the hospital for this measure; (6) Fewer than 100 patients completed the HCAHPS survey. Use these rates with caution, as the number of surveys may be too low to reliably assess hospital performance; (7) Survey results are based on less than 12 months of data; (8) Survey results are not available for this reporting period; (9) No or very few patients were eligible for the HCAHPS survey. The scores shown, if any, reflect a very small number of surveys; (10) A state average was not calculated because too few hospitals in the state submitted data; (11) There were discrepancies in the data collection process; Please refer to the User's Guide for a full explanation of data.

Lakes Region General Hospital[2]	Laconia	95%	199
Wentworth-Douglass Hospital[2]	Dover	95%	152
Southern Nh Medical Center	Nashua	94%	217
Concord Hospital[2]	Concord	92%	122
Frisbie Memorial Hospital	Rochester	92%	80
New London Hospital	New London	91%	35
Littleton Regional Hospital	Littleton	90%	61
Alice Peck Day Memorial Hospital[2]	Lebanon	89%	27

32. Urinary Catheter Removal

Hospital Name	City	Rate	Cases
Portsmouth Regional Hospital[2]	Portsmouth	100%	121
Speare Memorial Hospital	Plymouth	100%	31
Cheshire Medical Center	Keene	98%	82
Exeter Hospital	Exeter	98%	142
Frisbie Memorial Hospital	Rochester	97%	79
Catholic Medical Center[2]	Manchester	95%	140
Elliot Hospital[2]	Manchester	89%	76
Wentworth-Douglass Hospital[2]	Dover	88%	127
New London Hospital	New London	87%	30
Southern Nh Medical Center	Nashua	86%	136
Concord Hospital[2]	Concord	84%	111
Mary Hitchcock Memorial Hospital[2]	Lebanon	84%	230
Saint Joseph Hospital[2]	Nashua	83%	63
Valley Regional Hospital	Claremont	82%	34
Littleton Regional Hospital	Littleton	80%	65
Lakes Region General Hospital[2]	Laconia	78%	134

Use of Medical Imaging

36. Combination Abdominal CT Scan

Hospital Name	City	Ratio	Cases
Cheshire Medical Center	Keene	0.011	620
Franklin Regional Hospital	Franklin	0.013	156
Wentworth-Douglass Hospital	Dover	0.037	848
Mary Hitchcock Memorial Hospital	Lebanon	0.052	1772
Frisbie Memorial Hospital	Rochester	0.054	633
Speare Memorial Hospital	Plymouth	0.056	248
Monadnock Community Hospital	Peterborough	0.057	283
Lakes Region General Hospital	Laconia	0.061	727
Exeter Hospital	Exeter	0.068	841
Catholic Medical Center	Manchester	0.071	688
Parkland Medical Center	Derry	0.072	304
Saint Joseph Hospital	Nashua	0.078	703
Southern Nh Medical Center	Nashua	0.080	537
Portsmouth Regional Hospital	Portsmouth	0.081	595
Elliot Hospital	Manchester	0.091	950
New London Hospital	New London	0.095	221
Concord Hospital	Concord	0.139	743
Upper Connecticut Valley Hospital	Colebrook	0.213	80
Weeks Medical Center	Lancaster	0.594	175

37. Combination Chest CT Scan

Hospital Name	City	Ratio	Cases
Cheshire Medical Center	Keene	0.000	564
Elliot Hospital	Manchester	0.000	701
Franklin Regional Hospital	Franklin	0.000	141
Frisbie Memorial Hospital	Rochester	0.000	586
Lakes Region General Hospital	Laconia	0.000	623
New London Hospital	New London	0.000	145
Portsmouth Regional Hospital	Portsmouth	0.000	392
Saint Joseph Hospital	Nashua	0.000	583
Speare Memorial Hospital	Plymouth	0.000	182
Mary Hitchcock Memorial Hospital	Lebanon	0.001	1847
Wentworth-Douglass Hospital	Dover	0.001	725
Monadnock Community Hospital	Peterborough	0.004	246
Southern Nh Medical Center	Nashua	0.005	372
Catholic Medical Center	Manchester	0.008	487
Exeter Hospital	Exeter	0.016	825
Parkland Medical Center	Derry	0.021	191
Concord Hospital	Concord	0.046	439
Weeks Medical Center	Lancaster	0.133	83
Upper Connecticut Valley Hospital[1]	Colebrook	0.135	52

38. Follow-up Mammogram/Ultrasound

Hospital Name	City	Rate	Cases
Upper Connecticut Valley Hospital	Colebrook	2.8%	181
Weeks Medical Center	Lancaster	3.4%	294
Cheshire Medical Center	Keene	3.8%	1331
Exeter Hospital	Exeter	3.8%	1950
Elliot Hospital	Manchester	5.5%	1924
Lakes Region General Hospital	Laconia	6.1%	1315
Franklin Regional Hospital	Franklin	6.2%	307
Southern Nh Medical Center	Nashua	6.4%	1695
Mary Hitchcock Memorial Hospital	Lebanon	7.5%	2249
Speare Memorial Hospital	Plymouth	7.5%	571
Saint Joseph Hospital	Nashua	7.8%	1620
Concord Hospital	Concord	8.1%	713
Parkland Medical Center	Derry	8.7%	358
New London Hospital	New London	8.8%	909
Portsmouth Regional Hospital	Portsmouth	10.8%	1479
Monadnock Community Hospital	Peterborough	11.8%	621
Catholic Medical Center	Manchester	11.9%	1641

39. MRI for Low Back Pain

Hospital Name	City	Rate	Cases
Parkland Medical Center[1]	Derry	21.9%	32
Monadnock Community Hospital[1]	Peterborough	22.4%	58
Franklin Regional Hospital[1]	Franklin	24.1%	29
Exeter Hospital	Exeter	24.5%	192
Portsmouth Regional Hospital	Portsmouth	24.7%	194
Concord Hospital	Concord	27.3%	99
Mary Hitchcock Memorial Hospital	Lebanon	27.5%	454
Southern Nh Medical Center	Nashua	30.1%	173
Wentworth-Douglass Hospital	Dover	30.9%	178
Saint Joseph Hospital	Nashua	31.3%	144
Frisbie Memorial Hospital	Rochester	31.5%	92
Cheshire Medical Center	Keene	31.6%	206
Elliot Hospital	Manchester	32.9%	359
Catholic Medical Center	Manchester	33.0%	176
Lakes Region General Hospital	Laconia	35.6%	236
New London Hospital	New London	47.2%	53
Speare Memorial Hospital	Plymouth	49.0%	49
Weeks Medical Center[1]	Lancaster	65.9%	44

Survey of Patients' Hospital Experiences

40. Area Around Room 'Always' Quiet at Night

Hospital Name	City	Rate	Cases
Frisbie Memorial Hospital	Rochester	66%	300+
New London Hospital	New London	65%	(a)
Concord Hospital	Concord	62%	300+
Saint Joseph Hospital	Nashua	61%	300+
Parkland Medical Center	Derry	60%	300+
Monadnock Community Hospital	Peterborough	58%	300+
Southern Nh Medical Center	Nashua	58%	300+
Catholic Medical Center	Manchester	57%	300+
Franklin Regional Hospital	Franklin	57%	(a)
Speare Memorial Hospital	Plymouth	56%	300+
Wentworth-Douglass Hospital	Dover	56%	300+
Littleton Regional Hospital	Littleton	55%	(a)
Portsmouth Regional Hospital	Portsmouth	55%	300+
Exeter Hospital	Exeter	51%	300+
Huggins Hospital	Wolfeboro	51%	300+
Elliot Hospital	Manchester	50%	300+
Androscoggin Valley Hospital	Berlin	49%	(a)
Lakes Region General Hospital	Laconia	49%	300+
Cheshire Medical Center	Keene	47%	300+
Mary Hitchcock Memorial Hospital	Lebanon	40%	300+

41. Doctors 'Always' Communicated Well

Hospital Name	City	Rate	Cases
Monadnock Community Hospital	Peterborough	87%	300+
Speare Memorial Hospital	Plymouth	87%	300+
Littleton Regional Hospital	Littleton	84%	(a)
Concord Hospital	Concord	82%	300+
Exeter Hospital	Exeter	82%	300+
Androscoggin Valley Hospital	Berlin	81%	(a)
New London Hospital	New London	81%	(a)
Parkland Medical Center	Derry	81%	300+
Portsmouth Regional Hospital	Portsmouth	81%	300+
Cheshire Medical Center	Keene	80%	300+
Mary Hitchcock Memorial Hospital	Lebanon	80%	300+
Southern Nh Medical Center	Nashua	80%	300+
Catholic Medical Center	Manchester	79%	300+
Wentworth-Douglass Hospital	Dover	79%	300+
Frisbie Memorial Hospital	Rochester	78%	300+
Huggins Hospital	Wolfeboro	78%	300+
Elliot Hospital	Manchester	77%	300+
Saint Joseph Hospital	Nashua	77%	300+
Lakes Region General Hospital	Laconia	76%	300+
Franklin Regional Hospital	Franklin	71%	(a)

42. Home Recovery Information Given

Hospital Name	City	Rate	Cases
Wentworth-Douglass Hospital	Dover	93%	300+
Speare Memorial Hospital	Plymouth	91%	300+
Littleton Regional Hospital	Littleton	90%	(a)
Parkland Medical Center	Derry	90%	300+
Portsmouth Regional Hospital	Portsmouth	90%	300+
Exeter Hospital	Exeter	89%	300+
Southern Nh Medical Center	Nashua	89%	300+
Monadnock Community Hospital	Peterborough	88%	300+
Concord Hospital	Concord	87%	300+
Frisbie Memorial Hospital	Rochester	87%	300+
Mary Hitchcock Memorial Hospital	Lebanon	87%	300+
Catholic Medical Center	Manchester	86%	300+
Cheshire Medical Center	Keene	86%	300+
Lakes Region General Hospital	Laconia	86%	300+
Saint Joseph Hospital	Nashua	86%	300+
Elliot Hospital	Manchester	85%	300+
Huggins Hospital	Wolfeboro	84%	300+
Androscoggin Valley Hospital	Berlin	83%	(a)
Franklin Regional Hospital	Franklin	79%	(a)
New London Hospital	New London	79%	(a)

43. Hospital Given 9 or 10 on 10 Point Scale

Hospital Name	City	Rate	Cases
Monadnock Community Hospital	Peterborough	79%	300+
Concord Hospital	Concord	78%	300+
Mary Hitchcock Memorial Hospital	Lebanon	78%	300+
Exeter Hospital	Exeter	77%	300+
Speare Memorial Hospital	Plymouth	75%	300+
Southern Nh Medical Center	Nashua	74%	300+
Wentworth-Douglass Hospital	Dover	73%	300+
New London Hospital	New London	71%	(a)
Parkland Medical Center	Derry	71%	300+
Catholic Medical Center	Manchester	70%	300+
Saint Joseph Hospital	Nashua	70%	300+
Frisbie Memorial Hospital	Rochester	69%	300+
Littleton Regional Hospital	Littleton	69%	(a)
Elliot Hospital	Manchester	68%	300+
Portsmouth Regional Hospital	Portsmouth	68%	300+
Cheshire Medical Center	Keene	67%	300+
Franklin Regional Hospital	Franklin	63%	(a)
Lakes Region General Hospital	Laconia	63%	300+
Huggins Hospital	Wolfeboro	62%	300+
Androscoggin Valley Hospital	Berlin	61%	(a)

44. Meds 'Always' Explained Before Given

Hospital Name	City	Rate	Cases
Monadnock Community Hospital	Peterborough	71%	300+
Parkland Medical Center	Derry	68%	300+
Speare Memorial Hospital	Plymouth	68%	300+
Southern Nh Medical Center	Nashua	66%	300+
Concord Hospital	Concord	65%	300+
Frisbie Memorial Hospital	Rochester	65%	300+
Catholic Medical Center	Manchester	64%	300+
Wentworth-Douglass Hospital	Dover	64%	300+
Androscoggin Valley Hospital	Berlin	63%	(a)
Mary Hitchcock Memorial Hospital	Lebanon	63%	300+
Cheshire Medical Center	Keene	62%	300+
Elliot Hospital	Manchester	62%	300+
Exeter Hospital	Exeter	62%	300+
Littleton Regional Hospital	Littleton	62%	(a)
Saint Joseph Hospital	Nashua	62%	300+
Franklin Regional Hospital	Franklin	61%	(a)
Huggins Hospital	Wolfeboro	60%	300+
New London Hospital	New London	58%	(a)
Portsmouth Regional Hospital	Portsmouth	57%	300+
Lakes Region General Hospital	Laconia	55%	300+

45. Nurses 'Always' Communicated Well

Hospital Name	City	Rate	Cases
Monadnock Community Hospital	Peterborough	86%	300+
Speare Memorial Hospital	Plymouth	86%	300+
Concord Hospital	Concord	82%	300+
Parkland Medical Center	Derry	82%	300+
Catholic Medical Center	Manchester	81%	300+
Exeter Hospital	Exeter	81%	300+
Saint Joseph Hospital	Nashua	81%	300+
Wentworth-Douglass Hospital	Dover	81%	300+
Southern Nh Medical Center	Nashua	80%	300+
Frisbie Memorial Hospital	Rochester	79%	300+
Androscoggin Valley Hospital	Berlin	78%	(a)
Cheshire Medical Center	Keene	78%	300+
Mary Hitchcock Memorial Hospital	Lebanon	78%	300+
New London Hospital	New London	78%	(a)
Elliot Hospital	Manchester	77%	300+
Huggins Hospital	Wolfeboro	77%	300+
Portsmouth Regional Hospital	Portsmouth	75%	300+
Littleton Regional Hospital	Littleton	74%	(a)
Franklin Regional Hospital	Franklin	71%	(a)
Lakes Region General Hospital	Laconia	71%	300+

46. Pain 'Always' Well Controlled

Hospital Name	City	Rate	Cases
Speare Memorial Hospital	Plymouth	77%	300+
Monadnock Community Hospital	Peterborough	76%	300+
Exeter Hospital	Exeter	75%	300+
Huggins Hospital	Wolfeboro	75%	300+
Parkland Medical Center	Derry	75%	300+
Saint Joseph Hospital	Nashua	75%	300+
Wentworth-Douglass Hospital	Dover	75%	300+
Elliot Hospital	Manchester	72%	300+

NOTE: Hospital profiles are in alphabetical order by state, then city, then hospital within the city; Rankings exclude hospitals with less than 25 cases except for patient surveys which excludes hospitals with less than 100 cases; (a) 100–299 cases; (1) The number of cases is too small to be sure how well a hospital is performing; (2) The hospital indicated that the data submitted for this measure were based on a sample of cases; (3) Data was collected during a shorter time period (fewer quarters) than the maximum possible time for this measure; (4) Suppressed for one or more quarters by CMS; (5) No data is available from the hospital for this measure; (6) Fewer than 100 patients completed the HCAHPS survey. Use these rates with caution, as the number of surveys may be too low to reliably assess hospital performance; (7) Survey results are based on less than 12 months of data; (8) Survey results are not available for this reporting period; (9) No or very few patients were eligible for the HCAHPS survey. The scores shown, if any, reflect a very small number of surveys; (10) A state average was not calculated because too few hospitals in the state submitted data; (11) There were discrepancies in the data collection process; Please refer to the User's Guide for a full explanation of data.

Southern Nh Medical Center	Nashua	72%	300+
Concord Hospital	Concord	71%	300+
Frisbie Memorial Hospital	Rochester	71%	300+
Cheshire Medical Center	Keene	70%	300+
Littleton Regional Hospital	Littleton	70%	(a)
Catholic Medical Center	Manchester	69%	300+
New London Hospital	New London	69%	(a)
Portsmouth Regional Hospital	Portsmouth	69%	300+
Mary Hitchcock Memorial Hospital	Lebanon	68%	300+
Franklin Regional Hospital	Franklin	65%	(a)
Androscoggin Valley Hospital	Berlin	64%	(a)
Lakes Region General Hospital	Laconia	64%	300+

47. Room and Bathroom 'Always' Clean

Hospital Name	City	Rate	Cases
Speare Memorial Hospital	Plymouth	86%	300+
New London Hospital	New London	84%	(a)
Frisbie Memorial Hospital	Rochester	83%	300+
Monadnock Community Hospital	Peterborough	82%	300+
Parkland Medical Center	Derry	82%	300+
Wentworth-Douglass Hospital	Dover	81%	300+
Androscoggin Valley Hospital	Berlin	79%	(a)
Cheshire Medical Center	Keene	79%	300+
Franklin Regional Hospital	Franklin	79%	(a)
Littleton Regional Hospital	Littleton	77%	(a)
Concord Hospital	Concord	75%	300+
Saint Joseph Hospital	Nashua	75%	300+
Elliot Hospital	Manchester	73%	300+
Huggins Hospital	Wolfeboro	73%	300+
Exeter Hospital	Exeter	72%	300+
Portsmouth Regional Hospital	Portsmouth	72%	300+
Mary Hitchcock Memorial Hospital	Lebanon	71%	300+
Catholic Medical Center	Manchester	70%	300+
Southern Nh Medical Center	Nashua	70%	300+
Lakes Region General Hospital	Laconia	69%	300+

48. Timely Help 'Always' Received

Hospital Name	City	Rate	Cases
Monadnock Community Hospital	Peterborough	80%	300+
Speare Memorial Hospital	Plymouth	78%	300+
Parkland Medical Center	Derry	76%	300+
New London Hospital	New London	75%	(a)
Frisbie Memorial Hospital	Rochester	74%	300+
Mary Hitchcock Memorial Hospital	Lebanon	73%	300+
Androscoggin Valley Hospital	Berlin	72%	(a)
Exeter Hospital	Exeter	71%	300+
Concord Hospital	Concord	69%	300+
Wentworth-Douglass Hospital	Dover	69%	300+
Catholic Medical Center	Manchester	67%	300+
Littleton Regional Hospital	Littleton	67%	(a)
Cheshire Medical Center	Keene	64%	300+
Saint Joseph Hospital	Nashua	64%	300+
Southern Nh Medical Center	Nashua	64%	300+
Franklin Regional Hospital	Franklin	63%	(a)
Huggins Hospital	Wolfeboro	63%	300+
Elliot Hospital	Manchester	62%	300+
Portsmouth Regional Hospital	Portsmouth	62%	300+
Lakes Region General Hospital	Laconia	59%	300+

49. Would Definitely Recommend Hospital

Hospital Name	City	Rate	Cases
Mary Hitchcock Memorial Hospital	Lebanon	84%	300+
Concord Hospital	Concord	82%	300+
Monadnock Community Hospital	Peterborough	81%	300+
Speare Memorial Hospital	Plymouth	80%	300+
Wentworth-Douglass Hospital	Dover	80%	300+
Exeter Hospital	Exeter	79%	300+
Southern Nh Medical Center	Nashua	79%	300+
Catholic Medical Center	Manchester	76%	300+
Elliot Hospital	Manchester	76%	300+
New London Hospital	New London	75%	(a)
Saint Joseph Hospital	Nashua	75%	300+
Frisbie Memorial Hospital	Rochester	73%	300+
Portsmouth Regional Hospital	Portsmouth	72%	300+
Parkland Medical Center	Derry	71%	300+
Cheshire Medical Center	Keene	68%	300+
Littleton Regional Hospital	Littleton	68%	(a)
Huggins Hospital	Wolfeboro	64%	300+
Franklin Regional Hospital	Franklin	60%	(a)
Androscoggin Valley Hospital	Berlin	58%	(a)
Lakes Region General Hospital	Laconia	58%	300+

Androscoggin Valley Hospital

59 Page Hill Road
Berlin, NH 03570
Phone: 603-752-2200
Fax: 603-752-2376
E-mail: info@avhnh.com
URL: www.avhnh.com
Type: Critical Access Hospitals
Emergency Services: Yes
Ownership: Govt - Hospital Dist/Auth
Beds: 92

Key Personnel:

CEO/President. . . . . Russell G Keene
Chief of Medical Staff . . . . Grant Niskanen, MD
Infection Control. . . . . Thomas Marallo, MT
Operating Room. . . . . Suzie Holland, RN
Pediatric Ambulatory Care . . . . . . Brian Beals, MD
Pediatric In-Patient Care . . . . Brenda Aubin, RN, BSN
Quality Assurance . . . . John McDowell, MD
Radiology. . . . . Janet Sherman, RDMS, CT

Measure	Cases	This Hosp.	State Avg.	U.S. Avg.
Heart Attack Care				
ACE Inhibitor or ARB for LVSD[1]	2	100%	98%	96%
Aspirin at Arrival[1]	11	100%	100%	99%
Aspirin at Discharge[1]	8	100%	99%	98%
Beta Blocker at Discharge[1]	9	100%	100%	98%
Fibrinolytic Medication Timing	0	-	100%	55%
PCI Within 90 Minutes of Arrival[5]	0	-	89%	90%
Smoking Cessation Advice	0	-	99%	99%
Chest Pain/Possible Heart Attack Care				
Aspirin at Arrival	-	-	97%	95%
Median Time to ECG (minutes)	-	-	8	8
Median Time to Transfer (minutes)	-	-	41	61
Fibrinolytic Medication Timing	-	-	48%	54%
Heart Failure Care				
ACE Inhibitor or ARB for LVSD[1]	13	100%	96%	94%
Discharge Instructions	27	70%	92%	88%
Evaluation of LVS Function	41	98%	99%	98%
Smoking Cessation Advice[1]	2	100%	99%	98%
Pneumonia Care				
Appropriate Initial Antibiotic[1]	21	100%	95%	92%
Blood Culture Timing	37	100%	97%	96%
Influenza Vaccine[1]	20	100%	95%	91%
Initial Antibiotic Timing	36	100%	97%	95%
Pneumococcal Vaccine	44	95%	96%	93%
Smoking Cessation Advice[1]	10	100%	97%	97%
Surgical Care Improvement Project				
Appropriate VTP Within 24 Hours[1]	19	95%	96%	92%
Appropriate Hair Removal	44	100%	100%	99%
Appropriate Beta Blocker Usage[5]	0	-	95%	93%
Controlled Postoperative Blood Glucose[5]	0	-	95%	93%
Prophylactic Antibiotic Timing	35	94%	97%	97%
Prophylactic Antibiotic Timing (Outpatient)	-	-	96%	92%
Prophylactic Antibiotic Selection	35	91%	98%	97%
Prophylactic Antibiotic Select. (Outpatient)	-	-	97%	94%
Prophylactic Antibiotic Stopped	32	88%	97%	94%
Recommended VTP Ordered[1]	19	95%	97%	94%
Urinary Catheter Removal[5]	0	-	89%	90%
Children's Asthma Care				
Received Systemic Corticosteroids	-	-	-	100%
Received Home Management Plan	-	-	-	71%
Received Reliever Medication	-	-	-	100%
Use of Medical Imaging				
Combination Abdominal CT Scan	-	-	0.078	0.191
Combination Chest CT Scan	-	-	0.014	0.054
Follow-up Mammogram/Ultrasound	-	-	7.1%	8.4%
MRI for Low Back Pain	-	-	31.5%	32.7%
Survey of Patients' Hospital Experiences				
Area Around Room 'Always' Quiet at Night	(a)	49%	-	58%
Doctors 'Always' Communicated Well	(a)	81%	-	80%
Home Recovery Information Given	(a)	83%	-	82%
Hospital Given 9 or 10 on 10 Point Scale	(a)	61%	-	67%
Meds 'Always' Explained Before Given	(a)	63%	-	60%
Nurses 'Always' Communicated Well	(a)	78%	-	76%
Pain 'Always' Well Controlled	(a)	64%	-	69%
Room and Bathroom 'Always' Clean	(a)	79%	-	71%
Timely Help 'Always' Received	(a)	72%	-	64%
Would Definitely Recommend Hospital	(a)	58%	-	69%

Valley Regional Hospital

243 Elm Street
Claremont, NH 03743
Phone: 603-542-7771
Fax: 603-542-3403
URL: www.vrh.org
Type: Critical Access Hospitals
Emergency Services: Yes
Ownership: Voluntary Non-Profit - Private
Beds: 45

Key Personnel:

CEO/President. . . . . Claire Bowen
Chief of Medical Staff . . . . Roy M Barnes
Quality Assurance . . . . Sandy Gee
Radiology. . . . . Katherine F Gerke
Emergency Room . . . . Dr. Joseph Hagan

Measure	Cases	This Hosp.	State Avg.	U.S. Avg.
Heart Attack Care				
ACE Inhibitor or ARB for LVSD[1]	2	100%	98%	96%
Aspirin at Arrival[1]	9	100%	100%	99%
Aspirin at Discharge[1]	7	86%	99%	98%
Beta Blocker at Discharge[1]	6	100%	100%	98%
Fibrinolytic Medication Timing	0	-	100%	55%
PCI Within 90 Minutes of Arrival	0	-	89%	90%
Smoking Cessation Advice	0	-	99%	99%
Chest Pain/Possible Heart Attack Care				
Aspirin at Arrival	-	-	97%	95%
Median Time to ECG (minutes)	-	-	8	8
Median Time to Transfer (minutes)	-	-	41	61
Fibrinolytic Medication Timing	-	-	48%	54%
Heart Failure Care				
ACE Inhibitor or ARB for LVSD[1]	2	100%	96%	94%
Discharge Instructions[1]	11	91%	92%	88%
Evaluation of LVS Function[1]	20	100%	99%	98%
Smoking Cessation Advice[1]	3	100%	99%	98%
Pneumonia Care				
Appropriate Initial Antibiotic	26	100%	95%	92%
Blood Culture Timing	36	92%	97%	96%
Influenza Vaccine	27	89%	95%	91%
Initial Antibiotic Timing	31	100%	97%	95%
Pneumococcal Vaccine	32	88%	96%	93%
Smoking Cessation Advice[1]	11	100%	97%	97%
Surgical Care Improvement Project				
Appropriate VTP Within 24 Hours	49	100%	96%	92%
Appropriate Hair Removal	94	100%	100%	99%
Appropriate Beta Blocker Usage[5]	0	-	95%	93%
Controlled Postoperative Blood Glucose	0	-	95%	93%
Prophylactic Antibiotic Timing	82	98%	97%	97%
Prophylactic Antibiotic Timing (Outpatient)	-	-	96%	92%
Prophylactic Antibiotic Selection	81	98%	98%	97%
Prophylactic Antibiotic Select. (Outpatient)	-	-	97%	94%
Prophylactic Antibiotic Stopped	79	99%	97%	94%
Recommended VTP Ordered	49	100%	97%	94%
Urinary Catheter Removal	34	82%	89%	90%
Children's Asthma Care				
Received Systemic Corticosteroids	-	-	-	100%
Received Home Management Plan	-	-	-	71%
Received Reliever Medication	-	-	-	100%
Use of Medical Imaging				
Combination Abdominal CT Scan	-	-	0.078	0.191
Combination Chest CT Scan	-	-	0.014	0.054
Follow-up Mammogram/Ultrasound	-	-	7.1%	8.4%
MRI for Low Back Pain	-	-	31.5%	32.7%
Survey of Patients' Hospital Experiences				
Area Around Room 'Always' Quiet at Night[8]	-	-	-	58%
Doctors 'Always' Communicated Well[8]	-	-	-	80%
Home Recovery Information Given[8]	-	-	-	82%
Hospital Given 9 or 10 on 10 Point Scale[8]	-	-	-	67%
Meds 'Always' Explained Before Given[8]	-	-	-	60%
Nurses 'Always' Communicated Well[8]	-	-	-	76%
Pain 'Always' Well Controlled[8]	-	-	-	69%
Room and Bathroom 'Always' Clean[8]	-	-	-	71%
Timely Help 'Always' Received[8]	-	-	-	64%
Would Definitely Recommend Hospital[8]	-	-	-	69%

Upper Connecticut Valley Hospital

181 Corliss Lane
Colebrook, NH 03576
Phone: 603-237-4971
Fax: 603-237-4452
E-mail: ann.morrison@hitchcock.org
URL: www.dartmouth-hitchcock.org/ucvh
Type: Critical Access Hospitals
Emergency Services: Yes
Ownership: Voluntary Non-Profit - Private
Beds: 16

Key Personnel:

CEO/President. . . . . Louise A McCleery
Chief of Medical Staff . . . . Robert Soucy
Infection Control. . . . . Carol Bunnell, RN
Quality Assurance . . . . Irene Dodge
Anesthesiology. . . . . Dan McClenahan, CRNA
Emergency Room . . . . Sharon Curtis, MD

Measure	Cases	This Hosp.	State Avg.	U.S. Avg.
Heart Attack Care				
ACE Inhibitor or ARB for LVSD	0	-	98%	96%
Aspirin at Arrival[1]	6	100%	100%	99%
Aspirin at Discharge[1]	4	75%	99%	98%
Beta Blocker at Discharge[1]	5	100%	100%	98%
Fibrinolytic Medication Timing	0	-	100%	55%
PCI Within 90 Minutes of Arrival	0	-	89%	90%
Smoking Cessation Advice	0	-	99%	99%
Chest Pain/Possible Heart Attack Care				
Aspirin at Arrival	38	97%	97%	95%
Median Time to ECG (minutes)	38	10	8	8
Median Time to Transfer (minutes)[3]	0	-	41	61
Fibrinolytic Medication Timing[1]	4	25%	48%	54%
Heart Failure Care				
ACE Inhibitor or ARB for LVSD[1]	5	100%	96%	94%
Discharge Instructions[1]	15	100%	92%	88%
Evaluation of LVS Function[1]	23	91%	99%	98%
Smoking Cessation Advice[1]	4	100%	99%	98%
Pneumonia Care				
Appropriate Initial Antibiotic[1,2]	17	100%	95%	92%
Blood Culture Timing[1,2]	10	100%	97%	96%
Influenza Vaccine[1]	10	80%	95%	91%
Initial Antibiotic Timing[1,2]	21	100%	97%	95%
Pneumococcal Vaccine[1,2]	20	75%	96%	93%
Smoking Cessation Advice[1,2]	10	90%	97%	97%
Surgical Care Improvement Project				
Appropriate VTP Within 24 Hours[3]	0	-	96%	92%
Appropriate Hair Removal[1,3]	2	100%	100%	99%
Appropriate Beta Blocker Usage[1,3]	2	100%	95%	93%
Controlled Postoperative Blood Glucose[3]	0	-	95%	93%
Prophylactic Antibiotic Timing[1,3]	2	100%	97%	97%
Prophylactic Antibiotic Timing (Outpatient)[5]	0	-	96%	92%
Prophylactic Antibiotic Selection[1,3]	2	100%	98%	97%
Prophylactic Antibiotic Select. (Outpatient)[5]	0	-	97%	94%
Prophylactic Antibiotic Stopped[1,3]	2	100%	97%	94%
Recommended VTP Ordered[3]	0	-	97%	94%
Urinary Catheter Removal[5]	0	-	89%	90%
Children's Asthma Care				
Received Systemic Corticosteroids	-	-	-	100%
Received Home Management Plan	-	-	-	71%
Received Reliever Medication	-	-	-	100%
Use of Medical Imaging				
Combination Abdominal CT Scan	80	0.213	0.078	0.191
Combination Chest CT Scan[1]	52	0.135	0.014	0.054
Follow-up Mammogram/Ultrasound	181	2.8%	7.1%	8.4%
MRI for Low Back Pain[5]	0	-	31.5%	32.7%
Survey of Patients' Hospital Experiences				
Area Around Room 'Always' Quiet at Night[8]	-	-	-	58%
Doctors 'Always' Communicated Well[8]	-	-	-	80%
Home Recovery Information Given[8]	-	-	-	82%
Hospital Given 9 or 10 on 10 Point Scale[8]	-	-	-	67%
Meds 'Always' Explained Before Given[8]	-	-	-	60%
Nurses 'Always' Communicated Well[8]	-	-	-	76%
Pain 'Always' Well Controlled[8]	-	-	-	69%
Room and Bathroom 'Always' Clean[8]	-	-	-	71%
Timely Help 'Always' Received[8]	-	-	-	64%
Would Definitely Recommend Hospital[8]	-	-	-	69%

NOTE: Hospital profiles are in alphabetical order by state, then city, then hospital within the city; Rankings exclude hospitals with less than 25 cases except for patient surveys which excludes hospitals with less than 100 cases; (a) 100–299 cases; (1) The number of cases is too small to be sure how well a hospital is performing; (2) The hospital indicated that the data submitted for this measure were based on a sample of cases; (3) Data was collected during a shorter time period (fewer quarters) than the maximum possible time for this measure; (4) Suppressed for one or more quarters by CMS; (5) No data is available from the hospital for this measure; (6) Fewer than 100 patients completed the HCAHPS survey. Use these rates with caution, as the number of surveys may be too low to reliably assess hospital performance; (7) Survey results are based on less than 12 months of data; (8) Survey results are not available for this reporting period; (9) No or very few patients were eligible for the HCAHPS survey. The scores shown, if any, reflect a very small number of surveys; (10) A state average was not calculated because too few hospitals in the state submitted data; (11) There were discrepancies in the data collection process; Please refer to the User's Guide for a full explanation of data.

Concord Hospital

250 Pleasant St Phone: 603-225-2711
Concord, NH 03301 Fax: 603-228-7346
E-mail: karr@crhc.org
URL: www.concordhospital.org
Type: Acute Care Hospitals Emergency Services: Yes
Ownership: Voluntary Non-Profit - Private Beds: 295

Key Personnel:
CEO/President. . . . . Michael Green
Chief of Medical Staff . . . . David F Green, MD
Operating Room. . . . . Noreen Nixon
Quality Assurance . . . . Nancy Hacking
Radiology. . . . . Maureen Trombly
Emergency Room . . . . Leslie Mahoney

Measure	Cases	This Hosp.	State Avg.	U.S. Avg.
Heart Attack Care				
ACE Inhibitor or ARB for LVSD	29	100%	98%	96%
Aspirin at Arrival	165	100%	100%	99%
Aspirin at Discharge	228	100%	99%	98%
Beta Blocker at Discharge	226	100%	100%	98%
Fibrinolytic Medication Timing	0	-	100%	55%
PCI Within 90 Minutes of Arrival	48	96%	89%	90%
Smoking Cessation Advice	69	100%	99%	99%
Chest Pain/Possible Heart Attack Care				
Aspirin at Arrival[1]	1	100%	97%	95%
Median Time to ECG (minutes)[1]	2	4	8	8
Median Time to Transfer (minutes)[5]	0	-	41	61
Fibrinolytic Medication Timing[5]	0	-	48%	54%
Heart Failure Care				
ACE Inhibitor or ARB for LVSD	86	99%	96%	94%
Discharge Instructions	261	96%	92%	88%
Evaluation of LVS Function	343	100%	99%	98%
Smoking Cessation Advice	53	100%	99%	98%
Pneumonia Care				
Appropriate Initial Antibiotic	196	95%	95%	92%
Blood Culture Timing	285	96%	97%	96%
Influenza Vaccine	186	97%	95%	91%
Initial Antibiotic Timing	284	97%	97%	95%
Pneumococcal Vaccine	273	95%	96%	93%
Smoking Cessation Advice	104	97%	97%	97%
Surgical Care Improvement Project				
Appropriate VTP Within 24 Hours[2]	122	92%	96%	92%
Appropriate Hair Removal[2]	464	100%	100%	99%
Appropriate Beta Blocker Usage[2]	172	99%	95%	93%
Controlled Postoperative Blood Glucose[2]	106	95%	95%	93%
Prophylactic Antibiotic Timing[2]	360	96%	97%	97%
Prophylactic Antibiotic Timing (Outpatient)	406	98%	96%	92%
Prophylactic Antibiotic Selection[2]	369	97%	98%	97%
Prophylactic Antibiotic Select. (Outpatient)	402	96%	97%	94%
Prophylactic Antibiotic Stopped[2]	355	95%	97%	94%
Recommended VTP Ordered[2]	122	92%	97%	94%
Urinary Catheter Removal[2]	111	84%	89%	90%
Children's Asthma Care				
Received Systemic Corticosteroids	-	-	-	100%
Received Home Management Plan	-	-	-	71%
Received Reliever Medication	-	-	-	100%
Use of Medical Imaging				
Combination Abdominal CT Scan	743	0.139	0.078	0.191
Combination Chest CT Scan	439	0.046	0.014	0.054
Follow-up Mammogram/Ultrasound	713	8.1%	7.1%	8.4%
MRI for Low Back Pain	99	27.3%	31.5%	32.7%
Survey of Patients' Hospital Experiences				
Area Around Room 'Always' Quiet at Night	300+	62%	-	58%
Doctors 'Always' Communicated Well	300+	82%	-	80%
Home Recovery Information Given	300+	87%	-	82%
Hospital Given 9 or 10 on 10 Point Scale	300+	78%	-	67%
Meds 'Always' Explained Before Given	300+	65%	-	60%
Nurses 'Always' Communicated Well	300+	82%	-	76%
Pain 'Always' Well Controlled	300+	71%	-	69%
Room and Bathroom 'Always' Clean	300+	75%	-	71%
Timely Help 'Always' Received	300+	69%	-	64%
Would Definitely Recommend Hospital	300+	82%	-	69%

Parkland Medical Center

1 Parkland Drive Phone: 603-421-2100
Derry, NH 03038 Fax: 603-421-2111
URL: www.parklandmedicalcenter.com
Type: Acute Care Hospitals Emergency Services: Yes
Ownership: Proprietary Beds: 78

Key Personnel:
CEO/President. . . . . Anne Jamieson
Chief of Medical Staff . . . . Anne Loosmann, MD
Infection Control. . . . . Lynda Caine
Operating Room. . . . . Donald Colacchio, MD
Pediatric In-Patient Care . . . . Christopher Peterson, MD
Quality Assurance . . . . Anne Sands

Measure	Cases	This Hosp.	State Avg.	U.S. Avg.
Heart Attack Care				
ACE Inhibitor or ARB for LVSD[1]	15	100%	98%	96%
Aspirin at Arrival	85	100%	100%	99%
Aspirin at Discharge	73	100%	99%	98%
Beta Blocker at Discharge	74	100%	100%	98%
Fibrinolytic Medication Timing	0	-	100%	55%
PCI Within 90 Minutes of Arrival[1]	23	100%	89%	90%
Smoking Cessation Advice	25	100%	99%	99%
Chest Pain/Possible Heart Attack Care				
Aspirin at Arrival[1,3]	4	100%	97%	95%
Median Time to ECG (minutes)[1,3]	4	2	8	8
Median Time to Transfer (minutes)[5]	0	-	41	61
Fibrinolytic Medication Timing[3]	0	-	48%	54%
Heart Failure Care				
ACE Inhibitor or ARB for LVSD	27	100%	96%	94%
Discharge Instructions	104	98%	92%	88%
Evaluation of LVS Function	146	100%	99%	98%
Smoking Cessation Advice[1]	17	100%	99%	98%
Pneumonia Care				
Appropriate Initial Antibiotic	58	98%	95%	92%
Blood Culture Timing	96	99%	97%	96%
Influenza Vaccine	63	98%	95%	91%
Initial Antibiotic Timing	76	100%	97%	95%
Pneumococcal Vaccine	93	99%	96%	93%
Smoking Cessation Advice	33	100%	97%	97%
Surgical Care Improvement Project				
Appropriate VTP Within 24 Hours	70	94%	96%	92%
Appropriate Hair Removal	161	100%	100%	99%
Appropriate Beta Blocker Usage	41	100%	95%	93%
Controlled Postoperative Blood Glucose	0	-	95%	93%
Prophylactic Antibiotic Timing	56	98%	97%	97%
Prophylactic Antibiotic Timing (Outpatient)	80	100%	96%	92%
Prophylactic Antibiotic Selection	55	100%	98%	97%
Prophylactic Antibiotic Select. (Outpatient)	116	94%	97%	94%
Prophylactic Antibiotic Stopped	52	98%	97%	94%
Recommended VTP Ordered	70	100%	97%	94%
Urinary Catheter Removal[1]	15	80%	89%	90%
Children's Asthma Care				
Received Systemic Corticosteroids	-	-	-	100%
Received Home Management Plan	-	-	-	71%
Received Reliever Medication	-	-	-	100%
Use of Medical Imaging				
Combination Abdominal CT Scan	304	0.072	0.078	0.191
Combination Chest CT Scan	191	0.021	0.014	0.054
Follow-up Mammogram/Ultrasound	358	8.7%	7.1%	8.4%
MRI for Low Back Pain[1]	32	21.9%	31.5%	32.7%
Survey of Patients' Hospital Experiences				
Area Around Room 'Always' Quiet at Night	300+	60%	-	58%
Doctors 'Always' Communicated Well	300+	81%	-	80%
Home Recovery Information Given	300+	90%	-	82%
Hospital Given 9 or 10 on 10 Point Scale	300+	71%	-	67%
Meds 'Always' Explained Before Given	300+	68%	-	60%
Nurses 'Always' Communicated Well	300+	82%	-	76%
Pain 'Always' Well Controlled	300+	75%	-	69%
Room and Bathroom 'Always' Clean	300+	82%	-	71%
Timely Help 'Always' Received	300+	76%	-	64%
Would Definitely Recommend Hospital	300+	71%	-	69%

Wentworth-Douglass Hospital

789 Central Ave Phone: 603-740-2580
Dover, NH 03820 Fax: 603-740-2242
Type: Acute Care Hospitals Emergency Services: Yes
Ownership: Voluntary Non-Profit - Private Beds: 178

Key Personnel:
Chief of Medical Staff . . . . James McKenna, MD
Pediatric Ambulatory Care . . . . . . Andre Vanderzanden, MD
Pediatric In-Patient Care . . . . Andre Vanderzanden, MD
Radiology. . . . . Bernard M Casey, MD
Anesthesiology. . . . . James Tobin, MD
Emergency Room . . . . Owen MacCausland, MD

Measure	Cases	This Hosp.	State Avg.	U.S. Avg.
Heart Attack Care				
ACE Inhibitor or ARB for LVSD[1]	5	100%	98%	96%
Aspirin at Arrival	77	100%	100%	99%
Aspirin at Discharge	74	97%	99%	98%
Beta Blocker at Discharge	72	100%	100%	98%
Fibrinolytic Medication Timing	0	-	100%	55%
PCI Within 90 Minutes of Arrival[1]	21	71%	89%	90%
Smoking Cessation Advice	26	100%	99%	99%
Chest Pain/Possible Heart Attack Care				
Aspirin at Arrival[1,3]	2	100%	97%	95%
Median Time to ECG (minutes)[1,3]	2	12	8	8
Median Time to Transfer (minutes)[5]	0	-	41	61
Fibrinolytic Medication Timing[5]	0	-	48%	54%
Heart Failure Care				
ACE Inhibitor or ARB for LVSD	48	100%	96%	94%
Discharge Instructions	165	99%	92%	88%
Evaluation of LVS Function	203	99%	99%	98%
Smoking Cessation Advice[1]	18	100%	99%	98%
Pneumonia Care				
Appropriate Initial Antibiotic[2]	99	98%	95%	92%
Blood Culture Timing[2]	135	99%	97%	96%
Influenza Vaccine[2]	82	94%	95%	91%
Initial Antibiotic Timing[2]	139	96%	97%	95%
Pneumococcal Vaccine[2]	116	93%	96%	93%
Smoking Cessation Advice[2]	38	97%	97%	97%
Surgical Care Improvement Project				
Appropriate VTP Within 24 Hours[2]	152	93%	96%	92%
Appropriate Hair Removal[2]	448	100%	100%	99%
Appropriate Beta Blocker Usage[2]	119	92%	95%	93%
Controlled Postoperative Blood Glucose[2]	0	-	95%	93%
Prophylactic Antibiotic Timing[2]	307	100%	97%	97%
Prophylactic Antibiotic Timing (Outpatient)	346	99%	96%	92%
Prophylactic Antibiotic Selection[2]	310	99%	98%	97%
Prophylactic Antibiotic Select. (Outpatient)	345	98%	97%	94%
Prophylactic Antibiotic Stopped[2]	302	99%	97%	94%
Recommended VTP Ordered[2]	152	95%	97%	94%
Urinary Catheter Removal[2]	127	88%	89%	90%
Children's Asthma Care				
Received Systemic Corticosteroids	-	-	-	100%
Received Home Management Plan	-	-	-	71%
Received Reliever Medication	-	-	-	100%
Use of Medical Imaging				
Combination Abdominal CT Scan	848	0.037	0.078	0.191
Combination Chest CT Scan	725	0.001	0.014	0.054
Follow-up Mammogram/Ultrasound[5]	0	-	7.1%	8.4%
MRI for Low Back Pain	178	30.9%	31.5%	32.7%
Survey of Patients' Hospital Experiences				
Area Around Room 'Always' Quiet at Night	300+	56%	-	58%
Doctors 'Always' Communicated Well	300+	79%	-	80%
Home Recovery Information Given	300+	93%	-	82%
Hospital Given 9 or 10 on 10 Point Scale	300+	73%	-	67%
Meds 'Always' Explained Before Given	300+	64%	-	60%
Nurses 'Always' Communicated Well	300+	81%	-	76%
Pain 'Always' Well Controlled	300+	75%	-	69%
Room and Bathroom 'Always' Clean	300+	81%	-	71%
Timely Help 'Always' Received	300+	69%	-	64%
Would Definitely Recommend Hospital	300+	80%	-	69%

NOTE: Hospital profiles are in alphabetical order by state, then city, then hospital within the city; Rankings exclude hospitals with less than 25 cases except for patient surveys which excludes hospitals with less than 100 cases; (a) 100–299 cases; (1) The number of cases is too small to be sure how well a hospital is performing; (2) The hospital indicated that the data submitted for this measure were based on a sample of cases; (3) Data was collected during a shorter time period (fewer quarters) than the maximum possible time for this measure; (4) Suppressed for one or more quarters by CMS; (5) No data is available from the hospital for this measure; (6) Fewer than 100 patients completed the HCAHPS survey. Use these rates with caution, as the number of surveys may be too low to reliably assess hospital performance; (7) Survey results are based on less than 12 months of data; (8) Survey results are not available for this reporting period; (9) No or very few patients were eligible for the HCAHPS survey. The scores shown, if any, reflect a very small number of surveys; (10) A state average was not calculated because too few hospitals in the state submitted data; (11) There were discrepancies in the data collection process; Please refer to the User's Guide for a full explanation of data.

Exeter Hospital

5 Alumni Drive
Exeter, NH 03833
Type: Acute Care Hospitals
Ownership: Voluntary Non-Profit - Other

Phone: 603-778-7311
Fax: 603-778-6592
Emergency Services: Yes
Beds: 100

Key Personnel:

CEO/President. . . . . Kevin Callahan
Operating Room. . . . . Sheryl LaPlume
Pediatric Ambulatory Care . . . . . . Gregory Prazar, MD
Pediatric In-Patient Care . . . . Steve Loh, MD
Quality Assurance . . . . Lori Chabot
Emergency Room . . . . Mark Josephs, MD

Measure	Cases	This Hosp.	State Avg.	U.S. Avg.
Heart Attack Care				
ACE Inhibitor or ARB for LVSD[1]	8	100%	98%	96%
Aspirin at Arrival	118	100%	100%	99%
Aspirin at Discharge	96	99%	99%	98%
Beta Blocker at Discharge	88	100%	100%	98%
Fibrinolytic Medication Timing	0	-	100%	55%
PCI Within 90 Minutes of Arrival	32	94%	89%	90%
Smoking Cessation Advice	29	100%	99%	99%
Chest Pain/Possible Heart Attack Care				
Aspirin at Arrival[1]	5	100%	97%	95%
Median Time to ECG (minutes)[1]	5	15	8	8
Median Time to Transfer (minutes)[3,1]	3	48	41	61
Fibrinolytic Medication Timing[3]	0	-	48%	54%
Heart Failure Care				
ACE Inhibitor or ARB for LVSD	39	92%	96%	94%
Discharge Instructions	137	100%	92%	88%
Evaluation of LVS Function	185	100%	99%	98%
Smoking Cessation Advice[1]	17	100%	99%	98%
Pneumonia Care				
Appropriate Initial Antibiotic	123	94%	95%	92%
Blood Culture Timing	166	96%	97%	96%
Influenza Vaccine	111	95%	95%	91%
Initial Antibiotic Timing	182	95%	97%	95%
Pneumococcal Vaccine	165	94%	96%	93%
Smoking Cessation Advice	59	100%	97%	97%
Surgical Care Improvement Project				
Appropriate VTP Within 24 Hours	141	94%	96%	92%
Appropriate Hair Removal	543	100%	100%	99%
Appropriate Beta Blocker Usage	212	93%	95%	93%
Controlled Postoperative Blood Glucose	0	-	95%	93%
Prophylactic Antibiotic Timing	395	99%	97%	97%
Prophylactic Antibiotic Timing (Outpatient)	195	99%	96%	92%
Prophylactic Antibiotic Selection	399	98%	98%	97%
Prophylactic Antibiotic Select. (Outpatient)	194	96%	97%	94%
Prophylactic Antibiotic Stopped	386	97%	97%	94%
Recommended VTP Ordered	141	97%	97%	94%
Urinary Catheter Removal	142	98%	89%	90%
Children's Asthma Care				
Received Systemic Corticosteroids	-	-	-	100%
Received Home Management Plan	-	-	-	71%
Received Reliever Medication	-	-	-	100%
Use of Medical Imaging				
Combination Abdominal CT Scan	841	0.068	0.078	0.191
Combination Chest CT Scan	825	0.016	0.014	0.054
Follow-up Mammogram/Ultrasound	1,950	3.8%	7.1%	8.4%
MRI for Low Back Pain	192	24.5%	31.5%	32.7%
Survey of Patients' Hospital Experiences				
Area Around Room 'Always' Quiet at Night	300+	51%	-	58%
Doctors 'Always' Communicated Well	300+	82%	-	80%
Home Recovery Information Given	300+	89%	-	82%
Hospital Given 9 or 10 on 10 Point Scale	300+	77%	-	67%
Meds 'Always' Explained Before Given	300+	62%	-	60%
Nurses 'Always' Communicated Well	300+	81%	-	76%
Pain 'Always' Well Controlled	300+	75%	-	69%
Room and Bathroom 'Always' Clean	300+	72%	-	71%
Timely Help 'Always' Received	300+	71%	-	64%
Would Definitely Recommend Hospital	300+	79%	-	69%

Franklin Regional Hospital

15 Aiken Avenue
Franklin, NH 03235
E-mail: info@lrgh.org
URL: www.lrgh.org
Type: Critical Access Hospitals
Ownership: Voluntary Non-Profit - Private

Phone: 603-934-2060
Fax: 603-934-4616
Emergency Services: Yes
Beds: 25

Key Personnel:

CEO/President. . . . . Tom Clearmont
Chief of Medical Staff . . . . Peter Walkley
Infection Control. . . . . Marcia Hansen
Operating Room. . . . . Virginia McCabe-Crum, RN
Quality Assurance . . . . Kathy Fuller
Radiology. . . . . Robert C Andrews, MD
Emergency Room . . . . Paul Racicot, MD
Intensive Care Unit. . . . . Marilyn Minichiello, RN

Measure	Cases	This Hosp.	State Avg.	U.S. Avg.
Heart Attack Care				
ACE Inhibitor or ARB for LVSD	0	-	98%	96%
Aspirin at Arrival[1]	9	100%	100%	99%
Aspirin at Discharge[1]	6	100%	99%	98%
Beta Blocker at Discharge[1]	5	100%	100%	98%
Fibrinolytic Medication Timing	0	-	100%	55%
PCI Within 90 Minutes of Arrival	0	-	89%	90%
Smoking Cessation Advice	0	-	99%	99%
Chest Pain/Possible Heart Attack Care				
Aspirin at Arrival	31	100%	97%	95%
Median Time to ECG (minutes)	31	7	8	8
Median Time to Transfer (minutes)[1]	10	62	41	61
Fibrinolytic Medication Timing	0	-	48%	54%
Heart Failure Care				
ACE Inhibitor or ARB for LVSD[1]	6	83%	96%	94%
Discharge Instructions[1]	10	60%	92%	88%
Evaluation of LVS Function	30	87%	99%	98%
Smoking Cessation Advice[1]	2	100%	99%	98%
Pneumonia Care				
Appropriate Initial Antibiotic	44	98%	95%	92%
Blood Culture Timing	64	98%	97%	96%
Influenza Vaccine	53	91%	95%	91%
Initial Antibiotic Timing	68	93%	97%	95%
Pneumococcal Vaccine	80	100%	96%	93%
Smoking Cessation Advice[1]	17	94%	97%	97%
Surgical Care Improvement Project				
Appropriate VTP Within 24 Hours[1,2]	9	100%	96%	92%
Appropriate Hair Removal[2]	28	100%	100%	99%
Appropriate Beta Blocker Usage[5]	0	-	95%	93%
Controlled Postoperative Blood Glucose[2]	0	-	95%	93%
Prophylactic Antibiotic Timing[1,2]	16	100%	97%	97%
Prophylactic Antibiotic Timing (Outpatient)[1]	17	88%	96%	92%
Prophylactic Antibiotic Selection[1,2]	17	100%	98%	97%
Prophylactic Antibiotic Select. (Outpatient)[1]	16	100%	97%	94%
Prophylactic Antibiotic Stopped[1,2]	16	94%	97%	94%
Recommended VTP Ordered[1,2]	9	100%	97%	94%
Urinary Catheter Removal[1,2]	4	75%	89%	90%
Children's Asthma Care				
Received Systemic Corticosteroids	-	-	-	100%
Received Home Management Plan	-	-	-	71%
Received Reliever Medication	-	-	-	100%
Use of Medical Imaging				
Combination Abdominal CT Scan	156	0.013	0.078	0.191
Combination Chest CT Scan	141	0.000	0.014	0.054
Follow-up Mammogram/Ultrasound	307	6.2%	7.1%	8.4%
MRI for Low Back Pain[1]	29	24.1%	31.5%	32.7%
Survey of Patients' Hospital Experiences				
Area Around Room 'Always' Quiet at Night	(a)	57%	-	58%
Doctors 'Always' Communicated Well	(a)	71%	-	80%
Home Recovery Information Given	(a)	79%	-	82%
Hospital Given 9 or 10 on 10 Point Scale	(a)	63%	-	67%
Meds 'Always' Explained Before Given	(a)	61%	-	60%
Nurses 'Always' Communicated Well	(a)	71%	-	76%
Pain 'Always' Well Controlled	(a)	65%	-	69%
Room and Bathroom 'Always' Clean	(a)	79%	-	71%
Timely Help 'Always' Received	(a)	63%	-	64%
Would Definitely Recommend Hospital	(a)	60%	-	69%

Cheshire Medical Center

580 Court Street
Keene, NH 03431
URL: www.cheshire-med.com
Type: Acute Care Hospitals
Ownership: Voluntary Non-Profit - Private

Phone: 603-354-5400
Fax: 603-354-6519
Emergency Services: No
Beds: 169

Key Personnel:

CEO/President. . . . . Arthur Nichols
Chief of Medical Staff. . . . . William Toms
Coronary Care . . . . Carl Szot
Operating Room. . . . . James Bowden
Emergency Room . . . . Cheryl Pinney

Measure	Cases	This Hosp.	State Avg.	U.S. Avg.
Heart Attack Care				
ACE Inhibitor or ARB for LVSD[1]	3	100%	98%	96%
Aspirin at Arrival	31	100%	100%	99%
Aspirin at Discharge[1]	19	100%	99%	98%
Beta Blocker at Discharge[1]	17	100%	100%	98%
Fibrinolytic Medication Timing	0	-	100%	55%
PCI Within 90 Minutes of Arrival	0	-	89%	90%
Smoking Cessation Advice[1]	3	100%	99%	99%
Chest Pain/Possible Heart Attack Care				
Aspirin at Arrival	98	99%	97%	95%
Median Time to ECG (minutes)	99	5	8	8
Median Time to Transfer (minutes)[1,3]	2	181	41	61
Fibrinolytic Medication Timing[1]	7	57%	48%	54%
Heart Failure Care				
ACE Inhibitor or ARB for LVSD[1]	21	95%	96%	94%
Discharge Instructions	70	90%	92%	88%
Evaluation of LVS Function	97	100%	99%	98%
Smoking Cessation Advice[1]	14	100%	99%	98%
Pneumonia Care				
Appropriate Initial Antibiotic[2]	87	95%	95%	92%
Blood Culture Timing[2]	144	97%	97%	96%
Influenza Vaccine[2]	81	98%	95%	91%
Initial Antibiotic Timing[2]	146	97%	97%	95%
Pneumococcal Vaccine[2]	123	99%	96%	93%
Smoking Cessation Advice[2]	50	98%	97%	97%
Surgical Care Improvement Project				
Appropriate VTP Within 24 Hours	110	95%	96%	92%
Appropriate Hair Removal	263	100%	100%	99%
Appropriate Beta Blocker Usage	69	99%	95%	93%
Controlled Postoperative Blood Glucose	0	-	95%	93%
Prophylactic Antibiotic Timing	194	98%	97%	97%
Prophylactic Antibiotic Timing (Outpatient)	110	96%	96%	92%
Prophylactic Antibiotic Selection	194	99%	98%	97%
Prophylactic Antibiotic Select. (Outpatient)	109	96%	97%	94%
Prophylactic Antibiotic Stopped	191	99%	97%	94%
Recommended VTP Ordered	110	97%	97%	94%
Urinary Catheter Removal	82	98%	89%	90%
Children's Asthma Care				
Received Systemic Corticosteroids	-	-	-	100%
Received Home Management Plan	-	-	-	71%
Received Reliever Medication	-	-	-	100%
Use of Medical Imaging				
Combination Abdominal CT Scan	620	0.011	0.078	0.191
Combination Chest CT Scan	564	0.000	0.014	0.054
Follow-up Mammogram/Ultrasound	1,331	3.8%	7.1%	8.4%
MRI for Low Back Pain	206	31.6%	31.5%	32.7%
Survey of Patients' Hospital Experiences				
Area Around Room 'Always' Quiet at Night	300+	47%	-	58%
Doctors 'Always' Communicated Well	300+	80%	-	80%
Home Recovery Information Given	300+	86%	-	82%
Hospital Given 9 or 10 on 10 Point Scale	300+	67%	-	67%
Meds 'Always' Explained Before Given	300+	62%	-	60%
Nurses 'Always' Communicated Well	300+	78%	-	76%
Pain 'Always' Well Controlled	300+	70%	-	69%
Room and Bathroom 'Always' Clean	300+	79%	-	71%
Timely Help 'Always' Received	300+	64%	-	64%
Would Definitely Recommend Hospital	300+	68%	-	69%

NOTE: Hospital profiles are in alphabetical order by state, then city, then hospital within the city; Rankings exclude hospitals with less than 25 cases except for patient surveys which excludes hospitals with less than 100 cases; (a) 100–299 cases; (1) The number of cases is too small to be sure how well a hospital is performing; (2) The hospital indicated that the data submitted for this measure were based on a sample of cases; (3) Data was collected during a shorter time period (fewer quarters) than the maximum possible time for this measure; (4) Suppressed for one or more quarters by CMS; (5) No data is available from the hospital for this measure; (6) Fewer than 100 patients completed the HCAHPS survey. Use these rates with caution, as the number of surveys may be too low to reliably assess hospital performance; (7) Survey results are based on less than 12 months of data; (8) Survey results are not available for this reporting period; (9) No or very few patients were eligible for the HCAHPS survey. The scores shown, if any, reflect a very small number of surveys; (10) A state average was not calculated because too few hospitals in the state submitted data; (11) There were discrepancies in the data collection process; Please refer to the User's Guide for a full explanation of data.

Lakes Region General Hospital

80 Highland St Phone: 603-524-3211
Laconia, NH 03246 Fax: 603-527-2887
URL: www.lrgh.org
Type: Acute Care Hospitals Emergency Services: Yes
Ownership: Voluntary Non-Profit - Private Beds: 143

Key Personnel:
CEO/President . . . . Thomas Clairmont
Chief of Medical Staff . . . . Peter Walkley, MD
Infection Control . . . . Darlene Burrows, RN
Operating Room . . . . Alan Awrich, RN
Radiology . . . . Robert C Andrews
Emergency Room . . . . Andre Beauboeuf

Measure	Cases	This Hosp.	State Avg.	U.S. Avg.
Heart Attack Care				
ACE Inhibitor or ARB for LVSD[1]	6	83%	98%	96%
Aspirin at Arrival	44	98%	100%	99%
Aspirin at Discharge	26	100%	99%	98%
Beta Blocker at Discharge[1]	24	100%	100%	98%
Fibrinolytic Medication Timing	0	-	100%	55%
PCI Within 90 Minutes of Arrival	0	-	89%	90%
Smoking Cessation Advice[1]	2	50%	99%	99%
Chest Pain/Possible Heart Attack Care				
Aspirin at Arrival	135	97%	97%	95%
Median Time to ECG (minutes)	137	7	8	8
Median Time to Transfer (minutes)	34	36	41	61
Fibrinolytic Medication Timing	0	-	48%	54%
Heart Failure Care				
ACE Inhibitor or ARB for LVSD[1]	24	83%	96%	94%
Discharge Instructions	62	65%	92%	88%
Evaluation of LVS Function	90	97%	99%	98%
Smoking Cessation Advice[1]	19	100%	99%	98%
Pneumonia Care				
Appropriate Initial Antibiotic[2]	79	91%	95%	92%
Blood Culture Timing[2]	87	97%	97%	96%
Influenza Vaccine[2]	78	87%	95%	91%
Initial Antibiotic Timing[2]	120	98%	97%	95%
Pneumococcal Vaccine[2]	107	93%	96%	93%
Smoking Cessation Advice[2]	36	97%	97%	97%
Surgical Care Improvement Project				
Appropriate VTP Within 24 Hours[2]	199	94%	96%	92%
Appropriate Hair Removal[2]	448	100%	100%	99%
Appropriate Beta Blocker Usage[2]	133	94%	95%	93%
Controlled Postoperative Blood Glucose[2]	0	-	95%	93%
Prophylactic Antibiotic Timing[2]	311	96%	97%	97%
Prophylactic Antibiotic Timing (Outpatient)	182	93%	96%	92%
Prophylactic Antibiotic Selection[2]	314	97%	98%	97%
Prophylactic Antibiotic Select. (Outpatient)	175	95%	97%	94%
Prophylactic Antibiotic Stopped[2]	301	95%	97%	94%
Recommended VTP Ordered[2]	199	95%	97%	94%
Urinary Catheter Removal[2]	134	78%	89%	90%
Children's Asthma Care				
Received Systemic Corticosteroids	-	-	-	100%
Received Home Management Plan	-	-	-	71%
Received Reliever Medication	-	-	-	100%
Use of Medical Imaging				
Combination Abdominal CT Scan	727	0.061	0.078	0.191
Combination Chest CT Scan	623	0.000	0.014	0.054
Follow-up Mammogram/Ultrasound	1,315	6.1%	7.1%	8.4%
MRI for Low Back Pain	236	35.6%	31.5%	32.7%
Survey of Patients' Hospital Experiences				
Area Around Room 'Always' Quiet at Night	300+	49%	-	58%
Doctors 'Always' Communicated Well	300+	76%	-	80%
Home Recovery Information Given	300+	86%	-	82%
Hospital Given 9 or 10 on 10 Point Scale	300+	63%	-	67%
Meds 'Always' Explained Before Given	300+	55%	-	60%
Nurses 'Always' Communicated Well	300+	71%	-	76%
Pain 'Always' Well Controlled	300+	64%	-	69%
Room and Bathroom 'Always' Clean	300+	69%	-	71%
Timely Help 'Always' Received	300+	59%	-	64%
Would Definitely Recommend Hospital	300+	58%	-	69%

Weeks Medical Center

173 Middle Street Phone: 603-788-4911
Lancaster, NH 03584 Fax: 603-788-5027
URL: www.weeks.hitchcock.org
Type: Critical Access Hospitals Emergency Services: Yes
Ownership: Voluntary Non-Profit - Private Beds: 25

Key Personnel:
CEO/President . . . . Scott W Howe
Chief of Medical Staff . . . . Jeffrey Johnson, MD
Radiology . . . . Russel S Williams
Anesthesiology . . . . Donna Walker, CNE
Emergency Room . . . . John Dege, MD
Intensive Care Unit . . . . Chandre Engelbert

Measure	Cases	This Hosp.	State Avg.	U.S. Avg.
Heart Attack Care				
ACE Inhibitor or ARB for LVSD[1]	4	100%	98%	96%
Aspirin at Arrival[1]	14	100%	100%	99%
Aspirin at Discharge[1]	13	100%	99%	98%
Beta Blocker at Discharge[1]	11	91%	100%	98%
Fibrinolytic Medication Timing	0	-	100%	55%
PCI Within 90 Minutes of Arrival	0	-	89%	90%
Smoking Cessation Advice[1]	4	100%	99%	99%
Chest Pain/Possible Heart Attack Care				
Aspirin at Arrival	60	98%	97%	95%
Median Time to ECG (minutes)	65	11	8	8
Median Time to Transfer (minutes)[5]	0	-	41	61
Fibrinolytic Medication Timing[5]	0	-	48%	54%
Heart Failure Care				
ACE Inhibitor or ARB for LVSD[1]	14	93%	96%	94%
Discharge Instructions[1]	6	83%	92%	88%
Evaluation of LVS Function	34	100%	99%	98%
Smoking Cessation Advice[1]	1	100%	99%	98%
Pneumonia Care				
Appropriate Initial Antibiotic	28	100%	95%	92%
Blood Culture Timing	46	98%	97%	96%
Influenza Vaccine	34	100%	95%	91%
Initial Antibiotic Timing	55	98%	97%	95%
Pneumococcal Vaccine	49	98%	96%	93%
Smoking Cessation Advice[1]	10	100%	97%	97%
Surgical Care Improvement Project				
Appropriate VTP Within 24 Hours[1]	18	100%	96%	92%
Appropriate Hair Removal	29	100%	100%	99%
Appropriate Beta Blocker Usage[5]	0	-	95%	93%
Controlled Postoperative Blood Glucose	0	-	95%	93%
Prophylactic Antibiotic Timing	26	92%	97%	97%
Prophylactic Antibiotic Timing (Outpatient)[5]	0	-	96%	92%
Prophylactic Antibiotic Selection	26	100%	98%	97%
Prophylactic Antibiotic Select. (Outpatient)[5]	0	-	97%	94%
Prophylactic Antibiotic Stopped	25	96%	97%	94%
Recommended VTP Ordered[1]	18	100%	97%	94%
Urinary Catheter Removal[1]	11	55%	89%	90%
Children's Asthma Care				
Received Systemic Corticosteroids	-	-	-	100%
Received Home Management Plan	-	-	-	71%
Received Reliever Medication	-	-	-	100%
Use of Medical Imaging				
Combination Abdominal CT Scan	175	0.594	0.078	0.191
Combination Chest CT Scan	83	0.133	0.014	0.054
Follow-up Mammogram/Ultrasound	294	3.4%	7.1%	8.4%
MRI for Low Back Pain[1]	44	65.9%	31.5%	32.7%
Survey of Patients' Hospital Experiences				
Area Around Room 'Always' Quiet at Night[8]	-	-	-	58%
Doctors 'Always' Communicated Well[8]	-	-	-	80%
Home Recovery Information Given[8]	-	-	-	82%
Hospital Given 9 or 10 on 10 Point Scale[8]	-	-	-	67%
Meds 'Always' Explained Before Given[8]	-	-	-	60%
Nurses 'Always' Communicated Well[8]	-	-	-	76%
Pain 'Always' Well Controlled[8]	-	-	-	69%
Room and Bathroom 'Always' Clean[8]	-	-	-	71%
Timely Help 'Always' Received[8]	-	-	-	64%
Would Definitely Recommend Hospital[8]	-	-	-	69%

Alice Peck Day Memorial Hospital

125 Mascoma St Phone: 603-448-3121
Lebanon, NH 03766 Fax: 603-443-9620
Type: Critical Access Hospitals Emergency Services: Yes
Ownership: Voluntary Non-Profit - Other Beds: 82

Key Personnel:
CEO/President . . . . Harry G Dorman III
Chief of Medical Staff . . . . Brian Lombard
Infection Control . . . . Thom Goodwin
Operating Room . . . . David Kroner
Pediatric Ambulatory Care . . . . . . Douglas Williamson, MD
Quality Assurance . . . . Lora Smith
Radiology . . . . Katherine Gerke, RI

Measure	Cases	This Hosp.	State Avg.	U.S. Avg.
Heart Attack Care				
ACE Inhibitor or ARB for LVSD[5]	0	-	98%	96%
Aspirin at Arrival[5]	0	-	100%	99%
Aspirin at Discharge[5]	0	-	99%	98%
Beta Blocker at Discharge[5]	0	-	100%	98%
Fibrinolytic Medication Timing[5]	0	-	100%	55%
PCI Within 90 Minutes of Arrival[5]	0	-	89%	90%
Smoking Cessation Advice[5]	0	-	99%	99%
Chest Pain/Possible Heart Attack Care				
Aspirin at Arrival	-	-	97%	95%
Median Time to ECG (minutes)	-	-	8	8
Median Time to Transfer (minutes)	-	-	41	61
Fibrinolytic Medication Timing	-	-	48%	54%
Heart Failure Care				
ACE Inhibitor or ARB for LVSD[1,3]	3	100%	96%	94%
Discharge Instructions[1,3]	4	50%	92%	88%
Evaluation of LVS Function[1,3]	6	100%	99%	98%
Smoking Cessation Advice[1,3]	2	100%	99%	98%
Pneumonia Care				
Appropriate Initial Antibiotic[1]	18	94%	95%	92%
Blood Culture Timing[1]	20	90%	97%	96%
Influenza Vaccine[1]	10	100%	95%	91%
Initial Antibiotic Timing[1]	20	100%	97%	95%
Pneumococcal Vaccine[1]	11	100%	96%	93%
Smoking Cessation Advice[1]	7	100%	97%	97%
Surgical Care Improvement Project				
Appropriate VTP Within 24 Hours[2]	27	89%	96%	92%
Appropriate Hair Removal[2]	62	90%	100%	99%
Appropriate Beta Blocker Usage[5]	0	-	95%	93%
Controlled Postoperative Blood Glucose[2]	0	-	95%	93%
Prophylactic Antibiotic Timing[2]	48	98%	97%	97%
Prophylactic Antibiotic Timing (Outpatient)	-	-	96%	92%
Prophylactic Antibiotic Selection[2]	48	96%	98%	97%
Prophylactic Antibiotic Select. (Outpatient)	-	-	97%	94%
Prophylactic Antibiotic Stopped[2]	48	100%	97%	94%
Recommended VTP Ordered[2]	27	89%	97%	94%
Urinary Catheter Removal[1,2]	19	89%	89%	90%
Children's Asthma Care				
Received Systemic Corticosteroids	-	-	-	100%
Received Home Management Plan	-	-	-	71%
Received Reliever Medication	-	-	-	100%
Use of Medical Imaging				
Combination Abdominal CT Scan	-	-	0.078	0.191
Combination Chest CT Scan	-	-	0.014	0.054
Follow-up Mammogram/Ultrasound	-	-	7.1%	8.4%
MRI for Low Back Pain	-	-	31.5%	32.7%
Survey of Patients' Hospital Experiences				
Area Around Room 'Always' Quiet at Night[8]	-	-	-	58%
Doctors 'Always' Communicated Well[8]	-	-	-	80%
Home Recovery Information Given[8]	-	-	-	82%
Hospital Given 9 or 10 on 10 Point Scale[8]	-	-	-	67%
Meds 'Always' Explained Before Given[8]	-	-	-	60%
Nurses 'Always' Communicated Well[8]	-	-	-	76%
Pain 'Always' Well Controlled[8]	-	-	-	69%
Room and Bathroom 'Always' Clean[8]	-	-	-	71%
Timely Help 'Always' Received[8]	-	-	-	64%
Would Definitely Recommend Hospital[8]	-	-	-	69%

NOTE: Hospital profiles are in alphabetical order by state, then city, then hospital within the city; Rankings exclude hospitals with less than 25 cases except for patient surveys which excludes hospitals with less than 100 cases; (a) 100–299 cases; (1) The number of cases is too small to be sure how well a hospital is performing; (2) The hospital indicated that the data submitted for this measure were based on a sample of cases; (3) Data was collected during a shorter time period (fewer quarters) than the maximum possible time for this measure; (4) Suppressed for one or more quarters by CMS; (5) No data is available from the hospital for this measure; (6) Fewer than 100 patients completed the HCAHPS survey. Use these rates with caution, as the number of surveys may be too low to reliably assess hospital performance; (7) Survey results are based on less than 12 months of data; (8) Survey results are not available for this reporting period; (9) No or very few patients were eligible for the HCAHPS survey. The scores shown, if any, reflect a very small number of surveys; (10) A state average was not calculated because too few hospitals in the state submitted data; (11) There were discrepancies in the data collection process; Please refer to the User's Guide for a full explanation of data.

Mary Hitchcock Memorial Hospital

1 Medical Center Drive
Lebanon, NH 03756
URL: www.dhmc.org
Type: Acute Care Hospitals
Ownership: Voluntary Non-Profit - Other

Phone: 603-650-5000
Fax: 603-653-1906
Emergency Services: Yes
Beds: 400

Key Personnel:
CEO/President. . . . . James W Varnum
Chief of Medical Staff. . . . . Thomas Colacchio, MD
Infection Control. . . . . Judy Ptak
Operating Room. . . . . Doug Heavisides
Pediatric In-Patient Care . . . . Aden Henry
Quality Assurance . . . . Sally Trombly
Radiology. . . . . Monte Clinton

Measure	Cases	This Hosp.	State Avg.	U.S. Avg.
Heart Attack Care				
ACE Inhibitor or ARB for LVSD[2]	51	94%	98%	96%
Aspirin at Arrival[2]	88	100%	100%	99%
Aspirin at Discharge[2]	510	99%	99%	98%
Beta Blocker at Discharge[2]	498	99%	100%	98%
Fibrinolytic Medication Timing[2]	0	-	100%	55%
PCI Within 90 Minutes of Arrival[1,2]	21	86%	89%	90%
Smoking Cessation Advice[2]	152	95%	99%	99%
Chest Pain/Possible Heart Attack Care				
Aspirin at Arrival[5]	0	-	97%	95%
Median Time to ECG (minutes)[5]	0	-	8	8
Median Time to Transfer (minutes)[5]	0	-	41	61
Fibrinolytic Medication Timing[5]	0	-	48%	54%
Heart Failure Care				
ACE Inhibitor or ARB for LVSD	104	93%	96%	94%
Discharge Instructions	239	84%	92%	88%
Evaluation of LVS Function	281	100%	99%	98%
Smoking Cessation Advice	46	98%	99%	98%
Pneumonia Care				
Appropriate Initial Antibiotic[2]	74	88%	95%	92%
Blood Culture Timing[2]	128	95%	97%	96%
Influenza Vaccine[2]	147	98%	95%	91%
Initial Antibiotic Timing[2]	133	92%	97%	95%
Pneumococcal Vaccine[2]	159	96%	96%	93%
Smoking Cessation Advice[2]	77	87%	97%	97%
Surgical Care Improvement Project				
Appropriate VTP Within 24 Hours[2]	269	99%	96%	92%
Appropriate Hair Removal[2]	871	100%	100%	99%
Appropriate Beta Blocker Usage[2]	348	89%	95%	93%
Controlled Postoperative Blood Glucose[2]	207	96%	95%	93%
Prophylactic Antibiotic Timing[2]	633	97%	97%	97%
Prophylactic Antibiotic Timing (Outpatient)	608	97%	96%	92%
Prophylactic Antibiotic Selection[2]	647	99%	98%	97%
Prophylactic Antibiotic Select. (Outpatient)	640	98%	97%	94%
Prophylactic Antibiotic Stopped[2]	615	96%	97%	94%
Recommended VTP Ordered[2]	270	99%	97%	94%
Urinary Catheter Removal[2]	230	84%	89%	90%
Children's Asthma Care				
Received Systemic Corticosteroids	-	-	-	100%
Received Home Management Plan	-	-	-	71%
Received Reliever Medication	-	-	-	100%
Use of Medical Imaging				
Combination Abdominal CT Scan	1,772	0.052	0.078	0.191
Combination Chest CT Scan	1,847	0.001	0.014	0.054
Follow-up Mammogram/Ultrasound	2,249	7.5%	7.1%	8.4%
MRI for Low Back Pain	454	27.5%	31.5%	32.7%
Survey of Patients' Hospital Experiences				
Area Around Room 'Always' Quiet at Night	300+	40%	-	58%
Doctors 'Always' Communicated Well	300+	80%	-	80%
Home Recovery Information Given	300+	87%	-	82%
Hospital Given 9 or 10 on 10 Point Scale	300+	78%	-	67%
Meds 'Always' Explained Before Given	300+	63%	-	60%
Nurses 'Always' Communicated Well	300+	78%	-	76%
Pain 'Always' Well Controlled	300+	68%	-	69%
Room and Bathroom 'Always' Clean	300+	71%	-	71%
Timely Help 'Always' Received	300+	73%	-	64%
Would Definitely Recommend Hospital	300+	84%	-	69%

Littleton Regional Hospital

600 St Johnsbury Road
Littleton, NH 03561
URL: www.littletonhospital.org
Type: Critical Access Hospitals
Ownership: Voluntary Non-Profit - Private

Phone: 603-444-9000
Fax: 603-444-0443
Emergency Services: Yes

Key Personnel:
Chief of Medical Staff. . . . . Clare Wilmot
Infection Control. . . . . Kris Major
Operating Room. . . . . Jean Courteau
Pediatric Ambulatory Care . . . . . . William Lakey, MD
Quality Assurance . . . . Linda Gilmore
Emergency Room . . . . Edward Duffy, MD
Intensive Care Unit. . . . . Lois Peraino

Measure	Cases	This Hosp.	State Avg.	U.S. Avg.
Heart Attack Care				
ACE Inhibitor or ARB for LVSD[1,3]	1	100%	98%	96%
Aspirin at Arrival[1,3]	6	100%	100%	99%
Aspirin at Discharge[1,3]	6	100%	99%	98%
Beta Blocker at Discharge[1,3]	6	100%	100%	98%
Fibrinolytic Medication Timing[3]	0	-	100%	55%
PCI Within 90 Minutes of Arrival[3]	0	-	89%	90%
Smoking Cessation Advice[3]	0	-	99%	99%
Chest Pain/Possible Heart Attack Care				
Aspirin at Arrival	-	-	97%	95%
Median Time to ECG (minutes)	-	-	8	8
Median Time to Transfer (minutes)	-	-	41	61
Fibrinolytic Medication Timing	-	-	48%	54%
Heart Failure Care				
ACE Inhibitor or ARB for LVSD[1]	4	100%	96%	94%
Discharge Instructions[1]	15	53%	92%	88%
Evaluation of LVS Function[1]	20	75%	99%	98%
Smoking Cessation Advice[1]	5	80%	99%	98%
Pneumonia Care				
Appropriate Initial Antibiotic[1]	16	75%	95%	92%
Blood Culture Timing[1]	24	96%	97%	96%
Influenza Vaccine[1]	20	95%	95%	91%
Initial Antibiotic Timing	33	94%	97%	95%
Pneumococcal Vaccine	36	64%	96%	93%
Smoking Cessation Advice[1]	6	83%	97%	97%
Surgical Care Improvement Project				
Appropriate VTP Within 24 Hours	61	87%	96%	92%
Appropriate Hair Removal	204	100%	100%	99%
Appropriate Beta Blocker Usage	45	87%	95%	93%
Controlled Postoperative Blood Glucose	0	-	95%	93%
Prophylactic Antibiotic Timing	150	96%	97%	97%
Prophylactic Antibiotic Timing (Outpatient)	-	-	96%	92%
Prophylactic Antibiotic Selection	150	98%	98%	97%
Prophylactic Antibiotic Select. (Outpatient)	-	-	97%	94%
Prophylactic Antibiotic Stopped	150	95%	97%	94%
Recommended VTP Ordered	61	90%	97%	94%
Urinary Catheter Removal	65	80%	89%	90%
Children's Asthma Care				
Received Systemic Corticosteroids	-	-	-	100%
Received Home Management Plan	-	-	-	71%
Received Reliever Medication	-	-	-	100%
Use of Medical Imaging				
Combination Abdominal CT Scan	-	-	0.078	0.191
Combination Chest CT Scan	-	-	0.014	0.054
Follow-up Mammogram/Ultrasound	-	-	7.1%	8.4%
MRI for Low Back Pain	-	-	31.5%	32.7%
Survey of Patients' Hospital Experiences				
Area Around Room 'Always' Quiet at Night	(a)	55%	-	58%
Doctors 'Always' Communicated Well	(a)	84%	-	80%
Home Recovery Information Given	(a)	90%	-	82%
Hospital Given 9 or 10 on 10 Point Scale	(a)	69%	-	67%
Meds 'Always' Explained Before Given	(a)	62%	-	60%
Nurses 'Always' Communicated Well	(a)	74%	-	76%
Pain 'Always' Well Controlled	(a)	70%	-	69%
Room and Bathroom 'Always' Clean	(a)	77%	-	71%
Timely Help 'Always' Received	(a)	67%	-	64%
Would Definitely Recommend Hospital	(a)	68%	-	69%

Catholic Medical Center

100 Mcgregor Street
Manchester, NH 03102
URL: www.catholicmedicalcenter.org
Type: Acute Care Hospitals
Ownership: Voluntary Non-Profit - Other

Phone: 603-668-3545
Fax: 603-668-5348
Emergency Services: Yes
Beds: 224

Key Personnel:
CEO/President. . . . . Alyson Pitman Giles
Cardiac Laboratory. . . . . Louis A Fink, MD FACC
Chief of Medical Staff. . . . . William B Clutterbuck, MD FACS
Operating Room. . . . . Lisa Roux, MD FACS
Pediatric In-Patient Care . . . . Kevin Hodges, MD
Quality Assurance . . . . Diane Rogier
Emergency Room . . . . Kathleen Zaffino, MD
Patient Relations. . . . . Tina Legere

Measure	Cases	This Hosp.	State Avg.	U.S. Avg.
Heart Attack Care				
ACE Inhibitor or ARB for LVSD	76	100%	98%	96%
Aspirin at Arrival	213	100%	100%	99%
Aspirin at Discharge	460	100%	99%	98%
Beta Blocker at Discharge	451	100%	100%	98%
Fibrinolytic Medication Timing	0	-	100%	55%
PCI Within 90 Minutes of Arrival	43	95%	89%	90%
Smoking Cessation Advice	148	100%	99%	99%
Chest Pain/Possible Heart Attack Care				
Aspirin at Arrival[1,3]	4	25%	97%	95%
Median Time to ECG (minutes)[1,3]	4	6	8	8
Median Time to Transfer (minutes)[5]	0	-	41	61
Fibrinolytic Medication Timing[5]	0	-	48%	54%
Heart Failure Care				
ACE Inhibitor or ARB for LVSD[2]	102	100%	96%	94%
Discharge Instructions[2]	208	97%	92%	88%
Evaluation of LVS Function[2]	260	100%	99%	98%
Smoking Cessation Advice[2]	40	100%	99%	98%
Pneumonia Care				
Appropriate Initial Antibiotic[2]	80	100%	95%	92%
Blood Culture Timing[2]	139	98%	97%	96%
Influenza Vaccine[2]	93	99%	95%	91%
Initial Antibiotic Timing[2]	125	99%	97%	95%
Pneumococcal Vaccine[2]	130	100%	96%	93%
Smoking Cessation Advice[2]	50	100%	97%	97%
Surgical Care Improvement Project				
Appropriate VTP Within 24 Hours[2]	81	96%	96%	92%
Appropriate Hair Removal[2]	524	100%	100%	99%
Appropriate Beta Blocker Usage[2]	226	94%	95%	93%
Controlled Postoperative Blood Glucose[2]	131	98%	95%	93%
Prophylactic Antibiotic Timing[2]	376	98%	97%	97%
Prophylactic Antibiotic Timing (Outpatient)	316	95%	96%	92%
Prophylactic Antibiotic Selection[2]	383	98%	98%	97%
Prophylactic Antibiotic Select. (Outpatient)	320	98%	97%	94%
Prophylactic Antibiotic Stopped[2]	362	97%	97%	94%
Recommended VTP Ordered[2]	81	98%	97%	94%
Urinary Catheter Removal[2]	140	95%	89%	90%
Children's Asthma Care				
Received Systemic Corticosteroids	-	-	-	100%
Received Home Management Plan	-	-	-	71%
Received Reliever Medication	-	-	-	100%
Use of Medical Imaging				
Combination Abdominal CT Scan	688	0.071	0.078	0.191
Combination Chest CT Scan	487	0.008	0.014	0.054
Follow-up Mammogram/Ultrasound	1,641	11.9%	7.1%	8.4%
MRI for Low Back Pain	176	33.0%	31.5%	32.7%
Survey of Patients' Hospital Experiences				
Area Around Room 'Always' Quiet at Night	300+	57%	-	58%
Doctors 'Always' Communicated Well	300+	79%	-	80%
Home Recovery Information Given	300+	86%	-	82%
Hospital Given 9 or 10 on 10 Point Scale	300+	70%	-	67%
Meds 'Always' Explained Before Given	300+	64%	-	60%
Nurses 'Always' Communicated Well	300+	81%	-	76%
Pain 'Always' Well Controlled	300+	69%	-	69%
Room and Bathroom 'Always' Clean	300+	70%	-	71%
Timely Help 'Always' Received	300+	67%	-	64%
Would Definitely Recommend Hospital	300+	76%	-	69%

NOTE: Hospital profiles are in alphabetical order by state, then city, then hospital within the city; Rankings exclude hospitals with less than 25 cases except for patient surveys which excludes hospitals with less than 100 cases; (a) 100–299 cases; (1) The number of cases is too small to be sure how well a hospital is performing; (2) The hospital indicated that the data submitted for this measure were based on a sample of cases; (3) Data was collected during a shorter time period (fewer quarters) than the maximum possible time for this measure; (4) Suppressed for one or more quarters by CMS; (5) No data is available from the hospital for this measure; (6) Fewer than 100 patients completed the HCAHPS survey. Use these rates with caution, as the number of surveys may be too low to reliably assess hospital performance; (7) Survey results are based on less than 12 months of data; (8) Survey results are not available for this reporting period; (9) No or very few patients were eligible for the HCAHPS survey. The scores shown, if any, reflect a very small number of surveys; (10) A state average was not calculated because too few hospitals in the state submitted data; (11) There were discrepancies in the data collection process; Please refer to the User's Guide for a full explanation of data.

Elliot Hospital

1 Elliot Way
Manchester, NH 03103
Phone: 603-669-5300
Fax: 603-627-0561
URL: www.elliothospital.org
Type: Acute Care Hospitals
Emergency Services: Yes
Ownership: Voluntary Non-Profit - Private
Beds: 296

Key Personnel:
CEO/President. . . . . Douglas Dean
Cardiac Laboratory. . . . . Laurie King
Chief of Medical Staff . . . . Dr Mark Myers
Infection Control. . . . . Lynda Caine
Operating Room. . . . . Laurie York
Pediatric In-Patient Care . . . . Liz Castrogiovanni
Quality Assurance . . . . MaryAnn McEntee
Radiology. . . . . Richard Frechette

Measure	Cases	This Hosp.	State Avg.	U.S. Avg.
Heart Attack Care				
ACE Inhibitor or ARB for LVSD[1]	20	100%	98%	96%
Aspirin at Arrival	139	100%	100%	99%
Aspirin at Discharge	118	100%	99%	98%
Beta Blocker at Discharge	104	100%	100%	98%
Fibrinolytic Medication Timing[1]	1	100%	100%	55%
PCI Within 90 Minutes of Arrival[1]	16	75%	89%	90%
Smoking Cessation Advice	37	100%	99%	99%
Chest Pain/Possible Heart Attack Care				
Aspirin at Arrival[1]	20	90%	97%	95%
Median Time to ECG (minutes)[1]	21	10	8	8
Median Time to Transfer (minutes)[5]	0	-	41	61
Fibrinolytic Medication Timing[3]	0	-	48%	54%
Heart Failure Care				
ACE Inhibitor or ARB for LVSD	56	98%	96%	94%
Discharge Instructions	135	91%	92%	88%
Evaluation of LVS Function	195	99%	99%	98%
Smoking Cessation Advice[1]	21	100%	99%	98%
Pneumonia Care				
Appropriate Initial Antibiotic[2]	88	93%	95%	92%
Blood Culture Timing[2]	127	90%	97%	96%
Influenza Vaccine[2]	77	84%	95%	91%
Initial Antibiotic Timing[2]	135	99%	97%	95%
Pneumococcal Vaccine[2]	119	99%	96%	93%
Smoking Cessation Advice[2]	42	93%	97%	97%
Surgical Care Improvement Project				
Appropriate VTP Within 24 Hours[2]	131	100%	96%	92%
Appropriate Hair Removal[2]	377	100%	100%	99%
Appropriate Beta Blocker Usage[2]	86	86%	95%	93%
Controlled Postoperative Blood Glucose[2]	0	-	95%	93%
Prophylactic Antibiotic Timing[2]	255	98%	97%	97%
Prophylactic Antibiotic Timing (Outpatient)	466	96%	96%	92%
Prophylactic Antibiotic Selection[2]	257	99%	98%	97%
Prophylactic Antibiotic Select. (Outpatient)	463	98%	97%	94%
Prophylactic Antibiotic Stopped[2]	244	96%	97%	94%
Recommended VTP Ordered[2]	131	100%	97%	94%
Urinary Catheter Removal[2]	76	89%	89%	90%
Children's Asthma Care				
Received Systemic Corticosteroids	-	-	-	100%
Received Home Management Plan	-	-	-	71%
Received Reliever Medication	-	-	-	100%
Use of Medical Imaging				
Combination Abdominal CT Scan	950	0.091	0.078	0.191
Combination Chest CT Scan	701	0.000	0.014	0.054
Follow-up Mammogram/Ultrasound	1,924	5.5%	7.1%	8.4%
MRI for Low Back Pain	359	32.9%	31.5%	32.7%
Survey of Patients' Hospital Experiences				
Area Around Room 'Always' Quiet at Night	300+	50%	-	58%
Doctors 'Always' Communicated Well	300+	77%	-	80%
Home Recovery Information Given	300+	85%	-	82%
Hospital Given 9 or 10 on 10 Point Scale	300+	68%	-	67%
Meds 'Always' Explained Before Given	300+	62%	-	60%
Nurses 'Always' Communicated Well	300+	77%	-	76%
Pain 'Always' Well Controlled	300+	72%	-	69%
Room and Bathroom 'Always' Clean	300+	73%	-	71%
Timely Help 'Always' Received	300+	62%	-	64%
Would Definitely Recommend Hospital	300+	76%	-	69%

Saint Joseph Hospital

172 Kinsley St
Nashua, NH 03060
Phone: 603-882-3000
Fax: 603-889-1651
URL: www.stjosephhospital.com
Type: Acute Care Hospitals
Emergency Services: Yes
Ownership: Voluntary Non-Profit - Other
Beds: 208

Key Personnel:
CEO/President. . . . . Peter B Davis
Chief of Medical Staff . . . . John Posner, MD
Pediatric Ambulatory Care . . . . . . Ann Dobbins, MD
Pediatric In-Patient Care . . . . Ann Dobbins, MD
Quality Assurance . . . . Barbara Dotson
Radiology. . . . . Don Wiess, MD

Measure	Cases	This Hosp.	State Avg.	U.S. Avg.
Heart Attack Care				
ACE Inhibitor or ARB for LVSD[1,2]	8	100%	98%	96%
Aspirin at Arrival[2]	65	100%	100%	99%
Aspirin at Discharge[2]	46	100%	99%	98%
Beta Blocker at Discharge[2]	44	100%	100%	98%
Fibrinolytic Medication Timing[2]	0	-	100%	55%
PCI Within 90 Minutes of Arrival[1,2]	2	50%	89%	90%
Smoking Cessation Advice[1,2]	5	100%	99%	99%
Chest Pain/Possible Heart Attack Care				
Aspirin at Arrival	31	100%	97%	95%
Median Time to ECG (minutes)	32	8	8	8
Median Time to Transfer (minutes)[1]	14	37	41	61
Fibrinolytic Medication Timing	0	-	48%	54%
Heart Failure Care				
ACE Inhibitor or ARB for LVSD[2]	59	100%	96%	94%
Discharge Instructions[2]	123	84%	92%	88%
Evaluation of LVS Function[2]	201	100%	99%	98%
Smoking Cessation Advice[1,2]	15	100%	99%	98%
Pneumonia Care				
Appropriate Initial Antibiotic[2]	84	89%	95%	92%
Blood Culture Timing[2]	114	100%	97%	96%
Influenza Vaccine[2]	78	99%	95%	91%
Initial Antibiotic Timing[2]	131	92%	97%	95%
Pneumococcal Vaccine[2]	125	97%	96%	93%
Smoking Cessation Advice[2]	27	100%	97%	97%
Surgical Care Improvement Project				
Appropriate VTP Within 24 Hours[2]	151	99%	96%	92%
Appropriate Hair Removal[2]	312	100%	100%	99%
Appropriate Beta Blocker Usage[2]	82	98%	95%	93%
Controlled Postoperative Blood Glucose[2]	0	-	95%	93%
Prophylactic Antibiotic Timing[2]	218	96%	97%	97%
Prophylactic Antibiotic Timing (Outpatient)	140	94%	96%	92%
Prophylactic Antibiotic Selection[2]	219	99%	98%	97%
Prophylactic Antibiotic Select. (Outpatient)	139	96%	97%	94%
Prophylactic Antibiotic Stopped[2]	211	96%	97%	94%
Recommended VTP Ordered[2]	151	99%	97%	94%
Urinary Catheter Removal[2]	63	83%	89%	90%
Children's Asthma Care				
Received Systemic Corticosteroids	-	-	-	100%
Received Home Management Plan	-	-	-	71%
Received Reliever Medication	-	-	-	100%
Use of Medical Imaging				
Combination Abdominal CT Scan	703	0.078	0.078	0.191
Combination Chest CT Scan	583	0.000	0.014	0.054
Follow-up Mammogram/Ultrasound	1,620	7.8%	7.1%	8.4%
MRI for Low Back Pain	144	31.3%	31.5%	32.7%
Survey of Patients' Hospital Experiences				
Area Around Room 'Always' Quiet at Night	300+	61%	-	58%
Doctors 'Always' Communicated Well	300+	77%	-	80%
Home Recovery Information Given	300+	86%	-	82%
Hospital Given 9 or 10 on 10 Point Scale	300+	70%	-	67%
Meds 'Always' Explained Before Given	300+	62%	-	60%
Nurses 'Always' Communicated Well	300+	81%	-	76%
Pain 'Always' Well Controlled	300+	75%	-	69%
Room and Bathroom 'Always' Clean	300+	75%	-	71%
Timely Help 'Always' Received	300+	64%	-	64%
Would Definitely Recommend Hospital	300+	75%	-	69%

Southern Nh Medical Center

8 Prospect Street
Nashua, NH 03060
Phone: 603-577-2000
URL: www.snhmc.org
Type: Acute Care Hospitals
Emergency Services: Yes
Ownership: Voluntary Non-Profit - Private
Beds: 188

Key Personnel:
CEO/President. . . . . Thomas E. Wilhelmsen
Chief of Medical Staff . . . . Sean W. Fitzpatrick

Measure	Cases	This Hosp.	State Avg.	U.S. Avg.
Heart Attack Care				
ACE Inhibitor or ARB for LVSD	28	96%	98%	96%
Aspirin at Arrival	148	100%	100%	99%
Aspirin at Discharge	123	98%	99%	98%
Beta Blocker at Discharge	122	100%	100%	98%
Fibrinolytic Medication Timing	0	-	100%	55%
PCI Within 90 Minutes of Arrival[1]	18	72%	89%	90%
Smoking Cessation Advice	34	100%	99%	99%
Chest Pain/Possible Heart Attack Care				
Aspirin at Arrival[1]	13	100%	97%	95%
Median Time to ECG (minutes)[1]	12	11	8	8
Median Time to Transfer (minutes)[3]	0	-	41	61
Fibrinolytic Medication Timing[3]	0	-	48%	54%
Heart Failure Care				
ACE Inhibitor or ARB for LVSD	42	98%	96%	94%
Discharge Instructions	189	99%	92%	88%
Evaluation of LVS Function	227	100%	99%	98%
Smoking Cessation Advice	37	100%	99%	98%
Pneumonia Care				
Appropriate Initial Antibiotic	86	99%	95%	92%
Blood Culture Timing	167	98%	97%	96%
Influenza Vaccine	116	97%	95%	91%
Initial Antibiotic Timing	174	97%	97%	95%
Pneumococcal Vaccine	144	95%	96%	93%
Smoking Cessation Advice	67	100%	97%	97%
Surgical Care Improvement Project				
Appropriate VTP Within 24 Hours	215	94%	96%	92%
Appropriate Hair Removal	589	100%	100%	99%
Appropriate Beta Blocker Usage	137	98%	95%	93%
Controlled Postoperative Blood Glucose	0	-	95%	93%
Prophylactic Antibiotic Timing	422	100%	97%	97%
Prophylactic Antibiotic Timing (Outpatient)	224	96%	96%	92%
Prophylactic Antibiotic Selection	428	99%	98%	97%
Prophylactic Antibiotic Select. (Outpatient)	216	99%	97%	94%
Prophylactic Antibiotic Stopped	419	98%	97%	94%
Recommended VTP Ordered	217	94%	97%	94%
Urinary Catheter Removal	136	86%	89%	90%
Children's Asthma Care				
Received Systemic Corticosteroids	-	-	-	100%
Received Home Management Plan	-	-	-	71%
Received Reliever Medication	-	-	-	100%
Use of Medical Imaging				
Combination Abdominal CT Scan	537	0.080	0.078	0.191
Combination Chest CT Scan	372	0.005	0.014	0.054
Follow-up Mammogram/Ultrasound	1,695	6.4%	7.1%	8.4%
MRI for Low Back Pain	173	30.1%	31.5%	32.7%
Survey of Patients' Hospital Experiences				
Area Around Room 'Always' Quiet at Night	300+	58%	-	58%
Doctors 'Always' Communicated Well	300+	80%	-	80%
Home Recovery Information Given	300+	89%	-	82%
Hospital Given 9 or 10 on 10 Point Scale	300+	74%	-	67%
Meds 'Always' Explained Before Given	300+	66%	-	60%
Nurses 'Always' Communicated Well	300+	80%	-	76%
Pain 'Always' Well Controlled	300+	72%	-	69%
Room and Bathroom 'Always' Clean	300+	70%	-	71%
Timely Help 'Always' Received	300+	64%	-	64%
Would Definitely Recommend Hospital	300+	79%	-	69%

NOTE: Hospital profiles are in alphabetical order by state, then city, then hospital within the city; Rankings exclude hospitals with less than 25 cases except for patient surveys which excludes hospitals with less than 100 cases; (a) 100–299 cases; (1) The number of cases is too small to be sure how well a hospital is performing; (2) The hospital indicated that the data submitted for this measure were based on a sample of cases; (3) Data was collected during a shorter time period (fewer quarters) than the maximum possible time for this measure; (4) Suppressed for one or more quarters by CMS; (5) No data is available from the hospital for this measure; (6) Fewer than 100 patients completed the HCAHPS survey. Use these rates with caution, as the number of surveys may be too low to reliably assess hospital performance; (7) Survey results are based on less than 12 months of data; (8) Survey results are not available for this reporting period; (9) No or very few patients were eligible for the HCAHPS survey. The scores shown, if any, reflect a very small number of surveys; (10) A state average was not calculated because too few hospitals in the state submitted data; (11) There were discrepancies in the data collection process; Please refer to the User's Guide for a full explanation of data.

New London Hospital

273 County Road
New London, NH 03257
URL: www.newlondonhospital.org
Type: Critical Access Hospitals
Ownership: Voluntary Non-Profit - Private
Phone: 603-526-2911
Fax: 603-526-2990
Emergency Services: Yes
Beds: 25

Key Personnel:
CEO/President. . . . . Bruce King
Chief of Medical Staff. . . . . Douglas Moran, MD
Infection Control. . . . . Jean Hughes Dowe
Operating Room. . . . . Patricia Miller, RN
Quality Assurance . . . . Kieran Kays
Radiology. . . . . Debra Wilson
Anesthesiology. . . . . Thomas Lucas, MD
Emergency Room . . . . Kent Wheeler

Measure	Cases	This Hosp.	State Avg.	U.S. Avg.
Heart Attack Care				
ACE Inhibitor or ARB for LVSD[1]	1	100%	98%	96%
Aspirin at Arrival[1]	8	88%	100%	99%
Aspirin at Discharge[1]	5	100%	99%	98%
Beta Blocker at Discharge[1]	5	80%	100%	98%
Fibrinolytic Medication Timing[5]	0	-	100%	55%
PCI Within 90 Minutes of Arrival[5]	0	-	89%	90%
Smoking Cessation Advice	0	-	99%	99%
Chest Pain/Possible Heart Attack Care				
Aspirin at Arrival	37	95%	97%	95%
Median Time to ECG (minutes)	38	10	8	8
Median Time to Transfer (minutes)[1,3]	6	78	41	61
Fibrinolytic Medication Timing[1]	1	0%	48%	54%
Heart Failure Care				
ACE Inhibitor or ARB for LVSD[1]	4	100%	96%	94%
Discharge Instructions	32	97%	92%	88%
Evaluation of LVS Function	38	100%	99%	98%
Smoking Cessation Advice[1]	3	100%	99%	98%
Pneumonia Care				
Appropriate Initial Antibiotic	29	97%	95%	92%
Blood Culture Timing	36	97%	97%	96%
Influenza Vaccine	31	97%	95%	91%
Initial Antibiotic Timing	33	97%	97%	95%
Pneumococcal Vaccine	46	98%	96%	93%
Smoking Cessation Advice[1]	3	67%	97%	97%
Surgical Care Improvement Project				
Appropriate VTP Within 24 Hours	35	91%	96%	92%
Appropriate Hair Removal	112	100%	100%	99%
Appropriate Beta Blocker Usage	27	100%	95%	93%
Controlled Postoperative Blood Glucose	0	-	95%	93%
Prophylactic Antibiotic Timing	97	76%	97%	97%
Prophylactic Antibiotic Timing (Outpatient)	83	75%	96%	92%
Prophylactic Antibiotic Selection	98	99%	98%	97%
Prophylactic Antibiotic Select. (Outpatient)	81	99%	97%	94%
Prophylactic Antibiotic Stopped	96	99%	97%	94%
Recommended VTP Ordered	35	91%	97%	94%
Urinary Catheter Removal	30	87%	89%	90%
Children's Asthma Care				
Received Systemic Corticosteroids	-	-	-	100%
Received Home Management Plan	-	-	-	71%
Received Reliever Medication	-	-	-	100%
Use of Medical Imaging				
Combination Abdominal CT Scan	221	0.095	0.078	0.191
Combination Chest CT Scan	145	0.000	0.014	0.054
Follow-up Mammogram/Ultrasound	909	8.8%	7.1%	8.4%
MRI for Low Back Pain	53	47.2%	31.5%	32.7%
Survey of Patients' Hospital Experiences				
Area Around Room 'Always' Quiet at Night	(a)	65%	-	58%
Doctors 'Always' Communicated Well	(a)	81%	-	80%
Home Recovery Information Given	(a)	79%	-	82%
Hospital Given 9 or 10 on 10 Point Scale	(a)	71%	-	67%
Meds 'Always' Explained Before Given	(a)	58%	-	60%
Nurses 'Always' Communicated Well	(a)	78%	-	76%
Pain 'Always' Well Controlled	(a)	69%	-	69%
Room and Bathroom 'Always' Clean	(a)	84%	-	71%
Timely Help 'Always' Received	(a)	75%	-	64%
Would Definitely Recommend Hospital	(a)	75%	-	69%

The Memorial Hospital

3073 White Mountain Highway
North Conway, NH 03860
Type: Critical Access Hospitals
Ownership: Voluntary Non-Profit - Private
Phone: 603-356-5461
Fax: 603-356-9121
Emergency Services: Yes
Beds: 35

Key Personnel:
CEO/President. . . . . Gary Poquette
Chief of Medical Staff . . . . Diane Snow
Infection Control. . . . . Andrea Murphy, RN
Quality Assurance . . . . Susan Perrault
Radiology. . . . . Ray H VanWyngarden

Measure	Cases	This Hosp.	State Avg.	U.S. Avg.
Heart Attack Care				
ACE Inhibitor or ARB for LVSD[1]	1	0%	98%	96%
Aspirin at Arrival[1]	10	100%	100%	99%
Aspirin at Discharge[1]	6	100%	99%	98%
Beta Blocker at Discharge[1]	6	83%	100%	98%
Fibrinolytic Medication Timing	0	-	100%	55%
PCI Within 90 Minutes of Arrival	0	-	89%	90%
Smoking Cessation Advice[1]	1	100%	99%	99%
Chest Pain/Possible Heart Attack Care				
Aspirin at Arrival	-	-	97%	95%
Median Time to ECG (minutes)	-	-	8	8
Median Time to Transfer (minutes)	-	-	41	61
Fibrinolytic Medication Timing	-	-	48%	54%
Heart Failure Care				
ACE Inhibitor or ARB for LVSD[1]	15	87%	96%	94%
Discharge Instructions	30	97%	92%	88%
Evaluation of LVS Function	43	88%	99%	98%
Smoking Cessation Advice[1]	5	100%	99%	98%
Pneumonia Care				
Appropriate Initial Antibiotic[2]	27	89%	95%	92%
Blood Culture Timing[2]	29	93%	97%	96%
Influenza Vaccine[1,2]	18	67%	95%	91%
Initial Antibiotic Timing[2]	29	97%	97%	95%
Pneumococcal Vaccine[2]	29	97%	96%	93%
Smoking Cessation Advice[1,2]	9	78%	97%	97%
Surgical Care Improvement Project				
Appropriate VTP Within 24 Hours	29	100%	96%	92%
Appropriate Hair Removal	62	100%	100%	99%
Appropriate Beta Blocker Usage[5]	0	-	95%	93%
Controlled Postoperative Blood Glucose	0	-	95%	93%
Prophylactic Antibiotic Timing	59	95%	97%	97%
Prophylactic Antibiotic Timing (Outpatient)	-	-	96%	92%
Prophylactic Antibiotic Selection	58	98%	98%	97%
Prophylactic Antibiotic Select. (Outpatient)	-	-	97%	94%
Prophylactic Antibiotic Stopped	57	86%	97%	94%
Recommended VTP Ordered	29	100%	97%	94%
Urinary Catheter Removal[1]	21	100%	89%	90%
Children's Asthma Care				
Received Systemic Corticosteroids	-	-	-	100%
Received Home Management Plan	-	-	-	71%
Received Reliever Medication	-	-	-	100%
Use of Medical Imaging				
Combination Abdominal CT Scan	-	-	0.078	0.191
Combination Chest CT Scan	-	-	0.014	0.054
Follow-up Mammogram/Ultrasound	-	-	7.1%	8.4%
MRI for Low Back Pain	-	-	31.5%	32.7%
Survey of Patients' Hospital Experiences				
Area Around Room 'Always' Quiet at Night[8]	-	-	-	58%
Doctors 'Always' Communicated Well[8]	-	-	-	80%
Home Recovery Information Given[8]	-	-	-	82%
Hospital Given 9 or 10 on 10 Point Scale[8]	-	-	-	67%
Meds 'Always' Explained Before Given[8]	-	-	-	60%
Nurses 'Always' Communicated Well[8]	-	-	-	76%
Pain 'Always' Well Controlled[8]	-	-	-	69%
Room and Bathroom 'Always' Clean[8]	-	-	-	71%
Timely Help 'Always' Received[8]	-	-	-	64%
Would Definitely Recommend Hospital[8]	-	-	-	69%

Monadnock Community Hospital

452 Old Street Road
Peterborough, NH 03458
E-mail: info@monadnockhospital.org
URL: www.monadnockhospital.org
Type: Critical Access Hospitals
Ownership: Voluntary Non-Profit - Other
Phone: 603-924-7191
Fax: 603-924-9586
Emergency Services: Yes
Beds: 62

Key Personnel:
CEO/President. . . . . Peter Gosline
Chief of Medical Staff . . . . Peter Forssell, MD
Infection Control. . . . . Diana Clang
Operating Room. . . . . Edwin S Menor, RN
Pediatric In-Patient Care . . . . . . Jeffrey Boxer, MD
Quality Assurance . . . . Margaret Viverito
Radiology. . . . . Bhojwani Rajesh, MD
Intensive Care Unit. . . . . Dianne Bolton

Measure	Cases	This Hosp.	State Avg.	U.S. Avg.
Heart Attack Care				
ACE Inhibitor or ARB for LVSD[1]	5	100%	98%	96%
Aspirin at Arrival[1]	10	100%	100%	99%
Aspirin at Discharge[1]	8	100%	99%	98%
Beta Blocker at Discharge[1]	8	100%	100%	98%
Fibrinolytic Medication Timing	0	-	100%	55%
PCI Within 90 Minutes of Arrival[5]	0	-	89%	90%
Smoking Cessation Advice	0	-	99%	99%
Chest Pain/Possible Heart Attack Care				
Aspirin at Arrival	33	94%	97%	95%
Median Time to ECG (minutes)	35	11	8	8
Median Time to Transfer (minutes)[1,3]	2	66	41	61
Fibrinolytic Medication Timing[1]	3	33%	48%	54%
Heart Failure Care				
ACE Inhibitor or ARB for LVSD[1]	4	100%	96%	94%
Discharge Instructions[1]	18	89%	92%	88%
Evaluation of LVS Function	29	97%	99%	98%
Smoking Cessation Advice[1]	5	100%	99%	98%
Pneumonia Care				
Appropriate Initial Antibiotic	52	96%	95%	92%
Blood Culture Timing	96	99%	97%	96%
Influenza Vaccine	52	94%	95%	91%
Initial Antibiotic Timing	84	99%	97%	95%
Pneumococcal Vaccine	71	97%	96%	93%
Smoking Cessation Advice	26	92%	97%	97%
Surgical Care Improvement Project				
Appropriate VTP Within 24 Hours	36	97%	96%	92%
Appropriate Hair Removal	128	100%	100%	99%
Appropriate Beta Blocker Usage[5]	0	-	95%	93%
Controlled Postoperative Blood Glucose	0	-	95%	93%
Prophylactic Antibiotic Timing	111	97%	97%	97%
Prophylactic Antibiotic Timing (Outpatient)	45	98%	96%	92%
Prophylactic Antibiotic Selection	115	96%	98%	97%
Prophylactic Antibiotic Select. (Outpatient)	45	96%	97%	94%
Prophylactic Antibiotic Stopped	107	98%	97%	94%
Recommended VTP Ordered	36	100%	97%	94%
Urinary Catheter Removal[1]	8	50%	89%	90%
Children's Asthma Care				
Received Systemic Corticosteroids	-	-	-	100%
Received Home Management Plan	-	-	-	71%
Received Reliever Medication	-	-	-	100%
Use of Medical Imaging				
Combination Abdominal CT Scan	283	0.057	0.078	0.191
Combination Chest CT Scan	246	0.004	0.014	0.054
Follow-up Mammogram/Ultrasound	621	11.8%	7.1%	8.4%
MRI for Low Back Pain[1]	58	22.4%	31.5%	32.7%
Survey of Patients' Hospital Experiences				
Area Around Room 'Always' Quiet at Night	300+	58%	-	58%
Doctors 'Always' Communicated Well	300+	87%	-	80%
Home Recovery Information Given	300+	88%	-	82%
Hospital Given 9 or 10 on 10 Point Scale	300+	79%	-	67%
Meds 'Always' Explained Before Given	300+	71%	-	60%
Nurses 'Always' Communicated Well	300+	86%	-	76%
Pain 'Always' Well Controlled	300+	76%	-	69%
Room and Bathroom 'Always' Clean	300+	82%	-	71%
Timely Help 'Always' Received	300+	80%	-	64%
Would Definitely Recommend Hospital	300+	81%	-	69%

NOTE: Hospital profiles are in alphabetical order by state, then city, then hospital within the city; Rankings exclude hospitals with less than 25 cases except for patient surveys which excludes hospitals with less than 100 cases; (a) 100–299 cases; (1) The number of cases is too small to be sure how well a hospital is performing; (2) The hospital indicated that the data submitted for this measure were based on a sample of cases; (3) Data was collected during a shorter time period (fewer quarters) than the maximum possible time for this measure; (4) Suppressed for one or more quarters by CMS; (5) No data is available from the hospital for this measure; (6) Fewer than 100 patients completed the HCAHPS survey. Use these rates with caution, as the number of surveys may be too low to reliably assess hospital performance; (7) Survey results are based on less than 12 months of data; (8) Survey results are not available for this reporting period; (9) No or very few patients were eligible for the HCAHPS survey. The scores shown, if any, reflect a very small number of surveys; (10) A state average was not calculated because too few hospitals in the state submitted data; (11) There were discrepancies in the data collection process; Please refer to the User's Guide for a full explanation of data.

Speare Memorial Hospital

16 Hospital Road
Plymouth, NH 03264
Phone: 603-536-1120
Fax: 603-536-4828
URL: www.spearehospital.com
Type: Critical Access Hospitals
Emergency Services: Yes
Ownership: Voluntary Non-Profit - Private
Beds: 47

Key Personnel:

CEO/President. . . . . Michelle McEwen
Chief of Medical Staff. . . . . Joseph Ebner
Infection Control. . . . . Ann Graves
Operating Room. . . . . John Bentwood
Quality Assurance . . . . Priscilla Farrell
Radiology. . . . . Michael Beckerman
Emergency Room . . . . Alex Medlacot

Measure	Cases	This Hosp.	State Avg.	U.S. Avg.
Heart Attack Care				
ACE Inhibitor or ARB for LVSD	0	-	98%	96%
Aspirin at Arrival[1]	4	100%	100%	99%
Aspirin at Discharge[1]	2	100%	99%	98%
Beta Blocker at Discharge[1]	2	100%	100%	98%
Fibrinolytic Medication Timing	0	-	100%	55%
PCI Within 90 Minutes of Arrival[5]	0	-	89%	90%
Smoking Cessation Advice[1]	1	100%	99%	99%
Chest Pain/Possible Heart Attack Care				
Aspirin at Arrival	40	100%	97%	95%
Median Time to ECG (minutes)	40	14	8	8
Median Time to Transfer (minutes)[3]	0	-	41	61
Fibrinolytic Medication Timing[1]	6	67%	48%	54%
Heart Failure Care				
ACE Inhibitor or ARB for LVSD[1]	6	100%	96%	94%
Discharge Instructions	30	100%	92%	88%
Evaluation of LVS Function	33	100%	99%	98%
Smoking Cessation Advice[1]	1	100%	99%	98%
Pneumonia Care				
Appropriate Initial Antibiotic	27	100%	95%	92%
Blood Culture Timing	30	100%	97%	96%
Influenza Vaccine[1]	20	100%	95%	91%
Initial Antibiotic Timing	43	100%	97%	95%
Pneumococcal Vaccine	38	100%	96%	93%
Smoking Cessation Advice[1]	13	100%	97%	97%
Surgical Care Improvement Project				
Appropriate VTP Within 24 Hours[1]	22	100%	96%	92%
Appropriate Hair Removal	73	100%	100%	99%
Appropriate Beta Blocker Usage[1]	22	95%	95%	93%
Controlled Postoperative Blood Glucose	0	-	95%	93%
Prophylactic Antibiotic Timing	60	98%	97%	97%
Prophylactic Antibiotic Timing (Outpatient)	59	100%	96%	92%
Prophylactic Antibiotic Selection	59	100%	98%	97%
Prophylactic Antibiotic Select. (Outpatient)	59	97%	97%	94%
Prophylactic Antibiotic Stopped	57	95%	97%	94%
Recommended VTP Ordered[1]	22	100%	97%	94%
Urinary Catheter Removal	31	100%	89%	90%
Children's Asthma Care				
Received Systemic Corticosteroids	-	-	-	100%
Received Home Management Plan	-	-	-	71%
Received Reliever Medication	-	-	-	100%
Use of Medical Imaging				
Combination Abdominal CT Scan	248	0.056	0.078	0.191
Combination Chest CT Scan	182	0.000	0.014	0.054
Follow-up Mammogram/Ultrasound	571	7.5%	7.1%	8.4%
MRI for Low Back Pain	49	49.0%	31.5%	32.7%
Survey of Patients' Hospital Experiences				
Area Around Room 'Always' Quiet at Night	300+	56%	-	58%
Doctors 'Always' Communicated Well	300+	87%	-	80%
Home Recovery Information Given	300+	91%	-	82%
Hospital Given 9 or 10 on 10 Point Scale	300+	75%	-	67%
Meds 'Always' Explained Before Given	300+	68%	-	60%
Nurses 'Always' Communicated Well	300+	86%	-	76%
Pain 'Always' Well Controlled	300+	77%	-	69%
Room and Bathroom 'Always' Clean	300+	86%	-	71%
Timely Help 'Always' Received	300+	78%	-	64%
Would Definitely Recommend Hospital	300+	80%	-	69%

Portsmouth Regional Hospital

333 Borthwick Ave
Portsmouth, NH 03801
Phone: 603-436-5110
Fax: 603-433-5245
Type: Acute Care Hospitals
Emergency Services: No
Ownership: Proprietary
Beds: 209

Key Personnel:

CEO/President. . . . . William Schurer
Chief of Medical Staff . . . . Iva Schwartz, MD

Measure	Cases	This Hosp.	State Avg.	U.S. Avg.
Heart Attack Care				
ACE Inhibitor or ARB for LVSD	35	100%	98%	96%
Aspirin at Arrival	150	100%	100%	99%
Aspirin at Discharge	278	100%	99%	98%
Beta Blocker at Discharge	267	100%	100%	98%
Fibrinolytic Medication Timing	0	-	100%	55%
PCI Within 90 Minutes of Arrival	28	93%	89%	90%
Smoking Cessation Advice	81	100%	99%	99%
Chest Pain/Possible Heart Attack Care				
Aspirin at Arrival[1,3]	2	100%	97%	95%
Median Time to ECG (minutes)[1,3]	2	4	8	8
Median Time to Transfer (minutes)[5]	0	-	41	61
Fibrinolytic Medication Timing[5]	0	-	48%	54%
Heart Failure Care				
ACE Inhibitor or ARB for LVSD	29	100%	96%	94%
Discharge Instructions	78	90%	92%	88%
Evaluation of LVS Function	109	100%	99%	98%
Smoking Cessation Advice[1]	7	100%	99%	98%
Pneumonia Care				
Appropriate Initial Antibiotic	59	100%	95%	92%
Blood Culture Timing	111	98%	97%	96%
Influenza Vaccine	59	100%	95%	91%
Initial Antibiotic Timing	101	100%	97%	95%
Pneumococcal Vaccine	101	100%	96%	93%
Smoking Cessation Advice[1]	23	100%	97%	97%
Surgical Care Improvement Project				
Appropriate VTP Within 24 Hours[2]	166	97%	96%	92%
Appropriate Hair Removal[2]	595	100%	100%	99%
Appropriate Beta Blocker Usage[2]	256	100%	95%	93%
Controlled Postoperative Blood Glucose[2]	170	92%	95%	93%
Prophylactic Antibiotic Timing[2]	373	100%	97%	97%
Prophylactic Antibiotic Timing (Outpatient)	259	99%	96%	92%
Prophylactic Antibiotic Selection[2]	407	100%	98%	97%
Prophylactic Antibiotic Select. (Outpatient)	258	99%	97%	94%
Prophylactic Antibiotic Stopped[2]	348	98%	97%	94%
Recommended VTP Ordered[2]	166	99%	97%	94%
Urinary Catheter Removal[2]	121	100%	89%	90%
Children's Asthma Care				
Received Systemic Corticosteroids	-	-	-	100%
Received Home Management Plan	-	-	-	71%
Received Reliever Medication	-	-	-	100%
Use of Medical Imaging				
Combination Abdominal CT Scan	595	0.081	0.078	0.191
Combination Chest CT Scan	392	0.000	0.014	0.054
Follow-up Mammogram/Ultrasound	1,479	10.8%	7.1%	8.4%
MRI for Low Back Pain	194	24.7%	31.5%	32.7%
Survey of Patients' Hospital Experiences				
Area Around Room 'Always' Quiet at Night	300+	55%	-	58%
Doctors 'Always' Communicated Well	300+	81%	-	80%
Home Recovery Information Given	300+	90%	-	82%
Hospital Given 9 or 10 on 10 Point Scale	300+	68%	-	67%
Meds 'Always' Explained Before Given	300+	57%	-	60%
Nurses 'Always' Communicated Well	300+	75%	-	76%
Pain 'Always' Well Controlled	300+	69%	-	69%
Room and Bathroom 'Always' Clean	300+	72%	-	71%
Timely Help 'Always' Received	300+	62%	-	64%
Would Definitely Recommend Hospital	300+	72%	-	69%

Frisbie Memorial Hospital

11 Whitehall Road
Rochester, NH 03867
Phone: 603-332-5211
Fax: 603-332-2699
E-mail: fmh3666@rscs.net
URL: www.frisbiehospital.com
Type: Acute Care Hospitals
Emergency Services: No
Ownership: Voluntary Non-Profit - Private
Beds: 122

Key Personnel:

CEO/President. . . . . Alvin Felgar
Chief of Medical Staff . . . . Sara Stacey, MD
Operating Room. . . . . Joseph Shields
Pediatric In-Patient Care . . . . Wallace Hubbard, MD
Quality Assurance . . . . Ellen Littlefield
Radiology. . . . . Albert Chang
Intensive Care Unit. . . . . Sally Gallot
Patient Relations . . . . Karen Dutcher

Measure	Cases	This Hosp.	State Avg.	U.S. Avg.
Heart Attack Care				
ACE Inhibitor or ARB for LVSD	0	-	98%	96%
Aspirin at Arrival[1]	18	100%	100%	99%
Aspirin at Discharge[1]	4	100%	99%	98%
Beta Blocker at Discharge[1]	3	100%	100%	98%
Fibrinolytic Medication Timing	0	-	100%	55%
PCI Within 90 Minutes of Arrival	0	-	89%	90%
Smoking Cessation Advice[1]	2	100%	99%	99%
Chest Pain/Possible Heart Attack Care				
Aspirin at Arrival	37	89%	97%	95%
Median Time to ECG (minutes)	37	5	8	8
Median Time to Transfer (minutes)[1,3]	12	43	41	61
Fibrinolytic Medication Timing	0	-	48%	54%
Heart Failure Care				
ACE Inhibitor or ARB for LVSD[1]	17	94%	96%	94%
Discharge Instructions	81	95%	92%	88%
Evaluation of LVS Function	108	99%	99%	98%
Smoking Cessation Advice[1]	11	100%	99%	98%
Pneumonia Care				
Appropriate Initial Antibiotic	97	92%	95%	92%
Blood Culture Timing	122	96%	97%	96%
Influenza Vaccine	95	88%	95%	91%
Initial Antibiotic Timing	100	98%	97%	95%
Pneumococcal Vaccine	112	96%	96%	93%
Smoking Cessation Advice	59	100%	97%	97%
Surgical Care Improvement Project				
Appropriate VTP Within 24 Hours	80	92%	96%	92%
Appropriate Hair Removal	258	100%	100%	99%
Appropriate Beta Blocker Usage	92	100%	95%	93%
Controlled Postoperative Blood Glucose	0	-	95%	93%
Prophylactic Antibiotic Timing	174	97%	97%	97%
Prophylactic Antibiotic Timing (Outpatient)	78	94%	96%	92%
Prophylactic Antibiotic Selection	177	99%	98%	97%
Prophylactic Antibiotic Select. (Outpatient)	73	89%	97%	94%
Prophylactic Antibiotic Stopped	169	99%	97%	94%
Recommended VTP Ordered	80	92%	97%	94%
Urinary Catheter Removal	79	97%	89%	90%
Children's Asthma Care				
Received Systemic Corticosteroids	-	-	-	100%
Received Home Management Plan	-	-	-	71%
Received Reliever Medication	-	-	-	100%
Use of Medical Imaging				
Combination Abdominal CT Scan	633	0.054	0.078	0.191
Combination Chest CT Scan	586	0.000	0.014	0.054
Follow-up Mammogram/Ultrasound[5]	0	-	7.1%	8.4%
MRI for Low Back Pain	92	31.5%	31.5%	32.7%
Survey of Patients' Hospital Experiences				
Area Around Room 'Always' Quiet at Night	300+	66%	-	58%
Doctors 'Always' Communicated Well	300+	78%	-	80%
Home Recovery Information Given	300+	87%	-	82%
Hospital Given 9 or 10 on 10 Point Scale	300+	69%	-	67%
Meds 'Always' Explained Before Given	300+	65%	-	60%
Nurses 'Always' Communicated Well	300+	79%	-	76%
Pain 'Always' Well Controlled	300+	71%	-	69%
Room and Bathroom 'Always' Clean	300+	83%	-	71%
Timely Help 'Always' Received	300+	74%	-	64%
Would Definitely Recommend Hospital	300+	73%	-	69%

NOTE: Hospital profiles are in alphabetical order by state, then city, then hospital within the city; Rankings exclude hospitals with less than 25 cases except for patient surveys which excludes hospitals with less than 100 cases; (a) 100–299 cases; (1) The number of cases is too small to be sure how well a hospital is performing; (2) The hospital indicated that the data submitted for this measure were based on a sample of cases; (3) Data was collected during a shorter time period (fewer quarters) than the maximum possible time for this measure; (4) Suppressed for one or more quarters by CMS; (5) No data is available from the hospital for this measure; (6) Fewer than 100 patients completed the HCAHPS survey. Use these rates with caution, as the number of surveys may be too low to reliably assess hospital performance; (7) Survey results are based on less than 12 months of data; (8) Survey results are not available for this reporting period; (9) No or very few patients were eligible for the HCAHPS survey. The scores shown, if any, reflect a very small number of surveys; (10) A state average was not calculated because too few hospitals in the state submitted data; (11) There were discrepancies in the data collection process; Please refer to the User's Guide for a full explanation of data.

Huggins Hospital

240 South Main Street
Wolfeboro, NH 03894
E-mail: askhuggins@hugginshospital.org
URL: www.hugginshospital.org
Type: Critical Access Hospitals
Ownership: Voluntary Non-Profit - Private

Phone: 603-569-7500
Fax: 603-569-7509

Emergency Services: Yes
Beds: 55

Key Personnel:
CEO/President. . . . . David W Tower, FACHE
Chief of Medical Staff. . . . . Stephen Fleet, MD
Infection Control. . . . . Linda Brookes
Pediatric In-Patient Care . . . . . . Harley W Heath, MD
Quality Assurance . . . . Rebecca Mason
Emergency Room . . . . Sandi McKenzie

Measure	Cases	This Hosp.	State Avg.	U.S. Avg.
Heart Attack Care				
ACE Inhibitor or ARB for LVSD[1]	3	100%	98%	96%
Aspirin at Arrival[1]	15	100%	100%	99%
Aspirin at Discharge[1]	10	100%	99%	98%
Beta Blocker at Discharge[1]	11	100%	100%	98%
Fibrinolytic Medication Timing	0	-	100%	55%
PCI Within 90 Minutes of Arrival	0	-	89%	90%
Smoking Cessation Advice	0	-	99%	99%
Chest Pain/Possible Heart Attack Care				
Aspirin at Arrival	-	-	97%	95%
Median Time to ECG (minutes)	-	-	8	8
Median Time to Transfer (minutes)	-	-	41	61
Fibrinolytic Medication Timing	-	-	48%	54%
Heart Failure Care				
ACE Inhibitor or ARB for LVSD[1]	20	75%	96%	94%
Discharge Instructions[1]	21	57%	92%	88%
Evaluation of LVS Function	41	98%	99%	98%
Smoking Cessation Advice[1]	4	100%	99%	98%
Pneumonia Care				
Appropriate Initial Antibiotic	34	94%	95%	92%
Blood Culture Timing	55	96%	97%	96%
Influenza Vaccine[1]	18	89%	95%	91%
Initial Antibiotic Timing	54	98%	97%	95%
Pneumococcal Vaccine	44	100%	96%	93%
Smoking Cessation Advice[1]	10	100%	97%	97%
Surgical Care Improvement Project				
Appropriate VTP Within 24 Hours	41	100%	96%	92%
Appropriate Hair Removal	91	99%	100%	99%
Appropriate Beta Blocker Usage	30	100%	95%	93%
Controlled Postoperative Blood Glucose	0	-	95%	93%
Prophylactic Antibiotic Timing	56	98%	97%	97%
Prophylactic Antibiotic Timing (Outpatient)	-	-	96%	92%
Prophylactic Antibiotic Selection	56	91%	98%	97%
Prophylactic Antibiotic Select. (Outpatient)	-	-	97%	94%
Prophylactic Antibiotic Stopped	55	98%	97%	94%
Recommended VTP Ordered	41	100%	97%	94%
Urinary Catheter Removal[1]	19	95%	89%	90%
Children's Asthma Care				
Received Systemic Corticosteroids	-	-	-	100%
Received Home Management Plan	-	-	-	71%
Received Reliever Medication	-	-	-	100%
Use of Medical Imaging				
Combination Abdominal CT Scan	-	-	0.078	0.191
Combination Chest CT Scan	-	-	0.014	0.054
Follow-up Mammogram/Ultrasound	-	-	7.1%	8.4%
MRI for Low Back Pain	-	-	31.5%	32.7%
Survey of Patients' Hospital Experiences				
Area Around Room 'Always' Quiet at Night	300+	51%	-	58%
Doctors 'Always' Communicated Well	300+	78%	-	80%
Home Recovery Information Given	300+	84%	-	82%
Hospital Given 9 or 10 on 10 Point Scale	300+	62%	-	67%
Meds 'Always' Explained Before Given	300+	60%	-	60%
Nurses 'Always' Communicated Well	300+	77%	-	76%
Pain 'Always' Well Controlled	300+	75%	-	69%
Room and Bathroom 'Always' Clean	300+	73%	-	71%
Timely Help 'Always' Received	300+	63%	-	64%
Would Definitely Recommend Hospital	300+	64%	-	69%

Cottage Hospital

90 Swiftwater Rd
Woodsville, NH 03785
E-mail: myhospital@cottagehospital.org
URL: www.cottagehospital.org
Type: Critical Access Hospitals
Ownership: Voluntary Non-Profit - Private

Phone: 603-747-9000
Fax: 603-747-3310

Emergency Services: Yes
Beds: 25

Key Personnel:
CEO/President. . . . . Maria Ryan, PhD
Cardiac Laboratory. . . . . Lori Taylor
Chief of Medical Staff. . . . . Mealanie Lawrence, MD
Infection Control. . . . . Mary Ruppert, RN
Operating Room. . . . . Patricia Thaver, RN
Quality Assurance . . . . Laurie Hughes
Radiology. . . . . Marcy Rushford, RT

Measure	Cases	This Hosp.	State Avg.	U.S. Avg.
Heart Attack Care				
ACE Inhibitor or ARB for LVSD	0	-	98%	96%
Aspirin at Arrival[1]	3	100%	100%	99%
Aspirin at Discharge[1]	2	100%	99%	98%
Beta Blocker at Discharge[1]	2	100%	100%	98%
Fibrinolytic Medication Timing	0	-	100%	55%
PCI Within 90 Minutes of Arrival	0	-	89%	90%
Smoking Cessation Advice	0	-	99%	99%
Chest Pain/Possible Heart Attack Care				
Aspirin at Arrival	-	-	97%	95%
Median Time to ECG (minutes)	-	-	8	8
Median Time to Transfer (minutes)	-	-	41	61
Fibrinolytic Medication Timing	-	-	48%	54%
Heart Failure Care				
ACE Inhibitor or ARB for LVSD	0	-	96%	94%
Discharge Instructions[1]	12	92%	92%	88%
Evaluation of LVS Function[1]	15	93%	99%	98%
Smoking Cessation Advice	0	-	99%	98%
Pneumonia Care				
Appropriate Initial Antibiotic[1]	14	93%	95%	92%
Blood Culture Timing	30	97%	97%	96%
Influenza Vaccine[1]	19	100%	95%	91%
Initial Antibiotic Timing	32	100%	97%	95%
Pneumococcal Vaccine	32	100%	96%	93%
Smoking Cessation Advice[1]	6	83%	97%	97%
Surgical Care Improvement Project				
Appropriate VTP Within 24 Hours[1]	13	92%	96%	92%
Appropriate Hair Removal	58	100%	100%	99%
Appropriate Beta Blocker Usage[5]	0	-	95%	93%
Controlled Postoperative Blood Glucose	0	-	95%	93%
Prophylactic Antibiotic Timing	42	93%	97%	97%
Prophylactic Antibiotic Timing (Outpatient)	-	-	96%	92%
Prophylactic Antibiotic Selection	42	98%	98%	97%
Prophylactic Antibiotic Select. (Outpatient)	-	-	97%	94%
Prophylactic Antibiotic Stopped	42	90%	97%	94%
Recommended VTP Ordered[1]	13	92%	97%	94%
Urinary Catheter Removal[1]	20	100%	89%	90%
Children's Asthma Care				
Received Systemic Corticosteroids	-	-	-	100%
Received Home Management Plan	-	-	-	71%
Received Reliever Medication	-	-	-	100%
Use of Medical Imaging				
Combination Abdominal CT Scan	-	-	0.078	0.191
Combination Chest CT Scan	-	-	0.014	0.054
Follow-up Mammogram/Ultrasound	-	-	7.1%	8.4%
MRI for Low Back Pain	-	-	31.5%	32.7%
Survey of Patients' Hospital Experiences				
Area Around Room 'Always' Quiet at Night[8]	-	-	-	58%
Doctors 'Always' Communicated Well[8]	-	-	-	80%
Home Recovery Information Given[8]	-	-	-	82%
Hospital Given 9 or 10 on 10 Point Scale[8]	-	-	-	67%
Meds 'Always' Explained Before Given[8]	-	-	-	60%
Nurses 'Always' Communicated Well[8]	-	-	-	76%
Pain 'Always' Well Controlled[8]	-	-	-	69%
Room and Bathroom 'Always' Clean[8]	-	-	-	71%
Timely Help 'Always' Received[8]	-	-	-	64%
Would Definitely Recommend Hospital[8]	-	-	-	69%

NOTE: Hospital profiles are in alphabetical order by state, then city, then hospital within the city; Rankings exclude hospitals with less than 25 cases except for patient surveys which excludes hospitals with less than 100 cases; (a) 100–299 cases; (1) The number of cases is too small to be sure how well a hospital is performing; (2) The hospital indicated that the data submitted for this measure were based on a sample of cases; (3) Data was collected during a shorter time period (fewer quarters) than the maximum possible time for this measure; (4) Suppressed for one or more quarters by CMS; (5) No data is available from the hospital for this measure; (6) Fewer than 100 patients completed the HCAHPS survey. Use these rates with caution, as the number of surveys may be too low to reliably assess hospital performance; (7) Survey results are based on less than 12 months of data; (8) Survey results are not available for this reporting period; (9) No or very few patients were eligible for the HCAHPS survey. The scores shown, if any, reflect a very small number of surveys; (10) A state average was not calculated because too few hospitals in the state submitted data; (11) There were discrepancies in the data collection process; Please refer to the User's Guide for a full explanation of data.

Heart Attack Care

1. ACE Inhibitor or ARB for LVSD

Hospital Name	City	Rate	Cases
Bayonne Hospital Center	Bayonne	100%	29
Chilton Hospital	Pompton Plains	100%	29
Clara Maass Medical Center[2]	Belleville	100%	28
Community Medical Center[2]	Toms River	100%	41
Hackensack University Medical Center	Hackensack	100%	165
Holy Name Medical Center	Teaneck	100%	27
Libertyhealth-Jersey City Med Ctr Campus	Jersey City	100%	49
Newark Beth Israel Medical Center[2]	Newark	100%	69
Raritan Bay Medical Center	Perth Amboy	100%	30
Saint Barnabas Medical Center	Livingston	100%	64
Saint Francis Medical Center	Trenton	100%	48
Trinitas Regional Medical Center	Elizabeth	100%	35
UMDNJ University Hospital	Newark	100%	29
Virtua West Jersey Hospitals Berlin	Berlin	100%	45
Robert Wood Johnson University Hospital	New Brunswick	99%	108
Atlanticare Reg Med Ctr-City Division[2]	Atlantic City	98%	66
Cooper University Hospital	Camden	98%	100
Deborah Heart and Lung Center	Browns Mills	98%	55
Englewood Hospital and Medical Center[2]	Englewood	98%	55
Our Lady of Lourdes Medical Center[2]	Camden	98%	51
Jersey Shore University Medical Center[2]	Neptune	97%	60
Virtua Mem Hosp of Burlington County	Mount Holly	97%	29
Somerset Medical Center[2]	Somerville	96%	25
Saint Michael's Medical Center[2]	Newark	95%	78
Saint Joseph's Regional Medical Center	Paterson	94%	64
Valley Hospital[2]	Ridgewood	93%	46
Morristown Memorial Hospital[2]	Morristown	92%	52
Overlook Hospital	Summit	91%	32
JFK Medical Center	Edison	87%	39

2. Aspirin at Arrival

Hospital Name	City	Rate	Cases
Atlanticare Reg Med Ctr-City Division[2]	Atlantic City	100%	238
Bayonne Hospital Center	Bayonne	100%	139
Bayshore Community Hospital	Holmdel	100%	152
Cape Regional Medical Center	Cape May CH	100%	50
Centrastate Medical Center	Freehold	100%	111
Clara Maass Medical Center[2]	Belleville	100%	240
Community Medical Center[2]	Toms River	100%	467
East Orange General Hospital	East Orange	100%	70
Englewood Hospital and Medical Center[2]	Englewood	100%	248
Hackensack University Medical Center	Hackensack	100%	524
Hackettstown Regional Medical Center	Hackettstown	100%	61
Holy Name Medical Center	Teaneck	100%	200
Hunterdon Medical Center	Flemington	100%	117
Libertyhealth-Jersey City Med Ctr Campus	Jersey City	100%	189
Meadowlands Hospital Medical Center	Secaucus	100%	29
Memorial Hospital of Salem County	Salem	100%	30
Mountainside Hospital	Montclair	100%	165
Newark Beth Israel Medical Center[2]	Newark	100%	200
Newton Memorial Hospital	Newton	100%	66
Ocean Medical Center	Brick	100%	215
Riverview Medical Center	Red Bank	100%	187
Robert W Johnson Univ Hosp-Rahway	Rahway	100%	106
Saint Barnabas Medical Center	Livingston	100%	271
Saint Clare's Hospital	Denville	100%	169
Saint Francis Medical Center	Trenton	100%	118
Saint Peter's University Hospital	New Brunswick	100%	103
Somerset Medical Center[2]	Somerville	100%	252
South Jersey Healthcare-Elmer Hospital	Elmer	100%	39
UMDNJ University Hospital	Newark	100%	97
University Medical Center at Princeton	Princeton	100%	129
Virtua Mem Hosp of Burlington County	Mount Holly	100%	247
Virtua West Jersey Hospitals Berlin	Berlin	100%	356
Chilton Hospital	Pompton Plains	99%	172
Cooper University Hospital	Camden	99%	151
Jersey Shore University Medical Center[2]	Neptune	99%	159
Kimball Medical Center	Lakewood	99%	149
Lourdes Medical Center of Burlington County	Willingboro	99%	71
Monmouth Medical Center	Long Branch	99%	127
Our Lady of Lourdes Medical Center[2]	Camden	99%	116
Robert Wood Johnson University Hospital	New Brunswick	99%	419
Saint Joseph's Regional Medical Center	Paterson	99%	379
Saint Mary's Hospital - Passaic	Passaic	99%	84
Saint Michael's Medical Center[2]	Newark	99%	97
Shore Memorial Hospital	Somers Point	99%	89
South Jersey Healthcare Reg Med Ctr	Vineland	99%	125
Southern Ocean Medical Center	Manahawkin	99%	95
Underwood Memorial Hospital	Woodbury	99%	228
Raritan Bay Medical Center	Perth Amboy	98%	204
Valley Hospital[2]	Ridgewood	98%	289
Capital Health System - Mercer Campus	Trenton	97%	61
JFK Medical Center	Edison	97%	263
Overlook Hospital	Summit	97%	192
Palisades Medical Center	North Bergen	97%	88
Warren Hospital	Phillipsburg	97%	29

Christ Hospital	Jersey City	96%	161
Kennedy University Hospital	Stratford	96%	238
Morristown Memorial Hospital[2]	Morristown	96%	161
Trinitas Regional Medical Center	Elizabeth	96%	163
Hoboken University Medical Center	Hoboken	95%	43
Robert Wood Johnson Univ Hosp Hamilton	Hamilton	94%	161
Capital Health System-Fuld Campus	Trenton	92%	37

3. Aspirin at Discharge

Hospital Name	City	Rate	Cases
Atlanticare Reg Med Ctr-City Division[2]	Atlantic City	100%	330
Bayonne Hospital Center	Bayonne	100%	100
Bayshore Community Hospital	Holmdel	100%	59
Centrastate Medical Center	Freehold	100%	38
Clara Maass Medical Center[2]	Belleville	100%	123
Community Medical Center[2]	Toms River	100%	251
Deborah Heart and Lung Center	Browns Mills	100%	355
East Orange General Hospital	East Orange	100%	42
Englewood Hospital and Medical Center[2]	Englewood	100%	268
Hackensack University Medical Center	Hackensack	100%	741
Hackettstown Regional Medical Center	Hackettstown	100%	32
Holy Name Medical Center	Teaneck	100%	140
Hunterdon Medical Center	Flemington	100%	75
Mountainside Hospital	Montclair	100%	97
Newark Beth Israel Medical Center[2]	Newark	100%	284
Newton Memorial Hospital	Newton	100%	26
Our Lady of Lourdes Medical Center[2]	Camden	100%	293
Palisades Medical Center	North Bergen	100%	33
Riverview Medical Center	Red Bank	100%	113
Robert Wood Johnson University Hospital	New Brunswick	100%	859
Robert W Johnson Univ Hosp-Rahway	Rahway	100%	38
Saint Barnabas Medical Center	Livingston	100%	351
Saint Clare's Hospital	Denville	100%	123
Saint Francis Medical Center	Trenton	100%	291
Shore Memorial Hospital	Somers Point	100%	43
South Jersey Healthcare Reg Med Ctr	Vineland	100%	56
Southern Ocean Medical Center	Manahawkin	100%	53
UMDNJ University Hospital	Newark	100%	112
University Medical Center at Princeton	Princeton	100%	80
Valley Hospital[2]	Ridgewood	100%	291
Virtua West Jersey Hospitals Berlin	Berlin	100%	277
Cooper University Hospital	Camden	99%	437
Jersey Shore University Medical Center[2]	Neptune	99%	486
Libertyhealth-Jersey City Med Ctr Campus	Jersey City	99%	220
Monmouth Medical Center	Long Branch	99%	70
Morristown Memorial Hospital[2]	Morristown	99%	334
Somerset Medical Center[2]	Somerville	99%	175
Capital Health System - Mercer Campus	Trenton	98%	46
Chilton Hospital	Pompton Plains	98%	102
Christ Hospital	Jersey City	98%	81
JFK Medical Center	Edison	98%	163
Kimball Medical Center	Lakewood	98%	58
Ocean Medical Center	Brick	98%	111
Saint Peter's University Hospital	New Brunswick	98%	56
Underwood Memorial Hospital	Woodbury	98%	142
Overlook Hospital	Summit	97%	151
Saint Joseph's Regional Medical Center	Paterson	97%	377
Saint Mary's Hospital - Passaic	Passaic	97%	73
Virtua Mem Hosp of Burlington County	Mount Holly	97%	146
Kennedy University Hospital	Stratford	96%	120
Raritan Bay Medical Center	Perth Amboy	96%	134
Saint Michael's Medical Center[2]	Newark	96%	315
Trinitas Regional Medical Center	Elizabeth	95%	109
Robert Wood Johnson Univ Hosp Hamilton	Hamilton	93%	89
Lourdes Medical Center of Burlington County	Willingboro	92%	39

4. Beta Blocker at Discharge

Hospital Name	City	Rate	Cases
Atlanticare Reg Med Ctr-City Division[2]	Atlantic City	100%	325
Bayonne Hospital Center	Bayonne	100%	109
Bayshore Community Hospital	Holmdel	100%	67
Capital Health System - Mercer Campus	Trenton	100%	46
Centrastate Medical Center	Freehold	100%	38
Clara Maass Medical Center[2]	Belleville	100%	121
Community Medical Center[2]	Toms River	100%	264
Cooper University Hospital	Camden	100%	422
Deborah Heart and Lung Center	Browns Mills	100%	343
East Orange General Hospital	East Orange	100%	48
Hackensack University Medical Center	Hackensack	100%	731
Hackettstown Regional Medical Center	Hackettstown	100%	35
Holy Name Medical Center	Teaneck	100%	146
Hunterdon Medical Center	Flemington	100%	75
Kimball Medical Center	Lakewood	100%	60
Mountainside Hospital	Montclair	100%	105
Newark Beth Israel Medical Center[2]	Newark	100%	276
Newton Memorial Hospital	Newton	100%	32
Ocean Medical Center	Brick	100%	110
Palisades Medical Center	North Bergen	100%	35
Riverview Medical Center	Red Bank	100%	116
Robert Wood Johnson University Hospital	New Brunswick	100%	814

Robert W Johnson Univ Hosp-Rahway	Rahway	100%	44
Saint Barnabas Medical Center	Livingston	100%	350
Saint Clare's Hospital	Denville	100%	121
Saint Peter's University Hospital	New Brunswick	100%	59
Shore Memorial Hospital	Somers Point	100%	49
South Jersey Healthcare Reg Med Ctr	Vineland	100%	57
Southern Ocean Medical Center	Manahawkin	100%	54
UMDNJ University Hospital	Newark	100%	105
University Medical Center at Princeton	Princeton	100%	85
Libertyhealth-Jersey City Med Ctr Campus	Jersey City	99%	219
Morristown Memorial Hospital[2]	Morristown	99%	324
Saint Francis Medical Center	Trenton	99%	270
Saint Mary's Hospital - Passaic	Passaic	99%	78
Somerset Medical Center[2]	Somerville	99%	175
Underwood Memorial Hospital	Woodbury	99%	144
Valley Hospital[2]	Ridgewood	99%	296
Virtua Mem Hosp of Burlington County	Mount Holly	99%	155
Virtua West Jersey Hospitals Berlin	Berlin	99%	271
Chilton Hospital	Pompton Plains	98%	106
Christ Hospital	Jersey City	98%	87
Englewood Hospital and Medical Center[2]	Englewood	98%	261
Jersey Shore University Medical Center[2]	Neptune	98%	465
Monmouth Medical Center	Long Branch	98%	65
Our Lady of Lourdes Medical Center[2]	Camden	98%	278
Overlook Hospital	Summit	98%	151
Raritan Bay Medical Center	Perth Amboy	98%	132
Robert Wood Johnson Univ Hosp Hamilton	Hamilton	98%	86
JFK Medical Center	Edison	97%	172
Saint Michael's Medical Center[2]	Newark	97%	317
Kennedy University Hospital	Stratford	96%	113
Saint Joseph's Regional Medical Center	Paterson	96%	358
Trinitas Regional Medical Center	Elizabeth	96%	114
Lourdes Medical Center of Burlington County	Willingboro	95%	44

6. PCI Within 90 Minutes of Arrival

Hospital Name	City	Rate	Cases
Community Medical Center[2]	Toms River	100%	72
Holy Name Medical Center	Teaneck	100%	29
Hackensack University Medical Center	Hackensack	98%	88
Saint Clare's Hospital	Denville	98%	43
Saint Barnabas Medical Center	Livingston	97%	29
Saint Joseph's Regional Medical Center	Paterson	97%	79
Valley Hospital[2]	Ridgewood	96%	46
Hunterdon Medical Center	Flemington	95%	42
Riverview Medical Center	Red Bank	95%	39
Christ Hospital	Jersey City	94%	31
Libertyhealth-Jersey City Med Ctr Campus	Jersey City	92%	37
Underwood Memorial Hospital	Woodbury	92%	64
Chilton Hospital	Pompton Plains	90%	49
Ocean Medical Center	Brick	90%	42
Morristown Memorial Hospital[2]	Morristown	89%	35
Jersey Shore University Medical Center[2]	Neptune	88%	41
Englewood Hospital and Medical Center[2]	Englewood	87%	39
Raritan Bay Medical Center	Perth Amboy	87%	31
Somerset Medical Center[2]	Somerville	86%	64
Mountainside Hospital	Montclair	85%	40
Atlanticare Reg Med Ctr-City Division[2]	Atlantic City	83%	60
UMDNJ University Hospital	Newark	82%	28
Robert Wood Johnson University Hospital	New Brunswick	80%	103
Trinitas Regional Medical Center	Elizabeth	80%	35
Virtua West Jersey Hospitals Berlin	Berlin	80%	45
Overlook Hospital	Summit	78%	41
Cooper University Hospital	Camden	77%	30
JFK Medical Center	Edison	75%	61
Robert Wood Johnson Univ Hosp Hamilton	Hamilton	61%	36
Saint Francis Medical Center	Trenton	59%	34

7. Smoking Cessation Advice

Hospital Name	City	Rate	Cases
Atlanticare Reg Med Ctr-City Division[2]	Atlantic City	100%	114
Bayonne Hospital Center	Bayonne	100%	37
Clara Maass Medical Center[2]	Belleville	100%	29
Community Medical Center[2]	Toms River	100%	57
Cooper University Hospital	Camden	100%	198
Deborah Heart and Lung Center	Browns Mills	100%	100
Englewood Hospital and Medical Center[2]	Englewood	100%	42
Hackensack University Medical Center	Hackensack	100%	165
Holy Name Medical Center	Teaneck	100%	33
Hunterdon Medical Center	Flemington	100%	25
Jersey Shore University Medical Center[2]	Neptune	100%	161
JFK Medical Center	Edison	100%	26
Libertyhealth-Jersey City Med Ctr Campus	Jersey City	100%	67
Morristown Memorial Hospital[2]	Morristown	100%	84
Newark Beth Israel Medical Center[2]	Newark	100%	81
Our Lady of Lourdes Medical Center[2]	Camden	100%	79
Raritan Bay Medical Center	Perth Amboy	100%	42
Riverview Medical Center	Red Bank	100%	25
Robert Wood Johnson University Hospital	New Brunswick	100%	199
Robert Wood Johnson Univ Hosp Hamilton	Hamilton	100%	26
Saint Barnabas Medical Center	Livingston	100%	73

NOTE: Hospital profiles are in alphabetical order by state, then city, then hospital within the city; Rankings exclude hospitals with less than 25 cases except for patient surveys which excludes hospitals with less than 100 cases; (a) 100–299 cases; (1) The number of cases is too small to be sure how well a hospital is performing; (2) The hospital indicated that the data submitted for this measure were based on a sample of cases; (3) Data was collected during a shorter time period (fewer quarters) than the maximum possible time for this measure; (4) Suppressed for one or more quarters by CMS; (5) No data is available from the hospital for this measure; (6) Fewer than 100 patients completed the HCAHPS survey. Use these rates with caution, as the number of surveys may be too low to reliably assess hospital performance; (7) Survey results are based on less than 12 months of data; (8) Survey results are not available for this reporting period; (9) No or very few patients were eligible for the HCAHPS survey. The scores shown, if any, reflect a very small number of surveys; (10) A state average was not calculated because too few hospitals in the state submitted data; (11) There were discrepancies in the data collection process; Please refer to the User's Guide for a full explanation of data.

Saint Clare's Hospital	Denville	100%	30
Saint Francis Medical Center	Trenton	100%	99
Saint Joseph's Regional Medical Center	Paterson	100%	115
Saint Mary's Hospital - Passaic	Passaic	100%	26
Saint Michael's Medical Center[2]	Newark	100%	93
Somerset Medical Center[2]	Somerville	100%	50
Trinitas Regional Medical Center	Elizabeth	100%	35
UMDNJ University Hospital	Newark	100%	49
Underwood Memorial Hospital	Woodbury	100%	55
Valley Hospital[2]	Ridgewood	100%	56
Virtua Mem Hosp of Burlington County	Mount Holly	100%	28
Virtua West Jersey Hospitals Berlin	Berlin	100%	67

Chest Pain/Possible Heart Attack Care

8. Aspirin at Arrival

Hospital Name	City	Rate	Cases
Bayshore Community Hospital	Holmdel	100%	40
Community Medical Center	Toms River	100%	46
Hackettstown Regional Medical Center	Hackettstown	100%	33
Kimball Medical Center	Lakewood	100%	27
Newton Memorial Hospital	Newton	100%	31
Saint Clare's Hospital	Denville	100%	26
Shore Memorial Hospital	Somers Point	100%	68
Southern Ocean Medical Center	Manahawkin	100%	134
Warren Hospital	Phillipsburg	100%	34
Virtua Mem Hosp of Burlington County	Mount Holly	99%	143
Cape Regional Medical Center	Cape May CH	98%	83
South Jersey Healthcare Reg Med Ctr	Vineland	98%	96
Kennedy University Hospital	Stratford	97%	179
Virtua West Jersey Hospitals Berlin	Berlin	97%	119
Centrastate Medical Center	Freehold	96%	81
Lourdes Medical Center of Burlington County	Willingboro	95%	306
Hackensack University Medical Center	Hackensack	94%	33

9. Median Time to ECG (minutes)

Hospital Name	City	Min.	Cases
Centrastate Medical Center	Freehold	5	83
Newton Memorial Hospital	Newton	5	34
South Jersey Healthcare Reg Med Ctr	Vineland	5	99
Hackensack University Medical Center	Hackensack	6	37
Warren Hospital	Phillipsburg	6	36
Southern Ocean Medical Center	Manahawkin	7	136
Bayshore Community Hospital	Holmdel	8	38
Cape Regional Medical Center	Cape May CH	8	85
Shore Memorial Hospital	Somers Point	8	70
Community Medical Center	Toms River	9	46
Kennedy University Hospital	Stratford	9	183
Lourdes Medical Center of Burlington County	Willingboro	9	309
Kimball Medical Center	Lakewood	10	27
Virtua West Jersey Hospitals Berlin	Berlin	10	124
Saint Clare's Hospital	Denville	11	26
Virtua Mem Hosp of Burlington County	Mount Holly	11	149
Hackettstown Regional Medical Center	Hackettstown	15	37

10. Median Time to Transfer (minutes)

Hospital Name	City	Min.	Cases
Virtua Mem Hosp of Burlington County	Mount Holly	49	30

11. Fibrinolytic Medication Timing

Hospital Name	City	Rate	Cases
South Jersey Healthcare Reg Med Ctr	Vineland	75%	28

Heart Failure Care

12. ACE Inhibitor or ARB for LVSD

Hospital Name	City	Rate	Cases
Atlanticare Reg Med Ctr-City Division[2]	Atlantic City	100%	229
Bayshore Community Hospital	Holmdel	100%	67
Clara Maass Medical Center[2]	Belleville	100%	91
Community Medical Center[2]	Toms River	100%	78
Hackettstown Regional Medical Center	Hackettstown	100%	34
Hoboken University Medical Center[2]	Hoboken	100%	95
Holy Name Medical Center[2]	Teaneck	100%	79
Hunterdon Medical Center	Flemington	100%	57
Memorial Hospital of Salem County	Salem	100%	50
Monmouth Medical Center[2]	Long Branch	100%	53
Mountainside Hospital	Montclair	100%	121
Newark Beth Israel Medical Center[2]	Newark	100%	175
Our Lady of Lourdes Medical Center[2]	Camden	100%	90
Palisades Medical Center[2]	North Bergen	100%	79
Riverview Medical Center	Red Bank	100%	46
Somerset Medical Center[2]	Somerville	100%	78
South Jersey Healthcare Reg Med Ctr[2]	Vineland	100%	107
UMDNJ University Hospital	Newark	100%	269
University Medical Center at Princeton[2]	Princeton	100%	60
VA New Jersey Health Care System	East Orange	100%	60
Warren Hospital	Phillipsburg	100%	38
Cooper University Hospital	Camden	99%	200
Jersey Shore University Medical Center[2]	Neptune	99%	133
Kimball Medical Center	Lakewood	99%	90
Libertyhealth-Jersey City Med Ctr Campus[2]	Jersey City	99%	168
Ocean Medical Center[2]	Brick	99%	68
Raritan Bay Medical Center[2]	Perth Amboy	99%	193
Robert Wood Johnson University Hospital	New Brunswick	99%	378
Robert W Johnson Univ Hosp-Rahway	Rahway	99%	131
Saint Barnabas Medical Center[2]	Livingston	99%	113
Saint Clare's Hospital	Denville	99%	129
Virtua West Jersey Hospitals Berlin	Berlin	99%	172
Christ Hospital	Jersey City	98%	124
Englewood Hospital and Medical Center	Englewood	98%	166
Newton Memorial Hospital	Newton	98%	61
Saint Francis Medical Center	Trenton	98%	110
Saint Joseph's Regional Medical Center	Paterson	98%	335
Underwood Memorial Hospital	Woodbury	98%	133
East Orange General Hospital[2]	East Orange	97%	71
Meadowlands Hospital Medical Center	Secaucus	97%	39
Shore Memorial Hospital[2]	Somers Point	97%	64
Chilton Hospital	Pompton Plains	96%	81
Saint Peter's University Hospital	New Brunswick	96%	70
Cape Regional Medical Center	Cape May CH	95%	82
Saint Michael's Medical Center[2]	Newark	95%	174
Deborah Heart and Lung Center	Browns Mills	94%	68
Hackensack University Medical Center	Hackensack	94%	372
Morristown Memorial Hospital[2]	Morristown	94%	128
Robert Wood Johnson Univ Hosp Hamilton	Hamilton	94%	102
Saint Mary's Hospital - Passaic[2]	Passaic	94%	98
Southern Ocean Medical Center	Manahawkin	94%	86
Bayonne Hospital Center[2]	Bayonne	93%	60
Centrastate Medical Center	Freehold	93%	90
Capital Health System-Fuld Campus	Trenton	92%	87
Lourdes Medical Center of Burlington County	Willingboro	92%	116
South Jersey Healthcare-Elmer Hospital	Elmer	92%	36
Valley Hospital[2]	Ridgewood	92%	59
Virtua Mem Hosp of Burlington County	Mount Holly	92%	110
Capital Health System - Mercer Campus	Trenton	90%	83
JFK Medical Center	Edison	90%	178
Overlook Hospital[2]	Summit	89%	99
Kennedy University Hospital	Stratford	88%	170
Trinitas Regional Medical Center[2]	Elizabeth	85%	127

13. Discharge Instructions

Hospital Name	City	Rate	Cases
Atlanticare Reg Med Ctr-City Division[2]	Atlantic City	100%	468
Bayshore Community Hospital	Holmdel	100%	162
Christ Hospital	Jersey City	100%	312
Clara Maass Medical Center[2]	Belleville	100%	245
Community Medical Center[2]	Toms River	100%	190
Hoboken University Medical Center[2]	Hoboken	100%	176
Holy Name Medical Center[2]	Teaneck	100%	238
Monmouth Medical Center[2]	Long Branch	100%	182
Newark Beth Israel Medical Center[2]	Newark	100%	304
Newton Memorial Hospital	Newton	100%	151
Palisades Medical Center[2]	North Bergen	100%	169
Riverview Medical Center	Red Bank	100%	229
Saint Barnabas Medical Center[2]	Livingston	100%	268
Somerset Medical Center[2]	Somerville	100%	209
South Jersey Healthcare Reg Med Ctr[2]	Vineland	100%	253
South Jersey Healthcare-Elmer Hospital	Elmer	100%	98
UMDNJ University Hospital	Newark	100%	371
Underwood Memorial Hospital	Woodbury	100%	356
University Medical Center at Princeton[2]	Princeton	100%	164
Bayonne Hospital Center[2]	Bayonne	99%	156
Cooper University Hospital	Camden	99%	422
Deborah Heart and Lung Center	Browns Mills	99%	170
East Orange General Hospital[2]	East Orange	99%	176
Libertyhealth-Jersey City Med Ctr Campus[2]	Jersey City	99%	284
Lourdes Medical Center of Burlington County	Willingboro	99%	276
Memorial Hospital of Salem County	Salem	99%	151
Morristown Memorial Hospital[2]	Morristown	99%	249
Meadowlands Hospital Medical Center	Secaucus	98%	83
Our Lady of Lourdes Medical Center[2]	Camden	98%	245
Saint Joseph's Regional Medical Center	Paterson	98%	754
Warren Hospital	Phillipsburg	98%	111
Capital Health System-Fuld Campus	Trenton	96%	197
Hackettstown Regional Medical Center	Hackettstown	96%	117
Mountainside Hospital	Montclair	96%	255
Ocean Medical Center[2]	Brick	96%	223
Raritan Bay Medical Center[2]	Perth Amboy	96%	370
Shore Memorial Hospital[2]	Somers Point	96%	200
Capital Health System - Mercer Campus	Trenton	95%	197
Englewood Hospital and Medical Center	Englewood	94%	363
Saint Francis Medical Center	Trenton	94%	244
Hunterdon Medical Center	Flemington	93%	107
Chilton Hospital	Pompton Plains	92%	200
Overlook Hospital[2]	Summit	92%	247
Robert Wood Johnson Univ Hosp Hamilton	Hamilton	92%	314
Jersey Shore University Medical Center[2]	Neptune	91%	268
Trinitas Regional Medical Center[2]	Elizabeth	91%	235
Saint Clare's Hospital	Denville	90%	381
Saint Clare's Hospital - Sussex	Sussex	89%	46
Saint Mary's Hospital - Passaic[2]	Passaic	88%	247
Hackensack University Medical Center	Hackensack	87%	794
Robert Wood Johnson University Hospital	New Brunswick	87%	771
Saint Michael's Medical Center[2]	Newark	87%	243
VA New Jersey Health Care System	East Orange	87%	103
Virtua West Jersey Hospitals Berlin	Berlin	87%	588
Cape Regional Medical Center	Cape May CH	86%	230
Kennedy University Hospital	Stratford	85%	672
Kimball Medical Center	Lakewood	85%	199
Southern Ocean Medical Center	Manahawkin	85%	142
Centrastate Medical Center	Freehold	83%	230
Robert W Johnson Univ Hosp-Rahway	Rahway	83%	259
Virtua Mem Hosp of Burlington County	Mount Holly	83%	336
Valley Hospital[2]	Ridgewood	77%	244
JFK Medical Center	Edison	74%	436
Saint Peter's University Hospital	New Brunswick	67%	246

14. Evaluation of LVS Function

Hospital Name	City	Rate	Cases
Atlanticare Reg Med Ctr-City Division[2]	Atlantic City	100%	618
Bayshore Community Hospital	Holmdel	100%	284
Cape Regional Medical Center	Cape May CH	100%	302
Clara Maass Medical Center[2]	Belleville	100%	329
Community Medical Center[2]	Toms River	100%	325
Cooper University Hospital	Camden	100%	491
Deborah Heart and Lung Center	Browns Mills	100%	195
East Orange General Hospital[2]	East Orange	100%	276
Hackensack University Medical Center	Hackensack	100%	1086
Hackettstown Regional Medical Center	Hackettstown	100%	204
Hoboken University Medical Center[2]	Hoboken	100%	215
Holy Name Medical Center[2]	Teaneck	100%	335
Libertyhealth-Jersey City Med Ctr Campus[2]	Jersey City	100%	338
Memorial Hospital of Salem County	Salem	100%	186
Monmouth Medical Center[2]	Long Branch	100%	268
Mountainside Hospital	Montclair	100%	385
Newark Beth Israel Medical Center[2]	Newark	100%	359
Newton Memorial Hospital	Newton	100%	251
Our Lady of Lourdes Medical Center[2]	Camden	100%	307
Raritan Bay Medical Center[2]	Perth Amboy	100%	542
Riverview Medical Center	Red Bank	100%	320
Robert Wood Johnson University Hospital	New Brunswick	100%	1029
Robert W Johnson Univ Hosp-Rahway	Rahway	100%	430
Robert Wood Johnson Univ Hosp Hamilton	Hamilton	100%	413
Saint Barnabas Medical Center[2]	Livingston	100%	332
Saint Clare's Hospital	Denville	100%	560
Saint Francis Medical Center	Trenton	100%	297
Saint Mary's Hospital - Passaic[2]	Passaic	100%	335
Saint Michael's Medical Center[2]	Newark	100%	342
Shore Memorial Hospital[2]	Somers Point	100%	268
South Jersey Healthcare Reg Med Ctr[2]	Vineland	100%	322
South Jersey Healthcare-Elmer Hospital	Elmer	100%	122
UMDNJ University Hospital	Newark	100%	412
Underwood Memorial Hospital	Woodbury	100%	470
University Medical Center at Princeton[2]	Princeton	100%	255
VA New Jersey Health Care System	East Orange	100%	115
Virtua West Jersey Hospitals Berlin	Berlin	100%	859
Warren Hospital	Phillipsburg	100%	176
Bayonne Hospital Center[2]	Bayonne	99%	259
Capital Health System-Fuld Campus	Trenton	99%	242
Centrastate Medical Center	Freehold	99%	356
Chilton Hospital	Pompton Plains	99%	328
Christ Hospital	Jersey City	99%	430
Englewood Hospital and Medical Center	Englewood	99%	498
Hunterdon Medical Center	Flemington	99%	146
Jersey Shore University Medical Center[2]	Neptune	99%	362
JFK Medical Center	Edison	99%	650
Kennedy University Hospital	Stratford	99%	905
Kimball Medical Center	Lakewood	99%	329
Meadowlands Hospital Medical Center	Secaucus	99%	118
Palisades Medical Center[2]	North Bergen	99%	255
Saint Peter's University Hospital	New Brunswick	99%	328
Somerset Medical Center[2]	Somerville	99%	327
Southern Ocean Medical Center	Manahawkin	99%	234
Valley Hospital[2]	Ridgewood	99%	321
Lourdes Medical Center of Burlington County	Willingboro	98%	340
Morristown Memorial Hospital[2]	Morristown	98%	338
Ocean Medical Center[2]	Brick	98%	351
Saint Clare's Hospital - Sussex	Sussex	98%	53
Saint Joseph's Regional Medical Center	Paterson	98%	1003
Trinitas Regional Medical Center[2]	Elizabeth	98%	299
Virtua Mem Hosp of Burlington County	Mount Holly	98%	486
Overlook Hospital[2]	Summit	97%	360
Capital Health System - Mercer Campus	Trenton	95%	235

15. Smoking Cessation Advice

Hospital Name	City	Rate	Cases
Atlanticare Reg Med Ctr-City Division[2]	Atlantic City	100%	138

NOTE: Hospital profiles are in alphabetical order by state, then city, then hospital within the city; Rankings exclude hospitals with less than 25 cases except for patient surveys which excludes hospitals with less than 100 cases; (a) 100–299 cases; (1) The number of cases is too small to be sure how well a hospital is performing; (2) The hospital indicated that the data submitted for this measure were based on a sample of cases; (3) Data was collected during a shorter time period (fewer quarters) than the maximum possible time for this measure; (4) Suppressed for one or more quarters by CMS; (5) No data is available from the hospital for this measure; (6) Fewer than 100 patients completed the HCAHPS survey. Use these rates with caution, as the number of surveys may be too low to reliably assess hospital performance; (7) Survey results are based on less than 12 months of data; (8) Survey results are not available for this reporting period; (9) No or very few patients were eligible for the HCAHPS survey. The scores shown, if any, reflect a very small number of surveys; (10) A state average was not calculated because too few hospitals in the state submitted data; (11) There were discrepancies in the data collection process; Please refer to the User's Guide for a full explanation of data.

Bayshore Community Hospital	Holmdel	100%	26
Cape Regional Medical Center	Cape May CH	100%	46
Capital Health System - Mercer Campus	Trenton	100%	51
Capital Health System-Fuld Campus	Trenton	100%	56
Chilton Hospital	Pompton Plains	100%	38
Christ Hospital	Jersey City	100%	62
Clara Maass Medical Center[2]	Belleville	100%	37
Community Medical Center[2]	Toms River	100%	28
Cooper University Hospital	Camden	100%	140
Deborah Heart and Lung Center	Browns Mills	100%	36
East Orange General Hospital[2]	East Orange	100%	44
Englewood Hospital and Medical Center	Englewood	100%	40
Hackensack University Medical Center	Hackensack	100%	100
Hoboken University Medical Center[2]	Hoboken	100%	37
Holy Name Medical Center[2]	Teaneck	100%	26
Jersey Shore University Medical Center[2]	Neptune	100%	52
Kimball Medical Center	Lakewood	100%	34
Lourdes Medical Center of Burlington County	Willingboro	100%	41
Memorial Hospital of Salem County	Salem	100%	36
Monmouth Medical Center[2]	Long Branch	100%	31
Morristown Memorial Hospital[2]	Morristown	100%	36
Newark Beth Israel Medical Center[2]	Newark	100%	59
Our Lady of Lourdes Medical Center[2]	Camden	100%	61
Raritan Bay Medical Center[2]	Perth Amboy	100%	54
Riverview Medical Center	Red Bank	100%	31
Robert Wood Johnson University Hospital	New Brunswick	100%	117
Robert W Johnson Univ Hosp-Rahway	Rahway	100%	41
Robert Wood Johnson Univ Hosp Hamilton	Hamilton	100%	41
Saint Clare's Hospital	Denville	100%	51
Saint Francis Medical Center	Trenton	100%	65
Saint Joseph's Regional Medical Center	Paterson	100%	175
Saint Mary's Hospital - Passaic[2]	Passaic	100%	33
Saint Peter's University Hospital	New Brunswick	100%	39
Shore Memorial Hospital[2]	Somers Point	100%	32
South Jersey Healthcare Reg Med Ctr[2]	Vineland	100%	47
Southern Ocean Medical Center	Manahawkin	100%	48
Trinitas Regional Medical Center[2]	Elizabeth	100%	57
UMDNJ University Hospital	Newark	100%	164
Underwood Memorial Hospital	Woodbury	100%	70
VA New Jersey Health Care System	East Orange	100%	29
Virtua Mem Hosp of Burlington County	Mount Holly	100%	71
Virtua West Jersey Hospitals Berlin	Berlin	100%	113
Warren Hospital	Phillipsburg	100%	25
Kennedy University Hospital	Stratford	99%	141
Libertyhealth-Jersey City Med Ctr Campus[2]	Jersey City	99%	78
Saint Michael's Medical Center[2]	Newark	99%	67
JFK Medical Center	Edison	98%	59
Somerset Medical Center[2]	Somerville	97%	34

Pneumonia Care

16. Appropriate Initial Antibiotic

Hospital Name	City	Rate	Cases
Clara Maass Medical Center[2]	Belleville	100%	124
Mountainside Hospital	Montclair	100%	138
Newark Beth Israel Medical Center[2]	Newark	100%	70
Englewood Hospital and Medical Center	Englewood	99%	119
Hackensack University Medical Center	Hackensack	99%	270
Kimball Medical Center	Lakewood	99%	156
Lourdes Medical Center of Burlington County	Willingboro	99%	87
Our Lady of Lourdes Medical Center[2]	Camden	99%	87
Saint Clare's Hospital	Denville	99%	176
Saint Francis Medical Center	Trenton	99%	91
South Jersey Healthcare Reg Med Ctr[2]	Vineland	99%	93
Hackettstown Regional Medical Center	Hackettstown	98%	66
Libertyhealth-Jersey City Med Ctr Campus[2]	Jersey City	98%	59
Warren Hospital	Phillipsburg	98%	100
Community Medical Center[2]	Toms River	97%	124
Hunterdon Medical Center[2]	Flemington	97%	90
Kennedy University Hospital	Stratford	97%	520
Shore Memorial Hospital[2]	Somers Point	97%	120
South Jersey Healthcare-Elmer Hospital[2]	Elmer	97%	79
University Medical Center at Princeton[2]	Princeton	97%	102
Cape Regional Medical Center	Cape May CH	96%	289
Cooper University Hospital	Camden	96%	113
Monmouth Medical Center[2]	Long Branch	96%	116
Morristown Memorial Hospital[2]	Morristown	96%	78
Ocean Medical Center[2]	Brick	96%	95
Raritan Bay Medical Center[2]	Perth Amboy	96%	183
Robert W Johnson Univ Hosp-Rahway	Rahway	96%	141
Atlanticare Reg Med Ctr-City Division[2]	Atlantic City	95%	195
Bayshore Community Hospital	Holmdel	95%	133
Christ Hospital	Jersey City	95%	173
Holy Name Medical Center[2]	Teaneck	95%	96
Jersey Shore University Medical Center	Neptune	95%	146
Meadowlands Hospital Medical Center[2]	Secaucus	95%	75
Palisades Medical Center[2]	North Bergen	95%	80
Riverview Medical Center	Red Bank	95%	142
Saint Clare's Hospital - Sussex	Sussex	95%	40
Virtua West Jersey Hospitals Berlin	Berlin	95%	490
Saint Barnabas Medical Center[2]	Livingston	94%	87
Valley Hospital[2]	Ridgewood	94%	96
Capital Health System - Mercer Campus	Trenton	93%	95
Capital Health System-Fuld Campus	Trenton	93%	88
Centrastate Medical Center	Freehold	93%	193
JFK Medical Center	Edison	93%	262
Newton Memorial Hospital[2]	Newton	93%	84
Saint Mary's Hospital - Passaic[2]	Passaic	93%	95
Somerset Medical Center[2]	Somerville	93%	100
Southern Ocean Medical Center	Manahawkin	93%	103
VA New Jersey Health Care System	East Orange	93%	29
Virtua Mem Hosp of Burlington County	Mount Holly	93%	241
Bayonne Hospital Center[2]	Bayonne	92%	86
Bergen Regional Medical Center	Paramus	92%	38
Saint Michael's Medical Center[2]	Newark	92%	62
UMDNJ University Hospital[2]	Newark	92%	100
Underwood Memorial Hospital	Woodbury	92%	181
Memorial Hospital of Salem County	Salem	91%	110
Robert Wood Johnson University Hospital	New Brunswick	91%	185
Robert Wood Johnson Univ Hosp Hamilton	Hamilton	90%	203
Chilton Hospital[2]	Pompton Plains	89%	84
Overlook Hospital[2]	Summit	88%	162
Saint Joseph's Regional Medical Center	Paterson	86%	321
East Orange General Hospital[2]	East Orange	85%	41
Hoboken University Medical Center	Hoboken	85%	86
Trinitas Regional Medical Center[2]	Elizabeth	84%	94
Saint Peter's University Hospital[2]	New Brunswick	79%	179

17. Blood Culture Timing

Hospital Name	City	Rate	Cases
Bayshore Community Hospital	Holmdel	100%	228
Clara Maass Medical Center[2]	Belleville	100%	241
Community Medical Center[2]	Toms River	100%	216
Kimball Medical Center	Lakewood	100%	306
Saint Clare's Hospital	Denville	100%	278
Atlanticare Reg Med Ctr-City Division[2]	Atlantic City	99%	358
Jersey Shore University Medical Center	Neptune	99%	209
Monmouth Medical Center[2]	Long Branch	99%	175
Mountainside Hospital	Montclair	99%	243
Newark Beth Israel Medical Center[2]	Newark	99%	131
Newton Memorial Hospital[2]	Newton	99%	187
Ocean Medical Center[2]	Brick	99%	169
Riverview Medical Center	Red Bank	99%	219
Shore Memorial Hospital[2]	Somers Point	99%	168
Somerset Medical Center[2]	Somerville	99%	126
South Jersey Healthcare-Elmer Hospital[2]	Elmer	99%	99
Underwood Memorial Hospital	Woodbury	99%	267
Valley Hospital[2]	Ridgewood	99%	163
Virtua West Jersey Hospitals Berlin	Berlin	99%	818
Warren Hospital	Phillipsburg	99%	155
Bayonne Hospital Center[2]	Bayonne	98%	151
Christ Hospital	Jersey City	98%	234
East Orange General Hospital[2]	East Orange	98%	184
Hackensack University Medical Center	Hackensack	98%	258
Hackettstown Regional Medical Center	Hackettstown	98%	102
Holy Name Medical Center[2]	Teaneck	98%	188
Hunterdon Medical Center[2]	Flemington	98%	197
JFK Medical Center	Edison	98%	384
Meadowlands Hospital Medical Center[2]	Secaucus	98%	120
Memorial Hospital of Salem County	Salem	98%	105
Morristown Memorial Hospital[2]	Morristown	98%	168
Our Lady of Lourdes Medical Center[2]	Camden	98%	140
Robert Wood Johnson Univ Hosp Hamilton	Hamilton	98%	367
Saint Clare's Hospital - Sussex	Sussex	98%	53
Saint Francis Medical Center	Trenton	98%	132
Saint Michael's Medical Center[2]	Newark	98%	124
Trinitas Regional Medical Center[2]	Elizabeth	98%	131
Centrastate Medical Center	Freehold	97%	356
Chilton Hospital[2]	Pompton Plains	97%	154
Englewood Hospital and Medical Center	Englewood	97%	197
Kennedy University Hospital	Stratford	97%	1002
Lourdes Medical Center of Burlington County	Willingboro	97%	155
Raritan Bay Medical Center[2]	Perth Amboy	97%	343
Saint Barnabas Medical Center[2]	Livingston	97%	94
Saint Joseph's Regional Medical Center	Paterson	97%	521
Saint Mary's Hospital - Passaic[2]	Passaic	97%	180
South Jersey Healthcare Reg Med Ctr[2]	Vineland	97%	123
University Medical Center at Princeton[2]	Princeton	97%	68
Bergen Regional Medical Center	Paramus	96%	78
Libertyhealth-Jersey City Med Ctr Campus[2]	Jersey City	96%	74
Overlook Hospital[2]	Summit	96%	213
Robert W Johnson Univ Hosp-Rahway	Rahway	96%	254
Cooper University Hospital	Camden	95%	183
VA New Jersey Health Care System	East Orange	95%	56
Virtua Mem Hosp of Burlington County	Mount Holly	95%	351
Cape Regional Medical Center	Cape May CH	94%	482
Capital Health System - Mercer Campus	Trenton	94%	144
Palisades Medical Center[2]	North Bergen	93%	110
Robert Wood Johnson University Hospital	New Brunswick	92%	431
Capital Health System-Fuld Campus	Trenton	91%	162
Hoboken University Medical Center	Hoboken	90%	112
Southern Ocean Medical Center	Manahawkin	90%	248
UMDNJ University Hospital[2]	Newark	89%	250
Saint Peter's University Hospital[2]	New Brunswick	80%	204

18. Influenza Vaccine

Hospital Name	City	Rate	Cases
Atlanticare Reg Med Ctr-City Division[2]	Atlantic City	100%	166
Clara Maass Medical Center[2]	Belleville	100%	125
Community Medical Center[2]	Toms River	100%	120
Holy Name Medical Center[2]	Teaneck	100%	94
Newark Beth Israel Medical Center[2]	Newark	100%	88
Riverview Medical Center	Red Bank	100%	133
Saint Clare's Hospital - Sussex	Sussex	100%	30
South Jersey Healthcare Reg Med Ctr[2]	Vineland	100%	65
Valley Hospital[2]	Ridgewood	100%	92
Bayshore Community Hospital	Holmdel	99%	159
Ocean Medical Center[2]	Brick	99%	91
Our Lady of Lourdes Medical Center[2]	Camden	99%	85
Saint Clare's Hospital	Denville	99%	160
Saint Mary's Hospital - Passaic[2]	Passaic	99%	112
Shore Memorial Hospital[2]	Somers Point	99%	77
University Medical Center at Princeton[2]	Princeton	99%	97
Overlook Hospital[2]	Summit	98%	133
Robert W Johnson Univ Hosp-Rahway	Rahway	98%	157
Somerset Medical Center[2]	Somerville	98%	83
South Jersey Healthcare-Elmer Hospital	Elmer	98%	66
Bayonne Hospital Center[2]	Bayonne	97%	72
Hunterdon Medical Center[2]	Flemington	97%	94
Kimball Medical Center	Lakewood	97%	202
Palisades Medical Center[2]	North Bergen	97%	65
Saint Barnabas Medical Center[2]	Livingston	97%	95
VA New Jersey Health Care System	East Orange	97%	30
Warren Hospital	Phillipsburg	97%	130
Capital Health System - Mercer Campus	Trenton	96%	70
Englewood Hospital and Medical Center	Englewood	96%	170
Hackensack University Medical Center	Hackensack	96%	339
Hackettstown Regional Medical Center	Hackettstown	96%	51
Libertyhealth-Jersey City Med Ctr Campus[2]	Jersey City	96%	75
UMDNJ University Hospital	Newark	96%	101
Virtua West Jersey Hospitals Berlin	Berlin	96%	363
Bergen Regional Medical Center	Paramus	95%	42
Centrastate Medical Center	Freehold	95%	214
Raritan Bay Medical Center[2]	Perth Amboy	95%	156
Trinitas Regional Medical Center[2]	Elizabeth	94%	89
Jersey Shore University Medical Center	Neptune	93%	180
Kennedy University Hospital	Stratford	93%	417
Meadowlands Hospital Medical Center	Secaucus	93%	60
Robert Wood Johnson Univ Hosp Hamilton	Hamilton	93%	195
Saint Peter's University Hospital[2]	New Brunswick	93%	151
Capital Health System-Fuld Campus	Trenton	92%	77
East Orange General Hospital[2]	East Orange	92%	92
Monmouth Medical Center[2]	Long Branch	92%	93
Mountainside Hospital	Montclair	92%	142
Underwood Memorial Hospital	Woodbury	92%	167
Chilton Hospital[2]	Pompton Plains	91%	92
JFK Medical Center	Edison	91%	250
Memorial Hospital of Salem County	Salem	91%	125
Southern Ocean Medical Center	Manahawkin	91%	121
Newton Memorial Hospital[2]	Newton	90%	105
Virtua Mem Hosp of Burlington County	Mount Holly	90%	156
Morristown Memorial Hospital[2]	Morristown	89%	93
Christ Hospital	Jersey City	88%	124
Saint Francis Medical Center	Trenton	88%	75
Saint Michael's Medical Center[2]	Newark	88%	67
Cape Regional Medical Center	Cape May CH	87%	253
Robert Wood Johnson University Hospital	New Brunswick	87%	279
Lourdes Medical Center of Burlington County	Willingboro	86%	87
Saint Joseph's Regional Medical Center	Paterson	85%	344
Hoboken University Medical Center	Hoboken	82%	80

19. Initial Antibiotic Timing

Hospital Name	City	Rate	Cases
Hackettstown Regional Medical Center	Hackettstown	100%	82
Libertyhealth-Jersey City Med Ctr Campus[2]	Jersey City	100%	73
Memorial Hospital of Salem County	Salem	100%	180
Newark Beth Israel Medical Center[2]	Newark	100%	110
Newton Memorial Hospital[2]	Newton	100%	169
Palisades Medical Center[2]	North Bergen	100%	100
Saint Clare's Hospital - Sussex	Sussex	100%	49
Bayshore Community Hospital	Holmdel	99%	229
Clara Maass Medical Center[2]	Belleville	99%	203
Community Medical Center[2]	Toms River	99%	193
East Orange General Hospital[2]	East Orange	99%	168
Englewood Hospital and Medical Center	Englewood	99%	185
Kimball Medical Center	Lakewood	99%	274
Lourdes Medical Center of Burlington County	Willingboro	99%	147
Ocean Medical Center[2]	Brick	99%	154
Overlook Hospital[2]	Summit	99%	174
Saint Barnabas Medical Center[2]	Livingston	99%	132

NOTE: Hospital profiles are in alphabetical order by state, then city, then hospital within the city; Rankings exclude hospitals with less than 25 cases except for patient surveys which excludes hospitals with less than 100 cases; (a) 100–299 cases; (1) The number of cases is too small to be sure how well a hospital is performing; (2) The hospital indicated that the data submitted for this measure were based on a sample of cases; (3) Data was collected during a shorter time period (fewer quarters) than the maximum possible time for this measure; (4) Suppressed for one or more quarters by CMS; (5) No data is available from the hospital for this measure; (6) Fewer than 100 patients completed the HCAHPS survey. Use these rates with caution, as the number of surveys may be too low to reliably assess hospital performance; (7) Survey results are based on less than 12 months of data; (8) Survey results are not available for this reporting period; (9) No or very few patients were eligible for the HCAHPS survey. The scores shown, if any, reflect a very small number of surveys; (10) A state average was not calculated because too few hospitals in the state submitted data; (11) There were discrepancies in the data collection process; Please refer to the User's Guide for a full explanation of data.

Saint Clare's Hospital	Denville	99%	237
Somerset Medical Center[2]	Somerville	99%	139
University Medical Center at Princeton[2]	Princeton	99%	138
Virtua Mem Hosp of Burlington County	Mount Holly	99%	319
Virtua West Jersey Hospitals Berlin	Berlin	99%	741
Bayonne Hospital Center[2]	Bayonne	98%	135
Cape Regional Medical Center	Cape May CH	98%	454
Capital Health System - Mercer Campus	Trenton	98%	129
Hunterdon Medical Center[2]	Flemington	98%	149
Meadowlands Hospital Medical Center[2]	Secaucus	98%	103
Monmouth Medical Center[2]	Long Branch	98%	157
Our Lady of Lourdes Medical Center[2]	Camden	98%	122
Valley Hospital[2]	Ridgewood	98%	158
Warren Hospital	Phillipsburg	98%	153
Centrastate Medical Center	Freehold	97%	339
Christ Hospital	Jersey City	97%	184
Hackensack University Medical Center	Hackensack	97%	384
Jersey Shore University Medical Center	Neptune	97%	206
Kennedy University Hospital	Stratford	97%	860
Mountainside Hospital	Montclair	97%	215
Riverview Medical Center	Red Bank	97%	183
Robert Wood Johnson University Hospital	New Brunswick	97%	377
Robert Wood Johnson Univ Hosp Hamilton	Hamilton	97%	322
Saint Mary's Hospital - Passaic[2]	Passaic	97%	159
Shore Memorial Hospital[2]	Somers Point	97%	136
Bergen Regional Medical Center	Paramus	96%	46
Chilton Hospital[2]	Pompton Plains	96%	139
Cooper University Hospital	Camden	96%	160
Holy Name Medical Center[2]	Teaneck	96%	198
Robert W Johnson Univ Hosp-Rahway	Rahway	96%	230
VA New Jersey Health Care System	East Orange	96%	55
Atlanticare Reg Med Ctr-City Division[2]	Atlantic City	95%	313
Raritan Bay Medical Center[2]	Perth Amboy	95%	306
Saint Joseph's Regional Medical Center	Paterson	95%	540
South Jersey Healthcare-Elmer Hospital[2]	Elmer	95%	110
Southern Ocean Medical Center	Manahawkin	95%	210
Underwood Memorial Hospital	Woodbury	95%	255
Saint Francis Medical Center	Trenton	94%	134
Capital Health System-Fuld Campus	Trenton	93%	153
Morristown Memorial Hospital[2]	Morristown	93%	148
South Jersey Healthcare Reg Med Ctr[2]	Vineland	92%	177
JFK Medical Center	Edison	91%	418
Trinitas Regional Medical Center[2]	Elizabeth	91%	172
Hoboken University Medical Center	Hoboken	89%	132
UMDNJ University Hospital[2]	Newark	88%	239
Saint Michael's Medical Center[2]	Newark	87%	128
Saint Peter's University Hospital[2]	New Brunswick	82%	215

20. Pneumococcal Vaccine

Hospital Name	City	Rate	Cases
Atlanticare Reg Med Ctr-City Division[2]	Atlantic City	100%	234
Bayshore Community Hospital	Holmdel	100%	222
Clara Maass Medical Center[2]	Belleville	100%	189
Community Medical Center[2]	Toms River	100%	202
Hackettstown Regional Medical Center	Hackettstown	100%	85
Holy Name Medical Center[2]	Teaneck	100%	175
Kimball Medical Center	Lakewood	100%	309
Newark Beth Israel Medical Center[2]	Newark	100%	98
Palisades Medical Center[2]	North Bergen	100%	134
Saint Clare's Hospital	Denville	100%	243
Saint Clare's Hospital - Sussex	Sussex	100%	40
South Jersey Healthcare Reg Med Ctr[2]	Vineland	100%	108
Bergen Regional Medical Center	Paramus	99%	68
East Orange General Hospital[2]	East Orange	99%	141
Riverview Medical Center	Red Bank	99%	204
Shore Memorial Hospital[2]	Somers Point	99%	114
South Jersey Healthcare-Elmer Hospital[2]	Elmer	99%	98
Valley Hospital[2]	Ridgewood	99%	172
Ocean Medical Center[2]	Brick	98%	165
Our Lady of Lourdes Medical Center[2]	Camden	98%	118
Raritan Bay Medical Center[2]	Perth Amboy	98%	261
Robert W Johnson Univ Hosp-Rahway	Rahway	98%	241
Somerset Medical Center[2]	Somerville	98%	164
Trinitas Regional Medical Center[2]	Elizabeth	98%	126
University Medical Center at Princeton[2]	Princeton	98%	142
Virtua West Jersey Hospitals Berlin	Berlin	98%	677
Warren Hospital	Phillipsburg	98%	192
Englewood Hospital and Medical Center	Englewood	97%	264
Hunterdon Medical Center[2]	Flemington	97%	138
Overlook Hospital[2]	Summit	97%	228
Saint Mary's Hospital - Passaic[2]	Passaic	97%	186
Underwood Memorial Hospital	Woodbury	97%	249
Centrastate Medical Center	Freehold	96%	352
Hackensack University Medical Center	Hackensack	96%	482
Kennedy University Hospital	Stratford	96%	662
Memorial Hospital of Salem County	Salem	96%	132
Newton Memorial Hospital[2]	Newton	96%	178
Robert Wood Johnson University Hospital	New Brunswick	96%	411
Bayonne Hospital Center[2]	Bayonne	95%	138
Chilton Hospital[2]	Pompton Plains	95%	157
Meadowlands Hospital Medical Center[2]	Secaucus	95%	78
Saint Barnabas Medical Center[2]	Livingston	95%	130
UMDNJ University Hospital[2]	Newark	95%	60
Jersey Shore University Medical Center	Neptune	94%	246
JFK Medical Center	Edison	94%	346
Monmouth Medical Center[2]	Long Branch	94%	131
Robert Wood Johnson Univ Hosp Hamilton	Hamilton	94%	268
Saint Peter's University Hospital[2]	New Brunswick	94%	209
Hoboken University Medical Center	Hoboken	93%	120
Libertyhealth-Jersey City Med Ctr Campus[2]	Jersey City	93%	69
Morristown Memorial Hospital[2]	Morristown	93%	149
Saint Francis Medical Center	Trenton	93%	99
Cape Regional Medical Center	Cape May CH	91%	375
Capital Health System - Mercer Campus	Trenton	91%	81
Mountainside Hospital	Montclair	91%	233
VA New Jersey Health Care System	East Orange	91%	35
Capital Health System-Fuld Campus	Trenton	90%	98
Christ Hospital	Jersey City	89%	166
Lourdes Medical Center of Burlington County	Willingboro	89%	124
Southern Ocean Medical Center	Manahawkin	89%	225
Saint Michael's Medical Center[2]	Newark	88%	112
Virtua Mem Hosp of Burlington County	Mount Holly	88%	290
Saint Joseph's Regional Medical Center	Paterson	87%	444
Cooper University Hospital	Camden	85%	110

21. Smoking Cessation Advice

Hospital Name	City	Rate	Cases
Atlanticare Reg Med Ctr-City Division[2]	Atlantic City	100%	138
Bayonne Hospital Center[2]	Bayonne	100%	49
Bayshore Community Hospital	Holmdel	100%	97
Capital Health System - Mercer Campus	Trenton	100%	59
Capital Health System-Fuld Campus	Trenton	100%	65
Centrastate Medical Center	Freehold	100%	71
Chilton Hospital[2]	Pompton Plains	100%	37
Christ Hospital	Jersey City	100%	33
Clara Maass Medical Center[2]	Belleville	100%	61
Community Medical Center[2]	Toms River	100%	55
Cooper University Hospital	Camden	100%	88
East Orange General Hospital[2]	East Orange	100%	34
Englewood Hospital and Medical Center	Englewood	100%	32
Hackensack University Medical Center	Hackensack	100%	103
Holy Name Medical Center[2]	Teaneck	100%	30
Kennedy University Hospital	Stratford	100%	307
Kimball Medical Center	Lakewood	100%	80
Libertyhealth-Jersey City Med Ctr Campus[2]	Jersey City	100%	49
Lourdes Medical Center of Burlington County	Willingboro	100%	55
Memorial Hospital of Salem County	Salem	100%	91
Monmouth Medical Center[2]	Long Branch	100%	49
Morristown Memorial Hospital[2]	Morristown	100%	34
Newark Beth Israel Medical Center[2]	Newark	100%	45
Newton Memorial Hospital[2]	Newton	100%	44
Ocean Medical Center[2]	Brick	100%	46
Our Lady of Lourdes Medical Center[2]	Camden	100%	54
Riverview Medical Center	Red Bank	100%	59
Robert Wood Johnson University Hospital	New Brunswick	100%	82
Saint Barnabas Medical Center[2]	Livingston	100%	29
Saint Clare's Hospital	Denville	100%	71
Saint Clare's Hospital - Sussex	Sussex	100%	27
Saint Francis Medical Center	Trenton	100%	60
Saint Joseph's Regional Medical Center	Paterson	100%	103
Saint Mary's Hospital - Passaic[2]	Passaic	100%	41
Saint Peter's University Hospital[2]	New Brunswick	100%	67
Shore Memorial Hospital[2]	Somers Point	100%	56
Somerset Medical Center[2]	Somerville	100%	26
South Jersey Healthcare Reg Med Ctr[2]	Vineland	100%	59
South Jersey Healthcare-Elmer Hospital[2]	Elmer	100%	34
Southern Ocean Medical Center	Manahawkin	100%	55
Trinitas Regional Medical Center[2]	Elizabeth	100%	57
Underwood Memorial Hospital	Woodbury	100%	105
University Medical Center at Princeton[2]	Princeton	100%	29
Virtua Mem Hosp of Burlington County	Mount Holly	100%	95
Virtua West Jersey Hospitals Berlin	Berlin	100%	222
Warren Hospital	Phillipsburg	100%	71
Cape Regional Medical Center	Cape May CH	99%	155
Jersey Shore University Medical Center	Neptune	99%	93
JFK Medical Center	Edison	99%	90
Raritan Bay Medical Center[2]	Perth Amboy	99%	92
Robert Wood Johnson Univ Hosp Hamilton	Hamilton	99%	88
Saint Michael's Medical Center[2]	Newark	98%	42
UMDNJ University Hospital[2]	Newark	97%	173
Mountainside Hospital	Montclair	95%	61
Robert W Johnson Univ Hosp-Rahway	Rahway	95%	42
Overlook Hospital[2]	Summit	92%	37

Surgical Care Improvement Project

22. Appropriate VTP Within 24 Hours

Hospital Name	City	Rate	Cases
Clara Maass Medical Center[2]	Belleville	100%	259
Community Medical Center[2]	Toms River	100%	230
Our Lady of Lourdes Medical Center[2]	Camden	100%	152
Palisades Medical Center[2]	North Bergen	100%	83
Bayshore Community Hospital[2]	Holmdel	99%	123
Ocean Medical Center[2]	Brick	99%	222
Robert Wood Johnson University Hospital[2]	New Brunswick	99%	494
Cooper University Hospital[2]	Camden	98%	374
East Orange General Hospital	East Orange	98%	82
Holy Name Medical Center[2]	Teaneck	98%	238
Kennedy University Hospital[2]	Stratford	98%	383
Libertyhealth-Jersey City Med Ctr Campus[2]	Jersey City	98%	163
Memorial Hospital of Salem County[2]	Salem	98%	62
Overlook Hospital[2]	Summit	98%	208
Saint Francis Medical Center	Trenton	98%	117
University Medical Center at Princeton[2]	Princeton	98%	180
Virtua Mem Hosp of Burlington County[2]	Mount Holly	98%	427
Kimball Medical Center	Lakewood	97%	87
Monmouth Medical Center[2]	Long Branch	97%	192
Morristown Memorial Hospital[2]	Morristown	97%	209
Newark Beth Israel Medical Center[2]	Newark	97%	169
Shore Memorial Hospital[2]	Somers Point	97%	198
Somerset Medical Center[2]	Somerville	97%	220
Warren Hospital[2]	Phillipsburg	97%	93
Bergen Regional Medical Center	Paramus	96%	25
Lourdes Medical Center of Burlington County[2]	Willingboro	96%	138
Robert W Johnson Univ Hosp-Rahway	Rahway	96%	145
Saint Clare's Hospital	Denville	96%	376
Underwood Memorial Hospital[2]	Woodbury	96%	290
Virtua West Jersey Hospitals Berlin[2]	Berlin	96%	778
Capital Health System-Fuld Campus[2]	Trenton	95%	116
Hackettstown Regional Medical Center	Hackettstown	95%	76
Jersey Shore University Medical Center[2]	Neptune	95%	254
Riverview Medical Center[2]	Red Bank	95%	317
Saint Peter's University Hospital[2]	New Brunswick	95%	190
Atlanticare Reg Med Ctr-City Division[2]	Atlantic City	94%	285
Englewood Hospital and Medical Center[2]	Englewood	94%	311
Newton Memorial Hospital[2]	Newton	94%	152
UMDNJ University Hospital[2]	Newark	94%	194
Bayonne Hospital Center[2]	Bayonne	93%	97
Raritan Bay Medical Center[2]	Perth Amboy	93%	164
Hunterdon Medical Center[2]	Flemington	92%	139
Saint Barnabas Medical Center[2]	Livingston	91%	199
Saint Joseph's Regional Medical Center[2]	Paterson	91%	339
South Jersey Healthcare-Elmer Hospital[2]	Elmer	91%	67
VA New Jersey Health Care System[2]	East Orange	91%	119
Hoboken University Medical Center	Hoboken	90%	89
JFK Medical Center[2]	Edison	90%	408
Cape Regional Medical Center[2]	Cape May CH	89%	161
Chilton Hospital[2]	Pompton Plains	89%	186
Robert Wood Johnson Univ Hosp Hamilton[2]	Hamilton	89%	312
Southern Ocean Medical Center	Manahawkin	88%	163
Saint Michael's Medical Center[2]	Newark	87%	135
Valley Hospital[2]	Ridgewood	87%	219
Hackensack University Medical Center[2]	Hackensack	86%	148
Mountainside Hospital	Montclair	85%	206
South Jersey Healthcare Reg Med Ctr[2]	Vineland	84%	202
Deborah Heart and Lung Center	Browns Mills	83%	29
Christ Hospital[2]	Jersey City	82%	191
Trinitas Regional Medical Center[2]	Elizabeth	82%	186
Capital Health System - Mercer Campus[2]	Trenton	81%	157
Saint Mary's Hospital - Passaic[2]	Passaic	81%	171
Centrastate Medical Center[2]	Freehold	80%	284
Meadowlands Hospital Medical Center[2]	Secaucus	62%	47

23. Appropriate Hair Removal

Hospital Name	City	Rate	Cases
Atlanticare Reg Med Ctr-City Division[2]	Atlantic City	100%	1054
Bayonne Hospital Center[2]	Bayonne	100%	141
Bayshore Community Hospital[2]	Holmdel	100%	216
Bergen Regional Medical Center	Paramus	100%	33
Cape Regional Medical Center[2]	Cape May CH	100%	427
Capital Health System - Mercer Campus[2]	Trenton	100%	498
Capital Health System-Fuld Campus[2]	Trenton	100%	253
Chilton Hospital[2]	Pompton Plains	100%	438
Christ Hospital[2]	Jersey City	100%	400
Clara Maass Medical Center[2]	Belleville	100%	659
Community Medical Center[2]	Toms River	100%	601
Cooper University Hospital[2]	Camden	100%	1414
Deborah Heart and Lung Center	Browns Mills	100%	440
East Orange General Hospital	East Orange	100%	131
Englewood Hospital and Medical Center[2]	Englewood	100%	1154
Hackensack University Medical Center[2]	Hackensack	100%	658
Hackettstown Regional Medical Center	Hackettstown	100%	257
Hoboken University Medical Center	Hoboken	100%	187
Holy Name Medical Center[2]	Teaneck	100%	518
Hunterdon Medical Center[2]	Flemington	100%	418
Jersey Shore University Medical Center[2]	Neptune	100%	1179
Kimball Medical Center	Lakewood	100%	172
Libertyhealth-Jersey City Med Ctr Campus[2]	Jersey City	100%	472
Lourdes Medical Center of Burlington County[2]	Willingboro	100%	287
Meadowlands Hospital Medical Center[2]	Secaucus	100%	165

NOTE: Hospital profiles are in alphabetical order by state, then city, then hospital within the city; Rankings exclude hospitals with less than 25 cases except for patient surveys which excludes hospitals with less than 100 cases; (a) 100–299 cases; (1) The number of cases is too small to be sure how well a hospital is performing; (2) The hospital indicated that the data submitted for this measure were based on a sample of cases; (3) Data was collected during a shorter time period (fewer quarters) than the maximum possible time for this measure; (4) Suppressed for one or more quarters by CMS; (5) No data is available from the hospital for this measure; (6) Fewer than 100 patients completed the HCAHPS survey. Use these rates with caution, as the number of surveys may be too low to reliably assess hospital performance; (7) Survey results are based on less than 12 months of data; (8) Survey results are not available for this reporting period; (9) No or very few patients were eligible for the HCAHPS survey. The scores shown, if any, reflect a very small number of surveys; (10) A state average was not calculated because too few hospitals in the state submitted data; (11) There were discrepancies in the data collection process; Please refer to the User's Guide for a full explanation of data.

Memorial Hospital of Salem County[2]	Salem	100%	169
Monmouth Medical Center[2]	Long Branch	100%	523
Morristown Memorial Hospital[2]	Morristown	100%	840
Mountainside Hospital	Montclair	100%	522
Newark Beth Israel Medical Center[2]	Newark	100%	624
Newton Memorial Hospital[2]	Newton	100%	272
Ocean Medical Center[2]	Brick	100%	558
Our Lady of Lourdes Medical Center[2]	Camden	100%	516
Overlook Hospital[2]	Summit	100%	577
Palisades Medical Center[2]	North Bergen	100%	192
Raritan Bay Medical Center[2]	Perth Amboy	100%	330
Riverview Medical Center[2]	Red Bank	100%	990
Robert Wood Johnson University Hospital[2]	New Brunswick	100%	2018
Robert W Johnson Univ Hosp-Rahway	Rahway	100%	321
Robert Wood Johnson Univ Hosp Hamilton[2]	Hamilton	100%	782
Saint Barnabas Medical Center[2]	Livingston	100%	805
Saint Clare's Hospital	Denville	100%	872
Saint Clare's Hospital - Sussex	Sussex	100%	29
Saint Francis Medical Center	Trenton	100%	332
Saint Joseph's Regional Medical Center[2]	Paterson	100%	1127
Saint Michael's Medical Center[2]	Newark	100%	563
Shore Memorial Hospital[2]	Somers Point	100%	577
Somerset Medical Center[2]	Somerville	100%	541
South Jersey Healthcare-Elmer Hospital[2]	Elmer	100%	216
Southern Ocean Medical Center	Manahawkin	100%	313
UMDNJ University Hospital[2]	Newark	100%	435
Underwood Memorial Hospital[2]	Woodbury	100%	637
VA New Jersey Health Care System[2]	East Orange	100%	154
Valley Hospital[2]	Ridgewood	100%	807
Virtua Mem Hosp of Burlington County[2]	Mount Holly	100%	1517
Virtua West Jersey Hospitals Berlin[2]	Berlin	100%	1856
Warren Hospital[2]	Phillipsburg	100%	270
Centrastate Medical Center[2]	Freehold	99%	716
Kennedy University Hospital[2]	Stratford	99%	969
Saint Mary's Hospital - Passaic[2]	Passaic	99%	499
South Jersey Healthcare Reg Med Ctr[2]	Vineland	99%	515
Trinitas Regional Medical Center[2]	Elizabeth	99%	454
University Medical Center at Princeton[2]	Princeton	99%	507
JFK Medical Center[2]	Edison	98%	959
Saint Peter's University Hospital[2]	New Brunswick	81%	549

24. Appropriate Beta Blocker Usage

Hospital Name	City	Rate	Cases
Bayshore Community Hospital[2]	Holmdel	100%	53
Clara Maass Medical Center[2]	Belleville	100%	141
Community Medical Center[2]	Toms River	100%	178
Englewood Hospital and Medical Center[2]	Englewood	100%	429
Libertyhealth-Jersey City Med Ctr Campus[2]	Jersey City	100%	96
Newark Beth Israel Medical Center[2]	Newark	100%	192
Saint Barnabas Medical Center[2]	Livingston	100%	258
UMDNJ University Hospital[2]	Newark	100%	91
Capital Health System-Fuld Campus[2]	Trenton	99%	77
Hackettstown Regional Medical Center	Hackettstown	99%	75
Monmouth Medical Center[2]	Long Branch	99%	120
Riverview Medical Center[2]	Red Bank	99%	240
Robert Wood Johnson University Hospital[2]	New Brunswick	99%	746
Saint Joseph's Regional Medical Center[2]	Paterson	99%	365
University Medical Center at Princeton[2]	Princeton	99%	126
Jersey Shore University Medical Center[2]	Neptune	98%	496
Saint Francis Medical Center	Trenton	98%	158
Saint Michael's Medical Center[2]	Newark	98%	216
Trinitas Regional Medical Center[2]	Elizabeth	98%	129
VA New Jersey Health Care System[2]	East Orange	98%	45
Deborah Heart and Lung Center	Browns Mills	97%	267
Palisades Medical Center[2]	North Bergen	97%	64
Shore Memorial Hospital[2]	Somers Point	97%	206
Holy Name Medical Center[2]	Teaneck	96%	151
Kennedy University Hospital[2]	Stratford	96%	283
Overlook Hospital[2]	Summit	96%	124
Virtua West Jersey Hospitals Berlin[2]	Berlin	96%	507
Warren Hospital[2]	Phillipsburg	96%	76
Capital Health System - Mercer Campus[2]	Trenton	95%	139
Cooper University Hospital[2]	Camden	95%	460
Kimball Medical Center	Lakewood	95%	41
Lourdes Medical Center of Burlington County[2]	Willingboro	95%	74
Newton Memorial Hospital[2]	Newton	95%	93
Our Lady of Lourdes Medical Center[2]	Camden	95%	207
Robert W Johnson Univ Hosp-Rahway	Rahway	95%	110
Saint Clare's Hospital	Denville	95%	217
South Jersey Healthcare-Elmer Hospital[2]	Elmer	95%	73
Ocean Medical Center[2]	Brick	94%	154
Underwood Memorial Hospital[2]	Woodbury	94%	141
Virtua Mem Hosp of Burlington County[2]	Mount Holly	94%	506
Cape Regional Medical Center[2]	Cape May CH	93%	135
Chilton Hospital[2]	Pompton Plains	93%	122
Hackensack University Medical Center[2]	Hackensack	93%	247
Hunterdon Medical Center[2]	Flemington	93%	100
Somerset Medical Center[2]	Somerville	93%	161
East Orange General Hospital	East Orange	92%	25
Mountainside Hospital	Montclair	92%	113
Raritan Bay Medical Center[2]	Perth Amboy	92%	106
Robert Wood Johnson Univ Hosp Hamilton[2]	Hamilton	92%	289
Morristown Memorial Hospital[2]	Morristown	91%	287
Saint Mary's Hospital - Passaic[2]	Passaic	91%	155
Saint Peter's University Hospital[2]	New Brunswick	91%	173
Valley Hospital[2]	Ridgewood	90%	286
South Jersey Healthcare Reg Med Ctr[2]	Vineland	89%	117
Atlanticare Reg Med Ctr-City Division[2]	Atlantic City	88%	361
Southern Ocean Medical Center	Manahawkin	88%	110
Bayonne Hospital Center[2]	Bayonne	84%	38
Christ Hospital[2]	Jersey City	84%	75
JFK Medical Center[2]	Edison	84%	276
Hoboken University Medical Center	Hoboken	82%	44
Memorial Hospital of Salem County[2]	Salem	82%	38
Centrastate Medical Center[2]	Freehold	74%	200

25. Controlled Postoperative Blood Glucose

Hospital Name	City	Rate	Cases
Libertyhealth-Jersey City Med Ctr Campus[2]	Jersey City	100%	79
Saint Barnabas Medical Center[2]	Livingston	99%	168
Our Lady of Lourdes Medical Center[2]	Camden	98%	173
Atlanticare Reg Med Ctr-City Division[2]	Atlantic City	97%	143
Englewood Hospital and Medical Center[2]	Englewood	97%	259
Saint Michael's Medical Center[2]	Newark	97%	166
Valley Hospital[2]	Ridgewood	97%	169
Newark Beth Israel Medical Center[2]	Newark	96%	180
Hackensack University Medical Center[2]	Hackensack	95%	136
Jersey Shore University Medical Center[2]	Neptune	95%	402
Morristown Memorial Hospital[2]	Morristown	95%	168
Saint Joseph's Regional Medical Center[2]	Paterson	95%	253
UMDNJ University Hospital[2]	Newark	95%	74
Cooper University Hospital[2]	Camden	94%	394
Robert Wood Johnson University Hospital[2]	New Brunswick	88%	728
Deborah Heart and Lung Center	Browns Mills	86%	325
Saint Francis Medical Center	Trenton	80%	139
Saint Mary's Hospital - Passaic[2]	Passaic	80%	96

26. Prophylactic Antibiotic Timing

Hospital Name	City	Rate	Cases
Bayshore Community Hospital[2]	Holmdel	100%	117
Holy Name Medical Center[2]	Teaneck	100%	290
Libertyhealth-Jersey City Med Ctr Campus[2]	Jersey City	100%	211
Newark Beth Israel Medical Center[2]	Newark	100%	452
Riverview Medical Center[2]	Red Bank	100%	689
Robert W Johnson Univ Hosp-Rahway	Rahway	100%	161
Saint Clare's Hospital	Denville	100%	475
Saint Michael's Medical Center[2]	Newark	100%	367
Shore Memorial Hospital[2]	Somers Point	100%	359
Somerset Medical Center[2]	Somerville	100%	338
Cape Regional Medical Center[2]	Cape May CH	99%	272
Capital Health System - Mercer Campus[2]	Trenton	99%	344
Chilton Hospital[2]	Pompton Plains	99%	256
Clara Maass Medical Center[2]	Belleville	99%	386
Community Medical Center[2]	Toms River	99%	325
Englewood Hospital and Medical Center[2]	Englewood	99%	869
Hackensack University Medical Center[2]	Hackensack	99%	454
Hackettstown Regional Medical Center	Hackettstown	99%	176
Hoboken University Medical Center	Hoboken	99%	110
Jersey Shore University Medical Center[2]	Neptune	99%	826
Kennedy University Hospital[2]	Stratford	99%	562
Kimball Medical Center	Lakewood	99%	77
Monmouth Medical Center[2]	Long Branch	99%	326
Ocean Medical Center[2]	Brick	99%	301
Our Lady of Lourdes Medical Center[2]	Camden	99%	317
Overlook Hospital[2]	Summit	99%	371
Raritan Bay Medical Center[2]	Perth Amboy	99%	164
Saint Barnabas Medical Center[2]	Livingston	99%	537
Saint Mary's Hospital - Passaic[2]	Passaic	99%	271
Saint Peter's University Hospital[2]	New Brunswick	99%	338
South Jersey Healthcare-Elmer Hospital[2]	Elmer	99%	140
Trinitas Regional Medical Center[2]	Elizabeth	99%	210
University Medical Center at Princeton[2]	Princeton	99%	265
Warren Hospital[2]	Phillipsburg	99%	151
Capital Health System-Fuld Campus[2]	Trenton	98%	130
Deborah Heart and Lung Center	Browns Mills	98%	342
East Orange General Hospital	East Orange	98%	49
Hunterdon Medical Center[2]	Flemington	98%	291
Mountainside Hospital	Montclair	98%	249
Newton Memorial Hospital[2]	Newton	98%	164
Palisades Medical Center[2]	North Bergen	98%	103
Southern Ocean Medical Center	Manahawkin	98%	173
UMDNJ University Hospital[2]	Newark	98%	300
Valley Hospital[2]	Ridgewood	98%	538
Virtua West Jersey Hospitals Berlin[2]	Berlin	98%	1248
Atlanticare Reg Med Ctr-City Division[2]	Atlantic City	97%	546
Bayonne Hospital Center[2]	Bayonne	97%	35
Centrastate Medical Center[2]	Freehold	97%	415
Lourdes Medical Center of Burlington County[2]	Willingboro	97%	159
Meadowlands Hospital Medical Center[2]	Secaucus	97%	89
Memorial Hospital of Salem County[2]	Salem	97%	89
Robert Wood Johnson Univ Hosp Hamilton[2]	Hamilton	97%	515
Saint Joseph's Regional Medical Center[2]	Paterson	97%	878
Virtua Mem Hosp of Burlington County[2]	Mount Holly	97%	1155
Bergen Regional Medical Center	Paramus	96%	26
Cooper University Hospital[2]	Camden	96%	1148
JFK Medical Center[2]	Edison	96%	762
Robert Wood Johnson University Hospital[2]	New Brunswick	96%	1494
Saint Francis Medical Center	Trenton	96%	167
South Jersey Healthcare Reg Med Ctr[2]	Vineland	95%	290
Christ Hospital[2]	Jersey City	94%	224
Underwood Memorial Hospital[2]	Woodbury	94%	373
Morristown Memorial Hospital[2]	Morristown	93%	566
VA New Jersey Health Care System	East Orange	91%	93

27. Prophylactic Antibiotic Timing (Outpatient)

Hospital Name	City	Rate	Cases
Our Lady of Lourdes Medical Center	Camden	100%	446
Saint Michael's Medical Center	Newark	100%	150
Kimball Medical Center	Lakewood	99%	136
Newark Beth Israel Medical Center	Newark	99%	371
Shore Memorial Hospital	Somers Point	99%	146
Jersey Shore University Medical Center	Neptune	98%	703
Meadowlands Hospital Medical Center	Secaucus	98%	90
Newton Memorial Hospital	Newton	98%	50
Overlook Hospital	Summit	98%	462
Riverview Medical Center	Red Bank	98%	200
Robert W Johnson Univ Hosp-Rahway	Rahway	98%	121
Saint Clare's Hospital	Denville	98%	230
South Jersey Healthcare Reg Med Ctr	Vineland	98%	240
Trinitas Regional Medical Center	Elizabeth	98%	274
Community Medical Center	Toms River	97%	418
Englewood Hospital and Medical Center	Englewood	96%	334
Hackensack University Medical Center	Hackensack	96%	668
Hackettstown Regional Medical Center	Hackettstown	96%	52
Monmouth Medical Center	Long Branch	96%	294
South Jersey Healthcare-Elmer Hospital	Elmer	96%	49
Bayshore Community Hospital	Holmdel	95%	59
Virtua Mem Hosp of Burlington County	Mount Holly	95%	210
Warren Hospital	Phillipsburg	95%	107
Cooper University Hospital	Camden	94%	407
Saint Barnabas Medical Center	Livingston	94%	780
Saint Francis Medical Center	Trenton	94%	306
Virtua West Jersey Hospitals Berlin	Berlin	94%	361
Chilton Hospital	Pompton Plains	93%	174
Lourdes Medical Center of Burlington County	Willingboro	93%	92
Morristown Memorial Hospital	Morristown	93%	531
Atlanticare Reg Med Ctr-City Division	Atlantic City	92%	293
Capital Health System-Fuld Campus	Trenton	92%	92
Ocean Medical Center	Brick	92%	195
Somerset Medical Center	Somerville	92%	106
Valley Hospital	Ridgewood	92%	458
Clara Maass Medical Center	Belleville	91%	138
Kennedy University Hospital	Stratford	91%	267
Saint Mary's Hospital - Passaic	Passaic	91%	275
University Medical Center at Princeton	Princeton	91%	246
Hoboken University Medical Center	Hoboken	90%	143
Mountainside Hospital	Montclair	90%	192
Centrastate Medical Center	Freehold	89%	65
Memorial Hospital of Salem County	Salem	89%	38
Raritan Bay Medical Center	Perth Amboy	89%	130
Deborah Heart and Lung Center	Browns Mills	88%	260
Robert Wood Johnson University Hospital	New Brunswick	88%	793
Holy Name Medical Center	Teaneck	87%	193
Hunterdon Medical Center	Flemington	87%	180
JFK Medical Center	Edison	87%	400
Saint Joseph's Regional Medical Center	Paterson	87%	144
Cape Regional Medical Center	Cape May CH	86%	73
Southern Ocean Medical Center	Manahawkin	86%	69
Underwood Memorial Hospital	Woodbury	86%	105
Capital Health System - Mercer Campus	Trenton	85%	95
East Orange General Hospital	East Orange	84%	63
UMDNJ University Hospital	Newark	84%	160
Saint Peter's University Hospital	New Brunswick	79%	91
Christ Hospital	Jersey City	77%	204
Robert Wood Johnson Univ Hosp Hamilton	Hamilton	77%	131
Libertyhealth-Jersey City Med Ctr Campus	Jersey City	70%	43
Palisades Medical Center	North Bergen	70%	37

28. Prophylactic Antibiotic Selection

Hospital Name	City	Rate	Cases
Bayonne Hospital Center[2]	Bayonne	100%	36
Deborah Heart and Lung Center	Browns Mills	100%	354
Newark Beth Israel Medical Center[2]	Newark	100%	466
Community Medical Center[2]	Toms River	99%	323
Englewood Hospital and Medical Center[2]	Englewood	99%	871
Holy Name Medical Center[2]	Teaneck	99%	296
Hunterdon Medical Center[2]	Flemington	99%	289
Kennedy University Hospital[2]	Stratford	99%	565
Kimball Medical Center	Lakewood	99%	77
Robert W Johnson Univ Hosp-Rahway	Rahway	99%	162

NOTE: Hospital profiles are in alphabetical order by state, then city, then hospital within the city; Rankings exclude hospitals with less than 25 cases except for patient surveys which excludes hospitals with less than 100 cases; (a) 100–299 cases; (1) The number of cases is too small to be sure how well a hospital is performing; (2) The hospital indicated that the data submitted for this measure were based on a sample of cases; (3) Data was collected during a shorter time period (fewer quarters) than the maximum possible time for this measure; (4) Suppressed for one or more quarters by CMS; (5) No data is available from the hospital for this measure; (6) Fewer than 100 patients completed the HCAHPS survey. Use these rates with caution, as the number of surveys may be too low to reliably assess hospital performance; (7) Survey results are based on less than 12 months of data; (8) Survey results are not available for this reporting period; (9) No or very few patients were eligible for the HCAHPS survey. The scores shown, if any, reflect a very small number of surveys; (10) A state average was not calculated because too few hospitals in the state submitted data; (11) There were discrepancies in the data collection process; Please refer to the User's Guide for a full explanation of data.

Shore Memorial Hospital[2]	Somers Point	99%	360
Warren Hospital[2]	Phillipsburg	99%	151
Atlanticare Reg Med Ctr-City Division[2]	Atlantic City	98%	560
Bayshore Community Hospital[2]	Holmdel	98%	117
Clara Maass Medical Center[2]	Belleville	98%	386
East Orange General Hospital	East Orange	98%	51
Hoboken University Medical Center	Hoboken	98%	113
Jersey Shore University Medical Center[2]	Neptune	98%	846
Libertyhealth-Jersey City Med Ctr Campus[2]	Jersey City	98%	214
Memorial Hospital of Salem County[2]	Salem	98%	90
Morristown Memorial Hospital[2]	Morristown	98%	582
Ocean Medical Center[2]	Brick	98%	301
Our Lady of Lourdes Medical Center[2]	Camden	98%	324
Riverview Medical Center[2]	Red Bank	98%	693
Robert Wood Johnson University Hospital[2]	New Brunswick	98%	1520
Saint Francis Medical Center	Trenton	98%	175
Saint Michael's Medical Center[2]	Newark	98%	377
Saint Peter's University Hospital[2]	New Brunswick	98%	339
Somerset Medical Center[2]	Somerville	98%	339
South Jersey Healthcare-Elmer Hospital[2]	Elmer	98%	140
University Medical Center at Princeton[2]	Princeton	98%	266
Virtua Mem Hosp of Burlington County[2]	Mount Holly	98%	1155
Virtua West Jersey Hospitals Berlin[2]	Berlin	98%	1268
Chilton Hospital[2]	Pompton Plains	97%	257
Hackensack University Medical Center[2]	Hackensack	97%	462
Monmouth Medical Center[2]	Long Branch	97%	328
Overlook Hospital[2]	Summit	97%	378
Saint Barnabas Medical Center[2]	Livingston	97%	550
Saint Clare's Hospital	Denville	97%	478
Saint Joseph's Regional Medical Center[2]	Paterson	97%	878
UMDNJ University Hospital[2]	Newark	97%	320
Valley Hospital[2]	Ridgewood	97%	549
Cape Regional Medical Center[2]	Cape May CH	96%	274
Capital Health System - Mercer Campus[2]	Trenton	96%	345
Christ Hospital[2]	Jersey City	96%	226
Cooper University Hospital[2]	Camden	96%	1174
JFK Medical Center[2]	Edison	96%	763
Lourdes Medical Center of Burlington County[2]	Willingboro	96%	159
Mountainside Hospital	Montclair	96%	255
Robert Wood Johnson Univ Hosp Hamilton[2]	Hamilton	96%	520
Underwood Memorial Hospital[2]	Woodbury	96%	376
VA New Jersey Health Care System	East Orange	96%	92
Capital Health System-Fuld Campus[2]	Trenton	95%	127
Hackettstown Regional Medical Center	Hackettstown	95%	177
Newton Memorial Hospital[2]	Newton	95%	165
Saint Mary's Hospital - Passaic[2]	Passaic	95%	280
Southern Ocean Medical Center	Manahawkin	95%	172
Trinitas Regional Medical Center[2]	Elizabeth	95%	211
Raritan Bay Medical Center[2]	Perth Amboy	94%	164
South Jersey Healthcare Reg Med Ctr[2]	Vineland	94%	290
Centrastate Medical Center[2]	Freehold	93%	418
Palisades Medical Center[2]	North Bergen	93%	105
Bergen Regional Medical Center	Paramus	92%	26
Meadowlands Hospital Medical Center[2]	Secaucus	91%	90

29. Prophylactic Antibiotic Selection (Outpatient)

Hospital Name	City	Rate	Cases
Deborah Heart and Lung Center	Browns Mills	100%	254
Jersey Shore University Medical Center	Neptune	100%	692
Our Lady of Lourdes Medical Center	Camden	100%	445
Shore Memorial Hospital	Somers Point	100%	145
Bayshore Community Hospital	Holmdel	98%	57
Community Medical Center	Toms River	98%	417
Holy Name Medical Center	Teaneck	98%	181
Lourdes Medical Center of Burlington County	Willingboro	98%	88
Morristown Memorial Hospital	Morristown	98%	524
Newark Beth Israel Medical Center	Newark	98%	368
Newton Memorial Hospital	Newton	98%	52
Riverview Medical Center	Red Bank	98%	199
Robert W Johnson Univ Hosp-Rahway	Rahway	98%	120
Saint Francis Medical Center	Trenton	98%	291
Saint Michael's Medical Center	Newark	98%	150
South Jersey Healthcare-Elmer Hospital	Elmer	98%	47
Southern Ocean Medical Center	Manahawkin	98%	64
Clara Maass Medical Center	Belleville	97%	127
Kimball Medical Center	Lakewood	97%	135
Meadowlands Hospital Medical Center	Secaucus	97%	89
Monmouth Medical Center	Long Branch	97%	295
Raritan Bay Medical Center	Perth Amboy	97%	117
Cape Regional Medical Center	Cape May CH	96%	69
Hoboken University Medical Center	Hoboken	96%	137
Ocean Medical Center	Brick	96%	181
Palisades Medical Center	North Bergen	96%	26
Saint Barnabas Medical Center	Livingston	96%	762
Somerset Medical Center	Somerville	96%	97
Trinitas Regional Medical Center	Elizabeth	96%	271
University Medical Center at Princeton	Princeton	96%	228
Warren Hospital	Phillipsburg	96%	105
Atlanticare Reg Med Ctr-City Division	Atlantic City	95%	293
Capital Health System - Mercer Campus	Trenton	95%	83
Cooper University Hospital	Camden	95%	425
East Orange General Hospital	East Orange	95%	58
Valley Hospital	Ridgewood	95%	441
Centrastate Medical Center	Freehold	94%	192
Hackensack University Medical Center	Hackensack	94%	662
Hackettstown Regional Medical Center	Hackettstown	94%	52
JFK Medical Center	Edison	94%	373
Overlook Hospital	Summit	94%	459
Virtua West Jersey Hospitals Berlin	Berlin	94%	355
Saint Clare's Hospital	Denville	93%	229
South Jersey Healthcare Reg Med Ctr	Vineland	93%	237
Kennedy University Hospital	Stratford	92%	251
Underwood Memorial Hospital	Woodbury	92%	98
Chilton Hospital	Pompton Plains	91%	164
Libertyhealth-Jersey City Med Ctr Campus	Jersey City	91%	34
Memorial Hospital of Salem County	Salem	91%	34
Robert Wood Johnson University Hospital	New Brunswick	91%	777
Saint Mary's Hospital - Passaic	Passaic	91%	263
Englewood Hospital and Medical Center	Englewood	90%	338
Mountainside Hospital	Montclair	89%	178
Robert Wood Johnson Univ Hosp Hamilton	Hamilton	89%	109
Capital Health System-Fuld Campus	Trenton	87%	91
Hunterdon Medical Center	Flemington	86%	176
Christ Hospital	Jersey City	82%	206
UMDNJ University Hospital	Newark	81%	139
Saint Joseph's Regional Medical Center	Paterson	80%	128
Virtua Mem Hosp of Burlington County	Mount Holly	76%	209
Saint Peter's University Hospital	New Brunswick	75%	81

30. Prophylactic Antibiotic Stopped

Hospital Name	City	Rate	Cases
Bergen Regional Medical Center	Paramus	100%	26
Deborah Heart and Lung Center	Browns Mills	100%	317
Newark Beth Israel Medical Center[2]	Newark	100%	430
Holy Name Medical Center[2]	Teaneck	99%	270
Kennedy University Hospital[2]	Stratford	99%	549
Kimball Medical Center	Lakewood	99%	67
Robert W Johnson Univ Hosp-Rahway	Rahway	99%	154
Saint Michael's Medical Center[2]	Newark	99%	346
Shore Memorial Hospital[2]	Somers Point	99%	334
Virtua Mem Hosp of Burlington County[2]	Mount Holly	99%	1098
Clara Maass Medical Center[2]	Belleville	98%	363
Community Medical Center[2]	Toms River	98%	300
Cooper University Hospital[2]	Camden	98%	1112
Englewood Hospital and Medical Center[2]	Englewood	98%	839
University Medical Center at Princeton[2]	Princeton	98%	261
Bayshore Community Hospital[2]	Holmdel	97%	106
Hunterdon Medical Center[2]	Flemington	97%	286
Libertyhealth-Jersey City Med Ctr Campus[2]	Jersey City	97%	201
Monmouth Medical Center[2]	Long Branch	97%	312
Morristown Memorial Hospital[2]	Morristown	97%	521
Ocean Medical Center[2]	Brick	97%	283
Palisades Medical Center[2]	North Bergen	97%	88
Raritan Bay Medical Center[2]	Perth Amboy	97%	151
Riverview Medical Center[2]	Red Bank	97%	658
Virtua West Jersey Hospitals Berlin[2]	Berlin	97%	1208
Hackettstown Regional Medical Center	Hackettstown	96%	168
Jersey Shore University Medical Center[2]	Neptune	96%	774
Lourdes Medical Center of Burlington County[2]	Willingboro	96%	156
Overlook Hospital[2]	Summit	96%	364
Saint Clare's Hospital	Denville	96%	465
Saint Joseph's Regional Medical Center[2]	Paterson	96%	848
Somerset Medical Center[2]	Somerville	96%	322
Cape Regional Medical Center[2]	Cape May CH	95%	262
Chilton Hospital[2]	Pompton Plains	95%	229
Hackensack University Medical Center[2]	Hackensack	95%	433
Memorial Hospital of Salem County[2]	Salem	95%	82
Saint Barnabas Medical Center[2]	Livingston	95%	515
Saint Peter's University Hospital[2]	New Brunswick	95%	312
South Jersey Healthcare Reg Med Ctr[2]	Vineland	95%	281
South Jersey Healthcare-Elmer Hospital[2]	Elmer	95%	139
UMDNJ University Hospital[2]	Newark	95%	284
Valley Hospital[2]	Ridgewood	95%	519
Our Lady of Lourdes Medical Center[2]	Camden	94%	292
Robert Wood Johnson University Hospital[2]	New Brunswick	94%	1447
Robert Wood Johnson Univ Hosp Hamilton[2]	Hamilton	94%	484
Trinitas Regional Medical Center[2]	Elizabeth	94%	205
Underwood Memorial Hospital[2]	Woodbury	94%	359
Warren Hospital[2]	Phillipsburg	94%	145
Capital Health System - Mercer Campus[2]	Trenton	93%	331
East Orange General Hospital	East Orange	93%	44
Hoboken University Medical Center	Hoboken	93%	104
Southern Ocean Medical Center	Manahawkin	93%	161
Atlanticare Reg Med Ctr-City Division[2]	Atlantic City	92%	502
Centrastate Medical Center[2]	Freehold	92%	402
JFK Medical Center[2]	Edison	92%	747
VA New Jersey Health Care System	East Orange	92%	89
Christ Hospital[2]	Jersey City	91%	210
Mountainside Hospital	Montclair	91%	233
Capital Health System-Fuld Campus[2]	Trenton	90%	124
Newton Memorial Hospital[2]	Newton	88%	143
Saint Francis Medical Center	Trenton	87%	152
Meadowlands Hospital Medical Center[2]	Secaucus	86%	86
Saint Mary's Hospital - Passaic[2]	Passaic	84%	250
Bayonne Hospital Center[2]	Bayonne	82%	28

31. Recommended VTP Ordered

Hospital Name	City	Rate	Cases
Bayshore Community Hospital[2]	Holmdel	100%	123
Clara Maass Medical Center[2]	Belleville	100%	259
Community Medical Center[2]	Toms River	100%	230
Our Lady of Lourdes Medical Center[2]	Camden	100%	152
Palisades Medical Center[2]	North Bergen	100%	83
Cooper University Hospital[2]	Camden	99%	374
East Orange General Hospital	East Orange	99%	82
Kennedy University Hospital[2]	Stratford	99%	383
Libertyhealth-Jersey City Med Ctr Campus[2]	Jersey City	99%	163
Lourdes Medical Center of Burlington County[2]	Willingboro	99%	138
Ocean Medical Center[2]	Brick	99%	222
Overlook Hospital[2]	Summit	99%	209
Robert Wood Johnson University Hospital[2]	New Brunswick	99%	495
Somerset Medical Center[2]	Somerville	99%	220
Virtua Mem Hosp of Burlington County[2]	Mount Holly	99%	427
Holy Name Medical Center[2]	Teaneck	98%	238
Kimball Medical Center	Lakewood	98%	87
Memorial Hospital of Salem County[2]	Salem	98%	62
Monmouth Medical Center[2]	Long Branch	98%	192
Newark Beth Israel Medical Center[2]	Newark	98%	169
Saint Francis Medical Center	Trenton	98%	117
Shore Memorial Hospital[2]	Somers Point	98%	199
Underwood Memorial Hospital[2]	Woodbury	98%	290
University Medical Center at Princeton[2]	Princeton	98%	170
Warren Hospital[2]	Phillipsburg	98%	93
Atlanticare Reg Med Ctr-City Division[2]	Atlantic City	97%	285
Morristown Memorial Hospital[2]	Morristown	97%	209
Robert W Johnson Univ Hosp-Rahway	Rahway	97%	145
Saint Clare's Hospital	Denville	97%	376
Virtua West Jersey Hospitals Berlin[2]	Berlin	97%	780
Bayonne Hospital Center[2]	Bayonne	96%	97
Bergen Regional Medical Center	Paramus	96%	25
Englewood Hospital and Medical Center[2]	Englewood	96%	313
Hunterdon Medical Center[2]	Flemington	96%	139
Jersey Shore University Medical Center[2]	Neptune	96%	254
Riverview Medical Center[2]	Red Bank	96%	317
Saint Peter's University Hospital[2]	New Brunswick	96%	190
Southern Ocean Medical Center	Manahawkin	96%	163
UMDNJ University Hospital[2]	Newark	96%	194
Hoboken University Medical Center	Hoboken	95%	91
Raritan Bay Medical Center[2]	Perth Amboy	95%	165
VA New Jersey Health Care System[2]	East Orange	95%	120
Capital Health System-Fuld Campus[2]	Trenton	94%	117
Hackettstown Regional Medical Center	Hackettstown	94%	77
Newton Memorial Hospital[2]	Newton	94%	153
Saint Joseph's Regional Medical Center[2]	Paterson	94%	341
Valley Hospital[2]	Ridgewood	94%	219
Chilton Hospital[2]	Pompton Plains	93%	186
Robert Wood Johnson Univ Hosp Hamilton[2]	Hamilton	93%	312
Saint Barnabas Medical Center[2]	Livingston	93%	199
Cape Regional Medical Center[2]	Cape May CH	91%	164
JFK Medical Center[2]	Edison	91%	413
South Jersey Healthcare-Elmer Hospital[2]	Elmer	91%	67
Mountainside Hospital	Montclair	90%	207
Saint Michael's Medical Center[2]	Newark	90%	135
Hackensack University Medical Center[2]	Hackensack	87%	149
Capital Health System - Mercer Campus[2]	Trenton	84%	158
Christ Hospital[2]	Jersey City	83%	192
Deborah Heart and Lung Center	Browns Mills	83%	29
Saint Mary's Hospital - Passaic[2]	Passaic	83%	172
South Jersey Healthcare Reg Med Ctr[2]	Vineland	83%	204
Trinitas Regional Medical Center[2]	Elizabeth	83%	189
Centrastate Medical Center[2]	Freehold	81%	284
Meadowlands Hospital Medical Center[2]	Secaucus	62%	47

32. Urinary Catheter Removal

Hospital Name	City	Rate	Cases
Hackettstown Regional Medical Center	Hackettstown	100%	41
Libertyhealth-Jersey City Med Ctr Campus[2]	Jersey City	100%	63
Deborah Heart and Lung Center	Browns Mills	99%	91
Holy Name Medical Center[2]	Teaneck	99%	102
Saint Francis Medical Center	Trenton	99%	68
Jersey Shore University Medical Center[2]	Neptune	98%	260
Newark Beth Israel Medical Center[2]	Newark	98%	60
Shore Memorial Hospital[2]	Somers Point	98%	47
University Medical Center at Princeton[2]	Princeton	98%	133
Bayshore Community Hospital[2]	Holmdel	97%	39
Clara Maass Medical Center[2]	Belleville	97%	115
Riverview Medical Center[2]	Red Bank	97%	278
Robert W Johnson Univ Hosp-Rahway	Rahway	97%	32
Southern Ocean Medical Center	Manahawkin	97%	65
Christ Hospital[2]	Jersey City	96%	57

NOTE: Hospital profiles are in alphabetical order by state, then city, then hospital within the city; Rankings exclude hospitals with less than 25 cases except for patient surveys which excludes hospitals with less than 100 cases; (a) 100–299 cases; (1) The number of cases is too small to be sure how well a hospital is performing; (2) The hospital indicated that the data submitted for this measure were based on a sample of cases; (3) Data was collected during a shorter time period (fewer quarters) than the maximum possible time for this measure; (4) Suppressed for one or more quarters by CMS; (5) No data is available from the hospital for this measure; (6) Fewer than 100 patients completed the HCAHPS survey. Use these rates with caution, as the number of surveys may be too low to reliably assess hospital performance; (7) Survey results are based on less than 12 months of data; (8) Survey results are not available for this reporting period; (9) No or very few patients were eligible for the HCAHPS survey. The scores shown, if any, reflect a very small number of surveys; (10) A state average was not calculated because too few hospitals in the state submitted data; (11) There were discrepancies in the data collection process; Please refer to the User's Guide for a full explanation of data.

Englewood Hospital and Medical Center[2]	Englewood	96%	297
Hackensack University Medical Center[2]	Hackensack	96%	187
Monmouth Medical Center[2]	Long Branch	96%	130
Overlook Hospital[2]	Summit	96%	95
Virtua Mem Hosp of Burlington County[2]	Mount Holly	96%	457
Kennedy University Hospital[2]	Stratford	95%	164
Morristown Memorial Hospital[2]	Morristown	95%	168
Saint Michael's Medical Center[2]	Newark	95%	80
UMDNJ University Hospital[2]	Newark	95%	75
Atlanticare Reg Med Ctr-City Division[2]	Atlantic City	94%	217
Cape Regional Medical Center[2]	Cape May CH	94%	77
Cooper University Hospital[2]	Camden	94%	318
Saint Joseph's Regional Medical Center[2]	Paterson	94%	307
South Jersey Healthcare Reg Med Ctr[2]	Vineland	94%	113
Warren Hospital[2]	Phillipsburg	94%	71
Ocean Medical Center[2]	Brick	93%	130
Robert Wood Johnson Univ Hosp Hamilton	Hamilton	93%	242
Saint Barnabas Medical Center[2]	Livingston	93%	95
Saint Peter's University Hospital[2]	New Brunswick	93%	60
Valley Hospital[2]	Ridgewood	93%	209
Virtua West Jersey Hospitals Berlin[2]	Berlin	93%	401
Mountainside Hospital	Montclair	91%	97
Saint Mary's Hospital - Passaic[2]	Passaic	91%	86
Chilton Hospital[2]	Pompton Plains	90%	86
Raritan Bay Medical Center	Perth Amboy	90%	31
Saint Clare's Hospital	Denville	90%	168
Trinitas Regional Medical Center[2]	Elizabeth	90%	48
Our Lady of Lourdes Medical Center[2]	Camden	89%	94
Robert Wood Johnson University Hospital[2]	New Brunswick	89%	497
South Jersey Healthcare-Elmer Hospital[2]	Elmer	89%	84
Underwood Memorial Hospital[2]	Woodbury	89%	44
Centrastate Medical Center[2]	Freehold	87%	130
Hunterdon Medical Center[2]	Flemington	87%	90
Newton Memorial Hospital[2]	Newton	86%	56
Palisades Medical Center[2]	North Bergen	86%	35
Somerset Medical Center[2]	Somerville	85%	71
VA New Jersey Health Care System[2]	East Orange	84%	57
Lourdes Medical Center of Burlington County[2]	Willingboro	82%	61
Capital Health System-Fuld Campus[2]	Trenton	80%	51
Hoboken University Medical Center	Hoboken	80%	40
Capital Health System - Mercer Campus[2]	Trenton	76%	93
JFK Medical Center[2]	Edison	65%	118

Use of Medical Imaging

36. Combination Abdominal CT Scan

Hospital Name	City	Ratio	Cases
Lourdes Medical Center of Burlington County	Willingboro	0.014	576
Libertyhealth-Jersey City Med Ctr Campus	Jersey City	0.015	199
Virtua Mem Hosp of Burlington County	Mount Holly	0.016	808
Saint Peter's University Hospital	New Brunswick	0.017	348
Robert Wood Johnson University Hospital	New Brunswick	0.018	709
Saint Clare's Hospital - Sussex	Sussex	0.018	166
Morristown Memorial Hospital	Morristown	0.020	1618
Trinitas Regional Medical Center	Elizabeth	0.032	563
Community Medical Center	Toms River	0.036	1131
Newton Memorial Hospital	Newton	0.038	653
Atlanticare Reg Med Ctr-City Division	Atlantic City	0.040	805
Robert Wood Johnson Univ Hosp Hamilton	Hamilton	0.042	983
Deborah Heart and Lung Center	Browns Mills	0.043	47
Cooper University Hospital	Camden	0.045	1051
Kennedy University Hospital	Stratford	0.047	1770
Raritan Bay Medical Center	Perth Amboy	0.047	761
Virtua West Jersey Hospitals Berlin	Berlin	0.050	966
Bayshore Community Hospital	Holmdel	0.058	866
Southern Ocean Medical Center	Manahawkin	0.058	712
Saint Michael's Medical Center	Newark	0.060	500
Jersey Shore University Medical Center	Neptune	0.061	1271
Underwood Memorial Hospital	Woodbury	0.061	589
Warren Hospital	Phillipsburg	0.068	799
Hunterdon Medical Center	Flemington	0.069	737
Saint Barnabas Medical Center	Livingston	0.071	764
Memorial Hospital of Salem County	Salem	0.072	359
Centrastate Medical Center	Freehold	0.073	757
Riverview Medical Center	Red Bank	0.073	1238
Christ Hospital	Jersey City	0.078	709
Capital Health System-Fuld Campus	Trenton	0.079	430
Overlook Hospital	Summit	0.079	1249
Palisades Medical Center	North Bergen	0.081	492
Saint Francis Medical Center	Trenton	0.081	347
Hackettstown Regional Medical Center	Hackettstown	0.083	493
Saint Clare's Hospital	Denville	0.087	1911
Hackensack University Medical Center	Hackensack	0.088	2096
Monmouth Medical Center	Long Branch	0.094	757
Bayonne Hospital Center	Bayonne	0.099	779
Clara Maass Medical Center	Belleville	0.101	526
Hoboken University Medical Center	Hoboken	0.101	367
Robert W Johnson Univ Hosp-Rahway	Rahway	0.101	513
Saint Joseph's Regional Medical Center	Paterson	0.105	1029
Ocean Medical Center	Brick	0.106	1172
Valley Hospital	Ridgewood	0.106	2036
Saint Mary's Hospital - Passaic	Passaic	0.107	626
Capital Health System - Mercer Campus	Trenton	0.108	623
Mountainside Hospital	Montclair	0.109	724
Holy Name Medical Center	Teaneck	0.110	1103
South Jersey Healthcare-Elmer Hospital	Elmer	0.132	349
South Jersey Healthcare Reg Med Ctr	Vineland	0.138	898
Our Lady of Lourdes Medical Center	Camden	0.139	592
University Medical Center at Princeton	Princeton	0.140	769
Bergen Regional Medical Center[1]	Paramus	0.167	48
Englewood Hospital and Medical Center	Englewood	0.183	1560
Meadowlands Hospital Medical Center	Secaucus	0.196	107
UMDNJ University Hospital	Newark	0.332	617
Somerset Medical Center	Somerville	0.381	788
Kimball Medical Center	Lakewood	0.383	686
Cape Regional Medical Center	Cape May CH	0.433	559
Newark Beth Israel Medical Center	Newark	0.444	532
East Orange General Hospital	East Orange	0.483	203
Shore Memorial Hospital	Somers Point	0.512	484
Chilton Hospital	Pompton Plains	0.569	1053
JFK Medical Center	Edison	0.618	1192

37. Combination Chest CT Scan

Hospital Name	City	Ratio	Cases
Libertyhealth-Jersey City Med Ctr Campus	Jersey City	0.000	94
Lourdes Medical Center of Burlington County	Willingboro	0.000	281
Palisades Medical Center	North Bergen	0.000	291
Raritan Bay Medical Center	Perth Amboy	0.000	409
Saint Clare's Hospital - Sussex	Sussex	0.000	83
Saint Peter's University Hospital	New Brunswick	0.000	184
Virtua Mem Hosp of Burlington County	Mount Holly	0.000	321
JFK Medical Center	Edison	0.002	1081
Robert Wood Johnson University Hospital	New Brunswick	0.002	473
Centrastate Medical Center	Freehold	0.003	591
Christ Hospital	Jersey City	0.003	343
Jersey Shore University Medical Center	Neptune	0.003	1053
Saint Mary's Hospital - Passaic	Passaic	0.003	384
Cape Regional Medical Center	Cape May CH	0.004	242
Community Medical Center	Toms River	0.005	635
Chilton Hospital	Pompton Plains	0.006	780
Ocean Medical Center	Brick	0.006	927
Kennedy University Hospital	Stratford	0.007	995
Cooper University Hospital	Camden	0.008	914
Englewood Hospital and Medical Center	Englewood	0.008	1105
Somerset Medical Center	Somerville	0.008	634
Bayshore Community Hospital	Holmdel	0.010	629
Newton Memorial Hospital	Newton	0.010	419
Saint Michael's Medical Center	Newark	0.010	305
Saint Clare's Hospital	Denville	0.011	1398
Hackettstown Regional Medical Center	Hackettstown	0.012	253
Memorial Hospital of Salem County	Salem	0.012	258
Deborah Heart and Lung Center	Browns Mills	0.013	635
Riverview Medical Center	Red Bank	0.014	915
University Medical Center at Princeton	Princeton	0.014	499
Valley Hospital	Ridgewood	0.016	2050
Robert Wood Johnson Univ Hosp Hamilton	Hamilton	0.017	783
South Jersey Healthcare-Elmer Hospital	Elmer	0.017	299
Trinitas Regional Medical Center	Elizabeth	0.017	475
Hunterdon Medical Center	Flemington	0.018	832
Newark Beth Israel Medical Center	Newark	0.020	547
Saint Francis Medical Center	Trenton	0.022	225
Robert W Johnson Univ Hosp-Rahway	Rahway	0.023	440
Meadowlands Hospital Medical Center	Secaucus	0.027	75
Morristown Memorial Hospital	Morristown	0.030	1505
East Orange General Hospital	East Orange	0.033	121
Clara Maass Medical Center	Belleville	0.034	232
Bayonne Hospital Center	Bayonne	0.037	813
Virtua West Jersey Hospitals Berlin	Berlin	0.038	529
Saint Joseph's Regional Medical Center	Paterson	0.041	582
South Jersey Healthcare Reg Med Ctr	Vineland	0.041	559
Warren Hospital	Phillipsburg	0.042	520
Shore Memorial Hospital	Somers Point	0.043	278
Capital Health System - Mercer Campus	Trenton	0.044	520
Hoboken University Medical Center	Hoboken	0.046	217
UMDNJ University Hospital	Newark	0.046	261
Monmouth Medical Center	Long Branch	0.047	770
Bergen Regional Medical Center[1]	Paramus	0.051	39
Hackensack University Medical Center	Hackensack	0.051	2549
Overlook Hospital	Summit	0.055	1183
Southern Ocean Medical Center	Manahawkin	0.055	343
Holy Name Medical Center	Teaneck	0.059	828
Mountainside Hospital	Montclair	0.061	410
Saint Barnabas Medical Center	Livingston	0.071	324
Capital Health System-Fuld Campus	Trenton	0.083	314
Underwood Memorial Hospital	Woodbury	0.083	278
Kimball Medical Center	Lakewood	0.088	669
Our Lady of Lourdes Medical Center	Camden	0.098	224
Atlanticare Reg Med Ctr-City Division	Atlantic City	0.100	329

38. Follow-up Mammogram/Ultrasound

Hospital Name	City	Rate	Cases
Raritan Bay Medical Center	Perth Amboy	4.1%	880
Saint Joseph's Regional Medical Center	Paterson	5.2%	1132
Atlanticare Reg Med Ctr-City Division	Atlantic City	5.3%	891
Meadowlands Hospital Medical Center	Secaucus	5.6%	125
Bayonne Hospital Center	Bayonne	5.7%	795
Capital Health System - Mercer Campus	Trenton	5.9%	1215
South Jersey Healthcare Reg Med Ctr	Vineland	6.1%	1487
Trinitas Regional Medical Center	Elizabeth	6.1%	1048
Saint Francis Medical Center	Trenton	6.3%	457
Capital Health System-Fuld Campus	Trenton	6.4%	251
Newark Beth Israel Medical Center	Newark	6.7%	741
Warren Hospital	Phillipsburg	6.7%	1082
South Jersey Healthcare-Elmer Hospital	Elmer	6.8%	657
Monmouth Medical Center	Long Branch	7.2%	2020
Memorial Hospital of Salem County	Salem	7.3%	357
Community Medical Center	Toms River	7.8%	902
Bergen Regional Medical Center	Paramus	8.0%	87
East Orange General Hospital	East Orange	8.1%	395
Hackensack University Medical Center	Hackensack	8.4%	2174
Saint Michael's Medical Center	Newark	8.4%	645
Valley Hospital	Ridgewood	8.7%	1605
Saint Mary's Hospital - Passaic	Passaic	9.1%	729
Palisades Medical Center	North Bergen	9.3%	421
Robert W Johnson Univ Hosp-Rahway	Rahway	9.4%	266
Hoboken University Medical Center	Hoboken	9.6%	374
JFK Medical Center	Edison	9.6%	1516
Saint Clare's Hospital - Sussex	Sussex	9.7%	155
Centrastate Medical Center	Freehold	9.8%	784
Jersey Shore University Medical Center	Neptune	10.3%	545
Newton Memorial Hospital	Newton	10.3%	398
Robert Wood Johnson Univ Hosp Hamilton	Hamilton	10.7%	1096
UMDNJ University Hospital	Newark	10.7%	513
Somerset Medical Center	Somerville	10.8%	800
Kennedy University Hospital	Stratford	11.0%	836
Bayshore Community Hospital	Holmdel	11.1%	948
Lourdes Medical Center of Burlington County	Willingboro	11.1%	587
Virtua Mem Hosp of Burlington County	Mount Holly	11.2%	322
Mountainside Hospital	Montclair	11.8%	415
Chilton Hospital	Pompton Plains	12.0%	1959
Cooper University Hospital	Camden	12.1%	1293
Southern Ocean Medical Center	Manahawkin	12.1%	2049
Christ Hospital	Jersey City	12.5%	184
Hunterdon Medical Center	Flemington	12.5%	576
Saint Clare's Hospital	Denville	12.5%	2620
Cape Regional Medical Center	Cape May CH	12.9%	326
University Medical Center at Princeton	Princeton	12.9%	528
Ocean Medical Center	Brick	13.2%	816
Clara Maass Medical Center	Belleville	13.9%	374
Englewood Hospital and Medical Center	Englewood	13.9%	2429
Hackettstown Regional Medical Center	Hackettstown	14.5%	512
Virtua West Jersey Hospitals Berlin	Berlin	14.5%	152
Riverview Medical Center	Red Bank	16.2%	582
Shore Memorial Hospital	Somers Point	16.5%	704
Robert Wood Johnson University Hospital	New Brunswick	17.7%	379
Saint Peter's University Hospital	New Brunswick	18.0%	294
Underwood Memorial Hospital	Woodbury	18.6%	161
Our Lady of Lourdes Medical Center	Camden	19.0%	210
Overlook Hospital	Summit	20.0%	828
Morristown Memorial Hospital	Morristown	20.1%	648
Holy Name Medical Center	Teaneck	26.0%	1067

39. MRI for Low Back Pain

Hospital Name	City	Rate	Cases
UMDNJ University Hospital[1]	Newark	8.9%	56
Saint Michael's Medical Center[1]	Newark	13.6%	44
Robert W Johnson Univ Hosp-Rahway	Rahway	14.0%	86
Shore Memorial Hospital[1]	Somers Point	17.1%	41
Capital Health System-Fuld Campus	Trenton	18.2%	66
Atlanticare Reg Med Ctr-City Division	Atlantic City	19.2%	73
Riverview Medical Center	Red Bank	19.3%	83
Ocean Medical Center	Brick	19.5%	82
JFK Medical Center	Edison	20.4%	147
Morristown Memorial Hospital[1]	Morristown	21.2%	52
Virtua West Jersey Hospitals Berlin[1]	Berlin	21.3%	61
Hoboken University Medical Center[1]	Hoboken	22.2%	36
Hackensack University Medical Center	Hackensack	23.2%	95
Englewood Hospital and Medical Center	Englewood	23.4%	231
Chilton Hospital	Pompton Plains	23.7%	207
Kennedy University Hospital	Stratford	24.4%	90
Trinitas Regional Medical Center	Elizabeth	25.0%	64
Holy Name Medical Center	Teaneck	25.3%	312
University Medical Center at Princeton[1]	Princeton	25.5%	55
Hackettstown Regional Medical Center[1]	Hackettstown	25.9%	54
Overlook Hospital	Summit	25.9%	85
Bayonne Hospital Center	Bayonne	26.2%	141
Jersey Shore University Medical Center	Neptune	27.3%	88
Saint Joseph's Regional Medical Center	Paterson	27.6%	196
Kimball Medical Center	Lakewood	28.3%	106

NOTE: Hospital profiles are in alphabetical order by state, then city, then hospital within the city; Rankings exclude hospitals with less than 25 cases except for patient surveys which excludes hospitals with less than 100 cases; (a) 100–299 cases; (1) The number of cases is too small to be sure how well a hospital is performing; (2) The hospital indicated that the data submitted for this measure were based on a sample of cases; (3) Data was collected during a shorter time period (fewer quarters) than the maximum possible time for this measure; (4) Suppressed for one or more quarters by CMS; (5) No data is available from the hospital for this measure; (6) Fewer than 100 patients completed the HCAHPS survey. Use these rates with caution, as the number of surveys may be too low to reliably assess hospital performance; (7) Survey results are based on less than 12 months of data; (8) Survey results are not available for this reporting period; (9) No or very few patients were eligible for the HCAHPS survey. The scores shown, if any, reflect a very small number of surveys; (10) A state average was not calculated because too few hospitals in the state submitted data; (11) There were discrepancies in the data collection process; Please refer to the User's Guide for a full explanation of data.

Virtua Mem Hosp of Burlington County[1]	Mount Holly	28.3%	46
Somerset Medical Center	Somerville	28.4%	116
Valley Hospital	Ridgewood	28.4%	211
Bayshore Community Hospital	Holmdel	29.0%	100
Robert Wood Johnson Univ Hosp Hamilton	Hamilton	29.6%	108
Monmouth Medical Center	Long Branch	29.9%	87
Capital Health System - Mercer Campus[1]	Trenton	30.8%	26
Cape Regional Medical Center[1]	Cape May CH	31.9%	47
Southern Ocean Medical Center	Manahawkin	32.7%	55
Warren Hospital	Phillipsburg	32.9%	143
Memorial Hospital of Salem County	Salem	33.3%	69
Robert Wood Johnson University Hospital[1]	New Brunswick	33.3%	27
Palisades Medical Center	North Bergen	33.8%	65
South Jersey Healthcare Reg Med Ctr	Vineland	33.9%	115
Cooper University Hospital	Camden	34.6%	127
Saint Mary's Hospital - Passaic	Passaic	35.2%	54
Raritan Bay Medical Center[1]	Perth Amboy	35.5%	31
Mountainside Hospital	Montclair	38.3%	47
Community Medical Center	Toms River	41.1%	56
Newark Beth Israel Medical Center	Newark	41.3%	63

Survey of Patients' Hospital Experiences

40. Area Around Room 'Always' Quiet at Night

Hospital Name	City	Rate	Cases
Deborah Heart and Lung Center	Browns Mills	62%	300+
Meadowlands Hospital Medical Center	Secaucus	62%	300+
Capital Health System - Mercer Campus	Trenton	61%	300+
Newark Beth Israel Medical Center	Newark	60%	300+
South Jersey Healthcare Reg Med Ctr	Vineland	59%	300+
Christ Hospital	Jersey City	58%	(a)
Jersey Shore University Medical Center	Neptune	58%	300+
Memorial Hospital of Salem County	Salem	58%	300+
East Orange General Hospital	East Orange	57%	300+
Libertyhealth-Jersey City Med Ctr Campus	Jersey City	57%	300+
Robert Wood Johnson Univ Hosp Hamilton	Hamilton	56%	300+
Trinitas Regional Medical Center	Elizabeth	56%	300+
Morristown Memorial Hospital	Morristown	55%	300+
Saint Michael's Medical Center	Newark	55%	300+
Saint Peter's University Hospital	New Brunswick	55%	300+
South Jersey Healthcare-Elmer Hospital	Elmer	55%	300+
UMDNJ University Hospital	Newark	55%	300+
Saint Clare's Hospital - Sussex	Sussex	54%	(a)
Valley Hospital	Ridgewood	54%	300+
Cooper University Hospital	Camden	53%	300+
Centrastate Medical Center	Freehold	52%	300+
Englewood Hospital and Medical Center	Englewood	52%	300+
Holy Name Medical Center	Teaneck	52%	300+
Ocean Medical Center	Brick	52%	300+
Raritan Bay Medical Center	Perth Amboy	52%	300+
Riverview Medical Center	Red Bank	52%	300+
Southern Ocean Medical Center	Manahawkin	52%	300+
Mountainside Hospital	Montclair	51%	300+
Overlook Hospital	Summit	51%	300+
Shore Memorial Hospital	Somers Point	51%	300+
Underwood Memorial Hospital	Woodbury	51%	300+
Clara Maass Medical Center	Belleville	50%	300+
Kimball Medical Center	Lakewood	50%	300+
Saint Clare's Hospital	Denville	50%	300+
Virtua Mem Hosp of Burlington County	Mount Holly	50%	300+
Warren Hospital	Phillipsburg	50%	300+
Bayonne Hospital Center	Bayonne	49%	300+
Cape Regional Medical Center	Cape May CH	49%	300+
Hackensack University Medical Center	Hackensack	49%	300+
Hackettstown Regional Medical Center	Hackettstown	49%	300+
Lourdes Medical Center of Burlington County	Willingboro	49%	300+
Robert Wood Johnson University Hospital	New Brunswick	49%	300+
Saint Barnabas Medical Center	Livingston	49%	300+
Atlanticare Reg Med Ctr-City Division	Atlantic City	48%	300+
Bayshore Community Hospital	Holmdel	48%	300+
Community Medical Center	Toms River	48%	300+
Robert W Johnson Univ Hosp-Rahway	Rahway	48%	300+
Saint Mary's Hospital - Passaic	Passaic	48%	300+
University Medical Center at Princeton	Princeton	48%	300+
Hoboken University Medical Center	Hoboken	47%	300+
Hunterdon Medical Center	Flemington	47%	300+
Virtua West Jersey Hospitals Berlin	Berlin	47%	300+
Monmouth Medical Center	Long Branch	46%	300+
Somerset Medical Center	Somerville	46%	300+
Capital Health System-Fuld Campus	Trenton	45%	300+
Chilton Hospital	Pompton Plains	45%	300+
Kennedy University Hospital	Stratford	45%	300+
Our Lady of Lourdes Medical Center	Camden	45%	300+
Palisades Medical Center	North Bergen	45%	300+
Saint Joseph's Regional Medical Center	Paterson	45%	300+
Newton Memorial Hospital[11]	Newton	44%	300+
Saint Francis Medical Center	Trenton	44%	300+
JFK Medical Center	Edison	43%	300+
Bergen Regional Medical Center	Paramus	38%	(a)

41. Doctors 'Always' Communicated Well

Hospital Name	City	Rate	Cases
Capital Health System - Mercer Campus	Trenton	82%	300+
Deborah Heart and Lung Center	Browns Mills	81%	300+
Hoboken University Medical Center	Hoboken	81%	300+
Newark Beth Israel Medical Center	Newark	81%	300+
Saint Clare's Hospital - Sussex	Sussex	81%	(a)
South Jersey Healthcare-Elmer Hospital	Elmer	81%	300+
Holy Name Medical Center	Teaneck	80%	300+
Hunterdon Medical Center	Flemington	80%	300+
Meadowlands Hospital Medical Center	Secaucus	80%	300+
Mountainside Hospital	Montclair	80%	300+
Shore Memorial Hospital	Somers Point	80%	300+
Southern Ocean Medical Center	Manahawkin	80%	300+
Trinitas Regional Medical Center	Elizabeth	80%	300+
Valley Hospital	Ridgewood	80%	300+
Englewood Hospital and Medical Center	Englewood	79%	300+
Riverview Medical Center	Red Bank	79%	300+
Clara Maass Medical Center	Belleville	78%	300+
Hackensack University Medical Center	Hackensack	78%	300+
Hackettstown Regional Medical Center	Hackettstown	78%	300+
Jersey Shore University Medical Center	Neptune	78%	300+
JFK Medical Center	Edison	78%	300+
Robert Wood Johnson University Hospital	New Brunswick	78%	300+
Robert Wood Johnson Univ Hosp Hamilton	Hamilton	78%	300+
Saint Mary's Hospital - Passaic	Passaic	78%	300+
Saint Peter's University Hospital	New Brunswick	78%	300+
UMDNJ University Hospital	Newark	78%	300+
Virtua Mem Hosp of Burlington County	Mount Holly	78%	300+
Cape Regional Medical Center	Cape May CH	77%	300+
Capital Health System-Fuld Campus	Trenton	77%	300+
Chilton Hospital	Pompton Plains	77%	300+
Cooper University Hospital	Camden	77%	300+
Libertyhealth-Jersey City Med Ctr Campus	Jersey City	77%	300+
Morristown Memorial Hospital	Morristown	77%	300+
Overlook Hospital	Summit	77%	300+
Saint Barnabas Medical Center	Livingston	77%	300+
Saint Clare's Hospital	Denville	77%	300+
Somerset Medical Center	Somerville	77%	300+
South Jersey Healthcare Reg Med Ctr	Vineland	77%	300+
University Medical Center at Princeton	Princeton	77%	300+
Warren Hospital	Phillipsburg	77%	300+
Bayonne Hospital Center	Bayonne	76%	300+
Bayshore Community Hospital	Holmdel	76%	300+
Centrastate Medical Center	Freehold	76%	300+
Community Medical Center	Toms River	76%	300+
East Orange General Hospital	East Orange	76%	300+
Kimball Medical Center	Lakewood	76%	300+
Palisades Medical Center	North Bergen	76%	300+
Raritan Bay Medical Center	Perth Amboy	76%	300+
Atlanticare Reg Med Ctr-City Division	Atlantic City	75%	300+
Memorial Hospital of Salem County	Salem	75%	300+
Monmouth Medical Center	Long Branch	75%	300+
Robert W Johnson Univ Hosp-Rahway	Rahway	75%	300+
Saint Francis Medical Center	Trenton	75%	300+
Saint Michael's Medical Center	Newark	75%	300+
Underwood Memorial Hospital	Woodbury	75%	300+
Virtua West Jersey Hospitals Berlin	Berlin	75%	300+
Christ Hospital	Jersey City	74%	(a)
Kennedy University Hospital	Stratford	74%	300+
Ocean Medical Center	Brick	73%	300+
Saint Joseph's Regional Medical Center	Paterson	73%	300+
Newton Memorial Hospital[11]	Newton	72%	300+
Our Lady of Lourdes Medical Center	Camden	71%	300+
Lourdes Medical Center of Burlington County	Willingboro	68%	300+
Bergen Regional Medical Center	Paramus	55%	(a)

42. Home Recovery Information Given

Hospital Name	City	Rate	Cases
Atlanticare Reg Med Ctr-City Division	Atlantic City	89%	300+
Deborah Heart and Lung Center	Browns Mills	88%	300+
South Jersey Healthcare-Elmer Hospital	Elmer	86%	300+
Hunterdon Medical Center	Flemington	84%	300+
Hackettstown Regional Medical Center	Hackettstown	83%	300+
Robert Wood Johnson Univ Hosp Hamilton	Hamilton	83%	300+
South Jersey Healthcare Reg Med Ctr	Vineland	83%	300+
Cooper University Hospital	Camden	82%	300+
Shore Memorial Hospital	Somers Point	82%	300+
Southern Ocean Medical Center	Manahawkin	82%	300+
Virtua Mem Hosp of Burlington County	Mount Holly	82%	300+
Hackensack University Medical Center	Hackensack	81%	300+
Hoboken University Medical Center	Hoboken	81%	300+
Holy Name Medical Center	Teaneck	81%	300+
Kimball Medical Center	Lakewood	81%	300+
Morristown Memorial Hospital	Morristown	81%	300+
Overlook Hospital	Summit	81%	300+
Riverview Medical Center	Red Bank	81%	300+
Robert Wood Johnson University Hospital	New Brunswick	81%	300+
Centrastate Medical Center	Freehold	80%	300+
Community Medical Center	Toms River	80%	300+
Newton Memorial Hospital[11]	Newton	80%	300+
Saint Joseph's Regional Medical Center	Paterson	80%	300+
Valley Hospital	Ridgewood	80%	300+
Bayonne Hospital Center	Bayonne	79%	300+
Bayshore Community Hospital	Holmdel	79%	300+
Cape Regional Medical Center	Cape May CH	79%	300+
Memorial Hospital of Salem County	Salem	79%	300+
Newark Beth Israel Medical Center	Newark	79%	300+
Ocean Medical Center	Brick	79%	300+
Underwood Memorial Hospital	Woodbury	79%	300+
University Medical Center at Princeton	Princeton	79%	300+
Robert W Johnson Univ Hosp-Rahway	Rahway	78%	300+
Saint Clare's Hospital	Denville	78%	300+
UMDNJ University Hospital	Newark	78%	300+
Virtua West Jersey Hospitals Berlin	Berlin	78%	300+
Warren Hospital	Phillipsburg	78%	300+
Capital Health System - Mercer Campus	Trenton	77%	300+
Jersey Shore University Medical Center	Neptune	77%	300+
Kennedy University Hospital	Stratford	77%	300+
Raritan Bay Medical Center	Perth Amboy	77%	300+
Saint Clare's Hospital - Sussex	Sussex	77%	(a)
Saint Francis Medical Center	Trenton	77%	300+
Chilton Hospital	Pompton Plains	76%	300+
JFK Medical Center	Edison	76%	300+
Libertyhealth-Jersey City Med Ctr Campus	Jersey City	76%	300+
Saint Barnabas Medical Center	Livingston	76%	300+
Saint Peter's University Hospital	New Brunswick	76%	300+
Meadowlands Hospital Medical Center	Secaucus	75%	300+
Our Lady of Lourdes Medical Center	Camden	75%	300+
Capital Health System-Fuld Campus	Trenton	74%	300+
East Orange General Hospital	East Orange	74%	300+
Englewood Hospital and Medical Center	Englewood	74%	300+
Palisades Medical Center	North Bergen	74%	300+
Trinitas Regional Medical Center	Elizabeth	74%	300+
Saint Mary's Hospital - Passaic	Passaic	73%	300+
Somerset Medical Center	Somerville	73%	300+
Christ Hospital	Jersey City	72%	(a)
Clara Maass Medical Center	Belleville	72%	300+
Monmouth Medical Center	Long Branch	72%	300+
Mountainside Hospital	Montclair	71%	300+
Lourdes Medical Center of Burlington County	Willingboro	70%	300+
Saint Michael's Medical Center	Newark	69%	300+
Bergen Regional Medical Center	Paramus	63%	(a)

43. Hospital Given 9 or 10 on 10 Point Scale

Hospital Name	City	Rate	Cases
Deborah Heart and Lung Center	Browns Mills	82%	300+
Valley Hospital	Ridgewood	76%	300+
Morristown Memorial Hospital	Morristown	75%	300+
South Jersey Healthcare-Elmer Hospital	Elmer	73%	300+
Hackensack University Medical Center	Hackensack	72%	300+
Hunterdon Medical Center	Flemington	71%	300+
Centrastate Medical Center	Freehold	69%	300+
Jersey Shore University Medical Center	Neptune	69%	300+
Saint Clare's Hospital - Sussex	Sussex	69%	(a)
Robert Wood Johnson University Hospital	New Brunswick	68%	300+
Saint Peter's University Hospital	New Brunswick	68%	300+
Virtua Mem Hosp of Burlington County	Mount Holly	68%	300+
Englewood Hospital and Medical Center	Englewood	67%	300+
Hackettstown Regional Medical Center	Hackettstown	67%	300+
Holy Name Medical Center	Teaneck	67%	300+
Shore Memorial Hospital	Somers Point	67%	300+
Atlanticare Reg Med Ctr-City Division	Atlantic City	66%	300+
Ocean Medical Center	Brick	66%	300+
Overlook Hospital	Summit	66%	300+
Virtua West Jersey Hospitals Berlin	Berlin	66%	300+
Cooper University Hospital	Camden	65%	300+
South Jersey Healthcare Reg Med Ctr	Vineland	65%	300+
Robert Wood Johnson Univ Hosp Hamilton	Hamilton	64%	300+
Saint Barnabas Medical Center	Livingston	64%	300+
Southern Ocean Medical Center	Manahawkin	64%	300+
Cape Regional Medical Center	Cape May CH	63%	300+
Capital Health System - Mercer Campus	Trenton	63%	300+
Newton Memorial Hospital[11]	Newton	63%	300+
Riverview Medical Center	Red Bank	63%	300+
Libertyhealth-Jersey City Med Ctr Campus	Jersey City	62%	300+
Meadowlands Hospital Medical Center	Secaucus	62%	300+
Newark Beth Israel Medical Center	Newark	62%	300+
Our Lady of Lourdes Medical Center	Camden	62%	300+
Trinitas Regional Medical Center	Elizabeth	62%	300+
Chilton Hospital	Pompton Plains	61%	300+
Hoboken University Medical Center	Hoboken	61%	300+
Mountainside Hospital	Montclair	60%	300+
Saint Clare's Hospital	Denville	60%	300+
Somerset Medical Center	Somerville	60%	300+
Underwood Memorial Hospital	Woodbury	60%	300+
University Medical Center at Princeton	Princeton	60%	300+
Capital Health System-Fuld Campus	Trenton	58%	300+
UMDNJ University Hospital	Newark	58%	300+
Community Medical Center	Toms River	57%	300+

NOTE: Hospital profiles are in alphabetical order by state, then city, then hospital within the city; Rankings exclude hospitals with less than 25 cases except for patient surveys which excludes hospitals with less than 100 cases; (a) 100–299 cases; (1) The number of cases is too small to be sure how well a hospital is performing; (2) The hospital indicated that the data submitted for this measure were based on a sample of cases; (3) Data was collected during a shorter time period (fewer quarters) than the maximum possible time for this measure; (4) Suppressed for one or more quarters by CMS; (5) No data is available from the hospital for this measure; (6) Fewer than 100 patients completed the HCAHPS survey. Use these rates with caution, as the number of surveys may be too low to reliably assess hospital performance; (7) Survey results are based on less than 12 months of data; (8) Survey results are not available for this reporting period; (9) No or very few patients were eligible for the HCAHPS survey. The scores shown, if any, reflect a very small number of surveys; (10) A state average was not calculated because too few hospitals in the state submitted data; (11) There were discrepancies in the data collection process; Please refer to the User's Guide for a full explanation of data.

Raritan Bay Medical Center	Perth Amboy	57%	300+
Saint Joseph's Regional Medical Center	Paterson	57%	300+
Warren Hospital	Phillipsburg	57%	300+
Kennedy University Hospital	Stratford	56%	300+
Robert W Johnson Univ Hosp-Rahway	Rahway	56%	300+
Saint Francis Medical Center	Trenton	56%	300+
Christ Hospital	Jersey City	54%	(a)
Clara Maass Medical Center	Belleville	54%	300+
JFK Medical Center	Edison	54%	300+
Kimball Medical Center	Lakewood	54%	300+
Monmouth Medical Center	Long Branch	54%	300+
Bayshore Community Hospital	Holmdel	53%	300+
Saint Michael's Medical Center	Newark	53%	300+
Memorial Hospital of Salem County	Salem	52%	300+
East Orange General Hospital	East Orange	51%	300+
Palisades Medical Center	North Bergen	50%	300+
Bayonne Hospital Center	Bayonne	47%	300+
Saint Mary's Hospital - Passaic	Passaic	47%	300+
Lourdes Medical Center of Burlington County	Willingboro	46%	300+
Bergen Regional Medical Center	Paramus	32%	(a)

44. Meds 'Always' Explained Before Given

Hospital Name	City	Rate	Cases
Deborah Heart and Lung Center	Browns Mills	63%	300+
Southern Ocean Medical Center	Manahawkin	63%	300+
Cape Regional Medical Center	Cape May CH	62%	300+
Saint Peter's University Hospital	New Brunswick	62%	300+
Capital Health System - Mercer Campus	Trenton	61%	300+
Hunterdon Medical Center	Flemington	61%	300+
Riverview Medical Center	Red Bank	61%	300+
Saint Clare's Hospital - Sussex	Sussex	61%	(a)
South Jersey Healthcare-Elmer Hospital	Elmer	61%	300+
Underwood Memorial Hospital	Woodbury	61%	300+
Virtua Mem Hosp of Burlington County	Mount Holly	61%	300+
Centrastate Medical Center	Freehold	60%	300+
Community Medical Center	Toms River	60%	300+
Jersey Shore University Medical Center	Neptune	60%	300+
Saint Barnabas Medical Center	Livingston	60%	300+
Hackensack University Medical Center	Hackensack	59%	300+
Meadowlands Hospital Medical Center	Secaucus	59%	300+
Morristown Memorial Hospital	Morristown	59%	300+
Newark Beth Israel Medical Center	Newark	59%	300+
Robert Wood Johnson University Hospital	New Brunswick	59%	300+
Atlanticare Reg Med Ctr-City Division	Atlantic City	58%	300+
Ocean Medical Center	Brick	58%	300+
Robert Wood Johnson Univ Hosp Hamilton	Hamilton	58%	300+
Shore Memorial Hospital	Somers Point	58%	300+
Valley Hospital	Ridgewood	58%	300+
Virtua West Jersey Hospitals Berlin	Berlin	58%	300+
Capital Health System-Fuld Campus	Trenton	57%	300+
Clara Maass Medical Center	Belleville	57%	300+
Cooper University Hospital	Camden	57%	300+
Memorial Hospital of Salem County	Salem	57%	300+
Mountainside Hospital	Montclair	57%	300+
South Jersey Healthcare Reg Med Ctr	Vineland	57%	300+
Trinitas Regional Medical Center	Elizabeth	57%	300+
University Medical Center at Princeton	Princeton	57%	300+
Warren Hospital	Phillipsburg	57%	300+
Englewood Hospital and Medical Center	Englewood	56%	300+
Kennedy University Hospital	Stratford	56%	300+
Libertyhealth-Jersey City Med Ctr Campus	Jersey City	56%	300+
Robert W Johnson Univ Hosp-Rahway	Rahway	56%	300+
Somerset Medical Center	Somerville	56%	300+
Chilton Hospital	Pompton Plains	55%	300+
Holy Name Medical Center	Teaneck	55%	300+
JFK Medical Center	Edison	55%	300+
Monmouth Medical Center	Long Branch	55%	300+
UMDNJ University Hospital	Newark	55%	300+
East Orange General Hospital	East Orange	54%	300+
Hoboken University Medical Center	Hoboken	54%	300+
Our Lady of Lourdes Medical Center	Camden	54%	300+
Overlook Hospital	Summit	54%	300+
Raritan Bay Medical Center	Perth Amboy	54%	300+
Saint Clare's Hospital	Denville	54%	300+
Hackettstown Regional Medical Center	Hackettstown	53%	300+
Newton Memorial Hospital[11]	Newton	52%	300+
Saint Francis Medical Center	Trenton	52%	300+
Saint Joseph's Regional Medical Center	Paterson	52%	300+
Bayonne Hospital Center	Bayonne	51%	300+
Kimball Medical Center	Lakewood	51%	300+
Christ Hospital	Jersey City	49%	(a)
Saint Mary's Hospital - Passaic	Passaic	49%	300+
Saint Michael's Medical Center	Newark	49%	300+
Lourdes Medical Center of Burlington County	Willingboro	48%	300+
Palisades Medical Center	North Bergen	46%	300+
Bayshore Community Hospital	Holmdel	43%	300+
Bergen Regional Medical Center	Paramus	43%	(a)

45. Nurses 'Always' Communicated Well

Hospital Name	City	Rate	Cases
Deborah Heart and Lung Center	Browns Mills	82%	300+
Valley Hospital	Ridgewood	82%	300+
Southern Ocean Medical Center	Manahawkin	81%	300+
South Jersey Healthcare-Elmer Hospital	Elmer	80%	300+
Hunterdon Medical Center	Flemington	79%	300+
Jersey Shore University Medical Center	Neptune	79%	300+
Virtua West Jersey Hospitals Berlin	Berlin	79%	300+
Cape Regional Medical Center	Cape May CH	78%	300+
Underwood Memorial Hospital	Woodbury	78%	300+
Virtua Mem Hosp of Burlington County	Mount Holly	78%	300+
Capital Health System - Mercer Campus	Trenton	77%	300+
Hackensack University Medical Center	Hackensack	77%	300+
Ocean Medical Center	Brick	77%	300+
Saint Clare's Hospital - Sussex	Sussex	77%	(a)
Saint Peter's University Hospital	New Brunswick	77%	300+
Chilton Hospital	Pompton Plains	76%	300+
Meadowlands Hospital Medical Center	Secaucus	76%	300+
Morristown Memorial Hospital	Morristown	76%	300+
Newton Memorial Hospital[11]	Newton	76%	300+
Riverview Medical Center	Red Bank	76%	300+
Robert Wood Johnson University Hospital	New Brunswick	76%	300+
Warren Hospital	Phillipsburg	76%	300+
Atlanticare Reg Med Ctr-City Division	Atlantic City	75%	300+
Community Medical Center	Toms River	75%	300+
Hackettstown Regional Medical Center	Hackettstown	75%	300+
Kennedy University Hospital	Stratford	75%	300+
Overlook Hospital	Summit	75%	300+
Shore Memorial Hospital	Somers Point	75%	300+
Trinitas Regional Medical Center	Elizabeth	75%	300+
Centrastate Medical Center	Freehold	74%	300+
Englewood Hospital and Medical Center	Englewood	74%	300+
Holy Name Medical Center	Teaneck	74%	300+
Newark Beth Israel Medical Center	Newark	74%	300+
Raritan Bay Medical Center	Perth Amboy	74%	300+
Robert Wood Johnson Univ Hosp Hamilton	Hamilton	74%	300+
Saint Barnabas Medical Center	Livingston	74%	300+
Somerset Medical Center	Somerville	74%	300+
Capital Health System-Fuld Campus	Trenton	73%	300+
Mountainside Hospital	Montclair	73%	300+
Saint Clare's Hospital	Denville	73%	300+
South Jersey Healthcare Reg Med Ctr	Vineland	73%	300+
Clara Maass Medical Center	Belleville	72%	300+
Hoboken University Medical Center	Hoboken	72%	300+
JFK Medical Center	Edison	72%	300+
Saint Francis Medical Center	Trenton	72%	300+
Cooper University Hospital	Camden	71%	300+
Kimball Medical Center	Lakewood	71%	300+
Our Lady of Lourdes Medical Center	Camden	71%	300+
Robert W Johnson Univ Hosp-Rahway	Rahway	71%	300+
University Medical Center at Princeton	Princeton	71%	300+
Libertyhealth-Jersey City Med Ctr Campus	Jersey City	70%	300+
Memorial Hospital of Salem County	Salem	70%	300+
Bayshore Community Hospital	Holmdel	69%	300+
East Orange General Hospital	East Orange	69%	300+
Monmouth Medical Center	Long Branch	69%	300+
Bayonne Hospital Center	Bayonne	67%	300+
Saint Joseph's Regional Medical Center	Paterson	67%	300+
Saint Mary's Hospital - Passaic	Passaic	67%	300+
UMDNJ University Hospital	Newark	67%	300+
Christ Hospital	Jersey City	66%	(a)
Lourdes Medical Center of Burlington County	Willingboro	65%	300+
Saint Michael's Medical Center	Newark	62%	300+
Palisades Medical Center	North Bergen	60%	300+
Bergen Regional Medical Center	Paramus	48%	(a)

46. Pain 'Always' Well Controlled

Hospital Name	City	Rate	Cases
Meadowlands Hospital Medical Center	Secaucus	74%	300+
Southern Ocean Medical Center	Manahawkin	74%	300+
Valley Hospital	Ridgewood	74%	300+
Deborah Heart and Lung Center	Browns Mills	73%	300+
Shore Memorial Hospital	Somers Point	73%	300+
South Jersey Healthcare-Elmer Hospital	Elmer	73%	300+
Hunterdon Medical Center	Flemington	72%	300+
Jersey Shore University Medical Center	Neptune	72%	300+
Ocean Medical Center	Brick	72%	300+
Somerset Medical Center	Somerville	72%	300+
Cape Regional Medical Center	Cape May CH	71%	300+
Virtua West Jersey Hospitals Berlin	Berlin	71%	300+
Chilton Hospital	Pompton Plains	70%	300+
Morristown Memorial Hospital	Morristown	70%	300+
Riverview Medical Center	Red Bank	70%	300+
Saint Peter's University Hospital	New Brunswick	70%	300+
Virtua Mem Hosp of Burlington County	Mount Holly	70%	300+
Warren Hospital	Phillipsburg	70%	300+
Community Medical Center	Toms River	69%	300+
Hackensack University Medical Center	Hackensack	69%	300+
Kimball Medical Center	Lakewood	69%	300+
Saint Clare's Hospital - Sussex	Sussex	69%	(a)
Englewood Hospital and Medical Center	Englewood	68%	300+
Hoboken University Medical Center	Hoboken	68%	300+
Newark Beth Israel Medical Center	Newark	68%	300+
Newton Memorial Hospital[11]	Newton	68%	300+
Robert Wood Johnson University Hospital	New Brunswick	68%	300+
Underwood Memorial Hospital	Woodbury	68%	300+
Clara Maass Medical Center	Belleville	67%	300+
Holy Name Medical Center	Teaneck	67%	300+
Overlook Hospital	Summit	67%	300+
Robert Wood Johnson Univ Hosp Hamilton	Hamilton	67%	300+
Saint Barnabas Medical Center	Livingston	67%	300+
South Jersey Healthcare Reg Med Ctr	Vineland	67%	300+
University Medical Center at Princeton	Princeton	67%	300+
Capital Health System - Mercer Campus	Trenton	66%	300+
JFK Medical Center	Edison	66%	300+
Kennedy University Hospital	Stratford	66%	300+
Mountainside Hospital	Montclair	66%	300+
Robert W Johnson Univ Hosp-Rahway	Rahway	66%	300+
Capital Health System-Fuld Campus	Trenton	65%	300+
Centrastate Medical Center	Freehold	65%	300+
Libertyhealth-Jersey City Med Ctr Campus	Jersey City	65%	300+
Raritan Bay Medical Center	Perth Amboy	65%	300+
Saint Clare's Hospital	Denville	65%	300+
Saint Francis Medical Center	Trenton	65%	300+
Saint Mary's Hospital - Passaic	Passaic	65%	300+
UMDNJ University Hospital	Newark	65%	300+
Atlanticare Reg Med Ctr-City Division	Atlantic City	64%	300+
Bayshore Community Hospital	Holmdel	64%	300+
Cooper University Hospital	Camden	64%	300+
East Orange General Hospital	East Orange	64%	300+
Hackettstown Regional Medical Center	Hackettstown	64%	300+
Trinitas Regional Medical Center	Elizabeth	64%	300+
Lourdes Medical Center of Burlington County	Willingboro	63%	300+
Memorial Hospital of Salem County	Salem	63%	300+
Bayonne Hospital Center	Bayonne	62%	300+
Christ Hospital	Jersey City	62%	(a)
Saint Joseph's Regional Medical Center	Paterson	62%	300+
Monmouth Medical Center	Long Branch	61%	300+
Our Lady of Lourdes Medical Center	Camden	61%	300+
Palisades Medical Center	North Bergen	56%	300+
Saint Michael's Medical Center	Newark	56%	300+
Bergen Regional Medical Center	Paramus	47%	(a)

47. Room and Bathroom 'Always' Clean

Hospital Name	City	Rate	Cases
Valley Hospital	Ridgewood	80%	300+
Meadowlands Hospital Medical Center	Secaucus	78%	300+
Saint Peter's University Hospital	New Brunswick	77%	300+
South Jersey Healthcare-Elmer Hospital	Elmer	77%	300+
Deborah Heart and Lung Center	Browns Mills	76%	300+
Newton Memorial Hospital[11]	Newton	76%	300+
Saint Clare's Hospital - Sussex	Sussex	76%	(a)
Englewood Hospital and Medical Center	Englewood	74%	300+
Hunterdon Medical Center	Flemington	73%	300+
Morristown Memorial Hospital	Morristown	73%	300+
Trinitas Regional Medical Center	Elizabeth	73%	300+
Centrastate Medical Center	Freehold	72%	300+
Hackensack University Medical Center	Hackensack	72%	300+
Capital Health System - Mercer Campus	Trenton	71%	300+
Ocean Medical Center	Brick	71%	300+
Somerset Medical Center	Somerville	71%	300+
South Jersey Healthcare Reg Med Ctr	Vineland	71%	300+
Cape Regional Medical Center	Cape May CH	70%	300+
Libertyhealth-Jersey City Med Ctr Campus	Jersey City	70%	300+
Riverview Medical Center	Red Bank	70%	300+
Southern Ocean Medical Center	Manahawkin	70%	300+
Underwood Memorial Hospital	Woodbury	70%	300+
Virtua West Jersey Hospitals Berlin	Berlin	70%	300+
Warren Hospital	Phillipsburg	70%	300+
Capital Health System-Fuld Campus	Trenton	69%	300+
Jersey Shore University Medical Center	Neptune	69%	300+
JFK Medical Center	Edison	69%	300+
Robert W Johnson Univ Hosp-Rahway	Rahway	69%	300+
Robert Wood Johnson Univ Hosp Hamilton	Hamilton	69%	300+
Hackettstown Regional Medical Center	Hackettstown	67%	300+
Holy Name Medical Center	Teaneck	67%	300+
Kennedy University Hospital	Stratford	67%	300+
Shore Memorial Hospital	Somers Point	67%	300+
Atlanticare Reg Med Ctr-City Division	Atlantic City	66%	300+
Clara Maass Medical Center	Belleville	66%	300+
Overlook Hospital	Summit	66%	300+
Saint Francis Medical Center	Trenton	66%	300+
East Orange General Hospital	East Orange	65%	300+
Kimball Medical Center	Lakewood	65%	300+
Mountainside Hospital	Montclair	65%	300+
Newark Beth Israel Medical Center	Newark	65%	300+
Raritan Bay Medical Center	Perth Amboy	65%	300+
Robert Wood Johnson University Hospital	New Brunswick	65%	300+
Saint Joseph's Regional Medical Center	Paterson	65%	300+

NOTE: Hospital profiles are in alphabetical order by state, then city, then hospital within the city; Rankings exclude hospitals with less than 25 cases except for patient surveys which excludes hospitals with less than 100 cases; (a) 100–299 cases; (1) The number of cases is too small to be sure how well a hospital is performing; (2) The hospital indicated that the data submitted for this measure were based on a sample of cases; (3) Data was collected during a shorter time period (fewer quarters) than the maximum possible time for this measure; (4) Suppressed for one or more quarters by CMS; (5) No data is available from the hospital for this measure; (6) Fewer than 100 patients completed the HCAHPS survey. Use these rates with caution, as the number of surveys may be too low to reliably assess hospital performance; (7) Survey results are based on less than 12 months of data; (8) Survey results are not available for this reporting period; (9) No or very few patients were eligible for the HCAHPS survey. The scores shown, if any, reflect a very small number of surveys; (10) A state average was not calculated because too few hospitals in the state submitted data; (11) There were discrepancies in the data collection process; Please refer to the User's Guide for a full explanation of data.

Hospital Name	City	Rate	Cases
Cooper University Hospital	Camden	64%	300+
Saint Barnabas Medical Center	Livingston	64%	300+
Saint Mary's Hospital - Passaic	Passaic	64%	300+
Virtua Mem Hosp of Burlington County	Mount Holly	64%	300+
Community Medical Center	Toms River	63%	300+
Saint Clare's Hospital	Denville	63%	300+
Chilton Hospital	Pompton Plains	62%	300+
Christ Hospital	Jersey City	62%	(a)
Hoboken University Medical Center	Hoboken	62%	300+
Palisades Medical Center	North Bergen	62%	300+
Saint Michael's Medical Center	Newark	62%	300+
UMDNJ University Hospital	Newark	62%	300+
University Medical Center at Princeton	Princeton	61%	300+
Bayonne Hospital Center	Bayonne	60%	300+
Lourdes Medical Center of Burlington County	Willingboro	59%	300+
Memorial Hospital of Salem County	Salem	59%	300+
Bayshore Community Hospital	Holmdel	58%	300+
Monmouth Medical Center	Long Branch	58%	300+
Our Lady of Lourdes Medical Center	Camden	56%	300+
Bergen Regional Medical Center	Paramus	50%	(a)

48. Timely Help 'Always' Received

Hospital Name	City	Rate	Cases
Southern Ocean Medical Center	Manahawkin	71%	300+
Deborah Heart and Lung Center	Browns Mills	69%	300+
South Jersey Healthcare-Elmer Hospital	Elmer	69%	300+
Saint Clare's Hospital - Sussex	Sussex	67%	(a)
Valley Hospital	Ridgewood	65%	300+
Hunterdon Medical Center	Flemington	64%	300+
Jersey Shore University Medical Center	Neptune	64%	300+
Meadowlands Hospital Medical Center	Secaucus	64%	300+
Saint Peter's University Hospital	New Brunswick	64%	300+
Cape Regional Medical Center	Cape May CH	63%	300+
Chilton Hospital	Pompton Plains	63%	300+
Underwood Memorial Hospital	Woodbury	63%	300+
Robert Wood Johnson University Hospital	New Brunswick	62%	300+
South Jersey Healthcare Reg Med Ctr	Vineland	62%	300+
Virtua West Jersey Hospitals Berlin	Berlin	62%	300+
Centrastate Medical Center	Freehold	61%	300+
Community Medical Center	Toms River	61%	300+
Riverview Medical Center	Red Bank	61%	300+
Shore Memorial Hospital	Somers Point	61%	300+
Newton Memorial Hospital[11]	Newton	60%	300+
Atlanticare Reg Med Ctr-City Division	Atlantic City	59%	300+
Hackensack University Medical Center	Hackensack	59%	300+
Hackettstown Regional Medical Center	Hackettstown	59%	300+
Hoboken University Medical Center	Hoboken	59%	300+
Robert Wood Johnson Univ Hosp Hamilton	Hamilton	59%	300+
Trinitas Regional Medical Center	Elizabeth	59%	300+
Clara Maass Medical Center	Belleville	58%	300+
Newark Beth Israel Medical Center	Newark	58%	300+
Ocean Medical Center	Brick	58%	300+
Raritan Bay Medical Center	Perth Amboy	58%	300+
Virtua Mem Hosp of Burlington County	Mount Holly	58%	300+
Capital Health System-Fuld Campus	Trenton	57%	300+
Cooper University Hospital	Camden	57%	300+
Kennedy University Hospital	Stratford	57%	300+
Capital Health System - Mercer Campus	Trenton	56%	300+
Morristown Memorial Hospital	Morristown	56%	300+
Saint Clare's Hospital	Denville	56%	300+
Saint Francis Medical Center	Trenton	56%	300+
Somerset Medical Center	Somerville	56%	300+
Warren Hospital	Phillipsburg	56%	300+
Lourdes Medical Center of Burlington County	Willingboro	55%	300+
Mountainside Hospital	Montclair	55%	300+
Overlook Hospital	Summit	55%	300+
Robert W Johnson Univ Hosp-Rahway	Rahway	55%	300+
East Orange General Hospital	East Orange	54%	300+
Englewood Hospital and Medical Center	Englewood	54%	300+
Kimball Medical Center	Lakewood	54%	300+
Saint Barnabas Medical Center	Livingston	54%	300+
University Medical Center at Princeton	Princeton	54%	300+
Christ Hospital	Jersey City	53%	(a)
Holy Name Medical Center	Teaneck	53%	300+
Libertyhealth-Jersey City Med Ctr Campus	Jersey City	53%	300+
Memorial Hospital of Salem County	Salem	53%	300+
UMDNJ University Hospital	Newark	53%	300+
Bayonne Hospital Center	Bayonne	52%	300+
JFK Medical Center	Edison	51%	300+
Bayshore Community Hospital	Holmdel	50%	300+
Monmouth Medical Center	Long Branch	50%	300+
Our Lady of Lourdes Medical Center	Camden	50%	300+
Saint Mary's Hospital - Passaic	Passaic	50%	300+
Saint Michael's Medical Center	Newark	50%	300+
Saint Joseph's Regional Medical Center	Paterson	49%	300+
Palisades Medical Center	North Bergen	44%	300+
Bergen Regional Medical Center	Paramus	35%	(a)

49. Would Definitely Recommend Hospital

Hospital Name	City	Rate	Cases
Deborah Heart and Lung Center	Browns Mills	87%	300+
Valley Hospital	Ridgewood	82%	300+
Morristown Memorial Hospital	Morristown	81%	300+
Hackensack University Medical Center	Hackensack	80%	300+
South Jersey Healthcare-Elmer Hospital	Elmer	80%	300+
Saint Peter's University Hospital	New Brunswick	76%	300+
Holy Name Medical Center	Teaneck	75%	300+
Hunterdon Medical Center	Flemington	75%	300+
Jersey Shore University Medical Center	Neptune	75%	300+
Robert Wood Johnson University Hospital	New Brunswick	75%	300+
Shore Memorial Hospital	Somers Point	74%	300+
Englewood Hospital and Medical Center	Englewood	73%	300+
Overlook Hospital	Summit	73%	300+
Atlanticare Reg Med Ctr-City Division	Atlantic City	72%	300+
Centrastate Medical Center	Freehold	72%	300+
Saint Barnabas Medical Center	Livingston	72%	300+
Virtua West Jersey Hospitals Berlin	Berlin	72%	300+
Riverview Medical Center	Red Bank	71%	300+
Virtua Mem Hosp of Burlington County	Mount Holly	71%	300+
Cooper University Hospital	Camden	70%	300+
Hackettstown Regional Medical Center	Hackettstown	69%	300+
Meadowlands Hospital Medical Center	Secaucus	68%	300+
Ocean Medical Center	Brick	68%	300+
Robert Wood Johnson Univ Hosp Hamilton	Hamilton	68%	300+
Libertyhealth-Jersey City Med Ctr Campus	Jersey City	67%	300+
Saint Clare's Hospital - Sussex	Sussex	67%	(a)
Somerset Medical Center	Somerville	67%	300+
University Medical Center at Princeton	Princeton	67%	300+
Cape Regional Medical Center	Cape May CH	66%	300+
Chilton Hospital	Pompton Plains	66%	300+
Hoboken University Medical Center	Hoboken	66%	300+
Newark Beth Israel Medical Center	Newark	66%	300+
Newton Memorial Hospital[11]	Newton	66%	300+
Saint Clare's Hospital	Denville	66%	300+
Capital Health System - Mercer Campus	Trenton	65%	300+
Our Lady of Lourdes Medical Center	Camden	65%	300+
Southern Ocean Medical Center	Manahawkin	65%	300+
Saint Joseph's Regional Medical Center	Paterson	64%	300+
South Jersey Healthcare Reg Med Ctr	Vineland	64%	300+
Capital Health System-Fuld Campus	Trenton	63%	300+
Monmouth Medical Center	Long Branch	62%	300+
Mountainside Hospital	Montclair	62%	300+
Christ Hospital	Jersey City	61%	(a)
Community Medical Center	Toms River	61%	300+
UMDNJ University Hospital	Newark	61%	300+
Raritan Bay Medical Center	Perth Amboy	60%	300+
Clara Maass Medical Center	Belleville	59%	300+
Kennedy University Hospital	Stratford	59%	300+
Trinitas Regional Medical Center	Elizabeth	59%	300+
Underwood Memorial Hospital	Woodbury	59%	300+
Robert W Johnson Univ Hosp-Rahway	Rahway	58%	300+
Saint Francis Medical Center	Trenton	58%	300+
JFK Medical Center	Edison	56%	300+
Warren Hospital	Phillipsburg	55%	300+
Bayshore Community Hospital	Holmdel	54%	300+
Saint Michael's Medical Center	Newark	54%	300+
Palisades Medical Center	North Bergen	53%	300+
Kimball Medical Center	Lakewood	52%	300+
East Orange General Hospital	East Orange	50%	300+
Saint Mary's Hospital - Passaic	Passaic	49%	300+
Lourdes Medical Center of Burlington County	Willingboro	47%	300+
Memorial Hospital of Salem County	Salem	46%	300+
Bergen Regional Medical Center	Paramus	41%	(a)
Bayonne Hospital Center	Bayonne	38%	300+

Atlanticare Regional Medical Center - City Division

1925 Pacific Ave
Atlantic City, NJ 08401
Phone: 609-441-8020
Fax: 609-441-2108
URL: www.atlanticare.org/acmc/index.html
Type: Acute Care Hospitals
Emergency Services: Yes
Ownership: Voluntary Non-Profit - Other
Beds: 442

Key Personnel:
CEO/President. . . . . David P Tilton

Measure	Cases	This Hosp.	State Avg.	U.S. Avg.
Heart Attack Care				
ACE Inhibitor or ARB for LVSD[2]	66	98%	98%	96%
Aspirin at Arrival[2]	238	100%	99%	99%
Aspirin at Discharge[2]	330	100%	99%	98%
Beta Blocker at Discharge[2]	325	100%	99%	98%
Fibrinolytic Medication Timing[2]	0	-	65%	55%
PCI Within 90 Minutes of Arrival[2]	60	83%	87%	90%
Smoking Cessation Advice[2]	114	100%	100%	99%
Chest Pain/Possible Heart Attack Care				
Aspirin at Arrival[1]	6	67%	97%	95%
Median Time to ECG (minutes)[1]	7	29	8	8
Median Time to Transfer (minutes)[5]	0	-	81	61
Fibrinolytic Medication Timing[5]	0	-	65%	54%
Heart Failure Care				
ACE Inhibitor or ARB for LVSD[2]	229	100%	97%	94%
Discharge Instructions[2]	468	100%	93%	88%
Evaluation of LVS Function[2]	618	100%	99%	98%
Smoking Cessation Advice[2]	138	100%	100%	98%
Pneumonia Care				
Appropriate Initial Antibiotic[2]	195	95%	94%	92%
Blood Culture Timing[2]	358	99%	97%	96%
Influenza Vaccine[2]	166	100%	94%	91%
Initial Antibiotic Timing[2]	313	95%	96%	95%
Pneumococcal Vaccine[2]	234	100%	96%	93%
Smoking Cessation Advice[2]	138	100%	99%	97%
Surgical Care Improvement Project				
Appropriate VTP Within 24 Hours[2]	285	94%	94%	92%
Appropriate Hair Removal[2]	1,054	100%	100%	99%
Appropriate Beta Blocker Usage[2]	361	88%	95%	93%
Controlled Postoperative Blood Glucose[2]	143	97%	93%	93%
Prophylactic Antibiotic Timing[2]	546	97%	98%	97%
Prophylactic Antibiotic Timing (Outpatient)	293	92%	93%	92%
Prophylactic Antibiotic Selection[2]	560	98%	97%	97%
Prophylactic Antibiotic Select. (Outpatient)	293	95%	94%	94%
Prophylactic Antibiotic Stopped[2]	502	92%	96%	94%
Recommended VTP Ordered[2]	285	97%	95%	94%
Urinary Catheter Removal[2]	217	94%	93%	90%
Children's Asthma Care				
Received Systemic Corticosteroids	-	-	-	100%
Received Home Management Plan	-	-	-	71%
Received Reliever Medication	-	-	-	100%
Use of Medical Imaging				
Combination Abdominal CT Scan	805	0.040	0.126	0.191
Combination Chest CT Scan	329	0.100	0.026	0.054
Follow-up Mammogram/Ultrasound	891	5.3%	10.6%	8.4%
MRI for Low Back Pain	73	19.2%	26.4%	32.7%
Survey of Patients' Hospital Experiences				
Area Around Room 'Always' Quiet at Night	300+	48%	-	58%
Doctors 'Always' Communicated Well	300+	75%	-	80%
Home Recovery Information Given	300+	89%	-	82%
Hospital Given 9 or 10 on 10 Point Scale	300+	66%	-	67%
Meds 'Always' Explained Before Given	300+	58%	-	60%
Nurses 'Always' Communicated Well	300+	75%	-	76%
Pain 'Always' Well Controlled	300+	64%	-	69%
Room and Bathroom 'Always' Clean	300+	66%	-	71%
Timely Help 'Always' Received	300+	59%	-	64%
Would Definitely Recommend Hospital	300+	72%	-	69%

Bayonne Hospital Center

29 East 29th St
Bayonne, NJ 07002
Phone: 201-858-5000
Fax: 201-858-7355
URL: www.bayonnemedicalcenter.org
Type: Acute Care Hospitals
Emergency Services: Yes
Ownership: Voluntary Non-Profit - Private
Beds: 278

Key Personnel:
CEO/President. . . . . Robert Evans
Pediatric In-Patient Care . . . . S Aly, MD
Quality Assurance . . . . Eileen Konecko
Radiology. . . . . Q Chew, MD

Measure	Cases	This Hosp.	State Avg.	U.S. Avg.
Heart Attack Care				
ACE Inhibitor or ARB for LVSD	29	100%	98%	96%
Aspirin at Arrival	139	100%	99%	99%
Aspirin at Discharge	100	100%	99%	98%
Beta Blocker at Discharge	109	100%	99%	98%
Fibrinolytic Medication Timing	0	-	65%	55%
PCI Within 90 Minutes of Arrival[1]	18	83%	87%	90%
Smoking Cessation Advice	37	100%	100%	99%
Chest Pain/Possible Heart Attack Care				
Aspirin at Arrival[1,3]	1	100%	97%	95%
Median Time to ECG (minutes)[1,3]	1	3	8	8
Median Time to Transfer (minutes)[5]	0	-	81	61
Fibrinolytic Medication Timing[5]	0	-	65%	54%
Heart Failure Care				
ACE Inhibitor or ARB for LVSD[2]	60	93%	97%	94%
Discharge Instructions[2]	156	99%	93%	88%
Evaluation of LVS Function[2]	259	99%	99%	98%
Smoking Cessation Advice[1,2]	19	100%	100%	98%
Pneumonia Care				
Appropriate Initial Antibiotic[2]	86	92%	94%	92%
Blood Culture Timing[2]	151	98%	97%	96%
Influenza Vaccine[2]	72	97%	94%	91%
Initial Antibiotic Timing[2]	135	98%	96%	95%
Pneumococcal Vaccine[2]	138	95%	96%	93%
Smoking Cessation Advice[2]	49	100%	99%	97%
Surgical Care Improvement Project				
Appropriate VTP Within 24 Hours[2]	97	93%	94%	92%
Appropriate Hair Removal[2]	141	100%	100%	99%
Appropriate Beta Blocker Usage[2]	38	84%	95%	93%
Controlled Postoperative Blood Glucose[2]	0	-	93%	93%
Prophylactic Antibiotic Timing[2]	35	97%	98%	97%
Prophylactic Antibiotic Timing (Outpatient)[1]	22	91%	93%	92%
Prophylactic Antibiotic Selection[2]	36	100%	97%	97%
Prophylactic Antibiotic Select. (Outpatient)[1]	20	95%	94%	94%
Prophylactic Antibiotic Stopped[2]	28	82%	96%	94%
Recommended VTP Ordered[2]	97	96%	95%	94%
Urinary Catheter Removal[1]	7	100%	93%	90%
Children's Asthma Care				
Received Systemic Corticosteroids	-	-	-	100%
Received Home Management Plan	-	-	-	71%
Received Reliever Medication	-	-	-	100%
Use of Medical Imaging				
Combination Abdominal CT Scan	779	0.099	0.126	0.191
Combination Chest CT Scan	813	0.037	0.026	0.054
Follow-up Mammogram/Ultrasound	795	5.7%	10.6%	8.4%
MRI for Low Back Pain	141	26.2%	26.4%	32.7%
Survey of Patients' Hospital Experiences				
Area Around Room 'Always' Quiet at Night	300+	49%	-	58%
Doctors 'Always' Communicated Well	300+	76%	-	80%
Home Recovery Information Given	300+	79%	-	82%
Hospital Given 9 or 10 on 10 Point Scale	300+	47%	-	67%
Meds 'Always' Explained Before Given	300+	51%	-	60%
Nurses 'Always' Communicated Well	300+	67%	-	76%
Pain 'Always' Well Controlled	300+	62%	-	69%
Room and Bathroom 'Always' Clean	300+	60%	-	71%
Timely Help 'Always' Received	300+	52%	-	64%
Would Definitely Recommend Hospital	300+	38%	-	69%

Clara Maass Medical Center

One Clara Maas Drive
Belleville, NJ 07109
Phone: 973-450-2002
Fax: 973-450-0181
E-mail: info@sbhcs.com
URL: www.sbhcs.com/hospitals
Type: Acute Care Hospitals
Emergency Services: Yes
Ownership: Voluntary Non-Profit - Private
Beds: 445

Key Personnel:
Cardiac Laboratory. . . . . Michelle Witwick
Infection Control. . . . . Edward S Johnson
Operating Room. . . . . Sue Gallina
Quality Assurance . . . . Margaret Nielson
Radiology. . . . . James A. Heimann
Anesthesiology. . . . . Jose A. Dtetres-Palacio, MD
Emergency Room . . . . Karen Palletello, MD
Intensive Care Unit. . . . . Ronnie Castro

Measure	Cases	This Hosp.	State Avg.	U.S. Avg.
Heart Attack Care				
ACE Inhibitor or ARB for LVSD[2]	28	100%	98%	96%
Aspirin at Arrival[2]	240	100%	99%	99%
Aspirin at Discharge[2]	123	100%	99%	98%
Beta Blocker at Discharge[2]	121	100%	99%	98%
Fibrinolytic Medication Timing[2]	0	-	65%	55%
PCI Within 90 Minutes of Arrival[1,2]	24	100%	87%	90%
Smoking Cessation Advice[2]	29	100%	100%	99%
Chest Pain/Possible Heart Attack Care				
Aspirin at Arrival[1,3]	9	100%	97%	95%
Median Time to ECG (minutes)[1,3]	9	11	8	8
Median Time to Transfer (minutes)[3]	0	-	81	61
Fibrinolytic Medication Timing[3]	0	-	65%	54%
Heart Failure Care				
ACE Inhibitor or ARB for LVSD[2]	91	100%	97%	94%
Discharge Instructions[2]	245	100%	93%	88%
Evaluation of LVS Function[2]	329	100%	99%	98%
Smoking Cessation Advice[2]	37	100%	100%	98%
Pneumonia Care				
Appropriate Initial Antibiotic[2]	124	100%	94%	92%
Blood Culture Timing[2]	241	100%	97%	96%
Influenza Vaccine[2]	125	100%	94%	91%
Initial Antibiotic Timing[2]	203	99%	96%	95%
Pneumococcal Vaccine[2]	189	100%	96%	93%
Smoking Cessation Advice[2]	61	100%	99%	97%
Surgical Care Improvement Project				
Appropriate VTP Within 24 Hours[2]	259	100%	94%	92%
Appropriate Hair Removal[2]	659	100%	100%	99%
Appropriate Beta Blocker Usage[2]	141	100%	95%	93%
Controlled Postoperative Blood Glucose[1,2]	1	100%	93%	93%
Prophylactic Antibiotic Timing[2]	386	99%	98%	97%
Prophylactic Antibiotic Timing (Outpatient)	138	91%	93%	92%
Prophylactic Antibiotic Selection[2]	386	98%	97%	97%
Prophylactic Antibiotic Select. (Outpatient)	127	97%	94%	94%
Prophylactic Antibiotic Stopped[2]	363	98%	96%	94%
Recommended VTP Ordered[2]	259	100%	95%	94%
Urinary Catheter Removal[2]	115	97%	93%	90%
Children's Asthma Care				
Received Systemic Corticosteroids	-	-	-	100%
Received Home Management Plan	-	-	-	71%
Received Reliever Medication	-	-	-	100%
Use of Medical Imaging				
Combination Abdominal CT Scan	526	0.101	0.126	0.191
Combination Chest CT Scan	232	0.034	0.026	0.054
Follow-up Mammogram/Ultrasound	374	13.9%	10.6%	8.4%
MRI for Low Back Pain[1]	5	0.0%	26.4%	32.7%
Survey of Patients' Hospital Experiences				
Area Around Room 'Always' Quiet at Night	300+	50%	-	58%
Doctors 'Always' Communicated Well	300+	78%	-	80%
Home Recovery Information Given	300+	72%	-	82%
Hospital Given 9 or 10 on 10 Point Scale	300+	54%	-	67%
Meds 'Always' Explained Before Given	300+	57%	-	60%
Nurses 'Always' Communicated Well	300+	72%	-	76%
Pain 'Always' Well Controlled	300+	67%	-	69%
Room and Bathroom 'Always' Clean	300+	66%	-	71%
Timely Help 'Always' Received	300+	58%	-	64%
Would Definitely Recommend Hospital	300+	59%	-	69%

NOTE: Hospital profiles are in alphabetical order by state, then city, then hospital within the city; Rankings exclude hospitals with less than 25 cases except for patient surveys which excludes hospitals with less than 100 cases; (a) 100–299 cases; (1) The number of cases is too small to be sure how well a hospital is performing; (2) The hospital indicated that the data submitted for this measure were based on a sample of cases; (3) Data was collected during a shorter time period (fewer quarters) than the maximum possible time for this measure; (4) Suppressed for one or more quarters by CMS; (5) No data is available from the hospital for this measure; (6) Fewer than 100 patients completed the HCAHPS survey. Use these rates with caution, as the number of surveys may be too low to reliably assess hospital performance; (7) Survey results are based on less than 12 months of data; (8) Survey results are not available for this reporting period; (9) No or very few patients were eligible for the HCAHPS survey. The scores shown, if any, reflect a very small number of surveys; (10) A state average was not calculated because too few hospitals in the state submitted data; (11) There were discrepancies in the data collection process; Please refer to the User's Guide for a full explanation of data.

Virtua West Jersey Hospitals Berlin

100 Townsend Avenue — Phone: 856-322-3200
Berlin, NJ 08009 — Fax: 609-265-9514
Type: Acute Care Hospitals — Emergency Services: Yes
Ownership: Voluntary Non-Profit - Private — Beds: 92

Key Personnel:
CEO/President. . . . . Gary Long
Emergency Room . . . . Eileen Singer

Measure	Cases	This Hosp.	State Avg.	U.S. Avg.
Heart Attack Care				
ACE Inhibitor or ARB for LVSD	45	100%	98%	96%
Aspirin at Arrival	356	100%	99%	99%
Aspirin at Discharge	277	100%	99%	98%
Beta Blocker at Discharge	271	99%	99%	98%
Fibrinolytic Medication Timing[1]	4	50%	65%	55%
PCI Within 90 Minutes of Arrival	45	80%	87%	90%
Smoking Cessation Advice	67	100%	100%	99%
Chest Pain/Possible Heart Attack Care				
Aspirin at Arrival	119	97%	97%	95%
Median Time to ECG (minutes)	124	10	8	8
Median Time to Transfer (minutes)[1]	11	124	81	61
Fibrinolytic Medication Timing[1]	2	50%	65%	54%
Heart Failure Care				
ACE Inhibitor or ARB for LVSD	172	99%	97%	94%
Discharge Instructions	588	87%	93%	88%
Evaluation of LVS Function	859	100%	99%	98%
Smoking Cessation Advice	113	100%	100%	98%
Pneumonia Care				
Appropriate Initial Antibiotic	490	95%	94%	92%
Blood Culture Timing	818	99%	97%	96%
Influenza Vaccine	363	96%	94%	91%
Initial Antibiotic Timing	741	99%	96%	95%
Pneumococcal Vaccine	677	98%	96%	93%
Smoking Cessation Advice	222	100%	99%	97%
Surgical Care Improvement Project				
Appropriate VTP Within 24 Hours[2]	778	96%	94%	92%
Appropriate Hair Removal[2]	1,856	100%	100%	99%
Appropriate Beta Blocker Usage[2]	507	96%	95%	93%
Controlled Postoperative Blood Glucose[2]	0	-	93%	93%
Prophylactic Antibiotic Timing[2]	1,248	98%	98%	97%
Prophylactic Antibiotic Timing (Outpatient)	361	94%	93%	92%
Prophylactic Antibiotic Selection[2]	1,268	98%	97%	97%
Prophylactic Antibiotic Select. (Outpatient)	355	94%	94%	94%
Prophylactic Antibiotic Stopped[2]	1,208	97%	96%	94%
Recommended VTP Ordered[2]	780	97%	95%	94%
Urinary Catheter Removal[2]	401	93%	93%	90%
Children's Asthma Care				
Received Systemic Corticosteroids	-	-	-	100%
Received Home Management Plan	-	-	-	71%
Received Reliever Medication	-	-	-	100%
Use of Medical Imaging				
Combination Abdominal CT Scan	966	0.050	0.126	0.191
Combination Chest CT Scan	529	0.038	0.026	0.054
Follow-up Mammogram/Ultrasound	152	14.5%	10.6%	8.4%
MRI for Low Back Pain[1]	61	21.3%	26.4%	32.7%
Survey of Patients' Hospital Experiences				
Area Around Room 'Always' Quiet at Night	300+	47%	-	58%
Doctors 'Always' Communicated Well	300+	75%	-	80%
Home Recovery Information Given	300+	78%	-	82%
Hospital Given 9 or 10 on 10 Point Scale	300+	66%	-	67%
Meds 'Always' Explained Before Given	300+	58%	-	60%
Nurses 'Always' Communicated Well	300+	79%	-	76%
Pain 'Always' Well Controlled	300+	71%	-	69%
Room and Bathroom 'Always' Clean	300+	70%	-	71%
Timely Help 'Always' Received	300+	62%	-	64%
Would Definitely Recommend Hospital	300+	72%	-	69%

Ocean Medical Center

425 Jack Martin Blvd — Phone: 732-840-2200
Brick, NJ 08724 — Fax: 732-840-3284
URL: www.meridianhealth.com/mcoc.cfm/ind
Type: Acute Care Hospitals — Emergency Services: Yes
Ownership: Voluntary Non-Profit - Other — Beds: 281

Key Personnel:
CEO/President. . . . . W Peter Daniels, FACHE
Cardiac Laboratory. . . . . P Insantolino
Chief of Medical Staff . . . . David Neckritz, DO
Infection Control. . . . . Nancy Wagner, RN
Operating Room. . . . . Patricia Tharp, RN
Pediatric In-Patient Care . . . . Jacquie Stanley, RN
Quality Assurance . . . . Carole Page
Radiology. . . . . Regina Mulholland

Measure	Cases	This Hosp.	State Avg.	U.S. Avg.
Heart Attack Care				
ACE Inhibitor or ARB for LVSD[1]	10	90%	98%	96%
Aspirin at Arrival	215	100%	99%	99%
Aspirin at Discharge	111	98%	99%	98%
Beta Blocker at Discharge	110	100%	99%	98%
Fibrinolytic Medication Timing[1]	1	100%	65%	55%
PCI Within 90 Minutes of Arrival	42	90%	87%	90%
Smoking Cessation Advice[1]	17	100%	100%	99%
Chest Pain/Possible Heart Attack Care				
Aspirin at Arrival[1]	14	93%	97%	95%
Median Time to ECG (minutes)[1]	14	9	8	8
Median Time to Transfer (minutes)[1,3]	3	57	81	61
Fibrinolytic Medication Timing[1]	1	0%	65%	54%
Heart Failure Care				
ACE Inhibitor or ARB for LVSD[2]	68	99%	97%	94%
Discharge Instructions[2]	223	96%	93%	88%
Evaluation of LVS Function[2]	351	98%	99%	98%
Smoking Cessation Advice[1,2]	23	100%	100%	98%
Pneumonia Care				
Appropriate Initial Antibiotic[2]	95	96%	94%	92%
Blood Culture Timing[2]	169	99%	97%	96%
Influenza Vaccine[2]	91	99%	94%	91%
Initial Antibiotic Timing[2]	154	99%	96%	95%
Pneumococcal Vaccine[2]	165	98%	96%	93%
Smoking Cessation Advice[2]	46	100%	99%	97%
Surgical Care Improvement Project				
Appropriate VTP Within 24 Hours[2]	222	99%	94%	92%
Appropriate Hair Removal[2]	558	100%	100%	99%
Appropriate Beta Blocker Usage[2]	154	94%	95%	93%
Controlled Postoperative Blood Glucose[2]	0	-	93%	93%
Prophylactic Antibiotic Timing[2]	301	99%	98%	97%
Prophylactic Antibiotic Timing (Outpatient)	195	92%	93%	92%
Prophylactic Antibiotic Selection[2]	301	98%	97%	97%
Prophylactic Antibiotic Select. (Outpatient)	181	96%	94%	94%
Prophylactic Antibiotic Stopped[2]	283	97%	96%	94%
Recommended VTP Ordered[2]	222	99%	95%	94%
Urinary Catheter Removal[2]	130	93%	93%	90%
Children's Asthma Care				
Received Systemic Corticosteroids	-	-	-	100%
Received Home Management Plan	-	-	-	71%
Received Reliever Medication	-	-	-	100%
Use of Medical Imaging				
Combination Abdominal CT Scan	1,172	0.106	0.126	0.191
Combination Chest CT Scan	927	0.006	0.026	0.054
Follow-up Mammogram/Ultrasound	816	13.2%	10.6%	8.4%
MRI for Low Back Pain	82	19.5%	26.4%	32.7%
Survey of Patients' Hospital Experiences				
Area Around Room 'Always' Quiet at Night	300+	52%	-	58%
Doctors 'Always' Communicated Well	300+	73%	-	80%
Home Recovery Information Given	300+	79%	-	82%
Hospital Given 9 or 10 on 10 Point Scale	300+	66%	-	67%
Meds 'Always' Explained Before Given	300+	58%	-	60%
Nurses 'Always' Communicated Well	300+	77%	-	76%
Pain 'Always' Well Controlled	300+	72%	-	69%
Room and Bathroom 'Always' Clean	300+	71%	-	71%
Timely Help 'Always' Received	300+	58%	-	64%
Would Definitely Recommend Hospital	300+	68%	-	69%

Deborah Heart and Lung Center

200 Trenton Road — Phone: 609-893-6611
Browns Mills, NJ 08015 — Fax: 609-893-0626
Type: Acute Care Hospitals — Emergency Services: No
Ownership: Voluntary Non-Profit - Private — Beds: 161

Key Personnel:
CEO/President. . . . . John Ernest
Radiology. . . . . Thomas C Gallagher

Measure	Cases	This Hosp.	State Avg.	U.S. Avg.
Heart Attack Care				
ACE Inhibitor or ARB for LVSD	55	98%	98%	96%
Aspirin at Arrival[1]	17	100%	99%	99%
Aspirin at Discharge	355	100%	99%	98%
Beta Blocker at Discharge	343	100%	99%	98%
Fibrinolytic Medication Timing	0	-	65%	55%
PCI Within 90 Minutes of Arrival	0	-	87%	90%
Smoking Cessation Advice	100	100%	100%	99%
Chest Pain/Possible Heart Attack Care				
Aspirin at Arrival[5]	0	-	97%	95%
Median Time to ECG (minutes)[5]	0	-	8	8
Median Time to Transfer (minutes)[5]	0	-	81	61
Fibrinolytic Medication Timing[5]	0	-	65%	54%
Heart Failure Care				
ACE Inhibitor or ARB for LVSD	68	94%	97%	94%
Discharge Instructions	170	99%	93%	88%
Evaluation of LVS Function	195	100%	99%	98%
Smoking Cessation Advice	36	100%	100%	98%
Pneumonia Care				
Appropriate Initial Antibiotic	0	-	94%	92%
Blood Culture Timing	0	-	97%	96%
Influenza Vaccine[1]	6	100%	94%	91%
Initial Antibiotic Timing[1]	6	83%	96%	95%
Pneumococcal Vaccine[1]	12	83%	96%	93%
Smoking Cessation Advice[1]	11	100%	99%	97%
Surgical Care Improvement Project				
Appropriate VTP Within 24 Hours	29	83%	94%	92%
Appropriate Hair Removal	440	100%	100%	99%
Appropriate Beta Blocker Usage	267	97%	95%	93%
Controlled Postoperative Blood Glucose	325	86%	93%	93%
Prophylactic Antibiotic Timing	342	98%	98%	97%
Prophylactic Antibiotic Timing (Outpatient)	260	88%	93%	92%
Prophylactic Antibiotic Selection	354	100%	97%	97%
Prophylactic Antibiotic Select. (Outpatient)	254	100%	94%	94%
Prophylactic Antibiotic Stopped	317	100%	96%	94%
Recommended VTP Ordered	29	83%	95%	94%
Urinary Catheter Removal	91	99%	93%	90%
Children's Asthma Care				
Received Systemic Corticosteroids	-	-	-	100%
Received Home Management Plan	-	-	-	71%
Received Reliever Medication	-	-	-	100%
Use of Medical Imaging				
Combination Abdominal CT Scan	47	0.043	0.126	0.191
Combination Chest CT Scan	635	0.013	0.026	0.054
Follow-up Mammogram/Ultrasound[5]	0	-	10.6%	8.4%
MRI for Low Back Pain[5]	0	-	26.4%	32.7%
Survey of Patients' Hospital Experiences				
Area Around Room 'Always' Quiet at Night	300+	62%	-	58%
Doctors 'Always' Communicated Well	300+	81%	-	80%
Home Recovery Information Given	300+	88%	-	82%
Hospital Given 9 or 10 on 10 Point Scale	300+	82%	-	67%
Meds 'Always' Explained Before Given	300+	63%	-	60%
Nurses 'Always' Communicated Well	300+	82%	-	76%
Pain 'Always' Well Controlled	300+	73%	-	69%
Room and Bathroom 'Always' Clean	300+	76%	-	71%
Timely Help 'Always' Received	300+	69%	-	64%
Would Definitely Recommend Hospital	300+	87%	-	69%

NOTE: Hospital profiles are in alphabetical order by state, then city, then hospital within the city; Rankings exclude hospitals with less than 25 cases except for patient surveys which excludes hospitals with less than 100 cases; (a) 100–299 cases; (1) The number of cases is too small to be sure how well a hospital is performing; (2) The hospital indicated that the data submitted for this measure were based on a sample of cases; (3) Data was collected during a shorter time period (fewer quarters) than the maximum possible time for this measure; (4) Suppressed for one or more quarters by CMS; (5) No data is available from the hospital for this measure; (6) Fewer than 100 patients completed the HCAHPS survey. Use these rates with caution, as the number of surveys may be too low to reliably assess hospital performance; (7) Survey results are based on less than 12 months of data; (8) Survey results are not available for this reporting period; (9) No or very few patients were eligible for the HCAHPS survey. The scores shown, if any, reflect a very small number of surveys; (10) A state average was not calculated because too few hospitals in the state submitted data; (11) There were discrepancies in the data collection process; Please refer to the User's Guide for a full explanation of data.

Cooper University Hospital

1 Cooper Plaza
Camden, NJ 08103
Phone: 856-342-2000
Fax: 856-342-3299
URL: www.cooperhealth.org
Type: Acute Care Hospitals
Emergency Services: Yes
Ownership: Voluntary Non-Profit - Private
Key Personnel:
CEO/President. . . . . Christopher T Olivia, MD
Chief of Medical Staff. . . . . Raymond L Baraldi
Radiology. . . . . Eriberto T David

Measure	Cases	This Hosp.	State Avg.	U.S. Avg.
Heart Attack Care				
ACE Inhibitor or ARB for LVSD	100	98%	98%	96%
Aspirin at Arrival	151	99%	99%	99%
Aspirin at Discharge	437	99%	99%	98%
Beta Blocker at Discharge	422	100%	99%	98%
Fibrinolytic Medication Timing	0	-	65%	55%
PCI Within 90 Minutes of Arrival	30	77%	87%	90%
Smoking Cessation Advice	198	100%	100%	99%
Chest Pain/Possible Heart Attack Care				
Aspirin at Arrival[1,3]	1	100%	97%	95%
Median Time to ECG (minutes)[1,3]	1	4	8	8
Median Time to Transfer (minutes)[5]	0	-	81	61
Fibrinolytic Medication Timing[5]	0	-	65%	54%
Heart Failure Care				
ACE Inhibitor or ARB for LVSD	200	99%	97%	94%
Discharge Instructions	422	99%	93%	88%
Evaluation of LVS Function	491	100%	99%	98%
Smoking Cessation Advice	140	100%	100%	98%
Pneumonia Care				
Appropriate Initial Antibiotic	113	96%	94%	92%
Blood Culture Timing	183	95%	97%	96%
Influenza Vaccine[1]	23	100%	94%	91%
Initial Antibiotic Timing	160	96%	96%	95%
Pneumococcal Vaccine	110	85%	96%	93%
Smoking Cessation Advice	88	100%	99%	97%
Surgical Care Improvement Project				
Appropriate VTP Within 24 Hours[2]	374	98%	94%	92%
Appropriate Hair Removal[2]	1,414	100%	100%	99%
Appropriate Beta Blocker Usage[2]	460	95%	95%	93%
Controlled Postoperative Blood Glucose[2]	394	94%	93%	93%
Prophylactic Antibiotic Timing[2]	1,148	96%	98%	97%
Prophylactic Antibiotic Timing (Outpatient)	407	94%	93%	92%
Prophylactic Antibiotic Selection[2]	1,174	96%	97%	97%
Prophylactic Antibiotic Select. (Outpatient)	425	95%	94%	94%
Prophylactic Antibiotic Stopped[2]	1,112	98%	96%	94%
Recommended VTP Ordered[2]	374	99%	95%	94%
Urinary Catheter Removal[2]	318	94%	93%	90%
Children's Asthma Care				
Received Systemic Corticosteroids	-	-	-	100%
Received Home Management Plan	-	-	-	71%
Received Reliever Medication	-	-	-	100%
Use of Medical Imaging				
Combination Abdominal CT Scan	1,051	0.045	0.126	0.191
Combination Chest CT Scan	914	0.008	0.026	0.054
Follow-up Mammogram/Ultrasound	1,293	12.1%	10.6%	8.4%
MRI for Low Back Pain	127	34.6%	26.4%	32.7%
Survey of Patients' Hospital Experiences				
Area Around Room 'Always' Quiet at Night	300+	53%	-	58%
Doctors 'Always' Communicated Well	300+	77%	-	80%
Home Recovery Information Given	300+	82%	-	82%
Hospital Given 9 or 10 on 10 Point Scale	300+	65%	-	67%
Meds 'Always' Explained Before Given	300+	57%	-	60%
Nurses 'Always' Communicated Well	300+	71%	-	76%
Pain 'Always' Well Controlled	300+	64%	-	69%
Room and Bathroom 'Always' Clean	300+	64%	-	71%
Timely Help 'Always' Received	300+	57%	-	64%
Would Definitely Recommend Hospital	300+	70%	-	69%

Our Lady of Lourdes Medical Center

1600 Haddon Avenue
Camden, NJ 08103
Phone: 856-757-3500
E-mail: info@lourdesnet.org
URL: www.lourdesnet.org
Type: Acute Care Hospitals
Emergency Services: Yes
Ownership: Voluntary Non-Profit - Private
Beds: 410
Key Personnel:
CEO/President. . . . . Mark T. Bateman
Chief of Medical Staff . . . . John P. Capelli, M.D.

Measure	Cases	This Hosp.	State Avg.	U.S. Avg.
Heart Attack Care				
ACE Inhibitor or ARB for LVSD[2]	51	98%	98%	96%
Aspirin at Arrival[2]	116	99%	99%	99%
Aspirin at Discharge[2]	293	100%	99%	98%
Beta Blocker at Discharge[2]	278	98%	99%	98%
Fibrinolytic Medication Timing[2]	0	-	65%	55%
PCI Within 90 Minutes of Arrival[1,2]	22	86%	87%	90%
Smoking Cessation Advice[2]	79	100%	100%	99%
Chest Pain/Possible Heart Attack Care				
Aspirin at Arrival[1,3]	2	100%	97%	95%
Median Time to ECG (minutes)[1,3]	2	11	8	8
Median Time to Transfer (minutes)[5]	0	-	81	61
Fibrinolytic Medication Timing[5]	0	-	65%	54%
Heart Failure Care				
ACE Inhibitor or ARB for LVSD[2]	90	100%	97%	94%
Discharge Instructions[2]	245	98%	93%	88%
Evaluation of LVS Function[2]	307	100%	99%	98%
Smoking Cessation Advice[2]	61	100%	100%	98%
Pneumonia Care				
Appropriate Initial Antibiotic[2]	87	99%	94%	92%
Blood Culture Timing[2]	140	98%	97%	96%
Influenza Vaccine[2]	85	99%	94%	91%
Initial Antibiotic Timing[2]	122	98%	96%	95%
Pneumococcal Vaccine[2]	118	98%	96%	93%
Smoking Cessation Advice[2]	54	100%	99%	97%
Surgical Care Improvement Project				
Appropriate VTP Within 24 Hours[2]	152	100%	94%	92%
Appropriate Hair Removal[2]	516	100%	100%	99%
Appropriate Beta Blocker Usage[2]	207	95%	95%	93%
Controlled Postoperative Blood Glucose[2]	173	98%	93%	93%
Prophylactic Antibiotic Timing[2]	317	99%	98%	97%
Prophylactic Antibiotic Timing (Outpatient)	446	100%	93%	92%
Prophylactic Antibiotic Selection[2]	324	98%	97%	97%
Prophylactic Antibiotic Select. (Outpatient)	445	100%	94%	94%
Prophylactic Antibiotic Stopped[2]	292	94%	96%	94%
Recommended VTP Ordered[2]	152	100%	95%	94%
Urinary Catheter Removal[2]	94	89%	93%	90%
Children's Asthma Care				
Received Systemic Corticosteroids	-	-	-	100%
Received Home Management Plan	-	-	-	71%
Received Reliever Medication	-	-	-	100%
Use of Medical Imaging				
Combination Abdominal CT Scan	592	0.139	0.126	0.191
Combination Chest CT Scan	224	0.098	0.026	0.054
Follow-up Mammogram/Ultrasound	210	19.0%	10.6%	8.4%
MRI for Low Back Pain[1]	21	33.3%	26.4%	32.7%
Survey of Patients' Hospital Experiences				
Area Around Room 'Always' Quiet at Night	300+	45%	-	58%
Doctors 'Always' Communicated Well	300+	71%	-	80%
Home Recovery Information Given	300+	75%	-	82%
Hospital Given 9 or 10 on 10 Point Scale	300+	62%	-	67%
Meds 'Always' Explained Before Given	300+	54%	-	60%
Nurses 'Always' Communicated Well	300+	71%	-	76%
Pain 'Always' Well Controlled	300+	61%	-	69%
Room and Bathroom 'Always' Clean	300+	56%	-	71%
Timely Help 'Always' Received	300+	50%	-	64%
Would Definitely Recommend Hospital	300+	65%	-	69%

Cape Regional Medical Center

Two Stone Harbor Blvd
Cape May Court House, NJ 08210
Phone: 609-463-2000
Fax: 609-463-2379
URL: www.caperegional.com
Type: Acute Care Hospitals
Emergency Services: Yes
Ownership: Voluntary Non-Profit - Private
Beds: 272
Key Personnel:
CEO/President. . . . . Thomas L Scott
Chief of Medical Staff . . . . Robert Slating
Operating Room. . . . . Shirley Lathbury
Quality Assurance . . . . Mary Fay
Emergency Room . . . . Michael Dudnick, MD
Intensive Care Unit. . . . . Betsy Holz

Measure	Cases	This Hosp.	State Avg.	U.S. Avg.
Heart Attack Care				
ACE Inhibitor or ARB for LVSD[1]	3	100%	98%	96%
Aspirin at Arrival	50	100%	99%	99%
Aspirin at Discharge[1]	16	94%	99%	98%
Beta Blocker at Discharge[1]	18	100%	99%	98%
Fibrinolytic Medication Timing	0	-	65%	55%
PCI Within 90 Minutes of Arrival	0	-	87%	90%
Smoking Cessation Advice[1]	2	100%	100%	99%
Chest Pain/Possible Heart Attack Care				
Aspirin at Arrival	83	98%	97%	95%
Median Time to ECG (minutes)	85	8	8	8
Median Time to Transfer (minutes)[1]	9	78	81	61
Fibrinolytic Medication Timing[1]	17	53%	65%	54%
Heart Failure Care				
ACE Inhibitor or ARB for LVSD	82	95%	97%	94%
Discharge Instructions	230	86%	93%	88%
Evaluation of LVS Function	302	100%	99%	98%
Smoking Cessation Advice	46	100%	100%	98%
Pneumonia Care				
Appropriate Initial Antibiotic	289	96%	94%	92%
Blood Culture Timing	482	94%	97%	96%
Influenza Vaccine	253	87%	94%	91%
Initial Antibiotic Timing	454	98%	96%	95%
Pneumococcal Vaccine	375	91%	96%	93%
Smoking Cessation Advice	155	99%	99%	97%
Surgical Care Improvement Project				
Appropriate VTP Within 24 Hours[2]	161	89%	94%	92%
Appropriate Hair Removal[2]	427	100%	100%	99%
Appropriate Beta Blocker Usage[2]	135	93%	95%	93%
Controlled Postoperative Blood Glucose[2]	0	-	93%	93%
Prophylactic Antibiotic Timing[2]	272	99%	98%	97%
Prophylactic Antibiotic Timing (Outpatient)	73	86%	93%	92%
Prophylactic Antibiotic Selection[2]	274	96%	97%	97%
Prophylactic Antibiotic Select. (Outpatient)	69	96%	94%	94%
Prophylactic Antibiotic Stopped[2]	262	95%	96%	94%
Recommended VTP Ordered[2]	164	91%	95%	94%
Urinary Catheter Removal[2]	77	94%	93%	90%
Children's Asthma Care				
Received Systemic Corticosteroids	-	-	-	100%
Received Home Management Plan	-	-	-	71%
Received Reliever Medication	-	-	-	100%
Use of Medical Imaging				
Combination Abdominal CT Scan	559	0.433	0.126	0.191
Combination Chest CT Scan	242	0.004	0.026	0.054
Follow-up Mammogram/Ultrasound	326	12.9%	10.6%	8.4%
MRI for Low Back Pain[1]	47	31.9%	26.4%	32.7%
Survey of Patients' Hospital Experiences				
Area Around Room 'Always' Quiet at Night	300+	49%	-	58%
Doctors 'Always' Communicated Well	300+	77%	-	80%
Home Recovery Information Given	300+	79%	-	82%
Hospital Given 9 or 10 on 10 Point Scale	300+	63%	-	67%
Meds 'Always' Explained Before Given	300+	62%	-	60%
Nurses 'Always' Communicated Well	300+	78%	-	76%
Pain 'Always' Well Controlled	300+	71%	-	69%
Room and Bathroom 'Always' Clean	300+	70%	-	71%
Timely Help 'Always' Received	300+	63%	-	64%
Would Definitely Recommend Hospital	300+	66%	-	69%

NOTE: Hospital profiles are in alphabetical order by state, then city, then hospital within the city; Rankings exclude hospitals with less than 25 cases except for patient surveys which excludes hospitals with less than 100 cases; (a) 100–299 cases; (1) The number of cases is too small to be sure how well a hospital is performing; (2) The hospital indicated that the data submitted for this measure were based on a sample of cases; (3) Data was collected during a shorter time period (fewer quarters) than the maximum possible time for this measure; (4) Suppressed for one or more quarters by CMS; (5) No data is available from the hospital for this measure; (6) Fewer than 100 patients completed the HCAHPS survey. Use these rates with caution, as the number of surveys may be too low to reliably assess hospital performance; (7) Survey results are based on less than 12 months of data; (8) Survey results are not available for this reporting period; (9) No or very few patients were eligible for the HCAHPS survey. The scores shown, if any, reflect a very small number of surveys; (10) A state average was not calculated because too few hospitals in the state submitted data; (11) There were discrepancies in the data collection process; Please refer to the User's Guide for a full explanation of data.

Saint Clare's Hospital

25 Pocono Road
Denville, NJ 07834
Phone: 973-625-6000
Fax: 973-537-3959
URL: www.saintclares.org
Type: Acute Care Hospitals
Emergency Services: Yes
Ownership: Voluntary Non-Profit - Church
Beds: 331

Key Personnel:
CEO/President. . . . . Gary J Blan
Chief of Medical Staff. . . . . Stephen Papish

Measure	Cases	This Hosp.	State Avg.	U.S. Avg.
Heart Attack Care				
ACE Inhibitor or ARB for LVSD[1]	16	100%	98%	96%
Aspirin at Arrival	169	100%	99%	99%
Aspirin at Discharge	123	100%	99%	98%
Beta Blocker at Discharge	121	100%	99%	98%
Fibrinolytic Medication Timing	0	-	65%	55%
PCI Within 90 Minutes of Arrival	43	98%	87%	90%
Smoking Cessation Advice	30	100%	100%	99%
Chest Pain/Possible Heart Attack Care				
Aspirin at Arrival	26	100%	97%	95%
Median Time to ECG (minutes)	26	11	8	8
Median Time to Transfer (minutes)[1]	5	60	81	61
Fibrinolytic Medication Timing[1]	3	67%	65%	54%
Heart Failure Care				
ACE Inhibitor or ARB for LVSD	129	99%	97%	94%
Discharge Instructions	381	90%	93%	88%
Evaluation of LVS Function	560	100%	99%	98%
Smoking Cessation Advice	51	100%	100%	98%
Pneumonia Care				
Appropriate Initial Antibiotic	176	99%	94%	92%
Blood Culture Timing	278	100%	97%	96%
Influenza Vaccine	160	99%	94%	91%
Initial Antibiotic Timing	237	99%	96%	95%
Pneumococcal Vaccine	243	100%	96%	93%
Smoking Cessation Advice	71	100%	99%	97%
Surgical Care Improvement Project				
Appropriate VTP Within 24 Hours	376	96%	94%	92%
Appropriate Hair Removal	872	100%	100%	99%
Appropriate Beta Blocker Usage	217	95%	95%	93%
Controlled Postoperative Blood Glucose[1]	1	0%	93%	93%
Prophylactic Antibiotic Timing	475	100%	98%	97%
Prophylactic Antibiotic Timing (Outpatient)	230	98%	93%	92%
Prophylactic Antibiotic Selection	478	97%	97%	97%
Prophylactic Antibiotic Select. (Outpatient)	229	93%	94%	94%
Prophylactic Antibiotic Stopped	465	96%	96%	94%
Recommended VTP Ordered	376	97%	95%	94%
Urinary Catheter Removal	168	90%	93%	90%
Children's Asthma Care				
Received Systemic Corticosteroids	-	-	-	100%
Received Home Management Plan	-	-	-	71%
Received Reliever Medication	-	-	-	100%
Use of Medical Imaging				
Combination Abdominal CT Scan	1,911	0.087	0.126	0.191
Combination Chest CT Scan	1,398	0.011	0.026	0.054
Follow-up Mammogram/Ultrasound	2,620	12.5%	10.6%	8.4%
MRI for Low Back Pain[5]	0	-	26.4%	32.7%
Survey of Patients' Hospital Experiences				
Area Around Room 'Always' Quiet at Night	300+	50%	-	58%
Doctors 'Always' Communicated Well	300+	77%	-	80%
Home Recovery Information Given	300+	78%	-	82%
Hospital Given 9 or 10 on 10 Point Scale	300+	60%	-	67%
Meds 'Always' Explained Before Given	300+	54%	-	60%
Nurses 'Always' Communicated Well	300+	73%	-	76%
Pain 'Always' Well Controlled	300+	65%	-	69%
Room and Bathroom 'Always' Clean	300+	63%	-	71%
Timely Help 'Always' Received	300+	56%	-	64%
Would Definitely Recommend Hospital	300+	66%	-	69%

East Orange General Hospital

300 Central Ave
East Orange, NJ 07018
Phone: 973-266-4401
Fax: 973-266-8488
URL: www.evh.org
Type: Acute Care Hospitals
Emergency Services: Yes
Ownership: Voluntary Non-Profit - Private
Beds: 211

Key Personnel:
CEO/President. . . . . Kevin J Slavin
Chief of Medical Staff. . . . . Nelaton Zephirin, MD
Infection Control. . . . . Aldyth Stanford, RN C
Quality Assurance . . . . Blach Campbell
Radiology. . . . . Jose P Barba
Anesthesiology. . . . . Dr Owen Rhhman
Emergency Room . . . . Eduardo Tinio, MSN RN
Intensive Care Unit. . . . . Nancy Naspo, RN

Measure	Cases	This Hosp.	State Avg.	U.S. Avg.
Heart Attack Care				
ACE Inhibitor or ARB for LVSD[1]	4	100%	98%	96%
Aspirin at Arrival	70	100%	99%	99%
Aspirin at Discharge	42	100%	99%	98%
Beta Blocker at Discharge	48	100%	99%	98%
Fibrinolytic Medication Timing	0	-	65%	55%
PCI Within 90 Minutes of Arrival	0	-	87%	90%
Smoking Cessation Advice[1]	8	100%	100%	99%
Chest Pain/Possible Heart Attack Care				
Aspirin at Arrival[5]	0	-	97%	95%
Median Time to ECG (minutes)[5]	0	-	8	8
Median Time to Transfer (minutes)[5]	0	-	81	61
Fibrinolytic Medication Timing[5]	0	-	65%	54%
Heart Failure Care				
ACE Inhibitor or ARB for LVSD[2]	71	97%	97%	94%
Discharge Instructions[2]	176	99%	93%	88%
Evaluation of LVS Function[2]	276	100%	99%	98%
Smoking Cessation Advice[2]	44	100%	100%	98%
Pneumonia Care				
Appropriate Initial Antibiotic[2]	41	85%	94%	92%
Blood Culture Timing[2]	184	98%	97%	96%
Influenza Vaccine[2]	92	92%	94%	91%
Initial Antibiotic Timing[2]	168	99%	96%	95%
Pneumococcal Vaccine[2]	141	99%	96%	93%
Smoking Cessation Advice[2]	34	100%	99%	97%
Surgical Care Improvement Project				
Appropriate VTP Within 24 Hours	82	98%	94%	92%
Appropriate Hair Removal	131	100%	100%	99%
Appropriate Beta Blocker Usage	25	92%	95%	93%
Controlled Postoperative Blood Glucose	0	-	93%	93%
Prophylactic Antibiotic Timing	49	98%	98%	97%
Prophylactic Antibiotic Timing (Outpatient)	63	84%	93%	92%
Prophylactic Antibiotic Selection	51	98%	97%	97%
Prophylactic Antibiotic Select. (Outpatient)	58	95%	94%	94%
Prophylactic Antibiotic Stopped	44	93%	96%	94%
Recommended VTP Ordered	82	99%	95%	94%
Urinary Catheter Removal[1]	22	91%	93%	90%
Children's Asthma Care				
Received Systemic Corticosteroids	-	-	-	100%
Received Home Management Plan	-	-	-	71%
Received Reliever Medication	-	-	-	100%
Use of Medical Imaging				
Combination Abdominal CT Scan	203	0.483	0.126	0.191
Combination Chest CT Scan	121	0.033	0.026	0.054
Follow-up Mammogram/Ultrasound	395	8.1%	10.6%	8.4%
MRI for Low Back Pain[5]	0	-	26.4%	32.7%
Survey of Patients' Hospital Experiences				
Area Around Room 'Always' Quiet at Night	300+	57%	-	58%
Doctors 'Always' Communicated Well	300+	76%	-	80%
Home Recovery Information Given	300+	74%	-	82%
Hospital Given 9 or 10 on 10 Point Scale	300+	51%	-	67%
Meds 'Always' Explained Before Given	300+	54%	-	60%
Nurses 'Always' Communicated Well	300+	69%	-	76%
Pain 'Always' Well Controlled	300+	64%	-	69%
Room and Bathroom 'Always' Clean	300+	65%	-	71%
Timely Help 'Always' Received	300+	54%	-	64%
Would Definitely Recommend Hospital	300+	50%	-	69%

VA New Jersey Health Care System

385 Tremont Avenue
East Orange, NJ 07018
Phone: 973-676-1000
Fax: 973-395-7062
URL: www1.va.gov/visns/visn03/eorginfo.asp
Type: Acute Care-Veterans Administration
Emergency Services: No
Ownership: Government - Federal
Beds: 791

Key Personnel:
CEO/President. . . . . Kenneth H. Mizrach
Cardiac Laboratory. . . . . Steve Binenbaum, MD
Chief of Medical Staff. . . . . Steven L. Lieberman, MD
Infection Control. . . . . Robert Eng, MD
Operating Room. . . . . George Machiedo, RN
Quality Assurance . . . . Linda Mowad, RN, PhD
Radiology. . . . . Jyoti Shah, MD

Measure	Cases	This Hosp.	State Avg.	U.S. Avg.
Heart Attack Care				
ACE Inhibitor or ARB for LVSD[5]	0	-	98%	96%
Aspirin at Arrival[5]	0	-	99%	99%
Aspirin at Discharge[5]	0	-	99%	98%
Beta Blocker at Discharge[5]	0	-	99%	98%
Fibrinolytic Medication Timing[5]	0	-	65%	55%
PCI Within 90 Minutes of Arrival[5]	0	-	87%	90%
Smoking Cessation Advice[5]	0	-	100%	99%
Chest Pain/Possible Heart Attack Care				
Aspirin at Arrival	-	-	97%	95%
Median Time to ECG (minutes)	-	-	8	8
Median Time to Transfer (minutes)	-	-	81	61
Fibrinolytic Medication Timing	-	-	65%	54%
Heart Failure Care				
ACE Inhibitor or ARB for LVSD	60	100%	97%	94%
Discharge Instructions	103	87%	93%	88%
Evaluation of LVS Function	115	100%	99%	98%
Smoking Cessation Advice	29	100%	100%	98%
Pneumonia Care				
Appropriate Initial Antibiotic	29	93%	94%	92%
Blood Culture Timing	56	95%	97%	96%
Influenza Vaccine	30	97%	94%	91%
Initial Antibiotic Timing	55	96%	96%	95%
Pneumococcal Vaccine	35	91%	96%	93%
Smoking Cessation Advice[1]	22	100%	99%	97%
Surgical Care Improvement Project				
Appropriate VTP Within 24 Hours[2]	119	91%	94%	92%
Appropriate Hair Removal[2]	154	100%	100%	99%
Appropriate Beta Blocker Usage[2]	45	98%	95%	93%
Controlled Postoperative Blood Glucose[1,2]	1	100%	93%	93%
Prophylactic Antibiotic Timing	93	91%	98%	97%
Prophylactic Antibiotic Timing (Outpatient)	-	-	93%	92%
Prophylactic Antibiotic Selection	92	96%	97%	97%
Prophylactic Antibiotic Select. (Outpatient)	-	-	94%	94%
Prophylactic Antibiotic Stopped	89	92%	96%	94%
Recommended VTP Ordered[2]	120	95%	95%	94%
Urinary Catheter Removal[2]	57	84%	93%	90%
Children's Asthma Care				
Received Systemic Corticosteroids	-	-	-	100%
Received Home Management Plan	-	-	-	71%
Received Reliever Medication	-	-	-	100%
Use of Medical Imaging				
Combination Abdominal CT Scan	-	-	0.126	0.191
Combination Chest CT Scan	-	-	0.026	0.054
Follow-up Mammogram/Ultrasound	-	-	10.6%	8.4%
MRI for Low Back Pain	-	-	26.4%	32.7%
Survey of Patients' Hospital Experiences				
Area Around Room 'Always' Quiet at Night	-	-	-	58%
Doctors 'Always' Communicated Well	-	-	-	80%
Home Recovery Information Given	-	-	-	82%
Hospital Given 9 or 10 on 10 Point Scale	-	-	-	67%
Meds 'Always' Explained Before Given	-	-	-	60%
Nurses 'Always' Communicated Well	-	-	-	76%
Pain 'Always' Well Controlled	-	-	-	69%
Room and Bathroom 'Always' Clean	-	-	-	71%
Timely Help 'Always' Received	-	-	-	64%
Would Definitely Recommend Hospital	-	-	-	69%

NOTE: Hospital profiles are in alphabetical order by state, then city, then hospital within the city; Rankings exclude hospitals with less than 25 cases except for patient surveys which excludes hospitals with less than 100 cases; (a) 100–299 cases; (1) The number of cases is too small to be sure how well a hospital is performing; (2) The hospital indicated that the data submitted for this measure were based on a sample of cases; (3) Data was collected during a shorter time period (fewer quarters) than the maximum possible time for this measure; (4) Suppressed for one or more quarters by CMS; (5) No data is available from the hospital for this measure; (6) Fewer than 100 patients completed the HCAHPS survey. Use these rates with caution, as the number of surveys may be too low to reliably assess hospital performance; (7) Survey results are based on less than 12 months of data; (8) Survey results are not available for this reporting period; (9) No or very few patients were eligible for the HCAHPS survey. The scores shown, if any, reflect a very small number of surveys; (10) A state average was not calculated because too few hospitals in the state submitted data; (11) There were discrepancies in the data collection process; Please refer to the User's Guide for a full explanation of data.

JFK Medical Center

65 James Street Phone: 732-321-7000
Edison, NJ 08818 Fax: 732-549 8532
URL: www.jfkmc.org
Type: Acute Care Hospitals Emergency Services: Yes
Ownership: Voluntary Non-Profit - Private

Key Personnel:
CEO/President. . . . . John P McGee
Chief of Medical Staff. . . . . Williams Oser
Infection Control. . . . . John Sensokovic, MD
Operating Room. . . . . Tushar R Patel, RN
Pediatric Ambulatory Care . . . . . . Anthony Santor, MD
Pediatric In-Patient Care . . . . Anthony Santor, MD
Quality Assurance . . . . Lucy Gall
Radiology. . . . . Robert A Friedman, MD

Measure	Cases	This Hosp.	State Avg.	U.S. Avg.
Heart Attack Care				
ACE Inhibitor or ARB for LVSD	39	87%	98%	96%
Aspirin at Arrival	263	97%	99%	99%
Aspirin at Discharge	163	98%	99%	98%
Beta Blocker at Discharge	172	97%	99%	98%
Fibrinolytic Medication Timing	0	-	65%	55%
PCI Within 90 Minutes of Arrival	61	75%	87%	90%
Smoking Cessation Advice	26	100%	100%	99%
Chest Pain/Possible Heart Attack Care				
Aspirin at Arrival[1]	7	57%	97%	95%
Median Time to ECG (minutes)[1]	8	18	8	8
Median Time to Transfer (minutes)[5]	0	-	81	61
Fibrinolytic Medication Timing[5]	0	-	65%	54%
Heart Failure Care				
ACE Inhibitor or ARB for LVSD	178	90%	97%	94%
Discharge Instructions	436	74%	93%	88%
Evaluation of LVS Function	650	99%	99%	98%
Smoking Cessation Advice	59	98%	100%	98%
Pneumonia Care				
Appropriate Initial Antibiotic	262	93%	94%	92%
Blood Culture Timing	384	98%	97%	96%
Influenza Vaccine	250	91%	94%	91%
Initial Antibiotic Timing	418	91%	96%	95%
Pneumococcal Vaccine	346	94%	96%	93%
Smoking Cessation Advice	90	99%	99%	97%
Surgical Care Improvement Project				
Appropriate VTP Within 24 Hours[2]	408	90%	94%	92%
Appropriate Hair Removal[2]	959	98%	100%	99%
Appropriate Beta Blocker Usage[2]	276	84%	95%	93%
Controlled Postoperative Blood Glucose[2]	0	-	93%	93%
Prophylactic Antibiotic Timing[2]	762	96%	98%	97%
Prophylactic Antibiotic Timing (Outpatient)	400	87%	93%	92%
Prophylactic Antibiotic Selection[2]	763	96%	97%	97%
Prophylactic Antibiotic Select. (Outpatient)	373	94%	94%	94%
Prophylactic Antibiotic Stopped[2]	747	92%	96%	94%
Recommended VTP Ordered[2]	413	91%	95%	94%
Urinary Catheter Removal[2]	118	65%	93%	90%
Children's Asthma Care				
Received Systemic Corticosteroids	-	-	-	100%
Received Home Management Plan	-	-	-	71%
Received Reliever Medication	-	-	-	100%
Use of Medical Imaging				
Combination Abdominal CT Scan	1,192	0.618	0.126	0.191
Combination Chest CT Scan	1,081	0.002	0.026	0.054
Follow-up Mammogram/Ultrasound	1,516	9.6%	10.6%	8.4%
MRI for Low Back Pain	147	20.4%	26.4%	32.7%
Survey of Patients' Hospital Experiences				
Area Around Room 'Always' Quiet at Night	300+	43%	-	58%
Doctors 'Always' Communicated Well	300+	78%	-	80%
Home Recovery Information Given	300+	76%	-	82%
Hospital Given 9 or 10 on 10 Point Scale	300+	54%	-	67%
Meds 'Always' Explained Before Given	300+	55%	-	60%
Nurses 'Always' Communicated Well	300+	72%	-	76%
Pain 'Always' Well Controlled	300+	66%	-	69%
Room and Bathroom 'Always' Clean	300+	69%	-	71%
Timely Help 'Always' Received	300+	51%	-	64%
Would Definitely Recommend Hospital	300+	56%	-	69%

Trinitas Regional Medical Center

225 Williamson Street Phone: 908-994-5000
Elizabeth, NJ 07207 Fax: 908-994-5727
URL: www.trinitashospital.org
Type: Acute Care Hospitals Emergency Services: Yes
Ownership: Voluntary Non-Profit - Private Beds: 531

Key Personnel:
Cardiac Laboratory. . . . . Arthur Millman, MD
Chief of Medical Staff . . . . William McHugh, MD
Infection Control. . . . . Uwe Schmidt, MD
Pediatric In-Patient Care . . . . Cheryl Dickson, MD
Radiology. . . . . David Wirtshafter, MD
Anesthesiology. . . . . Leon Pirak, MD
Emergency Room . . . . Maribeth Santillo, RN MS
Hemotology Center . . . . Stanley Pomerantz, MD

Measure	Cases	This Hosp.	State Avg.	U.S. Avg.
Heart Attack Care				
ACE Inhibitor or ARB for LVSD	35	100%	98%	96%
Aspirin at Arrival	163	96%	99%	99%
Aspirin at Discharge	109	95%	99%	98%
Beta Blocker at Discharge	114	96%	99%	98%
Fibrinolytic Medication Timing	0	-	65%	55%
PCI Within 90 Minutes of Arrival	35	80%	87%	90%
Smoking Cessation Advice	35	100%	100%	99%
Chest Pain/Possible Heart Attack Care				
Aspirin at Arrival[1,3]	2	100%	97%	95%
Median Time to ECG (minutes)[1,3]	2	4	8	8
Median Time to Transfer (minutes)[5]	0	-	81	61
Fibrinolytic Medication Timing[5]	0	-	65%	54%
Heart Failure Care				
ACE Inhibitor or ARB for LVSD[2]	127	85%	97%	94%
Discharge Instructions[2]	235	91%	93%	88%
Evaluation of LVS Function[2]	299	98%	99%	98%
Smoking Cessation Advice[2]	57	100%	100%	98%
Pneumonia Care				
Appropriate Initial Antibiotic[2]	94	84%	94%	92%
Blood Culture Timing[2]	131	98%	97%	96%
Influenza Vaccine[2]	89	94%	94%	91%
Initial Antibiotic Timing[2]	172	91%	96%	95%
Pneumococcal Vaccine[2]	126	98%	96%	93%
Smoking Cessation Advice[2]	57	100%	99%	97%
Surgical Care Improvement Project				
Appropriate VTP Within 24 Hours[2]	186	82%	94%	92%
Appropriate Hair Removal[2]	454	99%	100%	99%
Appropriate Beta Blocker Usage[2]	129	98%	95%	93%
Controlled Postoperative Blood Glucose[2]	0	-	93%	93%
Prophylactic Antibiotic Timing[2]	210	99%	98%	97%
Prophylactic Antibiotic Timing (Outpatient)	274	98%	93%	92%
Prophylactic Antibiotic Selection[2]	211	95%	97%	97%
Prophylactic Antibiotic Select. (Outpatient)	271	96%	94%	94%
Prophylactic Antibiotic Stopped[2]	205	94%	96%	94%
Recommended VTP Ordered[2]	189	83%	95%	94%
Urinary Catheter Removal[2]	48	90%	93%	90%
Children's Asthma Care				
Received Systemic Corticosteroids	-	-	-	100%
Received Home Management Plan	-	-	-	71%
Received Reliever Medication	-	-	-	100%
Use of Medical Imaging				
Combination Abdominal CT Scan	563	0.032	0.126	0.191
Combination Chest CT Scan	475	0.017	0.026	0.054
Follow-up Mammogram/Ultrasound	1,048	6.1%	10.6%	8.4%
MRI for Low Back Pain	64	25.0%	26.4%	32.7%
Survey of Patients' Hospital Experiences				
Area Around Room 'Always' Quiet at Night	300+	56%	-	58%
Doctors 'Always' Communicated Well	300+	80%	-	80%
Home Recovery Information Given	300+	74%	-	82%
Hospital Given 9 or 10 on 10 Point Scale	300+	62%	-	67%
Meds 'Always' Explained Before Given	300+	57%	-	60%
Nurses 'Always' Communicated Well	300+	75%	-	76%
Pain 'Always' Well Controlled	300+	64%	-	69%
Room and Bathroom 'Always' Clean	300+	73%	-	71%
Timely Help 'Always' Received	300+	59%	-	64%
Would Definitely Recommend Hospital	300+	59%	-	69%

South Jersey Healthcare-Elmer Hospital

501 West Front Street Phone: 856-363-1000
Elmer, NJ 08318 Fax: 856-358-3248
URL: www.sjhs.com/content/SJHElmerHospit
Type: Acute Care Hospitals Emergency Services: Yes
Ownership: Voluntary Non-Profit - Private Beds: 88

Key Personnel:
CEO/President. . . . . Chet Kaletkowski
Chief of Medical Staff . . . . William Mills
Quality Assurance . . . . Donna Cross
Emergency Room . . . . Stanley Zoyac

Measure	Cases	This Hosp.	State Avg.	U.S. Avg.
Heart Attack Care				
ACE Inhibitor or ARB for LVSD[1]	6	83%	98%	96%
Aspirin at Arrival	39	100%	99%	99%
Aspirin at Discharge[1]	17	94%	99%	98%
Beta Blocker at Discharge[1]	19	100%	99%	98%
Fibrinolytic Medication Timing	0	-	65%	55%
PCI Within 90 Minutes of Arrival	0	-	87%	90%
Smoking Cessation Advice[1]	1	100%	100%	99%
Chest Pain/Possible Heart Attack Care				
Aspirin at Arrival[1]	22	100%	97%	95%
Median Time to ECG (minutes)[1]	21	10	8	8
Median Time to Transfer (minutes)[1,3]	1	140	81	61
Fibrinolytic Medication Timing[1]	5	60%	65%	54%
Heart Failure Care				
ACE Inhibitor or ARB for LVSD	36	92%	97%	94%
Discharge Instructions	98	100%	93%	88%
Evaluation of LVS Function	122	100%	99%	98%
Smoking Cessation Advice[1]	10	100%	100%	98%
Pneumonia Care				
Appropriate Initial Antibiotic[2]	79	97%	94%	92%
Blood Culture Timing[2]	99	99%	97%	96%
Influenza Vaccine	66	98%	94%	91%
Initial Antibiotic Timing[2]	110	95%	96%	95%
Pneumococcal Vaccine[2]	98	99%	96%	93%
Smoking Cessation Advice[2]	34	100%	99%	97%
Surgical Care Improvement Project				
Appropriate VTP Within 24 Hours[2]	67	91%	94%	92%
Appropriate Hair Removal[2]	216	100%	100%	99%
Appropriate Beta Blocker Usage[2]	73	95%	95%	93%
Controlled Postoperative Blood Glucose[2]	0	-	93%	93%
Prophylactic Antibiotic Timing[2]	140	99%	98%	97%
Prophylactic Antibiotic Timing (Outpatient)	49	96%	93%	92%
Prophylactic Antibiotic Selection[2]	140	98%	97%	97%
Prophylactic Antibiotic Select. (Outpatient)	47	98%	94%	94%
Prophylactic Antibiotic Stopped[2]	139	95%	96%	94%
Recommended VTP Ordered[2]	67	91%	95%	94%
Urinary Catheter Removal[2]	84	89%	93%	90%
Children's Asthma Care				
Received Systemic Corticosteroids	-	-	-	100%
Received Home Management Plan	-	-	-	71%
Received Reliever Medication	-	-	-	100%
Use of Medical Imaging				
Combination Abdominal CT Scan	349	0.132	0.126	0.191
Combination Chest CT Scan	299	0.017	0.026	0.054
Follow-up Mammogram/Ultrasound	657	6.8%	10.6%	8.4%
MRI for Low Back Pain[1]	12	33.3%	26.4%	32.7%
Survey of Patients' Hospital Experiences				
Area Around Room 'Always' Quiet at Night	300+	55%	-	58%
Doctors 'Always' Communicated Well	300+	81%	-	80%
Home Recovery Information Given	300+	86%	-	82%
Hospital Given 9 or 10 on 10 Point Scale	300+	73%	-	67%
Meds 'Always' Explained Before Given	300+	61%	-	60%
Nurses 'Always' Communicated Well	300+	80%	-	76%
Pain 'Always' Well Controlled	300+	73%	-	69%
Room and Bathroom 'Always' Clean	300+	77%	-	71%
Timely Help 'Always' Received	300+	69%	-	64%
Would Definitely Recommend Hospital	300+	80%	-	69%

NOTE: Hospital profiles are in alphabetical order by state, then city, then hospital within the city; Rankings exclude hospitals with less than 25 cases except for patient surveys which excludes hospitals with less than 100 cases; (a) 100–299 cases; (1) The number of cases is too small to be sure how well a hospital is performing; (2) The hospital indicated that the data submitted for this measure were based on a sample of cases; (3) Data was collected during a shorter time period (fewer quarters) than the maximum possible time for this measure; (4) Suppressed for one or more quarters by CMS; (5) No data is available from the hospital for this measure; (6) Fewer than 100 patients completed the HCAHPS survey. Use these rates with caution, as the number of surveys may be too low to reliably assess hospital performance; (7) Survey results are based on less than 12 months of data; (8) Survey results are not available for this reporting period; (9) No or very few patients were eligible for the HCAHPS survey. The scores shown, if any, reflect a very small number of surveys; (10) A state average was not calculated because too few hospitals in the state submitted data; (11) There were discrepancies in the data collection process; Please refer to the User's Guide for a full explanation of data.

Englewood Hospital and Medical Center

350 Engle St
Englewood, NJ 07631
URL: www.englewoodhospital.com
Type: Acute Care Hospitals
Ownership: Voluntary Non-Profit - Other

Phone: 201-894-3000
Fax: 201-894-4791

Emergency Services: Yes
Beds: 547

Key Personnel:
CEO/President . . . . Douglas A Duchak
Chief of Medical Staff . . . . Robert Adair
Radiology. . . . . Marina Gutwein
Hemotology Center . . . . Michael Schleider, MD

Measure	Cases	This Hosp.	State Avg.	U.S. Avg.
Heart Attack Care				
ACE Inhibitor or ARB for LVSD[2]	55	98%	98%	96%
Aspirin at Arrival[2]	248	100%	99%	99%
Aspirin at Discharge[2]	268	100%	99%	98%
Beta Blocker at Discharge[2]	261	98%	99%	98%
Fibrinolytic Medication Timing[2]	0	-	65%	55%
PCI Within 90 Minutes of Arrival[2]	39	87%	87%	90%
Smoking Cessation Advice[2]	42	100%	100%	99%
Chest Pain/Possible Heart Attack Care				
Aspirin at Arrival[1,3]	1	100%	97%	95%
Median Time to ECG (minutes)[1,3]	1	0	8	8
Median Time to Transfer (minutes)[5]	0	-	81	61
Fibrinolytic Medication Timing[5]	0	-	65%	54%
Heart Failure Care				
ACE Inhibitor or ARB for LVSD	166	98%	97%	94%
Discharge Instructions	363	94%	93%	88%
Evaluation of LVS Function	498	99%	99%	98%
Smoking Cessation Advice	40	100%	100%	98%
Pneumonia Care				
Appropriate Initial Antibiotic	119	99%	94%	92%
Blood Culture Timing	197	97%	97%	96%
Influenza Vaccine	170	96%	94%	91%
Initial Antibiotic Timing	185	99%	96%	95%
Pneumococcal Vaccine	264	97%	96%	93%
Smoking Cessation Advice	32	100%	99%	97%
Surgical Care Improvement Project				
Appropriate VTP Within 24 Hours[2]	311	94%	94%	92%
Appropriate Hair Removal[2]	1,154	100%	100%	99%
Appropriate Beta Blocker Usage[2]	429	100%	95%	93%
Controlled Postoperative Blood Glucose[2]	259	97%	93%	93%
Prophylactic Antibiotic Timing[2]	869	99%	98%	97%
Prophylactic Antibiotic Timing (Outpatient)	334	96%	93%	92%
Prophylactic Antibiotic Selection[2]	871	99%	97%	97%
Prophylactic Antibiotic Select. (Outpatient)	338	90%	94%	94%
Prophylactic Antibiotic Stopped[2]	839	98%	96%	94%
Recommended VTP Ordered[2]	313	96%	95%	94%
Urinary Catheter Removal[2]	297	96%	93%	90%
Children's Asthma Care				
Received Systemic Corticosteroids	-	-	-	100%
Received Home Management Plan	-	-	-	71%
Received Reliever Medication	-	-	-	100%
Use of Medical Imaging				
Combination Abdominal CT Scan	1,560	0.183	0.126	0.191
Combination Chest CT Scan	1,105	0.008	0.026	0.054
Follow-up Mammogram/Ultrasound	2,429	13.9%	10.6%	8.4%
MRI for Low Back Pain	231	23.4%	26.4%	32.7%
Survey of Patients' Hospital Experiences				
Area Around Room 'Always' Quiet at Night	300+	52%	-	58%
Doctors 'Always' Communicated Well	300+	79%	-	80%
Home Recovery Information Given	300+	74%	-	82%
Hospital Given 9 or 10 on 10 Point Scale	300+	67%	-	67%
Meds 'Always' Explained Before Given	300+	56%	-	60%
Nurses 'Always' Communicated Well	300+	74%	-	76%
Pain 'Always' Well Controlled	300+	68%	-	69%
Room and Bathroom 'Always' Clean	300+	74%	-	71%
Timely Help 'Always' Received	300+	54%	-	64%
Would Definitely Recommend Hospital	300+	73%	-	69%

Hunterdon Medical Center

2100 Wescott Drive
Flemington, NJ 08822
URL: www.hunterdonhealthcare.org
Type: Acute Care Hospitals
Ownership: Voluntary Non-Profit - Private

Phone: 908-788-6100
Fax: 908-788-6111

Emergency Services: Yes
Beds: 176

Key Personnel:
CEO/President. . . . . Robert P Wise
Chief of Medical Staff . . . . Robert Pickoff, MD
Infection Control . . . . Kathy Roye, RN
Operating Room . . . . Donna Cole, RN
Pediatric Ambulatory Care . . . . . Wayne Fellmeth, MD
Pediatric In-Patient Care . . . . . . Wayne Fellmeth, MD
Quality Assurance . . . . Stephanie Dougherty
Radiology. . . . . Brian Donnelly, MD

Measure	Cases	This Hosp.	State Avg.	U.S. Avg.
Heart Attack Care				
ACE Inhibitor or ARB for LVSD[1]	17	100%	98%	96%
Aspirin at Arrival	117	100%	99%	99%
Aspirin at Discharge	75	100%	99%	98%
Beta Blocker at Discharge	75	100%	99%	98%
Fibrinolytic Medication Timing	0	-	65%	55%
PCI Within 90 Minutes of Arrival	42	95%	87%	90%
Smoking Cessation Advice	25	100%	100%	99%
Chest Pain/Possible Heart Attack Care				
Aspirin at Arrival[1]	11	91%	97%	95%
Median Time to ECG (minutes)[1]	11	9	8	8
Median Time to Transfer (minutes)[1,3]	1	184	81	61
Fibrinolytic Medication Timing	0	-	65%	54%
Heart Failure Care				
ACE Inhibitor or ARB for LVSD	57	100%	97%	94%
Discharge Instructions	107	93%	93%	88%
Evaluation of LVS Function	146	99%	99%	98%
Smoking Cessation Advice[1]	14	100%	100%	98%
Pneumonia Care				
Appropriate Initial Antibiotic[2]	90	97%	94%	92%
Blood Culture Timing[2]	197	98%	97%	96%
Influenza Vaccine[2]	94	97%	94%	91%
Initial Antibiotic Timing[2]	149	98%	96%	95%
Pneumococcal Vaccine[2]	138	97%	96%	93%
Smoking Cessation Advice[1,2]	23	96%	99%	97%
Surgical Care Improvement Project				
Appropriate VTP Within 24 Hours[2]	139	92%	94%	92%
Appropriate Hair Removal[2]	418	100%	100%	99%
Appropriate Beta Blocker Usage[2]	100	93%	95%	93%
Controlled Postoperative Blood Glucose[2]	0	-	93%	93%
Prophylactic Antibiotic Timing[2]	291	98%	98%	97%
Prophylactic Antibiotic Timing (Outpatient)	180	87%	93%	92%
Prophylactic Antibiotic Selection[2]	289	99%	97%	97%
Prophylactic Antibiotic Select. (Outpatient)	176	86%	94%	94%
Prophylactic Antibiotic Stopped[2]	286	97%	96%	94%
Recommended VTP Ordered[2]	139	96%	95%	94%
Urinary Catheter Removal[2]	90	87%	93%	90%
Children's Asthma Care				
Received Systemic Corticosteroids	-	-	-	100%
Received Home Management Plan	-	-	-	71%
Received Reliever Medication	-	-	-	100%
Use of Medical Imaging				
Combination Abdominal CT Scan	737	0.069	0.126	0.191
Combination Chest CT Scan	832	0.018	0.026	0.054
Follow-up Mammogram/Ultrasound	576	12.5%	10.6%	8.4%
MRI for Low Back Pain[5]	0	-	26.4%	32.7%
Survey of Patients' Hospital Experiences				
Area Around Room 'Always' Quiet at Night	300+	47%	-	58%
Doctors 'Always' Communicated Well	300+	80%	-	80%
Home Recovery Information Given	300+	84%	-	82%
Hospital Given 9 or 10 on 10 Point Scale	300+	71%	-	67%
Meds 'Always' Explained Before Given	300+	61%	-	60%
Nurses 'Always' Communicated Well	300+	79%	-	76%
Pain 'Always' Well Controlled	300+	72%	-	69%
Room and Bathroom 'Always' Clean	300+	73%	-	71%
Timely Help 'Always' Received	300+	64%	-	64%
Would Definitely Recommend Hospital	300+	75%	-	69%

Centrastate Medical Center

901 West Main Street
Freehold, NJ 07728
URL: www.centrastate.com
Type: Acute Care Hospitals
Ownership: Voluntary Non-Profit - Private

Phone: 732-431-2000
Fax: 732-462-5129

Emergency Services: Yes
Beds: 271

Key Personnel:
CEO/President . . . . John T Gribbin, FACHE
Quality Assurance . . . . Janice De Young Breen, RN, APRN
Patient Relations . . . . Laura Geisler, RN

Measure	Cases	This Hosp.	State Avg.	U.S. Avg.
Heart Attack Care				
ACE Inhibitor or ARB for LVSD[1]	8	88%	98%	96%
Aspirin at Arrival	111	100%	99%	99%
Aspirin at Discharge	38	100%	99%	98%
Beta Blocker at Discharge	38	100%	99%	98%
Fibrinolytic Medication Timing[1]	2	100%	65%	55%
PCI Within 90 Minutes of Arrival	0	-	87%	90%
Smoking Cessation Advice[1]	3	100%	100%	99%
Chest Pain/Possible Heart Attack Care				
Aspirin at Arrival	81	96%	97%	95%
Median Time to ECG (minutes)	83	5	8	8
Median Time to Transfer (minutes)[1]	6	98	81	61
Fibrinolytic Medication Timing[1]	16	62%	65%	54%
Heart Failure Care				
ACE Inhibitor or ARB for LVSD	90	93%	97%	94%
Discharge Instructions	230	83%	93%	88%
Evaluation of LVS Function	356	99%	99%	98%
Smoking Cessation Advice[1]	22	100%	100%	98%
Pneumonia Care				
Appropriate Initial Antibiotic	193	93%	94%	92%
Blood Culture Timing	356	97%	97%	96%
Influenza Vaccine	214	95%	94%	91%
Initial Antibiotic Timing	339	97%	96%	95%
Pneumococcal Vaccine	352	96%	96%	93%
Smoking Cessation Advice	71	100%	99%	97%
Surgical Care Improvement Project				
Appropriate VTP Within 24 Hours[2]	284	80%	94%	92%
Appropriate Hair Removal[2]	716	99%	100%	99%
Appropriate Beta Blocker Usage[2]	200	74%	95%	93%
Controlled Postoperative Blood Glucose[2]	0	-	93%	93%
Prophylactic Antibiotic Timing[2]	415	97%	98%	97%
Prophylactic Antibiotic Timing (Outpatient)	65	89%	93%	92%
Prophylactic Antibiotic Selection[2]	418	93%	97%	97%
Prophylactic Antibiotic Select. (Outpatient)	192	94%	94%	94%
Prophylactic Antibiotic Stopped[2]	402	92%	96%	94%
Recommended VTP Ordered[2]	284	81%	95%	94%
Urinary Catheter Removal[2]	130	87%	93%	90%
Children's Asthma Care				
Received Systemic Corticosteroids	-	-	-	100%
Received Home Management Plan	-	-	-	71%
Received Reliever Medication	-	-	-	100%
Use of Medical Imaging				
Combination Abdominal CT Scan	757	0.073	0.126	0.191
Combination Chest CT Scan	591	0.003	0.026	0.054
Follow-up Mammogram/Ultrasound	784	9.8%	10.6%	8.4%
MRI for Low Back Pain[1]	1	0.0%	26.4%	32.7%
Survey of Patients' Hospital Experiences				
Area Around Room 'Always' Quiet at Night	300+	52%	-	58%
Doctors 'Always' Communicated Well	300+	76%	-	80%
Home Recovery Information Given	300+	80%	-	82%
Hospital Given 9 or 10 on 10 Point Scale	300+	69%	-	67%
Meds 'Always' Explained Before Given	300+	60%	-	60%
Nurses 'Always' Communicated Well	300+	74%	-	76%
Pain 'Always' Well Controlled	300+	65%	-	69%
Room and Bathroom 'Always' Clean	300+	72%	-	71%
Timely Help 'Always' Received	300+	61%	-	64%
Would Definitely Recommend Hospital	300+	72%	-	69%

NOTE: Hospital profiles are in alphabetical order by state, then city, then hospital within the city; Rankings exclude hospitals with less than 25 cases except for patient surveys which excludes hospitals with less than 100 cases; (a) 100–299 cases; (1) The number of cases is too small to be sure how well a hospital is performing; (2) The hospital indicated that the data submitted for this measure were based on a sample of cases; (3) Data was collected during a shorter time period (fewer quarters) than the maximum possible time for this measure; (4) Suppressed for one or more quarters by CMS; (5) No data is available from the hospital for this measure; (6) Fewer than 100 patients completed the HCAHPS survey. Use these rates with caution, as the number of surveys may be too low to reliably assess hospital performance; (7) Survey results are based on less than 12 months of data; (8) Survey results are not available for this reporting period; (9) No or very few patients were eligible for the HCAHPS survey. The scores shown, if any, reflect a very small number of surveys; (10) A state average was not calculated because too few hospitals in the state submitted data; (11) There were discrepancies in the data collection process; Please refer to the User's Guide for a full explanation of data.

Hackensack University Medical Center

30 Prospect Ave | Phone: 201-996-2000
Hackensack, NJ 07601 | Fax: 201-996-3452
URL: www.humed.com
Type: Acute Care Hospitals | Emergency Services: Yes
Ownership: Voluntary Non-Profit - Private | Beds: 614

Key Personnel:
CEO/President.............. Robert C. Garrett
Chief of Medical Staff.......... Jeanne Aversa
Infection Control.............. Nancy Nelsen, RN
Operating Room.............. Doreen Santora, RN
Pediatric In-Patient Care .... Donald Stark
Quality Assurance .... Audrey Murphy
Radiology................... Helen Chimel

Measure	Cases	This Hosp.	State Avg.	U.S. Avg.
Heart Attack Care				
ACE Inhibitor or ARB for LVSD	165	100%	98%	96%
Aspirin at Arrival	524	100%	99%	99%
Aspirin at Discharge	741	100%	99%	98%
Beta Blocker at Discharge	731	100%	99%	98%
Fibrinolytic Medication Timing	0	-	65%	55%
PCI Within 90 Minutes of Arrival	88	98%	87%	90%
Smoking Cessation Advice	165	100%	100%	99%
Chest Pain/Possible Heart Attack Care				
Aspirin at Arrival	33	94%	97%	95%
Median Time to ECG (minutes)	37	6	8	8
Median Time to Transfer (minutes)[5]	0	-	81	61
Fibrinolytic Medication Timing[3]	0	-	65%	54%
Heart Failure Care				
ACE Inhibitor or ARB for LVSD	372	94%	97%	94%
Discharge Instructions	794	87%	93%	88%
Evaluation of LVS Function	1,086	100%	99%	98%
Smoking Cessation Advice	100	100%	100%	98%
Pneumonia Care				
Appropriate Initial Antibiotic	270	99%	94%	92%
Blood Culture Timing	258	98%	97%	96%
Influenza Vaccine	339	96%	94%	91%
Initial Antibiotic Timing	384	97%	96%	95%
Pneumococcal Vaccine	482	96%	96%	93%
Smoking Cessation Advice	103	100%	99%	97%
Surgical Care Improvement Project				
Appropriate VTP Within 24 Hours[2]	148	86%	94%	92%
Appropriate Hair Removal[2]	658	100%	100%	99%
Appropriate Beta Blocker Usage[2]	247	93%	95%	93%
Controlled Postoperative Blood Glucose[2]	136	95%	93%	93%
Prophylactic Antibiotic Timing[2]	454	99%	98%	97%
Prophylactic Antibiotic Timing (Outpatient)	668	96%	93%	92%
Prophylactic Antibiotic Selection[2]	462	97%	97%	97%
Prophylactic Antibiotic Select. (Outpatient)	662	94%	94%	94%
Prophylactic Antibiotic Stopped[2]	433	95%	96%	94%
Recommended VTP Ordered[2]	149	87%	95%	94%
Urinary Catheter Removal[2]	187	96%	93%	90%
Children's Asthma Care				
Received Systemic Corticosteroids	-	-	-	100%
Received Home Management Plan	-	-	-	71%
Received Reliever Medication	-	-	-	100%
Use of Medical Imaging				
Combination Abdominal CT Scan	2,096	0.088	0.126	0.191
Combination Chest CT Scan	2,549	0.051	0.026	0.054
Follow-up Mammogram/Ultrasound	2,174	8.4%	10.6%	8.4%
MRI for Low Back Pain	95	23.2%	26.4%	32.7%
Survey of Patients' Hospital Experiences				
Area Around Room 'Always' Quiet at Night	300+	49%	-	58%
Doctors 'Always' Communicated Well	300+	78%	-	80%
Home Recovery Information Given	300+	81%	-	82%
Hospital Given 9 or 10 on 10 Point Scale	300+	72%	-	67%
Meds 'Always' Explained Before Given	300+	59%	-	60%
Nurses 'Always' Communicated Well	300+	77%	-	76%
Pain 'Always' Well Controlled	300+	69%	-	69%
Room and Bathroom 'Always' Clean	300+	72%	-	71%
Timely Help 'Always' Received	300+	59%	-	64%
Would Definitely Recommend Hospital	300+	80%	-	69%

Hackettstown Regional Medical Center

651 Willow Grove St | Phone: 908-852-5100
Hackettstown, NJ 07840 | Fax: 908-850-6822
URL: www.hrmcnj.org
Type: Acute Care Hospitals | Emergency Services: Yes
Ownership: Voluntary Non-Profit - Church | Beds: 99

Key Personnel:
CEO/President.............. Gene C Milton, FACHE
Chief of Medical Staff.......... Leong-Hean Tan
Pediatric In-Patient Care .... Adam Dick, MD
Quality Assurance .... Kim Foreman
Anesthesiology.............. Arnold Bodner, MD
Emergency Room .... Chester Skiba
Intensive Care Unit........... Cathy Richardson

Measure	Cases	This Hosp.	State Avg.	U.S. Avg.
Heart Attack Care				
ACE Inhibitor or ARB for LVSD[1]	8	100%	98%	96%
Aspirin at Arrival	61	100%	99%	99%
Aspirin at Discharge	32	100%	99%	98%
Beta Blocker at Discharge	35	100%	99%	98%
Fibrinolytic Medication Timing	0	-	65%	55%
PCI Within 90 Minutes of Arrival	0	-	87%	90%
Smoking Cessation Advice[1]	5	100%	100%	99%
Chest Pain/Possible Heart Attack Care				
Aspirin at Arrival	33	100%	97%	95%
Median Time to ECG (minutes)	37	15	8	8
Median Time to Transfer (minutes)[3]	0	-	81	61
Fibrinolytic Medication Timing[1]	7	71%	65%	54%
Heart Failure Care				
ACE Inhibitor or ARB for LVSD	34	100%	97%	94%
Discharge Instructions	117	96%	93%	88%
Evaluation of LVS Function	204	100%	99%	98%
Smoking Cessation Advice[1]	13	100%	100%	98%
Pneumonia Care				
Appropriate Initial Antibiotic	66	98%	94%	92%
Blood Culture Timing	102	98%	97%	96%
Influenza Vaccine	51	96%	94%	91%
Initial Antibiotic Timing	82	100%	96%	95%
Pneumococcal Vaccine	85	100%	96%	93%
Smoking Cessation Advice[1]	21	95%	99%	97%
Surgical Care Improvement Project				
Appropriate VTP Within 24 Hours	76	95%	94%	92%
Appropriate Hair Removal	257	100%	100%	99%
Appropriate Beta Blocker Usage	75	99%	95%	93%
Controlled Postoperative Blood Glucose	0	-	93%	93%
Prophylactic Antibiotic Timing	176	99%	98%	97%
Prophylactic Antibiotic Timing (Outpatient)	52	96%	93%	92%
Prophylactic Antibiotic Selection	177	95%	97%	97%
Prophylactic Antibiotic Select. (Outpatient)	52	94%	94%	94%
Prophylactic Antibiotic Stopped	168	96%	96%	94%
Recommended VTP Ordered	77	94%	95%	94%
Urinary Catheter Removal	41	100%	93%	90%
Children's Asthma Care				
Received Systemic Corticosteroids	-	-	-	100%
Received Home Management Plan	-	-	-	71%
Received Reliever Medication	-	-	-	100%
Use of Medical Imaging				
Combination Abdominal CT Scan	493	0.083	0.126	0.191
Combination Chest CT Scan	253	0.012	0.026	0.054
Follow-up Mammogram/Ultrasound	512	14.5%	10.6%	8.4%
MRI for Low Back Pain[1]	54	25.9%	26.4%	32.7%
Survey of Patients' Hospital Experiences				
Area Around Room 'Always' Quiet at Night	300+	49%	-	58%
Doctors 'Always' Communicated Well	300+	78%	-	80%
Home Recovery Information Given	300+	83%	-	82%
Hospital Given 9 or 10 on 10 Point Scale	300+	67%	-	67%
Meds 'Always' Explained Before Given	300+	53%	-	60%
Nurses 'Always' Communicated Well	300+	75%	-	76%
Pain 'Always' Well Controlled	300+	64%	-	69%
Room and Bathroom 'Always' Clean	300+	67%	-	71%
Timely Help 'Always' Received	300+	59%	-	64%
Would Definitely Recommend Hospital	300+	69%	-	69%

Robert Wood Johnson University Hospital Hamilton

One Hamilton Health Place | Phone: 609-586-7900
Hamilton, NJ 08690 | Fax: 609-584-6429
URL: www.rwjhamilton.org
Type: Acute Care Hospitals | Emergency Services: Yes
Ownership: Voluntary Non-Profit - Private | Beds: 200

Key Personnel:
CEO/President.............. Anthony Cimino
Chief of Medical Staff.......... Mahmoud Ghusson
Infection Control............. Anne Dikon
Operating Room.............. Louis G Fares II
Pediatric Ambulatory Care ...... David H Carver, MD
Pediatric In-Patient Care .... Dennis M. Baiser
Quality Assurance .... Jan Stout
Radiology.................. Hae W Won Shin

Measure	Cases	This Hosp.	State Avg.	U.S. Avg.
Heart Attack Care				
ACE Inhibitor or ARB for LVSD[1]	11	91%	98%	96%
Aspirin at Arrival	161	94%	99%	99%
Aspirin at Discharge	89	93%	99%	98%
Beta Blocker at Discharge	86	98%	99%	98%
Fibrinolytic Medication Timing	0	-	65%	55%
PCI Within 90 Minutes of Arrival	36	61%	87%	90%
Smoking Cessation Advice	26	100%	100%	99%
Chest Pain/Possible Heart Attack Care				
Aspirin at Arrival[5]	0	-	97%	95%
Median Time to ECG (minutes)[5]	0	-	8	8
Median Time to Transfer (minutes)[5]	0	-	81	61
Fibrinolytic Medication Timing[5]	0	-	65%	54%
Heart Failure Care				
ACE Inhibitor or ARB for LVSD	102	94%	97%	94%
Discharge Instructions	314	92%	93%	88%
Evaluation of LVS Function	413	100%	99%	98%
Smoking Cessation Advice	41	100%	100%	98%
Pneumonia Care				
Appropriate Initial Antibiotic	203	90%	94%	92%
Blood Culture Timing	367	98%	97%	96%
Influenza Vaccine	195	93%	94%	91%
Initial Antibiotic Timing	322	97%	96%	95%
Pneumococcal Vaccine	268	94%	96%	93%
Smoking Cessation Advice	88	99%	99%	97%
Surgical Care Improvement Project				
Appropriate VTP Within 24 Hours[2]	312	89%	94%	92%
Appropriate Hair Removal[2]	782	100%	100%	99%
Appropriate Beta Blocker Usage[2]	289	92%	95%	93%
Controlled Postoperative Blood Glucose[2]	0	-	93%	93%
Prophylactic Antibiotic Timing[2]	515	97%	98%	97%
Prophylactic Antibiotic Timing (Outpatient)	131	77%	93%	92%
Prophylactic Antibiotic Selection[2]	520	96%	97%	97%
Prophylactic Antibiotic Select. (Outpatient)	109	89%	94%	94%
Prophylactic Antibiotic Stopped[2]	484	94%	96%	94%
Recommended VTP Ordered[2]	312	93%	95%	94%
Urinary Catheter Removal	242	93%	93%	90%
Children's Asthma Care				
Received Systemic Corticosteroids	-	-	-	100%
Received Home Management Plan	-	-	-	71%
Received Reliever Medication	-	-	-	100%
Use of Medical Imaging				
Combination Abdominal CT Scan	983	0.042	0.126	0.191
Combination Chest CT Scan	783	0.017	0.026	0.054
Follow-up Mammogram/Ultrasound	1,096	10.7%	10.6%	8.4%
MRI for Low Back Pain	108	29.6%	26.4%	32.7%
Survey of Patients' Hospital Experiences				
Area Around Room 'Always' Quiet at Night	300+	56%	-	58%
Doctors 'Always' Communicated Well	300+	78%	-	80%
Home Recovery Information Given	300+	83%	-	82%
Hospital Given 9 or 10 on 10 Point Scale	300+	64%	-	67%
Meds 'Always' Explained Before Given	300+	58%	-	60%
Nurses 'Always' Communicated Well	300+	74%	-	76%
Pain 'Always' Well Controlled	300+	67%	-	69%
Room and Bathroom 'Always' Clean	300+	69%	-	71%
Timely Help 'Always' Received	300+	59%	-	64%
Would Definitely Recommend Hospital	300+	68%	-	69%

NOTE: Hospital profiles are in alphabetical order by state, then city, then hospital within the city; Rankings exclude hospitals with less than 25 cases except for patient surveys which excludes hospitals with less than 100 cases; (a) 100–299 cases; (1) The number of cases is too small to be sure how well a hospital is performing; (2) The hospital indicated that the data submitted for this measure were based on a sample of cases; (3) Data was collected during a shorter time period (fewer quarters) than the maximum possible time for this measure; (4) Suppressed for one or more quarters by CMS; (5) No data is available from the hospital for this measure; (6) Fewer than 100 patients completed the HCAHPS survey. Use these rates with caution, as the number of surveys may be too low to reliably assess hospital performance; (7) Survey results are based on less than 12 months of data; (8) Survey results are not available for this reporting period; (9) No or very few patients were eligible for the HCAHPS survey. The scores shown, if any, reflect a very small number of surveys; (10) A state average was not calculated because too few hospitals in the state submitted data; (11) There were discrepancies in the data collection process; Please refer to the User's Guide for a full explanation of data.

Hoboken University Medical Center

308 Willow Ave
Hoboken, NJ 07030
Phone: 201-418-1004
Fax: 201-418-1011
URL: www.bonsecoursnj.com
Type: Acute Care Hospitals
Emergency Services: Yes
Ownership: Voluntary Non-Profit - Church
Beds: 266

Key Personnel:
CEO/President. . . . . Richard J Statuto
Operating Room. . . . . Ira Jacobs, MD
Pediatric In-Patient Care . . . . Ruth Braddock

Measure	Cases	This Hosp.	State Avg.	U.S. Avg.
Heart Attack Care				
ACE Inhibitor or ARB for LVSD[1]	2	100%	98%	96%
Aspirin at Arrival	43	95%	99%	99%
Aspirin at Discharge[1]	17	100%	99%	98%
Beta Blocker at Discharge[1]	16	100%	99%	98%
Fibrinolytic Medication Timing[1]	1	0%	65%	55%
PCI Within 90 Minutes of Arrival	0	-	87%	90%
Smoking Cessation Advice[1]	1	100%	100%	99%
Chest Pain/Possible Heart Attack Care				
Aspirin at Arrival[1,3]	4	100%	97%	95%
Median Time to ECG (minutes)[1,3]	4	6	8	8
Median Time to Transfer (minutes)[5]	0	-	81	61
Fibrinolytic Medication Timing[1,3]	1	0%	65%	54%
Heart Failure Care				
ACE Inhibitor or ARB for LVSD[2]	95	100%	97%	94%
Discharge Instructions[2]	176	100%	93%	88%
Evaluation of LVS Function[2]	215	100%	99%	98%
Smoking Cessation Advice[2]	37	100%	100%	98%
Pneumonia Care				
Appropriate Initial Antibiotic	86	85%	94%	92%
Blood Culture Timing	112	90%	97%	96%
Influenza Vaccine	80	82%	94%	91%
Initial Antibiotic Timing	132	89%	96%	95%
Pneumococcal Vaccine	120	93%	96%	93%
Smoking Cessation Advice[1]	24	100%	99%	97%
Surgical Care Improvement Project				
Appropriate VTP Within 24 Hours	89	90%	94%	92%
Appropriate Hair Removal	187	100%	100%	99%
Appropriate Beta Blocker Usage	44	82%	95%	93%
Controlled Postoperative Blood Glucose	0	-	93%	93%
Prophylactic Antibiotic Timing	110	99%	98%	97%
Prophylactic Antibiotic Timing (Outpatient)	143	90%	93%	92%
Prophylactic Antibiotic Selection	113	98%	97%	97%
Prophylactic Antibiotic Select. (Outpatient)	137	96%	94%	94%
Prophylactic Antibiotic Stopped	104	93%	96%	94%
Recommended VTP Ordered	91	95%	95%	94%
Urinary Catheter Removal	40	80%	93%	90%
Children's Asthma Care				
Received Systemic Corticosteroids	-	-	-	100%
Received Home Management Plan	-	-	-	71%
Received Reliever Medication	-	-	-	100%
Use of Medical Imaging				
Combination Abdominal CT Scan	367	0.101	0.126	0.191
Combination Chest CT Scan	217	0.046	0.026	0.054
Follow-up Mammogram/Ultrasound	374	9.6%	10.6%	8.4%
MRI for Low Back Pain[1]	36	22.2%	26.4%	32.7%
Survey of Patients' Hospital Experiences				
Area Around Room 'Always' Quiet at Night	300+	47%	-	58%
Doctors 'Always' Communicated Well	300+	81%	-	80%
Home Recovery Information Given	300+	81%	-	82%
Hospital Given 9 or 10 on 10 Point Scale	300+	61%	-	67%
Meds 'Always' Explained Before Given	300+	54%	-	60%
Nurses 'Always' Communicated Well	300+	72%	-	76%
Pain 'Always' Well Controlled	300+	68%	-	69%
Room and Bathroom 'Always' Clean	300+	62%	-	71%
Timely Help 'Always' Received	300+	59%	-	64%
Would Definitely Recommend Hospital	300+	66%	-	69%

Bayshore Community Hospital

727 N Beers St
Holmdel, NJ 07733
Phone: 732-739-5900
Fax: 732-739-5887
E-mail: pr@bchs.com
URL: www.bchs.com
Type: Acute Care Hospitals
Emergency Services: Yes
Ownership: Voluntary Non-Profit - Private
Beds: 174

Key Personnel:
CEO/President. . . . . Raimonda Clark
Cardiac Laboratory. . . . . Greg Sabo, RN
Chief of Medical Staff . . . . Gerald V Costa, MD
Infection Control. . . . . Genevieve Anderson
Pediatric In-Patient Care . . . . Sharon Haskins, RN
Quality Assurance . . . . Carolina Nowaczyk
Radiology. . . . . David Chun

Measure	Cases	This Hosp.	State Avg.	U.S. Avg.
Heart Attack Care				
ACE Inhibitor or ARB for LVSD[1]	11	100%	98%	96%
Aspirin at Arrival	152	100%	99%	99%
Aspirin at Discharge	59	100%	99%	98%
Beta Blocker at Discharge	67	100%	99%	98%
Fibrinolytic Medication Timing	0	-	65%	55%
PCI Within 90 Minutes of Arrival	0	-	87%	90%
Smoking Cessation Advice[1]	16	100%	100%	99%
Chest Pain/Possible Heart Attack Care				
Aspirin at Arrival	40	100%	97%	95%
Median Time to ECG (minutes)	38	8	8	8
Median Time to Transfer (minutes)[3]	0	-	81	61
Fibrinolytic Medication Timing[1]	6	83%	65%	54%
Heart Failure Care				
ACE Inhibitor or ARB for LVSD	67	100%	97%	94%
Discharge Instructions	162	100%	93%	88%
Evaluation of LVS Function	284	100%	99%	98%
Smoking Cessation Advice	26	100%	100%	98%
Pneumonia Care				
Appropriate Initial Antibiotic	133	95%	94%	92%
Blood Culture Timing	228	100%	97%	96%
Influenza Vaccine	159	99%	94%	91%
Initial Antibiotic Timing	229	99%	96%	95%
Pneumococcal Vaccine	222	100%	96%	93%
Smoking Cessation Advice	97	100%	99%	97%
Surgical Care Improvement Project				
Appropriate VTP Within 24 Hours[2]	123	99%	94%	92%
Appropriate Hair Removal[2]	216	100%	100%	99%
Appropriate Beta Blocker Usage[2]	53	100%	95%	93%
Controlled Postoperative Blood Glucose[2]	0	-	93%	93%
Prophylactic Antibiotic Timing[2]	117	100%	98%	97%
Prophylactic Antibiotic Timing (Outpatient)	59	95%	93%	92%
Prophylactic Antibiotic Selection[2]	117	98%	97%	97%
Prophylactic Antibiotic Select. (Outpatient)	57	98%	94%	94%
Prophylactic Antibiotic Stopped[2]	106	97%	96%	94%
Recommended VTP Ordered[2]	123	100%	95%	94%
Urinary Catheter Removal[2]	39	97%	93%	90%
Children's Asthma Care				
Received Systemic Corticosteroids	-	-	-	100%
Received Home Management Plan	-	-	-	71%
Received Reliever Medication	-	-	-	100%
Use of Medical Imaging				
Combination Abdominal CT Scan	866	0.058	0.126	0.191
Combination Chest CT Scan	629	0.010	0.026	0.054
Follow-up Mammogram/Ultrasound	948	11.1%	10.6%	8.4%
MRI for Low Back Pain	100	29.0%	26.4%	32.7%
Survey of Patients' Hospital Experiences				
Area Around Room 'Always' Quiet at Night	300+	48%	-	58%
Doctors 'Always' Communicated Well	300+	76%	-	80%
Home Recovery Information Given	300+	79%	-	82%
Hospital Given 9 or 10 on 10 Point Scale	300+	53%	-	67%
Meds 'Always' Explained Before Given	300+	43%	-	60%
Nurses 'Always' Communicated Well	300+	69%	-	76%
Pain 'Always' Well Controlled	300+	64%	-	69%
Room and Bathroom 'Always' Clean	300+	58%	-	71%
Timely Help 'Always' Received	300+	50%	-	64%
Would Definitely Recommend Hospital	300+	54%	-	69%

Christ Hospital

176 Palisade Ave
Jersey City, NJ 07306
Phone: 201-795-8200
Fax: 201-795-8796
URL: www.christhospital.org
Type: Acute Care Hospitals
Emergency Services: Yes
Ownership: Voluntary Non-Profit - Church
Beds: 381

Key Personnel:
CEO/President. . . . . Peter Kelly
Chief of Medical Staff . . . . Anthony C Antonacci, MD
Infection Control. . . . . Marguerite Morgan
Operating Room. . . . . Mohamed Al-Bashir, RN
Pediatric Ambulatory Care . . . . . Miriam McKinney, MD
Pediatric In-Patient Care . . . . . . Carolyn Amato
Quality Assurance . . . . Barbara Vicari
Radiology. . . . . Eileen Concannon

Measure	Cases	This Hosp.	State Avg.	U.S. Avg.
Heart Attack Care				
ACE Inhibitor or ARB for LVSD[1]	18	100%	98%	96%
Aspirin at Arrival	161	96%	99%	99%
Aspirin at Discharge	81	98%	99%	98%
Beta Blocker at Discharge	87	98%	99%	98%
Fibrinolytic Medication Timing	0	-	65%	55%
PCI Within 90 Minutes of Arrival	31	94%	87%	90%
Smoking Cessation Advice[1]	18	100%	100%	99%
Chest Pain/Possible Heart Attack Care				
Aspirin at Arrival[1,3]	3	100%	97%	95%
Median Time to ECG (minutes)[1,3]	3	9	8	8
Median Time to Transfer (minutes)[1,3]	1	160	81	61
Fibrinolytic Medication Timing[1,3]	1	0%	65%	54%
Heart Failure Care				
ACE Inhibitor or ARB for LVSD	124	98%	97%	94%
Discharge Instructions	312	100%	93%	88%
Evaluation of LVS Function	430	99%	99%	98%
Smoking Cessation Advice	62	100%	100%	98%
Pneumonia Care				
Appropriate Initial Antibiotic	173	95%	94%	92%
Blood Culture Timing	234	98%	97%	96%
Influenza Vaccine	124	88%	94%	91%
Initial Antibiotic Timing	184	97%	96%	95%
Pneumococcal Vaccine	166	89%	96%	93%
Smoking Cessation Advice	33	100%	99%	97%
Surgical Care Improvement Project				
Appropriate VTP Within 24 Hours[2]	191	82%	94%	92%
Appropriate Hair Removal[2]	400	100%	100%	99%
Appropriate Beta Blocker Usage[2]	75	84%	95%	93%
Controlled Postoperative Blood Glucose[2]	0	-	93%	93%
Prophylactic Antibiotic Timing[2]	224	94%	98%	97%
Prophylactic Antibiotic Timing (Outpatient)	204	77%	93%	92%
Prophylactic Antibiotic Selection[2]	226	96%	97%	97%
Prophylactic Antibiotic Select. (Outpatient)	206	82%	94%	94%
Prophylactic Antibiotic Stopped[2]	210	91%	96%	94%
Recommended VTP Ordered[2]	192	83%	95%	94%
Urinary Catheter Removal[2]	57	96%	93%	90%
Children's Asthma Care				
Received Systemic Corticosteroids	-	-	-	100%
Received Home Management Plan	-	-	-	71%
Received Reliever Medication	-	-	-	100%
Use of Medical Imaging				
Combination Abdominal CT Scan	709	0.078	0.126	0.191
Combination Chest CT Scan	343	0.003	0.026	0.054
Follow-up Mammogram/Ultrasound	184	12.5%	10.6%	8.4%
MRI for Low Back Pain[1]	1	0.0%	26.4%	32.7%
Survey of Patients' Hospital Experiences				
Area Around Room 'Always' Quiet at Night	(a)	58%	-	58%
Doctors 'Always' Communicated Well	(a)	74%	-	80%
Home Recovery Information Given	(a)	72%	-	82%
Hospital Given 9 or 10 on 10 Point Scale	(a)	54%	-	67%
Meds 'Always' Explained Before Given	(a)	49%	-	60%
Nurses 'Always' Communicated Well	(a)	66%	-	76%
Pain 'Always' Well Controlled	(a)	62%	-	69%
Room and Bathroom 'Always' Clean	(a)	62%	-	71%
Timely Help 'Always' Received	(a)	53%	-	64%
Would Definitely Recommend Hospital	(a)	61%	-	69%

NOTE: Hospital profiles are in alphabetical order by state, then city, then hospital within the city; Rankings exclude hospitals with less than 25 cases except for patient surveys which excludes hospitals with less than 100 cases; (a) 100–299 cases; (1) The number of cases is too small to be sure how well a hospital is performing; (2) The hospital indicated that the data submitted for this measure were based on a sample of cases; (3) Data was collected during a shorter time period (fewer quarters) than the maximum possible time for this measure; (4) Suppressed for one or more quarters by CMS; (5) No data is available from the hospital for this measure; (6) Fewer than 100 patients completed the HCAHPS survey. Use these rates with caution, as the number of surveys may be too low to reliably assess hospital performance; (7) Survey results are based on less than 12 months of data; (8) Survey results are not available for this reporting period; (9) No or very few patients were eligible for the HCAHPS survey. The scores shown, if any, reflect a very small number of surveys; (10) A state average was not calculated because too few hospitals in the state submitted data; (11) There were discrepancies in the data collection process; Please refer to the User's Guide for a full explanation of data.

Libertyhealth-Jersey City Medical Center Campus

355 Grand Street
Jersey City, NJ 07302
E-mail: news@libertyhcs.org
URL: www.libertyhcs.org
Type: Acute Care Hospitals
Ownership: Voluntary Non-Profit - Private
Phone: 201-915-2000
Fax: 201-915-2038
Emergency Services: Yes
Beds: 609

Key Personnel:

CEO/President. . . . . Josephan M Scott
Chief of Medical Staff . . . . James Maguire, MD
Operating Room. . . . . Judy Neumeyer, RN
Pediatric Ambulatory Care . . . . . . Richard Bonforte
Quality Assurance . . . . Kathleen Locklear
Radiology. . . . . John Cholankeril, MD
Anesthesiology. . . . . Ion Pancu, MD
Patient Relations . . . . Rita Smith

Measure	Cases	This Hosp.	State Avg.	U.S. Avg.
Heart Attack Care				
ACE Inhibitor or ARB for LVSD	49	100%	98%	96%
Aspirin at Arrival	189	100%	99%	99%
Aspirin at Discharge	220	99%	99%	98%
Beta Blocker at Discharge	219	99%	99%	98%
Fibrinolytic Medication Timing	0	-	65%	55%
PCI Within 90 Minutes of Arrival	37	92%	87%	90%
Smoking Cessation Advice	67	100%	100%	99%
Chest Pain/Possible Heart Attack Care				
Aspirin at Arrival[1]	4	100%	97%	95%
Median Time to ECG (minutes)[1]	6	30	8	8
Median Time to Transfer (minutes)[5]	0	-	81	61
Fibrinolytic Medication Timing[5]	0	-	65%	54%
Heart Failure Care				
ACE Inhibitor or ARB for LVSD[2]	168	99%	97%	94%
Discharge Instructions[2]	284	99%	93%	88%
Evaluation of LVS Function[2]	338	100%	99%	98%
Smoking Cessation Advice[2]	78	99%	100%	98%
Pneumonia Care				
Appropriate Initial Antibiotic[2]	59	98%	94%	92%
Blood Culture Timing[2]	74	96%	97%	96%
Influenza Vaccine[2]	75	96%	94%	91%
Initial Antibiotic Timing[2]	73	100%	96%	95%
Pneumococcal Vaccine[2]	69	93%	96%	93%
Smoking Cessation Advice[2]	49	100%	99%	97%
Surgical Care Improvement Project				
Appropriate VTP Within 24 Hours[2]	163	98%	94%	92%
Appropriate Hair Removal[2]	472	100%	100%	99%
Appropriate Beta Blocker Usage[2]	96	100%	95%	93%
Controlled Postoperative Blood Glucose[2]	79	100%	93%	93%
Prophylactic Antibiotic Timing[2]	211	100%	98%	97%
Prophylactic Antibiotic Timing (Outpatient)	43	70%	93%	92%
Prophylactic Antibiotic Selection[2]	214	98%	97%	97%
Prophylactic Antibiotic Select. (Outpatient)	34	91%	94%	94%
Prophylactic Antibiotic Stopped[2]	201	97%	96%	94%
Recommended VTP Ordered[2]	163	99%	95%	94%
Urinary Catheter Removal[2]	63	100%	93%	90%
Children's Asthma Care				
Received Systemic Corticosteroids	-	-	-	100%
Received Home Management Plan	-	-	-	71%
Received Reliever Medication	-	-	-	100%
Use of Medical Imaging				
Combination Abdominal CT Scan	199	0.015	0.126	0.191
Combination Chest CT Scan	94	0.000	0.026	0.054
Follow-up Mammogram/Ultrasound[5]	0	-	10.6%	8.4%
MRI for Low Back Pain[1]	24	25.0%	26.4%	32.7%
Survey of Patients' Hospital Experiences				
Area Around Room 'Always' Quiet at Night	300+	57%	-	58%
Doctors 'Always' Communicated Well	300+	77%	-	80%
Home Recovery Information Given	300+	76%	-	82%
Hospital Given 9 or 10 on 10 Point Scale	300+	62%	-	67%
Meds 'Always' Explained Before Given	300+	56%	-	60%
Nurses 'Always' Communicated Well	300+	70%	-	76%
Pain 'Always' Well Controlled	300+	65%	-	69%
Room and Bathroom 'Always' Clean	300+	70%	-	71%
Timely Help 'Always' Received	300+	53%	-	64%
Would Definitely Recommend Hospital	300+	67%	-	69%

Kimball Medical Center

600 River Ave
Lakewood, NJ 08701
URL: www.sbhcs.com
Type: Acute Care Hospitals
Ownership: Voluntary Non-Profit - Private
Phone: 732-363-1900
Fax: 732-886-4406
Emergency Services: Yes
Beds: 350

Key Personnel:

CEO/President. . . . . Joe Hick
Chief of Medical Staff . . . . Eric Lennes MD
Infection Control. . . . . Carolyn Cox
Pediatric Ambulatory Care . . . . . . Norman Indich MD
Quality Assurance . . . . Joan Ruane
Radiology. . . . . Robert Cranley MD
Anesthesiology. . . . . Jitendra Jadav MD
Emergency Room . . . . William Dalsey MD

Measure	Cases	This Hosp.	State Avg.	U.S. Avg.
Heart Attack Care				
ACE Inhibitor or ARB for LVSD[1]	10	90%	98%	96%
Aspirin at Arrival	149	99%	99%	99%
Aspirin at Discharge	58	98%	99%	98%
Beta Blocker at Discharge	60	100%	99%	98%
Fibrinolytic Medication Timing[1]	5	100%	65%	55%
PCI Within 90 Minutes of Arrival	0	-	87%	90%
Smoking Cessation Advice[1]	3	100%	100%	99%
Chest Pain/Possible Heart Attack Care				
Aspirin at Arrival	27	100%	97%	95%
Median Time to ECG (minutes)	27	10	8	8
Median Time to Transfer (minutes)[3]	0	-	81	61
Fibrinolytic Medication Timing[1]	2	100%	65%	54%
Heart Failure Care				
ACE Inhibitor or ARB for LVSD	90	99%	97%	94%
Discharge Instructions	199	85%	93%	88%
Evaluation of LVS Function	329	99%	99%	98%
Smoking Cessation Advice	34	100%	100%	98%
Pneumonia Care				
Appropriate Initial Antibiotic	156	99%	94%	92%
Blood Culture Timing	306	100%	97%	96%
Influenza Vaccine	202	97%	94%	91%
Initial Antibiotic Timing	274	99%	96%	95%
Pneumococcal Vaccine	309	100%	96%	93%
Smoking Cessation Advice	80	100%	99%	97%
Surgical Care Improvement Project				
Appropriate VTP Within 24 Hours	87	97%	94%	92%
Appropriate Hair Removal	172	100%	100%	99%
Appropriate Beta Blocker Usage	41	95%	95%	93%
Controlled Postoperative Blood Glucose	0	-	93%	93%
Prophylactic Antibiotic Timing	77	99%	98%	97%
Prophylactic Antibiotic Timing (Outpatient)	136	99%	93%	92%
Prophylactic Antibiotic Selection	77	99%	97%	97%
Prophylactic Antibiotic Select. (Outpatient)	135	97%	94%	94%
Prophylactic Antibiotic Stopped	67	99%	96%	94%
Recommended VTP Ordered	87	98%	95%	94%
Urinary Catheter Removal[1]	13	85%	93%	90%
Children's Asthma Care				
Received Systemic Corticosteroids	-	-	-	100%
Received Home Management Plan	-	-	-	71%
Received Reliever Medication	-	-	-	100%
Use of Medical Imaging				
Combination Abdominal CT Scan	686	0.383	0.126	0.191
Combination Chest CT Scan	669	0.088	0.026	0.054
Follow-up Mammogram/Ultrasound[5]	0	-	10.6%	8.4%
MRI for Low Back Pain	106	28.3%	26.4%	32.7%
Survey of Patients' Hospital Experiences				
Area Around Room 'Always' Quiet at Night	300+	50%	-	58%
Doctors 'Always' Communicated Well	300+	76%	-	80%
Home Recovery Information Given	300+	81%	-	82%
Hospital Given 9 or 10 on 10 Point Scale	300+	54%	-	67%
Meds 'Always' Explained Before Given	300+	51%	-	60%
Nurses 'Always' Communicated Well	300+	71%	-	76%
Pain 'Always' Well Controlled	300+	69%	-	69%
Room and Bathroom 'Always' Clean	300+	65%	-	71%
Timely Help 'Always' Received	300+	54%	-	64%
Would Definitely Recommend Hospital	300+	52%	-	69%

Saint Barnabas Medical Center

94 Old Short Hills Road
Livingston, NJ 07039
E-mail: info@sbhcs.com
URL: www.saintbarnabas.com
Type: Acute Care Hospitals
Ownership: Voluntary Non-Profit - Other
Phone: 973-322-5000
Fax: 973-322-4346
Emergency Services: Yes
Beds: 597

Key Personnel:

CEO/President. . . . . Ronald J Del Mauro
Cardiac Laboratory. . . . . Maggie Lundberg
Chief of Medical Staff . . . . Gregory Rokoszt DO JD
Pediatric Ambulatory Care . . . . . . Agnes Hilbert
Pediatric In-Patient Care . . . . Susan Margolin MD
Radiology. . . . . Robert L Goodman MD
Intensive Care Unit. . . . . Chris Ruhren
Patient Relations . . . . Heather Veltra

Measure	Cases	This Hosp.	State Avg.	U.S. Avg.
Heart Attack Care				
ACE Inhibitor or ARB for LVSD	64	100%	98%	96%
Aspirin at Arrival	271	100%	99%	99%
Aspirin at Discharge	351	100%	99%	98%
Beta Blocker at Discharge	350	100%	99%	98%
Fibrinolytic Medication Timing	0	-	65%	55%
PCI Within 90 Minutes of Arrival	29	97%	87%	90%
Smoking Cessation Advice	73	100%	100%	99%
Chest Pain/Possible Heart Attack Care				
Aspirin at Arrival[1,3]	1	100%	97%	95%
Median Time to ECG (minutes)[1,3]	1	9	8	8
Median Time to Transfer (minutes)[5]	0	-	81	61
Fibrinolytic Medication Timing[5]	0	-	65%	54%
Heart Failure Care				
ACE Inhibitor or ARB for LVSD[2]	113	99%	97%	94%
Discharge Instructions[2]	268	100%	93%	88%
Evaluation of LVS Function[2]	332	100%	99%	98%
Smoking Cessation Advice[1,2]	21	100%	100%	98%
Pneumonia Care				
Appropriate Initial Antibiotic[2]	87	94%	94%	92%
Blood Culture Timing[2]	94	97%	97%	96%
Influenza Vaccine[2]	95	97%	94%	91%
Initial Antibiotic Timing[2]	132	99%	96%	95%
Pneumococcal Vaccine[2]	130	95%	96%	93%
Smoking Cessation Advice[2]	29	100%	99%	97%
Surgical Care Improvement Project				
Appropriate VTP Within 24 Hours[2]	199	91%	94%	92%
Appropriate Hair Removal[2]	805	100%	100%	99%
Appropriate Beta Blocker Usage[2]	258	100%	95%	93%
Controlled Postoperative Blood Glucose[2]	168	99%	93%	93%
Prophylactic Antibiotic Timing[2]	537	99%	98%	97%
Prophylactic Antibiotic Timing (Outpatient)	780	94%	93%	92%
Prophylactic Antibiotic Selection[2]	550	97%	97%	97%
Prophylactic Antibiotic Select. (Outpatient)	762	96%	94%	94%
Prophylactic Antibiotic Stopped[2]	515	95%	96%	94%
Recommended VTP Ordered[2]	199	93%	95%	94%
Urinary Catheter Removal[2]	95	93%	93%	90%
Children's Asthma Care				
Received Systemic Corticosteroids	-	-	-	100%
Received Home Management Plan	-	-	-	71%
Received Reliever Medication	-	-	-	100%
Use of Medical Imaging				
Combination Abdominal CT Scan	764	0.071	0.126	0.191
Combination Chest CT Scan	324	0.071	0.026	0.054
Follow-up Mammogram/Ultrasound[5]	0	-	10.6%	8.4%
MRI for Low Back Pain[1]	24	20.8%	26.4%	32.7%
Survey of Patients' Hospital Experiences				
Area Around Room 'Always' Quiet at Night	300+	49%	-	58%
Doctors 'Always' Communicated Well	300+	77%	-	80%
Home Recovery Information Given	300+	76%	-	82%
Hospital Given 9 or 10 on 10 Point Scale	300+	64%	-	67%
Meds 'Always' Explained Before Given	300+	60%	-	60%
Nurses 'Always' Communicated Well	300+	74%	-	76%
Pain 'Always' Well Controlled	300+	67%	-	69%
Room and Bathroom 'Always' Clean	300+	64%	-	71%
Timely Help 'Always' Received	300+	54%	-	64%
Would Definitely Recommend Hospital	300+	72%	-	69%

NOTE: Hospital profiles are in alphabetical order by state, then city, then hospital within the city; Rankings exclude hospitals with less than 25 cases except for patient surveys which excludes hospitals with less than 100 cases; (a) 100–299 cases; (1) The number of cases is too small to be sure how well a hospital is performing; (2) The hospital indicated that the data submitted for this measure were based on a sample of cases; (3) Data was collected during a shorter time period (fewer quarters) than the maximum possible time for this measure; (4) Suppressed for one or more quarters by CMS; (5) No data is available from the hospital for this measure; (6) Fewer than 100 patients completed the HCAHPS survey. Use these rates with caution, as the number of surveys may be too low to reliably assess hospital performance; (7) Survey results are based on less than 12 months of data; (8) Survey results are not available for this reporting period; (9) No or very few patients were eligible for the HCAHPS survey. The scores shown, if any, reflect a very small number of surveys; (10) A state average was not calculated because too few hospitals in the state submitted data; (11) There were discrepancies in the data collection process; Please refer to the User's Guide for a full explanation of data.

Monmouth Medical Center

300 Second Avenue
Long Branch, NJ 07740
E-mail: info@sbhcs.com
URL: www.sbhcs.com
Phone: 732-222-5200
Fax: 732-923-6633
Type: Acute Care Hospitals
Emergency Services: Yes
Ownership: Voluntary Non-Profit - Private
Beds: 526

Key Personnel:
CEO/President. . . . . David Wallace, MD
Chief of Medical Staff. . . . . Daniel Shine, MD
Infection Control. . . . . Nancy Nelsen
Operating Room. . . . . Jadd W Koury
Pediatric Ambulatory Care . . . . . Howard Fox, MD
Pediatric In-Patient Care . . . . . . Howard Fox, MD
Quality Assurance . . . . Pat Keating
Radiology. . . . . Soliman Rabbani, MD

Measure	Cases	This Hosp.	State Avg.	U.S. Avg.
Heart Attack Care				
ACE Inhibitor or ARB for LVSD[1]	8	100%	98%	96%
Aspirin at Arrival	127	99%	99%	99%
Aspirin at Discharge	70	99%	99%	98%
Beta Blocker at Discharge	65	98%	99%	98%
Fibrinolytic Medication Timing	0	-	65%	55%
PCI Within 90 Minutes of Arrival[1]	14	100%	87%	90%
Smoking Cessation Advice[1]	14	100%	100%	99%
Chest Pain/Possible Heart Attack Care				
Aspirin at Arrival[1,3]	8	88%	97%	95%
Median Time to ECG (minutes)[1,3]	9	4	8	8
Median Time to Transfer (minutes)[1,3]	2	75	81	61
Fibrinolytic Medication Timing[3]	0	-	65%	54%
Heart Failure Care				
ACE Inhibitor or ARB for LVSD[2]	53	100%	97%	94%
Discharge Instructions[2]	182	100%	93%	88%
Evaluation of LVS Function[2]	268	100%	99%	98%
Smoking Cessation Advice[2]	31	100%	100%	98%
Pneumonia Care				
Appropriate Initial Antibiotic[2]	116	96%	94%	92%
Blood Culture Timing[2]	175	99%	97%	96%
Influenza Vaccine[2]	93	92%	94%	91%
Initial Antibiotic Timing[2]	157	98%	96%	95%
Pneumococcal Vaccine[2]	131	94%	96%	93%
Smoking Cessation Advice[2]	49	100%	99%	97%
Surgical Care Improvement Project				
Appropriate VTP Within 24 Hours[2]	192	97%	94%	92%
Appropriate Hair Removal[2]	523	100%	100%	99%
Appropriate Beta Blocker Usage[2]	120	99%	95%	93%
Controlled Postoperative Blood Glucose[2]	0	-	93%	93%
Prophylactic Antibiotic Timing[2]	326	99%	98%	97%
Prophylactic Antibiotic Timing (Outpatient)	294	96%	93%	92%
Prophylactic Antibiotic Selection[2]	328	97%	97%	97%
Prophylactic Antibiotic Select. (Outpatient)	295	97%	94%	94%
Prophylactic Antibiotic Stopped[2]	312	97%	96%	94%
Recommended VTP Ordered[2]	192	98%	95%	94%
Urinary Catheter Removal[2]	130	96%	93%	90%
Children's Asthma Care				
Received Systemic Corticosteroids	-	-	-	100%
Received Home Management Plan	-	-	-	71%
Received Reliever Medication	-	-	-	100%
Use of Medical Imaging				
Combination Abdominal CT Scan	757	0.094	0.126	0.191
Combination Chest CT Scan	770	0.047	0.026	0.054
Follow-up Mammogram/Ultrasound	2,020	7.2%	10.6%	8.4%
MRI for Low Back Pain	87	29.9%	26.4%	32.7%
Survey of Patients' Hospital Experiences				
Area Around Room 'Always' Quiet at Night	300+	46%	-	58%
Doctors 'Always' Communicated Well	300+	75%	-	80%
Home Recovery Information Given	300+	72%	-	82%
Hospital Given 9 or 10 on 10 Point Scale	300+	54%	-	67%
Meds 'Always' Explained Before Given	300+	55%	-	60%
Nurses 'Always' Communicated Well	300+	69%	-	76%
Pain 'Always' Well Controlled	300+	61%	-	69%
Room and Bathroom 'Always' Clean	300+	58%	-	71%
Timely Help 'Always' Received	300+	50%	-	64%
Would Definitely Recommend Hospital	300+	62%	-	69%

Southern Ocean Medical Center

1140 Rt 72 W
Manahawkin, NJ 08050
E-mail: info@soch.com
URL: www.soch.com
Phone: 609-597-6011
Fax: 609-978-8920
Type: Acute Care Hospitals
Emergency Services: Yes
Ownership: Voluntary Non-Profit - Private
Beds: 144

Key Personnel:
CEO/President. . . . . Joseph P Coyle
Cardiac Laboratory. . . . . Jenny Stump
Chief of Medical Staff . . . . Walter Miller
Infection Control. . . . . Marsha Prato
Radiology. . . . . John Swidryk, MD
Anesthesiology. . . . . James Loftus, MD
Emergency Room . . . . William Wild

Measure	Cases	This Hosp.	State Avg.	U.S. Avg.
Heart Attack Care				
ACE Inhibitor or ARB for LVSD[1]	17	100%	98%	96%
Aspirin at Arrival	95	99%	99%	99%
Aspirin at Discharge	53	100%	99%	98%
Beta Blocker at Discharge	54	100%	99%	98%
Fibrinolytic Medication Timing	0	-	65%	55%
PCI Within 90 Minutes of Arrival	0	-	87%	90%
Smoking Cessation Advice[1]	8	100%	100%	99%
Chest Pain/Possible Heart Attack Care				
Aspirin at Arrival	134	100%	97%	95%
Median Time to ECG (minutes)	136	7	8	8
Median Time to Transfer (minutes)[1]	13	89	81	61
Fibrinolytic Medication Timing[1]	10	20%	65%	54%
Heart Failure Care				
ACE Inhibitor or ARB for LVSD	86	94%	97%	94%
Discharge Instructions	142	85%	93%	88%
Evaluation of LVS Function	234	99%	99%	98%
Smoking Cessation Advice	48	100%	100%	98%
Pneumonia Care				
Appropriate Initial Antibiotic	103	93%	94%	92%
Blood Culture Timing	248	90%	97%	96%
Influenza Vaccine	121	91%	94%	91%
Initial Antibiotic Timing	210	95%	96%	95%
Pneumococcal Vaccine	225	89%	96%	93%
Smoking Cessation Advice	55	100%	99%	97%
Surgical Care Improvement Project				
Appropriate VTP Within 24 Hours	163	88%	94%	92%
Appropriate Hair Removal	313	100%	100%	99%
Appropriate Beta Blocker Usage	110	88%	95%	93%
Controlled Postoperative Blood Glucose	0	-	93%	93%
Prophylactic Antibiotic Timing	173	98%	98%	97%
Prophylactic Antibiotic Timing (Outpatient)	69	86%	93%	92%
Prophylactic Antibiotic Selection	172	95%	97%	97%
Prophylactic Antibiotic Select. (Outpatient)	64	98%	94%	94%
Prophylactic Antibiotic Stopped	161	93%	96%	94%
Recommended VTP Ordered	163	96%	95%	94%
Urinary Catheter Removal	65	97%	93%	90%
Children's Asthma Care				
Received Systemic Corticosteroids	-	-	-	100%
Received Home Management Plan	-	-	-	71%
Received Reliever Medication	-	-	-	100%
Use of Medical Imaging				
Combination Abdominal CT Scan	712	0.058	0.126	0.191
Combination Chest CT Scan	343	0.055	0.026	0.054
Follow-up Mammogram/Ultrasound	2,049	12.1%	10.6%	8.4%
MRI for Low Back Pain	55	32.7%	26.4%	32.7%
Survey of Patients' Hospital Experiences				
Area Around Room 'Always' Quiet at Night	300+	52%	-	58%
Doctors 'Always' Communicated Well	300+	80%	-	80%
Home Recovery Information Given	300+	82%	-	82%
Hospital Given 9 or 10 on 10 Point Scale	300+	64%	-	67%
Meds 'Always' Explained Before Given	300+	63%	-	60%
Nurses 'Always' Communicated Well	300+	81%	-	76%
Pain 'Always' Well Controlled	300+	74%	-	69%
Room and Bathroom 'Always' Clean	300+	70%	-	71%
Timely Help 'Always' Received	300+	71%	-	64%
Would Definitely Recommend Hospital	300+	65%	-	69%

Mountainside Hospital

Bay and Highland Ave
Montclair, NJ 07042
E-mail: info@mountainsidehosp.com
URL: www.mountainsidenow.org
Phone: 973-429-6000
Fax: 973-429-6001
Type: Acute Care Hospitals
Emergency Services: Yes
Ownership: Voluntary Non-Profit - Private
Beds: 365

Key Personnel:
CEO/President. . . . . John Fromhold
Chief of Medical Staff. . . . . Theresa Soroko MD
Pediatric In-Patient Care . . . . . . Ragheda Saba

Measure	Cases	This Hosp.	State Avg.	U.S. Avg.
Heart Attack Care				
ACE Inhibitor or ARB for LVSD[1]	19	100%	98%	96%
Aspirin at Arrival	165	100%	99%	99%
Aspirin at Discharge	97	100%	99%	98%
Beta Blocker at Discharge	105	100%	99%	98%
Fibrinolytic Medication Timing	0	-	65%	55%
PCI Within 90 Minutes of Arrival	40	85%	87%	90%
Smoking Cessation Advice[1]	13	100%	100%	99%
Chest Pain/Possible Heart Attack Care				
Aspirin at Arrival[5]	0	-	97%	95%
Median Time to ECG (minutes)[5]	0	-	8	8
Median Time to Transfer (minutes)[5]	0	-	81	61
Fibrinolytic Medication Timing[5]	0	-	65%	54%
Heart Failure Care				
ACE Inhibitor or ARB for LVSD	121	100%	97%	94%
Discharge Instructions	255	96%	93%	88%
Evaluation of LVS Function	385	100%	99%	98%
Smoking Cessation Advice[1]	19	100%	100%	98%
Pneumonia Care				
Appropriate Initial Antibiotic	138	100%	94%	92%
Blood Culture Timing	243	99%	97%	96%
Influenza Vaccine	142	92%	94%	91%
Initial Antibiotic Timing	215	97%	96%	95%
Pneumococcal Vaccine	233	91%	96%	93%
Smoking Cessation Advice	61	95%	99%	97%
Surgical Care Improvement Project				
Appropriate VTP Within 24 Hours	206	85%	94%	92%
Appropriate Hair Removal	522	100%	100%	99%
Appropriate Beta Blocker Usage	113	92%	95%	93%
Controlled Postoperative Blood Glucose[1]	1	0%	93%	93%
Prophylactic Antibiotic Timing	249	98%	98%	97%
Prophylactic Antibiotic Timing (Outpatient)	192	90%	93%	92%
Prophylactic Antibiotic Selection	255	96%	97%	97%
Prophylactic Antibiotic Select. (Outpatient)	178	89%	94%	94%
Prophylactic Antibiotic Stopped	233	91%	96%	94%
Recommended VTP Ordered	207	90%	95%	94%
Urinary Catheter Removal	97	91%	93%	90%
Children's Asthma Care				
Received Systemic Corticosteroids	-	-	-	100%
Received Home Management Plan	-	-	-	71%
Received Reliever Medication	-	-	-	100%
Use of Medical Imaging				
Combination Abdominal CT Scan	724	0.109	0.126	0.191
Combination Chest CT Scan	410	0.061	0.026	0.054
Follow-up Mammogram/Ultrasound	415	11.8%	10.6%	8.4%
MRI for Low Back Pain	47	38.3%	26.4%	32.7%
Survey of Patients' Hospital Experiences				
Area Around Room 'Always' Quiet at Night	300+	51%	-	58%
Doctors 'Always' Communicated Well	300+	80%	-	80%
Home Recovery Information Given	300+	71%	-	82%
Hospital Given 9 or 10 on 10 Point Scale	300+	60%	-	67%
Meds 'Always' Explained Before Given	300+	57%	-	60%
Nurses 'Always' Communicated Well	300+	73%	-	76%
Pain 'Always' Well Controlled	300+	66%	-	69%
Room and Bathroom 'Always' Clean	300+	65%	-	71%
Timely Help 'Always' Received	300+	55%	-	64%
Would Definitely Recommend Hospital	300+	62%	-	69%

NOTE: Hospital profiles are in alphabetical order by state, then city, then hospital within the city; Rankings exclude hospitals with less than 25 cases except for patient surveys which excludes hospitals with less than 100 cases; (a) 100–299 cases; (1) The number of cases is too small to be sure how well a hospital is performing; (2) The hospital indicated that the data submitted for this measure were based on a sample of cases; (3) Data was collected during a shorter time period (fewer quarters) than the maximum possible time for this measure; (4) Suppressed for one or more quarters by CMS; (5) No data is available from the hospital for this measure; (6) Fewer than 100 patients completed the HCAHPS survey. Use these rates with caution, as the number of surveys may be too low to reliably assess hospital performance; (7) Survey results are based on less than 12 months of data; (8) Survey results are not available for this reporting period; (9) No or very few patients were eligible for the HCAHPS survey. The scores shown, if any, reflect a very small number of surveys; (10) A state average was not calculated because too few hospitals in the state submitted data; (11) There were discrepancies in the data collection process; Please refer to the User's Guide for a full explanation of data.

Morristown Memorial Hospital

100 Madison Ave
Morristown, NJ 07962
Phone: 973-660-3270
Fax: 973-290-7259
URL: www.morristownmemorialhospital.org
Type: Acute Care Hospitals
Emergency Services: Yes
Ownership: Voluntary Non-Profit - Private
Beds: 629

Key Personnel:
CEO/President.............. Joseph A Trunfio, PhD
Infection Control.............. Albert Klainer, MD
Operating Room.............. Liz Wein
Pediatric In-Patient Care .... Leonard Feld, MD
Radiology.................. Harry Stein
Anesthesiology.............. John T Lapchak, MD
Emergency Room .... John M Kealey, MD

Measure	Cases	This Hosp.	State Avg.	U.S. Avg.
Heart Attack Care				
ACE Inhibitor or ARB for LVSD[2]	52	92%	98%	96%
Aspirin at Arrival[2]	161	96%	99%	99%
Aspirin at Discharge[2]	334	99%	99%	98%
Beta Blocker at Discharge[2]	324	99%	99%	98%
Fibrinolytic Medication Timing[2]	0	-	65%	55%
PCI Within 90 Minutes of Arrival[2]	35	89%	87%	90%
Smoking Cessation Advice[2]	84	100%	100%	99%
Chest Pain/Possible Heart Attack Care				
Aspirin at Arrival[5]	0	-	97%	95%
Median Time to ECG (minutes)[5]	0	-	8	8
Median Time to Transfer (minutes)[5]	0	-	81	61
Fibrinolytic Medication Timing[5]	0	-	65%	54%
Heart Failure Care				
ACE Inhibitor or ARB for LVSD[2]	128	94%	97%	94%
Discharge Instructions[2]	249	99%	93%	88%
Evaluation of LVS Function[2]	338	98%	99%	98%
Smoking Cessation Advice[2]	36	100%	100%	98%
Pneumonia Care				
Appropriate Initial Antibiotic[2]	78	96%	94%	92%
Blood Culture Timing[2]	168	98%	97%	96%
Influenza Vaccine[2]	93	89%	94%	91%
Initial Antibiotic Timing[2]	148	93%	96%	95%
Pneumococcal Vaccine[2]	149	93%	96%	93%
Smoking Cessation Advice[2]	34	100%	99%	97%
Surgical Care Improvement Project				
Appropriate VTP Within 24 Hours[2]	209	97%	94%	92%
Appropriate Hair Removal[2]	840	100%	100%	99%
Appropriate Beta Blocker Usage[2]	287	91%	95%	93%
Controlled Postoperative Blood Glucose[2]	168	95%	93%	93%
Prophylactic Antibiotic Timing[2]	566	93%	98%	97%
Prophylactic Antibiotic Timing (Outpatient)	531	93%	93%	92%
Prophylactic Antibiotic Selection[2]	582	98%	97%	97%
Prophylactic Antibiotic Select. (Outpatient)	524	98%	94%	94%
Prophylactic Antibiotic Stopped[2]	521	97%	96%	94%
Recommended VTP Ordered[2]	209	97%	95%	94%
Urinary Catheter Removal[2]	168	95%	93%	90%
Children's Asthma Care				
Received Systemic Corticosteroids	-	-	-	100%
Received Home Management Plan	-	-	-	71%
Received Reliever Medication	-	-	-	100%
Use of Medical Imaging				
Combination Abdominal CT Scan	1,618	0.020	0.126	0.191
Combination Chest CT Scan	1,505	0.030	0.026	0.054
Follow-up Mammogram/Ultrasound	648	20.1%	10.6%	8.4%
MRI for Low Back Pain[1]	52	21.2%	26.4%	32.7%
Survey of Patients' Hospital Experiences				
Area Around Room 'Always' Quiet at Night	300+	55%	-	58%
Doctors 'Always' Communicated Well	300+	77%	-	80%
Home Recovery Information Given	300+	81%	-	82%
Hospital Given 9 or 10 on 10 Point Scale	300+	75%	-	67%
Meds 'Always' Explained Before Given	300+	59%	-	60%
Nurses 'Always' Communicated Well	300+	76%	-	76%
Pain 'Always' Well Controlled	300+	70%	-	69%
Room and Bathroom 'Always' Clean	300+	73%	-	71%
Timely Help 'Always' Received	300+	56%	-	64%
Would Definitely Recommend Hospital	300+	81%	-	69%

Virtua Memorial Hospital of Burlington County

175 Madison Ave
Mount Holly, NJ 08060
Phone: 609-914-6200
URL: www.virtua.org
Type: Acute Care Hospitals
Emergency Services: Yes
Ownership: Voluntary Non-Profit - Private
Beds: 433

Key Personnel:
CEO/President.............. Richard P. Miller

Measure	Cases	This Hosp.	State Avg.	U.S. Avg.
Heart Attack Care				
ACE Inhibitor or ARB for LVSD	29	97%	98%	96%
Aspirin at Arrival	247	100%	99%	99%
Aspirin at Discharge	146	97%	99%	98%
Beta Blocker at Discharge	155	99%	99%	98%
Fibrinolytic Medication Timing	0	-	65%	55%
PCI Within 90 Minutes of Arrival[1]	20	45%	87%	90%
Smoking Cessation Advice	28	100%	100%	99%
Chest Pain/Possible Heart Attack Care				
Aspirin at Arrival	143	99%	97%	95%
Median Time to ECG (minutes)	149	11	8	8
Median Time to Transfer (minutes)	30	49	81	61
Fibrinolytic Medication Timing[1]	1	100%	65%	54%
Heart Failure Care				
ACE Inhibitor or ARB for LVSD	110	92%	97%	94%
Discharge Instructions	336	83%	93%	88%
Evaluation of LVS Function	486	98%	99%	98%
Smoking Cessation Advice	71	100%	100%	98%
Pneumonia Care				
Appropriate Initial Antibiotic	241	93%	94%	92%
Blood Culture Timing	351	95%	97%	96%
Influenza Vaccine	156	90%	94%	91%
Initial Antibiotic Timing	319	99%	96%	95%
Pneumococcal Vaccine	290	88%	96%	93%
Smoking Cessation Advice	95	100%	99%	97%
Surgical Care Improvement Project				
Appropriate VTP Within 24 Hours[2]	427	98%	94%	92%
Appropriate Hair Removal[2]	1,517	100%	100%	99%
Appropriate Beta Blocker Usage[2]	506	94%	95%	93%
Controlled Postoperative Blood Glucose[2]	0	-	93%	93%
Prophylactic Antibiotic Timing[2]	1,155	97%	98%	97%
Prophylactic Antibiotic Timing (Outpatient)	210	95%	93%	92%
Prophylactic Antibiotic Selection[2]	1,155	98%	97%	97%
Prophylactic Antibiotic Select. (Outpatient)	209	76%	94%	94%
Prophylactic Antibiotic Stopped[2]	1,098	99%	96%	94%
Recommended VTP Ordered[2]	427	99%	95%	94%
Urinary Catheter Removal[2]	457	96%	93%	90%
Children's Asthma Care				
Received Systemic Corticosteroids	-	-	-	100%
Received Home Management Plan	-	-	-	71%
Received Reliever Medication	-	-	-	100%
Use of Medical Imaging				
Combination Abdominal CT Scan	808	0.016	0.126	0.191
Combination Chest CT Scan	321	0.000	0.026	0.054
Follow-up Mammogram/Ultrasound	322	11.2%	10.6%	8.4%
MRI for Low Back Pain[1]	46	28.3%	26.4%	32.7%
Survey of Patients' Hospital Experiences				
Area Around Room 'Always' Quiet at Night	300+	50%	-	58%
Doctors 'Always' Communicated Well	300+	78%	-	80%
Home Recovery Information Given	300+	82%	-	82%
Hospital Given 9 or 10 on 10 Point Scale	300+	68%	-	67%
Meds 'Always' Explained Before Given	300+	61%	-	60%
Nurses 'Always' Communicated Well	300+	78%	-	76%
Pain 'Always' Well Controlled	300+	70%	-	69%
Room and Bathroom 'Always' Clean	300+	64%	-	71%
Timely Help 'Always' Received	300+	58%	-	64%
Would Definitely Recommend Hospital	300+	71%	-	69%

Jersey Shore University Medical Center

1945 Rte 33
Neptune, NJ 07754
Phone: 732-775-5500
Fax: 732-776-4583
URL: www.meridianhealth.com
Type: Acute Care Hospitals
Emergency Services: Yes
Ownership: Voluntary Non-Profit - Private
Beds: 529

Key Personnel:
CEO/President.............. Steven G Littleson, FACHE
Chief of Medical Staff.......... John Crocco, MD
Infection Control.............. Elliott Frank, MD
Pediatric Ambulatory Care ...... Joseph Bogdan, MD
Pediatric In-Patient Care .... Joseph Bogdan, MD
Radiology.................. Rajiv Biswal, MD
Emergency Room .... Robert Sweeney, DO
Intensive Care Unit........... Richard Hayder, RN

Measure	Cases	This Hosp.	State Avg.	U.S. Avg.
Heart Attack Care				
ACE Inhibitor or ARB for LVSD[2]	60	97%	98%	96%
Aspirin at Arrival[2]	159	99%	99%	99%
Aspirin at Discharge[2]	486	99%	99%	98%
Beta Blocker at Discharge[2]	465	98%	99%	98%
Fibrinolytic Medication Timing[2]	0	-	65%	55%
PCI Within 90 Minutes of Arrival[2]	41	88%	87%	90%
Smoking Cessation Advice[2]	161	100%	100%	99%
Chest Pain/Possible Heart Attack Care				
Aspirin at Arrival[1,3]	1	100%	97%	95%
Median Time to ECG (minutes)[1,3]	1	21	8	8
Median Time to Transfer (minutes)[5]	0	-	81	61
Fibrinolytic Medication Timing[5]	0	-	65%	54%
Heart Failure Care				
ACE Inhibitor or ARB for LVSD[2]	133	99%	97%	94%
Discharge Instructions[2]	268	91%	93%	88%
Evaluation of LVS Function[2]	362	99%	99%	98%
Smoking Cessation Advice[2]	52	100%	100%	98%
Pneumonia Care				
Appropriate Initial Antibiotic	146	95%	94%	92%
Blood Culture Timing	209	99%	97%	96%
Influenza Vaccine	180	93%	94%	91%
Initial Antibiotic Timing	206	97%	96%	95%
Pneumococcal Vaccine	246	94%	96%	93%
Smoking Cessation Advice	93	99%	99%	97%
Surgical Care Improvement Project				
Appropriate VTP Within 24 Hours[2]	254	95%	94%	92%
Appropriate Hair Removal[2]	1,179	100%	100%	99%
Appropriate Beta Blocker Usage[2]	496	98%	95%	93%
Controlled Postoperative Blood Glucose[2]	402	95%	93%	93%
Prophylactic Antibiotic Timing[2]	826	99%	98%	97%
Prophylactic Antibiotic Timing (Outpatient)	703	98%	93%	92%
Prophylactic Antibiotic Selection[2]	846	98%	97%	97%
Prophylactic Antibiotic Select. (Outpatient)	692	100%	94%	94%
Prophylactic Antibiotic Stopped[2]	774	96%	96%	94%
Recommended VTP Ordered[2]	254	96%	95%	94%
Urinary Catheter Removal[2]	260	98%	93%	90%
Children's Asthma Care				
Received Systemic Corticosteroids	-	-	-	100%
Received Home Management Plan	-	-	-	71%
Received Reliever Medication	-	-	-	100%
Use of Medical Imaging				
Combination Abdominal CT Scan	1,271	0.061	0.126	0.191
Combination Chest CT Scan	1,053	0.003	0.026	0.054
Follow-up Mammogram/Ultrasound	545	10.3%	10.6%	8.4%
MRI for Low Back Pain	88	27.3%	26.4%	32.7%
Survey of Patients' Hospital Experiences				
Area Around Room 'Always' Quiet at Night	300+	58%	-	58%
Doctors 'Always' Communicated Well	300+	78%	-	80%
Home Recovery Information Given	300+	77%	-	82%
Hospital Given 9 or 10 on 10 Point Scale	300+	69%	-	67%
Meds 'Always' Explained Before Given	300+	60%	-	60%
Nurses 'Always' Communicated Well	300+	79%	-	76%
Pain 'Always' Well Controlled	300+	72%	-	69%
Room and Bathroom 'Always' Clean	300+	69%	-	71%
Timely Help 'Always' Received	300+	64%	-	64%
Would Definitely Recommend Hospital	300+	75%	-	69%

NOTE: Hospital profiles are in alphabetical order by state, then city, then hospital within the city; Rankings exclude hospitals with less than 25 cases except for patient surveys which excludes hospitals with less than 100 cases; (a) 100–299 cases; (1) The number of cases is too small to be sure how well a hospital is performing; (2) The hospital indicated that the data submitted for this measure were based on a sample of cases; (3) Data was collected during a shorter time period (fewer quarters) than the maximum possible time for this measure; (4) Suppressed for one or more quarters by CMS; (5) No data is available from the hospital for this measure; (6) Fewer than 100 patients completed the HCAHPS survey. Use these rates with caution, as the number of surveys may be too low to reliably assess hospital performance; (7) Survey results are based on less than 12 months of data; (8) Survey results are not available for this reporting period; (9) No or very few patients were eligible for the HCAHPS survey. The scores shown, if any, reflect a very small number of surveys; (10) A state average was not calculated because too few hospitals in the state submitted data; (11) There were discrepancies in the data collection process; Please refer to the User's Guide for a full explanation of data.

Robert Wood Johnson University Hospital

One Robert Wood Johnson Pl — Phone: 732-828-3000
New Brunswick, NJ 08901 — Fax: 732-937-8837
URL: www.rwjuh.edu
Type: Acute Care Hospitals — Emergency Services: Yes
Ownership: Voluntary Non-Profit - Private — Beds: 160

Key Personnel:
CEO/President. . . . . Clifton R Lacy
Cardiac Laboratory. . . . . Peter Scholz, MD
Chief of Medical Staff . . . . Peter Amenta, MD
Radiology. . . . . Leonard Bodner

Measure	Cases	This Hosp.	State Avg.	U.S. Avg.
Heart Attack Care				
ACE Inhibitor or ARB for LVSD	108	99%	98%	96%
Aspirin at Arrival	419	99%	99%	99%
Aspirin at Discharge	859	100%	99%	98%
Beta Blocker at Discharge	814	100%	99%	98%
Fibrinolytic Medication Timing	0	-	65%	55%
PCI Within 90 Minutes of Arrival	103	80%	87%	90%
Smoking Cessation Advice	199	100%	100%	99%
Chest Pain/Possible Heart Attack Care				
Aspirin at Arrival[5]	0	-	97%	95%
Median Time to ECG (minutes)[5]	0	-	8	8
Median Time to Transfer (minutes)[5]	0	-	81	61
Fibrinolytic Medication Timing[5]	0	-	65%	54%
Heart Failure Care				
ACE Inhibitor or ARB for LVSD	378	99%	97%	94%
Discharge Instructions	771	87%	93%	88%
Evaluation of LVS Function	1,029	100%	99%	98%
Smoking Cessation Advice	117	100%	100%	98%
Pneumonia Care				
Appropriate Initial Antibiotic	185	91%	94%	92%
Blood Culture Timing	431	92%	97%	96%
Influenza Vaccine	279	87%	94%	91%
Initial Antibiotic Timing	377	97%	96%	95%
Pneumococcal Vaccine	411	96%	96%	93%
Smoking Cessation Advice	82	100%	99%	97%
Surgical Care Improvement Project				
Appropriate VTP Within 24 Hours[2]	494	99%	94%	92%
Appropriate Hair Removal[2]	2,018	100%	100%	99%
Appropriate Beta Blocker Usage[2]	746	99%	95%	93%
Controlled Postoperative Blood Glucose[2]	728	88%	93%	93%
Prophylactic Antibiotic Timing[2]	1,494	96%	98%	97%
Prophylactic Antibiotic Timing (Outpatient)	793	88%	93%	92%
Prophylactic Antibiotic Selection[2]	1,520	98%	97%	97%
Prophylactic Antibiotic Select. (Outpatient)	777	91%	94%	94%
Prophylactic Antibiotic Stopped[2]	1,447	94%	96%	94%
Recommended VTP Ordered[2]	495	99%	95%	94%
Urinary Catheter Removal[2]	497	89%	93%	90%
Children's Asthma Care				
Received Systemic Corticosteroids	-	-	-	100%
Received Home Management Plan	-	-	-	71%
Received Reliever Medication	-	-	-	100%
Use of Medical Imaging				
Combination Abdominal CT Scan	709	0.018	0.126	0.191
Combination Chest CT Scan	473	0.002	0.026	0.054
Follow-up Mammogram/Ultrasound	379	17.7%	10.6%	8.4%
MRI for Low Back Pain[1]	27	33.3%	26.4%	32.7%
Survey of Patients' Hospital Experiences				
Area Around Room 'Always' Quiet at Night	300+	49%	-	58%
Doctors 'Always' Communicated Well	300+	78%	-	80%
Home Recovery Information Given	300+	81%	-	82%
Hospital Given 9 or 10 on 10 Point Scale	300+	68%	-	67%
Meds 'Always' Explained Before Given	300+	59%	-	60%
Nurses 'Always' Communicated Well	300+	76%	-	76%
Pain 'Always' Well Controlled	300+	68%	-	69%
Room and Bathroom 'Always' Clean	300+	65%	-	71%
Timely Help 'Always' Received	300+	62%	-	64%
Would Definitely Recommend Hospital	300+	75%	-	69%

Saint Peter's University Hospital

254 Easton Ave — Phone: 732-745-7944
New Brunswick, NJ 08901 — Fax: 732-220-8046
E-mail: info@saintpetersuh.com
URL: www.saintpetersuh.com
Type: Acute Care Hospitals — Emergency Services: Yes
Ownership: Voluntary Non-Profit - Church — Beds: 422

Key Personnel:
CEO/President. . . . . Sheryl Slanim
Coronary Care . . . . Lois Hobratschk, RN
Infection Control. . . . . Amy Gram
Operating Room. . . . . Jackie Carey, RN
Pediatric Ambulatory Care . . . . . . William Bernstein, MD
Pediatric In-Patient Care . . . . . . Bipin Patel, MD
Quality Assurance . . . . Jan Lichtenberger, RN
Radiology. . . . . Steven Schonfeld, MD

Measure	Cases	This Hosp.	State Avg.	U.S. Avg.
Heart Attack Care				
ACE Inhibitor or ARB for LVSD[1]	11	100%	98%	96%
Aspirin at Arrival	103	100%	99%	99%
Aspirin at Discharge	56	98%	99%	98%
Beta Blocker at Discharge	59	100%	99%	98%
Fibrinolytic Medication Timing	0	-	65%	55%
PCI Within 90 Minutes of Arrival[1]	19	79%	87%	90%
Smoking Cessation Advice[1]	16	100%	100%	99%
Chest Pain/Possible Heart Attack Care				
Aspirin at Arrival[1,3]	3	100%	97%	95%
Median Time to ECG (minutes)[1,3]	3	46	8	8
Median Time to Transfer (minutes)[5]	0	-	81	61
Fibrinolytic Medication Timing[5]	0	-	65%	54%
Heart Failure Care				
ACE Inhibitor or ARB for LVSD	70	96%	97%	94%
Discharge Instructions	246	67%	93%	88%
Evaluation of LVS Function	328	99%	99%	98%
Smoking Cessation Advice	39	100%	100%	98%
Pneumonia Care				
Appropriate Initial Antibiotic[2]	179	79%	94%	92%
Blood Culture Timing[2]	204	80%	97%	96%
Influenza Vaccine[2]	151	93%	94%	91%
Initial Antibiotic Timing[2]	215	82%	96%	95%
Pneumococcal Vaccine[2]	209	94%	96%	93%
Smoking Cessation Advice[2]	67	100%	99%	97%
Surgical Care Improvement Project				
Appropriate VTP Within 24 Hours[2]	190	95%	94%	92%
Appropriate Hair Removal[2]	549	81%	100%	99%
Appropriate Beta Blocker Usage[2]	173	91%	95%	93%
Controlled Postoperative Blood Glucose[2]	0	-	93%	93%
Prophylactic Antibiotic Timing[2]	338	99%	98%	97%
Prophylactic Antibiotic Timing (Outpatient)	91	79%	93%	92%
Prophylactic Antibiotic Selection[2]	339	98%	97%	97%
Prophylactic Antibiotic Select. (Outpatient)	81	75%	94%	94%
Prophylactic Antibiotic Stopped[2]	312	95%	96%	94%
Recommended VTP Ordered[2]	190	96%	95%	94%
Urinary Catheter Removal[2]	60	93%	93%	90%
Children's Asthma Care				
Received Systemic Corticosteroids	-	-	-	100%
Received Home Management Plan	-	-	-	71%
Received Reliever Medication	-	-	-	100%
Use of Medical Imaging				
Combination Abdominal CT Scan	348	0.017	0.126	0.191
Combination Chest CT Scan	184	0.000	0.026	0.054
Follow-up Mammogram/Ultrasound	294	18.0%	10.6%	8.4%
MRI for Low Back Pain[1]	18	22.2%	26.4%	32.7%
Survey of Patients' Hospital Experiences				
Area Around Room 'Always' Quiet at Night	300+	55%	-	58%
Doctors 'Always' Communicated Well	300+	78%	-	80%
Home Recovery Information Given	300+	76%	-	82%
Hospital Given 9 or 10 on 10 Point Scale	300+	68%	-	67%
Meds 'Always' Explained Before Given	300+	62%	-	60%
Nurses 'Always' Communicated Well	300+	77%	-	76%
Pain 'Always' Well Controlled	300+	70%	-	69%
Room and Bathroom 'Always' Clean	300+	77%	-	71%
Timely Help 'Always' Received	300+	64%	-	64%
Would Definitely Recommend Hospital	300+	76%	-	69%

Newark Beth Israel Medical Center

201 Lyons Ave — Phone: 973-926-7850
Newark, NJ 07112 — Fax: 973-926-8371
E-mail: info@sbhcs.com
URL: www.sbhcs.com
Type: Acute Care Hospitals — Emergency Services: Yes
Ownership: Voluntary Non-Profit - Private — Beds: 673

Key Personnel:
CEO/President. . . . . Paul A Mertz
Cardiac Laboratory. . . . . Marc Cohen
Chief of Medical Staff . . . . Donald Greenfield
Infection Control. . . . . Jeremias Murillo, MD
Pediatric In-Patient Care . . . . . . Jules A Titelbaum, MD
Quality Assurance . . . . Howard Previllile
Radiology. . . . . Richard Shoenfeld, MD
Hemotology Center . . . . Alice Cohen, MD

Measure	Cases	This Hosp.	State Avg.	U.S. Avg.
Heart Attack Care				
ACE Inhibitor or ARB for LVSD[2]	69	100%	98%	96%
Aspirin at Arrival[2]	200	100%	99%	99%
Aspirin at Discharge[2]	284	100%	99%	98%
Beta Blocker at Discharge[2]	276	100%	99%	98%
Fibrinolytic Medication Timing[2]	0	-	65%	55%
PCI Within 90 Minutes of Arrival[1,2]	24	100%	87%	90%
Smoking Cessation Advice[2]	81	100%	100%	99%
Chest Pain/Possible Heart Attack Care				
Aspirin at Arrival[1]	1	100%	97%	95%
Median Time to ECG (minutes)[1]	3	24	8	8
Median Time to Transfer (minutes)[5]	0	-	81	61
Fibrinolytic Medication Timing[5]	0	-	65%	54%
Heart Failure Care				
ACE Inhibitor or ARB for LVSD[2]	175	100%	97%	94%
Discharge Instructions[2]	304	100%	93%	88%
Evaluation of LVS Function[2]	359	100%	99%	98%
Smoking Cessation Advice[2]	59	100%	100%	98%
Pneumonia Care				
Appropriate Initial Antibiotic[2]	70	100%	94%	92%
Blood Culture Timing[2]	131	99%	97%	96%
Influenza Vaccine[2]	88	100%	94%	91%
Initial Antibiotic Timing[2]	110	100%	96%	95%
Pneumococcal Vaccine[2]	98	100%	96%	93%
Smoking Cessation Advice[2]	45	100%	99%	97%
Surgical Care Improvement Project				
Appropriate VTP Within 24 Hours[2]	169	97%	94%	92%
Appropriate Hair Removal[2]	624	100%	100%	99%
Appropriate Beta Blocker Usage[2]	192	100%	95%	93%
Controlled Postoperative Blood Glucose[2]	180	96%	93%	93%
Prophylactic Antibiotic Timing[2]	452	100%	98%	97%
Prophylactic Antibiotic Timing (Outpatient)	371	99%	93%	92%
Prophylactic Antibiotic Selection[2]	466	100%	97%	97%
Prophylactic Antibiotic Select. (Outpatient)	368	98%	94%	94%
Prophylactic Antibiotic Stopped[2]	430	100%	96%	94%
Recommended VTP Ordered[2]	169	98%	95%	94%
Urinary Catheter Removal[2]	60	98%	93%	90%
Children's Asthma Care				
Received Systemic Corticosteroids	-	-	-	100%
Received Home Management Plan	-	-	-	71%
Received Reliever Medication	-	-	-	100%
Use of Medical Imaging				
Combination Abdominal CT Scan	532	0.444	0.126	0.191
Combination Chest CT Scan	547	0.020	0.026	0.054
Follow-up Mammogram/Ultrasound	741	6.7%	10.6%	8.4%
MRI for Low Back Pain	63	41.3%	26.4%	32.7%
Survey of Patients' Hospital Experiences				
Area Around Room 'Always' Quiet at Night	300+	60%	-	58%
Doctors 'Always' Communicated Well	300+	81%	-	80%
Home Recovery Information Given	300+	79%	-	82%
Hospital Given 9 or 10 on 10 Point Scale	300+	62%	-	67%
Meds 'Always' Explained Before Given	300+	59%	-	60%
Nurses 'Always' Communicated Well	300+	74%	-	76%
Pain 'Always' Well Controlled	300+	68%	-	69%
Room and Bathroom 'Always' Clean	300+	65%	-	71%
Timely Help 'Always' Received	300+	58%	-	64%
Would Definitely Recommend Hospital	300+	66%	-	69%

NOTE: Hospital profiles are in alphabetical order by state, then city, then hospital within the city; Rankings exclude hospitals with less than 25 cases except for patient surveys which excludes hospitals with less than 100 cases; (a) 100–299 cases; (1) The number of cases is too small to be sure how well a hospital is performing; (2) The hospital indicated that the data submitted for this measure were based on a sample of cases; (3) Data was collected during a shorter time period (fewer quarters) than the maximum possible time for this measure; (4) Suppressed for one or more quarters by CMS; (5) No data is available from the hospital for this measure; (6) Fewer than 100 patients completed the HCAHPS survey. Use these rates with caution, as the number of surveys may be too low to reliably assess hospital performance; (7) Survey results are based on less than 12 months of data; (8) Survey results are not available for this reporting period; (9) No or very few patients were eligible for the HCAHPS survey. The scores shown, if any, reflect a very small number of surveys; (10) A state average was not calculated because too few hospitals in the state submitted data; (11) There were discrepancies in the data collection process; Please refer to the User's Guide for a full explanation of data.

Saint Michael's Medical Center

111 Central Avenue
Newark, NJ 07102
URL: www.cathedralhealth.org
Type: Acute Care Hospitals
Ownership: Voluntary Non-Profit - Private
Phone: 973-877-5350
Fax: 973-877-5635
Emergency Services: Yes
Beds: 337

Key Personnel:
CEO/President............... Henry Amoroso
Chief of Medical Staff.......... Nicholas Baranetsky, MD
Quality Assurance .... Adel Natividad, RN
Radiology.................. Suresh Mody, MD
Emergency Room .... Dr. Dwight Lee

Measure	Cases	This Hosp.	State Avg.	U.S. Avg.
Heart Attack Care				
ACE Inhibitor or ARB for LVSD[2]	78	95%	98%	96%
Aspirin at Arrival[2]	97	99%	99%	99%
Aspirin at Discharge[2]	315	96%	99%	98%
Beta Blocker at Discharge[2]	317	97%	99%	98%
Fibrinolytic Medication Timing[2]	0	-	65%	55%
PCI Within 90 Minutes of Arrival[1,2]	10	80%	87%	90%
Smoking Cessation Advice[2]	93	100%	100%	99%
Chest Pain/Possible Heart Attack Care				
Aspirin at Arrival[5]	0	-	97%	95%
Median Time to ECG (minutes)[5]	0	-	8	8
Median Time to Transfer (minutes)[5]	0	-	81	61
Fibrinolytic Medication Timing[5]	0	-	65%	54%
Heart Failure Care				
ACE Inhibitor or ARB for LVSD[2]	174	95%	97%	94%
Discharge Instructions[2]	243	87%	93%	88%
Evaluation of LVS Function[2]	342	100%	99%	98%
Smoking Cessation Advice[2]	67	99%	100%	98%
Pneumonia Care				
Appropriate Initial Antibiotic[2]	62	92%	94%	92%
Blood Culture Timing[2]	124	98%	97%	96%
Influenza Vaccine[2]	67	88%	94%	91%
Initial Antibiotic Timing[2]	128	87%	96%	95%
Pneumococcal Vaccine[2]	112	88%	96%	93%
Smoking Cessation Advice[2]	42	98%	99%	97%
Surgical Care Improvement Project				
Appropriate VTP Within 24 Hours[2]	135	87%	94%	92%
Appropriate Hair Removal[2]	563	100%	100%	99%
Appropriate Beta Blocker Usage[2]	216	98%	95%	93%
Controlled Postoperative Blood Glucose[2]	166	97%	93%	93%
Prophylactic Antibiotic Timing[2]	367	100%	98%	97%
Prophylactic Antibiotic Timing (Outpatient)	150	100%	93%	92%
Prophylactic Antibiotic Selection[2]	377	98%	97%	97%
Prophylactic Antibiotic Select. (Outpatient)	150	98%	94%	94%
Prophylactic Antibiotic Stopped[2]	346	99%	96%	94%
Recommended VTP Ordered[2]	135	90%	95%	94%
Urinary Catheter Removal[2]	80	95%	93%	90%
Children's Asthma Care				
Received Systemic Corticosteroids	-	-	-	100%
Received Home Management Plan	-	-	-	71%
Received Reliever Medication	-	-	-	100%
Use of Medical Imaging				
Combination Abdominal CT Scan	500	0.060	0.126	0.191
Combination Chest CT Scan	305	0.010	0.026	0.054
Follow-up Mammogram/Ultrasound	645	8.4%	10.6%	8.4%
MRI for Low Back Pain[1]	44	13.6%	26.4%	32.7%
Survey of Patients' Hospital Experiences				
Area Around Room 'Always' Quiet at Night	300+	55%	-	58%
Doctors 'Always' Communicated Well	300+	75%	-	80%
Home Recovery Information Given	300+	69%	-	82%
Hospital Given 9 or 10 on 10 Point Scale	300+	53%	-	67%
Meds 'Always' Explained Before Given	300+	49%	-	60%
Nurses 'Always' Communicated Well	300+	62%	-	76%
Pain 'Always' Well Controlled	300+	56%	-	69%
Room and Bathroom 'Always' Clean	300+	62%	-	71%
Timely Help 'Always' Received	300+	50%	-	64%
Would Definitely Recommend Hospital	300+	54%	-	69%

UMDNJ University Hospital

150 Bergen St
Newark, NJ 07103
E-mail: uhcontact@umdnj.edu
URL: www.theuniversityhospital.com
Type: Acute Care Hospitals
Ownership: Government - State
Phone: 973-972-5658
Fax: 973-972-6943
Emergency Services: Yes
Beds: 519

Key Personnel:
CEO/President............... Robin D Wittenstein
Chief of Medical Staff.......... WG Johanson
Infection Control.............. Steve Udem, MD
Pediatric Ambulatory Care ...... Frank Desposito, MD
Pediatric In-Patient Care .... Frank Desposito, MD
Quality Assurance .... Ronald DeVos
Radiology.................... Stephen Baker, MD

Measure	Cases	This Hosp.	State Avg.	U.S. Avg.
Heart Attack Care				
ACE Inhibitor or ARB for LVSD	29	100%	98%	96%
Aspirin at Arrival	97	100%	99%	99%
Aspirin at Discharge	112	100%	99%	98%
Beta Blocker at Discharge	105	100%	99%	98%
Fibrinolytic Medication Timing	0	-	65%	55%
PCI Within 90 Minutes of Arrival	28	82%	87%	90%
Smoking Cessation Advice	49	100%	100%	99%
Chest Pain/Possible Heart Attack Care				
Aspirin at Arrival[5]	0	-	97%	95%
Median Time to ECG (minutes)[5]	0	-	8	8
Median Time to Transfer (minutes)[5]	0	-	81	61
Fibrinolytic Medication Timing[5]	0	-	65%	54%
Heart Failure Care				
ACE Inhibitor or ARB for LVSD	269	100%	97%	94%
Discharge Instructions	371	100%	93%	88%
Evaluation of LVS Function	412	100%	99%	98%
Smoking Cessation Advice	164	100%	100%	98%
Pneumonia Care				
Appropriate Initial Antibiotic[2]	100	92%	94%	92%
Blood Culture Timing[2]	250	89%	97%	96%
Influenza Vaccine	101	96%	94%	91%
Initial Antibiotic Timing[2]	239	88%	96%	95%
Pneumococcal Vaccine[2]	60	95%	96%	93%
Smoking Cessation Advice[2]	173	97%	99%	97%
Surgical Care Improvement Project				
Appropriate VTP Within 24 Hours[2]	194	94%	94%	92%
Appropriate Hair Removal[2]	435	100%	100%	99%
Appropriate Beta Blocker Usage[2]	91	100%	95%	93%
Controlled Postoperative Blood Glucose[2]	74	95%	93%	93%
Prophylactic Antibiotic Timing[2]	300	98%	98%	97%
Prophylactic Antibiotic Timing (Outpatient)	160	84%	93%	92%
Prophylactic Antibiotic Selection[2]	320	97%	97%	97%
Prophylactic Antibiotic Select. (Outpatient)	139	81%	94%	94%
Prophylactic Antibiotic Stopped[2]	284	95%	96%	94%
Recommended VTP Ordered[2]	194	96%	95%	94%
Urinary Catheter Removal[2]	75	95%	93%	90%
Children's Asthma Care				
Received Systemic Corticosteroids	-	-	-	100%
Received Home Management Plan	-	-	-	71%
Received Reliever Medication	-	-	-	100%
Use of Medical Imaging				
Combination Abdominal CT Scan	617	0.332	0.126	0.191
Combination Chest CT Scan	261	0.046	0.026	0.054
Follow-up Mammogram/Ultrasound	513	10.7%	10.6%	8.4%
MRI for Low Back Pain[1]	56	8.9%	26.4%	32.7%
Survey of Patients' Hospital Experiences				
Area Around Room 'Always' Quiet at Night	300+	55%	-	58%
Doctors 'Always' Communicated Well	300+	78%	-	80%
Home Recovery Information Given	300+	78%	-	82%
Hospital Given 9 or 10 on 10 Point Scale	300+	58%	-	67%
Meds 'Always' Explained Before Given	300+	55%	-	60%
Nurses 'Always' Communicated Well	300+	67%	-	76%
Pain 'Always' Well Controlled	300+	65%	-	69%
Room and Bathroom 'Always' Clean	300+	62%	-	71%
Timely Help 'Always' Received	300+	53%	-	64%
Would Definitely Recommend Hospital	300+	61%	-	69%

Newton Memorial Hospital

175 High St
Newton, NJ 07860
E-mail: bgrace@itsyourlife.com
URL: www.itsyourlife.com
Type: Acute Care Hospitals
Ownership: Voluntary Non-Profit - Private
Phone: 973-383-2121
Fax: 973-383-8973
Emergency Services: Yes
Beds: 162

Key Personnel:
CEO/President............... Dennis Collette
Chief of Medical Staff.......... David Mattes
Operating Room.............. Donna Oregan
Quality Assurance .... Jean Jones
Radiology.................. Harmar D Brereton

Measure	Cases	This Hosp.	State Avg.	U.S. Avg.
Heart Attack Care				
ACE Inhibitor or ARB for LVSD[1]	5	100%	98%	96%
Aspirin at Arrival	66	100%	99%	99%
Aspirin at Discharge	26	100%	99%	98%
Beta Blocker at Discharge	32	100%	99%	98%
Fibrinolytic Medication Timing[1]	1	0%	65%	55%
PCI Within 90 Minutes of Arrival	0	-	87%	90%
Smoking Cessation Advice[1]	5	100%	100%	99%
Chest Pain/Possible Heart Attack Care				
Aspirin at Arrival	31	100%	97%	95%
Median Time to ECG (minutes)	34	5	8	8
Median Time to Transfer (minutes)[1]	5	90	81	61
Fibrinolytic Medication Timing[1]	4	75%	65%	54%
Heart Failure Care				
ACE Inhibitor or ARB for LVSD	61	98%	97%	94%
Discharge Instructions	151	100%	93%	88%
Evaluation of LVS Function	251	100%	99%	98%
Smoking Cessation Advice[1]	23	100%	100%	98%
Pneumonia Care				
Appropriate Initial Antibiotic[2]	84	93%	94%	92%
Blood Culture Timing[2]	187	99%	97%	96%
Influenza Vaccine[2]	105	90%	94%	91%
Initial Antibiotic Timing[2]	169	100%	96%	95%
Pneumococcal Vaccine[2]	178	96%	96%	93%
Smoking Cessation Advice[2]	44	100%	99%	97%
Surgical Care Improvement Project				
Appropriate VTP Within 24 Hours[2]	152	94%	94%	92%
Appropriate Hair Removal[2]	272	100%	100%	99%
Appropriate Beta Blocker Usage[2]	93	95%	95%	93%
Controlled Postoperative Blood Glucose[2]	0	-	93%	93%
Prophylactic Antibiotic Timing[2]	164	98%	98%	97%
Prophylactic Antibiotic Timing (Outpatient)	50	98%	93%	92%
Prophylactic Antibiotic Selection[2]	165	95%	97%	97%
Prophylactic Antibiotic Select. (Outpatient)	52	98%	94%	94%
Prophylactic Antibiotic Stopped[2]	143	88%	96%	94%
Recommended VTP Ordered[2]	153	94%	95%	94%
Urinary Catheter Removal[2]	56	86%	93%	90%
Children's Asthma Care				
Received Systemic Corticosteroids	-	-	-	100%
Received Home Management Plan	-	-	-	71%
Received Reliever Medication	-	-	-	100%
Use of Medical Imaging				
Combination Abdominal CT Scan	653	0.038	0.126	0.191
Combination Chest CT Scan	419	0.010	0.026	0.054
Follow-up Mammogram/Ultrasound	398	10.3%	10.6%	8.4%
MRI for Low Back Pain[5]	0	-	26.4%	32.7%
Survey of Patients' Hospital Experiences				
Area Around Room 'Always' Quiet at Night[11]	300+	44%	-	58%
Doctors 'Always' Communicated Well[11]	300+	72%	-	80%
Home Recovery Information Given[11]	300+	80%	-	82%
Hospital Given 9 or 10 on 10 Point Scale[11]	300+	63%	-	67%
Meds 'Always' Explained Before Given[11]	300+	52%	-	60%
Nurses 'Always' Communicated Well[11]	300+	76%	-	76%
Pain 'Always' Well Controlled[11]	300+	68%	-	69%
Room and Bathroom 'Always' Clean[11]	300+	76%	-	71%
Timely Help 'Always' Received[11]	300+	60%	-	64%
Would Definitely Recommend Hospital[11]	300+	66%	-	69%

NOTE: Hospital profiles are in alphabetical order by state, then city, then hospital within the city; Rankings exclude hospitals with less than 25 cases except for patient surveys which excludes hospitals with less than 100 cases; (a) 100–299 cases; (1) The number of cases is too small to be sure how well a hospital is performing; (2) The hospital indicated that the data submitted for this measure were based on a sample of cases; (3) Data was collected during a shorter time period (fewer quarters) than the maximum possible time for this measure; (4) Suppressed for one or more quarters by CMS; (5) No data is available from the hospital for this measure; (6) Fewer than 100 patients completed the HCAHPS survey. Use these rates with caution, as the number of surveys may be too low to reliably assess hospital performance; (7) Survey results are based on less than 12 months of data; (8) Survey results are not available for this reporting period; (9) No or very few patients were eligible for the HCAHPS survey. The scores shown, if any, reflect a very small number of surveys; (10) A state average was not calculated because too few hospitals in the state submitted data; (11) There were discrepancies in the data collection process; Please refer to the User's Guide for a full explanation of data.

Palisades Medical Center - NY Presbyterian Healthcare System

7600 River Rd
North Bergen, NJ 07047
Phone: 201-854-5000
Fax: 201-854-5036
URL: www.palisadesmedical.org
Type: Acute Care Hospitals
Emergency Services: Yes
Ownership: Voluntary Non-Profit - Private
Beds: 202

Key Personnel:

CEO/President . . . . Bruce J Markowitz
Chief of Medical Staff . . . . Maria Bornia, MD
Infection Control . . . . Doreen McSharry
Operating Room. . . . . Donna Vaglio, RN
Pediatric In-Patient Care . . . . Chitra Sethi, MD
Anesthesiology. . . . . Veena Sharma, MD
Intensive Care Unit. . . . . Adel Namour

Measure	Cases	This Hosp.	State Avg.	U.S. Avg.
Heart Attack Care				
ACE Inhibitor or ARB for LVSD[1]	10	100%	98%	96%
Aspirin at Arrival	88	97%	99%	99%
Aspirin at Discharge	33	100%	99%	98%
Beta Blocker at Discharge	35	100%	99%	98%
Fibrinolytic Medication Timing[1]	1	0%	65%	55%
PCI Within 90 Minutes of Arrival	0	-	87%	90%
Smoking Cessation Advice[1]	2	100%	100%	99%
Chest Pain/Possible Heart Attack Care				
Aspirin at Arrival[5]	0	-	97%	95%
Median Time to ECG (minutes)[5]	0	-	8	8
Median Time to Transfer (minutes)[5]	0	-	81	61
Fibrinolytic Medication Timing[5]	0	-	65%	54%
Heart Failure Care				
ACE Inhibitor or ARB for LVSD[2]	79	100%	97%	94%
Discharge Instructions[2]	169	100%	93%	88%
Evaluation of LVS Function[2]	255	99%	99%	98%
Smoking Cessation Advice[1,2]	17	100%	100%	98%
Pneumonia Care				
Appropriate Initial Antibiotic[2]	80	95%	94%	92%
Blood Culture Timing[2]	110	93%	97%	96%
Influenza Vaccine[2]	65	97%	94%	91%
Initial Antibiotic Timing[2]	100	100%	96%	95%
Pneumococcal Vaccine[2]	134	100%	96%	93%
Smoking Cessation Advice[1,2]	15	100%	99%	97%
Surgical Care Improvement Project				
Appropriate VTP Within 24 Hours[2]	83	100%	94%	92%
Appropriate Hair Removal[2]	192	100%	100%	99%
Appropriate Beta Blocker Usage[2]	64	97%	95%	93%
Controlled Postoperative Blood Glucose[2]	0	-	93%	93%
Prophylactic Antibiotic Timing[2]	103	98%	98%	97%
Prophylactic Antibiotic Timing (Outpatient)	37	70%	93%	92%
Prophylactic Antibiotic Selection[2]	105	93%	97%	97%
Prophylactic Antibiotic Select. (Outpatient)	26	96%	94%	94%
Prophylactic Antibiotic Stopped[2]	88	97%	96%	94%
Recommended VTP Ordered[2]	83	100%	95%	94%
Urinary Catheter Removal[2]	35	86%	93%	90%
Children's Asthma Care				
Received Systemic Corticosteroids	-	-	-	100%
Received Home Management Plan	-	-	-	71%
Received Reliever Medication	-	-	-	100%
Use of Medical Imaging				
Combination Abdominal CT Scan	492	0.081	0.126	0.191
Combination Chest CT Scan	291	0.000	0.026	0.054
Follow-up Mammogram/Ultrasound	421	9.3%	10.6%	8.4%
MRI for Low Back Pain	65	33.8%	26.4%	32.7%
Survey of Patients' Hospital Experiences				
Area Around Room 'Always' Quiet at Night	300+	45%	-	58%
Doctors 'Always' Communicated Well	300+	76%	-	80%
Home Recovery Information Given	300+	74%	-	82%
Hospital Given 9 or 10 on 10 Point Scale	300+	50%	-	67%
Meds 'Always' Explained Before Given	300+	46%	-	60%
Nurses 'Always' Communicated Well	300+	60%	-	76%
Pain 'Always' Well Controlled	300+	56%	-	69%
Room and Bathroom 'Always' Clean	300+	62%	-	71%
Timely Help 'Always' Received	300+	44%	-	64%
Would Definitely Recommend Hospital	300+	53%	-	69%

Bergen Regional Medical Center

230 East Ridgewood Ave
Paramus, NJ 07652
Phone: 201-967-4000
Fax: 201-967-4109
E-mail: webmaster@bergenregional.com
URL: www.bergenregional.com
Type: Acute Care Hospitals
Emergency Services: Yes
Ownership: Government - Local
Beds: 1,185

Key Personnel:

CEO/President. . . . . Joseph Gallagher
Radiology. . . . . Andrew S Lasser

Measure	Cases	This Hosp.	State Avg.	U.S. Avg.
Heart Attack Care				
ACE Inhibitor or ARB for LVSD[1]	4	100%	98%	96%
Aspirin at Arrival[1]	10	100%	99%	99%
Aspirin at Discharge[1]	11	100%	99%	98%
Beta Blocker at Discharge[1]	9	89%	99%	98%
Fibrinolytic Medication Timing	0	-	65%	55%
PCI Within 90 Minutes of Arrival	0	-	87%	90%
Smoking Cessation Advice[1]	2	100%	100%	99%
Chest Pain/Possible Heart Attack Care				
Aspirin at Arrival[1,3]	2	100%	97%	95%
Median Time to ECG (minutes)[1,3]	2	6	8	8
Median Time to Transfer (minutes)[3]	0	-	81	61
Fibrinolytic Medication Timing[3]	0	-	65%	54%
Heart Failure Care				
ACE Inhibitor or ARB for LVSD[1]	12	100%	97%	94%
Discharge Instructions[1]	10	100%	93%	88%
Evaluation of LVS Function[1]	23	100%	99%	98%
Smoking Cessation Advice[1]	6	100%	100%	98%
Pneumonia Care				
Appropriate Initial Antibiotic	38	92%	94%	92%
Blood Culture Timing	78	96%	97%	96%
Influenza Vaccine	42	95%	94%	91%
Initial Antibiotic Timing	46	96%	96%	95%
Pneumococcal Vaccine	68	99%	96%	93%
Smoking Cessation Advice[1]	14	100%	99%	97%
Surgical Care Improvement Project				
Appropriate VTP Within 24 Hours	25	96%	94%	92%
Appropriate Hair Removal	33	100%	100%	99%
Appropriate Beta Blocker Usage[1]	2	50%	95%	93%
Controlled Postoperative Blood Glucose	0	-	93%	93%
Prophylactic Antibiotic Timing	26	96%	98%	97%
Prophylactic Antibiotic Timing (Outpatient)[1,3]	4	50%	93%	92%
Prophylactic Antibiotic Selection	26	92%	97%	97%
Prophylactic Antibiotic Select. (Outpatient)[1,3]	2	50%	94%	94%
Prophylactic Antibiotic Stopped	26	100%	96%	94%
Recommended VTP Ordered	25	96%	95%	94%
Urinary Catheter Removal[1]	7	100%	93%	90%
Children's Asthma Care				
Received Systemic Corticosteroids	-	-	-	100%
Received Home Management Plan	-	-	-	71%
Received Reliever Medication	-	-	-	100%
Use of Medical Imaging				
Combination Abdominal CT Scan[1]	48	0.167	0.126	0.191
Combination Chest CT Scan[1]	39	0.051	0.026	0.054
Follow-up Mammogram/Ultrasound	87	8.0%	10.6%	8.4%
MRI for Low Back Pain[1]	7	42.9%	26.4%	32.7%
Survey of Patients' Hospital Experiences				
Area Around Room 'Always' Quiet at Night	(a)	38%	-	58%
Doctors 'Always' Communicated Well	(a)	55%	-	80%
Home Recovery Information Given	(a)	63%	-	82%
Hospital Given 9 or 10 on 10 Point Scale	(a)	32%	-	67%
Meds 'Always' Explained Before Given	(a)	43%	-	60%
Nurses 'Always' Communicated Well	(a)	48%	-	76%
Pain 'Always' Well Controlled	(a)	47%	-	69%
Room and Bathroom 'Always' Clean	(a)	50%	-	71%
Timely Help 'Always' Received	(a)	35%	-	64%
Would Definitely Recommend Hospital	(a)	41%	-	69%

Saint Mary's Hospital - Passaic

350 Boulevard
Passaic, NJ 07055
Phone: 973-365-4300
Fax: 973-471-5531
URL: www.smh-nj.com
Type: Acute Care Hospitals
Emergency Services: Yes
Ownership: Voluntary Non-Profit - Church
Beds: 264

Measure	Cases	This Hosp.	State Avg.	U.S. Avg.
Heart Attack Care				
ACE Inhibitor or ARB for LVSD[1]	18	100%	98%	96%
Aspirin at Arrival	84	99%	99%	99%
Aspirin at Discharge	73	97%	99%	98%
Beta Blocker at Discharge	78	99%	99%	98%
Fibrinolytic Medication Timing	0	-	65%	55%
PCI Within 90 Minutes of Arrival[1]	23	65%	87%	90%
Smoking Cessation Advice	26	100%	100%	99%
Chest Pain/Possible Heart Attack Care				
Aspirin at Arrival[3]	0	-	97%	95%
Median Time to ECG (minutes)[3]	0	-	8	8
Median Time to Transfer (minutes)[5]	0	-	81	61
Fibrinolytic Medication Timing[5]	0	-	65%	54%
Heart Failure Care				
ACE Inhibitor or ARB for LVSD[2]	98	94%	97%	94%
Discharge Instructions[2]	247	88%	93%	88%
Evaluation of LVS Function[2]	335	100%	99%	98%
Smoking Cessation Advice[2]	33	100%	100%	98%
Pneumonia Care				
Appropriate Initial Antibiotic[2]	95	93%	94%	92%
Blood Culture Timing[2]	180	97%	97%	96%
Influenza Vaccine[2]	112	99%	94%	91%
Initial Antibiotic Timing[2]	159	97%	96%	95%
Pneumococcal Vaccine[2]	186	97%	96%	93%
Smoking Cessation Advice[2]	41	100%	99%	97%
Surgical Care Improvement Project				
Appropriate VTP Within 24 Hours[2]	171	81%	94%	92%
Appropriate Hair Removal[2]	499	99%	100%	99%
Appropriate Beta Blocker Usage[2]	155	91%	95%	93%
Controlled Postoperative Blood Glucose[2]	96	80%	93%	93%
Prophylactic Antibiotic Timing[2]	271	99%	98%	97%
Prophylactic Antibiotic Timing (Outpatient)	275	91%	93%	92%
Prophylactic Antibiotic Selection[2]	280	95%	97%	97%
Prophylactic Antibiotic Select. (Outpatient)	263	91%	94%	94%
Prophylactic Antibiotic Stopped[2]	250	84%	96%	94%
Recommended VTP Ordered[2]	172	83%	95%	94%
Urinary Catheter Removal[2]	86	91%	93%	90%
Children's Asthma Care				
Received Systemic Corticosteroids	-	-	-	100%
Received Home Management Plan	-	-	-	71%
Received Reliever Medication	-	-	-	100%
Use of Medical Imaging				
Combination Abdominal CT Scan	626	0.107	0.126	0.191
Combination Chest CT Scan	384	0.003	0.026	0.054
Follow-up Mammogram/Ultrasound	729	9.1%	10.6%	8.4%
MRI for Low Back Pain	54	35.2%	26.4%	32.7%
Survey of Patients' Hospital Experiences				
Area Around Room 'Always' Quiet at Night	300+	48%	-	58%
Doctors 'Always' Communicated Well	300+	78%	-	80%
Home Recovery Information Given	300+	73%	-	82%
Hospital Given 9 or 10 on 10 Point Scale	300+	47%	-	67%
Meds 'Always' Explained Before Given	300+	49%	-	60%
Nurses 'Always' Communicated Well	300+	67%	-	76%
Pain 'Always' Well Controlled	300+	65%	-	69%
Room and Bathroom 'Always' Clean	300+	64%	-	71%
Timely Help 'Always' Received	300+	50%	-	64%
Would Definitely Recommend Hospital	300+	49%	-	69%

NOTE: Hospital profiles are in alphabetical order by state, then city, then hospital within the city; Rankings exclude hospitals with less than 25 cases except for patient surveys which excludes hospitals with less than 100 cases; (a) 100–299 cases; (1) The number of cases is too small to be sure how well a hospital is performing; (2) The hospital indicated that the data submitted for this measure were based on a sample of cases; (3) Data was collected during a shorter time period (fewer quarters) than the maximum possible time for this measure; (4) Suppressed for one or more quarters by CMS; (5) No data is available from the hospital for this measure; (6) Fewer than 100 patients completed the HCAHPS survey. Use these rates with caution, as the number of surveys may be too low to reliably assess hospital performance; (7) Survey results are based on less than 12 months of data; (8) Survey results are not available for this reporting period; (9) No or very few patients were eligible for the HCAHPS survey. The scores shown, if any, reflect a very small number of surveys; (10) A state average was not calculated because too few hospitals in the state submitted data; (11) There were discrepancies in the data collection process; Please refer to the User's Guide for a full explanation of data.

Saint Joseph's Regional Medical Center

703 Main St — Phone: 973-754-2000
Paterson, NJ 07503 — Fax: 973-754-3900
URL: www.sjhmc.org
Type: Acute Care Hospitals — Emergency Services: Yes
Ownership: Voluntary Non-Profit - Church — Beds: 642

Key Personnel:
CEO/President. . . . . William A McDonald
Infection Control. . . . . Marie Rella
Operating Room. . . . . Alan Sori, MD
Pediatric Ambulatory Care . . . . . . Albert Sanz, MD
Pediatric In-Patient Care . . . . . . Thomas Daley, MD
Radiology. . . . . Thomas M Herskovic, MD
Patient Relations . . . . Maureen Eisner

Measure	Cases	This Hosp.	State Avg.	U.S. Avg.
Heart Attack Care				
ACE Inhibitor or ARB for LVSD	64	94%	98%	96%
Aspirin at Arrival	379	99%	99%	99%
Aspirin at Discharge	377	97%	99%	98%
Beta Blocker at Discharge	358	96%	99%	98%
Fibrinolytic Medication Timing[1]	4	100%	65%	55%
PCI Within 90 Minutes of Arrival	79	97%	87%	90%
Smoking Cessation Advice	115	100%	100%	99%
Chest Pain/Possible Heart Attack Care				
Aspirin at Arrival[5]	0	-	97%	95%
Median Time to ECG (minutes)[5]	0	-	8	8
Median Time to Transfer (minutes)[5]	0	-	81	61
Fibrinolytic Medication Timing[5]	0	-	65%	54%
Heart Failure Care				
ACE Inhibitor or ARB for LVSD	335	98%	97%	94%
Discharge Instructions	754	98%	93%	88%
Evaluation of LVS Function	1,003	98%	99%	98%
Smoking Cessation Advice	175	100%	100%	98%
Pneumonia Care				
Appropriate Initial Antibiotic	321	86%	94%	92%
Blood Culture Timing	521	97%	97%	96%
Influenza Vaccine	344	85%	94%	91%
Initial Antibiotic Timing	540	95%	96%	95%
Pneumococcal Vaccine	444	87%	96%	93%
Smoking Cessation Advice	103	100%	99%	97%
Surgical Care Improvement Project				
Appropriate VTP Within 24 Hours[2]	339	91%	94%	92%
Appropriate Hair Removal[2]	1,127	100%	100%	99%
Appropriate Beta Blocker Usage[2]	365	99%	95%	93%
Controlled Postoperative Blood Glucose[2]	253	95%	93%	93%
Prophylactic Antibiotic Timing[2]	878	97%	98%	97%
Prophylactic Antibiotic Timing (Outpatient)	144	87%	93%	92%
Prophylactic Antibiotic Selection[2]	878	97%	97%	97%
Prophylactic Antibiotic Select. (Outpatient)	128	80%	94%	94%
Prophylactic Antibiotic Stopped[2]	848	96%	96%	94%
Recommended VTP Ordered[2]	341	94%	95%	94%
Urinary Catheter Removal[2]	307	94%	93%	90%
Children's Asthma Care				
Received Systemic Corticosteroids	-	-	-	100%
Received Home Management Plan	-	-	-	71%
Received Reliever Medication	-	-	-	100%
Use of Medical Imaging				
Combination Abdominal CT Scan	1,029	0.105	0.126	0.191
Combination Chest CT Scan	582	0.041	0.026	0.054
Follow-up Mammogram/Ultrasound	1,132	5.2%	10.6%	8.4%
MRI for Low Back Pain	196	27.6%	26.4%	32.7%
Survey of Patients' Hospital Experiences				
Area Around Room 'Always' Quiet at Night	300+	45%	-	58%
Doctors 'Always' Communicated Well	300+	73%	-	80%
Home Recovery Information Given	300+	80%	-	82%
Hospital Given 9 or 10 on 10 Point Scale	300+	57%	-	67%
Meds 'Always' Explained Before Given	300+	52%	-	60%
Nurses 'Always' Communicated Well	300+	67%	-	76%
Pain 'Always' Well Controlled	300+	62%	-	69%
Room and Bathroom 'Always' Clean	300+	65%	-	71%
Timely Help 'Always' Received	300+	49%	-	64%
Would Definitely Recommend Hospital	300+	64%	-	69%

Raritan Bay Medical Center

530 New Brunswick Ave — Phone: 732-442-3700
Perth Amboy, NJ 08861 — Fax: 732-324-4994
Type: Acute Care Hospitals — Emergency Services: Yes
Ownership: Voluntary Non-Profit - Private — Beds: 522

Key Personnel:
CEO/President. . . . . Michael D'Agnes
Chief of Medical Staff. . . . . John Middleton, MD
Infection Control. . . . . John R Middleton, MD
Operating Room. . . . . Geraldine DiGiovanni, RN
Pediatric Ambulatory Care . . . . . . Norman Barofsky, MD
Pediatric In-Patient Care . . . . . . Norman Barofsky, MD
Quality Assurance . . . . Erich Kreher
Radiology. . . . . Alvin Kravet, MD

Measure	Cases	This Hosp.	State Avg.	U.S. Avg.
Heart Attack Care				
ACE Inhibitor or ARB for LVSD	30	100%	98%	96%
Aspirin at Arrival	204	98%	99%	99%
Aspirin at Discharge	134	96%	99%	98%
Beta Blocker at Discharge	132	98%	99%	98%
Fibrinolytic Medication Timing	0	-	65%	55%
PCI Within 90 Minutes of Arrival	31	87%	87%	90%
Smoking Cessation Advice	42	100%	100%	99%
Chest Pain/Possible Heart Attack Care				
Aspirin at Arrival[1,3]	7	100%	97%	95%
Median Time to ECG (minutes)[1,3]	7	12	8	8
Median Time to Transfer (minutes)[5]	0	-	81	61
Fibrinolytic Medication Timing[3]	0	-	65%	54%
Heart Failure Care				
ACE Inhibitor or ARB for LVSD[2]	193	99%	97%	94%
Discharge Instructions[2]	370	96%	93%	88%
Evaluation of LVS Function[2]	542	100%	99%	98%
Smoking Cessation Advice[2]	54	100%	100%	98%
Pneumonia Care				
Appropriate Initial Antibiotic[2]	183	96%	94%	92%
Blood Culture Timing[2]	343	97%	97%	96%
Influenza Vaccine[2]	156	95%	94%	91%
Initial Antibiotic Timing[2]	306	95%	96%	95%
Pneumococcal Vaccine[2]	261	98%	96%	93%
Smoking Cessation Advice[2]	92	99%	99%	97%
Surgical Care Improvement Project				
Appropriate VTP Within 24 Hours[2]	164	93%	94%	92%
Appropriate Hair Removal[2]	330	100%	100%	99%
Appropriate Beta Blocker Usage[2]	106	92%	95%	93%
Controlled Postoperative Blood Glucose[2]	0	-	93%	93%
Prophylactic Antibiotic Timing[2]	164	99%	98%	97%
Prophylactic Antibiotic Timing (Outpatient)	130	89%	93%	92%
Prophylactic Antibiotic Selection[2]	164	94%	97%	97%
Prophylactic Antibiotic Select. (Outpatient)	117	97%	94%	94%
Prophylactic Antibiotic Stopped[2]	151	97%	96%	94%
Recommended VTP Ordered[2]	165	95%	95%	94%
Urinary Catheter Removal	31	90%	93%	90%
Children's Asthma Care				
Received Systemic Corticosteroids	-	-	-	100%
Received Home Management Plan	-	-	-	71%
Received Reliever Medication	-	-	-	100%
Use of Medical Imaging				
Combination Abdominal CT Scan	761	0.047	0.126	0.191
Combination Chest CT Scan	409	0.000	0.026	0.054
Follow-up Mammogram/Ultrasound	880	4.1%	10.6%	8.4%
MRI for Low Back Pain[1]	31	35.5%	26.4%	32.7%
Survey of Patients' Hospital Experiences				
Area Around Room 'Always' Quiet at Night	300+	52%	-	58%
Doctors 'Always' Communicated Well	300+	76%	-	80%
Home Recovery Information Given	300+	77%	-	82%
Hospital Given 9 or 10 on 10 Point Scale	300+	57%	-	67%
Meds 'Always' Explained Before Given	300+	54%	-	60%
Nurses 'Always' Communicated Well	300+	74%	-	76%
Pain 'Always' Well Controlled	300+	65%	-	69%
Room and Bathroom 'Always' Clean	300+	65%	-	71%
Timely Help 'Always' Received	300+	58%	-	64%
Would Definitely Recommend Hospital	300+	60%	-	69%

Warren Hospital

185 Roseberry St — Phone: 908-859-6700
Phillipsburg, NJ 08865 — Fax: 908-859-4546
URL: www.warrenhospital.org
Type: Acute Care Hospitals — Emergency Services: Yes
Ownership: Voluntary Non-Profit - Other — Beds: 214

Key Personnel:
CEO/President. . . . . Jeffrey C Goodwin
Chief of Medical Staff. . . . . Frank Gilley, MD
Quality Assurance . . . . Barbara Balas
Emergency Room . . . . Howard Swidler, MD

Measure	Cases	This Hosp.	State Avg.	U.S. Avg.
Heart Attack Care				
ACE Inhibitor or ARB for LVSD[1]	7	100%	98%	96%
Aspirin at Arrival	29	97%	99%	99%
Aspirin at Discharge[1]	20	100%	99%	98%
Beta Blocker at Discharge[1]	23	96%	99%	98%
Fibrinolytic Medication Timing	0	-	65%	55%
PCI Within 90 Minutes of Arrival	0	-	87%	90%
Smoking Cessation Advice[1]	3	100%	100%	99%
Chest Pain/Possible Heart Attack Care				
Aspirin at Arrival	34	100%	97%	95%
Median Time to ECG (minutes)	36	6	8	8
Median Time to Transfer (minutes)[1]	13	50	81	61
Fibrinolytic Medication Timing	0	-	65%	54%
Heart Failure Care				
ACE Inhibitor or ARB for LVSD	38	100%	97%	94%
Discharge Instructions	111	98%	93%	88%
Evaluation of LVS Function	176	100%	99%	98%
Smoking Cessation Advice	25	100%	100%	98%
Pneumonia Care				
Appropriate Initial Antibiotic	100	98%	94%	92%
Blood Culture Timing	155	99%	97%	96%
Influenza Vaccine	130	97%	94%	91%
Initial Antibiotic Timing	153	98%	96%	95%
Pneumococcal Vaccine	192	98%	96%	93%
Smoking Cessation Advice	71	100%	99%	97%
Surgical Care Improvement Project				
Appropriate VTP Within 24 Hours[2]	93	97%	94%	92%
Appropriate Hair Removal[2]	270	100%	100%	99%
Appropriate Beta Blocker Usage[2]	76	96%	95%	93%
Controlled Postoperative Blood Glucose[2]	0	-	93%	93%
Prophylactic Antibiotic Timing[2]	151	99%	98%	97%
Prophylactic Antibiotic Timing (Outpatient)	107	95%	93%	92%
Prophylactic Antibiotic Selection[2]	151	99%	97%	97%
Prophylactic Antibiotic Select. (Outpatient)	105	96%	94%	94%
Prophylactic Antibiotic Stopped[2]	145	94%	96%	94%
Recommended VTP Ordered[2]	93	98%	95%	94%
Urinary Catheter Removal[2]	71	94%	93%	90%
Children's Asthma Care				
Received Systemic Corticosteroids	-	-	-	100%
Received Home Management Plan	-	-	-	71%
Received Reliever Medication	-	-	-	100%
Use of Medical Imaging				
Combination Abdominal CT Scan	799	0.068	0.126	0.191
Combination Chest CT Scan	520	0.042	0.026	0.054
Follow-up Mammogram/Ultrasound	1,082	6.7%	10.6%	8.4%
MRI for Low Back Pain	143	32.9%	26.4%	32.7%
Survey of Patients' Hospital Experiences				
Area Around Room 'Always' Quiet at Night	300+	50%	-	58%
Doctors 'Always' Communicated Well	300+	77%	-	80%
Home Recovery Information Given	300+	78%	-	82%
Hospital Given 9 or 10 on 10 Point Scale	300+	57%	-	67%
Meds 'Always' Explained Before Given	300+	57%	-	60%
Nurses 'Always' Communicated Well	300+	76%	-	76%
Pain 'Always' Well Controlled	300+	70%	-	69%
Room and Bathroom 'Always' Clean	300+	70%	-	71%
Timely Help 'Always' Received	300+	56%	-	64%
Would Definitely Recommend Hospital	300+	55%	-	69%

NOTE: Hospital profiles are in alphabetical order by state, then city, then hospital within the city; Rankings exclude hospitals with less than 25 cases except for patient surveys which excludes hospitals with less than 100 cases; (a) 100–299 cases; (1) The number of cases is too small to be sure how well a hospital is performing; (2) The hospital indicated that the data submitted for this measure were based on a sample of cases; (3) Data was collected during a shorter time period (fewer quarters) than the maximum possible time for this measure; (4) Suppressed for one or more quarters by CMS; (5) No data is available from the hospital for this measure; (6) Fewer than 100 patients completed the HCAHPS survey. Use these rates with caution, as the number of surveys may be too low to reliably assess hospital performance; (7) Survey results are based on less than 12 months of data; (8) Survey results are not available for this reporting period; (9) No or very few patients were eligible for the HCAHPS survey. The scores shown, if any, reflect a very small number of surveys; (10) A state average was not calculated because too few hospitals in the state submitted data; (11) There were discrepancies in the data collection process; Please refer to the User's Guide for a full explanation of data.

Chilton Hospital

97 West Parkway
Pompton Plains, NJ 07444
URL: www.chiltonmemorial.org
Type: Acute Care Hospitals
Ownership: Voluntary Non-Profit - Private

Phone: 973-831-5000
Fax: 973-831-5516
Emergency Services: Yes
Beds: 256

Key Personnel:

CEO/President. . . . . Deborah K Zastocki
Cardiac Laboratory. . . . . Dina Tortorelli
Chief of Medical Staff . . . . Joel Nizon, MD
Operating Room. . . . . Donna Kirby
Quality Assurance . . . . John Browne
Ambulatory Care . . . . Donna Kirby
Emergency Room . . . . Amelia Bortelloni
Intensive Care Unit. . . . . Cindy O'Banks

Measure	Cases	This Hosp.	State Avg.	U.S. Avg.
Heart Attack Care				
ACE Inhibitor or ARB for LVSD	29	100%	98%	96%
Aspirin at Arrival	172	99%	99%	99%
Aspirin at Discharge	102	98%	99%	98%
Beta Blocker at Discharge	106	98%	99%	98%
Fibrinolytic Medication Timing	0	-	65%	55%
PCI Within 90 Minutes of Arrival	49	90%	87%	90%
Smoking Cessation Advice[1]	19	100%	100%	99%
Chest Pain/Possible Heart Attack Care				
Aspirin at Arrival[1,3]	1	100%	97%	95%
Median Time to ECG (minutes)[1,3]	1	4	8	8
Median Time to Transfer (minutes)[5]	0	-	81	61
Fibrinolytic Medication Timing[5]	0	-	65%	54%
Heart Failure Care				
ACE Inhibitor or ARB for LVSD	81	96%	97%	94%
Discharge Instructions	200	92%	93%	88%
Evaluation of LVS Function	328	99%	99%	98%
Smoking Cessation Advice	38	100%	100%	98%
Pneumonia Care				
Appropriate Initial Antibiotic[2]	84	89%	94%	92%
Blood Culture Timing[2]	154	97%	97%	96%
Influenza Vaccine[2]	92	91%	94%	91%
Initial Antibiotic Timing[2]	139	96%	96%	95%
Pneumococcal Vaccine[2]	157	95%	96%	93%
Smoking Cessation Advice[2]	37	100%	99%	97%
Surgical Care Improvement Project				
Appropriate VTP Within 24 Hours[2]	186	89%	94%	92%
Appropriate Hair Removal[2]	438	100%	100%	99%
Appropriate Beta Blocker Usage[2]	122	93%	95%	93%
Controlled Postoperative Blood Glucose[2]	0	-	93%	93%
Prophylactic Antibiotic Timing[2]	256	99%	98%	97%
Prophylactic Antibiotic Timing (Outpatient)	174	93%	93%	92%
Prophylactic Antibiotic Selection[2]	257	97%	97%	97%
Prophylactic Antibiotic Select. (Outpatient)	164	91%	94%	94%
Prophylactic Antibiotic Stopped[2]	229	95%	96%	94%
Recommended VTP Ordered[2]	186	93%	95%	94%
Urinary Catheter Removal[2]	86	90%	93%	90%
Children's Asthma Care				
Received Systemic Corticosteroids	-	-	-	100%
Received Home Management Plan	-	-	-	71%
Received Reliever Medication	-	-	-	100%
Use of Medical Imaging				
Combination Abdominal CT Scan	1,053	0.569	0.126	0.191
Combination Chest CT Scan	780	0.006	0.026	0.054
Follow-up Mammogram/Ultrasound	1,959	12.0%	10.6%	8.4%
MRI for Low Back Pain	207	23.7%	26.4%	32.7%
Survey of Patients' Hospital Experiences				
Area Around Room 'Always' Quiet at Night	300+	45%	-	58%
Doctors 'Always' Communicated Well	300+	77%	-	80%
Home Recovery Information Given	300+	76%	-	82%
Hospital Given 9 or 10 on 10 Point Scale	300+	61%	-	67%
Meds 'Always' Explained Before Given	300+	55%	-	60%
Nurses 'Always' Communicated Well	300+	76%	-	76%
Pain 'Always' Well Controlled	300+	70%	-	69%
Room and Bathroom 'Always' Clean	300+	62%	-	71%
Timely Help 'Always' Received	300+	63%	-	64%
Would Definitely Recommend Hospital	300+	66%	-	69%

University Medical Center at Princeton

253 Witherspoon St
Princeton, NJ 08540
URL: www.princetonhcs.org
Type: Acute Care Hospitals
Ownership: Voluntary Non-Profit - Private

Phone: 609-497-4000
Fax: 609-497-4991
Emergency Services: No
Beds: 396

Key Personnel:

CEO/President. . . . . Mark Jones
Chief of Medical Staff . . . . Henry Davison MD, JR
Infection Control. . . . . Dr Alexander Ackley
Operating Room. . . . . Kathy Raney
Pediatric In-Patient Care . . . . Stephen E Hefler MD
Quality Assurance . . . . Debbie Lloyd
Radiology. . . . . Donald Denny MD

Measure	Cases	This Hosp.	State Avg.	U.S. Avg.
Heart Attack Care				
ACE Inhibitor or ARB for LVSD[1]	16	100%	98%	96%
Aspirin at Arrival	129	100%	99%	99%
Aspirin at Discharge	80	100%	99%	98%
Beta Blocker at Discharge	85	100%	99%	98%
Fibrinolytic Medication Timing	0	-	65%	55%
PCI Within 90 Minutes of Arrival[1]	20	100%	87%	90%
Smoking Cessation Advice[1]	8	100%	100%	99%
Chest Pain/Possible Heart Attack Care				
Aspirin at Arrival[1]	7	100%	97%	95%
Median Time to ECG (minutes)[1]	7	0	8	8
Median Time to Transfer (minutes)[1,3]	1	167	81	61
Fibrinolytic Medication Timing[3]	0	-	65%	54%
Heart Failure Care				
ACE Inhibitor or ARB for LVSD[2]	60	100%	97%	94%
Discharge Instructions[2]	164	100%	93%	88%
Evaluation of LVS Function[2]	255	100%	99%	98%
Smoking Cessation Advice[1,2]	19	100%	100%	98%
Pneumonia Care				
Appropriate Initial Antibiotic[2]	102	97%	94%	92%
Blood Culture Timing[2]	68	97%	97%	96%
Influenza Vaccine[2]	97	99%	94%	91%
Initial Antibiotic Timing[2]	138	99%	96%	95%
Pneumococcal Vaccine[2]	142	98%	96%	93%
Smoking Cessation Advice[2]	29	100%	99%	97%
Surgical Care Improvement Project				
Appropriate VTP Within 24 Hours[2]	180	98%	94%	92%
Appropriate Hair Removal[2]	507	99%	100%	99%
Appropriate Beta Blocker Usage[2]	126	99%	95%	93%
Controlled Postoperative Blood Glucose[1,2]	1	0%	93%	93%
Prophylactic Antibiotic Timing[2]	265	99%	98%	97%
Prophylactic Antibiotic Timing (Outpatient)	246	91%	93%	92%
Prophylactic Antibiotic Selection[2]	266	98%	97%	97%
Prophylactic Antibiotic Select. (Outpatient)	228	96%	94%	94%
Prophylactic Antibiotic Stopped[2]	261	98%	96%	94%
Recommended VTP Ordered[2]	180	98%	95%	94%
Urinary Catheter Removal[2]	133	98%	93%	90%
Children's Asthma Care				
Received Systemic Corticosteroids	-	-	-	100%
Received Home Management Plan	-	-	-	71%
Received Reliever Medication	-	-	-	100%
Use of Medical Imaging				
Combination Abdominal CT Scan	769	0.140	0.126	0.191
Combination Chest CT Scan	499	0.014	0.026	0.054
Follow-up Mammogram/Ultrasound	528	12.9%	10.6%	8.4%
MRI for Low Back Pain[1]	55	25.5%	26.4%	32.7%
Survey of Patients' Hospital Experiences				
Area Around Room 'Always' Quiet at Night	300+	48%	-	58%
Doctors 'Always' Communicated Well	300+	77%	-	80%
Home Recovery Information Given	300+	79%	-	82%
Hospital Given 9 or 10 on 10 Point Scale	300+	60%	-	67%
Meds 'Always' Explained Before Given	300+	57%	-	60%
Nurses 'Always' Communicated Well	300+	71%	-	76%
Pain 'Always' Well Controlled	300+	67%	-	69%
Room and Bathroom 'Always' Clean	300+	61%	-	71%
Timely Help 'Always' Received	300+	54%	-	64%
Would Definitely Recommend Hospital	300+	67%	-	69%

Robert Wood Johnson University Hospital at Rahway

865 Stone St
Rahway, NJ 07065
URL: www.rwjuhr.com/about/history.html
Type: Acute Care Hospitals
Ownership: Voluntary Non-Profit - Private

Phone: 732-381-4200
Fax: 732-499-6337
Emergency Services: Yes
Beds: 311

Key Personnel:

CEO/President. . . . . Kirk C Tice
Chief of Medical Staff . . . . Barry Benisch
Infection Control. . . . . Bessie Boyant
Operating Room. . . . . Connie Saquing
Quality Assurance . . . . Lucinda Glynn
Radiology. . . . . Robert White
Emergency Room . . . . Lynn Keaoey

Measure	Cases	This Hosp.	State Avg.	U.S. Avg.
Heart Attack Care				
ACE Inhibitor or ARB for LVSD[1]	12	100%	98%	96%
Aspirin at Arrival	106	100%	99%	99%
Aspirin at Discharge	38	100%	99%	98%
Beta Blocker at Discharge	44	100%	99%	98%
Fibrinolytic Medication Timing[1]	9	44%	65%	55%
PCI Within 90 Minutes of Arrival	0	-	87%	90%
Smoking Cessation Advice[1]	4	100%	100%	99%
Chest Pain/Possible Heart Attack Care				
Aspirin at Arrival[1]	20	95%	97%	95%
Median Time to ECG (minutes)[1]	21	7	8	8
Median Time to Transfer (minutes)[1,3]	2	136	81	61
Fibrinolytic Medication Timing[1,3]	3	67%	65%	54%
Heart Failure Care				
ACE Inhibitor or ARB for LVSD	131	99%	97%	94%
Discharge Instructions	259	83%	93%	88%
Evaluation of LVS Function	430	100%	99%	98%
Smoking Cessation Advice	41	100%	100%	98%
Pneumonia Care				
Appropriate Initial Antibiotic	141	96%	94%	92%
Blood Culture Timing	254	96%	97%	96%
Influenza Vaccine	157	98%	94%	91%
Initial Antibiotic Timing	230	96%	96%	95%
Pneumococcal Vaccine	241	98%	96%	93%
Smoking Cessation Advice	42	95%	99%	97%
Surgical Care Improvement Project				
Appropriate VTP Within 24 Hours	145	96%	94%	92%
Appropriate Hair Removal	321	100%	100%	99%
Appropriate Beta Blocker Usage	110	95%	95%	93%
Controlled Postoperative Blood Glucose	0	-	93%	93%
Prophylactic Antibiotic Timing	161	100%	98%	97%
Prophylactic Antibiotic Timing (Outpatient)	121	98%	93%	92%
Prophylactic Antibiotic Selection	162	99%	97%	97%
Prophylactic Antibiotic Select. (Outpatient)	120	98%	94%	94%
Prophylactic Antibiotic Stopped	154	99%	96%	94%
Recommended VTP Ordered	145	97%	95%	94%
Urinary Catheter Removal	32	97%	93%	90%
Children's Asthma Care				
Received Systemic Corticosteroids	-	-	-	100%
Received Home Management Plan	-	-	-	71%
Received Reliever Medication	-	-	-	100%
Use of Medical Imaging				
Combination Abdominal CT Scan	513	0.101	0.126	0.191
Combination Chest CT Scan	440	0.023	0.026	0.054
Follow-up Mammogram/Ultrasound	266	9.4%	10.6%	8.4%
MRI for Low Back Pain	86	14.0%	26.4%	32.7%
Survey of Patients' Hospital Experiences				
Area Around Room 'Always' Quiet at Night	300+	48%	-	58%
Doctors 'Always' Communicated Well	300+	75%	-	80%
Home Recovery Information Given	300+	78%	-	82%
Hospital Given 9 or 10 on 10 Point Scale	300+	56%	-	67%
Meds 'Always' Explained Before Given	300+	56%	-	60%
Nurses 'Always' Communicated Well	300+	71%	-	76%
Pain 'Always' Well Controlled	300+	66%	-	69%
Room and Bathroom 'Always' Clean	300+	69%	-	71%
Timely Help 'Always' Received	300+	55%	-	64%
Would Definitely Recommend Hospital	300+	58%	-	69%

NOTE: Hospital profiles are in alphabetical order by state, then city, then hospital within the city; Rankings exclude hospitals with less than 25 cases except for patient surveys which excludes hospitals with less than 100 cases; (a) 100–299 cases; (1) The number of cases is too small to be sure how well a hospital is performing; (2) The hospital indicated that the data submitted for this measure were based on a sample of cases; (3) Data was collected during a shorter time period (fewer quarters) than the maximum possible time for this measure; (4) Suppressed for one or more quarters by CMS; (5) No data is available from the hospital for this measure; (6) Fewer than 100 patients completed the HCAHPS survey. Use these rates with caution, as the number of surveys may be too low to reliably assess hospital performance; (7) Survey results are based on less than 12 months of data; (8) Survey results are not available for this reporting period; (9) No or very few patients were eligible for the HCAHPS survey. The scores shown, if any, reflect a very small number of surveys; (10) A state average was not calculated because too few hospitals in the state submitted data; (11) There were discrepancies in the data collection process; Please refer to the User's Guide for a full explanation of data.

Riverview Medical Center

One Riverview Plaza Phone: 732-741-2700
Red Bank, NJ 07701 Fax: 732-224-8408
URL: www.meridianhealth.com
Type: Acute Care Hospitals Emergency Services: Yes
Ownership: Voluntary Non-Profit - Private Beds: 476

Key Personnel:
CEO/President............... Timothy J Hogan, FACHE
Chief of Medical Staff.......... Richard Scott, MD
Pediatric Ambulatory Care .... Robert Morgan, MD
Pediatric In-Patient Care .... Robert Morgan, MD
Radiology.................... John Parrella
Emergency Room .... James Cameron

Measure	Cases	This Hosp.	State Avg.	U.S. Avg.
Heart Attack Care				
ACE Inhibitor or ARB for LVSD[1]	9	100%	98%	96%
Aspirin at Arrival	187	100%	99%	99%
Aspirin at Discharge	113	100%	99%	98%
Beta Blocker at Discharge	116	100%	99%	98%
Fibrinolytic Medication Timing	0	-	65%	55%
PCI Within 90 Minutes of Arrival	39	95%	87%	90%
Smoking Cessation Advice	25	100%	100%	99%
Chest Pain/Possible Heart Attack Care				
Aspirin at Arrival[1]	10	100%	97%	95%
Median Time to ECG (minutes)[1]	11	11	8	8
Median Time to Transfer (minutes)[1,3]	1	103	81	61
Fibrinolytic Medication Timing[1]	1	100%	65%	54%
Heart Failure Care				
ACE Inhibitor or ARB for LVSD	46	100%	97%	94%
Discharge Instructions	229	100%	93%	88%
Evaluation of LVS Function	320	100%	99%	98%
Smoking Cessation Advice	31	100%	100%	98%
Pneumonia Care				
Appropriate Initial Antibiotic	142	95%	94%	92%
Blood Culture Timing	219	99%	97%	96%
Influenza Vaccine	133	100%	94%	91%
Initial Antibiotic Timing	183	97%	96%	95%
Pneumococcal Vaccine	204	99%	96%	93%
Smoking Cessation Advice	59	100%	99%	97%
Surgical Care Improvement Project				
Appropriate VTP Within 24 Hours[2]	317	95%	94%	92%
Appropriate Hair Removal[2]	990	100%	100%	99%
Appropriate Beta Blocker Usage[2]	240	99%	95%	93%
Controlled Postoperative Blood Glucose[1,2]	1	100%	93%	93%
Prophylactic Antibiotic Timing[2]	689	100%	98%	97%
Prophylactic Antibiotic Timing (Outpatient)	200	98%	93%	92%
Prophylactic Antibiotic Selection[2]	693	98%	97%	97%
Prophylactic Antibiotic Select. (Outpatient)	199	98%	94%	94%
Prophylactic Antibiotic Stopped[2]	658	97%	96%	94%
Recommended VTP Ordered[2]	317	96%	95%	94%
Urinary Catheter Removal[2]	278	97%	93%	90%
Children's Asthma Care				
Received Systemic Corticosteroids	-	-	-	100%
Received Home Management Plan	-	-	-	71%
Received Reliever Medication	-	-	-	100%
Use of Medical Imaging				
Combination Abdominal CT Scan	1,238	0.073	0.126	0.191
Combination Chest CT Scan	915	0.014	0.026	0.054
Follow-up Mammogram/Ultrasound	582	16.2%	10.6%	8.4%
MRI for Low Back Pain	83	19.3%	26.4%	32.7%
Survey of Patients' Hospital Experiences				
Area Around Room 'Always' Quiet at Night	300+	52%	-	58%
Doctors 'Always' Communicated Well	300+	79%	-	80%
Home Recovery Information Given	300+	81%	-	82%
Hospital Given 9 or 10 on 10 Point Scale	300+	63%	-	67%
Meds 'Always' Explained Before Given	300+	61%	-	60%
Nurses 'Always' Communicated Well	300+	76%	-	76%
Pain 'Always' Well Controlled	300+	70%	-	69%
Room and Bathroom 'Always' Clean	300+	70%	-	71%
Timely Help 'Always' Received	300+	61%	-	64%
Would Definitely Recommend Hospital	300+	71%	-	69%

Valley Hospital

223 N Van Dien Avenue Phone: 201-447-8000
Ridgewood, NJ 07450 Fax: 201-447-8732
E-mail: tvanmar@valleyhealth.com
URL: www.valleyhealth.com
Type: Acute Care Hospitals Emergency Services: Yes
Ownership: Voluntary Non-Profit - Private Beds: 442

Key Personnel:
CEO/President.............. Audrey Meyers
Chief of Medical Staff.......... Marc S Melamed, MD
Infection Control............. Terry Dannels, RN
Operating Room............. Lorraine Butler, RN
Pediatric Ambulatory Care ...... Joseph A Cannaliato, MD
Pediatric In-Patient Care .... Joseph A Cannaliato, MD
Quality Assurance .... Virginia O'Malley, RN
Radiology................... Louis Rambler, MD

Measure	Cases	This Hosp.	State Avg.	U.S. Avg.
Heart Attack Care				
ACE Inhibitor or ARB for LVSD[2]	46	93%	98%	96%
Aspirin at Arrival[2]	289	98%	99%	99%
Aspirin at Discharge[2]	291	100%	99%	98%
Beta Blocker at Discharge[2]	296	99%	99%	98%
Fibrinolytic Medication Timing[2]	0	-	65%	55%
PCI Within 90 Minutes of Arrival[2]	46	96%	87%	90%
Smoking Cessation Advice[2]	56	100%	100%	99%
Chest Pain/Possible Heart Attack Care				
Aspirin at Arrival[1,3]	1	100%	97%	95%
Median Time to ECG (minutes)[1,3]	1	9	8	8
Median Time to Transfer (minutes)[5]	0	-	81	61
Fibrinolytic Medication Timing[5]	0	-	65%	54%
Heart Failure Care				
ACE Inhibitor or ARB for LVSD[2]	59	92%	97%	94%
Discharge Instructions[2]	244	77%	93%	88%
Evaluation of LVS Function[2]	321	99%	99%	98%
Smoking Cessation Advice[1,2]	24	100%	100%	98%
Pneumonia Care				
Appropriate Initial Antibiotic[2]	96	94%	94%	92%
Blood Culture Timing[2]	163	99%	97%	96%
Influenza Vaccine[2]	92	100%	94%	91%
Initial Antibiotic Timing[2]	158	98%	96%	95%
Pneumococcal Vaccine[2]	172	99%	96%	93%
Smoking Cessation Advice[1,2]	22	100%	99%	97%
Surgical Care Improvement Project				
Appropriate VTP Within 24 Hours[2]	219	87%	94%	92%
Appropriate Hair Removal[2]	807	100%	100%	99%
Appropriate Beta Blocker Usage[2]	286	90%	95%	93%
Controlled Postoperative Blood Glucose[2]	169	97%	93%	93%
Prophylactic Antibiotic Timing[2]	538	98%	98%	97%
Prophylactic Antibiotic Timing (Outpatient)	458	92%	93%	92%
Prophylactic Antibiotic Selection[2]	549	97%	97%	97%
Prophylactic Antibiotic Select. (Outpatient)	441	95%	94%	94%
Prophylactic Antibiotic Stopped[2]	519	95%	96%	94%
Recommended VTP Ordered[2]	219	94%	95%	94%
Urinary Catheter Removal[2]	209	93%	93%	90%
Children's Asthma Care				
Received Systemic Corticosteroids	-	-	-	100%
Received Home Management Plan	-	-	-	71%
Received Reliever Medication	-	-	-	100%
Use of Medical Imaging				
Combination Abdominal CT Scan	2,036	0.106	0.126	0.191
Combination Chest CT Scan	2,050	0.016	0.026	0.054
Follow-up Mammogram/Ultrasound	1,605	8.7%	10.6%	8.4%
MRI for Low Back Pain	211	28.4%	26.4%	32.7%
Survey of Patients' Hospital Experiences				
Area Around Room 'Always' Quiet at Night	300+	54%	-	58%
Doctors 'Always' Communicated Well	300+	80%	-	80%
Home Recovery Information Given	300+	80%	-	82%
Hospital Given 9 or 10 on 10 Point Scale	300+	76%	-	67%
Meds 'Always' Explained Before Given	300+	58%	-	60%
Nurses 'Always' Communicated Well	300+	82%	-	76%
Pain 'Always' Well Controlled	300+	74%	-	69%
Room and Bathroom 'Always' Clean	300+	80%	-	71%
Timely Help 'Always' Received	300+	65%	-	64%
Would Definitely Recommend Hospital	300+	82%	-	69%

Memorial Hospital of Salem County

310 Woodstown Road Phone: 856-935-1000
Salem, NJ 08079 Fax: 856-935-3175
URL: www.mhshealth.com
Type: Acute Care Hospitals Emergency Services: Yes
Ownership: Voluntary Non-Profit - Private Beds: 140

Key Personnel:
CEO/President.............. Robert Allen
Chief of Medical Staff.......... John Amrien, MD
Emergency Room .... Dr. Jane Fleurantin

Measure	Cases	This Hosp.	State Avg.	U.S. Avg.
Heart Attack Care				
ACE Inhibitor or ARB for LVSD[1]	5	100%	98%	96%
Aspirin at Arrival	30	100%	99%	99%
Aspirin at Discharge[1]	10	100%	99%	98%
Beta Blocker at Discharge[1]	13	100%	99%	98%
Fibrinolytic Medication Timing	0	-	65%	55%
PCI Within 90 Minutes of Arrival	0	-	87%	90%
Smoking Cessation Advice[1]	3	100%	100%	99%
Chest Pain/Possible Heart Attack Care				
Aspirin at Arrival[1]	19	95%	97%	95%
Median Time to ECG (minutes)[1]	21	8	8	8
Median Time to Transfer (minutes)[1,3]	1	68	81	61
Fibrinolytic Medication Timing[1]	7	100%	65%	54%
Heart Failure Care				
ACE Inhibitor or ARB for LVSD	50	100%	97%	94%
Discharge Instructions	151	99%	93%	88%
Evaluation of LVS Function	186	100%	99%	98%
Smoking Cessation Advice	36	100%	100%	98%
Pneumonia Care				
Appropriate Initial Antibiotic	110	91%	94%	92%
Blood Culture Timing	105	98%	97%	96%
Influenza Vaccine	125	91%	94%	91%
Initial Antibiotic Timing	180	100%	96%	95%
Pneumococcal Vaccine	132	96%	96%	93%
Smoking Cessation Advice	91	100%	99%	97%
Surgical Care Improvement Project				
Appropriate VTP Within 24 Hours[2]	62	98%	94%	92%
Appropriate Hair Removal[2]	169	100%	100%	99%
Appropriate Beta Blocker Usage[2]	38	82%	95%	93%
Controlled Postoperative Blood Glucose[2]	0	-	93%	93%
Prophylactic Antibiotic Timing[2]	89	97%	98%	97%
Prophylactic Antibiotic Timing (Outpatient)	38	89%	93%	92%
Prophylactic Antibiotic Selection[2]	90	98%	97%	97%
Prophylactic Antibiotic Select. (Outpatient)	34	91%	94%	94%
Prophylactic Antibiotic Stopped[2]	82	95%	96%	94%
Recommended VTP Ordered[2]	62	98%	95%	94%
Urinary Catheter Removal[1]	23	87%	93%	90%
Children's Asthma Care				
Received Systemic Corticosteroids	-	-	-	100%
Received Home Management Plan	-	-	-	71%
Received Reliever Medication	-	-	-	100%
Use of Medical Imaging				
Combination Abdominal CT Scan	359	0.072	0.126	0.191
Combination Chest CT Scan	258	0.012	0.026	0.054
Follow-up Mammogram/Ultrasound	357	7.3%	10.6%	8.4%
MRI for Low Back Pain	69	33.3%	26.4%	32.7%
Survey of Patients' Hospital Experiences				
Area Around Room 'Always' Quiet at Night	300+	58%	-	58%
Doctors 'Always' Communicated Well	300+	75%	-	80%
Home Recovery Information Given	300+	79%	-	82%
Hospital Given 9 or 10 on 10 Point Scale	300+	52%	-	67%
Meds 'Always' Explained Before Given	300+	57%	-	60%
Nurses 'Always' Communicated Well	300+	70%	-	76%
Pain 'Always' Well Controlled	300+	63%	-	69%
Room and Bathroom 'Always' Clean	300+	59%	-	71%
Timely Help 'Always' Received	300+	53%	-	64%
Would Definitely Recommend Hospital	300+	46%	-	69%

NOTE: Hospital profiles are in alphabetical order by state, then city, then hospital within the city; Rankings exclude hospitals with less than 25 cases except for patient surveys which excludes hospitals with less than 100 cases; (a) 100–299 cases; (1) The number of cases is too small to be sure how well a hospital is performing; (2) The hospital indicated that the data submitted for this measure were based on a sample of cases; (3) Data was collected during a shorter time period (fewer quarters) than the maximum possible time for this measure; (4) Suppressed for one or more quarters by CMS; (5) No data is available from the hospital for this measure; (6) Fewer than 100 patients completed the HCAHPS survey. Use these rates with caution, as the number of surveys may be too low to reliably assess hospital performance; (7) Survey results are based on less than 12 months of data; (8) Survey results are not available for this reporting period; (9) No or very few patients were eligible for the HCAHPS survey. The scores shown, if any, reflect a very small number of surveys; (10) A state average was not calculated because too few hospitals in the state submitted data; (11) There were discrepancies in the data collection process; Please refer to the User's Guide for a full explanation of data.

Meadowlands Hospital Medical Center

55 Meadowlands Pkwy
Secaucus, NJ 07094
E-mail: news@libertyhcs.org
URL: www.libertyhcs.org/meadowlands
Type: Acute Care Hospitals
Ownership: Voluntary Non-Profit - Private
Phone: 201-392-3100
Fax: 201-392-3527
Emergency Services: Yes
Beds: 230

Key Personnel:
Operating Room. . . . . Denise Desouza
Pediatric Ambulatory Care . . . . . . Azzam Baker, MD
Pediatric In-Patient Care . . . . . . Azzam Baker, MD
Quality Assurance . . . . Kathleen Locklear
Emergency Room . . . . Liz Ramirez

Measure	Cases	This Hosp.	State Avg.	U.S. Avg.
Heart Attack Care				
ACE Inhibitor or ARB for LVSD[1]	4	100%	98%	96%
Aspirin at Arrival	29	100%	99%	99%
Aspirin at Discharge[1]	10	100%	99%	98%
Beta Blocker at Discharge[1]	9	100%	99%	98%
Fibrinolytic Medication Timing	0	-	65%	55%
PCI Within 90 Minutes of Arrival	0	-	87%	90%
Smoking Cessation Advice	0	-	100%	99%
Chest Pain/Possible Heart Attack Care				
Aspirin at Arrival[1]	5	100%	97%	95%
Median Time to ECG (minutes)[1]	5	10	8	8
Median Time to Transfer (minutes)[5]	0	-	81	61
Fibrinolytic Medication Timing[1,3]	1	100%	65%	54%
Heart Failure Care				
ACE Inhibitor or ARB for LVSD	39	97%	97%	94%
Discharge Instructions	83	98%	93%	88%
Evaluation of LVS Function	118	99%	99%	98%
Smoking Cessation Advice[1]	9	100%	100%	98%
Pneumonia Care				
Appropriate Initial Antibiotic[2]	75	95%	94%	92%
Blood Culture Timing[2]	120	98%	97%	96%
Influenza Vaccine	60	93%	94%	91%
Initial Antibiotic Timing[2]	103	98%	96%	95%
Pneumococcal Vaccine[2]	78	95%	96%	93%
Smoking Cessation Advice[1,2]	18	100%	99%	97%
Surgical Care Improvement Project				
Appropriate VTP Within 24 Hours[2]	47	62%	94%	92%
Appropriate Hair Removal[2]	165	100%	100%	99%
Appropriate Beta Blocker Usage[1,2]	18	100%	95%	93%
Controlled Postoperative Blood Glucose[2]	0	-	93%	93%
Prophylactic Antibiotic Timing[2]	89	97%	98%	97%
Prophylactic Antibiotic Timing (Outpatient)	90	98%	93%	92%
Prophylactic Antibiotic Selection[2]	90	91%	97%	97%
Prophylactic Antibiotic Select. (Outpatient)	89	97%	94%	94%
Prophylactic Antibiotic Stopped[2]	86	86%	96%	94%
Recommended VTP Ordered[2]	47	62%	95%	94%
Urinary Catheter Removal[1]	7	100%	93%	90%
Children's Asthma Care				
Received Systemic Corticosteroids	-	-	-	100%
Received Home Management Plan	-	-	-	71%
Received Reliever Medication	-	-	-	100%
Use of Medical Imaging				
Combination Abdominal CT Scan	107	0.196	0.126	0.191
Combination Chest CT Scan	75	0.027	0.026	0.054
Follow-up Mammogram/Ultrasound	125	5.6%	10.6%	8.4%
MRI for Low Back Pain[5]	0	-	26.4%	32.7%
Survey of Patients' Hospital Experiences				
Area Around Room 'Always' Quiet at Night	300+	62%	-	58%
Doctors 'Always' Communicated Well	300+	80%	-	80%
Home Recovery Information Given	300+	75%	-	82%
Hospital Given 9 or 10 on 10 Point Scale	300+	62%	-	67%
Meds 'Always' Explained Before Given	300+	59%	-	60%
Nurses 'Always' Communicated Well	300+	76%	-	76%
Pain 'Always' Well Controlled	300+	74%	-	69%
Room and Bathroom 'Always' Clean	300+	78%	-	71%
Timely Help 'Always' Received	300+	64%	-	64%
Would Definitely Recommend Hospital	300+	68%	-	69%

Shore Memorial Hospital

1 East New York Ave
Somers Point, NJ 08244
URL: www.shorememorial.org
Type: Acute Care Hospitals
Ownership: Voluntary Non-Profit - Private
Phone: 609-653-3545
Fax: 609-926-1987
Emergency Services: Yes
Beds: 296

Key Personnel:
CEO/President. . . . . Albert L Gutierrez
Operating Room. . . . . Cynthia Leggett, RN
Quality Assurance . . . . Angelo Sparagna
Emergency Room . . . . Mark Liwoch

Measure	Cases	This Hosp.	State Avg.	U.S. Avg.
Heart Attack Care				
ACE Inhibitor or ARB for LVSD[1]	11	100%	98%	96%
Aspirin at Arrival	89	99%	99%	99%
Aspirin at Discharge	43	100%	99%	98%
Beta Blocker at Discharge	49	100%	99%	98%
Fibrinolytic Medication Timing	0	-	65%	55%
PCI Within 90 Minutes of Arrival	0	-	87%	90%
Smoking Cessation Advice[1]	8	100%	100%	99%
Chest Pain/Possible Heart Attack Care				
Aspirin at Arrival	68	100%	97%	95%
Median Time to ECG (minutes)	70	8	8	8
Median Time to Transfer (minutes)[1]	20	82	81	61
Fibrinolytic Medication Timing	0	-	65%	54%
Heart Failure Care				
ACE Inhibitor or ARB for LVSD[2]	64	97%	97%	94%
Discharge Instructions[2]	200	96%	93%	88%
Evaluation of LVS Function[2]	268	100%	99%	98%
Smoking Cessation Advice[2]	32	100%	100%	98%
Pneumonia Care				
Appropriate Initial Antibiotic[2]	120	97%	94%	92%
Blood Culture Timing[2]	168	99%	97%	96%
Influenza Vaccine[2]	77	99%	94%	91%
Initial Antibiotic Timing[2]	136	97%	96%	95%
Pneumococcal Vaccine[2]	114	99%	96%	93%
Smoking Cessation Advice[2]	56	100%	99%	97%
Surgical Care Improvement Project				
Appropriate VTP Within 24 Hours[2]	198	97%	94%	92%
Appropriate Hair Removal[2]	577	100%	100%	99%
Appropriate Beta Blocker Usage[2]	206	97%	95%	93%
Controlled Postoperative Blood Glucose[2]	0	-	93%	93%
Prophylactic Antibiotic Timing[2]	359	100%	98%	97%
Prophylactic Antibiotic Timing (Outpatient)	146	99%	93%	92%
Prophylactic Antibiotic Selection[2]	360	99%	97%	97%
Prophylactic Antibiotic Select. (Outpatient)	145	100%	94%	94%
Prophylactic Antibiotic Stopped[2]	334	99%	96%	94%
Recommended VTP Ordered[2]	199	98%	95%	94%
Urinary Catheter Removal[2]	47	98%	93%	90%
Children's Asthma Care				
Received Systemic Corticosteroids	-	-	-	100%
Received Home Management Plan	-	-	-	71%
Received Reliever Medication	-	-	-	100%
Use of Medical Imaging				
Combination Abdominal CT Scan	484	0.512	0.126	0.191
Combination Chest CT Scan	278	0.043	0.026	0.054
Follow-up Mammogram/Ultrasound	704	16.5%	10.6%	8.4%
MRI for Low Back Pain[1]	41	17.1%	26.4%	32.7%
Survey of Patients' Hospital Experiences				
Area Around Room 'Always' Quiet at Night	300+	51%	-	58%
Doctors 'Always' Communicated Well	300+	80%	-	80%
Home Recovery Information Given	300+	82%	-	82%
Hospital Given 9 or 10 on 10 Point Scale	300+	67%	-	67%
Meds 'Always' Explained Before Given	300+	58%	-	60%
Nurses 'Always' Communicated Well	300+	75%	-	76%
Pain 'Always' Well Controlled	300+	73%	-	69%
Room and Bathroom 'Always' Clean	300+	67%	-	71%
Timely Help 'Always' Received	300+	61%	-	64%
Would Definitely Recommend Hospital	300+	74%	-	69%

Somerset Medical Center

110 Rehill Ave
Somerville, NJ 08876
URL: www.somersetmedicalcenter.com
Type: Acute Care Hospitals
Ownership: Voluntary Non-Profit - Private
Phone: 908-685-2200
Fax: 908-685-2894
Emergency Services: Yes
Beds: 364

Key Personnel:
CEO/President. . . . . Kenneth Batemen CPA
Chief of Medical Staff. . . . . Richard Todd Paris MD
Infection Control. . . . . Patricia Lafaro RN
Operating Room. . . . . Kristin Peterson
Quality Assurance . . . . Mary Lund
Radiology. . . . . Lawrence Gross MD
Emergency Room . . . . Dennis McGill MD
Patient Relations . . . . Steve Dean

Measure	Cases	This Hosp.	State Avg.	U.S. Avg.
Heart Attack Care				
ACE Inhibitor or ARB for LVSD[2]	25	96%	98%	96%
Aspirin at Arrival[2]	252	100%	99%	99%
Aspirin at Discharge[2]	175	99%	99%	98%
Beta Blocker at Discharge[2]	175	99%	99%	98%
Fibrinolytic Medication Timing[2]	0	-	65%	55%
PCI Within 90 Minutes of Arrival[2]	64	86%	87%	90%
Smoking Cessation Advice[2]	50	100%	100%	99%
Chest Pain/Possible Heart Attack Care				
Aspirin at Arrival[1,3]	1	0%	97%	95%
Median Time to ECG (minutes)[1,3]	4	14	8	8
Median Time to Transfer (minutes)[3]	0	-	81	61
Fibrinolytic Medication Timing[3]	0	-	65%	54%
Heart Failure Care				
ACE Inhibitor or ARB for LVSD[2]	78	100%	97%	94%
Discharge Instructions[2]	209	100%	93%	88%
Evaluation of LVS Function[2]	327	99%	99%	98%
Smoking Cessation Advice[2]	34	97%	100%	98%
Pneumonia Care				
Appropriate Initial Antibiotic[2]	100	93%	94%	92%
Blood Culture Timing[2]	126	99%	97%	96%
Influenza Vaccine[2]	83	98%	94%	91%
Initial Antibiotic Timing[2]	139	99%	96%	95%
Pneumococcal Vaccine[2]	164	98%	96%	93%
Smoking Cessation Advice[2]	26	100%	99%	97%
Surgical Care Improvement Project				
Appropriate VTP Within 24 Hours[2]	220	97%	94%	92%
Appropriate Hair Removal[2]	541	100%	100%	99%
Appropriate Beta Blocker Usage[2]	161	93%	95%	93%
Controlled Postoperative Blood Glucose[2]	0	-	93%	93%
Prophylactic Antibiotic Timing[2]	338	100%	98%	97%
Prophylactic Antibiotic Timing (Outpatient)	106	92%	93%	92%
Prophylactic Antibiotic Selection[2]	339	98%	97%	97%
Prophylactic Antibiotic Select. (Outpatient)	97	96%	94%	94%
Prophylactic Antibiotic Stopped[2]	322	96%	96%	94%
Recommended VTP Ordered[2]	220	99%	95%	94%
Urinary Catheter Removal[2]	71	85%	93%	90%
Children's Asthma Care				
Received Systemic Corticosteroids	-	-	-	100%
Received Home Management Plan	-	-	-	71%
Received Reliever Medication	-	-	-	100%
Use of Medical Imaging				
Combination Abdominal CT Scan	788	0.381	0.126	0.191
Combination Chest CT Scan	634	0.008	0.026	0.054
Follow-up Mammogram/Ultrasound	800	10.8%	10.6%	8.4%
MRI for Low Back Pain	116	28.4%	26.4%	32.7%
Survey of Patients' Hospital Experiences				
Area Around Room 'Always' Quiet at Night	300+	46%	-	58%
Doctors 'Always' Communicated Well	300+	77%	-	80%
Home Recovery Information Given	300+	73%	-	82%
Hospital Given 9 or 10 on 10 Point Scale	300+	60%	-	67%
Meds 'Always' Explained Before Given	300+	56%	-	60%
Nurses 'Always' Communicated Well	300+	74%	-	76%
Pain 'Always' Well Controlled	300+	72%	-	69%
Room and Bathroom 'Always' Clean	300+	71%	-	71%
Timely Help 'Always' Received	300+	56%	-	64%
Would Definitely Recommend Hospital	300+	67%	-	69%

NOTE: Hospital profiles are in alphabetical order by state, then city, then hospital within the city; Rankings exclude hospitals with less than 25 cases except for patient surveys which excludes hospitals with less than 100 cases; (a) 100–299 cases; (1) The number of cases is too small to be sure how well a hospital is performing; (2) The hospital indicated that the data submitted for this measure were based on a sample of cases; (3) Data was collected during a shorter time period (fewer quarters) than the maximum possible time for this measure; (4) Suppressed for one or more quarters by CMS; (5) No data is available from the hospital for this measure; (6) Fewer than 100 patients completed the HCAHPS survey. Use these rates with caution, as the number of surveys may be too low to reliably assess hospital performance; (7) Survey results are based on less than 12 months of data; (8) Survey results are not available for this reporting period; (9) No or very few patients were eligible for the HCAHPS survey. The scores shown, if any, reflect a very small number of surveys; (10) A state average was not calculated because too few hospitals in the state submitted data; (11) There were discrepancies in the data collection process; Please refer to the User's Guide for a full explanation of data.

Kennedy University Hospital

18 East Laurel Road
Stratford, NJ 08084
URL: www.kennedyhealth.org
Type: Acute Care Hospitals
Ownership: Voluntary Non-Profit - Private

Phone: 856-346-6000
Fax: 856-346-6005

Emergency Services: Yes
Beds: 236

Key Personnel:
CEO/President . . . . Richard E Murray
Chief of Medical Staff . . . . Daniel Herriman, MD, JD
Quality Assurance . . . . Dennis L Bush
Ambulatory Care . . . . Richard Koss

Measure	Cases	This Hosp.	State Avg.	U.S. Avg.
Heart Attack Care				
ACE Inhibitor or ARB for LVSD[1]	14	100%	98%	96%
Aspirin at Arrival	238	96%	99%	99%
Aspirin at Discharge	120	96%	99%	98%
Beta Blocker at Discharge	113	96%	99%	98%
Fibrinolytic Medication Timing[1]	3	33%	65%	55%
PCI Within 90 Minutes of Arrival	0	-	87%	90%
Smoking Cessation Advice[1]	14	100%	100%	99%
Chest Pain/Possible Heart Attack Care				
Aspirin at Arrival	179	97%	97%	95%
Median Time to ECG (minutes)	183	9	8	8
Median Time to Transfer (minutes)[1]	22	108	81	61
Fibrinolytic Medication Timing[1]	18	56%	65%	54%
Heart Failure Care				
ACE Inhibitor or ARB for LVSD	170	88%	97%	94%
Discharge Instructions	672	85%	93%	88%
Evaluation of LVS Function	905	99%	99%	98%
Smoking Cessation Advice	141	99%	100%	98%
Pneumonia Care				
Appropriate Initial Antibiotic	520	97%	94%	92%
Blood Culture Timing	1,002	97%	97%	96%
Influenza Vaccine	417	93%	94%	91%
Initial Antibiotic Timing	860	97%	96%	95%
Pneumococcal Vaccine	662	96%	96%	93%
Smoking Cessation Advice	307	100%	99%	97%
Surgical Care Improvement Project				
Appropriate VTP Within 24 Hours[2]	383	98%	94%	92%
Appropriate Hair Removal[2]	969	99%	100%	99%
Appropriate Beta Blocker Usage[2]	283	96%	95%	93%
Controlled Postoperative Blood Glucose[2]	0	-	93%	93%
Prophylactic Antibiotic Timing[2]	562	99%	98%	97%
Prophylactic Antibiotic Timing (Outpatient)	267	91%	93%	92%
Prophylactic Antibiotic Selection[2]	565	99%	97%	97%
Prophylactic Antibiotic Select. (Outpatient)	251	92%	94%	94%
Prophylactic Antibiotic Stopped[2]	549	99%	96%	94%
Recommended VTP Ordered[2]	383	99%	95%	94%
Urinary Catheter Removal[2]	164	95%	93%	90%
Children's Asthma Care				
Received Systemic Corticosteroids	-	-	-	100%
Received Home Management Plan	-	-	-	71%
Received Reliever Medication	-	-	-	100%
Use of Medical Imaging				
Combination Abdominal CT Scan	1,770	0.047	0.126	0.191
Combination Chest CT Scan	995	0.007	0.026	0.054
Follow-up Mammogram/Ultrasound	836	11.0%	10.6%	8.4%
MRI for Low Back Pain	90	24.4%	26.4%	32.7%
Survey of Patients' Hospital Experiences				
Area Around Room 'Always' Quiet at Night	300+	45%	-	58%
Doctors 'Always' Communicated Well	300+	74%	-	80%
Home Recovery Information Given	300+	77%	-	82%
Hospital Given 9 or 10 on 10 Point Scale	300+	56%	-	67%
Meds 'Always' Explained Before Given	300+	56%	-	60%
Nurses 'Always' Communicated Well	300+	75%	-	76%
Pain 'Always' Well Controlled	300+	66%	-	69%
Room and Bathroom 'Always' Clean	300+	67%	-	71%
Timely Help 'Always' Received	300+	57%	-	64%
Would Definitely Recommend Hospital	300+	59%	-	69%

Overlook Hospital

99 Beauvoir Ave
Summit, NJ 07902
URL: www.atlantichealth.org
Type: Acute Care Hospitals
Ownership: Voluntary Non-Profit - Other

Phone: 908-522-2000
Fax: 908-273-5134

Emergency Services: Yes
Beds: 504

Key Personnel:
CEO/President . . . . Alan Lieber
Chief of Medical Staff . . . . Susan Cantor, MD
Infection Control . . . . Sonia McGaugh, MD
Operating Room . . . . Dawn Petronio
Pediatric Ambulatory Care . . . . . Leonard Feid, MD
Pediatric In-Patient Care . . . . . . Leonard Feid, MD
Quality Assurance . . . . Jennifer Athens
Radiology . . . . William Matuozzi, MD

Measure	Cases	This Hosp.	State Avg.	U.S. Avg.
Heart Attack Care				
ACE Inhibitor or ARB for LVSD	32	91%	98%	96%
Aspirin at Arrival	192	97%	99%	99%
Aspirin at Discharge	151	97%	99%	98%
Beta Blocker at Discharge	151	98%	99%	98%
Fibrinolytic Medication Timing	0	-	65%	55%
PCI Within 90 Minutes of Arrival	41	78%	87%	90%
Smoking Cessation Advice[1]	15	80%	100%	99%
Chest Pain/Possible Heart Attack Care				
Aspirin at Arrival[5]	0	-	97%	95%
Median Time to ECG (minutes)[5]	0	-	8	8
Median Time to Transfer (minutes)[5]	0	-	81	61
Fibrinolytic Medication Timing[5]	0	-	65%	54%
Heart Failure Care				
ACE Inhibitor or ARB for LVSD[2]	99	89%	97%	94%
Discharge Instructions[2]	247	92%	93%	88%
Evaluation of LVS Function[2]	360	97%	99%	98%
Smoking Cessation Advice[1,2]	24	96%	100%	98%
Pneumonia Care				
Appropriate Initial Antibiotic[2]	162	88%	94%	92%
Blood Culture Timing[2]	213	96%	97%	96%
Influenza Vaccine[2]	133	98%	94%	91%
Initial Antibiotic Timing[2]	174	99%	96%	95%
Pneumococcal Vaccine[2]	228	97%	96%	93%
Smoking Cessation Advice[2]	37	92%	99%	97%
Surgical Care Improvement Project				
Appropriate VTP Within 24 Hours[2]	208	98%	94%	92%
Appropriate Hair Removal[2]	577	100%	100%	99%
Appropriate Beta Blocker Usage[2]	124	96%	95%	93%
Controlled Postoperative Blood Glucose[2]	0	-	93%	93%
Prophylactic Antibiotic Timing[2]	371	99%	98%	97%
Prophylactic Antibiotic Timing (Outpatient)	462	98%	93%	92%
Prophylactic Antibiotic Selection[2]	378	97%	97%	97%
Prophylactic Antibiotic Select. (Outpatient)	459	94%	94%	94%
Prophylactic Antibiotic Stopped[2]	364	96%	96%	94%
Recommended VTP Ordered[2]	209	99%	95%	94%
Urinary Catheter Removal[2]	95	96%	93%	90%
Children's Asthma Care				
Received Systemic Corticosteroids	-	-	-	100%
Received Home Management Plan	-	-	-	71%
Received Reliever Medication	-	-	-	100%
Use of Medical Imaging				
Combination Abdominal CT Scan	1,249	0.079	0.126	0.191
Combination Chest CT Scan	1,183	0.055	0.026	0.054
Follow-up Mammogram/Ultrasound	828	20.0%	10.6%	8.4%
MRI for Low Back Pain	85	25.9%	26.4%	32.7%
Survey of Patients' Hospital Experiences				
Area Around Room 'Always' Quiet at Night	300+	51%	-	58%
Doctors 'Always' Communicated Well	300+	77%	-	80%
Home Recovery Information Given	300+	81%	-	82%
Hospital Given 9 or 10 on 10 Point Scale	300+	66%	-	67%
Meds 'Always' Explained Before Given	300+	54%	-	60%
Nurses 'Always' Communicated Well	300+	75%	-	76%
Pain 'Always' Well Controlled	300+	67%	-	69%
Room and Bathroom 'Always' Clean	300+	66%	-	71%
Timely Help 'Always' Received	300+	55%	-	64%
Would Definitely Recommend Hospital	300+	73%	-	69%

Saint Clare's Hospital - Sussex

20 Walnut St
Sussex, NJ 07461
URL: www.saintclares.org
Type: Acute Care Hospitals
Ownership: Voluntary Non-Profit - Church

Phone: 973-702-2200
Fax: 973-989-3137

Emergency Services: Yes
Beds: 106

Key Personnel:
CEO/President . . . . Gary J Blan
Chief of Medical Staff . . . . Stephen Papish
Radiology . . . . Loucia Barton

Measure	Cases	This Hosp.	State Avg.	U.S. Avg.
Heart Attack Care				
ACE Inhibitor or ARB for LVSD[1]	1	100%	98%	96%
Aspirin at Arrival[1]	8	100%	99%	99%
Aspirin at Discharge[1]	3	100%	99%	98%
Beta Blocker at Discharge[1]	3	100%	99%	98%
Fibrinolytic Medication Timing	0	-	65%	55%
PCI Within 90 Minutes of Arrival	0	-	87%	90%
Smoking Cessation Advice[1]	1	100%	100%	99%
Chest Pain/Possible Heart Attack Care				
Aspirin at Arrival[1]	10	100%	97%	95%
Median Time to ECG (minutes)[1]	10	10	8	8
Median Time to Transfer (minutes)[1,3]	1	74	81	61
Fibrinolytic Medication Timing[1]	1	100%	65%	54%
Heart Failure Care				
ACE Inhibitor or ARB for LVSD[1]	8	100%	97%	94%
Discharge Instructions	46	89%	93%	88%
Evaluation of LVS Function	53	98%	99%	98%
Smoking Cessation Advice[1]	6	100%	100%	98%
Pneumonia Care				
Appropriate Initial Antibiotic	40	95%	94%	92%
Blood Culture Timing	53	98%	97%	96%
Influenza Vaccine	30	100%	94%	91%
Initial Antibiotic Timing	49	100%	96%	95%
Pneumococcal Vaccine	40	100%	96%	93%
Smoking Cessation Advice	27	100%	99%	97%
Surgical Care Improvement Project				
Appropriate VTP Within 24 Hours[1]	24	96%	94%	92%
Appropriate Hair Removal	29	100%	100%	99%
Appropriate Beta Blocker Usage[1]	9	67%	95%	93%
Controlled Postoperative Blood Glucose	0	-	93%	93%
Prophylactic Antibiotic Timing[1]	3	100%	98%	97%
Prophylactic Antibiotic Timing (Outpatient)[1,3]	3	100%	93%	92%
Prophylactic Antibiotic Selection[1]	3	67%	97%	97%
Prophylactic Antibiotic Select. (Outpatient)[1,3]	3	100%	94%	94%
Prophylactic Antibiotic Stopped[1]	3	100%	96%	94%
Recommended VTP Ordered[1]	24	100%	95%	94%
Urinary Catheter Removal[1]	4	100%	93%	90%
Children's Asthma Care				
Received Systemic Corticosteroids	-	-	-	100%
Received Home Management Plan	-	-	-	71%
Received Reliever Medication	-	-	-	100%
Use of Medical Imaging				
Combination Abdominal CT Scan	166	0.018	0.126	0.191
Combination Chest CT Scan	83	0.000	0.026	0.054
Follow-up Mammogram/Ultrasound	155	9.7%	10.6%	8.4%
MRI for Low Back Pain[5]	-	-	26.4%	32.7%
Survey of Patients' Hospital Experiences				
Area Around Room 'Always' Quiet at Night	(a)	54%	-	58%
Doctors 'Always' Communicated Well	(a)	81%	-	80%
Home Recovery Information Given	(a)	77%	-	82%
Hospital Given 9 or 10 on 10 Point Scale	(a)	69%	-	67%
Meds 'Always' Explained Before Given	(a)	61%	-	60%
Nurses 'Always' Communicated Well	(a)	77%	-	76%
Pain 'Always' Well Controlled	(a)	69%	-	69%
Room and Bathroom 'Always' Clean	(a)	76%	-	71%
Timely Help 'Always' Received	(a)	67%	-	64%
Would Definitely Recommend Hospital	(a)	67%	-	69%

Holy Name Medical Center

718 Teaneck Rd
Teaneck, NJ 07666
URL: www.holyname.org
Type: Acute Care Hospitals
Ownership: Voluntary Non-Profit - Other

Phone: 201-833-3000
Fax: 201-833-3230
Emergency Services: Yes
Beds: 361

Key Personnel:
Chief of Medical Staff.......... Pauln Mendelowitz, MD
Infection Control.............. Rosemary Perry, RN
Operating Room.............. Frank Chase
Pediatric Ambulatory Care...... Larysa Dyrszka, MD
Pediatric In-Patient Care...... Larysa Dyrszka, MD
Quality Assurance............ Paul Mendelowitz, MD
Radiology.................... Jacqueline Brunetti, MD
Emergency Room............ Richard Schwab, MD

Measure	Cases	This Hosp.	State Avg.	U.S. Avg.
Heart Attack Care				
ACE Inhibitor or ARB for LVSD	27	100%	98%	96%
Aspirin at Arrival	200	100%	99%	99%
Aspirin at Discharge	140	100%	99%	98%
Beta Blocker at Discharge	146	100%	99%	98%
Fibrinolytic Medication Timing	0	-	65%	55%
PCI Within 90 Minutes of Arrival	29	100%	87%	90%
Smoking Cessation Advice	33	100%	100%	99%
Chest Pain/Possible Heart Attack Care				
Aspirin at Arrival[1,3]	1	100%	97%	95%
Median Time to ECG (minutes)[1,3]	1	14	8	8
Median Time to Transfer (minutes)[5]	0	-	81	61
Fibrinolytic Medication Timing[5]	0	-	65%	54%
Heart Failure Care				
ACE Inhibitor or ARB for LVSD[2]	79	100%	97%	94%
Discharge Instructions[2]	238	100%	93%	88%
Evaluation of LVS Function[2]	335	100%	99%	98%
Smoking Cessation Advice[2]	26	100%	100%	98%
Pneumonia Care				
Appropriate Initial Antibiotic[2]	96	95%	94%	92%
Blood Culture Timing[2]	188	98%	97%	96%
Influenza Vaccine[2]	94	100%	94%	91%
Initial Antibiotic Timing[2]	198	96%	96%	95%
Pneumococcal Vaccine[2]	175	100%	96%	93%
Smoking Cessation Advice[2]	30	100%	99%	97%
Surgical Care Improvement Project				
Appropriate VTP Within 24 Hours[2]	238	98%	94%	92%
Appropriate Hair Removal[2]	518	100%	100%	99%
Appropriate Beta Blocker Usage[2]	151	96%	95%	93%
Controlled Postoperative Blood Glucose[2]	0	-	93%	93%
Prophylactic Antibiotic Timing[2]	290	100%	98%	97%
Prophylactic Antibiotic Timing (Outpatient)	193	87%	93%	92%
Prophylactic Antibiotic Selection[2]	296	99%	97%	97%
Prophylactic Antibiotic Select. (Outpatient)	181	98%	94%	94%
Prophylactic Antibiotic Stopped[2]	270	99%	96%	94%
Recommended VTP Ordered[2]	238	98%	95%	94%
Urinary Catheter Removal[2]	102	99%	93%	90%
Children's Asthma Care				
Received Systemic Corticosteroids	-	-	-	100%
Received Home Management Plan	-	-	-	71%
Received Reliever Medication	-	-	-	100%
Use of Medical Imaging				
Combination Abdominal CT Scan	1,103	0.110	0.126	0.191
Combination Chest CT Scan	828	0.059	0.026	0.054
Follow-up Mammogram/Ultrasound	1,067	26.0%	10.6%	8.4%
MRI for Low Back Pain	312	25.3%	26.4%	32.7%
Survey of Patients' Hospital Experiences				
Area Around Room 'Always' Quiet at Night	300+	52%	-	58%
Doctors 'Always' Communicated Well	300+	80%	-	80%
Home Recovery Information Given	300+	81%	-	82%
Hospital Given 9 or 10 on 10 Point Scale	300+	67%	-	67%
Meds 'Always' Explained Before Given	300+	55%	-	60%
Nurses 'Always' Communicated Well	300+	74%	-	76%
Pain 'Always' Well Controlled	300+	67%	-	69%
Room and Bathroom 'Always' Clean	300+	67%	-	71%
Timely Help 'Always' Received	300+	53%	-	64%
Would Definitely Recommend Hospital	300+	75%	-	69%

Community Medical Center

99 Rt 37 West
Toms River, NJ 08755
E-mail: info@sbhcs.com
URL: www.sbhcs.com
Type: Acute Care Hospitals
Ownership: Voluntary Non-Profit - Private

Phone: 732-557-8000
Fax: 732-286-7066
Emergency Services: Yes
Beds: 587

Key Personnel:
CEO/President.............. Nancy Woolen
Chief of Medical Staff.......... Frank Kelly, MD
Coronary Care.............. R Saunders Craig
Operating Room.............. Elyce Milgazo
Anesthesiology.............. Sang Kim
Emergency Room............ William Valfey

Measure	Cases	This Hosp.	State Avg.	U.S. Avg.
Heart Attack Care				
ACE Inhibitor or ARB for LVSD[2]	41	100%	98%	96%
Aspirin at Arrival[2]	467	100%	99%	99%
Aspirin at Discharge[2]	251	100%	99%	98%
Beta Blocker at Discharge[2]	264	100%	99%	98%
Fibrinolytic Medication Timing[1,2]	1	100%	65%	55%
PCI Within 90 Minutes of Arrival[2]	72	100%	87%	90%
Smoking Cessation Advice[2]	57	100%	100%	99%
Chest Pain/Possible Heart Attack Care				
Aspirin at Arrival	46	100%	97%	95%
Median Time to ECG (minutes)	46	9	8	8
Median Time to Transfer (minutes)[1]	6	110	81	61
Fibrinolytic Medication Timing	0	-	65%	54%
Heart Failure Care				
ACE Inhibitor or ARB for LVSD[2]	78	100%	97%	94%
Discharge Instructions[2]	190	100%	93%	88%
Evaluation of LVS Function[2]	325	100%	99%	98%
Smoking Cessation Advice[2]	28	100%	100%	98%
Pneumonia Care				
Appropriate Initial Antibiotic[2]	124	97%	94%	92%
Blood Culture Timing[2]	216	100%	97%	96%
Influenza Vaccine[2]	120	100%	94%	91%
Initial Antibiotic Timing[2]	193	99%	96%	95%
Pneumococcal Vaccine[2]	202	100%	96%	93%
Smoking Cessation Advice[2]	55	100%	99%	97%
Surgical Care Improvement Project				
Appropriate VTP Within 24 Hours[2]	230	100%	94%	92%
Appropriate Hair Removal[2]	601	100%	100%	99%
Appropriate Beta Blocker Usage[2]	178	100%	95%	93%
Controlled Postoperative Blood Glucose[1,2]	1	100%	93%	93%
Prophylactic Antibiotic Timing[2]	325	99%	98%	97%
Prophylactic Antibiotic Timing (Outpatient)	418	97%	93%	92%
Prophylactic Antibiotic Selection[2]	323	99%	97%	97%
Prophylactic Antibiotic Select. (Outpatient)	417	98%	94%	94%
Prophylactic Antibiotic Stopped[2]	300	98%	96%	94%
Recommended VTP Ordered[2]	230	100%	95%	94%
Urinary Catheter Removal[1,2]	23	91%	93%	90%
Children's Asthma Care				
Received Systemic Corticosteroids	-	-	-	100%
Received Home Management Plan	-	-	-	71%
Received Reliever Medication	-	-	-	100%
Use of Medical Imaging				
Combination Abdominal CT Scan	1,131	0.036	0.126	0.191
Combination Chest CT Scan	635	0.005	0.026	0.054
Follow-up Mammogram/Ultrasound	902	7.8%	10.6%	8.4%
MRI for Low Back Pain	56	41.1%	26.4%	32.7%
Survey of Patients' Hospital Experiences				
Area Around Room 'Always' Quiet at Night	300+	48%	-	58%
Doctors 'Always' Communicated Well	300+	76%	-	80%
Home Recovery Information Given	300+	80%	-	82%
Hospital Given 9 or 10 on 10 Point Scale	300+	57%	-	67%
Meds 'Always' Explained Before Given	300+	60%	-	60%
Nurses 'Always' Communicated Well	300+	75%	-	76%
Pain 'Always' Well Controlled	300+	69%	-	69%
Room and Bathroom 'Always' Clean	300+	63%	-	71%
Timely Help 'Always' Received	300+	61%	-	64%
Would Definitely Recommend Hospital	300+	61%	-	69%

Capital Health System - Mercer Campus

446 Bellevue Ave
Trenton, NJ 08618
URL: www.capitalhealth.org
Type: Acute Care Hospitals
Ownership: Voluntary Non-Profit - Private

Phone: 609-394-4000
Fax: 609-695-8865
Emergency Services: Yes
Beds: 589

Key Personnel:
CEO/President.................. Joseph Jingoli
Chief of Medical Staff.......... Robert Remstein, DO
Infection Control.............. Dawn Rumovitz
Operating Room.............. Ann Lando
Pediatric Ambulatory Care...... Randi Axelrod, MD
Pediatric In-Patient Care...... Randi Axelrod, MD
Quality Assurance............ Molly Sullivan
Radiology.................... Robert Collins, MD

Measure	Cases	This Hosp.	State Avg.	U.S. Avg.
Heart Attack Care				
ACE Inhibitor or ARB for LVSD[1]	15	100%	98%	96%
Aspirin at Arrival	61	97%	99%	99%
Aspirin at Discharge	46	98%	99%	98%
Beta Blocker at Discharge	46	100%	99%	98%
Fibrinolytic Medication Timing	0	-	65%	55%
PCI Within 90 Minutes of Arrival[1]	14	79%	87%	90%
Smoking Cessation Advice[1]	19	100%	100%	99%
Chest Pain/Possible Heart Attack Care				
Aspirin at Arrival[1,3]	4	100%	97%	95%
Median Time to ECG (minutes)[1,3]	4	2	8	8
Median Time to Transfer (minutes)[5]	0	-	81	61
Fibrinolytic Medication Timing[3]	0	-	65%	54%
Heart Failure Care				
ACE Inhibitor or ARB for LVSD	83	90%	97%	94%
Discharge Instructions	197	95%	93%	88%
Evaluation of LVS Function	235	95%	99%	98%
Smoking Cessation Advice	51	100%	100%	98%
Pneumonia Care				
Appropriate Initial Antibiotic	95	93%	94%	92%
Blood Culture Timing	144	94%	97%	96%
Influenza Vaccine	70	96%	94%	91%
Initial Antibiotic Timing	129	98%	96%	95%
Pneumococcal Vaccine	81	91%	96%	93%
Smoking Cessation Advice	59	100%	99%	97%
Surgical Care Improvement Project				
Appropriate VTP Within 24 Hours[2]	157	81%	94%	92%
Appropriate Hair Removal[2]	498	100%	100%	99%
Appropriate Beta Blocker Usage[2]	139	95%	95%	93%
Controlled Postoperative Blood Glucose[2]	0	-	93%	93%
Prophylactic Antibiotic Timing[2]	344	99%	98%	97%
Prophylactic Antibiotic Timing (Outpatient)	95	85%	93%	92%
Prophylactic Antibiotic Selection[2]	345	96%	97%	97%
Prophylactic Antibiotic Select. (Outpatient)	83	95%	94%	94%
Prophylactic Antibiotic Stopped[2]	331	93%	96%	94%
Recommended VTP Ordered[2]	158	84%	95%	94%
Urinary Catheter Removal[2]	93	76%	93%	90%
Children's Asthma Care				
Received Systemic Corticosteroids	-	-	-	100%
Received Home Management Plan	-	-	-	71%
Received Reliever Medication	-	-	-	100%
Use of Medical Imaging				
Combination Abdominal CT Scan	623	0.108	0.126	0.191
Combination Chest CT Scan	520	0.044	0.026	0.054
Follow-up Mammogram/Ultrasound	1,215	5.9%	10.6%	8.4%
MRI for Low Back Pain[1]	26	30.8%	26.4%	32.7%
Survey of Patients' Hospital Experiences				
Area Around Room 'Always' Quiet at Night	300+	61%	-	58%
Doctors 'Always' Communicated Well	300+	82%	-	80%
Home Recovery Information Given	300+	77%	-	82%
Hospital Given 9 or 10 on 10 Point Scale	300+	63%	-	67%
Meds 'Always' Explained Before Given	300+	61%	-	60%
Nurses 'Always' Communicated Well	300+	77%	-	76%
Pain 'Always' Well Controlled	300+	66%	-	69%
Room and Bathroom 'Always' Clean	300+	71%	-	71%
Timely Help 'Always' Received	300+	56%	-	64%
Would Definitely Recommend Hospital	300+	65%	-	69%

NOTE: Hospital profiles are in alphabetical order by state, then city, then hospital within the city; Rankings exclude hospitals with less than 25 cases except for patient surveys which excludes hospitals with less than 100 cases; (a) 100–299 cases; (1) The number of cases is too small to be sure how well a hospital is performing; (2) The hospital indicated that the data submitted for this measure were based on a sample of cases; (3) Data was collected during a shorter time period (fewer quarters) than the maximum possible time for this measure; (4) Suppressed for one or more quarters by CMS; (5) No data is available from the hospital for this measure; (6) Fewer than 100 patients completed the HCAHPS survey. Use these rates with caution, as the number of surveys may be too low to reliably assess hospital performance; (7) Survey results are based on less than 12 months of data; (8) Survey results are not available for this reporting period; (9) No or very few patients were eligible for the HCAHPS survey. The scores shown, if any, reflect a very small number of surveys; (10) A state average was not calculated because too few hospitals in the state submitted data; (11) There were discrepancies in the data collection process; Please refer to the User's Guide for a full explanation of data.

Capital Health System-Fuld Campus

750 Brunswick Ave   Phone: 609-394-6000
Trenton, NJ 08638
URL: www.capitalhealth.org
Type: Acute Care Hospitals   Emergency Services: Yes
Ownership: Voluntary Non-Profit - Private   Beds: 589
Key Personnel:
CEO/President . . . . Al Maghazehe PhD
Cardiac Laboratory . . . . Rita Brooks
Chief of Medical Staff . . . . Robert Remstein DO
Quality Assurance . . . . Molly Sullivan
Ambulatory Care . . . . Nathan Bosk
Emergency Room . . . . Robert Fine MD
Hemotology Center . . . . Shirnett Williamson MD
Intensive Care Unit . . . . Mary Wilcox

Measure	Cases	This Hosp.	State Avg.	U.S. Avg.
Heart Attack Care				
ACE Inhibitor or ARB for LVSD[1]	3	67%	98%	96%
Aspirin at Arrival	37	92%	99%	99%
Aspirin at Discharge[1]	14	100%	99%	98%
Beta Blocker at Discharge[1]	14	100%	99%	98%
Fibrinolytic Medication Timing	0	-	65%	55%
PCI Within 90 Minutes of Arrival	0	-	87%	90%
Smoking Cessation Advice[1]	2	100%	100%	99%
Chest Pain/Possible Heart Attack Care				
Aspirin at Arrival[1]	21	90%	97%	95%
Median Time to ECG (minutes)[1]	22	2	8	8
Median Time to Transfer (minutes)[1]	10	64	81	61
Fibrinolytic Medication Timing	0	-	65%	54%
Heart Failure Care				
ACE Inhibitor or ARB for LVSD	87	92%	97%	94%
Discharge Instructions	197	96%	93%	88%
Evaluation of LVS Function	242	99%	99%	98%
Smoking Cessation Advice	56	100%	100%	98%
Pneumonia Care				
Appropriate Initial Antibiotic	88	93%	94%	92%
Blood Culture Timing	162	91%	97%	96%
Influenza Vaccine	77	92%	94%	91%
Initial Antibiotic Timing	153	93%	96%	95%
Pneumococcal Vaccine	98	90%	96%	93%
Smoking Cessation Advice	65	100%	99%	97%
Surgical Care Improvement Project				
Appropriate VTP Within 24 Hours[2]	116	95%	94%	92%
Appropriate Hair Removal[2]	253	100%	100%	99%
Appropriate Beta Blocker Usage[2]	77	99%	95%	93%
Controlled Postoperative Blood Glucose[2]	0	-	93%	93%
Prophylactic Antibiotic Timing[2]	130	98%	98%	97%
Prophylactic Antibiotic Timing (Outpatient)	92	92%	93%	92%
Prophylactic Antibiotic Selection[2]	127	95%	97%	97%
Prophylactic Antibiotic Select. (Outpatient)	91	87%	94%	94%
Prophylactic Antibiotic Stopped[2]	124	90%	96%	94%
Recommended VTP Ordered[2]	117	94%	95%	94%
Urinary Catheter Removal[2]	51	80%	93%	90%
Children's Asthma Care				
Received Systemic Corticosteroids	-	-	-	100%
Received Home Management Plan	-	-	-	71%
Received Reliever Medication	-	-	-	100%
Use of Medical Imaging				
Combination Abdominal CT Scan	430	0.079	0.126	0.191
Combination Chest CT Scan	314	0.083	0.026	0.054
Follow-up Mammogram/Ultrasound	251	6.4%	10.6%	8.4%
MRI for Low Back Pain	66	18.2%	26.4%	32.7%
Survey of Patients' Hospital Experiences				
Area Around Room 'Always' Quiet at Night	300+	45%	-	58%
Doctors 'Always' Communicated Well	300+	77%	-	80%
Home Recovery Information Given	300+	74%	-	82%
Hospital Given 9 or 10 on 10 Point Scale	300+	58%	-	67%
Meds 'Always' Explained Before Given	300+	57%	-	60%
Nurses 'Always' Communicated Well	300+	73%	-	76%
Pain 'Always' Well Controlled	300+	65%	-	69%
Room and Bathroom 'Always' Clean	300+	69%	-	71%
Timely Help 'Always' Received	300+	57%	-	64%
Would Definitely Recommend Hospital	300+	62%	-	69%

Saint Francis Medical Center

601 Hamilton Ave   Phone: 609-599-5000
Trenton, NJ 08629   Fax: 609-599-6257
E-mail: info@stfrancismedical.com
URL: www.stfrancismedical.com
Type: Acute Care Hospitals   Emergency Services: Yes
Ownership: Voluntary Non-Profit - Private   Beds: 274
Key Personnel:
CEO/President . . . . Gerard J Jablonowski
Chief of Medical Staff . . . . C James Romano, MD
Infection Control . . . . Eileen Taylor
Operating Room . . . . Claude Abouchedid, RN
Quality Assurance . . . . Kathleen Vaccaro
Radiology . . . . Eric Bosworth
Anesthesiology . . . . Perry Loesberg, MD
Emergency Room . . . . Steven Katz, MD

Measure	Cases	This Hosp.	State Avg.	U.S. Avg.
Heart Attack Care				
ACE Inhibitor or ARB for LVSD	48	100%	98%	96%
Aspirin at Arrival	118	100%	99%	99%
Aspirin at Discharge	291	100%	99%	98%
Beta Blocker at Discharge	270	99%	99%	98%
Fibrinolytic Medication Timing	0	-	65%	55%
PCI Within 90 Minutes of Arrival	34	59%	87%	90%
Smoking Cessation Advice	99	100%	100%	99%
Chest Pain/Possible Heart Attack Care				
Aspirin at Arrival[3]	0	-	97%	95%
Median Time to ECG (minutes)[3]	0	-	8	8
Median Time to Transfer (minutes)[5]	0	-	81	61
Fibrinolytic Medication Timing[5]	0	-	65%	54%
Heart Failure Care				
ACE Inhibitor or ARB for LVSD	110	98%	97%	94%
Discharge Instructions	244	94%	93%	88%
Evaluation of LVS Function	297	100%	99%	98%
Smoking Cessation Advice	65	100%	100%	98%
Pneumonia Care				
Appropriate Initial Antibiotic	91	99%	94%	92%
Blood Culture Timing	132	98%	97%	96%
Influenza Vaccine	75	88%	94%	91%
Initial Antibiotic Timing	134	94%	96%	95%
Pneumococcal Vaccine	99	93%	96%	93%
Smoking Cessation Advice	60	100%	99%	97%
Surgical Care Improvement Project				
Appropriate VTP Within 24 Hours	117	98%	94%	92%
Appropriate Hair Removal	332	100%	100%	99%
Appropriate Beta Blocker Usage	158	98%	95%	93%
Controlled Postoperative Blood Glucose	139	80%	93%	93%
Prophylactic Antibiotic Timing	167	96%	98%	97%
Prophylactic Antibiotic Timing (Outpatient)	306	94%	93%	92%
Prophylactic Antibiotic Selection	175	98%	97%	97%
Prophylactic Antibiotic Select. (Outpatient)	291	98%	94%	94%
Prophylactic Antibiotic Stopped	152	87%	96%	94%
Recommended VTP Ordered	117	98%	95%	94%
Urinary Catheter Removal	68	99%	93%	90%
Children's Asthma Care				
Received Systemic Corticosteroids	-	-	-	100%
Received Home Management Plan	-	-	-	71%
Received Reliever Medication	-	-	-	100%
Use of Medical Imaging				
Combination Abdominal CT Scan	347	0.081	0.126	0.191
Combination Chest CT Scan	225	0.022	0.026	0.054
Follow-up Mammogram/Ultrasound	457	6.3%	10.6%	8.4%
MRI for Low Back Pain[1]	23	26.1%	26.4%	32.7%
Survey of Patients' Hospital Experiences				
Area Around Room 'Always' Quiet at Night	300+	44%	-	58%
Doctors 'Always' Communicated Well	300+	75%	-	80%
Home Recovery Information Given	300+	77%	-	82%
Hospital Given 9 or 10 on 10 Point Scale	300+	56%	-	67%
Meds 'Always' Explained Before Given	300+	52%	-	60%
Nurses 'Always' Communicated Well	300+	72%	-	76%
Pain 'Always' Well Controlled	300+	65%	-	69%
Room and Bathroom 'Always' Clean	300+	66%	-	71%
Timely Help 'Always' Received	300+	56%	-	64%
Would Definitely Recommend Hospital	300+	58%	-	69%

South Jersey Healthcare Regional Medical Center

1505 W Sherman Ave   Phone: 856-641-8000
Vineland, NJ 08360   Fax: 856-451-6998
URL: www.sjhs.com
Type: Acute Care Hospitals   Emergency Services: Yes
Ownership: Voluntary Non-Profit - Private   Beds: 262
Key Personnel:
CEO/President . . . . Chester B Kaletkowski

Measure	Cases	This Hosp.	State Avg.	U.S. Avg.
Heart Attack Care				
ACE Inhibitor or ARB for LVSD[1]	13	100%	98%	96%
Aspirin at Arrival	125	99%	99%	99%
Aspirin at Discharge	56	100%	99%	98%
Beta Blocker at Discharge	57	100%	99%	98%
Fibrinolytic Medication Timing[1]	2	100%	65%	55%
PCI Within 90 Minutes of Arrival	0	-	87%	90%
Smoking Cessation Advice[1]	11	100%	100%	99%
Chest Pain/Possible Heart Attack Care				
Aspirin at Arrival	96	98%	97%	95%
Median Time to ECG (minutes)	99	5	8	8
Median Time to Transfer (minutes)[1,3]	19	71	81	61
Fibrinolytic Medication Timing	28	75%	65%	54%
Heart Failure Care				
ACE Inhibitor or ARB for LVSD[2]	107	100%	97%	94%
Discharge Instructions[2]	253	100%	93%	88%
Evaluation of LVS Function[2]	322	100%	99%	98%
Smoking Cessation Advice[2]	47	100%	100%	98%
Pneumonia Care				
Appropriate Initial Antibiotic[2]	93	99%	94%	92%
Blood Culture Timing[2]	123	97%	97%	96%
Influenza Vaccine[2]	65	100%	94%	91%
Initial Antibiotic Timing[2]	177	92%	96%	95%
Pneumococcal Vaccine[2]	108	100%	96%	93%
Smoking Cessation Advice[2]	59	100%	99%	97%
Surgical Care Improvement Project				
Appropriate VTP Within 24 Hours[2]	202	84%	94%	92%
Appropriate Hair Removal[2]	515	99%	100%	99%
Appropriate Beta Blocker Usage[2]	117	89%	95%	93%
Controlled Postoperative Blood Glucose[2]	0	-	93%	93%
Prophylactic Antibiotic Timing[2]	290	95%	98%	97%
Prophylactic Antibiotic Timing (Outpatient)	240	98%	93%	92%
Prophylactic Antibiotic Selection[2]	290	94%	97%	97%
Prophylactic Antibiotic Select. (Outpatient)	237	93%	94%	94%
Prophylactic Antibiotic Stopped[2]	281	95%	96%	94%
Recommended VTP Ordered[2]	204	83%	95%	94%
Urinary Catheter Removal[2]	113	94%	93%	90%
Children's Asthma Care				
Received Systemic Corticosteroids	-	-	-	100%
Received Home Management Plan	-	-	-	71%
Received Reliever Medication	-	-	-	100%
Use of Medical Imaging				
Combination Abdominal CT Scan	898	0.138	0.126	0.191
Combination Chest CT Scan	559	0.041	0.026	0.054
Follow-up Mammogram/Ultrasound	1,487	6.1%	10.6%	8.4%
MRI for Low Back Pain	115	33.9%	26.4%	32.7%
Survey of Patients' Hospital Experiences				
Area Around Room 'Always' Quiet at Night	300+	59%	-	58%
Doctors 'Always' Communicated Well	300+	77%	-	80%
Home Recovery Information Given	300+	83%	-	82%
Hospital Given 9 or 10 on 10 Point Scale	300+	65%	-	67%
Meds 'Always' Explained Before Given	300+	57%	-	60%
Nurses 'Always' Communicated Well	300+	73%	-	76%
Pain 'Always' Well Controlled	300+	67%	-	69%
Room and Bathroom 'Always' Clean	300+	71%	-	71%
Timely Help 'Always' Received	300+	62%	-	64%
Would Definitely Recommend Hospital	300+	64%	-	69%

NOTE: Hospital profiles are in alphabetical order by state, then city, then hospital within the city; Rankings exclude hospitals with less than 25 cases except for patient surveys which excludes hospitals with less than 100 cases; (a) 100-299 cases; (1) The number of cases is too small to be sure how well a hospital is performing; (2) The hospital indicated that the data submitted for this measure were based on a sample of cases; (3) Data was collected during a shorter time period (fewer quarters) than the maximum possible time for this measure; (4) Suppressed for one or more quarters by CMS; (5) No data is available from the hospital for this measure; (6) Fewer than 100 patients completed the HCAHPS survey. Use these rates with caution, as the number of surveys may be too low to reliably assess hospital performance; (7) Survey results are based on less than 12 months of data; (8) Survey results are not available for this reporting period; (9) No or very few patients were eligible for the HCAHPS survey. The scores shown, if any, reflect a very small number of surveys; (10) A state average was not calculated because too few hospitals in the state submitted data; (11) There were discrepancies in the data collection process; Please refer to the User's Guide for a full explanation of data.

Saint Joseph's Wayne Hospital

224 Hamburg Tpke
Wayne, NJ 07470
Phone: 973-942-6900
Fax: 973-389-4046
Type: Acute Care Hospitals
Emergency Services: Yes
Ownership: Voluntary Non-Profit - Private
Beds: 225

Key Personnel:
CEO/President.............. William McDonnel
Cardiac Laboratory........... Zan Afribho
Chief of Medical Staff.......... SH Patel, MD
Operating Room.............. Kathleen Marcucilli, RN
Pediatric Ambulatory Care ...... N Nagahawatte
Pediatric In-Patient Care .... N Nagahawatte
Quality Assurance .... Bernice Hembrough, RN
Radiology.................. Tim Mullin

Measure	Cases	This Hosp.	State Avg.	U.S. Avg.
Heart Attack Care				
ACE Inhibitor or ARB for LVSD	-	-	98%	96%
Aspirin at Arrival	-	-	99%	99%
Aspirin at Discharge	-	-	99%	98%
Beta Blocker at Discharge	-	-	99%	98%
Fibrinolytic Medication Timing	-	-	65%	55%
PCI Within 90 Minutes of Arrival	-	-	87%	90%
Smoking Cessation Advice	-	-	100%	99%
Chest Pain/Possible Heart Attack Care				
Aspirin at Arrival	-	-	97%	95%
Median Time to ECG (minutes)	-	-	8	8
Median Time to Transfer (minutes)	-	-	81	61
Fibrinolytic Medication Timing	-	-	65%	54%
Heart Failure Care				
ACE Inhibitor or ARB for LVSD	-	-	97%	94%
Discharge Instructions	-	-	93%	88%
Evaluation of LVS Function	-	-	99%	98%
Smoking Cessation Advice	-	-	100%	98%
Pneumonia Care				
Appropriate Initial Antibiotic	-	-	94%	92%
Blood Culture Timing	-	-	97%	96%
Influenza Vaccine	-	-	94%	91%
Initial Antibiotic Timing	-	-	96%	95%
Pneumococcal Vaccine	-	-	96%	93%
Smoking Cessation Advice	-	-	99%	97%
Surgical Care Improvement Project				
Appropriate VTP Within 24 Hours	-	-	94%	92%
Appropriate Hair Removal	-	-	100%	99%
Appropriate Beta Blocker Usage	-	-	95%	93%
Controlled Postoperative Blood Glucose	-	-	93%	93%
Prophylactic Antibiotic Timing	-	-	98%	97%
Prophylactic Antibiotic Timing (Outpatient)	-	-	93%	92%
Prophylactic Antibiotic Selection	-	-	97%	97%
Prophylactic Antibiotic Select. (Outpatient)	-	-	94%	94%
Prophylactic Antibiotic Stopped	-	-	96%	94%
Recommended VTP Ordered	-	-	95%	94%
Urinary Catheter Removal	-	-	93%	90%
Children's Asthma Care				
Received Systemic Corticosteroids	-	-	-	100%
Received Home Management Plan	-	-	-	71%
Received Reliever Medication	-	-	-	100%
Use of Medical Imaging				
Combination Abdominal CT Scan	-	-	0.126	0.191
Combination Chest CT Scan	-	-	0.026	0.054
Follow-up Mammogram/Ultrasound	-	-	10.6%	8.4%
MRI for Low Back Pain	-	-	26.4%	32.7%
Survey of Patients' Hospital Experiences				
Area Around Room 'Always' Quiet at Night	-	-	-	58%
Doctors 'Always' Communicated Well	-	-	-	80%
Home Recovery Information Given	-	-	-	82%
Hospital Given 9 or 10 on 10 Point Scale	-	-	-	67%
Meds 'Always' Explained Before Given	-	-	-	60%
Nurses 'Always' Communicated Well	-	-	-	76%
Pain 'Always' Well Controlled	-	-	-	69%
Room and Bathroom 'Always' Clean	-	-	-	71%
Timely Help 'Always' Received	-	-	-	64%
Would Definitely Recommend Hospital	-	-	-	69%

Lourdes Medical Center of Burlington County

218a Sunset Road
Willingboro, NJ 08046
Phone: 609-835-2900
Fax: 865-635-2493
E-mail: info@lourdesnet.org
URL: www.lourdesnet.org/lourdes
Type: Acute Care Hospitals
Emergency Services: Yes
Ownership: Voluntary Non-Profit - Other
Beds: 410

Key Personnel:
CEO/President.............. Randall Maguire
Chief of Medical Staff.......... Alan Pope, MD
Coronary Care.............. Marianne Kraemer
Infection Control............. Peggy McDermott
Pediatric Ambulatory Care ...... Gerald Fendrick, MD
Pediatric In-Patient Care .... Gerald Fendrick, MD
Quality Assurance .... Ruthann Enriques
Radiology.................. Daniel Scott, MD

Measure	Cases	This Hosp.	State Avg.	U.S. Avg.
Heart Attack Care				
ACE Inhibitor or ARB for LVSD[1]	8	100%	98%	96%
Aspirin at Arrival	71	99%	99%	99%
Aspirin at Discharge	39	92%	99%	98%
Beta Blocker at Discharge	44	95%	99%	98%
Fibrinolytic Medication Timing	0	-	65%	55%
PCI Within 90 Minutes of Arrival	0	-	87%	90%
Smoking Cessation Advice[1]	4	100%	100%	99%
Chest Pain/Possible Heart Attack Care				
Aspirin at Arrival	306	95%	97%	95%
Median Time to ECG (minutes)	309	9	8	8
Median Time to Transfer (minutes)[1]	9	73	81	61
Fibrinolytic Medication Timing[1]	4	100%	65%	54%
Heart Failure Care				
ACE Inhibitor or ARB for LVSD	116	92%	97%	94%
Discharge Instructions	276	99%	93%	88%
Evaluation of LVS Function	340	98%	99%	98%
Smoking Cessation Advice	41	100%	100%	98%
Pneumonia Care				
Appropriate Initial Antibiotic	87	99%	94%	92%
Blood Culture Timing	155	97%	97%	96%
Influenza Vaccine	87	86%	94%	91%
Initial Antibiotic Timing	147	99%	96%	95%
Pneumococcal Vaccine	124	89%	96%	93%
Smoking Cessation Advice	55	100%	99%	97%
Surgical Care Improvement Project				
Appropriate VTP Within 24 Hours[2]	138	96%	94%	92%
Appropriate Hair Removal[2]	287	100%	100%	99%
Appropriate Beta Blocker Usage[2]	74	95%	95%	93%
Controlled Postoperative Blood Glucose[2]	0	-	93%	93%
Prophylactic Antibiotic Timing[2]	159	97%	98%	97%
Prophylactic Antibiotic Timing (Outpatient)	92	93%	93%	92%
Prophylactic Antibiotic Selection[2]	159	96%	97%	97%
Prophylactic Antibiotic Select. (Outpatient)	88	98%	94%	94%
Prophylactic Antibiotic Stopped[2]	156	96%	96%	94%
Recommended VTP Ordered[2]	138	99%	95%	94%
Urinary Catheter Removal[2]	61	82%	93%	90%
Children's Asthma Care				
Received Systemic Corticosteroids	-	-	-	100%
Received Home Management Plan	-	-	-	71%
Received Reliever Medication	-	-	-	100%
Use of Medical Imaging				
Combination Abdominal CT Scan	576	0.014	0.126	0.191
Combination Chest CT Scan	281	0.000	0.026	0.054
Follow-up Mammogram/Ultrasound	587	11.1%	10.6%	8.4%
MRI for Low Back Pain[1]	22	18.2%	26.4%	32.7%
Survey of Patients' Hospital Experiences				
Area Around Room 'Always' Quiet at Night	300+	49%	-	58%
Doctors 'Always' Communicated Well	300+	68%	-	80%
Home Recovery Information Given	300+	70%	-	82%
Hospital Given 9 or 10 on 10 Point Scale	300+	46%	-	67%
Meds 'Always' Explained Before Given	300+	48%	-	60%
Nurses 'Always' Communicated Well	300+	65%	-	76%
Pain 'Always' Well Controlled	300+	63%	-	69%
Room and Bathroom 'Always' Clean	300+	59%	-	71%
Timely Help 'Always' Received	300+	55%	-	64%
Would Definitely Recommend Hospital	300+	47%	-	69%

Underwood Memorial Hospital

509 N Broad St
Woodbury, NJ 08096
Phone: 856-845-0100
Fax: 856-251-0383
E-mail: humanresources@umhospital.org.
URL: www.umhospital.org
Type: Acute Care Hospitals
Emergency Services: Yes
Ownership: Voluntary Non-Profit - Private
Beds: 305

Key Personnel:
CEO/President.............. Eileen K Cardile RN, MS, CNA
Chief of Medical Staff.......... Jeffrey Bittner, MD
Infection Control............. Paula Simplot
Operating Room.............. Cindy Quint, RN
Pediatric In-Patient Care .... Lawrence Epple, MD
Quality Assurance .... Marla Maybrook
Radiology.................. Mary Welch
Intensive Care Unit........... Dennis Sacter

Measure	Cases	This Hosp.	State Avg.	U.S. Avg.
Heart Attack Care				
ACE Inhibitor or ARB for LVSD[1]	20	95%	98%	96%
Aspirin at Arrival	228	99%	99%	99%
Aspirin at Discharge	142	98%	99%	98%
Beta Blocker at Discharge	144	99%	99%	98%
Fibrinolytic Medication Timing	0	-	65%	55%
PCI Within 90 Minutes of Arrival	64	92%	87%	90%
Smoking Cessation Advice	55	100%	100%	99%
Chest Pain/Possible Heart Attack Care				
Aspirin at Arrival[1]	12	100%	97%	95%
Median Time to ECG (minutes)[1]	13	15	8	8
Median Time to Transfer (minutes)[1,3]	1	90	81	61
Fibrinolytic Medication Timing[3]	0	-	65%	54%
Heart Failure Care				
ACE Inhibitor or ARB for LVSD	133	98%	97%	94%
Discharge Instructions	356	100%	93%	88%
Evaluation of LVS Function	470	100%	99%	98%
Smoking Cessation Advice	70	100%	100%	98%
Pneumonia Care				
Appropriate Initial Antibiotic	181	92%	94%	92%
Blood Culture Timing	267	99%	97%	96%
Influenza Vaccine	167	92%	94%	91%
Initial Antibiotic Timing	255	95%	96%	95%
Pneumococcal Vaccine	249	97%	96%	93%
Smoking Cessation Advice	105	100%	99%	97%
Surgical Care Improvement Project				
Appropriate VTP Within 24 Hours[2]	290	96%	94%	92%
Appropriate Hair Removal[2]	637	100%	100%	99%
Appropriate Beta Blocker Usage[2]	141	94%	95%	93%
Controlled Postoperative Blood Glucose[2]	0	-	93%	93%
Prophylactic Antibiotic Timing[2]	373	94%	98%	97%
Prophylactic Antibiotic Timing (Outpatient)	105	86%	93%	92%
Prophylactic Antibiotic Selection[2]	376	96%	97%	97%
Prophylactic Antibiotic Select. (Outpatient)	98	92%	94%	94%
Prophylactic Antibiotic Stopped[2]	359	94%	96%	94%
Recommended VTP Ordered[2]	290	98%	95%	94%
Urinary Catheter Removal[2]	44	89%	93%	90%
Children's Asthma Care				
Received Systemic Corticosteroids	-	-	-	100%
Received Home Management Plan	-	-	-	71%
Received Reliever Medication	-	-	-	100%
Use of Medical Imaging				
Combination Abdominal CT Scan	589	0.061	0.126	0.191
Combination Chest CT Scan	278	0.083	0.026	0.054
Follow-up Mammogram/Ultrasound	161	18.6%	10.6%	8.4%
MRI for Low Back Pain[5]	0	-	26.4%	32.7%
Survey of Patients' Hospital Experiences				
Area Around Room 'Always' Quiet at Night	300+	51%	-	58%
Doctors 'Always' Communicated Well	300+	75%	-	80%
Home Recovery Information Given	300+	79%	-	82%
Hospital Given 9 or 10 on 10 Point Scale	300+	60%	-	67%
Meds 'Always' Explained Before Given	300+	61%	-	60%
Nurses 'Always' Communicated Well	300+	78%	-	76%
Pain 'Always' Well Controlled	300+	68%	-	69%
Room and Bathroom 'Always' Clean	300+	70%	-	71%
Timely Help 'Always' Received	300+	63%	-	64%
Would Definitely Recommend Hospital	300+	59%	-	69%

NOTE: Hospital profiles are in alphabetical order by state, then city, then hospital within the city; Rankings exclude hospitals with less than 25 cases except for patient surveys which excludes hospitals with less than 100 cases; (a) 100–299 cases; (1) The number of cases is too small to be sure how well a hospital is performing; (2) The hospital indicated that the data submitted for this measure were based on a sample of cases; (3) Data was collected during a shorter time period (fewer quarters) than the maximum possible time for this measure; (4) Suppressed for one or more quarters by CMS; (5) No data is available from the hospital for this measure; (6) Fewer than 100 patients completed the HCAHPS survey. Use these rates with caution, as the number of surveys may be too low to reliably assess hospital performance; (7) Survey results are based on less than 12 months of data; (8) Survey results are not available for this reporting period; (9) No or very few patients were eligible for the HCAHPS survey. The scores shown, if any, reflect a very small number of surveys; (10) A state average was not calculated because too few hospitals in the state submitted data; (11) There were discrepancies in the data collection process; Please refer to the User's Guide for a full explanation of data.

Heart Attack Care

1. ACE Inhibitor or ARB for LVSD

Hospital Name	City	Rate	Cases
Brookdale Hospital Medical Center	Brooklyn	100%	40
Ellis Hospital[2]	Schenectady	100%	71
Jamaica Hospital Medical Center[2]	Jamaica	100%	44
Long Island Jewish Medical Center[2]	New Hyde Park	100%	75
NYU Hospitals Center	New York	100%	47
Orange Regional Medical Center	Goshen	100%	28
Rochester General Hospital[2]	Rochester	100%	42
Saint Luke's Cornwall Hospital	Newburgh	100%	28
Staten Island University Hospital[2]	Staten Island	100%	42
Unity Hospital of Rochester[2]	Rochester	100%	39
Vassar Brothers Medical Center	Poughkeepsie	100%	62
Westchester Medical Center[2]	Valhalla	100%	73
Albany Medical Center Hospital	Albany	99%	82
Arnot Ogden Medical Center	Elmira	99%	94
Bellevue Hospital Center	New York	99%	137
Saint Peter's Hospital	Albany	99%	85
Strong Memorial Hospital	Rochester	99%	207
University Hospital of Brooklyn - Downstate[2]	Brooklyn	99%	81
Glens Falls Hospital	Glens Falls	98%	43
Mercy Hospital[2]	Buffalo	98%	43
North Shore University Hospital[2]	Manhasset	98%	53
Univ Hosp S U N Y Health Science Ctr	Syracuse	98%	53
Winthrop-University Hospital[2]	Mineola	98%	96
Champlain Valley Physicians Hospital	Plattsburgh	97%	38
Lenox Hill Hospital[2]	New York	97%	75
United Health Services Hospitals	Johnson City	97%	113
Crouse Hospital	Syracuse	96%	25
Saint Francis Hospital - Roslyn[2]	Roslyn	96%	79
University Hospital - Stony Brook[2]	Stony Brook	96%	92
Beth Israel Medical Center[2]	New York	95%	66
Elmhurst Hospital Center	Elmhurst	95%	61
Erie County Medical Center	Buffalo	95%	44
Saint Luke's Roosevelt Hospital[2]	New York	95%	88
Good Samaritan Hospital of Suffern	Suffern	94%	87
New York-Presbyterian Hospital[2]	New York	94%	158
Kaleida Health[2]	Buffalo	93%	116
Saint Elizabeth Medical Center	Utica	92%	107
Faxton-St Luke's Healthcare	Utica	91%	32
Lutheran Medical Center	Brooklyn	91%	32
Maimonides Medical Center[2]	Brooklyn	91%	87
New York Methodist Hospital	Brooklyn	91%	66
Mount Sinai Hospital[2]	New York	89%	57
South Nassau Communities Hospital	Oceanside	89%	38
New York Hospital Medical Center of Queens[2]	Flushing	88%	60
Mary Imogene Bassett Hospital	Cooperstown	86%	37
Long Island College Hospital[2]	Brooklyn	85%	41
Saint Joseph's Hospital Health Center	Syracuse	81%	114
Montefiore Medical Center[2]	Bronx	71%	63

2. Aspirin at Arrival

Hospital Name	City	Rate	Cases
Albany Medical Center Hospital	Albany	100%	188
Arnot Ogden Medical Center	Elmira	100%	193
Auburn Memorial Hospital	Auburn	100%	34
Bellevue Hospital Center	New York	100%	188
Bronx-Lebanon Hospital Center	Bronx	100%	194
Chenango Memorial Hospital	Norwich	100%	32
Claxton-Hepburn Medical Center	Ogdensburg	100%	32
Elmhurst Hospital Center	Elmhurst	100%	267
Geneva General Hospital	Geneva	100%	31
Glen Cove Hospital[2]	Glen Cove	100%	47
Glens Falls Hospital	Glens Falls	100%	268
Good Samaritan Hospital Medical Center	West Islip	100%	248
Harlem Hospital Center	New York	100%	38
Huntington Hospital[2]	Huntington	100%	159
Jamaica Hospital Medical Center[2]	Jamaica	100%	262
John T Mather Mem Hosp-Port Jefferson	Port Jefferson	100%	147
Kingston Hospital	Kingston	100%	56
Lakeside Memorial Hospital	Brockport	100%	28
Lincoln Medical & Mental Health Center	Bronx	100%	129
Mercy Medical Center	Rockville Centre	100%	59
Mount St Mary's Hospital and Health Center	Lewiston	100%	100
Nassau University Medical Center	East Meadow	100%	50
New York Westchester Square Medical Center	Bronx	100%	43
Niagara Falls Memorial Medical Center[2]	Niagara Falls	100%	49
Northern Westchester Hospital	Mount Kisco	100%	26
NYU Hospitals Center	New York	100%	223
Orange Regional Medical Center	Goshen	100%	211
Our Lady of Lourdes Memorial Hospital	Binghamton	100%	101
Phelps Memorial Hospital Assn	Sleepy Hollow	100%	57
Queens Hospital Center	Jamaica	100%	44
Saint Francis Hospital	Poughkeepsie	100%	25
St John's Episcopal Hosp-South Shore	Far Rockaway	100%	40
Saint Joseph Hospital	Bethpage	100%	47
Saint Mary's Hospital at Amsterdam	Amsterdam	100%	57
Saint Peter's Hospital	Albany	100%	383
Samaritan Hospital	Troy	100%	51
Saratoga Hospital	Saratoga Spgs	100%	62
Seton Health System-St Mary's Campus	Troy	100%	36
Sound Shore Medical Center of Westchester	New Rochelle	100%	108
Southside Hospital[2]	Bay Shore	100%	187
Staten Island University Hospital[2]	Staten Island	100%	260
Strong Memorial Hospital	Rochester	100%	350
Syracuse VA Medical Center	Syracuse	100%	37
University Hospital - Stony Brook[2]	Stony Brook	100%	224
University Hospital of Brooklyn - Downstate[2]	Brooklyn	100%	196
Univ Hosp S U N Y Health Science Ctr	Syracuse	100%	91
Upstate New York VA Healthcare System	Buffalo	100%	46
VA New York Harbor Healthcare System	New York	100%	86
Vassar Brothers Medical Center	Poughkeepsie	100%	292
Westchester Medical Center[2]	Valhalla	100%	57
Brookdale Hospital Medical Center	Brooklyn	99%	245
Brookhaven Memorial Hospital Med Ctr[2]	Patchogue	99%	185
Champlain Valley Physicians Hospital	Plattsburgh	99%	185
Coney Island Hospital	Brooklyn	99%	115
Good Samaritan Hospital of Suffern	Suffern	99%	251
Jacobi Medical Center	Bronx	99%	116
Kaleida Health[2]	Buffalo	99%	448
Lenox Hill Hospital[2]	New York	99%	136
Mercy Hospital[2]	Buffalo	99%	201
New York Community Hospital of Brooklyn	Brooklyn	99%	85
New York Methodist Hospital	Brooklyn	99%	203
New York-Presbyterian Hospital[2]	New York	99%	353
North Shore University Hospital[2]	Manhasset	99%	109
Nyack Hospital	Nyack	99%	67
Olean General Hospital	Olean	99%	80
Saint Elizabeth Medical Center	Utica	99%	194
Saint Joseph's Hospital Health Center	Syracuse	99%	507
Saint Luke's Cornwall Hospital	Newburgh	99%	190
Saint Luke's Roosevelt Hospital[2]	New York	99%	312
United Health Services Hospitals	Johnson City	99%	334
Cayuga Medical Center at Ithaca	Ithaca	98%	40
Crouse Hospital	Syracuse	98%	146
Ellis Hospital[2]	Schenectady	98%	409
Hudson Valley Hospital Center	Cortlandt Manor	98%	113
Kings County Hospital Center	Brooklyn	98%	97
Kingsbrook Jewish Medical Center	Brooklyn	98%	42
Long Island Jewish Medical Center[2]	New Hyde Park	98%	159
Lutheran Medical Center	Brooklyn	98%	256
New York Hospital Medical Center of Queens[2]	Flushing	98%	320
Newark-Wayne Community Hospital	Newark	98%	43
Peconic Bay Medical Center	Riverhead	98%	49
Plainview Hospital[2]	Plainview	98%	109
Putnam Hospital Center	Carmel	98%	43
Richmond University Medical Center[2]	Staten Island	98%	90
Rochester General Hospital[2]	Rochester	98%	213
Saint Barnabas Hospital	Bronx	98%	66
Saint Francis Hospital - Roslyn[2]	Roslyn	98%	132
Woman's Christian Association	Jamestown	98%	94
Woodhull Medical and Mental Health Center	Brooklyn	98%	52
Benedictine Hospital	Kingston	97%	38
Brooklyn Hospital Center at Downtown Campus	Brooklyn	97%	120
Highland Hospital	Rochester	97%	68
Kenmore Mercy Hospital	Kenmore	97%	91
Long Island College Hospital[2]	Brooklyn	97%	227
Metropolitan Hospital Center	New York	97%	39
Mount Sinai Hospital[2]	New York	97%	188
New York Downtown Hospital	New York	97%	36
North Central Bronx Hospital	Bronx	97%	39
Saint Catherine of Siena Hospital	Smithtown	97%	120
Sisters of Charity Hospital	Buffalo	97%	146
Unity Hospital of Rochester[2]	Rochester	97%	242
Winthrop-University Hospital[2]	Mineola	97%	282
Beth Israel Medical Center[2]	New York	96%	257
Erie County Medical Center	Buffalo	96%	131
Mary Imogene Bassett Hospital	Cooperstown	96%	114
Saint John's Riverside Hospital	Yonkers	96%	53
South Nassau Communities Hospital	Oceanside	96%	313
White Plains Hospital Center	White Plains	96%	81
Wyckoff Heights Medical Center	Brooklyn	96%	106
Faxton-St Luke's Healthcare	Utica	95%	119
Forest Hills Hospital[2]	Forest Hills	95%	111
Franklin Hospital[2]	Valley Stream	95%	56
Interfaith Medical Center	Brooklyn	95%	57
Lawrence Hospital Center	Bronxville	95%	38
Maimonides Medical Center[2]	Brooklyn	95%	284
Montefiore Medical Center[2]	Bronx	95%	281
Nathan Littauer Hospital	Gloversville	95%	43
Samaritan Medical Center	Watertown	95%	43
Albany Memorial Hospital	Albany	94%	33
Aurelia Osborn Fox Memorial Hospital	Oneonta	94%	51
Bon Secours Community Hospital	Port Jervis	94%	31
Oswego Hospital	Oswego	94%	63
Rome Memorial Hospital	Rome	94%	36
Comm-General Hosp of Greater Syracuse	Syracuse	93%	43
Medina Memorial Hospital	Medina	93%	27
Columbia Memorial Hospital	Hudson	92%	86
Eastern Niagara Hospital	Lockport	92%	37
Saint Joseph's Medical Center	Yonkers	92%	37
United Memorial Medical Center	Batavia	92%	26
Catskill Regional Medical Center	Harris	90%	41
F F Thompson Hospital	Canandaigua	89%	35
Flushing Hospital Medical Center	Flushing	89%	105
Mount Vernon Hospital	Mount Vernon	89%	45
Northern Dutchess Hospital	Rhinebeck	89%	28

3. Aspirin at Discharge

Hospital Name	City	Rate	Cases
Albany Medical Center Hospital	Albany	100%	484
Arnot Ogden Medical Center	Elmira	100%	293
Bellevue Hospital Center	New York	100%	520
Brookhaven Memorial Hospital Med Ctr[2]	Patchogue	100%	79
Brooklyn Hospital Center at Downtown Campus	Brooklyn	100%	45
Columbia Memorial Hospital	Hudson	100%	57
Coney Island Hospital	Brooklyn	100%	60
Elmhurst Hospital Center	Elmhurst	100%	268
Glens Falls Hospital	Glens Falls	100%	229
Good Samaritan Hospital Medical Center	West Islip	100%	202
Good Samaritan Hospital of Suffern	Suffern	100%	421
Highland Hospital	Rochester	100%	52
Hudson Valley Hospital Center	Cortlandt Manor	100%	65
Huntington Hospital[2]	Huntington	100%	103
Jamaica Hospital Medical Center[2]	Jamaica	100%	169
John T Mather Mem Hosp-Port Jefferson	Port Jefferson	100%	68
Kings County Hospital Center	Brooklyn	100%	58
Kingston Hospital	Kingston	100%	41
Lenox Hill Hospital[2]	New York	100%	331
Lincoln Medical & Mental Health Center	Bronx	100%	63
Mary Imogene Bassett Hospital	Cooperstown	100%	234
Mount St Mary's Hospital and Health Center	Lewiston	100%	62
Nassau University Medical Center	East Meadow	100%	31
New York Community Hospital of Brooklyn	Brooklyn	100%	42
Niagara Falls Memorial Medical Center[2]	Niagara Falls	100%	27
North Shore University Hospital[2]	Manhasset	100%	311
Nyack Hospital	Nyack	100%	41
NYU Hospitals Center	New York	100%	254
Orange Regional Medical Center	Goshen	100%	176
Our Lady of Lourdes Memorial Hospital	Binghamton	100%	73
Peconic Bay Medical Center	Riverhead	100%	25
Phelps Memorial Hospital Assn	Sleepy Hollow	100%	47
Putnam Hospital Center	Carmel	100%	25
Richmond University Medical Center[2]	Staten Island	100%	34
Rochester General Hospital[2]	Rochester	100%	308
Saint Barnabas Hospital	Bronx	100%	34
Saint Mary's Hospital at Amsterdam	Amsterdam	100%	30
Southside Hospital[2]	Bay Shore	100%	157
Staten Island University Hospital[2]	Staten Island	100%	280
Strong Memorial Hospital	Rochester	100%	684
United Health Services Hospitals	Johnson City	100%	463
Upstate New York VA Healthcare System	Buffalo	100%	46
Vassar Brothers Medical Center	Poughkeepsie	100%	378
White Plains Hospital Center	White Plains	100%	60
Woman's Christian Association	Jamestown	100%	59
Bronx-Lebanon Hospital Center	Bronx	99%	137
Brookdale Hospital Medical Center	Brooklyn	99%	185
Champlain Valley Physicians Hospital	Plattsburgh	99%	257
Crouse Hospital	Syracuse	99%	143
Ellis Hospital[2]	Schenectady	99%	510
Long Island Jewish Medical Center[2]	New Hyde Park	99%	301
New York Methodist Hospital	Brooklyn	99%	241
Saint Elizabeth Medical Center	Utica	99%	316
Saint Francis Hospital - Roslyn[2]	Roslyn	99%	337
Saint Joseph's Hospital Health Center	Syracuse	99%	945
Saint Luke's Cornwall Hospital	Newburgh	99%	168
Saint Peter's Hospital	Albany	99%	635
Unity Hospital of Rochester[2]	Rochester	99%	202
University Hospital of Brooklyn - Downstate[2]	Brooklyn	99%	237
Univ Hosp S U N Y Health Science Ctr	Syracuse	99%	183
VA New York Harbor Healthcare System	New York	99%	117
Westchester Medical Center[2]	Valhalla	99%	311
Winthrop-University Hospital[2]	Mineola	99%	387
Beth Israel Medical Center[2]	New York	98%	263
Erie County Medical Center	Buffalo	98%	214
Kenmore Mercy Hospital	Kenmore	98%	58
Mercy Hospital[2]	Buffalo	98%	320
Mount Sinai Hospital[2]	New York	98%	327
New York-Presbyterian Hospital[2]	New York	98%	744
Olean General Hospital	Olean	98%	43
Saint Luke's Roosevelt Hospital[2]	New York	98%	294
Sound Shore Medical Center of Westchester	New Rochelle	98%	62
University Hospital - Stony Brook[2]	Stony Brook	98%	532
Forest Hills Hospital[2]	Forest Hills	97%	61
Kaleida Health[2]	Buffalo	97%	854
Lutheran Medical Center	Brooklyn	97%	173
Glen Cove Hospital[2]	Glen Cove	96%	28
Jacobi Medical Center	Bronx	96%	70
Maimonides Medical Center[2]	Brooklyn	96%	302

NOTE: Hospital profiles are in alphabetical order by state, then city, then hospital within the city; Rankings exclude hospitals with less than 25 cases except for patient surveys which excludes hospitals with less than 100 cases; (a) 100–299 cases; (1) The number of cases is too small to be sure how well a hospital is performing; (2) The hospital indicated that the data submitted for this measure were based on a sample of cases; (3) Data was collected during a shorter time period (fewer quarters) than the maximum possible time for this measure; (4) Suppressed for one or more quarters by CMS; (5) No data is available from the hospital for this measure; (6) Fewer than 100 patients completed the HCAHPS survey. Use these rates with caution, as the number of surveys may be too low to reliably assess hospital performance; (7) Survey results are based on less than 12 months of data; (8) Survey results are not available for this reporting period; (9) No or very few patients were eligible for the HCAHPS survey. The scores shown, if any, reflect a very small number of surveys; (10) A state average was not calculated because too few hospitals in the state submitted data; (11) There were discrepancies in the data collection process; Please refer to the User's Guide for a full explanation of data.

Mercy Medical Center	Rockville Centre	96%	25
Montefiore Medical Center[2]	Bronx	96%	373
Mount Vernon Hospital	Mount Vernon	96%	26
Saint Catherine of Siena Hospital	Smithtown	96%	92
South Nassau Communities Hospital	Oceanside	96%	262
Faxton-St Luke's Healthcare	Utica	95%	110
New York Hospital Medical Center of Queens[2]	Flushing	95%	292
Plainview Hospital[2]	Plainview	95%	62
Saratoga Hospital	Saratoga Spgs	95%	37
Sisters of Charity Hospital	Buffalo	95%	79
Wyckoff Heights Medical Center	Brooklyn	95%	62
Long Island College Hospital[2]	Brooklyn	94%	176
Newark-Wayne Community Hospital	Newark	94%	32
Samaritan Hospital	Troy	94%	33
Seton Health System-St Mary's Campus	Troy	92%	25
Cayuga Medical Center at Ithaca	Ithaca	90%	29
Comm-General Hosp of Greater Syracuse	Syracuse	90%	30
Flushing Hospital Medical Center	Flushing	86%	64
Aurelia Osborn Fox Memorial Hospital	Oneonta	85%	39

4. Beta Blocker at Discharge

Hospital Name	City	Rate	Cases
Albany Medical Center Hospital	Albany	100%	480
Benedictine Hospital	Kingston	100%	25
Brookhaven Memorial Hospital Med Ctr[2]	Patchogue	100%	94
Ellis Hospital[2]	Schenectady	100%	506
Elmhurst Hospital Center	Elmhurst	100%	262
Glens Falls Hospital	Glens Falls	100%	235
Good Samaritan Hospital Medical Center	West Islip	100%	200
Good Samaritan Hospital of Suffern	Suffern	100%	418
Highland Hospital	Rochester	100%	49
Hudson Valley Hospital Center	Cortlandt Manor	100%	68
Huntington Hospital[2]	Huntington	100%	102
Jamaica Hospital Medical Center[2]	Jamaica	100%	169
Kingston Hospital	Kingston	100%	40
Lincoln Medical & Mental Health Center	Bronx	100%	64
Mary Imogene Bassett Hospital	Cooperstown	100%	233
Mount St Mary's Hospital and Health Center	Lewiston	100%	69
Nassau University Medical Center	East Meadow	100%	33
Nathan Littauer Hospital	Gloversville	100%	28
New York Community Hospital of Brooklyn	Brooklyn	100%	49
Newark-Wayne Community Hospital	Newark	100%	30
Niagara Falls Memorial Medical Center[2]	Niagara Falls	100%	30
North Shore University Hospital[2]	Manhasset	100%	294
Nyack Hospital	Nyack	100%	39
Orange Regional Medical Center	Goshen	100%	179
Peconic Bay Medical Center	Riverhead	100%	29
Phelps Memorial Hospital Assn	Sleepy Hollow	100%	46
Plainview Hospital[2]	Plainview	100%	61
Putnam Hospital Center	Carmel	100%	25
Rochester General Hospital[2]	Rochester	100%	309
Saint Luke's Cornwall Hospital	Newburgh	100%	164
Saint Mary's Hospital at Amsterdam	Amsterdam	100%	39
Samaritan Hospital	Troy	100%	38
Seton Health System-St Mary's Campus	Troy	100%	25
Southside Hospital[2]	Bay Shore	100%	155
Staten Island University Hospital[2]	Staten Island	100%	249
Strong Memorial Hospital	Rochester	100%	663
Unity Hospital of Rochester[2]	Rochester	100%	207
Upstate New York VA Healthcare System	Buffalo	100%	45
Vassar Brothers Medical Center	Poughkeepsie	100%	394
Winthrop-University Hospital[2]	Mineola	100%	378
Arnot Ogden Medical Center	Elmira	99%	313
Bellevue Hospital Center	New York	99%	491
Bronx-Lebanon Hospital Center	Bronx	99%	124
Brookdale Hospital Medical Center	Brooklyn	99%	187
Erie County Medical Center	Buffalo	99%	204
John T Mather Mem Hosp-Port Jefferson	Port Jefferson	99%	73
Lenox Hill Hospital[2]	New York	99%	321
Long Island Jewish Medical Center[2]	New Hyde Park	99%	294
NYU Hospitals Center	New York	99%	248
Our Lady of Lourdes Memorial Hospital	Binghamton	99%	76
Saint Francis Hospital - Roslyn[2]	Roslyn	99%	342
Saint Peter's Hospital	Albany	99%	646
Sisters of Charity Hospital	Buffalo	99%	84
Sound Shore Medical Center of Westschester	New Rochelle	99%	69
United Health Services Hospitals	Johnson City	99%	473
Univ Hosp S U N Y Health Science Ctr	Syracuse	99%	179
VA New York Harbor Healthcare System	New York	99%	107
Westchester Medical Center[2]	Valhalla	99%	305
Beth Israel Medical Center[2]	New York	98%	258
Coney Island Hospital	Brooklyn	98%	62
Kaleida Health[2]	Buffalo	98%	873
Kenmore Mercy Hospital	Kenmore	98%	60
Kings County Hospital Center	Brooklyn	98%	53
Mercy Hospital[2]	Buffalo	98%	319
New York Methodist Hospital	Brooklyn	98%	244
Olean General Hospital	Olean	98%	52
Saint Catherine of Siena Hospital	Smithtown	98%	97
Saint Elizabeth Medical Center	Utica	98%	309
Saint Joseph's Hospital Health Center	Syracuse	98%	913
Saratoga Hospital	Saratoga Spgs	98%	45
University Hospital - Stony Brook[2]	Stony Brook	98%	523
Woman's Christian Association	Jamestown	98%	66
Champlain Valley Physicians Hospital	Plattsburgh	97%	269
Crouse Hospital	Syracuse	97%	135
Faxton-St Luke's Healthcare	Utica	97%	115
Forest Hills Hospital[2]	Forest Hills	97%	67
Lutheran Medical Center	Brooklyn	97%	177
New York Hospital Medical Center of Queens[2]	Flushing	97%	289
South Nassau Communities Hospital	Oceanside	97%	263
Brooklyn Hospital Center at Downtown Campus	Brooklyn	96%	50
Columbia Memorial Hospital	Hudson	96%	56
Comm-General Hosp of Greater Syracuse	Syracuse	96%	28
Montefiore Medical Center[2]	Bronx	96%	366
Mount Sinai Hospital[2]	New York	96%	319
Saint Luke's Roosevelt Hospital[2]	New York	96%	290
University Hospital of Brooklyn - Downstate[2]	Brooklyn	96%	239
Jacobi Medical Center	Bronx	95%	64
Maimonides Medical Center[2]	Brooklyn	95%	307
New York-Presbyterian Hospital[2]	New York	95%	718
Richmond University Medical Center[2]	Staten Island	95%	37
White Plains Hospital Center	White Plains	95%	63
Long Island College Hospital[2]	Brooklyn	94%	177
Oswego Hospital	Oswego	94%	31
Saint Barnabas Hospital	Bronx	94%	34
Aurelia Osborn Fox Memorial Hospital	Oneonta	93%	42
Cayuga Medical Center at Ithaca	Ithaca	93%	30
F F Thompson Hospital	Canandaigua	93%	30
Wyckoff Heights Medical Center	Brooklyn	93%	60
Albany Memorial Hospital	Albany	92%	25
Interfaith Medical Center	Brooklyn	92%	26
Flushing Hospital Medical Center	Flushing	90%	70
Mount Vernon Hospital	Mount Vernon	80%	25
Eastern Niagara Hospital	Lockport	78%	27

6. PCI Within 90 Minutes of Arrival

Hospital Name	City	Rate	Cases
Good Samaritan Hospital Medical Center	West Islip	100%	35
Long Island Jewish Medical Center[2]	New Hyde Park	100%	33
New York Hospital Medical Center of Queens[2]	Flushing	100%	39
Orange Regional Medical Center	Goshen	100%	45
Crouse Hospital	Syracuse	98%	46
Staten Island University Hospital[2]	Staten Island	98%	45
Lutheran Medical Center	Brooklyn	97%	39
Albany Medical Center Hospital	Albany	96%	49
Glens Falls Hospital	Glens Falls	96%	47
Jamaica Hospital Medical Center[2]	Jamaica	96%	71
New York-Presbyterian Hospital[2]	New York	96%	46
Strong Memorial Hospital	Rochester	96%	77
Saint Joseph's Hospital Health Center	Syracuse	95%	126
University Hospital of Brooklyn - Downstate[2]	Brooklyn	95%	37
Ellis Hospital[2]	Schenectady	94%	65
Unity Hospital of Rochester[2]	Rochester	94%	47
Champlain Valley Physicians Hospital	Plattsburgh	93%	28
Southside Hospital[2]	Bay Shore	93%	41
South Nassau Communities Hospital	Oceanside	92%	40
Huntington Hospital[2]	Huntington	91%	47
Arnot Ogden Medical Center	Elmira	90%	40
NYU Hospitals Center	New York	90%	29
Saint Luke's Cornwall Hospital	Newburgh	90%	30
Vassar Brothers Medical Center	Poughkeepsie	90%	67
Bronx-Lebanon Hospital Center	Bronx	88%	33
Mercy Hospital[2]	Buffalo	88%	26
Good Samaritan Hospital of Suffern	Suffern	87%	69
University Hospital - Stony Brook[2]	Stony Brook	86%	57
Saint Elizabeth Medical Center	Utica	85%	65
United Health Services Hospitals	Johnson City	85%	60
Montefiore Medical Center[2]	Bronx	84%	51
Kaleida Health[2]	Buffalo	83%	36
Winthrop-University Hospital[2]	Mineola	83%	58
Brookdale Hospital Medical Center	Brooklyn	81%	36
Saint Peter's Hospital	Albany	81%	48
Erie County Medical Center	Buffalo	80%	35
New York Methodist Hospital	Brooklyn	78%	32
Rochester General Hospital[2]	Rochester	76%	33
Saint Luke's Roosevelt Hospital[2]	New York	70%	46
Maimonides Medical Center[2]	Brooklyn	69%	29
Elmhurst Hospital Center	Elmhurst	67%	90
Saint Catherine of Siena Hospital	Smithtown	62%	37

7. Smoking Cessation Advice

Hospital Name	City	Rate	Cases
Albany Medical Center Hospital	Albany	100%	204
Arnot Ogden Medical Center	Elmira	100%	119
Bellevue Hospital Center	New York	100%	183
Beth Israel Medical Center[2]	New York	100%	53
Bronx-Lebanon Hospital Center	Bronx	100%	55
Crouse Hospital	Syracuse	100%	51
Ellis Hospital[2]	Schenectady	100%	151
Elmhurst Hospital Center	Elmhurst	100%	91
Erie County Medical Center	Buffalo	100%	100
Glens Falls Hospital	Glens Falls	100%	73
Good Samaritan Hospital Medical Center	West Islip	100%	61
Jamaica Hospital Medical Center[2]	Jamaica	100%	58
Kaleida Health[2]	Buffalo	100%	250
Long Island College Hospital[2]	Brooklyn	100%	42
Long Island Jewish Medical Center[2]	New Hyde Park	100%	82
Lutheran Medical Center	Brooklyn	100%	33
Mary Imogene Bassett Hospital	Cooperstown	100%	78
Mercy Hospital[2]	Buffalo	100%	112
Mount Sinai Hospital[2]	New York	100%	80
New York Hospital Medical Center of Queens[2]	Flushing	100%	71
New York Methodist Hospital	Brooklyn	100%	65
North Shore University Hospital[2]	Manhasset	100%	67
NYU Hospitals Center	New York	100%	48
Orange Regional Medical Center	Goshen	100%	52
Rochester General Hospital[2]	Rochester	100%	113
Saint Elizabeth Medical Center	Utica	100%	125
Saint Francis Hospital - Roslyn[2]	Roslyn	100%	73
Saint Joseph's Hospital Health Center	Syracuse	100%	397
Saint Luke's Cornwall Hospital	Newburgh	100%	45
Saint Luke's Roosevelt Hospital[2]	New York	100%	98
Saint Peter's Hospital	Albany	100%	180
South Nassau Communities Hospital	Oceanside	100%	59
Southside Hospital[2]	Bay Shore	100%	50
Staten Island University Hospital[2]	Staten Island	100%	71
Strong Memorial Hospital	Rochester	100%	226
United Health Services Hospitals	Johnson City	100%	155
Unity Hospital of Rochester[2]	Rochester	100%	55
University Hospital - Stony Brook[2]	Stony Brook	100%	149
Univ Hosp S U N Y Health Science Ctr	Syracuse	100%	83
VA New York Harbor Healthcare System	New York	100%	31
Vassar Brothers Medical Center	Poughkeepsie	100%	121
Winthrop-University Hospital[2]	Mineola	100%	90
Good Samaritan Hospital of Suffern	Suffern	99%	120
Lenox Hill Hospital[2]	New York	99%	70
Maimonides Medical Center[2]	Brooklyn	99%	77
Montefiore Medical Center[2]	Bronx	99%	116
New York-Presbyterian Hospital[2]	New York	99%	152
Westchester Medical Center[2]	Valhalla	99%	81
Brookdale Hospital Medical Center	Brooklyn	98%	53
Champlain Valley Physicians Hospital	Plattsburgh	98%	92
University Hospital of Brooklyn - Downstate[2]	Brooklyn	97%	67
Faxton-St Luke's Healthcare	Utica	93%	27

Chest Pain/Possible Heart Attack Care

8. Aspirin at Arrival

Hospital Name	City	Rate	Cases
Adirondack Medical Center	Saranac Lake	100%	51
Bon Secours Community Hospital	Port Jervis	100%	55
Brooklyn Hospital Center at Downtown Campus	Brooklyn	100%	26
Community Memorial Hospital	Hamilton	100%	28
Elmhurst Hospital Center	Elmhurst	100%	192
Glen Cove Hospital	Glen Cove	100%	36
Huntington Hospital	Huntington	100%	25
John T Mather Mem Hosp-Port Jefferson	Port Jefferson	100%	118
Mercy Medical Center	Rockville Centre	100%	53
New York Westchester Square Medical Center	Bronx	100%	32
Northern Westchester Hospital	Mount Kisco	100%	108
Nyack Hospital	Nyack	100%	57
Our Lady of Lourdes Memorial Hospital	Binghamton	100%	42
Peconic Bay Medical Center	Riverhead	100%	121
Saint James Mercy Hospital	Hornell	100%	86
Sisters of Charity Hospital	Buffalo	100%	61
Wyckoff Heights Medical Center	Brooklyn	100%	31
Brookhaven Memorial Hospital Med Ctr	Patchogue	99%	105
Cobleskill Regional Hospital	Cobleskill	99%	114
Franklin Hospital	Valley Stream	99%	110
Saint Joseph Hospital	Bethpage	99%	138
United Memorial Medical Center	Batavia	99%	134
Westfield Memorial Hospital	Westfield	99%	128
Wyoming County Community Hospital	Warsaw	99%	95
Alice Hyde Medical Center	Malone	98%	84
Forest Hills Hospital	Forest Hills	98%	60
Geneva General Hospital	Geneva	98%	61
Hudson Valley Hospital Center	Cortlandt Manor	98%	62
Jones Memorial Hospital	Wellsville	98%	58
Long Beach Medical Center	Long Beach	98%	86
Massena Memorial Hospital	Massena	98%	49
Plainview Hospital	Plainview	98%	110
Rome Memorial Hospital	Rome	98%	50
Saint John's Riverside Hospital	Yonkers	98%	41
Sound Shore Medical Center of Westschester	New Rochelle	98%	54
Canton-Potsdam Hospital	Potsdam	97%	65
Claxton-Hepburn Medical Center	Ogdensburg	97%	59
Clifton Springs Hospital and Clinic	Clifton Springs	97%	63
Corning Hospital	Corning	97%	79
Kenmore Mercy Hospital	Kenmore	97%	36

NOTE: Hospital profiles are in alphabetical order by state, then city, then hospital within the city; Rankings exclude hospitals with less than 25 cases except for patient surveys which excludes hospitals with less than 100 cases; (a) 100–299 cases; (1) The number of cases is too small to be sure how well a hospital is performing; (2) The hospital indicated that the data submitted for this measure were based on a sample of cases; (3) Data was collected during a shorter time period (fewer quarters) than the maximum possible time for this measure; (4) Suppressed for one or more quarters by CMS; (5) No data is available from the hospital for this measure; (6) Fewer than 100 patients completed the HCAHPS survey. Use these rates with caution, as the number of surveys may be too low to reliably assess hospital performance; (7) Survey results are based on less than 12 months of data; (8) Survey results are not available for this reporting period; (9) No or very few patients were eligible for the HCAHPS survey. The scores shown, if any, reflect a very small number of surveys; (10) A state average was not calculated because too few hospitals in the state submitted data; (11) There were discrepancies in the data collection process; Please refer to the User's Guide for a full explanation of data.

Mount Sinai Hospital	New York	97%	61
Olean General Hospital	Olean	97%	348
Queens Hospital Center	Jamaica	97%	89
Saint Joseph's Medical Center	Yonkers	97%	32
White Plains Hospital Center	White Plains	97%	70
Brooks Memorial Hospital	Dunkirk	96%	147
Catskill Regional Medical Center	Harris	96%	51
Cayuga Medical Center at Ithaca	Ithaca	96%	72
F F Thompson Hospital	Canandaigua	96%	123
Lawrence Hospital Center	Bronxville	96%	55
Little Falls Hospital[3]	Little Falls	96%	51
Niagara Falls Memorial Medical Center	Niagara Falls	96%	46
Putnam Hospital Center	Carmel	96%	67
Saint Luke's Cornwall Hospital	Newburgh	96%	54
Saratoga Hospital	Saratoga Spgs	96%	27
Woman's Christian Association	Jamestown	96%	77
Auburn Memorial Hospital	Auburn	95%	137
Columbia Memorial Hospital	Hudson	95%	40
Kingston Hospital	Kingston	95%	37
Lakeside Memorial Hospital	Brockport	95%	106
Medina Memorial Hospital	Medina	95%	60
Oneida Healthcare Center	Oneida	95%	59
Southampton Hospital	Southampton	95%	65
Chenango Memorial Hospital	Norwich	94%	71
Eastern Niagara Hospital	Lockport	94%	151
Nathan Littauer Hospital	Gloversville	94%	54
Newark-Wayne Community Hospital	Newark	94%	145
Samaritan Hospital	Troy	94%	34
Samaritan Medical Center	Watertown	94%	101
Aurelia Osborn Fox Memorial Hospital	Oneonta	93%	46
Cortland Regional Medical Center	Cortland	93%	174
Carthage Area Hospital	Carthage	92%	40
New York Downtown Hospital	New York	92%	38
Soldiers and Sailors Mem Hosp of Yates	Penn Yan	91%	44
Saint Mary's Hospital at Amsterdam	Amsterdam	90%	70
Nicholas H Noyes Memorial Hospital	Dansville	89%	45
Oswego Hospital	Oswego	85%	66
Bertrand Chaffee Hospital	Springville	84%	93
TLC Health Network	Gowanda	83%	82

9. Median Time to ECG (minutes)

Hospital Name	City	Min.	Cases
Elmhurst Hospital Center	Elmhurst	0	198
Saint Luke's Cornwall Hospital	Newburgh	1	55
Community Memorial Hospital	Hamilton	4	30
Huntington Hospital	Huntington	4	26
Adirondack Medical Center	Saranac Lake	5	50
Kingston Hospital	Kingston	5	39
Nicholas H Noyes Memorial Hospital	Dansville	5	45
Northern Westchester Hospital	Mount Kisco	5	112
Oneida Healthcare Center	Oneida	5	65
Westfield Memorial Hospital	Westfield	5	130
Canton-Potsdam Hospital	Potsdam	6	67
Jones Memorial Hospital	Wellsville	6	63
Medina Memorial Hospital	Medina	6	62
Niagara Falls Memorial Medical Center	Niagara Falls	6	47
Nyack Hospital	Nyack	6	58
Our Lady of Lourdes Memorial Hospital	Binghamton	6	41
Rome Memorial Hospital	Rome	6	52
Samaritan Medical Center	Watertown	6	107
Carthage Area Hospital	Carthage	7	41
Hudson Valley Hospital Center	Cortlandt Manor	7	67
Saint Joseph Hospital	Bethpage	7	139
Chenango Memorial Hospital	Norwich	8	72
Claxton-Hepburn Medical Center	Ogdensburg	8	62
Glen Cove Hospital	Glen Cove	8	37
Mercy Medical Center	Rockville Centre	8	56
Nathan Littauer Hospital	Gloversville	8	56
Saratoga Hospital	Saratoga Spgs	8	27
Auburn Memorial Hospital	Auburn	9	140
Cayuga Medical Center at Ithaca	Ithaca	9	74
Cobleskill Regional Hospital	Cobleskill	9	118
Plainview Hospital	Plainview	9	112
Saint James Mercy Hospital	Hornell	9	88
Aurelia Osborn Fox Memorial Hospital	Oneonta	10	47
Columbia Memorial Hospital	Hudson	10	44
F F Thompson Hospital	Canandaigua	10	124
John T Mather Mem Hosp-Port Jefferson	Port Jefferson	10	120
Lakeside Memorial Hospital	Brockport	10	108
Long Beach Medical Center	Long Beach	10	95
Newark-Wayne Community Hospital	Newark	10	147
Peconic Bay Medical Center	Riverhead	10	126
TLC Health Network	Gowanda	10	79
Forest Hills Hospital	Forest Hills	11	62
Little Falls Hospital[3]	Little Falls	11	52
Queens Hospital Center	Jamaica	11	92
Saint Mary's Hospital at Amsterdam	Amsterdam	11	68
White Plains Hospital Center	White Plains	11	71
Bon Secours Community Hospital	Port Jervis	12	57
Mount Sinai Hospital	New York	12	64
Putnam Hospital Center	Carmel	12	67
Saint Joseph's Medical Center	Yonkers	12	35
Soldiers and Sailors Mem Hosp of Yates	Penn Yan	12	44
Woman's Christian Association	Jamestown	12	79
Alice Hyde Medical Center	Malone	13	89
Clifton Springs Hospital and Clinic	Clifton Springs	13	64
Cortland Regional Medical Center	Cortland	13	179
Kenmore Mercy Hospital	Kenmore	13	36
New York Westchester Square Medical Center	Bronx	13	32
United Memorial Medical Center	Batavia	13	139
Wyoming County Community Hospital	Warsaw	13	100
New York Downtown Hospital	New York	14	35
Saint John's Riverside Hospital	Yonkers	14	41
Samaritan Hospital	Troy	14	36
Sisters of Charity Hospital	Buffalo	14	64
Eastern Niagara Hospital	Lockport	15	154
Brookhaven Memorial Hospital Med Ctr	Patchogue	16	110
Franklin Hospital	Valley Stream	16	111
Brooks Memorial Hospital	Dunkirk	17	151
Lawrence Hospital Center	Bronxville	17	59
Oswego Hospital	Oswego	17	69
Southampton Hospital	Southampton	17	65
Bertrand Chaffee Hospital	Springville	18	97
Sound Shore Medical Center of Westchester	New Rochelle	18	55
Corning Hospital	Corning	19	82
Massena Memorial Hospital	Massena	19	50
Olean General Hospital	Olean	19	359
Geneva General Hospital	Geneva	20	64
Catskill Regional Medical Center	Harris	21	54
Highland Hospital	Rochester	22	25
Wyckoff Heights Medical Center	Brooklyn	32	30

10. Median Time to Transfer (minutes)

Hospital Name	City	Min.	Cases
F F Thompson Hospital	Canandaigua	44	28
Saint Joseph Hospital	Bethpage	45	51
Plainview Hospital	Plainview	58	32
Auburn Memorial Hospital	Auburn	60	27
John T Mather Mem Hosp-Port Jefferson	Port Jefferson	84	28
Franklin Hospital	Valley Stream	94	46
Mount Sinai Hospital	New York	120	28

Heart Failure Care

12. ACE Inhibitor or ARB for LVSD

Hospital Name	City	Rate	Cases
Bellevue Hospital Center	New York	100%	313
Clifton Springs Hospital and Clinic	Clifton Springs	100%	25
Good Samaritan Hospital Medical Center[2]	West Islip	100%	78
Jamaica Hospital Medical Center[2]	Jamaica	100%	132
Metropolitan Hospital Center	New York	100%	49
Mount St Mary's Hospital and Health Center	Lewiston	100%	55
Nassau University Medical Center	East Meadow	100%	86
Nathan Littauer Hospital	Gloversville	100%	36
New York Community Hospital of Brooklyn[2]	Brooklyn	100%	38
New York Westchester Square Medical Center	Bronx	100%	54
Niagara Falls Memorial Medical Center	Niagara Falls	100%	49
NYU Hospitals Center[2]	New York	100%	83
Phelps Memorial Hospital Assn	Sleepy Hollow	100%	39
Saint Joseph Hospital[2]	Bethpage	100%	34
Saint Mary's Hospital at Amsterdam[2]	Amsterdam	100%	53
Southside Hospital[2]	Bay Shore	100%	90
Staten Island University Hospital[2]	Staten Island	100%	95
Strong Memorial Hospital	Rochester	100%	232
Syracuse VA Medical Center	Syracuse	100%	47
Woodhull Medical and Mental Health Center	Brooklyn	100%	186
Ellis Hospital[2]	Schenectady	99%	99
Good Samaritan Hospital of Suffern	Suffern	99%	145
Kingsbrook Jewish Medical Center	Brooklyn	99%	107
Lawrence Hospital Center[2]	Bronxville	99%	77
Lincoln Medical & Mental Health Center	Bronx	99%	122
North Shore University Hospital[2]	Manhasset	99%	131
Westchester Medical Center	Valhalla	99%	135
Glens Falls Hospital[2]	Glens Falls	98%	112
Highland Hospital	Rochester	98%	59
Huntington Hospital[2]	Huntington	98%	65
Jacobi Medical Center	Bronx	98%	93
John T Mather Mem Hosp-Port Jefferson	Port Jefferson	98%	63
Kings County Hospital Center	Brooklyn	98%	306
North Central Bronx Hospital	Bronx	98%	61
Northern Westchester Hospital	Mount Kisco	98%	49
Orange Regional Medical Center	Goshen	98%	129
Our Lady of Lourdes Memorial Hospital	Binghamton	98%	55
Peconic Bay Medical Center	Riverhead	98%	54
Plainview Hospital[2]	Plainview	98%	51
Saratoga Hospital	Saratoga Spgs	98%	43
Unity Hospital of Rochester[2]	Rochester	98%	87
Winthrop-University Hospital[2]	Mineola	98%	130
Woman's Christian Association	Jamestown	98%	65
Benedictine Hospital	Kingston	97%	61
Bronx-Lebanon Hospital Center[2]	Bronx	97%	159
Canton-Potsdam Hospital	Potsdam	97%	34
Hudson Valley Hospital Center	Cortlandt Manor	97%	63
Interfaith Medical Center	Brooklyn	97%	88
Mercy Medical Center	Rockville Centre	97%	78
Northport VA Medical Center	Northport	97%	39
Olean General Hospital	Olean	97%	78
Peninsula Hospital Center	Far Rockaway	97%	61
Rochester General Hospital[2]	Rochester	97%	109
Saint Barnabas Hospital	Bronx	97%	175
Samaritan Hospital	Troy	97%	58
Seton Health System-St Mary's Campus	Troy	97%	32
Sound Shore Medical Center of Westchester	New Rochelle	97%	87
Wyckoff Heights Medical Center[2]	Brooklyn	97%	132
Wyoming County Community Hospital	Warsaw	97%	29
Brookdale Hospital Medical Center[2]	Brooklyn	96%	126
Brooklyn Hospital Center at Downtown Campus	Brooklyn	96%	145
Crouse Hospital	Syracuse	96%	97
Glen Cove Hospital[2]	Glen Cove	96%	28
Kaleida Health	Buffalo	96%	489
Kenmore Mercy Hospital[2]	Kenmore	96%	69
Lenox Hill Hospital[2]	New York	96%	192
Maimonides Medical Center[2]	Brooklyn	96%	114
Mercy Hospital[2]	Buffalo	96%	69
Newark-Wayne Community Hospital	Newark	96%	26
Nyack Hospital	Nyack	96%	80
Saint Joseph's Hospital	Elmira	96%	45
Samaritan Medical Center	Watertown	96%	28
Univ Hosp S U N Y Health Science Ctr	Syracuse	96%	100
Vassar Brothers Medical Center	Poughkeepsie	96%	176
Albany Medical Center Hospital	Albany	95%	172
Arnot Ogden Medical Center	Elmira	95%	74
Beth Israel Medical Center[2]	New York	95%	91
Brookhaven Memorial Hospital Med Ctr[2]	Patchogue	95%	106
Corning Hospital	Corning	95%	42
Franklin Hospital[2]	Valley Stream	95%	87
Long Island Jewish Medical Center[2]	New Hyde Park	95%	142
Mount Sinai Hospital[2]	New York	95%	215
New York Downtown Hospital	New York	95%	39
Saint Catherine of Siena Hospital[2]	Smithtown	95%	58
Saint Peter's Hospital	Albany	95%	132
United Health Services Hospitals	Johnson City	95%	141
University Hospital of Brooklyn - Downstate[2]	Brooklyn	95%	165
Elmhurst Hospital Center	Elmhurst	94%	141
Queens Hospital Center	Jamaica	94%	100
Saint Luke's Roosevelt Hospital[2]	New York	94%	166
United Memorial Medical Center	Batavia	94%	36
Aurelia Osborn Fox Memorial Hospital	Oneonta	93%	44
Bronx VA Medical Center	Bronx	93%	82
Catskill Regional Medical Center	Harris	93%	27
Coney Island Hospital	Brooklyn	93%	153
Harlem Hospital Center[2]	New York	93%	76
New York Methodist Hospital[2]	Brooklyn	93%	148
Rome Memorial Hospital	Rome	93%	55
Saint John's Riverside Hospital[2]	Yonkers	93%	70
Saint Luke's Cornwall Hospital	Newburgh	93%	119
South Nassau Communities Hospital	Oceanside	93%	179
VA New York Harbor Healthcare System	New York	93%	167
White Plains Hospital Center[2]	White Plains	93%	84
Mount Vernon Hospital	Mount Vernon	92%	38
St John's Episcopal Hosp-South Shore	Far Rockaway	92%	61
Saint Joseph's Medical Center	Yonkers	92%	51
Sisters of Charity Hospital[2]	Buffalo	92%	118
Auburn Memorial Hospital	Auburn	91%	54
Forest Hills Hospital[2]	Forest Hills	91%	65
Long Island College Hospital[2]	Brooklyn	91%	114
Mary Imogene Bassett Hospital	Cooperstown	91%	78
Putnam Hospital Center	Carmel	90%	62
Saint Francis Hospital - Roslyn[2]	Roslyn	90%	146
Richmond University Medical Center[2]	Staten Island	89%	57
University Hospital - Stony Brook[2]	Stony Brook	89%	107
Erie County Medical Center	Buffalo	88%	133
Kingston Hospital	Kingston	88%	69
New York Hospital Medical Center of Queens[2]	Flushing	88%	107
New York-Presbyterian Hospital[2]	New York	87%	452
Saint Joseph's Hospital Health Center	Syracuse	87%	254
Comm-General Hosp of Greater Syracuse	Syracuse	86%	43
Columbia Memorial Hospital	Hudson	85%	48
Faxton-St Luke's Healthcare	Utica	85%	103
Lutheran Medical Center	Brooklyn	84%	79
Saint Elizabeth Medical Center	Utica	84%	262
Champlain Valley Physicians Hospital	Plattsburgh	83%	78
F F Thompson Hospital	Canandaigua	82%	33
Upstate New York VA Healthcare System	Buffalo	82%	91
Flushing Hospital Medical Center[2]	Flushing	81%	68
Montefiore Medical Center[2]	Bronx	81%	251
Oswego Hospital	Oswego	81%	37
Adirondack Medical Center	Saranac Lake	80%	25
Cayuga Medical Center at Ithaca	Ithaca	79%	38
Eastern Niagara Hospital	Lockport	74%	38
Medina Memorial Hospital	Medina	73%	37

NOTE: Hospital profiles are in alphabetical order by state, then city, then hospital within the city; Rankings exclude hospitals with less than 25 cases except for patient surveys which excludes hospitals with less than 100 cases; (a) 100–299 cases; (1) The number of cases is too small to be sure how well a hospital is performing; (2) The hospital indicated that the data submitted for this measure were based on a sample of cases; (3) Data was collected during a shorter time period (fewer quarters) than the maximum possible time for this measure; (4) Suppressed for one or more quarters by CMS; (5) No data is available from the hospital for this measure; (6) Fewer than 100 patients completed the HCAHPS survey. Use these rates with caution, as the number of surveys may be too low to reliably assess hospital performance; (7) Survey results are based on less than 12 months of data; (8) Survey results are not available for this reporting period; (9) No or very few patients were eligible for the HCAHPS survey. The scores shown, if any, reflect a very small number of surveys; (10) A state average was not calculated because too few hospitals in the state submitted data; (11) There were discrepancies in the data collection process; Please refer to the User's Guide for a full explanation of data.

Nicholas H Noyes Memorial Hospital	Dansville	71%	51
Cortland Regional Medical Center	Cortland	66%	38

13. Discharge Instructions

Hospital Name	City	Rate	Cases
Albany VA Medical Center	Albany	100%	62
Bellevue Hospital Center	New York	100%	471
Elmhurst Hospital Center	Elmhurst	100%	315
Good Samaritan Hospital Medical Center[2]	West Islip	100%	259
Huntington Hospital[2]	Huntington	100%	220
Ira Davenport Memorial Hospital	Bath	100%	31
Jamaica Hospital Medical Center[2]	Jamaica	100%	271
Lincoln Medical & Mental Health Center	Bronx	100%	366
Saint Anthony Community Hospital	Warwick	100%	73
Saint Charles Hospital	Port Jefferson	100%	67
Saint Francis Hospital	Poughkeepsie	100%	42
St John's Episcopal Hosp-South Shore	Far Rockaway	100%	110
Benedictine Hospital	Kingston	99%	186
Bronx VA Medical Center	Bronx	99%	138
Bronx-Lebanon Hospital Center[2]	Bronx	99%	327
Ellis Hospital[2]	Schenectady	99%	440
Jacobi Medical Center	Bronx	99%	232
North Central Bronx Hospital	Bronx	99%	131
Richmond University Medical Center[2]	Staten Island	99%	105
Saint Catherine of Siena Hospital[2]	Smithtown	99%	195
Southampton Hospital	Southampton	99%	88
Good Samaritan Hospital of Suffern	Suffern	98%	263
John T Mather Mem Hosp-Port Jefferson	Port Jefferson	98%	250
Lakeside Memorial Hospital	Brockport	98%	96
Lawrence Hospital Center[2]	Bronxville	98%	195
North Shore University Hospital[2]	Manhasset	98%	313
Northport VA Medical Center	Northport	98%	115
Peconic Bay Medical Center	Riverhead	98%	177
Sound Shore Medical Center of Westchester	New Rochelle	98%	177
South Nassau Communities Hospital	Oceanside	98%	382
Southside Hospital[2]	Bay Shore	98%	228
Staten Island University Hospital[2]	Staten Island	98%	241
Strong Memorial Hospital	Rochester	98%	647
VA New York Harbor Healthcare System	New York	98%	353
Vassar Brothers Medical Center	Poughkeepsie	98%	466
Clifton Springs Hospital and Clinic	Clifton Springs	97%	72
Erie County Medical Center	Buffalo	97%	254
Highland Hospital	Rochester	97%	215
Long Island College Hospital[2]	Brooklyn	97%	272
Lutheran Medical Center	Brooklyn	97%	296
Massena Memorial Hospital	Massena	97%	75
Nassau University Medical Center	East Meadow	97%	198
New York Downtown Hospital	New York	97%	119
NYU Hospitals Center[2]	New York	97%	217
Saint Joseph Hospital[2]	Bethpage	97%	200
Soldiers and Sailors Mem Hosp of Yates	Penn Yan	97%	29
Unity Hospital of Rochester[2]	Rochester	97%	253
Wyckoff Heights Medical Center[2]	Brooklyn	97%	249
Glen Cove Hospital[2]	Glen Cove	96%	170
Nathan Littauer Hospital	Gloversville	96%	78
Peninsula Hospital Center	Far Rockaway	96%	114
Queens Hospital Center	Jamaica	96%	246
Saint Luke's Roosevelt Hospital[2]	New York	96%	282
Chenango Memorial Hospital	Norwich	95%	58
Franklin Hospital[2]	Valley Stream	95%	204
Kingston Hospital	Kingston	95%	167
New York Community Hospital of Brooklyn[2]	Brooklyn	95%	233
Northern Westchester Hospital	Mount Kisco	95%	156
Plainview Hospital[2]	Plainview	95%	192
Saratoga Hospital	Saratoga Spgs	95%	239
Upstate New York VA Healthcare System	Buffalo	95%	154
Cobleskill Regional Hospital	Cobleskill	94%	33
Phelps Memorial Hospital Assn	Sleepy Hollow	94%	98
Saint Joseph's Hospital	Elmira	94%	69
University Hospital of Brooklyn - Downstate[2]	Brooklyn	94%	282
Brookdale Hospital Medical Center[2]	Brooklyn	93%	286
Coney Island Hospital	Brooklyn	93%	406
New York Hospital Medical Center of Queens[2]	Flushing	93%	257
Niagara Falls Memorial Medical Center	Niagara Falls	93%	121
Saint Barnabas Hospital	Bronx	93%	324
Syracuse VA Medical Center	Syracuse	93%	152
Corning Hospital	Corning	92%	96
Mercy Medical Center	Rockville Centre	92%	160
Rochester General Hospital[2]	Rochester	92%	259
Saint Mary's Hospital at Amsterdam[2]	Amsterdam	92%	195
Saint Peter's Hospital	Albany	92%	399
Albany Medical Center Hospital	Albany	91%	324
Bertrand Chaffee Hospital	Springville	91%	32
Brooklyn Hospital Center at Downtown Campus	Brooklyn	91%	361
Claxton-Hepburn Medical Center	Ogdensburg	91%	45
Forest Hills Hospital[2]	Forest Hills	91%	191
Putnam Hospital Center	Carmel	91%	159
Saint Joseph's Medical Center	Yonkers	91%	135
United Memorial Medical Center	Batavia	91%	114
University Hospital - Stony Brook[2]	Stony Brook	91%	213
Westchester Medical Center	Valhalla	91%	257
Adirondack Medical Center	Saranac Lake	90%	62
Alice Hyde Medical Center	Malone	90%	50
Columbia Memorial Hospital	Hudson	90%	164
Hudson Valley Hospital Center	Cortlandt Manor	90%	157
Kingsbrook Jewish Medical Center	Brooklyn	90%	174
Mercy Hospital[2]	Buffalo	90%	244
New York Methodist Hospital[2]	Brooklyn	90%	277
Nyack Hospital	Nyack	90%	176
Seton Health System-St Mary's Campus	Troy	90%	139
TLC Health Network	Gowanda	90%	42
White Plains Hospital Center[2]	White Plains	90%	208
Flushing Hospital Medical Center[2]	Flushing	89%	124
Long Beach Medical Center[2]	Long Beach	89%	61
Long Island Jewish Medical Center[2]	New Hyde Park	89%	243
Mount St Mary's Hospital and Health Center	Lewiston	89%	190
Rome Memorial Hospital	Rome	89%	126
Saint Joseph's Hospital Health Center	Syracuse	89%	561
Brookhaven Memorial Hospital Med Ctr[2]	Patchogue	88%	302
Cortland Regional Medical Center	Cortland	88%	88
Lenox Hill Hospital[2]	New York	88%	365
Mount Vernon Hospital	Mount Vernon	88%	84
Orange Regional Medical Center	Goshen	88%	360
Saint Elizabeth Medical Center	Utica	88%	465
Canton-Potsdam Hospital	Potsdam	87%	85
Community Memorial Hospital	Hamilton	87%	30
Newark-Wayne Community Hospital	Newark	87%	78
Olean General Hospital	Olean	87%	171
Our Lady of Lourdes Memorial Hospital	Binghamton	87%	163
United Health Services Hospitals	Johnson City	87%	343
Winthrop-University Hospital[2]	Mineola	87%	284
Champlain Valley Physicians Hospital	Plattsburgh	86%	286
Kenmore Mercy Hospital[2]	Kenmore	86%	197
Maimonides Medical Center[2]	Brooklyn	86%	300
Montefiore Medical Center[2]	Bronx	86%	544
Saint Francis Hospital - Roslyn[2]	Roslyn	86%	310
Saint John's Riverside Hospital[2]	Yonkers	86%	191
Catskill Regional Medical Center	Harris	85%	55
Univ Hosp S U N Y Health Science Ctr	Syracuse	85%	212
Woodhull Medical and Mental Health Center	Brooklyn	85%	287
Aurelia Osborn Fox Memorial Hospital	Oneonta	84%	138
Bon Secours Community Hospital	Port Jervis	84%	77
Kaleida Health	Buffalo	84%	1265
Albany Memorial Hospital	Albany	83%	102
Mary Imogene Bassett Hospital	Cooperstown	83%	185
Metropolitan Hospital Center	New York	83%	128
Brooks Memorial Hospital	Dunkirk	82%	50
Interfaith Medical Center	Brooklyn	82%	188
Nicholas H Noyes Memorial Hospital	Dansville	82%	115
Arnot Ogden Medical Center	Elmira	81%	188
Eastern Long Island Hospital	Greenport	81%	36
Faxton-St Luke's Healthcare	Utica	81%	208
Medina Memorial Hospital	Medina	81%	63
Mount Sinai Hospital[2]	New York	81%	441
Oswego Hospital	Oswego	81%	99
Samaritan Medical Center	Watertown	81%	188
Woman's Christian Association	Jamestown	81%	224
Wyoming County Community Hospital	Warsaw	81%	57
New York Westchester Square Medical Center	Bronx	80%	159
Northern Dutchess Hospital	Rhinebeck	80%	51
Saint Luke's Cornwall Hospital	Newburgh	80%	337
Samaritan Hospital	Troy	80%	143
Auburn Memorial Hospital	Auburn	79%	155
Harlem Hospital Center[2]	New York	78%	206
Geneva General Hospital	Geneva	77%	109
Sisters of Charity Hospital[2]	Buffalo	77%	393
Cayuga Medical Center at Ithaca	Ithaca	75%	103
Glens Falls Hospital[2]	Glens Falls	75%	268
Jones Memorial Hospital	Wellsville	74%	54
Comm-General Hosp of Greater Syracuse	Syracuse	73%	121
Crouse Hospital	Syracuse	71%	331
Eastern Niagara Hospital	Lockport	71%	128
Carthage Area Hospital	Carthage	70%	54
New York-Presbyterian Hospital[2]	New York	70%	883
Kings County Hospital Center	Brooklyn	69%	577
F F Thompson Hospital	Canandaigua	66%	123
Beth Israel Medical Center[2]	New York	64%	260
Lewis County General Hospital	Lowville	48%	29
Edward John Noble Hospital of Gouverneur	Gouverneur	42%	40

14. Evaluation of LVS Function

Hospital Name	City	Rate	Cases
Albany Medical Center Hospital	Albany	100%	386
Albany VA Medical Center	Albany	100%	71
Arnot Ogden Medical Center	Elmira	100%	225
Bellevue Hospital Center	New York	100%	539
Bertrand Chaffee Hospital	Springville	100%	53
Bronx VA Medical Center	Bronx	100%	149
Catskill Regional Medical Center	Harris	100%	80
Champlain Valley Physicians Hospital	Plattsburgh	100%	356
Claxton-Hepburn Medical Center	Ogdensburg	100%	57
Clifton Springs Hospital and Clinic	Clifton Springs	100%	81
Corning Hospital	Corning	100%	137
Eastern Long Island Hospital	Greenport	100%	47
Elmhurst Hospital Center	Elmhurst	100%	339
Forest Hills Hospital[2]	Forest Hills	100%	267
Franklin Hospital[2]	Valley Stream	100%	273
Glen Cove Hospital[2]	Glen Cove	100%	249
Glens Falls Hospital[2]	Glens Falls	100%	338
Good Samaritan Hospital Medical Center[2]	West Islip	100%	344
Hudson Valley Hospital Center	Cortlandt Manor	100%	257
Huntington Hospital[2]	Huntington	100%	292
Interfaith Medical Center	Brooklyn	100%	209
Ira Davenport Memorial Hospital	Bath	100%	38
Jamaica Hospital Medical Center[2]	Jamaica	100%	310
John T Mather Mem Hosp-Port Jefferson	Port Jefferson	100%	389
Kings County Hospital Center	Brooklyn	100%	602
Kingsbrook Jewish Medical Center	Brooklyn	100%	265
Lenox Hill Hospital[2]	New York	100%	444
Lincoln Medical & Mental Health Center	Bronx	100%	396
Maimonides Medical Center[2]	Brooklyn	100%	359
Mary Imogene Bassett Hospital	Cooperstown	100%	216
Mercy Hospital[2]	Buffalo	100%	334
Mount St Mary's Hospital and Health Center	Lewiston	100%	241
Nassau University Medical Center	East Meadow	100%	245
New York Community Hospital of Brooklyn[2]	Brooklyn	100%	266
New York Downtown Hospital	New York	100%	133
New York Hospital Medical Center of Queens[2]	Flushing	100%	337
New York Methodist Hospital[2]	Brooklyn	100%	340
New York Westchester Square Medical Center	Bronx	100%	257
North Central Bronx Hospital	Bronx	100%	139
North Shore University Hospital[2]	Manhasset	100%	398
Northern Dutchess Hospital	Rhinebeck	100%	77
Northern Westchester Hospital	Mount Kisco	100%	198
Northport VA Medical Center	Northport	100%	131
NYU Hospitals Center[2]	New York	100%	283
Olean General Hospital	Olean	100%	261
Plainview Hospital[2]	Plainview	100%	270
Queens Hospital Center	Jamaica	100%	269
Saint Barnabas Hospital	Bronx	100%	354
Saint Francis Hospital	Poughkeepsie	100%	79
Saint Francis Hospital - Roslyn[2]	Roslyn	100%	357
Saint Joseph Hospital[2]	Bethpage	100%	251
Saint Joseph's Hospital	Elmira	100%	93
Saint Joseph's Medical Center	Yonkers	100%	200
Saint Luke's Cornwall Hospital	Newburgh	100%	429
Saint Mary's Hospital at Amsterdam[2]	Amsterdam	100%	244
Saratoga Hospital	Saratoga Spgs	100%	280
Schuyler Hospital	Montour Falls	100%	33
Sisters of Charity Hospital[2]	Buffalo	100%	516
Southside Hospital[2]	Bay Shore	100%	287
Staten Island University Hospital[2]	Staten Island	100%	301
Unity Hospital of Rochester[2]	Rochester	100%	322
Univ Hosp S U N Y Health Science Ctr	Syracuse	100%	266
Upstate New York VA Healthcare System	Buffalo	100%	184
VA Hudson Valley Healthcare System	Montrose	100%	26
VA New York Harbor Healthcare System	New York	100%	364
Vassar Brothers Medical Center	Poughkeepsie	100%	632
Westchester Medical Center	Valhalla	100%	293
White Plains Hospital Center[2]	White Plains	100%	277
Winthrop-University Hospital[2]	Mineola	100%	337
Woman's Christian Association	Jamestown	100%	273
Woodhull Medical and Mental Health Center	Brooklyn	100%	317
Wyckoff Heights Medical Center[2]	Brooklyn	100%	297
Wyoming County Community Hospital	Warsaw	100%	85
Bon Secours Community Hospital	Port Jervis	99%	97
Bronx-Lebanon Hospital Center[2]	Bronx	99%	371
Brookdale Hospital Medical Center[2]	Brooklyn	99%	327
Brookhaven Memorial Hospital Med Ctr[2]	Patchogue	99%	457
Coney Island Hospital	Brooklyn	99%	498
Crouse Hospital	Syracuse	99%	409
Erie County Medical Center	Buffalo	99%	311
F F Thompson Hospital	Canandaigua	99%	145
Good Samaritan Hospital of Suffern	Suffern	99%	375
Harlem Hospital Center[2]	New York	99%	219
Highland Hospital	Rochester	99%	309
Jacobi Medical Center	Bronx	99%	276
Kaleida Health	Buffalo	99%	1555
Kenmore Mercy Hospital[2]	Kenmore	99%	274
Kingston Hospital	Kingston	99%	208
Lawrence Hospital Center[2]	Bronxville	99%	256
Long Island Jewish Medical Center[2]	New Hyde Park	99%	306
Massena Memorial Hospital	Massena	99%	103
Mercy Medical Center	Rockville Centre	99%	226
Metropolitan Hospital Center	New York	99%	142
Newark-Wayne Community Hospital	Newark	99%	108
Nyack Hospital	Nyack	99%	249
Orange Regional Medical Center	Goshen	99%	485
Peninsula Hospital Center	Far Rockaway	99%	157
Phelps Memorial Hospital Assn	Sleepy Hollow	99%	152
Putnam Hospital Center	Carmel	99%	225

NOTE: Hospital profiles are in alphabetical order by state, then city, then hospital within the city; Rankings exclude hospitals with less than 25 cases except for patient surveys which excludes hospitals with less than 100 cases; (a) 100–299 cases; (1) The number of cases is too small to be sure how well a hospital is performing; (2) The hospital indicated that the data submitted for this measure were based on a sample of cases; (3) Data was collected during a shorter time period (fewer quarters) than the maximum possible time for this measure; (4) Suppressed for one or more quarters by CMS; (5) No data is available from the hospital for this measure; (6) Fewer than 100 patients completed the HCAHPS survey. Use these rates with caution, as the number of surveys may be too low to reliably assess hospital performance; (7) Survey results are based on less than 12 months of data; (8) Survey results are not available for this reporting period; (9) No or very few patients were eligible for the HCAHPS survey. The scores shown, if any, reflect a very small number of surveys; (10) A state average was not calculated because too few hospitals in the state submitted data; (11) There were discrepancies in the data collection process; Please refer to the User's Guide for a full explanation of data.

Richmond University Medical Center[2]	Staten Island	99%	158
Rochester General Hospital[2]	Rochester	99%	315
Saint Anthony Community Hospital	Warwick	99%	92
Saint Charles Hospital	Port Jefferson	99%	80
Samaritan Hospital	Troy	99%	183
Sound Shore Medical Center of Westschester	New Rochelle	99%	291
South Nassau Communities Hospital	Oceanside	99%	502
Southampton Hospital	Southampton	99%	113
Strong Memorial Hospital	Rochester	99%	738
Syracuse VA Medical Center	Syracuse	99%	167
United Health Services Hospitals	Johnson City	99%	451
United Memorial Medical Center	Batavia	99%	158
University Hospital - Stony Brook[2]	Stony Brook	99%	275
Benedictine Hospital	Kingston	98%	239
Beth Israel Medical Center[2]	New York	98%	307
Brooklyn Hospital Center at Downtown Campus	Brooklyn	98%	426
Ellis Hospital[2]	Schenectady	98%	572
Flushing Hospital Medical Center[2]	Flushing	98%	255
Lakeside Memorial Hospital	Brockport	98%	124
Lutheran Medical Center	Brooklyn	98%	402
Montefiore Medical Center[2]	Bronx	98%	679
Niagara Falls Memorial Medical Center	Niagara Falls	98%	145
Our Lady of Lourdes Memorial Hospital	Binghamton	98%	226
Saint Joseph's Hospital Health Center	Syracuse	98%	697
Samaritan Medical Center	Watertown	98%	216
Seton Health System-St Mary's Campus	Troy	98%	172
University Hospital of Brooklyn - Downstate[2]	Brooklyn	98%	292
Alice Hyde Medical Center	Malone	97%	59
Brooks Memorial Hospital	Dunkirk	97%	76
Canton-Potsdam Hospital	Potsdam	97%	99
Carthage Area Hospital	Carthage	97%	61
Mount Sinai Hospital[2]	New York	97%	555
New York-Presbyterian Hospital[2]	New York	97%	1062
Saint Luke's Roosevelt Hospital[2]	New York	97%	324
Saint Peter's Hospital	Albany	97%	490
Albany Memorial Hospital	Albany	96%	135
Auburn Memorial Hospital	Auburn	96%	196
Cayuga Medical Center at Ithaca	Ithaca	96%	130
Chenango Memorial Hospital	Norwich	96%	71
Comm-General Hosp of Greater Syracuse	Syracuse	96%	189
Long Island College Hospital[2]	Brooklyn	96%	311
Medina Memorial Hospital	Medina	96%	102
Peconic Bay Medical Center	Riverhead	96%	234
Rome Memorial Hospital	Rome	96%	204
Saint Elizabeth Medical Center	Utica	96%	607
St John's Episcopal Hosp-South Shore	Far Rockaway	96%	186
Cobleskill Regional Hospital	Cobleskill	95%	42
Columbia Memorial Hospital	Hudson	95%	226
Long Beach Medical Center[2]	Long Beach	95%	103
Saint Catherine of Siena Hospital[2]	Smithtown	95%	326
Aurelia Osborn Fox Memorial Hospital	Oneonta	94%	170
Geneva General Hospital	Geneva	94%	148
Jones Memorial Hospital	Wellsville	94%	63
Oswego Hospital	Oswego	94%	160
Faxton-St Luke's Healthcare	Utica	93%	309
Lewis County General Hospital	Lowville	93%	42
Saint James Mercy Hospital	Hornell	93%	29
Saint John's Riverside Hospital[2]	Yonkers	93%	260
Cortland Regional Medical Center	Cortland	92%	118
Adirondack Medical Center	Saranac Lake	91%	69
Community Memorial Hospital	Hamilton	91%	44
Nicholas H Noyes Memorial Hospital	Dansville	91%	148
Eastern Niagara Hospital	Lockport	90%	181
Delaware Valley Hospital[2]	Walton	89%	27
Mount Vernon Hospital	Mount Vernon	88%	122
Soldiers and Sailors Mem Hosp of Yates	Penn Yan	88%	34
TLC Health Network	Gowanda	88%	72
Nathan Littauer Hospital	Gloversville	87%	93
Oneida Healthcare Center	Oneida	87%	30
Edward John Noble Hospital of Gouverneur	Gouverneur	79%	53

15. Smoking Cessation Advice

Hospital Name	City	Rate	Cases
Albany Medical Center Hospital	Albany	100%	64
Arnot Ogden Medical Center	Elmira	100%	38
Bellevue Hospital Center	New York	100%	129
Benedictine Hospital	Kingston	100%	40
Brookhaven Memorial Hospital Med Ctr[2]	Patchogue	100%	48
Brooklyn Hospital Center at Downtown Campus	Brooklyn	100%	61
Columbia Memorial Hospital	Hudson	100%	34
Coney Island Hospital	Brooklyn	100%	96
Ellis Hospital[2]	Schenectady	100%	73
Elmhurst Hospital Center	Elmhurst	100%	61
Erie County Medical Center	Buffalo	100%	90
Franklin Hospital[2]	Valley Stream	100%	29
Glens Falls Hospital[2]	Glens Falls	100%	40
Good Samaritan Hospital Medical Center[2]	West Islip	100%	34
Good Samaritan Hospital of Suffern	Suffern	100%	52
Harlem Hospital Center[2]	New York	100%	69
Highland Hospital	Rochester	100%	43
Hudson Valley Hospital Center	Cortlandt Manor	100%	32
Jacobi Medical Center	Bronx	100%	64
Jamaica Hospital Medical Center[2]	Jamaica	100%	45
John T Mather Mem Hosp-Port Jefferson	Port Jefferson	100%	29
Kaleida Health	Buffalo	100%	274
Kingston Hospital	Kingston	100%	37
Lincoln Medical & Mental Health Center	Bronx	100%	69
Long Island College Hospital[2]	Brooklyn	100%	43
Maimonides Medical Center[2]	Brooklyn	100%	29
Mary Imogene Bassett Hospital	Cooperstown	100%	35
Montefiore Medical Center[2]	Bronx	100%	103
Mount Vernon Hospital	Mount Vernon	100%	27
Nassau University Medical Center	East Meadow	100%	54
New York Hospital Medical Center of Queens[2]	Flushing	100%	34
New York Methodist Hospital[2]	Brooklyn	100%	32
New York Westchester Square Medical Center	Bronx	100%	33
Niagara Falls Memorial Medical Center	Niagara Falls	100%	35
North Central Bronx Hospital	Bronx	100%	40
North Shore University Hospital[2]	Manhasset	100%	26
Olean General Hospital	Olean	100%	32
Orange Regional Medical Center	Goshen	100%	52
Peninsula Hospital Center	Far Rockaway	100%	26
Richmond University Medical Center[2]	Staten Island	100%	31
Rochester General Hospital[2]	Rochester	100%	48
Saint Francis Hospital - Roslyn[2]	Roslyn	100%	30
St John's Episcopal Hosp-South Shore	Far Rockaway	100%	39
Saint Joseph's Medical Center	Yonkers	100%	26
Saint Luke's Cornwall Hospital	Newburgh	100%	50
Saint Luke's Roosevelt Hospital[2]	New York	100%	70
Saint Mary's Hospital at Amsterdam[2]	Amsterdam	100%	30
Saint Peter's Hospital	Albany	100%	61
Samaritan Hospital	Troy	100%	29
Saratoga Hospital	Saratoga Spgs	100%	40
Seton Health System-St Mary's Campus	Troy	100%	25
Sound Shore Medical Center of Westchester	New Rochelle	100%	30
South Nassau Communities Hospital	Oceanside	100%	34
Southside Hospital[2]	Bay Shore	100%	47
Staten Island University Hospital[2]	Staten Island	100%	35
Syracuse VA Medical Center	Syracuse	100%	25
United Health Services Hospitals	Johnson City	100%	51
Unity Hospital of Rochester[2]	Rochester	100%	35
University Hospital - Stony Brook[2]	Stony Brook	100%	50
Univ Hosp S U N Y Health Science Ctr	Syracuse	100%	66
Upstate New York VA Healthcare System	Buffalo	100%	27
Vassar Brothers Medical Center	Poughkeepsie	100%	78
Westchester Medical Center	Valhalla	100%	47
Winthrop-University Hospital[2]	Mineola	100%	34
Woman's Christian Association	Jamestown	100%	39
Woodhull Medical and Mental Health Center	Brooklyn	100%	132
Wyckoff Heights Medical Center[2]	Brooklyn	100%	44
Bronx-Lebanon Hospital Center[2]	Bronx	99%	80
Saint Barnabas Hospital	Bronx	99%	123
Saint Elizabeth Medical Center	Utica	99%	89
Saint Joseph's Hospital Health Center	Syracuse	99%	163
Strong Memorial Hospital	Rochester	99%	124
Crouse Hospital	Syracuse	98%	56
VA New York Harbor Healthcare System	New York	98%	61
Beth Israel Medical Center[2]	New York	97%	33
Brookdale Hospital Medical Center[2]	Brooklyn	97%	61
Champlain Valley Physicians Hospital	Plattsburgh	97%	62
Faxton-St Luke's Healthcare	Utica	97%	34
Long Island Jewish Medical Center[2]	New Hyde Park	97%	39
Mount Sinai Hospital[2]	New York	97%	72
New York-Presbyterian Hospital[2]	New York	97%	87
Sisters of Charity Hospital[2]	Buffalo	97%	61
Kings County Hospital Center	Brooklyn	96%	105
White Plains Hospital Center[2]	White Plains	96%	25
Mercy Hospital[2]	Buffalo	95%	37
Queens Hospital Center	Jamaica	94%	35
University Hospital of Brooklyn - Downstate[2]	Brooklyn	92%	36
Interfaith Medical Center	Brooklyn	91%	82
Lenox Hill Hospital[2]	New York	91%	54

Pneumonia Care

16. Appropriate Initial Antibiotic

Hospital Name	City	Rate	Cases
Bath VA Medical Center	Bath	100%	41
Clifton Springs Hospital and Clinic	Clifton Springs	100%	85
Cobleskill Regional Hospital	Cobleskill	100%	61
Good Samaritan Hospital Medical Center[2]	West Islip	100%	73
Kingsbrook Jewish Medical Center	Brooklyn	100%	105
Lenox Hill Hospital[2]	New York	100%	88
Metropolitan Hospital Center	New York	100%	70
New York Community Hospital of Brooklyn[2]	Brooklyn	100%	81
NYU Hospitals Center[2]	New York	100%	74
Jamaica Hospital Medical Center[2]	Jamaica	99%	95
Saint Francis Hospital	Poughkeepsie	99%	67
Syracuse VA Medical Center	Syracuse	99%	82
Brooklyn Hospital Center at Downtown Campus	Brooklyn	98%	96
Claxton-Hepburn Medical Center	Ogdensburg	98%	48
Harlem Hospital Center[2]	New York	98%	47
Highland Hospital	Rochester	98%	167
Hudson Valley Hospital Center	Cortlandt Manor	98%	96
John T Mather Mem Hosp-Port Jefferson	Port Jefferson	98%	193
North Central Bronx Hospital	Bronx	98%	55
Northport VA Medical Center	Northport	98%	43
Saint Joseph's Hospital	Elmira	98%	95
Comm-General Hosp of Greater Syracuse[2]	Syracuse	97%	91
Kings County Hospital Center	Brooklyn	97%	117
Lutheran Medical Center	Brooklyn	97%	219
Niagara Falls Memorial Medical Center	Niagara Falls	97%	96
Saint Barnabas Hospital	Bronx	97%	150
Southside Hospital[2]	Bay Shore	97%	104
Unity Hospital of Rochester[2]	Rochester	97%	114
Albany Memorial Hospital[2]	Albany	96%	75
Ellis Hospital[2]	Schenectady	96%	171
Glen Cove Hospital[2]	Glen Cove	96%	71
Huntington Hospital[2]	Huntington	96%	82
Interfaith Medical Center	Brooklyn	96%	81
Kingston Hospital	Kingston	96%	135
Maimonides Medical Center[2]	Brooklyn	96%	74
New York Downtown Hospital[2]	New York	96%	107
Nyack Hospital[2]	Nyack	96%	105
Saint Charles Hospital	Port Jefferson	96%	73
Staten Island University Hospital[2]	Staten Island	96%	89
United Health Services Hospitals	Johnson City	96%	200
Univ Hosp S U N Y Health Science Ctr	Syracuse	96%	78
Woodhull Medical and Mental Health Center	Brooklyn	96%	124
Bertrand Chaffee Hospital	Springville	95%	88
Bon Secours Community Hospital	Port Jervis	95%	75
Corning Hospital	Corning	95%	81
Franklin Hospital[2]	Valley Stream	95%	94
Kaleida Health	Buffalo	95%	623
Lincoln Medical & Mental Health Center	Bronx	95%	257
Mary Imogene Bassett Hospital	Cooperstown	95%	57
Mercy Hospital[2]	Buffalo	95%	97
North Shore University Hospital[2]	Manhasset	95%	154
Plainview Hospital[2]	Plainview	95%	96
Queens Hospital Center	Jamaica	95%	103
Rochester General Hospital	Rochester	95%	369
Southampton Hospital	Southampton	95%	118
TLC Health Network	Gowanda	95%	63
VA New York Harbor Healthcare System	New York	95%	88
Benedictine Hospital	Kingston	94%	79
Community Memorial Hospital	Hamilton	94%	70
Kenmore Mercy Hospital[2]	Kenmore	94%	93
Mount Vernon Hospital	Mount Vernon	94%	52
New York-Presbyterian Hospital[2]	New York	94%	210
Northern Westchester Hospital[2]	Mount Kisco	94%	71
Oneida Healthcare Center	Oneida	94%	65
Putnam Hospital Center	Carmel	94%	107
Saint James Mercy Hospital	Hornell	94%	71
Saint Joseph's Medical Center	Yonkers	94%	84
Saint Mary's Hospital at Amsterdam[2]	Amsterdam	94%	81
Samaritan Medical Center	Watertown	94%	101
Saratoga Hospital	Saratoga Spgs	94%	162
Winthrop-University Hospital[2]	Mineola	94%	107
Albany VA Medical Center	Albany	93%	27
Alice Hyde Medical Center	Malone	93%	75
Arnot Ogden Medical Center	Elmira	93%	122
Beth Israel Medical Center[2]	New York	93%	108
Bronx VA Medical Center	Bronx	93%	58
Catskill Regional Medical Center	Harris	93%	83
Crouse Hospital	Syracuse	93%	180
Elmhurst Hospital Center	Elmhurst	93%	225
Flushing Hospital Medical Center[2]	Flushing	93%	42
Lawrence Hospital Center[2]	Bronxville	93%	105
Mount St Mary's Hospital and Health Center	Lewiston	93%	140
New York Hospital Medical Center of Queens[2]	Flushing	93%	90
New York Methodist Hospital[2]	Brooklyn	93%	90
New York Westchester Square Medical Center	Bronx	93%	114
Nicholas H Noyes Memorial Hospital	Dansville	93%	91
Oswego Hospital	Oswego	93%	130
Our Lady of Lourdes Memorial Hospital	Binghamton	93%	200
Saint Joseph Hospital[2]	Bethpage	93%	120
Samaritan Hospital[2]	Troy	93%	94
South Nassau Communities Hospital	Oceanside	93%	211
United Memorial Medical Center	Batavia	93%	83
Eastern Niagara Hospital	Lockport	92%	129
Jacobi Medical Center	Bronx	92%	86
Phelps Memorial Hospital Assn	Sleepy Hollow	92%	73
Saint Peter's Hospital[2]	Albany	92%	91
Vassar Brothers Medical Center[2]	Poughkeepsie	92%	142
Aurelia Osborn Fox Memorial Hospital	Oneonta	91%	74
Brookdale Hospital Medical Center[2]	Brooklyn	91%	79
Delaware Valley Hospital	Walton	91%	47
Long Beach Medical Center[2]	Long Beach	91%	58
Long Island College Hospital[2]	Brooklyn	91%	77
Mercy Medical Center	Rockville Centre	91%	113
Mount Sinai Hospital[2]	New York	91%	129

NOTE: Hospital profiles are in alphabetical order by state, then city, then hospital within the city; Rankings exclude hospitals with less than 25 cases except for patient surveys which excludes hospitals with less than 100 cases; (a) 100–299 cases; (1) The number of cases is too small to be sure how well a hospital is performing; (2) The hospital indicated that the data submitted for this measure were based on a sample of cases; (3) Data was collected during a shorter time period (fewer quarters) than the maximum possible time for this measure; (4) Suppressed for one or more quarters by CMS; (5) No data is available from the hospital for this measure; (6) Fewer than 100 patients completed the HCAHPS survey. Use these rates with caution, as the number of surveys may be too low to reliably assess hospital performance; (7) Survey results are based on less than 12 months of data; (8) Survey results are not available for this reporting period; (9) No or very few patients were eligible for the HCAHPS survey. The scores shown, if any, reflect a very small number of surveys; (10) A state average was not calculated because too few hospitals in the state submitted data; (11) There were discrepancies in the data collection process; Please refer to the User's Guide for a full explanation of data.

Orange Regional Medical Center	Goshen	91%	284
Saint Elizabeth Medical Center	Utica	91%	103
Saint Joseph's Hospital Health Center	Syracuse	91%	387
Saint Luke's Roosevelt Hospital[2]	New York	91%	115
Sisters of Charity Hospital[2]	Buffalo	91%	216
Sound Shore Medical Center of Westschester	New Rochelle	91%	117
Upstate New York VA Healthcare System	Buffalo	91%	57
Woman's Christian Association	Jamestown	91%	105
Columbia Memorial Hospital	Hudson	90%	126
Glens Falls Hospital[2]	Glens Falls	90%	132
Long Island Jewish Medical Center[2]	New Hyde Park	90%	92
Richmond University Medical Center[2]	Staten Island	90%	51
Schuyler Hospital	Montour Falls	90%	41
Seton Health System-St Mary's Campus	Troy	90%	94
Brookhaven Memorial Hospital Med Ctr[2]	Patchogue	89%	240
Brooks Memorial Hospital	Dunkirk	89%	62
Nathan Littauer Hospital	Gloversville	89%	66
Peconic Bay Medical Center	Riverhead	89%	82
Albany Medical Center Hospital	Albany	88%	123
Auburn Memorial Hospital	Auburn	88%	205
Coney Island Hospital	Brooklyn	88%	108
Erie County Medical Center	Buffalo	88%	93
Jones Memorial Hospital	Wellsville	88%	52
Olean General Hospital	Olean	88%	138
Peninsula Hospital Center	Far Rockaway	88%	84
Rome Memorial Hospital	Rome	88%	100
University Hospital - Stony Brook[2]	Stony Brook	88%	69
White Plains Hospital Center[2]	White Plains	88%	108
Wyckoff Heights Medical Center[2]	Brooklyn	88%	117
Bellevue Hospital Center	New York	87%	134
F F Thompson Hospital	Canandaigua	87%	163
Forest Hills Hospital[2]	Forest Hills	87%	77
Massena Memorial Hospital	Massena	87%	61
Saint John's Riverside Hospital[2]	Yonkers	87%	75
Canton-Potsdam Hospital	Potsdam	86%	74
Medina Memorial Hospital	Medina	86%	73
Saint Anthony Community Hospital	Warwick	86%	49
Saint Francis Hospital - Roslyn	Roslyn	86%	110
Saint Luke's Cornwall Hospital[2]	Newburgh	86%	115
University Hospital of Brooklyn - Downstate[2]	Brooklyn	86%	76
Champlain Valley Physicians Hospital	Plattsburgh	85%	187
Chenango Memorial Hospital	Norwich	85%	66
Geneva General Hospital[2]	Geneva	85%	73
Good Samaritan Hospital of Suffern	Suffern	85%	184
Nassau University Medical Center	East Meadow	85%	93
Newark-Wayne Community Hospital	Newark	85%	91
Cortland Regional Medical Center	Cortland	84%	170
Northern Dutchess Hospital	Rhinebeck	84%	38
Lakeside Memorial Hospital	Brockport	83%	98
Eastern Long Island Hospital	Greenport	82%	39
Strong Memorial Hospital[2]	Rochester	82%	74
Little Falls Hospital[3]	Little Falls	81%	42
Montefiore Medical Center[2]	Bronx	81%	190
Saint Catherine of Siena Hospital[2]	Smithtown	81%	110
Soldiers and Sailors Mem Hosp of Yates	Penn Yan	81%	36
Wyoming County Community Hospital	Warsaw	81%	54
Ira Davenport Memorial Hospital	Bath	80%	41
Adirondack Medical Center	Saranac Lake	78%	27
Cayuga Medical Center at Ithaca	Ithaca	78%	107
Westchester Medical Center	Valhalla	78%	32
Carthage Area Hospital	Carthage	77%	26
Lewis County General Hospital	Lowville	77%	43
Faxton-St Luke's Healthcare	Utica	76%	169
Bronx-Lebanon Hospital Center[2]	Bronx	74%	121

17. Blood Culture Timing

Hospital Name	City	Rate	Cases
Albany VA Medical Center	Albany	100%	60
Bath VA Medical Center	Bath	100%	71
Cobleskill Regional Hospital	Cobleskill	100%	55
Glen Cove Hospital[2]	Glen Cove	100%	126
Good Samaritan Hospital Medical Center[2]	West Islip	100%	135
Ira Davenport Memorial Hospital	Bath	100%	49
Mount Vernon Hospital	Mount Vernon	100%	107
Saint Charles Hospital	Port Jefferson	100%	130
Vassar Brothers Medical Center[2]	Poughkeepsie	100%	247
Beth Israel Medical Center[2]	New York	99%	172
Clifton Springs Hospital and Clinic	Clifton Springs	99%	114
Corning Hospital	Corning	99%	150
Eastern Niagara Hospital	Lockport	99%	155
Ellis Hospital[2]	Schenectady	99%	371
Flushing Hospital Medical Center[2]	Flushing	99%	160
Franklin Hospital[2]	Valley Stream	99%	154
John T Mather Mem Hosp-Port Jefferson	Port Jefferson	99%	352
Long Island College Hospital[2]	Brooklyn	99%	139
Long Island Jewish Medical Center[2]	New Hyde Park	99%	157
New York Downtown Hospital[2]	New York	99%	155
Niagara Falls Memorial Medical Center	Niagara Falls	99%	150
North Shore University Hospital[2]	Manhasset	99%	286
Plainview Hospital[2]	Plainview	99%	150
Rome Memorial Hospital	Rome	99%	207
Saint Francis Hospital	Poughkeepsie	99%	120
Samaritan Medical Center	Watertown	99%	189
Southside Hospital[2]	Bay Shore	99%	139
Staten Island University Hospital[2]	Staten Island	99%	209
Syracuse VA Medical Center	Syracuse	99%	132
Upstate New York VA Healthcare System	Buffalo	99%	107
Winthrop-University Hospital[2]	Mineola	99%	187
Benedictine Hospital	Kingston	98%	125
Bronx VA Medical Center	Bronx	98%	83
Community Memorial Hospital	Hamilton	98%	96
Delaware Valley Hospital	Walton	98%	56
Eastern Long Island Hospital	Greenport	98%	58
Highland Hospital	Rochester	98%	277
Kingsbrook Jewish Medical Center	Brooklyn	98%	299
Lenox Hill Hospital[2]	New York	98%	171
Mercy Hospital[2]	Buffalo	98%	133
Mount St Mary's Hospital and Health Center	Lewiston	98%	222
New York Hospital Medical Center of Queens[2]	Flushing	98%	187
New York Westchester Square Medical Center	Bronx	98%	236
Nicholas H Noyes Memorial Hospital	Dansville	98%	103
Nyack Hospital[2]	Nyack	98%	173
Putnam Hospital Center	Carmel	98%	157
Rochester General Hospital	Rochester	98%	514
St John's Episcopal Hosp-South Shore[2]	Far Rockaway	98%	124
Sound Shore Medical Center of Westschester	New Rochelle	98%	130
South Nassau Communities Hospital	Oceanside	98%	364
Unity Hospital of Rochester[2]	Rochester	98%	200
White Plains Hospital Center[2]	White Plains	98%	115
Woman's Christian Association	Jamestown	98%	180
Alice Hyde Medical Center	Malone	97%	90
Bertrand Chaffee Hospital	Springville	97%	116
Bon Secours Community Hospital	Port Jervis	97%	107
Chenango Memorial Hospital	Norwich	97%	117
Claxton-Hepburn Medical Center	Ogdensburg	97%	92
F F Thompson Hospital	Canandaigua	97%	221
Forest Hills Hospital[2]	Forest Hills	97%	141
Jamaica Hospital Medical Center[2]	Jamaica	97%	115
Kingston Hospital	Kingston	97%	232
Lakeside Memorial Hospital	Brockport	97%	143
Lawrence Hospital Center[2]	Bronxville	97%	88
Lincoln Medical & Mental Health Center	Bronx	97%	510
Mary Imogene Bassett Hospital	Cooperstown	97%	98
North Central Bronx Hospital	Bronx	97%	97
Olean General Hospital	Olean	97%	232
Oneida Healthcare Center	Oneida	97%	70
Oswego Hospital	Oswego	97%	218
Phelps Memorial Hospital Assn	Sleepy Hollow	97%	136
Saint Anthony Community Hospital	Warwick	97%	88
Saint James Mercy Hospital	Hornell	97%	106
Saint Luke's Roosevelt Hospital[2]	New York	97%	176
Saint Mary's Hospital at Amsterdam[2]	Amsterdam	97%	125
Schuyler Hospital	Montour Falls	97%	71
VA New York Harbor Healthcare System	New York	97%	157
Albany Memorial Hospital[2]	Albany	96%	177
Crouse Hospital	Syracuse	96%	310
Harlem Hospital Center[2]	New York	96%	147
Hudson Valley Hospital Center	Cortlandt Manor	96%	186
Kaleida Health	Buffalo	96%	951
Lutheran Medical Center	Brooklyn	96%	382
Maimonides Medical Center[2]	Brooklyn	96%	160
Medina Memorial Hospital	Medina	96%	107
Newark-Wayne Community Hospital	Newark	96%	121
Northern Westchester Hospital[2]	Mount Kisco	96%	175
NYU Hospitals Center[2]	New York	96%	140
Orange Regional Medical Center	Goshen	96%	547
Saint Joseph's Hospital Health Center	Syracuse	96%	615
Saratoga Hospital	Saratoga Spgs	96%	258
Sisters of Charity Hospital[2]	Buffalo	96%	263
TLC Health Network	Gowanda	96%	72
United Health Services Hospitals	Johnson City	96%	386
Univ Hosp S U N Y Health Science Ctr	Syracuse	96%	168
Arnot Ogden Medical Center	Elmira	95%	260
Aurelia Osborn Fox Memorial Hospital	Oneonta	95%	127
Catskill Regional Medical Center	Harris	95%	133
Huntington Hospital[2]	Huntington	95%	149
Lewis County General Hospital	Lowville	95%	60
Long Beach Medical Center[2]	Long Beach	95%	163
Massena Memorial Hospital	Massena	95%	116
Mount Sinai Hospital[2]	New York	95%	204
New York Community Hospital of Brooklyn[2]	Brooklyn	95%	110
Saint Barnabas Hospital	Bronx	95%	261
Saint Francis Hospital - Roslyn	Roslyn	95%	173
Saint Joseph's Hospital	Elmira	95%	158
Saint Joseph's Medical Center	Yonkers	95%	192
Albany Medical Center Hospital	Albany	94%	218
Brookhaven Memorial Hospital Med Ctr[2]	Patchogue	94%	454
Canton-Potsdam Hospital	Potsdam	94%	100
Columbia Memorial Hospital	Hudson	94%	266
Erie County Medical Center	Buffalo	94%	219
Good Samaritan Hospital of Suffern	Suffern	94%	278
Jones Memorial Hospital	Wellsville	94%	93
Kenmore Mercy Hospital[2]	Kenmore	94%	157
Mercy Medical Center	Rockville Centre	94%	207
Richmond University Medical Center[2]	Staten Island	94%	157
Saint Catherine of Siena Hospital[2]	Smithtown	94%	35
Samaritan Hospital[2]	Troy	94%	171
Seton Health System-St Mary's Campus	Troy	94%	108
Soldiers and Sailors Mem Hosp of Yates	Penn Yan	94%	54
Comm-General Hosp of Greater Syracuse[2]	Syracuse	93%	164
Saint Elizabeth Medical Center	Utica	93%	117
Saint Joseph Hospital[2]	Bethpage	93%	163
Cayuga Medical Center at Ithaca	Ithaca	92%	192
Champlain Valley Physicians Hospital	Plattsburgh	92%	322
Faxton-St Luke's Healthcare	Utica	92%	266
Jacobi Medical Center	Bronx	92%	174
Kings County Hospital Center	Brooklyn	92%	238
Metropolitan Hospital Center	New York	92%	112
Northern Dutchess Hospital	Rhinebeck	92%	71
Northport VA Medical Center	Northport	92%	93
Saint Luke's Cornwall Hospital[2]	Newburgh	92%	157
Saint Peter's Hospital[2]	Albany	92%	131
Southampton Hospital	Southampton	92%	194
Auburn Memorial Hospital	Auburn	91%	233
Coney Island Hospital	Brooklyn	91%	202
Geneva General Hospital[2]	Geneva	91%	138
New York-Presbyterian Hospital[2]	New York	91%	549
Brookdale Hospital Medical Center[2]	Brooklyn	90%	178
Our Lady of Lourdes Memorial Hospital	Binghamton	90%	383
University Hospital - Stony Brook[2]	Stony Brook	90%	132
Westchester Medical Center	Valhalla	90%	61
Brooklyn Hospital Center at Downtown Campus	Brooklyn	89%	303
Cortland Regional Medical Center	Cortland	89%	259
Elmhurst Hospital Center	Elmhurst	89%	228
Glens Falls Hospital[2]	Glens Falls	89%	170
United Memorial Medical Center	Batavia	89%	183
Wyckoff Heights Medical Center[2]	Brooklyn	89%	107
Wyoming County Community Hospital	Warsaw	89%	75
Bellevue Hospital Center	New York	88%	195
Moses-Ludington Hospital	Ticonderoga	88%	33
Strong Memorial Hospital[2]	Rochester	88%	157
Woodhull Medical and Mental Health Center	Brooklyn	87%	231
Brooks Memorial Hospital	Dunkirk	86%	114
Little Falls Hospital[3]	Little Falls	86%	51
Saint John's Riverside Hospital[2]	Yonkers	86%	165
Peconic Bay Medical Center	Riverhead	85%	124
University Hospital of Brooklyn - Downstate[2]	Brooklyn	85%	124
Peninsula Hospital Center	Far Rockaway	84%	171
Queens Hospital Center	Jamaica	84%	124
Adirondack Medical Center	Saranac Lake	82%	34
Montefiore Medical Center[2]	Bronx	82%	374
Nathan Littauer Hospital	Gloversville	80%	104
Carthage Area Hospital	Carthage	79%	29
Nassau University Medical Center	East Meadow	79%	92
Bronx-Lebanon Hospital Center[2]	Bronx	76%	139
Interfaith Medical Center	Brooklyn	76%	129
New York Methodist Hospital[2]	Brooklyn	69%	111

18. Influenza Vaccine

Hospital Name	City	Rate	Cases
Albany VA Medical Center	Albany	100%	41
Bon Secours Community Hospital	Port Jervis	100%	62
Eastern Long Island Hospital	Greenport	100%	26
Good Samaritan Hospital Medical Center[2]	West Islip	100%	100
Jamaica Hospital Medical Center[2]	Jamaica	100%	63
Lakeside Memorial Hospital	Brockport	100%	83
Long Island Jewish Medical Center[2]	New Hyde Park	100%	85
Nassau University Medical Center	East Meadow	100%	115
Saint Charles Hospital	Port Jefferson	100%	56
Saint Francis Hospital - Roslyn	Roslyn	100%	113
Southside Hospital[2]	Bay Shore	100%	84
VA Hudson Valley Healthcare System	Montrose	100%	26
Bronx-Lebanon Hospital Center[2]	Bronx	99%	92
Huntington Hospital[2]	Huntington	99%	93
North Shore University Hospital[2]	Manhasset	99%	148
Nyack Hospital[2]	Nyack	99%	108
Plainview Hospital[2]	Plainview	99%	93
Saint Catherine of Siena Hospital[2]	Smithtown	99%	139
Saint Francis Hospital	Poughkeepsie	99%	94
Saratoga Hospital	Saratoga Spgs	99%	167
Southampton Hospital	Southampton	99%	108
Syracuse VA Medical Center	Syracuse	99%	76
Catskill Regional Medical Center	Harris	98%	84
Metropolitan Hospital Center	New York	98%	54
NYU Hospitals Center[2]	New York	98%	84
Putnam Hospital Center	Carmel	98%	97
Queens Hospital Center	Jamaica	98%	88
Saint James Mercy Hospital	Hornell	98%	61
Schuyler Hospital	Montour Falls	98%	54
Vassar Brothers Medical Center[2]	Poughkeepsie	98%	204
Arnot Ogden Medical Center	Elmira	97%	179

NOTE: Hospital profiles are in alphabetical order by state, then city, then hospital within the city; Rankings exclude hospitals with less than 25 cases except for patient surveys which excludes hospitals with less than 100 cases; (a) 100–299 cases; (1) The number of cases is too small to be sure how well a hospital is performing; (2) The hospital indicated that the data submitted for this measure were based on a sample of cases; (3) Data was collected during a shorter time period (fewer quarters) than the maximum possible time for this measure; (4) Suppressed for one or more quarters by CMS; (5) No data is available from the hospital for this measure; (6) Fewer than 100 patients completed the HCAHPS survey. Use these rates with caution, as the number of surveys may be too low to reliably assess hospital performance; (7) Survey results are based on less than 12 months of data; (8) Survey results are not available for this reporting period; (9) No or very few patients were eligible for the HCAHPS survey. The scores shown, if any, reflect a very small number of surveys; (10) A state average was not calculated because too few hospitals in the state submitted data; (11) There were discrepancies in the data collection process; Please refer to the User's Guide for a full explanation of data.

Franklin Hospital[2]	Valley Stream	97%	89
Hudson Valley Hospital Center	Cortlandt Manor	97%	121
John T Mather Mem Hosp-Port Jefferson	Port Jefferson	97%	197
Kenmore Mercy Hospital[2]	Kenmore	97%	100
Mount St Mary's Hospital and Health Center	Lewiston	97%	117
Newark-Wayne Community Hospital	Newark	97%	75
Phelps Memorial Hospital Assn	Sleepy Hollow	97%	92
Saint Mary's Hospital at Amsterdam[2]	Amsterdam	97%	79
South Nassau Communities Hospital	Oceanside	97%	219
Winthrop-University Hospital[2]	Mineola	97%	101
Albany Medical Center Hospital	Albany	96%	105
Chenango Memorial Hospital	Norwich	96%	53
Clifton Springs Hospital and Clinic	Clifton Springs	96%	68
Community Memorial Hospital	Hamilton	96%	57
Forest Hills Hospital[2]	Forest Hills	96%	89
Highland Hospital	Rochester	96%	173
Lutheran Medical Center	Brooklyn	96%	246
Massena Memorial Hospital	Massena	96%	54
New York Community Hospital of Brooklyn[2]	Brooklyn	96%	70
New York Westchester Square Medical Center	Bronx	96%	108
Orange Regional Medical Center	Goshen	96%	302
Richmond University Medical Center[2]	Staten Island	96%	76
Sound Shore Medical Center of Westschester	New Rochelle	96%	122
Staten Island University Hospital[2]	Staten Island	96%	80
Ellis Hospital	Schenectady	95%	249
Long Beach Medical Center[2]	Long Beach	95%	80
Nathan Littauer Hospital	Gloversville	95%	73
Saint Joseph's Hospital	Elmira	95%	119
Saint Joseph's Hospital Health Center	Syracuse	95%	418
Samaritan Medical Center	Watertown	95%	120
United Health Services Hospitals	Johnson City	95%	232
Corning Hospital	Corning	94%	116
Glen Cove Hospital[2]	Glen Cove	94%	72
Kingston Hospital	Kingston	94%	123
Northport VA Medical Center	Northport	94%	47
Rome Memorial Hospital	Rome	94%	123
Seton Health System-St Mary's Campus	Troy	94%	88
Albany Memorial Hospital[2]	Albany	93%	92
Aurelia Osborn Fox Memorial Hospital	Oneonta	93%	69
Brookhaven Memorial Hospital Med Ctr[2]	Patchogue	93%	283
Kaleida Health	Buffalo	93%	551
Lawrence Hospital Center[2]	Bronxville	93%	96
Lenox Hill Hospital[2]	New York	93%	94
Lewis County General Hospital	Lowville	93%	30
New York Downtown Hospital[2]	New York	93%	84
Northern Westchester Hospital[2]	Mount Kisco	93%	95
St John's Episcopal Hosp-South Shore[2]	Far Rockaway	93%	75
Saint Joseph Hospital[2]	Bethpage	93%	73
United Memorial Medical Center	Batavia	93%	103
Unity Hospital of Rochester[2]	Rochester	93%	105
Bertrand Chaffee Hospital	Springville	92%	65
Champlain Valley Physicians Hospital	Plattsburgh	92%	184
Eastern Niagara Hospital	Lockport	92%	116
Glens Falls Hospital[2]	Glens Falls	92%	129
Good Samaritan Hospital of Suffern	Suffern	92%	220
Niagara Falls Memorial Medical Center	Niagara Falls	92%	106
Saint Joseph's Medical Center	Yonkers	92%	116
TLC Health Network	Gowanda	92%	61
Alice Hyde Medical Center	Malone	91%	53
Benedictine Hospital	Kingston	91%	87
Claxton-Hepburn Medical Center	Ogdensburg	91%	67
Cobleskill Regional Hospital	Cobleskill	91%	43
Ira Davenport Memorial Hospital	Bath	91%	32
Medina Memorial Hospital	Medina	91%	67
Mercy Medical Center	Rockville Centre	91%	118
New York-Presbyterian Hospital[2]	New York	91%	410
Olean General Hospital	Olean	91%	166
Bellevue Hospital Center	New York	90%	127
F F Thompson Hospital	Canandaigua	90%	124
Jacobi Medical Center	Bronx	90%	120
Mercy Hospital[2]	Buffalo	90%	79
New York Hospital Medical Center of Queens[2]	Flushing	90%	105
Coney Island Hospital	Brooklyn	89%	157
Lincoln Medical & Mental Health Center	Bronx	89%	179
New York Methodist Hospital[2]	Brooklyn	89%	94
Rochester General Hospital	Rochester	89%	348
Saint Peter's Hospital[2]	Albany	89%	100
Sisters of Charity Hospital[2]	Buffalo	89%	168
Bronx VA Medical Center	Bronx	88%	51
Canton-Potsdam Hospital	Potsdam	88%	69
Cortland Regional Medical Center	Cortland	88%	136
Oswego Hospital	Oswego	88%	142
Upstate New York VA Healthcare System	Buffalo	88%	59
Adirondack Medical Center	Saranac Lake	87%	45
Columbia Memorial Hospital	Hudson	87%	146
Our Lady of Lourdes Memorial Hospital	Binghamton	87%	222
Saint John's Riverside Hospital[2]	Yonkers	87%	69
Crouse Hospital	Syracuse	86%	182
Kings County Hospital Center	Brooklyn	86%	126
Nicholas H Noyes Memorial Hospital	Dansville	86%	81
Oneida Healthcare Center	Oneida	86%	50
Saint Elizabeth Medical Center	Utica	86%	168
Strong Memorial Hospital[2]	Rochester	86%	66
Wyckoff Heights Medical Center[2]	Brooklyn	86%	90
Auburn Memorial Hospital	Auburn	85%	149
Beth Israel Medical Center[2]	New York	85%	98
Comm-General Hosp of Greater Syracuse[2]	Syracuse	85%	97
Kingsbrook Jewish Medical Center	Brooklyn	85%	244
Saint Luke's Cornwall Hospital[2]	Newburgh	85%	106
Univ Hosp S U N Y Health Science Ctr	Syracuse	85%	134
Northern Dutchess Hospital	Rhinebeck	84%	56
Faxton-St Luke's Healthcare	Utica	83%	211
Long Island College Hospital[2]	Brooklyn	83%	75
Mount Sinai Hospital[2]	New York	83%	154
Peninsula Hospital Center	Far Rockaway	83%	112
Saint Barnabas Hospital	Bronx	83%	125
Woman's Christian Association	Jamestown	83%	115
Cayuga Medical Center at Ithaca	Ithaca	82%	91
Elmhurst Hospital Center	Elmhurst	82%	165
Mary Imogene Bassett Hospital	Cooperstown	82%	102
University Hospital of Brooklyn - Downstate[2]	Brooklyn	82%	71
White Plains Hospital Center[2]	White Plains	82%	98
Brooks Memorial Hospital	Dunkirk	81%	57
Soldiers and Sailors Mem Hosp of Yates	Penn Yan	81%	32
Woodhull Medical and Mental Health Center	Brooklyn	81%	101
Brooklyn Hospital Center at Downtown Campus	Brooklyn	80%	149
Harlem Hospital Center[2]	New York	80%	65
VA New York Harbor Healthcare System	New York	80%	98
Brookdale Hospital Medical Center[2]	Brooklyn	79%	70
Geneva General Hospital[2]	Geneva	79%	96
Jones Memorial Hospital	Wellsville	79%	47
Saint Anthony Community Hospital	Warwick	78%	60
Little Falls Hospital	Little Falls	77%	48
Montefiore Medical Center[2]	Bronx	77%	232
Samaritan Hospital[2]	Troy	77%	92
Wyoming County Community Hospital	Warsaw	77%	56
Flushing Hospital Medical Center[2]	Flushing	76%	100
Interfaith Medical Center	Brooklyn	75%	65
Peconic Bay Medical Center	Riverhead	73%	70
Westchester Medical Center	Valhalla	73%	59
Erie County Medical Center	Buffalo	71%	109
Mount Vernon Hospital	Mount Vernon	71%	45
North Central Bronx Hospital	Bronx	65%	49
University Hospital - Stony Brook[2]	Stony Brook	62%	65
Maimonides Medical Center[2]	Brooklyn	57%	96
Saint Luke's Roosevelt Hospital[2]	New York	52%	93

19. Initial Antibiotic Timing

Hospital Name	City	Rate	Cases
Benedictine Hospital	Kingston	100%	117
Delaware Valley Hospital	Walton	100%	49
Eastern Long Island Hospital	Greenport	100%	49
Good Samaritan Hospital Medical Center[2]	West Islip	100%	126
Ira Davenport Memorial Hospital	Bath	100%	52
Lakeside Memorial Hospital	Brockport	100%	148
Northern Westchester Hospital[2]	Mount Kisco	100%	159
Saint Charles Hospital	Port Jefferson	100%	98
VA Hudson Valley Healthcare System	Montrose	100%	25
Bronx VA Medical Center	Bronx	99%	79
Community Memorial Hospital	Hamilton	99%	97
Eastern Niagara Hospital	Lockport	99%	203
Glen Cove Hospital[2]	Glen Cove	99%	119
Highland Hospital	Rochester	99%	218
Kingston Hospital	Kingston	99%	206
Long Beach Medical Center[2]	Long Beach	99%	143
Massena Memorial Hospital	Massena	99%	125
New York Community Hospital of Brooklyn[2]	Brooklyn	99%	89
New York Westchester Square Medical Center	Bronx	99%	229
North Shore University Hospital[2]	Manhasset	99%	253
Plainview Hospital[2]	Plainview	99%	141
Putnam Hospital Center	Carmel	99%	148
Saint James Mercy Hospital	Hornell	99%	100
Southside Hospital[2]	Bay Shore	99%	160
Bath VA Medical Center	Bath	98%	56
Claxton-Hepburn Medical Center	Ogdensburg	98%	92
Flushing Hospital Medical Center[2]	Flushing	98%	130
John T Mather Mem Hosp-Port Jefferson	Port Jefferson	98%	281
Lenox Hill Hospital[2]	New York	98%	133
Mount St Mary's Hospital and Health Center	Lewiston	98%	214
Newark-Wayne Community Hospital	Newark	98%	136
Niagara Falls Memorial Medical Center	Niagara Falls	98%	106
North Central Bronx Hospital	Bronx	98%	95
NYU Hospitals Center[2]	New York	98%	129
Saint Anthony Community Hospital	Warwick	98%	83
Soldiers and Sailors Mem Hosp of Yates	Penn Yan	98%	41
Sound Shore Medical Center of Westschester	New Rochelle	98%	156
South Nassau Communities Hospital	Oceanside	98%	314
United Memorial Medical Center	Batavia	98%	167
Vassar Brothers Medical Center[2]	Poughkeepsie	98%	251
Bon Secours Community Hospital	Port Jervis	97%	93
F F Thompson Hospital	Canandaigua	97%	215
Franklin Hospital[2]	Valley Stream	97%	151
Hudson Valley Hospital Center	Cortlandt Manor	97%	197
Nyack Hospital[2]	Nyack	97%	165
Oneida Healthcare Center	Oneida	97%	76
Our Lady of Lourdes Memorial Hospital	Binghamton	97%	330
Richmond University Medical Center[2]	Staten Island	97%	130
Saint Francis Hospital	Poughkeepsie	97%	118
Saint Joseph's Medical Center	Yonkers	97%	190
Samaritan Hospital[2]	Troy	97%	171
Seton Health System-St Mary's Campus	Troy	97%	140
Westchester Medical Center	Valhalla	97%	59
Woman's Christian Association	Jamestown	97%	187
Albany Memorial Hospital[2]	Albany	96%	158
Arnot Ogden Medical Center	Elmira	96%	226
Bertrand Chaffee Hospital	Springville	96%	105
Chenango Memorial Hospital	Norwich	96%	111
Cobleskill Regional Hospital	Cobleskill	96%	71
Coney Island Hospital	Brooklyn	96%	186
Huntington Hospital[2]	Huntington	96%	132
Jamaica Hospital Medical Center[2]	Jamaica	96%	112
Metropolitan Hospital Center	New York	96%	104
New York Downtown Hospital[2]	New York	96%	139
Northern Dutchess Hospital	Rhinebeck	96%	70
Olean General Hospital	Olean	96%	221
Orange Regional Medical Center	Goshen	96%	524
Phelps Memorial Hospital Assn	Sleepy Hollow	96%	114
Rome Memorial Hospital	Rome	96%	192
Saint Elizabeth Medical Center	Utica	96%	176
Schuyler Hospital	Montour Falls	96%	76
Staten Island University Hospital[2]	Staten Island	96%	120
Winthrop-University Hospital[2]	Mineola	96%	157
Aurelia Osborn Fox Memorial Hospital	Oneonta	95%	132
Canton-Potsdam Hospital	Potsdam	95%	122
Ellis Hospital[2]	Schenectady	95%	309
Glens Falls Hospital[2]	Glens Falls	95%	197
Jones Memorial Hospital	Wellsville	95%	80
Kenmore Mercy Hospital[2]	Kenmore	95%	150
Kingsbrook Jewish Medical Center	Brooklyn	95%	280
Long Island Jewish Medical Center[2]	New Hyde Park	95%	151
Lutheran Medical Center	Brooklyn	95%	335
Medina Memorial Hospital	Medina	95%	116
Peconic Bay Medical Center	Riverhead	95%	115
Saint Barnabas Hospital	Bronx	95%	214
Saint Joseph's Hospital	Elmira	95%	156
White Plains Hospital Center[2]	White Plains	95%	163
Wyoming County Community Hospital	Warsaw	95%	82
Auburn Memorial Hospital	Auburn	94%	247
Brooks Memorial Hospital	Dunkirk	94%	118
Clifton Springs Hospital and Clinic	Clifton Springs	94%	108
Crouse Hospital	Syracuse	94%	307
Good Samaritan Hospital of Suffern	Suffern	94%	267
Harlem Hospital Center[2]	New York	94%	144
Lewis County General Hospital	Lowville	94%	67
Mercy Hospital[2]	Buffalo	94%	129
Mercy Medical Center	Rockville Centre	94%	203
Saint Mary's Hospital at Amsterdam[2]	Amsterdam	94%	148
Saratoga Hospital	Saratoga Spgs	94%	246
Sisters of Charity Hospital[2]	Buffalo	94%	285
Southampton Hospital	Southampton	94%	172
Syracuse VA Medical Center	Syracuse	94%	121
TLC Health Network	Gowanda	94%	89
Univ Hosp S U N Y Health Science Ctr	Syracuse	94%	145
VA New York Harbor Healthcare System	New York	94%	143
Albany VA Medical Center	Albany	93%	61
Alice Hyde Medical Center	Malone	93%	97
Columbia Memorial Hospital	Hudson	93%	246
Cortland Regional Medical Center	Cortland	93%	223
Elmhurst Hospital Center	Elmhurst	93%	252
Forest Hills Hospital[2]	Forest Hills	93%	122
Little Falls Hospital[3]	Little Falls	93%	59
Nathan Littauer Hospital	Gloversville	93%	114
Nicholas H Noyes Memorial Hospital	Dansville	93%	123
Saint Luke's Roosevelt Hospital[2]	New York	93%	178
Adirondack Medical Center	Saranac Lake	92%	49
Beth Israel Medical Center[2]	New York	92%	170
Brooklyn Hospital Center at Downtown Campus	Brooklyn	92%	305
Catskill Regional Medical Center	Harris	92%	126
Kaleida Health	Buffalo	92%	943
Mount Sinai Hospital[2]	New York	92%	237
Mount Vernon Hospital	Mount Vernon	92%	91
Nassau University Medical Center	East Meadow	92%	142
Saint Joseph Hospital[2]	Bethpage	92%	131
Samaritan Medical Center	Watertown	92%	176
United Health Services Hospitals	Johnson City	92%	350
Albany Medical Center Hospital	Albany	91%	166
Brookdale Hospital Medical Center[2]	Brooklyn	91%	161
Carthage Area Hospital	Carthage	91%	34
Cayuga Medical Center at Ithaca	Ithaca	91%	196
Corning Hospital	Corning	91%	137
Kings County Hospital Center	Brooklyn	91%	213
Lawrence Hospital Center[2]	Bronxville	91%	163

NOTE: Hospital profiles are in alphabetical order by state, then city, then hospital within the city; Rankings exclude hospitals with less than 25 cases except for patient surveys which excludes hospitals with less than 100 cases; (a) 100–299 cases; (1) The number of cases is too small to be sure how well a hospital is performing; (2) The hospital indicated that the data submitted for this measure were based on a sample of cases; (3) Data was collected during a shorter time period (fewer quarters) than the maximum possible time for this measure; (4) Suppressed for one or more quarters by CMS; (5) No data is available from the hospital for this measure; (6) Fewer than 100 patients completed the HCAHPS survey. Use these rates with caution, as the number of surveys may be too low to reliably assess hospital performance; (7) Survey results are based on less than 12 months of data; (8) Survey results are not available for this reporting period; (9) No or very few patients were eligible for the HCAHPS survey. The scores shown, if any, reflect a very small number of surveys; (10) A state average was not calculated because too few hospitals in the state submitted data; (11) There were discrepancies in the data collection process; Please refer to the User's Guide for a full explanation of data.

Lincoln Medical & Mental Health Center	Bronx	91%	464
Mary Imogene Bassett Hospital	Cooperstown	91%	104
Northport VA Medical Center	Northport	91%	87
Saint John's Riverside Hospital[2]	Yonkers	91%	142
Unity Hospital of Rochester[2]	Rochester	91%	190
University Hospital - Stony Brook[2]	Stony Brook	91%	135
Upstate New York VA Healthcare System	Buffalo	91%	95
Maimonides Medical Center[2]	Brooklyn	90%	134
New York Hospital Medical Center of Queens[2]	Flushing	90%	173
St John's Episcopal Hosp-South Shore[2]	Far Rockaway	90%	129
Saint Peter's Hospital[2]	Albany	90%	147
Brookhaven Memorial Hospital Med Ctr[2]	Patchogue	89%	428
Champlain Valley Physicians Hospital	Plattsburgh	89%	326
Edward John Noble Hospital of Gouverneur	Gouverneur	89%	28
Long Island College Hospital[2]	Brooklyn	89%	142
Oswego Hospital	Oswego	89%	223
Saint Catherine of Siena Hospital[2]	Smithtown	89%	228
Saint Luke's Cornwall Hospital[2]	Newburgh	89%	169
New York Methodist Hospital[2]	Brooklyn	88%	171
Rochester General Hospital	Rochester	88%	557
Saint Francis Hospital - Roslyn	Roslyn	88%	154
Bellevue Hospital Center	New York	87%	214
Woodhull Medical and Mental Health Center	Brooklyn	87%	193
Geneva General Hospital[2]	Geneva	86%	116
Faxton-St Luke's Healthcare	Utica	85%	311
New York-Presbyterian Hospital[2]	New York	83%	465
Peninsula Hospital Center	Far Rockaway	83%	195
Wyckoff Heights Medical Center[2]	Brooklyn	83%	173
Erie County Medical Center	Buffalo	82%	217
Saint Joseph's Hospital Health Center	Syracuse	82%	568
Bronx-Lebanon Hospital Center[2]	Bronx	81%	233
Jacobi Medical Center	Bronx	81%	186
Strong Memorial Hospital[2]	Rochester	81%	136
Comm-General Hosp of Greater Syracuse[2]	Syracuse	80%	155
University Hospital of Brooklyn - Downstate[2]	Brooklyn	80%	137
Montefiore Medical Center[2]	Bronx	79%	413
Queens Hospital Center	Jamaica	78%	161
Interfaith Medical Center	Brooklyn	77%	147

20. Pneumococcal Vaccine

Hospital Name	City	Rate	Cases
Albany VA Medical Center	Albany	100%	52
Bath VA Medical Center	Bath	100%	41
Catskill Regional Medical Center	Harris	100%	100
Chenango Memorial Hospital	Norwich	100%	64
Eastern Long Island Hospital	Greenport	100%	43
Good Samaritan Hospital Medical Center[2]	West Islip	100%	158
Jamaica Hospital Medical Center[2]	Jamaica	100%	86
Saint Catherine of Siena Hospital[2]	Smithtown	100%	219
Saint Charles Hospital	Port Jefferson	100%	62
Saint James Mercy Hospital	Hornell	100%	87
VA Hudson Valley Healthcare System	Montrose	100%	29
Bronx-Lebanon Hospital Center[2]	Bronx	99%	128
Harlem Hospital Center[2]	New York	99%	72
John T Mather Mem Hosp-Port Jefferson	Port Jefferson	99%	262
Nyack Hospital[2]	Nyack	99%	160
Saint Francis Hospital	Poughkeepsie	99%	115
Saint Francis Hospital - Roslyn	Roslyn	99%	203
Saint Mary's Hospital at Amsterdam[2]	Amsterdam	99%	116
Arnot Ogden Medical Center	Elmira	98%	255
Highland Hospital	Rochester	98%	249
Lakeside Memorial Hospital	Brockport	98%	123
New York Community Hospital of Brooklyn[2]	Brooklyn	98%	115
New York Methodist Hospital[2]	Brooklyn	98%	165
North Shore University Hospital[2]	Manhasset	98%	266
NYU Hospitals Center[2]	New York	98%	138
Plainview Hospital[2]	Plainview	98%	164
Richmond University Medical Center[2]	Staten Island	98%	122
Saratoga Hospital	Saratoga Spgs	98%	229
Southampton Hospital	Southampton	98%	181
Southside Hospital[2]	Bay Shore	98%	125
Staten Island University Hospital[2]	Staten Island	98%	117
Syracuse VA Medical Center	Syracuse	98%	115
Aurelia Osborn Fox Memorial Hospital	Oneonta	97%	103
Bellevue Hospital Center	New York	97%	121
Crouse Hospital	Syracuse	97%	259
Ellis Hospital[2]	Schenectady	97%	323
Glens Falls Hospital[2]	Glens Falls	97%	205
Hudson Valley Hospital Center	Cortlandt Manor	97%	246
Kenmore Mercy Hospital[2]	Kenmore	97%	154
Kingsbrook Jewish Medical Center	Brooklyn	97%	385
Mary Imogene Bassett Hospital	Cooperstown	97%	134
Massena Memorial Hospital	Massena	97%	77
Northport VA Medical Center	Northport	97%	77
Putnam Hospital Center	Carmel	97%	142
Queens Hospital Center	Jamaica	97%	94
Sound Shore Medical Center of Westchester	New Rochelle	97%	183
South Nassau Communities Hospital	Oceanside	97%	344
TLC Health Network	Gowanda	97%	78
VA New York Harbor Healthcare System	New York	97%	131
Vassar Brothers Medical Center[2]	Poughkeepsie	97%	302
Winthrop-University Hospital[2]	Mineola	97%	164
Benedictine Hospital	Kingston	96%	113
Corning Hospital	Corning	96%	155
Forest Hills Hospital[2]	Forest Hills	96%	162
Franklin Hospital[2]	Valley Stream	96%	135
Ira Davenport Memorial Hospital	Bath	96%	53
Kingston Hospital	Kingston	96%	157
Lawrence Hospital Center[2]	Bronxville	96%	160
Lewis County General Hospital	Lowville	96%	52
Lincoln Medical & Mental Health Center	Bronx	96%	159
Long Island Jewish Medical Center[2]	New Hyde Park	96%	119
Newark-Wayne Community Hospital	Newark	96%	105
Olean General Hospital	Olean	96%	227
Rome Memorial Hospital	Rome	96%	162
Schuyler Hospital	Montour Falls	96%	70
Bronx VA Medical Center	Bronx	95%	63
Canton-Potsdam Hospital	Potsdam	95%	103
Champlain Valley Physicians Hospital	Plattsburgh	95%	302
Eastern Niagara Hospital	Lockport	95%	185
Huntington Hospital[2]	Huntington	95%	152
Mercy Hospital[2]	Buffalo	95%	124
Mount St Mary's Hospital and Health Center	Lewiston	95%	188
New York Westchester Square Medical Center	Bronx	95%	187
Orange Regional Medical Center	Goshen	95%	490
Phelps Memorial Hospital Assn	Sleepy Hollow	95%	115
Saint Barnabas Hospital	Bronx	95%	122
Upstate New York VA Healthcare System	Buffalo	95%	92
Albany Medical Center Hospital	Albany	94%	129
Bon Secours Community Hospital	Port Jervis	94%	90
Claxton-Hepburn Medical Center	Ogdensburg	94%	88
Community Memorial Hospital	Hamilton	94%	78
Coney Island Hospital	Brooklyn	94%	260
Delaware Valley Hospital	Walton	94%	32
Niagara Falls Memorial Medical Center	Niagara Falls	94%	111
St John's Episcopal Hosp-South Shore[2]	Far Rockaway	94%	132
Saint Joseph Hospital[2]	Bethpage	94%	112
Saint Joseph's Hospital Health Center	Syracuse	94%	696
United Health Services Hospitals	Johnson City	94%	345
Adirondack Medical Center	Saranac Lake	93%	60
Alice Hyde Medical Center	Malone	93%	67
Good Samaritan Hospital of Suffern	Suffern	93%	317
Jones Memorial Hospital	Wellsville	93%	86
Lenox Hill Hospital[2]	New York	93%	141
Long Beach Medical Center[2]	Long Beach	93%	140
Moses-Ludington Hospital	Ticonderoga	93%	30
Nassau University Medical Center	East Meadow	93%	142
Northern Westchester Hospital[2]	Mount Kisco	93%	169
Saint Joseph's Hospital	Elmira	93%	179
Saint Peter's Hospital[2]	Albany	93%	150
United Memorial Medical Center	Batavia	93%	163
Unity Hospital of Rochester[2]	Rochester	93%	168
Cobleskill Regional Hospital	Cobleskill	92%	63
Glen Cove Hospital[2]	Glen Cove	92%	142
Jacobi Medical Center	Bronx	92%	133
Metropolitan Hospital Center	New York	92%	59
Mount Vernon Hospital	Mount Vernon	92%	59
Nicholas H Noyes Memorial Hospital	Dansville	92%	120
Oneida Healthcare Center	Oneida	92%	64
Saint Joseph's Medical Center	Yonkers	92%	162
Samaritan Medical Center	Watertown	92%	168
Sisters of Charity Hospital[2]	Buffalo	92%	248
Albany Memorial Hospital[2]	Albany	91%	137
Bertrand Chaffee Hospital	Springville	91%	102
Brookhaven Memorial Hospital Med Ctr[2]	Patchogue	91%	429
F F Thompson Hospital	Canandaigua	91%	194
Kings County Hospital Center	Brooklyn	91%	132
New York Downtown Hospital[2]	New York	91%	159
Saint John's Riverside Hospital[2]	Yonkers	91%	134
Clifton Springs Hospital and Clinic	Clifton Springs	90%	94
Lutheran Medical Center	Brooklyn	90%	344
Medina Memorial Hospital	Medina	90%	100
New York-Presbyterian Hospital[2]	New York	90%	590
Saint Elizabeth Medical Center	Utica	90%	236
Woman's Christian Association	Jamestown	90%	176
Woodhull Medical and Mental Health Center	Brooklyn	90%	117
Montefiore Medical Center[2]	Bronx	89%	340
North Central Bronx Hospital	Bronx	89%	37
Samaritan Hospital[2]	Troy	89%	155
Seton Health System-St Mary's Campus	Troy	89%	121
Wyckoff Heights Medical Center[2]	Brooklyn	89%	142
Brooks Memorial Hospital	Dunkirk	88%	95
Carthage Area Hospital	Carthage	88%	33
Oswego Hospital	Oswego	88%	224
Saint Luke's Cornwall Hospital[2]	Newburgh	88%	153
Auburn Memorial Hospital	Auburn	87%	208
Elmhurst Hospital Center	Elmhurst	87%	251
Geneva General Hospital[2]	Geneva	87%	122
Kaleida Health	Buffalo	87%	830
Strong Memorial Hospital[2]	Rochester	87%	77
Northern Dutchess Hospital	Rhinebeck	86%	73
Our Lady of Lourdes Memorial Hospital	Binghamton	86%	335
Peninsula Hospital Center	Far Rockaway	86%	192
Wyoming County Community Hospital	Warsaw	86%	70
Columbia Memorial Hospital	Hudson	85%	225
Faxton-St Luke's Healthcare	Utica	85%	301
Interfaith Medical Center	Brooklyn	85%	84
Mercy Medical Center	Rockville Centre	85%	215
New York Hospital Medical Center of Queens[2]	Flushing	85%	181
Rochester General Hospital	Rochester	85%	491
White Plains Hospital Center[2]	White Plains	85%	168
Flushing Hospital Medical Center[2]	Flushing	84%	161
Maimonides Medical Center[2]	Brooklyn	84%	174
Saint Anthony Community Hospital	Warwick	84%	91
Univ Hosp S U N Y Health Science Ctr	Syracuse	84%	126
Soldiers and Sailors Mem Hosp of Yates	Penn Yan	83%	47
Brooklyn Hospital Center at Downtown Campus	Brooklyn	82%	201
Cortland Regional Medical Center	Cortland	82%	192
University Hospital - Stony Brook[2]	Stony Brook	80%	94
Westchester Medical Center	Valhalla	80%	79
Cayuga Medical Center at Ithaca	Ithaca	79%	151
Comm-General Hosp of Greater Syracuse[2]	Syracuse	79%	150
Mount Sinai Hospital[2]	New York	79%	220
Beth Israel Medical Center[2]	New York	78%	165
Brookdale Hospital Medical Center[2]	Brooklyn	78%	85
Erie County Medical Center	Buffalo	74%	109
Peconic Bay Medical Center	Riverhead	70%	105
University Hospital of Brooklyn - Downstate[2]	Brooklyn	68%	95
Long Island College Hospital[2]	Brooklyn	67%	102
Little Falls Hospital[3]	Little Falls	66%	56
Saint Luke's Roosevelt Hospital[2]	New York	66%	129
Nathan Littauer Hospital	Gloversville	65%	108

21. Smoking Cessation Advice

Hospital Name	City	Rate	Cases
Albany Memorial Hospital[2]	Albany	100%	45
Albany VA Medical Center	Albany	100%	31
Alice Hyde Medical Center	Malone	100%	32
Aurelia Osborn Fox Memorial Hospital	Oneonta	100%	41
Benedictine Hospital	Kingston	100%	40
Bertrand Chaffee Hospital	Springville	100%	25
Beth Israel Medical Center[2]	New York	100%	53
Bon Secours Community Hospital	Port Jervis	100%	37
Bronx VA Medical Center	Bronx	100%	28
Bronx-Lebanon Hospital Center[2]	Bronx	100%	80
Brookhaven Memorial Hospital Med Ctr[2]	Patchogue	100%	163
Brooklyn Hospital Center at Downtown Campus	Brooklyn	100%	62
Catskill Regional Medical Center	Harris	100%	58
Clifton Springs Hospital and Clinic	Clifton Springs	100%	29
Comm-General Hosp of Greater Syracuse[2]	Syracuse	100%	31
Crouse Hospital	Syracuse	100%	90
Elmhurst Hospital Center	Elmhurst	100%	95
F F Thompson Hospital	Canandaigua	100%	63
Glens Falls Hospital[2]	Glens Falls	100%	75
Good Samaritan Hospital Medical Center[2]	West Islip	100%	36
Good Samaritan Hospital of Suffern	Suffern	100%	67
Highland Hospital	Rochester	100%	77
Hudson Valley Hospital Center	Cortlandt Manor	100%	63
Jamaica Hospital Medical Center[2]	Jamaica	100%	43
John T Mather Mem Hosp-Port Jefferson	Port Jefferson	100%	110
Kaleida Health	Buffalo	100%	240
Kingston Hospital	Kingston	100%	76
Lakeside Memorial Hospital	Brockport	100%	45
Lawrence Hospital Center[2]	Bronxville	100%	28
Lincoln Medical & Mental Health Center	Bronx	100%	156
Mercy Hospital[2]	Buffalo	100%	56
Mercy Medical Center	Rockville Centre	100%	34
Metropolitan Hospital Center	New York	100%	39
Montefiore Medical Center[2]	Bronx	100%	91
Mount Vernon Hospital	Mount Vernon	100%	31
Nassau University Medical Center	East Meadow	100%	55
New York Downtown Hospital[2]	New York	100%	35
New York Hospital Medical Center of Queens[2]	Flushing	100%	26
New York Methodist Hospital[2]	Brooklyn	100%	39
New York Westchester Square Medical Center	Bronx	100%	40
Newark-Wayne Community Hospital	Newark	100%	53
Niagara Falls Memorial Medical Center	Niagara Falls	100%	83
North Shore University Hospital[2]	Manhasset	100%	39
Nyack Hospital[2]	Nyack	100%	29
NYU Hospitals Center[2]	New York	100%	25
Olean General Hospital	Olean	100%	78
Our Lady of Lourdes Memorial Hospital	Binghamton	100%	100
Peconic Bay Medical Center	Riverhead	100%	35
Peninsula Hospital Center	Far Rockaway	100%	43
Plainview Hospital[2]	Plainview	100%	30
Putnam Hospital Center	Carmel	100%	38
Richmond University Medical Center[2]	Staten Island	100%	38
Rochester General Hospital	Rochester	100%	186
Saint Catherine of Siena Hospital[2]	Smithtown	100%	36
Saint Francis Hospital	Poughkeepsie	100%	56
Saint Joseph Hospital[2]	Bethpage	100%	38

NOTE: Hospital profiles are in alphabetical order by state, then city, then hospital within the city; Rankings exclude hospitals with less than 25 cases except for patient surveys which excludes hospitals with less than 100 cases; (a) 100–299 cases; (1) The number of cases is too small to be sure how well a hospital is performing; (2) The hospital indicated that the data submitted for this measure were based on a sample of cases; (3) Data was collected during a shorter time period (fewer quarters) than the maximum possible time for this measure; (4) Suppressed for one or more quarters by CMS; (5) No data is available from the hospital for this measure; (6) Fewer than 100 patients completed the HCAHPS survey. Use these rates with caution, as the number of surveys may be too low to reliably assess hospital performance; (7) Survey results are based on less than 12 months of data; (8) Survey results are not available for this reporting period; (9) No or very few patients were eligible for the HCAHPS survey. The scores shown, if any, reflect a very small number of surveys; (10) A state average was not calculated because too few hospitals in the state submitted data; (11) There were discrepancies in the data collection process; Please refer to the User's Guide for a full explanation of data.

Hospital Name	City	Rate	Cases
Saint Joseph's Hospital	Elmira	100%	56
Saint Joseph's Hospital Health Center	Syracuse	100%	314
Saint Luke's Roosevelt Hospital[2]	New York	100%	58
Saint Mary's Hospital at Amsterdam[2]	Amsterdam	100%	33
Saint Peter's Hospital[2]	Albany	100%	30
Seton Health System-St Mary's Campus	Troy	100%	39
Sound Shore Medical Center of Westchester	New Rochelle	100%	39
South Nassau Communities Hospital	Oceanside	100%	69
Southampton Hospital	Southampton	100%	34
Southside Hospital[2]	Bay Shore	100%	53
Staten Island University Hospital[2]	Staten Island	100%	40
Syracuse VA Medical Center	Syracuse	100%	43
United Health Services Hospitals	Johnson City	100%	144
Unity Hospital of Rochester[2]	Rochester	100%	52
University Hospital - Stony Brook[2]	Stony Brook	100%	55
Univ Hosp S U N Y Health Science Ctr	Syracuse	100%	90
Upstate New York VA Healthcare System	Buffalo	100%	26
VA New York Harbor Healthcare System	New York	100%	48
Vassar Brothers Medical Center[2]	Poughkeepsie	100%	64
Westchester Medical Center	Valhalla	100%	27
Winthrop-University Hospital[2]	Mineola	100%	32
Wyckoff Heights Medical Center[2]	Brooklyn	100%	36
Arnot Ogden Medical Center	Elmira	99%	67
Faxton-St Luke's Healthcare	Utica	99%	75
Harlem Hospital Center[2]	New York	99%	72
Jacobi Medical Center	Bronx	99%	69
Mount Sinai Hospital[2]	New York	99%	68
Orange Regional Medical Center	Goshen	99%	153
Saratoga Hospital	Saratoga Spgs	99%	90
Cayuga Medical Center at Ithaca	Ithaca	98%	52
Cortland Regional Medical Center	Cortland	98%	58
Ellis Hospital[2]	Schenectady	98%	108
Long Island College Hospital[2]	Brooklyn	98%	40
Sisters of Charity Hospital[2]	Buffalo	98%	104
Woman's Christian Association	Jamestown	98%	62
Brookdale Hospital Medical Center[2]	Brooklyn	97%	69
Kenmore Mercy Hospital[2]	Kenmore	97%	38
Massena Memorial Hospital	Massena	97%	35
Nathan Littauer Hospital	Gloversville	97%	33
North Central Bronx Hospital	Bronx	97%	35
Oneida Healthcare Center	Oneida	97%	34
Oswego Hospital	Oswego	97%	96
Saint Barnabas Hospital	Bronx	97%	110
Saint Charles Hospital	Port Jefferson	97%	30
Saint Elizabeth Medical Center	Utica	97%	74
Saint Joseph's Medical Center	Yonkers	97%	35
Woodhull Medical and Mental Health Center	Brooklyn	97%	108
Albany Medical Center Hospital	Albany	96%	80
Bellevue Hospital Center	New York	96%	96
Champlain Valley Physicians Hospital	Plattsburgh	96%	140
Coney Island Hospital	Brooklyn	96%	45
Kings County Hospital Center	Brooklyn	96%	101
Saint Luke's Cornwall Hospital[2]	Newburgh	96%	49
Samaritan Medical Center	Watertown	96%	57
Canton-Potsdam Hospital	Potsdam	95%	42
Erie County Medical Center	Buffalo	95%	98
New York-Presbyterian Hospital[2]	New York	95%	109
Columbia Memorial Hospital	Hudson	94%	64
Interfaith Medical Center	Brooklyn	94%	65
Queens Hospital Center	Jamaica	94%	32
Chenango Memorial Hospital	Norwich	93%	28
Lutheran Medical Center	Brooklyn	93%	60
Samaritan Hospital[2]	Troy	93%	58
Strong Memorial Hospital[2]	Rochester	93%	61
Kingsbrook Jewish Medical Center	Brooklyn	92%	49
Mary Imogene Bassett Hospital	Cooperstown	92%	63
Rome Memorial Hospital	Rome	92%	53
Corning Hospital	Corning	91%	54
Eastern Niagara Hospital	Lockport	91%	78
Mount St Mary's Hospital and Health Center	Lewiston	89%	56
White Plains Hospital Center[2]	White Plains	89%	28
Auburn Memorial Hospital	Auburn	88%	73
Geneva General Hospital[2]	Geneva	88%	32
United Memorial Medical Center	Batavia	88%	59
Saint John's Riverside Hospital[2]	Yonkers	86%	29
TLC Health Network	Gowanda	86%	29
Jones Memorial Hospital	Wellsville	83%	29
University Hospital of Brooklyn - Downstate[2]	Brooklyn	81%	31

Surgical Care Improvement Project

22. Appropriate VTP Within 24 Hours

Hospital Name	City	Rate	Cases
Albany VA Medical Center[2]	Albany	100%	62
Clifton Springs Hospital and Clinic	Clifton Springs	100%	52
Community Memorial Hospital	Hamilton	100%	183
Coney Island Hospital[2]	Brooklyn	100%	145
Lakeside Memorial Hospital	Brockport	100%	71
New York Community Hospital of Brooklyn[2]	Brooklyn	100%	85
New York-Presbyterian Hospital[2]	New York	100%	633
Saint Joseph's Hospital	Elmira	100%	49
Strong Memorial Hospital[2]	Rochester	100%	306
Syracuse VA Medical Center[2]	Syracuse	100%	107
TLC Health Network	Gowanda	100%	111
Bronx VA Medical Center[2]	Bronx	99%	118
Brooks Memorial Hospital	Dunkirk	99%	153
Canton-Potsdam Hospital	Potsdam	99%	139
Interfaith Medical Center	Brooklyn	99%	82
Long Island Jewish Medical Center[2]	New Hyde Park	99%	169
Metropolitan Hospital Center[2]	New York	99%	128
Nassau University Medical Center[2]	East Meadow	99%	178
New York Methodist Hospital[2]	Brooklyn	99%	334
North Shore University Hospital[2]	Manhasset	99%	352
Northport VA Medical Center[2]	Northport	99%	99
Olean General Hospital	Olean	99%	181
Oneida Healthcare Center	Oneida	99%	174
Phelps Memorial Hospital Assn[2]	Sleepy Hollow	99%	272
Plainview Hospital[2]	Plainview	99%	227
Saint Charles Hospital[2]	Port Jefferson	99%	269
Staten Island University Hospital[2]	Staten Island	99%	188
Unity Hospital of Rochester[2]	Rochester	99%	170
University Hospital - Stony Brook[2]	Stony Brook	99%	175
Univ Hosp S U N Y Health Science Ctr[2]	Syracuse	99%	171
VA New York Harbor Healthcare System[2]	New York	99%	108
Beth Israel Medical Center[2]	New York	98%	229
Elmhurst Hospital Center	Elmhurst	98%	323
Franklin Hospital[2]	Valley Stream	98%	205
Glen Cove Hospital[2]	Glen Cove	98%	183
Highland Hospital[2]	Rochester	98%	231
Huntington Hospital[2]	Huntington	98%	175
Lenox Hill Hospital[2]	New York	98%	245
Lincoln Medical & Mental Health Center[2]	Bronx	98%	166
Lutheran Medical Center[2]	Brooklyn	98%	482
New York Hospital Medical Center of Queens[2]	Flushing	98%	326
New York Westchester Square Medical Center	Bronx	98%	200
Nyack Hospital	Nyack	98%	255
NYU Hospitals Center[2]	New York	98%	274
Our Lady of Lourdes Memorial Hospital[2]	Binghamton	98%	122
Queens Hospital Center	Jamaica	98%	195
Richmond University Medical Center[2]	Staten Island	98%	183
Saint Catherine of Siena Hospital[2]	Smithtown	98%	232
Saint Joseph's Hospital Health Center[2]	Syracuse	98%	170
University Hospital of Brooklyn - Downstate[2]	Brooklyn	98%	184
Winthrop-University Hospital[2]	Mineola	98%	279
Albany Medical Center Hospital[2]	Albany	97%	135
Arnot Ogden Medical Center[2]	Elmira	97%	149
Bellevue Hospital Center[2]	New York	97%	298
Bon Secours Community Hospital	Port Jervis	97%	62
Ellis Hospital[2]	Schenectady	97%	225
Forest Hills Hospital[2]	Forest Hills	97%	191
Jamaica Hospital Medical Center[2]	Jamaica	97%	199
Kenmore Mercy Hospital[2]	Kenmore	97%	126
Kings County Hospital Center[2]	Brooklyn	97%	219
Kingsbrook Jewish Medical Center	Brooklyn	97%	126
Long Island College Hospital[2]	Brooklyn	97%	233
Mary Imogene Bassett Hospital[2]	Cooperstown	97%	237
Saint Francis Hospital - Roslyn[2]	Roslyn	97%	188
Saint Peter's Hospital[2]	Albany	97%	252
Southside Hospital[2]	Bay Shore	97%	236
Woodhull Medical and Mental Health Center[2]	Brooklyn	97%	145
Bronx-Lebanon Hospital Center[2]	Bronx	96%	185
Comm-General Hosp of Greater Syracuse[2]	Syracuse	96%	164
Flushing Hospital Medical Center[2]	Flushing	96%	229
Good Samaritan Hospital Medical Center[2]	West Islip	96%	281
Hospital for Special Surgery[2]	New York	96%	310
Mount St Mary's Hospital and Health Center[2]	Lewiston	96%	121
Newark-Wayne Community Hospital	Newark	96%	95
Rochester General Hospital[2]	Rochester	96%	553
Saint Francis Hospital[2]	Poughkeepsie	96%	136
Seton Health System-St Mary's Campus[2]	Troy	96%	203
South Nassau Communities Hospital[2]	Oceanside	96%	343
United Health Services Hospitals	Johnson City	96%	470
Crouse Hospital[2]	Syracuse	95%	141
Harlem Hospital Center[2]	New York	95%	77
Jacobi Medical Center	Bronx	95%	284
Kaleida Health[2]	Buffalo	95%	454
Lewis County General Hospital	Lowville	95%	58
Massena Memorial Hospital	Massena	95%	39
Mercy Hospital[2]	Buffalo	95%	152
Saint Barnabas Hospital[2]	Bronx	95%	132
Westchester Medical Center[2]	Valhalla	95%	348
Eastern Long Island Hospital	Greenport	94%	36
John T Mather Mem Hosp-Port Jefferson	Port Jefferson	94%	304
Maimonides Medical Center[2]	Brooklyn	94%	314
New York Downtown Hospital[2]	New York	94%	144
Niagara Falls Memorial Medical Center	Niagara Falls	94%	72
Northern Westchester Hospital[2]	Mount Kisco	94%	140
Orange Regional Medical Center[2]	Goshen	94%	409
Upstate New York VA Healthcare System[2]	Buffalo	94%	116
Wyckoff Heights Medical Center[2]	Brooklyn	94%	210
Aurelia Osborn Fox Memorial Hospital	Oneonta	93%	102
Catskill Regional Medical Center	Harris	93%	119
Hudson Valley Hospital Center	Cortlandt Manor	93%	239
Mount Sinai Hospital[2]	New York	93%	526
Putnam Hospital Center	Carmel	93%	424
Rome Memorial Hospital	Rome	93%	112
Saint Joseph's Medical Center	Yonkers	93%	85
Saint Mary's Hospital at Amsterdam[2]	Amsterdam	93%	122
Samaritan Medical Center	Watertown	93%	189
Saratoga Hospital	Saratoga Spgs	93%	345
Auburn Memorial Hospital	Auburn	92%	127
Chenango Memorial Hospital	Norwich	92%	89
Erie County Medical Center	Buffalo	92%	335
Oswego Hospital	Oswego	92%	97
Peconic Bay Medical Center	Riverhead	92%	229
Saint Anthony Community Hospital	Warwick	92%	76
Saint Luke's Roosevelt Hospital[2]	New York	92%	322
United Memorial Medical Center	Batavia	92%	150
Vassar Brothers Medical Center[2]	Poughkeepsie	92%	187
Cayuga Medical Center at Ithaca	Ithaca	91%	153
Cortland Regional Medical Center	Cortland	91%	74
Glens Falls Hospital[2]	Glens Falls	91%	268
Mercy Medical Center[2]	Rockville Centre	91%	274
Sisters of Charity Hospital[2]	Buffalo	91%	257
Albany Memorial Hospital[2]	Albany	90%	194
Columbia Memorial Hospital	Hudson	90%	163
F F Thompson Hospital	Canandaigua	90%	146
Long Beach Medical Center[2]	Long Beach	90%	39
Saint Luke's Cornwall Hospital[2]	Newburgh	90%	123
White Plains Hospital Center[2]	White Plains	90%	225
Faxton-St Luke's Healthcare[2]	Utica	89%	183
Northern Dutchess Hospital[2]	Rhinebeck	89%	101
Champlain Valley Physicians Hospital	Plattsburgh	88%	320
Corning Hospital	Corning	88%	98
Jones Memorial Hospital	Wellsville	88%	34
Montefiore Medical Center[2]	Bronx	88%	411
St John's Episcopal Hosp-South Shore[2]	Far Rockaway	88%	88
Saint Joseph Hospital[2]	Bethpage	88%	154
Sound Shore Medical Center of Westchester	New Rochelle	88%	282
Alice Hyde Medical Center	Malone	87%	97
Brookdale Hospital Medical Center[2]	Brooklyn	87%	189
Brookhaven Memorial Hospital Med Ctr[2]	Patchogue	87%	236
Brooklyn Hospital Center at Downtown Campus	Brooklyn	87%	254
Kingston Hospital	Kingston	87%	171
Saint James Mercy Hospital	Hornell	87%	60
Benedictine Hospital	Kingston	86%	138
Lawrence Hospital Center[2]	Bronxville	86%	141
Geneva General Hospital[2]	Geneva	85%	116
Medina Memorial Hospital	Medina	85%	34
Claxton-Hepburn Medical Center	Ogdensburg	84%	44
Southampton Hospital	Southampton	84%	70
Eastern Niagara Hospital	Lockport	83%	89
Nathan Littauer Hospital	Gloversville	83%	63
North Central Bronx Hospital	Bronx	83%	30
Woman's Christian Association	Jamestown	83%	126
Nicholas H Noyes Memorial Hospital	Dansville	82%	44
Saint John's Riverside Hospital[2]	Yonkers	77%	208
Saint Elizabeth Medical Center[2]	Utica	75%	173
Samaritan Hospital[2]	Troy	74%	152
Wyoming County Community Hospital	Warsaw	73%	82
Good Samaritan Hospital of Suffern[2]	Suffern	70%	158
Mount Vernon Hospital	Mount Vernon	68%	62
Peninsula Hospital Center	Far Rockaway	59%	54
Adirondack Medical Center	Saranac Lake	50%	150

23. Appropriate Hair Removal

Hospital Name	City	Rate	Cases
Adirondack Medical Center	Saranac Lake	100%	250
Albany VA Medical Center[2]	Albany	100%	122
Alice Hyde Medical Center	Malone	100%	159
Bellevue Hospital Center[2]	New York	100%	747
Bon Secours Community Hospital	Port Jervis	100%	109
Bronx VA Medical Center[2]	Bronx	100%	151
Bronx-Lebanon Hospital Center[2]	Bronx	100%	289
Brookhaven Memorial Hospital Med Ctr[2]	Patchogue	100%	392
Canton-Potsdam Hospital	Potsdam	100%	318
Carthage Area Hospital	Carthage	100%	45
Catskill Regional Medical Center	Harris	100%	235
Champlain Valley Physicians Hospital	Plattsburgh	100%	845
Chenango Memorial Hospital	Norwich	100%	183
Clifton Springs Hospital and Clinic	Clifton Springs	100%	331
Columbia Memorial Hospital	Hudson	100%	253
Community Memorial Hospital	Hamilton	100%	521
Comm-General Hosp of Greater Syracuse[2]	Syracuse	100%	412
Coney Island Hospital[2]	Brooklyn	100%	240
Eastern Long Island Hospital	Greenport	100%	45
Eastern Niagara Hospital	Lockport	100%	231
F F Thompson Hospital	Canandaigua	100%	464
Faxton-St Luke's Healthcare[2]	Utica	100%	499
Flushing Hospital Medical Center[2]	Flushing	100%	616
Forest Hills Hospital[2]	Forest Hills	100%	411

NOTE: Hospital profiles are in alphabetical order by state, then city, then hospital within the city; Rankings exclude hospitals with less than 25 cases except for patient surveys which excludes hospitals with less than 100 cases; (a) 100–299 cases; (1) The number of cases is too small to be sure how well a hospital is performing; (2) The hospital indicated that the data submitted for this measure were based on a sample of cases; (3) Data was collected during a shorter time period (fewer quarters) than the maximum possible time for this measure; (4) Suppressed for one or more quarters by CMS; (5) No data is available from the hospital for this measure; (6) Fewer than 100 patients completed the HCAHPS survey. Use these rates with caution, as the number of surveys may be too low to reliably assess hospital performance; (7) Survey results are based on less than 12 months of data; (8) Survey results are not available for this reporting period; (9) No or very few patients were eligible for the HCAHPS survey. The scores shown, if any, reflect a very small number of surveys; (10) A state average was not calculated because too few hospitals in the state submitted data; (11) There were discrepancies in the data collection process; Please refer to the User's Guide for a full explanation of data.

Franklin Hospital[2]	Valley Stream	100%	328
Geneva General Hospital[2]	Geneva	100%	238
Glen Cove Hospital[2]	Glen Cove	100%	299
Glens Falls Hospital[2]	Glens Falls	100%	655
Good Samaritan Hospital Medical Center[2]	West Islip	100%	500
Good Samaritan Hospital of Suffern[2]	Suffern	100%	540
Highland Hospital[2]	Rochester	100%	992
Hospital for Special Surgery[2]	New York	100%	566
Huntington Hospital[2]	Huntington	100%	397
Jamaica Hospital Medical Center[2]	Jamaica	100%	412
John T Mather Mem Hosp-Port Jefferson	Port Jefferson	100%	536
Kaleida Health[2]	Buffalo	100%	1365
Kenmore Mercy Hospital[2]	Kenmore	100%	384
Kings County Hospital Center[2]	Brooklyn	100%	330
Kingsbrook Jewish Medical Center	Brooklyn	100%	170
Lakeside Memorial Hospital	Brockport	100%	113
Lawrence Hospital Center[2]	Bronxville	100%	295
Lewis County General Hospital	Lowville	100%	132
Lincoln Medical & Mental Health Center[2]	Bronx	100%	276
Long Beach Medical Center[2]	Long Beach	100%	61
Long Island Jewish Medical Center[2]	New Hyde Park	100%	671
Maimonides Medical Center[2]	Brooklyn	100%	1231
Mary Imogene Bassett Hospital[2]	Cooperstown	100%	610
Massena Memorial Hospital	Massena	100%	105
Medina Memorial Hospital	Medina	100%	63
Mercy Hospital[2]	Buffalo	100%	701
Mercy Medical Center[2]	Rockville Centre	100%	497
Metropolitan Hospital Center[2]	New York	100%	257
Mount St Mary's Hospital and Health Center[2]	Lewiston	100%	385
Mount Vernon Hospital	Mount Vernon	100%	92
Nassau University Medical Center[2]	East Meadow	100%	326
New York Community Hospital of Brooklyn[2]	Brooklyn	100%	141
New York Downtown Hospital[2]	New York	100%	316
New York Hospital Medical Center of Queens[2]	Flushing	100%	771
New York Methodist Hospital[2]	Brooklyn	100%	791
New York Westchester Square Medical Center	Bronx	100%	321
New York-Presbyterian Hospital[2]	New York	100%	1737
Newark-Wayne Community Hospital	Newark	100%	259
Niagara Falls Memorial Medical Center	Niagara Falls	100%	134
Nicholas H Noyes Memorial Hospital	Dansville	100%	150
North Shore University Hospital[2]	Manhasset	100%	982
Northern Dutchess Hospital[2]	Rhinebeck	100%	320
Northern Westchester Hospital[2]	Mount Kisco	100%	371
Northport VA Medical Center[2]	Northport	100%	126
Nyack Hospital	Nyack	100%	664
NYU Hospitals Center[2]	New York	100%	710
Olean General Hospital	Olean	100%	399
Orange Regional Medical Center[2]	Goshen	100%	930
Oswego Hospital	Oswego	100%	190
Our Lady of Lourdes Memorial Hospital[2]	Binghamton	100%	349
Peconic Bay Medical Center	Riverhead	100%	463
Peninsula Hospital Center	Far Rockaway	100%	88
Phelps Memorial Hospital Assn[2]	Sleepy Hollow	100%	486
Plainview Hospital[2]	Plainview	100%	434
Putnam Hospital Center	Carmel	100%	708
Queens Hospital Center	Jamaica	100%	319
Richmond University Medical Center[2]	Staten Island	100%	434
Rochester General Hospital[2]	Rochester	100%	2308
Rome Memorial Hospital	Rome	100%	239
Saint Anthony Community Hospital	Warwick	100%	233
Saint Catherine of Siena Hospital[2]	Smithtown	100%	445
Saint Charles Hospital[2]	Port Jefferson	100%	691
Saint Francis Hospital[2]	Poughkeepsie	100%	367
Saint Francis Hospital - Roslyn[2]	Roslyn	100%	650
Saint James Mercy Hospital	Hornell	100%	117
St John's Episcopal Hosp-South Shore[2]	Far Rockaway	100%	148
Saint Joseph Hospital[2]	Bethpage	100%	262
Saint Joseph's Hospital	Elmira	100%	203
Saint Joseph's Hospital Health Center[2]	Syracuse	100%	752
Saint Joseph's Medical Center	Yonkers	100%	132
Saint Luke's Cornwall Hospital[2]	Newburgh	100%	360
Saint Mary's Hospital at Amsterdam[2]	Amsterdam	100%	297
Samaritan Medical Center	Watertown	100%	468
Saratoga Hospital	Saratoga Spgs	100%	713
Schuyler Hospital	Montour Falls	100%	60
Seton Health System-St Mary's Campus[2]	Troy	100%	383
Sisters of Charity Hospital[2]	Buffalo	100%	873
Sound Shore Medical Center of Westchester	New Rochelle	100%	473
South Nassau Communities Hospital[2]	Oceanside	100%	969
Southampton Hospital	Southampton	100%	168
Southside Hospital[2]	Bay Shore	100%	419
Staten Island University Hospital[2]	Staten Island	100%	536
Strong Memorial Hospital[2]	Rochester	100%	1282
Syracuse VA Medical Center[2]	Syracuse	100%	135
TLC Health Network	Gowanda	100%	159
United Health Services Hospitals	Johnson City	100%	1500
United Memorial Medical Center	Batavia	100%	268
University Hospital - Stony Brook[2]	Stony Brook	100%	542
University Hospital of Brooklyn - Downstate[2]	Brooklyn	100%	382
Univ Hosp S U N Y Health Science Ctr[2]	Syracuse	100%	588
Upstate New York VA Healthcare System[2]	Buffalo	100%	282
VA New York Harbor Healthcare System[2]	New York	100%	243
Westchester Medical Center[2]	Valhalla	100%	1026
White Plains Hospital Center[2]	White Plains	100%	429
Winthrop-University Hospital[2]	Mineola	100%	902
Woodhull Medical and Mental Health Center[2]	Brooklyn	100%	257
Wyoming County Community Hospital	Warsaw	100%	157
Auburn Memorial Hospital	Auburn	99%	255
Aurelia Osborn Fox Memorial Hospital	Oneonta	99%	191
Benedictine Hospital	Kingston	99%	373
Beth Israel Medical Center[2]	New York	99%	690
Brookdale Hospital Medical Center[2]	Brooklyn	99%	308
Brooklyn Hospital Center at Downtown Campus	Brooklyn	99%	438
Brooks Memorial Hospital	Dunkirk	99%	358
Cayuga Medical Center at Ithaca	Ithaca	99%	324
Corning Hospital	Corning	99%	264
Ellis Hospital[2]	Schenectady	99%	874
Erie County Medical Center	Buffalo	99%	741
Interfaith Medical Center	Brooklyn	99%	113
Jones Memorial Hospital	Wellsville	99%	114
Kingston Hospital	Kingston	99%	319
Lenox Hill Hospital[2]	New York	99%	741
Long Island College Hospital[2]	Brooklyn	99%	436
Lutheran Medical Center[2]	Brooklyn	99%	959
Mount Sinai Hospital[2]	New York	99%	1156
Nathan Littauer Hospital	Gloversville	99%	148
Saint Barnabas Hospital[2]	Bronx	99%	196
Saint Elizabeth Medical Center[2]	Utica	99%	1070
Saint John's Riverside Hospital[2]	Yonkers	99%	354
Saint Luke's Roosevelt Hospital[2]	New York	99%	768
Vassar Brothers Medical Center[2]	Poughkeepsie	99%	642
Woman's Christian Association	Jamestown	99%	429
Wyckoff Heights Medical Center[2]	Brooklyn	99%	329
Albany Medical Center Hospital[2]	Albany	98%	527
Albany Memorial Hospital[2]	Albany	98%	449
Arnot Ogden Medical Center[2]	Elmira	98%	732
Claxton-Hepburn Medical Center	Ogdensburg	98%	100
Cortland Regional Medical Center	Cortland	98%	153
Crouse Hospital[2]	Syracuse	98%	530
Hudson Valley Hospital Center	Cortlandt Manor	98%	389
Jacobi Medical Center	Bronx	98%	447
Oneida Healthcare Center	Oneida	98%	275
Saint Peter's Hospital[2]	Albany	98%	737
Unity Hospital of Rochester[2]	Rochester	98%	561
Elmhurst Hospital Center	Elmhurst	97%	436
Montefiore Medical Center[2]	Bronx	96%	1163
North Central Bronx Hospital	Bronx	96%	72
Samaritan Hospital[2]	Troy	96%	380
Harlem Hospital Center[2]	New York	94%	120

24. Appropriate Beta Blocker Usage

Hospital Name	City	Rate	Cases
Albany VA Medical Center[2]	Albany	100%	51
Arnot Ogden Medical Center[2]	Elmira	100%	293
Bronx VA Medical Center[2]	Bronx	100%	41
Clifton Springs Hospital and Clinic	Clifton Springs	100%	111
Community Memorial Hospital	Hamilton	100%	180
Coney Island Hospital[2]	Brooklyn	100%	53
Crouse Hospital[2]	Syracuse	100%	143
Elmhurst Hospital Center	Elmhurst	100%	74
Good Samaritan Hospital of Suffern[2]	Suffern	100%	221
Mercy Medical Center[2]	Rockville Centre	100%	216
Nassau University Medical Center[2]	East Meadow	100%	56
Nathan Littauer Hospital	Gloversville	100%	47
New York Community Hospital of Brooklyn[2]	Brooklyn	100%	53
Our Lady of Lourdes Memorial Hospital[2]	Binghamton	100%	77
Plainview Hospital[2]	Plainview	100%	159
Saint Catherine of Siena Hospital[2]	Smithtown	100%	151
Saint Charles Hospital[2]	Port Jefferson	100%	204
Saint James Mercy Hospital	Hornell	100%	29
St John's Episcopal Hosp-South Shore[2]	Far Rockaway	100%	38
Saint Mary's Hospital at Amsterdam[2]	Amsterdam	100%	100
United Memorial Medical Center	Batavia	100%	102
Bellevue Hospital Center[2]	New York	99%	190
Faxton-St Luke's Healthcare[2]	Utica	99%	146
Mount St Mary's Hospital and Health Center[2]	Lewiston	99%	101
New York-Presbyterian Hospital[2]	New York	99%	539
Nyack Hospital	Nyack	99%	138
Saint Joseph Hospital[2]	Bethpage	99%	85
Southside Hospital[2]	Bay Shore	99%	131
University Hospital of Brooklyn - Downstate[2]	Brooklyn	99%	110
VA New York Harbor Healthcare System[2]	New York	99%	128
Forest Hills Hospital[2]	Forest Hills	98%	110
Lenox Hill Hospital[2]	New York	98%	266
Lincoln Medical & Mental Health Center[2]	Bronx	98%	54
New York Westchester Square Medical Center	Bronx	98%	53
NYU Hospitals Center[2]	New York	98%	214
Phelps Memorial Hospital Assn[2]	Sleepy Hollow	98%	174
Saint Francis Hospital[2]	Poughkeepsie	98%	115
Saint Luke's Cornwall Hospital[2]	Newburgh	98%	95
Univ Hosp S U N Y Health Science Ctr[2]	Syracuse	98%	235
Albany Medical Center Hospital[2]	Albany	97%	195
Brooks Memorial Hospital	Dunkirk	97%	111
Glen Cove Hospital[2]	Glen Cove	97%	95
Good Samaritan Hospital Medical Center[2]	West Islip	97%	190
Hospital for Special Surgery[2]	New York	97%	147
John T Mather Mem Hosp-Port Jefferson	Port Jefferson	97%	191
Lakeside Memorial Hospital	Brockport	97%	33
Richmond University Medical Center[2]	Staten Island	97%	122
Saint Francis Hospital - Roslyn[2]	Roslyn	97%	331
Strong Memorial Hospital[2]	Rochester	97%	532
White Plains Hospital Center[2]	White Plains	97%	97
Chenango Memorial Hospital	Norwich	96%	47
Flushing Hospital Medical Center[2]	Flushing	96%	112
Huntington Hospital[2]	Huntington	96%	137
Jones Memorial Hospital	Wellsville	96%	27
Mount Sinai Hospital[2]	New York	96%	369
New York Hospital Medical Center of Queens[2]	Flushing	96%	230
North Shore University Hospital[2]	Manhasset	96%	297
Putnam Hospital Center	Carmel	96%	224
Seton Health System-St Mary's Campus[2]	Troy	96%	104
Upstate New York VA Healthcare System[2]	Buffalo	96%	129
Bon Secours Community Hospital	Port Jervis	95%	40
Franklin Hospital[2]	Valley Stream	95%	87
Geneva General Hospital[2]	Geneva	95%	55
Jacobi Medical Center	Bronx	95%	101
Kingsbrook Jewish Medical Center	Brooklyn	95%	43
Saint Barnabas Hospital[2]	Bronx	95%	40
Saint Joseph's Medical Center	Yonkers	95%	40
South Nassau Communities Hospital[2]	Oceanside	95%	333
Staten Island University Hospital[2]	Staten Island	95%	175
United Health Services Hospitals	Johnson City	95%	503
Vassar Brothers Medical Center[2]	Poughkeepsie	95%	274
Winthrop-University Hospital[2]	Mineola	95%	398
Canton-Potsdam Hospital	Potsdam	94%	86
Cayuga Medical Center at Ithaca	Ithaca	94%	80
Champlain Valley Physicians Hospital	Plattsburgh	94%	290
Mary Imogene Bassett Hospital[2]	Cooperstown	94%	263
Metropolitan Hospital Center[2]	New York	94%	48
Northern Westchester Hospital[2]	Mount Kisco	94%	83
Olean General Hospital	Olean	94%	97
Alice Hyde Medical Center	Malone	93%	42
Columbia Memorial Hospital	Hudson	93%	83
Cortland Regional Medical Center	Cortland	93%	30
Ellis Hospital[2]	Schenectady	93%	343
Glens Falls Hospital[2]	Glens Falls	93%	202
Long Island College Hospital[2]	Brooklyn	93%	100
Mercy Hospital[2]	Buffalo	93%	265
Niagara Falls Memorial Medical Center	Niagara Falls	93%	29
Orange Regional Medical Center[2]	Goshen	93%	304
Rochester General Hospital[2]	Rochester	93%	1057
Saint John's Riverside Hospital[2]	Yonkers	93%	100
Southampton Hospital	Southampton	93%	42
Wyoming County Community Hospital	Warsaw	93%	46
Benedictine Hospital	Kingston	92%	124
Kingston Hospital	Kingston	92%	83
Lawrence Hospital Center[2]	Bronxville	92%	77
New York Downtown Hospital[2]	New York	92%	65
Saint Joseph's Hospital	Elmira	92%	59
Westchester Medical Center[2]	Valhalla	92%	475
Kaleida Health[2]	Buffalo	91%	431
Kings County Hospital Center[2]	Brooklyn	91%	44
Saint Joseph's Hospital Health Center[2]	Syracuse	91%	292
Adirondack Medical Center	Saranac Lake	90%	69
Peconic Bay Medical Center	Riverhead	90%	146
Saint Anthony Community Hospital	Warwick	90%	50
Sisters of Charity Hospital[2]	Buffalo	90%	284
Auburn Memorial Hospital	Auburn	89%	71
Brooklyn Hospital Center at Downtown Campus	Brooklyn	89%	107
Maimonides Medical Center[2]	Brooklyn	89%	496
Rome Memorial Hospital	Rome	89%	35
Saint Elizabeth Medical Center[2]	Utica	89%	514
Samaritan Hospital[2]	Troy	89%	109
Woman's Christian Association	Jamestown	89%	154
Brookhaven Memorial Hospital Med Ctr[2]	Patchogue	88%	121
Kenmore Mercy Hospital[2]	Kenmore	88%	129
Long Island Jewish Medical Center[2]	New Hyde Park	88%	221
Northport VA Medical Center[2]	Northport	88%	43
Wyckoff Heights Medical Center[2]	Brooklyn	87%	79
Brookdale Hospital Medical Center[2]	Brooklyn	86%	71
Corning Hospital	Corning	86%	74
F F Thompson Hospital	Canandaigua	86%	125
Highland Hospital[2]	Rochester	86%	304
Lutheran Medical Center[2]	Brooklyn	86%	292
New York Methodist Hospital[2]	Brooklyn	86%	251
Oneida Healthcare Center	Oneida	86%	69
Saint Luke's Roosevelt Hospital[2]	New York	86%	181
Woodhull Medical and Mental Health Center[2]	Brooklyn	86%	28
Sound Shore Medical Center of Westchester	New Rochelle	85%	153
Syracuse VA Medical Center[2]	Syracuse	85%	62
Albany Memorial Hospital[2]	Albany	84%	133
Aurelia Osborn Fox Memorial Hospital	Oneonta	84%	44

NOTE: Hospital profiles are in alphabetical order by state, then city, then hospital within the city; Rankings exclude hospitals with less than 25 cases except for patient surveys which excludes hospitals with less than 100 cases; (a) 100–299 cases; (1) The number of cases is too small to be sure how well a hospital is performing; (2) The hospital indicated that the data submitted for this measure were based on a sample of cases; (3) Data was collected during a shorter time period (fewer quarters) than the maximum possible time for this measure; (4) Suppressed for one or more quarters by CMS; (5) No data is available from the hospital for this measure; (6) Fewer than 100 patients completed the HCAHPS survey. Use these rates with caution, as the number of surveys may be too low to reliably assess hospital performance; (7) Survey results are based on less than 12 months of data; (8) Survey results are not available for this reporting period; (9) No or very few patients were eligible for the HCAHPS survey. The scores shown, if any, reflect a very small number of surveys; (10) A state average was not calculated because too few hospitals in the state submitted data; (11) There were discrepancies in the data collection process; Please refer to the User's Guide for a full explanation of data.

Northern Dutchess Hospital[2]	Rhinebeck	84%	90
Catskill Regional Medical Center	Harris	83%	54
Jamaica Hospital Medical Center[2]	Jamaica	83%	75
Samaritan Medical Center	Watertown	83%	143
University Hospital - Stony Brook[2]	Stony Brook	82%	176
Nicholas H Noyes Memorial Hospital	Dansville	81%	54
Oswego Hospital	Oswego	81%	36
Unity Hospital of Rochester[2]	Rochester	81%	254
Saratoga Hospital	Saratoga Spgs	80%	205
Erie County Medical Center	Buffalo	79%	240
Newark-Wayne Community Hospital	Newark	79%	77
Beth Israel Medical Center[2]	New York	78%	222
Comm-General Hosp of Greater Syracuse[2]	Syracuse	78%	118
Hudson Valley Hospital Center	Cortlandt Manor	78%	101
Montefiore Medical Center[2]	Bronx	77%	415
Lewis County General Hospital	Lowville	73%	26
TLC Health Network	Gowanda	73%	51
Saint Peter's Hospital[2]	Albany	71%	210
Eastern Niagara Hospital	Lockport	70%	50
Queens Hospital Center	Jamaica	67%	52
Bronx-Lebanon Hospital Center[2]	Bronx	53%	58

25. Controlled Postoperative Blood Glucose

Hospital Name	City	Rate	Cases
Champlain Valley Physicians Hospital	Plattsburgh	99%	127
Good Samaritan Hospital of Suffern[2]	Suffern	99%	155
Long Island Jewish Medical Center[2]	New Hyde Park	99%	154
New York Hospital Medical Center of Queens[2]	Flushing	99%	107
NYU Hospitals Center[2]	New York	98%	131
Rochester General Hospital[2]	Rochester	98%	634
Saint Peter's Hospital[2]	Albany	98%	183
Bellevue Hospital Center[2]	New York	97%	192
New York Methodist Hospital[2]	Brooklyn	97%	118
North Shore University Hospital[2]	Manhasset	97%	159
Saint Francis Hospital - Roslyn[2]	Roslyn	97%	234
Univ Hosp S U N Y Health Science Ctr[2]	Syracuse	97%	198
Ellis Hospital[2]	Schenectady	96%	192
Saint Luke's Roosevelt Hospital[2]	New York	96%	144
Upstate New York VA Healthcare System[2]	Buffalo	96%	67
Vassar Brothers Medical Center[2]	Poughkeepsie	96%	171
Westchester Medical Center[2]	Valhalla	96%	335
Mercy Hospital[2]	Buffalo	95%	170
Saint Elizabeth Medical Center[2]	Utica	95%	350
United Health Services Hospitals	Johnson City	95%	285
Lenox Hill Hospital[2]	New York	93%	166
Maimonides Medical Center[2]	Brooklyn	93%	373
Kaleida Health[2]	Buffalo	92%	240
Staten Island University Hospital[2]	Staten Island	92%	128
Strong Memorial Hospital[2]	Rochester	92%	428
University Hospital - Stony Brook[2]	Stony Brook	92%	119
Erie County Medical Center	Buffalo	91%	127
Mount Sinai Hospital[2]	New York	91%	174
VA New York Harbor Healthcare System[2]	New York	91%	75
University Hospital of Brooklyn - Downstate[2]	Brooklyn	90%	60
Arnot Ogden Medical Center[2]	Elmira	89%	114
Mary Imogene Bassett Hospital[2]	Cooperstown	89%	109
Winthrop-University Hospital[2]	Mineola	89%	212
Beth Israel Medical Center[2]	New York	88%	141
New York-Presbyterian Hospital[2]	New York	87%	339
Saint Joseph's Hospital Health Center[2]	Syracuse	87%	180
Albany Medical Center Hospital[2]	Albany	85%	103
Montefiore Medical Center[2]	Bronx	83%	212

26. Prophylactic Antibiotic Timing

Hospital Name	City	Rate	Cases
Albany VA Medical Center	Albany	100%	68
Bon Secours Community Hospital	Port Jervis	100%	53
Community Memorial Hospital	Hamilton	100%	490
Ellis Hospital[2]	Schenectady	100%	668
Hudson Valley Hospital Center	Cortlandt Manor	100%	224
John T Mather Mem Hosp-Port Jefferson	Port Jefferson	100%	276
Lakeside Memorial Hospital	Brockport	100%	69
Long Beach Medical Center[2]	Long Beach	100%	28
Medina Memorial Hospital	Medina	100%	30
New York Downtown Hospital[2]	New York	100%	214
New York Hospital Medical Center of Queens[2]	Flushing	100%	496
Niagara Falls Memorial Medical Center	Niagara Falls	100%	65
Nyack Hospital	Nyack	100%	411
Olean General Hospital	Olean	100%	275
Saint Charles Hospital[2]	Port Jefferson	100%	488
Saint Francis Hospital[2]	Poughkeepsie	100%	233
Saint Luke's Cornwall Hospital[2]	Newburgh	100%	228
South Nassau Communities Hospital[2]	Oceanside	100%	707
VA New York Harbor Healthcare System	New York	100%	140
Arnot Ogden Medical Center[2]	Elmira	99%	572
Beth Israel Medical Center[2]	New York	99%	490
Bronx VA Medical Center	Bronx	99%	81
Canton-Potsdam Hospital	Potsdam	99%	220
Clifton Springs Hospital and Clinic	Clifton Springs	99%	255
Coney Island Hospital[2]	Brooklyn	99%	88
Elmhurst Hospital Center	Elmhurst	99%	127
Flushing Hospital Medical Center[2]	Flushing	99%	402
Forest Hills Hospital[2]	Forest Hills	99%	269
Kings County Hospital Center[2]	Brooklyn	99%	115
Kingsbrook Jewish Medical Center	Brooklyn	99%	78
Lutheran Medical Center[2]	Brooklyn	99%	665
Richmond University Medical Center[2]	Staten Island	99%	293
Rochester General Hospital[2]	Rochester	99%	1832
Saint Catherine of Siena Hospital[2]	Smithtown	99%	250
Saint Mary's Hospital at Amsterdam[2]	Amsterdam	99%	178
Strong Memorial Hospital[2]	Rochester	99%	847
University Hospital - Stony Brook[2]	Stony Brook	99%	358
White Plains Hospital Center[2]	White Plains	99%	296
Albany Medical Center Hospital[2]	Albany	98%	333
Brooks Memorial Hospital	Dunkirk	98%	313
Catskill Regional Medical Center	Harris	98%	157
Eastern Niagara Hospital	Lockport	98%	169
F F Thompson Hospital	Canandaigua	98%	401
Franklin Hospital[2]	Valley Stream	98%	209
Good Samaritan Hospital Medical Center[2]	West Islip	98%	296
Huntington Hospital[2]	Huntington	98%	249
Lenox Hill Hospital[2]	New York	98%	521
Long Island Jewish Medical Center[2]	New Hyde Park	98%	473
New York Methodist Hospital[2]	Brooklyn	98%	521
New York Westchester Square Medical Center	Bronx	98%	189
North Shore University Hospital[2]	Manhasset	98%	594
Northport VA Medical Center	Northport	98%	61
NYU Hospitals Center[2]	New York	98%	485
Orange Regional Medical Center[2]	Goshen	98%	682
Plainview Hospital[2]	Plainview	98%	265
Putnam Hospital Center	Carmel	98%	538
Saint Joseph's Hospital	Elmira	98%	173
Saratoga Hospital	Saratoga Spgs	98%	489
Southampton Hospital	Southampton	98%	85
Southside Hospital[2]	Bay Shore	98%	264
Staten Island University Hospital[2]	Staten Island	98%	381
United Health Services Hospitals	Johnson City	98%	967
Woman's Christian Association	Jamestown	98%	298
Bellevue Hospital Center[2]	New York	97%	410
Corning Hospital	Corning	97%	184
Erie County Medical Center	Buffalo	97%	364
Glen Cove Hospital[2]	Glen Cove	97%	194
Glens Falls Hospital[2]	Glens Falls	97%	442
Hospital for Special Surgery[2]	New York	97%	367
Jones Memorial Hospital	Wellsville	97%	76
Kingston Hospital	Kingston	97%	177
Lawrence Hospital Center[2]	Bronxville	97%	183
Lincoln Medical & Mental Health Center[2]	Bronx	97%	133
Mercy Medical Center[2]	Rockville Centre	97%	316
Mount Sinai Hospital[2]	New York	97%	710
Nassau University Medical Center[2]	East Meadow	97%	165
Newark-Wayne Community Hospital	Newark	97%	192
Northern Westchester Hospital[2]	Mount Kisco	97%	231
Phelps Memorial Hospital Assn[2]	Sleepy Hollow	97%	340
Saint Francis Hospital - Roslyn[2]	Roslyn	97%	399
Saint James Mercy Hospital	Hornell	97%	76
Saint Joseph Hospital[2]	Bethpage	97%	162
Seton Health System-St Mary's Campus[2]	Troy	97%	259
Sound Shore Medical Center of Westschester	New Rochelle	97%	298
Univ Hosp S U N Y Health Science Ctr[2]	Syracuse	97%	421
Vassar Brothers Medical Center[2]	Poughkeepsie	97%	442
Woodhull Medical and Mental Health Center[2]	Brooklyn	97%	94
Crouse Hospital[2]	Syracuse	96%	370
Geneva General Hospital[2]	Geneva	96%	166
Highland Hospital[2]	Rochester	96%	781
Mary Imogene Bassett Hospital[2]	Cooperstown	96%	449
Metropolitan Hospital Center[2]	New York	96%	163
Mount St Mary's Hospital and Health Center[2]	Lewiston	96%	289
Saint Anthony Community Hospital	Warwick	96%	155
Sisters of Charity Hospital[2]	Buffalo	96%	567
Syracuse VA Medical Center	Syracuse	96%	72
Upstate New York VA Healthcare System	Buffalo	96%	156
Alice Hyde Medical Center	Malone	95%	98
Benedictine Hospital	Kingston	95%	230
Cayuga Medical Center at Ithaca	Ithaca	95%	212
Claxton-Hepburn Medical Center	Ogdensburg	95%	59
Jamaica Hospital Medical Center[2]	Jamaica	95%	188
New York-Presbyterian Hospital[2]	New York	95%	811
Northern Dutchess Hospital[2]	Rhinebeck	95%	206
Our Lady of Lourdes Memorial Hospital[2]	Binghamton	95%	229
Peconic Bay Medical Center	Riverhead	95%	308
Queens Hospital Center	Jamaica	95%	133
Saint Peter's Hospital[2]	Albany	95%	547
Samaritan Medical Center	Watertown	95%	343
Winthrop-University Hospital[2]	Mineola	95%	642
Wyckoff Heights Medical Center[2]	Brooklyn	95%	143
Chenango Memorial Hospital	Norwich	94%	142
Cortland Regional Medical Center	Cortland	94%	63
Good Samaritan Hospital of Suffern[2]	Suffern	94%	338
Harlem Hospital Center[2]	New York	94%	34
Kaleida Health[2]	Buffalo	94%	907
Mercy Hospital[2]	Buffalo	94%	486
New York Community Hospital of Brooklyn[2]	Brooklyn	94%	63
North Central Bronx Hospital	Bronx	94%	35
Oneida Healthcare Center	Oneida	94%	181
Saint Barnabas Hospital[2]	Bronx	94%	100
Saint Joseph's Hospital Health Center[2]	Syracuse	94%	536
Saint Luke's Roosevelt Hospital[2]	New York	94%	571
TLC Health Network	Gowanda	94%	126
United Memorial Medical Center	Batavia	94%	217
Westchester Medical Center[2]	Valhalla	94%	588
Wyoming County Community Hospital	Warsaw	94%	119
Albany Memorial Hospital[2]	Albany	93%	300
Aurelia Osborn Fox Memorial Hospital	Oneonta	93%	89
Kenmore Mercy Hospital[2]	Kenmore	93%	250
Long Island College Hospital[2]	Brooklyn	93%	312
Maimonides Medical Center[2]	Brooklyn	93%	933
Massena Memorial Hospital	Massena	93%	89
Nicholas H Noyes Memorial Hospital	Dansville	93%	98
St John's Episcopal Hosp-South Shore[2]	Far Rockaway	93%	61
Unity Hospital of Rochester[2]	Rochester	93%	393
University Hospital of Brooklyn - Downstate[2]	Brooklyn	93%	256
Oswego Hospital	Oswego	92%	109
Peninsula Hospital Center	Far Rockaway	92%	36
Saint Elizabeth Medical Center[2]	Utica	92%	834
Samaritan Hospital[2]	Troy	92%	229
Bronx-Lebanon Hospital Center[2]	Bronx	91%	176
Brookdale Hospital Medical Center[2]	Brooklyn	91%	111
Brookhaven Memorial Hospital Med Ctr[2]	Patchogue	91%	237
Champlain Valley Physicians Hospital	Plattsburgh	91%	589
Comm-General Hosp of Greater Syracuse[2]	Syracuse	91%	267
Faxton-St Luke's Healthcare[2]	Utica	91%	333
Interfaith Medical Center	Brooklyn	91%	47
Lewis County General Hospital	Lowville	91%	103
Mount Vernon Hospital	Mount Vernon	91%	34
Rome Memorial Hospital	Rome	91%	116
Jacobi Medical Center	Bronx	90%	160
Columbia Memorial Hospital	Hudson	89%	125
Saint John's Riverside Hospital[2]	Yonkers	89%	218
Auburn Memorial Hospital	Auburn	88%	166
Saint Joseph's Medical Center	Yonkers	88%	69
Adirondack Medical Center	Saranac Lake	87%	157
Brooklyn Hospital Center at Downtown Campus	Brooklyn	87%	178
Carthage Area Hospital	Carthage	86%	29
Montefiore Medical Center[2]	Bronx	85%	750
Nathan Littauer Hospital	Gloversville	76%	46

27. Prophylactic Antibiotic Timing (Outpatient)

Hospital Name	City	Rate	Cases
Community Memorial Hospital	Hamilton	100%	98
Kings County Hospital Center	Brooklyn	100%	45
Saint Joseph's Hospital	Elmira	100%	94
Canton-Potsdam Hospital	Potsdam	99%	83
Good Samaritan Hospital Medical Center	West Islip	99%	352
NYU Hospitals Center	New York	99%	422
Southside Hospital	Bay Shore	99%	164
Bellevue Hospital Center	New York	98%	47
Jones Memorial Hospital	Wellsville	98%	43
Nyack Hospital	Nyack	98%	121
Saint Catherine of Siena Hospital	Smithtown	98%	387
Saint Charles Hospital	Port Jefferson	98%	46
South Nassau Communities Hospital	Oceanside	98%	378
Strong Memorial Hospital	Rochester	98%	572
United Health Services Hospitals	Johnson City	98%	1362
Arnot Ogden Medical Center	Elmira	97%	439
Hospital for Special Surgery	New York	97%	270
Hudson Valley Hospital Center	Cortlandt Manor	97%	97
John T Mather Mem Hosp-Port Jefferson	Port Jefferson	97%	165
Kenmore Mercy Hospital	Kenmore	97%	705
Mercy Hospital	Buffalo	97%	560
Northern Westchester Hospital	Mount Kisco	97%	336
Oswego Hospital	Oswego	97%	156
Saint Luke's Cornwall Hospital	Newburgh	97%	152
White Plains Hospital Center	White Plains	97%	354
Albany Medical Center Hospital	Albany	96%	594
Alice Hyde Medical Center	Malone	96%	82
Clifton Springs Hospital and Clinic	Clifton Springs	96%	71
Crouse Hospital	Syracuse	96%	870
F F Thompson Hospital	Canandaigua	96%	84
Forest Hills Hospital	Forest Hills	96%	122
Franklin Hospital	Valley Stream	96%	112
New York Westchester Square Medical Center	Bronx	96%	81
Saint Anthony Community Hospital	Warwick	96%	49
Saint Joseph's Medical Center	Yonkers	96%	83
Seton Health System-St Mary's Campus	Troy	96%	258
Winthrop-University Hospital	Mineola	96%	477
Beth Israel Medical Center	New York	95%	642
Glens Falls Hospital	Glens Falls	95%	424
Highland Hospital	Rochester	95%	203
Huntington Hospital	Huntington	95%	363
Lawrence Hospital Center	Bronxville	95%	110

NOTE: Hospital profiles are in alphabetical order by state, then city, then hospital within the city; Rankings exclude hospitals with less than 25 cases except for patient surveys which excludes hospitals with less than 100 cases; (a) 100–299 cases; (1) The number of cases is too small to be sure how well a hospital is performing; (2) The hospital indicated that the data submitted for this measure were based on a sample of cases; (3) Data was collected during a shorter time period (fewer quarters) than the maximum possible time for this measure; (4) Suppressed for one or more quarters by CMS; (5) No data is available from the hospital for this measure; (6) Fewer than 100 patients completed the HCAHPS survey. Use these rates with caution, as the number of surveys may be too low to reliably assess hospital performance; (7) Survey results are based on less than 12 months of data; (8) Survey results are not available for this reporting period; (9) No or very few patients were eligible for the HCAHPS survey. The scores shown, if any, reflect a very small number of surveys; (10) A state average was not calculated because too few hospitals in the state submitted data; (11) There were discrepancies in the data collection process; Please refer to the User's Guide for a full explanation of data.

Mercy Medical Center	Rockville Centre	95%	99
New York Methodist Hospital	Brooklyn	95%	186
Oneida Healthcare Center	Oneida	95%	219
Saint Francis Hospital - Roslyn	Roslyn	95%	340
Vassar Brothers Medical Center	Poughkeepsie	95%	637
Coney Island Hospital	Brooklyn	94%	50
Erie County Medical Center	Buffalo	94%	583
Metropolitan Hospital Center	New York	94%	65
Mount Vernon Hospital	Mount Vernon	94%	53
Our Lady of Lourdes Memorial Hospital	Binghamton	94%	422
Putnam Hospital Center	Carmel	94%	150
Saint Francis Hospital	Poughkeepsie	94%	181
Saint Joseph's Hospital Health Center	Syracuse	94%	794
University Hospital of Brooklyn - Downstate	Brooklyn	94%	108
Westchester Medical Center	Valhalla	94%	377
Auburn Memorial Hospital	Auburn	93%	116
Catskill Regional Medical Center	Harris	93%	41
Glen Cove Hospital	Glen Cove	93%	44
Kingsbrook Jewish Medical Center	Brooklyn	93%	61
Nassau University Medical Center	East Meadow	93%	59
New York Hospital Medical Center of Queens	Flushing	93%	312
Niagara Falls Memorial Medical Center	Niagara Falls	93%	89
Peconic Bay Medical Center	Riverhead	93%	67
Peninsula Hospital Center	Far Rockaway	93%	60
Unity Hospital of Rochester	Rochester	93%	423
Ellis Hospital	Schenectady	92%	538
Flushing Hospital Medical Center	Flushing	92%	166
Geneva General Hospital	Geneva	92%	72
Good Samaritan Hospital of Suffern	Suffern	92%	247
Ira Davenport Memorial Hospital	Bath	92%	25
Orange Regional Medical Center	Goshen	92%	314
Phelps Memorial Hospital Assn	Sleepy Hollow	92%	73
Rochester General Hospital	Rochester	92%	690
Saint Luke's Roosevelt Hospital	New York	92%	341
Albany Memorial Hospital	Albany	91%	190
Eastern Niagara Hospital	Lockport	91%	68
Kingston Hospital	Kingston	91%	126
North Shore University Hospital	Manhasset	91%	291
Richmond University Medical Center	Staten Island	91%	207
Saint Joseph Hospital	Bethpage	91%	58
Sisters of Charity Hospital	Buffalo	91%	614
Albany Med Ctr-South Clinical Campus	Albany	90%	154
Columbia Memorial Hospital	Hudson	90%	97
Comm-General Hosp of Greater Syracuse	Syracuse	90%	591
New York-Presbyterian Hospital	New York	90%	1187
Saint Peter's Hospital	Albany	90%	971
United Memorial Medical Center	Batavia	90%	60
Eastern Long Island Hospital	Greenport	89%	46
Kaleida Health	Buffalo	89%	1163
Lenox Hill Hospital	New York	89%	606
Mary Imogene Bassett Hospital	Cooperstown	89%	283
Mount Sinai Hospital	New York	89%	557
New York Downtown Hospital	New York	89%	76
Olean General Hospital	Olean	89%	151
Plainview Hospital	Plainview	89%	153
Sound Shore Medical Center of Westschester	New Rochelle	89%	97
Benedictine Hospital	Kingston	88%	115
Brooks Memorial Hospital	Dunkirk	88%	34
Harlem Hospital Center	New York	88%	26
Lakeside Memorial Hospital	Brockport	88%	51
Lincoln Medical & Mental Health Center	Bronx	88%	127
Nicholas H Noyes Memorial Hospital	Dansville	88%	40
Saratoga Hospital	Saratoga Spgs	88%	238
Southampton Hospital	Southampton	88%	50
University Hospital - Stony Brook	Stony Brook	88%	384
Adirondack Medical Center	Saranac Lake	87%	99
Claxton-Hepburn Medical Center	Ogdensburg	87%	45
Long Island Jewish Medical Center	New Hyde Park	87%	145
Lutheran Medical Center	Brooklyn	87%	118
Saint Barnabas Hospital	Bronx	87%	139
St John's Episcopal Hosp-South Shore	Far Rockaway	87%	69
Long Island College Hospital	Brooklyn	86%	176
Newark-Wayne Community Hospital	Newark	86%	76
Northern Dutchess Hospital	Rhinebeck	86%	110
Univ Hosp S U N Y Health Science Ctr	Syracuse	86%	269
Cayuga Medical Center at Ithaca	Ithaca	85%	109
Corning Hospital	Corning	85%	52
Maimonides Medical Center	Brooklyn	85%	176
Massena Memorial Hospital	Massena	84%	43
Samaritan Medical Center	Watertown	84%	443
Staten Island University Hospital	Staten Island	84%	233
Woodhull Medical and Mental Health Center	Brooklyn	84%	38
Saint John's Riverside Hospital	Yonkers	83%	83
Champlain Valley Physicians Hospital	Plattsburgh	82%	311
Cortland Regional Medical Center	Cortland	82%	60
Mount St Mary's Hospital and Health Center	Lewiston	82%	196
Queens Hospital Center	Jamaica	82%	38
Bronx-Lebanon Hospital Center	Bronx	81%	53
Brookhaven Memorial Hospital Med Ctr	Patchogue	81%	79
Saint Mary's Hospital at Amsterdam	Amsterdam	81%	91
Faxton-St Luke's Healthcare	Utica	80%	181
Nathan Littauer Hospital	Gloversville	80%	59
Rome Memorial Hospital	Rome	79%	53
Woman's Christian Association	Jamestown	79%	124
Saint Elizabeth Medical Center	Utica	77%	183
Wyckoff Heights Medical Center	Brooklyn	77%	132
Brookdale Hospital Medical Center	Brooklyn	76%	157
Jamaica Hospital Medical Center	Jamaica	74%	101
Montefiore Medical Center	Bronx	73%	681
Jacobi Medical Center	Bronx	71%	31
Samaritan Hospital	Troy	64%	85
Little Falls Hospital[3]	Little Falls	56%	25
Carthage Area Hospital	Carthage	55%	38
Brooklyn Hospital Center at Downtown Campus	Brooklyn	51%	164

28. Prophylactic Antibiotic Selection

Hospital Name	City	Rate	Cases
Albany VA Medical Center	Albany	100%	69
Benedictine Hospital	Kingston	100%	236
Clifton Springs Hospital and Clinic	Clifton Springs	100%	259
Columbia Memorial Hospital	Hudson	100%	124
Community Memorial Hospital	Hamilton	100%	489
Glen Cove Hospital[2]	Glen Cove	100%	194
Harlem Hospital Center[2]	New York	100%	34
Hospital for Special Surgery[2]	New York	100%	369
Saint Charles Hospital[2]	Port Jefferson	100%	490
Saint Luke's Cornwall Hospital[2]	Newburgh	100%	228
VA New York Harbor Healthcare System	New York	100%	149
Arnot Ogden Medical Center[2]	Elmira	99%	578
Brooks Memorial Hospital	Dunkirk	99%	313
Good Samaritan Hospital Medical Center[2]	West Islip	99%	298
Jacobi Medical Center	Bronx	99%	159
Jones Memorial Hospital	Wellsville	99%	77
Lenox Hill Hospital[2]	New York	99%	540
Lincoln Medical & Mental Health Center[2]	Bronx	99%	136
Newark-Wayne Community Hospital	Newark	99%	191
Nyack Hospital	Nyack	99%	412
Rochester General Hospital[2]	Rochester	99%	1874
Saint Francis Hospital[2]	Poughkeepsie	99%	231
Saint Francis Hospital - Roslyn[2]	Roslyn	99%	416
Saint Joseph's Hospital	Elmira	99%	174
Sound Shore Medical Center of Westschester	New Rochelle	99%	324
Southside Hospital[2]	Bay Shore	99%	266
Strong Memorial Hospital[2]	Rochester	99%	868
Univ Hosp S U N Y Health Science Ctr[2]	Syracuse	99%	427
Westchester Medical Center[2]	Valhalla	99%	614
Aurelia Osborn Fox Memorial Hospital	Oneonta	98%	89
Bellevue Hospital Center[2]	New York	98%	418
Cayuga Medical Center at Ithaca	Ithaca	98%	213
Elmhurst Hospital Center	Elmhurst	98%	129
Erie County Medical Center	Buffalo	98%	372
Forest Hills Hospital[2]	Forest Hills	98%	270
Huntington Hospital[2]	Huntington	98%	249
John T Mather Mem Hosp-Port Jefferson	Port Jefferson	98%	282
Kings County Hospital Center[2]	Brooklyn	98%	117
Kingsbrook Jewish Medical Center	Brooklyn	98%	81
Lawrence Hospital Center[2]	Bronxville	98%	184
Lutheran Medical Center[2]	Brooklyn	98%	665
Mary Imogene Bassett Hospital[2]	Cooperstown	98%	455
Mount Sinai Hospital[2]	New York	98%	721
New York Downtown Hospital[2]	New York	98%	213
New York Westchester Square Medical Center	Bronx	98%	190
North Shore University Hospital[2]	Manhasset	98%	603
Northern Dutchess Hospital[2]	Rhinebeck	98%	207
NYU Hospitals Center[2]	New York	98%	490
Orange Regional Medical Center[2]	Goshen	98%	687
Plainview Hospital[2]	Plainview	98%	265
Putnam Hospital Center	Carmel	98%	537
Saint Elizabeth Medical Center[2]	Utica	98%	851
Saint Joseph's Hospital Health Center[2]	Syracuse	98%	541
Saint Mary's Hospital at Amsterdam[2]	Amsterdam	98%	179
Samaritan Medical Center	Watertown	98%	348
United Memorial Medical Center	Batavia	98%	215
University Hospital - Stony Brook[2]	Stony Brook	98%	367
University Hospital of Brooklyn - Downstate[2]	Brooklyn	98%	261
Upstate New York VA Healthcare System	Buffalo	98%	163
Vassar Brothers Medical Center[2]	Poughkeepsie	98%	446
Winthrop-University Hospital[2]	Mineola	98%	648
Woman's Christian Association	Jamestown	98%	299
Albany Medical Center Hospital[2]	Albany	97%	352
Carthage Area Hospital	Carthage	97%	29
Claxton-Hepburn Medical Center	Ogdensburg	97%	60
Comm-General Hosp of Greater Syracuse[2]	Syracuse	97%	270
Cortland Regional Medical Center	Cortland	97%	63
Ellis Hospital[2]	Schenectady	97%	680
Highland Hospital[2]	Rochester	97%	777
Kaleida Health[2]	Buffalo	97%	922
Kenmore Mercy Hospital[2]	Kenmore	97%	253
Kingston Hospital	Kingston	97%	178
Maimonides Medical Center[2]	Brooklyn	97%	945
Mercy Hospital[2]	Buffalo	97%	506
Mercy Medical Center[2]	Rockville Centre	97%	317
Montefiore Medical Center[2]	Bronx	97%	749
Mount St Mary's Hospital and Health Center[2]	Lewiston	97%	289
New York Hospital Medical Center of Queens[2]	Flushing	97%	501
New York Methodist Hospital[2]	Brooklyn	97%	528
New York-Presbyterian Hospital[2]	New York	97%	954
Northern Westchester Hospital[2]	Mount Kisco	97%	245
Olean General Hospital	Olean	97%	276
Oneida Healthcare Center	Oneida	97%	181
Phelps Memorial Hospital Assn[2]	Sleepy Hollow	97%	341
Saint Peter's Hospital[2]	Albany	97%	548
Saratoga Hospital	Saratoga Spgs	97%	488
Seton Health System-St Mary's Campus[2]	Troy	97%	258
South Nassau Communities Hospital[2]	Oceanside	97%	708
Staten Island University Hospital[2]	Staten Island	97%	387
United Health Services Hospitals	Johnson City	97%	975
White Plains Hospital Center[2]	White Plains	97%	297
Woodhull Medical and Mental Health Center[2]	Brooklyn	97%	93
Wyoming County Community Hospital	Warsaw	97%	120
Adirondack Medical Center	Saranac Lake	96%	157
Alice Hyde Medical Center	Malone	96%	98
Beth Israel Medical Center[2]	New York	96%	490
Bon Secours Community Hospital	Port Jervis	96%	55
Bronx VA Medical Center	Bronx	96%	81
Bronx-Lebanon Hospital Center[2]	Bronx	96%	176
Brookhaven Memorial Hospital Med Ctr[2]	Patchogue	96%	238
Canton-Potsdam Hospital	Potsdam	96%	221
Corning Hospital	Corning	96%	186
F F Thompson Hospital	Canandaigua	96%	401
Jamaica Hospital Medical Center[2]	Jamaica	96%	190
Our Lady of Lourdes Memorial Hospital[2]	Binghamton	96%	230
Saint Barnabas Hospital[2]	Bronx	96%	98
Saint Catherine of Siena Hospital[2]	Smithtown	96%	252
Saint Joseph Hospital[2]	Bethpage	96%	162
Saint Luke's Roosevelt Hospital[2]	New York	96%	579
Brookdale Hospital Medical Center[2]	Brooklyn	95%	109
Champlain Valley Physicians Hospital	Plattsburgh	95%	591
Coney Island Hospital[2]	Brooklyn	95%	88
Flushing Hospital Medical Center[2]	Flushing	95%	404
Glens Falls Hospital[2]	Glens Falls	95%	447
Hudson Valley Hospital Center	Cortlandt Manor	95%	224
Northport VA Medical Center	Northport	95%	63
Queens Hospital Center	Jamaica	95%	132
Saint John's Riverside Hospital[2]	Yonkers	95%	220
Sisters of Charity Hospital[2]	Buffalo	95%	571
Brooklyn Hospital Center at Downtown Campus	Brooklyn	94%	179
Eastern Niagara Hospital	Lockport	94%	169
Franklin Hospital[2]	Valley Stream	94%	209
Geneva General Hospital[2]	Geneva	94%	153
Good Samaritan Hospital of Suffern[2]	Suffern	94%	375
Lakeside Memorial Hospital	Brockport	94%	69
Long Island College Hospital[2]	Brooklyn	94%	307
Long Island Jewish Medical Center[2]	New Hyde Park	94%	482
Metropolitan Hospital Center[2]	New York	94%	163
New York Community Hospital of Brooklyn[2]	Brooklyn	94%	63
Peninsula Hospital Center	Far Rockaway	94%	36
TLC Health Network	Gowanda	94%	126
Unity Hospital of Rochester[2]	Rochester	94%	391
Crouse Hospital[2]	Syracuse	93%	368
Faxton-St Luke's Healthcare[2]	Utica	93%	332
Interfaith Medical Center	Brooklyn	93%	46
Lewis County General Hospital	Lowville	93%	102
Medina Memorial Hospital	Medina	93%	30
Peconic Bay Medical Center	Riverhead	93%	308
Richmond University Medical Center[2]	Staten Island	93%	295
Niagara Falls Memorial Medical Center	Niagara Falls	92%	65
Nicholas H Noyes Memorial Hospital	Dansville	92%	96
Wyckoff Heights Medical Center[2]	Brooklyn	92%	146
Chenango Memorial Hospital	Norwich	91%	141
Nassau University Medical Center[2]	East Meadow	91%	164
Nathan Littauer Hospital	Gloversville	91%	46
Saint James Mercy Hospital	Hornell	90%	78
Saint Joseph's Medical Center	Yonkers	90%	71
Samaritan Hospital[2]	Troy	90%	231
Syracuse VA Medical Center	Syracuse	90%	72
Albany Memorial Hospital[2]	Albany	89%	298
Auburn Memorial Hospital	Auburn	89%	161
Oswego Hospital	Oswego	89%	112
Rome Memorial Hospital	Rome	89%	115
St John's Episcopal Hosp-South Shore[2]	Far Rockaway	89%	63
Saint Anthony Community Hospital	Warwick	88%	155
Southampton Hospital	Southampton	86%	85
Catskill Regional Medical Center	Harris	85%	158
Mount Vernon Hospital	Mount Vernon	85%	34
North Central Bronx Hospital	Bronx	85%	34
Long Beach Medical Center[2]	Long Beach	82%	28
Massena Memorial Hospital	Massena	81%	86

NOTE: Hospital profiles are in alphabetical order by state, then city, then hospital within the city; Rankings exclude hospitals with less than 25 cases except for patient surveys which excludes hospitals with less than 100 cases; (a) 100–299 cases; (1) The number of cases is too small to be sure how well a hospital is performing; (2) The hospital indicated that the data submitted for this measure were based on a sample of cases; (3) Data was collected during a shorter time period (fewer quarters) than the maximum possible time for this measure; (4) Suppressed for one or more quarters by CMS; (5) No data is available from the hospital for this measure; (6) Fewer than 100 patients completed the HCAHPS survey. Use these rates with caution, as the number of surveys may be too low to reliably assess hospital performance; (7) Survey results are based on less than 12 months of data; (8) Survey results are not available for this reporting period; (9) No or very few patients were eligible for the HCAHPS survey. The scores shown, if any, reflect a very small number of surveys; (10) A state average was not calculated because too few hospitals in the state submitted data; (11) There were discrepancies in the data collection process; Please refer to the User's Guide for a full explanation of data.

29. Prophylactic Antibiotic Selection (Outpatient)

Hospital Name	City	Rate	Cases
Brooks Memorial Hospital	Dunkirk	100%	31
Community Memorial Hospital	Hamilton	100%	98
Glen Cove Hospital	Glen Cove	100%	41
Hospital for Special Surgery	New York	100%	270
New York Downtown Hospital	New York	100%	69
Bellevue Hospital Center	New York	99%	164
Cayuga Medical Center at Ithaca	Ithaca	99%	99
F F Thompson Hospital	Canandaigua	99%	83
Good Samaritan Hospital Medical Center	West Islip	99%	351
Kenmore Mercy Hospital	Kenmore	99%	697
Kings County Hospital Center	Brooklyn	99%	126
Southside Hospital	Bay Shore	99%	163
Strong Memorial Hospital	Rochester	99%	572
White Plains Hospital Center	White Plains	99%	351
Arnot Ogden Medical Center	Elmira	98%	436
Bronx-Lebanon Hospital Center	Bronx	98%	46
Erie County Medical Center	Buffalo	98%	598
Geneva General Hospital	Geneva	98%	101
Harlem Hospital Center	New York	98%	43
Jones Memorial Hospital	Wellsville	98%	43
Lakeside Memorial Hospital	Brockport	98%	45
Mercy Hospital	Buffalo	98%	548
North Shore University Hospital	Manhasset	98%	281
Northern Dutchess Hospital	Rhinebeck	98%	103
Queens Hospital Center	Jamaica	98%	93
Saint Joseph's Hospital	Elmira	98%	94
Saint Joseph's Hospital Health Center	Syracuse	98%	789
Unity Hospital of Rochester	Rochester	98%	414
Univ Hosp S U N Y Health Science Ctr	Syracuse	98%	337
Woodhull Medical and Mental Health Center	Brooklyn	98%	117
Benedictine Hospital	Kingston	97%	110
Clifton Springs Hospital and Clinic	Clifton Springs	97%	71
Coney Island Hospital	Brooklyn	97%	99
Jacobi Medical Center	Bronx	97%	88
Metropolitan Hospital Center	New York	97%	63
Newark-Wayne Community Hospital	Newark	97%	67
Northern Westchester Hospital	Mount Kisco	97%	333
Peconic Bay Medical Center	Riverhead	97%	62
Saint Mary's Hospital at Amsterdam	Amsterdam	97%	116
Seton Health System-St Mary's Campus	Troy	97%	256
Sisters of Charity Hospital	Buffalo	97%	596
United Health Services Hospitals	Johnson City	97%	1361
Westchester Medical Center	Valhalla	97%	366
Albany Med Ctr-South Clinical Campus	Albany	96%	146
Albany Memorial Hospital	Albany	96%	181
Beth Israel Medical Center	New York	96%	649
Comm-General Hosp of Greater Syracuse	Syracuse	96%	581
Ellis Hospital	Schenectady	96%	515
Franklin Hospital	Valley Stream	96%	113
Highland Hospital	Rochester	96%	202
Kingston Hospital	Kingston	96%	122
New York Methodist Hospital	Brooklyn	96%	182
New York Westchester Square Medical Center	Bronx	96%	79
NYU Hospitals Center	New York	96%	422
Richmond University Medical Center	Staten Island	96%	199
Saint Charles Hospital	Port Jefferson	96%	45
Saint Francis Hospital - Roslyn	Roslyn	96%	341
Samaritan Medical Center	Watertown	96%	453
Saratoga Hospital	Saratoga Spgs	96%	214
University Hospital - Stony Brook	Stony Brook	96%	399
Woman's Christian Association	Jamestown	96%	112
Claxton-Hepburn Medical Center	Ogdensburg	95%	42
Eastern Long Island Hospital	Greenport	95%	43
Elmhurst Hospital Center	Elmhurst	95%	84
Good Samaritan Hospital of Suffern	Suffern	95%	231
Hudson Valley Hospital Center	Cortlandt Manor	95%	95
Lenox Hill Hospital	New York	95%	577
Mount Sinai Hospital	New York	95%	539
Oswego Hospital	Oswego	95%	155
Saint Barnabas Hospital	Bronx	95%	155
Saint Francis Hospital	Poughkeepsie	95%	176
Saint Joseph Hospital	Bethpage	95%	55
Vassar Brothers Medical Center	Poughkeepsie	95%	632
Albany Medical Center Hospital	Albany	94%	577
Brookhaven Memorial Hospital Med Ctr	Patchogue	94%	65
Glens Falls Hospital	Glens Falls	94%	413
Huntington Hospital	Huntington	94%	355
John T Mather Mem Hosp-Port Jefferson	Port Jefferson	94%	178
New York Hospital Medical Center of Queens	Flushing	94%	298
Niagara Falls Memorial Medical Center	Niagara Falls	94%	90
Phelps Memorial Hospital Assn	Sleepy Hollow	94%	104
Saint Elizabeth Medical Center	Utica	94%	150
South Nassau Communities Hospital	Oceanside	94%	379
Winthrop-University Hospital	Mineola	94%	475
Nyack Hospital	Nyack	93%	119
Saint Luke's Cornwall Hospital	Newburgh	93%	149
Saint Luke's Roosevelt Hospital	New York	93%	323
Samaritan Hospital	Troy	93%	67
Wyckoff Heights Medical Center	Brooklyn	93%	161
Champlain Valley Physicians Hospital	Plattsburgh	92%	283
Crouse Hospital	Syracuse	92%	862
Jamaica Hospital Medical Center	Jamaica	92%	87
Long Island College Hospital	Brooklyn	92%	162
Oneida Healthcare Center	Oneida	92%	216
Our Lady of Lourdes Memorial Hospital	Binghamton	92%	452
Putnam Hospital Center	Carmel	92%	148
Saint John's Riverside Hospital	Yonkers	92%	78
Adirondack Medical Center	Saranac Lake	91%	90
Eastern Niagara Hospital	Lockport	91%	64
Kaleida Health	Buffalo	91%	1122
Lawrence Hospital Center	Bronxville	91%	106
Mary Imogene Bassett Hospital	Cooperstown	91%	362
Sound Shore Medical Center of Westchester	New Rochelle	91%	88
University Hospital of Brooklyn - Downstate	Brooklyn	91%	103
Flushing Hospital Medical Center	Flushing	90%	162
New York-Presbyterian Hospital	New York	90%	1154
Rochester General Hospital	Rochester	90%	650
St John's Episcopal Hosp-South Shore	Far Rockaway	90%	62
Staten Island University Hospital	Staten Island	90%	253
Lincoln Medical & Mental Health Center	Bronx	89%	133
Saint Peter's Hospital	Albany	89%	952
Auburn Memorial Hospital	Auburn	88%	110
Catskill Regional Medical Center	Harris	88%	40
Corning Hospital	Corning	88%	48
Forest Hills Hospital	Forest Hills	88%	118
Maimonides Medical Center	Brooklyn	88%	158
Orange Regional Medical Center	Goshen	88%	297
Southampton Hospital	Southampton	87%	47
Kingsbrook Jewish Medical Center	Brooklyn	86%	58
Mercy Medical Center	Rockville Centre	86%	96
Mount Vernon Hospital	Mount Vernon	86%	51
Long Island Jewish Medical Center	New Hyde Park	85%	131
Massena Memorial Hospital	Massena	85%	40
Nathan Littauer Hospital	Gloversville	85%	52
Olean General Hospital	Olean	85%	139
Rome Memorial Hospital	Rome	85%	46
Brooklyn Hospital Center at Downtown Campus	Brooklyn	84%	179
Cortland Regional Medical Center	Cortland	84%	56
Saint Anthony Community Hospital	Warwick	84%	49
Saint Catherine of Siena Hospital	Smithtown	84%	383
United Memorial Medical Center	Batavia	84%	61
Lutheran Medical Center	Brooklyn	83%	103
Columbia Memorial Hospital	Hudson	80%	93
Brookdale Hospital Medical Center	Brooklyn	79%	135
Plainview Hospital	Plainview	79%	155
Faxton-St Luke's Healthcare	Utica	78%	156
Nassau University Medical Center	East Meadow	78%	90
Saint Joseph's Medical Center	Yonkers	76%	82
Medina Memorial Hospital	Medina	75%	32
Peninsula Hospital Center	Far Rockaway	73%	56
Alice Hyde Medical Center	Malone	72%	81
Mount St Mary's Hospital and Health Center	Lewiston	70%	186
Canton-Potsdam Hospital	Potsdam	67%	83
Montefiore Medical Center	Bronx	66%	624
Nicholas H Noyes Memorial Hospital	Dansville	61%	36
Carthage Area Hospital	Carthage	45%	31

30. Prophylactic Antibiotic Stopped

Hospital Name	City	Rate	Cases
Canton-Potsdam Hospital	Potsdam	100%	220
Claxton-Hepburn Medical Center	Ogdensburg	100%	56
Clifton Springs Hospital and Clinic	Clifton Springs	100%	254
Jones Memorial Hospital	Wellsville	100%	75
Saint Charles Hospital[2]	Port Jefferson	100%	483
Saint Luke's Cornwall Hospital[2]	Newburgh	100%	226
Aurelia Osborn Fox Memorial Hospital	Oneonta	99%	88
Bellevue Hospital Center[2]	New York	99%	401
Community Memorial Hospital	Hamilton	99%	486
Highland Hospital[2]	Rochester	99%	765
Rochester General Hospital[2]	Rochester	99%	1774
Saint Francis Hospital[2]	Poughkeepsie	99%	227
Saint Joseph's Hospital	Elmira	99%	168
Saint Mary's Hospital at Amsterdam[2]	Amsterdam	99%	174
Strong Memorial Hospital[2]	Rochester	99%	818
Winthrop-University Hospital[2]	Mineola	99%	605
Albany VA Medical Center	Albany	98%	66
Alice Hyde Medical Center	Malone	98%	93
Coney Island Hospital[2]	Brooklyn	98%	82
Ellis Hospital[2]	Schenectady	98%	647
F F Thompson Hospital	Canandaigua	98%	388
Franklin Hospital[2]	Valley Stream	98%	197
Glen Cove Hospital[2]	Glen Cove	98%	189
Lenox Hill Hospital[2]	New York	98%	503
Northern Dutchess Hospital[2]	Rhinebeck	98%	203
Nyack Hospital	Nyack	98%	394
NYU Hospitals Center[2]	New York	98%	462
Putnam Hospital Center	Carmel	98%	535
Saint Catherine of Siena Hospital[2]	Smithtown	98%	237
Saint Joseph Hospital[2]	Bethpage	98%	152
Seton Health System-St Mary's Campus[2]	Troy	98%	248
Sound Shore Medical Center of Westchester	New Rochelle	98%	291
Southside Hospital[2]	Bay Shore	98%	251
Arnot Ogden Medical Center[2]	Elmira	97%	547
Brooks Memorial Hospital	Dunkirk	97%	313
Geneva General Hospital[2]	Geneva	97%	150
Huntington Hospital[2]	Huntington	97%	234
John T Mather Mem Hosp-Port Jefferson	Port Jefferson	97%	266
Lewis County General Hospital	Lowville	97%	98
Mercy Hospital[2]	Buffalo	97%	459
Olean General Hospital	Olean	97%	248
Oneida Healthcare Center	Oneida	97%	179
Orange Regional Medical Center[2]	Goshen	97%	666
Our Lady of Lourdes Memorial Hospital[2]	Binghamton	97%	225
Saint Anthony Community Hospital	Warwick	97%	149
Saint Francis Hospital - Roslyn[2]	Roslyn	97%	381
Staten Island University Hospital[2]	Staten Island	97%	353
Vassar Brothers Medical Center[2]	Poughkeepsie	97%	409
Woodhull Medical and Mental Health Center[2]	Brooklyn	97%	89
Comm-General Hosp of Greater Syracuse[2]	Syracuse	96%	261
Corning Hospital	Corning	96%	177
Glens Falls Hospital[2]	Glens Falls	96%	428
Good Samaritan Hospital Medical Center[2]	West Islip	96%	277
Hudson Valley Hospital Center	Cortlandt Manor	96%	223
Long Island Jewish Medical Center[2]	New Hyde Park	96%	453
Nassau University Medical Center[2]	East Meadow	96%	161
New York Hospital Medical Center of Queens[2]	Flushing	96%	451
North Shore University Hospital[2]	Manhasset	96%	575
Northern Westchester Hospital[2]	Mount Kisco	96%	226
Plainview Hospital[2]	Plainview	96%	252
Saint Elizabeth Medical Center[2]	Utica	96%	818
Benedictine Hospital	Kingston	95%	227
Bronx VA Medical Center	Bronx	95%	79
Catskill Regional Medical Center	Harris	95%	151
Crouse Hospital[2]	Syracuse	95%	361
Kingsbrook Jewish Medical Center	Brooklyn	95%	65
Mercy Medical Center[2]	Rockville Centre	95%	298
Metropolitan Hospital Center[2]	New York	95%	149
New York Downtown Hospital[2]	New York	95%	208
Richmond University Medical Center[2]	Staten Island	95%	285
St John's Episcopal Hosp-South Shore[2]	Far Rockaway	95%	57
South Nassau Communities Hospital[2]	Oceanside	95%	687
United Health Services Hospitals	Johnson City	95%	933
Westchester Medical Center[2]	Valhalla	95%	537
Albany Medical Center Hospital[2]	Albany	94%	326
Auburn Memorial Hospital	Auburn	94%	152
Brookhaven Memorial Hospital Med Ctr[2]	Patchogue	94%	228
Chenango Memorial Hospital	Norwich	94%	137
Hospital for Special Surgery[2]	New York	94%	365
Kaleida Health[2]	Buffalo	94%	863
Lutheran Medical Center[2]	Brooklyn	94%	645
New York Community Hospital of Brooklyn[2]	Brooklyn	94%	50
Rome Memorial Hospital	Rome	94%	108
Saint Luke's Roosevelt Hospital[2]	New York	94%	549
Upstate New York VA Healthcare System	Buffalo	94%	151
Cayuga Medical Center at Ithaca	Ithaca	93%	210
Medina Memorial Hospital	Medina	93%	27
Mount Sinai Hospital[2]	New York	93%	675
Mount St Mary's Hospital and Health Center[2]	Lewiston	93%	289
New York-Presbyterian Hospital[2]	New York	93%	776
Saint Peter's Hospital[2]	Albany	93%	536
Unity Hospital of Rochester[2]	Rochester	93%	387
University Hospital - Stony Brook[2]	Stony Brook	93%	347
VA New York Harbor Healthcare System	New York	93%	136
Bon Secours Community Hospital	Port Jervis	92%	50
Champlain Valley Physicians Hospital	Plattsburgh	92%	581
Elmhurst Hospital Center	Elmhurst	92%	125
Erie County Medical Center	Buffalo	92%	345
Forest Hills Hospital[2]	Forest Hills	92%	257
Jamaica Hospital Medical Center[2]	Jamaica	92%	178
Mary Imogene Bassett Hospital[2]	Cooperstown	92%	418
Peconic Bay Medical Center	Riverhead	92%	298
Samaritan Medical Center	Watertown	92%	340
Sisters of Charity Hospital[2]	Buffalo	92%	545
Syracuse VA Medical Center	Syracuse	92%	72
University Hospital of Brooklyn - Downstate[2]	Brooklyn	92%	244
Woman's Christian Association	Jamestown	92%	283
Beth Israel Medical Center[2]	New York	91%	474
Kenmore Mercy Hospital[2]	Kenmore	91%	240
Lincoln Medical & Mental Health Center[2]	Bronx	91%	128
Maimonides Medical Center[2]	Brooklyn	91%	904
Newark-Wayne Community Hospital	Newark	91%	188
Nicholas H Noyes Memorial Hospital	Dansville	91%	96
Phelps Memorial Hospital Assn[2]	Sleepy Hollow	91%	327
Univ Hosp S U N Y Health Science Ctr[2]	Syracuse	91%	365
Bronx-Lebanon Hospital Center[2]	Bronx	90%	162
Carthage Area Hospital	Carthage	90%	29
Eastern Niagara Hospital	Lockport	90%	169
Flushing Hospital Medical Center[2]	Flushing	90%	391
Montefiore Medical Center[2]	Bronx	90%	711

NOTE: Hospital profiles are in alphabetical order by state, then city, then hospital within the city; Rankings exclude hospitals with less than 25 cases except for patient surveys which excludes hospitals with less than 100 cases; (a) 100–299 cases; (1) The number of cases is too small to be sure how well a hospital is performing; (2) The hospital indicated that the data submitted for this measure were based on a sample of cases; (3) Data was collected during a shorter time period (fewer quarters) than the maximum possible time for this measure; (4) Suppressed for one or more quarters by CMS; (5) No data is available from the hospital for this measure; (6) Fewer than 100 patients completed the HCAHPS survey. Use these rates with caution, as the number of surveys may be too low to reliably assess hospital performance; (7) Survey results are based on less than 12 months of data; (8) Survey results are not available for this reporting period; (9) No or very few patients were eligible for the HCAHPS survey. The scores shown, if any, reflect a very small number of surveys; (10) A state average was not calculated because too few hospitals in the state submitted data; (11) There were discrepancies in the data collection process; Please refer to the User's Guide for a full explanation of data.

New York Westchester Square Medical Center	Bronx	90%	186
Northport VA Medical Center	Northport	90%	60
Samaritan Hospital[2]	Troy	90%	221
Southampton Hospital	Southampton	90%	79
TLC Health Network	Gowanda	90%	122
Columbia Memorial Hospital	Hudson	89%	121
Harlem Hospital Center[2]	New York	89%	28
Jacobi Medical Center	Bronx	89%	155
Saint Joseph's Hospital Health Center[2]	Syracuse	89%	497
Good Samaritan Hospital of Suffern[2]	Suffern	88%	329
Kings County Hospital Center[2]	Brooklyn	88%	114
Lakeside Memorial Hospital	Brockport	88%	66
Queens Hospital Center	Jamaica	88%	125
Saint Barnabas Hospital[2]	Bronx	88%	91
Saint James Mercy Hospital	Hornell	88%	69
Cortland Regional Medical Center	Cortland	87%	63
Kingston Hospital	Kingston	87%	174
Massena Memorial Hospital	Massena	87%	85
Nathan Littauer Hospital	Gloversville	87%	45
Peninsula Hospital Center	Far Rockaway	87%	30
Wyoming County Community Hospital	Warsaw	87%	119
Long Island College Hospital[2]	Brooklyn	86%	300
Albany Memorial Hospital[2]	Albany	85%	296
Long Beach Medical Center[2]	Long Beach	85%	27
New York Methodist Hospital[2]	Brooklyn	85%	479
Niagara Falls Memorial Medical Center	Niagara Falls	85%	61
Saratoga Hospital	Saratoga Spgs	85%	472
Saint John's Riverside Hospital[2]	Yonkers	84%	214
Saint Joseph's Medical Center	Yonkers	83%	60
White Plains Hospital Center[2]	White Plains	83%	288
Lawrence Hospital Center[2]	Bronxville	80%	180
Wyckoff Heights Medical Center[2]	Brooklyn	80%	132
United Memorial Medical Center	Batavia	79%	211
Mount Vernon Hospital	Mount Vernon	78%	32
Oswego Hospital	Oswego	78%	102
Interfaith Medical Center	Brooklyn	76%	45
North Central Bronx Hospital	Bronx	76%	34
Faxton-St Luke's Healthcare[2]	Utica	75%	325
Brooklyn Hospital Center at Downtown Campus	Brooklyn	72%	164
Brookdale Hospital Medical Center[2]	Brooklyn	70%	107
Adirondack Medical Center	Saranac Lake	68%	155

31. Recommended VTP Ordered

Hospital Name	City	Rate	Cases
Albany VA Medical Center[2]	Albany	100%	62
Clifton Springs Hospital and Clinic	Clifton Springs	100%	52
Community Memorial Hospital	Hamilton	100%	183
Coney Island Hospital[2]	Brooklyn	100%	145
Ellis Hospital[2]	Schenectady	100%	225
Lakeside Memorial Hospital	Brockport	100%	71
New York Community Hospital of Brooklyn[2]	Brooklyn	100%	85
New York-Presbyterian Hospital[2]	New York	100%	635
Northport VA Medical Center[2]	Northport	100%	99
NYU Hospitals Center[2]	New York	100%	274
Phelps Memorial Hospital Assn[2]	Sleepy Hollow	100%	272
Plainview Hospital[2]	Plainview	100%	228
Saint Joseph's Hospital	Elmira	100%	49
Strong Memorial Hospital[2]	Rochester	100%	306
TLC Health Network	Gowanda	100%	111
Albany Medical Center Hospital[2]	Albany	99%	135
Brooks Memorial Hospital	Dunkirk	99%	154
Canton-Potsdam Hospital	Potsdam	99%	139
Forest Hills Hospital[2]	Forest Hills	99%	191
Franklin Hospital[2]	Valley Stream	99%	205
Glen Cove Hospital[2]	Glen Cove	99%	183
Highland Hospital[2]	Rochester	99%	231
Huntington Hospital[2]	Huntington	99%	175
Interfaith Medical Center	Brooklyn	99%	82
Lincoln Medical & Mental Health Center[2]	Bronx	99%	166
Lutheran Medical Center[2]	Brooklyn	99%	482
Mercy Hospital[2]	Buffalo	99%	152
Metropolitan Hospital Center[2]	New York	99%	128
Nassau University Medical Center[2]	East Meadow	99%	178
New York Methodist Hospital[2]	Brooklyn	99%	334
New York Westchester Square Medical Center	Bronx	99%	200
North Shore University Hospital[2]	Manhasset	99%	352
Oneida Healthcare Center	Oneida	99%	174
Saint Catherine of Siena Hospital[2]	Smithtown	99%	232
Saint Charles Hospital[2]	Port Jefferson	99%	269
Saint Francis Hospital[2]	Poughkeepsie	99%	136
Saint Joseph's Hospital Health Center[2]	Syracuse	99%	170
Saint Peter's Hospital[2]	Albany	99%	252
South Nassau Communities Hospital[2]	Oceanside	99%	343
Staten Island University Hospital[2]	Staten Island	99%	188
Syracuse VA Medical Center[2]	Syracuse	99%	108
Unity Hospital of Rochester[2]	Rochester	99%	170
University Hospital - Stony Brook[2]	Stony Brook	99%	176
Univ Hosp S U N Y Health Science Ctr[2]	Syracuse	99%	172
Winthrop-University Hospital[2]	Mineola	99%	279
Arnot Ogden Medical Center[2]	Elmira	98%	149
Beth Israel Medical Center[2]	New York	98%	229
Bon Secours Community Hospital	Port Jervis	98%	62
Bronx VA Medical Center[2]	Bronx	98%	120
Comm-General Hosp of Greater Syracuse[2]	Syracuse	98%	164
Elmhurst Hospital Center	Elmhurst	98%	323
Kingsbrook Jewish Medical Center	Brooklyn	98%	127
Lenox Hill Hospital[2]	New York	98%	247
Long Island Jewish Medical Center[2]	New Hyde Park	98%	171
New York Hospital Medical Center of Queens[2]	Flushing	98%	326
Nyack Hospital	Nyack	98%	255
Olean General Hospital	Olean	98%	183
Our Lady of Lourdes Memorial Hospital[2]	Binghamton	98%	122
Queens Hospital Center	Jamaica	98%	195
Richmond University Medical Center[2]	Staten Island	98%	183
Saint Francis Hospital - Roslyn[2]	Roslyn	98%	188
University Hospital of Brooklyn - Downstate[2]	Brooklyn	98%	184
VA New York Harbor Healthcare System[2]	New York	98%	109
Vassar Brothers Medical Center[2]	Poughkeepsie	98%	187
Bellevue Hospital Center[2]	New York	97%	298
Catskill Regional Medical Center	Harris	97%	119
Erie County Medical Center	Buffalo	97%	339
Geneva General Hospital[2]	Geneva	97%	116
Good Samaritan Hospital Medical Center[2]	West Islip	97%	281
Harlem Hospital Center[2]	New York	97%	77
Kaleida Health[2]	Buffalo	97%	454
Kings County Hospital Center[2]	Brooklyn	97%	219
Long Beach Medical Center[2]	Long Beach	97%	39
Long Island College Hospital[2]	Brooklyn	97%	233
Maimonides Medical Center[2]	Brooklyn	97%	321
Mary Imogene Bassett Hospital[2]	Cooperstown	97%	237
Mercy Medical Center[2]	Rockville Centre	97%	274
Mount Sinai Hospital[2]	New York	97%	526
Mount St Mary's Hospital and Health Center[2]	Lewiston	97%	121
Newark-Wayne Community Hospital	Newark	97%	95
Peconic Bay Medical Center	Riverhead	97%	229
Saint Barnabas Hospital[2]	Bronx	97%	132
Saint Joseph Hospital[2]	Bethpage	97%	154
Seton Health System-St Mary's Campus[2]	Troy	97%	203
Southside Hospital[2]	Bay Shore	97%	236
United Health Services Hospitals	Johnson City	97%	470
Woodhull Medical and Mental Health Center[2]	Brooklyn	97%	145
Aurelia Osborn Fox Memorial Hospital	Oneonta	96%	102
Bronx-Lebanon Hospital Center[2]	Bronx	96%	185
Flushing Hospital Medical Center[2]	Flushing	96%	231
Hospital for Special Surgery[2]	New York	96%	310
Hudson Valley Hospital Center	Cortlandt Manor	96%	239
Jacobi Medical Center	Bronx	96%	285
Kenmore Mercy Hospital[2]	Kenmore	96%	127
New York Downtown Hospital[2]	New York	96%	144
Northern Westchester Hospital[2]	Mount Kisco	96%	141
Orange Regional Medical Center[2]	Goshen	96%	409
Rochester General Hospital[2]	Rochester	96%	553
Westchester Medical Center[2]	Valhalla	96%	348
Wyckoff Heights Medical Center[2]	Brooklyn	96%	210
Brookhaven Memorial Hospital Med Ctr[2]	Patchogue	95%	237
Jamaica Hospital Medical Center[2]	Jamaica	95%	206
John T Mather Mem Hosp-Port Jefferson	Port Jefferson	95%	304
Lewis County General Hospital	Lowville	95%	58
Massena Memorial Hospital	Massena	95%	39
Putnam Hospital Center	Carmel	95%	424
Saint Anthony Community Hospital	Warwick	95%	76
United Memorial Medical Center	Batavia	95%	150
Auburn Memorial Hospital	Auburn	94%	129
Crouse Hospital[2]	Syracuse	94%	142
Eastern Long Island Hospital	Greenport	94%	36
Medina Memorial Hospital	Medina	94%	34
Niagara Falls Memorial Medical Center	Niagara Falls	94%	72
Northern Dutchess Hospital[2]	Rhinebeck	94%	101
Rome Memorial Hospital	Rome	94%	112
Saint Mary's Hospital at Amsterdam[2]	Amsterdam	94%	122
Samaritan Medical Center	Watertown	94%	189
Sound Shore Medical Center of Westschester	New Rochelle	94%	282
Upstate New York VA Healthcare System[2]	Buffalo	94%	116
Chenango Memorial Hospital	Norwich	93%	89
Saint Joseph's Medical Center	Yonkers	93%	85
Saint Luke's Cornwall Hospital[2]	Newburgh	93%	123
Saratoga Hospital	Saratoga Spgs	93%	349
Sisters of Charity Hospital[2]	Buffalo	93%	258
Albany Memorial Hospital[2]	Albany	92%	194
Glens Falls Hospital[2]	Glens Falls	92%	268
Oswego Hospital	Oswego	92%	97
Saint Luke's Roosevelt Hospital[2]	New York	92%	322
White Plains Hospital Center[2]	White Plains	92%	225
Benedictine Hospital	Kingston	91%	138
Champlain Valley Physicians Hospital	Plattsburgh	91%	320
Columbia Memorial Hospital	Hudson	91%	163
Cortland Regional Medical Center	Cortland	91%	74
Montefiore Medical Center[2]	Bronx	91%	416
Alice Hyde Medical Center	Malone	90%	97
Cayuga Medical Center at Ithaca	Ithaca	90%	155
F F Thompson Hospital	Canandaigua	90%	146
Faxton-St Luke's Healthcare[2]	Utica	90%	183
Kingston Hospital	Kingston	90%	174
Nathan Littauer Hospital	Gloversville	90%	63
Lawrence Hospital Center[2]	Bronxville	89%	142
Corning Hospital	Corning	88%	98
Jones Memorial Hospital	Wellsville	88%	34
Saint James Mercy Hospital	Hornell	88%	60
St John's Episcopal Hosp-South Shore[2]	Far Rockaway	88%	88
Brookdale Hospital Medical Center[2]	Brooklyn	87%	189
Brooklyn Hospital Center at Downtown Campus	Brooklyn	87%	254
Claxton-Hepburn Medical Center	Ogdensburg	87%	45
Eastern Niagara Hospital	Lockport	87%	89
North Central Bronx Hospital	Bronx	87%	30
Saint Elizabeth Medical Center[2]	Utica	86%	173
Southampton Hospital	Southampton	86%	70
Saint John's Riverside Hospital[2]	Yonkers	85%	208
Woman's Christian Association	Jamestown	85%	126
Samaritan Hospital[2]	Troy	84%	154
Nicholas H Noyes Memorial Hospital	Dansville	82%	44
Mount Vernon Hospital	Mount Vernon	76%	63
Good Samaritan Hospital of Suffern[2]	Suffern	74%	159
Wyoming County Community Hospital	Warsaw	73%	82
Peninsula Hospital Center	Far Rockaway	61%	54
Adirondack Medical Center	Saranac Lake	49%	154

32. Urinary Catheter Removal

Hospital Name	City	Rate	Cases
Albany VA Medical Center[2]	Albany	100%	47
Bronx VA Medical Center[2]	Bronx	100%	49
Clifton Springs Hospital and Clinic	Clifton Springs	100%	136
Corning Hospital	Corning	100%	46
Massena Memorial Hospital	Massena	100%	25
Metropolitan Hospital Center[2]	New York	100%	46
Nassau University Medical Center[2]	East Meadow	100%	39
Saint Catherine of Siena Hospital[2]	Smithtown	100%	89
Saint Charles Hospital	Port Jefferson	100%	248
Saint Francis Hospital[2]	Poughkeepsie	100%	32
Southside Hospital[2]	Bay Shore	100%	103
Syracuse VA Medical Center[2]	Syracuse	100%	66
VA New York Harbor Healthcare System[2]	New York	100%	55
Albany Medical Center Hospital[2]	Albany	99%	79
Forest Hills Hospital[2]	Forest Hills	99%	106
Good Samaritan Hospital Medical Center[2]	West Islip	99%	109
Mercy Medical Center[2]	Rockville Centre	99%	137
Nyack Hospital	Nyack	99%	168
Phelps Memorial Hospital Assn[2]	Sleepy Hollow	99%	159
Staten Island University Hospital[2]	Staten Island	99%	98
Canton-Potsdam Hospital	Potsdam	98%	55
Chenango Memorial Hospital	Norwich	98%	62
Coney Island Hospital[2]	Brooklyn	98%	44
Franklin Hospital[2]	Valley Stream	98%	103
Mount St Mary's Hospital and Health Center[2]	Lewiston	98%	86
Nicholas H Noyes Memorial Hospital	Dansville	98%	53
Orange Regional Medical Center[2]	Goshen	98%	265
Plainview Hospital[2]	Plainview	98%	52
Strong Memorial Hospital[2]	Rochester	98%	327
University Hospital of Brooklyn - Downstate[2]	Brooklyn	98%	90
Arnot Ogden Medical Center[2]	Elmira	97%	100
Benedictine Hospital	Kingston	97%	132
Community Memorial Hospital	Hamilton	97%	39
Lewis County General Hospital	Lowville	97%	32
Northern Westchester Hospital[2]	Mount Kisco	97%	108
Rochester General Hospital[2]	Rochester	97%	327
Seton Health System-St Mary's Campus[2]	Troy	97%	129
Peconic Bay Medical Center	Riverhead	96%	159
South Nassau Communities Hospital[2]	Oceanside	96%	290
Vassar Brothers Medical Center[2]	Poughkeepsie	96%	55
Aurelia Osborn Fox Memorial Hospital	Oneonta	95%	37
Highland Hospital[2]	Rochester	95%	287
Putnam Hospital Center	Carmel	95%	289
Sound Shore Medical Center of Westschester	New Rochelle	95%	152
Brooks Memorial Hospital	Dunkirk	94%	101
Crouse Hospital[2]	Syracuse	94%	115
Mercy Hospital[2]	Buffalo	94%	156
New York Downtown Hospital[2]	New York	94%	36
New York Hospital Medical Center of Queens[2]	Flushing	94%	156
F F Thompson Hospital	Canandaigua	93%	135
NYU Hospitals Center[2]	New York	93%	169
Saint Luke's Roosevelt Hospital[2]	New York	93%	178
Alice Hyde Medical Center	Malone	92%	40
Bellevue Hospital Center[2]	New York	92%	109
Champlain Valley Physicians Hospital	Plattsburgh	92%	234
Faxton-St Luke's Healthcare[2]	Utica	92%	85
Glen Cove Hospital[2]	Glen Cove	92%	105
Jamaica Hospital Medical Center[2]	Jamaica	92%	39
John T Mather Mem Hosp-Port Jefferson	Port Jefferson	92%	74
Lenox Hill Hospital[2]	New York	92%	118
Long Island Jewish Medical Center[2]	New Hyde Park	92%	153
United Health Services Hospitals	Johnson City	92%	406
Elmhurst Hospital Center	Elmhurst	91%	70

NOTE: Hospital profiles are in alphabetical order by state, then city, then hospital within the city; Rankings exclude hospitals with less than 25 cases except for patient surveys which excludes hospitals with less than 100 cases; (a) 100–299 cases; (1) The number of cases is too small to be sure how well a hospital is performing; (2) The hospital indicated that the data submitted for this measure were based on a sample of cases; (3) Data was collected during a shorter time period (fewer quarters) than the maximum possible time for this measure; (4) Suppressed for one or more quarters by CMS; (5) No data is available from the hospital for this measure; (6) Fewer than 100 patients completed the HCAHPS survey. Use these rates with caution, as the number of surveys may be too low to reliably assess hospital performance; (7) Survey results are based on less than 12 months of data; (8) Survey results are not available for this reporting period; (9) No or very few patients were eligible for the HCAHPS survey. The scores shown, if any, reflect a very small number of surveys; (10) A state average was not calculated because too few hospitals in the state submitted data; (11) There were discrepancies in the data collection process; Please refer to the User's Guide for a full explanation of data.

Long Island College Hospital[2]	Brooklyn	91%	101
New York Methodist Hospital[2]	Brooklyn	91%	180
New York-Presbyterian Hospital[2]	New York	91%	234
Saratoga Hospital	Saratoga Spgs	91%	225
Winthrop-University Hospital[2]	Mineola	91%	211
Adirondack Medical Center	Saranac Lake	90%	88
Ellis Hospital[2]	Schenectady	90%	106
Glens Falls Hospital[2]	Glens Falls	90%	60
Maimonides Medical Center[2]	Brooklyn	90%	256
Saint Francis Hospital - Roslyn[2]	Roslyn	90%	141
Unity Hospital of Rochester[2]	Rochester	90%	161
Columbia Memorial Hospital	Hudson	89%	65
Hudson Valley Hospital Center	Cortlandt Manor	89%	110
Kingsbrook Jewish Medical Center	Brooklyn	89%	36
Good Samaritan Hospital of Suffern[2]	Suffern	88%	110
Hospital for Special Surgery[2]	New York	88%	42
Lutheran Medical Center[2]	Brooklyn	88%	165
Sisters of Charity Hospital[2]	Buffalo	88%	215
Cayuga Medical Center at Ithaca	Ithaca	87%	82
University Hospital - Stony Brook[2]	Stony Brook	87%	134
Lawrence Hospital Center[2]	Bronxville	86%	42
Mary Imogene Bassett Hospital[2]	Cooperstown	86%	170
Northern Dutchess Hospital[2]	Rhinebeck	86%	123
Saint Joseph Hospital[2]	Bethpage	86%	28
Samaritan Medical Center	Watertown	86%	149
Westchester Medical Center[2]	Valhalla	86%	186
Erie County Medical Center	Buffalo	85%	155
Northport VA Medical Center[2]	Northport	85%	53
Saint Anthony Community Hospital	Warwick	85%	27
Geneva General Hospital[2]	Geneva	84%	67
Kaleida Health[2]	Buffalo	84%	321
Brooklyn Hospital Center at Downtown Campus	Brooklyn	83%	52
Lincoln Medical & Mental Health Center[2]	Bronx	83%	58
Olean General Hospital	Olean	83%	48
Brookhaven Memorial Hospital Med Ctr[2]	Patchogue	82%	121
Saint Peter's Hospital[2]	Albany	82%	112
Comm-General Hosp of Greater Syracuse[2]	Syracuse	81%	145
Beth Israel Medical Center[2]	New York	80%	196
Huntington Hospital[2]	Huntington	80%	30
Mount Sinai Hospital[2]	New York	80%	257
North Shore University Hospital[2]	Manhasset	80%	189
Auburn Memorial Hospital	Auburn	79%	38
Richmond University Medical Center[2]	Staten Island	78%	40
Univ Hosp S U N Y Health Science Ctr[2]	Syracuse	78%	124
Saint Joseph's Hospital Health Center[2]	Syracuse	77%	73
Jacobi Medical Center	Bronx	76%	67
Montefiore Medical Center[2]	Bronx	76%	210
Saint Mary's Hospital at Amsterdam[2]	Amsterdam	76%	78
Samaritan Hospital	Troy	76%	87
Albany Memorial Hospital[2]	Albany	75%	73
Flushing Hospital Medical Center	Flushing	75%	56
White Plains Hospital Center[2]	White Plains	72%	46
Saint John's Riverside Hospital[2]	Yonkers	71%	48
Cortland Regional Medical Center	Cortland	69%	36
Kings County Hospital Center[2]	Brooklyn	68%	31
Kenmore Mercy Hospital[2]	Kenmore	67%	30
United Memorial Medical Center	Batavia	66%	68
New York Westchester Square Medical Center	Bronx	65%	78
Upstate New York VA Healthcare System[2]	Buffalo	63%	86
Saint Elizabeth Medical Center[2]	Utica	62%	90
Wyckoff Heights Medical Center[2]	Brooklyn	57%	42
Brookdale Hospital Medical Center[2]	Brooklyn	42%	33

Children's Asthma Care

33. Received Systemic Corticosteroids

Hospital Name	City	Rate	Cases
New York-Presbyterian Hospital	New York	100%	412
Kaleida Health	Buffalo	98%	550

34. Received Home Management Plan of Care

Hospital Name	City	Rate	Cases
New York-Presbyterian Hospital[2]	New York	78%	410
Kaleida Health	Buffalo	16%	552

35. Received Reliever Medication

Hospital Name	City	Rate	Cases
Kaleida Health	Buffalo	100%	553
New York-Presbyterian Hospital	New York	100%	412

Use of Medical Imaging

36. Combination Abdominal CT Scan

Hospital Name	City	Ratio	Cases
Jamaica Hospital Medical Center	Jamaica	0.000	200
New York Westchester Square Medical Center	Bronx	0.000	47
St John's Episcopal Hosp-South Shore	Far Rockaway	0.000	183
Peninsula Hospital Center	Far Rockaway	0.002	415
Mount Vernon Hospital	Mount Vernon	0.005	212
Nassau University Medical Center	East Meadow	0.007	147
New York Community Hospital of Brooklyn	Brooklyn	0.009	110
River Hospital	Alexandria Bay	0.012	86
Winthrop-University Hospital	Mineola	0.014	284
Mercy Medical Center	Rockville Centre	0.016	607
Franklin Hospital	Valley Stream	0.018	276
Plainview Hospital	Plainview	0.019	324
Maimonides Medical Center	Brooklyn	0.021	751
Forest Hills Hospital	Forest Hills	0.022	228
Massena Memorial Hospital	Massena	0.022	464
Queens Hospital Center	Jamaica	0.022	180
Saint Joseph Hospital	Bethpage	0.022	228
Lutheran Medical Center	Brooklyn	0.023	400
Southside Hospital	Bay Shore	0.023	443
Interfaith Medical Center[1]	Brooklyn	0.024	41
Cayuga Medical Center at Ithaca	Ithaca	0.025	998
Ellis Hospital	Schenectady	0.026	1049
Claxton-Hepburn Medical Center	Ogdensburg	0.028	469
Comm-General Hosp of Greater Syracuse	Syracuse	0.031	710
Nyack Hospital	Nyack	0.031	508
White Plains Hospital Center	White Plains	0.031	1967
Woodhull Medical and Mental Health Center	Brooklyn	0.034	87
Wyckoff Heights Medical Center	Brooklyn	0.034	290
NYU Hospitals Center	New York	0.035	228
Saint Barnabas Hospital	Bronx	0.036	167
Albany Memorial Hospital	Albany	0.038	555
Good Samaritan Hospital Medical Center	West Islip	0.038	1058
Delaware Valley Hospital	Walton	0.040	100
Peconic Bay Medical Center	Riverhead	0.041	462
Richmond University Medical Center	Staten Island	0.041	49
Saratoga Hospital	Saratoga Spgs	0.042	990
Alice Hyde Medical Center	Malone	0.043	421
Saint Charles Hospital	Port Jefferson	0.043	328
Glens Falls Hospital	Glens Falls	0.044	1653
Sound Shore Medical Center of Westchester	New Rochelle	0.044	294
Nathan Littauer Hospital	Gloversville	0.045	464
Canton-Potsdam Hospital	Potsdam	0.046	459
Edward John Noble Hospital of Gouverneur	Gouverneur	0.046	109
Mount Sinai Hospital	New York	0.046	539
Samaritan Hospital	Troy	0.051	548
Sisters of Charity Hospital	Buffalo	0.051	292
Champlain Valley Physicians Hospital	Plattsburgh	0.052	956
Margaretville Memorial Hospital	Margaretville	0.052	97
Crouse Hospital	Syracuse	0.054	727
Faxton-St Luke's Healthcare	Utica	0.054	483
United Health Services Hospitals	Johnson City	0.055	1770
New York Hospital Medical Center of Queens	Flushing	0.057	1018
TLC Health Network	Gowanda	0.058	206
Southampton Hospital	Southampton	0.059	768
Brookhaven Memorial Hospital Med Ctr	Patchogue	0.061	759
Saint Anthony Community Hospital	Warwick	0.061	326
Benedictine Hospital	Kingston	0.062	601
John T Mather Mem Hosp-Port Jefferson	Port Jefferson	0.064	949
New York Methodist Hospital	Brooklyn	0.065	570
Seton Health System-St Mary's Campus	Troy	0.065	649
Bon Secours Community Hospital	Port Jervis	0.066	452
Chenango Memorial Hospital	Norwich	0.066	244
Huntington Hospital	Huntington	0.066	527
Ira Davenport Memorial Hospital	Bath	0.068	162
Cortland Regional Medical Center	Cortland	0.070	681
Montefiore Medical Center	Bronx	0.070	1769
Niagara Falls Memorial Medical Center	Niagara Falls	0.070	328
Saint Francis Hospital - Roslyn	Roslyn	0.070	428
Saint Peter's Hospital	Albany	0.070	1069
Brookdale Hospital Medical Center	Brooklyn	0.071	226
Staten Island University Hospital	Staten Island	0.071	608
Arnot Ogden Medical Center	Elmira	0.077	1141
Brooks Memorial Hospital	Dunkirk	0.077	287
Mount St Mary's Hospital and Health Center	Lewiston	0.079	356
Saint Luke's Roosevelt Hospital	New York	0.081	683
Auburn Memorial Hospital	Auburn	0.082	625
Mercy Hospital	Buffalo	0.084	692
University Hospital of Brooklyn - Downstate	Brooklyn	0.084	273
Long Island Jewish Medical Center	New Hyde Park	0.086	561
Good Samaritan Hospital of Suffern	Suffern	0.087	516
New York Downtown Hospital	New York	0.088	194
Saint Joseph's Hospital Health Center	Syracuse	0.088	774
Kingston Hospital	Kingston	0.089	541
Lenox Hill Hospital	New York	0.090	567
Saint John's Riverside Hospital	Yonkers	0.090	659
Aurelia Osborn Fox Memorial Hospital	Oneonta	0.092	393
Saint Luke's Cornwall Hospital	Newburgh	0.092	567
Lincoln Medical & Mental Health Center	Bronx	0.095	262
Bertrand Chaffee Hospital	Springville	0.098	92
North Shore University Hospital	Manhasset	0.098	2232
North Central Bronx Hospital[1]	Bronx	0.102	49
Cobleskill Regional Hospital	Cobleskill	0.103	312
Northern Westchester Hospital	Mount Kisco	0.105	382
Saint Joseph's Medical Center	Yonkers	0.106	340
Lawrence Hospital Center	Bronxville	0.108	584
Corning Hospital	Corning	0.114	753
Univ Hosp S U N Y Health Science Ctr	Syracuse	0.115	583
Orange Regional Medical Center	Goshen	0.116	1430
Bellevue Hospital Center	New York	0.118	245
Jones Memorial Hospital	Wellsville	0.119	218
Putnam Hospital Center	Carmel	0.120	566
Albany Medical Center Hospital	Albany	0.124	707
Elmhurst Hospital Center	Elmhurst	0.127	150
Coney Island Hospital	Brooklyn	0.139	245
Woman's Christian Association	Jamestown	0.144	563
Hudson Valley Hospital Center	Cortlandt Manor	0.146	670
Little Falls Hospital	Little Falls	0.146	301
Our Lady of Lourdes Memorial Hospital	Binghamton	0.146	1550
Community Memorial Hospital	Hamilton	0.147	191
Jacobi Medical Center	Bronx	0.150	240
Mary Imogene Bassett Hospital	Cooperstown	0.150	652
Catskill Regional Medical Center	Harris	0.153	491
Saint Francis Hospital	Poughkeepsie	0.153	444
University Hospital - Stony Brook	Stony Brook	0.156	1100
Oswego Hospital	Oswego	0.158	417
Kingsbrook Jewish Medical Center	Brooklyn	0.159	208
Medina Memorial Hospital	Medina	0.164	171
Beth Israel Medical Center	New York	0.165	872
South Nassau Communities Hospital	Oceanside	0.181	833
Soldiers and Sailors Mem Hosp of Yates	Penn Yan	0.189	122
Brooklyn Hospital Center at Downtown Campus	Brooklyn	0.195	307
Westfield Memorial Hospital	Westfield	0.206	170
Phelps Memorial Hospital Assn	Sleepy Hollow	0.216	1006
Vassar Brothers Medical Center	Poughkeepsie	0.216	709
Hospital for Special Surgery[1]	New York	0.237	38
Strong Memorial Hospital	Rochester	0.239	952
Albany Med Ctr-South Clinical Campus	Albany	0.252	246
Olean General Hospital	Olean	0.259	606
Oneida Healthcare Center	Oneida	0.259	464
Erie County Medical Center	Buffalo	0.260	415
Kings County Hospital Center	Brooklyn	0.263	133
Long Island College Hospital	Brooklyn	0.267	457
Bronx-Lebanon Hospital Center	Bronx	0.279	183
Metropolitan Hospital Center	New York	0.280	93
Saint James Mercy Hospital	Hornell	0.289	301
Clifton Springs Hospital and Clinic	Clifton Springs	0.304	316
Highland Hospital	Rochester	0.310	471
Saint Elizabeth Medical Center	Utica	0.315	515
Eastern Niagara Hospital	Lockport	0.316	244
Carthage Area Hospital	Carthage	0.331	169
Harlem Hospital Center	New York	0.348	115
Northern Dutchess Hospital	Rhinebeck	0.359	304
Westchester Medical Center	Valhalla	0.364	689
Kenmore Mercy Hospital	Kenmore	0.392	459
Columbia Memorial Hospital	Hudson	0.406	581
New York-Presbyterian Hospital	New York	0.415	2357
Saint Mary's Hospital at Amsterdam	Amsterdam	0.431	800
Geneva General Hospital	Geneva	0.440	361
Newark-Wayne Community Hospital	Newark	0.442	233
Glen Cove Hospital	Glen Cove	0.455	365
Lewis County General Hospital	Lowville	0.460	202
Saint Catherine of Siena Hospital	Smithtown	0.477	666
F F Thompson Hospital	Canandaigua	0.551	361
United Memorial Medical Center	Batavia	0.554	294
Samaritan Medical Center	Watertown	0.567	735
Wyoming County Community Hospital	Warsaw	0.568	132
Long Beach Medical Center	Long Beach	0.592	311
Rochester General Hospital	Rochester	0.592	596
Rome Memorial Hospital	Rome	0.592	591
Kaleida Health	Buffalo	0.600	1233
Unity Hospital of Rochester	Rochester	0.608	240
Adirondack Medical Center	Saranac Lake	0.674	344
Nicholas H Noyes Memorial Hospital	Dansville	0.683	243
Lakeside Memorial Hospital	Brockport	0.698	202

37. Combination Chest CT Scan

Hospital Name	City	Ratio	Cases
Albany Memorial Hospital	Albany	0.000	288
Auburn Memorial Hospital	Auburn	0.000	260
Brookdale Hospital Medical Center	Brooklyn	0.000	117
Chenango Memorial Hospital	Norwich	0.000	138
Comm-General Hosp of Greater Syracuse	Syracuse	0.000	293
Edward John Noble Hospital of Gouverneur	Gouverneur	0.000	84
Ellis Hospital	Schenectady	0.000	926
Faxton-St Luke's Healthcare	Utica	0.000	608
Flushing Hospital Medical Center	Flushing	0.000	54
Forest Hills Hospital	Forest Hills	0.000	103
Franklin Hospital	Valley Stream	0.000	112
Glen Cove Hospital	Glen Cove	0.000	279
Hospital for Special Surgery	New York	0.000	91
Huntington Hospital	Huntington	0.000	448
Ira Davenport Memorial Hospital	Bath	0.000	70
Jamaica Hospital Medical Center	Jamaica	0.000	136
Long Island Jewish Medical Center	New Hyde Park	0.000	278
Lutheran Medical Center	Brooklyn	0.000	177

NOTE: Hospital profiles are in alphabetical order by state, then city, then hospital within the city; Rankings exclude hospitals with less than 25 cases except for patient surveys which excludes hospitals with less than 100 cases; (a) 100–299 cases; (1) The number of cases is too small to be sure how well a hospital is performing; (2) The hospital indicated that the data submitted for this measure were based on a sample of cases; (3) Data was collected during a shorter time period (fewer quarters) than the maximum possible time for this measure; (4) Suppressed for one or more quarters by CMS; (5) No data is available from the hospital for this measure; (6) Fewer than 100 patients completed the HCAHPS survey. Use these rates with caution, as the number of surveys may be too low to reliably assess hospital performance; (7) Survey results are based on less than 12 months of data; (8) Survey results are not available for this reporting period; (9) No or very few patients were eligible for the HCAHPS survey. The scores shown, if any, reflect a very small number of surveys; (10) A state average was not calculated because too few hospitals in the state submitted data; (11) There were discrepancies in the data collection process; Please refer to the User's Guide for a full explanation of data.

Massena Memorial Hospital	Massena	0.000	307
Mercy Hospital	Buffalo	0.000	449
New York Community Hospital of Brooklyn[1]	Brooklyn	0.000	32
Northern Westchester Hospital	Mount Kisco	0.000	244
NYU Hospitals Center	New York	0.000	77
Peninsula Hospital Center	Far Rockaway	0.000	291
Phelps Memorial Hospital Assn	Sleepy Hollow	0.000	967
Plainview Hospital	Plainview	0.000	64
Richmond University Medical Center	Staten Island	0.000	65
River Hospital	Alexandria Bay	0.000	58
Saint Anthony Community Hospital	Warwick	0.000	227
St John's Episcopal Hosp-South Shore	Far Rockaway	0.000	122
Saint John's Riverside Hospital	Yonkers	0.000	748
Saint Joseph Hospital	Bethpage	0.000	73
Seton Health System-St Mary's Campus	Troy	0.000	329
Soldiers and Sailors Mem Hosp of Yates	Penn Yan	0.000	54
TLC Health Network	Gowanda	0.000	99
White Plains Hospital Center	White Plains	0.000	2229
Winthrop-University Hospital	Mineola	0.000	79
Cayuga Medical Center at Ithaca	Ithaca	0.001	672
Good Samaritan Hospital Medical Center	West Islip	0.001	785
Arnot Ogden Medical Center	Elmira	0.002	600
Glens Falls Hospital	Glens Falls	0.002	1383
Putnam Hospital Center	Carmel	0.002	463
Saratoga Hospital	Saratoga Spgs	0.002	570
South Nassau Communities Hospital	Oceanside	0.002	407
Southampton Hospital	Southampton	0.002	618
Alice Hyde Medical Center	Malone	0.003	322
Benedictine Hospital	Kingston	0.003	290
Canton-Potsdam Hospital	Potsdam	0.003	294
Woman's Christian Association	Jamestown	0.003	313
Albany Medical Center Hospital	Albany	0.004	512
Southside Hospital	Bay Shore	0.004	253
Corning Hospital	Corning	0.005	546
Long Beach Medical Center	Long Beach	0.005	195
New York Hospital Medical Center of Queens	Flushing	0.005	591
Crouse Hospital	Syracuse	0.006	524
Eastern Niagara Hospital	Lockport	0.006	173
Mount Vernon Hospital	Mount Vernon	0.006	173
Saint Joseph's Hospital Health Center	Syracuse	0.006	320
Albany Med Ctr-South Clinical Campus	Albany	0.007	137
John T Mather Mem Hosp-Port Jefferson	Port Jefferson	0.008	643
Long Island College Hospital	Brooklyn	0.008	239
Mercy Medical Center	Rockville Centre	0.008	492
Vassar Brothers Medical Center	Poughkeepsie	0.008	357
Lenox Hill Hospital	New York	0.009	434
North Shore University Hospital	Manhasset	0.009	2012
Queens Hospital Center	Jamaica	0.009	109
Samaritan Hospital	Troy	0.009	325
Clifton Springs Hospital and Clinic	Clifton Springs	0.010	206
Erie County Medical Center	Buffalo	0.010	197
Saint Joseph's Medical Center	Yonkers	0.010	208
Elmhurst Hospital Center	Elmhurst	0.011	87
Mount St Mary's Hospital and Health Center	Lewiston	0.011	357
Oneida Healthcare Center	Oneida	0.011	174
Saint Charles Hospital	Port Jefferson	0.011	261
Sound Shore Medical Center of Westschester	New Rochelle	0.011	88
New York Methodist Hospital	Brooklyn	0.012	409
Saint Luke's Roosevelt Hospital	New York	0.012	417
University Hospital - Stony Brook	Stony Brook	0.012	1186
Brookhaven Memorial Hospital Med Ctr	Patchogue	0.013	520
Kingston Hospital	Kingston	0.013	306
Montefiore Medical Center	Bronx	0.013	1222
Nassau University Medical Center	East Meadow	0.013	80
Peconic Bay Medical Center	Riverhead	0.013	391
Wyckoff Heights Medical Center	Brooklyn	0.013	150
Bellevue Hospital Center	New York	0.014	219
F F Thompson Hospital	Canandaigua	0.014	212
Little Falls Hospital	Little Falls	0.014	138
Orange Regional Medical Center	Goshen	0.014	1410
Saint Barnabas Hospital	Bronx	0.014	74
Kingsbrook Jewish Medical Center	Brooklyn	0.015	136
Columbia Memorial Hospital	Hudson	0.016	438
Geneva General Hospital	Geneva	0.017	173
Interfaith Medical Center	Brooklyn	0.017	60
Lawrence Hospital Center	Bronxville	0.017	476
Saint Francis Hospital - Roslyn	Roslyn	0.017	537
Claxton-Hepburn Medical Center	Ogdensburg	0.018	330
Cobleskill Regional Hospital	Cobleskill	0.018	166
Brooklyn Hospital Center at Downtown Campus	Brooklyn	0.019	214
Oswego Hospital	Oswego	0.020	344
Rome Memorial Hospital	Rome	0.020	343
Mary Imogene Bassett Hospital	Cooperstown	0.021	608
Cortland Regional Medical Center	Cortland	0.022	315
Maimonides Medical Center	Brooklyn	0.022	491
United Health Services Hospitals	Johnson City	0.022	1065
United Memorial Medical Center	Batavia	0.023	175
University Hospital of Brooklyn - Downstate	Brooklyn	0.023	129
Mount Sinai Hospital	New York	0.024	169
Margaretville Memorial Hospital[1]	Margaretville	0.025	40
New York-Presbyterian Hospital	New York	0.025	2332
Nyack Hospital	Nyack	0.025	365
Nathan Littauer Hospital	Gloversville	0.026	309
Saint Catherine of Siena Hospital	Smithtown	0.026	390
Samaritan Medical Center	Watertown	0.026	680
Saint James Mercy Hospital	Hornell	0.027	257
Woodhull Medical and Mental Health Center[1]	Brooklyn	0.029	35
Saint Luke's Cornwall Hospital	Newburgh	0.031	353
Bon Secours Community Hospital	Port Jervis	0.032	253
Catskill Regional Medical Center	Harris	0.032	282
Aurelia Osborn Fox Memorial Hospital	Oneonta	0.035	171
Good Samaritan Hospital of Suffern	Suffern	0.036	279
Saint Elizabeth Medical Center	Utica	0.039	357
Community Memorial Hospital	Hamilton	0.040	125
New York Downtown Hospital	New York	0.040	101
Saint Mary's Hospital at Amsterdam	Amsterdam	0.041	437
Coney Island Hospital	Brooklyn	0.043	92
Sisters of Charity Hospital	Buffalo	0.043	188
Lincoln Medical & Mental Health Center	Bronx	0.044	159
Brooks Memorial Hospital	Dunkirk	0.045	134
Saint Peter's Hospital	Albany	0.045	865
Lakeside Memorial Hospital	Brockport	0.047	107
Saint Francis Hospital	Poughkeepsie	0.048	312
Univ Hosp S U N Y Health Science Ctr	Syracuse	0.048	745
Delaware Valley Hospital[1]	Walton	0.050	40
Beth Israel Medical Center	New York	0.052	483
Metropolitan Hospital Center	New York	0.054	56
Northern Dutchess Hospital	Rhinebeck	0.054	168
Bertrand Chaffee Hospital[1]	Springville	0.056	36
Champlain Valley Physicians Hospital	Plattsburgh	0.056	694
North Central Bronx Hospital[1]	Bronx	0.059	34
Jacobi Medical Center	Bronx	0.061	164
Niagara Falls Memorial Medical Center	Niagara Falls	0.068	251
Staten Island University Hospital	Staten Island	0.069	232
Carthage Area Hospital	Carthage	0.077	130
Hudson Valley Hospital Center	Cortlandt Manor	0.084	547
Newark-Wayne Community Hospital	Newark	0.088	148
Kaleida Health	Buffalo	0.091	623
Our Lady of Lourdes Memorial Hospital	Binghamton	0.094	1151
Westchester Medical Center	Valhalla	0.094	479
Jones Memorial Hospital	Wellsville	0.096	115
Wyoming County Community Hospital	Warsaw	0.096	104
Kenmore Mercy Hospital	Kenmore	0.099	233
Lewis County General Hospital	Lowville	0.105	172
Strong Memorial Hospital	Rochester	0.123	788
Westfield Memorial Hospital	Westfield	0.154	78
Unity Hospital of Rochester[1]	Rochester	0.205	44
Harlem Hospital Center	New York	0.242	62
Medina Memorial Hospital	Medina	0.242	91
Kings County Hospital Center[1]	Brooklyn	0.256	43
Bronx-Lebanon Hospital Center	Bronx	0.284	116
Rochester General Hospital	Rochester	0.317	328
Highland Hospital	Rochester	0.337	338
Olean General Hospital	Olean	0.398	259
Nicholas H Noyes Memorial Hospital	Dansville	0.676	182
Adirondack Medical Center	Saranac Lake	0.677	303

38. Follow-up Mammogram/Ultrasound

Hospital Name	City	Rate	Cases
Eastern Niagara Hospital	Lockport	1.1%	528
North Central Bronx Hospital	Bronx	1.4%	220
University Hospital of Brooklyn - Downstate	Brooklyn	1.9%	480
Coney Island Hospital	Brooklyn	2.1%	94
Carthage Area Hospital	Carthage	2.3%	213
Crouse Hospital	Syracuse	2.7%	1161
Jacobi Medical Center	Bronx	2.7%	482
Cayuga Medical Center at Ithaca	Ithaca	3.2%	1676
Edward John Noble Hospital of Gouverneur	Gouverneur	3.2%	250
Benedictine Hospital	Kingston	3.4%	1029
Oswego Hospital	Oswego	3.5%	1327
Aurelia Osborn Fox Memorial Hospital	Oneonta	3.7%	938
Montefiore Medical Center	Bronx	3.7%	2215
Saint Luke's Cornwall Hospital	Newburgh	3.7%	323
Woodhull Medical and Mental Health Center	Brooklyn	3.8%	186
Elmhurst Hospital Center	Elmhurst	4.0%	175
Brookdale Hospital Medical Center	Brooklyn	4.1%	318
Brooks Memorial Hospital	Dunkirk	4.1%	390
Community Memorial Hospital	Hamilton	4.1%	266
Arnot Ogden Medical Center	Elmira	4.3%	1843
TLC Health Network	Gowanda	4.4%	364
F F Thompson Hospital	Canandaigua	4.5%	649
Ira Davenport Memorial Hospital	Bath	4.5%	243
Niagara Falls Memorial Medical Center	Niagara Falls	4.6%	918
Queens Hospital Center	Jamaica	4.7%	316
Saint Joseph's Hospital	Elmira	4.7%	741
New York Methodist Hospital	Brooklyn	4.8%	862
Saint Joseph's Medical Center	Yonkers	4.8%	518
Bertrand Chaffee Hospital	Springville	5.0%	200
Long Island College Hospital	Brooklyn	5.0%	519
University Hospital - Stony Brook	Stony Brook	5.0%	1177
Peconic Bay Medical Center	Riverhead	5.1%	59
Jones Memorial Hospital	Wellsville	5.2%	461
Woman's Christian Association	Jamestown	5.2%	1350
Jamaica Hospital Medical Center	Jamaica	5.3%	432
Saint Mary's Hospital at Amsterdam	Amsterdam	5.3%	904
Mercy Hospital	Buffalo	5.4%	1002
Oneida Healthcare Center	Oneida	5.4%	443
Saint Peter's Hospital	Albany	5.4%	2040
Newark-Wayne Community Hospital	Newark	5.5%	346
Saint James Mercy Hospital	Hornell	5.5%	309
Brooklyn Hospital Center at Downtown Campus	Brooklyn	5.6%	286
Canton-Potsdam Hospital	Potsdam	5.7%	978
Lewis County General Hospital	Lowville	5.7%	522
Saint Elizabeth Medical Center	Utica	5.7%	822
Sound Shore Medical Center of Westschester	New Rochelle	5.7%	175
Saratoga Hospital	Saratoga Spgs	5.8%	993
Cobleskill Regional Hospital	Cobleskill	5.9%	510
Sheehan Memorial Hospital[1]	Buffalo	5.9%	34
Saint Barnabas Hospital	Bronx	6.0%	133
Albany Memorial Hospital	Albany	6.2%	1097
Orange Regional Medical Center	Goshen	6.2%	1909
Catskill Regional Medical Center	Harris	6.4%	422
Mary Imogene Bassett Hospital	Cooperstown	6.4%	1829
Nathan Littauer Hospital	Gloversville	6.4%	754
Auburn Memorial Hospital	Auburn	6.5%	775
Medina Memorial Hospital	Medina	6.5%	245
Saint Luke's Roosevelt Hospital	New York	6.5%	246
Alice Hyde Medical Center	Malone	6.7%	993
Comm-General Hosp of Greater Syracuse	Syracuse	6.8%	1552
Ellis Hospital	Schenectady	6.9%	2387
Flushing Hospital Medical Center	Flushing	6.9%	131
Hudson Valley Hospital Center	Cortlandt Manor	6.9%	1007
United Memorial Medical Center	Batavia	7.0%	458
Bon Secours Community Hospital	Port Jervis	7.1%	603
Clifton Springs Hospital and Clinic	Clifton Springs	7.1%	562
Westfield Memorial Hospital	Westfield	7.2%	320
Kingston Hospital	Kingston	7.3%	877
Interfaith Medical Center	Brooklyn	7.4%	94
Lutheran Medical Center	Brooklyn	7.4%	243
Our Lady of Lourdes Memorial Hospital	Binghamton	7.5%	3113
Seton Health System-St Mary's Campus	Troy	7.6%	733
New York-Presbyterian Hospital	New York	7.7%	3236
Staten Island University Hospital	Staten Island	7.7%	2091
Wyckoff Heights Medical Center	Brooklyn	7.7%	404
Beth Israel Medical Center	New York	7.8%	884
Rochester General Hospital	Rochester	7.8%	232
Chenango Memorial Hospital	Norwich	7.9%	304
Southampton Hospital	Southampton	7.9%	1073
Phelps Memorial Hospital Assn	Sleepy Hollow	8.0%	1436
Harlem Hospital Center	New York	8.1%	136
Sisters of Charity Hospital	Buffalo	8.1%	372
Putnam Hospital Center	Carmel	8.3%	811
Strong Memorial Hospital	Rochester	8.3%	169
Northern Dutchess Hospital	Rhinebeck	8.8%	605
NYU Hospitals Center	New York	8.8%	1071
Glens Falls Hospital	Glens Falls	8.9%	1655
Champlain Valley Physicians Hospital	Plattsburgh	9.0%	2543
Margaretville Memorial Hospital	Margaretville	9.0%	133
Mercy Medical Center	Rockville Centre	9.0%	680
Bellevue Hospital Center[1]	New York	9.1%	44
Mount Sinai Hospital	New York	9.1%	165
River Hospital	Alexandria Bay	9.1%	132
Samaritan Medical Center	Watertown	9.2%	1354
Claxton-Hepburn Medical Center	Ogdensburg	9.3%	1085
Columbia Memorial Hospital	Hudson	9.5%	623
Mount Vernon Hospital	Mount Vernon	9.5%	367
Geneva General Hospital	Geneva	9.7%	677
Lincoln Medical & Mental Health Center	Bronx	9.7%	176
Highland Hospital	Rochester	10.0%	720
North Shore University Hospital	Manhasset	10.2%	1496
Little Falls Hospital	Little Falls	10.3%	300
United Health Services Hospitals	Johnson City	11.0%	2794
Brookhaven Memorial Hospital Med Ctr	Patchogue	11.3%	1189
Unity Hospital of Rochester	Rochester	11.3%	391
Massena Memorial Hospital	Massena	11.4%	519
St John's Episcopal Hosp-South Shore	Far Rockaway	11.5%	192
Kaleida Health	Buffalo	11.7%	1095
Samaritan Hospital	Troy	11.7%	538
Kenmore Mercy Hospital	Kenmore	11.8%	441
New York Hospital Medical Center of Queens	Flushing	11.9%	1525
Saint John's Riverside Hospital	Yonkers	12.0%	951
Delaware Valley Hospital	Walton	12.1%	206
Soldiers and Sailors Mem Hosp of Yates	Penn Yan	12.9%	357
Albany Med Ctr-South Clinical Campus	Albany	13.0%	693
Franklin Hospital	Valley Stream	13.0%	115
Westchester Medical Center	Valhalla	13.1%	359
Cortland Regional Medical Center	Cortland	13.2%	439
Lawrence Hospital Center	Bronxville	13.2%	642
Vassar Brothers Medical Center	Poughkeepsie	13.4%	679
Nyack Hospital	Nyack	13.5%	579
Erie County Medical Center	Buffalo	13.6%	360
Mount St Mary's Hospital and Health Center	Lewiston	13.7%	736

NOTE: Hospital profiles are in alphabetical order by state, then city, then hospital within the city; Rankings exclude hospitals with less than 25 cases except for patient surveys which excludes hospitals with less than 100 cases; (a) 100–299 cases; (1) The number of cases is too small to be sure how well a hospital is performing; (2) The hospital indicated that the data submitted for this measure were based on a sample of cases; (3) Data was collected during a shorter time period (fewer quarters) than the maximum possible time for this measure; (4) Suppressed for one or more quarters by CMS; (5) No data is available from the hospital for this measure; (6) Fewer than 100 patients completed the HCAHPS survey. Use these rates with caution, as the number of surveys may be too low to reliably assess hospital performance; (7) Survey results are based on less than 12 months of data; (8) Survey results are not available for this reporting period; (9) No or very few patients were eligible for the HCAHPS survey. The scores shown, if any, reflect a very small number of surveys; (10) A state average was not calculated because too few hospitals in the state submitted data; (11) There were discrepancies in the data collection process; Please refer to the User's Guide for a full explanation of data.

Saint Joseph's Hospital Health Center	Syracuse	13.9%	187
Saint Anthony Community Hospital	Warwick	14.1%	455
Corning Hospital	Corning	14.6%	858
Saint Francis Hospital	Poughkeepsie	15.0%	452
Glen Cove Hospital	Glen Cove	15.3%	235
Huntington Hospital	Huntington	15.3%	907
White Plains Hospital Center	White Plains	15.4%	1982
Lakeside Memorial Hospital	Brockport	15.6%	192
Olean General Hospital	Olean	15.6%	294
Good Samaritan Hospital Medical Center	West Islip	16.0%	1604
Winthrop-University Hospital	Mineola	17.0%	525
Wyoming County Community Hospital	Warsaw	17.8%	191
Faxton-St Luke's Healthcare	Utica	18.4%	1552
Adirondack Medical Center	Saranac Lake	18.5%	853
Peninsula Hospital Center	Far Rockaway	18.8%	458
Kingsbrook Jewish Medical Center	Brooklyn	19.8%	273
Nassau University Medical Center	East Meadow	20.9%	503
Good Samaritan Hospital of Suffern	Suffern	21.0%	362
Univ Hosp S U N Y Health Science Ctr	Syracuse	21.7%	506
Saint Catherine of Siena Hospital	Smithtown	23.2%	155
Saint Charles Hospital	Port Jefferson	24.2%	429
Rome Memorial Hospital	Rome	25.6%	425
Eastern Long Island Hospital	Greenport	26.2%	386
Northern Westchester Hospital[1]	Mount Kisco	28.6%	35
Richmond University Medical Center	Staten Island	29.4%	143
John T Mather Mem Hosp-Port Jefferson	Port Jefferson	33.7%	1724
Saint Francis Hospital - Roslyn	Roslyn	35.4%	577
Southside Hospital	Bay Shore	36.2%	58
Lenox Hill Hospital	New York	36.7%	196
New York Downtown Hospital	New York	37.7%	191
South Nassau Communities Hospital	Oceanside	39.4%	815
Forest Hills Hospital	Forest Hills	43.2%	88
New York Westchester Square Medical Center	Bronx	50.9%	108
Nicholas H Noyes Memorial Hospital	Dansville	56.6%	412

39. MRI for Low Back Pain

Hospital Name	City	Rate	Cases
Good Samaritan Hospital of Suffern[1]	Suffern	7.7%	26
Saint Charles Hospital[1]	Port Jefferson	10.3%	39
Univ Hosp S U N Y Health Science Ctr[1]	Syracuse	10.3%	29
Saint Anthony Community Hospital[1]	Warwick	10.9%	55
North Shore University Hospital	Manhasset	14.4%	118
Brooklyn Hospital Center at Downtown Campus[1]	Brooklyn	14.7%	34
Southside Hospital[1]	Bay Shore	16.7%	30
John T Mather Mem Hosp-Port Jefferson[1]	Port Jefferson	17.0%	53
University Hospital of Brooklyn - Downstate[1]	Brooklyn	17.2%	29
Lenox Hill Hospital	New York	17.9%	84
Long Island College Hospital[1]	Brooklyn	18.0%	50
Peconic Bay Medical Center	Riverhead	19.3%	88
Saint Catherine of Siena Hospital[1]	Smithtown	20.0%	45
Westchester Medical Center[1]	Valhalla	20.4%	54
Peninsula Hospital Center	Far Rockaway	20.6%	68
Saint John's Riverside Hospital[1]	Yonkers	21.3%	61
Mercy Medical Center[1]	Rockville Centre	21.8%	55
Lewis County General Hospital[1]	Lowville	22.2%	27
Hospital for Special Surgery	New York	22.5%	1071
Orange Regional Medical Center	Goshen	22.6%	133
Saint Peter's Hospital[1]	Albany	22.6%	31
Wyckoff Heights Medical Center[1]	Brooklyn	22.7%	44
Saint Joseph's Medical Center[1]	Yonkers	22.8%	57
Saint Luke's Roosevelt Hospital[1]	New York	22.8%	57
Albany Memorial Hospital	Albany	23.2%	95
Our Lady of Lourdes Memorial Hospital	Binghamton	23.6%	203
Lawrence Hospital Center	Bronxville	23.7%	139
Beth Israel Medical Center	New York	24.0%	96
Samaritan Medical Center	Watertown	24.0%	75
NYU Hospitals Center	New York	24.1%	87
Adirondack Medical Center[1]	Saranac Lake	24.2%	33
Good Samaritan Hospital Medical Center[1]	West Islip	24.2%	33
Southampton Hospital	Southampton	24.2%	165
Brookhaven Memorial Hospital Med Ctr[1]	Patchogue	24.4%	45
Canton-Potsdam Hospital	Potsdam	24.4%	135
Hudson Valley Hospital Center	Cortlandt Manor	24.4%	172
Maimonides Medical Center[1]	Brooklyn	24.4%	45
Eastern Long Island Hospital[1]	Greenport	24.5%	49
Cobleskill Regional Hospital	Cobleskill	25.0%	60
New York-Presbyterian Hospital	New York	25.0%	192
Kaleida Health	Buffalo	25.2%	111
University Hospital - Stony Brook	Stony Brook	25.5%	149
Staten Island University Hospital[1]	Staten Island	25.9%	27
Ellis Hospital	Schenectady	26.7%	101
Samaritan Hospital	Troy	27.7%	65
Kingsbrook Jewish Medical Center[1]	Brooklyn	28.0%	25
Bon Secours Community Hospital	Port Jervis	28.1%	96
Strong Memorial Hospital[1]	Rochester	28.3%	53
Alice Hyde Medical Center	Malone	28.8%	80
Saint Joseph's Hospital	Elmira	28.9%	76
Montefiore Medical Center	Bronx	29.2%	120
Columbia Memorial Hospital[1]	Hudson	29.3%	41
South Nassau Communities Hospital[1]	Oceanside	29.4%	34
New York Methodist Hospital	Brooklyn	29.7%	74
Northern Westchester Hospital	Mount Kisco	30.2%	53
Putnam Hospital Center	Carmel	30.2%	129
Catskill Regional Medical Center	Harris	30.4%	92
Niagara Falls Memorial Medical Center	Niagara Falls	30.5%	118
Claxton-Hepburn Medical Center	Ogdensburg	30.9%	81
Newark-Wayne Community Hospital[1]	Newark	31.4%	35
Saint Francis Hospital[1]	Poughkeepsie	31.6%	38
Mary Imogene Bassett Hospital	Cooperstown	31.7%	123
Northern Dutchess Hospital[1]	Rhinebeck	31.8%	44
Kingston Hospital	Kingston	31.9%	113
Vassar Brothers Medical Center[1]	Poughkeepsie	32.0%	25
Saratoga Hospital	Saratoga Spgs	32.3%	96
Jones Memorial Hospital[1]	Wellsville	32.4%	37
Oneida Healthcare Center[1]	Oneida	32.4%	37
Cayuga Medical Center at Ithaca	Ithaca	32.7%	223
Albany Medical Center Hospital	Albany	32.8%	58
Arnot Ogden Medical Center	Elmira	32.9%	143
New York Hospital Medical Center of Queens	Flushing	34.1%	91
Woman's Christian Association	Jamestown	34.2%	79
Clifton Springs Hospital and Clinic[1]	Clifton Springs	34.5%	29
Lakeside Memorial Hospital[1]	Brockport	35.3%	34
Massena Memorial Hospital	Massena	36.0%	50
Corning Hospital	Corning	36.1%	72
Mount St Mary's Hospital and Health Center	Lewiston	37.5%	136
Saint Mary's Hospital at Amsterdam	Amsterdam	37.5%	80
Olean General Hospital	Olean	37.6%	117
Community Memorial Hospital	Hamilton	38.9%	54
Brooks Memorial Hospital	Dunkirk	42.1%	38
Cortland Regional Medical Center[1]	Cortland	42.4%	33
Nathan Littauer Hospital	Gloversville	42.6%	47
Seton Health System-St Mary's Campus	Troy	43.5%	46
Aurelia Osborn Fox Memorial Hospital	Oneonta	45.2%	42
Champlain Valley Physicians Hospital	Plattsburgh	46.7%	45

Survey of Patients' Hospital Experiences

40. Area Around Room 'Always' Quiet at Night

Hospital Name	City	Rate	Cases
Westfield Memorial Hospital	Westfield	83%	(a)
Soldiers and Sailors Mem Hosp of Yates	Penn Yan	65%	(a)
NY Eye and Ear Infirmary	New York	63%	300+
Delaware Valley Hospital	Walton	61%	(a)
New York Westchester Square Medical Center[7]	Bronx	61%	(a)
Adirondack Medical Center	Saranac Lake	60%	300+
Kings County Hospital Center	Brooklyn	59%	300+
Lawrence Hospital Center	Bronxville	59%	300+
Mount Vernon Hospital	Mount Vernon	59%	300+
Saint James Mercy Hospital	Hornell	59%	300+
Bon Secours Community Hospital	Port Jervis	58%	300+
Harlem Hospital Center	New York	58%	300+
Nicholas H Noyes Memorial Hospital	Dansville	58%	300+
North Central Bronx Hospital	Bronx	58%	300+
Community Memorial Hospital	Hamilton	57%	300+
Northern Westchester Hospital	Mount Kisco	57%	300+
Interfaith Medical Center	Brooklyn	56%	300+
Corning Hospital	Corning	55%	300+
Geneva General Hospital	Geneva	55%	300+
Mount St Mary's Hospital and Health Center	Lewiston	55%	300+
Putnam Hospital Center	Carmel	55%	300+
Queens Hospital Center	Jamaica	55%	300+
Saint Anthony Community Hospital	Warwick	55%	300+
Cayuga Medical Center at Ithaca	Ithaca	54%	300+
Cobleskill Regional Hospital	Cobleskill	54%	(a)
Lincoln Medical & Mental Health Center	Bronx	54%	300+
Mercy Medical Center	Rockville Centre	54%	300+
Montefiore Medical Center	Bronx	54%	300+
Nathan Littauer Hospital	Gloversville	54%	300+
New York-Presbyterian Hospital	New York	54%	300+
Our Lady of Lourdes Memorial Hospital	Binghamton	54%	300+
Albany Memorial Hospital	Albany	53%	300+
Eastern Long Island Hospital	Greenport	53%	300+
Lewis County General Hospital	Lowville	53%	300+
Saint Francis Hospital - Roslyn	Roslyn	53%	300+
St John's Episcopal Hosp-South Shore	Far Rockaway	53%	300+
Seton Health System-St Mary's Campus	Troy	53%	300+
Vassar Brothers Medical Center[11]	Poughkeepsie	53%	300+
White Plains Hospital Center	White Plains	53%	300+
Bertrand Chaffee Hospital	Springville	52%	300+
Comm-General Hosp of Greater Syracuse	Syracuse	52%	300+
Long Island College Hospital	Brooklyn	52%	300+
Massena Memorial Hospital	Massena	52%	300+
Oneida Healthcare Center	Oneida	52%	300+
Hospital for Special Surgery	New York	51%	300+
Kingsbrook Jewish Medical Center	Brooklyn	51%	300+
Lakeside Memorial Hospital	Brockport	51%	300+
Northern Dutchess Hospital	Rhinebeck	51%	300+
Saint Joseph's Medical Center	Yonkers	51%	300+
University Hospital of Brooklyn - Downstate	Brooklyn	51%	300+
Beth Israel Medical Center	New York	50%	300+
Canton-Potsdam Hospital	Potsdam	50%	300+
Clifton Springs Hospital and Clinic	Clifton Springs	50%	300+
Glen Cove Hospital	Glen Cove	50%	300+
Hudson Valley Hospital Center	Cortlandt Manor	50%	300+
Jacobi Medical Center	Bronx	50%	300+
Niagara Falls Memorial Medical Center	Niagara Falls	50%	300+
Saint Barnabas Hospital	Bronx	50%	300+
Saint Charles Hospital	Port Jefferson	50%	300+
Aurelia Osborn Fox Memorial Hospital	Oneonta	49%	300+
Bronx-Lebanon Hospital Center	Bronx	49%	300+
Claxton-Hepburn Medical Center	Ogdensburg	49%	(a)
Coney Island Hospital	Brooklyn	49%	300+
Franklin Hospital	Valley Stream	49%	300+
John T Mather Mem Hosp-Port Jefferson	Port Jefferson	49%	300+
Jones Memorial Hospital	Wellsville	49%	300+
Lenox Hill Hospital[11]	New York	49%	300+
Little Falls Hospital	Little Falls	49%	300+
Mount Sinai Hospital	New York	49%	300+
Newark-Wayne Community Hospital	Newark	49%	300+
Saint Francis Hospital	Poughkeepsie	49%	300+
Saint Mary's Hospital at Amsterdam	Amsterdam	49%	300+
South Nassau Communities Hospital	Oceanside	49%	300+
Southampton Hospital	Southampton	49%	300+
Southside Hospital	Bay Shore	49%	300+
Woodhull Medical and Mental Health Center	Brooklyn	49%	300+
Benedictine Hospital	Kingston	48%	(a)
Catskill Regional Medical Center	Harris	48%	300+
Highland Hospital	Rochester	48%	300+
Metropolitan Hospital Center	New York	48%	300+
Saint Luke's Roosevelt Hospital	New York	48%	300+
Auburn Memorial Hospital	Auburn	47%	300+
Brooks Memorial Hospital	Dunkirk	47%	300+
Carthage Area Hospital	Carthage	47%	300+
Chenango Memorial Hospital	Norwich	47%	300+
F F Thompson Hospital	Canandaigua	47%	300+
Ira Davenport Memorial Hospital	Bath	47%	(a)
Nyack Hospital	Nyack	47%	300+
Saint John's Riverside Hospital	Yonkers	47%	300+
Saint Joseph's Hospital	Elmira	47%	300+
Saint Luke's Cornwall Hospital	Newburgh	47%	300+
Sisters of Charity Hospital	Buffalo	47%	300+
Unity Hospital of Rochester	Rochester	47%	300+
Woman's Christian Association	Jamestown	47%	300+
Brooklyn Hospital Center at Downtown Campus	Brooklyn	46%	300+
Glens Falls Hospital	Glens Falls	46%	300+
Good Samaritan Hospital of Suffern	Suffern	46%	300+
Huntington Hospital	Huntington	46%	300+
Long Island Jewish Medical Center	New Hyde Park	46%	300+
Medina Memorial Hospital	Medina	46%	300+
Samaritan Medical Center	Watertown	46%	300+
Univ Hosp S U N Y Health Science Ctr	Syracuse	46%	300+
Arnot Ogden Medical Center	Elmira	45%	300+
Brookdale Hospital Medical Center	Brooklyn	45%	300+
Edward John Noble Hospital of Gouverneur	Gouverneur	45%	300+
Maimonides Medical Center	Brooklyn	45%	300+
New York Methodist Hospital	Brooklyn	45%	300+
Olean General Hospital	Olean	45%	300+
Oswego Hospital	Oswego	45%	300+
Phelps Memorial Hospital Assn	Sleepy Hollow	45%	300+
Rome Memorial Hospital	Rome	45%	300+
Samaritan Hospital	Troy	45%	300+
United Memorial Medical Center	Batavia	45%	300+
Winthrop-University Hospital	Mineola	45%	300+
Albany Medical Center Hospital	Albany	44%	300+
Ellis Hospital	Schenectady	44%	300+
Forest Hills Hospital	Forest Hills	44%	300+
Kaleida Health	Buffalo	44%	300+
Mary Imogene Bassett Hospital	Cooperstown	44%	300+
New York Community Hospital of Brooklyn	Brooklyn	44%	300+
Saint Elizabeth Medical Center	Utica	44%	300+
Saint Joseph's Hospital Health Center	Syracuse	44%	300+
Sound Shore Medical Center of Westschester	New Rochelle	44%	300+
Staten Island University Hospital	Staten Island	44%	300+
University Hospital - Stony Brook	Stony Brook	44%	300+
Champlain Valley Physicians Hospital	Plattsburgh	43%	300+
Crouse Hospital	Syracuse	43%	300+
Eastern Niagara Hospital	Lockport	43%	300+
Good Samaritan Hospital Medical Center	West Islip	43%	300+
Kenmore Mercy Hospital	Kenmore	43%	300+
NYU Hospitals Center[11]	New York	43%	300+
Saint Joseph Hospital	Bethpage	43%	300+
Alice Hyde Medical Center	Malone	42%	300+
Bellevue Hospital Center	New York	42%	300+
Faxton-St Luke's Healthcare	Utica	42%	300+
Long Beach Medical Center	Long Beach	42%	300+
Nassau University Medical Center	East Meadow	42%	300+
New York Hospital Medical Center of Queens	Flushing	42%	300+
Rochester General Hospital	Rochester	42%	300+
Brookhaven Memorial Hospital Med Ctr	Patchogue	41%	300+
Cortland Regional Medical Center	Cortland	41%	300+
Elmhurst Hospital Center	Elmhurst	41%	300+

NOTE: Hospital profiles are in alphabetical order by state, then city, then hospital within the city; Rankings exclude hospitals with less than 25 cases except for patient surveys which excludes hospitals with less than 100 cases; (a) 100–299 cases; (1) The number of cases is too small to be sure how well a hospital is performing; (2) The hospital indicated that the data submitted for this measure were based on a sample of cases; (3) Data was collected during a shorter time period (fewer quarters) than the maximum possible time for this measure; (4) Suppressed for one or more quarters by CMS; (5) No data is available from the hospital for this measure; (6) Fewer than 100 patients completed the HCAHPS survey. Use these rates with caution, as the number of surveys may be too low to reliably assess hospital performance; (7) Survey results are based on less than 12 months of data; (8) Survey results are not available for this reporting period; (9) No or very few patients were eligible for the HCAHPS survey. The scores shown, if any, reflect a very small number of surveys; (10) A state average was not calculated because too few hospitals in the state submitted data; (11) There were discrepancies in the data collection process; Please refer to the User's Guide for a full explanation of data.

Orange Regional Medical Center	Goshen	41%	300+
Peninsula Hospital Center	Far Rockaway	41%	300+
Richmond University Medical Center	Staten Island	41%	300+
TLC Health Network	Gowanda	41%	300+
Erie County Medical Center	Buffalo	40%	300+
Jamaica Hospital Medical Center	Jamaica	40%	300+
North Shore University Hospital	Manhasset	40%	300+
Saint Catherine of Siena Hospital	Smithtown	40%	300+
Kingston Hospital	Kingston	39%	300+
Mercy Hospital	Buffalo	39%	300+
Peconic Bay Medical Center	Riverhead	39%	300+
Saratoga Hospital	Saratoga Spgs	39%	300+
United Health Services Hospitals	Johnson City	39%	300+
Wyckoff Heights Medical Center	Brooklyn	39%	300+
Columbia Memorial Hospital	Hudson	38%	300+
Flushing Hospital Medical Center	Flushing	38%	300+
Saint Peter's Hospital	Albany	38%	300+
Wyoming County Community Hospital	Warsaw	38%	300+
New York Downtown Hospital	New York	37%	300+
Strong Memorial Hospital	Rochester	37%	300+
Plainview Hospital	Plainview	36%	300+
Westchester Medical Center	Valhalla	35%	300+
Lutheran Medical Center	Brooklyn	34%	300+

41. Doctors 'Always' Communicated Well

Hospital Name	City	Rate	Cases
Westfield Memorial Hospital	Westfield	88%	(a)
Bertrand Chaffee Hospital	Springville	87%	300+
Clifton Springs Hospital and Clinic	Clifton Springs	86%	300+
Delaware Valley Hospital	Walton	86%	(a)
Claxton-Hepburn Medical Center	Ogdensburg	85%	(a)
Eastern Long Island Hospital	Greenport	85%	300+
Cobleskill Regional Hospital	Cobleskill	84%	(a)
Lewis County General Hospital	Lowville	84%	300+
Community Memorial Hospital	Hamilton	83%	300+
Hospital for Special Surgery	New York	83%	300+
Little Falls Hospital	Little Falls	83%	300+
Mount Vernon Hospital	Mount Vernon	83%	300+
Northern Westchester Hospital	Mount Kisco	83%	300+
Oneida Healthcare Center	Oneida	83%	300+
Putnam Hospital Center	Carmel	83%	300+
Adirondack Medical Center	Saranac Lake	82%	300+
Edward John Noble Hospital of Gouverneur	Gouverneur	82%	300+
Massena Memorial Hospital	Massena	82%	300+
Canton-Potsdam Hospital	Potsdam	81%	300+
Saint Charles Hospital	Port Jefferson	81%	300+
Saint Francis Hospital - Roslyn	Roslyn	81%	300+
Alice Hyde Medical Center	Malone	80%	300+
Comm-General Hosp of Greater Syracuse	Syracuse	80%	300+
F F Thompson Hospital	Canandaigua	80%	300+
Lawrence Hospital Center	Bronxville	80%	300+
Newark-Wayne Community Hospital	Newark	80%	300+
Northern Dutchess Hospital	Rhinebeck	80%	300+
Rochester General Hospital	Rochester	80%	300+
Saratoga Hospital	Saratoga Spgs	80%	300+
Seton Health System-St Mary's Campus	Troy	80%	300+
Arnot Ogden Medical Center	Elmira	79%	300+
Auburn Memorial Hospital	Auburn	79%	300+
Glen Cove Hospital	Glen Cove	79%	300+
Glens Falls Hospital	Glens Falls	79%	300+
Highland Hospital	Rochester	79%	300+
Hudson Valley Hospital Center	Cortlandt Manor	79%	300+
John T Mather Mem Hosp-Port Jefferson	Port Jefferson	79%	300+
Lenox Hill Hospital[11]	New York	79%	300+
Queens Hospital Center	Jamaica	79%	300+
Saint Anthony Community Hospital	Warwick	79%	300+
Saint John's Riverside Hospital	Yonkers	79%	300+
Southampton Hospital	Southampton	79%	300+
Vassar Brothers Medical Center[11]	Poughkeepsie	79%	300+
White Plains Hospital Center	White Plains	79%	300+
Cayuga Medical Center at Ithaca	Ithaca	78%	300+
Eastern Niagara Hospital	Lockport	78%	300+
Huntington Hospital	Huntington	78%	300+
Kings County Hospital Center	Brooklyn	78%	300+
Lakeside Memorial Hospital	Brockport	78%	300+
Mary Imogene Bassett Hospital	Cooperstown	78%	300+
Mercy Medical Center	Rockville Centre	78%	300+
Mount Sinai Hospital	New York	78%	300+
Mount St Mary's Hospital and Health Center	Lewiston	78%	300+
New York-Presbyterian Hospital	New York	78%	300+
Nicholas H Noyes Memorial Hospital	Dansville	78%	300+
Phelps Memorial Hospital Assn	Sleepy Hollow	78%	300+
Saint Mary's Hospital at Amsterdam	Amsterdam	78%	300+
Unity Hospital of Rochester	Rochester	78%	300+
Woman's Christian Association	Jamestown	78%	300+
Benedictine Hospital	Kingston	77%	(a)
Bon Secours Community Hospital	Port Jervis	77%	300+
Brooks Memorial Hospital	Dunkirk	77%	300+
Champlain Valley Physicians Hospital	Plattsburgh	77%	300+
Jacobi Medical Center	Bronx	77%	300+
Jones Memorial Hospital	Wellsville	77%	300+
Maimonides Medical Center	Brooklyn	77%	300+
Medina Memorial Hospital	Medina	77%	300+
Montefiore Medical Center	Bronx	77%	300+
Nathan Littauer Hospital	Gloversville	77%	300+
North Central Bronx Hospital	Bronx	77%	300+
Saint Catherine of Siena Hospital	Smithtown	77%	300+
Saint James Mercy Hospital	Hornell	77%	300+
Southside Hospital	Bay Shore	77%	300+
TLC Health Network	Gowanda	77%	300+
United Memorial Medical Center	Batavia	77%	300+
University Hospital of Brooklyn - Downstate	Brooklyn	77%	300+
Winthrop-University Hospital	Mineola	77%	300+
Albany Memorial Hospital	Albany	76%	300+
Chenango Memorial Hospital	Norwich	76%	300+
Columbia Memorial Hospital	Hudson	76%	300+
Good Samaritan Hospital Medical Center	West Islip	76%	300+
Harlem Hospital Center	New York	76%	300+
Lincoln Medical & Mental Health Center	Bronx	76%	300+
Oswego Hospital	Oswego	76%	300+
Our Lady of Lourdes Memorial Hospital	Binghamton	76%	300+
Samaritan Medical Center	Watertown	76%	300+
South Nassau Communities Hospital	Oceanside	76%	300+
Aurelia Osborn Fox Memorial Hospital	Oneonta	75%	300+
Bellevue Hospital Center	New York	75%	300+
Brookhaven Memorial Hospital Med Ctr	Patchogue	75%	300+
Franklin Hospital	Valley Stream	75%	300+
Geneva General Hospital	Geneva	75%	300+
Good Samaritan Hospital of Suffern	Suffern	75%	300+
Kenmore Mercy Hospital	Kenmore	75%	300+
Kingsbrook Jewish Medical Center	Brooklyn	75%	300+
Metropolitan Hospital Center	New York	75%	300+
North Shore University Hospital	Manhasset	75%	300+
NY Eye and Ear Infirmary	New York	75%	300+
NYU Hospitals Center[11]	New York	75%	300+
Olean General Hospital	Olean	75%	300+
Saint Barnabas Hospital	Bronx	75%	300+
Saint Joseph's Hospital Health Center	Syracuse	75%	300+
Saint Luke's Cornwall Hospital	Newburgh	75%	300+
Soldiers and Sailors Mem Hosp of Yates	Penn Yan	75%	(a)
Strong Memorial Hospital	Rochester	75%	300+
United Health Services Hospitals	Johnson City	75%	300+
Carthage Area Hospital	Carthage	74%	300+
Corning Hospital	Corning	74%	300+
Elmhurst Hospital Center	Elmhurst	74%	300+
Faxton-St Luke's Healthcare	Utica	74%	300+
Ira Davenport Memorial Hospital	Bath	74%	(a)
Kaleida Health	Buffalo	74%	300+
Long Island Jewish Medical Center	New Hyde Park	74%	300+
New York Westchester Square Medical Center[7]	Bronx	74%	(a)
Plainview Hospital	Plainview	74%	300+
Saint Elizabeth Medical Center	Utica	74%	300+
Saint Francis Hospital	Poughkeepsie	74%	300+
Saint Joseph's Hospital	Elmira	74%	300+
Sound Shore Medical Center of Westschester	New Rochelle	74%	300+
Woodhull Medical and Mental Health Center	Brooklyn	74%	300+
Wyoming County Community Hospital	Warsaw	74%	300+
Beth Israel Medical Center	New York	73%	300+
Crouse Hospital	Syracuse	73%	300+
Nyack Hospital	Nyack	73%	300+
Peconic Bay Medical Center	Riverhead	73%	300+
St John's Episcopal Hosp-South Shore	Far Rockaway	73%	300+
Saint Joseph Hospital	Bethpage	73%	300+
Saint Joseph's Medical Center	Yonkers	73%	300+
Saint Luke's Roosevelt Hospital	New York	73%	300+
Samaritan Hospital	Troy	73%	300+
Sisters of Charity Hospital	Buffalo	73%	300+
University Hospital - Stony Brook	Stony Brook	73%	300+
Univ Hosp S U N Y Health Science Ctr	Syracuse	73%	300+
Brooklyn Hospital Center at Downtown Campus	Brooklyn	72%	300+
Coney Island Hospital	Brooklyn	72%	300+
Cortland Regional Medical Center	Cortland	72%	300+
Ellis Hospital	Schenectady	72%	300+
Erie County Medical Center	Buffalo	72%	300+
Kingston Hospital	Kingston	72%	300+
Lutheran Medical Center	Brooklyn	72%	300+
Mercy Hospital	Buffalo	72%	300+
Orange Regional Medical Center	Goshen	72%	300+
Rome Memorial Hospital	Rome	72%	300+
Saint Peter's Hospital	Albany	72%	300+
Staten Island University Hospital	Staten Island	72%	300+
Catskill Regional Medical Center	Harris	71%	300+
Long Beach Medical Center	Long Beach	71%	300+
Long Island College Hospital	Brooklyn	71%	300+
New York Methodist Hospital	Brooklyn	71%	300+
Westchester Medical Center	Valhalla	71%	300+
Forest Hills Hospital	Forest Hills	70%	300+
New York Community Hospital of Brooklyn	Brooklyn	70%	300+
Niagara Falls Memorial Medical Center	Niagara Falls	70%	300+
Richmond University Medical Center	Staten Island	70%	300+
New York Hospital Medical Center of Queens	Flushing	69%	300+
Albany Medical Center Hospital	Albany	67%	300+
Bronx-Lebanon Hospital Center	Bronx	67%	300+
Brookdale Hospital Medical Center	Brooklyn	67%	300+
Interfaith Medical Center	Brooklyn	67%	300+
Jamaica Hospital Medical Center	Jamaica	66%	300+
New York Downtown Hospital	New York	66%	300+
Peninsula Hospital Center	Far Rockaway	66%	300+
Wyckoff Heights Medical Center	Brooklyn	66%	300+
Flushing Hospital Medical Center	Flushing	65%	300+
Nassau University Medical Center	East Meadow	65%	300+

42. Home Recovery Information Given

Hospital Name	City	Rate	Cases
Bertrand Chaffee Hospital	Springville	92%	300+
Clifton Springs Hospital and Clinic	Clifton Springs	91%	300+
Rochester General Hospital	Rochester	91%	300+
Saratoga Hospital	Saratoga Spgs	91%	300+
Lakeside Memorial Hospital	Brockport	89%	300+
Canton-Potsdam Hospital	Potsdam	88%	300+
Community Memorial Hospital	Hamilton	88%	300+
Hospital for Special Surgery	New York	88%	300+
Mary Imogene Bassett Hospital	Cooperstown	88%	300+
Saint Joseph's Hospital Health Center	Syracuse	88%	300+
TLC Health Network	Gowanda	88%	300+
Unity Hospital of Rochester	Rochester	88%	300+
Auburn Memorial Hospital	Auburn	87%	300+
Claxton-Hepburn Medical Center	Ogdensburg	87%	(a)
F F Thompson Hospital	Canandaigua	87%	300+
Geneva General Hospital	Geneva	87%	300+
John T Mather Mem Hosp-Port Jefferson	Port Jefferson	87%	300+
Newark-Wayne Community Hospital	Newark	87%	300+
Saint Francis Hospital - Roslyn	Roslyn	87%	300+
Saint James Mercy Hospital	Hornell	87%	300+
Saint Mary's Hospital at Amsterdam	Amsterdam	87%	300+
Strong Memorial Hospital	Rochester	87%	300+
Woman's Christian Association	Jamestown	87%	300+
Crouse Hospital	Syracuse	86%	300+
Delaware Valley Hospital	Walton	86%	(a)
Highland Hospital	Rochester	86%	300+
Lewis County General Hospital	Lowville	86%	300+
Our Lady of Lourdes Memorial Hospital	Binghamton	86%	300+
Saint Charles Hospital	Port Jefferson	86%	300+
Soldiers and Sailors Mem Hosp of Yates	Penn Yan	86%	(a)
United Memorial Medical Center	Batavia	86%	300+
Westfield Memorial Hospital	Westfield	86%	(a)
Albany Memorial Hospital	Albany	85%	300+
Arnot Ogden Medical Center	Elmira	85%	300+
Aurelia Osborn Fox Memorial Hospital	Oneonta	85%	300+
Cobleskill Regional Hospital	Cobleskill	85%	(a)
Ellis Hospital	Schenectady	85%	300+
Glens Falls Hospital	Glens Falls	85%	300+
Kenmore Mercy Hospital	Kenmore	85%	300+
Rome Memorial Hospital	Rome	85%	300+
Saint Anthony Community Hospital	Warwick	85%	300+
Saint Francis Hospital	Poughkeepsie	85%	300+
United Health Services Hospitals	Johnson City	85%	300+
Eastern Long Island Hospital	Greenport	84%	300+
Edward John Noble Hospital of Gouverneur	Gouverneur	84%	300+
Medina Memorial Hospital	Medina	84%	300+
Northern Dutchess Hospital	Rhinebeck	84%	300+
Oneida Healthcare Center	Oneida	84%	300+
Oswego Hospital	Oswego	84%	300+
Saint Peter's Hospital	Albany	84%	300+
Samaritan Medical Center	Watertown	84%	300+
Seton Health System-St Mary's Campus	Troy	84%	300+
Sisters of Charity Hospital	Buffalo	84%	300+
Wyoming County Community Hospital	Warsaw	84%	300+
Benedictine Hospital	Kingston	83%	(a)
Carthage Area Hospital	Carthage	83%	300+
Cayuga Medical Center at Ithaca	Ithaca	83%	300+
Comm-General Hosp of Greater Syracuse	Syracuse	83%	300+
Cortland Regional Medical Center	Cortland	83%	300+
Good Samaritan Hospital Medical Center	West Islip	83%	300+
Little Falls Hospital	Little Falls	83%	300+
Metropolitan Hospital Center	New York	83%	300+
Nathan Littauer Hospital	Gloversville	83%	300+
Univ Hosp S U N Y Health Science Ctr	Syracuse	83%	300+
Vassar Brothers Medical Center[11]	Poughkeepsie	83%	300+
Winthrop-University Hospital	Mineola	83%	300+
Adirondack Medical Center	Saranac Lake	82%	300+
Alice Hyde Medical Center	Malone	82%	300+
Corning Hospital	Corning	82%	300+
Kaleida Health	Buffalo	82%	300+
Massena Memorial Hospital	Massena	82%	300+
Mount St Mary's Hospital and Health Center	Lewiston	82%	300+
Mount Vernon Hospital	Mount Vernon	82%	300+
Samaritan Hospital	Troy	82%	300+
Woodhull Medical and Mental Health Center	Brooklyn	82%	300+
Albany Medical Center Hospital	Albany	81%	300+
Brookhaven Memorial Hospital Med Ctr	Patchogue	81%	300+

NOTE: Hospital profiles are in alphabetical order by state, then city, then hospital within the city; Rankings exclude hospitals with less than 25 cases except for patient surveys which excludes hospitals with less than 100 cases; (a) 100–299 cases; (1) The number of cases is too small to be sure how well a hospital is performing; (2) The hospital indicated that the data submitted for this measure were based on a sample of cases; (3) Data was collected during a shorter time period (fewer quarters) than the maximum possible time for this measure; (4) Suppressed for one or more quarters by CMS; (5) No data is available from the hospital for this measure; (6) Fewer than 100 patients completed the HCAHPS survey. Use these rates with caution, as the number of surveys may be too low to reliably assess hospital performance; (7) Survey results are based on less than 12 months of data; (8) Survey results are not available for this reporting period; (9) No or very few patients were eligible for the HCAHPS survey. The scores shown, if any, reflect a very small number of surveys; (10) A state average was not calculated because too few hospitals in the state submitted data; (11) There were discrepancies in the data collection process; Please refer to the User's Guide for a full explanation of data.

Champlain Valley Physicians Hospital	Plattsburgh	81%	300+
Chenango Memorial Hospital	Norwich	81%	300+
Elmhurst Hospital Center	Elmhurst	81%	300+
Mercy Medical Center	Rockville Centre	81%	300+
Nicholas H Noyes Memorial Hospital	Dansville	81%	300+
Olean General Hospital	Olean	81%	300+
Putnam Hospital Center	Carmel	81%	300+
Saint Catherine of Siena Hospital	Smithtown	81%	300+
Saint Elizabeth Medical Center	Utica	81%	300+
Saint Joseph's Hospital	Elmira	81%	300+
Saint Luke's Cornwall Hospital	Newburgh	81%	300+
Brooks Memorial Hospital	Dunkirk	80%	300+
Faxton-St Luke's Healthcare	Utica	80%	300+
Hudson Valley Hospital Center	Cortlandt Manor	80%	300+
Mercy Hospital	Buffalo	80%	300+
Orange Regional Medical Center	Goshen	80%	300+
Peconic Bay Medical Center	Riverhead	80%	300+
Saint Joseph Hospital	Bethpage	80%	300+
South Nassau Communities Hospital	Oceanside	80%	300+
Catskill Regional Medical Center	Harris	79%	300+
Columbia Memorial Hospital	Hudson	79%	300+
Erie County Medical Center	Buffalo	79%	300+
Kings County Hospital Center	Brooklyn	79%	300+
Phelps Memorial Hospital Assn	Sleepy Hollow	79%	300+
Southside Hospital	Bay Shore	79%	300+
University Hospital - Stony Brook	Stony Brook	79%	300+
Bellevue Hospital Center	New York	78%	300+
Bon Secours Community Hospital	Port Jervis	78%	300+
Eastern Niagara Hospital	Lockport	78%	300+
Glen Cove Hospital	Glen Cove	78%	300+
Good Samaritan Hospital of Suffern	Suffern	78%	300+
Harlem Hospital Center	New York	78%	300+
Jacobi Medical Center	Bronx	78%	300+
Jones Memorial Hospital	Wellsville	78%	300+
New York-Presbyterian Hospital	New York	78%	300+
Northern Westchester Hospital	Mount Kisco	78%	300+
NYU Hospitals Center[11]	New York	78%	300+
Queens Hospital Center	Jamaica	78%	300+
Coney Island Hospital	Brooklyn	77%	300+
Kingston Hospital	Kingston	77%	300+
Maimonides Medical Center	Brooklyn	77%	300+
Mount Sinai Hospital	New York	77%	300+
Niagara Falls Memorial Medical Center	Niagara Falls	77%	300+
Beth Israel Medical Center	New York	76%	300+
Kingsbrook Jewish Medical Center	Brooklyn	76%	300+
Lutheran Medical Center	Brooklyn	76%	300+
Montefiore Medical Center	Bronx	76%	300+
New York Community Hospital of Brooklyn	Brooklyn	76%	300+
North Central Bronx Hospital	Bronx	76%	300+
North Shore University Hospital	Manhasset	76%	300+
St John's Episcopal Hosp-South Shore	Far Rockaway	76%	300+
Staten Island University Hospital	Staten Island	76%	300+
Huntington Hospital	Huntington	75%	300+
Ira Davenport Memorial Hospital	Bath	75%	(a)
Lenox Hill Hospital[11]	New York	75%	300+
Long Island Jewish Medical Center	New Hyde Park	75%	300+
New York Hospital Medical Center of Queens	Flushing	75%	300+
New York Methodist Hospital	Brooklyn	75%	300+
NY Eye and Ear Infirmary	New York	75%	300+
Saint Joseph's Medical Center	Yonkers	75%	300+
Sound Shore Medical Center of Westschester	New Rochelle	75%	300+
New York Westchester Square Medical Center[7]	Bronx	74%	(a)
University Hospital of Brooklyn - Downstate	Brooklyn	74%	300+
Westchester Medical Center	Valhalla	74%	300+
Franklin Hospital	Valley Stream	73%	300+
Lawrence Hospital Center	Bronxville	73%	300+
Lincoln Medical & Mental Health Center	Bronx	73%	300+
Long Beach Medical Center	Long Beach	73%	300+
New York Downtown Hospital	New York	73%	300+
Plainview Hospital	Plainview	73%	300+
Southampton Hospital	Southampton	73%	300+
Forest Hills Hospital	Forest Hills	72%	300+
Saint John's Riverside Hospital	Yonkers	72%	300+
Saint Luke's Roosevelt Hospital	New York	72%	300+
White Plains Hospital Center	White Plains	72%	300+
Bronx-Lebanon Hospital Center	Bronx	70%	300+
Flushing Hospital Medical Center	Flushing	70%	300+
Jamaica Hospital Medical Center	Jamaica	70%	300+
Nassau University Medical Center	East Meadow	70%	300+
Peninsula Hospital Center	Far Rockaway	70%	300+
Richmond University Medical Center	Staten Island	70%	300+
Saint Barnabas Hospital	Bronx	70%	300+
Wyckoff Heights Medical Center	Brooklyn	70%	300+
Nyack Hospital	Nyack	68%	300+
Brookdale Hospital Medical Center	Brooklyn	66%	300+
Long Island College Hospital	Brooklyn	66%	300+
Brooklyn Hospital Center at Downtown Campus	Brooklyn	64%	300+
Interfaith Medical Center	Brooklyn	64%	300+

43. Hospital Given 9 or 10 on 10 Point Scale

Hospital Name	City	Rate	Cases
Westfield Memorial Hospital	Westfield	91%	(a)
Hospital for Special Surgery	New York	85%	300+
Saint Francis Hospital - Roslyn	Roslyn	82%	300+
Clifton Springs Hospital and Clinic	Clifton Springs	79%	300+
Eastern Long Island Hospital	Greenport	78%	300+
Bertrand Chaffee Hospital	Springville	74%	300+
Northern Westchester Hospital	Mount Kisco	74%	300+
Putnam Hospital Center	Carmel	74%	300+
Community Memorial Hospital	Hamilton	73%	300+
Delaware Valley Hospital	Walton	73%	(a)
New York-Presbyterian Hospital	New York	73%	300+
Northern Dutchess Hospital	Rhinebeck	73%	300+
Saint Anthony Community Hospital	Warwick	72%	300+
Rochester General Hospital	Rochester	71%	300+
Saint Joseph's Hospital Health Center	Syracuse	71%	300+
Vassar Brothers Medical Center[11]	Poughkeepsie	71%	300+
Cobleskill Regional Hospital	Cobleskill	70%	(a)
John T Mather Mem Hosp-Port Jefferson	Port Jefferson	70%	300+
Nicholas H Noyes Memorial Hospital	Dansville	70%	300+
Saint Charles Hospital	Port Jefferson	70%	300+
Adirondack Medical Center	Saranac Lake	69%	300+
F F Thompson Hospital	Canandaigua	69%	300+
Highland Hospital	Rochester	69%	300+
Lewis County General Hospital	Lowville	69%	300+
Mount St Mary's Hospital and Health Center	Lewiston	69%	300+
Saint Mary's Hospital at Amsterdam	Amsterdam	69%	300+
Our Lady of Lourdes Memorial Hospital	Binghamton	68%	300+
Seton Health System-St Mary's Campus	Troy	68%	300+
White Plains Hospital Center	White Plains	68%	300+
Arnot Ogden Medical Center	Elmira	67%	300+
Benedictine Hospital	Kingston	67%	(a)
Glen Cove Hospital	Glen Cove	67%	300+
Winthrop-University Hospital	Mineola	67%	300+
Albany Memorial Hospital	Albany	66%	300+
Cayuga Medical Center at Ithaca	Ithaca	66%	300+
Lawrence Hospital Center	Bronxville	66%	300+
Oneida Healthcare Center	Oneida	66%	300+
Phelps Memorial Hospital Assn	Sleepy Hollow	66%	300+
Saratoga Hospital	Saratoga Spgs	66%	300+
Soldiers and Sailors Mem Hosp of Yates	Penn Yan	66%	(a)
Canton-Potsdam Hospital	Potsdam	65%	300+
Hudson Valley Hospital Center	Cortlandt Manor	65%	300+
Lakeside Memorial Hospital	Brockport	65%	300+
South Nassau Communities Hospital	Oceanside	65%	300+
Strong Memorial Hospital	Rochester	65%	300+
Unity Hospital of Rochester	Rochester	65%	300+
Univ Hosp S U N Y Health Science Ctr	Syracuse	65%	300+
Kenmore Mercy Hospital	Kenmore	64%	300+
Little Falls Hospital	Little Falls	64%	300+
Mary Imogene Bassett Hospital	Cooperstown	64%	300+
Saint Elizabeth Medical Center	Utica	64%	300+
Sisters of Charity Hospital	Buffalo	64%	300+
United Health Services Hospitals	Johnson City	64%	300+
Claxton-Hepburn Medical Center	Ogdensburg	63%	(a)
Newark-Wayne Community Hospital	Newark	63%	300+
North Shore University Hospital	Manhasset	63%	300+
Saint Peter's Hospital	Albany	63%	300+
University Hospital - Stony Brook	Stony Brook	63%	300+
Good Samaritan Hospital Medical Center	West Islip	62%	300+
Metropolitan Hospital Center	New York	62%	300+
Mount Sinai Hospital	New York	62%	300+
North Central Bronx Hospital	Bronx	62%	300+
Comm-General Hosp of Greater Syracuse	Syracuse	61%	300+
Crouse Hospital	Syracuse	61%	300+
Lenox Hill Hospital[11]	New York	61%	300+
Massena Memorial Hospital	Massena	61%	300+
Medina Memorial Hospital	Medina	61%	300+
Nathan Littauer Hospital	Gloversville	61%	300+
NYU Hospitals Center[11]	New York	61%	300+
Queens Hospital Center	Jamaica	61%	300+
Saint Francis Hospital	Poughkeepsie	61%	300+
Southside Hospital	Bay Shore	61%	300+
Bon Secours Community Hospital	Port Jervis	60%	300+
Chenango Memorial Hospital	Norwich	60%	300+
Glens Falls Hospital	Glens Falls	60%	300+
Huntington Hospital	Huntington	60%	300+
Kaleida Health	Buffalo	60%	300+
NY Eye and Ear Infirmary	New York	60%	300+
Saint Catherine of Siena Hospital	Smithtown	60%	300+
Samaritan Hospital	Troy	60%	300+
Southampton Hospital	Southampton	60%	300+
United Memorial Medical Center	Batavia	60%	300+
Alice Hyde Medical Center	Malone	59%	300+
Auburn Memorial Hospital	Auburn	59%	300+
Eastern Niagara Hospital	Lockport	59%	300+
Ellis Hospital	Schenectady	59%	300+
Mercy Medical Center	Rockville Centre	59%	300+
Montefiore Medical Center	Bronx	59%	300+
Saint John's Riverside Hospital	Yonkers	59%	300+
Long Island Jewish Medical Center	New Hyde Park	58%	300+
Olean General Hospital	Olean	58%	300+
TLC Health Network	Gowanda	58%	300+
Albany Medical Center Hospital	Albany	57%	300+
Carthage Area Hospital	Carthage	57%	300+
Champlain Valley Physicians Hospital	Plattsburgh	57%	300+
Faxton-St Luke's Healthcare	Utica	57%	300+
Geneva General Hospital	Geneva	57%	300+
Kings County Hospital Center	Brooklyn	57%	300+
Staten Island University Hospital	Staten Island	57%	300+
Beth Israel Medical Center	New York	56%	300+
Corning Hospital	Corning	56%	300+
Elmhurst Hospital Center	Elmhurst	56%	300+
Franklin Hospital	Valley Stream	56%	300+
Good Samaritan Hospital of Suffern	Suffern	56%	300+
Mount Vernon Hospital	Mount Vernon	56%	300+
Westchester Medical Center	Valhalla	56%	300+
Aurelia Osborn Fox Memorial Hospital	Oneonta	55%	300+
Coney Island Hospital	Brooklyn	55%	300+
Jacobi Medical Center	Bronx	55%	300+
Jones Memorial Hospital	Wellsville	55%	300+
Rome Memorial Hospital	Rome	55%	300+
Saint Joseph's Hospital	Elmira	55%	300+
Wyoming County Community Hospital	Warsaw	55%	300+
Saint Luke's Cornwall Hospital	Newburgh	54%	300+
Woman's Christian Association	Jamestown	54%	300+
Brooks Memorial Hospital	Dunkirk	53%	300+
Erie County Medical Center	Buffalo	53%	300+
Kingston Hospital	Kingston	53%	300+
Niagara Falls Memorial Medical Center	Niagara Falls	53%	300+
Nyack Hospital	Nyack	53%	300+
Plainview Hospital	Plainview	53%	300+
Bellevue Hospital Center	New York	52%	300+
Cortland Regional Medical Center	Cortland	52%	300+
Lincoln Medical & Mental Health Center	Bronx	52%	300+
New York Hospital Medical Center of Queens	Flushing	52%	300+
New York Methodist Hospital	Brooklyn	52%	300+
Forest Hills Hospital	Forest Hills	51%	300+
Kingsbrook Jewish Medical Center	Brooklyn	51%	300+
Saint James Mercy Hospital	Hornell	51%	300+
Samaritan Medical Center	Watertown	51%	300+
Woodhull Medical and Mental Health Center	Brooklyn	51%	300+
Edward John Noble Hospital of Gouverneur	Gouverneur	50%	300+
Maimonides Medical Center	Brooklyn	50%	300+
New York Westchester Square Medical Center[7]	Bronx	50%	(a)
Oswego Hospital	Oswego	50%	300+
Peconic Bay Medical Center	Riverhead	50%	300+
Saint Luke's Roosevelt Hospital	New York	50%	300+
Lutheran Medical Center	Brooklyn	49%	300+
Orange Regional Medical Center	Goshen	49%	300+
Saint Joseph Hospital	Bethpage	49%	300+
Brookhaven Memorial Hospital Med Ctr	Patchogue	48%	300+
Brooklyn Hospital Center at Downtown Campus	Brooklyn	48%	300+
Mercy Hospital	Buffalo	48%	300+
St John's Episcopal Hosp-South Shore	Far Rockaway	48%	300+
Saint Joseph's Medical Center	Yonkers	48%	300+
Columbia Memorial Hospital	Hudson	47%	300+
New York Community Hospital of Brooklyn	Brooklyn	47%	300+
University Hospital of Brooklyn - Downstate	Brooklyn	47%	300+
Ira Davenport Memorial Hospital	Bath	46%	(a)
Harlem Hospital Center	New York	45%	300+
Interfaith Medical Center	Brooklyn	45%	300+
Sound Shore Medical Center of Westschester	New Rochelle	45%	300+
Long Island College Hospital	Brooklyn	44%	300+
Richmond University Medical Center	Staten Island	44%	300+
Bronx-Lebanon Hospital Center	Bronx	43%	300+
Flushing Hospital Medical Center	Flushing	43%	300+
Jamaica Hospital Medical Center	Jamaica	43%	300+
Nassau University Medical Center	East Meadow	43%	300+
Saint Barnabas Hospital	Bronx	42%	300+
Long Beach Medical Center	Long Beach	41%	300+
Catskill Regional Medical Center	Harris	40%	300+
Wyckoff Heights Medical Center	Brooklyn	39%	300+
Brookdale Hospital Medical Center	Brooklyn	37%	300+
New York Downtown Hospital	New York	37%	300+
Peninsula Hospital Center	Far Rockaway	33%	300+

44. Meds 'Always' Explained Before Given

Hospital Name	City	Rate	Cases
Westfield Memorial Hospital	Westfield	82%	(a)
Lewis County General Hospital	Lowville	67%	300+
Adirondack Medical Center	Saranac Lake	66%	300+
Claxton-Hepburn Medical Center	Ogdensburg	66%	(a)
Community Memorial Hospital	Hamilton	66%	300+
Oneida Healthcare Center	Oneida	66%	300+
Bertrand Chaffee Hospital	Springville	65%	300+
Little Falls Hospital	Little Falls	65%	300+
Mary Imogene Bassett Hospital	Cooperstown	65%	300+
Canton-Potsdam Hospital	Potsdam	64%	300+

NOTE: Hospital profiles are in alphabetical order by state, then city, then hospital within the city; Rankings exclude hospitals with less than 25 cases except for patient surveys which excludes hospitals with less than 100 cases; (a) 100–299 cases; (1) The number of cases is too small to be sure how well a hospital is performing; (2) The hospital indicated that the data submitted for this measure were based on a sample of cases; (3) Data was collected during a shorter time period (fewer quarters) than the maximum possible time for this measure; (4) Suppressed for one or more quarters by CMS; (5) No data is available from the hospital for this measure; (6) Fewer than 100 patients completed the HCAHPS survey. Use these rates with caution, as the number of surveys may be too low to reliably assess hospital performance; (7) Survey results are based on less than 12 months of data; (8) Survey results are not available for this reporting period; (9) No or very few patients were eligible for the HCAHPS survey. The scores shown, if any, reflect a very small number of surveys; (10) A state average was not calculated because too few hospitals in the state submitted data; (11) There were discrepancies in the data collection process; Please refer to the User's Guide for a full explanation of data.

Clifton Springs Hospital and Clinic	Clifton Springs	64%	300+
Northern Dutchess Hospital	Rhinebeck	64%	300+
Saratoga Hospital	Saratoga Spgs	64%	300+
Northern Westchester Hospital	Mount Kisco	63%	300+
Rochester General Hospital	Rochester	63%	300+
Saint Anthony Community Hospital	Warwick	63%	300+
United Memorial Medical Center	Batavia	63%	300+
Nathan Littauer Hospital	Gloversville	62%	300+
Newark-Wayne Community Hospital	Newark	62%	300+
Vassar Brothers Medical Center[11]	Poughkeepsie	62%	300+
White Plains Hospital Center	White Plains	62%	300+
Auburn Memorial Hospital	Auburn	61%	300+
Cayuga Medical Center at Ithaca	Ithaca	61%	300+
Edward John Noble Hospital of Gouverneur	Gouverneur	61%	300+
F F Thompson Hospital	Canandaigua	61%	300+
Highland Hospital	Rochester	61%	300+
Hudson Valley Hospital Center	Cortlandt Manor	61%	300+
John T Mather Mem Hosp-Port Jefferson	Port Jefferson	61%	300+
Kings County Hospital Center	Brooklyn	61%	300+
Massena Memorial Hospital	Massena	61%	300+
Saint Francis Hospital - Roslyn	Roslyn	61%	300+
Saint Mary's Hospital at Amsterdam	Amsterdam	61%	300+
Corning Hospital	Corning	60%	300+
Delaware Valley Hospital	Walton	60%	(a)
Hospital for Special Surgery	New York	60%	300+
Lakeside Memorial Hospital	Brockport	60%	300+
Our Lady of Lourdes Memorial Hospital	Binghamton	60%	300+
Putnam Hospital Center	Carmel	60%	300+
Strong Memorial Hospital	Rochester	60%	300+
Arnot Ogden Medical Center	Elmira	59%	300+
Bon Secours Community Hospital	Port Jervis	59%	300+
Carthage Area Hospital	Carthage	59%	300+
Champlain Valley Physicians Hospital	Plattsburgh	59%	300+
Comm-General Hosp of Greater Syracuse	Syracuse	59%	300+
Cortland Regional Medical Center	Cortland	59%	300+
Geneva General Hospital	Geneva	59%	300+
Glen Cove Hospital	Glen Cove	59%	300+
Lawrence Hospital Center	Bronxville	59%	300+
Phelps Memorial Hospital Assn	Sleepy Hollow	59%	300+
Saint James Mercy Hospital	Hornell	59%	300+
Saint Joseph's Hospital Health Center	Syracuse	59%	300+
Seton Health System-St Mary's Campus	Troy	59%	300+
Southampton Hospital	Southampton	59%	300+
Univ Hosp S U N Y Health Science Ctr	Syracuse	59%	300+
Cobleskill Regional Hospital	Cobleskill	58%	(a)
Ira Davenport Memorial Hospital	Bath	58%	(a)
Kenmore Mercy Hospital	Kenmore	58%	300+
New York-Presbyterian Hospital	New York	58%	300+
North Central Bronx Hospital	Bronx	58%	300+
NYU Hospitals Center[11]	New York	58%	300+
Queens Hospital Center	Jamaica	58%	300+
Rome Memorial Hospital	Rome	58%	300+
Saint Francis Hospital	Poughkeepsie	58%	300+
Southside Hospital	Bay Shore	58%	300+
United Health Services Hospitals	Johnson City	58%	300+
Alice Hyde Medical Center	Malone	57%	300+
Benedictine Hospital	Kingston	57%	(a)
Eastern Long Island Hospital	Greenport	57%	300+
Montefiore Medical Center	Bronx	57%	300+
Mount St Mary's Hospital and Health Center	Lewiston	57%	300+
Nicholas H Noyes Memorial Hospital	Dansville	57%	300+
Nyack Hospital	Nyack	57%	300+
Oswego Hospital	Oswego	57%	300+
Saint Charles Hospital	Port Jefferson	57%	300+
Saint Luke's Cornwall Hospital	Newburgh	57%	300+
Saint Peter's Hospital	Albany	57%	300+
Samaritan Medical Center	Watertown	57%	300+
South Nassau Communities Hospital	Oceanside	57%	300+
TLC Health Network	Gowanda	57%	300+
Winthrop-University Hospital	Mineola	57%	300+
Aurelia Osborn Fox Memorial Hospital	Oneonta	56%	300+
Glens Falls Hospital	Glens Falls	56%	300+
Good Samaritan Hospital Medical Center	West Islip	56%	300+
North Shore University Hospital	Manhasset	56%	300+
Richmond University Medical Center	Staten Island	56%	300+
Columbia Memorial Hospital	Hudson	55%	300+
Crouse Hospital	Syracuse	55%	300+
Huntington Hospital	Huntington	55%	300+
Long Island Jewish Medical Center	New Hyde Park	55%	300+
Medina Memorial Hospital	Medina	55%	300+
Sisters of Charity Hospital	Buffalo	55%	300+
Soldiers and Sailors Mem Hosp of Yates	Penn Yan	55%	(a)
Staten Island University Hospital	Staten Island	55%	300+
Unity Hospital of Rochester	Rochester	55%	300+
Wyoming County Community Hospital	Warsaw	55%	300+
Albany Memorial Hospital	Albany	54%	300+
Eastern Niagara Hospital	Lockport	54%	300+
Good Samaritan Hospital of Suffern	Suffern	54%	300+
Harlem Hospital Center	New York	54%	300+
Jones Memorial Hospital	Wellsville	54%	300+
Kaleida Health	Buffalo	54%	300+
Kingsbrook Jewish Medical Center	Brooklyn	54%	300+
Lenox Hill Hospital[11]	New York	54%	300+
Mercy Medical Center	Rockville Centre	54%	300+
Mount Vernon Hospital	Mount Vernon	54%	300+
NY Eye and Ear Infirmary	New York	54%	300+
Olean General Hospital	Olean	54%	300+
University Hospital - Stony Brook	Stony Brook	54%	300+
Albany Medical Center Hospital	Albany	53%	300+
Chenango Memorial Hospital	Norwich	53%	300+
Ellis Hospital	Schenectady	53%	300+
Faxton-St Luke's Healthcare	Utica	53%	300+
Kingston Hospital	Kingston	53%	300+
Maimonides Medical Center	Brooklyn	53%	300+
Metropolitan Hospital Center	New York	53%	300+
Mount Sinai Hospital	New York	53%	300+
Niagara Falls Memorial Medical Center	Niagara Falls	53%	300+
Plainview Hospital	Plainview	53%	300+
Saint Catherine of Siena Hospital	Smithtown	53%	300+
Saint Elizabeth Medical Center	Utica	53%	300+
Saint John's Riverside Hospital	Yonkers	53%	300+
Saint Joseph Hospital	Bethpage	53%	300+
Saint Joseph's Hospital	Elmira	53%	300+
Samaritan Hospital	Troy	53%	300+
Woman's Christian Association	Jamestown	53%	300+
Beth Israel Medical Center	New York	52%	300+
Franklin Hospital	Valley Stream	52%	300+
New York Community Hospital of Brooklyn	Brooklyn	52%	300+
Orange Regional Medical Center	Goshen	52%	300+
Peconic Bay Medical Center	Riverhead	52%	300+
St John's Episcopal Hosp-South Shore	Far Rockaway	52%	300+
Woodhull Medical and Mental Health Center	Brooklyn	52%	300+
Brookhaven Memorial Hospital Med Ctr	Patchogue	51%	300+
Erie County Medical Center	Buffalo	51%	300+
Forest Hills Hospital	Forest Hills	51%	300+
Interfaith Medical Center	Brooklyn	51%	300+
Saint Luke's Roosevelt Hospital	New York	51%	300+
Sound Shore Medical Center of Westchester	New Rochelle	51%	300+
University Hospital of Brooklyn - Downstate	Brooklyn	51%	300+
Brookdale Hospital Medical Center	Brooklyn	50%	300+
Coney Island Hospital	Brooklyn	50%	300+
Lincoln Medical & Mental Health Center	Bronx	50%	300+
New York Hospital Medical Center of Queens	Flushing	50%	300+
Saint Joseph's Medical Center	Yonkers	50%	300+
Bellevue Hospital Center	New York	49%	300+
Brooklyn Hospital Center at Downtown Campus	Brooklyn	49%	300+
Catskill Regional Medical Center	Harris	49%	300+
Jacobi Medical Center	Bronx	49%	300+
Long Beach Medical Center	Long Beach	49%	300+
Elmhurst Hospital Center	Elmhurst	48%	300+
Long Island College Hospital	Brooklyn	48%	300+
New York Downtown Hospital	New York	48%	300+
Westchester Medical Center	Valhalla	48%	300+
Brooks Memorial Hospital	Dunkirk	47%	300+
Mercy Hospital	Buffalo	47%	300+
Saint Barnabas Hospital	Bronx	47%	300+
Lutheran Medical Center	Brooklyn	46%	300+
Nassau University Medical Center	East Meadow	46%	300+
Wyckoff Heights Medical Center	Brooklyn	45%	300+
Bronx-Lebanon Hospital Center	Bronx	44%	300+
New York Methodist Hospital	Brooklyn	44%	300+
Jamaica Hospital Medical Center	Jamaica	43%	300+
Flushing Hospital Medical Center	Flushing	42%	300+
Peninsula Hospital Center	Far Rockaway	42%	300+
New York Westchester Square Medical Center[7]	Bronx	39%	(a)

45. Nurses 'Always' Communicated Well

Hospital Name	City	Rate	Cases
Westfield Memorial Hospital	Westfield	93%	(a)
Delaware Valley Hospital	Walton	85%	(a)
Bertrand Chaffee Hospital	Springville	84%	300+
Northern Westchester Hospital	Mount Kisco	82%	300+
Saint Francis Hospital - Roslyn	Roslyn	81%	300+
Vassar Brothers Medical Center[11]	Poughkeepsie	81%	300+
Clifton Springs Hospital and Clinic	Clifton Springs	80%	300+
Eastern Long Island Hospital	Greenport	80%	300+
Northern Dutchess Hospital	Rhinebeck	80%	300+
Saint Anthony Community Hospital	Warwick	80%	300+
Saint Mary's Hospital at Amsterdam	Amsterdam	80%	300+
Seton Health System-St Mary's Campus	Troy	80%	300+
Arnot Ogden Medical Center	Elmira	79%	300+
Community Memorial Hospital	Hamilton	79%	300+
Hospital for Special Surgery	New York	79%	300+
Putnam Hospital Center	Carmel	79%	300+
Rochester General Hospital	Rochester	79%	300+
Saratoga Hospital	Saratoga Spgs	79%	300+
White Plains Hospital Center	White Plains	79%	300+
Cobleskill Regional Hospital	Cobleskill	78%	(a)
Glen Cove Hospital	Glen Cove	78%	300+
John T Mather Mem Hosp-Port Jefferson	Port Jefferson	78%	300+
Newark-Wayne Community Hospital	Newark	78%	300+
United Memorial Medical Center	Batavia	78%	300+
Adirondack Medical Center	Saranac Lake	77%	300+
Claxton-Hepburn Medical Center	Ogdensburg	77%	(a)
F F Thompson Hospital	Canandaigua	77%	300+
Massena Memorial Hospital	Massena	77%	300+
Mount St Mary's Hospital and Health Center	Lewiston	77%	300+
Nicholas H Noyes Memorial Hospital	Dansville	77%	300+
Saint Elizabeth Medical Center	Utica	77%	300+
Southside Hospital	Bay Shore	77%	300+
Auburn Memorial Hospital	Auburn	76%	300+
Bon Secours Community Hospital	Port Jervis	76%	300+
Highland Hospital	Rochester	76%	300+
Hudson Valley Hospital Center	Cortlandt Manor	76%	300+
Lakeside Memorial Hospital	Brockport	76%	300+
Little Falls Hospital	Little Falls	76%	300+
Soldiers and Sailors Mem Hosp of Yates	Penn Yan	76%	(a)
Winthrop-University Hospital	Mineola	76%	300+
Canton-Potsdam Hospital	Potsdam	75%	300+
Huntington Hospital	Huntington	75%	300+
Lawrence Hospital Center	Bronxville	75%	300+
Lewis County General Hospital	Lowville	75%	300+
Nathan Littauer Hospital	Gloversville	75%	300+
Oneida Healthcare Center	Oneida	75%	300+
Our Lady of Lourdes Memorial Hospital	Binghamton	75%	300+
Saint Charles Hospital	Port Jefferson	75%	300+
Saint Joseph's Hospital Health Center	Syracuse	75%	300+
Strong Memorial Hospital	Rochester	75%	300+
United Health Services Hospitals	Johnson City	75%	300+
Unity Hospital of Rochester	Rochester	75%	300+
Albany Memorial Hospital	Albany	74%	300+
Benedictine Hospital	Kingston	74%	(a)
Cayuga Medical Center at Ithaca	Ithaca	74%	300+
Comm-General Hosp of Greater Syracuse	Syracuse	74%	300+
Corning Hospital	Corning	74%	300+
Mary Imogene Bassett Hospital	Cooperstown	74%	300+
Medina Memorial Hospital	Medina	74%	300+
Southampton Hospital	Southampton	74%	300+
Alice Hyde Medical Center	Malone	73%	300+
Champlain Valley Physicians Hospital	Plattsburgh	73%	300+
Edward John Noble Hospital of Gouverneur	Gouverneur	73%	300+
Good Samaritan Hospital Medical Center	West Islip	73%	300+
Kenmore Mercy Hospital	Kenmore	73%	300+
Mount Vernon Hospital	Mount Vernon	73%	300+
Olean General Hospital	Olean	73%	300+
Rome Memorial Hospital	Rome	73%	300+
Samaritan Medical Center	Watertown	73%	300+
Sisters of Charity Hospital	Buffalo	73%	300+
South Nassau Communities Hospital	Oceanside	73%	300+
University Hospital - Stony Brook	Stony Brook	73%	300+
Crouse Hospital	Syracuse	72%	300+
Geneva General Hospital	Geneva	72%	300+
Jones Memorial Hospital	Wellsville	72%	300+
Montefiore Medical Center	Bronx	72%	300+
New York-Presbyterian Hospital	New York	72%	300+
Saint Francis Hospital	Poughkeepsie	72%	300+
Saint John's Riverside Hospital	Yonkers	72%	300+
Staten Island University Hospital	Staten Island	72%	300+
TLC Health Network	Gowanda	72%	300+
Univ Hosp S U N Y Health Science Ctr	Syracuse	72%	300+
Wyoming County Community Hospital	Warsaw	72%	300+
Cortland Regional Medical Center	Cortland	71%	300+
Eastern Niagara Hospital	Lockport	71%	300+
Faxton-St Luke's Healthcare	Utica	71%	300+
Kaleida Health	Buffalo	71%	300+
Mercy Medical Center	Rockville Centre	71%	300+
Mount Sinai Hospital	New York	71%	300+
North Shore University Hospital	Manhasset	71%	300+
NYU Hospitals Center[11]	New York	71%	300+
Oswego Hospital	Oswego	71%	300+
Phelps Memorial Hospital Assn	Sleepy Hollow	71%	300+
Plainview Hospital	Plainview	71%	300+
Saint Catherine of Siena Hospital	Smithtown	71%	300+
Woman's Christian Association	Jamestown	71%	300+
Chenango Memorial Hospital	Norwich	70%	300+
Glens Falls Hospital	Glens Falls	70%	300+
Kingston Hospital	Kingston	70%	300+
Lenox Hill Hospital[11]	New York	70%	300+
Saint James Mercy Hospital	Hornell	70%	300+
Aurelia Osborn Fox Memorial Hospital	Oneonta	69%	300+
Brooks Memorial Hospital	Dunkirk	69%	300+
Carthage Area Hospital	Carthage	69%	300+
Columbia Memorial Hospital	Hudson	69%	300+
Ellis Hospital	Schenectady	69%	300+
Franklin Hospital	Valley Stream	69%	300+
Kingsbrook Jewish Medical Center	Brooklyn	69%	300+
Long Island Jewish Medical Center	New Hyde Park	69%	300+
Nyack Hospital	Nyack	69%	300+
Peconic Bay Medical Center	Riverhead	69%	300+
Richmond University Medical Center	Staten Island	69%	300+
Saint Joseph Hospital	Bethpage	69%	300+
Saint Luke's Cornwall Hospital	Newburgh	69%	300+

NOTE: Hospital profiles are in alphabetical order by state, then city, then hospital within the city; Rankings exclude hospitals with less than 25 cases except for patient surveys which excludes hospitals with less than 100 cases; (a) 100–299 cases; (1) The number of cases is too small to be sure how well a hospital is performing; (2) The hospital indicated that the data submitted for this measure were based on a sample of cases; (3) Data was collected during a shorter time period (fewer quarters) than the maximum possible time for this measure; (4) Suppressed for one or more quarters by CMS; (5) No data is available from the hospital for this measure; (6) Fewer than 100 patients completed the HCAHPS survey. Use these rates with caution, as the number of surveys may be too low to reliably assess hospital performance; (7) Survey results are based on less than 12 months of data; (8) Survey results are not available for this reporting period; (9) No or very few patients were eligible for the HCAHPS survey. The scores shown, if any, reflect a very small number of surveys; (10) A state average was not calculated because too few hospitals in the state submitted data; (11) There were discrepancies in the data collection process; Please refer to the User's Guide for a full explanation of data.

Saint Peter's Hospital	Albany	69%	300+
Samaritan Hospital	Troy	69%	300+
Good Samaritan Hospital of Suffern	Suffern	68%	300+
Ira Davenport Memorial Hospital	Bath	68%	(a)
Mercy Hospital	Buffalo	68%	300+
New York Westchester Square Medical Center[7]	Bronx	68%	(a)
Niagara Falls Memorial Medical Center	Niagara Falls	68%	300+
NY Eye and Ear Infirmary	New York	68%	300+
Orange Regional Medical Center	Goshen	68%	300+
Saint Joseph's Hospital	Elmira	68%	300+
Albany Medical Center Hospital	Albany	67%	300+
Brookhaven Memorial Hospital Med Ctr	Patchogue	67%	300+
Kings County Hospital Center	Brooklyn	67%	300+
Beth Israel Medical Center	New York	66%	300+
Erie County Medical Center	Buffalo	66%	300+
Maimonides Medical Center	Brooklyn	66%	300+
North Central Bronx Hospital	Bronx	66%	300+
Queens Hospital Center	Jamaica	66%	300+
St John's Episcopal Hosp-South Shore	Far Rockaway	66%	300+
Elmhurst Hospital Center	Elmhurst	65%	300+
New York Community Hospital of Brooklyn	Brooklyn	65%	300+
Saint Joseph's Medical Center	Yonkers	65%	300+
University Hospital of Brooklyn - Downstate	Brooklyn	65%	300+
Catskill Regional Medical Center	Harris	64%	300+
Coney Island Hospital	Brooklyn	64%	300+
Forest Hills Hospital	Forest Hills	64%	300+
Jacobi Medical Center	Bronx	64%	300+
Lincoln Medical & Mental Health Center	Bronx	64%	300+
Lutheran Medical Center	Brooklyn	64%	300+
New York Hospital Medical Center of Queens	Flushing	64%	300+
Sound Shore Medical Center of Westschester	New Rochelle	64%	300+
Westchester Medical Center	Valhalla	64%	300+
Brooklyn Hospital Center at Downtown Campus	Brooklyn	63%	300+
Interfaith Medical Center	Brooklyn	63%	300+
Woodhull Medical and Mental Health Center	Brooklyn	63%	300+
Metropolitan Hospital Center	New York	62%	300+
New York Methodist Hospital	Brooklyn	62%	300+
Saint Luke's Roosevelt Hospital	New York	62%	300+
Bellevue Hospital Center	New York	61%	300+
Harlem Hospital Center	New York	61%	300+
Long Beach Medical Center	Long Beach	61%	300+
Saint Barnabas Hospital	Bronx	61%	300+
Long Island College Hospital	Brooklyn	59%	300+
Bronx-Lebanon Hospital Center	Bronx	57%	300+
Brookdale Hospital Medical Center	Brooklyn	57%	300+
Flushing Hospital Medical Center	Flushing	57%	300+
New York Downtown Hospital	New York	57%	300+
Jamaica Hospital Medical Center	Jamaica	56%	300+
Nassau University Medical Center	East Meadow	56%	300+
Peninsula Hospital Center	Far Rockaway	54%	300+
Wyckoff Heights Medical Center	Brooklyn	54%	300+

46. Pain 'Always' Well Controlled

Hospital Name	City	Rate	Cases
Westfield Memorial Hospital	Westfield	82%	(a)
Eastern Long Island Hospital	Greenport	78%	300+
Delaware Valley Hospital	Walton	76%	(a)
Northern Westchester Hospital	Mount Kisco	75%	300+
Vassar Brothers Medical Center[11]	Poughkeepsie	75%	300+
Bertrand Chaffee Hospital	Springville	74%	300+
Hospital for Special Surgery	New York	74%	300+
Saint Anthony Community Hospital	Warwick	74%	300+
Lewis County General Hospital	Lowville	73%	300+
Putnam Hospital Center	Carmel	73%	300+
Adirondack Medical Center	Saranac Lake	72%	300+
Bon Secours Community Hospital	Port Jervis	72%	300+
Clifton Springs Hospital and Clinic	Clifton Springs	72%	300+
Community Memorial Hospital	Hamilton	72%	300+
Hudson Valley Hospital Center	Cortlandt Manor	72%	300+
John T Mather Mem Hosp-Port Jefferson	Port Jefferson	72%	300+
Massena Memorial Hospital	Massena	72%	300+
Northern Dutchess Hospital	Rhinebeck	72%	300+
Saratoga Hospital	Saratoga Spgs	72%	300+
Arnot Ogden Medical Center	Elmira	71%	300+
Little Falls Hospital	Little Falls	71%	300+
Mount St Mary's Hospital and Health Center	Lewiston	71%	300+
Oneida Healthcare Center	Oneida	71%	300+
Saint Francis Hospital - Roslyn	Roslyn	71%	300+
Saint Joseph's Hospital Health Center	Syracuse	71%	300+
Saint Mary's Hospital at Amsterdam	Amsterdam	71%	300+
White Plains Hospital Center	White Plains	71%	300+
Albany Memorial Hospital	Albany	70%	300+
Benedictine Hospital	Kingston	70%	(a)
Huntington Hospital	Huntington	70%	300+
Kenmore Mercy Hospital	Kenmore	70%	300+
Nathan Littauer Hospital	Gloversville	70%	300+
Newark-Wayne Community Hospital	Newark	70%	300+
Nicholas H Noyes Memorial Hospital	Dansville	70%	300+
Rochester General Hospital	Rochester	70%	300+
Claxton-Hepburn Medical Center	Ogdensburg	69%	(a)
Cobleskill Regional Hospital	Cobleskill	69%	(a)
Comm-General Hosp of Greater Syracuse	Syracuse	69%	300+
Corning Hospital	Corning	69%	300+
Good Samaritan Hospital Medical Center	West Islip	69%	300+
Lawrence Hospital Center	Bronxville	69%	300+
Lenox Hill Hospital[11]	New York	69%	300+
United Health Services Hospitals	Johnson City	69%	300+
Auburn Memorial Hospital	Auburn	68%	300+
Canton-Potsdam Hospital	Potsdam	68%	300+
F F Thompson Hospital	Canandaigua	68%	300+
Highland Hospital	Rochester	68%	300+
Rome Memorial Hospital	Rome	68%	300+
Saint Elizabeth Medical Center	Utica	68%	300+
Seton Health System-St Mary's Campus	Troy	68%	300+
Cayuga Medical Center at Ithaca	Ithaca	67%	300+
Glens Falls Hospital	Glens Falls	67%	300+
Lakeside Memorial Hospital	Brockport	67%	300+
Mary Imogene Bassett Hospital	Cooperstown	67%	300+
Mount Vernon Hospital	Mount Vernon	67%	300+
Our Lady of Lourdes Memorial Hospital	Binghamton	67%	300+
Saint Charles Hospital	Port Jefferson	67%	300+
Saint Francis Hospital	Poughkeepsie	67%	300+
South Nassau Communities Hospital	Oceanside	67%	300+
Southside Hospital	Bay Shore	67%	300+
TLC Health Network	Gowanda	67%	300+
United Memorial Medical Center	Batavia	67%	300+
University Hospital - Stony Brook	Stony Brook	67%	300+
Univ Hosp S U N Y Health Science Ctr	Syracuse	67%	300+
Winthrop-University Hospital	Mineola	67%	300+
Wyoming County Community Hospital	Warsaw	67%	300+
Alice Hyde Medical Center	Malone	66%	300+
Aurelia Osborn Fox Memorial Hospital	Oneonta	66%	300+
Champlain Valley Physicians Hospital	Plattsburgh	66%	300+
Glen Cove Hospital	Glen Cove	66%	300+
Mercy Medical Center	Rockville Centre	66%	300+
New York Westchester Square Medical Center[7]	Bronx	66%	(a)
Phelps Memorial Hospital Assn	Sleepy Hollow	66%	300+
Saint John's Riverside Hospital	Yonkers	66%	300+
Saint Joseph's Hospital	Elmira	66%	300+
Sisters of Charity Hospital	Buffalo	66%	300+
Southampton Hospital	Southampton	66%	300+
Eastern Niagara Hospital	Lockport	65%	300+
Edward John Noble Hospital of Gouverneur	Gouverneur	65%	300+
Faxton-St Luke's Healthcare	Utica	65%	300+
Geneva General Hospital	Geneva	65%	300+
Mount Sinai Hospital	New York	65%	300+
New York-Presbyterian Hospital	New York	65%	300+
Olean General Hospital	Olean	65%	300+
Plainview Hospital	Plainview	65%	300+
Saint Catherine of Siena Hospital	Smithtown	65%	300+
Saint Joseph Hospital	Bethpage	65%	300+
Samaritan Medical Center	Watertown	65%	300+
Staten Island University Hospital	Staten Island	65%	300+
Strong Memorial Hospital	Rochester	65%	300+
Unity Hospital of Rochester	Rochester	65%	300+
Albany Medical Center Hospital	Albany	64%	300+
Catskill Regional Medical Center	Harris	64%	300+
Chenango Memorial Hospital	Norwich	64%	300+
Columbia Memorial Hospital	Hudson	64%	300+
Crouse Hospital	Syracuse	64%	300+
Franklin Hospital	Valley Stream	64%	300+
Kaleida Health	Buffalo	64%	300+
Medina Memorial Hospital	Medina	64%	300+
Nyack Hospital	Nyack	64%	300+
NYU Hospitals Center[11]	New York	64%	300+
Saint Luke's Cornwall Hospital	Newburgh	64%	300+
Samaritan Hospital	Troy	64%	300+
Ellis Hospital	Schenectady	63%	300+
Montefiore Medical Center	Bronx	63%	300+
Niagara Falls Memorial Medical Center	Niagara Falls	63%	300+
North Central Bronx Hospital	Bronx	63%	300+
Richmond University Medical Center	Staten Island	63%	300+
Saint James Mercy Hospital	Hornell	63%	300+
Brookhaven Memorial Hospital Med Ctr	Patchogue	62%	300+
Carthage Area Hospital	Carthage	62%	300+
Jones Memorial Hospital	Wellsville	62%	300+
North Shore University Hospital	Manhasset	62%	300+
NY Eye and Ear Infirmary	New York	62%	300+
Queens Hospital Center	Jamaica	62%	300+
Woman's Christian Association	Jamestown	62%	300+
Beth Israel Medical Center	New York	61%	300+
Brooklyn Hospital Center at Downtown Campus	Brooklyn	61%	300+
Brooks Memorial Hospital	Dunkirk	61%	300+
Cortland Regional Medical Center	Cortland	61%	300+
Forest Hills Hospital	Forest Hills	61%	300+
Kingston Hospital	Kingston	61%	300+
Long Island Jewish Medical Center	New Hyde Park	61%	300+
Mercy Hospital	Buffalo	61%	300+
Orange Regional Medical Center	Goshen	61%	300+
Oswego Hospital	Oswego	61%	300+
Peconic Bay Medical Center	Riverhead	61%	300+
Saint Peter's Hospital	Albany	61%	300+
University Hospital of Brooklyn - Downstate	Brooklyn	61%	300+
Coney Island Hospital	Brooklyn	60%	300+
Erie County Medical Center	Buffalo	60%	300+
Long Beach Medical Center	Long Beach	60%	300+
Maimonides Medical Center	Brooklyn	60%	300+
St John's Episcopal Hosp-South Shore	Far Rockaway	60%	300+
Soldiers and Sailors Mem Hosp of Yates	Penn Yan	60%	(a)
Good Samaritan Hospital of Suffern	Suffern	59%	300+
Kings County Hospital Center	Brooklyn	59%	300+
Lutheran Medical Center	Brooklyn	59%	300+
Sound Shore Medical Center of Westschester	New Rochelle	59%	300+
Westchester Medical Center	Valhalla	59%	300+
Bellevue Hospital Center	New York	58%	300+
Elmhurst Hospital Center	Elmhurst	58%	300+
Saint Joseph's Medical Center	Yonkers	58%	300+
Saint Luke's Roosevelt Hospital	New York	58%	300+
Harlem Hospital Center	New York	57%	300+
Jacobi Medical Center	Bronx	57%	300+
New York Community Hospital of Brooklyn	Brooklyn	57%	300+
Woodhull Medical and Mental Health Center	Brooklyn	57%	300+
Ira Davenport Memorial Hospital	Bath	56%	(a)
Kingsbrook Jewish Medical Center	Brooklyn	56%	300+
Nassau University Medical Center	East Meadow	56%	300+
New York Methodist Hospital	Brooklyn	56%	300+
New York Hospital Medical Center of Queens	Flushing	55%	300+
Saint Barnabas Hospital	Bronx	54%	300+
Interfaith Medical Center	Brooklyn	53%	300+
Lincoln Medical & Mental Health Center	Bronx	53%	300+
Long Island College Hospital	Brooklyn	53%	300+
Metropolitan Hospital Center	New York	52%	300+
New York Downtown Hospital	New York	52%	300+
Jamaica Hospital Medical Center	Jamaica	51%	300+
Peninsula Hospital Center	Far Rockaway	51%	300+
Bronx-Lebanon Hospital Center	Bronx	50%	300+
Flushing Hospital Medical Center	Flushing	50%	300+
Wyckoff Heights Medical Center	Brooklyn	46%	300+
Brookdale Hospital Medical Center	Brooklyn	45%	300+

47. Room and Bathroom 'Always' Clean

Hospital Name	City	Rate	Cases
Delaware Valley Hospital	Walton	87%	(a)
Westfield Memorial Hospital	Westfield	87%	(a)
Bertrand Chaffee Hospital	Springville	79%	300+
Hospital for Special Surgery	New York	78%	300+
Canton-Potsdam Hospital	Potsdam	77%	300+
Community Memorial Hospital	Hamilton	77%	300+
Nathan Littauer Hospital	Gloversville	77%	300+
Saint Francis Hospital - Roslyn	Roslyn	77%	300+
Cobleskill Regional Hospital	Cobleskill	76%	(a)
Lewis County General Hospital	Lowville	76%	300+
Saint John's Riverside Hospital	Yonkers	76%	300+
Alice Hyde Medical Center	Malone	75%	300+
Little Falls Hospital	Little Falls	75%	300+
Massena Memorial Hospital	Massena	75%	300+
Mount St Mary's Hospital and Health Center	Lewiston	75%	300+
Saint Mary's Hospital at Amsterdam	Amsterdam	75%	300+
Eastern Long Island Hospital	Greenport	74%	300+
Glen Cove Hospital	Glen Cove	74%	300+
Kings County Hospital Center	Brooklyn	74%	300+
New York Westchester Square Medical Center[7]	Bronx	74%	(a)
Olean General Hospital	Olean	74%	300+
Putnam Hospital Center	Carmel	74%	300+
Southampton Hospital	Southampton	74%	300+
Adirondack Medical Center	Saranac Lake	73%	300+
Claxton-Hepburn Medical Center	Ogdensburg	73%	(a)
Clifton Springs Hospital and Clinic	Clifton Springs	73%	300+
Eastern Niagara Hospital	Lockport	73%	300+
Nyack Hospital	Nyack	73%	300+
Oneida Healthcare Center	Oneida	73%	300+
Carthage Area Hospital	Carthage	72%	300+
Hudson Valley Hospital Center	Cortlandt Manor	72%	300+
Interfaith Medical Center	Brooklyn	72%	300+
Soldiers and Sailors Mem Hosp of Yates	Penn Yan	72%	(a)
Wyoming County Community Hospital	Warsaw	72%	300+
Good Samaritan Hospital Medical Center	West Islip	71%	300+
Lawrence Hospital Center	Bronxville	71%	300+
Saint Elizabeth Medical Center	Utica	71%	300+
Samaritan Medical Center	Watertown	71%	300+
Southside Hospital	Bay Shore	71%	300+
Vassar Brothers Medical Center[11]	Poughkeepsie	71%	300+
Albany Memorial Hospital	Albany	70%	300+
Aurelia Osborn Fox Memorial Hospital	Oneonta	70%	300+
Bon Secours Community Hospital	Port Jervis	70%	300+
Edward John Noble Hospital of Gouverneur	Gouverneur	70%	300+
John T Mather Mem Hosp-Port Jefferson	Port Jefferson	70%	300+
Medina Memorial Hospital	Medina	70%	300+
Northern Westchester Hospital	Mount Kisco	70%	300+
Phelps Memorial Hospital Assn	Sleepy Hollow	70%	300+
Rome Memorial Hospital	Rome	70%	300+

NOTE: Hospital profiles are in alphabetical order by state, then city, then hospital within the city; Rankings exclude hospitals with less than 25 cases except for patient surveys which excludes hospitals with less than 100 cases; (a) 100–299 cases; (1) The number of cases is too small to be sure how well a hospital is performing; (2) The hospital indicated that the data submitted for this measure were based on a sample of cases; (3) Data was collected during a shorter time period (fewer quarters) than the maximum possible time for this measure; (4) Suppressed for one or more quarters by CMS; (5) No data is available from the hospital for this measure; (6) Fewer than 100 patients completed the HCAHPS survey. Use these rates with caution, as the number of surveys may be too low to reliably assess hospital performance; (7) Survey results are based on less than 12 months of data; (8) Survey results are not available for this reporting period; (9) No or very few patients were eligible for the HCAHPS survey. The scores shown, if any, reflect a very small number of surveys; (10) A state average was not calculated because too few hospitals in the state submitted data; (11) There were discrepancies in the data collection process; Please refer to the User's Guide for a full explanation of data.

Saint Charles Hospital	Port Jefferson	70%	300+
Saratoga Hospital	Saratoga Spgs	70%	300+
Winthrop-University Hospital	Mineola	70%	300+
Arnot Ogden Medical Center	Elmira	69%	300+
Cayuga Medical Center at Ithaca	Ithaca	69%	300+
F F Thompson Hospital	Canandaigua	69%	300+
Glens Falls Hospital	Glens Falls	69%	300+
Lakeside Memorial Hospital	Brockport	69%	300+
Newark-Wayne Community Hospital	Newark	69%	300+
Saint James Mercy Hospital	Hornell	69%	300+
University Hospital - Stony Brook	Stony Brook	69%	300+
Huntington Hospital	Huntington	68%	300+
Montefiore Medical Center	Bronx	68%	300+
NY Eye and Ear Infirmary	New York	68%	300+
Queens Hospital Center	Jamaica	68%	300+
Saint Catherine of Siena Hospital	Smithtown	68%	300+
United Memorial Medical Center	Batavia	68%	300+
White Plains Hospital Center	White Plains	68%	300+
Auburn Memorial Hospital	Auburn	67%	300+
Champlain Valley Physicians Hospital	Plattsburgh	67%	300+
Corning Hospital	Corning	67%	300+
Kingsbrook Jewish Medical Center	Brooklyn	67%	300+
Mary Imogene Bassett Hospital	Cooperstown	67%	300+
Mount Vernon Hospital	Mount Vernon	67%	300+
New York Community Hospital of Brooklyn	Brooklyn	67%	300+
Nicholas H Noyes Memorial Hospital	Dansville	67%	300+
Northern Dutchess Hospital	Rhinebeck	67%	300+
Our Lady of Lourdes Memorial Hospital	Binghamton	67%	300+
Saint Francis Hospital	Poughkeepsie	67%	300+
United Health Services Hospitals	Johnson City	67%	300+
Univ Hosp S U N Y Health Science Ctr	Syracuse	67%	300+
Brooks Memorial Hospital	Dunkirk	66%	300+
Chenango Memorial Hospital	Norwich	66%	300+
Cortland Regional Medical Center	Cortland	66%	300+
Forest Hills Hospital	Forest Hills	66%	300+
Franklin Hospital	Valley Stream	66%	300+
North Shore University Hospital	Manhasset	66%	300+
Oswego Hospital	Oswego	66%	300+
Rochester General Hospital	Rochester	66%	300+
Samaritan Hospital	Troy	66%	300+
South Nassau Communities Hospital	Oceanside	66%	300+
Highland Hospital	Rochester	65%	300+
Jacobi Medical Center	Bronx	65%	300+
Jones Memorial Hospital	Wellsville	65%	300+
St John's Episcopal Hosp-South Shore	Far Rockaway	65%	300+
Saint Joseph's Medical Center	Yonkers	65%	300+
Woman's Christian Association	Jamestown	65%	300+
Albany Medical Center Hospital	Albany	64%	300+
Beth Israel Medical Center	New York	64%	300+
Crouse Hospital	Syracuse	64%	300+
Ira Davenport Memorial Hospital	Bath	64%	(a)
New York-Presbyterian Hospital	New York	64%	300+
Saint Joseph's Hospital Health Center	Syracuse	64%	300+
Seton Health System-St Mary's Campus	Troy	64%	300+
Staten Island University Hospital	Staten Island	64%	300+
Coney Island Hospital	Brooklyn	63%	300+
Geneva General Hospital	Geneva	63%	300+
Mercy Medical Center	Rockville Centre	63%	300+
New York Hospital Medical Center of Queens	Flushing	63%	300+
Saint Barnabas Hospital	Bronx	63%	300+
Saint Luke's Cornwall Hospital	Newburgh	63%	300+
Saint Peter's Hospital	Albany	63%	300+
Woodhull Medical and Mental Health Center	Brooklyn	63%	300+
Benedictine Hospital	Kingston	62%	(a)
Columbia Memorial Hospital	Hudson	62%	300+
Ellis Hospital	Schenectady	62%	300+
Mount Sinai Hospital	New York	62%	300+
Plainview Hospital	Plainview	62%	300+
Saint Joseph's Hospital	Elmira	62%	300+
TLC Health Network	Gowanda	62%	300+
Brooklyn Hospital Center at Downtown Campus	Brooklyn	61%	300+
Kingston Hospital	Kingston	61%	300+
Long Beach Medical Center	Long Beach	61%	300+
Niagara Falls Memorial Medical Center	Niagara Falls	61%	300+
Saint Anthony Community Hospital	Warwick	61%	300+
Saint Joseph Hospital	Bethpage	61%	300+
Sisters of Charity Hospital	Buffalo	61%	300+
Strong Memorial Hospital	Rochester	61%	300+
Brookdale Hospital Medical Center	Brooklyn	60%	300+
Flushing Hospital Medical Center	Flushing	60%	300+
Lincoln Medical & Mental Health Center	Bronx	60%	300+
Long Island Jewish Medical Center	New Hyde Park	60%	300+
North Central Bronx Hospital	Bronx	60%	300+
NYU Hospitals Center[11]	New York	60%	300+
Orange Regional Medical Center	Goshen	60%	300+
Brookhaven Memorial Hospital Med Ctr	Patchogue	59%	300+
Metropolitan Hospital Center	New York	59%	300+
Peninsula Hospital Center	Far Rockaway	59%	300+
Elmhurst Hospital Center	Elmhurst	58%	300+
Good Samaritan Hospital of Suffern	Suffern	58%	300+
Harlem Hospital Center	New York	58%	300+
Kenmore Mercy Hospital	Kenmore	58%	300+
Maimonides Medical Center	Brooklyn	58%	300+
Peconic Bay Medical Center	Riverhead	58%	300+
Richmond University Medical Center	Staten Island	58%	300+
Unity Hospital of Rochester	Rochester	58%	300+
University Hospital of Brooklyn - Downstate	Brooklyn	58%	300+
Comm-General Hosp of Greater Syracuse	Syracuse	57%	300+
Kaleida Health	Buffalo	57%	300+
New York Downtown Hospital	New York	57%	300+
Jamaica Hospital Medical Center	Jamaica	56%	300+
New York Methodist Hospital	Brooklyn	56%	300+
Bellevue Hospital Center	New York	55%	300+
Lenox Hill Hospital[11]	New York	55%	300+
Wyckoff Heights Medical Center	Brooklyn	55%	300+
Saint Luke's Roosevelt Hospital	New York	54%	300+
Catskill Regional Medical Center	Harris	53%	300+
Long Island College Hospital	Brooklyn	53%	300+
Lutheran Medical Center	Brooklyn	53%	300+
Mercy Hospital	Buffalo	53%	300+
Sound Shore Medical Center of Westschester	New Rochelle	53%	300+
Westchester Medical Center	Valhalla	53%	300+
Faxton-St Luke's Healthcare	Utica	52%	300+
Bronx-Lebanon Hospital Center	Bronx	51%	300+
Nassau University Medical Center	East Meadow	51%	300+
Erie County Medical Center	Buffalo	49%	300+

48. Timely Help 'Always' Received

Hospital Name	City	Rate	Cases
Westfield Memorial Hospital	Westfield	90%	(a)
Bertrand Chaffee Hospital	Springville	78%	300+
Delaware Valley Hospital	Walton	77%	(a)
Adirondack Medical Center	Saranac Lake	72%	300+
Clifton Springs Hospital and Clinic	Clifton Springs	72%	300+
Newark-Wayne Community Hospital	Newark	69%	300+
Edward John Noble Hospital of Gouverneur	Gouverneur	68%	300+
F F Thompson Hospital	Canandaigua	68%	300+
Nicholas H Noyes Memorial Hospital	Dansville	68%	300+
Claxton-Hepburn Medical Center	Ogdensburg	67%	(a)
Community Memorial Hospital	Hamilton	67%	300+
Massena Memorial Hospital	Massena	67%	300+
Northern Westchester Hospital	Mount Kisco	66%	300+
Putnam Hospital Center	Carmel	66%	300+
Saint Anthony Community Hospital	Warwick	66%	300+
Saint Elizabeth Medical Center	Utica	66%	300+
Saint Mary's Hospital at Amsterdam	Amsterdam	66%	300+
Eastern Long Island Hospital	Greenport	65%	300+
John T Mather Mem Hosp-Port Jefferson	Port Jefferson	65%	300+
Saint Francis Hospital - Roslyn	Roslyn	65%	300+
Saint James Mercy Hospital	Hornell	65%	300+
Saratoga Hospital	Saratoga Spgs	65%	300+
Seton Health System-St Mary's Campus	Troy	65%	300+
Bon Secours Community Hospital	Port Jervis	64%	300+
Canton-Potsdam Hospital	Potsdam	64%	300+
Cayuga Medical Center at Ithaca	Ithaca	64%	300+
Lewis County General Hospital	Lowville	64%	300+
Northern Dutchess Hospital	Rhinebeck	64%	300+
Soldiers and Sailors Mem Hosp of Yates	Penn Yan	64%	(a)
Arnot Ogden Medical Center	Elmira	63%	300+
Hospital for Special Surgery	New York	63%	300+
Nathan Littauer Hospital	Gloversville	63%	300+
Oneida Healthcare Center	Oneida	63%	300+
Our Lady of Lourdes Memorial Hospital	Binghamton	63%	300+
Saint Francis Hospital	Poughkeepsie	63%	300+
United Health Services Hospitals	Johnson City	63%	300+
United Memorial Medical Center	Batavia	63%	300+
Vassar Brothers Medical Center[11]	Poughkeepsie	63%	300+
White Plains Hospital Center	White Plains	63%	300+
Glen Cove Hospital	Glen Cove	62%	300+
Hudson Valley Hospital Center	Cortlandt Manor	62%	300+
Rochester General Hospital	Rochester	62%	300+
Samaritan Medical Center	Watertown	62%	300+
Chenango Memorial Hospital	Norwich	61%	300+
Medina Memorial Hospital	Medina	61%	300+
Mount Vernon Hospital	Mount Vernon	61%	300+
Cobleskill Regional Hospital	Cobleskill	60%	(a)
Lawrence Hospital Center	Bronxville	60%	300+
NY Eye and Ear Infirmary	New York	60%	300+
Olean General Hospital	Olean	60%	300+
Albany Memorial Hospital	Albany	59%	300+
Auburn Memorial Hospital	Auburn	59%	300+
Champlain Valley Physicians Hospital	Plattsburgh	59%	300+
Comm-General Hosp of Greater Syracuse	Syracuse	59%	300+
Corning Hospital	Corning	59%	300+
Mount St Mary's Hospital and Health Center	Lewiston	59%	300+
New York Westchester Square Medical Center[7]	Bronx	59%	(a)
Nyack Hospital	Nyack	59%	300+
Saint Charles Hospital	Port Jefferson	59%	300+
Saint Joseph's Hospital Health Center	Syracuse	59%	300+
Southampton Hospital	Southampton	59%	300+
Aurelia Osborn Fox Memorial Hospital	Oneonta	58%	300+
Benedictine Hospital	Kingston	58%	(a)
Jones Memorial Hospital	Wellsville	58%	300+
Lakeside Memorial Hospital	Brockport	58%	300+
Mary Imogene Bassett Hospital	Cooperstown	58%	300+
University Hospital - Stony Brook	Stony Brook	58%	300+
Alice Hyde Medical Center	Malone	57%	300+
Beth Israel Medical Center	New York	57%	300+
Faxton-St Luke's Healthcare	Utica	57%	300+
Glens Falls Hospital	Glens Falls	57%	300+
Huntington Hospital	Huntington	57%	300+
Ira Davenport Memorial Hospital	Bath	57%	(a)
Little Falls Hospital	Little Falls	57%	300+
South Nassau Communities Hospital	Oceanside	57%	300+
TLC Health Network	Gowanda	57%	300+
Winthrop-University Hospital	Mineola	57%	300+
Wyoming County Community Hospital	Warsaw	57%	300+
Eastern Niagara Hospital	Lockport	56%	300+
Geneva General Hospital	Geneva	56%	300+
Good Samaritan Hospital Medical Center	West Islip	56%	300+
Highland Hospital	Rochester	56%	300+
Kenmore Mercy Hospital	Kenmore	56%	300+
Long Island Jewish Medical Center	New Hyde Park	56%	300+
Plainview Hospital	Plainview	56%	300+
Queens Hospital Center	Jamaica	56%	300+
Richmond University Medical Center	Staten Island	56%	300+
Samaritan Hospital	Troy	56%	300+
Sisters of Charity Hospital	Buffalo	56%	300+
Southside Hospital	Bay Shore	56%	300+
Staten Island University Hospital	Staten Island	56%	300+
Strong Memorial Hospital	Rochester	56%	300+
Unity Hospital of Rochester	Rochester	56%	300+
Catskill Regional Medical Center	Harris	55%	300+
Mercy Medical Center	Rockville Centre	55%	300+
New York-Presbyterian Hospital	New York	55%	300+
Phelps Memorial Hospital Assn	Sleepy Hollow	55%	300+
Univ Hosp S U N Y Health Science Ctr	Syracuse	55%	300+
Woman's Christian Association	Jamestown	55%	300+
Carthage Area Hospital	Carthage	54%	300+
Coney Island Hospital	Brooklyn	54%	300+
Cortland Regional Medical Center	Cortland	54%	300+
Kaleida Health	Buffalo	54%	300+
Oswego Hospital	Oswego	54%	300+
Rome Memorial Hospital	Rome	54%	300+
Saint John's Riverside Hospital	Yonkers	54%	300+
Westchester Medical Center	Valhalla	54%	300+
Albany Medical Center Hospital	Albany	53%	300+
Columbia Memorial Hospital	Hudson	53%	300+
Crouse Hospital	Syracuse	53%	300+
Ellis Hospital	Schenectady	53%	300+
Franklin Hospital	Valley Stream	53%	300+
Lenox Hill Hospital[11]	New York	53%	300+
Maimonides Medical Center	Brooklyn	53%	300+
Niagara Falls Memorial Medical Center	Niagara Falls	53%	300+
NYU Hospitals Center[11]	New York	53%	300+
Saint Joseph's Hospital	Elmira	53%	300+
Brooks Memorial Hospital	Dunkirk	52%	300+
Forest Hills Hospital	Forest Hills	52%	300+
Saint Catherine of Siena Hospital	Smithtown	52%	300+
Elmhurst Hospital Center	Elmhurst	51%	300+
Mount Sinai Hospital	New York	51%	300+
New York Community Hospital of Brooklyn	Brooklyn	51%	300+
Orange Regional Medical Center	Goshen	51%	300+
Saint Luke's Cornwall Hospital	Newburgh	51%	300+
Jacobi Medical Center	Bronx	50%	300+
Kingston Hospital	Kingston	50%	300+
Lutheran Medical Center	Brooklyn	50%	300+
Brookhaven Memorial Hospital Med Ctr	Patchogue	49%	300+
Lincoln Medical & Mental Health Center	Bronx	49%	300+
North Central Bronx Hospital	Bronx	49%	300+
North Shore University Hospital	Manhasset	49%	300+
Saint Joseph Hospital	Bethpage	49%	300+
Saint Peter's Hospital	Albany	49%	300+
Bellevue Hospital Center	New York	48%	300+
Long Beach Medical Center	Long Beach	48%	300+
Metropolitan Hospital Center	New York	48%	300+
Montefiore Medical Center	Bronx	48%	300+
St John's Episcopal Hosp-South Shore	Far Rockaway	48%	300+
University Hospital of Brooklyn - Downstate	Brooklyn	48%	300+
Good Samaritan Hospital of Suffern	Suffern	47%	300+
Harlem Hospital Center	New York	47%	300+
Mercy Hospital	Buffalo	47%	300+
Peconic Bay Medical Center	Riverhead	47%	300+
Saint Luke's Roosevelt Hospital	New York	47%	300+
Sound Shore Medical Center of Westschester	New Rochelle	47%	300+
New York Downtown Hospital	New York	46%	300+
New York Hospital Medical Center of Queens	Flushing	46%	300+
Kings County Hospital Center	Brooklyn	45%	300+
Kingsbrook Jewish Medical Center	Brooklyn	45%	300+
Long Island College Hospital	Brooklyn	45%	300+
Woodhull Medical and Mental Health Center	Brooklyn	45%	300+
Erie County Medical Center	Buffalo	44%	300+

NOTE: Hospital profiles are in alphabetical order by state, then city, then hospital within the city; Rankings exclude hospitals with less than 25 cases except for patient surveys which excludes hospitals with less than 100 cases; (a) 100–299 cases; (1) The number of cases is too small to be sure how well a hospital is performing; (2) The hospital indicated that the data submitted for this measure were based on a sample of cases; (3) Data was collected during a shorter time period (fewer quarters) than the maximum possible time for this measure; (4) Suppressed for one or more quarters by CMS; (5) No data is available from the hospital for this measure; (6) Fewer than 100 patients completed the HCAHPS survey. Use these rates with caution, as the number of surveys may be too low to reliably assess hospital performance; (7) Survey results are based on less than 12 months of data; (8) Survey results are not available for this reporting period; (9) No or very few patients were eligible for the HCAHPS survey. The scores shown, if any, reflect a very small number of surveys; (10) A state average was not calculated because too few hospitals in the state submitted data; (11) There were discrepancies in the data collection process; Please refer to the User's Guide for a full explanation of data.

Flushing Hospital Medical Center	Flushing	44%	300+
Nassau University Medical Center	East Meadow	44%	300+
Saint Joseph's Medical Center	Yonkers	43%	300+
New York Methodist Hospital	Brooklyn	42%	300+
Saint Barnabas Hospital	Bronx	42%	300+
Jamaica Hospital Medical Center	Jamaica	40%	300+
Brooklyn Hospital Center at Downtown Campus	Brooklyn	39%	300+
Peninsula Hospital Center	Far Rockaway	39%	300+
Interfaith Medical Center	Brooklyn	38%	300+
Bronx-Lebanon Hospital Center	Bronx	37%	300+
Brookdale Hospital Medical Center	Brooklyn	36%	300+
Wyckoff Heights Medical Center	Brooklyn	33%	300+

49. Would Definitely Recommend Hospital

Hospital Name	City	Rate	Cases
Westfield Memorial Hospital	Westfield	92%	(a)
Hospital for Special Surgery	New York	89%	300+
Saint Francis Hospital - Roslyn	Roslyn	86%	300+
Clifton Springs Hospital and Clinic	Clifton Springs	84%	300+
Eastern Long Island Hospital	Greenport	84%	300+
Northern Westchester Hospital	Mount Kisco	81%	300+
New York-Presbyterian Hospital	New York	80%	300+
Vassar Brothers Medical Center[11]	Poughkeepsie	80%	300+
Northern Dutchess Hospital	Rhinebeck	79%	300+
White Plains Hospital Center	White Plains	79%	300+
Community Memorial Hospital	Hamilton	78%	300+
Rochester General Hospital	Rochester	78%	300+
Lewis County General Hospital	Lowville	77%	300+
Saint Joseph's Hospital Health Center	Syracuse	77%	300+
Delaware Valley Hospital	Walton	76%	(a)
F F Thompson Hospital	Canandaigua	76%	300+
Highland Hospital	Rochester	76%	300+
John T Mather Mem Hosp-Port Jefferson	Port Jefferson	76%	300+
Putnam Hospital Center	Carmel	76%	300+
Adirondack Medical Center	Saranac Lake	75%	300+
Arnot Ogden Medical Center	Elmira	75%	300+
Mary Imogene Bassett Hospital	Cooperstown	75%	300+
Saint Charles Hospital	Port Jefferson	75%	300+
Bertrand Chaffee Hospital	Springville	74%	300+
Lawrence Hospital Center	Bronxville	74%	300+
North Shore University Hospital	Manhasset	74%	300+
Our Lady of Lourdes Memorial Hospital	Binghamton	74%	300+
Strong Memorial Hospital	Rochester	74%	300+
Crouse Hospital	Syracuse	73%	300+
Mount St Mary's Hospital and Health Center	Lewiston	73%	300+
Saint Anthony Community Hospital	Warwick	73%	300+
Winthrop-University Hospital	Mineola	73%	300+
NY Eye and Ear Infirmary	New York	72%	300+
Saint Mary's Hospital at Amsterdam	Amsterdam	72%	300+
United Health Services Hospitals	Johnson City	72%	300+
Unity Hospital of Rochester	Rochester	72%	300+
Albany Memorial Hospital	Albany	71%	300+
Benedictine Hospital	Kingston	71%	(a)
Cayuga Medical Center at Ithaca	Ithaca	71%	300+
Lenox Hill Hospital[11]	New York	71%	300+
Mount Sinai Hospital	New York	71%	300+
NYU Hospitals Center[11]	New York	71%	300+
Saint Peter's Hospital	Albany	71%	300+
Saratoga Hospital	Saratoga Spgs	71%	300+
Canton-Potsdam Hospital	Potsdam	70%	300+
Glen Cove Hospital	Glen Cove	70%	300+
Nicholas H Noyes Memorial Hospital	Dansville	70%	300+
Queens Hospital Center	Jamaica	70%	300+
Saint Elizabeth Medical Center	Utica	70%	300+
Soldiers and Sailors Mem Hosp of Yates	Penn Yan	70%	(a)
South Nassau Communities Hospital	Oceanside	70%	300+
University Hospital - Stony Brook	Stony Brook	70%	300+
Kenmore Mercy Hospital	Kenmore	69%	300+
Oneida Healthcare Center	Oneida	69%	300+
Phelps Memorial Hospital Assn	Sleepy Hollow	69%	300+
Univ Hosp S U N Y Health Science Ctr	Syracuse	69%	300+
Claxton-Hepburn Medical Center	Ogdensburg	68%	(a)
Good Samaritan Hospital Medical Center	West Islip	68%	300+
Hudson Valley Hospital Center	Cortlandt Manor	68%	300+
Huntington Hospital	Huntington	68%	300+
Lakeside Memorial Hospital	Brockport	68%	300+
Sisters of Charity Hospital	Buffalo	68%	300+
Albany Medical Center Hospital	Albany	67%	300+
Cobleskill Regional Hospital	Cobleskill	67%	(a)
Montefiore Medical Center	Bronx	67%	300+
Saint Francis Hospital	Poughkeepsie	67%	300+
Seton Health System-St Mary's Campus	Troy	67%	300+
Southside Hospital	Bay Shore	67%	300+
Comm-General Hosp of Greater Syracuse	Syracuse	66%	300+
Long Island Jewish Medical Center	New Hyde Park	66%	300+
Saint John's Riverside Hospital	Yonkers	66%	300+
Glens Falls Hospital	Glens Falls	65%	300+
Mercy Medical Center	Rockville Centre	65%	300+
Ellis Hospital	Schenectady	64%	300+
Kaleida Health	Buffalo	64%	300+
Medina Memorial Hospital	Medina	64%	300+
New York Westchester Square Medical Center[7]	Bronx	64%	(a)
Champlain Valley Physicians Hospital	Plattsburgh	63%	300+
Faxton-St Luke's Healthcare	Utica	63%	300+
Kings County Hospital Center	Brooklyn	63%	300+
North Central Bronx Hospital	Bronx	63%	300+
Samaritan Hospital	Troy	63%	300+
Southampton Hospital	Southampton	63%	300+
Auburn Memorial Hospital	Auburn	62%	300+
Bellevue Hospital Center	New York	62%	300+
Carthage Area Hospital	Carthage	62%	300+
Eastern Niagara Hospital	Lockport	62%	300+
Maimonides Medical Center	Brooklyn	62%	300+
TLC Health Network	Gowanda	62%	300+
Beth Israel Medical Center	New York	61%	300+
Geneva General Hospital	Geneva	61%	300+
Good Samaritan Hospital of Suffern	Suffern	61%	300+
Kingsbrook Jewish Medical Center	Brooklyn	61%	300+
Little Falls Hospital	Little Falls	61%	300+
Nathan Littauer Hospital	Gloversville	61%	300+
New York Hospital Medical Center of Queens	Flushing	61%	300+
New York Methodist Hospital	Brooklyn	61%	300+
Newark-Wayne Community Hospital	Newark	61%	300+
Saint Catherine of Siena Hospital	Smithtown	61%	300+
Staten Island University Hospital	Staten Island	61%	300+
Westchester Medical Center	Valhalla	61%	300+
Bon Secours Community Hospital	Port Jervis	60%	300+
Elmhurst Hospital Center	Elmhurst	60%	300+
Jacobi Medical Center	Bronx	60%	300+
Metropolitan Hospital Center	New York	60%	300+
Plainview Hospital	Plainview	60%	300+
Saint Luke's Roosevelt Hospital	New York	60%	300+
Alice Hyde Medical Center	Malone	59%	300+
Franklin Hospital	Valley Stream	59%	300+
Massena Memorial Hospital	Massena	59%	300+
Mount Vernon Hospital	Mount Vernon	59%	300+
Nyack Hospital	Nyack	59%	300+
Saint Joseph's Hospital	Elmira	59%	300+
Aurelia Osborn Fox Memorial Hospital	Oneonta	58%	300+
Erie County Medical Center	Buffalo	58%	300+
Forest Hills Hospital	Forest Hills	58%	300+
Kingston Hospital	Kingston	58%	300+
Rome Memorial Hospital	Rome	58%	300+
Niagara Falls Memorial Medical Center	Niagara Falls	57%	300+
Saint Luke's Cornwall Hospital	Newburgh	57%	300+
University Hospital of Brooklyn - Downstate	Brooklyn	57%	300+
Brooks Memorial Hospital	Dunkirk	56%	300+
Coney Island Hospital	Brooklyn	56%	300+
Corning Hospital	Corning	56%	300+
Jones Memorial Hospital	Wellsville	56%	300+
Olean General Hospital	Olean	56%	300+
United Memorial Medical Center	Batavia	56%	300+
Woman's Christian Association	Jamestown	56%	300+
Long Island College Hospital	Brooklyn	55%	300+
Lutheran Medical Center	Brooklyn	54%	300+
Saint Joseph Hospital	Bethpage	54%	300+
Samaritan Medical Center	Watertown	54%	300+
Wyoming County Community Hospital	Warsaw	54%	300+
Chenango Memorial Hospital	Norwich	53%	300+
Lincoln Medical & Mental Health Center	Bronx	53%	300+
Peconic Bay Medical Center	Riverhead	53%	300+
Woodhull Medical and Mental Health Center	Brooklyn	53%	300+
Harlem Hospital Center	New York	52%	300+
Orange Regional Medical Center	Goshen	52%	300+
Saint Joseph's Medical Center	Yonkers	52%	300+
Columbia Memorial Hospital	Hudson	51%	300+
New York Community Hospital of Brooklyn	Brooklyn	51%	300+
Richmond University Medical Center	Staten Island	51%	300+
Saint James Mercy Hospital	Hornell	51%	300+
Brookhaven Memorial Hospital Med Ctr	Patchogue	50%	300+
Brooklyn Hospital Center at Downtown Campus	Brooklyn	50%	300+
Cortland Regional Medical Center	Cortland	50%	300+
Oswego Hospital	Oswego	50%	300+
Jamaica Hospital Medical Center	Jamaica	49%	300+
Mercy Hospital	Buffalo	49%	300+
Saint Barnabas Hospital	Bronx	49%	300+
St John's Episcopal Hosp-South Shore	Far Rockaway	49%	300+
Sound Shore Medical Center of Westchester	New Rochelle	49%	300+
Flushing Hospital Medical Center	Flushing	47%	300+
Catskill Regional Medical Center	Harris	46%	300+
Interfaith Medical Center	Brooklyn	45%	300+
Long Beach Medical Center	Long Beach	45%	300+
Bronx-Lebanon Hospital Center	Bronx	44%	300+
Wyckoff Heights Medical Center	Brooklyn	44%	300+
New York Downtown Hospital	New York	43%	300+
Edward John Noble Hospital of Gouverneur	Gouverneur	42%	300+
Ira Davenport Memorial Hospital	Bath	42%	(a)
Nassau University Medical Center	East Meadow	42%	300+
Peninsula Hospital Center	Far Rockaway	41%	300+
Brookdale Hospital Medical Center	Brooklyn	37%	300+

NOTE: Hospital profiles are in alphabetical order by state, then city, then within the city; Rankings exclude hospitals with less than 25 cases except for patient surveys which excludes hospitals with less than 100 cases; (a) 100–299 cases; (1) The number of cases is too small to be sure how well a hospital is performing; (2) The hospital indicated that the data submitted for this measure were based on a sample of cases; (3) Data was collected during a shorter time period (fewer quarters) than the maximum possible time for this measure; (4) Suppressed for one or more quarters by CMS; (5) No data is available from the hospital for this measure; (6) Fewer than 100 patients completed the HCAHPS survey. Use these rates with caution, as the number of surveys may be too low to reliably assess hospital performance; (7) Survey results are based on less than 12 months of data; (8) Survey results are not available for this reporting period; (9) No or very few patients were eligible for the HCAHPS survey. The scores shown, if any, reflect a very small number of surveys; (10) A state average was not calculated because too few hospitals in the state submitted data; (11) There were discrepancies in the data collection process; Please refer to the User's Guide for a full explanation of data.

Albany Medical Center - South Clinical Campus

25 Hackett Boulevard
Albany, NY 12208
Type: Acute Care Hospitals
Ownership: Voluntary Non-Profit - Private

Phone: 518-242-1461
Emergency Services: No
Beds: 20

Key Personnel:
CEO/President . . . . Timothy Duffy

Measure	Cases	This Hosp.	State Avg.	U.S. Avg.
Heart Attack Care				
ACE Inhibitor or ARB for LVSD[5]	0	-	95%	96%
Aspirin at Arrival[5]	0	-	98%	99%
Aspirin at Discharge[5]	0	-	98%	98%
Beta Blocker at Discharge[5]	0	-	98%	98%
Fibrinolytic Medication Timing[5]	0	-	50%	55%
PCI Within 90 Minutes of Arrival[5]	0	-	88%	90%
Smoking Cessation Advice[5]	0	-	100%	99%
Chest Pain/Possible Heart Attack Care				
Aspirin at Arrival[5]	0	-	96%	95%
Median Time to ECG (minutes)[5]	0	-	11	8
Median Time to Transfer (minutes)[5]	0	-	75	61
Fibrinolytic Medication Timing[5]	0	-	55%	54%
Heart Failure Care				
ACE Inhibitor or ARB for LVSD[5]	0	-	94%	94%
Discharge Instructions[5]	0	-	89%	88%
Evaluation of LVS Function[5]	0	-	98%	98%
Smoking Cessation Advice[5]	0	-	98%	98%
Pneumonia Care				
Appropriate Initial Antibiotic[5]	0	-	92%	92%
Blood Culture Timing[5]	0	-	95%	96%
Influenza Vaccine[5]	0	-	90%	91%
Initial Antibiotic Timing[5]	0	-	93%	95%
Pneumococcal Vaccine[5]	0	-	92%	93%
Smoking Cessation Advice[5]	0	-	98%	97%
Surgical Care Improvement Project				
Appropriate VTP Within 24 Hours[2,3]	0	-	94%	92%
Appropriate Hair Removal[1,2,3]	7	100%	100%	99%
Appropriate Beta Blocker Usage[2,3]	0	-	92%	93%
Controlled Postoperative Blood Glucose[2,3]	0	-	94%	93%
Prophylactic Antibiotic Timing[1,2,3]	4	100%	96%	97%
Prophylactic Antibiotic Timing (Outpatient)	154	90%	92%	92%
Prophylactic Antibiotic Selection[1,2,3]	4	100%	97%	97%
Prophylactic Antibiotic Select. (Outpatient)	146	96%	93%	94%
Prophylactic Antibiotic Stopped[1,2,3]	4	100%	94%	94%
Recommended VTP Ordered[2,3]	0	-	96%	94%
Urinary Catheter Removal[2,3]	0	-	90%	90%
Children's Asthma Care				
Received Systemic Corticosteroids	-	-		100%
Received Home Management Plan	-	-		71%
Received Reliever Medication	-	-		100%
Use of Medical Imaging				
Combination Abdominal CT Scan	246	0.252	0.141	0.191
Combination Chest CT Scan	137	0.007	0.024	0.054
Follow-up Mammogram/Ultrasound	693	13.0%	9.8%	8.4%
MRI for Low Back Pain[1]	22	36.4%	26.9%	32.7%
Survey of Patients' Hospital Experiences				
Area Around Room 'Always' Quiet at Night[9]	-	-		58%
Doctors 'Always' Communicated Well[9]	-	-		80%
Home Recovery Information Given[9]	-	-		82%
Hospital Given 9 or 10 on 10 Point Scale[9]	-	-		67%
Meds 'Always' Explained Before Given[9]	-	-		60%
Nurses 'Always' Communicated Well[9]	-	-		76%
Pain 'Always' Well Controlled[9]	-	-		69%
Room and Bathroom 'Always' Clean[9]	-	-		71%
Timely Help 'Always' Received[9]	-	-		64%
Would Definitely Recommend Hospital[9]	-	-		69%

Albany Medical Center Hospital

43 New Scotland Avenue
Albany, NY 12208
Type: Acute Care Hospitals
Ownership: Voluntary Non-Profit - Private

Phone: 518-262-3125
Fax: 518-262-3398
Emergency Services: Yes
Beds: 651

Key Personnel:
CEO/President . . . . James J Barba
Chief of Medical Staff . . . . James Hoehn, MD
Quality Assurance . . . . Vickey Masta
Emergency Room . . . . Vincent Verdial, MD

Measure	Cases	This Hosp.	State Avg.	U.S. Avg.
Heart Attack Care				
ACE Inhibitor or ARB for LVSD	82	99%	95%	96%
Aspirin at Arrival	188	100%	98%	99%
Aspirin at Discharge	484	100%	98%	98%
Beta Blocker at Discharge	480	100%	98%	98%
Fibrinolytic Medication Timing[1]	1	0%	50%	55%
PCI Within 90 Minutes of Arrival	49	96%	88%	90%
Smoking Cessation Advice	204	100%	100%	99%
Chest Pain/Possible Heart Attack Care				
Aspirin at Arrival[5]	0	-	96%	95%
Median Time to ECG (minutes)[5]	0	-	11	8
Median Time to Transfer (minutes)[5]	0	-	75	61
Fibrinolytic Medication Timing[5]	0	-	55%	54%
Heart Failure Care				
ACE Inhibitor or ARB for LVSD	172	95%	94%	94%
Discharge Instructions	324	91%	89%	88%
Evaluation of LVS Function	386	100%	98%	98%
Smoking Cessation Advice	64	100%	98%	98%
Pneumonia Care				
Appropriate Initial Antibiotic	123	88%	92%	92%
Blood Culture Timing	218	94%	95%	96%
Influenza Vaccine	105	96%	90%	91%
Initial Antibiotic Timing	166	91%	93%	95%
Pneumococcal Vaccine	129	94%	92%	93%
Smoking Cessation Advice	80	94%	98%	97%
Surgical Care Improvement Project				
Appropriate VTP Within 24 Hours[2]	135	97%	94%	92%
Appropriate Hair Removal[2]	527	98%	100%	99%
Appropriate Beta Blocker Usage[2]	195	97%	92%	93%
Controlled Postoperative Blood Glucose[2]	103	85%	94%	93%
Prophylactic Antibiotic Timing[2]	333	98%	96%	97%
Prophylactic Antibiotic Timing (Outpatient)	594	96%	92%	92%
Prophylactic Antibiotic Selection[2]	352	97%	97%	97%
Prophylactic Antibiotic Select. (Outpatient)	577	94%	93%	94%
Prophylactic Antibiotic Stopped[2]	326	94%	94%	94%
Recommended VTP Ordered[2]	135	99%	96%	94%
Urinary Catheter Removal[2]	79	99%	90%	90%
Children's Asthma Care				
Received Systemic Corticosteroids	-	-		100%
Received Home Management Plan	-	-		71%
Received Reliever Medication	-	-		100%
Use of Medical Imaging				
Combination Abdominal CT Scan	707	0.124	0.141	0.191
Combination Chest CT Scan	512	0.004	0.024	0.054
Follow-up Mammogram/Ultrasound[5]	0		9.8%	8.4%
MRI for Low Back Pain	58	32.8%	26.9%	32.7%
Survey of Patients' Hospital Experiences				
Area Around Room 'Always' Quiet at Night	300+	44%	-	58%
Doctors 'Always' Communicated Well	300+	67%	-	80%
Home Recovery Information Given	300+	81%	-	82%
Hospital Given 9 or 10 on 10 Point Scale	300+	57%	-	67%
Meds 'Always' Explained Before Given	300+	53%	-	60%
Nurses 'Always' Communicated Well	300+	67%	-	76%
Pain 'Always' Well Controlled	300+	64%	-	69%
Room and Bathroom 'Always' Clean	300+	64%	-	71%
Timely Help 'Always' Received	300+	53%	-	64%
Would Definitely Recommend Hospital	300+	67%	-	69%

Albany Memorial Hospital

600 Northern Boulevard
Albany, NY 12204
URL: www.nehealth.com
Type: Acute Care Hospitals
Ownership: Voluntary Non-Profit - Private

Phone: 518-471-3221
Fax: 518-449-4410

Emergency Services: Yes
Beds: 165

Key Personnel:
CEO/President . . . . Norman Dascher
Cardiac Laboratory . . . . John Bennett
Infection Control . . . . Anna McClane
Quality Assurance . . . . Robert Allen
Radiology . . . . Michael P. Gaber
Ambulatory Care . . . . Nanci Lombard
Hemotology Center . . . . Marianne Roberto

Measure	Cases	This Hosp.	State Avg.	U.S. Avg.
Heart Attack Care				
ACE Inhibitor or ARB for LVSD[1]	5	100%	95%	96%
Aspirin at Arrival	33	94%	98%	99%
Aspirin at Discharge[1]	23	96%	98%	98%
Beta Blocker at Discharge	25	92%	98%	98%
Fibrinolytic Medication Timing	0	-	50%	55%
PCI Within 90 Minutes of Arrival	0	-	88%	90%
Smoking Cessation Advice[1]	2	100%	100%	99%
Chest Pain/Possible Heart Attack Care				
Aspirin at Arrival[1]	22	95%	96%	95%
Median Time to ECG (minutes)[1]	22	12	11	8
Median Time to Transfer (minutes)[1]	10	55	75	61
Fibrinolytic Medication Timing	0	-	55%	54%
Heart Failure Care				
ACE Inhibitor or ARB for LVSD[1]	22	100%	94%	94%
Discharge Instructions	102	83%	89%	88%
Evaluation of LVS Function	135	96%	98%	98%
Smoking Cessation Advice[1]	22	91%	98%	98%
Pneumonia Care				
Appropriate Initial Antibiotic[2]	75	96%	92%	92%
Blood Culture Timing[2]	177	96%	95%	96%
Influenza Vaccine[2]	92	93%	90%	91%
Initial Antibiotic Timing[2]	158	96%	93%	95%
Pneumococcal Vaccine[2]	137	91%	92%	93%
Smoking Cessation Advice[2]	45	100%	98%	97%
Surgical Care Improvement Project				
Appropriate VTP Within 24 Hours[2]	194	90%	94%	92%
Appropriate Hair Removal[2]	449	98%	100%	99%
Appropriate Beta Blocker Usage[2]	133	84%	92%	93%
Controlled Postoperative Blood Glucose[2]	0	-	94%	93%
Prophylactic Antibiotic Timing[2]	300	93%	96%	97%
Prophylactic Antibiotic Timing (Outpatient)	190	91%	92%	92%
Prophylactic Antibiotic Selection[2]	298	89%	97%	97%
Prophylactic Antibiotic Select. (Outpatient)	181	96%	93%	94%
Prophylactic Antibiotic Stopped[2]	296	85%	94%	94%
Recommended VTP Ordered[2]	194	92%	96%	94%
Urinary Catheter Removal[2]	73	75%	90%	90%
Children's Asthma Care				
Received Systemic Corticosteroids	-	-		100%
Received Home Management Plan	-	-		71%
Received Reliever Medication	-	-		100%
Use of Medical Imaging				
Combination Abdominal CT Scan	555	0.038	0.141	0.191
Combination Chest CT Scan	288	0.000	0.024	0.054
Follow-up Mammogram/Ultrasound	1,097	6.2%	9.8%	8.4%
MRI for Low Back Pain	95	23.2%	26.9%	32.7%
Survey of Patients' Hospital Experiences				
Area Around Room 'Always' Quiet at Night	300+	53%	-	58%
Doctors 'Always' Communicated Well	300+	76%	-	80%
Home Recovery Information Given	300+	85%	-	82%
Hospital Given 9 or 10 on 10 Point Scale	300+	66%	-	67%
Meds 'Always' Explained Before Given	300+	54%	-	60%
Nurses 'Always' Communicated Well	300+	74%	-	76%
Pain 'Always' Well Controlled	300+	70%	-	69%
Room and Bathroom 'Always' Clean	300+	70%	-	71%
Timely Help 'Always' Received	300+	59%	-	64%
Would Definitely Recommend Hospital	300+	71%	-	69%

Albany VA Medical Center

113 Holland Avenue Phone: 518-626-5000
Albany, NY 12208 Fax: 518-626-5500
URL: www1.va.gov/visns/visn02/albany.cfm
Type: Acute Care-Veterans Administration Emergency Services: No
Ownership: Government - Federal Beds: 156

Key Personnel:
Chief of Medical Staff. . . . . Lourdes Irizarry, MD
Operating Room. . . . . Kathy Kovarik
Quality Assurance . . . . Barbara Parker
Radiology. Vernon King
Patient Relations . . . . Deborah Spath

Measure	Cases	This Hosp.	State Avg.	U.S. Avg.
Heart Attack Care				
ACE Inhibitor or ARB for LVSD[1]	2	100%	95%	96%
Aspirin at Arrival[1]	21	100%	98%	99%
Aspirin at Discharge[1]	16	100%	98%	98%
Beta Blocker at Discharge[1]	15	100%	98%	98%
Fibrinolytic Medication Timing[5]	0	-	50%	55%
PCI Within 90 Minutes of Arrival[5]	0	-	88%	90%
Smoking Cessation Advice[1]	1	100%	100%	99%
Chest Pain/Possible Heart Attack Care				
Aspirin at Arrival	-	-	96%	95%
Median Time to ECG (minutes)	-	-	11	8
Median Time to Transfer (minutes)	-	-	75	61
Fibrinolytic Medication Timing	-	-	55%	54%
Heart Failure Care				
ACE Inhibitor or ARB for LVSD[1]	22	100%	94%	94%
Discharge Instructions	62	100%	89%	88%
Evaluation of LVS Function	71	100%	98%	98%
Smoking Cessation Advice[1]	13	100%	98%	98%
Pneumonia Care				
Appropriate Initial Antibiotic	27	93%	92%	92%
Blood Culture Timing	60	100%	95%	96%
Influenza Vaccine	41	100%	90%	91%
Initial Antibiotic Timing	61	93%	93%	95%
Pneumococcal Vaccine	52	100%	92%	93%
Smoking Cessation Advice	31	100%	98%	97%
Surgical Care Improvement Project				
Appropriate VTP Within 24 Hours[2]	62	100%	94%	92%
Appropriate Hair Removal[2]	122	100%	100%	99%
Appropriate Beta Blocker Usage[2]	51	100%	92%	93%
Controlled Postoperative Blood Glucose[2,5]	0	-	94%	93%
Prophylactic Antibiotic Timing	68	100%	96%	97%
Prophylactic Antibiotic Timing (Outpatient)	-	-	92%	92%
Prophylactic Antibiotic Selection	69	100%	97%	97%
Prophylactic Antibiotic Select. (Outpatient)	-	-	93%	94%
Prophylactic Antibiotic Stopped	66	98%	94%	94%
Recommended VTP Ordered[2]	62	100%	96%	94%
Urinary Catheter Removal[2]	47	100%	90%	90%
Children's Asthma Care				
Received Systemic Corticosteroids	-	-	-	100%
Received Home Management Plan	-	-	-	71%
Received Reliever Medication	-	-	-	100%
Use of Medical Imaging				
Combination Abdominal CT Scan	-	-	0.141	0.191
Combination Chest CT Scan	-	-	0.024	0.054
Follow-up Mammogram/Ultrasound	-	-	9.8%	8.4%
MRI for Low Back Pain	-	-	26.9%	32.7%
Survey of Patients' Hospital Experiences				
Area Around Room 'Always' Quiet at Night	-	-	-	58%
Doctors 'Always' Communicated Well	-	-	-	80%
Home Recovery Information Given	-	-	-	82%
Hospital Given 9 or 10 on 10 Point Scale	-	-	-	67%
Meds 'Always' Explained Before Given	-	-	-	60%
Nurses 'Always' Communicated Well	-	-	-	76%
Pain 'Always' Well Controlled	-	-	-	69%
Room and Bathroom 'Always' Clean	-	-	-	71%
Timely Help 'Always' Received	-	-	-	64%
Would Definitely Recommend Hospital	-	-	-	69%

Saint Peter's Hospital

315 South Manning Boulevard Phone: 518-525-1550
Albany, NY 12208 Fax: 518-525-1961
URL: www.stpetershealthcare.org
Type: Acute Care Hospitals Emergency Services: Yes
Ownership: Voluntary Non-Profit - Church Beds: 442

Key Personnel:
CEO/President. . . . . Steven P Boyle
Cardiac Laboratory. . . . . David Jacob
Chief of Medical Staff. . . . . Robert Cella, MD
Infection Control. . . . . Amy R Gram
Quality Assurance . . . . Judy Phaff
Radiology. . . . . Edward Vining
Intensive Care Unit. . . . . Steven Richards

Measure	Cases	This Hosp.	State Avg.	U.S. Avg.
Heart Attack Care				
ACE Inhibitor or ARB for LVSD	85	99%	95%	96%
Aspirin at Arrival	383	100%	98%	99%
Aspirin at Discharge	635	99%	98%	98%
Beta Blocker at Discharge	646	99%	98%	98%
Fibrinolytic Medication Timing	0	-	50%	55%
PCI Within 90 Minutes of Arrival	48	81%	88%	90%
Smoking Cessation Advice	180	100%	100%	99%
Chest Pain/Possible Heart Attack Care				
Aspirin at Arrival[5]	0	-	96%	95%
Median Time to ECG (minutes)[5]	0	-	11	8
Median Time to Transfer (minutes)[5]	0	-	75	61
Fibrinolytic Medication Timing[5]	0	-	55%	54%
Heart Failure Care				
ACE Inhibitor or ARB for LVSD	132	95%	94%	94%
Discharge Instructions	399	92%	89%	88%
Evaluation of LVS Function	490	97%	98%	98%
Smoking Cessation Advice	61	100%	98%	98%
Pneumonia Care				
Appropriate Initial Antibiotic[2]	91	92%	92%	92%
Blood Culture Timing[2]	131	92%	95%	96%
Influenza Vaccine[2]	100	89%	90%	91%
Initial Antibiotic Timing[2]	147	90%	93%	95%
Pneumococcal Vaccine[2]	150	93%	92%	93%
Smoking Cessation Advice[2]	30	100%	98%	97%
Surgical Care Improvement Project				
Appropriate VTP Within 24 Hours[2]	252	97%	94%	92%
Appropriate Hair Removal[2]	737	98%	100%	99%
Appropriate Beta Blocker Usage[2]	210	71%	92%	93%
Controlled Postoperative Blood Glucose[2]	183	98%	94%	93%
Prophylactic Antibiotic Timing[2]	547	95%	96%	97%
Prophylactic Antibiotic Timing (Outpatient)	971	90%	92%	92%
Prophylactic Antibiotic Selection[2]	548	97%	97%	97%
Prophylactic Antibiotic Select. (Outpatient)	952	89%	93%	94%
Prophylactic Antibiotic Stopped[2]	536	93%	94%	94%
Recommended VTP Ordered[2]	252	99%	96%	94%
Urinary Catheter Removal[2]	112	82%	90%	90%
Children's Asthma Care				
Received Systemic Corticosteroids	-	-	-	100%
Received Home Management Plan	-	-	-	71%
Received Reliever Medication	-	-	-	100%
Use of Medical Imaging				
Combination Abdominal CT Scan	1,069	0.070	0.141	0.191
Combination Chest CT Scan	865	0.045	0.024	0.054
Follow-up Mammogram/Ultrasound	2,040	5.4%	9.8%	8.4%
MRI for Low Back Pain[1]	31	22.6%	26.9%	32.7%
Survey of Patients' Hospital Experiences				
Area Around Room 'Always' Quiet at Night	300+	38%	-	58%
Doctors 'Always' Communicated Well	300+	72%	-	80%
Home Recovery Information Given	300+	84%	-	82%
Hospital Given 9 or 10 on 10 Point Scale	300+	63%	-	67%
Meds 'Always' Explained Before Given	300+	57%	-	60%
Nurses 'Always' Communicated Well	300+	69%	-	76%
Pain 'Always' Well Controlled	300+	61%	-	69%
Room and Bathroom 'Always' Clean	300+	63%	-	71%
Timely Help 'Always' Received	300+	49%	-	64%
Would Definitely Recommend Hospital	300+	71%	-	69%

River Hospital

4 Fuller Street Phone: 315-482-2511
Alexandria Bay, NY 13607 Fax: 315-482-6308
URL: www.samaritanhealth.com
Type: Critical Access Hospitals Emergency Services: Yes
Ownership: Voluntary Non-Profit - Private Beds: 52

Key Personnel:
CEO/President. . . . . David Tinker
Chief of Medical Staff. . . . . Stephen Grybowski
Emergency Room . . . . Philip A Chafe

Measure	Cases	This Hosp.	State Avg.	U.S. Avg.
Heart Attack Care				
ACE Inhibitor or ARB for LVSD[5]	0	-	95%	96%
Aspirin at Arrival[5]	0	-	98%	99%
Aspirin at Discharge[5]	0	-	98%	98%
Beta Blocker at Discharge[5]	0	-	98%	98%
Fibrinolytic Medication Timing[5]	0	-	50%	55%
PCI Within 90 Minutes of Arrival[5]	0	-	88%	90%
Smoking Cessation Advice[5]	0	-	100%	99%
Chest Pain/Possible Heart Attack Care				
Aspirin at Arrival[5]	0	-	96%	95%
Median Time to ECG (minutes)[5]	0	-	11	8
Median Time to Transfer (minutes)[5]	0	-	75	61
Fibrinolytic Medication Timing[5]	0	-	55%	54%
Heart Failure Care				
ACE Inhibitor or ARB for LVSD[3]	0	-	94%	94%
Discharge Instructions[3]	0	-	89%	88%
Evaluation of LVS Function[1,3]	1	0%	98%	98%
Smoking Cessation Advice[3]	0	-	98%	98%
Pneumonia Care				
Appropriate Initial Antibiotic[1,3]	1	0%	92%	92%
Blood Culture Timing[3]	0	-	95%	96%
Influenza Vaccine[5]	0	-	90%	91%
Initial Antibiotic Timing[1,3]	2	100%	93%	95%
Pneumococcal Vaccine[1,3]	6	67%	92%	93%
Smoking Cessation Advice[1,3]	1	0%	98%	97%
Surgical Care Improvement Project				
Appropriate VTP Within 24 Hours[5]	0	-	94%	92%
Appropriate Hair Removal[5]	0	-	100%	99%
Appropriate Beta Blocker Usage[5]	0	-	92%	93%
Controlled Postoperative Blood Glucose[5]	0	-	94%	93%
Prophylactic Antibiotic Timing[5]	0	-	96%	97%
Prophylactic Antibiotic Timing (Outpatient)[5]	0	-	92%	92%
Prophylactic Antibiotic Selection[5]	0	-	97%	97%
Prophylactic Antibiotic Select. (Outpatient)[5]	0	-	93%	94%
Prophylactic Antibiotic Stopped[5]	0	-	94%	94%
Recommended VTP Ordered[5]	0	-	96%	94%
Urinary Catheter Removal[5]	0	-	90%	90%
Children's Asthma Care				
Received Systemic Corticosteroids	-	-	-	100%
Received Home Management Plan	-	-	-	71%
Received Reliever Medication	-	-	-	100%
Use of Medical Imaging				
Combination Abdominal CT Scan	86	0.012	0.141	0.191
Combination Chest CT Scan	58	0.000	0.024	0.054
Follow-up Mammogram/Ultrasound	132	9.1%	9.8%	8.4%
MRI for Low Back Pain[5]	0	-	26.9%	32.7%
Survey of Patients' Hospital Experiences				
Area Around Room 'Always' Quiet at Night[6]	<100	59%	-	58%
Doctors 'Always' Communicated Well[6]	<100	85%	-	80%
Home Recovery Information Given[6]	<100	81%	-	82%
Hospital Given 9 or 10 on 10 Point Scale[6]	<100	82%	-	67%
Meds 'Always' Explained Before Given[6]	<100	71%	-	60%
Nurses 'Always' Communicated Well[6]	<100	82%	-	76%
Pain 'Always' Well Controlled[6]	<100	73%	-	69%
Room and Bathroom 'Always' Clean[6]	<100	87%	-	71%
Timely Help 'Always' Received[6]	<100	78%	-	64%
Would Definitely Recommend Hospital	<100	86%	-	69%

NOTE: Hospital profiles are in alphabetical order by state, then city, then hospital within the city; Rankings exclude hospitals with less than 25 cases except for patient surveys which excludes hospitals with less than 100 cases; (a) 100–299 cases; (1) The number of cases is too small to be sure how well a hospital is performing; (2) The hospital indicated that the data submitted for this measure were based on a sample of cases; (3) Data was collected during a shorter time period (fewer quarters) than the maximum possible time for this measure; (4) Suppressed for one or more quarters by CMS; (5) No data is available from the hospital for this measure; (6) Fewer than 100 patients completed the HCAHPS survey. Use these rates with caution, as the number of surveys may be too low to reliably assess hospital performance; (7) Survey results are based on less than 12 months of data; (8) Survey results are not available for this reporting period; (9) No or very few patients were eligible for the HCAHPS survey. The scores shown, if any, reflect a very small number of surveys; (10) A state average was not calculated because too few hospitals in the state submitted data; (11) There were discrepancies in the data collection process; Please refer to the User's Guide for a full explanation of data.

Saint Mary's Hospital at Amsterdam

427 Guy Park Avenue Phone: 518-842-1900
Amsterdam, NY 12010 Fax: 518-842-0107
E-mail: info@smha.org
URL: www.smha.org
Type: Acute Care Hospitals Emergency Services: Yes
Ownership: Voluntary Non-Profit - Private Beds: 143

Key Personnel:
CEO/President. . . . . Victor Giulianelli
Chief of Medical Staff . . . . Tim Shoen, MD
Infection Control . . . . Phyllis MacMillon
Operating Room. . . . . Theresa Moore, RN
Quality Assurance . . . . Kathleen Picciocca
Emergency Room . . . . Steve Okhravi
Intensive Care Unit. . . . . Nancy Mead

Measure	Cases	This Hosp.	State Avg.	U.S. Avg.
Heart Attack Care				
ACE Inhibitor or ARB for LVSD[1]	6	100%	95%	96%
Aspirin at Arrival	57	100%	98%	99%
Aspirin at Discharge	30	100%	98%	98%
Beta Blocker at Discharge	39	100%	98%	98%
Fibrinolytic Medication Timing	0	-	50%	55%
PCI Within 90 Minutes of Arrival	0	-	88%	90%
Smoking Cessation Advice[1]	7	100%	100%	99%
Chest Pain/Possible Heart Attack Care				
Aspirin at Arrival	70	90%	96%	95%
Median Time to ECG (minutes)	68	11	11	8
Median Time to Transfer (minutes)[1]	22	66	75	61
Fibrinolytic Medication Timing	0	-	55%	54%
Heart Failure Care				
ACE Inhibitor or ARB for LVSD[2]	53	100%	94%	94%
Discharge Instructions[2]	195	92%	89%	88%
Evaluation of LVS Function[2]	244	100%	98%	98%
Smoking Cessation Advice[2]	30	100%	98%	98%
Pneumonia Care				
Appropriate Initial Antibiotic[2]	81	94%	92%	92%
Blood Culture Timing[2]	125	97%	95%	96%
Influenza Vaccine[2]	79	97%	90%	91%
Initial Antibiotic Timing[2]	148	94%	93%	95%
Pneumococcal Vaccine[2]	116	99%	92%	93%
Smoking Cessation Advice[2]	33	100%	98%	97%
Surgical Care Improvement Project				
Appropriate VTP Within 24 Hours[2]	122	93%	94%	92%
Appropriate Hair Removal[2]	297	100%	100%	99%
Appropriate Beta Blocker Usage[2]	100	100%	92%	93%
Controlled Postoperative Blood Glucose[2]	0	-	94%	93%
Prophylactic Antibiotic Timing[2]	178	99%	96%	97%
Prophylactic Antibiotic Timing (Outpatient)	91	81%	92%	92%
Prophylactic Antibiotic Selection[2]	179	98%	97%	97%
Prophylactic Antibiotic Select. (Outpatient)	116	97%	93%	94%
Prophylactic Antibiotic Stopped[2]	174	99%	94%	94%
Recommended VTP Ordered[2]	122	94%	96%	94%
Urinary Catheter Removal[2]	78	76%	90%	90%
Children's Asthma Care				
Received Systemic Corticosteroids	-	-	-	100%
Received Home Management Plan	-	-	-	71%
Received Reliever Medication	-	-	-	100%
Use of Medical Imaging				
Combination Abdominal CT Scan	800	0.431	0.141	0.191
Combination Chest CT Scan	437	0.041	0.024	0.054
Follow-up Mammogram/Ultrasound	904	5.3%	9.8%	8.4%
MRI for Low Back Pain	80	37.5%	26.9%	32.7%
Survey of Patients' Hospital Experiences				
Area Around Room 'Always' Quiet at Night	300+	49%	-	58%
Doctors 'Always' Communicated Well	300+	78%	-	80%
Home Recovery Information Given	300+	87%	-	82%
Hospital Given 9 or 10 on 10 Point Scale	300+	63%	-	67%
Meds 'Always' Explained Before Given	300+	61%	-	60%
Nurses 'Always' Communicated Well	300+	80%	-	76%
Pain 'Always' Well Controlled	300+	71%	-	69%
Room and Bathroom 'Always' Clean	300+	75%	-	71%
Timely Help 'Always' Received	300+	66%	-	64%
Would Definitely Recommend Hospital	300+	72%	-	69%

Auburn Memorial Hospital

17 Lansing Street Phone: 315-255-7011
Auburn, NY 13021 Fax: 315-255-7018
E-mail: amhinput@auburnhospital.org
URL: www.auburnhospital.org
Type: Acute Care Hospitals Emergency Services: Yes
Ownership: Voluntary Non-Profit - Private Beds: 99

Key Personnel:
CEO/President. . . . . Scott Berlucchi
Chief of Medical Staff . . . . James F Blute III, MD
Infection Control. . . . . Donna Wrobel
Pediatric In-Patient Care . . . . Farokkh Nawer, MD
Radiology. . . . . G. Palmer
Ambulatory Care . . . . Lorissa Plis
Anesthesiology. . . . . Anthony Ascioti
Emergency Room . . . . Kathy Kendrick

Measure	Cases	This Hosp.	State Avg.	U.S. Avg.
Heart Attack Care				
ACE Inhibitor or ARB for LVSD[1]	6	83%	95%	96%
Aspirin at Arrival	34	100%	98%	99%
Aspirin at Discharge[1]	20	100%	98%	98%
Beta Blocker at Discharge[1]	22	100%	98%	98%
Fibrinolytic Medication Timing	0	-	50%	55%
PCI Within 90 Minutes of Arrival	0	-	88%	90%
Smoking Cessation Advice	0	-	100%	99%
Chest Pain/Possible Heart Attack Care				
Aspirin at Arrival	137	95%	96%	95%
Median Time to ECG (minutes)	140	9	11	8
Median Time to Transfer (minutes)	27	60	75	61
Fibrinolytic Medication Timing	0	-	55%	54%
Heart Failure Care				
ACE Inhibitor or ARB for LVSD	54	91%	94%	94%
Discharge Instructions	155	79%	89%	88%
Evaluation of LVS Function	196	96%	98%	98%
Smoking Cessation Advice[1]	18	83%	98%	98%
Pneumonia Care				
Appropriate Initial Antibiotic	205	88%	92%	92%
Blood Culture Timing	233	91%	95%	96%
Influenza Vaccine	149	85%	90%	91%
Initial Antibiotic Timing	247	94%	93%	95%
Pneumococcal Vaccine	208	87%	92%	93%
Smoking Cessation Advice	73	88%	98%	97%
Surgical Care Improvement Project				
Appropriate VTP Within 24 Hours	127	92%	94%	92%
Appropriate Hair Removal	255	99%	100%	99%
Appropriate Beta Blocker Usage	71	89%	92%	93%
Controlled Postoperative Blood Glucose	0	-	94%	93%
Prophylactic Antibiotic Timing	166	88%	96%	97%
Prophylactic Antibiotic Timing (Outpatient)	116	93%	92%	92%
Prophylactic Antibiotic Selection	161	89%	97%	97%
Prophylactic Antibiotic Select. (Outpatient)	110	88%	93%	94%
Prophylactic Antibiotic Stopped	152	94%	94%	94%
Recommended VTP Ordered	129	94%	96%	94%
Urinary Catheter Removal	38	79%	90%	90%
Children's Asthma Care				
Received Systemic Corticosteroids	-	-	-	100%
Received Home Management Plan	-	-	-	71%
Received Reliever Medication	-	-	-	100%
Use of Medical Imaging				
Combination Abdominal CT Scan	625	0.082	0.141	0.191
Combination Chest CT Scan	260	0.000	0.024	0.054
Follow-up Mammogram/Ultrasound	775	6.5%	9.8%	8.4%
MRI for Low Back Pain[5]	0	-	26.9%	32.7%
Survey of Patients' Hospital Experiences				
Area Around Room 'Always' Quiet at Night	300+	47%	-	58%
Doctors 'Always' Communicated Well	300+	79%	-	80%
Home Recovery Information Given	300+	87%	-	82%
Hospital Given 9 or 10 on 10 Point Scale	300+	59%	-	67%
Meds 'Always' Explained Before Given	300+	61%	-	60%
Nurses 'Always' Communicated Well	300+	76%	-	76%
Pain 'Always' Well Controlled	300+	68%	-	69%
Room and Bathroom 'Always' Clean	300+	67%	-	71%
Timely Help 'Always' Received	300+	59%	-	64%
Would Definitely Recommend Hospital	300+	62%	-	69%

United Memorial Medical Center

127 North Street Phone: 585-343-6030
Batavia, NY 14020 Fax: 585-344-7345
URL: www.ummc.org
Type: Acute Care Hospitals Emergency Services: Yes
Ownership: Voluntary Non-Profit - Private Beds: 126

Key Personnel:
CEO/President. . . . . Mark C Schoell
Chief of Medical Staff . . . . Jin Yoi Chang, MD
Infection Control . . . . Lorraine Goergen
Operating Room. . . . . Debbie Vick
Quality Assurance . . . . Carole Wujcik
Emergency Room . . . . Esther Natla, RN

Measure	Cases	This Hosp.	State Avg.	U.S. Avg.
Heart Attack Care				
ACE Inhibitor or ARB for LVSD[1]	5	80%	95%	96%
Aspirin at Arrival	26	92%	98%	99%
Aspirin at Discharge[1]	15	93%	98%	98%
Beta Blocker at Discharge[1]	16	100%	98%	98%
Fibrinolytic Medication Timing	0	-	50%	55%
PCI Within 90 Minutes of Arrival	0	-	88%	90%
Smoking Cessation Advice	0	-	100%	99%
Chest Pain/Possible Heart Attack Care				
Aspirin at Arrival	134	99%	96%	95%
Median Time to ECG (minutes)	139	13	11	8
Median Time to Transfer (minutes)[1]	7	127	75	61
Fibrinolytic Medication Timing[1]	13	38%	55%	54%
Heart Failure Care				
ACE Inhibitor or ARB for LVSD	36	94%	94%	94%
Discharge Instructions	114	91%	89%	88%
Evaluation of LVS Function	158	99%	98%	98%
Smoking Cessation Advice[1]	19	68%	98%	98%
Pneumonia Care				
Appropriate Initial Antibiotic	83	93%	92%	92%
Blood Culture Timing	183	89%	95%	96%
Influenza Vaccine	103	93%	90%	91%
Initial Antibiotic Timing	167	98%	93%	95%
Pneumococcal Vaccine	163	93%	92%	93%
Smoking Cessation Advice	59	88%	98%	97%
Surgical Care Improvement Project				
Appropriate VTP Within 24 Hours	150	92%	94%	92%
Appropriate Hair Removal	268	100%	100%	99%
Appropriate Beta Blocker Usage	102	100%	92%	93%
Controlled Postoperative Blood Glucose	0	-	94%	93%
Prophylactic Antibiotic Timing	217	94%	96%	97%
Prophylactic Antibiotic Timing (Outpatient)	60	90%	92%	92%
Prophylactic Antibiotic Selection	215	98%	97%	97%
Prophylactic Antibiotic Select. (Outpatient)	61	84%	93%	94%
Prophylactic Antibiotic Stopped	211	79%	94%	94%
Recommended VTP Ordered	150	95%	96%	94%
Urinary Catheter Removal	68	66%	90%	90%
Children's Asthma Care				
Received Systemic Corticosteroids	-	-	-	100%
Received Home Management Plan	-	-	-	71%
Received Reliever Medication	-	-	-	100%
Use of Medical Imaging				
Combination Abdominal CT Scan	294	0.554	0.141	0.191
Combination Chest CT Scan	175	0.023	0.024	0.054
Follow-up Mammogram/Ultrasound	458	7.0%	9.8%	8.4%
MRI for Low Back Pain[1]	18	27.8%	26.9%	32.7%
Survey of Patients' Hospital Experiences				
Area Around Room 'Always' Quiet at Night	300+	45%	-	58%
Doctors 'Always' Communicated Well	300+	77%	-	80%
Home Recovery Information Given	300+	86%	-	82%
Hospital Given 9 or 10 on 10 Point Scale	300+	60%	-	67%
Meds 'Always' Explained Before Given	300+	63%	-	60%
Nurses 'Always' Communicated Well	300+	78%	-	76%
Pain 'Always' Well Controlled	300+	67%	-	69%
Room and Bathroom 'Always' Clean	300+	68%	-	71%
Timely Help 'Always' Received	300+	63%	-	64%
Would Definitely Recommend Hospital	300+	56%	-	69%

NOTE: Hospital profiles are in alphabetical order by state, then city, then hospital within the city; Rankings exclude hospitals with less than 25 cases except for patient surveys which excludes hospitals with less than 100 cases; (a) 100–299 cases; (1) The number of cases is too small to be sure how well a hospital is performing; (2) The hospital indicated that the data submitted for this measure were based on a sample of cases; (3) Data was collected during a shorter time period (fewer quarters) than the maximum possible time for this measure; (4) Suppressed for one or more quarters by CMS; (5) No data is available from the hospital for this measure; (6) Fewer than 100 patients completed the HCAHPS survey. Use these rates with caution, as the number of surveys may be too low to reliably assess hospital performance; (7) Survey results are based on less than 12 months of data; (8) Survey results are not available for this reporting period; (9) No or very few patients were eligible for the HCAHPS survey. The scores shown, if any, reflect a very small number of surveys; (10) A state average was not calculated because too few hospitals in the state submitted data; (11) There were discrepancies in the data collection process; Please refer to the User's Guide for a full explanation of data.

Bath VA Medical Center

76 Veterans Ave.
Bath, NY 14810
URL: www1.va.gov/visns/visn02/bath.cfm
Type: Acute Care-Veterans Administration
Ownership: Government - Federal

Phone: 607-664-4000
Fax: 607-664-4756
Emergency Services: No
Beds: 440

Key Personnel:
Chief of Medical Staff . . . . Alan Fantuzzo, DO
Quality Assurance . . . . Judy Harris, RN
Radiology. . . . . Richard White
Emergency Room . . . . Anthony Gerbasi, DO
Intensive Care Unit. . . . . Alfred A Bibawy, MD
Patient Relations . . . . Shirley A Pikula, MSN

Measure	Cases	This Hosp.	State Avg.	U.S. Avg.
Heart Attack Care				
ACE Inhibitor or ARB for LVSD[5]	0	-	95%	96%
Aspirin at Arrival[5]	0	-	98%	99%
Aspirin at Discharge[5]	0	-	98%	98%
Beta Blocker at Discharge[5]	0	-	98%	98%
Fibrinolytic Medication Timing[5]	0	-	50%	55%
PCI Within 90 Minutes of Arrival[5]	0	-	88%	90%
Smoking Cessation Advice[5]	0	-	100%	99%
Chest Pain/Possible Heart Attack Care				
Aspirin at Arrival	-	-	96%	95%
Median Time to ECG (minutes)	-	-	11	8
Median Time to Transfer (minutes)	-	-	75	61
Fibrinolytic Medication Timing	-	-	55%	54%
Heart Failure Care				
ACE Inhibitor or ARB for LVSD[1]	7	100%	94%	94%
Discharge Instructions[1]	21	95%	89%	88%
Evaluation of LVS Function[1]	23	100%	98%	98%
Smoking Cessation Advice[1]	5	100%	98%	98%
Pneumonia Care				
Appropriate Initial Antibiotic	41	100%	92%	92%
Blood Culture Timing	71	100%	95%	96%
Influenza Vaccine[1]	24	100%	90%	91%
Initial Antibiotic Timing	56	98%	93%	95%
Pneumococcal Vaccine	41	100%	92%	93%
Smoking Cessation Advice[1]	17	94%	98%	97%
Surgical Care Improvement Project				
Appropriate VTP Within 24 Hours[2,5]	0	-	94%	92%
Appropriate Hair Removal[2,5]	0	-	100%	99%
Appropriate Beta Blocker Usage[2,5]	0	-	92%	93%
Controlled Postoperative Blood Glucose[2,5]	0	-	94%	93%
Prophylactic Antibiotic Timing[5]	-	-	96%	97%
Prophylactic Antibiotic Timing (Outpatient)	-	-	92%	92%
Prophylactic Antibiotic Selection[5]	-	-	97%	97%
Prophylactic Antibiotic Select. (Outpatient)	-	-	93%	94%
Prophylactic Antibiotic Stopped[5]	0	-	94%	94%
Recommended VTP Ordered[2,5]	0	-	96%	94%
Urinary Catheter Removal[2,5]	0	-	90%	90%
Children's Asthma Care				
Received Systemic Corticosteroids	-	-	-	100%
Received Home Management Plan	-	-	-	71%
Received Reliever Medication	-	-	-	100%
Use of Medical Imaging				
Combination Abdominal CT Scan	-	-	0.141	0.191
Combination Chest CT Scan	-	-	0.024	0.054
Follow-up Mammogram/Ultrasound	-	-	9.8%	8.4%
MRI for Low Back Pain	-	-	26.9%	32.7%
Survey of Patients' Hospital Experiences				
Area Around Room 'Always' Quiet at Night	-	-	-	58%
Doctors 'Always' Communicated Well	-	-	-	80%
Home Recovery Information Given	-	-	-	82%
Hospital Given 9 or 10 on 10 Point Scale	-	-	-	67%
Meds 'Always' Explained Before Given	-	-	-	60%
Nurses 'Always' Communicated Well	-	-	-	76%
Pain 'Always' Well Controlled	-	-	-	69%
Room and Bathroom 'Always' Clean	-	-	-	71%
Timely Help 'Always' Received	-	-	-	64%
Would Definitely Recommend Hospital	-	-	-	69%

Ira Davenport Memorial Hospital

7571 State Route 54
Bath, NY 14810
E-mail: prflb@idmh.org
URL: www.davenportandtaylor.org
Type: Acute Care Hospitals
Ownership: Voluntary Non-Profit - Other

Phone: 607-776-8500
Fax: 607-776-8817
Emergency Services: Yes
Beds: 66

Key Personnel:
CEO/President. . . . . James Watson
Radiology. . . . . Wendy Baker

Measure	Cases	This Hosp.	State Avg.	U.S. Avg.
Heart Attack Care				
ACE Inhibitor or ARB for LVSD[1]	2	100%	95%	96%
Aspirin at Arrival[1]	6	100%	98%	99%
Aspirin at Discharge[1]	6	83%	98%	98%
Beta Blocker at Discharge[1]	5	100%	98%	98%
Fibrinolytic Medication Timing	0	-	50%	55%
PCI Within 90 Minutes of Arrival	0	-	88%	90%
Smoking Cessation Advice[1]	2	50%	100%	99%
Chest Pain/Possible Heart Attack Care				
Aspirin at Arrival[1]	19	100%	96%	95%
Median Time to ECG (minutes)[1]	19	14	11	8
Median Time to Transfer (minutes)[5]	0	-	75	61
Fibrinolytic Medication Timing[1,3]	1	100%	55%	54%
Heart Failure Care				
ACE Inhibitor or ARB for LVSD[1]	9	89%	94%	94%
Discharge Instructions[1]	31	100%	89%	88%
Evaluation of LVS Function[1]	38	100%	98%	98%
Smoking Cessation Advice[1]	4	75%	98%	98%
Pneumonia Care				
Appropriate Initial Antibiotic	41	80%	92%	92%
Blood Culture Timing	49	100%	95%	96%
Influenza Vaccine	32	91%	90%	91%
Initial Antibiotic Timing	52	100%	93%	95%
Pneumococcal Vaccine	53	96%	92%	93%
Smoking Cessation Advice[1]	19	95%	98%	97%
Surgical Care Improvement Project				
Appropriate VTP Within 24 Hours[1,3]	3	100%	94%	92%
Appropriate Hair Removal[1,3]	5	100%	100%	99%
Appropriate Beta Blocker Usage[1,3]	2	100%	92%	93%
Controlled Postoperative Blood Glucose[3]	0	-	94%	93%
Prophylactic Antibiotic Timing[1,3]	4	100%	96%	97%
Prophylactic Antibiotic Timing (Outpatient)	25	92%	92%	92%
Prophylactic Antibiotic Selection[1,3]	4	100%	97%	97%
Prophylactic Antibiotic Select. (Outpatient)[1]	23	100%	93%	94%
Prophylactic Antibiotic Stopped[1,3]	4	100%	94%	94%
Recommended VTP Ordered[1,3]	3	100%	96%	94%
Urinary Catheter Removal	0	-	90%	90%
Children's Asthma Care				
Received Systemic Corticosteroids	-	-	-	100%
Received Home Management Plan	-	-	-	71%
Received Reliever Medication	-	-	-	100%
Use of Medical Imaging				
Combination Abdominal CT Scan	162	0.068	0.141	0.191
Combination Chest CT Scan	70	0.000	0.024	0.054
Follow-up Mammogram/Ultrasound	243	4.5%	9.8%	8.4%
MRI for Low Back Pain[1]	24	29.2%	26.9%	32.7%
Survey of Patients' Hospital Experiences				
Area Around Room 'Always' Quiet at Night	(a)	47%	-	58%
Doctors 'Always' Communicated Well	(a)	74%	-	80%
Home Recovery Information Given	(a)	75%	-	82%
Hospital Given 9 or 10 on 10 Point Scale	(a)	46%	-	67%
Meds 'Always' Explained Before Given	(a)	58%	-	60%
Nurses 'Always' Communicated Well	(a)	68%	-	76%
Pain 'Always' Well Controlled	(a)	56%	-	69%
Room and Bathroom 'Always' Clean	(a)	64%	-	71%
Timely Help 'Always' Received	(a)	57%	-	64%
Would Definitely Recommend Hospital	(a)	42%	-	69%

Southside Hospital

301 East Main Street
Bay Shore, NY 11706
URL: www.northshorelij.com
Type: Acute Care Hospitals
Ownership: Voluntary Non-Profit - Private

Phone: 631-968-3000
Fax: 631-968-3315
Emergency Services: Yes
Beds: 377

Key Personnel:
CEO/President. . . . . Michael J Dowling
Chief of Medical Staff . . . . Lawrence G Smith, MD
Coronary Care. . . . . Kathy Mann, RN
Infection Control. . . . . Bruce Farber, MD
Operating Room. . . . . Linda Olander, RN
Pediatric Ambulatory Care . . . . . . James Fagin, MD
Quality Assurance . . . . Donn Haber
Radiology. . . . . Mitchell Goldman, MD

Measure	Cases	This Hosp.	State Avg.	U.S. Avg.
Heart Attack Care				
ACE Inhibitor or ARB for LVSD[1,2]	19	100%	95%	96%
Aspirin at Arrival[2]	187	100%	98%	99%
Aspirin at Discharge[2]	157	100%	98%	98%
Beta Blocker at Discharge[2]	155	100%	98%	98%
Fibrinolytic Medication Timing[1,2]	1	0%	50%	55%
PCI Within 90 Minutes of Arrival[2]	41	93%	88%	90%
Smoking Cessation Advice[2]	50	100%	100%	99%
Chest Pain/Possible Heart Attack Care				
Aspirin at Arrival[1,3]	8	100%	96%	95%
Median Time to ECG (minutes)[1,3]	9	11	11	8
Median Time to Transfer (minutes)[5]	0	-	75	61
Fibrinolytic Medication Timing[3]	0	-	55%	54%
Heart Failure Care				
ACE Inhibitor or ARB for LVSD[2]	90	100%	94%	94%
Discharge Instructions[2]	228	98%	89%	88%
Evaluation of LVS Function[2]	287	100%	98%	98%
Smoking Cessation Advice[2]	47	100%	98%	98%
Pneumonia Care				
Appropriate Initial Antibiotic[2]	104	97%	92%	92%
Blood Culture Timing[2]	139	99%	95%	96%
Influenza Vaccine[2]	84	100%	90%	91%
Initial Antibiotic Timing[2]	160	99%	93%	95%
Pneumococcal Vaccine[2]	125	98%	92%	93%
Smoking Cessation Advice[2]	53	100%	98%	97%
Surgical Care Improvement Project				
Appropriate VTP Within 24 Hours[2]	236	97%	94%	92%
Appropriate Hair Removal[2]	419	100%	100%	99%
Appropriate Beta Blocker Usage[2]	131	99%	92%	93%
Controlled Postoperative Blood Glucose[2]	0	-	94%	93%
Prophylactic Antibiotic Timing[2]	264	98%	96%	97%
Prophylactic Antibiotic Timing (Outpatient)	164	99%	92%	92%
Prophylactic Antibiotic Selection[2]	266	99%	97%	97%
Prophylactic Antibiotic Select. (Outpatient)	163	99%	93%	94%
Prophylactic Antibiotic Stopped[2]	251	98%	94%	94%
Recommended VTP Ordered[2]	236	97%	96%	94%
Urinary Catheter Removal[2]	103	100%	90%	90%
Children's Asthma Care				
Received Systemic Corticosteroids	-	-	-	100%
Received Home Management Plan	-	-	-	71%
Received Reliever Medication	-	-	-	100%
Use of Medical Imaging				
Combination Abdominal CT Scan	443	0.023	0.141	0.191
Combination Chest CT Scan	253	0.004	0.024	0.054
Follow-up Mammogram/Ultrasound	58	36.2%	9.8%	8.4%
MRI for Low Back Pain[1]	30	16.7%	26.9%	32.7%
Survey of Patients' Hospital Experiences				
Area Around Room 'Always' Quiet at Night	300+	49%	-	58%
Doctors 'Always' Communicated Well	300+	77%	-	80%
Home Recovery Information Given	300+	79%	-	82%
Hospital Given 9 or 10 on 10 Point Scale	300+	61%	-	67%
Meds 'Always' Explained Before Given	300+	58%	-	60%
Nurses 'Always' Communicated Well	300+	77%	-	76%
Pain 'Always' Well Controlled	300+	67%	-	69%
Room and Bathroom 'Always' Clean	300+	71%	-	71%
Timely Help 'Always' Received	300+	56%	-	64%
Would Definitely Recommend Hospital	300+	67%	-	69%

Saint Joseph Hospital

4295 Hempstead Turnpike Phone: 516-579-6000
Bethpage, NY 11714 Fax: 516-579-0739
URL: www.newislandhospital.org
Type: Acute Care Hospitals Emergency Services: Yes
Ownership: Voluntary Non-Profit - Private Beds: 223

Key Personnel:

CEO/President. . . . . Aaron E Glatt, MD
Chief of Medical Staff. . . . . Vincent P Anzalone, MD
Coronary Care. . . . . Alan Scheinbach, DO
Infection Control. . . . . Vijay Shah, MD
Operating Room. . . . . Robert Sunshine, MD
Pediatric Ambulatory Care . . . . . . Behved Talebian
Quality Assurance . . . . Kathy Ambrose, RN
Radiology. . . . . Scott J Sherman, MD

Measure	Cases	This Hosp.	State Avg.	U.S. Avg.
Heart Attack Care				
ACE Inhibitor or ARB for LVSD[1]	2	50%	95%	96%
Aspirin at Arrival	47	100%	98%	99%
Aspirin at Discharge[1]	16	100%	98%	98%
Beta Blocker at Discharge[1]	17	100%	98%	98%
Fibrinolytic Medication Timing[1]	1	0%	50%	55%
PCI Within 90 Minutes of Arrival	0	-	88%	90%
Smoking Cessation Advice[1]	1	100%	100%	99%
Chest Pain/Possible Heart Attack Care				
Aspirin at Arrival	138	99%	96%	95%
Median Time to ECG (minutes)	139	7	11	8
Median Time to Transfer (minutes)	51	45	75	61
Fibrinolytic Medication Timing[1]	6	100%	55%	54%
Heart Failure Care				
ACE Inhibitor or ARB for LVSD[2]	34	100%	94%	94%
Discharge Instructions[2]	200	97%	89%	88%
Evaluation of LVS Function[2]	251	100%	98%	98%
Smoking Cessation Advice[1,2]	16	100%	98%	98%
Pneumonia Care				
Appropriate Initial Antibiotic[2]	120	93%	92%	92%
Blood Culture Timing[2]	163	93%	95%	96%
Influenza Vaccine[2]	73	93%	90%	91%
Initial Antibiotic Timing[2]	131	92%	93%	95%
Pneumococcal Vaccine[2]	112	94%	92%	93%
Smoking Cessation Advice[2]	38	100%	98%	97%
Surgical Care Improvement Project				
Appropriate VTP Within 24 Hours[2]	154	88%	94%	92%
Appropriate Hair Removal[2]	262	100%	100%	99%
Appropriate Beta Blocker Usage[2]	85	99%	92%	93%
Controlled Postoperative Blood Glucose[2]	0	-	94%	93%
Prophylactic Antibiotic Timing[2]	162	97%	96%	97%
Prophylactic Antibiotic Timing (Outpatient)	58	91%	92%	92%
Prophylactic Antibiotic Selection[2]	162	96%	97%	97%
Prophylactic Antibiotic Select. (Outpatient)	55	95%	93%	94%
Prophylactic Antibiotic Stopped[2]	152	98%	94%	94%
Recommended VTP Ordered[2]	154	97%	96%	94%
Urinary Catheter Removal[2]	28	86%	90%	90%
Children's Asthma Care				
Received Systemic Corticosteroids	-	-	-	100%
Received Home Management Plan	-	-	-	71%
Received Reliever Medication	-	-	-	100%
Use of Medical Imaging				
Combination Abdominal CT Scan	228	0.022	0.141	0.191
Combination Chest CT Scan	73	0.000	0.024	0.054
Follow-up Mammogram/Ultrasound[1]	13	46.2%	9.8%	8.4%
MRI for Low Back Pain[5]	0	-	26.9%	32.7%
Survey of Patients' Hospital Experiences				
Area Around Room 'Always' Quiet at Night	300+	43%	-	58%
Doctors 'Always' Communicated Well	300+	73%	-	80%
Home Recovery Information Given	300+	80%	-	82%
Hospital Given 9 or 10 on 10 Point Scale	300+	49%	-	67%
Meds 'Always' Explained Before Given	300+	53%	-	60%
Nurses 'Always' Communicated Well	300+	69%	-	76%
Pain 'Always' Well Controlled	300+	65%	-	69%
Room and Bathroom 'Always' Clean	300+	61%	-	71%
Timely Help 'Always' Received	300+	49%	-	64%
Would Definitely Recommend Hospital	300+	54%	-	69%

Our Lady of Lourdes Memorial Hospital

169 Riverside Drive Phone: 607-798-5111
Binghamton, NY 13905 Fax: 607-798-7681
E-mail: info@lourdes.com
URL: www.lourdes.com
Type: Acute Care Hospitals Emergency Services: Yes
Ownership: Voluntary Non-Profit - Private Beds: 161

Key Personnel:

CEO/President. . . . . John O'Neil
Chief of Medical Staff . . . . Robert Taylor III
Operating Room. . . . . Michael W Barrett
Pediatric In-Patient Care . . . . Suzanne Parsons
Quality Assurance . . . . Kathy Connerton
Radiology. . . . . Mike Shevach
Emergency Room . . . . Debra Hackett

Measure	Cases	This Hosp.	State Avg.	U.S. Avg.
Heart Attack Care				
ACE Inhibitor or ARB for LVSD[1]	10	100%	95%	96%
Aspirin at Arrival	101	100%	98%	99%
Aspirin at Discharge	73	100%	98%	98%
Beta Blocker at Discharge	76	99%	98%	98%
Fibrinolytic Medication Timing[1]	1	0%	50%	55%
PCI Within 90 Minutes of Arrival	0	-	88%	90%
Smoking Cessation Advice[1]	7	100%	100%	99%
Chest Pain/Possible Heart Attack Care				
Aspirin at Arrival	42	100%	96%	95%
Median Time to ECG (minutes)	41	6	11	8
Median Time to Transfer (minutes)[1]	15	54	75	61
Fibrinolytic Medication Timing[1]	1	0%	55%	54%
Heart Failure Care				
ACE Inhibitor or ARB for LVSD	55	98%	94%	94%
Discharge Instructions	163	87%	89%	88%
Evaluation of LVS Function	226	98%	98%	98%
Smoking Cessation Advice[1]	24	100%	98%	98%
Pneumonia Care				
Appropriate Initial Antibiotic	200	93%	92%	92%
Blood Culture Timing	383	90%	95%	96%
Influenza Vaccine	222	87%	90%	91%
Initial Antibiotic Timing	330	97%	93%	95%
Pneumococcal Vaccine	335	86%	92%	93%
Smoking Cessation Advice	100	100%	98%	97%
Surgical Care Improvement Project				
Appropriate VTP Within 24 Hours[2]	122	98%	94%	92%
Appropriate Hair Removal[2]	349	100%	100%	99%
Appropriate Beta Blocker Usage[2]	77	100%	92%	93%
Controlled Postoperative Blood Glucose[2]	0	-	94%	93%
Prophylactic Antibiotic Timing[2]	229	95%	96%	97%
Prophylactic Antibiotic Timing (Outpatient)	422	94%	92%	92%
Prophylactic Antibiotic Selection[2]	230	96%	97%	97%
Prophylactic Antibiotic Select. (Outpatient)	452	92%	93%	94%
Prophylactic Antibiotic Stopped[2]	225	97%	94%	94%
Recommended VTP Ordered[2]	122	98%	96%	94%
Urinary Catheter Removal[1,2]	24	100%	90%	90%
Children's Asthma Care				
Received Systemic Corticosteroids	-	-	-	100%
Received Home Management Plan	-	-	-	71%
Received Reliever Medication	-	-	-	100%
Use of Medical Imaging				
Combination Abdominal CT Scan	1,550	0.146	0.141	0.191
Combination Chest CT Scan	1,151	0.094	0.024	0.054
Follow-up Mammogram/Ultrasound	3,113	7.5%	9.8%	8.4%
MRI for Low Back Pain	203	23.6%	26.9%	32.7%
Survey of Patients' Hospital Experiences				
Area Around Room 'Always' Quiet at Night	300+	54%	-	58%
Doctors 'Always' Communicated Well	300+	76%	-	80%
Home Recovery Information Given	300+	86%	-	82%
Hospital Given 9 or 10 on 10 Point Scale	300+	68%	-	67%
Meds 'Always' Explained Before Given	300+	60%	-	60%
Nurses 'Always' Communicated Well	300+	75%	-	76%
Pain 'Always' Well Controlled	300+	67%	-	69%
Room and Bathroom 'Always' Clean	300+	67%	-	71%
Timely Help 'Always' Received	300+	63%	-	64%
Would Definitely Recommend Hospital	300+	74%	-	69%

Lakeside Memorial Hospital

156 West Avenue Phone: 585-637-3131
Brockport, NY 14420 Fax: 585-395-6036
URL: www.lakesidehealth.com
Type: Acute Care Hospitals Emergency Services: Yes
Ownership: Voluntary Non-Profit - Other Beds: 61

Key Personnel:

CEO/President. . . . . Robert W Harris
Radiology. . . . . William R Hampton

Measure	Cases	This Hosp.	State Avg.	U.S. Avg.
Heart Attack Care				
ACE Inhibitor or ARB for LVSD[1]	3	100%	95%	96%
Aspirin at Arrival	28	100%	98%	99%
Aspirin at Discharge[1]	20	100%	98%	98%
Beta Blocker at Discharge[1]	21	100%	98%	98%
Fibrinolytic Medication Timing	0	-	50%	55%
PCI Within 90 Minutes of Arrival	0	-	88%	90%
Smoking Cessation Advice	0	-	100%	99%
Chest Pain/Possible Heart Attack Care				
Aspirin at Arrival	106	95%	96%	95%
Median Time to ECG (minutes)	108	10	11	8
Median Time to Transfer (minutes)[1]	23	81	75	61
Fibrinolytic Medication Timing	0	-	55%	54%
Heart Failure Care				
ACE Inhibitor or ARB for LVSD[1]	22	100%	94%	94%
Discharge Instructions	96	98%	89%	88%
Evaluation of LVS Function	124	98%	98%	98%
Smoking Cessation Advice[1]	11	100%	98%	98%
Pneumonia Care				
Appropriate Initial Antibiotic	98	83%	92%	92%
Blood Culture Timing	143	97%	95%	96%
Influenza Vaccine	83	100%	90%	91%
Initial Antibiotic Timing	148	100%	93%	95%
Pneumococcal Vaccine	123	98%	92%	93%
Smoking Cessation Advice	45	100%	98%	97%
Surgical Care Improvement Project				
Appropriate VTP Within 24 Hours	71	100%	94%	92%
Appropriate Hair Removal	113	100%	100%	99%
Appropriate Beta Blocker Usage	33	97%	92%	93%
Controlled Postoperative Blood Glucose	0	-	94%	93%
Prophylactic Antibiotic Timing	69	100%	96%	97%
Prophylactic Antibiotic Timing (Outpatient)	51	88%	92%	92%
Prophylactic Antibiotic Selection	69	94%	97%	97%
Prophylactic Antibiotic Select. (Outpatient)	45	98%	93%	94%
Prophylactic Antibiotic Stopped	66	88%	94%	94%
Recommended VTP Ordered	71	100%	96%	94%
Urinary Catheter Removal[1]	13	85%	90%	90%
Children's Asthma Care				
Received Systemic Corticosteroids	-	-	-	100%
Received Home Management Plan	-	-	-	71%
Received Reliever Medication	-	-	-	100%
Use of Medical Imaging				
Combination Abdominal CT Scan	202	0.698	0.141	0.191
Combination Chest CT Scan	107	0.047	0.024	0.054
Follow-up Mammogram/Ultrasound	192	15.6%	9.8%	8.4%
MRI for Low Back Pain[1]	34	35.3%	26.9%	32.7%
Survey of Patients' Hospital Experiences				
Area Around Room 'Always' Quiet at Night	300+	51%	-	58%
Doctors 'Always' Communicated Well	300+	78%	-	80%
Home Recovery Information Given	300+	89%	-	82%
Hospital Given 9 or 10 on 10 Point Scale	300+	65%	-	67%
Meds 'Always' Explained Before Given	300+	60%	-	60%
Nurses 'Always' Communicated Well	300+	76%	-	76%
Pain 'Always' Well Controlled	300+	67%	-	69%
Room and Bathroom 'Always' Clean	300+	69%	-	71%
Timely Help 'Always' Received	300+	58%	-	64%
Would Definitely Recommend Hospital	300+	68%	-	69%

NOTE: Hospital profiles are in alphabetical order by state, then city, then hospital within the city; Rankings exclude hospitals with less than 25 cases except for patient surveys which excludes hospitals with less than 100 cases; (a) 100–299 cases; (1) The number of cases is too small to be sure how well a hospital is performing; (2) The hospital indicated that the data submitted for this measure were based on a sample of cases; (3) Data was collected during a shorter time period (fewer quarters) than the maximum possible time for this measure; (4) Suppressed for one or more quarters by CMS; (5) No data is available from the hospital for this measure; (6) Fewer than 100 patients completed the HCAHPS survey. Use these rates with caution, as the number of surveys may be too low to reliably assess hospital performance; (7) Survey results are based on less than 12 months of data; (8) Survey results are not available for this reporting period; (9) No or very few patients were eligible for the HCAHPS survey. The scores shown, if any, reflect a very small number of surveys; (10) A state average was not calculated because too few hospitals in the state submitted data; (11) There were discrepancies in the data collection process; Please refer to the User's Guide for a full explanation of data.

Bronx VA Medical Center

130 West Kingsbridge Road Phone: 718-584-9000
Bronx, NY 10468 Fax: 718-741-4491
URL: www.med.va.gov
Type: Acute Care-Veterans Administration Emergency Services: No
Ownership: Government - Federal Beds: 459

Key Personnel:
Chief of Medical Staff.......... Dr Erik Langnoff
Coronary Care.............. Yvonne Burrus
Infection Control.............. Sheldon Brown
Operating Room.............. Avrora Alconaba
Radiology.................. In Sook Song MD
Anesthesiology.............. Thomas Tagliente
Emergency Room .... Steve Pastores MD
Intensive Care Unit............ R Siegel MD

Measure	Cases	This Hosp.	State Avg.	U.S. Avg.
Heart Attack Care				
ACE Inhibitor or ARB for LVSD[1]	1	100%	95%	96%
Aspirin at Arrival[1]	11	100%	98%	99%
Aspirin at Discharge[1]	5	100%	98%	98%
Beta Blocker at Discharge[1]	5	100%	98%	98%
Fibrinolytic Medication Timing[5]	0	-	50%	55%
PCI Within 90 Minutes of Arrival[5]	0	-	88%	90%
Smoking Cessation Advice[1]	2	100%	100%	99%
Chest Pain/Possible Heart Attack Care				
Aspirin at Arrival	-	-	96%	95%
Median Time to ECG (minutes)	-	-	11	8
Median Time to Transfer (minutes)	-	-	75	61
Fibrinolytic Medication Timing	-	-	55%	54%
Heart Failure Care				
ACE Inhibitor or ARB for LVSD	82	93%	94%	94%
Discharge Instructions	138	99%	89%	88%
Evaluation of LVS Function	149	100%	98%	98%
Smoking Cessation Advice[1]	22	100%	98%	98%
Pneumonia Care				
Appropriate Initial Antibiotic	58	93%	92%	92%
Blood Culture Timing	83	98%	95%	96%
Influenza Vaccine	51	88%	90%	91%
Initial Antibiotic Timing	79	99%	93%	95%
Pneumococcal Vaccine	63	95%	92%	93%
Smoking Cessation Advice	28	100%	98%	97%
Surgical Care Improvement Project				
Appropriate VTP Within 24 Hours[2]	118	99%	94%	92%
Appropriate Hair Removal[2]	151	100%	100%	99%
Appropriate Beta Blocker Usage[2]	41	100%	92%	93%
Controlled Postoperative Blood Glucose[2,5]	0	-	94%	93%
Prophylactic Antibiotic Timing	81	99%	96%	97%
Prophylactic Antibiotic Timing (Outpatient)	-	-	92%	92%
Prophylactic Antibiotic Selection	81	96%	97%	97%
Prophylactic Antibiotic Select. (Outpatient)	-	-	93%	94%
Prophylactic Antibiotic Stopped	79	95%	94%	94%
Recommended VTP Ordered[2]	120	98%	96%	94%
Urinary Catheter Removal[2]	49	100%	90%	90%
Children's Asthma Care				
Received Systemic Corticosteroids	-	-	-	100%
Received Home Management Plan	-	-	-	71%
Received Reliever Medication	-	-	-	100%
Use of Medical Imaging				
Combination Abdominal CT Scan	-	-	0.141	0.191
Combination Chest CT Scan	-	-	0.024	0.054
Follow-up Mammogram/Ultrasound	-	-	9.8%	8.4%
MRI for Low Back Pain	-	-	26.9%	32.7%
Survey of Patients' Hospital Experiences				
Area Around Room 'Always' Quiet at Night	-	-	-	58%
Doctors 'Always' Communicated Well	-	-	-	80%
Home Recovery Information Given	-	-	-	82%
Hospital Given 9 or 10 on 10 Point Scale	-	-	-	67%
Meds 'Always' Explained Before Given	-	-	-	60%
Nurses 'Always' Communicated Well	-	-	-	76%
Pain 'Always' Well Controlled	-	-	-	69%
Room and Bathroom 'Always' Clean	-	-	-	71%
Timely Help 'Always' Received	-	-	-	64%
Would Definitely Recommend Hospital	-	-	-	69%

Bronx-Lebanon Hospital Center

1276 Fulton Avenue Phone: 212-588-7000
Bronx, NY 10456 Fax: 718-299-5447
URL: www.bronx-leb.org
Type: Acute Care Hospitals Emergency Services: Yes
Ownership: Proprietary Beds: 847

Key Personnel:
CEO/President.............. Miguel Fuentes
Cardiac Laboratory........... Jonathan N. Bella MD
Chief of Medical Staff.......... Jonathan Gold MD
Infection Control............. Victor Lorian MD
Operating Room............. John M. Cosgrove MD
Pediatric Ambulatory Care .... Ram Kairam, MD
Pediatric In-Patient Care .... Ram Kairam, MD
Radiology.................. Harvey Stern MD

Measure	Cases	This Hosp.	State Avg.	U.S. Avg.
Heart Attack Care				
ACE Inhibitor or ARB for LVSD[1]	23	100%	95%	96%
Aspirin at Arrival	194	100%	98%	99%
Aspirin at Discharge	137	99%	98%	98%
Beta Blocker at Discharge	124	99%	98%	98%
Fibrinolytic Medication Timing	0	-	50%	55%
PCI Within 90 Minutes of Arrival	33	88%	88%	90%
Smoking Cessation Advice	55	100%	100%	99%
Chest Pain/Possible Heart Attack Care				
Aspirin at Arrival[1,3]	1	100%	96%	95%
Median Time to ECG (minutes)[1,3]	1	1354	11	8
Median Time to Transfer (minutes)[5]	0	-	75	61
Fibrinolytic Medication Timing[5]	0	-	55%	54%
Heart Failure Care				
ACE Inhibitor or ARB for LVSD[2]	159	97%	94%	94%
Discharge Instructions[2]	327	99%	89%	88%
Evaluation of LVS Function[2]	371	99%	98%	98%
Smoking Cessation Advice[2]	80	99%	98%	98%
Pneumonia Care				
Appropriate Initial Antibiotic[2]	121	74%	92%	92%
Blood Culture Timing[2]	139	76%	95%	96%
Influenza Vaccine[2]	92	99%	90%	91%
Initial Antibiotic Timing[2]	233	81%	93%	95%
Pneumococcal Vaccine[2]	128	99%	92%	93%
Smoking Cessation Advice[2]	80	100%	98%	97%
Surgical Care Improvement Project				
Appropriate VTP Within 24 Hours[2]	185	96%	94%	92%
Appropriate Hair Removal[2]	289	100%	100%	99%
Appropriate Beta Blocker Usage[2]	58	53%	92%	93%
Controlled Postoperative Blood Glucose[2]	0	-	94%	93%
Prophylactic Antibiotic Timing[2]	176	91%	96%	97%
Prophylactic Antibiotic Timing (Outpatient)	53	81%	92%	92%
Prophylactic Antibiotic Selection[2]	176	96%	97%	97%
Prophylactic Antibiotic Select. (Outpatient)	46	98%	93%	94%
Prophylactic Antibiotic Stopped[2]	162	90%	94%	94%
Recommended VTP Ordered[2]	185	96%	96%	94%
Urinary Catheter Removal[1,2]	14	57%	90%	90%
Children's Asthma Care				
Received Systemic Corticosteroids	-	-	-	100%
Received Home Management Plan	-	-	-	71%
Received Reliever Medication	-	-	-	100%
Use of Medical Imaging				
Combination Abdominal CT Scan	183	0.279	0.141	0.191
Combination Chest CT Scan	116	0.284	0.024	0.054
Follow-up Mammogram/Ultrasound[1]	4	0.0%	9.8%	8.4%
MRI for Low Back Pain[1]	5	60.0%	26.9%	32.7%
Survey of Patients' Hospital Experiences				
Area Around Room 'Always' Quiet at Night	300+	49%	-	58%
Doctors 'Always' Communicated Well	300+	67%	-	80%
Home Recovery Information Given	300+	70%	-	82%
Hospital Given 9 or 10 on 10 Point Scale	300+	43%	-	67%
Meds 'Always' Explained Before Given	300+	44%	-	60%
Nurses 'Always' Communicated Well	300+	57%	-	76%
Pain 'Always' Well Controlled	300+	50%	-	69%
Room and Bathroom 'Always' Clean	300+	51%	-	71%
Timely Help 'Always' Received	300+	37%	-	64%
Would Definitely Recommend Hospital	300+	44%	-	69%

Jacobi Medical Center

1400 Pelham Parkway South Phone: 718-918-5000
Bronx, NY 10461 Fax: 718-918-4607
URL: www.ci.nyc.ny.us/html/hhc
Type: Acute Care Hospitals Emergency Services: Yes
Ownership: Government - Local Beds: 527

Key Personnel:
CEO/President............... Joseph Orlando
Emergency Room .... Paul Gennis, MD

Measure	Cases	This Hosp.	State Avg.	U.S. Avg.
Heart Attack Care				
ACE Inhibitor or ARB for LVSD[1]	18	94%	95%	96%
Aspirin at Arrival	116	99%	98%	99%
Aspirin at Discharge	70	96%	98%	98%
Beta Blocker at Discharge	64	95%	98%	98%
Fibrinolytic Medication Timing	0	-	50%	55%
PCI Within 90 Minutes of Arrival	0	-	88%	90%
Smoking Cessation Advice[1]	16	100%	100%	99%
Chest Pain/Possible Heart Attack Care				
Aspirin at Arrival[1]	18	100%	96%	95%
Median Time to ECG (minutes)[1]	19	4	11	8
Median Time to Transfer (minutes)[1]	7	85	75	61
Fibrinolytic Medication Timing	0	-	55%	54%
Heart Failure Care				
ACE Inhibitor or ARB for LVSD	93	98%	94%	94%
Discharge Instructions	232	99%	89%	88%
Evaluation of LVS Function	276	99%	98%	98%
Smoking Cessation Advice	64	100%	98%	98%
Pneumonia Care				
Appropriate Initial Antibiotic	86	92%	92%	92%
Blood Culture Timing	174	92%	95%	96%
Influenza Vaccine	120	90%	90%	91%
Initial Antibiotic Timing	186	81%	93%	95%
Pneumococcal Vaccine	133	92%	92%	93%
Smoking Cessation Advice	69	99%	98%	97%
Surgical Care Improvement Project				
Appropriate VTP Within 24 Hours	284	95%	94%	92%
Appropriate Hair Removal	447	98%	100%	99%
Appropriate Beta Blocker Usage	101	95%	92%	93%
Controlled Postoperative Blood Glucose[1]	2	50%	94%	93%
Prophylactic Antibiotic Timing	160	90%	96%	97%
Prophylactic Antibiotic Timing (Outpatient)	31	71%	92%	92%
Prophylactic Antibiotic Selection	159	99%	97%	97%
Prophylactic Antibiotic Select. (Outpatient)	88	97%	93%	94%
Prophylactic Antibiotic Stopped	155	89%	94%	94%
Recommended VTP Ordered	285	96%	96%	94%
Urinary Catheter Removal	67	76%	90%	90%
Children's Asthma Care				
Received Systemic Corticosteroids	-	-	-	100%
Received Home Management Plan	-	-	-	71%
Received Reliever Medication	-	-	-	100%
Use of Medical Imaging				
Combination Abdominal CT Scan	240	0.150	0.141	0.191
Combination Chest CT Scan	164	0.061	0.024	0.054
Follow-up Mammogram/Ultrasound	482	2.7%	9.8%	8.4%
MRI for Low Back Pain[1]	12	33.3%	26.9%	32.7%
Survey of Patients' Hospital Experiences				
Area Around Room 'Always' Quiet at Night	300+	50%	-	58%
Doctors 'Always' Communicated Well	300+	77%	-	80%
Home Recovery Information Given	300+	78%	-	82%
Hospital Given 9 or 10 on 10 Point Scale	300+	55%	-	67%
Meds 'Always' Explained Before Given	300+	49%	-	60%
Nurses 'Always' Communicated Well	300+	64%	-	76%
Pain 'Always' Well Controlled	300+	57%	-	69%
Room and Bathroom 'Always' Clean	300+	65%	-	71%
Timely Help 'Always' Received	300+	50%	-	64%
Would Definitely Recommend Hospital	300+	60%	-	69%

NOTE: Hospital profiles are in alphabetical order by state, then city, then hospital within the city; Rankings exclude hospitals with less than 25 cases except for patient surveys which excludes hospitals with less than 100 cases; (a) 100–299 cases; (1) The number of cases is too small to be sure how well a hospital is performing; (2) The hospital indicated that the data submitted for this measure were based on a sample of cases; (3) Data was collected during a shorter time period (fewer quarters) than the maximum possible time for this measure; (4) Suppressed for one or more quarters by CMS; (5) No data is available from the hospital for this measure; (6) Fewer than 100 patients completed the HCAHPS survey. Use these rates with caution, as the number of surveys may be too low to reliably assess hospital performance; (7) Survey results are based on less than 12 months of data; (8) Survey results are not available for this reporting period; (9) No or very few patients were eligible for the HCAHPS survey. The scores shown, if any, reflect a very small number of surveys; (10) A state average was not calculated because too few hospitals in the state submitted data; (11) There were discrepancies in the data collection process; Please refer to the User's Guide for a full explanation of data.

Lincoln Medical & Mental Health Center

234 East 149th Street
Bronx, NY 10451
Phone: 718-579-5000
Fax: 718-579-5319
Type: Acute Care Hospitals
Emergency Services: Yes
Ownership: Government - Local
Beds: 595

Key Personnel:

- CEO/President. . . . . Roberto Rodriguez
- Chief of Medical Staff. . . . . D Shine, MD
- Infection Control. . . . . D Hewlett, MD
- Operating Room. . . . . Barbara Booker, RN
- Pediatric Ambulatory Care . . . . . R Kairam, MD
- Pediatric In-Patient Care . . . . . . R Kairam, MD
- Quality Assurance . . . . David DeJesus
- Radiology. . . . . Y Fayemi, MD

Measure	Cases	This Hosp.	State Avg.	U.S. Avg.
Heart Attack Care				
ACE Inhibitor or ARB for LVSD[1]	14	100%	95%	96%
Aspirin at Arrival	129	100%	98%	99%
Aspirin at Discharge	63	100%	98%	98%
Beta Blocker at Discharge	64	100%	98%	98%
Fibrinolytic Medication Timing[1]	13	69%	50%	55%
PCI Within 90 Minutes of Arrival	0	-	88%	90%
Smoking Cessation Advice[1]	16	100%	100%	99%
Chest Pain/Possible Heart Attack Care				
Aspirin at Arrival[1]	7	100%	96%	95%
Median Time to ECG (minutes)[1]	7	5	11	8
Median Time to Transfer (minutes)[5]	0	-	75	61
Fibrinolytic Medication Timing[1]	5	100%	55%	54%
Heart Failure Care				
ACE Inhibitor or ARB for LVSD	122	99%	94%	94%
Discharge Instructions	366	100%	89%	88%
Evaluation of LVS Function	396	100%	98%	98%
Smoking Cessation Advice	69	100%	98%	98%
Pneumonia Care				
Appropriate Initial Antibiotic	257	95%	92%	92%
Blood Culture Timing	510	97%	95%	96%
Influenza Vaccine	179	89%	90%	91%
Initial Antibiotic Timing	464	91%	93%	95%
Pneumococcal Vaccine	159	96%	92%	93%
Smoking Cessation Advice	156	100%	98%	97%
Surgical Care Improvement Project				
Appropriate VTP Within 24 Hours[2]	166	98%	94%	92%
Appropriate Hair Removal[2]	276	100%	100%	99%
Appropriate Beta Blocker Usage[2]	54	98%	92%	93%
Controlled Postoperative Blood Glucose[2]	0	-	94%	93%
Prophylactic Antibiotic Timing[2]	133	97%	96%	97%
Prophylactic Antibiotic Timing (Outpatient)	127	88%	92%	92%
Prophylactic Antibiotic Selection[2]	136	99%	97%	97%
Prophylactic Antibiotic Select. (Outpatient)	133	89%	93%	94%
Prophylactic Antibiotic Stopped[2]	128	91%	94%	94%
Recommended VTP Ordered[2]	166	99%	96%	94%
Urinary Catheter Removal[2]	58	83%	90%	90%
Children's Asthma Care				
Received Systemic Corticosteroids	-	-	-	100%
Received Home Management Plan	-	-	-	71%
Received Reliever Medication	-	-	-	100%
Use of Medical Imaging				
Combination Abdominal CT Scan	262	0.095	0.141	0.191
Combination Chest CT Scan	159	0.044	0.024	0.054
Follow-up Mammogram/Ultrasound	176	9.7%	9.8%	8.4%
MRI for Low Back Pain[5]	0	-	26.9%	32.7%
Survey of Patients' Hospital Experiences				
Area Around Room 'Always' Quiet at Night	300+	54%	-	58%
Doctors 'Always' Communicated Well	300+	76%	-	80%
Home Recovery Information Given	300+	73%	-	82%
Hospital Given 9 or 10 on 10 Point Scale	300+	52%	-	67%
Meds 'Always' Explained Before Given	300+	50%	-	60%
Nurses 'Always' Communicated Well	300+	64%	-	76%
Pain 'Always' Well Controlled	300+	53%	-	69%
Room and Bathroom 'Always' Clean	300+	60%	-	71%
Timely Help 'Always' Received	300+	49%	-	64%
Would Definitely Recommend Hospital	300+	53%	-	69%

Montefiore Medical Center

111 East 210th Street
Bronx, NY 10467
Phone: 718-920-4321
Fax: 718-920-2242
URL: www.montefiore.org
Type: Acute Care Hospitals
Emergency Services: Yes
Ownership: Voluntary Non-Profit - Private
Beds: 1,062

Key Personnel:

- CEO/President. . . . . Steven M Safyer MD
- Chief of Medical Staff. . . . . Gary Kalkut MD MPH
- Operating Room. . . . . Arnold Berlin MD
- Pediatric Ambulatory Care . . . . . . Philip O Ozuah MD PhD
- Radiology. . . . . E Stephen Amis MD
- Anesthesiology. . . . . Albert J Saubermann MD
- Hemotology Center . . . . Roman Perez-Soler MD

Measure	Cases	This Hosp.	State Avg.	U.S. Avg.
Heart Attack Care				
ACE Inhibitor or ARB for LVSD[2]	63	71%	95%	96%
Aspirin at Arrival[2]	281	95%	98%	99%
Aspirin at Discharge[2]	373	96%	98%	98%
Beta Blocker at Discharge[2]	366	96%	98%	98%
Fibrinolytic Medication Timing[2]	0	-	50%	55%
PCI Within 90 Minutes of Arrival[2]	51	84%	88%	90%
Smoking Cessation Advice[2]	116	99%	100%	99%
Chest Pain/Possible Heart Attack Care				
Aspirin at Arrival[1,3]	2	100%	96%	95%
Median Time to ECG (minutes)[1,3]	2	10	11	8
Median Time to Transfer (minutes)[5]	0	-	75	61
Fibrinolytic Medication Timing[5]	0	-	55%	54%
Heart Failure Care				
ACE Inhibitor or ARB for LVSD[2]	251	81%	94%	94%
Discharge Instructions[2]	544	86%	89%	88%
Evaluation of LVS Function[2]	679	98%	98%	98%
Smoking Cessation Advice[2]	103	100%	98%	98%
Pneumonia Care				
Appropriate Initial Antibiotic[2]	190	81%	92%	92%
Blood Culture Timing[2]	374	82%	95%	96%
Influenza Vaccine[2]	232	77%	90%	91%
Initial Antibiotic Timing[2]	413	79%	93%	95%
Pneumococcal Vaccine[2]	340	89%	92%	93%
Smoking Cessation Advice[2]	91	100%	98%	97%
Surgical Care Improvement Project				
Appropriate VTP Within 24 Hours[2]	411	88%	94%	92%
Appropriate Hair Removal[2]	1,163	96%	100%	99%
Appropriate Beta Blocker Usage[2]	415	77%	92%	93%
Controlled Postoperative Blood Glucose[2]	212	83%	94%	93%
Prophylactic Antibiotic Timing[2]	750	85%	96%	97%
Prophylactic Antibiotic Timing (Outpatient)	681	73%	92%	92%
Prophylactic Antibiotic Selection[2]	749	97%	97%	97%
Prophylactic Antibiotic Select. (Outpatient)	624	66%	93%	94%
Prophylactic Antibiotic Stopped[2]	711	90%	94%	94%
Recommended VTP Ordered[2]	416	91%	96%	94%
Urinary Catheter Removal[2]	210	76%	90%	90%
Children's Asthma Care				
Received Systemic Corticosteroids	-	-	-	100%
Received Home Management Plan	-	-	-	71%
Received Reliever Medication	-	-	-	100%
Use of Medical Imaging				
Combination Abdominal CT Scan	1,769	0.070	0.141	0.191
Combination Chest CT Scan	1,222	0.013	0.024	0.054
Follow-up Mammogram/Ultrasound	2,215	3.7%	9.8%	8.4%
MRI for Low Back Pain	120	29.2%	26.9%	32.7%
Survey of Patients' Hospital Experiences				
Area Around Room 'Always' Quiet at Night	300+	54%	-	58%
Doctors 'Always' Communicated Well	300+	77%	-	80%
Home Recovery Information Given	300+	76%	-	82%
Hospital Given 9 or 10 on 10 Point Scale	300+	59%	-	67%
Meds 'Always' Explained Before Given	300+	57%	-	60%
Nurses 'Always' Communicated Well	300+	72%	-	76%
Pain 'Always' Well Controlled	300+	63%	-	69%
Room and Bathroom 'Always' Clean	300+	68%	-	71%
Timely Help 'Always' Received	300+	48%	-	64%
Would Definitely Recommend Hospital	300+	67%	-	69%

New York Westchester Square Medical Center

2475 St Raymond Avenue
Bronx, NY 10461
Phone: 718-430-7300
Fax: 718-518-7838
E-mail: contactus@nywsmc.org
URL: www.nywsmc.org
Type: Acute Care Hospitals
Emergency Services: Yes
Ownership: Voluntary Non-Profit - Private
Beds: 205

Key Personnel:

- CEO/President. . . . . Alan Kopman
- Chief of Medical Staff . . . . Rudolph Nisi, MD
- Operating Room. . . . . Albert Adu, RN
- Quality Assurance . . . . Henry Molinari, MD
- Radiology. . . . . Jack Baldassare, MD
- Emergency Room . . . . Theresa Mandarino, RN

Measure	Cases	This Hosp.	State Avg.	U.S. Avg.
Heart Attack Care				
ACE Inhibitor or ARB for LVSD[1]	3	100%	95%	96%
Aspirin at Arrival	43	100%	98%	99%
Aspirin at Discharge[1]	14	100%	98%	98%
Beta Blocker at Discharge[1]	20	95%	98%	98%
Fibrinolytic Medication Timing	0	-	50%	55%
PCI Within 90 Minutes of Arrival	0	-	88%	90%
Smoking Cessation Advice[1]	1	100%	100%	99%
Chest Pain/Possible Heart Attack Care				
Aspirin at Arrival	32	100%	96%	95%
Median Time to ECG (minutes)	32	13	11	8
Median Time to Transfer (minutes)[1,3]	1	353	75	61
Fibrinolytic Medication Timing[1]	5	40%	55%	54%
Heart Failure Care				
ACE Inhibitor or ARB for LVSD	54	100%	94%	94%
Discharge Instructions	159	80%	89%	88%
Evaluation of LVS Function	257	100%	98%	98%
Smoking Cessation Advice	33	100%	98%	98%
Pneumonia Care				
Appropriate Initial Antibiotic	114	93%	92%	92%
Blood Culture Timing	236	98%	95%	96%
Influenza Vaccine	108	96%	90%	91%
Initial Antibiotic Timing	229	99%	93%	95%
Pneumococcal Vaccine	187	95%	92%	93%
Smoking Cessation Advice	40	100%	98%	97%
Surgical Care Improvement Project				
Appropriate VTP Within 24 Hours	200	98%	94%	92%
Appropriate Hair Removal	321	100%	100%	99%
Appropriate Beta Blocker Usage	53	98%	92%	93%
Controlled Postoperative Blood Glucose	0	-	94%	93%
Prophylactic Antibiotic Timing	189	98%	96%	97%
Prophylactic Antibiotic Timing (Outpatient)	81	96%	92%	92%
Prophylactic Antibiotic Selection	190	98%	97%	97%
Prophylactic Antibiotic Select. (Outpatient)	79	96%	93%	94%
Prophylactic Antibiotic Stopped	186	90%	94%	94%
Recommended VTP Ordered	200	99%	96%	94%
Urinary Catheter Removal	78	65%	90%	90%
Children's Asthma Care				
Received Systemic Corticosteroids	-	-	-	100%
Received Home Management Plan	-	-	-	71%
Received Reliever Medication	-	-	-	100%
Use of Medical Imaging				
Combination Abdominal CT Scan	47	0.000	0.141	0.191
Combination Chest CT Scan[1]	3	0.000	0.024	0.054
Follow-up Mammogram/Ultrasound	108	50.9%	9.8%	8.4%
MRI for Low Back Pain[5]	0	-	26.9%	32.7%
Survey of Patients' Hospital Experiences				
Area Around Room 'Always' Quiet at Night[7]	(a)	61%	-	58%
Doctors 'Always' Communicated Well[7]	(a)	74%	-	80%
Home Recovery Information Given[7]	(a)	74%	-	82%
Hospital Given 9 or 10 on 10 Point Scale[7]	(a)	50%	-	67%
Meds 'Always' Explained Before Given[7]	(a)	39%	-	60%
Nurses 'Always' Communicated Well[7]	(a)	68%	-	76%
Pain 'Always' Well Controlled[7]	(a)	66%	-	69%
Room and Bathroom 'Always' Clean[7]	(a)	74%	-	71%
Timely Help 'Always' Received[7]	(a)	59%	-	64%
Would Definitely Recommend Hospital[7]	(a)	64%	-	69%

NOTE: Hospital profiles are in alphabetical order by state, then city, then hospital within the city; Rankings exclude hospitals with less than 25 cases except for patient surveys which excludes hospitals with less than 100 cases; (a) 100–299 cases; (1) The number of cases is too small to be sure how well a hospital is performing; (2) The hospital indicated that the data submitted for this measure were based on a sample of cases; (3) Data was collected during a shorter time period (fewer quarters) than the maximum possible time for this measure; (4) Suppressed for one or more quarters by CMS; (5) No data is available from the hospital for this measure; (6) Fewer than 100 patients completed the HCAHPS survey. Use these rates with caution, as the number of surveys may be too low to reliably assess hospital performance; (7) Survey results are based on less than 12 months of data; (8) Survey results are not available for this reporting period; (9) No or very few patients were eligible for the HCAHPS survey. The scores shown, if any, reflect a very small number of surveys; (10) A state average was not calculated because too few hospitals in the state submitted data; (11) There were discrepancies in the data collection process; Please refer to the User's Guide for a full explanation of data.

North Central Bronx Hospital

3424 Kossuth Avenue & 210th Street Phone: 212-519-5000
Bronx, NY 10467
URL: www.nyc.gov/html/hhc/ncbh/home.html
Type: Acute Care Hospitals Emergency Services: Yes
Ownership: Government - Local Beds: 202

Measure	Cases	This Hosp.	State Avg.	U.S. Avg.
Heart Attack Care				
ACE Inhibitor or ARB for LVSD[1]	7	100%	95%	96%
Aspirin at Arrival	39	97%	98%	99%
Aspirin at Discharge[1]	20	100%	98%	98%
Beta Blocker at Discharge[1]	19	100%	98%	98%
Fibrinolytic Medication Timing	0	-	50%	55%
PCI Within 90 Minutes of Arrival	0	-	88%	90%
Smoking Cessation Advice[1]	7	100%	100%	99%
Chest Pain/Possible Heart Attack Care				
Aspirin at Arrival[1,3]	8	100%	96%	95%
Median Time to ECG (minutes)[1,3]	7	6	11	8
Median Time to Transfer (minutes)[1,3]	4	67	75	61
Fibrinolytic Medication Timing[3]	0	-	55%	54%
Heart Failure Care				
ACE Inhibitor or ARB for LVSD	61	98%	94%	94%
Discharge Instructions	131	99%	89%	88%
Evaluation of LVS Function	139	100%	98%	98%
Smoking Cessation Advice	40	100%	98%	98%
Pneumonia Care				
Appropriate Initial Antibiotic	55	98%	92%	92%
Blood Culture Timing	97	97%	95%	96%
Influenza Vaccine	49	65%	90%	91%
Initial Antibiotic Timing	95	98%	93%	95%
Pneumococcal Vaccine	37	89%	92%	93%
Smoking Cessation Advice	35	97%	98%	97%
Surgical Care Improvement Project				
Appropriate VTP Within 24 Hours	30	83%	94%	92%
Appropriate Hair Removal	72	96%	100%	99%
Appropriate Beta Blocker Usage[1]	6	100%	92%	93%
Controlled Postoperative Blood Glucose	0	-	94%	93%
Prophylactic Antibiotic Timing	35	94%	96%	97%
Prophylactic Antibiotic Timing (Outpatient)[1]	13	69%	92%	92%
Prophylactic Antibiotic Selection	34	85%	97%	97%
Prophylactic Antibiotic Select. (Outpatient)[1]	24	100%	93%	94%
Prophylactic Antibiotic Stopped	34	76%	94%	94%
Recommended VTP Ordered	30	87%	96%	94%
Urinary Catheter Removal[1]	4	25%	90%	90%
Children's Asthma Care				
Received Systemic Corticosteroids	-	-	-	100%
Received Home Management Plan	-	-	-	71%
Received Reliever Medication	-	-	-	100%
Use of Medical Imaging				
Combination Abdominal CT Scan[1]	49	0.102	0.141	0.191
Combination Chest CT Scan[1]	34	0.059	0.024	0.054
Follow-up Mammogram/Ultrasound	220	1.4%	9.8%	8.4%
MRI for Low Back Pain[1]	4	50.0%	26.9%	32.7%
Survey of Patients' Hospital Experiences				
Area Around Room 'Always' Quiet at Night	300+	58%	-	58%
Doctors 'Always' Communicated Well	300+	77%	-	80%
Home Recovery Information Given	300+	76%	-	82%
Hospital Given 9 or 10 on 10 Point Scale	300+	62%	-	67%
Meds 'Always' Explained Before Given	300+	58%	-	60%
Nurses 'Always' Communicated Well	300+	66%	-	76%
Pain 'Always' Well Controlled	300+	63%	-	69%
Room and Bathroom 'Always' Clean	300+	60%	-	71%
Timely Help 'Always' Received	300+	49%	-	64%
Would Definitely Recommend Hospital	300+	63%	-	69%

Saint Barnabas Hospital

4422 Third Avenue Phone: 212-960-9000
Bronx, NY 10457 Fax: 718-960-6615
URL: www.stbarnabashospital.org
Type: Acute Care Hospitals Emergency Services: Yes
Ownership: Voluntary Non-Profit - Private Beds: 461

Key Personnel:
CEO/President. . . . . Scott Cooper, MD
Chief of Medical Staff. . . . . Jerry Balentine
Infection Control. . . . . Judith Berger, MD
Operating Room. . . . . Stephen Di Russo, MD
Pediatric In-Patient Care . . . . David Rubin, MD
Quality Assurance . . . . Toni Armada
Radiology. . . . . Rocco Ducchille, MD

Measure	Cases	This Hosp.	State Avg.	U.S. Avg.
Heart Attack Care				
ACE Inhibitor or ARB for LVSD[1]	8	88%	95%	96%
Aspirin at Arrival	66	98%	98%	99%
Aspirin at Discharge	34	100%	98%	98%
Beta Blocker at Discharge	34	94%	98%	98%
Fibrinolytic Medication Timing	0	-	50%	55%
PCI Within 90 Minutes of Arrival	0	-	88%	90%
Smoking Cessation Advice[1]	9	100%	100%	99%
Chest Pain/Possible Heart Attack Care				
Aspirin at Arrival[5]	0	-	96%	95%
Median Time to ECG (minutes)[5]	0	-	11	8
Median Time to Transfer (minutes)[5]	0	-	75	61
Fibrinolytic Medication Timing[5]	0	-	55%	54%
Heart Failure Care				
ACE Inhibitor or ARB for LVSD	175	97%	94%	94%
Discharge Instructions	324	93%	89%	88%
Evaluation of LVS Function	354	100%	98%	98%
Smoking Cessation Advice	123	99%	98%	98%
Pneumonia Care				
Appropriate Initial Antibiotic	150	97%	92%	92%
Blood Culture Timing	261	95%	95%	96%
Influenza Vaccine	125	83%	90%	91%
Initial Antibiotic Timing	214	95%	93%	95%
Pneumococcal Vaccine	122	95%	92%	93%
Smoking Cessation Advice	110	97%	98%	97%
Surgical Care Improvement Project				
Appropriate VTP Within 24 Hours[2]	132	95%	94%	92%
Appropriate Hair Removal[2]	196	99%	100%	99%
Appropriate Beta Blocker Usage[2]	40	95%	92%	93%
Controlled Postoperative Blood Glucose[2]	0	-	94%	93%
Prophylactic Antibiotic Timing[2]	100	94%	96%	97%
Prophylactic Antibiotic Timing (Outpatient)	139	87%	92%	92%
Prophylactic Antibiotic Selection[2]	98	96%	97%	97%
Prophylactic Antibiotic Select. (Outpatient)	155	95%	93%	94%
Prophylactic Antibiotic Stopped[2]	91	88%	94%	94%
Recommended VTP Ordered[2]	132	97%	96%	94%
Urinary Catheter Removal[1,2]	17	94%	90%	90%
Children's Asthma Care				
Received Systemic Corticosteroids	-	-	-	100%
Received Home Management Plan	-	-	-	71%
Received Reliever Medication	-	-	-	100%
Use of Medical Imaging				
Combination Abdominal CT Scan	167	0.036	0.141	0.191
Combination Chest CT Scan	74	0.014	0.024	0.054
Follow-up Mammogram/Ultrasound	133	6.0%	9.8%	8.4%
MRI for Low Back Pain[1]	9	55.6%	26.9%	32.7%
Survey of Patients' Hospital Experiences				
Area Around Room 'Always' Quiet at Night	300+	50%	-	58%
Doctors 'Always' Communicated Well	300+	75%	-	80%
Home Recovery Information Given	300+	70%	-	82%
Hospital Given 9 or 10 on 10 Point Scale	300+	42%	-	67%
Meds 'Always' Explained Before Given	300+	47%	-	60%
Nurses 'Always' Communicated Well	300+	61%	-	76%
Pain 'Always' Well Controlled	300+	54%	-	69%
Room and Bathroom 'Always' Clean	300+	63%	-	71%
Timely Help 'Always' Received	300+	42%	-	64%
Would Definitely Recommend Hospital	300+	49%	-	69%

Lawrence Hospital Center

55 Palmer Avenue Phone: 914-787-1000
Bronxville, NY 10708 Fax: 914-787-5154
URL: www.lawrencehealth.org
Type: Acute Care Hospitals Emergency Services: Yes
Ownership: Voluntary Non-Profit - Other Beds: 281

Key Personnel:
CEO/President. . . . . Edward Mdinan
Pediatric In-Patient Care . . . . M Levitt, MD
Quality Assurance . . . . Diane Lango
Radiology. . . . . Louis Perez, MD
Emergency Room . . . . Nicholas Crimarco, RN

Measure	Cases	This Hosp.	State Avg.	U.S. Avg.
Heart Attack Care				
ACE Inhibitor or ARB for LVSD[1]	5	100%	95%	96%
Aspirin at Arrival	38	95%	98%	99%
Aspirin at Discharge[1]	14	86%	98%	98%
Beta Blocker at Discharge[1]	19	95%	98%	98%
Fibrinolytic Medication Timing[1]	2	0%	50%	55%
PCI Within 90 Minutes of Arrival	0	-	88%	90%
Smoking Cessation Advice[1]	2	100%	100%	99%
Chest Pain/Possible Heart Attack Care				
Aspirin at Arrival	55	96%	96%	95%
Median Time to ECG (minutes)	59	17	11	8
Median Time to Transfer (minutes)[1]	3	82	75	61
Fibrinolytic Medication Timing[1]	20	35%	55%	54%
Heart Failure Care				
ACE Inhibitor or ARB for LVSD[2]	77	99%	94%	94%
Discharge Instructions[2]	195	98%	89%	88%
Evaluation of LVS Function[2]	256	99%	98%	98%
Smoking Cessation Advice[1,2]	9	89%	98%	98%
Pneumonia Care				
Appropriate Initial Antibiotic[2]	105	93%	92%	92%
Blood Culture Timing[2]	88	97%	95%	96%
Influenza Vaccine[2]	96	93%	90%	91%
Initial Antibiotic Timing[2]	163	91%	93%	95%
Pneumococcal Vaccine[2]	160	96%	92%	93%
Smoking Cessation Advice[2]	28	100%	98%	97%
Surgical Care Improvement Project				
Appropriate VTP Within 24 Hours[2]	141	86%	94%	92%
Appropriate Hair Removal[2]	295	100%	100%	99%
Appropriate Beta Blocker Usage[2]	77	92%	92%	93%
Controlled Postoperative Blood Glucose[2]	0	-	94%	93%
Prophylactic Antibiotic Timing[2]	183	97%	96%	97%
Prophylactic Antibiotic Timing (Outpatient)	110	95%	92%	92%
Prophylactic Antibiotic Selection[2]	184	98%	97%	97%
Prophylactic Antibiotic Select. (Outpatient)	106	91%	93%	94%
Prophylactic Antibiotic Stopped[2]	180	80%	94%	94%
Recommended VTP Ordered[2]	142	89%	96%	94%
Urinary Catheter Removal[2]	42	86%	90%	90%
Children's Asthma Care				
Received Systemic Corticosteroids	-	-	-	100%
Received Home Management Plan	-	-	-	71%
Received Reliever Medication	-	-	-	100%
Use of Medical Imaging				
Combination Abdominal CT Scan	584	0.108	0.141	0.191
Combination Chest CT Scan	476	0.017	0.024	0.054
Follow-up Mammogram/Ultrasound	642	13.2%	9.8%	8.4%
MRI for Low Back Pain	139	23.7%	26.9%	32.7%
Survey of Patients' Hospital Experiences				
Area Around Room 'Always' Quiet at Night	300+	59%	-	58%
Doctors 'Always' Communicated Well	300+	80%	-	80%
Home Recovery Information Given	300+	73%	-	82%
Hospital Given 9 or 10 on 10 Point Scale	300+	66%	-	67%
Meds 'Always' Explained Before Given	300+	59%	-	60%
Nurses 'Always' Communicated Well	300+	75%	-	76%
Pain 'Always' Well Controlled	300+	69%	-	69%
Room and Bathroom 'Always' Clean	300+	71%	-	71%
Timely Help 'Always' Received	300+	60%	-	64%
Would Definitely Recommend Hospital	300+	74%	-	69%

NOTE: Hospital profiles are in alphabetical order by state, then city, then hospital within the city; Rankings exclude hospitals with less than 25 cases except for patient surveys which excludes hospitals with less than 100 cases; (a) 100–299 cases; (1) The number of cases is too small to be sure how well a hospital is performing; (2) The hospital indicated that the data submitted for this measure were based on a sample of cases; (3) Data was collected during a shorter time period (fewer quarters) than the maximum possible time for this measure; (4) Suppressed for one or more quarters by CMS; (5) No data is available from the hospital for this measure; (6) Fewer than 100 patients completed the HCAHPS survey. Use these rates with caution, as the number of surveys may be too low to reliably assess hospital performance; (7) Survey results are based on less than 12 months of data; (8) Survey results are not available for this reporting period; (9) No or very few patients were eligible for the HCAHPS survey. The scores shown, if any, reflect a very small number of surveys; (10) A state average was not calculated because too few hospitals in the state submitted data; (11) There were discrepancies in the data collection process; Please refer to the User's Guide for a full explanation of data.

Brookdale Hospital Medical Center

Linden Boulevard at Brookdale Plaza
Brooklyn, NY 11212
E-mail: info@brookdale.edu
URL: www.brookdalehospital.org
Type: Acute Care Hospitals
Ownership: Govt - Hospital Dist/Auth

Phone: 718-240-5966
Fax: 718-240-6496

Emergency Services: Yes
Beds: 529

Key Personnel:
CEO/President . . . . David P Rosen
Chief of Medical Staff . . . . Richard J Fogler, MD
Coronary Care . . . . Trevor Grazette, RN
Infection Control . . . . Linda Jendresky
Operating Room . . . . Socorro Lucas, RN
Pediatric Ambulatory Care . . . . . Myron Sokal, MD
Quality Assurance . . . . Louise Falet, RN
Radiology . . . . I Akiva Wulkan, MD

Measure	Cases	This Hosp.	State Avg.	U.S. Avg.
Heart Attack Care				
ACE Inhibitor or ARB for LVSD	40	100%	95%	96%
Aspirin at Arrival	245	99%	98%	99%
Aspirin at Discharge	185	99%	98%	98%
Beta Blocker at Discharge	187	99%	98%	98%
Fibrinolytic Medication Timing	0	-	50%	55%
PCI Within 90 Minutes of Arrival	36	81%	88%	90%
Smoking Cessation Advice	53	98%	100%	99%
Chest Pain/Possible Heart Attack Care				
Aspirin at Arrival[5]	0	-	96%	95%
Median Time to ECG (minutes)[5]	0	-	11	8
Median Time to Transfer (minutes)[5]	0	-	75	61
Fibrinolytic Medication Timing[5]	0	-	55%	54%
Heart Failure Care				
ACE Inhibitor or ARB for LVSD[2]	126	96%	94%	94%
Discharge Instructions[2]	286	93%	89%	88%
Evaluation of LVS Function[2]	327	99%	98%	98%
Smoking Cessation Advice[2]	61	97%	98%	98%
Pneumonia Care				
Appropriate Initial Antibiotic[2]	79	91%	92%	92%
Blood Culture Timing[2]	178	90%	95%	96%
Influenza Vaccine[2]	70	79%	90%	91%
Initial Antibiotic Timing[2]	161	91%	93%	95%
Pneumococcal Vaccine[2]	85	78%	92%	93%
Smoking Cessation Advice[2]	69	97%	98%	97%
Surgical Care Improvement Project				
Appropriate VTP Within 24 Hours[2]	189	87%	94%	92%
Appropriate Hair Removal[2]	308	99%	100%	99%
Appropriate Beta Blocker Usage[2]	71	86%	92%	93%
Controlled Postoperative Blood Glucose[2]	0	-	94%	93%
Prophylactic Antibiotic Timing[2]	111	91%	96%	97%
Prophylactic Antibiotic Timing (Outpatient)	157	76%	92%	92%
Prophylactic Antibiotic Selection[2]	109	95%	97%	97%
Prophylactic Antibiotic Select. (Outpatient)	135	79%	93%	94%
Prophylactic Antibiotic Stopped[2]	107	70%	94%	94%
Recommended VTP Ordered[2]	189	87%	96%	94%
Urinary Catheter Removal[2]	33	42%	90%	90%
Children's Asthma Care				
Received Systemic Corticosteroids	-	-	-	100%
Received Home Management Plan	-	-	-	71%
Received Reliever Medication	-	-	-	100%
Use of Medical Imaging				
Combination Abdominal CT Scan	226	0.071	0.141	0.191
Combination Chest CT Scan	117	0.000	0.024	0.054
Follow-up Mammogram/Ultrasound	318	4.1%	9.8%	8.4%
MRI for Low Back Pain[1]	20	40.0%	26.9%	32.7%
Survey of Patients' Hospital Experiences				
Area Around Room 'Always' Quiet at Night	300+	45%	-	58%
Doctors 'Always' Communicated Well	300+	67%	-	80%
Home Recovery Information Given	300+	66%	-	82%
Hospital Given 9 or 10 on 10 Point Scale	300+	37%	-	67%
Meds 'Always' Explained Before Given	300+	50%	-	60%
Nurses 'Always' Communicated Well	300+	57%	-	76%
Pain 'Always' Well Controlled	300+	45%	-	69%
Room and Bathroom 'Always' Clean	300+	60%	-	71%
Timely Help 'Always' Received	300+	36%	-	64%
Would Definitely Recommend Hospital	300+	37%	-	69%

Brooklyn Hospital Center at Downtown Campus

121 Dekalb Avenue
Brooklyn, NY 11201
URL: www.tbh.org
Type: Acute Care Hospitals
Ownership: Voluntary Non-Profit - Private

Phone: 718-250-8000
Fax: 718-260-2730

Emergency Services: Yes
Beds: 416

Key Personnel:
CEO/President . . . . Richard Becker
Chief of Medical Staff . . . . Vincent Tricomi, MD
Infection Control . . . . Anne Goonan
Pediatric In-Patient Care . . . . . . Michael LaCorte, MD
Quality Assurance . . . . Robert Rosati
Radiology . . . . Mohsen Samii, MD
Intensive Care Unit . . . . Reynaldo Rivera
Patient Relations . . . . Suzanne Nicolettie-Kras

Measure	Cases	This Hosp.	State Avg.	U.S. Avg.
Heart Attack Care				
ACE Inhibitor or ARB for LVSD[1]	9	89%	95%	96%
Aspirin at Arrival	120	97%	98%	99%
Aspirin at Discharge	45	100%	98%	98%
Beta Blocker at Discharge	50	96%	98%	98%
Fibrinolytic Medication Timing	0	-	50%	55%
PCI Within 90 Minutes of Arrival	0	-	88%	90%
Smoking Cessation Advice[1]	2	100%	100%	99%
Chest Pain/Possible Heart Attack Care				
Aspirin at Arrival	26	100%	96%	95%
Median Time to ECG (minutes)[1]	23	31	11	8
Median Time to Transfer (minutes)[1,3]	3	208	75	61
Fibrinolytic Medication Timing	0	-	55%	54%
Heart Failure Care				
ACE Inhibitor or ARB for LVSD	145	96%	94%	94%
Discharge Instructions	361	91%	89%	88%
Evaluation of LVS Function	426	98%	98%	98%
Smoking Cessation Advice	61	100%	98%	98%
Pneumonia Care				
Appropriate Initial Antibiotic	96	98%	92%	92%
Blood Culture Timing	303	89%	95%	96%
Influenza Vaccine	149	80%	90%	91%
Initial Antibiotic Timing	305	92%	93%	95%
Pneumococcal Vaccine	201	82%	92%	93%
Smoking Cessation Advice	62	100%	98%	97%
Surgical Care Improvement Project				
Appropriate VTP Within 24 Hours	254	87%	94%	92%
Appropriate Hair Removal	438	99%	100%	99%
Appropriate Beta Blocker Usage	107	89%	92%	93%
Controlled Postoperative Blood Glucose	0	-	94%	93%
Prophylactic Antibiotic Timing	178	87%	96%	97%
Prophylactic Antibiotic Timing (Outpatient)	164	51%	92%	92%
Prophylactic Antibiotic Selection	179	94%	97%	97%
Prophylactic Antibiotic Select. (Outpatient)	179	84%	93%	94%
Prophylactic Antibiotic Stopped	164	72%	94%	94%
Recommended VTP Ordered	254	87%	96%	94%
Urinary Catheter Removal	52	83%	90%	90%
Children's Asthma Care				
Received Systemic Corticosteroids	-	-	-	100%
Received Home Management Plan	-	-	-	71%
Received Reliever Medication	-	-	-	100%
Use of Medical Imaging				
Combination Abdominal CT Scan	307	0.195	0.141	0.191
Combination Chest CT Scan	214	0.019	0.024	0.054
Follow-up Mammogram/Ultrasound	286	5.6%	9.8%	8.4%
MRI for Low Back Pain[1]	34	14.7%	26.9%	32.7%
Survey of Patients' Hospital Experiences				
Area Around Room 'Always' Quiet at Night	300+	46%	-	58%
Doctors 'Always' Communicated Well	300+	72%	-	80%
Home Recovery Information Given	300+	64%	-	82%
Hospital Given 9 or 10 on 10 Point Scale	300+	48%	-	67%
Meds 'Always' Explained Before Given	300+	49%	-	60%
Nurses 'Always' Communicated Well	300+	63%	-	76%
Pain 'Always' Well Controlled	300+	61%	-	69%
Room and Bathroom 'Always' Clean	300+	61%	-	71%
Timely Help 'Always' Received	300+	39%	-	64%
Would Definitely Recommend Hospital	300+	50%	-	69%

Coney Island Hospital

2601 Ocean Parkway
Brooklyn, NY 11235
Type: Acute Care Hospitals
Ownership: Government - Local

Phone: 718-616-3000
Fax: 718-616-4448
Emergency Services: Yes
Beds: 450

Key Personnel:
CEO/President . . . . Arthur Wagner, CEO
Chief of Medical Staff . . . . Sandor Friedman, MD
Coronary Care . . . . Jennifer Mitchener, RN
Infection Control . . . . Rose Recco, MD
Pediatric Ambulatory Care . . . . . Warren Seigel, MD
Pediatric In-Patient Care . . . . . . Warren Seigel, MD
Quality Assurance . . . . Betsy Lograno
Radiology . . . . B Khurana, MD

Measure	Cases	This Hosp.	State Avg.	U.S. Avg.
Heart Attack Care				
ACE Inhibitor or ARB for LVSD[1]	17	94%	95%	96%
Aspirin at Arrival	115	99%	98%	99%
Aspirin at Discharge	60	100%	98%	98%
Beta Blocker at Discharge	62	98%	98%	98%
Fibrinolytic Medication Timing[1]	14	50%	50%	55%
PCI Within 90 Minutes of Arrival	0	-	88%	90%
Smoking Cessation Advice[1]	8	100%	100%	99%
Chest Pain/Possible Heart Attack Care				
Aspirin at Arrival[1,3]	5	100%	96%	95%
Median Time to ECG (minutes)[1,3]	5	14	11	8
Median Time to Transfer (minutes)[3]	0	-	75	61
Fibrinolytic Medication Timing[3]	0	-	55%	54%
Heart Failure Care				
ACE Inhibitor or ARB for LVSD	153	93%	94%	94%
Discharge Instructions	406	93%	89%	88%
Evaluation of LVS Function	498	99%	98%	98%
Smoking Cessation Advice	96	100%	98%	98%
Pneumonia Care				
Appropriate Initial Antibiotic	108	88%	92%	92%
Blood Culture Timing	202	91%	95%	96%
Influenza Vaccine	157	89%	90%	91%
Initial Antibiotic Timing	186	96%	93%	95%
Pneumococcal Vaccine	260	94%	92%	93%
Smoking Cessation Advice	45	96%	98%	97%
Surgical Care Improvement Project				
Appropriate VTP Within 24 Hours[2]	145	100%	94%	92%
Appropriate Hair Removal[2]	240	100%	100%	99%
Appropriate Beta Blocker Usage[2]	53	100%	92%	93%
Controlled Postoperative Blood Glucose[2]	0	-	94%	93%
Prophylactic Antibiotic Timing[2]	88	99%	96%	97%
Prophylactic Antibiotic Timing (Outpatient)	50	94%	92%	92%
Prophylactic Antibiotic Selection[2]	88	95%	97%	97%
Prophylactic Antibiotic Select. (Outpatient)	99	97%	93%	94%
Prophylactic Antibiotic Stopped[2]	82	98%	94%	94%
Recommended VTP Ordered[2]	145	100%	96%	94%
Urinary Catheter Removal[2]	44	98%	90%	90%
Children's Asthma Care				
Received Systemic Corticosteroids	-	-	-	100%
Received Home Management Plan	-	-	-	71%
Received Reliever Medication	-	-	-	100%
Use of Medical Imaging				
Combination Abdominal CT Scan	245	0.139	0.141	0.191
Combination Chest CT Scan	92	0.043	0.024	0.054
Follow-up Mammogram/Ultrasound	94	2.1%	9.8%	8.4%
MRI for Low Back Pain[1]	14	21.4%	26.9%	32.7%
Survey of Patients' Hospital Experiences				
Area Around Room 'Always' Quiet at Night	300+	49%	-	58%
Doctors 'Always' Communicated Well	300+	72%	-	80%
Home Recovery Information Given	300+	77%	-	82%
Hospital Given 9 or 10 on 10 Point Scale	300+	55%	-	67%
Meds 'Always' Explained Before Given	300+	50%	-	60%
Nurses 'Always' Communicated Well	300+	64%	-	76%
Pain 'Always' Well Controlled	300+	60%	-	69%
Room and Bathroom 'Always' Clean	300+	63%	-	71%
Timely Help 'Always' Received	300+	54%	-	64%
Would Definitely Recommend Hospital	300+	56%	-	69%

NOTE: Hospital profiles are in alphabetical order by state, then city, then hospital within the city; Rankings exclude hospitals with less than 25 cases except for patient surveys which excludes hospitals with less than 100 cases; (a) 100–299 cases; (1) The number of cases is too small to be sure how well a hospital is performing; (2) The hospital indicated that the data submitted for this measure were based on a sample of cases; (3) Data was collected during a shorter time period (fewer quarters) than the maximum possible time for this measure; (4) Suppressed for one or more quarters by CMS; (5) No data is available from the hospital for this measure; (6) Fewer than 100 patients completed the HCAHPS survey. Use these rates with caution, as the number of surveys may be too low to reliably assess hospital performance; (7) Survey results are based on less than 12 months of data; (8) Survey results are not available for this reporting period; (9) No or very few patients were eligible for the HCAHPS survey. The scores shown, if any, reflect a very small number of surveys; (10) A state average was not calculated because too few hospitals in the state submitted data; (11) There were discrepancies in the data collection process; Please refer to the User's Guide for a full explanation of data.

Interfaith Medical Center

1545 Atlantic Avenue Phone: 718-613-4000
Brooklyn, NY 11213 Fax: 718-613-4101
URL: www.interfaithmedical.com
Type: Acute Care Hospitals Emergency Services: Yes
Ownership: Voluntary Non-Profit - Private Beds: 287

Key Personnel:

CEO/President. . . . . Michael S Kaminski
Chief of Medical Staff . . . . Franklin Marsh, MD
Infection Control . . . . Paul Dobre, PharmD
Pediatric In-Patient Care . . . . . . Mary Bastawros, MD
Quality Assurance . . . . Virginia Baron
Radiology. . . . . Richard Heiden, MD
Emergency Room . . . . K Chandramohan, MD
Intensive Care Unit. . . . . Joseph Quist, MD

Measure	Cases	This Hosp.	State Avg.	U.S. Avg.
Heart Attack Care				
ACE Inhibitor or ARB for LVSD[1]	8	100%	95%	96%
Aspirin at Arrival	57	95%	98%	99%
Aspirin at Discharge[1]	22	91%	98%	98%
Beta Blocker at Discharge	26	92%	98%	98%
Fibrinolytic Medication Timing[1]	1	0%	50%	55%
PCI Within 90 Minutes of Arrival	0	-	88%	90%
Smoking Cessation Advice[1]	10	90%	100%	99%
Chest Pain/Possible Heart Attack Care				
Aspirin at Arrival[5]	0	-	96%	95%
Median Time to ECG (minutes)[5]	0	-	11	8
Median Time to Transfer (minutes)[5]	0	-	75	61
Fibrinolytic Medication Timing[5]	0	-	55%	54%
Heart Failure Care				
ACE Inhibitor or ARB for LVSD	88	97%	94%	94%
Discharge Instructions	188	82%	89%	88%
Evaluation of LVS Function	209	100%	98%	98%
Smoking Cessation Advice	82	91%	98%	98%
Pneumonia Care				
Appropriate Initial Antibiotic	81	96%	92%	92%
Blood Culture Timing	129	76%	95%	96%
Influenza Vaccine	65	75%	90%	91%
Initial Antibiotic Timing	147	77%	93%	95%
Pneumococcal Vaccine	84	85%	92%	93%
Smoking Cessation Advice	65	94%	98%	97%
Surgical Care Improvement Project				
Appropriate VTP Within 24 Hours	82	99%	94%	92%
Appropriate Hair Removal	113	99%	100%	99%
Appropriate Beta Blocker Usage[1]	9	44%	92%	93%
Controlled Postoperative Blood Glucose	0	-	94%	93%
Prophylactic Antibiotic Timing	47	91%	96%	97%
Prophylactic Antibiotic Timing (Outpatient)[1,3]	21	76%	92%	92%
Prophylactic Antibiotic Selection	46	93%	97%	97%
Prophylactic Antibiotic Select. (Outpatient)[1,3]	17	100%	93%	94%
Prophylactic Antibiotic Stopped	45	76%	94%	94%
Recommended VTP Ordered	82	99%	96%	94%
Urinary Catheter Removal[1]	8	88%	90%	90%
Children's Asthma Care				
Received Systemic Corticosteroids	-	-	-	100%
Received Home Management Plan	-	-	-	71%
Received Reliever Medication	-	-	-	100%
Use of Medical Imaging				
Combination Abdominal CT Scan[1]	41	0.024	0.141	0.191
Combination Chest CT Scan	60	0.017	0.024	0.054
Follow-up Mammogram/Ultrasound	94	7.4%	9.8%	8.4%
MRI for Low Back Pain[1]	4	25.0%	26.9%	32.7%
Survey of Patients' Hospital Experiences				
Area Around Room 'Always' Quiet at Night	300+	56%	-	58%
Doctors 'Always' Communicated Well	300+	67%	-	80%
Home Recovery Information Given	300+	64%	-	82%
Hospital Given 9 or 10 on 10 Point Scale	300+	45%	-	67%
Meds 'Always' Explained Before Given	300+	51%	-	60%
Nurses 'Always' Communicated Well	300+	63%	-	76%
Pain 'Always' Well Controlled	300+	53%	-	69%
Room and Bathroom 'Always' Clean	300+	72%	-	71%
Timely Help 'Always' Received	300+	38%	-	64%
Would Definitely Recommend Hospital	300+	45%	-	69%

Kings County Hospital Center

451 Clarkson Avenue Phone: 718-245-3901
Brooklyn, NY 11203 Fax: 718-245-3019
URL: www.nyc.gov/html/hhc/html/facilities/kings.shtml
Type: Acute Care Hospitals Emergency Services: Yes
Ownership: Government - Local Beds: 627

Key Personnel:

CEO/President. . . . . Alan D Aviles
Chief of Medical Staff . . . . Stephan Kamholz, MD
Infection Control . . . . Stephen Seligman, MD
Operating Room. . . . . Connie Thomas
Pediatric In-Patient Care . . . . . . Leonard Glass, MD
Quality Assurance . . . . Audrey Phillips-Caesar
Radiology. . . . . Joshua Becker, MD

Measure	Cases	This Hosp.	State Avg.	U.S. Avg.
Heart Attack Care				
ACE Inhibitor or ARB for LVSD[1]	9	89%	95%	96%
Aspirin at Arrival	97	98%	98%	99%
Aspirin at Discharge	58	100%	98%	98%
Beta Blocker at Discharge	53	98%	98%	98%
Fibrinolytic Medication Timing	0	-	50%	55%
PCI Within 90 Minutes of Arrival	0	-	88%	90%
Smoking Cessation Advice[1]	8	100%	100%	99%
Chest Pain/Possible Heart Attack Care				
Aspirin at Arrival[1,3]	3	100%	96%	95%
Median Time to ECG (minutes)[1,3]	3	12	11	8
Median Time to Transfer (minutes)[1,3]	3	129	75	61
Fibrinolytic Medication Timing[3]	0	-	55%	54%
Heart Failure Care				
ACE Inhibitor or ARB for LVSD	306	98%	94%	94%
Discharge Instructions	577	69%	89%	88%
Evaluation of LVS Function	602	100%	98%	98%
Smoking Cessation Advice	105	96%	98%	98%
Pneumonia Care				
Appropriate Initial Antibiotic	117	97%	92%	92%
Blood Culture Timing	238	92%	95%	96%
Influenza Vaccine	126	86%	90%	91%
Initial Antibiotic Timing	213	91%	93%	95%
Pneumococcal Vaccine	132	91%	92%	93%
Smoking Cessation Advice	101	96%	98%	97%
Surgical Care Improvement Project				
Appropriate VTP Within 24 Hours[2]	219	97%	94%	92%
Appropriate Hair Removal[2]	330	100%	100%	99%
Appropriate Beta Blocker Usage[2]	44	91%	92%	93%
Controlled Postoperative Blood Glucose[1,2]	1	100%	94%	93%
Prophylactic Antibiotic Timing[2]	115	99%	96%	97%
Prophylactic Antibiotic Timing (Outpatient)	45	100%	92%	92%
Prophylactic Antibiotic Selection[2]	117	98%	97%	97%
Prophylactic Antibiotic Select. (Outpatient)	126	99%	93%	94%
Prophylactic Antibiotic Stopped[2]	114	88%	94%	94%
Recommended VTP Ordered[2]	219	97%	96%	94%
Urinary Catheter Removal[2]	31	68%	90%	90%
Children's Asthma Care				
Received Systemic Corticosteroids	-	-	-	100%
Received Home Management Plan	-	-	-	71%
Received Reliever Medication	-	-	-	100%
Use of Medical Imaging				
Combination Abdominal CT Scan	133	0.263	0.141	0.191
Combination Chest CT Scan[1]	43	0.256	0.024	0.054
Follow-up Mammogram/Ultrasound[1]	10	0.0%	9.8%	8.4%
MRI for Low Back Pain[1]	8	0.0%	26.9%	32.7%
Survey of Patients' Hospital Experiences				
Area Around Room 'Always' Quiet at Night	300+	59%	-	58%
Doctors 'Always' Communicated Well	300+	78%	-	80%
Home Recovery Information Given	300+	79%	-	82%
Hospital Given 9 or 10 on 10 Point Scale	300+	57%	-	67%
Meds 'Always' Explained Before Given	300+	61%	-	60%
Nurses 'Always' Communicated Well	300+	67%	-	76%
Pain 'Always' Well Controlled	300+	59%	-	69%
Room and Bathroom 'Always' Clean	300+	74%	-	71%
Timely Help 'Always' Received	300+	45%	-	64%
Would Definitely Recommend Hospital	300+	63%	-	69%

Kingsbrook Jewish Medical Center

585 Schenectady Avenue Phone: 718-604-5789
Brooklyn, NY 11203 Fax: 718-604-5243
E-mail: info@kjmc.org
URL: www.kingsbrook.org
Type: Acute Care Hospitals Emergency Services: Yes
Ownership: Voluntary Non-Profit - Private Beds: 864

Key Personnel:

CEO/President. . . . . Linda Brady, MD
Chief of Medical Staff . . . . Akbarali Virani, MD
Infection Control . . . . Rizwanullah Hameed, MD
Operating Room. . . . . William A Lois, MD
Pediatric In-Patient Care . . . . . . Hua-Chin Chen, MD
Quality Assurance . . . . Mary Marshall
Radiology. . . . . Kenneth Schwartz, MD

Measure	Cases	This Hosp.	State Avg.	U.S. Avg.
Heart Attack Care				
ACE Inhibitor or ARB for LVSD[1]	3	100%	95%	96%
Aspirin at Arrival	42	98%	98%	99%
Aspirin at Discharge[1]	15	100%	98%	98%
Beta Blocker at Discharge[1]	17	100%	98%	98%
Fibrinolytic Medication Timing	0	-	50%	55%
PCI Within 90 Minutes of Arrival	0	-	88%	90%
Smoking Cessation Advice[1]	2	100%	100%	99%
Chest Pain/Possible Heart Attack Care				
Aspirin at Arrival[1]	20	100%	96%	95%
Median Time to ECG (minutes)[1]	20	12	11	8
Median Time to Transfer (minutes)[1,3]	1	200	75	61
Fibrinolytic Medication Timing	0	-	55%	54%
Heart Failure Care				
ACE Inhibitor or ARB for LVSD	107	99%	94%	94%
Discharge Instructions	174	90%	89%	88%
Evaluation of LVS Function	265	100%	98%	98%
Smoking Cessation Advice[1]	21	100%	98%	98%
Pneumonia Care				
Appropriate Initial Antibiotic	105	100%	92%	92%
Blood Culture Timing	299	98%	95%	96%
Influenza Vaccine	244	85%	90%	91%
Initial Antibiotic Timing	280	95%	93%	95%
Pneumococcal Vaccine	385	97%	92%	93%
Smoking Cessation Advice	49	92%	98%	97%
Surgical Care Improvement Project				
Appropriate VTP Within 24 Hours	126	97%	94%	92%
Appropriate Hair Removal	170	100%	100%	99%
Appropriate Beta Blocker Usage	43	95%	92%	93%
Controlled Postoperative Blood Glucose	0	-	94%	93%
Prophylactic Antibiotic Timing	78	99%	96%	97%
Prophylactic Antibiotic Timing (Outpatient)	61	93%	92%	92%
Prophylactic Antibiotic Selection	81	98%	97%	97%
Prophylactic Antibiotic Select. (Outpatient)	58	86%	93%	94%
Prophylactic Antibiotic Stopped	65	95%	94%	94%
Recommended VTP Ordered	127	98%	96%	94%
Urinary Catheter Removal	36	89%	90%	90%
Children's Asthma Care				
Received Systemic Corticosteroids	-	-	-	100%
Received Home Management Plan	-	-	-	71%
Received Reliever Medication	-	-	-	100%
Use of Medical Imaging				
Combination Abdominal CT Scan	208	0.159	0.141	0.191
Combination Chest CT Scan	136	0.015	0.024	0.054
Follow-up Mammogram/Ultrasound	273	19.8%	9.8%	8.4%
MRI for Low Back Pain[1]	25	28.0%	26.9%	32.7%
Survey of Patients' Hospital Experiences				
Area Around Room 'Always' Quiet at Night	300+	51%	-	58%
Doctors 'Always' Communicated Well	300+	75%	-	80%
Home Recovery Information Given	300+	76%	-	82%
Hospital Given 9 or 10 on 10 Point Scale	300+	51%	-	67%
Meds 'Always' Explained Before Given	300+	54%	-	60%
Nurses 'Always' Communicated Well	300+	69%	-	76%
Pain 'Always' Well Controlled	300+	56%	-	69%
Room and Bathroom 'Always' Clean	300+	67%	-	71%
Timely Help 'Always' Received	300+	45%	-	64%
Would Definitely Recommend Hospital	300+	61%	-	69%

NOTE: Hospital profiles are in alphabetical order by state, then city, then hospital within the city; Rankings exclude hospitals with less than 25 cases except for patient surveys which excludes hospitals with less than 100 cases; (a) 100–299 cases; (1) The number of cases is too small to be sure how well a hospital is performing; (2) The hospital indicated that the data submitted for this measure were based on a sample of cases; (3) Data was collected during a shorter time period (fewer quarters) than the maximum possible time for this measure; (4) Suppressed for one or more quarters by CMS; (5) No data is available from the hospital for this measure; (6) Fewer than 100 patients completed the HCAHPS survey. Use these rates with caution, as the number of surveys may be too low to reliably assess hospital performance; (7) Survey results are based on less than 12 months of data; (8) Survey results are not available for this reporting period; (9) No or very few patients were eligible for the HCAHPS survey. The scores shown, if any, reflect a very small number of surveys; (10) A state average was not calculated because too few hospitals in the state submitted data; (11) There were discrepancies in the data collection process; Please refer to the User's Guide for a full explanation of data.

Long Island College Hospital

339 Hicks Street
Brooklyn, NY 11201
Phone: 718-780-4651
Fax: 718-780-1365
URL: www.wehealny.org
Type: Acute Care Hospitals
Emergency Services: Yes
Ownership: Voluntary Non-Profit - Private
Beds: 506

Key Personnel:
CEO/President. . . . . Dominick Stanzione
Cardiac Laboratory. . . . . Balendu Vasavada, MD
Infection Control. . . . . Douglas Sepkowitz, MD
Operating Room. . . . . Antonio E Alfonso, MD
Pediatric Ambulatory Care . . . . . Steven Schwarz, MD
Quality Assurance . . . . Tina Sernick, ESQ
Radiology. . . . . Michael M Abiri, MD

Measure	Cases	This Hosp.	State Avg.	U.S. Avg.
Heart Attack Care				
ACE Inhibitor or ARB for LVSD[2]	41	85%	95%	96%
Aspirin at Arrival[2]	227	97%	98%	99%
Aspirin at Discharge[2]	176	94%	98%	98%
Beta Blocker at Discharge[2]	177	94%	98%	98%
Fibrinolytic Medication Timing[1,2]	1	0%	50%	55%
PCI Within 90 Minutes of Arrival[1,2]	13	62%	88%	90%
Smoking Cessation Advice[2]	42	100%	100%	99%
Chest Pain/Possible Heart Attack Care				
Aspirin at Arrival[1,3]	5	80%	96%	95%
Median Time to ECG (minutes)[1,3]	5	28	11	8
Median Time to Transfer (minutes)[5]	0	-	75	61
Fibrinolytic Medication Timing[5]	0	-	55%	54%
Heart Failure Care				
ACE Inhibitor or ARB for LVSD[2]	114	91%	94%	94%
Discharge Instructions[2]	272	97%	89%	88%
Evaluation of LVS Function[2]	311	96%	98%	98%
Smoking Cessation Advice[2]	43	100%	98%	98%
Pneumonia Care				
Appropriate Initial Antibiotic[2]	77	91%	92%	92%
Blood Culture Timing[2]	139	99%	95%	96%
Influenza Vaccine[2]	75	83%	90%	91%
Initial Antibiotic Timing[2]	142	89%	93%	95%
Pneumococcal Vaccine[2]	102	67%	92%	93%
Smoking Cessation Advice[2]	40	98%	98%	97%
Surgical Care Improvement Project				
Appropriate VTP Within 24 Hours[2]	233	97%	94%	92%
Appropriate Hair Removal[2]	436	99%	100%	99%
Appropriate Beta Blocker Usage[2]	100	93%	92%	93%
Controlled Postoperative Blood Glucose[2]	0	-	94%	93%
Prophylactic Antibiotic Timing[2]	312	93%	96%	97%
Prophylactic Antibiotic Timing (Outpatient)	176	86%	92%	92%
Prophylactic Antibiotic Selection[2]	307	94%	97%	97%
Prophylactic Antibiotic Select. (Outpatient)	162	92%	93%	94%
Prophylactic Antibiotic Stopped[2]	300	86%	94%	94%
Recommended VTP Ordered[2]	233	97%	96%	94%
Urinary Catheter Removal[2]	101	91%	90%	90%
Children's Asthma Care				
Received Systemic Corticosteroids	-	-	-	100%
Received Home Management Plan	-	-	-	71%
Received Reliever Medication	-	-	-	100%
Use of Medical Imaging				
Combination Abdominal CT Scan	457	0.267	0.141	0.191
Combination Chest CT Scan	239	0.008	0.024	0.054
Follow-up Mammogram/Ultrasound	519	5.0%	9.8%	8.4%
MRI for Low Back Pain[1]	50	18.0%	26.9%	32.7%
Survey of Patients' Hospital Experiences				
Area Around Room 'Always' Quiet at Night	300+	52%	-	58%
Doctors 'Always' Communicated Well	300+	71%	-	80%
Home Recovery Information Given	300+	66%	-	82%
Hospital Given 9 or 10 on 10 Point Scale	300+	44%	-	67%
Meds 'Always' Explained Before Given	300+	48%	-	60%
Nurses 'Always' Communicated Well	300+	59%	-	76%
Pain 'Always' Well Controlled	300+	53%	-	69%
Room and Bathroom 'Always' Clean	300+	53%	-	71%
Timely Help 'Always' Received	300+	45%	-	64%
Would Definitely Recommend Hospital	300+	55%	-	69%

Lutheran Medical Center

150 55th Street
Brooklyn, NY 11220
Phone: 718-630-8000
Fax: 718-630-8653
URL: www.lmcmc.com
Type: Acute Care Hospitals
Emergency Services: Yes
Ownership: Voluntary Non-Profit - Private
Beds: 476

Key Personnel:
CEO/President. . . . . Wendy Z Goldstein
Chief of Medical Staff . . . . Beth Raucher, MD
Infection Control. . . . . Ernest Visconti, MD
Operating Room. . . . . George Ferzli, MD
Pediatric Ambulatory Care . . . . . Steven Shelov, MD
Radiology. . . . . Jayanth Rao, MD
Emergency Room . . . . Bonnie Simmons, DO
Patient Relations . . . . Sheldon Rock

Measure	Cases	This Hosp.	State Avg.	U.S. Avg.
Heart Attack Care				
ACE Inhibitor or ARB for LVSD	32	91%	95%	96%
Aspirin at Arrival	256	98%	98%	99%
Aspirin at Discharge	173	97%	98%	98%
Beta Blocker at Discharge	177	97%	98%	98%
Fibrinolytic Medication Timing	0	-	50%	55%
PCI Within 90 Minutes of Arrival	39	97%	88%	90%
Smoking Cessation Advice	33	100%	100%	99%
Chest Pain/Possible Heart Attack Care				
Aspirin at Arrival[1,3]	17	88%	96%	95%
Median Time to ECG (minutes)[1,3]	17	8	11	8
Median Time to Transfer (minutes)[1,3]	3	109	75	61
Fibrinolytic Medication Timing[3]	0	-	55%	54%
Heart Failure Care				
ACE Inhibitor or ARB for LVSD	79	84%	94%	94%
Discharge Instructions	296	97%	89%	88%
Evaluation of LVS Function	402	98%	98%	98%
Smoking Cessation Advice[1]	21	95%	98%	98%
Pneumonia Care				
Appropriate Initial Antibiotic	219	97%	92%	92%
Blood Culture Timing	382	96%	95%	96%
Influenza Vaccine	246	96%	90%	91%
Initial Antibiotic Timing	335	95%	93%	95%
Pneumococcal Vaccine	344	90%	92%	93%
Smoking Cessation Advice	60	93%	98%	97%
Surgical Care Improvement Project				
Appropriate VTP Within 24 Hours[2]	482	98%	94%	92%
Appropriate Hair Removal[2]	959	99%	100%	99%
Appropriate Beta Blocker Usage[2]	292	86%	92%	93%
Controlled Postoperative Blood Glucose[2]	0	-	94%	93%
Prophylactic Antibiotic Timing[2]	665	99%	96%	97%
Prophylactic Antibiotic Timing (Outpatient)	118	87%	92%	92%
Prophylactic Antibiotic Selection[2]	665	98%	97%	97%
Prophylactic Antibiotic Select. (Outpatient)	103	83%	93%	94%
Prophylactic Antibiotic Stopped[2]	645	94%	94%	94%
Recommended VTP Ordered[2]	482	99%	96%	94%
Urinary Catheter Removal[2]	165	88%	90%	90%
Children's Asthma Care				
Received Systemic Corticosteroids	-	-	-	100%
Received Home Management Plan	-	-	-	71%
Received Reliever Medication	-	-	-	100%
Use of Medical Imaging				
Combination Abdominal CT Scan	400	0.023	0.141	0.191
Combination Chest CT Scan	177	0.000	0.024	0.054
Follow-up Mammogram/Ultrasound	243	7.4%	9.8%	8.4%
MRI for Low Back Pain[1]	11	18.2%	26.9%	32.7%
Survey of Patients' Hospital Experiences				
Area Around Room 'Always' Quiet at Night	300+	34%	-	58%
Doctors 'Always' Communicated Well	300+	72%	-	80%
Home Recovery Information Given	300+	76%	-	82%
Hospital Given 9 or 10 on 10 Point Scale	300+	49%	-	67%
Meds 'Always' Explained Before Given	300+	46%	-	60%
Nurses 'Always' Communicated Well	300+	64%	-	76%
Pain 'Always' Well Controlled	300+	59%	-	69%
Room and Bathroom 'Always' Clean	300+	53%	-	71%
Timely Help 'Always' Received	300+	50%	-	64%
Would Definitely Recommend Hospital	300+	54%	-	69%

Maimonides Medical Center

4802 Tenth Avenue
Brooklyn, NY 11219
Phone: 718-283-6000
Fax: 718-283-8553
E-mail: info@maimonidesmed.org
URL: www.maimonidesmed.org
Type: Acute Care Hospitals
Emergency Services: Yes
Ownership: Voluntary Non-Profit - Private
Beds: 705

Key Personnel:
CEO/President. . . . . Pamela S Brier
Chief of Medical Staff . . . . Samuel Kopel, MD
Operating Room. . . . . Patrick I Borgen, MD
Pediatric Ambulatory Care . . . . . Steven P Shelov, MD
Radiology. . . . . Javier Beltran, MD
Anesthesiology. . . . . Steven Konstadt, MD
Emergency Room . . . . Steven J Davidson, MD

Measure	Cases	This Hosp.	State Avg.	U.S. Avg.
Heart Attack Care				
ACE Inhibitor or ARB for LVSD[2]	87	91%	95%	96%
Aspirin at Arrival[2]	284	95%	98%	99%
Aspirin at Discharge[2]	302	96%	98%	98%
Beta Blocker at Discharge[2]	307	95%	98%	98%
Fibrinolytic Medication Timing[1,2]	1	100%	50%	55%
PCI Within 90 Minutes of Arrival[2]	29	69%	88%	90%
Smoking Cessation Advice[2]	77	99%	100%	99%
Chest Pain/Possible Heart Attack Care				
Aspirin at Arrival[5]	0	-	96%	95%
Median Time to ECG (minutes)[5]	0	-	11	8
Median Time to Transfer (minutes)[5]	0	-	75	61
Fibrinolytic Medication Timing[5]	0	-	55%	54%
Heart Failure Care				
ACE Inhibitor or ARB for LVSD[2]	114	96%	94%	94%
Discharge Instructions[2]	300	86%	89%	88%
Evaluation of LVS Function[2]	359	100%	98%	98%
Smoking Cessation Advice[2]	29	100%	98%	98%
Pneumonia Care				
Appropriate Initial Antibiotic[2]	74	96%	92%	92%
Blood Culture Timing[2]	160	96%	95%	96%
Influenza Vaccine[2]	96	57%	90%	91%
Initial Antibiotic Timing[2]	134	90%	93%	95%
Pneumococcal Vaccine[2]	174	84%	92%	93%
Smoking Cessation Advice[1,2]	19	100%	98%	97%
Surgical Care Improvement Project				
Appropriate VTP Within 24 Hours[2]	314	94%	94%	92%
Appropriate Hair Removal[2]	1,231	100%	100%	99%
Appropriate Beta Blocker Usage[2]	496	89%	92%	93%
Controlled Postoperative Blood Glucose[2]	373	93%	94%	93%
Prophylactic Antibiotic Timing[2]	933	93%	96%	97%
Prophylactic Antibiotic Timing (Outpatient)	176	85%	92%	92%
Prophylactic Antibiotic Selection[2]	945	97%	97%	97%
Prophylactic Antibiotic Select. (Outpatient)	158	88%	93%	94%
Prophylactic Antibiotic Stopped[2]	904	91%	94%	94%
Recommended VTP Ordered[2]	321	97%	96%	94%
Urinary Catheter Removal[2]	256	90%	90%	90%
Children's Asthma Care				
Received Systemic Corticosteroids	-	-	-	100%
Received Home Management Plan	-	-	-	71%
Received Reliever Medication	-	-	-	100%
Use of Medical Imaging				
Combination Abdominal CT Scan	751	0.021	0.141	0.191
Combination Chest CT Scan	491	0.022	0.024	0.054
Follow-up Mammogram/Ultrasound[5]	0	-	9.8%	8.4%
MRI for Low Back Pain[1]	45	24.4%	26.9%	32.7%
Survey of Patients' Hospital Experiences				
Area Around Room 'Always' Quiet at Night	300+	45%	-	58%
Doctors 'Always' Communicated Well	300+	77%	-	80%
Home Recovery Information Given	300+	77%	-	82%
Hospital Given 9 or 10 on 10 Point Scale	300+	50%	-	67%
Meds 'Always' Explained Before Given	300+	53%	-	60%
Nurses 'Always' Communicated Well	300+	66%	-	76%
Pain 'Always' Well Controlled	300+	60%	-	69%
Room and Bathroom 'Always' Clean	300+	58%	-	71%
Timely Help 'Always' Received	300+	53%	-	64%
Would Definitely Recommend Hospital	300+	62%	-	69%

NOTE: Hospital profiles are in alphabetical order by state, then city, then hospital within the city; Rankings exclude hospitals with less than 25 cases except for patient surveys which excludes hospitals with less than 100 cases; (a) 100–299 cases; (1) The number of cases is too small to be sure how well a hospital is performing; (2) The hospital indicated that the data submitted for this measure were based on a sample of cases; (3) Data was collected during a shorter time period (fewer quarters) than the maximum possible time for this measure; (4) Suppressed for one or more quarters by CMS; (5) No data is available from the hospital for this measure; (6) Fewer than 100 patients completed the HCAHPS survey. Use these rates with caution, as the number of surveys may be too low to reliably assess hospital performance; (7) Survey results are based on less than 12 months of data; (8) Survey results are not available for this reporting period; (9) No or very few patients were eligible for the HCAHPS survey. The scores shown, if any, reflect a very small number of surveys; (10) A state average was not calculated because too few hospitals in the state submitted data; (11) There were discrepancies in the data collection process; Please refer to the User's Guide for a full explanation of data.

New York Community Hospital of Brooklyn

2525 Kings Highway　Phone: 718-692-5302
Brooklyn, NY 11229　Fax: 718-692-5368
URL: www.nych.com
Type: Acute Care Hospitals　Emergency Services: Yes
Ownership: Voluntary Non-Profit - Private　Beds: 134

Key Personnel:
CEO/President. . . . . Lin H Mo
Emergency Room . . . . Nermard Yonk, MD

Measure	Cases	This Hosp.	State Avg.	U.S. Avg.
Heart Attack Care				
ACE Inhibitor or ARB for LVSD[1]	5	100%	95%	96%
Aspirin at Arrival	85	99%	98%	99%
Aspirin at Discharge	42	100%	98%	98%
Beta Blocker at Discharge	49	100%	98%	98%
Fibrinolytic Medication Timing[1]	1	100%	50%	55%
PCI Within 90 Minutes of Arrival	0	-	88%	90%
Smoking Cessation Advice[1]	1	100%	100%	99%
Chest Pain/Possible Heart Attack Care				
Aspirin at Arrival[5]	0	-	96%	95%
Median Time to ECG (minutes)[5]	0	-	11	8
Median Time to Transfer (minutes)[5]	0	-	75	61
Fibrinolytic Medication Timing[5]	0	-	55%	54%
Heart Failure Care				
ACE Inhibitor or ARB for LVSD[2]	38	100%	94%	94%
Discharge Instructions[2]	233	95%	89%	88%
Evaluation of LVS Function[2]	266	100%	98%	98%
Smoking Cessation Advice[1,2]	12	100%	98%	98%
Pneumonia Care				
Appropriate Initial Antibiotic[2]	81	100%	92%	92%
Blood Culture Timing[2]	110	95%	95%	96%
Influenza Vaccine[2]	70	96%	90%	91%
Initial Antibiotic Timing[2]	89	99%	93%	95%
Pneumococcal Vaccine[2]	115	98%	92%	93%
Smoking Cessation Advice[1,2]	14	100%	98%	97%
Surgical Care Improvement Project				
Appropriate VTP Within 24 Hours[2]	85	100%	94%	92%
Appropriate Hair Removal[2]	141	100%	100%	99%
Appropriate Beta Blocker Usage[2]	53	100%	92%	93%
Controlled Postoperative Blood Glucose[1,2]	1	100%	94%	93%
Prophylactic Antibiotic Timing[2]	63	94%	96%	97%
Prophylactic Antibiotic Timing (Outpatient)[1]	22	100%	92%	92%
Prophylactic Antibiotic Selection[2]	63	94%	97%	97%
Prophylactic Antibiotic Select. (Outpatient)[1]	22	82%	93%	94%
Prophylactic Antibiotic Stopped[2]	50	94%	94%	94%
Recommended VTP Ordered[2]	85	100%	96%	94%
Urinary Catheter Removal[1,2]	16	94%	90%	90%
Children's Asthma Care				
Received Systemic Corticosteroids	-	-	-	100%
Received Home Management Plan	-	-	-	71%
Received Reliever Medication	-	-	-	100%
Use of Medical Imaging				
Combination Abdominal CT Scan	110	0.009	0.141	0.191
Combination Chest CT Scan[1]	32	0.000	0.024	0.054
Follow-up Mammogram/Ultrasound[1]	3	0.0%	9.8%	8.4%
MRI for Low Back Pain[5]	0	-	26.9%	32.7%
Survey of Patients' Hospital Experiences				
Area Around Room 'Always' Quiet at Night	300+	44%	-	58%
Doctors 'Always' Communicated Well	300+	70%	-	80%
Home Recovery Information Given	300+	76%	-	82%
Hospital Given 9 or 10 on 10 Point Scale	300+	47%	-	67%
Meds 'Always' Explained Before Given	300+	52%	-	60%
Nurses 'Always' Communicated Well	300+	65%	-	76%
Pain 'Always' Well Controlled	300+	57%	-	69%
Room and Bathroom 'Always' Clean	300+	67%	-	71%
Timely Help 'Always' Received	300+	51%	-	64%
Would Definitely Recommend Hospital	300+	51%	-	69%

New York Methodist Hospital

506 Sixth Street　Phone: 718-780-3000
Brooklyn, NY 11215　Fax: 718-780-3770
E-mail: lyn9001@nyp.org
URL: www.nym.org
Type: Acute Care Hospitals　Emergency Services: Yes
Ownership: Voluntary Non-Profit - Private　Beds: 576

Key Personnel:
CEO/President. . . . . Mark J Mundy
Chief of Medical Staff. . . . . Anthony Saleh, MD
Infection Control. . . . . Kathleen McNamara, RN
Operating Room. . . . . Joanne Lagnes, RN
Pediatric In-Patient Care . . . . Pramod Narula
Quality Assurance . . . . Pamela Monastero
Radiology. . . . . Pina Pureddy

Measure	Cases	This Hosp.	State Avg.	U.S. Avg.
Heart Attack Care				
ACE Inhibitor or ARB for LVSD	66	91%	95%	96%
Aspirin at Arrival	203	99%	98%	99%
Aspirin at Discharge	241	99%	98%	98%
Beta Blocker at Discharge	244	98%	98%	98%
Fibrinolytic Medication Timing	0	-	50%	55%
PCI Within 90 Minutes of Arrival	32	78%	88%	90%
Smoking Cessation Advice	65	100%	100%	99%
Chest Pain/Possible Heart Attack Care				
Aspirin at Arrival[5]	0	-	96%	95%
Median Time to ECG (minutes)[5]	0	-	11	8
Median Time to Transfer (minutes)[5]	0	-	75	61
Fibrinolytic Medication Timing[5]	0	-	55%	54%
Heart Failure Care				
ACE Inhibitor or ARB for LVSD[2]	148	93%	94%	94%
Discharge Instructions[2]	277	90%	89%	88%
Evaluation of LVS Function[2]	340	100%	98%	98%
Smoking Cessation Advice[2]	32	100%	98%	98%
Pneumonia Care				
Appropriate Initial Antibiotic[2]	90	93%	92%	92%
Blood Culture Timing[2]	111	69%	95%	96%
Influenza Vaccine[2]	94	89%	90%	91%
Initial Antibiotic Timing[2]	171	88%	93%	95%
Pneumococcal Vaccine[2]	165	98%	92%	93%
Smoking Cessation Advice[2]	39	100%	98%	97%
Surgical Care Improvement Project				
Appropriate VTP Within 24 Hours[2]	334	99%	94%	92%
Appropriate Hair Removal[2]	791	100%	100%	99%
Appropriate Beta Blocker Usage[2]	251	86%	92%	93%
Controlled Postoperative Blood Glucose[2]	118	97%	94%	93%
Prophylactic Antibiotic Timing[2]	521	98%	96%	97%
Prophylactic Antibiotic Timing (Outpatient)	186	95%	92%	92%
Prophylactic Antibiotic Selection[2]	528	97%	97%	97%
Prophylactic Antibiotic Select. (Outpatient)	182	96%	93%	94%
Prophylactic Antibiotic Stopped[2]	479	85%	94%	94%
Recommended VTP Ordered[2]	334	99%	96%	94%
Urinary Catheter Removal[2]	180	91%	90%	90%
Children's Asthma Care				
Received Systemic Corticosteroids	-	-	-	100%
Received Home Management Plan	-	-	-	71%
Received Reliever Medication	-	-	-	100%
Use of Medical Imaging				
Combination Abdominal CT Scan	570	0.065	0.141	0.191
Combination Chest CT Scan	409	0.012	0.024	0.054
Follow-up Mammogram/Ultrasound	862	4.8%	9.8%	8.4%
MRI for Low Back Pain	74	29.7%	26.9%	32.7%
Survey of Patients' Hospital Experiences				
Area Around Room 'Always' Quiet at Night	300+	45%	-	58%
Doctors 'Always' Communicated Well	300+	71%	-	80%
Home Recovery Information Given	300+	75%	-	82%
Hospital Given 9 or 10 on 10 Point Scale	300+	52%	-	67%
Meds 'Always' Explained Before Given	300+	44%	-	60%
Nurses 'Always' Communicated Well	300+	62%	-	76%
Pain 'Always' Well Controlled	300+	56%	-	69%
Room and Bathroom 'Always' Clean	300+	56%	-	71%
Timely Help 'Always' Received	300+	42%	-	64%
Would Definitely Recommend Hospital	300+	61%	-	69%

University Hospital of Brooklyn - Downstate

445 Lenox Road　Phone: 718-270-1000
Brooklyn, NY 11203　Fax: 718-270-1815
URL: www.downstate.edu
Type: Acute Care Hospitals　Emergency Services: Yes
Ownership: Government - State　Beds: 406

Key Personnel:
CEO/President. . . . . Debra Carey, MS
Cardiac Laboratory. . . . . Luther Clark, MD
Chief of Medical Staff. . . . . Michael Lucchesi, MD
Infection Control. . . . . Michael Augenbraun, MD
Operating Room. . . . . Edward Serio, MBA
Pediatric In-Patient Care . . . . Stanley Fisher, MD
Quality Assurance . . . . True Samms
Radiology. . . . . David Stark, MD

Measure	Cases	This Hosp.	State Avg.	U.S. Avg.
Heart Attack Care				
ACE Inhibitor or ARB for LVSD[2]	81	99%	95%	96%
Aspirin at Arrival[2]	196	100%	98%	99%
Aspirin at Discharge[2]	237	99%	98%	98%
Beta Blocker at Discharge[2]	239	96%	98%	98%
Fibrinolytic Medication Timing[2]	0	-	50%	55%
PCI Within 90 Minutes of Arrival[2]	37	95%	88%	90%
Smoking Cessation Advice[2]	67	97%	100%	99%
Chest Pain/Possible Heart Attack Care				
Aspirin at Arrival[1]	15	93%	96%	95%
Median Time to ECG (minutes)[1]	16	28	11	8
Median Time to Transfer (minutes)[5]	0	-	75	61
Fibrinolytic Medication Timing[3]	0	-	55%	54%
Heart Failure Care				
ACE Inhibitor or ARB for LVSD[2]	165	95%	94%	94%
Discharge Instructions[2]	282	94%	89%	88%
Evaluation of LVS Function[2]	292	98%	98%	98%
Smoking Cessation Advice[2]	36	92%	98%	98%
Pneumonia Care				
Appropriate Initial Antibiotic[2]	76	86%	92%	92%
Blood Culture Timing[2]	124	85%	95%	96%
Influenza Vaccine[2]	71	82%	90%	91%
Initial Antibiotic Timing[2]	137	80%	93%	95%
Pneumococcal Vaccine[2]	95	68%	92%	93%
Smoking Cessation Advice[2]	31	81%	98%	97%
Surgical Care Improvement Project				
Appropriate VTP Within 24 Hours[2]	184	98%	94%	92%
Appropriate Hair Removal[2]	382	100%	100%	99%
Appropriate Beta Blocker Usage[2]	110	99%	92%	93%
Controlled Postoperative Blood Glucose[2]	60	90%	94%	93%
Prophylactic Antibiotic Timing[2]	256	93%	96%	97%
Prophylactic Antibiotic Timing (Outpatient)	108	94%	92%	92%
Prophylactic Antibiotic Selection[2]	261	98%	97%	97%
Prophylactic Antibiotic Select. (Outpatient)	103	91%	93%	94%
Prophylactic Antibiotic Stopped[2]	244	92%	94%	94%
Recommended VTP Ordered[2]	184	98%	96%	94%
Urinary Catheter Removal[2]	90	98%	90%	90%
Children's Asthma Care				
Received Systemic Corticosteroids	-	-	-	100%
Received Home Management Plan	-	-	-	71%
Received Reliever Medication	-	-	-	100%
Use of Medical Imaging				
Combination Abdominal CT Scan	273	0.084	0.141	0.191
Combination Chest CT Scan	129	0.023	0.024	0.054
Follow-up Mammogram/Ultrasound	480	1.9%	9.8%	8.4%
MRI for Low Back Pain[1]	29	17.2%	26.9%	32.7%
Survey of Patients' Hospital Experiences				
Area Around Room 'Always' Quiet at Night	300+	51%	-	58%
Doctors 'Always' Communicated Well	300+	77%	-	80%
Home Recovery Information Given	300+	74%	-	82%
Hospital Given 9 or 10 on 10 Point Scale	300+	47%	-	67%
Meds 'Always' Explained Before Given	300+	51%	-	60%
Nurses 'Always' Communicated Well	300+	65%	-	76%
Pain 'Always' Well Controlled	300+	61%	-	69%
Room and Bathroom 'Always' Clean	300+	58%	-	71%
Timely Help 'Always' Received	300+	48%	-	64%
Would Definitely Recommend Hospital	300+	57%	-	69%

NOTE: Hospital profiles are in alphabetical order by state, then city, then hospital within the city; Rankings exclude hospitals with less than 25 cases except for patient surveys which excludes hospitals with less than 100 cases; (a) 100–299 cases; (1) The number of cases is too small to be sure how well a hospital is performing; (2) The hospital indicated that the data submitted for this measure were based on a sample of cases; (3) Data was collected during a shorter time period (fewer quarters) than the maximum possible time for this measure; (4) Suppressed for one or more quarters by CMS; (5) No data is available from the hospital for this measure; (6) Fewer than 100 patients completed the HCAHPS survey. Use these rates with caution, as the number of surveys may be too low to reliably assess hospital performance; (7) Survey results are based on less than 12 months of data; (8) Survey results are not available for this reporting period; (9) No or very few patients were eligible for the HCAHPS survey. The scores shown, if any, reflect a very small number of surveys; (10) A state average was not calculated because too few hospitals in the state submitted data; (11) There were discrepancies in the data collection process; Please refer to the User's Guide for a full explanation of data.

Woodhull Medical and Mental Health Center

760 Broadway Phone: 718-963-8100
Brooklyn, NY 11206 Fax: 718-963-8501
URL: www.ci.nyc.ny.us
Type: Acute Care Hospitals Emergency Services: Yes
Ownership: Government - Local

Key Personnel:

Chief of Medical Staff. . . . . Edward Fishkin
Infection Control. . . . . Rosalie Giardina
Anesthesiology. . . . . Stephan Petranker
Intensive Care Unit. . . . . Stacie Stewart

Measure	Cases	This Hosp.	State Avg.	U.S. Avg.
Heart Attack Care				
ACE Inhibitor or ARB for LVSD[1]	4	100%	95%	96%
Aspirin at Arrival	52	98%	98%	99%
Aspirin at Discharge[1]	7	71%	98%	98%
Beta Blocker at Discharge[1]	8	75%	98%	98%
Fibrinolytic Medication Timing[1]	2	100%	50%	55%
PCI Within 90 Minutes of Arrival	0	-	88%	90%
Smoking Cessation Advice[1]	2	100%	100%	99%
Chest Pain/Possible Heart Attack Care				
Aspirin at Arrival[1]	9	100%	96%	95%
Median Time to ECG (minutes)[1]	10	13	11	8
Median Time to Transfer (minutes)[1,3]	1	340	75	61
Fibrinolytic Medication Timing[1]	4	25%	55%	54%
Heart Failure Care				
ACE Inhibitor or ARB for LVSD	186	100%	94%	94%
Discharge Instructions	287	85%	89%	88%
Evaluation of LVS Function	317	100%	98%	98%
Smoking Cessation Advice	132	100%	98%	98%
Pneumonia Care				
Appropriate Initial Antibiotic	124	96%	92%	92%
Blood Culture Timing	231	87%	95%	96%
Influenza Vaccine	101	81%	90%	91%
Initial Antibiotic Timing	193	87%	93%	95%
Pneumococcal Vaccine	117	90%	92%	93%
Smoking Cessation Advice	108	97%	98%	97%
Surgical Care Improvement Project				
Appropriate VTP Within 24 Hours[2]	145	97%	94%	92%
Appropriate Hair Removal[2]	257	100%	100%	99%
Appropriate Beta Blocker Usage[2]	28	86%	92%	93%
Controlled Postoperative Blood Glucose[2]	0	-	94%	93%
Prophylactic Antibiotic Timing[2]	94	97%	96%	97%
Prophylactic Antibiotic Timing (Outpatient)	38	84%	92%	92%
Prophylactic Antibiotic Selection[2]	93	97%	97%	97%
Prophylactic Antibiotic Select. (Outpatient)	117	98%	93%	94%
Prophylactic Antibiotic Stopped[2]	89	97%	94%	94%
Recommended VTP Ordered[2]	145	97%	96%	94%
Urinary Catheter Removal[1,2]	22	73%	90%	90%
Children's Asthma Care				
Received Systemic Corticosteroids	-	-	-	100%
Received Home Management Plan	-	-	-	71%
Received Reliever Medication	-	-	-	100%
Use of Medical Imaging				
Combination Abdominal CT Scan	87	0.034	0.141	0.191
Combination Chest CT Scan[1]	35	0.029	0.024	0.054
Follow-up Mammogram/Ultrasound	186	3.8%	9.8%	8.4%
MRI for Low Back Pain[1]	7	14.3%	26.9%	32.7%
Survey of Patients' Hospital Experiences				
Area Around Room 'Always' Quiet at Night	300+	49%	-	58%
Doctors 'Always' Communicated Well	300+	74%	-	80%
Home Recovery Information Given	300+	82%	-	82%
Hospital Given 9 or 10 on 10 Point Scale	300+	51%	-	67%
Meds 'Always' Explained Before Given	300+	52%	-	60%
Nurses 'Always' Communicated Well	300+	63%	-	76%
Pain 'Always' Well Controlled	300+	57%	-	69%
Room and Bathroom 'Always' Clean	300+	63%	-	71%
Timely Help 'Always' Received	300+	45%	-	64%
Would Definitely Recommend Hospital	300+	53%	-	69%

Wyckoff Heights Medical Center

374 Stockholm Street Phone: 718-963-7272
Brooklyn, NY 11237 Fax: 718-963-7752
URL: www.wyckoffhospital.org
Type: Acute Care Hospitals Emergency Services: Yes
Ownership: Voluntary Non-Profit - Other Beds: 305

Key Personnel:

CEO/President. . . . . Dominick J Gio
Chief of Medical Staff . . . . Dr Nirmal Mattoo
Infection Control. . . . . John Vernaloo, MD
Operating Room. . . . . Vivian Jager, RN
Pediatric Ambulatory Care . . . . . . Sol Gourji, MD
Pediatric In-Patient Care . . . . Alvin Eden, MD
Quality Assurance . . . . Ruth Krauthamer, RN
Radiology. . . . . Mohsen Sanui

Measure	Cases	This Hosp.	State Avg.	U.S. Avg.
Heart Attack Care				
ACE Inhibitor or ARB for LVSD[1]	10	70%	95%	96%
Aspirin at Arrival	106	96%	98%	99%
Aspirin at Discharge	62	95%	98%	98%
Beta Blocker at Discharge	60	93%	98%	98%
Fibrinolytic Medication Timing	0	-	50%	55%
PCI Within 90 Minutes of Arrival	0	-	88%	90%
Smoking Cessation Advice[1]	7	86%	100%	99%
Chest Pain/Possible Heart Attack Care				
Aspirin at Arrival	31	100%	96%	95%
Median Time to ECG (minutes)	30	32	11	8
Median Time to Transfer (minutes)[1,3]	1	179	75	61
Fibrinolytic Medication Timing[1]	4	25%	55%	54%
Heart Failure Care				
ACE Inhibitor or ARB for LVSD[2]	132	97%	94%	94%
Discharge Instructions[2]	249	97%	89%	88%
Evaluation of LVS Function[2]	297	100%	98%	98%
Smoking Cessation Advice[2]	44	100%	98%	98%
Pneumonia Care				
Appropriate Initial Antibiotic[2]	117	88%	92%	92%
Blood Culture Timing[2]	107	89%	95%	96%
Influenza Vaccine[2]	90	86%	90%	91%
Initial Antibiotic Timing[2]	173	83%	93%	95%
Pneumococcal Vaccine[2]	142	89%	92%	93%
Smoking Cessation Advice[2]	36	100%	98%	97%
Surgical Care Improvement Project				
Appropriate VTP Within 24 Hours[2]	210	94%	94%	92%
Appropriate Hair Removal[2]	329	99%	100%	99%
Appropriate Beta Blocker Usage[2]	79	87%	92%	93%
Controlled Postoperative Blood Glucose[2]	0	-	94%	93%
Prophylactic Antibiotic Timing[2]	143	95%	96%	97%
Prophylactic Antibiotic Timing (Outpatient)	132	77%	92%	92%
Prophylactic Antibiotic Selection[2]	146	92%	97%	97%
Prophylactic Antibiotic Select. (Outpatient)	161	93%	93%	94%
Prophylactic Antibiotic Stopped[2]	132	80%	94%	94%
Recommended VTP Ordered[2]	210	96%	96%	94%
Urinary Catheter Removal[2]	42	57%	90%	90%
Children's Asthma Care				
Received Systemic Corticosteroids	-	-	-	100%
Received Home Management Plan	-	-	-	71%
Received Reliever Medication	-	-	-	100%
Use of Medical Imaging				
Combination Abdominal CT Scan	290	0.034	0.141	0.191
Combination Chest CT Scan	150	0.013	0.024	0.054
Follow-up Mammogram/Ultrasound	404	7.7%	9.8%	8.4%
MRI for Low Back Pain[1]	44	22.7%	26.9%	32.7%
Survey of Patients' Hospital Experiences				
Area Around Room 'Always' Quiet at Night	300+	39%	-	58%
Doctors 'Always' Communicated Well	300+	66%	-	80%
Home Recovery Information Given	300+	70%	-	82%
Hospital Given 9 or 10 on 10 Point Scale	300+	39%	-	67%
Meds 'Always' Explained Before Given	300+	45%	-	60%
Nurses 'Always' Communicated Well	300+	54%	-	76%
Pain 'Always' Well Controlled	300+	46%	-	69%
Room and Bathroom 'Always' Clean	300+	55%	-	71%
Timely Help 'Always' Received	300+	33%	-	64%
Would Definitely Recommend Hospital	300+	44%	-	69%

Erie County Medical Center

462 Grider Street Phone: 716-898-3936
Buffalo, NY 14215 Fax: 716-898-5178
URL: www.ecmc.edu
Type: Acute Care Hospitals Emergency Services: Yes
Ownership: Government - Local Beds: 550

Key Personnel:

CEO/President. . . . . Mark C Barabas, MHA
Chief of Medical Staff. . . . . John Fudyma, MD
Infection Control. . . . . Charlene Lulow
Operating Room. . . . . Jim Turner
Pediatric Ambulatory Care . . . . . . Melinda Cameron, MD
Quality Assurance . . . . Kitty Gazda
Radiology. . . . . Robert R Conti

Measure	Cases	This Hosp.	State Avg.	U.S. Avg.
Heart Attack Care				
ACE Inhibitor or ARB for LVSD	44	95%	95%	96%
Aspirin at Arrival	131	96%	98%	99%
Aspirin at Discharge	214	98%	98%	98%
Beta Blocker at Discharge	204	99%	98%	98%
Fibrinolytic Medication Timing	0	-	50%	55%
PCI Within 90 Minutes of Arrival	35	80%	88%	90%
Smoking Cessation Advice	100	100%	100%	99%
Chest Pain/Possible Heart Attack Care				
Aspirin at Arrival[5]	0	-	96%	95%
Median Time to ECG (minutes)[5]	0	-	11	8
Median Time to Transfer (minutes)[5]	0	-	75	61
Fibrinolytic Medication Timing[5]	0	-	55%	54%
Heart Failure Care				
ACE Inhibitor or ARB for LVSD	133	88%	94%	94%
Discharge Instructions	254	97%	89%	88%
Evaluation of LVS Function	311	99%	98%	98%
Smoking Cessation Advice	90	100%	98%	98%
Pneumonia Care				
Appropriate Initial Antibiotic	93	88%	92%	92%
Blood Culture Timing	219	94%	95%	96%
Influenza Vaccine	109	71%	90%	91%
Initial Antibiotic Timing	217	82%	93%	95%
Pneumococcal Vaccine	109	74%	92%	93%
Smoking Cessation Advice	98	95%	98%	97%
Surgical Care Improvement Project				
Appropriate VTP Within 24 Hours	335	92%	94%	92%
Appropriate Hair Removal	741	99%	100%	99%
Appropriate Beta Blocker Usage	240	79%	92%	93%
Controlled Postoperative Blood Glucose	127	91%	94%	93%
Prophylactic Antibiotic Timing	364	97%	96%	97%
Prophylactic Antibiotic Timing (Outpatient)	583	94%	92%	92%
Prophylactic Antibiotic Selection	372	98%	97%	97%
Prophylactic Antibiotic Select. (Outpatient)	598	98%	93%	94%
Prophylactic Antibiotic Stopped	345	92%	94%	94%
Recommended VTP Ordered	339	97%	96%	94%
Urinary Catheter Removal	155	85%	90%	90%
Children's Asthma Care				
Received Systemic Corticosteroids	-	-	-	100%
Received Home Management Plan	-	-	-	71%
Received Reliever Medication	-	-	-	100%
Use of Medical Imaging				
Combination Abdominal CT Scan	415	0.260	0.141	0.191
Combination Chest CT Scan	197	0.010	0.024	0.054
Follow-up Mammogram/Ultrasound	360	13.6%	9.8%	8.4%
MRI for Low Back Pain[5]	0	-	26.9%	32.7%
Survey of Patients' Hospital Experiences				
Area Around Room 'Always' Quiet at Night	300+	40%	-	58%
Doctors 'Always' Communicated Well	300+	72%	-	80%
Home Recovery Information Given	300+	79%	-	82%
Hospital Given 9 or 10 on 10 Point Scale	300+	53%	-	67%
Meds 'Always' Explained Before Given	300+	51%	-	60%
Nurses 'Always' Communicated Well	300+	66%	-	76%
Pain 'Always' Well Controlled	300+	60%	-	69%
Room and Bathroom 'Always' Clean	300+	49%	-	71%
Timely Help 'Always' Received	300+	44%	-	64%
Would Definitely Recommend Hospital	300+	58%	-	69%

NOTE: Hospital profiles are in alphabetical order by state, then city, then hospital within the city; Rankings exclude hospitals with less than 25 cases except for patient surveys which excludes hospitals with less than 100 cases; (a) 100–299 cases; (1) The number of cases is too small to be sure how well a hospital is performing; (2) The hospital indicated that the data submitted for this measure were based on a sample of cases; (3) Data was collected during a shorter time period (fewer quarters) than the maximum possible time for this measure; (4) Suppressed for one or more quarters by CMS; (5) No data is available from the hospital for this measure; (6) Fewer than 100 patients completed the HCAHPS survey. Use these rates with caution, as the number of surveys may be too low to reliably assess hospital performance; (7) Survey results are based on less than 12 months of data; (8) Survey results are not available for this reporting period; (9) No or very few patients were eligible for the HCAHPS survey. The scores shown, if any, reflect a very small number of surveys; (10) A state average was not calculated because too few hospitals in the state submitted data; (11) There were discrepancies in the data collection process; Please refer to the User's Guide for a full explanation of data.

Kaleida Health

726 Exchange Street, Suite 522
Buffalo, NY 14210
Phone: 716-859-8620
URL: kaleidahealth.org
Type: Acute Care Hospitals
Emergency Services: Yes
Ownership: Voluntary Non-Profit - Private

Key Personnel:
President/CEO . . . . James R Kaskie

Measure	Cases	This Hosp.	State Avg.	U.S. Avg.
Heart Attack Care				
ACE Inhibitor or ARB for LVSD[2]	116	93%	95%	96%
Aspirin at Arrival[2]	448	99%	98%	99%
Aspirin at Discharge[2]	854	97%	98%	98%
Beta Blocker at Discharge[2]	873	98%	98%	98%
Fibrinolytic Medication Timing[1,2]	6	83%	50%	55%
PCI Within 90 Minutes of Arrival[2]	36	83%	88%	90%
Smoking Cessation Advice[2]	250	100%	100%	99%
Chest Pain/Possible Heart Attack Care				
Aspirin at Arrival[1]	9	78%	96%	95%
Median Time to ECG (minutes)[1]	10	11	11	8
Median Time to Transfer (minutes)[5]	0	-	75	61
Fibrinolytic Medication Timing[3]	0	-	55%	54%
Heart Failure Care				
ACE Inhibitor or ARB for LVSD	489	96%	94%	94%
Discharge Instructions	1,265	84%	89%	88%
Evaluation of LVS Function	1,555	99%	98%	98%
Smoking Cessation Advice	274	100%	98%	98%
Pneumonia Care				
Appropriate Initial Antibiotic	623	95%	92%	92%
Blood Culture Timing	951	96%	95%	96%
Influenza Vaccine	551	93%	90%	91%
Initial Antibiotic Timing	943	92%	93%	95%
Pneumococcal Vaccine	830	87%	92%	93%
Smoking Cessation Advice	240	100%	98%	97%
Surgical Care Improvement Project				
Appropriate VTP Within 24 Hours[2]	454	95%	94%	92%
Appropriate Hair Removal[2]	1,365	100%	100%	99%
Appropriate Beta Blocker Usage[2]	431	91%	92%	93%
Controlled Postoperative Blood Glucose[2]	240	92%	94%	93%
Prophylactic Antibiotic Timing[2]	907	94%	96%	97%
Prophylactic Antibiotic Timing (Outpatient)	1,163	89%	92%	92%
Prophylactic Antibiotic Selection[2]	922	97%	97%	97%
Prophylactic Antibiotic Select. (Outpatient)	1,122	91%	93%	94%
Prophylactic Antibiotic Stopped[2]	863	94%	94%	94%
Recommended VTP Ordered[2]	454	97%	96%	94%
Urinary Catheter Removal[2]	321	84%	90%	90%
Children's Asthma Care				
Received Systemic Corticosteroids	550	98%	-	100%
Received Home Management Plan	552	16%	-	71%
Received Reliever Medication	553	100%	-	100%
Use of Medical Imaging				
Combination Abdominal CT Scan	1,233	0.600	0.141	0.191
Combination Chest CT Scan	623	0.091	0.024	0.054
Follow-up Mammogram/Ultrasound	1,095	11.7%	9.8%	8.4%
MRI for Low Back Pain	111	25.2%	26.9%	32.7%
Survey of Patients' Hospital Experiences				
Area Around Room 'Always' Quiet at Night	300+	44%	-	58%
Doctors 'Always' Communicated Well	300+	74%	-	80%
Home Recovery Information Given	300+	82%	-	82%
Hospital Given 9 or 10 on 10 Point Scale	300+	60%	-	67%
Meds 'Always' Explained Before Given	300+	54%	-	60%
Nurses 'Always' Communicated Well	300+	71%	-	76%
Pain 'Always' Well Controlled	300+	64%	-	69%
Room and Bathroom 'Always' Clean	300+	57%	-	71%
Timely Help 'Always' Received	300+	54%	-	64%
Would Definitely Recommend Hospital	300+	64%	-	69%

Mercy Hospital

565 Abbott Road
Buffalo, NY 14220
Phone: 716-826-7000
Fax: 716-828-2700
URL: www.chsbuffalo.org
Type: Acute Care Hospitals
Emergency Services: Yes
Ownership: Voluntary Non-Profit - Church
Beds: 349

Key Personnel:
CEO/President. . . . . John Davanzo
Chief of Medical Staff . . . . Richard Ruh, MD
Infection Control. . . . . Carole McCann
Operating Room. . . . . Sharon Kimaid
Quality Assurance . . . . Nancy Sheehan
Radiology. . . . . Margaret Jetter

Measure	Cases	This Hosp.	State Avg.	U.S. Avg.
Heart Attack Care				
ACE Inhibitor or ARB for LVSD[2]	43	98%	95%	96%
Aspirin at Arrival[2]	201	99%	98%	99%
Aspirin at Discharge[2]	320	98%	98%	98%
Beta Blocker at Discharge[2]	319	98%	98%	98%
Fibrinolytic Medication Timing[1,2]	3	67%	50%	55%
PCI Within 90 Minutes of Arrival[2]	26	88%	88%	90%
Smoking Cessation Advice[2]	112	100%	100%	99%
Chest Pain/Possible Heart Attack Care				
Aspirin at Arrival[1,3]	19	84%	96%	95%
Median Time to ECG (minutes)[1,3]	19	20	11	8
Median Time to Transfer (minutes)[1,3]	1	80	75	61
Fibrinolytic Medication Timing[3]	0	-	55%	54%
Heart Failure Care				
ACE Inhibitor or ARB for LVSD[2]	69	96%	94%	94%
Discharge Instructions[2]	244	90%	89%	88%
Evaluation of LVS Function[2]	334	100%	98%	98%
Smoking Cessation Advice[2]	37	95%	98%	98%
Pneumonia Care				
Appropriate Initial Antibiotic[2]	97	95%	92%	92%
Blood Culture Timing[2]	133	98%	95%	96%
Influenza Vaccine[2]	79	90%	90%	91%
Initial Antibiotic Timing[2]	129	94%	93%	95%
Pneumococcal Vaccine[2]	124	95%	92%	93%
Smoking Cessation Advice[2]	56	100%	98%	97%
Surgical Care Improvement Project				
Appropriate VTP Within 24 Hours[2]	152	95%	94%	92%
Appropriate Hair Removal[2]	701	100%	100%	99%
Appropriate Beta Blocker Usage[2]	265	93%	92%	93%
Controlled Postoperative Blood Glucose[2]	170	95%	94%	93%
Prophylactic Antibiotic Timing[2]	486	94%	96%	97%
Prophylactic Antibiotic Timing (Outpatient)	560	97%	92%	92%
Prophylactic Antibiotic Selection[2]	506	97%	97%	97%
Prophylactic Antibiotic Select. (Outpatient)	548	98%	93%	94%
Prophylactic Antibiotic Stopped[2]	459	97%	94%	94%
Recommended VTP Ordered[2]	152	99%	96%	94%
Urinary Catheter Removal[2]	156	94%	90%	90%
Children's Asthma Care				
Received Systemic Corticosteroids	-	-	-	100%
Received Home Management Plan	-	-	-	71%
Received Reliever Medication	-	-	-	100%
Use of Medical Imaging				
Combination Abdominal CT Scan	692	0.084	0.141	0.191
Combination Chest CT Scan	449	0.000	0.024	0.054
Follow-up Mammogram/Ultrasound	1,002	5.4%	9.8%	8.4%
MRI for Low Back Pain[1]	14	28.6%	26.9%	32.7%
Survey of Patients' Hospital Experiences				
Area Around Room 'Always' Quiet at Night	300+	39%	-	58%
Doctors 'Always' Communicated Well	300+	72%	-	80%
Home Recovery Information Given	300+	80%	-	82%
Hospital Given 9 or 10 on 10 Point Scale	300+	48%	-	67%
Meds 'Always' Explained Before Given	300+	47%	-	60%
Nurses 'Always' Communicated Well	300+	68%	-	76%
Pain 'Always' Well Controlled	300+	61%	-	69%
Room and Bathroom 'Always' Clean	300+	53%	-	71%
Timely Help 'Always' Received	300+	47%	-	64%
Would Definitely Recommend Hospital	300+	49%	-	69%

Sheehan Memorial Hospital

425 Michigan Avenue
Buffalo, NY 14203
Phone: 716-848-2000
Fax: 716-848-2125
E-mail: info@smhhealth.org
URL: www.smhhealth.org
Type: Acute Care Hospitals
Emergency Services: No
Ownership: Voluntary Non-Profit - Private
Beds: 109

Key Personnel:
CEO/President. . . . . Sheila Kee
Chief of Medical Staff . . . . Nathaniel Webster
Emergency Room . . . . Jospeh L Maddi
Intensive Care Unit. . . . . Petricia Mitchell

Measure	Cases	This Hosp.	State Avg.	U.S. Avg.
Heart Attack Care				
ACE Inhibitor or ARB for LVSD[5]	0	-	95%	96%
Aspirin at Arrival[5]	0	-	98%	99%
Aspirin at Discharge[5]	0	-	98%	98%
Beta Blocker at Discharge[5]	0	-	98%	98%
Fibrinolytic Medication Timing[5]	0	-	50%	55%
PCI Within 90 Minutes of Arrival[5]	0	-	88%	90%
Smoking Cessation Advice[5]	0	-	100%	99%
Chest Pain/Possible Heart Attack Care				
Aspirin at Arrival[5]	0	-	96%	95%
Median Time to ECG (minutes)[5]	0	-	11	8
Median Time to Transfer (minutes)[5]	0	-	75	61
Fibrinolytic Medication Timing[5]	0	-	55%	54%
Heart Failure Care				
ACE Inhibitor or ARB for LVSD[5]	0	-	94%	94%
Discharge Instructions[5]	0	-	89%	88%
Evaluation of LVS Function[5]	0	-	98%	98%
Smoking Cessation Advice[5]	0	-	98%	98%
Pneumonia Care				
Appropriate Initial Antibiotic[5]	0	-	92%	92%
Blood Culture Timing[5]	0	-	95%	96%
Influenza Vaccine[5]	0	-	90%	91%
Initial Antibiotic Timing[5]	0	-	93%	95%
Pneumococcal Vaccine[5]	0	-	92%	93%
Smoking Cessation Advice[5]	0	-	98%	97%
Surgical Care Improvement Project				
Appropriate VTP Within 24 Hours[5]	0	-	94%	92%
Appropriate Hair Removal[5]	0	-	100%	99%
Appropriate Beta Blocker Usage[5]	0	-	92%	93%
Controlled Postoperative Blood Glucose[5]	0	-	94%	93%
Prophylactic Antibiotic Timing[5]	0	-	96%	97%
Prophylactic Antibiotic Timing (Outpatient)[5]	0	-	92%	92%
Prophylactic Antibiotic Selection[5]	0	-	97%	97%
Prophylactic Antibiotic Select. (Outpatient)[5]	0	-	93%	94%
Prophylactic Antibiotic Stopped[5]	0	-	94%	94%
Recommended VTP Ordered[5]	0	-	96%	94%
Urinary Catheter Removal[5]	0	-	90%	90%
Children's Asthma Care				
Received Systemic Corticosteroids	-	-	-	100%
Received Home Management Plan	-	-	-	71%
Received Reliever Medication	-	-	-	100%
Use of Medical Imaging				
Combination Abdominal CT Scan[1]	6	0.000	0.141	0.191
Combination Chest CT Scan[1]	9	0.000	0.024	0.054
Follow-up Mammogram/Ultrasound[1]	34	5.9%	9.8%	8.4%
MRI for Low Back Pain[5]	0	-	26.9%	32.7%
Survey of Patients' Hospital Experiences				
Area Around Room 'Always' Quiet at Night[9]	-	-	-	58%
Doctors 'Always' Communicated Well[9]	-	-	-	80%
Home Recovery Information Given[9]	-	-	-	82%
Hospital Given 9 or 10 on 10 Point Scale[9]	-	-	-	67%
Meds 'Always' Explained Before Given[9]	-	-	-	60%
Nurses 'Always' Communicated Well[9]	-	-	-	76%
Pain 'Always' Well Controlled[9]	-	-	-	69%
Room and Bathroom 'Always' Clean[9]	-	-	-	71%
Timely Help 'Always' Received[9]	-	-	-	64%
Would Definitely Recommend Hospital[9]	-	-	-	69%

NOTE: Hospital profiles are in alphabetical order by state, then city, then hospital within the city; Rankings exclude hospitals with less than 25 cases except for patient surveys which excludes hospitals with less than 100 cases; (a) 100–299 cases; (1) The number of cases is too small to be sure how well a hospital is performing; (2) The hospital indicated that the data submitted for this measure were based on a sample of cases; (3) Data was collected during a shorter time period (fewer quarters) than the maximum possible time for this measure; (4) Suppressed for one or more quarters by CMS; (5) No data is available from the hospital for this measure; (6) Fewer than 100 patients completed the HCAHPS survey. Use these rates with caution, as the number of surveys may be too low to reliably assess hospital performance; (7) Survey results are based on less than 12 months of data; (8) Survey results are not available for this reporting period; (9) No or very few patients were eligible for the HCAHPS survey. The scores shown, if any, reflect a very small number of surveys; (10) A state average was not calculated because too few hospitals in the state submitted data; (11) There were discrepancies in the data collection process; Please refer to the User's Guide for a full explanation of data.

Sisters of Charity Hospital

2157 Main Street
Buffalo, NY 14214
Phone: 716-862-1000
Fax: 716-862-1809
URL: www.chsbuffalo.org
Type: Acute Care Hospitals
Emergency Services: Yes
Ownership: Voluntary Non-Profit - Church
Beds: 413

Key Personnel:
CEO/President.............. Peter Bergmann
Chief of Medical Staff.......... Nady Shehata MD
Coronary Care............ Susan Cirbus
Infection Control............ Patricia Jones
Pediatric Ambulatory Care...... Frank Giacobbe MD
Pediatric In-Patient Care...... Frank Giacobbe MD
Quality Assurance........... Carolyn Yeates
Radiology................. Michael Reilly

Measure	Cases	This Hosp.	State Avg.	U.S. Avg.
Heart Attack Care				
ACE Inhibitor or ARB for LVSD[1]	15	93%	95%	96%
Aspirin at Arrival	146	97%	98%	99%
Aspirin at Discharge	79	95%	98%	98%
Beta Blocker at Discharge	84	99%	98%	98%
Fibrinolytic Medication Timing[1]	1	100%	50%	55%
PCI Within 90 Minutes of Arrival	0	-	88%	90%
Smoking Cessation Advice[1]	11	100%	100%	99%
Chest Pain/Possible Heart Attack Care				
Aspirin at Arrival	61	100%	96%	95%
Median Time to ECG (minutes)	64	14	11	8
Median Time to Transfer (minutes)[1]	5	108	75	61
Fibrinolytic Medication Timing[1]	3	67%	55%	54%
Heart Failure Care				
ACE Inhibitor or ARB for LVSD[2]	118	92%	94%	94%
Discharge Instructions[2]	393	77%	89%	88%
Evaluation of LVS Function[2]	516	100%	98%	98%
Smoking Cessation Advice[2]	61	97%	98%	98%
Pneumonia Care				
Appropriate Initial Antibiotic[2]	216	91%	92%	92%
Blood Culture Timing[2]	263	96%	95%	96%
Influenza Vaccine[2]	168	89%	90%	91%
Initial Antibiotic Timing[2]	285	94%	93%	95%
Pneumococcal Vaccine[2]	248	92%	92%	93%
Smoking Cessation Advice[2]	104	98%	98%	97%
Surgical Care Improvement Project				
Appropriate VTP Within 24 Hours[2]	257	91%	94%	92%
Appropriate Hair Removal[2]	873	100%	100%	99%
Appropriate Beta Blocker Usage[2]	284	90%	92%	93%
Controlled Postoperative Blood Glucose[2]	0	-	94%	93%
Prophylactic Antibiotic Timing[2]	567	96%	96%	97%
Prophylactic Antibiotic Timing (Outpatient)	614	91%	92%	92%
Prophylactic Antibiotic Selection[2]	571	95%	97%	97%
Prophylactic Antibiotic Select. (Outpatient)	596	97%	93%	94%
Prophylactic Antibiotic Stopped[2]	545	92%	94%	94%
Recommended VTP Ordered[2]	258	93%	96%	94%
Urinary Catheter Removal[2]	215	88%	90%	90%
Children's Asthma Care				
Received Systemic Corticosteroids	-	-	-	100%
Received Home Management Plan	-	-	-	71%
Received Reliever Medication	-	-	-	100%
Use of Medical Imaging				
Combination Abdominal CT Scan	292	0.051	0.141	0.191
Combination Chest CT Scan	188	0.043	0.024	0.054
Follow-up Mammogram/Ultrasound	372	8.1%	9.8%	8.4%
MRI for Low Back Pain[1]	11	18.2%	26.9%	32.7%
Survey of Patients' Hospital Experiences				
Area Around Room 'Always' Quiet at Night	300+	47%	-	58%
Doctors 'Always' Communicated Well	300+	73%	-	80%
Home Recovery Information Given	300+	84%	-	82%
Hospital Given 9 or 10 on 10 Point Scale	300+	64%	-	67%
Meds 'Always' Explained Before Given	300+	55%	-	60%
Nurses 'Always' Communicated Well	300+	73%	-	76%
Pain 'Always' Well Controlled	300+	66%	-	69%
Room and Bathroom 'Always' Clean	300+	61%	-	71%
Timely Help 'Always' Received	300+	56%	-	64%
Would Definitely Recommend Hospital	300+	68%	-	69%

Upstate New York VA Healthcare System

3495 Bailey Avenue
Buffalo, NY 14215
Phone: 716-862-3611
Fax: 716-862-8759
URL: www.buffalo.va.gov
Type: Acute Care-Veterans Administration
Emergency Services: No
Ownership: Government - Federal
Beds: 288

Key Personnel:
Chief of Medical Staff.......... Miguel Rainstein, MD
Infection Control............ John Sellick, MD
Operating Room............. Israel Ziv, MD
Quality Assurance........... Kathryn Varkonda
Emergency Room............ Mukesh Nangia, MD
Patient Relations............ Lizabeth M Weiss, RN, CNA

Measure	Cases	This Hosp.	State Avg.	U.S. Avg.
Heart Attack Care				
ACE Inhibitor or ARB for LVSD[1]	14	71%	95%	96%
Aspirin at Arrival	46	100%	98%	99%
Aspirin at Discharge	46	100%	98%	98%
Beta Blocker at Discharge	45	100%	98%	98%
Fibrinolytic Medication Timing[1]	1	0%	50%	55%
PCI Within 90 Minutes of Arrival[1]	6	83%	88%	90%
Smoking Cessation Advice[1]	15	100%	100%	99%
Chest Pain/Possible Heart Attack Care				
Aspirin at Arrival	-	-	96%	95%
Median Time to ECG (minutes)	-	-	11	8
Median Time to Transfer (minutes)	-	-	75	61
Fibrinolytic Medication Timing	-	-	55%	54%
Heart Failure Care				
ACE Inhibitor or ARB for LVSD	91	82%	94%	94%
Discharge Instructions	154	95%	89%	88%
Evaluation of LVS Function	184	100%	98%	98%
Smoking Cessation Advice	27	100%	98%	98%
Pneumonia Care				
Appropriate Initial Antibiotic	57	91%	92%	92%
Blood Culture Timing	107	99%	95%	96%
Influenza Vaccine	59	88%	90%	91%
Initial Antibiotic Timing	95	91%	93%	95%
Pneumococcal Vaccine	92	95%	92%	93%
Smoking Cessation Advice	26	100%	98%	97%
Surgical Care Improvement Project				
Appropriate VTP Within 24 Hours[2]	116	94%	94%	92%
Appropriate Hair Removal[2]	282	100%	100%	99%
Appropriate Beta Blocker Usage[2]	129	96%	92%	93%
Controlled Postoperative Blood Glucose[2]	67	96%	94%	93%
Prophylactic Antibiotic Timing	156	96%	96%	97%
Prophylactic Antibiotic Timing (Outpatient)	-	-	92%	92%
Prophylactic Antibiotic Selection	163	98%	97%	97%
Prophylactic Antibiotic Select. (Outpatient)	-	-	93%	94%
Prophylactic Antibiotic Stopped	151	94%	94%	94%
Recommended VTP Ordered[2]	116	94%	96%	94%
Urinary Catheter Removal[2]	86	63%	90%	90%
Children's Asthma Care				
Received Systemic Corticosteroids	-	-	-	100%
Received Home Management Plan	-	-	-	71%
Received Reliever Medication	-	-	-	100%
Use of Medical Imaging				
Combination Abdominal CT Scan	-	-	0.141	0.191
Combination Chest CT Scan	-	-	0.024	0.054
Follow-up Mammogram/Ultrasound	-	-	9.8%	8.4%
MRI for Low Back Pain	-	-	26.9%	32.7%
Survey of Patients' Hospital Experiences				
Area Around Room 'Always' Quiet at Night	-	-	-	58%
Doctors 'Always' Communicated Well	-	-	-	80%
Home Recovery Information Given	-	-	-	82%
Hospital Given 9 or 10 on 10 Point Scale	-	-	-	67%
Meds 'Always' Explained Before Given	-	-	-	60%
Nurses 'Always' Communicated Well	-	-	-	76%
Pain 'Always' Well Controlled	-	-	-	69%
Room and Bathroom 'Always' Clean	-	-	-	71%
Timely Help 'Always' Received	-	-	-	64%
Would Definitely Recommend Hospital	-	-	-	69%

Canandaigua VA Medical Center

400 Foot Hill Ave.
Canandaigua, NY 14424
Phone: 585-394-2000
Fax: 585-393-8328
URL: www.va.gov
Type: Acute Care-Veterans Administration
Emergency Services: No
Ownership: Government - Federal
Beds: 251

Key Personnel:
Chief of Medical Staff.......... Robert Babcock, MD
Infection Control............ Marguerite Sutton
Quality Assurance........... Doug Nather, RN
Ambulatory Care............ Richard Beninegna, MD
Patient Relations............ Laurie Guererri

Measure	Cases	This Hosp.	State Avg.	U.S. Avg.
Heart Attack Care				
ACE Inhibitor or ARB for LVSD[5]	0	-	95%	96%
Aspirin at Arrival[5]	0	-	98%	99%
Aspirin at Discharge[5]	0	-	98%	98%
Beta Blocker at Discharge[5]	0	-	98%	98%
Fibrinolytic Medication Timing[5]	0	-	50%	55%
PCI Within 90 Minutes of Arrival[5]	0	-	88%	90%
Smoking Cessation Advice[5]	0	-	100%	99%
Chest Pain/Possible Heart Attack Care				
Aspirin at Arrival	-	-	96%	95%
Median Time to ECG (minutes)	-	-	11	8
Median Time to Transfer (minutes)	-	-	75	61
Fibrinolytic Medication Timing	-	-	55%	54%
Heart Failure Care				
ACE Inhibitor or ARB for LVSD[5]	0	-	94%	94%
Discharge Instructions[5]	0	-	89%	88%
Evaluation of LVS Function[5]	0	-	98%	98%
Smoking Cessation Advice[5]	0	-	98%	98%
Pneumonia Care				
Appropriate Initial Antibiotic[5]	0	-	92%	92%
Blood Culture Timing[5]	0	-	95%	96%
Influenza Vaccine[5]	0	-	90%	91%
Initial Antibiotic Timing[5]	0	-	93%	95%
Pneumococcal Vaccine[5]	0	-	92%	93%
Smoking Cessation Advice[5]	0	-	98%	97%
Surgical Care Improvement Project				
Appropriate VTP Within 24 Hours[2,5]	0	-	94%	92%
Appropriate Hair Removal[2,5]	0	-	100%	99%
Appropriate Beta Blocker Usage[2,5]	0	-	92%	93%
Controlled Postoperative Blood Glucose[2,5]	0	-	94%	93%
Prophylactic Antibiotic Timing[5]	0	-	96%	97%
Prophylactic Antibiotic Timing (Outpatient)	-	-	92%	92%
Prophylactic Antibiotic Selection[5]	0	-	97%	97%
Prophylactic Antibiotic Select. (Outpatient)	-	-	93%	94%
Prophylactic Antibiotic Stopped[5]	0	-	94%	94%
Recommended VTP Ordered[2,5]	0	-	96%	94%
Urinary Catheter Removal[2,5]	0	-	90%	90%
Children's Asthma Care				
Received Systemic Corticosteroids	-	-	-	100%
Received Home Management Plan	-	-	-	71%
Received Reliever Medication	-	-	-	100%
Use of Medical Imaging				
Combination Abdominal CT Scan	-	-	0.141	0.191
Combination Chest CT Scan	-	-	0.024	0.054
Follow-up Mammogram/Ultrasound	-	-	9.8%	8.4%
MRI for Low Back Pain	-	-	26.9%	32.7%
Survey of Patients' Hospital Experiences				
Area Around Room 'Always' Quiet at Night	-	-	-	58%
Doctors 'Always' Communicated Well	-	-	-	80%
Home Recovery Information Given	-	-	-	82%
Hospital Given 9 or 10 on 10 Point Scale	-	-	-	67%
Meds 'Always' Explained Before Given	-	-	-	60%
Nurses 'Always' Communicated Well	-	-	-	76%
Pain 'Always' Well Controlled	-	-	-	69%
Room and Bathroom 'Always' Clean	-	-	-	71%
Timely Help 'Always' Received	-	-	-	64%
Would Definitely Recommend Hospital	-	-	-	69%

NOTE: Hospital profiles are in alphabetical order by state, then city, then hospital within the city; Rankings exclude hospitals with less than 25 cases except for patient surveys which excludes hospitals with less than 100 cases; (a) 100–299 cases; (1) The number of cases is too small to be sure how well a hospital is performing; (2) The hospital indicated that the data submitted for this measure were based on a sample of cases; (3) Data was collected during a shorter time period (fewer quarters) than the maximum possible time for this measure; (4) Suppressed for one or more quarters by CMS; (5) No data is available from the hospital for this measure; (6) Fewer than 100 patients completed the HCAHPS survey. Use these rates with caution, as the number of surveys may be too low to reliably assess hospital performance; (7) Survey results are based on less than 12 months of data; (8) Survey results are not available for this reporting period; (9) No or very few patients were eligible for the HCAHPS survey. The scores shown, if any, reflect a very small number of surveys; (10) A state average was not calculated because too few hospitals in the state submitted data; (11) There were discrepancies in the data collection process; Please refer to the User's Guide for a full explanation of data.

F F Thompson Hospital

350 Parrish Street Phone: 585-396-6000
Canandaigua, NY 14424 Fax: 585-396-6477
URL: www.thompsonhealth.com
Type: Acute Care Hospitals Emergency Services: Yes
Ownership: Voluntary Non-Profit - Private Beds: 113

Key Personnel:
CEO/President. . . . . Linda M Farchione
Chief of Medical Staff. . . . . R Douglas Alling, MD
Infection Control. . . . . Gloria Karr
Operating Room. . . . . Donna Fulmer
Pediatric In-Patient Care . . . . Diana Ellison
Quality Assurance . . . . Linda Neva
Hemotology Center . . . . Susan Bonanni
Intensive Care Unit. . . . . Donna Fulmer

Measure	Cases	This Hosp.	State Avg.	U.S. Avg.
Heart Attack Care				
ACE Inhibitor or ARB for LVSD[1]	5	100%	95%	96%
Aspirin at Arrival	35	89%	98%	99%
Aspirin at Discharge[1]	24	92%	98%	98%
Beta Blocker at Discharge	30	93%	98%	98%
Fibrinolytic Medication Timing	0	-	50%	55%
PCI Within 90 Minutes of Arrival	0	-	88%	90%
Smoking Cessation Advice[1]	3	100%	100%	99%
Chest Pain/Possible Heart Attack Care				
Aspirin at Arrival	123	96%	96%	95%
Median Time to ECG (minutes)	124	10	11	8
Median Time to Transfer (minutes)	28	44	75	61
Fibrinolytic Medication Timing	0	-	55%	54%
Heart Failure Care				
ACE Inhibitor or ARB for LVSD	33	82%	94%	94%
Discharge Instructions	123	66%	89%	88%
Evaluation of LVS Function	145	99%	98%	98%
Smoking Cessation Advice[1]	4	100%	98%	98%
Pneumonia Care				
Appropriate Initial Antibiotic	163	87%	92%	92%
Blood Culture Timing	221	97%	95%	96%
Influenza Vaccine	124	90%	90%	91%
Initial Antibiotic Timing	215	97%	93%	95%
Pneumococcal Vaccine	194	91%	92%	93%
Smoking Cessation Advice	63	100%	98%	97%
Surgical Care Improvement Project				
Appropriate VTP Within 24 Hours	146	90%	94%	92%
Appropriate Hair Removal	464	100%	100%	99%
Appropriate Beta Blocker Usage	125	86%	92%	93%
Controlled Postoperative Blood Glucose	0	-	94%	93%
Prophylactic Antibiotic Timing	401	98%	96%	97%
Prophylactic Antibiotic Timing (Outpatient)	84	96%	92%	92%
Prophylactic Antibiotic Selection	401	96%	97%	97%
Prophylactic Antibiotic Select. (Outpatient)	83	99%	93%	94%
Prophylactic Antibiotic Stopped	388	98%	94%	94%
Recommended VTP Ordered	146	90%	96%	94%
Urinary Catheter Removal	135	93%	90%	90%
Children's Asthma Care				
Received Systemic Corticosteroids	-	-	-	100%
Received Home Management Plan	-	-	-	71%
Received Reliever Medication	-	-	-	100%
Use of Medical Imaging				
Combination Abdominal CT Scan	361	0.551	0.141	0.191
Combination Chest CT Scan	212	0.014	0.024	0.054
Follow-up Mammogram/Ultrasound	649	4.5%	9.8%	8.4%
MRI for Low Back Pain[5]	0	-	26.9%	32.7%
Survey of Patients' Hospital Experiences				
Area Around Room 'Always' Quiet at Night	300+	47%	-	58%
Doctors 'Always' Communicated Well	300+	80%	-	80%
Home Recovery Information Given	300+	87%	-	82%
Hospital Given 9 or 10 on 10 Point Scale	300+	69%	-	67%
Meds 'Always' Explained Before Given	300+	61%	-	60%
Nurses 'Always' Communicated Well	300+	77%	-	76%
Pain 'Always' Well Controlled	300+	68%	-	69%
Room and Bathroom 'Always' Clean	300+	69%	-	71%
Timely Help 'Always' Received	300+	68%	-	64%
Would Definitely Recommend Hospital	300+	76%	-	69%

Putnam Hospital Center

670 Stoneleigh Avenue Phone: 914-279-5711
Carmel, NY 10512 Fax: 845-279-7482
E-mail: info@putnamhospital.org
URL: www.putnamhospital.org
Type: Acute Care Hospitals Emergency Services: Yes
Ownership: Voluntary Non-Profit - Private Beds: 164

Key Personnel:
Radiology. . . . . Philip Amatulle

Measure	Cases	This Hosp.	State Avg.	U.S. Avg.
Heart Attack Care				
ACE Inhibitor or ARB for LVSD[1]	6	83%	95%	96%
Aspirin at Arrival	43	98%	98%	99%
Aspirin at Discharge	25	100%	98%	98%
Beta Blocker at Discharge	25	100%	98%	98%
Fibrinolytic Medication Timing	0	-	50%	55%
PCI Within 90 Minutes of Arrival	0	-	88%	90%
Smoking Cessation Advice[1]	3	100%	100%	99%
Chest Pain/Possible Heart Attack Care				
Aspirin at Arrival	67	96%	96%	95%
Median Time to ECG (minutes)	67	12	11	8
Median Time to Transfer (minutes)[1,3]	3	198	75	61
Fibrinolytic Medication Timing[1]	14	43%	55%	54%
Heart Failure Care				
ACE Inhibitor or ARB for LVSD	62	90%	94%	94%
Discharge Instructions	159	91%	89%	88%
Evaluation of LVS Function	225	99%	98%	98%
Smoking Cessation Advice[1]	20	100%	98%	98%
Pneumonia Care				
Appropriate Initial Antibiotic	107	94%	92%	92%
Blood Culture Timing	157	98%	95%	96%
Influenza Vaccine	97	98%	90%	91%
Initial Antibiotic Timing	148	99%	93%	95%
Pneumococcal Vaccine	142	97%	92%	93%
Smoking Cessation Advice	38	100%	98%	97%
Surgical Care Improvement Project				
Appropriate VTP Within 24 Hours	424	93%	94%	92%
Appropriate Hair Removal	708	100%	100%	99%
Appropriate Beta Blocker Usage	224	96%	92%	93%
Controlled Postoperative Blood Glucose	0	-	94%	93%
Prophylactic Antibiotic Timing	538	98%	96%	97%
Prophylactic Antibiotic Timing (Outpatient)	150	94%	92%	92%
Prophylactic Antibiotic Selection	537	98%	97%	97%
Prophylactic Antibiotic Select. (Outpatient)	148	92%	93%	94%
Prophylactic Antibiotic Stopped	535	98%	94%	94%
Recommended VTP Ordered	424	95%	96%	94%
Urinary Catheter Removal	289	95%	90%	90%
Children's Asthma Care				
Received Systemic Corticosteroids	-	-	-	100%
Received Home Management Plan	-	-	-	71%
Received Reliever Medication	-	-	-	100%
Use of Medical Imaging				
Combination Abdominal CT Scan	566	0.120	0.141	0.191
Combination Chest CT Scan	463	0.002	0.024	0.054
Follow-up Mammogram/Ultrasound	811	8.3%	9.8%	8.4%
MRI for Low Back Pain	129	30.2%	26.9%	32.7%
Survey of Patients' Hospital Experiences				
Area Around Room 'Always' Quiet at Night	300+	55%	-	58%
Doctors 'Always' Communicated Well	300+	83%	-	80%
Home Recovery Information Given	300+	81%	-	82%
Hospital Given 9 or 10 on 10 Point Scale	300+	74%	-	67%
Meds 'Always' Explained Before Given	300+	60%	-	60%
Nurses 'Always' Communicated Well	300+	79%	-	76%
Pain 'Always' Well Controlled	300+	73%	-	69%
Room and Bathroom 'Always' Clean	300+	74%	-	71%
Timely Help 'Always' Received	300+	66%	-	64%
Would Definitely Recommend Hospital	300+	76%	-	69%

Carthage Area Hospital

1001 West Street Phone: 315-493-1000
Carthage, NY 13619 Fax: 315-493-4231
E-mail: cahadmin@carthageareahospital.com
URL: www.carthagehospital.com
Type: Acute Care Hospitals Emergency Services: Yes
Ownership: Voluntary Non-Profit - Private Beds: 78

Key Personnel:
CEO/President. . . . . Walter Becker
Cardiac Laboratory. . . . . Mirza Ashraf, MD
Chief of Medical Staff . . . . Kenneth Fish, DO
Infection Control. . . . . Patti Jahnke
Operating Room. . . . . Belinda Pearson, RN
Quality Assurance . . . . Jan Widrick
Radiology. . . . . Daniel Gray
Intensive Care Unit. . . . . Paula Bigelow, RN

Measure	Cases	This Hosp.	State Avg.	U.S. Avg.
Heart Attack Care				
ACE Inhibitor or ARB for LVSD[3]	0	-	95%	96%
Aspirin at Arrival[1,3]	7	100%	98%	99%
Aspirin at Discharge[1,3]	2	50%	98%	98%
Beta Blocker at Discharge[1,3]	2	100%	98%	98%
Fibrinolytic Medication Timing[3]	0	-	50%	55%
PCI Within 90 Minutes of Arrival[3]	0	-	88%	90%
Smoking Cessation Advice[1,3]	1	0%	100%	99%
Chest Pain/Possible Heart Attack Care				
Aspirin at Arrival	40	92%	96%	95%
Median Time to ECG (minutes)	41	7	11	8
Median Time to Transfer (minutes)[1,3]	3	320	75	61
Fibrinolytic Medication Timing	0	-	55%	54%
Heart Failure Care				
ACE Inhibitor or ARB for LVSD[1]	15	80%	94%	94%
Discharge Instructions	54	70%	89%	88%
Evaluation of LVS Function	61	97%	98%	98%
Smoking Cessation Advice[1]	7	86%	98%	98%
Pneumonia Care				
Appropriate Initial Antibiotic	26	77%	92%	92%
Blood Culture Timing	29	79%	95%	96%
Influenza Vaccine[1]	24	79%	90%	91%
Initial Antibiotic Timing	34	91%	93%	95%
Pneumococcal Vaccine	33	88%	92%	93%
Smoking Cessation Advice[1]	12	100%	98%	97%
Surgical Care Improvement Project				
Appropriate VTP Within 24 Hours[1]	10	40%	94%	92%
Appropriate Hair Removal	45	100%	100%	99%
Appropriate Beta Blocker Usage[1]	4	75%	92%	93%
Controlled Postoperative Blood Glucose	0	-	94%	93%
Prophylactic Antibiotic Timing	29	86%	96%	97%
Prophylactic Antibiotic Timing (Outpatient)	38	55%	92%	92%
Prophylactic Antibiotic Selection	29	97%	97%	97%
Prophylactic Antibiotic Select. (Outpatient)	31	45%	93%	94%
Prophylactic Antibiotic Stopped	29	90%	94%	94%
Recommended VTP Ordered[1]	10	50%	96%	94%
Urinary Catheter Removal[1]	1	100%	90%	90%
Children's Asthma Care				
Received Systemic Corticosteroids	-	-	-	100%
Received Home Management Plan	-	-	-	71%
Received Reliever Medication	-	-	-	100%
Use of Medical Imaging				
Combination Abdominal CT Scan	169	0.331	0.141	0.191
Combination Chest CT Scan	130	0.077	0.024	0.054
Follow-up Mammogram/Ultrasound	213	2.3%	9.8%	8.4%
MRI for Low Back Pain[1]	23	26.1%	26.9%	32.7%
Survey of Patients' Hospital Experiences				
Area Around Room 'Always' Quiet at Night	300+	47%	-	58%
Doctors 'Always' Communicated Well	300+	74%	-	80%
Home Recovery Information Given	300+	83%	-	82%
Hospital Given 9 or 10 on 10 Point Scale	300+	57%	-	67%
Meds 'Always' Explained Before Given	300+	59%	-	60%
Nurses 'Always' Communicated Well	300+	69%	-	76%
Pain 'Always' Well Controlled	300+	62%	-	69%
Room and Bathroom 'Always' Clean	300+	72%	-	71%
Timely Help 'Always' Received	300+	54%	-	64%
Would Definitely Recommend Hospital	300+	62%	-	69%

NOTE: Hospital profiles are in alphabetical order by state, then city, then hospital within the city; Rankings exclude hospitals with less than 25 cases except for patient surveys which excludes hospitals with less than 100 cases; (a) 100–299 cases; (1) The number of cases is too small to be sure how well a hospital is performing; (2) The hospital indicated that the data submitted for this measure were based on a sample of cases; (3) Data was collected during a shorter time period (fewer quarters) than the maximum possible time for this measure; (4) Suppressed for one or more quarters by CMS; (5) No data is available from the hospital for this measure; (6) Fewer than 100 patients completed the HCAHPS survey. Use these rates with caution, as the number of surveys may be too low to reliably assess hospital performance; (7) Survey results are based on less than 12 months of data; (8) Survey results are not available for this reporting period; (9) No or very few patients were eligible for the HCAHPS survey. The scores shown, if any, reflect a very small number of surveys; (10) A state average was not calculated because too few hospitals in the state submitted data; (11) There were discrepancies in the data collection process; Please refer to the User's Guide for a full explanation of data.

Clifton Springs Hospital and Clinic

2 Coulter Road Phone: 315-462-9561
Clifton Springs, NY 14432 Fax: 315-462-3492
Type: Acute Care Hospitals Emergency Services: Yes
Ownership: Voluntary Non-Profit - Private Beds: 262

Key Personnel:
CEO/President. . . . . John Galati
Cardiac Laboratory. . . . . Karen Pyle
Chief of Medical Staff. . . . . Lewis Zwich, MD
Operating Room. . . . . Betsy Kearney
Quality Assurance . . . . Sue Pettis
Radiology. . . . . John Severins

Measure	Cases	This Hosp.	State Avg.	U.S. Avg.
Heart Attack Care				
ACE Inhibitor or ARB for LVSD[1,2]	3	100%	95%	96%
Aspirin at Arrival[1,2]	15	100%	98%	99%
Aspirin at Discharge[1,2]	6	100%	98%	98%
Beta Blocker at Discharge[1,2]	9	100%	98%	98%
Fibrinolytic Medication Timing[2]	0	-	50%	55%
PCI Within 90 Minutes of Arrival[2]	0	-	88%	90%
Smoking Cessation Advice[2]	0	-	100%	99%
Chest Pain/Possible Heart Attack Care				
Aspirin at Arrival	63	97%	96%	95%
Median Time to ECG (minutes)	64	13	11	8
Median Time to Transfer (minutes)[1]	6	80	75	61
Fibrinolytic Medication Timing[1]	2	0%	55%	54%
Heart Failure Care				
ACE Inhibitor or ARB for LVSD	25	100%	94%	94%
Discharge Instructions	72	97%	89%	88%
Evaluation of LVS Function	81	100%	98%	98%
Smoking Cessation Advice[1]	7	100%	98%	98%
Pneumonia Care				
Appropriate Initial Antibiotic	85	100%	92%	92%
Blood Culture Timing	114	99%	95%	96%
Influenza Vaccine	68	96%	90%	91%
Initial Antibiotic Timing	108	94%	93%	95%
Pneumococcal Vaccine	94	90%	92%	93%
Smoking Cessation Advice	29	100%	98%	97%
Surgical Care Improvement Project				
Appropriate VTP Within 24 Hours	52	100%	94%	92%
Appropriate Hair Removal	331	100%	100%	99%
Appropriate Beta Blocker Usage	111	100%	92%	93%
Controlled Postoperative Blood Glucose	0	-	94%	93%
Prophylactic Antibiotic Timing	255	99%	96%	97%
Prophylactic Antibiotic Timing (Outpatient)	71	96%	92%	92%
Prophylactic Antibiotic Selection	259	100%	97%	97%
Prophylactic Antibiotic Select. (Outpatient)	71	97%	93%	94%
Prophylactic Antibiotic Stopped	254	100%	94%	94%
Recommended VTP Ordered	52	100%	96%	94%
Urinary Catheter Removal	136	100%	90%	90%
Children's Asthma Care				
Received Systemic Corticosteroids	-	-	-	100%
Received Home Management Plan	-	-	-	71%
Received Reliever Medication	-	-	-	100%
Use of Medical Imaging				
Combination Abdominal CT Scan	316	0.304	0.141	0.191
Combination Chest CT Scan	206	0.010	0.024	0.054
Follow-up Mammogram/Ultrasound	562	7.1%	9.8%	8.4%
MRI for Low Back Pain[1]	29	34.5%	26.9%	32.7%
Survey of Patients' Hospital Experiences				
Area Around Room 'Always' Quiet at Night	300+	50%	-	58%
Doctors 'Always' Communicated Well	300+	86%	-	80%
Home Recovery Information Given	300+	91%	-	82%
Hospital Given 9 or 10 on 10 Point Scale	300+	79%	-	67%
Meds 'Always' Explained Before Given	300+	64%	-	60%
Nurses 'Always' Communicated Well	300+	80%	-	76%
Pain 'Always' Well Controlled	300+	72%	-	69%
Room and Bathroom 'Always' Clean	300+	73%	-	71%
Timely Help 'Always' Received	300+	72%	-	64%
Would Definitely Recommend Hospital	300+	84%	-	69%

Cobleskill Regional Hospital

178 Grandview Drive Phone: 518-254-3270
Cobleskill, NY 12043 Fax: 518-234-4839
E-mail: customer.service@bassett.org.
URL: www.bassett.org
Type: Acute Care Hospitals Emergency Services: Yes
Ownership: Voluntary Non-Profit - Private Beds: 40

Key Personnel:
CEO/President. . . . . William F Streck
Chief of Medical Staff. . . . . Bertine C McKenna, MD
Infection Control. . . . . Irene Abbott
Operating Room. . . . . Nancy Simmons-Dawley
Pediatric In-Patient Care . . . . Linda Rodriguez
Quality Assurance . . . . Janet Gorton
Radiology. . . . . Lawrence Barnowsky

Measure	Cases	This Hosp.	State Avg.	U.S. Avg.
Heart Attack Care				
ACE Inhibitor or ARB for LVSD[1]	2	100%	95%	96%
Aspirin at Arrival[1]	4	100%	98%	99%
Aspirin at Discharge[1]	4	100%	98%	98%
Beta Blocker at Discharge[1]	4	100%	98%	98%
Fibrinolytic Medication Timing	0	-	50%	55%
PCI Within 90 Minutes of Arrival	0	-	88%	90%
Smoking Cessation Advice[1]	2	100%	100%	99%
Chest Pain/Possible Heart Attack Care				
Aspirin at Arrival	114	99%	96%	95%
Median Time to ECG (minutes)	118	9	11	8
Median Time to Transfer (minutes)[1]	10	73	75	61
Fibrinolytic Medication Timing	0	-	55%	54%
Heart Failure Care				
ACE Inhibitor or ARB for LVSD[1]	11	100%	94%	94%
Discharge Instructions	33	94%	89%	88%
Evaluation of LVS Function	42	95%	98%	98%
Smoking Cessation Advice[1]	5	100%	98%	98%
Pneumonia Care				
Appropriate Initial Antibiotic	61	100%	92%	92%
Blood Culture Timing	55	100%	95%	96%
Influenza Vaccine	43	91%	90%	91%
Initial Antibiotic Timing	71	96%	93%	95%
Pneumococcal Vaccine	63	92%	92%	93%
Smoking Cessation Advice[1]	21	95%	98%	97%
Surgical Care Improvement Project				
Appropriate VTP Within 24 Hours[5]	0	-	94%	92%
Appropriate Hair Removal[5]	0	-	100%	99%
Appropriate Beta Blocker Usage[5]	0	-	92%	93%
Controlled Postoperative Blood Glucose[5]	0	-	94%	93%
Prophylactic Antibiotic Timing[5]	0	-	96%	97%
Prophylactic Antibiotic Timing (Outpatient)[1]	4	100%	92%	92%
Prophylactic Antibiotic Selection[5]	0	-	97%	97%
Prophylactic Antibiotic Select. (Outpatient)[1]	18	94%	93%	94%
Prophylactic Antibiotic Stopped[5]	0	-	94%	94%
Recommended VTP Ordered[5]	0	-	96%	94%
Urinary Catheter Removal[5]	0	-	90%	90%
Children's Asthma Care				
Received Systemic Corticosteroids	-	-	-	100%
Received Home Management Plan	-	-	-	71%
Received Reliever Medication	-	-	-	100%
Use of Medical Imaging				
Combination Abdominal CT Scan	312	0.103	0.141	0.191
Combination Chest CT Scan	166	0.018	0.024	0.054
Follow-up Mammogram/Ultrasound	510	5.9%	9.8%	8.4%
MRI for Low Back Pain	60	25.0%	26.9%	32.7%
Survey of Patients' Hospital Experiences				
Area Around Room 'Always' Quiet at Night	(a)	54%	-	58%
Doctors 'Always' Communicated Well	(a)	84%	-	80%
Home Recovery Information Given	(a)	85%	-	82%
Hospital Given 9 or 10 on 10 Point Scale	(a)	70%	-	67%
Meds 'Always' Explained Before Given	(a)	58%	-	60%
Nurses 'Always' Communicated Well	(a)	78%	-	76%
Pain 'Always' Well Controlled	(a)	69%	-	69%
Room and Bathroom 'Always' Clean	(a)	76%	-	71%
Timely Help 'Always' Received	(a)	60%	-	64%
Would Definitely Recommend Hospital	(a)	67%	-	69%

Mary Imogene Bassett Hospital

One Atwell Road Phone: 607-547-3456
Cooperstown, NY 13326 Fax: 607-547-3921
Type: Acute Care Hospitals Emergency Services: Yes
Ownership: Voluntary Non-Profit - Private Beds: 180

Key Personnel:
CEO/President. . . . . William F Streck, MD
Emergency Room . . . . Timothy J Barrett

Measure	Cases	This Hosp.	State Avg.	U.S. Avg.
Heart Attack Care				
ACE Inhibitor or ARB for LVSD	37	86%	95%	96%
Aspirin at Arrival	114	96%	98%	99%
Aspirin at Discharge	234	100%	98%	98%
Beta Blocker at Discharge	233	100%	98%	98%
Fibrinolytic Medication Timing	0	-	50%	55%
PCI Within 90 Minutes of Arrival[1]	21	76%	88%	90%
Smoking Cessation Advice	78	100%	100%	99%
Chest Pain/Possible Heart Attack Care				
Aspirin at Arrival[3]	0	-	96%	95%
Median Time to ECG (minutes)[3]	0	-	11	8
Median Time to Transfer (minutes)[5]	0	-	75	61
Fibrinolytic Medication Timing[5]	0	-	55%	54%
Heart Failure Care				
ACE Inhibitor or ARB for LVSD	78	91%	94%	94%
Discharge Instructions	185	83%	89%	88%
Evaluation of LVS Function	216	100%	98%	98%
Smoking Cessation Advice	35	100%	98%	98%
Pneumonia Care				
Appropriate Initial Antibiotic	57	95%	92%	92%
Blood Culture Timing	98	97%	95%	96%
Influenza Vaccine	102	82%	90%	91%
Initial Antibiotic Timing	104	91%	93%	95%
Pneumococcal Vaccine	134	97%	92%	93%
Smoking Cessation Advice	63	92%	98%	97%
Surgical Care Improvement Project				
Appropriate VTP Within 24 Hours[2]	237	97%	94%	92%
Appropriate Hair Removal[2]	610	100%	100%	99%
Appropriate Beta Blocker Usage[2]	263	94%	92%	93%
Controlled Postoperative Blood Glucose[2]	109	89%	94%	93%
Prophylactic Antibiotic Timing[2]	449	96%	96%	97%
Prophylactic Antibiotic Timing (Outpatient)	283	89%	92%	92%
Prophylactic Antibiotic Selection[2]	455	98%	97%	97%
Prophylactic Antibiotic Select. (Outpatient)	362	91%	93%	94%
Prophylactic Antibiotic Stopped[2]	418	92%	94%	94%
Recommended VTP Ordered[2]	237	97%	96%	94%
Urinary Catheter Removal[2]	170	86%	90%	90%
Children's Asthma Care				
Received Systemic Corticosteroids	-	-	-	100%
Received Home Management Plan	-	-	-	71%
Received Reliever Medication	-	-	-	100%
Use of Medical Imaging				
Combination Abdominal CT Scan	652	0.150	0.141	0.191
Combination Chest CT Scan	608	0.021	0.024	0.054
Follow-up Mammogram/Ultrasound	1,829	6.4%	9.8%	8.4%
MRI for Low Back Pain	123	31.7%	26.9%	32.7%
Survey of Patients' Hospital Experiences				
Area Around Room 'Always' Quiet at Night	300+	44%	-	58%
Doctors 'Always' Communicated Well	300+	78%	-	80%
Home Recovery Information Given	300+	88%	-	82%
Hospital Given 9 or 10 on 10 Point Scale	300+	64%	-	67%
Meds 'Always' Explained Before Given	300+	65%	-	60%
Nurses 'Always' Communicated Well	300+	74%	-	76%
Pain 'Always' Well Controlled	300+	67%	-	69%
Room and Bathroom 'Always' Clean	300+	67%	-	71%
Timely Help 'Always' Received	300+	58%	-	64%
Would Definitely Recommend Hospital	300+	75%	-	69%

NOTE: Hospital profiles are in alphabetical order by state, then city, then hospital within the city; Rankings exclude hospitals with less than 25 cases except for patient surveys which excludes hospitals with less than 100 cases; (a) 100–299 cases; (1) The number of cases is too small to be sure how well a hospital is performing; (2) The hospital indicated that the data submitted for this measure were based on a sample of cases; (3) Data was collected during a shorter time period (fewer quarters) than the maximum possible time for this measure; (4) Suppressed for one or more quarters by CMS; (5) No data is available from the hospital for this measure; (6) Fewer than 100 patients completed the HCAHPS survey. Use these rates with caution, as the number of surveys may be too low to reliably assess hospital performance; (7) Survey results are based on less than 12 months of data; (8) Survey results are not available for this reporting period; (9) No or very few patients were eligible for the HCAHPS survey. The scores shown, if any, reflect a very small number of surveys; (10) A state average was not calculated because too few hospitals in the state submitted data; (11) There were discrepancies in the data collection process; Please refer to the User's Guide for a full explanation of data.

Corning Hospital

176 Denison Parkway East   Phone: 607-937-7200
Corning, NY 14830
URL: www.corninghospital.org
Type: Acute Care Hospitals   Emergency Services: Yes
Ownership: Voluntary Non-Profit - Private   Beds: 99
Key Personnel:
CEO/President . . . . Shirley Magana
Chief of Medical Staff . . . . William Sorber MD PhD
Operating Room . . . . John Olmstead MD
Pediatric Ambulatory Care . . . . . . Rowshanul Khan MD
Radiology . . . . Joseph Bifano MD
Anesthesiology . . . . Chris Wentzel MD
Emergency Room . . . . Gary Enders MD

Measure	Cases	This Hosp.	State Avg.	U.S. Avg.
Heart Attack Care				
ACE Inhibitor or ARB for LVSD[1]	2	100%	95%	96%
Aspirin at Arrival[1]	13	100%	98%	99%
Aspirin at Discharge[1]	8	100%	98%	98%
Beta Blocker at Discharge[1]	8	100%	98%	98%
Fibrinolytic Medication Timing	0	-	50%	55%
PCI Within 90 Minutes of Arrival	0	-	88%	90%
Smoking Cessation Advice[1]	1	100%	100%	99%
Chest Pain/Possible Heart Attack Care				
Aspirin at Arrival	79	97%	96%	95%
Median Time to ECG (minutes)	82	19	11	8
Median Time to Transfer (minutes)[1]	6	52	75	61
Fibrinolytic Medication Timing[1]	1	100%	55%	54%
Heart Failure Care				
ACE Inhibitor or ARB for LVSD	42	95%	94%	94%
Discharge Instructions	96	92%	89%	88%
Evaluation of LVS Function	137	100%	98%	98%
Smoking Cessation Advice[1]	15	87%	98%	98%
Pneumonia Care				
Appropriate Initial Antibiotic	81	95%	92%	92%
Blood Culture Timing	150	99%	95%	96%
Influenza Vaccine	116	94%	90%	91%
Initial Antibiotic Timing	137	91%	93%	95%
Pneumococcal Vaccine	155	96%	92%	93%
Smoking Cessation Advice	54	91%	98%	97%
Surgical Care Improvement Project				
Appropriate VTP Within 24 Hours	98	88%	94%	92%
Appropriate Hair Removal	264	99%	100%	99%
Appropriate Beta Blocker Usage	74	86%	92%	93%
Controlled Postoperative Blood Glucose	0	-	94%	93%
Prophylactic Antibiotic Timing	184	97%	96%	97%
Prophylactic Antibiotic Timing (Outpatient)	52	85%	92%	92%
Prophylactic Antibiotic Selection	186	96%	97%	97%
Prophylactic Antibiotic Select. (Outpatient)	48	88%	93%	94%
Prophylactic Antibiotic Stopped	177	96%	94%	94%
Recommended VTP Ordered	98	88%	96%	94%
Urinary Catheter Removal	46	100%	90%	90%
Children's Asthma Care				
Received Systemic Corticosteroids	-	-	-	100%
Received Home Management Plan	-	-	-	71%
Received Reliever Medication	-	-	-	100%
Use of Medical Imaging				
Combination Abdominal CT Scan	753	0.114	0.141	0.191
Combination Chest CT Scan	546	0.005	0.024	0.054
Follow-up Mammogram/Ultrasound	858	14.6%	9.8%	8.4%
MRI for Low Back Pain	72	36.1%	26.9%	32.7%
Survey of Patients' Hospital Experiences				
Area Around Room 'Always' Quiet at Night	300+	55%	-	58%
Doctors 'Always' Communicated Well	300+	74%	-	80%
Home Recovery Information Given	300+	82%	-	82%
Hospital Given 9 or 10 on 10 Point Scale	300+	56%	-	67%
Meds 'Always' Explained Before Given	300+	60%	-	60%
Nurses 'Always' Communicated Well	300+	74%	-	76%
Pain 'Always' Well Controlled	300+	69%	-	69%
Room and Bathroom 'Always' Clean	300+	67%	-	71%
Timely Help 'Always' Received	300+	59%	-	64%
Would Definitely Recommend Hospital	300+	56%	-	69%

Cortland Regional Medical Center

134 Homer Avenue   Phone: 607-756-3500
Cortland, NY 13045   Fax: 607-756-3590
URL: www.cortlandhospitals.org
Type: Acute Care Hospitals   Emergency Services: Yes
Ownership: Voluntary Non-Profit - Private   Beds: 181
Key Personnel:
CEO/President . . . . Brian Mitteer
Chief of Medical Staff . . . . Peter Martin
Emergency Room . . . . Ralph Battles, MD

Measure	Cases	This Hosp.	State Avg.	U.S. Avg.
Heart Attack Care				
ACE Inhibitor or ARB for LVSD[1]	1	100%	95%	96%
Aspirin at Arrival[1]	21	100%	98%	99%
Aspirin at Discharge[1]	9	100%	98%	98%
Beta Blocker at Discharge[1]	7	100%	98%	98%
Fibrinolytic Medication Timing	0	-	50%	55%
PCI Within 90 Minutes of Arrival	0	-	88%	90%
Smoking Cessation Advice[1]	1	100%	100%	99%
Chest Pain/Possible Heart Attack Care				
Aspirin at Arrival	174	93%	96%	95%
Median Time to ECG (minutes)	179	13	11	8
Median Time to Transfer (minutes)	0	-	75	61
Fibrinolytic Medication Timing[1]	2	0%	55%	54%
Heart Failure Care				
ACE Inhibitor or ARB for LVSD	38	66%	94%	94%
Discharge Instructions	88	88%	89%	88%
Evaluation of LVS Function	118	92%	98%	98%
Smoking Cessation Advice[1]	19	95%	98%	98%
Pneumonia Care				
Appropriate Initial Antibiotic	170	84%	92%	92%
Blood Culture Timing	259	89%	95%	96%
Influenza Vaccine	136	88%	90%	91%
Initial Antibiotic Timing	223	93%	93%	95%
Pneumococcal Vaccine	192	82%	92%	93%
Smoking Cessation Advice	58	98%	98%	97%
Surgical Care Improvement Project				
Appropriate VTP Within 24 Hours	74	91%	94%	92%
Appropriate Hair Removal	153	98%	100%	99%
Appropriate Beta Blocker Usage	30	93%	92%	93%
Controlled Postoperative Blood Glucose	0	-	94%	93%
Prophylactic Antibiotic Timing	63	94%	96%	97%
Prophylactic Antibiotic Timing (Outpatient)	60	82%	92%	92%
Prophylactic Antibiotic Selection	63	97%	97%	97%
Prophylactic Antibiotic Select. (Outpatient)	56	84%	93%	94%
Prophylactic Antibiotic Stopped	63	87%	94%	94%
Recommended VTP Ordered	74	91%	96%	94%
Urinary Catheter Removal	36	69%	90%	90%
Children's Asthma Care				
Received Systemic Corticosteroids	-	-	-	100%
Received Home Management Plan	-	-	-	71%
Received Reliever Medication	-	-	-	100%
Use of Medical Imaging				
Combination Abdominal CT Scan	681	0.070	0.141	0.191
Combination Chest CT Scan	315	0.022	0.024	0.054
Follow-up Mammogram/Ultrasound	439	13.2%	9.8%	8.4%
MRI for Low Back Pain[1]	33	42.4%	26.9%	32.7%
Survey of Patients' Hospital Experiences				
Area Around Room 'Always' Quiet at Night	300+	41%	-	58%
Doctors 'Always' Communicated Well	300+	72%	-	80%
Home Recovery Information Given	300+	83%	-	82%
Hospital Given 9 or 10 on 10 Point Scale	300+	52%	-	67%
Meds 'Always' Explained Before Given	300+	59%	-	60%
Nurses 'Always' Communicated Well	300+	71%	-	76%
Pain 'Always' Well Controlled	300+	61%	-	69%
Room and Bathroom 'Always' Clean	300+	66%	-	71%
Timely Help 'Always' Received	300+	54%	-	64%
Would Definitely Recommend Hospital	300+	50%	-	69%

Hudson Valley Hospital Center

1980 Crompond Road   Phone: 914-734-3611
Cortlandt Manor, NY 10567   Fax: 914-736-3459
E-mail: hvhc@hvhc.org
URL: www.hvhc.org
Type: Acute Care Hospitals   Emergency Services: Yes
Ownership: Voluntary Non-Profit - Private   Beds: 120
Key Personnel:
CEO/President . . . . John C Federspiel
Chief of Medical Staff . . . . Valerie Zarcone, MD
Radiology . . . . Maurice R Poplausky
Emergency Room . . . . Lindsay Aarstad, MD

Measure	Cases	This Hosp.	State Avg.	U.S. Avg.
Heart Attack Care				
ACE Inhibitor or ARB for LVSD[1]	12	100%	95%	96%
Aspirin at Arrival	113	98%	98%	99%
Aspirin at Discharge	65	100%	98%	98%
Beta Blocker at Discharge	68	100%	98%	98%
Fibrinolytic Medication Timing[1]	6	83%	50%	55%
PCI Within 90 Minutes of Arrival	0	-	88%	90%
Smoking Cessation Advice[1]	4	100%	100%	99%
Chest Pain/Possible Heart Attack Care				
Aspirin at Arrival	62	98%	96%	95%
Median Time to ECG (minutes)	67	7	11	8
Median Time to Transfer (minutes)[1]	8	99	75	61
Fibrinolytic Medication Timing[1]	6	83%	55%	54%
Heart Failure Care				
ACE Inhibitor or ARB for LVSD	63	97%	94%	94%
Discharge Instructions	157	90%	89%	88%
Evaluation of LVS Function	257	100%	98%	98%
Smoking Cessation Advice	32	100%	98%	98%
Pneumonia Care				
Appropriate Initial Antibiotic	96	98%	92%	92%
Blood Culture Timing	186	96%	95%	96%
Influenza Vaccine	121	97%	90%	91%
Initial Antibiotic Timing	197	97%	93%	95%
Pneumococcal Vaccine	246	97%	92%	93%
Smoking Cessation Advice	63	100%	98%	97%
Surgical Care Improvement Project				
Appropriate VTP Within 24 Hours	239	93%	94%	92%
Appropriate Hair Removal	389	98%	100%	99%
Appropriate Beta Blocker Usage	101	78%	92%	93%
Controlled Postoperative Blood Glucose	0	-	94%	93%
Prophylactic Antibiotic Timing	224	100%	96%	97%
Prophylactic Antibiotic Timing (Outpatient)	97	97%	92%	92%
Prophylactic Antibiotic Selection	224	95%	97%	97%
Prophylactic Antibiotic Select. (Outpatient)	95	95%	93%	94%
Prophylactic Antibiotic Stopped	223	96%	94%	94%
Recommended VTP Ordered	239	96%	96%	94%
Urinary Catheter Removal	110	89%	90%	90%
Children's Asthma Care				
Received Systemic Corticosteroids	-	-	-	100%
Received Home Management Plan	-	-	-	71%
Received Reliever Medication	-	-	-	100%
Use of Medical Imaging				
Combination Abdominal CT Scan	670	0.146	0.141	0.191
Combination Chest CT Scan	547	0.084	0.024	0.054
Follow-up Mammogram/Ultrasound	1,007	6.9%	9.8%	8.4%
MRI for Low Back Pain	172	24.4%	26.9%	32.7%
Survey of Patients' Hospital Experiences				
Area Around Room 'Always' Quiet at Night	300+	50%	-	58%
Doctors 'Always' Communicated Well	300+	79%	-	80%
Home Recovery Information Given	300+	80%	-	82%
Hospital Given 9 or 10 on 10 Point Scale	300+	65%	-	67%
Meds 'Always' Explained Before Given	300+	61%	-	60%
Nurses 'Always' Communicated Well	300+	76%	-	76%
Pain 'Always' Well Controlled	300+	72%	-	69%
Room and Bathroom 'Always' Clean	300+	72%	-	71%
Timely Help 'Always' Received	300+	62%	-	64%
Would Definitely Recommend Hospital	300+	68%	-	69%

Nicholas H Noyes Memorial Hospital

111 Clara Barton Street Phone: 585-335-6001
Dansville, NY 14437 Fax: 585-335-2769
E-mail: tingram@noyes-hospital.org
URL: www.noyes-health.org
Type: Acute Care Hospitals Emergency Services: Yes
Ownership: Voluntary Non-Profit - Private Beds: 72

Key Personnel:

CEO/President. . . . . James Wissler
Cardiac Laboratory. . . . . Syed Igbal, MD
Chief of Medical Staff . . . . Tony Witte, MD
Infection Control. . . . . Mary Stewart
Operating Room. . . . . Andree Brasser
Radiology. . . . . Omar Qureshi
Emergency Room . . . . Douglas Mayhle, MD

Measure	Cases	This Hosp.	State Avg.	U.S. Avg.
Heart Attack Care				
ACE Inhibitor or ARB for LVSD[1]	3	67%	95%	96%
Aspirin at Arrival[1]	13	92%	98%	99%
Aspirin at Discharge[1]	8	88%	98%	98%
Beta Blocker at Discharge[1]	8	88%	98%	98%
Fibrinolytic Medication Timing	0	-	50%	55%
PCI Within 90 Minutes of Arrival	0	-	88%	90%
Smoking Cessation Advice[1]	2	100%	100%	99%
Chest Pain/Possible Heart Attack Care				
Aspirin at Arrival	45	89%	96%	95%
Median Time to ECG (minutes)	45	5	11	8
Median Time to Transfer (minutes)[1,3]	3	77	75	61
Fibrinolytic Medication Timing[1]	8	50%	55%	54%
Heart Failure Care				
ACE Inhibitor or ARB for LVSD	51	71%	94%	94%
Discharge Instructions	115	82%	89%	88%
Evaluation of LVS Function	148	91%	98%	98%
Smoking Cessation Advice[1]	18	83%	98%	98%
Pneumonia Care				
Appropriate Initial Antibiotic	91	93%	92%	92%
Blood Culture Timing	103	98%	95%	96%
Influenza Vaccine	81	86%	90%	91%
Initial Antibiotic Timing	123	93%	93%	95%
Pneumococcal Vaccine	120	92%	92%	93%
Smoking Cessation Advice[1]	21	95%	98%	97%
Surgical Care Improvement Project				
Appropriate VTP Within 24 Hours	44	82%	94%	92%
Appropriate Hair Removal	150	100%	100%	99%
Appropriate Beta Blocker Usage	54	81%	92%	93%
Controlled Postoperative Blood Glucose	0	-	94%	93%
Prophylactic Antibiotic Timing	98	93%	96%	97%
Prophylactic Antibiotic Timing (Outpatient)	40	88%	92%	92%
Prophylactic Antibiotic Selection	96	92%	97%	97%
Prophylactic Antibiotic Select. (Outpatient)	36	61%	93%	94%
Prophylactic Antibiotic Stopped	96	91%	94%	94%
Recommended VTP Ordered	44	82%	96%	94%
Urinary Catheter Removal	53	98%	90%	90%
Children's Asthma Care				
Received Systemic Corticosteroids	-	-	-	100%
Received Home Management Plan	-	-	-	71%
Received Reliever Medication	-	-	-	100%
Use of Medical Imaging				
Combination Abdominal CT Scan	243	0.683	0.141	0.191
Combination Chest CT Scan	182	0.676	0.024	0.054
Follow-up Mammogram/Ultrasound	412	56.6%	9.8%	8.4%
MRI for Low Back Pain[5]	0	-	26.9%	32.7%
Survey of Patients' Hospital Experiences				
Area Around Room 'Always' Quiet at Night	300+	58%	-	58%
Doctors 'Always' Communicated Well	300+	78%	-	80%
Home Recovery Information Given	300+	81%	-	82%
Hospital Given 9 or 10 on 10 Point Scale	300+	70%	-	67%
Meds 'Always' Explained Before Given	300+	57%	-	60%
Nurses 'Always' Communicated Well	300+	77%	-	76%
Pain 'Always' Well Controlled	300+	70%	-	69%
Room and Bathroom 'Always' Clean	300+	67%	-	71%
Timely Help 'Always' Received	300+	68%	-	64%
Would Definitely Recommend Hospital	300+	70%	-	69%

O'Connor Hospital

460 Andes Road Phone: 607-746-0300
Delhi, NY 13753 Fax: 607-746-0347
E-mail: pvogt@catskill.net
URL: www.oconnorhospital.org
Type: Critical Access Hospitals Emergency Services: Yes
Ownership: Voluntary Non-Profit - Private Beds: 28

Key Personnel:

CEO/President. . . . . Ronald J Galonsky Jr
Chief of Medical Staff . . . . George Block
Operating Room. . . . . Betsy Morales
Quality Assurance . . . . Jean Krzyston
Radiology. . . . . Richard Kaplan

Measure	Cases	This Hosp.	State Avg.	U.S. Avg.
Heart Attack Care				
ACE Inhibitor or ARB for LVSD[5]	0	-	95%	96%
Aspirin at Arrival[5]	0	-	98%	99%
Aspirin at Discharge[5]	0	-	98%	98%
Beta Blocker at Discharge[5]	0	-	98%	98%
Fibrinolytic Medication Timing[5]	0	-	50%	55%
PCI Within 90 Minutes of Arrival[5]	0	-	88%	90%
Smoking Cessation Advice[5]	0	-	100%	99%
Chest Pain/Possible Heart Attack Care				
Aspirin at Arrival	-	-	96%	95%
Median Time to ECG (minutes)	-	-	11	8
Median Time to Transfer (minutes)	-	-	75	61
Fibrinolytic Medication Timing	-	-	55%	54%
Heart Failure Care				
ACE Inhibitor or ARB for LVSD[1,3]	4	100%	94%	94%
Discharge Instructions[1,3]	12	75%	89%	88%
Evaluation of LVS Function[1,3]	15	93%	98%	98%
Smoking Cessation Advice[3]	0	-	98%	98%
Pneumonia Care				
Appropriate Initial Antibiotic[1,3]	6	100%	92%	92%
Blood Culture Timing[1,3]	4	100%	95%	96%
Influenza Vaccine[1,3]	3	100%	90%	91%
Initial Antibiotic Timing[1,3]	3	100%	93%	95%
Pneumococcal Vaccine[1,3]	8	100%	92%	93%
Smoking Cessation Advice[3]	0	-	98%	97%
Surgical Care Improvement Project				
Appropriate VTP Within 24 Hours[5]	0	-	94%	92%
Appropriate Hair Removal[5]	0	-	100%	99%
Appropriate Beta Blocker Usage[5]	0	-	92%	93%
Controlled Postoperative Blood Glucose[5]	0	-	94%	93%
Prophylactic Antibiotic Timing[5]	0	-	96%	97%
Prophylactic Antibiotic Timing (Outpatient)	-	-	92%	92%
Prophylactic Antibiotic Selection[5]	0	-	97%	97%
Prophylactic Antibiotic Select. (Outpatient)	-	-	93%	94%
Prophylactic Antibiotic Stopped[5]	0	-	94%	94%
Recommended VTP Ordered[5]	0	-	96%	94%
Urinary Catheter Removal[5]	0	-	90%	90%
Children's Asthma Care				
Received Systemic Corticosteroids	-	-	-	100%
Received Home Management Plan	-	-	-	71%
Received Reliever Medication	-	-	-	100%
Use of Medical Imaging				
Combination Abdominal CT Scan	-	-	0.141	0.191
Combination Chest CT Scan	-	-	0.024	0.054
Follow-up Mammogram/Ultrasound	-	-	9.8%	8.4%
MRI for Low Back Pain	-	-	26.9%	32.7%
Survey of Patients' Hospital Experiences				
Area Around Room 'Always' Quiet at Night[8]	-	-	-	58%
Doctors 'Always' Communicated Well[8]	-	-	-	80%
Home Recovery Information Given[8]	-	-	-	82%
Hospital Given 9 or 10 on 10 Point Scale[8]	-	-	-	67%
Meds 'Always' Explained Before Given[8]	-	-	-	60%
Nurses 'Always' Communicated Well[8]	-	-	-	76%
Pain 'Always' Well Controlled[8]	-	-	-	69%
Room and Bathroom 'Always' Clean[8]	-	-	-	71%
Timely Help 'Always' Received[8]	-	-	-	64%
Would Definitely Recommend Hospital[8]	-	-	-	69%

Brooks Memorial Hospital

529 Central Avenue Phone: 716-366-1111
Dunkirk, NY 14048 Fax: 716-363-7288
URL: www.brookshospital.org
Type: Acute Care Hospitals Emergency Services: Yes
Ownership: Voluntary Non-Profit - Private Beds: 99

Key Personnel:

CEO/President. . . . . Richard H Ketcham
Chief of Medical Staff . . . . G Jay Bishop, MD
Infection Control. . . . . Susan Lis, RN
Operating Room. . . . . Sallie Piazza, RN
Quality Assurance . . . . Teresa Larson
Radiology. . . . . Sharon Muntz
Emergency Room . . . . John Radford, MD
Intensive Care Unit. . . . . Karen Hurlacher

Measure	Cases	This Hosp.	State Avg.	U.S. Avg.
Heart Attack Care				
ACE Inhibitor or ARB for LVSD[1]	3	67%	95%	96%
Aspirin at Arrival[1]	11	91%	98%	99%
Aspirin at Discharge[1]	7	86%	98%	98%
Beta Blocker at Discharge[1]	9	89%	98%	98%
Fibrinolytic Medication Timing	0	-	50%	55%
PCI Within 90 Minutes of Arrival	0	-	88%	90%
Smoking Cessation Advice[1]	4	100%	100%	99%
Chest Pain/Possible Heart Attack Care				
Aspirin at Arrival	147	96%	96%	95%
Median Time to ECG (minutes)	151	17	11	8
Median Time to Transfer (minutes)[1]	1	78	75	61
Fibrinolytic Medication Timing[1]	9	67%	55%	54%
Heart Failure Care				
ACE Inhibitor or ARB for LVSD[1]	18	89%	94%	94%
Discharge Instructions	50	82%	89%	88%
Evaluation of LVS Function	76	97%	98%	98%
Smoking Cessation Advice[1]	12	75%	98%	98%
Pneumonia Care				
Appropriate Initial Antibiotic	62	89%	92%	92%
Blood Culture Timing	114	86%	95%	96%
Influenza Vaccine	57	81%	90%	91%
Initial Antibiotic Timing	118	94%	93%	95%
Pneumococcal Vaccine	95	88%	92%	93%
Smoking Cessation Advice[1]	24	75%	98%	97%
Surgical Care Improvement Project				
Appropriate VTP Within 24 Hours	153	99%	94%	92%
Appropriate Hair Removal	358	99%	100%	99%
Appropriate Beta Blocker Usage	111	97%	92%	93%
Controlled Postoperative Blood Glucose	0	-	94%	93%
Prophylactic Antibiotic Timing	313	98%	96%	97%
Prophylactic Antibiotic Timing (Outpatient)	34	88%	92%	92%
Prophylactic Antibiotic Selection	313	99%	97%	97%
Prophylactic Antibiotic Select. (Outpatient)	31	100%	93%	94%
Prophylactic Antibiotic Stopped	313	97%	94%	94%
Recommended VTP Ordered	154	99%	96%	94%
Urinary Catheter Removal	101	94%	90%	90%
Children's Asthma Care				
Received Systemic Corticosteroids	-	-	-	100%
Received Home Management Plan	-	-	-	71%
Received Reliever Medication	-	-	-	100%
Use of Medical Imaging				
Combination Abdominal CT Scan	287	0.077	0.141	0.191
Combination Chest CT Scan	134	0.045	0.024	0.054
Follow-up Mammogram/Ultrasound	390	4.1%	9.8%	8.4%
MRI for Low Back Pain	38	42.1%	26.9%	32.7%
Survey of Patients' Hospital Experiences				
Area Around Room 'Always' Quiet at Night	300+	47%	-	58%
Doctors 'Always' Communicated Well	300+	77%	-	80%
Home Recovery Information Given	300+	80%	-	82%
Hospital Given 9 or 10 on 10 Point Scale	300+	53%	-	67%
Meds 'Always' Explained Before Given	300+	47%	-	60%
Nurses 'Always' Communicated Well	300+	69%	-	76%
Pain 'Always' Well Controlled	300+	61%	-	69%
Room and Bathroom 'Always' Clean	300+	66%	-	71%
Timely Help 'Always' Received	300+	52%	-	64%
Would Definitely Recommend Hospital	300+	56%	-	69%

NOTE: Hospital profiles are in alphabetical order by state, then city, then hospital within the city; Rankings exclude hospitals with less than 25 cases except for patient surveys which excludes hospitals with less than 100 cases; (a) 100–299 cases; (1) The number of cases is too small to be sure how well a hospital is performing; (2) The hospital indicated that the data submitted for this measure were based on a sample of cases; (3) Data was collected during a shorter time period (fewer quarters) than the maximum possible time for this measure; (4) Suppressed for one or more quarters by CMS; (5) No data is available from the hospital for this measure; (6) Fewer than 100 patients completed the HCAHPS survey. Use these rates with caution, as the number of surveys may be too low to reliably assess hospital performance; (7) Survey results are based on less than 12 months of data; (8) Survey results are not available for this reporting period; (9) No or very few patients were eligible for the HCAHPS survey. The scores shown, if any, reflect a very small number of surveys; (10) A state average was not calculated because too few hospitals in the state submitted data; (11) There were discrepancies in the data collection process; Please refer to the User's Guide for a full explanation of data.

Nassau University Medical Center

2201 Hempstead Turnpike Phone: 516-572-0123
East Meadow, NY 11554 Fax: 516-572-5792
URL: www.numc.edu
Type: Acute Care Hospitals Emergency Services: Yes
Ownership: Government - State Beds: 1,500

Key Personnel:

CEO/President. . . . . Arthur Gianelli
Chief of Medical Staff. . . . . Steven J Walerstein MD
Infection Control. . . . . Joanne Selva MD
Operating Room. . . . . LD George Angus, MD
Pediatric In-Patient Care . . . . Bella Silecchia, MD
Quality Assurance . . . . Maureen P Shannon, RN MHA
Radiology. . . . . Paul Moh, MD

Measure	Cases	This Hosp.	State Avg.	U.S. Avg.
Heart Attack Care				
ACE Inhibitor or ARB for LVSD[1]	10	100%	95%	96%
Aspirin at Arrival	50	100%	98%	99%
Aspirin at Discharge	31	100%	98%	98%
Beta Blocker at Discharge	33	100%	98%	98%
Fibrinolytic Medication Timing	0	-	50%	55%
PCI Within 90 Minutes of Arrival	0	-	88%	90%
Smoking Cessation Advice[1]	6	100%	100%	99%
Chest Pain/Possible Heart Attack Care				
Aspirin at Arrival[1,3]	4	100%	96%	95%
Median Time to ECG (minutes)[1,3]	4	22	11	8
Median Time to Transfer (minutes)[3]	0	-	75	61
Fibrinolytic Medication Timing[3]	0	-	55%	54%
Heart Failure Care				
ACE Inhibitor or ARB for LVSD	86	100%	94%	94%
Discharge Instructions	198	97%	89%	88%
Evaluation of LVS Function	245	100%	98%	98%
Smoking Cessation Advice	54	100%	98%	98%
Pneumonia Care				
Appropriate Initial Antibiotic	93	85%	92%	92%
Blood Culture Timing	92	79%	95%	96%
Influenza Vaccine	115	100%	90%	91%
Initial Antibiotic Timing	142	92%	93%	95%
Pneumococcal Vaccine	142	93%	92%	93%
Smoking Cessation Advice	55	100%	98%	97%
Surgical Care Improvement Project				
Appropriate VTP Within 24 Hours[2]	178	99%	94%	92%
Appropriate Hair Removal[2]	326	100%	100%	99%
Appropriate Beta Blocker Usage[2]	56	100%	92%	93%
Controlled Postoperative Blood Glucose[2]	0	-	94%	93%
Prophylactic Antibiotic Timing[2]	165	97%	96%	97%
Prophylactic Antibiotic Timing (Outpatient)	59	93%	92%	92%
Prophylactic Antibiotic Selection[2]	164	91%	97%	97%
Prophylactic Antibiotic Select. (Outpatient)	90	78%	93%	94%
Prophylactic Antibiotic Stopped[2]	161	96%	94%	94%
Recommended VTP Ordered[2]	178	99%	96%	94%
Urinary Catheter Removal[2]	39	100%	90%	90%
Children's Asthma Care				
Received Systemic Corticosteroids	-	-	-	100%
Received Home Management Plan	-	-	-	71%
Received Reliever Medication	-	-	-	100%
Use of Medical Imaging				
Combination Abdominal CT Scan	147	0.007	0.141	0.191
Combination Chest CT Scan	80	0.013	0.024	0.054
Follow-up Mammogram/Ultrasound	503	20.9%	9.8%	8.4%
MRI for Low Back Pain[1]	18	22.2%	26.9%	32.7%
Survey of Patients' Hospital Experiences				
Area Around Room 'Always' Quiet at Night	300+	42%	-	58%
Doctors 'Always' Communicated Well	300+	65%	-	80%
Home Recovery Information Given	300+	70%	-	82%
Hospital Given 9 or 10 on 10 Point Scale	300+	43%	-	67%
Meds 'Always' Explained Before Given	300+	46%	-	60%
Nurses 'Always' Communicated Well	300+	56%	-	76%
Pain 'Always' Well Controlled	300+	56%	-	69%
Room and Bathroom 'Always' Clean	300+	51%	-	71%
Timely Help 'Always' Received	300+	44%	-	64%
Would Definitely Recommend Hospital	300+	42%	-	69%

Elizabethtown Community Hospital

75 Park Street Phone: 518-873-6377
Elizabethtown, NY 12932 Fax: 518-873-2005
URL: www.ech.org
Type: Critical Access Hospitals Emergency Services: Yes
Ownership: Voluntary Non-Profit - Private Beds: 25

Key Personnel:

CEO/President. . . . . Rod Boula
Emergency Room . . . . Rob DeMuro, MD

Measure	Cases	This Hosp.	State Avg.	U.S. Avg.
Heart Attack Care				
ACE Inhibitor or ARB for LVSD[1]	1	100%	95%	96%
Aspirin at Arrival[1]	2	100%	98%	99%
Aspirin at Discharge[1]	2	50%	98%	98%
Beta Blocker at Discharge[1]	3	100%	98%	98%
Fibrinolytic Medication Timing	0	-	50%	55%
PCI Within 90 Minutes of Arrival[5]	0	-	88%	90%
Smoking Cessation Advice	0	-	100%	99%
Chest Pain/Possible Heart Attack Care				
Aspirin at Arrival	-	-	96%	95%
Median Time to ECG (minutes)	-	-	11	8
Median Time to Transfer (minutes)	-	-	75	61
Fibrinolytic Medication Timing	-	-	55%	54%
Heart Failure Care				
ACE Inhibitor or ARB for LVSD[1]	2	100%	94%	94%
Discharge Instructions[1]	7	86%	89%	88%
Evaluation of LVS Function[1]	12	92%	98%	98%
Smoking Cessation Advice[1]	1	100%	98%	98%
Pneumonia Care				
Appropriate Initial Antibiotic[1]	22	91%	92%	92%
Blood Culture Timing[1]	23	91%	95%	96%
Influenza Vaccine[1]	16	94%	90%	91%
Initial Antibiotic Timing[1]	23	96%	93%	95%
Pneumococcal Vaccine[1]	23	87%	92%	93%
Smoking Cessation Advice[1]	2	100%	98%	97%
Surgical Care Improvement Project				
Appropriate VTP Within 24 Hours[5]	0	-	94%	92%
Appropriate Hair Removal[5]	0	-	100%	99%
Appropriate Beta Blocker Usage[5]	0	-	92%	93%
Controlled Postoperative Blood Glucose[5]	0	-	94%	93%
Prophylactic Antibiotic Timing[5]	0	-	96%	97%
Prophylactic Antibiotic Timing (Outpatient)	-	-	92%	92%
Prophylactic Antibiotic Selection[5]	0	-	97%	97%
Prophylactic Antibiotic Select. (Outpatient)	-	-	93%	94%
Prophylactic Antibiotic Stopped[5]	0	-	94%	94%
Recommended VTP Ordered[5]	0	-	96%	94%
Urinary Catheter Removal[5]	0	-	90%	90%
Children's Asthma Care				
Received Systemic Corticosteroids	-	-	-	100%
Received Home Management Plan	-	-	-	71%
Received Reliever Medication	-	-	-	100%
Use of Medical Imaging				
Combination Abdominal CT Scan	-	-	0.141	0.191
Combination Chest CT Scan	-	-	0.024	0.054
Follow-up Mammogram/Ultrasound	-	-	9.8%	8.4%
MRI for Low Back Pain	-	-	26.9%	32.7%
Survey of Patients' Hospital Experiences				
Area Around Room 'Always' Quiet at Night[8]	-	-	-	58%
Doctors 'Always' Communicated Well[8]	-	-	-	80%
Home Recovery Information Given[8]	-	-	-	82%
Hospital Given 9 or 10 on 10 Point Scale[8]	-	-	-	67%
Meds 'Always' Explained Before Given[8]	-	-	-	60%
Nurses 'Always' Communicated Well[8]	-	-	-	76%
Pain 'Always' Well Controlled[8]	-	-	-	69%
Room and Bathroom 'Always' Clean[8]	-	-	-	71%
Timely Help 'Always' Received[8]	-	-	-	64%
Would Definitely Recommend Hospital[8]	-	-	-	69%

Ellenville Regional Hospital

10 Healthy Way Phone: 845-647-6400
Ellenville, NY 12428 Fax: 845-647-6450
URL: www.ellenvilleregional.org
Type: Critical Access Hospitals Emergency Services: Yes
Ownership: Voluntary Non-Profit - Private Beds: 35

Key Personnel:

CEO/President. . . . . Michael Mazzarello
Chief of Medical Staff. . . . . Charles Johnson
Infection Control. . . . . Kathy Guido
Pediatric Ambulatory Care . . . . . . Kathy Guido
Quality Assurance . . . . Kathy Guido
Emergency Room . . . . Cathy Quinn, RN
Hemotology Center . . . . Eva Edwards, RN
Patient Relations . . . . Cecelia Krom

Measure	Cases	This Hosp.	State Avg.	U.S. Avg.
Heart Attack Care				
ACE Inhibitor or ARB for LVSD[5]	0	-	95%	96%
Aspirin at Arrival[5]	0	-	98%	99%
Aspirin at Discharge[5]	0	-	98%	98%
Beta Blocker at Discharge[5]	0	-	98%	98%
Fibrinolytic Medication Timing[5]	0	-	50%	55%
PCI Within 90 Minutes of Arrival[5]	0	-	88%	90%
Smoking Cessation Advice[5]	0	-	100%	99%
Chest Pain/Possible Heart Attack Care				
Aspirin at Arrival	-	-	96%	95%
Median Time to ECG (minutes)	-	-	11	8
Median Time to Transfer (minutes)	-	-	75	61
Fibrinolytic Medication Timing	-	-	55%	54%
Heart Failure Care				
ACE Inhibitor or ARB for LVSD[1,3]	1	100%	94%	94%
Discharge Instructions[1,3]	8	75%	89%	88%
Evaluation of LVS Function[1,3]	9	100%	98%	98%
Smoking Cessation Advice[3]	0	-	98%	98%
Pneumonia Care				
Appropriate Initial Antibiotic[1,3]	3	33%	92%	92%
Blood Culture Timing[1,3]	7	100%	95%	96%
Influenza Vaccine[1,3]	2	50%	90%	91%
Initial Antibiotic Timing[1,3]	3	100%	93%	95%
Pneumococcal Vaccine[1,3]	7	86%	92%	93%
Smoking Cessation Advice[1,3]	1	100%	98%	97%
Surgical Care Improvement Project				
Appropriate VTP Within 24 Hours[5]	0	-	94%	92%
Appropriate Hair Removal[5]	0	-	100%	99%
Appropriate Beta Blocker Usage[5]	0	-	92%	93%
Controlled Postoperative Blood Glucose[5]	0	-	94%	93%
Prophylactic Antibiotic Timing[5]	0	-	96%	97%
Prophylactic Antibiotic Timing (Outpatient)	-	-	92%	92%
Prophylactic Antibiotic Selection[5]	0	-	97%	97%
Prophylactic Antibiotic Select. (Outpatient)	-	-	93%	94%
Prophylactic Antibiotic Stopped[5]	0	-	94%	94%
Recommended VTP Ordered[5]	0	-	96%	94%
Urinary Catheter Removal[5]	0	-	90%	90%
Children's Asthma Care				
Received Systemic Corticosteroids	-	-	-	100%
Received Home Management Plan	-	-	-	71%
Received Reliever Medication	-	-	-	100%
Use of Medical Imaging				
Combination Abdominal CT Scan	-	-	0.141	0.191
Combination Chest CT Scan	-	-	0.024	0.054
Follow-up Mammogram/Ultrasound	-	-	9.8%	8.4%
MRI for Low Back Pain	-	-	26.9%	32.7%
Survey of Patients' Hospital Experiences				
Area Around Room 'Always' Quiet at Night[8]	-	-	-	58%
Doctors 'Always' Communicated Well[8]	-	-	-	80%
Home Recovery Information Given[8]	-	-	-	82%
Hospital Given 9 or 10 on 10 Point Scale[8]	-	-	-	67%
Meds 'Always' Explained Before Given[8]	-	-	-	60%
Nurses 'Always' Communicated Well[8]	-	-	-	76%
Pain 'Always' Well Controlled[8]	-	-	-	69%
Room and Bathroom 'Always' Clean[8]	-	-	-	71%
Timely Help 'Always' Received[8]	-	-	-	64%
Would Definitely Recommend Hospital[8]	-	-	-	69%

NOTE: Hospital profiles are in alphabetical order by state, then city, then hospital within the city; Rankings exclude hospitals with less than 25 cases except for patient surveys which excludes hospitals with less than 100 cases; (a) 100–299 cases; (1) The number of cases is too small to be sure how well a hospital is performing; (2) The hospital indicated that the data submitted for this measure were based on a sample of cases; (3) Data was collected during a shorter time period (fewer quarters) than the maximum possible time for this measure; (4) Suppressed for one or more quarters by CMS; (5) No data is available from the hospital for this measure; (6) Fewer than 100 patients completed the HCAHPS survey. Use these rates with caution, as the number of surveys may be too low to reliably assess hospital performance; (7) Survey results are based on less than 12 months of data; (8) Survey results are not available for this reporting period; (9) No or very few patients were eligible for the HCAHPS survey. The scores shown, if any, reflect a very small number of surveys; (10) A state average was not calculated because too few hospitals in the state submitted data; (11) There were discrepancies in the data collection process; Please refer to the User's Guide for a full explanation of data.

Elmhurst Hospital Center

79-01 Broadway
Elmhurst, NY 11373
Phone: 718-334-1141
Fax: 718-334-1810
URL: nyc.gov
Type: Acute Care Hospitals
Emergency Services: Yes
Ownership: Government - Local
Beds: 525

Key Personnel:
Operating Room. . . . . Anne McGann, RN
Pediatric Ambulatory Care . . . . . . Melvin Gertner, MD
Pediatric In-Patient Care . . . . Melvin Gertner, MD
Quality Assurance . . . . Beverly Carroll
Radiology. . . . . David Hayt, MD
Anesthesiology. . . . . Kenneth Abrams, MD
Emergency Room . . . . Stuart Kessler, MD
Intensive Care Unit. . . . . JoAnn Gull, RN

Measure	Cases	This Hosp.	State Avg.	U.S. Avg.
Heart Attack Care				
ACE Inhibitor or ARB for LVSD	61	95%	95%	96%
Aspirin at Arrival	267	100%	98%	99%
Aspirin at Discharge	268	100%	98%	98%
Beta Blocker at Discharge	262	100%	98%	98%
Fibrinolytic Medication Timing	0	-	50%	55%
PCI Within 90 Minutes of Arrival	90	67%	88%	90%
Smoking Cessation Advice	91	100%	100%	99%
Chest Pain/Possible Heart Attack Care				
Aspirin at Arrival	192	100%	96%	95%
Median Time to ECG (minutes)	198	0	11	8
Median Time to Transfer (minutes)[5]	0	-	75	61
Fibrinolytic Medication Timing[5]	0	-	55%	54%
Heart Failure Care				
ACE Inhibitor or ARB for LVSD	141	94%	94%	94%
Discharge Instructions	315	100%	89%	88%
Evaluation of LVS Function	339	100%	98%	98%
Smoking Cessation Advice	61	100%	98%	98%
Pneumonia Care				
Appropriate Initial Antibiotic	225	93%	92%	92%
Blood Culture Timing	228	89%	95%	96%
Influenza Vaccine	165	82%	90%	91%
Initial Antibiotic Timing	252	93%	93%	95%
Pneumococcal Vaccine	251	87%	92%	93%
Smoking Cessation Advice	95	100%	98%	97%
Surgical Care Improvement Project				
Appropriate VTP Within 24 Hours	323	98%	94%	92%
Appropriate Hair Removal	436	97%	100%	99%
Appropriate Beta Blocker Usage	74	100%	92%	93%
Controlled Postoperative Blood Glucose[1]	1	100%	94%	93%
Prophylactic Antibiotic Timing	127	99%	96%	97%
Prophylactic Antibiotic Timing (Outpatient)[1]	21	86%	92%	92%
Prophylactic Antibiotic Selection	129	98%	97%	97%
Prophylactic Antibiotic Select. (Outpatient)	84	95%	93%	94%
Prophylactic Antibiotic Stopped	125	92%	94%	94%
Recommended VTP Ordered	323	98%	96%	94%
Urinary Catheter Removal	70	91%	90%	90%
Children's Asthma Care				
Received Systemic Corticosteroids	-	-	-	100%
Received Home Management Plan	-	-	-	71%
Received Reliever Medication	-	-	-	100%
Use of Medical Imaging				
Combination Abdominal CT Scan	150	0.127	0.141	0.191
Combination Chest CT Scan	87	0.011	0.024	0.054
Follow-up Mammogram/Ultrasound	175	4.0%	9.8%	8.4%
MRI for Low Back Pain[1]	8	12.5%	26.9%	32.7%
Survey of Patients' Hospital Experiences				
Area Around Room 'Always' Quiet at Night	300+	41%	-	58%
Doctors 'Always' Communicated Well	300+	74%	-	80%
Home Recovery Information Given	300+	81%	-	82%
Hospital Given 9 or 10 on 10 Point Scale	300+	56%	-	67%
Meds 'Always' Explained Before Given	300+	48%	-	60%
Nurses 'Always' Communicated Well	300+	65%	-	76%
Pain 'Always' Well Controlled	300+	58%	-	69%
Room and Bathroom 'Always' Clean	300+	58%	-	71%
Timely Help 'Always' Received	300+	51%	-	64%
Would Definitely Recommend Hospital	300+	60%	-	69%

Arnot Ogden Medical Center

600 Roe Avenue
Elmira, NY 14905
Phone: 607-737-4100
Fax: 607-737-4447
E-mail: chandrick@aomc.org
URL: www.arnothealth.org
Type: Acute Care Hospitals
Emergency Services: Yes
Ownership: Voluntary Non-Profit - Private
Beds: 256

Key Personnel:
CEO/President. . . . . Anthony J Cooper
Chief of Medical Staff . . . . Luis Tapia, MD
Operating Room. . . . . Beverly Hulslander
Pediatric Ambulatory Care . . . . . . Kurt Kraus, MD
Pediatric In-Patient Care . . . . Kurt Kraus, MD
Quality Assurance . . . . Rita McCabe, RN
Radiology. . . . . Edwin Hutsal, MD
Patient Relations . . . . Elaine Sherhood

Measure	Cases	This Hosp.	State Avg.	U.S. Avg.
Heart Attack Care				
ACE Inhibitor or ARB for LVSD	94	99%	95%	96%
Aspirin at Arrival	193	100%	98%	99%
Aspirin at Discharge	293	100%	98%	98%
Beta Blocker at Discharge	313	99%	98%	98%
Fibrinolytic Medication Timing	0	-	50%	55%
PCI Within 90 Minutes of Arrival	40	90%	88%	90%
Smoking Cessation Advice	119	100%	100%	99%
Chest Pain/Possible Heart Attack Care				
Aspirin at Arrival[5]	0	-	96%	95%
Median Time to ECG (minutes)[5]	0	-	11	8
Median Time to Transfer (minutes)[5]	0	-	75	61
Fibrinolytic Medication Timing[5]	0	-	55%	54%
Heart Failure Care				
ACE Inhibitor or ARB for LVSD	74	95%	94%	94%
Discharge Instructions	188	81%	89%	88%
Evaluation of LVS Function	225	100%	98%	98%
Smoking Cessation Advice	38	100%	98%	98%
Pneumonia Care				
Appropriate Initial Antibiotic	122	93%	92%	92%
Blood Culture Timing	260	95%	95%	96%
Influenza Vaccine	179	97%	90%	91%
Initial Antibiotic Timing	226	96%	93%	95%
Pneumococcal Vaccine	255	98%	92%	93%
Smoking Cessation Advice	67	99%	98%	97%
Surgical Care Improvement Project				
Appropriate VTP Within 24 Hours[2]	149	97%	94%	92%
Appropriate Hair Removal[2]	732	98%	100%	99%
Appropriate Beta Blocker Usage[2]	293	100%	92%	93%
Controlled Postoperative Blood Glucose[2]	114	89%	94%	93%
Prophylactic Antibiotic Timing[2]	572	99%	96%	97%
Prophylactic Antibiotic Timing (Outpatient)	439	97%	92%	92%
Prophylactic Antibiotic Selection[2]	578	99%	97%	97%
Prophylactic Antibiotic Select. (Outpatient)	436	98%	93%	94%
Prophylactic Antibiotic Stopped[2]	547	97%	94%	94%
Recommended VTP Ordered[2]	149	98%	96%	94%
Urinary Catheter Removal[2]	100	97%	90%	90%
Children's Asthma Care				
Received Systemic Corticosteroids	-	-	-	100%
Received Home Management Plan	-	-	-	71%
Received Reliever Medication	-	-	-	100%
Use of Medical Imaging				
Combination Abdominal CT Scan	1,141	0.077	0.141	0.191
Combination Chest CT Scan	600	0.002	0.024	0.054
Follow-up Mammogram/Ultrasound	1,843	4.3%	9.8%	8.4%
MRI for Low Back Pain	143	32.9%	26.9%	32.7%
Survey of Patients' Hospital Experiences				
Area Around Room 'Always' Quiet at Night	300+	45%	-	58%
Doctors 'Always' Communicated Well	300+	79%	-	80%
Home Recovery Information Given	300+	85%	-	82%
Hospital Given 9 or 10 on 10 Point Scale	300+	67%	-	67%
Meds 'Always' Explained Before Given	300+	59%	-	60%
Nurses 'Always' Communicated Well	300+	79%	-	76%
Pain 'Always' Well Controlled	300+	71%	-	69%
Room and Bathroom 'Always' Clean	300+	69%	-	71%
Timely Help 'Always' Received	300+	63%	-	64%
Would Definitely Recommend Hospital	300+	75%	-	69%

Saint Joseph's Hospital

555 East Market Street
Elmira, NY 14902
Phone: 607-733-6541
Fax: 607-737-7837
URL: www.stjosephs.org
Type: Acute Care Hospitals
Emergency Services: Yes
Ownership: Voluntary Non-Profit - Private
Beds: 295

Key Personnel:
CEO/President. . . . . Marie Castagnaro SSJ
Infection Control. . . . . Deb Woodard
Operating Room. . . . . Lori Youmans RN
Quality Assurance . . . . Diane Giantiso
Intensive Care Unit. . . . . Antoinette Shields

Measure	Cases	This Hosp.	State Avg.	U.S. Avg.
Heart Attack Care				
ACE Inhibitor or ARB for LVSD[1]	5	100%	95%	96%
Aspirin at Arrival[1]	19	95%	98%	99%
Aspirin at Discharge[1]	15	100%	98%	98%
Beta Blocker at Discharge[1]	17	100%	98%	98%
Fibrinolytic Medication Timing	0	-	50%	55%
PCI Within 90 Minutes of Arrival	0	-	88%	90%
Smoking Cessation Advice[1]	4	100%	100%	99%
Chest Pain/Possible Heart Attack Care				
Aspirin at Arrival[1]	17	88%	96%	95%
Median Time to ECG (minutes)[1]	18	13	11	8
Median Time to Transfer (minutes)[1,3]	3	42	75	61
Fibrinolytic Medication Timing	0	-	55%	54%
Heart Failure Care				
ACE Inhibitor or ARB for LVSD	45	96%	94%	94%
Discharge Instructions	69	94%	89%	88%
Evaluation of LVS Function	93	100%	98%	98%
Smoking Cessation Advice[1]	20	100%	98%	98%
Pneumonia Care				
Appropriate Initial Antibiotic	95	98%	92%	92%
Blood Culture Timing	158	95%	95%	96%
Influenza Vaccine	119	95%	90%	91%
Initial Antibiotic Timing	156	95%	93%	95%
Pneumococcal Vaccine	179	93%	92%	93%
Smoking Cessation Advice	56	100%	98%	97%
Surgical Care Improvement Project				
Appropriate VTP Within 24 Hours	49	100%	94%	92%
Appropriate Hair Removal	203	100%	100%	99%
Appropriate Beta Blocker Usage	59	92%	92%	93%
Controlled Postoperative Blood Glucose	0	-	94%	93%
Prophylactic Antibiotic Timing	173	98%	96%	97%
Prophylactic Antibiotic Timing (Outpatient)	94	100%	92%	92%
Prophylactic Antibiotic Selection	174	99%	97%	97%
Prophylactic Antibiotic Select. (Outpatient)	94	98%	93%	94%
Prophylactic Antibiotic Stopped	168	99%	94%	94%
Recommended VTP Ordered	49	100%	96%	94%
Urinary Catheter Removal[1]	21	95%	90%	90%
Children's Asthma Care				
Received Systemic Corticosteroids	-	-	-	100%
Received Home Management Plan	-	-	-	71%
Received Reliever Medication	-	-	-	100%
Use of Medical Imaging				
Combination Abdominal CT Scan[1]	1	0.000	0.141	0.191
Combination Chest CT Scan[5]	0	-	0.024	0.054
Follow-up Mammogram/Ultrasound	741	4.7%	9.8%	8.4%
MRI for Low Back Pain	76	28.9%	26.9%	32.7%
Survey of Patients' Hospital Experiences				
Area Around Room 'Always' Quiet at Night	300+	47%	-	58%
Doctors 'Always' Communicated Well	300+	74%	-	80%
Home Recovery Information Given	300+	81%	-	82%
Hospital Given 9 or 10 on 10 Point Scale	300+	55%	-	67%
Meds 'Always' Explained Before Given	300+	53%	-	60%
Nurses 'Always' Communicated Well	300+	68%	-	76%
Pain 'Always' Well Controlled	300+	66%	-	69%
Room and Bathroom 'Always' Clean	300+	62%	-	71%
Timely Help 'Always' Received	300+	53%	-	64%
Would Definitely Recommend Hospital	300+	59%	-	69%

NOTE: Hospital profiles are in alphabetical order by state, then city, then hospital within the city; Rankings exclude hospitals with less than 25 cases except for patient surveys which excludes hospitals with less than 100 cases; (a) 100–299 cases; (1) The number of cases is too small to be sure how well a hospital is performing; (2) The hospital indicated that the data submitted for this measure were based on a sample of cases; (3) Data was collected during a shorter time period (fewer quarters) than the maximum possible time for this measure; (4) Suppressed for one or more quarters by CMS; (5) No data is available from the hospital for this measure; (6) Fewer than 100 patients completed the HCAHPS survey. Use these rates with caution, as the number of surveys may be too low to reliably assess hospital performance; (7) Survey results are based on less than 12 months of data; (8) Survey results are not available for this reporting period; (9) No or very few patients were eligible for the HCAHPS survey. The scores shown, if any, reflect a very small number of surveys; (10) A state average was not calculated because too few hospitals in the state submitted data; (11) There were discrepancies in the data collection process; Please refer to the User's Guide for a full explanation of data.

Peninsula Hospital Center

51-15 Beach Channel Drive Phone: 718-734-2000
Far Rockaway, NY 11691 Fax: 718-734-2993
URL: www.peninsulahospital.org
Type: Acute Care Hospitals Emergency Services: Yes
Ownership: Voluntary Non-Profit - Private Beds: 272

Key Personnel:
CEO/President. . . . . Peter Galwin
Chief of Medical Staff . . . . Peter A Galvin, MD
Infection Control. . . . . Alice Peele, RN
Operating Room. . . . . Edwin Jovellanos, RN
Quality Assurance . . . . Linda Dascher
Radiology. . . . . James Martinez
Emergency Room . . . . Vicki Backus, RN
Patient Relations . . . . Carol Breem

Measure	Cases	This Hosp.	State Avg.	U.S. Avg.
Heart Attack Care				
ACE Inhibitor or ARB for LVSD[1]	1	100%	95%	96%
Aspirin at Arrival[1]	14	100%	98%	99%
Aspirin at Discharge[1]	4	75%	98%	98%
Beta Blocker at Discharge[1]	6	100%	98%	98%
Fibrinolytic Medication Timing[1]	2	0%	50%	55%
PCI Within 90 Minutes of Arrival	0	-	88%	90%
Smoking Cessation Advice	0	-	100%	99%
Chest Pain/Possible Heart Attack Care				
Aspirin at Arrival[1,3]	5	100%	96%	95%
Median Time to ECG (minutes)[1,3]	5	21	11	8
Median Time to Transfer (minutes)[3]	0	-	75	61
Fibrinolytic Medication Timing[1,3]	2	50%	55%	54%
Heart Failure Care				
ACE Inhibitor or ARB for LVSD	61	97%	94%	94%
Discharge Instructions	114	96%	89%	88%
Evaluation of LVS Function	157	99%	98%	98%
Smoking Cessation Advice	26	100%	98%	98%
Pneumonia Care				
Appropriate Initial Antibiotic	84	88%	92%	92%
Blood Culture Timing	171	84%	95%	96%
Influenza Vaccine	112	83%	90%	91%
Initial Antibiotic Timing	195	83%	93%	95%
Pneumococcal Vaccine	192	86%	92%	93%
Smoking Cessation Advice	43	100%	98%	97%
Surgical Care Improvement Project				
Appropriate VTP Within 24 Hours	54	59%	94%	92%
Appropriate Hair Removal	88	100%	100%	99%
Appropriate Beta Blocker Usage[1]	20	90%	92%	93%
Controlled Postoperative Blood Glucose[1]	1	100%	94%	93%
Prophylactic Antibiotic Timing	36	92%	96%	97%
Prophylactic Antibiotic Timing (Outpatient)	60	93%	92%	92%
Prophylactic Antibiotic Selection	36	94%	97%	97%
Prophylactic Antibiotic Select. (Outpatient)	56	73%	93%	94%
Prophylactic Antibiotic Stopped	30	87%	94%	94%
Recommended VTP Ordered	54	61%	96%	94%
Urinary Catheter Removal[1]	11	82%	90%	90%
Children's Asthma Care				
Received Systemic Corticosteroids	-	-	-	100%
Received Home Management Plan	-	-	-	71%
Received Reliever Medication	-	-	-	100%
Use of Medical Imaging				
Combination Abdominal CT Scan	415	0.002	0.141	0.191
Combination Chest CT Scan	291	0.000	0.024	0.054
Follow-up Mammogram/Ultrasound	458	18.8%	9.8%	8.4%
MRI for Low Back Pain	68	20.6%	26.9%	32.7%
Survey of Patients' Hospital Experiences				
Area Around Room 'Always' Quiet at Night	300+	41%	-	58%
Doctors 'Always' Communicated Well	300+	66%	-	80%
Home Recovery Information Given	300+	70%	-	82%
Hospital Given 9 or 10 on 10 Point Scale	300+	33%	-	67%
Meds 'Always' Explained Before Given	300+	42%	-	60%
Nurses 'Always' Communicated Well	300+	54%	-	76%
Pain 'Always' Well Controlled	300+	51%	-	69%
Room and Bathroom 'Always' Clean	300+	59%	-	71%
Timely Help 'Always' Received	300+	39%	-	64%
Would Definitely Recommend Hospital	300+	41%	-	69%

Saint John's Episcopal Hospital at South Shore

327 Beach 19th Street Phone: 718-869-7000
Far Rockaway, NY 11691 Fax: 718-869-8507
Type: Acute Care Hospitals Emergency Services: Yes
Ownership: Voluntary Non-Profit - Church Beds: 332

Key Personnel:
CEO/President. . . . . Louis A Hernandez
Chief of Medical Staff . . . . Raymond Pastore, MD
Coronary Care . . . . Lynore Dupiton
Infection Control. . . . . Mary Anne Hauff
Operating Room. . . . . Gilbert Makabali, MD
Pediatric In-Patient Care . . . . Allan Steinberg, MD
Quality Assurance . . . . Carol Seaman
Radiology. . . . . Dennis Rossi, MD

Measure	Cases	This Hosp.	State Avg.	U.S. Avg.
Heart Attack Care				
ACE Inhibitor or ARB for LVSD[1]	6	100%	95%	96%
Aspirin at Arrival	40	100%	98%	99%
Aspirin at Discharge[1]	23	100%	98%	98%
Beta Blocker at Discharge[1]	22	100%	98%	98%
Fibrinolytic Medication Timing	0	-	50%	55%
PCI Within 90 Minutes of Arrival	0	-	88%	90%
Smoking Cessation Advice[1]	1	100%	100%	99%
Chest Pain/Possible Heart Attack Care				
Aspirin at Arrival[1]	12	100%	96%	95%
Median Time to ECG (minutes)[1]	12	10	11	8
Median Time to Transfer (minutes)	0	-	75	61
Fibrinolytic Medication Timing	0	-	55%	54%
Heart Failure Care				
ACE Inhibitor or ARB for LVSD	61	92%	94%	94%
Discharge Instructions	110	100%	89%	88%
Evaluation of LVS Function	186	96%	98%	98%
Smoking Cessation Advice	39	100%	98%	98%
Pneumonia Care				
Appropriate Initial Antibiotic[1,2]	24	92%	92%	92%
Blood Culture Timing[2]	124	98%	95%	96%
Influenza Vaccine[2]	75	93%	90%	91%
Initial Antibiotic Timing[2]	129	90%	93%	95%
Pneumococcal Vaccine[2]	132	94%	92%	93%
Smoking Cessation Advice[1,2]	18	100%	98%	97%
Surgical Care Improvement Project				
Appropriate VTP Within 24 Hours[2]	88	88%	94%	92%
Appropriate Hair Removal[2]	148	100%	100%	99%
Appropriate Beta Blocker Usage[2]	38	100%	92%	93%
Controlled Postoperative Blood Glucose[2]	0	-	94%	93%
Prophylactic Antibiotic Timing[2]	61	93%	96%	97%
Prophylactic Antibiotic Timing (Outpatient)	69	87%	92%	92%
Prophylactic Antibiotic Selection[2]	63	89%	97%	97%
Prophylactic Antibiotic Select. (Outpatient)	62	90%	93%	94%
Prophylactic Antibiotic Stopped[2]	57	95%	94%	94%
Recommended VTP Ordered[2]	88	88%	96%	94%
Urinary Catheter Removal[1,2]	17	94%	90%	90%
Children's Asthma Care				
Received Systemic Corticosteroids	-	-	-	100%
Received Home Management Plan	-	-	-	71%
Received Reliever Medication	-	-	-	100%
Use of Medical Imaging				
Combination Abdominal CT Scan	183	0.000	0.141	0.191
Combination Chest CT Scan	122	0.000	0.024	0.054
Follow-up Mammogram/Ultrasound	192	11.5%	9.8%	8.4%
MRI for Low Back Pain[1]	1	0.0%	26.9%	32.7%
Survey of Patients' Hospital Experiences				
Area Around Room 'Always' Quiet at Night	300+	53%	-	58%
Doctors 'Always' Communicated Well	300+	73%	-	80%
Home Recovery Information Given	300+	76%	-	82%
Hospital Given 9 or 10 on 10 Point Scale	300+	48%	-	67%
Meds 'Always' Explained Before Given	300+	52%	-	60%
Nurses 'Always' Communicated Well	300+	66%	-	76%
Pain 'Always' Well Controlled	300+	60%	-	69%
Room and Bathroom 'Always' Clean	300+	65%	-	71%
Timely Help 'Always' Received	300+	48%	-	64%
Would Definitely Recommend Hospital	300+	49%	-	69%

Flushing Hospital Medical Center

45th Avenue and Parsons Boulevard Phone: 718-670-5000
Flushing, NY 11355 Fax: 718-670-3077
URL: www.flushinghospital.org
Type: Acute Care Hospitals Emergency Services: Yes
Ownership: Voluntary Non-Profit - Private Beds: 293

Key Personnel:
CEO/President. . . . . Frederick I Weinbaum
Pediatric In-Patient Care . . . . Susana Rapaport, MD
Quality Assurance . . . . Dawn Lewis
Radiology. . . . . Glenn Schwartz, MD

Measure	Cases	This Hosp.	State Avg.	U.S. Avg.
Heart Attack Care				
ACE Inhibitor or ARB for LVSD[1]	15	93%	95%	96%
Aspirin at Arrival	105	89%	98%	99%
Aspirin at Discharge	64	86%	98%	98%
Beta Blocker at Discharge	70	90%	98%	98%
Fibrinolytic Medication Timing	0	-	50%	55%
PCI Within 90 Minutes of Arrival	0	-	88%	90%
Smoking Cessation Advice[1]	7	86%	100%	99%
Chest Pain/Possible Heart Attack Care				
Aspirin at Arrival[1]	23	100%	96%	95%
Median Time to ECG (minutes)[1]	23	13	11	8
Median Time to Transfer (minutes)[1,3]	5	139	75	61
Fibrinolytic Medication Timing[1]	2	100%	55%	54%
Heart Failure Care				
ACE Inhibitor or ARB for LVSD[2]	68	81%	94%	94%
Discharge Instructions[2]	124	89%	89%	88%
Evaluation of LVS Function[2]	255	98%	98%	98%
Smoking Cessation Advice[1,2]	14	86%	98%	98%
Pneumonia Care				
Appropriate Initial Antibiotic[2]	42	93%	92%	92%
Blood Culture Timing[2]	160	99%	95%	96%
Influenza Vaccine[2]	100	76%	90%	91%
Initial Antibiotic Timing[2]	130	98%	93%	95%
Pneumococcal Vaccine[2]	161	84%	92%	93%
Smoking Cessation Advice[1,2]	13	92%	98%	97%
Surgical Care Improvement Project				
Appropriate VTP Within 24 Hours[2]	229	96%	94%	92%
Appropriate Hair Removal[2]	616	100%	100%	99%
Appropriate Beta Blocker Usage[2]	112	96%	92%	93%
Controlled Postoperative Blood Glucose[1,2]	1	100%	94%	93%
Prophylactic Antibiotic Timing[2]	402	99%	96%	97%
Prophylactic Antibiotic Timing (Outpatient)	166	92%	92%	92%
Prophylactic Antibiotic Selection[2]	404	95%	97%	97%
Prophylactic Antibiotic Select. (Outpatient)	162	90%	93%	94%
Prophylactic Antibiotic Stopped[2]	391	90%	94%	94%
Recommended VTP Ordered[2]	231	96%	96%	94%
Urinary Catheter Removal	56	75%	90%	90%
Children's Asthma Care				
Received Systemic Corticosteroids	-	-	-	100%
Received Home Management Plan	-	-	-	71%
Received Reliever Medication	-	-	-	100%
Use of Medical Imaging				
Combination Abdominal CT Scan[1]	3	0.000	0.141	0.191
Combination Chest CT Scan	54	0.000	0.024	0.054
Follow-up Mammogram/Ultrasound	131	6.9%	9.8%	8.4%
MRI for Low Back Pain[1]	1	0.0%	26.9%	32.7%
Survey of Patients' Hospital Experiences				
Area Around Room 'Always' Quiet at Night	300+	38%	-	58%
Doctors 'Always' Communicated Well	300+	65%	-	80%
Home Recovery Information Given	300+	70%	-	82%
Hospital Given 9 or 10 on 10 Point Scale	300+	43%	-	67%
Meds 'Always' Explained Before Given	300+	42%	-	60%
Nurses 'Always' Communicated Well	300+	57%	-	76%
Pain 'Always' Well Controlled	300+	50%	-	69%
Room and Bathroom 'Always' Clean	300+	60%	-	71%
Timely Help 'Always' Received	300+	44%	-	64%
Would Definitely Recommend Hospital	300+	47%	-	69%

NOTE: Hospital profiles are in alphabetical order by state, then city, then hospital within the city; Rankings exclude hospitals with less than 25 cases except for patient surveys which excludes hospitals with less than 100 cases; (a) 100–299 cases; (1) The number of cases is too small to be sure how well a hospital is performing; (2) The hospital indicated that the data submitted for this measure were based on a sample of cases; (3) Data was collected during a shorter time period (fewer quarters) than the maximum possible time for this measure; (4) Suppressed for one or more quarters by CMS; (5) No data is available from the hospital for this measure; (6) Fewer than 100 patients completed the HCAHPS survey. Use these rates with caution, as the number of surveys may be too low to reliably assess hospital performance; (7) Survey results are based on less than 12 months of data; (8) Survey results are not available for this reporting period; (9) No or very few patients were eligible for the HCAHPS survey. The scores shown, if any, reflect a very small number of surveys; (10) A state average was not calculated because too few hospitals in the state submitted data; (11) There were discrepancies in the data collection process; Please refer to the User's Guide for a full explanation of data.

New York Hospital Medical Center of Queens

56-45 Main Street
Flushing, NY 11355
Phone: 718-670-1231
Fax: 718-661-7976
URL: www.nyhq.org
Type: Acute Care Hospitals
Emergency Services: Yes
Ownership: Voluntary Non-Profit - Other
Beds: 439

Key Personnel:

Chief of Medical Staff.......... Stephen Rimar
Infection Control............. James J Rahal, MD
Pediatric In-Patient Care....... Joe Abularrage
Radiology.................. William Wolff
Anesthesiology............... Peter Silverberg
Emergency Room............ Diane Sixsmith, MD
Patient Relations............ Michael Grady, MD

Measure	Cases	This Hosp.	State Avg.	U.S. Avg.
Heart Attack Care				
ACE Inhibitor or ARB for LVSD[2]	60	88%	95%	96%
Aspirin at Arrival[2]	320	98%	98%	99%
Aspirin at Discharge[2]	292	95%	98%	98%
Beta Blocker at Discharge[2]	289	97%	98%	98%
Fibrinolytic Medication Timing[1,2]	1	100%	50%	55%
PCI Within 90 Minutes of Arrival[2]	39	100%	88%	90%
Smoking Cessation Advice[2]	71	100%	100%	99%
Chest Pain/Possible Heart Attack Care				
Aspirin at Arrival[5]	0	-	96%	95%
Median Time to ECG (minutes)[5]	0	-	11	8
Median Time to Transfer (minutes)[5]	0	-	75	61
Fibrinolytic Medication Timing[5]	0	-	55%	54%
Heart Failure Care				
ACE Inhibitor or ARB for LVSD[2]	107	88%	94%	94%
Discharge Instructions[2]	257	93%	89%	88%
Evaluation of LVS Function[2]	337	100%	98%	98%
Smoking Cessation Advice[2]	34	100%	98%	98%
Pneumonia Care				
Appropriate Initial Antibiotic[2]	90	93%	92%	92%
Blood Culture Timing[2]	187	98%	95%	96%
Influenza Vaccine[2]	105	90%	90%	91%
Initial Antibiotic Timing[2]	173	90%	93%	95%
Pneumococcal Vaccine[2]	181	85%	92%	93%
Smoking Cessation Advice[2]	26	100%	98%	97%
Surgical Care Improvement Project				
Appropriate VTP Within 24 Hours[2]	326	98%	94%	92%
Appropriate Hair Removal[2]	771	100%	100%	99%
Appropriate Beta Blocker Usage[2]	230	96%	92%	93%
Controlled Postoperative Blood Glucose[2]	107	99%	94%	93%
Prophylactic Antibiotic Timing[2]	496	100%	96%	97%
Prophylactic Antibiotic Timing (Outpatient)	312	93%	92%	92%
Prophylactic Antibiotic Selection[2]	501	97%	97%	97%
Prophylactic Antibiotic Select. (Outpatient)	298	94%	93%	94%
Prophylactic Antibiotic Stopped[2]	451	96%	94%	94%
Recommended VTP Ordered[2]	326	98%	96%	94%
Urinary Catheter Removal[2]	156	94%	90%	90%
Children's Asthma Care				
Received Systemic Corticosteroids	-	-	-	100%
Received Home Management Plan	-	-	-	71%
Received Reliever Medication	-	-	-	100%
Use of Medical Imaging				
Combination Abdominal CT Scan	1,018	0.057	0.141	0.191
Combination Chest CT Scan	591	0.005	0.024	0.054
Follow-up Mammogram/Ultrasound	1,525	11.9%	9.8%	8.4%
MRI for Low Back Pain	91	34.1%	26.9%	32.7%
Survey of Patients' Hospital Experiences				
Area Around Room 'Always' Quiet at Night	300+	42%	-	58%
Doctors 'Always' Communicated Well	300+	69%	-	80%
Home Recovery Information Given	300+	75%	-	82%
Hospital Given 9 or 10 on 10 Point Scale	300+	52%	-	67%
Meds 'Always' Explained Before Given	300+	50%	-	60%
Nurses 'Always' Communicated Well	300+	64%	-	76%
Pain 'Always' Well Controlled	300+	55%	-	69%
Room and Bathroom 'Always' Clean	300+	63%	-	71%
Timely Help 'Always' Received	300+	46%	-	64%
Would Definitely Recommend Hospital	300+	61%	-	69%

Forest Hills Hospital

102-01 66th Road
Forest Hills, NY 11375
Phone: 718-830-4000
Fax: 718-275-0950
URL: www.northshorelij.com
Type: Acute Care Hospitals
Emergency Services: Yes
Ownership: Voluntary Non-Profit - Other
Beds: 309

Key Personnel:

CEO/President............... Geralyn Randazzo
Chief of Medical Staff.......... Gerard Brogan MD
Infection Control.............. Cecilia Wilfingon
Operating Room............. Moises Tenembaum
Pediatric Ambulatory Care...... Reginald McLaughlin MD
Pediatric In-Patient Care....... Reginald McLaughlin MD
Quality Assurance............ Linda Dascher
Radiology.................. Kenneth Schwartz MD

Measure	Cases	This Hosp.	State Avg.	U.S. Avg.
Heart Attack Care				
ACE Inhibitor or ARB for LVSD[1,2]	12	100%	95%	96%
Aspirin at Arrival[2]	111	95%	98%	99%
Aspirin at Discharge[2]	61	97%	98%	98%
Beta Blocker at Discharge[2]	67	97%	98%	98%
Fibrinolytic Medication Timing[2]	0	-	50%	55%
PCI Within 90 Minutes of Arrival[2]	0	-	88%	90%
Smoking Cessation Advice[1,2]	6	100%	100%	99%
Chest Pain/Possible Heart Attack Care				
Aspirin at Arrival	60	98%	96%	95%
Median Time to ECG (minutes)	62	11	11	8
Median Time to Transfer (minutes)[1]	19	80	75	61
Fibrinolytic Medication Timing	0	-	55%	54%
Heart Failure Care				
ACE Inhibitor or ARB for LVSD[2]	65	91%	94%	94%
Discharge Instructions[2]	191	91%	89%	88%
Evaluation of LVS Function[2]	267	100%	98%	98%
Smoking Cessation Advice[1,2]	22	100%	98%	98%
Pneumonia Care				
Appropriate Initial Antibiotic[2]	77	87%	92%	92%
Blood Culture Timing[2]	141	97%	95%	96%
Influenza Vaccine[2]	89	96%	90%	91%
Initial Antibiotic Timing[2]	122	93%	93%	95%
Pneumococcal Vaccine[2]	162	96%	92%	93%
Smoking Cessation Advice[1,2]	21	95%	98%	97%
Surgical Care Improvement Project				
Appropriate VTP Within 24 Hours[2]	191	97%	94%	92%
Appropriate Hair Removal[2]	411	100%	100%	99%
Appropriate Beta Blocker Usage[2]	110	98%	92%	93%
Controlled Postoperative Blood Glucose[2]	0	-	94%	93%
Prophylactic Antibiotic Timing[2]	269	99%	96%	97%
Prophylactic Antibiotic Timing (Outpatient)	122	96%	92%	92%
Prophylactic Antibiotic Selection[2]	270	98%	97%	97%
Prophylactic Antibiotic Select. (Outpatient)	118	88%	93%	94%
Prophylactic Antibiotic Stopped[2]	257	92%	94%	94%
Recommended VTP Ordered[2]	191	99%	96%	94%
Urinary Catheter Removal[2]	106	99%	90%	90%
Children's Asthma Care				
Received Systemic Corticosteroids	-	-	-	100%
Received Home Management Plan	-	-	-	71%
Received Reliever Medication	-	-	-	100%
Use of Medical Imaging				
Combination Abdominal CT Scan	228	0.022	0.141	0.191
Combination Chest CT Scan	103	0.000	0.024	0.054
Follow-up Mammogram/Ultrasound	88	43.2%	9.8%	8.4%
MRI for Low Back Pain[1]	12	41.7%	26.9%	32.7%
Survey of Patients' Hospital Experiences				
Area Around Room 'Always' Quiet at Night	300+	44%	-	58%
Doctors 'Always' Communicated Well	300+	70%	-	80%
Home Recovery Information Given	300+	72%	-	82%
Hospital Given 9 or 10 on 10 Point Scale	300+	51%	-	67%
Meds 'Always' Explained Before Given	300+	51%	-	60%
Nurses 'Always' Communicated Well	300+	64%	-	76%
Pain 'Always' Well Controlled	300+	61%	-	69%
Room and Bathroom 'Always' Clean	300+	66%	-	71%
Timely Help 'Always' Received	300+	52%	-	64%
Would Definitely Recommend Hospital	300+	58%	-	69%

Geneva General Hospital

196 -198 North Street
Geneva, NY 14456
Phone: 315-787-4175
Fax: 315-787-4009
URL: www.flhealth.org
Type: Acute Care Hospitals
Emergency Services: Yes
Ownership: Voluntary Non-Profit - Private
Beds: 136

Key Personnel:

CEO/President............... James Dooley
Chief of Medical Staff.......... Jane McCaffrey, MD
Infection Control............. Marge Brinn
Operating Room............. Rose Leo
Pediatric In-Patient Care....... Mary Jo Olmstead
Quality Assurance............ Betty Scarnati
Radiology.................. Rodolfo Queiroz
Intensive Care Unit............ Barb Weinberg

Measure	Cases	This Hosp.	State Avg.	U.S. Avg.
Heart Attack Care				
ACE Inhibitor or ARB for LVSD[1]	4	100%	95%	96%
Aspirin at Arrival	31	100%	98%	99%
Aspirin at Discharge[1]	20	100%	98%	98%
Beta Blocker at Discharge[1]	20	90%	98%	98%
Fibrinolytic Medication Timing	0	-	50%	55%
PCI Within 90 Minutes of Arrival	0	-	88%	90%
Smoking Cessation Advice[1]	1	100%	100%	99%
Chest Pain/Possible Heart Attack Care				
Aspirin at Arrival	61	98%	96%	95%
Median Time to ECG (minutes)	64	20	11	8
Median Time to Transfer (minutes)[1]	3	74	75	61
Fibrinolytic Medication Timing[1]	4	75%	55%	54%
Heart Failure Care				
ACE Inhibitor or ARB for LVSD[1]	20	100%	94%	94%
Discharge Instructions	109	77%	89%	88%
Evaluation of LVS Function	148	94%	98%	98%
Smoking Cessation Advice[1]	16	100%	98%	98%
Pneumonia Care				
Appropriate Initial Antibiotic[2]	73	85%	92%	92%
Blood Culture Timing[2]	138	91%	95%	96%
Influenza Vaccine[2]	96	79%	90%	91%
Initial Antibiotic Timing[2]	116	86%	93%	95%
Pneumococcal Vaccine[2]	122	87%	92%	93%
Smoking Cessation Advice[2]	32	88%	98%	97%
Surgical Care Improvement Project				
Appropriate VTP Within 24 Hours[2]	116	85%	94%	92%
Appropriate Hair Removal[2]	238	100%	100%	99%
Appropriate Beta Blocker Usage[2]	55	95%	92%	93%
Controlled Postoperative Blood Glucose[2]	0	-	94%	93%
Prophylactic Antibiotic Timing[2]	166	96%	96%	97%
Prophylactic Antibiotic Timing (Outpatient)	72	92%	92%	92%
Prophylactic Antibiotic Selection[2]	153	94%	97%	97%
Prophylactic Antibiotic Select. (Outpatient)	101	98%	93%	94%
Prophylactic Antibiotic Stopped[2]	150	97%	94%	94%
Recommended VTP Ordered[2]	116	97%	96%	94%
Urinary Catheter Removal[2]	67	84%	90%	90%
Children's Asthma Care				
Received Systemic Corticosteroids	-	-	-	100%
Received Home Management Plan	-	-	-	71%
Received Reliever Medication	-	-	-	100%
Use of Medical Imaging				
Combination Abdominal CT Scan	361	0.440	0.141	0.191
Combination Chest CT Scan	173	0.017	0.024	0.054
Follow-up Mammogram/Ultrasound	677	9.7%	9.8%	8.4%
MRI for Low Back Pain[5]	0	-	26.9%	32.7%
Survey of Patients' Hospital Experiences				
Area Around Room 'Always' Quiet at Night	300+	55%	-	58%
Doctors 'Always' Communicated Well	300+	75%	-	80%
Home Recovery Information Given	300+	87%	-	82%
Hospital Given 9 or 10 on 10 Point Scale	300+	57%	-	67%
Meds 'Always' Explained Before Given	300+	59%	-	60%
Nurses 'Always' Communicated Well	300+	72%	-	76%
Pain 'Always' Well Controlled	300+	65%	-	69%
Room and Bathroom 'Always' Clean	300+	63%	-	71%
Timely Help 'Always' Received	300+	56%	-	64%
Would Definitely Recommend Hospital	300+	61%	-	69%

NOTE: Hospital profiles are in alphabetical order by state, then city, then hospital within the city; Rankings exclude hospitals with less than 25 cases except for patient surveys which excludes hospitals with less than 100 cases; (a) 100–299 cases; (1) The number of cases is too small to be sure how well a hospital is performing; (2) The hospital indicated that the data submitted for this measure were based on a sample of cases; (3) Data was collected during a shorter time period (fewer quarters) than the maximum possible time for this measure; (4) Suppressed for one or more quarters by CMS; (5) No data is available from the hospital for this measure; (6) Fewer than 100 patients completed the HCAHPS survey. Use these rates with caution, as the number of surveys may be too low to reliably assess hospital performance; (7) Survey results are based on less than 12 months of data; (8) Survey results are not available for this reporting period; (9) No or very few patients were eligible for the HCAHPS survey. The scores shown, if any, reflect a very small number of surveys; (10) A state average was not calculated because too few hospitals in the state submitted data; (11) There were discrepancies in the data collection process; Please refer to the User's Guide for a full explanation of data.

Glen Cove Hospital

101 St Andrews Lane Phone: 516-674-7300
Glen Cove, NY 11542 Fax: 516-674-7670
URL: www.northshorelij.com
Type: Acute Care Hospitals Emergency Services: Yes
Ownership: Voluntary Non-Profit - Private Beds: 265

Key Personnel:
CEO/President. . . . . John ST Gallagher
Chief of Medical Staff. . . . . Jon R Cohen, MD
Coronary Care. . . . . Kathy Mann, RN
Infection Control. . . . . Bruce Farber, MD
Operating Room. . . . . Linda Olander, RN
Pediatric Ambulatory Care . . . . . . James Fagin, MD
Quality Assurance . . . . Donn Haber
Radiology. . . . . Mitchell Goldman, MD

Measure	Cases	This Hosp.	State Avg.	U.S. Avg.
Heart Attack Care				
ACE Inhibitor or ARB for LVSD[1,2]	7	100%	95%	96%
Aspirin at Arrival[2]	47	100%	98%	99%
Aspirin at Discharge[2]	28	96%	98%	98%
Beta Blocker at Discharge[1,2]	24	100%	98%	98%
Fibrinolytic Medication Timing[2]	0	-	50%	55%
PCI Within 90 Minutes of Arrival[2]	0	-	88%	90%
Smoking Cessation Advice[1,2]	2	100%	100%	99%
Chest Pain/Possible Heart Attack Care				
Aspirin at Arrival	36	100%	96%	95%
Median Time to ECG (minutes)	37	8	11	8
Median Time to Transfer (minutes)[1]	18	78	75	61
Fibrinolytic Medication Timing	0	-	55%	54%
Heart Failure Care				
ACE Inhibitor or ARB for LVSD[2]	28	96%	94%	94%
Discharge Instructions[2]	170	96%	89%	88%
Evaluation of LVS Function[2]	249	100%	98%	98%
Smoking Cessation Advice[1,2]	7	100%	98%	98%
Pneumonia Care				
Appropriate Initial Antibiotic[2]	71	96%	92%	92%
Blood Culture Timing[2]	126	100%	95%	96%
Influenza Vaccine[2]	72	94%	90%	91%
Initial Antibiotic Timing[2]	119	99%	93%	95%
Pneumococcal Vaccine[2]	142	92%	92%	93%
Smoking Cessation Advice[1,2]	15	100%	98%	97%
Surgical Care Improvement Project				
Appropriate VTP Within 24 Hours[2]	183	98%	94%	92%
Appropriate Hair Removal[2]	299	100%	100%	99%
Appropriate Beta Blocker Usage[2]	95	97%	92%	93%
Controlled Postoperative Blood Glucose[2]	0	-	94%	93%
Prophylactic Antibiotic Timing[2]	194	97%	96%	97%
Prophylactic Antibiotic Timing (Outpatient)	44	93%	92%	92%
Prophylactic Antibiotic Selection[2]	194	100%	97%	97%
Prophylactic Antibiotic Select. (Outpatient)	41	100%	93%	94%
Prophylactic Antibiotic Stopped[2]	189	98%	94%	94%
Recommended VTP Ordered[2]	183	99%	96%	94%
Urinary Catheter Removal[2]	105	92%	90%	90%
Children's Asthma Care				
Received Systemic Corticosteroids	-	-	-	100%
Received Home Management Plan	-	-	-	71%
Received Reliever Medication	-	-	-	100%
Use of Medical Imaging				
Combination Abdominal CT Scan	365	0.455	0.141	0.191
Combination Chest CT Scan	279	0.000	0.024	0.054
Follow-up Mammogram/Ultrasound	235	15.3%	9.8%	8.4%
MRI for Low Back Pain[5]	0	-	26.9%	32.7%
Survey of Patients' Hospital Experiences				
Area Around Room 'Always' Quiet at Night	300+	50%	-	58%
Doctors 'Always' Communicated Well	300+	79%	-	80%
Home Recovery Information Given	300+	78%	-	82%
Hospital Given 9 or 10 on 10 Point Scale	300+	67%	-	67%
Meds 'Always' Explained Before Given	300+	59%	-	60%
Nurses 'Always' Communicated Well	300+	78%	-	76%
Pain 'Always' Well Controlled	300+	66%	-	69%
Room and Bathroom 'Always' Clean	300+	74%	-	71%
Timely Help 'Always' Received	300+	62%	-	64%
Would Definitely Recommend Hospital	300+	70%	-	69%

Glens Falls Hospital

100 Park Street Phone: 518-926-1000
Glens Falls, NY 12801 Fax: 518-926-1919
E-mail: mail@glensfallshosp.org
URL: www.glensfallshospital.org
Type: Acute Care Hospitals Emergency Services: Yes
Ownership: Voluntary Non-Profit - Private Beds: 410

Key Personnel:
CEO/President. . . . . David G Kruczlnicki
Chief of Medical Staff. . . . . John Bulova, MD
Coronary Care. . . . . Carol Forman
Infection Control. . . . . Kathkeen Sposato
Operating Room. . . . . Nancy Lombard
Pediatric Ambulatory Care . . . . . . Guy Lehine, MD
Quality Assurance . . . . Phyllis Western
Radiology. . . . . Ed Hanchett

Measure	Cases	This Hosp.	State Avg.	U.S. Avg.
Heart Attack Care				
ACE Inhibitor or ARB for LVSD	43	98%	95%	96%
Aspirin at Arrival	268	100%	98%	99%
Aspirin at Discharge	229	100%	98%	98%
Beta Blocker at Discharge	235	100%	98%	98%
Fibrinolytic Medication Timing	0	-	50%	55%
PCI Within 90 Minutes of Arrival	47	96%	88%	90%
Smoking Cessation Advice	73	100%	100%	99%
Chest Pain/Possible Heart Attack Care				
Aspirin at Arrival[1,3]	3	100%	96%	95%
Median Time to ECG (minutes)[1,3]	3	5	11	8
Median Time to Transfer (minutes)[5]	0	-	75	61
Fibrinolytic Medication Timing[5]	0	-	55%	54%
Heart Failure Care				
ACE Inhibitor or ARB for LVSD[2]	112	98%	94%	94%
Discharge Instructions[2]	268	75%	89%	88%
Evaluation of LVS Function[2]	338	100%	98%	98%
Smoking Cessation Advice[2]	40	100%	98%	98%
Pneumonia Care				
Appropriate Initial Antibiotic[2]	132	90%	92%	92%
Blood Culture Timing[2]	170	89%	95%	96%
Influenza Vaccine[2]	129	92%	90%	91%
Initial Antibiotic Timing[2]	197	95%	93%	95%
Pneumococcal Vaccine[2]	205	97%	92%	93%
Smoking Cessation Advice[2]	75	100%	98%	97%
Surgical Care Improvement Project				
Appropriate VTP Within 24 Hours[2]	268	91%	94%	92%
Appropriate Hair Removal[2]	655	100%	100%	99%
Appropriate Beta Blocker Usage[2]	202	93%	92%	93%
Controlled Postoperative Blood Glucose[2]	0	-	94%	93%
Prophylactic Antibiotic Timing[2]	442	97%	96%	97%
Prophylactic Antibiotic Timing (Outpatient)	424	95%	92%	92%
Prophylactic Antibiotic Selection[2]	447	95%	97%	97%
Prophylactic Antibiotic Select. (Outpatient)	413	94%	93%	94%
Prophylactic Antibiotic Stopped[2]	428	96%	94%	94%
Recommended VTP Ordered[2]	268	92%	96%	94%
Urinary Catheter Removal[2]	60	90%	90%	90%
Children's Asthma Care				
Received Systemic Corticosteroids	-	-	-	100%
Received Home Management Plan	-	-	-	71%
Received Reliever Medication	-	-	-	100%
Use of Medical Imaging				
Combination Abdominal CT Scan	1,653	0.044	0.141	0.191
Combination Chest CT Scan	1,383	0.002	0.024	0.054
Follow-up Mammogram/Ultrasound	1,655	8.9%	9.8%	8.4%
MRI for Low Back Pain[5]	0	-	26.9%	32.7%
Survey of Patients' Hospital Experiences				
Area Around Room 'Always' Quiet at Night	300+	46%	-	58%
Doctors 'Always' Communicated Well	300+	79%	-	80%
Home Recovery Information Given	300+	85%	-	82%
Hospital Given 9 or 10 on 10 Point Scale	300+	60%	-	67%
Meds 'Always' Explained Before Given	300+	56%	-	60%
Nurses 'Always' Communicated Well	300+	70%	-	76%
Pain 'Always' Well Controlled	300+	67%	-	69%
Room and Bathroom 'Always' Clean	300+	69%	-	71%
Timely Help 'Always' Received	300+	57%	-	64%
Would Definitely Recommend Hospital	300+	65%	-	69%

Nathan Littauer Hospital

99 East State Street Phone: 518-725-8621
Gloversville, NY 12078 Fax: 518-773-5757
E-mail: info@nlh.org
URL: www.nlh.org
Type: Acute Care Hospitals Emergency Services: Yes
Ownership: Voluntary Non-Profit - Private Beds: 208

Key Personnel:
CEO/President. . . . . Laurence E Kelly
Chief of Medical Staff. . . . . George Disney, MD
Infection Control. . . . . Melissa Bown, RN
Operating Room. . . . . John Fox, DDS
Quality Assurance . . . . Diane Swartz
Radiology. . . . . Jerome Brustein, MD
Emergency Room . . . . Marie Born, RN
Intensive Care Unit. . . . . Nancy Hisert, RN

Measure	Cases	This Hosp.	State Avg.	U.S. Avg.
Heart Attack Care				
ACE Inhibitor or ARB for LVSD[1]	1	100%	95%	96%
Aspirin at Arrival	43	95%	98%	99%
Aspirin at Discharge[1]	24	92%	98%	98%
Beta Blocker at Discharge	28	100%	98%	98%
Fibrinolytic Medication Timing	0	-	50%	55%
PCI Within 90 Minutes of Arrival	0	-	88%	90%
Smoking Cessation Advice[1]	4	75%	100%	99%
Chest Pain/Possible Heart Attack Care				
Aspirin at Arrival	54	94%	96%	95%
Median Time to ECG (minutes)	56	8	11	8
Median Time to Transfer (minutes)[1]	10	56	75	61
Fibrinolytic Medication Timing	0	-	55%	54%
Heart Failure Care				
ACE Inhibitor or ARB for LVSD	36	100%	94%	94%
Discharge Instructions	78	96%	89%	88%
Evaluation of LVS Function	93	87%	98%	98%
Smoking Cessation Advice[1]	17	71%	98%	98%
Pneumonia Care				
Appropriate Initial Antibiotic	66	89%	92%	92%
Blood Culture Timing	104	80%	95%	96%
Influenza Vaccine	73	95%	90%	91%
Initial Antibiotic Timing	114	93%	93%	95%
Pneumococcal Vaccine	108	65%	92%	93%
Smoking Cessation Advice	33	97%	98%	97%
Surgical Care Improvement Project				
Appropriate VTP Within 24 Hours	63	83%	94%	92%
Appropriate Hair Removal	148	99%	100%	99%
Appropriate Beta Blocker Usage	47	100%	92%	93%
Controlled Postoperative Blood Glucose	0	-	94%	93%
Prophylactic Antibiotic Timing	46	76%	96%	97%
Prophylactic Antibiotic Timing (Outpatient)	59	80%	92%	92%
Prophylactic Antibiotic Selection	46	91%	97%	97%
Prophylactic Antibiotic Select. (Outpatient)	52	85%	93%	94%
Prophylactic Antibiotic Stopped	45	87%	94%	94%
Recommended VTP Ordered	63	90%	96%	94%
Urinary Catheter Removal[1]	3	100%	90%	90%
Children's Asthma Care				
Received Systemic Corticosteroids	-	-	-	100%
Received Home Management Plan	-	-	-	71%
Received Reliever Medication	-	-	-	100%
Use of Medical Imaging				
Combination Abdominal CT Scan	464	0.045	0.141	0.191
Combination Chest CT Scan	309	0.026	0.024	0.054
Follow-up Mammogram/Ultrasound	754	6.4%	9.8%	8.4%
MRI for Low Back Pain	47	42.6%	26.9%	32.7%
Survey of Patients' Hospital Experiences				
Area Around Room 'Always' Quiet at Night	300+	54%	-	58%
Doctors 'Always' Communicated Well	300+	77%	-	80%
Home Recovery Information Given	300+	83%	-	82%
Hospital Given 9 or 10 on 10 Point Scale	300+	61%	-	67%
Meds 'Always' Explained Before Given	300+	62%	-	60%
Nurses 'Always' Communicated Well	300+	75%	-	76%
Pain 'Always' Well Controlled	300+	70%	-	69%
Room and Bathroom 'Always' Clean	300+	77%	-	71%
Timely Help 'Always' Received	300+	63%	-	64%
Would Definitely Recommend Hospital	300+	61%	-	69%

NOTE: Hospital profiles are in alphabetical order by state, then city, then hospital within the city; Rankings exclude hospitals with less than 25 cases except for patient surveys which excludes hospitals with less than 100 cases; (a) 100–299 cases; (1) The number of cases is too small to be sure how well a hospital is performing; (2) The hospital indicated that the data submitted for this measure were based on a sample of cases; (3) Data was collected during a shorter time period (fewer quarters) than the maximum possible time for this measure; (4) Suppressed for one or more quarters by CMS; (5) No data is available from the hospital for this measure; (6) Fewer than 100 patients completed the HCAHPS survey. Use these rates with caution, as the number of surveys may be too low to reliably assess hospital performance; (7) Survey results are based on less than 12 months of data; (8) Survey results are not available for this reporting period; (9) No or very few patients were eligible for the HCAHPS survey. The scores shown, if any, reflect a very small number of surveys; (10) A state average was not calculated because too few hospitals in the state submitted data; (11) There were discrepancies in the data collection process; Please refer to the User's Guide for a full explanation of data.

Orange Regional Medical Center

4 Harriman Drive
Goshen, NY 10924
Phone: 845-343-2424
Fax: 845-294-2105
Type: Acute Care Hospitals
Emergency Services: Yes
Ownership: Voluntary Non-Profit - Other
Beds: 174

Key Personnel:
CEO/President. . . . . Scott Batulis
Chief of Medical Staff. . . . . Olanrewaju O Somorin, MD
Radiology. . . . . Susan M Beatty

Measure	Cases	This Hosp.	State Avg.	U.S. Avg.
Heart Attack Care				
ACE Inhibitor or ARB for LVSD	28	100%	95%	96%
Aspirin at Arrival	211	100%	98%	99%
Aspirin at Discharge	176	100%	98%	98%
Beta Blocker at Discharge	179	100%	98%	98%
Fibrinolytic Medication Timing	0	-	50%	55%
PCI Within 90 Minutes of Arrival	45	100%	88%	90%
Smoking Cessation Advice	52	100%	100%	99%
Chest Pain/Possible Heart Attack Care				
Aspirin at Arrival[1]	13	92%	96%	95%
Median Time to ECG (minutes)[1]	14	10	11	8
Median Time to Transfer (minutes)[1,3]	1	81	75	61
Fibrinolytic Medication Timing[3]	0	-	55%	54%
Heart Failure Care				
ACE Inhibitor or ARB for LVSD	129	98%	94%	94%
Discharge Instructions	360	88%	89%	88%
Evaluation of LVS Function	485	99%	98%	98%
Smoking Cessation Advice	52	100%	98%	98%
Pneumonia Care				
Appropriate Initial Antibiotic	284	91%	92%	92%
Blood Culture Timing	547	96%	95%	96%
Influenza Vaccine	302	96%	90%	91%
Initial Antibiotic Timing	524	96%	93%	95%
Pneumococcal Vaccine	490	95%	92%	93%
Smoking Cessation Advice	153	99%	98%	97%
Surgical Care Improvement Project				
Appropriate VTP Within 24 Hours[2]	409	94%	94%	92%
Appropriate Hair Removal[2]	930	100%	100%	99%
Appropriate Beta Blocker Usage[2]	304	93%	92%	93%
Controlled Postoperative Blood Glucose[1,2]	1	100%	94%	93%
Prophylactic Antibiotic Timing[2]	682	98%	96%	97%
Prophylactic Antibiotic Timing (Outpatient)	314	92%	92%	92%
Prophylactic Antibiotic Selection[2]	687	98%	97%	97%
Prophylactic Antibiotic Select. (Outpatient)	297	88%	93%	94%
Prophylactic Antibiotic Stopped[2]	666	97%	94%	94%
Recommended VTP Ordered[2]	409	96%	96%	94%
Urinary Catheter Removal[2]	265	98%	90%	90%
Children's Asthma Care				
Received Systemic Corticosteroids	-	-	-	100%
Received Home Management Plan	-	-	-	71%
Received Reliever Medication	-	-	-	100%
Use of Medical Imaging				
Combination Abdominal CT Scan	1,430	0.116	0.141	0.191
Combination Chest CT Scan	1,410	0.014	0.024	0.054
Follow-up Mammogram/Ultrasound	1,909	6.2%	9.8%	8.4%
MRI for Low Back Pain	133	22.6%	26.9%	32.7%
Survey of Patients' Hospital Experiences				
Area Around Room 'Always' Quiet at Night	300+	41%	-	58%
Doctors 'Always' Communicated Well	300+	72%	-	80%
Home Recovery Information Given	300+	80%	-	82%
Hospital Given 9 or 10 on 10 Point Scale	300+	49%	-	67%
Meds 'Always' Explained Before Given	300+	52%	-	60%
Nurses 'Always' Communicated Well	300+	68%	-	76%
Pain 'Always' Well Controlled	300+	61%	-	69%
Room and Bathroom 'Always' Clean	300+	60%	-	71%
Timely Help 'Always' Received	300+	51%	-	64%
Would Definitely Recommend Hospital	300+	52%	-	69%

Edward John Noble Hospital of Gouverneur

77 West Barney Street
Gouverneur, NY 13642
Phone: 315-287-1000
Fax: 315-535-9313
E-mail: bporter@ejnoble.org
URL: www.ejnoble.com
Type: Acute Care Hospitals
Emergency Services: No
Ownership: Voluntary Non-Profit - Private
Beds: 87

Key Personnel:
CEO/President. . . . . Timothy Monroe, DVM
Chief of Medical Staff. . . . . Marlene Heyal, MD
Coronary Care . . . . Nadel Makreal, MD
Infection Control. . . . . Chris Thompson, RN
Operating Room. . . . . Vijaykumar Mandalayw, MD
Quality Assurance . . . . Alice Finnerty
Radiology. . . . . Michael G Maresca, MD

Measure	Cases	This Hosp.	State Avg.	U.S. Avg.
Heart Attack Care				
ACE Inhibitor or ARB for LVSD	0	-	95%	96%
Aspirin at Arrival[1]	4	100%	98%	99%
Aspirin at Discharge[1]	1	100%	98%	98%
Beta Blocker at Discharge[1]	1	100%	98%	98%
Fibrinolytic Medication Timing	0	-	50%	55%
PCI Within 90 Minutes of Arrival	0	-	88%	90%
Smoking Cessation Advice	0	-	100%	99%
Chest Pain/Possible Heart Attack Care				
Aspirin at Arrival[1]	20	95%	96%	95%
Median Time to ECG (minutes)[1]	20	7	11	8
Median Time to Transfer (minutes)[1,3]	1	255	75	61
Fibrinolytic Medication Timing[1,3]	3	33%	55%	54%
Heart Failure Care				
ACE Inhibitor or ARB for LVSD[1]	6	83%	94%	94%
Discharge Instructions	40	42%	89%	88%
Evaluation of LVS Function	53	79%	98%	98%
Smoking Cessation Advice[1]	7	86%	98%	98%
Pneumonia Care				
Appropriate Initial Antibiotic[1]	15	93%	92%	92%
Blood Culture Timing[1]	23	100%	95%	96%
Influenza Vaccine[1]	15	73%	90%	91%
Initial Antibiotic Timing	28	89%	93%	95%
Pneumococcal Vaccine[1]	19	58%	92%	93%
Smoking Cessation Advice[1]	7	100%	98%	97%
Surgical Care Improvement Project				
Appropriate VTP Within 24 Hours[1]	3	33%	94%	92%
Appropriate Hair Removal[1]	21	90%	100%	99%
Appropriate Beta Blocker Usage[1]	3	67%	92%	93%
Controlled Postoperative Blood Glucose	0	-	94%	93%
Prophylactic Antibiotic Timing[1]	18	67%	96%	97%
Prophylactic Antibiotic Timing (Outpatient)[1,3]	5	40%	92%	92%
Prophylactic Antibiotic Selection[1]	18	94%	97%	97%
Prophylactic Antibiotic Select. (Outpatient)[1,3]	5	100%	93%	94%
Prophylactic Antibiotic Stopped[1]	18	83%	94%	94%
Recommended VTP Ordered[1]	3	33%	96%	94%
Urinary Catheter Removal[1]	2	100%	90%	90%
Children's Asthma Care				
Received Systemic Corticosteroids	-	-	-	100%
Received Home Management Plan	-	-	-	71%
Received Reliever Medication	-	-	-	100%
Use of Medical Imaging				
Combination Abdominal CT Scan	109	0.046	0.141	0.191
Combination Chest CT Scan	84	0.000	0.024	0.054
Follow-up Mammogram/Ultrasound	250	3.2%	9.8%	8.4%
MRI for Low Back Pain[1]	14	21.4%	26.9%	32.7%
Survey of Patients' Hospital Experiences				
Area Around Room 'Always' Quiet at Night	300+	45%	-	58%
Doctors 'Always' Communicated Well	300+	82%	-	80%
Home Recovery Information Given	300+	84%	-	82%
Hospital Given 9 or 10 on 10 Point Scale	300+	50%	-	67%
Meds 'Always' Explained Before Given	300+	61%	-	60%
Nurses 'Always' Communicated Well	300+	73%	-	76%
Pain 'Always' Well Controlled	300+	65%	-	69%
Room and Bathroom 'Always' Clean	300+	70%	-	71%
Timely Help 'Always' Received	300+	68%	-	64%
Would Definitely Recommend Hospital	300+	42%	-	69%

TLC Health Network

100 Memorial Drive
Gowanda, NY 14070
Phone: 716-532-3377
Fax: 716-532-3774
E-mail: wssmith@kaleidahealth.org
Type: Acute Care Hospitals
Emergency Services: Yes
Ownership: Voluntary Non-Profit - Private
Beds: 65

Key Personnel:
CEO/President. . . . . James H Campbell
Cardiac Laboratory. . . . . Ellen Franz, RN
Chief of Medical Staff. . . . . Ramiah Sathananthan, MD
Infection Control. . . . . Ellen Franz, RN
Operating Room. . . . . Cindy Lille
Quality Assurance . . . . Karen Volk, RN
Radiology. . . . . Noel Chiantella

Measure	Cases	This Hosp.	State Avg.	U.S. Avg.
Heart Attack Care				
ACE Inhibitor or ARB for LVSD[1]	1	100%	95%	96%
Aspirin at Arrival[1]	16	94%	98%	99%
Aspirin at Discharge[1]	8	88%	98%	98%
Beta Blocker at Discharge[1]	9	100%	98%	98%
Fibrinolytic Medication Timing	0	-	50%	55%
PCI Within 90 Minutes of Arrival	0	-	88%	90%
Smoking Cessation Advice	0	-	100%	99%
Chest Pain/Possible Heart Attack Care				
Aspirin at Arrival	82	83%	96%	95%
Median Time to ECG (minutes)	79	10	11	8
Median Time to Transfer (minutes)[1,3]	1	315	75	61
Fibrinolytic Medication Timing[1]	9	56%	55%	54%
Heart Failure Care				
ACE Inhibitor or ARB for LVSD[1]	18	72%	94%	94%
Discharge Instructions	42	90%	89%	88%
Evaluation of LVS Function	72	88%	98%	98%
Smoking Cessation Advice[1]	9	89%	98%	98%
Pneumonia Care				
Appropriate Initial Antibiotic	63	95%	92%	92%
Blood Culture Timing	72	96%	95%	96%
Influenza Vaccine	61	92%	90%	91%
Initial Antibiotic Timing	89	94%	93%	95%
Pneumococcal Vaccine	78	97%	92%	93%
Smoking Cessation Advice	29	86%	98%	97%
Surgical Care Improvement Project				
Appropriate VTP Within 24 Hours	111	100%	94%	92%
Appropriate Hair Removal	159	100%	100%	99%
Appropriate Beta Blocker Usage	51	73%	92%	93%
Controlled Postoperative Blood Glucose	0	-	94%	93%
Prophylactic Antibiotic Timing	126	94%	96%	97%
Prophylactic Antibiotic Timing (Outpatient)[1]	19	89%	92%	92%
Prophylactic Antibiotic Selection	126	94%	97%	97%
Prophylactic Antibiotic Select. (Outpatient)[1]	19	100%	93%	94%
Prophylactic Antibiotic Stopped	122	90%	94%	94%
Recommended VTP Ordered	111	100%	96%	94%
Urinary Catheter Removal[1]	12	50%	90%	90%
Children's Asthma Care				
Received Systemic Corticosteroids	-	-	-	100%
Received Home Management Plan	-	-	-	71%
Received Reliever Medication	-	-	-	100%
Use of Medical Imaging				
Combination Abdominal CT Scan	206	0.058	0.141	0.191
Combination Chest CT Scan	99	0.000	0.024	0.054
Follow-up Mammogram/Ultrasound	364	4.4%	9.8%	8.4%
MRI for Low Back Pain[5]	0	-	26.9%	32.7%
Survey of Patients' Hospital Experiences				
Area Around Room 'Always' Quiet at Night	300+	41%	-	58%
Doctors 'Always' Communicated Well	300+	77%	-	80%
Home Recovery Information Given	300+	88%	-	82%
Hospital Given 9 or 10 on 10 Point Scale	300+	58%	-	67%
Meds 'Always' Explained Before Given	300+	57%	-	60%
Nurses 'Always' Communicated Well	300+	72%	-	76%
Pain 'Always' Well Controlled	300+	67%	-	69%
Room and Bathroom 'Always' Clean	300+	62%	-	71%
Timely Help 'Always' Received	300+	57%	-	64%
Would Definitely Recommend Hospital	300+	62%	-	69%

NOTE: Hospital profiles are in alphabetical order by state, then city, then hospital within the city; Rankings exclude hospitals with less than 25 cases except for patient surveys which excludes hospitals with less than 100 cases; (a) 100–299 cases; (1) The number of cases is too small to be sure how well a hospital is performing; (2) The hospital indicated that the data submitted for this measure were based on a sample of cases; (3) Data was collected during a shorter time period (fewer quarters) than the maximum possible time for this measure; (4) Suppressed for one or more quarters by CMS; (5) No data is available from the hospital for this measure; (6) Fewer than 100 patients completed the HCAHPS survey. Use these rates with caution, as the number of surveys may be too low to reliably assess hospital performance; (7) Survey results are based on less than 12 months of data; (8) Survey results are not available for this reporting period; (9) No or very few patients were eligible for the HCAHPS survey. The scores shown, if any, reflect a very small number of surveys; (10) A state average was not calculated because too few hospitals in the state submitted data; (11) There were discrepancies in the data collection process; Please refer to the User's Guide for a full explanation of data.

Eastern Long Island Hospital

201 Manor Place Phone: 631-477-1000
Greenport, NY 11944 Fax: 631-477-1746
URL: www.elih.org
Type: Acute Care Hospitals Emergency Services: Yes
Ownership: Voluntary Non-Profit - Private Beds: 90

Key Personnel:
CEO/President. . . . . Paul J Connor III, III
Chief of Medical Staff. . . . . Frank J Adipietro, MD
Operating Room. . . . . Joanne Rutkowsi
Quality Assurance . . . . Tara Kraemer
Radiology. . . . . Anthony Mitarotondo
Anesthesiology. . . . . Frank J Adipietro MD

Measure	Cases	This Hosp.	State Avg.	U.S. Avg.
Heart Attack Care				
ACE Inhibitor or ARB for LVSD[1]	1	100%	95%	96%
Aspirin at Arrival[1]	12	100%	98%	99%
Aspirin at Discharge[1]	9	100%	98%	98%
Beta Blocker at Discharge[1]	11	100%	98%	98%
Fibrinolytic Medication Timing	0	-	50%	55%
PCI Within 90 Minutes of Arrival	0	-	88%	90%
Smoking Cessation Advice	0	-	100%	99%
Chest Pain/Possible Heart Attack Care				
Aspirin at Arrival[1]	20	100%	96%	95%
Median Time to ECG (minutes)[1]	19	9	11	8
Median Time to Transfer (minutes)[1,3]	1	82	75	61
Fibrinolytic Medication Timing[1]	1	100%	55%	54%
Heart Failure Care				
ACE Inhibitor or ARB for LVSD[1]	11	91%	94%	94%
Discharge Instructions	36	81%	89%	88%
Evaluation of LVS Function	47	100%	98%	98%
Smoking Cessation Advice[1]	3	100%	98%	98%
Pneumonia Care				
Appropriate Initial Antibiotic	39	82%	92%	92%
Blood Culture Timing	58	98%	95%	96%
Influenza Vaccine	26	100%	90%	91%
Initial Antibiotic Timing	49	100%	93%	95%
Pneumococcal Vaccine	43	100%	92%	93%
Smoking Cessation Advice[1]	5	100%	98%	97%
Surgical Care Improvement Project				
Appropriate VTP Within 24 Hours	36	94%	94%	92%
Appropriate Hair Removal	45	100%	100%	99%
Appropriate Beta Blocker Usage[1]	13	100%	92%	93%
Controlled Postoperative Blood Glucose	0	-	94%	93%
Prophylactic Antibiotic Timing[1]	24	100%	96%	97%
Prophylactic Antibiotic Timing (Outpatient)	46	89%	92%	92%
Prophylactic Antibiotic Selection[1]	24	100%	97%	97%
Prophylactic Antibiotic Select. (Outpatient)	43	95%	93%	94%
Prophylactic Antibiotic Stopped[1]	24	88%	94%	94%
Recommended VTP Ordered	36	94%	96%	94%
Urinary Catheter Removal[1]	2	50%	90%	90%
Children's Asthma Care				
Received Systemic Corticosteroids	-	-	-	100%
Received Home Management Plan	-	-	-	71%
Received Reliever Medication	-	-	-	100%
Use of Medical Imaging				
Combination Abdominal CT Scan[1]	1	0.000	0.141	0.191
Combination Chest CT Scan[5]	0	-	0.024	0.054
Follow-up Mammogram/Ultrasound	386	26.2%	9.8%	8.4%
MRI for Low Back Pain[1]	49	24.5%	26.9%	32.7%
Survey of Patients' Hospital Experiences				
Area Around Room 'Always' Quiet at Night	300+	53%	-	58%
Doctors 'Always' Communicated Well	300+	85%	-	80%
Home Recovery Information Given	300+	84%	-	82%
Hospital Given 9 or 10 on 10 Point Scale	300+	78%	-	67%
Meds 'Always' Explained Before Given	300+	57%	-	60%
Nurses 'Always' Communicated Well	300+	80%	-	76%
Pain 'Always' Well Controlled	300+	78%	-	69%
Room and Bathroom 'Always' Clean	300+	74%	-	71%
Timely Help 'Always' Received	300+	65%	-	64%
Would Definitely Recommend Hospital	300+	84%	-	69%

Community Memorial Hospital

150 Broad Street Phone: 315-824-1100
Hamilton, NY 13346 Fax: 315-824-3182
URL: www.communitymemorial.org
Type: Acute Care Hospitals Emergency Services: Yes
Ownership: Voluntary Non-Profit - Private Beds: 88

Key Personnel:
CEO/President. . . . . David Felton
Chief of Medical Staff. . . . . Michael Jastremski
Radiology. . . . . Paul J Badami
Emergency Room . . . . Michael Jastremski
Intensive Care Unit. . . . . Diana Banalphulis

Measure	Cases	This Hosp.	State Avg.	U.S. Avg.
Heart Attack Care				
ACE Inhibitor or ARB for LVSD[1]	1	100%	95%	96%
Aspirin at Arrival[1]	7	100%	98%	99%
Aspirin at Discharge[1]	4	100%	98%	98%
Beta Blocker at Discharge[1]	6	100%	98%	98%
Fibrinolytic Medication Timing	0	-	50%	55%
PCI Within 90 Minutes of Arrival	0	-	88%	90%
Smoking Cessation Advice[1]	1	100%	100%	99%
Chest Pain/Possible Heart Attack Care				
Aspirin at Arrival	28	100%	96%	95%
Median Time to ECG (minutes)	30	4	11	8
Median Time to Transfer (minutes)[1,3]	1	49	75	61
Fibrinolytic Medication Timing[3]	0	-	55%	54%
Heart Failure Care				
ACE Inhibitor or ARB for LVSD[1]	12	100%	94%	94%
Discharge Instructions	30	87%	89%	88%
Evaluation of LVS Function	44	91%	98%	98%
Smoking Cessation Advice[1]	1	100%	98%	98%
Pneumonia Care				
Appropriate Initial Antibiotic	70	94%	92%	92%
Blood Culture Timing	96	98%	95%	96%
Influenza Vaccine	57	96%	90%	91%
Initial Antibiotic Timing	97	99%	93%	95%
Pneumococcal Vaccine	78	94%	92%	93%
Smoking Cessation Advice[1]	11	91%	98%	97%
Surgical Care Improvement Project				
Appropriate VTP Within 24 Hours	183	100%	94%	92%
Appropriate Hair Removal	521	100%	100%	99%
Appropriate Beta Blocker Usage	180	100%	92%	93%
Controlled Postoperative Blood Glucose	0	-	94%	93%
Prophylactic Antibiotic Timing	490	100%	96%	97%
Prophylactic Antibiotic Timing (Outpatient)	98	100%	92%	92%
Prophylactic Antibiotic Selection	489	100%	97%	97%
Prophylactic Antibiotic Select. (Outpatient)	98	100%	93%	94%
Prophylactic Antibiotic Stopped	486	99%	94%	94%
Recommended VTP Ordered	183	100%	96%	94%
Urinary Catheter Removal	39	97%	90%	90%
Children's Asthma Care				
Received Systemic Corticosteroids	-	-	-	100%
Received Home Management Plan	-	-	-	71%
Received Reliever Medication	-	-	-	100%
Use of Medical Imaging				
Combination Abdominal CT Scan	191	0.147	0.141	0.191
Combination Chest CT Scan	125	0.040	0.024	0.054
Follow-up Mammogram/Ultrasound	266	4.1%	9.8%	8.4%
MRI for Low Back Pain	54	38.9%	26.9%	32.7%
Survey of Patients' Hospital Experiences				
Area Around Room 'Always' Quiet at Night	300+	57%	-	58%
Doctors 'Always' Communicated Well	300+	83%	-	80%
Home Recovery Information Given	300+	88%	-	82%
Hospital Given 9 or 10 on 10 Point Scale	300+	73%	-	67%
Meds 'Always' Explained Before Given	300+	66%	-	60%
Nurses 'Always' Communicated Well	300+	79%	-	76%
Pain 'Always' Well Controlled	300+	72%	-	69%
Room and Bathroom 'Always' Clean	300+	77%	-	71%
Timely Help 'Always' Received	300+	67%	-	64%
Would Definitely Recommend Hospital	300+	78%	-	69%

Catskill Regional Medical Center

68 Harris Bushville Road Phone: 845-794-3300
Harris, NY 12742 Fax: 845-794-3240
URL: www.crmcny.org
Type: Acute Care Hospitals Emergency Services: Yes
Ownership: Voluntary Non-Profit - Other Beds: 263

Key Personnel:
CEO/President. . . . . Arthur L Briens
Chief of Medical Staff. . . . . Gary Good, MD
Operating Room. . . . . Dotty Schultz, RN
Pediatric In-Patient Care . . . . Amarjit Gill, MD
Quality Assurance . . . . Debra DeJesus
Radiology. . . . . George Osmur

Measure	Cases	This Hosp.	State Avg.	U.S. Avg.
Heart Attack Care				
ACE Inhibitor or ARB for LVSD[1]	2	100%	95%	96%
Aspirin at Arrival	41	90%	98%	99%
Aspirin at Discharge[1]	14	100%	98%	98%
Beta Blocker at Discharge[1]	13	100%	98%	98%
Fibrinolytic Medication Timing	0	-	50%	55%
PCI Within 90 Minutes of Arrival	0	-	88%	90%
Smoking Cessation Advice[1]	2	100%	100%	99%
Chest Pain/Possible Heart Attack Care				
Aspirin at Arrival	51	96%	96%	95%
Median Time to ECG (minutes)	54	21	11	8
Median Time to Transfer (minutes)[1]	5	95	75	61
Fibrinolytic Medication Timing	0	-	55%	54%
Heart Failure Care				
ACE Inhibitor or ARB for LVSD	27	93%	94%	94%
Discharge Instructions	55	85%	89%	88%
Evaluation of LVS Function	80	100%	98%	98%
Smoking Cessation Advice[1]	19	100%	98%	98%
Pneumonia Care				
Appropriate Initial Antibiotic	83	93%	92%	92%
Blood Culture Timing	133	95%	95%	96%
Influenza Vaccine	84	98%	90%	91%
Initial Antibiotic Timing	126	92%	93%	95%
Pneumococcal Vaccine	100	100%	92%	93%
Smoking Cessation Advice	58	100%	98%	97%
Surgical Care Improvement Project				
Appropriate VTP Within 24 Hours	119	93%	94%	92%
Appropriate Hair Removal	235	100%	100%	99%
Appropriate Beta Blocker Usage	54	83%	92%	93%
Controlled Postoperative Blood Glucose	0	-	94%	93%
Prophylactic Antibiotic Timing	157	98%	96%	97%
Prophylactic Antibiotic Timing (Outpatient)	41	93%	92%	92%
Prophylactic Antibiotic Selection	158	85%	97%	97%
Prophylactic Antibiotic Select. (Outpatient)	40	88%	93%	94%
Prophylactic Antibiotic Stopped	151	95%	94%	94%
Recommended VTP Ordered	119	97%	96%	94%
Urinary Catheter Removal[1]	24	92%	90%	90%
Children's Asthma Care				
Received Systemic Corticosteroids	-	-	-	100%
Received Home Management Plan	-	-	-	71%
Received Reliever Medication	-	-	-	100%
Use of Medical Imaging				
Combination Abdominal CT Scan	491	0.153	0.141	0.191
Combination Chest CT Scan	282	0.032	0.024	0.054
Follow-up Mammogram/Ultrasound	422	6.4%	9.8%	8.4%
MRI for Low Back Pain	92	30.4%	26.9%	32.7%
Survey of Patients' Hospital Experiences				
Area Around Room 'Always' Quiet at Night	300+	48%	-	58%
Doctors 'Always' Communicated Well	300+	71%	-	80%
Home Recovery Information Given	300+	79%	-	82%
Hospital Given 9 or 10 on 10 Point Scale	300+	40%	-	67%
Meds 'Always' Explained Before Given	300+	49%	-	60%
Nurses 'Always' Communicated Well	300+	64%	-	76%
Pain 'Always' Well Controlled	300+	64%	-	69%
Room and Bathroom 'Always' Clean	300+	53%	-	71%
Timely Help 'Always' Received	300+	55%	-	64%
Would Definitely Recommend Hospital	300+	46%	-	69%

NOTE: Hospital profiles are in alphabetical order by state, then city, then hospital within the city; Rankings exclude hospitals with less than 25 cases except for patient surveys which excludes hospitals with less than 100 cases; (a) 100–299 cases; (1) The number of cases is too small to be sure how well a hospital is performing; (2) The hospital indicated that the data submitted for this measure were based on a sample of cases; (3) Data was collected during a shorter time period (fewer quarters) than the maximum possible time for this measure; (4) Suppressed for one or more quarters by CMS; (5) No data is available from the hospital for this measure; (6) Fewer than 100 patients completed the HCAHPS survey. Use these rates with caution, as the number of surveys may be too low to reliably assess hospital performance; (7) Survey results are based on less than 12 months of data; (8) Survey results are not available for this reporting period; (9) No or very few patients were eligible for the HCAHPS survey. The scores shown, if any, reflect a very small number of surveys; (10) A state average was not calculated because too few hospitals in the state submitted data; (11) There were discrepancies in the data collection process; Please refer to the User's Guide for a full explanation of data.

Saint James Mercy Hospital

411 Canisteo Street
Hornell, NY 14843
Phone: 607-324-8000
Fax: 607-324-8115
E-mail: Info@StJamesMercy.org
URL: www.stjamesmercy.org

Type: Acute Care Hospitals
Emergency Services: Yes
Ownership: Voluntary Non-Profit - Church
Beds: 297

Key Personnel:

CEO/President. . . . . Mary LaRowe
Operating Room. . . . . Mary Jo Foreman
Quality Assurance . . . . Linda Henshaw
Radiology. . . . . Anne Konopa
Patient Relations . . . . Kim Meacham

Measure	Cases	This Hosp.	State Avg.	U.S. Avg.
Heart Attack Care				
ACE Inhibitor or ARB for LVSD	0	-	95%	96%
Aspirin at Arrival[1]	15	93%	98%	99%
Aspirin at Discharge[1]	11	91%	98%	98%
Beta Blocker at Discharge[1]	12	100%	98%	98%
Fibrinolytic Medication Timing	0	-	50%	55%
PCI Within 90 Minutes of Arrival	0	-	88%	90%
Smoking Cessation Advice[1]	2	100%	100%	99%
Chest Pain/Possible Heart Attack Care				
Aspirin at Arrival	86	100%	96%	95%
Median Time to ECG (minutes)	88	9	11	8
Median Time to Transfer (minutes)[1,3]	2	72	75	61
Fibrinolytic Medication Timing[1]	6	17%	55%	54%
Heart Failure Care				
ACE Inhibitor or ARB for LVSD[1]	2	100%	94%	94%
Discharge Instructions[1]	22	95%	89%	88%
Evaluation of LVS Function	29	93%	98%	98%
Smoking Cessation Advice[1]	2	100%	98%	98%
Pneumonia Care				
Appropriate Initial Antibiotic	71	94%	92%	92%
Blood Culture Timing	106	97%	95%	96%
Influenza Vaccine	61	98%	90%	91%
Initial Antibiotic Timing	100	99%	93%	95%
Pneumococcal Vaccine	87	100%	92%	93%
Smoking Cessation Advice[1]	23	87%	98%	97%
Surgical Care Improvement Project				
Appropriate VTP Within 24 Hours	60	87%	94%	92%
Appropriate Hair Removal	117	100%	100%	99%
Appropriate Beta Blocker Usage	29	100%	92%	93%
Controlled Postoperative Blood Glucose	0	-	94%	93%
Prophylactic Antibiotic Timing	76	97%	96%	97%
Prophylactic Antibiotic Timing (Outpatient)[1]	15	100%	92%	92%
Prophylactic Antibiotic Selection	78	90%	97%	97%
Prophylactic Antibiotic Select. (Outpatient)[1]	15	93%	93%	94%
Prophylactic Antibiotic Stopped	69	88%	94%	94%
Recommended VTP Ordered	60	88%	96%	94%
Urinary Catheter Removal[1]	19	100%	90%	90%
Children's Asthma Care				
Received Systemic Corticosteroids	-	-	-	100%
Received Home Management Plan	-	-	-	71%
Received Reliever Medication	-	-	-	100%
Use of Medical Imaging				
Combination Abdominal CT Scan	301	0.289	0.141	0.191
Combination Chest CT Scan	257	0.027	0.024	0.054
Follow-up Mammogram/Ultrasound	309	5.5%	9.8%	8.4%
MRI for Low Back Pain[5]	0	-	26.9%	32.7%
Survey of Patients' Hospital Experiences				
Area Around Room 'Always' Quiet at Night	300+	59%	-	58%
Doctors 'Always' Communicated Well	300+	77%	-	80%
Home Recovery Information Given	300+	87%	-	82%
Hospital Given 9 or 10 on 10 Point Scale	300+	51%	-	67%
Meds 'Always' Explained Before Given	300+	59%	-	60%
Nurses 'Always' Communicated Well	300+	70%	-	76%
Pain 'Always' Well Controlled	300+	63%	-	69%
Room and Bathroom 'Always' Clean	300+	69%	-	71%
Timely Help 'Always' Received	300+	65%	-	64%
Would Definitely Recommend Hospital	300+	51%	-	69%

Columbia Memorial Hospital

71 Prospect Avenue
Hudson, NY 12534
Phone: 518-828-7601
Fax: 518-828-8243
E-mail: info@columbiamemorial.com
URL: www.columbiamemorial.com

Type: Acute Care Hospitals
Emergency Services: Yes
Ownership: Voluntary Non-Profit - Private
Beds: 103

Key Personnel:

CEO/President. . . . . Brian Rogoz
Cardiac Laboratory. . . . . H L Clinton
Infection Control. . . . . Sherri Meyer, MD
Operating Room. . . . . Barbara Brady, MD
Pediatric In-Patient Care . . . . . . Sara Friess
Radiology. . . . . Tariq Gill
Emergency Room . . . . Barbara Brady, RN
Intensive Care Unit. . . . . Donald Tessitore

Measure	Cases	This Hosp.	State Avg.	U.S. Avg.
Heart Attack Care				
ACE Inhibitor or ARB for LVSD[1]	10	100%	95%	96%
Aspirin at Arrival	86	92%	98%	99%
Aspirin at Discharge	57	100%	98%	98%
Beta Blocker at Discharge	56	96%	98%	98%
Fibrinolytic Medication Timing	0	-	50%	55%
PCI Within 90 Minutes of Arrival	0	-	88%	90%
Smoking Cessation Advice[1]	9	89%	100%	99%
Chest Pain/Possible Heart Attack Care				
Aspirin at Arrival	40	95%	96%	95%
Median Time to ECG (minutes)	44	10	11	8
Median Time to Transfer (minutes)[1]	4	120	75	61
Fibrinolytic Medication Timing[1]	3	0%	55%	54%
Heart Failure Care				
ACE Inhibitor or ARB for LVSD	48	85%	94%	94%
Discharge Instructions	164	90%	89%	88%
Evaluation of LVS Function	226	95%	98%	98%
Smoking Cessation Advice	34	100%	98%	98%
Pneumonia Care				
Appropriate Initial Antibiotic	126	90%	92%	92%
Blood Culture Timing	266	94%	95%	96%
Influenza Vaccine	146	87%	90%	91%
Initial Antibiotic Timing	246	93%	93%	95%
Pneumococcal Vaccine	225	85%	92%	93%
Smoking Cessation Advice	64	94%	98%	97%
Surgical Care Improvement Project				
Appropriate VTP Within 24 Hours	163	90%	94%	92%
Appropriate Hair Removal	253	100%	100%	99%
Appropriate Beta Blocker Usage	83	93%	92%	93%
Controlled Postoperative Blood Glucose	0	-	94%	93%
Prophylactic Antibiotic Timing	125	89%	96%	97%
Prophylactic Antibiotic Timing (Outpatient)	97	90%	92%	92%
Prophylactic Antibiotic Selection	124	100%	97%	97%
Prophylactic Antibiotic Select. (Outpatient)	93	80%	93%	94%
Prophylactic Antibiotic Stopped	121	89%	94%	94%
Recommended VTP Ordered	163	91%	96%	94%
Urinary Catheter Removal	65	89%	90%	90%
Children's Asthma Care				
Received Systemic Corticosteroids	-	-	-	100%
Received Home Management Plan	-	-	-	71%
Received Reliever Medication	-	-	-	100%
Use of Medical Imaging				
Combination Abdominal CT Scan	581	0.406	0.141	0.191
Combination Chest CT Scan	438	0.016	0.024	0.054
Follow-up Mammogram/Ultrasound	623	9.5%	9.8%	8.4%
MRI for Low Back Pain[1]	41	29.3%	26.9%	32.7%
Survey of Patients' Hospital Experiences				
Area Around Room 'Always' Quiet at Night	300+	38%	-	58%
Doctors 'Always' Communicated Well	300+	76%	-	80%
Home Recovery Information Given	300+	79%	-	82%
Hospital Given 9 or 10 on 10 Point Scale	300+	47%	-	67%
Meds 'Always' Explained Before Given	300+	55%	-	60%
Nurses 'Always' Communicated Well	300+	69%	-	76%
Pain 'Always' Well Controlled	300+	64%	-	69%
Room and Bathroom 'Always' Clean	300+	62%	-	71%
Timely Help 'Always' Received	300+	53%	-	64%
Would Definitely Recommend Hospital	300+	51%	-	69%

Huntington Hospital

270 Park Avenue
Huntington, NY 11743
Phone: 631-351-2000
Fax: 631-351-2586
E-mail: staff@hunthosp.org
URL: www.hunthosp.org

Type: Acute Care Hospitals
Emergency Services: Yes
Ownership: Voluntary Non-Profit - Private
Beds: 396

Key Personnel:

CEO/President. . . . . J Ronald Gaudreault
Chief of Medical Staff . . . . Noah Finkel, MD
Coronary Care . . . . Kathy Mann, RN
Infection Control. . . . . Bruce Farber, MD
Operating Room. . . . . Linda Olander, RN
Pediatric Ambulatory Care . . . . . James Fagin, MD
Quality Assurance . . . . Donn Haber
Radiology. . . . . Mitchell Goldman, MD

Measure	Cases	This Hosp.	State Avg.	U.S. Avg.
Heart Attack Care				
ACE Inhibitor or ARB for LVSD[1,2]	15	100%	95%	96%
Aspirin at Arrival[2]	159	100%	98%	99%
Aspirin at Discharge[2]	103	100%	98%	98%
Beta Blocker at Discharge[2]	102	100%	98%	98%
Fibrinolytic Medication Timing[2]	0	-	50%	55%
PCI Within 90 Minutes of Arrival[2]	47	91%	88%	90%
Smoking Cessation Advice[1,2]	24	100%	100%	99%
Chest Pain/Possible Heart Attack Care				
Aspirin at Arrival	25	100%	96%	95%
Median Time to ECG (minutes)	26	4	11	8
Median Time to Transfer (minutes)[1,3]	3	61	75	61
Fibrinolytic Medication Timing[3]	0	-	55%	54%
Heart Failure Care				
ACE Inhibitor or ARB for LVSD[2]	65	98%	94%	94%
Discharge Instructions[2]	220	100%	89%	88%
Evaluation of LVS Function[2]	292	100%	98%	98%
Smoking Cessation Advice[1,2]	21	100%	98%	98%
Pneumonia Care				
Appropriate Initial Antibiotic[2]	82	96%	92%	92%
Blood Culture Timing[2]	149	95%	95%	96%
Influenza Vaccine[2]	93	99%	90%	91%
Initial Antibiotic Timing[2]	132	96%	93%	95%
Pneumococcal Vaccine[2]	152	95%	92%	93%
Smoking Cessation Advice[1,2]	24	100%	98%	97%
Surgical Care Improvement Project				
Appropriate VTP Within 24 Hours[2]	175	98%	94%	92%
Appropriate Hair Removal[2]	397	100%	100%	99%
Appropriate Beta Blocker Usage[2]	137	96%	92%	93%
Controlled Postoperative Blood Glucose[2]	0	-	94%	93%
Prophylactic Antibiotic Timing[2]	249	98%	96%	97%
Prophylactic Antibiotic Timing (Outpatient)	363	95%	92%	92%
Prophylactic Antibiotic Selection[2]	249	98%	97%	97%
Prophylactic Antibiotic Select. (Outpatient)	355	94%	93%	94%
Prophylactic Antibiotic Stopped[2]	234	97%	94%	94%
Recommended VTP Ordered[2]	175	99%	96%	94%
Urinary Catheter Removal[2]	30	80%	90%	90%
Children's Asthma Care				
Received Systemic Corticosteroids	-	-	-	100%
Received Home Management Plan	-	-	-	71%
Received Reliever Medication	-	-	-	100%
Use of Medical Imaging				
Combination Abdominal CT Scan	527	0.066	0.141	0.191
Combination Chest CT Scan	448	0.000	0.024	0.054
Follow-up Mammogram/Ultrasound	907	15.3%	9.8%	8.4%
MRI for Low Back Pain[1]	20	30.0%	26.9%	32.7%
Survey of Patients' Hospital Experiences				
Area Around Room 'Always' Quiet at Night	300+	46%	-	58%
Doctors 'Always' Communicated Well	300+	78%	-	80%
Home Recovery Information Given	300+	75%	-	82%
Hospital Given 9 or 10 on 10 Point Scale	300+	60%	-	67%
Meds 'Always' Explained Before Given	300+	55%	-	60%
Nurses 'Always' Communicated Well	300+	75%	-	76%
Pain 'Always' Well Controlled	300+	70%	-	69%
Room and Bathroom 'Always' Clean	300+	68%	-	71%
Timely Help 'Always' Received	300+	57%	-	64%
Would Definitely Recommend Hospital	300+	68%	-	69%

NOTE: Hospital profiles are in alphabetical order by state, then city, then hospital within the city; Rankings exclude hospitals with less than 25 cases except for patient surveys which excludes hospitals with less than 100 cases; (a) 100–299 cases; (1) The number of cases is too small to be sure how well a hospital is performing; (2) The hospital indicated that the data submitted for this measure were based on a sample of cases; (3) Data was collected during a shorter time period (fewer quarters) than the maximum possible time for this measure; (4) Suppressed for one or more quarters by CMS; (5) No data is available from the hospital for this measure; (6) Fewer than 100 patients completed the HCAHPS survey. Use these rates with caution, as the number of surveys may be too low to reliably assess hospital performance; (7) Survey results are based on less than 12 months of data; (8) Survey results are not available for this reporting period; (9) No or very few patients were eligible for the HCAHPS survey. The scores shown, if any, reflect a very small number of surveys; (10) A state average was not calculated because too few hospitals in the state submitted data; (11) There were discrepancies in the data collection process; Please refer to the User's Guide for a full explanation of data.

Cayuga Medical Center at Ithaca

101 Dates Drive Phone: 607-274-4401
Ithaca, NY 14850 Fax: 607-274-4527
E-mail: bconner@cayugamed.org
URL: www.cayugamed.org
Type: Acute Care Hospitals Emergency Services: Yes
Ownership: Voluntary Non-Profit - Private Beds: 204

Key Personnel:
CEO/President. . . . . Rob Mackenzie, MD
Chief of Medical Staff. . . . . Dr. Jeffrey Snedecker, MD
Coronary Care. . . . . Sue McKelvey
Infection Control. . . . . Sandra Coaley, RN
Pediatric Ambulatory Care . . . . . . Terri Koski
Pediatric In-Patient Care . . . . Terri Koski
Quality Assurance . . . . Carol LaBorie
Radiology. . . . . William Caroll

Measure	Cases	This Hosp.	State Avg.	U.S. Avg.
Heart Attack Care				
ACE Inhibitor or ARB for LVSD[1]	6	50%	95%	96%
Aspirin at Arrival	40	98%	98%	99%
Aspirin at Discharge	29	90%	98%	98%
Beta Blocker at Discharge	30	93%	98%	98%
Fibrinolytic Medication Timing[1]	4	25%	50%	55%
PCI Within 90 Minutes of Arrival	0	-	88%	90%
Smoking Cessation Advice[1]	5	100%	100%	99%
Chest Pain/Possible Heart Attack Care				
Aspirin at Arrival	72	96%	96%	95%
Median Time to ECG (minutes)	74	9	11	8
Median Time to Transfer (minutes)[3]	0	-	75	61
Fibrinolytic Medication Timing[1]	24	79%	55%	54%
Heart Failure Care				
ACE Inhibitor or ARB for LVSD	38	79%	94%	94%
Discharge Instructions	103	75%	89%	88%
Evaluation of LVS Function	130	96%	98%	98%
Smoking Cessation Advice[1]	17	100%	98%	98%
Pneumonia Care				
Appropriate Initial Antibiotic	107	78%	92%	92%
Blood Culture Timing	192	92%	95%	96%
Influenza Vaccine	91	82%	90%	91%
Initial Antibiotic Timing	196	91%	93%	95%
Pneumococcal Vaccine	151	79%	92%	93%
Smoking Cessation Advice	52	98%	98%	97%
Surgical Care Improvement Project				
Appropriate VTP Within 24 Hours	153	91%	94%	92%
Appropriate Hair Removal	324	99%	100%	99%
Appropriate Beta Blocker Usage	80	94%	92%	93%
Controlled Postoperative Blood Glucose	0	-	94%	93%
Prophylactic Antibiotic Timing	212	95%	96%	97%
Prophylactic Antibiotic Timing (Outpatient)	109	85%	92%	92%
Prophylactic Antibiotic Selection	213	98%	97%	97%
Prophylactic Antibiotic Select. (Outpatient)	99	99%	93%	94%
Prophylactic Antibiotic Stopped	210	93%	94%	94%
Recommended VTP Ordered	155	90%	96%	94%
Urinary Catheter Removal	82	87%	90%	90%
Children's Asthma Care				
Received Systemic Corticosteroids	-	-	-	100%
Received Home Management Plan	-	-	-	71%
Received Reliever Medication	-	-	-	100%
Use of Medical Imaging				
Combination Abdominal CT Scan	998	0.025	0.141	0.191
Combination Chest CT Scan	672	0.001	0.024	0.054
Follow-up Mammogram/Ultrasound	1,676	3.2%	9.8%	8.4%
MRI for Low Back Pain	223	32.7%	26.9%	32.7%
Survey of Patients' Hospital Experiences				
Area Around Room 'Always' Quiet at Night	300+	54%	-	58%
Doctors 'Always' Communicated Well	300+	78%	-	80%
Home Recovery Information Given	300+	83%	-	82%
Hospital Given 9 or 10 on 10 Point Scale	300+	66%	-	67%
Meds 'Always' Explained Before Given	300+	61%	-	60%
Nurses 'Always' Communicated Well	300+	74%	-	76%
Pain 'Always' Well Controlled	300+	67%	-	69%
Room and Bathroom 'Always' Clean	300+	69%	-	71%
Timely Help 'Always' Received	300+	64%	-	64%
Would Definitely Recommend Hospital	300+	71%	-	69%

Jamaica Hospital Medical Center

8900 Van Wyck Expressway Phone: 718-262-6000
Jamaica, NY 11418 Fax: 718-657-0545
URL: www.jamaicahospital.org
Type: Acute Care Hospitals Emergency Services: Yes
Ownership: Government - Federal Beds: 387

Key Personnel:
CEO/President. . . . . David P Rosen
Cardiac Laboratory. . . . . Robert Mendelson
Chief of Medical Staff. . . . . Antonietta Morisca, MD
Infection Control. . . . . Judy Fine
Operating Room. . . . . Doreen Voda
Pediatric Ambulatory Care . . . . . . Susan Rapaport, MD
Pediatric In-Patient Care . . . . Phyllis Weiner, MD

Measure	Cases	This Hosp.	State Avg.	U.S. Avg.
Heart Attack Care				
ACE Inhibitor or ARB for LVSD[2]	44	100%	95%	96%
Aspirin at Arrival[2]	262	100%	98%	99%
Aspirin at Discharge[2]	169	100%	98%	98%
Beta Blocker at Discharge[2]	169	100%	98%	98%
Fibrinolytic Medication Timing[2]	0	-	50%	55%
PCI Within 90 Minutes of Arrival[2]	71	96%	88%	90%
Smoking Cessation Advice[2]	58	100%	100%	99%
Chest Pain/Possible Heart Attack Care				
Aspirin at Arrival[1]	19	95%	96%	95%
Median Time to ECG (minutes)[1]	20	16	11	8
Median Time to Transfer (minutes)[1,3]	1	176	75	61
Fibrinolytic Medication Timing[3]	0	-	55%	54%
Heart Failure Care				
ACE Inhibitor or ARB for LVSD[2]	132	100%	94%	94%
Discharge Instructions[2]	271	100%	89%	88%
Evaluation of LVS Function[2]	310	100%	98%	98%
Smoking Cessation Advice[2]	45	100%	98%	98%
Pneumonia Care				
Appropriate Initial Antibiotic[2]	95	99%	92%	92%
Blood Culture Timing[2]	115	97%	95%	96%
Influenza Vaccine[2]	63	100%	90%	91%
Initial Antibiotic Timing[2]	112	96%	93%	95%
Pneumococcal Vaccine[2]	86	100%	92%	93%
Smoking Cessation Advice[2]	43	100%	98%	97%
Surgical Care Improvement Project				
Appropriate VTP Within 24 Hours[2]	199	97%	94%	92%
Appropriate Hair Removal[2]	412	100%	100%	99%
Appropriate Beta Blocker Usage[2]	75	83%	92%	93%
Controlled Postoperative Blood Glucose[1,2]	1	0%	94%	93%
Prophylactic Antibiotic Timing[2]	188	95%	96%	97%
Prophylactic Antibiotic Timing (Outpatient)	101	74%	92%	92%
Prophylactic Antibiotic Selection[2]	190	96%	97%	97%
Prophylactic Antibiotic Select. (Outpatient)	87	92%	93%	94%
Prophylactic Antibiotic Stopped[2]	178	92%	94%	94%
Recommended VTP Ordered[2]	206	95%	96%	94%
Urinary Catheter Removal[2]	39	92%	90%	90%
Children's Asthma Care				
Received Systemic Corticosteroids	-	-	-	100%
Received Home Management Plan	-	-	-	71%
Received Reliever Medication	-	-	-	100%
Use of Medical Imaging				
Combination Abdominal CT Scan	200	0.000	0.141	0.191
Combination Chest CT Scan	136	0.000	0.024	0.054
Follow-up Mammogram/Ultrasound	432	5.3%	9.8%	8.4%
MRI for Low Back Pain[1]	17	29.4%	26.9%	32.7%
Survey of Patients' Hospital Experiences				
Area Around Room 'Always' Quiet at Night	300+	40%	-	58%
Doctors 'Always' Communicated Well	300+	66%	-	80%
Home Recovery Information Given	300+	70%	-	82%
Hospital Given 9 or 10 on 10 Point Scale	300+	43%	-	67%
Meds 'Always' Explained Before Given	300+	43%	-	60%
Nurses 'Always' Communicated Well	300+	56%	-	76%
Pain 'Always' Well Controlled	300+	51%	-	69%
Room and Bathroom 'Always' Clean	300+	56%	-	71%
Timely Help 'Always' Received	300+	40%	-	64%
Would Definitely Recommend Hospital	300+	49%	-	69%

Queens Hospital Center

82-68 164th Street Phone: 718-883-3000
Jamaica, NY 11432
URL: www.nyc.gov/html/hhc/qhn/home.html
Type: Acute Care Hospitals Emergency Services: Yes
Ownership: Government - Local Beds: 408

Key Personnel:
CEO/President. . . . . Antonio Martin
Chief of Medical Staff. . . . . Jean Bernard-Poulard, MD
Pediatric Ambulatory Care . . . . . . Hedda Acs, MD
Pediatric In-Patient Care . . . . Hedda Acs, MD
Patient Relations . . . . Joan Gabriele, RN

Measure	Cases	This Hosp.	State Avg.	U.S. Avg.
Heart Attack Care				
ACE Inhibitor or ARB for LVSD[1]	5	80%	95%	96%
Aspirin at Arrival	44	100%	98%	99%
Aspirin at Discharge[1]	13	100%	98%	98%
Beta Blocker at Discharge[1]	9	100%	98%	98%
Fibrinolytic Medication Timing	0	-	50%	55%
PCI Within 90 Minutes of Arrival	0	-	88%	90%
Smoking Cessation Advice	0	-	100%	99%
Chest Pain/Possible Heart Attack Care				
Aspirin at Arrival	89	97%	96%	95%
Median Time to ECG (minutes)	92	11	11	8
Median Time to Transfer (minutes)[1]	23	66	75	61
Fibrinolytic Medication Timing	0	-	55%	54%
Heart Failure Care				
ACE Inhibitor or ARB for LVSD	100	94%	94%	94%
Discharge Instructions	246	96%	89%	88%
Evaluation of LVS Function	269	100%	98%	98%
Smoking Cessation Advice	35	94%	98%	98%
Pneumonia Care				
Appropriate Initial Antibiotic	103	95%	92%	92%
Blood Culture Timing	124	84%	95%	96%
Influenza Vaccine	88	98%	90%	91%
Initial Antibiotic Timing	161	78%	93%	95%
Pneumococcal Vaccine	94	97%	92%	93%
Smoking Cessation Advice	32	94%	98%	97%
Surgical Care Improvement Project				
Appropriate VTP Within 24 Hours	195	98%	94%	92%
Appropriate Hair Removal	319	100%	100%	99%
Appropriate Beta Blocker Usage	52	67%	92%	93%
Controlled Postoperative Blood Glucose	0	-	94%	93%
Prophylactic Antibiotic Timing	133	95%	96%	97%
Prophylactic Antibiotic Timing (Outpatient)	38	82%	92%	92%
Prophylactic Antibiotic Selection	132	95%	97%	97%
Prophylactic Antibiotic Select. (Outpatient)	93	98%	93%	94%
Prophylactic Antibiotic Stopped	125	88%	94%	94%
Recommended VTP Ordered	195	98%	96%	94%
Urinary Catheter Removal[1]	13	92%	90%	90%
Children's Asthma Care				
Received Systemic Corticosteroids	-	-	-	100%
Received Home Management Plan	-	-	-	71%
Received Reliever Medication	-	-	-	100%
Use of Medical Imaging				
Combination Abdominal CT Scan	180	0.022	0.141	0.191
Combination Chest CT Scan	109	0.009	0.024	0.054
Follow-up Mammogram/Ultrasound	316	4.7%	9.8%	8.4%
MRI for Low Back Pain[1]	6	16.7%	26.9%	32.7%
Survey of Patients' Hospital Experiences				
Area Around Room 'Always' Quiet at Night	300+	55%	-	58%
Doctors 'Always' Communicated Well	300+	79%	-	80%
Home Recovery Information Given	300+	78%	-	82%
Hospital Given 9 or 10 on 10 Point Scale	300+	61%	-	67%
Meds 'Always' Explained Before Given	300+	58%	-	60%
Nurses 'Always' Communicated Well	300+	66%	-	76%
Pain 'Always' Well Controlled	300+	62%	-	69%
Room and Bathroom 'Always' Clean	300+	68%	-	71%
Timely Help 'Always' Received	300+	56%	-	64%
Would Definitely Recommend Hospital	300+	70%	-	69%

NOTE: Hospital profiles are in alphabetical order by state, then city, then hospital within the city; Rankings exclude hospitals with less than 25 cases except for patient surveys which excludes hospitals with less than 100 cases; (a) 100–299 cases; (1) The number of cases is too small to be sure how well a hospital is performing; (2) The hospital indicated that the data submitted for this measure were based on a sample of cases; (3) Data was collected during a shorter time period (fewer quarters) than the maximum possible time for this measure; (4) Suppressed for one or more quarters by CMS; (5) No data is available from the hospital for this measure; (6) Fewer than 100 patients completed the HCAHPS survey. Use these rates with caution, as the number of surveys may be too low to reliably assess hospital performance; (7) Survey results are based on less than 12 months of data; (8) Survey results are not available for this reporting period; (9) No or very few patients were eligible for the HCAHPS survey. The scores shown, if any, reflect a very small number of surveys; (10) A state average was not calculated because too few hospitals in the state submitted data; (11) There were discrepancies in the data collection process; Please refer to the User's Guide for a full explanation of data.

Woman's Christian Association

207 Foote Avenue Phone: 716-487-0141
Jamestown, NY 14701 Fax: 716-664-8336
URL: www.wcahospital.org
Type: Acute Care Hospitals Emergency Services: Yes
Ownership: Voluntary Non-Profit - Private Beds: 342

Key Personnel:
CEO/President. . . . . RonaldT Klizek, MD
Pediatric In-Patient Care . . . . Virginia Campion, MD
Quality Assurance . . . . Betsy Wright
Radiology. . . . . Eugene Graham
Emergency Room . . . . Bonnie Stockwell
Patient Relations . . . . Diana Buttafarro

Measure	Cases	This Hosp.	State Avg.	U.S. Avg.
Heart Attack Care				
ACE Inhibitor or ARB for LVSD[1]	15	100%	95%	96%
Aspirin at Arrival	94	98%	98%	99%
Aspirin at Discharge	59	100%	98%	98%
Beta Blocker at Discharge	66	98%	98%	98%
Fibrinolytic Medication Timing	0	-	50%	55%
PCI Within 90 Minutes of Arrival	0	-	88%	90%
Smoking Cessation Advice[1]	7	100%	100%	99%
Chest Pain/Possible Heart Attack Care				
Aspirin at Arrival	77	96%	96%	95%
Median Time to ECG (minutes)	79	12	11	8
Median Time to Transfer (minutes)[1,3]	2	121	75	61
Fibrinolytic Medication Timing[1]	3	67%	55%	54%
Heart Failure Care				
ACE Inhibitor or ARB for LVSD	65	98%	94%	94%
Discharge Instructions	224	81%	89%	88%
Evaluation of LVS Function	273	100%	98%	98%
Smoking Cessation Advice	39	100%	98%	98%
Pneumonia Care				
Appropriate Initial Antibiotic	105	91%	92%	92%
Blood Culture Timing	180	98%	95%	96%
Influenza Vaccine	115	83%	90%	91%
Initial Antibiotic Timing	187	97%	93%	95%
Pneumococcal Vaccine	176	90%	92%	93%
Smoking Cessation Advice	62	98%	98%	97%
Surgical Care Improvement Project				
Appropriate VTP Within 24 Hours	126	83%	94%	92%
Appropriate Hair Removal	429	99%	100%	99%
Appropriate Beta Blocker Usage	154	89%	92%	93%
Controlled Postoperative Blood Glucose	0	-	94%	93%
Prophylactic Antibiotic Timing	298	98%	96%	97%
Prophylactic Antibiotic Timing (Outpatient)	124	79%	92%	92%
Prophylactic Antibiotic Selection	299	98%	97%	97%
Prophylactic Antibiotic Select. (Outpatient)	112	96%	93%	94%
Prophylactic Antibiotic Stopped	283	92%	94%	94%
Recommended VTP Ordered	126	85%	96%	94%
Urinary Catheter Removal[1]	18	50%	90%	90%
Children's Asthma Care				
Received Systemic Corticosteroids	-	-	-	100%
Received Home Management Plan	-	-	-	71%
Received Reliever Medication	-	-	-	100%
Use of Medical Imaging				
Combination Abdominal CT Scan	563	0.144	0.141	0.191
Combination Chest CT Scan	313	0.003	0.024	0.054
Follow-up Mammogram/Ultrasound	1,350	5.2%	9.8%	8.4%
MRI for Low Back Pain	79	34.2%	26.9%	32.7%
Survey of Patients' Hospital Experiences				
Area Around Room 'Always' Quiet at Night	300+	47%	-	58%
Doctors 'Always' Communicated Well	300+	78%	-	80%
Home Recovery Information Given	300+	87%	-	82%
Hospital Given 9 or 10 on 10 Point Scale	300+	54%	-	67%
Meds 'Always' Explained Before Given	300+	53%	-	60%
Nurses 'Always' Communicated Well	300+	71%	-	76%
Pain 'Always' Well Controlled	300+	62%	-	69%
Room and Bathroom 'Always' Clean	300+	65%	-	71%
Timely Help 'Always' Received	300+	55%	-	64%
Would Definitely Recommend Hospital	300+	56%	-	69%

United Health Services Hospitals

33-57 Harrison Street Phone: 607-763-6000
Johnson City, NY 13790 Fax: 607-763-6789
URL: www.vhs.ent
Type: Acute Care Hospitals Emergency Services: No
Ownership: Voluntary Non-Profit - Private Beds: 516

Key Personnel:
CEO/President. . . . . Matthew J Salanger
Chief of Medical Staff . . . . Rajesh Dave, MD
Infection Control. . . . . Debbie Mack
Operating Room. . . . . Michael Aronis
Quality Assurance . . . . Roberta Rivero

Measure	Cases	This Hosp.	State Avg.	U.S. Avg.
Heart Attack Care				
ACE Inhibitor or ARB for LVSD	113	97%	95%	96%
Aspirin at Arrival	334	99%	98%	99%
Aspirin at Discharge	463	100%	98%	98%
Beta Blocker at Discharge	473	99%	98%	98%
Fibrinolytic Medication Timing	0	-	50%	55%
PCI Within 90 Minutes of Arrival	60	85%	88%	90%
Smoking Cessation Advice	155	100%	100%	99%
Chest Pain/Possible Heart Attack Care				
Aspirin at Arrival[5]	0	-	96%	95%
Median Time to ECG (minutes)[5]	0	-	11	8
Median Time to Transfer (minutes)[5]	0	-	75	61
Fibrinolytic Medication Timing[5]	0	-	55%	54%
Heart Failure Care				
ACE Inhibitor or ARB for LVSD	141	95%	94%	94%
Discharge Instructions	343	87%	89%	88%
Evaluation of LVS Function	451	99%	98%	98%
Smoking Cessation Advice	51	100%	98%	98%
Pneumonia Care				
Appropriate Initial Antibiotic	200	96%	92%	92%
Blood Culture Timing	386	96%	95%	96%
Influenza Vaccine	232	95%	90%	91%
Initial Antibiotic Timing	350	92%	93%	95%
Pneumococcal Vaccine	345	94%	92%	93%
Smoking Cessation Advice	144	100%	98%	97%
Surgical Care Improvement Project				
Appropriate VTP Within 24 Hours	470	96%	94%	92%
Appropriate Hair Removal	1,500	100%	100%	99%
Appropriate Beta Blocker Usage	503	95%	92%	93%
Controlled Postoperative Blood Glucose	285	95%	94%	93%
Prophylactic Antibiotic Timing	967	98%	96%	97%
Prophylactic Antibiotic Timing (Outpatient)	1,362	98%	92%	92%
Prophylactic Antibiotic Selection	975	97%	97%	97%
Prophylactic Antibiotic Select. (Outpatient)	1,361	97%	93%	94%
Prophylactic Antibiotic Stopped	933	95%	94%	94%
Recommended VTP Ordered	470	97%	96%	94%
Urinary Catheter Removal	406	92%	90%	90%
Children's Asthma Care				
Received Systemic Corticosteroids	-	-	-	100%
Received Home Management Plan	-	-	-	71%
Received Reliever Medication	-	-	-	100%
Use of Medical Imaging				
Combination Abdominal CT Scan	1,770	0.055	0.141	0.191
Combination Chest CT Scan	1,065	0.022	0.024	0.054
Follow-up Mammogram/Ultrasound	2,794	11.0%	9.8%	8.4%
MRI for Low Back Pain[5]	0	-	26.9%	32.7%
Survey of Patients' Hospital Experiences				
Area Around Room 'Always' Quiet at Night	300+	39%	-	58%
Doctors 'Always' Communicated Well	300+	75%	-	80%
Home Recovery Information Given	300+	85%	-	82%
Hospital Given 9 or 10 on 10 Point Scale	300+	64%	-	67%
Meds 'Always' Explained Before Given	300+	58%	-	60%
Nurses 'Always' Communicated Well	300+	75%	-	76%
Pain 'Always' Well Controlled	300+	69%	-	69%
Room and Bathroom 'Always' Clean	300+	67%	-	71%
Timely Help 'Always' Received	300+	63%	-	64%
Would Definitely Recommend Hospital	300+	72%	-	69%

Kenmore Mercy Hospital

2950 Elmwood Avenue Phone: 716-447-6100
Kenmore, NY 14217 Fax: 716-447-6090
URL: www.chsbuffalo.org
Type: Acute Care Hospitals Emergency Services: Yes
Ownership: Voluntary Non-Profit - Church Beds: 184

Key Personnel:
CEO/President. . . . . James Millard
Chief of Medical Staff . . . . James Fitzpatrick
Radiology. . . . . Amina Akhtar
Patient Relations . . . . Cheryl Haynes, RN

Measure	Cases	This Hosp.	State Avg.	U.S. Avg.
Heart Attack Care				
ACE Inhibitor or ARB for LVSD[1]	19	100%	95%	96%
Aspirin at Arrival	91	97%	98%	99%
Aspirin at Discharge	58	98%	98%	98%
Beta Blocker at Discharge	60	98%	98%	98%
Fibrinolytic Medication Timing	0	-	50%	55%
PCI Within 90 Minutes of Arrival	0	-	88%	90%
Smoking Cessation Advice[1]	9	100%	100%	99%
Chest Pain/Possible Heart Attack Care				
Aspirin at Arrival	36	97%	96%	95%
Median Time to ECG (minutes)	36	13	11	8
Median Time to Transfer (minutes)[1,3]	2	55	75	61
Fibrinolytic Medication Timing[1]	5	80%	55%	54%
Heart Failure Care				
ACE Inhibitor or ARB for LVSD[2]	69	96%	94%	94%
Discharge Instructions[2]	197	86%	89%	88%
Evaluation of LVS Function[2]	274	99%	98%	98%
Smoking Cessation Advice[1,2]	22	100%	98%	98%
Pneumonia Care				
Appropriate Initial Antibiotic[2]	93	94%	92%	92%
Blood Culture Timing[2]	157	94%	95%	96%
Influenza Vaccine[2]	100	97%	90%	91%
Initial Antibiotic Timing[2]	150	95%	93%	95%
Pneumococcal Vaccine[2]	154	97%	92%	93%
Smoking Cessation Advice[2]	38	97%	98%	97%
Surgical Care Improvement Project				
Appropriate VTP Within 24 Hours[2]	126	97%	94%	92%
Appropriate Hair Removal[2]	384	100%	100%	99%
Appropriate Beta Blocker Usage[2]	129	88%	92%	93%
Controlled Postoperative Blood Glucose[2]	0	-	94%	93%
Prophylactic Antibiotic Timing[2]	250	93%	96%	97%
Prophylactic Antibiotic Timing (Outpatient)	705	97%	92%	92%
Prophylactic Antibiotic Selection[2]	253	97%	97%	97%
Prophylactic Antibiotic Select. (Outpatient)	697	99%	93%	94%
Prophylactic Antibiotic Stopped[2]	240	91%	94%	94%
Recommended VTP Ordered[2]	127	96%	96%	94%
Urinary Catheter Removal[2]	30	67%	90%	90%
Children's Asthma Care				
Received Systemic Corticosteroids	-	-	-	100%
Received Home Management Plan	-	-	-	71%
Received Reliever Medication	-	-	-	100%
Use of Medical Imaging				
Combination Abdominal CT Scan	459	0.392	0.141	0.191
Combination Chest CT Scan	233	0.099	0.024	0.054
Follow-up Mammogram/Ultrasound	441	11.8%	9.8%	8.4%
MRI for Low Back Pain[5]	0	-	26.9%	32.7%
Survey of Patients' Hospital Experiences				
Area Around Room 'Always' Quiet at Night	300+	43%	-	58%
Doctors 'Always' Communicated Well	300+	75%	-	80%
Home Recovery Information Given	300+	85%	-	82%
Hospital Given 9 or 10 on 10 Point Scale	300+	64%	-	67%
Meds 'Always' Explained Before Given	300+	58%	-	60%
Nurses 'Always' Communicated Well	300+	73%	-	76%
Pain 'Always' Well Controlled	300+	70%	-	69%
Room and Bathroom 'Always' Clean	300+	58%	-	71%
Timely Help 'Always' Received	300+	56%	-	64%
Would Definitely Recommend Hospital	300+	69%	-	69%

NOTE: Hospital profiles are in alphabetical order by state, then city, then hospital within the city; Rankings exclude hospitals with less than 25 cases except for patient surveys which excludes hospitals with less than 100 cases; (a) 100–299 cases; (1) The number of cases is too small to be sure how well a hospital is performing; (2) The hospital indicated that the data submitted for this measure were based on a sample of cases; (3) Data was collected during a shorter time period (fewer quarters) than the maximum possible time for this measure; (4) Suppressed for one or more quarters by CMS; (5) No data is available from the hospital for this measure; (6) Fewer than 100 patients completed the HCAHPS survey. Use these rates with caution, as the number of surveys may be too low to reliably assess hospital performance; (7) Survey results are based on less than 12 months of data; (8) Survey results are not available for this reporting period; (9) No or very few patients were eligible for the HCAHPS survey. The scores shown, if any, reflect a very small number of surveys; (10) A state average was not calculated because too few hospitals in the state submitted data; (11) There were discrepancies in the data collection process; Please refer to the User's Guide for a full explanation of data.

Benedictine Hospital

105 Mary's Avenue   Phone: 845-338-2500
Kingston, NY 12401   Fax: 845-334-3149
E-mail: webmaster@benedictine.org
URL: www.benedictine.org
Type: Acute Care Hospitals   Emergency Services: Yes
Ownership: Voluntary Non-Profit - Church   Beds: 222

Key Personnel:
CEO/President. . . . . Thomas A Dee
Chief of Medical Staff . . . . Rafael Olazagasti, MD
Infection Control. . . . . Lorna DeGrazia, RN
Quality Assurance . . . . Jim Hansen, RN
Radiology. . . . . Laurie Abrams
Anesthesiology. . . . . Martin Cascio, MD
Emergency Room . . . . Mamie Caton
Intensive Care Unit. . . . . Marcie Truesdale, RN

Measure	Cases	This Hosp.	State Avg.	U.S. Avg.
Heart Attack Care				
ACE Inhibitor or ARB for LVSD[1]	5	100%	95%	96%
Aspirin at Arrival	38	97%	98%	99%
Aspirin at Discharge[1]	22	95%	98%	98%
Beta Blocker at Discharge	25	100%	98%	98%
Fibrinolytic Medication Timing[1]	7	43%	50%	55%
PCI Within 90 Minutes of Arrival	0	-	88%	90%
Smoking Cessation Advice[1]	9	100%	100%	99%
Chest Pain/Possible Heart Attack Care				
Aspirin at Arrival[1]	18	89%	96%	95%
Median Time to ECG (minutes)[1]	21	8	11	8
Median Time to Transfer (minutes)[3]	0	-	75	61
Fibrinolytic Medication Timing[1]	7	43%	55%	54%
Heart Failure Care				
ACE Inhibitor or ARB for LVSD	61	97%	94%	94%
Discharge Instructions	186	99%	89%	88%
Evaluation of LVS Function	239	98%	98%	98%
Smoking Cessation Advice	40	100%	98%	98%
Pneumonia Care				
Appropriate Initial Antibiotic	79	94%	92%	92%
Blood Culture Timing	125	98%	95%	96%
Influenza Vaccine	87	91%	90%	91%
Initial Antibiotic Timing	117	100%	93%	95%
Pneumococcal Vaccine	113	96%	92%	93%
Smoking Cessation Advice	40	100%	98%	97%
Surgical Care Improvement Project				
Appropriate VTP Within 24 Hours	138	86%	94%	92%
Appropriate Hair Removal	373	99%	100%	99%
Appropriate Beta Blocker Usage	124	92%	92%	93%
Controlled Postoperative Blood Glucose	0	-	94%	93%
Prophylactic Antibiotic Timing	230	95%	96%	97%
Prophylactic Antibiotic Timing (Outpatient)	115	88%	92%	92%
Prophylactic Antibiotic Selection	236	100%	97%	97%
Prophylactic Antibiotic Select. (Outpatient)	110	97%	93%	94%
Prophylactic Antibiotic Stopped	227	95%	94%	94%
Recommended VTP Ordered	138	91%	96%	94%
Urinary Catheter Removal	132	97%	90%	90%
Children's Asthma Care				
Received Systemic Corticosteroids	-	-	-	100%
Received Home Management Plan	-	-	-	71%
Received Reliever Medication	-	-	-	100%
Use of Medical Imaging				
Combination Abdominal CT Scan	601	0.062	0.141	0.191
Combination Chest CT Scan	290	0.003	0.024	0.054
Follow-up Mammogram/Ultrasound	1,029	3.4%	9.8%	8.4%
MRI for Low Back Pain[5]	0	-	26.9%	32.7%
Survey of Patients' Hospital Experiences				
Area Around Room 'Always' Quiet at Night	(a)	48%	-	58%
Doctors 'Always' Communicated Well	(a)	77%	-	80%
Home Recovery Information Given	(a)	83%	-	82%
Hospital Given 9 or 10 on 10 Point Scale	(a)	67%	-	67%
Meds 'Always' Explained Before Given	(a)	57%	-	60%
Nurses 'Always' Communicated Well	(a)	74%	-	76%
Pain 'Always' Well Controlled	(a)	70%	-	69%
Room and Bathroom 'Always' Clean	(a)	62%	-	71%
Timely Help 'Always' Received	(a)	58%	-	64%
Would Definitely Recommend Hospital	(a)	71%	-	69%

Kingston Hospital

396 Broadway   Phone: 914-331-3131
Kingston, NY 12401   Fax: 845-331-3238
URL: www.kingstonregionalhealth.org
Type: Acute Care Hospitals   Emergency Services: Yes
Ownership: Voluntary Non-Profit - Private   Beds: 150

Key Personnel:
CEO/President. . . . . Michael Kaminski
Operating Room. . . . . Jane Lucente
Quality Assurance . . . . Sherie Ashdawn
Radiology. . . . . Steven Schwartz, MD
Anesthesiology. . . . . James Kikuoka, MD
Emergency Room . . . . Marc A. Borenstein, MD

Measure	Cases	This Hosp.	State Avg.	U.S. Avg.
Heart Attack Care				
ACE Inhibitor or ARB for LVSD[1]	14	100%	95%	96%
Aspirin at Arrival	56	100%	98%	99%
Aspirin at Discharge	41	100%	98%	98%
Beta Blocker at Discharge	40	100%	98%	98%
Fibrinolytic Medication Timing[1]	4	50%	50%	55%
PCI Within 90 Minutes of Arrival	0	-	88%	90%
Smoking Cessation Advice[1]	8	100%	100%	99%
Chest Pain/Possible Heart Attack Care				
Aspirin at Arrival	37	95%	96%	95%
Median Time to ECG (minutes)	39	5	11	8
Median Time to Transfer (minutes)[1,3]	1	94	75	61
Fibrinolytic Medication Timing[1]	14	79%	55%	54%
Heart Failure Care				
ACE Inhibitor or ARB for LVSD	69	88%	94%	94%
Discharge Instructions	167	95%	89%	88%
Evaluation of LVS Function	208	99%	98%	98%
Smoking Cessation Advice	37	100%	98%	98%
Pneumonia Care				
Appropriate Initial Antibiotic	135	96%	92%	92%
Blood Culture Timing	232	97%	95%	96%
Influenza Vaccine	123	94%	90%	91%
Initial Antibiotic Timing	206	99%	93%	95%
Pneumococcal Vaccine	157	96%	92%	93%
Smoking Cessation Advice	76	100%	98%	97%
Surgical Care Improvement Project				
Appropriate VTP Within 24 Hours	171	87%	94%	92%
Appropriate Hair Removal	319	99%	100%	99%
Appropriate Beta Blocker Usage	83	92%	92%	93%
Controlled Postoperative Blood Glucose	0	-	94%	93%
Prophylactic Antibiotic Timing	177	97%	96%	97%
Prophylactic Antibiotic Timing (Outpatient)	126	91%	92%	92%
Prophylactic Antibiotic Selection	178	97%	97%	97%
Prophylactic Antibiotic Select. (Outpatient)	122	96%	93%	94%
Prophylactic Antibiotic Stopped	174	87%	94%	94%
Recommended VTP Ordered	174	90%	96%	94%
Urinary Catheter Removal[1]	19	84%	90%	90%
Children's Asthma Care				
Received Systemic Corticosteroids	-	-	-	100%
Received Home Management Plan	-	-	-	71%
Received Reliever Medication	-	-	-	100%
Use of Medical Imaging				
Combination Abdominal CT Scan	541	0.089	0.141	0.191
Combination Chest CT Scan	306	0.013	0.024	0.054
Follow-up Mammogram/Ultrasound	877	7.3%	9.8%	8.4%
MRI for Low Back Pain	113	31.9%	26.9%	32.7%
Survey of Patients' Hospital Experiences				
Area Around Room 'Always' Quiet at Night	300+	39%	-	58%
Doctors 'Always' Communicated Well	300+	72%	-	80%
Home Recovery Information Given	300+	77%	-	82%
Hospital Given 9 or 10 on 10 Point Scale	300+	53%	-	67%
Meds 'Always' Explained Before Given	300+	53%	-	60%
Nurses 'Always' Communicated Well	300+	70%	-	76%
Pain 'Always' Well Controlled	300+	61%	-	69%
Room and Bathroom 'Always' Clean	300+	61%	-	71%
Timely Help 'Always' Received	300+	50%	-	64%
Would Definitely Recommend Hospital	300+	58%	-	69%

Mount St Mary's Hospital and Health Center

5300 Military Road   Phone: 716-297-4800
Lewiston, NY 14092   Fax: 716-298-2091
URL: www.msmh.org
Type: Acute Care Hospitals   Emergency Services: Yes
Ownership: Voluntary Non-Profit - Church   Beds: 179

Key Personnel:
CEO/President. . . . . Judith A Maness
Cardiac Laboratory. . . . . John Macklasuo, MD
Chief of Medical Staff . . . . Domonic F Falsetti, MD
Pediatric Ambulatory Care . . . . . . T Kaul, MD
Quality Assurance . . . . Laurie Merletti
Emergency Room . . . . Linda Dattaglia, MD
Patient Relations . . . . Barbara Bucci

Measure	Cases	This Hosp.	State Avg.	U.S. Avg.
Heart Attack Care				
ACE Inhibitor or ARB for LVSD[1]	13	100%	95%	96%
Aspirin at Arrival	100	100%	98%	99%
Aspirin at Discharge	62	100%	98%	98%
Beta Blocker at Discharge	69	100%	98%	98%
Fibrinolytic Medication Timing[1]	3	33%	50%	55%
PCI Within 90 Minutes of Arrival	0	-	88%	90%
Smoking Cessation Advice[1]	12	100%	100%	99%
Chest Pain/Possible Heart Attack Care				
Aspirin at Arrival[1]	13	92%	96%	95%
Median Time to ECG (minutes)[1]	13	15	11	8
Median Time to Transfer (minutes)[3]	0	-	75	61
Fibrinolytic Medication Timing[3]	0	-	55%	54%
Heart Failure Care				
ACE Inhibitor or ARB for LVSD	55	100%	94%	94%
Discharge Instructions	190	89%	89%	88%
Evaluation of LVS Function	241	100%	98%	98%
Smoking Cessation Advice[1]	15	100%	98%	98%
Pneumonia Care				
Appropriate Initial Antibiotic	140	93%	92%	92%
Blood Culture Timing	222	98%	95%	96%
Influenza Vaccine	117	97%	90%	91%
Initial Antibiotic Timing	214	98%	93%	95%
Pneumococcal Vaccine	188	95%	92%	93%
Smoking Cessation Advice	56	89%	98%	97%
Surgical Care Improvement Project				
Appropriate VTP Within 24 Hours[2]	121	96%	94%	92%
Appropriate Hair Removal[2]	385	100%	100%	99%
Appropriate Beta Blocker Usage[2]	101	99%	92%	93%
Controlled Postoperative Blood Glucose[2]	0	-	94%	93%
Prophylactic Antibiotic Timing[2]	289	96%	96%	97%
Prophylactic Antibiotic Timing (Outpatient)	196	82%	92%	92%
Prophylactic Antibiotic Selection[2]	289	97%	97%	97%
Prophylactic Antibiotic Select. (Outpatient)	186	70%	93%	94%
Prophylactic Antibiotic Stopped[2]	289	93%	94%	94%
Recommended VTP Ordered[2]	121	97%	96%	94%
Urinary Catheter Removal[2]	86	98%	90%	90%
Children's Asthma Care				
Received Systemic Corticosteroids	-	-	-	100%
Received Home Management Plan	-	-	-	71%
Received Reliever Medication	-	-	-	100%
Use of Medical Imaging				
Combination Abdominal CT Scan	356	0.079	0.141	0.191
Combination Chest CT Scan	357	0.011	0.024	0.054
Follow-up Mammogram/Ultrasound	736	13.7%	9.8%	8.4%
MRI for Low Back Pain	136	37.5%	26.9%	32.7%
Survey of Patients' Hospital Experiences				
Area Around Room 'Always' Quiet at Night	300+	55%	-	58%
Doctors 'Always' Communicated Well	300+	78%	-	80%
Home Recovery Information Given	300+	82%	-	82%
Hospital Given 9 or 10 on 10 Point Scale	300+	69%	-	67%
Meds 'Always' Explained Before Given	300+	57%	-	60%
Nurses 'Always' Communicated Well	300+	77%	-	76%
Pain 'Always' Well Controlled	300+	71%	-	69%
Room and Bathroom 'Always' Clean	300+	75%	-	71%
Timely Help 'Always' Received	300+	59%	-	64%
Would Definitely Recommend Hospital	300+	73%	-	69%

NOTE: Hospital profiles are in alphabetical order by state, then city, then hospital within the city; Rankings exclude hospitals with less than 25 cases except for patient surveys which excludes hospitals with less than 100 cases; (a) 100–299 cases; (1) The number of cases is too small to be sure how well a hospital is performing; (2) The hospital indicated that the data submitted for this measure were based on a sample of cases; (3) Data was collected during a shorter time period (fewer quarters) than the maximum possible time for this measure; (4) Suppressed for one or more quarters by CMS; (5) No data is available from the hospital for this measure; (6) Fewer than 100 patients completed the HCAHPS survey. Use these rates with caution, as the number of surveys may be too low to reliably assess hospital performance; (7) Survey results are based on less than 12 months of data; (8) Survey results are not available for this reporting period; (9) No or very few patients were eligible for the HCAHPS survey. The scores shown, if any, reflect a very small number of surveys; (10) A state average was not calculated because too few hospitals in the state submitted data; (11) There were discrepancies in the data collection process; Please refer to the User's Guide for a full explanation of data.

Little Falls Hospital

140 Burwell Street
Little Falls, NY 13365
Phone: 315-823-5261
Fax: 315-823-5383
E-mail: c.mowers@lfny.org
URL: www.lfhny.org
Type: Critical Access Hospitals
Emergency Services: Yes
Ownership: Voluntary Non-Profit - Private
Beds: 59

Key Personnel:

CEO/President. . . . . Michael L. Ogden
Chief of Medical Staff . . . . L.Andrew Rauscher, MD
Infection Control. . . . . Patty Seifried, RUN
Operating Room. . . . . Tammy Hedrick, RN
Quality Assurance . . . . Catherine Kunz, RN, CPHQ
Emergency Room . . . . Rebecca Akers, RN, BSN
Intensive Care Unit. . . . . Heidi Camardello, BSN, CNOR
Patient Relations . . . . Catherine Kunz, MS, CPHQ

Measure	Cases	This Hosp.	State Avg.	U.S. Avg.
Heart Attack Care				
ACE Inhibitor or ARB for LVSD[1,3]	1	0%	95%	96%
Aspirin at Arrival[1,3]	10	90%	98%	99%
Aspirin at Discharge[1,3]	9	100%	98%	98%
Beta Blocker at Discharge[1,3]	8	100%	98%	98%
Fibrinolytic Medication Timing[3]	0	-	50%	55%
PCI Within 90 Minutes of Arrival[3]	0	-	88%	90%
Smoking Cessation Advice[3]	0	-	100%	99%
Chest Pain/Possible Heart Attack Care				
Aspirin at Arrival[3]	51	96%	96%	95%
Median Time to ECG (minutes)[3]	52	11	11	8
Median Time to Transfer (minutes)[1,3]	5	74	75	61
Fibrinolytic Medication Timing[3]	0	-	55%	54%
Heart Failure Care				
ACE Inhibitor or ARB for LVSD[1,3]	5	60%	94%	94%
Discharge Instructions[1,3]	13	77%	89%	88%
Evaluation of LVS Function[1,3]	24	96%	98%	98%
Smoking Cessation Advice[1,3]	2	0%	98%	98%
Pneumonia Care				
Appropriate Initial Antibiotic[3]	42	81%	92%	92%
Blood Culture Timing[3]	51	86%	95%	96%
Influenza Vaccine	48	77%	90%	91%
Initial Antibiotic Timing[3]	59	93%	93%	95%
Pneumococcal Vaccine[3]	56	66%	92%	93%
Smoking Cessation Advice[1,3]	12	75%	98%	97%
Surgical Care Improvement Project				
Appropriate VTP Within 24 Hours[5]	0	-	94%	92%
Appropriate Hair Removal[5]	0	-	100%	99%
Appropriate Beta Blocker Usage[5]	0	-	92%	93%
Controlled Postoperative Blood Glucose[5]	0	-	94%	93%
Prophylactic Antibiotic Timing[5]	0	-	96%	97%
Prophylactic Antibiotic Timing (Outpatient)[3]	25	56%	92%	92%
Prophylactic Antibiotic Selection[5]	0	-	97%	97%
Prophylactic Antibiotic Select. (Outpatient)[1,3]	22	77%	93%	94%
Prophylactic Antibiotic Stopped[5]	0	-	94%	94%
Recommended VTP Ordered[5]	0	-	96%	94%
Urinary Catheter Removal[5]	0	-	90%	90%
Children's Asthma Care				
Received Systemic Corticosteroids	-	-	-	100%
Received Home Management Plan	-	-	-	71%
Received Reliever Medication	-	-	-	100%
Use of Medical Imaging				
Combination Abdominal CT Scan	301	0.146	0.141	0.191
Combination Chest CT Scan	138	0.014	0.024	0.054
Follow-up Mammogram/Ultrasound	300	10.3%	9.8%	8.4%
MRI for Low Back Pain[5]	0	-	26.9%	32.7%
Survey of Patients' Hospital Experiences				
Area Around Room 'Always' Quiet at Night	300+	49%	-	58%
Doctors 'Always' Communicated Well	300+	83%	-	80%
Home Recovery Information Given	300+	83%	-	82%
Hospital Given 9 or 10 on 10 Point Scale	300+	64%	-	67%
Meds 'Always' Explained Before Given	300+	65%	-	60%
Nurses 'Always' Communicated Well	300+	76%	-	76%
Pain 'Always' Well Controlled	300+	71%	-	69%
Room and Bathroom 'Always' Clean	300+	75%	-	71%
Timely Help 'Always' Received	300+	57%	-	64%
Would Definitely Recommend Hospital	300+	61%	-	69%

Eastern Niagara Hospital

521 East Avenue
Lockport, NY 14094
Phone: 716-514-5700
Fax: 716-514-5587
Type: Acute Care Hospitals
Emergency Services: Yes
Ownership: Voluntary Non-Profit - Private
Beds: 134

Key Personnel:

CEO/President. . . . . Clare A Haar
Emergency Room . . . . Michael Torres, MD

Measure	Cases	This Hosp.	State Avg.	U.S. Avg.
Heart Attack Care				
ACE Inhibitor or ARB for LVSD[1]	1	0%	95%	96%
Aspirin at Arrival	37	92%	98%	99%
Aspirin at Discharge[1]	23	74%	98%	98%
Beta Blocker at Discharge	27	78%	98%	98%
Fibrinolytic Medication Timing	0	-	50%	55%
PCI Within 90 Minutes of Arrival	0	-	88%	90%
Smoking Cessation Advice[1]	4	100%	100%	99%
Chest Pain/Possible Heart Attack Care				
Aspirin at Arrival	151	94%	96%	95%
Median Time to ECG (minutes)	154	15	11	8
Median Time to Transfer (minutes)[1,3]	1	413	75	61
Fibrinolytic Medication Timing[1]	15	33%	55%	54%
Heart Failure Care				
ACE Inhibitor or ARB for LVSD	38	74%	94%	94%
Discharge Instructions	128	71%	89%	88%
Evaluation of LVS Function	181	90%	98%	98%
Smoking Cessation Advice[1]	18	83%	98%	98%
Pneumonia Care				
Appropriate Initial Antibiotic	129	92%	92%	92%
Blood Culture Timing	155	99%	95%	96%
Influenza Vaccine	116	92%	90%	91%
Initial Antibiotic Timing	203	99%	93%	95%
Pneumococcal Vaccine	185	95%	92%	93%
Smoking Cessation Advice	78	91%	98%	97%
Surgical Care Improvement Project				
Appropriate VTP Within 24 Hours	89	83%	94%	92%
Appropriate Hair Removal	231	100%	100%	99%
Appropriate Beta Blocker Usage	50	70%	92%	93%
Controlled Postoperative Blood Glucose	0	-	94%	93%
Prophylactic Antibiotic Timing	169	98%	96%	97%
Prophylactic Antibiotic Timing (Outpatient)	68	91%	92%	92%
Prophylactic Antibiotic Selection	169	94%	97%	97%
Prophylactic Antibiotic Select. (Outpatient)	64	91%	93%	94%
Prophylactic Antibiotic Stopped	169	90%	94%	94%
Recommended VTP Ordered	89	87%	96%	94%
Urinary Catheter Removal[1]	19	58%	90%	90%
Children's Asthma Care				
Received Systemic Corticosteroids	-	-	-	100%
Received Home Management Plan	-	-	-	71%
Received Reliever Medication	-	-	-	100%
Use of Medical Imaging				
Combination Abdominal CT Scan	244	0.316	0.141	0.191
Combination Chest CT Scan	173	0.006	0.024	0.054
Follow-up Mammogram/Ultrasound	528	1.1%	9.8%	8.4%
MRI for Low Back Pain[1]	7	0.0%	26.9%	32.7%
Survey of Patients' Hospital Experiences				
Area Around Room 'Always' Quiet at Night	300+	43%	-	58%
Doctors 'Always' Communicated Well	300+	78%	-	80%
Home Recovery Information Given	300+	78%	-	82%
Hospital Given 9 or 10 on 10 Point Scale	300+	59%	-	67%
Meds 'Always' Explained Before Given	300+	54%	-	60%
Nurses 'Always' Communicated Well	300+	71%	-	76%
Pain 'Always' Well Controlled	300+	65%	-	69%
Room and Bathroom 'Always' Clean	300+	73%	-	71%
Timely Help 'Always' Received	300+	56%	-	64%
Would Definitely Recommend Hospital	300+	62%	-	69%

Long Beach Medical Center

455 East Bay Drive
Long Beach, NY 11561
Phone: 516-897-1000
Fax: 516-897-1214
URL: www.lbmc.org
Type: Acute Care Hospitals
Emergency Services: Yes
Ownership: Voluntary Non-Profit - Private
Beds: 203

Key Personnel:

CEO/President. . . . . Douglas L Melzer
Chief of Medical Staff . . . . Iqbal Jangda

Measure	Cases	This Hosp.	State Avg.	U.S. Avg.
Heart Attack Care				
ACE Inhibitor or ARB for LVSD[1]	1	100%	95%	96%
Aspirin at Arrival[1]	8	100%	98%	99%
Aspirin at Discharge[1]	8	100%	98%	98%
Beta Blocker at Discharge[1]	5	80%	98%	98%
Fibrinolytic Medication Timing	0	-	50%	55%
PCI Within 90 Minutes of Arrival	0	-	88%	90%
Smoking Cessation Advice	0	-	100%	99%
Chest Pain/Possible Heart Attack Care				
Aspirin at Arrival	86	98%	96%	95%
Median Time to ECG (minutes)	95	10	11	8
Median Time to Transfer (minutes)[1]	9	99	75	61
Fibrinolytic Medication Timing	0	-	55%	54%
Heart Failure Care				
ACE Inhibitor or ARB for LVSD[1,2]	21	90%	94%	94%
Discharge Instructions[2]	61	89%	89%	88%
Evaluation of LVS Function[2]	103	95%	98%	98%
Smoking Cessation Advice[1,2]	10	100%	98%	98%
Pneumonia Care				
Appropriate Initial Antibiotic[2]	58	91%	92%	92%
Blood Culture Timing[2]	163	95%	95%	96%
Influenza Vaccine[2]	80	95%	90%	91%
Initial Antibiotic Timing[2]	143	99%	93%	95%
Pneumococcal Vaccine[2]	140	93%	92%	93%
Smoking Cessation Advice[1,2]	24	88%	98%	97%
Surgical Care Improvement Project				
Appropriate VTP Within 24 Hours[2]	39	90%	94%	92%
Appropriate Hair Removal[2]	61	100%	100%	99%
Appropriate Beta Blocker Usage[1,2]	16	94%	92%	93%
Controlled Postoperative Blood Glucose[2]	0	-	94%	93%
Prophylactic Antibiotic Timing[2]	28	100%	96%	97%
Prophylactic Antibiotic Timing (Outpatient)[1]	20	95%	92%	92%
Prophylactic Antibiotic Selection[2]	28	82%	97%	97%
Prophylactic Antibiotic Select. (Outpatient)[1]	19	100%	93%	94%
Prophylactic Antibiotic Stopped[2]	27	85%	94%	94%
Recommended VTP Ordered[2]	39	97%	96%	94%
Urinary Catheter Removal[1,2]	7	86%	90%	90%
Children's Asthma Care				
Received Systemic Corticosteroids	-	-	-	100%
Received Home Management Plan	-	-	-	71%
Received Reliever Medication	-	-	-	100%
Use of Medical Imaging				
Combination Abdominal CT Scan	311	0.592	0.141	0.191
Combination Chest CT Scan	195	0.005	0.024	0.054
Follow-up Mammogram/Ultrasound[1]	3	66.7%	9.8%	8.4%
MRI for Low Back Pain[1]	15	26.7%	26.9%	32.7%
Survey of Patients' Hospital Experiences				
Area Around Room 'Always' Quiet at Night	300+	42%	-	58%
Doctors 'Always' Communicated Well	300+	71%	-	80%
Home Recovery Information Given	300+	73%	-	82%
Hospital Given 9 or 10 on 10 Point Scale	300+	41%	-	67%
Meds 'Always' Explained Before Given	300+	49%	-	60%
Nurses 'Always' Communicated Well	300+	61%	-	76%
Pain 'Always' Well Controlled	300+	60%	-	69%
Room and Bathroom 'Always' Clean	300+	61%	-	71%
Timely Help 'Always' Received	300+	48%	-	64%
Would Definitely Recommend Hospital	300+	45%	-	69%

NOTE: Hospital profiles are in alphabetical order by state, then city, then hospital within the city; Rankings exclude hospitals with less than 25 cases except for patient surveys which excludes hospitals with less than 100 cases; (a) 100–299 cases; (1) The number of cases is too small to be sure how well a hospital is performing; (2) The hospital indicated that the data submitted for this measure were based on a sample of cases; (3) Data was collected during a shorter time period (fewer quarters) than the maximum possible time for this measure; (4) Suppressed for one or more quarters by CMS; (5) No data is available from the hospital for this measure; (6) Fewer than 100 patients completed the HCAHPS survey. Use these rates with caution, as the number of surveys may be too low to reliably assess hospital performance; (7) Survey results are based on less than 12 months of data; (8) Survey results are not available for this reporting period; (9) No or very few patients were eligible for the HCAHPS survey. The scores shown, if any, reflect a very small number of surveys; (10) A state average was not calculated because too few hospitals in the state submitted data; (11) There were discrepancies in the data collection process; Please refer to the User's Guide for a full explanation of data.

Lewis County General Hospital

7785 North State Street Phone: 315-376-5200
Lowville, NY 13367 Fax: 315-376-9317
URL: www.lcgh.net
Type: Acute Care Hospitals Emergency Services: Yes
Ownership: Government - Local Beds: 160

Key Personnel:

CEO/President. . . . . Charles Truax
Cardiac Laboratory. . . . . Dr Manoj Vera
Chief of Medical Staff. . . . . Dr Daniel Pisaniello
Infection Control. . . . . Christopher Cole
Operating Room. . . . . Earl Der
Quality Assurance . . . . Pamela Mc Cain
Radiology. . . . . Cindy Sirois
Intensive Care Unit. . . . . Fern Lynclecker, RN

Measure	Cases	This Hosp.	State Avg.	U.S. Avg.
Heart Attack Care				
ACE Inhibitor or ARB for LVSD[1]	2	100%	95%	96%
Aspirin at Arrival[1]	8	100%	98%	99%
Aspirin at Discharge[1]	7	71%	98%	98%
Beta Blocker at Discharge[1]	7	100%	98%	98%
Fibrinolytic Medication Timing[1]	1	100%	50%	55%
PCI Within 90 Minutes of Arrival	0	-	88%	90%
Smoking Cessation Advice[1]	1	100%	100%	99%
Chest Pain/Possible Heart Attack Care				
Aspirin at Arrival[1]	20	100%	96%	95%
Median Time to ECG (minutes)[1]	19	10	11	8
Median Time to Transfer (minutes)[3]	0	-	75	61
Fibrinolytic Medication Timing[1]	3	33%	55%	54%
Heart Failure Care				
ACE Inhibitor or ARB for LVSD[1]	15	67%	94%	94%
Discharge Instructions	29	48%	89%	88%
Evaluation of LVS Function	42	93%	98%	98%
Smoking Cessation Advice[1]	6	50%	98%	98%
Pneumonia Care				
Appropriate Initial Antibiotic	43	77%	92%	92%
Blood Culture Timing	60	95%	95%	96%
Influenza Vaccine	30	93%	90%	91%
Initial Antibiotic Timing	67	94%	93%	95%
Pneumococcal Vaccine	52	96%	92%	93%
Smoking Cessation Advice[1]	10	80%	98%	97%
Surgical Care Improvement Project				
Appropriate VTP Within 24 Hours	58	95%	94%	92%
Appropriate Hair Removal	132	100%	100%	99%
Appropriate Beta Blocker Usage	26	73%	92%	93%
Controlled Postoperative Blood Glucose	0	-	94%	93%
Prophylactic Antibiotic Timing	103	91%	96%	97%
Prophylactic Antibiotic Timing (Outpatient)[1,3]	2	50%	92%	92%
Prophylactic Antibiotic Selection	102	93%	97%	97%
Prophylactic Antibiotic Select. (Outpatient)[1,3]	2	100%	93%	94%
Prophylactic Antibiotic Stopped	98	97%	94%	94%
Recommended VTP Ordered	58	95%	96%	94%
Urinary Catheter Removal	32	97%	90%	90%
Children's Asthma Care				
Received Systemic Corticosteroids	-	-	-	100%
Received Home Management Plan	-	-	-	71%
Received Reliever Medication	-	-	-	100%
Use of Medical Imaging				
Combination Abdominal CT Scan	202	0.460	0.141	0.191
Combination Chest CT Scan	172	0.105	0.024	0.054
Follow-up Mammogram/Ultrasound	522	5.7%	9.8%	8.4%
MRI for Low Back Pain[1]	27	22.2%	26.9%	32.7%
Survey of Patients' Hospital Experiences				
Area Around Room 'Always' Quiet at Night	300+	53%	-	58%
Doctors 'Always' Communicated Well	300+	84%	-	80%
Home Recovery Information Given	300+	86%	-	82%
Hospital Given 9 or 10 on 10 Point Scale	300+	69%	-	67%
Meds 'Always' Explained Before Given	300+	67%	-	60%
Nurses 'Always' Communicated Well	300+	75%	-	76%
Pain 'Always' Well Controlled	300+	73%	-	69%
Room and Bathroom 'Always' Clean	300+	76%	-	71%
Timely Help 'Always' Received	300+	64%	-	64%
Would Definitely Recommend Hospital	300+	77%	-	69%

Alice Hyde Medical Center

133 Park Street Phone: 518-483-3000
Malone, NY 12953 Fax: 518-481-2598
E-mail: support@alicehyde.com
URL: www.alicehyde.com
Type: Acute Care Hospitals Emergency Services: Yes
Ownership: Voluntary Non-Profit - Other Beds: 151

Key Personnel:

CEO/President. . . . . John W Johnson
Chief of Medical Staff. . . . . Leonardo Dishman, MD
Coronary Care . . . . Sharon Martin, RN
Infection Control. . . . . Sandi Pfaff
Operating Room. . . . . Barb LaBombard
Pediatric In-Patient Care . . . . Ira Weissman, MD
Quality Assurance . . . . Jeanette Snell, RN
Radiology. . . . . Morris Brownman, RTR

Measure	Cases	This Hosp.	State Avg.	U.S. Avg.
Heart Attack Care				
ACE Inhibitor or ARB for LVSD[1]	2	100%	95%	96%
Aspirin at Arrival[1]	9	100%	98%	99%
Aspirin at Discharge[1]	6	100%	98%	98%
Beta Blocker at Discharge[1]	6	100%	98%	98%
Fibrinolytic Medication Timing	0	-	50%	55%
PCI Within 90 Minutes of Arrival	0	-	88%	90%
Smoking Cessation Advice	0	-	100%	99%
Chest Pain/Possible Heart Attack Care				
Aspirin at Arrival	84	98%	96%	95%
Median Time to ECG (minutes)	89	13	11	8
Median Time to Transfer (minutes)[1,3]	2	106	75	61
Fibrinolytic Medication Timing[1]	10	60%	55%	54%
Heart Failure Care				
ACE Inhibitor or ARB for LVSD[1]	16	100%	94%	94%
Discharge Instructions	50	90%	89%	88%
Evaluation of LVS Function	59	97%	98%	98%
Smoking Cessation Advice[1]	6	100%	98%	98%
Pneumonia Care				
Appropriate Initial Antibiotic	75	93%	92%	92%
Blood Culture Timing	90	97%	95%	96%
Influenza Vaccine	53	91%	90%	91%
Initial Antibiotic Timing	97	93%	93%	95%
Pneumococcal Vaccine	67	93%	92%	93%
Smoking Cessation Advice	32	100%	98%	97%
Surgical Care Improvement Project				
Appropriate VTP Within 24 Hours	97	87%	94%	92%
Appropriate Hair Removal	159	100%	100%	99%
Appropriate Beta Blocker Usage	42	93%	92%	93%
Controlled Postoperative Blood Glucose	0	-	94%	93%
Prophylactic Antibiotic Timing	98	95%	96%	97%
Prophylactic Antibiotic Timing (Outpatient)	82	96%	92%	92%
Prophylactic Antibiotic Selection	98	96%	97%	97%
Prophylactic Antibiotic Select. (Outpatient)	81	72%	93%	94%
Prophylactic Antibiotic Stopped	93	98%	94%	94%
Recommended VTP Ordered	97	90%	96%	94%
Urinary Catheter Removal	40	92%	90%	90%
Children's Asthma Care				
Received Systemic Corticosteroids	-	-	-	100%
Received Home Management Plan	-	-	-	71%
Received Reliever Medication	-	-	-	100%
Use of Medical Imaging				
Combination Abdominal CT Scan	421	0.043	0.141	0.191
Combination Chest CT Scan	322	0.003	0.024	0.054
Follow-up Mammogram/Ultrasound	993	6.7%	9.8%	8.4%
MRI for Low Back Pain	80	28.8%	26.9%	32.7%
Survey of Patients' Hospital Experiences				
Area Around Room 'Always' Quiet at Night	300+	42%	-	58%
Doctors 'Always' Communicated Well	300+	80%	-	80%
Home Recovery Information Given	300+	82%	-	82%
Hospital Given 9 or 10 on 10 Point Scale	300+	59%	-	67%
Meds 'Always' Explained Before Given	300+	57%	-	60%
Nurses 'Always' Communicated Well	300+	73%	-	76%
Pain 'Always' Well Controlled	300+	66%	-	69%
Room and Bathroom 'Always' Clean	300+	75%	-	71%
Timely Help 'Always' Received	300+	57%	-	64%
Would Definitely Recommend Hospital	300+	59%	-	69%

North Shore University Hospital

300 Community Drive Phone: 516-562-0100
Manhasset, NY 11030 Fax: 516-562-1395
URL: www.northshorelij.com
Type: Acute Care Hospitals Emergency Services: Yes
Ownership: Voluntary Non-Profit - Private Beds: 900

Key Personnel:

CEO/President. . . . . Susan Somerville RN
Cardiac Laboratory. . . . . Stanley Katz MD
Chief of Medical Staff. . . . . Lawrence G Smith MD
Infection Control. . . . . Bruce Farber MD
Operating Room. . . . . George DeNoto MD
Pediatric Ambulatory Care . . . . . . James Fagin MD
Quality Assurance . . . . Donn Haber
Radiology. . . . . Mitchell Goldman MD

Measure	Cases	This Hosp.	State Avg.	U.S. Avg.
Heart Attack Care				
ACE Inhibitor or ARB for LVSD[2]	53	98%	95%	96%
Aspirin at Arrival[2]	109	99%	98%	99%
Aspirin at Discharge[2]	311	100%	98%	98%
Beta Blocker at Discharge[2]	294	100%	98%	98%
Fibrinolytic Medication Timing[2]	0	-	50%	55%
PCI Within 90 Minutes of Arrival[1,2]	21	90%	88%	90%
Smoking Cessation Advice[2]	67	100%	100%	99%
Chest Pain/Possible Heart Attack Care				
Aspirin at Arrival[1,3]	4	100%	96%	95%
Median Time to ECG (minutes)[1,3]	4	16	11	8
Median Time to Transfer (minutes)[1,3]	1	48	75	61
Fibrinolytic Medication Timing[3]	0	-	55%	54%
Heart Failure Care				
ACE Inhibitor or ARB for LVSD[2]	131	99%	94%	94%
Discharge Instructions[2]	313	98%	89%	88%
Evaluation of LVS Function[2]	398	100%	98%	98%
Smoking Cessation Advice[2]	26	100%	98%	98%
Pneumonia Care				
Appropriate Initial Antibiotic[2]	154	95%	92%	92%
Blood Culture Timing[2]	286	99%	95%	96%
Influenza Vaccine[2]	148	99%	90%	91%
Initial Antibiotic Timing[2]	253	99%	93%	95%
Pneumococcal Vaccine[2]	266	98%	92%	93%
Smoking Cessation Advice[2]	39	100%	98%	97%
Surgical Care Improvement Project				
Appropriate VTP Within 24 Hours[2]	352	99%	94%	92%
Appropriate Hair Removal[2]	982	100%	100%	99%
Appropriate Beta Blocker Usage[2]	297	96%	92%	93%
Controlled Postoperative Blood Glucose[2]	159	97%	94%	93%
Prophylactic Antibiotic Timing[2]	594	98%	96%	97%
Prophylactic Antibiotic Timing (Outpatient)	291	91%	92%	92%
Prophylactic Antibiotic Selection[2]	603	98%	97%	97%
Prophylactic Antibiotic Select. (Outpatient)	281	98%	93%	94%
Prophylactic Antibiotic Stopped[2]	575	96%	94%	94%
Recommended VTP Ordered[2]	352	99%	96%	94%
Urinary Catheter Removal[2]	189	80%	90%	90%
Children's Asthma Care				
Received Systemic Corticosteroids	-	-	-	100%
Received Home Management Plan	-	-	-	71%
Received Reliever Medication	-	-	-	100%
Use of Medical Imaging				
Combination Abdominal CT Scan	2,232	0.098	0.141	0.191
Combination Chest CT Scan	2,012	0.009	0.024	0.054
Follow-up Mammogram/Ultrasound	1,496	10.2%	9.8%	8.4%
MRI for Low Back Pain	118	14.4%	26.9%	32.7%
Survey of Patients' Hospital Experiences				
Area Around Room 'Always' Quiet at Night	300+	40%	-	58%
Doctors 'Always' Communicated Well	300+	75%	-	80%
Home Recovery Information Given	300+	76%	-	82%
Hospital Given 9 or 10 on 10 Point Scale	300+	63%	-	67%
Meds 'Always' Explained Before Given	300+	56%	-	60%
Nurses 'Always' Communicated Well	300+	71%	-	76%
Pain 'Always' Well Controlled	300+	62%	-	69%
Room and Bathroom 'Always' Clean	300+	66%	-	71%
Timely Help 'Always' Received	300+	49%	-	64%
Would Definitely Recommend Hospital	300+	74%	-	69%

NOTE: Hospital profiles are in alphabetical order by state, then city, then hospital within the city; Rankings exclude hospitals with less than 25 cases except for patient surveys which excludes hospitals with less than 100 cases; (a) 100–299 cases; (1) The number of cases is too small to be sure how well a hospital is performing; (2) The hospital indicated that the data submitted for this measure were based on a sample of cases; (3) Data was collected during a shorter time period (fewer quarters) than the maximum possible time for this measure; (4) Suppressed for one or more quarters by CMS; (5) No data is available from the hospital for this measure; (6) Fewer than 100 patients completed the HCAHPS survey. Use these rates with caution, as the number of surveys may be too low to reliably assess hospital performance; (7) Survey results are based on less than 12 months of data; (8) Survey results are not available for this reporting period; (9) No or very few patients were eligible for the HCAHPS survey. The scores shown, if any, reflect a very small number of surveys; (10) A state average was not calculated because too few hospitals in the state submitted data; (11) There were discrepancies in the data collection process; Please refer to the User's Guide for a full explanation of data.

Margaretville Memorial Hospital

42084 State Highway 28
Margaretville, NY 12455
Phone: 845-586-5631
Fax: 845-586-1638
Type: Critical Access Hospitals
Emergency Services: Yes
Ownership: Voluntary Non-Profit - Private
Beds: 15

Key Personnel:
CEO/President. . . . . Edmond Morache
Chief of Medical Staff . . . . Susan Fiore, MD
Infection Control. . . . . Nora Todd, RN
Operating Room. . . . . Marilyn Donnelly, RN
Radiology. . . . . Tony Allen

Measure	Cases	This Hosp.	State Avg.	U.S. Avg.
Heart Attack Care				
ACE Inhibitor or ARB for LVSD[3]	0	-	95%	96%
Aspirin at Arrival[3]	0	-	98%	99%
Aspirin at Discharge[3]	0	-	98%	98%
Beta Blocker at Discharge[3]	0	-	98%	98%
Fibrinolytic Medication Timing[3]	0	-	50%	55%
PCI Within 90 Minutes of Arrival[3]	0	-	88%	90%
Smoking Cessation Advice[3]	0	-	100%	99%
Chest Pain/Possible Heart Attack Care				
Aspirin at Arrival[5]	0	-	96%	95%
Median Time to ECG (minutes)[5]	0	-	11	8
Median Time to Transfer (minutes)[5]	0	-	75	61
Fibrinolytic Medication Timing[5]	0	-	55%	54%
Heart Failure Care				
ACE Inhibitor or ARB for LVSD[1,3]	2	100%	94%	94%
Discharge Instructions[1,3]	8	88%	89%	88%
Evaluation of LVS Function[1,3]	8	88%	98%	98%
Smoking Cessation Advice[1,3]	1	100%	98%	98%
Pneumonia Care				
Appropriate Initial Antibiotic[1,3]	12	83%	92%	92%
Blood Culture Timing[1,3]	19	84%	95%	96%
Influenza Vaccine[1]	8	100%	90%	91%
Initial Antibiotic Timing[3]	0	-	93%	95%
Pneumococcal Vaccine[1,3]	18	100%	92%	93%
Smoking Cessation Advice[1,3]	1	100%	98%	97%
Surgical Care Improvement Project				
Appropriate VTP Within 24 Hours[5]	0	-	94%	92%
Appropriate Hair Removal[5]	0	-	100%	99%
Appropriate Beta Blocker Usage[5]	0	-	92%	93%
Controlled Postoperative Blood Glucose[5]	0	-	94%	93%
Prophylactic Antibiotic Timing[5]	0	-	96%	97%
Prophylactic Antibiotic Timing (Outpatient)[5]	0	-	92%	92%
Prophylactic Antibiotic Selection[5]	0	-	97%	97%
Prophylactic Antibiotic Select. (Outpatient)[5]	0	-	93%	94%
Prophylactic Antibiotic Stopped[5]	0	-	94%	94%
Recommended VTP Ordered[5]	0	-	96%	94%
Urinary Catheter Removal[5]	0	-	90%	90%
Children's Asthma Care				
Received Systemic Corticosteroids	-	-	-	100%
Received Home Management Plan	-	-	-	71%
Received Reliever Medication	-	-	-	100%
Use of Medical Imaging				
Combination Abdominal CT Scan	97	0.052	0.141	0.191
Combination Chest CT Scan[1]	40	0.025	0.024	0.054
Follow-up Mammogram/Ultrasound	133	9.0%	9.8%	8.4%
MRI for Low Back Pain[5]	0	-	26.9%	32.7%
Survey of Patients' Hospital Experiences				
Area Around Room 'Always' Quiet at Night[6]	<100	63%	-	58%
Doctors 'Always' Communicated Well[6]	<100	82%	-	80%
Home Recovery Information Given[6]	<100	81%	-	82%
Hospital Given 9 or 10 on 10 Point Scale[6]	<100	77%	-	67%
Meds 'Always' Explained Before Given[6]	<100	66%	-	60%
Nurses 'Always' Communicated Well[6]	<100	83%	-	76%
Pain 'Always' Well Controlled[6]	<100	75%	-	69%
Room and Bathroom 'Always' Clean[6]	<100	84%	-	71%
Timely Help 'Always' Received[6]	<100	79%	-	64%
Would Definitely Recommend Hospital	<100	66%	-	69%

Massena Memorial Hospital

1 Hospital Drive
Massena, NY 13662
Phone: 315-764-1711
Fax: 315-769-4344
E-mail: mmh@northnet.org
URL: www.massenahospital.org
Type: Acute Care Hospitals
Emergency Services: Yes
Ownership: Government - Local
Beds: 50

Key Personnel:
CEO/President. . . . . Charles F Fahd, II
Chief of Medical Staff . . . . Nimesh Desai, MD
Infection Control. . . . . Denille Dillabough, RN
Operating Room. . . . . Karen Wilkins, RN
Quality Assurance . . . . Betty MacDonald
Emergency Room . . . . Judy Markell, RN, BSN
Hemotology Center . . . . Marcia Cox, RN
Intensive Care Unit. . . . . Judy Markell, RN, BSN

Measure	Cases	This Hosp.	State Avg.	U.S. Avg.
Heart Attack Care				
ACE Inhibitor or ARB for LVSD	0	-	95%	96%
Aspirin at Arrival[1]	11	91%	98%	99%
Aspirin at Discharge[1]	3	100%	98%	98%
Beta Blocker at Discharge[1]	3	100%	98%	98%
Fibrinolytic Medication Timing[1]	1	100%	50%	55%
PCI Within 90 Minutes of Arrival	0	-	88%	90%
Smoking Cessation Advice[1]	1	100%	100%	99%
Chest Pain/Possible Heart Attack Care				
Aspirin at Arrival	49	98%	96%	95%
Median Time to ECG (minutes)	50	19	11	8
Median Time to Transfer (minutes)[3]	0	-	75	61
Fibrinolytic Medication Timing[1]	21	95%	55%	54%
Heart Failure Care				
ACE Inhibitor or ARB for LVSD[1]	19	95%	94%	94%
Discharge Instructions	75	97%	89%	88%
Evaluation of LVS Function	103	99%	98%	98%
Smoking Cessation Advice[1]	13	85%	98%	98%
Pneumonia Care				
Appropriate Initial Antibiotic	61	87%	92%	92%
Blood Culture Timing	116	95%	95%	96%
Influenza Vaccine	54	96%	90%	91%
Initial Antibiotic Timing	125	99%	93%	95%
Pneumococcal Vaccine	77	97%	92%	93%
Smoking Cessation Advice	35	97%	98%	97%
Surgical Care Improvement Project				
Appropriate VTP Within 24 Hours	39	95%	94%	92%
Appropriate Hair Removal	105	100%	100%	99%
Appropriate Beta Blocker Usage[1]	24	96%	92%	93%
Controlled Postoperative Blood Glucose	0	-	94%	93%
Prophylactic Antibiotic Timing	89	93%	96%	97%
Prophylactic Antibiotic Timing (Outpatient)	43	84%	92%	92%
Prophylactic Antibiotic Selection	86	81%	97%	97%
Prophylactic Antibiotic Select. (Outpatient)	40	85%	93%	94%
Prophylactic Antibiotic Stopped	85	87%	94%	94%
Recommended VTP Ordered	39	95%	96%	94%
Urinary Catheter Removal	25	100%	90%	90%
Children's Asthma Care				
Received Systemic Corticosteroids	-	-	-	100%
Received Home Management Plan	-	-	-	71%
Received Reliever Medication	-	-	-	100%
Use of Medical Imaging				
Combination Abdominal CT Scan	464	0.022	0.141	0.191
Combination Chest CT Scan	307	0.000	0.024	0.054
Follow-up Mammogram/Ultrasound	519	11.4%	9.8%	8.4%
MRI for Low Back Pain	50	36.0%	26.9%	32.7%
Survey of Patients' Hospital Experiences				
Area Around Room 'Always' Quiet at Night	300+	52%	-	58%
Doctors 'Always' Communicated Well	300+	82%	-	80%
Home Recovery Information Given	300+	82%	-	82%
Hospital Given 9 or 10 on 10 Point Scale	300+	61%	-	67%
Meds 'Always' Explained Before Given	300+	61%	-	60%
Nurses 'Always' Communicated Well	300+	77%	-	76%
Pain 'Always' Well Controlled	300+	72%	-	69%
Room and Bathroom 'Always' Clean	300+	75%	-	71%
Timely Help 'Always' Received	300+	67%	-	64%
Would Definitely Recommend Hospital	300+	59%	-	69%

Medina Memorial Hospital

200 Ohio Street
Medina, NY 14103
Phone: 585-798-8111
Fax: 585-798-8107
E-mail: info@medinamemorial.org
URL: www.medinahospital.com
Type: Acute Care Hospitals
Emergency Services: Yes
Ownership: Government - Federal
Beds: 101

Key Personnel:
CEO/President. . . . . James Sinner
Emergency Room . . . . C Jay Ellie Jr, MD

Measure	Cases	This Hosp.	State Avg.	U.S. Avg.
Heart Attack Care				
ACE Inhibitor or ARB for LVSD[1]	3	33%	95%	96%
Aspirin at Arrival	27	93%	98%	99%
Aspirin at Discharge[1]	20	85%	98%	98%
Beta Blocker at Discharge[1]	22	82%	98%	98%
Fibrinolytic Medication Timing[1]	1	0%	50%	55%
PCI Within 90 Minutes of Arrival	0	-	88%	90%
Smoking Cessation Advice[1]	7	100%	100%	99%
Chest Pain/Possible Heart Attack Care				
Aspirin at Arrival	60	95%	96%	95%
Median Time to ECG (minutes)	62	6	11	8
Median Time to Transfer (minutes)[1,3]	3	60	75	61
Fibrinolytic Medication Timing[1]	6	67%	55%	54%
Heart Failure Care				
ACE Inhibitor or ARB for LVSD	37	73%	94%	94%
Discharge Instructions	63	81%	89%	88%
Evaluation of LVS Function	102	96%	98%	98%
Smoking Cessation Advice[1]	12	100%	98%	98%
Pneumonia Care				
Appropriate Initial Antibiotic	73	86%	92%	92%
Blood Culture Timing	107	96%	95%	96%
Influenza Vaccine	67	91%	90%	91%
Initial Antibiotic Timing	116	95%	93%	95%
Pneumococcal Vaccine	100	90%	92%	93%
Smoking Cessation Advice[1]	21	100%	98%	97%
Surgical Care Improvement Project				
Appropriate VTP Within 24 Hours	34	85%	94%	92%
Appropriate Hair Removal	63	100%	100%	99%
Appropriate Beta Blocker Usage[1]	24	83%	92%	93%
Controlled Postoperative Blood Glucose	0	-	94%	93%
Prophylactic Antibiotic Timing	30	100%	96%	97%
Prophylactic Antibiotic Timing (Outpatient)[1]	15	53%	92%	92%
Prophylactic Antibiotic Selection	30	93%	97%	97%
Prophylactic Antibiotic Select. (Outpatient)	32	75%	93%	94%
Prophylactic Antibiotic Stopped	27	93%	94%	94%
Recommended VTP Ordered	34	94%	96%	94%
Urinary Catheter Removal[1]	8	75%	90%	90%
Children's Asthma Care				
Received Systemic Corticosteroids	-	-	-	100%
Received Home Management Plan	-	-	-	71%
Received Reliever Medication	-	-	-	100%
Use of Medical Imaging				
Combination Abdominal CT Scan	171	0.164	0.141	0.191
Combination Chest CT Scan	91	0.242	0.024	0.054
Follow-up Mammogram/Ultrasound	245	6.5%	9.8%	8.4%
MRI for Low Back Pain[5]	0	-	26.9%	32.7%
Survey of Patients' Hospital Experiences				
Area Around Room 'Always' Quiet at Night	300+	46%	-	58%
Doctors 'Always' Communicated Well	300+	77%	-	80%
Home Recovery Information Given	300+	84%	-	82%
Hospital Given 9 or 10 on 10 Point Scale	300+	61%	-	67%
Meds 'Always' Explained Before Given	300+	55%	-	60%
Nurses 'Always' Communicated Well	300+	74%	-	76%
Pain 'Always' Well Controlled	300+	64%	-	69%
Room and Bathroom 'Always' Clean	300+	70%	-	71%
Timely Help 'Always' Received	300+	61%	-	64%
Would Definitely Recommend Hospital	300+	64%	-	69%

NOTE: Hospital profiles are in alphabetical order by state, then city, then hospital within the city; Rankings exclude hospitals with less than 25 cases except for patient surveys which excludes hospitals with less than 100 cases; (a) 100–299 cases; (1) The number of cases is too small to be sure how well a hospital is performing; (2) The hospital indicated that the data submitted for this measure were based on a sample of cases; (3) Data was collected during a shorter time period (fewer quarters) than the maximum possible time for this measure; (4) Suppressed for one or more quarters by CMS; (5) No data is available from the hospital for this measure; (6) Fewer than 100 patients completed the HCAHPS survey. Use these rates with caution, as the number of surveys may be too low to reliably assess hospital performance; (7) Survey results are based on less than 12 months of data; (8) Survey results are not available for this reporting period; (9) No or very few patients were eligible for the HCAHPS survey. The scores shown, if any, reflect a very small number of surveys; (10) A state average was not calculated because too few hospitals in the state submitted data; (11) There were discrepancies in the data collection process; Please refer to the User's Guide for a full explanation of data.

Winthrop-University Hospital

259 First Street Phone: 516-663-0333
Mineola, NY 11501 Fax: 516-663-2953
URL: www.winthrop.org
Type: Acute Care Hospitals Emergency Services: Yes
Ownership: Voluntary Non-Profit - Private Beds: 591

Key Personnel:
CEO/President. . . . . John F Collins
Chief of Medical Staff . . . . Joseph Greensher MD
Infection Control. . . . . Burke Cunha MD
Pediatric Ambulatory Care . . . . . . Warren Rosenfeld MD
Pediatric In-Patient Care . . . . Warren Rosenfeld MD
Quality Assurance . . . . Bruce Cohn
Radiology. . . . . Orlando Ortiz
Emergency Room . . . . Barry Rosenthal MD

Measure	Cases	This Hosp.	State Avg.	U.S. Avg.
Heart Attack Care				
ACE Inhibitor or ARB for LVSD[2]	96	98%	95%	96%
Aspirin at Arrival[2]	282	97%	98%	99%
Aspirin at Discharge[2]	387	99%	98%	98%
Beta Blocker at Discharge[2]	378	100%	98%	98%
Fibrinolytic Medication Timing[2]	0	-	50%	55%
PCI Within 90 Minutes of Arrival[2]	58	83%	88%	90%
Smoking Cessation Advice[2]	90	100%	100%	99%
Chest Pain/Possible Heart Attack Care				
Aspirin at Arrival[5]	0	-	96%	95%
Median Time to ECG (minutes)[5]	0	-	11	8
Median Time to Transfer (minutes)[5]	0	-	75	61
Fibrinolytic Medication Timing[5]	0	-	55%	54%
Heart Failure Care				
ACE Inhibitor or ARB for LVSD[2]	130	98%	94%	94%
Discharge Instructions[2]	284	87%	89%	88%
Evaluation of LVS Function[2]	337	100%	98%	98%
Smoking Cessation Advice[2]	34	100%	98%	98%
Pneumonia Care				
Appropriate Initial Antibiotic[2]	107	94%	92%	92%
Blood Culture Timing[2]	187	99%	95%	96%
Influenza Vaccine[2]	101	97%	90%	91%
Initial Antibiotic Timing[2]	157	96%	93%	95%
Pneumococcal Vaccine[2]	164	97%	92%	93%
Smoking Cessation Advice[2]	32	100%	98%	97%
Surgical Care Improvement Project				
Appropriate VTP Within 24 Hours[2]	279	98%	94%	92%
Appropriate Hair Removal[2]	902	100%	100%	99%
Appropriate Beta Blocker Usage[2]	398	95%	92%	93%
Controlled Postoperative Blood Glucose[2]	212	89%	94%	93%
Prophylactic Antibiotic Timing[2]	642	95%	96%	97%
Prophylactic Antibiotic Timing (Outpatient)	477	96%	92%	92%
Prophylactic Antibiotic Selection[2]	648	98%	97%	97%
Prophylactic Antibiotic Select. (Outpatient)	475	94%	93%	94%
Prophylactic Antibiotic Stopped[2]	605	99%	94%	94%
Recommended VTP Ordered[2]	279	99%	96%	94%
Urinary Catheter Removal[2]	211	91%	90%	90%
Children's Asthma Care				
Received Systemic Corticosteroids	-	-	-	100%
Received Home Management Plan	-	-	-	71%
Received Reliever Medication	-	-	-	100%
Use of Medical Imaging				
Combination Abdominal CT Scan	284	0.014	0.141	0.191
Combination Chest CT Scan	79	0.000	0.024	0.054
Follow-up Mammogram/Ultrasound	525	17.0%	9.8%	8.4%
MRI for Low Back Pain[1]	10	20.0%	26.9%	32.7%
Survey of Patients' Hospital Experiences				
Area Around Room 'Always' Quiet at Night	300+	45%	-	58%
Doctors 'Always' Communicated Well	300+	77%	-	80%
Home Recovery Information Given	300+	83%	-	82%
Hospital Given 9 or 10 on 10 Point Scale	300+	67%	-	67%
Meds 'Always' Explained Before Given	300+	57%	-	60%
Nurses 'Always' Communicated Well	300+	76%	-	76%
Pain 'Always' Well Controlled	300+	67%	-	69%
Room and Bathroom 'Always' Clean	300+	70%	-	71%
Timely Help 'Always' Received	300+	57%	-	64%
Would Definitely Recommend Hospital	300+	73%	-	69%

Schuyler Hospital

220 Steuben Street Phone: 607-530-7121
Montour Falls, NY 14865 Fax: 607-535-2433
URL: www.schuylerhospital.org
Type: Critical Access Hospitals Emergency Services: Yes
Ownership: Voluntary Non-Profit - Private Beds: 169

Key Personnel:
CEO/President. . . . . Richard Stelzer
Chief of Medical Staff . . . . Dr Willaim Saks
Coronary Care . . . . Jonathon Laurence
Infection Control. . . . . Dr Irene Alexandraki
Pediatric Ambulatory Care . . . . . . Dr Manuel Castellanos
Pediatric In-Patient Care . . . . Dr Manuel Castellanos
Quality Assurance . . . . Rita Tague
Radiology. . . . . Edwin Acosta

Measure	Cases	This Hosp.	State Avg.	U.S. Avg.
Heart Attack Care				
ACE Inhibitor or ARB for LVSD[1,3]	1	100%	95%	96%
Aspirin at Arrival[1,3]	4	100%	98%	99%
Aspirin at Discharge[1,3]	3	100%	98%	98%
Beta Blocker at Discharge[1,3]	4	75%	98%	98%
Fibrinolytic Medication Timing[5]	0	-	50%	55%
PCI Within 90 Minutes of Arrival[5]	0	-	88%	90%
Smoking Cessation Advice[3]	0	-	100%	99%
Chest Pain/Possible Heart Attack Care				
Aspirin at Arrival	-	-	96%	95%
Median Time to ECG (minutes)	-	-	11	8
Median Time to Transfer (minutes)			75	61
Fibrinolytic Medication Timing	-	-	55%	54%
Heart Failure Care				
ACE Inhibitor or ARB for LVSD[1]	5	80%	94%	94%
Discharge Instructions[1]	18	100%	89%	88%
Evaluation of LVS Function	33	100%	98%	98%
Smoking Cessation Advice[1]	2	100%	98%	98%
Pneumonia Care				
Appropriate Initial Antibiotic	41	90%	92%	92%
Blood Culture Timing	71	97%	95%	96%
Influenza Vaccine	54	98%	90%	91%
Initial Antibiotic Timing	76	96%	93%	95%
Pneumococcal Vaccine	70	96%	92%	93%
Smoking Cessation Advice[1]	15	100%	98%	97%
Surgical Care Improvement Project				
Appropriate VTP Within 24 Hours[5]	0	-	94%	92%
Appropriate Hair Removal	60	100%	100%	99%
Appropriate Beta Blocker Usage[5]	0	-	92%	93%
Controlled Postoperative Blood Glucose	0	-	94%	93%
Prophylactic Antibiotic Timing[5]	0	-	96%	97%
Prophylactic Antibiotic Timing (Outpatient)	-	-	92%	92%
Prophylactic Antibiotic Selection[5]	0	-	97%	97%
Prophylactic Antibiotic Select. (Outpatient)	-	-	93%	94%
Prophylactic Antibiotic Stopped[5]	0	-	94%	94%
Recommended VTP Ordered[5]	0	-	96%	94%
Urinary Catheter Removal[1]	7	100%	90%	90%
Children's Asthma Care				
Received Systemic Corticosteroids	-	-	-	100%
Received Home Management Plan	-	-	-	71%
Received Reliever Medication	-	-	-	100%
Use of Medical Imaging				
Combination Abdominal CT Scan	-	-	0.141	0.191
Combination Chest CT Scan	-	-	0.024	0.054
Follow-up Mammogram/Ultrasound	-	-	9.8%	8.4%
MRI for Low Back Pain	-	-	26.9%	32.7%
Survey of Patients' Hospital Experiences				
Area Around Room 'Always' Quiet at Night[8]	-	-	-	58%
Doctors 'Always' Communicated Well[8]	-	-	-	80%
Home Recovery Information Given[8]	-	-	-	82%
Hospital Given 9 or 10 on 10 Point Scale[8]	-	-	-	67%
Meds 'Always' Explained Before Given[8]	-	-	-	60%
Nurses 'Always' Communicated Well[8]	-	-	-	76%
Pain 'Always' Well Controlled[8]	-	-	-	69%
Room and Bathroom 'Always' Clean[8]	-	-	-	71%
Timely Help 'Always' Received[8]	-	-	-	64%
Would Definitely Recommend Hospital[8]	-	-	-	69%

VA Hudson Valley Healthcare System

2094 Albany Post Road Phone: 914-737-4400
Montrose, NY 10548 Fax: 914-788-4244
URL: www.va.gov
Type: Acute Care-Veterans Administration Emergency Services: No
Ownership: Government - Federal

Key Personnel:
CEO/President. . . . . Michael A Sabo
Chief of Medical Staff . . . . Malati Kollali, MD
Quality Assurance . . . . Mary Ann Tyner

Measure	Cases	This Hosp.	State Avg.	U.S. Avg.
Heart Attack Care				
ACE Inhibitor or ARB for LVSD[5]	0	-	95%	96%
Aspirin at Arrival[5]	0	-	98%	99%
Aspirin at Discharge[5]	0	-	98%	98%
Beta Blocker at Discharge[5]	0	-	98%	98%
Fibrinolytic Medication Timing[5]	0	-	50%	55%
PCI Within 90 Minutes of Arrival[5]	0	-	88%	90%
Smoking Cessation Advice[5]	0	-	100%	99%
Chest Pain/Possible Heart Attack Care				
Aspirin at Arrival	-	-	96%	95%
Median Time to ECG (minutes)	-	-	11	8
Median Time to Transfer (minutes)	-	-	75	61
Fibrinolytic Medication Timing	-	-	55%	54%
Heart Failure Care				
ACE Inhibitor or ARB for LVSD[1]	5	100%	94%	94%
Discharge Instructions[1]	21	100%	89%	88%
Evaluation of LVS Function	26	100%	98%	98%
Smoking Cessation Advice[5]	0	-	98%	98%
Pneumonia Care				
Appropriate Initial Antibiotic[1]	8	100%	92%	92%
Blood Culture Timing[1]	21	100%	95%	96%
Influenza Vaccine	26	100%	90%	91%
Initial Antibiotic Timing	25	100%	93%	95%
Pneumococcal Vaccine	29	100%	92%	93%
Smoking Cessation Advice[1]	9	100%	98%	97%
Surgical Care Improvement Project				
Appropriate VTP Within 24 Hours[2,5]	0	-	94%	92%
Appropriate Hair Removal[2,5]	0	-	100%	99%
Appropriate Beta Blocker Usage[2,5]	0	-	92%	93%
Controlled Postoperative Blood Glucose[2,5]	0	-	94%	93%
Prophylactic Antibiotic Timing[5]	0	-	96%	97%
Prophylactic Antibiotic Timing (Outpatient)	-	-	92%	92%
Prophylactic Antibiotic Selection[5]	0	-	97%	97%
Prophylactic Antibiotic Select. (Outpatient)	-	-	93%	94%
Prophylactic Antibiotic Stopped[5]	0	-	94%	94%
Recommended VTP Ordered[2,5]	0	-	96%	94%
Urinary Catheter Removal[2,5]	0	-	90%	90%
Children's Asthma Care				
Received Systemic Corticosteroids	-	-	-	100%
Received Home Management Plan	-	-	-	71%
Received Reliever Medication	-	-	-	100%
Use of Medical Imaging				
Combination Abdominal CT Scan	-	-	0.141	0.191
Combination Chest CT Scan	-	-	0.024	0.054
Follow-up Mammogram/Ultrasound	-	-	9.8%	8.4%
MRI for Low Back Pain	-	-	26.9%	32.7%
Survey of Patients' Hospital Experiences				
Area Around Room 'Always' Quiet at Night	-	-	-	58%
Doctors 'Always' Communicated Well	-	-	-	80%
Home Recovery Information Given	-	-	-	82%
Hospital Given 9 or 10 on 10 Point Scale	-	-	-	67%
Meds 'Always' Explained Before Given	-	-	-	60%
Nurses 'Always' Communicated Well	-	-	-	76%
Pain 'Always' Well Controlled	-	-	-	69%
Room and Bathroom 'Always' Clean	-	-	-	71%
Timely Help 'Always' Received	-	-	-	64%
Would Definitely Recommend Hospital	-	-	-	69%

NOTE: Hospital profiles are in alphabetical order by state, then city, then hospital within the city; Rankings exclude hospitals with less than 25 cases except for patient surveys which excludes hospitals with less than 100 cases; (a) 100–299 cases; (1) The number of cases is too small to be sure how well a hospital is performing; (2) The hospital indicated that the data submitted for this measure were based on a sample of cases; (3) Data was collected during a shorter time period (fewer quarters) than the maximum possible time for this measure; (4) Suppressed for one or more quarters by CMS; (5) No data is available from the hospital for this measure; (6) Fewer than 100 patients completed the HCAHPS survey. Use these rates with caution, as the number of surveys may be too low to reliably assess hospital performance; (7) Survey results are based on less than 12 months of data; (8) Survey results are not available for this reporting period; (9) No or very few patients were eligible for the HCAHPS survey. The scores shown, if any, reflect a very small number of surveys; (10) A state average was not calculated because too few hospitals in the state submitted data; (11) There were discrepancies in the data collection process; Please refer to the User's Guide for a full explanation of data.

Northern Westchester Hospital

400 East Main Street
Mount Kisco, NY 10549
Phone: 914-666-1200
Fax: 914-666-1163
E-mail: nwhmarketing@nwhc.net
URL: www.nwhc.net
Type: Acute Care Hospitals
Emergency Services: Yes
Ownership: Voluntary Non-Profit - Private
Beds: 233

Key Personnel:
CEO/President. . . . . Joel Seligman
Chief of Medical Staff . . . . Marla Koroly, MD
Coronary Care . . . . Judy Kinkel, RN
Infection Control. . . . . Sonia Appel
Operating Room. . . . . Susan Roy
Pediatric In-Patient Care . . . . Jill Ratner, MD
Quality Assurance . . . . Lisa Hanrahan
Radiology. . . . . Peter Khouri, MD

Measure	Cases	This Hosp.	State Avg.	U.S. Avg.
Heart Attack Care				
ACE Inhibitor or ARB for LVSD[1]	4	100%	95%	96%
Aspirin at Arrival	26	100%	98%	99%
Aspirin at Discharge[1]	12	100%	98%	98%
Beta Blocker at Discharge[1]	16	100%	98%	98%
Fibrinolytic Medication Timing[1]	1	0%	50%	55%
PCI Within 90 Minutes of Arrival	0	-	88%	90%
Smoking Cessation Advice	0	-	100%	99%
Chest Pain/Possible Heart Attack Care				
Aspirin at Arrival	108	100%	96%	95%
Median Time to ECG (minutes)	112	5	11	8
Median Time to Transfer (minutes)[1]	12	72	75	61
Fibrinolytic Medication Timing[1]	4	100%	55%	54%
Heart Failure Care				
ACE Inhibitor or ARB for LVSD	49	98%	94%	94%
Discharge Instructions	156	95%	89%	88%
Evaluation of LVS Function	198	100%	98%	98%
Smoking Cessation Advice[1]	12	92%	98%	98%
Pneumonia Care				
Appropriate Initial Antibiotic[2]	71	94%	92%	92%
Blood Culture Timing[2]	175	96%	95%	96%
Influenza Vaccine[2]	95	93%	90%	91%
Initial Antibiotic Timing[2]	159	100%	93%	95%
Pneumococcal Vaccine[2]	169	93%	92%	93%
Smoking Cessation Advice[1,2]	21	95%	98%	97%
Surgical Care Improvement Project				
Appropriate VTP Within 24 Hours[2]	140	94%	94%	92%
Appropriate Hair Removal[2]	371	100%	100%	99%
Appropriate Beta Blocker Usage[2]	83	94%	92%	93%
Controlled Postoperative Blood Glucose[2]	0	-	94%	93%
Prophylactic Antibiotic Timing[2]	231	97%	96%	97%
Prophylactic Antibiotic Timing (Outpatient)	336	97%	92%	92%
Prophylactic Antibiotic Selection[2]	245	97%	97%	97%
Prophylactic Antibiotic Select. (Outpatient)	333	97%	93%	94%
Prophylactic Antibiotic Stopped[2]	226	96%	94%	94%
Recommended VTP Ordered[2]	141	96%	96%	94%
Urinary Catheter Removal[2]	108	97%	90%	90%
Children's Asthma Care				
Received Systemic Corticosteroids	-	-	-	100%
Received Home Management Plan	-	-	-	71%
Received Reliever Medication	-	-	-	100%
Use of Medical Imaging				
Combination Abdominal CT Scan	382	0.105	0.141	0.191
Combination Chest CT Scan	244	0.000	0.024	0.054
Follow-up Mammogram/Ultrasound[1]	35	28.6%	9.8%	8.4%
MRI for Low Back Pain	53	30.2%	26.9%	32.7%
Survey of Patients' Hospital Experiences				
Area Around Room 'Always' Quiet at Night	300+	57%	-	58%
Doctors 'Always' Communicated Well	300+	83%	-	80%
Home Recovery Information Given	300+	78%	-	82%
Hospital Given 9 or 10 on 10 Point Scale	300+	74%	-	67%
Meds 'Always' Explained Before Given	300+	63%	-	60%
Nurses 'Always' Communicated Well	300+	82%	-	76%
Pain 'Always' Well Controlled	300+	75%	-	69%
Room and Bathroom 'Always' Clean	300+	70%	-	71%
Timely Help 'Always' Received	300+	66%	-	64%
Would Definitely Recommend Hospital	300+	81%	-	69%

Mount Vernon Hospital

12 North 7th Avenue
Mount Vernon, NY 10550
Phone: 914-664-8000
Fax: 914-664-1569
URL: www.sshsw.org
Type: Acute Care Hospitals
Emergency Services: Yes
Ownership: Voluntary Non-Profit - Private
Beds: 228

Key Personnel:
CEO/President. . . . . George Haskins
Cardiac Laboratory. . . . . Gariush Alaie, MD
Chief of Medical Staff . . . . Richard Petrillo, MD
Operating Room. . . . . Vicky Reed
Pediatric Ambulatory Care . . . . . . Lori Semel, MD
Pediatric In-Patient Care . . . . Lori Semel, MD
Quality Assurance . . . . Janice Mule
Radiology. . . . . Mark Armstrong, MD

Measure	Cases	This Hosp.	State Avg.	U.S. Avg.
Heart Attack Care				
ACE Inhibitor or ARB for LVSD[1]	5	80%	95%	96%
Aspirin at Arrival	45	89%	98%	99%
Aspirin at Discharge	26	96%	98%	98%
Beta Blocker at Discharge	25	80%	98%	98%
Fibrinolytic Medication Timing[1]	1	0%	50%	55%
PCI Within 90 Minutes of Arrival	0	-	88%	90%
Smoking Cessation Advice[1]	4	100%	100%	99%
Chest Pain/Possible Heart Attack Care				
Aspirin at Arrival[1,3]	5	100%	96%	95%
Median Time to ECG (minutes)[1,3]	5	58	11	8
Median Time to Transfer (minutes)[3]	0	-	75	61
Fibrinolytic Medication Timing[1,3]	1	0%	55%	54%
Heart Failure Care				
ACE Inhibitor or ARB for LVSD	38	92%	94%	94%
Discharge Instructions	84	88%	89%	88%
Evaluation of LVS Function	122	88%	98%	98%
Smoking Cessation Advice	27	100%	98%	98%
Pneumonia Care				
Appropriate Initial Antibiotic	52	94%	92%	92%
Blood Culture Timing	107	100%	95%	96%
Influenza Vaccine	45	71%	90%	91%
Initial Antibiotic Timing	91	92%	93%	95%
Pneumococcal Vaccine	59	92%	92%	93%
Smoking Cessation Advice	31	100%	98%	97%
Surgical Care Improvement Project				
Appropriate VTP Within 24 Hours	62	68%	94%	92%
Appropriate Hair Removal	92	100%	100%	99%
Appropriate Beta Blocker Usage[1]	19	63%	92%	93%
Controlled Postoperative Blood Glucose	0	-	94%	93%
Prophylactic Antibiotic Timing	34	91%	96%	97%
Prophylactic Antibiotic Timing (Outpatient)	53	94%	92%	92%
Prophylactic Antibiotic Selection	34	85%	97%	97%
Prophylactic Antibiotic Select. (Outpatient)	51	86%	93%	94%
Prophylactic Antibiotic Stopped	32	78%	94%	94%
Recommended VTP Ordered	63	76%	96%	94%
Urinary Catheter Removal[1]	23	91%	90%	90%
Children's Asthma Care				
Received Systemic Corticosteroids	-	-	-	100%
Received Home Management Plan	-	-	-	71%
Received Reliever Medication	-	-	-	100%
Use of Medical Imaging				
Combination Abdominal CT Scan	212	0.005	0.141	0.191
Combination Chest CT Scan	173	0.006	0.024	0.054
Follow-up Mammogram/Ultrasound	367	9.5%	9.8%	8.4%
MRI for Low Back Pain[1]	21	38.1%	26.9%	32.7%
Survey of Patients' Hospital Experiences				
Area Around Room 'Always' Quiet at Night	300+	59%	-	58%
Doctors 'Always' Communicated Well	300+	83%	-	80%
Home Recovery Information Given	300+	82%	-	82%
Hospital Given 9 or 10 on 10 Point Scale	300+	56%	-	67%
Meds 'Always' Explained Before Given	300+	54%	-	60%
Nurses 'Always' Communicated Well	300+	73%	-	76%
Pain 'Always' Well Controlled	300+	67%	-	69%
Room and Bathroom 'Always' Clean	300+	67%	-	71%
Timely Help 'Always' Received	300+	61%	-	64%
Would Definitely Recommend Hospital	300+	59%	-	69%

Long Island Jewish Medical Center

270 - 05 76th Avenue
New Hyde Park, NY 11040
Phone: 718-470-7000
Fax: 516-465-2650
URL: www.northshoreLIJ.com
Type: Acute Care Hospitals
Emergency Services: Yes
Ownership: Voluntary Non-Profit - Private
Beds: 452

Key Personnel:
Cardiac Laboratory. . . . . Stacy E Rosen, MD FACC
Chief of Medical Staff . . . . Jeremy Roal
Coronary Care . . . . Denise Maye, RN
Infection Control. . . . . Carol Singer, MD
Operating Room. . . . . Diane Simmons, RN
Pediatric Ambulatory Care . . . . . . Arthor Klein, MD
Quality Assurance . . . . Dorothy Feildman
Radiology. . . . . Lawrence Davis, MD

Measure	Cases	This Hosp.	State Avg.	U.S. Avg.
Heart Attack Care				
ACE Inhibitor or ARB for LVSD[2]	75	100%	95%	96%
Aspirin at Arrival[2]	159	98%	98%	99%
Aspirin at Discharge[2]	301	99%	98%	98%
Beta Blocker at Discharge[2]	294	99%	98%	98%
Fibrinolytic Medication Timing[2]	0	-	50%	55%
PCI Within 90 Minutes of Arrival[2]	33	100%	88%	90%
Smoking Cessation Advice[2]	82	100%	100%	99%
Chest Pain/Possible Heart Attack Care				
Aspirin at Arrival[3]	0	-	96%	95%
Median Time to ECG (minutes)[1,3]	1	14	11	8
Median Time to Transfer (minutes)[5]	0	-	75	61
Fibrinolytic Medication Timing[5]	0	-	55%	54%
Heart Failure Care				
ACE Inhibitor or ARB for LVSD[2]	142	95%	94%	94%
Discharge Instructions[2]	243	89%	89%	88%
Evaluation of LVS Function[2]	306	99%	98%	98%
Smoking Cessation Advice[2]	39	97%	98%	98%
Pneumonia Care				
Appropriate Initial Antibiotic[2]	92	90%	92%	92%
Blood Culture Timing[2]	157	99%	95%	96%
Influenza Vaccine[2]	85	100%	90%	91%
Initial Antibiotic Timing[2]	151	95%	93%	95%
Pneumococcal Vaccine[2]	119	96%	92%	93%
Smoking Cessation Advice[1,2]	23	100%	98%	97%
Surgical Care Improvement Project				
Appropriate VTP Within 24 Hours[2]	169	99%	94%	92%
Appropriate Hair Removal[2]	671	100%	100%	99%
Appropriate Beta Blocker Usage[2]	221	88%	92%	93%
Controlled Postoperative Blood Glucose[2]	154	99%	94%	93%
Prophylactic Antibiotic Timing[2]	473	98%	96%	97%
Prophylactic Antibiotic Timing (Outpatient)	145	87%	92%	92%
Prophylactic Antibiotic Selection[2]	482	94%	97%	97%
Prophylactic Antibiotic Select. (Outpatient)	131	85%	93%	94%
Prophylactic Antibiotic Stopped[2]	453	96%	94%	94%
Recommended VTP Ordered[2]	171	98%	96%	94%
Urinary Catheter Removal[2]	153	92%	90%	90%
Children's Asthma Care				
Received Systemic Corticosteroids	-	-	-	100%
Received Home Management Plan	-	-	-	71%
Received Reliever Medication	-	-	-	100%
Use of Medical Imaging				
Combination Abdominal CT Scan	561	0.086	0.141	0.191
Combination Chest CT Scan	278	0.000	0.024	0.054
Follow-up Mammogram/Ultrasound[5]	0	-	9.8%	8.4%
MRI for Low Back Pain[1]	24	37.5%	26.9%	32.7%
Survey of Patients' Hospital Experiences				
Area Around Room 'Always' Quiet at Night	300+	46%	-	58%
Doctors 'Always' Communicated Well	300+	74%	-	80%
Home Recovery Information Given	300+	75%	-	82%
Hospital Given 9 or 10 on 10 Point Scale	300+	58%	-	67%
Meds 'Always' Explained Before Given	300+	55%	-	60%
Nurses 'Always' Communicated Well	300+	69%	-	76%
Pain 'Always' Well Controlled	300+	61%	-	69%
Room and Bathroom 'Always' Clean	300+	60%	-	71%
Timely Help 'Always' Received	300+	56%	-	64%
Would Definitely Recommend Hospital	300+	66%	-	69%

NOTE: Hospital profiles are in alphabetical order by state, then city, then hospital within the city; Rankings exclude hospitals with less than 25 cases except for patient surveys which excludes hospitals with less than 100 cases; (a) 100–299 cases; (1) The number of cases is too small to be sure how well a hospital is performing; (2) The hospital indicated that the data submitted for this measure were based on a sample of cases; (3) Data was collected during a shorter time period (fewer quarters) than the maximum possible time for this measure; (4) Suppressed for one or more quarters by CMS; (5) No data is available from the hospital for this measure; (6) Fewer than 100 patients completed the HCAHPS survey. Use these rates with caution, as the number of surveys may be too low to reliably assess hospital performance; (7) Survey results are based on less than 12 months of data; (8) Survey results are not available for this reporting period; (9) No or very few patients were eligible for the HCAHPS survey. The scores shown, if any, reflect a very small number of surveys; (10) A state average was not calculated because too few hospitals in the state submitted data; (11) There were discrepancies in the data collection process; Please refer to the User's Guide for a full explanation of data.

Sound Shore Medical Center of Westschester

16 Guion Place Phone: 914-632-5000
New Rochelle, NY 10802 Fax: 914-637-1203
URL: www.ssmc.org
Type: Acute Care Hospitals Emergency Services: Yes
Ownership: Voluntary Non-Profit - Private Beds: 476

Key Personnel:
CEO/President. . . . . John R Spicer
Operating Room. . . . . Irene Giarolo
Pediatric In-Patient Care . . . . Mark Glassman, MD
Ambulatory Care . . . . Ann Reyna

Measure	Cases	This Hosp.	State Avg.	U.S. Avg.
Heart Attack Care				
ACE Inhibitor or ARB for LVSD[1]	12	100%	95%	96%
Aspirin at Arrival	108	100%	98%	99%
Aspirin at Discharge	62	98%	98%	98%
Beta Blocker at Discharge	69	99%	98%	98%
Fibrinolytic Medication Timing[1]	7	29%	50%	55%
PCI Within 90 Minutes of Arrival	0	-	88%	90%
Smoking Cessation Advice[1]	5	100%	100%	99%
Chest Pain/Possible Heart Attack Care				
Aspirin at Arrival	54	98%	96%	95%
Median Time to ECG (minutes)	55	18	11	8
Median Time to Transfer (minutes)[3]	0	-	75	61
Fibrinolytic Medication Timing[1]	9	67%	55%	54%
Heart Failure Care				
ACE Inhibitor or ARB for LVSD	87	97%	94%	94%
Discharge Instructions	177	98%	89%	88%
Evaluation of LVS Function	291	99%	98%	98%
Smoking Cessation Advice	30	100%	98%	98%
Pneumonia Care				
Appropriate Initial Antibiotic	117	91%	92%	92%
Blood Culture Timing	130	98%	95%	96%
Influenza Vaccine	122	96%	90%	91%
Initial Antibiotic Timing	156	98%	93%	95%
Pneumococcal Vaccine	183	97%	92%	93%
Smoking Cessation Advice	39	100%	98%	97%
Surgical Care Improvement Project				
Appropriate VTP Within 24 Hours	282	88%	94%	92%
Appropriate Hair Removal	473	100%	100%	99%
Appropriate Beta Blocker Usage	153	85%	92%	93%
Controlled Postoperative Blood Glucose	0	-	94%	93%
Prophylactic Antibiotic Timing	298	97%	96%	97%
Prophylactic Antibiotic Timing (Outpatient)	97	89%	92%	92%
Prophylactic Antibiotic Selection	324	99%	97%	97%
Prophylactic Antibiotic Select. (Outpatient)	88	91%	93%	94%
Prophylactic Antibiotic Stopped	291	98%	94%	94%
Recommended VTP Ordered	282	94%	96%	94%
Urinary Catheter Removal	152	95%	90%	90%
Children's Asthma Care				
Received Systemic Corticosteroids	-	-	-	100%
Received Home Management Plan	-	-	-	71%
Received Reliever Medication	-	-	-	100%
Use of Medical Imaging				
Combination Abdominal CT Scan	294	0.044	0.141	0.191
Combination Chest CT Scan	88	0.011	0.024	0.054
Follow-up Mammogram/Ultrasound	175	5.7%	9.8%	8.4%
MRI for Low Back Pain[5]	0	-	26.9%	32.7%
Survey of Patients' Hospital Experiences				
Area Around Room 'Always' Quiet at Night	300+	44%	-	58%
Doctors 'Always' Communicated Well	300+	74%	-	80%
Home Recovery Information Given	300+	75%	-	82%
Hospital Given 9 or 10 on 10 Point Scale	300+	45%	-	67%
Meds 'Always' Explained Before Given	300+	51%	-	60%
Nurses 'Always' Communicated Well	300+	64%	-	76%
Pain 'Always' Well Controlled	300+	59%	-	69%
Room and Bathroom 'Always' Clean	300+	53%	-	71%
Timely Help 'Always' Received	300+	47%	-	64%
Would Definitely Recommend Hospital	300+	49%	-	69%

Bellevue Hospital Center

First Avenue at 27th Street Phone: 212-561-4132
New York, NY 10016 Fax: 212-562-4009
URL: www.nyc.gov/html/hhc/html/facilities/bellevue.shtml
Type: Acute Care Hospitals Emergency Services: Yes
Ownership: Government - Local Beds: 809

Key Personnel:
CEO/President. . . . . Alan D. Aviles
Chief of Medical Staff. . . . . Joe Schickmer
Infection Control. . . . . Robert Holzman, MD
Operating Room. . . . . Alex Stone, MD
Pediatric Ambulatory Care . . . . . . Wade Parks, MD
Pediatric In-Patient Care . . . . Wade Parks, MD
Quality Assurance . . . . Susan Schnall, RN, CPHQ
Radiology. . . . . Albert Keegan, MD

Measure	Cases	This Hosp.	State Avg.	U.S. Avg.
Heart Attack Care				
ACE Inhibitor or ARB for LVSD	137	99%	95%	96%
Aspirin at Arrival	188	100%	98%	99%
Aspirin at Discharge	520	100%	98%	98%
Beta Blocker at Discharge	491	99%	98%	98%
Fibrinolytic Medication Timing	0	-	50%	55%
PCI Within 90 Minutes of Arrival[1]	24	96%	88%	90%
Smoking Cessation Advice	183	100%	100%	99%
Chest Pain/Possible Heart Attack Care				
Aspirin at Arrival[5]	0	-	96%	95%
Median Time to ECG (minutes)[5]	0	-	11	8
Median Time to Transfer (minutes)[5]	0	-	75	61
Fibrinolytic Medication Timing[5]	0	-	55%	54%
Heart Failure Care				
ACE Inhibitor or ARB for LVSD	313	100%	94%	94%
Discharge Instructions	471	100%	89%	88%
Evaluation of LVS Function	539	100%	98%	98%
Smoking Cessation Advice	129	100%	98%	98%
Pneumonia Care				
Appropriate Initial Antibiotic	134	87%	92%	92%
Blood Culture Timing	195	88%	95%	96%
Influenza Vaccine	127	90%	90%	91%
Initial Antibiotic Timing	214	87%	93%	95%
Pneumococcal Vaccine	121	97%	92%	93%
Smoking Cessation Advice	96	96%	98%	97%
Surgical Care Improvement Project				
Appropriate VTP Within 24 Hours[2]	298	97%	94%	92%
Appropriate Hair Removal[2]	747	100%	100%	99%
Appropriate Beta Blocker Usage[2]	190	99%	92%	93%
Controlled Postoperative Blood Glucose[2]	192	97%	94%	93%
Prophylactic Antibiotic Timing[2]	410	97%	96%	97%
Prophylactic Antibiotic Timing (Outpatient)	47	98%	92%	92%
Prophylactic Antibiotic Selection[2]	418	98%	97%	97%
Prophylactic Antibiotic Select. (Outpatient)	164	99%	93%	94%
Prophylactic Antibiotic Stopped[2]	401	99%	94%	94%
Recommended VTP Ordered[2]	298	97%	96%	94%
Urinary Catheter Removal[2]	109	92%	90%	90%
Children's Asthma Care				
Received Systemic Corticosteroids	-	-	-	100%
Received Home Management Plan	-	-	-	71%
Received Reliever Medication	-	-	-	100%
Use of Medical Imaging				
Combination Abdominal CT Scan	245	0.118	0.141	0.191
Combination Chest CT Scan	219	0.014	0.024	0.054
Follow-up Mammogram/Ultrasound[1]	44	9.1%	9.8%	8.4%
MRI for Low Back Pain[1]	9	44.4%	26.9%	32.7%
Survey of Patients' Hospital Experiences				
Area Around Room 'Always' Quiet at Night	300+	42%	-	58%
Doctors 'Always' Communicated Well	300+	75%	-	80%
Home Recovery Information Given	300+	78%	-	82%
Hospital Given 9 or 10 on 10 Point Scale	300+	52%	-	67%
Meds 'Always' Explained Before Given	300+	49%	-	60%
Nurses 'Always' Communicated Well	300+	61%	-	76%
Pain 'Always' Well Controlled	300+	58%	-	69%
Room and Bathroom 'Always' Clean	300+	55%	-	71%
Timely Help 'Always' Received	300+	48%	-	64%
Would Definitely Recommend Hospital	300+	62%	-	69%

Beth Israel Medical Center

First Avenue at 16th Street Phone: 212-420-2000
New York, NY 10003
URL: www.wehealny.org
Type: Acute Care Hospitals Emergency Services: Yes
Ownership: Voluntary Non-Profit - Private Beds: 1,368

Key Personnel:
CEO/President. . . . . Harris Nagler, MD FACS
Chief of Medical Staff . . . . David B Bernard, MD
Operating Room. . . . . George J Todd, MD FACS
Pediatric Ambulatory Care . . . . . . Richard Bonforte, MD
Pediatric In-Patient Care . . . . Richard Bonforte, MD
Quality Assurance . . . . Barb Challan
Patient Relations . . . . Kathryn Davis

Measure	Cases	This Hosp.	State Avg.	U.S. Avg.
Heart Attack Care				
ACE Inhibitor or ARB for LVSD[2]	66	95%	95%	96%
Aspirin at Arrival[2]	257	96%	98%	99%
Aspirin at Discharge[2]	263	98%	98%	98%
Beta Blocker at Discharge[2]	258	98%	98%	98%
Fibrinolytic Medication Timing[2]	0	-	50%	55%
PCI Within 90 Minutes of Arrival[1,2]	24	71%	88%	90%
Smoking Cessation Advice[2]	53	100%	100%	99%
Chest Pain/Possible Heart Attack Care				
Aspirin at Arrival[5]	0	-	96%	95%
Median Time to ECG (minutes)[5]	0	-	11	8
Median Time to Transfer (minutes)[5]	0	-	75	61
Fibrinolytic Medication Timing[5]	0	-	55%	54%
Heart Failure Care				
ACE Inhibitor or ARB for LVSD[2]	91	95%	94%	94%
Discharge Instructions[2]	260	64%	89%	88%
Evaluation of LVS Function[2]	307	98%	98%	98%
Smoking Cessation Advice[2]	33	97%	98%	98%
Pneumonia Care				
Appropriate Initial Antibiotic[2]	108	93%	92%	92%
Blood Culture Timing[2]	172	99%	95%	96%
Influenza Vaccine[2]	98	85%	90%	91%
Initial Antibiotic Timing[2]	170	92%	93%	95%
Pneumococcal Vaccine[2]	165	78%	92%	93%
Smoking Cessation Advice[2]	53	100%	98%	97%
Surgical Care Improvement Project				
Appropriate VTP Within 24 Hours[2]	229	98%	94%	92%
Appropriate Hair Removal[2]	690	99%	100%	99%
Appropriate Beta Blocker Usage[2]	222	78%	92%	93%
Controlled Postoperative Blood Glucose[2]	141	88%	94%	93%
Prophylactic Antibiotic Timing[2]	490	99%	96%	97%
Prophylactic Antibiotic Timing (Outpatient)	642	95%	92%	92%
Prophylactic Antibiotic Selection[2]	490	96%	97%	97%
Prophylactic Antibiotic Select. (Outpatient)	649	96%	93%	94%
Prophylactic Antibiotic Stopped[2]	474	91%	94%	94%
Recommended VTP Ordered[2]	229	98%	96%	94%
Urinary Catheter Removal[2]	196	80%	90%	90%
Children's Asthma Care				
Received Systemic Corticosteroids	-	-	-	100%
Received Home Management Plan	-	-	-	71%
Received Reliever Medication	-	-	-	100%
Use of Medical Imaging				
Combination Abdominal CT Scan	872	0.165	0.141	0.191
Combination Chest CT Scan	483	0.052	0.024	0.054
Follow-up Mammogram/Ultrasound	884	7.8%	9.8%	8.4%
MRI for Low Back Pain	96	24.0%	26.9%	32.7%
Survey of Patients' Hospital Experiences				
Area Around Room 'Always' Quiet at Night	300+	50%	-	58%
Doctors 'Always' Communicated Well	300+	73%	-	80%
Home Recovery Information Given	300+	76%	-	82%
Hospital Given 9 or 10 on 10 Point Scale	300+	56%	-	67%
Meds 'Always' Explained Before Given	300+	52%	-	60%
Nurses 'Always' Communicated Well	300+	66%	-	76%
Pain 'Always' Well Controlled	300+	61%	-	69%
Room and Bathroom 'Always' Clean	300+	64%	-	71%
Timely Help 'Always' Received	300+	57%	-	64%
Would Definitely Recommend Hospital	300+	61%	-	69%

NOTE: Hospital profiles are in alphabetical order by state, then city, then hospital within the city; Rankings exclude hospitals with less than 25 cases except for patient surveys which excludes hospitals with less than 100 cases; (a) 100–299 cases; (1) The number of cases is too small to be sure how well a hospital is performing; (2) The hospital indicated that the data submitted for this measure were based on a sample of cases; (3) Data was collected during a shorter time period (fewer quarters) than the maximum possible time for this measure; (4) Suppressed for one or more quarters by CMS; (5) No data is available from the hospital for this measure; (6) Fewer than 100 patients completed the HCAHPS survey. Use these rates with caution, as the number of surveys may be too low to reliably assess hospital performance; (7) Survey results are based on less than 12 months of data; (8) Survey results are not available for this reporting period; (9) No or very few patients were eligible for the HCAHPS survey. The scores shown, if any, reflect a very small number of surveys; (10) A state average was not calculated because too few hospitals in the state submitted data; (11) There were discrepancies in the data collection process; Please refer to the User's Guide for a full explanation of data.

Harlem Hospital Center

506 Lenox Avenue — Phone: 212-491-8400
New York, NY 10037
URL: www.nyc.gov/hhc
Type: Acute Care Hospitals — Emergency Services: Yes
Ownership: Government - Local — Beds: 7,560

Key Personnel:
CEO/President. . . . . Alan Aviles

Measure	Cases	This Hosp.	State Avg.	U.S. Avg.
Heart Attack Care				
ACE Inhibitor or ARB for LVSD[1]	9	100%	95%	96%
Aspirin at Arrival	38	100%	98%	99%
Aspirin at Discharge[1]	20	100%	98%	98%
Beta Blocker at Discharge[1]	19	100%	98%	98%
Fibrinolytic Medication Timing[1]	1	0%	50%	55%
PCI Within 90 Minutes of Arrival	0	-	88%	90%
Smoking Cessation Advice[1]	7	100%	100%	99%
Chest Pain/Possible Heart Attack Care				
Aspirin at Arrival[1]	6	100%	96%	95%
Median Time to ECG (minutes)[1]	6	26	11	8
Median Time to Transfer (minutes)[5]	0	-	75	61
Fibrinolytic Medication Timing[1,3]	1	0%	55%	54%
Heart Failure Care				
ACE Inhibitor or ARB for LVSD[2]	76	93%	94%	94%
Discharge Instructions[2]	206	78%	89%	88%
Evaluation of LVS Function[2]	219	99%	98%	98%
Smoking Cessation Advice[2]	69	100%	98%	98%
Pneumonia Care				
Appropriate Initial Antibiotic[2]	47	98%	92%	92%
Blood Culture Timing[2]	147	96%	95%	96%
Influenza Vaccine[2]	65	80%	90%	91%
Initial Antibiotic Timing[2]	144	94%	93%	95%
Pneumococcal Vaccine[2]	72	99%	92%	93%
Smoking Cessation Advice[2]	72	99%	98%	97%
Surgical Care Improvement Project				
Appropriate VTP Within 24 Hours[2]	77	95%	94%	92%
Appropriate Hair Removal[2]	120	94%	100%	99%
Appropriate Beta Blocker Usage[1,2]	12	83%	92%	93%
Controlled Postoperative Blood Glucose[2]	0	-	94%	93%
Prophylactic Antibiotic Timing[2]	34	94%	96%	97%
Prophylactic Antibiotic Timing (Outpatient)	26	88%	92%	92%
Prophylactic Antibiotic Selection[2]	34	100%	97%	97%
Prophylactic Antibiotic Select. (Outpatient)	43	98%	93%	94%
Prophylactic Antibiotic Stopped[2]	28	89%	94%	94%
Recommended VTP Ordered[2]	77	97%	96%	94%
Urinary Catheter Removal[1,2]	3	100%	90%	90%
Children's Asthma Care				
Received Systemic Corticosteroids	-	-	-	100%
Received Home Management Plan	-	-	-	71%
Received Reliever Medication	-	-	-	100%
Use of Medical Imaging				
Combination Abdominal CT Scan	115	0.348	0.141	0.191
Combination Chest CT Scan	62	0.242	0.024	0.054
Follow-up Mammogram/Ultrasound	136	8.1%	9.8%	8.4%
MRI for Low Back Pain[1]	6	33.3%	26.9%	32.7%
Survey of Patients' Hospital Experiences				
Area Around Room 'Always' Quiet at Night	300+	58%	-	58%
Doctors 'Always' Communicated Well	300+	76%	-	80%
Home Recovery Information Given	300+	78%	-	82%
Hospital Given 9 or 10 on 10 Point Scale	300+	45%	-	67%
Meds 'Always' Explained Before Given	300+	54%	-	60%
Nurses 'Always' Communicated Well	300+	61%	-	76%
Pain 'Always' Well Controlled	300+	57%	-	69%
Room and Bathroom 'Always' Clean	300+	58%	-	71%
Timely Help 'Always' Received	300+	47%	-	64%
Would Definitely Recommend Hospital	300+	52%	-	69%

Hospital for Special Surgery

535 East 70th Street — Phone: 212-606-1000
New York, NY 10021 — Fax: 212-606-1961
URL: www.hss.edu
Type: Acute Care Hospitals — Emergency Services: Yes
Ownership: Voluntary Non-Profit - Private — Beds: 160

Key Personnel:
CEO/President. . . . . John Reynolds
Chief of Medical Staff . . . . Thomas P Sculco, MD
Quality Assurance . . . . Susan Flics
Radiology. . . . . Ronald S Adler

Measure	Cases	This Hosp.	State Avg.	U.S. Avg.
Heart Attack Care				
ACE Inhibitor or ARB for LVSD[5]	0	-	95%	96%
Aspirin at Arrival[5]	0	-	98%	99%
Aspirin at Discharge[5]	0	-	98%	98%
Beta Blocker at Discharge[5]	0	-	98%	98%
Fibrinolytic Medication Timing[5]	0	-	50%	55%
PCI Within 90 Minutes of Arrival[5]	0	-	88%	90%
Smoking Cessation Advice[5]	0	-	100%	99%
Chest Pain/Possible Heart Attack Care				
Aspirin at Arrival[5]	0	-	96%	95%
Median Time to ECG (minutes)[5]	0	-	11	8
Median Time to Transfer (minutes)[5]	0	-	75	61
Fibrinolytic Medication Timing[5]	0	-	55%	54%
Heart Failure Care				
ACE Inhibitor or ARB for LVSD[5]	0	-	94%	94%
Discharge Instructions[5]	0	-	89%	88%
Evaluation of LVS Function[5]	0	-	98%	98%
Smoking Cessation Advice[5]	0	-	98%	98%
Pneumonia Care				
Appropriate Initial Antibiotic[5]	0	-	92%	92%
Blood Culture Timing[5]	0	-	95%	96%
Influenza Vaccine[5]	0	-	90%	91%
Initial Antibiotic Timing[5]	0	-	93%	95%
Pneumococcal Vaccine[5]	0	-	92%	93%
Smoking Cessation Advice[5]	0	-	98%	97%
Surgical Care Improvement Project				
Appropriate VTP Within 24 Hours[2]	310	96%	94%	92%
Appropriate Hair Removal[2]	566	100%	100%	99%
Appropriate Beta Blocker Usage[2]	147	97%	92%	93%
Controlled Postoperative Blood Glucose[2]	0	-	94%	93%
Prophylactic Antibiotic Timing[2]	367	97%	96%	97%
Prophylactic Antibiotic Timing (Outpatient)	270	97%	92%	92%
Prophylactic Antibiotic Selection[2]	369	100%	97%	97%
Prophylactic Antibiotic Select. (Outpatient)	270	100%	93%	94%
Prophylactic Antibiotic Stopped[2]	365	94%	94%	94%
Recommended VTP Ordered[2]	310	96%	96%	94%
Urinary Catheter Removal[2]	42	88%	90%	90%
Children's Asthma Care				
Received Systemic Corticosteroids	-	-	-	100%
Received Home Management Plan	-	-	-	71%
Received Reliever Medication	-	-	-	100%
Use of Medical Imaging				
Combination Abdominal CT Scan[1]	38	0.237	0.141	0.191
Combination Chest CT Scan	91	0.000	0.024	0.054
Follow-up Mammogram/Ultrasound[5]	0	-	9.8%	8.4%
MRI for Low Back Pain	1,071	22.5%	26.9%	32.7%
Survey of Patients' Hospital Experiences				
Area Around Room 'Always' Quiet at Night	300+	51%	-	58%
Doctors 'Always' Communicated Well	300+	83%	-	80%
Home Recovery Information Given	300+	88%	-	82%
Hospital Given 9 or 10 on 10 Point Scale	300+	85%	-	67%
Meds 'Always' Explained Before Given	300+	60%	-	60%
Nurses 'Always' Communicated Well	300+	79%	-	76%
Pain 'Always' Well Controlled	300+	74%	-	69%
Room and Bathroom 'Always' Clean	300+	78%	-	71%
Timely Help 'Always' Received	300+	63%	-	64%
Would Definitely Recommend Hospital	300+	89%	-	69%

Lenox Hill Hospital

100 East 77th Street — Phone: 212-439-2345
New York, NY 10021
URL: www.lenoxhillhospital.org
Type: Acute Care Hospitals — Emergency Services: Yes
Ownership: Voluntary Non-Profit - Private — Beds: 652

Key Personnel:
Infection Control. . . . . Sarah Petrello
Operating Room. . . . . Richard Green, RN
Pediatric Ambulatory Care . . . . . . Armand Grassi, MD
Quality Assurance . . . . Janice Fajardo
Radiology. . . . . Eric L. Charles
Anesthesiology. . . . . James Richter, MD
Patient Relations . . . . Michael Conroy

Measure	Cases	This Hosp.	State Avg.	U.S. Avg.
Heart Attack Care				
ACE Inhibitor or ARB for LVSD[2]	75	97%	95%	96%
Aspirin at Arrival[2]	136	99%	98%	99%
Aspirin at Discharge[2]	331	100%	98%	98%
Beta Blocker at Discharge[2]	321	99%	98%	98%
Fibrinolytic Medication Timing[2]	0	-	50%	55%
PCI Within 90 Minutes of Arrival[1,2]	15	100%	88%	90%
Smoking Cessation Advice[2]	70	99%	100%	99%
Chest Pain/Possible Heart Attack Care				
Aspirin at Arrival[5]	0	-	96%	95%
Median Time to ECG (minutes)[5]	0	-	11	8
Median Time to Transfer (minutes)[5]	0	-	75	61
Fibrinolytic Medication Timing[5]	0	-	55%	54%
Heart Failure Care				
ACE Inhibitor or ARB for LVSD[2]	192	96%	94%	94%
Discharge Instructions[2]	365	88%	89%	88%
Evaluation of LVS Function[2]	444	100%	98%	98%
Smoking Cessation Advice[2]	54	91%	98%	98%
Pneumonia Care				
Appropriate Initial Antibiotic[2]	88	100%	92%	92%
Blood Culture Timing[2]	171	98%	95%	96%
Influenza Vaccine[2]	94	93%	90%	91%
Initial Antibiotic Timing[2]	133	98%	93%	95%
Pneumococcal Vaccine[2]	141	93%	92%	93%
Smoking Cessation Advice[1,2]	22	100%	98%	97%
Surgical Care Improvement Project				
Appropriate VTP Within 24 Hours[2]	245	98%	94%	92%
Appropriate Hair Removal[2]	741	99%	100%	99%
Appropriate Beta Blocker Usage[2]	266	98%	92%	93%
Controlled Postoperative Blood Glucose[2]	166	93%	94%	93%
Prophylactic Antibiotic Timing[2]	521	98%	96%	97%
Prophylactic Antibiotic Timing (Outpatient)	606	89%	92%	92%
Prophylactic Antibiotic Selection[2]	540	99%	97%	97%
Prophylactic Antibiotic Select. (Outpatient)	577	95%	93%	94%
Prophylactic Antibiotic Stopped[2]	503	98%	94%	94%
Recommended VTP Ordered[2]	247	98%	96%	94%
Urinary Catheter Removal[2]	118	92%	90%	90%
Children's Asthma Care				
Received Systemic Corticosteroids	-	-	-	100%
Received Home Management Plan	-	-	-	71%
Received Reliever Medication	-	-	-	100%
Use of Medical Imaging				
Combination Abdominal CT Scan	567	0.090	0.141	0.191
Combination Chest CT Scan	434	0.009	0.024	0.054
Follow-up Mammogram/Ultrasound	196	36.7%	9.8%	8.4%
MRI for Low Back Pain	84	17.9%	26.9%	32.7%
Survey of Patients' Hospital Experiences				
Area Around Room 'Always' Quiet at Night[11]	300+	49%	-	58%
Doctors 'Always' Communicated Well[11]	300+	79%	-	80%
Home Recovery Information Given[11]	300+	75%	-	82%
Hospital Given 9 or 10 on 10 Point Scale[11]	300+	61%	-	67%
Meds 'Always' Explained Before Given[11]	300+	54%	-	60%
Nurses 'Always' Communicated Well[11]	300+	70%	-	76%
Pain 'Always' Well Controlled[11]	300+	69%	-	69%
Room and Bathroom 'Always' Clean[11]	300+	55%	-	71%
Timely Help 'Always' Received[11]	300+	53%	-	64%
Would Definitely Recommend Hospital[11]	300+	71%	-	69%

NOTE: Hospital profiles are in alphabetical order by state, then city, then hospital within the city; Rankings exclude hospitals with less than 25 cases except for patient surveys which excludes hospitals with less than 100 cases; (a) 100–299 cases; (1) The number of cases is too small to be sure how well a hospital is performing; (2) The hospital indicated that the data submitted for this measure were based on a sample of cases; (3) Data was collected during a shorter time period (fewer quarters) than the maximum possible time for this measure; (4) Suppressed for one or more quarters by CMS; (5) No data is available from the hospital for this measure; (6) Fewer than 100 patients completed the HCAHPS survey. Use these rates with caution, as the number of surveys may be too low to reliably assess hospital performance; (7) Survey results are based on less than 12 months of data; (8) Survey results are not available for this reporting period; (9) No or very few patients were eligible for the HCAHPS survey. The scores shown, if any, reflect a very small number of surveys; (10) A state average was not calculated because too few hospitals in the state submitted data; (11) There were discrepancies in the data collection process; Please refer to the User's Guide for a full explanation of data.

Metropolitan Hospital Center

1901 First Avenue Phone: 212-423-7554
New York, NY 10029 Fax: 212-423-6180
URL: www.nymc.edu/metres/mhc
Type: Acute Care Hospitals Emergency Services: Yes
Ownership: Government - Local Beds: 341

Key Personnel:

Chief of Medical Staff.......... Choi Chang-Shik, MD
Infection Control.............. Joyce Luther
Pediatric Ambulatory Care ...... Sarla Inamdar, MD
Pediatric In-Patient Care .... Sarla Inamdar, MD
Quality Assurance .... Sandy Bezacqua
Radiology.................. Matari Hussein, MD
Anesthesiology............... Joseph Lopez, MD
Emergency Room .... Greg Almond, MD

Measure	Cases	This Hosp.	State Avg.	U.S. Avg.
Heart Attack Care				
ACE Inhibitor or ARB for LVSD[1]	6	100%	95%	96%
Aspirin at Arrival	39	97%	98%	99%
Aspirin at Discharge[1]	18	100%	98%	98%
Beta Blocker at Discharge[1]	17	100%	98%	98%
Fibrinolytic Medication Timing	0	-	50%	55%
PCI Within 90 Minutes of Arrival	0	-	88%	90%
Smoking Cessation Advice[1]	3	100%	100%	99%
Chest Pain/Possible Heart Attack Care				
Aspirin at Arrival[1,3]	1	100%	96%	95%
Median Time to ECG (minutes)[1,3]	2	82	11	8
Median Time to Transfer (minutes)[3]	0	-	75	61
Fibrinolytic Medication Timing[3]	0	-	55%	54%
Heart Failure Care				
ACE Inhibitor or ARB for LVSD	49	100%	94%	94%
Discharge Instructions	128	83%	89%	88%
Evaluation of LVS Function	142	99%	98%	98%
Smoking Cessation Advice[1]	15	100%	98%	98%
Pneumonia Care				
Appropriate Initial Antibiotic	70	100%	92%	92%
Blood Culture Timing	112	92%	95%	96%
Influenza Vaccine	54	98%	90%	91%
Initial Antibiotic Timing	104	96%	93%	95%
Pneumococcal Vaccine	59	92%	92%	93%
Smoking Cessation Advice	39	100%	98%	97%
Surgical Care Improvement Project				
Appropriate VTP Within 24 Hours[2]	128	99%	94%	92%
Appropriate Hair Removal[2]	257	100%	100%	99%
Appropriate Beta Blocker Usage[2]	48	94%	92%	93%
Controlled Postoperative Blood Glucose[2]	0	-	94%	93%
Prophylactic Antibiotic Timing[2]	163	96%	96%	97%
Prophylactic Antibiotic Timing (Outpatient)	65	94%	92%	92%
Prophylactic Antibiotic Selection[2]	163	94%	97%	97%
Prophylactic Antibiotic Select. (Outpatient)	63	97%	93%	94%
Prophylactic Antibiotic Stopped[2]	149	95%	94%	94%
Recommended VTP Ordered[2]	128	99%	96%	94%
Urinary Catheter Removal[2]	46	100%	90%	90%
Children's Asthma Care				
Received Systemic Corticosteroids	-	-	-	100%
Received Home Management Plan	-	-	-	71%
Received Reliever Medication	-	-	-	100%
Use of Medical Imaging				
Combination Abdominal CT Scan	93	0.280	0.141	0.191
Combination Chest CT Scan	56	0.054	0.024	0.054
Follow-up Mammogram/Ultrasound[1]	17	0.0%	9.8%	8.4%
MRI for Low Back Pain[5]	0	-	26.9%	32.7%
Survey of Patients' Hospital Experiences				
Area Around Room 'Always' Quiet at Night	300+	48%	-	58%
Doctors 'Always' Communicated Well	300+	75%	-	80%
Home Recovery Information Given	300+	83%	-	82%
Hospital Given 9 or 10 on 10 Point Scale	300+	62%	-	67%
Meds 'Always' Explained Before Given	300+	53%	-	60%
Nurses 'Always' Communicated Well	300+	62%	-	76%
Pain 'Always' Well Controlled	300+	52%	-	69%
Room and Bathroom 'Always' Clean	300+	59%	-	71%
Timely Help 'Always' Received	300+	48%	-	64%
Would Definitely Recommend Hospital	300+	60%	-	69%

Mount Sinai Hospital

One Gustave L Levy Place Phone: 212-241-7981
New York, NY 10029 Fax: 212-987-1763
URL: www.mountsinai.org
Type: Acute Care Hospitals Emergency Services: Yes
Ownership: Voluntary Non-Profit - Private Beds: 1,171

Key Personnel:

CEO/President............... Judith Willner
Cardiac Laboratory............ Valentin Fuster Md, PhD
Chief of Medical Staff.......... Ira S Nash MD
Operating Room.............. Michael McCarry RN, BS
Quality Assurance .... Vivian Hammer
Radiology.................. Burton P Drayer, MD
Emergency Room .... Andy S Jagoda, MD

Measure	Cases	This Hosp.	State Avg.	U.S. Avg.
Heart Attack Care				
ACE Inhibitor or ARB for LVSD[2]	57	89%	95%	96%
Aspirin at Arrival[2]	188	97%	98%	99%
Aspirin at Discharge[2]	327	98%	98%	98%
Beta Blocker at Discharge[2]	319	96%	98%	98%
Fibrinolytic Medication Timing[2]	0	-	50%	55%
PCI Within 90 Minutes of Arrival[1,2]	11	100%	88%	90%
Smoking Cessation Advice[2]	80	100%	100%	99%
Chest Pain/Possible Heart Attack Care				
Aspirin at Arrival	61	97%	96%	95%
Median Time to ECG (minutes)	64	12	11	8
Median Time to Transfer (minutes)	28	120	75	61
Fibrinolytic Medication Timing	0	-	55%	54%
Heart Failure Care				
ACE Inhibitor or ARB for LVSD[2]	215	95%	94%	94%
Discharge Instructions[2]	441	81%	89%	88%
Evaluation of LVS Function[2]	555	97%	98%	98%
Smoking Cessation Advice[2]	72	97%	98%	98%
Pneumonia Care				
Appropriate Initial Antibiotic[2]	129	91%	92%	92%
Blood Culture Timing[2]	204	95%	95%	96%
Influenza Vaccine[2]	154	83%	90%	91%
Initial Antibiotic Timing[2]	237	92%	93%	95%
Pneumococcal Vaccine[2]	220	79%	92%	93%
Smoking Cessation Advice[2]	68	99%	98%	97%
Surgical Care Improvement Project				
Appropriate VTP Within 24 Hours[2]	526	93%	94%	92%
Appropriate Hair Removal[2]	1,156	99%	100%	99%
Appropriate Beta Blocker Usage[2]	369	96%	92%	93%
Controlled Postoperative Blood Glucose[2]	174	91%	94%	93%
Prophylactic Antibiotic Timing[2]	710	97%	96%	97%
Prophylactic Antibiotic Timing (Outpatient)	557	89%	92%	92%
Prophylactic Antibiotic Selection[2]	721	98%	97%	97%
Prophylactic Antibiotic Select. (Outpatient)	539	95%	93%	94%
Prophylactic Antibiotic Stopped[2]	675	93%	94%	94%
Recommended VTP Ordered[2]	526	97%	96%	94%
Urinary Catheter Removal[2]	257	80%	90%	90%
Children's Asthma Care				
Received Systemic Corticosteroids	-	-	-	100%
Received Home Management Plan	-	-	-	71%
Received Reliever Medication	-	-	-	100%
Use of Medical Imaging				
Combination Abdominal CT Scan	539	0.046	0.141	0.191
Combination Chest CT Scan	169	0.024	0.024	0.054
Follow-up Mammogram/Ultrasound	165	9.1%	9.8%	8.4%
MRI for Low Back Pain[1]	22	27.3%	26.9%	32.7%
Survey of Patients' Hospital Experiences				
Area Around Room 'Always' Quiet at Night	300+	49%	-	58%
Doctors 'Always' Communicated Well	300+	78%	-	80%
Home Recovery Information Given	300+	77%	-	82%
Hospital Given 9 or 10 on 10 Point Scale	300+	62%	-	67%
Meds 'Always' Explained Before Given	300+	53%	-	60%
Nurses 'Always' Communicated Well	300+	71%	-	76%
Pain 'Always' Well Controlled	300+	65%	-	69%
Room and Bathroom 'Always' Clean	300+	62%	-	71%
Timely Help 'Always' Received	300+	51%	-	64%
Would Definitely Recommend Hospital	300+	71%	-	69%

New York Downtown Hospital

170 William Street Phone: 212-312-5000
New York, NY 10038 Fax: 646-292-9588
URL: www.downtownhospital.org
Type: Acute Care Hospitals Emergency Services: Yes
Ownership: Voluntary Non-Profit - Private Beds: 155

Key Personnel:

CEO/President............... Jeffrey Menkes
Chief of Medical Staff.......... Warren Licht, MD
Operating Room.............. Steven Friedman, MD
Pediatric In-Patient Care .... Federic Bajhahr, MD
Quality Assurance .... Marie Cavanough
Anesthesiology............... Lee Winter, MD
Emergency Room .... Antonio Dajer, MD

Measure	Cases	This Hosp.	State Avg.	U.S. Avg.
Heart Attack Care				
ACE Inhibitor or ARB for LVSD[1]	2	100%	95%	96%
Aspirin at Arrival	36	97%	98%	99%
Aspirin at Discharge[1]	8	100%	98%	98%
Beta Blocker at Discharge[1]	7	100%	98%	98%
Fibrinolytic Medication Timing	0	-	50%	55%
PCI Within 90 Minutes of Arrival	0	-	88%	90%
Smoking Cessation Advice[1]	1	100%	100%	99%
Chest Pain/Possible Heart Attack Care				
Aspirin at Arrival	38	92%	96%	95%
Median Time to ECG (minutes)	35	14	11	8
Median Time to Transfer (minutes)[1]	12	120	75	61
Fibrinolytic Medication Timing[1]	1	0%	55%	54%
Heart Failure Care				
ACE Inhibitor or ARB for LVSD	39	95%	94%	94%
Discharge Instructions	119	97%	89%	88%
Evaluation of LVS Function	133	100%	98%	98%
Smoking Cessation Advice[1]	23	100%	98%	98%
Pneumonia Care				
Appropriate Initial Antibiotic[2]	107	96%	92%	92%
Blood Culture Timing[2]	155	99%	95%	96%
Influenza Vaccine[2]	84	93%	90%	91%
Initial Antibiotic Timing[2]	139	96%	93%	95%
Pneumococcal Vaccine[2]	159	91%	92%	93%
Smoking Cessation Advice[2]	35	100%	98%	97%
Surgical Care Improvement Project				
Appropriate VTP Within 24 Hours[2]	144	94%	94%	92%
Appropriate Hair Removal[2]	316	100%	100%	99%
Appropriate Beta Blocker Usage[2]	65	92%	92%	93%
Controlled Postoperative Blood Glucose[2]	0	-	94%	93%
Prophylactic Antibiotic Timing[2]	214	100%	96%	97%
Prophylactic Antibiotic Timing (Outpatient)	76	89%	92%	92%
Prophylactic Antibiotic Selection[2]	213	98%	97%	97%
Prophylactic Antibiotic Select. (Outpatient)	69	100%	93%	94%
Prophylactic Antibiotic Stopped[2]	208	95%	94%	94%
Recommended VTP Ordered[2]	144	96%	96%	94%
Urinary Catheter Removal[2]	36	94%	90%	90%
Children's Asthma Care				
Received Systemic Corticosteroids	-	-	-	100%
Received Home Management Plan	-	-	-	71%
Received Reliever Medication	-	-	-	100%
Use of Medical Imaging				
Combination Abdominal CT Scan	194	0.088	0.141	0.191
Combination Chest CT Scan	101	0.040	0.024	0.054
Follow-up Mammogram/Ultrasound	191	37.7%	9.8%	8.4%
MRI for Low Back Pain[5]	0	-	26.9%	32.7%
Survey of Patients' Hospital Experiences				
Area Around Room 'Always' Quiet at Night	300+	37%	-	58%
Doctors 'Always' Communicated Well	300+	66%	-	80%
Home Recovery Information Given	300+	73%	-	82%
Hospital Given 9 or 10 on 10 Point Scale	300+	37%	-	67%
Meds 'Always' Explained Before Given	300+	48%	-	60%
Nurses 'Always' Communicated Well	300+	57%	-	76%
Pain 'Always' Well Controlled	300+	52%	-	69%
Room and Bathroom 'Always' Clean	300+	57%	-	71%
Timely Help 'Always' Received	300+	46%	-	64%
Would Definitely Recommend Hospital	300+	43%	-	69%

NOTE: Hospital profiles are in alphabetical order by state, then city, then hospital within the city; Rankings exclude hospitals with less than 25 cases except for patient surveys which excludes hospitals with less than 100 cases; (a) 100–299 cases; (1) The number of cases is too small to be sure how well a hospital is performing; (2) The hospital indicated that the data submitted for this measure were based on a sample of cases; (3) Data was collected during a shorter time period (fewer quarters) than the maximum possible time for this measure; (4) Suppressed for one or more quarters by CMS; (5) No data is available from the hospital for this measure; (6) Fewer than 100 patients completed the HCAHPS survey. Use these rates with caution, as the number of surveys may be too low to reliably assess hospital performance; (7) Survey results are based on less than 12 months of data; (8) Survey results are not available for this reporting period; (9) No or very few patients were eligible for the HCAHPS survey. The scores shown, if any, reflect a very small number of surveys; (10) A state average was not calculated because too few hospitals in the state submitted data; (11) There were discrepancies in the data collection process; Please refer to the User's Guide for a full explanation of data.

New York-Presbyterian Hospital

525 East 68th Street
New York, NY 10021
E-mail: publicaffairs@med.cornell.edu
URL: www.nyp.org
Type: Acute Care Hospitals
Ownership: Voluntary Non-Profit - Private
Phone: 212-746-4189
Fax: 212-821-0576
Emergency Services: Yes
Beds: 2,344

Key Personnel:
CEO/President. . . . . Herbert Pardes, MD
Chief of Medical Staff . . . . Laura L Forese, MD
Operating Room. . . . . Robert L Jones, MD
Pediatric In-Patient Care . . . . . . Lawrence Stanberry, MD
Quality Assurance . . . . John V Campano, Esq
Radiology. . . . . Lawrence Schwartz, MD
Anesthesiology. . . . . Magaret Wood, MD
Patient Relations . . . . Andrea Colon

Measure	Cases	This Hosp.	State Avg.	U.S. Avg.
Heart Attack Care				
ACE Inhibitor or ARB for LVSD[2]	158	94%	95%	96%
Aspirin at Arrival[2]	353	99%	98%	99%
Aspirin at Discharge[2]	744	98%	98%	98%
Beta Blocker at Discharge[2]	718	95%	98%	98%
Fibrinolytic Medication Timing[2]	0	-	50%	55%
PCI Within 90 Minutes of Arrival[2]	46	96%	88%	90%
Smoking Cessation Advice[2]	152	99%	100%	99%
Chest Pain/Possible Heart Attack Care				
Aspirin at Arrival[5]	0	-	96%	95%
Median Time to ECG (minutes)[5]	0	-	11	8
Median Time to Transfer (minutes)[5]	0	-	75	61
Fibrinolytic Medication Timing[5]	0	-	55%	54%
Heart Failure Care				
ACE Inhibitor or ARB for LVSD[2]	452	87%	94%	94%
Discharge Instructions[2]	883	70%	89%	88%
Evaluation of LVS Function[2]	1,062	97%	98%	98%
Smoking Cessation Advice[2]	87	97%	98%	98%
Pneumonia Care				
Appropriate Initial Antibiotic[2]	210	94%	92%	92%
Blood Culture Timing[2]	549	91%	95%	96%
Influenza Vaccine[2]	410	91%	90%	91%
Initial Antibiotic Timing[2]	465	83%	93%	95%
Pneumococcal Vaccine[2]	590	90%	92%	93%
Smoking Cessation Advice[2]	109	95%	98%	97%
Surgical Care Improvement Project				
Appropriate VTP Within 24 Hours[2]	633	100%	94%	92%
Appropriate Hair Removal[2]	1,737	100%	100%	99%
Appropriate Beta Blocker Usage[2]	539	99%	92%	93%
Controlled Postoperative Blood Glucose[2]	339	87%	94%	93%
Prophylactic Antibiotic Timing[2]	811	95%	96%	97%
Prophylactic Antibiotic Timing (Outpatient)	1,187	90%	92%	92%
Prophylactic Antibiotic Selection[2]	954	97%	97%	97%
Prophylactic Antibiotic Select. (Outpatient)	1,154	90%	93%	94%
Prophylactic Antibiotic Stopped[2]	776	93%	94%	94%
Recommended VTP Ordered[2]	635	100%	96%	94%
Urinary Catheter Removal[2]	234	91%	90%	90%
Children's Asthma Care				
Received Systemic Corticosteroids	412	100%	-	100%
Received Home Management Plan[2]	410	78%	-	71%
Received Reliever Medication	412	100%	-	100%
Use of Medical Imaging				
Combination Abdominal CT Scan	2,357	0.415	0.141	0.191
Combination Chest CT Scan	2,332	0.025	0.024	0.054
Follow-up Mammogram/Ultrasound	3,236	7.7%	9.8%	8.4%
MRI for Low Back Pain	192	25.0%	26.9%	32.7%
Survey of Patients' Hospital Experiences				
Area Around Room 'Always' Quiet at Night	300+	54%	-	58%
Doctors 'Always' Communicated Well	300+	78%	-	80%
Home Recovery Information Given	300+	78%	-	82%
Hospital Given 9 or 10 on 10 Point Scale	300+	73%	-	67%
Meds 'Always' Explained Before Given	300+	58%	-	60%
Nurses 'Always' Communicated Well	300+	72%	-	76%
Pain 'Always' Well Controlled	300+	65%	-	69%
Room and Bathroom 'Always' Clean	300+	64%	-	71%
Timely Help 'Always' Received	300+	55%	-	64%
Would Definitely Recommend Hospital	300+	80%	-	69%

North General Hospital

1879 Madison Avenue
New York, NY 10035
Type: Acute Care Hospitals
Ownership: Voluntary Non-Profit - Private
Phone: 212-650-4000
Emergency Services: Yes

Measure	Cases	This Hosp.	State Avg.	U.S. Avg.
Heart Attack Care				
ACE Inhibitor or ARB for LVSD	-	-	95%	96%
Aspirin at Arrival	-	-	98%	99%
Aspirin at Discharge	-	-	98%	98%
Beta Blocker at Discharge	-	-	98%	98%
Fibrinolytic Medication Timing	-	-	50%	55%
PCI Within 90 Minutes of Arrival	-	-	88%	90%
Smoking Cessation Advice	-	-	100%	99%
Chest Pain/Possible Heart Attack Care				
Aspirin at Arrival	-	-	96%	95%
Median Time to ECG (minutes)	-	-	11	8
Median Time to Transfer (minutes)	-	-	75	61
Fibrinolytic Medication Timing	-	-	55%	54%
Heart Failure Care				
ACE Inhibitor or ARB for LVSD	-	-	94%	94%
Discharge Instructions	-	-	89%	88%
Evaluation of LVS Function	-	-	98%	98%
Smoking Cessation Advice	-	-	98%	98%
Pneumonia Care				
Appropriate Initial Antibiotic	-	-	92%	92%
Blood Culture Timing	-	-	95%	96%
Influenza Vaccine	-	-	90%	91%
Initial Antibiotic Timing	-	-	93%	95%
Pneumococcal Vaccine	-	-	92%	93%
Smoking Cessation Advice	-	-	98%	97%
Surgical Care Improvement Project				
Appropriate VTP Within 24 Hours	-	-	94%	92%
Appropriate Hair Removal	-	-	100%	99%
Appropriate Beta Blocker Usage	-	-	92%	93%
Controlled Postoperative Blood Glucose	-	-	94%	93%
Prophylactic Antibiotic Timing	-	-	96%	97%
Prophylactic Antibiotic Timing (Outpatient)	-	-	92%	92%
Prophylactic Antibiotic Selection	-	-	97%	97%
Prophylactic Antibiotic Select. (Outpatient)	-	-	93%	94%
Prophylactic Antibiotic Stopped	-	-	94%	94%
Recommended VTP Ordered	-	-	96%	94%
Urinary Catheter Removal	-	-	90%	90%
Children's Asthma Care				
Received Systemic Corticosteroids	-	-	-	100%
Received Home Management Plan	-	-	-	71%
Received Reliever Medication	-	-	-	100%
Use of Medical Imaging				
Combination Abdominal CT Scan	-	-	0.141	0.191
Combination Chest CT Scan	-	-	0.024	0.054
Follow-up Mammogram/Ultrasound	-	-	9.8%	8.4%
MRI for Low Back Pain	-	-	26.9%	32.7%
Survey of Patients' Hospital Experiences				
Area Around Room 'Always' Quiet at Night	-	-	-	58%
Doctors 'Always' Communicated Well	-	-	-	80%
Home Recovery Information Given	-	-	-	82%
Hospital Given 9 or 10 on 10 Point Scale	-	-	-	67%
Meds 'Always' Explained Before Given	-	-	-	60%
Nurses 'Always' Communicated Well	-	-	-	76%
Pain 'Always' Well Controlled	-	-	-	69%
Room and Bathroom 'Always' Clean	-	-	-	71%
Timely Help 'Always' Received	-	-	-	64%
Would Definitely Recommend Hospital	-	-	-	69%

NY Eye and Ear Infirmary

310 East 14th Street
New York, NY 10003
URL: www.nyee.edu
Type: Acute Care Hospitals
Ownership: Voluntary Non-Profit - Private
Phone: 212-979-4000
Fax: 212-228-0664
Emergency Services: No
Beds: 103

Key Personnel:
Infection Control. . . . . Mercy Nelson, RN
Operating Room. . . . . Nitin Sheth, RN
Quality Assurance . . . . Linda Klingos, RN
Radiology. . . . . Roy Holliday, MD
Ambulatory Care . . . . Ann Marie Palladino
Anesthesiology. . . . . Robert Durell, MD

Measure	Cases	This Hosp.	State Avg.	U.S. Avg.
Heart Attack Care				
ACE Inhibitor or ARB for LVSD[5]	0	-	95%	96%
Aspirin at Arrival[5]	0	-	98%	99%
Aspirin at Discharge[5]	0	-	98%	98%
Beta Blocker at Discharge[5]	0	-	98%	98%
Fibrinolytic Medication Timing[5]	0	-	50%	55%
PCI Within 90 Minutes of Arrival[5]	0	-	88%	90%
Smoking Cessation Advice[5]	0	-	100%	99%
Chest Pain/Possible Heart Attack Care				
Aspirin at Arrival[5]	0	-	96%	95%
Median Time to ECG (minutes)[5]	0	-	11	8
Median Time to Transfer (minutes)[5]	0	-	75	61
Fibrinolytic Medication Timing[5]	0	-	55%	54%
Heart Failure Care				
ACE Inhibitor or ARB for LVSD[5]	0	-	94%	94%
Discharge Instructions[5]	0	-	89%	88%
Evaluation of LVS Function[5]	0	-	98%	98%
Smoking Cessation Advice[5]	0	-	98%	98%
Pneumonia Care				
Appropriate Initial Antibiotic[5]	0	-	92%	92%
Blood Culture Timing[5]	0	-	95%	96%
Influenza Vaccine[5]	0	-	90%	91%
Initial Antibiotic Timing[5]	0	-	93%	95%
Pneumococcal Vaccine[5]	0	-	92%	93%
Smoking Cessation Advice[5]	0	-	98%	97%
Surgical Care Improvement Project				
Appropriate VTP Within 24 Hours[5]	0	-	94%	92%
Appropriate Hair Removal[5]	0	-	100%	99%
Appropriate Beta Blocker Usage[5]	0	-	92%	93%
Controlled Postoperative Blood Glucose[5]	0	-	94%	93%
Prophylactic Antibiotic Timing[5]	0	-	96%	97%
Prophylactic Antibiotic Timing (Outpatient)[5]	0	-	92%	92%
Prophylactic Antibiotic Selection[5]	0	-	97%	97%
Prophylactic Antibiotic Select. (Outpatient)[5]	0	-	93%	94%
Prophylactic Antibiotic Stopped[5]	0	-	94%	94%
Recommended VTP Ordered[5]	0	-	96%	94%
Urinary Catheter Removal[5]	0	-	90%	90%
Children's Asthma Care				
Received Systemic Corticosteroids	-	-	-	100%
Received Home Management Plan	-	-	-	71%
Received Reliever Medication	-	-	-	100%
Use of Medical Imaging				
Combination Abdominal CT Scan[1]	6	0.667	0.141	0.191
Combination Chest CT Scan[1]	16	0.000	0.024	0.054
Follow-up Mammogram/Ultrasound[5]	0	-	9.8%	8.4%
MRI for Low Back Pain[5]	0	-	26.9%	32.7%
Survey of Patients' Hospital Experiences				
Area Around Room 'Always' Quiet at Night	300+	63%	-	58%
Doctors 'Always' Communicated Well	300+	75%	-	80%
Home Recovery Information Given	300+	75%	-	82%
Hospital Given 9 or 10 on 10 Point Scale	300+	60%	-	67%
Meds 'Always' Explained Before Given	300+	54%	-	60%
Nurses 'Always' Communicated Well	300+	68%	-	76%
Pain 'Always' Well Controlled	300+	62%	-	69%
Room and Bathroom 'Always' Clean	300+	68%	-	71%
Timely Help 'Always' Received	300+	60%	-	64%
Would Definitely Recommend Hospital	300+	72%	-	69%

NOTE: Hospital profiles are in alphabetical order by state, then city, then hospital within the city; Rankings exclude hospitals with less than 25 cases except for patient surveys which excludes hospitals with less than 100 cases; (a) 100–299 cases; (1) The number of cases is too small to be sure how well a hospital is performing; (2) The hospital indicated that the data submitted for this measure were based on a sample of cases; (3) Data was collected during a shorter time period (fewer quarters) than the maximum possible time for this measure; (4) Suppressed for one or more quarters by CMS; (5) No data is available from the hospital for this measure; (6) Fewer than 100 patients completed the HCAHPS survey. Use these rates with caution, as the number of surveys may be too low to reliably assess hospital performance; (7) Survey results are based on less than 12 months of data; (8) Survey results are not available for this reporting period; (9) No or very few patients were eligible for the HCAHPS survey. The scores shown, if any, reflect a very small number of surveys; (10) A state average was not calculated because too few hospitals in the state submitted data; (11) There were discrepancies in the data collection process; Please refer to the User's Guide for a full explanation of data.

NYU Hospitals Center

550 First Avenue Phone: 212-263-7300
New York, NY 10016 Fax: 212-263-6690
URL: www.med.nyu.edu
Type: Acute Care Hospitals Emergency Services: Yes
Ownership: Voluntary Non-Profit - Private Beds: 1,069

Key Personnel:

CEO/President. . . . . Robert I Grossman, MD
Chief of Medical Staff. . . . . Andrew W Litt, MD
Infection Control. . . . . Roger Wetherbee, MD
Operating Room. . . . . H Leon Patcher, RN
Pediatric In-Patient Care . . . . Catherin Scott Manno, MD
Quality Assurance . . . . John Bittoni
Radiology. . . . . Michael Recht, MD

Measure	Cases	This Hosp.	State Avg.	U.S. Avg.
Heart Attack Care				
ACE Inhibitor or ARB for LVSD	47	100%	95%	96%
Aspirin at Arrival	223	100%	98%	99%
Aspirin at Discharge	254	100%	98%	98%
Beta Blocker at Discharge	248	99%	98%	98%
Fibrinolytic Medication Timing	0	-	50%	55%
PCI Within 90 Minutes of Arrival	29	90%	88%	90%
Smoking Cessation Advice	48	100%	100%	99%
Chest Pain/Possible Heart Attack Care				
Aspirin at Arrival[5]	0	-	96%	95%
Median Time to ECG (minutes)[5]	0	-	11	8
Median Time to Transfer (minutes)[5]	0	-	75	61
Fibrinolytic Medication Timing[5]	0	-	55%	54%
Heart Failure Care				
ACE Inhibitor or ARB for LVSD[2]	83	100%	94%	94%
Discharge Instructions[2]	217	97%	89%	88%
Evaluation of LVS Function[2]	283	100%	98%	98%
Smoking Cessation Advice[1,2]	23	100%	98%	98%
Pneumonia Care				
Appropriate Initial Antibiotic[2]	74	100%	92%	92%
Blood Culture Timing[2]	140	96%	95%	96%
Influenza Vaccine[2]	84	98%	90%	91%
Initial Antibiotic Timing[2]	129	98%	93%	95%
Pneumococcal Vaccine[2]	138	98%	92%	93%
Smoking Cessation Advice[2]	25	100%	98%	97%
Surgical Care Improvement Project				
Appropriate VTP Within 24 Hours[2]	274	98%	94%	92%
Appropriate Hair Removal[2]	710	100%	100%	99%
Appropriate Beta Blocker Usage[2]	214	98%	92%	93%
Controlled Postoperative Blood Glucose[2]	131	98%	94%	93%
Prophylactic Antibiotic Timing[2]	485	98%	96%	97%
Prophylactic Antibiotic Timing (Outpatient)	422	99%	92%	92%
Prophylactic Antibiotic Selection[2]	490	98%	97%	97%
Prophylactic Antibiotic Select. (Outpatient)	422	96%	93%	94%
Prophylactic Antibiotic Stopped[2]	462	98%	94%	94%
Recommended VTP Ordered[2]	274	100%	96%	94%
Urinary Catheter Removal[2]	169	93%	90%	90%
Children's Asthma Care				
Received Systemic Corticosteroids[1,2]	19	100%	-	100%
Received Home Management Plan[1]	19	0%	-	71%
Received Reliever Medication[1,2]	19	100%	-	100%
Use of Medical Imaging				
Combination Abdominal CT Scan	228	0.035	0.141	0.191
Combination Chest CT Scan	77	0.000	0.024	0.054
Follow-up Mammogram/Ultrasound	1,071	8.8%	9.8%	8.4%
MRI for Low Back Pain	87	24.1%	26.9%	32.7%
Survey of Patients' Hospital Experiences				
Area Around Room 'Always' Quiet at Night[11]	300+	43%	-	58%
Doctors 'Always' Communicated Well[11]	300+	75%	-	80%
Home Recovery Information Given[11]	300+	78%	-	82%
Hospital Given 9 or 10 on 10 Point Scale[11]	300+	61%	-	67%
Meds 'Always' Explained Before Given[11]	300+	58%	-	60%
Nurses 'Always' Communicated Well[11]	300+	71%	-	76%
Pain 'Always' Well Controlled[11]	300+	64%	-	69%
Room and Bathroom 'Always' Clean[11]	300+	60%	-	71%
Timely Help 'Always' Received[11]	300+	53%	-	64%
Would Definitely Recommend Hospital[11]	300+	71%	-	69%

Saint Luke's Roosevelt Hospital

1111 Amsterdam Avenue Phone: 212-523-4000
New York, NY 10025 Fax: 212-523-2617
URL: www.wehealny.org
Type: Acute Care Hospitals Emergency Services: Yes
Ownership: Voluntary Non-Profit - Private Beds: 1,354

Key Personnel:

CEO/President. . . . . Frank J. Cracolici
Chief of Medical Staff. . . . . Robert Catalano
Infection Control. . . . . Bruce Polsky, MD
Operating Room. . . . . George J Todd, MD/FACS
Quality Assurance . . . . Timothy Day
Anesthesiology. . . . . Joanne Miller, MD
Emergency Room . . . . Richard G Lanoix, MD

Measure	Cases	This Hosp.	State Avg.	U.S. Avg.
Heart Attack Care				
ACE Inhibitor or ARB for LVSD[2]	88	95%	95%	96%
Aspirin at Arrival[2]	312	99%	98%	99%
Aspirin at Discharge[2]	294	98%	98%	98%
Beta Blocker at Discharge[2]	290	96%	98%	98%
Fibrinolytic Medication Timing[2]	0	-	50%	55%
PCI Within 90 Minutes of Arrival[2]	46	70%	88%	90%
Smoking Cessation Advice[2]	98	100%	100%	99%
Chest Pain/Possible Heart Attack Care				
Aspirin at Arrival[5]	0	-	96%	95%
Median Time to ECG (minutes)[5]	0	-	11	8
Median Time to Transfer (minutes)[5]	0	-	75	61
Fibrinolytic Medication Timing[5]	0	-	55%	54%
Heart Failure Care				
ACE Inhibitor or ARB for LVSD[2]	166	94%	94%	94%
Discharge Instructions[2]	282	96%	89%	88%
Evaluation of LVS Function[2]	324	97%	98%	98%
Smoking Cessation Advice[2]	70	100%	98%	98%
Pneumonia Care				
Appropriate Initial Antibiotic[2]	115	91%	92%	92%
Blood Culture Timing[2]	176	97%	95%	96%
Influenza Vaccine[2]	93	52%	90%	91%
Initial Antibiotic Timing[2]	178	93%	93%	95%
Pneumococcal Vaccine[2]	129	66%	92%	93%
Smoking Cessation Advice[2]	58	100%	98%	97%
Surgical Care Improvement Project				
Appropriate VTP Within 24 Hours[2]	322	92%	94%	92%
Appropriate Hair Removal[2]	768	99%	100%	99%
Appropriate Beta Blocker Usage[2]	181	86%	92%	93%
Controlled Postoperative Blood Glucose[2]	144	96%	94%	93%
Prophylactic Antibiotic Timing[2]	571	94%	96%	97%
Prophylactic Antibiotic Timing (Outpatient)	341	92%	92%	92%
Prophylactic Antibiotic Selection[2]	579	96%	97%	97%
Prophylactic Antibiotic Select. (Outpatient)	323	93%	93%	94%
Prophylactic Antibiotic Stopped[2]	549	94%	94%	94%
Recommended VTP Ordered[2]	322	92%	96%	94%
Urinary Catheter Removal[2]	178	93%	90%	90%
Children's Asthma Care				
Received Systemic Corticosteroids	-	-	-	100%
Received Home Management Plan	-	-	-	71%
Received Reliever Medication	-	-	-	100%
Use of Medical Imaging				
Combination Abdominal CT Scan	683	0.081	0.141	0.191
Combination Chest CT Scan	417	0.012	0.024	0.054
Follow-up Mammogram/Ultrasound	246	6.5%	9.8%	8.4%
MRI for Low Back Pain[1]	57	22.8%	26.9%	32.7%
Survey of Patients' Hospital Experiences				
Area Around Room 'Always' Quiet at Night	300+	48%	-	58%
Doctors 'Always' Communicated Well	300+	73%	-	80%
Home Recovery Information Given	300+	72%	-	82%
Hospital Given 9 or 10 on 10 Point Scale	300+	50%	-	67%
Meds 'Always' Explained Before Given	300+	51%	-	60%
Nurses 'Always' Communicated Well	300+	62%	-	76%
Pain 'Always' Well Controlled	300+	58%	-	69%
Room and Bathroom 'Always' Clean	300+	54%	-	71%
Timely Help 'Always' Received	300+	47%	-	64%
Would Definitely Recommend Hospital	300+	60%	-	69%

VA New York Harbor Healthcare System

423 East 23rd Street Phone: 212-686-7500
New York, NY 10010 Fax: 212-951-3375
URL: www.nyharbor.va.gov
Type: Acute Care-Veterans Administration Emergency Services: No
Ownership: Government - Federal Beds: 350

Key Personnel:

Chief of Medical Staff. . . . . Michael Simberkoff
Infection Control. . . . . Michael Simberkoff, MD
Operating Room. . . . . Doris Richardson, RN
Quality Assurance . . . . May Mayor, RN
Radiology. . . . . Norma Ettenger, MD
Anesthesiology. . . . . Patrick Annello, MD
Intensive Care Unit. . . . . Elvira Miller

Measure	Cases	This Hosp.	State Avg.	U.S. Avg.
Heart Attack Care				
ACE Inhibitor or ARB for LVSD[1]	23	96%	95%	96%
Aspirin at Arrival	86	100%	98%	99%
Aspirin at Discharge	117	99%	98%	98%
Beta Blocker at Discharge	107	99%	98%	98%
Fibrinolytic Medication Timing[1]	4	75%	50%	55%
PCI Within 90 Minutes of Arrival[1]	5	60%	88%	90%
Smoking Cessation Advice	31	100%	100%	99%
Chest Pain/Possible Heart Attack Care				
Aspirin at Arrival	-	-	96%	95%
Median Time to ECG (minutes)	-	-	11	8
Median Time to Transfer (minutes)	-	-	75	61
Fibrinolytic Medication Timing	-	-	55%	54%
Heart Failure Care				
ACE Inhibitor or ARB for LVSD	167	93%	94%	94%
Discharge Instructions	353	98%	89%	88%
Evaluation of LVS Function	364	100%	98%	98%
Smoking Cessation Advice	61	98%	98%	98%
Pneumonia Care				
Appropriate Initial Antibiotic	88	95%	92%	92%
Blood Culture Timing	157	97%	95%	96%
Influenza Vaccine	98	80%	90%	91%
Initial Antibiotic Timing	143	94%	93%	95%
Pneumococcal Vaccine	131	97%	92%	93%
Smoking Cessation Advice	48	100%	98%	97%
Surgical Care Improvement Project				
Appropriate VTP Within 24 Hours[2]	108	99%	94%	92%
Appropriate Hair Removal[2]	243	100%	100%	99%
Appropriate Beta Blocker Usage[2]	128	99%	92%	93%
Controlled Postoperative Blood Glucose[2]	75	91%	94%	93%
Prophylactic Antibiotic Timing	140	100%	96%	97%
Prophylactic Antibiotic Timing (Outpatient)	-	-	92%	92%
Prophylactic Antibiotic Selection	149	100%	97%	97%
Prophylactic Antibiotic Select. (Outpatient)	-	-	93%	94%
Prophylactic Antibiotic Stopped	136	93%	94%	94%
Recommended VTP Ordered[2]	109	98%	96%	94%
Urinary Catheter Removal[2]	55	100%	90%	90%
Children's Asthma Care				
Received Systemic Corticosteroids	-	-	-	100%
Received Home Management Plan	-	-	-	71%
Received Reliever Medication	-	-	-	100%
Use of Medical Imaging				
Combination Abdominal CT Scan	-	-	0.141	0.191
Combination Chest CT Scan	-	-	0.024	0.054
Follow-up Mammogram/Ultrasound	-	-	9.8%	8.4%
MRI for Low Back Pain	-	-	26.9%	32.7%
Survey of Patients' Hospital Experiences				
Area Around Room 'Always' Quiet at Night	-	-	-	58%
Doctors 'Always' Communicated Well	-	-	-	80%
Home Recovery Information Given	-	-	-	82%
Hospital Given 9 or 10 on 10 Point Scale	-	-	-	67%
Meds 'Always' Explained Before Given	-	-	-	60%
Nurses 'Always' Communicated Well	-	-	-	76%
Pain 'Always' Well Controlled	-	-	-	69%
Room and Bathroom 'Always' Clean	-	-	-	71%
Timely Help 'Always' Received	-	-	-	64%
Would Definitely Recommend Hospital	-	-	-	69%

NOTE: Hospital profiles are in alphabetical order by state, then city, then hospital within the city; Rankings exclude hospitals with less than 25 cases except for patient surveys which excludes hospitals with less than 100 cases; (a) 100–299 cases; (1) The number of cases is too small to be sure how well a hospital is performing; (2) The hospital indicated that the data submitted for this measure were based on a sample of cases; (3) Data was collected during a shorter time period (fewer quarters) than the maximum possible time for this measure; (4) Suppressed for one or more quarters by CMS; (5) No data is available from the hospital for this measure; (6) Fewer than 100 patients completed the HCAHPS survey. Use these rates with caution, as the number of surveys may be too low to reliably assess hospital performance; (7) Survey results are based on less than 12 months of data; (8) Survey results are not available for this reporting period; (9) No or very few patients were eligible for the HCAHPS survey. The scores shown, if any, reflect a very small number of surveys; (10) A state average was not calculated because too few hospitals in the state submitted data; (11) There were discrepancies in the data collection process; Please refer to the User's Guide for a full explanation of data.

Newark-Wayne Community Hospital

111 Driving Park Avenue Phone: 315-332-2022
Newark, NY 14513
URL: www.viahealth.org/home_newarkwayne.cfm
Type: Acute Care Hospitals Emergency Services: Yes
Ownership: Voluntary Non-Profit - Private
Key Personnel:
CEO/President. . . . . Annette Leahy
Chief of Medical Staff . . . . Arun Nagpaul MD
Emergency Room . . . . Frank Edwards

Measure	Cases	This Hosp.	State Avg.	U.S. Avg.
Heart Attack Care				
ACE Inhibitor or ARB for LVSD[1]	3	100%	95%	96%
Aspirin at Arrival	43	98%	98%	99%
Aspirin at Discharge	32	94%	98%	98%
Beta Blocker at Discharge	30	100%	98%	98%
Fibrinolytic Medication Timing	0	-	50%	55%
PCI Within 90 Minutes of Arrival	0	-	88%	90%
Smoking Cessation Advice[1]	5	100%	100%	99%
Chest Pain/Possible Heart Attack Care				
Aspirin at Arrival	145	94%	96%	95%
Median Time to ECG (minutes)	147	10	11	8
Median Time to Transfer (minutes)[1]	18	93	75	61
Fibrinolytic Medication Timing	0	-	55%	54%
Heart Failure Care				
ACE Inhibitor or ARB for LVSD	26	96%	94%	94%
Discharge Instructions	78	87%	89%	88%
Evaluation of LVS Function	108	99%	98%	98%
Smoking Cessation Advice[1]	13	100%	98%	98%
Pneumonia Care				
Appropriate Initial Antibiotic	91	85%	92%	92%
Blood Culture Timing	121	96%	95%	96%
Influenza Vaccine	75	97%	90%	91%
Initial Antibiotic Timing	136	98%	93%	95%
Pneumococcal Vaccine	105	96%	92%	93%
Smoking Cessation Advice	53	100%	98%	97%
Surgical Care Improvement Project				
Appropriate VTP Within 24 Hours	95	96%	94%	92%
Appropriate Hair Removal	259	100%	100%	99%
Appropriate Beta Blocker Usage	77	79%	92%	93%
Controlled Postoperative Blood Glucose	0	-	94%	93%
Prophylactic Antibiotic Timing	192	97%	96%	97%
Prophylactic Antibiotic Timing (Outpatient)	76	86%	92%	92%
Prophylactic Antibiotic Selection	191	99%	97%	97%
Prophylactic Antibiotic Select. (Outpatient)	67	97%	93%	94%
Prophylactic Antibiotic Stopped	188	91%	94%	94%
Recommended VTP Ordered	95	97%	96%	94%
Urinary Catheter Removal[1]	18	100%	90%	90%
Children's Asthma Care				
Received Systemic Corticosteroids	-	-	-	100%
Received Home Management Plan	-	-	-	71%
Received Reliever Medication	-	-	-	100%
Use of Medical Imaging				
Combination Abdominal CT Scan	233	0.442	0.141	0.191
Combination Chest CT Scan	148	0.088	0.024	0.054
Follow-up Mammogram/Ultrasound	346	5.5%	9.8%	8.4%
MRI for Low Back Pain[1]	35	31.4%	26.9%	32.7%
Survey of Patients' Hospital Experiences				
Area Around Room 'Always' Quiet at Night	300+	49%	-	58%
Doctors 'Always' Communicated Well	300+	80%	-	80%
Home Recovery Information Given	300+	87%	-	82%
Hospital Given 9 or 10 on 10 Point Scale	300+	63%	-	67%
Meds 'Always' Explained Before Given	300+	62%	-	60%
Nurses 'Always' Communicated Well	300+	78%	-	76%
Pain 'Always' Well Controlled	300+	70%	-	69%
Room and Bathroom 'Always' Clean	300+	69%	-	71%
Timely Help 'Always' Received	300+	69%	-	64%
Would Definitely Recommend Hospital	300+	61%	-	69%

Saint Luke's Cornwall Hospital

70 Dubois Street Phone: 845-561-4400
Newburgh, NY 12550 Fax: 845-568-2902
URL: www.stlukeshospital.org
Type: Acute Care Hospitals Emergency Services: No
Ownership: Voluntary Non-Profit - Other Beds: 259
Key Personnel:
CEO/President. . . . . Allan E. Atzrott
Cardiac Laboratory. . . . . Nirav D. Shah, MD
Operating Room. . . . . Jackie Veerboom
Pediatric In-Patient Care . . . . . . Kathy Sellick
Quality Assurance . . . . Patty Smith
Radiology. . . . . Clifford Barker, MD
Hemotology Center . . . . Kathy Sellick
Patient Relations . . . . Renita McGuiness

Measure	Cases	This Hosp.	State Avg.	U.S. Avg.
Heart Attack Care				
ACE Inhibitor or ARB for LVSD	28	100%	95%	96%
Aspirin at Arrival	190	99%	98%	99%
Aspirin at Discharge	168	99%	98%	98%
Beta Blocker at Discharge	164	100%	98%	98%
Fibrinolytic Medication Timing	0	-	50%	55%
PCI Within 90 Minutes of Arrival	30	90%	88%	90%
Smoking Cessation Advice	45	100%	100%	99%
Chest Pain/Possible Heart Attack Care				
Aspirin at Arrival	54	96%	96%	95%
Median Time to ECG (minutes)	55	1	11	8
Median Time to Transfer (minutes)[5]	0	-	75	61
Fibrinolytic Medication Timing[3]	0	-	55%	54%
Heart Failure Care				
ACE Inhibitor or ARB for LVSD	119	93%	94%	94%
Discharge Instructions	337	80%	89%	88%
Evaluation of LVS Function	429	100%	98%	98%
Smoking Cessation Advice	50	100%	98%	98%
Pneumonia Care				
Appropriate Initial Antibiotic[2]	115	86%	92%	92%
Blood Culture Timing[2]	157	92%	95%	96%
Influenza Vaccine[2]	106	85%	90%	91%
Initial Antibiotic Timing[2]	169	89%	93%	95%
Pneumococcal Vaccine[2]	153	88%	92%	93%
Smoking Cessation Advice[2]	49	96%	98%	97%
Surgical Care Improvement Project				
Appropriate VTP Within 24 Hours[2]	123	90%	94%	92%
Appropriate Hair Removal[2]	360	100%	100%	99%
Appropriate Beta Blocker Usage[2]	95	98%	92%	93%
Controlled Postoperative Blood Glucose[1,2]	1	100%	94%	93%
Prophylactic Antibiotic Timing[2]	228	100%	96%	97%
Prophylactic Antibiotic Timing (Outpatient)	152	97%	92%	92%
Prophylactic Antibiotic Selection[2]	228	100%	97%	97%
Prophylactic Antibiotic Select. (Outpatient)	149	93%	93%	94%
Prophylactic Antibiotic Stopped[2]	226	100%	94%	94%
Recommended VTP Ordered[2]	123	93%	96%	94%
Urinary Catheter Removal[1,2]	23	96%	90%	90%
Children's Asthma Care				
Received Systemic Corticosteroids	-	-	-	100%
Received Home Management Plan	-	-	-	71%
Received Reliever Medication	-	-	-	100%
Use of Medical Imaging				
Combination Abdominal CT Scan	567	0.092	0.141	0.191
Combination Chest CT Scan	353	0.031	0.024	0.054
Follow-up Mammogram/Ultrasound	323	3.7%	9.8%	8.4%
MRI for Low Back Pain[5]	0	-	26.9%	32.7%
Survey of Patients' Hospital Experiences				
Area Around Room 'Always' Quiet at Night	300+	47%	-	58%
Doctors 'Always' Communicated Well	300+	75%	-	80%
Home Recovery Information Given	300+	81%	-	82%
Hospital Given 9 or 10 on 10 Point Scale	300+	54%	-	67%
Meds 'Always' Explained Before Given	300+	57%	-	60%
Nurses 'Always' Communicated Well	300+	69%	-	76%
Pain 'Always' Well Controlled	300+	64%	-	69%
Room and Bathroom 'Always' Clean	300+	63%	-	71%
Timely Help 'Always' Received	300+	51%	-	64%
Would Definitely Recommend Hospital	300+	57%	-	69%

Niagara Falls Memorial Medical Center

621 Tenth Street Phone: 716-278-4000
Niagara Falls, NY 14302 Fax: 716-278-4054
E-mail: healthbeat@nfmmc.org
URL: www.nfmmc.org
Type: Acute Care Hospitals Emergency Services: No
Ownership: Voluntary Non-Profit - Other
Key Personnel:
CEO/President. . . . . Joseph A Ruffolo
Chief of Medical Staff. . . . . Vijay Bojedla, MD
Infection Control. . . . . Lorrianne Duthe
Quality Assurance . . . . Karen Tunis-Manny
Radiology. . . . . Mark Perry
Emergency Room . . . . Laura Hickey, RN
Hemotology Center . . . . Joseph F Gioia, MD

Measure	Cases	This Hosp.	State Avg.	U.S. Avg.
Heart Attack Care				
ACE Inhibitor or ARB for LVSD[1,2]	2	100%	95%	96%
Aspirin at Arrival[2]	49	100%	98%	99%
Aspirin at Discharge[2]	27	100%	98%	98%
Beta Blocker at Discharge[2]	30	100%	98%	98%
Fibrinolytic Medication Timing[2]	0	-	50%	55%
PCI Within 90 Minutes of Arrival[2]	0	-	88%	90%
Smoking Cessation Advice[1,2]	6	100%	100%	99%
Chest Pain/Possible Heart Attack Care				
Aspirin at Arrival	46	96%	96%	95%
Median Time to ECG (minutes)	47	6	11	8
Median Time to Transfer (minutes)[1]	1	68	75	61
Fibrinolytic Medication Timing[1]	12	42%	55%	54%
Heart Failure Care				
ACE Inhibitor or ARB for LVSD	49	100%	94%	94%
Discharge Instructions	121	93%	89%	88%
Evaluation of LVS Function	145	98%	98%	98%
Smoking Cessation Advice	35	100%	98%	98%
Pneumonia Care				
Appropriate Initial Antibiotic	96	97%	92%	92%
Blood Culture Timing	150	99%	95%	96%
Influenza Vaccine	106	92%	90%	91%
Initial Antibiotic Timing	106	98%	93%	95%
Pneumococcal Vaccine	111	94%	92%	93%
Smoking Cessation Advice	83	100%	98%	97%
Surgical Care Improvement Project				
Appropriate VTP Within 24 Hours	72	94%	94%	92%
Appropriate Hair Removal	134	100%	100%	99%
Appropriate Beta Blocker Usage	29	93%	92%	93%
Controlled Postoperative Blood Glucose	0	-	94%	93%
Prophylactic Antibiotic Timing	65	100%	96%	97%
Prophylactic Antibiotic Timing (Outpatient)	89	93%	92%	92%
Prophylactic Antibiotic Selection	65	92%	97%	97%
Prophylactic Antibiotic Select. (Outpatient)	90	94%	93%	94%
Prophylactic Antibiotic Stopped	61	85%	94%	94%
Recommended VTP Ordered	72	94%	96%	94%
Urinary Catheter Removal[1]	11	100%	90%	90%
Children's Asthma Care				
Received Systemic Corticosteroids	-	-	-	100%
Received Home Management Plan	-	-	-	71%
Received Reliever Medication	-	-	-	100%
Use of Medical Imaging				
Combination Abdominal CT Scan	328	0.070	0.141	0.191
Combination Chest CT Scan	251	0.068	0.024	0.054
Follow-up Mammogram/Ultrasound	918	4.6%	9.8%	8.4%
MRI for Low Back Pain	118	30.5%	26.9%	32.7%
Survey of Patients' Hospital Experiences				
Area Around Room 'Always' Quiet at Night	300+	50%	-	58%
Doctors 'Always' Communicated Well	300+	70%	-	80%
Home Recovery Information Given	300+	77%	-	82%
Hospital Given 9 or 10 on 10 Point Scale	300+	53%	-	67%
Meds 'Always' Explained Before Given	300+	53%	-	60%
Nurses 'Always' Communicated Well	300+	68%	-	76%
Pain 'Always' Well Controlled	300+	63%	-	69%
Room and Bathroom 'Always' Clean	300+	61%	-	71%
Timely Help 'Always' Received	300+	53%	-	64%
Would Definitely Recommend Hospital	300+	57%	-	69%

NOTE: Hospital profiles are in alphabetical order by state, then city, then hospital within the city; Rankings exclude hospitals with less than 25 cases except for patient surveys which excludes hospitals with less than 100 cases; (a) 100–299 cases; (1) The number of cases is too small to be sure how well a hospital is performing; (2) The hospital indicated that the data submitted for this measure were based on a sample of cases; (3) Data was collected during a shorter time period (fewer quarters) than the maximum possible time for this measure; (4) Suppressed for one or more quarters by CMS; (5) No data is available from the hospital for this measure; (6) Fewer than 100 patients completed the HCAHPS survey. Use these rates with caution, as the number of surveys may be too low to reliably assess hospital performance; (7) Survey results are based on less than 12 months of data; (8) Survey results are not available for this reporting period; (9) No or very few patients were eligible for the HCAHPS survey. The scores shown, if any, reflect a very small number of surveys; (10) A state average was not calculated because too few hospitals in the state submitted data; (11) There were discrepancies in the data collection process; Please refer to the User's Guide for a full explanation of data.

Northport VA Medical Center

79 Middleville Road
Northport, NY 11768
Phone: 516-261-4400
Fax: 631-754-7933
URL: www.va.gov
Type: Acute Care-Veterans Administration
Emergency Services: No
Ownership: Government - Federal
Beds: 524

Key Personnel:

CEO/President. . . . . James A Clark
Chief of Medical Staff. . . . . Mark Graber, MD
Operating Room. . . . . Mary Ann Loh, RN
Radiology. . . . . Margaret Johnstone, MD
Emergency Room . . . . Shirley Tansiongco, MD

Measure	Cases	This Hosp.	State Avg.	U.S. Avg.
Heart Attack Care				
ACE Inhibitor or ARB for LVSD[5]	0	-	95%	96%
Aspirin at Arrival[5]	0	-	98%	99%
Aspirin at Discharge[5]	0	-	98%	98%
Beta Blocker at Discharge[5]	0	-	98%	98%
Fibrinolytic Medication Timing[5]	0	-	50%	55%
PCI Within 90 Minutes of Arrival[5]	0	-	88%	90%
Smoking Cessation Advice[5]	0	-	100%	99%
Chest Pain/Possible Heart Attack Care				
Aspirin at Arrival	-	-	96%	95%
Median Time to ECG (minutes)	-	-	11	8
Median Time to Transfer (minutes)	-	-	75	61
Fibrinolytic Medication Timing	-	-	55%	54%
Heart Failure Care				
ACE Inhibitor or ARB for LVSD	39	97%	94%	94%
Discharge Instructions	115	98%	89%	88%
Evaluation of LVS Function	131	100%	98%	98%
Smoking Cessation Advice[1]	15	100%	98%	98%
Pneumonia Care				
Appropriate Initial Antibiotic	43	98%	92%	92%
Blood Culture Timing	93	92%	95%	96%
Influenza Vaccine	47	94%	90%	91%
Initial Antibiotic Timing	87	91%	93%	95%
Pneumococcal Vaccine	77	97%	92%	93%
Smoking Cessation Advice[1]	23	100%	98%	97%
Surgical Care Improvement Project				
Appropriate VTP Within 24 Hours[2]	99	99%	94%	92%
Appropriate Hair Removal[2]	126	100%	100%	99%
Appropriate Beta Blocker Usage[2]	43	88%	92%	93%
Controlled Postoperative Blood Glucose[2,5]	0	-	94%	93%
Prophylactic Antibiotic Timing	61	98%	96%	97%
Prophylactic Antibiotic Timing (Outpatient)	-	-	92%	92%
Prophylactic Antibiotic Selection	63	95%	97%	97%
Prophylactic Antibiotic Select. (Outpatient)	-	-	93%	94%
Prophylactic Antibiotic Stopped	60	90%	94%	94%
Recommended VTP Ordered[2]	99	100%	96%	94%
Urinary Catheter Removal[2]	53	85%	90%	90%
Children's Asthma Care				
Received Systemic Corticosteroids	-	-	-	100%
Received Home Management Plan	-	-	-	71%
Received Reliever Medication	-	-	-	100%
Use of Medical Imaging				
Combination Abdominal CT Scan	-	-	0.141	0.191
Combination Chest CT Scan	-	-	0.024	0.054
Follow-up Mammogram/Ultrasound	-	-	9.8%	8.4%
MRI for Low Back Pain	-	-	26.9%	32.7%
Survey of Patients' Hospital Experiences				
Area Around Room 'Always' Quiet at Night	-	-	-	58%
Doctors 'Always' Communicated Well	-	-	-	80%
Home Recovery Information Given	-	-	-	82%
Hospital Given 9 or 10 on 10 Point Scale	-	-	-	67%
Meds 'Always' Explained Before Given	-	-	-	60%
Nurses 'Always' Communicated Well	-	-	-	76%
Pain 'Always' Well Controlled	-	-	-	69%
Room and Bathroom 'Always' Clean	-	-	-	71%
Timely Help 'Always' Received	-	-	-	64%
Would Definitely Recommend Hospital	-	-	-	69%

Chenango Memorial Hospital

179 North Broad Street
Norwich, NY 13815
Phone: 607-335-4111
Fax: 607-337-4284
URL: www.uhs.net
Type: Acute Care Hospitals
Emergency Services: Yes
Ownership: Voluntary Non-Profit - Private
Beds: 139

Key Personnel:

CEO/President. . . . . Frank Mirabito
Chief of Medical Staff. . . . . David Race, MD
Infection Control. . . . . Dottie VanVliet, RN
Operating Room. . . . . Patty Roma
Quality Assurance . . . . Shirley Caezza, RN, BSN
Emergency Room . . . . William Boudreau, MD
Patient Relations . . . . Julie Briggs, RN

Measure	Cases	This Hosp.	State Avg.	U.S. Avg.
Heart Attack Care				
ACE Inhibitor or ARB for LVSD[1]	2	50%	95%	96%
Aspirin at Arrival	32	100%	98%	99%
Aspirin at Discharge[1]	19	100%	98%	98%
Beta Blocker at Discharge[1]	17	100%	98%	98%
Fibrinolytic Medication Timing	0	-	50%	55%
PCI Within 90 Minutes of Arrival	0	-	88%	90%
Smoking Cessation Advice[1]	2	100%	100%	99%
Chest Pain/Possible Heart Attack Care				
Aspirin at Arrival	71	94%	96%	95%
Median Time to ECG (minutes)	72	8	11	8
Median Time to Transfer (minutes)[1]	5	82	75	61
Fibrinolytic Medication Timing[1]	1	100%	55%	54%
Heart Failure Care				
ACE Inhibitor or ARB for LVSD[1]	10	90%	94%	94%
Discharge Instructions	58	95%	89%	88%
Evaluation of LVS Function	71	96%	98%	98%
Smoking Cessation Advice[1]	12	100%	98%	98%
Pneumonia Care				
Appropriate Initial Antibiotic	66	85%	92%	92%
Blood Culture Timing	117	97%	95%	96%
Influenza Vaccine	53	96%	90%	91%
Initial Antibiotic Timing	111	96%	93%	95%
Pneumococcal Vaccine	64	100%	92%	93%
Smoking Cessation Advice	28	93%	98%	97%
Surgical Care Improvement Project				
Appropriate VTP Within 24 Hours	89	92%	94%	92%
Appropriate Hair Removal	183	100%	100%	99%
Appropriate Beta Blocker Usage	47	96%	92%	93%
Controlled Postoperative Blood Glucose	0	-	94%	93%
Prophylactic Antibiotic Timing	142	94%	96%	97%
Prophylactic Antibiotic Timing (Outpatient)[1,3]	6	83%	92%	92%
Prophylactic Antibiotic Selection	141	91%	97%	97%
Prophylactic Antibiotic Select. (Outpatient)[1,3]	6	100%	93%	94%
Prophylactic Antibiotic Stopped	137	94%	94%	94%
Recommended VTP Ordered	89	93%	96%	94%
Urinary Catheter Removal	62	98%	90%	90%
Children's Asthma Care				
Received Systemic Corticosteroids	-	-	-	100%
Received Home Management Plan	-	-	-	71%
Received Reliever Medication	-	-	-	100%
Use of Medical Imaging				
Combination Abdominal CT Scan	244	0.066	0.141	0.191
Combination Chest CT Scan	138	0.000	0.024	0.054
Follow-up Mammogram/Ultrasound	304	7.9%	9.8%	8.4%
MRI for Low Back Pain[5]	0	-	26.9%	32.7%
Survey of Patients' Hospital Experiences				
Area Around Room 'Always' Quiet at Night	300+	47%	-	58%
Doctors 'Always' Communicated Well	300+	76%	-	80%
Home Recovery Information Given	300+	81%	-	82%
Hospital Given 9 or 10 on 10 Point Scale	300+	60%	-	67%
Meds 'Always' Explained Before Given	300+	53%	-	60%
Nurses 'Always' Communicated Well	300+	70%	-	76%
Pain 'Always' Well Controlled	300+	64%	-	69%
Room and Bathroom 'Always' Clean	300+	66%	-	71%
Timely Help 'Always' Received	300+	61%	-	64%
Would Definitely Recommend Hospital	300+	53%	-	69%

Nyack Hospital

160 North Midland Avenue
Nyack, NY 10960
Phone: 845-348-2000
Fax: 845-348-2160
URL: www.nyackhospital.org
Type: Acute Care Hospitals
Emergency Services: Yes
Ownership: Voluntary Non-Profit - Other
Beds: 375

Key Personnel:

CEO/President. . . . . David H Freed, DHA
Chief of Medical Staff. . . . . Michael Rader, MD
Coronary Care . . . . Mary Ortiz
Infection Control. . . . . Joan Graham-Rauscher, BSN RN
Operating Room. . . . . Nancy Madura, RN
Pediatric Ambulatory Care . . . . . . Mary Ann Clay, RN
Quality Assurance . . . . Kathleen O'Keefe, CFNP
Radiology. . . . . Mark Geller, MD

Measure	Cases	This Hosp.	State Avg.	U.S. Avg.
Heart Attack Care				
ACE Inhibitor or ARB for LVSD[1]	11	100%	95%	96%
Aspirin at Arrival	67	99%	98%	99%
Aspirin at Discharge	41	100%	98%	98%
Beta Blocker at Discharge	39	100%	98%	98%
Fibrinolytic Medication Timing	0	-	50%	55%
PCI Within 90 Minutes of Arrival	0	-	88%	90%
Smoking Cessation Advice[1]	1	100%	100%	99%
Chest Pain/Possible Heart Attack Care				
Aspirin at Arrival	57	100%	96%	95%
Median Time to ECG (minutes)	58	6	11	8
Median Time to Transfer (minutes)[1]	17	53	75	61
Fibrinolytic Medication Timing	0	-	55%	54%
Heart Failure Care				
ACE Inhibitor or ARB for LVSD	80	96%	94%	94%
Discharge Instructions	176	90%	89%	88%
Evaluation of LVS Function	249	99%	98%	98%
Smoking Cessation Advice[1]	14	100%	98%	98%
Pneumonia Care				
Appropriate Initial Antibiotic[2]	105	96%	92%	92%
Blood Culture Timing[2]	173	98%	95%	96%
Influenza Vaccine[2]	108	99%	90%	91%
Initial Antibiotic Timing[2]	165	97%	93%	95%
Pneumococcal Vaccine[2]	160	99%	92%	93%
Smoking Cessation Advice[2]	29	100%	98%	97%
Surgical Care Improvement Project				
Appropriate VTP Within 24 Hours	255	98%	94%	92%
Appropriate Hair Removal	664	100%	100%	99%
Appropriate Beta Blocker Usage	138	99%	92%	93%
Controlled Postoperative Blood Glucose	0	-	94%	93%
Prophylactic Antibiotic Timing	411	100%	96%	97%
Prophylactic Antibiotic Timing (Outpatient)	121	98%	92%	92%
Prophylactic Antibiotic Selection	412	99%	97%	97%
Prophylactic Antibiotic Select. (Outpatient)	119	93%	93%	94%
Prophylactic Antibiotic Stopped	394	98%	94%	94%
Recommended VTP Ordered	255	98%	96%	94%
Urinary Catheter Removal	168	99%	90%	90%
Children's Asthma Care				
Received Systemic Corticosteroids	-	-	-	100%
Received Home Management Plan	-	-	-	71%
Received Reliever Medication	-	-	-	100%
Use of Medical Imaging				
Combination Abdominal CT Scan	508	0.031	0.141	0.191
Combination Chest CT Scan	365	0.025	0.024	0.054
Follow-up Mammogram/Ultrasound	579	13.5%	9.8%	8.4%
MRI for Low Back Pain[5]	0	-	26.9%	32.7%
Survey of Patients' Hospital Experiences				
Area Around Room 'Always' Quiet at Night	300+	47%	-	58%
Doctors 'Always' Communicated Well	300+	73%	-	80%
Home Recovery Information Given	300+	68%	-	82%
Hospital Given 9 or 10 on 10 Point Scale	300+	53%	-	67%
Meds 'Always' Explained Before Given	300+	57%	-	60%
Nurses 'Always' Communicated Well	300+	69%	-	76%
Pain 'Always' Well Controlled	300+	64%	-	69%
Room and Bathroom 'Always' Clean	300+	73%	-	71%
Timely Help 'Always' Received	300+	59%	-	64%
Would Definitely Recommend Hospital	300+	59%	-	69%

NOTE: Hospital profiles are in alphabetical order by state, then city, then hospital within the city; Rankings exclude hospitals with less than 25 cases except for patient surveys which excludes hospitals with less than 100 cases; (a) 100–299 cases; (1) The number of cases is too small to be sure how well a hospital is performing; (2) The hospital indicated that the data submitted for this measure were based on a sample of cases; (3) Data was collected during a shorter time period (fewer quarters) than the maximum possible time for this measure; (4) Suppressed for one or more quarters by CMS; (5) No data is available from the hospital for this measure; (6) Fewer than 100 patients completed the HCAHPS survey. Use these rates with caution, as the number of surveys may be too low to reliably assess hospital performance; (7) Survey results are based on less than 12 months of data; (8) Survey results are not available for this reporting period; (9) No or very few patients were eligible for the HCAHPS survey. The scores shown, if any, reflect a very small number of surveys; (10) A state average was not calculated because too few hospitals in the state submitted data; (11) There were discrepancies in the data collection process; Please refer to the User's Guide for a full explanation of data.

South Nassau Communities Hospital

One Healthy Way
Oceanside, NY 11572
Phone: 516-632-3000
Fax: 516-632-3981
URL: www.southnassau.org
Type: Acute Care Hospitals
Emergency Services: Yes
Ownership: Voluntary Non-Profit - Private
Beds: 435

Key Personnel:
CEO/President. . . . . Joseph Quegliata
Cardiac Laboratory. . . . . Robert Kramer, MD
Chief of Medical Staff . . . . Akram Boutros, MD
Infection Control. . . . . Judith Goldstein, MD
Operating Room. . . . . Mary Weiner
Quality Assurance . . . . Ruth Ragusa
Radiology. . . . . Michael Burghardt

Measure	Cases	This Hosp.	State Avg.	U.S. Avg.
Heart Attack Care				
ACE Inhibitor or ARB for LVSD	38	89%	95%	96%
Aspirin at Arrival	313	96%	98%	99%
Aspirin at Discharge	262	96%	98%	98%
Beta Blocker at Discharge	263	97%	98%	98%
Fibrinolytic Medication Timing	0	-	50%	55%
PCI Within 90 Minutes of Arrival	40	92%	88%	90%
Smoking Cessation Advice	59	100%	100%	99%
Chest Pain/Possible Heart Attack Care				
Aspirin at Arrival[1]	13	92%	96%	95%
Median Time to ECG (minutes)[1]	12	5	11	8
Median Time to Transfer (minutes)[5]	0	-	75	61
Fibrinolytic Medication Timing[3]	0	-	55%	54%
Heart Failure Care				
ACE Inhibitor or ARB for LVSD	179	93%	94%	94%
Discharge Instructions	382	98%	89%	88%
Evaluation of LVS Function	502	99%	98%	98%
Smoking Cessation Advice	34	100%	98%	98%
Pneumonia Care				
Appropriate Initial Antibiotic	211	93%	92%	92%
Blood Culture Timing	364	98%	95%	96%
Influenza Vaccine	219	97%	90%	91%
Initial Antibiotic Timing	314	98%	93%	95%
Pneumococcal Vaccine	344	97%	92%	93%
Smoking Cessation Advice	69	100%	98%	97%
Surgical Care Improvement Project				
Appropriate VTP Within 24 Hours[2]	343	96%	94%	92%
Appropriate Hair Removal[2]	969	100%	100%	99%
Appropriate Beta Blocker Usage[2]	333	95%	92%	93%
Controlled Postoperative Blood Glucose[2]	0	-	94%	93%
Prophylactic Antibiotic Timing[2]	707	100%	96%	97%
Prophylactic Antibiotic Timing (Outpatient)	378	98%	92%	92%
Prophylactic Antibiotic Selection[2]	708	97%	97%	97%
Prophylactic Antibiotic Select. (Outpatient)	379	94%	93%	94%
Prophylactic Antibiotic Stopped[2]	687	95%	94%	94%
Recommended VTP Ordered[2]	343	99%	96%	94%
Urinary Catheter Removal[2]	290	96%	90%	90%
Children's Asthma Care				
Received Systemic Corticosteroids	-	-	-	100%
Received Home Management Plan	-	-	-	71%
Received Reliever Medication	-	-	-	100%
Use of Medical Imaging				
Combination Abdominal CT Scan	833	0.181	0.141	0.191
Combination Chest CT Scan	407	0.002	0.024	0.054
Follow-up Mammogram/Ultrasound	815	39.4%	9.8%	8.4%
MRI for Low Back Pain[1]	34	29.4%	26.9%	32.7%
Survey of Patients' Hospital Experiences				
Area Around Room 'Always' Quiet at Night	300+	49%	-	58%
Doctors 'Always' Communicated Well	300+	76%	-	80%
Home Recovery Information Given	300+	80%	-	82%
Hospital Given 9 or 10 on 10 Point Scale	300+	65%	-	67%
Meds 'Always' Explained Before Given	300+	57%	-	60%
Nurses 'Always' Communicated Well	300+	73%	-	76%
Pain 'Always' Well Controlled	300+	67%	-	69%
Room and Bathroom 'Always' Clean	300+	66%	-	71%
Timely Help 'Always' Received	300+	57%	-	64%
Would Definitely Recommend Hospital	300+	70%	-	69%

Claxton-Hepburn Medical Center

214 King Street
Ogdensburg, NY 13669
Phone: 315-393-3600
Fax: 315-393-8506
E-mail: info@chmed.org
URL: www.chmed.org
Type: Acute Care Hospitals
Emergency Services: Yes
Ownership: Voluntary Non-Profit - Private
Beds: 159

Key Personnel:
CEO/President. . . . . Mark Webster
Cardiac Laboratory. . . . . Keith Warren
Chief of Medical Staff . . . . Michael Roark, MD
Infection Control. . . . . Vicki Hockenbery, RN
Operating Room. . . . . Lenette Deloney
Quality Assurance . . . . Robin Wood
Radiology. . . . . Angela Klimaszewski

Measure	Cases	This Hosp.	State Avg.	U.S. Avg.
Heart Attack Care				
ACE Inhibitor or ARB for LVSD[1]	5	100%	95%	96%
Aspirin at Arrival	32	100%	98%	99%
Aspirin at Discharge[1]	22	95%	98%	98%
Beta Blocker at Discharge[1]	18	100%	98%	98%
Fibrinolytic Medication Timing[1]	1	100%	50%	55%
PCI Within 90 Minutes of Arrival	0	-	88%	90%
Smoking Cessation Advice[1]	6	100%	100%	99%
Chest Pain/Possible Heart Attack Care				
Aspirin at Arrival	59	97%	96%	95%
Median Time to ECG (minutes)	62	8	11	8
Median Time to Transfer (minutes)[1,3]	5	196	75	61
Fibrinolytic Medication Timing[1]	12	33%	55%	54%
Heart Failure Care				
ACE Inhibitor or ARB for LVSD[1]	11	100%	94%	94%
Discharge Instructions	45	91%	89%	88%
Evaluation of LVS Function	57	100%	98%	98%
Smoking Cessation Advice[1]	6	100%	98%	98%
Pneumonia Care				
Appropriate Initial Antibiotic	48	98%	92%	92%
Blood Culture Timing	92	97%	95%	96%
Influenza Vaccine	67	91%	90%	91%
Initial Antibiotic Timing	92	98%	93%	95%
Pneumococcal Vaccine	88	94%	92%	93%
Smoking Cessation Advice[1]	20	100%	98%	97%
Surgical Care Improvement Project				
Appropriate VTP Within 24 Hours	44	84%	94%	92%
Appropriate Hair Removal	100	98%	100%	99%
Appropriate Beta Blocker Usage[1]	24	88%	92%	93%
Controlled Postoperative Blood Glucose	0	-	94%	93%
Prophylactic Antibiotic Timing	59	95%	96%	97%
Prophylactic Antibiotic Timing (Outpatient)	45	87%	92%	92%
Prophylactic Antibiotic Selection	60	97%	97%	97%
Prophylactic Antibiotic Select. (Outpatient)	42	95%	93%	94%
Prophylactic Antibiotic Stopped	56	100%	94%	94%
Recommended VTP Ordered	45	87%	96%	94%
Urinary Catheter Removal[1]	11	91%	90%	90%
Children's Asthma Care				
Received Systemic Corticosteroids	-	-	-	100%
Received Home Management Plan	-	-	-	71%
Received Reliever Medication	-	-	-	100%
Use of Medical Imaging				
Combination Abdominal CT Scan	469	0.028	0.141	0.191
Combination Chest CT Scan	330	0.018	0.024	0.054
Follow-up Mammogram/Ultrasound	1,085	9.3%	9.8%	8.4%
MRI for Low Back Pain	81	30.9%	26.9%	32.7%
Survey of Patients' Hospital Experiences				
Area Around Room 'Always' Quiet at Night	(a)	49%	-	58%
Doctors 'Always' Communicated Well	(a)	85%	-	80%
Home Recovery Information Given	(a)	87%	-	82%
Hospital Given 9 or 10 on 10 Point Scale	(a)	63%	-	67%
Meds 'Always' Explained Before Given	(a)	66%	-	60%
Nurses 'Always' Communicated Well	(a)	77%	-	76%
Pain 'Always' Well Controlled	(a)	69%	-	69%
Room and Bathroom 'Always' Clean	(a)	73%	-	71%
Timely Help 'Always' Received	(a)	67%	-	64%
Would Definitely Recommend Hospital	(a)	68%	-	69%

Olean General Hospital

515 Main Street
Olean, NY 14760
Phone: 716-373-2600
Fax: 716-375-6380
URL: www.ogh.org
Type: Acute Care Hospitals
Emergency Services: Yes
Ownership: Proprietary
Beds: 217

Key Personnel:
CEO/President. . . . . Timothy Finan
Chief of Medical Staff . . . . Richard Decker, MD
Coronary Care . . . . Denise Fish
Infection Control. . . . . Cynthia Paxhia
Pediatric Ambulatory Care . . . . . . Pat Allen
Quality Assurance . . . . Donna Brenneman
Radiology. . . . . Helen Layman

Measure	Cases	This Hosp.	State Avg.	U.S. Avg.
Heart Attack Care				
ACE Inhibitor or ARB for LVSD[1]	16	100%	95%	96%
Aspirin at Arrival	80	99%	98%	99%
Aspirin at Discharge	43	98%	98%	98%
Beta Blocker at Discharge	52	98%	98%	98%
Fibrinolytic Medication Timing	0	-	50%	55%
PCI Within 90 Minutes of Arrival	0	-	88%	90%
Smoking Cessation Advice[1]	3	100%	100%	99%
Chest Pain/Possible Heart Attack Care				
Aspirin at Arrival	348	97%	96%	95%
Median Time to ECG (minutes)	359	19	11	8
Median Time to Transfer (minutes)[5]	0	-	75	61
Fibrinolytic Medication Timing[1]	13	38%	55%	54%
Heart Failure Care				
ACE Inhibitor or ARB for LVSD	78	97%	94%	94%
Discharge Instructions	171	87%	89%	88%
Evaluation of LVS Function	261	100%	98%	98%
Smoking Cessation Advice	32	100%	98%	98%
Pneumonia Care				
Appropriate Initial Antibiotic	138	88%	92%	92%
Blood Culture Timing	232	97%	95%	96%
Influenza Vaccine	166	91%	90%	91%
Initial Antibiotic Timing	221	96%	93%	95%
Pneumococcal Vaccine	227	96%	92%	93%
Smoking Cessation Advice	78	100%	98%	97%
Surgical Care Improvement Project				
Appropriate VTP Within 24 Hours	181	99%	94%	92%
Appropriate Hair Removal	399	100%	100%	99%
Appropriate Beta Blocker Usage	97	94%	92%	93%
Controlled Postoperative Blood Glucose	0	-	94%	93%
Prophylactic Antibiotic Timing	275	100%	96%	97%
Prophylactic Antibiotic Timing (Outpatient)	151	89%	92%	92%
Prophylactic Antibiotic Selection	276	97%	97%	97%
Prophylactic Antibiotic Select. (Outpatient)	139	85%	93%	94%
Prophylactic Antibiotic Stopped	248	97%	94%	94%
Recommended VTP Ordered	183	98%	96%	94%
Urinary Catheter Removal	48	83%	90%	90%
Children's Asthma Care				
Received Systemic Corticosteroids	-	-	-	100%
Received Home Management Plan	-	-	-	71%
Received Reliever Medication	-	-	-	100%
Use of Medical Imaging				
Combination Abdominal CT Scan	606	0.259	0.141	0.191
Combination Chest CT Scan	259	0.398	0.024	0.054
Follow-up Mammogram/Ultrasound	294	15.6%	9.8%	8.4%
MRI for Low Back Pain	117	37.6%	26.9%	32.7%
Survey of Patients' Hospital Experiences				
Area Around Room 'Always' Quiet at Night	300+	45%	-	58%
Doctors 'Always' Communicated Well	300+	75%	-	80%
Home Recovery Information Given	300+	81%	-	82%
Hospital Given 9 or 10 on 10 Point Scale	300+	58%	-	67%
Meds 'Always' Explained Before Given	300+	54%	-	60%
Nurses 'Always' Communicated Well	300+	73%	-	76%
Pain 'Always' Well Controlled	300+	65%	-	69%
Room and Bathroom 'Always' Clean	300+	74%	-	71%
Timely Help 'Always' Received	300+	60%	-	64%
Would Definitely Recommend Hospital	300+	56%	-	69%

NOTE: Hospital profiles are in alphabetical order by state, then city, then hospital within the city; Rankings exclude hospitals with less than 25 cases except for patient surveys which excludes hospitals with less than 100 cases; (a) 100–299 cases; (1) The number of cases is too small to be sure how well a hospital is performing; (2) The hospital indicated that the data submitted for this measure were based on a sample of cases; (3) Data was collected during a shorter time period (fewer quarters) than the maximum possible time for this measure; (4) Suppressed for one or more quarters by CMS; (5) No data is available from the hospital for this measure; (6) Fewer than 100 patients completed the HCAHPS survey. Use these rates with caution, as the number of surveys may be too low to reliably assess hospital performance; (7) Survey results are based on less than 12 months of data; (8) Survey results are not available for this reporting period; (9) No or very few patients were eligible for the HCAHPS survey. The scores shown, if any, reflect a very small number of surveys; (10) A state average was not calculated because too few hospitals in the state submitted data; (11) There were discrepancies in the data collection process; Please refer to the User's Guide for a full explanation of data.

Oneida Healthcare Center

321 Genesee Street
Oneida, NY 13421
E-mail: info@oneidahealthcare.org
URL: www.oneidahealthcare.org
Type: Acute Care Hospitals
Ownership: Voluntary Non-Profit - Other
Phone: 315-363-6000
Fax: 315-361-2043
Emergency Services: Yes
Beds: 101

Key Personnel:
CEO/President. . . . . Gene F Morreale
Chief of Medical Staff . . . . Leonard Argentine, MD
Operating Room. . . . . Jeanette Suchewski
Pediatric Ambulatory Care . . . . . . I Vanderhoof, MD
Pediatric In-Patient Care . . . . I Vanderhoof, MD
Quality Assurance . . . . Susan Daley
Radiology. . . . . Roberto Goldberg, MD
Hemotology Center . . . . Amy Ross

Measure	Cases	This Hosp.	State Avg.	U.S. Avg.
Heart Attack Care				
ACE Inhibitor or ARB for LVSD[1,3]	1	100%	95%	96%
Aspirin at Arrival[1,3]	8	100%	98%	99%
Aspirin at Discharge[1,3]	3	100%	98%	98%
Beta Blocker at Discharge[1,3]	3	100%	98%	98%
Fibrinolytic Medication Timing[3]	0	-	50%	55%
PCI Within 90 Minutes of Arrival[3]	0	-	88%	90%
Smoking Cessation Advice[3]	0	-	100%	99%
Chest Pain/Possible Heart Attack Care				
Aspirin at Arrival	59	95%	96%	95%
Median Time to ECG (minutes)	65	5	11	8
Median Time to Transfer (minutes)[1,3]	7	54	75	61
Fibrinolytic Medication Timing[1]	3	0%	55%	54%
Heart Failure Care				
ACE Inhibitor or ARB for LVSD[1]	11	73%	94%	94%
Discharge Instructions[1]	20	90%	89%	88%
Evaluation of LVS Function	30	87%	98%	98%
Smoking Cessation Advice	0	-	98%	98%
Pneumonia Care				
Appropriate Initial Antibiotic	65	94%	92%	92%
Blood Culture Timing	70	97%	95%	96%
Influenza Vaccine	50	86%	90%	91%
Initial Antibiotic Timing	76	97%	93%	95%
Pneumococcal Vaccine	64	92%	92%	93%
Smoking Cessation Advice	34	97%	98%	97%
Surgical Care Improvement Project				
Appropriate VTP Within 24 Hours	174	99%	94%	92%
Appropriate Hair Removal	275	98%	100%	99%
Appropriate Beta Blocker Usage	69	86%	92%	93%
Controlled Postoperative Blood Glucose	0	-	94%	93%
Prophylactic Antibiotic Timing	181	94%	96%	97%
Prophylactic Antibiotic Timing (Outpatient)	219	95%	92%	92%
Prophylactic Antibiotic Selection	181	97%	97%	97%
Prophylactic Antibiotic Select. (Outpatient)	216	92%	93%	94%
Prophylactic Antibiotic Stopped	179	97%	94%	94%
Recommended VTP Ordered	174	99%	96%	94%
Urinary Catheter Removal[1]	20	70%	90%	90%
Children's Asthma Care				
Received Systemic Corticosteroids	-	-	-	100%
Received Home Management Plan	-	-	-	71%
Received Reliever Medication	-	-	-	100%
Use of Medical Imaging				
Combination Abdominal CT Scan	464	0.259	0.141	0.191
Combination Chest CT Scan	174	0.011	0.024	0.054
Follow-up Mammogram/Ultrasound	443	5.4%	9.8%	8.4%
MRI for Low Back Pain[1]	37	32.4%	26.9%	32.7%
Survey of Patients' Hospital Experiences				
Area Around Room 'Always' Quiet at Night	300+	52%	-	58%
Doctors 'Always' Communicated Well	300+	83%	-	80%
Home Recovery Information Given	300+	84%	-	82%
Hospital Given 9 or 10 on 10 Point Scale	300+	66%	-	67%
Meds 'Always' Explained Before Given	300+	66%	-	60%
Nurses 'Always' Communicated Well	300+	75%	-	76%
Pain 'Always' Well Controlled	300+	71%	-	69%
Room and Bathroom 'Always' Clean	300+	73%	-	71%
Timely Help 'Always' Received	300+	63%	-	64%
Would Definitely Recommend Hospital	300+	69%	-	69%

Aurelia Osborn Fox Memorial Hospital

One Norton Avenue
Oneonta, NY 13820
E-mail: aofox@catskill.net
URL: www.foxcarenetwork.com
Type: Acute Care Hospitals
Ownership: Voluntary Non-Profit - Other
Phone: 607-423-2000
Fax: 607-431-5006
Emergency Services: Yes
Beds: 128

Key Personnel:
Cardiac Laboratory. . . . . Jeff Hewings
Chief of Medical Staff . . . . David G Evelyn, MD
Infection Control . . . . Ruth Sickler, RN
Operating Room. . . . . Nancy Mitchell, RN
Quality Assurance . . . . Donna L Schultes
Radiology. . . . . James McChesney
Emergency Room . . . . Francis Nolan, MD
Intensive Care Unit. . . . . James Wheeling, MD

Measure	Cases	This Hosp.	State Avg.	U.S. Avg.
Heart Attack Care				
ACE Inhibitor or ARB for LVSD[1]	4	100%	95%	96%
Aspirin at Arrival	51	94%	98%	99%
Aspirin at Discharge	39	85%	98%	98%
Beta Blocker at Discharge	42	93%	98%	98%
Fibrinolytic Medication Timing	0	-	50%	55%
PCI Within 90 Minutes of Arrival	0	-	88%	90%
Smoking Cessation Advice[1]	7	57%	100%	99%
Chest Pain/Possible Heart Attack Care				
Aspirin at Arrival	46	93%	96%	95%
Median Time to ECG (minutes)	47	10	11	8
Median Time to Transfer (minutes)[1]	13	75	75	61
Fibrinolytic Medication Timing[1]	1	0%	55%	54%
Heart Failure Care				
ACE Inhibitor or ARB for LVSD	44	93%	94%	94%
Discharge Instructions	138	84%	89%	88%
Evaluation of LVS Function	170	94%	98%	98%
Smoking Cessation Advice[1]	20	100%	98%	98%
Pneumonia Care				
Appropriate Initial Antibiotic	74	91%	92%	92%
Blood Culture Timing	127	95%	95%	96%
Influenza Vaccine	69	93%	90%	91%
Initial Antibiotic Timing	132	95%	93%	95%
Pneumococcal Vaccine	103	97%	92%	93%
Smoking Cessation Advice	41	100%	98%	97%
Surgical Care Improvement Project				
Appropriate VTP Within 24 Hours	102	93%	94%	92%
Appropriate Hair Removal	191	99%	100%	99%
Appropriate Beta Blocker Usage	44	84%	92%	93%
Controlled Postoperative Blood Glucose	0	-	94%	93%
Prophylactic Antibiotic Timing	89	93%	96%	97%
Prophylactic Antibiotic Timing (Outpatient)[1,3]	1	100%	92%	92%
Prophylactic Antibiotic Selection	89	98%	97%	97%
Prophylactic Antibiotic Select. (Outpatient)[1,3]	1	100%	93%	94%
Prophylactic Antibiotic Stopped	88	99%	94%	94%
Recommended VTP Ordered	102	96%	96%	94%
Urinary Catheter Removal	37	95%	90%	90%
Children's Asthma Care				
Received Systemic Corticosteroids	-	-	-	100%
Received Home Management Plan	-	-	-	71%
Received Reliever Medication	-	-	-	100%
Use of Medical Imaging				
Combination Abdominal CT Scan	393	0.092	0.141	0.191
Combination Chest CT Scan	171	0.035	0.024	0.054
Follow-up Mammogram/Ultrasound	938	3.7%	9.8%	8.4%
MRI for Low Back Pain	42	45.2%	26.9%	32.7%
Survey of Patients' Hospital Experiences				
Area Around Room 'Always' Quiet at Night	300+	49%	-	58%
Doctors 'Always' Communicated Well	300+	75%	-	80%
Home Recovery Information Given	300+	85%	-	82%
Hospital Given 9 or 10 on 10 Point Scale	300+	55%	-	67%
Meds 'Always' Explained Before Given	300+	56%	-	60%
Nurses 'Always' Communicated Well	300+	69%	-	76%
Pain 'Always' Well Controlled	300+	66%	-	69%
Room and Bathroom 'Always' Clean	300+	70%	-	71%
Timely Help 'Always' Received	300+	58%	-	64%
Would Definitely Recommend Hospital	300+	58%	-	69%

Oswego Hospital

110 West Sixth Street
Oswego, NY 13126
URL: www.oswegohealth.org
Type: Acute Care Hospitals
Ownership: Voluntary Non-Profit - Private
Phone: 315-349-5511
Fax: 315-349-5732
Emergency Services: Yes
Beds: 74

Key Personnel:
CEO/President. . . . . Ann C Gilpin
Chief of Medical Staff . . . . Patsy Iannolo, MD
Radiology. . . . . Sudhir Guthikonda
Anesthesiology. . . . . Stanley Lubinga, MD
Emergency Room . . . . Michael Russell

Measure	Cases	This Hosp.	State Avg.	U.S. Avg.
Heart Attack Care				
ACE Inhibitor or ARB for LVSD[1]	6	83%	95%	96%
Aspirin at Arrival	63	94%	98%	99%
Aspirin at Discharge[1]	23	96%	98%	98%
Beta Blocker at Discharge	31	94%	98%	98%
Fibrinolytic Medication Timing	0	-	50%	55%
PCI Within 90 Minutes of Arrival	0	-	88%	90%
Smoking Cessation Advice[1]	8	100%	100%	99%
Chest Pain/Possible Heart Attack Care				
Aspirin at Arrival	66	85%	96%	95%
Median Time to ECG (minutes)	69	17	11	8
Median Time to Transfer (minutes)[1]	19	80	75	61
Fibrinolytic Medication Timing	0	-	55%	54%
Heart Failure Care				
ACE Inhibitor or ARB for LVSD	37	81%	94%	94%
Discharge Instructions	99	81%	89%	88%
Evaluation of LVS Function	160	94%	98%	98%
Smoking Cessation Advice[1]	20	85%	98%	98%
Pneumonia Care				
Appropriate Initial Antibiotic	130	93%	92%	92%
Blood Culture Timing	218	97%	95%	96%
Influenza Vaccine	142	88%	90%	91%
Initial Antibiotic Timing	223	89%	93%	95%
Pneumococcal Vaccine	224	88%	92%	93%
Smoking Cessation Advice	96	97%	98%	97%
Surgical Care Improvement Project				
Appropriate VTP Within 24 Hours	97	92%	94%	92%
Appropriate Hair Removal	190	100%	100%	99%
Appropriate Beta Blocker Usage	36	81%	92%	93%
Controlled Postoperative Blood Glucose	0	-	94%	93%
Prophylactic Antibiotic Timing	109	92%	96%	97%
Prophylactic Antibiotic Timing (Outpatient)	156	97%	92%	92%
Prophylactic Antibiotic Selection	112	89%	97%	97%
Prophylactic Antibiotic Select. (Outpatient)	155	95%	93%	94%
Prophylactic Antibiotic Stopped	102	78%	94%	94%
Recommended VTP Ordered	97	92%	96%	94%
Urinary Catheter Removal[1]	11	91%	90%	90%
Children's Asthma Care				
Received Systemic Corticosteroids	-	-	-	100%
Received Home Management Plan	-	-	-	71%
Received Reliever Medication	-	-	-	100%
Use of Medical Imaging				
Combination Abdominal CT Scan	417	0.158	0.141	0.191
Combination Chest CT Scan	344	0.020	0.024	0.054
Follow-up Mammogram/Ultrasound	1,327	3.5%	9.8%	8.4%
MRI for Low Back Pain[1]	23	30.4%	26.9%	32.7%
Survey of Patients' Hospital Experiences				
Area Around Room 'Always' Quiet at Night	300+	45%	-	58%
Doctors 'Always' Communicated Well	300+	76%	-	80%
Home Recovery Information Given	300+	84%	-	82%
Hospital Given 9 or 10 on 10 Point Scale	300+	50%	-	67%
Meds 'Always' Explained Before Given	300+	57%	-	60%
Nurses 'Always' Communicated Well	300+	71%	-	76%
Pain 'Always' Well Controlled	300+	61%	-	69%
Room and Bathroom 'Always' Clean	300+	66%	-	71%
Timely Help 'Always' Received	300+	54%	-	64%
Would Definitely Recommend Hospital	300+	50%	-	69%

NOTE: Hospital profiles are in alphabetical order by state, then city, then hospital within the city; Rankings exclude hospitals with less than 25 cases except for patient surveys which excludes hospitals with less than 100 cases; (a) 100–299 cases; (1) The number of cases is too small to be sure how well a hospital is performing; (2) The hospital indicated that the data submitted for this measure were based on a sample of cases; (3) Data was collected during a shorter time period (fewer quarters) than the maximum possible time for this measure; (4) Suppressed for one or more quarters by CMS; (5) No data is available from the hospital for this measure; (6) Fewer than 100 patients completed the HCAHPS survey. Use these rates with caution, as the number of surveys may be too low to reliably assess hospital performance; (7) Survey results are based on less than 12 months of data; (8) Survey results are not available for this reporting period; (9) No or very few patients were eligible for the HCAHPS survey. The scores shown, if any, reflect a very small number of surveys; (10) A state average was not calculated because too few hospitals in the state submitted data; (11) There were discrepancies in the data collection process; Please refer to the User's Guide for a full explanation of data.

Brookhaven Memorial Hospital Medical Center

101 Hospital Road
Patchogue, NY 11772
Phone: 631-654-7100
Fax: 631-447-3714
E-mail: communityrelations@bmhmc.org
URL: www.brookhavenhospitalorg
Type: Acute Care Hospitals
Emergency Services: Yes
Ownership: Voluntary Non-Profit - Private
Beds: 321

Key Personnel:

CEO/President. . . . . Thomas Ockers
Chief of Medical Staff. . . . . Anthony J Shallash, MD
Infection Control. . . . . Doreen Virgil, RN
Operating Room. . . . . Philip Messina
Pediatric Ambulatory Care . . . . . . Kenneth Huml, MD
Pediatric In-Patient Care . . . . Kenneth Huml, MD
Quality Assurance . . . . Walter Metz
Radiology. . . . . Scott Coyner

Measure	Cases	This Hosp.	State Avg.	U.S. Avg.
Heart Attack Care				
ACE Inhibitor or ARB for LVSD[1,2]	18	94%	95%	96%
Aspirin at Arrival[2]	185	99%	98%	99%
Aspirin at Discharge[2]	79	100%	98%	98%
Beta Blocker at Discharge[2]	94	100%	98%	98%
Fibrinolytic Medication Timing[2]	0	-	50%	55%
PCI Within 90 Minutes of Arrival[2]	0	-	88%	90%
Smoking Cessation Advice[1,2]	12	100%	100%	99%
Chest Pain/Possible Heart Attack Care				
Aspirin at Arrival	105	99%	96%	95%
Median Time to ECG (minutes)	110	16	11	8
Median Time to Transfer (minutes)[1,3]	1	125	75	61
Fibrinolytic Medication Timing	0	-	55%	54%
Heart Failure Care				
ACE Inhibitor or ARB for LVSD[2]	106	95%	94%	94%
Discharge Instructions[2]	302	88%	89%	88%
Evaluation of LVS Function[2]	457	99%	98%	98%
Smoking Cessation Advice[2]	48	100%	98%	98%
Pneumonia Care				
Appropriate Initial Antibiotic[2]	240	89%	92%	92%
Blood Culture Timing[2]	454	94%	95%	96%
Influenza Vaccine[2]	283	93%	90%	91%
Initial Antibiotic Timing[2]	428	89%	93%	95%
Pneumococcal Vaccine[2]	429	91%	92%	93%
Smoking Cessation Advice[2]	163	100%	98%	97%
Surgical Care Improvement Project				
Appropriate VTP Within 24 Hours[2]	236	87%	94%	92%
Appropriate Hair Removal[2]	392	100%	100%	99%
Appropriate Beta Blocker Usage[2]	121	88%	92%	93%
Controlled Postoperative Blood Glucose[2]	0	-	94%	93%
Prophylactic Antibiotic Timing[2]	237	91%	96%	97%
Prophylactic Antibiotic Timing (Outpatient)	79	81%	92%	92%
Prophylactic Antibiotic Selection[2]	238	96%	97%	97%
Prophylactic Antibiotic Select. (Outpatient)	65	94%	93%	94%
Prophylactic Antibiotic Stopped[2]	228	94%	94%	94%
Recommended VTP Ordered[2]	237	95%	96%	94%
Urinary Catheter Removal[2]	121	82%	90%	90%
Children's Asthma Care				
Received Systemic Corticosteroids	-	-	-	100%
Received Home Management Plan	-	-	-	71%
Received Reliever Medication	-	-	-	100%
Use of Medical Imaging				
Combination Abdominal CT Scan	759	0.061	0.141	0.191
Combination Chest CT Scan	520	0.013	0.024	0.054
Follow-up Mammogram/Ultrasound	1,189	11.3%	9.8%	8.4%
MRI for Low Back Pain[1]	45	24.4%	26.9%	32.7%
Survey of Patients' Hospital Experiences				
Area Around Room 'Always' Quiet at Night	300+	41%	-	58%
Doctors 'Always' Communicated Well	300+	75%	-	80%
Home Recovery Information Given	300+	81%	-	82%
Hospital Given 9 or 10 on 10 Point Scale	300+	48%	-	67%
Meds 'Always' Explained Before Given	300+	51%	-	60%
Nurses 'Always' Communicated Well	300+	67%	-	76%
Pain 'Always' Well Controlled	300+	62%	-	69%
Room and Bathroom 'Always' Clean	300+	59%	-	71%
Timely Help 'Always' Received	300+	49%	-	64%
Would Definitely Recommend Hospital	300+	50%	-	69%

Soldiers and Sailors Memorial Hospital of Yates

418 North Main Street
Penn Yan, NY 14527
Phone: 315-787-4175
Fax: 315-531-2014
URL: www.flhealth.org
Type: Critical Access Hospitals
Emergency Services: Yes
Ownership: Voluntary Non-Profit - Private
Beds: 186

Key Personnel:

CEO/President. . . . . James J Dooley
Chief of Medical Staff . . . . Jose Acevedo, MD
Infection Control. . . . . Marge Brinn, RN
Operating Room. . . . . Cindy Presher
Quality Assurance . . . . Sally Bittner
Radiology. . . . . Rodolfo Queiroz
Emergency Room . . . . Deb McCaig, RN/BSN
Intensive Care Unit. . . . . Kelley Stout

Measure	Cases	This Hosp.	State Avg.	U.S. Avg.
Heart Attack Care				
ACE Inhibitor or ARB for LVSD[1]	1	100%	95%	96%
Aspirin at Arrival[1]	11	100%	98%	99%
Aspirin at Discharge[1]	6	100%	98%	98%
Beta Blocker at Discharge[1]	6	100%	98%	98%
Fibrinolytic Medication Timing	0	-	50%	55%
PCI Within 90 Minutes of Arrival	0	-	88%	90%
Smoking Cessation Advice	0	-	100%	99%
Chest Pain/Possible Heart Attack Care				
Aspirin at Arrival	44	91%	96%	95%
Median Time to ECG (minutes)	44	12	11	8
Median Time to Transfer (minutes)[3]	0	-	75	61
Fibrinolytic Medication Timing[1]	4	75%	55%	54%
Heart Failure Care				
ACE Inhibitor or ARB for LVSD[1]	7	100%	94%	94%
Discharge Instructions	29	97%	89%	88%
Evaluation of LVS Function	34	88%	98%	98%
Smoking Cessation Advice[1]	2	100%	98%	98%
Pneumonia Care				
Appropriate Initial Antibiotic	36	81%	92%	92%
Blood Culture Timing	54	94%	95%	96%
Influenza Vaccine	32	81%	90%	91%
Initial Antibiotic Timing	41	98%	93%	95%
Pneumococcal Vaccine	47	83%	92%	93%
Smoking Cessation Advice[1]	7	86%	98%	97%
Surgical Care Improvement Project				
Appropriate VTP Within 24 Hours[5]	0	-	94%	92%
Appropriate Hair Removal[5]	0	-	100%	99%
Appropriate Beta Blocker Usage[5]	0	-	92%	93%
Controlled Postoperative Blood Glucose[5]	0	-	94%	93%
Prophylactic Antibiotic Timing[5]	0	-	96%	97%
Prophylactic Antibiotic Timing (Outpatient)[5]	0	-	92%	92%
Prophylactic Antibiotic Selection[5]	0	-	97%	97%
Prophylactic Antibiotic Select. (Outpatient)[5]	0	-	93%	94%
Prophylactic Antibiotic Stopped[5]	0	-	94%	94%
Recommended VTP Ordered[5]	0	-	96%	94%
Urinary Catheter Removal[5]	0	-	90%	90%
Children's Asthma Care				
Received Systemic Corticosteroids	-	-	-	100%
Received Home Management Plan	-	-	-	71%
Received Reliever Medication	-	-	-	100%
Use of Medical Imaging				
Combination Abdominal CT Scan	122	0.189	0.141	0.191
Combination Chest CT Scan	54	0.000	0.024	0.054
Follow-up Mammogram/Ultrasound	357	12.9%	9.8%	8.4%
MRI for Low Back Pain[5]	0	-	26.9%	32.7%
Survey of Patients' Hospital Experiences				
Area Around Room 'Always' Quiet at Night	(a)	65%	-	58%
Doctors 'Always' Communicated Well	(a)	75%	-	80%
Home Recovery Information Given	(a)	86%	-	82%
Hospital Given 9 or 10 on 10 Point Scale	(a)	66%	-	67%
Meds 'Always' Explained Before Given	(a)	55%	-	60%
Nurses 'Always' Communicated Well	(a)	76%	-	76%
Pain 'Always' Well Controlled	(a)	60%	-	69%
Room and Bathroom 'Always' Clean	(a)	72%	-	71%
Timely Help 'Always' Received	(a)	64%	-	64%
Would Definitely Recommend Hospital	(a)	70%	-	69%

Plainview Hospital

888 Old Country Road
Plainview, NY 11803
Phone: 516-719-3000
Fax: 516-719-2729
URL: www.nslij.com
Type: Acute Care Hospitals
Emergency Services: Yes
Ownership: Voluntary Non-Profit - Private
Beds: 239

Key Personnel:

CEO/President. . . . . Michael J Dowling
Coronary Care . . . . Kathleen Gallo, RN PhD
Operating Room. . . . . Linda Olander, RN
Pediatric Ambulatory Care . . . . . . James Fagin, MD
Quality Assurance . . . . Jeffrey A Kraut
Radiology. . . . . Howard Heimowitz, MD
Patient Relations . . . . Sylvia Lester

Measure	Cases	This Hosp.	State Avg.	U.S. Avg.
Heart Attack Care				
ACE Inhibitor or ARB for LVSD[1,2]	12	100%	95%	96%
Aspirin at Arrival[2]	109	98%	98%	99%
Aspirin at Discharge[2]	62	95%	98%	98%
Beta Blocker at Discharge[2]	61	100%	98%	98%
Fibrinolytic Medication Timing[2]	0	-	50%	55%
PCI Within 90 Minutes of Arrival[2]	0	-	88%	90%
Smoking Cessation Advice[2]	0	-	100%	99%
Chest Pain/Possible Heart Attack Care				
Aspirin at Arrival	110	98%	96%	95%
Median Time to ECG (minutes)	112	9	11	8
Median Time to Transfer (minutes)	32	58	75	61
Fibrinolytic Medication Timing	0	-	55%	54%
Heart Failure Care				
ACE Inhibitor or ARB for LVSD[2]	51	98%	94%	94%
Discharge Instructions[2]	192	95%	89%	88%
Evaluation of LVS Function[2]	270	100%	98%	98%
Smoking Cessation Advice[1,2]	12	100%	98%	98%
Pneumonia Care				
Appropriate Initial Antibiotic[2]	96	95%	92%	92%
Blood Culture Timing[2]	150	99%	95%	96%
Influenza Vaccine[2]	93	99%	90%	91%
Initial Antibiotic Timing[2]	141	99%	93%	95%
Pneumococcal Vaccine[2]	164	98%	92%	93%
Smoking Cessation Advice[2]	30	100%	98%	97%
Surgical Care Improvement Project				
Appropriate VTP Within 24 Hours[2]	227	99%	94%	92%
Appropriate Hair Removal[2]	434	100%	100%	99%
Appropriate Beta Blocker Usage[2]	159	100%	92%	93%
Controlled Postoperative Blood Glucose[1,2]	1	100%	94%	93%
Prophylactic Antibiotic Timing[2]	265	98%	96%	97%
Prophylactic Antibiotic Timing (Outpatient)	153	89%	92%	92%
Prophylactic Antibiotic Selection[2]	265	98%	97%	97%
Prophylactic Antibiotic Select. (Outpatient)	155	93%	93%	94%
Prophylactic Antibiotic Stopped[2]	252	96%	94%	94%
Recommended VTP Ordered[2]	228	100%	96%	94%
Urinary Catheter Removal[2]	52	98%	90%	90%
Children's Asthma Care				
Received Systemic Corticosteroids	-	-	-	100%
Received Home Management Plan	-	-	-	71%
Received Reliever Medication	-	-	-	100%
Use of Medical Imaging				
Combination Abdominal CT Scan	324	0.019	0.141	0.191
Combination Chest CT Scan	64	0.000	0.024	0.054
Follow-up Mammogram/Ultrasound[5]	0	-	9.8%	8.4%
MRI for Low Back Pain[1]	3	66.7%	26.9%	32.7%
Survey of Patients' Hospital Experiences				
Area Around Room 'Always' Quiet at Night	300+	36%	-	58%
Doctors 'Always' Communicated Well	300+	74%	-	80%
Home Recovery Information Given	300+	73%	-	82%
Hospital Given 9 or 10 on 10 Point Scale	300+	53%	-	67%
Meds 'Always' Explained Before Given	300+	53%	-	60%
Nurses 'Always' Communicated Well	300+	71%	-	76%
Pain 'Always' Well Controlled	300+	65%	-	69%
Room and Bathroom 'Always' Clean	300+	62%	-	71%
Timely Help 'Always' Received	300+	56%	-	64%
Would Definitely Recommend Hospital	300+	60%	-	69%

NOTE: Hospital profiles are in alphabetical order by state, then city, then hospital within the city; Rankings exclude hospitals with less than 25 cases except for patient surveys which excludes hospitals with less than 100 cases; (a) 100–299 cases; (1) The number of cases is too small to be sure how well a hospital is performing; (2) The hospital indicated that the data submitted for this measure were based on a sample of cases; (3) Data was collected during a shorter time period (fewer quarters) than the maximum possible time for this measure; (4) Suppressed for one or more quarters by CMS; (5) No data is available from the hospital for this measure; (6) Fewer than 100 patients completed the HCAHPS survey. Use these rates with caution, as the number of surveys may be too low to reliably assess hospital performance; (7) Survey results are based on less than 12 months of data; (8) Survey results are not available for this reporting period; (9) No or very few patients were eligible for the HCAHPS survey. The scores shown, if any, reflect a very small number of surveys; (10) A state average was not calculated because too few hospitals in the state submitted data; (11) There were discrepancies in the data collection process; Please refer to the User's Guide for a full explanation of data.

Champlain Valley Physicians Hospital Medical Center

75 Beekman Street Phone: 518-561-2000
Plattsburgh, NY 12901 Fax: 518-562-7302
URL: www.cvph.org
Type: Acute Care Hospitals Emergency Services: Yes
Ownership: Voluntary Non-Profit - Private Beds: 405

Key Personnel:
CEO/President. . . . . Stephens M Mundy
Chief of Medical Staff. . . . . Albert Abbott Jr
Radiology. . . . . Gary King

Measure	Cases	This Hosp.	State Avg.	U.S. Avg.
Heart Attack Care				
ACE Inhibitor or ARB for LVSD	38	97%	95%	96%
Aspirin at Arrival	185	99%	98%	99%
Aspirin at Discharge	257	99%	98%	98%
Beta Blocker at Discharge	269	97%	98%	98%
Fibrinolytic Medication Timing	0	-	50%	55%
PCI Within 90 Minutes of Arrival	28	93%	88%	90%
Smoking Cessation Advice	92	98%	100%	99%
Chest Pain/Possible Heart Attack Care				
Aspirin at Arrival[1]	11	100%	96%	95%
Median Time to ECG (minutes)[1]	11	15	11	8
Median Time to Transfer (minutes)[5]	0	-	75	61
Fibrinolytic Medication Timing[5]	0	-	55%	54%
Heart Failure Care				
ACE Inhibitor or ARB for LVSD	78	83%	94%	94%
Discharge Instructions	286	86%	89%	88%
Evaluation of LVS Function	356	100%	98%	98%
Smoking Cessation Advice	62	97%	98%	98%
Pneumonia Care				
Appropriate Initial Antibiotic	187	85%	92%	92%
Blood Culture Timing	322	92%	95%	96%
Influenza Vaccine	184	92%	90%	91%
Initial Antibiotic Timing	326	89%	93%	95%
Pneumococcal Vaccine	302	95%	92%	93%
Smoking Cessation Advice	140	96%	98%	97%
Surgical Care Improvement Project				
Appropriate VTP Within 24 Hours	320	88%	94%	92%
Appropriate Hair Removal	845	100%	100%	99%
Appropriate Beta Blocker Usage	290	94%	92%	93%
Controlled Postoperative Blood Glucose	127	99%	94%	93%
Prophylactic Antibiotic Timing	589	91%	96%	97%
Prophylactic Antibiotic Timing (Outpatient)	311	82%	92%	92%
Prophylactic Antibiotic Selection	591	95%	97%	97%
Prophylactic Antibiotic Select. (Outpatient)	283	92%	93%	94%
Prophylactic Antibiotic Stopped	581	92%	94%	94%
Recommended VTP Ordered	320	91%	96%	94%
Urinary Catheter Removal	234	92%	90%	90%
Children's Asthma Care				
Received Systemic Corticosteroids	-	-	-	100%
Received Home Management Plan	-	-	-	71%
Received Reliever Medication	-	-	-	100%
Use of Medical Imaging				
Combination Abdominal CT Scan	956	0.052	0.141	0.191
Combination Chest CT Scan	694	0.056	0.024	0.054
Follow-up Mammogram/Ultrasound	2,543	9.0%	9.8%	8.4%
MRI for Low Back Pain	45	46.7%	26.9%	32.7%
Survey of Patients' Hospital Experiences				
Area Around Room 'Always' Quiet at Night	300+	43%	-	58%
Doctors 'Always' Communicated Well	300+	77%	-	80%
Home Recovery Information Given	300+	81%	-	82%
Hospital Given 9 or 10 on 10 Point Scale	300+	57%	-	67%
Meds 'Always' Explained Before Given	300+	59%	-	60%
Nurses 'Always' Communicated Well	300+	73%	-	76%
Pain 'Always' Well Controlled	300+	66%	-	69%
Room and Bathroom 'Always' Clean	300+	67%	-	71%
Timely Help 'Always' Received	300+	59%	-	64%
Would Definitely Recommend Hospital	300+	63%	-	69%

John T Mather Memorial Hospital of Port Jefferson

75 North Country Road Phone: 631-473-1320
Port Jefferson, NY 11777 Fax: 631-473-7367
E-mail: publicaffairs@matherhospital.org
URL: www.matherhospital.com
Type: Acute Care Hospitals Emergency Services: Yes
Ownership: Voluntary Non-Profit - Private Beds: 248

Key Personnel:
CEO/President. . . . . Kenneth Roberts
Chief of Medical Staff. . . . . Lloyd Lense, MD
Operating Room. . . . . Colleen McCloy
Pediatric Ambulatory Care . . . . . . Martin Kaplan, MD
Pediatric In-Patient Care . . . . Martin Kaplan, MD
Quality Assurance . . . . Kevin Murray
Radiology. . . . . Huntley Alper, MD
Emergency Room . . . . Mitchell Pollack

Measure	Cases	This Hosp.	State Avg.	U.S. Avg.
Heart Attack Care				
ACE Inhibitor or ARB for LVSD[1]	10	100%	95%	96%
Aspirin at Arrival	147	100%	98%	99%
Aspirin at Discharge	68	100%	98%	98%
Beta Blocker at Discharge	73	99%	98%	98%
Fibrinolytic Medication Timing	0	-	50%	55%
PCI Within 90 Minutes of Arrival	0	-	88%	90%
Smoking Cessation Advice[1]	2	100%	100%	99%
Chest Pain/Possible Heart Attack Care				
Aspirin at Arrival	118	100%	96%	95%
Median Time to ECG (minutes)	120	10	11	8
Median Time to Transfer (minutes)	28	84	75	61
Fibrinolytic Medication Timing	0	-	55%	54%
Heart Failure Care				
ACE Inhibitor or ARB for LVSD	63	98%	94%	94%
Discharge Instructions	250	98%	89%	88%
Evaluation of LVS Function	389	100%	98%	98%
Smoking Cessation Advice	29	100%	98%	98%
Pneumonia Care				
Appropriate Initial Antibiotic	193	98%	92%	92%
Blood Culture Timing	352	99%	95%	96%
Influenza Vaccine	197	97%	90%	91%
Initial Antibiotic Timing	281	98%	93%	95%
Pneumococcal Vaccine	262	99%	92%	93%
Smoking Cessation Advice	110	100%	98%	97%
Surgical Care Improvement Project				
Appropriate VTP Within 24 Hours	304	94%	94%	92%
Appropriate Hair Removal	536	100%	100%	99%
Appropriate Beta Blocker Usage	191	97%	92%	93%
Controlled Postoperative Blood Glucose	0	-	94%	93%
Prophylactic Antibiotic Timing	276	100%	96%	97%
Prophylactic Antibiotic Timing (Outpatient)	165	97%	92%	92%
Prophylactic Antibiotic Selection	282	98%	97%	97%
Prophylactic Antibiotic Select. (Outpatient)	178	94%	93%	94%
Prophylactic Antibiotic Stopped	266	97%	94%	94%
Recommended VTP Ordered	304	95%	96%	94%
Urinary Catheter Removal	74	92%	90%	90%
Children's Asthma Care				
Received Systemic Corticosteroids	-	-	-	100%
Received Home Management Plan	-	-	-	71%
Received Reliever Medication	-	-	-	100%
Use of Medical Imaging				
Combination Abdominal CT Scan	949	0.064	0.141	0.191
Combination Chest CT Scan	643	0.008	0.024	0.054
Follow-up Mammogram/Ultrasound	1,724	33.7%	9.8%	8.4%
MRI for Low Back Pain[1]	53	17.0%	26.9%	32.7%
Survey of Patients' Hospital Experiences				
Area Around Room 'Always' Quiet at Night	300+	49%	-	58%
Doctors 'Always' Communicated Well	300+	79%	-	80%
Home Recovery Information Given	300+	87%	-	82%
Hospital Given 9 or 10 on 10 Point Scale	300+	70%	-	67%
Meds 'Always' Explained Before Given	300+	61%	-	60%
Nurses 'Always' Communicated Well	300+	78%	-	76%
Pain 'Always' Well Controlled	300+	72%	-	69%
Room and Bathroom 'Always' Clean	300+	70%	-	71%
Timely Help 'Always' Received	300+	65%	-	64%
Would Definitely Recommend Hospital	300+	76%	-	69%

Saint Charles Hospital

200 Belle Terre Road Phone: 631-474-6000
Port Jefferson, NY 11777 Fax: 631-474-6824
URL: www.stcharles.org
Type: Acute Care Hospitals Emergency Services: Yes
Ownership: Voluntary Non-Profit - Church Beds: 289

Key Personnel:
CEO/President. . . . . David A Dibner
Operating Room. . . . . Margaret Fischer
Pediatric Ambulatory Care . . . . . . Harvey Kolker, MD
Pediatric In-Patient Care . . . . Harvey Kolker, MD
Quality Assurance . . . . Dante Latorre
Radiology. . . . . Albert Trachtenberg, MD
Patient Relations . . . . Debra Vion

Measure	Cases	This Hosp.	State Avg.	U.S. Avg.
Heart Attack Care				
ACE Inhibitor or ARB for LVSD[1]	1	100%	95%	96%
Aspirin at Arrival[1]	21	100%	98%	99%
Aspirin at Discharge[1]	7	100%	98%	98%
Beta Blocker at Discharge[1]	8	100%	98%	98%
Fibrinolytic Medication Timing	0	-	50%	55%
PCI Within 90 Minutes of Arrival	0	-	88%	90%
Smoking Cessation Advice[1]	1	100%	100%	99%
Chest Pain/Possible Heart Attack Care				
Aspirin at Arrival[1]	10	100%	96%	95%
Median Time to ECG (minutes)[1]	11	9	11	8
Median Time to Transfer (minutes)[1,3]	5	80	75	61
Fibrinolytic Medication Timing[3]	0	-	55%	54%
Heart Failure Care				
ACE Inhibitor or ARB for LVSD[1]	16	100%	94%	94%
Discharge Instructions	67	100%	89%	88%
Evaluation of LVS Function	80	99%	98%	98%
Smoking Cessation Advice[1]	10	100%	98%	98%
Pneumonia Care				
Appropriate Initial Antibiotic	73	96%	92%	92%
Blood Culture Timing	130	100%	95%	96%
Influenza Vaccine	56	100%	90%	91%
Initial Antibiotic Timing	98	100%	93%	95%
Pneumococcal Vaccine	62	100%	92%	93%
Smoking Cessation Advice	30	97%	98%	97%
Surgical Care Improvement Project				
Appropriate VTP Within 24 Hours[2]	269	99%	94%	92%
Appropriate Hair Removal[2]	691	100%	100%	99%
Appropriate Beta Blocker Usage[2]	204	100%	92%	93%
Controlled Postoperative Blood Glucose[2]	0	-	94%	93%
Prophylactic Antibiotic Timing[2]	488	100%	96%	97%
Prophylactic Antibiotic Timing (Outpatient)	46	98%	92%	92%
Prophylactic Antibiotic Selection[2]	490	100%	97%	97%
Prophylactic Antibiotic Select. (Outpatient)	45	96%	93%	94%
Prophylactic Antibiotic Stopped[2]	483	100%	94%	94%
Recommended VTP Ordered[2]	269	99%	96%	94%
Urinary Catheter Removal	248	100%	90%	90%
Children's Asthma Care				
Received Systemic Corticosteroids	-	-	-	100%
Received Home Management Plan	-	-	-	71%
Received Reliever Medication	-	-	-	100%
Use of Medical Imaging				
Combination Abdominal CT Scan	328	0.043	0.141	0.191
Combination Chest CT Scan	261	0.011	0.024	0.054
Follow-up Mammogram/Ultrasound	429	24.2%	9.8%	8.4%
MRI for Low Back Pain[1]	39	10.3%	26.9%	32.7%
Survey of Patients' Hospital Experiences				
Area Around Room 'Always' Quiet at Night	300+	50%	-	58%
Doctors 'Always' Communicated Well	300+	81%	-	80%
Home Recovery Information Given	300+	86%	-	82%
Hospital Given 9 or 10 on 10 Point Scale	300+	70%	-	67%
Meds 'Always' Explained Before Given	300+	57%	-	60%
Nurses 'Always' Communicated Well	300+	75%	-	76%
Pain 'Always' Well Controlled	300+	67%	-	69%
Room and Bathroom 'Always' Clean	300+	70%	-	71%
Timely Help 'Always' Received	300+	59%	-	64%
Would Definitely Recommend Hospital	300+	75%	-	69%

NOTE: Hospital profiles are in alphabetical order by state, then city, then hospital within the city; Rankings exclude hospitals with less than 25 cases except for patient surveys which excludes hospitals with less than 100 cases; (a) 100–299 cases; (1) The number of cases is too small to be sure how well a hospital is performing; (2) The hospital indicated that the data submitted for this measure were based on a sample of cases; (3) Data was collected during a shorter time period (fewer quarters) than the maximum possible time for this measure; (4) Suppressed for one or more quarters by CMS; (5) No data is available from the hospital for this measure; (6) Fewer than 100 patients completed the HCAHPS survey. Use these rates with caution, as the number of surveys may be too low to reliably assess hospital performance; (7) Survey results are based on less than 12 months of data; (8) Survey results are not available for this reporting period; (9) No or very few patients were eligible for the HCAHPS survey. The scores shown, if any, reflect a very small number of surveys; (10) A state average was not calculated because too few hospitals in the state submitted data; (11) There were discrepancies in the data collection process; Please refer to the User's Guide for a full explanation of data.

Bon Secours Community Hospital

160 East Main Street Phone: 845-856-5351
Port Jervis, NY 12771 Fax: 845-858-7415
URL: www.bonsecourscommunityhosp.com
Type: Acute Care Hospitals Emergency Services: Yes
Ownership: Voluntary Non-Profit - Church Beds: 183

Key Personnel:

CEO/President. . . . . Dominick Stanzione
Cardiac Laboratory. . . . . Fradrick Ayers
Chief of Medical Staff . . . . Richard J Daboul
Radiology. . . . . Rachael Braunstein
Emergency Room . . . . David Israel

Measure	Cases	This Hosp.	State Avg.	U.S. Avg.
Heart Attack Care				
ACE Inhibitor or ARB for LVSD[1]	4	100%	95%	96%
Aspirin at Arrival	31	94%	98%	99%
Aspirin at Discharge[1]	19	100%	98%	98%
Beta Blocker at Discharge[1]	22	95%	98%	98%
Fibrinolytic Medication Timing	0	-	50%	55%
PCI Within 90 Minutes of Arrival	0	-	88%	90%
Smoking Cessation Advice[1]	4	100%	100%	99%
Chest Pain/Possible Heart Attack Care				
Aspirin at Arrival	55	100%	96%	95%
Median Time to ECG (minutes)	57	12	11	8
Median Time to Transfer (minutes)[1]	8	68	75	61
Fibrinolytic Medication Timing[1]	6	50%	55%	54%
Heart Failure Care				
ACE Inhibitor or ARB for LVSD[1]	23	100%	94%	94%
Discharge Instructions	77	84%	89%	88%
Evaluation of LVS Function	97	99%	98%	98%
Smoking Cessation Advice[1]	23	100%	98%	98%
Pneumonia Care				
Appropriate Initial Antibiotic	75	95%	92%	92%
Blood Culture Timing	107	97%	95%	96%
Influenza Vaccine	62	100%	90%	91%
Initial Antibiotic Timing	93	97%	93%	95%
Pneumococcal Vaccine	90	94%	92%	93%
Smoking Cessation Advice	37	100%	98%	97%
Surgical Care Improvement Project				
Appropriate VTP Within 24 Hours	62	97%	94%	92%
Appropriate Hair Removal	109	100%	100%	99%
Appropriate Beta Blocker Usage	40	95%	92%	93%
Controlled Postoperative Blood Glucose	0	-	94%	93%
Prophylactic Antibiotic Timing	53	100%	96%	97%
Prophylactic Antibiotic Timing (Outpatient)[1]	16	88%	92%	92%
Prophylactic Antibiotic Selection	55	96%	97%	97%
Prophylactic Antibiotic Select. (Outpatient)[1]	16	94%	93%	94%
Prophylactic Antibiotic Stopped	50	92%	94%	94%
Recommended VTP Ordered	62	98%	96%	94%
Urinary Catheter Removal[1]	14	64%	90%	90%
Children's Asthma Care				
Received Systemic Corticosteroids	-	-	-	100%
Received Home Management Plan	-	-	-	71%
Received Reliever Medication	-	-	-	100%
Use of Medical Imaging				
Combination Abdominal CT Scan	452	0.066	0.141	0.191
Combination Chest CT Scan	253	0.032	0.024	0.054
Follow-up Mammogram/Ultrasound	603	7.1%	9.8%	8.4%
MRI for Low Back Pain	96	28.1%	26.9%	32.7%
Survey of Patients' Hospital Experiences				
Area Around Room 'Always' Quiet at Night	300+	58%	-	58%
Doctors 'Always' Communicated Well	300+	77%	-	80%
Home Recovery Information Given	300+	78%	-	82%
Hospital Given 9 or 10 on 10 Point Scale	300+	60%	-	67%
Meds 'Always' Explained Before Given	300+	59%	-	60%
Nurses 'Always' Communicated Well	300+	76%	-	76%
Pain 'Always' Well Controlled	300+	72%	-	69%
Room and Bathroom 'Always' Clean	300+	70%	-	71%
Timely Help 'Always' Received	300+	64%	-	64%
Would Definitely Recommend Hospital	300+	60%	-	69%

Canton-Potsdam Hospital

50 Leroy Street Phone: 315-265-3300
Potsdam, NY 13676 Fax: 315-265-2056
URL: www.cphospital.org
Type: Acute Care Hospitals Emergency Services: Yes
Ownership: Voluntary Non-Profit - Private Beds: 94

Key Personnel:

CEO/President. . . . . David B Acker, FACHE
Cardiac Laboratory. . . . . Alexandru Stoian, MD
Chief of Medical Staff . . . . G Michael Maresca, MD
Infection Control . . . . Nancy Wood
Operating Room. . . . . Marion Vandenheuvel
Radiology. . . . . Mark Morales

Measure	Cases	This Hosp.	State Avg.	U.S. Avg.
Heart Attack Care				
ACE Inhibitor or ARB for LVSD	0	-	95%	96%
Aspirin at Arrival[1]	11	100%	98%	99%
Aspirin at Discharge[1]	4	100%	98%	98%
Beta Blocker at Discharge[1]	5	80%	98%	98%
Fibrinolytic Medication Timing	0	-	50%	55%
PCI Within 90 Minutes of Arrival	0	-	88%	90%
Smoking Cessation Advice	0	-	100%	99%
Chest Pain/Possible Heart Attack Care				
Aspirin at Arrival	65	97%	96%	95%
Median Time to ECG (minutes)	67	6	11	8
Median Time to Transfer (minutes)[1,3]	1	255	75	61
Fibrinolytic Medication Timing[1]	21	62%	55%	54%
Heart Failure Care				
ACE Inhibitor or ARB for LVSD	34	97%	94%	94%
Discharge Instructions	85	87%	89%	88%
Evaluation of LVS Function	99	97%	98%	98%
Smoking Cessation Advice[1]	20	95%	98%	98%
Pneumonia Care				
Appropriate Initial Antibiotic	74	86%	92%	92%
Blood Culture Timing	100	94%	95%	96%
Influenza Vaccine	69	88%	90%	91%
Initial Antibiotic Timing	122	95%	93%	95%
Pneumococcal Vaccine	103	95%	92%	93%
Smoking Cessation Advice	42	95%	98%	97%
Surgical Care Improvement Project				
Appropriate VTP Within 24 Hours	139	99%	94%	92%
Appropriate Hair Removal	318	100%	100%	99%
Appropriate Beta Blocker Usage	86	94%	92%	93%
Controlled Postoperative Blood Glucose	0	-	94%	93%
Prophylactic Antibiotic Timing	220	99%	96%	97%
Prophylactic Antibiotic Timing (Outpatient)	83	99%	92%	92%
Prophylactic Antibiotic Selection	221	96%	97%	97%
Prophylactic Antibiotic Select. (Outpatient)	83	67%	93%	94%
Prophylactic Antibiotic Stopped	220	100%	94%	94%
Recommended VTP Ordered	139	99%	96%	94%
Urinary Catheter Removal	55	98%	90%	90%
Children's Asthma Care				
Received Systemic Corticosteroids	-	-	-	100%
Received Home Management Plan	-	-	-	71%
Received Reliever Medication	-	-	-	100%
Use of Medical Imaging				
Combination Abdominal CT Scan	459	0.046	0.141	0.191
Combination Chest CT Scan	294	0.003	0.024	0.054
Follow-up Mammogram/Ultrasound	978	5.7%	9.8%	8.4%
MRI for Low Back Pain	135	24.4%	26.9%	32.7%
Survey of Patients' Hospital Experiences				
Area Around Room 'Always' Quiet at Night	300+	50%	-	58%
Doctors 'Always' Communicated Well	300+	81%	-	80%
Home Recovery Information Given	300+	88%	-	82%
Hospital Given 9 or 10 on 10 Point Scale	300+	65%	-	67%
Meds 'Always' Explained Before Given	300+	64%	-	60%
Nurses 'Always' Communicated Well	300+	75%	-	76%
Pain 'Always' Well Controlled	300+	68%	-	69%
Room and Bathroom 'Always' Clean	300+	77%	-	71%
Timely Help 'Always' Received	300+	64%	-	64%
Would Definitely Recommend Hospital	300+	70%	-	69%

Saint Francis Hospital

241 North Road Phone: 845-483-5000
Poughkeepsie, NY 12601 Fax: 845-485-3762
URL: www.sfhhc.org
Type: Acute Care Hospitals Emergency Services: Yes
Ownership: Voluntary Non-Profit - Private Beds: 400

Key Personnel:

CEO/President. . . . . Robert Savage
Cardiac Laboratory. . . . . Lisa LaFalce
Chief of Medical Staff . . . . J Keith Fasta, MD
Infection Control . . . . Kathy Hollister
Operating Room. . . . . Terri Egitto
Quality Assurance . . . . Patricia Smith
Radiology. . . . . Lisa LaFalce

Measure	Cases	This Hosp.	State Avg.	U.S. Avg.
Heart Attack Care				
ACE Inhibitor or ARB for LVSD[1]	1	100%	95%	96%
Aspirin at Arrival	25	100%	98%	99%
Aspirin at Discharge[1]	17	100%	98%	98%
Beta Blocker at Discharge[1]	15	100%	98%	98%
Fibrinolytic Medication Timing	0	-	50%	55%
PCI Within 90 Minutes of Arrival	0	-	88%	90%
Smoking Cessation Advice[1]	6	100%	100%	99%
Chest Pain/Possible Heart Attack Care				
Aspirin at Arrival[1]	10	100%	96%	95%
Median Time to ECG (minutes)[1]	10	16	11	8
Median Time to Transfer (minutes)[1,3]	5	48	75	61
Fibrinolytic Medication Timing	0	-	55%	54%
Heart Failure Care				
ACE Inhibitor or ARB for LVSD[1]	20	100%	94%	94%
Discharge Instructions	42	100%	89%	88%
Evaluation of LVS Function	79	100%	98%	98%
Smoking Cessation Advice[1]	15	100%	98%	98%
Pneumonia Care				
Appropriate Initial Antibiotic	67	99%	92%	92%
Blood Culture Timing	120	99%	95%	96%
Influenza Vaccine	94	99%	90%	91%
Initial Antibiotic Timing	118	97%	93%	95%
Pneumococcal Vaccine	115	99%	92%	93%
Smoking Cessation Advice	56	100%	98%	97%
Surgical Care Improvement Project				
Appropriate VTP Within 24 Hours[2]	136	96%	94%	92%
Appropriate Hair Removal[2]	367	100%	100%	99%
Appropriate Beta Blocker Usage[2]	115	98%	92%	93%
Controlled Postoperative Blood Glucose[2]	0	-	94%	93%
Prophylactic Antibiotic Timing[2]	233	100%	96%	97%
Prophylactic Antibiotic Timing (Outpatient)	181	94%	92%	92%
Prophylactic Antibiotic Selection[2]	231	99%	97%	97%
Prophylactic Antibiotic Select. (Outpatient)	176	95%	93%	94%
Prophylactic Antibiotic Stopped[2]	227	99%	94%	94%
Recommended VTP Ordered[2]	136	99%	96%	94%
Urinary Catheter Removal[2]	32	100%	90%	90%
Children's Asthma Care				
Received Systemic Corticosteroids	-	-	-	100%
Received Home Management Plan	-	-	-	71%
Received Reliever Medication	-	-	-	100%
Use of Medical Imaging				
Combination Abdominal CT Scan	444	0.153	0.141	0.191
Combination Chest CT Scan	312	0.048	0.024	0.054
Follow-up Mammogram/Ultrasound	452	15.0%	9.8%	8.4%
MRI for Low Back Pain[1]	38	31.6%	26.9%	32.7%
Survey of Patients' Hospital Experiences				
Area Around Room 'Always' Quiet at Night	300+	49%	-	58%
Doctors 'Always' Communicated Well	300+	74%	-	80%
Home Recovery Information Given	300+	85%	-	82%
Hospital Given 9 or 10 on 10 Point Scale	300+	61%	-	67%
Meds 'Always' Explained Before Given	300+	58%	-	60%
Nurses 'Always' Communicated Well	300+	72%	-	76%
Pain 'Always' Well Controlled	300+	67%	-	69%
Room and Bathroom 'Always' Clean	300+	67%	-	71%
Timely Help 'Always' Received	300+	63%	-	64%
Would Definitely Recommend Hospital	300+	67%	-	69%

NOTE: Hospital profiles are in alphabetical order by state, then city, then hospital within the city; Rankings exclude hospitals with less than 25 cases except for patient surveys which excludes hospitals with less than 100 cases; (a) 100–299 cases; (1) The number of cases is too small to be sure how well a hospital is performing; (2) The hospital indicated that the data submitted for this measure were based on a sample of cases; (3) Data was collected during a shorter time period (fewer quarters) than the maximum possible time for this measure; (4) Suppressed for one or more quarters by CMS; (5) No data is available from the hospital for this measure; (6) Fewer than 100 patients completed the HCAHPS survey. Use these rates with caution, as the number of surveys may be too low to reliably assess hospital performance; (7) Survey results are based on less than 12 months of data; (8) Survey results are not available for this reporting period; (9) No or very few patients were eligible for the HCAHPS survey. The scores shown, if any, reflect a very small number of surveys; (10) A state average was not calculated because too few hospitals in the state submitted data; (11) There were discrepancies in the data collection process; Please refer to the User's Guide for a full explanation of data.

Vassar Brothers Medical Center

45 Reade Place Phone: 845-454-8500
Poughkeepsie, NY 12601 Fax: 845-437-3120
URL: www.vasserbrothers.org
Type: Acute Care Hospitals Emergency Services: Yes
Ownership: Voluntary Non-Profit - Other Beds: 365

Key Personnel:
Chief of Medical Staff.......... Lawrence Scheck, MD
Infection Control.............. Mary Ann Magerl
Pediatric In-Patient Care .... Lawrence Schaeffer, MD
Radiology.................... Bryan Yen
Anesthesiology............... Richard Goldmann, MD
Emergency Room .... David Weinreich
Intensive Care Unit........... Carol Wilson

Measure	Cases	This Hosp.	State Avg.	U.S. Avg.
Heart Attack Care				
ACE Inhibitor or ARB for LVSD	62	100%	95%	96%
Aspirin at Arrival	292	100%	98%	99%
Aspirin at Discharge	378	100%	98%	98%
Beta Blocker at Discharge	394	100%	98%	98%
Fibrinolytic Medication Timing[1]	1	0%	50%	55%
PCI Within 90 Minutes of Arrival	67	90%	88%	90%
Smoking Cessation Advice	121	100%	100%	99%
Chest Pain/Possible Heart Attack Care				
Aspirin at Arrival[5]	0	-	96%	95%
Median Time to ECG (minutes)[5]	0	-	11	8
Median Time to Transfer (minutes)[5]	0	-	75	61
Fibrinolytic Medication Timing[5]	0	-	55%	54%
Heart Failure Care				
ACE Inhibitor or ARB for LVSD	176	96%	94%	94%
Discharge Instructions	466	98%	89%	88%
Evaluation of LVS Function	632	100%	98%	98%
Smoking Cessation Advice	78	100%	98%	98%
Pneumonia Care				
Appropriate Initial Antibiotic[2]	142	92%	92%	92%
Blood Culture Timing[2]	247	100%	95%	96%
Influenza Vaccine[2]	204	98%	90%	91%
Initial Antibiotic Timing[2]	251	98%	93%	95%
Pneumococcal Vaccine[2]	302	97%	92%	93%
Smoking Cessation Advice[2]	64	100%	98%	97%
Surgical Care Improvement Project				
Appropriate VTP Within 24 Hours[2]	187	92%	94%	92%
Appropriate Hair Removal[2]	642	99%	100%	99%
Appropriate Beta Blocker Usage[2]	274	95%	92%	93%
Controlled Postoperative Blood Glucose[2]	171	96%	94%	93%
Prophylactic Antibiotic Timing[2]	442	97%	96%	97%
Prophylactic Antibiotic Timing (Outpatient)	637	95%	92%	92%
Prophylactic Antibiotic Selection[2]	446	98%	97%	97%
Prophylactic Antibiotic Select. (Outpatient)	632	95%	93%	94%
Prophylactic Antibiotic Stopped[2]	409	97%	94%	94%
Recommended VTP Ordered[2]	187	98%	96%	94%
Urinary Catheter Removal[2]	55	96%	90%	90%
Children's Asthma Care				
Received Systemic Corticosteroids	-	-	-	100%
Received Home Management Plan	-	-	-	71%
Received Reliever Medication	-	-	-	100%
Use of Medical Imaging				
Combination Abdominal CT Scan	709	0.216	0.141	0.191
Combination Chest CT Scan	357	0.008	0.024	0.054
Follow-up Mammogram/Ultrasound	679	13.4%	9.8%	8.4%
MRI for Low Back Pain[1]	25	32.0%	26.9%	32.7%
Survey of Patients' Hospital Experiences				
Area Around Room 'Always' Quiet at Night[11]	300+	53%	-	58%
Doctors 'Always' Communicated Well[11]	300+	79%	-	80%
Home Recovery Information Given[11]	300+	83%	-	82%
Hospital Given 9 or 10 on 10 Point Scale[11]	300+	71%	-	67%
Meds 'Always' Explained Before Given[11]	300+	62%	-	60%
Nurses 'Always' Communicated Well[11]	300+	81%	-	76%
Pain 'Always' Well Controlled[11]	300+	75%	-	69%
Room and Bathroom 'Always' Clean[11]	300+	71%	-	71%
Timely Help 'Always' Received[11]	300+	63%	-	64%
Would Definitely Recommend Hospital[11]	300+	80%	-	69%

Northern Dutchess Hospital

6511 Springbrook Avenue Phone: 845-871-3391
Rhinebeck, NY 12572 Fax: 845-876-7195
E-mail: ndinfo@health-quest.org
URL: www.health-quest.org
Type: Acute Care Hospitals Emergency Services: Yes
Ownership: Voluntary Non-Profit - Other Beds: 68

Key Personnel:
CEO/President............... Denise George
Chief of Medical Staff.......... Robert Rosenzweig, MD
Infection Control.............. Maija Wheeler
Operating Room.............. Gailri Richardson
Pediatric In-Patient Care .... Jane Ferguson
Radiology................... Judy Zaho
Intensive Care Unit........... Kathleen Liston-Scott, RN
Patient Relations .... Jean Clarke

Measure	Cases	This Hosp.	State Avg.	U.S. Avg.
Heart Attack Care				
ACE Inhibitor or ARB for LVSD[1]	4	100%	95%	96%
Aspirin at Arrival	28	89%	98%	99%
Aspirin at Discharge[1]	16	100%	98%	98%
Beta Blocker at Discharge[1]	17	100%	98%	98%
Fibrinolytic Medication Timing	0	-	50%	55%
PCI Within 90 Minutes of Arrival	0	-	88%	90%
Smoking Cessation Advice[1]	1	100%	100%	99%
Chest Pain/Possible Heart Attack Care				
Aspirin at Arrival[1]	17	100%	96%	95%
Median Time to ECG (minutes)[1]	19	14	11	8
Median Time to Transfer (minutes)[1]	4	70	75	61
Fibrinolytic Medication Timing	0	-	55%	54%
Heart Failure Care				
ACE Inhibitor or ARB for LVSD[1]	22	95%	94%	94%
Discharge Instructions	51	80%	89%	88%
Evaluation of LVS Function	77	100%	98%	98%
Smoking Cessation Advice[1]	7	43%	98%	98%
Pneumonia Care				
Appropriate Initial Antibiotic	38	84%	92%	92%
Blood Culture Timing	71	92%	95%	96%
Influenza Vaccine	56	84%	90%	91%
Initial Antibiotic Timing	70	96%	93%	95%
Pneumococcal Vaccine	73	86%	92%	93%
Smoking Cessation Advice[1]	18	72%	98%	97%
Surgical Care Improvement Project				
Appropriate VTP Within 24 Hours[2]	101	89%	94%	92%
Appropriate Hair Removal[2]	320	100%	100%	99%
Appropriate Beta Blocker Usage[2]	90	84%	92%	93%
Controlled Postoperative Blood Glucose[2]	0	-	94%	93%
Prophylactic Antibiotic Timing[2]	206	95%	96%	97%
Prophylactic Antibiotic Timing (Outpatient)	110	86%	92%	92%
Prophylactic Antibiotic Selection[2]	207	98%	97%	97%
Prophylactic Antibiotic Select. (Outpatient)	103	98%	93%	94%
Prophylactic Antibiotic Stopped[2]	203	98%	94%	94%
Recommended VTP Ordered[2]	101	94%	96%	94%
Urinary Catheter Removal[2]	123	86%	90%	90%
Children's Asthma Care				
Received Systemic Corticosteroids	-	-	-	100%
Received Home Management Plan	-	-	-	71%
Received Reliever Medication	-	-	-	100%
Use of Medical Imaging				
Combination Abdominal CT Scan	304	0.359	0.141	0.191
Combination Chest CT Scan	168	0.054	0.024	0.054
Follow-up Mammogram/Ultrasound	605	8.8%	9.8%	8.4%
MRI for Low Back Pain[1]	44	31.8%	26.9%	32.7%
Survey of Patients' Hospital Experiences				
Area Around Room 'Always' Quiet at Night	300+	51%	-	58%
Doctors 'Always' Communicated Well	300+	80%	-	80%
Home Recovery Information Given	300+	84%	-	82%
Hospital Given 9 or 10 on 10 Point Scale	300+	73%	-	67%
Meds 'Always' Explained Before Given	300+	64%	-	60%
Nurses 'Always' Communicated Well	300+	80%	-	76%
Pain 'Always' Well Controlled	300+	72%	-	69%
Room and Bathroom 'Always' Clean	300+	67%	-	71%
Timely Help 'Always' Received	300+	64%	-	64%
Would Definitely Recommend Hospital	300+	79%	-	69%

Peconic Bay Medical Center

1300 Roanoke Avenue Phone: 631-548-6000
Riverhead, NY 11901 Fax: 631-548-6048
E-mail: info@pbmedicalcenter.org
URL: www.pbmedicalcenter.org
Type: Acute Care Hospitals Emergency Services: Yes
Ownership: Voluntary Non-Profit - Private Beds: 214

Key Personnel:
CEO/President............... Andrew J Mitchell
Chief of Medical Staff.......... Samir Bute
Radiology................... James Badia

Measure	Cases	This Hosp.	State Avg.	U.S. Avg.
Heart Attack Care				
ACE Inhibitor or ARB for LVSD[1]	5	80%	95%	96%
Aspirin at Arrival	49	98%	98%	99%
Aspirin at Discharge	25	100%	98%	98%
Beta Blocker at Discharge	29	100%	98%	98%
Fibrinolytic Medication Timing	0	-	50%	55%
PCI Within 90 Minutes of Arrival	0	-	88%	90%
Smoking Cessation Advice[1]	3	100%	100%	99%
Chest Pain/Possible Heart Attack Care				
Aspirin at Arrival	121	100%	96%	95%
Median Time to ECG (minutes)	126	10	11	8
Median Time to Transfer (minutes)[1]	18	50	75	61
Fibrinolytic Medication Timing[1]	2	100%	55%	54%
Heart Failure Care				
ACE Inhibitor or ARB for LVSD	54	98%	94%	94%
Discharge Instructions	177	98%	89%	88%
Evaluation of LVS Function	234	96%	98%	98%
Smoking Cessation Advice[1]	13	100%	98%	98%
Pneumonia Care				
Appropriate Initial Antibiotic	82	89%	92%	92%
Blood Culture Timing	124	85%	95%	96%
Influenza Vaccine	70	73%	90%	91%
Initial Antibiotic Timing	115	95%	93%	95%
Pneumococcal Vaccine	105	70%	92%	93%
Smoking Cessation Advice	35	100%	98%	97%
Surgical Care Improvement Project				
Appropriate VTP Within 24 Hours	229	92%	94%	92%
Appropriate Hair Removal	463	100%	100%	99%
Appropriate Beta Blocker Usage	146	90%	92%	93%
Controlled Postoperative Blood Glucose	0	-	94%	93%
Prophylactic Antibiotic Timing	308	95%	96%	97%
Prophylactic Antibiotic Timing (Outpatient)	67	93%	92%	92%
Prophylactic Antibiotic Selection	308	93%	97%	97%
Prophylactic Antibiotic Select. (Outpatient)	62	97%	93%	94%
Prophylactic Antibiotic Stopped	298	92%	94%	94%
Recommended VTP Ordered	229	97%	96%	94%
Urinary Catheter Removal	159	96%	90%	90%
Children's Asthma Care				
Received Systemic Corticosteroids	-	-	-	100%
Received Home Management Plan	-	-	-	71%
Received Reliever Medication	-	-	-	100%
Use of Medical Imaging				
Combination Abdominal CT Scan	462	0.041	0.141	0.191
Combination Chest CT Scan	391	0.013	0.024	0.054
Follow-up Mammogram/Ultrasound	59	5.1%	9.8%	8.4%
MRI for Low Back Pain	88	19.3%	26.9%	32.7%
Survey of Patients' Hospital Experiences				
Area Around Room 'Always' Quiet at Night	300+	39%	-	58%
Doctors 'Always' Communicated Well	300+	73%	-	80%
Home Recovery Information Given	300+	80%	-	82%
Hospital Given 9 or 10 on 10 Point Scale	300+	50%	-	67%
Meds 'Always' Explained Before Given	300+	52%	-	60%
Nurses 'Always' Communicated Well	300+	69%	-	76%
Pain 'Always' Well Controlled	300+	61%	-	69%
Room and Bathroom 'Always' Clean	300+	58%	-	71%
Timely Help 'Always' Received	300+	47%	-	64%
Would Definitely Recommend Hospital	300+	53%	-	69%

NOTE: Hospital profiles are in alphabetical order by state, then city, then hospital within the city; Rankings exclude hospitals with less than 25 cases except for patient surveys which excludes hospitals with less than 100 cases; (a) 100–299 cases; (1) The number of cases is too small to be sure how well a hospital is performing; (2) The hospital indicated that the data submitted for this measure were based on a sample of cases; (3) Data was collected during a shorter time period (fewer quarters) than the maximum possible time for this measure; (4) Suppressed for one or more quarters by CMS; (5) No data is available from the hospital for this measure; (6) Fewer than 100 patients completed the HCAHPS survey. Use these rates with caution, as the number of surveys may be too low to reliably assess hospital performance; (7) Survey results are based on less than 12 months of data; (8) Survey results are not available for this reporting period; (9) No or very few patients were eligible for the HCAHPS survey. The scores shown, if any, reflect a very small number of surveys; (10) A state average was not calculated because too few hospitals in the state submitted data; (11) There were discrepancies in the data collection process; Please refer to the User's Guide for a full explanation of data.

Highland Hospital

1000 South Avenue
Rochester, NY 14620
URL: www.urmc.rochester.edu
Type: Acute Care Hospitals
Ownership: Voluntary Non-Profit - Private

Phone: 585-473-2200
Fax: 585-341-6703

Emergency Services: Yes
Beds: 272

Key Personnel:
CEO/President . . . . William Remizowski
Chief of Medical Staff . . . . Howard Beckman, MD
Infection Control . . . . Ann Marie Pettis, RN
Operating Room . . . . Amy Matroniano, RN
Pediatric Ambulatory Care . . . . . Veronica Guillet, MD
Pediatric In-Patient Care . . . . . . Veronica Guillet, MD
Quality Assurance . . . . Donna Johnston
Radiology . . . . Francis Kelley, MD

Measure	Cases	This Hosp.	State Avg.	U.S. Avg.
Heart Attack Care				
ACE Inhibitor or ARB for LVSD[1]	13	92%	95%	96%
Aspirin at Arrival	68	97%	98%	99%
Aspirin at Discharge	52	100%	98%	98%
Beta Blocker at Discharge	49	100%	98%	98%
Fibrinolytic Medication Timing	0	-	50%	55%
PCI Within 90 Minutes of Arrival	0	-	88%	90%
Smoking Cessation Advice[1]	7	100%	100%	99%
Chest Pain/Possible Heart Attack Care				
Aspirin at Arrival[1]	24	96%	96%	95%
Median Time to ECG (minutes)	25	22	11	8
Median Time to Transfer (minutes)[1]	5	45	75	61
Fibrinolytic Medication Timing	0	-	55%	54%
Heart Failure Care				
ACE Inhibitor or ARB for LVSD	59	98%	94%	94%
Discharge Instructions	215	97%	89%	88%
Evaluation of LVS Function	309	99%	98%	98%
Smoking Cessation Advice	43	100%	98%	98%
Pneumonia Care				
Appropriate Initial Antibiotic	167	98%	92%	92%
Blood Culture Timing	277	98%	95%	96%
Influenza Vaccine	173	96%	90%	91%
Initial Antibiotic Timing	218	99%	93%	95%
Pneumococcal Vaccine	249	98%	92%	93%
Smoking Cessation Advice	77	100%	98%	97%
Surgical Care Improvement Project				
Appropriate VTP Within 24 Hours[2]	231	98%	94%	92%
Appropriate Hair Removal[2]	992	100%	100%	99%
Appropriate Beta Blocker Usage[2]	304	86%	92%	93%
Controlled Postoperative Blood Glucose[2]	0	-	94%	93%
Prophylactic Antibiotic Timing[2]	781	96%	96%	97%
Prophylactic Antibiotic Timing (Outpatient)	203	95%	92%	92%
Prophylactic Antibiotic Selection[2]	777	97%	97%	97%
Prophylactic Antibiotic Select. (Outpatient)	202	96%	93%	94%
Prophylactic Antibiotic Stopped[2]	765	99%	94%	94%
Recommended VTP Ordered[2]	231	99%	96%	94%
Urinary Catheter Removal[2]	287	95%	90%	90%
Children's Asthma Care				
Received Systemic Corticosteroids	-	-	-	100%
Received Home Management Plan	-	-	-	71%
Received Reliever Medication	-	-	-	100%
Use of Medical Imaging				
Combination Abdominal CT Scan	471	0.310	0.141	0.191
Combination Chest CT Scan	338	0.337	0.024	0.054
Follow-up Mammogram/Ultrasound	720	10.0%	9.8%	8.4%
MRI for Low Back Pain[5]	0	-	26.9%	32.7%
Survey of Patients' Hospital Experiences				
Area Around Room 'Always' Quiet at Night	300+	48%	-	58%
Doctors 'Always' Communicated Well	300+	79%	-	80%
Home Recovery Information Given	300+	86%	-	82%
Hospital Given 9 or 10 on 10 Point Scale	300+	69%	-	67%
Meds 'Always' Explained Before Given	300+	61%	-	60%
Nurses 'Always' Communicated Well	300+	76%	-	76%
Pain 'Always' Well Controlled	300+	68%	-	69%
Room and Bathroom 'Always' Clean	300+	65%	-	71%
Timely Help 'Always' Received	300+	56%	-	64%
Would Definitely Recommend Hospital	300+	76%	-	69%

Monroe Community Hospital

435 East Henrietta Road
Rochester, NY 14620
E-mail: info@monroehosp.org
URL: www.monroehosp.org
Type: Acute Care Hospitals
Ownership: Government - Local

Phone: 585-760-6500
Fax: 585-760-6066

Emergency Services: No
Beds: 566

Key Personnel:
Chief of Medical Staff . . . . Paul Katz
Infection Control . . . . Paul Graman
Quality Assurance . . . . Tom Yale
Radiology . . . . Antoinette Cavalieri

Measure	Cases	This Hosp.	State Avg.	U.S. Avg.
Heart Attack Care				
ACE Inhibitor or ARB for LVSD[5]	0	-	95%	96%
Aspirin at Arrival[5]	0	-	98%	99%
Aspirin at Discharge[5]	0	-	98%	98%
Beta Blocker at Discharge[5]	0	-	98%	98%
Fibrinolytic Medication Timing[5]	0	-	50%	55%
PCI Within 90 Minutes of Arrival[5]	0	-	88%	90%
Smoking Cessation Advice[5]	0	-	100%	99%
Chest Pain/Possible Heart Attack Care				
Aspirin at Arrival	-	-	96%	95%
Median Time to ECG (minutes)	-	-	11	8
Median Time to Transfer (minutes)	-	-	75	61
Fibrinolytic Medication Timing	-	-	55%	54%
Heart Failure Care				
ACE Inhibitor or ARB for LVSD[5]	0	-	94%	94%
Discharge Instructions[5]	0	-	89%	88%
Evaluation of LVS Function[5]	0	-	98%	98%
Smoking Cessation Advice[5]	0	-	98%	98%
Pneumonia Care				
Appropriate Initial Antibiotic[5]	0	-	92%	92%
Blood Culture Timing[5]	0	-	95%	96%
Influenza Vaccine[5]	0	-	90%	91%
Initial Antibiotic Timing[5]	0	-	93%	95%
Pneumococcal Vaccine[5]	0	-	92%	93%
Smoking Cessation Advice[5]	0	-	98%	97%
Surgical Care Improvement Project				
Appropriate VTP Within 24 Hours[5]	0	-	94%	92%
Appropriate Hair Removal[5]	0	-	100%	99%
Appropriate Beta Blocker Usage[5]	0	-	92%	93%
Controlled Postoperative Blood Glucose[5]	0	-	94%	93%
Prophylactic Antibiotic Timing[5]	0	-	96%	97%
Prophylactic Antibiotic Timing (Outpatient)	-	-	92%	92%
Prophylactic Antibiotic Selection[5]	-	-	97%	97%
Prophylactic Antibiotic Select. (Outpatient)	-	-	93%	94%
Prophylactic Antibiotic Stopped[5]	0	-	94%	94%
Recommended VTP Ordered[5]	-	-	96%	94%
Urinary Catheter Removal[5]	0	-	90%	90%
Children's Asthma Care				
Received Systemic Corticosteroids	-	-	-	100%
Received Home Management Plan	-	-	-	71%
Received Reliever Medication	-	-	-	100%
Use of Medical Imaging				
Combination Abdominal CT Scan	-	-	0.141	0.191
Combination Chest CT Scan	-	-	0.024	0.054
Follow-up Mammogram/Ultrasound	-	-	9.8%	8.4%
MRI for Low Back Pain	-	-	26.9%	32.7%
Survey of Patients' Hospital Experiences				
Area Around Room 'Always' Quiet at Night[9]	-	-	-	58%
Doctors 'Always' Communicated Well[9]	-	-	-	80%
Home Recovery Information Given[9]	-	-	-	82%
Hospital Given 9 or 10 on 10 Point Scale[9]	-	-	-	67%
Meds 'Always' Explained Before Given[9]	-	-	-	60%
Nurses 'Always' Communicated Well[9]	-	-	-	76%
Pain 'Always' Well Controlled[9]	-	-	-	69%
Room and Bathroom 'Always' Clean[9]	-	-	-	71%
Timely Help 'Always' Received[9]	-	-	-	64%
Would Definitely Recommend Hospital[9]	-	-	-	69%

Rochester General Hospital

1425 Portland Avenue
Rochester, NY 14621
URL: www.rochestergeneral.org
Type: Acute Care Hospitals
Ownership: Voluntary Non-Profit - Private

Phone: 585-922-4000
Fax: 585-922-4290

Emergency Services: Yes
Beds: 528

Key Personnel:
CEO/President . . . . Mark Clement
Chief of Medical Staff . . . . Georgianne Zigarowicz, MD
Coronary Care . . . . Ronald Kirshner, MD
Infection Control . . . . Edward Walsh, MD
Pediatric Ambulatory Care . . . . . David Siegal, MD
Pediatric In-Patient Care . . . . . . David Siegal, MD
Quality Assurance . . . . Mary Tribuzzi
Radiology . . . . Jonathan Broder, MD

Measure	Cases	This Hosp.	State Avg.	U.S. Avg.
Heart Attack Care				
ACE Inhibitor or ARB for LVSD[2]	42	100%	95%	96%
Aspirin at Arrival[2]	213	98%	98%	99%
Aspirin at Discharge[2]	308	100%	98%	98%
Beta Blocker at Discharge[2]	309	100%	98%	98%
Fibrinolytic Medication Timing[2]	0	-	50%	55%
PCI Within 90 Minutes of Arrival[2]	33	76%	88%	90%
Smoking Cessation Advice[2]	113	100%	100%	99%
Chest Pain/Possible Heart Attack Care				
Aspirin at Arrival[1,3]	11	82%	96%	95%
Median Time to ECG (minutes)[1,3]	11	27	11	8
Median Time to Transfer (minutes)[5]	-	-	75	61
Fibrinolytic Medication Timing[2]	0	-	55%	54%
Heart Failure Care				
ACE Inhibitor or ARB for LVSD[2]	109	97%	94%	94%
Discharge Instructions[2]	259	92%	89%	88%
Evaluation of LVS Function[2]	315	99%	98%	98%
Smoking Cessation Advice[2]	48	100%	98%	98%
Pneumonia Care				
Appropriate Initial Antibiotic	369	95%	92%	92%
Blood Culture Timing	514	98%	95%	96%
Influenza Vaccine	348	89%	90%	91%
Initial Antibiotic Timing	557	88%	93%	95%
Pneumococcal Vaccine	491	85%	92%	93%
Smoking Cessation Advice	186	100%	98%	97%
Surgical Care Improvement Project				
Appropriate VTP Within 24 Hours[2]	553	96%	94%	92%
Appropriate Hair Removal[2]	2,308	100%	100%	99%
Appropriate Beta Blocker Usage[2]	1,057	93%	92%	93%
Controlled Postoperative Blood Glucose[2]	634	98%	94%	93%
Prophylactic Antibiotic Timing[2]	1,832	99%	96%	97%
Prophylactic Antibiotic Timing (Outpatient)	690	92%	92%	92%
Prophylactic Antibiotic Selection[2]	1,874	99%	97%	97%
Prophylactic Antibiotic Select. (Outpatient)	650	90%	93%	94%
Prophylactic Antibiotic Stopped[2]	1,774	99%	94%	94%
Recommended VTP Ordered[2]	553	96%	96%	94%
Urinary Catheter Removal[2]	327	97%	90%	90%
Children's Asthma Care				
Received Systemic Corticosteroids	-	-	-	100%
Received Home Management Plan	-	-	-	71%
Received Reliever Medication	-	-	-	100%
Use of Medical Imaging				
Combination Abdominal CT Scan	596	0.592	0.141	0.191
Combination Chest CT Scan	328	0.317	0.024	0.054
Follow-up Mammogram/Ultrasound	232	7.8%	9.8%	8.4%
MRI for Low Back Pain[1]	19	42.1%	26.9%	32.7%
Survey of Patients' Hospital Experiences				
Area Around Room 'Always' Quiet at Night	300+	42%	-	58%
Doctors 'Always' Communicated Well	300+	80%	-	80%
Home Recovery Information Given	300+	91%	-	82%
Hospital Given 9 or 10 on 10 Point Scale	300+	71%	-	67%
Meds 'Always' Explained Before Given	300+	63%	-	60%
Nurses 'Always' Communicated Well	300+	79%	-	76%
Pain 'Always' Well Controlled	300+	70%	-	69%
Room and Bathroom 'Always' Clean	300+	66%	-	71%
Timely Help 'Always' Received	300+	62%	-	64%
Would Definitely Recommend Hospital	300+	78%	-	69%

NOTE: Hospital profiles are in alphabetical order by state, then city, then hospital within the city; Rankings exclude hospitals with less than 25 cases except for patient surveys which excludes hospitals with less than 100 cases; (a) 100–299 cases; (1) The number of cases is too small to be sure how well a hospital is performing; (2) The hospital indicated that the data submitted for this measure were based on a sample of cases; (3) Data was collected during a shorter time period (fewer quarters) than the maximum possible time for this measure; (4) Suppressed for one or more quarters by CMS; (5) No data is available from the hospital for this measure; (6) Fewer than 100 patients completed the HCAHPS survey. Use these rates with caution, as the number of surveys may be too low to reliably assess hospital performance; (7) Survey results are based on less than 12 months of data; (8) Survey results are not available for this reporting period; (9) No or very few patients were eligible for the HCAHPS survey. The scores shown, if any, reflect a very small number of surveys; (10) A state average was not calculated because too few hospitals in the state submitted data; (11) There were discrepancies in the data collection process; Please refer to the User's Guide for a full explanation of data.

Strong Memorial Hospital

601 Elmwood Ave Phone: 585-275-2121
Rochester, NY 14642 Fax: 585-256-3805
URL: www.urmc.rochester.edu
Type: Acute Care Hospitals Emergency Services: Yes
Ownership: Voluntary Non-Profit - Private Beds: 750

Key Personnel:
CEO/President. . . . . Steven I Goldstein
Chief of Medical Staff . . . . Mark Utell, MD
Infection Control. . . . . John J. Treanorn, MD
Operating Room. . . . . Sandra Monacelli
Pediatric Ambulatory Care . . . . . . Nina F. Schor, MD, PhD
Pediatric In-Patient Care . . . . Nina F. Schor, MD, PhD
Quality Assurance . . . . Ted Case
Radiology. . . . . David Waldman, MD

Measure	Cases	This Hosp.	State Avg.	U.S. Avg.
Heart Attack Care				
ACE Inhibitor or ARB for LVSD	207	99%	95%	96%
Aspirin at Arrival	350	100%	98%	99%
Aspirin at Discharge	684	100%	98%	98%
Beta Blocker at Discharge	663	100%	98%	98%
Fibrinolytic Medication Timing	0	-	50%	55%
PCI Within 90 Minutes of Arrival	77	96%	88%	90%
Smoking Cessation Advice	226	100%	100%	99%
Chest Pain/Possible Heart Attack Care				
Aspirin at Arrival[5]	0	-	96%	95%
Median Time to ECG (minutes)[5]	0	-	11	8
Median Time to Transfer (minutes)[5]	0	-	75	61
Fibrinolytic Medication Timing[5]	0	-	55%	54%
Heart Failure Care				
ACE Inhibitor or ARB for LVSD	232	100%	94%	94%
Discharge Instructions	647	98%	89%	88%
Evaluation of LVS Function	738	99%	98%	98%
Smoking Cessation Advice	124	99%	98%	98%
Pneumonia Care				
Appropriate Initial Antibiotic[2]	74	82%	92%	92%
Blood Culture Timing[2]	157	88%	95%	96%
Influenza Vaccine[2]	66	86%	90%	91%
Initial Antibiotic Timing[2]	136	81%	93%	95%
Pneumococcal Vaccine[2]	77	87%	92%	93%
Smoking Cessation Advice[2]	61	93%	98%	97%
Surgical Care Improvement Project				
Appropriate VTP Within 24 Hours[2]	306	100%	94%	92%
Appropriate Hair Removal[2]	1,282	100%	100%	99%
Appropriate Beta Blocker Usage[2]	532	97%	92%	93%
Controlled Postoperative Blood Glucose[2]	428	92%	94%	93%
Prophylactic Antibiotic Timing[2]	847	99%	96%	97%
Prophylactic Antibiotic Timing (Outpatient)	572	98%	92%	92%
Prophylactic Antibiotic Selection[2]	868	99%	97%	97%
Prophylactic Antibiotic Select. (Outpatient)	572	99%	93%	94%
Prophylactic Antibiotic Stopped[2]	818	99%	94%	94%
Recommended VTP Ordered[2]	306	100%	96%	94%
Urinary Catheter Removal[2]	327	98%	90%	90%
Children's Asthma Care				
Received Systemic Corticosteroids	-	-	-	100%
Received Home Management Plan	-	-	-	71%
Received Reliever Medication	-	-	-	100%
Use of Medical Imaging				
Combination Abdominal CT Scan	952	0.239	0.141	0.191
Combination Chest CT Scan	788	0.123	0.024	0.054
Follow-up Mammogram/Ultrasound	169	8.3%	9.8%	8.4%
MRI for Low Back Pain[1]	53	28.3%	26.9%	32.7%
Survey of Patients' Hospital Experiences				
Area Around Room 'Always' Quiet at Night	300+	37%	-	58%
Doctors 'Always' Communicated Well	300+	75%	-	80%
Home Recovery Information Given	300+	87%	-	82%
Hospital Given 9 or 10 on 10 Point Scale	300+	65%	-	67%
Meds 'Always' Explained Before Given	300+	60%	-	60%
Nurses 'Always' Communicated Well	300+	75%	-	76%
Pain 'Always' Well Controlled	300+	65%	-	69%
Room and Bathroom 'Always' Clean	300+	61%	-	71%
Timely Help 'Always' Received	300+	56%	-	64%
Would Definitely Recommend Hospital	300+	74%	-	69%

Unity Hospital of Rochester

1555 Long Pond Road Phone: 585-723-7000
Rochester, NY 14626
URL: www.unityhealth.org
Type: Acute Care Hospitals Emergency Services: Yes
Ownership: Voluntary Non-Profit - Private Beds: 681

Measure	Cases	This Hosp.	State Avg.	U.S. Avg.
Heart Attack Care				
ACE Inhibitor or ARB for LVSD[2]	39	100%	95%	96%
Aspirin at Arrival[2]	242	97%	98%	99%
Aspirin at Discharge[2]	202	99%	98%	98%
Beta Blocker at Discharge[2]	207	100%	98%	98%
Fibrinolytic Medication Timing[2]	0	-	50%	55%
PCI Within 90 Minutes of Arrival[2]	47	94%	88%	90%
Smoking Cessation Advice[2]	55	100%	100%	99%
Chest Pain/Possible Heart Attack Care				
Aspirin at Arrival[1]	23	96%	96%	95%
Median Time to ECG (minutes)[1]	24	12	11	8
Median Time to Transfer (minutes)[5]	0	-	75	61
Fibrinolytic Medication Timing[3]	0	-	55%	54%
Heart Failure Care				
ACE Inhibitor or ARB for LVSD[2]	87	98%	94%	94%
Discharge Instructions[2]	253	97%	89%	88%
Evaluation of LVS Function[2]	322	100%	98%	98%
Smoking Cessation Advice[2]	35	100%	98%	98%
Pneumonia Care				
Appropriate Initial Antibiotic[2]	114	97%	92%	92%
Blood Culture Timing[2]	200	98%	95%	96%
Influenza Vaccine[2]	105	93%	90%	91%
Initial Antibiotic Timing[2]	190	91%	93%	95%
Pneumococcal Vaccine[2]	168	93%	92%	93%
Smoking Cessation Advice[2]	52	100%	98%	97%
Surgical Care Improvement Project				
Appropriate VTP Within 24 Hours[2]	170	99%	94%	92%
Appropriate Hair Removal[2]	561	98%	100%	99%
Appropriate Beta Blocker Usage[2]	254	81%	92%	93%
Controlled Postoperative Blood Glucose[2]	0	-	94%	93%
Prophylactic Antibiotic Timing[2]	393	93%	96%	97%
Prophylactic Antibiotic Timing (Outpatient)	423	93%	92%	92%
Prophylactic Antibiotic Selection[2]	391	94%	97%	97%
Prophylactic Antibiotic Select. (Outpatient)	414	98%	93%	94%
Prophylactic Antibiotic Stopped[2]	387	93%	94%	94%
Recommended VTP Ordered[2]	170	99%	96%	94%
Urinary Catheter Removal[2]	161	90%	90%	90%
Children's Asthma Care				
Received Systemic Corticosteroids	-	-	-	100%
Received Home Management Plan	-	-	-	71%
Received Reliever Medication	-	-	-	100%
Use of Medical Imaging				
Combination Abdominal CT Scan	240	0.608	0.141	0.191
Combination Chest CT Scan[1]	44	0.205	0.024	0.054
Follow-up Mammogram/Ultrasound	391	11.3%	9.8%	8.4%
MRI for Low Back Pain[5]	0	-	26.9%	32.7%
Survey of Patients' Hospital Experiences				
Area Around Room 'Always' Quiet at Night	300+	47%	-	58%
Doctors 'Always' Communicated Well	300+	78%	-	80%
Home Recovery Information Given	300+	88%	-	82%
Hospital Given 9 or 10 on 10 Point Scale	300+	65%	-	67%
Meds 'Always' Explained Before Given	300+	55%	-	60%
Nurses 'Always' Communicated Well	300+	75%	-	76%
Pain 'Always' Well Controlled	300+	65%	-	69%
Room and Bathroom 'Always' Clean	300+	58%	-	71%
Timely Help 'Always' Received	300+	56%	-	64%
Would Definitely Recommend Hospital	300+	72%	-	69%

Mercy Medical Center

1000 North Village Avenue Phone: 516-705-2525
Rockville Centre, NY 11570 Fax: 516-705-2584
URL: www.mercymedicalcenter.info
Type: Acute Care Hospitals Emergency Services: Yes
Ownership: Voluntary Non-Profit - Church Beds: 375

Key Personnel:
CEO/President. . . . . Alan D Guerci MD
Chief of Medical Staff . . . . John P Reilly MD
Quality Assurance . . . . Catherine Magoone RN

Measure	Cases	This Hosp.	State Avg.	U.S. Avg.
Heart Attack Care				
ACE Inhibitor or ARB for LVSD[1]	5	80%	95%	96%
Aspirin at Arrival	59	100%	98%	99%
Aspirin at Discharge	25	96%	98%	98%
Beta Blocker at Discharge[1]	24	100%	98%	98%
Fibrinolytic Medication Timing	0	-	50%	55%
PCI Within 90 Minutes of Arrival	0	-	88%	90%
Smoking Cessation Advice[1]	2	100%	100%	99%
Chest Pain/Possible Heart Attack Care				
Aspirin at Arrival	53	100%	96%	95%
Median Time to ECG (minutes)	56	8	11	8
Median Time to Transfer (minutes)[1]	21	45	75	61
Fibrinolytic Medication Timing	0	-	55%	54%
Heart Failure Care				
ACE Inhibitor or ARB for LVSD	78	97%	94%	94%
Discharge Instructions	160	92%	89%	88%
Evaluation of LVS Function	226	99%	98%	98%
Smoking Cessation Advice[1]	18	100%	98%	98%
Pneumonia Care				
Appropriate Initial Antibiotic	113	91%	92%	92%
Blood Culture Timing	207	94%	95%	96%
Influenza Vaccine	118	91%	90%	91%
Initial Antibiotic Timing	203	94%	93%	95%
Pneumococcal Vaccine	215	85%	92%	93%
Smoking Cessation Advice	34	100%	98%	97%
Surgical Care Improvement Project				
Appropriate VTP Within 24 Hours[2]	274	91%	94%	92%
Appropriate Hair Removal[2]	497	100%	100%	99%
Appropriate Beta Blocker Usage[2]	216	100%	92%	93%
Controlled Postoperative Blood Glucose[1,2]	1	100%	94%	93%
Prophylactic Antibiotic Timing[2]	316	97%	96%	97%
Prophylactic Antibiotic Timing (Outpatient)	99	95%	92%	92%
Prophylactic Antibiotic Selection[2]	317	97%	97%	97%
Prophylactic Antibiotic Select. (Outpatient)	96	86%	93%	94%
Prophylactic Antibiotic Stopped[2]	298	95%	94%	94%
Recommended VTP Ordered[2]	274	97%	96%	94%
Urinary Catheter Removal[2]	137	99%	90%	90%
Children's Asthma Care				
Received Systemic Corticosteroids	-	-	-	100%
Received Home Management Plan	-	-	-	71%
Received Reliever Medication	-	-	-	100%
Use of Medical Imaging				
Combination Abdominal CT Scan	607	0.016	0.141	0.191
Combination Chest CT Scan	492	0.008	0.024	0.054
Follow-up Mammogram/Ultrasound	680	9.0%	9.8%	8.4%
MRI for Low Back Pain[1]	55	21.8%	26.9%	32.7%
Survey of Patients' Hospital Experiences				
Area Around Room 'Always' Quiet at Night	300+	54%	-	58%
Doctors 'Always' Communicated Well	300+	78%	-	80%
Home Recovery Information Given	300+	81%	-	82%
Hospital Given 9 or 10 on 10 Point Scale	300+	59%	-	67%
Meds 'Always' Explained Before Given	300+	54%	-	60%
Nurses 'Always' Communicated Well	300+	71%	-	76%
Pain 'Always' Well Controlled	300+	66%	-	69%
Room and Bathroom 'Always' Clean	300+	63%	-	71%
Timely Help 'Always' Received	300+	55%	-	64%
Would Definitely Recommend Hospital	300+	65%	-	69%

NOTE: Hospital profiles are in alphabetical order by state, then city, then hospital within the city; Rankings exclude hospitals with less than 25 cases except for patient surveys which excludes hospitals with less than 100 cases; (a) 100–299 cases; (1) The number of cases is too small to be sure how well a hospital is performing; (2) The hospital indicated that the data submitted for this measure were based on a sample of cases; (3) Data was collected during a shorter time period (fewer quarters) than the maximum possible time for this measure; (4) Suppressed for one or more quarters by CMS; (5) No data is available from the hospital for this measure; (6) Fewer than 100 patients completed the HCAHPS survey. Use these rates with caution, as the number of surveys may be too low to reliably assess hospital performance; (7) Survey results are based on less than 12 months of data; (8) Survey results are not available for this reporting period; (9) No or very few patients were eligible for the HCAHPS survey. The scores shown, if any, reflect a very small number of surveys; (10) A state average was not calculated because too few hospitals in the state submitted data; (11) There were discrepancies in the data collection process; Please refer to the User's Guide for a full explanation of data.

Rome Memorial Hospital

1500 North James Street
Rome, NY 13440
Phone: 315-338-7000
Fax: 315-338-7072
URL: www.romehosp.org
Type: Acute Care Hospitals
Emergency Services: Yes
Ownership: Voluntary Non-Profit - Private
Beds: 129

Key Personnel:
CEO/President. . . . . Darlene A Burns
Chief of Medical Staff. . . . . Marybeth McCall, MD
Infection Control. . . . . LeAnna Grace
Operating Room. . . . . Teresa Bell
Pediatric Ambulatory Care . . . . . . Laurie Elwell, DO
Pediatric In-Patient Care . . . . Laurie Elwell, DO
Quality Assurance . . . . Kathleen Ulrich
Radiology. . . . . Amy Weakley

Measure	Cases	This Hosp.	State Avg.	U.S. Avg.
Heart Attack Care				
ACE Inhibitor or ARB for LVSD[1]	6	100%	95%	96%
Aspirin at Arrival	36	94%	98%	99%
Aspirin at Discharge[1]	20	95%	98%	98%
Beta Blocker at Discharge[1]	19	95%	98%	98%
Fibrinolytic Medication Timing	0	-	50%	55%
PCI Within 90 Minutes of Arrival	0	-	88%	90%
Smoking Cessation Advice[1]	2	100%	100%	99%
Chest Pain/Possible Heart Attack Care				
Aspirin at Arrival	50	98%	96%	95%
Median Time to ECG (minutes)	52	6	11	8
Median Time to Transfer (minutes)[1,3]	4	70	75	61
Fibrinolytic Medication Timing[1]	1	100%	55%	54%
Heart Failure Care				
ACE Inhibitor or ARB for LVSD	55	93%	94%	94%
Discharge Instructions	126	89%	89%	88%
Evaluation of LVS Function	204	96%	98%	98%
Smoking Cessation Advice[1]	23	91%	98%	98%
Pneumonia Care				
Appropriate Initial Antibiotic	100	88%	92%	92%
Blood Culture Timing	207	99%	95%	96%
Influenza Vaccine	123	94%	90%	91%
Initial Antibiotic Timing	192	96%	93%	95%
Pneumococcal Vaccine	162	96%	92%	93%
Smoking Cessation Advice	53	92%	98%	97%
Surgical Care Improvement Project				
Appropriate VTP Within 24 Hours	112	93%	94%	92%
Appropriate Hair Removal	239	100%	100%	99%
Appropriate Beta Blocker Usage	35	89%	92%	93%
Controlled Postoperative Blood Glucose	0	-	94%	93%
Prophylactic Antibiotic Timing	116	91%	96%	97%
Prophylactic Antibiotic Timing (Outpatient)	53	79%	92%	92%
Prophylactic Antibiotic Selection	115	89%	97%	97%
Prophylactic Antibiotic Select. (Outpatient)	46	85%	93%	94%
Prophylactic Antibiotic Stopped	108	94%	94%	94%
Recommended VTP Ordered	112	94%	96%	94%
Urinary Catheter Removal[1]	20	95%	90%	90%
Children's Asthma Care				
Received Systemic Corticosteroids	-	-	-	100%
Received Home Management Plan	-	-	-	71%
Received Reliever Medication	-	-	-	100%
Use of Medical Imaging				
Combination Abdominal CT Scan	591	0.592	0.141	0.191
Combination Chest CT Scan	343	0.020	0.024	0.054
Follow-up Mammogram/Ultrasound	425	25.6%	9.8%	8.4%
MRI for Low Back Pain[5]	0	-	26.9%	32.7%
Survey of Patients' Hospital Experiences				
Area Around Room 'Always' Quiet at Night	300+	45%	-	58%
Doctors 'Always' Communicated Well	300+	72%	-	80%
Home Recovery Information Given	300+	85%	-	82%
Hospital Given 9 or 10 on 10 Point Scale	300+	55%	-	67%
Meds 'Always' Explained Before Given	300+	58%	-	60%
Nurses 'Always' Communicated Well	300+	73%	-	76%
Pain 'Always' Well Controlled	300+	68%	-	69%
Room and Bathroom 'Always' Clean	300+	70%	-	71%
Timely Help 'Always' Received	300+	54%	-	64%
Would Definitely Recommend Hospital	300+	58%	-	69%

Saint Francis Hospital - Roslyn

100 Port Washington Boulevard
Roslyn, NY 11576
Phone: 516-562-6000
Fax: 516-705-6661
URL: www.stfrancisheartcenter.com
Type: Acute Care Hospitals
Emergency Services: Yes
Ownership: Voluntary Non-Profit - Church
Beds: 279

Key Personnel:
CEO/President. . . . . Alan D Guerci, MD
Chief of Medical Staff . . . . Lawrence A Reduto, MD
Coronary Care . . . . Susan Knoeffler, RN NCC
Infection Control. . . . . Marylou Solliday, RN
Pediatric Ambulatory Care . . . . . . Donna Rebelo, RN NCC
Pediatric In-Patient Care . . . . Donna Rebelo, RN NCC
Quality Assurance . . . . Nonette Schafer, RN
Radiology. . . . . Ken Goodman, MD

Measure	Cases	This Hosp.	State Avg.	U.S. Avg.
Heart Attack Care				
ACE Inhibitor or ARB for LVSD[2]	79	96%	95%	96%
Aspirin at Arrival[2]	132	98%	98%	99%
Aspirin at Discharge[2]	337	99%	98%	98%
Beta Blocker at Discharge[2]	342	99%	98%	98%
Fibrinolytic Medication Timing[2]	0	-	50%	55%
PCI Within 90 Minutes of Arrival[1,2]	9	89%	88%	90%
Smoking Cessation Advice[2]	73	100%	100%	99%
Chest Pain/Possible Heart Attack Care				
Aspirin at Arrival[5]	0	-	96%	95%
Median Time to ECG (minutes)[5]	0	-	11	8
Median Time to Transfer (minutes)[5]	0	-	75	61
Fibrinolytic Medication Timing[5]	0	-	55%	54%
Heart Failure Care				
ACE Inhibitor or ARB for LVSD[2]	146	90%	94%	94%
Discharge Instructions[2]	310	86%	89%	88%
Evaluation of LVS Function[2]	357	100%	98%	98%
Smoking Cessation Advice[2]	30	100%	98%	98%
Pneumonia Care				
Appropriate Initial Antibiotic	110	86%	92%	92%
Blood Culture Timing	173	95%	95%	96%
Influenza Vaccine	113	100%	90%	91%
Initial Antibiotic Timing	154	88%	93%	95%
Pneumococcal Vaccine	203	99%	92%	93%
Smoking Cessation Advice[1]	21	100%	98%	97%
Surgical Care Improvement Project				
Appropriate VTP Within 24 Hours[2]	188	97%	94%	92%
Appropriate Hair Removal[2]	650	100%	100%	99%
Appropriate Beta Blocker Usage[2]	331	97%	92%	93%
Controlled Postoperative Blood Glucose[2]	234	97%	94%	93%
Prophylactic Antibiotic Timing[2]	399	97%	96%	97%
Prophylactic Antibiotic Timing (Outpatient)	340	95%	92%	92%
Prophylactic Antibiotic Selection[2]	416	99%	97%	97%
Prophylactic Antibiotic Select. (Outpatient)	341	96%	93%	94%
Prophylactic Antibiotic Stopped[2]	381	97%	94%	94%
Recommended VTP Ordered[2]	188	98%	96%	94%
Urinary Catheter Removal[2]	141	90%	90%	90%
Children's Asthma Care				
Received Systemic Corticosteroids	-	-	-	100%
Received Home Management Plan	-	-	-	71%
Received Reliever Medication	-	-	-	100%
Use of Medical Imaging				
Combination Abdominal CT Scan	428	0.070	0.141	0.191
Combination Chest CT Scan	537	0.017	0.024	0.054
Follow-up Mammogram/Ultrasound	577	35.4%	9.8%	8.4%
MRI for Low Back Pain[1]	22	27.3%	26.9%	32.7%
Survey of Patients' Hospital Experiences				
Area Around Room 'Always' Quiet at Night	300+	53%	-	58%
Doctors 'Always' Communicated Well	300+	81%	-	80%
Home Recovery Information Given	300+	87%	-	82%
Hospital Given 9 or 10 on 10 Point Scale	300+	82%	-	67%
Meds 'Always' Explained Before Given	300+	61%	-	60%
Nurses 'Always' Communicated Well	300+	81%	-	76%
Pain 'Always' Well Controlled	300+	71%	-	69%
Room and Bathroom 'Always' Clean	300+	77%	-	71%
Timely Help 'Always' Received	300+	65%	-	64%
Would Definitely Recommend Hospital	300+	86%	-	69%

Adirondack Medical Center

2233 State Route 86
Saranac Lake, NY 12983
Phone: 518-891-4141
Fax: 518-891-1191
URL: www.amccares.org
Type: Acute Care Hospitals
Emergency Services: Yes
Ownership: Voluntary Non-Profit - Private
Beds: 97

Key Personnel:
CEO/President. . . . . Chandler M Ralph
Chief of Medical Staff. . . . . W Roy Slanowhite, MD
Infection Control. . . . . Mim Tracy, RN
Quality Assurance . . . . Doug Sarr, RN
Ambulatory Care . . . . Barbara Dukett, RN
Anesthesiology. . . . . Richard Rowell, MD
Emergency Room . . . . Mary O'Connor, RN
Hemotology Center . . . . Michael Randolph

Measure	Cases	This Hosp.	State Avg.	U.S. Avg.
Heart Attack Care				
ACE Inhibitor or ARB for LVSD[1]	4	100%	95%	96%
Aspirin at Arrival[1]	22	91%	98%	99%
Aspirin at Discharge[1]	14	86%	98%	98%
Beta Blocker at Discharge[1]	16	88%	98%	98%
Fibrinolytic Medication Timing	0	-	50%	55%
PCI Within 90 Minutes of Arrival	0	-	88%	90%
Smoking Cessation Advice[1]	3	100%	100%	99%
Chest Pain/Possible Heart Attack Care				
Aspirin at Arrival	51	100%	96%	95%
Median Time to ECG (minutes)	50	5	11	8
Median Time to Transfer (minutes)[5]	0	-	75	61
Fibrinolytic Medication Timing[1]	5	20%	55%	54%
Heart Failure Care				
ACE Inhibitor or ARB for LVSD	25	80%	94%	94%
Discharge Instructions	62	90%	89%	88%
Evaluation of LVS Function	69	91%	98%	98%
Smoking Cessation Advice[1]	9	100%	98%	98%
Pneumonia Care				
Appropriate Initial Antibiotic	27	78%	92%	92%
Blood Culture Timing	34	82%	95%	96%
Influenza Vaccine	45	87%	90%	91%
Initial Antibiotic Timing	49	92%	93%	95%
Pneumococcal Vaccine	60	93%	92%	93%
Smoking Cessation Advice[1]	13	92%	98%	97%
Surgical Care Improvement Project				
Appropriate VTP Within 24 Hours	150	50%	94%	92%
Appropriate Hair Removal	250	100%	100%	99%
Appropriate Beta Blocker Usage	69	90%	92%	93%
Controlled Postoperative Blood Glucose	0	-	94%	93%
Prophylactic Antibiotic Timing	157	87%	96%	97%
Prophylactic Antibiotic Timing (Outpatient)	99	87%	92%	92%
Prophylactic Antibiotic Selection	157	96%	97%	97%
Prophylactic Antibiotic Select. (Outpatient)	90	91%	93%	94%
Prophylactic Antibiotic Stopped	155	68%	94%	94%
Recommended VTP Ordered	154	49%	96%	94%
Urinary Catheter Removal	88	90%	90%	90%
Children's Asthma Care				
Received Systemic Corticosteroids	-	-	-	100%
Received Home Management Plan	-	-	-	71%
Received Reliever Medication	-	-	-	100%
Use of Medical Imaging				
Combination Abdominal CT Scan	344	0.674	0.141	0.191
Combination Chest CT Scan	303	0.677	0.024	0.054
Follow-up Mammogram/Ultrasound	853	18.5%	9.8%	8.4%
MRI for Low Back Pain[1]	33	24.2%	26.9%	32.7%
Survey of Patients' Hospital Experiences				
Area Around Room 'Always' Quiet at Night	300+	60%	-	58%
Doctors 'Always' Communicated Well	300+	82%	-	80%
Home Recovery Information Given	300+	82%	-	82%
Hospital Given 9 or 10 on 10 Point Scale	300+	69%	-	67%
Meds 'Always' Explained Before Given	300+	66%	-	60%
Nurses 'Always' Communicated Well	300+	77%	-	76%
Pain 'Always' Well Controlled	300+	72%	-	69%
Room and Bathroom 'Always' Clean	300+	73%	-	71%
Timely Help 'Always' Received	300+	72%	-	64%
Would Definitely Recommend Hospital	300+	75%	-	69%

NOTE: Hospital profiles are in alphabetical order by state, then city, then hospital within the city; Rankings exclude hospitals with less than 25 cases except for patient surveys which excludes hospitals with less than 100 cases; (a) 100–299 cases; (1) The number of cases is too small to be sure how well a hospital is performing; (2) The hospital indicated that the data submitted for this measure were based on a sample of cases; (3) Data was collected during a shorter time period (fewer quarters) than the maximum possible time for this measure; (4) Suppressed for one or more quarters by CMS; (5) No data is available from the hospital for this measure; (6) Fewer than 100 patients completed the HCAHPS survey. Use these rates with caution, as the number of surveys may be too low to reliably assess hospital performance; (7) Survey results are based on less than 12 months of data; (8) Survey results are not available for this reporting period; (9) No or very few patients were eligible for the HCAHPS survey. The scores shown, if any, reflect a very small number of surveys; (10) A state average was not calculated because too few hospitals in the state submitted data; (11) There were discrepancies in the data collection process; Please refer to the User's Guide for a full explanation of data.

Saratoga Hospital

211 Church Street Phone: 518-587-3222
Saratoga Springs, NY 12866 Fax: 518-583-8428
URL: www.saratogacare.org
Type: Acute Care Hospitals Emergency Services: Yes
Ownership: Voluntary Non-Profit - Private Beds: 243

Key Personnel:
CEO/President. . . . . Angelo Calbone
Chief of Medical Staff. . . . . Joyce L Peabody, MD
Operating Room. . . . . Cathleen Hamel
Quality Assurance . . . . Kim Hedley
Emergency Room . . . . Timothy Brooks
Intensive Care Unit. . . . . Diane Bartos
Patient Relations . . . . Noel Cook

Measure	Cases	This Hosp.	State Avg.	U.S. Avg.
Heart Attack Care				
ACE Inhibitor or ARB for LVSD[1]	10	80%	95%	96%
Aspirin at Arrival	62	100%	98%	99%
Aspirin at Discharge	37	95%	98%	98%
Beta Blocker at Discharge	45	98%	98%	98%
Fibrinolytic Medication Timing[1]	2	50%	50%	55%
PCI Within 90 Minutes of Arrival	0	-	88%	90%
Smoking Cessation Advice[1]	7	100%	100%	99%
Chest Pain/Possible Heart Attack Care				
Aspirin at Arrival	27	96%	96%	95%
Median Time to ECG (minutes)	27	8	11	8
Median Time to Transfer (minutes)[1,3]	2	199	75	61
Fibrinolytic Medication Timing[1]	14	36%	55%	54%
Heart Failure Care				
ACE Inhibitor or ARB for LVSD	43	98%	94%	94%
Discharge Instructions	239	95%	89%	88%
Evaluation of LVS Function	280	100%	98%	98%
Smoking Cessation Advice	40	100%	98%	98%
Pneumonia Care				
Appropriate Initial Antibiotic	162	94%	92%	92%
Blood Culture Timing	258	96%	95%	96%
Influenza Vaccine	167	99%	90%	91%
Initial Antibiotic Timing	246	94%	93%	95%
Pneumococcal Vaccine	229	98%	92%	93%
Smoking Cessation Advice	90	99%	98%	97%
Surgical Care Improvement Project				
Appropriate VTP Within 24 Hours	345	93%	94%	92%
Appropriate Hair Removal	713	100%	100%	99%
Appropriate Beta Blocker Usage	205	80%	92%	93%
Controlled Postoperative Blood Glucose	0	-	94%	93%
Prophylactic Antibiotic Timing	489	98%	96%	97%
Prophylactic Antibiotic Timing (Outpatient)	238	88%	92%	92%
Prophylactic Antibiotic Selection	488	97%	97%	97%
Prophylactic Antibiotic Select. (Outpatient)	214	96%	93%	94%
Prophylactic Antibiotic Stopped	472	85%	94%	94%
Recommended VTP Ordered	349	93%	96%	94%
Urinary Catheter Removal	225	91%	90%	90%
Children's Asthma Care				
Received Systemic Corticosteroids	-	-	-	100%
Received Home Management Plan	-	-	-	71%
Received Reliever Medication	-	-	-	100%
Use of Medical Imaging				
Combination Abdominal CT Scan	990	0.042	0.141	0.191
Combination Chest CT Scan	570	0.002	0.024	0.054
Follow-up Mammogram/Ultrasound	993	5.8%	9.8%	8.4%
MRI for Low Back Pain	96	32.3%	26.9%	32.7%
Survey of Patients' Hospital Experiences				
Area Around Room 'Always' Quiet at Night	300+	39%	-	58%
Doctors 'Always' Communicated Well	300+	80%	-	80%
Home Recovery Information Given	300+	91%	-	82%
Hospital Given 9 or 10 on 10 Point Scale	300+	66%	-	67%
Meds 'Always' Explained Before Given	300+	64%	-	60%
Nurses 'Always' Communicated Well	300+	79%	-	76%
Pain 'Always' Well Controlled	300+	72%	-	69%
Room and Bathroom 'Always' Clean	300+	70%	-	71%
Timely Help 'Always' Received	300+	65%	-	64%
Would Definitely Recommend Hospital	300+	71%	-	69%

Ellis Hospital

1101 Nott Street Phone: 518-243-4196
Schenectady, NY 12308 Fax: 518-243-4668
E-mail: webmaster@ellishospital.org
URL: www.ellishospital.org
Type: Acute Care Hospitals Emergency Services: Yes
Ownership: Proprietary Beds: 368

Key Personnel:
CEO/President. . . . . James W Connolly
Cardiac Laboratory. . . . . Lewis Bergman
Chief of Medical Staff. . . . . Michael Jakubowski, MD
Infection Control. . . . . Peg Wyant
Operating Room. . . . . Carmen Hercules, RN
Pediatric Ambulatory Care . . . . . . Pashu Pati Kumar, MD
Radiology. . . . . Gary Wood, MD

Measure	Cases	This Hosp.	State Avg.	U.S. Avg.
Heart Attack Care				
ACE Inhibitor or ARB for LVSD[2]	71	100%	95%	96%
Aspirin at Arrival[2]	409	98%	98%	99%
Aspirin at Discharge[2]	510	99%	98%	98%
Beta Blocker at Discharge[2]	506	100%	98%	98%
Fibrinolytic Medication Timing[2]	0	-	50%	55%
PCI Within 90 Minutes of Arrival[2]	65	94%	88%	90%
Smoking Cessation Advice[2]	151	100%	100%	99%
Chest Pain/Possible Heart Attack Care				
Aspirin at Arrival[1,3]	1	100%	96%	95%
Median Time to ECG (minutes)[1,3]	1	5	11	8
Median Time to Transfer (minutes)[5]	0	-	75	61
Fibrinolytic Medication Timing[5]	0	-	55%	54%
Heart Failure Care				
ACE Inhibitor or ARB for LVSD[2]	99	99%	94%	94%
Discharge Instructions[2]	440	99%	89%	88%
Evaluation of LVS Function[2]	572	98%	98%	98%
Smoking Cessation Advice[2]	73	100%	98%	98%
Pneumonia Care				
Appropriate Initial Antibiotic[2]	171	96%	92%	92%
Blood Culture Timing[2]	371	99%	95%	96%
Influenza Vaccine	249	95%	90%	91%
Initial Antibiotic Timing[2]	309	95%	93%	95%
Pneumococcal Vaccine[2]	323	97%	92%	93%
Smoking Cessation Advice[2]	108	98%	98%	97%
Surgical Care Improvement Project				
Appropriate VTP Within 24 Hours[2]	225	97%	94%	92%
Appropriate Hair Removal[2]	874	99%	100%	99%
Appropriate Beta Blocker Usage[2]	343	93%	92%	93%
Controlled Postoperative Blood Glucose[2]	192	96%	94%	93%
Prophylactic Antibiotic Timing[2]	668	100%	96%	97%
Prophylactic Antibiotic Timing (Outpatient)	538	92%	92%	92%
Prophylactic Antibiotic Selection[2]	680	97%	97%	97%
Prophylactic Antibiotic Select. (Outpatient)	515	96%	93%	94%
Prophylactic Antibiotic Stopped[2]	647	98%	94%	94%
Recommended VTP Ordered[2]	225	100%	96%	94%
Urinary Catheter Removal[2]	106	90%	90%	90%
Children's Asthma Care				
Received Systemic Corticosteroids	-	-	-	100%
Received Home Management Plan	-	-	-	71%
Received Reliever Medication	-	-	-	100%
Use of Medical Imaging				
Combination Abdominal CT Scan	1,049	0.026	0.141	0.191
Combination Chest CT Scan	926	0.000	0.024	0.054
Follow-up Mammogram/Ultrasound	2,387	6.9%	9.8%	8.4%
MRI for Low Back Pain	101	26.7%	26.9%	32.7%
Survey of Patients' Hospital Experiences				
Area Around Room 'Always' Quiet at Night	300+	44%	-	58%
Doctors 'Always' Communicated Well	300+	72%	-	80%
Home Recovery Information Given	300+	85%	-	82%
Hospital Given 9 or 10 on 10 Point Scale	300+	59%	-	67%
Meds 'Always' Explained Before Given	300+	53%	-	60%
Nurses 'Always' Communicated Well	300+	69%	-	76%
Pain 'Always' Well Controlled	300+	63%	-	69%
Room and Bathroom 'Always' Clean	300+	62%	-	71%
Timely Help 'Always' Received	300+	53%	-	64%
Would Definitely Recommend Hospital	300+	64%	-	69%

Sunnyview Hospital and Rehabilitation Center

1270 Belmont Avenue Phone: 518-386-3580
Schenectady, NY 12308 Fax: 518-382-4533
URL: www.sunnyview.org
Type: Acute Care Hospitals Emergency Services: No
Ownership: Voluntary Non-Profit - Private Beds: 104

Key Personnel:
CEO/President. . . . . Robert Bylancik
Chief of Medical Staff. . . . . Gary Williams, MD
Pediatric In-Patient Care . . . . George W Crawl, MD
Quality Assurance . . . . John Mackey

Measure	Cases	This Hosp.	State Avg.	U.S. Avg.
Heart Attack Care				
ACE Inhibitor or ARB for LVSD[5]	0	-	95%	96%
Aspirin at Arrival[5]	0	-	98%	99%
Aspirin at Discharge[5]	0	-	98%	98%
Beta Blocker at Discharge[5]	0	-	98%	98%
Fibrinolytic Medication Timing[5]	0	-	50%	55%
PCI Within 90 Minutes of Arrival[5]	0	-	88%	90%
Smoking Cessation Advice[5]	0	-	100%	99%
Chest Pain/Possible Heart Attack Care				
Aspirin at Arrival[5]	0	-	96%	95%
Median Time to ECG (minutes)[5]	0	-	11	8
Median Time to Transfer (minutes)[5]	0	-	75	61
Fibrinolytic Medication Timing[5]	0	-	55%	54%
Heart Failure Care				
ACE Inhibitor or ARB for LVSD[5]	0	-	94%	94%
Discharge Instructions[5]	0	-	89%	88%
Evaluation of LVS Function[5]	0	-	98%	98%
Smoking Cessation Advice[5]	0	-	98%	98%
Pneumonia Care				
Appropriate Initial Antibiotic[5]	0	-	92%	92%
Blood Culture Timing[5]	0	-	95%	96%
Influenza Vaccine[5]	0	-	90%	91%
Initial Antibiotic Timing[5]	0	-	93%	95%
Pneumococcal Vaccine[5]	0	-	92%	93%
Smoking Cessation Advice[5]	0	-	98%	97%
Surgical Care Improvement Project				
Appropriate VTP Within 24 Hours[5]	0	-	94%	92%
Appropriate Hair Removal[5]	0	-	100%	99%
Appropriate Beta Blocker Usage[5]	0	-	92%	93%
Controlled Postoperative Blood Glucose[5]	0	-	94%	93%
Prophylactic Antibiotic Timing[5]	0	-	96%	97%
Prophylactic Antibiotic Timing (Outpatient)[5]	0	-	92%	92%
Prophylactic Antibiotic Selection[5]	0	-	97%	97%
Prophylactic Antibiotic Select. (Outpatient)[5]	0	-	93%	94%
Prophylactic Antibiotic Stopped[5]	0	-	94%	94%
Recommended VTP Ordered[5]	0	-	96%	94%
Urinary Catheter Removal[5]	0	-	90%	90%
Children's Asthma Care				
Received Systemic Corticosteroids	-	-	-	100%
Received Home Management Plan	-	-	-	71%
Received Reliever Medication	-	-	-	100%
Use of Medical Imaging				
Combination Abdominal CT Scan[5]	0	-	0.141	0.191
Combination Chest CT Scan[5]	0	-	0.024	0.054
Follow-up Mammogram/Ultrasound[5]	0	-	9.8%	8.4%
MRI for Low Back Pain[5]	0	-	26.9%	32.7%
Survey of Patients' Hospital Experiences				
Area Around Room 'Always' Quiet at Night[9]	-	-	-	58%
Doctors 'Always' Communicated Well[9]	-	-	-	80%
Home Recovery Information Given[9]	-	-	-	82%
Hospital Given 9 or 10 on 10 Point Scale[9]	-	-	-	67%
Meds 'Always' Explained Before Given[9]	-	-	-	60%
Nurses 'Always' Communicated Well[9]	-	-	-	76%
Pain 'Always' Well Controlled[9]	-	-	-	69%
Room and Bathroom 'Always' Clean[9]	-	-	-	71%
Timely Help 'Always' Received[9]	-	-	-	64%
Would Definitely Recommend Hospital[9]	-	-	-	69%

NOTE: Hospital profiles are in alphabetical order by state, then city, then hospital within the city; Rankings exclude hospitals with less than 25 cases except for patient surveys which excludes hospitals with less than 100 cases; (a) 100–299 cases; (1) The number of cases is too small to be sure how well a hospital is performing; (2) The hospital indicated that the data submitted for this measure were based on a sample of cases; (3) Data was collected during a shorter time period (fewer quarters) than the maximum possible time for this measure; (4) Suppressed for one or more quarters by CMS; (5) No data is available from the hospital for this measure; (6) Fewer than 100 patients completed the HCAHPS survey. Use these rates with caution, as the number of surveys may be too low to reliably assess hospital performance; (7) Survey results are based on less than 12 months of data; (8) Survey results are not available for this reporting period; (9) No or very few patients were eligible for the HCAHPS survey. The scores shown, if any, reflect a very small number of surveys; (10) A state average was not calculated because too few hospitals in the state submitted data; (11) There were discrepancies in the data collection process; Please refer to the User's Guide for a full explanation of data.

Phelps Memorial Hospital Assn

701 North Broadway
Sleepy Hollow, NY 10591
E-mail: msematinger@pmhc.us
URL: www.phelpshospital.org
Type: Acute Care Hospitals
Ownership: Voluntary Non-Profit - Other
Phone: 914-366-3000
Fax: 914-366-1308
Emergency Services: Yes
Beds: 235

Key Personnel:
CEO/President. . . . . Keith F Safian
Cardiac Laboratory. . . . . Kenneth Kaplan, MD
Chief of Medical Staff . . . . Elio Ippolito, MD
Infection Control . . . . Anita Watson
Operating Room. . . . . Robert Raniolo
Pediatric In-Patient Care . . . . Margaret Stillman, MD
Quality Assurance . . . . Eileen Egan
Radiology. . . . . Robert Perelman, MD

Measure	Cases	This Hosp.	State Avg.	U.S. Avg.
Heart Attack Care				
ACE Inhibitor or ARB for LVSD[1]	8	100%	95%	96%
Aspirin at Arrival	57	100%	98%	99%
Aspirin at Discharge	47	100%	98%	98%
Beta Blocker at Discharge	46	100%	98%	98%
Fibrinolytic Medication Timing[1]	2	100%	50%	55%
PCI Within 90 Minutes of Arrival	0	-	88%	90%
Smoking Cessation Advice[1]	5	100%	100%	99%
Chest Pain/Possible Heart Attack Care				
Aspirin at Arrival[1]	10	100%	96%	95%
Median Time to ECG (minutes)[1]	10	12	11	8
Median Time to Transfer (minutes)[1,3]	1	130	75	61
Fibrinolytic Medication Timing[1,3]	1	100%	55%	54%
Heart Failure Care				
ACE Inhibitor or ARB for LVSD	39	100%	94%	94%
Discharge Instructions	98	94%	89%	88%
Evaluation of LVS Function	152	99%	98%	98%
Smoking Cessation Advice[1]	10	100%	98%	98%
Pneumonia Care				
Appropriate Initial Antibiotic	73	92%	92%	92%
Blood Culture Timing	136	97%	95%	96%
Influenza Vaccine	92	97%	90%	91%
Initial Antibiotic Timing	114	96%	93%	95%
Pneumococcal Vaccine	115	95%	92%	93%
Smoking Cessation Advice[1]	23	100%	98%	97%
Surgical Care Improvement Project				
Appropriate VTP Within 24 Hours[2]	272	99%	94%	92%
Appropriate Hair Removal[2]	486	100%	100%	99%
Appropriate Beta Blocker Usage[2]	174	98%	92%	93%
Controlled Postoperative Blood Glucose[2]	0	-	94%	93%
Prophylactic Antibiotic Timing[2]	340	97%	96%	97%
Prophylactic Antibiotic Timing (Outpatient)	73	92%	92%	92%
Prophylactic Antibiotic Selection[2]	341	97%	97%	97%
Prophylactic Antibiotic Select. (Outpatient)	104	94%	93%	94%
Prophylactic Antibiotic Stopped[2]	327	91%	94%	94%
Recommended VTP Ordered[2]	272	100%	96%	94%
Urinary Catheter Removal[2]	159	99%	90%	90%
Children's Asthma Care				
Received Systemic Corticosteroids	-	-	-	100%
Received Home Management Plan	-	-	-	71%
Received Reliever Medication	-	-	-	100%
Use of Medical Imaging				
Combination Abdominal CT Scan	1,006	0.216	0.141	0.191
Combination Chest CT Scan	967	0.000	0.024	0.054
Follow-up Mammogram/Ultrasound	1,436	8.0%	9.8%	8.4%
MRI for Low Back Pain[1]	3	33.3%	26.9%	32.7%
Survey of Patients' Hospital Experiences				
Area Around Room 'Always' Quiet at Night	300+	45%	-	58%
Doctors 'Always' Communicated Well	300+	78%	-	80%
Home Recovery Information Given	300+	79%	-	82%
Hospital Given 9 or 10 on 10 Point Scale	300+	66%	-	67%
Meds 'Always' Explained Before Given	300+	59%	-	60%
Nurses 'Always' Communicated Well	300+	71%	-	76%
Pain 'Always' Well Controlled	300+	66%	-	69%
Room and Bathroom 'Always' Clean	300+	70%	-	71%
Timely Help 'Always' Received	300+	55%	-	64%
Would Definitely Recommend Hospital	300+	69%	-	69%

Saint Catherine of Siena Hospital

50 Route 25a
Smithtown, NY 11787
URL: www.stcatherines.chsli.org
Type: Acute Care Hospitals
Ownership: Voluntary Non-Profit - Church
Phone: 631-862-3000
Fax: 631-862-3768
Emergency Services: Yes
Beds: 311

Key Personnel:
CEO/President. . . . . Vincent DiRubbio
Chief of Medical Staff . . . . Augustusd Mantia, MD
Infection Control. . . . . Catherine Shannon
Operating Room. . . . . Patrice Kelly
Radiology. . . . . Scott Coyne, MD
Anesthesiology. . . . . Anthony Bonono, MD
Emergency Room . . . . Michael Kennedy, DO
Patient Relations . . . . Gana Edelstein

Measure	Cases	This Hosp.	State Avg.	U.S. Avg.
Heart Attack Care				
ACE Inhibitor or ARB for LVSD[1]	14	79%	95%	96%
Aspirin at Arrival	120	97%	98%	99%
Aspirin at Discharge	92	96%	98%	98%
Beta Blocker at Discharge	97	98%	98%	98%
Fibrinolytic Medication Timing	0	-	50%	55%
PCI Within 90 Minutes of Arrival	37	62%	88%	90%
Smoking Cessation Advice[1]	18	100%	100%	99%
Chest Pain/Possible Heart Attack Care				
Aspirin at Arrival[1]	22	86%	96%	95%
Median Time to ECG (minutes)[1]	24	14	11	8
Median Time to Transfer (minutes)[1,3]	2	137	75	61
Fibrinolytic Medication Timing[3]	0	-	55%	54%
Heart Failure Care				
ACE Inhibitor or ARB for LVSD[2]	58	95%	94%	94%
Discharge Instructions[2]	195	99%	89%	88%
Evaluation of LVS Function[2]	326	95%	98%	98%
Smoking Cessation Advice[1,2]	11	100%	98%	98%
Pneumonia Care				
Appropriate Initial Antibiotic[2]	110	81%	92%	92%
Blood Culture Timing[2]	35	94%	95%	96%
Influenza Vaccine[2]	139	99%	90%	91%
Initial Antibiotic Timing[2]	228	89%	93%	95%
Pneumococcal Vaccine[2]	219	100%	92%	93%
Smoking Cessation Advice[2]	36	100%	98%	97%
Surgical Care Improvement Project				
Appropriate VTP Within 24 Hours[2]	232	98%	94%	92%
Appropriate Hair Removal[2]	445	100%	100%	99%
Appropriate Beta Blocker Usage[2]	151	100%	92%	93%
Controlled Postoperative Blood Glucose[2]	0	-	94%	93%
Prophylactic Antibiotic Timing[2]	250	99%	96%	97%
Prophylactic Antibiotic Timing (Outpatient)	387	98%	92%	92%
Prophylactic Antibiotic Selection[2]	252	96%	97%	97%
Prophylactic Antibiotic Select. (Outpatient)	383	84%	93%	94%
Prophylactic Antibiotic Stopped[2]	237	98%	94%	94%
Recommended VTP Ordered[2]	232	99%	96%	94%
Urinary Catheter Removal[2]	89	100%	90%	90%
Children's Asthma Care				
Received Systemic Corticosteroids	-	-	-	100%
Received Home Management Plan	-	-	-	71%
Received Reliever Medication	-	-	-	100%
Use of Medical Imaging				
Combination Abdominal CT Scan	666	0.477	0.141	0.191
Combination Chest CT Scan	390	0.026	0.024	0.054
Follow-up Mammogram/Ultrasound	155	23.2%	9.8%	8.4%
MRI for Low Back Pain[1]	45	20.0%	26.9%	32.7%
Survey of Patients' Hospital Experiences				
Area Around Room 'Always' Quiet at Night	300+	40%	-	58%
Doctors 'Always' Communicated Well	300+	77%	-	80%
Home Recovery Information Given	300+	81%	-	82%
Hospital Given 9 or 10 on 10 Point Scale	300+	60%	-	67%
Meds 'Always' Explained Before Given	300+	53%	-	60%
Nurses 'Always' Communicated Well	300+	71%	-	76%
Pain 'Always' Well Controlled	300+	65%	-	69%
Room and Bathroom 'Always' Clean	300+	68%	-	71%
Timely Help 'Always' Received	300+	52%	-	64%
Would Definitely Recommend Hospital	300+	61%	-	69%

Southampton Hospital

240 Meeting House Lane
Southampton, NY 11968
URL: www.southamptonhospital.org
Type: Acute Care Hospitals
Ownership: Voluntary Non-Profit - Private
Phone: 516-726-8200
Fax: 631-283-2842
Emergency Services: Yes
Beds: 168

Key Personnel:
CEO/President. . . . . John N Kastanis
Chief of Medical Staff . . . . Alan N DeCarlo, MD
Infection Control. . . . . Karen D'John
Operating Room. . . . . John Hubbell, RN
Quality Assurance . . . . Jeanne Salerno
Radiology. . . . . William R Brancaccio
Emergency Room . . . . Dr Darren Wiggins

Measure	Cases	This Hosp.	State Avg.	U.S. Avg.
Heart Attack Care				
ACE Inhibitor or ARB for LVSD[1]	1	100%	95%	96%
Aspirin at Arrival[1]	12	100%	98%	99%
Aspirin at Discharge[1]	6	100%	98%	98%
Beta Blocker at Discharge[1]	7	100%	98%	98%
Fibrinolytic Medication Timing	0	-	50%	55%
PCI Within 90 Minutes of Arrival	0	-	88%	90%
Smoking Cessation Advice	0	-	100%	99%
Chest Pain/Possible Heart Attack Care				
Aspirin at Arrival	65	95%	96%	95%
Median Time to ECG (minutes)	65	17	11	8
Median Time to Transfer (minutes)[1,3]	7	75	75	61
Fibrinolytic Medication Timing[1]	10	80%	55%	54%
Heart Failure Care				
ACE Inhibitor or ARB for LVSD[1]	20	100%	94%	94%
Discharge Instructions	88	99%	89%	88%
Evaluation of LVS Function	113	99%	98%	98%
Smoking Cessation Advice[1]	14	100%	98%	98%
Pneumonia Care				
Appropriate Initial Antibiotic	118	95%	92%	92%
Blood Culture Timing	194	92%	95%	96%
Influenza Vaccine	108	99%	90%	91%
Initial Antibiotic Timing	172	94%	93%	95%
Pneumococcal Vaccine	181	98%	92%	93%
Smoking Cessation Advice	34	100%	98%	97%
Surgical Care Improvement Project				
Appropriate VTP Within 24 Hours	70	84%	94%	92%
Appropriate Hair Removal	168	100%	100%	99%
Appropriate Beta Blocker Usage	42	93%	92%	93%
Controlled Postoperative Blood Glucose	0	-	94%	93%
Prophylactic Antibiotic Timing	85	98%	96%	97%
Prophylactic Antibiotic Timing (Outpatient)	50	88%	92%	92%
Prophylactic Antibiotic Selection	85	86%	97%	97%
Prophylactic Antibiotic Select. (Outpatient)	47	87%	93%	94%
Prophylactic Antibiotic Stopped	79	90%	94%	94%
Recommended VTP Ordered	70	86%	96%	94%
Urinary Catheter Removal[1]	11	82%	90%	90%
Children's Asthma Care				
Received Systemic Corticosteroids	-	-	-	100%
Received Home Management Plan	-	-	-	71%
Received Reliever Medication	-	-	-	100%
Use of Medical Imaging				
Combination Abdominal CT Scan	768	0.059	0.141	0.191
Combination Chest CT Scan	618	0.002	0.024	0.054
Follow-up Mammogram/Ultrasound	1,073	7.9%	9.8%	8.4%
MRI for Low Back Pain	165	24.2%	26.9%	32.7%
Survey of Patients' Hospital Experiences				
Area Around Room 'Always' Quiet at Night	300+	49%	-	58%
Doctors 'Always' Communicated Well	300+	79%	-	80%
Home Recovery Information Given	300+	73%	-	82%
Hospital Given 9 or 10 on 10 Point Scale	300+	60%	-	67%
Meds 'Always' Explained Before Given	300+	59%	-	60%
Nurses 'Always' Communicated Well	300+	74%	-	76%
Pain 'Always' Well Controlled	300+	66%	-	69%
Room and Bathroom 'Always' Clean	300+	74%	-	71%
Timely Help 'Always' Received	300+	59%	-	64%
Would Definitely Recommend Hospital	300+	63%	-	69%

NOTE: Hospital profiles are in alphabetical order by state, then city, then hospital within the city; Rankings exclude hospitals with less than 25 cases except for patient surveys which excludes hospitals with less than 100 cases; (a) 100–299 cases; (1) The number of cases is too small to be sure how well a hospital is performing; (2) The hospital indicated that the data submitted for this measure were based on a sample of cases; (3) Data was collected during a shorter time period (fewer quarters) than the maximum possible time for this measure; (4) Suppressed for one or more quarters by CMS; (5) No data is available from the hospital for this measure; (6) Fewer than 100 patients completed the HCAHPS survey. Use these rates with caution, as the number of surveys may be too low to reliably assess hospital performance; (7) Survey results are based on less than 12 months of data; (8) Survey results are not available for this reporting period; (9) No or very few patients were eligible for the HCAHPS survey. The scores shown, if any, reflect a very small number of surveys; (10) A state average was not calculated because too few hospitals in the state submitted data; (11) There were discrepancies in the data collection process; Please refer to the User's Guide for a full explanation of data.

Bertrand Chaffee Hospital

224 East Main Street | Phone: 716-592-2871
Springville, NY 14141 | Fax: 716-592-8105
Type: Acute Care Hospitals | Emergency Services: Yes
Ownership: Voluntary Non-Profit - Private | Beds: 49

Key Personnel:
CEO/President. . . . . Steven Krisiak
Chief of Medical Staff. . . . . Edwin Heidelberger
Infection Control. . . . . Barbara Whittemore
Operating Room. . . . . Barbara Appleby
Pediatric Ambulatory Care . . . . . Robbin Hansen
Quality Assurance . . . . Linda Reehling
Radiology. . . . . Steven Christen

Measure	Cases	This Hosp.	State Avg.	U.S. Avg.
Heart Attack Care				
ACE Inhibitor or ARB for LVSD[1]	5	40%	95%	96%
Aspirin at Arrival[1]	17	88%	98%	99%
Aspirin at Discharge[1]	7	86%	98%	98%
Beta Blocker at Discharge[1]	10	80%	98%	98%
Fibrinolytic Medication Timing	0	-	50%	55%
PCI Within 90 Minutes of Arrival	0	-	88%	90%
Smoking Cessation Advice	0	-	100%	99%
Chest Pain/Possible Heart Attack Care				
Aspirin at Arrival	93	84%	96%	95%
Median Time to ECG (minutes)	97	18	11	8
Median Time to Transfer (minutes)[1,3]	1	228	75	61
Fibrinolytic Medication Timing[1]	6	67%	55%	54%
Heart Failure Care				
ACE Inhibitor or ARB for LVSD[1]	12	83%	94%	94%
Discharge Instructions	32	91%	89%	88%
Evaluation of LVS Function	53	100%	98%	98%
Smoking Cessation Advice[1]	6	100%	98%	98%
Pneumonia Care				
Appropriate Initial Antibiotic	88	95%	92%	92%
Blood Culture Timing	116	97%	95%	96%
Influenza Vaccine	65	92%	90%	91%
Initial Antibiotic Timing	105	96%	93%	95%
Pneumococcal Vaccine	102	91%	92%	93%
Smoking Cessation Advice	25	100%	98%	97%
Surgical Care Improvement Project				
Appropriate VTP Within 24 Hours[1]	7	71%	94%	92%
Appropriate Hair Removal[1]	8	88%	100%	99%
Appropriate Beta Blocker Usage[1]	1	0%	92%	93%
Controlled Postoperative Blood Glucose	0	-	94%	93%
Prophylactic Antibiotic Timing[1]	2	50%	96%	97%
Prophylactic Antibiotic Timing (Outpatient)[1,3]	14	93%	92%	92%
Prophylactic Antibiotic Selection[1]	2	100%	97%	97%
Prophylactic Antibiotic Select. (Outpatient)[1,3]	14	64%	93%	94%
Prophylactic Antibiotic Stopped[1]	2	100%	94%	94%
Recommended VTP Ordered[1]	7	71%	96%	94%
Urinary Catheter Removal[1]	1	100%	90%	90%
Children's Asthma Care				
Received Systemic Corticosteroids	-	-	-	100%
Received Home Management Plan	-	-	-	71%
Received Reliever Medication	-	-	-	100%
Use of Medical Imaging				
Combination Abdominal CT Scan	92	0.098	0.141	0.191
Combination Chest CT Scan[1]	36	0.056	0.024	0.054
Follow-up Mammogram/Ultrasound	200	5.0%	9.8%	8.4%
MRI for Low Back Pain[5]	0	-	26.9%	32.7%
Survey of Patients' Hospital Experiences				
Area Around Room 'Always' Quiet at Night	300+	52%	-	58%
Doctors 'Always' Communicated Well	300+	87%	-	80%
Home Recovery Information Given	300+	92%	-	82%
Hospital Given 9 or 10 on 10 Point Scale	300+	74%	-	67%
Meds 'Always' Explained Before Given	300+	65%	-	60%
Nurses 'Always' Communicated Well	300+	84%	-	76%
Pain 'Always' Well Controlled	300+	74%	-	69%
Room and Bathroom 'Always' Clean	300+	79%	-	71%
Timely Help 'Always' Received	300+	78%	-	64%
Would Definitely Recommend Hospital	300+	74%	-	69%

Richmond University Medical Center

355 Bard Avenue | Phone: 718-818-1234
Staten Island, NY 10304
URL: www.rumcsi.org
Type: Acute Care Hospitals | Emergency Services: Yes
Ownership: Voluntary Non-Profit - Private

Key Personnel:
CEO/President. . . . . Richard J. Murphy
Chief of Medical Staff. . . . . Edward Arsura
Pediatric In-Patient Care . . . . Simon Rabinowitz

Measure	Cases	This Hosp.	State Avg.	U.S. Avg.
Heart Attack Care				
ACE Inhibitor or ARB for LVSD[1,2]	8	88%	95%	96%
Aspirin at Arrival[2]	90	98%	98%	99%
Aspirin at Discharge[2]	34	100%	98%	98%
Beta Blocker at Discharge[2]	37	95%	98%	98%
Fibrinolytic Medication Timing[2]	0	-	50%	55%
PCI Within 90 Minutes of Arrival[2]	0	-	88%	90%
Smoking Cessation Advice[1,2]	16	100%	100%	99%
Chest Pain/Possible Heart Attack Care				
Aspirin at Arrival[1]	19	100%	96%	95%
Median Time to ECG (minutes)[1]	20	25	11	8
Median Time to Transfer (minutes)[1]	7	71	75	61
Fibrinolytic Medication Timing	0	-	55%	54%
Heart Failure Care				
ACE Inhibitor or ARB for LVSD[2]	57	89%	94%	94%
Discharge Instructions[2]	105	99%	89%	88%
Evaluation of LVS Function[2]	158	99%	98%	98%
Smoking Cessation Advice[2]	31	100%	98%	98%
Pneumonia Care				
Appropriate Initial Antibiotic[2]	51	90%	92%	92%
Blood Culture Timing[2]	157	94%	95%	96%
Influenza Vaccine[2]	76	96%	90%	91%
Initial Antibiotic Timing[2]	130	97%	93%	95%
Pneumococcal Vaccine[2]	122	98%	92%	93%
Smoking Cessation Advice[2]	38	100%	98%	97%
Surgical Care Improvement Project				
Appropriate VTP Within 24 Hours[2]	183	98%	94%	92%
Appropriate Hair Removal[2]	434	100%	100%	99%
Appropriate Beta Blocker Usage[2]	122	97%	92%	93%
Controlled Postoperative Blood Glucose[1,2]	1	100%	94%	93%
Prophylactic Antibiotic Timing[2]	293	99%	96%	97%
Prophylactic Antibiotic Timing (Outpatient)	207	91%	92%	92%
Prophylactic Antibiotic Selection[2]	295	93%	97%	97%
Prophylactic Antibiotic Select. (Outpatient)	199	96%	93%	94%
Prophylactic Antibiotic Stopped[2]	285	95%	94%	94%
Recommended VTP Ordered[2]	183	98%	96%	94%
Urinary Catheter Removal[2]	40	78%	90%	90%
Children's Asthma Care				
Received Systemic Corticosteroids	-	-	-	100%
Received Home Management Plan	-	-	-	71%
Received Reliever Medication	-	-	-	100%
Use of Medical Imaging				
Combination Abdominal CT Scan	49	0.041	0.141	0.191
Combination Chest CT Scan	65	0.000	0.024	0.054
Follow-up Mammogram/Ultrasound	143	29.4%	9.8%	8.4%
MRI for Low Back Pain[5]	0	-	26.9%	32.7%
Survey of Patients' Hospital Experiences				
Area Around Room 'Always' Quiet at Night	300+	41%	-	58%
Doctors 'Always' Communicated Well	300+	70%	-	80%
Home Recovery Information Given	300+	70%	-	82%
Hospital Given 9 or 10 on 10 Point Scale	300+	44%	-	67%
Meds 'Always' Explained Before Given	300+	56%	-	60%
Nurses 'Always' Communicated Well	300+	69%	-	76%
Pain 'Always' Well Controlled	300+	63%	-	69%
Room and Bathroom 'Always' Clean	300+	58%	-	71%
Timely Help 'Always' Received	300+	56%	-	64%
Would Definitely Recommend Hospital	300+	51%	-	69%

Staten Island University Hospital

475 Seaview Avenue | Phone: 718-226-9000
Staten Island, NY 10305 | Fax: 718-226-8966
E-mail: webmaster@siuh.edu
URL: www.siuh.edu
Type: Acute Care Hospitals | Emergency Services: Yes
Ownership: Voluntary Non-Profit - Private | Beds: 813

Key Personnel:
CEO/President. . . . . John ST Gallagher
Chief of Medical Staff. . . . . Jon R Cohen, MD
Coronary Care . . . . Kathy Mann, RN
Infection Control. . . . . Jordan b. Glaser, MD
Operating Room. . . . . Joseph T. McGinn, RN
Pediatric Ambulatory Care . . . . . Lawrence Bodenstein, MD
Quality Assurance . . . . Donn Haber
Radiology. . . . . Mark Raden, MD

Measure	Cases	This Hosp.	State Avg.	U.S. Avg.
Heart Attack Care				
ACE Inhibitor or ARB for LVSD[2]	42	100%	95%	96%
Aspirin at Arrival[2]	260	100%	98%	99%
Aspirin at Discharge[2]	280	100%	98%	98%
Beta Blocker at Discharge[2]	249	100%	98%	98%
Fibrinolytic Medication Timing[2]	0	-	50%	55%
PCI Within 90 Minutes of Arrival[2]	45	98%	88%	90%
Smoking Cessation Advice[2]	71	100%	100%	99%
Chest Pain/Possible Heart Attack Care				
Aspirin at Arrival[1,3]	1	100%	96%	95%
Median Time to ECG (minutes)[1,3]	1	11	11	8
Median Time to Transfer (minutes)[5]	0	-	75	61
Fibrinolytic Medication Timing[3]	0	-	55%	54%
Heart Failure Care				
ACE Inhibitor or ARB for LVSD[2]	95	100%	94%	94%
Discharge Instructions[2]	241	98%	89%	88%
Evaluation of LVS Function[2]	301	100%	98%	98%
Smoking Cessation Advice[2]	35	100%	98%	98%
Pneumonia Care				
Appropriate Initial Antibiotic[2]	89	96%	92%	92%
Blood Culture Timing[2]	209	99%	95%	96%
Influenza Vaccine[2]	80	96%	90%	91%
Initial Antibiotic Timing[2]	120	96%	93%	95%
Pneumococcal Vaccine[2]	117	98%	92%	93%
Smoking Cessation Advice[2]	40	100%	98%	97%
Surgical Care Improvement Project				
Appropriate VTP Within 24 Hours[2]	188	99%	94%	92%
Appropriate Hair Removal[2]	536	100%	100%	99%
Appropriate Beta Blocker Usage[2]	175	95%	92%	93%
Controlled Postoperative Blood Glucose[2]	128	92%	94%	93%
Prophylactic Antibiotic Timing[2]	381	98%	96%	97%
Prophylactic Antibiotic Timing (Outpatient)	233	84%	92%	92%
Prophylactic Antibiotic Selection[2]	387	97%	97%	97%
Prophylactic Antibiotic Select. (Outpatient)	253	90%	93%	94%
Prophylactic Antibiotic Stopped[2]	353	97%	94%	94%
Recommended VTP Ordered[2]	188	99%	96%	94%
Urinary Catheter Removal[2]	98	99%	90%	90%
Children's Asthma Care				
Received Systemic Corticosteroids	-	-	-	100%
Received Home Management Plan	-	-	-	71%
Received Reliever Medication	-	-	-	100%
Use of Medical Imaging				
Combination Abdominal CT Scan	608	0.071	0.141	0.191
Combination Chest CT Scan	232	0.069	0.024	0.054
Follow-up Mammogram/Ultrasound	2,091	7.7%	9.8%	8.4%
MRI for Low Back Pain[1]	27	25.9%	26.9%	32.7%
Survey of Patients' Hospital Experiences				
Area Around Room 'Always' Quiet at Night	300+	44%	-	58%
Doctors 'Always' Communicated Well	300+	72%	-	80%
Home Recovery Information Given	300+	76%	-	82%
Hospital Given 9 or 10 on 10 Point Scale	300+	57%	-	67%
Meds 'Always' Explained Before Given	300+	55%	-	60%
Nurses 'Always' Communicated Well	300+	72%	-	76%
Pain 'Always' Well Controlled	300+	65%	-	69%
Room and Bathroom 'Always' Clean	300+	64%	-	71%
Timely Help 'Always' Received	300+	56%	-	64%
Would Definitely Recommend Hospital	300+	61%	-	69%

NOTE: Hospital profiles are in alphabetical order by state, then city, then hospital within the city; Rankings exclude hospitals with less than 25 cases except for patient surveys which excludes hospitals with less than 100 cases; (a) 100–299 cases; (1) The number of cases is too small to be sure how well a hospital is performing; (2) The hospital indicated that the data submitted for this measure were based on a sample of cases; (3) Data was collected during a shorter time period (fewer quarters) than the maximum possible time for this measure; (4) Suppressed for one or more quarters by CMS; (5) No data is available from the hospital for this measure; (6) Fewer than 100 patients completed the HCAHPS survey. Use these rates with caution, as the number of surveys may be too low to reliably assess hospital performance; (7) Survey results are based on less than 12 months of data; (8) Survey results are not available for this reporting period; (9) No or very few patients were eligible for the HCAHPS survey. The scores shown, if any, reflect a very small number of surveys; (10) A state average was not calculated because too few hospitals in the state submitted data; (11) There were discrepancies in the data collection process; Please refer to the User's Guide for a full explanation of data.

University Hospital - Stony Brook

Health Sciences Center Suny
Stony Brook, NY 11794
Phone: 631-444-4000
Fax: 631-444-4724
URL: www.stonybrookmedicalcenter.org
Type: Acute Care Hospitals
Emergency Services: Yes
Ownership: Government - State
Beds: 540

Key Personnel:
CEO/President............... Steven Strongwater MD
Chief of Medical Staff.......... Dr. Norman Edelman
Infection Control............. Francina Sing
Operating Room............. Faith Buck
Pediatric Ambulatory Care ...... Richard Fine, MD
Pediatric In-Patient Care .... Richard Fine, MD
Quality Assurance .... Carol Comes
Radiology.................. Donald Harrington, MD

Measure	Cases	This Hosp.	State Avg.	U.S. Avg.
Heart Attack Care				
ACE Inhibitor or ARB for LVSD[2]	92	96%	95%	96%
Aspirin at Arrival[2]	224	100%	98%	99%
Aspirin at Discharge[2]	532	98%	98%	98%
Beta Blocker at Discharge[2]	523	98%	98%	98%
Fibrinolytic Medication Timing[2]	0	-	50%	55%
PCI Within 90 Minutes of Arrival[2]	57	86%	88%	90%
Smoking Cessation Advice[2]	149	100%	100%	99%
Chest Pain/Possible Heart Attack Care				
Aspirin at Arrival[5]	0	-	96%	95%
Median Time to ECG (minutes)[5]	0	-	11	8
Median Time to Transfer (minutes)[5]	0	-	75	61
Fibrinolytic Medication Timing[5]	0	-	55%	54%
Heart Failure Care				
ACE Inhibitor or ARB for LVSD[2]	107	89%	94%	94%
Discharge Instructions[2]	213	91%	89%	88%
Evaluation of LVS Function[2]	275	99%	98%	98%
Smoking Cessation Advice[2]	50	100%	98%	98%
Pneumonia Care				
Appropriate Initial Antibiotic[2]	69	88%	92%	92%
Blood Culture Timing[2]	132	90%	95%	96%
Influenza Vaccine[2]	65	62%	90%	91%
Initial Antibiotic Timing[2]	135	91%	93%	95%
Pneumococcal Vaccine[2]	94	80%	92%	93%
Smoking Cessation Advice[2]	55	100%	98%	97%
Surgical Care Improvement Project				
Appropriate VTP Within 24 Hours[2]	175	99%	94%	92%
Appropriate Hair Removal[2]	542	100%	100%	99%
Appropriate Beta Blocker Usage[2]	176	82%	92%	93%
Controlled Postoperative Blood Glucose[2]	119	92%	94%	93%
Prophylactic Antibiotic Timing[2]	358	99%	96%	97%
Prophylactic Antibiotic Timing (Outpatient)	384	88%	92%	92%
Prophylactic Antibiotic Selection[2]	367	98%	97%	97%
Prophylactic Antibiotic Select. (Outpatient)	399	96%	93%	94%
Prophylactic Antibiotic Stopped[2]	347	93%	94%	94%
Recommended VTP Ordered[2]	176	99%	96%	94%
Urinary Catheter Removal[2]	134	87%	90%	90%
Children's Asthma Care				
Received Systemic Corticosteroids[1,2]	20	95%	-	100%
Received Home Management Plan[1]	20	45%	-	71%
Received Reliever Medication[1,2]	20	100%	-	100%
Use of Medical Imaging				
Combination Abdominal CT Scan	1,100	0.156	0.141	0.191
Combination Chest CT Scan	1,186	0.012	0.024	0.054
Follow-up Mammogram/Ultrasound	1,177	5.0%	9.8%	8.4%
MRI for Low Back Pain	149	25.5%	26.9%	32.7%
Survey of Patients' Hospital Experiences				
Area Around Room 'Always' Quiet at Night	300+	44%	-	58%
Doctors 'Always' Communicated Well	300+	73%	-	80%
Home Recovery Information Given	300+	79%	-	82%
Hospital Given 9 or 10 on 10 Point Scale	300+	63%	-	67%
Meds 'Always' Explained Before Given	300+	54%	-	60%
Nurses 'Always' Communicated Well	300+	73%	-	76%
Pain 'Always' Well Controlled	300+	67%	-	69%
Room and Bathroom 'Always' Clean	300+	69%	-	71%
Timely Help 'Always' Received	300+	58%	-	64%
Would Definitely Recommend Hospital	300+	70%	-	69%

Good Samaritan Hospital of Suffern

255 Lafayette Avenue
Suffern, NY 10901
Phone: 914-368-5000
Fax: 845-368-5430
URL: www.goodsamhosp.org
Type: Acute Care Hospitals
Emergency Services: Yes
Ownership: Voluntary Non-Profit - Church
Beds: 370

Key Personnel:
Chief of Medical Staff.......... William Cors, MD
Infection Control............. Eileen Englebracht
Operating Room............. Nancy Berger
Pediatric Ambulatory Care ...... Richard Snop
Pediatric In-Patient Care .... Richard Snop
Quality Assurance .... Maureen Reynolds
Radiology.................. Scott G Luchs, MD

Measure	Cases	This Hosp.	State Avg.	U.S. Avg.
Heart Attack Care				
ACE Inhibitor or ARB for LVSD	87	94%	95%	96%
Aspirin at Arrival	251	99%	98%	99%
Aspirin at Discharge	421	100%	98%	98%
Beta Blocker at Discharge	418	100%	98%	98%
Fibrinolytic Medication Timing	0	-	50%	55%
PCI Within 90 Minutes of Arrival	69	87%	88%	90%
Smoking Cessation Advice	120	99%	100%	99%
Chest Pain/Possible Heart Attack Care				
Aspirin at Arrival[1,3]	2	100%	96%	95%
Median Time to ECG (minutes)[1,3]	1	8	11	8
Median Time to Transfer (minutes)[5]	0	-	75	61
Fibrinolytic Medication Timing[5]	0	-	55%	54%
Heart Failure Care				
ACE Inhibitor or ARB for LVSD	145	99%	94%	94%
Discharge Instructions	263	98%	89%	88%
Evaluation of LVS Function	375	99%	98%	98%
Smoking Cessation Advice	52	100%	98%	98%
Pneumonia Care				
Appropriate Initial Antibiotic	184	85%	92%	92%
Blood Culture Timing	278	94%	95%	96%
Influenza Vaccine	220	92%	90%	91%
Initial Antibiotic Timing	267	94%	93%	95%
Pneumococcal Vaccine	317	93%	92%	93%
Smoking Cessation Advice	67	100%	98%	97%
Surgical Care Improvement Project				
Appropriate VTP Within 24 Hours[2]	158	70%	94%	92%
Appropriate Hair Removal[2]	540	100%	100%	99%
Appropriate Beta Blocker Usage[2]	221	100%	92%	93%
Controlled Postoperative Blood Glucose[2]	155	99%	94%	93%
Prophylactic Antibiotic Timing[2]	338	94%	96%	97%
Prophylactic Antibiotic Timing (Outpatient)	247	92%	92%	92%
Prophylactic Antibiotic Selection[2]	375	94%	97%	97%
Prophylactic Antibiotic Select. (Outpatient)	231	95%	93%	94%
Prophylactic Antibiotic Stopped[2]	329	88%	94%	94%
Recommended VTP Ordered[2]	159	74%	96%	94%
Urinary Catheter Removal[2]	110	88%	90%	90%
Children's Asthma Care				
Received Systemic Corticosteroids	-	-	-	100%
Received Home Management Plan	-	-	-	71%
Received Reliever Medication	-	-	-	100%
Use of Medical Imaging				
Combination Abdominal CT Scan	516	0.087	0.141	0.191
Combination Chest CT Scan	279	0.036	0.024	0.054
Follow-up Mammogram/Ultrasound	362	21.0%	9.8%	8.4%
MRI for Low Back Pain[1]	26	7.7%	26.9%	32.7%
Survey of Patients' Hospital Experiences				
Area Around Room 'Always' Quiet at Night	300+	46%	-	58%
Doctors 'Always' Communicated Well	300+	75%	-	80%
Home Recovery Information Given	300+	78%	-	82%
Hospital Given 9 or 10 on 10 Point Scale	300+	56%	-	67%
Meds 'Always' Explained Before Given	300+	54%	-	60%
Nurses 'Always' Communicated Well	300+	68%	-	76%
Pain 'Always' Well Controlled	300+	59%	-	69%
Room and Bathroom 'Always' Clean	300+	58%	-	71%
Timely Help 'Always' Received	300+	47%	-	64%
Would Definitely Recommend Hospital	300+	61%	-	69%

Community-General Hospital of Greater Syracuse

4900 Broad Road
Syracuse, NY 13215
Phone: 315-492-5011
Fax: 315-492-5993
URL: www.cgh.org
Type: Acute Care Hospitals
Emergency Services: Yes
Ownership: Voluntary Non-Profit - Private
Beds: 356

Key Personnel:
CEO/President............... Thomas Quinn
Chief of Medical Staff.......... Frederick Goldberg MD
Infection Control............. Sue Chamberlain, RN CIC
Pediatric In-Patient Care .... Leonard Ledy MD
Quality Assurance .... Sally Ramsden
Radiology.................. David Wang MD
Emergency Room .... Melissa Martin
Intensive Care Unit............ Sue Kompf

Measure	Cases	This Hosp.	State Avg.	U.S. Avg.
Heart Attack Care				
ACE Inhibitor or ARB for LVSD[1]	7	86%	95%	96%
Aspirin at Arrival	43	93%	98%	99%
Aspirin at Discharge	30	90%	98%	98%
Beta Blocker at Discharge	28	96%	98%	98%
Fibrinolytic Medication Timing[1]	2	0%	50%	55%
PCI Within 90 Minutes of Arrival	0	-	88%	90%
Smoking Cessation Advice[1]	3	100%	100%	99%
Chest Pain/Possible Heart Attack Care				
Aspirin at Arrival[1]	17	82%	96%	95%
Median Time to ECG (minutes)[1]	17	19	11	8
Median Time to Transfer (minutes)[1]	6	86	75	61
Fibrinolytic Medication Timing[1]	3	33%	55%	54%
Heart Failure Care				
ACE Inhibitor or ARB for LVSD	43	86%	94%	94%
Discharge Instructions	121	73%	89%	88%
Evaluation of LVS Function	189	96%	98%	98%
Smoking Cessation Advice[1]	15	100%	98%	98%
Pneumonia Care				
Appropriate Initial Antibiotic[2]	91	97%	92%	92%
Blood Culture Timing[2]	164	93%	95%	96%
Influenza Vaccine[2]	97	85%	90%	91%
Initial Antibiotic Timing[2]	155	80%	93%	95%
Pneumococcal Vaccine[2]	150	79%	92%	93%
Smoking Cessation Advice[2]	31	100%	98%	97%
Surgical Care Improvement Project				
Appropriate VTP Within 24 Hours[2]	164	96%	94%	92%
Appropriate Hair Removal[2]	412	100%	100%	99%
Appropriate Beta Blocker Usage[2]	118	78%	92%	93%
Controlled Postoperative Blood Glucose[2]	0	-	94%	93%
Prophylactic Antibiotic Timing[2]	267	91%	96%	97%
Prophylactic Antibiotic Timing (Outpatient)	591	90%	92%	92%
Prophylactic Antibiotic Selection[2]	270	97%	97%	97%
Prophylactic Antibiotic Select. (Outpatient)	581	96%	93%	94%
Prophylactic Antibiotic Stopped[2]	261	96%	94%	94%
Recommended VTP Ordered[2]	164	98%	96%	94%
Urinary Catheter Removal[2]	145	81%	90%	90%
Children's Asthma Care				
Received Systemic Corticosteroids	-	-	-	100%
Received Home Management Plan	-	-	-	71%
Received Reliever Medication	-	-	-	100%
Use of Medical Imaging				
Combination Abdominal CT Scan	710	0.031	0.141	0.191
Combination Chest CT Scan	293	0.000	0.024	0.054
Follow-up Mammogram/Ultrasound	1,552	6.8%	9.8%	8.4%
MRI for Low Back Pain[5]	0	-	26.9%	32.7%
Survey of Patients' Hospital Experiences				
Area Around Room 'Always' Quiet at Night	300+	52%	-	58%
Doctors 'Always' Communicated Well	300+	80%	-	80%
Home Recovery Information Given	300+	83%	-	82%
Hospital Given 9 or 10 on 10 Point Scale	300+	61%	-	67%
Meds 'Always' Explained Before Given	300+	59%	-	60%
Nurses 'Always' Communicated Well	300+	74%	-	76%
Pain 'Always' Well Controlled	300+	69%	-	69%
Room and Bathroom 'Always' Clean	300+	57%	-	71%
Timely Help 'Always' Received	300+	59%	-	64%
Would Definitely Recommend Hospital	300+	66%	-	69%

NOTE: Hospital profiles are in alphabetical order by state, then city, then hospital within the city; Rankings exclude hospitals with less than 25 cases except for patient surveys which excludes hospitals with less than 100 cases; (a) 100–299 cases; (1) The number of cases is too small to be sure how well a hospital is performing; (2) The hospital indicated that the data submitted for this measure were based on a sample of cases; (3) Data was collected during a shorter time period (fewer quarters) than the maximum possible time for this measure; (4) Suppressed for one or more quarters by CMS; (5) No data is available from the hospital for this measure; (6) Fewer than 100 patients completed the HCAHPS survey. Use these rates with caution, as the number of surveys may be too low to reliably assess hospital performance; (7) Survey results are based on less than 12 months of data; (8) Survey results are not available for this reporting period; (9) No or very few patients were eligible for the HCAHPS survey. The scores shown, if any, reflect a very small number of surveys; (10) A state average was not calculated because too few hospitals in the state submitted data; (11) There were discrepancies in the data collection process; Please refer to the User's Guide for a full explanation of data.

Crouse Hospital

736 Irving Avenue
Syracuse, NY 13210
Phone: 315-470-7449
Fax: 315-470-7232
URL: www.crouse.org
Type: Acute Care Hospitals
Emergency Services: Yes
Ownership: Voluntary Non-Profit - Private
Beds: 566

Key Personnel:

CEO/President. . . . . Maud White
Chief of Medical Staff. . . . . Paul Kronenberg, MD
Infection Control. . . . . James Turchik, MD
Operating Room. . . . . Tammy Tenerovicz
Pediatric Ambulatory Care . . . . . . Winston Gaum, MD
Pediatric In-Patient Care . . . . Winston Gaum, MD
Quality Assurance . . . . Ron Press
Radiology. . . . . Stuart Singer

Measure	Cases	This Hosp.	State Avg.	U.S. Avg.
Heart Attack Care				
ACE Inhibitor or ARB for LVSD	25	96%	95%	96%
Aspirin at Arrival	146	98%	98%	99%
Aspirin at Discharge	143	99%	98%	98%
Beta Blocker at Discharge	135	97%	98%	98%
Fibrinolytic Medication Timing	0	-	50%	55%
PCI Within 90 Minutes of Arrival	46	98%	88%	90%
Smoking Cessation Advice	51	100%	100%	99%
Chest Pain/Possible Heart Attack Care				
Aspirin at Arrival[1]	1	100%	96%	95%
Median Time to ECG (minutes)[1]	2	8	11	8
Median Time to Transfer (minutes)[5]	0	-	75	61
Fibrinolytic Medication Timing[5]	0	-	55%	54%
Heart Failure Care				
ACE Inhibitor or ARB for LVSD	97	96%	94%	94%
Discharge Instructions	331	71%	89%	88%
Evaluation of LVS Function	409	99%	98%	98%
Smoking Cessation Advice	56	98%	98%	98%
Pneumonia Care				
Appropriate Initial Antibiotic	180	93%	92%	92%
Blood Culture Timing	310	96%	95%	96%
Influenza Vaccine	182	86%	90%	91%
Initial Antibiotic Timing	307	94%	93%	95%
Pneumococcal Vaccine	259	97%	92%	93%
Smoking Cessation Advice	90	100%	98%	97%
Surgical Care Improvement Project				
Appropriate VTP Within 24 Hours[2]	141	95%	94%	92%
Appropriate Hair Removal[2]	530	98%	100%	99%
Appropriate Beta Blocker Usage[2]	143	100%	92%	93%
Controlled Postoperative Blood Glucose[2]	0	-	94%	93%
Prophylactic Antibiotic Timing[2]	370	96%	96%	97%
Prophylactic Antibiotic Timing (Outpatient)	870	96%	92%	92%
Prophylactic Antibiotic Selection[2]	368	93%	97%	97%
Prophylactic Antibiotic Select. (Outpatient)	862	92%	93%	94%
Prophylactic Antibiotic Stopped[2]	361	95%	94%	94%
Recommended VTP Ordered[2]	142	94%	96%	94%
Urinary Catheter Removal[2]	115	94%	90%	90%
Children's Asthma Care				
Received Systemic Corticosteroids	-	-	-	100%
Received Home Management Plan	-	-	-	71%
Received Reliever Medication	-	-	-	100%
Use of Medical Imaging				
Combination Abdominal CT Scan	727	0.054	0.141	0.191
Combination Chest CT Scan	524	0.006	0.024	0.054
Follow-up Mammogram/Ultrasound	1,161	2.7%	9.8%	8.4%
MRI for Low Back Pain[5]	0	-	26.9%	32.7%
Survey of Patients' Hospital Experiences				
Area Around Room 'Always' Quiet at Night	300+	43%	-	58%
Doctors 'Always' Communicated Well	300+	73%	-	80%
Home Recovery Information Given	300+	86%	-	82%
Hospital Given 9 or 10 on 10 Point Scale	300+	61%	-	67%
Meds 'Always' Explained Before Given	300+	55%	-	60%
Nurses 'Always' Communicated Well	300+	72%	-	76%
Pain 'Always' Well Controlled	300+	64%	-	69%
Room and Bathroom 'Always' Clean	300+	64%	-	71%
Timely Help 'Always' Received	300+	53%	-	64%
Would Definitely Recommend Hospital	300+	73%	-	69%

Saint Joseph's Hospital Health Center

301 Prospect Avenue
Syracuse, NY 13203
Phone: 315-448-5111
Fax: 315-703-2129
E-mail: community.relations@sjhsyr.org
URL: www.sjhsyr.org
Type: Acute Care Hospitals
Emergency Services: Yes
Ownership: Voluntary Non-Profit - Church
Beds: 431

Key Personnel:

CEO/President. . . . . Theodore M Pasinski
Chief of Medical Staff. . . . . Sandra Sulik MD
Coronary Care . . . . AnneMarie Czyz RN
Operating Room. . . . . Kim Murray RN
Radiology. . . . . Robert Whitmarsh
Emergency Room . . . . Sarah Tubbert RN

Measure	Cases	This Hosp.	State Avg.	U.S. Avg.
Heart Attack Care				
ACE Inhibitor or ARB for LVSD	114	81%	95%	96%
Aspirin at Arrival	507	99%	98%	99%
Aspirin at Discharge	945	99%	98%	98%
Beta Blocker at Discharge	913	98%	98%	98%
Fibrinolytic Medication Timing	0	-	50%	55%
PCI Within 90 Minutes of Arrival	126	95%	88%	90%
Smoking Cessation Advice	397	100%	100%	99%
Chest Pain/Possible Heart Attack Care				
Aspirin at Arrival[3]	0	-	96%	95%
Median Time to ECG (minutes)[1,3]	1	174	11	8
Median Time to Transfer (minutes)[5]	0	-	75	61
Fibrinolytic Medication Timing[5]	0	-	55%	54%
Heart Failure Care				
ACE Inhibitor or ARB for LVSD	254	87%	94%	94%
Discharge Instructions	561	89%	89%	88%
Evaluation of LVS Function	697	98%	98%	98%
Smoking Cessation Advice	163	99%	98%	98%
Pneumonia Care				
Appropriate Initial Antibiotic	387	91%	92%	92%
Blood Culture Timing	615	96%	95%	96%
Influenza Vaccine	418	95%	90%	91%
Initial Antibiotic Timing	568	82%	93%	95%
Pneumococcal Vaccine	696	94%	92%	93%
Smoking Cessation Advice	314	100%	98%	97%
Surgical Care Improvement Project				
Appropriate VTP Within 24 Hours[2]	170	98%	94%	92%
Appropriate Hair Removal[2]	752	100%	100%	99%
Appropriate Beta Blocker Usage[2]	292	91%	92%	93%
Controlled Postoperative Blood Glucose[2]	180	87%	94%	93%
Prophylactic Antibiotic Timing[2]	536	94%	96%	97%
Prophylactic Antibiotic Timing (Outpatient)	794	94%	92%	92%
Prophylactic Antibiotic Selection[2]	541	98%	97%	97%
Prophylactic Antibiotic Select. (Outpatient)	789	98%	93%	94%
Prophylactic Antibiotic Stopped[2]	497	89%	94%	94%
Recommended VTP Ordered[2]	170	99%	96%	94%
Urinary Catheter Removal[2]	73	77%	90%	90%
Children's Asthma Care				
Received Systemic Corticosteroids	-	-	-	100%
Received Home Management Plan	-	-	-	71%
Received Reliever Medication	-	-	-	100%
Use of Medical Imaging				
Combination Abdominal CT Scan	774	0.088	0.141	0.191
Combination Chest CT Scan	320	0.006	0.024	0.054
Follow-up Mammogram/Ultrasound	187	13.9%	9.8%	8.4%
MRI for Low Back Pain[1]	1	0.0%	26.9%	32.7%
Survey of Patients' Hospital Experiences				
Area Around Room 'Always' Quiet at Night	300+	44%	-	58%
Doctors 'Always' Communicated Well	300+	75%	-	80%
Home Recovery Information Given	300+	88%	-	82%
Hospital Given 9 or 10 on 10 Point Scale	300+	71%	-	67%
Meds 'Always' Explained Before Given	300+	59%	-	60%
Nurses 'Always' Communicated Well	300+	75%	-	76%
Pain 'Always' Well Controlled	300+	71%	-	69%
Room and Bathroom 'Always' Clean	300+	64%	-	71%
Timely Help 'Always' Received	300+	59%	-	64%
Would Definitely Recommend Hospital	300+	77%	-	69%

Syracuse VA Medical Center

800 Irving Ave.
Syracuse, NY 13210
Phone: 315-425-4400
Fax: 315-425-4375
URL: www1.va.gov/visns/visn02
Type: Acute Care-Veterans Administration
Emergency Services: No
Ownership: Government - Federal
Beds: 164

Key Personnel:

Chief of Medical Staff. . . . . William H Marx, DO, FACS
Operating Room. . . . . Brenda Rudy
Quality Assurance . . . . Marcia Dawley
Patient Relations . . . . Kerry Grant

Measure	Cases	This Hosp.	State Avg.	U.S. Avg.
Heart Attack Care				
ACE Inhibitor or ARB for LVSD[1]	7	100%	95%	96%
Aspirin at Arrival	37	100%	98%	99%
Aspirin at Discharge[1]	24	100%	98%	98%
Beta Blocker at Discharge[1]	22	95%	98%	98%
Fibrinolytic Medication Timing[5]	0	-	50%	55%
PCI Within 90 Minutes of Arrival[1]	2	0%	88%	90%
Smoking Cessation Advice[1]	8	100%	100%	99%
Chest Pain/Possible Heart Attack Care				
Aspirin at Arrival	-	-	96%	95%
Median Time to ECG (minutes)	-	-	11	8
Median Time to Transfer (minutes)	-	-	75	61
Fibrinolytic Medication Timing	-	-	55%	54%
Heart Failure Care				
ACE Inhibitor or ARB for LVSD	47	100%	94%	94%
Discharge Instructions	152	93%	89%	88%
Evaluation of LVS Function	167	99%	98%	98%
Smoking Cessation Advice	25	100%	98%	98%
Pneumonia Care				
Appropriate Initial Antibiotic	82	99%	92%	92%
Blood Culture Timing	132	99%	95%	96%
Influenza Vaccine	76	99%	90%	91%
Initial Antibiotic Timing	121	94%	93%	95%
Pneumococcal Vaccine	115	98%	92%	93%
Smoking Cessation Advice	43	100%	98%	97%
Surgical Care Improvement Project				
Appropriate VTP Within 24 Hours[2]	107	100%	94%	92%
Appropriate Hair Removal[2]	135	100%	100%	99%
Appropriate Beta Blocker Usage[2]	62	85%	92%	93%
Controlled Postoperative Blood Glucose[2,5]	0	-	94%	93%
Prophylactic Antibiotic Timing	72	96%	96%	97%
Prophylactic Antibiotic Timing (Outpatient)	-	-	92%	92%
Prophylactic Antibiotic Selection	72	90%	97%	97%
Prophylactic Antibiotic Select. (Outpatient)	-	-	93%	94%
Prophylactic Antibiotic Stopped	72	92%	94%	94%
Recommended VTP Ordered[2]	108	99%	96%	94%
Urinary Catheter Removal[2]	66	100%	90%	90%
Children's Asthma Care				
Received Systemic Corticosteroids	-	-	-	100%
Received Home Management Plan	-	-	-	71%
Received Reliever Medication	-	-	-	100%
Use of Medical Imaging				
Combination Abdominal CT Scan	-	-	0.141	0.191
Combination Chest CT Scan	-	-	0.024	0.054
Follow-up Mammogram/Ultrasound	-	-	9.8%	8.4%
MRI for Low Back Pain	-	-	26.9%	32.7%
Survey of Patients' Hospital Experiences				
Area Around Room 'Always' Quiet at Night	-	-	-	58%
Doctors 'Always' Communicated Well	-	-	-	80%
Home Recovery Information Given	-	-	-	82%
Hospital Given 9 or 10 on 10 Point Scale	-	-	-	67%
Meds 'Always' Explained Before Given	-	-	-	60%
Nurses 'Always' Communicated Well	-	-	-	76%
Pain 'Always' Well Controlled	-	-	-	69%
Room and Bathroom 'Always' Clean	-	-	-	71%
Timely Help 'Always' Received	-	-	-	64%
Would Definitely Recommend Hospital	-	-	-	69%

NOTE: Hospital profiles are in alphabetical order by state, then city, then hospital within the city; Rankings exclude hospitals with less than 25 cases except for patient surveys which excludes hospitals with less than 100 cases; (a) 100–299 cases; (1) The number of cases is too small to be sure how well a hospital is performing; (2) The hospital indicated that the data submitted for this measure were based on a sample of cases; (3) Data was collected during a shorter time period (fewer quarters) than the maximum possible time for this measure; (4) Suppressed for one or more quarters by CMS; (5) No data is available from the hospital for this measure; (6) Fewer than 100 patients completed the HCAHPS survey. Use these rates with caution, as the number of surveys may be too low to reliably assess hospital performance; (7) Survey results are based on less than 12 months of data; (8) Survey results are not available for this reporting period; (9) No or very few patients were eligible for the HCAHPS survey. The scores shown, if any, reflect a very small number of surveys; (10) A state average was not calculated because too few hospitals in the state submitted data; (11) There were discrepancies in the data collection process; Please refer to the User's Guide for a full explanation of data.

University Hospital S U N Y Health Science Center

750 East Adams Street
Syracuse, NY 13210
URL: www.upstate.edu
Type: Acute Care Hospitals
Ownership: Government - State

Phone: 315-473-4240
Fax: 315-464-4838
Emergency Services: Yes
Beds: 356

Key Personnel:
CEO/President. . . . . David R Smith, MBA JD
Chief of Medical Staff. . . . . Steven J Scheinman
Infection Control. . . . . Fred Rose, MD
Operating Room. . . . . Paul Cunningham, MD
Quality Assurance . . . . Theresa Gagnon
Emergency Room . . . . Richard Hunt, MD

Measure	Cases	This Hosp.	State Avg.	U.S. Avg.
Heart Attack Care				
ACE Inhibitor or ARB for LVSD	53	98%	95%	96%
Aspirin at Arrival	91	100%	98%	99%
Aspirin at Discharge	183	99%	98%	98%
Beta Blocker at Discharge	179	99%	98%	98%
Fibrinolytic Medication Timing	0	-	50%	55%
PCI Within 90 Minutes of Arrival[1]	24	88%	88%	90%
Smoking Cessation Advice	83	100%	100%	99%
Chest Pain/Possible Heart Attack Care				
Aspirin at Arrival[5]	0	-	96%	95%
Median Time to ECG (minutes)[5]	0	-	11	8
Median Time to Transfer (minutes)[5]	0	-	75	61
Fibrinolytic Medication Timing[5]	0	-	55%	54%
Heart Failure Care				
ACE Inhibitor or ARB for LVSD	100	96%	94%	94%
Discharge Instructions	212	85%	89%	88%
Evaluation of LVS Function	266	100%	98%	98%
Smoking Cessation Advice	66	100%	98%	98%
Pneumonia Care				
Appropriate Initial Antibiotic	78	96%	92%	92%
Blood Culture Timing	168	96%	95%	96%
Influenza Vaccine	134	85%	90%	91%
Initial Antibiotic Timing	145	94%	93%	95%
Pneumococcal Vaccine	126	84%	92%	93%
Smoking Cessation Advice	90	100%	98%	97%
Surgical Care Improvement Project				
Appropriate VTP Within 24 Hours[2]	171	99%	94%	92%
Appropriate Hair Removal[2]	588	100%	100%	99%
Appropriate Beta Blocker Usage[2]	235	98%	92%	93%
Controlled Postoperative Blood Glucose[2]	198	97%	94%	93%
Prophylactic Antibiotic Timing[2]	421	97%	96%	97%
Prophylactic Antibiotic Timing (Outpatient)	269	86%	92%	92%
Prophylactic Antibiotic Selection[2]	427	99%	97%	97%
Prophylactic Antibiotic Select. (Outpatient)	337	98%	93%	94%
Prophylactic Antibiotic Stopped[2]	365	91%	94%	94%
Recommended VTP Ordered[2]	172	99%	96%	94%
Urinary Catheter Removal[2]	124	78%	90%	90%
Children's Asthma Care				
Received Systemic Corticosteroids	-	-	-	100%
Received Home Management Plan	-	-	-	71%
Received Reliever Medication	-	-	-	100%
Use of Medical Imaging				
Combination Abdominal CT Scan	583	0.115	0.141	0.191
Combination Chest CT Scan	745	0.048	0.024	0.054
Follow-up Mammogram/Ultrasound	506	21.7%	9.8%	8.4%
MRI for Low Back Pain[1]	29	10.3%	26.9%	32.7%
Survey of Patients' Hospital Experiences				
Area Around Room 'Always' Quiet at Night	300+	46%	-	58%
Doctors 'Always' Communicated Well	300+	73%	-	80%
Home Recovery Information Given	300+	83%	-	82%
Hospital Given 9 or 10 on 10 Point Scale	300+	65%	-	67%
Meds 'Always' Explained Before Given	300+	59%	-	60%
Nurses 'Always' Communicated Well	300+	72%	-	76%
Pain 'Always' Well Controlled	300+	67%	-	69%
Room and Bathroom 'Always' Clean	300+	67%	-	71%
Timely Help 'Always' Received	300+	55%	-	64%
Would Definitely Recommend Hospital	300+	69%	-	69%

Moses-Ludington Hospital

1019 Wicker Street
Ticonderoga, NY 12883
E-mail: catherine.larsen@tenethealth.com
URL: www.tenethealth.com/dmcmodesto
Type: Critical Access Hospitals
Ownership: Voluntary Non-Profit - Private

Phone: 518-585-2831
Fax: 518-585-2576
Emergency Services: Yes
Beds: 99

Key Personnel:
CEO/President. . . . . Diane Hart
Chief of Medical Staff. . . . . Robert Holterman, MD
Infection Control. . . . . Pat Chamberlain, DON
Operating Room. . . . . Nancy LaTour
Quality Assurance . . . . Lynne Reale
Radiology. . . . . Valerie Brace

Measure	Cases	This Hosp.	State Avg.	U.S. Avg.
Heart Attack Care				
ACE Inhibitor or ARB for LVSD[3]	0	-	95%	96%
Aspirin at Arrival[1,3]	1	100%	98%	99%
Aspirin at Discharge[3]	0	-	98%	98%
Beta Blocker at Discharge[3]	0	-	98%	98%
Fibrinolytic Medication Timing[3]	0	-	50%	55%
PCI Within 90 Minutes of Arrival[3]	0	-	88%	90%
Smoking Cessation Advice[3]	0	-	100%	99%
Chest Pain/Possible Heart Attack Care				
Aspirin at Arrival	-	-	96%	95%
Median Time to ECG (minutes)	-	-	11	8
Median Time to Transfer (minutes)	-	-	75	61
Fibrinolytic Medication Timing	-	-	55%	54%
Heart Failure Care				
ACE Inhibitor or ARB for LVSD[1]	2	100%	94%	94%
Discharge Instructions[1]	4	75%	89%	88%
Evaluation of LVS Function[1]	8	88%	98%	98%
Smoking Cessation Advice[1]	1	100%	98%	98%
Pneumonia Care				
Appropriate Initial Antibiotic[1]	24	79%	92%	92%
Blood Culture Timing	33	88%	95%	96%
Influenza Vaccine[1]	23	87%	90%	91%
Initial Antibiotic Timing[1]	2	50%	93%	95%
Pneumococcal Vaccine	30	93%	92%	93%
Smoking Cessation Advice[1]	6	100%	98%	97%
Surgical Care Improvement Project				
Appropriate VTP Within 24 Hours[5]	0	-	94%	92%
Appropriate Hair Removal[5]	0	-	100%	99%
Appropriate Beta Blocker Usage[5]	0	-	92%	93%
Controlled Postoperative Blood Glucose[5]	0	-	94%	93%
Prophylactic Antibiotic Timing[5]	0	-	96%	97%
Prophylactic Antibiotic Timing (Outpatient)	-	-	92%	92%
Prophylactic Antibiotic Selection[5]	0	-	97%	97%
Prophylactic Antibiotic Select. (Outpatient)	-	-	93%	94%
Prophylactic Antibiotic Stopped[5]	0	-	94%	94%
Recommended VTP Ordered[5]	0	-	96%	94%
Urinary Catheter Removal[5]	0	-	90%	90%
Children's Asthma Care				
Received Systemic Corticosteroids	-	-	-	100%
Received Home Management Plan	-	-	-	71%
Received Reliever Medication	-	-	-	100%
Use of Medical Imaging				
Combination Abdominal CT Scan	-	-	0.141	0.191
Combination Chest CT Scan	-	-	0.024	0.054
Follow-up Mammogram/Ultrasound	-	-	9.8%	8.4%
MRI for Low Back Pain	-	-	26.9%	32.7%
Survey of Patients' Hospital Experiences				
Area Around Room 'Always' Quiet at Night[8]	-	-	-	58%
Doctors 'Always' Communicated Well[8]	-	-	-	80%
Home Recovery Information Given[8]	-	-	-	82%
Hospital Given 9 or 10 on 10 Point Scale[8]	-	-	-	67%
Meds 'Always' Explained Before Given[8]	-	-	-	60%
Nurses 'Always' Communicated Well[8]	-	-	-	76%
Pain 'Always' Well Controlled[8]	-	-	-	69%
Room and Bathroom 'Always' Clean[8]	-	-	-	71%
Timely Help 'Always' Received[8]	-	-	-	64%
Would Definitely Recommend Hospital[8]	-	-	-	69%

Samaritan Hospital

2215 Burdett Avenue
Troy, NY 12180
URL: www.nehealth.com
Type: Acute Care Hospitals
Ownership: Voluntary Non-Profit - Private

Phone: 518-271-3225
Fax: 518-271-3781
Emergency Services: Yes
Beds: 238

Key Personnel:
CEO/President. . . . . James K Reed, MD
Chief of Medical Staff . . . . John A Collins
Patient Relations . . . . Norman E Dascher, Jr, CHE

Measure	Cases	This Hosp.	State Avg.	U.S. Avg.
Heart Attack Care				
ACE Inhibitor or ARB for LVSD[1]	5	80%	95%	96%
Aspirin at Arrival	51	100%	98%	99%
Aspirin at Discharge	33	94%	98%	98%
Beta Blocker at Discharge	38	100%	98%	98%
Fibrinolytic Medication Timing	0	-	50%	55%
PCI Within 90 Minutes of Arrival	0	-	88%	90%
Smoking Cessation Advice[1]	8	100%	100%	99%
Chest Pain/Possible Heart Attack Care				
Aspirin at Arrival	34	94%	96%	95%
Median Time to ECG (minutes)	36	14	11	8
Median Time to Transfer (minutes)[1,3]	13	86	75	61
Fibrinolytic Medication Timing	0	-	55%	54%
Heart Failure Care				
ACE Inhibitor or ARB for LVSD	58	97%	94%	94%
Discharge Instructions	143	80%	89%	88%
Evaluation of LVS Function	183	99%	98%	98%
Smoking Cessation Advice	29	100%	98%	98%
Pneumonia Care				
Appropriate Initial Antibiotic[2]	94	93%	92%	92%
Blood Culture Timing[2]	171	94%	95%	96%
Influenza Vaccine[2]	92	77%	90%	91%
Initial Antibiotic Timing[2]	171	97%	93%	95%
Pneumococcal Vaccine[2]	155	89%	92%	93%
Smoking Cessation Advice[2]	58	93%	98%	97%
Surgical Care Improvement Project				
Appropriate VTP Within 24 Hours[2]	152	74%	94%	92%
Appropriate Hair Removal[2]	380	96%	100%	99%
Appropriate Beta Blocker Usage[2]	109	89%	92%	93%
Controlled Postoperative Blood Glucose[2]	0	-	94%	93%
Prophylactic Antibiotic Timing[2]	229	92%	96%	97%
Prophylactic Antibiotic Timing (Outpatient)	85	64%	92%	92%
Prophylactic Antibiotic Selection[2]	231	90%	97%	97%
Prophylactic Antibiotic Select. (Outpatient)	67	93%	93%	94%
Prophylactic Antibiotic Stopped[2]	221	90%	94%	94%
Recommended VTP Ordered[2]	154	84%	96%	94%
Urinary Catheter Removal	87	76%	90%	90%
Children's Asthma Care				
Received Systemic Corticosteroids	-	-	-	100%
Received Home Management Plan	-	-	-	71%
Received Reliever Medication	-	-	-	100%
Use of Medical Imaging				
Combination Abdominal CT Scan	548	0.051	0.141	0.191
Combination Chest CT Scan	325	0.009	0.024	0.054
Follow-up Mammogram/Ultrasound	538	11.7%	9.8%	8.4%
MRI for Low Back Pain	65	27.7%	26.9%	32.7%
Survey of Patients' Hospital Experiences				
Area Around Room 'Always' Quiet at Night	300+	45%	-	58%
Doctors 'Always' Communicated Well	300+	73%	-	80%
Home Recovery Information Given	300+	82%	-	82%
Hospital Given 9 or 10 on 10 Point Scale	300+	60%	-	67%
Meds 'Always' Explained Before Given	300+	53%	-	60%
Nurses 'Always' Communicated Well	300+	69%	-	76%
Pain 'Always' Well Controlled	300+	64%	-	69%
Room and Bathroom 'Always' Clean	300+	66%	-	71%
Timely Help 'Always' Received	300+	56%	-	64%
Would Definitely Recommend Hospital	300+	63%	-	69%

NOTE: Hospital profiles are in alphabetical order by state, then city, then hospital within the city; Rankings exclude hospitals with less than 25 cases except for patient surveys which excludes hospitals with less than 100 cases; (a) 100–299 cases; (1) The number of cases is too small to be sure how well a hospital is performing; (2) The hospital indicated that the data submitted for this measure were based on a sample of cases; (3) Data was collected during a shorter time period (fewer quarters) than the maximum possible time for this measure; (4) Suppressed for one or more quarters by CMS; (5) No data is available from the hospital for this measure; (6) Fewer than 100 patients completed the HCAHPS survey. Use these rates with caution, as the number of surveys may be too low to reliably assess hospital performance; (7) Survey results are based on less than 12 months of data; (8) Survey results are not available for this reporting period; (9) No or very few patients were eligible for the HCAHPS survey. The scores shown, if any, reflect a very small number of surveys; (10) A state average was not calculated because too few hospitals in the state submitted data; (11) There were discrepancies in the data collection process; Please refer to the User's Guide for a full explanation of data.

Seton Health System-St Mary's Campus

1300 Massachusetts Avenue
Troy, NY 12180
Phone: 518-272-5000
Fax: 518-268-5257
E-mail: info@setonhealth.org
URL: www.setonhealth.org
Type: Acute Care Hospitals
Emergency Services: Yes
Ownership: Voluntary Non-Profit - Church
Beds: 201

Key Personnel:
CEO/President. . . . . Scott St. George
Chief of Medical Staff . . . . Richard Rubin, MD
Infection Control. . . . . Mary Beth Farley
Operating Room. . . . . Debra Shumelda
Pediatric In-Patient Care . . . . Colleen Hatman, RN
Quality Assurance . . . . Carol Crucetti
Radiology. . . . . Patti Nazarko

Measure	Cases	This Hosp.	State Avg.	U.S. Avg.
Heart Attack Care				
ACE Inhibitor or ARB for LVSD[1]	3	100%	95%	96%
Aspirin at Arrival	36	100%	98%	99%
Aspirin at Discharge	25	92%	98%	98%
Beta Blocker at Discharge	25	100%	98%	98%
Fibrinolytic Medication Timing	0	-	50%	55%
PCI Within 90 Minutes of Arrival	0	-	88%	90%
Smoking Cessation Advice[1]	8	100%	100%	99%
Chest Pain/Possible Heart Attack Care				
Aspirin at Arrival[5]	0	-	96%	95%
Median Time to ECG (minutes)[5]	0	-	11	8
Median Time to Transfer (minutes)[5]	0	-	75	61
Fibrinolytic Medication Timing[5]	0	-	55%	54%
Heart Failure Care				
ACE Inhibitor or ARB for LVSD	32	97%	94%	94%
Discharge Instructions	139	90%	89%	88%
Evaluation of LVS Function	172	98%	98%	98%
Smoking Cessation Advice	25	100%	98%	98%
Pneumonia Care				
Appropriate Initial Antibiotic	94	90%	92%	92%
Blood Culture Timing	108	94%	95%	96%
Influenza Vaccine	88	94%	90%	91%
Initial Antibiotic Timing	140	97%	93%	95%
Pneumococcal Vaccine	121	89%	92%	93%
Smoking Cessation Advice	39	100%	98%	97%
Surgical Care Improvement Project				
Appropriate VTP Within 24 Hours[2]	203	96%	94%	92%
Appropriate Hair Removal[2]	383	100%	100%	99%
Appropriate Beta Blocker Usage[2]	104	96%	92%	93%
Controlled Postoperative Blood Glucose[2]	0	-	94%	93%
Prophylactic Antibiotic Timing[2]	259	97%	96%	97%
Prophylactic Antibiotic Timing (Outpatient)	258	96%	92%	92%
Prophylactic Antibiotic Selection[2]	258	97%	97%	97%
Prophylactic Antibiotic Select. (Outpatient)	256	97%	93%	94%
Prophylactic Antibiotic Stopped[2]	248	98%	94%	94%
Recommended VTP Ordered[2]	203	97%	96%	94%
Urinary Catheter Removal[2]	129	97%	90%	90%
Children's Asthma Care				
Received Systemic Corticosteroids	-	-	-	100%
Received Home Management Plan	-	-	-	71%
Received Reliever Medication	-	-	-	100%
Use of Medical Imaging				
Combination Abdominal CT Scan	649	0.065	0.141	0.191
Combination Chest CT Scan	329	0.000	0.024	0.054
Follow-up Mammogram/Ultrasound	733	7.6%	9.8%	8.4%
MRI for Low Back Pain	46	43.5%	26.9%	32.7%
Survey of Patients' Hospital Experiences				
Area Around Room 'Always' Quiet at Night	300+	53%	-	58%
Doctors 'Always' Communicated Well	300+	80%	-	80%
Home Recovery Information Given	300+	84%	-	82%
Hospital Given 9 or 10 on 10 Point Scale	300+	68%	-	67%
Meds 'Always' Explained Before Given	300+	59%	-	60%
Nurses 'Always' Communicated Well	300+	80%	-	76%
Pain 'Always' Well Controlled	300+	68%	-	69%
Room and Bathroom 'Always' Clean	300+	64%	-	71%
Timely Help 'Always' Received	300+	65%	-	64%
Would Definitely Recommend Hospital	300+	67%	-	69%

Faxton-St Luke's Healthcare

1656 Champlin Avenue
Utica, NY 13503
Phone: 315-798-6000
Type: Acute Care Hospitals
Emergency Services: Yes
Ownership: Voluntary Non-Profit - Other

Measure	Cases	This Hosp.	State Avg.	U.S. Avg.
Heart Attack Care				
ACE Inhibitor or ARB for LVSD	32	91%	95%	96%
Aspirin at Arrival	119	95%	98%	99%
Aspirin at Discharge	110	95%	98%	98%
Beta Blocker at Discharge	115	97%	98%	98%
Fibrinolytic Medication Timing	0	-	50%	55%
PCI Within 90 Minutes of Arrival[1]	12	58%	88%	90%
Smoking Cessation Advice	27	93%	100%	99%
Chest Pain/Possible Heart Attack Care				
Aspirin at Arrival[1,3]	1	100%	96%	95%
Median Time to ECG (minutes)[1,3]	1	0	11	8
Median Time to Transfer (minutes)[5]	0	-	75	61
Fibrinolytic Medication Timing[5]	0	-	55%	54%
Heart Failure Care				
ACE Inhibitor or ARB for LVSD	103	85%	94%	94%
Discharge Instructions	208	81%	89%	88%
Evaluation of LVS Function	309	93%	98%	98%
Smoking Cessation Advice	34	97%	98%	98%
Pneumonia Care				
Appropriate Initial Antibiotic	169	76%	92%	92%
Blood Culture Timing	266	92%	95%	96%
Influenza Vaccine	211	83%	90%	91%
Initial Antibiotic Timing	311	85%	93%	95%
Pneumococcal Vaccine	301	85%	92%	93%
Smoking Cessation Advice	75	99%	98%	97%
Surgical Care Improvement Project				
Appropriate VTP Within 24 Hours[2]	183	89%	94%	92%
Appropriate Hair Removal[2]	499	100%	100%	99%
Appropriate Beta Blocker Usage[2]	146	99%	92%	93%
Controlled Postoperative Blood Glucose[2]	0	-	94%	93%
Prophylactic Antibiotic Timing[2]	333	91%	96%	97%
Prophylactic Antibiotic Timing (Outpatient)	181	80%	92%	92%
Prophylactic Antibiotic Selection[2]	332	93%	97%	97%
Prophylactic Antibiotic Select. (Outpatient)	156	78%	93%	94%
Prophylactic Antibiotic Stopped[2]	325	75%	94%	94%
Recommended VTP Ordered[2]	183	90%	96%	94%
Urinary Catheter Removal[2]	85	92%	90%	90%
Children's Asthma Care				
Received Systemic Corticosteroids	-	-	-	100%
Received Home Management Plan	-	-	-	71%
Received Reliever Medication	-	-	-	100%
Use of Medical Imaging				
Combination Abdominal CT Scan	483	0.054	0.141	0.191
Combination Chest CT Scan	608	0.000	0.024	0.054
Follow-up Mammogram/Ultrasound	1,552	18.4%	9.8%	8.4%
MRI for Low Back Pain[5]	0	-	26.9%	32.7%
Survey of Patients' Hospital Experiences				
Area Around Room 'Always' Quiet at Night	300+	42%	-	58%
Doctors 'Always' Communicated Well	300+	74%	-	80%
Home Recovery Information Given	300+	80%	-	82%
Hospital Given 9 or 10 on 10 Point Scale	300+	57%	-	67%
Meds 'Always' Explained Before Given	300+	53%	-	60%
Nurses 'Always' Communicated Well	300+	71%	-	76%
Pain 'Always' Well Controlled	300+	65%	-	69%
Room and Bathroom 'Always' Clean	300+	52%	-	71%
Timely Help 'Always' Received	300+	57%	-	64%
Would Definitely Recommend Hospital	300+	63%	-	69%

Saint Elizabeth Medical Center

2209 Genesee Street
Utica, NY 13501
Phone: 315-798-8100
Fax: 315-734-3008
E-mail: marketing@stemc.org
URL: www.stemc.org
Type: Acute Care Hospitals
Emergency Services: Yes
Ownership: Voluntary Non-Profit - Private
Beds: 201

Key Personnel:
CEO/President. . . . . Sister M Johanna
Chief of Medical Staff . . . . Fred Talarico, MD
Pediatric Ambulatory Care . . . . . . Waleed Kaashmire
Quality Assurance . . . . Christine Holehan, RN
Emergency Room . . . . Anna Giannico

Measure	Cases	This Hosp.	State Avg.	U.S. Avg.
Heart Attack Care				
ACE Inhibitor or ARB for LVSD	107	92%	95%	96%
Aspirin at Arrival	194	99%	98%	99%
Aspirin at Discharge	316	99%	98%	98%
Beta Blocker at Discharge	309	98%	98%	98%
Fibrinolytic Medication Timing	0	-	50%	55%
PCI Within 90 Minutes of Arrival	65	85%	88%	90%
Smoking Cessation Advice	125	100%	100%	99%
Chest Pain/Possible Heart Attack Care				
Aspirin at Arrival[5]	0	-	96%	95%
Median Time to ECG (minutes)[5]	0	-	11	8
Median Time to Transfer (minutes)[5]	0	-	75	61
Fibrinolytic Medication Timing[5]	0	-	55%	54%
Heart Failure Care				
ACE Inhibitor or ARB for LVSD	262	84%	94%	94%
Discharge Instructions	465	88%	89%	88%
Evaluation of LVS Function	607	96%	98%	98%
Smoking Cessation Advice	89	99%	98%	98%
Pneumonia Care				
Appropriate Initial Antibiotic	103	91%	92%	92%
Blood Culture Timing	117	93%	95%	96%
Influenza Vaccine	168	86%	90%	91%
Initial Antibiotic Timing	176	96%	93%	95%
Pneumococcal Vaccine	236	90%	92%	93%
Smoking Cessation Advice	74	97%	98%	97%
Surgical Care Improvement Project				
Appropriate VTP Within 24 Hours[2]	173	75%	94%	92%
Appropriate Hair Removal[2]	1,070	99%	100%	99%
Appropriate Beta Blocker Usage[2]	514	89%	92%	93%
Controlled Postoperative Blood Glucose[2]	350	95%	94%	93%
Prophylactic Antibiotic Timing[2]	834	92%	96%	97%
Prophylactic Antibiotic Timing (Outpatient)	183	77%	92%	92%
Prophylactic Antibiotic Selection[2]	851	98%	97%	97%
Prophylactic Antibiotic Select. (Outpatient)	150	94%	93%	94%
Prophylactic Antibiotic Stopped[2]	818	96%	94%	94%
Recommended VTP Ordered[2]	173	86%	96%	94%
Urinary Catheter Removal[2]	90	62%	90%	90%
Children's Asthma Care				
Received Systemic Corticosteroids	-	-	-	100%
Received Home Management Plan	-	-	-	71%
Received Reliever Medication	-	-	-	100%
Use of Medical Imaging				
Combination Abdominal CT Scan	515	0.315	0.141	0.191
Combination Chest CT Scan	357	0.039	0.024	0.054
Follow-up Mammogram/Ultrasound	822	5.7%	9.8%	8.4%
MRI for Low Back Pain[5]	0	-	26.9%	32.7%
Survey of Patients' Hospital Experiences				
Area Around Room 'Always' Quiet at Night	300+	44%	-	58%
Doctors 'Always' Communicated Well	300+	74%	-	80%
Home Recovery Information Given	300+	81%	-	82%
Hospital Given 9 or 10 on 10 Point Scale	300+	64%	-	67%
Meds 'Always' Explained Before Given	300+	53%	-	60%
Nurses 'Always' Communicated Well	300+	77%	-	76%
Pain 'Always' Well Controlled	300+	68%	-	69%
Room and Bathroom 'Always' Clean	300+	71%	-	71%
Timely Help 'Always' Received	300+	66%	-	64%
Would Definitely Recommend Hospital	300+	70%	-	69%

NOTE: Hospital profiles are in alphabetical order by state, then city, then hospital within the city; Rankings exclude hospitals with less than 25 cases except for patient surveys which excludes hospitals with less than 100 cases; (a) 100–299 cases; (1) The number of cases is too small to be sure how well a hospital is performing; (2) The hospital indicated that the data submitted for this measure were based on a sample of cases; (3) Data was collected during a shorter time period (fewer quarters) than the maximum possible time for this measure; (4) Suppressed for one or more quarters by CMS; (5) No data is available from the hospital for this measure; (6) Fewer than 100 patients completed the HCAHPS survey. Use these rates with caution, as the number of surveys may be too low to reliably assess hospital performance; (7) Survey results are based on less than 12 months of data; (8) Survey results are not available for this reporting period; (9) No or very few patients were eligible for the HCAHPS survey. The scores shown, if any, reflect a very small number of surveys; (10) A state average was not calculated because too few hospitals in the state submitted data; (11) There were discrepancies in the data collection process; Please refer to the User's Guide for a full explanation of data.

Westchester Medical Center

100 Woods Rd
Valhalla, NY 10595
URL: www.wcmc.com
Phone: 914-285-7017
Type: Acute Care Hospitals
Emergency Services: Yes
Ownership: Voluntary Non-Profit - Other
Beds: 635

Key Personnel:

CEO/President. . . . . Michael D Israel
Chief of Medical Staff. . . . . Michael Gewitz, MD
Infection Control. . . . . Gary Wormser, MD
Operating Room. . . . . John Savino, MD
Pediatric Ambulatory Care . . . . . . Michael Gerwitz, MD
Quality Assurance . . . . Michael Lauria
Radiology. . . . . Chitti R Moorthy, MD

Measure	Cases	This Hosp.	State Avg.	U.S. Avg.
Heart Attack Care				
ACE Inhibitor or ARB for LVSD[2]	73	100%	95%	96%
Aspirin at Arrival[2]	57	100%	98%	99%
Aspirin at Discharge[2]	311	99%	98%	98%
Beta Blocker at Discharge[2]	305	99%	98%	98%
Fibrinolytic Medication Timing[2]	0	-	50%	55%
PCI Within 90 Minutes of Arrival[1,2]	17	94%	88%	90%
Smoking Cessation Advice[2]	81	99%	100%	99%
Chest Pain/Possible Heart Attack Care				
Aspirin at Arrival[5]	0	-	96%	95%
Median Time to ECG (minutes)[5]	0	-	11	8
Median Time to Transfer (minutes)[5]	0	-	75	61
Fibrinolytic Medication Timing[5]	0	-	55%	54%
Heart Failure Care				
ACE Inhibitor or ARB for LVSD	135	99%	94%	94%
Discharge Instructions	257	91%	89%	88%
Evaluation of LVS Function	293	100%	98%	98%
Smoking Cessation Advice	47	100%	98%	98%
Pneumonia Care				
Appropriate Initial Antibiotic	32	78%	92%	92%
Blood Culture Timing	61	90%	95%	96%
Influenza Vaccine	59	73%	90%	91%
Initial Antibiotic Timing	59	97%	93%	95%
Pneumococcal Vaccine	79	80%	92%	93%
Smoking Cessation Advice	27	100%	98%	97%
Surgical Care Improvement Project				
Appropriate VTP Within 24 Hours[2]	348	95%	94%	92%
Appropriate Hair Removal[2]	1,026	100%	100%	99%
Appropriate Beta Blocker Usage[2]	475	92%	92%	93%
Controlled Postoperative Blood Glucose[2]	335	96%	94%	93%
Prophylactic Antibiotic Timing[2]	588	94%	96%	97%
Prophylactic Antibiotic Timing (Outpatient)	377	94%	92%	92%
Prophylactic Antibiotic Selection[2]	614	99%	97%	97%
Prophylactic Antibiotic Select. (Outpatient)	366	97%	93%	94%
Prophylactic Antibiotic Stopped[2]	537	95%	94%	94%
Recommended VTP Ordered[2]	348	96%	96%	94%
Urinary Catheter Removal[2]	186	86%	90%	90%
Children's Asthma Care				
Received Systemic Corticosteroids	-	-	-	100%
Received Home Management Plan	-	-	-	71%
Received Reliever Medication	-	-	-	100%
Use of Medical Imaging				
Combination Abdominal CT Scan	689	0.364	0.141	0.191
Combination Chest CT Scan	479	0.094	0.024	0.054
Follow-up Mammogram/Ultrasound	359	13.1%	9.8%	8.4%
MRI for Low Back Pain[1]	54	20.4%	26.9%	32.7%
Survey of Patients' Hospital Experiences				
Area Around Room 'Always' Quiet at Night	300+	35%	-	58%
Doctors 'Always' Communicated Well	300+	71%	-	80%
Home Recovery Information Given	300+	74%	-	82%
Hospital Given 9 or 10 on 10 Point Scale	300+	56%	-	67%
Meds 'Always' Explained Before Given	300+	48%	-	60%
Nurses 'Always' Communicated Well	300+	64%	-	76%
Pain 'Always' Well Controlled	300+	59%	-	69%
Room and Bathroom 'Always' Clean	300+	53%	-	71%
Timely Help 'Always' Received	300+	54%	-	64%
Would Definitely Recommend Hospital	300+	61%	-	69%

Franklin Hospital

900 Franklin Avenue
Valley Stream, NY 11580
URL: www.northshorelij.com
Phone: 516-256-6000
Fax: 516-256-6053
Type: Acute Care Hospitals
Emergency Services: Yes
Ownership: Voluntary Non-Profit - Private
Beds: 305

Key Personnel:

CEO/President. . . . . Michael J Dowling
Chief of Medical Staff . . . . Leonard Timpone, MD
Coronary Care . . . . Kathy Mann, RN
Infection Control. . . . . Bruce Farber, MD
Operating Room. . . . . Linda Olander, RN
Pediatric Ambulatory Care . . . . . . James Fagin, MD
Quality Assurance . . . . Roberta Dixon, RN
Radiology. . . . . Mitchell Goldman, MD

Measure	Cases	This Hosp.	State Avg.	U.S. Avg.
Heart Attack Care				
ACE Inhibitor or ARB for LVSD[1,2]	5	80%	95%	96%
Aspirin at Arrival[2]	56	95%	98%	99%
Aspirin at Discharge[1,2]	20	95%	98%	98%
Beta Blocker at Discharge[1,2]	20	90%	98%	98%
Fibrinolytic Medication Timing[2]	0	-	50%	55%
PCI Within 90 Minutes of Arrival[2]	0	-	88%	90%
Smoking Cessation Advice[2]	0	-	100%	99%
Chest Pain/Possible Heart Attack Care				
Aspirin at Arrival	110	99%	96%	95%
Median Time to ECG (minutes)	111	16	11	8
Median Time to Transfer (minutes)	46	94	75	61
Fibrinolytic Medication Timing	0	-	55%	54%
Heart Failure Care				
ACE Inhibitor or ARB for LVSD[2]	87	95%	94%	94%
Discharge Instructions[2]	204	95%	89%	88%
Evaluation of LVS Function[2]	273	100%	98%	98%
Smoking Cessation Advice[2]	29	100%	98%	98%
Pneumonia Care				
Appropriate Initial Antibiotic[2]	94	95%	92%	92%
Blood Culture Timing[2]	154	99%	95%	96%
Influenza Vaccine[2]	89	97%	90%	91%
Initial Antibiotic Timing[2]	151	97%	93%	95%
Pneumococcal Vaccine[2]	135	96%	92%	93%
Smoking Cessation Advice[1,2]	17	100%	98%	97%
Surgical Care Improvement Project				
Appropriate VTP Within 24 Hours[2]	205	98%	94%	92%
Appropriate Hair Removal[2]	328	100%	100%	99%
Appropriate Beta Blocker Usage[2]	87	95%	92%	93%
Controlled Postoperative Blood Glucose[2]	0	-	94%	93%
Prophylactic Antibiotic Timing[2]	209	98%	96%	97%
Prophylactic Antibiotic Timing (Outpatient)	112	96%	92%	92%
Prophylactic Antibiotic Selection[2]	209	94%	97%	97%
Prophylactic Antibiotic Select. (Outpatient)	113	96%	93%	94%
Prophylactic Antibiotic Stopped[2]	197	98%	94%	94%
Recommended VTP Ordered[2]	205	99%	96%	94%
Urinary Catheter Removal[2]	103	98%	90%	90%
Children's Asthma Care				
Received Systemic Corticosteroids	-	-	-	100%
Received Home Management Plan	-	-	-	71%
Received Reliever Medication	-	-	-	100%
Use of Medical Imaging				
Combination Abdominal CT Scan	276	0.018	0.141	0.191
Combination Chest CT Scan	112	0.000	0.024	0.054
Follow-up Mammogram/Ultrasound	115	13.0%	9.8%	8.4%
MRI for Low Back Pain[1]	10	30.0%	26.9%	32.7%
Survey of Patients' Hospital Experiences				
Area Around Room 'Always' Quiet at Night	300+	49%	-	58%
Doctors 'Always' Communicated Well	300+	75%	-	80%
Home Recovery Information Given	300+	73%	-	82%
Hospital Given 9 or 10 on 10 Point Scale	300+	56%	-	67%
Meds 'Always' Explained Before Given	300+	52%	-	60%
Nurses 'Always' Communicated Well	300+	69%	-	76%
Pain 'Always' Well Controlled	300+	64%	-	69%
Room and Bathroom 'Always' Clean	300+	66%	-	71%
Timely Help 'Always' Received	300+	53%	-	64%
Would Definitely Recommend Hospital	300+	59%	-	69%

Delaware Valley Hospital

1 Titus Place
Walton, NY 13856
URL: www.uhs.net
Phone: 607-865-2100
Fax: 607-865-8482
Type: Critical Access Hospitals
Emergency Services: Yes
Ownership: Voluntary Non-Profit - Private
Beds: 42

Key Personnel:

CEO/President. . . . . David Polge
Chief of Medical Staff . . . . Michael J Freeman
Infection Control. . . . . Christina Jones, RN
Operating Room. . . . . Cathy Phraner, RN
Quality Assurance . . . . Deborah Hitt
Anesthesiology. . . . . Michael Branigan, CRIIA
Emergency Room . . . . Mary Doig, RN

Measure	Cases	This Hosp.	State Avg.	U.S. Avg.
Heart Attack Care				
ACE Inhibitor or ARB for LVSD[1]	1	100%	95%	96%
Aspirin at Arrival[1]	2	100%	98%	99%
Aspirin at Discharge[1]	2	100%	98%	98%
Beta Blocker at Discharge[1]	2	100%	98%	98%
Fibrinolytic Medication Timing	0	-	50%	55%
PCI Within 90 Minutes of Arrival	0	-	88%	90%
Smoking Cessation Advice	0	-	100%	99%
Chest Pain/Possible Heart Attack Care				
Aspirin at Arrival[1,3]	23	100%	96%	95%
Median Time to ECG (minutes)[1,3]	24	7	11	8
Median Time to Transfer (minutes)[1,3]	1	155	75	61
Fibrinolytic Medication Timing[3]	0	-	55%	54%
Heart Failure Care				
ACE Inhibitor or ARB for LVSD[1,2]	7	86%	94%	94%
Discharge Instructions[1,2]	21	95%	89%	88%
Evaluation of LVS Function[2]	27	89%	98%	98%
Smoking Cessation Advice[1,2]	4	100%	98%	98%
Pneumonia Care				
Appropriate Initial Antibiotic	47	91%	92%	92%
Blood Culture Timing	56	98%	95%	96%
Influenza Vaccine[1]	22	100%	90%	91%
Initial Antibiotic Timing	49	100%	93%	95%
Pneumococcal Vaccine	32	94%	92%	93%
Smoking Cessation Advice[1]	8	88%	98%	97%
Surgical Care Improvement Project				
Appropriate VTP Within 24 Hours[5]	0	-	94%	92%
Appropriate Hair Removal[5]	0	-	100%	99%
Appropriate Beta Blocker Usage[5]	0	-	92%	93%
Controlled Postoperative Blood Glucose[5]	0	-	94%	93%
Prophylactic Antibiotic Timing[5]	0	-	96%	97%
Prophylactic Antibiotic Timing (Outpatient)[5]	0	-	92%	92%
Prophylactic Antibiotic Selection[5]	0	-	97%	97%
Prophylactic Antibiotic Select. (Outpatient)[5]	0	-	93%	94%
Prophylactic Antibiotic Stopped[5]	0	-	94%	94%
Recommended VTP Ordered[5]	0	-	96%	94%
Urinary Catheter Removal[5]	0	-	90%	90%
Children's Asthma Care				
Received Systemic Corticosteroids	-	-	-	100%
Received Home Management Plan	-	-	-	71%
Received Reliever Medication	-	-	-	100%
Use of Medical Imaging				
Combination Abdominal CT Scan	100	0.040	0.141	0.191
Combination Chest CT Scan[1]	40	0.050	0.024	0.054
Follow-up Mammogram/Ultrasound	206	12.1%	9.8%	8.4%
MRI for Low Back Pain[5]	0	-	26.9%	32.7%
Survey of Patients' Hospital Experiences				
Area Around Room 'Always' Quiet at Night	(a)	61%	-	58%
Doctors 'Always' Communicated Well	(a)	86%	-	80%
Home Recovery Information Given	(a)	86%	-	82%
Hospital Given 9 or 10 on 10 Point Scale	(a)	73%	-	67%
Meds 'Always' Explained Before Given	(a)	60%	-	60%
Nurses 'Always' Communicated Well	(a)	85%	-	76%
Pain 'Always' Well Controlled	(a)	76%	-	69%
Room and Bathroom 'Always' Clean	(a)	87%	-	71%
Timely Help 'Always' Received	(a)	77%	-	64%
Would Definitely Recommend Hospital	(a)	76%	-	69%

NOTE: Hospital profiles are in alphabetical order by state, then city, then hospital within the city; Rankings exclude hospitals with less than 25 cases except for patient surveys which excludes hospitals with less than 100 cases; (a) 100–299 cases; (1) The number of cases is too small to be sure how well a hospital is performing; (2) The hospital indicated that the data submitted for this measure were based on a sample of cases; (3) Data was collected during a shorter time period (fewer quarters) than the maximum possible time for this measure; (4) Suppressed for one or more quarters by CMS; (5) No data is available from the hospital for this measure; (6) Fewer than 100 patients completed the HCAHPS survey. Use these rates with caution, as the number of surveys may be too low to reliably assess hospital performance; (7) Survey results are based on less than 12 months of data; (8) Survey results are not available for this reporting period; (9) No or very few patients were eligible for the HCAHPS survey. The scores shown, if any, reflect a very small number of surveys; (10) A state average was not calculated because too few hospitals in the state submitted data; (11) There were discrepancies in the data collection process; Please refer to the User's Guide for a full explanation of data.

Wyoming County Community Hospital

400 North Main Street Phone: 585-786-2233
Warsaw, NY 14569 Fax: 585-786-1222
URL: www.wccns.net
Type: Acute Care Hospitals Emergency Services: Yes
Ownership: Government - Local Beds: 264

Key Personnel:
CEO/President. . . . . Ronald Krawiec
Cardiac Laboratory. . . . . Lori Merrill
Chief of Medical Staff . . . . Greig Collins, MD
Infection Control. . . . . Connie Almeter
Operating Room. . . . . Cynthia Elbow
Quality Assurance . . . . Peg Cunningham
Radiology. . . . . Margaret Morgan Hise

Measure	Cases	This Hosp.	State Avg.	U.S. Avg.
Heart Attack Care				
ACE Inhibitor or ARB for LVSD[1]	1	100%	95%	96%
Aspirin at Arrival[1]	12	92%	98%	99%
Aspirin at Discharge[1]	5	80%	98%	98%
Beta Blocker at Discharge[1]	5	100%	98%	98%
Fibrinolytic Medication Timing[1]	1	100%	50%	55%
PCI Within 90 Minutes of Arrival	0	-	88%	90%
Smoking Cessation Advice	0	-	100%	99%
Chest Pain/Possible Heart Attack Care				
Aspirin at Arrival	95	99%	96%	95%
Median Time to ECG (minutes)	100	13	11	8
Median Time to Transfer (minutes)[3]	0	-	75	61
Fibrinolytic Medication Timing[1]	8	38%	55%	54%
Heart Failure Care				
ACE Inhibitor or ARB for LVSD	29	97%	94%	94%
Discharge Instructions	57	81%	89%	88%
Evaluation of LVS Function	85	100%	98%	98%
Smoking Cessation Advice[1]	17	82%	98%	98%
Pneumonia Care				
Appropriate Initial Antibiotic	54	81%	92%	92%
Blood Culture Timing	75	89%	95%	96%
Influenza Vaccine	56	77%	90%	91%
Initial Antibiotic Timing	82	95%	93%	95%
Pneumococcal Vaccine	70	86%	92%	93%
Smoking Cessation Advice[1]	22	91%	98%	97%
Surgical Care Improvement Project				
Appropriate VTP Within 24 Hours	82	73%	94%	92%
Appropriate Hair Removal	157	100%	100%	99%
Appropriate Beta Blocker Usage	46	93%	92%	93%
Controlled Postoperative Blood Glucose	0	-	94%	93%
Prophylactic Antibiotic Timing	119	94%	96%	97%
Prophylactic Antibiotic Timing (Outpatient)[1]	23	78%	92%	92%
Prophylactic Antibiotic Selection	120	97%	97%	97%
Prophylactic Antibiotic Select. (Outpatient)[1]	19	74%	93%	94%
Prophylactic Antibiotic Stopped	119	87%	94%	94%
Recommended VTP Ordered	82	73%	96%	94%
Urinary Catheter Removal[1]	6	100%	90%	90%
Children's Asthma Care				
Received Systemic Corticosteroids	-	-	-	100%
Received Home Management Plan	-	-	-	71%
Received Reliever Medication	-	-	-	100%
Use of Medical Imaging				
Combination Abdominal CT Scan	132	0.568	0.141	0.191
Combination Chest CT Scan	104	0.096	0.024	0.054
Follow-up Mammogram/Ultrasound	191	17.8%	9.8%	8.4%
MRI for Low Back Pain[1]	9	11.1%	26.9%	32.7%
Survey of Patients' Hospital Experiences				
Area Around Room 'Always' Quiet at Night	300+	38%	-	58%
Doctors 'Always' Communicated Well	300+	74%	-	80%
Home Recovery Information Given	300+	84%	-	82%
Hospital Given 9 or 10 on 10 Point Scale	300+	55%	-	67%
Meds 'Always' Explained Before Given	300+	55%	-	60%
Nurses 'Always' Communicated Well	300+	72%	-	76%
Pain 'Always' Well Controlled	300+	67%	-	69%
Room and Bathroom 'Always' Clean	300+	72%	-	71%
Timely Help 'Always' Received	300+	57%	-	64%
Would Definitely Recommend Hospital	300+	54%	-	69%

Saint Anthony Community Hospital

15 - 19 Maple Avenue Phone: 845-986-2276
Warwick, NY 10990 Fax: 845-986-2687
URL: www.stanthonycommunityhosp.org
Type: Acute Care Hospitals Emergency Services: Yes
Ownership: Voluntary Non-Profit - Church Beds: 73

Key Personnel:
CEO/President. . . . . Stephen Majetich, SC
Radiology. . . . . Patricia Barnes

Measure	Cases	This Hosp.	State Avg.	U.S. Avg.
Heart Attack Care				
ACE Inhibitor or ARB for LVSD[1]	4	100%	95%	96%
Aspirin at Arrival[1]	23	100%	98%	99%
Aspirin at Discharge[1]	12	100%	98%	98%
Beta Blocker at Discharge[1]	11	100%	98%	98%
Fibrinolytic Medication Timing	0	-	50%	55%
PCI Within 90 Minutes of Arrival	0	-	88%	90%
Smoking Cessation Advice[1]	2	100%	100%	99%
Chest Pain/Possible Heart Attack Care				
Aspirin at Arrival[1]	21	95%	96%	95%
Median Time to ECG (minutes)[1]	19	5	11	8
Median Time to Transfer (minutes)[1,3]	1	332	75	61
Fibrinolytic Medication Timing	0	-	55%	54%
Heart Failure Care				
ACE Inhibitor or ARB for LVSD[1]	21	95%	94%	94%
Discharge Instructions	73	100%	89%	88%
Evaluation of LVS Function	92	99%	98%	98%
Smoking Cessation Advice[1]	11	100%	98%	98%
Pneumonia Care				
Appropriate Initial Antibiotic	49	86%	92%	92%
Blood Culture Timing	88	97%	95%	96%
Influenza Vaccine	60	78%	90%	91%
Initial Antibiotic Timing	83	98%	93%	95%
Pneumococcal Vaccine	91	84%	92%	93%
Smoking Cessation Advice[1]	22	100%	98%	97%
Surgical Care Improvement Project				
Appropriate VTP Within 24 Hours	76	92%	94%	92%
Appropriate Hair Removal	233	100%	100%	99%
Appropriate Beta Blocker Usage	50	90%	92%	93%
Controlled Postoperative Blood Glucose	0	-	94%	93%
Prophylactic Antibiotic Timing	155	96%	96%	97%
Prophylactic Antibiotic Timing (Outpatient)	49	96%	92%	92%
Prophylactic Antibiotic Selection	155	88%	97%	97%
Prophylactic Antibiotic Select. (Outpatient)	49	84%	93%	94%
Prophylactic Antibiotic Stopped	149	97%	94%	94%
Recommended VTP Ordered	76	95%	96%	94%
Urinary Catheter Removal	27	85%	90%	90%
Children's Asthma Care				
Received Systemic Corticosteroids	-	-	-	100%
Received Home Management Plan	-	-	-	71%
Received Reliever Medication	-	-	-	100%
Use of Medical Imaging				
Combination Abdominal CT Scan	326	0.061	0.141	0.191
Combination Chest CT Scan	227	0.000	0.024	0.054
Follow-up Mammogram/Ultrasound	455	14.1%	9.8%	8.4%
MRI for Low Back Pain[1]	55	10.9%	26.9%	32.7%
Survey of Patients' Hospital Experiences				
Area Around Room 'Always' Quiet at Night	300+	55%	-	58%
Doctors 'Always' Communicated Well	300+	79%	-	80%
Home Recovery Information Given	300+	85%	-	82%
Hospital Given 9 or 10 on 10 Point Scale	300+	72%	-	67%
Meds 'Always' Explained Before Given	300+	63%	-	60%
Nurses 'Always' Communicated Well	300+	80%	-	76%
Pain 'Always' Well Controlled	300+	74%	-	69%
Room and Bathroom 'Always' Clean	300+	61%	-	71%
Timely Help 'Always' Received	300+	66%	-	64%
Would Definitely Recommend Hospital	300+	73%	-	69%

Samaritan Medical Center

830 Washington Street Phone: 315-785-4121
Watertown, NY 13601 Fax: 315-785-4343
URL: www.samaritanhealth.com
Type: Acute Care Hospitals Emergency Services: Yes
Ownership: Voluntary Non-Profit - Other Beds: 287

Key Personnel:
CEO/President. . . . . Thomas H Carman
Chief of Medical Staff . . . . Leverne R. Vandewall, MD
Operating Room. . . . . Bonnie Trudeau
Pediatric In-Patient Care . . . . Robert Bacsik, MD
Radiology. . . . . Gary L Robbins, MD

Measure	Cases	This Hosp.	State Avg.	U.S. Avg.
Heart Attack Care				
ACE Inhibitor or ARB for LVSD[1]	2	100%	95%	96%
Aspirin at Arrival	43	95%	98%	99%
Aspirin at Discharge[1]	23	96%	98%	98%
Beta Blocker at Discharge[1]	21	95%	98%	98%
Fibrinolytic Medication Timing[1]	1	0%	50%	55%
PCI Within 90 Minutes of Arrival	0	-	88%	90%
Smoking Cessation Advice[1]	2	100%	100%	99%
Chest Pain/Possible Heart Attack Care				
Aspirin at Arrival	101	94%	96%	95%
Median Time to ECG (minutes)	107	6	11	8
Median Time to Transfer (minutes)[1,3]	5	130	75	61
Fibrinolytic Medication Timing[1]	16	44%	55%	54%
Heart Failure Care				
ACE Inhibitor or ARB for LVSD	28	96%	94%	94%
Discharge Instructions	188	81%	89%	88%
Evaluation of LVS Function	216	98%	98%	98%
Smoking Cessation Advice[1]	23	100%	98%	98%
Pneumonia Care				
Appropriate Initial Antibiotic	101	94%	92%	92%
Blood Culture Timing	189	99%	95%	96%
Influenza Vaccine	120	95%	90%	91%
Initial Antibiotic Timing	176	92%	93%	95%
Pneumococcal Vaccine	168	92%	92%	93%
Smoking Cessation Advice	57	96%	98%	97%
Surgical Care Improvement Project				
Appropriate VTP Within 24 Hours	189	93%	94%	92%
Appropriate Hair Removal	468	100%	100%	99%
Appropriate Beta Blocker Usage	143	83%	92%	93%
Controlled Postoperative Blood Glucose	0	-	94%	93%
Prophylactic Antibiotic Timing	343	95%	96%	97%
Prophylactic Antibiotic Timing (Outpatient)	443	84%	92%	92%
Prophylactic Antibiotic Selection	348	98%	97%	97%
Prophylactic Antibiotic Select. (Outpatient)	453	96%	93%	94%
Prophylactic Antibiotic Stopped	340	92%	94%	94%
Recommended VTP Ordered	189	94%	96%	94%
Urinary Catheter Removal	149	86%	90%	90%
Children's Asthma Care				
Received Systemic Corticosteroids	-	-	-	100%
Received Home Management Plan	-	-	-	71%
Received Reliever Medication	-	-	-	100%
Use of Medical Imaging				
Combination Abdominal CT Scan	735	0.567	0.141	0.191
Combination Chest CT Scan	680	0.026	0.024	0.054
Follow-up Mammogram/Ultrasound	1,354	9.2%	9.8%	8.4%
MRI for Low Back Pain	75	24.0%	26.9%	32.7%
Survey of Patients' Hospital Experiences				
Area Around Room 'Always' Quiet at Night	300+	46%	-	58%
Doctors 'Always' Communicated Well	300+	76%	-	80%
Home Recovery Information Given	300+	84%	-	82%
Hospital Given 9 or 10 on 10 Point Scale	300+	51%	-	67%
Meds 'Always' Explained Before Given	300+	57%	-	60%
Nurses 'Always' Communicated Well	300+	73%	-	76%
Pain 'Always' Well Controlled	300+	65%	-	69%
Room and Bathroom 'Always' Clean	300+	71%	-	71%
Timely Help 'Always' Received	300+	62%	-	64%
Would Definitely Recommend Hospital	300+	54%	-	69%

NOTE: Hospital profiles are in alphabetical order by state, then city, then hospital within the city; Rankings exclude hospitals with less than 25 cases except for patient surveys which excludes hospitals with less than 100 cases; (a) 100–299 cases; (1) The number of cases is too small to be sure how well a hospital is performing; (2) The hospital indicated that the data submitted for this measure were based on a sample of cases; (3) Data was collected during a shorter time period (fewer quarters) than the maximum possible time for this measure; (4) Suppressed for one or more quarters by CMS; (5) No data is available from the hospital for this measure; (6) Fewer than 100 patients completed the HCAHPS survey. Use these rates with caution, as the number of surveys may be too low to reliably assess hospital performance; (7) Survey results are based on less than 12 months of data; (8) Survey results are not available for this reporting period; (9) No or very few patients were eligible for the HCAHPS survey. The scores shown, if any, reflect a very small number of surveys; (10) A state average was not calculated because too few hospitals in the state submitted data; (11) There were discrepancies in the data collection process; Please refer to the User's Guide for a full explanation of data.

Jones Memorial Hospital

191 North Main Street
Wellsville, NY 14895
Phone: 585-593-1100
Fax: 585-596-4005
URL: www.jmhny.org
Type: Acute Care Hospitals
Emergency Services: Yes
Ownership: Voluntary Non-Profit - Private
Beds: 70

Key Personnel:
CEO/President. . . . . Ann Gilpin
Chief of Medical Staff . . . . William Coach, MD
Infection Control. . . . . Lisa Lang, RN
Operating Room. . . . . James H Edmonston, RN
Quality Assurance . . . . Cheryl Macafee

Measure	Cases	This Hosp.	State Avg.	U.S. Avg.
Heart Attack Care				
ACE Inhibitor or ARB for LVSD[1]	2	100%	95%	96%
Aspirin at Arrival[1]	13	92%	98%	99%
Aspirin at Discharge[1]	7	71%	98%	98%
Beta Blocker at Discharge[1]	8	100%	98%	98%
Fibrinolytic Medication Timing	0	-	50%	55%
PCI Within 90 Minutes of Arrival	0	-	88%	90%
Smoking Cessation Advice[1]	1	100%	100%	99%
Chest Pain/Possible Heart Attack Care				
Aspirin at Arrival	58	98%	96%	95%
Median Time to ECG (minutes)	63	6	11	8
Median Time to Transfer (minutes)[1,3]	1	181	75	61
Fibrinolytic Medication Timing[1]	8	75%	55%	54%
Heart Failure Care				
ACE Inhibitor or ARB for LVSD[1]	15	87%	94%	94%
Discharge Instructions	54	74%	89%	88%
Evaluation of LVS Function	63	94%	98%	98%
Smoking Cessation Advice[1]	14	100%	98%	98%
Pneumonia Care				
Appropriate Initial Antibiotic	52	88%	92%	92%
Blood Culture Timing	93	94%	95%	96%
Influenza Vaccine	47	79%	90%	91%
Initial Antibiotic Timing	80	95%	93%	95%
Pneumococcal Vaccine	86	93%	92%	93%
Smoking Cessation Advice	29	83%	98%	97%
Surgical Care Improvement Project				
Appropriate VTP Within 24 Hours	34	88%	94%	92%
Appropriate Hair Removal	114	99%	100%	99%
Appropriate Beta Blocker Usage	27	96%	92%	93%
Controlled Postoperative Blood Glucose	0	-	94%	93%
Prophylactic Antibiotic Timing	76	97%	96%	97%
Prophylactic Antibiotic Timing (Outpatient)	43	98%	92%	92%
Prophylactic Antibiotic Selection	77	99%	97%	97%
Prophylactic Antibiotic Select. (Outpatient)	43	98%	93%	94%
Prophylactic Antibiotic Stopped	75	100%	94%	94%
Recommended VTP Ordered	34	88%	96%	94%
Urinary Catheter Removal[1]	7	86%	90%	90%
Children's Asthma Care				
Received Systemic Corticosteroids	-	-	-	100%
Received Home Management Plan	-	-	-	71%
Received Reliever Medication	-	-	-	100%
Use of Medical Imaging				
Combination Abdominal CT Scan	218	0.119	0.141	0.191
Combination Chest CT Scan	115	0.096	0.024	0.054
Follow-up Mammogram/Ultrasound	461	5.2%	9.8%	8.4%
MRI for Low Back Pain[1]	37	32.4%	26.9%	32.7%
Survey of Patients' Hospital Experiences				
Area Around Room 'Always' Quiet at Night	300+	49%	-	58%
Doctors 'Always' Communicated Well	300+	77%	-	80%
Home Recovery Information Given	300+	78%	-	82%
Hospital Given 9 or 10 on 10 Point Scale	300+	55%	-	67%
Meds 'Always' Explained Before Given	300+	54%	-	60%
Nurses 'Always' Communicated Well	300+	72%	-	76%
Pain 'Always' Well Controlled	300+	62%	-	69%
Room and Bathroom 'Always' Clean	300+	65%	-	71%
Timely Help 'Always' Received	300+	58%	-	64%
Would Definitely Recommend Hospital	300+	56%	-	69%

Helen Hayes Hospital

51 North Route 9w
West Haverstraw, NY 10993
Phone: 845-786-4000
Fax: 845-947-3097
E-mail: info@helenhayeshospital.org
URL: www.helenhayeshospital.org
Type: Acute Care Hospitals
Emergency Services: No
Ownership: Government - Local
Beds: 155

Key Personnel:
CEO/President. . . . . Val S Gray
Chief of Medical Staff . . . . John Pellicone, MD
Infection Control. . . . . Liz Brown, RN
Ambulatory Care . . . . Bruce Marshall
Patient Relations . . . . Mary Bianco

Measure	Cases	This Hosp.	State Avg.	U.S. Avg.
Heart Attack Care				
ACE Inhibitor or ARB for LVSD[5]	0	-	95%	96%
Aspirin at Arrival[5]	0	-	98%	99%
Aspirin at Discharge[5]	0	-	98%	98%
Beta Blocker at Discharge[5]	0	-	98%	98%
Fibrinolytic Medication Timing[5]	0	-	50%	55%
PCI Within 90 Minutes of Arrival[5]	0	-	88%	90%
Smoking Cessation Advice[5]	0	-	100%	99%
Chest Pain/Possible Heart Attack Care				
Aspirin at Arrival[5]	0	-	96%	95%
Median Time to ECG (minutes)[5]	0	-	11	8
Median Time to Transfer (minutes)[5]	0	-	75	61
Fibrinolytic Medication Timing[5]	0	-	55%	54%
Heart Failure Care				
ACE Inhibitor or ARB for LVSD[5]	0	-	94%	94%
Discharge Instructions[5]	0	-	89%	88%
Evaluation of LVS Function[5]	0	-	98%	98%
Smoking Cessation Advice[5]	0	-	98%	98%
Pneumonia Care				
Appropriate Initial Antibiotic[5]	0	-	92%	92%
Blood Culture Timing[5]	0	-	95%	96%
Influenza Vaccine[5]	0	-	90%	91%
Initial Antibiotic Timing[5]	0	-	93%	95%
Pneumococcal Vaccine[5]	0	-	92%	93%
Smoking Cessation Advice[5]	0	-	98%	97%
Surgical Care Improvement Project				
Appropriate VTP Within 24 Hours[5]	0	-	94%	92%
Appropriate Hair Removal[5]	0	-	100%	99%
Appropriate Beta Blocker Usage[5]	0	-	92%	93%
Controlled Postoperative Blood Glucose[5]	0	-	94%	93%
Prophylactic Antibiotic Timing[5]	0	-	96%	97%
Prophylactic Antibiotic Timing (Outpatient)[5]	0	-	92%	92%
Prophylactic Antibiotic Selection[5]	0	-	97%	97%
Prophylactic Antibiotic Select. (Outpatient)[5]	0	-	93%	94%
Prophylactic Antibiotic Stopped[5]	0	-	94%	94%
Recommended VTP Ordered[5]	0	-	96%	94%
Urinary Catheter Removal[5]	0	-	90%	90%
Children's Asthma Care				
Received Systemic Corticosteroids	-	-	-	100%
Received Home Management Plan	-	-	-	71%
Received Reliever Medication	-	-	-	100%
Use of Medical Imaging				
Combination Abdominal CT Scan[5]	0	-	0.141	0.191
Combination Chest CT Scan[5]	0	-	0.024	0.054
Follow-up Mammogram/Ultrasound[5]	0	-	9.8%	8.4%
MRI for Low Back Pain[5]	0	-	26.9%	32.7%
Survey of Patients' Hospital Experiences				
Area Around Room 'Always' Quiet at Night[9]	-	-	-	58%
Doctors 'Always' Communicated Well[9]	-	-	-	80%
Home Recovery Information Given[9]	-	-	-	82%
Hospital Given 9 or 10 on 10 Point Scale[9]	-	-	-	67%
Meds 'Always' Explained Before Given[9]	-	-	-	60%
Nurses 'Always' Communicated Well[9]	-	-	-	76%
Pain 'Always' Well Controlled[9]	-	-	-	69%
Room and Bathroom 'Always' Clean[9]	-	-	-	71%
Timely Help 'Always' Received[9]	-	-	-	64%
Would Definitely Recommend Hospital[9]	-	-	-	69%

Good Samaritan Hospital Medical Center

1000 Montauk Highway
West Islip, NY 11795
Phone: 631-376-3000
Fax: 631-376-3893
URL: www.good-samaritan-hospital.org
Type: Acute Care Hospitals
Emergency Services: Yes
Ownership: Voluntary Non-Profit - Church
Beds: 437

Key Personnel:
CEO/President. . . . . William Allison
Chief of Medical Staff . . . . Kenneth Long
Infection Control. . . . . Franes Edwards RN
Operating Room. . . . . John W Francfort MD
Pediatric Ambulatory Care . . . . . . Barry Goldberg MD
Quality Assurance . . . . Fred B Landon
Radiology. . . . . Matthew Rifkin MD

Measure	Cases	This Hosp.	State Avg.	U.S. Avg.
Heart Attack Care				
ACE Inhibitor or ARB for LVSD[1]	23	100%	95%	96%
Aspirin at Arrival	248	100%	98%	99%
Aspirin at Discharge	202	100%	98%	98%
Beta Blocker at Discharge	200	100%	98%	98%
Fibrinolytic Medication Timing	0	-	50%	55%
PCI Within 90 Minutes of Arrival	35	100%	88%	90%
Smoking Cessation Advice	61	100%	100%	99%
Chest Pain/Possible Heart Attack Care				
Aspirin at Arrival[1]	6	100%	96%	95%
Median Time to ECG (minutes)[1]	7	3	11	8
Median Time to Transfer (minutes)[5]	0	-	75	61
Fibrinolytic Medication Timing[5]	0	-	55%	54%
Heart Failure Care				
ACE Inhibitor or ARB for LVSD[2]	78	100%	94%	94%
Discharge Instructions[2]	259	100%	89%	88%
Evaluation of LVS Function[2]	344	100%	98%	98%
Smoking Cessation Advice[2]	34	100%	98%	98%
Pneumonia Care				
Appropriate Initial Antibiotic[2]	73	100%	92%	92%
Blood Culture Timing[2]	135	100%	95%	96%
Influenza Vaccine[2]	100	100%	90%	91%
Initial Antibiotic Timing[2]	126	100%	93%	95%
Pneumococcal Vaccine[2]	158	100%	92%	93%
Smoking Cessation Advice[2]	36	100%	98%	97%
Surgical Care Improvement Project				
Appropriate VTP Within 24 Hours[2]	281	96%	94%	92%
Appropriate Hair Removal[2]	500	100%	100%	99%
Appropriate Beta Blocker Usage[2]	190	97%	92%	93%
Controlled Postoperative Blood Glucose[2]	0	-	94%	93%
Prophylactic Antibiotic Timing[2]	296	98%	96%	97%
Prophylactic Antibiotic Timing (Outpatient)	352	99%	92%	92%
Prophylactic Antibiotic Selection[2]	298	99%	97%	97%
Prophylactic Antibiotic Select. (Outpatient)	351	99%	93%	94%
Prophylactic Antibiotic Stopped[2]	277	96%	94%	94%
Recommended VTP Ordered[2]	281	97%	96%	94%
Urinary Catheter Removal[2]	109	99%	90%	90%
Children's Asthma Care				
Received Systemic Corticosteroids	-	-	-	100%
Received Home Management Plan	-	-	-	71%
Received Reliever Medication	-	-	-	100%
Use of Medical Imaging				
Combination Abdominal CT Scan	1,058	0.038	0.141	0.191
Combination Chest CT Scan	785	0.001	0.024	0.054
Follow-up Mammogram/Ultrasound	1,604	16.0%	9.8%	8.4%
MRI for Low Back Pain[1]	33	24.2%	26.9%	32.7%
Survey of Patients' Hospital Experiences				
Area Around Room 'Always' Quiet at Night	300+	43%	-	58%
Doctors 'Always' Communicated Well	300+	76%	-	80%
Home Recovery Information Given	300+	83%	-	82%
Hospital Given 9 or 10 on 10 Point Scale	300+	62%	-	67%
Meds 'Always' Explained Before Given	300+	56%	-	60%
Nurses 'Always' Communicated Well	300+	73%	-	76%
Pain 'Always' Well Controlled	300+	69%	-	69%
Room and Bathroom 'Always' Clean	300+	71%	-	71%
Timely Help 'Always' Received	300+	56%	-	64%
Would Definitely Recommend Hospital	300+	68%	-	69%

NOTE: Hospital profiles are in alphabetical order by state, then city, then hospital within the city; Rankings exclude hospitals with less than 25 cases except for patient surveys which excludes hospitals with less than 100 cases; (a) 100–299 cases; (1) The number of cases is too small to be sure how well a hospital is performing; (2) The hospital indicated that the data submitted for this measure were based on a sample of cases; (3) Data was collected during a shorter time period (fewer quarters) than the maximum possible time for this measure; (4) Suppressed for one or more quarters by CMS; (5) No data is available from the hospital for this measure; (6) Fewer than 100 patients completed the HCAHPS survey. Use these rates with caution, as the number of surveys may be too low to reliably assess hospital performance; (7) Survey results are based on less than 12 months of data; (8) Survey results are not available for this reporting period; (9) No or very few patients were eligible for the HCAHPS survey. The scores shown, if any, reflect a very small number of surveys; (10) A state average was not calculated because too few hospitals in the state submitted data; (11) There were discrepancies in the data collection process; Please refer to the User's Guide for a full explanation of data.

Westfield Memorial Hospital

189 East Main Street Phone: 716-326-4921
Westfield, NY 14787 Fax: 716-326-3802
URL: www.wmhinc.org
Type: Acute Care Hospitals Emergency Services: No
Ownership: Voluntary Non-Profit - Private Beds: 32

Key Personnel:
CEO/President. . . . . Mary Larowe
Chief of Medical Staff . . . . Russell Ellwell, MD
Infection Control. . . . . Gail Hiddell
Operating Room. . . . . Kathy Petroff
Quality Assurance . . . . Patricia Uldrich
Radiology. . . . . Zhengming Gu
Anesthesiology. . . . . Russell Elwell, MD
Emergency Room . . . . Grant Stephenson, MD

Measure	Cases	This Hosp.	State Avg.	U.S. Avg.
Heart Attack Care				
ACE Inhibitor or ARB for LVSD[3]	0	-	95%	96%
Aspirin at Arrival[3]	0	-	98%	99%
Aspirin at Discharge[3]	0	-	98%	98%
Beta Blocker at Discharge[3]	0	-	98%	98%
Fibrinolytic Medication Timing[3]	0	-	50%	55%
PCI Within 90 Minutes of Arrival[3]	0	-	88%	90%
Smoking Cessation Advice[3]	0	-	100%	99%
Chest Pain/Possible Heart Attack Care				
Aspirin at Arrival	128	99%	96%	95%
Median Time to ECG (minutes)	130	5	11	8
Median Time to Transfer (minutes)[3]	0	-	75	61
Fibrinolytic Medication Timing[3]	0	-	55%	54%
Heart Failure Care				
ACE Inhibitor or ARB for LVSD[3]	0	-	94%	94%
Discharge Instructions[3]	0	-	89%	88%
Evaluation of LVS Function[1,3]	1	100%	98%	98%
Smoking Cessation Advice[3]	0	-	98%	98%
Pneumonia Care				
Appropriate Initial Antibiotic[1,2]	5	60%	92%	92%
Blood Culture Timing[1,2]	3	100%	95%	96%
Influenza Vaccine[1,2]	3	100%	90%	91%
Initial Antibiotic Timing[1,2]	3	100%	93%	95%
Pneumococcal Vaccine[1,2]	4	100%	92%	93%
Smoking Cessation Advice[1,2]	2	100%	98%	97%
Surgical Care Improvement Project				
Appropriate VTP Within 24 Hours	0	-	94%	92%
Appropriate Hair Removal[1]	9	100%	100%	99%
Appropriate Beta Blocker Usage[1]	1	100%	92%	93%
Controlled Postoperative Blood Glucose	0	-	94%	93%
Prophylactic Antibiotic Timing[1]	8	100%	96%	97%
Prophylactic Antibiotic Timing (Outpatient)[5]	0	-	92%	92%
Prophylactic Antibiotic Selection[1]	8	100%	97%	97%
Prophylactic Antibiotic Select. (Outpatient)[5]	0	-	93%	94%
Prophylactic Antibiotic Stopped[1]	8	100%	94%	94%
Recommended VTP Ordered	0	-	96%	94%
Urinary Catheter Removal	0	-	90%	90%
Children's Asthma Care				
Received Systemic Corticosteroids	-	-	-	100%
Received Home Management Plan	-	-	-	71%
Received Reliever Medication	-	-	-	100%
Use of Medical Imaging				
Combination Abdominal CT Scan	170	0.206	0.141	0.191
Combination Chest CT Scan	78	0.154	0.024	0.054
Follow-up Mammogram/Ultrasound	320	7.2%	9.8%	8.4%
MRI for Low Back Pain[5]	0	-	26.9%	32.7%
Survey of Patients' Hospital Experiences				
Area Around Room 'Always' Quiet at Night	(a)	83%	-	58%
Doctors 'Always' Communicated Well	(a)	88%	-	80%
Home Recovery Information Given	(a)	86%	-	82%
Hospital Given 9 or 10 on 10 Point Scale	(a)	91%	-	67%
Meds 'Always' Explained Before Given	(a)	82%	-	60%
Nurses 'Always' Communicated Well	(a)	93%	-	76%
Pain 'Always' Well Controlled	(a)	82%	-	69%
Room and Bathroom 'Always' Clean	(a)	87%	-	71%
Timely Help 'Always' Received	(a)	90%	-	64%
Would Definitely Recommend Hospital	(a)	92%	-	69%

White Plains Hospital Center

41 East Post R0ad Phone: 914-681-0600
White Plains, NY 10601 Fax: 914-681-2902
E-mail: wphcmail@wphospital.org
URL: www.wphospital.org
Type: Acute Care Hospitals Emergency Services: Yes
Ownership: Voluntary Non-Profit - Private Beds: 307

Key Personnel:
CEO/President. . . . . Jon B Schandler
Chief of Medical Staff . . . . Michael Palumbo, MD
Infection Control. . . . . Arthur L Forni, MD
Operating Room. . . . . Lynn G Josephson, MD
Pediatric Ambulatory Care . . . . . . Scott D Bookner, MD
Quality Assurance . . . . Ellen Perlman
Radiology. . . . . Paul T Khoury, MD

Measure	Cases	This Hosp.	State Avg.	U.S. Avg.
Heart Attack Care				
ACE Inhibitor or ARB for LVSD[1]	16	100%	95%	96%
Aspirin at Arrival	81	96%	98%	99%
Aspirin at Discharge	60	100%	98%	98%
Beta Blocker at Discharge	63	95%	98%	98%
Fibrinolytic Medication Timing[1]	1	0%	50%	55%
PCI Within 90 Minutes of Arrival[1]	11	82%	88%	90%
Smoking Cessation Advice[1]	12	100%	100%	99%
Chest Pain/Possible Heart Attack Care				
Aspirin at Arrival	70	97%	96%	95%
Median Time to ECG (minutes)	71	11	11	8
Median Time to Transfer (minutes)[1,3]	13	98	75	61
Fibrinolytic Medication Timing[1]	12	42%	55%	54%
Heart Failure Care				
ACE Inhibitor or ARB for LVSD[2]	84	93%	94%	94%
Discharge Instructions[2]	208	90%	89%	88%
Evaluation of LVS Function[2]	277	100%	98%	98%
Smoking Cessation Advice[2]	25	96%	98%	98%
Pneumonia Care				
Appropriate Initial Antibiotic[2]	108	88%	92%	92%
Blood Culture Timing[2]	115	98%	95%	96%
Influenza Vaccine[2]	98	82%	90%	91%
Initial Antibiotic Timing[2]	163	95%	93%	95%
Pneumococcal Vaccine[2]	168	85%	92%	93%
Smoking Cessation Advice[2]	28	89%	98%	97%
Surgical Care Improvement Project				
Appropriate VTP Within 24 Hours[2]	225	90%	94%	92%
Appropriate Hair Removal[2]	429	100%	100%	99%
Appropriate Beta Blocker Usage[2]	97	97%	92%	93%
Controlled Postoperative Blood Glucose[2]	0	-	94%	93%
Prophylactic Antibiotic Timing[2]	296	99%	96%	97%
Prophylactic Antibiotic Timing (Outpatient)	354	97%	92%	92%
Prophylactic Antibiotic Selection[2]	297	97%	97%	97%
Prophylactic Antibiotic Select. (Outpatient)	351	99%	93%	94%
Prophylactic Antibiotic Stopped[2]	288	83%	94%	94%
Recommended VTP Ordered[2]	225	92%	96%	94%
Urinary Catheter Removal[2]	46	72%	90%	90%
Children's Asthma Care				
Received Systemic Corticosteroids	-	-	-	100%
Received Home Management Plan	-	-	-	71%
Received Reliever Medication	-	-	-	100%
Use of Medical Imaging				
Combination Abdominal CT Scan	1,967	0.031	0.141	0.191
Combination Chest CT Scan	2,229	0.000	0.024	0.054
Follow-up Mammogram/Ultrasound	1,982	15.4%	9.8%	8.4%
MRI for Low Back Pain[5]	0	-	26.9%	32.7%
Survey of Patients' Hospital Experiences				
Area Around Room 'Always' Quiet at Night	300+	53%	-	58%
Doctors 'Always' Communicated Well	300+	79%	-	80%
Home Recovery Information Given	300+	72%	-	82%
Hospital Given 9 or 10 on 10 Point Scale	300+	68%	-	67%
Meds 'Always' Explained Before Given	300+	62%	-	60%
Nurses 'Always' Communicated Well	300+	79%	-	76%
Pain 'Always' Well Controlled	300+	71%	-	69%
Room and Bathroom 'Always' Clean	300+	68%	-	71%
Timely Help 'Always' Received	300+	63%	-	64%
Would Definitely Recommend Hospital	300+	79%	-	69%

Winifred Masterson Burke Rehab Hospital

785 Mamaroneck Avenue Phone: 914-597-2232
White Plains, NY 10605 Fax: 914-597-2757
E-mail: web@burke.org
URL: www.burke.org
Type: Acute Care Hospitals Emergency Services: No
Ownership: Voluntary Non-Profit - Private Beds: 150

Key Personnel:
CEO/President. . . . . Mary Beth Walsh, MD
Chief of Medical Staff . . . . Mary Beth Walsh, MD
Infection Control. . . . . Lois Van Fleet
Quality Assurance . . . . Christine Reicke

Measure	Cases	This Hosp.	State Avg.	U.S. Avg.
Heart Attack Care				
ACE Inhibitor or ARB for LVSD[5]	0	-	95%	96%
Aspirin at Arrival[5]	0	-	98%	99%
Aspirin at Discharge[5]	0	-	98%	98%
Beta Blocker at Discharge[5]	0	-	98%	98%
Fibrinolytic Medication Timing[5]	0	-	50%	55%
PCI Within 90 Minutes of Arrival[5]	0	-	88%	90%
Smoking Cessation Advice[5]	0	-	100%	99%
Chest Pain/Possible Heart Attack Care				
Aspirin at Arrival[5]	0	-	96%	95%
Median Time to ECG (minutes)[5]	0	-	11	8
Median Time to Transfer (minutes)[5]	0	-	75	61
Fibrinolytic Medication Timing[5]	0	-	55%	54%
Heart Failure Care				
ACE Inhibitor or ARB for LVSD[5]	0	-	94%	94%
Discharge Instructions[5]	0	-	89%	88%
Evaluation of LVS Function[5]	0	-	98%	98%
Smoking Cessation Advice[5]	0	-	98%	98%
Pneumonia Care				
Appropriate Initial Antibiotic[5]	0	-	92%	92%
Blood Culture Timing[5]	0	-	95%	96%
Influenza Vaccine[5]	0	-	90%	91%
Initial Antibiotic Timing[5]	0	-	93%	95%
Pneumococcal Vaccine[5]	0	-	92%	93%
Smoking Cessation Advice[5]	0	-	98%	97%
Surgical Care Improvement Project				
Appropriate VTP Within 24 Hours[5]	0	-	94%	92%
Appropriate Hair Removal[5]	0	-	100%	99%
Appropriate Beta Blocker Usage[5]	0	-	92%	93%
Controlled Postoperative Blood Glucose[5]	0	-	94%	93%
Prophylactic Antibiotic Timing[5]	0	-	96%	97%
Prophylactic Antibiotic Timing (Outpatient)[5]	0	-	92%	92%
Prophylactic Antibiotic Selection[5]	0	-	97%	97%
Prophylactic Antibiotic Select. (Outpatient)[5]	0	-	93%	94%
Prophylactic Antibiotic Stopped[5]	0	-	94%	94%
Recommended VTP Ordered[5]	0	-	96%	94%
Urinary Catheter Removal[5]	0	-	90%	90%
Children's Asthma Care				
Received Systemic Corticosteroids	-	-	-	100%
Received Home Management Plan	-	-	-	71%
Received Reliever Medication	-	-	-	100%
Use of Medical Imaging				
Combination Abdominal CT Scan[5]	0	-	0.141	0.191
Combination Chest CT Scan[5]	0	-	0.024	0.054
Follow-up Mammogram/Ultrasound[5]	0	-	9.8%	8.4%
MRI for Low Back Pain[5]	0	-	26.9%	32.7%
Survey of Patients' Hospital Experiences				
Area Around Room 'Always' Quiet at Night[9]	-	-	-	58%
Doctors 'Always' Communicated Well[9]	-	-	-	80%
Home Recovery Information Given[9]	-	-	-	82%
Hospital Given 9 or 10 on 10 Point Scale[9]	-	-	-	67%
Meds 'Always' Explained Before Given[9]	-	-	-	60%
Nurses 'Always' Communicated Well[9]	-	-	-	76%
Pain 'Always' Well Controlled[9]	-	-	-	69%
Room and Bathroom 'Always' Clean[9]	-	-	-	71%
Timely Help 'Always' Received[9]	-	-	-	64%
Would Definitely Recommend Hospital[9]	-	-	-	69%

NOTE: Hospital profiles are in alphabetical order by state, then city, then hospital within the city; Rankings exclude hospitals with less than 25 cases except for patient surveys which excludes hospitals with less than 100 cases; (a) 100–299 cases; (1) The number of cases is too small to be sure how well a hospital is performing; (2) The hospital indicated that the data submitted for this measure were based on a sample of cases; (3) Data was collected during a shorter time period (fewer quarters) than the maximum possible time for this measure; (4) Suppressed for one or more quarters by CMS; (5) No data is available from the hospital for this measure; (6) Fewer than 100 patients completed the HCAHPS survey. Use these rates with caution, as the number of surveys may be too low to reliably assess hospital performance; (7) Survey results are based on less than 12 months of data; (8) Survey results are not available for this reporting period; (9) No or very few patients were eligible for the HCAHPS survey. The scores shown, if any, reflect a very small number of surveys; (10) A state average was not calculated because too few hospitals in the state submitted data; (11) There were discrepancies in the data collection process; Please refer to the User's Guide for a full explanation of data.

Saint John's Riverside Hospital

976 North Broadway
Yonkers, NY 10701
URL: www.riversidehealth.org
Type: Acute Care Hospitals
Ownership: Voluntary Non-Profit - Private

Phone: 914-964-4444

Emergency Services: Yes
Beds: 407

Measure	Cases	This Hosp.	State Avg.	U.S. Avg.
Heart Attack Care				
ACE Inhibitor or ARB for LVSD[1]	2	100%	95%	96%
Aspirin at Arrival	53	96%	98%	99%
Aspirin at Discharge[1]	23	91%	98%	98%
Beta Blocker at Discharge[1]	24	92%	98%	98%
Fibrinolytic Medication Timing[1]	1	0%	50%	55%
PCI Within 90 Minutes of Arrival	0	-	88%	90%
Smoking Cessation Advice[1]	1	100%	100%	99%
Chest Pain/Possible Heart Attack Care				
Aspirin at Arrival	41	98%	96%	95%
Median Time to ECG (minutes)	41	14	11	8
Median Time to Transfer (minutes)[1]	8	152	75	61
Fibrinolytic Medication Timing[1]	4	50%	55%	54%
Heart Failure Care				
ACE Inhibitor or ARB for LVSD[2]	70	93%	94%	94%
Discharge Instructions[2]	191	86%	89%	88%
Evaluation of LVS Function[2]	260	93%	98%	98%
Smoking Cessation Advice[1,2]	19	74%	98%	98%
Pneumonia Care				
Appropriate Initial Antibiotic[2]	75	87%	92%	92%
Blood Culture Timing[2]	165	86%	95%	96%
Influenza Vaccine[2]	69	87%	90%	91%
Initial Antibiotic Timing[2]	142	91%	93%	95%
Pneumococcal Vaccine[2]	134	91%	92%	93%
Smoking Cessation Advice[2]	29	86%	98%	97%
Surgical Care Improvement Project				
Appropriate VTP Within 24 Hours[2]	208	77%	94%	92%
Appropriate Hair Removal[2]	354	99%	100%	99%
Appropriate Beta Blocker Usage[2]	100	93%	92%	93%
Controlled Postoperative Blood Glucose[2]	0	-	94%	93%
Prophylactic Antibiotic Timing[2]	218	89%	96%	97%
Prophylactic Antibiotic Timing (Outpatient)	83	83%	92%	92%
Prophylactic Antibiotic Selection[2]	220	95%	97%	97%
Prophylactic Antibiotic Select. (Outpatient)	78	92%	93%	94%
Prophylactic Antibiotic Stopped[2]	214	84%	94%	94%
Recommended VTP Ordered[2]	208	85%	96%	94%
Urinary Catheter Removal[2]	48	71%	90%	90%
Children's Asthma Care				
Received Systemic Corticosteroids	-	-	-	100%
Received Home Management Plan	-	-	-	71%
Received Reliever Medication	-	-	-	100%
Use of Medical Imaging				
Combination Abdominal CT Scan	659	0.090	0.141	0.191
Combination Chest CT Scan	748	0.000	0.024	0.054
Follow-up Mammogram/Ultrasound	951	12.0%	9.8%	8.4%
MRI for Low Back Pain[1]	61	21.3%	26.9%	32.7%
Survey of Patients' Hospital Experiences				
Area Around Room 'Always' Quiet at Night	300+	47%	-	58%
Doctors 'Always' Communicated Well	300+	79%	-	80%
Home Recovery Information Given	300+	72%	-	82%
Hospital Given 9 or 10 on 10 Point Scale	300+	59%	-	67%
Meds 'Always' Explained Before Given	300+	53%	-	60%
Nurses 'Always' Communicated Well	300+	72%	-	76%
Pain 'Always' Well Controlled	300+	66%	-	69%
Room and Bathroom 'Always' Clean	300+	76%	-	71%
Timely Help 'Always' Received	300+	54%	-	64%
Would Definitely Recommend Hospital	300+	66%	-	69%

Saint Joseph's Medical Center

127 South Broadway
Yonkers, NY 10701
URL: www.saintjosephs.org
Type: Acute Care Hospitals
Ownership: Voluntary Non-Profit - Other

Phone: 914-378-7000
Fax: 914-965-4838

Emergency Services: Yes
Beds: 194

Key Personnel:
CEO/President . . . . Michael J Spicer, FACHE
Chief of Medical Staff . . . . Nicholas E DeRobertis
Coronary Care . . . . Melvyn Pleiberg
Pediatric Ambulatory Care . . . . . . Sami E Sayegh, MD
Pediatric In-Patient Care . . . . Sami E Sayegh, MD
Quality Assurance . . . . Francis Casola

Measure	Cases	This Hosp.	State Avg.	U.S. Avg.
Heart Attack Care				
ACE Inhibitor or ARB for LVSD[1]	5	100%	95%	96%
Aspirin at Arrival	37	92%	98%	99%
Aspirin at Discharge[1]	19	84%	98%	98%
Beta Blocker at Discharge[1]	20	90%	98%	98%
Fibrinolytic Medication Timing	0	-	50%	55%
PCI Within 90 Minutes of Arrival	0	-	88%	90%
Smoking Cessation Advice[1]	4	100%	100%	99%
Chest Pain/Possible Heart Attack Care				
Aspirin at Arrival	32	97%	96%	95%
Median Time to ECG (minutes)	35	12	11	8
Median Time to Transfer (minutes)[1]	6	115	75	61
Fibrinolytic Medication Timing	0	-	55%	54%
Heart Failure Care				
ACE Inhibitor or ARB for LVSD	51	92%	94%	94%
Discharge Instructions	135	91%	89%	88%
Evaluation of LVS Function	200	100%	98%	98%
Smoking Cessation Advice	26	100%	98%	98%
Pneumonia Care				
Appropriate Initial Antibiotic	84	94%	92%	92%
Blood Culture Timing	192	95%	95%	96%
Influenza Vaccine	116	92%	90%	91%
Initial Antibiotic Timing	190	97%	93%	95%
Pneumococcal Vaccine	162	92%	92%	93%
Smoking Cessation Advice	35	97%	98%	97%
Surgical Care Improvement Project				
Appropriate VTP Within 24 Hours	85	93%	94%	92%
Appropriate Hair Removal	132	100%	100%	99%
Appropriate Beta Blocker Usage	40	95%	92%	93%
Controlled Postoperative Blood Glucose	0	-	94%	93%
Prophylactic Antibiotic Timing	69	88%	96%	97%
Prophylactic Antibiotic Timing (Outpatient)	83	96%	92%	92%
Prophylactic Antibiotic Selection	71	90%	97%	97%
Prophylactic Antibiotic Select. (Outpatient)	82	76%	93%	94%
Prophylactic Antibiotic Stopped	60	83%	94%	94%
Recommended VTP Ordered	85	93%	96%	94%
Urinary Catheter Removal[1]	6	50%	90%	90%
Children's Asthma Care				
Received Systemic Corticosteroids	-	-	-	100%
Received Home Management Plan	-	-	-	71%
Received Reliever Medication	-	-	-	100%
Use of Medical Imaging				
Combination Abdominal CT Scan	340	0.106	0.141	0.191
Combination Chest CT Scan	208	0.010	0.024	0.054
Follow-up Mammogram/Ultrasound	518	4.8%	9.8%	8.4%
MRI for Low Back Pain[1]	57	22.8%	26.9%	32.7%
Survey of Patients' Hospital Experiences				
Area Around Room 'Always' Quiet at Night	300+	51%	-	58%
Doctors 'Always' Communicated Well	300+	73%	-	80%
Home Recovery Information Given	300+	75%	-	82%
Hospital Given 9 or 10 on 10 Point Scale	300+	48%	-	67%
Meds 'Always' Explained Before Given	300+	50%	-	60%
Nurses 'Always' Communicated Well	300+	65%	-	76%
Pain 'Always' Well Controlled	300+	58%	-	69%
Room and Bathroom 'Always' Clean	300+	65%	-	71%
Timely Help 'Always' Received	300+	43%	-	64%
Would Definitely Recommend Hospital	300+	52%	-	69%

NOTE: Hospital profiles are in alphabetical order by state, then city, then hospital within the city; Rankings exclude hospitals with less than 25 cases except for patient surveys which excludes hospitals with less than 100 cases; (a) 100–299 cases; (1) The number of cases is too small to be sure how well a hospital is performing; (2) The hospital indicated that the data submitted for this measure were based on a sample of cases; (3) Data was collected during a shorter time period (fewer quarters) than the maximum possible time for this measure; (4) Suppressed for one or more quarters by CMS; (5) No data is available from the hospital for this measure; (6) Fewer than 100 patients completed the HCAHPS survey. Use these rates with caution, as the number of surveys may be too low to reliably assess hospital performance; (7) Survey results are based on less than 12 months of data; (8) Survey results are not available for this reporting period; (9) No or very few patients are eligible for the HCAHPS survey. The scores shown, if any, reflect a very small number of surveys; (10) A state average was not calculated because too few hospitals in the state submitted data; (11) There were discrepancies in the data collection process; Please refer to the User's Guide for a full explanation of data.

Heart Attack Care

1. ACE Inhibitor or ARB for LVSD

Hospital Name	City	Rate	Cases
Carolinas Medical Center-Mercy	Charlotte	100%	51
Duke University Hospital	Durham	100%	127
Forsyth Memorial Hospital	Winston-Salem	100%	120
Gaston Memorial Hospital	Gastonia	100%	96
Memorial Mission Hospital	Asheville	100%	310
The Moses H Cone Memorial Hospital[2]	Greensboro	100%	38
Presbyterian Hospital	Charlotte	100%	115
Rex Hospital[2]	Raleigh	100%	42
Carolinas Medical Center-Northeast	Concord	99%	105
Carolinas Medical Center-Behavioral Health	Charlotte	98%	220
Durham Regional Hospital	Durham	98%	52
High Point Regional Hospital	High Point	98%	91
University of North Carolina Hospital[2]	Chapel Hill	98%	42
North Carolina Baptist Hospital	Winston-Salem	97%	119
Cape Fear Valley Medical Center	Fayetteville	96%	102
Firsthealth Moore Regional Hospital[2]	Pinehurst	96%	94
Pitt County Memorial Hospital	Greenville	95%	276
Wakemed - Raleigh Campus	Raleigh	95%	234
Alamance Regional Medical Center	Burlington	94%	32
Carolina East Medical Center	New Bern	93%	83
Frye Regional Medical Center	Hickory	93%	57
Southeastern Regional Medical Center	Lumberton	92%	26
Nash General Hospital	Rocky Mount	90%	50
New Hanover Regional Medical Center[2]	Wilmington	84%	55

2. Aspirin at Arrival

Hospital Name	City	Rate	Cases
Asheville-Oteen VA Medical Center	Asheville	100%	46
Carolinas Medical Center-Mercy	Charlotte	100%	85
Carolinas Medical Center-Union	Monroe	100%	70
Carolinas Medical Center-University	Charlotte	100%	29
Central Carolina Hospital	Sanford	100%	33
Duke Health Raleigh Hospital	Raleigh	100%	71
Durham Regional Hospital	Durham	100%	247
Forsyth Memorial Hospital	Winston-Salem	100%	608
Gaston Memorial Hospital	Gastonia	100%	523
High Point Regional Hospital	High Point	100%	368
Hugh Chatham Memorial Hospital	Elkin	100%	63
Iredell Memorial Hospital	Statesville	100%	59
Lake Norman Regional Medical Center	Mooresville	100%	76
Margaret R Pardee Memorial Hospital	Hendersonville	100%	58
Memorial Mission Hospital	Asheville	100%	696
North Carolina Baptist Hospital	Winston-Salem	100%	239
Presbyterian Hospital	Charlotte	100%	295
Presbyterian Hospital Matthews	Matthews	100%	57
Rex Hospital[2]	Raleigh	100%	298
Thomasville Medical Center	Thomasville	100%	32
University of North Carolina Hospital[2]	Chapel Hill	100%	165
Wakemed - Cary Hospital	Cary	100%	62
Wakemed - Raleigh Campus	Raleigh	100%	530
Wayne Memorial Hospital	Goldsboro	100%	50
Alamance Regional Medical Center	Burlington	99%	196
Cape Fear Valley Medical Center	Fayetteville	99%	499
Carolina East Medical Center	New Bern	99%	315
Carolinas Medical Center-Behavioral Health	Charlotte	99%	319
Carteret General Hospital	Morehead City	99%	117
Cleveland Regional Medical Center	Shelby	99%	79
Duke University Hospital	Durham	99%	338
Firsthealth Moore Regional Hospital[2]	Pinehurst	99%	309
Frye Regional Medical Center	Hickory	99%	308
The Moses H Cone Memorial Hospital[2]	Greensboro	99%	200
New Hanover Regional Medical Center[2]	Wilmington	99%	160
Rowan Regional Medical Center	Salisbury	99%	141
Carolinas Medical Center-Northeast	Concord	98%	439
Catawba Valley Medical Center	Hickory	98%	95
Durham VA Medical Center	Durham	98%	43
Grace Hospital	Morganton	98%	51
Maria Parham Hospital	Henderson	98%	45
Pitt County Memorial Hospital	Greenville	98%	400
Watauga Medical Center	Boone	98%	61
Johnston Memorial Hospital	Smithfield	97%	109
Randolph Hospital	Asheboro	97%	59
Rutherford Hospital	Rutherfordton	97%	35
Sandhills Regional Medical Center	Hamlet	97%	36
Scotland Memorial Hospital	Laurinburg	97%	72
Southeastern Regional Medical Center	Lumberton	97%	207
Albemarle Hospital Authority[2]	Elizabeth City	95%	38
Nash General Hospital	Rocky Mount	95%	309
Stanly Regional Medical Center	Albemarle	95%	41
Lenoir Memorial Hospital	Kinston	94%	133
Lexington Memorial Hospital	Lexington	94%	50
Wilson Medical Center	Wilson	94%	63
Caldwell Memorial Hospital	Lenoir	92%	25
Morehead Memorial Hospital	Eden	92%	38
Halifax Regional Medical Center	Roanoke Rapids	90%	52

3. Aspirin at Discharge

Hospital Name	City	Rate	Cases
Albemarle Hospital Authority[2]	Elizabeth City	100%	27
Cape Fear Valley Medical Center	Fayetteville	100%	542
Carolinas Medical Center-Union	Monroe	100%	40
Catawba Valley Medical Center	Hickory	100%	73
Duke Health Raleigh Hospital	Raleigh	100%	63
Duke University Hospital	Durham	100%	622
Durham Regional Hospital	Durham	100%	228
Firsthealth Moore Regional Hospital[2]	Pinehurst	100%	467
Forsyth Memorial Hospital	Winston-Salem	100%	834
Gaston Memorial Hospital	Gastonia	100%	503
Grace Hospital	Morganton	100%	34
Iredell Memorial Hospital	Statesville	100%	39
Lake Norman Regional Medical Center	Mooresville	100%	55
Memorial Mission Hospital	Asheville	100%	1297
New Hanover Regional Medical Center[2]	Wilmington	100%	283
Presbyterian Hospital	Charlotte	100%	593
Presbyterian Hospital Matthews	Matthews	100%	36
Rex Hospital[2]	Raleigh	100%	312
Rowan Regional Medical Center	Salisbury	100%	104
Scotland Memorial Hospital	Laurinburg	100%	41
Stanly Regional Medical Center	Albemarle	100%	26
Wakemed - Cary Hospital	Cary	100%	35
Wayne Memorial Hospital	Goldsboro	100%	28
Alamance Regional Medical Center	Burlington	99%	154
Carolina East Medical Center	New Bern	99%	399
Carolinas Medical Center-Northeast	Concord	99%	483
High Point Regional Hospital	High Point	99%	516
The Moses H Cone Memorial Hospital[2]	Greensboro	99%	288
North Carolina Baptist Hospital	Winston-Salem	99%	571
University of North Carolina Hospital[2]	Chapel Hill	99%	236
Wakemed - Raleigh Campus	Raleigh	99%	1539
Carolinas Medical Center-Behavioral Health	Charlotte	98%	1058
Carolinas Medical Center-Mercy	Charlotte	98%	213
Durham VA Medical Center	Durham	98%	45
Frye Regional Medical Center	Hickory	98%	487
Hugh Chatham Memorial Hospital	Elkin	98%	45
Pitt County Memorial Hospital	Greenville	98%	1326
Southeastern Regional Medical Center	Lumberton	98%	171
Margaret R Pardee Memorial Hospital	Hendersonville	97%	32
Maria Parham Hospital	Henderson	97%	31
Asheville-Oteen VA Medical Center	Asheville	95%	41
Cleveland Regional Medical Center	Shelby	95%	42
Wilson Medical Center	Wilson	95%	37
Carteret General Hospital	Morehead City	93%	55
Lenoir Memorial Hospital	Kinston	93%	82
Nash General Hospital	Rocky Mount	90%	210
Watauga Medical Center	Boone	89%	38
Johnston Memorial Hospital	Smithfield	88%	33
Randolph Hospital	Asheboro	88%	32
Lexington Memorial Hospital	Lexington	79%	29
Morehead Memorial Hospital	Eden	79%	29

4. Beta Blocker at Discharge

Hospital Name	City	Rate	Cases
Carolinas Medical Center-Northeast	Concord	100%	479
Carolinas Medical Center-Union	Monroe	100%	42
Duke Health Raleigh Hospital	Raleigh	100%	62
Duke University Hospital	Durham	100%	583
Durham VA Medical Center	Durham	100%	45
Forsyth Memorial Hospital	Winston-Salem	100%	792
Gaston Memorial Hospital	Gastonia	100%	467
Grace Hospital	Morganton	100%	37
High Point Regional Hospital	High Point	100%	521
Lake Norman Regional Medical Center	Mooresville	100%	54
Memorial Mission Hospital	Asheville	100%	1273
North Carolina Baptist Hospital	Winston-Salem	100%	541
Pitt County Memorial Hospital	Greenville	100%	1293
Presbyterian Hospital	Charlotte	100%	583
Presbyterian Hospital Matthews	Matthews	100%	37
Randolph Hospital	Asheboro	100%	36
Rowan Regional Medical Center	Salisbury	100%	87
Scotland Memorial Hospital	Laurinburg	100%	39
University of North Carolina Hospital[2]	Chapel Hill	100%	219
Wakemed - Cary Hospital	Cary	100%	34
Wayne Memorial Hospital	Goldsboro	100%	35
Carolinas Medical Center-Behavioral Health	Charlotte	99%	1010
Durham Regional Hospital	Durham	99%	219
Frye Regional Medical Center	Hickory	99%	481
The Moses H Cone Memorial Hospital[2]	Greensboro	99%	266
Rex Hospital[2]	Raleigh	99%	297
Southeastern Regional Medical Center	Lumberton	99%	171
Wakemed - Raleigh Campus	Raleigh	99%	1432
Asheville-Oteen VA Medical Center	Asheville	98%	41
Albemarle Hospital Authority[2]	Elizabeth City	97%	32
Cape Fear Valley Medical Center	Fayetteville	97%	517
Carolinas Medical Center-Mercy	Charlotte	97%	201
Catawba Valley Medical Center	Hickory	97%	70
Firsthealth Moore Regional Hospital[2]	Pinehurst	97%	451
Iredell Memorial Hospital	Statesville	97%	37
Lexington Memorial Hospital	Lexington	97%	30
Margaret R Pardee Memorial Hospital	Hendersonville	97%	32
New Hanover Regional Medical Center[2]	Wilmington	97%	275
Carolina East Medical Center	New Bern	96%	365
Alamance Regional Medical Center	Burlington	94%	151
Hugh Chatham Memorial Hospital	Elkin	94%	47
Johnston Memorial Hospital	Smithfield	94%	33
Watauga Medical Center	Boone	94%	33
Wilson Medical Center	Wilson	94%	34
Nash General Hospital	Rocky Mount	92%	215
Carteret General Hospital	Morehead City	91%	53
Lenoir Memorial Hospital	Kinston	91%	85
Cleveland Regional Medical Center	Shelby	90%	41
Morehead Memorial Hospital	Eden	90%	29
Maria Parham Hospital	Henderson	89%	35
Stanly Regional Medical Center	Albemarle	89%	27

6. PCI Within 90 Minutes of Arrival

Hospital Name	City	Rate	Cases
Gaston Memorial Hospital	Gastonia	100%	107
North Carolina Baptist Hospital	Winston-Salem	100%	49
Wakemed - Raleigh Campus	Raleigh	100%	105
Forsyth Memorial Hospital	Winston-Salem	99%	151
High Point Regional Hospital	High Point	99%	88
Presbyterian Hospital	Charlotte	98%	88
Carolinas Medical Center-Behavioral Health	Charlotte	97%	88
Frye Regional Medical Center	Hickory	97%	134
Carolinas Medical Center-Northeast	Concord	95%	85
Firsthealth Moore Regional Hospital[2]	Pinehurst	95%	38
Memorial Mission Hospital	Asheville	95%	109
Duke University Hospital	Durham	94%	79
Carolina East Medical Center	New Bern	93%	75
Rex Hospital[2]	Raleigh	93%	67
University of North Carolina Hospital[2]	Chapel Hill	93%	29
Alamance Regional Medical Center	Burlington	92%	25
Pitt County Memorial Hospital	Greenville	92%	39
The Moses H Cone Memorial Hospital[2]	Greensboro	86%	37
New Hanover Regional Medical Center[2]	Wilmington	85%	39
Cape Fear Valley Medical Center	Fayetteville	84%	92
Durham Regional Hospital	Durham	83%	30

7. Smoking Cessation Advice

Hospital Name	City	Rate	Cases
Alamance Regional Medical Center	Burlington	100%	55
Cape Fear Valley Medical Center	Fayetteville	100%	235
Carolina East Medical Center	New Bern	100%	146
Carolinas Medical Center-Behavioral Health	Charlotte	100%	423
Carolinas Medical Center-Mercy	Charlotte	100%	74
Catawba Valley Medical Center	Hickory	100%	32
Duke University Hospital	Durham	100%	237
Durham Regional Hospital	Durham	100%	85
Firsthealth Moore Regional Hospital[2]	Pinehurst	100%	163
Forsyth Memorial Hospital	Winston-Salem	100%	337
Frye Regional Medical Center	Hickory	100%	218
Gaston Memorial Hospital	Gastonia	100%	211
High Point Regional Hospital	High Point	100%	205
Memorial Mission Hospital	Asheville	100%	455
The Moses H Cone Memorial Hospital[2]	Greensboro	100%	119
Nash General Hospital	Rocky Mount	100%	66
North Carolina Baptist Hospital	Winston-Salem	100%	268
Pitt County Memorial Hospital	Greenville	100%	581
Presbyterian Hospital	Charlotte	100%	186
Rex Hospital[2]	Raleigh	100%	67
Rowan Regional Medical Center	Salisbury	100%	32
Southeastern Regional Medical Center	Lumberton	100%	84
University of North Carolina Hospital[2]	Chapel Hill	100%	84
Wakemed - Raleigh Campus	Raleigh	100%	622
Carolinas Medical Center-Northeast	Concord	99%	184
New Hanover Regional Medical Center[2]	Wilmington	97%	107

Chest Pain/Possible Heart Attack Care

8. Aspirin at Arrival

Hospital Name	City	Rate	Cases
Carolinas Medical Center-University	Charlotte	100%	106
Cleveland Regional Medical Center	Shelby	100%	127
Davis Regional Medical Center	Statesville	100%	40
Duplin General Hospital	Kenansville	100%	82
Granville Medical Center	Oxford	100%	79
Heritage Hospital	Tarboro	100%	51
Lake Norman Regional Medical Center	Mooresville	100%	61
Presbyterian Hospital Matthews	Matthews	100%	73
Roanoke Chowan Hospital	Ahoskie	100%	61
Thomasville Medical Center	Thomasville	100%	52
Washington County Hospital	Plymouth	100%	25
Watauga Medical Center	Boone	100%	77
Carolinas Medical Center-Mercy	Charlotte	99%	118
Central Carolina Hospital	Sanford	99%	99

NOTE: Hospital profiles are in alphabetical order by state, then city, then hospital within the city; Rankings exclude hospitals with less than 25 cases except for patient surveys which excludes hospitals with less than 100 cases; (a) 100–299 cases; (1) The number of cases is too small to be sure how well a hospital is performing; (2) The hospital indicated that the data submitted for this measure were based on a sample of cases; (3) Data was collected during a shorter time period (fewer quarters) than the maximum possible time for this measure; (4) Suppressed for one or more quarters by CMS; (5) No data is available from the hospital for this measure; (6) Fewer than 100 patients completed the HCAHPS survey. Use these rates with caution, as the number of surveys may be too low to reliably assess hospital performance; (7) Survey results are based on less than 12 months of data; (8) Survey results are not available for this reporting period; (9) No or very few patients were eligible for the HCAHPS survey. The scores shown, if any, reflect a very small number of surveys; (10) A state average was not calculated because too few hospitals in the state submitted data; (11) There were discrepancies in the data collection process; Please refer to the User's Guide for a full explanation of data.

Franklin Regional Medical Center	Louisburg	99%	95
Hugh Chatham Memorial Hospital	Elkin	99%	152
Iredell Memorial Hospital	Statesville	99%	88
Margaret R Pardee Memorial Hospital	Hendersonville	99%	89
The Moses H Cone Memorial Hospital	Greensboro	99%	76
Presbyterian Hospital Huntersville	Huntersville	99%	87
Rowan Regional Medical Center	Salisbury	99%	88
Wayne Memorial Hospital	Goldsboro	99%	295
Wilkes Regional Medical Center	N Wilkesboro	99%	284
Angel Medical Center	Franklin	98%	99
Morehead Memorial Hospital	Eden	98%	103
Northern Hospital of Surry County	Mount Airy	98%	255
Scotland Memorial Hospital	Laurinburg	98%	46
Ashe Memorial Hospital	Jefferson	97%	90
Brunswick Community Hospital	Supply	97%	87
C J Harris Community Hospital	Sylva	97%	34
Carteret General Hospital	Morehead City	97%	111
Kings Mountain Hospital	Kings Mountain	97%	87
Lexington Memorial Hospital	Lexington	97%	64
Stanly Regional Medical Center	Albemarle	97%	92
Wakemed - Cary Hospital	Cary	97%	31
Wakemed - Raleigh Campus	Raleigh	97%	32
Wilson Medical Center	Wilson	97%	96
Caldwell Memorial Hospital	Lenoir	96%	54
Carolinas Medical Center-Lincoln	Lincolnton	96%	89
Carolinas Medical Center-Union	Monroe	96%	147
The Mcdowell Hospital	Marion	96%	84
Columbus Regional Healthcare System	Whiteville	95%	118
Halifax Regional Medical Center	Roanoke Rapids	95%	186
Martin General Hospital	Williamston	95%	40
Rutherford Hospital	Rutherfordton	95%	165
Albemarle Hospital Authority	Elizabeth City	94%	69
Beaufort County Medical Center	Washington	94%	173
Grace Hospital	Morganton	94%	72
Lenoir Memorial Hospital	Kinston	94%	94
Maria Parham Hospital	Henderson	94%	145
Murphy Medical Center	Murphy	94%	127
Randolph Hospital	Asheboro	94%	178
Cape Fear Valley Medical Center	Fayetteville	92%	63
J Arthur Dosher Memorial Hospital	Southport	92%	72
Johnston Memorial Hospital	Smithfield	92%	257
Person Memorial Hospital	Roxboro	92%	132
Betsy Johnson Regional Hospital	Dunn	91%	261
Spruce Pine Community Hospital	Spruce Pine	91%	58
Valdese General Hospital	Valdese	91%	35
Catawba Valley Medical Center	Hickory	90%	48
Sampson Regional Medical Center	Clinton	90%	418
Nash General Hospital	Rocky Mount	89%	264
Alamance Regional Medical Center	Burlington	88%	73
Anson Community Hospital	Wadesboro	88%	210
Onslow Memorial Hospital	Jacksonville	87%	173
Haywood Regional Medical Center	Clyde	85%	75
Southeastern Regional Medical Center	Lumberton	83%	36

9. Median Time to ECG (minutes)

Hospital Name	City	Min.	Cases
Carolinas Medical Center-Lincoln	Lincolnton	2	89
Wakemed - Raleigh Campus	Raleigh	2	33
Brunswick Community Hospital	Supply	3	86
Cleveland Regional Medical Center	Shelby	3	129
Davis Regional Medical Center	Statesville	3	40
Kings Mountain Hospital	Kings Mountain	4	89
Lake Norman Regional Medical Center	Mooresville	4	62
Presbyterian Hospital Matthews	Matthews	4	77
Thomasville Medical Center	Thomasville	4	52
Franklin Regional Medical Center	Louisburg	5	96
Hugh Chatham Memorial Hospital	Elkin	5	157
Washington County Hospital	Plymouth	5	28
Alamance Regional Medical Center	Burlington	6	74
Anson Community Hospital	Wadesboro	6	221
Beaufort County Medical Center	Washington	6	176
Carolinas Medical Center-Mercy	Charlotte	6	117
Central Carolina Hospital	Sanford	6	102
Granville Medical Center	Oxford	6	86
Halifax Regional Medical Center	Roanoke Rapids	6	194
Presbyterian Hospital Huntersville	Huntersville	6	91
Rowan Regional Medical Center	Salisbury	6	92
Stanly Regional Medical Center	Albemarle	6	90
Wakemed - Cary Hospital	Cary	6	32
Wilkes Regional Medical Center	N Wilkesboro	6	291
Iredell Memorial Hospital	Statesville	7	89
The Mcdowell Hospital	Marion	7	87
Person Memorial Hospital	Roxboro	7	139
Wayne Memorial Hospital	Goldsboro	7	304
Caldwell Memorial Hospital	Lenoir	8	56
Duplin General Hospital	Kenansville	8	87
Haywood Regional Medical Center	Clyde	8	78
Lenoir Memorial Hospital	Kinston	8	97
Margaret R Pardee Memorial Hospital	Hendersonville	8	92
Martin General Hospital	Williamston	8	39
Randolph Hospital	Asheboro	8	185
Roanoke Chowan Hospital	Ahoskie	8	64
Spruce Pine Community Hospital	Spruce Pine	8	61
Ashe Memorial Hospital	Jefferson	9	97
Betsy Johnson Regional Hospital	Dunn	9	275
Carolinas Medical Center-Union	Monroe	9	145
Carolinas Medical Center-University	Charlotte	9	106
Heritage Hospital	Tarboro	9	51
Lexington Memorial Hospital	Lexington	9	65
Morehead Memorial Hospital	Eden	9	85
Murphy Medical Center	Murphy	9	133
Nash General Hospital	Rocky Mount	9	268
Valdese General Hospital	Valdese	9	37
Angel Medical Center	Franklin	10	102
C J Harris Community Hospital	Sylva	10	33
The Moses H Cone Memorial Hospital	Greensboro	10	78
Sampson Regional Medical Center	Clinton	10	442
Scotland Memorial Hospital	Laurinburg	10	46
Carteret General Hospital	Morehead City	11	113
Catawba Valley Medical Center	Hickory	11	48
Columbus Regional Healthcare System	Whiteville	11	123
Grace Hospital	Morganton	12	78
Maria Parham Hospital	Henderson	12	143
Northern Hospital of Surry County	Mount Airy	12	264
Rutherford Hospital	Rutherfordton	12	168
Watauga Medical Center	Boone	12	79
Johnston Memorial Hospital	Smithfield	13	268
Onslow Memorial Hospital	Jacksonville	13	172
Wilson Medical Center	Wilson	15	88
Albemarle Hospital Authority	Elizabeth City	17	72
J Arthur Dosher Memorial Hospital	Southport	17	73
Cape Fear Valley Medical Center	Fayetteville	18	69
Southeastern Regional Medical Center	Lumberton	23	35

10. Median Time to Transfer (minutes)

Hospital Name	City	Min.	Cases
Presbyterian Hospital Huntersville	Huntersville	32	25
Presbyterian Hospital Matthews	Matthews	34	36
Carolinas Medical Center-Lincoln	Lincolnton	35	28
Carolinas Medical Center-Union	Monroe	41	43
Rowan Regional Medical Center	Salisbury	42	42
Grace Hospital	Morganton	46	29
Margaret R Pardee Memorial Hospital	Hendersonville	55	35
Iredell Memorial Hospital	Statesville	58	33
Randolph Hospital	Asheboro	58	40

11. Fibrinolytic Medication Timing

Hospital Name	City	Rate	Cases
Wayne Memorial Hospital	Goldsboro	71%	34

Heart Failure Care

12. ACE Inhibitor or ARB for LVSD

Hospital Name	City	Rate	Cases
Betsy Johnson Regional Hospital	Dunn	100%	44
Brunswick Community Hospital	Supply	100%	47
Carolinas Medical Center-Lincoln	Lincolnton	100%	28
Carolinas Medical Center-University	Charlotte	100%	77
Central Carolina Hospital	Sanford	100%	73
Davis Regional Medical Center	Statesville	100%	31
Duke Health Raleigh Hospital	Raleigh	100%	64
Forsyth Memorial Hospital	Winston-Salem	100%	254
Iredell Memorial Hospital	Statesville	100%	62
Lake Norman Regional Medical Center	Mooresville	100%	41
Presbyterian Hospital	Charlotte	100%	207
Presbyterian Hospital Huntersville	Huntersville	100%	36
Presbyterian Hospital Matthews	Matthews	100%	43
Rowan Regional Medical Center	Salisbury	100%	114
Thomasville Medical Center	Thomasville	100%	32
Watauga Medical Center	Boone	100%	36
Carolinas Medical Center-Behavioral Health	Charlotte	99%	383
Gaston Memorial Hospital	Gastonia	99%	236
Heritage Hospital	Tarboro	99%	75
High Point Regional Hospital	High Point	99%	155
University of North Carolina Hospital[2]	Chapel Hill	99%	118
C J Harris Community Hospital	Sylva	98%	42
Carolinas Medical Center-Mercy	Charlotte	98%	133
Carolinas Medical Center-Union	Monroe	98%	133
Duke University Hospital	Durham	98%	362
Fayetteville North Carolina VA Med Ctr	Fayetteville	98%	47
Memorial Mission Hospital[2]	Asheville	98%	314
Onslow Memorial Hospital	Jacksonville	98%	55
Wakemed - Raleigh Campus[2]	Raleigh	98%	123
Cape Fear Valley Medical Center	Fayetteville	97%	396
North Carolina Baptist Hospital	Winston-Salem	97%	257
Sandhills Regional Medical Center	Hamlet	97%	78
Wilkes Regional Medical Center	N Wilkesboro	97%	32
Durham VA Medical Center	Durham	96%	68
Margaret R Pardee Memorial Hospital	Hendersonville	96%	67
Roanoke Chowan Hospital	Ahoskie	96%	50
Wayne Memorial Hospital	Goldsboro	96%	176
Alamance Regional Medical Center	Burlington	95%	112
Durham Regional Hospital	Durham	95%	166
Lexington Memorial Hospital	Lexington	95%	37
The Moses H Cone Memorial Hospital[2]	Greensboro	95%	132
New Hanover Regional Medical Center[2]	Wilmington	95%	198
Northern Hospital of Surry County	Mount Airy	95%	40
Southeastern Regional Medical Center	Lumberton	95%	155
Carolinas Medical Center-Northeast	Concord	94%	233
Firsthealth Moore Regional Hospital[2]	Pinehurst	94%	221
Pitt County Memorial Hospital	Greenville	94%	537
Stanly Regional Medical Center	Albemarle	94%	54
Grace Hospital	Morganton	93%	44
Wakemed - Cary Hospital	Cary	93%	57
Martin General Hospital	Williamston	92%	36
Rex Hospital[2]	Raleigh	92%	106
Albemarle Hospital Authority[2]	Elizabeth City	91%	86
Carteret General Hospital	Morehead City	91%	74
Catawba Valley Medical Center	Hickory	91%	46
Frye Regional Medical Center	Hickory	91%	79
Granville Medical Center	Oxford	91%	35
Nash General Hospital	Rocky Mount	91%	156
Cleveland Regional Medical Center	Shelby	90%	63
Halifax Regional Medical Center	Roanoke Rapids	90%	91
Rutherford Hospital	Rutherfordton	89%	37
Maria Parham Hospital	Henderson	88%	88
Murphy Medical Center	Murphy	88%	25
Lenoir Memorial Hospital	Kinston	87%	143
Scotland Memorial Hospital	Laurinburg	87%	116
Wilson Medical Center	Wilson	87%	94
Asheville-Oteen VA Medical Center	Asheville	86%	51
Carolina East Medical Center	New Bern	86%	173
Sampson Regional Medical Center	Clinton	86%	72
Columbus Regional Healthcare System	Whiteville	83%	30
Caldwell Memorial Hospital	Lenoir	81%	31
Randolph Hospital[2]	Asheboro	81%	59
Haywood Regional Medical Center	Clyde	80%	25
Morehead Memorial Hospital	Eden	80%	66
Johnston Memorial Hospital	Smithfield	67%	85

13. Discharge Instructions

Hospital Name	City	Rate	Cases
Alleghany County Memorial Hospital	Sparta	100%	27
Central Carolina Hospital	Sanford	100%	225
Charles A Cannon Jr Memorial Hospital	Linville	100%	52
Davis Regional Medical Center	Statesville	100%	159
Fayetteville North Carolina VA Med Ctr	Fayetteville	100%	116
Forsyth Memorial Hospital	Winston-Salem	100%	814
Carolinas Medical Center-Lincoln	Lincolnton	99%	101
Durham VA Medical Center	Durham	99%	160
Granville Medical Center	Oxford	99%	94
Presbyterian Hospital	Charlotte	99%	491
Brunswick Community Hospital	Supply	98%	92
Carolinas Medical Center-Behavioral Health	Charlotte	98%	681
Carolinas Medical Center-Union	Monroe	98%	323
Duke Health Raleigh Hospital	Raleigh	98%	134
Duke University Hospital	Durham	98%	776
Heritage Hospital	Tarboro	98%	151
Lexington Memorial Hospital	Lexington	98%	117
Carolinas Medical Center-University	Charlotte	97%	150
Duplin General Hospital	Kenansville	97%	59
Grace Hospital	Morganton	97%	97
Nash General Hospital	Rocky Mount	97%	387
Northern Hospital of Surry County	Mount Airy	97%	145
Presbyterian Hospital Huntersville	Huntersville	97%	97
Roanoke Chowan Hospital	Ahoskie	97%	155
Rowan Regional Medical Center	Salisbury	97%	237
Sandhills Regional Medical Center	Hamlet	97%	174
Thomasville Medical Center	Thomasville	97%	90
Chowan Hospital	Edenton	96%	49
North Carolina Baptist Hospital	Winston-Salem	96%	602
Person Memorial Hospital	Roxboro	96%	71
Presbyterian Hospital Matthews	Matthews	96%	142
Pungo District Hospital	Belhaven	96%	26
Carolinas Medical Center-Mercy	Charlotte	94%	327
Gaston Memorial Hospital	Gastonia	94%	654
Iredell Memorial Hospital	Statesville	94%	250
The Mcdowell Hospital	Marion	94%	47
Spruce Pine Community Hospital	Spruce Pine	94%	48
Watauga Medical Center	Boone	94%	102
Wilson Medical Center	Wilson	94%	222
Ashe Memorial Hospital	Jefferson	93%	28
Frye Regional Medical Center	Hickory	93%	251
High Point Regional Hospital	High Point	93%	384
Anson Community Hospital	Wadesboro	92%	39
Durham Regional Hospital	Durham	92%	317
Lake Norman Regional Medical Center	Mooresville	92%	115
W G (Bill) Hefner Salisbury VA Med Ctr	Salisbury	92%	48
Wilkes Regional Medical Center	N Wilkesboro	92%	86

NOTE: Hospital profiles are in alphabetical order by state, then city, then hospital within the city; Rankings exclude hospitals with less than 25 cases except for patient surveys which excludes hospitals with less than 100 cases; (a) 100–299 cases; (1) The number of cases is too small to be sure how well a hospital is performing; (2) The hospital indicated that the data submitted for this measure were based on a sample of cases; (3) Data was collected during a shorter time period (fewer quarters) than the maximum possible time for this measure; (4) Suppressed for one or more quarters by CMS; (5) No data is available from the hospital for this measure; (6) Fewer than 100 patients completed the HCAHPS survey. Use these rates with caution, as the number of surveys may be too low to reliably assess hospital performance; (7) Survey results are based on less than 12 months of data; (8) Survey results are not available for this reporting period; (9) No or very few patients were eligible for the HCAHPS survey. The scores shown, if any, reflect a very small number of surveys; (10) A state average was not calculated because too few hospitals in the state submitted data; (11) There were discrepancies in the data collection process; Please refer to the User's Guide for a full explanation of data.

Cape Fear Valley Medical Center	Fayetteville	91%	899
Columbus Regional Healthcare System	Whiteville	91%	121
Memorial Mission Hospital[2]	Asheville	91%	665
University of North Carolina Hospital[2]	Chapel Hill	91%	242
Valdese General Hospital	Valdese	91%	54
Halifax Regional Medical Center	Roanoke Rapids	90%	263
Kings Mountain Hospital	Kings Mountain	90%	40
Rutherford Hospital	Rutherfordton	90%	126
Wayne Memorial Hospital	Goldsboro	90%	389
Carteret General Hospital	Morehead City	89%	193
Sampson Regional Medical Center	Clinton	89%	139
Carolinas Medical Center-Northeast	Concord	88%	559
Bertie Memorial Hospital	Windsor	87%	30
Cleveland Regional Medical Center	Shelby	87%	211
Alamance Regional Medical Center	Burlington	86%	294
Angel Medical Center	Franklin	86%	49
Franklin Regional Medical Center	Louisburg	86%	58
Johnston Memorial Hospital	Smithfield	86%	253
Asheville-Oteen VA Medical Center	Asheville	85%	96
Hugh Chatham Memorial Hospital	Elkin	85%	142
Martin General Hospital	Williamston	85%	82
Park Ridge Hospital	Fletcher	85%	39
Southeastern Regional Medical Center	Lumberton	85%	525
Catawba Valley Medical Center	Hickory	84%	107
The Moses H Cone Memorial Hospital[2]	Greensboro	84%	330
Washington County Hospital	Plymouth	84%	31
Rex Hospital[2]	Raleigh	83%	257
Wakemed - Raleigh Campus[2]	Raleigh	83%	278
Firsthealth Moore Regional Hospital[2]	Pinehurst	82%	511
Onslow Memorial Hospital	Jacksonville	82%	166
Scotland Memorial Hospital	Laurinburg	82%	320
Wakemed - Cary Hospital	Cary	82%	209
Beaufort County Medical Center	Washington	81%	91
Albemarle Hospital Authority[2]	Elizabeth City	80%	163
Pitt County Memorial Hospital	Greenville	80%	941
Haywood Regional Medical Center	Clyde	79%	77
New Hanover Regional Medical Center[2]	Wilmington	79%	542
C J Harris Community Hospital	Sylva	78%	73
Lenoir Memorial Hospital	Kinston	76%	404
Maria Parham Hospital	Henderson	76%	150
Margaret R Pardee Memorial Hospital	Hendersonville	73%	144
Transylvania Regional Hospital	Brevard	71%	28
Morehead Memorial Hospital	Eden	70%	209
Murphy Medical Center	Murphy	70%	54
Stanly Regional Medical Center	Albemarle	70%	135
Chatham Hospital	Siler City	67%	27
Randolph Hospital[2]	Asheboro	66%	219
Caldwell Memorial Hospital	Lenoir	65%	95
Betsy Johnson Regional Hospital	Dunn	63%	150
Carolina East Medical Center	New Bern	59%	483

14. Evaluation of LVS Function

Hospital Name	City	Rate	Cases
Anson Community Hospital	Wadesboro	100%	52
Bertie Memorial Hospital	Windsor	100%	39
Brunswick Community Hospital	Supply	100%	117
Cape Fear Valley Medical Center	Fayetteville	100%	1036
Carolinas Medical Center-Behavioral Health	Charlotte	100%	766
Carolinas Medical Center-Lincoln	Lincolnton	100%	120
Carolinas Medical Center-Northeast	Concord	100%	635
Carolinas Medical Center-Union	Monroe	100%	356
Cleveland Regional Medical Center	Shelby	100%	263
Davis Regional Medical Center	Statesville	100%	180
Duke University Hospital	Durham	100%	853
Duplin General Hospital	Kenansville	100%	66
Durham Regional Hospital	Durham	100%	394
Durham VA Medical Center	Durham	100%	173
Fayetteville North Carolina VA Med Ctr	Fayetteville	100%	118
Forsyth Memorial Hospital	Winston-Salem	100%	989
Franklin Regional Medical Center	Louisburg	100%	73
Gaston Memorial Hospital	Gastonia	100%	735
Heritage Hospital	Tarboro	100%	196
Hugh Chatham Memorial Hospital	Elkin	100%	175
Iredell Memorial Hospital	Statesville	100%	316
Johnston Memorial Hospital	Smithfield	100%	310
Kings Mountain Hospital	Kings Mountain	100%	50
The Mcdowell Hospital	Marion	100%	52
Memorial Mission Hospital[2]	Asheville	100%	791
The Moses H Cone Memorial Hospital[2]	Greensboro	100%	390
North Carolina Baptist Hospital	Winston-Salem	100%	652
Presbyterian Hospital	Charlotte	100%	584
Presbyterian Hospital Huntersville	Huntersville	100%	110
Presbyterian Hospital Matthews	Matthews	100%	180
Roanoke Chowan Hospital	Ahoskie	100%	175
Rowan Regional Medical Center	Salisbury	100%	289
Rutherford Hospital	Rutherfordton	100%	168
Southeastern Regional Medical Center	Lumberton	100%	572
Thomasville Medical Center	Thomasville	100%	101
Transylvania Regional Hospital	Brevard	100%	42
University of North Carolina Hospital[2]	Chapel Hill	100%	272
W G (Bill) Hefner Salisbury VA Med Ctr	Salisbury	100%	53
Wakemed - Cary Hospital	Cary	100%	265
Wakemed - Raleigh Campus[2]	Raleigh	100%	328
Watauga Medical Center	Boone	100%	127
Alamance Regional Medical Center	Burlington	99%	365
Caldwell Memorial Hospital	Lenoir	99%	117
Carolinas Medical Center-Mercy	Charlotte	99%	398
Carteret General Hospital	Morehead City	99%	251
Catawba Valley Medical Center	Hickory	99%	141
Central Carolina Hospital	Sanford	99%	266
Duke Health Raleigh Hospital	Raleigh	99%	158
Firsthealth Moore Regional Hospital[2]	Pinehurst	99%	583
Lake Norman Regional Medical Center	Mooresville	99%	161
Nash General Hospital	Rocky Mount	99%	447
Northern Hospital of Surry County	Mount Airy	99%	167
Onslow Memorial Hospital	Jacksonville	99%	202
Person Memorial Hospital	Roxboro	99%	88
Pitt County Memorial Hospital	Greenville	99%	1057
Sampson Regional Medical Center	Clinton	99%	196
Sandhills Regional Medical Center	Hamlet	99%	188
Scotland Memorial Hospital	Laurinburg	99%	345
Valdese General Hospital	Valdese	99%	81
Wayne Memorial Hospital	Goldsboro	99%	456
Wilkes Regional Medical Center	N Wilkesboro	99%	117
Asheville-Oteen VA Medical Center	Asheville	98%	117
Carolina East Medical Center	New Bern	98%	529
Carolinas Medical Center-University	Charlotte	98%	169
Frye Regional Medical Center	Hickory	98%	294
Granville Medical Center	Oxford	98%	122
High Point Regional Hospital	High Point	98%	460
Lexington Memorial Hospital	Lexington	98%	142
Margaret R Pardee Memorial Hospital	Hendersonville	98%	195
Park Ridge Hospital	Fletcher	98%	52
Rex Hospital[2]	Raleigh	98%	325
Albemarle Hospital Authority[2]	Elizabeth City	97%	197
C J Harris Community Hospital	Sylva	97%	87
Chatham Hospital	Siler City	97%	30
Chowan Hospital	Edenton	97%	65
Grace Hospital	Morganton	97%	124
Halifax Regional Medical Center	Roanoke Rapids	97%	303
Maria Parham Hospital	Henderson	97%	180
Martin General Hospital	Williamston	97%	108
Murphy Medical Center	Murphy	97%	78
New Hanover Regional Medical Center[2]	Wilmington	97%	652
Randolph Hospital[2]	Asheboro	97%	284
Columbus Regional Healthcare System	Whiteville	96%	157
Haywood Regional Medical Center	Clyde	96%	99
Lenoir Memorial Hospital	Kinston	96%	479
Wilson Medical Center	Wilson	96%	275
Stanly Regional Medical Center	Albemarle	95%	184
Beaufort County Medical Center	Washington	93%	98
Betsy Johnson Regional Hospital	Dunn	93%	201
Charles A Cannon Jr Memorial Hospital	Linville	93%	76
Washington County Hospital	Plymouth	92%	39
Alleghany County Memorial Hospital	Sparta	91%	33
Saint Lukes Hospital	Columbus	90%	49
Ashe Memorial Hospital	Jefferson	89%	35
Cape Fear Valley-Bladen County Hospital	Elizabethtown	88%	26
Angel Medical Center	Franklin	87%	54
Morehead Memorial Hospital	Eden	84%	258
Spruce Pine Community Hospital	Spruce Pine	78%	64

15. Smoking Cessation Advice

Hospital Name	City	Rate	Cases
Alamance Regional Medical Center	Burlington	100%	86
Asheville-Oteen VA Medical Center	Asheville	100%	25
Brunswick Community Hospital	Supply	100%	26
Cape Fear Valley Medical Center	Fayetteville	100%	220
Carolina East Medical Center	New Bern	100%	102
Carolinas Medical Center-Behavioral Health	Charlotte	100%	196
Carolinas Medical Center-Mercy	Charlotte	100%	65
Carolinas Medical Center-Northeast	Concord	100%	130
Carolinas Medical Center-Union	Monroe	100%	68
Carolinas Medical Center-University	Charlotte	100%	46
Carteret General Hospital	Morehead City	100%	40
Catawba Valley Medical Center	Hickory	100%	36
Central Carolina Hospital	Sanford	100%	62
Cleveland Regional Medical Center	Shelby	100%	66
Davis Regional Medical Center	Statesville	100%	71
Duke Health Raleigh Hospital	Raleigh	100%	30
Duke University Hospital	Durham	100%	135
Durham Regional Hospital	Durham	100%	84
Fayetteville North Carolina VA Med Ctr	Fayetteville	100%	31
Firsthealth Moore Regional Hospital[2]	Pinehurst	100%	101
Forsyth Memorial Hospital	Winston-Salem	100%	142
Frye Regional Medical Center	Hickory	100%	57
Gaston Memorial Hospital	Gastonia	100%	152
Grace Hospital	Morganton	100%	30
Halifax Regional Medical Center	Roanoke Rapids	100%	61
Heritage Hospital	Tarboro	100%	36
High Point Regional Hospital	High Point	100%	110
Hugh Chatham Memorial Hospital	Elkin	100%	30
Iredell Memorial Hospital	Statesville	100%	70
Johnston Memorial Hospital	Smithfield	100%	54
Lake Norman Regional Medical Center	Mooresville	100%	27
Lenoir Memorial Hospital	Kinston	100%	86
Lexington Memorial Hospital	Lexington	100%	30
Margaret R Pardee Memorial Hospital	Hendersonville	100%	25
Maria Parham Hospital	Henderson	100%	48
Memorial Mission Hospital[2]	Asheville	100%	131
The Moses H Cone Memorial Hospital[2]	Greensboro	100%	108
Nash General Hospital	Rocky Mount	100%	114
North Carolina Baptist Hospital	Winston-Salem	100%	161
Onslow Memorial Hospital	Jacksonville	100%	40
Pitt County Memorial Hospital	Greenville	100%	247
Presbyterian Hospital	Charlotte	100%	106
Randolph Hospital[2]	Asheboro	100%	59
Rex Hospital[2]	Raleigh	100%	46
Roanoke Chowan Hospital	Ahoskie	100%	36
Rowan Regional Medical Center	Salisbury	100%	75
Rutherford Hospital	Rutherfordton	100%	32
Sampson Regional Medical Center	Clinton	100%	38
Sandhills Regional Medical Center	Hamlet	100%	69
Scotland Memorial Hospital	Laurinburg	100%	96
Southeastern Regional Medical Center	Lumberton	100%	138
Stanly Regional Medical Center	Albemarle	100%	29
University of North Carolina Hospital[2]	Chapel Hill	100%	65
Wakemed - Cary Hospital	Cary	100%	51
Wakemed - Raleigh Campus[2]	Raleigh	100%	86
Wilson Medical Center	Wilson	100%	65
Wayne Memorial Hospital	Goldsboro	99%	98
Albemarle Hospital Authority[2]	Elizabeth City	98%	40
Betsy Johnson Regional Hospital	Dunn	96%	26
Northern Hospital of Surry County	Mount Airy	96%	28
New Hanover Regional Medical Center[2]	Wilmington	94%	134
Morehead Memorial Hospital	Eden	88%	43

Pneumonia Care

16. Appropriate Initial Antibiotic

Hospital Name	City	Rate	Cases
Gaston Memorial Hospital	Gastonia	100%	359
Columbus Regional Healthcare System	Whiteville	99%	68
Lake Norman Regional Medical Center	Mooresville	99%	69
Presbyterian Hospital	Charlotte	99%	202
Carolinas Medical Center-Lincoln	Lincolnton	98%	109
Carolinas Medical Center-Northeast	Concord	98%	431
Central Carolina Hospital	Sanford	98%	123
Duke University Hospital	Durham	98%	90
Duplin General Hospital	Kenansville	98%	65
Forsyth Memorial Hospital	Winston-Salem	98%	418
Hugh Chatham Memorial Hospital	Elkin	98%	127
Presbyterian Hospital Huntersville	Huntersville	98%	129
Rowan Regional Medical Center	Salisbury	98%	206
Presbyterian Hospital Matthews	Matthews	97%	193
Wakemed - Cary Hospital	Cary	97%	74
Wayne Memorial Hospital	Goldsboro	97%	96
Ashe Memorial Hospital	Jefferson	96%	99
Rex Hospital[2]	Raleigh	96%	129
Saint Lukes Hospital	Columbus	96%	47
Thomasville Medical Center	Thomasville	96%	75
Cape Fear Valley Medical Center	Fayetteville	95%	377
Carolinas Medical Center-Mercy	Charlotte	95%	177
Carolinas Medical Center-University	Charlotte	95%	112
Davis Regional Medical Center	Statesville	95%	78
Durham Regional Hospital	Durham	95%	195
Franklin Regional Medical Center	Louisburg	95%	37
Frye Regional Medical Center	Hickory	95%	221
Margaret R Pardee Memorial Hospital	Hendersonville	95%	139
The Outer Banks Hospital	Nags Head	95%	39
Transylvania Regional Hospital	Brevard	95%	57
Wakemed - Raleigh Campus	Raleigh	95%	152
Anson Community Hospital	Wadesboro	94%	47
C J Harris Community Hospital	Sylva	94%	141
Carolinas Medical Center-Union[2]	Monroe	94%	89
The Mcdowell Hospital	Marion	94%	31
The Moses H Cone Memorial Hospital[2]	Greensboro	94%	141
North Carolina Baptist Hospital	Winston-Salem	94%	171
Northern Hospital of Surry County	Mount Airy	94%	119
W G (Bill) Hefner Salisbury VA Med Ctr	Salisbury	94%	35
Watauga Medical Center	Boone	94%	88
Brunswick Community Hospital	Supply	93%	74
Carolina East Medical Center	New Bern	93%	147
Duke Health Raleigh Hospital	Raleigh	93%	103
Firsthealth Moore Regional Hospital[2]	Pinehurst	93%	180
Heritage Hospital	Tarboro	93%	44
Lenoir Memorial Hospital	Kinston	93%	136
Kings Mountain Hospital	Kings Mountain	92%	51
Maria Parham Hospital	Henderson	92%	85
Sandhills Regional Medical Center	Hamlet	92%	48

NOTE: Hospital profiles are in alphabetical order by state, then city, then hospital within the city; Rankings exclude hospitals with less than 25 cases except for patient surveys which excludes hospitals with less than 100 cases; (a) 100–299 cases; (1) The number of cases is too small to be sure how well a hospital is performing; (2) The hospital indicated that the data submitted for this measure were based on a sample of cases; (3) Data was collected during a shorter time period (fewer quarters) than the maximum possible time for this measure; (4) Suppressed for one or more quarters by CMS; (5) No data is available from the hospital for this measure; (6) Fewer than 100 patients completed the HCAHPS survey. Use these rates with caution, as the number of surveys may be too low to reliably assess hospital performance; (7) Survey results are based on less than 12 months of data; (8) Survey results are not available for this reporting period; (9) No or very few patients were eligible for the HCAHPS survey. The scores shown, if any, reflect a very small number of surveys; (10) A state average was not calculated because too few hospitals in the state submitted data; (11) There were discrepancies in the data collection process; Please refer to the User's Guide for a full explanation of data.

High Point Regional Hospital	High Point	91%	220
Southeastern Regional Medical Center	Lumberton	91%	242
Carolinas Medical Center-Behavioral Health	Charlotte	90%	145
Catawba Valley Medical Center	Hickory	90%	156
Chowan Hospital	Edenton	90%	31
Granville Medical Center	Oxford	90%	59
Iredell Memorial Hospital	Statesville	90%	175
Onslow Memorial Hospital	Jacksonville	90%	126
Sampson Regional Medical Center	Clinton	90%	86
Scotland Memorial Hospital	Laurinburg	90%	72
Fayetteville North Carolina VA Med Ctr	Fayetteville	89%	46
Murphy Medical Center	Murphy	89%	88
Randolph Hospital[2]	Asheboro	89%	116
Wilkes Regional Medical Center	N Wilkesboro	89%	139
Angel Medical Center	Franklin	88%	50
Carteret General Hospital	Morehead City	88%	95
Chatham Hospital	Siler City	88%	42
New Hanover Regional Medical Center[2]	Wilmington	88%	75
Park Ridge Hospital	Fletcher	88%	73
University of North Carolina Hospital[2]	Chapel Hill	88%	49
Alamance Regional Medical Center	Burlington	87%	115
Betsy Johnson Regional Hospital	Dunn	87%	159
Grace Hospital	Morganton	87%	112
Lexington Memorial Hospital	Lexington	87%	126
Morehead Memorial Hospital	Eden	87%	182
Roanoke Chowan Hospital	Ahoskie	87%	62
Stanly Regional Medical Center	Albemarle	87%	124
Valdese General Hospital	Valdese	87%	55
Alleghany County Memorial Hospital	Sparta	86%	51
Memorial Mission Hospital[2]	Asheville	86%	146
Nash General Hospital[2]	Rocky Mount	86%	114
Cleveland Regional Medical Center	Shelby	85%	169
Durham VA Medical Center	Durham	85%	26
Halifax Regional Medical Center	Roanoke Rapids	85%	104
Johnston Memorial Hospital	Smithfield	84%	171
Person Memorial Hospital	Roxboro	84%	61
Albemarle Hospital Authority[2]	Elizabeth City	83%	66
Haywood Regional Medical Center	Clyde	83%	135
Asheville-Oteen VA Medical Center	Asheville	82%	106
Beaufort County Medical Center	Washington	82%	49
Caldwell Memorial Hospital	Lenoir	82%	74
Pitt County Memorial Hospital	Greenville	82%	181
Rutherford Hospital	Rutherfordton	81%	116
Martin General Hospital	Williamston	80%	55
Spruce Pine Community Hospital	Spruce Pine	80%	112
Wilson Medical Center	Wilson	79%	121
Charles A Cannon Jr Memorial Hospital	Linville	73%	37
Cherokee Indian Hospital Authority[2]	Cherokee	65%	26

17. Blood Culture Timing

Hospital Name	City	Rate	Cases
Carolinas Medical Center-Northeast	Concord	100%	635
Fayetteville North Carolina VA Med Ctr	Fayetteville	100%	52
Forsyth Memorial Hospital	Winston-Salem	100%	694
Gaston Memorial Hospital	Gastonia	100%	842
Lake Norman Regional Medical Center	Mooresville	100%	97
Martin General Hospital	Williamston	100%	58
The Mcdowell Hospital	Marion	100%	64
Presbyterian Hospital	Charlotte	100%	277
Presbyterian Hospital Huntersville	Huntersville	100%	167
Presbyterian Hospital Matthews	Matthews	100%	258
Rowan Regional Medical Center	Salisbury	100%	303
Thomasville Medical Center	Thomasville	100%	135
W G (Bill) Hefner Salisbury VA Med Ctr	Salisbury	100%	61
Asheville-Oteen VA Medical Center	Asheville	99%	127
Brunswick Community Hospital	Supply	99%	106
Duplin General Hospital	Kenansville	99%	102
Scotland Memorial Hospital	Laurinburg	99%	121
Transylvania Regional Hospital	Brevard	99%	70
Wakemed - Raleigh Campus	Raleigh	99%	276
Ashe Memorial Hospital	Jefferson	98%	53
Caldwell Memorial Hospital	Lenoir	98%	140
Carolinas Medical Center-Lincoln	Lincolnton	98%	139
Carolinas Medical Center-Union[2]	Monroe	98%	137
Carolinas Medical Center-University	Charlotte	98%	158
Charles A Cannon Jr Memorial Hospital	Linville	98%	46
Chatham Hospital	Siler City	98%	51
Columbus Regional Healthcare System	Whiteville	98%	137
Duke Health Raleigh Hospital	Raleigh	98%	148
Duke University Hospital	Durham	98%	240
Durham Regional Hospital	Durham	98%	321
Grace Hospital	Morganton	98%	204
Hugh Chatham Memorial Hospital	Elkin	98%	155
Kings Mountain Hospital	Kings Mountain	98%	51
Valdese General Hospital	Valdese	98%	97
Wilkes Regional Medical Center	N Wilkesboro	98%	217
Cape Fear Valley Medical Center	Fayetteville	97%	634
Carteret General Hospital	Morehead City	97%	129
Central Carolina Hospital	Sanford	97%	157
Davis Regional Medical Center	Statesville	97%	116
Firsthealth Moore Regional Hospital[2]	Pinehurst	97%	262
Heritage Hospital	Tarboro	97%	76
Iredell Memorial Hospital	Statesville	97%	200
Lenoir Memorial Hospital	Kinston	97%	206
Lexington Memorial Hospital	Lexington	97%	185
North Carolina Baptist Hospital	Winston-Salem	97%	453
Wakemed - Cary Hospital	Cary	97%	134
Watauga Medical Center	Boone	97%	137
C J Harris Community Hospital	Sylva	96%	158
Carolinas Medical Center-Mercy	Charlotte	96%	235
Durham VA Medical Center	Durham	96%	57
Franklin Regional Medical Center	Louisburg	96%	68
Frye Regional Medical Center	Hickory	96%	335
Haywood Regional Medical Center	Clyde	96%	159
Margaret R Pardee Memorial Hospital	Hendersonville	96%	186
Morehead Memorial Hospital	Eden	96%	129
Northern Hospital of Surry County	Mount Airy	96%	216
Rex Hospital[2]	Raleigh	96%	227
Wayne Memorial Hospital	Goldsboro	96%	112
Carolina East Medical Center	New Bern	95%	300
Chowan Hospital	Edenton	95%	41
Granville Medical Center	Oxford	95%	66
The Moses H Cone Memorial Hospital[2]	Greensboro	95%	131
Murphy Medical Center	Murphy	95%	129
Person Memorial Hospital	Roxboro	95%	95
Randolph Hospital[2]	Asheboro	95%	140
Roanoke Chowan Hospital	Ahoskie	95%	99
Stanly Regional Medical Center	Albemarle	95%	203
University of North Carolina Hospital[2]	Chapel Hill	95%	99
Anson Community Hospital	Wadesboro	94%	89
Carolinas Medical Center-Behavioral Health	Charlotte	94%	174
Memorial Mission Hospital[2]	Asheville	94%	256
The Outer Banks Hospital	Nags Head	94%	48
Park Ridge Hospital	Fletcher	94%	101
Rutherford Hospital	Rutherfordton	94%	183
Alamance Regional Medical Center	Burlington	93%	149
Betsy Johnson Regional Hospital	Dunn	93%	188
High Point Regional Hospital	High Point	93%	397
Onslow Memorial Hospital	Jacksonville	93%	176
Saint Lukes Hospital	Columbus	93%	76
Sandhills Regional Medical Center	Hamlet	93%	60
Southeastern Regional Medical Center	Lumberton	93%	307
Catawba Valley Medical Center	Hickory	92%	253
Halifax Regional Medical Center	Roanoke Rapids	92%	132
Nash General Hospital[2]	Rocky Mount	92%	259
Pitt County Memorial Hospital	Greenville	92%	272
Alleghany County Memorial Hospital	Sparta	91%	55
Angel Medical Center	Franklin	91%	47
Johnston Memorial Hospital	Smithfield	91%	213
Cleveland Regional Medical Center	Shelby	90%	202
Maria Parham Hospital	Henderson	90%	102
Sampson Regional Medical Center	Clinton	90%	133
Washington County Hospital	Plymouth	89%	27
Albemarle Hospital Authority[2]	Elizabeth City	88%	94
Beaufort County Medical Center	Washington	88%	67
New Hanover Regional Medical Center[2]	Wilmington	86%	81
Cape Fear Valley-Bladen County Hospital	Elizabethtown	85%	34
Spruce Pine Community Hospital	Spruce Pine	82%	114
Wilson Medical Center	Wilson	82%	191

18. Influenza Vaccine

Hospital Name	City	Rate	Cases
Anson Community Hospital	Wadesboro	100%	56
Brunswick Community Hospital	Supply	100%	68
Davis Regional Medical Center	Statesville	100%	62
Forsyth Memorial Hospital	Winston-Salem	100%	531
Gaston Memorial Hospital	Gastonia	100%	555
Granville Medical Center	Oxford	100%	56
Lake Norman Regional Medical Center	Mooresville	100%	68
Rowan Regional Medical Center	Salisbury	100%	236
Sandhills Regional Medical Center	Hamlet	100%	29
Scotland Memorial Hospital	Laurinburg	100%	77
W G (Bill) Hefner Salisbury VA Med Ctr	Salisbury	100%	35
Carolinas Medical Center-Lincoln	Lincolnton	99%	82
Carolinas Medical Center-University	Charlotte	99%	86
Columbus Regional Healthcare System	Whiteville	99%	76
Duke Health Raleigh Hospital	Raleigh	99%	90
Grace Hospital	Morganton	99%	129
Iredell Memorial Hospital	Statesville	99%	142
Presbyterian Hospital Matthews	Matthews	99%	160
University of North Carolina Hospital[2]	Chapel Hill	99%	68
Valdese General Hospital	Valdese	99%	76
Carolinas Medical Center-Behavioral Health	Charlotte	98%	204
Carolinas Medical Center-Northeast	Concord	98%	392
Central Carolina Hospital	Sanford	98%	111
Chatham Hospital	Siler City	98%	47
Duke University Hospital	Durham	98%	232
Duplin General Hospital	Kenansville	98%	51
Durham Regional Hospital	Durham	98%	199
Franklin Regional Medical Center	Louisburg	98%	48
Kings Mountain Hospital	Kings Mountain	98%	43
Onslow Memorial Hospital	Jacksonville	98%	126
Presbyterian Hospital	Charlotte	98%	225
Presbyterian Hospital Huntersville	Huntersville	98%	89
Carolinas Medical Center-Mercy	Charlotte	97%	184
Charles A Cannon Jr Memorial Hospital	Linville	97%	34
Durham VA Medical Center	Durham	97%	60
Fayetteville North Carolina VA Med Ctr	Fayetteville	97%	32
Firsthealth Moore Regional Hospital[2]	Pinehurst	97%	268
The Moses H Cone Memorial Hospital[2]	Greensboro	97%	163
Roanoke Chowan Hospital	Ahoskie	97%	66
Saint Lukes Hospital	Columbus	97%	38
Transylvania Regional Hospital	Brevard	97%	37
C J Harris Community Hospital	Sylva	96%	130
Frye Regional Medical Center	Hickory	96%	209
Thomasville Medical Center	Thomasville	96%	51
Cape Fear Valley Medical Center	Fayetteville	95%	447
Carolinas Medical Center-Union[2]	Monroe	95%	83
Cleveland Regional Medical Center	Shelby	95%	169
Lexington Memorial Hospital	Lexington	95%	105
Person Memorial Hospital	Roxboro	95%	61
Pitt County Memorial Hospital	Greenville	95%	312
Wakemed - Cary Hospital	Cary	95%	122
Alamance Regional Medical Center	Burlington	94%	130
Carteret General Hospital	Morehead City	94%	94
The Mcdowell Hospital	Marion	94%	54
Wilkes Regional Medical Center	N Wilkesboro	94%	126
Hugh Chatham Memorial Hospital	Elkin	93%	112
Martin General Hospital	Williamston	93%	44
Murphy Medical Center	Murphy	93%	83
Park Ridge Hospital	Fletcher	93%	58
Wakemed - Raleigh Campus	Raleigh	93%	274
Chowan Hospital	Edenton	92%	25
Nash General Hospital	Rocky Mount	92%	194
North Carolina Baptist Hospital	Winston-Salem	92%	142
Northern Hospital of Surry County	Mount Airy	92%	146
Randolph Hospital[2]	Asheboro	92%	89
Southeastern Regional Medical Center	Lumberton	92%	220
Beaufort County Medical Center	Washington	91%	54
Halifax Regional Medical Center	Roanoke Rapids	91%	111
Heritage Hospital	Tarboro	91%	53
Morehead Memorial Hospital	Eden	91%	149
Rex Hospital[2]	Raleigh	91%	127
Stanly Regional Medical Center	Albemarle	91%	137
Alleghany County Memorial Hospital	Sparta	90%	48
Asheville-Oteen VA Medical Center	Asheville	90%	87
Haywood Regional Medical Center	Clyde	89%	146
Maria Parham Hospital	Henderson	89%	82
Sampson Regional Medical Center	Clinton	88%	85
Spruce Pine Community Hospital	Spruce Pine	88%	74
Betsy Johnson Regional Hospital	Dunn	87%	162
Margaret R Pardee Memorial Hospital	Hendersonville	87%	126
Memorial Mission Hospital[2]	Asheville	87%	416
Catawba Valley Medical Center	Hickory	86%	108
Rutherford Hospital	Rutherfordton	86%	118
Angel Medical Center	Franklin	85%	41
Watauga Medical Center	Boone	85%	153
New Hanover Regional Medical Center[2]	Wilmington	83%	87
Wilson Medical Center	Wilson	83%	162
Albemarle Hospital Authority[2]	Elizabeth City	82%	88
Caldwell Memorial Hospital	Lenoir	81%	97
Carolina East Medical Center	New Bern	78%	204
Lenoir Memorial Hospital	Kinston	74%	151
Ashe Memorial Hospital	Jefferson	73%	85
High Point Regional Hospital	High Point	73%	249
Johnston Memorial Hospital	Smithfield	67%	163
Wayne Memorial Hospital	Goldsboro	57%	155

19. Initial Antibiotic Timing

Hospital Name	City	Rate	Cases
Brunswick Community Hospital	Supply	100%	105
Central Carolina Hospital	Sanford	100%	157
Chowan Hospital	Edenton	100%	39
Duke Health Raleigh Hospital	Raleigh	100%	125
Duplin General Hospital	Kenansville	100%	85
Forsyth Memorial Hospital	Winston-Salem	100%	624
Heritage Hospital	Tarboro	100%	72
Martin General Hospital	Williamston	100%	70
The Mcdowell Hospital	Marion	100%	65
The Outer Banks Hospital	Nags Head	100%	32
Washington County Hospital	Plymouth	100%	30
Anson Community Hospital	Wadesboro	99%	88
Carolinas Medical Center-University	Charlotte	99%	155
Gaston Memorial Hospital	Gastonia	99%	706
Iredell Memorial Hospital	Statesville	99%	253
Kings Mountain Hospital	Kings Mountain	99%	68
Lexington Memorial Hospital	Lexington	99%	175
Presbyterian Hospital	Charlotte	99%	314
Presbyterian Hospital Matthews	Matthews	99%	236
Rowan Regional Medical Center	Salisbury	99%	348

NOTE: Hospital profiles are in alphabetical order by state, then city, then hospital within the city; Rankings exclude hospitals with less than 25 cases except for patient surveys which excludes hospitals with less than 100 cases; (a) 100–299 cases; (1) The number of cases is too small to be sure how well a hospital is performing; (2) The hospital indicated that the data submitted for this measure were based on a sample of cases; (3) Data was collected during a shorter time period (fewer quarters) than the maximum possible time for this measure; (4) Suppressed for one or more quarters by CMS; (5) No data is available from the hospital for this measure; (6) Fewer than 100 patients completed the HCAHPS survey. Use these rates with caution, as the number of surveys may be too low to reliably assess hospital performance; (7) Survey results are based on less than 12 months of data; (8) Survey results are not available for this reporting period; (9) No or very few patients were eligible for the HCAHPS survey. The scores shown, if any, reflect a very small number of surveys; (10) A state average was not calculated because too few hospitals in the state submitted data; (11) There were discrepancies in the data collection process; Please refer to the User's Guide for a full explanation of data.

Thomasville Medical Center	Thomasville	99%	110
Wilkes Regional Medical Center	N Wilkesboro	99%	195
Angel Medical Center	Franklin	98%	64
Carolinas Medical Center-Union[2]	Monroe	98%	128
Davis Regional Medical Center	Statesville	98%	94
Frye Regional Medical Center	Hickory	98%	291
Hugh Chatham Memorial Hospital	Elkin	98%	155
North Carolina Baptist Hospital	Winston-Salem	98%	413
Person Memorial Hospital	Roxboro	98%	85
Presbyterian Hospital Huntersville	Huntersville	98%	156
Roanoke Chowan Hospital	Ahoskie	98%	94
Scotland Memorial Hospital	Laurinburg	98%	113
W G (Bill) Hefner Salisbury VA Med Ctr	Salisbury	98%	49
Wakemed - Cary Hospital	Cary	98%	122
Carolinas Medical Center-Northeast	Concord	97%	606
Grace Hospital	Morganton	97%	181
Margaret R Pardee Memorial Hospital	Hendersonville	97%	184
The Moses H Cone Memorial Hospital[2]	Greensboro	97%	244
Park Ridge Hospital	Fletcher	97%	94
Saint Lukes Hospital	Columbus	97%	59
Transylvania Regional Hospital	Brevard	97%	67
Watauga Medical Center	Boone	97%	145
Carolinas Medical Center-Lincoln	Lincolnton	96%	135
Firsthealth Moore Regional Hospital[2]	Pinehurst	96%	281
High Point Regional Hospital	High Point	96%	421
Lake Norman Regional Medical Center	Mooresville	96%	103
Lenoir Memorial Hospital	Kinston	96%	241
Sampson Regional Medical Center	Clinton	96%	113
Sandhills Regional Medical Center	Hamlet	96%	54
University of North Carolina Hospital[2]	Chapel Hill	96%	93
Ashe Memorial Hospital	Jefferson	95%	111
Betsy Johnson Regional Hospital	Dunn	95%	206
Carolina East Medical Center	New Bern	95%	283
Franklin Regional Medical Center	Louisburg	95%	59
Granville Medical Center	Oxford	95%	76
Northern Hospital of Surry County	Mount Airy	95%	203
Stanly Regional Medical Center	Albemarle	95%	191
C J Harris Community Hospital	Sylva	94%	179
Cape Fear Valley Medical Center	Fayetteville	94%	593
Carolinas Medical Center-Mercy	Charlotte	94%	266
Catawba Valley Medical Center	Hickory	94%	217
Charles A Cannon Jr Memorial Hospital	Linville	94%	72
Durham Regional Hospital	Durham	94%	297
Morehead Memorial Hospital	Eden	94%	227
Nash General Hospital[2]	Rocky Mount	94%	233
Randolph Hospital[2]	Asheboro	94%	108
Southeastern Regional Medical Center	Lumberton	94%	314
Alamance Regional Medical Center	Burlington	93%	166
Asheville-Oteen VA Medical Center	Asheville	93%	129
Beaufort County Medical Center	Washington	93%	76
Cleveland Regional Medical Center	Shelby	93%	214
Murphy Medical Center	Murphy	93%	138
Rex Hospital[2]	Raleigh	93%	189
Rutherford Hospital	Rutherfordton	93%	168
Wakemed - Raleigh Campus	Raleigh	93%	204
Alleghany County Memorial Hospital	Sparta	92%	65
Carolinas Medical Center-Behavioral Health	Charlotte	92%	236
Carteret General Hospital	Morehead City	92%	142
Halifax Regional Medical Center	Roanoke Rapids	92%	155
Memorial Mission Hospital[2]	Asheville	92%	275
Caldwell Memorial Hospital	Lenoir	91%	125
Duke University Hospital	Durham	91%	233
Johnston Memorial Hospital	Smithfield	91%	253
Wayne Memorial Hospital	Goldsboro	90%	160
Maria Parham Hospital	Henderson	89%	121
Wilson Medical Center	Wilson	89%	230
Albemarle Hospital Authority[2]	Elizabeth City	88%	101
Chatham Hospital	Siler City	88%	49
Columbus Regional Healthcare System	Whiteville	88%	136
Durham VA Medical Center	Durham	88%	60
New Hanover Regional Medical Center[2]	Wilmington	88%	104
Valdese General Hospital	Valdese	88%	90
Haywood Regional Medical Center	Clyde	87%	191
Pitt County Memorial Hospital	Greenville	87%	271
Davie County Hospital	Mocksville	85%	27
Spruce Pine Community Hospital	Spruce Pine	85%	139
Onslow Memorial Hospital	Jacksonville	83%	180

20. Pneumococcal Vaccine

Hospital Name	City	Rate	Cases
Anson Community Hospital	Wadesboro	100%	88
Davis Regional Medical Center	Statesville	100%	68
Fayetteville North Carolina VA Med Ctr	Fayetteville	100%	33
Forsyth Memorial Hospital	Winston-Salem	100%	710
Gaston Memorial Hospital	Gastonia	100%	603
Granville Medical Center	Oxford	100%	52
Kings Mountain Hospital	Kings Mountain	100%	46
Lake Norman Regional Medical Center	Mooresville	100%	87
The Outer Banks Hospital	Nags Head	100%	39
Pungo District Hospital	Belhaven	100%	25
Rowan Regional Medical Center	Salisbury	100%	276
Sandhills Regional Medical Center	Hamlet	100%	28
Scotland Memorial Hospital	Laurinburg	100%	107
Transylvania Regional Hospital	Brevard	100%	59
W G (Bill) Hefner Salisbury VA Med Ctr	Salisbury	100%	40
Brunswick Community Hospital	Supply	99%	94
C J Harris Community Hospital	Sylva	99%	193
Duke University Hospital	Durham	99%	251
Grace Hospital	Morganton	99%	162
Iredell Memorial Hospital	Statesville	99%	238
Onslow Memorial Hospital	Jacksonville	99%	142
Presbyterian Hospital	Charlotte	99%	268
Presbyterian Hospital Matthews	Matthews	99%	197
Thomasville Medical Center	Thomasville	99%	90
University of North Carolina Hospital[2]	Chapel Hill	99%	89
Carolinas Medical Center-Behavioral Health	Charlotte	98%	244
Carolinas Medical Center-Lincoln	Lincolnton	98%	80
Carolinas Medical Center-Mercy	Charlotte	98%	217
Carolinas Medical Center-University	Charlotte	98%	86
Central Carolina Hospital	Sanford	98%	133
Charles A Cannon Jr Memorial Hospital	Linville	98%	61
Durham VA Medical Center	Durham	98%	59
Lexington Memorial Hospital	Lexington	98%	158
The Mcdowell Hospital	Marion	98%	65
Person Memorial Hospital	Roxboro	98%	82
Presbyterian Hospital Huntersville	Huntersville	98%	129
Roanoke Chowan Hospital	Ahoskie	98%	80
Valdese General Hospital	Valdese	98%	107
Cape Fear Valley Medical Center	Fayetteville	97%	512
Cleveland Regional Medical Center	Shelby	97%	188
Duplin General Hospital	Kenansville	97%	70
Durham Regional Hospital	Durham	97%	274
Firsthealth Moore Regional Hospital[2]	Pinehurst	97%	300
Franklin Regional Medical Center	Louisburg	97%	63
Lenoir Memorial Hospital	Kinston	97%	229
The Moses H Cone Memorial Hospital[2]	Greensboro	97%	228
Wilkes Regional Medical Center	N Wilkesboro	97%	198
Betsy Johnson Regional Hospital	Dunn	96%	173
Carolinas Medical Center-Northeast	Concord	96%	483
Carolinas Medical Center-Union[2]	Monroe	96%	109
Carteret General Hospital	Morehead City	96%	110
Chatham Hospital	Siler City	96%	54
Columbus Regional Healthcare System	Whiteville	96%	108
Duke Health Raleigh Hospital	Raleigh	96%	121
Rex Hospital[2]	Raleigh	96%	213
Southeastern Regional Medical Center	Lumberton	96%	253
Wakemed - Raleigh Campus	Raleigh	96%	315
Watauga Medical Center	Boone	96%	200
Alamance Regional Medical Center	Burlington	95%	173
Albemarle Hospital Authority[2]	Elizabeth City	95%	112
Alleghany County Memorial Hospital	Sparta	95%	61
Chowan Hospital	Edenton	95%	37
Frye Regional Medical Center	Hickory	95%	276
Heritage Hospital	Tarboro	95%	58
Nash General Hospital[2]	Rocky Mount	95%	213
Park Ridge Hospital	Fletcher	95%	83
Martin General Hospital	Williamston	94%	66
Memorial Mission Hospital[2]	Asheville	94%	532
Pitt County Memorial Hospital	Greenville	94%	371
Sampson Regional Medical Center	Clinton	94%	143
Spruce Pine Community Hospital	Spruce Pine	94%	129
Wakemed - Cary Hospital	Cary	94%	144
Caldwell Memorial Hospital	Lenoir	93%	120
Maria Parham Hospital	Henderson	93%	103
Stanly Regional Medical Center	Albemarle	93%	191
Asheville-Oteen VA Medical Center	Asheville	92%	126
Davie County Hospital	Mocksville	92%	25
Haywood Regional Medical Center	Clyde	92%	182
Hugh Chatham Memorial Hospital	Elkin	92%	130
North Carolina Baptist Hospital	Winston-Salem	92%	283
Angel Medical Center	Franklin	91%	67
Catawba Valley Medical Center	Hickory	91%	154
Halifax Regional Medical Center	Roanoke Rapids	91%	134
Margaret R Pardee Memorial Hospital	Hendersonville	91%	162
Rutherford Hospital	Rutherfordton	91%	167
Saint Lukes Hospital	Columbus	91%	58
Beaufort County Medical Center	Washington	90%	61
Morehead Memorial Hospital	Eden	90%	197
Ashe Memorial Hospital	Jefferson	88%	136
New Hanover Regional Medical Center[2]	Wilmington	88%	113
Northern Hospital of Surry County	Mount Airy	88%	190
Cape Fear Valley-Bladen County Hospital	Elizabethtown	87%	30
High Point Regional Hospital	High Point	87%	347
Murphy Medical Center	Murphy	87%	116
Randolph Hospital[2]	Asheboro	85%	109
Carolina East Medical Center	New Bern	82%	258
Wayne Memorial Hospital	Goldsboro	81%	180
Wilson Medical Center	Wilson	81%	203
Johnston Memorial Hospital	Smithfield	70%	222

21. Smoking Cessation Advice

Hospital Name	City	Rate	Cases
Alamance Regional Medical Center	Burlington	100%	59
Asheville-Oteen VA Medical Center	Asheville	100%	40
Brunswick Community Hospital	Supply	100%	56
C J Harris Community Hospital	Sylva	100%	81
Cape Fear Valley Medical Center	Fayetteville	100%	296
Carolinas Medical Center-Lincoln	Lincolnton	100%	82
Carolinas Medical Center-Mercy	Charlotte	100%	99
Carolinas Medical Center-Northeast	Concord	100%	245
Carolinas Medical Center-Union[2]	Monroe	100%	75
Carolinas Medical Center-University	Charlotte	100%	73
Central Carolina Hospital	Sanford	100%	53
Columbus Regional Healthcare System	Whiteville	100%	53
Davis Regional Medical Center	Statesville	100%	59
Duke University Hospital	Durham	100%	78
Duplin General Hospital	Kenansville	100%	29
Durham VA Medical Center	Durham	100%	29
Firsthealth Moore Regional Hospital[2]	Pinehurst	100%	142
Forsyth Memorial Hospital	Winston-Salem	100%	323
Franklin Regional Medical Center	Louisburg	100%	26
Gaston Memorial Hospital	Gastonia	100%	375
Granville Medical Center	Oxford	100%	35
Halifax Regional Medical Center	Roanoke Rapids	100%	66
High Point Regional Hospital	High Point	100%	196
Hugh Chatham Memorial Hospital	Elkin	100%	87
Iredell Memorial Hospital	Statesville	100%	93
Johnston Memorial Hospital	Smithfield	100%	82
Kings Mountain Hospital	Kings Mountain	100%	35
Lake Norman Regional Medical Center	Mooresville	100%	50
Lenoir Memorial Hospital	Kinston	100%	68
Lexington Memorial Hospital	Lexington	100%	55
Maria Parham Hospital	Henderson	100%	47
The Mcdowell Hospital	Marion	100%	36
Memorial Mission Hospital[2]	Asheville	100%	244
The Moses H Cone Memorial Hospital[2]	Greensboro	100%	106
North Carolina Baptist Hospital	Winston-Salem	100%	264
Onslow Memorial Hospital	Jacksonville	100%	82
Park Ridge Hospital	Fletcher	100%	42
Person Memorial Hospital	Roxboro	100%	28
Pitt County Memorial Hospital	Greenville	100%	200
Presbyterian Hospital	Charlotte	100%	149
Presbyterian Hospital Huntersville	Huntersville	100%	46
Presbyterian Hospital Matthews	Matthews	100%	70
Randolph Hospital[2]	Asheboro	100%	75
Roanoke Chowan Hospital	Ahoskie	100%	30
Rowan Regional Medical Center	Salisbury	100%	143
Rutherford Hospital	Rutherfordton	100%	60
Sampson Regional Medical Center	Clinton	100%	36
Sandhills Regional Medical Center	Hamlet	100%	33
Scotland Memorial Hospital	Laurinburg	100%	63
Thomasville Medical Center	Thomasville	100%	45
University of North Carolina Hospital[2]	Chapel Hill	100%	48
Valdese General Hospital	Valdese	100%	50
Wakemed - Cary Hospital	Cary	100%	55
Wayne Memorial Hospital	Goldsboro	100%	105
Betsy Johnson Regional Hospital	Dunn	99%	78
Carolina East Medical Center	New Bern	99%	142
Catawba Valley Medical Center	Hickory	99%	74
Cleveland Regional Medical Center	Shelby	99%	109
Durham Regional Hospital	Durham	99%	145
Grace Hospital	Morganton	99%	84
Northern Hospital of Surry County	Mount Airy	99%	92
Southeastern Regional Medical Center	Lumberton	99%	174
Wakemed - Raleigh Campus	Raleigh	99%	206
Carolinas Medical Center-Behavioral Health	Charlotte	98%	178
Carteret General Hospital	Morehead City	98%	54
Duke Health Raleigh Hospital	Raleigh	98%	42
Frye Regional Medical Center	Hickory	98%	100
Margaret R Pardee Memorial Hospital	Hendersonville	98%	63
Murphy Medical Center	Murphy	98%	51
Nash General Hospital[2]	Rocky Mount	98%	128
Rex Hospital[2]	Raleigh	98%	43
Stanly Regional Medical Center	Albemarle	98%	81
Albemarle Hospital Authority[2]	Elizabeth City	97%	39
Caldwell Memorial Hospital	Lenoir	97%	72
Watauga Medical Center	Boone	97%	66
Beaufort County Medical Center	Washington	96%	26
Wilson Medical Center	Wilson	96%	89
Ashe Memorial Hospital	Jefferson	95%	42
Wilkes Regional Medical Center	N Wilkesboro	95%	77
W G (Bill) Hefner Salisbury VA Med Ctr	Salisbury	93%	27
Haywood Regional Medical Center	Clyde	92%	103
New Hanover Regional Medical Center[2]	Wilmington	91%	66
Morehead Memorial Hospital	Eden	89%	89
Spruce Pine Community Hospital	Spruce Pine	74%	46

NOTE: Hospital profiles are in alphabetical order by state, then city, then hospital within the city; Rankings exclude hospitals with less than 25 cases except for patient surveys which excludes hospitals with less than 100 cases; (a) 100–299 cases; (1) The number of cases is too small to be sure how well a hospital is performing; (2) The hospital indicated that the data submitted for this measure were based on a sample of cases; (3) Data was collected during a shorter time period (fewer quarters) than the maximum possible time for this measure; (4) Suppressed for one or more quarters by CMS; (5) No data is available from the hospital for this measure; (6) Fewer than 100 patients completed the HCAHPS survey. Use these rates with caution, as the number of surveys may be too low to reliably assess hospital performance; (7) Survey results are based on less than 12 months of data; (8) Survey results are not available for this reporting period; (9) No or very few patients were eligible for the HCAHPS survey. The scores shown, if any, reflect a very small number of surveys; (10) A state average was not calculated because too few hospitals in the state submitted data; (11) There were discrepancies in the data collection process; Please refer to the User's Guide for a full explanation of data.

Surgical Care Improvement Project

22. Appropriate VTP Within 24 Hours

Hospital Name	City	Rate	Cases
Duke University Hospital[2]	Durham	100%	202
North Carolina Specialty Hospital[2]	Durham	100%	47
The Outer Banks Hospital	Nags Head	100%	37
Presbyterian-Orthopaedic Hospital[2]	Charlotte	100%	616
Roanoke Chowan Hospital	Ahoskie	100%	66
Brunswick Community Hospital	Supply	99%	134
Davis Regional Medical Center	Statesville	99%	135
Gaston Memorial Hospital	Gastonia	99%	393
Granville Medical Center	Oxford	99%	88
High Point Regional Hospital[2]	High Point	99%	131
Hugh Chatham Memorial Hospital	Elkin	99%	118
Carolinas Medical Center-Mercy[2]	Charlotte	98%	725
Chowan Hospital	Edenton	98%	65
Scotland Memorial Hospital	Laurinburg	98%	195
Asheville-Oteen VA Medical Center[2]	Asheville	97%	87
Carolinas Medical Center-Union[2]	Monroe	97%	212
Forsyth Memorial Hospital[2]	Winston-Salem	97%	1018
Memorial Mission Hospital[2]	Asheville	97%	906
North Carolina Baptist Hospital[2]	Winston-Salem	97%	363
Presbyterian Hospital[2]	Charlotte	97%	499
Rowan Regional Medical Center[2]	Salisbury	97%	241
Transylvania Regional Hospital	Brevard	97%	58
Albemarle Hospital Authority[2]	Elizabeth City	96%	124
Lake Norman Regional Medical Center	Mooresville	96%	171
Medical Park Hospital[2]	Winston-Salem	96%	179
Presbyterian Hospital Matthews[2]	Matthews	96%	216
Alamance Regional Medical Center	Burlington	95%	427
Carolinas Medical Center-Behavioral Health[2]	Charlotte	95%	571
Carolinas Medical Center-Lincoln	Lincolnton	95%	39
Carolinas Medical Center-University[2]	Charlotte	95%	154
Durham Regional Hospital[2]	Durham	95%	196
New Hanover Regional Medical Center[2]	Wilmington	95%	345
Pitt County Memorial Hospital[2]	Greenville	95%	700
Rutherford Hospital	Rutherfordton	95%	113
University of North Carolina Hospital[2]	Chapel Hill	95%	286
Valdese General Hospital	Valdese	95%	66
Catawba Valley Medical Center	Hickory	94%	263
Cleveland Regional Medical Center[2]	Shelby	94%	170
Iredell Memorial Hospital[2]	Statesville	94%	242
Wakemed - Cary Hospital[2]	Cary	94%	145
Carolina East Medical Center	New Bern	93%	665
Carolinas Medical Center-Northeast[2]	Concord	93%	455
Haywood Regional Medical Center	Clyde	93%	110
Heritage Hospital	Tarboro	93%	75
Presbyterian Hospital Huntersville[2]	Huntersville	93%	201
Thomasville Medical Center[2]	Thomasville	93%	90
Wayne Memorial Hospital[2]	Goldsboro	93%	299
Durham VA Medical Center[2]	Durham	92%	111
Firsthealth Moore Regional Hospital[2]	Pinehurst	92%	376
Maria Parham Hospital	Henderson	92%	77
The Mcdowell Hospital	Marion	92%	63
Northern Hospital of Surry County	Mount Airy	92%	126
Park Ridge Hospital	Fletcher	92%	112
Wakemed - Raleigh Campus[2]	Raleigh	92%	241
Angel Medical Center	Franklin	91%	45
Central Carolina Hospital[2]	Sanford	91%	123
Duke Health Raleigh Hospital	Raleigh	91%	414
Frye Regional Medical Center[2]	Hickory	91%	149
Cape Fear Valley Medical Center[2]	Fayetteville	90%	199
Columbus Regional Healthcare System	Whiteville	90%	170
Margaret R Pardee Memorial Hospital[2]	Hendersonville	90%	245
Nash General Hospital[2]	Rocky Mount	90%	146
Person Memorial Hospital	Roxboro	90%	105
Southeastern Regional Medical Center	Lumberton	90%	185
Caldwell Memorial Hospital	Lenoir	89%	113
Lexington Memorial Hospital	Lexington	89%	80
Rex Hospital[2]	Raleigh	89%	287
Spruce Pine Community Hospital	Spruce Pine	89%	57
Wilkes Regional Medical Center	N Wilkesboro	89%	83
Onslow Memorial Hospital	Jacksonville	88%	136
Stanly Regional Medical Center	Albemarle	88%	90
W G (Bill) Hefner Salisbury VA Med Ctr[2]	Salisbury	88%	40
The Moses H Cone Memorial Hospital[2]	Greensboro	87%	415
Kings Mountain Hospital	Kings Mountain	86%	28
Martin General Hospital[2]	Williamston	86%	50
Morehead Memorial Hospital	Eden	86%	103
Saint Lukes Hospital	Columbus	86%	36
Beaufort County Medical Center	Washington	85%	106
C J Harris Community Hospital[2]	Sylva	85%	152
Murphy Medical Center	Murphy	84%	64
Randolph Hospital[2]	Asheboro	83%	125
Watauga Medical Center	Boone	82%	136
Wilson Medical Center[2]	Wilson	78%	167
Johnston Memorial Hospital	Smithfield	77%	195
Grace Hospital	Morganton	76%	136
Betsy Johnson Regional Hospital	Dunn	75%	102
Carteret General Hospital	Morehead City	72%	155
Halifax Regional Medical Center[2]	Roanoke Rapids	72%	74
Lenoir Memorial Hospital	Kinston	66%	217
Sampson Regional Medical Center	Clinton	62%	60

23. Appropriate Hair Removal

Hospital Name	City	Rate	Cases
Alamance Regional Medical Center	Burlington	100%	755
Albemarle Hospital Authority[2]	Elizabeth City	100%	232
Ashe Memorial Hospital	Jefferson	100%	29
Asheville-Oteen VA Medical Center[2]	Asheville	100%	477
Beaufort County Medical Center	Washington	100%	275
Brunswick Community Hospital	Supply	100%	307
C J Harris Community Hospital[2]	Sylva	100%	274
Caldwell Memorial Hospital	Lenoir	100%	308
Cape Fear Valley Medical Center[2]	Fayetteville	100%	615
Carolina East Medical Center	New Bern	100%	1419
Carolinas Medical Center-Behavioral Health[2]	Charlotte	100%	2153
Carolinas Medical Center-Lincoln	Lincolnton	100%	113
Carolinas Medical Center-Mercy[2]	Charlotte	100%	2101
Carolinas Medical Center-Northeast[2]	Concord	100%	1225
Carolinas Medical Center-Union[2]	Monroe	100%	359
Carolinas Medical Center-University[2]	Charlotte	100%	328
Carteret General Hospital	Morehead City	100%	497
Catawba Valley Medical Center	Hickory	100%	671
Central Carolina Hospital[2]	Sanford	100%	201
Cleveland Regional Medical Center[2]	Shelby	100%	587
Columbus Regional Healthcare System	Whiteville	100%	256
Davis Regional Medical Center	Statesville	100%	192
Duplin General Hospital	Kenansville	100%	47
Durham Regional Hospital[2]	Durham	100%	935
Durham VA Medical Center[2]	Durham	100%	276
Forsyth Memorial Hospital[2]	Winston-Salem	100%	2869
Frye Regional Medical Center[2]	Hickory	100%	1462
Gaston Memorial Hospital	Gastonia	100%	1384
Grace Hospital	Morganton	100%	240
Granville Medical Center	Oxford	100%	218
Halifax Regional Medical Center[2]	Roanoke Rapids	100%	423
Haywood Regional Medical Center	Clyde	100%	472
Heritage Hospital	Tarboro	100%	130
High Point Regional Hospital[2]	High Point	100%	506
Hugh Chatham Memorial Hospital	Elkin	100%	344
Iredell Memorial Hospital[2]	Statesville	100%	389
Johnston Memorial Hospital	Smithfield	100%	450
Kings Mountain Hospital	Kings Mountain	100%	37
Lake Norman Regional Medical Center	Mooresville	100%	377
Lenoir Memorial Hospital	Kinston	100%	461
Margaret R Pardee Memorial Hospital[2]	Hendersonville	100%	408
Maria Parham Hospital	Henderson	100%	180
Martin General Hospital[2]	Williamston	100%	97
The Mcdowell Hospital	Marion	100%	111
Medical Park Hospital[2]	Winston-Salem	100%	412
Memorial Mission Hospital[2]	Asheville	100%	3005
Morehead Memorial Hospital	Eden	100%	176
The Moses H Cone Memorial Hospital[2]	Greensboro	100%	1088
Murphy Medical Center	Murphy	100%	168
Nash General Hospital[2]	Rocky Mount	100%	698
North Carolina Baptist Hospital[2]	Winston-Salem	100%	954
North Carolina Specialty Hospital[2]	Durham	100%	265
Northern Hospital of Surry County	Mount Airy	100%	337
Onslow Memorial Hospital	Jacksonville	100%	294
The Outer Banks Hospital	Nags Head	100%	109
Park Ridge Hospital	Fletcher	100%	231
Person Memorial Hospital	Roxboro	100%	200
Presbyterian Hospital[2]	Charlotte	100%	1515
Presbyterian Hospital Huntersville[2]	Huntersville	100%	540
Presbyterian Hospital Matthews[2]	Matthews	100%	468
Presbyterian-Orthopaedic Hospital[2]	Charlotte	100%	1497
Roanoke Chowan Hospital	Ahoskie	100%	189
Rowan Regional Medical Center[2]	Salisbury	100%	779
Rutherford Hospital	Rutherfordton	100%	340
Saint Lukes Hospital	Columbus	100%	174
Sampson Regional Medical Center	Clinton	100%	146
Sandhills Regional Medical Center	Hamlet	100%	52
Scotland Memorial Hospital	Laurinburg	100%	318
Southeastern Regional Medical Center	Lumberton	100%	389
Spruce Pine Community Hospital	Spruce Pine	100%	137
Thomasville Medical Center[2]	Thomasville	100%	178
Transylvania Regional Hospital	Brevard	100%	126
University of North Carolina Hospital[2]	Chapel Hill	100%	568
Valdese General Hospital	Valdese	100%	148
W G (Bill) Hefner Salisbury VA Med Ctr[2]	Salisbury	100%	77
Wakemed - Cary Hospital[2]	Cary	100%	383
Wakemed - Raleigh Campus[2]	Raleigh	100%	751
Watauga Medical Center	Boone	100%	308
Wilkes Regional Medical Center	N Wilkesboro	100%	168
Betsy Johnson Regional Hospital	Dunn	99%	206
Duke Health Raleigh Hospital	Raleigh	99%	1098
Firsthealth Moore Regional Hospital[2]	Pinehurst	99%	1626
Randolph Hospital[2]	Asheboro	99%	229
Rex Hospital[2]	Raleigh	99%	947
Stanly Regional Medical Center	Albemarle	99%	222
Wayne Memorial Hospital[2]	Goldsboro	99%	571
Wilson Medical Center[2]	Wilson	99%	539
Chowan Hospital	Edenton	98%	177
Duke University Hospital[2]	Durham	98%	634
Lexington Memorial Hospital	Lexington	98%	298
New Hanover Regional Medical Center[2]	Wilmington	98%	961
Pitt County Memorial Hospital[2]	Greenville	98%	2790
Angel Medical Center	Franklin	97%	69

24. Appropriate Beta Blocker Usage

Hospital Name	City	Rate	Cases
Asheville-Oteen VA Medical Center[2]	Asheville	100%	263
Brunswick Community Hospital	Supply	100%	73
C J Harris Community Hospital[2]	Sylva	100%	47
Central Carolina Hospital[2]	Sanford	100%	45
Davis Regional Medical Center	Statesville	100%	48
Durham VA Medical Center[2]	Durham	100%	80
Gaston Memorial Hospital	Gastonia	100%	404
Hugh Chatham Memorial Hospital	Elkin	100%	112
North Carolina Specialty Hospital[2]	Durham	100%	57
Park Ridge Hospital	Fletcher	100%	42
Presbyterian Hospital[2]	Charlotte	100%	430
Roanoke Chowan Hospital	Ahoskie	100%	39
Rowan Regional Medical Center[2]	Salisbury	100%	204
Transylvania Regional Hospital	Brevard	100%	30
Wilkes Regional Medical Center	N Wilkesboro	100%	35
Catawba Valley Medical Center	Hickory	99%	164
Lake Norman Regional Medical Center	Mooresville	99%	74
Medical Park Hospital[2]	Winston-Salem	99%	85
Cape Fear Valley Medical Center[2]	Fayetteville	98%	187
Carolinas Medical Center-University[2]	Charlotte	98%	59
Chowan Hospital	Edenton	98%	52
Margaret R Pardee Memorial Hospital[2]	Hendersonville	98%	102
Memorial Mission Hospital[2]	Asheville	98%	999
Presbyterian Hospital Matthews[2]	Matthews	98%	85
Scotland Memorial Hospital	Laurinburg	98%	102
Valdese General Hospital	Valdese	98%	49
Carolinas Medical Center-Mercy[2]	Charlotte	97%	483
Duke University Hospital[2]	Durham	97%	160
Firsthealth Moore Regional Hospital[2]	Pinehurst	97%	579
Forsyth Memorial Hospital[2]	Winston-Salem	97%	1006
Lexington Memorial Hospital	Lexington	97%	70
Presbyterian-Orthopaedic Hospital[2]	Charlotte	97%	384
Thomasville Medical Center[2]	Thomasville	97%	29
Watauga Medical Center	Boone	97%	75
Caldwell Memorial Hospital	Lenoir	96%	56
Carolinas Medical Center-Behavioral Health[2]	Charlotte	96%	650
Carolinas Medical Center-Northeast[2]	Concord	96%	398
Carolinas Medical Center-Union[2]	Monroe	96%	69
Iredell Memorial Hospital[2]	Statesville	96%	117
Nash General Hospital[2]	Rocky Mount	96%	180
North Carolina Baptist Hospital[2]	Winston-Salem	96%	328
Rutherford Hospital	Rutherfordton	96%	71
Wakemed - Raleigh Campus[2]	Raleigh	96%	268
Wilson Medical Center[2]	Wilson	96%	136
Albemarle Hospital Authority[2]	Elizabeth City	95%	62
Cleveland Regional Medical Center[2]	Shelby	95%	130
Durham Regional Hospital[2]	Durham	95%	253
Presbyterian Hospital Huntersville[2]	Huntersville	95%	128
Wakemed - Cary Hospital[2]	Cary	95%	78
Carteret General Hospital	Morehead City	94%	118
Granville Medical Center	Oxford	94%	50
Rex Hospital[2]	Raleigh	94%	329
University of North Carolina Hospital[2]	Chapel Hill	94%	174
Columbus Regional Healthcare System	Whiteville	93%	73
Frye Regional Medical Center[2]	Hickory	93%	215
Pitt County Memorial Hospital[2]	Greenville	93%	1105
Stanly Regional Medical Center	Albemarle	93%	59
Haywood Regional Medical Center	Clyde	92%	123
Person Memorial Hospital	Roxboro	92%	77
Saint Lukes Hospital	Columbus	92%	52
Sampson Regional Medical Center	Clinton	92%	40
Southeastern Regional Medical Center	Lumberton	92%	110
Alamance Regional Medical Center	Burlington	90%	208
Grace Hospital	Morganton	89%	47
Johnston Memorial Hospital	Smithfield	89%	160
New Hanover Regional Medical Center[2]	Wilmington	89%	317
Duke Health Raleigh Hospital	Raleigh	88%	294
Spruce Pine Community Hospital	Spruce Pine	88%	33
Wayne Memorial Hospital[2]	Goldsboro	88%	162
The Moses H Cone Memorial Hospital[2]	Greensboro	87%	337
Halifax Regional Medical Center[2]	Roanoke Rapids	86%	129
Murphy Medical Center	Murphy	85%	40
Carolina East Medical Center	New Bern	83%	383
Maria Parham Hospital	Henderson	82%	40
Beaufort County Medical Center	Washington	81%	53
High Point Regional Hospital[2]	High Point	81%	167
Onslow Memorial Hospital	Jacksonville	80%	74
Randolph Hospital[2]	Asheboro	79%	70

NOTE: Hospital profiles are in alphabetical order by state, then city, then hospital within the city; Rankings exclude hospitals with less than 25 cases except for patient surveys which excludes hospitals with less than 100 cases; (a) 100–299 cases; (1) The number of cases is too small to be sure how well a hospital is performing; (2) The hospital indicated that the data submitted for this measure were based on a sample of cases; (3) Data was collected during a shorter time period (fewer quarters) than the maximum possible time for this measure; (4) Suppressed for one or more quarters by CMS; (5) No data is available from the hospital for this measure; (6) Fewer than 100 patients completed the HCAHPS survey. Use these rates with caution, as the number of surveys may be too low to reliably assess hospital performance; (7) Survey results are based on less than 12 months of data; (8) Survey results are not available for this reporting period; (9) No or very few patients were eligible for the HCAHPS survey. The scores shown, if any, reflect a very small number of surveys; (10) A state average was not calculated because too few hospitals in the state submitted data; (11) There were discrepancies in the data collection process; Please refer to the User's Guide for a full explanation of data.

Morehead Memorial Hospital	Eden	78%	40
Northern Hospital of Surry County	Mount Airy	78%	101
Betsy Johnson Regional Hospital	Dunn	71%	51
Lenoir Memorial Hospital	Kinston	58%	125

25. Controlled Postoperative Blood Glucose

Hospital Name	City	Rate	Cases
Presbyterian Hospital[2]	Charlotte	100%	408
Southeastern Regional Medical Center	Lumberton	100%	33
Forsyth Memorial Hospital[2]	Winston-Salem	99%	483
Memorial Mission Hospital[2]	Asheville	99%	611
Wakemed - Raleigh Campus[2]	Raleigh	99%	170
Duke University Hospital[2]	Durham	98%	126
Asheville-Oteen VA Medical Center[2]	Asheville	97%	194
Gaston Memorial Hospital	Gastonia	97%	142
Firsthealth Moore Regional Hospital[2]	Pinehurst	96%	306
North Carolina Baptist Hospital[2]	Winston-Salem	96%	187
University of North Carolina Hospital[2]	Chapel Hill	96%	71
Durham VA Medical Center[2]	Durham	95%	111
High Point Regional Hospital[2]	High Point	95%	102
New Hanover Regional Medical Center[2]	Wilmington	95%	134
Cape Fear Valley Medical Center[2]	Fayetteville	94%	101
Durham Regional Hospital[2]	Durham	94%	51
The Moses H Cone Memorial Hospital[2]	Greensboro	94%	160
Rex Hospital[2]	Raleigh	94%	176
Carolinas Medical Center-Behavioral Health[2]	Charlotte	92%	520
Carolinas Medical Center-Northeast[2]	Concord	91%	190
Pitt County Memorial Hospital[2]	Greenville	90%	786
Frye Regional Medical Center[2]	Hickory	86%	261
Carolinas Medical Center-Mercy[2]	Charlotte	83%	30
Carolina East Medical Center	New Bern	74%	198

26. Prophylactic Antibiotic Timing

Hospital Name	City	Rate	Cases
Albemarle Hospital Authority[2]	Elizabeth City	100%	141
Brunswick Community Hospital	Supply	100%	233
Carolinas Medical Center-Union[2]	Monroe	100%	235
Duplin General Hospital	Kenansville	100%	34
Forsyth Memorial Hospital[2]	Winston-Salem	100%	2078
Heritage Hospital	Tarboro	100%	64
Hugh Chatham Memorial Hospital	Elkin	100%	313
Medical Park Hospital[2]	Winston-Salem	100%	230
Presbyterian Hospital[2]	Charlotte	100%	1096
Presbyterian-Orthopaedic Hospital[2]	Charlotte	100%	1255
Rowan Regional Medical Center[2]	Salisbury	100%	582
Sandhills Regional Medical Center	Hamlet	100%	37
Thomasville Medical Center[2]	Thomasville	100%	97
Transylvania Regional Hospital	Brevard	100%	84
Asheville-Oteen VA Medical Center	Asheville	99%	387
Beaufort County Medical Center	Washington	99%	181
Carolinas Medical Center-Northeast[2]	Concord	99%	965
Carolinas Medical Center-University[2]	Charlotte	99%	239
Central Carolina Hospital[2]	Sanford	99%	101
Durham Regional Hospital[2]	Durham	99%	781
Durham VA Medical Center	Durham	99%	176
Gaston Memorial Hospital	Gastonia	99%	897
Lake Norman Regional Medical Center	Mooresville	99%	225
Martin General Hospital[2]	Williamston	99%	91
North Carolina Baptist Hospital[2]	Winston-Salem	99%	619
North Carolina Specialty Hospital[2]	Durham	99%	187
Presbyterian Hospital Huntersville[2]	Huntersville	99%	396
Rutherford Hospital	Rutherfordton	99%	244
Saint Lukes Hospital	Columbus	99%	136
Southeastern Regional Medical Center	Lumberton	99%	251
Valdese General Hospital	Valdese	99%	108
Angel Medical Center	Franklin	98%	47
Cape Fear Valley Medical Center[2]	Fayetteville	98%	444
Carolinas Medical Center-Behavioral Health[2]	Charlotte	98%	1653
Carolinas Medical Center-Lincoln	Lincolnton	98%	81
Carteret General Hospital	Morehead City	98%	306
Chowan Hospital	Edenton	98%	140
Cleveland Regional Medical Center[2]	Shelby	98%	438
Davis Regional Medical Center	Statesville	98%	119
Firsthealth Moore Regional Hospital[2]	Pinehurst	98%	1129
High Point Regional Hospital[2]	High Point	98%	344
Iredell Memorial Hospital[2]	Statesville	98%	238
Johnston Memorial Hospital	Smithfield	98%	285
Margaret R Pardee Memorial Hospital[2]	Hendersonville	98%	284
Memorial Mission Hospital[2]	Asheville	98%	2378
The Outer Banks Hospital	Nags Head	98%	85
Presbyterian Hospital Matthews[2]	Matthews	98%	303
Rex Hospital[2]	Raleigh	98%	674
Scotland Memorial Hospital	Laurinburg	98%	204
University of North Carolina Hospital[2]	Chapel Hill	98%	309
W G (Bill) Hefner Salisbury VA Med Ctr	Salisbury	98%	44
Wakemed - Raleigh Campus[2]	Raleigh	98%	511
Watauga Medical Center	Boone	98%	224
Wilkes Regional Medical Center	N Wilkesboro	98%	111
Alamance Regional Medical Center	Burlington	97%	519
Carolinas Medical Center-Mercy[2]	Charlotte	97%	1774
Columbus Regional Healthcare System	Whiteville	97%	138
Duke University Hospital[2]	Durham	97%	396
Halifax Regional Medical Center[2]	Roanoke Rapids	97%	285
Lenoir Memorial Hospital	Kinston	97%	317
Maria Parham Hospital	Henderson	97%	95
Murphy Medical Center	Murphy	97%	117
Onslow Memorial Hospital	Jacksonville	97%	194
Park Ridge Hospital	Fletcher	97%	141
Pitt County Memorial Hospital[2]	Greenville	97%	1919
Roanoke Chowan Hospital	Ahoskie	97%	143
Stanly Regional Medical Center	Albemarle	97%	121
Wayne Memorial Hospital[2]	Goldsboro	97%	386
Wilson Medical Center[2]	Wilson	97%	397
Carolina East Medical Center	New Bern	96%	1028
Catawba Valley Medical Center	Hickory	96%	472
Frye Regional Medical Center[2]	Hickory	96%	517
The Moses H Cone Memorial Hospital[2]	Greensboro	96%	753
Nash General Hospital[2]	Rocky Mount	96%	564
Northern Hospital of Surry County	Mount Airy	96%	235
Person Memorial Hospital	Roxboro	96%	144
Wakemed - Cary Hospital[2]	Cary	96%	208
Betsy Johnson Regional Hospital	Dunn	95%	125
C J Harris Community Hospital[2]	Sylva	95%	212
Caldwell Memorial Hospital	Lenoir	95%	199
Grace Hospital	Morganton	95%	129
Granville Medical Center	Oxford	95%	147
Lexington Memorial Hospital	Lexington	95%	236
The Mcdowell Hospital	Marion	95%	64
Morehead Memorial Hospital	Eden	95%	112
New Hanover Regional Medical Center[2]	Wilmington	95%	622
Randolph Hospital[2]	Asheboro	95%	125
Spruce Pine Community Hospital	Spruce Pine	95%	104
Haywood Regional Medical Center	Clyde	94%	341
Duke Health Raleigh Hospital	Raleigh	93%	799
Sampson Regional Medical Center	Clinton	91%	79

27. Prophylactic Antibiotic Timing (Outpatient)

Hospital Name	City	Rate	Cases
Cleveland Regional Medical Center	Shelby	100%	249
Davis Regional Medical Center	Statesville	100%	308
Hugh Chatham Memorial Hospital	Elkin	100%	99
Lake Norman Regional Medical Center	Mooresville	100%	469
Spruce Pine Community Hospital	Spruce Pine	100%	25
Carolinas Medical Center-Northeast	Concord	99%	565
Carteret General Hospital	Morehead City	99%	152
Gaston Memorial Hospital	Gastonia	99%	750
Heritage Hospital	Tarboro	99%	154
Medical Park Hospital	Winston-Salem	99%	434
Presbyterian-Orthopaedic Hospital	Charlotte	99%	692
Rowan Regional Medical Center	Salisbury	99%	526
Carolinas Medical Center-University	Charlotte	98%	362
Forsyth Memorial Hospital	Winston-Salem	98%	1706
Martin General Hospital	Williamston	98%	54
Presbyterian Hospital Matthews	Matthews	98%	336
Albemarle Hospital Authority	Elizabeth City	97%	256
Catawba Valley Medical Center	Hickory	97%	649
Durham Regional Hospital	Durham	97%	560
Frye Regional Medical Center	Hickory	97%	693
Memorial Mission Hospital	Asheville	97%	1003
North Carolina Baptist Hospital	Winston-Salem	97%	672
North Carolina Specialty Hospital	Durham	97%	95
Presbyterian Hospital	Charlotte	97%	1140
Presbyterian Hospital Huntersville	Huntersville	97%	162
Sandhills Regional Medical Center	Hamlet	97%	37
Wakemed - Cary Hospital	Cary	97%	366
Brunswick Community Hospital	Supply	96%	98
Grace Hospital	Morganton	96%	333
Johnston Memorial Hospital	Smithfield	96%	252
The Moses H Cone Memorial Hospital	Greensboro	96%	969
Thomasville Medical Center	Thomasville	96%	211
Wakemed - Raleigh Campus	Raleigh	96%	955
Wilson Medical Center	Wilson	96%	93
Carolinas Medical Center-Union	Monroe	95%	170
Maria Parham Hospital	Henderson	95%	81
The Mcdowell Hospital	Marion	95%	57
Park Ridge Hospital	Fletcher	95%	126
Randolph Hospital	Asheboro	95%	193
Scotland Memorial Hospital	Laurinburg	95%	153
Southeastern Regional Medical Center	Lumberton	95%	357
Caldwell Memorial Hospital	Lenoir	94%	105
Central Carolina Hospital	Sanford	94%	200
Margaret R Pardee Memorial Hospital	Hendersonville	94%	223
Nash General Hospital	Rocky Mount	94%	400
Rex Hospital	Raleigh	94%	1091
University of North Carolina Hospital	Chapel Hill	94%	688
Alamance Regional Medical Center	Burlington	93%	283
Granville Medical Center	Oxford	93%	43
New Hanover Regional Medical Center	Wilmington	93%	751
Pitt County Memorial Hospital	Greenville	93%	1400
Watauga Medical Center	Boone	93%	128
Cape Fear Valley Medical Center	Fayetteville	92%	486
Carolina East Medical Center	New Bern	92%	589
Carolinas Medical Center-Mercy	Charlotte	92%	1223
Halifax Regional Medical Center	Roanoke Rapids	92%	135
Iredell Memorial Hospital	Statesville	92%	200
Valdese General Hospital	Valdese	92%	87
Wayne Memorial Hospital	Goldsboro	92%	344
Beaufort County Medical Center	Washington	91%	160
Lexington Memorial Hospital	Lexington	91%	205
Onslow Memorial Hospital	Jacksonville	91%	233
C J Harris Community Hospital	Sylva	90%	144
High Point Regional Hospital	High Point	90%	489
Rutherford Hospital	Rutherfordton	90%	117
Morehead Memorial Hospital	Eden	89%	72
Murphy Medical Center	Murphy	89%	27
Northern Hospital of Surry County	Mount Airy	89%	70
Duke University Hospital	Durham	88%	749
Carolinas Medical Center-Behavioral Health	Charlotte	87%	1148
Duke Health Raleigh Hospital	Raleigh	87%	515
Betsy Johnson Regional Hospital	Dunn	86%	157
Haywood Regional Medical Center	Clyde	86%	266
Firsthealth Moore Regional Hospital	Pinehurst	84%	614
Roanoke Chowan Hospital	Ahoskie	84%	37
Columbus Regional Healthcare System	Whiteville	80%	40
Stanly Regional Medical Center	Albemarle	80%	127
Lenoir Memorial Hospital	Kinston	73%	142

28. Prophylactic Antibiotic Selection

Hospital Name	City	Rate	Cases
Angel Medical Center	Franklin	100%	47
Asheville-Oteen VA Medical Center	Asheville	100%	389
Brunswick Community Hospital	Supply	100%	233
Carolinas Medical Center-Northeast[2]	Concord	100%	978
Carteret General Hospital	Morehead City	100%	306
Chowan Hospital	Edenton	100%	139
Duplin General Hospital	Kenansville	100%	35
Forsyth Memorial Hospital[2]	Winston-Salem	100%	2095
Martin General Hospital[2]	Williamston	100%	91
Medical Park Hospital[2]	Winston-Salem	100%	230
Memorial Mission Hospital[2]	Asheville	100%	2405
North Carolina Specialty Hospital[2]	Durham	100%	187
Presbyterian Hospital Huntersville[2]	Huntersville	100%	396
Presbyterian-Orthopaedic Hospital[2]	Charlotte	100%	1256
Saint Lukes Hospital	Columbus	100%	137
Sandhills Regional Medical Center	Hamlet	100%	39
Transylvania Regional Hospital	Brevard	100%	87
Caldwell Memorial Hospital	Lenoir	99%	202
Carolinas Medical Center-Lincoln	Lincolnton	99%	83
Carolinas Medical Center-Mercy[2]	Charlotte	99%	1780
Carolinas Medical Center-Union[2]	Monroe	99%	235
Catawba Valley Medical Center	Hickory	99%	476
Durham Regional Hospital[2]	Durham	99%	781
Frye Regional Medical Center[2]	Hickory	99%	522
Gaston Memorial Hospital	Gastonia	99%	902
Granville Medical Center	Oxford	99%	148
Halifax Regional Medical Center[2]	Roanoke Rapids	99%	290
The Moses H Cone Memorial Hospital[2]	Greensboro	99%	754
Nash General Hospital[2]	Rocky Mount	99%	565
North Carolina Baptist Hospital[2]	Winston-Salem	99%	633
Northern Hospital of Surry County	Mount Airy	99%	235
The Outer Banks Hospital	Nags Head	99%	85
Person Memorial Hospital	Roxboro	99%	146
Presbyterian Hospital[2]	Charlotte	99%	1124
Presbyterian Hospital Matthews[2]	Matthews	99%	303
Rowan Regional Medical Center[2]	Salisbury	99%	585
Spruce Pine Community Hospital	Spruce Pine	99%	103
Valdese General Hospital	Valdese	99%	108
Wilson Medical Center[2]	Wilson	99%	421
Albemarle Hospital Authority[2]	Elizabeth City	98%	146
Betsy Johnson Regional Hospital	Dunn	98%	125
C J Harris Community Hospital[2]	Sylva	98%	214
Carolinas Medical Center-University[2]	Charlotte	98%	239
Davis Regional Medical Center	Statesville	98%	120
Duke Health Raleigh Hospital	Raleigh	98%	801
Durham VA Medical Center	Durham	98%	180
Firsthealth Moore Regional Hospital[2]	Pinehurst	98%	1140
Grace Hospital	Morganton	98%	128
Haywood Regional Medical Center	Clyde	98%	340
Heritage Hospital	Tarboro	98%	64
Hugh Chatham Memorial Hospital	Elkin	98%	312
Lake Norman Regional Medical Center	Mooresville	98%	227
Lexington Memorial Hospital	Lexington	98%	235
Margaret R Pardee Memorial Hospital[2]	Hendersonville	98%	285
Morehead Memorial Hospital	Eden	98%	109
Pitt County Memorial Hospital[2]	Greenville	98%	1950
Rutherford Hospital	Rutherfordton	98%	245
Scotland Memorial Hospital	Laurinburg	98%	205
Thomasville Medical Center[2]	Thomasville	98%	99
University of North Carolina Hospital[2]	Chapel Hill	98%	313
W G (Bill) Hefner Salisbury VA Med Ctr	Salisbury	98%	43

NOTE: Hospital profiles are in alphabetical order by state, then city, then hospital within the city; Rankings exclude hospitals with less than 25 cases except for patient surveys which excludes hospitals with less than 100 cases; (a) 100–299 cases; (1) The number of cases is too small to be sure how well a hospital is performing; (2) The hospital indicated that the data submitted for this measure were based on a sample of cases; (3) Data was collected during a shorter time period (fewer quarters) than the maximum possible time for this measure; (4) Suppressed for one or more quarters by CMS; (5) No data is available from the hospital for this measure; (6) Fewer than 100 patients completed the HCAHPS survey. Use these rates with caution, as the number of surveys may be too low to reliably assess hospital performance; (7) Survey results are based on less than 12 months of data; (8) Survey results are not available for this reporting period; (9) No or very few patients were eligible for the HCAHPS survey. The scores shown, if any, reflect a very small number of surveys; (10) A state average was not calculated because too few hospitals in the state submitted data; (11) There were discrepancies in the data collection process; Please refer to the User's Guide for a full explanation of data.

Wakemed - Raleigh Campus[2]	Raleigh	98%	523
Cape Fear Valley Medical Center[2]	Fayetteville	97%	451
Carolina East Medical Center	New Bern	97%	1031
Carolinas Medical Center-Behavioral Health[2]	Charlotte	97%	1675
Duke University Hospital[2]	Durham	97%	405
High Point Regional Hospital[2]	High Point	97%	348
Randolph Hospital[2]	Asheboro	97%	126
Rex Hospital[2]	Raleigh	97%	675
Roanoke Chowan Hospital	Ahoskie	97%	143
Sampson Regional Medical Center	Clinton	97%	79
Southeastern Regional Medical Center	Lumberton	97%	251
Stanly Regional Medical Center	Albemarle	97%	121
Wakemed - Cary Hospital[2]	Cary	97%	212
Wayne Memorial Hospital[2]	Goldsboro	97%	386
Columbus Regional Healthcare System	Whiteville	96%	138
Iredell Memorial Hospital[2]	Statesville	96%	240
New Hanover Regional Medical Center[2]	Wilmington	96%	633
Onslow Memorial Hospital	Jacksonville	96%	197
Watauga Medical Center	Boone	96%	226
Beaufort County Medical Center	Washington	95%	182
Lenoir Memorial Hospital	Kinston	95%	320
Park Ridge Hospital	Fletcher	95%	148
Alamance Regional Medical Center	Burlington	94%	520
Cleveland Regional Medical Center[2]	Shelby	94%	441
Maria Parham Hospital	Henderson	94%	96
Murphy Medical Center	Murphy	93%	119
The Mcdowell Hospital	Marion	91%	64
Central Carolina Hospital[2]	Sanford	90%	101
Johnston Memorial Hospital	Smithfield	89%	287
Wilkes Regional Medical Center	N Wilkesboro	88%	110

29. Prophylactic Antibiotic Selection (Outpatient)

Hospital Name	City	Rate	Cases
Presbyterian-Orthopaedic Hospital	Charlotte	100%	687
Beaufort County Medical Center	Washington	99%	163
Davis Regional Medical Center	Statesville	99%	308
Durham Regional Hospital	Durham	99%	556
Forsyth Memorial Hospital	Winston-Salem	99%	1702
Hugh Chatham Memorial Hospital	Elkin	99%	100
Medical Park Hospital	Winston-Salem	99%	434
Rowan Regional Medical Center	Salisbury	99%	526
Wakemed - Raleigh Campus	Raleigh	99%	933
Carolinas Medical Center-Mercy	Charlotte	98%	1174
Catawba Valley Medical Center	Hickory	98%	638
Duke Health Raleigh Hospital	Raleigh	98%	508
Frye Regional Medical Center	Hickory	98%	684
Memorial Mission Hospital	Asheville	98%	1003
North Carolina Baptist Hospital	Winston-Salem	98%	680
Presbyterian Hospital	Charlotte	98%	1141
Presbyterian Hospital Matthews	Matthews	98%	336
Wayne Memorial Hospital	Goldsboro	98%	333
Wilson Medical Center	Wilson	98%	93
Carolinas Medical Center-Northeast	Concord	97%	563
Gaston Memorial Hospital	Gastonia	97%	749
Lake Norman Regional Medical Center	Mooresville	97%	468
North Carolina Specialty Hospital	Durham	97%	95
Betsy Johnson Regional Hospital	Dunn	96%	142
Carolinas Medical Center-Behavioral Health	Charlotte	96%	1168
Carolinas Medical Center-Union	Monroe	96%	166
Carolinas Medical Center-University	Charlotte	96%	362
Firsthealth Moore Regional Hospital	Pinehurst	96%	599
Haywood Regional Medical Center	Clyde	96%	266
Martin General Hospital	Williamston	96%	55
The Mcdowell Hospital	Marion	96%	54
The Moses H Cone Memorial Hospital	Greensboro	96%	948
Alamance Regional Medical Center	Burlington	95%	273
Caldwell Memorial Hospital	Lenoir	95%	104
Carteret General Hospital	Morehead City	95%	152
Granville Medical Center	Oxford	95%	42
Halifax Regional Medical Center	Roanoke Rapids	95%	129
Margaret R Pardee Memorial Hospital	Hendersonville	95%	214
Park Ridge Hospital	Fletcher	95%	131
Roanoke Chowan Hospital	Ahoskie	95%	43
Southeastern Regional Medical Center	Lumberton	95%	344
Wakemed - Cary Hospital	Cary	95%	365
Carolina East Medical Center	New Bern	94%	571
Maria Parham Hospital	Henderson	94%	81
Nash General Hospital	Rocky Mount	94%	409
Onslow Memorial Hospital	Jacksonville	94%	228
Pitt County Memorial Hospital	Greenville	94%	1374
Presbyterian Hospital Huntersville	Huntersville	94%	161
University of North Carolina Hospital	Chapel Hill	94%	685
Heritage Hospital	Tarboro	93%	153
Iredell Memorial Hospital	Statesville	93%	192
Morehead Memorial Hospital	Eden	93%	68
New Hanover Regional Medical Center	Wilmington	93%	733
Thomasville Medical Center	Thomasville	93%	204
Albemarle Hospital Authority	Elizabeth City	92%	252
Grace Hospital	Morganton	92%	324
Murphy Medical Center	Murphy	92%	25
Rex Hospital	Raleigh	92%	1060
Rutherford Hospital	Rutherfordton	92%	111
Sandhills Regional Medical Center	Hamlet	92%	37
Spruce Pine Community Hospital	Spruce Pine	92%	25
C J Harris Community Hospital	Sylva	91%	139
Cleveland Regional Medical Center	Shelby	91%	249
Lenoir Memorial Hospital	Kinston	91%	112
Lexington Memorial Hospital	Lexington	91%	201
Randolph Hospital	Asheboro	91%	191
Valdese General Hospital	Valdese	90%	82
Central Carolina Hospital	Sanford	89%	194
Brunswick Community Hospital	Supply	88%	95
Johnston Memorial Hospital	Smithfield	88%	247
Northern Hospital of Surry County	Mount Airy	88%	68
Scotland Memorial Hospital	Laurinburg	88%	153
Stanly Regional Medical Center	Albemarle	88%	129
Duke University Hospital	Durham	87%	832
Columbus Regional Healthcare System	Whiteville	84%	32
Cape Fear Valley Medical Center	Fayetteville	83%	471
Watauga Medical Center	Boone	79%	123
High Point Regional Hospital	High Point	68%	470

30. Prophylactic Antibiotic Stopped

Hospital Name	City	Rate	Cases
Forsyth Memorial Hospital[2]	Winston-Salem	100%	1984
Gaston Memorial Hospital	Gastonia	100%	846
Martin General Hospital[2]	Williamston	100%	91
Medical Park Hospital[2]	Winston-Salem	100%	220
The Outer Banks Hospital	Nags Head	100%	80
W G (Bill) Hefner Salisbury VA Med Ctr	Salisbury	100%	42
Asheville-Oteen VA Medical Center	Asheville	99%	369
Chowan Hospital	Edenton	99%	136
Duke University Hospital[2]	Durham	99%	371
Lake Norman Regional Medical Center	Mooresville	99%	201
North Carolina Specialty Hospital[2]	Durham	99%	186
Person Memorial Hospital[2]	Roxboro	99%	143
Presbyterian Hospital[2]	Charlotte	99%	1037
Presbyterian-Orthopaedic Hospital[2]	Charlotte	99%	1234
Rowan Regional Medical Center[2]	Salisbury	99%	553
Thomasville Medical Center[2]	Thomasville	99%	81
Transylvania Regional Hospital	Brevard	99%	83
Beaufort County Medical Center	Washington	98%	173
Brunswick Community Hospital	Supply	98%	220
Carolinas Medical Center-Northeast[2]	Concord	98%	921
Carteret General Hospital	Morehead City	98%	297
Duke Health Raleigh Hospital	Raleigh	98%	789
Firsthealth Moore Regional Hospital[2]	Pinehurst	98%	1095
Halifax Regional Medical Center[2]	Roanoke Rapids	98%	274
Haywood Regional Medical Center	Clyde	98%	329
Hugh Chatham Memorial Hospital	Elkin	98%	299
Lexington Memorial Hospital	Lexington	98%	229
Margaret R Pardee Memorial Hospital[2]	Hendersonville	98%	273
Northern Hospital of Surry County	Mount Airy	98%	231
Presbyterian Hospital Huntersville[2]	Huntersville	98%	387
Presbyterian Hospital Matthews[2]	Matthews	98%	290
Saint Lukes Hospital	Columbus	98%	129
Scotland Memorial Hospital	Laurinburg	98%	198
Wakemed - Raleigh Campus[2]	Raleigh	98%	484
Albemarle Hospital Authority[2]	Elizabeth City	97%	128
Carolinas Medical Center-Behavioral Health[2]	Charlotte	97%	1581
Carolinas Medical Center-Mercy[2]	Charlotte	97%	1747
Carolinas Medical Center-Union[2]	Monroe	97%	216
Carolinas Medical Center-University[2]	Charlotte	97%	227
Durham Regional Hospital[2]	Durham	97%	747
Memorial Mission Hospital[2]	Asheville	97%	2258
The Moses H Cone Memorial Hospital[2]	Greensboro	97%	712
North Carolina Baptist Hospital[2]	Winston-Salem	97%	599
Roanoke Chowan Hospital	Ahoskie	97%	136
C J Harris Community Hospital[2]	Sylva	96%	193
Carolinas Medical Center-Lincoln	Lincolnton	96%	68
High Point Regional Hospital[2]	High Point	96%	288
Murphy Medical Center	Murphy	96%	116
Rutherford Hospital	Rutherfordton	96%	233
Southeastern Regional Medical Center	Lumberton	96%	239
Spruce Pine Community Hospital	Spruce Pine	96%	100
Catawba Valley Medical Center	Hickory	95%	463
Heritage Hospital	Tarboro	95%	62
Iredell Memorial Hospital[2]	Statesville	95%	228
Nash General Hospital[2]	Rocky Mount	95%	550
Park Ridge Hospital	Fletcher	95%	125
Rex Hospital[2]	Raleigh	95%	654
Central Carolina Hospital[2]	Sanford	94%	97
Duplin General Hospital	Kenansville	94%	31
Granville Medical Center	Oxford	94%	133
Onslow Memorial Hospital	Jacksonville	94%	186
Pitt County Memorial Hospital[2]	Greenville	94%	1822
Stanly Regional Medical Center	Albemarle	94%	108
University of North Carolina Hospital[2]	Chapel Hill	94%	294
Alamance Regional Medical Center	Burlington	93%	506
Cleveland Regional Medical Center[2]	Shelby	93%	432
Columbus Regional Healthcare System	Whiteville	93%	128
Davis Regional Medical Center	Statesville	93%	114
Maria Parham Hospital	Henderson	93%	91
New Hanover Regional Medical Center[2]	Wilmington	93%	579
Valdese General Hospital	Valdese	93%	103
Wakemed - Cary Hospital[2]	Cary	93%	198
Wayne Memorial Hospital[2]	Goldsboro	93%	378
Durham VA Medical Center	Durham	92%	174
Grace Hospital	Morganton	92%	117
Lenoir Memorial Hospital	Kinston	92%	305
Wilkes Regional Medical Center	N Wilkesboro	92%	102
Betsy Johnson Regional Hospital	Dunn	91%	121
Cape Fear Valley Medical Center[2]	Fayetteville	91%	434
Frye Regional Medical Center[2]	Hickory	91%	495
Randolph Hospital[2]	Asheboro	91%	116
Sandhills Regional Medical Center	Hamlet	91%	35
Caldwell Memorial Hospital	Lenoir	90%	187
Watauga Medical Center	Boone	90%	212
The Mcdowell Hospital	Marion	89%	57
Wilson Medical Center[2]	Wilson	89%	394
Carolina East Medical Center	New Bern	88%	1004
Johnston Memorial Hospital	Smithfield	88%	277
Sampson Regional Medical Center	Clinton	87%	75
Angel Medical Center	Franklin	85%	46
Morehead Memorial Hospital	Eden	78%	99

31. Recommended VTP Ordered

Hospital Name	City	Rate	Cases
Duke University Hospital[2]	Durham	100%	202
North Carolina Specialty Hospital[2]	Durham	100%	47
The Outer Banks Hospital	Nags Head	100%	37
Presbyterian-Orthopaedic Hospital[2]	Charlotte	100%	616
Roanoke Chowan Hospital	Ahoskie	100%	66
Rowan Regional Medical Center[2]	Salisbury	100%	241
Brunswick Community Hospital	Supply	99%	134
Davis Regional Medical Center	Statesville	99%	135
Gaston Memorial Hospital	Gastonia	99%	394
Granville Medical Center	Oxford	99%	88
High Point Regional Hospital[2]	High Point	99%	131
Hugh Chatham Memorial Hospital	Elkin	99%	118
Northern Hospital of Surry County	Mount Airy	99%	126
Scotland Memorial Hospital	Laurinburg	99%	195
Albemarle Hospital Authority[2]	Elizabeth City	98%	124
Carolinas Medical Center-Behavioral Health[2]	Charlotte	98%	572
Carolinas Medical Center-Mercy[2]	Charlotte	98%	726
Carolinas Medical Center-Union[2]	Monroe	98%	212
Carolinas Medical Center-University[2]	Charlotte	98%	154
Chowan Hospital	Edenton	98%	65
Durham Regional Hospital[2]	Durham	98%	196
Forsyth Memorial Hospital[2]	Winston-Salem	98%	1018
Medical Park Hospital[2]	Winston-Salem	98%	179
Memorial Mission Hospital[2]	Asheville	98%	906
Presbyterian Hospital[2]	Charlotte	98%	499
Rutherford Hospital	Rutherfordton	98%	113
Asheville-Oteen VA Medical Center[2]	Asheville	97%	87
Lake Norman Regional Medical Center	Mooresville	97%	172
New Hanover Regional Medical Center[2]	Wilmington	97%	347
North Carolina Baptist Hospital[2]	Winston-Salem	97%	363
Pitt County Memorial Hospital[2]	Greenville	97%	701
Presbyterian Hospital Matthews[2]	Matthews	97%	216
Southeastern Regional Medical Center	Lumberton	97%	185
University of North Carolina Hospital[2]	Chapel Hill	97%	287
Wakemed - Cary Hospital[2]	Cary	97%	145
Carolinas Medical Center-Northeast[2]	Concord	96%	455
Iredell Memorial Hospital[2]	Statesville	96%	245
Park Ridge Hospital	Fletcher	96%	112
Spruce Pine Community Hospital	Spruce Pine	96%	57
Valdese General Hospital	Valdese	96%	68
Alamance Regional Medical Center	Burlington	95%	431
C J Harris Community Hospital[2]	Sylva	95%	152
Catawba Valley Medical Center	Hickory	95%	263
Cleveland Regional Medical Center[2]	Shelby	95%	170
Firsthealth Moore Regional Hospital[2]	Pinehurst	95%	380
Haywood Regional Medical Center	Clyde	95%	111
Margaret R Pardee Memorial Hospital[2]	Hendersonville	95%	245
Maria Parham Hospital	Henderson	95%	77
Nash General Hospital[2]	Rocky Mount	95%	146
Transylvania Regional Hospital	Brevard	95%	59
Cape Fear Valley Medical Center[2]	Fayetteville	94%	199
The Mcdowell Hospital	Marion	94%	63
Presbyterian Hospital Huntersville[2]	Huntersville	94%	201
Thomasville Medical Center[2]	Thomasville	94%	90
Wayne Memorial Hospital[2]	Goldsboro	94%	303
Angel Medical Center	Franklin	93%	45
Carolina East Medical Center	New Bern	93%	667
Duke Health Raleigh Hospital	Raleigh	93%	414
W G (Bill) Hefner Salisbury VA Med Ctr[2]	Salisbury	93%	40
Wakemed - Raleigh Campus[2]	Raleigh	93%	242
Carolinas Medical Center-Lincoln	Lincolnton	92%	40
Central Carolina Hospital[2]	Sanford	92%	123

NOTE: Hospital profiles are in alphabetical order by state, then city, then hospital within the city; Rankings exclude hospitals with less than 25 cases except for patient surveys which excludes hospitals with less than 100 cases; (a) 100–299 cases; (1) The number of cases is too small to be sure how well a hospital is performing; (2) The hospital indicated that the data submitted for this measure were based on a sample of cases; (3) Data was collected during a shorter time period (fewer quarters) than the maximum possible time for this measure; (4) Suppressed for one or more quarters by CMS; (5) No data is available from the hospital for this measure; (6) Fewer than 100 patients completed the HCAHPS survey. Use these rates with caution, as the number of surveys may be too low to reliably assess hospital performance; (7) Survey results are based on less than 12 months of data; (8) Survey results are not available for this reporting period; (9) No or very few patients were eligible for the HCAHPS survey. The scores shown, if any, reflect a very small number of surveys; (10) A state average was not calculated because too few hospitals in the state submitted data; (11) There were discrepancies in the data collection process; Please refer to the User's Guide for a full explanation of data.

Heritage Hospital	Tarboro	92%	76
Martin General Hospital[2]	Williamston	92%	50
The Moses H Cone Memorial Hospital[2]	Greensboro	92%	416
Caldwell Memorial Hospital	Lenoir	91%	113
Columbus Regional Healthcare System	Whiteville	91%	170
Durham VA Medical Center[2]	Durham	91%	112
Frye Regional Medical Center[2]	Hickory	91%	149
Stanly Regional Medical Center	Albemarle	90%	91
Wilkes Regional Medical Center	N Wilkesboro	90%	83
Kings Mountain Hospital	Kings Mountain	89%	28
Person Memorial Hospital	Roxboro	89%	108
Rex Hospital[2]	Raleigh	89%	288
Morehead Memorial Hospital	Eden	88%	104
Onslow Memorial Hospital	Jacksonville	88%	137
Randolph Hospital[2]	Asheboro	88%	125
Wilson Medical Center[2]	Wilson	88%	169
Lexington Memorial Hospital	Lexington	87%	82
Saint Lukes Hospital	Columbus	86%	36
Watauga Medical Center	Boone	85%	136
Murphy Medical Center	Murphy	84%	64
Beaufort County Medical Center	Washington	83%	108
Betsy Johnson Regional Hospital	Dunn	82%	102
Johnston Memorial Hospital	Smithfield	81%	200
Carteret General Hospital	Morehead City	77%	155
Grace Hospital	Morganton	77%	139
Halifax Regional Medical Center[2]	Roanoke Rapids	76%	76
Lenoir Memorial Hospital	Kinston	70%	221
Sampson Regional Medical Center	Clinton	68%	60

32. Urinary Catheter Removal

Hospital Name	City	Rate	Cases
Asheville-Oteen VA Medical Center[2]	Asheville	100%	297
Gaston Memorial Hospital	Gastonia	100%	358
The Outer Banks Hospital	Nags Head	100%	48
Randolph Hospital[2]	Asheboro	100%	25
Lake Norman Regional Medical Center	Mooresville	99%	70
Rowan Regional Medical Center[2]	Salisbury	99%	166
Davis Regional Medical Center	Statesville	98%	48
Forsyth Memorial Hospital[2]	Winston-Salem	98%	921
Valdese General Hospital	Valdese	98%	45
Wakemed - Raleigh Campus[2]	Raleigh	98%	130
North Carolina Specialty Hospital[2]	Durham	97%	118
Presbyterian Hospital Matthews[2]	Matthews	97%	119
Scotland Memorial Hospital	Laurinburg	97%	93
Wakemed - Cary Hospital[2]	Cary	97%	78
Carolinas Medical Center-Mercy[2]	Charlotte	96%	829
Catawba Valley Medical Center	Hickory	96%	197
Grace Hospital	Morganton	96%	50
Lexington Memorial Hospital	Lexington	96%	81
Presbyterian-Orthopaedic Hospital[2]	Charlotte	96%	604
Southeastern Regional Medical Center	Lumberton	96%	97
Wilson Medical Center[2]	Wilson	96%	186
Brunswick Community Hospital	Supply	95%	82
Durham Regional Hospital[2]	Durham	95%	357
Durham VA Medical Center[2]	Durham	95%	97
Iredell Memorial Hospital[2]	Statesville	95%	61
Memorial Mission Hospital[2]	Asheville	95%	544
Presbyterian Hospital Huntersville[2]	Huntersville	95%	143
Chowan Hospital	Edenton	94%	69
Granville Medical Center	Oxford	94%	68
Maria Parham Hospital	Henderson	94%	32
Nash General Hospital[2]	Rocky Mount	94%	180
Person Memorial Hospital	Roxboro	93%	74
C J Harris Community Hospital[2]	Sylva	92%	74
Columbus Regional Healthcare System	Whiteville	92%	39
Duke University Hospital[2]	Durham	92%	160
Firsthealth Moore Regional Hospital[2]	Pinehurst	92%	244
High Point Regional Hospital[2]	High Point	92%	106
Park Ridge Hospital	Fletcher	92%	49
University of North Carolina Hospital[2]	Chapel Hill	92%	138
Duke Health Raleigh Hospital	Raleigh	91%	447
Frye Regional Medical Center[2]	Hickory	91%	187
Margaret R Pardee Memorial Hospital[2]	Hendersonville	91%	85
Murphy Medical Center	Murphy	91%	33
Saint Lukes Hospital	Columbus	91%	44
Wilkes Regional Medical Center	N Wilkesboro	91%	43
Carolinas Medical Center-Northeast[2]	Concord	90%	398
New Hanover Regional Medical Center[2]	Wilmington	90%	211
Caldwell Memorial Hospital	Lenoir	89%	73
Carolinas Medical Center-Union[2]	Monroe	89%	71
Rex Hospital[2]	Raleigh	89%	245
Beaufort County Medical Center	Washington	88%	93
Medical Park Hospital[2]	Winston-Salem	88%	60
The Moses H Cone Memorial Hospital[2]	Greensboro	88%	280
North Carolina Baptist Hospital[2]	Winston-Salem	88%	229
Presbyterian Hospital[2]	Charlotte	88%	263
Transylvania Regional Hospital	Brevard	88%	25
Cape Fear Valley Medical Center[2]	Fayetteville	87%	127
Onslow Memorial Hospital	Jacksonville	87%	45
Pitt County Memorial Hospital[2]	Greenville	87%	438
Central Carolina Hospital[2]	Sanford	85%	34
Alamance Regional Medical Center	Burlington	84%	199
Watauga Medical Center	Boone	84%	25
Wayne Memorial Hospital[2]	Goldsboro	84%	122
Betsy Johnson Regional Hospital	Dunn	82%	50
Sampson Regional Medical Center	Clinton	82%	40
Cleveland Regional Medical Center[2]	Shelby	81%	91
Stanly Regional Medical Center	Albemarle	81%	27
Johnston Memorial Hospital	Smithfield	80%	110
Carolina East Medical Center	New Bern	76%	422
Lenoir Memorial Hospital	Kinston	73%	62
Morehead Memorial Hospital	Eden	73%	26
Albemarle Hospital Authority[2]	Elizabeth City	68%	37
Northern Hospital of Surry County	Mount Airy	68%	25
Carolinas Medical Center-Behavioral Health[2]	Charlotte	65%	337
Carteret General Hospital	Morehead City	60%	30

Children's Asthma Care

33. Received Systemic Corticosteroids

Hospital Name	City	Rate	Cases
Carolinas Medical Center-Behavioral Health	Charlotte	100%	429
Carolinas Medical Center-Northeast	Concord	100%	44
Davis Regional Medical Center	Statesville	100%	29
Firsthealth Moore Regional Hospital	Pinehurst	100%	55
Lake Norman Regional Medical Center	Mooresville	100%	25
Memorial Mission Hospital	Asheville	100%	36
North Carolina Baptist Hospital[2]	Winston-Salem	100%	72
Presbyterian Hospital	Charlotte	100%	173
Wilson Medical Center	Wilson	97%	30

34. Received Home Management Plan of Care

Hospital Name	City	Rate	Cases
Davis Regional Medical Center	Statesville	97%	29
Wilson Medical Center	Wilson	90%	30
Carolinas Medical Center-Behavioral Health	Charlotte	87%	427
Carolinas Medical Center-Northeast	Concord	82%	45
Presbyterian Hospital	Charlotte	82%	172
North Carolina Baptist Hospital[2]	Winston-Salem	68%	72
Firsthealth Moore Regional Hospital	Pinehurst	22%	54
Memorial Mission Hospital	Asheville	19%	36

35. Received Reliever Medication

Hospital Name	City	Rate	Cases
Carolinas Medical Center-Behavioral Health	Charlotte	100%	430
Carolinas Medical Center-Northeast	Concord	100%	45
Davis Regional Medical Center	Statesville	100%	29
Firsthealth Moore Regional Hospital	Pinehurst	100%	55
Lake Norman Regional Medical Center	Mooresville	100%	25
Memorial Mission Hospital	Asheville	100%	36
North Carolina Baptist Hospital[2]	Winston-Salem	100%	72
Presbyterian Hospital	Charlotte	100%	173
Wilson Medical Center	Wilson	97%	30

Use of Medical Imaging

36. Combination Abdominal CT Scan

Hospital Name	City	Ratio	Cases
Forsyth Memorial Hospital	Winston-Salem	0.001	991
High Point Regional Hospital	High Point	0.013	748
Memorial Mission Hospital	Asheville	0.013	1109
Durham Regional Hospital	Durham	0.020	744
Thomasville Medical Center	Thomasville	0.021	387
Presbyterian Hospital	Charlotte	0.024	829
Cape Fear Valley-Bladen County Hospital	Elizabethtown	0.025	278
Wayne Memorial Hospital	Goldsboro	0.026	495
Anson Community Hospital	Wadesboro	0.027	222
The Mcdowell Hospital	Marion	0.028	464
Iredell Memorial Hospital	Statesville	0.029	756
Maria Parham Hospital	Henderson	0.029	653
Carolinas Medical Center-Lincoln	Lincolnton	0.030	467
Randolph Hospital	Asheboro	0.032	727
The Moses H Cone Memorial Hospital	Greensboro	0.033	1813
Presbyterian Hospital Huntersville	Huntersville	0.033	850
Albemarle Hospital Authority	Elizabeth City	0.037	730
Southeastern Regional Medical Center	Lumberton	0.037	970
Granville Medical Center	Oxford	0.038	286
Rutherford Hospital	Rutherfordton	0.039	837
Nash General Hospital	Rocky Mount	0.040	970
Carolinas Medical Center-Northeast	Concord	0.042	2369
Lexington Memorial Hospital	Lexington	0.045	514
Presbyterian-Orthopaedic Hospital	Charlotte	0.045	156
Gaston Memorial Hospital	Gastonia	0.046	1769
Wakemed - Raleigh Campus	Raleigh	0.049	835
Brunswick Community Hospital	Supply	0.050	516
Wakemed - Cary Hospital	Cary	0.050	619
Presbyterian Hospital Matthews	Matthews	0.051	1365
New Hanover Regional Medical Center	Wilmington	0.053	1836
Catawba Valley Medical Center	Hickory	0.055	875
Caldwell Memorial Hospital	Lenoir	0.059	438
Carteret General Hospital	Morehead City	0.059	909
University of North Carolina Hospital	Chapel Hill	0.059	1762
Heritage Hospital	Tarboro	0.066	304
Carolina East Medical Center	New Bern	0.069	598
Davis Regional Medical Center	Statesville	0.070	329
Frye Regional Medical Center	Hickory	0.070	952
Franklin Regional Medical Center	Louisburg	0.075	255
Person Memorial Hospital	Roxboro	0.075	227
Stanly Regional Medical Center	Albemarle	0.079	828
Lake Norman Regional Medical Center	Mooresville	0.080	858
Carolinas Medical Center-Mercy	Charlotte	0.081	1763
Haywood Regional Medical Center	Clyde	0.084	370
Carolinas Medical Center-University	Charlotte	0.085	845
Pitt County Memorial Hospital	Greenville	0.088	1155
Alamance Regional Medical Center	Burlington	0.090	1037
Beaufort County Medical Center	Washington	0.090	633
Carolinas Medical Center-Union	Monroe	0.090	1185
Firsthealth Moore Regional Hospital	Pinehurst	0.090	1089
Park Ridge Hospital	Fletcher	0.091	463
Duke University Hospital	Durham	0.092	3829
Halifax Regional Medical Center	Roanoke Rapids	0.092	606
Hugh Chatham Memorial Hospital	Elkin	0.093	518
Roanoke Chowan Hospital	Ahoskie	0.094	448
Columbus Regional Healthcare System	Whiteville	0.098	500
Scotland Memorial Hospital	Laurinburg	0.099	1048
Johnston Memorial Hospital	Smithfield	0.105	553
Wilkes Regional Medical Center	N Wilkesboro	0.105	743
Onslow Memorial Hospital	Jacksonville	0.107	579
Northern Hospital of Surry County	Mount Airy	0.108	986
Carolinas Medical Center-Behavioral Health	Charlotte	0.109	1772
Grace Hospital	Morganton	0.116	302
Duplin General Hospital	Kenansville	0.117	264
Saint Lukes Hospital	Columbus	0.125	305
Central Carolina Hospital	Sanford	0.126	525
Wilson Medical Center	Wilson	0.126	1007
Margaret R Pardee Memorial Hospital	Hendersonville	0.127	1234
Morehead Memorial Hospital	Eden	0.127	503
Duke Health Raleigh Hospital	Raleigh	0.129	775
Valdese General Hospital	Valdese	0.137	263
Cape Fear Valley Medical Center	Fayetteville	0.140	1359
Rowan Regional Medical Center	Salisbury	0.170	949
Rex Hospital	Raleigh	0.173	1430
Watauga Medical Center	Boone	0.210	572
Betsy Johnson Regional Hospital	Dunn	0.228	707
North Carolina Baptist Hospital	Winston-Salem	0.293	3253
Lenoir Memorial Hospital	Kinston	0.324	565
Murphy Medical Center	Murphy	0.366	755
Sampson Regional Medical Center	Clinton	0.395	588
Alleghany County Memorial Hospital	Sparta	0.469	81
Sandhills Regional Medical Center	Hamlet	0.545	132
C J Harris Community Hospital	Sylva	0.583	544
Kings Mountain Hospital	Kings Mountain	0.585	205
Cleveland Regional Medical Center	Shelby	0.655	1011
Martin General Hospital	Williamston	0.689	135
Ashe Memorial Hospital	Jefferson	0.710	279
Spruce Pine Community Hospital	Spruce Pine	0.790	315
Washington County Hospital	Plymouth	0.881	67

37. Combination Chest CT Scan

Hospital Name	City	Ratio	Cases
Alamance Regional Medical Center	Burlington	0.000	942
Alleghany County Memorial Hospital[1]	Sparta	0.000	33
Caldwell Memorial Hospital	Lenoir	0.000	327
Carolinas Medical Center-Behavioral Health	Charlotte	0.000	1593
Carteret General Hospital	Morehead City	0.000	658
Duplin General Hospital	Kenansville	0.000	166
Forsyth Memorial Hospital	Winston-Salem	0.000	204
Halifax Regional Medical Center	Roanoke Rapids	0.000	458
Kings Mountain Hospital	Kings Mountain	0.000	92
Lenoir Memorial Hospital	Kinston	0.000	400
Martin General Hospital	Williamston	0.000	101
Memorial Mission Hospital	Asheville	0.000	407
Northern Hospital of Surry County	Mount Airy	0.000	786
Presbyterian Hospital Huntersville	Huntersville	0.000	695
Presbyterian Hospital Matthews	Matthews	0.000	907
Presbyterian-Orthopaedic Hospital	Charlotte	0.000	107
University of North Carolina Hospital	Chapel Hill	0.000	1929
Valdese General Hospital	Valdese	0.000	272
Washington County Hospital[1]	Plymouth	0.000	35
Albemarle Hospital Authority	Elizabeth City	0.001	679
The Moses H Cone Memorial Hospital	Greensboro	0.001	1623
Cleveland Regional Medical Center	Shelby	0.002	896
Rutherford Hospital	Rutherfordton	0.002	412
Carolinas Medical Center-University	Charlotte	0.003	372
Lexington Memorial Hospital	Lexington	0.003	349
The Mcdowell Hospital	Marion	0.003	291
Presbyterian Hospital	Charlotte	0.003	380
Heritage Hospital	Tarboro	0.005	201

NOTE: Hospital profiles are in alphabetical order by state, then city, then hospital within the city; Rankings exclude hospitals with less than 25 cases except for patient surveys which excludes hospitals with less than 100 cases; (a) 100–299 cases; (1) The number of cases is too small to be sure how well a hospital is performing; (2) The hospital indicated that the data submitted for this measure were based on a sample of cases; (3) Data was collected during a shorter time period (fewer quarters) than the maximum possible time for this measure; (4) Suppressed for one or more quarters by CMS; (5) No data is available from the hospital for this measure; (6) Fewer than 100 patients completed the HCAHPS survey. Use these rates with caution, as the number of surveys may be too low to reliably assess hospital performance; (7) Survey results are based on less than 12 months of data; (8) Survey results are not available for this reporting period; (9) No or very few patients were eligible for the HCAHPS survey. The scores shown, if any, reflect a very small number of surveys; (10) A state average was not calculated because too few hospitals in the state submitted data; (11) There were discrepancies in the data collection process; Please refer to the User's Guide for a full explanation of data.

Iredell Memorial Hospital	Statesville	0.005	366
Roanoke Chowan Hospital	Ahoskie	0.005	200
Murphy Medical Center	Murphy	0.006	473
New Hanover Regional Medical Center	Wilmington	0.006	1150
North Carolina Baptist Hospital	Winston-Salem	0.006	3046
Gaston Memorial Hospital	Gastonia	0.008	1005
Granville Medical Center	Oxford	0.008	126
Onslow Memorial Hospital	Jacksonville	0.008	374
High Point Regional Hospital	High Point	0.009	223
Beaufort County Medical Center	Washington	0.010	492
Hugh Chatham Memorial Hospital	Elkin	0.010	315
Lake Norman Regional Medical Center	Mooresville	0.010	620
Davis Regional Medical Center	Statesville	0.011	89
Grace Hospital	Morganton	0.011	271
Durham Regional Hospital	Durham	0.012	432
Nash General Hospital	Rocky Mount	0.012	490
Cape Fear Valley-Bladen County Hospital	Elizabethtown	0.013	75
Columbus Regional Healthcare System	Whiteville	0.013	237
Pitt County Memorial Hospital	Greenville	0.014	694
Betsy Johnson Regional Hospital	Dunn	0.015	327
Carolinas Medical Center-Mercy	Charlotte	0.016	1267
Catawba Valley Medical Center	Hickory	0.016	708
Person Memorial Hospital	Roxboro	0.016	187
Southeastern Regional Medical Center	Lumberton	0.016	708
Thomasville Medical Center	Thomasville	0.016	190
Maria Parham Hospital	Henderson	0.017	468
Wakemed - Cary Hospital	Cary	0.017	424
Brunswick Community Hospital	Supply	0.018	337
Carolinas Medical Center-Lincoln	Lincolnton	0.020	307
Stanly Regional Medical Center	Albemarle	0.020	543
Anson Community Hospital	Wadesboro	0.023	88
Wayne Memorial Hospital	Goldsboro	0.023	310
Frye Regional Medical Center	Hickory	0.025	849
Firsthealth Moore Regional Hospital	Pinehurst	0.026	926
Haywood Regional Medical Center	Clyde	0.026	308
Carolina East Medical Center	New Bern	0.029	244
Carolinas Medical Center-Northeast	Concord	0.031	2438
Wakemed - Raleigh Campus	Raleigh	0.033	599
Duke University Hospital	Durham	0.034	5860
Johnston Memorial Hospital	Smithfield	0.041	591
Watauga Medical Center	Boone	0.041	462
Margaret R Pardee Memorial Hospital	Hendersonville	0.043	792
Ashe Memorial Hospital	Jefferson	0.050	159
Rex Hospital	Raleigh	0.056	1014
Wilkes Regional Medical Center	N Wilkesboro	0.063	334
Franklin Regional Medical Center	Louisburg	0.070	200
Sampson Regional Medical Center	Clinton	0.081	369
Cape Fear Valley Medical Center	Fayetteville	0.082	944
Park Ridge Hospital	Fletcher	0.092	305
Morehead Memorial Hospital	Eden	0.094	469
Central Carolina Hospital	Sanford	0.099	333
Scotland Memorial Hospital	Laurinburg	0.115	399
Duke Health Raleigh Hospital	Raleigh	0.119	899
C J Harris Community Hospital	Sylva	0.125	655
Randolph Hospital	Asheboro	0.130	532
Saint Lukes Hospital	Columbus	0.144	132
Carolinas Medical Center-Union	Monroe	0.148	896
Rowan Regional Medical Center	Salisbury	0.202	575
Wilson Medical Center	Wilson	0.325	787
Sandhills Regional Medical Center	Hamlet	0.371	97
Spruce Pine Community Hospital	Spruce Pine	0.890	200

38. Follow-up Mammogram/Ultrasound

Hospital Name	City	Rate	Cases
Columbus Regional Healthcare System	Whiteville	2.9%	1328
Alleghany County Memorial Hospital	Sparta	3.0%	298
Iredell Memorial Hospital	Statesville	3.1%	1783
Murphy Medical Center	Murphy	3.1%	786
Hugh Chatham Memorial Hospital	Elkin	3.3%	848
Central Carolina Hospital	Sanford	3.4%	1508
Ashe Memorial Hospital	Jefferson	3.6%	753
Spruce Pine Community Hospital	Spruce Pine	3.7%	574
Wakemed - Cary Hospital	Cary	4.1%	458
Sampson Regional Medical Center	Clinton	4.7%	993
Duplin General Hospital	Kenansville	4.8%	482
The Mcdowell Hospital	Marion	5.0%	707
Stanly Regional Medical Center	Albemarle	5.1%	1442
Wayne Memorial Hospital	Goldsboro	5.1%	292
Carolinas Medical Center-Northeast	Concord	5.4%	3964
Morehead Memorial Hospital	Eden	5.4%	745
Brunswick Community Hospital	Supply	5.5%	1086
High Point Regional Hospital	High Point	5.5%	289
Person Memorial Hospital	Roxboro	5.5%	685
Presbyterian Hospital Matthews	Matthews	5.8%	1153
Rex Hospital	Raleigh	5.8%	1895
Wakemed - Raleigh Campus	Raleigh	5.8%	1184
Heritage Hospital	Tarboro	6.0%	1019
Scotland Memorial Hospital	Laurinburg	6.2%	1181
Martin General Hospital	Williamston	6.4%	515
Northern Hospital of Surry County	Mount Airy	6.5%	1137
Cape Fear Valley Medical Center	Fayetteville	6.6%	1006
Thomasville Medical Center	Thomasville	6.6%	588
Alamance Regional Medical Center	Burlington	6.9%	2443
The Moses H Cone Memorial Hospital	Greensboro	7.1%	1837
Frye Regional Medical Center	Hickory	7.5%	2322
University of North Carolina Hospital	Chapel Hill	7.5%	1715
Cape Fear Valley-Bladen County Hospital	Elizabethtown	7.6%	409
Wilson Medical Center	Wilson	7.6%	1520
Duke University Hospital	Durham	7.7%	2854
Haywood Regional Medical Center	Clyde	7.7%	673
Lexington Memorial Hospital	Lexington	7.8%	857
Lake Norman Regional Medical Center	Mooresville	7.9%	1339
Catawba Valley Medical Center	Hickory	8.3%	2280
Maria Parham Hospital	Henderson	8.4%	1250
North Carolina Baptist Hospital	Winston-Salem	8.5%	1443
Firsthealth Moore Regional Hospital	Pinehurst	8.8%	272
Franklin Regional Medical Center	Louisburg	8.8%	546
Carolina East Medical Center	New Bern	8.9%	1119
Gaston Memorial Hospital	Gastonia	9.0%	3801
New Hanover Regional Medical Center	Wilmington	9.0%	1355
Saint Lukes Hospital	Columbus	9.3%	536
Washington County Hospital	Plymouth	9.3%	225
Wilkes Regional Medical Center	N Wilkesboro	9.3%	1388
Margaret R Pardee Memorial Hospital	Hendersonville	9.4%	2610
Durham Regional Hospital	Durham	9.5%	526
Rutherford Hospital	Rutherfordton	9.5%	1637
Carteret General Hospital	Morehead City	9.6%	1516
Johnston Memorial Hospital	Smithfield	9.7%	1057
Sandhills Regional Medical Center	Hamlet	9.7%	258
Randolph Hospital	Asheboro	10.0%	928
Albemarle Hospital Authority	Elizabeth City	10.1%	1849
Park Ridge Hospital	Fletcher	10.4%	597
Kings Mountain Hospital	Kings Mountain	10.6%	378
Roanoke Chowan Hospital	Ahoskie	10.6%	1225
Watauga Medical Center	Boone	10.6%	1171
Anson Community Hospital	Wadesboro	10.7%	419
Davis Regional Medical Center	Statesville	10.7%	103
Carolinas Medical Center-Lincoln	Lincolnton	10.8%	720
Caldwell Memorial Hospital	Lenoir	11.1%	1333
Pitt County Memorial Hospital	Greenville	11.3%	71
Halifax Regional Medical Center	Roanoke Rapids	11.4%	1381
Betsy Johnson Regional Hospital	Dunn	11.6%	715
Onslow Memorial Hospital	Jacksonville	11.9%	732
Cleveland Regional Medical Center	Shelby	12.1%	741
C J Harris Community Hospital	Sylva	12.4%	956
Nash General Hospital	Rocky Mount	12.5%	1224
Duke Health Raleigh Hospital	Raleigh	13.8%	232
Granville Medical Center	Oxford	13.9%	525
Grace Hospital	Morganton	16.2%	499
Rowan Regional Medical Center	Salisbury	17.6%	771
Valdese General Hospital	Valdese	18.0%	372

39. MRI for Low Back Pain

Hospital Name	City	Rate	Cases
Onslow Memorial Hospital[1]	Jacksonville	22.8%	57
University of North Carolina Hospital	Chapel Hill	23.0%	200
Granville Medical Center	Oxford	23.3%	116
Cape Fear Valley Medical Center[1]	Fayetteville	23.6%	55
New Hanover Regional Medical Center	Wilmington	23.7%	558
Heritage Hospital	Tarboro	24.1%	141
Gaston Memorial Hospital	Gastonia	24.6%	780
Presbyterian Hospital	Charlotte	25.4%	71
Firsthealth Moore Regional Hospital	Pinehurst	25.5%	756
Lake Norman Regional Medical Center	Mooresville	25.7%	140
Valdese General Hospital	Valdese	26.2%	84
Duke Health Raleigh Hospital	Raleigh	26.5%	98
Watauga Medical Center	Boone	26.5%	170
Park Ridge Hospital	Fletcher	26.6%	188
Presbyterian Hospital Matthews	Matthews	26.7%	243
Frye Regional Medical Center	Hickory	27.3%	432
Haywood Regional Medical Center	Clyde	27.6%	283
Betsy Johnson Regional Hospital	Dunn	27.7%	155
Central Carolina Hospital	Sanford	27.7%	137
Columbus Regional Healthcare System	Whiteville	27.7%	141
Davis Regional Medical Center	Statesville	27.7%	166
Carolinas Medical Center-Northeast	Concord	27.8%	837
Wakemed - Cary Hospital	Cary	27.8%	115
Saint Lukes Hospital	Columbus	27.9%	68
Presbyterian-Orthopaedic Hospital	Charlotte	28.1%	114
Brunswick Community Hospital	Supply	28.3%	106
North Carolina Baptist Hospital	Winston-Salem	28.3%	219
Iredell Memorial Hospital	Statesville	28.6%	175
C J Harris Community Hospital	Sylva	28.7%	223
Lenoir Memorial Hospital	Kinston	28.7%	157
Carolinas Medical Center-Union	Monroe	28.9%	232
Murphy Medical Center	Murphy	29.1%	151
Lexington Memorial Hospital	Lexington	29.3%	133
Margaret R Pardee Memorial Hospital	Hendersonville	29.3%	451
Randolph Hospital	Asheboro	29.3%	157
Rutherford Hospital	Rutherfordton	29.4%	211
Carteret General Hospital	Morehead City	29.5%	166
Rowan Regional Medical Center	Salisbury	29.7%	438
Sandhills Regional Medical Center	Hamlet	29.7%	64
High Point Regional Hospital	High Point	30.1%	186
Catawba Valley Medical Center	Hickory	30.2%	305
Johnston Memorial Hospital	Smithfield	30.2%	139
Scotland Memorial Hospital	Laurinburg	30.5%	164
Presbyterian Hospital Huntersville	Huntersville	30.6%	170
Rex Hospital	Raleigh	30.7%	316
Ashe Memorial Hospital	Jefferson	30.8%	65
The Moses H Cone Memorial Hospital	Greensboro	30.8%	312
Pitt County Memorial Hospital	Greenville	30.9%	123
Forsyth Memorial Hospital[1]	Winston-Salem	31.0%	42
Northern Hospital of Surry County	Mount Airy	31.1%	164
Southeastern Regional Medical Center	Lumberton	31.1%	338
Duke University Hospital	Durham	32.1%	446
Grace Hospital	Morganton	32.1%	106
Carolina East Medical Center	New Bern	32.4%	176
Carolinas Medical Center-Mercy	Charlotte	32.5%	338
Nash General Hospital	Rocky Mount	32.6%	427
Durham Regional Hospital	Durham	33.0%	100
Alamance Regional Medical Center	Burlington	33.6%	318
Caldwell Memorial Hospital	Lenoir	34.1%	132
Hugh Chatham Memorial Hospital	Elkin	34.2%	155
Carolinas Medical Center-Behavioral Health	Charlotte	34.6%	188
Stanly Regional Medical Center	Albemarle	34.6%	156
Wilkes Regional Medical Center	N Wilkesboro	34.7%	176
Albemarle Hospital Authority	Elizabeth City	35.9%	206
Cleveland Regional Medical Center	Shelby	35.9%	295
Martin General Hospital	Williamston	35.9%	64
Maria Parham Hospital	Henderson	36.1%	97
Memorial Mission Hospital	Asheville	36.4%	151
Person Memorial Hospital	Roxboro	36.9%	65
Franklin Regional Medical Center	Louisburg	37.1%	62
Wayne Memorial Hospital	Goldsboro	37.2%	406
Cape Fear Valley-Bladen County Hospital[1]	Elizabethtown	37.8%	37
Wilson Medical Center	Wilson	38.1%	181
Carolinas Medical Center-Lincoln	Lincolnton	38.2%	123
Carolinas Medical Center-University	Charlotte	38.3%	128
Wakemed - Raleigh Campus	Raleigh	38.3%	149
Beaufort County Medical Center	Washington	38.7%	155
Thomasville Medical Center	Thomasville	39.0%	77
Halifax Regional Medical Center	Roanoke Rapids	39.4%	94
Spruce Pine Community Hospital	Spruce Pine	40.7%	81
Sampson Regional Medical Center	Clinton	41.0%	134
Morehead Memorial Hospital	Eden	42.0%	119
Washington County Hospital[1]	Plymouth	42.3%	26
Roanoke Chowan Hospital	Ahoskie	45.6%	57
Kings Mountain Hospital	Kings Mountain	49.4%	81
Duplin General Hospital	Kenansville	50.0%	54

Survey of Patients' Hospital Experiences

40. Area Around Room 'Always' Quiet at Night

Hospital Name	City	Rate	Cases
North Carolina Specialty Hospital	Durham	83%	300+
Bertie Memorial Hospital	Windsor	81%	(a)
Cleveland Regional Medical Center	Shelby	72%	300+
Granville Medical Center	Oxford	72%	300+
Sandhills Regional Medical Center	Hamlet	72%	300+
Southeastern Regional Medical Center	Lumberton	72%	300+
Kings Mountain Hospital	Kings Mountain	71%	(a)
Medical Park Hospital	Winston-Salem	71%	300+
Wilkes Regional Medical Center	N Wilkesboro	71%	300+
Chatham Hospital	Siler City	70%	(a)
Duplin General Hospital	Kenansville	69%	300+
Sampson Regional Medical Center	Clinton	69%	300+
Valdese General Hospital	Valdese	69%	300+
Maria Parham Hospital	Henderson	68%	300+
Martin General Hospital	Williamston	68%	300+
Spruce Pine Community Hospital	Spruce Pine	68%	300+
Transylvania Regional Hospital	Brevard	68%	300+
Wilson Medical Center	Wilson	68%	300+
Anson Community Hospital	Wadesboro	67%	(a)
Carolinas Medical Center-Mercy	Charlotte	67%	300+
Cherokee Indian Hospital Authority	Cherokee	67%	(a)
Davis Regional Medical Center	Statesville	67%	300+
Franklin Regional Medical Center	Louisburg	67%	(a)
Grace Hospital	Morganton	67%	300+
Heritage Hospital	Tarboro	67%	300+
Hugh Chatham Memorial Hospital	Elkin	67%	300+
Person Memorial Hospital	Roxboro	67%	300+
Rowan Regional Medical Center	Salisbury	67%	300+
Scotland Memorial Hospital	Laurinburg	67%	300+
Iredell Memorial Hospital	Statesville	66%	300+
North Carolina Baptist Hospital	Winston-Salem	66%	300+
The Outer Banks Hospital	Nags Head	66%	300+
Rutherford Hospital	Rutherfordton	65%	300+
Betsy Johnson Regional Hospital	Dunn	64%	300+
Carolinas Medical Center-Behavioral Health	Charlotte	64%	300+

NOTE: Hospital profiles are in alphabetical order by state, then city, then hospital within the city; Rankings exclude hospitals with less than 25 cases except for patient surveys which excludes hospitals with less than 100 cases; (a) 100–299 cases; (1) The number of cases is too small to be sure how well a hospital is performing; (2) The hospital indicated that the data submitted for this measure were based on a sample of cases; (3) Data was collected during a shorter time period (fewer quarters) than the maximum possible time for this measure; (4) Suppressed for one or more quarters by CMS; (5) No data is available from the hospital for this measure; (6) Fewer than 100 patients completed the HCAHPS survey. Use these rates with caution, as the number of surveys may be too low to reliably assess hospital performance; (7) Survey results are based on less than 12 months of data; (8) Survey results are not available for this reporting period; (9) No or very few patients were eligible for the HCAHPS survey. The scores shown, if any, reflect a very small number of surveys; (10) A state average was not calculated because too few hospitals in the state submitted data; (11) There were discrepancies in the data collection process; Please refer to the User's Guide for a full explanation of data.

Johnston Memorial Hospital	Smithfield	64%	300+
The Mcdowell Hospital	Marion	64%	300+
Roanoke Chowan Hospital	Ahoskie	64%	300+
University of North Carolina Hospital	Chapel Hill	64%	300+
Wayne Memorial Hospital	Goldsboro	64%	300+
Angel Medical Center	Franklin	63%	300+
Carolinas Medical Center-Union	Monroe	63%	300+
Carolinas Medical Center-University	Charlotte	63%	300+
Chowan Hospital	Edenton	63%	300+
Halifax Regional Medical Center	Roanoke Rapids	63%	300+
Thomasville Medical Center	Thomasville	63%	300+
Duke Health Raleigh Hospital	Raleigh	62%	300+
New Hanover Regional Medical Center	Wilmington	62%	300+
Presbyterian Hospital Matthews	Matthews	62%	300+
Saint Lukes Hospital	Columbus	62%	(a)
C J Harris Community Hospital	Sylva	61%	300+
Carolinas Medical Center-Northeast	Concord	61%	300+
Carteret General Hospital	Morehead City	61%	300+
Columbus Regional Healthcare System	Whiteville	61%	300+
Firsthealth Moore Regional Hospital	Pinehurst	61%	300+
Presbyterian Hospital	Charlotte	61%	300+
Presbyterian Hospital Huntersville	Huntersville	61%	300+
Albemarle Hospital Authority	Elizabeth City	60%	300+
Frye Regional Medical Center	Hickory	60%	300+
Memorial Mission Hospital	Asheville	60%	300+
Pitt County Memorial Hospital	Greenville	60%	300+
Wakemed - Raleigh Campus	Raleigh	60%	300+
Watauga Medical Center	Boone	60%	300+
Caldwell Memorial Hospital	Lenoir	59%	300+
The Moses H Cone Memorial Hospital	Greensboro	59%	300+
Stanly Regional Medical Center	Albemarle	59%	300+
High Point Regional Hospital	High Point	58%	300+
Lake Norman Regional Medical Center	Mooresville	58%	300+
Lexington Memorial Hospital	Lexington	58%	300+
Northern Hospital of Surry County	Mount Airy	58%	300+
Park Ridge Hospital	Fletcher	58%	300+
Randolph Hospital	Asheboro	58%	300+
Ashe Memorial Hospital	Jefferson	57%	300+
Presbyterian-Orthopaedic Hospital	Charlotte	57%	300+
Wakemed - Cary Hospital	Cary	57%	300+
Carolina East Medical Center	New Bern	56%	300+
Catawba Valley Medical Center	Hickory	56%	300+
Central Carolina Hospital	Sanford	56%	300+
Forsyth Memorial Hospital	Winston-Salem	56%	300+
Gaston Memorial Hospital	Gastonia	56%	300+
Onslow Memorial Hospital	Jacksonville	56%	300+
Beaufort County Medical Center	Washington	55%	300+
Duke University Hospital	Durham	55%	300+
Haywood Regional Medical Center	Clyde	55%	300+
Lenoir Memorial Hospital	Kinston	55%	300+
Carolinas Medical Center-Lincoln	Lincolnton	54%	300+
Nash General Hospital	Rocky Mount	54%	300+
Cape Fear Valley Medical Center	Fayetteville	53%	300+
Margaret R Pardee Memorial Hospital	Hendersonville	53%	300+
Murphy Medical Center	Murphy	53%	300+
Rex Hospital	Raleigh	52%	300+
Alamance Regional Medical Center	Burlington	51%	300+
Alleghany County Memorial Hospital	Sparta	50%	(a)
Brunswick Community Hospital	Supply	50%	300+
Morehead Memorial Hospital	Eden	48%	300+
Durham Regional Hospital	Durham	45%	300+

41. Doctors 'Always' Communicated Well

Hospital Name	City	Rate	Cases
Bertie Memorial Hospital	Windsor	93%	(a)
North Carolina Specialty Hospital	Durham	91%	300+
Chatham Hospital	Siler City	90%	(a)
Angel Medical Center	Franklin	88%	300+
Chowan Hospital	Edenton	88%	300+
Anson Community Hospital	Wadesboro	86%	(a)
Ashe Memorial Hospital	Jefferson	86%	300+
Cleveland Regional Medical Center	Shelby	86%	300+
Iredell Memorial Hospital	Statesville	86%	300+
Kings Mountain Hospital	Kings Mountain	86%	(a)
Medical Park Hospital	Winston-Salem	86%	300+
Rutherford Hospital	Rutherfordton	86%	300+
Thomasville Medical Center	Thomasville	86%	300+
Watauga Medical Center	Boone	86%	300+
Carolinas Medical Center-Northeast	Concord	85%	300+
Firsthealth Moore Regional Hospital	Pinehurst	85%	300+
Heritage Hospital	Tarboro	85%	300+
Hugh Chatham Memorial Hospital	Elkin	85%	300+
The Outer Banks Hospital	Nags Head	85%	300+
Roanoke Chowan Hospital	Ahoskie	85%	300+
Valdese General Hospital	Valdese	85%	300+
Wilkes Regional Medical Center	N Wilkesboro	85%	300+
Carolinas Medical Center-Mercy	Charlotte	84%	300+
Carolinas Medical Center-University	Charlotte	84%	300+
Duke Health Raleigh Hospital	Raleigh	84%	300+
Frye Regional Medical Center	Hickory	84%	300+
Granville Medical Center	Oxford	84%	300+
Haywood Regional Medical Center	Clyde	84%	300+
Lake Norman Regional Medical Center	Mooresville	84%	300+
Morehead Memorial Hospital	Eden	84%	300+
Person Memorial Hospital	Roxboro	84%	300+
Presbyterian Hospital	Charlotte	84%	300+
Presbyterian-Orthopaedic Hospital	Charlotte	84%	300+
Sampson Regional Medical Center	Clinton	84%	300+
Scotland Memorial Hospital	Laurinburg	84%	300+
Southeastern Regional Medical Center	Lumberton	84%	300+
Spruce Pine Community Hospital	Spruce Pine	84%	300+
Wilson Medical Center	Wilson	84%	300+
Alleghany County Memorial Hospital	Sparta	83%	(a)
Beaufort County Medical Center	Washington	83%	300+
C J Harris Community Hospital	Sylva	83%	300+
Caldwell Memorial Hospital	Lenoir	83%	300+
Carolinas Medical Center-Union	Monroe	83%	300+
Central Carolina Hospital	Sanford	83%	300+
Forsyth Memorial Hospital	Winston-Salem	83%	300+
Grace Hospital	Morganton	83%	300+
Maria Parham Hospital	Henderson	83%	300+
Martin General Hospital	Williamston	83%	300+
Memorial Mission Hospital	Asheville	83%	300+
Murphy Medical Center	Murphy	83%	300+
Presbyterian Hospital Huntersville	Huntersville	83%	300+
Rowan Regional Medical Center	Salisbury	83%	300+
Wayne Memorial Hospital	Goldsboro	83%	300+
Alamance Regional Medical Center	Burlington	82%	300+
Brunswick Community Hospital	Supply	82%	300+
Carolinas Medical Center-Behavioral Health	Charlotte	82%	300+
Davis Regional Medical Center	Statesville	82%	300+
Gaston Memorial Hospital	Gastonia	82%	300+
Lexington Memorial Hospital	Lexington	82%	300+
Nash General Hospital	Rocky Mount	82%	300+
New Hanover Regional Medical Center	Wilmington	82%	300+
Pitt County Memorial Hospital	Greenville	82%	300+
Rex Hospital	Raleigh	82%	300+
Saint Lukes Hospital	Columbus	82%	(a)
University of North Carolina Hospital	Chapel Hill	82%	300+
Carolinas Medical Center-Lincoln	Lincolnton	81%	300+
Carteret General Hospital	Morehead City	81%	300+
Columbus Regional Healthcare System	Whiteville	81%	300+
Duplin General Hospital	Kenansville	81%	300+
Halifax Regional Medical Center	Roanoke Rapids	81%	300+
Johnston Memorial Hospital	Smithfield	81%	300+
The Mcdowell Hospital	Marion	81%	300+
Park Ridge Hospital	Fletcher	81%	300+
Sandhills Regional Medical Center	Hamlet	81%	300+
Stanly Regional Medical Center	Albemarle	81%	300+
Albemarle Hospital Authority	Elizabeth City	80%	300+
Catawba Valley Medical Center	Hickory	80%	300+
Duke University Hospital	Durham	80%	300+
Margaret R Pardee Memorial Hospital	Hendersonville	80%	300+
North Carolina Baptist Hospital	Winston-Salem	80%	300+
Randolph Hospital	Asheboro	80%	300+
Transylvania Regional Hospital	Brevard	80%	300+
Wakemed - Cary Hospital	Cary	80%	300+
Franklin Regional Medical Center	Louisburg	79%	(a)
Wakemed - Raleigh Campus	Raleigh	79%	300+
Durham Regional Hospital	Durham	78%	300+
High Point Regional Hospital	High Point	78%	300+
The Moses H Cone Memorial Hospital	Greensboro	78%	300+
Northern Hospital of Surry County	Mount Airy	78%	300+
Presbyterian Hospital Matthews	Matthews	78%	300+
Lenoir Memorial Hospital	Kinston	77%	300+
Onslow Memorial Hospital	Jacksonville	77%	300+
Cape Fear Valley Medical Center	Fayetteville	76%	300+
Betsy Johnson Regional Hospital	Dunn	75%	300+
Carolina East Medical Center	New Bern	75%	300+
Cherokee Indian Hospital Authority	Cherokee	71%	(a)

42. Home Recovery Information Given

Hospital Name	City	Rate	Cases
North Carolina Specialty Hospital	Durham	91%	300+
Valdese General Hospital	Valdese	91%	300+
Bertie Memorial Hospital	Windsor	89%	(a)
Presbyterian-Orthopaedic Hospital	Charlotte	89%	300+
Carolinas Medical Center-Mercy	Charlotte	88%	300+
Chowan Hospital	Edenton	88%	300+
Duke Health Raleigh Hospital	Raleigh	88%	300+
Duke University Hospital	Durham	88%	300+
Frye Regional Medical Center	Hickory	88%	300+
The Outer Banks Hospital	Nags Head	88%	300+
Pitt County Memorial Hospital	Greenville	88%	300+
University of North Carolina Hospital	Chapel Hill	88%	300+
Cleveland Regional Medical Center	Shelby	87%	300+
Franklin Regional Medical Center	Louisburg	87%	(a)
Heritage Hospital	Tarboro	87%	300+
Rex Hospital	Raleigh	87%	300+
Transylvania Regional Hospital	Brevard	87%	300+
Wilson Medical Center	Wilson	87%	300+
Carolinas Medical Center-Lincoln	Lincolnton	86%	300+
Carolinas Medical Center-Northeast	Concord	86%	300+
Carolinas Medical Center-Union	Monroe	86%	300+
Carolinas Medical Center-University	Charlotte	86%	300+
Lake Norman Regional Medical Center	Mooresville	86%	300+
Presbyterian Hospital Huntersville	Huntersville	86%	300+
Albemarle Hospital Authority	Elizabeth City	85%	300+
Beaufort County Medical Center	Washington	85%	300+
Caldwell Memorial Hospital	Lenoir	85%	300+
Carolinas Medical Center-Behavioral Health	Charlotte	85%	300+
Columbus Regional Healthcare System	Whiteville	85%	300+
Grace Hospital	Morganton	85%	300+
Kings Mountain Hospital	Kings Mountain	85%	(a)
Memorial Mission Hospital	Asheville	85%	300+
New Hanover Regional Medical Center	Wilmington	85%	300+
Onslow Memorial Hospital	Jacksonville	85%	300+
Presbyterian Hospital Matthews	Matthews	85%	300+
Rowan Regional Medical Center	Salisbury	85%	300+
Sampson Regional Medical Center	Clinton	85%	300+
Thomasville Medical Center	Thomasville	85%	300+
Wakemed - Raleigh Campus	Raleigh	85%	300+
Ashe Memorial Hospital	Jefferson	84%	300+
Brunswick Community Hospital	Supply	84%	300+
Catawba Valley Medical Center	Hickory	84%	300+
Iredell Memorial Hospital	Statesville	84%	300+
The Mcdowell Hospital	Marion	84%	300+
Roanoke Chowan Hospital	Ahoskie	84%	300+
Saint Lukes Hospital	Columbus	84%	(a)
Southeastern Regional Medical Center	Lumberton	84%	300+
Alleghany County Memorial Hospital	Sparta	83%	(a)
C J Harris Community Hospital	Sylva	83%	300+
Central Carolina Hospital	Sanford	83%	300+
Firsthealth Moore Regional Hospital	Pinehurst	83%	300+
Forsyth Memorial Hospital	Winston-Salem	83%	300+
Gaston Memorial Hospital	Gastonia	83%	300+
Hugh Chatham Memorial Hospital	Elkin	83%	300+
Johnston Memorial Hospital	Smithfield	83%	300+
Lexington Memorial Hospital	Lexington	83%	300+
Maria Parham Hospital	Henderson	83%	300+
Presbyterian Hospital	Charlotte	83%	300+
Watauga Medical Center	Boone	83%	300+
Angel Medical Center	Franklin	82%	300+
Carolina East Medical Center	New Bern	82%	300+
Martin General Hospital	Williamston	82%	300+
Medical Park Hospital	Winston-Salem	82%	300+
Murphy Medical Center	Murphy	82%	300+
North Carolina Baptist Hospital	Winston-Salem	82%	300+
Northern Hospital of Surry County	Mount Airy	82%	300+
Rutherford Hospital	Rutherfordton	82%	300+
Wakemed - Cary Hospital	Cary	82%	300+
Wayne Memorial Hospital	Goldsboro	82%	300+
Alamance Regional Medical Center	Burlington	81%	300+
Davis Regional Medical Center	Statesville	81%	300+
Duplin General Hospital	Kenansville	81%	300+
Haywood Regional Medical Center	Clyde	81%	300+
Margaret R Pardee Memorial Hospital	Hendersonville	81%	300+
Nash General Hospital	Rocky Mount	81%	300+
Park Ridge Hospital	Fletcher	81%	300+
Wilkes Regional Medical Center	N Wilkesboro	81%	300+
Granville Medical Center	Oxford	80%	300+
High Point Regional Hospital	High Point	80%	300+
Morehead Memorial Hospital	Eden	80%	300+
The Moses H Cone Memorial Hospital	Greensboro	80%	300+
Scotland Memorial Hospital	Laurinburg	80%	300+
Stanly Regional Medical Center	Albemarle	80%	300+
Anson Community Hospital	Wadesboro	79%	(a)
Carteret General Hospital	Morehead City	79%	300+
Halifax Regional Medical Center	Roanoke Rapids	79%	300+
Randolph Hospital	Asheboro	79%	300+
Spruce Pine Community Hospital	Spruce Pine	79%	300+
Lenoir Memorial Hospital	Kinston	78%	300+
Person Memorial Hospital	Roxboro	78%	300+
Sandhills Regional Medical Center	Hamlet	78%	300+
Cape Fear Valley Medical Center	Fayetteville	77%	300+
Durham Regional Hospital	Durham	77%	300+
Betsy Johnson Regional Hospital	Dunn	75%	300+
Chatham Hospital	Siler City	75%	(a)
Cherokee Indian Hospital Authority	Cherokee	71%	(a)

43. Hospital Given 9 or 10 on 10 Point Scale

Hospital Name	City	Rate	Cases
North Carolina Specialty Hospital	Durham	89%	300+
Medical Park Hospital	Winston-Salem	84%	300+
Bertie Memorial Hospital	Windsor	81%	(a)
University of North Carolina Hospital	Chapel Hill	81%	300+
Firsthealth Moore Regional Hospital	Pinehurst	79%	300+
Hugh Chatham Memorial Hospital	Elkin	79%	300+
Carolinas Medical Center-Mercy	Charlotte	78%	300+
The Outer Banks Hospital	Nags Head	78%	300+

NOTE: Hospital profiles are in alphabetical order by state, then city, then hospital within the city; Rankings exclude hospitals with less than 25 cases except for patient surveys which excludes hospitals with less than 100 cases; (a) 100–299 cases; (1) The number of cases is too small to be sure how well a hospital is performing; (2) The hospital indicated that the data submitted for this measure were based on a sample of cases; (3) Data was collected during a shorter time period (fewer quarters) than the maximum possible time for this measure; (4) Suppressed for one or more quarters by CMS; (5) No data is available from the hospital for this measure; (6) Fewer than 100 patients completed the HCAHPS survey. Use these rates with caution, as the number of surveys may be too low to reliably assess hospital performance; (7) Survey results are based on less than 12 months of data; (8) Survey results are not available for this reporting period; (9) No or very few patients were eligible for the HCAHPS survey. The scores shown, if any, reflect a very small number of surveys; (10) A state average was not calculated because too few hospitals in the state submitted data; (11) There were discrepancies in the data collection process; Please refer to the User's Guide for a full explanation of data.

Pitt County Memorial Hospital	Greenville	78%	300+
Chatham Hospital	Siler City	77%	(a)
Heritage Hospital	Tarboro	77%	300+
Kings Mountain Hospital	Kings Mountain	77%	(a)
Presbyterian Hospital	Charlotte	77%	300+
Presbyterian Hospital Huntersville	Huntersville	77%	300+
Angel Medical Center	Franklin	76%	300+
Cleveland Regional Medical Center	Shelby	76%	300+
North Carolina Baptist Hospital	Winston-Salem	76%	300+
Spruce Pine Community Hospital	Spruce Pine	76%	300+
Transylvania Regional Hospital	Brevard	76%	300+
Forsyth Memorial Hospital	Winston-Salem	75%	300+
Rex Hospital	Raleigh	75%	300+
Valdese General Hospital	Valdese	75%	300+
C J Harris Community Hospital	Sylva	74%	300+
Davis Regional Medical Center	Statesville	74%	300+
Duke University Hospital	Durham	74%	300+
Iredell Memorial Hospital	Statesville	74%	300+
New Hanover Regional Medical Center	Wilmington	74%	300+
Saint Lukes Hospital	Columbus	74%	(a)
Wakemed - Raleigh Campus	Raleigh	74%	300+
Chowan Hospital	Edenton	73%	300+
Thomasville Medical Center	Thomasville	73%	300+
Carolinas Medical Center-Northeast	Concord	72%	300+
Carolinas Medical Center-Union	Monroe	72%	300+
Carolinas Medical Center-University	Charlotte	72%	300+
Ashe Memorial Hospital	Jefferson	71%	300+
Carolinas Medical Center-Behavioral Health	Charlotte	71%	300+
Duke Health Raleigh Hospital	Raleigh	71%	300+
Memorial Mission Hospital	Asheville	71%	300+
Park Ridge Hospital	Fletcher	71%	300+
Watauga Medical Center	Boone	71%	300+
Anson Community Hospital	Wadesboro	70%	(a)
Catawba Valley Medical Center	Hickory	70%	300+
Franklin Regional Medical Center	Louisburg	70%	(a)
Lake Norman Regional Medical Center	Mooresville	70%	300+
Presbyterian Hospital Matthews	Matthews	70%	300+
Rutherford Hospital	Rutherfordton	70%	300+
Wilkes Regional Medical Center	N Wilkesboro	70%	300+
Wilson Medical Center	Wilson	70%	300+
Carolinas Medical Center-Lincoln	Lincolnton	69%	300+
Duplin General Hospital	Kenansville	69%	300+
The Mcdowell Hospital	Marion	69%	300+
Roanoke Chowan Hospital	Ahoskie	69%	300+
Rowan Regional Medical Center	Salisbury	69%	300+
Wayne Memorial Hospital	Goldsboro	69%	300+
Carteret General Hospital	Morehead City	68%	300+
Gaston Memorial Hospital	Gastonia	68%	300+
High Point Regional Hospital	High Point	68%	300+
Presbyterian-Orthopaedic Hospital	Charlotte	68%	300+
Wakemed - Cary Hospital	Cary	68%	300+
Alleghany County Memorial Hospital	Sparta	67%	(a)
Granville Medical Center	Oxford	67%	300+
Randolph Hospital	Asheboro	67%	300+
Southeastern Regional Medical Center	Lumberton	67%	300+
Albemarle Hospital Authority	Elizabeth City	66%	300+
Columbus Regional Healthcare System	Whiteville	66%	300+
Frye Regional Medical Center	Hickory	66%	300+
Grace Hospital	Morganton	66%	300+
Lexington Memorial Hospital	Lexington	66%	300+
Morehead Memorial Hospital	Eden	66%	300+
Sampson Regional Medical Center	Clinton	65%	300+
Beaufort County Medical Center	Washington	64%	300+
Margaret R Pardee Memorial Hospital	Hendersonville	64%	300+
Person Memorial Hospital	Roxboro	64%	300+
Scotland Memorial Hospital	Laurinburg	64%	300+
Caldwell Memorial Hospital	Lenoir	63%	300+
Maria Parham Hospital	Henderson	63%	300+
The Moses H Cone Memorial Hospital	Greensboro	63%	300+
Murphy Medical Center	Murphy	63%	300+
Onslow Memorial Hospital	Jacksonville	63%	300+
Stanly Regional Medical Center	Albemarle	63%	300+
Alamance Regional Medical Center	Burlington	62%	300+
Brunswick Community Hospital	Supply	62%	300+
Halifax Regional Medical Center	Roanoke Rapids	62%	300+
Johnston Memorial Hospital	Smithfield	62%	300+
Lenoir Memorial Hospital	Kinston	62%	300+
Haywood Regional Medical Center	Clyde	61%	300+
Northern Hospital of Surry County	Mount Airy	61%	300+
Central Carolina Hospital	Sanford	60%	300+
Martin General Hospital	Williamston	60%	300+
Nash General Hospital	Rocky Mount	60%	300+
Carolina East Medical Center	New Bern	59%	300+
Cape Fear Valley Medical Center	Fayetteville	58%	300+
Cherokee Indian Hospital Authority	Cherokee	58%	(a)
Durham Regional Hospital	Durham	58%	300+
Sandhills Regional Medical Center	Hamlet	58%	300+
Betsy Johnson Regional Hospital	Dunn	56%	300+

44. Meds 'Always' Explained Before Given

Hospital Name	City	Rate	Cases
Bertie Memorial Hospital	Windsor	76%	(a)
Anson Community Hospital	Wadesboro	74%	(a)
Cleveland Regional Medical Center	Shelby	74%	300+
Roanoke Chowan Hospital	Ahoskie	74%	300+
Chatham Hospital	Siler City	73%	(a)
North Carolina Specialty Hospital	Durham	73%	300+
Heritage Hospital	Tarboro	72%	300+
Kings Mountain Hospital	Kings Mountain	71%	(a)
The Outer Banks Hospital	Nags Head	70%	300+
Southeastern Regional Medical Center	Lumberton	70%	300+
Duplin General Hospital	Kenansville	69%	300+
Iredell Memorial Hospital	Statesville	68%	300+
University of North Carolina Hospital	Chapel Hill	68%	300+
Carolinas Medical Center-University	Charlotte	67%	300+
Columbus Regional Healthcare System	Whiteville	67%	300+
Lexington Memorial Hospital	Lexington	67%	300+
Ashe Memorial Hospital	Jefferson	66%	300+
Carolinas Medical Center-Northeast	Concord	66%	300+
Duke Health Raleigh Hospital	Raleigh	66%	300+
Franklin Regional Medical Center	Louisburg	66%	(a)
Hugh Chatham Memorial Hospital	Elkin	66%	300+
Pitt County Memorial Hospital	Greenville	66%	300+
Spruce Pine Community Hospital	Spruce Pine	66%	300+
Wilkes Regional Medical Center	N Wilkesboro	66%	300+
Alamance Regional Medical Center	Burlington	65%	300+
Beaufort County Medical Center	Washington	65%	300+
Carolinas Medical Center-Union	Monroe	65%	300+
Chowan Hospital	Edenton	65%	300+
Grace Hospital	Morganton	65%	300+
Maria Parham Hospital	Henderson	65%	300+
Nash General Hospital	Rocky Mount	65%	300+
Sampson Regional Medical Center	Clinton	65%	300+
Scotland Memorial Hospital	Laurinburg	65%	300+
Valdese General Hospital	Valdese	65%	300+
Carolinas Medical Center-Mercy	Charlotte	64%	300+
Davis Regional Medical Center	Statesville	64%	300+
Duke University Hospital	Durham	64%	300+
Firsthealth Moore Regional Hospital	Pinehurst	64%	300+
Forsyth Memorial Hospital	Winston-Salem	64%	300+
Frye Regional Medical Center	Hickory	64%	300+
Johnston Memorial Hospital	Smithfield	64%	300+
The Mcdowell Hospital	Marion	64%	300+
Medical Park Hospital	Winston-Salem	64%	300+
New Hanover Regional Medical Center	Wilmington	64%	300+
Rutherford Hospital	Rutherfordton	64%	300+
C J Harris Community Hospital	Sylva	63%	300+
Carteret General Hospital	Morehead City	63%	300+
Haywood Regional Medical Center	Clyde	63%	300+
Presbyterian Hospital	Charlotte	63%	300+
Rowan Regional Medical Center	Salisbury	63%	300+
Watauga Medical Center	Boone	63%	300+
Wayne Memorial Hospital	Goldsboro	63%	300+
Caldwell Memorial Hospital	Lenoir	62%	300+
Catawba Valley Medical Center	Hickory	62%	300+
Gaston Memorial Hospital	Gastonia	62%	300+
Halifax Regional Medical Center	Roanoke Rapids	62%	300+
Lake Norman Regional Medical Center	Mooresville	62%	300+
Randolph Hospital	Asheboro	62%	300+
Rex Hospital	Raleigh	62%	300+
Transylvania Regional Hospital	Brevard	62%	300+
Wakemed - Raleigh Campus	Raleigh	62%	300+
Carolinas Medical Center-Behavioral Health	Charlotte	61%	300+
Martin General Hospital	Williamston	61%	300+
North Carolina Baptist Hospital	Winston-Salem	61%	300+
Presbyterian-Orthopaedic Hospital	Charlotte	61%	300+
Wilson Medical Center	Wilson	61%	300+
Angel Medical Center	Franklin	60%	300+
Cape Fear Valley Medical Center	Fayetteville	60%	300+
Central Carolina Hospital	Sanford	60%	300+
Margaret R Pardee Memorial Hospital	Hendersonville	60%	300+
Morehead Memorial Hospital	Eden	60%	300+
Onslow Memorial Hospital	Jacksonville	60%	300+
Stanly Regional Medical Center	Albemarle	60%	300+
Thomasville Medical Center	Thomasville	60%	300+
Wakemed - Cary Hospital	Cary	60%	300+
Granville Medical Center	Oxford	59%	300+
Memorial Mission Hospital	Asheville	59%	300+
Presbyterian Hospital Huntersville	Huntersville	59%	300+
Saint Lukes Hospital	Columbus	59%	(a)
Sandhills Regional Medical Center	Hamlet	59%	300+
Carolinas Medical Center-Lincoln	Lincolnton	58%	300+
High Point Regional Hospital	High Point	58%	300+
Murphy Medical Center	Murphy	58%	300+
Albemarle Hospital Authority	Elizabeth City	57%	300+
Alleghany County Memorial Hospital	Sparta	57%	(a)
Betsy Johnson Regional Hospital	Dunn	57%	300+
Person Memorial Hospital	Roxboro	57%	300+
Presbyterian Hospital Matthews	Matthews	57%	300+
Lenoir Memorial Hospital	Kinston	56%	300+
The Moses H Cone Memorial Hospital	Greensboro	56%	300+
Park Ridge Hospital	Fletcher	56%	300+
Brunswick Community Hospital	Supply	55%	300+
Carolina East Medical Center	New Bern	55%	300+
Durham Regional Hospital	Durham	55%	300+
Northern Hospital of Surry County	Mount Airy	54%	300+
Cherokee Indian Hospital Authority	Cherokee	52%	(a)

45. Nurses 'Always' Communicated Well

Hospital Name	City	Rate	Cases
Bertie Memorial Hospital	Windsor	90%	(a)
North Carolina Specialty Hospital	Durham	87%	300+
Chatham Hospital	Siler City	86%	(a)
Chowan Hospital	Edenton	84%	300+
Cleveland Regional Medical Center	Shelby	84%	300+
Hugh Chatham Memorial Hospital	Elkin	84%	300+
Kings Mountain Hospital	Kings Mountain	84%	(a)
Ashe Memorial Hospital	Jefferson	83%	300+
Carolinas Medical Center-Union	Monroe	83%	300+
Heritage Hospital	Tarboro	83%	300+
Medical Park Hospital	Winston-Salem	83%	300+
New Hanover Regional Medical Center	Wilmington	83%	300+
Valdese General Hospital	Valdese	83%	300+
Angel Medical Center	Franklin	82%	300+
Iredell Memorial Hospital	Statesville	82%	300+
Presbyterian Hospital	Charlotte	82%	300+
Roanoke Chowan Hospital	Ahoskie	82%	300+
Spruce Pine Community Hospital	Spruce Pine	82%	300+
Wilkes Regional Medical Center	N Wilkesboro	82%	300+
C J Harris Community Hospital	Sylva	81%	300+
Carolinas Medical Center-Mercy	Charlotte	81%	300+
Firsthealth Moore Regional Hospital	Pinehurst	81%	300+
The Outer Banks Hospital	Nags Head	81%	300+
Pitt County Memorial Hospital	Greenville	81%	300+
Southeastern Regional Medical Center	Lumberton	81%	300+
Transylvania Regional Hospital	Brevard	81%	300+
Carolinas Medical Center-Northeast	Concord	80%	300+
Carolinas Medical Center-University	Charlotte	80%	300+
Carteret General Hospital	Morehead City	80%	300+
Gaston Memorial Hospital	Gastonia	80%	300+
Maria Parham Hospital	Henderson	80%	300+
The Mcdowell Hospital	Marion	80%	300+
Randolph Hospital	Asheboro	80%	300+
Rowan Regional Medical Center	Salisbury	80%	300+
Rutherford Hospital	Rutherfordton	80%	300+
Thomasville Medical Center	Thomasville	80%	300+
University of North Carolina Hospital	Chapel Hill	80%	300+
Wayne Memorial Hospital	Goldsboro	80%	300+
Wilson Medical Center	Wilson	80%	300+
Anson Community Hospital	Wadesboro	79%	(a)
Carolinas Medical Center-Lincoln	Lincolnton	79%	300+
Columbus Regional Healthcare System	Whiteville	79%	300+
Duplin General Hospital	Kenansville	79%	300+
Forsyth Memorial Hospital	Winston-Salem	79%	300+
Franklin Regional Medical Center	Louisburg	79%	(a)
Granville Medical Center	Oxford	79%	300+
Haywood Regional Medical Center	Clyde	79%	300+
Lexington Memorial Hospital	Lexington	79%	300+
Memorial Mission Hospital	Asheville	79%	300+
Saint Lukes Hospital	Columbus	79%	(a)
Sampson Regional Medical Center	Clinton	79%	300+
Watauga Medical Center	Boone	79%	300+
Alleghany County Memorial Hospital	Sparta	78%	(a)
Beaufort County Medical Center	Washington	78%	300+
Duke Health Raleigh Hospital	Raleigh	78%	300+
Grace Hospital	Morganton	78%	300+
Johnston Memorial Hospital	Smithfield	78%	300+
Morehead Memorial Hospital	Eden	78%	300+
Nash General Hospital	Rocky Mount	78%	300+
Onslow Memorial Hospital	Jacksonville	78%	300+
Scotland Memorial Hospital	Laurinburg	78%	300+
Alamance Regional Medical Center	Burlington	77%	300+
Catawba Valley Medical Center	Hickory	77%	300+
Davis Regional Medical Center	Statesville	77%	300+
Duke University Hospital	Durham	77%	300+
Murphy Medical Center	Murphy	77%	300+
Person Memorial Hospital	Roxboro	77%	300+
Presbyterian Hospital Huntersville	Huntersville	77%	300+
Rex Hospital	Raleigh	77%	300+
Albemarle Hospital Authority	Elizabeth City	76%	300+
Brunswick Community Hospital	Supply	76%	300+
Caldwell Memorial Hospital	Lenoir	76%	300+
Carolinas Medical Center-Behavioral Health	Charlotte	76%	300+
Central Carolina Hospital	Sanford	76%	300+
Frye Regional Medical Center	Hickory	76%	300+
High Point Regional Hospital	High Point	76%	300+
Lake Norman Regional Medical Center	Mooresville	76%	300+
Martin General Hospital	Williamston	76%	300+
Stanly Regional Medical Center	Albemarle	76%	300+

NOTE: Hospital profiles are in alphabetical order by state, then city, then hospital within the city; Rankings exclude hospitals with less than 25 cases except for patient surveys which excludes hospitals with less than 100 cases; (a) 100–299 cases; (1) The number of cases is too small to be sure how well a hospital is performing; (2) The hospital indicated that the data submitted for this measure were based on a sample of cases; (3) Data was collected during a shorter time period (fewer quarters) than the maximum possible time for this measure; (4) Suppressed for one or more quarters by CMS; (5) No data is available from the hospital for this measure; (6) Fewer than 100 patients completed the HCAHPS survey. Use these rates with caution, as the number of surveys may be too low to reliably assess hospital performance; (7) Survey results are based on less than 12 months of data; (8) Survey results are not available for this reporting period; (9) No or very few patients were eligible for the HCAHPS survey. The scores shown, if any, reflect a very small number of surveys; (10) A state average was not calculated because too few hospitals in the state submitted data; (11) There were discrepancies in the data collection process; Please refer to the User's Guide for a full explanation of data.

Wakemed - Raleigh Campus	Raleigh	76%	300+
Lenoir Memorial Hospital	Kinston	75%	300+
Margaret R Pardee Memorial Hospital	Hendersonville	75%	300+
North Carolina Baptist Hospital	Winston-Salem	75%	300+
Northern Hospital of Surry County	Mount Airy	75%	300+
Park Ridge Hospital	Fletcher	75%	300+
Wakemed - Cary Hospital	Cary	75%	300+
Halifax Regional Medical Center	Roanoke Rapids	74%	300+
Sandhills Regional Medical Center	Hamlet	74%	300+
Cape Fear Valley Medical Center	Fayetteville	73%	300+
Carolina East Medical Center	New Bern	73%	300+
Presbyterian Hospital Matthews	Matthews	73%	300+
Betsy Johnson Regional Hospital	Dunn	72%	300+
The Moses H Cone Memorial Hospital	Greensboro	72%	300+
Presbyterian-Orthopaedic Hospital	Charlotte	71%	300+
Cherokee Indian Hospital Authority	Cherokee	70%	(a)
Durham Regional Hospital	Durham	70%	300+

46. Pain 'Always' Well Controlled

Hospital Name	City	Rate	Cases
Bertie Memorial Hospital	Windsor	85%	(a)
Cleveland Regional Medical Center	Shelby	79%	300+
North Carolina Specialty Hospital	Durham	79%	300+
Columbus Regional Healthcare System	Whiteville	77%	300+
Kings Mountain Hospital	Kings Mountain	77%	(a)
Valdese General Hospital	Valdese	77%	300+
Angel Medical Center	Franklin	76%	300+
Chowan Hospital	Edenton	76%	300+
Firsthealth Moore Regional Hospital	Pinehurst	76%	300+
Presbyterian Hospital	Charlotte	76%	300+
Heritage Hospital	Tarboro	75%	300+
Medical Park Hospital	Winston-Salem	75%	300+
Spruce Pine Community Hospital	Spruce Pine	75%	300+
Wilson Medical Center	Wilson	75%	300+
Duke Health Raleigh Hospital	Raleigh	74%	300+
Maria Parham Hospital	Henderson	74%	300+
The Outer Banks Hospital	Nags Head	74%	300+
Roanoke Chowan Hospital	Ahoskie	74%	300+
C J Harris Community Hospital	Sylva	73%	300+
Carolinas Medical Center-Mercy	Charlotte	73%	300+
Carolinas Medical Center-Union	Monroe	73%	300+
Franklin Regional Medical Center	Louisburg	73%	(a)
Hugh Chatham Memorial Hospital	Elkin	73%	300+
Iredell Memorial Hospital	Statesville	73%	300+
New Hanover Regional Medical Center	Wilmington	73%	300+
Pitt County Memorial Hospital	Greenville	73%	300+
Rowan Regional Medical Center	Salisbury	73%	300+
University of North Carolina Hospital	Chapel Hill	73%	300+
Watauga Medical Center	Boone	73%	300+
Carolinas Medical Center-Behavioral Health	Charlotte	72%	300+
Carteret General Hospital	Morehead City	72%	300+
Gaston Memorial Hospital	Gastonia	72%	300+
The Mcdowell Hospital	Marion	72%	300+
Memorial Mission Hospital	Asheville	72%	300+
Presbyterian Hospital Huntersville	Huntersville	72%	300+
Wilkes Regional Medical Center	N Wilkesboro	72%	300+
Carolinas Medical Center-University	Charlotte	71%	300+
Catawba Valley Medical Center	Hickory	71%	300+
Chatham Hospital	Siler City	71%	(a)
Forsyth Memorial Hospital	Winston-Salem	71%	300+
Haywood Regional Medical Center	Clyde	71%	300+
Lake Norman Regional Medical Center	Mooresville	71%	300+
Lexington Memorial Hospital	Lexington	71%	300+
Nash General Hospital	Rocky Mount	71%	300+
Saint Lukes Hospital	Columbus	71%	(a)
Sampson Regional Medical Center	Clinton	71%	300+
Scotland Memorial Hospital	Laurinburg	71%	300+
Transylvania Regional Hospital	Brevard	71%	300+
Wakemed - Raleigh Campus	Raleigh	71%	300+
Albemarle Hospital Authority	Elizabeth City	70%	300+
Anson Community Hospital	Wadesboro	70%	(a)
Ashe Memorial Hospital	Jefferson	70%	300+
Caldwell Memorial Hospital	Lenoir	70%	300+
Central Carolina Hospital	Sanford	70%	300+
Johnston Memorial Hospital	Smithfield	70%	300+
Martin General Hospital	Williamston	70%	300+
Sandhills Regional Medical Center	Hamlet	70%	300+
Southeastern Regional Medical Center	Lumberton	70%	300+
Wayne Memorial Hospital	Goldsboro	70%	300+
Alamance Regional Medical Center	Burlington	69%	300+
Brunswick Community Hospital	Supply	69%	300+
Carolinas Medical Center-Northeast	Concord	69%	300+
Frye Regional Medical Center	Hickory	69%	300+
Granville Medical Center	Oxford	69%	300+
High Point Regional Hospital	High Point	69%	300+
Morehead Memorial Hospital	Eden	69%	300+
Murphy Medical Center	Murphy	69%	300+
Rex Hospital	Raleigh	69%	300+
Rutherford Hospital	Rutherfordton	69%	300+
Thomasville Medical Center	Thomasville	69%	300+
Carolinas Medical Center-Lincoln	Lincolnton	68%	300+
Grace Hospital	Morganton	68%	300+
Lenoir Memorial Hospital	Kinston	68%	300+
North Carolina Baptist Hospital	Winston-Salem	68%	300+
Northern Hospital of Surry County	Mount Airy	68%	300+
Onslow Memorial Hospital	Jacksonville	68%	300+
Park Ridge Hospital	Fletcher	68%	300+
Person Memorial Hospital	Roxboro	68%	300+
Randolph Hospital	Asheboro	68%	300+
Stanly Regional Medical Center	Albemarle	68%	300+
Alleghany County Memorial Hospital	Sparta	67%	(a)
Beaufort County Medical Center	Washington	67%	300+
Carolina East Medical Center	New Bern	67%	300+
Duplin General Hospital	Kenansville	67%	300+
Halifax Regional Medical Center	Roanoke Rapids	67%	300+
The Moses H Cone Memorial Hospital	Greensboro	67%	300+
Presbyterian Hospital Matthews	Matthews	67%	300+
Wakemed - Cary Hospital	Cary	67%	300+
Presbyterian-Orthopaedic Hospital	Charlotte	66%	300+
Cape Fear Valley Medical Center	Fayetteville	65%	300+
Davis Regional Medical Center	Statesville	65%	300+
Duke University Hospital	Durham	65%	300+
Betsy Johnson Regional Hospital	Dunn	64%	300+
Margaret R Pardee Memorial Hospital	Hendersonville	64%	300+
Durham Regional Hospital	Durham	63%	300+
Cherokee Indian Hospital Authority	Cherokee	51%	(a)

47. Room and Bathroom 'Always' Clean

Hospital Name	City	Rate	Cases
Bertie Memorial Hospital	Windsor	89%	(a)
North Carolina Specialty Hospital	Durham	88%	300+
Chatham Hospital	Siler City	82%	(a)
Hugh Chatham Memorial Hospital	Elkin	82%	300+
Ashe Memorial Hospital	Jefferson	80%	300+
Northern Hospital of Surry County	Mount Airy	78%	300+
Thomasville Medical Center	Thomasville	78%	300+
Transylvania Regional Hospital	Brevard	78%	300+
The Mcdowell Hospital	Marion	77%	300+
Rutherford Hospital	Rutherfordton	77%	300+
Spruce Pine Community Hospital	Spruce Pine	77%	300+
Davis Regional Medical Center	Statesville	76%	300+
Morehead Memorial Hospital	Eden	76%	300+
The Outer Banks Hospital	Nags Head	76%	300+
Valdese General Hospital	Valdese	76%	300+
Lexington Memorial Hospital	Lexington	75%	300+
Medical Park Hospital	Winston-Salem	75%	300+
New Hanover Regional Medical Center	Wilmington	75%	300+
Wayne Memorial Hospital	Goldsboro	75%	300+
Albemarle Hospital Authority	Elizabeth City	74%	300+
Chowan Hospital	Edenton	74%	300+
Firsthealth Moore Regional Hospital	Pinehurst	74%	300+
Margaret R Pardee Memorial Hospital	Hendersonville	74%	300+
Maria Parham Hospital	Henderson	74%	300+
Watauga Medical Center	Boone	74%	300+
Wilkes Regional Medical Center	N Wilkesboro	74%	300+
Alamance Regional Medical Center	Burlington	73%	300+
Heritage Hospital	Tarboro	73%	300+
Iredell Memorial Hospital	Statesville	73%	300+
Lake Norman Regional Medical Center	Mooresville	73%	300+
Randolph Hospital	Asheboro	73%	300+
Saint Lukes Hospital	Columbus	73%	(a)
Carolinas Medical Center-Lincoln	Lincolnton	72%	300+
Carteret General Hospital	Morehead City	72%	300+
Duplin General Hospital	Kenansville	72%	300+
Grace Hospital	Morganton	72%	300+
Murphy Medical Center	Murphy	72%	300+
Pitt County Memorial Hospital	Greenville	72%	300+
University of North Carolina Hospital	Chapel Hill	72%	300+
Angel Medical Center	Franklin	71%	300+
Beaufort County Medical Center	Washington	71%	300+
Carolinas Medical Center-Northeast	Concord	71%	300+
Carolinas Medical Center-Union	Monroe	71%	300+
Franklin Regional Medical Center	Louisburg	71%	(a)
Presbyterian Hospital	Charlotte	71%	300+
Stanly Regional Medical Center	Albemarle	71%	300+
Lenoir Memorial Hospital	Kinston	70%	300+
Presbyterian Hospital Matthews	Matthews	70%	300+
Rowan Regional Medical Center	Salisbury	70%	300+
Southeastern Regional Medical Center	Lumberton	70%	300+
Anson Community Hospital	Wadesboro	69%	(a)
Carolinas Medical Center-University	Charlotte	69%	300+
Cleveland Regional Medical Center	Shelby	69%	300+
Granville Medical Center	Oxford	69%	300+
North Carolina Baptist Hospital	Winston-Salem	69%	300+
Roanoke Chowan Hospital	Ahoskie	69%	300+
Central Carolina Hospital	Sanford	68%	300+
Duke Health Raleigh Hospital	Raleigh	68%	300+
Gaston Memorial Hospital	Gastonia	68%	300+
High Point Regional Hospital	High Point	68%	300+
Johnston Memorial Hospital	Smithfield	68%	300+
Kings Mountain Hospital	Kings Mountain	68%	(a)
Park Ridge Hospital	Fletcher	68%	300+
Sampson Regional Medical Center	Clinton	68%	300+
Catawba Valley Medical Center	Hickory	67%	300+
Cherokee Indian Hospital Authority	Cherokee	67%	(a)
Nash General Hospital	Rocky Mount	67%	300+
Wakemed - Cary Hospital	Cary	67%	300+
Wilson Medical Center	Wilson	67%	300+
Cape Fear Valley Medical Center	Fayetteville	66%	300+
Columbus Regional Healthcare System	Whiteville	66%	300+
Onslow Memorial Hospital	Jacksonville	66%	300+
Person Memorial Hospital	Roxboro	66%	300+
Sandhills Regional Medical Center	Hamlet	66%	300+
Alleghany County Memorial Hospital	Sparta	65%	(a)
Betsy Johnson Regional Hospital	Dunn	65%	300+
C J Harris Community Hospital	Sylva	65%	300+
Forsyth Memorial Hospital	Winston-Salem	65%	300+
Presbyterian Hospital Huntersville	Huntersville	65%	300+
Presbyterian-Orthopaedic Hospital	Charlotte	65%	300+
Carolinas Medical Center-Mercy	Charlotte	64%	300+
Rex Hospital	Raleigh	64%	300+
Brunswick Community Hospital	Supply	63%	300+
Caldwell Memorial Hospital	Lenoir	63%	300+
Memorial Mission Hospital	Asheville	63%	300+
The Moses H Cone Memorial Hospital	Greensboro	63%	300+
Scotland Memorial Hospital	Laurinburg	63%	300+
Frye Regional Medical Center	Hickory	62%	300+
Halifax Regional Medical Center	Roanoke Rapids	62%	300+
Wakemed - Raleigh Campus	Raleigh	62%	300+
Carolinas Medical Center-Behavioral Health	Charlotte	60%	300+
Durham Regional Hospital	Durham	59%	300+
Haywood Regional Medical Center	Clyde	59%	300+
Martin General Hospital	Williamston	58%	300+
Carolina East Medical Center	New Bern	57%	300+
Duke University Hospital	Durham	56%	300+

48. Timely Help 'Always' Received

Hospital Name	City	Rate	Cases
Bertie Memorial Hospital	Windsor	85%	(a)
North Carolina Specialty Hospital	Durham	82%	300+
Chatham Hospital	Siler City	79%	(a)
The Outer Banks Hospital	Nags Head	79%	300+
Cleveland Regional Medical Center	Shelby	77%	300+
Medical Park Hospital	Winston-Salem	76%	300+
Kings Mountain Hospital	Kings Mountain	75%	(a)
Saint Lukes Hospital	Columbus	75%	(a)
Angel Medical Center	Franklin	74%	300+
Heritage Hospital	Tarboro	74%	300+
Wilkes Regional Medical Center	N Wilkesboro	74%	300+
Chowan Hospital	Edenton	73%	300+
Rutherford Hospital	Rutherfordton	73%	300+
Valdese General Hospital	Valdese	73%	300+
Carteret General Hospital	Morehead City	72%	300+
Firsthealth Moore Regional Hospital	Pinehurst	72%	300+
Frye Regional Medical Center	Hickory	72%	300+
Spruce Pine Community Hospital	Spruce Pine	72%	300+
Carolinas Medical Center-Union	Monroe	71%	300+
Franklin Regional Medical Center	Louisburg	71%	(a)
Hugh Chatham Memorial Hospital	Elkin	71%	300+
Roanoke Chowan Hospital	Ahoskie	71%	300+
Thomasville Medical Center	Thomasville	71%	300+
Brunswick Community Hospital	Supply	70%	300+
C J Harris Community Hospital	Sylva	70%	300+
The Mcdowell Hospital	Marion	70%	300+
Southeastern Regional Medical Center	Lumberton	70%	300+
Ashe Memorial Hospital	Jefferson	69%	300+
Carolinas Medical Center-Mercy	Charlotte	69%	300+
Duplin General Hospital	Kenansville	69%	300+
Gaston Memorial Hospital	Gastonia	69%	300+
Onslow Memorial Hospital	Jacksonville	69%	300+
Lexington Memorial Hospital	Lexington	68%	300+
Maria Parham Hospital	Henderson	68%	300+
Presbyterian Hospital	Charlotte	68%	300+
Randolph Hospital	Asheboro	68%	300+
Rowan Regional Medical Center	Salisbury	68%	300+
Scotland Memorial Hospital	Laurinburg	68%	300+
Transylvania Regional Hospital	Brevard	68%	300+
Anson Community Hospital	Wadesboro	67%	(a)
Carolinas Medical Center-Lincoln	Lincolnton	67%	300+
Davis Regional Medical Center	Statesville	67%	300+
Granville Medical Center	Oxford	67%	300+
Haywood Regional Medical Center	Clyde	67%	300+
Iredell Memorial Hospital	Statesville	67%	300+
Memorial Mission Hospital	Asheville	67%	300+
Morehead Memorial Hospital	Eden	67%	300+
New Hanover Regional Medical Center	Wilmington	67%	300+
Presbyterian Hospital Huntersville	Huntersville	67%	300+
Carolinas Medical Center-Northeast	Concord	66%	300+
Pitt County Memorial Hospital	Greenville	66%	300+
Stanly Regional Medical Center	Albemarle	66%	300+

NOTE: Hospital profiles are in alphabetical order by state, then city, then hospital within the city; Rankings exclude hospitals with less than 25 cases except for patient surveys which excludes hospitals with less than 100 cases; (a) 100–299 cases; (1) The number of cases is too small to be sure how well a hospital is performing; (2) The hospital indicated that the data submitted for this measure were based on a sample of cases; (3) Data was collected during a shorter time period (fewer quarters) than the maximum possible time for this measure; (4) Suppressed for one or more quarters by CMS; (5) No data is available from the hospital for this measure; (6) Fewer than 100 patients completed the HCAHPS survey. Use these rates with caution, as the number of surveys may be too low to reliably assess hospital performance; (7) Survey results are based on less than 12 months of data; (8) Survey results are not available for this reporting period; (9) No or very few patients were eligible for the HCAHPS survey. The scores shown, if any, reflect a very small number of surveys; (10) A state average was not calculated because too few hospitals in the state submitted data; (11) There were discrepancies in the data collection process; Please refer to the User's Guide for a full explanation of data.

Hospital Name	City	Rate	Cases
Wilson Medical Center	Wilson	66%	300+
Alamance Regional Medical Center	Burlington	65%	300+
Beaufort County Medical Center	Washington	65%	300+
Carolinas Medical Center-Behavioral Health	Charlotte	65%	300+
Columbus Regional Healthcare System	Whiteville	65%	300+
Forsyth Memorial Hospital	Winston-Salem	65%	300+
Lake Norman Regional Medical Center	Mooresville	65%	300+
Murphy Medical Center	Murphy	65%	300+
Northern Hospital of Surry County	Mount Airy	65%	300+
Sampson Regional Medical Center	Clinton	65%	300+
University of North Carolina Hospital	Chapel Hill	65%	300+
Catawba Valley Medical Center	Hickory	64%	300+
Halifax Regional Medical Center	Roanoke Rapids	64%	300+
Nash General Hospital	Rocky Mount	64%	300+
Rex Hospital	Raleigh	64%	300+
Wakemed - Raleigh Campus	Raleigh	64%	300+
Watauga Medical Center	Boone	64%	300+
Albemarle Hospital Authority	Elizabeth City	63%	300+
Alleghany County Memorial Hospital	Sparta	63%	(a)
Carolina East Medical Center	New Bern	63%	300+
Carolinas Medical Center-University	Charlotte	63%	300+
Cherokee Indian Hospital Authority	Cherokee	63%	(a)
Grace Hospital	Morganton	63%	300+
High Point Regional Hospital	High Point	63%	300+
Johnston Memorial Hospital	Smithfield	63%	300+
Park Ridge Hospital	Fletcher	63%	300+
Wayne Memorial Hospital	Goldsboro	63%	300+
Caldwell Memorial Hospital	Lenoir	62%	300+
Duke Health Raleigh Hospital	Raleigh	62%	300+
Margaret R Pardee Memorial Hospital	Hendersonville	62%	300+
Wakemed - Cary Hospital	Cary	61%	300+
Person Memorial Hospital	Roxboro	60%	300+
Presbyterian Hospital Matthews	Matthews	60%	300+
Sandhills Regional Medical Center	Hamlet	60%	300+
Central Carolina Hospital	Sanford	59%	300+
North Carolina Baptist Hospital	Winston-Salem	59%	300+
Lenoir Memorial Hospital	Kinston	58%	300+
The Moses H Cone Memorial Hospital	Greensboro	58%	300+
Martin General Hospital	Williamston	57%	300+
Cape Fear Valley Medical Center	Fayetteville	56%	300+
Durham Regional Hospital	Durham	55%	300+
Betsy Johnson Regional Hospital	Dunn	54%	300+
Duke University Hospital	Durham	54%	300+
Presbyterian-Orthopaedic Hospital	Charlotte	49%	300+
Frye Regional Medical Center	Hickory	72%	300+
Gaston Memorial Hospital	Gastonia	72%	300+
High Point Regional Hospital	High Point	72%	300+
Lake Norman Regional Medical Center	Mooresville	72%	300+
Carteret General Hospital	Morehead City	71%	300+
Chatham Hospital	Siler City	71%	(a)
Carolinas Medical Center-Union	Monroe	70%	300+
Granville Medical Center	Oxford	70%	300+
Margaret R Pardee Memorial Hospital	Hendersonville	70%	300+
Person Memorial Hospital	Roxboro	70%	300+
Alleghany County Memorial Hospital	Sparta	69%	(a)
Durham Regional Hospital	Durham	69%	300+
Ashe Memorial Hospital	Jefferson	68%	300+
The Mcdowell Hospital	Marion	68%	300+
Randolph Hospital	Asheboro	68%	300+
Rutherford Hospital	Rutherfordton	68%	300+
Beaufort County Medical Center	Washington	67%	300+
Haywood Regional Medical Center	Clyde	67%	300+
Murphy Medical Center	Murphy	67%	300+
Rowan Regional Medical Center	Salisbury	67%	300+
Wayne Memorial Hospital	Goldsboro	67%	300+
Wilson Medical Center	Wilson	67%	300+
Carolina East Medical Center	New Bern	66%	300+
Franklin Regional Medical Center	Louisburg	66%	(a)
Grace Hospital	Morganton	66%	300+
Albemarle Hospital Authority	Elizabeth City	65%	300+
Wilkes Regional Medical Center	N Wilkesboro	65%	300+
Maria Parham Hospital	Henderson	64%	300+
Roanoke Chowan Hospital	Ahoskie	64%	300+
Southeastern Regional Medical Center	Lumberton	64%	300+
Carolinas Medical Center-Lincoln	Lincolnton	63%	300+
Columbus Regional Healthcare System	Whiteville	63%	300+
Johnston Memorial Hospital	Smithfield	63%	300+
Lexington Memorial Hospital	Lexington	63%	300+
Alamance Regional Medical Center	Burlington	62%	300+
Brunswick Community Hospital	Supply	62%	300+
Caldwell Memorial Hospital	Lenoir	62%	300+
Duplin General Hospital	Kenansville	62%	300+
Scotland Memorial Hospital	Laurinburg	62%	300+
Lenoir Memorial Hospital	Kinston	61%	300+
Martin General Hospital	Williamston	61%	300+
Sampson Regional Medical Center	Clinton	61%	300+
Northern Hospital of Surry County	Mount Airy	60%	300+
Onslow Memorial Hospital	Jacksonville	60%	300+
Stanly Regional Medical Center	Albemarle	60%	300+
Anson Community Hospital	Wadesboro	59%	(a)
Cape Fear Valley Medical Center	Fayetteville	59%	300+
Central Carolina Hospital	Sanford	59%	300+
Halifax Regional Medical Center	Roanoke Rapids	59%	300+
Sandhills Regional Medical Center	Hamlet	59%	300+
Nash General Hospital	Rocky Mount	57%	300+
Cherokee Indian Hospital Authority	Cherokee	55%	(a)
Betsy Johnson Regional Hospital	Dunn	53%	300+

49. Would Definitely Recommend Hospital

Hospital Name	City	Rate	Cases
North Carolina Specialty Hospital	Durham	92%	300+
Medical Park Hospital	Winston-Salem	88%	300+
Bertie Memorial Hospital	Windsor	85%	(a)
University of North Carolina Hospital	Chapel Hill	85%	300+
Memorial Mission Hospital	Asheville	84%	300+
Rex Hospital	Raleigh	84%	300+
Firsthealth Moore Regional Hospital	Pinehurst	83%	300+
Angel Medical Center	Franklin	82%	300+
Forsyth Memorial Hospital	Winston-Salem	82%	300+
North Carolina Baptist Hospital	Winston-Salem	82%	300+
Pitt County Memorial Hospital	Greenville	82%	300+
Presbyterian Hospital Huntersville	Huntersville	82%	300+
Carolinas Medical Center-Mercy	Charlotte	81%	300+
Presbyterian Hospital	Charlotte	81%	300+
Duke University Hospital	Durham	80%	300+
New Hanover Regional Medical Center	Wilmington	80%	300+
Iredell Memorial Hospital	Statesville	79%	300+
Hugh Chatham Memorial Hospital	Elkin	78%	300+
Cleveland Regional Medical Center	Shelby	77%	300+
Duke Health Raleigh Hospital	Raleigh	77%	300+
Presbyterian Hospital Matthews	Matthews	77%	300+
Saint Lukes Hospital	Columbus	77%	(a)
Valdese General Hospital	Valdese	77%	300+
Watauga Medical Center	Boone	77%	300+
C J Harris Community Hospital	Sylva	76%	300+
Carolinas Medical Center-Behavioral Health	Charlotte	76%	300+
Carolinas Medical Center-Northeast	Concord	76%	300+
Presbyterian-Orthopaedic Hospital	Charlotte	76%	300+
Carolinas Medical Center-University	Charlotte	75%	300+
Catawba Valley Medical Center	Hickory	75%	300+
Davis Regional Medical Center	Statesville	75%	300+
Heritage Hospital	Tarboro	75%	300+
The Outer Banks Hospital	Nags Head	75%	300+
Spruce Pine Community Hospital	Spruce Pine	75%	300+
Transylvania Regional Hospital	Brevard	75%	300+
Wakemed - Cary Hospital	Cary	75%	300+
Wakemed - Raleigh Campus	Raleigh	75%	300+
Chowan Hospital	Edenton	74%	300+
Kings Mountain Hospital	Kings Mountain	74%	(a)
Morehead Memorial Hospital	Eden	74%	300+
Thomasville Medical Center	Thomasville	74%	300+
The Moses H Cone Memorial Hospital	Greensboro	73%	300+
Park Ridge Hospital	Fletcher	73%	300+

NOTE: Hospital profiles are in alphabetical order by state, then city, then hospital within the city; Rankings exclude hospitals with less than 25 cases except for patient surveys which excludes hospitals with less than 100 cases; (a) 100–299 cases (1) The number of cases is too small to be sure how well a hospital is performing; (2) The hospital indicated that the data submitted for this measure were based on a sample of cases; (3) Data was collected during a shorter time period (fewer quarters) than the maximum possible time for this measure; (4) Suppressed for one or more quarters by CMS; (5) No data is available from the hospital for this measure; (6) Fewer than 100 patients completed the HCAHPS survey. Use these rates with caution, as the number of surveys may be too low to reliably assess hospital performance; (7) Survey results are based on less than 12 months of data; (8) Survey results are not available for this reporting period; (9) No or very few patients were eligible for the HCAHPS survey. The scores shown, if any, reflect a very small number of surveys; (10) A state average was not calculated because too few hospitals in the state submitted data; (11) There were discrepancies in the data collection process; Please refer to the User's Guide for a full explanation of data.

Roanoke Chowan Hospital

500 S Academy St Phone: 252-209-3000
Ahoskie, NC 27910 Fax: 252-209-3049
E-mail: lnewsome@uhseast.com
URL: www.uhseast.com
Type: Acute Care Hospitals Emergency Services: Yes
Ownership: Voluntary Non-Profit - Private Beds: 105
Key Personnel:
CEO/President. . . . . Susan S Lassiter
Chief of Medical Staff . . . . Robert Kahn
Radiology. . . . . Mark Adkins

Measure	Cases	This Hosp.	State Avg.	U.S. Avg.
Heart Attack Care				
ACE Inhibitor or ARB for LVSD[1]	2	100%	97%	96%
Aspirin at Arrival[1]	19	100%	99%	99%
Aspirin at Discharge[1]	18	100%	99%	98%
Beta Blocker at Discharge[1]	18	94%	99%	98%
Fibrinolytic Medication Timing	0	-	38%	55%
PCI Within 90 Minutes of Arrival	0	-	95%	90%
Smoking Cessation Advice[1]	9	100%	100%	99%
Chest Pain/Possible Heart Attack Care				
Aspirin at Arrival	61	100%	95%	95%
Median Time to ECG (minutes)	64	8	8	8
Median Time to Transfer (minutes)[3]	0	-	48	61
Fibrinolytic Medication Timing[1]	3	67%	53%	54%
Heart Failure Care				
ACE Inhibitor or ARB for LVSD	50	96%	95%	94%
Discharge Instructions	155	97%	89%	88%
Evaluation of LVS Function	175	100%	99%	98%
Smoking Cessation Advice	36	100%	99%	98%
Pneumonia Care				
Appropriate Initial Antibiotic	62	87%	92%	92%
Blood Culture Timing	99	95%	96%	96%
Influenza Vaccine	66	97%	93%	91%
Initial Antibiotic Timing	94	98%	95%	95%
Pneumococcal Vaccine	80	98%	95%	93%
Smoking Cessation Advice	30	100%	99%	97%
Surgical Care Improvement Project				
Appropriate VTP Within 24 Hours	66	100%	93%	92%
Appropriate Hair Removal	189	100%	100%	99%
Appropriate Beta Blocker Usage	39	100%	94%	93%
Controlled Postoperative Blood Glucose	0	-	94%	93%
Prophylactic Antibiotic Timing	143	97%	98%	97%
Prophylactic Antibiotic Timing (Outpatient)	37	84%	94%	92%
Prophylactic Antibiotic Selection	143	97%	98%	97%
Prophylactic Antibiotic Select. (Outpatient)	43	95%	95%	94%
Prophylactic Antibiotic Stopped	136	97%	96%	94%
Recommended VTP Ordered	66	100%	95%	94%
Urinary Catheter Removal[1]	23	100%	91%	90%
Children's Asthma Care				
Received Systemic Corticosteroids	-	-	100%	100%
Received Home Management Plan	-	-	75%	71%
Received Reliever Medication	-	-	100%	100%
Use of Medical Imaging				
Combination Abdominal CT Scan	448	0.094	0.115	0.191
Combination Chest CT Scan	200	0.005	0.037	0.054
Follow-up Mammogram/Ultrasound	1,225	10.6%	7.9%	8.4%
MRI for Low Back Pain	57	45.6%	30.6%	32.7%
Survey of Patients' Hospital Experiences				
Area Around Room 'Always' Quiet at Night	300+	64%	-	58%
Doctors 'Always' Communicated Well	300+	85%	-	80%
Home Recovery Information Given	300+	84%	-	82%
Hospital Given 9 or 10 on 10 Point Scale	300+	69%	-	67%
Meds 'Always' Explained Before Given	300+	74%	-	60%
Nurses 'Always' Communicated Well	300+	82%	-	76%
Pain 'Always' Well Controlled	300+	74%	-	69%
Room and Bathroom 'Always' Clean	300+	69%	-	71%
Timely Help 'Always' Received	300+	71%	-	64%
Would Definitely Recommend Hospital	300+	64%	-	69%

Stanly Regional Medical Center

301 Yadkin St Phone: 704-984-4000
Albemarle, NC 28001 Fax: 704-983-3562
URL: www.stanly.org
Type: Acute Care Hospitals Emergency Services: Yes
Ownership: Voluntary Non-Profit - Private Beds: 119
Key Personnel:
CEO/President. . . . . Roy Hinson
Chief of Medical Staff . . . . Eric Johnsen
Radiology. . . . . Peter Gusmer
Emergency Room . . . . Judy Moore

Measure	Cases	This Hosp.	State Avg.	U.S. Avg.
Heart Attack Care				
ACE Inhibitor or ARB for LVSD[1]	13	92%	97%	96%
Aspirin at Arrival	41	95%	99%	99%
Aspirin at Discharge	26	100%	99%	98%
Beta Blocker at Discharge	27	89%	99%	98%
Fibrinolytic Medication Timing[1]	1	0%	38%	55%
PCI Within 90 Minutes of Arrival	0	-	95%	90%
Smoking Cessation Advice[1]	3	100%	100%	99%
Chest Pain/Possible Heart Attack Care				
Aspirin at Arrival	92	97%	95%	95%
Median Time to ECG (minutes)	90	6	8	8
Median Time to Transfer (minutes)[1,3]	2	42	48	61
Fibrinolytic Medication Timing[1]	6	67%	53%	54%
Heart Failure Care				
ACE Inhibitor or ARB for LVSD	54	94%	95%	94%
Discharge Instructions	135	70%	89%	88%
Evaluation of LVS Function	184	95%	99%	98%
Smoking Cessation Advice	29	100%	99%	98%
Pneumonia Care				
Appropriate Initial Antibiotic	124	87%	92%	92%
Blood Culture Timing	203	95%	96%	96%
Influenza Vaccine	137	91%	93%	91%
Initial Antibiotic Timing	191	95%	95%	95%
Pneumococcal Vaccine	191	93%	95%	93%
Smoking Cessation Advice	81	98%	99%	97%
Surgical Care Improvement Project				
Appropriate VTP Within 24 Hours	90	88%	93%	92%
Appropriate Hair Removal	222	99%	100%	99%
Appropriate Beta Blocker Usage	59	93%	94%	93%
Controlled Postoperative Blood Glucose	0	-	94%	93%
Prophylactic Antibiotic Timing	121	97%	98%	97%
Prophylactic Antibiotic Timing (Outpatient)	127	80%	94%	92%
Prophylactic Antibiotic Selection	121	97%	98%	97%
Prophylactic Antibiotic Select. (Outpatient)	129	88%	95%	94%
Prophylactic Antibiotic Stopped	108	94%	96%	94%
Recommended VTP Ordered	91	90%	95%	94%
Urinary Catheter Removal	27	81%	91%	90%
Children's Asthma Care				
Received Systemic Corticosteroids	-	-	100%	100%
Received Home Management Plan	-	-	75%	71%
Received Reliever Medication	-	-	100%	100%
Use of Medical Imaging				
Combination Abdominal CT Scan	828	0.079	0.115	0.191
Combination Chest CT Scan	543	0.020	0.037	0.054
Follow-up Mammogram/Ultrasound	1,442	5.1%	7.9%	8.4%
MRI for Low Back Pain	156	34.6%	30.6%	32.7%
Survey of Patients' Hospital Experiences				
Area Around Room 'Always' Quiet at Night	300+	59%	-	58%
Doctors 'Always' Communicated Well	300+	81%	-	80%
Home Recovery Information Given	300+	80%	-	82%
Hospital Given 9 or 10 on 10 Point Scale	300+	63%	-	67%
Meds 'Always' Explained Before Given	300+	60%	-	60%
Nurses 'Always' Communicated Well	300+	76%	-	76%
Pain 'Always' Well Controlled	300+	68%	-	69%
Room and Bathroom 'Always' Clean	300+	71%	-	71%
Timely Help 'Always' Received	300+	66%	-	64%
Would Definitely Recommend Hospital	300+	60%	-	69%

Randolph Hospital

364 White Oak Street Phone: 336-625-5151
Asheboro, NC 27204 Fax: 336-626-7664
E-mail: amt@randolphhospital.org
URL: www.randolphhospital.org
Type: Acute Care Hospitals Emergency Services: Yes
Ownership: Voluntary Non-Profit - Private Beds: 145
Key Personnel:
CEO/President. . . . . Robert E Morrison
Chief of Medical Staff . . . . Charles B West, MD
Radiology. . . . . Paul D Barry

Measure	Cases	This Hosp.	State Avg.	U.S. Avg.
Heart Attack Care				
ACE Inhibitor or ARB for LVSD[1]	6	100%	97%	96%
Aspirin at Arrival	59	97%	99%	99%
Aspirin at Discharge	32	88%	99%	98%
Beta Blocker at Discharge	36	100%	99%	98%
Fibrinolytic Medication Timing	0	-	38%	55%
PCI Within 90 Minutes of Arrival	0	-	95%	90%
Smoking Cessation Advice[1]	7	100%	100%	99%
Chest Pain/Possible Heart Attack Care				
Aspirin at Arrival	178	94%	95%	95%
Median Time to ECG (minutes)	185	8	8	8
Median Time to Transfer (minutes)	40	58	48	61
Fibrinolytic Medication Timing	0	-	53%	54%
Heart Failure Care				
ACE Inhibitor or ARB for LVSD[2]	59	81%	95%	94%
Discharge Instructions[2]	219	66%	89%	88%
Evaluation of LVS Function[2]	284	97%	99%	98%
Smoking Cessation Advice[2]	59	100%	99%	98%
Pneumonia Care				
Appropriate Initial Antibiotic[2]	116	89%	92%	92%
Blood Culture Timing[2]	140	95%	96%	96%
Influenza Vaccine[2]	89	92%	93%	91%
Initial Antibiotic Timing[2]	108	94%	95%	95%
Pneumococcal Vaccine[2]	109	85%	95%	93%
Smoking Cessation Advice[2]	75	100%	99%	97%
Surgical Care Improvement Project				
Appropriate VTP Within 24 Hours[2]	125	83%	93%	92%
Appropriate Hair Removal[2]	229	99%	100%	99%
Appropriate Beta Blocker Usage[2]	70	79%	94%	93%
Controlled Postoperative Blood Glucose[2]	0	-	94%	93%
Prophylactic Antibiotic Timing[2]	125	95%	98%	97%
Prophylactic Antibiotic Timing (Outpatient)	193	95%	94%	92%
Prophylactic Antibiotic Selection[2]	126	97%	98%	97%
Prophylactic Antibiotic Select. (Outpatient)	191	91%	95%	94%
Prophylactic Antibiotic Stopped[2]	116	91%	96%	94%
Recommended VTP Ordered[2]	125	88%	95%	94%
Urinary Catheter Removal[2]	25	100%	91%	90%
Children's Asthma Care				
Received Systemic Corticosteroids	-	-	100%	100%
Received Home Management Plan	-	-	75%	71%
Received Reliever Medication	-	-	100%	100%
Use of Medical Imaging				
Combination Abdominal CT Scan	727	0.032	0.115	0.191
Combination Chest CT Scan	532	0.130	0.037	0.054
Follow-up Mammogram/Ultrasound	928	10.0%	7.9%	8.4%
MRI for Low Back Pain	157	29.3%	30.6%	32.7%
Survey of Patients' Hospital Experiences				
Area Around Room 'Always' Quiet at Night	300+	58%	-	58%
Doctors 'Always' Communicated Well	300+	80%	-	80%
Home Recovery Information Given	300+	79%	-	82%
Hospital Given 9 or 10 on 10 Point Scale	300+	67%	-	67%
Meds 'Always' Explained Before Given	300+	62%	-	60%
Nurses 'Always' Communicated Well	300+	80%	-	76%
Pain 'Always' Well Controlled	300+	68%	-	69%
Room and Bathroom 'Always' Clean	300+	73%	-	71%
Timely Help 'Always' Received	300+	68%	-	64%
Would Definitely Recommend Hospital	300+	68%	-	69%

NOTE: Hospital profiles are in alphabetical order by state, then city, then hospital within the city; Rankings exclude hospitals with less than 25 cases except for patient surveys which excludes hospitals with less than 100 cases; (a) 100–299 cases; (1) The number of cases is too small to be sure how well a hospital is performing; (2) The hospital indicated that the data submitted for this measure were based on a sample of cases; (3) Data was collected during a shorter time period (fewer quarters) than the maximum possible time for this measure; (4) Suppressed for one or more quarters by CMS; (5) No data is available from the hospital for this measure; (6) Fewer than 100 patients completed the HCAHPS survey. Use these rates with caution, as the number of surveys may be too low to reliably assess hospital performance; (7) Survey results are based on less than 12 months of data; (8) Survey results are not available for this reporting period; (9) No or very few patients were eligible for the HCAHPS survey. The scores shown, if any, reflect a very small number of surveys; (10) A state average was not calculated because too few hospitals in the state submitted data; (11) There were discrepancies in the data collection process; Please refer to the User's Guide for a full explanation of data.

Asheville-Oteen VA Medical Center

1100 Tunnel Road
Asheville, NC 28805
Phone: 828-298-7911
Fax: 828-299-2501
URL: www.asheville.va.gov
Type: Acute Care-Veterans Administration
Emergency Services: No
Ownership: Government - Federal

Key Personnel:
CEO/President. . . . . Susan Pendergrass
Chief of Medical Staff. . . . . MaryAnn Curl MD
Radiology. . . . . Keith Kohatsu MD
Emergency Room . . . . James Johnson MD

Measure	Cases	This Hosp.	State Avg.	U.S. Avg.
Heart Attack Care				
ACE Inhibitor or ARB for LVSD[1]	10	90%	97%	96%
Aspirin at Arrival	46	100%	99%	99%
Aspirin at Discharge	41	95%	99%	98%
Beta Blocker at Discharge	41	98%	99%	98%
Fibrinolytic Medication Timing[5]	0	-	38%	55%
PCI Within 90 Minutes of Arrival[1]	4	25%	95%	90%
Smoking Cessation Advice[1]	16	100%	100%	99%
Chest Pain/Possible Heart Attack Care				
Aspirin at Arrival	-	-	95%	95%
Median Time to ECG (minutes)	-	-	8	8
Median Time to Transfer (minutes)	-	-	48	61
Fibrinolytic Medication Timing	-	-	53%	54%
Heart Failure Care				
ACE Inhibitor or ARB for LVSD	51	86%	95%	94%
Discharge Instructions	96	85%	89%	88%
Evaluation of LVS Function	117	98%	99%	98%
Smoking Cessation Advice	25	100%	99%	98%
Pneumonia Care				
Appropriate Initial Antibiotic	106	82%	92%	92%
Blood Culture Timing	127	99%	96%	96%
Influenza Vaccine	87	90%	93%	91%
Initial Antibiotic Timing	129	93%	95%	95%
Pneumococcal Vaccine	126	92%	95%	93%
Smoking Cessation Advice	40	100%	99%	97%
Surgical Care Improvement Project				
Appropriate VTP Within 24 Hours[2]	87	97%	93%	92%
Appropriate Hair Removal[2]	477	100%	100%	99%
Appropriate Beta Blocker Usage[2]	263	100%	94%	93%
Controlled Postoperative Blood Glucose[2]	194	97%	94%	93%
Prophylactic Antibiotic Timing	387	99%	98%	97%
Prophylactic Antibiotic Timing (Outpatient)	-	-	94%	92%
Prophylactic Antibiotic Selection	389	100%	98%	97%
Prophylactic Antibiotic Select. (Outpatient)	-	-	95%	94%
Prophylactic Antibiotic Stopped	369	99%	96%	94%
Recommended VTP Ordered[2]	87	97%	95%	94%
Urinary Catheter Removal[2]	297	100%	91%	90%
Children's Asthma Care				
Received Systemic Corticosteroids	-	-	100%	100%
Received Home Management Plan	-	-	75%	71%
Received Reliever Medication	-	-	100%	100%
Use of Medical Imaging				
Combination Abdominal CT Scan	-	-	0.115	0.191
Combination Chest CT Scan	-	-	0.037	0.054
Follow-up Mammogram/Ultrasound	-	-	7.9%	8.4%
MRI for Low Back Pain	-	-	30.6%	32.7%
Survey of Patients' Hospital Experiences				
Area Around Room 'Always' Quiet at Night	-	-	-	58%
Doctors 'Always' Communicated Well	-	-	-	80%
Home Recovery Information Given	-	-	-	82%
Hospital Given 9 or 10 on 10 Point Scale	-	-	-	67%
Meds 'Always' Explained Before Given	-	-	-	60%
Nurses 'Always' Communicated Well	-	-	-	76%
Pain 'Always' Well Controlled	-	-	-	69%
Room and Bathroom 'Always' Clean	-	-	-	71%
Timely Help 'Always' Received	-	-	-	64%
Would Definitely Recommend Hospital	-	-	-	69%

Memorial Mission Hospital and Asheville Surgery Center

509 Biltmore Ave
Asheville, NC 28801
Phone: 828-213-1111
Fax: 828-213-4404
URL: www.missionhospitals.org
Type: Acute Care Hospitals
Emergency Services: Yes
Ownership: Voluntary Non-Profit - Private
Beds: 800

Key Personnel:
CEO/President. . . . . Carlton T. Rider
Cardiac Laboratory. . . . . Karen Lemieux
Chief of Medical Staff. . . . . Alan S. Baumgarten, MD
Ambulatory Care . . . . Kristi Sink
Anesthesiology. . . . . Ann Young, JD

Measure	Cases	This Hosp.	State Avg.	U.S. Avg.
Heart Attack Care				
ACE Inhibitor or ARB for LVSD	310	100%	97%	96%
Aspirin at Arrival	696	100%	99%	99%
Aspirin at Discharge	1,297	100%	99%	98%
Beta Blocker at Discharge	1,273	100%	99%	98%
Fibrinolytic Medication Timing	0	-	38%	55%
PCI Within 90 Minutes of Arrival	109	95%	95%	90%
Smoking Cessation Advice	455	100%	100%	99%
Chest Pain/Possible Heart Attack Care				
Aspirin at Arrival[1]	4	100%	95%	95%
Median Time to ECG (minutes)[1]	4	18	8	8
Median Time to Transfer (minutes)[5]	0	-	48	61
Fibrinolytic Medication Timing[3]	0	-	53%	54%
Heart Failure Care				
ACE Inhibitor or ARB for LVSD[2]	314	98%	95%	94%
Discharge Instructions[2]	665	91%	89%	88%
Evaluation of LVS Function[2]	791	100%	99%	98%
Smoking Cessation Advice[2]	131	100%	99%	98%
Pneumonia Care				
Appropriate Initial Antibiotic[2]	146	86%	92%	92%
Blood Culture Timing[2]	256	94%	96%	96%
Influenza Vaccine[2]	416	87%	93%	91%
Initial Antibiotic Timing[2]	275	92%	95%	95%
Pneumococcal Vaccine[2]	532	94%	95%	93%
Smoking Cessation Advice[2]	244	100%	99%	97%
Surgical Care Improvement Project				
Appropriate VTP Within 24 Hours[2]	906	97%	93%	92%
Appropriate Hair Removal[2]	3,005	100%	100%	99%
Appropriate Beta Blocker Usage[2]	999	98%	94%	93%
Controlled Postoperative Blood Glucose[2]	611	99%	94%	93%
Prophylactic Antibiotic Timing[2]	2,378	98%	98%	97%
Prophylactic Antibiotic Timing (Outpatient)	1,003	97%	94%	92%
Prophylactic Antibiotic Selection[2]	2,405	100%	98%	97%
Prophylactic Antibiotic Select. (Outpatient)	1,003	98%	95%	94%
Prophylactic Antibiotic Stopped[2]	2,258	97%	96%	94%
Recommended VTP Ordered[2]	906	98%	95%	94%
Urinary Catheter Removal[2]	544	95%	91%	90%
Children's Asthma Care				
Received Systemic Corticosteroids	36	100%	100%	100%
Received Home Management Plan	36	19%	75%	71%
Received Reliever Medication	36	100%	100%	100%
Use of Medical Imaging				
Combination Abdominal CT Scan	1,109	0.013	0.115	0.191
Combination Chest CT Scan	407	0.000	0.037	0.054
Follow-up Mammogram/Ultrasound[5]	0	-	7.9%	8.4%
MRI for Low Back Pain	151	36.4%	30.6%	32.7%
Survey of Patients' Hospital Experiences				
Area Around Room 'Always' Quiet at Night	300+	60%	-	58%
Doctors 'Always' Communicated Well	300+	83%	-	80%
Home Recovery Information Given	300+	85%	-	82%
Hospital Given 9 or 10 on 10 Point Scale	300+	71%	-	67%
Meds 'Always' Explained Before Given	300+	59%	-	60%
Nurses 'Always' Communicated Well	300+	79%	-	76%
Pain 'Always' Well Controlled	300+	72%	-	69%
Room and Bathroom 'Always' Clean	300+	63%	-	71%
Timely Help 'Always' Received	300+	67%	-	64%
Would Definitely Recommend Hospital	300+	84%	-	69%

Pungo District Hospital

210 East Water St
Belhaven, NC 27810
Phone: 252-943-2111
Fax: 252-944-2236
Type: Critical Access Hospitals
Emergency Services: Yes
Ownership: Voluntary Non-Profit - Private
Beds: 49

Key Personnel:
CEO/President. . . . . Kenneth Ragland
Chief of Medical Staff. . . . . Mark Beamer, MD

Measure	Cases	This Hosp.	State Avg.	U.S. Avg.
Heart Attack Care				
ACE Inhibitor or ARB for LVSD[5]	0	-	97%	96%
Aspirin at Arrival[5]	0	-	99%	99%
Aspirin at Discharge[5]	0	-	99%	98%
Beta Blocker at Discharge[5]	0	-	99%	98%
Fibrinolytic Medication Timing[5]	0	-	38%	55%
PCI Within 90 Minutes of Arrival[5]	0	-	95%	90%
Smoking Cessation Advice[5]	0	-	100%	99%
Chest Pain/Possible Heart Attack Care				
Aspirin at Arrival	-	-	95%	95%
Median Time to ECG (minutes)	-	-	8	8
Median Time to Transfer (minutes)	-	-	48	61
Fibrinolytic Medication Timing	-	-	53%	54%
Heart Failure Care				
ACE Inhibitor or ARB for LVSD[1]	7	100%	95%	94%
Discharge Instructions	26	96%	89%	88%
Evaluation of LVS Function[1]	24	100%	99%	98%
Smoking Cessation Advice[1]	5	100%	99%	98%
Pneumonia Care				
Appropriate Initial Antibiotic[1]	18	61%	92%	92%
Blood Culture Timing[1]	19	74%	96%	96%
Influenza Vaccine[1]	16	100%	93%	91%
Initial Antibiotic Timing[1]	22	86%	95%	95%
Pneumococcal Vaccine	25	100%	95%	93%
Smoking Cessation Advice[1]	7	100%	99%	97%
Surgical Care Improvement Project				
Appropriate VTP Within 24 Hours[5]	0	-	93%	92%
Appropriate Hair Removal[5]	0	-	100%	99%
Appropriate Beta Blocker Usage[5]	0	-	94%	93%
Controlled Postoperative Blood Glucose[5]	0	-	94%	93%
Prophylactic Antibiotic Timing[5]	0	-	98%	97%
Prophylactic Antibiotic Timing (Outpatient)	-	-	94%	92%
Prophylactic Antibiotic Selection[5]	0	-	98%	97%
Prophylactic Antibiotic Select. (Outpatient)	-	-	95%	94%
Prophylactic Antibiotic Stopped[5]	0	-	96%	94%
Recommended VTP Ordered[5]	0	-	95%	94%
Urinary Catheter Removal[5]	0	-	91%	90%
Children's Asthma Care				
Received Systemic Corticosteroids	-	-	100%	100%
Received Home Management Plan	-	-	75%	71%
Received Reliever Medication	-	-	100%	100%
Use of Medical Imaging				
Combination Abdominal CT Scan	-	-	0.115	0.191
Combination Chest CT Scan	-	-	0.037	0.054
Follow-up Mammogram/Ultrasound	-	-	7.9%	8.4%
MRI for Low Back Pain	-	-	30.6%	32.7%
Survey of Patients' Hospital Experiences				
Area Around Room 'Always' Quiet at Night[8]	-	-	-	58%
Doctors 'Always' Communicated Well[8]	-	-	-	80%
Home Recovery Information Given[8]	-	-	-	82%
Hospital Given 9 or 10 on 10 Point Scale[8]	-	-	-	67%
Meds 'Always' Explained Before Given[8]	-	-	-	60%
Nurses 'Always' Communicated Well[8]	-	-	-	76%
Pain 'Always' Well Controlled[8]	-	-	-	69%
Room and Bathroom 'Always' Clean[8]	-	-	-	71%
Timely Help 'Always' Received[8]	-	-	-	64%
Would Definitely Recommend Hospital[8]	-	-	-	69%

NOTE: Hospital profiles are in alphabetical order by state, then city, then hospital within the city; Rankings exclude hospitals with less than 25 cases except for patient surveys which excludes hospitals with less than 100 cases; (a) 100–299 cases; (1) The number of cases is too small to be sure how well a hospital is performing; (2) The hospital indicated that the data submitted for this measure were based on a sample of cases; (3) Data was collected during a shorter time period (fewer quarters) than the maximum possible time for this measure; (4) Suppressed for one or more quarters by CMS; (5) No data is available from the hospital for this measure; (6) Fewer than 100 patients completed the HCAHPS survey. Use these rates with caution, as the number of surveys may be too low to reliably assess hospital performance; (7) Survey results are based on less than 12 months of data; (8) Survey results are not available for this reporting period; (9) No or very few patients were eligible for the HCAHPS survey. The scores shown, if any, reflect a very small number of surveys; (10) A state average was not calculated because too few hospitals in the state submitted data; (11) There were discrepancies in the data collection process; Please refer to the User's Guide for a full explanation of data.

Blowing Rock Hospital

418 Chestnut Drive
Blowing Rock, NC 28605
Phone: 828-295-3136
Fax: 828-295-6698
URL: www.blowingrockhospital.org
Type: Critical Access Hospitals
Emergency Services: Yes
Ownership: Voluntary Non-Profit - Private
Beds: 100

Key Personnel:
CEO/President. . . . . Alice Salthouse
Chief of Medical Staff. . . . . Dr. Charles Davant, III

Measure	Cases	This Hosp.	State Avg.	U.S. Avg.
Heart Attack Care				
ACE Inhibitor or ARB for LVSD[5]	0	-	97%	96%
Aspirin at Arrival[5]	0	-	99%	99%
Aspirin at Discharge[5]	0	-	99%	98%
Beta Blocker at Discharge[5]	0	-	99%	98%
Fibrinolytic Medication Timing[5]	0	-	38%	55%
PCI Within 90 Minutes of Arrival[5]	0	-	95%	90%
Smoking Cessation Advice[5]	0	-	100%	99%
Chest Pain/Possible Heart Attack Care				
Aspirin at Arrival	-	-	95%	95%
Median Time to ECG (minutes)	-	-	8	8
Median Time to Transfer (minutes)	-	-	48	61
Fibrinolytic Medication Timing	-	-	53%	54%
Heart Failure Care				
ACE Inhibitor or ARB for LVSD[5]	0	-	95%	94%
Discharge Instructions[5]	0	-	89%	88%
Evaluation of LVS Function[5]	0	-	99%	98%
Smoking Cessation Advice[5]	0	-	99%	98%
Pneumonia Care				
Appropriate Initial Antibiotic[5]	0	-	92%	92%
Blood Culture Timing[5]	0	-	96%	96%
Influenza Vaccine[5]	0	-	93%	91%
Initial Antibiotic Timing[5]	0	-	95%	95%
Pneumococcal Vaccine[5]	0	-	95%	93%
Smoking Cessation Advice[5]	0	-	99%	97%
Surgical Care Improvement Project				
Appropriate VTP Within 24 Hours[5]	0	-	93%	92%
Appropriate Hair Removal[5]	0	-	100%	99%
Appropriate Beta Blocker Usage[5]	0	-	94%	93%
Controlled Postoperative Blood Glucose[5]	0	-	94%	93%
Prophylactic Antibiotic Timing[5]	0	-	98%	97%
Prophylactic Antibiotic Timing (Outpatient)	-	-	94%	92%
Prophylactic Antibiotic Selection[5]	0	-	98%	97%
Prophylactic Antibiotic Select. (Outpatient)	-	-	95%	94%
Prophylactic Antibiotic Stopped[5]	0	-	96%	94%
Recommended VTP Ordered[5]	0	-	95%	94%
Urinary Catheter Removal[5]	0	-	91%	90%
Children's Asthma Care				
Received Systemic Corticosteroids	-	-	100%	100%
Received Home Management Plan	-	-	75%	71%
Received Reliever Medication	-	-	100%	100%
Use of Medical Imaging				
Combination Abdominal CT Scan	-	-	0.115	0.191
Combination Chest CT Scan	-	-	0.037	0.054
Follow-up Mammogram/Ultrasound	-	-	7.9%	8.4%
MRI for Low Back Pain	-	-	30.6%	32.7%
Survey of Patients' Hospital Experiences				
Area Around Room 'Always' Quiet at Night[8]	-	-	-	58%
Doctors 'Always' Communicated Well[8]	-	-	-	80%
Home Recovery Information Given[8]	-	-	-	82%
Hospital Given 9 or 10 on 10 Point Scale[8]	-	-	-	67%
Meds 'Always' Explained Before Given[8]	-	-	-	60%
Nurses 'Always' Communicated Well[8]	-	-	-	76%
Pain 'Always' Well Controlled[8]	-	-	-	69%
Room and Bathroom 'Always' Clean[8]	-	-	-	71%
Timely Help 'Always' Received[8]	-	-	-	64%
Would Definitely Recommend Hospital[8]	-	-	-	69%

Watauga Medical Center

336 Deerfield Road
Boone, NC 28607
Phone: 828-262-4100
Fax: 828-262-4103
URL: www.wataugamc.org
Type: Acute Care Hospitals
Emergency Services: Yes
Ownership: Government - Local
Beds: 127

Key Personnel:
CEO/President. . . . . Richard G Sparks
Infection Control. . . . . Anne Brown
Operating Room. . . . . Peggy Burdiss
Quality Assurance . . . . Maran Sigmon
Emergency Room . . . . Allen Brandon, MD
Intensive Care Unit. . . . . Terry McGuire

Measure	Cases	This Hosp.	State Avg.	U.S. Avg.
Heart Attack Care				
ACE Inhibitor or ARB for LVSD[1]	4	100%	97%	96%
Aspirin at Arrival	61	98%	99%	99%
Aspirin at Discharge	38	89%	99%	98%
Beta Blocker at Discharge	33	94%	99%	98%
Fibrinolytic Medication Timing	0	-	38%	55%
PCI Within 90 Minutes of Arrival	0	-	95%	90%
Smoking Cessation Advice[1]	5	100%	100%	99%
Chest Pain/Possible Heart Attack Care				
Aspirin at Arrival	77	100%	95%	95%
Median Time to ECG (minutes)	79	12	8	8
Median Time to Transfer (minutes)[1,3]	1	81	48	61
Fibrinolytic Medication Timing[1]	9	67%	53%	54%
Heart Failure Care				
ACE Inhibitor or ARB for LVSD	36	100%	95%	94%
Discharge Instructions	102	94%	89%	88%
Evaluation of LVS Function	127	100%	99%	98%
Smoking Cessation Advice[1]	10	100%	99%	98%
Pneumonia Care				
Appropriate Initial Antibiotic	88	94%	92%	92%
Blood Culture Timing	137	97%	96%	96%
Influenza Vaccine	153	85%	93%	91%
Initial Antibiotic Timing	145	97%	95%	95%
Pneumococcal Vaccine	200	96%	95%	93%
Smoking Cessation Advice	66	97%	99%	97%
Surgical Care Improvement Project				
Appropriate VTP Within 24 Hours	136	82%	93%	92%
Appropriate Hair Removal	308	100%	100%	99%
Appropriate Beta Blocker Usage	75	97%	94%	93%
Controlled Postoperative Blood Glucose	0	-	94%	93%
Prophylactic Antibiotic Timing	224	98%	98%	97%
Prophylactic Antibiotic Timing (Outpatient)	128	93%	94%	92%
Prophylactic Antibiotic Selection	226	96%	98%	97%
Prophylactic Antibiotic Select. (Outpatient)	123	79%	95%	94%
Prophylactic Antibiotic Stopped	212	90%	96%	94%
Recommended VTP Ordered	136	85%	95%	94%
Urinary Catheter Removal	25	84%	91%	90%
Children's Asthma Care				
Received Systemic Corticosteroids	-	-	100%	100%
Received Home Management Plan	-	-	75%	71%
Received Reliever Medication	-	-	100%	100%
Use of Medical Imaging				
Combination Abdominal CT Scan	572	0.210	0.115	0.191
Combination Chest CT Scan	462	0.041	0.037	0.054
Follow-up Mammogram/Ultrasound	1,171	10.6%	7.9%	8.4%
MRI for Low Back Pain	170	26.5%	30.6%	32.7%
Survey of Patients' Hospital Experiences				
Area Around Room 'Always' Quiet at Night	300+	60%	-	58%
Doctors 'Always' Communicated Well	300+	86%	-	80%
Home Recovery Information Given	300+	83%	-	82%
Hospital Given 9 or 10 on 10 Point Scale	300+	71%	-	67%
Meds 'Always' Explained Before Given	300+	63%	-	60%
Nurses 'Always' Communicated Well	300+	79%	-	76%
Pain 'Always' Well Controlled	300+	73%	-	69%
Room and Bathroom 'Always' Clean	300+	74%	-	71%
Timely Help 'Always' Received	300+	64%	-	64%
Would Definitely Recommend Hospital	300+	77%	-	69%

Transylvania Regional Hospital

90 Hospital Drive
Brevard, NC 28712
Phone: 828-883-5302
Fax: 828-883-5370
URL: www.tchospital.org
Type: Critical Access Hospitals
Emergency Services: Yes
Ownership: Voluntary Non-Profit - Private
Beds: 88

Key Personnel:
Chief of Medical Staff. . . . . Carmelo Hernandez
Radiology. . . . . Timothy P Desmond

Measure	Cases	This Hosp.	State Avg.	U.S. Avg.
Heart Attack Care				
ACE Inhibitor or ARB for LVSD	0	-	97%	96%
Aspirin at Arrival[1]	7	86%	99%	99%
Aspirin at Discharge[1]	5	100%	99%	98%
Beta Blocker at Discharge[1]	5	100%	99%	98%
Fibrinolytic Medication Timing	0	-	38%	55%
PCI Within 90 Minutes of Arrival	0	-	95%	90%
Smoking Cessation Advice	0	-	100%	99%
Chest Pain/Possible Heart Attack Care				
Aspirin at Arrival	-	-	95%	95%
Median Time to ECG (minutes)	-	-	8	8
Median Time to Transfer (minutes)	-	-	48	61
Fibrinolytic Medication Timing	-	-	53%	54%
Heart Failure Care				
ACE Inhibitor or ARB for LVSD[1]	16	100%	95%	94%
Discharge Instructions	28	71%	89%	88%
Evaluation of LVS Function	42	100%	99%	98%
Smoking Cessation Advice[1]	10	100%	99%	98%
Pneumonia Care				
Appropriate Initial Antibiotic	57	95%	92%	92%
Blood Culture Timing	70	99%	96%	96%
Influenza Vaccine	37	97%	93%	91%
Initial Antibiotic Timing	67	97%	95%	95%
Pneumococcal Vaccine	59	100%	95%	93%
Smoking Cessation Advice[1]	24	92%	99%	97%
Surgical Care Improvement Project				
Appropriate VTP Within 24 Hours	58	97%	93%	92%
Appropriate Hair Removal	126	100%	100%	99%
Appropriate Beta Blocker Usage	30	100%	94%	93%
Controlled Postoperative Blood Glucose	0	-	94%	93%
Prophylactic Antibiotic Timing	84	100%	98%	97%
Prophylactic Antibiotic Timing (Outpatient)	-	-	94%	92%
Prophylactic Antibiotic Selection	87	100%	98%	97%
Prophylactic Antibiotic Select. (Outpatient)	-	-	95%	94%
Prophylactic Antibiotic Stopped	83	99%	96%	94%
Recommended VTP Ordered	59	95%	95%	94%
Urinary Catheter Removal	25	88%	91%	90%
Children's Asthma Care				
Received Systemic Corticosteroids	-	-	100%	100%
Received Home Management Plan	-	-	75%	71%
Received Reliever Medication	-	-	100%	100%
Use of Medical Imaging				
Combination Abdominal CT Scan	-	-	0.115	0.191
Combination Chest CT Scan	-	-	0.037	0.054
Follow-up Mammogram/Ultrasound	-	-	7.9%	8.4%
MRI for Low Back Pain	-	-	30.6%	32.7%
Survey of Patients' Hospital Experiences				
Area Around Room 'Always' Quiet at Night	300+	68%	-	58%
Doctors 'Always' Communicated Well	300+	80%	-	80%
Home Recovery Information Given	300+	87%	-	82%
Hospital Given 9 or 10 on 10 Point Scale	300+	76%	-	67%
Meds 'Always' Explained Before Given	300+	62%	-	60%
Nurses 'Always' Communicated Well	300+	81%	-	76%
Pain 'Always' Well Controlled	300+	71%	-	69%
Room and Bathroom 'Always' Clean	300+	78%	-	71%
Timely Help 'Always' Received	300+	68%	-	64%
Would Definitely Recommend Hospital	300+	75%	-	69%

NOTE: Hospital profiles are in alphabetical order by state, then city, then hospital within the city; Rankings exclude hospitals with less than 25 cases except for patient surveys which excludes hospitals with less than 100 cases; (a) 100–299 cases; (1) The number of cases is too small to be sure how well a hospital is performing; (2) The hospital indicated that the data submitted for this measure were based on a sample of cases; (3) Data was collected during a shorter time period (fewer quarters) than the maximum possible time for this measure; (4) Suppressed for one or more quarters by CMS; (5) No data is available from the hospital for this measure; (6) Fewer than 100 patients completed the HCAHPS survey. Use these rates with caution, as the number of surveys may be too low to reliably assess hospital performance; (7) Survey results are based on less than 12 months of data; (8) Survey results are not available for this reporting period; (9) No or very few patients were eligible for the HCAHPS survey. The scores shown, if any, reflect a very small number of surveys; (10) A state average was not calculated because too few hospitals in the state submitted data; (11) There were discrepancies in the data collection process; Please refer to the User's Guide for a full explanation of data.

Pender Memorial Hospital

507 E Fremont St
Burgaw, NC 28425
URL: www.nhhn.org
Type: Critical Access Hospitals
Ownership: Government - Local

Phone: 910-259-5451
Fax: 910-259-7136

Emergency Services: Yes
Beds: 68

Key Personnel:

Chief of Medical Staff	Naseem Nasrallah, MD
Operating Room	Karenie Schaller
Quality Assurance	Verna Walkins
Radiology	Walter C Whitehurst, Jr
Anesthesiology	Don Shinoskie

Measure	Cases	This Hosp.	State Avg.	U.S. Avg.
Heart Attack Care				
ACE Inhibitor or ARB for LVSD[5]	0	-	97%	96%
Aspirin at Arrival[5]	0	-	99%	99%
Aspirin at Discharge[5]	0	-	99%	98%
Beta Blocker at Discharge[5]	0	-	99%	98%
Fibrinolytic Medication Timing[5]	0	-	38%	55%
PCI Within 90 Minutes of Arrival[5]	0	-	95%	90%
Smoking Cessation Advice[5]	0	-	100%	99%
Chest Pain/Possible Heart Attack Care				
Aspirin at Arrival	-	-	95%	95%
Median Time to ECG (minutes)	-	-	8	8
Median Time to Transfer (minutes)	-	-	48	61
Fibrinolytic Medication Timing	-	-	53%	54%
Heart Failure Care				
ACE Inhibitor or ARB for LVSD[1,3]	3	100%	95%	94%
Discharge Instructions[1,3]	11	100%	89%	88%
Evaluation of LVS Function[1,3]	13	92%	99%	98%
Smoking Cessation Advice[1,3]	6	83%	99%	98%
Pneumonia Care				
Appropriate Initial Antibiotic[3]	0	-	92%	92%
Blood Culture Timing[1,3]	17	100%	96%	96%
Influenza Vaccine[1,3]	7	86%	93%	91%
Initial Antibiotic Timing[1,3]	23	96%	95%	95%
Pneumococcal Vaccine[1,3]	15	80%	95%	93%
Smoking Cessation Advice[1,3]	7	100%	99%	97%
Surgical Care Improvement Project				
Appropriate VTP Within 24 Hours[1,3]	1	0%	93%	92%
Appropriate Hair Removal[1,3]	4	100%	100%	99%
Appropriate Beta Blocker Usage[5]	0	-	94%	93%
Controlled Postoperative Blood Glucose[3]	0	-	94%	93%
Prophylactic Antibiotic Timing[1,3]	1	100%	98%	97%
Prophylactic Antibiotic Timing (Outpatient)	-	-	94%	92%
Prophylactic Antibiotic Selection[1,3]	1	100%	98%	97%
Prophylactic Antibiotic Select. (Outpatient)	-	-	95%	94%
Prophylactic Antibiotic Stopped[1,3]	1	100%	96%	94%
Recommended VTP Ordered[1,3]	1	0%	95%	94%
Urinary Catheter Removal[5]	0	-	91%	90%
Children's Asthma Care				
Received Systemic Corticosteroids	-	-	100%	100%
Received Home Management Plan	-	-	75%	71%
Received Reliever Medication	-	-	100%	100%
Use of Medical Imaging				
Combination Abdominal CT Scan	-	-	0.115	0.191
Combination Chest CT Scan	-	-	0.037	0.054
Follow-up Mammogram/Ultrasound	-	-	7.9%	8.4%
MRI for Low Back Pain	-	-	30.6%	32.7%
Survey of Patients' Hospital Experiences				
Area Around Room 'Always' Quiet at Night[8]	-	-	-	58%
Doctors 'Always' Communicated Well[8]	-	-	-	80%
Home Recovery Information Given[8]	-	-	-	82%
Hospital Given 9 or 10 on 10 Point Scale[8]	-	-	-	67%
Meds 'Always' Explained Before Given[8]	-	-	-	60%
Nurses 'Always' Communicated Well[8]	-	-	-	76%
Pain 'Always' Well Controlled[8]	-	-	-	69%
Room and Bathroom 'Always' Clean[8]	-	-	-	71%
Timely Help 'Always' Received[8]	-	-	-	64%
Would Definitely Recommend Hospital[8]	-	-	-	69%

Alamance Regional Medical Center

1240 Huffman Mill Rd
Burlington, NC 27216
E-mail: info@armc.com
URL: www.armc.com
Type: Acute Care Hospitals
Ownership: Voluntary Non-Profit - Private

Phone: 336-538-7000
Fax: 336-538-7425

Emergency Services: Yes
Beds: 298

Key Personnel:

CEO/President	John G Currin Jr
Chief of Medical Staff	Barbara Aldridge
Radiology	Geoffrey H Browne
Emergency Room	Linda Lawter

Measure	Cases	This Hosp.	State Avg.	U.S. Avg.
Heart Attack Care				
ACE Inhibitor or ARB for LVSD	32	94%	97%	96%
Aspirin at Arrival	196	99%	99%	99%
Aspirin at Discharge	154	99%	99%	98%
Beta Blocker at Discharge	151	94%	99%	98%
Fibrinolytic Medication Timing	0	-	38%	55%
PCI Within 90 Minutes of Arrival	25	92%	95%	90%
Smoking Cessation Advice	55	100%	100%	99%
Chest Pain/Possible Heart Attack Care				
Aspirin at Arrival	73	88%	95%	95%
Median Time to ECG (minutes)	74	6	8	8
Median Time to Transfer (minutes)[1]	23	32	48	61
Fibrinolytic Medication Timing	0	-	53%	54%
Heart Failure Care				
ACE Inhibitor or ARB for LVSD	112	95%	95%	94%
Discharge Instructions	294	86%	89%	88%
Evaluation of LVS Function	365	99%	99%	98%
Smoking Cessation Advice	86	100%	99%	98%
Pneumonia Care				
Appropriate Initial Antibiotic	115	87%	92%	92%
Blood Culture Timing	149	93%	96%	96%
Influenza Vaccine	130	94%	93%	91%
Initial Antibiotic Timing	166	93%	95%	95%
Pneumococcal Vaccine	173	95%	95%	93%
Smoking Cessation Advice	59	100%	99%	97%
Surgical Care Improvement Project				
Appropriate VTP Within 24 Hours	427	95%	93%	92%
Appropriate Hair Removal	755	100%	100%	99%
Appropriate Beta Blocker Usage	208	90%	94%	93%
Controlled Postoperative Blood Glucose	0	-	94%	93%
Prophylactic Antibiotic Timing	519	97%	98%	97%
Prophylactic Antibiotic Timing (Outpatient)	283	93%	94%	92%
Prophylactic Antibiotic Selection	520	94%	98%	97%
Prophylactic Antibiotic Select. (Outpatient)	273	95%	95%	94%
Prophylactic Antibiotic Stopped	506	93%	96%	94%
Recommended VTP Ordered	431	95%	95%	94%
Urinary Catheter Removal	199	84%	91%	90%
Children's Asthma Care				
Received Systemic Corticosteroids	-	-	100%	100%
Received Home Management Plan	-	-	75%	71%
Received Reliever Medication	-	-	100%	100%
Use of Medical Imaging				
Combination Abdominal CT Scan	1,037	0.090	0.115	0.191
Combination Chest CT Scan	942	0.000	0.037	0.054
Follow-up Mammogram/Ultrasound	2,443	6.9%	7.9%	8.4%
MRI for Low Back Pain	318	33.6%	30.6%	32.7%
Survey of Patients' Hospital Experiences				
Area Around Room 'Always' Quiet at Night	300+	51%	-	58%
Doctors 'Always' Communicated Well	300+	82%	-	80%
Home Recovery Information Given	300+	81%	-	82%
Hospital Given 9 or 10 on 10 Point Scale	300+	62%	-	67%
Meds 'Always' Explained Before Given	300+	65%	-	60%
Nurses 'Always' Communicated Well	300+	77%	-	76%
Pain 'Always' Well Controlled	300+	69%	-	69%
Room and Bathroom 'Always' Clean	300+	73%	-	71%
Timely Help 'Always' Received	300+	65%	-	64%
Would Definitely Recommend Hospital	300+	62%	-	69%

Wakemed - Cary Hospital

1900 Kildare Farm Road
Cary, NC 27511
URL: www.wakemed.org
Type: Acute Care Hospitals
Ownership: Voluntary Non-Profit - Private

Phone: 919-350-2550
Fax: 919-233-2555

Emergency Services: Yes
Beds: 156

Key Personnel:

CEO/President	Michael D DeVaughn, MD
Chief of Medical Staff	H West Lawson
Infection Control	Robin Carver
Operating Room	Maria Maag
Quality Assurance	Maggie Driscol
Radiology	Libby Dove

Measure	Cases	This Hosp.	State Avg.	U.S. Avg.
Heart Attack Care				
ACE Inhibitor or ARB for LVSD[1]	2	100%	97%	96%
Aspirin at Arrival	62	100%	99%	99%
Aspirin at Discharge	35	100%	99%	98%
Beta Blocker at Discharge	34	100%	99%	98%
Fibrinolytic Medication Timing	0	-	38%	55%
PCI Within 90 Minutes of Arrival	0	-	95%	90%
Smoking Cessation Advice[1]	6	100%	100%	99%
Chest Pain/Possible Heart Attack Care				
Aspirin at Arrival	31	97%	95%	95%
Median Time to ECG (minutes)	32	6	8	8
Median Time to Transfer (minutes)[1,3]	5	31	48	61
Fibrinolytic Medication Timing	0	-	53%	54%
Heart Failure Care				
ACE Inhibitor or ARB for LVSD	57	93%	95%	94%
Discharge Instructions	209	82%	89%	88%
Evaluation of LVS Function	265	100%	99%	98%
Smoking Cessation Advice	51	100%	99%	98%
Pneumonia Care				
Appropriate Initial Antibiotic	74	97%	92%	92%
Blood Culture Timing	134	97%	96%	96%
Influenza Vaccine	122	95%	93%	91%
Initial Antibiotic Timing	122	98%	95%	95%
Pneumococcal Vaccine	144	94%	95%	93%
Smoking Cessation Advice	55	100%	99%	97%
Surgical Care Improvement Project				
Appropriate VTP Within 24 Hours[2]	145	94%	93%	92%
Appropriate Hair Removal[2]	383	100%	100%	99%
Appropriate Beta Blocker Usage[2]	78	95%	94%	93%
Controlled Postoperative Blood Glucose[2]	0	-	94%	93%
Prophylactic Antibiotic Timing[2]	208	96%	98%	97%
Prophylactic Antibiotic Timing (Outpatient)	366	97%	94%	92%
Prophylactic Antibiotic Selection[2]	212	97%	98%	97%
Prophylactic Antibiotic Select. (Outpatient)	365	95%	95%	94%
Prophylactic Antibiotic Stopped[2]	198	93%	96%	94%
Recommended VTP Ordered[2]	145	97%	95%	94%
Urinary Catheter Removal[2]	78	97%	91%	90%
Children's Asthma Care				
Received Systemic Corticosteroids	-	-	100%	100%
Received Home Management Plan	-	-	75%	71%
Received Reliever Medication	-	-	100%	100%
Use of Medical Imaging				
Combination Abdominal CT Scan	619	0.050	0.115	0.191
Combination Chest CT Scan	424	0.017	0.037	0.054
Follow-up Mammogram/Ultrasound	458	4.1%	7.9%	8.4%
MRI for Low Back Pain	115	27.8%	30.6%	32.7%
Survey of Patients' Hospital Experiences				
Area Around Room 'Always' Quiet at Night	300+	57%	-	58%
Doctors 'Always' Communicated Well	300+	80%	-	80%
Home Recovery Information Given	300+	82%	-	82%
Hospital Given 9 or 10 on 10 Point Scale	300+	68%	-	67%
Meds 'Always' Explained Before Given	300+	60%	-	60%
Nurses 'Always' Communicated Well	300+	75%	-	76%
Pain 'Always' Well Controlled	300+	67%	-	69%
Room and Bathroom 'Always' Clean	300+	67%	-	71%
Timely Help 'Always' Received	300+	61%	-	64%
Would Definitely Recommend Hospital	300+	75%	-	69%

NOTE: Hospital profiles are in alphabetical order by state, then city, then hospital within the city; Rankings exclude hospitals with less than 25 cases except for patient surveys which excludes hospitals with less than 100 cases; (a) 100–299 cases; (1) The number of cases is too small to be sure how well a hospital is performing; (2) The hospital indicated that the data submitted for this measure were based on a sample of cases; (3) Data was collected during a shorter time period (fewer quarters) than the maximum possible time for this measure; (4) Suppressed for one or more quarters by CMS; (5) No data is available from the hospital for this measure; (6) Fewer than 100 patients completed the HCAHPS survey. Use these rates with caution, as the number of surveys may be too low to reliably assess hospital performance; (7) Survey results are based on less than 12 months of data; (8) Survey results are not available for this reporting period; (9) No or very few patients were eligible for the HCAHPS survey. The scores shown, if any, reflect a very small number of surveys; (10) A state average was not calculated because too few hospitals in the state submitted data; (11) There were discrepancies in the data collection process; Please refer to the User's Guide for a full explanation of data.

University of North Carolina Hospital

101 Manning Drive Phone: 919-966-4131
Chapel Hill, NC 27514 Fax: 919-966-3709
URL: www.unchealthcare.org
Type: Acute Care Hospitals Emergency Services: Yes
Ownership: Government - State Beds: 760

Key Personnel:
CEO/President. . . . . Gary L Park
Chief of Medical Staff . . . . Brian Goldstein, MD
Infection Control. . . . . William Rutala
Pediatric Ambulatory Care . . . . . . Roberta Williams, MD
Pediatric In-Patient Care . . . . Roberta Williams, MD
Quality Assurance . . . . Bette Brotherton
Radiology. . . . . Joseph KT Lee, MD

Measure	Cases	This Hosp.	State Avg.	U.S. Avg.
Heart Attack Care				
ACE Inhibitor or ARB for LVSD[2]	42	98%	97%	96%
Aspirin at Arrival[2]	165	100%	99%	99%
Aspirin at Discharge[2]	236	99%	99%	98%
Beta Blocker at Discharge[2]	219	100%	99%	98%
Fibrinolytic Medication Timing[2]	0	-	38%	55%
PCI Within 90 Minutes of Arrival[2]	29	93%	95%	90%
Smoking Cessation Advice[2]	84	100%	100%	99%
Chest Pain/Possible Heart Attack Care				
Aspirin at Arrival[5]	0	-	95%	95%
Median Time to ECG (minutes)[5]	0	-	8	8
Median Time to Transfer (minutes)[5]	0	-	48	61
Fibrinolytic Medication Timing[5]	0	-	53%	54%
Heart Failure Care				
ACE Inhibitor or ARB for LVSD[2]	118	99%	95%	94%
Discharge Instructions[2]	242	91%	89%	88%
Evaluation of LVS Function[2]	272	100%	99%	98%
Smoking Cessation Advice[2]	65	100%	99%	98%
Pneumonia Care				
Appropriate Initial Antibiotic[2]	49	88%	92%	92%
Blood Culture Timing[2]	99	95%	96%	96%
Influenza Vaccine[2]	68	99%	93%	91%
Initial Antibiotic Timing[2]	93	96%	95%	95%
Pneumococcal Vaccine[2]	89	99%	95%	93%
Smoking Cessation Advice[2]	48	100%	99%	97%
Surgical Care Improvement Project				
Appropriate VTP Within 24 Hours[2]	286	95%	93%	92%
Appropriate Hair Removal[2]	568	100%	100%	99%
Appropriate Beta Blocker Usage[2]	174	94%	94%	93%
Controlled Postoperative Blood Glucose[2]	71	96%	94%	93%
Prophylactic Antibiotic Timing[2]	309	98%	98%	97%
Prophylactic Antibiotic Timing (Outpatient)	688	94%	94%	92%
Prophylactic Antibiotic Selection[2]	313	98%	98%	97%
Prophylactic Antibiotic Select. (Outpatient)	685	94%	95%	94%
Prophylactic Antibiotic Stopped[2]	294	94%	96%	94%
Recommended VTP Ordered[2]	287	97%	95%	94%
Urinary Catheter Removal[2]	138	92%	91%	90%
Children's Asthma Care				
Received Systemic Corticosteroids	-	-	100%	100%
Received Home Management Plan	-	-	75%	71%
Received Reliever Medication	-	-	100%	100%
Use of Medical Imaging				
Combination Abdominal CT Scan	1,762	0.059	0.115	0.191
Combination Chest CT Scan	1,929	0.000	0.037	0.054
Follow-up Mammogram/Ultrasound	1,715	7.5%	7.9%	8.4%
MRI for Low Back Pain	200	23.0%	30.6%	32.7%
Survey of Patients' Hospital Experiences				
Area Around Room 'Always' Quiet at Night	300+	64%	-	58%
Doctors 'Always' Communicated Well	300+	82%	-	80%
Home Recovery Information Given	300+	88%	-	82%
Hospital Given 9 or 10 on 10 Point Scale	300+	81%	-	67%
Meds 'Always' Explained Before Given	300+	68%	-	60%
Nurses 'Always' Communicated Well	300+	80%	-	76%
Pain 'Always' Well Controlled	300+	73%	-	69%
Room and Bathroom 'Always' Clean	300+	72%	-	71%
Timely Help 'Always' Received	300+	65%	-	64%
Would Definitely Recommend Hospital	300+	85%	-	69%

Carolinas Medical Center-Behavioral Health

1000 Blythe Blvd Phone: 704-355-2000
Charlotte, NC 28203 Fax: 704-355-4084
URL: www.carolinasmedicalcenter.org
Type: Acute Care Hospitals Emergency Services: Yes
Ownership: Voluntary Non-Profit - Other Beds: 874

Key Personnel:
CEO/President. . . . . Suzanne H. Freeman
Infection Control. . . . . James M Horton, MD
Operating Room. . . . . Frederick L. Greene, MD, FACS
Pediatric Ambulatory Care . . . . . . Leonard G. Feld MD, PhD, MMM, FAAP
Pediatric In-Patient Care . . . . Leonard G. Feld MD, PhD, MMM, FAAP
Quality Assurance . . . . Edward E Bethea
Radiology. . . . . John Baumann
Emergency Room . . . . John A. Watts, PhD

Measure	Cases	This Hosp.	State Avg.	U.S. Avg.
Heart Attack Care				
ACE Inhibitor or ARB for LVSD	220	98%	97%	96%
Aspirin at Arrival	319	99%	99%	99%
Aspirin at Discharge	1,058	98%	99%	98%
Beta Blocker at Discharge	1,010	99%	99%	98%
Fibrinolytic Medication Timing	0	-	38%	55%
PCI Within 90 Minutes of Arrival	88	97%	95%	90%
Smoking Cessation Advice	423	100%	100%	99%
Chest Pain/Possible Heart Attack Care				
Aspirin at Arrival[1,3]	1	100%	95%	95%
Median Time to ECG (minutes)[1,3]	1	10	8	8
Median Time to Transfer (minutes)[5]	0	-	48	61
Fibrinolytic Medication Timing[5]	0	-	53%	54%
Heart Failure Care				
ACE Inhibitor or ARB for LVSD	383	99%	95%	94%
Discharge Instructions	681	98%	89%	88%
Evaluation of LVS Function	766	100%	99%	98%
Smoking Cessation Advice	196	100%	99%	98%
Pneumonia Care				
Appropriate Initial Antibiotic	145	90%	92%	92%
Blood Culture Timing	174	94%	96%	96%
Influenza Vaccine	204	98%	93%	91%
Initial Antibiotic Timing	236	92%	95%	95%
Pneumococcal Vaccine	244	98%	95%	93%
Smoking Cessation Advice	178	98%	99%	97%
Surgical Care Improvement Project				
Appropriate VTP Within 24 Hours[2]	571	95%	93%	92%
Appropriate Hair Removal[2]	2,153	100%	100%	99%
Appropriate Beta Blocker Usage[2]	650	96%	94%	93%
Controlled Postoperative Blood Glucose[2]	520	92%	94%	93%
Prophylactic Antibiotic Timing[2]	1,653	98%	98%	97%
Prophylactic Antibiotic Timing (Outpatient)	1,148	87%	94%	92%
Prophylactic Antibiotic Selection[2]	1,675	97%	98%	97%
Prophylactic Antibiotic Select. (Outpatient)	1,168	96%	95%	94%
Prophylactic Antibiotic Stopped[2]	1,581	97%	96%	94%
Recommended VTP Ordered[2]	572	98%	95%	94%
Urinary Catheter Removal[2]	337	65%	91%	90%
Children's Asthma Care				
Received Systemic Corticosteroids	429	100%	100%	100%
Received Home Management Plan	427	87%	75%	71%
Received Reliever Medication	430	100%	100%	100%
Use of Medical Imaging				
Combination Abdominal CT Scan	1,772	0.109	0.115	0.191
Combination Chest CT Scan	1,593	0.000	0.037	0.054
Follow-up Mammogram/Ultrasound[5]	0	-	7.9%	8.4%
MRI for Low Back Pain	188	34.6%	30.6%	32.7%
Survey of Patients' Hospital Experiences				
Area Around Room 'Always' Quiet at Night	300+	64%	-	58%
Doctors 'Always' Communicated Well	300+	82%	-	80%
Home Recovery Information Given	300+	85%	-	82%
Hospital Given 9 or 10 on 10 Point Scale	300+	71%	-	67%
Meds 'Always' Explained Before Given	300+	61%	-	60%
Nurses 'Always' Communicated Well	300+	76%	-	76%
Pain 'Always' Well Controlled	300+	72%	-	69%
Room and Bathroom 'Always' Clean	300+	60%	-	71%
Timely Help 'Always' Received	300+	65%	-	64%
Would Definitely Recommend Hospital	300+	76%	-	69%

Carolinas Medical Center-Mercy

2001 Vail Ave Phone: 704-379-5000
Charlotte, NC 28207 Fax: 704-379-5695
URL: www.carolinashealthcare.org
Type: Acute Care Hospitals Emergency Services: Yes
Ownership: Govt - Hospital Dist/Auth Beds: 224

Key Personnel:
Chief of Medical Staff . . . . Fred Vermeulen
Infection Control. . . . . Dona Haney
Operating Room. . . . . Carol Puckett
Quality Assurance . . . . Pat Presley
Anesthesiology. . . . . Carter Keith, MD
Emergency Room . . . . Stacey Gouzenne
Intensive Care Unit. . . . . Anne Focht, RN

Measure	Cases	This Hosp.	State Avg.	U.S. Avg.
Heart Attack Care				
ACE Inhibitor or ARB for LVSD	51	100%	97%	96%
Aspirin at Arrival	85	100%	99%	99%
Aspirin at Discharge	213	98%	99%	98%
Beta Blocker at Discharge	201	97%	99%	98%
Fibrinolytic Medication Timing	0	-	38%	55%
PCI Within 90 Minutes of Arrival[1]	24	100%	95%	90%
Smoking Cessation Advice	74	100%	100%	99%
Chest Pain/Possible Heart Attack Care				
Aspirin at Arrival	118	99%	95%	95%
Median Time to ECG (minutes)	117	6	8	8
Median Time to Transfer (minutes)[1]	13	40	48	61
Fibrinolytic Medication Timing	0	-	53%	54%
Heart Failure Care				
ACE Inhibitor or ARB for LVSD	133	98%	95%	94%
Discharge Instructions	327	94%	89%	88%
Evaluation of LVS Function	398	99%	99%	98%
Smoking Cessation Advice	65	100%	99%	98%
Pneumonia Care				
Appropriate Initial Antibiotic	177	95%	92%	92%
Blood Culture Timing	235	96%	96%	96%
Influenza Vaccine	184	97%	93%	91%
Initial Antibiotic Timing	266	94%	95%	95%
Pneumococcal Vaccine	217	98%	95%	93%
Smoking Cessation Advice	99	100%	99%	97%
Surgical Care Improvement Project				
Appropriate VTP Within 24 Hours[2]	725	98%	93%	92%
Appropriate Hair Removal[2]	2,101	100%	100%	99%
Appropriate Beta Blocker Usage[2]	483	97%	94%	93%
Controlled Postoperative Blood Glucose[2]	30	83%	94%	93%
Prophylactic Antibiotic Timing[2]	1,774	97%	98%	97%
Prophylactic Antibiotic Timing (Outpatient)	1,223	92%	94%	92%
Prophylactic Antibiotic Selection[2]	1,780	99%	98%	97%
Prophylactic Antibiotic Select. (Outpatient)	1,174	98%	95%	94%
Prophylactic Antibiotic Stopped[2]	1,747	97%	96%	94%
Recommended VTP Ordered[2]	726	98%	95%	94%
Urinary Catheter Removal[2]	829	96%	91%	90%
Children's Asthma Care				
Received Systemic Corticosteroids	-	-	100%	100%
Received Home Management Plan	-	-	75%	71%
Received Reliever Medication	-	-	100%	100%
Use of Medical Imaging				
Combination Abdominal CT Scan	1,763	0.081	0.115	0.191
Combination Chest CT Scan	1,267	0.016	0.037	0.054
Follow-up Mammogram/Ultrasound[5]	0	-	7.9%	8.4%
MRI for Low Back Pain	338	32.5%	30.6%	32.7%
Survey of Patients' Hospital Experiences				
Area Around Room 'Always' Quiet at Night	300+	67%	-	58%
Doctors 'Always' Communicated Well	300+	84%	-	80%
Home Recovery Information Given	300+	88%	-	82%
Hospital Given 9 or 10 on 10 Point Scale	300+	78%	-	67%
Meds 'Always' Explained Before Given	300+	64%	-	60%
Nurses 'Always' Communicated Well	300+	81%	-	76%
Pain 'Always' Well Controlled	300+	73%	-	69%
Room and Bathroom 'Always' Clean	300+	64%	-	71%
Timely Help 'Always' Received	300+	69%	-	64%
Would Definitely Recommend Hospital	300+	81%	-	69%

NOTE: Hospital profiles are in alphabetical order by state, then city, then hospital within the city; Rankings exclude hospitals with less than 25 cases except for patient surveys which excludes hospitals with less than 100 cases; (a) 100–299 cases; (1) The number of cases is too small to be sure how well a hospital is performing; (2) The hospital indicated that the data submitted for this measure were based on a sample of cases; (3) Data was collected during a shorter time period (fewer quarters) than the maximum possible time for this measure; (4) Suppressed for one or more quarters by CMS; (5) No data is available from the hospital for this measure; (6) Fewer than 100 patients completed the HCAHPS survey. Use these rates with caution, as the number of surveys may be too low to reliably assess hospital performance; (7) Survey results are based on less than 12 months of data; (8) Survey results are not available for this reporting period; (9) No or very few patients were eligible for the HCAHPS survey. The scores shown, if any, reflect a very small number of surveys; (10) A state average was not calculated because too few hospitals in the state submitted data; (11) There were discrepancies in the data collection process; Please refer to the User's Guide for a full explanation of data.

Carolinas Medical Center-University

8800 North Tyron Street — Phone: 704-548-6000
Charlotte, NC 28262
Type: Acute Care Hospitals — Emergency Services: Yes
Ownership: Govt - Hospital Dist/Auth

Measure	Cases	This Hosp.	State Avg.	U.S. Avg.
Heart Attack Care				
ACE Inhibitor or ARB for LVSD[1]	7	100%	97%	96%
Aspirin at Arrival	29	100%	99%	99%
Aspirin at Discharge[1]	19	100%	99%	98%
Beta Blocker at Discharge[1]	19	100%	99%	98%
Fibrinolytic Medication Timing	0	-	38%	55%
PCI Within 90 Minutes of Arrival	0	-	95%	90%
Smoking Cessation Advice[1]	8	100%	100%	99%
Chest Pain/Possible Heart Attack Care				
Aspirin at Arrival	106	100%	95%	95%
Median Time to ECG (minutes)	106	9	8	8
Median Time to Transfer (minutes)[1]	22	42	48	61
Fibrinolytic Medication Timing	0	-	53%	54%
Heart Failure Care				
ACE Inhibitor or ARB for LVSD	77	100%	95%	94%
Discharge Instructions	150	97%	89%	88%
Evaluation of LVS Function	169	98%	99%	98%
Smoking Cessation Advice	46	100%	99%	98%
Pneumonia Care				
Appropriate Initial Antibiotic	112	95%	92%	92%
Blood Culture Timing	158	98%	96%	96%
Influenza Vaccine	85	99%	93%	91%
Initial Antibiotic Timing	155	99%	95%	95%
Pneumococcal Vaccine	86	98%	95%	93%
Smoking Cessation Advice	73	100%	99%	97%
Surgical Care Improvement Project				
Appropriate VTP Within 24 Hours[2]	154	95%	93%	92%
Appropriate Hair Removal[2]	328	100%	100%	99%
Appropriate Beta Blocker Usage[2]	59	98%	94%	93%
Controlled Postoperative Blood Glucose[2]	0	-	94%	93%
Prophylactic Antibiotic Timing[2]	239	99%	98%	97%
Prophylactic Antibiotic Timing (Outpatient)	362	98%	94%	92%
Prophylactic Antibiotic Selection[2]	239	98%	98%	97%
Prophylactic Antibiotic Select. (Outpatient)	362	96%	95%	94%
Prophylactic Antibiotic Stopped[2]	227	97%	96%	94%
Recommended VTP Ordered[2]	154	98%	95%	94%
Urinary Catheter Removal[1,2]	17	76%	91%	90%
Children's Asthma Care				
Received Systemic Corticosteroids	-	-	100%	100%
Received Home Management Plan	-	-	75%	71%
Received Reliever Medication	-	-	100%	100%
Use of Medical Imaging				
Combination Abdominal CT Scan	845	0.085	0.115	0.191
Combination Chest CT Scan	372	0.003	0.037	0.054
Follow-up Mammogram/Ultrasound[5]	0	-	7.9%	8.4%
MRI for Low Back Pain	128	38.3%	30.6%	32.7%
Survey of Patients' Hospital Experiences				
Area Around Room 'Always' Quiet at Night	300+	63%	-	58%
Doctors 'Always' Communicated Well	300+	84%	-	80%
Home Recovery Information Given	300+	86%	-	82%
Hospital Given 9 or 10 on 10 Point Scale	300+	72%	-	67%
Meds 'Always' Explained Before Given	300+	67%	-	60%
Nurses 'Always' Communicated Well	300+	80%	-	76%
Pain 'Always' Well Controlled	300+	71%	-	69%
Room and Bathroom 'Always' Clean	300+	69%	-	71%
Timely Help 'Always' Received	300+	63%	-	64%
Would Definitely Recommend Hospital	300+	75%	-	69%

Presbyterian Hospital

200 Hawthorne Lane Box 33549 — Phone: 704-384-4000
Charlotte, NC 28233 — Fax: 704-384-4296
URL: www.presbyterian.org
Type: Acute Care Hospitals — Emergency Services: Yes
Ownership: Voluntary Non-Profit - Other — Beds: 547

Key Personnel:
CEO/President. . . . . Mark Billings
Chief of Medical Staff . . . . Paul Blake, MD
Coronary Care . . . . Mary Hopin
Infection Control. . . . . Sandy Cox
Pediatric Ambulatory Care . . . . . . Pat Campbell
Pediatric In-Patient Care . . . . Pat Campbell
Quality Assurance . . . . Carol Mault
Radiology. . . . . Shelly Hall

Measure	Cases	This Hosp.	State Avg.	U.S. Avg.
Heart Attack Care				
ACE Inhibitor or ARB for LVSD	115	100%	97%	96%
Aspirin at Arrival	295	100%	99%	99%
Aspirin at Discharge	593	100%	99%	98%
Beta Blocker at Discharge	583	100%	99%	98%
Fibrinolytic Medication Timing	0	-	38%	55%
PCI Within 90 Minutes of Arrival	88	98%	95%	90%
Smoking Cessation Advice	186	100%	100%	99%
Chest Pain/Possible Heart Attack Care				
Aspirin at Arrival[3]	0	-	95%	95%
Median Time to ECG (minutes)[3]	0	-	8	8
Median Time to Transfer (minutes)[5]	0	-	48	61
Fibrinolytic Medication Timing[5]	0	-	53%	54%
Heart Failure Care				
ACE Inhibitor or ARB for LVSD	207	100%	95%	94%
Discharge Instructions	491	99%	89%	88%
Evaluation of LVS Function	584	100%	99%	98%
Smoking Cessation Advice	106	100%	99%	98%
Pneumonia Care				
Appropriate Initial Antibiotic	202	99%	92%	92%
Blood Culture Timing	277	100%	96%	96%
Influenza Vaccine	225	98%	93%	91%
Initial Antibiotic Timing	314	99%	95%	95%
Pneumococcal Vaccine	268	99%	95%	93%
Smoking Cessation Advice	149	100%	99%	97%
Surgical Care Improvement Project				
Appropriate VTP Within 24 Hours[2]	499	97%	93%	92%
Appropriate Hair Removal[2]	1,515	100%	100%	99%
Appropriate Beta Blocker Usage[2]	430	100%	94%	93%
Controlled Postoperative Blood Glucose[2]	408	100%	94%	93%
Prophylactic Antibiotic Timing[2]	1,096	100%	98%	97%
Prophylactic Antibiotic Timing (Outpatient)	1,140	97%	94%	92%
Prophylactic Antibiotic Selection[2]	1,124	99%	98%	97%
Prophylactic Antibiotic Select. (Outpatient)	1,141	98%	95%	94%
Prophylactic Antibiotic Stopped[2]	1,037	99%	96%	94%
Recommended VTP Ordered[2]	499	98%	95%	94%
Urinary Catheter Removal[2]	263	88%	91%	90%
Children's Asthma Care				
Received Systemic Corticosteroids	173	100%	100%	100%
Received Home Management Plan	172	82%	75%	71%
Received Reliever Medication	173	100%	100%	100%
Use of Medical Imaging				
Combination Abdominal CT Scan	829	0.024	0.115	0.191
Combination Chest CT Scan	380	0.003	0.037	0.054
Follow-up Mammogram/Ultrasound[5]	0	-	7.9%	8.4%
MRI for Low Back Pain	71	25.4%	30.6%	32.7%
Survey of Patients' Hospital Experiences				
Area Around Room 'Always' Quiet at Night	300+	61%	-	58%
Doctors 'Always' Communicated Well	300+	84%	-	80%
Home Recovery Information Given	300+	83%	-	82%
Hospital Given 9 or 10 on 10 Point Scale	300+	77%	-	67%
Meds 'Always' Explained Before Given	300+	63%	-	60%
Nurses 'Always' Communicated Well	300+	82%	-	76%
Pain 'Always' Well Controlled	300+	76%	-	69%
Room and Bathroom 'Always' Clean	300+	71%	-	71%
Timely Help 'Always' Received	300+	68%	-	64%
Would Definitely Recommend Hospital	300+	81%	-	69%

Presbyterian-Orthopaedic Hospital

1901 Randolph Rd — Phone: 704-316-2000
Charlotte, NC 28207
URL: www.presbyterian.org
Type: Acute Care Hospitals — Emergency Services: Yes
Ownership: Voluntary Non-Profit - Other

Key Personnel:
CEO/President. . . . . Paul M. Wiles
Chief of Medical Staff . . . . Stephen L. Wallenhaupt
Ambulatory Care . . . . Dean Swindle

Measure	Cases	This Hosp.	State Avg.	U.S. Avg.
Heart Attack Care				
ACE Inhibitor or ARB for LVSD[5]	0	-	97%	96%
Aspirin at Arrival[5]	0	-	99%	99%
Aspirin at Discharge[5]	0	-	99%	98%
Beta Blocker at Discharge[5]	0	-	99%	98%
Fibrinolytic Medication Timing[5]	0	-	38%	55%
PCI Within 90 Minutes of Arrival[5]	0	-	95%	90%
Smoking Cessation Advice[5]	0	-	100%	99%
Chest Pain/Possible Heart Attack Care				
Aspirin at Arrival[5]	0	-	95%	95%
Median Time to ECG (minutes)[5]	0	-	8	8
Median Time to Transfer (minutes)[5]	0	-	48	61
Fibrinolytic Medication Timing[5]	0	-	53%	54%
Heart Failure Care				
ACE Inhibitor or ARB for LVSD[5]	0	-	95%	94%
Discharge Instructions[5]	0	-	89%	88%
Evaluation of LVS Function[5]	0	-	99%	98%
Smoking Cessation Advice[5]	0	-	99%	98%
Pneumonia Care				
Appropriate Initial Antibiotic[5]	0	-	92%	92%
Blood Culture Timing[5]	0	-	96%	96%
Influenza Vaccine[5]	0	-	93%	91%
Initial Antibiotic Timing[5]	0	-	95%	95%
Pneumococcal Vaccine[5]	0	-	95%	93%
Smoking Cessation Advice[5]	0	-	99%	97%
Surgical Care Improvement Project				
Appropriate VTP Within 24 Hours[2]	616	100%	93%	92%
Appropriate Hair Removal[2]	1,497	100%	100%	99%
Appropriate Beta Blocker Usage[2]	384	97%	94%	93%
Controlled Postoperative Blood Glucose[2]	0	-	94%	93%
Prophylactic Antibiotic Timing[2]	1,255	100%	98%	97%
Prophylactic Antibiotic Timing (Outpatient)	692	99%	94%	92%
Prophylactic Antibiotic Selection[2]	1,256	100%	98%	97%
Prophylactic Antibiotic Select. (Outpatient)	687	100%	95%	94%
Prophylactic Antibiotic Stopped[2]	1,234	99%	96%	94%
Recommended VTP Ordered[2]	616	100%	95%	94%
Urinary Catheter Removal[2]	604	96%	91%	90%
Children's Asthma Care				
Received Systemic Corticosteroids	-	-	100%	100%
Received Home Management Plan	-	-	75%	71%
Received Reliever Medication	-	-	100%	100%
Use of Medical Imaging				
Combination Abdominal CT Scan	156	0.045	0.115	0.191
Combination Chest CT Scan	107	0.000	0.037	0.054
Follow-up Mammogram/Ultrasound[5]	0	-	7.9%	8.4%
MRI for Low Back Pain	114	28.1%	30.6%	32.7%
Survey of Patients' Hospital Experiences				
Area Around Room 'Always' Quiet at Night	300+	57%	-	58%
Doctors 'Always' Communicated Well	300+	84%	-	80%
Home Recovery Information Given	300+	89%	-	82%
Hospital Given 9 or 10 on 10 Point Scale	300+	68%	-	67%
Meds 'Always' Explained Before Given	300+	61%	-	60%
Nurses 'Always' Communicated Well	300+	71%	-	76%
Pain 'Always' Well Controlled	300+	66%	-	69%
Room and Bathroom 'Always' Clean	300+	65%	-	71%
Timely Help 'Always' Received	300+	49%	-	64%
Would Definitely Recommend Hospital	300+	76%	-	69%

NOTE: Hospital profiles are in alphabetical order by state, then city, then hospital within the city; Rankings exclude hospitals with less than 25 cases except for patient surveys which excludes hospitals with less than 100 cases; (a) 100–299 cases; (1) The number of cases is too small to be sure how well a hospital is performing; (2) The hospital indicated that the data submitted for this measure were based on a sample of cases; (3) Data was collected during a shorter time period (fewer quarters) than the maximum possible time for this measure; (4) Suppressed for one or more quarters by CMS; (5) No data is available from the hospital for this measure; (6) Fewer than 100 patients completed the HCAHPS survey. Use these rates with caution, as the number of surveys may be too low to reliably assess hospital performance; (7) Survey results are based on less than 12 months of data; (8) Survey results are not available for this reporting period; (9) No or very few patients were eligible for the HCAHPS survey. The scores shown, if any, reflect a very small number of surveys; (10) A state average was not calculated because too few hospitals in the state submitted data; (11) There were discrepancies in the data collection process; Please refer to the User's Guide for a full explanation of data.

Cherokee Indian Hospital Authority

Caller Box C268 Phone: 704-497-9163
Cherokee, NC 28719 Fax: 828-497-5343
Type: Acute Care Hospitals Emergency Services: Yes
Ownership: Government - Federal Beds: 32

Measure	Cases	This Hosp.	State Avg.	U.S. Avg.
Heart Attack Care				
ACE Inhibitor or ARB for LVSD[5]	0	-	97%	96%
Aspirin at Arrival[5]	0	-	99%	99%
Aspirin at Discharge[5]	0	-	99%	98%
Beta Blocker at Discharge[5]	0	-	99%	98%
Fibrinolytic Medication Timing[5]	0	-	38%	55%
PCI Within 90 Minutes of Arrival[5]	0	-	95%	90%
Smoking Cessation Advice[5]	0	-	100%	99%
Chest Pain/Possible Heart Attack Care				
Aspirin at Arrival	-	-	95%	95%
Median Time to ECG (minutes)	-	-	8	8
Median Time to Transfer (minutes)	-	-	48	61
Fibrinolytic Medication Timing	-	-	53%	54%
Heart Failure Care				
ACE Inhibitor or ARB for LVSD[1,2]	3	100%	95%	94%
Discharge Instructions[1,2]	4	50%	89%	88%
Evaluation of LVS Function[1,2]	5	80%	99%	98%
Smoking Cessation Advice[2]	0	-	99%	98%
Pneumonia Care				
Appropriate Initial Antibiotic[2]	26	65%	92%	92%
Blood Culture Timing[1,2]	15	80%	96%	96%
Influenza Vaccine[1]	20	80%	93%	91%
Initial Antibiotic Timing[1,2]	6	83%	95%	95%
Pneumococcal Vaccine[1,2]	20	100%	95%	93%
Smoking Cessation Advice[1,2]	17	88%	99%	97%
Surgical Care Improvement Project				
Appropriate VTP Within 24 Hours[5]	0	-	93%	92%
Appropriate Hair Removal[5]	0	-	100%	99%
Appropriate Beta Blocker Usage[5]	0	-	94%	93%
Controlled Postoperative Blood Glucose[5]	0	-	94%	93%
Prophylactic Antibiotic Timing[5]	0	-	98%	97%
Prophylactic Antibiotic Timing (Outpatient)	-	-	94%	92%
Prophylactic Antibiotic Selection[5]	0	-	98%	97%
Prophylactic Antibiotic Select. (Outpatient)	-	-	95%	94%
Prophylactic Antibiotic Stopped[5]	0	-	96%	94%
Recommended VTP Ordered[5]	0	-	95%	94%
Urinary Catheter Removal[5]	0	-	91%	90%
Children's Asthma Care				
Received Systemic Corticosteroids	-	-	100%	100%
Received Home Management Plan	-	-	75%	71%
Received Reliever Medication	-	-	100%	100%
Use of Medical Imaging				
Combination Abdominal CT Scan	-	-	0.115	0.191
Combination Chest CT Scan	-	-	0.037	0.054
Follow-up Mammogram/Ultrasound	-	-	7.9%	8.4%
MRI for Low Back Pain	-	-	30.6%	32.7%
Survey of Patients' Hospital Experiences				
Area Around Room 'Always' Quiet at Night	(a)	67%	-	58%
Doctors 'Always' Communicated Well	(a)	71%	-	80%
Home Recovery Information Given	(a)	71%	-	82%
Hospital Given 9 or 10 on 10 Point Scale	(a)	58%	-	67%
Meds 'Always' Explained Before Given	(a)	52%	-	60%
Nurses 'Always' Communicated Well	(a)	70%	-	76%
Pain 'Always' Well Controlled	(a)	51%	-	69%
Room and Bathroom 'Always' Clean	(a)	67%	-	71%
Timely Help 'Always' Received	(a)	63%	-	64%
Would Definitely Recommend Hospital	(a)	55%	-	69%

Sampson Regional Medical Center

607 Beaman St Phone: 910-592-8511
Clinton, NC 28328 Fax: 910-590-2321
URL: www.sampsonrmc.org
Type: Acute Care Hospitals Emergency Services: Yes
Ownership: Government - Local Beds: 146

Key Personnel:
CEO/President. . . . . Larry H Chewning
Operating Room. . . . . Lisa King
Pediatric Ambulatory Care . . . . . . Sara Hesketh
Quality Assurance . . . . Rebecca Mahler
Radiology. . . . . Verlon Salley
Emergency Room . . . . Laurie Smith
Intensive Care Unit. . . . . Heidi Jackson
Patient Relations . . . . Ann Butler

Measure	Cases	This Hosp.	State Avg.	U.S. Avg.
Heart Attack Care				
ACE Inhibitor or ARB for LVSD[1]	3	100%	97%	96%
Aspirin at Arrival[1]	13	100%	99%	99%
Aspirin at Discharge[1]	6	100%	99%	98%
Beta Blocker at Discharge[1]	6	83%	99%	98%
Fibrinolytic Medication Timing	0	-	38%	55%
PCI Within 90 Minutes of Arrival	0	-	95%	90%
Smoking Cessation Advice	0	-	100%	99%
Chest Pain/Possible Heart Attack Care				
Aspirin at Arrival	418	90%	95%	95%
Median Time to ECG (minutes)	442	10	8	8
Median Time to Transfer (minutes)[1,3]	6	118	48	61
Fibrinolytic Medication Timing[1]	21	67%	53%	54%
Heart Failure Care				
ACE Inhibitor or ARB for LVSD	72	86%	95%	94%
Discharge Instructions	139	89%	89%	88%
Evaluation of LVS Function	196	99%	99%	98%
Smoking Cessation Advice	38	100%	99%	98%
Pneumonia Care				
Appropriate Initial Antibiotic	86	90%	92%	92%
Blood Culture Timing	133	90%	96%	96%
Influenza Vaccine	85	88%	93%	91%
Initial Antibiotic Timing	113	96%	95%	95%
Pneumococcal Vaccine	143	94%	95%	93%
Smoking Cessation Advice	36	100%	99%	97%
Surgical Care Improvement Project				
Appropriate VTP Within 24 Hours	60	62%	93%	92%
Appropriate Hair Removal	146	100%	100%	99%
Appropriate Beta Blocker Usage	40	92%	94%	93%
Controlled Postoperative Blood Glucose	0	-	94%	93%
Prophylactic Antibiotic Timing	79	91%	98%	97%
Prophylactic Antibiotic Timing (Outpatient)[1]	13	77%	94%	92%
Prophylactic Antibiotic Selection	79	97%	98%	97%
Prophylactic Antibiotic Select. (Outpatient)[1]	11	73%	95%	94%
Prophylactic Antibiotic Stopped	75	87%	96%	94%
Recommended VTP Ordered	60	68%	95%	94%
Urinary Catheter Removal	40	82%	91%	90%
Children's Asthma Care				
Received Systemic Corticosteroids	-	-	100%	100%
Received Home Management Plan	-	-	75%	71%
Received Reliever Medication	-	-	100%	100%
Use of Medical Imaging				
Combination Abdominal CT Scan	588	0.395	0.115	0.191
Combination Chest CT Scan	369	0.081	0.037	0.054
Follow-up Mammogram/Ultrasound	993	4.7%	7.9%	8.4%
MRI for Low Back Pain	134	41.0%	30.6%	32.7%
Survey of Patients' Hospital Experiences				
Area Around Room 'Always' Quiet at Night	300+	69%	-	58%
Doctors 'Always' Communicated Well	300+	84%	-	80%
Home Recovery Information Given	300+	85%	-	82%
Hospital Given 9 or 10 on 10 Point Scale	300+	65%	-	67%
Meds 'Always' Explained Before Given	300+	65%	-	60%
Nurses 'Always' Communicated Well	300+	79%	-	76%
Pain 'Always' Well Controlled	300+	71%	-	69%
Room and Bathroom 'Always' Clean	300+	68%	-	71%
Timely Help 'Always' Received	300+	65%	-	64%
Would Definitely Recommend Hospital	300+	61%	-	69%

Haywood Regional Medical Center

262 Leroy George Drive Phone: 828-456-7311
Clyde, NC 28721 Fax: 828-452-8294
URL: www.haymed.org
Type: Acute Care Hospitals Emergency Services: Yes
Ownership: Govt - Hospital Dist/Auth Beds: 200

Key Personnel:
CEO/President. . . . . Mike Poore
Chief of Medical Staff . . . . Keturah C Bell, MD
Infection Control. . . . . Dianne Warren
Operating Room. . . . . Alfred Mina, RN
Quality Assurance . . . . David Love, MD
Radiology. . . . . Debera L Huderly
Emergency Room . . . . Ryan Davis
Patient Relations . . . . Nancy Burleson

Measure	Cases	This Hosp.	State Avg.	U.S. Avg.
Heart Attack Care				
ACE Inhibitor or ARB for LVSD[1]	2	100%	97%	96%
Aspirin at Arrival[1]	21	100%	99%	99%
Aspirin at Discharge[1]	10	100%	99%	98%
Beta Blocker at Discharge[1]	8	100%	99%	98%
Fibrinolytic Medication Timing	0	-	38%	55%
PCI Within 90 Minutes of Arrival	0	-	95%	90%
Smoking Cessation Advice[1]	2	50%	100%	99%
Chest Pain/Possible Heart Attack Care				
Aspirin at Arrival	75	85%	95%	95%
Median Time to ECG (minutes)	78	8	8	8
Median Time to Transfer (minutes)[1]	16	64	48	61
Fibrinolytic Medication Timing	0	-	53%	54%
Heart Failure Care				
ACE Inhibitor or ARB for LVSD	25	80%	95%	94%
Discharge Instructions	77	79%	89%	88%
Evaluation of LVS Function	99	96%	99%	98%
Smoking Cessation Advice[1]	11	91%	99%	98%
Pneumonia Care				
Appropriate Initial Antibiotic	135	83%	92%	92%
Blood Culture Timing	159	96%	96%	96%
Influenza Vaccine	146	89%	93%	91%
Initial Antibiotic Timing	191	87%	95%	95%
Pneumococcal Vaccine	182	92%	95%	93%
Smoking Cessation Advice	103	92%	99%	97%
Surgical Care Improvement Project				
Appropriate VTP Within 24 Hours	110	93%	93%	92%
Appropriate Hair Removal	472	100%	100%	99%
Appropriate Beta Blocker Usage	123	92%	94%	93%
Controlled Postoperative Blood Glucose	0	-	94%	93%
Prophylactic Antibiotic Timing	341	94%	98%	97%
Prophylactic Antibiotic Timing (Outpatient)	266	86%	94%	92%
Prophylactic Antibiotic Selection	340	98%	98%	97%
Prophylactic Antibiotic Select. (Outpatient)	266	96%	95%	94%
Prophylactic Antibiotic Stopped	329	98%	96%	94%
Recommended VTP Ordered	111	95%	95%	94%
Urinary Catheter Removal[1]	18	94%	91%	90%
Children's Asthma Care				
Received Systemic Corticosteroids	-	-	100%	100%
Received Home Management Plan	-	-	75%	71%
Received Reliever Medication	-	-	100%	100%
Use of Medical Imaging				
Combination Abdominal CT Scan	370	0.084	0.115	0.191
Combination Chest CT Scan	308	0.026	0.037	0.054
Follow-up Mammogram/Ultrasound	673	7.7%	7.9%	8.4%
MRI for Low Back Pain	283	27.6%	30.6%	32.7%
Survey of Patients' Hospital Experiences				
Area Around Room 'Always' Quiet at Night	300+	55%	-	58%
Doctors 'Always' Communicated Well	300+	84%	-	80%
Home Recovery Information Given	300+	81%	-	82%
Hospital Given 9 or 10 on 10 Point Scale	300+	61%	-	67%
Meds 'Always' Explained Before Given	300+	63%	-	60%
Nurses 'Always' Communicated Well	300+	79%	-	76%
Pain 'Always' Well Controlled	300+	71%	-	69%
Room and Bathroom 'Always' Clean	300+	59%	-	71%
Timely Help 'Always' Received	300+	67%	-	64%
Would Definitely Recommend Hospital	300+	67%	-	69%

NOTE: Hospital profiles are in alphabetical order by state, then city, then hospital within the city; Rankings exclude hospitals with less than 25 cases except for patient surveys which excludes hospitals with less than 100 cases; (a) 100–299 cases; (1) The number of cases is too small to be sure how well a hospital is performing; (2) The hospital indicated that the data submitted for this measure were based on a sample of cases; (3) Data was collected during a shorter time period (fewer quarters) than the maximum possible time for this measure; (4) Suppressed for one or more quarters by CMS; (5) No data is available from the hospital for this measure; (6) Fewer than 100 patients completed the HCAHPS survey. Use these rates with caution, as the number of surveys may be too low to reliably assess hospital performance; (7) Survey results are based on less than 12 months of data; (8) Survey results are not available for this reporting period; (9) No or very few patients were eligible for the HCAHPS survey. The scores shown, if any, reflect a very small number of surveys; (10) A state average was not calculated because too few hospitals in the state submitted data; (11) There were discrepancies in the data collection process; Please refer to the User's Guide for a full explanation of data.

Saint Lukes Hospital

101 Hospital Drive
Columbus, NC 28722
URL: www.saintlukeshospital.com
Type: Critical Access Hospitals
Ownership: Voluntary Non-Profit - Private

Phone: 828-894-3311
Fax: 828-894-2155

Emergency Services: Yes
Beds: 73

Key Personnel:
CEO/President . . . . Cameron Highsmith
Chief of Medical Staff . . . . Todd Colson, MD
Operating Room . . . . Laurann Adams
Radiology . . . . Martin Black
Emergency Room . . . . Lori Oliver
Patient Relations . . . . Sandra Page

Measure	Cases	This Hosp.	State Avg.	U.S. Avg.
Heart Attack Care				
ACE Inhibitor or ARB for LVSD[5]	0	-	97%	96%
Aspirin at Arrival[5]	0	-	99%	99%
Aspirin at Discharge[5]	0	-	99%	98%
Beta Blocker at Discharge[5]	0	-	99%	98%
Fibrinolytic Medication Timing[5]	0	-	38%	55%
PCI Within 90 Minutes of Arrival[5]	0	-	95%	90%
Smoking Cessation Advice[5]	0	-	100%	99%
Chest Pain/Possible Heart Attack Care				
Aspirin at Arrival[5]	0	-	95%	95%
Median Time to ECG (minutes)[5]	0	-	8	8
Median Time to Transfer (minutes)[5]	0	-	48	61
Fibrinolytic Medication Timing[5]	0	-	53%	54%
Heart Failure Care				
ACE Inhibitor or ARB for LVSD[1]	7	100%	95%	94%
Discharge Instructions[1]	21	95%	89%	88%
Evaluation of LVS Function	49	90%	99%	98%
Smoking Cessation Advice[1]	5	60%	99%	98%
Pneumonia Care				
Appropriate Initial Antibiotic	47	96%	92%	92%
Blood Culture Timing	76	93%	96%	96%
Influenza Vaccine	38	97%	93%	91%
Initial Antibiotic Timing	59	97%	95%	95%
Pneumococcal Vaccine	58	91%	95%	93%
Smoking Cessation Advice[1]	12	100%	99%	97%
Surgical Care Improvement Project				
Appropriate VTP Within 24 Hours	36	86%	93%	92%
Appropriate Hair Removal	174	100%	100%	99%
Appropriate Beta Blocker Usage	52	92%	94%	93%
Controlled Postoperative Blood Glucose	0	-	94%	93%
Prophylactic Antibiotic Timing	136	99%	98%	97%
Prophylactic Antibiotic Timing (Outpatient)[5]	0	-	94%	92%
Prophylactic Antibiotic Selection	137	100%	98%	97%
Prophylactic Antibiotic Select. (Outpatient)[5]	0	-	95%	94%
Prophylactic Antibiotic Stopped	129	98%	96%	94%
Recommended VTP Ordered	36	86%	95%	94%
Urinary Catheter Removal	44	91%	91%	90%
Children's Asthma Care				
Received Systemic Corticosteroids	-	-	100%	100%
Received Home Management Plan	-	-	75%	71%
Received Reliever Medication	-	-	100%	100%
Use of Medical Imaging				
Combination Abdominal CT Scan	305	0.125	0.115	0.191
Combination Chest CT Scan	132	0.144	0.037	0.054
Follow-up Mammogram/Ultrasound	536	9.3%	7.9%	8.4%
MRI for Low Back Pain	68	27.9%	30.6%	32.7%
Survey of Patients' Hospital Experiences				
Area Around Room 'Always' Quiet at Night	(a)	62%	-	58%
Doctors 'Always' Communicated Well	(a)	82%	-	80%
Home Recovery Information Given	(a)	84%	-	82%
Hospital Given 9 or 10 on 10 Point Scale	(a)	74%	-	67%
Meds 'Always' Explained Before Given	(a)	59%	-	60%
Nurses 'Always' Communicated Well	(a)	79%	-	76%
Pain 'Always' Well Controlled	(a)	71%	-	69%
Room and Bathroom 'Always' Clean	(a)	73%	-	71%
Timely Help 'Always' Received	(a)	75%	-	64%
Would Definitely Recommend Hospital	(a)	77%	-	69%

Carolinas Medical Center-Northeast

920 Church St N
Concord, NC 28025
URL: www.northeastmedical.org
Type: Acute Care Hospitals
Ownership: Govt - Hospital Dist/Auth

Phone: 704-783-3000
Fax: 704-783-3579

Emergency Services: Yes
Beds: 457

Key Personnel:
Infection Control . . . . Pat Hinson
Quality Assurance . . . . Leesa Bain
Radiology . . . . Timothy O Jenkins, MD

Measure	Cases	This Hosp.	State Avg.	U.S. Avg.
Heart Attack Care				
ACE Inhibitor or ARB for LVSD	105	99%	97%	96%
Aspirin at Arrival	439	98%	99%	99%
Aspirin at Discharge	483	99%	99%	98%
Beta Blocker at Discharge	479	100%	99%	98%
Fibrinolytic Medication Timing	0	-	38%	55%
PCI Within 90 Minutes of Arrival	85	95%	95%	90%
Smoking Cessation Advice	184	99%	100%	99%
Chest Pain/Possible Heart Attack Care				
Aspirin at Arrival[1,3]	4	75%	95%	95%
Median Time to ECG (minutes)[1,3]	4	14	8	8
Median Time to Transfer (minutes)[5]	0	-	48	61
Fibrinolytic Medication Timing[3]	0	-	53%	54%
Heart Failure Care				
ACE Inhibitor or ARB for LVSD	233	94%	95%	94%
Discharge Instructions	559	88%	89%	88%
Evaluation of LVS Function	635	100%	99%	98%
Smoking Cessation Advice	130	100%	99%	98%
Pneumonia Care				
Appropriate Initial Antibiotic	431	98%	92%	92%
Blood Culture Timing	635	100%	96%	96%
Influenza Vaccine	392	98%	93%	91%
Initial Antibiotic Timing	606	97%	95%	95%
Pneumococcal Vaccine	483	96%	95%	93%
Smoking Cessation Advice	245	100%	99%	97%
Surgical Care Improvement Project				
Appropriate VTP Within 24 Hours[2]	455	93%	93%	92%
Appropriate Hair Removal[2]	1,225	100%	100%	99%
Appropriate Beta Blocker Usage[2]	398	96%	94%	93%
Controlled Postoperative Blood Glucose[2]	190	91%	94%	93%
Prophylactic Antibiotic Timing[2]	965	99%	98%	97%
Prophylactic Antibiotic Timing (Outpatient)	565	99%	94%	92%
Prophylactic Antibiotic Selection[2]	978	100%	98%	97%
Prophylactic Antibiotic Select. (Outpatient)	563	97%	95%	94%
Prophylactic Antibiotic Stopped	921	98%	96%	94%
Recommended VTP Ordered[2]	455	96%	95%	94%
Urinary Catheter Removal[2]	398	90%	91%	90%
Children's Asthma Care				
Received Systemic Corticosteroids	44	100%	100%	100%
Received Home Management Plan	45	82%	75%	71%
Received Reliever Medication	45	100%	100%	100%
Use of Medical Imaging				
Combination Abdominal CT Scan	2,369	0.042	0.115	0.191
Combination Chest CT Scan	2,438	0.031	0.037	0.054
Follow-up Mammogram/Ultrasound	3,964	5.4%	7.9%	8.4%
MRI for Low Back Pain	837	27.8%	30.6%	32.7%
Survey of Patients' Hospital Experiences				
Area Around Room 'Always' Quiet at Night	300+	61%	-	58%
Doctors 'Always' Communicated Well	300+	85%	-	80%
Home Recovery Information Given	300+	86%	-	82%
Hospital Given 9 or 10 on 10 Point Scale	300+	72%	-	67%
Meds 'Always' Explained Before Given	300+	66%	-	60%
Nurses 'Always' Communicated Well	300+	80%	-	76%
Pain 'Always' Well Controlled	300+	69%	-	69%
Room and Bathroom 'Always' Clean	300+	71%	-	71%
Timely Help 'Always' Received	300+	66%	-	64%
Would Definitely Recommend Hospital	300+	76%	-	69%

Stokes-Reynolds Memorial Hospital

1570 Nc 8 & 89 Hwy North
Danbury, NC 27016
E-mail: llabine@wfubmc.edu
URL: www.wfubmc.edu/stokes
Type: Critical Access Hospitals
Ownership: Voluntary Non-Profit - Private

Phone: 336-593-2831
Fax: 336-593-5350

Emergency Services: Yes
Beds: 93

Key Personnel:
CEO/President . . . . Sandra Priddy
Chief of Medical Staff . . . . Samuel C Newsome
Infection Control . . . . Pam Boyles
Operating Room . . . . Dana Mabe
Anesthesiology . . . . Bill Sawyer, CRNA
Emergency Room . . . . Wendy Tachardson

Measure	Cases	This Hosp.	State Avg.	U.S. Avg.
Heart Attack Care				
ACE Inhibitor or ARB for LVSD[5]	0	-	97%	96%
Aspirin at Arrival[5]	0	-	99%	99%
Aspirin at Discharge[5]	0	-	99%	98%
Beta Blocker at Discharge[5]	0	-	99%	98%
Fibrinolytic Medication Timing[5]	0	-	38%	55%
PCI Within 90 Minutes of Arrival[5]	0	-	95%	90%
Smoking Cessation Advice[5]	0	-	100%	99%
Chest Pain/Possible Heart Attack Care				
Aspirin at Arrival	-	-	95%	95%
Median Time to ECG (minutes)	-	-	8	8
Median Time to Transfer (minutes)	-	-	48	61
Fibrinolytic Medication Timing	-	-	53%	54%
Heart Failure Care				
ACE Inhibitor or ARB for LVSD[1,3]	1	100%	95%	94%
Discharge Instructions[1,3]	4	75%	89%	88%
Evaluation of LVS Function[1,3]	3	33%	99%	98%
Smoking Cessation Advice[1,3]	2	100%	99%	98%
Pneumonia Care				
Appropriate Initial Antibiotic[5]	0	-	92%	92%
Blood Culture Timing[1]	6	100%	96%	96%
Influenza Vaccine[1]	2	50%	93%	91%
Initial Antibiotic Timing[1]	10	100%	95%	95%
Pneumococcal Vaccine[1]	6	50%	95%	93%
Smoking Cessation Advice[1]	4	100%	99%	97%
Surgical Care Improvement Project				
Appropriate VTP Within 24 Hours[5]	0	-	93%	92%
Appropriate Hair Removal[5]	0	-	100%	99%
Appropriate Beta Blocker Usage[5]	0	-	94%	93%
Controlled Postoperative Blood Glucose[5]	0	-	94%	93%
Prophylactic Antibiotic Timing[5]	0	-	98%	97%
Prophylactic Antibiotic Timing (Outpatient)	-	-	94%	92%
Prophylactic Antibiotic Selection[5]	0	-	98%	97%
Prophylactic Antibiotic Select. (Outpatient)	-	-	95%	94%
Prophylactic Antibiotic Stopped[5]	0	-	96%	94%
Recommended VTP Ordered[5]	0	-	95%	94%
Urinary Catheter Removal[5]	0	-	91%	90%
Children's Asthma Care				
Received Systemic Corticosteroids	-	-	100%	100%
Received Home Management Plan	-	-	75%	71%
Received Reliever Medication	-	-	100%	100%
Use of Medical Imaging				
Combination Abdominal CT Scan	-	-	0.115	0.191
Combination Chest CT Scan	-	-	0.037	0.054
Follow-up Mammogram/Ultrasound	-	-	7.9%	8.4%
MRI for Low Back Pain	-	-	30.6%	32.7%
Survey of Patients' Hospital Experiences				
Area Around Room 'Always' Quiet at Night[8]	-	-	-	58%
Doctors 'Always' Communicated Well[8]	-	-	-	80%
Home Recovery Information Given[8]	-	-	-	82%
Hospital Given 9 or 10 on 10 Point Scale[8]	-	-	-	67%
Meds 'Always' Explained Before Given[8]	-	-	-	60%
Nurses 'Always' Communicated Well[8]	-	-	-	76%
Pain 'Always' Well Controlled[8]	-	-	-	69%
Room and Bathroom 'Always' Clean[8]	-	-	-	71%
Timely Help 'Always' Received[8]	-	-	-	64%
Would Definitely Recommend Hospital[8]	-	-	-	69%

NOTE: Hospital profiles are in alphabetical order by state, then city, then hospital within the city; Rankings exclude hospitals with less than 25 cases except for patient surveys which excludes hospitals with less than 100 cases; (a) 100–299 cases; (1) The number of cases is too small to be sure how well a hospital is performing; (2) The hospital indicated that the data submitted for this measure were based on a sample of data; (3) Data was collected during a shorter time period (fewer quarters) than the maximum possible time for this measure; (4) Suppressed for one or more quarters by CMS; (5) No data is available from the hospital for this measure; (6) Fewer than 100 patients completed the HCAHPS survey. Use these rates with caution, as the number of surveys may be too low to reliably assess hospital performance; (7) Survey results are based on less than 12 months of data; (8) Survey results are not available for this reporting period; (9) No or very few patients were eligible for the HCAHPS survey. The scores shown, if any, reflect a very small number of surveys; (10) A state average was not calculated because too few hospitals in the state submitted data; (11) There were discrepancies in the data collection process; Please refer to the User's Guide for a full explanation of data.

Betsy Johnson Regional Hospital

800 Tilghman Dr
Dunn, NC 28334
E-mail: bjrh@bjrh.org
URL: www.bjrh.org
Type: Acute Care Hospitals
Ownership: Voluntary Non-Profit - Private
Phone: 910-892-7161
Fax: 910-892-5032
Emergency Services: Yes
Beds: 101

Key Personnel:
CEO/President. . . . . Kenneth E Bryan, FACHE
Cardiac Laboratory. . . . . Betsy Johnson
Chief of Medical Staff . . . . Patrick Gray
Radiology. . . . . David J Allison

Measure	Cases	This Hosp.	State Avg.	U.S. Avg.
Heart Attack Care				
ACE Inhibitor or ARB for LVSD[1]	1	100%	97%	96%
Aspirin at Arrival[1]	14	79%	99%	99%
Aspirin at Discharge[1]	7	86%	99%	98%
Beta Blocker at Discharge[1]	7	100%	99%	98%
Fibrinolytic Medication Timing	0	-	38%	55%
PCI Within 90 Minutes of Arrival	0	-	95%	90%
Smoking Cessation Advice	0	-	100%	99%
Chest Pain/Possible Heart Attack Care				
Aspirin at Arrival	261	91%	95%	95%
Median Time to ECG (minutes)	275	9	8	8
Median Time to Transfer (minutes)[1,3]	1	61	48	61
Fibrinolytic Medication Timing[1]	6	33%	53%	54%
Heart Failure Care				
ACE Inhibitor or ARB for LVSD	44	100%	95%	94%
Discharge Instructions	150	63%	89%	88%
Evaluation of LVS Function	201	93%	99%	98%
Smoking Cessation Advice	26	96%	99%	98%
Pneumonia Care				
Appropriate Initial Antibiotic	159	87%	92%	92%
Blood Culture Timing	188	93%	96%	96%
Influenza Vaccine	162	87%	93%	91%
Initial Antibiotic Timing	206	95%	95%	95%
Pneumococcal Vaccine	173	96%	95%	93%
Smoking Cessation Advice	78	99%	99%	97%
Surgical Care Improvement Project				
Appropriate VTP Within 24 Hours	102	75%	93%	92%
Appropriate Hair Removal	206	99%	100%	99%
Appropriate Beta Blocker Usage	51	71%	94%	93%
Controlled Postoperative Blood Glucose	0	-	94%	93%
Prophylactic Antibiotic Timing	125	95%	98%	97%
Prophylactic Antibiotic Timing (Outpatient)	157	86%	94%	92%
Prophylactic Antibiotic Selection	125	98%	98%	97%
Prophylactic Antibiotic Select. (Outpatient)	142	96%	95%	94%
Prophylactic Antibiotic Stopped	121	91%	96%	94%
Recommended VTP Ordered	102	82%	95%	94%
Urinary Catheter Removal	50	82%	91%	90%
Children's Asthma Care				
Received Systemic Corticosteroids	-	-	100%	100%
Received Home Management Plan	-	-	75%	71%
Received Reliever Medication	-	-	100%	100%
Use of Medical Imaging				
Combination Abdominal CT Scan	707	0.228	0.115	0.191
Combination Chest CT Scan	327	0.015	0.037	0.054
Follow-up Mammogram/Ultrasound	715	11.6%	7.9%	8.4%
MRI for Low Back Pain	155	27.7%	30.6%	32.7%
Survey of Patients' Hospital Experiences				
Area Around Room 'Always' Quiet at Night	300+	64%	-	58%
Doctors 'Always' Communicated Well	300+	75%	-	80%
Home Recovery Information Given	300+	75%	-	82%
Hospital Given 9 or 10 on 10 Point Scale	300+	56%	-	67%
Meds 'Always' Explained Before Given	300+	57%	-	60%
Nurses 'Always' Communicated Well	300+	72%	-	76%
Pain 'Always' Well Controlled	300+	64%	-	69%
Room and Bathroom 'Always' Clean	300+	65%	-	71%
Timely Help 'Always' Received	300+	54%	-	64%
Would Definitely Recommend Hospital	300+	53%	-	69%

Duke University Hospital

2301 Erwin Road
Durham, NC 27710
URL: www.dukehealth.org
Type: Acute Care Hospitals
Ownership: Voluntary Non-Profit - Private
Phone: 919-684-8111
Fax: 919-470-7376
Emergency Services: Yes
Beds: 1,019

Key Personnel:
CEO/President. . . . . Kevin Sowers RN, MSN
Chief of Medical Staff . . . . Ian Greenwald MD
Coronary Care . . . . Christopher B. Granger, MD
Pediatric Ambulatory Care . . . . . . Clay Bordley, MD
Radiology. . . . . Diana Voorhees, MD
Ambulatory Care . . . . Paul Newman
Anesthesiology. . . . . Anthony M. Roche, MD
Emergency Room . . . . Michael B. Hocker MD, MHS-CL

Measure	Cases	This Hosp.	State Avg.	U.S. Avg.
Heart Attack Care				
ACE Inhibitor or ARB for LVSD	127	100%	97%	96%
Aspirin at Arrival	338	99%	99%	99%
Aspirin at Discharge	622	100%	99%	98%
Beta Blocker at Discharge	583	100%	99%	98%
Fibrinolytic Medication Timing[1]	2	50%	38%	55%
PCI Within 90 Minutes of Arrival	79	94%	95%	90%
Smoking Cessation Advice	237	100%	100%	99%
Chest Pain/Possible Heart Attack Care				
Aspirin at Arrival[5]	0	-	95%	95%
Median Time to ECG (minutes)[5]	0	-	8	8
Median Time to Transfer (minutes)[5]	0	-	48	61
Fibrinolytic Medication Timing[5]	0	-	53%	54%
Heart Failure Care				
ACE Inhibitor or ARB for LVSD	362	98%	95%	94%
Discharge Instructions	776	98%	89%	88%
Evaluation of LVS Function	853	100%	99%	98%
Smoking Cessation Advice	135	100%	99%	98%
Pneumonia Care				
Appropriate Initial Antibiotic	90	98%	92%	92%
Blood Culture Timing	240	98%	96%	96%
Influenza Vaccine	232	98%	93%	91%
Initial Antibiotic Timing	233	91%	95%	95%
Pneumococcal Vaccine	251	99%	95%	93%
Smoking Cessation Advice	78	100%	99%	97%
Surgical Care Improvement Project				
Appropriate VTP Within 24 Hours[2]	202	100%	93%	92%
Appropriate Hair Removal[2]	634	98%	100%	99%
Appropriate Beta Blocker Usage[2]	160	97%	94%	93%
Controlled Postoperative Blood Glucose[2]	126	98%	94%	93%
Prophylactic Antibiotic Timing[2]	396	97%	98%	97%
Prophylactic Antibiotic Timing (Outpatient)	749	88%	94%	92%
Prophylactic Antibiotic Selection[2]	405	97%	98%	97%
Prophylactic Antibiotic Select. (Outpatient)	832	87%	95%	94%
Prophylactic Antibiotic Stopped[2]	371	99%	96%	94%
Recommended VTP Ordered[2]	202	100%	95%	94%
Urinary Catheter Removal[2]	160	92%	91%	90%
Children's Asthma Care				
Received Systemic Corticosteroids	-	-	100%	100%
Received Home Management Plan	-	-	75%	71%
Received Reliever Medication	-	-	100%	100%
Use of Medical Imaging				
Combination Abdominal CT Scan	3,829	0.092	0.115	0.191
Combination Chest CT Scan	5,860	0.034	0.037	0.054
Follow-up Mammogram/Ultrasound	2,854	7.7%	7.9%	8.4%
MRI for Low Back Pain	446	32.1%	30.6%	32.7%
Survey of Patients' Hospital Experiences				
Area Around Room 'Always' Quiet at Night	300+	55%	-	58%
Doctors 'Always' Communicated Well	300+	80%	-	80%
Home Recovery Information Given	300+	88%	-	82%
Hospital Given 9 or 10 on 10 Point Scale	300+	74%	-	67%
Meds 'Always' Explained Before Given	300+	64%	-	60%
Nurses 'Always' Communicated Well	300+	77%	-	76%
Pain 'Always' Well Controlled	300+	65%	-	69%
Room and Bathroom 'Always' Clean	300+	56%	-	71%
Timely Help 'Always' Received	300+	54%	-	64%
Would Definitely Recommend Hospital	300+	80%	-	69%

Durham Regional Hospital

3643 N Roxboro Road
Durham, NC 27704
URL: durhamregional.org
Type: Acute Care Hospitals
Ownership: Government - Local
Phone: 919-620-1078
Fax: 919-681-7925
Emergency Services: Yes
Beds: 369

Key Personnel:
CEO/President. . . . . David McQuaid
Chief of Medical Staff . . . . Lisa Clark Pickett MD
Operating Room. . . . . Ralph Randal Bollinger
Radiology. . . . . Mitchell Steven Anscher
Emergency Room . . . . Sarah A. Stahmer, MD
Intensive Care Unit. . . . . Betty Hinshaw

Measure	Cases	This Hosp.	State Avg.	U.S. Avg.
Heart Attack Care				
ACE Inhibitor or ARB for LVSD	52	98%	97%	96%
Aspirin at Arrival	247	100%	99%	99%
Aspirin at Discharge	228	100%	99%	98%
Beta Blocker at Discharge	219	99%	99%	98%
Fibrinolytic Medication Timing	0	-	38%	55%
PCI Within 90 Minutes of Arrival	30	83%	95%	90%
Smoking Cessation Advice	85	100%	100%	99%
Chest Pain/Possible Heart Attack Care				
Aspirin at Arrival[1,3]	2	100%	95%	95%
Median Time to ECG (minutes)[1,3]	4	34	8	8
Median Time to Transfer (minutes)[3]	0	-	48	61
Fibrinolytic Medication Timing[3]	0	-	53%	54%
Heart Failure Care				
ACE Inhibitor or ARB for LVSD	166	95%	95%	94%
Discharge Instructions	317	92%	89%	88%
Evaluation of LVS Function	394	100%	99%	98%
Smoking Cessation Advice	84	100%	99%	98%
Pneumonia Care				
Appropriate Initial Antibiotic	195	95%	92%	92%
Blood Culture Timing	321	98%	96%	96%
Influenza Vaccine	199	98%	93%	91%
Initial Antibiotic Timing	297	94%	95%	95%
Pneumococcal Vaccine	274	97%	95%	93%
Smoking Cessation Advice	145	99%	99%	97%
Surgical Care Improvement Project				
Appropriate VTP Within 24 Hours[2]	196	95%	93%	92%
Appropriate Hair Removal[2]	935	100%	100%	99%
Appropriate Beta Blocker Usage[2]	253	95%	94%	93%
Controlled Postoperative Blood Glucose[2]	51	94%	94%	93%
Prophylactic Antibiotic Timing[2]	781	99%	98%	97%
Prophylactic Antibiotic Timing (Outpatient)	560	97%	94%	92%
Prophylactic Antibiotic Selection[2]	781	99%	98%	97%
Prophylactic Antibiotic Select. (Outpatient)	556	99%	95%	94%
Prophylactic Antibiotic Stopped[2]	747	97%	96%	94%
Recommended VTP Ordered[2]	196	98%	95%	94%
Urinary Catheter Removal[2]	357	95%	91%	90%
Children's Asthma Care				
Received Systemic Corticosteroids	-	-	100%	100%
Received Home Management Plan	-	-	75%	71%
Received Reliever Medication	-	-	100%	100%
Use of Medical Imaging				
Combination Abdominal CT Scan	744	0.020	0.115	0.191
Combination Chest CT Scan	432	0.012	0.037	0.054
Follow-up Mammogram/Ultrasound	526	9.5%	7.9%	8.4%
MRI for Low Back Pain	100	33.0%	30.6%	32.7%
Survey of Patients' Hospital Experiences				
Area Around Room 'Always' Quiet at Night	300+	45%	-	58%
Doctors 'Always' Communicated Well	300+	78%	-	80%
Home Recovery Information Given	300+	77%	-	82%
Hospital Given 9 or 10 on 10 Point Scale	300+	58%	-	67%
Meds 'Always' Explained Before Given	300+	55%	-	60%
Nurses 'Always' Communicated Well	300+	70%	-	76%
Pain 'Always' Well Controlled	300+	63%	-	69%
Room and Bathroom 'Always' Clean	300+	59%	-	71%
Timely Help 'Always' Received	300+	55%	-	64%
Would Definitely Recommend Hospital	300+	69%	-	69%

NOTE: Hospital profiles are in alphabetical order by state, then city, then hospital within the city; Rankings exclude hospitals with less than 25 cases except for patient surveys which excludes hospitals with less than 100 cases; (a) 100–299 cases; (1) The number of cases is too small to be sure how well a hospital is performing; (2) The hospital indicated that the data submitted for this measure were based on a sample of cases; (3) Data was collected during a shorter time period (fewer quarters) than the maximum possible time for this measure; (4) Suppressed for one or more quarters by CMS; (5) No data is available from the hospital for this measure; (6) Fewer than 100 patients completed the HCAHPS survey. Use these rates with caution, as the number of surveys may be too low to reliably assess hospital performance; (7) Survey results are based on less than 12 months of data; (8) Survey results are not available for this reporting period; (9) No or very few patients were eligible for the HCAHPS survey. The scores shown, if any, reflect a very small number of surveys; (10) A state average was not calculated because too few hospitals in the state submitted data; (11) There were discrepancies in the data collection process; Please refer to the User's Guide for a full explanation of data.

Durham VA Medical Center

508 Fulton Street
Durham, NC 27705
URL: www.va.gov/sta/guide/facility.asp?id=43
Type: Acute Care-Veterans Administration
Ownership: Government - Federal

Phone: 919-286-0411
Fax: 919-286-6825

Emergency Services: No
Beds: 232

Key Personnel:
CEO/President . . . . Ralph T Gigliotti
Chief of Medical Staff . . . . John Shelburne, MD
Coronary Care . . . . David Holzer, RN
Infection Control . . . . Kenneth R Wilson, MD
Operating Room . . . . Lael Jackson, RN
Quality Assurance . . . . Rose Burk
Emergency Room . . . . Paul Matson, MD
Intensive Care Unit . . . . Charles S. Brudney MD, BCh

Measure	Cases	This Hosp.	State Avg.	U.S. Avg.
Heart Attack Care				
ACE Inhibitor or ARB for LVSD[1]	10	90%	97%	96%
Aspirin at Arrival	43	98%	99%	99%
Aspirin at Discharge	45	98%	99%	98%
Beta Blocker at Discharge	45	100%	99%	98%
Fibrinolytic Medication Timing[5]	0	-	38%	55%
PCI Within 90 Minutes of Arrival[1]	4	50%	95%	90%
Smoking Cessation Advice[1]	16	100%	100%	99%
Chest Pain/Possible Heart Attack Care				
Aspirin at Arrival	-	-	95%	95%
Median Time to ECG (minutes)	-	-	8	8
Median Time to Transfer (minutes)	-	-	48	61
Fibrinolytic Medication Timing	-	-	53%	54%
Heart Failure Care				
ACE Inhibitor or ARB for LVSD	68	96%	95%	94%
Discharge Instructions	160	99%	89%	88%
Evaluation of LVS Function	173	100%	99%	98%
Smoking Cessation Advice[1]	24	96%	99%	98%
Pneumonia Care				
Appropriate Initial Antibiotic	26	85%	92%	92%
Blood Culture Timing	57	96%	96%	96%
Influenza Vaccine	60	97%	93%	91%
Initial Antibiotic Timing	60	88%	95%	95%
Pneumococcal Vaccine	59	98%	95%	93%
Smoking Cessation Advice	29	100%	99%	97%
Surgical Care Improvement Project				
Appropriate VTP Within 24 Hours[2]	111	92%	93%	92%
Appropriate Hair Removal[2]	276	100%	100%	99%
Appropriate Beta Blocker Usage[2]	80	100%	94%	93%
Controlled Postoperative Blood Glucose[2]	111	95%	94%	93%
Prophylactic Antibiotic Timing	176	99%	98%	97%
Prophylactic Antibiotic Timing (Outpatient)	-	-	94%	92%
Prophylactic Antibiotic Selection	180	98%	98%	97%
Prophylactic Antibiotic Select. (Outpatient)	-	-	95%	94%
Prophylactic Antibiotic Stopped	174	92%	96%	94%
Recommended VTP Ordered[2]	112	91%	95%	94%
Urinary Catheter Removal[2]	97	95%	91%	90%
Children's Asthma Care				
Received Systemic Corticosteroids	-	-	100%	100%
Received Home Management Plan	-	-	75%	71%
Received Reliever Medication	-	-	100%	100%
Use of Medical Imaging				
Combination Abdominal CT Scan	-	-	0.115	0.191
Combination Chest CT Scan	-	-	0.037	0.054
Follow-up Mammogram/Ultrasound	-	-	7.9%	8.4%
MRI for Low Back Pain	-	-	30.6%	32.7%
Survey of Patients' Hospital Experiences				
Area Around Room 'Always' Quiet at Night	-	-	-	58%
Doctors 'Always' Communicated Well	-	-	-	80%
Home Recovery Information Given	-	-	-	82%
Hospital Given 9 or 10 on 10 Point Scale	-	-	-	67%
Meds 'Always' Explained Before Given	-	-	-	60%
Nurses 'Always' Communicated Well	-	-	-	76%
Pain 'Always' Well Controlled	-	-	-	69%
Room and Bathroom 'Always' Clean	-	-	-	71%
Timely Help 'Always' Received	-	-	-	64%
Would Definitely Recommend Hospital	-	-	-	69%

North Carolina Specialty Hospital

3916 Ben Franklin Boulevard
Durham, NC 27704
Type: Acute Care Hospitals
Ownership: Proprietary

Phone: 919-956-9300
Fax: 919-287-3237
Emergency Services: No
Beds: 14

Key Personnel:
CEO/President . . . . Randi Pisko
Chief of Medical Staff . . . . Dr David Dellaero
Infection Control . . . . Donna Lockamy

Measure	Cases	This Hosp.	State Avg.	U.S. Avg.
Heart Attack Care				
ACE Inhibitor or ARB for LVSD[5]	0	-	97%	96%
Aspirin at Arrival[5]	0	-	99%	99%
Aspirin at Discharge[5]	0	-	99%	98%
Beta Blocker at Discharge[5]	0	-	99%	98%
Fibrinolytic Medication Timing[5]	0	-	38%	55%
PCI Within 90 Minutes of Arrival[5]	0	-	95%	90%
Smoking Cessation Advice[5]	0	-	100%	99%
Chest Pain/Possible Heart Attack Care				
Aspirin at Arrival[5]	0	-	95%	95%
Median Time to ECG (minutes)[5]	0	-	8	8
Median Time to Transfer (minutes)[5]	0	-	48	61
Fibrinolytic Medication Timing[5]	0	-	53%	54%
Heart Failure Care				
ACE Inhibitor or ARB for LVSD[5]	0	-	95%	94%
Discharge Instructions[5]	0	-	89%	88%
Evaluation of LVS Function[5]	0	-	99%	98%
Smoking Cessation Advice[5]	0	-	99%	98%
Pneumonia Care				
Appropriate Initial Antibiotic[5]	0	-	92%	92%
Blood Culture Timing[5]	0	-	96%	96%
Influenza Vaccine[5]	0	-	93%	91%
Initial Antibiotic Timing[5]	0	-	95%	95%
Pneumococcal Vaccine[5]	0	-	95%	93%
Smoking Cessation Advice[5]	0	-	99%	97%
Surgical Care Improvement Project				
Appropriate VTP Within 24 Hours[2]	47	100%	93%	92%
Appropriate Hair Removal[2]	265	100%	100%	99%
Appropriate Beta Blocker Usage[2]	57	100%	94%	93%
Controlled Postoperative Blood Glucose[2]	0	-	94%	93%
Prophylactic Antibiotic Timing[2]	187	99%	98%	97%
Prophylactic Antibiotic Timing (Outpatient)	95	97%	94%	92%
Prophylactic Antibiotic Selection[2]	187	100%	98%	97%
Prophylactic Antibiotic Select. (Outpatient)	95	97%	95%	94%
Prophylactic Antibiotic Stopped[2]	186	99%	96%	94%
Recommended VTP Ordered[2]	47	100%	95%	94%
Urinary Catheter Removal[2]	118	97%	91%	90%
Children's Asthma Care				
Received Systemic Corticosteroids	-	-	100%	100%
Received Home Management Plan	-	-	75%	71%
Received Reliever Medication	-	-	100%	100%
Use of Medical Imaging				
Combination Abdominal CT Scan[5]	0	-	0.115	0.191
Combination Chest CT Scan[5]	0	-	0.037	0.054
Follow-up Mammogram/Ultrasound[5]	0	-	7.9%	8.4%
MRI for Low Back Pain[5]	0	-	30.6%	32.7%
Survey of Patients' Hospital Experiences				
Area Around Room 'Always' Quiet at Night	300+	83%	-	58%
Doctors 'Always' Communicated Well	300+	91%	-	80%
Home Recovery Information Given	300+	91%	-	82%
Hospital Given 9 or 10 on 10 Point Scale	300+	89%	-	67%
Meds 'Always' Explained Before Given	300+	73%	-	60%
Nurses 'Always' Communicated Well	300+	87%	-	76%
Pain 'Always' Well Controlled	300+	79%	-	69%
Room and Bathroom 'Always' Clean	300+	88%	-	71%
Timely Help 'Always' Received	300+	82%	-	64%
Would Definitely Recommend Hospital	300+	92%	-	69%

Morehead Memorial Hospital

117 E Kings Highway
Eden, NC 27288
URL: www.morehead.org
Type: Acute Care Hospitals
Ownership: Voluntary Non-Profit - Private

Phone: 336-623-9711
Fax: 336-623-6182

Emergency Services: Yes
Beds: 108

Key Personnel:
CEO/President . . . . Robert A Enders Jr
Chief of Medical Staff . . . . Daphyne Anderson
Quality Assurance . . . . Susan Netherland
Radiology . . . . David L Call
Emergency Room . . . . Anne Mills
Intensive Care Unit . . . . Rose Cullom
Patient Relations . . . . Linda Chambers

Measure	Cases	This Hosp.	State Avg.	U.S. Avg.
Heart Attack Care				
ACE Inhibitor or ARB for LVSD[1]	5	80%	97%	96%
Aspirin at Arrival	38	92%	99%	99%
Aspirin at Discharge	29	79%	99%	98%
Beta Blocker at Discharge	29	90%	99%	98%
Fibrinolytic Medication Timing	0	-	38%	55%
PCI Within 90 Minutes of Arrival	0	-	95%	90%
Smoking Cessation Advice[1]	4	75%	100%	99%
Chest Pain/Possible Heart Attack Care				
Aspirin at Arrival	103	98%	95%	95%
Median Time to ECG (minutes)	95	9	8	8
Median Time to Transfer (minutes)[1]	21	47	48	61
Fibrinolytic Medication Timing	0	-	53%	54%
Heart Failure Care				
ACE Inhibitor or ARB for LVSD	66	80%	95%	94%
Discharge Instructions	209	70%	89%	88%
Evaluation of LVS Function	258	84%	99%	98%
Smoking Cessation Advice	43	88%	99%	98%
Pneumonia Care				
Appropriate Initial Antibiotic	182	87%	92%	92%
Blood Culture Timing	129	96%	96%	96%
Influenza Vaccine	149	91%	93%	91%
Initial Antibiotic Timing	227	94%	95%	95%
Pneumococcal Vaccine	197	90%	95%	93%
Smoking Cessation Advice	89	89%	99%	97%
Surgical Care Improvement Project				
Appropriate VTP Within 24 Hours	103	86%	93%	92%
Appropriate Hair Removal	176	100%	100%	99%
Appropriate Beta Blocker Usage	40	78%	94%	93%
Controlled Postoperative Blood Glucose	0	-	94%	93%
Prophylactic Antibiotic Timing	112	95%	98%	97%
Prophylactic Antibiotic Timing (Outpatient)	72	89%	94%	92%
Prophylactic Antibiotic Selection	109	98%	98%	97%
Prophylactic Antibiotic Select. (Outpatient)	68	93%	95%	94%
Prophylactic Antibiotic Stopped	99	78%	96%	94%
Recommended VTP Ordered	104	88%	95%	94%
Urinary Catheter Removal	26	73%	91%	90%
Children's Asthma Care				
Received Systemic Corticosteroids	-	-	100%	100%
Received Home Management Plan	-	-	75%	71%
Received Reliever Medication	-	-	100%	100%
Use of Medical Imaging				
Combination Abdominal CT Scan	503	0.127	0.115	0.191
Combination Chest CT Scan	469	0.094	0.037	0.054
Follow-up Mammogram/Ultrasound	745	5.4%	7.9%	8.4%
MRI for Low Back Pain	119	42.0%	30.6%	32.7%
Survey of Patients' Hospital Experiences				
Area Around Room 'Always' Quiet at Night	300+	48%	-	58%
Doctors 'Always' Communicated Well	300+	84%	-	80%
Home Recovery Information Given	300+	80%	-	82%
Hospital Given 9 or 10 on 10 Point Scale	300+	66%	-	67%
Meds 'Always' Explained Before Given	300+	60%	-	60%
Nurses 'Always' Communicated Well	300+	78%	-	76%
Pain 'Always' Well Controlled	300+	69%	-	69%
Room and Bathroom 'Always' Clean	300+	76%	-	71%
Timely Help 'Always' Received	300+	67%	-	64%
Would Definitely Recommend Hospital	300+	74%	-	69%

Chowan Hospital

211 Virginia Rd
Edenton, NC 27932
Phone: 252-482-8451
Fax: 252-482-6224
URL: www.uhseast.com
Type: Critical Access Hospitals
Emergency Services: Yes
Ownership: Government - Local
Beds: 111

Key Personnel:
CEO/President. . . . . Jeffrey N Sackrison
Chief of Medical Staff. . . . . Robin Adams
Radiology. . . . . Mark Adkins

Measure	Cases	This Hosp.	State Avg.	U.S. Avg.
Heart Attack Care				
ACE Inhibitor or ARB for LVSD[1,3]	1	100%	97%	96%
Aspirin at Arrival[1,3]	4	100%	99%	99%
Aspirin at Discharge[1,3]	1	100%	99%	98%
Beta Blocker at Discharge[1,3]	3	67%	99%	98%
Fibrinolytic Medication Timing[3]	0	-	38%	55%
PCI Within 90 Minutes of Arrival[3]	0	-	95%	90%
Smoking Cessation Advice[1,3]	1	100%	100%	99%
Chest Pain/Possible Heart Attack Care				
Aspirin at Arrival	-	-	95%	95%
Median Time to ECG (minutes)	-	-	8	8
Median Time to Transfer (minutes)	-	-	48	61
Fibrinolytic Medication Timing	-	-	53%	54%
Heart Failure Care				
ACE Inhibitor or ARB for LVSD[1]	20	95%	95%	94%
Discharge Instructions	49	96%	89%	88%
Evaluation of LVS Function	65	97%	99%	98%
Smoking Cessation Advice[1]	13	100%	99%	98%
Pneumonia Care				
Appropriate Initial Antibiotic	31	90%	92%	92%
Blood Culture Timing	41	95%	96%	96%
Influenza Vaccine	25	92%	93%	91%
Initial Antibiotic Timing	39	100%	95%	95%
Pneumococcal Vaccine	37	95%	95%	93%
Smoking Cessation Advice[1]	19	100%	99%	97%
Surgical Care Improvement Project				
Appropriate VTP Within 24 Hours	65	98%	93%	92%
Appropriate Hair Removal	177	98%	100%	99%
Appropriate Beta Blocker Usage	52	98%	94%	93%
Controlled Postoperative Blood Glucose	0	-	94%	93%
Prophylactic Antibiotic Timing	140	98%	98%	97%
Prophylactic Antibiotic Timing (Outpatient)	-	-	94%	92%
Prophylactic Antibiotic Selection	139	100%	98%	97%
Prophylactic Antibiotic Select. (Outpatient)	-	-	95%	94%
Prophylactic Antibiotic Stopped	136	99%	96%	94%
Recommended VTP Ordered	65	98%	95%	94%
Urinary Catheter Removal	69	94%	91%	90%
Children's Asthma Care				
Received Systemic Corticosteroids	-	-	100%	100%
Received Home Management Plan	-	-	75%	71%
Received Reliever Medication	-	-	100%	100%
Use of Medical Imaging				
Combination Abdominal CT Scan	-	-	0.115	0.191
Combination Chest CT Scan	-	-	0.037	0.054
Follow-up Mammogram/Ultrasound	-	-	7.9%	8.4%
MRI for Low Back Pain	-	-	30.6%	32.7%
Survey of Patients' Hospital Experiences				
Area Around Room 'Always' Quiet at Night	300+	63%	-	58%
Doctors 'Always' Communicated Well	300+	88%	-	80%
Home Recovery Information Given	300+	88%	-	82%
Hospital Given 9 or 10 on 10 Point Scale	300+	73%	-	67%
Meds 'Always' Explained Before Given	300+	65%	-	60%
Nurses 'Always' Communicated Well	300+	84%	-	76%
Pain 'Always' Well Controlled	300+	76%	-	69%
Room and Bathroom 'Always' Clean	300+	74%	-	71%
Timely Help 'Always' Received	300+	73%	-	64%
Would Definitely Recommend Hospital	300+	74%	-	69%

Albemarle Hospital Authority

1144 N Road St
Elizabeth City, NC 27909
Phone: 252-335-0531
Fax: 252-384-4637
URL: www.albemarlehealth.org
Type: Acute Care Hospitals
Emergency Services: Yes
Ownership: Govt - Hospital Dist/Auth
Beds: 182

Key Personnel:
CEO/President. . . . . Janet Jarrett
Chief of Medical Staff. . . . . Victor Sonnino
Pediatric In-Patient Care . . . . Connie Swartz, MD
Quality Assurance . . . . Richard Thompson
Radiology. . . . . Annapurna C Rao, MD

Measure	Cases	This Hosp.	State Avg.	U.S. Avg.
Heart Attack Care				
ACE Inhibitor or ARB for LVSD[1,2]	8	75%	97%	96%
Aspirin at Arrival[2]	38	95%	99%	99%
Aspirin at Discharge[2]	27	100%	99%	98%
Beta Blocker at Discharge[2]	32	97%	99%	98%
Fibrinolytic Medication Timing[2]	0	-	38%	55%
PCI Within 90 Minutes of Arrival[2]	0	-	95%	90%
Smoking Cessation Advice[1,2]	8	100%	100%	99%
Chest Pain/Possible Heart Attack Care				
Aspirin at Arrival	69	94%	95%	95%
Median Time to ECG (minutes)	72	17	8	8
Median Time to Transfer (minutes)[1]	15	118	48	61
Fibrinolytic Medication Timing[1]	10	20%	53%	54%
Heart Failure Care				
ACE Inhibitor or ARB for LVSD[2]	86	91%	95%	94%
Discharge Instructions[2]	163	80%	89%	88%
Evaluation of LVS Function[2]	197	97%	99%	98%
Smoking Cessation Advice[2]	40	98%	99%	98%
Pneumonia Care				
Appropriate Initial Antibiotic[2]	66	83%	92%	92%
Blood Culture Timing[2]	94	88%	96%	96%
Influenza Vaccine[2]	88	82%	93%	91%
Initial Antibiotic Timing[2]	101	88%	95%	95%
Pneumococcal Vaccine[2]	112	95%	95%	93%
Smoking Cessation Advice[2]	39	97%	99%	97%
Surgical Care Improvement Project				
Appropriate VTP Within 24 Hours[2]	124	96%	93%	92%
Appropriate Hair Removal[2]	232	100%	100%	99%
Appropriate Beta Blocker Usage[2]	62	95%	94%	93%
Controlled Postoperative Blood Glucose[2]	0	-	94%	93%
Prophylactic Antibiotic Timing[2]	141	100%	98%	97%
Prophylactic Antibiotic Timing (Outpatient)	256	97%	94%	92%
Prophylactic Antibiotic Selection[2]	146	98%	98%	97%
Prophylactic Antibiotic Select. (Outpatient)	252	92%	95%	94%
Prophylactic Antibiotic Stopped[2]	128	97%	96%	94%
Recommended VTP Ordered[2]	124	98%	95%	94%
Urinary Catheter Removal[2]	37	68%	91%	90%
Children's Asthma Care				
Received Systemic Corticosteroids	-	-	100%	100%
Received Home Management Plan	-	-	75%	71%
Received Reliever Medication	-	-	100%	100%
Use of Medical Imaging				
Combination Abdominal CT Scan	730	0.037	0.115	0.191
Combination Chest CT Scan	679	0.001	0.037	0.054
Follow-up Mammogram/Ultrasound	1,849	10.1%	7.9%	8.4%
MRI for Low Back Pain	206	35.9%	30.6%	32.7%
Survey of Patients' Hospital Experiences				
Area Around Room 'Always' Quiet at Night	300+	60%	-	58%
Doctors 'Always' Communicated Well	300+	80%	-	80%
Home Recovery Information Given	300+	85%	-	82%
Hospital Given 9 or 10 on 10 Point Scale	300+	66%	-	67%
Meds 'Always' Explained Before Given	300+	57%	-	60%
Nurses 'Always' Communicated Well	300+	76%	-	76%
Pain 'Always' Well Controlled	300+	70%	-	69%
Room and Bathroom 'Always' Clean	300+	74%	-	71%
Timely Help 'Always' Received	300+	63%	-	64%
Would Definitely Recommend Hospital	300+	65%	-	69%

Cape Fear Valley-Bladen County Hospital

501 South Poplar Street
Elizabethtown, NC 28337
Phone: 910-862-5100
Fax: 910-862-1241
URL: www.bchn.org
Type: Critical Access Hospitals
Emergency Services: Yes
Ownership: Voluntary Non-Profit - Private
Beds: 35

Key Personnel:
CEO/President. . . . . David Masterson, Jr
Cardiac Laboratory. . . . . Brenda McLamb
Chief of Medical Staff. . . . . Vicki Lanier, MD
Infection Control. . . . . Sandra Taylor, RN
Operating Room. . . . . Jennifer Dove
Pediatric In-Patient Care . . . . Martha Gooden
Quality Assurance . . . . Jim Burney
Radiology. . . . . Betty Carroll

Measure	Cases	This Hosp.	State Avg.	U.S. Avg.
Heart Attack Care				
ACE Inhibitor or ARB for LVSD[3]	0	-	97%	96%
Aspirin at Arrival[3]	0	-	99%	99%
Aspirin at Discharge[3]	0	-	99%	98%
Beta Blocker at Discharge[3]	0	-	99%	98%
Fibrinolytic Medication Timing[3]	0	-	38%	55%
PCI Within 90 Minutes of Arrival[3]	0	-	95%	90%
Smoking Cessation Advice[3]	0	-	100%	99%
Chest Pain/Possible Heart Attack Care				
Aspirin at Arrival[5]	0	-	95%	95%
Median Time to ECG (minutes)[5]	0	-	8	8
Median Time to Transfer (minutes)[5]	0	-	48	61
Fibrinolytic Medication Timing[5]	0	-	53%	54%
Heart Failure Care				
ACE Inhibitor or ARB for LVSD[1]	10	100%	95%	94%
Discharge Instructions[1]	15	80%	89%	88%
Evaluation of LVS Function	26	88%	99%	98%
Smoking Cessation Advice[1]	4	75%	99%	98%
Pneumonia Care				
Appropriate Initial Antibiotic[1]	24	92%	92%	92%
Blood Culture Timing	34	85%	96%	96%
Influenza Vaccine[1]	24	92%	93%	91%
Initial Antibiotic Timing[1]	23	87%	95%	95%
Pneumococcal Vaccine	30	87%	95%	93%
Smoking Cessation Advice[1]	7	71%	99%	97%
Surgical Care Improvement Project				
Appropriate VTP Within 24 Hours[1]	6	67%	93%	92%
Appropriate Hair Removal[1]	24	100%	100%	99%
Appropriate Beta Blocker Usage[5]	0	-	94%	93%
Controlled Postoperative Blood Glucose	0	-	94%	93%
Prophylactic Antibiotic Timing[1]	17	88%	98%	97%
Prophylactic Antibiotic Timing (Outpatient)[5]	0	-	94%	92%
Prophylactic Antibiotic Selection[1]	17	100%	98%	97%
Prophylactic Antibiotic Select. (Outpatient)[5]	0	-	95%	94%
Prophylactic Antibiotic Stopped[1]	16	100%	96%	94%
Recommended VTP Ordered[1]	6	67%	95%	94%
Urinary Catheter Removal	0	-	91%	90%
Children's Asthma Care				
Received Systemic Corticosteroids	-	-	100%	100%
Received Home Management Plan	-	-	75%	71%
Received Reliever Medication	-	-	100%	100%
Use of Medical Imaging				
Combination Abdominal CT Scan	278	0.025	0.115	0.191
Combination Chest CT Scan	75	0.013	0.037	0.054
Follow-up Mammogram/Ultrasound	409	7.6%	7.9%	8.4%
MRI for Low Back Pain[1]	37	37.8%	30.6%	32.7%
Survey of Patients' Hospital Experiences				
Area Around Room 'Always' Quiet at Night[8]	-	-	-	58%
Doctors 'Always' Communicated Well[8]	-	-	-	80%
Home Recovery Information Given[8]	-	-	-	82%
Hospital Given 9 or 10 on 10 Point Scale[8]	-	-	-	67%
Meds 'Always' Explained Before Given[8]	-	-	-	60%
Nurses 'Always' Communicated Well[8]	-	-	-	76%
Pain 'Always' Well Controlled[8]	-	-	-	69%
Room and Bathroom 'Always' Clean[8]	-	-	-	71%
Timely Help 'Always' Received[8]	-	-	-	64%
Would Definitely Recommend Hospital[8]	-	-	-	69%

NOTE: Hospital profiles are in alphabetical order by state, then city, then hospital within the city; Rankings exclude hospitals with less than 25 cases except for patient surveys which excludes hospitals with less than 100 cases; (a) 100–299 cases; (1) The number of cases is too small to be sure how well a hospital is performing; (2) The hospital indicated that the data submitted for this measure were based on a sample of cases; (3) Data was collected during a shorter time period (fewer quarters) than the maximum possible time for this measure; (4) Suppressed for one or more quarters by CMS; (5) No data is available from the hospital for this measure; (6) Fewer than 100 patients completed the HCAHPS survey. Use these rates with caution, as the number of surveys may be too low to reliably assess hospital performance; (7) Survey results are based on less than 12 months of data; (8) Survey results are not available for this reporting period; (9) No or very few patients were eligible for the HCAHPS survey. The scores shown, if any, reflect a very small number of surveys; (10) A state average was not calculated because too few hospitals in the state submitted data; (11) There were discrepancies in the data collection process; Please refer to the User's Guide for a full explanation of data.

Hugh Chatham Memorial Hospital

180 Parkwood Dr
Elkin, NC 28621
Phone: 336-527-7000
Fax: 336-835-9262
E-mail: info@hughchatham.org
URL: www.hughchatham.org
Type: Acute Care Hospitals
Emergency Services: Yes
Ownership: Voluntary Non-Profit - Private
Beds: 222

Key Personnel:
CEO/President. . . . . Richard Osmus
Chief of Medical Staff. . . . . Evan Ballard
Radiology. . . . . Paul Beerman

Measure	Cases	This Hosp.	State Avg.	U.S. Avg.
Heart Attack Care				
ACE Inhibitor or ARB for LVSD[1]	7	100%	97%	96%
Aspirin at Arrival	63	100%	99%	99%
Aspirin at Discharge	45	98%	99%	98%
Beta Blocker at Discharge	47	94%	99%	98%
Fibrinolytic Medication Timing	0	-	38%	55%
PCI Within 90 Minutes of Arrival	0	-	95%	90%
Smoking Cessation Advice[1]	10	100%	100%	99%
Chest Pain/Possible Heart Attack Care				
Aspirin at Arrival	152	99%	95%	95%
Median Time to ECG (minutes)	157	5	8	8
Median Time to Transfer (minutes)[1]	4	46	48	61
Fibrinolytic Medication Timing[1]	5	60%	53%	54%
Heart Failure Care				
ACE Inhibitor or ARB for LVSD[1]	21	95%	95%	94%
Discharge Instructions	142	85%	89%	88%
Evaluation of LVS Function	175	100%	99%	98%
Smoking Cessation Advice	30	100%	99%	98%
Pneumonia Care				
Appropriate Initial Antibiotic	127	98%	92%	92%
Blood Culture Timing	155	98%	96%	96%
Influenza Vaccine	112	93%	93%	91%
Initial Antibiotic Timing	155	98%	95%	95%
Pneumococcal Vaccine	130	92%	95%	93%
Smoking Cessation Advice	87	100%	99%	97%
Surgical Care Improvement Project				
Appropriate VTP Within 24 Hours	118	99%	93%	92%
Appropriate Hair Removal	344	100%	100%	99%
Appropriate Beta Blocker Usage	112	100%	94%	93%
Controlled Postoperative Blood Glucose	0	-	94%	93%
Prophylactic Antibiotic Timing	313	100%	98%	97%
Prophylactic Antibiotic Timing (Outpatient)	99	100%	94%	92%
Prophylactic Antibiotic Selection	312	98%	98%	97%
Prophylactic Antibiotic Select. (Outpatient)	100	99%	95%	94%
Prophylactic Antibiotic Stopped	299	98%	96%	94%
Recommended VTP Ordered	118	99%	95%	94%
Urinary Catheter Removal[1]	19	84%	91%	90%
Children's Asthma Care				
Received Systemic Corticosteroids	-	-	100%	100%
Received Home Management Plan	-	-	75%	71%
Received Reliever Medication	-	-	100%	100%
Use of Medical Imaging				
Combination Abdominal CT Scan	518	0.093	0.115	0.191
Combination Chest CT Scan	315	0.010	0.037	0.054
Follow-up Mammogram/Ultrasound	848	3.3%	7.9%	8.4%
MRI for Low Back Pain	155	34.2%	30.6%	32.7%
Survey of Patients' Hospital Experiences				
Area Around Room 'Always' Quiet at Night	300+	67%	-	58%
Doctors 'Always' Communicated Well	300+	85%	-	80%
Home Recovery Information Given	300+	83%	-	82%
Hospital Given 9 or 10 on 10 Point Scale	300+	79%	-	67%
Meds 'Always' Explained Before Given	300+	66%	-	60%
Nurses 'Always' Communicated Well	300+	84%	-	76%
Pain 'Always' Well Controlled	300+	73%	-	69%
Room and Bathroom 'Always' Clean	300+	82%	-	71%
Timely Help 'Always' Received	300+	71%	-	64%
Would Definitely Recommend Hospital	300+	78%	-	69%

Cape Fear Valley Medical Center

1638 Owen Drive
Fayetteville, NC 28302
Phone: 910-609-4000
Fax: 910-609-6160
URL: www.capefearvalley.com
Type: Acute Care Hospitals
Emergency Services: Yes
Ownership: Voluntary Non-Profit - Private
Beds: 616

Key Personnel:
CEO/President. . . . . Michael Nagowski
Chief of Medical Staff . . . . Eugene Wright
Infection Control. . . . . Kathy Butler
Operating Room. . . . . Ravinder K Annamaneni, RN
Pediatric In-Patient Care . . . . Clarito Pang
Quality Assurance . . . . Harold Mayner
Radiology. . . . . David J Allison

Measure	Cases	This Hosp.	State Avg.	U.S. Avg.
Heart Attack Care				
ACE Inhibitor or ARB for LVSD	102	96%	97%	96%
Aspirin at Arrival	499	99%	99%	99%
Aspirin at Discharge	542	100%	99%	98%
Beta Blocker at Discharge	517	97%	99%	98%
Fibrinolytic Medication Timing	0	-	38%	55%
PCI Within 90 Minutes of Arrival	92	84%	95%	90%
Smoking Cessation Advice	235	100%	100%	99%
Chest Pain/Possible Heart Attack Care				
Aspirin at Arrival	63	92%	95%	95%
Median Time to ECG (minutes)	69	18	8	8
Median Time to Transfer (minutes)[1,3]	1	44	48	61
Fibrinolytic Medication Timing[3]	0	-	53%	54%
Heart Failure Care				
ACE Inhibitor or ARB for LVSD	396	97%	95%	94%
Discharge Instructions	899	91%	89%	88%
Evaluation of LVS Function	1,036	100%	99%	98%
Smoking Cessation Advice	220	100%	99%	98%
Pneumonia Care				
Appropriate Initial Antibiotic	377	95%	92%	92%
Blood Culture Timing	634	97%	96%	96%
Influenza Vaccine	447	95%	93%	91%
Initial Antibiotic Timing	593	94%	95%	95%
Pneumococcal Vaccine	512	97%	95%	93%
Smoking Cessation Advice	296	100%	99%	97%
Surgical Care Improvement Project				
Appropriate VTP Within 24 Hours[2]	199	90%	93%	92%
Appropriate Hair Removal[2]	615	100%	100%	99%
Appropriate Beta Blocker Usage[2]	187	98%	94%	93%
Controlled Postoperative Blood Glucose[2]	101	94%	94%	93%
Prophylactic Antibiotic Timing[2]	444	98%	98%	97%
Prophylactic Antibiotic Timing (Outpatient)	486	92%	94%	92%
Prophylactic Antibiotic Selection[2]	451	97%	98%	97%
Prophylactic Antibiotic Select. (Outpatient)	471	83%	95%	94%
Prophylactic Antibiotic Stopped[2]	434	91%	96%	94%
Recommended VTP Ordered[2]	199	94%	95%	94%
Urinary Catheter Removal[2]	127	87%	91%	90%
Children's Asthma Care				
Received Systemic Corticosteroids	-	-	100%	100%
Received Home Management Plan	-	-	75%	71%
Received Reliever Medication	-	-	100%	100%
Use of Medical Imaging				
Combination Abdominal CT Scan	1,359	0.140	0.115	0.191
Combination Chest CT Scan	944	0.082	0.037	0.054
Follow-up Mammogram/Ultrasound	1,006	6.6%	7.9%	8.4%
MRI for Low Back Pain[1]	55	23.6%	30.6%	32.7%
Survey of Patients' Hospital Experiences				
Area Around Room 'Always' Quiet at Night	300+	53%	-	58%
Doctors 'Always' Communicated Well	300+	76%	-	80%
Home Recovery Information Given	300+	77%	-	82%
Hospital Given 9 or 10 on 10 Point Scale	300+	58%	-	67%
Meds 'Always' Explained Before Given	300+	60%	-	60%
Nurses 'Always' Communicated Well	300+	73%	-	76%
Pain 'Always' Well Controlled	300+	65%	-	69%
Room and Bathroom 'Always' Clean	300+	66%	-	71%
Timely Help 'Always' Received	300+	56%	-	64%
Would Definitely Recommend Hospital	300+	59%	-	69%

Fayetteville North Carolina VA Medical Center

2300 Ramsey Street
Fayetteville, NC 28301
Phone: 910-488-2120
Fax: 910-822-7927
URL: www.va.gov/sta/guide/home.asp
Type: Acute Care-Veterans Administration
Emergency Services: No
Ownership: Government - Federal
Beds: 159

Key Personnel:
CEO/President. . . . . Bruce C Triplett
Chief of Medical Staff . . . . Kanan Chatterje MD, MD
Quality Assurance . . . . Beatrice Olack, RN

Measure	Cases	This Hosp.	State Avg.	U.S. Avg.
Heart Attack Care				
ACE Inhibitor or ARB for LVSD[5]	0	-	97%	96%
Aspirin at Arrival[5]	0	-	99%	99%
Aspirin at Discharge[5]	0	-	99%	98%
Beta Blocker at Discharge[5]	0	-	99%	98%
Fibrinolytic Medication Timing[5]	0	-	38%	55%
PCI Within 90 Minutes of Arrival[5]	0	-	95%	90%
Smoking Cessation Advice[5]	0	-	100%	99%
Chest Pain/Possible Heart Attack Care				
Aspirin at Arrival	-	-	95%	95%
Median Time to ECG (minutes)	-	-	8	8
Median Time to Transfer (minutes)	-	-	48	61
Fibrinolytic Medication Timing	-	-	53%	54%
Heart Failure Care				
ACE Inhibitor or ARB for LVSD	47	98%	95%	94%
Discharge Instructions	116	100%	89%	88%
Evaluation of LVS Function	118	100%	99%	98%
Smoking Cessation Advice	31	100%	99%	98%
Pneumonia Care				
Appropriate Initial Antibiotic	46	89%	92%	92%
Blood Culture Timing	52	100%	96%	96%
Influenza Vaccine	32	97%	93%	91%
Initial Antibiotic Timing[1]	4	75%	95%	95%
Pneumococcal Vaccine	33	100%	95%	93%
Smoking Cessation Advice[1]	23	100%	99%	97%
Surgical Care Improvement Project				
Appropriate VTP Within 24 Hours[2,5]	0	-	93%	92%
Appropriate Hair Removal[2,5]	0	-	100%	99%
Appropriate Beta Blocker Usage[2,5]	0	-	94%	93%
Controlled Postoperative Blood Glucose[2,5]	0	-	94%	93%
Prophylactic Antibiotic Timing[5]	0	-	98%	97%
Prophylactic Antibiotic Timing (Outpatient)	-	-	94%	92%
Prophylactic Antibiotic Selection[5]	0	-	98%	97%
Prophylactic Antibiotic Select. (Outpatient)	-	-	95%	94%
Prophylactic Antibiotic Stopped[5]	0	-	96%	94%
Recommended VTP Ordered[2,5]	0	-	95%	94%
Urinary Catheter Removal[2,5]	0	-	91%	90%
Children's Asthma Care				
Received Systemic Corticosteroids	-	-	100%	100%
Received Home Management Plan	-	-	75%	71%
Received Reliever Medication	-	-	100%	100%
Use of Medical Imaging				
Combination Abdominal CT Scan	-	-	0.115	0.191
Combination Chest CT Scan	-	-	0.037	0.054
Follow-up Mammogram/Ultrasound	-	-	7.9%	8.4%
MRI for Low Back Pain	-	-	30.6%	32.7%
Survey of Patients' Hospital Experiences				
Area Around Room 'Always' Quiet at Night	-	-	-	58%
Doctors 'Always' Communicated Well	-	-	-	80%
Home Recovery Information Given	-	-	-	82%
Hospital Given 9 or 10 on 10 Point Scale	-	-	-	67%
Meds 'Always' Explained Before Given	-	-	-	60%
Nurses 'Always' Communicated Well	-	-	-	76%
Pain 'Always' Well Controlled	-	-	-	69%
Room and Bathroom 'Always' Clean	-	-	-	71%
Timely Help 'Always' Received	-	-	-	64%
Would Definitely Recommend Hospital	-	-	-	69%

NOTE: Hospital profiles are in alphabetical order by state, then city, then hospital within the city; Rankings exclude hospitals with less than 25 cases except for patient surveys which excludes hospitals with less than 100 cases; (a) 100–299 cases; (1) The number of cases is too small to be sure how well a hospital is performing; (2) The hospital indicated that the data submitted for this measure were based on a sample of cases; (3) Data was collected during a shorter time period (fewer quarters) than the maximum possible time for this measure; (4) Suppressed for one or more quarters by CMS; (5) No data is available from the hospital for this measure; (6) Fewer than 100 patients completed the HCAHPS survey. Use these rates with caution, as the number of surveys may be too low to reliably assess hospital performance; (7) Survey results are based on less than 12 months of data; (8) Survey results are not available for this reporting period; (9) No or very few patients were eligible for the HCAHPS survey. The scores shown, if any, reflect a very small number of surveys; (10) A state average was not calculated because too few hospitals in the state submitted data; (11) There were discrepancies in the data collection process; Please refer to the User's Guide for a full explanation of data.

Park Ridge Hospital

Naples Rd Box 1569 Phone: 828-684-8501
Fletcher, NC 28732 Fax: 828-681-2770
E-mail: Parkridge@ahss.org
URL: www.parkridgehospital.org
Type: Acute Care Hospitals Emergency Services: Yes
Ownership: Voluntary Non-Profit - Other Beds: 103

Key Personnel:
CEO/President. . . . . Jimm Bunch
Cardiac Laboratory. . . . . Melissa Byrd
Chief of Medical Staff. . . . . Clive Possinger, Jr, MD
Infection Control. . . . . Paula Thum
Quality Assurance . . . . Duane Price
Anesthesiology. . . . . Jeff Coston, MD
Emergency Room . . . . DeWayne Butcher, MD
Intensive Care Unit. . . . . Lora Harris

Measure	Cases	This Hosp.	State Avg.	U.S. Avg.
Heart Attack Care				
ACE Inhibitor or ARB for LVSD[1]	1	100%	97%	96%
Aspirin at Arrival[1]	21	95%	99%	99%
Aspirin at Discharge[1]	11	100%	99%	98%
Beta Blocker at Discharge[1]	12	92%	99%	98%
Fibrinolytic Medication Timing	0	-	38%	55%
PCI Within 90 Minutes of Arrival	0	-	95%	90%
Smoking Cessation Advice[1]	1	100%	100%	99%
Chest Pain/Possible Heart Attack Care				
Aspirin at Arrival[1]	18	89%	95%	95%
Median Time to ECG (minutes)[1]	19	23	8	8
Median Time to Transfer (minutes)[5]	0	-	48	61
Fibrinolytic Medication Timing[3]	0	-	53%	54%
Heart Failure Care				
ACE Inhibitor or ARB for LVSD[1]	9	78%	95%	94%
Discharge Instructions	39	85%	89%	88%
Evaluation of LVS Function	52	98%	99%	98%
Smoking Cessation Advice[1]	5	100%	99%	98%
Pneumonia Care				
Appropriate Initial Antibiotic	73	88%	92%	92%
Blood Culture Timing	101	94%	96%	96%
Influenza Vaccine	58	93%	93%	91%
Initial Antibiotic Timing	94	97%	95%	95%
Pneumococcal Vaccine	83	95%	95%	93%
Smoking Cessation Advice	42	100%	99%	97%
Surgical Care Improvement Project				
Appropriate VTP Within 24 Hours	112	92%	93%	92%
Appropriate Hair Removal	231	100%	100%	99%
Appropriate Beta Blocker Usage	42	100%	94%	93%
Controlled Postoperative Blood Glucose	0	-	94%	93%
Prophylactic Antibiotic Timing	141	97%	98%	97%
Prophylactic Antibiotic Timing (Outpatient)	126	95%	94%	92%
Prophylactic Antibiotic Selection	148	95%	98%	97%
Prophylactic Antibiotic Select. (Outpatient)	131	95%	95%	94%
Prophylactic Antibiotic Stopped	125	95%	96%	94%
Recommended VTP Ordered	112	96%	95%	94%
Urinary Catheter Removal	49	92%	91%	90%
Children's Asthma Care				
Received Systemic Corticosteroids	-	-	100%	100%
Received Home Management Plan	-	-	75%	71%
Received Reliever Medication	-	-	100%	100%
Use of Medical Imaging				
Combination Abdominal CT Scan	463	0.091	0.115	0.191
Combination Chest CT Scan	305	0.092	0.037	0.054
Follow-up Mammogram/Ultrasound	597	10.4%	7.9%	8.4%
MRI for Low Back Pain	188	26.6%	30.6%	32.7%
Survey of Patients' Hospital Experiences				
Area Around Room 'Always' Quiet at Night	300+	58%	-	58%
Doctors 'Always' Communicated Well	300+	81%	-	80%
Home Recovery Information Given	300+	81%	-	82%
Hospital Given 9 or 10 on 10 Point Scale	300+	71%	-	67%
Meds 'Always' Explained Before Given	300+	56%	-	60%
Nurses 'Always' Communicated Well	300+	75%	-	76%
Pain 'Always' Well Controlled	300+	68%	-	69%
Room and Bathroom 'Always' Clean	300+	68%	-	71%
Timely Help 'Always' Received	300+	63%	-	64%
Would Definitely Recommend Hospital	300+	73%	-	69%

Angel Medical Center

120 Riverview St Phone: 828-524-8411
Franklin, NC 28734 Fax: 828-369-4162
E-mail: amc@angelmed.org
URL: www.angelmed.org
Type: Critical Access Hospitals Emergency Services: Yes
Ownership: Voluntary Non-Profit - Private Beds: 52

Key Personnel:
CEO/President. . . . . Tim Hubbs
Cardiac Laboratory. . . . . Michael J Kegan, MD
Radiology. . . . . Robert Berger, MD

Measure	Cases	This Hosp.	State Avg.	U.S. Avg.
Heart Attack Care				
ACE Inhibitor or ARB for LVSD[1]	1	100%	97%	96%
Aspirin at Arrival[1]	6	100%	99%	99%
Aspirin at Discharge[1]	5	100%	99%	98%
Beta Blocker at Discharge[1]	4	100%	99%	98%
Fibrinolytic Medication Timing	0	-	38%	55%
PCI Within 90 Minutes of Arrival	0	-	95%	90%
Smoking Cessation Advice	0	-	100%	99%
Chest Pain/Possible Heart Attack Care				
Aspirin at Arrival	99	98%	95%	95%
Median Time to ECG (minutes)	102	10	8	8
Median Time to Transfer (minutes)[1]	7	105	48	61
Fibrinolytic Medication Timing[1]	3	67%	53%	54%
Heart Failure Care				
ACE Inhibitor or ARB for LVSD[1]	20	95%	95%	94%
Discharge Instructions	49	86%	89%	88%
Evaluation of LVS Function	54	87%	99%	98%
Smoking Cessation Advice[1]	11	73%	99%	98%
Pneumonia Care				
Appropriate Initial Antibiotic	50	88%	92%	92%
Blood Culture Timing	47	91%	96%	96%
Influenza Vaccine	41	85%	93%	91%
Initial Antibiotic Timing	64	98%	95%	95%
Pneumococcal Vaccine	67	91%	95%	93%
Smoking Cessation Advice[1]	15	100%	99%	97%
Surgical Care Improvement Project				
Appropriate VTP Within 24 Hours	45	91%	93%	92%
Appropriate Hair Removal	69	97%	100%	99%
Appropriate Beta Blocker Usage[1]	15	100%	94%	93%
Controlled Postoperative Blood Glucose	0	-	94%	93%
Prophylactic Antibiotic Timing	47	98%	98%	97%
Prophylactic Antibiotic Timing (Outpatient)[1]	19	95%	94%	92%
Prophylactic Antibiotic Selection	47	100%	98%	97%
Prophylactic Antibiotic Select. (Outpatient)[1]	19	95%	95%	94%
Prophylactic Antibiotic Stopped	46	85%	96%	94%
Recommended VTP Ordered	45	93%	95%	94%
Urinary Catheter Removal[1]	11	91%	91%	90%
Children's Asthma Care				
Received Systemic Corticosteroids	-	-	100%	100%
Received Home Management Plan	-	-	75%	71%
Received Reliever Medication	-	-	100%	100%
Use of Medical Imaging				
Combination Abdominal CT Scan[5]	0	-	0.115	0.191
Combination Chest CT Scan[5]	0	-	0.037	0.054
Follow-up Mammogram/Ultrasound[5]	0	-	7.9%	8.4%
MRI for Low Back Pain[5]	0	-	30.6%	32.7%
Survey of Patients' Hospital Experiences				
Area Around Room 'Always' Quiet at Night	300+	63%	-	58%
Doctors 'Always' Communicated Well	300+	88%	-	80%
Home Recovery Information Given	300+	82%	-	82%
Hospital Given 9 or 10 on 10 Point Scale	300+	76%	-	67%
Meds 'Always' Explained Before Given	300+	60%	-	60%
Nurses 'Always' Communicated Well	300+	82%	-	76%
Pain 'Always' Well Controlled	300+	76%	-	69%
Room and Bathroom 'Always' Clean	300+	71%	-	71%
Timely Help 'Always' Received	300+	74%	-	64%
Would Definitely Recommend Hospital	300+	82%	-	69%

Gaston Memorial Hospital

2525 Court Dr Phone: 704-834-2000
Gastonia, NC 28052 Fax: 704-834-2068
URL: www.caromont.org
Type: Acute Care Hospitals Emergency Services: Yes
Ownership: Government - Local Beds: 435

Key Personnel:
Chief of Medical Staff. . . . . H Thomason, MD
Infection Control. . . . . Connie Ford
Operating Room. . . . . Rose O'Neill
Quality Assurance . . . . Martha Rockett
Radiology. . . . . Gerald W Arney, MD
Anesthesiology. . . . . Thomas W Wingfield, MD
Emergency Room . . . . Carol Dare
Intensive Care Unit. . . . . Kathy Abrams

Measure	Cases	This Hosp.	State Avg.	U.S. Avg.
Heart Attack Care				
ACE Inhibitor or ARB for LVSD	96	100%	97%	96%
Aspirin at Arrival	523	100%	99%	99%
Aspirin at Discharge	503	100%	99%	98%
Beta Blocker at Discharge	467	100%	99%	98%
Fibrinolytic Medication Timing[1]	1	100%	38%	55%
PCI Within 90 Minutes of Arrival	107	100%	95%	90%
Smoking Cessation Advice	211	100%	100%	99%
Chest Pain/Possible Heart Attack Care				
Aspirin at Arrival[5]	0	-	95%	95%
Median Time to ECG (minutes)[5]	0	-	8	8
Median Time to Transfer (minutes)[5]	0	-	48	61
Fibrinolytic Medication Timing[5]	0	-	53%	54%
Heart Failure Care				
ACE Inhibitor or ARB for LVSD	236	99%	95%	94%
Discharge Instructions	654	94%	89%	88%
Evaluation of LVS Function	735	100%	99%	98%
Smoking Cessation Advice	152	100%	99%	98%
Pneumonia Care				
Appropriate Initial Antibiotic	359	100%	92%	92%
Blood Culture Timing	842	100%	96%	96%
Influenza Vaccine	555	100%	93%	91%
Initial Antibiotic Timing	706	99%	95%	95%
Pneumococcal Vaccine	603	100%	95%	93%
Smoking Cessation Advice	375	100%	99%	97%
Surgical Care Improvement Project				
Appropriate VTP Within 24 Hours	393	99%	93%	92%
Appropriate Hair Removal	1,384	100%	100%	99%
Appropriate Beta Blocker Usage	404	100%	94%	93%
Controlled Postoperative Blood Glucose	142	97%	94%	93%
Prophylactic Antibiotic Timing	897	99%	98%	97%
Prophylactic Antibiotic Timing (Outpatient)	750	99%	94%	92%
Prophylactic Antibiotic Selection	902	99%	98%	97%
Prophylactic Antibiotic Select. (Outpatient)	749	97%	95%	94%
Prophylactic Antibiotic Stopped	846	100%	96%	94%
Recommended VTP Ordered	394	99%	95%	94%
Urinary Catheter Removal	358	100%	91%	90%
Children's Asthma Care				
Received Systemic Corticosteroids	-	-	100%	100%
Received Home Management Plan	-	-	75%	71%
Received Reliever Medication	-	-	100%	100%
Use of Medical Imaging				
Combination Abdominal CT Scan	1,769	0.046	0.115	0.191
Combination Chest CT Scan	1,005	0.008	0.037	0.054
Follow-up Mammogram/Ultrasound	3,801	9.0%	7.9%	8.4%
MRI for Low Back Pain	780	24.6%	30.6%	32.7%
Survey of Patients' Hospital Experiences				
Area Around Room 'Always' Quiet at Night	300+	56%	-	58%
Doctors 'Always' Communicated Well	300+	82%	-	80%
Home Recovery Information Given	300+	83%	-	82%
Hospital Given 9 or 10 on 10 Point Scale	300+	68%	-	67%
Meds 'Always' Explained Before Given	300+	62%	-	60%
Nurses 'Always' Communicated Well	300+	80%	-	76%
Pain 'Always' Well Controlled	300+	72%	-	69%
Room and Bathroom 'Always' Clean	300+	68%	-	71%
Timely Help 'Always' Received	300+	69%	-	64%
Would Definitely Recommend Hospital	300+	72%	-	69%

NOTE: Hospital profiles are in alphabetical order by state, then city, then hospital within the city; Rankings exclude hospitals with less than 25 cases except for patient surveys which excludes hospitals with less than 100 cases; (a) 100–299 cases; (1) The number of cases is too small to be sure how well a hospital is performing; (2) The hospital indicated that the data submitted for this measure were based on a sample of cases; (3) Data was collected during a shorter time period (fewer quarters) than the maximum possible time for this measure; (4) Suppressed for one or more quarters by CMS; (5) No data is available from the hospital for this measure; (6) Fewer than 100 patients completed the HCAHPS survey. Use these rates with caution, as the number of surveys may be too low to reliably assess hospital performance; (7) Survey results are based on less than 12 months of data; (8) Survey results are not available for this reporting period; (9) No or very few patients were eligible for the HCAHPS survey. The scores shown, if any, reflect a very small number of surveys; (10) A state average was not calculated because too few hospitals in the state submitted data; (11) There were discrepancies in the data collection process; Please refer to the User's Guide for a full explanation of data.

Wayne Memorial Hospital

2700 Wayne Memorial Dr Phone: 919-736-1110
Goldsboro, NC 27534 Fax: 919-731-6966
URL: www.waynehealth.org
Type: Acute Care Hospitals Emergency Services: Yes
Ownership: Voluntary Non-Profit - Private Beds: 316

Key Personnel:
CEO/President. . . . . J William Paugh
Chief of Medical Staff. . . . . Michael Johnson
Radiology. . . . . Lance Arnder

Measure	Cases	This Hosp.	State Avg.	U.S. Avg.
Heart Attack Care				
ACE Inhibitor or ARB for LVSD[1]	12	100%	97%	96%
Aspirin at Arrival	50	100%	99%	99%
Aspirin at Discharge	28	100%	99%	98%
Beta Blocker at Discharge	35	100%	99%	98%
Fibrinolytic Medication Timing	0	-	38%	55%
PCI Within 90 Minutes of Arrival	0	-	95%	90%
Smoking Cessation Advice[1]	5	100%	100%	99%
Chest Pain/Possible Heart Attack Care				
Aspirin at Arrival	295	99%	95%	95%
Median Time to ECG (minutes)	304	7	8	8
Median Time to Transfer (minutes)[1]	1	46	48	61
Fibrinolytic Medication Timing	34	71%	53%	54%
Heart Failure Care				
ACE Inhibitor or ARB for LVSD	176	96%	95%	94%
Discharge Instructions	389	90%	89%	88%
Evaluation of LVS Function	456	99%	99%	98%
Smoking Cessation Advice	98	99%	99%	98%
Pneumonia Care				
Appropriate Initial Antibiotic	96	97%	92%	92%
Blood Culture Timing	112	96%	96%	96%
Influenza Vaccine	155	57%	93%	91%
Initial Antibiotic Timing	160	90%	95%	95%
Pneumococcal Vaccine	180	81%	95%	93%
Smoking Cessation Advice	105	100%	99%	97%
Surgical Care Improvement Project				
Appropriate VTP Within 24 Hours[2]	299	93%	93%	92%
Appropriate Hair Removal[2]	571	99%	100%	99%
Appropriate Beta Blocker Usage[2]	162	88%	94%	93%
Controlled Postoperative Blood Glucose[2]	0	-	94%	93%
Prophylactic Antibiotic Timing[2]	386	97%	98%	97%
Prophylactic Antibiotic Timing (Outpatient)	344	92%	94%	92%
Prophylactic Antibiotic Selection[2]	386	97%	98%	97%
Prophylactic Antibiotic Select. (Outpatient)	333	98%	95%	94%
Prophylactic Antibiotic Stopped[2]	378	93%	96%	94%
Recommended VTP Ordered[2]	303	94%	95%	94%
Urinary Catheter Removal[2]	122	84%	91%	90%
Children's Asthma Care				
Received Systemic Corticosteroids	-	-	100%	100%
Received Home Management Plan	-	-	75%	71%
Received Reliever Medication	-	-	100%	100%
Use of Medical Imaging				
Combination Abdominal CT Scan	495	0.026	0.115	0.191
Combination Chest CT Scan	310	0.023	0.037	0.054
Follow-up Mammogram/Ultrasound	292	5.1%	7.9%	8.4%
MRI for Low Back Pain	406	37.2%	30.6%	32.7%
Survey of Patients' Hospital Experiences				
Area Around Room 'Always' Quiet at Night	300+	64%	-	58%
Doctors 'Always' Communicated Well	300+	83%	-	80%
Home Recovery Information Given	300+	82%	-	82%
Hospital Given 9 or 10 on 10 Point Scale	300+	69%	-	67%
Meds 'Always' Explained Before Given	300+	63%	-	60%
Nurses 'Always' Communicated Well	300+	80%	-	76%
Pain 'Always' Well Controlled	300+	70%	-	69%
Room and Bathroom 'Always' Clean	300+	75%	-	71%
Timely Help 'Always' Received	300+	63%	-	64%
Would Definitely Recommend Hospital	300+	67%	-	69%

The Moses H Cone Memorial Hospital

1200 N Elm St Phone: 336-832-7000
Greensboro, NC 27401 Fax: 336-832-6630
E-mail: comments@mosescone.com
URL: www.mosescone.com
Type: Acute Care Hospitals Emergency Services: Yes
Ownership: Voluntary Non-Profit - Private Beds: 529

Key Personnel:
CEO/President. . . . . Tim Rice
Cardiac Laboratory. . . . . Tony Petrillo
Chief of Medical Staff . . . . Glenn Visbeen
Infection Control. . . . . Debbie Houston
Quality Assurance . . . . Ken Boggs
Radiology. . . . . Judy Grzyva
Anesthesiology. . . . . Franklin Hatchett Jr, MD
Emergency Room . . . . Robert Beaton

Measure	Cases	This Hosp.	State Avg.	U.S. Avg.
Heart Attack Care				
ACE Inhibitor or ARB for LVSD[2]	38	100%	97%	96%
Aspirin at Arrival[2]	200	99%	99%	99%
Aspirin at Discharge[2]	288	99%	99%	98%
Beta Blocker at Discharge[2]	266	99%	99%	98%
Fibrinolytic Medication Timing[2]	0	-	38%	55%
PCI Within 90 Minutes of Arrival[2]	37	86%	95%	90%
Smoking Cessation Advice[2]	119	100%	100%	99%
Chest Pain/Possible Heart Attack Care				
Aspirin at Arrival	76	99%	95%	95%
Median Time to ECG (minutes)	78	10	8	8
Median Time to Transfer (minutes)[5]	0	-	48	61
Fibrinolytic Medication Timing[3]	0	-	53%	54%
Heart Failure Care				
ACE Inhibitor or ARB for LVSD[2]	132	95%	95%	94%
Discharge Instructions[2]	330	84%	89%	88%
Evaluation of LVS Function[2]	390	100%	99%	98%
Smoking Cessation Advice[2]	108	100%	99%	98%
Pneumonia Care				
Appropriate Initial Antibiotic[2]	141	94%	92%	92%
Blood Culture Timing[2]	131	95%	96%	96%
Influenza Vaccine[2]	163	97%	93%	91%
Initial Antibiotic Timing[2]	244	97%	95%	95%
Pneumococcal Vaccine[2]	228	97%	95%	93%
Smoking Cessation Advice[2]	106	100%	99%	97%
Surgical Care Improvement Project				
Appropriate VTP Within 24 Hours[2]	415	87%	93%	92%
Appropriate Hair Removal[2]	1,088	100%	100%	99%
Appropriate Beta Blocker Usage[2]	337	87%	94%	93%
Controlled Postoperative Blood Glucose[2]	160	94%	94%	93%
Prophylactic Antibiotic Timing[2]	753	96%	98%	97%
Prophylactic Antibiotic Timing (Outpatient)	969	96%	94%	92%
Prophylactic Antibiotic Selection[2]	754	99%	98%	97%
Prophylactic Antibiotic Select. (Outpatient)	948	96%	95%	94%
Prophylactic Antibiotic Stopped[2]	712	97%	96%	94%
Recommended VTP Ordered[2]	416	92%	95%	94%
Urinary Catheter Removal[2]	280	88%	91%	90%
Children's Asthma Care				
Received Systemic Corticosteroids	-	-	100%	100%
Received Home Management Plan	-	-	75%	71%
Received Reliever Medication	-	-	100%	100%
Use of Medical Imaging				
Combination Abdominal CT Scan	1,813	0.033	0.115	0.191
Combination Chest CT Scan	1,623	0.001	0.037	0.054
Follow-up Mammogram/Ultrasound	1,837	7.1%	7.9%	8.4%
MRI for Low Back Pain	312	30.8%	30.6%	32.7%
Survey of Patients' Hospital Experiences				
Area Around Room 'Always' Quiet at Night	300+	59%	-	58%
Doctors 'Always' Communicated Well	300+	78%	-	80%
Home Recovery Information Given	300+	80%	-	82%
Hospital Given 9 or 10 on 10 Point Scale	300+	63%	-	67%
Meds 'Always' Explained Before Given	300+	56%	-	60%
Nurses 'Always' Communicated Well	300+	72%	-	76%
Pain 'Always' Well Controlled	300+	67%	-	69%
Room and Bathroom 'Always' Clean	300+	63%	-	71%
Timely Help 'Always' Received	300+	58%	-	64%
Would Definitely Recommend Hospital	300+	73%	-	69%

Pitt County Memorial Hospital

2100 Stantonsburg Rd Phone: 252-847-4100
Greenville, NC 27835 Fax: 252-847-8170
URL: www.uhseast.com
Type: Acute Care Hospitals Emergency Services: Yes
Ownership: Voluntary Non-Profit - Private Beds: 745

Key Personnel:
CEO/President. . . . . Steve Lawler
Chief of Medical Staff . . . . Ernest Larkin, MD
Operating Room. . . . . Sanjay Saha
Pediatric In-Patient Care . . . . . . Ron Perkin, MD
Quality Assurance . . . . Nancy Aycock
Radiology. . . . . Michael Weaver, MD
Anesthesiology. . . . . Joshua Schwartz, MD
Emergency Room . . . . Nick Benson, MD

Measure	Cases	This Hosp.	State Avg.	U.S. Avg.
Heart Attack Care				
ACE Inhibitor or ARB for LVSD	276	95%	97%	96%
Aspirin at Arrival	400	98%	99%	99%
Aspirin at Discharge	1,326	98%	99%	98%
Beta Blocker at Discharge	1,293	100%	99%	98%
Fibrinolytic Medication Timing	0	-	38%	55%
PCI Within 90 Minutes of Arrival	39	92%	95%	90%
Smoking Cessation Advice	581	100%	100%	99%
Chest Pain/Possible Heart Attack Care				
Aspirin at Arrival[5]	0	-	95%	95%
Median Time to ECG (minutes)[5]	0	-	8	8
Median Time to Transfer (minutes)[5]	0	-	48	61
Fibrinolytic Medication Timing[5]	0	-	53%	54%
Heart Failure Care				
ACE Inhibitor or ARB for LVSD	537	94%	95%	94%
Discharge Instructions	941	80%	89%	88%
Evaluation of LVS Function	1,057	99%	99%	98%
Smoking Cessation Advice	247	100%	99%	98%
Pneumonia Care				
Appropriate Initial Antibiotic	181	82%	92%	92%
Blood Culture Timing	272	92%	96%	96%
Influenza Vaccine	312	95%	93%	91%
Initial Antibiotic Timing	271	87%	95%	95%
Pneumococcal Vaccine	371	94%	95%	93%
Smoking Cessation Advice	200	100%	99%	97%
Surgical Care Improvement Project				
Appropriate VTP Within 24 Hours[2]	700	95%	93%	92%
Appropriate Hair Removal[2]	2,790	98%	100%	99%
Appropriate Beta Blocker Usage[2]	1,105	93%	94%	93%
Controlled Postoperative Blood Glucose[2]	786	90%	94%	93%
Prophylactic Antibiotic Timing[2]	1,919	97%	98%	97%
Prophylactic Antibiotic Timing (Outpatient)	1,400	93%	94%	92%
Prophylactic Antibiotic Selection[2]	1,950	98%	98%	97%
Prophylactic Antibiotic Select. (Outpatient)	1,374	94%	95%	94%
Prophylactic Antibiotic Stopped[2]	1,822	94%	96%	94%
Recommended VTP Ordered[2]	701	97%	95%	94%
Urinary Catheter Removal[2]	438	87%	91%	90%
Children's Asthma Care				
Received Systemic Corticosteroids	-	-	100%	100%
Received Home Management Plan	-	-	75%	71%
Received Reliever Medication	-	-	100%	100%
Use of Medical Imaging				
Combination Abdominal CT Scan	1,155	0.088	0.115	0.191
Combination Chest CT Scan	694	0.014	0.037	0.054
Follow-up Mammogram/Ultrasound	71	11.3%	7.9%	8.4%
MRI for Low Back Pain	123	30.9%	30.6%	32.7%
Survey of Patients' Hospital Experiences				
Area Around Room 'Always' Quiet at Night	300+	60%	-	58%
Doctors 'Always' Communicated Well	300+	82%	-	80%
Home Recovery Information Given	300+	88%	-	82%
Hospital Given 9 or 10 on 10 Point Scale	300+	78%	-	67%
Meds 'Always' Explained Before Given	300+	66%	-	60%
Nurses 'Always' Communicated Well	300+	81%	-	76%
Pain 'Always' Well Controlled	300+	73%	-	69%
Room and Bathroom 'Always' Clean	300+	72%	-	71%
Timely Help 'Always' Received	300+	66%	-	64%
Would Definitely Recommend Hospital	300+	82%	-	69%

NOTE: Hospital profiles are in alphabetical order by state, then city, then hospital within the city; Rankings exclude hospitals with less than 25 cases except for patient surveys which excludes hospitals with less than 100 cases; (a) 100–299 cases; (1) The number of cases is too small to be sure how well a hospital is performing; (2) The hospital indicated that the data submitted for this measure were based on a sample of cases; (3) Data was collected during a shorter time period (fewer quarters) than the maximum possible time for this measure; (4) Suppressed for one or more quarters by CMS; (5) No data is available from the hospital for this measure; (6) Fewer than 100 patients completed the HCAHPS survey. Use these rates with caution, as the number of surveys may be too low to reliably assess hospital performance; (7) Survey results are based on less than 12 months of data; (8) Survey results are not available for this reporting period; (9) No or very few patients were eligible for the HCAHPS survey. The scores shown, if any, reflect a very small number of surveys; (10) A state average was not calculated because too few hospitals in the state submitted data; (11) There were discrepancies in the data collection process; Please refer to the User's Guide for a full explanation of data.

Sandhills Regional Medical Center

1000 West Hamlet Avenue — Phone: 910-958-2361
Hamlet, NC 28345 — Fax: 910-205-8117
URL: www.hma-corp.com
Type: Acute Care Hospitals — Emergency Services: Yes
Ownership: Proprietary — Beds: 64

Key Personnel:
CEO/President. . . . . Andy Davis
Chief of Medical Staff. . . . . Gilbert D Arenas
Radiology. . . . . Robert B Groves

Measure	Cases	This Hosp.	State Avg.	U.S. Avg.
Heart Attack Care				
ACE Inhibitor or ARB for LVSD[1]	4	100%	97%	96%
Aspirin at Arrival	36	97%	99%	99%
Aspirin at Discharge[1]	22	95%	99%	98%
Beta Blocker at Discharge[1]	22	95%	99%	98%
Fibrinolytic Medication Timing	0	-	38%	55%
PCI Within 90 Minutes of Arrival	0	-	95%	90%
Smoking Cessation Advice[1]	10	100%	100%	99%
Chest Pain/Possible Heart Attack Care				
Aspirin at Arrival[1]	12	83%	95%	95%
Median Time to ECG (minutes)[1]	12	11	8	8
Median Time to Transfer (minutes)[1,3]	1	67	48	61
Fibrinolytic Medication Timing[3]	0	-	53%	54%
Heart Failure Care				
ACE Inhibitor or ARB for LVSD	78	97%	95%	94%
Discharge Instructions	174	97%	89%	88%
Evaluation of LVS Function	188	99%	99%	98%
Smoking Cessation Advice	69	100%	99%	98%
Pneumonia Care				
Appropriate Initial Antibiotic	48	92%	92%	92%
Blood Culture Timing	60	93%	96%	96%
Influenza Vaccine	29	100%	93%	91%
Initial Antibiotic Timing	54	96%	95%	95%
Pneumococcal Vaccine	28	100%	95%	93%
Smoking Cessation Advice	33	100%	99%	97%
Surgical Care Improvement Project				
Appropriate VTP Within 24 Hours[1]	22	95%	93%	92%
Appropriate Hair Removal	52	100%	100%	99%
Appropriate Beta Blocker Usage[1]	12	83%	94%	93%
Controlled Postoperative Blood Glucose	0	-	94%	93%
Prophylactic Antibiotic Timing	37	100%	98%	97%
Prophylactic Antibiotic Timing (Outpatient)	37	97%	94%	92%
Prophylactic Antibiotic Selection	39	100%	98%	97%
Prophylactic Antibiotic Select. (Outpatient)	37	92%	95%	94%
Prophylactic Antibiotic Stopped	35	91%	96%	94%
Recommended VTP Ordered[1]	23	91%	95%	94%
Urinary Catheter Removal[1]	1	100%	91%	90%
Children's Asthma Care				
Received Systemic Corticosteroids	-	-	100%	100%
Received Home Management Plan	-	-	75%	71%
Received Reliever Medication	-	-	100%	100%
Use of Medical Imaging				
Combination Abdominal CT Scan	132	0.545	0.115	0.191
Combination Chest CT Scan	97	0.371	0.037	0.054
Follow-up Mammogram/Ultrasound	258	9.7%	7.9%	8.4%
MRI for Low Back Pain	64	29.7%	30.6%	32.7%
Survey of Patients' Hospital Experiences				
Area Around Room 'Always' Quiet at Night	300+	72%	-	58%
Doctors 'Always' Communicated Well	300+	81%	-	80%
Home Recovery Information Given	300+	78%	-	82%
Hospital Given 9 or 10 on 10 Point Scale	300+	58%	-	67%
Meds 'Always' Explained Before Given	300+	59%	-	60%
Nurses 'Always' Communicated Well	300+	74%	-	76%
Pain 'Always' Well Controlled	300+	70%	-	69%
Room and Bathroom 'Always' Clean	300+	66%	-	71%
Timely Help 'Always' Received	300+	60%	-	64%
Would Definitely Recommend Hospital	300+	59%	-	69%

Maria Parham Hospital

Po Drawer 59 Ruin Creek Rd — Phone: 252-438-4143
Henderson, NC 27536 — Fax: 252-436-1114
E-mail: information@mphosp.org
URL: www.mphosp.org
Type: Acute Care Hospitals — Emergency Services: Yes
Ownership: Voluntary Non-Profit - Other — Beds: 102

Key Personnel:
CEO/President. . . . . Bob Singletary
Chief of Medical Staff. . . . . Rhonda Boyd
Infection Control. . . . . Patsy Stainback, RN
Radiology. . . . . Rober Mintz
Emergency Room . . . . Jan Ryan
Intensive Care Unit. . . . . Debby Pearce

Measure	Cases	This Hosp.	State Avg.	U.S. Avg.
Heart Attack Care				
ACE Inhibitor or ARB for LVSD[1]	13	92%	97%	96%
Aspirin at Arrival	45	98%	99%	99%
Aspirin at Discharge	31	97%	99%	98%
Beta Blocker at Discharge	35	89%	99%	98%
Fibrinolytic Medication Timing	0	-	38%	55%
PCI Within 90 Minutes of Arrival	0	-	95%	90%
Smoking Cessation Advice[1]	7	100%	100%	99%
Chest Pain/Possible Heart Attack Care				
Aspirin at Arrival	145	94%	95%	95%
Median Time to ECG (minutes)	143	12	8	8
Median Time to Transfer (minutes)[1]	15	49	48	61
Fibrinolytic Medication Timing	0	-	53%	54%
Heart Failure Care				
ACE Inhibitor or ARB for LVSD	88	88%	95%	94%
Discharge Instructions	150	76%	89%	88%
Evaluation of LVS Function	180	97%	99%	98%
Smoking Cessation Advice	48	100%	99%	98%
Pneumonia Care				
Appropriate Initial Antibiotic	85	92%	92%	92%
Blood Culture Timing	102	90%	96%	96%
Influenza Vaccine	82	89%	93%	91%
Initial Antibiotic Timing	121	89%	95%	95%
Pneumococcal Vaccine	103	93%	95%	93%
Smoking Cessation Advice	47	100%	99%	97%
Surgical Care Improvement Project				
Appropriate VTP Within 24 Hours	77	92%	93%	92%
Appropriate Hair Removal	180	100%	100%	99%
Appropriate Beta Blocker Usage	40	82%	94%	93%
Controlled Postoperative Blood Glucose	0	-	94%	93%
Prophylactic Antibiotic Timing	95	97%	98%	97%
Prophylactic Antibiotic Timing (Outpatient)	81	95%	94%	92%
Prophylactic Antibiotic Selection	96	94%	98%	97%
Prophylactic Antibiotic Select. (Outpatient)	81	94%	95%	94%
Prophylactic Antibiotic Stopped	91	93%	96%	94%
Recommended VTP Ordered	77	95%	95%	94%
Urinary Catheter Removal	32	94%	91%	90%
Children's Asthma Care				
Received Systemic Corticosteroids	-	-	100%	100%
Received Home Management Plan	-	-	75%	71%
Received Reliever Medication	-	-	100%	100%
Use of Medical Imaging				
Combination Abdominal CT Scan	653	0.029	0.115	0.191
Combination Chest CT Scan	468	0.017	0.037	0.054
Follow-up Mammogram/Ultrasound	1,250	8.4%	7.9%	8.4%
MRI for Low Back Pain	97	36.1%	30.6%	32.7%
Survey of Patients' Hospital Experiences				
Area Around Room 'Always' Quiet at Night	300+	68%	-	58%
Doctors 'Always' Communicated Well	300+	83%	-	80%
Home Recovery Information Given	300+	83%	-	82%
Hospital Given 9 or 10 on 10 Point Scale	300+	63%	-	67%
Meds 'Always' Explained Before Given	300+	65%	-	60%
Nurses 'Always' Communicated Well	300+	80%	-	76%
Pain 'Always' Well Controlled	300+	74%	-	69%
Room and Bathroom 'Always' Clean	300+	74%	-	71%
Timely Help 'Always' Received	300+	68%	-	64%
Would Definitely Recommend Hospital	300+	64%	-	69%

Margaret R Pardee Memorial Hospital

800 N Justice St — Phone: 828-696-1000
Hendersonville, NC 28791 — Fax: 828-696-1128
E-mail: tiffany.ervin@pardeehospital.org
URL: www.pardeehospital.org
Type: Acute Care Hospitals — Emergency Services: Yes
Ownership: Government - Local — Beds: 282

Key Personnel:
CEO/President. . . . . Jon Schurmeier
Chief of Medical Staff. . . . . David Ellis, MD

Measure	Cases	This Hosp.	State Avg.	U.S. Avg.
Heart Attack Care				
ACE Inhibitor or ARB for LVSD[1]	6	100%	97%	96%
Aspirin at Arrival	58	100%	99%	99%
Aspirin at Discharge	32	97%	99%	98%
Beta Blocker at Discharge	32	97%	99%	98%
Fibrinolytic Medication Timing	0	-	38%	55%
PCI Within 90 Minutes of Arrival	0	-	95%	90%
Smoking Cessation Advice[1]	5	100%	100%	99%
Chest Pain/Possible Heart Attack Care				
Aspirin at Arrival	89	99%	95%	95%
Median Time to ECG (minutes)	92	8	8	8
Median Time to Transfer (minutes)	35	55	48	61
Fibrinolytic Medication Timing	0	-	53%	54%
Heart Failure Care				
ACE Inhibitor or ARB for LVSD	67	96%	95%	94%
Discharge Instructions	144	73%	89%	88%
Evaluation of LVS Function	195	98%	99%	98%
Smoking Cessation Advice	25	100%	99%	98%
Pneumonia Care				
Appropriate Initial Antibiotic	139	95%	92%	92%
Blood Culture Timing	186	96%	96%	96%
Influenza Vaccine	126	87%	93%	91%
Initial Antibiotic Timing	184	97%	95%	95%
Pneumococcal Vaccine	162	91%	95%	93%
Smoking Cessation Advice	63	98%	99%	97%
Surgical Care Improvement Project				
Appropriate VTP Within 24 Hours[2]	245	90%	93%	92%
Appropriate Hair Removal[2]	408	100%	100%	99%
Appropriate Beta Blocker Usage[2]	102	98%	94%	93%
Controlled Postoperative Blood Glucose[2]	0	-	94%	93%
Prophylactic Antibiotic Timing[2]	284	98%	98%	97%
Prophylactic Antibiotic Timing (Outpatient)	223	94%	94%	92%
Prophylactic Antibiotic Selection[2]	285	98%	98%	97%
Prophylactic Antibiotic Select. (Outpatient)	214	95%	95%	94%
Prophylactic Antibiotic Stopped[2]	273	98%	96%	94%
Recommended VTP Ordered[2]	245	95%	95%	94%
Urinary Catheter Removal[2]	85	91%	91%	90%
Children's Asthma Care				
Received Systemic Corticosteroids	-	-	100%	100%
Received Home Management Plan	-	-	75%	71%
Received Reliever Medication	-	-	100%	100%
Use of Medical Imaging				
Combination Abdominal CT Scan	1,234	0.127	0.115	0.191
Combination Chest CT Scan	792	0.043	0.037	0.054
Follow-up Mammogram/Ultrasound	2,610	9.4%	7.9%	8.4%
MRI for Low Back Pain	451	29.3%	30.6%	32.7%
Survey of Patients' Hospital Experiences				
Area Around Room 'Always' Quiet at Night	300+	53%	-	58%
Doctors 'Always' Communicated Well	300+	80%	-	80%
Home Recovery Information Given	300+	81%	-	82%
Hospital Given 9 or 10 on 10 Point Scale	300+	64%	-	67%
Meds 'Always' Explained Before Given	300+	60%	-	60%
Nurses 'Always' Communicated Well	300+	75%	-	76%
Pain 'Always' Well Controlled	300+	64%	-	69%
Room and Bathroom 'Always' Clean	300+	74%	-	71%
Timely Help 'Always' Received	300+	62%	-	64%
Would Definitely Recommend Hospital	300+	70%	-	69%

NOTE: Hospital profiles are in alphabetical order by state, then city, then hospital within the city; Rankings exclude hospitals with less than 25 cases except for patient surveys which excludes hospitals with less than 100 cases; (a) 100–299 cases; (1) The number of cases is too small to be sure how well a hospital is performing; (2) The hospital indicated that the data submitted for this measure were based on a sample of cases; (3) Data was collected during a shorter time period (fewer quarters) than the maximum possible time for this measure; (4) Suppressed for one or more quarters by CMS; (5) No data is available from the hospital for this measure; (6) Fewer than 100 patients completed the HCAHPS survey. Use these rates with caution, as the number of surveys may be too low to reliably assess hospital performance; (7) Survey results are based on less than 12 months of data; (8) Survey results are not available for this reporting period; (9) No or very few patients were eligible for the HCAHPS survey. The scores shown, if any, reflect a very small number of surveys; (10) A state average was not calculated because too few hospitals in the state submitted data; (11) There were discrepancies in the data collection process; Please refer to the User's Guide for a full explanation of data.

Catawba Valley Medical Center

810 Fairgrove Church Rd
Hickory, NC 28602
Phone: 828-326-3809
Fax: 828-326-3371
URL: www.catawbavalleymc.org
Type: Acute Care Hospitals
Emergency Services: Yes
Ownership: Voluntary Non-Profit - Other
Beds: 213

Key Personnel:

CEO/President. . . . . J Anthony Rose
Chief of Medical Staff . . . . I Shenoy, MD
Infection Control. . . . . Dorothea Wyant
Operating Room. . . . . Peter Bradshaw, RN
Pediatric Ambulatory Care . . . . . . David Berry, MD
Quality Assurance . . . . Sarah Bailey, RN
Radiology. . . . . Parks J Booker, MD

Measure	Cases	This Hosp.	State Avg.	U.S. Avg.
Heart Attack Care				
ACE Inhibitor or ARB for LVSD[1]	15	100%	97%	96%
Aspirin at Arrival	95	98%	99%	99%
Aspirin at Discharge	73	100%	99%	98%
Beta Blocker at Discharge	70	97%	99%	98%
Fibrinolytic Medication Timing	0	-	38%	55%
PCI Within 90 Minutes of Arrival[1]	4	50%	95%	90%
Smoking Cessation Advice	32	100%	100%	99%
Chest Pain/Possible Heart Attack Care				
Aspirin at Arrival	48	90%	95%	95%
Median Time to ECG (minutes)	48	11	8	8
Median Time to Transfer (minutes)[1]	15	79	48	61
Fibrinolytic Medication Timing	0	-	53%	54%
Heart Failure Care				
ACE Inhibitor or ARB for LVSD	46	91%	95%	94%
Discharge Instructions	107	84%	89%	88%
Evaluation of LVS Function	141	99%	99%	98%
Smoking Cessation Advice	36	100%	99%	98%
Pneumonia Care				
Appropriate Initial Antibiotic	156	90%	92%	92%
Blood Culture Timing	253	92%	96%	96%
Influenza Vaccine	108	86%	93%	91%
Initial Antibiotic Timing	217	94%	95%	95%
Pneumococcal Vaccine	154	91%	95%	93%
Smoking Cessation Advice	74	99%	99%	97%
Surgical Care Improvement Project				
Appropriate VTP Within 24 Hours	263	94%	93%	92%
Appropriate Hair Removal	671	100%	100%	99%
Appropriate Beta Blocker Usage	164	99%	94%	93%
Controlled Postoperative Blood Glucose	0	-	94%	93%
Prophylactic Antibiotic Timing	472	96%	98%	97%
Prophylactic Antibiotic Timing (Outpatient)	649	97%	94%	92%
Prophylactic Antibiotic Selection	476	99%	98%	97%
Prophylactic Antibiotic Select. (Outpatient)	638	98%	95%	94%
Prophylactic Antibiotic Stopped	463	95%	96%	94%
Recommended VTP Ordered	263	95%	95%	94%
Urinary Catheter Removal	197	96%	91%	90%
Children's Asthma Care				
Received Systemic Corticosteroids	-	-	100%	100%
Received Home Management Plan	-	-	75%	71%
Received Reliever Medication	-	-	100%	100%
Use of Medical Imaging				
Combination Abdominal CT Scan	875	0.055	0.115	0.191
Combination Chest CT Scan	708	0.016	0.037	0.054
Follow-up Mammogram/Ultrasound	2,280	8.3%	7.9%	8.4%
MRI for Low Back Pain	305	30.2%	30.6%	32.7%
Survey of Patients' Hospital Experiences				
Area Around Room 'Always' Quiet at Night	300+	56%	-	58%
Doctors 'Always' Communicated Well	300+	80%	-	80%
Home Recovery Information Given	300+	84%	-	82%
Hospital Given 9 or 10 on 10 Point Scale	300+	70%	-	67%
Meds 'Always' Explained Before Given	300+	62%	-	60%
Nurses 'Always' Communicated Well	300+	77%	-	76%
Pain 'Always' Well Controlled	300+	71%	-	69%
Room and Bathroom 'Always' Clean	300+	67%	-	71%
Timely Help 'Always' Received	300+	64%	-	64%
Would Definitely Recommend Hospital	300+	75%	-	69%

Frye Regional Medical Center

420 N Center St
Hickory, NC 28601
Phone: 828-322-6070
Fax: 828-345-5755
URL: www.fryemedctr.com
Type: Acute Care Hospitals
Emergency Services: Yes
Ownership: Proprietary
Beds: 355

Key Personnel:

CEO/President. . . . . Dennis Phillips
Chief of Medical Staff . . . . Mark Anderson
Operating Room. . . . . Jan Fisk
Quality Assurance . . . . Linda Drum
Radiology. . . . . Charles Scheil

Measure	Cases	This Hosp.	State Avg.	U.S. Avg.
Heart Attack Care				
ACE Inhibitor or ARB for LVSD	57	93%	97%	96%
Aspirin at Arrival	308	99%	99%	99%
Aspirin at Discharge	487	98%	99%	98%
Beta Blocker at Discharge	481	99%	99%	98%
Fibrinolytic Medication Timing	0	-	38%	55%
PCI Within 90 Minutes of Arrival	134	97%	95%	90%
Smoking Cessation Advice	218	100%	100%	99%
Chest Pain/Possible Heart Attack Care				
Aspirin at Arrival[1]	7	86%	95%	95%
Median Time to ECG (minutes)[1]	7	1	8	8
Median Time to Transfer (minutes)[5]	0	-	48	61
Fibrinolytic Medication Timing[5]	0	-	53%	54%
Heart Failure Care				
ACE Inhibitor or ARB for LVSD	79	91%	95%	94%
Discharge Instructions	251	93%	89%	88%
Evaluation of LVS Function	294	98%	99%	98%
Smoking Cessation Advice	57	100%	99%	98%
Pneumonia Care				
Appropriate Initial Antibiotic	221	95%	92%	92%
Blood Culture Timing	335	96%	96%	96%
Influenza Vaccine	209	96%	93%	91%
Initial Antibiotic Timing	291	98%	95%	95%
Pneumococcal Vaccine	276	95%	95%	93%
Smoking Cessation Advice	100	98%	99%	97%
Surgical Care Improvement Project				
Appropriate VTP Within 24 Hours[2]	149	91%	93%	92%
Appropriate Hair Removal[2]	662	100%	100%	99%
Appropriate Beta Blocker Usage[2]	215	93%	94%	93%
Controlled Postoperative Blood Glucose[2]	261	86%	94%	93%
Prophylactic Antibiotic Timing[2]	517	96%	98%	97%
Prophylactic Antibiotic Timing (Outpatient)	693	97%	94%	92%
Prophylactic Antibiotic Selection[2]	522	99%	98%	97%
Prophylactic Antibiotic Select. (Outpatient)	684	98%	95%	94%
Prophylactic Antibiotic Stopped[2]	495	91%	96%	94%
Recommended VTP Ordered[2]	149	91%	95%	94%
Urinary Catheter Removal[2]	187	91%	91%	90%
Children's Asthma Care				
Received Systemic Corticosteroids	-	-	100%	100%
Received Home Management Plan	-	-	75%	71%
Received Reliever Medication	-	-	100%	100%
Use of Medical Imaging				
Combination Abdominal CT Scan	952	0.070	0.115	0.191
Combination Chest CT Scan	849	0.025	0.037	0.054
Follow-up Mammogram/Ultrasound	2,322	7.5%	7.9%	8.4%
MRI for Low Back Pain	432	27.3%	30.6%	32.7%
Survey of Patients' Hospital Experiences				
Area Around Room 'Always' Quiet at Night	300+	60%	-	58%
Doctors 'Always' Communicated Well	300+	84%	-	80%
Home Recovery Information Given	300+	88%	-	82%
Hospital Given 9 or 10 on 10 Point Scale	300+	66%	-	67%
Meds 'Always' Explained Before Given	300+	64%	-	60%
Nurses 'Always' Communicated Well	300+	76%	-	76%
Pain 'Always' Well Controlled	300+	69%	-	69%
Room and Bathroom 'Always' Clean	300+	62%	-	71%
Timely Help 'Always' Received	300+	72%	-	64%
Would Definitely Recommend Hospital	300+	72%	-	69%

High Point Regional Hospital

601 N Elm St
High Point, NC 27261
Phone: 336-878-6000
Fax: 336-878-6709
URL: www.highpointregional.com
Type: Acute Care Hospitals
Emergency Services: Yes
Ownership: Voluntary Non-Profit - Private
Beds: 400

Key Personnel:

CEO/President. . . . . Jeffrey S Miller
Chief of Medical Staff . . . . Greg Taylor
Infection Control. . . . . Vicki Tutor
Operating Room. . . . . Denise Rhew
Pediatric Ambulatory Care . . . . . . Allison Poston, MD
Radiology. . . . . Diane O'Connell, MD
Anesthesiology. . . . . Kevin Speight, MD
Emergency Room . . . . Karen Olsen

Measure	Cases	This Hosp.	State Avg.	U.S. Avg.
Heart Attack Care				
ACE Inhibitor or ARB for LVSD	91	98%	97%	96%
Aspirin at Arrival	368	100%	99%	99%
Aspirin at Discharge	516	99%	99%	98%
Beta Blocker at Discharge	521	100%	99%	98%
Fibrinolytic Medication Timing	0	-	38%	55%
PCI Within 90 Minutes of Arrival	88	99%	95%	90%
Smoking Cessation Advice	205	100%	100%	99%
Chest Pain/Possible Heart Attack Care				
Aspirin at Arrival[1]	2	100%	95%	95%
Median Time to ECG (minutes)[1]	3	1	8	8
Median Time to Transfer (minutes)[5]	0	-	48	61
Fibrinolytic Medication Timing[5]	0	-	53%	54%
Heart Failure Care				
ACE Inhibitor or ARB for LVSD	155	99%	95%	94%
Discharge Instructions	384	93%	89%	88%
Evaluation of LVS Function	460	98%	99%	98%
Smoking Cessation Advice	110	100%	99%	98%
Pneumonia Care				
Appropriate Initial Antibiotic	220	91%	92%	92%
Blood Culture Timing	397	93%	96%	96%
Influenza Vaccine	249	73%	93%	91%
Initial Antibiotic Timing	421	96%	95%	95%
Pneumococcal Vaccine	347	87%	95%	93%
Smoking Cessation Advice	196	100%	99%	97%
Surgical Care Improvement Project				
Appropriate VTP Within 24 Hours[2]	131	99%	93%	92%
Appropriate Hair Removal[2]	506	100%	100%	99%
Appropriate Beta Blocker Usage[2]	167	81%	94%	93%
Controlled Postoperative Blood Glucose[2]	102	95%	94%	93%
Prophylactic Antibiotic Timing[2]	344	98%	98%	97%
Prophylactic Antibiotic Timing (Outpatient)	489	90%	94%	92%
Prophylactic Antibiotic Selection[2]	348	97%	98%	97%
Prophylactic Antibiotic Select. (Outpatient)	470	68%	95%	94%
Prophylactic Antibiotic Stopped[2]	288	96%	96%	94%
Recommended VTP Ordered[2]	131	99%	95%	94%
Urinary Catheter Removal[2]	106	92%	91%	90%
Children's Asthma Care				
Received Systemic Corticosteroids	-	-	100%	100%
Received Home Management Plan	-	-	75%	71%
Received Reliever Medication	-	-	100%	100%
Use of Medical Imaging				
Combination Abdominal CT Scan	748	0.013	0.115	0.191
Combination Chest CT Scan	223	0.009	0.037	0.054
Follow-up Mammogram/Ultrasound	289	5.5%	7.9%	8.4%
MRI for Low Back Pain	186	30.1%	30.6%	32.7%
Survey of Patients' Hospital Experiences				
Area Around Room 'Always' Quiet at Night	300+	58%	-	58%
Doctors 'Always' Communicated Well	300+	78%	-	80%
Home Recovery Information Given	300+	80%	-	82%
Hospital Given 9 or 10 on 10 Point Scale	300+	68%	-	67%
Meds 'Always' Explained Before Given	300+	58%	-	60%
Nurses 'Always' Communicated Well	300+	76%	-	76%
Pain 'Always' Well Controlled	300+	69%	-	69%
Room and Bathroom 'Always' Clean	300+	68%	-	71%
Timely Help 'Always' Received	300+	63%	-	64%
Would Definitely Recommend Hospital	300+	72%	-	69%

NOTE: Hospital profiles are in alphabetical order by state, then city, then hospital within the city; Rankings exclude hospitals with less than 25 cases except for patient surveys which excludes hospitals with less than 100 cases; (a) 100–299 cases; (1) The number of cases is too small to be sure how well a hospital is performing; (2) The hospital indicated that the data submitted for this measure were based on a sample of cases; (3) Data was collected during a shorter time period (fewer quarters) than the maximum possible time for this measure; (4) Suppressed for one or more quarters by CMS; (5) No data is available from the hospital for this measure; (6) Fewer than 100 patients completed the HCAHPS survey. Use these rates with caution, as the number of surveys may be too low to reliably assess hospital performance; (7) Survey results are based on less than 12 months of data; (8) Survey results are not available for this reporting period; (9) No or very few patients were eligible for the HCAHPS survey. The scores shown, if any, reflect a very small number of surveys; (10) A state average was not calculated because too few hospitals in the state submitted data; (11) There were discrepancies in the data collection process; Please refer to the User's Guide for a full explanation of data.

Highlands Cashiers Hospital

190 Hospital Drive
Highlands, NC 28741
Phone: 828-526-1200
Fax: 828-526-1230
E-mail: ftaylor@hchospital.org
URL: www.hchospital.org
Type: Critical Access Hospitals
Emergency Services: Yes
Ownership: Voluntary Non-Profit - Other
Beds: 104

Key Personnel:
CEO/President. . . . . Kenneth A Shull
Chief of Medical Staff . . . . David M Wheeler
Radiology. . . . . Rodney Stinnett

Measure	Cases	This Hosp.	State Avg.	U.S. Avg.
Heart Attack Care				
ACE Inhibitor or ARB for LVSD[5]	0	-	97%	96%
Aspirin at Arrival[5]	0	-	99%	99%
Aspirin at Discharge[5]	0	-	99%	98%
Beta Blocker at Discharge[5]	0	-	99%	98%
Fibrinolytic Medication Timing[5]	0	-	38%	55%
PCI Within 90 Minutes of Arrival[5]	0	-	95%	90%
Smoking Cessation Advice[5]	0	-	100%	99%
Chest Pain/Possible Heart Attack Care				
Aspirin at Arrival	-	-	95%	95%
Median Time to ECG (minutes)	-	-	8	8
Median Time to Transfer (minutes)	-	-	48	61
Fibrinolytic Medication Timing	-	-	53%	54%
Heart Failure Care				
ACE Inhibitor or ARB for LVSD[1,3]	1	100%	95%	94%
Discharge Instructions[1,3]	4	0%	89%	88%
Evaluation of LVS Function[1,3]	5	40%	99%	98%
Smoking Cessation Advice[1,3]	2	50%	99%	98%
Pneumonia Care				
Appropriate Initial Antibiotic[1,3]	4	75%	92%	92%
Blood Culture Timing[1,3]	6	83%	96%	96%
Influenza Vaccine[1]	5	80%	93%	91%
Initial Antibiotic Timing[1,3]	1	0%	95%	95%
Pneumococcal Vaccine[1,3]	13	46%	95%	93%
Smoking Cessation Advice[1,3]	1	100%	99%	97%
Surgical Care Improvement Project				
Appropriate VTP Within 24 Hours[5]	0	-	93%	92%
Appropriate Hair Removal[5]	0	-	100%	99%
Appropriate Beta Blocker Usage[5]	0	-	94%	93%
Controlled Postoperative Blood Glucose[5]	0	-	94%	93%
Prophylactic Antibiotic Timing[5]	0	-	98%	97%
Prophylactic Antibiotic Timing (Outpatient)	-	-	94%	92%
Prophylactic Antibiotic Selection[5]	0	-	98%	97%
Prophylactic Antibiotic Select. (Outpatient)	-	-	95%	94%
Prophylactic Antibiotic Stopped[5]	0	-	96%	94%
Recommended VTP Ordered[5]	0	-	95%	94%
Urinary Catheter Removal[5]	0	-	91%	90%
Children's Asthma Care				
Received Systemic Corticosteroids	-	-	100%	100%
Received Home Management Plan	-	-	75%	71%
Received Reliever Medication	-	-	100%	100%
Use of Medical Imaging				
Combination Abdominal CT Scan	-	-	0.115	0.191
Combination Chest CT Scan	-	-	0.037	0.054
Follow-up Mammogram/Ultrasound	-	-	7.9%	8.4%
MRI for Low Back Pain	-	-	30.6%	32.7%
Survey of Patients' Hospital Experiences				
Area Around Room 'Always' Quiet at Night[8]	-	-	-	58%
Doctors 'Always' Communicated Well[8]	-	-	-	80%
Home Recovery Information Given[8]	-	-	-	82%
Hospital Given 9 or 10 on 10 Point Scale[8]	-	-	-	67%
Meds 'Always' Explained Before Given[8]	-	-	-	60%
Nurses 'Always' Communicated Well[8]	-	-	-	76%
Pain 'Always' Well Controlled[8]	-	-	-	69%
Room and Bathroom 'Always' Clean[8]	-	-	-	71%
Timely Help 'Always' Received[8]	-	-	-	64%
Would Definitely Recommend Hospital[8]	-	-	-	69%

Presbyterian Hospital Huntersville

10030 Gilead Road
Huntersville, NC 28078
Phone: 704-316-4000
E-mail: hic@novanthealth.org
URL: www.presbyterian.org
Type: Acute Care Hospitals
Emergency Services: No
Ownership: Voluntary Non-Profit - Private

Key Personnel:
CEO/President. . . . . Melissa Robson
Chief of Medical Staff . . . . David Cook
Operating Room. . . . . Rohit Bhasin
Pediatric In-Patient Care . . . . William Flannery
Radiology. . . . . John Black
Anesthesiology. . . . . Jeffrey Welna
Emergency Room . . . . Joshua Sarett

Measure	Cases	This Hosp.	State Avg.	U.S. Avg.
Heart Attack Care				
ACE Inhibitor or ARB for LVSD[1]	4	100%	97%	96%
Aspirin at Arrival[1]	22	100%	99%	99%
Aspirin at Discharge[1]	10	100%	99%	98%
Beta Blocker at Discharge[1]	9	100%	99%	98%
Fibrinolytic Medication Timing	0	-	38%	55%
PCI Within 90 Minutes of Arrival	0	-	95%	90%
Smoking Cessation Advice	0	-	100%	99%
Chest Pain/Possible Heart Attack Care				
Aspirin at Arrival	87	99%	95%	95%
Median Time to ECG (minutes)	91	6	8	8
Median Time to Transfer (minutes)	25	32	48	61
Fibrinolytic Medication Timing	0	-	53%	54%
Heart Failure Care				
ACE Inhibitor or ARB for LVSD	36	100%	95%	94%
Discharge Instructions	97	97%	89%	88%
Evaluation of LVS Function	110	100%	99%	98%
Smoking Cessation Advice[1]	12	100%	99%	98%
Pneumonia Care				
Appropriate Initial Antibiotic	129	98%	92%	92%
Blood Culture Timing	167	100%	96%	96%
Influenza Vaccine	89	98%	93%	91%
Initial Antibiotic Timing	156	98%	95%	95%
Pneumococcal Vaccine	129	98%	95%	93%
Smoking Cessation Advice	46	100%	99%	97%
Surgical Care Improvement Project				
Appropriate VTP Within 24 Hours[2]	201	93%	93%	92%
Appropriate Hair Removal[2]	540	100%	100%	99%
Appropriate Beta Blocker Usage[2]	128	95%	94%	93%
Controlled Postoperative Blood Glucose[2]	0	-	94%	93%
Prophylactic Antibiotic Timing[2]	396	99%	98%	97%
Prophylactic Antibiotic Timing (Outpatient)	162	97%	94%	92%
Prophylactic Antibiotic Selection[2]	396	100%	98%	97%
Prophylactic Antibiotic Select. (Outpatient)	161	94%	95%	94%
Prophylactic Antibiotic Stopped[2]	387	98%	96%	94%
Recommended VTP Ordered[2]	201	94%	95%	94%
Urinary Catheter Removal[2]	143	95%	91%	90%
Children's Asthma Care				
Received Systemic Corticosteroids	-	-	100%	100%
Received Home Management Plan	-	-	75%	71%
Received Reliever Medication	-	-	100%	100%
Use of Medical Imaging				
Combination Abdominal CT Scan	850	0.033	0.115	0.191
Combination Chest CT Scan	695	0.000	0.037	0.054
Follow-up Mammogram/Ultrasound[5]	0	-	7.9%	8.4%
MRI for Low Back Pain	170	30.6%	30.6%	32.7%
Survey of Patients' Hospital Experiences				
Area Around Room 'Always' Quiet at Night	300+	61%	-	58%
Doctors 'Always' Communicated Well	300+	83%	-	80%
Home Recovery Information Given	300+	86%	-	82%
Hospital Given 9 or 10 on 10 Point Scale	300+	77%	-	67%
Meds 'Always' Explained Before Given	300+	59%	-	60%
Nurses 'Always' Communicated Well	300+	77%	-	76%
Pain 'Always' Well Controlled	300+	72%	-	69%
Room and Bathroom 'Always' Clean	300+	65%	-	71%
Timely Help 'Always' Received	300+	67%	-	64%
Would Definitely Recommend Hospital	300+	82%	-	69%

Onslow Memorial Hospital

317 Western Boulevard
Jacksonville, NC 28540
Phone: 910-577-2345
Fax: 910-577-2858
URL: www.onslowmemorial.org
Type: Acute Care Hospitals
Emergency Services: Yes
Ownership: Govt - Hospital Dist/Auth
Beds: 162

Key Personnel:
Cardiac Laboratory. . . . . Jean Brazell, RN
Chief of Medical Staff . . . . Scott Johnson, MD
Infection Control. . . . . Gloria Horne, RN
Operating Room. . . . . Kathy Schumacker, RN
Pediatric In-Patient Care . . . . Angela Pollack, RN
Quality Assurance . . . . Richard Thompson
Radiology. . . . . Joanne Offult

Measure	Cases	This Hosp.	State Avg.	U.S. Avg.
Heart Attack Care				
ACE Inhibitor or ARB for LVSD	0	-	97%	96%
Aspirin at Arrival[1]	23	87%	99%	99%
Aspirin at Discharge[1]	15	87%	99%	98%
Beta Blocker at Discharge[1]	15	87%	99%	98%
Fibrinolytic Medication Timing	0	-	38%	55%
PCI Within 90 Minutes of Arrival	0	-	95%	90%
Smoking Cessation Advice[1]	2	100%	100%	99%
Chest Pain/Possible Heart Attack Care				
Aspirin at Arrival	173	87%	95%	95%
Median Time to ECG (minutes)	172	13	8	8
Median Time to Transfer (minutes)[1,3]	7	363	48	61
Fibrinolytic Medication Timing[1]	16	44%	53%	54%
Heart Failure Care				
ACE Inhibitor or ARB for LVSD	55	98%	95%	94%
Discharge Instructions	166	82%	89%	88%
Evaluation of LVS Function	202	99%	99%	98%
Smoking Cessation Advice	40	100%	99%	98%
Pneumonia Care				
Appropriate Initial Antibiotic	126	90%	92%	92%
Blood Culture Timing	176	93%	96%	96%
Influenza Vaccine	126	98%	93%	91%
Initial Antibiotic Timing	180	83%	95%	95%
Pneumococcal Vaccine	142	99%	95%	93%
Smoking Cessation Advice	82	100%	99%	97%
Surgical Care Improvement Project				
Appropriate VTP Within 24 Hours	136	88%	93%	92%
Appropriate Hair Removal	294	100%	100%	99%
Appropriate Beta Blocker Usage	74	80%	94%	93%
Controlled Postoperative Blood Glucose	0	-	94%	93%
Prophylactic Antibiotic Timing	194	97%	98%	97%
Prophylactic Antibiotic Timing (Outpatient)	233	91%	94%	92%
Prophylactic Antibiotic Selection	197	96%	98%	97%
Prophylactic Antibiotic Select. (Outpatient)	228	94%	95%	94%
Prophylactic Antibiotic Stopped	186	94%	96%	94%
Recommended VTP Ordered	137	88%	95%	94%
Urinary Catheter Removal	45	87%	91%	90%
Children's Asthma Care				
Received Systemic Corticosteroids	-	-	100%	100%
Received Home Management Plan	-	-	75%	71%
Received Reliever Medication	-	-	100%	100%
Use of Medical Imaging				
Combination Abdominal CT Scan	579	0.107	0.115	0.191
Combination Chest CT Scan	374	0.008	0.037	0.054
Follow-up Mammogram/Ultrasound	732	11.9%	7.9%	8.4%
MRI for Low Back Pain[1]	57	22.8%	30.6%	32.7%
Survey of Patients' Hospital Experiences				
Area Around Room 'Always' Quiet at Night	300+	56%	-	58%
Doctors 'Always' Communicated Well	300+	77%	-	80%
Home Recovery Information Given	300+	85%	-	82%
Hospital Given 9 or 10 on 10 Point Scale	300+	63%	-	67%
Meds 'Always' Explained Before Given	300+	60%	-	60%
Nurses 'Always' Communicated Well	300+	78%	-	76%
Pain 'Always' Well Controlled	300+	68%	-	69%
Room and Bathroom 'Always' Clean	300+	66%	-	71%
Timely Help 'Always' Received	300+	69%	-	64%
Would Definitely Recommend Hospital	300+	60%	-	69%

NOTE: Hospital profiles are in alphabetical order by state, then city, then hospital within the city; Rankings exclude hospitals with less than 25 cases except for patient surveys which excludes hospitals with less than 100 cases; (a) 100–299 cases; (1) The number of cases is too small to be sure how well a hospital is performing; (2) The hospital indicated that the data submitted for this measure were based on a sample of cases; (3) Data was collected during a shorter time period (fewer quarters) than the maximum possible time for this measure; (4) Suppressed for one or more quarters by CMS; (5) No data is available from the hospital for this measure; (6) Fewer than 100 patients completed the HCAHPS survey. Use these rates with caution, as the number of surveys may be too low to reliably assess hospital performance; (7) Survey results are based on less than 12 months of data; (8) Survey results are not available for this reporting period; (9) No or very few patients were eligible for the HCAHPS survey. The scores shown, if any, reflect a very small number of surveys; (10) A state average was not calculated because too few hospitals in the state submitted data; (11) There were discrepancies in the data collection process; Please refer to the User's Guide for a full explanation of data.

Ashe Memorial Hospital

200 Hospital Ave Phone: 336-246-7101
Jefferson, NC 28640 Fax: 336-846-0746
E-mail: info@ashememorial.org
URL: www.ashememorial.org
Type: Critical Access Hospitals Emergency Services: Yes
Ownership: Voluntary Non-Profit - Private

Key Personnel:
CEO/President. . . . . RD Williams
Chief of Medical Staff. . . . . Norma Gross
Infection Control. . . . . Shirlene Widner, RN
Operating Room. . . . . Charles W Jones
Quality Assurance . . . . Leisa Powell
Radiology. . . . . David McCune
Emergency Room . . . . Kina Jones, RN
Intensive Care Unit. . . . . Polly Osowitt, RN

Measure	Cases	This Hosp.	State Avg.	U.S. Avg.
Heart Attack Care				
ACE Inhibitor or ARB for LVSD[1]	1	0%	97%	96%
Aspirin at Arrival[1]	7	100%	99%	99%
Aspirin at Discharge[1]	5	100%	99%	98%
Beta Blocker at Discharge[1]	5	60%	99%	98%
Fibrinolytic Medication Timing	0	-	38%	55%
PCI Within 90 Minutes of Arrival	0	-	95%	90%
Smoking Cessation Advice	0	-	100%	99%
Chest Pain/Possible Heart Attack Care				
Aspirin at Arrival	90	97%	95%	95%
Median Time to ECG (minutes)	97	9	8	8
Median Time to Transfer (minutes)[1,3]	1	43	48	61
Fibrinolytic Medication Timing[1]	6	100%	53%	54%
Heart Failure Care				
ACE Inhibitor or ARB for LVSD[1]	9	44%	95%	94%
Discharge Instructions	28	93%	89%	88%
Evaluation of LVS Function	35	89%	99%	98%
Smoking Cessation Advice[1]	4	75%	99%	98%
Pneumonia Care				
Appropriate Initial Antibiotic	99	96%	92%	92%
Blood Culture Timing	53	98%	96%	96%
Influenza Vaccine	85	73%	93%	91%
Initial Antibiotic Timing	111	95%	95%	95%
Pneumococcal Vaccine	136	88%	95%	93%
Smoking Cessation Advice	42	95%	99%	97%
Surgical Care Improvement Project				
Appropriate VTP Within 24 Hours[1]	22	100%	93%	92%
Appropriate Hair Removal	29	100%	100%	99%
Appropriate Beta Blocker Usage[1]	5	60%	94%	93%
Controlled Postoperative Blood Glucose	0	-	94%	93%
Prophylactic Antibiotic Timing[1]	8	100%	98%	97%
Prophylactic Antibiotic Timing (Outpatient)[1,3]	9	100%	94%	92%
Prophylactic Antibiotic Selection[1]	8	88%	98%	97%
Prophylactic Antibiotic Select. (Outpatient)[1,3]	9	100%	95%	94%
Prophylactic Antibiotic Stopped[1]	8	100%	96%	94%
Recommended VTP Ordered[1]	22	100%	95%	94%
Urinary Catheter Removal[1]	2	100%	91%	90%
Children's Asthma Care				
Received Systemic Corticosteroids	-	-	100%	100%
Received Home Management Plan	-	-	75%	71%
Received Reliever Medication	-	-	100%	100%
Use of Medical Imaging				
Combination Abdominal CT Scan	279	0.710	0.115	0.191
Combination Chest CT Scan	159	0.050	0.037	0.054
Follow-up Mammogram/Ultrasound	753	3.6%	7.9%	8.4%
MRI for Low Back Pain	65	30.8%	30.6%	32.7%
Survey of Patients' Hospital Experiences				
Area Around Room 'Always' Quiet at Night	300+	57%	-	58%
Doctors 'Always' Communicated Well	300+	86%	-	80%
Home Recovery Information Given	300+	84%	-	82%
Hospital Given 9 or 10 on 10 Point Scale	300+	71%	-	67%
Meds 'Always' Explained Before Given	300+	66%	-	60%
Nurses 'Always' Communicated Well	300+	83%	-	76%
Pain 'Always' Well Controlled	300+	70%	-	69%
Room and Bathroom 'Always' Clean	300+	80%	-	71%
Timely Help 'Always' Received	300+	69%	-	64%
Would Definitely Recommend Hospital	300+	68%	-	69%

Duplin General Hospital

401 N Main St Phone: 910-296-0941
Kenansville, NC 28349 Fax: 910-296-2951
URL: www.dgh.org
Type: Acute Care Hospitals Emergency Services: Yes
Ownership: Government - Local Beds: 89

Key Personnel:
CEO/President. . . . . Harvey Case
Chief of Medical Staff . . . . C Daniel Pate, Jr
Operating Room. . . . . Dyrek Miller
Quality Assurance . . . . Margaret Broadhurst
Radiology. . . . . Barry Powers
Anesthesiology. . . . . Elizabeth Brayton, MD
Emergency Room . . . . Brenda Grubbs
Intensive Care Unit. . . . . Deborah Coombs

Measure	Cases	This Hosp.	State Avg.	U.S. Avg.
Heart Attack Care				
ACE Inhibitor or ARB for LVSD	0	-	97%	96%
Aspirin at Arrival[1]	9	100%	99%	99%
Aspirin at Discharge[1]	7	86%	99%	98%
Beta Blocker at Discharge[1]	8	100%	99%	98%
Fibrinolytic Medication Timing	0	-	38%	55%
PCI Within 90 Minutes of Arrival	0	-	95%	90%
Smoking Cessation Advice	0	-	100%	99%
Chest Pain/Possible Heart Attack Care				
Aspirin at Arrival	82	100%	95%	95%
Median Time to ECG (minutes)	87	8	8	8
Median Time to Transfer (minutes)[1,3]	2	364	48	61
Fibrinolytic Medication Timing[1]	4	0%	53%	54%
Heart Failure Care				
ACE Inhibitor or ARB for LVSD[1]	23	100%	95%	94%
Discharge Instructions	59	97%	89%	88%
Evaluation of LVS Function	66	100%	99%	98%
Smoking Cessation Advice[1]	14	100%	99%	98%
Pneumonia Care				
Appropriate Initial Antibiotic	65	98%	92%	92%
Blood Culture Timing	102	99%	96%	96%
Influenza Vaccine	51	98%	93%	91%
Initial Antibiotic Timing	85	100%	95%	95%
Pneumococcal Vaccine	70	97%	95%	93%
Smoking Cessation Advice	29	100%	99%	97%
Surgical Care Improvement Project				
Appropriate VTP Within 24 Hours[1]	10	70%	93%	92%
Appropriate Hair Removal	47	100%	100%	99%
Appropriate Beta Blocker Usage[1]	7	100%	94%	93%
Controlled Postoperative Blood Glucose	0	-	94%	93%
Prophylactic Antibiotic Timing	34	100%	98%	97%
Prophylactic Antibiotic Timing (Outpatient)[1]	7	71%	94%	92%
Prophylactic Antibiotic Selection	35	100%	98%	97%
Prophylactic Antibiotic Select. (Outpatient)[1]	7	86%	95%	94%
Prophylactic Antibiotic Stopped	31	94%	96%	94%
Recommended VTP Ordered[1]	10	80%	95%	94%
Urinary Catheter Removal[1]	2	100%	91%	90%
Children's Asthma Care				
Received Systemic Corticosteroids	-	-	100%	100%
Received Home Management Plan	-	-	75%	71%
Received Reliever Medication	-	-	100%	100%
Use of Medical Imaging				
Combination Abdominal CT Scan	264	0.117	0.115	0.191
Combination Chest CT Scan	166	0.000	0.037	0.054
Follow-up Mammogram/Ultrasound	482	4.8%	7.9%	8.4%
MRI for Low Back Pain	54	50.0%	30.6%	32.7%
Survey of Patients' Hospital Experiences				
Area Around Room 'Always' Quiet at Night	300+	69%	-	58%
Doctors 'Always' Communicated Well	300+	81%	-	80%
Home Recovery Information Given	300+	81%	-	82%
Hospital Given 9 or 10 on 10 Point Scale	300+	69%	-	67%
Meds 'Always' Explained Before Given	300+	69%	-	60%
Nurses 'Always' Communicated Well	300+	79%	-	76%
Pain 'Always' Well Controlled	300+	67%	-	69%
Room and Bathroom 'Always' Clean	300+	72%	-	71%
Timely Help 'Always' Received	300+	69%	-	64%
Would Definitely Recommend Hospital	300+	62%	-	69%

Kings Mountain Hospital

706 W King St Phone: 704-739-3601
Kings Mountain, NC 28086 Fax: 704-739-0800
Type: Acute Care Hospitals Emergency Services: Yes
Ownership: Govt - Hospital Dist/Auth Beds: 102

Key Personnel:
CEO/President. . . . . John Young
Chief of Medical Staff . . . . Austin Osemeka, MD
Operating Room. . . . . Jama Hammond, RN
Quality Assurance . . . . Nadine Harris
Anesthesiology. . . . . Gene Tom, MD
Emergency Room . . . . Lisa Rice

Measure	Cases	This Hosp.	State Avg.	U.S. Avg.
Heart Attack Care				
ACE Inhibitor or ARB for LVSD[1]	1	100%	97%	96%
Aspirin at Arrival[1]	15	93%	99%	99%
Aspirin at Discharge[1]	6	83%	99%	98%
Beta Blocker at Discharge[1]	7	86%	99%	98%
Fibrinolytic Medication Timing	0	-	38%	55%
PCI Within 90 Minutes of Arrival	0	-	95%	90%
Smoking Cessation Advice[1]	4	100%	100%	99%
Chest Pain/Possible Heart Attack Care				
Aspirin at Arrival	87	97%	95%	95%
Median Time to ECG (minutes)	89	4	8	8
Median Time to Transfer (minutes)[1]	4	64	48	61
Fibrinolytic Medication Timing[1]	1	0%	53%	54%
Heart Failure Care				
ACE Inhibitor or ARB for LVSD[1]	14	79%	95%	94%
Discharge Instructions	40	90%	89%	88%
Evaluation of LVS Function	50	100%	99%	98%
Smoking Cessation Advice[1]	18	100%	99%	98%
Pneumonia Care				
Appropriate Initial Antibiotic	51	92%	92%	92%
Blood Culture Timing	51	98%	96%	96%
Influenza Vaccine	43	98%	93%	91%
Initial Antibiotic Timing	68	99%	95%	95%
Pneumococcal Vaccine	46	100%	95%	93%
Smoking Cessation Advice	35	100%	99%	97%
Surgical Care Improvement Project				
Appropriate VTP Within 24 Hours	28	86%	93%	92%
Appropriate Hair Removal	37	100%	100%	99%
Appropriate Beta Blocker Usage[1]	9	67%	94%	93%
Controlled Postoperative Blood Glucose	0	-	94%	93%
Prophylactic Antibiotic Timing[1]	15	93%	98%	97%
Prophylactic Antibiotic Timing (Outpatient)[1,3]	4	100%	94%	92%
Prophylactic Antibiotic Selection[1]	16	75%	98%	97%
Prophylactic Antibiotic Select. (Outpatient)[1,3]	4	75%	95%	94%
Prophylactic Antibiotic Stopped[1]	13	92%	96%	94%
Recommended VTP Ordered	28	89%	95%	94%
Urinary Catheter Removal[1]	9	89%	91%	90%
Children's Asthma Care				
Received Systemic Corticosteroids	-	-	100%	100%
Received Home Management Plan	-	-	75%	71%
Received Reliever Medication	-	-	100%	100%
Use of Medical Imaging				
Combination Abdominal CT Scan	205	0.585	0.115	0.191
Combination Chest CT Scan	92	0.000	0.037	0.054
Follow-up Mammogram/Ultrasound	378	10.6%	7.9%	8.4%
MRI for Low Back Pain	81	49.4%	30.6%	32.7%
Survey of Patients' Hospital Experiences				
Area Around Room 'Always' Quiet at Night	(a)	71%	-	58%
Doctors 'Always' Communicated Well	(a)	86%	-	80%
Home Recovery Information Given	(a)	85%	-	82%
Hospital Given 9 or 10 on 10 Point Scale	(a)	77%	-	67%
Meds 'Always' Explained Before Given	(a)	71%	-	60%
Nurses 'Always' Communicated Well	(a)	84%	-	76%
Pain 'Always' Well Controlled	(a)	77%	-	69%
Room and Bathroom 'Always' Clean	(a)	68%	-	71%
Timely Help 'Always' Received	(a)	75%	-	64%
Would Definitely Recommend Hospital	(a)	74%	-	69%

NOTE: Hospital profiles are in alphabetical order by state, then city, then hospital within the city; Rankings exclude hospitals with less than 25 cases except for patient surveys which excludes hospitals with less than 100 cases; (a) 100–299 cases; (1) The number of cases is too small to be sure how well a hospital is performing; (2) The hospital indicated that the data submitted for this measure were based on a sample of cases; (3) Data was collected during a shorter time period (fewer quarters) than the maximum possible time for this measure; (4) Suppressed for one or more quarters by CMS; (5) No data is available from the hospital for this measure; (6) Fewer than 100 patients completed the HCAHPS survey. Use these rates with caution, as the number of surveys may be too low to reliably assess hospital performance; (7) Survey results are based on less than 12 months of data; (8) Survey results are not available for this reporting period; (9) No or very few patients were eligible for the HCAHPS survey. The scores shown, if any, reflect a very small number of surveys; (10) A state average was not calculated because too few hospitals in the state submitted data; (11) There were discrepancies in the data collection process; Please refer to the User's Guide for a full explanation of data.

Lenoir Memorial Hospital

100 Airport Rd
Kinston, NC 28501
Phone: 252-522-7000
Fax: 252-522-7007
E-mail: hr@lenoir.org
URL: www.lenoirmemorial.org
Type: Acute Care Hospitals
Emergency Services: No
Ownership: Voluntary Non-Profit - Private
Beds: 261

Key Personnel:
CEO/President.............. Gary E Black
Chief of Medical Staff.......... Donald Riddle MD, MD
Coronary Care.............. Jessica Baker RN
Infection Control.............. Jody Robbins RN
Operating Room.............. Gisela Stroud
Pediatric In-Patient Care....... Nanci Hood RN
Quality Assurance............ Donna Floyd
Radiology................... Jeff Cartwright

Measure	Cases	This Hosp.	State Avg.	U.S. Avg.
Heart Attack Care				
ACE Inhibitor or ARB for LVSD[1]	13	92%	97%	96%
Aspirin at Arrival	133	94%	99%	99%
Aspirin at Discharge	82	93%	99%	98%
Beta Blocker at Discharge	85	91%	99%	98%
Fibrinolytic Medication Timing	0	-	38%	55%
PCI Within 90 Minutes of Arrival	0	-	95%	90%
Smoking Cessation Advice[1]	11	100%	100%	99%
Chest Pain/Possible Heart Attack Care				
Aspirin at Arrival	94	94%	95%	95%
Median Time to ECG (minutes)	97	8	8	8
Median Time to Transfer (minutes)[1]	5	101	48	61
Fibrinolytic Medication Timing[1]	20	60%	53%	54%
Heart Failure Care				
ACE Inhibitor or ARB for LVSD	143	87%	95%	94%
Discharge Instructions	404	76%	89%	88%
Evaluation of LVS Function	479	96%	99%	98%
Smoking Cessation Advice	86	100%	99%	98%
Pneumonia Care				
Appropriate Initial Antibiotic	136	93%	92%	92%
Blood Culture Timing	206	97%	96%	96%
Influenza Vaccine	151	74%	93%	91%
Initial Antibiotic Timing	241	96%	95%	95%
Pneumococcal Vaccine	229	97%	95%	93%
Smoking Cessation Advice	68	100%	99%	97%
Surgical Care Improvement Project				
Appropriate VTP Within 24 Hours	217	66%	93%	92%
Appropriate Hair Removal	461	100%	100%	99%
Appropriate Beta Blocker Usage	125	58%	94%	93%
Controlled Postoperative Blood Glucose	0	-	94%	93%
Prophylactic Antibiotic Timing	317	97%	98%	97%
Prophylactic Antibiotic Timing (Outpatient)	142	73%	94%	92%
Prophylactic Antibiotic Selection	320	95%	98%	97%
Prophylactic Antibiotic Select. (Outpatient)	112	91%	95%	94%
Prophylactic Antibiotic Stopped	305	92%	96%	94%
Recommended VTP Ordered	221	70%	95%	94%
Urinary Catheter Removal	62	73%	91%	90%
Children's Asthma Care				
Received Systemic Corticosteroids	-	-	100%	100%
Received Home Management Plan	-	-	75%	71%
Received Reliever Medication	-	-	100%	100%
Use of Medical Imaging				
Combination Abdominal CT Scan	565	0.324	0.115	0.191
Combination Chest CT Scan	400	0.000	0.037	0.054
Follow-up Mammogram/Ultrasound[5]	0	-	7.9%	8.4%
MRI for Low Back Pain	157	28.7%	30.6%	32.7%
Survey of Patients' Hospital Experiences				
Area Around Room 'Always' Quiet at Night	300+	55%	-	58%
Doctors 'Always' Communicated Well	300+	77%	-	80%
Home Recovery Information Given	300+	78%	-	82%
Hospital Given 9 or 10 on 10 Point Scale	300+	62%	-	67%
Meds 'Always' Explained Before Given	300+	56%	-	60%
Nurses 'Always' Communicated Well	300+	75%	-	76%
Pain 'Always' Well Controlled	300+	68%	-	69%
Room and Bathroom 'Always' Clean	300+	70%	-	71%
Timely Help 'Always' Received	300+	58%	-	64%
Would Definitely Recommend Hospital	300+	61%	-	69%

Scotland Memorial Hospital

500 Lauchwood Dr
Laurinburg, NC 28352
Phone: 910-291-7000
Fax: 910-291-7499
URL: www.scotlandhealth.org
Type: Acute Care Hospitals
Emergency Services: Yes
Ownership: Voluntary Non-Profit - Private
Beds: 154

Key Personnel:
CEO/President............... Gregory C Wood
Chief of Medical Staff.......... Paul Rash, MD
Operating Room.............. Patricia Decker
Pediatric Ambulatory Care...... Laura Gailey
Quality Assurance............ Lori Dove, RN
Radiology................... Zim Townsend
Hemotology Center........... Camille Utter, RN
Patient Relations............. Ronnie Norton

Measure	Cases	This Hosp.	State Avg.	U.S. Avg.
Heart Attack Care				
ACE Inhibitor or ARB for LVSD[1]	9	100%	97%	96%
Aspirin at Arrival	72	97%	99%	99%
Aspirin at Discharge	41	100%	99%	98%
Beta Blocker at Discharge	39	100%	99%	98%
Fibrinolytic Medication Timing	0	-	38%	55%
PCI Within 90 Minutes of Arrival	0	-	95%	90%
Smoking Cessation Advice[1]	13	100%	100%	99%
Chest Pain/Possible Heart Attack Care				
Aspirin at Arrival	46	98%	95%	95%
Median Time to ECG (minutes)	46	10	8	8
Median Time to Transfer (minutes)[1,3]	19	84	48	61
Fibrinolytic Medication Timing[1]	2	50%	53%	54%
Heart Failure Care				
ACE Inhibitor or ARB for LVSD	116	87%	95%	94%
Discharge Instructions	320	82%	89%	88%
Evaluation of LVS Function	345	99%	99%	98%
Smoking Cessation Advice	96	100%	99%	98%
Pneumonia Care				
Appropriate Initial Antibiotic	72	90%	92%	92%
Blood Culture Timing	121	99%	96%	96%
Influenza Vaccine	77	100%	93%	91%
Initial Antibiotic Timing	113	98%	95%	95%
Pneumococcal Vaccine	107	100%	95%	93%
Smoking Cessation Advice	63	100%	99%	97%
Surgical Care Improvement Project				
Appropriate VTP Within 24 Hours	195	98%	93%	92%
Appropriate Hair Removal	318	100%	100%	99%
Appropriate Beta Blocker Usage	102	98%	94%	93%
Controlled Postoperative Blood Glucose	0	-	94%	93%
Prophylactic Antibiotic Timing	204	98%	98%	97%
Prophylactic Antibiotic Timing (Outpatient)	153	95%	94%	92%
Prophylactic Antibiotic Selection	205	98%	98%	97%
Prophylactic Antibiotic Select. (Outpatient)	153	88%	95%	94%
Prophylactic Antibiotic Stopped	198	98%	96%	94%
Recommended VTP Ordered	195	99%	95%	94%
Urinary Catheter Removal	93	97%	91%	90%
Children's Asthma Care				
Received Systemic Corticosteroids	-	-	100%	100%
Received Home Management Plan	-	-	75%	71%
Received Reliever Medication	-	-	100%	100%
Use of Medical Imaging				
Combination Abdominal CT Scan	1,048	0.099	0.115	0.191
Combination Chest CT Scan	399	0.115	0.037	0.054
Follow-up Mammogram/Ultrasound	1,181	6.2%	7.9%	8.4%
MRI for Low Back Pain	164	30.5%	30.6%	32.7%
Survey of Patients' Hospital Experiences				
Area Around Room 'Always' Quiet at Night	300+	67%	-	58%
Doctors 'Always' Communicated Well	300+	84%	-	80%
Home Recovery Information Given	300+	80%	-	82%
Hospital Given 9 or 10 on 10 Point Scale	300+	64%	-	67%
Meds 'Always' Explained Before Given	300+	65%	-	60%
Nurses 'Always' Communicated Well	300+	78%	-	76%
Pain 'Always' Well Controlled	300+	71%	-	69%
Room and Bathroom 'Always' Clean	300+	63%	-	71%
Timely Help 'Always' Received	300+	68%	-	64%
Would Definitely Recommend Hospital	300+	62%	-	69%

Caldwell Memorial Hospital

321 Mulberry St SW
Lenoir, NC 28645
Phone: 828-757-5100
Fax: 828-757-5512
E-mail: lsmith@caldwell_mem.org
URL: www.caldwellmemorial.org
Type: Acute Care Hospitals
Emergency Services: Yes
Ownership: Voluntary Non-Profit - Other
Beds: 110

Key Personnel:
CEO/President............... Laura Easton, RN, MSN
Chief of Medical Staff.......... John D Powell
Infection Control............. Patricia Hicks, RN
Operating Room.............. Thomas A Pezzi, RN
Quality Assurance............ Kathy Proffitt
Radiology................... Ed Pearce, RRT

Measure	Cases	This Hosp.	State Avg.	U.S. Avg.
Heart Attack Care				
ACE Inhibitor or ARB for LVSD[1]	1	0%	97%	96%
Aspirin at Arrival	25	92%	99%	99%
Aspirin at Discharge[1]	12	92%	99%	98%
Beta Blocker at Discharge[1]	12	100%	99%	98%
Fibrinolytic Medication Timing	0	-	38%	55%
PCI Within 90 Minutes of Arrival	0	-	95%	90%
Smoking Cessation Advice[1]	5	100%	100%	99%
Chest Pain/Possible Heart Attack Care				
Aspirin at Arrival	54	96%	95%	95%
Median Time to ECG (minutes)	56	8	8	8
Median Time to Transfer (minutes)[1]	13	35	48	61
Fibrinolytic Medication Timing	0	-	53%	54%
Heart Failure Care				
ACE Inhibitor or ARB for LVSD	31	81%	95%	94%
Discharge Instructions	95	65%	89%	88%
Evaluation of LVS Function	117	99%	99%	98%
Smoking Cessation Advice[1]	21	95%	99%	98%
Pneumonia Care				
Appropriate Initial Antibiotic	74	82%	92%	92%
Blood Culture Timing	140	98%	96%	96%
Influenza Vaccine	97	81%	93%	91%
Initial Antibiotic Timing	125	91%	95%	95%
Pneumococcal Vaccine	120	93%	95%	93%
Smoking Cessation Advice	72	97%	99%	97%
Surgical Care Improvement Project				
Appropriate VTP Within 24 Hours	113	89%	93%	92%
Appropriate Hair Removal	308	100%	100%	99%
Appropriate Beta Blocker Usage	56	96%	94%	93%
Controlled Postoperative Blood Glucose	0	-	94%	93%
Prophylactic Antibiotic Timing	199	95%	98%	97%
Prophylactic Antibiotic Timing (Outpatient)	105	94%	94%	92%
Prophylactic Antibiotic Selection	202	99%	98%	97%
Prophylactic Antibiotic Select. (Outpatient)	104	95%	95%	94%
Prophylactic Antibiotic Stopped	187	90%	96%	94%
Recommended VTP Ordered	113	91%	95%	94%
Urinary Catheter Removal	73	89%	91%	90%
Children's Asthma Care				
Received Systemic Corticosteroids	-	-	100%	100%
Received Home Management Plan	-	-	75%	71%
Received Reliever Medication	-	-	100%	100%
Use of Medical Imaging				
Combination Abdominal CT Scan	438	0.059	0.115	0.191
Combination Chest CT Scan	327	0.000	0.037	0.054
Follow-up Mammogram/Ultrasound	1,333	11.1%	7.9%	8.4%
MRI for Low Back Pain	132	34.1%	30.6%	32.7%
Survey of Patients' Hospital Experiences				
Area Around Room 'Always' Quiet at Night	300+	59%	-	58%
Doctors 'Always' Communicated Well	300+	83%	-	80%
Home Recovery Information Given	300+	85%	-	82%
Hospital Given 9 or 10 on 10 Point Scale	300+	63%	-	67%
Meds 'Always' Explained Before Given	300+	62%	-	60%
Nurses 'Always' Communicated Well	300+	76%	-	76%
Pain 'Always' Well Controlled	300+	70%	-	69%
Room and Bathroom 'Always' Clean	300+	63%	-	71%
Timely Help 'Always' Received	300+	62%	-	64%
Would Definitely Recommend Hospital	300+	62%	-	69%

NOTE: Hospital profiles are in alphabetical order by state, then city, then hospital within the city; Rankings exclude hospitals with less than 25 cases except for patient surveys which excludes hospitals with less than 100 cases; (a) 100–299 cases; (1) The number of cases is too small to be sure how well a hospital is performing; (2) The hospital indicated that the data submitted for this measure were based on a sample of cases; (3) Data was collected during a shorter time period (fewer quarters) than the maximum possible time for this measure; (4) Suppressed for one or more quarters by CMS; (5) No data is available from the hospital for this measure; (6) Fewer than 100 patients completed the HCAHPS survey. Use these rates with caution, as the number of surveys may be too low to reliably assess hospital performance; (7) Survey results are based on less than 12 months of data; (8) Survey results are not available for this reporting period; (9) No or very few patients were eligible for the HCAHPS survey. The scores shown, if any, reflect a very small number of surveys; (10) A state average was not calculated because too few hospitals in the state submitted data; (11) There were discrepancies in the data collection process; Please refer to the User's Guide for a full explanation of data.

Lexington Memorial Hospital

250 Hospital Drive Phone: 336-248-5161
Lexington, NC 27293 Fax: 336-248-4711
E-mail: info@lmh.cc
URL: www.lexingtonmemorial.com
Type: Acute Care Hospitals Emergency Services: Yes
Ownership: Voluntary Non-Profit - Private Beds: 94

Key Personnel:
CEO/President. . . . . John Cashion
Chief of Medical Staff. . . . . Malin Sadler
Coronary Care. . . . . Kathryn A McFarland
Radiology. . . . . Ira E Bell, III
Emergency Room . . . . Mark Bardou

Measure	Cases	This Hosp.	State Avg.	U.S. Avg.
Heart Attack Care				
ACE Inhibitor or ARB for LVSD[1]	6	83%	97%	96%
Aspirin at Arrival	50	94%	99%	99%
Aspirin at Discharge	29	79%	99%	98%
Beta Blocker at Discharge	30	97%	99%	98%
Fibrinolytic Medication Timing	0	-	38%	55%
PCI Within 90 Minutes of Arrival	0	-	95%	90%
Smoking Cessation Advice[1]	4	100%	100%	99%
Chest Pain/Possible Heart Attack Care				
Aspirin at Arrival	64	97%	95%	95%
Median Time to ECG (minutes)	65	9	8	8
Median Time to Transfer (minutes)[1]	21	46	48	61
Fibrinolytic Medication Timing	0	-	53%	54%
Heart Failure Care				
ACE Inhibitor or ARB for LVSD	37	95%	95%	94%
Discharge Instructions	117	98%	89%	88%
Evaluation of LVS Function	142	98%	99%	98%
Smoking Cessation Advice	30	100%	99%	98%
Pneumonia Care				
Appropriate Initial Antibiotic	126	87%	92%	92%
Blood Culture Timing	185	97%	96%	96%
Influenza Vaccine	105	95%	93%	91%
Initial Antibiotic Timing	175	99%	95%	95%
Pneumococcal Vaccine	158	98%	95%	93%
Smoking Cessation Advice	55	100%	99%	97%
Surgical Care Improvement Project				
Appropriate VTP Within 24 Hours	80	89%	93%	92%
Appropriate Hair Removal	298	98%	100%	99%
Appropriate Beta Blocker Usage	70	97%	94%	93%
Controlled Postoperative Blood Glucose	0	-	94%	93%
Prophylactic Antibiotic Timing	236	95%	98%	97%
Prophylactic Antibiotic Timing (Outpatient)	205	91%	94%	92%
Prophylactic Antibiotic Selection	235	98%	98%	97%
Prophylactic Antibiotic Select. (Outpatient)	201	91%	95%	94%
Prophylactic Antibiotic Stopped	229	98%	96%	94%
Recommended VTP Ordered	82	87%	95%	94%
Urinary Catheter Removal	81	96%	91%	90%
Children's Asthma Care				
Received Systemic Corticosteroids	-	-	100%	100%
Received Home Management Plan	-	-	75%	71%
Received Reliever Medication	-	-	100%	100%
Use of Medical Imaging				
Combination Abdominal CT Scan	514	0.045	0.115	0.191
Combination Chest CT Scan	349	0.003	0.037	0.054
Follow-up Mammogram/Ultrasound	857	7.8%	7.9%	8.4%
MRI for Low Back Pain	133	29.3%	30.6%	32.7%
Survey of Patients' Hospital Experiences				
Area Around Room 'Always' Quiet at Night	300+	58%	-	58%
Doctors 'Always' Communicated Well	300+	82%	-	80%
Home Recovery Information Given	300+	83%	-	82%
Hospital Given 9 or 10 on 10 Point Scale	300+	66%	-	67%
Meds 'Always' Explained Before Given	300+	67%	-	60%
Nurses 'Always' Communicated Well	300+	79%	-	76%
Pain 'Always' Well Controlled	300+	71%	-	69%
Room and Bathroom 'Always' Clean	300+	75%	-	71%
Timely Help 'Always' Received	300+	68%	-	64%
Would Definitely Recommend Hospital	300+	63%	-	69%

Carolinas Medical Center-Lincoln

200 Gamble Dr Phone: 704-735-3071
Lincolnton, NC 28092 Fax: 704-732-5494
URL: www.lincolnmedical.org
Type: Acute Care Hospitals Emergency Services: No
Ownership: Govt - Hospital Dist/Auth Beds: 87

Key Personnel:
CEO/President. . . . . Peter W Acker
Chief of Medical Staff. . . . . Larry Weems, MD
Infection Control. . . . . Suzanne Gazzaway, RN
Operating Room. . . . . William Beutel, RN
Quality Assurance . . . . Beth King
Radiology. . . . . Deborah Agisim
Emergency Room . . . . V Washington, MD
Intensive Care Unit. . . . . Anne Parker, RN

Measure	Cases	This Hosp.	State Avg.	U.S. Avg.
Heart Attack Care				
ACE Inhibitor or ARB for LVSD[1]	2	100%	97%	96%
Aspirin at Arrival[1]	16	100%	99%	99%
Aspirin at Discharge[1]	3	100%	99%	98%
Beta Blocker at Discharge[1]	5	100%	99%	98%
Fibrinolytic Medication Timing	0	-	38%	55%
PCI Within 90 Minutes of Arrival	0	-	95%	90%
Smoking Cessation Advice[1]	1	100%	100%	99%
Chest Pain/Possible Heart Attack Care				
Aspirin at Arrival	89	96%	95%	95%
Median Time to ECG (minutes)	89	2	8	8
Median Time to Transfer (minutes)	28	35	48	61
Fibrinolytic Medication Timing	0	-	53%	54%
Heart Failure Care				
ACE Inhibitor or ARB for LVSD	28	100%	95%	94%
Discharge Instructions	101	99%	89%	88%
Evaluation of LVS Function	120	100%	99%	98%
Smoking Cessation Advice[1]	23	100%	99%	98%
Pneumonia Care				
Appropriate Initial Antibiotic	109	98%	92%	92%
Blood Culture Timing	139	98%	96%	96%
Influenza Vaccine	82	99%	93%	91%
Initial Antibiotic Timing	135	96%	95%	95%
Pneumococcal Vaccine	80	98%	95%	93%
Smoking Cessation Advice	82	100%	99%	97%
Surgical Care Improvement Project				
Appropriate VTP Within 24 Hours	39	95%	93%	92%
Appropriate Hair Removal	113	100%	100%	99%
Appropriate Beta Blocker Usage[1]	19	100%	94%	93%
Controlled Postoperative Blood Glucose	0	-	94%	93%
Prophylactic Antibiotic Timing	81	98%	98%	97%
Prophylactic Antibiotic Timing (Outpatient)[1,3]	19	89%	94%	92%
Prophylactic Antibiotic Selection	83	99%	98%	97%
Prophylactic Antibiotic Select. (Outpatient)[1,3]	17	100%	95%	94%
Prophylactic Antibiotic Stopped	68	96%	96%	94%
Recommended VTP Ordered	40	92%	95%	94%
Urinary Catheter Removal[1]	8	75%	91%	90%
Children's Asthma Care				
Received Systemic Corticosteroids	-	-	100%	100%
Received Home Management Plan	-	-	75%	71%
Received Reliever Medication	-	-	100%	100%
Use of Medical Imaging				
Combination Abdominal CT Scan	467	0.030	0.115	0.191
Combination Chest CT Scan	307	0.020	0.037	0.054
Follow-up Mammogram/Ultrasound	720	10.8%	7.9%	8.4%
MRI for Low Back Pain	123	38.2%	30.6%	32.7%
Survey of Patients' Hospital Experiences				
Area Around Room 'Always' Quiet at Night	300+	54%	-	58%
Doctors 'Always' Communicated Well	300+	81%	-	80%
Home Recovery Information Given	300+	86%	-	82%
Hospital Given 9 or 10 on 10 Point Scale	300+	69%	-	67%
Meds 'Always' Explained Before Given	300+	58%	-	60%
Nurses 'Always' Communicated Well	300+	79%	-	76%
Pain 'Always' Well Controlled	300+	68%	-	69%
Room and Bathroom 'Always' Clean	300+	72%	-	71%
Timely Help 'Always' Received	300+	67%	-	64%
Would Definitely Recommend Hospital	300+	63%	-	69%

Charles A Cannon Jr Memorial Hospital

434 Hospital Drive Phone: 828-737-7000
Linville, NC 28646 Fax: 828-737-7491
URL: www.cannonmh.org
Type: Critical Access Hospitals Emergency Services: Yes
Ownership: Voluntary Non-Profit - Private Beds: 70

Key Personnel:
CEO/President. . . . . Chuck Montooth
Chief of Medical Staff. . . . . Thomas Haizlip Jr, MD
Infection Control. . . . . Elizabeth Kress
Operating Room. . . . . Elizabeth Kress, RN
Quality Assurance . . . . Carmen Lacey
Emergency Room . . . . Terri Yoder
Intensive Care Unit. . . . . Terri Yoder

Measure	Cases	This Hosp.	State Avg.	U.S. Avg.
Heart Attack Care				
ACE Inhibitor or ARB for LVSD[5]	0	-	97%	96%
Aspirin at Arrival[5]	0	-	99%	99%
Aspirin at Discharge[5]	0	-	99%	98%
Beta Blocker at Discharge[5]	0	-	99%	98%
Fibrinolytic Medication Timing[5]	0	-	38%	55%
PCI Within 90 Minutes of Arrival[5]	0	-	95%	90%
Smoking Cessation Advice[5]	0	-	100%	99%
Chest Pain/Possible Heart Attack Care				
Aspirin at Arrival	-	-	95%	95%
Median Time to ECG (minutes)	-	-	8	8
Median Time to Transfer (minutes)	-	-	48	61
Fibrinolytic Medication Timing	-	-	53%	54%
Heart Failure Care				
ACE Inhibitor or ARB for LVSD[1]	5	100%	95%	94%
Discharge Instructions	52	100%	89%	88%
Evaluation of LVS Function	76	93%	99%	98%
Smoking Cessation Advice[1]	10	100%	99%	98%
Pneumonia Care				
Appropriate Initial Antibiotic	37	73%	92%	92%
Blood Culture Timing	46	98%	96%	96%
Influenza Vaccine	34	97%	93%	91%
Initial Antibiotic Timing	72	94%	95%	95%
Pneumococcal Vaccine	61	98%	95%	93%
Smoking Cessation Advice[1]	14	100%	99%	97%
Surgical Care Improvement Project				
Appropriate VTP Within 24 Hours[5]	0	-	93%	92%
Appropriate Hair Removal[5]	0	-	100%	99%
Appropriate Beta Blocker Usage[5]	0	-	94%	93%
Controlled Postoperative Blood Glucose[5]	0	-	94%	93%
Prophylactic Antibiotic Timing[5]	0	-	98%	97%
Prophylactic Antibiotic Timing (Outpatient)	-	-	94%	92%
Prophylactic Antibiotic Selection[5]	0	-	98%	97%
Prophylactic Antibiotic Select. (Outpatient)	-	-	95%	94%
Prophylactic Antibiotic Stopped[5]	0	-	96%	94%
Recommended VTP Ordered[5]	0	-	95%	94%
Urinary Catheter Removal[5]	0	-	91%	90%
Children's Asthma Care				
Received Systemic Corticosteroids	-	-	100%	100%
Received Home Management Plan	-	-	75%	71%
Received Reliever Medication	-	-	100%	100%
Use of Medical Imaging				
Combination Abdominal CT Scan	-	-	0.115	0.191
Combination Chest CT Scan	-	-	0.037	0.054
Follow-up Mammogram/Ultrasound	-	-	7.9%	8.4%
MRI for Low Back Pain	-	-	30.6%	32.7%
Survey of Patients' Hospital Experiences				
Area Around Room 'Always' Quiet at Night[8]	-	-	-	58%
Doctors 'Always' Communicated Well[8]	-	-	-	80%
Home Recovery Information Given[8]	-	-	-	82%
Hospital Given 9 or 10 on 10 Point Scale[8]	-	-	-	67%
Meds 'Always' Explained Before Given[8]	-	-	-	60%
Nurses 'Always' Communicated Well[8]	-	-	-	76%
Pain 'Always' Well Controlled[8]	-	-	-	69%
Room and Bathroom 'Always' Clean[8]	-	-	-	71%
Timely Help 'Always' Received[8]	-	-	-	64%
Would Definitely Recommend Hospital[8]	-	-	-	69%

NOTE: Hospital profiles are in alphabetical order by state, then city, then hospital within the city; Rankings exclude hospitals with less than 25 cases except for patient surveys which excludes hospitals with less than 100 cases; (a) 100–299 cases; (1) The number of cases is too small to be sure how well a hospital is performing; (2) The hospital indicated that the data submitted for this measure were based on a sample of cases; (3) Data was collected during a shorter time period (fewer quarters) than the maximum possible time for this measure; (4) Suppressed for one or more quarters by CMS; (5) No data is available from the hospital for this measure; (6) Fewer than 100 patients completed the HCAHPS survey. Use these rates with caution, as the number of surveys may be too low to reliably assess hospital performance; (7) Survey results are based on less than 12 months of data; (8) Survey results are not available for this reporting period; (9) No or very few patients were eligible for the HCAHPS survey. The scores shown, if any, reflect a very small number of surveys; (10) A state average was not calculated because too few hospitals in the state submitted data; (11) There were discrepancies in the data collection process; Please refer to the User's Guide for a full explanation of data.

Franklin Regional Medical Center

100 Hospital Dr Box 609 Phone: 919-496-5131
Louisburg, NC 27549 Fax: 919-497-8018
URL: www.franklinregionalmedicalctr.com
Type: Acute Care Hospitals Emergency Services: No
Ownership: Voluntary Non-Profit - Private Beds: 85

Key Personnel:
CEO/President. . . . . Mike McNair
Chief of Medical Staff. . . . . Grant Jenkins
Infection Control. . . . . Betty Bernette
Operating Room. . . . . Chad D Caldwell
Quality Assurance . . . . Betty Bernette
Radiology. . . . . Paul C D'Angelo
Anesthesiology. . . . . Steve Ziegler
Emergency Room . . . . Andrew Pacos

Measure	Cases	This Hosp.	State Avg.	U.S. Avg.
Heart Attack Care				
ACE Inhibitor or ARB for LVSD[3]	0	-	97%	96%
Aspirin at Arrival[1,3]	2	100%	99%	99%
Aspirin at Discharge[3]	0	-	99%	98%
Beta Blocker at Discharge[3]	0	-	99%	98%
Fibrinolytic Medication Timing[3]	0	-	38%	55%
PCI Within 90 Minutes of Arrival[3]	0	-	95%	90%
Smoking Cessation Advice[3]	0	-	100%	99%
Chest Pain/Possible Heart Attack Care				
Aspirin at Arrival	95	99%	95%	95%
Median Time to ECG (minutes)	96	5	8	8
Median Time to Transfer (minutes)[1]	15	50	48	61
Fibrinolytic Medication Timing	0	-	53%	54%
Heart Failure Care				
ACE Inhibitor or ARB for LVSD[1]	22	91%	95%	94%
Discharge Instructions	58	86%	89%	88%
Evaluation of LVS Function	73	100%	99%	98%
Smoking Cessation Advice[1]	17	100%	99%	98%
Pneumonia Care				
Appropriate Initial Antibiotic	37	95%	92%	92%
Blood Culture Timing	68	96%	96%	96%
Influenza Vaccine	48	98%	93%	91%
Initial Antibiotic Timing	59	95%	95%	95%
Pneumococcal Vaccine	63	97%	95%	93%
Smoking Cessation Advice	26	100%	99%	97%
Surgical Care Improvement Project				
Appropriate VTP Within 24 Hours[1]	12	75%	93%	92%
Appropriate Hair Removal[1]	14	100%	100%	99%
Appropriate Beta Blocker Usage[1]	4	100%	94%	93%
Controlled Postoperative Blood Glucose	0	-	94%	93%
Prophylactic Antibiotic Timing[1]	5	100%	98%	97%
Prophylactic Antibiotic Timing (Outpatient)[1,3]	1	100%	94%	92%
Prophylactic Antibiotic Selection[1]	5	100%	98%	97%
Prophylactic Antibiotic Select. (Outpatient)[1,3]	1	100%	95%	94%
Prophylactic Antibiotic Stopped[1]	4	100%	96%	94%
Recommended VTP Ordered[1]	12	75%	95%	94%
Urinary Catheter Removal[1]	5	40%	91%	90%
Children's Asthma Care				
Received Systemic Corticosteroids	-	-	100%	100%
Received Home Management Plan	-	-	75%	71%
Received Reliever Medication	-	-	100%	100%
Use of Medical Imaging				
Combination Abdominal CT Scan	255	0.075	0.115	0.191
Combination Chest CT Scan	200	0.070	0.037	0.054
Follow-up Mammogram/Ultrasound	546	8.8%	7.9%	8.4%
MRI for Low Back Pain	62	37.1%	30.6%	32.7%
Survey of Patients' Hospital Experiences				
Area Around Room 'Always' Quiet at Night	(a)	67%	-	58%
Doctors 'Always' Communicated Well	(a)	79%	-	80%
Home Recovery Information Given	(a)	87%	-	82%
Hospital Given 9 or 10 on 10 Point Scale	(a)	70%	-	67%
Meds 'Always' Explained Before Given	(a)	66%	-	60%
Nurses 'Always' Communicated Well	(a)	79%	-	76%
Pain 'Always' Well Controlled	(a)	73%	-	69%
Room and Bathroom 'Always' Clean	(a)	71%	-	71%
Timely Help 'Always' Received	(a)	71%	-	64%
Would Definitely Recommend Hospital	(a)	66%	-	69%

Southeastern Regional Medical Center

300 W 27 St Phone: 910-671-5000
Lumberton, NC 28359 Fax: 910-671-5200
URL: www.srmc.org
Type: Acute Care Hospitals Emergency Services: Yes
Ownership: Voluntary Non-Profit - Private Beds: 403

Key Personnel:
CEO/President. . . . . Joann Anderson
Cardiac Laboratory. . . . . Amy Kessenich
Coronary Care . . . . Renee Hester
Infection Control. . . . . Dale Gifford
Operating Room. . . . . Anette Dial
Quality Assurance . . . . Elizabeth Kirschling
Radiology. . . . . Jon Thorsten

Measure	Cases	This Hosp.	State Avg.	U.S. Avg.
Heart Attack Care				
ACE Inhibitor or ARB for LVSD	26	92%	97%	96%
Aspirin at Arrival	207	97%	99%	99%
Aspirin at Discharge	171	98%	99%	98%
Beta Blocker at Discharge	171	99%	99%	98%
Fibrinolytic Medication Timing	0	-	38%	55%
PCI Within 90 Minutes of Arrival[1]	10	60%	95%	90%
Smoking Cessation Advice	84	100%	100%	99%
Chest Pain/Possible Heart Attack Care				
Aspirin at Arrival	36	83%	95%	95%
Median Time to ECG (minutes)	35	23	8	8
Median Time to Transfer (minutes)[1,3]	4	185	48	61
Fibrinolytic Medication Timing[1]	6	17%	53%	54%
Heart Failure Care				
ACE Inhibitor or ARB for LVSD	155	95%	95%	94%
Discharge Instructions	525	85%	89%	88%
Evaluation of LVS Function	572	100%	99%	98%
Smoking Cessation Advice	138	100%	99%	98%
Pneumonia Care				
Appropriate Initial Antibiotic	242	91%	92%	92%
Blood Culture Timing	307	93%	96%	96%
Influenza Vaccine	220	92%	93%	91%
Initial Antibiotic Timing	314	94%	95%	95%
Pneumococcal Vaccine	253	96%	95%	93%
Smoking Cessation Advice	174	99%	99%	97%
Surgical Care Improvement Project				
Appropriate VTP Within 24 Hours	185	90%	93%	92%
Appropriate Hair Removal	389	100%	100%	99%
Appropriate Beta Blocker Usage	110	92%	94%	93%
Controlled Postoperative Blood Glucose	33	100%	94%	93%
Prophylactic Antibiotic Timing	251	99%	98%	97%
Prophylactic Antibiotic Timing (Outpatient)	357	95%	94%	92%
Prophylactic Antibiotic Selection	251	97%	98%	97%
Prophylactic Antibiotic Select. (Outpatient)	344	95%	95%	94%
Prophylactic Antibiotic Stopped	239	96%	96%	94%
Recommended VTP Ordered	185	97%	95%	94%
Urinary Catheter Removal	97	96%	91%	90%
Children's Asthma Care				
Received Systemic Corticosteroids	-	-	100%	100%
Received Home Management Plan	-	-	75%	71%
Received Reliever Medication	-	-	100%	100%
Use of Medical Imaging				
Combination Abdominal CT Scan	970	0.037	0.115	0.191
Combination Chest CT Scan	708	0.016	0.037	0.054
Follow-up Mammogram/Ultrasound[5]	0	-	7.9%	8.4%
MRI for Low Back Pain	338	31.1%	30.6%	32.7%
Survey of Patients' Hospital Experiences				
Area Around Room 'Always' Quiet at Night	300+	72%	-	58%
Doctors 'Always' Communicated Well	300+	84%	-	80%
Home Recovery Information Given	300+	84%	-	82%
Hospital Given 9 or 10 on 10 Point Scale	300+	67%	-	67%
Meds 'Always' Explained Before Given	300+	70%	-	60%
Nurses 'Always' Communicated Well	300+	81%	-	76%
Pain 'Always' Well Controlled	300+	70%	-	69%
Room and Bathroom 'Always' Clean	300+	70%	-	71%
Timely Help 'Always' Received	300+	70%	-	64%
Would Definitely Recommend Hospital	300+	64%	-	69%

The Mcdowell Hospital

430 Rankin Drive Phone: 828-659-5000
Marion, NC 28752 Fax: 828-652-1626
URL: www.mcdhospital.org
Type: Acute Care Hospitals Emergency Services: Yes
Ownership: Voluntary Non-Profit - Private Beds: 65

Key Personnel:
CEO/President. . . . . Ed Hannon
Operating Room. . . . . Lori Elam
Pediatric Ambulatory Care . . . . . . Teresa Wall
Pediatric In-Patient Care . . . . Teresa Wall
Radiology. . . . . Kelly McFarland
Emergency Room . . . . Karen English, RN
Intensive Care Unit. . . . . Keisha Hastings

Measure	Cases	This Hosp.	State Avg.	U.S. Avg.
Heart Attack Care				
ACE Inhibitor or ARB for LVSD[1]	2	50%	97%	96%
Aspirin at Arrival[1]	6	100%	99%	99%
Aspirin at Discharge[1]	3	100%	99%	98%
Beta Blocker at Discharge[1]	3	100%	99%	98%
Fibrinolytic Medication Timing	0	-	38%	55%
PCI Within 90 Minutes of Arrival	0	-	95%	90%
Smoking Cessation Advice[1]	1	100%	100%	99%
Chest Pain/Possible Heart Attack Care				
Aspirin at Arrival	84	96%	95%	95%
Median Time to ECG (minutes)	87	7	8	8
Median Time to Transfer (minutes)[1]	9	32	48	61
Fibrinolytic Medication Timing	0	-	53%	54%
Heart Failure Care				
ACE Inhibitor or ARB for LVSD[1]	24	96%	95%	94%
Discharge Instructions	47	94%	89%	88%
Evaluation of LVS Function	52	100%	99%	98%
Smoking Cessation Advice[1]	11	100%	99%	98%
Pneumonia Care				
Appropriate Initial Antibiotic	31	94%	92%	92%
Blood Culture Timing	64	100%	96%	96%
Influenza Vaccine	54	94%	93%	91%
Initial Antibiotic Timing	65	100%	95%	95%
Pneumococcal Vaccine	65	98%	95%	93%
Smoking Cessation Advice	36	100%	99%	97%
Surgical Care Improvement Project				
Appropriate VTP Within 24 Hours	63	92%	93%	92%
Appropriate Hair Removal	111	100%	100%	99%
Appropriate Beta Blocker Usage[1]	20	75%	94%	93%
Controlled Postoperative Blood Glucose	0	-	94%	93%
Prophylactic Antibiotic Timing	64	95%	98%	97%
Prophylactic Antibiotic Timing (Outpatient)	57	95%	94%	92%
Prophylactic Antibiotic Selection	64	91%	98%	97%
Prophylactic Antibiotic Select. (Outpatient)	54	96%	95%	94%
Prophylactic Antibiotic Stopped	57	89%	96%	94%
Recommended VTP Ordered	63	94%	95%	94%
Urinary Catheter Removal[1]	16	81%	91%	90%
Children's Asthma Care				
Received Systemic Corticosteroids	-	-	100%	100%
Received Home Management Plan	-	-	75%	71%
Received Reliever Medication	-	-	100%	100%
Use of Medical Imaging				
Combination Abdominal CT Scan	464	0.028	0.115	0.191
Combination Chest CT Scan	291	0.003	0.037	0.054
Follow-up Mammogram/Ultrasound	707	5.0%	7.9%	8.4%
MRI for Low Back Pain[5]	0	-	30.6%	32.7%
Survey of Patients' Hospital Experiences				
Area Around Room 'Always' Quiet at Night	300+	64%	-	58%
Doctors 'Always' Communicated Well	300+	81%	-	80%
Home Recovery Information Given	300+	84%	-	82%
Hospital Given 9 or 10 on 10 Point Scale	300+	69%	-	67%
Meds 'Always' Explained Before Given	300+	64%	-	60%
Nurses 'Always' Communicated Well	300+	80%	-	76%
Pain 'Always' Well Controlled	300+	72%	-	69%
Room and Bathroom 'Always' Clean	300+	77%	-	71%
Timely Help 'Always' Received	300+	70%	-	64%
Would Definitely Recommend Hospital	300+	68%	-	69%

NOTE: Hospital profiles are in alphabetical order by state, then city, then hospital within the city; Rankings exclude hospitals with less than 25 cases except for patient surveys which excludes hospitals with less than 100 cases; (a) 100–299 cases; (1) The number of cases is too small to be sure how well a hospital is performing; (2) The hospital indicated that the data submitted for this measure were based on a sample of cases; (3) Data was collected during a shorter time period (fewer quarters) than the maximum possible time for this measure; (4) Suppressed for one or more quarters by CMS; (5) No data is available from the hospital for this measure; (6) Fewer than 100 patients completed the HCAHPS survey. Use these rates with caution, as the number of surveys may be too low to reliably assess hospital performance; (7) Survey results are based on less than 12 months of data; (8) Survey results are not available for this reporting period; (9) No or very few patients were eligible for the HCAHPS survey. The scores shown, if any, reflect a very small number of surveys; (10) A state average was not calculated because too few hospitals in the state submitted data; (11) There were discrepancies in the data collection process; Please refer to the User's Guide for a full explanation of data.

Presbyterian Hospital Matthews

1500 Matthews Twp Pkwy
Matthews, NC 28106
Phone: 704-384-6500
Fax: 704-384-6515
E-mail: tcthompson@ph.novanthealth.org
URL: www.presbyterian.org
Type: Acute Care Hospitals
Emergency Services: Yes
Ownership: Voluntary Non-Profit - Other
Beds: 94

Key Personnel:
Chief of Medical Staff.......... Thomas H Phillips
Radiology.................. Steven M Genkins

Measure	Cases	This Hosp.	State Avg.	U.S. Avg.
Heart Attack Care				
ACE Inhibitor or ARB for LVSD[1]	4	100%	97%	96%
Aspirin at Arrival	57	100%	99%	99%
Aspirin at Discharge	36	100%	99%	98%
Beta Blocker at Discharge	37	100%	99%	98%
Fibrinolytic Medication Timing	0	-	38%	55%
PCI Within 90 Minutes of Arrival	0	-	95%	90%
Smoking Cessation Advice[1]	8	100%	100%	99%
Chest Pain/Possible Heart Attack Care				
Aspirin at Arrival	73	100%	95%	95%
Median Time to ECG (minutes)	77	4	8	8
Median Time to Transfer (minutes)	36	34	48	61
Fibrinolytic Medication Timing	0	-	53%	54%
Heart Failure Care				
ACE Inhibitor or ARB for LVSD	43	100%	95%	94%
Discharge Instructions	142	96%	89%	88%
Evaluation of LVS Function	180	100%	99%	98%
Smoking Cessation Advice[1]	16	100%	99%	98%
Pneumonia Care				
Appropriate Initial Antibiotic	193	97%	92%	92%
Blood Culture Timing	258	100%	96%	96%
Influenza Vaccine	160	99%	93%	91%
Initial Antibiotic Timing	236	99%	95%	95%
Pneumococcal Vaccine	197	99%	95%	93%
Smoking Cessation Advice	70	100%	99%	97%
Surgical Care Improvement Project				
Appropriate VTP Within 24 Hours[2]	216	96%	93%	92%
Appropriate Hair Removal[2]	468	100%	100%	99%
Appropriate Beta Blocker Usage[2]	85	98%	94%	93%
Controlled Postoperative Blood Glucose[2]	0	-	94%	93%
Prophylactic Antibiotic Timing[2]	303	98%	98%	97%
Prophylactic Antibiotic Timing (Outpatient)	336	98%	94%	92%
Prophylactic Antibiotic Selection[2]	303	99%	98%	97%
Prophylactic Antibiotic Select. (Outpatient)	336	98%	95%	94%
Prophylactic Antibiotic Stopped[2]	290	98%	96%	94%
Recommended VTP Ordered[2]	216	97%	95%	94%
Urinary Catheter Removal[2]	119	97%	91%	90%
Children's Asthma Care				
Received Systemic Corticosteroids	-	-	100%	100%
Received Home Management Plan	-	-	75%	71%
Received Reliever Medication	-	-	100%	100%
Use of Medical Imaging				
Combination Abdominal CT Scan	1,365	0.051	0.115	0.191
Combination Chest CT Scan	907	0.000	0.037	0.054
Follow-up Mammogram/Ultrasound	1,153	5.8%	7.9%	8.4%
MRI for Low Back Pain	243	26.7%	30.6%	32.7%
Survey of Patients' Hospital Experiences				
Area Around Room 'Always' Quiet at Night	300+	62%	-	58%
Doctors 'Always' Communicated Well	300+	78%	-	80%
Home Recovery Information Given	300+	85%	-	82%
Hospital Given 9 or 10 on 10 Point Scale	300+	70%	-	67%
Meds 'Always' Explained Before Given	300+	57%	-	60%
Nurses 'Always' Communicated Well	300+	73%	-	76%
Pain 'Always' Well Controlled	300+	67%	-	69%
Room and Bathroom 'Always' Clean	300+	70%	-	71%
Timely Help 'Always' Received	300+	60%	-	64%
Would Definitely Recommend Hospital	300+	77%	-	69%

Davie County Hospital

223 Hospital St
Mocksville, NC 27028
Phone: 336-751-8100
Fax: 336-751-8402
URL: www.daviehospital.org
Type: Critical Access Hospitals
Emergency Services: Yes
Ownership: Voluntary Non-Profit - Other
Beds: 81

Key Personnel:
CEO/President.............. Donny Lambath

Measure	Cases	This Hosp.	State Avg.	U.S. Avg.
Heart Attack Care				
ACE Inhibitor or ARB for LVSD[5]	0	-	97%	96%
Aspirin at Arrival[5]	0	-	99%	99%
Aspirin at Discharge[5]	0	-	99%	98%
Beta Blocker at Discharge[5]	0	-	99%	98%
Fibrinolytic Medication Timing[5]	0	-	38%	55%
PCI Within 90 Minutes of Arrival[5]	0	-	95%	90%
Smoking Cessation Advice[5]	0	-	100%	99%
Chest Pain/Possible Heart Attack Care				
Aspirin at Arrival	-	-	95%	95%
Median Time to ECG (minutes)	-	-	8	8
Median Time to Transfer (minutes)	-	-	48	61
Fibrinolytic Medication Timing	-	-	53%	54%
Heart Failure Care				
ACE Inhibitor or ARB for LVSD	0	-	95%	94%
Discharge Instructions[1]	4	100%	89%	88%
Evaluation of LVS Function[1]	6	17%	99%	98%
Smoking Cessation Advice	0	-	99%	98%
Pneumonia Care				
Appropriate Initial Antibiotic[1]	21	71%	92%	92%
Blood Culture Timing[1]	22	95%	96%	96%
Influenza Vaccine[1]	14	71%	93%	91%
Initial Antibiotic Timing	27	85%	95%	95%
Pneumococcal Vaccine	25	92%	95%	93%
Smoking Cessation Advice[1]	8	62%	99%	97%
Surgical Care Improvement Project				
Appropriate VTP Within 24 Hours[5]	0	-	93%	92%
Appropriate Hair Removal[5]	0	-	100%	99%
Appropriate Beta Blocker Usage[5]	0	-	94%	93%
Controlled Postoperative Blood Glucose[5]	0	-	94%	93%
Prophylactic Antibiotic Timing[5]	0	-	98%	97%
Prophylactic Antibiotic Timing (Outpatient)	-	-	94%	92%
Prophylactic Antibiotic Selection[5]	0	-	98%	97%
Prophylactic Antibiotic Select. (Outpatient)	-	-	95%	94%
Prophylactic Antibiotic Stopped[5]	0	-	96%	94%
Recommended VTP Ordered[5]	0	-	95%	94%
Urinary Catheter Removal[5]	0	-	91%	90%
Children's Asthma Care				
Received Systemic Corticosteroids	-	-	100%	100%
Received Home Management Plan	-	-	75%	71%
Received Reliever Medication	-	-	100%	100%
Use of Medical Imaging				
Combination Abdominal CT Scan	-	-	0.115	0.191
Combination Chest CT Scan	-	-	0.037	0.054
Follow-up Mammogram/Ultrasound	-	-	7.9%	8.4%
MRI for Low Back Pain	-	-	30.6%	32.7%
Survey of Patients' Hospital Experiences				
Area Around Room 'Always' Quiet at Night[6]	<100	68%	-	58%
Doctors 'Always' Communicated Well[6]	<100	79%	-	80%
Home Recovery Information Given[6]	<100	68%	-	82%
Hospital Given 9 or 10 on 10 Point Scale[6]	<100	54%	-	67%
Meds 'Always' Explained Before Given[6]	<100	46%	-	60%
Nurses 'Always' Communicated Well[6]	<100	74%	-	76%
Pain 'Always' Well Controlled[6]	<100	62%	-	69%
Room and Bathroom 'Always' Clean[6]	<100	69%	-	71%
Timely Help 'Always' Received[6]	<100	60%	-	64%
Would Definitely Recommend Hospital	<100	60%	-	69%

Carolinas Medical Center-Union

600 Hospital Dr
Monroe, NC 28110
Phone: 704-283-3100
Fax: 704-296-4175
Type: Acute Care Hospitals
Emergency Services: Yes
Ownership: Govt - Hospital Dist/Auth
Beds: 157

Key Personnel:
CEO/President.............. Michael Lutes
Cardiac Laboratory............ Steve Dence
Chief of Medical Staff.......... Dan Hagler
Coronary Care................ Steve Dence
Infection Control............. Janet Little
Operating Room.............. Edward Bower
Radiology.................. John Adams

Measure	Cases	This Hosp.	State Avg.	U.S. Avg.
Heart Attack Care				
ACE Inhibitor or ARB for LVSD[1]	6	100%	97%	96%
Aspirin at Arrival	70	100%	99%	99%
Aspirin at Discharge	40	100%	99%	98%
Beta Blocker at Discharge	42	100%	99%	98%
Fibrinolytic Medication Timing	0	-	38%	55%
PCI Within 90 Minutes of Arrival	0	-	95%	90%
Smoking Cessation Advice[1]	10	100%	100%	99%
Chest Pain/Possible Heart Attack Care				
Aspirin at Arrival	147	96%	95%	95%
Median Time to ECG (minutes)	145	9	8	8
Median Time to Transfer (minutes)	43	41	48	61
Fibrinolytic Medication Timing	0	-	53%	54%
Heart Failure Care				
ACE Inhibitor or ARB for LVSD	133	98%	95%	94%
Discharge Instructions	323	98%	89%	88%
Evaluation of LVS Function	356	100%	99%	98%
Smoking Cessation Advice	68	100%	99%	98%
Pneumonia Care				
Appropriate Initial Antibiotic[2]	89	94%	92%	92%
Blood Culture Timing[2]	137	98%	96%	96%
Influenza Vaccine[2]	83	95%	93%	91%
Initial Antibiotic Timing[2]	128	98%	95%	95%
Pneumococcal Vaccine[2]	109	96%	95%	93%
Smoking Cessation Advice[2]	75	100%	99%	97%
Surgical Care Improvement Project				
Appropriate VTP Within 24 Hours[2]	212	97%	93%	92%
Appropriate Hair Removal[2]	359	100%	100%	99%
Appropriate Beta Blocker Usage[2]	69	96%	94%	93%
Controlled Postoperative Blood Glucose[2]	0	-	94%	93%
Prophylactic Antibiotic Timing[2]	235	100%	98%	97%
Prophylactic Antibiotic Timing (Outpatient)	170	95%	94%	92%
Prophylactic Antibiotic Selection[2]	235	99%	98%	97%
Prophylactic Antibiotic Select. (Outpatient)	166	96%	95%	94%
Prophylactic Antibiotic Stopped[2]	216	97%	96%	94%
Recommended VTP Ordered[2]	212	98%	95%	94%
Urinary Catheter Removal[2]	71	89%	91%	90%
Children's Asthma Care				
Received Systemic Corticosteroids	-	-	100%	100%
Received Home Management Plan	-	-	75%	71%
Received Reliever Medication	-	-	100%	100%
Use of Medical Imaging				
Combination Abdominal CT Scan	1,185	0.090	0.115	0.191
Combination Chest CT Scan	896	0.148	0.037	0.054
Follow-up Mammogram/Ultrasound[1]	9	0.0%	7.9%	8.4%
MRI for Low Back Pain	232	28.9%	30.6%	32.7%
Survey of Patients' Hospital Experiences				
Area Around Room 'Always' Quiet at Night	300+	63%	-	58%
Doctors 'Always' Communicated Well	300+	83%	-	80%
Home Recovery Information Given	300+	86%	-	82%
Hospital Given 9 or 10 on 10 Point Scale	300+	72%	-	67%
Meds 'Always' Explained Before Given	300+	65%	-	60%
Nurses 'Always' Communicated Well	300+	83%	-	76%
Pain 'Always' Well Controlled	300+	73%	-	69%
Room and Bathroom 'Always' Clean	300+	71%	-	71%
Timely Help 'Always' Received	300+	71%	-	64%
Would Definitely Recommend Hospital	300+	70%	-	69%

NOTE: Hospital profiles are in alphabetical order by state, then city, then hospital within the city; Rankings exclude hospitals with less than 25 cases except for patient surveys which excludes hospitals with less than 100 cases; (a) 100–299 cases; (1) The number of cases is too small to be sure how well a hospital is performing; (2) The hospital indicated that the data submitted for this measure were based on a sample of cases; (3) Data was collected during a shorter time period (fewer quarters) than the maximum possible time for this measure; (4) Suppressed for one or more quarters by CMS; (5) No data is available from the hospital for this measure; (6) Fewer than 100 patients completed the HCAHPS survey. Use these rates with caution, as the number of surveys may be too low to reliably assess hospital performance; (7) Survey results are based on less than 12 months of data; (8) Survey results are not available for this reporting period; (9) No or very few patients were eligible for the HCAHPS survey. The scores shown, if any, reflect a very small number of surveys; (10) A state average was not calculated because too few hospitals in the state submitted data; (11) There were discrepancies in the data collection process; Please refer to the User's Guide for a full explanation of data.

Lake Norman Regional Medical Center

171 Fairview Road Phone: 704-660-4000
Mooresville, NC 28117 Fax: 704-660-4005
E-mail: information@lnrmc.hma-corp.com
URL: www.lnrmc.com
Type: Acute Care Hospitals Emergency Services: Yes
Ownership: Proprietary Beds: 117

Key Personnel:
Chief of Medical Staff. . . . . Steven Bradley, MD
Coronary Care. . . . . Deborah Dickens
Infection Control. . . . . Brynne Beaver
Operating Room. . . . . Michelle Bertsch
Pediatric In-Patient Care . . . . . . Kristy Miller
Quality Assurance . . . . Ann Allen
Radiology. . . . . Teresa Lother

Measure	Cases	This Hosp.	State Avg.	U.S. Avg.
Heart Attack Care				
ACE Inhibitor or ARB for LVSD[1]	14	100%	97%	96%
Aspirin at Arrival	76	100%	99%	99%
Aspirin at Discharge	55	100%	99%	98%
Beta Blocker at Discharge	54	100%	99%	98%
Fibrinolytic Medication Timing[1]	1	100%	38%	55%
PCI Within 90 Minutes of Arrival	0	-	95%	90%
Smoking Cessation Advice[1]	17	100%	100%	99%
Chest Pain/Possible Heart Attack Care				
Aspirin at Arrival	61	100%	95%	95%
Median Time to ECG (minutes)	62	4	8	8
Median Time to Transfer (minutes)[1]	23	26	48	61
Fibrinolytic Medication Timing	0	-	53%	54%
Heart Failure Care				
ACE Inhibitor or ARB for LVSD	41	100%	95%	94%
Discharge Instructions	115	92%	89%	88%
Evaluation of LVS Function	161	99%	99%	98%
Smoking Cessation Advice	27	100%	99%	98%
Pneumonia Care				
Appropriate Initial Antibiotic	69	99%	92%	92%
Blood Culture Timing	97	100%	96%	96%
Influenza Vaccine	68	100%	93%	91%
Initial Antibiotic Timing	103	96%	95%	95%
Pneumococcal Vaccine	87	100%	95%	93%
Smoking Cessation Advice	50	100%	99%	97%
Surgical Care Improvement Project				
Appropriate VTP Within 24 Hours	171	96%	93%	92%
Appropriate Hair Removal	377	100%	100%	99%
Appropriate Beta Blocker Usage	74	99%	94%	93%
Controlled Postoperative Blood Glucose	0	-	94%	93%
Prophylactic Antibiotic Timing	225	99%	98%	97%
Prophylactic Antibiotic Timing (Outpatient)	469	100%	94%	92%
Prophylactic Antibiotic Selection	227	98%	98%	97%
Prophylactic Antibiotic Select. (Outpatient)	468	97%	95%	94%
Prophylactic Antibiotic Stopped	201	99%	96%	94%
Recommended VTP Ordered	172	97%	95%	94%
Urinary Catheter Removal	70	99%	91%	90%
Children's Asthma Care				
Received Systemic Corticosteroids	25	100%	100%	100%
Received Home Management Plan[1]	23	100%	75%	71%
Received Reliever Medication	25	100%	100%	100%
Use of Medical Imaging				
Combination Abdominal CT Scan	858	0.080	0.115	0.191
Combination Chest CT Scan	620	0.010	0.037	0.054
Follow-up Mammogram/Ultrasound	1,339	7.9%	7.9%	8.4%
MRI for Low Back Pain	140	25.7%	30.6%	32.7%
Survey of Patients' Hospital Experiences				
Area Around Room 'Always' Quiet at Night	300+	58%	-	58%
Doctors 'Always' Communicated Well	300+	84%	-	80%
Home Recovery Information Given	300+	86%	-	82%
Hospital Given 9 or 10 on 10 Point Scale	300+	70%	-	67%
Meds 'Always' Explained Before Given	300+	62%	-	60%
Nurses 'Always' Communicated Well	300+	76%	-	76%
Pain 'Always' Well Controlled	300+	71%	-	69%
Room and Bathroom 'Always' Clean	300+	73%	-	71%
Timely Help 'Always' Received	300+	65%	-	64%
Would Definitely Recommend Hospital	300+	72%	-	69%

Carteret General Hospital

3500 Arendell St Phone: 252-808-6000
Morehead City, NC 28557 Fax: 252-808-6916
E-mail: PR@ccgh.org
URL: www.ccgh.org
Type: Acute Care Hospitals Emergency Services: Yes
Ownership: Government - Local Beds: 117

Key Personnel:
CEO/President. . . . . Fred A Odell, III, III
Cardiac Laboratory. . . . . John Gould, MD
Chief of Medical Staff . . . . Leon Morrison, MD
Infection Control. . . . . Elaine Crittonton
Operating Room. . . . . Michael Bell
Pediatric In-Patient Care . . . . . . Callie Young
Quality Assurance . . . . Martha Kenworthy, RN
Radiology. . . . . S Joseph Buff

Measure	Cases	This Hosp.	State Avg.	U.S. Avg.
Heart Attack Care				
ACE Inhibitor or ARB for LVSD[1]	12	100%	97%	96%
Aspirin at Arrival	117	99%	99%	99%
Aspirin at Discharge	55	93%	99%	98%
Beta Blocker at Discharge	53	91%	99%	98%
Fibrinolytic Medication Timing[1]	1	0%	38%	55%
PCI Within 90 Minutes of Arrival	0	-	95%	90%
Smoking Cessation Advice[1]	13	100%	100%	99%
Chest Pain/Possible Heart Attack Care				
Aspirin at Arrival	111	97%	95%	95%
Median Time to ECG (minutes)	113	11	8	8
Median Time to Transfer (minutes)[1]	5	169	48	61
Fibrinolytic Medication Timing[1]	19	32%	53%	54%
Heart Failure Care				
ACE Inhibitor or ARB for LVSD	74	91%	95%	94%
Discharge Instructions	193	89%	89%	88%
Evaluation of LVS Function	251	99%	99%	98%
Smoking Cessation Advice	40	100%	99%	98%
Pneumonia Care				
Appropriate Initial Antibiotic	95	88%	92%	92%
Blood Culture Timing	129	97%	96%	96%
Influenza Vaccine	94	94%	93%	91%
Initial Antibiotic Timing	142	92%	95%	95%
Pneumococcal Vaccine	110	96%	95%	93%
Smoking Cessation Advice	54	98%	99%	97%
Surgical Care Improvement Project				
Appropriate VTP Within 24 Hours	155	72%	93%	92%
Appropriate Hair Removal	497	100%	100%	99%
Appropriate Beta Blocker Usage	118	94%	94%	93%
Controlled Postoperative Blood Glucose	0	-	94%	93%
Prophylactic Antibiotic Timing	306	98%	98%	97%
Prophylactic Antibiotic Timing (Outpatient)	152	99%	94%	92%
Prophylactic Antibiotic Selection	306	100%	98%	97%
Prophylactic Antibiotic Select. (Outpatient)	152	95%	95%	94%
Prophylactic Antibiotic Stopped	297	98%	96%	94%
Recommended VTP Ordered	155	77%	95%	94%
Urinary Catheter Removal	30	60%	91%	90%
Children's Asthma Care				
Received Systemic Corticosteroids	-	-	100%	100%
Received Home Management Plan	-	-	75%	71%
Received Reliever Medication	-	-	100%	100%
Use of Medical Imaging				
Combination Abdominal CT Scan	909	0.059	0.115	0.191
Combination Chest CT Scan	658	0.000	0.037	0.054
Follow-up Mammogram/Ultrasound	1,516	9.6%	7.9%	8.4%
MRI for Low Back Pain	166	29.5%	30.6%	32.7%
Survey of Patients' Hospital Experiences				
Area Around Room 'Always' Quiet at Night	300+	61%	-	58%
Doctors 'Always' Communicated Well	300+	81%	-	80%
Home Recovery Information Given	300+	79%	-	82%
Hospital Given 9 or 10 on 10 Point Scale	300+	68%	-	67%
Meds 'Always' Explained Before Given	300+	63%	-	60%
Nurses 'Always' Communicated Well	300+	80%	-	76%
Pain 'Always' Well Controlled	300+	72%	-	69%
Room and Bathroom 'Always' Clean	300+	72%	-	71%
Timely Help 'Always' Received	300+	72%	-	64%
Would Definitely Recommend Hospital	300+	71%	-	69%

Grace Hospital

2201 S Sterling St Phone: 828-580-5000
Morganton, NC 28655 Fax: 828-580-5509
URL: www.gracehcs.org
Type: Acute Care Hospitals Emergency Services: Yes
Ownership: Proprietary Beds: 269

Key Personnel:
CEO/President. . . . . Kenneth W Wood

Measure	Cases	This Hosp.	State Avg.	U.S. Avg.
Heart Attack Care				
ACE Inhibitor or ARB for LVSD[1]	8	100%	97%	96%
Aspirin at Arrival	51	98%	99%	99%
Aspirin at Discharge	34	100%	99%	98%
Beta Blocker at Discharge	37	100%	99%	98%
Fibrinolytic Medication Timing	0	-	38%	55%
PCI Within 90 Minutes of Arrival	0	-	95%	90%
Smoking Cessation Advice[1]	12	100%	100%	99%
Chest Pain/Possible Heart Attack Care				
Aspirin at Arrival	72	94%	95%	95%
Median Time to ECG (minutes)	78	12	8	8
Median Time to Transfer (minutes)	29	46	48	61
Fibrinolytic Medication Timing	0	-	53%	54%
Heart Failure Care				
ACE Inhibitor or ARB for LVSD	44	93%	95%	94%
Discharge Instructions	97	97%	89%	88%
Evaluation of LVS Function	124	97%	99%	98%
Smoking Cessation Advice	30	100%	99%	98%
Pneumonia Care				
Appropriate Initial Antibiotic	112	87%	92%	92%
Blood Culture Timing	204	98%	96%	96%
Influenza Vaccine	129	99%	93%	91%
Initial Antibiotic Timing	181	97%	95%	95%
Pneumococcal Vaccine	162	99%	95%	93%
Smoking Cessation Advice	84	99%	99%	97%
Surgical Care Improvement Project				
Appropriate VTP Within 24 Hours	136	76%	93%	92%
Appropriate Hair Removal	240	100%	100%	99%
Appropriate Beta Blocker Usage	47	89%	94%	93%
Controlled Postoperative Blood Glucose	0	-	94%	93%
Prophylactic Antibiotic Timing	129	95%	98%	97%
Prophylactic Antibiotic Timing (Outpatient)	333	96%	94%	92%
Prophylactic Antibiotic Selection	128	98%	98%	97%
Prophylactic Antibiotic Select. (Outpatient)	324	92%	95%	94%
Prophylactic Antibiotic Stopped	117	92%	96%	94%
Recommended VTP Ordered	139	77%	95%	94%
Urinary Catheter Removal	50	96%	91%	90%
Children's Asthma Care				
Received Systemic Corticosteroids	-	-	100%	100%
Received Home Management Plan	-	-	75%	71%
Received Reliever Medication	-	-	100%	100%
Use of Medical Imaging				
Combination Abdominal CT Scan	302	0.116	0.115	0.191
Combination Chest CT Scan	271	0.011	0.037	0.054
Follow-up Mammogram/Ultrasound	499	16.2%	7.9%	8.4%
MRI for Low Back Pain	106	32.1%	30.6%	32.7%
Survey of Patients' Hospital Experiences				
Area Around Room 'Always' Quiet at Night	300+	67%	-	58%
Doctors 'Always' Communicated Well	300+	83%	-	80%
Home Recovery Information Given	300+	85%	-	82%
Hospital Given 9 or 10 on 10 Point Scale	300+	66%	-	67%
Meds 'Always' Explained Before Given	300+	65%	-	60%
Nurses 'Always' Communicated Well	300+	78%	-	76%
Pain 'Always' Well Controlled	300+	68%	-	69%
Room and Bathroom 'Always' Clean	300+	72%	-	71%
Timely Help 'Always' Received	300+	63%	-	64%
Would Definitely Recommend Hospital	300+	66%	-	69%

NOTE: Hospital profiles are in alphabetical order by state, then city, then hospital within the city; Rankings exclude hospitals with less than 25 cases except for patient surveys which excludes hospitals with less than 100 cases; (a) 100–299 cases; (1) The number of cases is too small to be sure how well a hospital is performing; (2) The hospital indicated that the data submitted for this measure were based on a sample of cases; (3) Data was collected during a shorter time period (fewer quarters) than the maximum possible time for this measure; (4) Suppressed for one or more quarters by CMS; (5) No data is available from the hospital for this measure; (6) Fewer than 100 patients completed the HCAHPS survey. Use these rates with caution, as the number of surveys may be too low to reliably assess hospital performance; (7) Survey results are based on less than 12 months of data; (8) Survey results are not available for this reporting period; (9) No or very few patients were eligible for the HCAHPS survey. The scores shown, if any, reflect a very small number of surveys; (10) A state average was not calculated because too few hospitals in the state submitted data; (11) There were discrepancies in the data collection process; Please refer to the User's Guide for a full explanation of data.

Northern Hospital of Surry County

830 Rockford St Phone: 336-719-7000
Mount Airy, NC 27030 Fax: 336-789-3470
URL: www.northernhospital.com
Type: Acute Care Hospitals Emergency Services: Yes
Ownership: Govt - Hospital Dist/Auth Beds: 113

Key Personnel:
CEO/President.............. William James
Chief of Medical Staff.......... Bill Refvem, MD
Coronary Care.............. Randy Collins, RN
Infection Control.............. Debbie Borawski, RN
Operating Room.............. Terri Grace, RN
Quality Assurance........... Deborah Borawski
Radiology.................. Eric S Scharling

Measure	Cases	This Hosp.	State Avg.	U.S. Avg.
Heart Attack Care				
ACE Inhibitor or ARB for LVSD[1]	6	100%	97%	96%
Aspirin at Arrival[1]	15	100%	99%	99%
Aspirin at Discharge[1]	8	100%	99%	98%
Beta Blocker at Discharge[1]	12	100%	99%	98%
Fibrinolytic Medication Timing	0	-	38%	55%
PCI Within 90 Minutes of Arrival	0	-	95%	90%
Smoking Cessation Advice[1]	4	100%	100%	99%
Chest Pain/Possible Heart Attack Care				
Aspirin at Arrival	255	98%	95%	95%
Median Time to ECG (minutes)	264	12	8	8
Median Time to Transfer (minutes)[1]	9	40	48	61
Fibrinolytic Medication Timing[1]	4	100%	53%	54%
Heart Failure Care				
ACE Inhibitor or ARB for LVSD	40	95%	95%	94%
Discharge Instructions	145	97%	89%	88%
Evaluation of LVS Function	167	99%	99%	98%
Smoking Cessation Advice	28	96%	99%	98%
Pneumonia Care				
Appropriate Initial Antibiotic	119	94%	92%	92%
Blood Culture Timing	216	96%	96%	96%
Influenza Vaccine	146	92%	93%	91%
Initial Antibiotic Timing	203	95%	95%	95%
Pneumococcal Vaccine	190	88%	95%	93%
Smoking Cessation Advice	92	99%	99%	97%
Surgical Care Improvement Project				
Appropriate VTP Within 24 Hours	126	92%	93%	92%
Appropriate Hair Removal	337	100%	100%	99%
Appropriate Beta Blocker Usage	101	78%	94%	93%
Controlled Postoperative Blood Glucose	0	-	94%	93%
Prophylactic Antibiotic Timing	235	96%	98%	97%
Prophylactic Antibiotic Timing (Outpatient)	70	89%	94%	92%
Prophylactic Antibiotic Selection	235	99%	98%	97%
Prophylactic Antibiotic Select. (Outpatient)	68	88%	95%	94%
Prophylactic Antibiotic Stopped	231	98%	96%	94%
Recommended VTP Ordered	126	99%	95%	94%
Urinary Catheter Removal	25	68%	91%	90%
Children's Asthma Care				
Received Systemic Corticosteroids	-	-	100%	100%
Received Home Management Plan	-	-	75%	71%
Received Reliever Medication	-	-	100%	100%
Use of Medical Imaging				
Combination Abdominal CT Scan	986	0.108	0.115	0.191
Combination Chest CT Scan	786	0.000	0.037	0.054
Follow-up Mammogram/Ultrasound	1,137	6.5%	7.9%	8.4%
MRI for Low Back Pain	164	31.1%	30.6%	32.7%
Survey of Patients' Hospital Experiences				
Area Around Room 'Always' Quiet at Night	300+	58%	-	58%
Doctors 'Always' Communicated Well	300+	78%	-	80%
Home Recovery Information Given	300+	82%	-	82%
Hospital Given 9 or 10 on 10 Point Scale	300+	61%	-	67%
Meds 'Always' Explained Before Given	300+	54%	-	60%
Nurses 'Always' Communicated Well	300+	75%	-	76%
Pain 'Always' Well Controlled	300+	68%	-	69%
Room and Bathroom 'Always' Clean	300+	78%	-	71%
Timely Help 'Always' Received	300+	65%	-	64%
Would Definitely Recommend Hospital	300+	60%	-	69%

Murphy Medical Center

3990 East Us Highway 64 Alt Phone: 828-837-8161
Murphy, NC 28906 Fax: 828-835-7507
Type: Acute Care Hospitals Emergency Services: Yes
Ownership: Voluntary Non-Profit - Private Beds: 184

Key Personnel:
CEO/President.............. Mark Stevenson
Chief of Medical Staff.......... Steven Zimmer, MD
Quality Assurance........... Sherrie Maze
Emergency Room........... Dr. Mark Walters

Measure	Cases	This Hosp.	State Avg.	U.S. Avg.
Heart Attack Care				
ACE Inhibitor or ARB for LVSD[1]	2	50%	97%	96%
Aspirin at Arrival[1]	20	100%	99%	99%
Aspirin at Discharge[1]	8	100%	99%	98%
Beta Blocker at Discharge[1]	6	83%	99%	98%
Fibrinolytic Medication Timing[1]	1	100%	38%	55%
PCI Within 90 Minutes of Arrival	0	-	95%	90%
Smoking Cessation Advice[1]	1	100%	100%	99%
Chest Pain/Possible Heart Attack Care				
Aspirin at Arrival	127	94%	95%	95%
Median Time to ECG (minutes)	133	9	8	8
Median Time to Transfer (minutes)[3]	0	-	48	61
Fibrinolytic Medication Timing[1]	14	50%	53%	54%
Heart Failure Care				
ACE Inhibitor or ARB for LVSD	25	88%	95%	94%
Discharge Instructions	54	70%	89%	88%
Evaluation of LVS Function	78	97%	99%	98%
Smoking Cessation Advice[1]	5	100%	99%	98%
Pneumonia Care				
Appropriate Initial Antibiotic	88	89%	92%	92%
Blood Culture Timing	129	95%	96%	96%
Influenza Vaccine	83	93%	93%	91%
Initial Antibiotic Timing	138	93%	95%	95%
Pneumococcal Vaccine	116	87%	95%	93%
Smoking Cessation Advice	51	98%	99%	97%
Surgical Care Improvement Project				
Appropriate VTP Within 24 Hours	64	84%	93%	92%
Appropriate Hair Removal	168	100%	100%	99%
Appropriate Beta Blocker Usage	40	85%	94%	93%
Controlled Postoperative Blood Glucose	0	-	94%	93%
Prophylactic Antibiotic Timing	117	97%	98%	97%
Prophylactic Antibiotic Timing (Outpatient)	27	89%	94%	92%
Prophylactic Antibiotic Selection	119	93%	98%	97%
Prophylactic Antibiotic Select. (Outpatient)	25	92%	95%	94%
Prophylactic Antibiotic Stopped	116	96%	96%	94%
Recommended VTP Ordered	64	84%	95%	94%
Urinary Catheter Removal	33	91%	91%	90%
Children's Asthma Care				
Received Systemic Corticosteroids	-	-	100%	100%
Received Home Management Plan	-	-	75%	71%
Received Reliever Medication	-	-	100%	100%
Use of Medical Imaging				
Combination Abdominal CT Scan	755	0.366	0.115	0.191
Combination Chest CT Scan	473	0.006	0.037	0.054
Follow-up Mammogram/Ultrasound	786	3.1%	7.9%	8.4%
MRI for Low Back Pain	151	29.1%	30.6%	32.7%
Survey of Patients' Hospital Experiences				
Area Around Room 'Always' Quiet at Night	300+	53%	-	58%
Doctors 'Always' Communicated Well	300+	83%	-	80%
Home Recovery Information Given	300+	82%	-	82%
Hospital Given 9 or 10 on 10 Point Scale	300+	63%	-	67%
Meds 'Always' Explained Before Given	300+	58%	-	60%
Nurses 'Always' Communicated Well	300+	77%	-	76%
Pain 'Always' Well Controlled	300+	69%	-	69%
Room and Bathroom 'Always' Clean	300+	72%	-	71%
Timely Help 'Always' Received	300+	65%	-	64%
Would Definitely Recommend Hospital	300+	67%	-	69%

The Outer Banks Hospital

4800 South Croatan Highway Phone: 252-449-4500
Nags Head, NC 27959
URL: www.theouterbankshospital.com
Type: Critical Access Hospitals Emergency Services: Yes
Ownership: Voluntary Non-Profit - Private Beds: 19

Key Personnel:
CEO/President.............. D. Van Smith, Jr.

Measure	Cases	This Hosp.	State Avg.	U.S. Avg.
Heart Attack Care				
ACE Inhibitor or ARB for LVSD[3]	0	-	97%	96%
Aspirin at Arrival[3]	0	-	99%	99%
Aspirin at Discharge[3]	0	-	99%	98%
Beta Blocker at Discharge[3]	0	-	99%	98%
Fibrinolytic Medication Timing[3]	0	-	38%	55%
PCI Within 90 Minutes of Arrival[3]	0	-	95%	90%
Smoking Cessation Advice[3]	0	-	100%	99%
Chest Pain/Possible Heart Attack Care				
Aspirin at Arrival	-	-	95%	95%
Median Time to ECG (minutes)	-	-	8	8
Median Time to Transfer (minutes)	-	-	48	61
Fibrinolytic Medication Timing	-	-	53%	54%
Heart Failure Care				
ACE Inhibitor or ARB for LVSD[1]	4	100%	95%	94%
Discharge Instructions[1]	7	100%	89%	88%
Evaluation of LVS Function[1]	11	100%	99%	98%
Smoking Cessation Advice[1]	2	100%	99%	98%
Pneumonia Care				
Appropriate Initial Antibiotic	39	95%	92%	92%
Blood Culture Timing	48	94%	96%	96%
Influenza Vaccine[1]	18	100%	93%	91%
Initial Antibiotic Timing	32	100%	95%	95%
Pneumococcal Vaccine	39	100%	95%	93%
Smoking Cessation Advice[1]	18	100%	99%	97%
Surgical Care Improvement Project				
Appropriate VTP Within 24 Hours	37	100%	93%	92%
Appropriate Hair Removal	109	100%	100%	99%
Appropriate Beta Blocker Usage[1]	21	81%	94%	93%
Controlled Postoperative Blood Glucose	0	-	94%	93%
Prophylactic Antibiotic Timing	85	98%	98%	97%
Prophylactic Antibiotic Timing (Outpatient)	-	-	94%	92%
Prophylactic Antibiotic Selection	85	99%	98%	97%
Prophylactic Antibiotic Select. (Outpatient)	-	-	95%	94%
Prophylactic Antibiotic Stopped	80	100%	96%	94%
Recommended VTP Ordered	37	100%	95%	94%
Urinary Catheter Removal	48	100%	91%	90%
Children's Asthma Care				
Received Systemic Corticosteroids	-	-	100%	100%
Received Home Management Plan	-	-	75%	71%
Received Reliever Medication	-	-	100%	100%
Use of Medical Imaging				
Combination Abdominal CT Scan	-	-	0.115	0.191
Combination Chest CT Scan	-	-	0.037	0.054
Follow-up Mammogram/Ultrasound	-	-	7.9%	8.4%
MRI for Low Back Pain	-	-	30.6%	32.7%
Survey of Patients' Hospital Experiences				
Area Around Room 'Always' Quiet at Night	300+	66%	-	58%
Doctors 'Always' Communicated Well	300+	85%	-	80%
Home Recovery Information Given	300+	88%	-	82%
Hospital Given 9 or 10 on 10 Point Scale	300+	78%	-	67%
Meds 'Always' Explained Before Given	300+	70%	-	60%
Nurses 'Always' Communicated Well	300+	81%	-	76%
Pain 'Always' Well Controlled	300+	74%	-	69%
Room and Bathroom 'Always' Clean	300+	76%	-	71%
Timely Help 'Always' Received	300+	79%	-	64%
Would Definitely Recommend Hospital	300+	75%	-	69%

NOTE: Hospital profiles are in alphabetical order by state, then city, then hospital within the city; Rankings exclude hospitals with less than 25 cases except for patient surveys which excludes hospitals with less than 100 cases; (a) 100–299 cases; (1) The number of cases is too small to be sure how well a hospital is performing; (2) The hospital indicated that the data submitted for this measure were based on a sample of cases; (3) Data was collected during a shorter time period (fewer quarters) than the maximum possible time for this measure; (4) Suppressed for one or more quarters by CMS; (5) No data is available from the hospital for this measure; (6) Fewer than 100 patients completed the HCAHPS survey. Use these rates with caution, as the number of surveys may be too low to reliably assess hospital performance; (7) Survey results are based on less than 12 months of data; (8) Survey results are not available for this reporting period; (9) No or very few patients were eligible for the HCAHPS survey. The scores shown, if any, reflect a very small number of surveys; (10) A state average was not calculated because too few hospitals in the state submitted data; (11) There were discrepancies in the data collection process; Please refer to the User's Guide for a full explanation of data.

Carolina East Medical Center

2000 Neuse Blvd
New Bern, NC 28560
URL: www.cravenhealthcare.org
Type: Acute Care Hospitals
Ownership: Govt - Hospital Dist/Auth

Phone: 252-633-8640
Fax: 252-633-8144

Emergency Services: Yes
Beds: 350

Key Personnel:
CEO/President. . . . . G Raymond Leggett
Chief of Medical Staff. . . . . Ron May MD
Infection Control. . . . . Cathy Fischer
Operating Room. . . . . Robin Schaefer
Pediatric In-Patient Care . . . . Cyndi Morton RN
Quality Assurance . . . . Pam Burkett
Radiology. . . . . David Williams
Patient Relations . . . . Leslie Pittman

Measure	Cases	This Hosp.	State Avg.	U.S. Avg.
Heart Attack Care				
ACE Inhibitor or ARB for LVSD	83	93%	97%	96%
Aspirin at Arrival	315	99%	99%	99%
Aspirin at Discharge	399	99%	99%	98%
Beta Blocker at Discharge	365	96%	99%	98%
Fibrinolytic Medication Timing	0	-	38%	55%
PCI Within 90 Minutes of Arrival	75	93%	95%	90%
Smoking Cessation Advice	146	100%	100%	99%
Chest Pain/Possible Heart Attack Care				
Aspirin at Arrival[1,3]	10	90%	95%	95%
Median Time to ECG (minutes)[1,3]	11	6	8	8
Median Time to Transfer (minutes)[1,3]	1	447	48	61
Fibrinolytic Medication Timing[3]	0	-	53%	54%
Heart Failure Care				
ACE Inhibitor or ARB for LVSD	173	86%	95%	94%
Discharge Instructions	483	59%	89%	88%
Evaluation of LVS Function	529	98%	99%	98%
Smoking Cessation Advice	102	100%	99%	98%
Pneumonia Care				
Appropriate Initial Antibiotic	147	93%	92%	92%
Blood Culture Timing	300	95%	96%	96%
Influenza Vaccine	204	78%	93%	91%
Initial Antibiotic Timing	283	95%	95%	95%
Pneumococcal Vaccine	258	82%	95%	93%
Smoking Cessation Advice	142	99%	99%	97%
Surgical Care Improvement Project				
Appropriate VTP Within 24 Hours	665	93%	93%	92%
Appropriate Hair Removal	1,419	100%	100%	99%
Appropriate Beta Blocker Usage	383	83%	94%	93%
Controlled Postoperative Blood Glucose	198	74%	94%	93%
Prophylactic Antibiotic Timing	1,028	96%	98%	97%
Prophylactic Antibiotic Timing (Outpatient)	589	92%	94%	92%
Prophylactic Antibiotic Selection	1,031	97%	98%	97%
Prophylactic Antibiotic Select. (Outpatient)	571	94%	95%	94%
Prophylactic Antibiotic Stopped	1,004	88%	96%	94%
Recommended VTP Ordered	667	93%	95%	94%
Urinary Catheter Removal	422	76%	91%	90%
Children's Asthma Care				
Received Systemic Corticosteroids	-	-	100%	100%
Received Home Management Plan			75%	71%
Received Reliever Medication			100%	100%
Use of Medical Imaging				
Combination Abdominal CT Scan	598	0.069	0.115	0.191
Combination Chest CT Scan	244	0.029	0.037	0.054
Follow-up Mammogram/Ultrasound	1,119	8.9%	7.9%	8.4%
MRI for Low Back Pain	176	32.4%	30.6%	32.7%
Survey of Patients' Hospital Experiences				
Area Around Room 'Always' Quiet at Night	300+	56%	-	58%
Doctors 'Always' Communicated Well	300+	75%	-	80%
Home Recovery Information Given	300+	82%	-	82%
Hospital Given 9 or 10 on 10 Point Scale	300+	59%	-	67%
Meds 'Always' Explained Before Given	300+	55%	-	60%
Nurses 'Always' Communicated Well	300+	73%	-	76%
Pain 'Always' Well Controlled	300+	67%	-	69%
Room and Bathroom 'Always' Clean	300+	57%	-	71%
Timely Help 'Always' Received	300+	63%	-	64%
Would Definitely Recommend Hospital	300+	66%	-	69%

Wilkes Regional Medical Center

1370 West D St
North Wilkesboro, NC 28659
URL: www.wilkesregional.com
Type: Acute Care Hospitals
Ownership: Government - Local

Phone: 336-651-8100
Fax: 336-651-8196

Emergency Services: Yes
Beds: 120

Key Personnel:
CEO/President. . . . . David Henson
Chief of Medical Staff. . . . . Susan Albert
Radiology. . . . . Gregory Evans

Measure	Cases	This Hosp.	State Avg.	U.S. Avg.
Heart Attack Care				
ACE Inhibitor or ARB for LVSD	0	-	97%	96%
Aspirin at Arrival[1]	14	93%	99%	99%
Aspirin at Discharge[1]	8	100%	99%	98%
Beta Blocker at Discharge[1]	6	100%	99%	98%
Fibrinolytic Medication Timing	0	-	38%	55%
PCI Within 90 Minutes of Arrival	0	-	95%	90%
Smoking Cessation Advice[1]	1	100%	100%	99%
Chest Pain/Possible Heart Attack Care				
Aspirin at Arrival	284	99%	95%	95%
Median Time to ECG (minutes)	291	6	8	8
Median Time to Transfer (minutes)[1]	2	31	48	61
Fibrinolytic Medication Timing[1]	4	75%	53%	54%
Heart Failure Care				
ACE Inhibitor or ARB for LVSD	32	97%	95%	94%
Discharge Instructions	86	92%	89%	88%
Evaluation of LVS Function	117	99%	99%	98%
Smoking Cessation Advice[1]	18	100%	99%	98%
Pneumonia Care				
Appropriate Initial Antibiotic	139	89%	92%	92%
Blood Culture Timing	217	98%	96%	96%
Influenza Vaccine	126	94%	93%	91%
Initial Antibiotic Timing	195	99%	95%	95%
Pneumococcal Vaccine	198	97%	95%	93%
Smoking Cessation Advice	77	95%	99%	97%
Surgical Care Improvement Project				
Appropriate VTP Within 24 Hours	83	89%	93%	92%
Appropriate Hair Removal	168	100%	100%	99%
Appropriate Beta Blocker Usage	35	100%	94%	93%
Controlled Postoperative Blood Glucose	0	-	94%	93%
Prophylactic Antibiotic Timing	111	98%	98%	97%
Prophylactic Antibiotic Timing (Outpatient)[1]	20	80%	94%	92%
Prophylactic Antibiotic Selection	110	88%	98%	97%
Prophylactic Antibiotic Select. (Outpatient)[1]	16	88%	95%	94%
Prophylactic Antibiotic Stopped	102	92%	96%	94%
Recommended VTP Ordered	83	90%	95%	94%
Urinary Catheter Removal	43	91%	91%	90%
Children's Asthma Care				
Received Systemic Corticosteroids	-	-	100%	100%
Received Home Management Plan	-	-	75%	71%
Received Reliever Medication	-	-	100%	100%
Use of Medical Imaging				
Combination Abdominal CT Scan	743	0.105	0.115	0.191
Combination Chest CT Scan	334	0.063	0.037	0.054
Follow-up Mammogram/Ultrasound	1,388	9.3%	7.9%	8.4%
MRI for Low Back Pain	176	34.7%	30.6%	32.7%
Survey of Patients' Hospital Experiences				
Area Around Room 'Always' Quiet at Night	300+	71%	-	58%
Doctors 'Always' Communicated Well	300+	85%	-	80%
Home Recovery Information Given	300+	81%	-	82%
Hospital Given 9 or 10 on 10 Point Scale	300+	70%	-	67%
Meds 'Always' Explained Before Given	300+	66%	-	60%
Nurses 'Always' Communicated Well	300+	82%	-	76%
Pain 'Always' Well Controlled	300+	72%	-	69%
Room and Bathroom 'Always' Clean	300+	74%	-	71%
Timely Help 'Always' Received	300+	74%	-	64%
Would Definitely Recommend Hospital	300+	65%	-	69%

Granville Medical Center

College St Box 947
Oxford, NC 27565
Type: Acute Care Hospitals
Ownership: Government - Local

Phone: 919-690-3000
Fax: 919-690-1430

Emergency Services: Yes
Beds: 142

Key Personnel:
CEO/President. . . . . Joe Pollard
Chief of Medical Staff. . . . . Francine Chavis, MD
Infection Control . . . . Jeanette Briggs, RN
Quality Assurance . . . . Ann Barnes
Radiology. . . . . Michael P Stoll, MD
Anesthesiology. . . . . Allen Ng, MD
Emergency Room . . . . Robert Walston, MD
Intensive Care Unit. . . . . Stephen Ertischeck, MD

Measure	Cases	This Hosp.	State Avg.	U.S. Avg.
Heart Attack Care				
ACE Inhibitor or ARB for LVSD	0	-	97%	96%
Aspirin at Arrival[1]	17	94%	99%	99%
Aspirin at Discharge[1]	11	100%	99%	98%
Beta Blocker at Discharge[1]	10	100%	99%	98%
Fibrinolytic Medication Timing	0	-	38%	55%
PCI Within 90 Minutes of Arrival	0	-	95%	90%
Smoking Cessation Advice[1]	1	100%	100%	99%
Chest Pain/Possible Heart Attack Care				
Aspirin at Arrival	79	100%	95%	95%
Median Time to ECG (minutes)	86	6	8	8
Median Time to Transfer (minutes)[1,3]	3	29	48	61
Fibrinolytic Medication Timing	0	-	53%	54%
Heart Failure Care				
ACE Inhibitor or ARB for LVSD	35	91%	95%	94%
Discharge Instructions	94	99%	89%	88%
Evaluation of LVS Function	122	98%	99%	98%
Smoking Cessation Advice[1]	17	100%	99%	98%
Pneumonia Care				
Appropriate Initial Antibiotic	59	90%	92%	92%
Blood Culture Timing	66	95%	96%	96%
Influenza Vaccine	56	100%	93%	91%
Initial Antibiotic Timing	76	95%	95%	95%
Pneumococcal Vaccine	52	100%	95%	93%
Smoking Cessation Advice	35	100%	99%	97%
Surgical Care Improvement Project				
Appropriate VTP Within 24 Hours	88	99%	93%	92%
Appropriate Hair Removal	218	100%	100%	99%
Appropriate Beta Blocker Usage	50	94%	94%	93%
Controlled Postoperative Blood Glucose	0	-	94%	93%
Prophylactic Antibiotic Timing	147	95%	98%	97%
Prophylactic Antibiotic Timing (Outpatient)	43	93%	94%	92%
Prophylactic Antibiotic Selection	148	99%	98%	97%
Prophylactic Antibiotic Select. (Outpatient)	42	95%	95%	94%
Prophylactic Antibiotic Stopped	133	94%	96%	94%
Recommended VTP Ordered	88	99%	95%	94%
Urinary Catheter Removal	68	94%	91%	90%
Children's Asthma Care				
Received Systemic Corticosteroids	-	-	100%	100%
Received Home Management Plan	-	-	75%	71%
Received Reliever Medication	-	-	100%	100%
Use of Medical Imaging				
Combination Abdominal CT Scan	286	0.038	0.115	0.191
Combination Chest CT Scan	126	0.008	0.037	0.054
Follow-up Mammogram/Ultrasound	525	13.9%	7.9%	8.4%
MRI for Low Back Pain	116	23.3%	30.6%	32.7%
Survey of Patients' Hospital Experiences				
Area Around Room 'Always' Quiet at Night	300+	72%	-	58%
Doctors 'Always' Communicated Well	300+	84%	-	80%
Home Recovery Information Given	300+	80%	-	82%
Hospital Given 9 or 10 on 10 Point Scale	300+	67%	-	67%
Meds 'Always' Explained Before Given	300+	59%	-	60%
Nurses 'Always' Communicated Well	300+	79%	-	76%
Pain 'Always' Well Controlled	300+	69%	-	69%
Room and Bathroom 'Always' Clean	300+	69%	-	71%
Timely Help 'Always' Received	300+	67%	-	64%
Would Definitely Recommend Hospital	300+	70%	-	69%

NOTE: Hospital profiles are in alphabetical order by state, then city, then hospital within the city; Rankings exclude hospitals with less than 25 cases except for patient surveys which excludes hospitals with less than 100 cases; (a) 100–299 cases; (1) The number of cases is too small to be sure how well a hospital is performing; (2) The hospital indicated that the data submitted for this measure were based on a sample of cases; (3) Data was collected during a shorter time period (fewer quarters) than the maximum possible time for this measure; (4) Suppressed for one or more quarters by CMS; (5) No data is available from the hospital for this measure; (6) Fewer than 100 patients completed the HCAHPS survey. Use these rates with caution, as the number of surveys may be too low to reliably assess hospital performance; (7) Survey results are based on less than 12 months of data; (8) Survey results are not available for this reporting period; (9) No or very few patients were eligible for the HCAHPS survey. The scores shown, if any, reflect a very small number of surveys; (10) A state average was not calculated because too few hospitals in the state submitted data; (11) There were discrepancies in the data collection process; Please refer to the User's Guide for a full explanation of data.

Firsthealth Moore Regional Hospital

155 Memorial Drive Phone: 910-715-1000
Pinehurst, NC 28374 Fax: 910-715-1444
URL: www.firsthealth.org
Type: Acute Care Hospitals Emergency Services: Yes
Ownership: Voluntary Non-Profit - Private Beds: 385

Key Personnel:
CEO/President. . . . . Charles T Frock
Cardiac Laboratory. . . . . Roger Noble
Chief of Medical Staff . . . . Ward S Oakley
Coronary Care . . . . Beverly Alphin
Infection Control. . . . . Jayne Lee
Operating Room. . . . . Ken Schwann
Quality Assurance . . . . Barbara Bennett
Radiology. . . . . Ole S Aassar

Measure	Cases	This Hosp.	State Avg.	U.S. Avg.
Heart Attack Care				
ACE Inhibitor or ARB for LVSD[2]	94	96%	97%	96%
Aspirin at Arrival[2]	309	99%	99%	99%
Aspirin at Discharge[2]	467	100%	99%	98%
Beta Blocker at Discharge[2]	451	97%	99%	98%
Fibrinolytic Medication Timing[2]	0	-	38%	55%
PCI Within 90 Minutes of Arrival[2]	38	95%	95%	90%
Smoking Cessation Advice[2]	163	100%	100%	99%
Chest Pain/Possible Heart Attack Care				
Aspirin at Arrival[1,3]	3	100%	95%	95%
Median Time to ECG (minutes)[1,3]	6	10	8	8
Median Time to Transfer (minutes)[5]	0	-	48	61
Fibrinolytic Medication Timing[3]	0	-	53%	54%
Heart Failure Care				
ACE Inhibitor or ARB for LVSD[2]	221	94%	95%	94%
Discharge Instructions[2]	511	82%	89%	88%
Evaluation of LVS Function[2]	583	99%	99%	98%
Smoking Cessation Advice[2]	101	100%	99%	98%
Pneumonia Care				
Appropriate Initial Antibiotic[2]	180	93%	92%	92%
Blood Culture Timing[2]	262	97%	96%	96%
Influenza Vaccine[2]	268	97%	93%	91%
Initial Antibiotic Timing[2]	281	96%	95%	95%
Pneumococcal Vaccine[2]	300	97%	95%	93%
Smoking Cessation Advice[2]	142	100%	99%	97%
Surgical Care Improvement Project				
Appropriate VTP Within 24 Hours[2]	376	92%	93%	92%
Appropriate Hair Removal[2]	1,626	99%	100%	99%
Appropriate Beta Blocker Usage[2]	579	97%	94%	93%
Controlled Postoperative Blood Glucose[2]	306	96%	94%	93%
Prophylactic Antibiotic Timing[2]	1,129	98%	98%	97%
Prophylactic Antibiotic Timing (Outpatient)	614	84%	94%	92%
Prophylactic Antibiotic Selection[2]	1,140	98%	98%	97%
Prophylactic Antibiotic Select. (Outpatient)	599	96%	95%	94%
Prophylactic Antibiotic Stopped[2]	1,095	98%	96%	94%
Recommended VTP Ordered[2]	380	95%	95%	94%
Urinary Catheter Removal[2]	244	92%	91%	90%
Children's Asthma Care				
Received Systemic Corticosteroids	55	100%	100%	100%
Received Home Management Plan	54	22%	75%	71%
Received Reliever Medication	55	100%	100%	100%
Use of Medical Imaging				
Combination Abdominal CT Scan	1,089	0.090	0.115	0.191
Combination Chest CT Scan	926	0.026	0.037	0.054
Follow-up Mammogram/Ultrasound	272	8.8%	7.9%	8.4%
MRI for Low Back Pain	756	25.5%	30.6%	32.7%
Survey of Patients' Hospital Experiences				
Area Around Room 'Always' Quiet at Night	300+	61%	-	58%
Doctors 'Always' Communicated Well	300+	85%	-	80%
Home Recovery Information Given	300+	83%	-	82%
Hospital Given 9 or 10 on 10 Point Scale	300+	79%	-	67%
Meds 'Always' Explained Before Given	300+	64%	-	60%
Nurses 'Always' Communicated Well	300+	81%	-	76%
Pain 'Always' Well Controlled	300+	76%	-	69%
Room and Bathroom 'Always' Clean	300+	74%	-	71%
Timely Help 'Always' Received	300+	72%	-	64%
Would Definitely Recommend Hospital	300+	83%	-	69%

Washington County Hospital

958 Us Hwy 64 East Phone: 252-793-4135
Plymouth, NC 27962 Fax: 252-793-1530
URL: www.wchonline.com
Type: Critical Access Hospitals Emergency Services: Yes
Ownership: Voluntary Non-Profit - Private Beds: 49

Key Personnel:
CEO/President. . . . . Betty Bowen
Chief of Medical Staff . . . . Robert Benadale
Coronary Care . . . . Sandy Downs
Quality Assurance . . . . Deborah Raebuck
Emergency Room . . . . Ann Davenport

Measure	Cases	This Hosp.	State Avg.	U.S. Avg.
Heart Attack Care				
ACE Inhibitor or ARB for LVSD[1]	2	100%	97%	96%
Aspirin at Arrival[1]	3	100%	99%	99%
Aspirin at Discharge[1]	3	100%	99%	98%
Beta Blocker at Discharge[1]	3	100%	99%	98%
Fibrinolytic Medication Timing	0	-	38%	55%
PCI Within 90 Minutes of Arrival	0	-	95%	90%
Smoking Cessation Advice	0	-	100%	99%
Chest Pain/Possible Heart Attack Care				
Aspirin at Arrival	25	100%	95%	95%
Median Time to ECG (minutes)	28	5	8	8
Median Time to Transfer (minutes)[1,3]	3	139	48	61
Fibrinolytic Medication Timing[1,3]	2	100%	53%	54%
Heart Failure Care				
ACE Inhibitor or ARB for LVSD[1]	19	100%	95%	94%
Discharge Instructions	31	84%	89%	88%
Evaluation of LVS Function	39	92%	99%	98%
Smoking Cessation Advice[1]	10	70%	99%	98%
Pneumonia Care				
Appropriate Initial Antibiotic[1]	20	80%	92%	92%
Blood Culture Timing	27	89%	96%	96%
Influenza Vaccine[1]	12	92%	93%	91%
Initial Antibiotic Timing	30	100%	95%	95%
Pneumococcal Vaccine[1]	21	95%	95%	93%
Smoking Cessation Advice[1]	2	50%	99%	97%
Surgical Care Improvement Project				
Appropriate VTP Within 24 Hours[5]	0	-	93%	92%
Appropriate Hair Removal[5]	0	-	100%	99%
Appropriate Beta Blocker Usage[5]	0	-	94%	93%
Controlled Postoperative Blood Glucose[5]	0	-	94%	93%
Prophylactic Antibiotic Timing[5]	0	-	98%	97%
Prophylactic Antibiotic Timing (Outpatient)[5]	0	-	94%	92%
Prophylactic Antibiotic Selection[5]	0	-	98%	97%
Prophylactic Antibiotic Select. (Outpatient)[5]	0	-	95%	94%
Prophylactic Antibiotic Stopped[5]	0	-	96%	94%
Recommended VTP Ordered[5]	0	-	95%	94%
Urinary Catheter Removal[5]	0	-	91%	90%
Children's Asthma Care				
Received Systemic Corticosteroids	-	-	100%	100%
Received Home Management Plan	-	-	75%	71%
Received Reliever Medication	-	-	100%	100%
Use of Medical Imaging				
Combination Abdominal CT Scan	67	0.881	0.115	0.191
Combination Chest CT Scan[1]	35	0.000	0.037	0.054
Follow-up Mammogram/Ultrasound	225	9.3%	7.9%	8.4%
MRI for Low Back Pain[1]	26	42.3%	30.6%	32.7%
Survey of Patients' Hospital Experiences				
Area Around Room 'Always' Quiet at Night[8]	-	-	-	58%
Doctors 'Always' Communicated Well[8]	-	-	-	80%
Home Recovery Information Given[8]	-	-	-	82%
Hospital Given 9 or 10 on 10 Point Scale[8]	-	-	-	67%
Meds 'Always' Explained Before Given[8]	-	-	-	60%
Nurses 'Always' Communicated Well[8]	-	-	-	76%
Pain 'Always' Well Controlled[8]	-	-	-	69%
Room and Bathroom 'Always' Clean[8]	-	-	-	71%
Timely Help 'Always' Received[8]	-	-	-	64%
Would Definitely Recommend Hospital[8]	-	-	-	69%

Duke Health Raleigh Hospital

3400 Wake Forest Rd Phone: 919-954-3000
Raleigh, NC 27609 Fax: 919-954-3900
URL: www.raleighcommunityhospital.com
Type: Acute Care Hospitals Emergency Services: No
Ownership: Voluntary Non-Profit - Private Beds: 222

Key Personnel:
CEO/President. . . . . Doug Vinsel
Chief of Medical Staff . . . . Ted Kunstling
Infection Control. . . . . Polly Patget
Quality Assurance . . . . Cindy Nordlund
Radiology. . . . . Tedric Dale Boyse
Anesthesiology. . . . . Randy Efird, MD
Emergency Room . . . . Marc Calabrese

Measure	Cases	This Hosp.	State Avg.	U.S. Avg.
Heart Attack Care				
ACE Inhibitor or ARB for LVSD[1]	6	100%	97%	96%
Aspirin at Arrival	71	100%	99%	99%
Aspirin at Discharge	63	100%	99%	98%
Beta Blocker at Discharge	62	100%	99%	98%
Fibrinolytic Medication Timing	0	-	38%	55%
PCI Within 90 Minutes of Arrival[1]	3	100%	95%	90%
Smoking Cessation Advice[1]	14	100%	100%	99%
Chest Pain/Possible Heart Attack Care				
Aspirin at Arrival[1]	20	95%	95%	95%
Median Time to ECG (minutes)[1]	18	16	8	8
Median Time to Transfer (minutes)[1,3]	5	49	48	61
Fibrinolytic Medication Timing[3]	0	-	53%	54%
Heart Failure Care				
ACE Inhibitor or ARB for LVSD	64	100%	95%	94%
Discharge Instructions	134	98%	89%	88%
Evaluation of LVS Function	158	99%	99%	98%
Smoking Cessation Advice	30	100%	99%	98%
Pneumonia Care				
Appropriate Initial Antibiotic	103	93%	92%	92%
Blood Culture Timing	148	98%	96%	96%
Influenza Vaccine	90	99%	93%	91%
Initial Antibiotic Timing	125	100%	95%	95%
Pneumococcal Vaccine	121	96%	95%	93%
Smoking Cessation Advice	42	98%	99%	97%
Surgical Care Improvement Project				
Appropriate VTP Within 24 Hours	414	91%	93%	92%
Appropriate Hair Removal	1,098	99%	100%	99%
Appropriate Beta Blocker Usage	294	88%	94%	93%
Controlled Postoperative Blood Glucose	0	-	94%	93%
Prophylactic Antibiotic Timing	799	93%	98%	97%
Prophylactic Antibiotic Timing (Outpatient)	515	87%	94%	92%
Prophylactic Antibiotic Selection	801	98%	98%	97%
Prophylactic Antibiotic Select. (Outpatient)	508	98%	95%	94%
Prophylactic Antibiotic Stopped	789	98%	96%	94%
Recommended VTP Ordered	414	93%	95%	94%
Urinary Catheter Removal	447	91%	91%	90%
Children's Asthma Care				
Received Systemic Corticosteroids	-	-	100%	100%
Received Home Management Plan	-	-	75%	71%
Received Reliever Medication	-	-	100%	100%
Use of Medical Imaging				
Combination Abdominal CT Scan	775	0.129	0.115	0.191
Combination Chest CT Scan	899	0.119	0.037	0.054
Follow-up Mammogram/Ultrasound	232	13.8%	7.9%	8.4%
MRI for Low Back Pain	98	26.5%	30.6%	32.7%
Survey of Patients' Hospital Experiences				
Area Around Room 'Always' Quiet at Night	300+	62%	-	58%
Doctors 'Always' Communicated Well	300+	84%	-	80%
Home Recovery Information Given	300+	88%	-	82%
Hospital Given 9 or 10 on 10 Point Scale	300+	71%	-	67%
Meds 'Always' Explained Before Given	300+	66%	-	60%
Nurses 'Always' Communicated Well	300+	78%	-	76%
Pain 'Always' Well Controlled	300+	74%	-	69%
Room and Bathroom 'Always' Clean	300+	68%	-	71%
Timely Help 'Always' Received	300+	62%	-	64%
Would Definitely Recommend Hospital	300+	77%	-	69%

NOTE: Hospital profiles are in alphabetical order by state, then city, then hospital within the city; Rankings exclude hospitals with less than 25 cases except for patient surveys which excludes hospitals with less than 100 cases; (a) 100–299 cases; (1) The number of cases is too small to be sure how well a hospital is performing; (2) The hospital indicated that the data submitted for this measure were based on a sample of cases; (3) Data was collected during a shorter time period (fewer quarters) than the maximum possible time for this measure; (4) Suppressed for one or more quarters by CMS; (5) No data is available from the hospital for this measure; (6) Fewer than 100 patients completed the HCAHPS survey. Use these rates with caution, as the number of surveys may be too low to reliably assess hospital performance; (7) Survey results are based on less than 12 months of data; (8) Survey results are not available for this reporting period; (9) No or very few patients were eligible for the HCAHPS survey. The scores shown, if any, reflect a very small number of surveys; (10) A state average was not calculated because too few hospitals in the state submitted data; (11) There were discrepancies in the data collection process; Please refer to the User's Guide for a full explanation of data.

Rex Hospital

4420 Lake Boone Trail Phone: 919-784-3100
Raleigh, NC 27607 Fax: 919-784-3336
E-mail: healthnet@rexhealth.com
URL: www.rexhealth.com
Type: Acute Care Hospitals Emergency Services: Yes
Ownership: Voluntary Non-Profit - Private Beds: 394

Key Personnel:
CEO/President. . . . . David Strong
Infection Control. . . . . Linda Calderone
Operating Room. . . . . Jayne Byrd
Quality Assurance . . . . Sue Sherman
Radiology. . . . . John Contrael
Emergency Room . . . . Pat Nelson, RN

Measure	Cases	This Hosp.	State Avg.	U.S. Avg.
Heart Attack Care				
ACE Inhibitor or ARB for LVSD[2]	42	100%	97%	96%
Aspirin at Arrival[2]	298	100%	99%	99%
Aspirin at Discharge[2]	312	100%	99%	98%
Beta Blocker at Discharge[2]	297	99%	99%	98%
Fibrinolytic Medication Timing[2]	0	-	38%	55%
PCI Within 90 Minutes of Arrival[2]	67	93%	95%	90%
Smoking Cessation Advice[2]	67	100%	100%	99%
Chest Pain/Possible Heart Attack Care				
Aspirin at Arrival[5]	0	-	95%	95%
Median Time to ECG (minutes)[5]	0	-	8	8
Median Time to Transfer (minutes)[5]	0	-	48	61
Fibrinolytic Medication Timing[5]	0	-	53%	54%
Heart Failure Care				
ACE Inhibitor or ARB for LVSD[2]	106	92%	95%	94%
Discharge Instructions[2]	257	83%	89%	88%
Evaluation of LVS Function[2]	325	98%	99%	98%
Smoking Cessation Advice[2]	46	100%	99%	98%
Pneumonia Care				
Appropriate Initial Antibiotic[2]	129	96%	92%	92%
Blood Culture Timing[2]	227	96%	96%	96%
Influenza Vaccine[2]	127	91%	93%	91%
Initial Antibiotic Timing[2]	189	93%	95%	95%
Pneumococcal Vaccine[2]	213	96%	95%	93%
Smoking Cessation Advice[2]	43	98%	99%	97%
Surgical Care Improvement Project				
Appropriate VTP Within 24 Hours[2]	287	89%	93%	92%
Appropriate Hair Removal[2]	947	99%	100%	99%
Appropriate Beta Blocker Usage[2]	329	94%	94%	93%
Controlled Postoperative Blood Glucose[2]	176	94%	94%	93%
Prophylactic Antibiotic Timing[2]	674	98%	98%	97%
Prophylactic Antibiotic Timing (Outpatient)	1,091	94%	94%	92%
Prophylactic Antibiotic Selection[2]	675	97%	98%	97%
Prophylactic Antibiotic Select. (Outpatient)	1,060	92%	95%	94%
Prophylactic Antibiotic Stopped[2]	654	95%	96%	94%
Recommended VTP Ordered[2]	288	89%	95%	94%
Urinary Catheter Removal[2]	245	89%	91%	90%
Children's Asthma Care				
Received Systemic Corticosteroids	-	-	100%	100%
Received Home Management Plan	-	-	75%	71%
Received Reliever Medication	-	-	100%	100%
Use of Medical Imaging				
Combination Abdominal CT Scan	1,430	0.173	0.115	0.191
Combination Chest CT Scan	1,014	0.056	0.037	0.054
Follow-up Mammogram/Ultrasound	1,895	5.8%	7.9%	8.4%
MRI for Low Back Pain	316	30.7%	30.6%	32.7%
Survey of Patients' Hospital Experiences				
Area Around Room 'Always' Quiet at Night	300+	52%	-	58%
Doctors 'Always' Communicated Well	300+	82%	-	80%
Home Recovery Information Given	300+	87%	-	82%
Hospital Given 9 or 10 on 10 Point Scale	300+	75%	-	67%
Meds 'Always' Explained Before Given	300+	62%	-	60%
Nurses 'Always' Communicated Well	300+	77%	-	76%
Pain 'Always' Well Controlled	300+	69%	-	69%
Room and Bathroom 'Always' Clean	300+	64%	-	71%
Timely Help 'Always' Received	300+	64%	-	64%
Would Definitely Recommend Hospital	300+	84%	-	69%

Wakemed - Raleigh Campus

3000 New Bern Ave Phone: 919-350-8000
Raleigh, NC 27610 Fax: 919-350-8868
E-mail: staylor@wakemed.org
URL: www.wakemed.org
Type: Acute Care Hospitals Emergency Services: Yes
Ownership: Voluntary Non-Profit - Private Beds: 515

Key Personnel:
CEO/President. . . . . William Atkinson, PhD, MPH
Chief of Medical Staff . . . . H West Lawson, MD

Measure	Cases	This Hosp.	State Avg.	U.S. Avg.
Heart Attack Care				
ACE Inhibitor or ARB for LVSD	234	95%	97%	96%
Aspirin at Arrival	530	100%	99%	99%
Aspirin at Discharge	1,539	99%	99%	98%
Beta Blocker at Discharge	1,432	99%	99%	98%
Fibrinolytic Medication Timing	0	-	38%	55%
PCI Within 90 Minutes of Arrival	105	100%	95%	90%
Smoking Cessation Advice	622	100%	100%	99%
Chest Pain/Possible Heart Attack Care				
Aspirin at Arrival	32	97%	95%	95%
Median Time to ECG (minutes)	33	2	8	8
Median Time to Transfer (minutes)[5]	0	-	48	61
Fibrinolytic Medication Timing[5]	0	-	53%	54%
Heart Failure Care				
ACE Inhibitor or ARB for LVSD[2]	123	98%	95%	94%
Discharge Instructions[2]	278	83%	89%	88%
Evaluation of LVS Function[2]	328	100%	99%	98%
Smoking Cessation Advice[2]	86	100%	99%	98%
Pneumonia Care				
Appropriate Initial Antibiotic	152	95%	92%	92%
Blood Culture Timing	276	99%	96%	96%
Influenza Vaccine	274	93%	93%	91%
Initial Antibiotic Timing	204	93%	95%	95%
Pneumococcal Vaccine	315	96%	95%	93%
Smoking Cessation Advice	206	99%	99%	97%
Surgical Care Improvement Project				
Appropriate VTP Within 24 Hours[2]	241	92%	93%	92%
Appropriate Hair Removal[2]	751	100%	100%	99%
Appropriate Beta Blocker Usage[2]	268	96%	94%	93%
Controlled Postoperative Blood Glucose[2]	170	99%	94%	93%
Prophylactic Antibiotic Timing[2]	511	98%	98%	97%
Prophylactic Antibiotic Timing (Outpatient)	955	96%	94%	92%
Prophylactic Antibiotic Selection[2]	523	98%	98%	97%
Prophylactic Antibiotic Select. (Outpatient)	933	99%	95%	94%
Prophylactic Antibiotic Stopped[2]	484	98%	96%	94%
Recommended VTP Ordered[2]	242	93%	95%	94%
Urinary Catheter Removal[2]	130	98%	91%	90%
Children's Asthma Care				
Received Systemic Corticosteroids	-	-	100%	100%
Received Home Management Plan	-	-	75%	71%
Received Reliever Medication	-	-	100%	100%
Use of Medical Imaging				
Combination Abdominal CT Scan	835	0.049	0.115	0.191
Combination Chest CT Scan	599	0.033	0.037	0.054
Follow-up Mammogram/Ultrasound	1,184	5.8%	7.9%	8.4%
MRI for Low Back Pain	149	38.3%	30.6%	32.7%
Survey of Patients' Hospital Experiences				
Area Around Room 'Always' Quiet at Night	300+	60%	-	58%
Doctors 'Always' Communicated Well	300+	79%	-	80%
Home Recovery Information Given	300+	85%	-	82%
Hospital Given 9 or 10 on 10 Point Scale	300+	74%	-	67%
Meds 'Always' Explained Before Given	300+	62%	-	60%
Nurses 'Always' Communicated Well	300+	76%	-	76%
Pain 'Always' Well Controlled	300+	71%	-	69%
Room and Bathroom 'Always' Clean	300+	62%	-	71%
Timely Help 'Always' Received	300+	64%	-	64%
Would Definitely Recommend Hospital	300+	75%	-	69%

Halifax Regional Medical Center

250 Smith Church Rd Phone: 252-535-8005
Roanoke Rapids, NC 27870 Fax: 252-535-8466
URL: www.halifaxmedicalcenter.org
Type: Acute Care Hospitals Emergency Services: Yes
Ownership: Voluntary Non-Profit - Private Beds: 206

Key Personnel:
CEO/President. . . . . William Mahone V
Chief of Medical Staff . . . . N Manikham
Infection Control. . . . . Sarah Pulley
Pediatric Ambulatory Care . . . . . . Paulette Ingram, MD
Pediatric In-Patient Care . . . . Paulette Ingram, MD
Quality Assurance . . . . Margaret Rose
Emergency Room . . . . Mark MD
Intensive Care Unit. . . . . Merrie Bischoff, RN

Measure	Cases	This Hosp.	State Avg.	U.S. Avg.
Heart Attack Care				
ACE Inhibitor or ARB for LVSD[1]	6	83%	97%	96%
Aspirin at Arrival	52	90%	99%	99%
Aspirin at Discharge[1]	22	91%	99%	98%
Beta Blocker at Discharge[1]	24	100%	99%	98%
Fibrinolytic Medication Timing	0	-	38%	55%
PCI Within 90 Minutes of Arrival	0	-	95%	90%
Smoking Cessation Advice[1]	2	100%	100%	99%
Chest Pain/Possible Heart Attack Care				
Aspirin at Arrival	186	95%	95%	95%
Median Time to ECG (minutes)	194	6	8	8
Median Time to Transfer (minutes)[1,3]	1	57	48	61
Fibrinolytic Medication Timing[1]	12	75%	53%	54%
Heart Failure Care				
ACE Inhibitor or ARB for LVSD	91	90%	95%	94%
Discharge Instructions	263	90%	89%	88%
Evaluation of LVS Function	303	97%	99%	98%
Smoking Cessation Advice	61	100%	99%	98%
Pneumonia Care				
Appropriate Initial Antibiotic	104	85%	92%	92%
Blood Culture Timing	132	92%	96%	96%
Influenza Vaccine	111	91%	93%	91%
Initial Antibiotic Timing	155	92%	95%	95%
Pneumococcal Vaccine	134	91%	95%	93%
Smoking Cessation Advice	66	100%	99%	97%
Surgical Care Improvement Project				
Appropriate VTP Within 24 Hours[2]	74	72%	93%	92%
Appropriate Hair Removal[2]	423	100%	100%	99%
Appropriate Beta Blocker Usage[2]	129	86%	94%	93%
Controlled Postoperative Blood Glucose[2]	0	-	94%	93%
Prophylactic Antibiotic Timing[2]	285	97%	98%	97%
Prophylactic Antibiotic Timing (Outpatient)	135	92%	94%	92%
Prophylactic Antibiotic Selection[2]	290	99%	98%	97%
Prophylactic Antibiotic Select. (Outpatient)	129	95%	95%	94%
Prophylactic Antibiotic Stopped[2]	274	98%	96%	94%
Recommended VTP Ordered[2]	76	76%	95%	94%
Urinary Catheter Removal[1,2]	9	67%	91%	90%
Children's Asthma Care				
Received Systemic Corticosteroids	-	-	100%	100%
Received Home Management Plan	-	-	75%	71%
Received Reliever Medication	-	-	100%	100%
Use of Medical Imaging				
Combination Abdominal CT Scan	606	0.092	0.115	0.191
Combination Chest CT Scan	458	0.000	0.037	0.054
Follow-up Mammogram/Ultrasound	1,381	11.4%	7.9%	8.4%
MRI for Low Back Pain	94	39.4%	30.6%	32.7%
Survey of Patients' Hospital Experiences				
Area Around Room 'Always' Quiet at Night	300+	63%	-	58%
Doctors 'Always' Communicated Well	300+	81%	-	80%
Home Recovery Information Given	300+	79%	-	82%
Hospital Given 9 or 10 on 10 Point Scale	300+	62%	-	67%
Meds 'Always' Explained Before Given	300+	62%	-	60%
Nurses 'Always' Communicated Well	300+	74%	-	76%
Pain 'Always' Well Controlled	300+	67%	-	69%
Room and Bathroom 'Always' Clean	300+	62%	-	71%
Timely Help 'Always' Received	300+	64%	-	64%
Would Definitely Recommend Hospital	300+	59%	-	69%

NOTE: Hospital profiles are in alphabetical order by state, then city, then hospital within the city; Rankings exclude hospitals with less than 25 cases except for patient surveys which excludes hospitals with less than 100 cases; (a) 100–299 cases; (1) The number of cases is too small to be sure how well a hospital is performing; (2) The hospital indicated that the data submitted for this measure were based on a sample of cases; (3) Data was collected during a shorter time period (fewer quarters) than the maximum possible time for this measure; (4) Suppressed for one or more quarters by CMS; (5) No data is available from the hospital for this measure; (6) Fewer than 100 patients completed the HCAHPS survey. Use these rates with caution, as the number of surveys may be too low to reliably assess hospital performance; (7) Survey results are based on less than 12 months of data; (8) Survey results are not available for this reporting period; (9) No or very few patients were eligible for the HCAHPS survey. The scores shown, if any, reflect a very small number of surveys; (10) A state average was not calculated because too few hospitals in the state submitted data; (11) There were discrepancies in the data collection process; Please refer to the User's Guide for a full explanation of data.

Firsthealth Richmond Memorial Hospital

925 Long Dr Phone: 910-417-3000
Rockingham, NC 28379 Fax: 910-417-3658
URL: www.firsthealth.org
Type: Acute Care Hospitals Emergency Services: Yes
Ownership: Voluntary Non-Profit - Private Beds: 150

Key Personnel:
Chief of Medical Staff.......... Gilbert D Arenas
Radiology.................. John Adams
Hemotology Center .... Ellen M Willard, MD

Measure	Cases	This Hosp.	State Avg.	U.S. Avg.
Heart Attack Care				
ACE Inhibitor or ARB for LVSD	-	-	97%	96%
Aspirin at Arrival	-	-	99%	99%
Aspirin at Discharge	-	-	99%	98%
Beta Blocker at Discharge	-	-	99%	98%
Fibrinolytic Medication Timing	-	-	38%	55%
PCI Within 90 Minutes of Arrival	-	-	95%	90%
Smoking Cessation Advice	-	-	100%	99%
Chest Pain/Possible Heart Attack Care				
Aspirin at Arrival	-	-	95%	95%
Median Time to ECG (minutes)	-	-	8	8
Median Time to Transfer (minutes)	-	-	48	61
Fibrinolytic Medication Timing	-	-	53%	54%
Heart Failure Care				
ACE Inhibitor or ARB for LVSD	-	-	95%	94%
Discharge Instructions	-	-	89%	88%
Evaluation of LVS Function	-	-	99%	98%
Smoking Cessation Advice	-	-	99%	98%
Pneumonia Care				
Appropriate Initial Antibiotic	-	-	92%	92%
Blood Culture Timing	-	-	96%	96%
Influenza Vaccine	-	-	93%	91%
Initial Antibiotic Timing	-	-	95%	95%
Pneumococcal Vaccine	-	-	95%	93%
Smoking Cessation Advice	-	-	99%	97%
Surgical Care Improvement Project				
Appropriate VTP Within 24 Hours	-	-	93%	92%
Appropriate Hair Removal	-	-	100%	99%
Appropriate Beta Blocker Usage	-	-	94%	93%
Controlled Postoperative Blood Glucose	-	-	94%	93%
Prophylactic Antibiotic Timing	-	-	98%	97%
Prophylactic Antibiotic Timing (Outpatient)	-	-	94%	92%
Prophylactic Antibiotic Selection	-	-	98%	97%
Prophylactic Antibiotic Select. (Outpatient)	-	-	95%	94%
Prophylactic Antibiotic Stopped	-	-	96%	94%
Recommended VTP Ordered	-	-	95%	94%
Urinary Catheter Removal	-	-	91%	90%
Children's Asthma Care				
Received Systemic Corticosteroids	-	-	100%	100%
Received Home Management Plan	-	-	75%	71%
Received Reliever Medication	-	-	100%	100%
Use of Medical Imaging				
Combination Abdominal CT Scan	-	-	0.115	0.191
Combination Chest CT Scan	-	-	0.037	0.054
Follow-up Mammogram/Ultrasound	-	-	7.9%	8.4%
MRI for Low Back Pain	-	-	30.6%	32.7%
Survey of Patients' Hospital Experiences				
Area Around Room 'Always' Quiet at Night	-	-	-	58%
Doctors 'Always' Communicated Well	-	-	-	80%
Home Recovery Information Given	-	-	-	82%
Hospital Given 9 or 10 on 10 Point Scale	-	-	-	67%
Meds 'Always' Explained Before Given	-	-	-	60%
Nurses 'Always' Communicated Well	-	-	-	76%
Pain 'Always' Well Controlled	-	-	-	69%
Room and Bathroom 'Always' Clean	-	-	-	71%
Timely Help 'Always' Received	-	-	-	64%
Would Definitely Recommend Hospital	-	-	-	69%

Nash General Hospital

2460 Curtis Ellis Drive Phone: 252-443-8000
Rocky Mount, NC 27804 Fax: 252-443-8067
URL: www.nhcs.org
Type: Acute Care Hospitals Emergency Services: Yes
Ownership: Govt - Hospital Dist/Auth Beds: 280

Key Personnel:
CEO/President............... Michael D Crawford
Chief of Medical Staff.......... Robert K Schellenberg, MD
Infection Control............. Wanda Lamm
Operating Room............. Tom Jenkins
Quality Assurance .... Sandi Paige
Radiology.................. Gerald Capps
Emergency Room .... Jamie Parsons
Patient Relations .... Lita Watson

Measure	Cases	This Hosp.	State Avg.	U.S. Avg.
Heart Attack Care				
ACE Inhibitor or ARB for LVSD	50	90%	97%	96%
Aspirin at Arrival	309	95%	99%	99%
Aspirin at Discharge	210	90%	99%	98%
Beta Blocker at Discharge	215	92%	99%	98%
Fibrinolytic Medication Timing	0	-	38%	55%
PCI Within 90 Minutes of Arrival	0	-	95%	90%
Smoking Cessation Advice	66	100%	100%	99%
Chest Pain/Possible Heart Attack Care				
Aspirin at Arrival	264	89%	95%	95%
Median Time to ECG (minutes)	268	9	8	8
Median Time to Transfer (minutes)[1]	1	90	48	61
Fibrinolytic Medication Timing[1]	21	33%	53%	54%
Heart Failure Care				
ACE Inhibitor or ARB for LVSD	156	91%	95%	94%
Discharge Instructions	387	97%	89%	88%
Evaluation of LVS Function	447	99%	99%	98%
Smoking Cessation Advice	114	100%	99%	98%
Pneumonia Care				
Appropriate Initial Antibiotic[2]	114	86%	92%	92%
Blood Culture Timing[2]	259	92%	96%	96%
Influenza Vaccine	194	92%	93%	91%
Initial Antibiotic Timing[2]	233	94%	95%	95%
Pneumococcal Vaccine[2]	213	95%	95%	93%
Smoking Cessation Advice[2]	128	98%	99%	97%
Surgical Care Improvement Project				
Appropriate VTP Within 24 Hours[2]	146	90%	93%	92%
Appropriate Hair Removal[2]	698	100%	100%	99%
Appropriate Beta Blocker Usage[2]	180	96%	94%	93%
Controlled Postoperative Blood Glucose[2]	0	-	94%	93%
Prophylactic Antibiotic Timing[2]	564	96%	98%	97%
Prophylactic Antibiotic Timing (Outpatient)	400	94%	94%	92%
Prophylactic Antibiotic Selection[2]	565	99%	98%	97%
Prophylactic Antibiotic Select. (Outpatient)	409	94%	95%	94%
Prophylactic Antibiotic Stopped[2]	550	95%	96%	94%
Recommended VTP Ordered[2]	146	95%	95%	94%
Urinary Catheter Removal[2]	180	94%	91%	90%
Children's Asthma Care				
Received Systemic Corticosteroids	-	-	100%	100%
Received Home Management Plan	-	-	75%	71%
Received Reliever Medication	-	-	100%	100%
Use of Medical Imaging				
Combination Abdominal CT Scan	970	0.040	0.115	0.191
Combination Chest CT Scan	490	0.012	0.037	0.054
Follow-up Mammogram/Ultrasound	1,224	12.5%	7.9%	8.4%
MRI for Low Back Pain	427	32.6%	30.6%	32.7%
Survey of Patients' Hospital Experiences				
Area Around Room 'Always' Quiet at Night	300+	54%	-	58%
Doctors 'Always' Communicated Well	300+	82%	-	80%
Home Recovery Information Given	300+	81%	-	82%
Hospital Given 9 or 10 on 10 Point Scale	300+	60%	-	67%
Meds 'Always' Explained Before Given	300+	65%	-	60%
Nurses 'Always' Communicated Well	300+	78%	-	76%
Pain 'Always' Well Controlled	300+	71%	-	69%
Room and Bathroom 'Always' Clean	300+	67%	-	71%
Timely Help 'Always' Received	300+	64%	-	64%
Would Definitely Recommend Hospital	300+	57%	-	69%

Person Memorial Hospital

615 Ridge Rd Phone: 336-599-2121
Roxboro, NC 27573 Fax: 336-503-5765
E-mail: c_brigham98@yahoo.com
URL: www.personhospital.com
Type: Acute Care Hospitals Emergency Services: Yes
Ownership: Voluntary Non-Profit - Private Beds: 110

Key Personnel:
CEO/President............... Craig James
Chief of Medical Staff.......... Jeffrey C Kafer, MD
Infection Control............. Donna Lungford
Operating Room............. Ginny Campbell
Quality Assurance .... Linda Braunstein
Radiology.................. William L Hall
Anesthesiology.............. Rick Jacobs, MD
Emergency Room .... Margaret Bowen

Measure	Cases	This Hosp.	State Avg.	U.S. Avg.
Heart Attack Care				
ACE Inhibitor or ARB for LVSD	0	-	97%	96%
Aspirin at Arrival[1]	7	100%	99%	99%
Aspirin at Discharge[1]	4	100%	99%	98%
Beta Blocker at Discharge[1]	3	33%	99%	98%
Fibrinolytic Medication Timing	0	-	38%	55%
PCI Within 90 Minutes of Arrival	0	-	95%	90%
Smoking Cessation Advice	0	-	100%	99%
Chest Pain/Possible Heart Attack Care				
Aspirin at Arrival	132	92%	95%	95%
Median Time to ECG (minutes)	139	7	8	8
Median Time to Transfer (minutes)[1]	15	32	48	61
Fibrinolytic Medication Timing	0	-	53%	54%
Heart Failure Care				
ACE Inhibitor or ARB for LVSD[1]	21	86%	95%	94%
Discharge Instructions	71	96%	89%	88%
Evaluation of LVS Function	88	99%	99%	98%
Smoking Cessation Advice[1]	7	86%	99%	98%
Pneumonia Care				
Appropriate Initial Antibiotic	61	84%	92%	92%
Blood Culture Timing	95	95%	96%	96%
Influenza Vaccine	61	95%	93%	91%
Initial Antibiotic Timing	85	98%	95%	95%
Pneumococcal Vaccine	82	98%	95%	93%
Smoking Cessation Advice	28	100%	99%	97%
Surgical Care Improvement Project				
Appropriate VTP Within 24 Hours	105	90%	93%	92%
Appropriate Hair Removal	200	100%	100%	99%
Appropriate Beta Blocker Usage	77	92%	94%	93%
Controlled Postoperative Blood Glucose	0	-	94%	93%
Prophylactic Antibiotic Timing	144	96%	98%	97%
Prophylactic Antibiotic Timing (Outpatient)[1]	16	75%	94%	92%
Prophylactic Antibiotic Selection	146	99%	98%	97%
Prophylactic Antibiotic Select. (Outpatient)[1]	14	100%	95%	94%
Prophylactic Antibiotic Stopped	143	99%	96%	94%
Recommended VTP Ordered	108	89%	95%	94%
Urinary Catheter Removal	74	93%	91%	90%
Children's Asthma Care				
Received Systemic Corticosteroids	-	-	100%	100%
Received Home Management Plan	-	-	75%	71%
Received Reliever Medication	-	-	100%	100%
Use of Medical Imaging				
Combination Abdominal CT Scan	227	0.075	0.115	0.191
Combination Chest CT Scan	187	0.016	0.037	0.054
Follow-up Mammogram/Ultrasound	685	5.5%	7.9%	8.4%
MRI for Low Back Pain	65	36.9%	30.6%	32.7%
Survey of Patients' Hospital Experiences				
Area Around Room 'Always' Quiet at Night	300+	67%	-	58%
Doctors 'Always' Communicated Well	300+	84%	-	80%
Home Recovery Information Given	300+	78%	-	82%
Hospital Given 9 or 10 on 10 Point Scale	300+	64%	-	67%
Meds 'Always' Explained Before Given	300+	57%	-	60%
Nurses 'Always' Communicated Well	300+	77%	-	76%
Pain 'Always' Well Controlled	300+	68%	-	69%
Room and Bathroom 'Always' Clean	300+	66%	-	71%
Timely Help 'Always' Received	300+	60%	-	64%
Would Definitely Recommend Hospital	300+	70%	-	69%

NOTE: Hospital profiles are in alphabetical order by state, then city, then hospital within the city; Rankings exclude hospitals with less than 25 cases except for patient surveys which excludes hospitals with less than 100 cases; (a) 100–299 cases; (1) The number of cases is too small to be sure how well a hospital is performing; (2) The hospital indicated that the data submitted for this measure were based on a sample of cases; (3) Data was collected during a shorter time period (fewer quarters) than the maximum possible time for this measure; (4) Suppressed for one or more quarters by CMS; (5) No data is available from the hospital for this measure; (6) Fewer than 100 patients completed the HCAHPS survey. Use these rates with caution, as the number of surveys may be too low to reliably assess hospital performance; (7) Survey results are based on less than 12 months of data; (8) Survey results are not available for this reporting period; (9) No or very few patients were eligible for the HCAHPS survey. The scores shown, if any, reflect a very small number of surveys; (10) A state average was not calculated because too few hospitals in the state submitted data; (11) There were discrepancies in the data collection process; Please refer to the User's Guide for a full explanation of data.

Rutherford Hospital

288 South Ridgecrest Ave
Rutherfordton, NC 28139
URL: www.rutherfordhosp.org
Type: Acute Care Hospitals
Ownership: Voluntary Non-Profit - Private

Phone: 828-286-5000
Fax: 828-286-5207

Emergency Services: Yes
Beds: 143

Key Personnel:
CEO/President . . . . David Bixler
Chief of Medical Staff . . . . Dean Beckstrom
Radiology. . . . . Edward K Grishaw
Patient Relations . . . . Nancy Boffemmyer

Measure	Cases	This Hosp.	State Avg.	U.S. Avg.
Heart Attack Care				
ACE Inhibitor or ARB for LVSD[1]	3	100%	97%	96%
Aspirin at Arrival	35	97%	99%	99%
Aspirin at Discharge[1]	17	100%	99%	98%
Beta Blocker at Discharge[1]	22	100%	99%	98%
Fibrinolytic Medication Timing	0	-	38%	55%
PCI Within 90 Minutes of Arrival	0	-	95%	90%
Smoking Cessation Advice[1]	5	100%	100%	99%
Chest Pain/Possible Heart Attack Care				
Aspirin at Arrival	165	95%	95%	95%
Median Time to ECG (minutes)	168	12	8	8
Median Time to Transfer (minutes)[1]	18	73	48	61
Fibrinolytic Medication Timing[1]	13	15%	53%	54%
Heart Failure Care				
ACE Inhibitor or ARB for LVSD	37	89%	95%	94%
Discharge Instructions	126	90%	89%	88%
Evaluation of LVS Function	168	100%	99%	98%
Smoking Cessation Advice	32	100%	99%	98%
Pneumonia Care				
Appropriate Initial Antibiotic	116	81%	92%	92%
Blood Culture Timing	183	94%	96%	96%
Influenza Vaccine	118	86%	93%	91%
Initial Antibiotic Timing	168	93%	95%	95%
Pneumococcal Vaccine	167	91%	95%	93%
Smoking Cessation Advice	60	100%	99%	97%
Surgical Care Improvement Project				
Appropriate VTP Within 24 Hours	113	95%	93%	92%
Appropriate Hair Removal	340	100%	100%	99%
Appropriate Beta Blocker Usage	71	96%	94%	93%
Controlled Postoperative Blood Glucose	0	-	94%	93%
Prophylactic Antibiotic Timing	244	99%	98%	97%
Prophylactic Antibiotic Timing (Outpatient)	117	90%	94%	92%
Prophylactic Antibiotic Selection	245	98%	98%	97%
Prophylactic Antibiotic Select. (Outpatient)	111	92%	95%	94%
Prophylactic Antibiotic Stopped	233	96%	96%	94%
Recommended VTP Ordered	113	98%	95%	94%
Urinary Catheter Removal[1]	19	79%	91%	90%
Children's Asthma Care				
Received Systemic Corticosteroids	-	-	100%	100%
Received Home Management Plan	-	-	75%	71%
Received Reliever Medication	-	-	100%	100%
Use of Medical Imaging				
Combination Abdominal CT Scan	837	0.039	0.115	0.191
Combination Chest CT Scan	412	0.002	0.037	0.054
Follow-up Mammogram/Ultrasound	1,637	9.5%	7.9%	8.4%
MRI for Low Back Pain	211	29.4%	30.6%	32.7%
Survey of Patients' Hospital Experiences				
Area Around Room 'Always' Quiet at Night	300+	65%	-	58%
Doctors 'Always' Communicated Well	300+	86%	-	80%
Home Recovery Information Given	300+	82%	-	82%
Hospital Given 9 or 10 on 10 Point Scale	300+	70%	-	67%
Meds 'Always' Explained Before Given	300+	64%	-	60%
Nurses 'Always' Communicated Well	300+	80%	-	76%
Pain 'Always' Well Controlled	300+	69%	-	69%
Room and Bathroom 'Always' Clean	300+	77%	-	71%
Timely Help 'Always' Received	300+	73%	-	64%
Would Definitely Recommend Hospital	300+	68%	-	69%

Rowan Regional Medical Center

612 Mocksville Ave
Salisbury, NC 28144
E-mail: webdoctor@rowan.org
URL: www.rowan.org
Type: Acute Care Hospitals
Ownership: Voluntary Non-Profit - Private

Phone: 704-210-5000
Fax: 704-210-5631

Emergency Services: Yes
Beds: 188

Key Personnel:
CEO/President . . . . Jeff Lindsay
Chief of Medical Staff . . . . David Smith
Coronary Care . . . . Sabrina Adkins
Operating Room. . . . . William Birmingham
Quality Assurance . . . . David Cook
Radiology. . . . . Marvin Abdalah
Patient Relations . . . . Julie Gainer

Measure	Cases	This Hosp.	State Avg.	U.S. Avg.
Heart Attack Care				
ACE Inhibitor or ARB for LVSD[1]	21	100%	97%	96%
Aspirin at Arrival	141	99%	99%	99%
Aspirin at Discharge	104	100%	99%	98%
Beta Blocker at Discharge	87	100%	99%	98%
Fibrinolytic Medication Timing	0	-	38%	55%
PCI Within 90 Minutes of Arrival[1]	8	88%	95%	90%
Smoking Cessation Advice	32	100%	100%	99%
Chest Pain/Possible Heart Attack Care				
Aspirin at Arrival	88	99%	95%	95%
Median Time to ECG (minutes)	92	6	8	8
Median Time to Transfer (minutes)	42	42	48	61
Fibrinolytic Medication Timing	0	-	53%	54%
Heart Failure Care				
ACE Inhibitor or ARB for LVSD	114	100%	95%	94%
Discharge Instructions	237	97%	89%	88%
Evaluation of LVS Function	289	100%	99%	98%
Smoking Cessation Advice	75	100%	99%	98%
Pneumonia Care				
Appropriate Initial Antibiotic	206	98%	92%	92%
Blood Culture Timing	303	100%	96%	96%
Influenza Vaccine	236	100%	93%	91%
Initial Antibiotic Timing	348	99%	95%	95%
Pneumococcal Vaccine	276	100%	95%	93%
Smoking Cessation Advice	143	100%	99%	97%
Surgical Care Improvement Project				
Appropriate VTP Within 24 Hours[2]	241	97%	93%	92%
Appropriate Hair Removal[2]	779	100%	100%	99%
Appropriate Beta Blocker Usage[2]	204	100%	94%	93%
Controlled Postoperative Blood Glucose[2]	0	-	94%	93%
Prophylactic Antibiotic Timing[2]	582	100%	98%	97%
Prophylactic Antibiotic Timing (Outpatient)	526	100%	94%	92%
Prophylactic Antibiotic Selection[2]	585	100%	98%	97%
Prophylactic Antibiotic Select. (Outpatient)	526	99%	95%	94%
Prophylactic Antibiotic Stopped[2]	553	99%	96%	94%
Recommended VTP Ordered[2]	241	100%	95%	94%
Urinary Catheter Removal[2]	166	99%	91%	90%
Children's Asthma Care				
Received Systemic Corticosteroids[1]	18	100%	100%	100%
Received Home Management Plan[1]	18	100%	75%	71%
Received Reliever Medication[1]	18	100%	100%	100%
Use of Medical Imaging				
Combination Abdominal CT Scan	949	0.170	0.115	0.191
Combination Chest CT Scan	575	0.202	0.037	0.054
Follow-up Mammogram/Ultrasound	771	17.6%	7.9%	8.4%
MRI for Low Back Pain	438	29.7%	30.6%	32.7%
Survey of Patients' Hospital Experiences				
Area Around Room 'Always' Quiet at Night	300+	67%	-	58%
Doctors 'Always' Communicated Well	300+	83%	-	80%
Home Recovery Information Given	300+	85%	-	82%
Hospital Given 9 or 10 on 10 Point Scale	300+	69%	-	67%
Meds 'Always' Explained Before Given	300+	63%	-	60%
Nurses 'Always' Communicated Well	300+	80%	-	76%
Pain 'Always' Well Controlled	300+	73%	-	69%
Room and Bathroom 'Always' Clean	300+	70%	-	71%
Timely Help 'Always' Received	300+	68%	-	64%
Would Definitely Recommend Hospital	300+	67%	-	69%

W G (Bill) Hefner Salisbury VA Medical Center

1601 Brenner Avenue
Salisbury, NC 28144
URL: www.va.gov/sta/guide/home.asp
Type: Acute Care-Veterans Administration
Ownership: Government - Federal

Phone: 704-638-9000
Fax: 704-638-3395

Emergency Services: No
Beds: 429

Key Personnel:
Chief of Medical Staff . . . . Robin Hurley
Infection Control. . . . . Charles A De Comarmond
Operating Room. . . . . Charles Graham
Quality Assurance . . . . Beverly Hartsell
Radiology. . . . . Paul Karmin, MD

Measure	Cases	This Hosp.	State Avg.	U.S. Avg.
Heart Attack Care				
ACE Inhibitor or ARB for LVSD[5]	0	-	97%	96%
Aspirin at Arrival[5]	0	-	99%	99%
Aspirin at Discharge[5]	0	-	99%	98%
Beta Blocker at Discharge[5]	0	-	99%	98%
Fibrinolytic Medication Timing[5]	0	-	38%	55%
PCI Within 90 Minutes of Arrival[5]	0	-	95%	90%
Smoking Cessation Advice[5]	0	-	100%	99%
Chest Pain/Possible Heart Attack Care				
Aspirin at Arrival	-	-	95%	95%
Median Time to ECG (minutes)	-	-	8	8
Median Time to Transfer (minutes)	-	-	48	61
Fibrinolytic Medication Timing	-	-	53%	54%
Heart Failure Care				
ACE Inhibitor or ARB for LVSD[1]	17	94%	95%	94%
Discharge Instructions	48	92%	89%	88%
Evaluation of LVS Function	53	100%	99%	98%
Smoking Cessation Advice[1]	5	100%	99%	98%
Pneumonia Care				
Appropriate Initial Antibiotic	35	94%	92%	92%
Blood Culture Timing	61	100%	96%	96%
Influenza Vaccine	35	100%	93%	91%
Initial Antibiotic Timing	49	98%	95%	95%
Pneumococcal Vaccine	40	100%	95%	93%
Smoking Cessation Advice	27	93%	99%	97%
Surgical Care Improvement Project				
Appropriate VTP Within 24 Hours[2]	40	88%	93%	92%
Appropriate Hair Removal[2]	77	100%	100%	99%
Appropriate Beta Blocker Usage[1,2]	14	93%	94%	93%
Controlled Postoperative Blood Glucose[2,5]	0	-	94%	93%
Prophylactic Antibiotic Timing	44	98%	98%	97%
Prophylactic Antibiotic Timing (Outpatient)	-	-	94%	92%
Prophylactic Antibiotic Selection	43	98%	98%	97%
Prophylactic Antibiotic Select. (Outpatient)	-	-	95%	94%
Prophylactic Antibiotic Stopped	42	100%	96%	94%
Recommended VTP Ordered[2]	40	93%	95%	94%
Urinary Catheter Removal[1,2]	14	86%	91%	90%
Children's Asthma Care				
Received Systemic Corticosteroids	-	-	100%	100%
Received Home Management Plan	-	-	75%	71%
Received Reliever Medication	-	-	100%	100%
Use of Medical Imaging				
Combination Abdominal CT Scan	-	-	0.115	0.191
Combination Chest CT Scan	-	-	0.037	0.054
Follow-up Mammogram/Ultrasound	-	-	7.9%	8.4%
MRI for Low Back Pain	-	-	30.6%	32.7%
Survey of Patients' Hospital Experiences				
Area Around Room 'Always' Quiet at Night	-	-	-	58%
Doctors 'Always' Communicated Well	-	-	-	80%
Home Recovery Information Given	-	-	-	82%
Hospital Given 9 or 10 on 10 Point Scale	-	-	-	67%
Meds 'Always' Explained Before Given	-	-	-	60%
Nurses 'Always' Communicated Well	-	-	-	76%
Pain 'Always' Well Controlled	-	-	-	69%
Room and Bathroom 'Always' Clean	-	-	-	71%
Timely Help 'Always' Received	-	-	-	64%
Would Definitely Recommend Hospital	-	-	-	69%

Central Carolina Hospital

1135 Carthage St
Sanford, NC 27330
Phone: 919-774-2100
Fax: 919-774-2295
URL: www.centralcarolinahosp.com
Type: Acute Care Hospitals
Emergency Services: Yes
Ownership: Proprietary
Beds: 137

Key Personnel:

CEO/President.............. Doug Dorris
Chief of Medical Staff.......... Joseph Tozi, MD
Infection Control............. Tawny Ramsperburger
Operating Room.............. James B Collins III
Radiology.................. Douglas Dacko
Anesthesiology.............. Jill Hilburger, MD
Emergency Room............ Dean Flynn
Intensive Care Unit........... Phyllis Poe, RN

Measure	Cases	This Hosp.	State Avg.	U.S. Avg.
Heart Attack Care				
ACE Inhibitor or ARB for LVSD[1]	2	100%	97%	96%
Aspirin at Arrival	33	100%	99%	99%
Aspirin at Discharge[1]	12	100%	99%	98%
Beta Blocker at Discharge[1]	14	100%	99%	98%
Fibrinolytic Medication Timing	0	-	38%	55%
PCI Within 90 Minutes of Arrival	0	-	95%	90%
Smoking Cessation Advice[1]	2	100%	100%	99%
Chest Pain/Possible Heart Attack Care				
Aspirin at Arrival	99	99%	95%	95%
Median Time to ECG (minutes)	102	6	8	8
Median Time to Transfer (minutes)[1]	7	37	48	61
Fibrinolytic Medication Timing	0	-	53%	54%
Heart Failure Care				
ACE Inhibitor or ARB for LVSD	73	100%	95%	94%
Discharge Instructions	225	100%	89%	88%
Evaluation of LVS Function	266	99%	99%	98%
Smoking Cessation Advice	62	100%	99%	98%
Pneumonia Care				
Appropriate Initial Antibiotic	123	98%	92%	92%
Blood Culture Timing	157	97%	96%	96%
Influenza Vaccine	111	98%	93%	91%
Initial Antibiotic Timing	157	100%	95%	95%
Pneumococcal Vaccine	133	98%	95%	93%
Smoking Cessation Advice	53	100%	99%	97%
Surgical Care Improvement Project				
Appropriate VTP Within 24 Hours[2]	123	91%	93%	92%
Appropriate Hair Removal[2]	201	100%	100%	99%
Appropriate Beta Blocker Usage[2]	45	100%	94%	93%
Controlled Postoperative Blood Glucose[2]	0	-	94%	93%
Prophylactic Antibiotic Timing[2]	101	99%	98%	97%
Prophylactic Antibiotic Timing (Outpatient)	200	94%	94%	92%
Prophylactic Antibiotic Selection[2]	101	90%	98%	97%
Prophylactic Antibiotic Select. (Outpatient)	194	89%	95%	94%
Prophylactic Antibiotic Stopped[2]	97	94%	96%	94%
Recommended VTP Ordered[2]	123	92%	95%	94%
Urinary Catheter Removal[2]	34	85%	91%	90%
Children's Asthma Care				
Received Systemic Corticosteroids	-	-	100%	100%
Received Home Management Plan	-	-	75%	71%
Received Reliever Medication	-	-	100%	100%
Use of Medical Imaging				
Combination Abdominal CT Scan	525	0.126	0.115	0.191
Combination Chest CT Scan	333	0.099	0.037	0.054
Follow-up Mammogram/Ultrasound	1,508	3.4%	7.9%	8.4%
MRI for Low Back Pain	137	27.7%	30.6%	32.7%
Survey of Patients' Hospital Experiences				
Area Around Room 'Always' Quiet at Night	300+	56%	-	58%
Doctors 'Always' Communicated Well	300+	83%	-	80%
Home Recovery Information Given	300+	83%	-	82%
Hospital Given 9 or 10 on 10 Point Scale	300+	60%	-	67%
Meds 'Always' Explained Before Given	300+	60%	-	60%
Nurses 'Always' Communicated Well	300+	76%	-	76%
Pain 'Always' Well Controlled	300+	70%	-	69%
Room and Bathroom 'Always' Clean	300+	68%	-	71%
Timely Help 'Always' Received	300+	59%	-	64%
Would Definitely Recommend Hospital	300+	59%	-	69%

Cleveland Regional Medical Center

201 E Grover St
Shelby, NC 28150
Phone: 704-487-3000
Fax: 704-487-3290
URL: www.clevelandregional.org
Type: Acute Care Hospitals
Emergency Services: Yes
Ownership: Govt - Hospital Dist/Auth
Beds: 261

Key Personnel:

CEO/President.............. Brian Gwyn
Chief of Medical Staff.......... Thomas Davis, MD
Infection Control............. Brian Hudson
Pediatric In-Patient Care .... Nancy Porter
Quality Assurance .... Pat Hartsoe

Measure	Cases	This Hosp.	State Avg.	U.S. Avg.
Heart Attack Care				
ACE Inhibitor or ARB for LVSD[1]	7	100%	97%	96%
Aspirin at Arrival	79	99%	99%	99%
Aspirin at Discharge	42	95%	99%	98%
Beta Blocker at Discharge	41	90%	99%	98%
Fibrinolytic Medication Timing	0	-	38%	55%
PCI Within 90 Minutes of Arrival	0	-	95%	90%
Smoking Cessation Advice[1]	8	100%	100%	99%
Chest Pain/Possible Heart Attack Care				
Aspirin at Arrival	127	100%	95%	95%
Median Time to ECG (minutes)	129	3	8	8
Median Time to Transfer (minutes)	0	-	48	61
Fibrinolytic Medication Timing[1]	5	60%	53%	54%
Heart Failure Care				
ACE Inhibitor or ARB for LVSD	63	90%	95%	94%
Discharge Instructions	211	87%	89%	88%
Evaluation of LVS Function	263	100%	99%	98%
Smoking Cessation Advice	66	100%	99%	98%
Pneumonia Care				
Appropriate Initial Antibiotic	169	85%	92%	92%
Blood Culture Timing	202	90%	96%	96%
Influenza Vaccine	169	95%	93%	91%
Initial Antibiotic Timing	214	93%	95%	95%
Pneumococcal Vaccine	188	97%	95%	93%
Smoking Cessation Advice	109	99%	99%	97%
Surgical Care Improvement Project				
Appropriate VTP Within 24 Hours[2]	170	94%	93%	92%
Appropriate Hair Removal[2]	587	100%	100%	99%
Appropriate Beta Blocker Usage[2]	130	95%	94%	93%
Controlled Postoperative Blood Glucose[2]	0	-	94%	93%
Prophylactic Antibiotic Timing[2]	438	98%	98%	97%
Prophylactic Antibiotic Timing (Outpatient)	249	100%	94%	92%
Prophylactic Antibiotic Selection[2]	441	94%	98%	97%
Prophylactic Antibiotic Select. (Outpatient)	249	91%	95%	94%
Prophylactic Antibiotic Stopped[2]	432	93%	96%	94%
Recommended VTP Ordered[2]	170	95%	95%	94%
Urinary Catheter Removal[2]	91	81%	91%	90%
Children's Asthma Care				
Received Systemic Corticosteroids	-	-	100%	100%
Received Home Management Plan	-	-	75%	71%
Received Reliever Medication	-	-	100%	100%
Use of Medical Imaging				
Combination Abdominal CT Scan	1,011	0.655	0.115	0.191
Combination Chest CT Scan	896	0.002	0.037	0.054
Follow-up Mammogram/Ultrasound	741	12.1%	7.9%	8.4%
MRI for Low Back Pain	295	35.9%	30.6%	32.7%
Survey of Patients' Hospital Experiences				
Area Around Room 'Always' Quiet at Night	300+	72%	-	58%
Doctors 'Always' Communicated Well	300+	86%	-	80%
Home Recovery Information Given	300+	87%	-	82%
Hospital Given 9 or 10 on 10 Point Scale	300+	76%	-	67%
Meds 'Always' Explained Before Given	300+	74%	-	60%
Nurses 'Always' Communicated Well	300+	84%	-	76%
Pain 'Always' Well Controlled	300+	79%	-	69%
Room and Bathroom 'Always' Clean	300+	69%	-	71%
Timely Help 'Always' Received	300+	77%	-	64%
Would Definitely Recommend Hospital	300+	77%	-	69%

Chatham Hospital

475 Progress Blvd
Siler City, NC 27344
Phone: 919-663-2113
Fax: 919-663-2343
URL: www.chathamhospital.org
Type: Critical Access Hospitals
Emergency Services: Yes
Ownership: Voluntary Non-Profit - Private
Beds: 68

Key Personnel:

CEO/President.............. Carol Straight
Chief of Medical Staff.......... David Gibson
Operating Room.............. Donna Sessoms
Radiology.................. Kenneth Winter
Anesthesiology.............. Daniel Caraher, CRNA
Emergency Room............ Wilbur Carter

Measure	Cases	This Hosp.	State Avg.	U.S. Avg.
Heart Attack Care				
ACE Inhibitor or ARB for LVSD	0	-	97%	96%
Aspirin at Arrival[1]	8	100%	99%	99%
Aspirin at Discharge[1]	5	80%	99%	98%
Beta Blocker at Discharge[1]	5	80%	99%	98%
Fibrinolytic Medication Timing	0	-	38%	55%
PCI Within 90 Minutes of Arrival	0	-	95%	90%
Smoking Cessation Advice[1]	1	100%	100%	99%
Chest Pain/Possible Heart Attack Care				
Aspirin at Arrival	-	-	95%	95%
Median Time to ECG (minutes)	-	-	8	8
Median Time to Transfer (minutes)	-	-	48	61
Fibrinolytic Medication Timing	-	-	53%	54%
Heart Failure Care				
ACE Inhibitor or ARB for LVSD[1]	8	100%	95%	94%
Discharge Instructions	27	67%	89%	88%
Evaluation of LVS Function	30	97%	99%	98%
Smoking Cessation Advice[1]	9	89%	99%	98%
Pneumonia Care				
Appropriate Initial Antibiotic	42	88%	92%	92%
Blood Culture Timing	51	98%	96%	96%
Influenza Vaccine	47	98%	93%	91%
Initial Antibiotic Timing	49	88%	95%	95%
Pneumococcal Vaccine	54	96%	95%	93%
Smoking Cessation Advice[1]	16	94%	99%	97%
Surgical Care Improvement Project				
Appropriate VTP Within 24 Hours[1]	11	55%	93%	92%
Appropriate Hair Removal[1]	13	100%	100%	99%
Appropriate Beta Blocker Usage[5]	0	-	94%	93%
Controlled Postoperative Blood Glucose	0	-	94%	93%
Prophylactic Antibiotic Timing[1]	4	100%	98%	97%
Prophylactic Antibiotic Timing (Outpatient)	-	-	94%	92%
Prophylactic Antibiotic Selection[1]	4	100%	98%	97%
Prophylactic Antibiotic Select. (Outpatient)	-	-	95%	94%
Prophylactic Antibiotic Stopped[1]	4	100%	96%	94%
Recommended VTP Ordered[1]	11	55%	95%	94%
Urinary Catheter Removal[1]	5	100%	91%	90%
Children's Asthma Care				
Received Systemic Corticosteroids	-	-	100%	100%
Received Home Management Plan	-	-	75%	71%
Received Reliever Medication	-	-	100%	100%
Use of Medical Imaging				
Combination Abdominal CT Scan	-	-	0.115	0.191
Combination Chest CT Scan	-	-	0.037	0.054
Follow-up Mammogram/Ultrasound	-	-	7.9%	8.4%
MRI for Low Back Pain	-	-	30.6%	32.7%
Survey of Patients' Hospital Experiences				
Area Around Room 'Always' Quiet at Night	(a)	70%	-	58%
Doctors 'Always' Communicated Well	(a)	90%	-	80%
Home Recovery Information Given	(a)	75%	-	82%
Hospital Given 9 or 10 on 10 Point Scale	(a)	77%	-	67%
Meds 'Always' Explained Before Given	(a)	73%	-	60%
Nurses 'Always' Communicated Well	(a)	86%	-	76%
Pain 'Always' Well Controlled	(a)	71%	-	69%
Room and Bathroom 'Always' Clean	(a)	82%	-	71%
Timely Help 'Always' Received	(a)	79%	-	64%
Would Definitely Recommend Hospital	(a)	71%	-	69%

NOTE: Hospital profiles are in alphabetical order by state, then city, then hospital within the city; Rankings exclude hospitals with less than 25 cases except for patient surveys which excludes hospitals with less than 100 cases; (a) 100–299 cases; (1) The number of cases is too small to be sure how well a hospital is performing; (2) The hospital indicated that the data submitted for this measure were based on a sample of cases; (3) Data was collected during a shorter time period (fewer quarters) than the maximum possible time for this measure; (4) Suppressed for one or more quarters by CMS; (5) No data is available from the hospital for this measure; (6) Fewer than 100 patients completed the HCAHPS survey. Use these rates with caution, as the number of surveys may be too low to reliably assess hospital performance; (7) Survey results are based on less than 12 months of data; (8) Survey results are not available for this reporting period; (9) No or very few patients were eligible for the HCAHPS survey. The scores shown, if any, reflect a very small number of surveys; (10) A state average was not calculated because too few hospitals in the state submitted data; (11) There were discrepancies in the data collection process; Please refer to the User's Guide for a full explanation of data.

Johnston Memorial Hospital

509 Bright Leaf Blvd Phone: 919-934-8171
Smithfield, NC 27577 Fax: 919-989-7297
URL: www.johnstanmemorial.org
Type: Acute Care Hospitals Emergency Services: Yes
Ownership: Govt - Hospital Dist/Auth Beds: 175

Key Personnel:
CEO/President. . . . . Kevin L Rogols
Chief of Medical Staff. . . . . Dr Eric Gloss

Measure	Cases	This Hosp.	State Avg.	U.S. Avg.
Heart Attack Care				
ACE Inhibitor or ARB for LVSD[1]	2	100%	97%	96%
Aspirin at Arrival	109	97%	99%	99%
Aspirin at Discharge	33	88%	99%	98%
Beta Blocker at Discharge	33	94%	99%	98%
Fibrinolytic Medication Timing[1]	4	25%	38%	55%
PCI Within 90 Minutes of Arrival	0	-	95%	90%
Smoking Cessation Advice[1]	8	100%	100%	99%
Chest Pain/Possible Heart Attack Care				
Aspirin at Arrival	257	92%	95%	95%
Median Time to ECG (minutes)	268	13	8	8
Median Time to Transfer (minutes)[1]	12	80	48	61
Fibrinolytic Medication Timing[1]	4	75%	53%	54%
Heart Failure Care				
ACE Inhibitor or ARB for LVSD	85	67%	95%	94%
Discharge Instructions	253	86%	89%	88%
Evaluation of LVS Function	310	100%	99%	98%
Smoking Cessation Advice	54	100%	99%	98%
Pneumonia Care				
Appropriate Initial Antibiotic	171	84%	92%	92%
Blood Culture Timing	213	91%	96%	96%
Influenza Vaccine	163	67%	93%	91%
Initial Antibiotic Timing	253	91%	95%	95%
Pneumococcal Vaccine	222	70%	95%	93%
Smoking Cessation Advice	82	100%	99%	97%
Surgical Care Improvement Project				
Appropriate VTP Within 24 Hours	195	77%	93%	92%
Appropriate Hair Removal	450	100%	100%	99%
Appropriate Beta Blocker Usage	160	89%	94%	93%
Controlled Postoperative Blood Glucose	0	-	94%	93%
Prophylactic Antibiotic Timing	285	98%	98%	97%
Prophylactic Antibiotic Timing (Outpatient)	252	96%	94%	92%
Prophylactic Antibiotic Selection	287	89%	98%	97%
Prophylactic Antibiotic Select. (Outpatient)	247	88%	95%	94%
Prophylactic Antibiotic Stopped	277	88%	96%	94%
Recommended VTP Ordered	200	81%	95%	94%
Urinary Catheter Removal	110	80%	91%	90%
Children's Asthma Care				
Received Systemic Corticosteroids	-	-	100%	100%
Received Home Management Plan	-	-	75%	71%
Received Reliever Medication	-	-	100%	100%
Use of Medical Imaging				
Combination Abdominal CT Scan	553	0.105	0.115	0.191
Combination Chest CT Scan	591	0.041	0.037	0.054
Follow-up Mammogram/Ultrasound	1,057	9.7%	7.9%	8.4%
MRI for Low Back Pain	139	30.2%	30.6%	32.7%
Survey of Patients' Hospital Experiences				
Area Around Room 'Always' Quiet at Night	300+	64%	-	58%
Doctors 'Always' Communicated Well	300+	81%	-	80%
Home Recovery Information Given	300+	83%	-	82%
Hospital Given 9 or 10 on 10 Point Scale	300+	62%	-	67%
Meds 'Always' Explained Before Given	300+	64%	-	60%
Nurses 'Always' Communicated Well	300+	78%	-	76%
Pain 'Always' Well Controlled	300+	70%	-	69%
Room and Bathroom 'Always' Clean	300+	68%	-	71%
Timely Help 'Always' Received	300+	63%	-	64%
Would Definitely Recommend Hospital	300+	63%	-	69%

J Arthur Dosher Memorial Hospital

924 Howe St Phone: 910-457-3800
Southport, NC 28461 Fax: 910-457-3908
URL: www.dosher.org
Type: Critical Access Hospitals Emergency Services: Yes
Ownership: Voluntary Non-Profit - Other Beds: 64

Key Personnel:
CEO/President. . . . . Edgar Haywood, III
Quality Assurance . . . . Connie Shea
Radiology. . . . . Gail M Capel

Measure	Cases	This Hosp.	State Avg.	U.S. Avg.
Heart Attack Care				
ACE Inhibitor or ARB for LVSD	-	-	97%	96%
Aspirin at Arrival	-	-	99%	99%
Aspirin at Discharge	-	-	99%	98%
Beta Blocker at Discharge	-	-	99%	98%
Fibrinolytic Medication Timing	-	-	38%	55%
PCI Within 90 Minutes of Arrival	-	-	95%	90%
Smoking Cessation Advice	-	-	100%	99%
Chest Pain/Possible Heart Attack Care				
Aspirin at Arrival	72	92%	95%	95%
Median Time to ECG (minutes)	73	17	8	8
Median Time to Transfer (minutes)[5]	0	-	48	61
Fibrinolytic Medication Timing[3]	0	-	53%	54%
Heart Failure Care				
ACE Inhibitor or ARB for LVSD	-	-	95%	94%
Discharge Instructions	-	-	89%	88%
Evaluation of LVS Function	-	-	99%	98%
Smoking Cessation Advice	-	-	99%	98%
Pneumonia Care				
Appropriate Initial Antibiotic	-	-	92%	92%
Blood Culture Timing	-	-	96%	96%
Influenza Vaccine	-	-	93%	91%
Initial Antibiotic Timing	-	-	95%	95%
Pneumococcal Vaccine	-	-	95%	93%
Smoking Cessation Advice	-	-	99%	97%
Surgical Care Improvement Project				
Appropriate VTP Within 24 Hours	-	-	93%	92%
Appropriate Hair Removal	-	-	100%	99%
Appropriate Beta Blocker Usage	-	-	94%	93%
Controlled Postoperative Blood Glucose	-	-	94%	93%
Prophylactic Antibiotic Timing	-	-	98%	97%
Prophylactic Antibiotic Timing (Outpatient)[5]	0	-	94%	92%
Prophylactic Antibiotic Selection	-	-	98%	97%
Prophylactic Antibiotic Select. (Outpatient)[5]	0	-	95%	94%
Prophylactic Antibiotic Stopped	-	-	96%	94%
Recommended VTP Ordered	-	-	95%	94%
Urinary Catheter Removal	-	-	91%	90%
Children's Asthma Care				
Received Systemic Corticosteroids	-	-	100%	100%
Received Home Management Plan	-	-	75%	71%
Received Reliever Medication	-	-	100%	100%
Use of Medical Imaging				
Combination Abdominal CT Scan	-	-	0.115	0.191
Combination Chest CT Scan	-	-	0.037	0.054
Follow-up Mammogram/Ultrasound	-	-	7.9%	8.4%
MRI for Low Back Pain	-	-	30.6%	32.7%
Survey of Patients' Hospital Experiences				
Area Around Room 'Always' Quiet at Night	-	-	-	58%
Doctors 'Always' Communicated Well	-	-	-	80%
Home Recovery Information Given	-	-	-	82%
Hospital Given 9 or 10 on 10 Point Scale	-	-	-	67%
Meds 'Always' Explained Before Given	-	-	-	60%
Nurses 'Always' Communicated Well	-	-	-	76%
Pain 'Always' Well Controlled	-	-	-	69%
Room and Bathroom 'Always' Clean	-	-	-	71%
Timely Help 'Always' Received	-	-	-	64%
Would Definitely Recommend Hospital	-	-	-	69%

Alleghany County Memorial Hospital

617 Doctors Street Phone: 336-372-5511
Sparta, NC 28675 Fax: 336-372-8451
URL: www.amhsparta.org
Type: Critical Access Hospitals Emergency Services: Yes
Ownership: Voluntary Non-Profit - Private Beds: 25

Key Personnel:
CEO/President. . . . . Kevin W Harlan
Chief of Medical Staff. . . . . Jeffrey Ray, MD
Infection Control. . . . . Mary Jones, RN
Operating Room. . . . . Pam Moss
Quality Assurance . . . . Jayne Phipps-Boger
Radiology. . . . . Paul Beerman, RT
Emergency Room . . . . Jeff Ray, MD
Patient Relations . . . . Miranda Miller

Measure	Cases	This Hosp.	State Avg.	U.S. Avg.
Heart Attack Care				
ACE Inhibitor or ARB for LVSD	0	-	97%	96%
Aspirin at Arrival[1]	12	83%	99%	99%
Aspirin at Discharge[1]	9	89%	99%	98%
Beta Blocker at Discharge[1]	9	100%	99%	98%
Fibrinolytic Medication Timing	0	-	38%	55%
PCI Within 90 Minutes of Arrival	0	-	95%	90%
Smoking Cessation Advice	0	-	100%	99%
Chest Pain/Possible Heart Attack Care				
Aspirin at Arrival[1,3]	11	91%	95%	95%
Median Time to ECG (minutes)[1,3]	12	46	8	8
Median Time to Transfer (minutes)[3]	0	-	48	61
Fibrinolytic Medication Timing[1,3]	4	0%	53%	54%
Heart Failure Care				
ACE Inhibitor or ARB for LVSD[1]	3	100%	95%	94%
Discharge Instructions	27	100%	89%	88%
Evaluation of LVS Function	33	91%	99%	98%
Smoking Cessation Advice[1]	2	50%	99%	98%
Pneumonia Care				
Appropriate Initial Antibiotic	51	86%	92%	92%
Blood Culture Timing	55	91%	96%	96%
Influenza Vaccine	48	90%	93%	91%
Initial Antibiotic Timing	65	92%	95%	95%
Pneumococcal Vaccine	61	95%	95%	93%
Smoking Cessation Advice[1]	23	96%	99%	97%
Surgical Care Improvement Project				
Appropriate VTP Within 24 Hours[5]	0	-	93%	92%
Appropriate Hair Removal[5]	0	-	100%	99%
Appropriate Beta Blocker Usage[5]	0	-	94%	93%
Controlled Postoperative Blood Glucose[5]	0	-	94%	93%
Prophylactic Antibiotic Timing[5]	0	-	98%	97%
Prophylactic Antibiotic Timing (Outpatient)[1,3]	3	67%	94%	92%
Prophylactic Antibiotic Selection[5]	0	-	98%	97%
Prophylactic Antibiotic Select. (Outpatient)[1,3]	2	100%	95%	94%
Prophylactic Antibiotic Stopped[5]	0	-	96%	94%
Recommended VTP Ordered[5]	0	-	95%	94%
Urinary Catheter Removal[5]	0	-	91%	90%
Children's Asthma Care				
Received Systemic Corticosteroids	-	-	100%	100%
Received Home Management Plan	-	-	75%	71%
Received Reliever Medication	-	-	100%	100%
Use of Medical Imaging				
Combination Abdominal CT Scan	81	0.469	0.115	0.191
Combination Chest CT Scan[1]	33	0.000	0.037	0.054
Follow-up Mammogram/Ultrasound	298	3.0%	7.9%	8.4%
MRI for Low Back Pain[5]	0	-	30.6%	32.7%
Survey of Patients' Hospital Experiences				
Area Around Room 'Always' Quiet at Night	(a)	50%	-	58%
Doctors 'Always' Communicated Well	(a)	83%	-	80%
Home Recovery Information Given	(a)	83%	-	82%
Hospital Given 9 or 10 on 10 Point Scale	(a)	67%	-	67%
Meds 'Always' Explained Before Given	(a)	57%	-	60%
Nurses 'Always' Communicated Well	(a)	78%	-	76%
Pain 'Always' Well Controlled	(a)	67%	-	69%
Room and Bathroom 'Always' Clean	(a)	65%	-	71%
Timely Help 'Always' Received	(a)	63%	-	64%
Would Definitely Recommend Hospital	(a)	69%	-	69%

NOTE: Hospital profiles are in alphabetical order by state, then city, then hospital within the city; Rankings exclude hospitals with less than 25 cases except for patient surveys which excludes hospitals with less than 100 cases; (a) 100–299 cases; (1) The number of cases is too small to be sure how well a hospital is performing; (2) The hospital indicated that the data submitted for this measure were based on a sample of cases; (3) Data was collected during a shorter time period (fewer quarters) than the maximum possible time for this measure; (4) Suppressed for one or more quarters by CMS; (5) No data is available from the hospital for this measure; (6) Fewer than 100 patients completed the HCAHPS survey. Use these rates with caution, as the number of surveys may be too low to reliably assess hospital performance; (7) Survey results are based on less than 12 months of data; (8) Survey results are not available for this reporting period; (9) No or very few patients were eligible for the HCAHPS survey. The scores shown, if any, reflect a very small number of surveys; (10) A state average was not calculated because too few hospitals in the state submitted data; (11) There were discrepancies in the data collection process; Please refer to the User's Guide for a full explanation of data.

Spruce Pine Community Hospital

125 Hospital Dr
Spruce Pine, NC 28777
URL: www.spchospital.org
Type: Acute Care Hospitals
Ownership: Voluntary Non-Profit - Other
Phone: 828-765-4201
Fax: 828-765-0824
Emergency Services: Yes
Beds: 40

Key Personnel:
CEO/President. . . . . Keith Holtsclaw
Chief of Medical Staff . . . . Jerry Cade, MD
Infection Control. . . . . Mary Ann Johnson, RN
Quality Assurance . . . . John Brazil
Anesthesiology. . . . . Andrea Hinson
Emergency Room . . . . Jerry Cade, MD
Intensive Care Unit. . . . . Vicky Tolley, RN
Patient Relations . . . . Jane Edwards

Measure	Cases	This Hosp.	State Avg.	U.S. Avg.
Heart Attack Care				
ACE Inhibitor or ARB for LVSD[1]	1	100%	97%	96%
Aspirin at Arrival[1]	10	100%	99%	99%
Aspirin at Discharge[1]	5	60%	99%	98%
Beta Blocker at Discharge[1]	5	100%	99%	98%
Fibrinolytic Medication Timing	0	-	38%	55%
PCI Within 90 Minutes of Arrival	0	-	95%	90%
Smoking Cessation Advice	0	-	100%	99%
Chest Pain/Possible Heart Attack Care				
Aspirin at Arrival	58	91%	95%	95%
Median Time to ECG (minutes)	61	8	8	8
Median Time to Transfer (minutes)[1,3]	5	108	48	61
Fibrinolytic Medication Timing[1]	2	0%	53%	54%
Heart Failure Care				
ACE Inhibitor or ARB for LVSD[1]	16	88%	95%	94%
Discharge Instructions	48	94%	89%	88%
Evaluation of LVS Function	64	78%	99%	98%
Smoking Cessation Advice[1]	11	82%	99%	98%
Pneumonia Care				
Appropriate Initial Antibiotic	112	80%	92%	92%
Blood Culture Timing	114	82%	96%	96%
Influenza Vaccine	74	88%	93%	91%
Initial Antibiotic Timing	139	85%	95%	95%
Pneumococcal Vaccine	129	94%	95%	93%
Smoking Cessation Advice	46	74%	99%	97%
Surgical Care Improvement Project				
Appropriate VTP Within 24 Hours	57	89%	93%	92%
Appropriate Hair Removal	137	100%	100%	99%
Appropriate Beta Blocker Usage	33	88%	94%	93%
Controlled Postoperative Blood Glucose	0	-	94%	93%
Prophylactic Antibiotic Timing	104	95%	98%	97%
Prophylactic Antibiotic Timing (Outpatient)	25	100%	94%	92%
Prophylactic Antibiotic Selection	103	99%	98%	97%
Prophylactic Antibiotic Select. (Outpatient)	25	92%	95%	94%
Prophylactic Antibiotic Stopped	100	96%	96%	94%
Recommended VTP Ordered	57	96%	95%	94%
Urinary Catheter Removal	0	-	91%	90%
Children's Asthma Care				
Received Systemic Corticosteroids	-	-	100%	100%
Received Home Management Plan	-	-	75%	71%
Received Reliever Medication	-	-	100%	100%
Use of Medical Imaging				
Combination Abdominal CT Scan	315	0.790	0.115	0.191
Combination Chest CT Scan	200	0.890	0.037	0.054
Follow-up Mammogram/Ultrasound	574	3.7%	7.9%	8.4%
MRI for Low Back Pain	81	40.7%	30.6%	32.7%
Survey of Patients' Hospital Experiences				
Area Around Room 'Always' Quiet at Night	300+	68%	-	58%
Doctors 'Always' Communicated Well	300+	84%	-	80%
Home Recovery Information Given	300+	79%	-	82%
Hospital Given 9 or 10 on 10 Point Scale	300+	76%	-	67%
Meds 'Always' Explained Before Given	300+	66%	-	60%
Nurses 'Always' Communicated Well	300+	82%	-	76%
Pain 'Always' Well Controlled	300+	75%	-	69%
Room and Bathroom 'Always' Clean	300+	77%	-	71%
Timely Help 'Always' Received	300+	72%	-	64%
Would Definitely Recommend Hospital	300+	75%	-	69%

Davis Regional Medical Center

218 Old Mocksville Rd
Statesville, NC 28687
Type: Acute Care Hospitals
Ownership: Proprietary
Phone: 704-873-0281
Fax: 704-838-7289
Emergency Services: No
Beds: 131

Key Personnel:
Cardiac Laboratory. . . . . Kimberly Harrell
Chief of Medical Staff . . . . Seema Garcha, MD
Infection Control. . . . . Amy Painter
Operating Room. . . . . Gary Robinson, MD
Radiology. . . . . Andrew M Schneider
Emergency Room . . . . Tammy Brooks, RN

Measure	Cases	This Hosp.	State Avg.	U.S. Avg.
Heart Attack Care				
ACE Inhibitor or ARB for LVSD[1]	1	100%	97%	96%
Aspirin at Arrival[1]	8	100%	99%	99%
Aspirin at Discharge[1]	4	100%	99%	98%
Beta Blocker at Discharge[1]	5	100%	99%	98%
Fibrinolytic Medication Timing	0	-	38%	55%
PCI Within 90 Minutes of Arrival	0	-	95%	90%
Smoking Cessation Advice[1]	2	100%	100%	99%
Chest Pain/Possible Heart Attack Care				
Aspirin at Arrival	40	100%	95%	95%
Median Time to ECG (minutes)	40	3	8	8
Median Time to Transfer (minutes)[1,3]	7	24	48	61
Fibrinolytic Medication Timing[1]	3	67%	53%	54%
Heart Failure Care				
ACE Inhibitor or ARB for LVSD	31	100%	95%	94%
Discharge Instructions	159	100%	89%	88%
Evaluation of LVS Function	180	100%	99%	98%
Smoking Cessation Advice	71	100%	99%	98%
Pneumonia Care				
Appropriate Initial Antibiotic	78	95%	92%	92%
Blood Culture Timing	116	97%	96%	96%
Influenza Vaccine	62	100%	93%	91%
Initial Antibiotic Timing	94	98%	95%	95%
Pneumococcal Vaccine	68	100%	95%	93%
Smoking Cessation Advice	59	100%	99%	97%
Surgical Care Improvement Project				
Appropriate VTP Within 24 Hours	135	99%	93%	92%
Appropriate Hair Removal	192	100%	100%	99%
Appropriate Beta Blocker Usage	48	100%	94%	93%
Controlled Postoperative Blood Glucose	0	-	94%	93%
Prophylactic Antibiotic Timing	119	98%	98%	97%
Prophylactic Antibiotic Timing (Outpatient)	308	100%	94%	92%
Prophylactic Antibiotic Selection	120	98%	98%	97%
Prophylactic Antibiotic Select. (Outpatient)	308	99%	95%	94%
Prophylactic Antibiotic Stopped	114	93%	96%	94%
Recommended VTP Ordered	135	99%	95%	94%
Urinary Catheter Removal	48	98%	91%	90%
Children's Asthma Care				
Received Systemic Corticosteroids	29	100%	100%	100%
Received Home Management Plan	29	97%	75%	71%
Received Reliever Medication	29	100%	100%	100%
Use of Medical Imaging				
Combination Abdominal CT Scan	329	0.070	0.115	0.191
Combination Chest CT Scan	89	0.011	0.037	0.054
Follow-up Mammogram/Ultrasound	103	10.7%	7.9%	8.4%
MRI for Low Back Pain	166	27.7%	30.6%	32.7%
Survey of Patients' Hospital Experiences				
Area Around Room 'Always' Quiet at Night	300+	67%	-	58%
Doctors 'Always' Communicated Well	300+	82%	-	80%
Home Recovery Information Given	300+	81%	-	82%
Hospital Given 9 or 10 on 10 Point Scale	300+	74%	-	67%
Meds 'Always' Explained Before Given	300+	64%	-	60%
Nurses 'Always' Communicated Well	300+	77%	-	76%
Pain 'Always' Well Controlled	300+	65%	-	69%
Room and Bathroom 'Always' Clean	300+	76%	-	71%
Timely Help 'Always' Received	300+	67%	-	64%
Would Definitely Recommend Hospital	300+	75%	-	69%

Iredell Memorial Hospital

557 Brookdale Dr
Statesville, NC 28677
URL: www.iredellmemorial.org
Type: Acute Care Hospitals
Ownership: Voluntary Non-Profit - Other
Phone: 704-873-5661
Fax: 704-872-7924
Emergency Services: Yes
Beds: 247

Key Personnel:
CEO/President. . . . . Ed Rush
Chief of Medical Staff . . . . Anthony Mebech
Infection Control. . . . . Sylvia Chapman
Operating Room. . . . . Cindy Miller
Quality Assurance . . . . Tracy Thomas
Radiology. . . . . Reid D Breckwoldt
Emergency Room . . . . James Bryant, MD
Intensive Care Unit. . . . . Eddie Bass, RN

Measure	Cases	This Hosp.	State Avg.	U.S. Avg.
Heart Attack Care				
ACE Inhibitor or ARB for LVSD[1]	2	100%	97%	96%
Aspirin at Arrival	59	100%	99%	99%
Aspirin at Discharge	39	100%	99%	98%
Beta Blocker at Discharge	37	97%	99%	98%
Fibrinolytic Medication Timing	0	-	38%	55%
PCI Within 90 Minutes of Arrival[1]	5	100%	95%	90%
Smoking Cessation Advice[1]	9	100%	100%	99%
Chest Pain/Possible Heart Attack Care				
Aspirin at Arrival	88	99%	95%	95%
Median Time to ECG (minutes)	89	7	8	8
Median Time to Transfer (minutes)	33	58	48	61
Fibrinolytic Medication Timing[1]	3	67%	53%	54%
Heart Failure Care				
ACE Inhibitor or ARB for LVSD	62	100%	95%	94%
Discharge Instructions	250	94%	89%	88%
Evaluation of LVS Function	316	100%	99%	98%
Smoking Cessation Advice	70	100%	99%	98%
Pneumonia Care				
Appropriate Initial Antibiotic	175	90%	92%	92%
Blood Culture Timing	200	97%	96%	96%
Influenza Vaccine	142	99%	93%	91%
Initial Antibiotic Timing	253	99%	95%	95%
Pneumococcal Vaccine	238	99%	95%	93%
Smoking Cessation Advice	93	100%	99%	97%
Surgical Care Improvement Project				
Appropriate VTP Within 24 Hours[2]	242	94%	93%	92%
Appropriate Hair Removal[2]	389	100%	100%	99%
Appropriate Beta Blocker Usage[2]	117	96%	94%	93%
Controlled Postoperative Blood Glucose[2]	0	-	94%	93%
Prophylactic Antibiotic Timing[2]	238	98%	98%	97%
Prophylactic Antibiotic Timing (Outpatient)	200	92%	94%	92%
Prophylactic Antibiotic Selection[2]	240	96%	98%	97%
Prophylactic Antibiotic Select. (Outpatient)	192	93%	95%	94%
Prophylactic Antibiotic Stopped[2]	228	95%	96%	94%
Recommended VTP Ordered[2]	245	96%	95%	94%
Urinary Catheter Removal[2]	61	95%	91%	90%
Children's Asthma Care				
Received Systemic Corticosteroids	-	-	100%	100%
Received Home Management Plan	-	-	75%	71%
Received Reliever Medication	-	-	100%	100%
Use of Medical Imaging				
Combination Abdominal CT Scan	756	0.029	0.115	0.191
Combination Chest CT Scan	366	0.005	0.037	0.054
Follow-up Mammogram/Ultrasound	1,783	3.1%	7.9%	8.4%
MRI for Low Back Pain	175	28.6%	30.6%	32.7%
Survey of Patients' Hospital Experiences				
Area Around Room 'Always' Quiet at Night	300+	66%	-	58%
Doctors 'Always' Communicated Well	300+	86%	-	80%
Home Recovery Information Given	300+	84%	-	82%
Hospital Given 9 or 10 on 10 Point Scale	300+	74%	-	67%
Meds 'Always' Explained Before Given	300+	68%	-	60%
Nurses 'Always' Communicated Well	300+	82%	-	76%
Pain 'Always' Well Controlled	300+	73%	-	69%
Room and Bathroom 'Always' Clean	300+	73%	-	71%
Timely Help 'Always' Received	300+	67%	-	64%
Would Definitely Recommend Hospital	300+	79%	-	69%

NOTE: Hospital profiles are in alphabetical order by state, then city, then hospital within the city; Rankings exclude hospitals with less than 25 cases except for patient surveys which excludes hospitals with less than 100 cases; (a) 100–299 cases; (1) The number of cases is too small to be sure how well a hospital is performing; (2) The hospital indicated that the data submitted for this measure were based on a sample of cases; (3) Data was collected during a shorter time period (fewer quarters) than the maximum possible time for this measure; (4) Suppressed for one or more quarters by CMS; (5) No data is available from the hospital for this measure; (6) Fewer than 100 patients completed the HCAHPS survey. Use these rates with caution, as the number of surveys may be too low to reliably assess hospital performance; (7) Survey results are based on less than 12 months of data; (8) Survey results are not available for this reporting period; (9) No or very few patients were eligible for the HCAHPS survey. The scores shown, if any, reflect a very small number of surveys; (10) A state average was not calculated because too few hospitals in the state submitted data; (11) There were discrepancies in the data collection process; Please refer to the User's Guide for a full explanation of data.

Brunswick Community Hospital

1 Medical Center Drive Phone: 910-755-8121
Supply, NC 28462 Fax: 910-755-1200
URL: www.brunswickcommunityhospital.com
Type: Acute Care Hospitals Emergency Services: Yes
Ownership: Voluntary Non-Profit - Other Beds: 60

Key Personnel:
CEO/President.............. Denise Mihal
Chief of Medical Staff.......... Robert Haffler
Quality Assurance .... Sherry Cappellino
Emergency Room .... Warren Faulk

Measure	Cases	This Hosp.	State Avg.	U.S. Avg.
Heart Attack Care				
ACE Inhibitor or ARB for LVSD[1]	1	100%	97%	96%
Aspirin at Arrival[1]	12	100%	99%	99%
Aspirin at Discharge[1]	3	100%	99%	98%
Beta Blocker at Discharge[1]	3	100%	99%	98%
Fibrinolytic Medication Timing	0	-	38%	55%
PCI Within 90 Minutes of Arrival	0	-	95%	90%
Smoking Cessation Advice	0	-	100%	99%
Chest Pain/Possible Heart Attack Care				
Aspirin at Arrival	87	97%	95%	95%
Median Time to ECG (minutes)	86	3	8	8
Median Time to Transfer (minutes)[1]	15	32	48	61
Fibrinolytic Medication Timing[1]	1	100%	53%	54%
Heart Failure Care				
ACE Inhibitor or ARB for LVSD	47	100%	95%	94%
Discharge Instructions	92	98%	89%	88%
Evaluation of LVS Function	117	100%	99%	98%
Smoking Cessation Advice	26	100%	99%	98%
Pneumonia Care				
Appropriate Initial Antibiotic	74	93%	92%	92%
Blood Culture Timing	106	99%	96%	96%
Influenza Vaccine	68	100%	93%	91%
Initial Antibiotic Timing	105	100%	95%	95%
Pneumococcal Vaccine	94	99%	95%	93%
Smoking Cessation Advice	56	100%	99%	97%
Surgical Care Improvement Project				
Appropriate VTP Within 24 Hours	134	99%	93%	92%
Appropriate Hair Removal	307	100%	100%	99%
Appropriate Beta Blocker Usage	73	100%	94%	93%
Controlled Postoperative Blood Glucose	0	-	94%	93%
Prophylactic Antibiotic Timing	233	100%	98%	97%
Prophylactic Antibiotic Timing (Outpatient)	98	96%	94%	92%
Prophylactic Antibiotic Selection	233	100%	98%	97%
Prophylactic Antibiotic Select. (Outpatient)	95	88%	95%	94%
Prophylactic Antibiotic Stopped	220	98%	96%	94%
Recommended VTP Ordered	134	99%	95%	94%
Urinary Catheter Removal	82	95%	91%	90%
Children's Asthma Care				
Received Systemic Corticosteroids	-	-	100%	100%
Received Home Management Plan	-	-	75%	71%
Received Reliever Medication	-	-	100%	100%
Use of Medical Imaging				
Combination Abdominal CT Scan	516	0.050	0.115	0.191
Combination Chest CT Scan	337	0.018	0.037	0.054
Follow-up Mammogram/Ultrasound	1,086	5.5%	7.9%	8.4%
MRI for Low Back Pain	106	28.3%	30.6%	32.7%
Survey of Patients' Hospital Experiences				
Area Around Room 'Always' Quiet at Night	300+	50%	-	58%
Doctors 'Always' Communicated Well	300+	82%	-	80%
Home Recovery Information Given	300+	84%	-	82%
Hospital Given 9 or 10 on 10 Point Scale	300+	62%	-	67%
Meds 'Always' Explained Before Given	300+	55%	-	60%
Nurses 'Always' Communicated Well	300+	76%	-	76%
Pain 'Always' Well Controlled	300+	69%	-	69%
Room and Bathroom 'Always' Clean	300+	63%	-	71%
Timely Help 'Always' Received	300+	70%	-	64%
Would Definitely Recommend Hospital	300+	62%	-	69%

C J Harris Community Hospital

68 Hospital Rd Phone: 828-586-7000
Sylva, NC 28779 Fax: 828-586-7467
URL: www.westcare.org
Type: Acute Care Hospitals Emergency Services: Yes
Ownership: Voluntary Non-Profit - Private Beds: 86

Key Personnel:
CEO/President.............. Mike Poore
Cardiac Laboratory............ Earl Haddock MD
Chief of Medical Staff.......... David Zimmerman
Infection Control.............. Alice Gibson
Operating Room.............. Nora Myers
Quality Assurance .... Debra Bennett
Radiology.................. Jacky Bradley
Emergency Room .... Katrina Coggins

Measure	Cases	This Hosp.	State Avg.	U.S. Avg.
Heart Attack Care				
ACE Inhibitor or ARB for LVSD	0	-	97%	96%
Aspirin at Arrival[1]	8	100%	99%	99%
Aspirin at Discharge[1]	2	100%	99%	98%
Beta Blocker at Discharge[1]	1	100%	99%	98%
Fibrinolytic Medication Timing	0	-	38%	55%
PCI Within 90 Minutes of Arrival	0	-	95%	90%
Smoking Cessation Advice	0	-	100%	99%
Chest Pain/Possible Heart Attack Care				
Aspirin at Arrival	34	97%	95%	95%
Median Time to ECG (minutes)	33	10	8	8
Median Time to Transfer (minutes)[1,3]	5	103	48	61
Fibrinolytic Medication Timing[3]	0	-	53%	54%
Heart Failure Care				
ACE Inhibitor or ARB for LVSD	42	98%	95%	94%
Discharge Instructions	73	78%	89%	88%
Evaluation of LVS Function	87	97%	99%	98%
Smoking Cessation Advice[1]	15	100%	99%	98%
Pneumonia Care				
Appropriate Initial Antibiotic	141	94%	92%	92%
Blood Culture Timing	158	96%	96%	96%
Influenza Vaccine	130	96%	93%	91%
Initial Antibiotic Timing	179	94%	95%	95%
Pneumococcal Vaccine	193	99%	95%	93%
Smoking Cessation Advice	81	100%	99%	97%
Surgical Care Improvement Project				
Appropriate VTP Within 24 Hours[2]	152	85%	93%	92%
Appropriate Hair Removal[2]	274	100%	100%	99%
Appropriate Beta Blocker Usage[2]	47	100%	94%	93%
Controlled Postoperative Blood Glucose[2]	0	-	94%	93%
Prophylactic Antibiotic Timing[2]	212	95%	98%	97%
Prophylactic Antibiotic Timing (Outpatient)	144	90%	94%	92%
Prophylactic Antibiotic Selection[2]	214	98%	98%	97%
Prophylactic Antibiotic Select. (Outpatient)	139	91%	95%	94%
Prophylactic Antibiotic Stopped[2]	193	96%	96%	94%
Recommended VTP Ordered[2]	152	95%	95%	94%
Urinary Catheter Removal[2]	74	92%	91%	90%
Children's Asthma Care				
Received Systemic Corticosteroids	-	-	100%	100%
Received Home Management Plan	-	-	75%	71%
Received Reliever Medication	-	-	100%	100%
Use of Medical Imaging				
Combination Abdominal CT Scan	544	0.583	0.115	0.191
Combination Chest CT Scan	655	0.125	0.037	0.054
Follow-up Mammogram/Ultrasound	956	12.4%	7.9%	8.4%
MRI for Low Back Pain	223	28.7%	30.6%	32.7%
Survey of Patients' Hospital Experiences				
Area Around Room 'Always' Quiet at Night	300+	61%	-	58%
Doctors 'Always' Communicated Well	300+	83%	-	80%
Home Recovery Information Given	300+	83%	-	82%
Hospital Given 9 or 10 on 10 Point Scale	300+	74%	-	67%
Meds 'Always' Explained Before Given	300+	63%	-	60%
Nurses 'Always' Communicated Well	300+	81%	-	76%
Pain 'Always' Well Controlled	300+	73%	-	69%
Room and Bathroom 'Always' Clean	300+	65%	-	71%
Timely Help 'Always' Received	300+	70%	-	64%
Would Definitely Recommend Hospital	300+	76%	-	69%

Heritage Hospital

111 Hospital Dr Phone: 252-641-7700
Tarboro, NC 27886
Type: Acute Care Hospitals Emergency Services: Yes
Ownership: Government - Local

Key Personnel:
CEO/President.............. Wick Baker
Radiology.................. Michael McLaughlin MD

Measure	Cases	This Hosp.	State Avg.	U.S. Avg.
Heart Attack Care				
ACE Inhibitor or ARB for LVSD[1]	1	100%	97%	96%
Aspirin at Arrival[1]	17	100%	99%	99%
Aspirin at Discharge[1]	8	88%	99%	98%
Beta Blocker at Discharge[1]	10	100%	99%	98%
Fibrinolytic Medication Timing	0	-	38%	55%
PCI Within 90 Minutes of Arrival	0	-	95%	90%
Smoking Cessation Advice[1]	2	100%	100%	99%
Chest Pain/Possible Heart Attack Care				
Aspirin at Arrival	51	100%	95%	95%
Median Time to ECG (minutes)	51	9	8	8
Median Time to Transfer (minutes)[5]	0	-	48	61
Fibrinolytic Medication Timing[1]	2	100%	53%	54%
Heart Failure Care				
ACE Inhibitor or ARB for LVSD	75	99%	95%	94%
Discharge Instructions	151	98%	89%	88%
Evaluation of LVS Function	196	100%	99%	98%
Smoking Cessation Advice	36	100%	99%	98%
Pneumonia Care				
Appropriate Initial Antibiotic	44	93%	92%	92%
Blood Culture Timing	76	97%	96%	96%
Influenza Vaccine	53	91%	93%	91%
Initial Antibiotic Timing	72	100%	95%	95%
Pneumococcal Vaccine	58	95%	95%	93%
Smoking Cessation Advice[1]	24	100%	99%	97%
Surgical Care Improvement Project				
Appropriate VTP Within 24 Hours	75	93%	93%	92%
Appropriate Hair Removal	130	100%	100%	99%
Appropriate Beta Blocker Usage[1]	24	96%	94%	93%
Controlled Postoperative Blood Glucose	0	-	94%	93%
Prophylactic Antibiotic Timing	64	100%	98%	97%
Prophylactic Antibiotic Timing (Outpatient)	154	99%	94%	92%
Prophylactic Antibiotic Selection	64	98%	98%	97%
Prophylactic Antibiotic Select. (Outpatient)	153	93%	95%	94%
Prophylactic Antibiotic Stopped	62	95%	96%	94%
Recommended VTP Ordered	76	92%	95%	94%
Urinary Catheter Removal[1]	22	95%	91%	90%
Children's Asthma Care				
Received Systemic Corticosteroids	-	-	100%	100%
Received Home Management Plan	-	-	75%	71%
Received Reliever Medication	-	-	100%	100%
Use of Medical Imaging				
Combination Abdominal CT Scan	304	0.066	0.115	0.191
Combination Chest CT Scan	201	0.005	0.037	0.054
Follow-up Mammogram/Ultrasound	1,019	6.0%	7.9%	8.4%
MRI for Low Back Pain	141	24.1%	30.6%	32.7%
Survey of Patients' Hospital Experiences				
Area Around Room 'Always' Quiet at Night	300+	67%	-	58%
Doctors 'Always' Communicated Well	300+	85%	-	80%
Home Recovery Information Given	300+	87%	-	82%
Hospital Given 9 or 10 on 10 Point Scale	300+	77%	-	67%
Meds 'Always' Explained Before Given	300+	72%	-	60%
Nurses 'Always' Communicated Well	300+	83%	-	76%
Pain 'Always' Well Controlled	300+	75%	-	69%
Room and Bathroom 'Always' Clean	300+	73%	-	71%
Timely Help 'Always' Received	300+	74%	-	64%
Would Definitely Recommend Hospital	300+	75%	-	69%

NOTE: Hospital profiles are in alphabetical order by state, then city, then hospital within the city; Rankings exclude hospitals with less than 25 cases except for patient surveys which excludes hospitals with less than 100 cases; (a) 100–299 cases; (1) The number of cases is too small to be sure how well a hospital is performing; (2) The hospital indicated that the data submitted for this measure were based on a sample of cases; (3) Data was collected during a shorter time period (fewer quarters) than the maximum possible time for this measure; (4) Suppressed for one or more quarters by CMS; (5) No data is available from the hospital for this measure; (6) Fewer than 100 patients completed the HCAHPS survey. Use these rates with caution, as the number of surveys may be too low to reliably assess hospital performance; (7) Survey results are based on less than 12 months of data; (8) Survey results are not available for this reporting period; (9) No or very few patients were eligible for the HCAHPS survey. The scores shown, if any, reflect a very small number of surveys; (10) A state average was not calculated because too few hospitals in the state submitted data; (11) There were discrepancies in the data collection process; Please refer to the User's Guide for a full explanation of data.

Thomasville Medical Center

207 Old Lexington Rd Box 789
Thomasville, NC 27360
Phone: 336-472-2000
Fax: 336-476-2534
URL: www.thomasvillemedicalcenter.org
Type: Acute Care Hospitals
Emergency Services: Yes
Ownership: Voluntary Non-Profit - Private
Beds: 81

Key Personnel:
CEO/President. . . . . Kathie Johnson
Chief of Medical Staff . . . . Richard Kirsch
Infection Control. . . . . Martha Musselman, RN
Operating Room. . . . . Lynn Maxwell
Quality Assurance . . . . Martha Musselman, RN
Radiology. . . . . Sam Thomas Auringer, MD

Measure	Cases	This Hosp.	State Avg.	U.S. Avg.
Heart Attack Care				
ACE Inhibitor or ARB for LVSD[1]	6	100%	97%	96%
Aspirin at Arrival	32	100%	99%	99%
Aspirin at Discharge[1]	15	100%	99%	98%
Beta Blocker at Discharge[1]	19	100%	99%	98%
Fibrinolytic Medication Timing	0	-	38%	55%
PCI Within 90 Minutes of Arrival	0	-	95%	90%
Smoking Cessation Advice[1]	5	100%	100%	99%
Chest Pain/Possible Heart Attack Care				
Aspirin at Arrival	52	100%	95%	95%
Median Time to ECG (minutes)	52	4	8	8
Median Time to Transfer (minutes)[1]	5	38	48	61
Fibrinolytic Medication Timing[1]	3	67%	53%	54%
Heart Failure Care				
ACE Inhibitor or ARB for LVSD	32	100%	95%	94%
Discharge Instructions	90	97%	89%	88%
Evaluation of LVS Function	101	100%	99%	98%
Smoking Cessation Advice[1]	19	100%	99%	98%
Pneumonia Care				
Appropriate Initial Antibiotic	75	96%	92%	92%
Blood Culture Timing	135	100%	96%	96%
Influenza Vaccine	51	96%	93%	91%
Initial Antibiotic Timing	110	99%	95%	95%
Pneumococcal Vaccine	90	99%	95%	93%
Smoking Cessation Advice	45	100%	99%	97%
Surgical Care Improvement Project				
Appropriate VTP Within 24 Hours[2]	90	93%	93%	92%
Appropriate Hair Removal[2]	178	100%	100%	99%
Appropriate Beta Blocker Usage[2]	29	97%	94%	93%
Controlled Postoperative Blood Glucose[2]	0	-	94%	93%
Prophylactic Antibiotic Timing[2]	97	100%	98%	97%
Prophylactic Antibiotic Timing (Outpatient)	211	96%	94%	92%
Prophylactic Antibiotic Selection[2]	99	98%	98%	97%
Prophylactic Antibiotic Select. (Outpatient)	204	93%	95%	94%
Prophylactic Antibiotic Stopped[2]	81	99%	96%	94%
Recommended VTP Ordered[2]	90	94%	95%	94%
Urinary Catheter Removal[1]	20	85%	91%	90%
Children's Asthma Care				
Received Systemic Corticosteroids[1]	9	100%	100%	100%
Received Home Management Plan[1]	9	33%	75%	71%
Received Reliever Medication[1]	9	100%	100%	100%
Use of Medical Imaging				
Combination Abdominal CT Scan	387	0.021	0.115	0.191
Combination Chest CT Scan	190	0.016	0.037	0.054
Follow-up Mammogram/Ultrasound	588	6.6%	7.9%	8.4%
MRI for Low Back Pain	77	39.0%	30.6%	32.7%
Survey of Patients' Hospital Experiences				
Area Around Room 'Always' Quiet at Night	300+	63%	-	58%
Doctors 'Always' Communicated Well	300+	86%	-	80%
Home Recovery Information Given	300+	85%	-	82%
Hospital Given 9 or 10 on 10 Point Scale	300+	73%	-	67%
Meds 'Always' Explained Before Given	300+	60%	-	60%
Nurses 'Always' Communicated Well	300+	80%	-	76%
Pain 'Always' Well Controlled	300+	69%	-	69%
Room and Bathroom 'Always' Clean	300+	78%	-	71%
Timely Help 'Always' Received	300+	71%	-	64%
Would Definitely Recommend Hospital	300+	74%	-	69%

Firsthealth Montgomery Memorial Hospital

520 Allen Street
Troy, NC 27371
Phone: 910-572-1301
Fax: 910-572-4140
URL: www.firsthealth.org
Type: Critical Access Hospitals
Emergency Services: Yes
Ownership: Voluntary Non-Profit - Private
Beds: 55

Key Personnel:
CEO/President. . . . . Kerry Hensley
Chief of Medical Staff . . . . Gilbert D Arenas
Radiology. . . . . Jacob Abraham

Measure	Cases	This Hosp.	State Avg.	U.S. Avg.
Heart Attack Care				
ACE Inhibitor or ARB for LVSD[3]	0	-	97%	96%
Aspirin at Arrival[1,3]	3	100%	99%	99%
Aspirin at Discharge[1,3]	2	100%	99%	98%
Beta Blocker at Discharge[1,3]	2	100%	99%	98%
Fibrinolytic Medication Timing[3]	0	-	38%	55%
PCI Within 90 Minutes of Arrival[3]	0	-	95%	90%
Smoking Cessation Advice[3]	0	-	100%	99%
Chest Pain/Possible Heart Attack Care				
Aspirin at Arrival	-	-	95%	95%
Median Time to ECG (minutes)	-	-	8	8
Median Time to Transfer (minutes)	-	-	48	61
Fibrinolytic Medication Timing	-	-	53%	54%
Heart Failure Care				
ACE Inhibitor or ARB for LVSD[1]	3	100%	95%	94%
Discharge Instructions[1]	16	94%	89%	88%
Evaluation of LVS Function[1]	18	100%	99%	98%
Smoking Cessation Advice[1]	5	100%	99%	98%
Pneumonia Care				
Appropriate Initial Antibiotic[1]	10	90%	92%	92%
Blood Culture Timing[1]	16	100%	96%	96%
Influenza Vaccine[1]	17	100%	93%	91%
Initial Antibiotic Timing[1]	17	100%	95%	95%
Pneumococcal Vaccine[1]	19	95%	95%	93%
Smoking Cessation Advice[1]	11	100%	99%	97%
Surgical Care Improvement Project				
Appropriate VTP Within 24 Hours[5]	0	-	93%	92%
Appropriate Hair Removal[5]	0	-	100%	99%
Appropriate Beta Blocker Usage[5]	0	-	94%	93%
Controlled Postoperative Blood Glucose[5]	0	-	94%	93%
Prophylactic Antibiotic Timing[5]	0	-	98%	97%
Prophylactic Antibiotic Timing (Outpatient)	-	-	94%	92%
Prophylactic Antibiotic Selection[5]	0	-	98%	97%
Prophylactic Antibiotic Select. (Outpatient)	-	-	95%	94%
Prophylactic Antibiotic Stopped[5]	0	-	96%	94%
Recommended VTP Ordered[5]	0	-	95%	94%
Urinary Catheter Removal[5]	0	-	91%	90%
Children's Asthma Care				
Received Systemic Corticosteroids	-	-	100%	100%
Received Home Management Plan	-	-	75%	71%
Received Reliever Medication	-	-	100%	100%
Use of Medical Imaging				
Combination Abdominal CT Scan	-	-	0.115	0.191
Combination Chest CT Scan	-	-	0.037	0.054
Follow-up Mammogram/Ultrasound	-	-	7.9%	8.4%
MRI for Low Back Pain	-	-	30.6%	32.7%
Survey of Patients' Hospital Experiences				
Area Around Room 'Always' Quiet at Night[8]	-	-	-	58%
Doctors 'Always' Communicated Well[8]	-	-	-	80%
Home Recovery Information Given[8]	-	-	-	82%
Hospital Given 9 or 10 on 10 Point Scale[8]	-	-	-	67%
Meds 'Always' Explained Before Given[8]	-	-	-	60%
Nurses 'Always' Communicated Well[8]	-	-	-	76%
Pain 'Always' Well Controlled[8]	-	-	-	69%
Room and Bathroom 'Always' Clean[8]	-	-	-	71%
Timely Help 'Always' Received[8]	-	-	-	64%
Would Definitely Recommend Hospital[8]	-	-	-	69%

Valdese General Hospital

720 Malcolm Blvd
Valdese, NC 28690
Phone: 828-874-2251
URL: www.carolinas.org/facilities/hospitals/valdese
Type: Acute Care Hospitals
Emergency Services: Yes
Ownership: Govt - Hospital Dist/Auth
Beds: 131

Key Personnel:
CEO/President. . . . . Ken Wood

Measure	Cases	This Hosp.	State Avg.	U.S. Avg.
Heart Attack Care				
ACE Inhibitor or ARB for LVSD[1]	3	67%	97%	96%
Aspirin at Arrival[1]	16	100%	99%	99%
Aspirin at Discharge[1]	8	100%	99%	98%
Beta Blocker at Discharge[1]	7	100%	99%	98%
Fibrinolytic Medication Timing	0	-	38%	55%
PCI Within 90 Minutes of Arrival	0	-	95%	90%
Smoking Cessation Advice[1]	2	100%	100%	99%
Chest Pain/Possible Heart Attack Care				
Aspirin at Arrival	35	91%	95%	95%
Median Time to ECG (minutes)	37	9	8	8
Median Time to Transfer (minutes)[1]	15	27	48	61
Fibrinolytic Medication Timing	0	-	53%	54%
Heart Failure Care				
ACE Inhibitor or ARB for LVSD[1]	19	79%	95%	94%
Discharge Instructions	54	91%	89%	88%
Evaluation of LVS Function	81	99%	99%	98%
Smoking Cessation Advice[1]	24	100%	99%	98%
Pneumonia Care				
Appropriate Initial Antibiotic	55	87%	92%	92%
Blood Culture Timing	97	98%	96%	96%
Influenza Vaccine	76	99%	93%	91%
Initial Antibiotic Timing	90	88%	95%	95%
Pneumococcal Vaccine	107	98%	95%	93%
Smoking Cessation Advice	50	100%	99%	97%
Surgical Care Improvement Project				
Appropriate VTP Within 24 Hours	66	95%	93%	92%
Appropriate Hair Removal	148	100%	100%	99%
Appropriate Beta Blocker Usage	48	98%	94%	93%
Controlled Postoperative Blood Glucose	0	-	94%	93%
Prophylactic Antibiotic Timing	108	99%	98%	97%
Prophylactic Antibiotic Timing (Outpatient)	87	92%	94%	92%
Prophylactic Antibiotic Selection	108	99%	98%	97%
Prophylactic Antibiotic Select. (Outpatient)	82	90%	95%	94%
Prophylactic Antibiotic Stopped	103	93%	96%	94%
Recommended VTP Ordered	68	96%	95%	94%
Urinary Catheter Removal	45	98%	91%	90%
Children's Asthma Care				
Received Systemic Corticosteroids	-	-	100%	100%
Received Home Management Plan	-	-	75%	71%
Received Reliever Medication	-	-	100%	100%
Use of Medical Imaging				
Combination Abdominal CT Scan	263	0.137	0.115	0.191
Combination Chest CT Scan	272	0.000	0.037	0.054
Follow-up Mammogram/Ultrasound	372	18.0%	7.9%	8.4%
MRI for Low Back Pain	84	26.2%	30.6%	32.7%
Survey of Patients' Hospital Experiences				
Area Around Room 'Always' Quiet at Night	300+	69%	-	58%
Doctors 'Always' Communicated Well	300+	85%	-	80%
Home Recovery Information Given	300+	91%	-	82%
Hospital Given 9 or 10 on 10 Point Scale	300+	75%	-	67%
Meds 'Always' Explained Before Given	300+	65%	-	60%
Nurses 'Always' Communicated Well	300+	83%	-	76%
Pain 'Always' Well Controlled	300+	77%	-	69%
Room and Bathroom 'Always' Clean	300+	76%	-	71%
Timely Help 'Always' Received	300+	73%	-	64%
Would Definitely Recommend Hospital	300+	77%	-	69%

NOTE: Hospital profiles are in alphabetical order by state, then city, then hospital within the city; Rankings exclude hospitals with less than 25 cases except for patient surveys which excludes hospitals with less than 100 cases; (a) 100–299 cases; (1) The number of cases is too small to be sure how well a hospital is performing; (2) The hospital indicated that the data submitted for this measure were based on a sample of cases; (3) Data was collected during a shorter time period (fewer quarters) than the maximum possible time for this measure; (4) Suppressed for one or more quarters by CMS; (5) No data is available from the hospital for this measure; (6) Fewer than 100 patients completed the HCAHPS survey. Use these rates with caution, as the number of surveys may be too low to reliably assess hospital performance; (7) Survey results are based on less than 12 months of data; (8) Survey results are not available for this reporting period; (9) No or very few patients were eligible for the HCAHPS survey. The scores shown, if any, reflect a very small number of surveys; (10) A state average was not calculated because too few hospitals in the state submitted data; (11) There were discrepancies in the data collection process; Please refer to the User's Guide for a full explanation of data.

Anson Community Hospital

500 Morven Road — Phone: 704-694-5131
Wadesboro, NC 28170 — Fax: 704-694-3900
URL: www.carolinashealthcare.org/facilities/hospitals/anson
Type: Acute Care Hospitals — Emergency Services: Yes
Ownership: Govt - Hospital Dist/Auth — Beds: 125

Key Personnel:
CEO/President . . . . Frederick G Thompson, PhD
Chief of Medical Staff . . . . Syed Haider, MD
Operating Room. . . . . Christie Grooms
Quality Assurance . . . . Carol Williams, RN
Emergency Room . . . . Maureen Lear

Measure	Cases	This Hosp.	State Avg.	U.S. Avg.
Heart Attack Care				
ACE Inhibitor or ARB for LVSD[1,3]	1	100%	97%	96%
Aspirin at Arrival[1,3]	1	100%	99%	99%
Aspirin at Discharge[3]	0	-	99%	98%
Beta Blocker at Discharge[1,3]	1	100%	99%	98%
Fibrinolytic Medication Timing[1,3]	1	0%	38%	55%
PCI Within 90 Minutes of Arrival[3]	0	-	95%	90%
Smoking Cessation Advice[3]	0	-	100%	99%
Chest Pain/Possible Heart Attack Care				
Aspirin at Arrival	210	88%	95%	95%
Median Time to ECG (minutes)	221	6	8	8
Median Time to Transfer (minutes)[1,3]	2	52	48	61
Fibrinolytic Medication Timing[1]	3	67%	53%	54%
Heart Failure Care				
ACE Inhibitor or ARB for LVSD[1]	20	100%	95%	94%
Discharge Instructions	39	92%	89%	88%
Evaluation of LVS Function	52	100%	99%	98%
Smoking Cessation Advice[1]	6	100%	99%	98%
Pneumonia Care				
Appropriate Initial Antibiotic	47	94%	92%	92%
Blood Culture Timing	89	94%	96%	96%
Influenza Vaccine	56	100%	93%	91%
Initial Antibiotic Timing	88	99%	95%	95%
Pneumococcal Vaccine	88	100%	95%	93%
Smoking Cessation Advice[1]	21	100%	99%	97%
Surgical Care Improvement Project				
Appropriate VTP Within 24 Hours[1]	8	100%	93%	92%
Appropriate Hair Removal[1]	20	100%	100%	99%
Appropriate Beta Blocker Usage[1]	2	50%	94%	93%
Controlled Postoperative Blood Glucose	0	-	94%	93%
Prophylactic Antibiotic Timing[1]	9	100%	98%	97%
Prophylactic Antibiotic Timing (Outpatient)[1]	8	88%	94%	92%
Prophylactic Antibiotic Selection[1]	9	100%	98%	97%
Prophylactic Antibiotic Select. (Outpatient)[1]	9	67%	95%	94%
Prophylactic Antibiotic Stopped[1]	8	100%	96%	94%
Recommended VTP Ordered[1]	8	100%	95%	94%
Urinary Catheter Removal[1]	2	50%	91%	90%
Children's Asthma Care				
Received Systemic Corticosteroids	-	-	100%	100%
Received Home Management Plan	-	-	75%	71%
Received Reliever Medication	-	-	100%	100%
Use of Medical Imaging				
Combination Abdominal CT Scan	222	0.027	0.115	0.191
Combination Chest CT Scan	88	0.023	0.037	0.054
Follow-up Mammogram/Ultrasound	419	10.7%	7.9%	8.4%
MRI for Low Back Pain[1]	5	40.0%	30.6%	32.7%
Survey of Patients' Hospital Experiences				
Area Around Room 'Always' Quiet at Night	(a)	67%	-	58%
Doctors 'Always' Communicated Well	(a)	86%	-	80%
Home Recovery Information Given	(a)	79%	-	82%
Hospital Given 9 or 10 on 10 Point Scale	(a)	70%	-	67%
Meds 'Always' Explained Before Given	(a)	74%	-	60%
Nurses 'Always' Communicated Well	(a)	79%	-	76%
Pain 'Always' Well Controlled	(a)	70%	-	69%
Room and Bathroom 'Always' Clean	(a)	69%	-	71%
Timely Help 'Always' Received	(a)	67%	-	64%
Would Definitely Recommend Hospital	(a)	59%	-	69%

Beaufort County Medical Center

628 E 12th St — Phone: 252-975-4100
Washington, NC 27889 — Fax: 252-975-4129
URL: www.beaufortcountyhospital.org
Type: Acute Care Hospitals — Emergency Services: Yes
Ownership: Govt - Hospital Dist/Auth — Beds: 142

Key Personnel:
CEO/President . . . . Bill R Bedsole
Chief of Medical Staff . . . . Fred Teixeira, MD
Operating Room. . . . . Betsy Hodges, RN
Anesthesiology. . . . . Patrick M Riley, MD
Intensive Care Unit. . . . . Linda Cox, RN

Measure	Cases	This Hosp.	State Avg.	U.S. Avg.
Heart Attack Care				
ACE Inhibitor or ARB for LVSD[1]	4	100%	97%	96%
Aspirin at Arrival[1]	16	94%	99%	99%
Aspirin at Discharge[1]	14	93%	99%	98%
Beta Blocker at Discharge[1]	14	100%	99%	98%
Fibrinolytic Medication Timing	0	-	38%	55%
PCI Within 90 Minutes of Arrival	0	-	95%	90%
Smoking Cessation Advice[1]	4	100%	100%	99%
Chest Pain/Possible Heart Attack Care				
Aspirin at Arrival	173	94%	95%	95%
Median Time to ECG (minutes)	176	6	8	8
Median Time to Transfer (minutes)[1,3]	1	45	48	61
Fibrinolytic Medication Timing[1]	15	67%	53%	54%
Heart Failure Care				
ACE Inhibitor or ARB for LVSD[1]	24	92%	95%	94%
Discharge Instructions	91	81%	89%	88%
Evaluation of LVS Function	98	93%	99%	98%
Smoking Cessation Advice[1]	17	100%	99%	98%
Pneumonia Care				
Appropriate Initial Antibiotic	49	82%	92%	92%
Blood Culture Timing	67	88%	96%	96%
Influenza Vaccine	54	91%	93%	91%
Initial Antibiotic Timing	76	93%	95%	95%
Pneumococcal Vaccine	61	90%	95%	93%
Smoking Cessation Advice	26	96%	99%	97%
Surgical Care Improvement Project				
Appropriate VTP Within 24 Hours	106	85%	93%	92%
Appropriate Hair Removal	275	100%	100%	99%
Appropriate Beta Blocker Usage	53	81%	94%	93%
Controlled Postoperative Blood Glucose	0	-	94%	93%
Prophylactic Antibiotic Timing	181	99%	98%	97%
Prophylactic Antibiotic Timing (Outpatient)	160	91%	94%	92%
Prophylactic Antibiotic Selection	182	95%	98%	97%
Prophylactic Antibiotic Select. (Outpatient)	163	99%	95%	94%
Prophylactic Antibiotic Stopped	173	98%	96%	94%
Recommended VTP Ordered	108	83%	95%	94%
Urinary Catheter Removal	93	88%	91%	90%
Children's Asthma Care				
Received Systemic Corticosteroids	-	-	100%	100%
Received Home Management Plan	-	-	75%	71%
Received Reliever Medication	-	-	100%	100%
Use of Medical Imaging				
Combination Abdominal CT Scan	633	0.090	0.115	0.191
Combination Chest CT Scan	492	0.010	0.037	0.054
Follow-up Mammogram/Ultrasound[5]	0	-	7.9%	8.4%
MRI for Low Back Pain	155	38.7%	30.6%	32.7%
Survey of Patients' Hospital Experiences				
Area Around Room 'Always' Quiet at Night	300+	55%	-	58%
Doctors 'Always' Communicated Well	300+	83%	-	80%
Home Recovery Information Given	300+	85%	-	82%
Hospital Given 9 or 10 on 10 Point Scale	300+	64%	-	67%
Meds 'Always' Explained Before Given	300+	65%	-	60%
Nurses 'Always' Communicated Well	300+	78%	-	76%
Pain 'Always' Well Controlled	300+	67%	-	69%
Room and Bathroom 'Always' Clean	300+	71%	-	71%
Timely Help 'Always' Received	300+	65%	-	64%
Would Definitely Recommend Hospital	300+	67%	-	69%

Columbus Regional Healthcare System

500 Jefferson St — Phone: 910-642-8011
Whiteville, NC 28472 — Fax: 910-640-9305
E-mail: tpriest@crhealthcare.org
URL: www.crhealthcare.org
Type: Acute Care Hospitals — Emergency Services: Yes
Ownership: Voluntary Non-Profit - Other — Beds: 154

Key Personnel:
CEO/President . . . . Henry Hawthorne III
Chief of Medical Staff . . . . V Wade Hash, MD
Infection Control. . . . . Miranda Dufour, RN
Operating Room. . . . . Luis E Donayre
Quality Assurance . . . . W Hardy Ledbetter
Radiology. . . . . Demir Bastug, MD
Anesthesiology. . . . . Robin Dimitrious, MD
Emergency Room . . . . Paul DO, MD

Measure	Cases	This Hosp.	State Avg.	U.S. Avg.
Heart Attack Care				
ACE Inhibitor or ARB for LVSD[1]	1	100%	97%	96%
Aspirin at Arrival[1]	8	88%	99%	99%
Aspirin at Discharge[1]	6	100%	99%	98%
Beta Blocker at Discharge[1]	6	100%	99%	98%
Fibrinolytic Medication Timing	0	-	38%	55%
PCI Within 90 Minutes of Arrival	0	-	95%	90%
Smoking Cessation Advice	0	-	100%	99%
Chest Pain/Possible Heart Attack Care				
Aspirin at Arrival	118	95%	95%	95%
Median Time to ECG (minutes)	123	11	8	8
Median Time to Transfer (minutes)[1,3]	7	63	48	61
Fibrinolytic Medication Timing[1]	7	29%	53%	54%
Heart Failure Care				
ACE Inhibitor or ARB for LVSD	30	83%	95%	94%
Discharge Instructions	121	91%	89%	88%
Evaluation of LVS Function	157	96%	99%	98%
Smoking Cessation Advice[1]	21	100%	99%	98%
Pneumonia Care				
Appropriate Initial Antibiotic	68	99%	92%	92%
Blood Culture Timing	137	98%	96%	96%
Influenza Vaccine	76	99%	93%	91%
Initial Antibiotic Timing	136	88%	95%	95%
Pneumococcal Vaccine	108	96%	95%	93%
Smoking Cessation Advice	53	100%	99%	97%
Surgical Care Improvement Project				
Appropriate VTP Within 24 Hours	170	90%	93%	92%
Appropriate Hair Removal	256	100%	100%	99%
Appropriate Beta Blocker Usage	73	93%	94%	93%
Controlled Postoperative Blood Glucose	0	-	94%	93%
Prophylactic Antibiotic Timing	138	97%	98%	97%
Prophylactic Antibiotic Timing (Outpatient)	40	80%	94%	92%
Prophylactic Antibiotic Selection	138	96%	98%	97%
Prophylactic Antibiotic Select. (Outpatient)	32	84%	95%	94%
Prophylactic Antibiotic Stopped	128	93%	96%	94%
Recommended VTP Ordered	170	91%	95%	94%
Urinary Catheter Removal	39	92%	91%	90%
Children's Asthma Care				
Received Systemic Corticosteroids	-	-	100%	100%
Received Home Management Plan	-	-	75%	71%
Received Reliever Medication	-	-	100%	100%
Use of Medical Imaging				
Combination Abdominal CT Scan	500	0.098	0.115	0.191
Combination Chest CT Scan	237	0.013	0.037	0.054
Follow-up Mammogram/Ultrasound	1,328	2.9%	7.9%	8.4%
MRI for Low Back Pain	141	27.7%	30.6%	32.7%
Survey of Patients' Hospital Experiences				
Area Around Room 'Always' Quiet at Night	300+	61%	-	58%
Doctors 'Always' Communicated Well	300+	81%	-	80%
Home Recovery Information Given	300+	85%	-	82%
Hospital Given 9 or 10 on 10 Point Scale	300+	66%	-	67%
Meds 'Always' Explained Before Given	300+	67%	-	60%
Nurses 'Always' Communicated Well	300+	79%	-	76%
Pain 'Always' Well Controlled	300+	77%	-	69%
Room and Bathroom 'Always' Clean	300+	66%	-	71%
Timely Help 'Always' Received	300+	65%	-	64%
Would Definitely Recommend Hospital	300+	63%	-	69%

NOTE: Hospital profiles are in alphabetical order by state, then city, then hospital within the city; Rankings exclude hospitals with less than 25 cases except for patient surveys which excludes hospitals with less than 100 cases; (a) 100–299 cases; (1) The number of cases is too small to be sure how well a hospital is performing; (2) The hospital indicated that the data submitted for this measure were based on a sample of cases; (3) Data was collected during a shorter time period (fewer quarters) than the maximum possible time for this measure; (4) Suppressed for one or more quarters by CMS; (5) No data is available from the hospital for this measure; (6) Fewer than 100 patients completed the HCAHPS survey. Use these rates with caution, as the number of surveys may be too low to reliably assess hospital performance; (7) Survey results are based on less than 12 months of data; (8) Survey results are not available for this reporting period; (9) No or very few patients were eligible for the HCAHPS survey. The scores shown, if any, reflect a very small number of surveys; (10) A state average was not calculated because too few hospitals in the state submitted data; (11) There were discrepancies in the data collection process; Please refer to the User's Guide for a full explanation of data.

Martin General Hospital

310 S Mccaskey Rd Phone: 252-809-6179
Williamston, NC 27892 Fax: 252-809-6283
E-mail: billi_wynn@chs.net
URL: www.martingeneral.com
Type: Acute Care Hospitals Emergency Services: Yes
Ownership: Government - Local Beds: 49

Key Personnel:
CEO/President. . . . . David Sanders
Cardiac Laboratory. . . . . Harold Finn
Chief of Medical Staff . . . . Domingo Cue, MD
Infection Control. . . . . Tonya Perry
Operating Room. . . . . Bonnie Speller, RN
Radiology. . . . . Raymond Hassett
Emergency Room . . . . Thomas Hunter

Measure	Cases	This Hosp.	State Avg.	U.S. Avg.
Heart Attack Care				
ACE Inhibitor or ARB for LVSD[1]	3	100%	97%	96%
Aspirin at Arrival[1]	20	95%	99%	99%
Aspirin at Discharge[1]	16	88%	99%	98%
Beta Blocker at Discharge[1]	17	94%	99%	98%
Fibrinolytic Medication Timing	0	-	38%	55%
PCI Within 90 Minutes of Arrival	0	-	95%	90%
Smoking Cessation Advice[1]	5	100%	100%	99%
Chest Pain/Possible Heart Attack Care				
Aspirin at Arrival	40	95%	95%	95%
Median Time to ECG (minutes)	39	8	8	8
Median Time to Transfer (minutes)[1,3]	4	168	48	61
Fibrinolytic Medication Timing[1]	9	33%	53%	54%
Heart Failure Care				
ACE Inhibitor or ARB for LVSD	36	92%	95%	94%
Discharge Instructions	82	85%	89%	88%
Evaluation of LVS Function	108	97%	99%	98%
Smoking Cessation Advice[1]	21	100%	99%	98%
Pneumonia Care				
Appropriate Initial Antibiotic	55	80%	92%	92%
Blood Culture Timing	58	100%	96%	96%
Influenza Vaccine	44	93%	93%	91%
Initial Antibiotic Timing	70	100%	95%	95%
Pneumococcal Vaccine	66	94%	95%	93%
Smoking Cessation Advice[1]	21	100%	99%	97%
Surgical Care Improvement Project				
Appropriate VTP Within 24 Hours[2]	50	86%	93%	92%
Appropriate Hair Removal[2]	97	100%	100%	99%
Appropriate Beta Blocker Usage[1,2]	20	90%	94%	93%
Controlled Postoperative Blood Glucose[2]	0	-	94%	93%
Prophylactic Antibiotic Timing[2]	91	99%	98%	97%
Prophylactic Antibiotic Timing (Outpatient)	54	98%	94%	92%
Prophylactic Antibiotic Selection[2]	91	100%	98%	97%
Prophylactic Antibiotic Select. (Outpatient)	55	96%	95%	94%
Prophylactic Antibiotic Stopped[2]	91	100%	96%	94%
Recommended VTP Ordered[2]	50	92%	95%	94%
Urinary Catheter Removal[1]	8	62%	91%	90%
Children's Asthma Care				
Received Systemic Corticosteroids	-	-	100%	100%
Received Home Management Plan	-	-	75%	71%
Received Reliever Medication	-	-	100%	100%
Use of Medical Imaging				
Combination Abdominal CT Scan	135	0.689	0.115	0.191
Combination Chest CT Scan	101	0.000	0.037	0.054
Follow-up Mammogram/Ultrasound	515	6.4%	7.9%	8.4%
MRI for Low Back Pain	64	35.9%	30.6%	32.7%
Survey of Patients' Hospital Experiences				
Area Around Room 'Always' Quiet at Night	300+	68%	-	58%
Doctors 'Always' Communicated Well	300+	83%	-	80%
Home Recovery Information Given	300+	82%	-	82%
Hospital Given 9 or 10 on 10 Point Scale	300+	60%	-	67%
Meds 'Always' Explained Before Given	300+	61%	-	60%
Nurses 'Always' Communicated Well	300+	76%	-	76%
Pain 'Always' Well Controlled	300+	70%	-	69%
Room and Bathroom 'Always' Clean	300+	58%	-	71%
Timely Help 'Always' Received	300+	57%	-	64%
Would Definitely Recommend Hospital	300+	61%	-	69%

New Hanover Regional Medical Center

2131 S 17th St Box 9000 Phone: 910-343-7000
Wilmington, NC 28402 Fax: 910-343-7220
URL: www.nhrmc.org
Type: Acute Care Hospitals Emergency Services: Yes
Ownership: Government - Local Beds: 628

Key Personnel:
CEO/President. . . . . Jack Barto
Chief of Medical Staff . . . . Pat Canover
Infection Control. . . . . Patricia Schlegel, RN
Operating Room. . . . . Carolyn Knaup
Pediatric Ambulatory Care . . . . . . Mary Forehand, MD
Pediatric In-Patient Care . . . . Mary Forehand, MD
Quality Assurance . . . . Patricia Wheeler
Radiology. . . . . Neal L Beard, MD

Measure	Cases	This Hosp.	State Avg.	U.S. Avg.
Heart Attack Care				
ACE Inhibitor or ARB for LVSD[2]	55	84%	97%	96%
Aspirin at Arrival[2]	160	99%	99%	99%
Aspirin at Discharge[2]	283	100%	99%	98%
Beta Blocker at Discharge[2]	275	97%	99%	98%
Fibrinolytic Medication Timing[1,2]	1	0%	38%	55%
PCI Within 90 Minutes of Arrival[2]	39	85%	95%	90%
Smoking Cessation Advice[2]	107	97%	100%	99%
Chest Pain/Possible Heart Attack Care				
Aspirin at Arrival[1,3]	1	100%	95%	95%
Median Time to ECG (minutes)[1,3]	1	4	8	8
Median Time to Transfer (minutes)[5]	0	-	48	61
Fibrinolytic Medication Timing[5]	0	-	53%	54%
Heart Failure Care				
ACE Inhibitor or ARB for LVSD[2]	198	95%	95%	94%
Discharge Instructions[2]	542	79%	89%	88%
Evaluation of LVS Function[2]	652	97%	99%	98%
Smoking Cessation Advice[2]	134	94%	99%	98%
Pneumonia Care				
Appropriate Initial Antibiotic[2]	75	88%	92%	92%
Blood Culture Timing[2]	81	86%	96%	96%
Influenza Vaccine[2]	87	83%	93%	91%
Initial Antibiotic Timing[2]	104	88%	95%	95%
Pneumococcal Vaccine[2]	113	88%	95%	93%
Smoking Cessation Advice[2]	66	91%	99%	97%
Surgical Care Improvement Project				
Appropriate VTP Within 24 Hours[2]	345	95%	93%	92%
Appropriate Hair Removal[2]	961	98%	100%	99%
Appropriate Beta Blocker Usage[2]	317	89%	94%	93%
Controlled Postoperative Blood Glucose[2]	134	95%	94%	93%
Prophylactic Antibiotic Timing[2]	622	95%	98%	97%
Prophylactic Antibiotic Timing (Outpatient)	751	93%	94%	92%
Prophylactic Antibiotic Selection[2]	633	96%	98%	97%
Prophylactic Antibiotic Select. (Outpatient)	733	93%	95%	94%
Prophylactic Antibiotic Stopped[2]	579	93%	96%	94%
Recommended VTP Ordered[2]	347	97%	95%	94%
Urinary Catheter Removal[2]	211	90%	91%	90%
Children's Asthma Care				
Received Systemic Corticosteroids	-	-	100%	100%
Received Home Management Plan	-	-	75%	71%
Received Reliever Medication	-	-	100%	100%
Use of Medical Imaging				
Combination Abdominal CT Scan	1,836	0.053	0.115	0.191
Combination Chest CT Scan	1,150	0.006	0.037	0.054
Follow-up Mammogram/Ultrasound	1,355	9.0%	7.9%	8.4%
MRI for Low Back Pain	558	23.7%	30.6%	32.7%
Survey of Patients' Hospital Experiences				
Area Around Room 'Always' Quiet at Night	300+	62%	-	58%
Doctors 'Always' Communicated Well	300+	82%	-	80%
Home Recovery Information Given	300+	85%	-	82%
Hospital Given 9 or 10 on 10 Point Scale	300+	74%	-	67%
Meds 'Always' Explained Before Given	300+	64%	-	60%
Nurses 'Always' Communicated Well	300+	83%	-	76%
Pain 'Always' Well Controlled	300+	73%	-	69%
Room and Bathroom 'Always' Clean	300+	75%	-	71%
Timely Help 'Always' Received	300+	67%	-	64%
Would Definitely Recommend Hospital	300+	80%	-	69%

Wilson Medical Center

1705 S Tarboro St Phone: 252-399-8040
Wilson, NC 27893 Fax: 252-399-8778
URL: www.wilmed.org/contact.asp
Type: Acute Care Hospitals Emergency Services: Yes
Ownership: Voluntary Non-Profit - Private Beds: 317

Key Personnel:
CEO/President. . . . . Christopher T Durrer
Chief of Medical Staff . . . . Roger Thurman, MD
Operating Room. . . . . Glenda Mitchell, RN
Pediatric Ambulatory Care . . . . . . Robert Pope, MD
Pediatric In-Patient Care . . . . Robert Pope, MD
Quality Assurance . . . . Jane Rosenmarkel
Radiology. . . . . Paul Guay, MD
Emergency Room . . . . Suzie Bass, RN

Measure	Cases	This Hosp.	State Avg.	U.S. Avg.
Heart Attack Care				
ACE Inhibitor or ARB for LVSD[1]	11	91%	97%	96%
Aspirin at Arrival	63	94%	99%	99%
Aspirin at Discharge	37	95%	99%	98%
Beta Blocker at Discharge	34	94%	99%	98%
Fibrinolytic Medication Timing	0	-	38%	55%
PCI Within 90 Minutes of Arrival	0	-	95%	90%
Smoking Cessation Advice[1]	5	100%	100%	99%
Chest Pain/Possible Heart Attack Care				
Aspirin at Arrival	96	97%	95%	95%
Median Time to ECG (minutes)	88	15	8	8
Median Time to Transfer (minutes)[1,3]	4	415	48	61
Fibrinolytic Medication Timing[1]	9	67%	53%	54%
Heart Failure Care				
ACE Inhibitor or ARB for LVSD	94	87%	95%	94%
Discharge Instructions	222	94%	89%	88%
Evaluation of LVS Function	275	96%	99%	98%
Smoking Cessation Advice	65	100%	99%	98%
Pneumonia Care				
Appropriate Initial Antibiotic	121	79%	92%	92%
Blood Culture Timing	191	82%	96%	96%
Influenza Vaccine	162	83%	93%	91%
Initial Antibiotic Timing	230	89%	95%	95%
Pneumococcal Vaccine	203	81%	95%	93%
Smoking Cessation Advice	89	96%	99%	97%
Surgical Care Improvement Project				
Appropriate VTP Within 24 Hours[2]	167	78%	93%	92%
Appropriate Hair Removal[2]	539	99%	100%	99%
Appropriate Beta Blocker Usage[2]	136	96%	94%	93%
Controlled Postoperative Blood Glucose[2]	0	-	94%	93%
Prophylactic Antibiotic Timing[2]	397	97%	98%	97%
Prophylactic Antibiotic Timing (Outpatient)	93	96%	94%	92%
Prophylactic Antibiotic Selection[2]	421	99%	98%	97%
Prophylactic Antibiotic Select. (Outpatient)	93	98%	95%	94%
Prophylactic Antibiotic Stopped[2]	394	89%	96%	94%
Recommended VTP Ordered[2]	169	88%	95%	94%
Urinary Catheter Removal[2]	186	96%	91%	90%
Children's Asthma Care				
Received Systemic Corticosteroids	30	97%	100%	100%
Received Home Management Plan	30	90%	75%	71%
Received Reliever Medication	30	97%	100%	100%
Use of Medical Imaging				
Combination Abdominal CT Scan	1,007	0.126	0.115	0.191
Combination Chest CT Scan	787	0.325	0.037	0.054
Follow-up Mammogram/Ultrasound	1,520	7.6%	7.9%	8.4%
MRI for Low Back Pain	181	38.1%	30.6%	32.7%
Survey of Patients' Hospital Experiences				
Area Around Room 'Always' Quiet at Night	300+	68%	-	58%
Doctors 'Always' Communicated Well	300+	84%	-	80%
Home Recovery Information Given	300+	87%	-	82%
Hospital Given 9 or 10 on 10 Point Scale	300+	70%	-	67%
Meds 'Always' Explained Before Given	300+	61%	-	60%
Nurses 'Always' Communicated Well	300+	80%	-	76%
Pain 'Always' Well Controlled	300+	75%	-	69%
Room and Bathroom 'Always' Clean	300+	67%	-	71%
Timely Help 'Always' Received	300+	66%	-	64%
Would Definitely Recommend Hospital	300+	67%	-	69%

NOTE: Hospital profiles are in alphabetical order by state, then city, then hospital within the city; Rankings exclude hospitals with less than 25 cases except for patient surveys which excludes hospitals with less than 100 cases; (a) 100–299 cases; (1) The number of cases is too small to be sure how well a hospital is performing; (2) The hospital indicated that the data submitted for this measure were based on a sample of cases; (3) Data was collected during a shorter time period (fewer quarters) than the maximum possible time for this measure; (4) Suppressed for one or more quarters by CMS; (5) No data is available from the hospital for this measure; (6) Fewer than 100 patients completed the HCAHPS survey. Use these rates with caution, as the number of surveys may be too low to reliably assess hospital performance; (7) Survey results are based on less than 12 months of data; (8) Survey results are not available for this reporting period; (9) No or very few patients were eligible for the HCAHPS survey. The scores shown, if any, reflect a very small number of surveys; (10) A state average was not calculated because too few hospitals in the state submitted data; (11) There were discrepancies in the data collection process; Please refer to the User's Guide for a full explanation of data.

Bertie Memorial Hospital

1403 South Kings Street Phone: 252-794-6600
Windsor, NC 27983 Fax: 252-794-6641
E-mail: tmullen@coastalnet.com
Type: Critical Access Hospitals Emergency Services: Yes
Ownership: Voluntary Non-Profit - Private Beds: 15

Key Personnel:
CEO/President. . . . . Jeffery Fackrison
Chief of Medical Staff . . . . V Ballance
Emergency Room . . . . Pat Taylor

Measure	Cases	This Hosp.	State Avg.	U.S. Avg.
Heart Attack Care				
ACE Inhibitor or ARB for LVSD[5]	0	-	97%	96%
Aspirin at Arrival[5]	0	-	99%	99%
Aspirin at Discharge[5]	0	-	99%	98%
Beta Blocker at Discharge[5]	0	-	99%	98%
Fibrinolytic Medication Timing[5]	0	-	38%	55%
PCI Within 90 Minutes of Arrival[5]	0	-	95%	90%
Smoking Cessation Advice[5]	0	-	100%	99%
Chest Pain/Possible Heart Attack Care				
Aspirin at Arrival	-	-	95%	95%
Median Time to ECG (minutes)	-	-	8	8
Median Time to Transfer (minutes)	-	-	48	61
Fibrinolytic Medication Timing	-	-	53%	54%
Heart Failure Care				
ACE Inhibitor or ARB for LVSD[1]	14	100%	95%	94%
Discharge Instructions	30	87%	89%	88%
Evaluation of LVS Function	39	100%	99%	98%
Smoking Cessation Advice[1]	5	100%	99%	98%
Pneumonia Care				
Appropriate Initial Antibiotic[1]	15	100%	92%	92%
Blood Culture Timing[1]	22	100%	96%	96%
Influenza Vaccine[1]	10	90%	93%	91%
Initial Antibiotic Timing[1]	23	100%	95%	95%
Pneumococcal Vaccine[1]	19	95%	95%	93%
Smoking Cessation Advice[1]	2	100%	99%	97%
Surgical Care Improvement Project				
Appropriate VTP Within 24 Hours[5]	0	-	93%	92%
Appropriate Hair Removal[5]	0	-	100%	99%
Appropriate Beta Blocker Usage[5]	0	-	94%	93%
Controlled Postoperative Blood Glucose[5]	0	-	94%	93%
Prophylactic Antibiotic Timing[5]	0	-	98%	97%
Prophylactic Antibiotic Timing (Outpatient)	-	-	94%	92%
Prophylactic Antibiotic Selection[5]	0	-	98%	97%
Prophylactic Antibiotic Select. (Outpatient)	-	-	95%	94%
Prophylactic Antibiotic Stopped[5]	0	-	96%	94%
Recommended VTP Ordered[5]	0	-	95%	94%
Urinary Catheter Removal[5]	0	-	91%	90%
Children's Asthma Care				
Received Systemic Corticosteroids	-	-	100%	100%
Received Home Management Plan	-	-	75%	71%
Received Reliever Medication	-	-	100%	100%
Use of Medical Imaging				
Combination Abdominal CT Scan	-	-	0.115	0.191
Combination Chest CT Scan	-	-	0.037	0.054
Follow-up Mammogram/Ultrasound	-	-	7.9%	8.4%
MRI for Low Back Pain	-	-	30.6%	32.7%
Survey of Patients' Hospital Experiences				
Area Around Room 'Always' Quiet at Night	(a)	81%	-	58%
Doctors 'Always' Communicated Well	(a)	93%	-	80%
Home Recovery Information Given	(a)	89%	-	82%
Hospital Given 9 or 10 on 10 Point Scale	(a)	81%	-	67%
Meds 'Always' Explained Before Given	(a)	76%	-	60%
Nurses 'Always' Communicated Well	(a)	90%	-	76%
Pain 'Always' Well Controlled	(a)	85%	-	69%
Room and Bathroom 'Always' Clean	(a)	89%	-	71%
Timely Help 'Always' Received	(a)	85%	-	64%
Would Definitely Recommend Hospital	(a)	85%	-	69%

Forsyth Memorial Hospital

3333 Silas Creek Parkway Phone: 336-718-5000
Winston-Salem, NC 27103 Fax: 336-718-9863
URL: www.forsythmedicalcenter.org
Type: Acute Care Hospitals Emergency Services: Yes
Ownership: Voluntary Non-Profit - Private Beds: 911

Key Personnel:
CEO/President. . . . . Gregory J Beier
Chief of Medical Staff . . . . Stephen L Wallenhaupt, MD
Quality Assurance . . . . Harold Whitt
Radiology. . . . . Sam Thomas Auringer
Anesthesiology. . . . . Suresh Penkar, MD
Emergency Room . . . . Paul Horton, MD

Measure	Cases	This Hosp.	State Avg.	U.S. Avg.
Heart Attack Care				
ACE Inhibitor or ARB for LVSD	120	100%	97%	96%
Aspirin at Arrival	608	100%	99%	99%
Aspirin at Discharge	834	100%	99%	98%
Beta Blocker at Discharge	792	100%	99%	98%
Fibrinolytic Medication Timing	0	-	38%	55%
PCI Within 90 Minutes of Arrival	151	99%	95%	90%
Smoking Cessation Advice	337	100%	100%	99%
Chest Pain/Possible Heart Attack Care				
Aspirin at Arrival[1,3]	1	100%	95%	95%
Median Time to ECG (minutes)[1,3]	1	29	8	8
Median Time to Transfer (minutes)[5]	0	-	48	61
Fibrinolytic Medication Timing[5]	0	-	53%	54%
Heart Failure Care				
ACE Inhibitor or ARB for LVSD	254	100%	95%	94%
Discharge Instructions	814	100%	89%	88%
Evaluation of LVS Function	989	100%	99%	98%
Smoking Cessation Advice	142	100%	99%	98%
Pneumonia Care				
Appropriate Initial Antibiotic	418	98%	92%	92%
Blood Culture Timing	694	100%	96%	96%
Influenza Vaccine	531	100%	93%	91%
Initial Antibiotic Timing	624	100%	95%	95%
Pneumococcal Vaccine	710	100%	95%	93%
Smoking Cessation Advice	323	100%	99%	97%
Surgical Care Improvement Project				
Appropriate VTP Within 24 Hours[2]	1,018	97%	93%	92%
Appropriate Hair Removal[2]	2,869	100%	100%	99%
Appropriate Beta Blocker Usage[2]	1,006	97%	94%	93%
Controlled Postoperative Blood Glucose[2]	483	99%	94%	93%
Prophylactic Antibiotic Timing[2]	2,078	100%	98%	97%
Prophylactic Antibiotic Timing (Outpatient)	1,706	98%	94%	92%
Prophylactic Antibiotic Selection[2]	2,095	100%	98%	97%
Prophylactic Antibiotic Select. (Outpatient)	1,702	99%	95%	94%
Prophylactic Antibiotic Stopped[2]	1,984	100%	96%	94%
Recommended VTP Ordered[2]	1,018	98%	95%	94%
Urinary Catheter Removal[2]	921	98%	91%	90%
Children's Asthma Care				
Received Systemic Corticosteroids	-	-	100%	100%
Received Home Management Plan	-	-	75%	71%
Received Reliever Medication	-	-	100%	100%
Use of Medical Imaging				
Combination Abdominal CT Scan	991	0.001	0.115	0.191
Combination Chest CT Scan	204	0.000	0.037	0.054
Follow-up Mammogram/Ultrasound[5]	0	-	7.9%	8.4%
MRI for Low Back Pain[1]	42	31.0%	30.6%	32.7%
Survey of Patients' Hospital Experiences				
Area Around Room 'Always' Quiet at Night	300+	56%	-	58%
Doctors 'Always' Communicated Well	300+	83%	-	80%
Home Recovery Information Given	300+	83%	-	82%
Hospital Given 9 or 10 on 10 Point Scale	300+	75%	-	67%
Meds 'Always' Explained Before Given	300+	64%	-	60%
Nurses 'Always' Communicated Well	300+	79%	-	76%
Pain 'Always' Well Controlled	300+	71%	-	69%
Room and Bathroom 'Always' Clean	300+	65%	-	71%
Timely Help 'Always' Received	300+	65%	-	64%
Would Definitely Recommend Hospital	300+	82%	-	69%

Medical Park Hospital

1950 S Hawthorne Rd Phone: 336-718-0600
Winston-Salem, NC 27103 Fax: 336-718-0384
URL: www.novanthealth.org
Type: Acute Care Hospitals Emergency Services: No
Ownership: Voluntary Non-Profit - Other Beds: 40

Key Personnel:
CEO/President. . . . . Timothy S Shelton, Jr

Measure	Cases	This Hosp.	State Avg.	U.S. Avg.
Heart Attack Care				
ACE Inhibitor or ARB for LVSD[5]	0	-	97%	96%
Aspirin at Arrival[5]	0	-	99%	99%
Aspirin at Discharge[5]	0	-	99%	98%
Beta Blocker at Discharge[5]	0	-	99%	98%
Fibrinolytic Medication Timing[5]	0	-	38%	55%
PCI Within 90 Minutes of Arrival[5]	0	-	95%	90%
Smoking Cessation Advice[5]	0	-	100%	99%
Chest Pain/Possible Heart Attack Care				
Aspirin at Arrival[5]	0	-	95%	95%
Median Time to ECG (minutes)[5]	0	-	8	8
Median Time to Transfer (minutes)[5]	0	-	48	61
Fibrinolytic Medication Timing[5]	0	-	53%	54%
Heart Failure Care				
ACE Inhibitor or ARB for LVSD[5]	0	-	95%	94%
Discharge Instructions[5]	0	-	89%	88%
Evaluation of LVS Function[5]	0	-	99%	98%
Smoking Cessation Advice[5]	0	-	99%	98%
Pneumonia Care				
Appropriate Initial Antibiotic[5]	0	-	92%	92%
Blood Culture Timing[5]	0	-	96%	96%
Influenza Vaccine[5]	0	-	93%	91%
Initial Antibiotic Timing[5]	0	-	95%	95%
Pneumococcal Vaccine[5]	0	-	95%	93%
Smoking Cessation Advice[5]	0	-	99%	97%
Surgical Care Improvement Project				
Appropriate VTP Within 24 Hours[2]	179	96%	93%	92%
Appropriate Hair Removal[2]	412	100%	100%	99%
Appropriate Beta Blocker Usage[2]	85	99%	94%	93%
Controlled Postoperative Blood Glucose[2]	0	-	94%	93%
Prophylactic Antibiotic Timing[2]	230	100%	98%	97%
Prophylactic Antibiotic Timing (Outpatient)	434	99%	94%	92%
Prophylactic Antibiotic Selection[2]	230	100%	98%	97%
Prophylactic Antibiotic Select. (Outpatient)	434	99%	95%	94%
Prophylactic Antibiotic Stopped[2]	220	100%	96%	94%
Recommended VTP Ordered[2]	179	98%	95%	94%
Urinary Catheter Removal[2]	60	88%	91%	90%
Children's Asthma Care				
Received Systemic Corticosteroids	-	-	100%	100%
Received Home Management Plan	-	-	75%	71%
Received Reliever Medication	-	-	100%	100%
Use of Medical Imaging				
Combination Abdominal CT Scan[5]	0	-	0.115	0.191
Combination Chest CT Scan[5]	0	-	0.037	0.054
Follow-up Mammogram/Ultrasound[5]	0	-	7.9%	8.4%
MRI for Low Back Pain[5]	0	-	30.6%	32.7%
Survey of Patients' Hospital Experiences				
Area Around Room 'Always' Quiet at Night	300+	71%	-	58%
Doctors 'Always' Communicated Well	300+	86%	-	80%
Home Recovery Information Given	300+	82%	-	82%
Hospital Given 9 or 10 on 10 Point Scale	300+	84%	-	67%
Meds 'Always' Explained Before Given	300+	64%	-	60%
Nurses 'Always' Communicated Well	300+	83%	-	76%
Pain 'Always' Well Controlled	300+	75%	-	69%
Room and Bathroom 'Always' Clean	300+	75%	-	71%
Timely Help 'Always' Received	300+	76%	-	64%
Would Definitely Recommend Hospital	300+	88%	-	69%

NOTE: Hospital profiles are in alphabetical order by state, then city, then hospital within the city; Rankings exclude hospitals with less than 25 cases except for patient surveys which excludes hospitals with less than 100 cases; (a) 100–299 cases; (1) The number of cases is too small to be sure how well a hospital is performing; (2) The hospital indicated that the data submitted for this measure were based on a sample of cases; (3) Data was collected during a shorter time period (fewer quarters) than the maximum possible time for this measure; (4) Suppressed for one or more quarters by CMS; (5) No data is available from the hospital for this measure; (6) Fewer than 100 patients completed the HCAHPS survey. Use these rates with caution, as the number of surveys may be too low to reliably assess hospital performance; (7) Survey results are based on less than 12 months of data; (8) Survey results are not available for this reporting period; (9) No or very few patients were eligible for the HCAHPS survey. The scores shown, if any, reflect a very small number of surveys; (10) A state average was not calculated because too few hospitals in the state submitted data; (11) There were discrepancies in the data collection process; Please refer to the User's Guide for a full explanation of data.

North Carolina Baptist Hospital

Medical Center Boulevard
Winston-Salem, NC 27157
URL: www.wfubmc.edu
Type: Acute Care Hospitals
Ownership: Voluntary Non-Profit - Private

Phone: 336-716-2011
Fax: 336-716-6841

Emergency Services: Yes
Beds: 1,238

Key Personnel:
CEO/President . . . . John D McConnell, Jr
Infection Control . . . . Robert Sherertz, MD
Operating Room . . . . Willa M Abbott
Quality Assurance . . . . Jerold Smith
Radiology . . . . Allen D Elster, MD
Anesthesiology . . . . Raymond Roy, MD
Emergency Room . . . . Patricia Johnson
Patient Relations . . . . Amanda F Smith

Measure	Cases	This Hosp.	State Avg.	U.S. Avg.
Heart Attack Care				
ACE Inhibitor or ARB for LVSD	119	97%	97%	96%
Aspirin at Arrival	239	100%	99%	99%
Aspirin at Discharge	571	99%	99%	98%
Beta Blocker at Discharge	541	100%	99%	98%
Fibrinolytic Medication Timing	0	-	38%	55%
PCI Within 90 Minutes of Arrival	49	100%	95%	90%
Smoking Cessation Advice	268	100%	100%	99%
Chest Pain/Possible Heart Attack Care				
Aspirin at Arrival[5]	0	-	95%	95%
Median Time to ECG (minutes)[5]	0	-	8	8
Median Time to Transfer (minutes)[5]	0	-	48	61
Fibrinolytic Medication Timing[5]	0	-	53%	54%
Heart Failure Care				
ACE Inhibitor or ARB for LVSD	257	97%	95%	94%
Discharge Instructions	602	96%	89%	88%
Evaluation of LVS Function	652	100%	99%	98%
Smoking Cessation Advice	161	100%	99%	98%
Pneumonia Care				
Appropriate Initial Antibiotic	171	94%	92%	92%
Blood Culture Timing	453	97%	96%	96%
Influenza Vaccine	142	92%	93%	91%
Initial Antibiotic Timing	413	98%	95%	95%
Pneumococcal Vaccine	283	92%	95%	93%
Smoking Cessation Advice	264	100%	99%	97%
Surgical Care Improvement Project				
Appropriate VTP Within 24 Hours[2]	363	97%	93%	92%
Appropriate Hair Removal[2]	954	100%	100%	99%
Appropriate Beta Blocker Usage[2]	328	96%	94%	93%
Controlled Postoperative Blood Glucose[2]	187	96%	94%	93%
Prophylactic Antibiotic Timing[2]	619	99%	98%	97%
Prophylactic Antibiotic Timing (Outpatient)	672	97%	94%	92%
Prophylactic Antibiotic Selection[2]	633	99%	98%	97%
Prophylactic Antibiotic Select. (Outpatient)	680	98%	95%	94%
Prophylactic Antibiotic Stopped[2]	599	97%	96%	94%
Recommended VTP Ordered[2]	363	97%	95%	94%
Urinary Catheter Removal[2]	229	88%	91%	90%
Children's Asthma Care				
Received Systemic Corticosteroids[2]	72	100%	100%	100%
Received Home Management Plan[2]	72	68%	75%	71%
Received Reliever Medication[2]	72	100%	100%	100%
Use of Medical Imaging				
Combination Abdominal CT Scan	3,253	0.293	0.115	0.191
Combination Chest CT Scan	3,046	0.006	0.037	0.054
Follow-up Mammogram/Ultrasound	1,443	8.5%	7.9%	8.4%
MRI for Low Back Pain	219	28.3%	30.6%	32.7%
Survey of Patients' Hospital Experiences				
Area Around Room 'Always' Quiet at Night	300+	66%	-	58%
Doctors 'Always' Communicated Well	300+	80%	-	80%
Home Recovery Information Given	300+	82%	-	82%
Hospital Given 9 or 10 on 10 Point Scale	300+	76%	-	67%
Meds 'Always' Explained Before Given	300+	61%	-	60%
Nurses 'Always' Communicated Well	300+	75%	-	76%
Pain 'Always' Well Controlled	300+	68%	-	69%
Room and Bathroom 'Always' Clean	300+	69%	-	71%
Timely Help 'Always' Received	300+	59%	-	64%
Would Definitely Recommend Hospital	300+	82%	-	69%

Yadkin Valley Community Hospital

624 West Main St
Yadkinville, NC 27055
E-mail: llabine@wfubmc.edu
Type: Critical Access Hospitals
Ownership: Voluntary Non-Profit - Other

Phone: 336-679-2041
Fax: 336-679-6717

Emergency Services: Yes
Beds: 22

Key Personnel:
CEO/President . . . . Ted Chapin
Chief of Medical Staff . . . . James S. McGrath
Infection Control . . . . Ellen Reece
Quality Assurance . . . . Lance Labine
Radiology . . . . Paul J. Beerman
Ambulatory Care . . . . Sharon Hill
Anesthesiology . . . . Elizabeth Randleman
Emergency Room . . . . Lisa Miller

Measure	Cases	This Hosp.	State Avg.	U.S. Avg.
Heart Attack Care				
ACE Inhibitor or ARB for LVSD[5]	0	-	97%	96%
Aspirin at Arrival[5]	0	-	99%	99%
Aspirin at Discharge[5]	0	-	99%	98%
Beta Blocker at Discharge[5]	0	-	99%	98%
Fibrinolytic Medication Timing[5]	0	-	38%	55%
PCI Within 90 Minutes of Arrival[5]	0	-	95%	90%
Smoking Cessation Advice[5]	0	-	100%	99%
Chest Pain/Possible Heart Attack Care				
Aspirin at Arrival	-	-	95%	95%
Median Time to ECG (minutes)	-	-	8	8
Median Time to Transfer (minutes)	-	-	48	61
Fibrinolytic Medication Timing	-	-	53%	54%
Heart Failure Care				
ACE Inhibitor or ARB for LVSD[1]	2	100%	95%	94%
Discharge Instructions[1]	1	100%	89%	88%
Evaluation of LVS Function[1]	3	100%	99%	98%
Smoking Cessation Advice	0	-	99%	98%
Pneumonia Care				
Appropriate Initial Antibiotic[1]	6	83%	92%	92%
Blood Culture Timing[1]	8	100%	96%	96%
Influenza Vaccine[1]	4	50%	93%	91%
Initial Antibiotic Timing[1]	7	100%	95%	95%
Pneumococcal Vaccine[1]	8	88%	95%	93%
Smoking Cessation Advice[1]	3	67%	99%	97%
Surgical Care Improvement Project				
Appropriate VTP Within 24 Hours[5]	0	-	93%	92%
Appropriate Hair Removal[5]	0	-	100%	99%
Appropriate Beta Blocker Usage[5]	0	-	94%	93%
Controlled Postoperative Blood Glucose[5]	0	-	94%	93%
Prophylactic Antibiotic Timing[5]	0	-	98%	97%
Prophylactic Antibiotic Timing (Outpatient)	-	-	94%	92%
Prophylactic Antibiotic Selection[5]	0	-	98%	97%
Prophylactic Antibiotic Select. (Outpatient)	-	-	95%	94%
Prophylactic Antibiotic Stopped[5]	0	-	96%	94%
Recommended VTP Ordered[5]	0	-	95%	94%
Urinary Catheter Removal[5]	0	-	91%	90%
Children's Asthma Care				
Received Systemic Corticosteroids	-	-	100%	100%
Received Home Management Plan	-	-	75%	71%
Received Reliever Medication	-	-	100%	100%
Use of Medical Imaging				
Combination Abdominal CT Scan	-	-	0.115	0.191
Combination Chest CT Scan	-	-	0.037	0.054
Follow-up Mammogram/Ultrasound	-	-	7.9%	8.4%
MRI for Low Back Pain	-	-	30.6%	32.7%
Survey of Patients' Hospital Experiences				
Area Around Room 'Always' Quiet at Night[8]	-	-	-	58%
Doctors 'Always' Communicated Well[8]	-	-	-	80%
Home Recovery Information Given[8]	-	-	-	82%
Hospital Given 9 or 10 on 10 Point Scale[8]	-	-	-	67%
Meds 'Always' Explained Before Given[8]	-	-	-	60%
Nurses 'Always' Communicated Well[8]	-	-	-	76%
Pain 'Always' Well Controlled[8]	-	-	-	69%
Room and Bathroom 'Always' Clean[8]	-	-	-	71%
Timely Help 'Always' Received[6]	-	-	-	64%
Would Definitely Recommend Hospital[8]	-	-	-	69%

NOTE: Hospital profiles are in alphabetical order by state, then city, then hospital within the city; Rankings exclude hospitals with less than 25 cases except for patient surveys which excludes hospitals with less than 100 cases; (a) 100–299 cases; (1) The number of cases is too small to be sure how well a hospital is performing; (2) The hospital indicated that the data submitted for this measure were based on a sample of cases; (3) Data was collected during a shorter time period (fewer quarters) than the maximum possible time for this measure; (4) Suppressed for one or more quarters by CMS; (5) No data is available from the hospital for this measure; (6) Fewer than 100 patients completed the HCAHPS survey. Use these rates with caution, as the number of surveys may be too low to reliably assess hospital performance; (7) Survey results are based on less than 12 months of data; (8) Survey results are not available for this reporting period; (9) No or very few patients were eligible for the HCAHPS survey. The scores shown, if any, reflect a very small number of surveys; (10) A state average was not calculated because too few hospitals in the state submitted data; (11) There were discrepancies in the data collection process; Please refer to the User's Guide for a full explanation of data.

Heart Attack Care

1. ACE Inhibitor or ARB for LVSD

Hospital Name	City	Rate	Cases
Atrium Medical Center[2]	Franklin	100%	42
Christ Hospital	Cincinnati	100%	101
Community Regional Medical Center	Lorain	100%	43
Firelands Regional Medical Center	Sandusky	100%	28
Grandview Hospital & Medical Center	Dayton	100%	28
Grant Medical Center	Columbus	100%	41
Hillcrest Hospital	Mayfield Heights	100%	68
Lake Health[2]	Concord	100%	51
Lima Memorial Health System	Lima	100%	29
Mercy Hospital Fairfield	Fairfield	100%	54
Mount Carmel Health	Columbus	100%	133
Saint Luke's Hospital	Maumee	100%	41
Summa Health Systems Hospitals[2]	Akron	100%	56
Trumbull Memorial Hospital	Warren	100%	35
University of Toledo Medical Center	Toledo	100%	32
Aultman Hospital	Canton	99%	105
Cleveland Clinic[2]	Cleveland	99%	180
Kettering Medical Center	Kettering	99%	86
Saint Rita's Medical Center	Lima	99%	71
Fairfield Medical Center	Lancaster	98%	53
Genesis Healthcare System	Zanesville	98%	63
Good Samaritan Hospital	Cincinnati	98%	49
Jewish Hospital	Cincinnati	98%	41
Mercy Hospital Anderson	Cincinnati	98%	63
Bethesda North Hospital	Cincinnati	97%	87
Doctors Hospital	Columbus	97%	32
Marion General Hospital	Marion	97%	35
Mercy St Vincent Medical Center	Toledo	97%	149
Ohio State University Hospitals[2]	Columbus	97%	66
Riverside Methodist Hospital[2]	Columbus	97%	125
Saint Elizabeth Health Center	Youngstown	97%	79
Southern Ohio Medical Center	Portsmouth	97%	39
The Toledo Hospital[2]	Toledo	97%	60
Adena Regional Medical Center	Chillicothe	96%	118
Fairview Hospital[2]	Cleveland	96%	28
Medcentral Health System[2]	Mansfield	96%	50
Springfield Regional Medical Center	Springfield	96%	71
Good Samaritan Hospital	Dayton	95%	74
Southwest General Health Center	Middleburg Hgts	95%	73
Akron General Medical Center[2]	Akron	94%	71
University Hospitals of Cleveland	Cleveland	94%	97
Metro Health Medical Center	Cleveland	93%	27
Parma Community General Hospital	Parma	93%	72
Trinity Medical Center East & West	Steubenville	93%	89
Miami Valley Hospital[2]	Dayton	92%	59
Emh Regional Medical Center[2]	Elyria	91%	58
Mercy Medical Center	Canton	90%	61
University Hospital	Cincinnati	89%	44

2. Aspirin at Arrival

Hospital Name	City	Rate	Cases
Ashtabula County Medical Center	Ashtabula	100%	26
Atrium Medical Center[2]	Franklin	100%	280
Blanchard Valley Hospital	Findlay	100%	124
Christ Hospital	Cincinnati	100%	196
Cincinnati VA Medical Center	Cincinnati	100%	52
Cleveland Clinic[2]	Cleveland	100%	156
Community Hospitals and Wellness Centers	Bryan	100%	52
Community Regional Medical Center	Lorain	100%	228
Doctors Hospital	Columbus	100%	175
Firelands Regional Medical Center	Sandusky	100%	89
Flower Hospital	Sylvania	100%	61
Good Samaritan Hospital	Dayton	100%	324
Grant Medical Center	Columbus	100%	179
Greene Memorial Hospital	Xenia	100%	29
Hillcrest Hospital	Mayfield Heights	100%	250
Jewish Hospital	Cincinnati	100%	165
Kettering Medical Center	Kettering	100%	260
Licking Memorial Hospital	Newark	100%	40
Lima Memorial Health System	Lima	100%	136
Marion General Hospital	Marion	100%	164
Mary Rutan Hospital	Bellefontaine	100%	46
Marymount Hospital	Garfield Heights	100%	62
Mercy Hospital Clermont	Batavia	100%	47
Metro Health Medical Center	Cleveland	100%	236
Miami Valley Hospital[2]	Dayton	100%	263
Mount Carmel Health	Columbus	100%	688
Mount Carmel St Ann's Hospital	Westerville	100%	118
Northside Medical Center	Youngstown	100%	101
Saint Elizabeth Boardman Health Center	Youngstown	100%	42
Saint Elizabeth Health Center	Youngstown	100%	274
Saint John Medical Center[2]	Westlake	100%	214
Saint Joseph Health Center	Warren	100%	46
Saint Rita's Medical Center	Lima	100%	252
South Pointe Hospital	Warrensville Hgts	100%	52
Southern Ohio Medical Center	Portsmouth	100%	203
Summa Barberton Hospital	Barberton	100%	88
Summa Health Systems Hospitals[2]	Akron	100%	198
Trumbull Memorial Hospital	Warren	100%	194
UH Geauga Medical Center	Chardon	100%	73
UHHS Richmond Heights Hospital	Richmond Hghts	100%	31
Union Hospital	Dover	100%	63
University Hospitals of Cleveland	Cleveland	100%	181
Akron General Medical Center[2]	Akron	99%	216
Aultman Hospital	Canton	99%	394
Fairfield Medical Center	Lancaster	99%	243
Fairview Hospital[2]	Cleveland	99%	225
Good Samaritan Hospital	Cincinnati	99%	221
Marietta Memorial Hospital	Marietta	99%	95
Mercy Franciscan Hospital Western Hills	Cincinnati	99%	71
Mercy Hospital Anderson	Cincinnati	99%	235
Mercy Hospital Fairfield	Fairfield	99%	268
Mercy St Vincent Medical Center	Toledo	99%	331
Ohio State University Hospitals[2]	Columbus	99%	120
The Toledo Hospital[2]	Toledo	99%	125
University Hospital	Cincinnati	99%	182
University of Toledo Medical Center	Toledo	99%	100
Upper Valley Medical Center	Troy	99%	85
Adena Regional Medical Center	Chillicothe	98%	347
Affinity Medical Center	Massillon	98%	82
Bethesda North Hospital	Cincinnati	98%	357
Fort Hamilton Hughes Memorial Hospital	Hamilton	98%	40
Genesis Healthcare System	Zanesville	98%	281
Grandview Hospital & Medical Center	Dayton	98%	132
Knox Community Hospital	Mount Vernon	98%	51
Lake Health[2]	Concord	98%	259
Medcentral Health System[2]	Mansfield	98%	266
Mercy Franciscan Hospital - Mt Airy	Cincinnati	98%	64
Parma Community General Hospital	Parma	98%	303
Riverside Methodist Hospital[2]	Columbus	98%	296
Saint Luke's Hospital	Maumee	98%	143
Saint Vincent Charity Medical Center	Cleveland	98%	66
Southwest General Health Center	Middleburg Hgts	98%	424
Cleveland-Wade Park VA Medical Center	Cleveland	97%	36
Emh Regional Medical Center[2]	Elyria	97%	244
Euclid Hospital	Euclid	97%	29
Lakewood Hospital	Lakewood	97%	96
Springfield Regional Medical Center	Springfield	97%	310
Holzer Medical Center	Gallipolis	96%	95
Mercy Medical Center	Canton	96%	317
Robinson Memorial Hospital	Ravenna	96%	81
Trinity Medical Center East & West	Steubenville	96%	251
Mercy St Anne Hospital	Toledo	95%	37
Salem Community Hospital	Salem	95%	44
UHHS Bedford Medical Center	Bedford	94%	35
Alliance Community Hospital	Alliance	93%	30
Mercy St Charles Hospital	Oregon	92%	40
Wooster Community Hospital	Wooster	88%	34
Medina Hospital	Medina	85%	34
East Ohio Regional Hospital	Martins Ferry	82%	51

3. Aspirin at Discharge

Hospital Name	City	Rate	Cases
Atrium Medical Center[2]	Franklin	100%	251
Aultman Hospital	Canton	100%	619
Bethesda North Hospital	Cincinnati	100%	471
Blanchard Valley Hospital	Findlay	100%	128
Christ Hospital	Cincinnati	100%	509
Cincinnati VA Medical Center	Cincinnati	100%	37
Cleveland Clinic[2]	Cleveland	100%	839
Cleveland-Wade Park VA Medical Center	Cleveland	100%	35
Community Regional Medical Center	Lorain	100%	228
Emh Regional Medical Center[2]	Elyria	100%	291
Firelands Regional Medical Center	Sandusky	100%	129
Good Samaritan Hospital	Cincinnati	100%	372
Grant Medical Center	Columbus	100%	306
Hillcrest Hospital	Mayfield Heights	100%	311
Lima Memorial Health System	Lima	100%	232
Marietta Memorial Hospital	Marietta	100%	81
Marion General Hospital	Marion	100%	169
Mary Rutan Hospital	Bellefontaine	100%	38
Marymount Hospital	Garfield Heights	100%	37
Mercy Franciscan Hospital - Mt Airy	Cincinnati	100%	27
Mercy Franciscan Hospital Western Hills	Cincinnati	100%	34
Mercy Hospital Anderson	Cincinnati	100%	255
Mercy Hospital Fairfield	Fairfield	100%	291
Mercy St Vincent Medical Center	Toledo	100%	645
Miami Valley Hospital[2]	Dayton	100%	321
Mount Carmel Health	Columbus	100%	855
Mount Carmel St Ann's Hospital	Westerville	100%	88
Northside Medical Center	Youngstown	100%	153
Saint Elizabeth Boardman Health Center	Youngstown	100%	25
Saint Elizabeth Health Center	Youngstown	100%	490
Saint John Medical Center[2]	Westlake	100%	190
Saint Rita's Medical Center	Lima	100%	301
Saint Vincent Charity Medical Center	Cleveland	100%	66
South Pointe Hospital	Warrensville Hgts	100%	28
Southern Ohio Medical Center	Portsmouth	100%	181
Summa Barberton Hospital	Barberton	100%	83
Trumbull Memorial Hospital	Warren	100%	180
UH Geauga Medical Center	Chardon	100%	59
Union Hospital	Dover	100%	42
Community Hospitals and Wellness Centers	Bryan	99%	72
Doctors Hospital	Columbus	99%	195
Genesis Healthcare System	Zanesville	99%	388
Grandview Hospital & Medical Center	Dayton	99%	177
Kettering Medical Center	Kettering	99%	372
Lake Health[2]	Concord	99%	271
Metro Health Medical Center	Cleveland	99%	226
Ohio State University Hospitals[2]	Columbus	99%	279
Parma Community General Hospital	Parma	99%	313
Riverside Methodist Hospital[2]	Columbus	99%	581
Saint Luke's Hospital	Maumee	99%	157
Summa Health Systems Hospitals[2]	Akron	99%	314
The Toledo Hospital[2]	Toledo	99%	300
University Hospitals of Cleveland	Cleveland	99%	439
University of Toledo Medical Center	Toledo	99%	178
Adena Regional Medical Center	Chillicothe	98%	442
Affinity Medical Center	Massillon	98%	85
Fairview Hospital[2]	Cleveland	98%	269
Good Samaritan Hospital	Dayton	98%	493
Knox Community Hospital	Mount Vernon	98%	40
Lakewood Hospital	Lakewood	98%	87
Robinson Memorial Hospital	Ravenna	98%	55
Springfield Regional Medical Center	Springfield	98%	348
Trinity Medical Center East & West	Steubenville	98%	317
University Hospital	Cincinnati	98%	217
Upper Valley Medical Center	Troy	98%	59
Akron General Medical Center[2]	Akron	97%	284
Fairfield Medical Center	Lancaster	97%	252
Mercy Medical Center	Canton	97%	352
Fort Hamilton Hughes Memorial Hospital	Hamilton	96%	26
Jewish Hospital	Cincinnati	96%	165
Southwest General Health Center	Middleburg Hgts	96%	410
Flower Hospital	Sylvania	95%	38
Medcentral Health System[2]	Mansfield	94%	377
Holzer Medical Center	Gallipolis	92%	95
Licking Memorial Hospital	Newark	91%	33

4. Beta Blocker at Discharge

Hospital Name	City	Rate	Cases
Atrium Medical Center[2]	Franklin	100%	240
Aultman Hospital	Canton	100%	603
Blanchard Valley Hospital	Findlay	100%	117
Christ Hospital	Cincinnati	100%	486
Cincinnati VA Medical Center	Cincinnati	100%	34
Cleveland Clinic[2]	Cleveland	100%	804
Cleveland-Wade Park VA Medical Center	Cleveland	100%	35
Community Regional Medical Center	Lorain	100%	228
Doctors Hospital	Columbus	100%	192
Fairfield Medical Center	Lancaster	100%	240
Flower Hospital	Sylvania	100%	41
Fort Hamilton Hughes Memorial Hospital	Hamilton	100%	25
Good Samaritan Hospital	Cincinnati	100%	364
Hillcrest Hospital	Mayfield Heights	100%	306
Lake Health[2]	Concord	100%	280
Licking Memorial Hospital	Newark	100%	32
Marietta Memorial Hospital	Marietta	100%	88
Marymount Hospital	Garfield Heights	100%	38
Mercy Franciscan Hospital - Mt Airy	Cincinnati	100%	31
Mercy Franciscan Hospital Western Hills	Cincinnati	100%	38
Mercy St Vincent Medical Center	Toledo	100%	632
Metro Health Medical Center	Cleveland	100%	227
Mount Carmel Health	Columbus	100%	819
Northside Medical Center	Youngstown	100%	154
Ohio State University Hospitals[2]	Columbus	100%	284
Saint Elizabeth Boardman Health Center	Youngstown	100%	30
Saint Elizabeth Health Center	Youngstown	100%	487
Saint John Medical Center[2]	Westlake	100%	194
Saint Rita's Medical Center	Lima	100%	302
South Pointe Hospital	Warrensville Hgts	100%	36
Southern Ohio Medical Center	Portsmouth	100%	189
Summa Barberton Hospital	Barberton	100%	79
Summa Health Systems Hospitals[2]	Akron	100%	292
The Toledo Hospital[2]	Toledo	100%	303
Trumbull Memorial Hospital	Warren	100%	177
UH Geauga Medical Center	Chardon	100%	66
UHHS Bedford Medical Center	Bedford	100%	28
UHHS Richmond Heights Hospital	Richmond Hghts	100%	25
University Hospitals of Cleveland	Cleveland	100%	424
University of Toledo Medical Center	Toledo	100%	172
Akron General Medical Center[2]	Akron	99%	270
Bethesda North Hospital	Cincinnati	99%	433
Emh Regional Medical Center[2]	Elyria	99%	292
Genesis Healthcare System	Zanesville	99%	379
Good Samaritan Hospital	Dayton	99%	474

NOTE: Hospital profiles are in alphabetical order by state, then city, then hospital within the city; Rankings exclude hospitals with less than 25 cases except for patient surveys which excludes hospitals with less than 100 cases; (a) 100–299 cases; (1) The number of cases is too small to be sure how well a hospital is performing; (2) The hospital indicated that the data submitted for this measure were based on a sample of cases; (3) Data was collected during a shorter time period (fewer quarters) than the maximum possible time for this measure; (4) Suppressed for one or more quarters by CMS; (5) No data is available from the hospital for this measure; (6) Fewer than 100 patients completed the HCAHPS survey. Use these rates with caution, as the number of surveys may be too low to reliably assess hospital performance; (7) Survey results are based on less than 12 months of data; (8) Survey results are not available for this reporting period; (9) No or very few patients were eligible for the HCAHPS survey. The scores shown, if any, reflect a very small number of surveys; (10) A state average was not calculated because too few hospitals in the state submitted data; (11) There were discrepancies in the data collection process; Please refer to the User's Guide for a full explanation of data.

Grandview Hospital & Medical Center	Dayton	99%	175
Grant Medical Center	Columbus	99%	306
Jewish Hospital	Cincinnati	99%	153
Kettering Medical Center	Kettering	99%	365
Lakewood Hospital	Lakewood	99%	89
Lima Memorial Health System	Lima	99%	210
Marion General Hospital	Marion	99%	169
Mercy Hospital Anderson	Cincinnati	99%	240
Mercy Hospital Fairfield	Fairfield	99%	273
Miami Valley Hospital[2]	Dayton	99%	318
Mount Carmel St Ann's Hospital	Westerville	99%	83
Saint Luke's Hospital	Maumee	99%	156
University Hospital	Cincinnati	99%	202
Adena Regional Medical Center	Chillicothe	98%	453
Firelands Regional Medical Center	Sandusky	98%	125
Mercy Medical Center	Canton	98%	350
Riverside Methodist Hospital[2]	Columbus	98%	572
Robinson Memorial Hospital	Ravenna	98%	56
Union Hospital	Dover	98%	44
Upper Valley Medical Center	Troy	98%	58
Community Hospitals and Wellness Centers	Bryan	97%	68
Fairview Hospital[2]	Cleveland	97%	268
Mary Rutan Hospital	Bellefontaine	97%	39
Medcentral Health System[2]	Mansfield	97%	397
Saint Vincent Charity Medical Center	Cleveland	97%	67
Springfield Regional Medical Center	Springfield	97%	339
Trinity Medical Center East & West	Steubenville	97%	324
Affinity Medical Center	Massillon	96%	90
Parma Community General Hospital	Parma	96%	305
Holzer Medical Center	Gallipolis	95%	98
Knox Community Hospital	Mount Vernon	95%	42
Southwest General Health Center	Middleburg Hgts	95%	409

6. PCI Within 90 Minutes of Arrival

Hospital Name	City	Rate	Cases
Christ Hospital	Cincinnati	100%	33
Saint John Medical Center[2]	Westlake	100%	44
Saint Rita's Medical Center	Lima	100%	49
Summa Health Systems Hospitals[2]	Akron	100%	59
Emh Regional Medical Center[2]	Elyria	98%	40
Good Samaritan Hospital	Cincinnati	98%	43
Marion General Hospital	Marion	98%	53
Riverside Methodist Hospital[2]	Columbus	98%	87
Southern Ohio Medical Center	Portsmouth	98%	46
Southwest General Health Center	Middleburg Hgts	98%	61
Bethesda North Hospital	Cincinnati	97%	75
Doctors Hospital	Columbus	97%	37
Mount Carmel St Ann's Hospital	Westerville	97%	33
Mount Carmel Health	Columbus	96%	170
Saint Elizabeth Health Center	Youngstown	95%	62
Blanchard Valley Hospital	Findlay	94%	50
Mercy Hospital Anderson	Cincinnati	94%	51
Mercy Hospital Fairfield	Fairfield	94%	48
Mercy Medical Center	Canton	94%	70
Grant Medical Center	Columbus	93%	42
Mercy St Vincent Medical Center	Toledo	93%	82
Parma Community General Hospital	Parma	93%	61
Aultman Hospital	Canton	92%	90
Fairview Hospital[2]	Cleveland	92%	49
Hillcrest Hospital	Mayfield Heights	92%	49
Kettering Medical Center	Kettering	92%	60
Miami Valley Hospital[2]	Dayton	92%	60
University of Toledo Medical Center	Toledo	92%	25
Genesis Healthcare System	Zanesville	91%	58
Good Samaritan Hospital	Dayton	91%	66
Metro Health Medical Center	Cleveland	91%	44
Lake Health[2]	Concord	90%	50
Jewish Hospital	Cincinnati	89%	28
Community Regional Medical Center	Lorain	88%	50
Saint Luke's Hospital	Maumee	88%	42
Springfield Regional Medical Center	Springfield	88%	49
University Hospital	Cincinnati	88%	40
Akron General Medical Center[2]	Akron	87%	47
University Hospitals of Cleveland	Cleveland	86%	28
Affinity Medical Center	Massillon	85%	27
Atrium Medical Center[2]	Franklin	85%	54
Grandview Hospital & Medical Center	Dayton	85%	34
Lakewood Hospital	Lakewood	82%	28
Fairfield Medical Center	Lancaster	81%	52
Medcentral Health System[2]	Mansfield	79%	39
Trumbull Memorial Hospital	Warren	76%	42
Adena Regional Medical Center	Chillicothe	74%	47
Trinity Medical Center East & West	Steubenville	73%	33

7. Smoking Cessation Advice

Hospital Name	City	Rate	Cases
Adena Regional Medical Center	Chillicothe	100%	175
Affinity Medical Center	Massillon	100%	35
Akron General Medical Center[2]	Akron	100%	104
Atrium Medical Center[2]	Franklin	100%	98
Aultman Hospital	Canton	100%	213
Bethesda North Hospital	Cincinnati	100%	153
Christ Hospital	Cincinnati	100%	200
Cleveland Clinic[2]	Cleveland	100%	288
Community Hospitals and Wellness Centers	Bryan	100%	25
Doctors Hospital	Columbus	100%	98
Emh Regional Medical Center[2]	Elyria	100%	106
Fairview Hospital[2]	Cleveland	100%	87
Firelands Regional Medical Center	Sandusky	100%	45
Good Samaritan Hospital	Cincinnati	100%	160
Grandview Hospital & Medical Center	Dayton	100%	74
Grant Medical Center	Columbus	100%	138
Hillcrest Hospital	Mayfield Heights	100%	81
Jewish Hospital	Cincinnati	100%	57
Kettering Medical Center	Kettering	100%	100
Lakewood Hospital	Lakewood	100%	38
Lima Memorial Health System	Lima	100%	81
Marietta Memorial Hospital	Marietta	100%	27
Marion General Hospital	Marion	100%	72
Medcentral Health System[2]	Mansfield	100%	165
Mercy Hospital Anderson	Cincinnati	100%	105
Mercy Hospital Fairfield	Fairfield	100%	110
Mercy Medical Center	Canton	100%	130
Mercy St Vincent Medical Center	Toledo	100%	283
Metro Health Medical Center	Cleveland	100%	126
Miami Valley Hospital[2]	Dayton	100%	149
Mount Carmel Health	Columbus	100%	355
Northside Medical Center	Youngstown	100%	51
Ohio State University Hospitals[2]	Columbus	100%	110
Riverside Methodist Hospital[2]	Columbus	100%	209
Saint John Medical Center[2]	Westlake	100%	70
Saint Rita's Medical Center	Lima	100%	121
Saint Vincent Charity Medical Center	Cleveland	100%	28
Southern Ohio Medical Center	Portsmouth	100%	86
Springfield Regional Medical Center	Springfield	100%	126
Summa Barberton Hospital	Barberton	100%	25
Trinity Medical Center East & West	Steubenville	100%	105
Trumbull Memorial Hospital	Warren	100%	61
University Hospital	Cincinnati	100%	114
University Hospitals of Cleveland	Cleveland	100%	154
University of Toledo Medical Center	Toledo	100%	75
Fairfield Medical Center	Lancaster	99%	93
Genesis Healthcare System	Zanesville	99%	149
Good Samaritan Hospital	Dayton	99%	175
Parma Community General Hospital	Parma	99%	85
Saint Elizabeth Health Center	Youngstown	99%	190
Summa Health Systems Hospitals[2]	Akron	99%	123
The Toledo Hospital[2]	Toledo	99%	123
Blanchard Valley Hospital	Findlay	98%	45
Community Regional Medical Center	Lorain	98%	98
Lake Health[2]	Concord	98%	97
Saint Luke's Hospital	Maumee	98%	55
Southwest General Health Center	Middleburg Hgts	98%	105
Holzer Medical Center	Gallipolis	97%	30

Chest Pain/Possible Heart Attack Care

8. Aspirin at Arrival

Hospital Name	City	Rate	Cases
Alliance Community Hospital	Alliance	100%	101
Atrium Medical Center	Franklin	100%	31
Bay Park Community Hospital	Oregon	100%	46
Fort Hamilton Hughes Memorial Hospital	Hamilton	100%	36
McCullough-Hyde Memorial Hospital	Oxford	100%	64
Mercer County Joint Twp Comm Hosp	Coldwater	100%	83
Mercy Franciscan Hospital - Mt Airy	Cincinnati	100%	41
Mercy St Anne Hospital	Toledo	100%	71
Mercy St Charles Hospital	Oregon	100%	83
Saint Rita's Medical Center	Lima	100%	58
Summa Barberton Hospital	Barberton	100%	25
UH Geauga Medical Center	Chardon	100%	68
UHHS Memorial Hospital of Geneva	Geneva	100%	222
Univ Hosps Conneaut Med Ctr	Conneaut	100%	56
Adena Regional Medical Center	Chillicothe	99%	118
Berger Hospital	Circleville	99%	179
Brown County Hospital	Georgetown	99%	87
Grady Memorial Hospital	Delaware	99%	123
Kettering Medical Center - Sycamore	Miamisburg	99%	97
Lodi Community Hospital	Lodi	99%	134
Marion General Hospital	Marion	99%	134
Saint Joseph Health Center	Warren	99%	134
Summa Wadsworth-Rittman Hospital	Wadsworth	99%	99
Wilson Memorial Hospital	Sidney	99%	99
Ashtabula County Medical Center	Ashtabula	98%	137
CMH Regional Health System	Wilmington	98%	97
Euclid Hospital	Euclid	98%	84
Fairview Hospital	Cleveland	98%	47
Greene Memorial Hospital	Xenia	98%	56
Mercy Hospital of Defiance	Defiance	98%	62
Robinson Memorial Hospital	Ravenna	98%	115
South Pointe Hospital	Warrensville Hgts	98%	398
West Chester Medical Center	West Chester	98%	46
Wooster Community Hospital	Wooster	98%	218
Fairfield Medical Center	Lancaster	97%	33
Fayette County Memorial Hospital	Washington CH	97%	143
Madison County Hospital	London	97%	115
Mary Rutan Hospital	Bellefontaine	97%	126
Saint Elizabeth Boardman Health Center	Youngstown	97%	119
Saint Elizabeth Health Center	Youngstown	97%	63
Saint John Medical Center	Westlake	97%	36
Saint Vincent Charity Medical Center	Cleveland	97%	159
Southeastern Ohio Regional Medical Center	Cambridge	97%	276
Southern Ohio Medical Center	Portsmouth	97%	104
Union Hospital	Dover	97%	185
Community Hospitals and Wellness Centers	Bryan	96%	46
Flower Hospital	Sylvania	96%	53
Joel Pomerene Memorial Hospital	Millersburg	96%	140
Marymount Hospital	Garfield Heights	96%	134
Memorial Hospital of Union County	Marysville	96%	196
Mercy Franciscan Hospital Western Hills	Cincinnati	96%	132
Mercy Hospital Clermont	Batavia	96%	106
Samaritan Hospital - Peoples Hospital	Ashland	96%	159
UHHS Bedford Medical Center	Bedford	96%	94
Upper Valley Medical Center	Troy	96%	124
Wood County Hospital	Bowling Green	96%	91
Fisher Titus Memorial Hospital	Norwalk	95%	74
Licking Memorial Hospital	Newark	95%	64
Parma Community General Hospital	Parma	95%	43
Van Wert County Hospital	Van Wert	95%	172
Bethesda North Hospital	Cincinnati	94%	48
Coshocton County Memorial Hospital	Coshocton	94%	228
East Ohio Regional Hospital	Martins Ferry	94%	47
Huron Hospital	Cleveland	94%	63
Joint Township District Memorial Hospital	Saint Marys	94%	136
Knox Community Hospital	Mount Vernon	94%	48
Lake Health	Concord	94%	48
Marietta Memorial Hospital	Marietta	94%	50
UHHS Richmond Heights Hospital	Richmond Hghts	94%	63
Bellevue Hospital	Bellevue	93%	72
Lakewood Hospital	Lakewood	93%	29
Mount Carmel St Ann's Hospital	Westerville	93%	30
O'Bleness Memorial Hospital	Athens	93%	312
Salem Community Hospital	Salem	93%	75
Wayne Hospital	Greenville	93%	134
Hillcrest Hospital	Mayfield Heights	92%	48
Summa Western Reserve Hospital	Cuyahoga Falls	92%	40
Dublin Methodist Hospital	Dublin	91%	120
Lutheran Hospital	Cleveland	91%	44
Medcentral Health System	Mansfield	91%	55
Medina Hospital	Medina	91%	123
Mercy Tiffin Hospital	Tiffin	91%	100
Morrow County Hospital[3]	Mount Gilead	90%	60
Memorial Hospital	Fremont	89%	98
Southwest General Health Center	Middleburg Hgts	89%	84
East Liverpool City Hospital	East Liverpool	85%	124
Emh Regional Medical Center	Elyria	85%	110
Amherst Hospital	Amherst	84%	121
Holzer Medical Center	Gallipolis	82%	33
Fulton County Health Center	Wauseon	74%	107

9. Median Time to ECG (minutes)

Hospital Name	City	Min.	Cases
Hillcrest Hospital	Mayfield Heights	0	52
Ashtabula County Medical Center	Ashtabula	2	146
Medina Hospital	Medina	2	122
Parma Community General Hospital	Parma	2	43
UH Geauga Medical Center	Chardon	2	68
Bellevue Hospital	Bellevue	3	74
Licking Memorial Hospital	Newark	3	65
Marion General Hospital	Marion	3	135
McCullough-Hyde Memorial Hospital	Oxford	3	65
Bay Park Community Hospital	Oregon	4	46
Fort Hamilton Hughes Memorial Hospital	Hamilton	4	38
Grady Memorial Hospital	Delaware	4	133
Joel Pomerene Memorial Hospital	Millersburg	4	142
Lutheran Hospital	Cleveland	4	48
Madison County Hospital	London	4	117
Memorial Hospital of Union County	Marysville	4	205
Mercy Hospital of Defiance	Defiance	4	66
Mercy St Charles Hospital	Oregon	4	85
Mount Carmel St Ann's Hospital	Westerville	4	30
Salem Community Hospital	Salem	4	75
Summa Wadsworth-Rittman Hospital	Wadsworth	4	102
UHHS Bedford Medical Center	Bedford	4	103
Bethesda North Hospital	Cincinnati	5	52
Euclid Hospital	Euclid	5	91
Firelands Regional Medical Center	Sandusky	5	25
Flower Hospital	Sylvania	5	57
Holzer Medical Center	Gallipolis	5	31
Knox Community Hospital	Mount Vernon	5	50

NOTE: Hospital profiles are in alphabetical order by state, then city, then hospital within the city; Rankings exclude hospitals with less than 25 cases except for patient surveys which excludes hospitals with less than 100 cases; (a) 100–299 cases; (1) The number of cases is too small to be sure how well a hospital is performing; (2) The hospital indicated that the data submitted for this measure were based on a sample of cases; (3) Data was collected during a shorter time period (fewer quarters) than the maximum possible time for this measure; (4) Suppressed for one or more quarters by CMS; (5) No data is available from the hospital for this measure; (6) Fewer than 100 patients completed the HCAHPS survey. Use these rates with caution, as the number of surveys may be too low to reliably assess hospital performance; (7) Survey results are based on less than 12 months of data; (8) Survey results are not available for this reporting period; (9) No or very few patients were eligible for the HCAHPS survey. The scores shown, if any, reflect a very small number of surveys; (10) A state average was not calculated because too few hospitals in the state submitted data; (11) There were discrepancies in the data collection process; Please refer to the User's Guide for a full explanation of data.

Lakewood Hospital	Lakewood	5	29
Saint John Medical Center	Westlake	5	38
Saint Joseph Health Center	Warren	5	139
Southern Ohio Medical Center	Portsmouth	5	113
UHHS Memorial Hospital of Geneva	Geneva	5	235
Wooster Community Hospital	Wooster	5	229
Adena Regional Medical Center	Chillicothe	6	121
Brown County Hospital	Georgetown	6	94
Community Hospitals and Wellness Centers	Bryan	6	48
Fayette County Memorial Hospital	Washington CH	6	153
Fisher Titus Memorial Hospital	Norwalk	6	76
Greene Memorial Hospital	Xenia	6	58
Kettering Medical Center - Sycamore	Miamisburg	6	99
Lake Health	Concord	6	49
Mary Rutan Hospital	Bellefontaine	6	132
Mercy Tiffin Hospital	Tiffin	6	105
Saint Elizabeth Boardman Health Center	Youngstown	6	125
Saint Elizabeth Health Center	Youngstown	6	64
Samaritan Hospital - Peoples Hospital	Ashland	6	172
Summa Barberton Hospital	Barberton	6	25
UHHS Richmond Heights Hospital	Richmond Hghts	6	68
Atrium Medical Center	Franklin	7	31
Berger Hospital	Circleville	7	180
Fairview Hospital	Cleveland	7	48
Joint Township District Memorial Hospital	Saint Marys	7	150
Lodi Community Hospital	Lodi	7	138
Marymount Hospital	Garfield Heights	7	137
Medcentral Health System	Mansfield	7	63
O'Bleness Memorial Hospital	Athens	7	315
Robinson Memorial Hospital	Ravenna	7	117
South Pointe Hospital	Warrensville Hgts	7	411
Univ Hosps Conneaut Med Ctr	Conneaut	7	60
Mercer County Joint Twp Comm Hosp	Coldwater	8	84
Mercy Franciscan Hospital Western Hills	Cincinnati	8	139
Saint Vincent Charity Medical Center	Cleveland	8	159
Southeastern Ohio Regional Medical Center	Cambridge	8	275
Southwest General Health Center	Middleburg Hgts	8	86
Upper Valley Medical Center	Troy	8	126
Alliance Community Hospital	Alliance	9	107
Dublin Methodist Hospital	Dublin	9	123
Emh Regional Medical Center	Elyria	9	120
Saint Rita's Medical Center	Lima	9	66
Amherst Hospital	Amherst	10	131
CMH Regional Health System	Wilmington	10	110
Huron Hospital	Cleveland	10	62
Marietta Memorial Hospital	Marietta	10	51
Wood County Hospital	Bowling Green	10	94
Bluffton Hospital	Bluffton	11	26
Fairfield Medical Center	Lancaster	11	37
Mercy Franciscan Hospital - Mt Airy	Cincinnati	11	42
Mercy Hospital Clermont	Batavia	11	114
Summa Western Reserve Hospital	Cuyahoga Falls	11	43
Union Hospital	Dover	11	195
West Chester Medical Center	West Chester	11	47
Coshocton County Memorial Hospital	Coshocton	12	236
Wilson Memorial Hospital	Sidney	12	100
Morrow County Hospital[3]	Mount Gilead	13	63
Van Wert County Hospital	Van Wert	13	176
East Ohio Regional Hospital	Martins Ferry	14	52
Memorial Hospital	Fremont	14	108
Fulton County Health Center	Wauseon	15	114
East Liverpool City Hospital	East Liverpool	20	126
Mercy St Anne Hospital	Toledo	21	75
Wayne Hospital	Greenville	22	150

10. Median Time to Transfer (minutes)

Hospital Name	City	Min.	Cases
Mary Rutan Hospital	Bellefontaine	40	35
Kettering Medical Center - Sycamore	Miamisburg	44	25
Saint Elizabeth Boardman Health Center	Youngstown	48	56
Union Hospital	Dover	48	42
Robinson Memorial Hospital	Ravenna	50	40
Marymount Hospital	Garfield Heights	55	33
South Pointe Hospital	Warrensville Hgts	60	29
Saint Joseph Health Center	Warren	62	46
Upper Valley Medical Center	Troy	65	57
Medina Hospital[3]	Medina	68	25
Fisher Titus Memorial Hospital	Norwalk	74	25
East Liverpool City Hospital	East Liverpool	77	28
Mercy Hospital Clermont	Batavia	128	29

Heart Failure Care

12. ACE Inhibitor or ARB for LVSD

Hospital Name	City	Rate	Cases
Bay Park Community Hospital	Oregon	100%	25
Blanchard Valley Hospital	Findlay	100%	47
CMH Regional Health System	Wilmington	100%	40
Firelands Regional Medical Center	Sandusky	100%	81
Flower Hospital	Sylvania	100%	41
Grandview Hospital & Medical Center	Dayton	100%	93
Mercy Franciscan Hospital - Mt Airy	Cincinnati	100%	69
Mercy Franciscan Hospital Western Hills	Cincinnati	100%	47
Mercy Hospital Clermont	Batavia	100%	32
Mount Carmel Health	Columbus	100%	411
Mount Carmel St Ann's Hospital	Westerville	100%	97
Saint Elizabeth Health Center[2]	Youngstown	100%	85
Southwest General Health Center	Middleburg Hgts	100%	141
Summa Barberton Hospital	Barberton	100%	54
Summa Western Reserve Hospital	Cuyahoga Falls	100%	27
Trumbull Memorial Hospital	Warren	100%	117
UH Geauga Medical Center	Chardon	100%	49
UHHS Bedford Medical Center	Bedford	100%	59
Union Hospital	Dover	100%	72
Upper Valley Medical Center	Troy	100%	44
Aultman Hospital	Canton	99%	163
Christ Hospital	Cincinnati	99%	396
Cincinnati VA Medical Center	Cincinnati	99%	93
Fort Hamilton Hughes Memorial Hospital	Hamilton	99%	69
Grant Medical Center[2]	Columbus	99%	129
Hillcrest Hospital	Mayfield Heights	99%	167
Kettering Medical Center	Kettering	99%	195
Lakewood Hospital	Lakewood	99%	67
Marietta Memorial Hospital	Marietta	99%	74
Mercy Hospital Fairfield	Fairfield	99%	138
Northside Medical Center	Youngstown	99%	71
Ohio State University Hospitals[2]	Columbus	99%	139
South Pointe Hospital	Warrensville Hgts	99%	137
Southern Ohio Medical Center	Portsmouth	99%	123
University of Toledo Medical Center[2]	Toledo	99%	85
Ashtabula County Medical Center	Ashtabula	98%	53
Atrium Medical Center	Franklin	98%	64
Cleveland Clinic	Cleveland	98%	487
Cleveland-Wade Park VA Medical Center	Cleveland	98%	174
Community Regional Medical Center	Lorain	98%	121
Euclid Hospital	Euclid	98%	84
Fairfield Medical Center	Lancaster	98%	92
Huron Hospital	Cleveland	98%	97
Knox Community Hospital	Mount Vernon	98%	55
Lima Memorial Health System	Lima	98%	63
Mercy Hospital Anderson	Cincinnati	98%	90
Mercy Medical Center	Canton	98%	146
Riverside Methodist Hospital[2]	Columbus	98%	252
Saint Luke's Hospital	Maumee	98%	97
University Hospital[2]	Cincinnati	98%	332
West Chester Medical Center	West Chester	98%	40
Bethesda North Hospital	Cincinnati	97%	251
Doctors Hospital	Columbus	97%	89
Licking Memorial Hospital	Newark	97%	73
Mercer County Joint Twp Comm Hosp	Coldwater	97%	29
Mercy St Vincent Medical Center	Toledo	97%	324
Saint Joseph Health Center[2]	Warren	97%	71
Saint Rita's Medical Center	Lima	97%	152
Springfield Regional Medical Center	Springfield	97%	180
Summa Health Systems Hospitals[2]	Akron	97%	110
University Hospitals of Cleveland	Cleveland	97%	308
Dayton VA Medical Center	Dayton	96%	70
East Liverpool City Hospital	East Liverpool	96%	48
Marion General Hospital	Marion	96%	126
Mary Rutan Hospital	Bellefontaine	96%	28
Jewish Hospital	Cincinnati	95%	139
Marymount Hospital	Garfield Heights	95%	178
Metro Health Medical Center	Cleveland	95%	261
Miami Valley Hospital[2]	Dayton	95%	106
Saint Vincent Charity Medical Center[2]	Cleveland	95%	118
The Toledo Hospital[2]	Toledo	95%	75
Affinity Medical Center	Massillon	94%	50
Grady Memorial Hospital	Delaware	94%	35
Joint Township District Memorial Hospital	Saint Marys	94%	48
McCullough-Hyde Memorial Hospital	Oxford	94%	34
Robinson Memorial Hospital	Ravenna	94%	78
Adena Regional Medical Center	Chillicothe	93%	134
Good Samaritan Hospital	Cincinnati	93%	202
Saint Elizabeth Boardman Health Center[2]	Youngstown	93%	58
Salem Community Hospital	Salem	93%	27
Community Hospitals and Wellness Centers	Bryan	92%	52
Good Samaritan Hospital[2]	Dayton	92%	100
Lutheran Hospital	Cleveland	92%	38
Medcentral Health System[2]	Mansfield	92%	86
UHHS Richmond Heights Hospital	Richmond Hghts	92%	63
Akron General Medical Center[2]	Akron	91%	102
Lake Health[2]	Concord	91%	119
Mercy St Anne Hospital	Toledo	91%	47
East Ohio Regional Hospital	Martins Ferry	90%	39
Genesis Healthcare System	Zanesville	90%	100
Mercy St Charles Hospital	Oregon	90%	67
Saint John Medical Center[2]	Westlake	90%	40
Southeastern Ohio Regional Medical Center	Cambridge	89%	28
Wooster Community Hospital	Wooster	89%	27
Greene Memorial Hospital	Xenia	88%	32
Alliance Community Hospital	Alliance	87%	45
Emh Regional Medical Center[2]	Elyria	87%	108
Fisher Titus Memorial Hospital	Norwalk	87%	39
Parma Community General Hospital	Parma	87%	208
Fairview Hospital	Cleveland	86%	200
Holzer Medical Center	Gallipolis	86%	84
Trinity Medical Center East & West	Steubenville	84%	205
Medina Hospital	Medina	82%	51
O'Bleness Memorial Hospital	Athens	69%	29

13. Discharge Instructions

Hospital Name	City	Rate	Cases
Bay Park Community Hospital	Oregon	100%	100
Berger Hospital	Circleville	100%	84
Cleveland-Wade Park VA Medical Center	Cleveland	100%	391
CMH Regional Health System	Wilmington	100%	130
Dublin Methodist Hospital	Dublin	100%	35
Grant Medical Center[2]	Columbus	100%	266
Hardin Memorial Hospital	Kenton	100%	29
Medcentral Health System[2]	Mansfield	100%	254
Memorial Hospital of Union County	Marysville	100%	37
Mercer County Joint Twp Comm Hosp	Coldwater	100%	33
Mercy Memorial Hospital	Urbana	100%	52
Mercy St Vincent Medical Center	Toledo	100%	565
Ohio State University Hospitals[2]	Columbus	100%	260
Riverside Methodist Hospital[2]	Columbus	100%	487
Robinson Memorial Hospital	Ravenna	100%	267
Saint Elizabeth Boardman Health Center[2]	Youngstown	100%	153
Saint Elizabeth Health Center[2]	Youngstown	100%	221
Saint John Medical Center[2]	Westlake	100%	143
Saint Joseph Health Center[2]	Warren	100%	209
Southern Ohio Medical Center	Portsmouth	100%	334
Summa Barberton Hospital	Barberton	100%	260
UH Geauga Medical Center	Chardon	100%	123
Univ Hosps Conneaut Med Ctr	Conneaut	100%	25
Christ Hospital	Cincinnati	99%	826
Fairfield Medical Center	Lancaster	99%	298
Huron Hospital	Cleveland	99%	192
McCullough-Hyde Memorial Hospital	Oxford	99%	70
South Pointe Hospital	Warrensville Hgts	99%	301
Doctors Hospital	Columbus	98%	180
Fort Hamilton Hughes Memorial Hospital	Hamilton	98%	211
Grady Memorial Hospital	Delaware	98%	95
Greene Memorial Hospital	Xenia	98%	127
Kettering Medical Center - Sycamore	Miamisburg	98%	96
Lakewood Hospital	Lakewood	98%	187
Lutheran Hospital	Cleveland	98%	84
Mercy St Charles Hospital	Oregon	98%	172
Southwest General Health Center	Middleburg Hgts	98%	374
Union Hospital	Dover	98%	210
Barnesville Hospital Association	Barnesville	97%	74
Fostoria Community Hospital	Fostoria	97%	29
Grandview Hospital & Medical Center	Dayton	97%	315
Joel Pomerene Memorial Hospital	Millersburg	97%	38
Mercy St Anne Hospital	Toledo	97%	157
Mercy Tiffin Hospital	Tiffin	97%	66
Saint Rita's Medical Center	Lima	97%	267
Samaritan Hospital - Peoples Hospital	Ashland	97%	69
UHHS Bedford Medical Center	Bedford	97%	146
Bethesda North Hospital	Cincinnati	96%	601
Blanchard Valley Hospital	Findlay	96%	70
Community Hospitals and Wellness Centers	Bryan	96%	92
Community Regional Medical Center	Lorain	96%	317
Defiance Regional Medical Center	Defiance	96%	27
Firelands Regional Medical Center	Sandusky	96%	183
Genesis Healthcare System	Zanesville	96%	331
Jewish Hospital	Cincinnati	96%	302
Marion General Hospital	Marion	96%	256
Mercy Franciscan Hospital Western Hills	Cincinnati	96%	160
Mercy Hospital Fairfield	Fairfield	96%	347
Mercy Hospital of Defiance	Defiance	96%	26
Northside Medical Center	Youngstown	96%	238
Saint Luke's Hospital	Maumee	96%	254
Cincinnati VA Medical Center	Cincinnati	95%	191
East Liverpool City Hospital	East Liverpool	95%	162
Fairview Hospital	Cleveland	95%	578
Kettering Medical Center	Kettering	95%	387
Mercy Hospital Clermont	Batavia	95%	76
West Chester Medical Center	West Chester	95%	64
Chillicothe VA Medical Center	Chillicothe	94%	99
Good Samaritan Hospital	Cincinnati	94%	472
Saint Vincent Charity Medical Center[2]	Cleveland	94%	236
Cleveland Clinic	Cleveland	93%	1009
Mercy Hospital Anderson	Cincinnati	93%	262
Summa Wadsworth-Rittman Hospital	Wadsworth	93%	69
UHHS Richmond Heights Hospital	Richmond Hghts	93%	148
University Hospitals of Cleveland	Cleveland	93%	667
University of Toledo Medical Center[2]	Toledo	93%	212
Henry County Hospital	Napoleon	92%	25
Licking Memorial Hospital	Newark	92%	188
Lima Memorial Health System	Lima	92%	158

NOTE: Hospital profiles are in alphabetical order by state, then city, then hospital within the city; Rankings exclude hospitals with less than 25 cases except for patient surveys which excludes hospitals with less than 100 cases; (a) 100–299 cases; (1) The number of cases is too small to be sure how well a hospital is performing; (2) The hospital indicated that the data submitted for this measure were based on a sample of cases; (3) Data was collected during a shorter time period (fewer quarters) than the maximum possible time for this measure; (4) Suppressed for one or more quarters by CMS; (5) No data is available from the hospital for this measure; (6) Fewer than 100 patients completed the HCAHPS survey. Use these rates with caution, as the number of surveys may be too low to reliably assess hospital performance; (7) Survey results are based on less than 12 months of data; (8) Survey results are not available for this reporting period; (9) No or very few patients were eligible for the HCAHPS survey. The scores shown, if any, reflect a very small number of surveys; (10) A state average was not calculated because too few hospitals in the state submitted data; (11) There were discrepancies in the data collection process; Please refer to the User's Guide for a full explanation of data.

Marymount Hospital	Garfield Heights	92%	439
Springfield Regional Medical Center	Springfield	92%	368
Summa Health Systems Hospitals[2]	Akron	92%	266
Trinity Medical Center East & West	Steubenville	92%	406
Upper Valley Medical Center	Troy	92%	173
Atrium Medical Center	Franklin	91%	290
Euclid Hospital	Euclid	91%	222
Good Samaritan Hospital[2]	Dayton	91%	248
Mount Carmel St Ann's Hospital	Westerville	91%	247
Salem Community Hospital	Salem	91%	122
Southeastern Ohio Regional Medical Center	Cambridge	91%	102
Alliance Community Hospital	Alliance	90%	99
Fisher Titus Memorial Hospital	Norwalk	90%	80
Dayton VA Medical Center	Dayton	89%	150
Wilson Memorial Hospital	Sidney	88%	41
Affinity Medical Center	Massillon	87%	119
Aultman Hospital	Canton	87%	445
Brown County Hospital	Georgetown	87%	39
Flower Hospital	Sylvania	87%	146
Medina Hospital	Medina	87%	163
Mercy Franciscan Hospital - Mt Airy	Cincinnati	87%	205
Ashtabula County Medical Center	Ashtabula	86%	142
Hillcrest Hospital	Mayfield Heights	86%	398
Mercy Medical Center	Canton	86%	333
Mount Carmel Health	Columbus	86%	956
Bellevue Hospital	Bellevue	85%	27
Holzer Medical Center	Gallipolis	85%	253
Lake Health[2]	Concord	85%	371
Marietta Memorial Hospital	Marietta	85%	217
Miami Valley Hospital[2]	Dayton	85%	253
Wooster Community Hospital	Wooster	85%	81
Adena Regional Medical Center	Chillicothe	84%	271
Summa Western Reserve Hospital	Cuyahoga Falls	84%	80
Mary Rutan Hospital	Bellefontaine	83%	47
Wood County Hospital	Bowling Green	83%	58
Parma Community General Hospital	Parma	81%	418
Holzer Medical Center Jackson	Jackson	80%	74
Joint Township District Memorial Hospital	Saint Marys	79%	99
Memorial Hospital	Fremont	79%	34
Van Wert County Hospital	Van Wert	79%	28
Akron General Medical Center[2]	Akron	77%	244
University Hospital[2]	Cincinnati	76%	489
Coshocton County Memorial Hospital	Coshocton	75%	36
Fayette County Memorial Hospital	Washington CH	74%	39
Madison County Hospital	London	74%	57
Trumbull Memorial Hospital	Warren	74%	408
East Ohio Regional Hospital	Martins Ferry	72%	137
Emh Regional Medical Center[2]	Elyria	72%	229
Knox Community Hospital	Mount Vernon	71%	132
Fulton County Health Center	Wauseon	69%	26
H B Magruder Memorial Hospital	Port Clinton	69%	26
Highland District Hospital	Hillsboro	66%	53
O'Bleness Memorial Hospital	Athens	64%	72
The Toledo Hospital[2]	Toledo	64%	224
Metro Health Medical Center	Cleveland	63%	589
Selby General Hospital	Marietta	60%	25
Wayne Hospital	Greenville	51%	84
Belmont Community Hospital	Bellaire	23%	43
Deaconess Hospital	Cincinnati	12%	33

14. Evaluation of LVS Function

Hospital Name	City	Rate	Cases
Adams County Regional Medical Center	Seaman	100%	26
Affinity Medical Center	Massillon	100%	174
Atrium Medical Center	Franklin	100%	358
Aultman Hospital	Canton	100%	593
Bay Park Community Hospital	Oregon	100%	139
Berger Hospital	Circleville	100%	108
Bethesda North Hospital	Cincinnati	100%	742
Blanchard Valley Hospital	Findlay	100%	105
Brown County Hospital	Georgetown	100%	62
Bucyrus Community Hospital	Bucyrus	100%	25
Christ Hospital	Cincinnati	100%	996
Cincinnati VA Medical Center	Cincinnati	100%	207
Cleveland Clinic	Cleveland	100%	1206
Cleveland-Wade Park VA Medical Center	Cleveland	100%	417
Community Hospitals and Wellness Centers	Bryan	100%	115
Community Regional Medical Center	Lorain	100%	402
Dayton VA Medical Center	Dayton	100%	174
Defiance Regional Medical Center	Defiance	100%	37
Doctors Hospital	Columbus	100%	158
East Ohio Regional Hospital	Martins Ferry	100%	204
Euclid Hospital	Euclid	100%	309
Fairfield Medical Center	Lancaster	100%	362
Fort Hamilton Hughes Memorial Hospital	Hamilton	100%	269
Fostoria Community Hospital	Fostoria	100%	32
Genesis Healthcare System	Zanesville	100%	392
Good Samaritan Hospital	Cincinnati	100%	555
Good Samaritan Hospital[2]	Dayton	100%	290
Grandview Hospital & Medical Center	Dayton	100%	410
Grant Medical Center[2]	Columbus	100%	306
Greene Memorial Hospital	Xenia	100%	157
H B Magruder Memorial Hospital	Port Clinton	100%	33
Hardin Memorial Hospital	Kenton	100%	42
Huron Hospital	Cleveland	100%	223
Jewish Hospital	Cincinnati	100%	405
Kettering Medical Center	Kettering	100%	500
Kettering Medical Center - Sycamore	Miamisburg	100%	127
Lima Memorial Health System	Lima	100%	191
Marietta Memorial Hospital	Marietta	100%	278
Memorial Hospital of Union County	Marysville	100%	51
Mercer County Joint Twp Comm Hosp	Coldwater	100%	54
Mercy Franciscan Hospital - Mt Airy	Cincinnati	100%	254
Mercy Hospital Clermont	Batavia	100%	90
Mercy Hospital of Defiance	Defiance	100%	36
Mercy Medical Center	Canton	100%	431
Mercy Memorial Hospital	Urbana	100%	64
Mercy St Charles Hospital	Oregon	100%	217
Mercy St Vincent Medical Center	Toledo	100%	657
Metro Health Medical Center	Cleveland	100%	660
Miami Valley Hospital[2]	Dayton	100%	317
Mount Carmel Health	Columbus	100%	1208
Mount Carmel St Ann's Hospital	Westerville	100%	337
O'Bleness Memorial Hospital	Athens	100%	90
Ohio State University Hospitals[2]	Columbus	100%	295
Riverside Methodist Hospital[2]	Columbus	100%	648
Saint Elizabeth Health Center[2]	Youngstown	100%	301
Saint John Medical Center[2]	Westlake	100%	206
Saint Joseph Health Center[2]	Warren	100%	254
Saint Vincent Charity Medical Center[2]	Cleveland	100%	287
South Pointe Hospital	Warrensville Hgts	100%	399
Southern Ohio Medical Center	Portsmouth	100%	419
Southwest General Health Center	Middleburg Hgts	100%	527
Summa Barberton Hospital	Barberton	100%	337
Trumbull Memorial Hospital	Warren	100%	519
UH Geauga Medical Center	Chardon	100%	175
UHHS Bedford Medical Center	Bedford	100%	200
UHHS Memorial Hospital of Geneva	Geneva	100%	44
UHHS Richmond Heights Hospital	Richmond Hghts	100%	215
Union Hospital	Dover	100%	301
Univ Hosps Conneaut Med Ctr	Conneaut	100%	38
University Hospitals of Cleveland	Cleveland	100%	795
University of Toledo Medical Center[2]	Toledo	100%	244
Upper Valley Medical Center	Troy	100%	221
Adena Regional Medical Center	Chillicothe	99%	344
Akron General Medical Center[2]	Akron	99%	302
Ashtabula County Medical Center	Ashtabula	99%	187
Barnesville Hospital Association	Barnesville	99%	90
Chillicothe VA Medical Center	Chillicothe	99%	105
CMH Regional Health System	Wilmington	99%	160
Fisher Titus Memorial Hospital	Norwalk	99%	109
Hillcrest Hospital	Mayfield Heights	99%	598
Joint Township District Memorial Hospital	Saint Marys	99%	121
Lakewood Hospital	Lakewood	99%	306
Licking Memorial Hospital	Newark	99%	239
Lutheran Hospital	Cleveland	99%	108
Marion General Hospital	Marion	99%	339
Marymount Hospital	Garfield Heights	99%	623
McCullough-Hyde Memorial Hospital	Oxford	99%	113
Medina Hospital	Medina	99%	225
Mercy Hospital Fairfield	Fairfield	99%	411
Mercy St Anne Hospital	Toledo	99%	195
Mercy Tiffin Hospital	Tiffin	99%	103
Northside Medical Center	Youngstown	99%	293
Parma Community General Hospital	Parma	99%	625
Robinson Memorial Hospital	Ravenna	99%	336
Saint Elizabeth Boardman Health Center[2]	Youngstown	99%	224
Saint Luke's Hospital	Maumee	99%	317
Saint Rita's Medical Center	Lima	99%	343
Salem Community Hospital	Salem	99%	165
Samaritan Hospital - Peoples Hospital	Ashland	99%	85
Springfield Regional Medical Center	Springfield	99%	470
Summa Wadsworth-Rittman Hospital	Wadsworth	99%	87
Trinity Medical Center East & West	Steubenville	99%	579
University Hospital[2]	Cincinnati	99%	559
West Chester Medical Center	West Chester	99%	102
Alliance Community Hospital	Alliance	98%	132
Belmont Community Hospital	Bellaire	98%	48
Dublin Methodist Hospital	Dublin	98%	46
Emh Regional Medical Center[2]	Elyria	98%	287
Firelands Regional Medical Center	Sandusky	98%	255
Grady Memorial Hospital	Delaware	98%	115
Joel Pomerene Memorial Hospital	Millersburg	98%	52
Knox Community Hospital	Mount Vernon	98%	184
Lake Health[2]	Concord	98%	511
Medcentral Health System[2]	Mansfield	98%	330
Mercy Franciscan Hospital Western Hills	Cincinnati	98%	212
Mercy Hospital Anderson	Cincinnati	98%	328
Summa Health Systems Hospitals[2]	Akron	98%	308
The Toledo Hospital[2]	Toledo	98%	286
Van Wert County Hospital	Van Wert	98%	53
Flower Hospital	Sylvania	97%	210
Holzer Medical Center	Gallipolis	97%	309
Coshocton County Memorial Hospital	Coshocton	96%	48
Mary Rutan Hospital	Bellefontaine	96%	70
Wyandot Memorial Hospital	Upper Sandusky	96%	26
Bellevue Hospital	Bellevue	95%	39
East Liverpool City Hospital	East Liverpool	95%	193
Memorial Hospital	Fremont	95%	44
Southeastern Ohio Regional Medical Center	Cambridge	95%	128
Wilson Memorial Hospital	Sidney	95%	73
Summa Western Reserve Hospital	Cuyahoga Falls	94%	95
Fairview Hospital	Cleveland	93%	805
Fayette County Memorial Hospital	Washington CH	93%	45
Henry County Hospital	Napoleon	92%	39
Wooster Community Hospital	Wooster	92%	104
Wood County Hospital	Bowling Green	90%	73
Morrow County Hospital[2]	Mount Gilead	89%	37
Deaconess Hospital	Cincinnati	87%	39
Wayne Hospital	Greenville	86%	120
Madison County Hospital	London	85%	67
Fulton County Health Center	Wauseon	81%	37
Highland District Hospital	Hillsboro	81%	70
Holzer Medical Center Jackson	Jackson	81%	108
Selby General Hospital	Marietta	75%	32
Pike Community Hospital	Waverly	44%	39

15. Smoking Cessation Advice

Hospital Name	City	Rate	Cases
Ashtabula County Medical Center	Ashtabula	100%	32
Atrium Medical Center	Franklin	100%	86
Aultman Hospital	Canton	100%	99
Bethesda North Hospital	Cincinnati	100%	101
Christ Hospital	Cincinnati	100%	194
Cincinnati VA Medical Center	Cincinnati	100%	64
Cleveland Clinic	Cleveland	100%	220
Cleveland-Wade Park VA Medical Center	Cleveland	100%	95
CMH Regional Health System	Wilmington	100%	25
Community Regional Medical Center	Lorain	100%	62
Doctors Hospital	Columbus	100%	44
Euclid Hospital	Euclid	100%	84
Fairfield Medical Center	Lancaster	100%	73
Fairview Hospital	Cleveland	100%	109
Fort Hamilton Hughes Memorial Hospital	Hamilton	100%	54
Genesis Healthcare System	Zanesville	100%	64
Good Samaritan Hospital	Cincinnati	100%	127
Good Samaritan Hospital[2]	Dayton	100%	54
Grandview Hospital & Medical Center	Dayton	100%	74
Grant Medical Center[2]	Columbus	100%	76
Greene Memorial Hospital	Xenia	100%	25
Hillcrest Hospital	Mayfield Heights	100%	51
Huron Hospital	Cleveland	100%	76
Jewish Hospital	Cincinnati	100%	65
Kettering Medical Center	Kettering	100%	61
Lakewood Hospital	Lakewood	100%	68
Licking Memorial Hospital	Newark	100%	58
Lima Memorial Health System	Lima	100%	26
Marietta Memorial Hospital	Marietta	100%	45
Marion General Hospital	Marion	100%	59
Mercy Franciscan Hospital - Mt Airy	Cincinnati	100%	44
Mercy Hospital Clermont	Batavia	100%	25
Mercy Hospital Fairfield	Fairfield	100%	68
Mercy St Charles Hospital	Oregon	100%	41
Mercy St Vincent Medical Center	Toledo	100%	190
Miami Valley Hospital[2]	Dayton	100%	84
Mount Carmel Health	Columbus	100%	194
Mount Carmel St Ann's Hospital	Westerville	100%	44
Northside Medical Center	Youngstown	100%	51
Ohio State University Hospitals[2]	Columbus	100%	76
Riverside Methodist Hospital[2]	Columbus	100%	100
Robinson Memorial Hospital	Ravenna	100%	52
Saint Elizabeth Boardman Health Center[2]	Youngstown	100%	25
Saint Elizabeth Health Center[2]	Youngstown	100%	55
Saint Joseph Health Center[2]	Warren	100%	61
Saint Rita's Medical Center	Lima	100%	62
South Pointe Hospital	Warrensville Hgts	100%	98
Southeastern Ohio Regional Medical Center	Cambridge	100%	26
Southern Ohio Medical Center	Portsmouth	100%	71
Summa Barberton Hospital	Barberton	100%	64
Summa Health Systems Hospitals[2]	Akron	100%	70
The Toledo Hospital[2]	Toledo	100%	44
Trinity Medical Center East & West	Steubenville	100%	85
Trumbull Memorial Hospital	Warren	100%	84
UHHS Bedford Medical Center	Bedford	100%	39
UHHS Richmond Heights Hospital	Richmond Hghts	100%	26
Union Hospital	Dover	100%	38
University Hospitals of Cleveland	Cleveland	100%	143
University of Toledo Medical Center[2]	Toledo	100%	43
Lake Health[2]	Concord	99%	82
Saint Vincent Charity Medical Center[2]	Cleveland	99%	86
Springfield Regional Medical Center	Springfield	99%	88

NOTE: Hospital profiles are in alphabetical order by state, then city, then hospital within the city; Rankings exclude hospitals with less than 25 cases except for patient surveys which excludes hospitals with less than 100 cases; (a) 100–299 cases; (1) The number of cases is too small to be sure how well a hospital is performing; (2) The hospital indicated that the data submitted for this measure were based on a sample of cases; (3) Data was collected during a shorter time period (fewer quarters) than the maximum possible time for this measure; (4) Suppressed for one or more quarters by CMS; (5) No data is available from the hospital for this measure; (6) Fewer than 100 patients completed the HCAHPS survey. Use these rates with caution, as the number of surveys may be too low to reliably assess hospital performance; (7) Survey results are based on less than 12 months of data; (8) Survey results are not available for this reporting period; (9) No or very few patients were eligible for the HCAHPS survey. The scores shown, if any, reflect a very small number of surveys; (10) A state average was not calculated because too few hospitals in the state submitted data; (11) There were discrepancies in the data collection process; Please refer to the User's Guide for a full explanation of data.

University Hospital[2]	Cincinnati	99%	202
Adena Regional Medical Center	Chillicothe	98%	62
Firelands Regional Medical Center	Sandusky	98%	42
Medcentral Health System[2]	Mansfield	98%	60
Mercy St Anne Hospital	Toledo	98%	43
Metro Health Medical Center	Cleveland	98%	225
Marymount Hospital	Garfield Heights	97%	98
Mercy Franciscan Hospital Western Hills	Cincinnati	97%	35
Mercy Hospital Anderson	Cincinnati	97%	30
Mercy Medical Center	Canton	97%	76
Akron General Medical Center[2]	Akron	96%	46
Emh Regional Medical Center[2]	Elyria	96%	49
Southwest General Health Center	Middleburg Hgts	96%	52
Dayton VA Medical Center	Dayton	94%	49
Saint Luke's Hospital	Maumee	94%	32
Holzer Medical Center	Gallipolis	93%	43
Chillicothe VA Medical Center	Chillicothe	92%	38
Parma Community General Hospital	Parma	91%	46
East Liverpool City Hospital	East Liverpool	90%	41
Alliance Community Hospital	Alliance	89%	27

Pneumonia Care

16. Appropriate Initial Antibiotic

Hospital Name	City	Rate	Cases
Bucyrus Community Hospital	Bucyrus	100%	31
Christ Hospital[2]	Cincinnati	100%	40
Cincinnati VA Medical Center	Cincinnati	100%	57
Doctors Hospital of Nelsonville	Nelsonville	100%	26
Fulton County Health Center	Wauseon	100%	40
Joel Pomerene Memorial Hospital	Millersburg	100%	29
Joint Township District Memorial Hospital	Saint Marys	100%	73
Mercy Memorial Hospital	Urbana	100%	57
Euclid Hospital	Euclid	99%	73
Good Samaritan Hospital[2]	Dayton	99%	78
Kettering Medical Center - Sycamore	Miamisburg	99%	114
Brown County Hospital[2]	Georgetown	98%	44
Good Samaritan Hospital	Cincinnati	98%	218
Grandview Hospital & Medical Center	Dayton	98%	165
Grant Medical Center[2]	Columbus	98%	91
Jewish Hospital[2]	Cincinnati	98%	63
Mercy Franciscan Hospital - Mt Airy	Cincinnati	98%	144
Mercy Hospital of Defiance	Defiance	98%	64
Saint Rita's Medical Center	Lima	98%	157
UHHS Bedford Medical Center	Bedford	98%	52
Affinity Medical Center	Massillon	97%	119
Doctors Hospital	Columbus	97%	182
Fostoria Community Hospital	Fostoria	97%	38
Genesis Healthcare System	Zanesville	97%	261
Huron Hospital	Cleveland	97%	39
Kettering Medical Center	Kettering	97%	189
Marion General Hospital	Marion	97%	156
Saint Elizabeth Health Center[2]	Youngstown	97%	58
Summa Barberton Hospital	Barberton	97%	120
Adena Regional Medical Center	Chillicothe	96%	162
Defiance Regional Medical Center	Defiance	96%	52
Fort Hamilton Hughes Memorial Hospital[2]	Hamilton	96%	73
Lutheran Hospital	Cleveland	96%	83
Mercy Hospital Anderson	Cincinnati	96%	216
Morrow County Hospital	Mount Gilead	96%	54
Mount Carmel St Ann's Hospital[2]	Westerville	96%	173
Ohio State University Hospitals[2]	Columbus	96%	51
Saint John Medical Center[2]	Westlake	96%	98
UHHS Richmond Heights Hospital	Richmond Hghts	96%	46
Aultman Hospital	Canton	95%	370
Berger Hospital	Circleville	95%	74
Cleveland-Wade Park VA Medical Center	Cleveland	95%	56
Dublin Methodist Hospital	Dublin	95%	87
Fisher Titus Memorial Hospital	Norwalk	95%	110
Mercy Franciscan Hospital Western Hills	Cincinnati	95%	188
Mercy St Anne Hospital	Toledo	95%	107
Metro Health Medical Center	Cleveland	95%	113
Mount Carmel Health[2]	Columbus	95%	240
Riverside Methodist Hospital[2]	Columbus	95%	212
Robinson Memorial Hospital[2]	Ravenna	95%	134
South Pointe Hospital	Warrensville Hgts	95%	118
Springfield Regional Medical Center	Springfield	95%	304
Union Hospital	Dover	95%	184
University Hospitals of Cleveland	Cleveland	95%	135
Akron General Medical Center[2]	Akron	94%	69
Bethesda North Hospital	Cincinnati	94%	363
Community Regional Medical Center	Lorain	94%	221
Fairview Hospital	Cleveland	94%	250
Hillcrest Hospital	Mayfield Heights	94%	204
Knox Community Hospital	Mount Vernon	94%	107
Marymount Hospital	Garfield Heights	94%	140
Mercy Tiffin Hospital	Tiffin	94%	62
Saint Joseph Health Center[2]	Warren	94%	90
Saint Luke's Hospital	Maumee	94%	137
Summa Health Systems Hospitals[2]	Akron	94%	71
Summa Western Reserve Hospital	Cuyahoga Falls	94%	111
UHHS Memorial Hospital of Geneva	Geneva	94%	49
Upper Valley Medical Center	Troy	94%	188
Alliance Community Hospital	Alliance	93%	92
Ashtabula County Medical Center	Ashtabula	93%	87
Atrium Medical Center	Franklin	93%	182
Bay Park Community Hospital	Oregon	93%	94
Flower Hospital	Sylvania	93%	120
Greene Memorial Hospital	Xenia	93%	151
Hardin Memorial Hospital	Kenton	93%	41
Lima Memorial Health System	Lima	93%	120
Madison County Hospital	London	93%	60
Mercer County Joint Twp Comm Hosp	Coldwater	93%	67
Mercy Hospital Clermont	Batavia	93%	151
Saint Elizabeth Boardman Health Center[2]	Youngstown	93%	76
Salem Community Hospital	Salem	93%	123
Samaritan Hospital - Peoples Hospital	Ashland	93%	70
Summa Wadsworth-Rittman Hospital	Wadsworth	93%	103
Trinity Medical Center East & West	Steubenville	93%	212
Univ Hosps Conneaut Med Ctr	Conneaut	93%	28
Chillicothe VA Medical Center	Chillicothe	92%	59
Cleveland Clinic[2]	Cleveland	92%	71
Fayette County Memorial Hospital	Washington CH	92%	37
Marietta Memorial Hospital[2]	Marietta	92%	40
Mercy Hospital Fairfield	Fairfield	92%	237
Mercy St Vincent Medical Center	Toledo	92%	97
Saint Vincent Charity Medical Center[2]	Cleveland	92%	53
Southwest General Health Center	Middleburg Hgts	92%	255
University Hospital[2]	Cincinnati	92%	49
Van Wert County Hospital	Van Wert	92%	65
Adams County Regional Medical Center	Seaman	91%	58
Allen Community Hospital	Oberlin	91%	35
Community Hospitals and Wellness Centers	Bryan	91%	68
Dayton VA Medical Center	Dayton	91%	79
Medcentral Health System[2]	Mansfield	91%	195
Firelands Regional Medical Center	Sandusky	90%	99
Mary Rutan Hospital	Bellefontaine	90%	78
Mercy St Charles Hospital	Oregon	90%	112
Wooster Community Hospital	Wooster	90%	120
Blanchard Valley Hospital	Findlay	89%	95
Emh Regional Medical Center[2]	Elyria	89%	79
Lakewood Hospital	Lakewood	89%	89
McCullough-Hyde Memorial Hospital	Oxford	89%	84
Memorial Hospital of Union County	Marysville	89%	64
Mercy Medical Center	Canton	89%	243
Southeastern Ohio Regional Medical Center[2]	Cambridge	89%	112
Trumbull Memorial Hospital[2]	Warren	89%	232
Barnesville Hospital Association	Barnesville	88%	91
Fairfield Medical Center	Lancaster	88%	140
Grady Memorial Hospital	Delaware	88%	77
Lake Health[2]	Concord	88%	284
CMH Regional Health System	Wilmington	87%	82
East Ohio Regional Hospital	Martins Ferry	87%	110
Miami Valley Hospital[2]	Dayton	87%	104
Parma Community General Hospital	Parma	87%	276
Southern Ohio Medical Center	Portsmouth	87%	252
Northside Medical Center	Youngstown	86%	100
The Toledo Hospital[2]	Toledo	86%	65
UH Geauga Medical Center	Chardon	86%	113
West Chester Medical Center	West Chester	86%	77
Holzer Medical Center[2]	Gallipolis	85%	115
Holzer Medical Center Jackson	Jackson	85%	108
Licking Memorial Hospital[2]	Newark	85%	166
Pike Community Hospital	Waverly	85%	40
Medina Hospital	Medina	84%	176
Hocking Valley Community Hospital	Logan	83%	58
Memorial Hospital	Fremont	82%	40
Wilson Memorial Hospital	Sidney	82%	78
H B Magruder Memorial Hospital	Port Clinton	81%	26
Medical Center of Newark	Newark	81%	26
O'Bleness Memorial Hospital	Athens	81%	67
Wayne Hospital	Greenville	81%	62
Highland District Hospital	Hillsboro	80%	90
Bellevue Hospital	Bellevue	77%	69
Amherst Hospital	Amherst	76%	25
Belmont Community Hospital	Bellaire	75%	32
University of Toledo Medical Center[2]	Toledo	75%	53
Coshocton County Memorial Hospital	Coshocton	73%	30
East Liverpool City Hospital[2]	East Liverpool	72%	114
Wood County Hospital	Bowling Green	67%	114

17. Blood Culture Timing

Hospital Name	City	Rate	Cases
Allen Community Hospital	Oberlin	100%	35
Bucyrus Community Hospital	Bucyrus	100%	49
Community Hospitals and Wellness Centers	Bryan	100%	61
Fostoria Community Hospital	Fostoria	100%	36
Joel Pomerene Memorial Hospital	Millersburg	100%	78
Kettering Medical Center	Kettering	100%	320
Marietta Memorial Hospital[2]	Marietta	100%	81
Saint Elizabeth Boardman Health Center[2]	Youngstown	100%	98
Summa Barberton Hospital	Barberton	100%	239
Univ Hosps Conneaut Med Ctr	Conneaut	100%	31
Akron General Medical Center[2]	Akron	99%	81
Bellevue Hospital	Bellevue	99%	73
Cincinnati VA Medical Center	Cincinnati	99%	97
Emh Regional Medical Center[2]	Elyria	99%	70
Fairview Hospital	Cleveland	99%	339
Good Samaritan Hospital	Cincinnati	99%	407
Grandview Hospital & Medical Center	Dayton	99%	280
Grant Medical Center[2]	Columbus	99%	105
Jewish Hospital[2]	Cincinnati	99%	123
Kettering Medical Center - Sycamore	Miamisburg	99%	171
Lima Memorial Health System	Lima	99%	160
Mercy Franciscan Hospital - Mt Airy	Cincinnati	99%	234
Mercy Franciscan Hospital Western Hills	Cincinnati	99%	272
Mercy Hospital Clermont	Batavia	99%	230
Mercy Hospital Fairfield	Fairfield	99%	388
Mercy Hospital of Defiance	Defiance	99%	83
Mercy Memorial Hospital	Urbana	99%	83
Mercy St Charles Hospital	Oregon	99%	174
Mercy Tiffin Hospital	Tiffin	99%	82
Parma Community General Hospital	Parma	99%	409
Riverside Methodist Hospital[2]	Columbus	99%	322
Saint Joseph Health Center[2]	Warren	99%	80
Saint Luke's Hospital	Maumee	99%	160
South Pointe Hospital	Warrensville Hgts	99%	137
Southeastern Ohio Regional Medical Center[2]	Cambridge	99%	144
Trumbull Memorial Hospital[2]	Warren	99%	236
UHHS Memorial Hospital of Geneva	Geneva	99%	90
Wilson Memorial Hospital	Sidney	99%	124
Barnesville Hospital Association	Barnesville	98%	53
Bay Park Community Hospital	Oregon	98%	121
Bethesda North Hospital	Cincinnati	98%	643
Blanchard Valley Hospital	Findlay	98%	120
Cleveland-Wade Park VA Medical Center	Cleveland	98%	91
Community Regional Medical Center	Lorain	98%	386
Dayton VA Medical Center	Dayton	98%	113
Dublin Methodist Hospital	Dublin	98%	109
Greene Memorial Hospital	Xenia	98%	239
Hillcrest Hospital	Mayfield Heights	98%	248
Licking Memorial Hospital[2]	Newark	98%	207
Madison County Hospital	London	98%	43
Marion General Hospital	Marion	98%	200
Mercy Medical Center	Canton	98%	305
Mercy St Anne Hospital	Toledo	98%	166
Saint Elizabeth Health Center[2]	Youngstown	98%	52
Springfield Regional Medical Center	Springfield	98%	455
Summa Wadsworth-Rittman Hospital	Wadsworth	98%	136
UHHS Bedford Medical Center	Bedford	98%	107
University Hospital[2]	Cincinnati	98%	123
Wooster Community Hospital	Wooster	98%	169
Atrium Medical Center	Franklin	97%	286
Aultman Hospital	Canton	97%	632
CMH Regional Health System	Wilmington	97%	130
Defiance Regional Medical Center	Defiance	97%	68
Doctors Hospital	Columbus	97%	183
Euclid Hospital	Euclid	97%	132
Firelands Regional Medical Center	Sandusky	97%	152
Fisher Titus Memorial Hospital	Norwalk	97%	167
Flower Hospital	Sylvania	97%	199
Fort Hamilton Hughes Memorial Hospital[2]	Hamilton	97%	113
Grady Memorial Hospital	Delaware	97%	68
Lakewood Hospital	Lakewood	97%	164
Lutheran Hospital	Cleveland	97%	123
Marymount Hospital	Garfield Heights	97%	293
Medina Hospital	Medina	97%	228
Memorial Hospital of Union County	Marysville	97%	75
Mercy Hospital Anderson	Cincinnati	97%	327
Mount Carmel St Ann's Hospital[2]	Westerville	97%	243
Southwest General Health Center	Middleburg Hgts	97%	456
Trinity Medical Center East & West	Steubenville	97%	309
UHHS Richmond Heights Hospital	Richmond Hghts	97%	73
Union Hospital	Dover	97%	231
West Chester Medical Center	West Chester	97%	128
Adams County Regional Medical Center	Seaman	96%	74
Ashtabula County Medical Center	Ashtabula	96%	164
Belmont Community Hospital	Bellaire	96%	27
Cleveland Clinic[2]	Cleveland	96%	106
Joint Township District Memorial Hospital	Saint Marys	96%	67
McCullough-Hyde Memorial Hospital	Oxford	96%	98
Morrow County Hospital	Mount Gilead	96%	75
Mount Carmel Health[2]	Columbus	96%	383
Saint John Medical Center[2]	Westlake	96%	137
Saint Rita's Medical Center	Lima	96%	321
Salem Community Hospital	Salem	96%	147
The Toledo Hospital[2]	Toledo	96%	106
University Hospitals of Cleveland	Cleveland	96%	246
Upper Valley Medical Center	Troy	96%	301
Berger Hospital	Circleville	95%	130
Fairfield Medical Center	Lancaster	95%	289

NOTE: Hospital profiles are in alphabetical order by state, then city, then hospital within the city; Rankings exclude hospitals with less than 25 cases except for patient surveys which excludes hospitals with less than 100 cases; (a) 100–299 cases; (1) The number of cases is too small to be sure how well a hospital is performing; (2) The hospital indicated that the data submitted for this measure were based on a sample of cases; (3) Data was collected during a shorter time period (fewer quarters) than the maximum possible time for this measure; (4) Suppressed for one or more quarters by CMS; (5) No data is available from the hospital for this measure; (6) Fewer than 100 patients completed the HCAHPS survey. Use these rates with caution, as the number of surveys may be too low to reliably assess hospital performance; (7) Survey results are based on less than 12 months of data; (8) Survey results are not available for this reporting period; (9) No or very few patients were eligible for the HCAHPS survey. The scores shown, if any, reflect a very small number of surveys; (10) A state average was not calculated because too few hospitals in the state submitted data; (11) There were discrepancies in the data collection process; Please refer to the User's Guide for a full explanation of data.

Genesis Healthcare System	Zanesville	95%	392
Mary Rutan Hospital	Bellefontaine	95%	79
Mercy St Vincent Medical Center	Toledo	95%	212
Pike Community Hospital	Waverly	95%	58
Saint Vincent Charity Medical Center[2]	Cleveland	95%	83
Summa Western Reserve Hospital	Cuyahoga Falls	95%	128
Brown County Hospital[2]	Georgetown	94%	112
Christ Hospital[2]	Cincinnati	94%	84
Medcentral Health System[2]	Mansfield	94%	328
Mercer County Joint Twp Comm Hosp	Coldwater	94%	78
Miami Valley Hospital[2]	Dayton	94%	174
Ohio State University Hospitals[2]	Columbus	94%	95
University of Toledo Medical Center[2]	Toledo	94%	83
Adena Regional Medical Center	Chillicothe	93%	120
Affinity Medical Center	Massillon	93%	198
Hardin Memorial Hospital	Kenton	93%	41
Holzer Medical Center Jackson	Jackson	93%	117
Huron Hospital	Cleveland	93%	83
Memorial Hospital	Fremont	93%	73
Southern Ohio Medical Center	Portsmouth	93%	293
Coshocton County Memorial Hospital	Coshocton	92%	37
East Ohio Regional Hospital	Martins Ferry	92%	149
H B Magruder Memorial Hospital	Port Clinton	92%	40
Northside Medical Center	Youngstown	92%	189
Summa Health Systems Hospitals[2]	Akron	92%	106
UH Geauga Medical Center	Chardon	92%	153
Lake Health[2]	Concord	91%	333
Samaritan Hospital - Peoples Hospital	Ashland	91%	90
Wayne Hospital	Greenville	91%	97
Alliance Community Hospital	Alliance	90%	156
Holzer Medical Center[2]	Gallipolis	90%	115
Robinson Memorial Hospital[2]	Ravenna	89%	157
Van Wert County Hospital	Van Wert	89%	54
Wood County Hospital	Bowling Green	89%	105
East Liverpool City Hospital[2]	East Liverpool	88%	103
Fayette County Memorial Hospital	Washington CH	88%	59
O'Bleness Memorial Hospital	Athens	88%	120
Metro Health Medical Center	Cleveland	86%	97
Fulton County Health Center	Wauseon	85%	39
Good Samaritan Hospital[2]	Dayton	85%	131
Hocking Valley Community Hospital	Logan	84%	43
Knox Community Hospital	Mount Vernon	84%	153
Highland District Hospital	Hillsboro	83%	98

18. Influenza Vaccine

Hospital Name	City	Rate	Cases
Cleveland Clinic[2]	Cleveland	100%	189
Jewish Hospital[2]	Cincinnati	100%	84
Joel Pomerene Memorial Hospital	Millersburg	100%	41
Lutheran Hospital	Cleveland	100%	83
Mary Rutan Hospital	Bellefontaine	100%	65
Mercy Hospital of Defiance	Defiance	100%	46
Mercy Memorial Hospital	Urbana	100%	48
Robinson Memorial Hospital[2]	Ravenna	100%	77
Saint Elizabeth Boardman Health Center[2]	Youngstown	100%	82
Saint Rita's Medical Center	Lima	100%	133
Summa Barberton Hospital	Barberton	100%	174
UH Geauga Medical Center	Chardon	100%	121
Bay Park Community Hospital	Oregon	99%	91
Berger Hospital	Circleville	99%	84
Blanchard Valley Hospital	Findlay	99%	90
Firelands Regional Medical Center	Sandusky	99%	100
Fort Hamilton Hughes Memorial Hospital[2]	Hamilton	99%	97
Grandview Hospital & Medical Center	Dayton	99%	175
Kettering Medical Center - Sycamore	Miamisburg	99%	143
Marion General Hospital	Marion	99%	145
Mercy Hospital Fairfield	Fairfield	99%	210
Adams County Regional Medical Center	Seaman	98%	42
Adena Regional Medical Center	Chillicothe	98%	250
Ashtabula County Medical Center	Ashtabula	98%	80
Atrium Medical Center	Franklin	98%	201
Christ Hospital[2]	Cincinnati	98%	87
Defiance Regional Medical Center	Defiance	98%	53
Grady Memorial Hospital	Delaware	98%	62
Lima Memorial Health System	Lima	98%	132
Marietta Memorial Hospital[2]	Marietta	98%	58
Mercer County Joint Twp Comm Hosp	Coldwater	98%	54
Mercy Franciscan Hospital - Mt Airy	Cincinnati	98%	132
Mercy Hospital Clermont	Batavia	98%	185
Mercy St Charles Hospital	Oregon	98%	120
Samaritan Hospital - Peoples Hospital	Ashland	98%	51
Southeastern Ohio Regional Medical Center[2]	Cambridge	98%	91
Springfield Regional Medical Center	Springfield	98%	277
Union Hospital	Dover	98%	220
Wooster Community Hospital	Wooster	98%	154
Greene Memorial Hospital	Xenia	97%	167
H B Magruder Memorial Hospital	Port Clinton	97%	30
Lake Health	Concord	97%	273
Lakewood Hospital	Lakewood	97%	88
Northside Medical Center	Youngstown	97%	130
South Pointe Hospital	Warrensville Hgts	97%	146
Bucyrus Community Hospital	Bucyrus	96%	28
CMH Regional Health System	Wilmington	96%	95
Community Regional Medical Center	Lorain	96%	225
Grant Medical Center[2]	Columbus	96%	68
Hillcrest Hospital	Mayfield Heights	96%	208
Kettering Medical Center	Kettering	96%	231
Memorial Hospital of Union County	Marysville	96%	51
Mercy Hospital Anderson	Cincinnati	96%	228
Mercy St Anne Hospital	Toledo	96%	80
Mercy St Vincent Medical Center	Toledo	96%	160
Summa Wadsworth-Rittman Hospital	Wadsworth	96%	70
Wayne Hospital	Greenville	96%	67
Affinity Medical Center	Massillon	95%	136
Dayton VA Medical Center	Dayton	95%	92
Licking Memorial Hospital[2]	Newark	95%	174
Mercy Franciscan Hospital Western Hills	Cincinnati	95%	166
Mercy Medical Center	Canton	95%	231
Saint John Medical Center[2]	Westlake	95%	62
Saint Joseph Health Center[2]	Warren	95%	83
Trumbull Memorial Hospital[2]	Warren	95%	196
UHHS Richmond Heights Hospital	Richmond Hghts	95%	60
Alliance Community Hospital	Alliance	94%	126
Aultman Hospital	Canton	94%	499
Brown County Hospital[2]	Georgetown	94%	65
Chillicothe VA Medical Center	Chillicothe	94%	54
Community Hospitals and Wellness Centers	Bryan	94%	66
Good Samaritan Hospital	Cincinnati	94%	277
Mercy Tiffin Hospital	Tiffin	94%	65
Saint Luke's Hospital	Maumee	94%	128
Southern Ohio Medical Center	Portsmouth	94%	103
Summa Western Reserve Hospital	Cuyahoga Falls	94%	93
Wilson Memorial Hospital	Sidney	94%	79
Bethesda North Hospital	Cincinnati	93%	469
Euclid Hospital	Euclid	93%	76
Fairfield Medical Center	Lancaster	93%	259
Good Samaritan Hospital[2]	Dayton	93%	59
Hocking Valley Community Hospital	Logan	93%	28
Marymount Hospital	Garfield Heights	93%	249
Riverside Methodist Hospital[2]	Columbus	93%	181
UHHS Memorial Hospital of Geneva	Geneva	93%	41
West Chester Medical Center	West Chester	93%	60
Flower Hospital	Sylvania	92%	146
Medcentral Health System	Mansfield	92%	284
Salem Community Hospital	Salem	92%	119
Cincinnati VA Medical Center	Cincinnati	91%	81
Fairview Hospital	Cleveland	91%	207
Fulton County Health Center	Wauseon	91%	34
McCullough-Hyde Memorial Hospital	Oxford	91%	69
Medina Hospital	Medina	91%	173
Saint Vincent Charity Medical Center[2]	Cleveland	91%	65
Upper Valley Medical Center	Troy	91%	141
Doctors Hospital	Columbus	90%	176
Fisher Titus Memorial Hospital	Norwalk	90%	101
Ohio State University Hospitals[2]	Columbus	90%	42
The Toledo Hospital[2]	Toledo	90%	73
Trinity Medical Center East & West	Steubenville	90%	208
Cleveland-Wade Park VA Medical Center	Cleveland	89%	118
Dublin Methodist Hospital	Dublin	89%	56
Barnesville Hospital Association	Barnesville	88%	59
Bellevue Hospital	Bellevue	88%	51
Fostoria Community Hospital	Fostoria	88%	25
Joint Township District Memorial Hospital	Saint Marys	88%	51
Madison County Hospital	London	88%	43
Van Wert County Hospital	Van Wert	88%	32
Coshocton County Memorial Hospital	Coshocton	87%	31
Genesis Healthcare System	Zanesville	87%	282
Parma Community General Hospital	Parma	87%	334
UHHS Bedford Medical Center	Bedford	87%	76
Holzer Medical Center[2]	Gallipolis	86%	91
Holzer Medical Center Jackson	Jackson	86%	49
Miami Valley Hospital[2]	Dayton	86%	102
Saint Elizabeth Health Center[2]	Youngstown	86%	78
Wood County Hospital	Bowling Green	86%	63
Akron General Medical Center[2]	Akron	85%	92
Huron Hospital	Cleveland	85%	55
Mount Carmel Health[2]	Columbus	85%	218
O'Bleness Memorial Hospital	Athens	85%	65
Knox Community Hospital	Mount Vernon	84%	87
Highland District Hospital	Hillsboro	83%	60
Southwest General Health Center	Middleburg Hgts	83%	236
University Hospital[2]	Cincinnati	82%	72
University Hospitals of Cleveland	Cleveland	82%	193
University of Toledo Medical Center[2]	Toledo	82%	78
Mount Carmel St Ann's Hospital[2]	Westerville	81%	111
Summa Health Systems Hospitals[2]	Akron	81%	107
Belmont Community Hospital	Bellaire	79%	34
Memorial Hospital	Fremont	78%	46
Morrow County Hospital	Mount Gilead	66%	41
East Liverpool City Hospital[2]	East Liverpool	65%	78
East Ohio Regional Hospital	Martins Ferry	64%	78
Metro Health Medical Center	Cleveland	59%	186
Emh Regional Medical Center[2]	Elyria	58%	100

19. Initial Antibiotic Timing

Hospital Name	City	Rate	Cases
Allen Community Hospital	Oberlin	100%	42
Berger Hospital	Circleville	100%	117
Bucyrus Community Hospital	Bucyrus	100%	42
Defiance Regional Medical Center	Defiance	100%	75
Doctors Hospital of Nelsonville	Nelsonville	100%	28
Dublin Methodist Hospital	Dublin	100%	110
Fostoria Community Hospital	Fostoria	100%	46
Grady Memorial Hospital	Delaware	100%	104
H B Magruder Memorial Hospital	Port Clinton	100%	39
Joel Pomerene Memorial Hospital	Millersburg	100%	64
Joint Township District Memorial Hospital	Saint Marys	100%	84
Kettering Medical Center - Sycamore	Miamisburg	100%	165
Mercer County Joint Twp Comm Hosp	Coldwater	100%	80
Mercy Tiffin Hospital	Tiffin	100%	84
Summa Western Reserve Hospital	Cuyahoga Falls	100%	149
UHHS Memorial Hospital of Geneva	Geneva	100%	69
Univ Hosps Conneaut Med Ctr	Conneaut	100%	30
Bay Park Community Hospital	Oregon	99%	138
Brown County Hospital[2]	Georgetown	99%	107
Cincinnati VA Medical Center	Cincinnati	99%	96
Community Hospitals and Wellness Centers	Bryan	99%	83
Fisher Titus Memorial Hospital	Norwalk	99%	158
Greene Memorial Hospital	Xenia	99%	173
Kettering Medical Center	Kettering	99%	287
Marion General Hospital	Marion	99%	220
Mercy Hospital of Defiance	Defiance	99%	84
Mercy Memorial Hospital	Urbana	99%	79
Mercy St Anne Hospital	Toledo	99%	140
Morrow County Hospital	Mount Gilead	99%	71
Summa Barberton Hospital	Barberton	99%	212
Upper Valley Medical Center	Troy	99%	263
Adams County Regional Medical Center	Seaman	98%	53
Alliance Community Hospital	Alliance	98%	144
Doctors Hospital	Columbus	98%	277
Euclid Hospital	Euclid	98%	144
Fairview Hospital	Cleveland	98%	322
Firelands Regional Medical Center	Sandusky	98%	166
Flower Hospital	Sylvania	98%	188
Fulton County Health Center	Wauseon	98%	51
Licking Memorial Hospital[2]	Newark	98%	229
McCullough-Hyde Memorial Hospital	Oxford	98%	101
Mercy Franciscan Hospital - Mt Airy	Cincinnati	98%	202
Mercy Hospital Clermont	Batavia	98%	257
Mercy Hospital Fairfield	Fairfield	98%	340
Saint John Medical Center[2]	Westlake	98%	142
Saint Rita's Medical Center	Lima	98%	217
South Pointe Hospital	Warrensville Hgts	98%	244
Summa Health Systems Hospitals[2]	Akron	98%	153
Trinity Medical Center East & West	Steubenville	98%	311
Union Hospital	Dover	98%	302
Van Wert County Hospital	Van Wert	98%	64
Wayne Hospital	Greenville	98%	91
Affinity Medical Center	Massillon	97%	197
Ashtabula County Medical Center	Ashtabula	97%	145
Atrium Medical Center	Franklin	97%	268
Barnesville Hospital Association	Barnesville	97%	100
Blanchard Valley Hospital	Findlay	97%	118
CMH Regional Health System	Wilmington	97%	121
Community Regional Medical Center	Lorain	97%	348
Good Samaritan Hospital[2]	Dayton	97%	123
Grandview Hospital & Medical Center	Dayton	97%	236
Grant Medical Center[2]	Columbus	97%	151
Henry County Hospital	Napoleon	97%	30
Knox Community Hospital	Mount Vernon	97%	114
Mary Rutan Hospital	Bellefontaine	97%	99
Mercy St Vincent Medical Center	Toledo	97%	183
Mount Carmel St Ann's Hospital[2]	Westerville	97%	231
Riverside Methodist Hospital[2]	Columbus	97%	288
Robinson Memorial Hospital[2]	Ravenna	97%	193
Saint Luke's Hospital	Maumee	97%	182
Summa Wadsworth-Rittman Hospital	Wadsworth	97%	118
Wilson Memorial Hospital	Sidney	97%	93
Wooster Community Hospital	Wooster	97%	212
Adena Regional Medical Center	Chillicothe	96%	249
Aultman Hospital	Canton	96%	609
Fayette County Memorial Hospital	Washington CH	96%	51
Genesis Healthcare System	Zanesville	96%	396
Good Samaritan Hospital	Cincinnati	96%	394
Hocking Valley Community Hospital	Logan	96%	52
Holzer Medical Center Jackson	Jackson	96%	113
Lima Memorial Health System	Lima	96%	140
Marymount Hospital	Garfield Heights	96%	280
Mercy Franciscan Hospital Western Hills	Cincinnati	96%	257
Miami Valley Hospital[2]	Dayton	96%	159
Saint Elizabeth Boardman Health Center[2]	Youngstown	96%	126

NOTE: Hospital profiles are in alphabetical order by state, then city, then hospital within the city; Rankings exclude hospitals with less than 25 cases except for patient surveys which excludes hospitals with less than 100 cases; (a) 100–299 cases; (1) The number of cases is too small to be sure how well a hospital is performing; (2) The hospital indicated that the data submitted for this measure were based on a sample of cases; (3) Data was collected during a shorter time period (fewer quarters) than the maximum possible time for this measure; (4) Suppressed for one or more quarters by CMS; (5) No data is available from the hospital for this measure; (6) Fewer than 100 patients completed the HCAHPS survey. Use these rates with caution, as the number of surveys may be too low to reliably assess hospital performance; (7) Survey results are based on less than 12 months of data; (8) Survey results are not available for this reporting period; (9) No or very few patients were eligible for the HCAHPS survey. The scores shown, if any, reflect a very small number of surveys; (10) A state average was not calculated because too few hospitals in the state submitted data; (11) There were discrepancies in the data collection process; Please refer to the User's Guide for a full explanation of data.

Saint Joseph Health Center[2]	Warren	96%	126
Southeastern Ohio Regional Medical Center[2]	Cambridge	96%	150
Southern Ohio Medical Center	Portsmouth	96%	311
Southwest General Health Center	Middleburg Hgts	96%	427
The Toledo Hospital[2]	Toledo	96%	103
UHHS Richmond Heights Hospital	Richmond Hghts	96%	89
University of Toledo Medical Center[2]	Toledo	96%	76
Belmont Community Hospital	Bellaire	95%	39
East Ohio Regional Hospital	Martins Ferry	95%	167
Fort Hamilton Hughes Memorial Hospital[2]	Hamilton	95%	126
Hardin Memorial Hospital	Kenton	95%	39
Holzer Medical Center[2]	Gallipolis	95%	136
Lakewood Hospital	Lakewood	95%	158
Lutheran Hospital	Cleveland	95%	152
Madison County Hospital	London	95%	62
Marietta Memorial Hospital[2]	Marietta	95%	110
Memorial Hospital of Union County	Marysville	95%	84
Mercy Hospital Anderson	Cincinnati	95%	381
Metro Health Medical Center	Cleveland	95%	241
Mount Carmel Health[2]	Columbus	95%	344
Ohio State University Hospitals[2]	Columbus	95%	97
Parma Community General Hospital	Parma	95%	438
Pike Community Hospital	Waverly	95%	61
Salem Community Hospital	Salem	95%	188
Samaritan Hospital - Peoples Hospital	Ashland	95%	87
Springfield Regional Medical Center	Springfield	95%	469
UHHS Bedford Medical Center	Bedford	95%	110
Bethesda North Hospital	Cincinnati	94%	564
Chillicothe VA Medical Center	Chillicothe	94%	54
Highland District Hospital	Hillsboro	94%	68
Hillcrest Hospital	Mayfield Heights	94%	316
Huron Hospital	Cleveland	94%	98
Jewish Hospital[2]	Cincinnati	94%	127
Mercy St Charles Hospital	Oregon	94%	180
West Chester Medical Center	West Chester	94%	85
Coshocton County Memorial Hospital	Coshocton	93%	42
Mercy Medical Center	Canton	93%	341
Northside Medical Center	Youngstown	93%	199
O'Bleness Memorial Hospital	Athens	93%	118
UH Geauga Medical Center	Chardon	93%	156
Christ Hospital[2]	Cincinnati	92%	74
Cleveland Clinic[2]	Cleveland	92%	142
East Liverpool City Hospital[2]	East Liverpool	92%	141
Fairfield Medical Center	Lancaster	92%	285
Lake Health[2]	Concord	92%	394
Medina Hospital	Medina	92%	238
Memorial Hospital	Fremont	92%	71
Bellevue Hospital	Bellevue	91%	74
Cleveland-Wade Park VA Medical Center	Cleveland	91%	93
Dayton VA Medical Center	Dayton	91%	119
Emh Regional Medical Center[2]	Elyria	91%	116
Medcentral Health System[2]	Mansfield	91%	371
Saint Elizabeth Health Center[2]	Youngstown	91%	90
Trumbull Memorial Hospital[2]	Warren	91%	280
Saint Vincent Charity Medical Center[2]	Cleveland	90%	99
Medical Center of Newark	Newark	89%	27
Deaconess Hospital[3]	Cincinnati	88%	33
University Hospitals of Cleveland	Cleveland	88%	284
Wood County Hospital	Bowling Green	88%	114
University Hospital[2]	Cincinnati	86%	115
Amherst Hospital	Amherst	82%	28
Akron General Medical Center[2]	Akron	76%	108

20. Pneumococcal Vaccine

Hospital Name	City	Rate	Cases
Adams County Regional Medical Center	Seaman	100%	48
Allen Community Hospital	Oberlin	100%	25
Bellevue Hospital	Bellevue	100%	71
Berger Hospital	Circleville	100%	98
Blanchard Valley Hospital	Findlay	100%	127
Bucyrus Community Hospital	Bucyrus	100%	30
Chillicothe VA Medical Center	Chillicothe	100%	39
Christ Hospital[2]	Cincinnati	100%	113
Fort Hamilton Hughes Memorial Hospital[2]	Hamilton	100%	134
Grandview Hospital & Medical Center	Dayton	100%	215
Grant Medical Center[2]	Columbus	100%	75
Lutheran Hospital	Cleveland	100%	82
Mercy Hospital Clermont	Batavia	100%	216
Mercy Hospital of Defiance	Defiance	100%	72
Summa Barberton Hospital	Barberton	100%	184
UH Geauga Medical Center	Chardon	100%	168
UHHS Memorial Hospital of Geneva	Geneva	100%	48
Cleveland-Wade Park VA Medical Center	Cleveland	99%	104
CMH Regional Health System	Wilmington	99%	115
Firelands Regional Medical Center	Sandusky	99%	135
Kettering Medical Center	Kettering	99%	260
Kettering Medical Center - Sycamore	Miamisburg	99%	173
Lakewood Hospital	Lakewood	99%	110
Marion General Hospital	Marion	99%	171
Mercy Franciscan Hospital - Mt Airy	Cincinnati	99%	179
Saint Elizabeth Boardman Health Center[2]	Youngstown	99%	126
Saint Rita's Medical Center	Lima	99%	229
Wooster Community Hospital	Wooster	99%	216
Atrium Medical Center	Franklin	98%	264
Bay Park Community Hospital	Oregon	98%	123
Cleveland Clinic[2]	Cleveland	98%	225
Dayton VA Medical Center	Dayton	98%	93
Defiance Regional Medical Center	Defiance	98%	62
Grady Memorial Hospital	Delaware	98%	85
Holzer Medical Center[2]	Gallipolis	98%	122
Joel Pomerene Memorial Hospital	Millersburg	98%	56
Licking Memorial Hospital[2]	Newark	98%	180
Lima Memorial Health System	Lima	98%	151
Mary Rutan Hospital	Bellefontaine	98%	90
Memorial Hospital of Union County	Marysville	98%	62
Mercy Hospital Anderson	Cincinnati	98%	325
Mercy Hospital Fairfield	Fairfield	98%	255
Mercy Memorial Hospital	Urbana	98%	59
Saint John Medical Center[2]	Westlake	98%	110
South Pointe Hospital	Warrensville Hgts	98%	200
Springfield Regional Medical Center	Springfield	98%	344
Summa Wadsworth-Rittman Hospital	Wadsworth	98%	87
Union Hospital	Dover	98%	303
Alliance Community Hospital	Alliance	97%	156
Aultman Hospital	Canton	97%	627
Brown County Hospital[2]	Georgetown	97%	93
Community Hospitals and Wellness Centers	Bryan	97%	69
Community Regional Medical Center	Lorain	97%	290
Doctors Hospital	Columbus	97%	177
Fisher Titus Memorial Hospital	Norwalk	97%	147
Fostoria Community Hospital	Fostoria	97%	35
Hocking Valley Community Hospital	Logan	97%	31
Huron Hospital	Cleveland	97%	72
Mercy St Anne Hospital	Toledo	97%	94
Northside Medical Center	Youngstown	97%	190
Robinson Memorial Hospital[2]	Ravenna	97%	151
Saint Elizabeth Health Center[2]	Youngstown	97%	94
Samaritan Hospital - Peoples Hospital	Ashland	97%	74
Southern Ohio Medical Center	Portsmouth	97%	262
Cincinnati VA Medical Center	Cincinnati	96%	79
Dublin Methodist Hospital	Dublin	96%	67
East Liverpool City Hospital[2]	East Liverpool	96%	90
Fairview Hospital	Cleveland	96%	296
Greene Memorial Hospital	Xenia	96%	208
Hardin Memorial Hospital	Kenton	96%	25
Medina Hospital	Medina	96%	222
Mercer County Joint Twp Comm Hosp	Coldwater	96%	74
Mercy Franciscan Hospital Western Hills	Cincinnati	96%	221
Mercy Medical Center	Canton	96%	264
Mercy St Vincent Medical Center	Toledo	96%	167
Parma Community General Hospital	Parma	96%	467
Saint Joseph Health Center[2]	Warren	96%	103
Southeastern Ohio Regional Medical Center[2]	Cambridge	96%	136
Trumbull Memorial Hospital[2]	Warren	96%	292
Wilson Memorial Hospital	Sidney	96%	108
Adena Regional Medical Center	Chillicothe	95%	318
Affinity Medical Center	Massillon	95%	180
Ashtabula County Medical Center	Ashtabula	95%	109
Fairfield Medical Center	Lancaster	95%	339
Jewish Hospital[2]	Cincinnati	95%	119
Joint Township District Memorial Hospital	Saint Marys	95%	84
Lake Health[2]	Concord	95%	388
Marietta Memorial Hospital[2]	Marietta	95%	100
Medcentral Health System[2]	Mansfield	95%	342
Mercy St Charles Hospital	Oregon	95%	154
Riverside Methodist Hospital[2]	Columbus	95%	307
Saint Luke's Hospital	Maumee	95%	155
UHHS Richmond Heights Hospital	Richmond Hghts	95%	79
Bethesda North Hospital	Cincinnati	94%	595
Coshocton County Memorial Hospital	Coshocton	94%	36
Flower Hospital	Sylvania	94%	181
Fulton County Health Center	Wauseon	94%	48
Good Samaritan Hospital	Cincinnati	94%	297
Marymount Hospital	Garfield Heights	94%	324
Saint Vincent Charity Medical Center[2]	Cleveland	94%	79
West Chester Medical Center	West Chester	94%	96
Euclid Hospital	Euclid	93%	125
Mercy Tiffin Hospital	Tiffin	93%	88
Ohio State University Hospitals[2]	Columbus	93%	56
Upper Valley Medical Center	Troy	93%	246
Belmont Community Hospital	Bellaire	92%	39
Good Samaritan Hospital[2]	Dayton	92%	100
Hillcrest Hospital	Mayfield Heights	92%	368
UHHS Bedford Medical Center	Bedford	92%	109
Wayne Hospital	Greenville	92%	86
H B Magruder Memorial Hospital	Port Clinton	91%	35
Knox Community Hospital	Mount Vernon	91%	122
The Toledo Hospital[2]	Toledo	91%	97
University Hospitals of Cleveland	Cleveland	91%	257
Wood County Hospital	Bowling Green	91%	69
Madison County Hospital	London	90%	50
Trinity Medical Center East & West	Steubenville	90%	261
Mount Carmel Health[2]	Columbus	89%	306
Mount Carmel St Ann's Hospital[2]	Westerville	89%	160
Salem Community Hospital	Salem	89%	164
Barnesville Hospital Association	Barnesville	88%	101
McCullough-Hyde Memorial Hospital	Oxford	88%	90
Memorial Hospital	Fremont	88%	56
Metro Health Medical Center	Cleveland	88%	161
O'Bleness Memorial Hospital	Athens	88%	78
Akron General Medical Center[2]	Akron	87%	127
Genesis Healthcare System	Zanesville	87%	343
Highland District Hospital	Hillsboro	87%	68
Miami Valley Hospital[2]	Dayton	87%	156
Summa Western Reserve Hospital	Cuyahoga Falls	87%	132
Van Wert County Hospital	Van Wert	87%	52
Holzer Medical Center Jackson	Jackson	86%	78
Amherst Hospital	Amherst	85%	26
Southwest General Health Center	Middleburg Hgts	85%	358
Fayette County Memorial Hospital	Washington CH	84%	37
University Hospital[2]	Cincinnati	82%	55
East Ohio Regional Hospital	Martins Ferry	81%	104
Emh Regional Medical Center[2]	Elyria	81%	143
Morrow County Hospital	Mount Gilead	80%	54
University of Toledo Medical Center[2]	Toledo	78%	87
Summa Health Systems Hospitals[2]	Akron	73%	128
Pike Community Hospital	Waverly	68%	41
Deaconess Hospital[3]	Cincinnati	52%	29

21. Smoking Cessation Advice

Hospital Name	City	Rate	Cases
Adams County Regional Medical Center	Seaman	100%	33
Affinity Medical Center	Massillon	100%	80
Ashtabula County Medical Center	Ashtabula	100%	72
Atrium Medical Center	Franklin	100%	181
Barnesville Hospital Association	Barnesville	100%	30
Bay Park Community Hospital	Oregon	100%	46
Berger Hospital	Circleville	100%	55
Bethesda North Hospital	Cincinnati	100%	231
Cincinnati VA Medical Center	Cincinnati	100%	59
Cleveland-Wade Park VA Medical Center	Cleveland	100%	83
Community Hospitals and Wellness Centers	Bryan	100%	28
Doctors Hospital	Columbus	100%	155
Dublin Methodist Hospital	Dublin	100%	29
Emh Regional Medical Center[2]	Elyria	100%	58
Euclid Hospital	Euclid	100%	69
Fairfield Medical Center	Lancaster	100%	155
Fairview Hospital	Cleveland	100%	104
Fort Hamilton Hughes Memorial Hospital[2]	Hamilton	100%	72
Good Samaritan Hospital	Cincinnati	100%	181
Grady Memorial Hospital	Delaware	100%	37
Grandview Hospital & Medical Center	Dayton	100%	115
Grant Medical Center[2]	Columbus	100%	102
Greene Memorial Hospital	Xenia	100%	83
Hillcrest Hospital	Mayfield Heights	100%	95
Holzer Medical Center Jackson	Jackson	100%	38
Jewish Hospital[2]	Cincinnati	100%	44
Joint Township District Memorial Hospital	Saint Marys	100%	25
Kettering Medical Center - Sycamore	Miamisburg	100%	61
Lima Memorial Health System	Lima	100%	66
Lutheran Hospital	Cleveland	100%	79
Marietta Memorial Hospital[2]	Marietta	100%	41
Marion General Hospital	Marion	100%	87
Mary Rutan Hospital	Bellefontaine	100%	27
Marymount Hospital	Garfield Heights	100%	125
Mercy Franciscan Hospital Western Hills	Cincinnati	100%	108
Mercy Hospital Clermont	Batavia	100%	170
Mercy Hospital Fairfield	Fairfield	100%	127
Mercy St Anne Hospital	Toledo	100%	75
Mercy St Vincent Medical Center	Toledo	100%	154
O'Bleness Memorial Hospital	Athens	100%	44
Ohio State University Hospitals[2]	Columbus	100%	86
Riverside Methodist Hospital[2]	Columbus	100%	153
Robinson Memorial Hospital[2]	Ravenna	100%	65
Saint Elizabeth Boardman Health Center[2]	Youngstown	100%	33
Saint Elizabeth Health Center[2]	Youngstown	100%	51
Saint John Medical Center[2]	Westlake	100%	41
Saint Joseph Health Center[2]	Warren	100%	67
Saint Luke's Hospital	Maumee	100%	56
Saint Rita's Medical Center	Lima	100%	132
Saint Vincent Charity Medical Center[2]	Cleveland	100%	42
South Pointe Hospital	Warrensville Hgts	100%	114
Southeastern Ohio Regional Medical Center[2]	Cambridge	100%	72
Summa Barberton Hospital	Barberton	100%	90
Summa Health Systems Hospitals[2]	Akron	100%	63
Summa Wadsworth-Rittman Hospital	Wadsworth	100%	49
Summa Western Reserve Hospital	Cuyahoga Falls	100%	40
Trinity Medical Center East & West	Steubenville	100%	111
UH Geauga Medical Center	Chardon	100%	31
UHHS Memorial Hospital of Geneva	Geneva	100%	28
University of Toledo Medical Center[2]	Toledo	100%	55

NOTE: Hospital profiles are in alphabetical order by state, then city, then hospital within the city; Rankings exclude hospitals with less than 25 cases except for patient surveys which excludes hospitals with less than 100 cases; (a) 100–299 cases; (1) The number of cases is too small to be sure how well a hospital is performing; (2) The hospital indicated that the data submitted for this measure were based on a sample of cases; (3) Data was collected during a shorter time period (fewer quarters) than the maximum possible time for this measure; (4) Suppressed for one or more quarters by CMS; (5) No data is available from the hospital for this measure; (6) Fewer than 100 patients completed the HCAHPS survey. Use these rates with caution, as the number of surveys may be too low to reliably assess hospital performance; (7) Survey results are based on less than 12 months of data; (8) Survey results are not available for this reporting period; (9) No or very few patients were eligible for the HCAHPS survey. The scores shown, if any, reflect a very small number of surveys; (10) A state average was not calculated because too few hospitals in the state submitted data; (11) There were discrepancies in the data collection process; Please refer to the User's Guide for a full explanation of data.

Wood County Hospital	Bowling Green	100%	28
Community Regional Medical Center	Lorain	99%	152
Genesis Healthcare System	Zanesville	99%	172
Kettering Medical Center	Kettering	99%	111
Lakewood Hospital	Lakewood	99%	68
Licking Memorial Hospital[2]	Newark	99%	136
Medcentral Health System[2]	Mansfield	99%	135
Mercy Medical Center	Canton	99%	148
Mercy St Charles Hospital	Oregon	99%	96
Mount Carmel Health[2]	Columbus	99%	150
Mount Carmel St Ann's Hospital[2]	Westerville	99%	96
Parma Community General Hospital	Parma	99%	114
Southern Ohio Medical Center	Portsmouth	99%	134
University Hospitals of Cleveland	Cleveland	99%	138
Wooster Community Hospital	Wooster	99%	67
Adena Regional Medical Center	Chillicothe	98%	187
Brown County Hospital[2]	Georgetown	98%	43
Christ Hospital[2]	Cincinnati	98%	48
Dayton VA Medical Center	Dayton	98%	53
East Ohio Regional Hospital	Martins Ferry	98%	48
Firelands Regional Medical Center	Sandusky	98%	53
Fisher Titus Memorial Hospital	Norwalk	98%	51
Good Samaritan Hospital[2]	Dayton	98%	63
Mercy Hospital Anderson	Cincinnati	98%	162
Metro Health Medical Center	Cleveland	98%	236
Miami Valley Hospital[2]	Dayton	98%	91
Springfield Regional Medical Center	Springfield	98%	179
Trumbull Memorial Hospital[2]	Warren	98%	101
University Hospital[2]	Cincinnati	98%	83
Upper Valley Medical Center	Troy	98%	87
Aultman Hospital	Canton	97%	240
Defiance Regional Medical Center	Defiance	97%	37
Flower Hospital	Sylvania	97%	65
Huron Hospital	Cleveland	97%	62
Mercy Franciscan Hospital - Mt Airy	Cincinnati	97%	104
Mercy Tiffin Hospital	Tiffin	97%	37
Union Hospital	Dover	97%	98
CMH Regional Health System	Wilmington	96%	26
McCullough-Hyde Memorial Hospital	Oxford	96%	48
Northside Medical Center	Youngstown	96%	77
Chillicothe VA Medical Center	Chillicothe	95%	64
Cleveland Clinic[2]	Cleveland	95%	110
Holzer Medical Center[2]	Gallipolis	95%	76
Medina Hospital	Medina	94%	66
UHHS Bedford Medical Center	Bedford	94%	35
Akron General Medical Center[2]	Akron	93%	59
Bellevue Hospital	Bellevue	93%	46
Blanchard Valley Hospital	Findlay	93%	44
Lake Health[2]	Concord	93%	147
East Liverpool City Hospital[2]	East Liverpool	92%	66
Highland District Hospital	Hillsboro	92%	26
West Chester Medical Center	West Chester	92%	39
Memorial Hospital of Union County	Marysville	91%	33
Alliance Community Hospital	Alliance	90%	67
The Toledo Hospital[2]	Toledo	90%	49
Memorial Hospital	Fremont	89%	28
Wayne Hospital	Greenville	89%	28
Knox Community Hospital	Mount Vernon	85%	41
Salem Community Hospital	Salem	80%	46
Southwest General Health Center	Middleburg Hgts	76%	89

Surgical Care Improvement Project

22. Appropriate VTP Within 24 Hours

Hospital Name	City	Rate	Cases
Kettering Medical Center[2]	Kettering	100%	617
Mount Carmel New Albany Surgical Hospital[2]	New Albany	100%	31
Ohio Valley Medical Center[3]	Springfield	100%	26
Selby General Hospital[3]	Marietta	100%	32
Affinity Medical Center	Massillon	99%	134
Cincinnati VA Medical Center[2]	Cincinnati	99%	139
Doctors Hospital[2]	Columbus	99%	137
Fort Hamilton Hughes Memorial Hospital[2]	Hamilton	99%	147
Kettering Medical Center - Sycamore[2]	Miamisburg	99%	215
Mercy Hospital Clermont[2]	Batavia	99%	158
University Hospitals of Cleveland[2]	Cleveland	99%	251
Christ Hospital[2]	Cincinnati	98%	148
Grady Memorial Hospital	Delaware	98%	96
Grant Medical Center[2]	Columbus	98%	188
Lutheran Hospital[2]	Cleveland	98%	130
Marion General Hospital[2]	Marion	98%	195
Mercy Hospital of Defiance	Defiance	98%	62
Metro Health Medical Center[2]	Cleveland	98%	219
Riverside Methodist Hospital[2]	Columbus	98%	880
Atrium Medical Center[2]	Franklin	97%	312
Bucyrus Community Hospital	Bucyrus	97%	33
CMH Regional Health System[2]	Wilmington	97%	66
Community Regional Medical Center[2]	Lorain	97%	258
Euclid Hospital[2]	Euclid	97%	214
Fairfield Medical Center[2]	Lancaster	97%	209
Huron Hospital	Cleveland	97%	127
McCullough-Hyde Memorial Hospital	Oxford	97%	120
Mercy Franciscan Hospital - Mt Airy[2]	Cincinnati	97%	130
Mercy Franciscan Hospital Western Hills[2]	Cincinnati	97%	156
Mount Carmel St Ann's Hospital[2]	Westerville	97%	150
Saint Elizabeth Health Center[2]	Youngstown	97%	174
Summa Barberton Hospital	Barberton	97%	279
University Hospital[2]	Cincinnati	97%	211
Amherst Hospital[2]	Amherst	96%	26
Cleveland Clinic[2]	Cleveland	96%	461
Grandview Hospital & Medical Center[2]	Dayton	96%	276
Hocking Valley Community Hospital	Logan	96%	25
Lakewood Hospital	Lakewood	96%	245
Marietta Memorial Hospital	Marietta	96%	214
Mary Rutan Hospital	Bellefontaine	96%	82
Mercy St Anne Hospital[2]	Toledo	96%	170
Saint Vincent Charity Medical Center[2]	Cleveland	96%	120
University of Toledo Medical Center[2]	Toledo	96%	152
Wilson Memorial Hospital	Sidney	96%	54
Dayton VA Medical Center[2]	Dayton	95%	40
Dublin Methodist Hospital	Dublin	95%	75
Good Samaritan Hospital[2]	Cincinnati	95%	119
Hillcrest Hospital[2]	Mayfield Heights	95%	307
Ohio State University Hospitals[2]	Columbus	95%	184
Summa Health Systems Hospitals[2]	Akron	95%	150
Summa Wadsworth-Rittman Hospital	Wadsworth	95%	57
Upper Valley Medical Center	Troy	95%	185
Ashtabula County Medical Center	Ashtabula	94%	77
Cleveland-Wade Park VA Medical Center[2]	Cleveland	94%	254
Emh Regional Medical Center[2]	Elyria	94%	193
Genesis Healthcare System[2]	Zanesville	94%	107
Northside Medical Center	Youngstown	94%	269
Akron General Medical Center[2]	Akron	93%	248
Flower Hospital[2]	Sylvania	93%	202
Jewish Hospital[2]	Cincinnati	93%	132
Saint Joseph Health Center[2]	Warren	93%	151
South Pointe Hospital	Warrensville Hgts	93%	141
UHHS Richmond Heights Hospital	Richmond Hghts	93%	75
Union Hospital[2]	Dover	93%	114
Bay Park Community Hospital	Oregon	92%	114
Bethesda North Hospital[2]	Cincinnati	92%	173
Mercer County Joint Twp Comm Hosp	Coldwater	92%	50
Mount Carmel Health[2]	Columbus	92%	208
Parma Community General Hospital	Parma	92%	320
Saint Elizabeth Boardman Health Center[2]	Youngstown	92%	157
Saint Luke's Hospital	Maumee	92%	203
Saint Rita's Medical Center	Lima	92%	388
Samaritan Hospital - Peoples Hospital	Ashland	92%	60
UH Geauga Medical Center[2]	Chardon	92%	155
West Chester Medical Center	West Chester	92%	130
Wood County Hospital	Bowling Green	92%	112
Fairview Hospital[2]	Cleveland	91%	285
Joel Pomerene Memorial Hospital	Millersburg	91%	45
Lima Memorial Health System[2]	Lima	91%	140
Mercy Hospital Fairfield[2]	Fairfield	91%	260
UHHS Bedford Medical Center	Bedford	91%	94
Community Hospitals and Wellness Centers	Bryan	90%	101
Firelands Regional Medical Center[2]	Sandusky	90%	144
Mercy Hospital Anderson[2]	Cincinnati	90%	207
Mercy St Vincent Medical Center[2]	Toledo	90%	175
Southern Ohio Medical Center	Portsmouth	90%	237
Trinity Medical Center East & West[2]	Steubenville	90%	138
Wayne Hospital	Greenville	90%	82
Aultman Hospital[2]	Canton	89%	205
Good Samaritan Hospital[2]	Dayton	89%	122
Greene Memorial Hospital	Xenia	89%	83
Mercy Medical Center[2]	Canton	89%	205
Mercy St Charles Hospital[2]	Oregon	89%	170
The Toledo Hospital[2]	Toledo	89%	152
Adena Regional Medical Center	Chillicothe	88%	266
Berger Hospital[2]	Circleville	88%	84
Defiance Regional Medical Center	Defiance	88%	48
Joint Township District Memorial Hospital	Saint Marys	88%	68
Medcentral Health System[2]	Mansfield	88%	288
Medina Hospital[2]	Medina	88%	152
Knox Community Hospital	Mount Vernon	87%	86
Marymount Hospital[2]	Garfield Heights	87%	182
Miami Valley Hospital[2]	Dayton	87%	206
Saint John Medical Center[2]	Westlake	87%	160
Southeastern Ohio Regional Medical Center[2]	Cambridge	87%	90
Blanchard Valley Hospital[2]	Findlay	86%	183
Holzer Medical Center	Gallipolis	86%	94
Robinson Memorial Hospital[2]	Ravenna	86%	175
Southwest General Health Center[2]	Middleburg Hgts	86%	160
Springfield Regional Medical Center	Springfield	86%	384
Trumbull Memorial Hospital[2]	Warren	85%	196
Madison County Hospital	London	84%	31
O'Bleness Memorial Hospital	Athens	83%	52
Fisher Titus Memorial Hospital	Norwalk	82%	82
Memorial Hospital of Union County	Marysville	82%	33
Memorial Hospital	Fremont	81%	62
Summa Western Reserve Hospital[2]	Cuyahoga Falls	81%	84
Van Wert County Hospital	Van Wert	81%	62
Licking Memorial Hospital[2]	Newark	80%	121
Mercy Tiffin Hospital	Tiffin	80%	50
Holzer Medical Center Jackson	Jackson	79%	34
Bellevue Hospital	Bellevue	78%	69
East Liverpool City Hospital	East Liverpool	77%	53
East Ohio Regional Hospital	Martins Ferry	77%	90
Alliance Community Hospital[2]	Alliance	76%	119
Salem Community Hospital[2]	Salem	76%	135
Coshocton County Memorial Hospital	Coshocton	72%	29
Medical Center of Newark	Newark	71%	42
Lake Health[2]	Concord	68%	146
Wooster Community Hospital	Wooster	68%	75
Fulton County Health Center	Wauseon	66%	50

23. Appropriate Hair Removal

Hospital Name	City	Rate	Cases
Adena Regional Medical Center	Chillicothe	100%	850
Affinity Medical Center	Massillon	100%	492
Akron General Medical Center[2]	Akron	100%	614
Allen Community Hospital	Oberlin	100%	118
Amherst Hospital[2]	Amherst	100%	217
Ashtabula County Medical Center	Ashtabula	100%	225
Atrium Medical Center[2]	Franklin	100%	894
Aultman Hospital[2]	Canton	100%	739
Bay Park Community Hospital	Oregon	100%	348
Bellevue Hospital	Bellevue	100%	201
Berger Hospital[2]	Circleville	100%	377
Bethesda North Hospital[2]	Cincinnati	100%	628
Blanchard Valley Hospital[2]	Findlay	100%	754
Brown County Hospital[2]	Georgetown	100%	39
Butler County Medical Center	Hamilton	100%	209
Christ Hospital[2]	Cincinnati	100%	734
Cincinnati VA Medical Center[2]	Cincinnati	100%	238
Cleveland-Wade Park VA Medical Center[2]	Cleveland	100%	559
CMH Regional Health System[2]	Wilmington	100%	254
Community Hospitals and Wellness Centers	Bryan	100%	237
Community Regional Medical Center[2]	Lorain	100%	621
Crystal Clinic Orthopaedic Center[2,3]	Akron	100%	139
Dayton VA Medical Center[2]	Dayton	100%	156
Doctors Hospital[2]	Columbus	100%	523
Dublin Methodist Hospital	Dublin	100%	166
East Liverpool City Hospital	East Liverpool	100%	141
East Ohio Regional Hospital	Martins Ferry	100%	353
Emh Regional Medical Center[2]	Elyria	100%	620
Euclid Hospital[2]	Euclid	100%	948
Evendale Medical Center	Cincinnati	100%	287
Fairview Hospital[2]	Cleveland	100%	616
Fayette County Memorial Hospital[2]	Washington CH	100%	28
Fisher Titus Memorial Hospital	Norwalk	100%	298
Fort Hamilton Hughes Memorial Hospital[2]	Hamilton	100%	353
Fostoria Community Hospital	Fostoria	100%	141
Fulton County Health Center	Wauseon	100%	263
Galion Community Hospital[3]	Galion	100%	123
Genesis Healthcare System[2]	Zanesville	100%	518
Good Samaritan Hospital[2]	Dayton	100%	650
Grady Memorial Hospital	Delaware	100%	221
Grandview Hospital & Medical Center[2]	Dayton	100%	1007
Grant Medical Center[2]	Columbus	100%	886
Greene Memorial Hospital	Xenia	100%	239
H B Magruder Memorial Hospital	Port Clinton	100%	57
Henry County Hospital	Napoleon	100%	48
Hillcrest Hospital[2]	Mayfield Heights	100%	837
Hocking Valley Community Hospital	Logan	100%	57
Huron Hospital	Cleveland	100%	208
Jewish Hospital[2]	Cincinnati	100%	523
Joel Pomerene Memorial Hospital	Millersburg	100%	113
Kettering Medical Center[2]	Kettering	100%	2599
Kettering Medical Center - Sycamore[2]	Miamisburg	100%	447
Knox Community Hospital	Mount Vernon	100%	447
Lakewood Hospital	Lakewood	100%	564
Lima Memorial Health System[2]	Lima	100%	580
Lutheran Hospital[2]	Cleveland	100%	343
Madison County Hospital	London	100%	105
Marietta Memorial Hospital	Marietta	100%	610
Marion General Hospital[2]	Marion	100%	486
Marymount Hospital[2]	Garfield Heights	100%	526
McCullough-Hyde Memorial Hospital	Oxford	100%	265
Medical Center at Elizabeth Place	Dayton	100%	160
Medina Hospital[2]	Medina	100%	426
Mercy Franciscan Hospital - Mt Airy[2]	Cincinnati	100%	493
Mercy Franciscan Hospital Western Hills[2]	Cincinnati	100%	331
Mercy Hospital Anderson[2]	Cincinnati	100%	908
Mercy Hospital Clermont[2]	Batavia	100%	388
Mercy Hospital Fairfield[2]	Fairfield	100%	963
Mercy Hospital of Defiance	Defiance	100%	113
Mercy Hospital of Willard	Willard	100%	42
Mercy Medical Center[2]	Canton	100%	788
Mercy St Anne Hospital[2]	Toledo	100%	412

NOTE: Hospital profiles are in alphabetical order by state, then city, then hospital within the city; Rankings exclude hospitals with less than 25 cases except for patient surveys which excludes hospitals with less than 100 cases; (a) 100–299 cases; (1) The number of cases is too small to be sure how well a hospital is performing; (2) The hospital indicated that the data submitted for this measure were based on a sample of cases; (3) Data was collected during a shorter time period (fewer quarters) than the maximum possible time for this measure; (4) Suppressed for one or more quarters by CMS; (5) No data is available from the hospital for this measure; (6) Fewer than 100 patients completed the HCAHPS survey. Use these rates with caution, as the number of surveys may be too low to reliably assess hospital performance; (7) Survey results are based on less than 12 months of data; (8) Survey results are not available for this reporting period; (9) No or very few patients were eligible for the HCAHPS survey. The scores shown, if any, reflect a very small number of surveys; (10) A state average was not calculated because too few hospitals in the state submitted data; (11) There were discrepancies in the data collection process; Please refer to the User's Guide for a full explanation of data.

Mercy St Charles Hospital[2]	Oregon	100%	489
Mercy St Vincent Medical Center[2]	Toledo	100%	872
Mercy Tiffin Hospital	Tiffin	100%	166
Metro Health Medical Center[2]	Cleveland	100%	662
Miami Valley Hospital[2]	Dayton	100%	729
Mount Carmel Health[2]	Columbus	100%	1104
Mount Carmel New Albany Surgical Hospital[2]	New Albany	100%	596
Mount Carmel St Ann's Hospital[2]	Westerville	100%	553
Northside Medical Center	Youngstown	100%	1070
O'Bleness Memorial Hospital	Athens	100%	89
Ohio State University Hospitals[2]	Columbus	100%	607
Ohio Valley Medical Center[3]	Springfield	100%	230
Parma Community General Hospital	Parma	100%	1136
Riverside Methodist Hospital[2]	Columbus	100%	3209
Robinson Memorial Hospital[2]	Ravenna	100%	451
Saint Elizabeth Boardman Health Center[2]	Youngstown	100%	363
Saint Elizabeth Health Center[2]	Youngstown	100%	660
Saint John Medical Center[2]	Westlake	100%	417
Saint Joseph Health Center[2]	Warren	100%	417
Saint Vincent Charity Medical Center[2]	Cleveland	100%	352
Salem Community Hospital[2]	Salem	100%	351
Samaritan Hospital - Peoples Hospital	Ashland	100%	535
South Pointe Hospital	Warrensville Hgts	100%	305
Southeastern Ohio Regional Medical Center[2]	Cambridge	100%	183
Southern Ohio Medical Center	Portsmouth	100%	867
Southwest General Health Center[2]	Middleburg Hgts	100%	1092
Springfield Regional Medical Center	Springfield	100%	1068
Summa Barberton Hospital	Barberton	100%	553
Summa Wadsworth-Rittman Hospital	Wadsworth	100%	172
Summa Western Reserve Hospital[2]	Cuyahoga Falls	100%	261
Surgical Hospital at Southwoods[2]	Youngstown	100%	289
The Toledo Hospital[2]	Toledo	100%	674
Trinity Medical Center East & West[2]	Steubenville	100%	547
UH Geauga Medical Center[2]	Chardon	100%	491
UHHS Bedford Medical Center	Bedford	100%	187
UHHS Memorial Hospital of Geneva	Geneva	100%	25
UHHS Richmond Heights Hospital	Richmond Hghts	100%	218
Union Hospital[2]	Dover	100%	404
University Hospital[2]	Cincinnati	100%	645
University of Toledo Medical Center[2]	Toledo	100%	477
Upper Valley Medical Center	Troy	100%	420
Van Wert County Hospital	Van Wert	100%	157
West Chester Medical Center	West Chester	100%	402
Wilson Memorial Hospital	Sidney	100%	165
Wyandot Memorial Hospital	Upper Sandusky	100%	31
Bucyrus Community Hospital	Bucyrus	99%	113
Coshocton County Memorial Hospital	Coshocton	99%	74
Defiance Regional Medical Center	Defiance	99%	162
Fairfield Medical Center[2]	Lancaster	99%	990
Firelands Regional Medical Center[2]	Sandusky	99%	517
Flower Hospital[2]	Sylvania	99%	473
Good Samaritan Hospital[2]	Cincinnati	99%	621
Holzer Medical Center	Gallipolis	99%	302
Holzer Medical Center Jackson	Jackson	99%	171
Institute for Orthopedic Surgery[2]	Lima	99%	214
Lake Health[2]	Concord	99%	530
Licking Memorial Hospital[2]	Newark	99%	444
Mary Rutan Hospital	Bellefontaine	99%	264
Memorial Hospital	Fremont	99%	220
Memorial Hospital of Union County	Marysville	99%	122
Mercer County Joint Twp Comm Hosp	Coldwater	99%	131
Saint Luke's Hospital	Maumee	99%	893
Saint Rita's Medical Center	Lima	99%	1164
Summa Health Systems Hospitals[2]	Akron	99%	495
Trumbull Memorial Hospital[2]	Warren	99%	699
Univ Hosps Conneaut Med Ctr[3]	Conneaut	99%	92
University Hospitals of Cleveland[2]	Cleveland	99%	785
Wood County Hospital	Bowling Green	99%	225
Wooster Community Hospital	Wooster	99%	465
Deaconess Hospital[2]	Cincinnati	98%	125
Medical Center of Newark	Newark	98%	104
Selby General Hospital[3]	Marietta	98%	82
Joint Township District Memorial Hospital	Saint Marys	97%	189
Medcentral Health System[2]	Mansfield	97%	930
Alliance Community Hospital[2]	Alliance	96%	344
Wayne Hospital	Greenville	96%	207
Cleveland Clinic[2]	Cleveland	91%	1487

24. Appropriate Beta Blocker Usage

Hospital Name	City	Rate	Cases
Atrium Medical Center[2]	Franklin	100%	256
Dublin Methodist Hospital	Dublin	100%	26
Grant Medical Center[2]	Columbus	100%	265
Marion General Hospital[2]	Marion	100%	217
Medical Center at Elizabeth Place	Dayton	100%	27
Summa Barberton Hospital	Barberton	100%	146
UHHS Bedford Medical Center	Bedford	100%	50
Univ Hosps Conneaut Med Ctr[3]	Conneaut	100%	26
Van Wert County Hospital	Van Wert	100%	56
Berger Hospital[2]	Circleville	99%	103
Cleveland-Wade Park VA Medical Center[2]	Cleveland	99%	298
Kettering Medical Center - Sycamore[2]	Miamisburg	99%	164
Lutheran Hospital[2]	Cleveland	99%	115
Mercy Franciscan Hospital Western Hills[2]	Cincinnati	99%	146
Samaritan Hospital - Peoples Hospital	Ashland	99%	169
University Hospitals of Cleveland[2]	Cleveland	99%	281
Christ Hospital[2]	Cincinnati	98%	229
Cincinnati VA Medical Center[2]	Cincinnati	98%	83
Community Regional Medical Center[2]	Lorain	98%	264
Dayton VA Medical Center[2]	Dayton	98%	64
Kettering Medical Center[2]	Kettering	98%	892
Mercy Franciscan Hospital - Mt Airy[2]	Cincinnati	98%	156
Mercy St Anne Hospital[2]	Toledo	98%	143
Mercy St Charles Hospital[2]	Oregon	98%	171
South Pointe Hospital	Warrensville Hgts	98%	102
Springfield Regional Medical Center	Springfield	98%	386
Summa Wadsworth-Rittman Hospital	Wadsworth	98%	53
Surgical Hospital at Southwoods[2]	Youngstown	98%	47
Ashtabula County Medical Center	Ashtabula	97%	63
CMH Regional Health System[2]	Wilmington	97%	69
Doctors Hospital[2]	Columbus	97%	146
Genesis Healthcare System[2]	Zanesville	97%	193
Grandview Hospital & Medical Center[2]	Dayton	97%	316
Huron Hospital	Cleveland	97%	35
Institute for Orthopedic Surgery[2]	Lima	97%	64
Riverside Methodist Hospital[2]	Columbus	97%	1072
Saint Elizabeth Health Center[2]	Youngstown	97%	249
Saint John Medical Center[2]	Westlake	97%	148
Saint Rita's Medical Center	Lima	97%	436
Southeastern Ohio Regional Medical Center[2]	Cambridge	97%	63
The Toledo Hospital[2]	Toledo	97%	268
UHHS Richmond Heights Hospital	Richmond Hghts	97%	67
Union Hospital[2]	Dover	97%	109
Aultman Hospital[2]	Canton	96%	289
Bethesda North Hospital[2]	Cincinnati	96%	198
Flower Hospital[2]	Sylvania	96%	152
Lakewood Hospital	Lakewood	96%	191
Medcentral Health System[2]	Mansfield	96%	380
Mount Carmel St Ann's Hospital[2]	Westerville	96%	193
Robinson Memorial Hospital[2]	Ravenna	96%	139
University of Toledo Medical Center[2]	Toledo	96%	200
Cleveland Clinic[2]	Cleveland	95%	538
Fort Hamilton Hughes Memorial Hospital[2]	Hamilton	95%	81
Good Samaritan Hospital[2]	Cincinnati	95%	185
Good Samaritan Hospital[2]	Dayton	95%	220
Greene Memorial Hospital	Xenia	95%	74
Jewish Hospital[2]	Cincinnati	95%	164
Lima Memorial Health System[2]	Lima	95%	185
Mercy Hospital Anderson[2]	Cincinnati	95%	283
Mercy Hospital Clermont[2]	Batavia	95%	112
Mercy St Vincent Medical Center[2]	Toledo	95%	319
Northside Medical Center	Youngstown	95%	352
Saint Elizabeth Boardman Health Center[2]	Youngstown	95%	105
Saint Joseph Health Center[2]	Warren	95%	111
Salem Community Hospital[2]	Salem	95%	100
Southwest General Health Center[2]	Middleburg Hgts	95%	429
Adena Regional Medical Center	Chillicothe	94%	348
Affinity Medical Center	Massillon	94%	177
Bay Park Community Hospital	Oregon	94%	121
East Ohio Regional Hospital	Martins Ferry	94%	144
Euclid Hospital[2]	Euclid	94%	264
Fairview Hospital[2]	Cleveland	94%	226
Mercy Hospital of Defiance	Defiance	94%	34
Mercy Tiffin Hospital	Tiffin	94%	52
Parma Community General Hospital	Parma	94%	423
Saint Luke's Hospital	Maumee	94%	295
Wayne Hospital	Greenville	94%	48
Community Hospitals and Wellness Centers	Bryan	93%	94
Hillcrest Hospital[2]	Mayfield Heights	93%	297
McCullough-Hyde Memorial Hospital	Oxford	93%	54
Mercer County Joint Twp Comm Hosp	Coldwater	93%	28
Mount Carmel Health[2]	Columbus	93%	427
Southern Ohio Medical Center	Portsmouth	93%	275
Upper Valley Medical Center	Troy	93%	105
Akron General Medical Center[2]	Akron	92%	180
Alliance Community Hospital[2]	Alliance	92%	101
Grady Memorial Hospital	Delaware	92%	64
Mercy Hospital Fairfield[2]	Fairfield	92%	268
Ohio State University Hospitals[2]	Columbus	92%	206
University Hospital[2]	Cincinnati	92%	181
Bellevue Hospital	Bellevue	91%	35
Marymount Hospital[2]	Garfield Heights	91%	173
Amherst Hospital[2]	Amherst	90%	62
Emh Regional Medical Center[2]	Elyria	90%	249
Evendale Medical Center	Cincinnati	90%	61
Fisher Titus Memorial Hospital	Norwalk	90%	121
Licking Memorial Hospital[2]	Newark	90%	140
Marietta Memorial Hospital	Marietta	90%	188
Mary Rutan Hospital	Bellefontaine	90%	80
Medina Hospital[2]	Medina	90%	127
Metro Health Medical Center[2]	Cleveland	90%	244
Miami Valley Hospital[2]	Dayton	90%	239
Mount Carmel New Albany Surgical Hospital[2]	New Albany	90%	178
Firelands Regional Medical Center[2]	Sandusky	89%	184
Knox Community Hospital	Mount Vernon	89%	117
Trumbull Memorial Hospital[2]	Warren	89%	201
West Chester Medical Center	West Chester	89%	111
Wilson Memorial Hospital	Sidney	89%	47
Deaconess Hospital[2]	Cincinnati	88%	60
Memorial Hospital of Union County	Marysville	88%	25
Trinity Medical Center East & West[2]	Steubenville	88%	206
UH Geauga Medical Center[2]	Chardon	88%	163
Blanchard Valley Hospital[2]	Findlay	87%	216
Holzer Medical Center	Gallipolis	87%	117
Fairfield Medical Center[2]	Lancaster	86%	312
Mercy Medical Center[2]	Canton	86%	258
Saint Vincent Charity Medical Center[2]	Cleveland	86%	123
Crystal Clinic Orthopaedic Center[2,3]	Akron	85%	41
Memorial Hospital	Fremont	85%	62
Joel Pomerene Memorial Hospital	Millersburg	84%	25
Wood County Hospital	Bowling Green	84%	69
Summa Western Reserve Hospital[2]	Cuyahoga Falls	82%	55
Lake Health[2]	Concord	81%	201
Ohio Valley Medical Center[3]	Springfield	81%	43
Galion Community Hospital[3]	Galion	80%	40
Joint Township District Memorial Hospital	Saint Marys	80%	60
Wooster Community Hospital	Wooster	80%	122
Fulton County Health Center	Wauseon	79%	92
Summa Health Systems Hospitals[2]	Akron	62%	178
Butler County Medical Center	Hamilton	61%	41
East Liverpool City Hospital	East Liverpool	60%	42

25. Controlled Postoperative Blood Glucose

Hospital Name	City	Rate	Cases
Bethesda North Hospital[2]	Cincinnati	100%	137
Marion General Hospital[2]	Marion	100%	59
Mercy St Vincent Medical Center[2]	Toledo	100%	314
Saint Luke's Hospital	Maumee	100%	121
Saint Rita's Medical Center	Lima	100%	163
Doctors Hospital[2]	Columbus	99%	94
Miami Valley Hospital[2]	Dayton	99%	135
Genesis Healthcare System[2]	Zanesville	98%	97
Mercy Hospital Anderson[2]	Cincinnati	98%	85
Ohio State University Hospitals[2]	Columbus	98%	129
Springfield Regional Medical Center	Springfield	98%	172
Akron General Medical Center[2]	Akron	97%	116
Grant Medical Center[2]	Columbus	97%	180
Kettering Medical Center[2]	Kettering	97%	355
Southwest General Health Center[2]	Middleburg Hgts	97%	71
Atrium Medical Center[2]	Franklin	96%	97
Blanchard Valley Hospital[2]	Findlay	96%	69
Cleveland-Wade Park VA Medical Center[2]	Cleveland	96%	157
Good Samaritan Hospital[2]	Cincinnati	96%	126
Hillcrest Hospital[2]	Mayfield Heights	96%	185
Lima Memorial Health System[2]	Lima	96%	240
Medcentral Health System[2]	Mansfield	96%	304
Mercy Hospital Fairfield[2]	Fairfield	96%	187
Mercy Medical Center[2]	Canton	96%	145
Mount Carmel Health[2]	Columbus	96%	206
Saint John Medical Center[2]	Westlake	96%	51
Community Regional Medical Center[2]	Lorain	95%	42
Good Samaritan Hospital[2]	Dayton	95%	162
Jewish Hospital[2]	Cincinnati	95%	88
Riverside Methodist Hospital[2]	Columbus	95%	527
Southern Ohio Medical Center	Portsmouth	95%	137
University Hospital[2]	Cincinnati	95%	106
University Hospitals of Cleveland[2]	Cleveland	95%	162
Aultman Hospital[2]	Canton	94%	182
Metro Health Medical Center[2]	Cleveland	94%	95
Affinity Medical Center	Massillon	93%	88
Christ Hospital[2]	Cincinnati	92%	152
Cleveland Clinic[2]	Cleveland	92%	407
Northside Medical Center	Youngstown	92%	98
Parma Community General Hospital	Parma	92%	97
Saint Elizabeth Health Center[2]	Youngstown	92%	144
Holzer Medical Center	Gallipolis	91%	35
Lake Health[2]	Concord	91%	99
Fairview Hospital[2]	Cleveland	90%	119
Firelands Regional Medical Center[2]	Sandusky	90%	31
The Toledo Hospital[2]	Toledo	90%	151
Trinity Medical Center East & West[2]	Steubenville	90%	109
University of Toledo Medical Center[2]	Toledo	90%	94
Grandview Hospital & Medical Center[2]	Dayton	89%	126
Adena Regional Medical Center	Chillicothe	88%	109
Deaconess Hospital[2]	Cincinnati	88%	80
Saint Vincent Charity Medical Center[2]	Cleveland	86%	50
Trumbull Memorial Hospital[2]	Warren	84%	86
Summa Barberton Hospital	Barberton	81%	37
Summa Health Systems Hospitals[2]	Akron	81%	149
Fairfield Medical Center[2]	Lancaster	78%	154
Emh Regional Medical Center[2]	Elyria	77%	117

NOTE: Hospital profiles are in alphabetical order by state, then city, then hospital within the city; Rankings exclude hospitals with less than 25 cases except for patient surveys which excludes hospitals with less than 100 cases; (a) 100–299 cases; (1) The number of cases is too small to be sure how well a hospital is performing; (2) The hospital indicated that the data submitted for this measure were based on a sample of cases; (3) Data was collected during a shorter time period (fewer quarters) than the maximum possible time for this measure; (4) Suppressed for one or more quarters by CMS; (5) No data is available from the hospital for this measure; (6) Fewer than 100 patients completed the HCAHPS survey. Use these rates with caution, as the number of surveys may be too low to reliably assess hospital performance; (7) Survey results are based on less than 12 months of data; (8) Survey results are not available for this reporting period; (9) No or very few patients were eligible for the HCAHPS survey. The scores shown, if any, reflect a very small number of surveys; (10) A state average was not calculated because too few hospitals in the state submitted data; (11) There were discrepancies in the data collection process; Please refer to the User's Guide for a full explanation of data.

26. Prophylactic Antibiotic Timing

Hospital Name	City	Rate	Cases
Allen Community Hospital	Oberlin	100%	99
Community Regional Medical Center[2]	Lorain	100%	481
Dublin Methodist Hospital	Dublin	100%	95
Fostoria Community Hospital	Fostoria	100%	135
Grant Medical Center[2]	Columbus	100%	693
Huron Hospital	Cleveland	100%	73
Institute for Orthopedic Surgery[2]	Lima	100%	191
Kettering Medical Center[2]	Kettering	100%	2258
Mercy Hospital Clermont[2]	Batavia	100%	267
Ohio Valley Medical Center[3]	Springfield	100%	202
Summa Barberton Hospital	Barberton	100%	333
Affinity Medical Center	Massillon	99%	378
Ashtabula County Medical Center	Ashtabula	99%	149
Atrium Medical Center[2]	Franklin	99%	508
Berger Hospital[2]	Circleville	99%	281
Bucyrus Community Hospital	Bucyrus	99%	94
Cincinnati VA Medical Center	Cincinnati	99%	152
Doctors Hospital[2]	Columbus	99%	387
Fairview Hospital[2]	Cleveland	99%	450
Grady Memorial Hospital	Delaware	99%	142
Grandview Hospital & Medical Center[2]	Dayton	99%	780
Greene Memorial Hospital	Xenia	99%	155
Kettering Medical Center - Sycamore[2]	Miamisburg	99%	304
Marion General Hospital[2]	Marion	99%	406
Marymount Hospital[2]	Garfield Heights	99%	363
Medina Hospital[2]	Medina	99%	303
Mercy Franciscan Hospital Western Hills[2]	Cincinnati	99%	194
Mercy St Charles Hospital[2]	Oregon	99%	331
Mercy Tiffin Hospital	Tiffin	99%	136
Mount Carmel New Albany Surgical Hospital[2]	New Albany	99%	466
Mount Carmel St Ann's Hospital[2]	Westerville	99%	380
Ohio State University Hospitals[2]	Columbus	99%	385
Riverside Methodist Hospital[2]	Columbus	99%	2123
Robinson Memorial Hospital[2]	Ravenna	99%	296
Saint Elizabeth Boardman Health Center[2]	Youngstown	99%	226
Southeastern Ohio Regional Medical Center[2]	Cambridge	99%	141
UHHS Bedford Medical Center	Bedford	99%	109
Union Hospital[2]	Dover	99%	266
Univ Hosps Conneaut Med Ctr[3]	Conneaut	99%	76
University Hospitals of Cleveland[2]	Cleveland	99%	518
Wayne Hospital	Greenville	99%	140
Amherst Hospital[2]	Amherst	98%	178
Blanchard Valley Hospital[2]	Findlay	98%	604
Cleveland Clinic[2]	Cleveland	98%	1019
Cleveland-Wade Park VA Medical Center	Cleveland	98%	401
Coshocton County Memorial Hospital	Coshocton	98%	43
Dayton VA Medical Center	Dayton	98%	111
Defiance Regional Medical Center	Defiance	98%	125
Emh Regional Medical Center[2]	Elyria	98%	449
Fort Hamilton Hughes Memorial Hospital[2]	Hamilton	98%	185
H B Magruder Memorial Hospital	Port Clinton	98%	41
Jewish Hospital[2]	Cincinnati	98%	338
Joel Pomerene Memorial Hospital	Millersburg	98%	64
Knox Community Hospital	Mount Vernon	98%	382
Lutheran Hospital[2]	Cleveland	98%	216
Mercy Hospital Anderson[2]	Cincinnati	98%	673
Mercy Hospital of Defiance	Defiance	98%	84
Mercy St Vincent Medical Center[2]	Toledo	98%	672
Metro Health Medical Center[2]	Cleveland	98%	483
Mount Carmel Health[2]	Columbus	98%	839
Saint Elizabeth Health Center[2]	Youngstown	98%	463
Saint Joseph Health Center[2]	Warren	98%	269
Saint Luke's Hospital	Maumee	98%	632
Saint Rita's Medical Center	Lima	98%	693
Samaritan Hospital - Peoples Hospital	Ashland	98%	473
Springfield Regional Medical Center	Springfield	98%	635
Summa Wadsworth-Rittman Hospital	Wadsworth	98%	127
UHHS Richmond Heights Hospital	Richmond Hghts	98%	146
West Chester Medical Center	West Chester	98%	297
Adena Regional Medical Center	Chillicothe	97%	736
Akron General Medical Center[2]	Akron	97%	442
Alliance Community Hospital[2]	Alliance	97%	221
Bay Park Community Hospital	Oregon	97%	263
Deaconess Hospital[2]	Cincinnati	97%	34
East Ohio Regional Hospital	Martins Ferry	97%	296
Flower Hospital[2]	Sylvania	97%	314
Henry County Hospital	Napoleon	97%	39
Hillcrest Hospital[2]	Mayfield Heights	97%	593
Holzer Medical Center	Gallipolis	97%	179
Medcentral Health System[2]	Mansfield	97%	639
Medical Center at Elizabeth Place	Dayton	97%	63
Mercy Franciscan Hospital - Mt Airy[2]	Cincinnati	97%	331
Northside Medical Center	Youngstown	97%	829
Saint Vincent Charity Medical Center[2]	Cleveland	97%	248
Southwest General Health Center[2]	Middleburg Hgts	97%	890
Trinity Medical Center East & West[2]	Steubenville	97%	410
University Hospital[2]	Cincinnati	97%	418
Aultman Hospital[2]	Canton	96%	554
Bethesda North Hospital[2]	Cincinnati	96%	440
CMH Regional Health System[2]	Wilmington	96%	190
Community Hospitals and Wellness Centers	Bryan	96%	180
Euclid Hospital[2]	Euclid	96%	765
Fisher Titus Memorial Hospital	Norwalk	96%	211
Fulton County Health Center	Wauseon	96%	208
Good Samaritan Hospital[2]	Cincinnati	96%	436
Good Samaritan Hospital[2]	Dayton	96%	488
Lakewood Hospital	Lakewood	96%	363
McCullough-Hyde Memorial Hospital	Oxford	96%	207
Mercy Hospital Fairfield[2]	Fairfield	96%	716
Mercy Medical Center[2]	Canton	96%	610
Miami Valley Hospital[2]	Dayton	96%	492
O'Bleness Memorial Hospital	Athens	96%	71
Parma Community General Hospital	Parma	96%	819
Salem Community Hospital[2]	Salem	96%	228
Southern Ohio Medical Center	Portsmouth	96%	600
The Toledo Hospital[2]	Toledo	96%	486
University of Toledo Medical Center[2]	Toledo	96%	337
Upper Valley Medical Center	Troy	96%	264
Christ Hospital[2]	Cincinnati	95%	492
Crystal Clinic Orthopaedic Center[2,3]	Akron	95%	98
Firelands Regional Medical Center[2]	Sandusky	95%	353
Licking Memorial Hospital[2]	Newark	95%	279
Lima Memorial Health System[2]	Lima	95%	406
Mary Rutan Hospital	Bellefontaine	95%	207
Mercy St Anne Hospital[2]	Toledo	95%	284
Saint John Medical Center[2]	Westlake	95%	285
Summa Western Reserve Hospital[2]	Cuyahoga Falls	95%	172
Trumbull Memorial Hospital[2]	Warren	95%	475
UH Geauga Medical Center[2]	Chardon	95%	363
Wilson Memorial Hospital	Sidney	95%	110
Bellevue Hospital	Bellevue	94%	138
Fairfield Medical Center[2]	Lancaster	94%	761
Galion Community Hospital[3]	Galion	94%	112
Hocking Valley Community Hospital	Logan	94%	51
Madison County Hospital	London	94%	62
Mercy Hospital of Willard	Willard	94%	35
Wooster Community Hospital	Wooster	94%	387
Butler County Medical Center	Hamilton	93%	190
Genesis Healthcare System[2]	Zanesville	93%	368
South Pointe Hospital	Warrensville Hgts	93%	176
Van Wert County Hospital	Van Wert	93%	113
Highland District Hospital	Hillsboro	92%	26
Joint Township District Memorial Hospital	Saint Marys	92%	146
Lake Health[2]	Concord	92%	377
Marietta Memorial Hospital	Marietta	92%	473
Memorial Hospital of Union County	Marysville	92%	93
Summa Health Systems Hospitals[2]	Akron	92%	343
Wood County Hospital	Bowling Green	92%	178
Mercer County Joint Twp Comm Hosp	Coldwater	91%	96
Surgical Hospital at Southwoods[2]	Youngstown	91%	267
Medical Center of Newark	Newark	90%	72
Evendale Medical Center	Cincinnati	89%	208
Selby General Hospital[3]	Marietta	89%	70
East Liverpool City Hospital	East Liverpool	87%	94
Holzer Medical Center Jackson	Jackson	84%	158
Memorial Hospital	Fremont	83%	173
Wyandot Memorial Hospital	Upper Sandusky	79%	29

27. Prophylactic Antibiotic Timing (Outpatient)

Hospital Name	City	Rate	Cases
Berger Hospital	Circleville	100%	40
Institute for Orthopedic Surgery	Lima	100%	83
Mount Carmel New Albany Surgical Hospital	New Albany	100%	503
UHHS Memorial Hospital of Geneva	Geneva	100%	51
Summa Barberton Hospital	Barberton	99%	114
Summa Wadsworth-Rittman Hospital	Wadsworth	99%	81
Blanchard Valley Hospital	Findlay	98%	545
Community Regional Medical Center	Lorain	98%	307
Crystal Clinic Orthopaedic Center[3]	Akron	98%	324
Dublin Methodist Hospital	Dublin	98%	541
Lutheran Hospital	Cleveland	98%	226
Grant Medical Center	Columbus	97%	627
Marion General Hospital	Marion	97%	198
Marymount Hospital	Garfield Heights	97%	254
Mercy St Anne Hospital	Toledo	97%	101
Mercy St Vincent Medical Center	Toledo	97%	474
Miami Valley Hospital	Dayton	97%	912
Mount Carmel Health	Columbus	97%	758
O'Bleness Memorial Hospital	Athens	97%	199
Ohio State University Hospitals	Columbus	97%	377
Saint Vincent Charity Medical Center	Cleveland	97%	145
Summa Western Reserve Hospital	Cuyahoga Falls	97%	122
The Toledo Hospital	Toledo	97%	588
University of Toledo Medical Center	Toledo	97%	196
Van Wert County Hospital	Van Wert	97%	88
Adena Regional Medical Center	Chillicothe	96%	314
Mercy Hospital Anderson	Cincinnati	96%	261
Saint John Medical Center	Westlake	96%	276
Akron General Medical Center	Akron	95%	698
Grandview Hospital & Medical Center	Dayton	95%	559
Kettering Medical Center	Kettering	95%	622
McCullough-Hyde Memorial Hospital	Oxford	95%	42
Mercy Franciscan Hospital - Mt Airy	Cincinnati	95%	104
Metro Health Medical Center	Cleveland	95%	599
Riverside Methodist Hospital	Columbus	95%	806
Saint Luke's Hospital	Maumee	95%	262
Summa Health Systems Hospitals	Akron	95%	529
Three Gables Surgery Center	Proctorville	95%	57
Upper Valley Medical Center	Troy	95%	100
Christ Hospital	Cincinnati	94%	815
Emh Regional Medical Center	Elyria	94%	459
Medical Center at Elizabeth Place	Dayton	94%	111
Ohio Valley Medical Center[3]	Springfield	94%	31
Robinson Memorial Hospital	Ravenna	94%	264
Southern Ohio Medical Center	Portsmouth	94%	161
Trumbull Memorial Hospital	Warren	94%	304
University Hospitals of Cleveland	Cleveland	94%	678
West Chester Medical Center	West Chester	94%	67
Bethesda North Hospital	Cincinnati	93%	655
Greene Memorial Hospital	Xenia	93%	72
Mercy St Charles Hospital	Oregon	93%	108
Northside Medical Center	Youngstown	93%	260
Southeastern Ohio Regional Medical Center	Cambridge	93%	155
Trinity Medical Center East & West	Steubenville	93%	270
Union Hospital	Dover	93%	143
Ashtabula County Medical Center	Ashtabula	92%	154
Aultman Hospital	Canton	92%	1067
Bay Park Community Hospital	Oregon	92%	78
Community Hospitals and Wellness Centers	Bryan	92%	85
Doctors Hospital	Columbus	92%	201
Euclid Hospital	Euclid	92%	90
Fairview Hospital	Cleveland	92%	626
Fayette County Memorial Hospital	Washington CH	92%	61
Fort Hamilton Hughes Memorial Hospital	Hamilton	92%	78
Good Samaritan Hospital	Cincinnati	92%	603
Grady Memorial Hospital	Delaware	92%	113
Kettering Medical Center - Sycamore	Miamisburg	92%	145
Mercy Franciscan Hospital Western Hills	Cincinnati	92%	59
Mercy Medical Center	Canton	92%	810
Atrium Medical Center	Franklin	91%	255
Bluffton Hospital	Bluffton	91%	106
Mercy Hospital Clermont	Batavia	91%	65
Saint Rita's Medical Center	Lima	91%	275
Wilson Memorial Hospital	Sidney	91%	115
Affinity Medical Center	Massillon	90%	144
CMH Regional Health System	Wilmington	90%	134
Hillcrest Hospital	Mayfield Heights	90%	648
Holzer Medical Center	Gallipolis	90%	59
Mary Rutan Hospital	Bellefontaine	90%	68
Medina Hospital	Medina	90%	214
Memorial Hospital of Union County	Marysville	90%	62
UHHS Richmond Heights Hospital	Richmond Hghts	90%	87
Flower Hospital	Sylvania	89%	179
Mercy Hospital Fairfield	Fairfield	89%	159
Saint Elizabeth Health Center	Youngstown	89%	528
Southwest General Health Center	Middleburg Hgts	89%	371
Firelands Regional Medical Center	Sandusky	88%	281
Lakewood Hospital	Lakewood	88%	151
Fairfield Medical Center	Lancaster	87%	427
Joint Township District Memorial Hospital	Saint Marys	87%	31
Lima Memorial Health System	Lima	87%	370
Springfield Regional Medical Center	Springfield	87%	197
UHHS Bedford Medical Center	Bedford	87%	79
Wooster Community Hospital	Wooster	87%	191
Fisher Titus Memorial Hospital	Norwalk	86%	93
Jewish Hospital	Cincinnati	86%	324
Wood County Hospital	Bowling Green	86%	110
Alliance Community Hospital	Alliance	85%	82
Good Samaritan Hospital	Dayton	85%	609
Lake Health	Concord	85%	377
Brown County Hospital	Georgetown	84%	38
Huron Hospital	Cleveland	84%	32
Medcentral Health System	Mansfield	84%	319
Samaritan Hospital - Peoples Hospital	Ashland	84%	88
University Hospital	Cincinnati	84%	395
Cleveland Clinic	Cleveland	83%	826
Saint Joseph Health Center	Warren	83%	249
Salem Community Hospital	Salem	83%	98
UH Geauga Medical Center	Chardon	83%	249
Butler County Medical Center	Hamilton	82%	90
East Ohio Regional Hospital	Martins Ferry	82%	66
Licking Memorial Hospital	Newark	79%	89
Saint Elizabeth Boardman Health Center	Youngstown	78%	135
Knox Community Hospital	Mount Vernon	76%	85
Bellevue Hospital	Bellevue	74%	73
Parma Community General Hospital	Parma	74%	263
Marietta Memorial Hospital	Marietta	71%	162
Mercer County Joint Twp Comm Hosp	Coldwater	71%	35
Fulton County Health Center	Wauseon	70%	141

NOTE: Hospital profiles are in alphabetical order by state, then city, then hospital within the city; Rankings exclude hospitals with less than 25 cases except for patient surveys which excludes hospitals with less than 100 cases; (a) 100–299 cases; (1) The number of cases is too small to be sure how well a hospital is performing; (2) The hospital indicated that the data submitted for this measure were based on a sample of cases; (3) Data was collected during a shorter time period (fewer quarters) than the maximum possible time for this measure; (4) Suppressed for one or more quarters by CMS; (5) No data is available from the hospital for this measure; (6) Fewer than 100 patients completed the HCAHPS survey. Use these rates with caution, as the number of surveys may be too low to reliably assess hospital performance; (7) Survey results are based on less than 12 months of data; (8) Survey results are not available for this reporting period; (9) No or very few patients were eligible for the HCAHPS survey. The scores shown, if any, reflect a very small number of surveys; (10) A state average was not calculated because too few hospitals in the state submitted data; (11) There were discrepancies in the data collection process; Please refer to the User's Guide for a full explanation of data.

Evendale Medical Center	Cincinnati	69%	232
Genesis Healthcare System	Zanesville	69%	188
South Pointe Hospital	Warrensville Hgts	69%	167
Surgical Hospital at Southwoods	Youngstown	66%	218
Memorial Hospital	Fremont	65%	79
Medical Center of Newark	Newark	63%	43
Amherst Hospital	Amherst	62%	29
Mount Carmel St Ann's Hospital	Westerville	61%	240
Mercy Tiffin Hospital	Tiffin	60%	43
Madison County Hospital	London	40%	40

28. Prophylactic Antibiotic Selection

Hospital Name	City	Rate	Cases
Affinity Medical Center	Massillon	100%	384
Alliance Community Hospital[2]	Alliance	100%	220
Amherst Hospital[2]	Amherst	100%	178
Cleveland-Wade Park VA Medical Center	Cleveland	100%	403
Crystal Clinic Orthopaedic Center[2,3]	Akron	100%	98
Dayton VA Medical Center	Dayton	100%	111
Euclid Hospital[2]	Euclid	100%	768
Evendale Medical Center	Cincinnati	100%	208
Grady Memorial Hospital	Delaware	100%	142
H B Magruder Memorial Hospital	Port Clinton	100%	41
Institute for Orthopedic Surgery[2]	Lima	100%	191
Kettering Medical Center[2]	Kettering	100%	2280
Kettering Medical Center - Sycamore[2]	Miamisburg	100%	305
Knox Community Hospital	Mount Vernon	100%	383
Medina Hospital[2]	Medina	100%	305
Mercy Franciscan Hospital - Mt Airy[2]	Cincinnati	100%	331
Mount Carmel New Albany Surgical Hospital[2]	New Albany	100%	469
Summa Western Reserve Hospital[2]	Cuyahoga Falls	100%	172
Univ Hosps Conneaut Med Ctr[3]	Conneaut	100%	76
Adena Regional Medical Center	Chillicothe	99%	744
Allen Community Hospital	Oberlin	99%	101
Ashtabula County Medical Center	Ashtabula	99%	149
Atrium Medical Center[2]	Franklin	99%	512
Berger Hospital[2]	Circleville	99%	284
Bucyrus Community Hospital	Bucyrus	99%	94
Community Hospitals and Wellness Centers	Bryan	99%	180
East Ohio Regional Hospital	Martins Ferry	99%	297
Fostoria Community Hospital	Fostoria	99%	135
Genesis Healthcare System[2]	Zanesville	99%	374
Grant Medical Center[2]	Columbus	99%	699
Holzer Medical Center Jackson	Jackson	99%	156
Jewish Hospital[2]	Cincinnati	99%	342
Lakewood Hospital	Lakewood	99%	364
Licking Memorial Hospital[2]	Newark	99%	278
Lima Memorial Health System[2]	Lima	99%	410
Lutheran Hospital[2]	Cleveland	99%	217
Marietta Memorial Hospital	Marietta	99%	476
Mercy Franciscan Hospital Western Hills[2]	Cincinnati	99%	194
Mercy Hospital Anderson[2]	Cincinnati	99%	695
Mercy Hospital Clermont[2]	Batavia	99%	269
Mercy Hospital of Defiance	Defiance	99%	85
Mercy St Charles Hospital[2]	Oregon	99%	345
Mercy St Vincent Medical Center[2]	Toledo	99%	681
Miami Valley Hospital[2]	Dayton	99%	499
Ohio Valley Medical Center[3]	Springfield	99%	202
Parma Community General Hospital	Parma	99%	822
Riverside Methodist Hospital[2]	Columbus	99%	2151
Saint Elizabeth Boardman Health Center[2]	Youngstown	99%	226
Saint John Medical Center[2]	Westlake	99%	289
Samaritan Hospital - Peoples Hospital	Ashland	99%	473
Summa Barberton Hospital	Barberton	99%	334
Summa Wadsworth-Rittman Hospital	Wadsworth	99%	127
UH Geauga Medical Center[2]	Chardon	99%	365
UHHS Bedford Medical Center	Bedford	99%	110
UHHS Richmond Heights Hospital	Richmond Hghts	99%	147
Union Hospital[2]	Dover	99%	268
Akron General Medical Center[2]	Akron	98%	448
Aultman Hospital[2]	Canton	98%	563
Bethesda North Hospital[2]	Cincinnati	98%	438
Blanchard Valley Hospital[2]	Findlay	98%	614
Christ Hospital[2]	Cincinnati	98%	504
Doctors Hospital[2]	Columbus	98%	391
Emh Regional Medical Center[2]	Elyria	98%	453
Fairfield Medical Center[2]	Lancaster	98%	769
Fisher Titus Memorial Hospital	Norwalk	98%	210
Flower Hospital[2]	Sylvania	98%	316
Fulton County Health Center	Wauseon	98%	208
Good Samaritan Hospital[2]	Dayton	98%	500
Hillcrest Hospital[2]	Mayfield Heights	98%	597
Madison County Hospital	London	98%	62
Marion General Hospital[2]	Marion	98%	409
McCullough-Hyde Memorial Hospital	Oxford	98%	208
Memorial Hospital of Union County	Marysville	98%	93
Mercy St Anne Hospital[2]	Toledo	98%	285
Mercy Tiffin Hospital	Tiffin	98%	136
Metro Health Medical Center[2]	Cleveland	98%	492
Mount Carmel Health[2]	Columbus	98%	851
Mount Carmel St Ann's Hospital[2]	Westerville	98%	380
Northside Medical Center	Youngstown	98%	836
Ohio State University Hospitals[2]	Columbus	98%	396
Saint Rita's Medical Center	Lima	98%	703
Southern Ohio Medical Center	Portsmouth	98%	610
Southwest General Health Center[2]	Middleburg Hgts	98%	895
Springfield Regional Medical Center	Springfield	98%	647
Trinity Medical Center East & West[2]	Steubenville	98%	415
University Hospitals of Cleveland[2]	Cleveland	98%	524
University of Toledo Medical Center[2]	Toledo	98%	345
West Chester Medical Center	West Chester	98%	300
Bay Park Community Hospital	Oregon	97%	264
Cincinnati VA Medical Center	Cincinnati	97%	152
Cleveland Clinic[2]	Cleveland	97%	1050
Community Regional Medical Center[2]	Lorain	97%	485
Good Samaritan Hospital[2]	Cincinnati	97%	446
Grandview Hospital & Medical Center[2]	Dayton	97%	786
Greene Memorial Hospital	Xenia	97%	155
Henry County Hospital	Napoleon	97%	39
Joel Pomerene Memorial Hospital	Millersburg	97%	64
Joint Township District Memorial Hospital	Saint Marys	97%	146
Mary Rutan Hospital	Bellefontaine	97%	208
Marymount Hospital[2]	Garfield Heights	97%	367
Memorial Hospital	Fremont	97%	174
Mercy Hospital Fairfield[2]	Fairfield	97%	716
Mercy Hospital of Willard	Willard	97%	36
Mercy Medical Center[2]	Canton	97%	617
The Toledo Hospital[2]	Toledo	97%	495
Trumbull Memorial Hospital[2]	Warren	97%	477
Wilson Memorial Hospital	Sidney	97%	108
Wyandot Memorial Hospital	Upper Sandusky	97%	29
CMH Regional Health System[2]	Wilmington	96%	188
Defiance Regional Medical Center	Defiance	96%	126
Galion Community Hospital[3]	Galion	96%	114
Hocking Valley Community Hospital	Logan	96%	51
Huron Hospital	Cleveland	96%	75
Lake Health[2]	Concord	96%	381
Medcentral Health System[2]	Mansfield	96%	647
O'Bleness Memorial Hospital	Athens	96%	71
Robinson Memorial Hospital[2]	Ravenna	96%	297
Saint Elizabeth Health Center[2]	Youngstown	96%	467
Saint Joseph Health Center[2]	Warren	96%	269
Saint Luke's Hospital	Maumee	96%	636
Saint Vincent Charity Medical Center[2]	Cleveland	96%	248
Selby General Hospital[3]	Marietta	96%	69
Upper Valley Medical Center	Troy	96%	266
Wood County Hospital	Bowling Green	96%	178
Butler County Medical Center	Hamilton	95%	186
Holzer Medical Center	Gallipolis	95%	179
Salem Community Hospital[2]	Salem	95%	228
South Pointe Hospital	Warrensville Hgts	95%	176
Summa Health Systems Hospitals[2]	Akron	95%	349
University Hospital[2]	Cincinnati	95%	435
Wooster Community Hospital	Wooster	95%	387
Bellevue Hospital	Bellevue	94%	140
Deaconess Hospital[2]	Cincinnati	94%	34
Medical Center of Newark	Newark	94%	72
Mercer County Joint Twp Comm Hosp	Coldwater	94%	96
Southeastern Ohio Regional Medical Center[2]	Cambridge	94%	143
Surgical Hospital at Southwoods[2]	Youngstown	94%	269
Coshocton County Memorial Hospital	Coshocton	93%	43
Dublin Methodist Hospital	Dublin	93%	95
East Liverpool City Hospital	East Liverpool	93%	94
Fairview Hospital[2]	Cleveland	93%	454
Fort Hamilton Hughes Memorial Hospital[2]	Hamilton	93%	184
Firelands Regional Medical Center[2]	Sandusky	91%	352
Van Wert County Hospital	Van Wert	89%	114
Highland District Hospital	Hillsboro	88%	25
Wayne Hospital	Greenville	88%	141
Medical Center at Elizabeth Place	Dayton	85%	65

29. Prophylactic Antibiotic Selection (Outpatient)

Hospital Name	City	Rate	Cases
Alliance Community Hospital	Alliance	100%	70
Crystal Clinic Orthopaedic Center[3]	Akron	100%	324
Dublin Methodist Hospital	Dublin	100%	536
Mount Carmel New Albany Surgical Hospital	New Albany	100%	502
UHHS Memorial Hospital of Geneva	Geneva	100%	51
West Chester Medical Center	West Chester	100%	65
Adena Regional Medical Center	Chillicothe	99%	307
Bay Park Community Hospital	Oregon	99%	73
Greene Memorial Hospital	Xenia	99%	70
Kettering Medical Center - Sycamore	Miamisburg	99%	169
Lima Memorial Health System	Lima	99%	359
Marion General Hospital	Marion	99%	197
Mercy Franciscan Hospital - Mt Airy	Cincinnati	99%	102
Summa Wadsworth-Rittman Hospital	Wadsworth	99%	80
Union Hospital	Dover	99%	139
Doctors Hospital	Columbus	98%	189
Euclid Hospital	Euclid	98%	86
Evendale Medical Center	Cincinnati	98%	165
Fayette County Memorial Hospital	Washington CH	98%	58
Holzer Medical Center	Gallipolis	98%	54
Institute for Orthopedic Surgery	Lima	98%	83
Mercy Medical Center	Canton	98%	767
Mercy St Charles Hospital	Oregon	98%	102
Riverside Methodist Hospital	Columbus	98%	780
Summa Barberton Hospital	Barberton	98%	113
Bethesda North Hospital	Cincinnati	97%	634
Blanchard Valley Hospital	Findlay	97%	538
Fort Hamilton Hughes Memorial Hospital	Hamilton	97%	78
Good Samaritan Hospital	Dayton	97%	593
Grant Medical Center	Columbus	97%	616
Kettering Medical Center	Kettering	97%	615
Mercy St Anne Hospital	Toledo	97%	99
Metro Health Medical Center	Cleveland	97%	687
Ohio State University Hospitals	Columbus	97%	370
Ohio Valley Medical Center[3]	Springfield	97%	31
UHHS Bedford Medical Center	Bedford	97%	70
Aultman Hospital	Canton	96%	1296
Bluffton Hospital	Bluffton	96%	104
Christ Hospital	Cincinnati	96%	825
Community Hospitals and Wellness Centers	Bryan	96%	79
Grandview Hospital & Medical Center	Dayton	96%	547
Joint Township District Memorial Hospital	Saint Marys	96%	28
Lake Health	Concord	96%	354
Lutheran Hospital	Cleveland	96%	222
Mercy Hospital Anderson	Cincinnati	96%	255
Miami Valley Hospital	Dayton	96%	913
Saint Luke's Hospital	Maumee	96%	254
Saint Rita's Medical Center	Lima	96%	266
Samaritan Hospital - Peoples Hospital	Ashland	96%	78
Atrium Medical Center	Franklin	95%	238
East Ohio Regional Hospital	Martins Ferry	95%	58
Emh Regional Medical Center	Elyria	95%	448
Mary Rutan Hospital	Bellefontaine	95%	63
Memorial Hospital of Union County	Marysville	95%	61
Robinson Memorial Hospital	Ravenna	95%	273
Saint Elizabeth Health Center	Youngstown	95%	511
Southern Ohio Medical Center	Portsmouth	95%	155
Trinity Medical Center East & West	Steubenville	95%	262
University of Toledo Medical Center	Toledo	95%	210
Wooster Community Hospital	Wooster	95%	170
Ashtabula County Medical Center	Ashtabula	94%	195
Community Regional Medical Center	Lorain	94%	307
Fairview Hospital	Cleveland	94%	666
Flower Hospital	Sylvania	94%	174
Grady Memorial Hospital	Delaware	94%	110
Hillcrest Hospital	Mayfield Heights	94%	619
Lakewood Hospital	Lakewood	94%	138
Marymount Hospital	Garfield Heights	94%	297
Northside Medical Center	Youngstown	94%	252
Salem Community Hospital	Salem	94%	82
Summa Western Reserve Hospital	Cuyahoga Falls	94%	118
Akron General Medical Center	Akron	93%	687
Butler County Medical Center	Hamilton	93%	75
Jewish Hospital	Cincinnati	93%	296
Marietta Memorial Hospital	Marietta	93%	126
Medina Hospital	Medina	93%	203
Memorial Hospital	Fremont	93%	54
Mount Carmel Health	Columbus	93%	746
The Toledo Hospital	Toledo	93%	581
UHHS Richmond Heights Hospital	Richmond Hghts	93%	90
University Hospital	Cincinnati	93%	375
Van Wert County Hospital	Van Wert	93%	88
Brown County Hospital	Georgetown	92%	36
Fairfield Medical Center	Lancaster	92%	388
Good Samaritan Hospital	Cincinnati	92%	586
Licking Memorial Hospital	Newark	92%	105
McCullough-Hyde Memorial Hospital	Oxford	92%	40
Saint Joseph Health Center	Warren	92%	226
Summa Health Systems Hospitals	Akron	92%	530
Fisher Titus Memorial Hospital	Norwalk	91%	88
Genesis Healthcare System	Zanesville	91%	182
Mount Carmel St Ann's Hospital	Westerville	91%	149
Saint Elizabeth Boardman Health Center	Youngstown	91%	119
Saint Vincent Charity Medical Center	Cleveland	91%	145
Southeastern Ohio Regional Medical Center	Cambridge	91%	145
Springfield Regional Medical Center	Springfield	91%	174
Upper Valley Medical Center	Troy	91%	96
Firelands Regional Medical Center	Sandusky	90%	254
Mercy Franciscan Hospital Western Hills	Cincinnati	90%	58
Mercy Hospital Fairfield	Fairfield	90%	181
Mercy St Vincent Medical Center	Toledo	90%	474
Affinity Medical Center	Massillon	89%	140
CMH Regional Health System	Wilmington	89%	122
Knox Community Hospital	Mount Vernon	89%	73
Southwest General Health Center	Middleburg Hgts	89%	349
Wayne Hospital	Greenville	89%	36
Wilson Memorial Hospital	Sidney	89%	113
Cleveland Clinic	Cleveland	88%	1336

NOTE: Hospital profiles are in alphabetical order by state, then city, then hospital within the city; Rankings exclude hospitals with less than 25 cases except for patient surveys which excludes hospitals with less than 100 cases; (a) 100–299 cases; (1) The number of cases is too small to be sure how well a hospital is performing; (2) The hospital indicated that the data submitted for this measure were based on a sample of cases; (3) Data was collected during a shorter time period (fewer quarters) than the maximum possible time for this measure; (4) Suppressed for one or more quarters by CMS; (5) No data is available from the hospital for this measure; (6) Fewer than 100 patients completed the HCAHPS survey. Use these rates with caution, as the number of surveys may be too low to reliably assess hospital performance; (7) Survey results are based on less than 12 months of data; (8) Survey results are not available for this reporting period; (9) No or very few patients were eligible for the HCAHPS survey. The scores shown, if any, reflect a very small number of surveys; (10) A state average was not calculated because too few hospitals in the state submitted data; (11) There were discrepancies in the data collection process; Please refer to the User's Guide for a full explanation of data.

Saint John Medical Center	Westlake	88%	269
University Hospitals of Cleveland	Cleveland	88%	670
Medcentral Health System	Mansfield	87%	275
O'Bleness Memorial Hospital	Athens	87%	197
Surgical Hospital at Southwoods	Youngstown	87%	182
Mercy Hospital Clermont	Batavia	86%	74
Berger Hospital	Circleville	85%	40
Medical Center of Newark	Newark	85%	27
Mercer County Joint Twp Comm Hosp	Coldwater	85%	27
Trumbull Memorial Hospital	Warren	85%	303
UH Geauga Medical Center	Chardon	85%	229
Medical Center at Elizabeth Place	Dayton	84%	109
South Pointe Hospital	Warrensville Hgts	82%	134
Fulton County Health Center	Wauseon	74%	121
Bellevue Hospital	Bellevue	71%	63
Parma Community General Hospital	Parma	70%	211
Mercy Tiffin Hospital	Tiffin	69%	62
Huron Hospital	Cleveland	54%	28
Wood County Hospital	Bowling Green	54%	104
Three Gables Surgery Center	Proctorville	22%	54

30. Prophylactic Antibiotic Stopped

Hospital Name	City	Rate	Cases
Allen Community Hospital	Oberlin	100%	99
Crystal Clinic Orthopaedic Center[2,3]	Akron	100%	98
Fostoria Community Hospital	Fostoria	100%	132
Highland District Hospital	Hillsboro	100%	25
Mercy Hospital of Willard	Willard	100%	33
Univ Hosps Conneaut Med Ctr[3]	Conneaut	100%	75
Akron General Medical Center[2]	Akron	99%	422
Cincinnati VA Medical Center	Cincinnati	99%	150
Community Regional Medical Center[2]	Lorain	99%	453
Dayton VA Medical Center	Dayton	99%	109
Doctors Hospital[2]	Columbus	99%	375
Euclid Hospital[2]	Euclid	99%	744
Grady Memorial Hospital	Delaware	99%	137
Grant Medical Center[2]	Columbus	99%	676
Kettering Medical Center[2]	Kettering	99%	2191
Kettering Medical Center - Sycamore[2]	Miamisburg	99%	294
Lakewood Hospital	Lakewood	99%	342
Lutheran Hospital[2]	Cleveland	99%	213
Mercy Franciscan Hospital Western Hills[2]	Cincinnati	99%	190
Mercy Hospital Anderson[2]	Cincinnati	99%	622
Mount Carmel New Albany Surgical Hospital[2]	New Albany	99%	462
Ohio Valley Medical Center[3]	Springfield	99%	200
Samaritan Hospital - Peoples Hospital	Ashland	99%	472
Summa Barberton Hospital	Barberton	99%	305
UHHS Bedford Medical Center	Bedford	99%	100
Atrium Medical Center[2]	Franklin	98%	483
Bucyrus Community Hospital	Bucyrus	98%	93
Dublin Methodist Hospital	Dublin	98%	94
Flower Hospital[2]	Sylvania	98%	295
Fulton County Health Center	Wauseon	98%	206
Huron Hospital	Cleveland	98%	64
Institute for Orthopedic Surgery[2]	Lima	98%	189
Jewish Hospital[2]	Cincinnati	98%	325
Marion General Hospital[2]	Marion	98%	397
Mary Rutan Hospital	Bellefontaine	98%	202
McCullough-Hyde Memorial Hospital	Oxford	98%	204
Mercy Hospital Clermont[2]	Batavia	98%	254
Mercy St Vincent Medical Center[2]	Toledo	98%	647
Mercy Tiffin Hospital	Tiffin	98%	134
Mount Carmel Health[2]	Columbus	98%	818
Ohio State University Hospitals[2]	Columbus	98%	371
Parma Community General Hospital	Parma	98%	790
Saint Elizabeth Boardman Health Center[2]	Youngstown	98%	219
Saint Joseph Health Center[2]	Warren	98%	253
Springfield Regional Medical Center	Springfield	98%	615
Union Hospital[2]	Dover	98%	254
West Chester Medical Center	West Chester	98%	288
Adena Regional Medical Center	Chillicothe	97%	704
Affinity Medical Center	Massillon	97%	355
Blanchard Valley Hospital[2]	Findlay	97%	585
Cleveland-Wade Park VA Medical Center	Cleveland	97%	379
CMH Regional Health System[2]	Wilmington	97%	187
Community Hospitals and Wellness Centers	Bryan	97%	175
Evendale Medical Center	Cincinnati	97%	206
Fairview Hospital[2]	Cleveland	97%	439
Genesis Healthcare System[2]	Zanesville	97%	359
Licking Memorial Hospital[2]	Newark	97%	266
Marymount Hospital[2]	Garfield Heights	97%	351
Medina Hospital[2]	Medina	97%	299
Mercy Franciscan Hospital - Mt Airy[2]	Cincinnati	97%	314
Mercy St Charles Hospital[2]	Oregon	97%	322
Riverside Methodist Hospital[2]	Columbus	97%	2064
Saint Elizabeth Health Center[2]	Youngstown	97%	445
Saint Luke's Hospital	Maumee	97%	609
Salem Community Hospital[2]	Salem	97%	222
Surgical Hospital at Southwoods[2]	Youngstown	97%	265
Trumbull Memorial Hospital[2]	Warren	97%	463
University of Toledo Medical Center[2]	Toledo	97%	295
Aultman Hospital[2]	Canton	96%	538
Bethesda North Hospital[2]	Cincinnati	96%	412
Christ Hospital[2]	Cincinnati	96%	456
Fairfield Medical Center[2]	Lancaster	96%	722
Fort Hamilton Hughes Memorial Hospital[2]	Hamilton	96%	155
Galion Community Hospital[3]	Galion	96%	112
Good Samaritan Hospital[2]	Cincinnati	96%	417
Grandview Hospital & Medical Center[2]	Dayton	96%	737
Marietta Memorial Hospital	Marietta	96%	451
Mercy Hospital of Defiance	Defiance	96%	83
Mount Carmel St Ann's Hospital[2]	Westerville	96%	364
South Pointe Hospital	Warrensville Hgts	96%	169
Southern Ohio Medical Center	Portsmouth	96%	565
Summa Wadsworth-Rittman Hospital	Wadsworth	96%	124
UHHS Richmond Heights Hospital	Richmond Hghts	96%	142
Berger Hospital[2]	Circleville	95%	274
Butler County Medical Center	Hamilton	95%	180
Defiance Regional Medical Center	Defiance	95%	114
Greene Memorial Hospital	Xenia	95%	150
Knox Community Hospital	Mount Vernon	95%	373
Mercy Hospital Fairfield[2]	Fairfield	95%	691
Robinson Memorial Hospital[2]	Ravenna	95%	279
Southeastern Ohio Regional Medical Center[2]	Cambridge	95%	131
Southwest General Health Center[2]	Middleburg Hgts	95%	879
Wooster Community Hospital	Wooster	95%	385
Bay Park Community Hospital	Oregon	94%	252
East Ohio Regional Hospital	Martins Ferry	94%	293
Hocking Valley Community Hospital	Logan	94%	51
Mercer County Joint Twp Comm Hosp	Coldwater	94%	95
Mercy St Anne Hospital[2]	Toledo	94%	267
Metro Health Medical Center[2]	Cleveland	94%	466
Northside Medical Center	Youngstown	94%	816
Saint John Medical Center[2]	Westlake	94%	265
Firelands Regional Medical Center[2]	Sandusky	93%	342
Joel Pomerene Memorial Hospital	Millersburg	93%	61
Lima Memorial Health System[2]	Lima	93%	382
Madison County Hospital	London	93%	59
Memorial Hospital of Union County	Marysville	93%	90
Summa Western Reserve Hospital[2]	Cuyahoga Falls	93%	165
University Hospital[2]	Cincinnati	93%	409
University Hospitals of Cleveland[2]	Cleveland	93%	502
Cleveland Clinic[2]	Cleveland	92%	989
Fisher Titus Memorial Hospital	Norwalk	92%	200
Good Samaritan Hospital[2]	Dayton	92%	464
H B Magruder Memorial Hospital	Port Clinton	92%	38
Hillcrest Hospital[2]	Mayfield Heights	92%	580
Holzer Medical Center Jackson	Jackson	92%	158
Joint Township District Memorial Hospital	Saint Marys	92%	142
Medcentral Health System[2]	Mansfield	92%	624
Medical Center at Elizabeth Place	Dayton	92%	63
Saint Rita's Medical Center	Lima	92%	669
UH Geauga Medical Center[2]	Chardon	92%	350
Ashtabula County Medical Center	Ashtabula	91%	135
Bellevue Hospital	Bellevue	91%	137
Deaconess Hospital[2]	Cincinnati	91%	33
Mercy Medical Center[2]	Canton	91%	594
Saint Vincent Charity Medical Center[2]	Cleveland	91%	238
Selby General Hospital[3]	Marietta	91%	67
The Toledo Hospital[2]	Toledo	91%	468
Trinity Medical Center East & West[2]	Steubenville	91%	400
Van Wert County Hospital	Van Wert	91%	107
Amherst Hospital[2]	Amherst	90%	173
Miami Valley Hospital[2]	Dayton	90%	465
Upper Valley Medical Center	Troy	90%	250
Wyandot Memorial Hospital	Upper Sandusky	90%	29
Summa Health Systems Hospitals[2]	Akron	88%	329
Wood County Hospital	Bowling Green	88%	171
Holzer Medical Center	Gallipolis	87%	175
Wilson Memorial Hospital	Sidney	87%	108
East Liverpool City Hospital	East Liverpool	85%	88
Henry County Hospital	Napoleon	85%	39
Alliance Community Hospital[2]	Alliance	84%	206
O'Bleness Memorial Hospital	Athens	83%	71
Lake Health[2]	Concord	82%	355
Wayne Hospital	Greenville	82%	137
Coshocton County Memorial Hospital	Coshocton	81%	42
Emh Regional Medical Center[2]	Elyria	79%	442
Medical Center of Newark	Newark	76%	71
Memorial Hospital	Fremont	71%	171

31. Recommended VTP Ordered

Hospital Name	City	Rate	Cases
Affinity Medical Center	Massillon	100%	134
Grant Medical Center[2]	Columbus	100%	188
Kettering Medical Center[2]	Kettering	100%	617
Kettering Medical Center - Sycamore[2]	Miamisburg	100%	215
Mercy Hospital Anderson[2]	Cincinnati	100%	207
Mount Carmel New Albany Surgical Hospital[2]	New Albany	100%	31
Ohio Valley Medical Center[3]	Springfield	100%	26
Selby General Hospital[3]	Marietta	100%	32
University of Toledo Medical Center[2]	Toledo	100%	152
Atrium Medical Center[2]	Franklin	99%	312
Cincinnati VA Medical Center[2]	Cincinnati	99%	139
Doctors Hospital[2]	Columbus	99%	137
Fort Hamilton Hughes Memorial Hospital[2]	Hamilton	99%	147
Grady Memorial Hospital	Delaware	99%	96
Mercy Hospital Clermont[2]	Batavia	99%	158
Mount Carmel St Ann's Hospital[2]	Westerville	99%	150
Riverside Methodist Hospital[2]	Columbus	99%	881
Union Hospital[2]	Dover	99%	114
University Hospitals of Cleveland[2]	Cleveland	99%	251
Akron General Medical Center[2]	Akron	98%	248
Christ Hospital[2]	Cincinnati	98%	148
Euclid Hospital[2]	Euclid	98%	214
Huron Hospital	Cleveland	98%	127
Lutheran Hospital[2]	Cleveland	98%	130
Marion General Hospital[2]	Marion	98%	195
Mercy Franciscan Hospital - Mt Airy[2]	Cincinnati	98%	130
Mercy Franciscan Hospital Western Hills[2]	Cincinnati	98%	156
Mercy Hospital of Defiance	Defiance	98%	62
Mercy Tiffin Hospital	Tiffin	98%	50
Metro Health Medical Center[2]	Cleveland	98%	219
Samaritan Hospital - Peoples Hospital	Ashland	98%	60
University Hospital[2]	Cincinnati	98%	214
Upper Valley Medical Center	Troy	98%	185
Wilson Memorial Hospital	Sidney	98%	54
Bay Park Community Hospital	Oregon	97%	114
Bucyrus Community Hospital	Bucyrus	97%	33
CMH Regional Health System[2]	Wilmington	97%	66
Community Hospitals and Wellness Centers	Bryan	97%	101
Community Regional Medical Center[2]	Lorain	97%	260
Dublin Methodist Hospital	Dublin	97%	75
Grandview Hospital & Medical Center[2]	Dayton	97%	277
Lakewood Hospital	Lakewood	97%	245
Marietta Memorial Hospital	Marietta	97%	215
Mercy St Anne Hospital[2]	Toledo	97%	170
Mercy St Vincent Medical Center[2]	Toledo	97%	175
Saint Elizabeth Health Center[2]	Youngstown	97%	175
Saint Luke's Hospital	Maumee	97%	203
Saint Vincent Charity Medical Center[2]	Cleveland	97%	120
Summa Barberton Hospital	Barberton	97%	279
UHHS Richmond Heights Hospital	Richmond Hghts	97%	75
Cleveland Clinic[2]	Cleveland	96%	462
Greene Memorial Hospital	Xenia	96%	83
Hillcrest Hospital[2]	Mayfield Heights	96%	307
Hocking Valley Community Hospital	Logan	96%	25
Joel Pomerene Memorial Hospital	Millersburg	96%	45
Lima Memorial Health System[2]	Lima	96%	141
Mary Rutan Hospital	Bellefontaine	96%	83
McCullough-Hyde Memorial Hospital	Oxford	96%	121
Mount Carmel Health[2]	Columbus	96%	209
Northside Medical Center	Youngstown	96%	269
Ohio State University Hospitals[2]	Columbus	96%	184
South Pointe Hospital	Warrensville Hgts	96%	141
Wayne Hospital	Greenville	96%	82
Ashtabula County Medical Center	Ashtabula	95%	77
Berger Hospital[2]	Circleville	95%	84
Bethesda North Hospital[2]	Cincinnati	95%	173
Dayton VA Medical Center[2]	Dayton	95%	40
Fairfield Medical Center[2]	Lancaster	95%	214
Fairview Hospital[2]	Cleveland	95%	286
Good Samaritan Hospital[2]	Cincinnati	95%	119
Saint Joseph Health Center[2]	Warren	95%	151
Saint Rita's Medical Center	Lima	95%	388
Summa Health Systems Hospitals[2]	Akron	95%	150
Summa Wadsworth-Rittman Hospital	Wadsworth	95%	57
West Chester Medical Center	West Chester	95%	130
Aultman Hospital[2]	Canton	94%	206
Cleveland-Wade Park VA Medical Center[2]	Cleveland	94%	254
Defiance Regional Medical Center	Defiance	94%	48
Flower Hospital[2]	Sylvania	94%	202
Genesis Healthcare System[2]	Zanesville	94%	108
Jewish Hospital[2]	Cincinnati	94%	132
Mercy Hospital Fairfield[2]	Fairfield	94%	260
Mercy Medical Center[2]	Canton	94%	205
O'Bleness Memorial Hospital	Athens	94%	52
Parma Community General Hospital	Parma	94%	321
Saint Elizabeth Boardman Health Center[2]	Youngstown	94%	157
UH Geauga Medical Center[2]	Chardon	94%	156
Amherst Hospital[2]	Amherst	93%	27
Emh Regional Medical Center[2]	Elyria	93%	199
Knox Community Hospital	Mount Vernon	93%	86
Firelands Regional Medical Center[2]	Sandusky	92%	145
Good Samaritan Hospital[2]	Dayton	92%	123
Medina Hospital[2]	Medina	92%	152
Mercer County Joint Twp Comm Hosp	Coldwater	92%	50
Mercy St Charles Hospital[2]	Oregon	92%	170
Miami Valley Hospital[2]	Dayton	92%	206
Southern Ohio Medical Center	Portsmouth	92%	238
Adena Regional Medical Center	Chillicothe	91%	268

NOTE: Hospital profiles are in alphabetical order by state, then city, then hospital within the city; Rankings exclude hospitals with less than 25 cases except for patient surveys which excludes hospitals with less than 100 cases; (a) 100–299 cases; (1) The number of cases is too small to be sure how well a hospital is performing; (2) The hospital indicated that the data submitted for this measure were based on a sample of cases; (3) Data was collected during a shorter time period (fewer quarters) than the maximum possible time for this measure; (4) Suppressed for one or more quarters by CMS; (5) No data is available from the hospital for this measure; (6) Fewer than 100 patients completed the HCAHPS survey. Use these rates with caution, as the number of surveys may be too low to reliably assess hospital performance; (7) Survey results are based on less than 12 months of data; (8) Survey results are not available for this reporting period; (9) No or very few patients were eligible for the HCAHPS survey. The scores shown, if any, reflect a very small number of surveys; (10) A state average was not calculated because too few hospitals in the state submitted data; (11) There were discrepancies in the data collection process; Please refer to the User's Guide for a full explanation of data.

Robinson Memorial Hospital[2]	Ravenna	91%	176
Southwest General Health Center[2]	Middleburg Hgts	91%	160
Springfield Regional Medical Center	Springfield	91%	386
The Toledo Hospital[2]	Toledo	91%	152
Trinity Medical Center East & West[2]	Steubenville	91%	139
UHHS Bedford Medical Center	Bedford	91%	94
Fisher Titus Memorial Hospital	Norwalk	90%	82
Medcentral Health System[2]	Mansfield	90%	289
Joint Township District Memorial Hospital	Saint Marys	89%	70
Trumbull Memorial Hospital[2]	Warren	89%	197
Blanchard Valley Hospital[2]	Findlay	88%	184
Summa Western Reserve Hospital[2]	Cuyahoga Falls	88%	84
Wood County Hospital	Bowling Green	88%	118
Licking Memorial Hospital[2]	Newark	87%	121
Marymount Hospital[2]	Garfield Heights	87%	182
Saint John Medical Center[2]	Westlake	87%	160
Southeastern Ohio Regional Medical Center[2]	Cambridge	87%	90
Holzer Medical Center	Gallipolis	86%	98
Bellevue Hospital	Bellevue	84%	69
Madison County Hospital	London	84%	32
East Liverpool City Hospital	East Liverpool	83%	53
Fulton County Health Center	Wauseon	82%	50
Memorial Hospital of Union County	Marysville	82%	33
Coshocton County Memorial Hospital	Coshocton	81%	31
Van Wert County Hospital	Van Wert	81%	62
Memorial Hospital	Fremont	80%	64
Holzer Medical Center Jackson	Jackson	79%	34
East Ohio Regional Hospital	Martins Ferry	77%	90
Alliance Community Hospital[2]	Alliance	76%	120
Salem Community Hospital[2]	Salem	76%	135
Wooster Community Hospital	Wooster	75%	75
Lake Health[2]	Concord	72%	146
Medical Center of Newark	Newark	70%	43

32. Urinary Catheter Removal

Hospital Name	City	Rate	Cases
Allen Community Hospital	Oberlin	100%	49
Berger Hospital[2]	Circleville	100%	103
Bucyrus Community Hospital	Bucyrus	100%	30
CMH Regional Health System[2]	Wilmington	100%	76
Mercy Franciscan Hospital Western Hills[2]	Cincinnati	100%	26
Mercy Hospital of Defiance	Defiance	100%	35
Mount Carmel New Albany Surgical Hospital[2]	New Albany	100%	183
Univ Hosps Conneaut Med Ctr	Conneaut	100%	74
Affinity Medical Center	Massillon	99%	147
Community Regional Medical Center[2]	Lorain	99%	156
Good Samaritan Hospital[2]	Cincinnati	99%	87
Kettering Medical Center[2]	Kettering	99%	683
Knox Community Hospital	Mount Vernon	99%	115
Lakewood Hospital	Lakewood	99%	175
Mercy St Anne Hospital[2]	Toledo	99%	103
Saint Elizabeth Health Center[2]	Youngstown	99%	143
Samaritan Hospital - Peoples Hospital	Ashland	99%	164
Southern Ohio Medical Center	Portsmouth	99%	214
Surgical Hospital at Southwoods[2]	Youngstown	99%	68
Atrium Medical Center	Franklin	98%	167
Deaconess Hospital[2]	Cincinnati	98%	41
Doctors Hospital[2]	Columbus	98%	122
Grant Medical Center[2]	Columbus	98%	218
Greene Memorial Hospital	Xenia	98%	63
Lutheran Hospital[2]	Cleveland	98%	126
Mercy St Charles Hospital[2]	Oregon	98%	142
Mercy St Vincent Medical Center[2]	Toledo	98%	172
Saint Elizabeth Boardman Health Center[2]	Youngstown	98%	103
University of Toledo Medical Center[2]	Toledo	98%	102
Adena Regional Medical Center	Chillicothe	97%	240
Community Hospitals and Wellness Centers	Bryan	97%	35
Evendale Medical Center	Cincinnati	97%	110
Holzer Medical Center Jackson	Jackson	97%	29
Parma Community General Hospital	Parma	97%	325
Saint Joseph Health Center[2]	Warren	97%	63
West Chester Medical Center	West Chester	97%	145
Fort Hamilton Hughes Memorial Hospital	Hamilton	96%	48
Kettering Medical Center - Sycamore[2]	Miamisburg	96%	50
Mercy Hospital Anderson[2]	Cincinnati	96%	204
Union Hospital	Dover	96%	69
Wilson Memorial Hospital	Sidney	96%	25
Fisher Titus Memorial Hospital	Norwalk	95%	113
Good Samaritan Hospital[2]	Dayton	95%	148
Mount Carmel Health[2]	Columbus	95%	344
Aultman Hospital[2]	Canton	94%	168
Flower Hospital[2]	Sylvania	94%	100
Memorial Hospital	Fremont	94%	62
UHHS Richmond Heights Hospital	Richmond Hghts	94%	71
Upper Valley Medical Center	Troy	94%	34
Cleveland-Wade Park VA Medical Center[2]	Cleveland	93%	215
Euclid Hospital[2]	Euclid	93%	369
Grady Memorial Hospital	Delaware	93%	60
Metro Health Medical Center[2]	Cleveland	93%	163
Riverside Methodist Hospital	Columbus	93%	1408
Southeastern Ohio Regional Medical Center[2]	Cambridge	93%	44
Grandview Hospital & Medical Center[2]	Dayton	92%	95
Marietta Memorial Hospital	Marietta	92%	131
McCullough-Hyde Memorial Hospital	Oxford	92%	77
Mount Carmel St Ann's Hospital[2]	Westerville	92%	104
Northside Medical Center	Youngstown	92%	177
Saint John Medical Center[2]	Westlake	92%	114
Jewish Hospital[2]	Cincinnati	91%	35
Mercy Hospital Fairfield[2]	Fairfield	91%	249
Ohio State University Hospitals[2]	Columbus	91%	145
Ohio Valley Medical Center	Springfield	91%	68
Saint Luke's Hospital	Maumee	91%	57
Christ Hospital[2]	Cincinnati	90%	156
East Ohio Regional Hospital	Martins Ferry	90%	113
Southwest General Health Center[2]	Middleburg Hgts	90%	317
Cleveland Clinic[2]	Cleveland	89%	313
Fairview Hospital[2]	Cleveland	89%	142
Firelands Regional Medical Center[2]	Sandusky	89%	135
Licking Memorial Hospital	Newark	89%	85
Marymount Hospital[2]	Garfield Heights	89%	139
Mercer County Joint Twp Comm Hosp	Coldwater	89%	28
Miami Valley Hospital[2]	Dayton	89%	137
Summa Western Reserve Hospital[2]	Cuyahoga Falls	89%	53
Amherst Hospital[2]	Amherst	88%	91
Mercy Medical Center[2]	Canton	88%	159
Summa Barberton Hospital	Barberton	88%	42
The Toledo Hospital[2]	Toledo	88%	153
Bay Park Community Hospital	Oregon	87%	127
Fairfield Medical Center[2]	Lancaster	87%	234
O'Bleness Memorial Hospital	Athens	87%	30
Trinity Medical Center East & West[2]	Steubenville	87%	110
UH Geauga Medical Center[2]	Chardon	87%	140
University Hospitals of Cleveland[2]	Cleveland	87%	210
Bellevue Hospital	Bellevue	86%	36
Springfield Regional Medical Center	Springfield	86%	99
Saint Vincent Charity Medical Center[2]	Cleveland	85%	143
Medical Center of Newark	Newark	84%	32
Mercy Hospital Clermont[2]	Batavia	84%	89
Robinson Memorial Hospital[2]	Ravenna	84%	89
Salem Community Hospital[2]	Salem	84%	91
South Pointe Hospital	Warrensville Hgts	84%	76
Bethesda North Hospital[2]	Cincinnati	83%	135
Mercy Franciscan Hospital - Mt Airy[2]	Cincinnati	83%	36
Akron General Medical Center[2]	Akron	82%	105
Blanchard Valley Hospital[2]	Findlay	82%	131
Saint Rita's Medical Center	Lima	82%	171
Mary Rutan Hospital	Bellefontaine	81%	67
Holzer Medical Center	Gallipolis	80%	44
Hillcrest Hospital[2]	Mayfield Heights	79%	160
Marion General Hospital[2]	Marion	79%	156
Medina Hospital	Medina	79%	123
Trumbull Memorial Hospital[2]	Warren	79%	57
University Hospital[2]	Cincinnati	79%	131
Emh Regional Medical Center[2]	Elyria	76%	142
Lake Health[2]	Concord	76%	97
Joint Township District Memorial Hospital	Saint Marys	75%	40
Medcentral Health System[2]	Mansfield	74%	213
Summa Health Systems Hospitals[2]	Akron	72%	90
Wayne Hospital	Greenville	65%	37
Alliance Community Hospital[2]	Alliance	64%	56
Lima Memorial Health System[2]	Lima	64%	78
Genesis Healthcare System[2]	Zanesville	60%	52
Wood County Hospital	Bowling Green	53%	70

Children's Asthma Care

33. Received Systemic Corticosteroids

Hospital Name	City	Rate	Cases
Cleveland Clinic	Cleveland	100%	30
Saint John Medical Center[2]	Westlake	100%	28
The Toledo Hospital	Toledo	100%	201
University Hospitals of Cleveland	Cleveland	99%	378

34. Received Home Management Plan of Care

Hospital Name	City	Rate	Cases
The Toledo Hospital	Toledo	95%	201
University Hospitals of Cleveland	Cleveland	95%	380
Cleveland Clinic	Cleveland	0%	29

35. Received Reliever Medication

Hospital Name	City	Rate	Cases
Cleveland Clinic	Cleveland	100%	30
Saint John Medical Center[2]	Westlake	100%	28
The Toledo Hospital	Toledo	100%	201
University Hospitals of Cleveland	Cleveland	100%	380

Use of Medical Imaging

36. Combination Abdominal CT Scan

Hospital Name	City	Ratio	Cases
Amherst Hospital	Amherst	0.000	97
Huron Hospital	Cleveland	0.019	158
Licking Memorial Hospital	Newark	0.019	1257
Mercy St Anne Hospital	Toledo	0.021	473
Flower Hospital	Sylvania	0.022	458
Mercy St Charles Hospital	Oregon	0.022	811
Mercy St Vincent Medical Center	Toledo	0.023	436
Wayne Hospital	Greenville	0.024	458
Ashtabula County Medical Center	Ashtabula	0.027	634
Greenfield Area Medical Center	Greenfield	0.027	110
Marion General Hospital	Marion	0.027	221
Ohio State University Hospitals	Columbus	0.028	1351
Saint Elizabeth Boardman Health Center	Youngstown	0.028	496
Grant Medical Center	Columbus	0.032	658
Dublin Methodist Hospital	Dublin	0.035	142
Medcentral Health System	Mansfield	0.035	1143
Adena Regional Medical Center	Chillicothe	0.039	1190
Grady Memorial Hospital	Delaware	0.040	346
Brown County Hospital	Georgetown	0.041	241
Holzer Medical Center Jackson	Jackson	0.041	416
Parma Community General Hospital	Parma	0.041	1159
Madison County Hospital	London	0.042	165
Fayette County Memorial Hospital	Washington CH	0.044	343
Bay Park Community Hospital	Oregon	0.045	246
Lake Health	Concord	0.045	1628
Mercy Hospital Fairfield	Fairfield	0.045	1221
Lima Memorial Health System	Lima	0.046	694
Mercy Hospital of Defiance	Defiance	0.046	151
Good Samaritan Hospital	Dayton	0.047	1102
Lakewood Hospital	Lakewood	0.047	444
Mary Rutan Hospital	Bellefontaine	0.048	504
Berger Hospital	Circleville	0.049	546
Community Hospitals and Wellness Centers	Bryan	0.049	246
Lutheran Hospital	Cleveland	0.049	243
Saint Vincent Charity Medical Center	Cleveland	0.049	288
The Toledo Hospital	Toledo	0.049	790
Mount Carmel Health	Columbus	0.050	2279
Community Regional Medical Center	Lorain	0.051	995
Emh Regional Medical Center	Elyria	0.053	1118
Metro Health Medical Center	Cleveland	0.054	782
Fort Hamilton Hughes Memorial Hospital	Hamilton	0.057	645
Northside Medical Center	Youngstown	0.057	530
Saint John Medical Center	Westlake	0.057	526
Southwest General Health Center	Middleburg Hgts	0.057	1359
McCullough-Hyde Memorial Hospital	Oxford	0.059	358
Mount Carmel St Ann's Hospital	Westerville	0.060	815
Bluffton Hospital	Bluffton	0.061	99
Holzer Medical Center	Gallipolis	0.061	294
Atrium Medical Center	Franklin	0.062	961
Medical Center at Elizabeth Place	Dayton	0.063	80
Euclid Hospital	Euclid	0.065	291
Upper Valley Medical Center	Troy	0.066	869
Affinity Medical Center	Massillon	0.067	478
South Pointe Hospital	Warrensville Hgts	0.067	869
Christ Hospital	Cincinnati	0.069	1411
Samaritan Hospital - Peoples Hospital	Ashland	0.069	506
Aultman Hospital	Canton	0.071	1864
Mercy Hospital Anderson	Cincinnati	0.072	1074
Fairview Hospital	Cleveland	0.073	926
Summa Barberton Hospital	Barberton	0.073	506
Doctors Hospital	Columbus	0.074	498
O'Bleness Memorial Hospital	Athens	0.074	350
Summa Western Reserve Hospital	Cuyahoga Falls	0.075	254
Lodi Community Hospital	Lodi	0.076	105
Miami Valley Hospital	Dayton	0.076	2133
Wood County Hospital	Bowling Green	0.077	469
University Hospital	Cincinnati	0.078	688
East Liverpool City Hospital	East Liverpool	0.079	390
Fairfield Medical Center	Lancaster	0.081	853
Good Samaritan Hospital	Cincinnati	0.082	939
Springfield Regional Medical Center	Springfield	0.083	1085
Genesis Healthcare System	Zanesville	0.085	756
Butler County Medical Center	Hamilton	0.087	286
Jewish Hospital	Cincinnati	0.087	1196
Kettering Medical Center - Sycamore	Miamisburg	0.088	922
Memorial Hospital of Union County	Marysville	0.088	306
Saint Luke's Hospital	Maumee	0.088	826
Saint Rita's Medical Center	Lima	0.091	1586
UH Geauga Medical Center	Chardon	0.096	500
Bethesda North Hospital	Cincinnati	0.098	1959
Coshocton County Memorial Hospital	Coshocton	0.098	315
Joel Pomerene Memorial Hospital	Millersburg	0.101	109
Summa Wadsworth-Rittman Hospital	Wadsworth	0.101	415
Union Hospital	Dover	0.101	759
Salem Community Hospital	Salem	0.102	811
Akron General Medical Center	Akron	0.105	1703
University Pointe Surgical Hospital	West Chester	0.105	267

NOTE: Hospital profiles are in alphabetical order by state, then city, then hospital within the city; Rankings exclude hospitals with less than 25 cases except for patient surveys which excludes hospitals with less than 100 cases; (a) 100–299 cases; (1) The number of cases is too small to be sure how well a hospital is performing; (2) The hospital indicated that the data submitted for this measure were based on a sample of cases; (3) Data was collected during a shorter time period (fewer quarters) than the maximum possible time for this measure; (4) Suppressed for one or more quarters by CMS; (5) No data is available from the hospital for this measure; (6) Fewer than 100 patients completed the HCAHPS survey. Use these rates with caution, as the number of surveys may be too low to reliably assess hospital performance; (7) Survey results are based on less than 12 months of data; (8) Survey results are not available for this reporting period; (9) No or very few patients were eligible for the HCAHPS survey. The scores shown, if any, reflect a very small number of surveys; (10) A state average was not calculated because too few hospitals in the state submitted data; (11) There were discrepancies in the data collection process; Please refer to the User's Guide for a full explanation of data.

Fisher Titus Memorial Hospital	Norwalk	0.106	395
Greene Memorial Hospital	Xenia	0.107	467
UHHS Bedford Medical Center	Bedford	0.107	262
Riverside Methodist Hospital	Columbus	0.113	2908
Summa Health Systems Hospitals	Akron	0.116	1395
Kettering Medical Center	Kettering	0.119	1540
Blanchard Valley Hospital	Findlay	0.121	1107
Mercy Medical Center	Canton	0.122	1174
Wooster Community Hospital	Wooster	0.124	507
Saint Elizabeth Health Center	Youngstown	0.131	883
Mercer County Joint Twp Comm Hosp	Coldwater	0.142	254
UHHS Memorial Hospital of Geneva	Geneva	0.142	431
Medical Center of Newark	Newark	0.145	276
Univ Hosps Conneaut Med Ctr	Conneaut	0.146	178
Mercy Franciscan Hospital - Mt Airy	Cincinnati	0.148	779
Robinson Memorial Hospital	Ravenna	0.148	751
Firelands Regional Medical Center	Sandusky	0.150	851
Belmont Community Hospital	Bellaire	0.152	79
Southeastern Ohio Regional Medical Center	Cambridge	0.156	598
Fulton County Health Center	Wauseon	0.173	387
Barnesville Hospital Association	Barnesville	0.181	177
Mercy Hospital Clermont	Batavia	0.187	646
Wilson Memorial Hospital	Sidney	0.236	364
Marymount Hospital	Garfield Heights	0.244	766
Morrow County Hospital	Mount Gilead	0.256	215
Grandview Hospital & Medical Center	Dayton	0.263	1413
Mercy Hospital of Willard	Willard	0.281	139
UHHS Richmond Heights Hospital	Richmond Hghts	0.294	272
Medina Hospital	Medina	0.310	675
Cleveland Clinic	Cleveland	0.311	3773
Mercy Franciscan Hospital Western Hills	Cincinnati	0.315	930
Bellevue Hospital	Bellevue	0.330	306
University of Toledo Medical Center	Toledo	0.341	505
Hillcrest Hospital	Mayfield Heights	0.403	1485
Deaconess Hospital	Cincinnati	0.484	215
Knox Community Hospital	Mount Vernon	0.540	611
Southern Ohio Medical Center	Portsmouth	0.547	1527
CMH Regional Health System	Wilmington	0.563	528
Joint Township District Memorial Hospital	Saint Marys	0.582	354
University Hospitals of Cleveland	Cleveland	0.604	2483
Highland District Hospital	Hillsboro	0.613	507
East Ohio Regional Hospital	Martins Ferry	0.632	277
Memorial Hospital	Fremont	0.639	468
Trumbull Memorial Hospital	Warren	0.648	1081
Trinity Medical Center East & West	Steubenville	0.659	543
Saint Joseph Health Center	Warren	0.662	749
Van Wert County Hospital	Van Wert	0.672	421
Alliance Community Hospital	Alliance	0.678	574
Mercy Tiffin Hospital	Tiffin	0.691	431
Selby General Hospital	Marietta	0.727	143
Marietta Memorial Hospital	Marietta	0.755	783

37. Combination Chest CT Scan

Hospital Name	City	Ratio	Cases
Amherst Hospital	Amherst	0.000	47
Belmont Community Hospital	Bellaire	0.000	100
Euclid Hospital	Euclid	0.000	248
Genesis Healthcare System	Zanesville	0.000	485
Hillcrest Hospital	Mayfield Heights	0.000	1074
Holzer Medical Center Jackson	Jackson	0.000	107
Joel Pomerene Memorial Hospital	Millersburg	0.000	99
Licking Memorial Hospital	Newark	0.000	666
Lutheran Hospital	Cleveland	0.000	123
Madison County Hospital	London	0.000	128
McCullough-Hyde Memorial Hospital	Oxford	0.000	273
Medical Center of Newark	Newark	0.000	165
Mercy Franciscan Hospital - Mt Airy	Cincinnati	0.000	664
Mercy St Anne Hospital	Toledo	0.000	315
O'Bleness Memorial Hospital	Athens	0.000	161
Robinson Memorial Hospital	Ravenna	0.000	437
Saint John Medical Center	Westlake	0.000	519
Saint Vincent Charity Medical Center	Cleveland	0.000	189
Selby General Hospital	Marietta	0.000	91
Wayne Hospital	Greenville	0.000	308
Emh Regional Medical Center	Elyria	0.001	722
Mercy Medical Center	Canton	0.001	814
Salem Community Hospital	Salem	0.001	710
Summa Health Systems Hospitals	Akron	0.001	1495
Cleveland Clinic	Cleveland	0.002	3973
Fairfield Medical Center	Lancaster	0.002	550
Fort Hamilton Hughes Memorial Hospital	Hamilton	0.002	441
Good Samaritan Hospital	Cincinnati	0.002	919
Mercy Hospital Anderson	Cincinnati	0.002	930
Mercy St Vincent Medical Center	Toledo	0.002	410
Fairview Hospital	Cleveland	0.003	641
Mercy Hospital Clermont	Batavia	0.003	633
Mercy St Charles Hospital	Oregon	0.003	667
Northside Medical Center	Youngstown	0.003	333
Ashtabula County Medical Center	Ashtabula	0.004	560
Bay Park Community Hospital	Oregon	0.004	254
Butler County Medical Center	Hamilton	0.004	244
Lake Health	Concord	0.004	1310
UHHS Memorial Hospital of Geneva	Geneva	0.004	508
Lima Memorial Health System	Lima	0.005	582
Summa Western Reserve Hospital	Cuyahoga Falls	0.005	205
Union Hospital	Dover	0.005	610
East Ohio Regional Hospital	Martins Ferry	0.006	340
Fayette County Memorial Hospital	Washington CH	0.006	176
Akron General Medical Center	Akron	0.007	1532
University Hospitals of Cleveland	Cleveland	0.007	2916
Marymount Hospital	Garfield Heights	0.008	502
Trumbull Memorial Hospital	Warren	0.008	846
Grant Medical Center	Columbus	0.009	441
Holzer Medical Center	Gallipolis	0.009	110
Univ Hosps Conneaut Med Ctr	Conneaut	0.009	108
University Pointe Surgical Hospital	West Chester	0.009	326
Bethesda North Hospital	Cincinnati	0.010	1878
Grady Memorial Hospital	Delaware	0.010	195
Jewish Hospital	Cincinnati	0.010	955
Mercy Franciscan Hospital Western Hills	Cincinnati	0.010	820
Summa Barberton Hospital	Barberton	0.010	311
Upper Valley Medical Center	Troy	0.010	711
Berger Hospital	Circleville	0.011	366
Christ Hospital	Cincinnati	0.011	1279
Good Samaritan Hospital	Dayton	0.011	1070
Mount Carmel St Ann's Hospital	Westerville	0.011	354
Doctors Hospital	Columbus	0.013	391
Mercer County Joint Twp Comm Hosp	Coldwater	0.013	154
Mercy Hospital of Defiance	Defiance	0.013	78
Fisher Titus Memorial Hospital	Norwalk	0.014	281
Kettering Medical Center - Sycamore	Miamisburg	0.014	507
Parma Community General Hospital	Parma	0.014	859
Lakewood Hospital	Lakewood	0.015	324
Saint Joseph Health Center	Warren	0.015	608
Saint Rita's Medical Center	Lima	0.015	952
Alliance Community Hospital	Alliance	0.016	377
Atrium Medical Center	Franklin	0.016	765
Flower Hospital	Sylvania	0.016	378
Miami Valley Hospital	Dayton	0.017	1834
Southwest General Health Center	Middleburg Hgts	0.017	1261
The Toledo Hospital	Toledo	0.017	654
Memorial Hospital of Union County	Marysville	0.018	222
Mount Carmel Health	Columbus	0.018	1181
Marion General Hospital	Marion	0.019	52
University Hospital	Cincinnati	0.020	649
Bluffton Hospital	Bluffton	0.022	45
Coshocton County Memorial Hospital	Coshocton	0.024	207
Metro Health Medical Center	Cleveland	0.024	830
CMH Regional Health System	Wilmington	0.025	447
Summa Wadsworth-Rittman Hospital	Wadsworth	0.025	276
Mercy Hospital Fairfield	Fairfield	0.026	820
UH Geauga Medical Center	Chardon	0.027	291
University of Toledo Medical Center	Toledo	0.027	366
Kettering Medical Center	Kettering	0.028	1350
Huron Hospital	Cleveland	0.029	139
Firelands Regional Medical Center	Sandusky	0.032	527
Mary Rutan Hospital	Bellefontaine	0.033	305
Blanchard Valley Hospital	Findlay	0.034	582
Saint Elizabeth Boardman Health Center	Youngstown	0.034	205
Dublin Methodist Hospital	Dublin	0.035	85
Springfield Regional Medical Center	Springfield	0.035	803
Saint Elizabeth Health Center	Youngstown	0.038	524
Medina Hospital	Medina	0.040	323
Fulton County Health Center	Wauseon	0.041	217
Lodi Community Hospital[1]	Lodi	0.045	44
UHHS Bedford Medical Center	Bedford	0.047	279
Ohio State University Hospitals	Columbus	0.048	1010
Brown County Hospital	Georgetown	0.053	132
Mercy Hospital of Willard	Willard	0.056	72
Riverside Methodist Hospital	Columbus	0.056	2735
Aultman Hospital	Canton	0.059	1474
Medcentral Health System	Mansfield	0.060	833
Medical Center at Elizabeth Place	Dayton	0.061	66
Van Wert County Hospital	Van Wert	0.065	214
East Liverpool City Hospital	East Liverpool	0.069	274
Community Hospitals and Wellness Centers	Bryan	0.073	219
Joint Township District Memorial Hospital	Saint Marys	0.074	257
Adena Regional Medical Center	Chillicothe	0.076	939
Mercy Tiffin Hospital	Tiffin	0.079	241
Samaritan Hospital - Peoples Hospital	Ashland	0.085	295
UHHS Richmond Heights Hospital	Richmond Hghts	0.087	195
Barnesville Hospital Association	Barnesville	0.101	138
Knox Community Hospital	Mount Vernon	0.101	337
Saint Luke's Hospital	Maumee	0.102	420
South Pointe Hospital	Warrensville Hgts	0.103	513
Southern Ohio Medical Center	Portsmouth	0.110	1359
Greenfield Area Medical Center[1]	Greenfield	0.111	63
Wood County Hospital	Bowling Green	0.130	330
Wooster Community Hospital	Wooster	0.131	496
Marietta Memorial Hospital	Marietta	0.137	942
Wilson Memorial Hospital	Sidney	0.158	298
Deaconess Hospital	Cincinnati	0.159	157
Affinity Medical Center	Massillon	0.160	324
Grandview Hospital & Medical Center	Dayton	0.171	643
Southeastern Ohio Regional Medical Center	Cambridge	0.183	436
Greene Memorial Hospital	Xenia	0.188	287
Memorial Hospital	Fremont	0.227	392
Community Regional Medical Center	Lorain	0.269	759
Morrow County Hospital	Mount Gilead	0.325	126
Highland District Hospital	Hillsboro	0.333	330
Bellevue Hospital	Bellevue	0.381	202
Trinity Medical Center East & West	Steubenville	0.708	411

38. Follow-up Mammogram/Ultrasound

Hospital Name	City	Rate	Cases
Licking Memorial Hospital	Newark	2.4%	2142
Summa Wadsworth-Rittman Hospital	Wadsworth	2.8%	639
Saint Elizabeth Boardman Health Center	Youngstown	2.9%	70
Mercy Hospital Fairfield	Fairfield	3.0%	1186
Van Wert County Hospital	Van Wert	3.0%	297
UHHS Richmond Heights Hospital	Richmond Hghts	3.5%	395
Fulton County Health Center	Wauseon	3.9%	512
O'Bleness Memorial Hospital	Athens	4.1%	736
University of Toledo Medical Center	Toledo	4.1%	536
Holzer Medical Center Jackson	Jackson	4.3%	70
Summa Health Systems Hospitals	Akron	4.3%	2614
Firelands Regional Medical Center	Sandusky	4.4%	1373
Lutheran Hospital	Cleveland	4.4%	321
Univ Hosps Conneaut Med Ctr	Conneaut	4.5%	221
Saint Elizabeth Health Center	Youngstown	4.8%	584
Saint Luke's Hospital	Maumee	4.8%	482
Marietta Memorial Hospital	Marietta	4.9%	1015
Morrow County Hospital	Mount Gilead	4.9%	244
Genesis Healthcare System	Zanesville	5.0%	101
Christ Hospital	Cincinnati	5.1%	2445
Southeastern Ohio Regional Medical Center	Cambridge	5.1%	901
Deaconess Hospital	Cincinnati	5.4%	332
Joint Township District Memorial Hospital	Saint Marys	5.4%	553
Knox Community Hospital	Mount Vernon	5.4%	736
Upper Valley Medical Center	Troy	5.4%	1622
Miami Valley Hospital	Dayton	5.6%	2588
Mercy Hospital of Willard	Willard	5.7%	261
Parma Community General Hospital	Parma	5.7%	1649
South Pointe Hospital	Warrensville Hgts	5.7%	945
Southern Ohio Medical Center	Portsmouth	5.7%	1356
Southwest General Health Center	Middleburg Hgts	5.8%	1435
Grandview Hospital & Medical Center	Dayton	5.9%	942
Selby General Hospital	Marietta	5.9%	135
Springfield Regional Medical Center	Springfield	5.9%	1449
Mercy Tiffin Hospital	Tiffin	6.0%	600
Emh Regional Medical Center	Elyria	6.1%	558
Akron General Medical Center	Akron	6.4%	4412
Mount Carmel Health	Columbus	6.4%	3959
Alliance Community Hospital	Alliance	6.5%	769
Madison County Hospital	London	6.6%	256
Samaritan Hospital - Peoples Hospital	Ashland	6.6%	699
Union Hospital	Dover	6.6%	776
Doctors Hospital	Columbus	6.7%	582
Lakewood Hospital	Lakewood	6.8%	717
Mercy St Anne Hospital	Toledo	6.8%	1406
Memorial Hospital	Fremont	6.9%	807
East Liverpool City Hospital	East Liverpool	7.2%	446
Lake Health	Concord	7.2%	2629
Community Hospitals and Wellness Centers	Bryan	7.3%	179
Community Regional Medical Center	Lorain	7.4%	2206
UH Geauga Medical Center	Chardon	7.4%	571
UHHS Bedford Medical Center	Bedford	7.4%	443
Mercy Hospital Anderson	Cincinnati	7.5%	1554
Ohio State University Hospitals	Columbus	7.6%	382
Robinson Memorial Hospital	Ravenna	7.6%	1328
Wood County Hospital	Bowling Green	7.7%	598
Salem Community Hospital	Salem	7.9%	1087
Marymount Hospital	Garfield Heights	8.0%	1116
Medina Hospital	Medina	8.0%	1232
CMH Regional Health System	Wilmington	8.1%	980
Huron Hospital	Cleveland	8.1%	186
Adena Regional Medical Center	Chillicothe	8.2%	1710
Jewish Hospital	Cincinnati	8.2%	3500
Joel Pomerene Memorial Hospital	Millersburg	8.2%	233
Saint Rita's Medical Center	Lima	8.2%	2427
Medcentral Health System	Mansfield	8.3%	1715
Mercy Medical Center	Canton	8.3%	1712
Flower Hospital	Sylvania	8.5%	661
Mercy St Vincent Medical Center	Toledo	8.5%	471
Riverside Methodist Hospital	Columbus	8.5%	5816
Trinity Medical Center East & West	Steubenville	8.5%	982
Aultman Hospital	Canton	8.6%	1705
Mercy Hospital Clermont	Batavia	8.6%	1039
Mount Carmel St Ann's Hospital	Westerville	8.7%	1369
Atrium Medical Center	Franklin	8.9%	1455
Bay Park Community Hospital	Oregon	8.9%	484

NOTE: Hospital profiles are in alphabetical order by state, then city, then hospital within the city; Rankings exclude hospitals with less than 25 cases except for patient surveys which excludes hospitals with less than 100 cases; (a) 100–299 cases; (1) The number of cases is too small to be sure how well a hospital is performing; (2) The hospital indicated that the data submitted for this measure were based on a sample of cases; (3) Data was collected during a shorter time period (fewer quarters) than the maximum possible time for this measure; (4) Suppressed for one or more quarters by CMS; (5) No data is available from the hospital for this measure; (6) Fewer than 100 patients completed the HCAHPS survey. Use these rates with caution, as the number of surveys may be too low to reliably assess hospital performance; (7) Survey results are based on less than 12 months of data; (8) Survey results are not available for this reporting period; (9) No or very few patients were eligible for the HCAHPS survey. The scores shown, if any, reflect a very small number of surveys; (10) A state average was not calculated because too few hospitals in the state submitted data; (11) There were discrepancies in the data collection process; Please refer to the User's Guide for a full explanation of data.

Greenfield Area Medical Center	Greenfield	8.9%	112
The Toledo Hospital	Toledo	9.0%	2091
Wayne Hospital	Greenville	9.0%	846
Coshocton County Memorial Hospital	Coshocton	9.2%	654
Fisher Titus Memorial Hospital	Norwalk	9.2%	661
Blanchard Valley Hospital	Findlay	9.3%	1414
Fort Hamilton Hughes Memorial Hospital	Hamilton	9.3%	983
Brown County Hospital	Georgetown	9.4%	299
Good Samaritan Hospital	Cincinnati	9.4%	1559
Trumbull Memorial Hospital	Warren	9.4%	2456
Fairfield Medical Center	Lancaster	9.6%	655
Euclid Hospital	Euclid	9.7%	422
Good Samaritan Hospital	Dayton	9.7%	2531
Grant Medical Center	Columbus	10.1%	485
Memorial Hospital of Union County	Marysville	10.1%	435
Northside Medical Center	Youngstown	10.1%	566
Mercy Franciscan Hospital - Mt Airy	Cincinnati	10.2%	1033
Saint John Medical Center	Westlake	10.2%	648
Bellevue Hospital	Bellevue	10.3%	390
Hillcrest Hospital	Mayfield Heights	10.3%	1692
Mercy Franciscan Hospital Western Hills	Cincinnati	10.3%	1184
Saint Joseph Health Center	Warren	10.4%	811
Berger Hospital	Circleville	10.5%	630
Fayette County Memorial Hospital	Washington CH	10.8%	344
Mary Rutan Hospital	Bellefontaine	10.9%	787
Affinity Medical Center	Massillon	11.1%	633
Greene Memorial Hospital	Xenia	11.1%	704
UHHS Memorial Hospital of Geneva	Geneva	11.2%	258
University Hospital	Cincinnati	11.4%	1540
Highland District Hospital	Hillsboro	11.9%	461
Mercy St Charles Hospital	Oregon	12.0%	1176
Cleveland Clinic	Cleveland	12.1%	1905
Grady Memorial Hospital	Delaware	12.1%	527
Lima Memorial Health System	Lima	12.1%	1360
East Ohio Regional Hospital	Martins Ferry	12.3%	471
Butler County Medical Center	Hamilton	12.7%	166
Saint Vincent Charity Medical Center	Cleveland	12.7%	314
University Pointe Surgical Hospital	West Chester	12.9%	139
Bluffton Hospital	Bluffton	13.0%	276
Wilson Memorial Hospital	Sidney	13.5%	645
Ashtabula County Medical Center	Ashtabula	13.9%	677
Fairview Hospital	Cleveland	13.9%	1415
Mercer County Joint Twp Comm Hosp	Coldwater	14.0%	435
Belmont Community Hospital	Bellaire	14.4%	180
McCullough-Hyde Memorial Hospital	Oxford	14.7%	421
University Hospitals of Cleveland	Cleveland	15.5%	1589
Bethesda North Hospital	Cincinnati	16.0%	2888
Summa Barberton Hospital	Barberton	16.0%	681
Lodi Community Hospital	Lodi	16.4%	134
Barnesville Hospital Association	Barnesville	17.6%	159
Wooster Community Hospital	Wooster	18.1%	602
Metro Health Medical Center	Cleveland	19.1%	1611

39. MRI for Low Back Pain

Hospital Name	City	Rate	Cases
Euclid Hospital[1]	Euclid	17.0%	47
Doctors Hospital	Columbus	17.7%	96
Deaconess Hospital[1]	Cincinnati	18.4%	49
Wood County Hospital	Bowling Green	19.5%	82
Community Hospitals and Wellness Centers	Bryan	20.7%	92
Medical Center at Elizabeth Place	Dayton	20.9%	110
Mount Carmel New Albany Surgical Hospital	New Albany	22.2%	63
Upper Valley Medical Center	Troy	22.4%	116
The Toledo Hospital	Toledo	22.8%	193
Mercy Franciscan Hospital Western Hills	Cincinnati	22.9%	83
Wooster Community Hospital	Wooster	22.9%	96
Grant Medical Center	Columbus	23.0%	122
Alliance Community Hospital	Alliance	23.3%	90
Grady Memorial Hospital	Delaware	23.4%	64
Greene Memorial Hospital	Xenia	23.8%	63
Joel Pomerene Memorial Hospital[1]	Millersburg	24.0%	25
Mercy Tiffin Hospital	Tiffin	24.0%	129
Saint Joseph Health Center	Warren	24.2%	153
UHHS Memorial Hospital of Geneva	Geneva	24.2%	62
Joint Township District Memorial Hospital	Saint Marys	24.4%	82
Cleveland Clinic	Cleveland	24.9%	205
Mercy Hospital Fairfield	Fairfield	25.1%	215
Ohio State University Hospitals	Columbus	25.3%	198
Fulton County Health Center[1]	Wauseon	25.5%	55
Affinity Medical Center	Massillon	25.8%	66
Medcentral Health System	Mansfield	25.8%	198
University Hospitals of Cleveland	Cleveland	25.8%	360
Huron Hospital[1]	Cleveland	25.9%	27
Saint Luke's Hospital	Maumee	26.0%	123
Memorial Hospital	Fremont	26.4%	125
Holzer Medical Center Jackson[1]	Jackson	26.5%	34
Robinson Memorial Hospital	Ravenna	26.6%	154
Trumbull Memorial Hospital	Warren	26.6%	218
Medical Center of Newark	Newark	26.7%	116
Blanchard Valley Hospital	Findlay	27.1%	339
Fairfield Medical Center	Lancaster	27.1%	96
University of Toledo Medical Center	Toledo	27.1%	181
Van Wert County Hospital	Van Wert	27.1%	70
Firelands Regional Medical Center	Sandusky	27.2%	173
Kettering Medical Center - Sycamore	Miamisburg	27.3%	99
Samaritan Hospital - Peoples Hospital	Ashland	27.3%	99
Community Regional Medical Center	Lorain	27.6%	246
Hillcrest Hospital	Mayfield Heights	27.6%	214
Coshocton County Memorial Hospital	Coshocton	27.9%	68
Good Samaritan Hospital	Cincinnati	28.1%	160
Saint Rita's Medical Center	Lima	28.1%	288
Emh Regional Medical Center	Elyria	28.2%	117
Adena Regional Medical Center	Chillicothe	28.7%	397
Mercy St Charles Hospital	Oregon	28.7%	167
Medina Hospital	Medina	28.9%	114
Miami Valley Hospital	Dayton	29.4%	350
Lima Memorial Health System	Lima	29.5%	173
Bethesda North Hospital	Cincinnati	29.7%	273
Summa Western Reserve Hospital	Cuyahoga Falls	29.7%	128
Grandview Hospital & Medical Center	Dayton	29.8%	235
Salem Community Hospital	Salem	29.8%	171
Atrium Medical Center	Franklin	29.9%	147
CMH Regional Health System	Wilmington	30.1%	113
Mary Rutan Hospital	Bellefontaine	30.1%	83
Mercy Medical Center	Canton	30.2%	159
Belmont Community Hospital	Bellaire	30.4%	56
Butler County Medical Center	Hamilton	30.4%	168
Riverside Methodist Hospital	Columbus	30.5%	537
Springfield Regional Medical Center	Springfield	30.5%	177
Trinity Medical Center East & West	Steubenville	30.5%	128
Fisher Titus Memorial Hospital	Norwalk	30.6%	85
Mercy Hospital Anderson	Cincinnati	30.9%	272
Summa Wadsworth-Rittman Hospital	Wadsworth	31.0%	71
Berger Hospital	Circleville	31.2%	77
East Ohio Regional Hospital[1]	Martins Ferry	31.3%	32
Metro Health Medical Center	Cleveland	31.3%	147
Bellevue Hospital	Bellevue	31.5%	73
Summa Barberton Hospital	Barberton	31.8%	88
Aultman Hospital	Canton	31.9%	389
South Pointe Hospital	Warrensville Hgts	31.9%	141
Flower Hospital	Sylvania	32.0%	97
Kettering Medical Center	Kettering	32.0%	172
Mercy St Vincent Medical Center	Toledo	32.0%	75
Mercy Franciscan Hospital - Mt Airy	Cincinnati	32.2%	174
Mercy Hospital Clermont	Batavia	32.2%	242
Licking Memorial Hospital	Newark	32.3%	158
Akron General Medical Center	Akron	32.5%	379
Wilson Memorial Hospital	Sidney	32.5%	80
East Liverpool City Hospital	East Liverpool	32.7%	98
Southwest General Health Center	Middleburg Hgts	32.7%	110
Mercy St Anne Hospital	Toledo	32.9%	73
Union Hospital	Dover	33.1%	139
Highland District Hospital	Hillsboro	33.3%	72
Lutheran Hospital	Cleveland	33.3%	54
Memorial Hospital of Union County	Marysville	33.3%	51
University Hospital	Cincinnati	33.3%	183
Good Samaritan Hospital	Dayton	33.5%	200
Mount Carmel St Ann's Hospital	Westerville	33.6%	122
Mount Carmel Health	Columbus	33.7%	439
Wayne Hospital	Greenville	33.7%	98
Summa Health Systems Hospitals	Akron	33.8%	361
Parma Community General Hospital	Parma	33.9%	115
Saint John Medical Center	Westlake	33.9%	62
Jewish Hospital	Cincinnati	34.3%	396
UHHS Richmond Heights Hospital	Richmond Hghts	34.4%	64
Ashtabula County Medical Center	Ashtabula	34.7%	95
McCullough-Hyde Memorial Hospital	Oxford	34.7%	98
Lakewood Hospital	Lakewood	35.5%	76
Christ Hospital	Cincinnati	35.7%	213
Mercer County Joint Twp Comm Hosp	Coldwater	35.8%	67
Fort Hamilton Hughes Memorial Hospital	Hamilton	36.1%	119
Southeastern Ohio Regional Medical Center[1]	Cambridge	36.1%	36
Bay Park Community Hospital	Oregon	36.2%	58
Fairview Hospital	Cleveland	36.4%	55
Saint Elizabeth Health Center	Youngstown	36.6%	71
Saint Vincent Charity Medical Center	Cleveland	36.7%	60
Marymount Hospital	Garfield Heights	37.1%	151
Southern Ohio Medical Center	Portsmouth	37.4%	257
Fayette County Memorial Hospital[1]	Washington CH	37.5%	32
Marietta Memorial Hospital	Marietta	37.7%	159
UH Geauga Medical Center	Chardon	37.9%	66
Lake Health	Concord	38.0%	171
O'Bleness Memorial Hospital	Athens	38.4%	73
Knox Community Hospital	Mount Vernon	39.8%	113
UHHS Bedford Medical Center	Bedford	40.7%	54
Genesis Healthcare System	Zanesville	42.1%	38
University Pointe Surgical Hospital	West Chester	42.9%	56
Brown County Hospital	Georgetown	50.0%	60

Survey of Patients' Hospital Experiences

40. Area Around Room 'Always' Quiet at Night

Hospital Name	City	Rate	Cases
Surgical Hospital at Southwoods	Youngstown	84%	(a)
Butler County Medical Center	Hamilton	80%	(a)
Evendale Medical Center	Cincinnati	80%	300+
Mount Carmel New Albany Surgical Hospital	New Albany	79%	300+
Dublin Methodist Hospital	Dublin	78%	300+
Institute for Orthopedic Surgery	Lima	78%	300+
Medical Center at Elizabeth Place	Dayton	78%	(a)
Bluffton Hospital	Bluffton	75%	(a)
Medical Center of Newark	Newark	73%	300+
Henry County Hospital	Napoleon	72%	(a)
Holzer Medical Center Jackson	Jackson	71%	300+
West Chester Medical Center	West Chester	71%	300+
Saint Vincent Charity Medical Center	Cleveland	70%	300+
Amherst Hospital	Amherst	67%	300+
H B Magruder Memorial Hospital	Port Clinton	66%	300+
Southern Ohio Medical Center	Portsmouth	65%	300+
Mercy St Anne Hospital	Toledo	64%	300+
Univ Hosps Conneaut Med Ctr[11]	Conneaut	64%	(a)
Defiance Regional Medical Center	Defiance	63%	300+
Bucyrus Community Hospital	Bucyrus	62%	(a)
Community Hospitals and Wellness Centers	Bryan	62%	300+
Hocking Valley Community Hospital	Logan	62%	300+
Memorial Hospital of Union County	Marysville	62%	300+
Mercy Hospital of Defiance	Defiance	62%	300+
Mercy Tiffin Hospital	Tiffin	62%	300+
Blanchard Valley Hospital	Findlay	61%	300+
Hardin Memorial Hospital	Kenton	61%	(a)
Lodi Community Hospital[11]	Lodi	61%	(a)
Summa Western Reserve Hospital	Cuyahoga Falls	61%	300+
Bay Park Community Hospital	Oregon	60%	300+
McCullough-Hyde Memorial Hospital	Oxford	60%	300+
Wilson Memorial Hospital	Sidney	60%	300+
Atrium Medical Center	Franklin	59%	300+
Bellevue Hospital	Bellevue	59%	300+
Fostoria Community Hospital	Fostoria	59%	300+
Joel Pomerene Memorial Hospital	Millersburg	59%	300+
Joint Township District Memorial Hospital	Saint Marys	59%	300+
Metro Health Medical Center	Cleveland	59%	300+
Doctors Hospital	Columbus	58%	300+
Licking Memorial Hospital	Newark	58%	300+
Fairview Hospital	Cleveland	57%	300+
Genesis Healthcare System	Zanesville	57%	300+
Holzer Medical Center	Gallipolis	57%	300+
Lima Memorial Health System	Lima	57%	300+
Mercy Hospital of Willard	Willard	57%	(a)
Southeastern Ohio Regional Medical Center	Cambridge	57%	300+
Allen Community Hospital	Oberlin	56%	300+
Huron Hospital	Cleveland	56%	300+
Madison County Hospital	London	56%	300+
Morrow County Hospital	Mount Gilead	56%	(a)
Saint Elizabeth Boardman Health Center	Youngstown	56%	300+
Saint John Medical Center	Westlake	56%	300+
Wood County Hospital	Bowling Green	56%	300+
Deaconess Hospital	Cincinnati	55%	(a)
Fisher Titus Memorial Hospital	Norwalk	55%	300+
Galion Community Hospital	Galion	55%	300+
Memorial Hospital	Fremont	55%	300+
Mercy St Vincent Medical Center	Toledo	55%	300+
Saint Rita's Medical Center	Lima	55%	300+
Samaritan Hospital - Peoples Hospital	Ashland	55%	300+
Christ Hospital	Cincinnati	54%	300+
CMH Regional Health System	Wilmington	54%	300+
Firelands Regional Medical Center	Sandusky	54%	300+
Mercy Hospital Clermont	Batavia	54%	300+
Mercy Hospital Fairfield	Fairfield	54%	300+
University Hospital	Cincinnati	54%	300+
Van Wert County Hospital	Van Wert	54%	300+
Fayette County Memorial Hospital	Washington CH	53%	(a)
Good Samaritan Hospital	Cincinnati	53%	300+
Grady Memorial Hospital	Delaware	53%	300+
Knox Community Hospital	Mount Vernon	53%	300+
Medcentral Health System Shelby Hospital	Shelby	53%	300+
Ohio State University Hospitals	Columbus	53%	300+
Wayne Hospital	Greenville	53%	300+
Wooster Community Hospital	Wooster	53%	300+
Aultman Hospital	Canton	52%	300+
Bethesda North Hospital	Cincinnati	52%	300+
Community Regional Medical Center	Lorain	52%	300+
Euclid Hospital	Euclid	52%	300+
Lutheran Hospital	Cleveland	52%	300+
Saint Luke's Hospital	Maumee	52%	300+
Barnesville Hospital Association	Barnesville	51%	300+
Cleveland Clinic	Cleveland	51%	300+
Grandview Hospital & Medical Center	Dayton	51%	300+
Grant Medical Center	Columbus	51%	300+
Jewish Hospital	Cincinnati	51%	300+
Trinity Medical Center East & West	Steubenville	51%	300+

NOTE: Hospital profiles are in alphabetical order by state, then city, then hospital within the city; Rankings exclude hospitals with less than 25 cases except for patient surveys which excludes hospitals with less than 100 cases; (a) 100–299 cases; (1) The number of cases is too small to be sure how well a hospital is performing; (2) The hospital indicated that the data submitted for this measure were based on a sample of cases; (3) Data was collected during a shorter time period (fewer quarters) than the maximum possible time for this measure; (4) Suppressed for one or more quarters by CMS; (5) No data is available from the hospital for this measure; (6) Fewer than 100 patients completed the HCAHPS survey. Use these rates with caution, as the number of surveys may be too low to reliably assess hospital performance; (7) Survey results are based on less than 12 months of data; (8) Survey results are not available for this reporting period; (9) No or very few patients were eligible for the HCAHPS survey. The scores shown, if any, reflect a very small number of surveys; (10) A state average was not calculated because too few hospitals in the state submitted data; (11) There were discrepancies in the data collection process; Please refer to the User's Guide for a full explanation of data.

East Liverpool City Hospital	East Liverpool	50%	300+
Flower Hospital	Sylvania	50%	300+
Fulton County Health Center	Wauseon	50%	300+
Good Samaritan Hospital	Dayton	50%	300+
Mercer County Joint Twp Comm Hosp	Coldwater	50%	(a)
Mercy Medical Center	Canton	50%	300+
Mount Carmel Health	Columbus	50%	300+
O'Bleness Memorial Hospital	Athens	50%	300+
South Pointe Hospital	Warrensville Hgts	50%	300+
Belmont Community Hospital	Bellaire	49%	(a)
Brown County Hospital	Georgetown	49%	300+
Fort Hamilton Hughes Memorial Hospital	Hamilton	49%	300+
Lake Health	Concord	49%	300+
Marion General Hospital	Marion	49%	300+
Mercy St Charles Hospital	Oregon	49%	300+
Mount Carmel St Ann's Hospital	Westerville	49%	300+
Alliance Community Hospital	Alliance	48%	300+
Kettering Medical Center - Sycamore	Miamisburg	48%	300+
Riverside Methodist Hospital	Columbus	48%	300+
The Toledo Hospital	Toledo	48%	300+
Coshocton County Memorial Hospital	Coshocton	47%	300+
UHHS Memorial Hospital of Geneva[11]	Geneva	47%	300+
University Hospitals of Cleveland	Cleveland	47%	300+
Upper Valley Medical Center	Troy	47%	300+
Affinity Medical Center	Massillon	46%	300+
Akron General Medical Center[11]	Akron	46%	300+
Greene Memorial Hospital	Xenia	46%	300+
Mary Rutan Hospital	Bellefontaine	46%	300+
Medina Hospital	Medina	46%	300+
Mercy Franciscan Hospital Western Hills	Cincinnati	46%	300+
Miami Valley Hospital	Dayton	46%	300+
Robinson Memorial Hospital	Ravenna	46%	300+
Summa Barberton Hospital	Barberton	46%	300+
UH Geauga Medical Center[11]	Chardon	46%	300+
Union Hospital	Dover	46%	300+
Emh Regional Medical Center	Elyria	45%	300+
Lakewood Hospital	Lakewood	45%	300+
Mercy Hospital Anderson	Cincinnati	45%	300+
Parma Community General Hospital	Parma	45%	300+
Southwest General Health Center	Middleburg Hgts	45%	300+
Summa Health Systems Hospitals	Akron	45%	300+
UHHS Bedford Medical Center[11]	Bedford	45%	300+
Kettering Medical Center	Kettering	44%	300+
Mercy Franciscan Hospital - Mt Airy	Cincinnati	44%	300+
Mercy Memorial Hospital	Urbana	44%	300+
UHHS Richmond Heights Hospital[11]	Richmond Hghts	43%	300+
Fairfield Medical Center	Lancaster	42%	300+
Saint Elizabeth Health Center	Youngstown	42%	300+
Saint Joseph Health Center	Warren	42%	300+
Adena Regional Medical Center	Chillicothe	41%	300+
Marymount Hospital	Garfield Heights	41%	300+
Trumbull Memorial Hospital	Warren	41%	300+
Marietta Memorial Hospital	Marietta	40%	300+
Northside Medical Center	Youngstown	40%	300+
Springfield Regional Medical Center	Springfield	40%	300+
Summa Wadsworth-Rittman Hospital	Wadsworth	40%	300+
Ashtabula County Medical Center	Ashtabula	39%	300+
Hillcrest Hospital	Mayfield Heights	39%	300+
Medcentral Health System	Mansfield	39%	300+
Berger Hospital	Circleville	37%	300+
East Ohio Regional Hospital	Martins Ferry	37%	300+
Salem Community Hospital	Salem	35%	300+
University of Toledo Medical Center	Toledo	35%	300+

41. Doctors 'Always' Communicated Well

Hospital Name	City	Rate	Cases
Surgical Hospital at Southwoods	Youngstown	98%	(a)
Butler County Medical Center	Hamilton	97%	(a)
Mercy Hospital of Willard	Willard	93%	(a)
Evendale Medical Center	Cincinnati	91%	300+
H B Magruder Memorial Hospital	Port Clinton	90%	300+
Institute for Orthopedic Surgery	Lima	90%	300+
Galion Community Hospital	Galion	88%	300+
Bluffton Hospital	Bluffton	87%	(a)
Henry County Hospital	Napoleon	87%	(a)
Univ Hosps Conneaut Med Ctr[11]	Conneaut	87%	(a)
Deaconess Hospital	Cincinnati	86%	(a)
Bellevue Hospital	Bellevue	85%	300+
Mount Carmel New Albany Surgical Hospital	New Albany	85%	300+
Allen Community Hospital	Oberlin	84%	300+
Mary Rutan Hospital	Bellefontaine	84%	300+
McCullough-Hyde Memorial Hospital	Oxford	84%	300+
Memorial Hospital	Fremont	84%	300+
Mercy Hospital of Defiance	Defiance	84%	300+
Mercy Tiffin Hospital	Tiffin	84%	300+
Morrow County Hospital	Mount Gilead	84%	(a)
Wilson Memorial Hospital	Sidney	84%	300+
Blanchard Valley Hospital	Findlay	83%	300+
Dublin Methodist Hospital	Dublin	83%	300+
Hocking Valley Community Hospital	Logan	83%	300+
Madison County Hospital	London	83%	300+
Memorial Hospital of Union County	Marysville	83%	300+
Southern Ohio Medical Center	Portsmouth	83%	300+
UHHS Memorial Hospital of Geneva[11]	Geneva	83%	300+
Barnesville Hospital Association	Barnesville	82%	300+
Christ Hospital	Cincinnati	82%	300+
Medcentral Health System Shelby Hospital	Shelby	82%	300+
Adena Regional Medical Center	Chillicothe	81%	300+
Grady Memorial Hospital	Delaware	81%	300+
Joint Township District Memorial Hospital	Saint Marys	81%	300+
Marion General Hospital	Marion	81%	300+
Medical Center of Newark	Newark	81%	300+
Southeastern Ohio Regional Medical Center	Cambridge	81%	300+
Van Wert County Hospital	Van Wert	81%	300+
Bucyrus Community Hospital	Bucyrus	80%	(a)
Fostoria Community Hospital	Fostoria	80%	300+
Fulton County Health Center	Wauseon	80%	300+
Holzer Medical Center	Gallipolis	80%	300+
Holzer Medical Center Jackson	Jackson	80%	300+
Joel Pomerene Memorial Hospital	Millersburg	80%	300+
Mercer County Joint Twp Comm Hosp	Coldwater	80%	(a)
Mount Carmel Health	Columbus	80%	300+
Saint Vincent Charity Medical Center	Cleveland	80%	300+
Union Hospital	Dover	80%	300+
Wooster Community Hospital	Wooster	80%	300+
Community Hospitals and Wellness Centers	Bryan	79%	300+
Doctors Hospital	Columbus	79%	300+
Grandview Hospital & Medical Center	Dayton	79%	300+
Grant Medical Center	Columbus	79%	300+
Licking Memorial Hospital	Newark	79%	300+
Lodi Community Hospital[11]	Lodi	79%	(a)
Medical Center at Elizabeth Place	Dayton	79%	(a)
O'Bleness Memorial Hospital	Athens	79%	300+
Riverside Methodist Hospital	Columbus	79%	300+
Trinity Medical Center East & West	Steubenville	79%	300+
West Chester Medical Center	West Chester	79%	300+
Aultman Hospital	Canton	78%	300+
East Liverpool City Hospital	East Liverpool	78%	300+
Firelands Regional Medical Center	Sandusky	78%	300+
Flower Hospital	Sylvania	78%	300+
Genesis Healthcare System	Zanesville	78%	300+
Hardin Memorial Hospital	Kenton	78%	(a)
Lima Memorial Health System	Lima	78%	300+
Medina Hospital	Medina	78%	300+
Mount Carmel St Ann's Hospital	Westerville	78%	300+
Robinson Memorial Hospital	Ravenna	78%	300+
Saint John Medical Center	Westlake	78%	300+
Saint Joseph Health Center	Warren	78%	300+
Saint Rita's Medical Center	Lima	78%	300+
Samaritan Hospital - Peoples Hospital	Ashland	78%	300+
Southwest General Health Center	Middleburg Hgts	78%	300+
UH Geauga Medical Center[11]	Chardon	78%	300+
Wood County Hospital	Bowling Green	78%	300+
Affinity Medical Center	Massillon	77%	300+
Amherst Hospital	Amherst	77%	300+
Belmont Community Hospital	Bellaire	77%	(a)
CMH Regional Health System	Wilmington	77%	300+
Community Regional Medical Center	Lorain	77%	300+
Defiance Regional Medical Center	Defiance	77%	300+
Fairview Hospital	Cleveland	77%	300+
Good Samaritan Hospital	Cincinnati	77%	300+
Greene Memorial Hospital	Xenia	77%	300+
Jewish Hospital	Cincinnati	77%	300+
Kettering Medical Center	Kettering	77%	300+
Mercy Franciscan Hospital Western Hills	Cincinnati	77%	300+
Mercy Memorial Hospital	Urbana	77%	300+
Parma Community General Hospital	Parma	77%	300+
Saint Elizabeth Boardman Health Center	Youngstown	77%	300+
Saint Elizabeth Health Center	Youngstown	77%	300+
Salem Community Hospital	Salem	77%	300+
Summa Western Reserve Hospital	Cuyahoga Falls	77%	300+
Trumbull Memorial Hospital	Warren	77%	300+
Wayne Hospital	Greenville	77%	300+
Akron General Medical Center[11]	Akron	76%	300+
Atrium Medical Center	Franklin	76%	300+
Cleveland Clinic	Cleveland	76%	300+
Coshocton County Memorial Hospital	Coshocton	76%	300+
Euclid Hospital	Euclid	76%	300+
Fairfield Medical Center	Lancaster	76%	300+
Knox Community Hospital	Mount Vernon	76%	300+
Mercy Hospital Clermont	Batavia	76%	300+
Mercy Hospital Fairfield	Fairfield	76%	300+
Mercy Medical Center	Canton	76%	300+
Metro Health Medical Center	Cleveland	76%	300+
Ohio State University Hospitals	Columbus	76%	300+
Saint Luke's Hospital	Maumee	76%	300+
Summa Barberton Hospital	Barberton	76%	300+
Summa Wadsworth-Rittman Hospital	Wadsworth	76%	300+
Upper Valley Medical Center	Troy	76%	300+
Alliance Community Hospital	Alliance	75%	300+
Bethesda North Hospital	Cincinnati	75%	300+
Fayette County Memorial Hospital	Washington CH	75%	(a)
Fort Hamilton Hughes Memorial Hospital	Hamilton	75%	300+
Mercy St Anne Hospital	Toledo	75%	300+
Springfield Regional Medical Center	Springfield	75%	300+
University Hospitals of Cleveland	Cleveland	75%	300+
Berger Hospital	Circleville	74%	300+
Fisher Titus Memorial Hospital	Norwalk	74%	300+
Kettering Medical Center - Sycamore	Miamisburg	74%	300+
Lake Health	Concord	74%	300+
Lutheran Hospital	Cleveland	74%	300+
Marietta Memorial Hospital	Marietta	74%	300+
Mercy Hospital Anderson	Cincinnati	74%	300+
Miami Valley Hospital	Dayton	74%	300+
Northside Medical Center	Youngstown	74%	300+
South Pointe Hospital	Warrensville Hgts	74%	300+
Summa Health Systems Hospitals	Akron	74%	300+
Ashtabula County Medical Center	Ashtabula	73%	300+
Bay Park Community Hospital	Oregon	73%	300+
Good Samaritan Hospital	Dayton	73%	300+
Hillcrest Hospital	Mayfield Heights	73%	300+
Lakewood Hospital	Lakewood	73%	300+
Mercy St Vincent Medical Center	Toledo	73%	300+
University Hospital	Cincinnati	73%	300+
Brown County Hospital	Georgetown	72%	300+
Huron Hospital	Cleveland	72%	300+
Marymount Hospital	Garfield Heights	72%	300+
Mercy Franciscan Hospital - Mt Airy	Cincinnati	72%	300+
Mercy St Charles Hospital	Oregon	72%	300+
Emh Regional Medical Center	Elyria	71%	300+
Medcentral Health System	Mansfield	71%	300+
UHHS Bedford Medical Center[11]	Bedford	71%	300+
East Ohio Regional Hospital	Martins Ferry	70%	300+
The Toledo Hospital	Toledo	70%	300+
UHHS Richmond Heights Hospital[11]	Richmond Hghts	70%	300+
University of Toledo Medical Center	Toledo	66%	300+

42. Home Recovery Information Given

Hospital Name	City	Rate	Cases
Institute for Orthopedic Surgery	Lima	95%	300+
Surgical Hospital at Southwoods	Youngstown	93%	(a)
Evendale Medical Center	Cincinnati	92%	300+
Butler County Medical Center	Hamilton	91%	(a)
Morrow County Hospital	Mount Gilead	91%	(a)
Bucyrus Community Hospital	Bucyrus	90%	(a)
Deaconess Hospital	Cincinnati	90%	(a)
Henry County Hospital	Napoleon	90%	(a)
Lodi Community Hospital[11]	Lodi	90%	(a)
Mercy Hospital of Willard	Willard	90%	(a)
Mount Carmel New Albany Surgical Hospital	New Albany	90%	300+
Galion Community Hospital	Galion	89%	300+
Lima Memorial Health System	Lima	89%	300+
Mercy Tiffin Hospital	Tiffin	89%	300+
Wood County Hospital	Bowling Green	89%	300+
Hocking Valley Community Hospital	Logan	88%	300+
Medcentral Health System Shelby Hospital	Shelby	88%	300+
Medical Center at Elizabeth Place	Dayton	88%	(a)
Mercy Hospital of Defiance	Defiance	88%	300+
Miami Valley Hospital	Dayton	88%	300+
Samaritan Hospital - Peoples Hospital	Ashland	88%	300+
Southern Ohio Medical Center	Portsmouth	88%	300+
Bethesda North Hospital	Cincinnati	87%	300+
Bluffton Hospital	Bluffton	87%	(a)
CMH Regional Health System	Wilmington	87%	300+
Flower Hospital	Sylvania	87%	300+
Fostoria Community Hospital	Fostoria	87%	300+
Good Samaritan Hospital	Cincinnati	87%	300+
Grant Medical Center	Columbus	87%	300+
Licking Memorial Hospital	Newark	87%	300+
Marietta Memorial Hospital	Marietta	87%	300+
Marion General Hospital	Marion	87%	300+
Memorial Hospital	Fremont	87%	300+
Van Wert County Hospital	Van Wert	87%	300+
Akron General Medical Center[11]	Akron	86%	300+
Bay Park Community Hospital	Oregon	86%	300+
Christ Hospital	Cincinnati	86%	300+
Fisher Titus Memorial Hospital	Norwalk	86%	300+
Kettering Medical Center	Kettering	86%	300+
Kettering Medical Center - Sycamore	Miamisburg	86%	300+
Memorial Hospital of Union County	Marysville	86%	300+
Saint John Medical Center	Westlake	86%	300+
Trinity Medical Center East & West	Steubenville	86%	300+
Univ Hosps Conneaut Med Ctr[11]	Conneaut	86%	(a)
Affinity Medical Center	Massillon	85%	300+
Amherst Hospital	Amherst	85%	300+
Bellevue Hospital	Bellevue	85%	300+
Community Regional Medical Center	Lorain	85%	300+
Defiance Regional Medical Center	Defiance	85%	300+
Fulton County Health Center	Wauseon	85%	300+
Good Samaritan Hospital	Dayton	85%	300+
Holzer Medical Center	Gallipolis	85%	300+

NOTE: Hospital profiles are in alphabetical order by state, then city, then hospital within the city; Rankings exclude hospitals with less than 25 cases except for patient surveys which excludes hospitals with less than 100 cases; (a) 100–299 cases; (1) The number of cases is too small to be sure how well a hospital is performing; (2) The hospital indicated that the data submitted for this measure were based on a sample of cases; (3) Data was collected during a shorter time period (fewer quarters) than the maximum possible time for this measure; (4) Suppressed for one or more quarters by CMS; (5) No data is available from the hospital for this measure; (6) Fewer than 100 patients completed the HCAHPS survey. Use these rates with caution, as the number of surveys may be too low to reliably assess hospital performance; (7) Survey results are based on less than 12 months of data; (8) Survey results are not available for this reporting period; (9) No or very few patients were eligible for the HCAHPS survey. The scores shown, if any, reflect a very small number of surveys; (10) A state average was not calculated because too few hospitals in the state submitted data; (11) There were discrepancies in the data collection process; Please refer to the User's Guide for a full explanation of data.

Holzer Medical Center Jackson	Jackson	85%	300+
Joint Township District Memorial Hospital	Saint Marys	85%	300+
Mercy St Anne Hospital	Toledo	85%	300+
Mercy St Vincent Medical Center	Toledo	85%	300+
Riverside Methodist Hospital	Columbus	85%	300+
Saint Rita's Medical Center	Lima	85%	300+
Saint Vincent Charity Medical Center	Cleveland	85%	300+
Summa Wadsworth-Rittman Hospital	Wadsworth	85%	300+
The Toledo Hospital	Toledo	85%	300+
West Chester Medical Center	West Chester	85%	300+
Alliance Community Hospital	Alliance	84%	300+
Community Hospitals and Wellness Centers	Bryan	84%	300+
Euclid Hospital	Euclid	84%	300+
Lake Health	Concord	84%	300+
Ohio State University Hospitals	Columbus	84%	300+
Wooster Community Hospital	Wooster	84%	300+
Allen Community Hospital	Oberlin	83%	300+
Berger Hospital	Circleville	83%	300+
Blanchard Valley Hospital	Findlay	83%	300+
Cleveland Clinic	Cleveland	83%	300+
Fairfield Medical Center	Lancaster	83%	300+
Firelands Regional Medical Center	Sandusky	83%	300+
Grady Memorial Hospital	Delaware	83%	300+
Grandview Hospital & Medical Center	Dayton	83%	300+
Joel Pomerene Memorial Hospital	Millersburg	83%	300+
Marymount Hospital	Garfield Heights	83%	300+
Medcentral Health System	Mansfield	83%	300+
Metro Health Medical Center	Cleveland	83%	300+
Mount Carmel Health	Columbus	83%	300+
Mount Carmel St Ann's Hospital	Westerville	83%	300+
Parma Community General Hospital	Parma	83%	300+
Southeastern Ohio Regional Medical Center	Cambridge	83%	300+
UHHS Memorial Hospital of Geneva[11]	Geneva	83%	300+
University Hospital	Cincinnati	83%	300+
Atrium Medical Center	Franklin	82%	300+
Doctors Hospital	Columbus	82%	300+
Genesis Healthcare System	Zanesville	82%	300+
H B Magruder Memorial Hospital	Port Clinton	82%	300+
Jewish Hospital	Cincinnati	82%	300+
Mary Rutan Hospital	Bellefontaine	82%	300+
McCullough-Hyde Memorial Hospital	Oxford	82%	300+
Mercer County Joint Twp Comm Hosp	Coldwater	82%	(a)
Mercy Hospital Clermont	Batavia	82%	300+
Saint Joseph Health Center	Warren	82%	300+
Saint Luke's Hospital	Maumee	82%	300+
Summa Health Systems Hospitals	Akron	82%	300+
Union Hospital	Dover	82%	300+
University Hospitals of Cleveland	Cleveland	82%	300+
Upper Valley Medical Center	Troy	82%	300+
Dublin Methodist Hospital	Dublin	81%	300+
Fairview Hospital	Cleveland	81%	300+
Fayette County Memorial Hospital	Washington CH	81%	(a)
Greene Memorial Hospital	Xenia	81%	300+
Lutheran Hospital	Cleveland	81%	300+
Mercy Medical Center	Canton	81%	300+
Mercy Memorial Hospital	Urbana	81%	300+
Mercy St Charles Hospital	Oregon	81%	300+
O'Bleness Memorial Hospital	Athens	81%	300+
Summa Western Reserve Hospital	Cuyahoga Falls	81%	300+
Wilson Memorial Hospital	Sidney	81%	300+
Brown County Hospital	Georgetown	80%	300+
Coshocton County Memorial Hospital	Coshocton	80%	300+
Mercy Hospital Anderson	Cincinnati	80%	300+
Mercy Hospital Fairfield	Fairfield	80%	300+
Northside Medical Center	Youngstown	80%	300+
Salem Community Hospital	Salem	80%	300+
South Pointe Hospital	Warrensville Hgts	80%	300+
Southwest General Health Center	Middleburg Hgts	80%	300+
Trumbull Memorial Hospital	Warren	80%	300+
University of Toledo Medical Center	Toledo	80%	300+
Wayne Hospital	Greenville	80%	300+
Aultman Hospital	Canton	79%	300+
Barnesville Hospital Association	Barnesville	79%	300+
Belmont Community Hospital	Bellaire	79%	(a)
Emh Regional Medical Center	Elyria	79%	300+
Huron Hospital	Cleveland	79%	300+
Knox Community Hospital	Mount Vernon	79%	300+
Lakewood Hospital	Lakewood	79%	300+
Madison County Hospital	London	79%	300+
Medical Center of Newark	Newark	79%	300+
Mercy Franciscan Hospital - Mt Airy	Cincinnati	79%	300+
Saint Elizabeth Boardman Health Center	Youngstown	79%	300+
UH Geauga Medical Center[11]	Chardon	79%	300+
Medina Hospital	Medina	78%	300+
Robinson Memorial Hospital	Ravenna	78%	300+
Saint Elizabeth Health Center	Youngstown	78%	300+
Adena Regional Medical Center	Chillicothe	77%	300+
East Liverpool City Hospital	East Liverpool	76%	300+
East Ohio Regional Hospital	Martins Ferry	76%	300+
Hardin Memorial Hospital	Kenton	76%	(a)
Hillcrest Hospital	Mayfield Heights	76%	300+
Mercy Franciscan Hospital Western Hills	Cincinnati	76%	300+
Summa Barberton Hospital	Barberton	76%	300+
Ashtabula County Medical Center	Ashtabula	75%	300+
Fort Hamilton Hughes Memorial Hospital	Hamilton	75%	300+
Springfield Regional Medical Center	Springfield	74%	300+
UHHS Richmond Heights Hospital[11]	Richmond Hghts	74%	300+
UHHS Bedford Medical Center[11]	Bedford	73%	300+

43. Hospital Given 9 or 10 on 10 Point Scale

Hospital Name	City	Rate	Cases
Surgical Hospital at Southwoods	Youngstown	100%	(a)
Butler County Medical Center	Hamilton	93%	(a)
Institute for Orthopedic Surgery	Lima	92%	300+
Bluffton Hospital	Bluffton	87%	(a)
Mount Carmel New Albany Surgical Hospital	New Albany	86%	300+
Mercy Hospital of Willard	Willard	85%	(a)
Henry County Hospital	Napoleon	84%	(a)
Lodi Community Hospital[11]	Lodi	84%	(a)
Evendale Medical Center	Cincinnati	83%	300+
Univ Hosps Conneaut Med Ctr[11]	Conneaut	83%	(a)
Bellevue Hospital	Bellevue	82%	300+
Dublin Methodist Hospital	Dublin	82%	300+
H B Magruder Memorial Hospital	Port Clinton	81%	300+
Amherst Hospital	Amherst	80%	300+
Christ Hospital	Cincinnati	80%	300+
Morrow County Hospital	Mount Gilead	80%	(a)
West Chester Medical Center	West Chester	80%	300+
Deaconess Hospital	Cincinnati	79%	(a)
Medical Center at Elizabeth Place	Dayton	79%	(a)
Saint Elizabeth Boardman Health Center	Youngstown	78%	300+
Barnesville Hospital Association	Barnesville	77%	300+
Mercy Hospital of Defiance	Defiance	77%	300+
Cleveland Clinic	Cleveland	76%	300+
Hocking Valley Community Hospital	Logan	76%	300+
Allen Community Hospital	Oberlin	75%	300+
Defiance Regional Medical Center	Defiance	75%	300+
McCullough-Hyde Memorial Hospital	Oxford	75%	300+
Southern Ohio Medical Center	Portsmouth	75%	300+
Wooster Community Hospital	Wooster	75%	300+
Aultman Hospital	Canton	74%	300+
Bay Park Community Hospital	Oregon	74%	300+
Medical Center of Newark	Newark	74%	300+
Mercy St Anne Hospital	Toledo	74%	300+
Riverside Methodist Hospital	Columbus	74%	300+
Community Hospitals and Wellness Centers	Bryan	73%	300+
Fairview Hospital	Cleveland	73%	300+
Fulton County Health Center	Wauseon	73%	300+
Galion Community Hospital	Galion	73%	300+
Good Samaritan Hospital	Cincinnati	73%	300+
Medcentral Health System Shelby Hospital	Shelby	73%	300+
Memorial Hospital of Union County	Marysville	73%	300+
Mercy Tiffin Hospital	Tiffin	73%	300+
Saint Rita's Medical Center	Lima	73%	300+
Bethesda North Hospital	Cincinnati	72%	300+
Blanchard Valley Hospital	Findlay	72%	300+
Doctors Hospital	Columbus	72%	300+
Joint Township District Memorial Hospital	Saint Marys	72%	300+
UHHS Memorial Hospital of Geneva[11]	Geneva	72%	300+
Fisher Titus Memorial Hospital	Norwalk	71%	300+
Mercer County Joint Twp Comm Hosp	Coldwater	71%	(a)
Mercy St Charles Hospital	Oregon	71%	300+
Ohio State University Hospitals	Columbus	71%	300+
Saint John Medical Center	Westlake	71%	300+
Flower Hospital	Sylvania	70%	300+
Fostoria Community Hospital	Fostoria	70%	300+
Holzer Medical Center Jackson	Jackson	70%	300+
Mercy Hospital Fairfield	Fairfield	70%	300+
Mercy Medical Center	Canton	70%	300+
Mercy Memorial Hospital	Urbana	70%	300+
Saint Luke's Hospital	Maumee	70%	300+
Saint Vincent Charity Medical Center	Cleveland	70%	300+
Summa Western Reserve Hospital	Cuyahoga Falls	70%	300+
Bucyrus Community Hospital	Bucyrus	69%	(a)
CMH Regional Health System	Wilmington	69%	300+
Genesis Healthcare System	Zanesville	69%	300+
Lima Memorial Health System	Lima	69%	300+
Mercy Hospital Clermont	Batavia	69%	300+
University Hospitals of Cleveland	Cleveland	69%	300+
Wilson Memorial Hospital	Sidney	69%	300+
Grandview Hospital & Medical Center	Dayton	68%	300+
Grant Medical Center	Columbus	68%	300+
Jewish Hospital	Cincinnati	68%	300+
Kettering Medical Center	Kettering	68%	300+
Kettering Medical Center - Sycamore	Miamisburg	68%	300+
Marion General Hospital	Marion	68%	300+
Mount Carmel Health	Columbus	68%	300+
Mount Carmel St Ann's Hospital	Westerville	68%	300+
Saint Joseph Health Center	Warren	68%	300+
Southeastern Ohio Regional Medical Center	Cambridge	68%	300+
Southwest General Health Center	Middleburg Hgts	68%	300+
Van Wert County Hospital	Van Wert	68%	300+
Grady Memorial Hospital	Delaware	67%	300+
Hardin Memorial Hospital	Kenton	67%	(a)
Joel Pomerene Memorial Hospital	Millersburg	67%	300+
Mercy St Vincent Medical Center	Toledo	67%	300+
Samaritan Hospital - Peoples Hospital	Ashland	67%	300+
Wood County Hospital	Bowling Green	67%	300+
Akron General Medical Center[11]	Akron	66%	300+
Alliance Community Hospital	Alliance	66%	300+
Licking Memorial Hospital	Newark	66%	300+
Madison County Hospital	London	66%	300+
Miami Valley Hospital	Dayton	66%	300+
Union Hospital	Dover	66%	300+
Firelands Regional Medical Center	Sandusky	65%	300+
Holzer Medical Center	Gallipolis	65%	300+
Memorial Hospital	Fremont	65%	300+
Summa Barberton Hospital	Barberton	65%	300+
UH Geauga Medical Center[11]	Chardon	65%	300+
Affinity Medical Center	Massillon	64%	300+
Atrium Medical Center	Franklin	64%	300+
Belmont Community Hospital	Bellaire	64%	(a)
Fairfield Medical Center	Lancaster	64%	300+
Metro Health Medical Center	Cleveland	64%	300+
Robinson Memorial Hospital	Ravenna	64%	300+
Summa Wadsworth-Rittman Hospital	Wadsworth	64%	300+
Trinity Medical Center East & West	Steubenville	64%	300+
Euclid Hospital	Euclid	63%	300+
Knox Community Hospital	Mount Vernon	63%	300+
Lake Health	Concord	63%	300+
Mercy Hospital Anderson	Cincinnati	63%	300+
The Toledo Hospital	Toledo	63%	300+
University Hospital	Cincinnati	63%	300+
Adena Regional Medical Center	Chillicothe	62%	300+
Good Samaritan Hospital	Dayton	62%	300+
Marietta Memorial Hospital	Marietta	62%	300+
Medcentral Health System	Mansfield	62%	300+
Summa Health Systems Hospitals	Akron	62%	300+
Mary Rutan Hospital	Bellefontaine	61%	300+
Mercy Franciscan Hospital Western Hills	Cincinnati	61%	300+
Community Regional Medical Center	Lorain	60%	300+
Emh Regional Medical Center	Elyria	60%	300+
Medina Hospital	Medina	60%	300+
Parma Community General Hospital	Parma	60%	300+
South Pointe Hospital	Warrensville Hgts	60%	300+
Fayette County Memorial Hospital	Washington CH	59%	(a)
Hillcrest Hospital	Mayfield Heights	59%	300+
Lakewood Hospital	Lakewood	59%	300+
Northside Medical Center	Youngstown	59%	300+
Saint Elizabeth Health Center	Youngstown	59%	300+
Upper Valley Medical Center	Troy	59%	300+
Wayne Hospital	Greenville	59%	300+
Coshocton County Memorial Hospital	Coshocton	58%	300+
O'Bleness Memorial Hospital	Athens	58%	300+
Salem Community Hospital	Salem	57%	300+
Berger Hospital	Circleville	56%	300+
Greene Memorial Hospital	Xenia	56%	300+
East Liverpool City Hospital	East Liverpool	55%	300+
Fort Hamilton Hughes Memorial Hospital	Hamilton	55%	300+
Marymount Hospital	Garfield Heights	55%	300+
UHHS Bedford Medical Center[11]	Bedford	55%	300+
Lutheran Hospital	Cleveland	54%	300+
Trumbull Memorial Hospital	Warren	54%	300+
UHHS Richmond Heights Hospital[11]	Richmond Hghts	54%	300+
Mercy Franciscan Hospital - Mt Airy	Cincinnati	53%	300+
University of Toledo Medical Center	Toledo	52%	300+
Brown County Hospital	Georgetown	51%	300+
Huron Hospital	Cleveland	50%	300+
Ashtabula County Medical Center	Ashtabula	49%	300+
East Ohio Regional Hospital	Martins Ferry	49%	300+
Springfield Regional Medical Center	Springfield	45%	300+

44. Meds 'Always' Explained Before Given

Hospital Name	City	Rate	Cases
Surgical Hospital at Southwoods	Youngstown	80%	(a)
Institute for Orthopedic Surgery	Lima	78%	300+
Butler County Medical Center	Hamilton	77%	(a)
Univ Hosps Conneaut Med Ctr[11]	Conneaut	74%	(a)
Henry County Hospital	Napoleon	73%	(a)
Mercy Hospital of Willard	Willard	73%	(a)
Evendale Medical Center	Cincinnati	71%	300+
H B Magruder Memorial Hospital	Port Clinton	71%	300+
Mount Carmel New Albany Surgical Hospital	New Albany	70%	300+
Bluffton Hospital	Bluffton	69%	(a)
Galion Community Hospital	Galion	69%	300+
Joint Township District Memorial Hospital	Saint Marys	68%	300+
Morrow County Hospital	Mount Gilead	68%	(a)
Barnesville Hospital Association	Barnesville	67%	300+
Memorial Hospital of Union County	Marysville	67%	300+
Mercy Tiffin Hospital	Tiffin	67%	300+
Allen Community Hospital	Oberlin	66%	300+

NOTE: Hospital profiles are in alphabetical order by state, then city, then hospital within the city; Rankings exclude hospitals with less than 25 cases except for patient surveys which excludes hospitals with less than 100 cases; (a) 100–299 cases; (1) The number of cases is too small to be sure how well a hospital is performing; (2) The hospital indicated that the data submitted for this measure were based on a sample of cases; (3) Data was collected during a shorter time period (fewer quarters) than the maximum possible time for this measure; (4) Suppressed for one or more quarters by CMS; (5) No data is available from the hospital for this measure; (6) Fewer than 100 patients completed the HCAHPS survey. Use these rates with caution, as the number of surveys may be too low to reliably assess hospital performance; (7) Survey results are based on less than 12 months of data; (8) Survey results are not available for this reporting period; (9) No or very few patients were eligible for the HCAHPS survey. The scores shown, if any, reflect a very small number of surveys; (10) A state average was not calculated because too few hospitals in the state submitted data; (11) There were discrepancies in the data collection process; Please refer to the User's Guide for a full explanation of data.

Deaconess Hospital	Cincinnati	66%	(a)
Marion General Hospital	Marion	66%	300+
Bucyrus Community Hospital	Bucyrus	65%	(a)
Dublin Methodist Hospital	Dublin	65%	300+
Holzer Medical Center Jackson	Jackson	65%	300+
McCullough-Hyde Memorial Hospital	Oxford	65%	300+
Van Wert County Hospital	Van Wert	65%	300+
Bellevue Hospital	Bellevue	64%	300+
CMH Regional Health System	Wilmington	64%	300+
Doctors Hospital	Columbus	64%	300+
Hocking Valley Community Hospital	Logan	64%	300+
Medcentral Health System Shelby Hospital	Shelby	64%	300+
Southeastern Ohio Regional Medical Center	Cambridge	64%	300+
Southern Ohio Medical Center	Portsmouth	64%	300+
Amherst Hospital	Amherst	63%	300+
Aultman Hospital	Canton	63%	300+
Community Hospitals and Wellness Centers	Bryan	63%	300+
Fisher Titus Memorial Hospital	Norwalk	63%	300+
Lodi Community Hospital[11]	Lodi	63%	(a)
Medical Center at Elizabeth Place	Dayton	63%	(a)
Mercy Hospital of Defiance	Defiance	63%	300+
UHHS Memorial Hospital of Geneva[11]	Geneva	63%	300+
Blanchard Valley Hospital	Findlay	62%	300+
Christ Hospital	Cincinnati	62%	300+
Hardin Memorial Hospital	Kenton	62%	(a)
Jewish Hospital	Cincinnati	62%	300+
Mary Rutan Hospital	Bellefontaine	62%	300+
Mercy Memorial Hospital	Urbana	62%	300+
Riverside Methodist Hospital	Columbus	62%	300+
Wilson Memorial Hospital	Sidney	62%	300+
Bay Park Community Hospital	Oregon	61%	300+
Fayette County Memorial Hospital	Washington CH	61%	(a)
Fostoria Community Hospital	Fostoria	61%	300+
Genesis Healthcare System	Zanesville	61%	300+
Grant Medical Center	Columbus	61%	300+
Holzer Medical Center	Gallipolis	61%	300+
Memorial Hospital	Fremont	61%	300+
Mercy Hospital Clermont	Batavia	61%	300+
Saint Luke's Hospital	Maumee	61%	300+
Southwest General Health Center	Middleburg Hgts	61%	300+
West Chester Medical Center	West Chester	61%	300+
Wood County Hospital	Bowling Green	61%	300+
Defiance Regional Medical Center	Defiance	60%	300+
Fairview Hospital	Cleveland	60%	300+
Madison County Hospital	London	60%	300+
Medical Center of Newark	Newark	60%	300+
Mercer County Joint Twp Comm Hosp	Coldwater	60%	(a)
Mercy Hospital Fairfield	Fairfield	60%	300+
Metro Health Medical Center	Cleveland	60%	300+
Saint Elizabeth Boardman Health Center	Youngstown	60%	300+
Saint Rita's Medical Center	Lima	60%	300+
Trinity Medical Center East & West	Steubenville	60%	300+
Wooster Community Hospital	Wooster	60%	300+
Akron General Medical Center[11]	Akron	59%	300+
Belmont Community Hospital	Bellaire	59%	(a)
Cleveland Clinic	Cleveland	59%	300+
Firelands Regional Medical Center	Sandusky	59%	300+
Good Samaritan Hospital	Cincinnati	59%	300+
Grady Memorial Hospital	Delaware	59%	300+
Licking Memorial Hospital	Newark	59%	300+
Mercy Medical Center	Canton	59%	300+
Mercy St Anne Hospital	Toledo	59%	300+
Ohio State University Hospitals	Columbus	59%	300+
Saint Vincent Charity Medical Center	Cleveland	59%	300+
Samaritan Hospital - Peoples Hospital	Ashland	59%	300+
University Hospitals of Cleveland	Cleveland	59%	300+
Wayne Hospital	Greenville	59%	300+
Adena Regional Medical Center	Chillicothe	58%	300+
Community Regional Medical Center	Lorain	58%	300+
Euclid Hospital	Euclid	58%	300+
Fulton County Health Center	Wauseon	58%	300+
Kettering Medical Center	Kettering	58%	300+
Atrium Medical Center	Franklin	57%	300+
East Liverpool City Hospital	East Liverpool	57%	300+
Flower Hospital	Sylvania	57%	300+
Greene Memorial Hospital	Xenia	57%	300+
Joel Pomerene Memorial Hospital	Millersburg	57%	300+
Knox Community Hospital	Mount Vernon	57%	300+
Lake Health	Concord	57%	300+
Lima Memorial Health System	Lima	57%	300+
Mercy St Vincent Medical Center	Toledo	57%	300+
Mount Carmel Health	Columbus	57%	300+
O'Bleness Memorial Hospital	Athens	57%	300+
Saint Joseph Health Center	Warren	57%	300+
Summa Barberton Hospital	Barberton	57%	300+
Summa Western Reserve Hospital	Cuyahoga Falls	57%	300+
Union Hospital	Dover	57%	300+
University Hospital	Cincinnati	57%	300+
Upper Valley Medical Center	Troy	57%	300+
Alliance Community Hospital	Alliance	56%	300+
Fairfield Medical Center	Lancaster	56%	300+
Lakewood Hospital	Lakewood	56%	300+
Medina Hospital	Medina	56%	300+
Miami Valley Hospital	Dayton	56%	300+
Mount Carmel St Ann's Hospital	Westerville	56%	300+
Robinson Memorial Hospital	Ravenna	56%	300+
Saint John Medical Center	Westlake	56%	300+
UH Geauga Medical Center[11]	Chardon	56%	300+
Affinity Medical Center	Massillon	55%	300+
Ashtabula County Medical Center	Ashtabula	55%	300+
Coshocton County Memorial Hospital	Coshocton	55%	300+
Emh Regional Medical Center	Elyria	55%	300+
Grandview Hospital & Medical Center	Dayton	55%	300+
Huron Hospital	Cleveland	55%	300+
Mercy Hospital Anderson	Cincinnati	55%	300+
Mercy St Charles Hospital	Oregon	55%	300+
Summa Health Systems Hospitals	Akron	55%	300+
Fort Hamilton Hughes Memorial Hospital	Hamilton	54%	300+
Good Samaritan Hospital	Dayton	54%	300+
Lutheran Hospital	Cleveland	54%	300+
Marietta Memorial Hospital	Marietta	54%	300+
Mercy Franciscan Hospital Western Hills	Cincinnati	54%	300+
South Pointe Hospital	Warrensville Hgts	54%	300+
Springfield Regional Medical Center	Springfield	54%	300+
Summa Wadsworth-Rittman Hospital	Wadsworth	54%	300+
Berger Hospital	Circleville	53%	300+
Kettering Medical Center - Sycamore	Miamisburg	53%	300+
Northside Medical Center	Youngstown	53%	300+
Parma Community General Hospital	Parma	53%	300+
Saint Elizabeth Health Center	Youngstown	53%	300+
Salem Community Hospital	Salem	53%	300+
UHHS Bedford Medical Center[11]	Bedford	53%	300+
University of Toledo Medical Center	Toledo	53%	300+
Bethesda North Hospital	Cincinnati	52%	300+
Hillcrest Hospital	Mayfield Heights	52%	300+
Marymount Hospital	Garfield Heights	52%	300+
Medcentral Health System	Mansfield	52%	300+
The Toledo Hospital	Toledo	52%	300+
UHHS Richmond Heights Hospital[11]	Richmond Hghts	52%	300+
Brown County Hospital	Georgetown	51%	300+
East Ohio Regional Hospital	Martins Ferry	51%	300+
Mercy Franciscan Hospital - Mt Airy	Cincinnati	50%	300+
Trumbull Memorial Hospital	Warren	50%	300+

45. Nurses 'Always' Communicated Well

Hospital Name	City	Rate	Cases
Surgical Hospital at Southwoods	Youngstown	97%	(a)
Butler County Medical Center	Hamilton	92%	(a)
Institute for Orthopedic Surgery	Lima	91%	300+
H B Magruder Memorial Hospital	Port Clinton	88%	300+
Lodi Community Hospital[11]	Lodi	87%	(a)
Mercy Hospital of Willard	Willard	87%	(a)
Univ Hosps Conneaut Med Ctr[11]	Conneaut	87%	(a)
Bluffton Hospital	Bluffton	86%	(a)
Henry County Hospital	Napoleon	86%	(a)
Barnesville Hospital Association	Barnesville	85%	300+
Medical Center at Elizabeth Place	Dayton	85%	(a)
Holzer Medical Center Jackson	Jackson	84%	300+
Medcentral Health System Shelby Hospital	Shelby	84%	300+
Morrow County Hospital	Mount Gilead	84%	(a)
Mount Carmel New Albany Surgical Hospital	New Albany	84%	300+
Amherst Hospital	Amherst	83%	300+
Christ Hospital	Cincinnati	83%	300+
Galion Community Hospital	Galion	83%	300+
Mercy Hospital of Defiance	Defiance	83%	300+
Southern Ohio Medical Center	Portsmouth	83%	300+
Allen Community Hospital	Oberlin	82%	300+
Evendale Medical Center	Cincinnati	82%	300+
Mercy Tiffin Hospital	Tiffin	82%	300+
Doctors Hospital	Columbus	81%	300+
Hocking Valley Community Hospital	Logan	81%	300+
Joint Township District Memorial Hospital	Saint Marys	81%	300+
McCullough-Hyde Memorial Hospital	Oxford	81%	300+
Memorial Hospital of Union County	Marysville	81%	300+
Mercer County Joint Twp Comm Hosp	Coldwater	81%	(a)
Mercy Memorial Hospital	Urbana	81%	300+
Southeastern Ohio Regional Medical Center	Cambridge	81%	300+
West Chester Medical Center	West Chester	81%	300+
Dublin Methodist Hospital	Dublin	80%	300+
Marion General Hospital	Marion	80%	300+
UHHS Memorial Hospital of Geneva[11]	Geneva	80%	300+
Wilson Memorial Hospital	Sidney	80%	300+
Wooster Community Hospital	Wooster	80%	300+
Bellevue Hospital	Bellevue	79%	300+
Fostoria Community Hospital	Fostoria	79%	300+
Genesis Healthcare System	Zanesville	79%	300+
Holzer Medical Center	Gallipolis	79%	300+
Madison County Hospital	London	79%	300+
Mary Rutan Hospital	Bellefontaine	79%	300+
Medical Center of Newark	Newark	79%	300+
Riverside Methodist Hospital	Columbus	79%	300+
Saint Elizabeth Boardman Health Center	Youngstown	79%	300+
Southwest General Health Center	Middleburg Hgts	79%	300+
Bay Park Community Hospital	Oregon	78%	300+
CMH Regional Health System	Wilmington	78%	300+
Community Hospitals and Wellness Centers	Bryan	78%	300+
Deaconess Hospital	Cincinnati	78%	(a)
Grant Medical Center	Columbus	78%	300+
Hardin Memorial Hospital	Kenton	78%	(a)
Jewish Hospital	Cincinnati	78%	300+
Knox Community Hospital	Mount Vernon	78%	300+
Memorial Hospital	Fremont	78%	300+
Mercy Hospital Clermont	Batavia	78%	300+
Mercy St Anne Hospital	Toledo	78%	300+
Mercy St Charles Hospital	Oregon	78%	300+
Saint Rita's Medical Center	Lima	78%	300+
Van Wert County Hospital	Van Wert	78%	300+
Aultman Hospital	Canton	77%	300+
Bucyrus Community Hospital	Bucyrus	77%	(a)
Defiance Regional Medical Center	Defiance	77%	300+
Firelands Regional Medical Center	Sandusky	77%	300+
Flower Hospital	Sylvania	77%	300+
Good Samaritan Hospital	Cincinnati	77%	300+
Licking Memorial Hospital	Newark	77%	300+
Mercy Hospital Fairfield	Fairfield	77%	300+
Mercy Medical Center	Canton	77%	300+
Ohio State University Hospitals	Columbus	77%	300+
Saint Luke's Hospital	Maumee	77%	300+
Summa Barberton Hospital	Barberton	77%	300+
Adena Regional Medical Center	Chillicothe	76%	300+
Akron General Medical Center[11]	Akron	76%	300+
Blanchard Valley Hospital	Findlay	76%	300+
Fairfield Medical Center	Lancaster	76%	300+
Fayette County Memorial Hospital	Washington CH	76%	(a)
Grady Memorial Hospital	Delaware	76%	300+
Joel Pomerene Memorial Hospital	Millersburg	76%	300+
Mercy St Vincent Medical Center	Toledo	76%	300+
Mount Carmel Health	Columbus	76%	300+
Robinson Memorial Hospital	Ravenna	76%	300+
Saint Vincent Charity Medical Center	Cleveland	76%	300+
Samaritan Hospital - Peoples Hospital	Ashland	76%	300+
Bethesda North Hospital	Cincinnati	75%	300+
Cleveland Clinic	Cleveland	75%	300+
Euclid Hospital	Euclid	75%	300+
Grandview Hospital & Medical Center	Dayton	75%	300+
Kettering Medical Center	Kettering	75%	300+
O'Bleness Memorial Hospital	Athens	75%	300+
Summa Western Reserve Hospital	Cuyahoga Falls	75%	300+
Trinity Medical Center East & West	Steubenville	75%	300+
UH Geauga Medical Center[11]	Chardon	75%	300+
University Hospitals of Cleveland	Cleveland	75%	300+
Coshocton County Memorial Hospital	Coshocton	74%	300+
Fairview Hospital	Cleveland	74%	300+
Fisher Titus Memorial Hospital	Norwalk	74%	300+
Fort Hamilton Hughes Memorial Hospital	Hamilton	74%	300+
Fulton County Health Center	Wauseon	74%	300+
Lakewood Hospital	Lakewood	74%	300+
Mercy Hospital Anderson	Cincinnati	74%	300+
Miami Valley Hospital	Dayton	74%	300+
Mount Carmel St Ann's Hospital	Westerville	74%	300+
Saint John Medical Center	Westlake	74%	300+
Summa Wadsworth-Rittman Hospital	Wadsworth	74%	300+
Upper Valley Medical Center	Troy	74%	300+
Wayne Hospital	Greenville	74%	300+
Alliance Community Hospital	Alliance	73%	300+
Atrium Medical Center	Franklin	73%	300+
Community Regional Medical Center	Lorain	73%	300+
Kettering Medical Center - Sycamore	Miamisburg	73%	300+
Lake Health	Concord	73%	300+
Marietta Memorial Hospital	Marietta	73%	300+
Mercy Franciscan Hospital Western Hills	Cincinnati	73%	300+
Summa Health Systems Hospitals	Akron	73%	300+
Union Hospital	Dover	73%	300+
Affinity Medical Center	Massillon	72%	300+
Ashtabula County Medical Center	Ashtabula	72%	300+
Berger Hospital	Circleville	72%	300+
Greene Memorial Hospital	Xenia	72%	300+
Lima Memorial Health System	Lima	72%	300+
Medcentral Health System	Mansfield	72%	300+
Medina Hospital	Medina	72%	300+
Metro Health Medical Center	Cleveland	72%	300+
Parma Community General Hospital	Parma	72%	300+
Saint Joseph Health Center	Warren	72%	300+
University Hospital	Cincinnati	72%	300+
Wood County Hospital	Bowling Green	72%	300+
Brown County Hospital	Georgetown	71%	300+
Emh Regional Medical Center	Elyria	71%	300+
Good Samaritan Hospital	Dayton	71%	300+
Northside Medical Center	Youngstown	71%	300+
UHHS Bedford Medical Center[11]	Bedford	71%	300+
Belmont Community Hospital	Bellaire	70%	(a)
East Liverpool City Hospital	East Liverpool	70%	300+

NOTE: Hospital profiles are in alphabetical order by state, then city, then hospital within the city; Rankings exclude hospitals with less than 25 cases except for patient surveys which excludes hospitals with less than 100 cases; (a) 100–299 cases; (1) The number of cases is too small to be sure how well a hospital is performing; (2) The hospital indicated that the data submitted for this measure were based on a sample of cases; (3) Data was collected during a shorter time period (fewer quarters) than the maximum possible time for this measure; (4) Suppressed for one or more quarters by CMS; (5) No data is available from the hospital for this measure; (6) Fewer than 100 patients completed the HCAHPS survey. Use these rates with caution, as the number of surveys may be too low to reliably assess hospital performance; (7) Survey results are based on less than 12 months of data; (8) Survey results are not available for this reporting period; (9) No or very few patients were eligible for the HCAHPS survey. The scores shown, if any, reflect a very small number of surveys; (10) A state average was not calculated because too few hospitals in the state submitted data; (11) There were discrepancies in the data collection process; Please refer to the User's Guide for a full explanation of data.

Huron Hospital	Cleveland	70%	300+
South Pointe Hospital	Warrensville Hgts	70%	300+
Marymount Hospital	Garfield Heights	69%	300+
Mercy Franciscan Hospital - Mt Airy	Cincinnati	69%	300+
Saint Elizabeth Health Center	Youngstown	69%	300+
Salem Community Hospital	Salem	69%	300+
Hillcrest Hospital	Mayfield Heights	68%	300+
Lutheran Hospital	Cleveland	68%	300+
The Toledo Hospital	Toledo	68%	300+
East Ohio Regional Hospital	Martins Ferry	67%	300+
Trumbull Memorial Hospital	Warren	67%	300+
Springfield Regional Medical Center	Springfield	66%	300+
UHHS Richmond Heights Hospital[11]	Richmond Hghts	66%	300+
University of Toledo Medical Center	Toledo	63%	300+

46. Pain 'Always' Well Controlled

Hospital Name	City	Rate	Cases
Surgical Hospital at Southwoods	Youngstown	90%	(a)
Butler County Medical Center	Hamilton	86%	(a)
Mercy Hospital of Willard	Willard	84%	(a)
Henry County Hospital	Napoleon	81%	(a)
Southern Ohio Medical Center	Portsmouth	81%	300+
Institute for Orthopedic Surgery	Lima	80%	300+
Mercy Hospital of Defiance	Defiance	80%	300+
Bluffton Hospital	Bluffton	79%	(a)
Galion Community Hospital	Galion	77%	300+
H B Magruder Memorial Hospital	Port Clinton	77%	300+
Medical Center at Elizabeth Place	Dayton	77%	(a)
Allen Community Hospital	Oberlin	76%	300+
Evendale Medical Center	Cincinnati	76%	300+
Hocking Valley Community Hospital	Logan	76%	300+
Mount Carmel New Albany Surgical Hospital	New Albany	76%	300+
Amherst Hospital	Amherst	75%	300+
Barnesville Hospital Association	Barnesville	75%	300+
Holzer Medical Center Jackson	Jackson	75%	300+
Lodi Community Hospital[11]	Lodi	75%	(a)
McCullough-Hyde Memorial Hospital	Oxford	75%	300+
Univ Hosps Conneaut Med Ctr[11]	Conneaut	75%	(a)
Madison County Hospital	London	74%	300+
Memorial Hospital of Union County	Marysville	74%	300+
West Chester Medical Center	West Chester	74%	300+
Wooster Community Hospital	Wooster	74%	300+
Christ Hospital	Cincinnati	73%	300+
Deaconess Hospital	Cincinnati	73%	(a)
Holzer Medical Center	Gallipolis	73%	300+
Joint Township District Memorial Hospital	Saint Marys	73%	300+
Medcentral Health System Shelby Hospital	Shelby	73%	300+
Mercer County Joint Twp Comm Hosp	Coldwater	73%	(a)
Mercy Medical Center	Canton	73%	300+
Van Wert County Hospital	Van Wert	73%	300+
Bucyrus Community Hospital	Bucyrus	72%	(a)
Community Hospitals and Wellness Centers	Bryan	72%	300+
Fostoria Community Hospital	Fostoria	72%	300+
Fulton County Health Center	Wauseon	72%	300+
Genesis Healthcare System	Zanesville	72%	300+
Bellevue Hospital	Bellevue	71%	300+
Blanchard Valley Hospital	Findlay	71%	300+
Dublin Methodist Hospital	Dublin	71%	300+
Good Samaritan Hospital	Cincinnati	71%	300+
Marion General Hospital	Marion	71%	300+
Mercy Hospital Fairfield	Fairfield	71%	300+
Mercy Tiffin Hospital	Tiffin	71%	300+
Riverside Methodist Hospital	Columbus	71%	300+
Aultman Hospital	Canton	70%	300+
Bay Park Community Hospital	Oregon	70%	300+
Grant Medical Center	Columbus	70%	300+
Memorial Hospital	Fremont	70%	300+
Mercy St Anne Hospital	Toledo	70%	300+
Ohio State University Hospitals	Columbus	70%	300+
Southwest General Health Center	Middleburg Hgts	70%	300+
UHHS Memorial Hospital of Geneva[11]	Geneva	70%	300+
Wilson Memorial Hospital	Sidney	70%	300+
Affinity Medical Center	Massillon	69%	300+
Akron General Medical Center[11]	Akron	69%	300+
Belmont Community Hospital	Bellaire	69%	(a)
Doctors Hospital	Columbus	69%	300+
Grady Memorial Hospital	Delaware	69%	300+
Jewish Hospital	Cincinnati	69%	300+
Medical Center of Newark	Newark	69%	300+
Mercy Hospital Clermont	Batavia	69%	300+
Mercy St Charles Hospital	Oregon	69%	300+
Mount Carmel Health	Columbus	69%	300+
Robinson Memorial Hospital	Ravenna	69%	300+
Saint John Medical Center	Westlake	69%	300+
Saint Rita's Medical Center	Lima	69%	300+
Saint Vincent Charity Medical Center	Cleveland	69%	300+
Summa Barberton Hospital	Barberton	69%	300+
Adena Regional Medical Center	Chillicothe	68%	300+
Atrium Medical Center	Franklin	68%	300+
Cleveland Clinic	Cleveland	68%	300+
Defiance Regional Medical Center	Defiance	68%	300+
Fairfield Medical Center	Lancaster	68%	300+
Fairview Hospital	Cleveland	68%	300+
Fisher Titus Memorial Hospital	Norwalk	68%	300+
Hardin Memorial Hospital	Kenton	68%	(a)
Knox Community Hospital	Mount Vernon	68%	300+
Marietta Memorial Hospital	Marietta	68%	300+
Mary Rutan Hospital	Bellefontaine	68%	300+
Mercy Memorial Hospital	Urbana	68%	300+
Miami Valley Hospital	Dayton	68%	300+
Mount Carmel St Ann's Hospital	Westerville	68%	300+
Saint Elizabeth Boardman Health Center	Youngstown	68%	300+
Southeastern Ohio Regional Medical Center	Cambridge	68%	300+
Trinity Medical Center East & West	Steubenville	68%	300+
Union Hospital	Dover	68%	300+
Wayne Hospital	Greenville	68%	300+
Euclid Hospital	Euclid	67%	300+
Firelands Regional Medical Center	Sandusky	67%	300+
Flower Hospital	Sylvania	67%	300+
Kettering Medical Center	Kettering	67%	300+
Licking Memorial Hospital	Newark	67%	300+
Lima Memorial Health System	Lima	67%	300+
O'Bleness Memorial Hospital	Athens	67%	300+
Parma Community General Hospital	Parma	67%	300+
Saint Luke's Hospital	Maumee	67%	300+
Summa Wadsworth-Rittman Hospital	Wadsworth	67%	300+
UH Geauga Medical Center[11]	Chardon	67%	300+
Wood County Hospital	Bowling Green	67%	300+
Bethesda North Hospital	Cincinnati	66%	300+
CMH Regional Health System	Wilmington	66%	300+
Fort Hamilton Hughes Memorial Hospital	Hamilton	66%	300+
Grandview Hospital & Medical Center	Dayton	66%	300+
Lake Health	Concord	66%	300+
Lakewood Hospital	Lakewood	66%	300+
Medina Hospital	Medina	66%	300+
Mercy Hospital Anderson	Cincinnati	66%	300+
Metro Health Medical Center	Cleveland	66%	300+
Northside Medical Center	Youngstown	66%	300+
South Pointe Hospital	Warrensville Hgts	66%	300+
Summa Health Systems Hospitals	Akron	66%	300+
Summa Western Reserve Hospital	Cuyahoga Falls	66%	300+
University Hospitals of Cleveland	Cleveland	66%	300+
Upper Valley Medical Center	Troy	66%	300+
Berger Hospital	Circleville	65%	300+
Community Regional Medical Center	Lorain	65%	300+
Coshocton County Memorial Hospital	Coshocton	65%	300+
Greene Memorial Hospital	Xenia	65%	300+
Joel Pomerene Memorial Hospital	Millersburg	65%	300+
Mercy Franciscan Hospital Western Hills	Cincinnati	65%	300+
Mercy St Vincent Medical Center	Toledo	65%	300+
Morrow County Hospital	Mount Gilead	65%	(a)
The Toledo Hospital	Toledo	65%	300+
Alliance Community Hospital	Alliance	64%	300+
Emh Regional Medical Center	Elyria	64%	300+
Good Samaritan Hospital	Dayton	64%	300+
Medcentral Health System	Mansfield	64%	300+
Mercy Franciscan Hospital - Mt Airy	Cincinnati	64%	300+
Saint Joseph Health Center	Warren	64%	300+
Samaritan Hospital - Peoples Hospital	Ashland	64%	300+
UHHS Bedford Medical Center[11]	Bedford	64%	300+
Ashtabula County Medical Center	Ashtabula	63%	300+
East Liverpool City Hospital	East Liverpool	63%	300+
Hillcrest Hospital	Mayfield Heights	63%	300+
University Hospital	Cincinnati	63%	300+
East Ohio Regional Hospital	Martins Ferry	62%	300+
Huron Hospital	Cleveland	62%	300+
Kettering Medical Center - Sycamore	Miamisburg	62%	300+
Lutheran Hospital	Cleveland	62%	300+
Marymount Hospital	Garfield Heights	62%	300+
UHHS Richmond Heights Hospital[11]	Richmond Hghts	62%	300+
Brown County Hospital	Georgetown	61%	300+
Fayette County Memorial Hospital	Washington CH	61%	(a)
Saint Elizabeth Health Center	Youngstown	61%	300+
Salem Community Hospital	Salem	60%	300+
Springfield Regional Medical Center	Springfield	60%	300+
University of Toledo Medical Center	Toledo	60%	300+
Trumbull Memorial Hospital	Warren	59%	300+

47. Room and Bathroom 'Always' Clean

Hospital Name	City	Rate	Cases
Henry County Hospital	Napoleon	90%	(a)
Morrow County Hospital	Mount Gilead	89%	(a)
Univ Hosps Conneaut Med Ctr[11]	Conneaut	89%	(a)
Butler County Medical Center	Hamilton	88%	(a)
Surgical Hospital at Southwoods	Youngstown	87%	(a)
H B Magruder Memorial Hospital	Port Clinton	85%	300+
Mercy Hospital of Willard	Willard	85%	(a)
Amherst Hospital	Amherst	84%	300+
Evendale Medical Center	Cincinnati	84%	300+
Fulton County Health Center	Wauseon	84%	300+
Lodi Community Hospital[11]	Lodi	84%	(a)
Mercy Hospital of Defiance	Defiance	84%	300+
Bellevue Hospital	Bellevue	83%	300+
CMH Regional Health System	Wilmington	83%	300+
Fairview Hospital	Cleveland	83%	300+
McCullough-Hyde Memorial Hospital	Oxford	83%	300+
Mercy Memorial Hospital	Urbana	83%	300+
Mercy Tiffin Hospital	Tiffin	83%	300+
Blanchard Valley Hospital	Findlay	82%	300+
Community Hospitals and Wellness Centers	Bryan	82%	300+
Firelands Regional Medical Center	Sandusky	82%	300+
Institute for Orthopedic Surgery	Lima	82%	300+
Joint Township District Memorial Hospital	Saint Marys	82%	300+
UHHS Memorial Hospital of Geneva[11]	Geneva	82%	300+
Bluffton Hospital	Bluffton	81%	(a)
Galion Community Hospital	Galion	81%	300+
Holzer Medical Center Jackson	Jackson	81%	300+
Mount Carmel New Albany Surgical Hospital	New Albany	81%	300+
Southern Ohio Medical Center	Portsmouth	81%	300+
Barnesville Hospital Association	Barnesville	80%	300+
Mercy St Charles Hospital	Oregon	80%	300+
Wilson Memorial Hospital	Sidney	80%	300+
Allen Community Hospital	Oberlin	79%	300+
Fisher Titus Memorial Hospital	Norwalk	79%	300+
Hardin Memorial Hospital	Kenton	79%	(a)
Mercer County Joint Twp Comm Hosp	Coldwater	79%	(a)
Van Wert County Hospital	Van Wert	79%	300+
Joel Pomerene Memorial Hospital	Millersburg	78%	300+
Medcentral Health System Shelby Hospital	Shelby	78%	300+
Mercy St Anne Hospital	Toledo	78%	300+
Fostoria Community Hospital	Fostoria	77%	300+
Holzer Medical Center	Gallipolis	77%	300+
Medical Center of Newark	Newark	77%	300+
Southeastern Ohio Regional Medical Center	Cambridge	77%	300+
Wooster Community Hospital	Wooster	77%	300+
Ashtabula County Medical Center	Ashtabula	76%	300+
Defiance Regional Medical Center	Defiance	76%	300+
Memorial Hospital of Union County	Marysville	76%	300+
Wood County Hospital	Bowling Green	76%	300+
Alliance Community Hospital	Alliance	75%	300+
Marion General Hospital	Marion	75%	300+
Medical Center at Elizabeth Place	Dayton	75%	(a)
Memorial Hospital	Fremont	75%	300+
Bay Park Community Hospital	Oregon	74%	300+
Fayette County Memorial Hospital	Washington CH	74%	(a)
Licking Memorial Hospital	Newark	74%	300+
Lima Memorial Health System	Lima	74%	300+
Atrium Medical Center	Franklin	73%	300+
Dublin Methodist Hospital	Dublin	73%	300+
Hocking Valley Community Hospital	Logan	73%	300+
Madison County Hospital	London	73%	300+
Mercy Medical Center	Canton	73%	300+
Mercy St Vincent Medical Center	Toledo	73%	300+
Wayne Hospital	Greenville	73%	300+
West Chester Medical Center	West Chester	73%	300+
Coshocton County Memorial Hospital	Coshocton	72%	300+
Fairfield Medical Center	Lancaster	72%	300+
Genesis Healthcare System	Zanesville	72%	300+
Grady Memorial Hospital	Delaware	72%	300+
Saint Elizabeth Boardman Health Center	Youngstown	72%	300+
Bethesda North Hospital	Cincinnati	71%	300+
Flower Hospital	Sylvania	71%	300+
Mercy Hospital Clermont	Batavia	71%	300+
Saint Luke's Hospital	Maumee	71%	300+
Union Hospital	Dover	71%	300+
Belmont Community Hospital	Bellaire	70%	(a)
Brown County Hospital	Georgetown	70%	300+
Community Regional Medical Center	Lorain	70%	300+
Fort Hamilton Hughes Memorial Hospital	Hamilton	70%	300+
Grant Medical Center	Columbus	70%	300+
Knox Community Hospital	Mount Vernon	70%	300+
Lake Health	Concord	70%	300+
Robinson Memorial Hospital	Ravenna	70%	300+
Trinity Medical Center East & West	Steubenville	70%	300+
East Liverpool City Hospital	East Liverpool	69%	300+
Jewish Hospital	Cincinnati	69%	300+
Mary Rutan Hospital	Bellefontaine	69%	300+
Saint Rita's Medical Center	Lima	69%	300+
Summa Wadsworth-Rittman Hospital	Wadsworth	69%	300+
Summa Western Reserve Hospital	Cuyahoga Falls	69%	300+
Bucyrus Community Hospital	Bucyrus	68%	(a)
Cleveland Clinic	Cleveland	68%	300+
Doctors Hospital	Columbus	68%	300+
Kettering Medical Center - Sycamore	Miamisburg	68%	300+
Lakewood Hospital	Lakewood	68%	300+
Medcentral Health System	Mansfield	68%	300+
Mercy Hospital Fairfield	Fairfield	68%	300+
Ohio State University Hospitals	Columbus	68%	300+
Saint Vincent Charity Medical Center	Cleveland	68%	300+
Samaritan Hospital - Peoples Hospital	Ashland	68%	300+
Summa Barberton Hospital	Barberton	68%	300+

NOTE: Hospital profiles are in alphabetical order by state, then city, then hospital within the city; Rankings exclude hospitals with less than 25 cases except for patient surveys which excludes hospitals with less than 100 cases; (a) 100–299 cases; (1) The number of cases is too small to be sure how well a hospital is performing; (2) The hospital indicated that the data submitted for this measure were based on a sample of cases; (3) Data was collected during a shorter time period (fewer quarters) than the maximum possible time for this measure; (4) Suppressed for one or more quarters by CMS; (5) No data is available from the hospital for this measure; (6) Fewer than 100 patients completed the HCAHPS survey. Use these rates with caution, as the number of surveys may be too low to reliably assess hospital performance; (7) Survey results are based on less than 12 months of data; (8) Survey results are not available for this reporting period; (9) No or very few patients were eligible for the HCAHPS survey. The scores shown, if any, reflect a very small number of surveys; (10) A state average was not calculated because too few hospitals in the state submitted data; (11) There were discrepancies in the data collection process; Please refer to the User's Guide for a full explanation of data.

The Toledo Hospital	Toledo	68%	300+
Affinity Medical Center	Massillon	67%	300+
Aultman Hospital	Canton	67%	300+
Grandview Hospital & Medical Center	Dayton	67%	300+
Marietta Memorial Hospital	Marietta	67%	300+
UH Geauga Medical Center[11]	Chardon	67%	300+
Upper Valley Medical Center	Troy	67%	300+
Good Samaritan Hospital	Cincinnati	66%	300+
Medina Hospital	Medina	66%	300+
Riverside Methodist Hospital	Columbus	66%	300+
Southwest General Health Center	Middleburg Hgts	66%	300+
Marymount Hospital	Garfield Heights	65%	300+
O'Bleness Memorial Hospital	Athens	65%	300+
Parma Community General Hospital	Parma	65%	300+
Saint John Medical Center	Westlake	65%	300+
Summa Health Systems Hospitals	Akron	65%	300+
Christ Hospital	Cincinnati	64%	300+
Greene Memorial Hospital	Xenia	64%	300+
Kettering Medical Center	Kettering	64%	300+
Mount Carmel Health	Columbus	64%	300+
Saint Joseph Health Center	Warren	64%	300+
Berger Hospital	Circleville	63%	300+
Euclid Hospital	Euclid	63%	300+
Hillcrest Hospital	Mayfield Heights	63%	300+
Mercy Hospital Anderson	Cincinnati	63%	300+
Mount Carmel St Ann's Hospital	Westerville	63%	300+
Northside Medical Center	Youngstown	63%	300+
Salem Community Hospital	Salem	63%	300+
South Pointe Hospital	Warrensville Hgts	63%	300+
UHHS Bedford Medical Center[11]	Bedford	63%	300+
Deaconess Hospital	Cincinnati	62%	(a)
Emh Regional Medical Center	Elyria	62%	300+
Huron Hospital	Cleveland	62%	300+
Mercy Franciscan Hospital Western Hills	Cincinnati	62%	300+
University Hospitals of Cleveland	Cleveland	62%	300+
Akron General Medical Center[11]	Akron	61%	300+
Metro Health Medical Center	Cleveland	61%	300+
Miami Valley Hospital	Dayton	61%	300+
Saint Elizabeth Health Center	Youngstown	61%	300+
University Hospital	Cincinnati	61%	300+
Adena Regional Medical Center	Chillicothe	60%	300+
East Ohio Regional Hospital	Martins Ferry	60%	300+
Lutheran Hospital	Cleveland	59%	300+
UHHS Richmond Heights Hospital[11]	Richmond Hghts	59%	300+
Good Samaritan Hospital	Dayton	58%	300+
Mercy Franciscan Hospital - Mt Airy	Cincinnati	58%	300+
Springfield Regional Medical Center	Springfield	56%	300+
Trumbull Memorial Hospital	Warren	56%	300+
University of Toledo Medical Center	Toledo	52%	300+

48. Timely Help 'Always' Received

Hospital Name	City	Rate	Cases
Surgical Hospital at Southwoods	Youngstown	92%	(a)
Butler County Medical Center	Hamilton	88%	(a)
Institute for Orthopedic Surgery	Lima	88%	300+
Univ Hosps Conneaut Med Ctr[11]	Conneaut	85%	(a)
Henry County Hospital	Napoleon	84%	(a)
Mercy Hospital of Willard	Willard	84%	(a)
Bluffton Hospital	Bluffton	83%	(a)
H B Magruder Memorial Hospital	Port Clinton	83%	300+
Barnesville Hospital Association	Barnesville	80%	300+
Galion Community Hospital	Galion	79%	300+
Medical Center at Elizabeth Place	Dayton	79%	(a)
Mercy Hospital of Defiance	Defiance	78%	300+
Evendale Medical Center	Cincinnati	77%	300+
Holzer Medical Center Jackson	Jackson	77%	300+
Medcentral Health System Shelby Hospital	Shelby	77%	300+
Morrow County Hospital	Mount Gilead	77%	(a)
Bucyrus Community Hospital	Bucyrus	76%	(a)
Memorial Hospital of Union County	Marysville	76%	300+
Amherst Hospital	Amherst	75%	300+
Mercer County Joint Twp Comm Hosp	Coldwater	75%	(a)
Community Hospitals and Wellness Centers	Bryan	74%	300+
Lodi Community Hospital[11]	Lodi	74%	(a)
Mercy Memorial Hospital	Urbana	73%	300+
UHHS Memorial Hospital of Geneva[11]	Geneva	73%	300+
Joint Township District Memorial Hospital	Saint Marys	72%	300+
Medical Center of Newark	Newark	72%	300+
Mount Carmel New Albany Surgical Hospital	New Albany	72%	300+
Allen Community Hospital	Oberlin	71%	300+
Fostoria Community Hospital	Fostoria	71%	300+
Genesis Healthcare System	Zanesville	71%	300+
Hocking Valley Community Hospital	Logan	71%	300+
Madison County Hospital	London	71%	300+
Mary Rutan Hospital	Bellefontaine	71%	300+
Fayette County Memorial Hospital	Washington CH	70%	(a)
Marion General Hospital	Marion	70%	300+
McCullough-Hyde Memorial Hospital	Oxford	70%	300+
Wood County Hospital	Bowling Green	70%	300+
CMH Regional Health System	Wilmington	69%	300+
Defiance Regional Medical Center	Defiance	69%	300+
Doctors Hospital	Columbus	69%	300+
Hardin Memorial Hospital	Kenton	69%	(a)
Saint Rita's Medical Center	Lima	69%	300+
Christ Hospital	Cincinnati	68%	300+
Deaconess Hospital	Cincinnati	68%	(a)
Fulton County Health Center	Wauseon	68%	300+
Holzer Medical Center	Gallipolis	68%	300+
Memorial Hospital	Fremont	68%	300+
Mercy Tiffin Hospital	Tiffin	68%	300+
Southeastern Ohio Regional Medical Center	Cambridge	68%	300+
Southern Ohio Medical Center	Portsmouth	68%	300+
Van Wert County Hospital	Van Wert	68%	300+
Wayne Hospital	Greenville	68%	300+
Wilson Memorial Hospital	Sidney	68%	300+
Bellevue Hospital	Bellevue	67%	300+
Blanchard Valley Hospital	Findlay	67%	300+
Dublin Methodist Hospital	Dublin	67%	300+
Mercy St Charles Hospital	Oregon	67%	300+
Summa Wadsworth-Rittman Hospital	Wadsworth	67%	300+
Bay Park Community Hospital	Oregon	66%	300+
Knox Community Hospital	Mount Vernon	66%	300+
Licking Memorial Hospital	Newark	66%	300+
Summa Barberton Hospital	Barberton	66%	300+
Coshocton County Memorial Hospital	Coshocton	65%	300+
Mercy Hospital Fairfield	Fairfield	65%	300+
Saint Luke's Hospital	Maumee	65%	300+
Southwest General Health Center	Middleburg Hgts	65%	300+
West Chester Medical Center	West Chester	65%	300+
Alliance Community Hospital	Alliance	64%	300+
Aultman Hospital	Canton	64%	300+
Berger Hospital	Circleville	64%	300+
Fairfield Medical Center	Lancaster	64%	300+
Mercy St Anne Hospital	Toledo	64%	300+
Union Hospital	Dover	64%	300+
Wooster Community Hospital	Wooster	64%	300+
Akron General Medical Center[11]	Akron	63%	300+
Belmont Community Hospital	Bellaire	63%	(a)
Firelands Regional Medical Center	Sandusky	63%	300+
Good Samaritan Hospital	Cincinnati	63%	300+
Mercy St Vincent Medical Center	Toledo	63%	300+
Summa Western Reserve Hospital	Cuyahoga Falls	63%	300+
Upper Valley Medical Center	Troy	63%	300+
Fairview Hospital	Cleveland	62%	300+
Grant Medical Center	Columbus	62%	300+
Jewish Hospital	Cincinnati	62%	300+
Joel Pomerene Memorial Hospital	Millersburg	62%	300+
Marietta Memorial Hospital	Marietta	62%	300+
Medcentral Health System	Mansfield	62%	300+
Mercy Hospital Clermont	Batavia	62%	300+
Mercy Medical Center	Canton	62%	300+
Ohio State University Hospitals	Columbus	62%	300+
Trinity Medical Center East & West	Steubenville	62%	300+
UH Geauga Medical Center[11]	Chardon	62%	300+
Bethesda North Hospital	Cincinnati	61%	300+
Fisher Titus Memorial Hospital	Norwalk	61%	300+
Flower Hospital	Sylvania	61%	300+
Mount Carmel St Ann's Hospital	Westerville	61%	300+
O'Bleness Memorial Hospital	Athens	61%	300+
Riverside Methodist Hospital	Columbus	61%	300+
Saint Vincent Charity Medical Center	Cleveland	61%	300+
Summa Health Systems Hospitals	Akron	61%	300+
East Liverpool City Hospital	East Liverpool	60%	300+
Emh Regional Medical Center	Elyria	60%	300+
Fort Hamilton Hughes Memorial Hospital	Hamilton	60%	300+
Grady Memorial Hospital	Delaware	60%	300+
Mercy Franciscan Hospital Western Hills	Cincinnati	60%	300+
Mount Carmel Health	Columbus	60%	300+
South Pointe Hospital	Warrensville Hgts	60%	300+
Brown County Hospital	Georgetown	59%	300+
Grandview Hospital & Medical Center	Dayton	59%	300+
Medina Hospital	Medina	59%	300+
Metro Health Medical Center	Cleveland	59%	300+
Robinson Memorial Hospital	Ravenna	59%	300+
Saint John Medical Center	Westlake	59%	300+
Samaritan Hospital - Peoples Hospital	Ashland	59%	300+
Adena Regional Medical Center	Chillicothe	58%	300+
Ashtabula County Medical Center	Ashtabula	58%	300+
Cleveland Clinic	Cleveland	58%	300+
Lake Health	Concord	58%	300+
Mercy Hospital Anderson	Cincinnati	58%	300+
Parma Community General Hospital	Parma	58%	300+
Salem Community Hospital	Salem	58%	300+
Affinity Medical Center	Massillon	57%	300+
Community Regional Medical Center	Lorain	57%	300+
Lakewood Hospital	Lakewood	57%	300+
Lima Memorial Health System	Lima	57%	300+
Saint Elizabeth Boardman Health Center	Youngstown	57%	300+
Saint Joseph Health Center	Warren	57%	300+
Euclid Hospital	Euclid	56%	300+
Greene Memorial Hospital	Xenia	56%	300+
Hillcrest Hospital	Mayfield Heights	56%	300+
Kettering Medical Center	Kettering	56%	300+
The Toledo Hospital	Toledo	56%	300+
Atrium Medical Center	Franklin	55%	300+
Marymount Hospital	Garfield Heights	55%	300+
Miami Valley Hospital	Dayton	55%	300+
Northside Medical Center	Youngstown	55%	300+
Trumbull Memorial Hospital	Warren	55%	300+
University Hospital	Cincinnati	55%	300+
University Hospitals of Cleveland	Cleveland	55%	300+
Mercy Franciscan Hospital - Mt Airy	Cincinnati	54%	300+
UHHS Bedford Medical Center[11]	Bedford	54%	300+
Good Samaritan Hospital	Dayton	53%	300+
Kettering Medical Center - Sycamore	Miamisburg	53%	300+
Saint Elizabeth Health Center	Youngstown	53%	300+
East Ohio Regional Hospital	Martins Ferry	51%	300+
Lutheran Hospital	Cleveland	51%	300+
University of Toledo Medical Center	Toledo	51%	300+
Springfield Regional Medical Center	Springfield	49%	300+
Huron Hospital	Cleveland	48%	300+
UHHS Richmond Heights Hospital[11]	Richmond Hghts	48%	300+

49. Would Definitely Recommend Hospital

Hospital Name	City	Rate	Cases
Surgical Hospital at Southwoods	Youngstown	97%	(a)
Institute for Orthopedic Surgery	Lima	94%	300+
Butler County Medical Center	Hamilton	90%	(a)
Bluffton Hospital	Bluffton	89%	(a)
Mount Carmel New Albany Surgical Hospital	New Albany	89%	300+
Dublin Methodist Hospital	Dublin	86%	300+
Lodi Community Hospital[11]	Lodi	86%	(a)
Christ Hospital	Cincinnati	85%	300+
West Chester Medical Center	West Chester	85%	300+
Mercy Hospital of Willard	Willard	84%	(a)
Riverside Methodist Hospital	Columbus	83%	300+
Amherst Hospital	Amherst	82%	300+
Cleveland Clinic	Cleveland	82%	300+
Saint Elizabeth Boardman Health Center	Youngstown	82%	300+
Univ Hosps Conneaut Med Ctr[11]	Conneaut	82%	(a)
Evendale Medical Center	Cincinnati	81%	300+
H B Magruder Memorial Hospital	Port Clinton	81%	300+
Bellevue Hospital	Bellevue	80%	300+
Aultman Hospital	Canton	79%	300+
Morrow County Hospital	Mount Gilead	79%	(a)
Bethesda North Hospital	Cincinnati	78%	300+
Henry County Hospital	Napoleon	78%	(a)
Medcentral Health System Shelby Hospital	Shelby	78%	300+
Medical Center of Newark	Newark	78%	300+
Mercy Hospital of Defiance	Defiance	78%	300+
Mercy St Anne Hospital	Toledo	78%	300+
Defiance Regional Medical Center	Defiance	77%	300+
Fairview Hospital	Cleveland	77%	300+
Bay Park Community Hospital	Oregon	76%	300+
Good Samaritan Hospital	Cincinnati	76%	300+
McCullough-Hyde Memorial Hospital	Oxford	76%	300+
Medical Center at Elizabeth Place	Dayton	76%	(a)
Memorial Hospital of Union County	Marysville	76%	300+
Saint Rita's Medical Center	Lima	76%	300+
UHHS Memorial Hospital of Geneva[11]	Geneva	76%	300+
University Hospitals of Cleveland	Cleveland	76%	300+
Wooster Community Hospital	Wooster	76%	300+
Allen Community Hospital	Oberlin	75%	300+
Barnesville Hospital Association	Barnesville	75%	300+
Jewish Hospital	Cincinnati	75%	300+
Kettering Medical Center	Kettering	75%	300+
Lima Memorial Health System	Lima	75%	300+
Mercer County Joint Twp Comm Hosp	Coldwater	75%	(a)
Mercy Hospital Fairfield	Fairfield	75%	300+
Summa Western Reserve Hospital	Cuyahoga Falls	75%	300+
Deaconess Hospital	Cincinnati	74%	(a)
Fisher Titus Memorial Hospital	Norwalk	74%	300+
Fostoria Community Hospital	Fostoria	74%	300+
Grant Medical Center	Columbus	74%	300+
Doctors Hospital	Columbus	73%	300+
Flower Hospital	Sylvania	73%	300+
Galion Community Hospital	Galion	73%	300+
Joint Township District Memorial Hospital	Saint Marys	73%	300+
Kettering Medical Center - Sycamore	Miamisburg	73%	300+
Mercy Medical Center	Canton	73%	300+
Mercy St Charles Hospital	Oregon	73%	300+
Mercy St Vincent Medical Center	Toledo	73%	300+
Metro Health Medical Center	Cleveland	73%	300+
Ohio State University Hospitals	Columbus	73%	300+
Saint Joseph Health Center	Warren	73%	300+
Saint Luke's Hospital	Maumee	73%	300+
Southern Ohio Medical Center	Portsmouth	73%	300+
Akron General Medical Center[11]	Akron	72%	300+
Blanchard Valley Hospital	Findlay	72%	300+
Fulton County Health Center	Wauseon	72%	300+
Mercy Hospital Clermont	Batavia	72%	300+

NOTE: Hospital profiles are in alphabetical order by state, then city, then hospital within the city; Rankings exclude hospitals with less than 25 cases except for patient surveys which excludes hospitals with less than 100 cases; (a) 100–299 cases; (1) The number of cases is too small to be sure how well a hospital is performing; (2) The hospital indicated that the data submitted for this measure were based on a sample of cases; (3) Data was collected during a shorter time period (fewer quarters) than the maximum possible time for this measure; (4) Suppressed for one or more quarters by CMS; (5) No data is available from the hospital for this measure; (6) Fewer than 100 patients completed the HCAHPS survey. Use these rates with caution, as the number of surveys may be too low to reliably assess hospital performance; (7) Survey results are based on less than 12 months of data; (8) Survey results are not available for this reporting period; (9) No or very few patients were eligible for the HCAHPS survey. The scores shown, if any, reflect a very small number of surveys; (10) A state average was not calculated because too few hospitals in the state submitted data; (11) There were discrepancies in the data collection process; Please refer to the User's Guide for a full explanation of data.

Miami Valley Hospital	Dayton	72%	300+
Mount Carmel Health	Columbus	72%	300+
Saint John Medical Center	Westlake	72%	300+
Grandview Hospital & Medical Center	Dayton	71%	300+
Mount Carmel St Ann's Hospital	Westerville	71%	300+
Saint Vincent Charity Medical Center	Cleveland	71%	300+
Southwest General Health Center	Middleburg Hgts	71%	300+
Community Hospitals and Wellness Centers	Bryan	70%	300+
Genesis Healthcare System	Zanesville	70%	300+
Holzer Medical Center Jackson	Jackson	70%	300+
Firelands Regional Medical Center	Sandusky	69%	300+
Marion General Hospital	Marion	69%	300+
Mercy Tiffin Hospital	Tiffin	69%	300+
Summa Health Systems Hospitals	Akron	69%	300+
Euclid Hospital	Euclid	68%	300+
Fairfield Medical Center	Lancaster	68%	300+
Grady Memorial Hospital	Delaware	68%	300+
Mercy Memorial Hospital	Urbana	68%	300+
CMH Regional Health System	Wilmington	67%	300+
Lake Health	Concord	67%	300+
Mercy Hospital Anderson	Cincinnati	67%	300+
Summa Barberton Hospital	Barberton	67%	300+
Summa Wadsworth-Rittman Hospital	Wadsworth	67%	300+
UH Geauga Medical Center[11]	Chardon	67%	300+
University Hospital	Cincinnati	67%	300+
Adena Regional Medical Center	Chillicothe	66%	300+
Hocking Valley Community Hospital	Logan	66%	300+
Lakewood Hospital	Lakewood	66%	300+
Madison County Hospital	London	66%	300+
The Toledo Hospital	Toledo	66%	300+
Trinity Medical Center East & West	Steubenville	66%	300+
Affinity Medical Center	Massillon	65%	300+
Atrium Medical Center	Franklin	65%	300+
Good Samaritan Hospital	Dayton	65%	300+
Hillcrest Hospital	Mayfield Heights	65%	300+
Van Wert County Hospital	Van Wert	65%	300+
Wood County Hospital	Bowling Green	65%	300+
Alliance Community Hospital	Alliance	64%	300+
Belmont Community Hospital	Bellaire	64%	(a)
Bucyrus Community Hospital	Bucyrus	64%	(a)
Marietta Memorial Hospital	Marietta	64%	300+
Northside Medical Center	Youngstown	64%	300+
Southeastern Ohio Regional Medical Center	Cambridge	64%	300+
Wilson Memorial Hospital	Sidney	64%	300+
Holzer Medical Center	Gallipolis	63%	300+
Knox Community Hospital	Mount Vernon	63%	300+
Samaritan Hospital - Peoples Hospital	Ashland	63%	300+
Union Hospital	Dover	63%	300+
Emh Regional Medical Center	Elyria	62%	300+
Medina Hospital	Medina	62%	300+
Memorial Hospital	Fremont	62%	300+
Parma Community General Hospital	Parma	62%	300+
Robinson Memorial Hospital	Ravenna	62%	300+
Licking Memorial Hospital	Newark	61%	300+
Medcentral Health System	Mansfield	61%	300+
Saint Elizabeth Health Center	Youngstown	61%	300+
Joel Pomerene Memorial Hospital	Millersburg	60%	300+
Upper Valley Medical Center	Troy	60%	300+
Community Regional Medical Center	Lorain	59%	300+
Greene Memorial Hospital	Xenia	59%	300+
Hardin Memorial Hospital	Kenton	59%	(a)
Lutheran Hospital	Cleveland	59%	300+
Mary Rutan Hospital	Bellefontaine	59%	300+
Salem Community Hospital	Salem	59%	300+
South Pointe Hospital	Warrensville Hgts	59%	300+
Berger Hospital	Circleville	58%	300+
Fort Hamilton Hughes Memorial Hospital	Hamilton	58%	300+
Marymount Hospital	Garfield Heights	57%	300+
Mercy Franciscan Hospital - Mt Airy	Cincinnati	57%	300+
Mercy Franciscan Hospital Western Hills	Cincinnati	57%	300+
Trumbull Memorial Hospital	Warren	57%	300+
Wayne Hospital	Greenville	57%	300+
O'Bleness Memorial Hospital	Athens	56%	300+
UHHS Richmond Heights Hospital[11]	Richmond Hghts	56%	300+
UHHS Bedford Medical Center[11]	Bedford	55%	300+
Fayette County Memorial Hospital	Washington CH	54%	(a)
University of Toledo Medical Center	Toledo	53%	300+
Brown County Hospital	Georgetown	51%	300+
Coshocton County Memorial Hospital	Coshocton	51%	300+
East Ohio Regional Hospital	Martins Ferry	51%	300+
East Liverpool City Hospital	East Liverpool	50%	300+
Ashtabula County Medical Center	Ashtabula	49%	300+
Huron Hospital	Cleveland	48%	300+
Springfield Regional Medical Center	Springfield	45%	300+

NOTE: Hospital profiles are in alphabetical order by state, then city, then hospital within the city; Rankings exclude hospitals with less than 25 cases except for patient surveys which excludes hospitals with less than 100 cases; (a) 100–299 cases; (1) The number of cases is too small to be sure how well a hospital is performing; (2) The hospital indicated that the data submitted for this measure were based on a sample of cases; (3) Data was collected during a shorter time period (fewer quarters) than the maximum possible time for this measure; (4) Suppressed for one or more quarters by CMS; (5) No data is available from the hospital for this measure; (6) Fewer than 100 patients completed the HCAHPS survey. Use these rates with caution, as the number of surveys may be too low to reliably assess hospital performance; (7) Survey results are based on a sample of cases; (3) Survey results are based on less than 12 months of data; (8) Survey results are not available for this reporting period; (9) No or very few patients were eligible for the HCAHPS survey. The scores shown, if any, reflect a very small number of surveys; (10) A state average was not calculated because too few hospitals in the state submitted data; (11) There were discrepancies in the data collection process; Please refer to the User's Guide for a full explanation of data.

Akron General Medical Center

400 Wabash Avenue
Akron, OH 44307
Phone: 330-344-6000
Fax: 330-376-4835
E-mail: jarmstrong@agmc.org
URL: www.akrongeneral.org
Type: Acute Care Hospitals
Emergency Services: Yes
Ownership: Voluntary Non-Profit - Private
Beds: 537

Key Personnel:
CEO/President. . . . . Alan Bleyer
Cardiac Laboratory. . . . . George I Litman, MD
Chief of Medical Staff. . . . . Richard J Streck, MD
Infection Control. . . . . Gary Bollin, MD
Operating Room. . . . . Gary Tomcho, RN
Quality Assurance . . . . Susan Carter
Radiology. . . . . Marilyn Schultz, MD

Measure	Cases	This Hosp.	State Avg.	U.S. Avg.
Heart Attack Care				
ACE Inhibitor or ARB for LVSD[2]	71	94%	97%	96%
Aspirin at Arrival[2]	216	99%	99%	99%
Aspirin at Discharge[2]	284	97%	99%	98%
Beta Blocker at Discharge[2]	270	99%	99%	98%
Fibrinolytic Medication Timing[2]	0	-	14%	55%
PCI Within 90 Minutes of Arrival[2]	47	87%	92%	90%
Smoking Cessation Advice[2]	104	100%	100%	99%
Chest Pain/Possible Heart Attack Care				
Aspirin at Arrival[1,3]	2	100%	96%	95%
Median Time to ECG (minutes)[1,3]	2	0	7	8
Median Time to Transfer (minutes)[5]	0	-	61	61
Fibrinolytic Medication Timing[5]	0	-	47%	54%
Heart Failure Care				
ACE Inhibitor or ARB for LVSD[2]	102	91%	96%	94%
Discharge Instructions[2]	244	77%	91%	88%
Evaluation of LVS Function[2]	302	99%	99%	98%
Smoking Cessation Advice[2]	46	96%	99%	98%
Pneumonia Care				
Appropriate Initial Antibiotic[2]	69	94%	92%	92%
Blood Culture Timing[2]	81	99%	96%	96%
Influenza Vaccine[2]	92	85%	93%	91%
Initial Antibiotic Timing[2]	108	76%	96%	95%
Pneumococcal Vaccine[2]	127	87%	95%	93%
Smoking Cessation Advice[2]	59	93%	98%	97%
Surgical Care Improvement Project				
Appropriate VTP Within 24 Hours[2]	248	93%	92%	92%
Appropriate Hair Removal[2]	614	100%	100%	99%
Appropriate Beta Blocker Usage[2]	180	92%	94%	93%
Controlled Postoperative Blood Glucose[2]	116	97%	94%	93%
Prophylactic Antibiotic Timing[2]	442	97%	97%	97%
Prophylactic Antibiotic Timing (Outpatient)	698	95%	91%	92%
Prophylactic Antibiotic Selection[2]	448	98%	98%	97%
Prophylactic Antibiotic Select. (Outpatient)	687	93%	94%	94%
Prophylactic Antibiotic Stopped[2]	422	99%	95%	94%
Recommended VTP Ordered[2]	248	98%	94%	94%
Urinary Catheter Removal[2]	105	82%	91%	90%
Children's Asthma Care				
Received Systemic Corticosteroids	-	-	-	100%
Received Home Management Plan	-	-	-	71%
Received Reliever Medication	-	-	-	100%
Use of Medical Imaging				
Combination Abdominal CT Scan	1,703	0.105	0.164	0.191
Combination Chest CT Scan	1,532	0.007	0.038	0.054
Follow-up Mammogram/Ultrasound	4,412	6.4%	8.4%	8.4%
MRI for Low Back Pain	379	32.5%	30.2%	32.7%
Survey of Patients' Hospital Experiences				
Area Around Room 'Always' Quiet at Night[11]	300+	46%	-	58%
Doctors 'Always' Communicated Well[11]	300+	76%	-	80%
Home Recovery Information Given[11]	300+	86%	-	82%
Hospital Given 9 or 10 on 10 Point Scale[11]	300+	66%	-	67%
Meds 'Always' Explained Before Given[11]	300+	59%	-	60%
Nurses 'Always' Communicated Well[11]	300+	76%	-	76%
Pain 'Always' Well Controlled[11]	300+	69%	-	69%
Room and Bathroom 'Always' Clean[11]	300+	61%	-	71%
Timely Help 'Always' Received[11]	300+	63%	-	64%
Would Definitely Recommend Hospital[11]	300+	72%	-	69%

Crystal Clinic Orthopaedic Center

444 North Main Street
Akron, OH 44310
Phone: 330-668-4040
URL: www.crystalclinic.com
Type: Acute Care Hospitals
Emergency Services: No
Ownership: Proprietary

Key Personnel:
President/CEO. . . . . Ronald R Sutken, EdD

Measure	Cases	This Hosp.	State Avg.	U.S. Avg.
Heart Attack Care				
ACE Inhibitor or ARB for LVSD[5]	0	-	97%	96%
Aspirin at Arrival[5]	0	-	99%	99%
Aspirin at Discharge[5]	0	-	99%	98%
Beta Blocker at Discharge[5]	0	-	99%	98%
Fibrinolytic Medication Timing[5]	0	-	14%	55%
PCI Within 90 Minutes of Arrival[5]	0	-	92%	90%
Smoking Cessation Advice[5]	0	-	100%	99%
Chest Pain/Possible Heart Attack Care				
Aspirin at Arrival[5]	0	-	96%	95%
Median Time to ECG (minutes)[5]	0	-	7	8
Median Time to Transfer (minutes)[5]	0	-	61	61
Fibrinolytic Medication Timing[5]	0	-	47%	54%
Heart Failure Care				
ACE Inhibitor or ARB for LVSD[5]	0	-	96%	94%
Discharge Instructions[5]	0	-	91%	88%
Evaluation of LVS Function[5]	0	-	99%	98%
Smoking Cessation Advice[5]	0	-	99%	98%
Pneumonia Care				
Appropriate Initial Antibiotic[5]	0	-	92%	92%
Blood Culture Timing[5]	0	-	96%	96%
Influenza Vaccine[5]	0	-	93%	91%
Initial Antibiotic Timing[5]	0	-	96%	95%
Pneumococcal Vaccine[5]	0	-	95%	93%
Smoking Cessation Advice[5]	0	-	98%	97%
Surgical Care Improvement Project				
Appropriate VTP Within 24 Hours[1,2,3]	24	100%	92%	92%
Appropriate Hair Removal[2,3]	139	100%	100%	99%
Appropriate Beta Blocker Usage[2,3]	41	85%	94%	93%
Controlled Postoperative Blood Glucose[2,3]	0	-	94%	93%
Prophylactic Antibiotic Timing[2,3]	98	95%	97%	97%
Prophylactic Antibiotic Timing (Outpatient)[3]	324	98%	91%	92%
Prophylactic Antibiotic Selection[2,3]	98	100%	98%	97%
Prophylactic Antibiotic Select. (Outpatient)[3]	324	100%	94%	94%
Prophylactic Antibiotic Stopped[2,3]	98	100%	95%	94%
Recommended VTP Ordered[1,2,3]	24	100%	94%	94%
Urinary Catheter Removal[1,2]	11	73%	91%	90%
Children's Asthma Care				
Received Systemic Corticosteroids	-	-	-	100%
Received Home Management Plan	-	-	-	71%
Received Reliever Medication	-	-	-	100%
Use of Medical Imaging				
Combination Abdominal CT Scan[5]	0	-	0.164	0.191
Combination Chest CT Scan[5]	0	-	0.038	0.054
Follow-up Mammogram/Ultrasound[5]	0	-	8.4%	8.4%
MRI for Low Back Pain[5]	0	-	30.2%	32.7%
Survey of Patients' Hospital Experiences				
Area Around Room 'Always' Quiet at Night[8]	-	-	-	58%
Doctors 'Always' Communicated Well[8]	-	-	-	80%
Home Recovery Information Given[8]	-	-	-	82%
Hospital Given 9 or 10 on 10 Point Scale[8]	-	-	-	67%
Meds 'Always' Explained Before Given[8]	-	-	-	60%
Nurses 'Always' Communicated Well[8]	-	-	-	76%
Pain 'Always' Well Controlled[8]	-	-	-	69%
Room and Bathroom 'Always' Clean[8]	-	-	-	71%
Timely Help 'Always' Received[8]	-	-	-	64%
Would Definitely Recommend Hospital[8]	-	-	-	69%

Summa Health Systems Hospitals

525 East Market Street
Akron, OH 44309
Phone: 330-375-3000
Fax: 330-375-7936
URL: www.summahealth.org
Type: Acute Care Hospitals
Emergency Services: Yes
Ownership: Voluntary Non-Profit - Other
Beds: 658

Key Personnel:
CEO/President. . . . . Thomas Strauss
Infection Control. . . . . Ginnie Abell
Radiology. . . . . Daniel Finelli

Measure	Cases	This Hosp.	State Avg.	U.S. Avg.
Heart Attack Care				
ACE Inhibitor or ARB for LVSD[2]	56	100%	97%	96%
Aspirin at Arrival[2]	198	100%	99%	99%
Aspirin at Discharge[2]	314	99%	99%	98%
Beta Blocker at Discharge[2]	292	100%	99%	98%
Fibrinolytic Medication Timing[2]	0	-	14%	55%
PCI Within 90 Minutes of Arrival[2]	59	100%	92%	90%
Smoking Cessation Advice[2]	123	99%	100%	99%
Chest Pain/Possible Heart Attack Care				
Aspirin at Arrival[1]	9	100%	96%	95%
Median Time to ECG (minutes)[1]	9	16	7	8
Median Time to Transfer (minutes)[5]	0	-	61	61
Fibrinolytic Medication Timing[5]	0	-	47%	54%
Heart Failure Care				
ACE Inhibitor or ARB for LVSD[2]	110	97%	96%	94%
Discharge Instructions[2]	266	92%	91%	88%
Evaluation of LVS Function[2]	308	98%	99%	98%
Smoking Cessation Advice[2]	70	100%	99%	98%
Pneumonia Care				
Appropriate Initial Antibiotic[2]	71	94%	92%	92%
Blood Culture Timing[2]	106	92%	96%	96%
Influenza Vaccine[2]	107	81%	93%	91%
Initial Antibiotic Timing[2]	153	98%	96%	95%
Pneumococcal Vaccine[2]	128	73%	95%	93%
Smoking Cessation Advice[2]	63	100%	98%	97%
Surgical Care Improvement Project				
Appropriate VTP Within 24 Hours[2]	150	95%	92%	92%
Appropriate Hair Removal[2]	495	99%	100%	99%
Appropriate Beta Blocker Usage[2]	178	62%	94%	93%
Controlled Postoperative Blood Glucose[2]	149	81%	94%	93%
Prophylactic Antibiotic Timing[2]	343	92%	97%	97%
Prophylactic Antibiotic Timing (Outpatient)	529	95%	91%	92%
Prophylactic Antibiotic Selection[2]	349	95%	98%	97%
Prophylactic Antibiotic Select. (Outpatient)	530	92%	94%	94%
Prophylactic Antibiotic Stopped[2]	329	88%	95%	94%
Recommended VTP Ordered[2]	150	95%	94%	94%
Urinary Catheter Removal[2]	90	72%	91%	90%
Children's Asthma Care				
Received Systemic Corticosteroids	-	-	-	100%
Received Home Management Plan	-	-	-	71%
Received Reliever Medication	-	-	-	100%
Use of Medical Imaging				
Combination Abdominal CT Scan	1,395	0.116	0.164	0.191
Combination Chest CT Scan	1,495	0.001	0.038	0.054
Follow-up Mammogram/Ultrasound	2,614	4.3%	8.4%	8.4%
MRI for Low Back Pain	361	33.8%	30.2%	32.7%
Survey of Patients' Hospital Experiences				
Area Around Room 'Always' Quiet at Night	300+	45%	-	58%
Doctors 'Always' Communicated Well	300+	74%	-	80%
Home Recovery Information Given	300+	82%	-	82%
Hospital Given 9 or 10 on 10 Point Scale	300+	62%	-	67%
Meds 'Always' Explained Before Given	300+	55%	-	60%
Nurses 'Always' Communicated Well	300+	73%	-	76%
Pain 'Always' Well Controlled	300+	66%	-	69%
Room and Bathroom 'Always' Clean	300+	65%	-	71%
Timely Help 'Always' Received	300+	61%	-	64%
Would Definitely Recommend Hospital	300+	69%	-	69%

NOTE: Hospital profiles are in alphabetical order by state, then city, then hospital within the city; Rankings exclude hospitals with less than 25 cases except for patient surveys which excludes hospitals with less than 100 cases; (a) 100–299 cases; (1) The number of cases is too small to be sure how well a hospital is performing; (2) The hospital indicated that the data submitted for this measure were based on a sample of cases; (3) Data was collected during a shorter time period (fewer quarters) than the maximum possible time for this measure; (4) Suppressed for one or more quarters by CMS; (5) No data is available from the hospital for this measure; (6) Fewer than 100 patients completed the HCAHPS survey. Use these rates with caution, as the number of surveys may be too low to reliably assess hospital performance; (7) Survey results are based on less than 12 months of data; (8) Survey results are not available for this reporting period; (9) No or very few patients were eligible for the HCAHPS survey. The scores shown, if any, reflect a very small number of surveys; (10) A state average was not calculated because too few hospitals in the state submitted data; (11) There were discrepancies in the data collection process; Please refer to the User's Guide for a full explanation of data.

Alliance Community Hospital

200 East State Street Phone: 330-596-7201
Alliance, OH 44601 Fax: 330-596-7117
E-mail: gayleb@achosp.org
URL: www.achosp.org
Type: Acute Care Hospitals Emergency Services: Yes
Ownership: Voluntary Non-Profit - Other Beds: 184

Key Personnel:
CEO/President. . . . . Stan W Jonas
Chief of Medical Staff . . . . Karen Gade-Pulido, MD
Infection Control. . . . . Tonia Martin
Operating Room. . . . . Debbie Percha
Quality Assurance . . . . Barb Dragomir
Radiology. . . . . Gary L Dier
Emergency Room . . . . Timothy Billups, RN
Intensive Care Unit. . . . . Joe Sealak, RN

Measure	Cases	This Hosp.	State Avg.	U.S. Avg.
Heart Attack Care				
ACE Inhibitor or ARB for LVSD[1]	7	100%	97%	96%
Aspirin at Arrival	30	93%	99%	99%
Aspirin at Discharge[1]	23	91%	99%	98%
Beta Blocker at Discharge[1]	23	96%	99%	98%
Fibrinolytic Medication Timing	0	-	14%	55%
PCI Within 90 Minutes of Arrival	0	-	92%	90%
Smoking Cessation Advice[1]	2	100%	100%	99%
Chest Pain/Possible Heart Attack Care				
Aspirin at Arrival	101	100%	96%	95%
Median Time to ECG (minutes)	107	9	7	8
Median Time to Transfer (minutes)[1]	14	46	61	61
Fibrinolytic Medication Timing	0	-	47%	54%
Heart Failure Care				
ACE Inhibitor or ARB for LVSD	45	87%	96%	94%
Discharge Instructions	99	90%	91%	88%
Evaluation of LVS Function	132	98%	99%	98%
Smoking Cessation Advice	27	89%	99%	98%
Pneumonia Care				
Appropriate Initial Antibiotic	92	93%	92%	92%
Blood Culture Timing	156	90%	96%	96%
Influenza Vaccine	126	94%	93%	91%
Initial Antibiotic Timing	144	98%	96%	95%
Pneumococcal Vaccine	156	97%	95%	93%
Smoking Cessation Advice	67	90%	98%	97%
Surgical Care Improvement Project				
Appropriate VTP Within 24 Hours[2]	119	76%	92%	92%
Appropriate Hair Removal[2]	344	96%	100%	99%
Appropriate Beta Blocker Usage[2]	101	92%	94%	93%
Controlled Postoperative Blood Glucose[2]	0	-	94%	93%
Prophylactic Antibiotic Timing[2]	221	97%	97%	97%
Prophylactic Antibiotic Timing (Outpatient)	82	85%	91%	92%
Prophylactic Antibiotic Selection[2]	220	100%	98%	97%
Prophylactic Antibiotic Select. (Outpatient)	70	100%	94%	94%
Prophylactic Antibiotic Stopped[2]	206	84%	95%	94%
Recommended VTP Ordered[2]	120	76%	94%	94%
Urinary Catheter Removal[2]	56	64%	91%	90%
Children's Asthma Care				
Received Systemic Corticosteroids	-	-	-	100%
Received Home Management Plan	-	-	-	71%
Received Reliever Medication	-	-	-	100%
Use of Medical Imaging				
Combination Abdominal CT Scan	574	0.678	0.164	0.191
Combination Chest CT Scan	377	0.016	0.038	0.054
Follow-up Mammogram/Ultrasound	769	6.5%	8.4%	8.4%
MRI for Low Back Pain	90	23.3%	30.2%	32.7%
Survey of Patients' Hospital Experiences				
Area Around Room 'Always' Quiet at Night	300+	48%	-	58%
Doctors 'Always' Communicated Well	300+	75%	-	80%
Home Recovery Information Given	300+	84%	-	82%
Hospital Given 9 or 10 on 10 Point Scale	300+	66%	-	67%
Meds 'Always' Explained Before Given	300+	56%	-	60%
Nurses 'Always' Communicated Well	300+	73%	-	76%
Pain 'Always' Well Controlled	300+	64%	-	69%
Room and Bathroom 'Always' Clean	300+	75%	-	71%
Timely Help 'Always' Received	300+	64%	-	64%
Would Definitely Recommend Hospital	300+	64%	-	69%

Amherst Hospital

254 Cleveland Avenue Phone: 440-988-6000
Amherst, OH 44001 Fax: 440-988-6016
Type: Acute Care Hospitals Emergency Services: Yes
Ownership: Voluntary Non-Profit - Private Beds: 71

Key Personnel:
CEO/President. . . . . Kevin Martin
Chief of Medical Staff . . . . S Palaker

Measure	Cases	This Hosp.	State Avg.	U.S. Avg.
Heart Attack Care				
ACE Inhibitor or ARB for LVSD[5]	0	-	97%	96%
Aspirin at Arrival[5]	0	-	99%	99%
Aspirin at Discharge[5]	0	-	99%	98%
Beta Blocker at Discharge[5]	0	-	99%	98%
Fibrinolytic Medication Timing[5]	0	-	14%	55%
PCI Within 90 Minutes of Arrival[5]	0	-	92%	90%
Smoking Cessation Advice[5]	0	-	100%	99%
Chest Pain/Possible Heart Attack Care				
Aspirin at Arrival	121	84%	96%	95%
Median Time to ECG (minutes)	131	10	7	8
Median Time to Transfer (minutes)[1,3]	2	29	61	61
Fibrinolytic Medication Timing[3]	0	-	47%	54%
Heart Failure Care				
ACE Inhibitor or ARB for LVSD[1]	4	100%	96%	94%
Discharge Instructions[1]	8	50%	91%	88%
Evaluation of LVS Function[1]	12	83%	99%	98%
Smoking Cessation Advice[1]	1	100%	99%	98%
Pneumonia Care				
Appropriate Initial Antibiotic	25	76%	92%	92%
Blood Culture Timing[1]	16	94%	96%	96%
Influenza Vaccine[1]	19	79%	93%	91%
Initial Antibiotic Timing	28	82%	96%	95%
Pneumococcal Vaccine	26	85%	95%	93%
Smoking Cessation Advice[1]	12	92%	98%	97%
Surgical Care Improvement Project				
Appropriate VTP Within 24 Hours[2]	26	96%	92%	92%
Appropriate Hair Removal[2]	217	100%	100%	99%
Appropriate Beta Blocker Usage[2]	62	90%	94%	93%
Controlled Postoperative Blood Glucose[2]	0	-	94%	93%
Prophylactic Antibiotic Timing[2]	178	98%	97%	97%
Prophylactic Antibiotic Timing (Outpatient)	29	62%	91%	92%
Prophylactic Antibiotic Selection[2]	178	100%	98%	97%
Prophylactic Antibiotic Select. (Outpatient)[1]	23	83%	94%	94%
Prophylactic Antibiotic Stopped[2]	173	90%	95%	94%
Recommended VTP Ordered[2]	27	93%	94%	94%
Urinary Catheter Removal[2]	91	88%	91%	90%
Children's Asthma Care				
Received Systemic Corticosteroids	-	-	-	100%
Received Home Management Plan	-	-	-	71%
Received Reliever Medication	-	-	-	100%
Use of Medical Imaging				
Combination Abdominal CT Scan	97	0.000	0.164	0.191
Combination Chest CT Scan	47	0.000	0.038	0.054
Follow-up Mammogram/Ultrasound[5]	0	-	8.4%	8.4%
MRI for Low Back Pain[5]	0	-	30.2%	32.7%
Survey of Patients' Hospital Experiences				
Area Around Room 'Always' Quiet at Night	300+	67%	-	58%
Doctors 'Always' Communicated Well	300+	77%	-	80%
Home Recovery Information Given	300+	85%	-	82%
Hospital Given 9 or 10 on 10 Point Scale	300+	80%	-	67%
Meds 'Always' Explained Before Given	300+	63%	-	60%
Nurses 'Always' Communicated Well	300+	83%	-	76%
Pain 'Always' Well Controlled	300+	75%	-	69%
Room and Bathroom 'Always' Clean	300+	84%	-	71%
Timely Help 'Always' Received	300+	75%	-	64%
Would Definitely Recommend Hospital	300+	82%	-	69%

Samaritan Hospital - Peoples Hospital

1025 Center St Phone: 419-289-0491
Ashland, OH 44805 Fax: 419-207-2608
URL: www.samho.org
Type: Acute Care Hospitals Emergency Services: Yes
Ownership: Voluntary Non-Profit - Other Beds: 110

Key Personnel:
CEO/President. . . . . Danny Boggs
Chief of Medical Staff . . . . Philip Myers
Radiology. . . . . Richard W Adams

Measure	Cases	This Hosp.	State Avg.	U.S. Avg.
Heart Attack Care				
ACE Inhibitor or ARB for LVSD[1]	2	100%	97%	96%
Aspirin at Arrival[1]	15	100%	99%	99%
Aspirin at Discharge[1]	9	100%	99%	98%
Beta Blocker at Discharge[1]	9	100%	99%	98%
Fibrinolytic Medication Timing	0	-	14%	55%
PCI Within 90 Minutes of Arrival	0	-	92%	90%
Smoking Cessation Advice[1]	2	100%	100%	99%
Chest Pain/Possible Heart Attack Care				
Aspirin at Arrival	159	96%	96%	95%
Median Time to ECG (minutes)	172	6	7	8
Median Time to Transfer (minutes)[1]	19	70	61	61
Fibrinolytic Medication Timing[1]	3	67%	47%	54%
Heart Failure Care				
ACE Inhibitor or ARB for LVSD[1]	23	100%	96%	94%
Discharge Instructions	69	97%	91%	88%
Evaluation of LVS Function	85	99%	99%	98%
Smoking Cessation Advice[1]	6	100%	99%	98%
Pneumonia Care				
Appropriate Initial Antibiotic	70	93%	92%	92%
Blood Culture Timing	90	91%	96%	96%
Influenza Vaccine	51	98%	93%	91%
Initial Antibiotic Timing	87	95%	96%	95%
Pneumococcal Vaccine	74	97%	95%	93%
Smoking Cessation Advice[1]	21	95%	98%	97%
Surgical Care Improvement Project				
Appropriate VTP Within 24 Hours	60	92%	92%	92%
Appropriate Hair Removal	535	100%	100%	99%
Appropriate Beta Blocker Usage	169	99%	94%	93%
Controlled Postoperative Blood Glucose	0	-	94%	93%
Prophylactic Antibiotic Timing	473	98%	97%	97%
Prophylactic Antibiotic Timing (Outpatient)	88	84%	91%	92%
Prophylactic Antibiotic Selection	473	99%	98%	97%
Prophylactic Antibiotic Select. (Outpatient)	78	96%	94%	94%
Prophylactic Antibiotic Stopped	472	99%	95%	94%
Recommended VTP Ordered	60	98%	94%	94%
Urinary Catheter Removal	164	99%	91%	90%
Children's Asthma Care				
Received Systemic Corticosteroids	-	-	-	100%
Received Home Management Plan	-	-	-	71%
Received Reliever Medication	-	-	-	100%
Use of Medical Imaging				
Combination Abdominal CT Scan	506	0.069	0.164	0.191
Combination Chest CT Scan	295	0.085	0.038	0.054
Follow-up Mammogram/Ultrasound	699	6.6%	8.4%	8.4%
MRI for Low Back Pain	99	27.3%	30.2%	32.7%
Survey of Patients' Hospital Experiences				
Area Around Room 'Always' Quiet at Night	300+	55%	-	58%
Doctors 'Always' Communicated Well	300+	78%	-	80%
Home Recovery Information Given	300+	88%	-	82%
Hospital Given 9 or 10 on 10 Point Scale	300+	67%	-	67%
Meds 'Always' Explained Before Given	300+	59%	-	60%
Nurses 'Always' Communicated Well	300+	76%	-	76%
Pain 'Always' Well Controlled	300+	64%	-	69%
Room and Bathroom 'Always' Clean	300+	68%	-	71%
Timely Help 'Always' Received	300+	59%	-	64%
Would Definitely Recommend Hospital	300+	63%	-	69%

NOTE: Hospital profiles are in alphabetical order by state, then city, then hospital within the city; Rankings exclude hospitals with less than 25 cases except for patient surveys which excludes hospitals with less than 100 cases; (a) 100–299 cases; (1) The number of cases is too small to be sure how well a hospital is performing; (2) The hospital indicated that the data submitted for this measure were based on a sample of cases; (3) Data was collected during a shorter time period (fewer quarters) than the maximum possible time for this measure; (4) Suppressed for one or more quarters by CMS; (5) No data is available from the hospital for this measure; (6) Fewer than 100 patients completed the HCAHPS survey. Use these rates with caution, as the number of surveys may be too low to reliably assess hospital performance; (7) Survey results are based on less than 12 months of data; (8) Survey results are not available for this reporting period; (9) No or very few patients were eligible for the HCAHPS survey. The scores shown, if any, reflect a very small number of surveys; (10) A state average was not calculated because too few hospitals in the state submitted data; (11) There were discrepancies in the data collection process; Please refer to the User's Guide for a full explanation of data.

Ashtabula County Medical Center

2420 Lake Avenue
Ashtabula, OH 44004
Phone: 440-997-2262
Fax: 440-997-6644
URL: www.acmchealth.org
Type: Acute Care Hospitals
Emergency Services: Yes
Ownership: Voluntary Non-Profit - Other
Beds: 234

Key Personnel:
CEO/President. . . . . Kevin J Miller
Cardiac Laboratory. . . . . James Cho, MD
Chief of Medical Staff . . . . Timothy D. O'Brien
Infection Control. . . . . Cindy Callahan
Operating Room. . . . . Lo Bruno
Radiology. . . . . Jack Thome

Measure	Cases	This Hosp.	State Avg.	U.S. Avg.
Heart Attack Care				
ACE Inhibitor or ARB for LVSD	0	-	97%	96%
Aspirin at Arrival	26	100%	99%	99%
Aspirin at Discharge[1]	11	100%	99%	98%
Beta Blocker at Discharge[1]	14	86%	99%	98%
Fibrinolytic Medication Timing	0	-	14%	55%
PCI Within 90 Minutes of Arrival	0	-	92%	90%
Smoking Cessation Advice[1]	5	100%	100%	99%
Chest Pain/Possible Heart Attack Care				
Aspirin at Arrival	137	98%	96%	95%
Median Time to ECG (minutes)	146	2	7	8
Median Time to Transfer (minutes)[1]	9	75	61	61
Fibrinolytic Medication Timing	0	-	47%	54%
Heart Failure Care				
ACE Inhibitor or ARB for LVSD	53	98%	96%	94%
Discharge Instructions	142	86%	91%	88%
Evaluation of LVS Function	187	99%	99%	98%
Smoking Cessation Advice	32	100%	99%	98%
Pneumonia Care				
Appropriate Initial Antibiotic	87	93%	92%	92%
Blood Culture Timing	164	96%	96%	96%
Influenza Vaccine	80	98%	93%	91%
Initial Antibiotic Timing	145	97%	96%	95%
Pneumococcal Vaccine	109	95%	95%	93%
Smoking Cessation Advice	72	100%	98%	97%
Surgical Care Improvement Project				
Appropriate VTP Within 24 Hours	77	94%	92%	92%
Appropriate Hair Removal	225	100%	100%	99%
Appropriate Beta Blocker Usage	63	97%	94%	93%
Controlled Postoperative Blood Glucose	0	-	94%	93%
Prophylactic Antibiotic Timing	149	99%	97%	97%
Prophylactic Antibiotic Timing (Outpatient)	154	92%	91%	92%
Prophylactic Antibiotic Selection	149	99%	98%	97%
Prophylactic Antibiotic Select. (Outpatient)	195	94%	94%	94%
Prophylactic Antibiotic Stopped	135	91%	95%	94%
Recommended VTP Ordered	77	95%	94%	94%
Urinary Catheter Removal[1]	18	83%	91%	90%
Children's Asthma Care				
Received Systemic Corticosteroids	-	-	-	100%
Received Home Management Plan	-	-	-	71%
Received Reliever Medication	-	-	-	100%
Use of Medical Imaging				
Combination Abdominal CT Scan	634	0.027	0.164	0.191
Combination Chest CT Scan	560	0.004	0.038	0.054
Follow-up Mammogram/Ultrasound	677	13.9%	8.4%	8.4%
MRI for Low Back Pain	95	34.7%	30.2%	32.7%
Survey of Patients' Hospital Experiences				
Area Around Room 'Always' Quiet at Night	300+	39%	-	58%
Doctors 'Always' Communicated Well	300+	73%	-	80%
Home Recovery Information Given	300+	75%	-	82%
Hospital Given 9 or 10 on 10 Point Scale	300+	49%	-	67%
Meds 'Always' Explained Before Given	300+	55%	-	60%
Nurses 'Always' Communicated Well	300+	72%	-	76%
Pain 'Always' Well Controlled	300+	63%	-	69%
Room and Bathroom 'Always' Clean	300+	76%	-	71%
Timely Help 'Always' Received	300+	58%	-	64%
Would Definitely Recommend Hospital	300+	49%	-	69%

O'Bleness Memorial Hospital

55 Hospital Drive
Athens, OH 45701
Phone: 740-593-5551
Fax: 740-592-9200
URL: www.obleness.org
Type: Acute Care Hospitals
Emergency Services: Yes
Ownership: Voluntary Non-Profit - Other
Beds: 114

Key Personnel:
CEO/President. . . . . Richard Castrop
Chief of Medical Staff . . . . J Phillip Jones, DO
Infection Control. . . . . Donna Lofgren
Operating Room. . . . . Shelly Cooper, RN
Pediatric Ambulatory Care . . . . . . Karen Montgomery-Reag, DO
Pediatric In-Patient Care . . . . Karen Montgomery-Reag, DO
Quality Assurance . . . . Judy U Moffitt, RN, B
Radiology. . . . . Jeffrey S Benseler, DO

Measure	Cases	This Hosp.	State Avg.	U.S. Avg.
Heart Attack Care				
ACE Inhibitor or ARB for LVSD[1]	4	100%	97%	96%
Aspirin at Arrival[1]	15	73%	99%	99%
Aspirin at Discharge[1]	10	90%	99%	98%
Beta Blocker at Discharge[1]	10	80%	99%	98%
Fibrinolytic Medication Timing	0	-	14%	55%
PCI Within 90 Minutes of Arrival	0	-	92%	90%
Smoking Cessation Advice[1]	2	100%	100%	99%
Chest Pain/Possible Heart Attack Care				
Aspirin at Arrival	312	93%	96%	95%
Median Time to ECG (minutes)	315	7	7	8
Median Time to Transfer (minutes)[1,3]	5	166	61	61
Fibrinolytic Medication Timing[1]	15	53%	47%	54%
Heart Failure Care				
ACE Inhibitor or ARB for LVSD	29	69%	96%	94%
Discharge Instructions	72	64%	91%	88%
Evaluation of LVS Function	90	100%	99%	98%
Smoking Cessation Advice[1]	21	100%	99%	98%
Pneumonia Care				
Appropriate Initial Antibiotic	67	81%	92%	92%
Blood Culture Timing	120	88%	96%	96%
Influenza Vaccine	65	85%	93%	91%
Initial Antibiotic Timing	118	93%	96%	95%
Pneumococcal Vaccine	78	88%	95%	93%
Smoking Cessation Advice	44	100%	98%	97%
Surgical Care Improvement Project				
Appropriate VTP Within 24 Hours	52	83%	92%	92%
Appropriate Hair Removal	89	100%	100%	99%
Appropriate Beta Blocker Usage[1]	21	67%	94%	93%
Controlled Postoperative Blood Glucose	0	-	94%	93%
Prophylactic Antibiotic Timing	71	96%	97%	97%
Prophylactic Antibiotic Timing (Outpatient)	199	97%	91%	92%
Prophylactic Antibiotic Selection	71	96%	98%	97%
Prophylactic Antibiotic Select. (Outpatient)	197	87%	94%	94%
Prophylactic Antibiotic Stopped	71	83%	95%	94%
Recommended VTP Ordered	52	94%	94%	94%
Urinary Catheter Removal	30	87%	91%	90%
Children's Asthma Care				
Received Systemic Corticosteroids	-	-	-	100%
Received Home Management Plan	-	-	-	71%
Received Reliever Medication	-	-	-	100%
Use of Medical Imaging				
Combination Abdominal CT Scan	350	0.074	0.164	0.191
Combination Chest CT Scan	161	0.000	0.038	0.054
Follow-up Mammogram/Ultrasound	736	4.1%	8.4%	8.4%
MRI for Low Back Pain	73	38.4%	30.2%	32.7%
Survey of Patients' Hospital Experiences				
Area Around Room 'Always' Quiet at Night	300+	50%	-	58%
Doctors 'Always' Communicated Well	300+	79%	-	80%
Home Recovery Information Given	300+	81%	-	82%
Hospital Given 9 or 10 on 10 Point Scale	300+	58%	-	67%
Meds 'Always' Explained Before Given	300+	57%	-	60%
Nurses 'Always' Communicated Well	300+	75%	-	76%
Pain 'Always' Well Controlled	300+	67%	-	69%
Room and Bathroom 'Always' Clean	300+	65%	-	71%
Timely Help 'Always' Received	300+	61%	-	64%
Would Definitely Recommend Hospital	300+	56%	-	69%

Summa Barberton Hospital

155 5th Street N E
Barberton, OH 44203
Phone: 330-615-3000
Fax: 330-615-3033
URL: www.barbhosp.com
Type: Acute Care Hospitals
Emergency Services: Yes
Ownership: Proprietary
Beds: 311

Key Personnel:
CEO/President. . . . . James W Pope MHHA FACHE
Chief of Medical Staff . . . . Robert Debski MD
Operating Room. . . . . Dean Majors, MD
Quality Assurance . . . . Mary Jo Goss
Radiology. . . . . Matthew Karlen MD
Anesthesiology. . . . . James Cantoni MD
Emergency Room . . . . Gregory Smith, MD

Measure	Cases	This Hosp.	State Avg.	U.S. Avg.
Heart Attack Care				
ACE Inhibitor or ARB for LVSD[1]	16	100%	97%	96%
Aspirin at Arrival	88	100%	99%	99%
Aspirin at Discharge	83	100%	99%	98%
Beta Blocker at Discharge	79	100%	99%	98%
Fibrinolytic Medication Timing	0	-	14%	55%
PCI Within 90 Minutes of Arrival[1]	17	100%	92%	90%
Smoking Cessation Advice	25	100%	100%	99%
Chest Pain/Possible Heart Attack Care				
Aspirin at Arrival	25	100%	96%	95%
Median Time to ECG (minutes)	25	6	7	8
Median Time to Transfer (minutes)[1,3]	2	35	61	61
Fibrinolytic Medication Timing[3]	0	-	47%	54%
Heart Failure Care				
ACE Inhibitor or ARB for LVSD	54	100%	96%	94%
Discharge Instructions	260	100%	91%	88%
Evaluation of LVS Function	337	100%	99%	98%
Smoking Cessation Advice	64	100%	99%	98%
Pneumonia Care				
Appropriate Initial Antibiotic	120	97%	92%	92%
Blood Culture Timing	239	100%	96%	96%
Influenza Vaccine	174	100%	93%	91%
Initial Antibiotic Timing	212	99%	96%	95%
Pneumococcal Vaccine	184	100%	95%	93%
Smoking Cessation Advice	90	100%	98%	97%
Surgical Care Improvement Project				
Appropriate VTP Within 24 Hours	279	97%	92%	92%
Appropriate Hair Removal	553	100%	100%	99%
Appropriate Beta Blocker Usage	146	100%	94%	93%
Controlled Postoperative Blood Glucose	37	81%	94%	93%
Prophylactic Antibiotic Timing	333	100%	97%	97%
Prophylactic Antibiotic Timing (Outpatient)	114	99%	91%	92%
Prophylactic Antibiotic Selection	334	99%	98%	97%
Prophylactic Antibiotic Select. (Outpatient)	113	98%	94%	94%
Prophylactic Antibiotic Stopped	305	99%	95%	94%
Recommended VTP Ordered	279	97%	94%	94%
Urinary Catheter Removal	42	88%	91%	90%
Children's Asthma Care				
Received Systemic Corticosteroids	-	-	-	100%
Received Home Management Plan	-	-	-	71%
Received Reliever Medication	-	-	-	100%
Use of Medical Imaging				
Combination Abdominal CT Scan	506	0.073	0.164	0.191
Combination Chest CT Scan	311	0.010	0.038	0.054
Follow-up Mammogram/Ultrasound	681	16.0%	8.4%	8.4%
MRI for Low Back Pain	88	31.8%	30.2%	32.7%
Survey of Patients' Hospital Experiences				
Area Around Room 'Always' Quiet at Night	300+	46%	-	58%
Doctors 'Always' Communicated Well	300+	76%	-	80%
Home Recovery Information Given	300+	76%	-	82%
Hospital Given 9 or 10 on 10 Point Scale	300+	65%	-	67%
Meds 'Always' Explained Before Given	300+	57%	-	60%
Nurses 'Always' Communicated Well	300+	77%	-	76%
Pain 'Always' Well Controlled	300+	69%	-	69%
Room and Bathroom 'Always' Clean	300+	68%	-	71%
Timely Help 'Always' Received	300+	66%	-	64%
Would Definitely Recommend Hospital	300+	67%	-	69%

NOTE: Hospital profiles are in alphabetical order by state, then city, then hospital within the city; Rankings exclude hospitals with less than 25 cases except for patient surveys which excludes hospitals with less than 100 cases; (a) 100–299 cases; (1) The number of cases is too small to be sure how well a hospital is performing; (2) The hospital indicated that the data submitted for this measure were based on a sample of cases; (3) Data was collected during a shorter time period (fewer quarters) than the maximum possible time for this measure; (4) Suppressed for one or more quarters by CMS; (5) No data is available from the hospital for this measure; (6) Fewer than 100 patients completed the HCAHPS survey. Use these rates with caution, as the number of surveys may be too low to reliably assess hospital performance; (7) Survey results are based on less than 12 months of data; (8) Survey results are not available for this reporting period; (9) No or very few patients were eligible for the HCAHPS survey. The scores shown, if any, reflect a very small number of surveys; (10) A state average was not calculated because too few hospitals in the state submitted data; (11) There were discrepancies in the data collection process; Please refer to the User's Guide for a full explanation of data.

Barnesville Hospital Association

639 West Main Street Phone: 740-425-5101
Barnesville, OH 43713 Fax: 740-425-9213
E-mail: dcarroll@barnesvillehospital.com
URL: www.barnesvillehospital.com
Type: Critical Access Hospitals Emergency Services: Yes
Ownership: Voluntary Non-Profit - Private Beds: 25

Key Personnel:
CEO/President. . . . . R Melvin Milburn
Chief of Medical Staff . . . . PK Souri, MD
Infection Control. . . . . JoAnn Barylak, RN
Operating Room. . . . . Barb Mcmahon, RN
Quality Assurance . . . . Jane Hall, RN
Radiology. . . . . Theresa Smith, DO
Emergency Room . . . . Michael Baum, MD
Intensive Care Unit. . . . . Joyce Weiss

Measure	Cases	This Hosp.	State Avg.	U.S. Avg.
Heart Attack Care				
ACE Inhibitor or ARB for LVSD[1]	5	100%	97%	96%
Aspirin at Arrival[1]	19	100%	99%	99%
Aspirin at Discharge[1]	14	93%	99%	98%
Beta Blocker at Discharge[1]	17	94%	99%	98%
Fibrinolytic Medication Timing	0	-	14%	55%
PCI Within 90 Minutes of Arrival	0	-	92%	90%
Smoking Cessation Advice[1]	1	100%	100%	99%
Chest Pain/Possible Heart Attack Care				
Aspirin at Arrival[5]	0	-	96%	95%
Median Time to ECG (minutes)[5]	0	-	7	8
Median Time to Transfer (minutes)[5]	0	-	61	61
Fibrinolytic Medication Timing[5]	0	-	47%	54%
Heart Failure Care				
ACE Inhibitor or ARB for LVSD[1]	20	95%	96%	94%
Discharge Instructions	74	97%	91%	88%
Evaluation of LVS Function	90	99%	99%	98%
Smoking Cessation Advice[1]	10	90%	99%	98%
Pneumonia Care				
Appropriate Initial Antibiotic	91	88%	92%	92%
Blood Culture Timing	53	98%	96%	96%
Influenza Vaccine	59	88%	93%	91%
Initial Antibiotic Timing	100	97%	96%	95%
Pneumococcal Vaccine	101	88%	95%	93%
Smoking Cessation Advice	30	100%	98%	97%
Surgical Care Improvement Project				
Appropriate VTP Within 24 Hours[5]	0	-	92%	92%
Appropriate Hair Removal[5]	0	-	100%	99%
Appropriate Beta Blocker Usage[5]	0	-	94%	93%
Controlled Postoperative Blood Glucose[5]	0	-	94%	93%
Prophylactic Antibiotic Timing[5]	0	-	97%	97%
Prophylactic Antibiotic Timing (Outpatient)[5]	0	-	91%	92%
Prophylactic Antibiotic Selection[5]	0	-	98%	97%
Prophylactic Antibiotic Select. (Outpatient)[5]	0	-	94%	94%
Prophylactic Antibiotic Stopped[5]	0	-	95%	94%
Recommended VTP Ordered[5]	0	-	94%	94%
Urinary Catheter Removal[5]	0	-	91%	90%
Children's Asthma Care				
Received Systemic Corticosteroids	-	-	-	100%
Received Home Management Plan	-	-	-	71%
Received Reliever Medication	-	-	-	100%
Use of Medical Imaging				
Combination Abdominal CT Scan	177	0.181	0.164	0.191
Combination Chest CT Scan	138	0.101	0.038	0.054
Follow-up Mammogram/Ultrasound	159	17.6%	8.4%	8.4%
MRI for Low Back Pain[1]	14	50.0%	30.2%	32.7%
Survey of Patients' Hospital Experiences				
Area Around Room 'Always' Quiet at Night	300+	51%	-	58%
Doctors 'Always' Communicated Well	300+	82%	-	80%
Home Recovery Information Given	300+	79%	-	82%
Hospital Given 9 or 10 on 10 Point Scale	300+	77%	-	67%
Meds 'Always' Explained Before Given	300+	67%	-	60%
Nurses 'Always' Communicated Well	300+	85%	-	76%
Pain 'Always' Well Controlled	300+	75%	-	69%
Room and Bathroom 'Always' Clean	300+	80%	-	71%
Timely Help 'Always' Received	300+	80%	-	64%
Would Definitely Recommend Hospital	300+	75%	-	69%

Mercy Hospital Clermont

3000 Hospital Drive Phone: 513-732-8278
Batavia, OH 45103 Fax: 513-732-8361
URL: www.e-mercy.com
Type: Acute Care Hospitals Emergency Services: Yes
Ownership: Voluntary Non-Profit - Church Beds: 114

Key Personnel:
CEO/President. . . . . Mark Shugarmn
Chief of Medical Staff . . . . Judy Stout
Quality Assurance . . . . Patti Schroer
Radiology. . . . . Richard G Cardella
Anesthesiology. . . . . Ben Lee
Emergency Room . . . . Gayle Heintzelman

Measure	Cases	This Hosp.	State Avg.	U.S. Avg.
Heart Attack Care				
ACE Inhibitor or ARB for LVSD[1]	3	100%	97%	96%
Aspirin at Arrival	47	100%	99%	99%
Aspirin at Discharge[1]	23	100%	99%	98%
Beta Blocker at Discharge[1]	19	100%	99%	98%
Fibrinolytic Medication Timing	0	-	14%	55%
PCI Within 90 Minutes of Arrival	0	-	92%	90%
Smoking Cessation Advice[1]	4	100%	100%	99%
Chest Pain/Possible Heart Attack Care				
Aspirin at Arrival	106	96%	96%	95%
Median Time to ECG (minutes)	114	11	7	8
Median Time to Transfer (minutes)	29	128	61	61
Fibrinolytic Medication Timing	0	-	47%	54%
Heart Failure Care				
ACE Inhibitor or ARB for LVSD	32	100%	96%	94%
Discharge Instructions	76	95%	91%	88%
Evaluation of LVS Function	90	100%	99%	98%
Smoking Cessation Advice	25	100%	99%	98%
Pneumonia Care				
Appropriate Initial Antibiotic	151	93%	92%	92%
Blood Culture Timing	230	99%	96%	96%
Influenza Vaccine	185	98%	93%	91%
Initial Antibiotic Timing	257	98%	96%	95%
Pneumococcal Vaccine	216	100%	95%	93%
Smoking Cessation Advice	170	100%	98%	97%
Surgical Care Improvement Project				
Appropriate VTP Within 24 Hours[2]	158	99%	92%	92%
Appropriate Hair Removal[2]	388	100%	100%	99%
Appropriate Beta Blocker Usage[2]	112	95%	94%	93%
Controlled Postoperative Blood Glucose[2]	0	-	94%	93%
Prophylactic Antibiotic Timing[2]	267	100%	97%	97%
Prophylactic Antibiotic Timing (Outpatient)	65	91%	91%	92%
Prophylactic Antibiotic Selection[2]	269	99%	98%	97%
Prophylactic Antibiotic Select. (Outpatient)	74	86%	94%	94%
Prophylactic Antibiotic Stopped[2]	254	98%	95%	94%
Recommended VTP Ordered[2]	158	99%	94%	94%
Urinary Catheter Removal[2]	89	84%	91%	90%
Children's Asthma Care				
Received Systemic Corticosteroids	-	-	-	100%
Received Home Management Plan	-	-	-	71%
Received Reliever Medication	-	-	-	100%
Use of Medical Imaging				
Combination Abdominal CT Scan	646	0.187	0.164	0.191
Combination Chest CT Scan	633	0.003	0.038	0.054
Follow-up Mammogram/Ultrasound	1,039	8.6%	8.4%	8.4%
MRI for Low Back Pain	242	32.2%	30.2%	32.7%
Survey of Patients' Hospital Experiences				
Area Around Room 'Always' Quiet at Night	300+	54%	-	58%
Doctors 'Always' Communicated Well	300+	76%	-	80%
Home Recovery Information Given	300+	82%	-	82%
Hospital Given 9 or 10 on 10 Point Scale	300+	69%	-	67%
Meds 'Always' Explained Before Given	300+	61%	-	60%
Nurses 'Always' Communicated Well	300+	78%	-	76%
Pain 'Always' Well Controlled	300+	69%	-	69%
Room and Bathroom 'Always' Clean	300+	71%	-	71%
Timely Help 'Always' Received	300+	62%	-	64%
Would Definitely Recommend Hospital	300+	72%	-	69%

UHHS Bedford Medical Center

44 Blaine Avenue Phone: 440-735-3628
Bedford, OH 44146 Fax: 440-735-3631
URL: www.uhhsbmc.com
Type: Acute Care Hospitals Emergency Services: Yes
Ownership: Voluntary Non-Profit - Private Beds: 110

Key Personnel:
CEO/President. . . . . Sean H McKibben
Cardiac Laboratory. . . . . Karla Balasko
Chief of Medical Staff. . . . . Dennis Grossman, MD
Infection Control. . . . . Chris Tusoch
Operating Room. . . . . Francina Edwards
Radiology. . . . . Baz DeBaz, MD
Emergency Room . . . . Eric Csernyik, MD

Measure	Cases	This Hosp.	State Avg.	U.S. Avg.
Heart Attack Care				
ACE Inhibitor or ARB for LVSD[1]	7	100%	97%	96%
Aspirin at Arrival	35	94%	99%	99%
Aspirin at Discharge[1]	23	96%	99%	98%
Beta Blocker at Discharge	28	100%	99%	98%
Fibrinolytic Medication Timing	0	-	14%	55%
PCI Within 90 Minutes of Arrival	0	-	92%	90%
Smoking Cessation Advice[1]	6	100%	100%	99%
Chest Pain/Possible Heart Attack Care				
Aspirin at Arrival	94	96%	96%	95%
Median Time to ECG (minutes)	103	4	7	8
Median Time to Transfer (minutes)[1]	18	42	61	61
Fibrinolytic Medication Timing	0	-	47%	54%
Heart Failure Care				
ACE Inhibitor or ARB for LVSD	59	100%	96%	94%
Discharge Instructions	146	97%	91%	88%
Evaluation of LVS Function	200	100%	99%	98%
Smoking Cessation Advice	39	100%	99%	98%
Pneumonia Care				
Appropriate Initial Antibiotic	52	98%	92%	92%
Blood Culture Timing	107	98%	96%	96%
Influenza Vaccine	76	87%	93%	91%
Initial Antibiotic Timing	110	95%	96%	95%
Pneumococcal Vaccine	109	92%	95%	93%
Smoking Cessation Advice	35	94%	98%	97%
Surgical Care Improvement Project				
Appropriate VTP Within 24 Hours	94	91%	92%	92%
Appropriate Hair Removal	187	100%	100%	99%
Appropriate Beta Blocker Usage	50	100%	94%	93%
Controlled Postoperative Blood Glucose	0	-	94%	93%
Prophylactic Antibiotic Timing	109	99%	97%	97%
Prophylactic Antibiotic Timing (Outpatient)	79	87%	91%	92%
Prophylactic Antibiotic Selection	110	99%	98%	97%
Prophylactic Antibiotic Select. (Outpatient)	70	97%	94%	94%
Prophylactic Antibiotic Stopped	100	99%	95%	94%
Recommended VTP Ordered	94	91%	94%	94%
Urinary Catheter Removal[1]	21	81%	91%	90%
Children's Asthma Care				
Received Systemic Corticosteroids	-	-	-	100%
Received Home Management Plan	-	-	-	71%
Received Reliever Medication	-	-	-	100%
Use of Medical Imaging				
Combination Abdominal CT Scan	262	0.107	0.164	0.191
Combination Chest CT Scan	279	0.047	0.038	0.054
Follow-up Mammogram/Ultrasound	443	7.4%	8.4%	8.4%
MRI for Low Back Pain	54	40.7%	30.2%	32.7%
Survey of Patients' Hospital Experiences				
Area Around Room 'Always' Quiet at Night[11]	300+	45%	-	58%
Doctors 'Always' Communicated Well[11]	300+	71%	-	80%
Home Recovery Information Given[11]	300+	73%	-	82%
Hospital Given 9 or 10 on 10 Point Scale[11]	300+	55%	-	67%
Meds 'Always' Explained Before Given[11]	300+	53%	-	60%
Nurses 'Always' Communicated Well[11]	300+	71%	-	76%
Pain 'Always' Well Controlled[11]	300+	64%	-	69%
Room and Bathroom 'Always' Clean[11]	300+	63%	-	71%
Timely Help 'Always' Received[11]	300+	54%	-	64%
Would Definitely Recommend Hospital[11]	300+	55%	-	69%

NOTE: Hospital profiles are in alphabetical order by state, then city, then hospital within the city; Rankings exclude hospitals with less than 25 cases except for patient surveys which excludes hospitals with less than 100 cases; (a) 100–299 cases; (1) The number of cases is too small to be sure how well a hospital is performing; (2) The hospital indicated that the data submitted for this measure were based on a sample of cases; (3) Data was collected during a shorter time period (fewer quarters) than the maximum possible time for this measure; (4) Suppressed for one or more quarters by CMS; (5) No data is available from the hospital for this measure; (6) Fewer than 100 patients completed the HCAHPS survey. Use these rates with caution, as the number of surveys may be too low to reliably assess hospital performance; (7) Survey results are based on less than 12 months of data; (8) Survey results are not available for this reporting period; (9) No or very few patients were eligible for the HCAHPS survey. The scores shown, if any, reflect a very small number of surveys; (10) A state average was not calculated because too few hospitals in the state submitted data; (11) There were discrepancies in the data collection process; Please refer to the User's Guide for a full explanation of data.

Belmont Community Hospital

4697 Harrison Street
Bellaire, OH 43906
Phone: 740-671-1200
Fax: 740-671-1210
E-mail: webmaster@wheelinghospital.com
URL: www.wheelinghospital.com
Type: Acute Care Hospitals
Emergency Services: Yes
Ownership: Voluntary Non-Profit - Other
Beds: 99

Key Personnel:
CEO/President. . . . . Gary Gold
Cardiac Laboratory. . . . . Catherine Stegman
Chief of Medical Staff . . . . Wilmer G Heceta, MD
Infection Control. . . . . Carolyn Skorich
Operating Room. . . . . Jean Thoburn
Quality Assurance . . . . Diane Patt
Radiology. . . . . Eric R Balzano

Measure	Cases	This Hosp.	State Avg.	U.S. Avg.
Heart Attack Care				
ACE Inhibitor or ARB for LVSD	0	-	97%	96%
Aspirin at Arrival[1]	11	82%	99%	99%
Aspirin at Discharge[1]	5	60%	99%	98%
Beta Blocker at Discharge[1]	4	100%	99%	98%
Fibrinolytic Medication Timing	0	-	14%	55%
PCI Within 90 Minutes of Arrival	0	-	92%	90%
Smoking Cessation Advice	0	-	100%	99%
Chest Pain/Possible Heart Attack Care				
Aspirin at Arrival[1,3]	3	100%	96%	95%
Median Time to ECG (minutes)[1,3]	3	3	7	8
Median Time to Transfer (minutes)[5]	0	-	61	61
Fibrinolytic Medication Timing[1,3]	1	0%	47%	54%
Heart Failure Care				
ACE Inhibitor or ARB for LVSD[1]	6	83%	96%	94%
Discharge Instructions	43	23%	91%	88%
Evaluation of LVS Function	48	98%	99%	98%
Smoking Cessation Advice[1]	11	91%	99%	98%
Pneumonia Care				
Appropriate Initial Antibiotic	32	75%	92%	92%
Blood Culture Timing	27	96%	96%	96%
Influenza Vaccine	34	79%	93%	91%
Initial Antibiotic Timing	39	95%	96%	95%
Pneumococcal Vaccine	39	92%	95%	93%
Smoking Cessation Advice[1]	16	100%	98%	97%
Surgical Care Improvement Project				
Appropriate VTP Within 24 Hours[3]	0	-	92%	92%
Appropriate Hair Removal[1,3]	3	100%	100%	99%
Appropriate Beta Blocker Usage[3]	0	-	94%	93%
Controlled Postoperative Blood Glucose[3]	0	-	94%	93%
Prophylactic Antibiotic Timing[1,3]	3	100%	97%	97%
Prophylactic Antibiotic Timing (Outpatient)[1]	5	0%	91%	92%
Prophylactic Antibiotic Selection[1,3]	3	100%	98%	97%
Prophylactic Antibiotic Select. (Outpatient)[1]	1	100%	94%	94%
Prophylactic Antibiotic Stopped[1,3]	3	67%	95%	94%
Recommended VTP Ordered[3]	0	-	94%	94%
Urinary Catheter Removal[3]	0	-	91%	90%
Children's Asthma Care				
Received Systemic Corticosteroids	-	-	-	100%
Received Home Management Plan	-	-	-	71%
Received Reliever Medication	-	-	-	100%
Use of Medical Imaging				
Combination Abdominal CT Scan	79	0.152	0.164	0.191
Combination Chest CT Scan	100	0.000	0.038	0.054
Follow-up Mammogram/Ultrasound	180	14.4%	8.4%	8.4%
MRI for Low Back Pain	56	30.4%	30.2%	32.7%
Survey of Patients' Hospital Experiences				
Area Around Room 'Always' Quiet at Night	(a)	49%	-	58%
Doctors 'Always' Communicated Well	(a)	77%	-	80%
Home Recovery Information Given	(a)	79%	-	82%
Hospital Given 9 or 10 on 10 Point Scale	(a)	64%	-	67%
Meds 'Always' Explained Before Given	(a)	59%	-	60%
Nurses 'Always' Communicated Well	(a)	70%	-	76%
Pain 'Always' Well Controlled	(a)	69%	-	69%
Room and Bathroom 'Always' Clean	(a)	70%	-	71%
Timely Help 'Always' Received	(a)	63%	-	64%
Would Definitely Recommend Hospital	(a)	64%	-	69%

Mary Rutan Hospital

205 Palmer Avenue
Bellefontaine, OH 43311
Phone: 937-592-4015
Fax: 937-592-7007
E-mail: pjmcbrien@maryrutan.org
Type: Acute Care Hospitals
Emergency Services: Yes
Ownership: Voluntary Non-Profit - Private
Beds: 105

Key Personnel:
CEO/President. . . . . Mandy Goble
Radiology. . . . . Therese Jones

Measure	Cases	This Hosp.	State Avg.	U.S. Avg.
Heart Attack Care				
ACE Inhibitor or ARB for LVSD[1]	10	100%	97%	96%
Aspirin at Arrival	46	100%	99%	99%
Aspirin at Discharge	38	100%	99%	98%
Beta Blocker at Discharge	39	97%	99%	98%
Fibrinolytic Medication Timing	0	-	14%	55%
PCI Within 90 Minutes of Arrival	0	-	92%	90%
Smoking Cessation Advice[1]	4	100%	100%	99%
Chest Pain/Possible Heart Attack Care				
Aspirin at Arrival	126	97%	96%	95%
Median Time to ECG (minutes)	132	6	7	8
Median Time to Transfer (minutes)	35	40	61	61
Fibrinolytic Medication Timing[1]	5	100%	47%	54%
Heart Failure Care				
ACE Inhibitor or ARB for LVSD	28	96%	96%	94%
Discharge Instructions	47	83%	91%	88%
Evaluation of LVS Function	70	96%	99%	98%
Smoking Cessation Advice[1]	9	100%	99%	98%
Pneumonia Care				
Appropriate Initial Antibiotic	78	90%	92%	92%
Blood Culture Timing	79	95%	96%	96%
Influenza Vaccine	65	100%	93%	91%
Initial Antibiotic Timing	99	97%	96%	95%
Pneumococcal Vaccine	90	98%	95%	93%
Smoking Cessation Advice	27	100%	98%	97%
Surgical Care Improvement Project				
Appropriate VTP Within 24 Hours	82	96%	92%	92%
Appropriate Hair Removal	264	99%	100%	99%
Appropriate Beta Blocker Usage	80	90%	94%	93%
Controlled Postoperative Blood Glucose	0	-	94%	93%
Prophylactic Antibiotic Timing	207	95%	97%	97%
Prophylactic Antibiotic Timing (Outpatient)	68	90%	91%	92%
Prophylactic Antibiotic Selection	208	97%	98%	97%
Prophylactic Antibiotic Select. (Outpatient)	63	95%	94%	94%
Prophylactic Antibiotic Stopped	202	98%	95%	94%
Recommended VTP Ordered	83	96%	94%	94%
Urinary Catheter Removal	67	81%	91%	90%
Children's Asthma Care				
Received Systemic Corticosteroids	-	-	-	100%
Received Home Management Plan	-	-	-	71%
Received Reliever Medication	-	-	-	100%
Use of Medical Imaging				
Combination Abdominal CT Scan	504	0.048	0.164	0.191
Combination Chest CT Scan	305	0.033	0.038	0.054
Follow-up Mammogram/Ultrasound	787	10.9%	8.4%	8.4%
MRI for Low Back Pain	83	30.1%	30.2%	32.7%
Survey of Patients' Hospital Experiences				
Area Around Room 'Always' Quiet at Night	300+	46%	-	58%
Doctors 'Always' Communicated Well	300+	84%	-	80%
Home Recovery Information Given	300+	82%	-	82%
Hospital Given 9 or 10 on 10 Point Scale	300+	61%	-	67%
Meds 'Always' Explained Before Given	300+	62%	-	60%
Nurses 'Always' Communicated Well	300+	79%	-	76%
Pain 'Always' Well Controlled	300+	68%	-	69%
Room and Bathroom 'Always' Clean	300+	69%	-	71%
Timely Help 'Always' Received	300+	71%	-	64%
Would Definitely Recommend Hospital	300+	59%	-	69%

Bellevue Hospital

1400 West Main Street
Bellevue, OH 44811
Phone: 419-483-4040
Fax: 419-483-9718
E-mail: webmaster@bellevuehospital.com
URL: www.bellevuehospital.com
Type: Acute Care Hospitals
Emergency Services: Yes
Ownership: Voluntary Non-Profit - Other
Beds: 64

Key Personnel:
Chief of Medical Staff . . . . Richard Kendall, MD
Infection Control. . . . . Susan Kistler
Operating Room. . . . . Tammi Lewis, RN
Quality Assurance . . . . Patricia Hetrick Semer
Anesthesiology. . . . . Joseph Colizoli, MD
Intensive Care Unit. . . . . Emily Wadsworth, RN

Measure	Cases	This Hosp.	State Avg.	U.S. Avg.
Heart Attack Care				
ACE Inhibitor or ARB for LVSD	0	-	97%	96%
Aspirin at Arrival[1]	10	100%	99%	99%
Aspirin at Discharge[1]	6	100%	99%	98%
Beta Blocker at Discharge[1]	9	100%	99%	98%
Fibrinolytic Medication Timing	0	-	14%	55%
PCI Within 90 Minutes of Arrival	0	-	92%	90%
Smoking Cessation Advice[1]	1	100%	100%	99%
Chest Pain/Possible Heart Attack Care				
Aspirin at Arrival	72	93%	96%	95%
Median Time to ECG (minutes)	74	3	7	8
Median Time to Transfer (minutes)[1]	9	67	61	61
Fibrinolytic Medication Timing[1]	4	25%	47%	54%
Heart Failure Care				
ACE Inhibitor or ARB for LVSD[1]	21	81%	96%	94%
Discharge Instructions	27	85%	91%	88%
Evaluation of LVS Function	39	95%	99%	98%
Smoking Cessation Advice[1]	4	100%	99%	98%
Pneumonia Care				
Appropriate Initial Antibiotic	69	77%	92%	92%
Blood Culture Timing	73	99%	96%	96%
Influenza Vaccine	51	88%	93%	91%
Initial Antibiotic Timing	74	91%	96%	95%
Pneumococcal Vaccine	71	100%	95%	93%
Smoking Cessation Advice	46	93%	98%	97%
Surgical Care Improvement Project				
Appropriate VTP Within 24 Hours	69	78%	92%	92%
Appropriate Hair Removal	201	100%	100%	99%
Appropriate Beta Blocker Usage	35	91%	94%	93%
Controlled Postoperative Blood Glucose	0	-	94%	93%
Prophylactic Antibiotic Timing	138	94%	97%	97%
Prophylactic Antibiotic Timing (Outpatient)	73	74%	91%	92%
Prophylactic Antibiotic Selection	140	94%	98%	97%
Prophylactic Antibiotic Select. (Outpatient)	63	71%	94%	94%
Prophylactic Antibiotic Stopped	137	91%	95%	94%
Recommended VTP Ordered	69	84%	94%	94%
Urinary Catheter Removal	36	86%	91%	90%
Children's Asthma Care				
Received Systemic Corticosteroids	-	-	-	100%
Received Home Management Plan	-	-	-	71%
Received Reliever Medication	-	-	-	100%
Use of Medical Imaging				
Combination Abdominal CT Scan	306	0.330	0.164	0.191
Combination Chest CT Scan	202	0.381	0.038	0.054
Follow-up Mammogram/Ultrasound	390	10.3%	8.4%	8.4%
MRI for Low Back Pain	73	31.5%	30.2%	32.7%
Survey of Patients' Hospital Experiences				
Area Around Room 'Always' Quiet at Night	300+	59%	-	58%
Doctors 'Always' Communicated Well	300+	85%	-	80%
Home Recovery Information Given	300+	85%	-	82%
Hospital Given 9 or 10 on 10 Point Scale	300+	82%	-	67%
Meds 'Always' Explained Before Given	300+	64%	-	60%
Nurses 'Always' Communicated Well	300+	79%	-	76%
Pain 'Always' Well Controlled	300+	71%	-	69%
Room and Bathroom 'Always' Clean	300+	83%	-	71%
Timely Help 'Always' Received	300+	67%	-	64%
Would Definitely Recommend Hospital	300+	80%	-	69%

NOTE: Hospital profiles are in alphabetical order by state, then city, then hospital within the city; Rankings exclude hospitals with less than 25 cases except for patient surveys which excludes hospitals with less than 100 cases; (a) 100–299 cases; (1) The number of cases is too small to be sure how well a hospital is performing; (2) The hospital indicated that the data submitted for this measure were based on a sample of cases; (3) Data was collected during a shorter time period (fewer quarters) than the maximum possible time for this measure; (4) Suppressed for one or more quarters by CMS; (5) No data is available from the hospital for this measure; (6) Fewer than 100 patients completed the HCAHPS survey. Use these rates with caution, as the number of surveys may be too low to reliably assess hospital performance; (7) Survey results are based on less than 12 months of data; (8) Survey results are not available for this reporting period; (9) No or very few patients were eligible for the HCAHPS survey. The scores shown, if any, reflect a very small number of surveys; (10) A state average was not calculated because too few hospitals in the state submitted data; (11) There were discrepancies in the data collection process; Please refer to the User's Guide for a full explanation of data.

Bluffton Hospital

139 Garau Street   Phone: 419-358-9010
Bluffton, OH 45817
URL: www.bvhealthsystem.org
Type: Critical Access Hospitals   Emergency Services: Yes
Ownership: Voluntary Non-Profit - Private   Beds: 25
Key Personnel:
Administrator . . . . Bill Watkins

Measure	Cases	This Hosp.	State Avg.	U.S. Avg.
Heart Attack Care				
ACE Inhibitor or ARB for LVSD[3]	0	-	97%	96%
Aspirin at Arrival[1,3]	1	100%	99%	99%
Aspirin at Discharge[1,3]	1	0%	99%	98%
Beta Blocker at Discharge[1,3]	1	0%	99%	98%
Fibrinolytic Medication Timing[3]	0	-	14%	55%
PCI Within 90 Minutes of Arrival[3]	0	-	92%	90%
Smoking Cessation Advice[3]	0	-	100%	99%
Chest Pain/Possible Heart Attack Care				
Aspirin at Arrival[1]	24	96%	96%	95%
Median Time to ECG (minutes)	26	11	7	8
Median Time to Transfer (minutes)[1,3]	3	54	61	61
Fibrinolytic Medication Timing[3]	0	-	47%	54%
Heart Failure Care				
ACE Inhibitor or ARB for LVSD	0	-	96%	94%
Discharge Instructions	0	-	91%	88%
Evaluation of LVS Function[1]	2	100%	99%	98%
Smoking Cessation Advice	0	-	99%	98%
Pneumonia Care				
Appropriate Initial Antibiotic[1]	6	100%	92%	92%
Blood Culture Timing[1]	12	100%	96%	96%
Influenza Vaccine[1]	9	100%	93%	91%
Initial Antibiotic Timing[1]	12	100%	96%	95%
Pneumococcal Vaccine[1]	13	100%	95%	93%
Smoking Cessation Advice[1]	2	100%	98%	97%
Surgical Care Improvement Project				
Appropriate VTP Within 24 Hours[1,2]	1	100%	92%	92%
Appropriate Hair Removal[1,2]	23	100%	100%	99%
Appropriate Beta Blocker Usage[1,2]	3	100%	94%	93%
Controlled Postoperative Blood Glucose[2]	0	-	94%	93%
Prophylactic Antibiotic Timing[1,2]	22	73%	97%	97%
Prophylactic Antibiotic Timing (Outpatient)	106	91%	91%	92%
Prophylactic Antibiotic Selection[1,2]	22	100%	98%	97%
Prophylactic Antibiotic Select. (Outpatient)	104	96%	94%	94%
Prophylactic Antibiotic Stopped[1,2]	22	100%	95%	94%
Recommended VTP Ordered[1,2]	1	100%	94%	94%
Urinary Catheter Removal[2]	0	-	91%	90%
Children's Asthma Care				
Received Systemic Corticosteroids	-	-	-	100%
Received Home Management Plan	-	-	-	71%
Received Reliever Medication	-	-	-	100%
Use of Medical Imaging				
Combination Abdominal CT Scan	99	0.061	0.164	0.191
Combination Chest CT Scan	45	0.022	0.038	0.054
Follow-up Mammogram/Ultrasound	276	13.0%	8.4%	8.4%
MRI for Low Back Pain[5]	0	-	30.2%	32.7%
Survey of Patients' Hospital Experiences				
Area Around Room 'Always' Quiet at Night	(a)	75%	-	58%
Doctors 'Always' Communicated Well	(a)	87%	-	80%
Home Recovery Information Given	(a)	87%	-	82%
Hospital Given 9 or 10 on 10 Point Scale	(a)	87%	-	67%
Meds 'Always' Explained Before Given	(a)	69%	-	60%
Nurses 'Always' Communicated Well	(a)	86%	-	76%
Pain 'Always' Well Controlled	(a)	79%	-	69%
Room and Bathroom 'Always' Clean	(a)	81%	-	71%
Timely Help 'Always' Received	(a)	83%	-	64%
Would Definitely Recommend Hospital	(a)	89%	-	69%

Wood County Hospital

950 West Wooster Street   Phone: 419-354-8900
Bowling Green, OH 43402   Fax: 419-354-8957
E-mail: woodhosp@wcnet.org
URL: www.wch.net
Type: Acute Care Hospitals   Emergency Services: Yes
Ownership: Voluntary Non-Profit - Private   Beds: 162
Key Personnel:
CEO/President. . . . . Stanley R Kordueki
Infection Control. . . . . Louise White
Pediatric In-Patient Care . . . . Lori Tuck
Quality Assurance . . . . Steve Hunter
Radiology. . . . . Sue Rayle
Intensive Care Unit. . . . . Alan Mintz

Measure	Cases	This Hosp.	State Avg.	U.S. Avg.
Heart Attack Care				
ACE Inhibitor or ARB for LVSD[1]	3	100%	97%	96%
Aspirin at Arrival[1]	11	100%	99%	99%
Aspirin at Discharge[1]	7	100%	99%	98%
Beta Blocker at Discharge[1]	7	100%	99%	98%
Fibrinolytic Medication Timing	0	-	14%	55%
PCI Within 90 Minutes of Arrival	0	-	92%	90%
Smoking Cessation Advice	0	-	100%	99%
Chest Pain/Possible Heart Attack Care				
Aspirin at Arrival	91	96%	96%	95%
Median Time to ECG (minutes)	94	10	7	8
Median Time to Transfer (minutes)[1]	8	72	61	61
Fibrinolytic Medication Timing[1]	3	33%	47%	54%
Heart Failure Care				
ACE Inhibitor or ARB for LVSD[1]	23	96%	96%	94%
Discharge Instructions	58	83%	91%	88%
Evaluation of LVS Function	73	90%	99%	98%
Smoking Cessation Advice[1]	10	100%	99%	98%
Pneumonia Care				
Appropriate Initial Antibiotic	114	67%	92%	92%
Blood Culture Timing	105	89%	96%	96%
Influenza Vaccine	63	86%	93%	91%
Initial Antibiotic Timing	114	88%	96%	95%
Pneumococcal Vaccine	69	91%	95%	93%
Smoking Cessation Advice	28	100%	98%	97%
Surgical Care Improvement Project				
Appropriate VTP Within 24 Hours	112	92%	92%	92%
Appropriate Hair Removal	225	99%	100%	99%
Appropriate Beta Blocker Usage	69	84%	94%	93%
Controlled Postoperative Blood Glucose	0	-	94%	93%
Prophylactic Antibiotic Timing	178	92%	97%	97%
Prophylactic Antibiotic Timing (Outpatient)	110	86%	91%	92%
Prophylactic Antibiotic Selection	178	96%	98%	97%
Prophylactic Antibiotic Select. (Outpatient)	104	54%	94%	94%
Prophylactic Antibiotic Stopped	171	88%	95%	94%
Recommended VTP Ordered	118	88%	94%	94%
Urinary Catheter Removal	70	53%	91%	90%
Children's Asthma Care				
Received Systemic Corticosteroids	-	-	-	100%
Received Home Management Plan	-	-	-	71%
Received Reliever Medication	-	-	-	100%
Use of Medical Imaging				
Combination Abdominal CT Scan	469	0.077	0.164	0.191
Combination Chest CT Scan	330	0.130	0.038	0.054
Follow-up Mammogram/Ultrasound	598	7.7%	8.4%	8.4%
MRI for Low Back Pain	82	19.5%	30.2%	32.7%
Survey of Patients' Hospital Experiences				
Area Around Room 'Always' Quiet at Night	300+	56%	-	58%
Doctors 'Always' Communicated Well	300+	78%	-	80%
Home Recovery Information Given	300+	89%	-	82%
Hospital Given 9 or 10 on 10 Point Scale	300+	67%	-	67%
Meds 'Always' Explained Before Given	300+	61%	-	60%
Nurses 'Always' Communicated Well	300+	72%	-	76%
Pain 'Always' Well Controlled	300+	67%	-	69%
Room and Bathroom 'Always' Clean	300+	76%	-	71%
Timely Help 'Always' Received	300+	70%	-	64%
Would Definitely Recommend Hospital	300+	65%	-	69%

Community Hospitals and Wellness Centers

433 West High Street   Phone: 419-636-1131
Bryan, OH 43506   Fax: 419-636-3100
URL: www.chwchospital.com
Type: Acute Care Hospitals   Emergency Services: Yes
Ownership: Voluntary Non-Profit - Other   Beds: 131
Key Personnel:
CEO/President. . . . . Philip L Ennen
Coronary Care . . . . Marilyn Frank, RN
Infection Control. . . . . Vickie Shaffer
Operating Room. . . . . Kathy Lienberger, RN
Quality Assurance . . . . Sharon Mesnard, RN
Radiology. . . . . Darren Chao
Patient Relations . . . . Jan David, RN

Measure	Cases	This Hosp.	State Avg.	U.S. Avg.
Heart Attack Care				
ACE Inhibitor or ARB for LVSD[1]	13	77%	97%	96%
Aspirin at Arrival	52	100%	99%	99%
Aspirin at Discharge	72	99%	99%	98%
Beta Blocker at Discharge	68	97%	99%	98%
Fibrinolytic Medication Timing	0	-	14%	55%
PCI Within 90 Minutes of Arrival[1]	16	69%	92%	90%
Smoking Cessation Advice	25	100%	100%	99%
Chest Pain/Possible Heart Attack Care				
Aspirin at Arrival	46	96%	96%	95%
Median Time to ECG (minutes)	48	6	7	8
Median Time to Transfer (minutes)[1,3]	3	57	61	61
Fibrinolytic Medication Timing[3]	0	-	47%	54%
Heart Failure Care				
ACE Inhibitor or ARB for LVSD	52	92%	96%	94%
Discharge Instructions	92	96%	91%	88%
Evaluation of LVS Function	115	100%	99%	98%
Smoking Cessation Advice[1]	12	100%	99%	98%
Pneumonia Care				
Appropriate Initial Antibiotic	68	91%	92%	92%
Blood Culture Timing	61	100%	96%	96%
Influenza Vaccine	66	94%	93%	91%
Initial Antibiotic Timing	83	99%	96%	95%
Pneumococcal Vaccine	69	97%	95%	93%
Smoking Cessation Advice	28	100%	98%	97%
Surgical Care Improvement Project				
Appropriate VTP Within 24 Hours	101	90%	92%	92%
Appropriate Hair Removal	237	100%	100%	99%
Appropriate Beta Blocker Usage	94	93%	94%	93%
Controlled Postoperative Blood Glucose	0	-	94%	93%
Prophylactic Antibiotic Timing	180	96%	97%	97%
Prophylactic Antibiotic Timing (Outpatient)	85	92%	91%	92%
Prophylactic Antibiotic Selection	180	99%	98%	97%
Prophylactic Antibiotic Select. (Outpatient)	79	96%	94%	94%
Prophylactic Antibiotic Stopped	175	97%	95%	94%
Recommended VTP Ordered	101	97%	94%	94%
Urinary Catheter Removal	35	97%	91%	90%
Children's Asthma Care				
Received Systemic Corticosteroids	-	-	-	100%
Received Home Management Plan	-	-	-	71%
Received Reliever Medication	-	-	-	100%
Use of Medical Imaging				
Combination Abdominal CT Scan	246	0.049	0.164	0.191
Combination Chest CT Scan	219	0.073	0.038	0.054
Follow-up Mammogram/Ultrasound	179	7.3%	8.4%	8.4%
MRI for Low Back Pain	92	20.7%	30.2%	32.7%
Survey of Patients' Hospital Experiences				
Area Around Room 'Always' Quiet at Night	300+	62%	-	58%
Doctors 'Always' Communicated Well	300+	79%	-	80%
Home Recovery Information Given	300+	84%	-	82%
Hospital Given 9 or 10 on 10 Point Scale	300+	73%	-	67%
Meds 'Always' Explained Before Given	300+	63%	-	60%
Nurses 'Always' Communicated Well	300+	78%	-	76%
Pain 'Always' Well Controlled	300+	72%	-	69%
Room and Bathroom 'Always' Clean	300+	82%	-	71%
Timely Help 'Always' Received	300+	74%	-	64%
Would Definitely Recommend Hospital	300+	70%	-	69%

NOTE: Hospital profiles are in alphabetical order by state, then city, then hospital within the city; Rankings exclude hospitals with less than 25 cases except for patient surveys which excludes hospitals with less than 100 cases; (a) 100–299 cases; (1) The number of cases is too small to be sure how well a hospital is performing; (2) The hospital indicated that the data submitted for this measure were based on a sample of cases; (3) Data was collected during a shorter time period (fewer quarters) than the maximum possible time for this measure; (4) Suppressed for one or more quarters by CMS; (5) No data is available from the hospital for this measure; (6) Fewer than 100 patients completed the HCAHPS survey. Use these rates with caution, as the number of surveys may be too low to reliably assess hospital performance; (7) Survey results are based on less than 12 months of data; (8) Survey results are not available for this reporting period; (9) No or very few patients were eligible for the HCAHPS survey. The scores shown, if any, reflect a very small number of surveys; (10) A state average was not calculated because too few hospitals in the state submitted data; (11) There were discrepancies in the data collection process; Please refer to the User's Guide for a full explanation of data.

Bucyrus Community Hospital

629 North Sandusky Avenue
Bucyrus, OH 44820
Phone: 419-562-4677
Fax: 419-562-6766
URL: www.bchonline.org
Type: Critical Access Hospitals
Emergency Services: Yes
Ownership: Voluntary Non-Profit - Other
Beds: 25

Key Personnel:
Cardiac Laboratory. . . . . Tammi Wolfe, RN
Chief of Medical Staff. . . . . Candy Christian
Infection Control. . . . . Joyce Weaver
Operating Room. . . . . Phyllis Crall
Quality Assurance . . . . Jeanne Perkins
Emergency Room . . . . Larry Tincher
Hemotology Center . . . . Joann Riedlinger

Measure	Cases	This Hosp.	State Avg.	U.S. Avg.
Heart Attack Care				
ACE Inhibitor or ARB for LVSD[1,3]	1	100%	97%	96%
Aspirin at Arrival[1,3]	1	100%	99%	99%
Aspirin at Discharge[1,3]	1	100%	99%	98%
Beta Blocker at Discharge[1,3]	1	0%	99%	98%
Fibrinolytic Medication Timing[3]	0	-	14%	55%
PCI Within 90 Minutes of Arrival[5]	0	-	92%	90%
Smoking Cessation Advice[3]	0	-	100%	99%
Chest Pain/Possible Heart Attack Care				
Aspirin at Arrival	-	-	96%	95%
Median Time to ECG (minutes)	-	-	7	8
Median Time to Transfer (minutes)	-	-	61	61
Fibrinolytic Medication Timing	-	-	47%	54%
Heart Failure Care				
ACE Inhibitor or ARB for LVSD[1]	6	83%	96%	94%
Discharge Instructions[1]	13	85%	91%	88%
Evaluation of LVS Function	25	100%	99%	98%
Smoking Cessation Advice[1]	3	100%	99%	98%
Pneumonia Care				
Appropriate Initial Antibiotic	31	100%	92%	92%
Blood Culture Timing	49	100%	96%	96%
Influenza Vaccine	28	96%	93%	91%
Initial Antibiotic Timing	42	100%	96%	95%
Pneumococcal Vaccine	30	100%	95%	93%
Smoking Cessation Advice[1]	13	100%	98%	97%
Surgical Care Improvement Project				
Appropriate VTP Within 24 Hours	33	97%	92%	92%
Appropriate Hair Removal	113	99%	100%	99%
Appropriate Beta Blocker Usage[5]	0	-	94%	93%
Controlled Postoperative Blood Glucose[3]	0	-	94%	93%
Prophylactic Antibiotic Timing	94	99%	97%	97%
Prophylactic Antibiotic Timing (Outpatient)	-	-	91%	92%
Prophylactic Antibiotic Selection	94	99%	98%	97%
Prophylactic Antibiotic Select. (Outpatient)	-	-	94%	94%
Prophylactic Antibiotic Stopped	93	98%	95%	94%
Recommended VTP Ordered	33	97%	94%	94%
Urinary Catheter Removal	30	100%	91%	90%
Children's Asthma Care				
Received Systemic Corticosteroids	-	-	-	100%
Received Home Management Plan	-	-	-	71%
Received Reliever Medication	-	-	-	100%
Use of Medical Imaging				
Combination Abdominal CT Scan	-	-	0.164	0.191
Combination Chest CT Scan	-	-	0.038	0.054
Follow-up Mammogram/Ultrasound	-	-	8.4%	8.4%
MRI for Low Back Pain	-	-	30.2%	32.7%
Survey of Patients' Hospital Experiences				
Area Around Room 'Always' Quiet at Night	(a)	62%	-	58%
Doctors 'Always' Communicated Well	(a)	80%	-	80%
Home Recovery Information Given	(a)	90%	-	82%
Hospital Given 9 or 10 on 10 Point Scale	(a)	69%	-	67%
Meds 'Always' Explained Before Given	(a)	65%	-	60%
Nurses 'Always' Communicated Well	(a)	77%	-	76%
Pain 'Always' Well Controlled	(a)	72%	-	69%
Room and Bathroom 'Always' Clean	(a)	68%	-	71%
Timely Help 'Always' Received	(a)	76%	-	64%
Would Definitely Recommend Hospital	(a)	64%	-	69%

Harrison Community Hospital

951 East Market Street
Cadiz, OH 43907
Phone: 740-942-4631
Fax: 740-942-2749
E-mail: hchosp@1st.net
URL: www.harrisoncommunity.com
Type: Critical Access Hospitals
Emergency Services: Yes
Ownership: Voluntary Non-Profit - Private
Beds: 48

Key Personnel:
CEO/President. . . . . Terry M Carson
Chief of Medical Staff . . . . Carole Patton
Operating Room. . . . . Anandhi Murthy
Anesthesiology. . . . . Shary Hillard
Emergency Room . . . . Ajit Modi, MD

Measure	Cases	This Hosp.	State Avg.	U.S. Avg.
Heart Attack Care				
ACE Inhibitor or ARB for LVSD[5]	0	-	97%	96%
Aspirin at Arrival[5]	0	-	99%	99%
Aspirin at Discharge[5]	0	-	99%	98%
Beta Blocker at Discharge[5]	0	-	99%	98%
Fibrinolytic Medication Timing[5]	0	-	14%	55%
PCI Within 90 Minutes of Arrival[5]	0	-	92%	90%
Smoking Cessation Advice[5]	0	-	100%	99%
Chest Pain/Possible Heart Attack Care				
Aspirin at Arrival	-	-	96%	95%
Median Time to ECG (minutes)	-	-	7	8
Median Time to Transfer (minutes)	-	-	61	61
Fibrinolytic Medication Timing	-	-	47%	54%
Heart Failure Care				
ACE Inhibitor or ARB for LVSD[1]	2	50%	96%	94%
Discharge Instructions[1]	3	67%	91%	88%
Evaluation of LVS Function[1]	10	90%	99%	98%
Smoking Cessation Advice[1]	3	100%	99%	98%
Pneumonia Care				
Appropriate Initial Antibiotic[1]	12	100%	92%	92%
Blood Culture Timing[1]	4	100%	96%	96%
Influenza Vaccine[1]	3	100%	93%	91%
Initial Antibiotic Timing[1]	14	93%	96%	95%
Pneumococcal Vaccine[1]	8	88%	95%	93%
Smoking Cessation Advice[1]	4	100%	98%	97%
Surgical Care Improvement Project				
Appropriate VTP Within 24 Hours[1]	3	67%	92%	92%
Appropriate Hair Removal[1]	7	100%	100%	99%
Appropriate Beta Blocker Usage[5]	0	-	94%	93%
Controlled Postoperative Blood Glucose[5]	0	-	94%	93%
Prophylactic Antibiotic Timing[1]	7	86%	97%	97%
Prophylactic Antibiotic Timing (Outpatient)	-	-	91%	92%
Prophylactic Antibiotic Selection[1]	7	86%	98%	97%
Prophylactic Antibiotic Select. (Outpatient)	-	-	94%	94%
Prophylactic Antibiotic Stopped[1]	7	100%	95%	94%
Recommended VTP Ordered[1]	3	67%	94%	94%
Urinary Catheter Removal	0	-	91%	90%
Children's Asthma Care				
Received Systemic Corticosteroids	-	-	-	100%
Received Home Management Plan	-	-	-	71%
Received Reliever Medication	-	-	-	100%
Use of Medical Imaging				
Combination Abdominal CT Scan	-	-	0.164	0.191
Combination Chest CT Scan	-	-	0.038	0.054
Follow-up Mammogram/Ultrasound	-	-	8.4%	8.4%
MRI for Low Back Pain	-	-	30.2%	32.7%
Survey of Patients' Hospital Experiences				
Area Around Room 'Always' Quiet at Night[8]	-	-	-	58%
Doctors 'Always' Communicated Well[8]	-	-	-	80%
Home Recovery Information Given[8]	-	-	-	82%
Hospital Given 9 or 10 on 10 Point Scale[8]	-	-	-	67%
Meds 'Always' Explained Before Given[8]	-	-	-	60%
Nurses 'Always' Communicated Well[8]	-	-	-	76%
Pain 'Always' Well Controlled[8]	-	-	-	69%
Room and Bathroom 'Always' Clean[8]	-	-	-	71%
Timely Help 'Always' Received[8]	-	-	-	64%
Would Definitely Recommend Hospital[8]	-	-	-	69%

Southeastern Ohio Regional Medical Center

1341 North Clark Street
Cambridge, OH 43725
Phone: 740-439-8111
Fax: 740-439-8175
URL: www.seormc.org
Type: Acute Care Hospitals
Emergency Services: Yes
Ownership: Voluntary Non-Profit - Private
Beds: 209

Key Personnel:
CEO/President. . . . . James Keller, MD
Cardiac Laboratory. . . . . Gilbert Kukielka, MD
Chief of Medical Staff . . . . Brady Stonen, MD
Infection Control. . . . . Christine Daugherty, RN
Operating Room. . . . . Cathy McIntire, RN
Quality Assurance . . . . James Keller, MD
Radiology. . . . . Shane Backus

Measure	Cases	This Hosp.	State Avg.	U.S. Avg.
Heart Attack Care				
ACE Inhibitor or ARB for LVSD[1]	1	100%	97%	96%
Aspirin at Arrival[1]	9	100%	99%	99%
Aspirin at Discharge[1]	4	100%	99%	98%
Beta Blocker at Discharge[1]	4	100%	99%	98%
Fibrinolytic Medication Timing	0	-	14%	55%
PCI Within 90 Minutes of Arrival	0	-	92%	90%
Smoking Cessation Advice[1]	1	100%	100%	99%
Chest Pain/Possible Heart Attack Care				
Aspirin at Arrival	276	97%	96%	95%
Median Time to ECG (minutes)	275	8	7	8
Median Time to Transfer (minutes)[1]	14	50	61	61
Fibrinolytic Medication Timing[1]	5	60%	47%	54%
Heart Failure Care				
ACE Inhibitor or ARB for LVSD	28	89%	96%	94%
Discharge Instructions	102	91%	91%	88%
Evaluation of LVS Function	128	95%	99%	98%
Smoking Cessation Advice	26	100%	99%	98%
Pneumonia Care				
Appropriate Initial Antibiotic[2]	112	89%	92%	92%
Blood Culture Timing[2]	144	99%	96%	96%
Influenza Vaccine[2]	91	98%	93%	91%
Initial Antibiotic Timing[2]	150	96%	96%	95%
Pneumococcal Vaccine[2]	136	96%	95%	93%
Smoking Cessation Advice[2]	72	100%	98%	97%
Surgical Care Improvement Project				
Appropriate VTP Within 24 Hours[2]	90	87%	92%	92%
Appropriate Hair Removal[2]	183	100%	100%	99%
Appropriate Beta Blocker Usage[2]	63	97%	94%	93%
Controlled Postoperative Blood Glucose[2]	0	-	94%	93%
Prophylactic Antibiotic Timing[2]	141	99%	97%	97%
Prophylactic Antibiotic Timing (Outpatient)	155	93%	91%	92%
Prophylactic Antibiotic Selection[2]	143	94%	98%	97%
Prophylactic Antibiotic Select. (Outpatient)	145	91%	94%	94%
Prophylactic Antibiotic Stopped[2]	131	95%	95%	94%
Recommended VTP Ordered[2]	90	87%	94%	94%
Urinary Catheter Removal[2]	44	93%	91%	90%
Children's Asthma Care				
Received Systemic Corticosteroids	-	-	-	100%
Received Home Management Plan	-	-	-	71%
Received Reliever Medication	-	-	-	100%
Use of Medical Imaging				
Combination Abdominal CT Scan	598	0.156	0.164	0.191
Combination Chest CT Scan	436	0.183	0.038	0.054
Follow-up Mammogram/Ultrasound	901	5.1%	8.4%	8.4%
MRI for Low Back Pain[1]	36	36.1%	30.2%	32.7%
Survey of Patients' Hospital Experiences				
Area Around Room 'Always' Quiet at Night	300+	57%	-	58%
Doctors 'Always' Communicated Well	300+	81%	-	80%
Home Recovery Information Given	300+	83%	-	82%
Hospital Given 9 or 10 on 10 Point Scale	300+	68%	-	67%
Meds 'Always' Explained Before Given	300+	64%	-	60%
Nurses 'Always' Communicated Well	300+	81%	-	76%
Pain 'Always' Well Controlled	300+	68%	-	69%
Room and Bathroom 'Always' Clean	300+	77%	-	71%
Timely Help 'Always' Received	300+	68%	-	64%
Would Definitely Recommend Hospital	300+	64%	-	69%

NOTE: Hospital profiles are in alphabetical order by state, then city, then hospital within the city; Rankings exclude hospitals with less than 25 cases except for patient surveys which excludes hospitals with less than 100 cases; (a) 100–299 cases; (1) The number of cases is too small to be sure how well a hospital is performing; (2) The hospital indicated that the data submitted for this measure were based on a sample of cases; (3) Data was collected during a shorter time period (fewer quarters) than the maximum possible time for this measure; (4) Suppressed for one or more quarters by CMS; (5) No data is available from the hospital for this measure; (6) Fewer than 100 patients completed the HCAHPS survey. Use these rates with caution, as the number of surveys may be too low to reliably assess hospital performance; (7) Survey results are based on less than 12 months of data; (8) Survey results are not available for this reporting period; (9) No or very few patients were eligible for the HCAHPS survey. The scores shown, if any, reflect a very small number of surveys; (10) A state average was not calculated because too few hospitals in the state submitted data; (11) There were discrepancies in the data collection process; Please refer to the User's Guide for a full explanation of data.

Diley Ridge Medical Center

7911 Diley Road
Canal Winchester, OH 43110
URL: www.dileyridgemedicalcenter.com
Type: Acute Care Hospitals
Ownership: Voluntary Non-Profit - Private

Phone: 614-838-7910

Emergency Services: Yes

Measure	Cases	This Hosp.	State Avg.	U.S. Avg.
Heart Attack Care				
ACE Inhibitor or ARB for LVSD[5]	0	-	97%	96%
Aspirin at Arrival[5]	0	-	99%	99%
Aspirin at Discharge[5]	0	-	99%	98%
Beta Blocker at Discharge[5]	0	-	99%	98%
Fibrinolytic Medication Timing[5]	0	-	14%	55%
PCI Within 90 Minutes of Arrival[5]	0	-	92%	90%
Smoking Cessation Advice[5]	0	-	100%	99%
Chest Pain/Possible Heart Attack Care				
Aspirin at Arrival	-	-	96%	95%
Median Time to ECG (minutes)	-	-	7	8
Median Time to Transfer (minutes)	-	-	61	61
Fibrinolytic Medication Timing	-	-	47%	54%
Heart Failure Care				
ACE Inhibitor or ARB for LVSD[5]	0	-	96%	94%
Discharge Instructions[5]	0	-	91%	88%
Evaluation of LVS Function[5]	0	-	99%	98%
Smoking Cessation Advice[5]	0	-	99%	98%
Pneumonia Care				
Appropriate Initial Antibiotic[1,3]	2	100%	92%	92%
Blood Culture Timing[1,3]	4	100%	96%	96%
Influenza Vaccine[5]	0	-	93%	91%
Initial Antibiotic Timing[1,3]	2	100%	96%	95%
Pneumococcal Vaccine[1,3]	2	50%	95%	93%
Smoking Cessation Advice[1,3]	2	50%	98%	97%
Surgical Care Improvement Project				
Appropriate VTP Within 24 Hours[5]	0	-	92%	92%
Appropriate Hair Removal[5]	0	-	100%	99%
Appropriate Beta Blocker Usage[5]	0	-	94%	93%
Controlled Postoperative Blood Glucose[5]	0	-	94%	93%
Prophylactic Antibiotic Timing[5]	0	-	97%	97%
Prophylactic Antibiotic Timing (Outpatient)	-	-	91%	92%
Prophylactic Antibiotic Selection[5]	0	-	98%	97%
Prophylactic Antibiotic Select. (Outpatient)	-	-	94%	94%
Prophylactic Antibiotic Stopped[5]	0	-	95%	94%
Recommended VTP Ordered[5]	0	-	94%	94%
Urinary Catheter Removal[5]	0	-	91%	90%
Children's Asthma Care				
Received Systemic Corticosteroids	-	-	-	100%
Received Home Management Plan	-	-	-	71%
Received Reliever Medication	-	-	-	100%
Use of Medical Imaging				
Combination Abdominal CT Scan	-	-	0.164	0.191
Combination Chest CT Scan	-	-	0.038	0.054
Follow-up Mammogram/Ultrasound	-	-	8.4%	8.4%
MRI for Low Back Pain	-	-	30.2%	32.7%
Survey of Patients' Hospital Experiences				
Area Around Room 'Always' Quiet at Night[8]	-	-	-	58%
Doctors 'Always' Communicated Well[8]	-	-	-	80%
Home Recovery Information Given[8]	-	-	-	82%
Hospital Given 9 or 10 on 10 Point Scale[8]	-	-	-	67%
Meds 'Always' Explained Before Given[8]	-	-	-	60%
Nurses 'Always' Communicated Well[8]	-	-	-	76%
Pain 'Always' Well Controlled[8]	-	-	-	69%
Room and Bathroom 'Always' Clean[8]	-	-	-	71%
Timely Help 'Always' Received[8]	-	-	-	64%
Would Definitely Recommend Hospital[8]	-	-	-	69%

Aultman Hospital

2600 Sixth Street SW
Canton, OH 44710
URL: www.aultman.com
Type: Acute Care Hospitals
Ownership: Voluntary Non-Profit - Other

Phone: 330-452-9911
Fax: 330-438-9811

Emergency Services: Yes
Beds: 814

Key Personnel:
CEO/President . . . . Edward Roth
Chief of Medical Staff . . . . Allen Rovner, MD
Infection Control . . . . Joan Pugnale
Operating Room . . . . Elizabeth Edmunds, RN
Radiology. . . . . Liz Getz
Anesthesiology. . . . . Milton P Midis, MD
Emergency Room . . . . Liz Edmunds, MD
Patient Relations . . . . Jennie Shisler

Measure	Cases	This Hosp.	State Avg.	U.S. Avg.
Heart Attack Care				
ACE Inhibitor or ARB for LVSD	105	99%	97%	96%
Aspirin at Arrival	394	99%	99%	99%
Aspirin at Discharge	619	100%	99%	98%
Beta Blocker at Discharge	603	100%	99%	98%
Fibrinolytic Medication Timing	0	-	14%	55%
PCI Within 90 Minutes of Arrival	90	92%	92%	90%
Smoking Cessation Advice	213	100%	100%	99%
Chest Pain/Possible Heart Attack Care				
Aspirin at Arrival[1]	17	82%	96%	95%
Median Time to ECG (minutes)[1]	18	6	7	8
Median Time to Transfer (minutes)[5]	0	-	61	61
Fibrinolytic Medication Timing[5]	0	-	47%	54%
Heart Failure Care				
ACE Inhibitor or ARB for LVSD	163	99%	96%	94%
Discharge Instructions	445	87%	91%	88%
Evaluation of LVS Function	593	100%	99%	98%
Smoking Cessation Advice	99	100%	99%	98%
Pneumonia Care				
Appropriate Initial Antibiotic	370	95%	92%	92%
Blood Culture Timing	632	97%	96%	96%
Influenza Vaccine	499	94%	93%	91%
Initial Antibiotic Timing	609	96%	96%	95%
Pneumococcal Vaccine	627	97%	95%	93%
Smoking Cessation Advice	240	97%	98%	97%
Surgical Care Improvement Project				
Appropriate VTP Within 24 Hours[2]	205	89%	92%	92%
Appropriate Hair Removal[2]	739	100%	100%	99%
Appropriate Beta Blocker Usage[2]	289	96%	94%	93%
Controlled Postoperative Blood Glucose[2]	182	94%	94%	93%
Prophylactic Antibiotic Timing[2]	554	96%	97%	97%
Prophylactic Antibiotic Timing (Outpatient)	1,067	92%	91%	92%
Prophylactic Antibiotic Selection[2]	563	98%	98%	97%
Prophylactic Antibiotic Select. (Outpatient)	1,296	96%	94%	94%
Prophylactic Antibiotic Stopped[2]	538	96%	95%	94%
Recommended VTP Ordered[2]	206	94%	94%	94%
Urinary Catheter Removal[2]	168	94%	91%	90%
Children's Asthma Care				
Received Systemic Corticosteroids[1]	13	100%	-	100%
Received Home Management Plan[1]	13	62%	-	71%
Received Reliever Medication[1]	14	100%	-	100%
Use of Medical Imaging				
Combination Abdominal CT Scan	1,864	0.071	0.164	0.191
Combination Chest CT Scan	1,474	0.059	0.038	0.054
Follow-up Mammogram/Ultrasound	1,705	8.6%	8.4%	8.4%
MRI for Low Back Pain	389	31.9%	30.2%	32.7%
Survey of Patients' Hospital Experiences				
Area Around Room 'Always' Quiet at Night	300+	52%	-	58%
Doctors 'Always' Communicated Well	300+	78%	-	80%
Home Recovery Information Given	300+	79%	-	82%
Hospital Given 9 or 10 on 10 Point Scale	300+	74%	-	67%
Meds 'Always' Explained Before Given	300+	63%	-	60%
Nurses 'Always' Communicated Well	300+	77%	-	76%
Pain 'Always' Well Controlled	300+	70%	-	69%
Room and Bathroom 'Always' Clean	300+	67%	-	71%
Timely Help 'Always' Received	300+	64%	-	64%
Would Definitely Recommend Hospital	300+	79%	-	69%

Mercy Medical Center

1320 Mercy Drive NW
Canton, OH 44708
URL: www.thequalityhospital.com
Type: Acute Care Hospitals
Ownership: Voluntary Non-Profit - Church

Phone: 330-489-1008
Fax: 330-489-1127

Emergency Services: Yes
Beds: 476

Key Personnel:
CEO/President . . . . Thomas E Cecconi
Chief of Medical Staff . . . . David L Gormsen, DO
Coronary Care . . . . Allyson Kelly
Infection Control . . . . Pat Nelson
Operating Room. . . . . Laurie Hartline, RN
Pediatric In-Patient Care . . . . . . Sally Frantz
Quality Assurance . . . . Tracey Majors, RN
Radiology. . . . . Judith Hadam

Measure	Cases	This Hosp.	State Avg.	U.S. Avg.
Heart Attack Care				
ACE Inhibitor or ARB for LVSD	61	90%	97%	96%
Aspirin at Arrival	317	96%	99%	99%
Aspirin at Discharge	352	97%	99%	98%
Beta Blocker at Discharge	350	98%	99%	98%
Fibrinolytic Medication Timing	0	-	14%	55%
PCI Within 90 Minutes of Arrival	70	94%	92%	90%
Smoking Cessation Advice	130	100%	100%	99%
Chest Pain/Possible Heart Attack Care				
Aspirin at Arrival[1]	21	100%	96%	95%
Median Time to ECG (minutes)[1]	21	7	7	8
Median Time to Transfer (minutes)[5]	0	-	61	61
Fibrinolytic Medication Timing[3]	0	-	47%	54%
Heart Failure Care				
ACE Inhibitor or ARB for LVSD	146	98%	96%	94%
Discharge Instructions	333	86%	91%	88%
Evaluation of LVS Function	431	100%	99%	98%
Smoking Cessation Advice	76	97%	99%	98%
Pneumonia Care				
Appropriate Initial Antibiotic	243	89%	92%	92%
Blood Culture Timing	305	98%	96%	96%
Influenza Vaccine	231	95%	93%	91%
Initial Antibiotic Timing	341	93%	96%	95%
Pneumococcal Vaccine	264	96%	95%	93%
Smoking Cessation Advice	148	99%	98%	97%
Surgical Care Improvement Project				
Appropriate VTP Within 24 Hours[2]	205	89%	92%	92%
Appropriate Hair Removal[2]	788	100%	100%	99%
Appropriate Beta Blocker Usage[2]	258	86%	94%	93%
Controlled Postoperative Blood Glucose[2]	145	96%	94%	93%
Prophylactic Antibiotic Timing[2]	610	96%	97%	97%
Prophylactic Antibiotic Timing (Outpatient)	810	92%	91%	92%
Prophylactic Antibiotic Selection[2]	617	97%	98%	97%
Prophylactic Antibiotic Select. (Outpatient)	767	98%	94%	94%
Prophylactic Antibiotic Stopped[2]	594	91%	95%	94%
Recommended VTP Ordered[2]	205	94%	94%	94%
Urinary Catheter Removal[2]	159	88%	91%	90%
Children's Asthma Care				
Received Systemic Corticosteroids	-	-	-	100%
Received Home Management Plan	-	-	-	71%
Received Reliever Medication	-	-	-	100%
Use of Medical Imaging				
Combination Abdominal CT Scan	1,174	0.122	0.164	0.191
Combination Chest CT Scan	814	0.001	0.038	0.054
Follow-up Mammogram/Ultrasound	1,712	8.3%	8.4%	8.4%
MRI for Low Back Pain	159	30.2%	30.2%	32.7%
Survey of Patients' Hospital Experiences				
Area Around Room 'Always' Quiet at Night	300+	50%	-	58%
Doctors 'Always' Communicated Well	300+	76%	-	80%
Home Recovery Information Given	300+	81%	-	82%
Hospital Given 9 or 10 on 10 Point Scale	300+	70%	-	67%
Meds 'Always' Explained Before Given	300+	59%	-	60%
Nurses 'Always' Communicated Well	300+	77%	-	76%
Pain 'Always' Well Controlled	300+	73%	-	69%
Room and Bathroom 'Always' Clean	300+	73%	-	71%
Timely Help 'Always' Received	300+	62%	-	64%
Would Definitely Recommend Hospital	300+	73%	-	69%

NOTE: Hospital profiles are in alphabetical order by state, then city, then hospital within the city; Rankings exclude hospitals with less than 25 cases except for patient surveys which excludes hospitals with less than 100 cases; (a) 100–299 cases; (1) The number of cases is too small to be sure how well a hospital is performing; (2) The hospital indicated that the data submitted for this measure were based on a sample of cases; (3) Data was collected during a shorter time period (fewer quarters) than the maximum possible time for this measure; (4) Suppressed for one or more quarters by CMS; (5) No data is available from the hospital for this measure; (6) Fewer than 100 patients completed the HCAHPS survey. Use these rates with caution, as the number of surveys may be too low to reliably assess hospital performance; (7) Survey results are based on less than 12 months of data; (8) Survey results are not available for this reporting period; (9) No or very few patients were eligible for the HCAHPS survey. The scores shown, if any, reflect a very small number of surveys; (10) A state average was not calculated because too few hospitals in the state submitted data; (11) There were discrepancies in the data collection process; Please refer to the User's Guide for a full explanation of data.

UH Geauga Medical Center

13207 Ravenna Rd Phone: 440-269-6000
Chardon, OH 44024
URL: www.uhgeauga.org
Type: Acute Care Hospitals Emergency Services: Yes
Ownership: Voluntary Non-Profit - Private
Key Personnel:
CEO/President. . . . . Richard J. Frenchie
Chief of Medical Staff . . . . Donald Goddard

Measure	Cases	This Hosp.	State Avg.	U.S. Avg.
Heart Attack Care				
ACE Inhibitor or ARB for LVSD[1]	13	100%	97%	96%
Aspirin at Arrival	73	100%	99%	99%
Aspirin at Discharge	59	100%	99%	98%
Beta Blocker at Discharge	66	100%	99%	98%
Fibrinolytic Medication Timing	0	-	14%	55%
PCI Within 90 Minutes of Arrival[1]	7	71%	92%	90%
Smoking Cessation Advice[1]	23	100%	100%	99%
Chest Pain/Possible Heart Attack Care				
Aspirin at Arrival	68	100%	96%	95%
Median Time to ECG (minutes)	68	2	7	8
Median Time to Transfer (minutes)[1]	10	40	61	61
Fibrinolytic Medication Timing	0	-	47%	54%
Heart Failure Care				
ACE Inhibitor or ARB for LVSD	49	100%	96%	94%
Discharge Instructions	123	100%	91%	88%
Evaluation of LVS Function	175	100%	99%	98%
Smoking Cessation Advice[1]	22	100%	99%	98%
Pneumonia Care				
Appropriate Initial Antibiotic	113	86%	92%	92%
Blood Culture Timing	153	92%	96%	96%
Influenza Vaccine	121	100%	93%	91%
Initial Antibiotic Timing	156	93%	96%	95%
Pneumococcal Vaccine	168	100%	95%	93%
Smoking Cessation Advice	31	100%	98%	97%
Surgical Care Improvement Project				
Appropriate VTP Within 24 Hours[2]	155	92%	92%	92%
Appropriate Hair Removal[2]	491	100%	100%	99%
Appropriate Beta Blocker Usage[2]	163	88%	94%	93%
Controlled Postoperative Blood Glucose[2]	0	-	94%	93%
Prophylactic Antibiotic Timing[2]	363	95%	97%	97%
Prophylactic Antibiotic Timing (Outpatient)	249	83%	91%	92%
Prophylactic Antibiotic Selection[2]	365	99%	98%	97%
Prophylactic Antibiotic Select. (Outpatient)	229	85%	94%	94%
Prophylactic Antibiotic Stopped[2]	350	92%	95%	94%
Recommended VTP Ordered[2]	156	94%	94%	94%
Urinary Catheter Removal[2]	140	87%	91%	90%
Children's Asthma Care				
Received Systemic Corticosteroids	-	-	-	100%
Received Home Management Plan	-	-	-	71%
Received Reliever Medication	-	-	-	100%
Use of Medical Imaging				
Combination Abdominal CT Scan	500	0.096	0.164	0.191
Combination Chest CT Scan	291	0.027	0.038	0.054
Follow-up Mammogram/Ultrasound	571	7.4%	8.4%	8.4%
MRI for Low Back Pain	66	37.9%	30.2%	32.7%
Survey of Patients' Hospital Experiences				
Area Around Room 'Always' Quiet at Night[11]	300+	46%	-	58%
Doctors 'Always' Communicated Well[11]	300+	78%	-	80%
Home Recovery Information Given[11]	300+	79%	-	82%
Hospital Given 9 or 10 on 10 Point Scale[11]	300+	65%	-	67%
Meds 'Always' Explained Before Given[11]	300+	56%	-	60%
Nurses 'Always' Communicated Well[11]	300+	75%	-	76%
Pain 'Always' Well Controlled[11]	300+	67%	-	69%
Room and Bathroom 'Always' Clean[11]	300+	67%	-	71%
Timely Help 'Always' Received[11]	300+	62%	-	64%
Would Definitely Recommend Hospital[11]	300+	67%	-	69%

Adena Regional Medical Center

272 Hospital Road Phone: 740-779-7778
Chillicothe, OH 45601 Fax: 740-779-7934
URL: www.adena.org
Type: Acute Care Hospitals Emergency Services: Yes
Ownership: Voluntary Non-Profit - Private Beds: 238
Key Personnel:
CEO/President. . . . . Mark Shuter FACHE
Cardiac Laboratory. . . . . Marla Weber
Chief of Medical Staff . . . . Alan Shaw MD
Infection Control. . . . . Julie McCray
Operating Room. . . . . Damien Benjamin
Quality Assurance . . . . Patti Lamphear
Radiology. . . . . Bryan I Borland

Measure	Cases	This Hosp.	State Avg.	U.S. Avg.
Heart Attack Care				
ACE Inhibitor or ARB for LVSD	118	96%	97%	96%
Aspirin at Arrival	347	98%	99%	99%
Aspirin at Discharge	442	98%	99%	98%
Beta Blocker at Discharge	453	98%	99%	98%
Fibrinolytic Medication Timing	0	-	14%	55%
PCI Within 90 Minutes of Arrival	47	74%	92%	90%
Smoking Cessation Advice	175	100%	100%	99%
Chest Pain/Possible Heart Attack Care				
Aspirin at Arrival	118	99%	96%	95%
Median Time to ECG (minutes)	121	6	7	8
Median Time to Transfer (minutes)[1,3]	3	51	61	61
Fibrinolytic Medication Timing[3]	0	-	47%	54%
Heart Failure Care				
ACE Inhibitor or ARB for LVSD	134	93%	96%	94%
Discharge Instructions	271	84%	91%	88%
Evaluation of LVS Function	344	99%	99%	98%
Smoking Cessation Advice	62	98%	99%	98%
Pneumonia Care				
Appropriate Initial Antibiotic	162	96%	92%	92%
Blood Culture Timing	120	93%	96%	96%
Influenza Vaccine	250	98%	93%	91%
Initial Antibiotic Timing	249	96%	96%	95%
Pneumococcal Vaccine	318	95%	95%	93%
Smoking Cessation Advice	187	98%	98%	97%
Surgical Care Improvement Project				
Appropriate VTP Within 24 Hours	266	88%	92%	92%
Appropriate Hair Removal	850	100%	100%	99%
Appropriate Beta Blocker Usage	348	94%	94%	93%
Controlled Postoperative Blood Glucose	109	88%	94%	93%
Prophylactic Antibiotic Timing	736	97%	97%	97%
Prophylactic Antibiotic Timing (Outpatient)	314	96%	91%	92%
Prophylactic Antibiotic Selection	744	99%	98%	97%
Prophylactic Antibiotic Select. (Outpatient)	307	99%	94%	94%
Prophylactic Antibiotic Stopped	704	97%	95%	94%
Recommended VTP Ordered	268	91%	94%	94%
Urinary Catheter Removal	240	97%	91%	90%
Children's Asthma Care				
Received Systemic Corticosteroids	-	-	-	100%
Received Home Management Plan	-	-	-	71%
Received Reliever Medication	-	-	-	100%
Use of Medical Imaging				
Combination Abdominal CT Scan	1,190	0.039	0.164	0.191
Combination Chest CT Scan	939	0.076	0.038	0.054
Follow-up Mammogram/Ultrasound	1,710	8.2%	8.4%	8.4%
MRI for Low Back Pain	397	28.7%	30.2%	32.7%
Survey of Patients' Hospital Experiences				
Area Around Room 'Always' Quiet at Night	300+	41%	-	58%
Doctors 'Always' Communicated Well	300+	81%	-	80%
Home Recovery Information Given	300+	77%	-	82%
Hospital Given 9 or 10 on 10 Point Scale	300+	62%	-	67%
Meds 'Always' Explained Before Given	300+	58%	-	60%
Nurses 'Always' Communicated Well	300+	76%	-	76%
Pain 'Always' Well Controlled	300+	68%	-	69%
Room and Bathroom 'Always' Clean	300+	60%	-	71%
Timely Help 'Always' Received	300+	58%	-	64%
Would Definitely Recommend Hospital	300+	66%	-	69%

Chillicothe VA Medical Center

17273 State Route 104 Phone: 740-773-1141
Chillicothe, OH 45601
URL: www.chillicothe.va.gov
Type: Acute Care-Veterans Administration Emergency Services: No
Ownership: Government - Federal Beds: 297
Key Personnel:
Chief of Medical Staff . . . . Deborah M Meesig, MD JD
Infection Control. . . . . Teresa Davis, RN
Emergency Room . . . . Thomas Oommen, MD

Measure	Cases	This Hosp.	State Avg.	U.S. Avg.
Heart Attack Care				
ACE Inhibitor or ARB for LVSD[5]	0	-	97%	96%
Aspirin at Arrival[5]	0	-	99%	99%
Aspirin at Discharge[5]	0	-	99%	98%
Beta Blocker at Discharge[5]	0	-	99%	98%
Fibrinolytic Medication Timing[5]	0	-	14%	55%
PCI Within 90 Minutes of Arrival[5]	0	-	92%	90%
Smoking Cessation Advice[5]	0	-	100%	99%
Chest Pain/Possible Heart Attack Care				
Aspirin at Arrival	-	-	96%	95%
Median Time to ECG (minutes)	-	-	7	8
Median Time to Transfer (minutes)	-	-	61	61
Fibrinolytic Medication Timing	-	-	47%	54%
Heart Failure Care				
ACE Inhibitor or ARB for LVSD[1]	23	96%	96%	94%
Discharge Instructions	99	94%	91%	88%
Evaluation of LVS Function	105	99%	99%	98%
Smoking Cessation Advice	38	92%	99%	98%
Pneumonia Care				
Appropriate Initial Antibiotic	59	92%	92%	92%
Blood Culture Timing[1]	13	92%	96%	96%
Influenza Vaccine	54	94%	93%	91%
Initial Antibiotic Timing	54	94%	96%	95%
Pneumococcal Vaccine	39	100%	95%	93%
Smoking Cessation Advice	64	95%	98%	97%
Surgical Care Improvement Project				
Appropriate VTP Within 24 Hours[2,5]	0	-	92%	92%
Appropriate Hair Removal[2,5]	0	-	100%	99%
Appropriate Beta Blocker Usage[2,5]	0	-	94%	93%
Controlled Postoperative Blood Glucose[2,5]	0	-	94%	93%
Prophylactic Antibiotic Timing[5]	0	-	97%	97%
Prophylactic Antibiotic Timing (Outpatient)	-	-	91%	92%
Prophylactic Antibiotic Selection[5]	0	-	98%	97%
Prophylactic Antibiotic Select. (Outpatient)	-	-	94%	94%
Prophylactic Antibiotic Stopped[5]	0	-	95%	94%
Recommended VTP Ordered[2,5]	0	-	94%	94%
Urinary Catheter Removal[2,5]	0	-	91%	90%
Children's Asthma Care				
Received Systemic Corticosteroids	-	-	-	100%
Received Home Management Plan	-	-	-	71%
Received Reliever Medication	-	-	-	100%
Use of Medical Imaging				
Combination Abdominal CT Scan	-	-	0.164	0.191
Combination Chest CT Scan	-	-	0.038	0.054
Follow-up Mammogram/Ultrasound	-	-	8.4%	8.4%
MRI for Low Back Pain	-	-	30.2%	32.7%
Survey of Patients' Hospital Experiences				
Area Around Room 'Always' Quiet at Night	-	-	-	58%
Doctors 'Always' Communicated Well	-	-	-	80%
Home Recovery Information Given	-	-	-	82%
Hospital Given 9 or 10 on 10 Point Scale	-	-	-	67%
Meds 'Always' Explained Before Given	-	-	-	60%
Nurses 'Always' Communicated Well	-	-	-	76%
Pain 'Always' Well Controlled	-	-	-	69%
Room and Bathroom 'Always' Clean	-	-	-	71%
Timely Help 'Always' Received	-	-	-	64%
Would Definitely Recommend Hospital	-	-	-	69%

NOTE: Hospital profiles are in alphabetical order by state, then city, then hospital within the city; Rankings exclude hospitals with less than 25 cases except for patient surveys which excludes hospitals with less than 100 cases; (a) 100–299 cases; (1) The number of cases is too small to be sure how well a hospital is performing; (2) The hospital indicated that the data submitted for this measure were based on a sample of cases; (3) Data was collected during a shorter time period (fewer quarters) than the maximum possible time for this measure; (4) Suppressed for one or more quarters by CMS; (5) No data is available from the hospital for this measure; (6) Fewer than 100 patients completed the HCAHPS survey. Use these rates with caution, as the number of surveys may be too low to reliably assess hospital performance; (7) Survey results are based on less than 12 months of data; (8) Survey results are not available for this reporting period; (9) No or very few patients were eligible for the HCAHPS survey. The scores shown, if any, reflect a very small number of surveys; (10) A state average was not calculated because too few hospitals in the state submitted data; (11) There were discrepancies in the data collection process; Please refer to the User's Guide for a full explanation of data.

Bethesda North Hospital

10500 Montgomery Road Phone: 513-569-6141
Cincinnati, OH 45242 Fax: 513-745-1441
Type: Acute Care Hospitals Emergency Services: Yes
Ownership: Voluntary Non-Profit - Church Beds: 314

Key Personnel:
CEO/President. . . . . John Prout
Cardiac Laboratory. . . . . Nancy Dallas
Chief of Medical Staff. . . . . Larry Johnsaw
Operating Room. . . . . Daniel Warmack
Quality Assurance . . . . Tim Walters
Emergency Room . . . . Bonnie Sheedy

Measure	Cases	This Hosp.	State Avg.	U.S. Avg.
Heart Attack Care				
ACE Inhibitor or ARB for LVSD	87	97%	97%	96%
Aspirin at Arrival	357	98%	99%	99%
Aspirin at Discharge	471	100%	99%	98%
Beta Blocker at Discharge	433	99%	99%	98%
Fibrinolytic Medication Timing	0	-	14%	55%
PCI Within 90 Minutes of Arrival	75	97%	92%	90%
Smoking Cessation Advice	153	100%	100%	99%
Chest Pain/Possible Heart Attack Care				
Aspirin at Arrival	48	94%	96%	95%
Median Time to ECG (minutes)	52	5	7	8
Median Time to Transfer (minutes)[1,3]	1	193	61	61
Fibrinolytic Medication Timing[1,3]	1	0%	47%	54%
Heart Failure Care				
ACE Inhibitor or ARB for LVSD	251	97%	96%	94%
Discharge Instructions	601	96%	91%	88%
Evaluation of LVS Function	742	100%	99%	98%
Smoking Cessation Advice	101	100%	99%	98%
Pneumonia Care				
Appropriate Initial Antibiotic	363	94%	92%	92%
Blood Culture Timing	643	98%	96%	96%
Influenza Vaccine	469	93%	93%	91%
Initial Antibiotic Timing	564	94%	96%	95%
Pneumococcal Vaccine	595	94%	95%	93%
Smoking Cessation Advice	231	100%	98%	97%
Surgical Care Improvement Project				
Appropriate VTP Within 24 Hours[2]	173	92%	92%	92%
Appropriate Hair Removal[2]	628	100%	100%	99%
Appropriate Beta Blocker Usage[2]	198	96%	94%	93%
Controlled Postoperative Blood Glucose[2]	137	100%	94%	93%
Prophylactic Antibiotic Timing[2]	440	96%	97%	97%
Prophylactic Antibiotic Timing (Outpatient)	655	93%	91%	92%
Prophylactic Antibiotic Selection[2]	438	98%	98%	97%
Prophylactic Antibiotic Select. (Outpatient)	634	97%	94%	94%
Prophylactic Antibiotic Stopped[2]	412	96%	95%	94%
Recommended VTP Ordered[2]	173	95%	94%	94%
Urinary Catheter Removal[2]	135	83%	91%	90%
Children's Asthma Care				
Received Systemic Corticosteroids	-	-	-	100%
Received Home Management Plan	-	-	-	71%
Received Reliever Medication	-	-	-	100%
Use of Medical Imaging				
Combination Abdominal CT Scan	1,959	0.098	0.164	0.191
Combination Chest CT Scan	1,878	0.010	0.038	0.054
Follow-up Mammogram/Ultrasound	2,888	16.0%	8.4%	8.4%
MRI for Low Back Pain	273	29.7%	30.2%	32.7%
Survey of Patients' Hospital Experiences				
Area Around Room 'Always' Quiet at Night	300+	52%	-	58%
Doctors 'Always' Communicated Well	300+	75%	-	80%
Home Recovery Information Given	300+	87%	-	82%
Hospital Given 9 or 10 on 10 Point Scale	300+	72%	-	67%
Meds 'Always' Explained Before Given	300+	52%	-	60%
Nurses 'Always' Communicated Well	300+	75%	-	76%
Pain 'Always' Well Controlled	300+	66%	-	69%
Room and Bathroom 'Always' Clean	300+	71%	-	71%
Timely Help 'Always' Received	300+	61%	-	64%
Would Definitely Recommend Hospital	300+	78%	-	69%

Christ Hospital

2139 Auburn Avenue Phone: 513-585-2771
Cincinnati, OH 45219 Fax: 513-585-4313
URL: www.thechristhospital.com
Type: Acute Care Hospitals Emergency Services: Yes
Ownership: Voluntary Non-Profit - Private

Key Personnel:
CEO/President. . . . . Susan Croushore
Chief of Medical Staff. . . . . Berc Gawne, MD
Infection Control. . . . . Corwin Dunn, MD
Operating Room. . . . . Jeff Morneanlt
Radiology. . . . . Richard Buddetein, MD
Emergency Room . . . . Steven Yamaguschi, MD
Patient Relations . . . . Kathy Zimmerman

Measure	Cases	This Hosp.	State Avg.	U.S. Avg.
Heart Attack Care				
ACE Inhibitor or ARB for LVSD	101	100%	97%	96%
Aspirin at Arrival	196	100%	99%	99%
Aspirin at Discharge	509	100%	99%	98%
Beta Blocker at Discharge	486	100%	99%	98%
Fibrinolytic Medication Timing	0	-	14%	55%
PCI Within 90 Minutes of Arrival	33	100%	92%	90%
Smoking Cessation Advice	200	100%	100%	99%
Chest Pain/Possible Heart Attack Care				
Aspirin at Arrival[3]	0	-	96%	95%
Median Time to ECG (minutes)[3]	0	-	7	8
Median Time to Transfer (minutes)[5]	0	-	61	61
Fibrinolytic Medication Timing[5]	0	-	47%	54%
Heart Failure Care				
ACE Inhibitor or ARB for LVSD	396	99%	96%	94%
Discharge Instructions	826	99%	91%	88%
Evaluation of LVS Function	996	100%	99%	98%
Smoking Cessation Advice	194	100%	99%	98%
Pneumonia Care				
Appropriate Initial Antibiotic[2]	40	100%	92%	92%
Blood Culture Timing[2]	84	94%	96%	96%
Influenza Vaccine[2]	87	98%	93%	91%
Initial Antibiotic Timing[2]	74	92%	96%	95%
Pneumococcal Vaccine[2]	113	100%	95%	93%
Smoking Cessation Advice[2]	48	98%	98%	97%
Surgical Care Improvement Project				
Appropriate VTP Within 24 Hours[2]	148	98%	92%	92%
Appropriate Hair Removal[2]	734	100%	100%	99%
Appropriate Beta Blocker Usage[2]	229	98%	94%	93%
Controlled Postoperative Blood Glucose[2]	152	92%	94%	93%
Prophylactic Antibiotic Timing[2]	492	95%	97%	97%
Prophylactic Antibiotic Timing (Outpatient)	815	94%	91%	92%
Prophylactic Antibiotic Selection[2]	504	98%	98%	97%
Prophylactic Antibiotic Select. (Outpatient)	825	96%	94%	94%
Prophylactic Antibiotic Stopped[2]	456	96%	95%	94%
Recommended VTP Ordered[2]	148	98%	94%	94%
Urinary Catheter Removal[2]	156	90%	91%	90%
Children's Asthma Care				
Received Systemic Corticosteroids	-	-	-	100%
Received Home Management Plan	-	-	-	71%
Received Reliever Medication	-	-	-	100%
Use of Medical Imaging				
Combination Abdominal CT Scan	1,411	0.069	0.164	0.191
Combination Chest CT Scan	1,279	0.011	0.038	0.054
Follow-up Mammogram/Ultrasound	2,445	5.1%	8.4%	8.4%
MRI for Low Back Pain	213	35.7%	30.2%	32.7%
Survey of Patients' Hospital Experiences				
Area Around Room 'Always' Quiet at Night	300+	54%	-	58%
Doctors 'Always' Communicated Well	300+	82%	-	80%
Home Recovery Information Given	300+	86%	-	82%
Hospital Given 9 or 10 on 10 Point Scale	300+	80%	-	67%
Meds 'Always' Explained Before Given	300+	62%	-	60%
Nurses 'Always' Communicated Well	300+	83%	-	76%
Pain 'Always' Well Controlled	300+	73%	-	69%
Room and Bathroom 'Always' Clean	300+	64%	-	71%
Timely Help 'Always' Received	300+	68%	-	64%
Would Definitely Recommend Hospital	300+	85%	-	69%

Cincinnati VA Medical Center

3200 Vine Street Phone: 513-861-3100
Cincinnati, OH 45220 Fax: 513-475-6525
URL: www.cincinnati.va.gov
Type: Acute Care-Veterans Administration Emergency Services: No
Ownership: Government - Federal Beds: 378

Key Personnel:
CEO/President. . . . . Carlos B Lott, Jr
Chief of Medical Staff. . . . . Sidney R Steinberg MD
Infection Control. . . . . Gary Roselle MD
Operating Room. . . . . Robert Bower
Quality Assurance . . . . Barbara Thomas RN
Emergency Room . . . . James Huey MD
Hemotology Center . . . . Albert Muhleman MD
Patient Relations . . . . Linda Dubois

Measure	Cases	This Hosp.	State Avg.	U.S. Avg.
Heart Attack Care				
ACE Inhibitor or ARB for LVSD[1]	7	100%	97%	96%
Aspirin at Arrival	52	100%	99%	99%
Aspirin at Discharge	37	100%	99%	98%
Beta Blocker at Discharge	34	100%	99%	98%
Fibrinolytic Medication Timing[5]	0	-	14%	55%
PCI Within 90 Minutes of Arrival[1]	1	100%	92%	90%
Smoking Cessation Advice[1]	18	100%	100%	99%
Chest Pain/Possible Heart Attack Care				
Aspirin at Arrival	-	-	96%	95%
Median Time to ECG (minutes)	-	-	7	8
Median Time to Transfer (minutes)	-	-	61	61
Fibrinolytic Medication Timing	-	-	47%	54%
Heart Failure Care				
ACE Inhibitor or ARB for LVSD	93	99%	96%	94%
Discharge Instructions	191	95%	91%	88%
Evaluation of LVS Function	207	100%	99%	98%
Smoking Cessation Advice	64	100%	99%	98%
Pneumonia Care				
Appropriate Initial Antibiotic	57	100%	92%	92%
Blood Culture Timing	97	99%	96%	96%
Influenza Vaccine	81	91%	93%	91%
Initial Antibiotic Timing	96	99%	96%	95%
Pneumococcal Vaccine	79	96%	95%	93%
Smoking Cessation Advice	59	100%	98%	97%
Surgical Care Improvement Project				
Appropriate VTP Within 24 Hours[2]	139	99%	92%	92%
Appropriate Hair Removal[2]	238	100%	100%	99%
Appropriate Beta Blocker Usage[2]	83	98%	94%	93%
Controlled Postoperative Blood Glucose[2,5]	0	-	94%	93%
Prophylactic Antibiotic Timing	152	99%	97%	97%
Prophylactic Antibiotic Timing (Outpatient)	-	-	91%	92%
Prophylactic Antibiotic Selection	152	97%	98%	97%
Prophylactic Antibiotic Select. (Outpatient)	-	-	94%	94%
Prophylactic Antibiotic Stopped	150	99%	95%	94%
Recommended VTP Ordered[2]	139	99%	94%	94%
Urinary Catheter Removal[1,2]	19	58%	91%	90%
Children's Asthma Care				
Received Systemic Corticosteroids	-	-	-	100%
Received Home Management Plan	-	-	-	71%
Received Reliever Medication	-	-	-	100%
Use of Medical Imaging				
Combination Abdominal CT Scan	-	-	0.164	0.191
Combination Chest CT Scan	-	-	0.038	0.054
Follow-up Mammogram/Ultrasound	-	-	8.4%	8.4%
MRI for Low Back Pain	-	-	30.2%	32.7%
Survey of Patients' Hospital Experiences				
Area Around Room 'Always' Quiet at Night	-	-	-	58%
Doctors 'Always' Communicated Well	-	-	-	80%
Home Recovery Information Given	-	-	-	82%
Hospital Given 9 or 10 on 10 Point Scale	-	-	-	67%
Meds 'Always' Explained Before Given	-	-	-	60%
Nurses 'Always' Communicated Well	-	-	-	76%
Pain 'Always' Well Controlled	-	-	-	69%
Room and Bathroom 'Always' Clean	-	-	-	71%
Timely Help 'Always' Received	-	-	-	64%
Would Definitely Recommend Hospital	-	-	-	69%

NOTE: Hospital profiles are in alphabetical order by state, then city, then hospital within the city; Rankings exclude hospitals with less than 25 cases except for patient surveys which excludes hospitals with less than 100 cases; (a) 100–299 cases; (1) The number of cases is too small to be sure how well a hospital is performing; (2) The hospital indicated that the data submitted for this measure were based on a sample of cases; (3) Data was collected during a shorter time period (fewer quarters) than the maximum possible time for this measure; (4) Suppressed for one or more quarters by CMS; (5) No data is available from the hospital for this measure; (6) Fewer than 100 patients completed the HCAHPS survey. Use these rates with caution, as the number of surveys may be too low to reliably assess hospital performance; (7) Survey results are based on less than 12 months of data; (8) Survey results are not available for this reporting period; (9) No or very few patients were eligible for the HCAHPS survey. The scores shown, if any, reflect a very small number of surveys; (10) A state average was not calculated because too few hospitals in the state submitted data; (11) There were discrepancies in the data collection process; Please refer to the User's Guide for a full explanation of data.

Deaconess Hospital

311 Straight Street
Cincinnati, OH 45219
URL: www.deaconess-healthcare.com
Type: Acute Care Hospitals
Ownership: Voluntary Non-Profit - Private

Phone: 513-559-2100
Fax: 513-475-5251
Emergency Services: Yes
Beds: 273

Key Personnel:
CEO/President. . . . . E Anthony Woods
Cardiac Laboratory. . . . . Brenda Arthur
Chief of Medical Staff . . . . James Hawkins, MD
Coronary Care . . . . Cathy Jones
Infection Control. . . . . Eileen Alexander
Quality Assurance . . . . Nancy Wilson
Radiology. . . . . Ronals Weitz

Measure	Cases	This Hosp.	State Avg.	U.S. Avg.
Heart Attack Care				
ACE Inhibitor or ARB for LVSD[3]	0	-	97%	96%
Aspirin at Arrival[1,3]	4	100%	99%	99%
Aspirin at Discharge[1,3]	2	100%	99%	98%
Beta Blocker at Discharge[1,3]	2	100%	99%	98%
Fibrinolytic Medication Timing[3]	0	-	14%	55%
PCI Within 90 Minutes of Arrival[3]	0	-	92%	90%
Smoking Cessation Advice[1,3]	1	100%	100%	99%
Chest Pain/Possible Heart Attack Care				
Aspirin at Arrival[1,3]	1	100%	96%	95%
Median Time to ECG (minutes)[1,3]	1	0	7	8
Median Time to Transfer (minutes)[5]	0	-	61	61
Fibrinolytic Medication Timing[5]	0	-	47%	54%
Heart Failure Care				
ACE Inhibitor or ARB for LVSD[1]	18	83%	96%	94%
Discharge Instructions	33	12%	91%	88%
Evaluation of LVS Function	39	87%	99%	98%
Smoking Cessation Advice[1]	10	40%	99%	98%
Pneumonia Care				
Appropriate Initial Antibiotic[1,3]	18	61%	92%	92%
Blood Culture Timing[1,3]	22	86%	96%	96%
Influenza Vaccine[1]	13	46%	93%	91%
Initial Antibiotic Timing[3]	33	88%	96%	95%
Pneumococcal Vaccine[3]	29	52%	95%	93%
Smoking Cessation Advice[1,3]	6	33%	98%	97%
Surgical Care Improvement Project				
Appropriate VTP Within 24 Hours[1,2]	21	90%	92%	92%
Appropriate Hair Removal[2]	125	98%	100%	99%
Appropriate Beta Blocker Usage[2]	60	88%	94%	93%
Controlled Postoperative Blood Glucose[2]	80	88%	94%	93%
Prophylactic Antibiotic Timing[2]	34	97%	97%	97%
Prophylactic Antibiotic Timing (Outpatient)[1,3]	3	67%	91%	92%
Prophylactic Antibiotic Selection[2]	34	94%	98%	97%
Prophylactic Antibiotic Select. (Outpatient)[1,3]	2	50%	94%	94%
Prophylactic Antibiotic Stopped[2]	33	91%	95%	94%
Recommended VTP Ordered[1,2]	21	90%	94%	94%
Urinary Catheter Removal[2]	41	98%	91%	90%
Children's Asthma Care				
Received Systemic Corticosteroids	-	-	-	100%
Received Home Management Plan	-	-	-	71%
Received Reliever Medication	-	-	-	100%
Use of Medical Imaging				
Combination Abdominal CT Scan	215	0.484	0.164	0.191
Combination Chest CT Scan	157	0.159	0.038	0.054
Follow-up Mammogram/Ultrasound	332	5.4%	8.4%	8.4%
MRI for Low Back Pain[1]	49	18.4%	30.2%	32.7%
Survey of Patients' Hospital Experiences				
Area Around Room 'Always' Quiet at Night	(a)	55%	-	58%
Doctors 'Always' Communicated Well	(a)	86%	-	80%
Home Recovery Information Given	(a)	90%	-	82%
Hospital Given 9 or 10 on 10 Point Scale	(a)	79%	-	67%
Meds 'Always' Explained Before Given	(a)	66%	-	60%
Nurses 'Always' Communicated Well	(a)	78%	-	76%
Pain 'Always' Well Controlled	(a)	73%	-	69%
Room and Bathroom 'Always' Clean	(a)	62%	-	71%
Timely Help 'Always' Received	(a)	68%	-	64%
Would Definitely Recommend Hospital	(a)	74%	-	69%

Evendale Medical Center

3155 Glendale-Milford Road
Cincinnati, OH 45241
Type: Acute Care Hospitals
Ownership: Proprietary

Phone: 513-454-2222
Emergency Services: No

Measure	Cases	This Hosp.	State Avg.	U.S. Avg.
Heart Attack Care				
ACE Inhibitor or ARB for LVSD[5]	0	-	97%	96%
Aspirin at Arrival[5]	0	-	99%	99%
Aspirin at Discharge[5]	0	-	99%	98%
Beta Blocker at Discharge[5]	0	-	99%	98%
Fibrinolytic Medication Timing[5]	0	-	14%	55%
PCI Within 90 Minutes of Arrival[5]	0	-	92%	90%
Smoking Cessation Advice[5]	0	-	100%	99%
Chest Pain/Possible Heart Attack Care				
Aspirin at Arrival[5]	0	-	96%	95%
Median Time to ECG (minutes)[5]	0	-	7	8
Median Time to Transfer (minutes)[5]	0	-	61	61
Fibrinolytic Medication Timing[5]	0	-	47%	54%
Heart Failure Care				
ACE Inhibitor or ARB for LVSD[5]	0	-	96%	94%
Discharge Instructions[5]	0	-	91%	88%
Evaluation of LVS Function[5]	0	-	99%	98%
Smoking Cessation Advice[5]	0	-	99%	98%
Pneumonia Care				
Appropriate Initial Antibiotic[5]	0	-	92%	92%
Blood Culture Timing[5]	0	-	96%	96%
Influenza Vaccine[5]	0	-	93%	91%
Initial Antibiotic Timing[5]	0	-	96%	95%
Pneumococcal Vaccine[5]	0	-	95%	93%
Smoking Cessation Advice[5]	0	-	98%	97%
Surgical Care Improvement Project				
Appropriate VTP Within 24 Hours[1]	8	100%	92%	92%
Appropriate Hair Removal	287	100%	100%	99%
Appropriate Beta Blocker Usage	61	90%	94%	93%
Controlled Postoperative Blood Glucose	0	-	94%	93%
Prophylactic Antibiotic Timing	208	89%	97%	97%
Prophylactic Antibiotic Timing (Outpatient)	232	69%	91%	92%
Prophylactic Antibiotic Selection	208	100%	98%	97%
Prophylactic Antibiotic Select. (Outpatient)	165	98%	94%	94%
Prophylactic Antibiotic Stopped	206	97%	95%	94%
Recommended VTP Ordered[1]	8	100%	94%	94%
Urinary Catheter Removal	110	97%	91%	90%
Children's Asthma Care				
Received Systemic Corticosteroids	-	-	-	100%
Received Home Management Plan	-	-	-	71%
Received Reliever Medication	-	-	-	100%
Use of Medical Imaging				
Combination Abdominal CT Scan[5]	0	-	0.164	0.191
Combination Chest CT Scan[5]	0	-	0.038	0.054
Follow-up Mammogram/Ultrasound[5]	0	-	8.4%	8.4%
MRI for Low Back Pain[5]	0	-	30.2%	32.7%
Survey of Patients' Hospital Experiences				
Area Around Room 'Always' Quiet at Night	300+	80%	-	58%
Doctors 'Always' Communicated Well	300+	91%	-	80%
Home Recovery Information Given	300+	92%	-	82%
Hospital Given 9 or 10 on 10 Point Scale	300+	83%	-	67%
Meds 'Always' Explained Before Given	300+	71%	-	60%
Nurses 'Always' Communicated Well	300+	82%	-	76%
Pain 'Always' Well Controlled	300+	76%	-	69%
Room and Bathroom 'Always' Clean	300+	84%	-	71%
Timely Help 'Always' Received	300+	77%	-	64%
Would Definitely Recommend Hospital	300+	81%	-	69%

Good Samaritan Hospital

375 Dixmyth Avenue
Cincinnati, OH 45220
URL: www.trihealth.com
Type: Acute Care Hospitals
Ownership: Voluntary Non-Profit - Church

Phone: 513-862-2601
Fax: 513-872-3435
Emergency Services: Yes
Beds: 700

Key Personnel:
CEO/President. . . . . John Prout
Chief of Medical Staff . . . . Larry Johnstone
Emergency Room . . . . Jim Owen

Measure	Cases	This Hosp.	State Avg.	U.S. Avg.
Heart Attack Care				
ACE Inhibitor or ARB for LVSD	49	98%	97%	96%
Aspirin at Arrival	221	99%	99%	99%
Aspirin at Discharge	372	100%	99%	98%
Beta Blocker at Discharge	364	100%	99%	98%
Fibrinolytic Medication Timing	0	-	14%	55%
PCI Within 90 Minutes of Arrival	43	98%	92%	90%
Smoking Cessation Advice	160	100%	100%	99%
Chest Pain/Possible Heart Attack Care				
Aspirin at Arrival[1,3]	1	100%	96%	95%
Median Time to ECG (minutes)[1,3]	1	36	7	8
Median Time to Transfer (minutes)[5]	0	-	61	61
Fibrinolytic Medication Timing[5]	0	-	47%	54%
Heart Failure Care				
ACE Inhibitor or ARB for LVSD	202	93%	96%	94%
Discharge Instructions	472	94%	91%	88%
Evaluation of LVS Function	555	100%	99%	98%
Smoking Cessation Advice	127	100%	99%	98%
Pneumonia Care				
Appropriate Initial Antibiotic	218	98%	92%	92%
Blood Culture Timing	407	99%	96%	96%
Influenza Vaccine	277	94%	93%	91%
Initial Antibiotic Timing	394	96%	96%	95%
Pneumococcal Vaccine	297	94%	95%	93%
Smoking Cessation Advice	181	100%	98%	97%
Surgical Care Improvement Project				
Appropriate VTP Within 24 Hours[2]	119	95%	92%	92%
Appropriate Hair Removal[2]	621	99%	100%	99%
Appropriate Beta Blocker Usage[2]	185	95%	94%	93%
Controlled Postoperative Blood Glucose[2]	126	96%	94%	93%
Prophylactic Antibiotic Timing[2]	436	96%	97%	97%
Prophylactic Antibiotic Timing (Outpatient)	603	92%	91%	92%
Prophylactic Antibiotic Selection[2]	446	97%	98%	97%
Prophylactic Antibiotic Select. (Outpatient)	586	92%	94%	94%
Prophylactic Antibiotic Stopped[2]	417	96%	95%	94%
Recommended VTP Ordered[2]	119	95%	94%	94%
Urinary Catheter Removal[2]	87	99%	91%	90%
Children's Asthma Care				
Received Systemic Corticosteroids	-	-	-	100%
Received Home Management Plan	-	-	-	71%
Received Reliever Medication	-	-	-	100%
Use of Medical Imaging				
Combination Abdominal CT Scan	939	0.082	0.164	0.191
Combination Chest CT Scan	919	0.002	0.038	0.054
Follow-up Mammogram/Ultrasound	1,559	9.4%	8.4%	8.4%
MRI for Low Back Pain	160	28.1%	30.2%	32.7%
Survey of Patients' Hospital Experiences				
Area Around Room 'Always' Quiet at Night	300+	53%	-	58%
Doctors 'Always' Communicated Well	300+	77%	-	80%
Home Recovery Information Given	300+	87%	-	82%
Hospital Given 9 or 10 on 10 Point Scale	300+	73%	-	67%
Meds 'Always' Explained Before Given	300+	59%	-	60%
Nurses 'Always' Communicated Well	300+	77%	-	76%
Pain 'Always' Well Controlled	300+	71%	-	69%
Room and Bathroom 'Always' Clean	300+	66%	-	71%
Timely Help 'Always' Received	300+	63%	-	64%
Would Definitely Recommend Hospital	300+	76%	-	69%

NOTE: Hospital profiles are in alphabetical order by state, then city, then hospital within the city; Rankings exclude hospitals with less than 25 cases except for patient surveys which excludes hospitals with less than 100 cases; (a) 100–299 cases; (1) The number of cases is too small to be sure how well a hospital is performing; (2) The hospital indicated that the data submitted for this measure were based on a sample of cases; (3) Data was collected during a shorter time period (fewer quarters) than the maximum possible time for this measure; (4) Suppressed for one or more quarters by CMS; (5) No data is available from the hospital for this measure; (6) Fewer than 100 patients completed the HCAHPS survey. Use these rates with caution, as the number of surveys may be too low to reliably assess hospital performance; (7) Survey results are based on less than 12 months of data; (8) Survey results are not available for this reporting period; (9) No or very few patients were eligible for the HCAHPS survey. The scores shown, if any, reflect a very small number of surveys; (10) A state average was not calculated because too few hospitals in the state submitted data; (11) There were discrepancies in the data collection process; Please refer to the User's Guide for a full explanation of data.

Jewish Hospital

4777 East Galbraith Road Phone: 513-686-3003
Cincinnati, OH 45236 Fax: 513-585-6168
URL: www.jewishhospitalcincinnati.com
Type: Acute Care Hospitals Emergency Services: Yes
Ownership: Voluntary Non-Profit - Private

Key Personnel:
CEO/President. . . . . Aurora Lambert
Chief of Medical Staff . . . . David Dort
Infection Control . . . . Marla Clifton
Operating Room. . . . . Pam Photiadis
Radiology. . . . . Robert Lenobel, MD
Emergency Room . . . . Richard Regan
Hemotology Center . . . . E Randolph Broun, MD
Intensive Care Unit. . . . . Linda Miller

Measure	Cases	This Hosp.	State Avg.	U.S. Avg.
Heart Attack Care				
ACE Inhibitor or ARB for LVSD	41	98%	97%	96%
Aspirin at Arrival	165	100%	99%	99%
Aspirin at Discharge	165	96%	99%	98%
Beta Blocker at Discharge	153	99%	99%	98%
Fibrinolytic Medication Timing	0	-	14%	55%
PCI Within 90 Minutes of Arrival	28	89%	92%	90%
Smoking Cessation Advice	57	100%	100%	99%
Chest Pain/Possible Heart Attack Care				
Aspirin at Arrival[1,3]	3	100%	96%	95%
Median Time to ECG (minutes)[1,3]	3	1	7	8
Median Time to Transfer (minutes)[5]	0	-	61	61
Fibrinolytic Medication Timing[5]	0	-	47%	54%
Heart Failure Care				
ACE Inhibitor or ARB for LVSD	139	95%	96%	94%
Discharge Instructions	302	96%	91%	88%
Evaluation of LVS Function	405	100%	99%	98%
Smoking Cessation Advice	65	100%	99%	98%
Pneumonia Care				
Appropriate Initial Antibiotic[2]	63	98%	92%	92%
Blood Culture Timing[2]	123	99%	96%	96%
Influenza Vaccine[2]	84	100%	93%	91%
Initial Antibiotic Timing[2]	127	94%	96%	95%
Pneumococcal Vaccine[2]	119	95%	95%	93%
Smoking Cessation Advice[2]	44	100%	98%	97%
Surgical Care Improvement Project				
Appropriate VTP Within 24 Hours[2]	132	93%	92%	92%
Appropriate Hair Removal[2]	523	100%	100%	99%
Appropriate Beta Blocker Usage[2]	164	95%	94%	93%
Controlled Postoperative Blood Glucose[2]	88	95%	94%	93%
Prophylactic Antibiotic Timing[2]	338	98%	97%	97%
Prophylactic Antibiotic Timing (Outpatient)	324	86%	91%	92%
Prophylactic Antibiotic Selection[2]	342	99%	98%	97%
Prophylactic Antibiotic Select. (Outpatient)	296	93%	94%	94%
Prophylactic Antibiotic Stopped[2]	325	98%	95%	94%
Recommended VTP Ordered[2]	132	94%	94%	94%
Urinary Catheter Removal[2]	35	91%	91%	90%
Children's Asthma Care				
Received Systemic Corticosteroids	-	-	-	100%
Received Home Management Plan	-	-	-	71%
Received Reliever Medication	-	-	-	100%
Use of Medical Imaging				
Combination Abdominal CT Scan	1,196	0.087	0.164	0.191
Combination Chest CT Scan	955	0.010	0.038	0.054
Follow-up Mammogram/Ultrasound	3,500	8.2%	8.4%	8.4%
MRI for Low Back Pain	396	34.3%	30.2%	32.7%
Survey of Patients' Hospital Experiences				
Area Around Room 'Always' Quiet at Night	300+	51%	-	58%
Doctors 'Always' Communicated Well	300+	77%	-	80%
Home Recovery Information Given	300+	82%	-	82%
Hospital Given 9 or 10 on 10 Point Scale	300+	68%	-	67%
Meds 'Always' Explained Before Given	300+	62%	-	60%
Nurses 'Always' Communicated Well	300+	78%	-	76%
Pain 'Always' Well Controlled	300+	69%	-	69%
Room and Bathroom 'Always' Clean	300+	69%	-	71%
Timely Help 'Always' Received	300+	62%	-	64%
Would Definitely Recommend Hospital	300+	75%	-	69%

Mercy Franciscan Hospital - Mt Airy

2446 Kipling Avenue Phone: 513-853-5000
Cincinnati, OH 45239 Fax: 513-853-5758
Type: Acute Care Hospitals Emergency Services: No
Ownership: Voluntary Non-Profit - Private Beds: 269

Key Personnel:
CEO/President. . . . . Paul Hiltz
Chief of Medical Staff . . . . Thomas Morand, MD

Measure	Cases	This Hosp.	State Avg.	U.S. Avg.
Heart Attack Care				
ACE Inhibitor or ARB for LVSD[1]	5	100%	97%	96%
Aspirin at Arrival	64	98%	99%	99%
Aspirin at Discharge	27	100%	99%	98%
Beta Blocker at Discharge	31	100%	99%	98%
Fibrinolytic Medication Timing	0	-	14%	55%
PCI Within 90 Minutes of Arrival	0	-	92%	90%
Smoking Cessation Advice[1]	6	100%	100%	99%
Chest Pain/Possible Heart Attack Care				
Aspirin at Arrival	41	100%	96%	95%
Median Time to ECG (minutes)	42	11	7	8
Median Time to Transfer (minutes)[1]	15	63	61	61
Fibrinolytic Medication Timing	0	-	47%	54%
Heart Failure Care				
ACE Inhibitor or ARB for LVSD	69	100%	96%	94%
Discharge Instructions	205	87%	91%	88%
Evaluation of LVS Function	254	100%	99%	98%
Smoking Cessation Advice	44	100%	99%	98%
Pneumonia Care				
Appropriate Initial Antibiotic	144	98%	92%	92%
Blood Culture Timing	234	99%	96%	96%
Influenza Vaccine	132	98%	93%	91%
Initial Antibiotic Timing	202	98%	96%	95%
Pneumococcal Vaccine	179	99%	95%	93%
Smoking Cessation Advice	104	97%	98%	97%
Surgical Care Improvement Project				
Appropriate VTP Within 24 Hours[2]	130	97%	92%	92%
Appropriate Hair Removal[2]	493	100%	100%	99%
Appropriate Beta Blocker Usage[2]	156	98%	94%	93%
Controlled Postoperative Blood Glucose[2]	0	-	94%	93%
Prophylactic Antibiotic Timing[2]	331	97%	97%	97%
Prophylactic Antibiotic Timing (Outpatient)	104	95%	91%	92%
Prophylactic Antibiotic Selection[2]	331	100%	98%	97%
Prophylactic Antibiotic Select. (Outpatient)	102	99%	94%	94%
Prophylactic Antibiotic Stopped[2]	314	97%	95%	94%
Recommended VTP Ordered[2]	130	98%	94%	94%
Urinary Catheter Removal[2]	36	83%	91%	90%
Children's Asthma Care				
Received Systemic Corticosteroids	-	-	-	100%
Received Home Management Plan	-	-	-	71%
Received Reliever Medication	-	-	-	100%
Use of Medical Imaging				
Combination Abdominal CT Scan	779	0.148	0.164	0.191
Combination Chest CT Scan	664	0.000	0.038	0.054
Follow-up Mammogram/Ultrasound	1,033	10.2%	8.4%	8.4%
MRI for Low Back Pain	174	32.2%	30.2%	32.7%
Survey of Patients' Hospital Experiences				
Area Around Room 'Always' Quiet at Night	300+	44%	-	58%
Doctors 'Always' Communicated Well	300+	72%	-	80%
Home Recovery Information Given	300+	79%	-	82%
Hospital Given 9 or 10 on 10 Point Scale	300+	53%	-	67%
Meds 'Always' Explained Before Given	300+	50%	-	60%
Nurses 'Always' Communicated Well	300+	69%	-	76%
Pain 'Always' Well Controlled	300+	64%	-	69%
Room and Bathroom 'Always' Clean	300+	58%	-	71%
Timely Help 'Always' Received	300+	54%	-	64%
Would Definitely Recommend Hospital	300+	57%	-	69%

Mercy Franciscan Hospital Western Hills

3131 Queen City Avenue Phone: 513-389-5915
Cincinnati, OH 45238 Fax: 513-389-5841
Type: Acute Care Hospitals Emergency Services: Yes
Ownership: Voluntary Non-Profit - Private Beds: 290

Key Personnel:
CEO/President. . . . . Patrick Kowalski
Chief of Medical Staff . . . . Prasad Chandra, MD
Quality Assurance . . . . Maria Markesbery

Measure	Cases	This Hosp.	State Avg.	U.S. Avg.
Heart Attack Care				
ACE Inhibitor or ARB for LVSD[1]	8	100%	97%	96%
Aspirin at Arrival	71	99%	99%	99%
Aspirin at Discharge	34	100%	99%	98%
Beta Blocker at Discharge	38	100%	99%	98%
Fibrinolytic Medication Timing	0	-	14%	55%
PCI Within 90 Minutes of Arrival	0	-	92%	90%
Smoking Cessation Advice[1]	9	100%	100%	99%
Chest Pain/Possible Heart Attack Care				
Aspirin at Arrival	132	96%	96%	95%
Median Time to ECG (minutes)	139	8	7	8
Median Time to Transfer (minutes)[1]	24	60	61	61
Fibrinolytic Medication Timing[1]	1	0%	47%	54%
Heart Failure Care				
ACE Inhibitor or ARB for LVSD	47	100%	96%	94%
Discharge Instructions	160	96%	91%	88%
Evaluation of LVS Function	212	98%	99%	98%
Smoking Cessation Advice	35	97%	99%	98%
Pneumonia Care				
Appropriate Initial Antibiotic	188	95%	92%	92%
Blood Culture Timing	272	99%	96%	96%
Influenza Vaccine	166	95%	93%	91%
Initial Antibiotic Timing	257	96%	96%	95%
Pneumococcal Vaccine	221	96%	95%	93%
Smoking Cessation Advice	108	100%	98%	97%
Surgical Care Improvement Project				
Appropriate VTP Within 24 Hours[2]	156	97%	92%	92%
Appropriate Hair Removal[2]	331	100%	100%	99%
Appropriate Beta Blocker Usage[2]	146	99%	94%	93%
Controlled Postoperative Blood Glucose[2]	0	-	94%	93%
Prophylactic Antibiotic Timing[2]	194	99%	97%	97%
Prophylactic Antibiotic Timing (Outpatient)	59	92%	91%	92%
Prophylactic Antibiotic Selection[2]	194	99%	98%	97%
Prophylactic Antibiotic Select. (Outpatient)	58	90%	94%	94%
Prophylactic Antibiotic Stopped[2]	190	99%	95%	94%
Recommended VTP Ordered[2]	156	98%	94%	94%
Urinary Catheter Removal[2]	26	100%	91%	90%
Children's Asthma Care				
Received Systemic Corticosteroids	-	-	-	100%
Received Home Management Plan	-	-	-	71%
Received Reliever Medication	-	-	-	100%
Use of Medical Imaging				
Combination Abdominal CT Scan	930	0.315	0.164	0.191
Combination Chest CT Scan	820	0.010	0.038	0.054
Follow-up Mammogram/Ultrasound	1,184	10.3%	8.4%	8.4%
MRI for Low Back Pain	83	22.9%	30.2%	32.7%
Survey of Patients' Hospital Experiences				
Area Around Room 'Always' Quiet at Night	300+	46%	-	58%
Doctors 'Always' Communicated Well	300+	77%	-	80%
Home Recovery Information Given	300+	76%	-	82%
Hospital Given 9 or 10 on 10 Point Scale	300+	61%	-	67%
Meds 'Always' Explained Before Given	300+	54%	-	60%
Nurses 'Always' Communicated Well	300+	73%	-	76%
Pain 'Always' Well Controlled	300+	65%	-	69%
Room and Bathroom 'Always' Clean	300+	62%	-	71%
Timely Help 'Always' Received	300+	60%	-	64%
Would Definitely Recommend Hospital	300+	57%	-	69%

NOTE: Hospital profiles are in alphabetical order by state, then city, then hospital within the city; Rankings exclude hospitals with less than 25 cases except for patient surveys which excludes hospitals with less than 100 cases; (a) 100–299 cases; (1) The number of cases is too small to be sure how well a hospital is performing; (2) The hospital indicated that the data submitted for this measure were based on a sample of cases; (3) Data was collected during a shorter time period (fewer quarters) than the maximum possible time for this measure; (4) Suppressed for one or more quarters by CMS; (5) No data is available from the hospital for this measure; (6) Fewer than 100 patients completed the HCAHPS survey. Use these rates with caution, as the number of surveys may be too low to reliably assess hospital performance; (7) Survey results are based on less than 12 months of data; (8) Survey results are not available for this reporting period; (9) No or very few patients were eligible for the HCAHPS survey. The scores shown, if any, reflect a very small number of surveys; (10) A state average was not calculated because too few hospitals in the state submitted data; (11) There were discrepancies in the data collection process; Please refer to the User's Guide for a full explanation of data.

Mercy Hospital Anderson

7500 State Road
Cincinnati, OH 45255
Phone: 513-624-4501
Fax: 513-624-3299
Type: Acute Care Hospitals
Emergency Services: Yes
Ownership: Voluntary Non-Profit - Church
Beds: 186

Key Personnel:

CEO/President. . . . . Patricia Ann Schroer
Cardiac Laboratory. . . . . Terri Martin
Chief of Medical Staff . . . . Denberg Stanfield
Infection Control. . . . . Kathy Puthoff
Operating Room. . . . . Pam Brinks
Quality Assurance . . . . Dani Hext
Emergency Room . . . . Harry Boyce

Measure	Cases	This Hosp.	State Avg.	U.S. Avg.
Heart Attack Care				
ACE Inhibitor or ARB for LVSD	63	98%	97%	96%
Aspirin at Arrival	235	99%	99%	99%
Aspirin at Discharge	255	100%	99%	98%
Beta Blocker at Discharge	240	99%	99%	98%
Fibrinolytic Medication Timing	0	-	14%	55%
PCI Within 90 Minutes of Arrival	51	94%	92%	90%
Smoking Cessation Advice	105	100%	100%	99%
Chest Pain/Possible Heart Attack Care				
Aspirin at Arrival[1]	8	100%	96%	95%
Median Time to ECG (minutes)[1]	10	6	7	8
Median Time to Transfer (minutes)[5]	0	-	61	61
Fibrinolytic Medication Timing[3]	0	-	47%	54%
Heart Failure Care				
ACE Inhibitor or ARB for LVSD	90	98%	96%	94%
Discharge Instructions	262	93%	91%	88%
Evaluation of LVS Function	328	98%	99%	98%
Smoking Cessation Advice	30	97%	99%	98%
Pneumonia Care				
Appropriate Initial Antibiotic	216	96%	92%	92%
Blood Culture Timing	327	97%	96%	96%
Influenza Vaccine	228	96%	93%	91%
Initial Antibiotic Timing	381	95%	96%	95%
Pneumococcal Vaccine	325	98%	95%	93%
Smoking Cessation Advice	162	98%	98%	97%
Surgical Care Improvement Project				
Appropriate VTP Within 24 Hours[2]	207	90%	92%	92%
Appropriate Hair Removal[2]	908	100%	100%	99%
Appropriate Beta Blocker Usage[2]	283	95%	94%	93%
Controlled Postoperative Blood Glucose[2]	85	98%	94%	93%
Prophylactic Antibiotic Timing[2]	673	98%	97%	97%
Prophylactic Antibiotic Timing (Outpatient)	261	96%	91%	92%
Prophylactic Antibiotic Selection[2]	695	99%	98%	97%
Prophylactic Antibiotic Select. (Outpatient)	255	96%	94%	94%
Prophylactic Antibiotic Stopped[2]	622	99%	95%	94%
Recommended VTP Ordered[2]	207	100%	94%	94%
Urinary Catheter Removal[2]	204	96%	91%	90%
Children's Asthma Care				
Received Systemic Corticosteroids	-	-	-	100%
Received Home Management Plan	-	-	-	71%
Received Reliever Medication	-	-	-	100%
Use of Medical Imaging				
Combination Abdominal CT Scan	1,074	0.072	0.164	0.191
Combination Chest CT Scan	930	0.002	0.038	0.054
Follow-up Mammogram/Ultrasound	1,554	7.5%	8.4%	8.4%
MRI for Low Back Pain	272	30.9%	30.2%	32.7%
Survey of Patients' Hospital Experiences				
Area Around Room 'Always' Quiet at Night	300+	45%	-	58%
Doctors 'Always' Communicated Well	300+	74%	-	80%
Home Recovery Information Given	300+	80%	-	82%
Hospital Given 9 or 10 on 10 Point Scale	300+	63%	-	67%
Meds 'Always' Explained Before Given	300+	55%	-	60%
Nurses 'Always' Communicated Well	300+	74%	-	76%
Pain 'Always' Well Controlled	300+	66%	-	69%
Room and Bathroom 'Always' Clean	300+	63%	-	71%
Timely Help 'Always' Received	300+	58%	-	64%
Would Definitely Recommend Hospital	300+	67%	-	69%

University Hospital

234 Goodman Street
Cincinnati, OH 45267
Phone: 513-584-1000
URL: www.universityhospitalcincinnati.com
Type: Acute Care Hospitals
Emergency Services: Yes
Ownership: Voluntary Non-Profit - Private

Key Personnel:

CEO/President. . . . . Lee Ann Liska

Measure	Cases	This Hosp.	State Avg.	U.S. Avg.
Heart Attack Care				
ACE Inhibitor or ARB for LVSD	44	89%	97%	96%
Aspirin at Arrival	182	99%	99%	99%
Aspirin at Discharge	217	98%	99%	98%
Beta Blocker at Discharge	202	99%	99%	98%
Fibrinolytic Medication Timing	0	-	14%	55%
PCI Within 90 Minutes of Arrival	40	88%	92%	90%
Smoking Cessation Advice	114	100%	100%	99%
Chest Pain/Possible Heart Attack Care				
Aspirin at Arrival[1,3]	3	100%	96%	95%
Median Time to ECG (minutes)[1,3]	3	14	7	8
Median Time to Transfer (minutes)[5]	0	-	61	61
Fibrinolytic Medication Timing[5]	0	-	47%	54%
Heart Failure Care				
ACE Inhibitor or ARB for LVSD[2]	332	98%	96%	94%
Discharge Instructions[2]	489	76%	91%	88%
Evaluation of LVS Function[2]	559	99%	99%	98%
Smoking Cessation Advice[2]	202	99%	99%	98%
Pneumonia Care				
Appropriate Initial Antibiotic[2]	49	92%	92%	92%
Blood Culture Timing[2]	123	98%	96%	96%
Influenza Vaccine[2]	72	82%	93%	91%
Initial Antibiotic Timing[2]	115	86%	96%	95%
Pneumococcal Vaccine[2]	55	82%	95%	93%
Smoking Cessation Advice[2]	83	98%	98%	97%
Surgical Care Improvement Project				
Appropriate VTP Within 24 Hours[2]	211	97%	92%	92%
Appropriate Hair Removal[2]	645	100%	100%	99%
Appropriate Beta Blocker Usage[2]	181	92%	94%	93%
Controlled Postoperative Blood Glucose[2]	106	95%	94%	93%
Prophylactic Antibiotic Timing[2]	418	97%	97%	97%
Prophylactic Antibiotic Timing (Outpatient)	395	84%	91%	92%
Prophylactic Antibiotic Selection[2]	435	95%	98%	97%
Prophylactic Antibiotic Select. (Outpatient)	375	93%	94%	94%
Prophylactic Antibiotic Stopped[2]	409	93%	95%	94%
Recommended VTP Ordered[2]	214	98%	94%	94%
Urinary Catheter Removal[2]	131	79%	91%	90%
Children's Asthma Care				
Received Systemic Corticosteroids	-	-	-	100%
Received Home Management Plan	-	-	-	71%
Received Reliever Medication	-	-	-	100%
Use of Medical Imaging				
Combination Abdominal CT Scan	688	0.078	0.164	0.191
Combination Chest CT Scan	649	0.020	0.038	0.054
Follow-up Mammogram/Ultrasound	1,540	11.4%	8.4%	8.4%
MRI for Low Back Pain	183	33.3%	30.2%	32.7%
Survey of Patients' Hospital Experiences				
Area Around Room 'Always' Quiet at Night	300+	54%	-	58%
Doctors 'Always' Communicated Well	300+	73%	-	80%
Home Recovery Information Given	300+	83%	-	82%
Hospital Given 9 or 10 on 10 Point Scale	300+	63%	-	67%
Meds 'Always' Explained Before Given	300+	57%	-	60%
Nurses 'Always' Communicated Well	300+	72%	-	76%
Pain 'Always' Well Controlled	300+	63%	-	69%
Room and Bathroom 'Always' Clean	300+	61%	-	71%
Timely Help 'Always' Received	300+	55%	-	64%
Would Definitely Recommend Hospital	300+	67%	-	69%

Berger Hospital

600 North Pickaway Street
Circleville, OH 43113
Phone: 740-420-8585
Fax: 740-474-1897
E-mail: pr@bergerhealth.com
URL: www.bergerhealth.com
Type: Acute Care Hospitals
Emergency Services: Yes
Ownership: Government - Local
Beds: 91

Key Personnel:

CEO/President. . . . . Larry W Thornhill
Chief of Medical Staff . . . . Charles Hedges, MD
Infection Control. . . . . Marilyn Frost, RN
Operating Room. . . . . Bobbin Peters, RN
Quality Assurance . . . . Paul Westbrock
Radiology. . . . . Laurian Dean, MD
Emergency Room . . . . Bobby Dale, MD
Intensive Care Unit. . . . . Joan King, RN

Measure	Cases	This Hosp.	State Avg.	U.S. Avg.
Heart Attack Care				
ACE Inhibitor or ARB for LVSD	0	-	97%	96%
Aspirin at Arrival[1]	11	100%	99%	99%
Aspirin at Discharge[1]	8	100%	99%	98%
Beta Blocker at Discharge[1]	9	100%	99%	98%
Fibrinolytic Medication Timing	0	-	14%	55%
PCI Within 90 Minutes of Arrival	0	-	92%	90%
Smoking Cessation Advice	0	-	100%	99%
Chest Pain/Possible Heart Attack Care				
Aspirin at Arrival	179	99%	96%	95%
Median Time to ECG (minutes)	180	7	7	8
Median Time to Transfer (minutes)[1]	13	66	61	61
Fibrinolytic Medication Timing[1]	10	80%	47%	54%
Heart Failure Care				
ACE Inhibitor or ARB for LVSD[1]	13	92%	96%	94%
Discharge Instructions	84	100%	91%	88%
Evaluation of LVS Function	108	100%	99%	98%
Smoking Cessation Advice[1]	22	100%	99%	98%
Pneumonia Care				
Appropriate Initial Antibiotic	74	95%	92%	92%
Blood Culture Timing	130	95%	96%	96%
Influenza Vaccine	84	99%	93%	91%
Initial Antibiotic Timing	117	100%	96%	95%
Pneumococcal Vaccine	98	100%	95%	93%
Smoking Cessation Advice	55	100%	98%	97%
Surgical Care Improvement Project				
Appropriate VTP Within 24 Hours[2]	84	88%	92%	92%
Appropriate Hair Removal[2]	377	100%	100%	99%
Appropriate Beta Blocker Usage[2]	103	99%	94%	93%
Controlled Postoperative Blood Glucose[2]	0	-	94%	93%
Prophylactic Antibiotic Timing[2]	281	99%	97%	97%
Prophylactic Antibiotic Timing (Outpatient)	40	100%	91%	92%
Prophylactic Antibiotic Selection[2]	284	99%	98%	97%
Prophylactic Antibiotic Select. (Outpatient)	40	85%	94%	94%
Prophylactic Antibiotic Stopped[2]	274	95%	95%	94%
Recommended VTP Ordered[2]	84	95%	94%	94%
Urinary Catheter Removal[2]	103	100%	91%	90%
Children's Asthma Care				
Received Systemic Corticosteroids	-	-	-	100%
Received Home Management Plan	-	-	-	71%
Received Reliever Medication	-	-	-	100%
Use of Medical Imaging				
Combination Abdominal CT Scan	546	0.049	0.164	0.191
Combination Chest CT Scan	366	0.011	0.038	0.054
Follow-up Mammogram/Ultrasound	630	10.5%	8.4%	8.4%
MRI for Low Back Pain	77	31.2%	30.2%	32.7%
Survey of Patients' Hospital Experiences				
Area Around Room 'Always' Quiet at Night	300+	37%	-	58%
Doctors 'Always' Communicated Well	300+	74%	-	80%
Home Recovery Information Given	300+	83%	-	82%
Hospital Given 9 or 10 on 10 Point Scale	300+	56%	-	67%
Meds 'Always' Explained Before Given	300+	53%	-	60%
Nurses 'Always' Communicated Well	300+	72%	-	76%
Pain 'Always' Well Controlled	300+	65%	-	69%
Room and Bathroom 'Always' Clean	300+	63%	-	71%
Timely Help 'Always' Received	300+	64%	-	64%
Would Definitely Recommend Hospital	300+	58%	-	69%

NOTE: Hospital profiles are in alphabetical order by state, then city, then hospital within the city; Rankings exclude hospitals with less than 25 cases except for patient surveys which excludes hospitals with less than 100 cases; (a) 100–299 cases; (1) The number of cases is too small to be sure how well a hospital is performing; (2) The hospital indicated that the data submitted for this measure were based on a sample of cases; (3) Data was collected during a shorter time period (fewer quarters) than the maximum possible time for this measure; (4) Suppressed for one or more quarters by CMS; (5) No data is available from the hospital for this measure; (6) Fewer than 100 patients completed the HCAHPS survey. Use these rates with caution, as the number of surveys may be too low to reliably assess hospital performance; (7) Survey results are based on less than 12 months of data; (8) Survey results are not available for this reporting period; (9) No or very few patients were eligible for the HCAHPS survey. The scores shown, if any, reflect a very small number of surveys; (10) A state average was not calculated because too few hospitals in the state submitted data; (11) There were discrepancies in the data collection process; Please refer to the User's Guide for a full explanation of data.

Cleveland Clinic

9500 Euclid Avenue Phone: 216-444-2200
Cleveland, OH 44195 Fax: 216-445-7758
URL: www.clevelandclinic.org
Type: Acute Care Hospitals Emergency Services: Yes
Ownership: Voluntary Non-Profit - Private Beds: 1,113

Key Personnel:
CEO/President. . . . . Delos M Cosgrove, MD
Chief of Medical Staff. . . . . Marc Harrison, MD
Infection Control. . . . . David L Longworth, MD
Operating Room. . . . . Allan Siperstein, MD
Pediatric Ambulatory Care . . . . . . Robert Wyllie, MD
Pediatric In-Patient Care . . . . . . Robert Wyllie, MD
Quality Assurance . . . . J Michael Henderson, MD
Radiology. . . . . Gregory P Borkowski, MD

Measure	Cases	This Hosp.	State Avg.	U.S. Avg.
Heart Attack Care				
ACE Inhibitor or ARB for LVSD[2]	180	99%	97%	96%
Aspirin at Arrival[2]	156	100%	99%	99%
Aspirin at Discharge[2]	839	100%	99%	98%
Beta Blocker at Discharge[2]	804	100%	99%	98%
Fibrinolytic Medication Timing[2]	0	-	14%	55%
PCI Within 90 Minutes of Arrival[1,2]	15	87%	92%	90%
Smoking Cessation Advice[2]	288	100%	100%	99%
Chest Pain/Possible Heart Attack Care				
Aspirin at Arrival[1]	4	100%	96%	95%
Median Time to ECG (minutes)[1]	4	2	7	8
Median Time to Transfer (minutes)[5]	0	-	61	61
Fibrinolytic Medication Timing[5]	0	-	47%	54%
Heart Failure Care				
ACE Inhibitor or ARB for LVSD	487	98%	96%	94%
Discharge Instructions	1,009	93%	91%	88%
Evaluation of LVS Function	1,206	100%	99%	98%
Smoking Cessation Advice	220	100%	99%	98%
Pneumonia Care				
Appropriate Initial Antibiotic[2]	71	92%	92%	92%
Blood Culture Timing[2]	106	96%	96%	96%
Influenza Vaccine[2]	189	100%	93%	91%
Initial Antibiotic Timing[2]	142	92%	96%	95%
Pneumococcal Vaccine[2]	225	98%	95%	93%
Smoking Cessation Advice[2]	110	95%	98%	97%
Surgical Care Improvement Project				
Appropriate VTP Within 24 Hours[2]	461	96%	92%	92%
Appropriate Hair Removal[2]	1,487	91%	100%	99%
Appropriate Beta Blocker Usage[2]	538	95%	94%	93%
Controlled Postoperative Blood Glucose[2]	407	92%	94%	93%
Prophylactic Antibiotic Timing[2]	1,019	98%	97%	97%
Prophylactic Antibiotic Timing (Outpatient)	826	83%	91%	92%
Prophylactic Antibiotic Selection[2]	1,050	97%	98%	97%
Prophylactic Antibiotic Select. (Outpatient)	1,336	88%	94%	94%
Prophylactic Antibiotic Stopped[2]	989	92%	95%	94%
Recommended VTP Ordered[2]	462	96%	94%	94%
Urinary Catheter Removal[2]	313	89%	91%	90%
Children's Asthma Care				
Received Systemic Corticosteroids	30	100%	-	100%
Received Home Management Plan	29	0%	-	71%
Received Reliever Medication	30	100%	-	100%
Use of Medical Imaging				
Combination Abdominal CT Scan	3,773	0.311	0.164	0.191
Combination Chest CT Scan	3,973	0.002	0.038	0.054
Follow-up Mammogram/Ultrasound	1,905	12.1%	8.4%	8.4%
MRI for Low Back Pain	205	24.9%	30.2%	32.7%
Survey of Patients' Hospital Experiences				
Area Around Room 'Always' Quiet at Night	300+	51%	-	58%
Doctors 'Always' Communicated Well	300+	76%	-	80%
Home Recovery Information Given	300+	83%	-	82%
Hospital Given 9 or 10 on 10 Point Scale	300+	76%	-	67%
Meds 'Always' Explained Before Given	300+	59%	-	60%
Nurses 'Always' Communicated Well	300+	75%	-	76%
Pain 'Always' Well Controlled	300+	68%	-	69%
Room and Bathroom 'Always' Clean	300+	68%	-	71%
Timely Help 'Always' Received	300+	58%	-	64%
Would Definitely Recommend Hospital	300+	82%	-	69%

Cleveland-Wade Park VA Medical Center

10701 East Blvd Phone: 216-791-3800
Cleveland, OH 44106 Fax: 440-838-6017
Type: Acute Care-Veterans Administration Emergency Services: No
Ownership: Government - Federal Beds: 688

Key Personnel:
CEO/President. . . . . William D Montatue
Chief of Medical Staff. . . . . Murray Altose, MD
Coronary Care. . . . . Verena Briley-Hudson, RN
Infection Control. . . . . Luis Rice
Operating Room. . . . . Donald Benson, MD
Quality Assurance . . . . Dora Rice, RN
Radiology. . . . . MH Naheedy, MD

Measure	Cases	This Hosp.	State Avg.	U.S. Avg.
Heart Attack Care				
ACE Inhibitor or ARB for LVSD[1]	4	100%	97%	96%
Aspirin at Arrival	36	97%	99%	99%
Aspirin at Discharge	35	100%	99%	98%
Beta Blocker at Discharge	35	100%	99%	98%
Fibrinolytic Medication Timing[5]	0	-	14%	55%
PCI Within 90 Minutes of Arrival[1]	3	100%	92%	90%
Smoking Cessation Advice[1]	11	100%	100%	99%
Chest Pain/Possible Heart Attack Care				
Aspirin at Arrival	-	-	96%	95%
Median Time to ECG (minutes)	-	-	7	8
Median Time to Transfer (minutes)	-	-	61	61
Fibrinolytic Medication Timing	-	-	47%	54%
Heart Failure Care				
ACE Inhibitor or ARB for LVSD	174	98%	96%	94%
Discharge Instructions	391	100%	91%	88%
Evaluation of LVS Function	417	100%	99%	98%
Smoking Cessation Advice	95	100%	99%	98%
Pneumonia Care				
Appropriate Initial Antibiotic	56	95%	92%	92%
Blood Culture Timing	91	98%	96%	96%
Influenza Vaccine	118	89%	93%	91%
Initial Antibiotic Timing	93	91%	96%	95%
Pneumococcal Vaccine	104	99%	95%	93%
Smoking Cessation Advice	83	100%	98%	97%
Surgical Care Improvement Project				
Appropriate VTP Within 24 Hours[2]	254	94%	92%	92%
Appropriate Hair Removal[2]	559	100%	100%	99%
Appropriate Beta Blocker Usage[2]	298	99%	94%	93%
Controlled Postoperative Blood Glucose[2]	157	96%	94%	93%
Prophylactic Antibiotic Timing	401	98%	97%	97%
Prophylactic Antibiotic Timing (Outpatient)	-	-	91%	92%
Prophylactic Antibiotic Selection	403	100%	98%	97%
Prophylactic Antibiotic Select. (Outpatient)	-	-	94%	94%
Prophylactic Antibiotic Stopped	379	97%	95%	94%
Recommended VTP Ordered[2]	254	94%	94%	94%
Urinary Catheter Removal[2]	215	93%	91%	90%
Children's Asthma Care				
Received Systemic Corticosteroids	-	-	-	100%
Received Home Management Plan	-	-	-	71%
Received Reliever Medication	-	-	-	100%
Use of Medical Imaging				
Combination Abdominal CT Scan	-	-	0.164	0.191
Combination Chest CT Scan	-	-	0.038	0.054
Follow-up Mammogram/Ultrasound	-	-	8.4%	8.4%
MRI for Low Back Pain	-	-	30.2%	32.7%
Survey of Patients' Hospital Experiences				
Area Around Room 'Always' Quiet at Night	-	-	-	58%
Doctors 'Always' Communicated Well	-	-	-	80%
Home Recovery Information Given	-	-	-	82%
Hospital Given 9 or 10 on 10 Point Scale	-	-	-	67%
Meds 'Always' Explained Before Given	-	-	-	60%
Nurses 'Always' Communicated Well	-	-	-	76%
Pain 'Always' Well Controlled	-	-	-	69%
Room and Bathroom 'Always' Clean	-	-	-	71%
Timely Help 'Always' Received	-	-	-	64%
Would Definitely Recommend Hospital	-	-	-	69%

Fairview Hospital

18101 Lorain Avenue Phone: 216-476-7000
Cleveland, OH 44111 Fax: 216-476-7017
URL: www.fairviewhospital.org
Type: Acute Care Hospitals Emergency Services: Yes
Ownership: Voluntary Non-Profit - Private Beds: 511

Key Personnel:
CEO/President. . . . . Janice Murphy
Chief of Medical Staff. . . . . Michael Waggoner, MD
Infection Control. . . . . KV Gopal, MD
Operating Room. . . . . Susan Keane, RN
Pediatric Ambulatory Care . . . . . . Sudhir Mehta, MD
Pediatric In-Patient Care . . . . . . Sudhir Mehta, MD
Quality Assurance . . . . Martha Mugford
Radiology. . . . . William Bishop, MD

Measure	Cases	This Hosp.	State Avg.	U.S. Avg.
Heart Attack Care				
ACE Inhibitor or ARB for LVSD[2]	28	96%	97%	96%
Aspirin at Arrival[2]	225	99%	99%	99%
Aspirin at Discharge[2]	269	98%	99%	98%
Beta Blocker at Discharge[2]	268	97%	99%	98%
Fibrinolytic Medication Timing[2]	0	-	14%	55%
PCI Within 90 Minutes of Arrival[2]	49	92%	92%	90%
Smoking Cessation Advice[2]	87	100%	100%	99%
Chest Pain/Possible Heart Attack Care				
Aspirin at Arrival	47	98%	96%	95%
Median Time to ECG (minutes)	48	7	7	8
Median Time to Transfer (minutes)[5]	0	-	61	61
Fibrinolytic Medication Timing[3]	0	-	47%	54%
Heart Failure Care				
ACE Inhibitor or ARB for LVSD	200	86%	96%	94%
Discharge Instructions	578	95%	91%	88%
Evaluation of LVS Function	805	93%	99%	98%
Smoking Cessation Advice	109	100%	99%	98%
Pneumonia Care				
Appropriate Initial Antibiotic	250	94%	92%	92%
Blood Culture Timing	339	99%	96%	96%
Influenza Vaccine	207	91%	93%	91%
Initial Antibiotic Timing	322	98%	96%	95%
Pneumococcal Vaccine	296	96%	95%	93%
Smoking Cessation Advice	104	100%	98%	97%
Surgical Care Improvement Project				
Appropriate VTP Within 24 Hours[2]	285	91%	92%	92%
Appropriate Hair Removal[2]	616	100%	100%	99%
Appropriate Beta Blocker Usage[2]	226	94%	94%	93%
Controlled Postoperative Blood Glucose[2]	119	90%	94%	93%
Prophylactic Antibiotic Timing[2]	450	99%	97%	97%
Prophylactic Antibiotic Timing (Outpatient)	626	92%	91%	92%
Prophylactic Antibiotic Selection[2]	454	93%	98%	97%
Prophylactic Antibiotic Select. (Outpatient)	666	94%	94%	94%
Prophylactic Antibiotic Stopped[2]	439	97%	95%	94%
Recommended VTP Ordered[2]	286	95%	94%	94%
Urinary Catheter Removal[2]	142	89%	91%	90%
Children's Asthma Care				
Received Systemic Corticosteroids	-	-	-	100%
Received Home Management Plan	-	-	-	71%
Received Reliever Medication	-	-	-	100%
Use of Medical Imaging				
Combination Abdominal CT Scan	926	0.073	0.164	0.191
Combination Chest CT Scan	641	0.003	0.038	0.054
Follow-up Mammogram/Ultrasound	1,415	13.9%	8.4%	8.4%
MRI for Low Back Pain	55	36.4%	30.2%	32.7%
Survey of Patients' Hospital Experiences				
Area Around Room 'Always' Quiet at Night	300+	57%	-	58%
Doctors 'Always' Communicated Well	300+	77%	-	80%
Home Recovery Information Given	300+	81%	-	82%
Hospital Given 9 or 10 on 10 Point Scale	300+	73%	-	67%
Meds 'Always' Explained Before Given	300+	60%	-	60%
Nurses 'Always' Communicated Well	300+	74%	-	76%
Pain 'Always' Well Controlled	300+	68%	-	69%
Room and Bathroom 'Always' Clean	300+	83%	-	71%
Timely Help 'Always' Received	300+	62%	-	64%
Would Definitely Recommend Hospital	300+	77%	-	69%

NOTE: Hospital profiles are in alphabetical order by state, then city, then hospital within the city; Rankings exclude hospitals with less than 25 cases except for patient surveys which excludes hospitals with less than 100 cases; (a) 100–299 cases; (1) The number of cases is too small to be sure how well a hospital is performing; (2) The hospital indicated that the data submitted for this measure were based on a sample of cases; (3) Data was collected during a shorter time period (fewer quarters) than the maximum possible time for this measure; (4) Suppressed for one or more quarters by CMS; (5) No data is available from the hospital for this measure; (6) Fewer than 100 patients completed the HCAHPS survey. Use these rates with caution, as the number of surveys may be too low to reliably assess hospital performance; (7) Survey results are based on less than 12 months of data; (8) Survey results are not available for this reporting period; (9) No or very few patients were eligible for the HCAHPS survey. The scores shown, if any, reflect a very small number of surveys; (10) A state average was not calculated because too few hospitals in the state submitted data; (11) There were discrepancies in the data collection process; Please refer to the User's Guide for a full explanation of data.

Huron Hospital

13951 Terrace Road
Cleveland, OH 44112
Type: Acute Care Hospitals
Ownership: Voluntary Non-Profit - Private
Phone: 216-761-3300
Fax: 216-761-7476
Emergency Services: Yes
Beds: 346

Key Personnel:
Chief of Medical Staff.......... Lori Slusarski
Infection Control.............. Richard Lyon
Operating Room.............. John Singleton
Quality Assurance .... Lynn Wolchovich
Radiology.................. Mervyn Thynne, MD

Measure	Cases	This Hosp.	State Avg.	U.S. Avg.
Heart Attack Care				
ACE Inhibitor or ARB for LVSD	0	-	97%	96%
Aspirin at Arrival[1]	13	100%	99%	99%
Aspirin at Discharge[1]	7	100%	99%	98%
Beta Blocker at Discharge[1]	9	100%	99%	98%
Fibrinolytic Medication Timing	0	-	14%	55%
PCI Within 90 Minutes of Arrival	0	-	92%	90%
Smoking Cessation Advice[1]	5	100%	100%	99%
Chest Pain/Possible Heart Attack Care				
Aspirin at Arrival	63	94%	96%	95%
Median Time to ECG (minutes)	62	10	7	8
Median Time to Transfer (minutes)[1]	8	68	61	61
Fibrinolytic Medication Timing[1]	1	100%	47%	54%
Heart Failure Care				
ACE Inhibitor or ARB for LVSD	97	98%	96%	94%
Discharge Instructions	192	99%	91%	88%
Evaluation of LVS Function	223	100%	99%	98%
Smoking Cessation Advice	76	100%	99%	98%
Pneumonia Care				
Appropriate Initial Antibiotic	39	97%	92%	92%
Blood Culture Timing	83	93%	96%	96%
Influenza Vaccine	55	85%	93%	91%
Initial Antibiotic Timing	98	94%	96%	95%
Pneumococcal Vaccine	72	97%	95%	93%
Smoking Cessation Advice	62	97%	98%	97%
Surgical Care Improvement Project				
Appropriate VTP Within 24 Hours	127	97%	92%	92%
Appropriate Hair Removal	208	100%	100%	99%
Appropriate Beta Blocker Usage	35	97%	94%	93%
Controlled Postoperative Blood Glucose	0	-	94%	93%
Prophylactic Antibiotic Timing	73	100%	97%	97%
Prophylactic Antibiotic Timing (Outpatient)	32	84%	91%	92%
Prophylactic Antibiotic Selection	75	96%	98%	97%
Prophylactic Antibiotic Select. (Outpatient)	28	54%	94%	94%
Prophylactic Antibiotic Stopped	64	98%	95%	94%
Recommended VTP Ordered	127	98%	94%	94%
Urinary Catheter Removal[1]	23	96%	91%	90%
Children's Asthma Care				
Received Systemic Corticosteroids	-	-	-	100%
Received Home Management Plan	-	-	-	71%
Received Reliever Medication	-	-	-	100%
Use of Medical Imaging				
Combination Abdominal CT Scan	158	0.019	0.164	0.191
Combination Chest CT Scan	139	0.029	0.038	0.054
Follow-up Mammogram/Ultrasound	186	8.1%	8.4%	8.4%
MRI for Low Back Pain[1]	27	25.9%	30.2%	32.7%
Survey of Patients' Hospital Experiences				
Area Around Room 'Always' Quiet at Night	300+	56%	-	58%
Doctors 'Always' Communicated Well	300+	72%	-	80%
Home Recovery Information Given	300+	79%	-	82%
Hospital Given 9 or 10 on 10 Point Scale	300+	50%	-	67%
Meds 'Always' Explained Before Given	300+	55%	-	60%
Nurses 'Always' Communicated Well	300+	70%	-	76%
Pain 'Always' Well Controlled	300+	62%	-	69%
Room and Bathroom 'Always' Clean	300+	62%	-	71%
Timely Help 'Always' Received	300+	48%	-	64%
Would Definitely Recommend Hospital	300+	48%	-	69%

Lutheran Hospital

1730 West 25th Street
Cleveland, OH 44113
URL: www.lutheranhospital.org
Type: Acute Care Hospitals
Ownership: Voluntary Non-Profit - Private
Phone: 216-696-4300
Fax: 216-696-7397
Emergency Services: Yes
Beds: 209

Key Personnel:
CEO/President............... David F Perse
Operating Room.............. Bernard M Stulberg, MD

Measure	Cases	This Hosp.	State Avg.	U.S. Avg.
Heart Attack Care				
ACE Inhibitor or ARB for LVSD	0	-	97%	96%
Aspirin at Arrival[1]	17	100%	99%	99%
Aspirin at Discharge[1]	9	100%	99%	98%
Beta Blocker at Discharge[1]	11	100%	99%	98%
Fibrinolytic Medication Timing	0	-	14%	55%
PCI Within 90 Minutes of Arrival	0	-	92%	90%
Smoking Cessation Advice[1]	1	100%	100%	99%
Chest Pain/Possible Heart Attack Care				
Aspirin at Arrival	44	91%	96%	95%
Median Time to ECG (minutes)	48	4	7	8
Median Time to Transfer (minutes)[1,3]	9	56	61	61
Fibrinolytic Medication Timing	0	-	47%	54%
Heart Failure Care				
ACE Inhibitor or ARB for LVSD	38	92%	96%	94%
Discharge Instructions	84	98%	91%	88%
Evaluation of LVS Function	108	99%	99%	98%
Smoking Cessation Advice[1]	23	100%	99%	98%
Pneumonia Care				
Appropriate Initial Antibiotic	83	96%	92%	92%
Blood Culture Timing	123	97%	96%	96%
Influenza Vaccine	83	100%	93%	91%
Initial Antibiotic Timing	152	95%	96%	95%
Pneumococcal Vaccine	82	100%	95%	93%
Smoking Cessation Advice	79	100%	98%	97%
Surgical Care Improvement Project				
Appropriate VTP Within 24 Hours[2]	130	98%	92%	92%
Appropriate Hair Removal[2]	343	100%	100%	99%
Appropriate Beta Blocker Usage[2]	115	99%	94%	93%
Controlled Postoperative Blood Glucose[2]	0	-	94%	93%
Prophylactic Antibiotic Timing[2]	216	98%	97%	97%
Prophylactic Antibiotic Timing (Outpatient)	226	98%	91%	92%
Prophylactic Antibiotic Selection[2]	217	99%	98%	97%
Prophylactic Antibiotic Select. (Outpatient)	222	96%	94%	94%
Prophylactic Antibiotic Stopped[2]	213	99%	95%	94%
Recommended VTP Ordered[2]	130	98%	94%	94%
Urinary Catheter Removal[2]	126	98%	91%	90%
Children's Asthma Care				
Received Systemic Corticosteroids	-	-	-	100%
Received Home Management Plan	-	-	-	71%
Received Reliever Medication	-	-	-	100%
Use of Medical Imaging				
Combination Abdominal CT Scan	243	0.049	0.164	0.191
Combination Chest CT Scan	123	0.000	0.038	0.054
Follow-up Mammogram/Ultrasound	321	4.4%	8.4%	8.4%
MRI for Low Back Pain	54	33.3%	30.2%	32.7%
Survey of Patients' Hospital Experiences				
Area Around Room 'Always' Quiet at Night	300+	52%	-	58%
Doctors 'Always' Communicated Well	300+	74%	-	80%
Home Recovery Information Given	300+	81%	-	82%
Hospital Given 9 or 10 on 10 Point Scale	300+	54%	-	67%
Meds 'Always' Explained Before Given	300+	54%	-	60%
Nurses 'Always' Communicated Well	300+	68%	-	76%
Pain 'Always' Well Controlled	300+	62%	-	69%
Room and Bathroom 'Always' Clean	300+	59%	-	71%
Timely Help 'Always' Received	300+	51%	-	64%
Would Definitely Recommend Hospital	300+	59%	-	69%

Metro Health Medical Center

2500 Metrohealth Drive
Cleveland, OH 44109
URL: www.metrohealth.org
Type: Acute Care Hospitals
Ownership: Government - Local
Phone: 216-778-5700
Fax: 216-368-4678
Emergency Services: Yes
Beds: 728

Key Personnel:
CEO/President............... John Sideras
Cardiac Laboratory............ Norman Snow, MD
Chief of Medical Staff.......... Gerald Oliphant
Infection Control.............. Richard Blinkhorn, MD
Operating Room.............. Mark A Malangoni, MD
Pediatric In-Patient Care .... Margaret Stager, MD
Quality Assurance .... Sandra Amin
Radiology.................. Robert Ferguson, MD

Measure	Cases	This Hosp.	State Avg.	U.S. Avg.
Heart Attack Care				
ACE Inhibitor or ARB for LVSD	27	93%	97%	96%
Aspirin at Arrival	236	100%	99%	99%
Aspirin at Discharge	226	99%	99%	98%
Beta Blocker at Discharge	227	100%	99%	98%
Fibrinolytic Medication Timing	0	-	14%	55%
PCI Within 90 Minutes of Arrival	44	91%	92%	90%
Smoking Cessation Advice	126	100%	100%	99%
Chest Pain/Possible Heart Attack Care				
Aspirin at Arrival[1]	15	93%	96%	95%
Median Time to ECG (minutes)[1]	16	12	7	8
Median Time to Transfer (minutes)[5]	0	-	61	61
Fibrinolytic Medication Timing[5]	0	-	47%	54%
Heart Failure Care				
ACE Inhibitor or ARB for LVSD	261	95%	96%	94%
Discharge Instructions	589	63%	91%	88%
Evaluation of LVS Function	660	100%	99%	98%
Smoking Cessation Advice	225	98%	99%	98%
Pneumonia Care				
Appropriate Initial Antibiotic	113	95%	92%	92%
Blood Culture Timing	97	86%	96%	96%
Influenza Vaccine	186	59%	93%	91%
Initial Antibiotic Timing	241	95%	96%	95%
Pneumococcal Vaccine	161	88%	95%	93%
Smoking Cessation Advice	236	98%	98%	97%
Surgical Care Improvement Project				
Appropriate VTP Within 24 Hours[2]	219	98%	92%	92%
Appropriate Hair Removal[2]	662	100%	100%	99%
Appropriate Beta Blocker Usage[2]	244	90%	94%	93%
Controlled Postoperative Blood Glucose[2]	95	94%	94%	93%
Prophylactic Antibiotic Timing[2]	483	98%	97%	97%
Prophylactic Antibiotic Timing (Outpatient)	599	95%	91%	92%
Prophylactic Antibiotic Selection[2]	492	98%	98%	97%
Prophylactic Antibiotic Select. (Outpatient)	687	97%	94%	94%
Prophylactic Antibiotic Stopped[2]	466	94%	95%	94%
Recommended VTP Ordered[2]	219	98%	94%	94%
Urinary Catheter Removal[2]	163	93%	91%	90%
Children's Asthma Care				
Received Systemic Corticosteroids	-	-	-	100%
Received Home Management Plan	-	-	-	71%
Received Reliever Medication	-	-	-	100%
Use of Medical Imaging				
Combination Abdominal CT Scan	782	0.054	0.164	0.191
Combination Chest CT Scan	830	0.024	0.038	0.054
Follow-up Mammogram/Ultrasound	1,611	19.1%	8.4%	8.4%
MRI for Low Back Pain	147	31.3%	30.2%	32.7%
Survey of Patients' Hospital Experiences				
Area Around Room 'Always' Quiet at Night	300+	59%	-	58%
Doctors 'Always' Communicated Well	300+	76%	-	80%
Home Recovery Information Given	300+	83%	-	82%
Hospital Given 9 or 10 on 10 Point Scale	300+	64%	-	67%
Meds 'Always' Explained Before Given	300+	60%	-	60%
Nurses 'Always' Communicated Well	300+	72%	-	76%
Pain 'Always' Well Controlled	300+	66%	-	69%
Room and Bathroom 'Always' Clean	300+	61%	-	71%
Timely Help 'Always' Received	300+	59%	-	64%
Would Definitely Recommend Hospital	300+	73%	-	69%

NOTE: Hospital profiles are in alphabetical order by state, then city, then hospital within the city; Rankings exclude hospitals with less than 25 cases except for patient surveys which excludes hospitals with less than 100 cases; (a) 100–299 cases; (1) The number of cases is too small to be sure how well a hospital is performing; (2) The hospital indicated that the data submitted for this measure were based on a sample of cases; (3) Data was collected during a shorter time period (fewer quarters) than the maximum possible time for this measure; (4) Suppressed for one or more quarters by CMS; (5) No data is available from the hospital for this measure; (6) Fewer than 100 patients completed the HCAHPS survey. Use these rates with caution, as the number of surveys may be too low to reliably assess hospital performance; (7) Survey results are based on less than 12 months of data; (8) Survey results are not available for this reporting period; (9) No or very few patients were eligible for the HCAHPS survey. The scores shown, if any, reflect a very small number of surveys; (10) A state average was not calculated because too few hospitals in the state submitted data; (11) There were discrepancies in the data collection process; Please refer to the User's Guide for a full explanation of data.

Saint Vincent Charity Medical Center

2351 East 22nd Street Phone: 216-861-6200
Cleveland, OH 44115 Fax: 216-363-2796
Type: Acute Care Hospitals Emergency Services: Yes
Ownership: Voluntary Non-Profit - Private Beds: 492

Key Personnel:
CEO/President. . . . . Jeffrey Jeney
Chief of Medical Staff. . . . . Charity Kankan, MD
Infection Control. . . . . Richard Chmielewski, MD
Operating Room. . . . . Jo Ellen Horn
Quality Assurance . . . . Jane Jones
Radiology. . . . . Robert Porter, MD
Anesthesiology. . . . . John Bastulli, MD
Emergency Room . . . . Gayle Galan, MD

Measure	Cases	This Hosp.	State Avg.	U.S. Avg.
Heart Attack Care				
ACE Inhibitor or ARB for LVSD[1]	14	93%	97%	96%
Aspirin at Arrival	66	98%	99%	99%
Aspirin at Discharge	66	100%	99%	98%
Beta Blocker at Discharge	67	97%	99%	98%
Fibrinolytic Medication Timing	0	-	14%	55%
PCI Within 90 Minutes of Arrival[1]	10	90%	92%	90%
Smoking Cessation Advice	28	100%	100%	99%
Chest Pain/Possible Heart Attack Care				
Aspirin at Arrival	159	97%	96%	95%
Median Time to ECG (minutes)	159	8	7	8
Median Time to Transfer (minutes)[1,3]	1	31	61	61
Fibrinolytic Medication Timing[3]	0	-	47%	54%
Heart Failure Care				
ACE Inhibitor or ARB for LVSD[2]	118	95%	96%	94%
Discharge Instructions[2]	236	94%	91%	88%
Evaluation of LVS Function[2]	287	100%	99%	98%
Smoking Cessation Advice[2]	86	99%	99%	98%
Pneumonia Care				
Appropriate Initial Antibiotic[2]	53	92%	92%	92%
Blood Culture Timing[2]	83	95%	96%	96%
Influenza Vaccine[2]	65	91%	93%	91%
Initial Antibiotic Timing[2]	99	90%	96%	95%
Pneumococcal Vaccine[2]	79	94%	95%	93%
Smoking Cessation Advice[2]	42	100%	98%	97%
Surgical Care Improvement Project				
Appropriate VTP Within 24 Hours[2]	120	96%	92%	92%
Appropriate Hair Removal[2]	352	100%	100%	99%
Appropriate Beta Blocker Usage[2]	123	86%	94%	93%
Controlled Postoperative Blood Glucose[2]	50	86%	94%	93%
Prophylactic Antibiotic Timing[2]	248	97%	97%	97%
Prophylactic Antibiotic Timing (Outpatient)	145	97%	91%	92%
Prophylactic Antibiotic Selection[2]	248	96%	98%	97%
Prophylactic Antibiotic Select. (Outpatient)	145	91%	94%	94%
Prophylactic Antibiotic Stopped[2]	238	91%	95%	94%
Recommended VTP Ordered[2]	120	97%	94%	94%
Urinary Catheter Removal[2]	143	85%	91%	90%
Children's Asthma Care				
Received Systemic Corticosteroids	-	-	-	100%
Received Home Management Plan	-	-	-	71%
Received Reliever Medication	-	-	-	100%
Use of Medical Imaging				
Combination Abdominal CT Scan	288	0.049	0.164	0.191
Combination Chest CT Scan	189	0.000	0.038	0.054
Follow-up Mammogram/Ultrasound	314	12.7%	8.4%	8.4%
MRI for Low Back Pain	60	36.7%	30.2%	32.7%
Survey of Patients' Hospital Experiences				
Area Around Room 'Always' Quiet at Night	300+	70%	-	58%
Doctors 'Always' Communicated Well	300+	80%	-	80%
Home Recovery Information Given	300+	85%	-	82%
Hospital Given 9 or 10 on 10 Point Scale	300+	70%	-	67%
Meds 'Always' Explained Before Given	300+	59%	-	60%
Nurses 'Always' Communicated Well	300+	76%	-	76%
Pain 'Always' Well Controlled	300+	69%	-	69%
Room and Bathroom 'Always' Clean	300+	68%	-	71%
Timely Help 'Always' Received	300+	61%	-	64%
Would Definitely Recommend Hospital	300+	71%	-	69%

University Hospitals of Cleveland

11100 Euclid Avenue Phone: 216-844-1000
Cleveland, OH 44106 Fax: 216-844-5805
URL: www.uhhs.com
Type: Acute Care Hospitals Emergency Services: Yes
Ownership: Voluntary Non-Profit - Private Beds: 1,032

Key Personnel:
CEO/President. . . . . Fred C. Rothstein, MD
Chief of Medical Staff. . . . . Pam Meyer
Infection Control. . . . . Michael Jacobs, MD
Operating Room. . . . . Cindy Danko
Pediatric Ambulatory Care . . . . . . Ellis Avner, MD
Pediatric In-Patient Care . . . . Ellis Avner, MD
Radiology. . . . . Baz Debaz, MD

Measure	Cases	This Hosp.	State Avg.	U.S. Avg.
Heart Attack Care				
ACE Inhibitor or ARB for LVSD	97	94%	97%	96%
Aspirin at Arrival	181	100%	99%	99%
Aspirin at Discharge	439	99%	99%	98%
Beta Blocker at Discharge	424	100%	99%	98%
Fibrinolytic Medication Timing	0	-	14%	55%
PCI Within 90 Minutes of Arrival	28	86%	92%	90%
Smoking Cessation Advice	154	100%	100%	99%
Chest Pain/Possible Heart Attack Care				
Aspirin at Arrival[1]	5	100%	96%	95%
Median Time to ECG (minutes)[1]	5	0	7	8
Median Time to Transfer (minutes)[5]	0	-	61	61
Fibrinolytic Medication Timing[5]	0	-	47%	54%
Heart Failure Care				
ACE Inhibitor or ARB for LVSD	308	97%	96%	94%
Discharge Instructions	667	93%	91%	88%
Evaluation of LVS Function	795	100%	99%	98%
Smoking Cessation Advice	143	100%	99%	98%
Pneumonia Care				
Appropriate Initial Antibiotic	135	95%	92%	92%
Blood Culture Timing	246	96%	96%	96%
Influenza Vaccine	193	82%	93%	91%
Initial Antibiotic Timing	284	88%	96%	95%
Pneumococcal Vaccine	257	91%	95%	93%
Smoking Cessation Advice	138	99%	98%	97%
Surgical Care Improvement Project				
Appropriate VTP Within 24 Hours[2]	251	99%	92%	92%
Appropriate Hair Removal[2]	785	99%	100%	99%
Appropriate Beta Blocker Usage[2]	281	99%	94%	93%
Controlled Postoperative Blood Glucose[2]	162	95%	94%	93%
Prophylactic Antibiotic Timing[2]	518	99%	97%	97%
Prophylactic Antibiotic Timing (Outpatient)	678	94%	91%	92%
Prophylactic Antibiotic Selection[2]	524	98%	98%	97%
Prophylactic Antibiotic Select. (Outpatient)	670	88%	94%	94%
Prophylactic Antibiotic Stopped[2]	502	93%	95%	94%
Recommended VTP Ordered[2]	251	99%	94%	94%
Urinary Catheter Removal[2]	210	87%	91%	90%
Children's Asthma Care				
Received Systemic Corticosteroids	378	99%	-	100%
Received Home Management Plan	380	95%	-	71%
Received Reliever Medication	380	100%	-	100%
Use of Medical Imaging				
Combination Abdominal CT Scan	2,483	0.604	0.164	0.191
Combination Chest CT Scan	2,916	0.007	0.038	0.054
Follow-up Mammogram/Ultrasound	1,589	15.5%	8.4%	8.4%
MRI for Low Back Pain	360	25.8%	30.2%	32.7%
Survey of Patients' Hospital Experiences				
Area Around Room 'Always' Quiet at Night	300+	47%	-	58%
Doctors 'Always' Communicated Well	300+	75%	-	80%
Home Recovery Information Given	300+	82%	-	82%
Hospital Given 9 or 10 on 10 Point Scale	300+	69%	-	67%
Meds 'Always' Explained Before Given	300+	59%	-	60%
Nurses 'Always' Communicated Well	300+	75%	-	76%
Pain 'Always' Well Controlled	300+	66%	-	69%
Room and Bathroom 'Always' Clean	300+	62%	-	71%
Timely Help 'Always' Received	300+	55%	-	64%
Would Definitely Recommend Hospital	300+	76%	-	69%

Mercer County Joint Township Community Hospital

800 West Main Street Phone: 419-678-4843
Coldwater, OH 45828 Fax: 419-678-3271
Type: Acute Care Hospitals Emergency Services: Yes
Ownership: Govt - Hospital Dist/Auth Beds: 76

Key Personnel:
CEO/President. . . . . Terrance Padden
Chief of Medical Staff . . . . Franklin Holzer
Quality Assurance . . . . Karen Smalley
Emergency Room . . . . Ross Warren, DO

Measure	Cases	This Hosp.	State Avg.	U.S. Avg.
Heart Attack Care				
ACE Inhibitor or ARB for LVSD	0	-	97%	96%
Aspirin at Arrival[1]	5	100%	99%	99%
Aspirin at Discharge[1]	4	75%	99%	98%
Beta Blocker at Discharge[1]	4	100%	99%	98%
Fibrinolytic Medication Timing	0	-	14%	55%
PCI Within 90 Minutes of Arrival	0	-	92%	90%
Smoking Cessation Advice[1]	1	100%	100%	99%
Chest Pain/Possible Heart Attack Care				
Aspirin at Arrival	83	100%	96%	95%
Median Time to ECG (minutes)	84	8	7	8
Median Time to Transfer (minutes)[1]	9	75	61	61
Fibrinolytic Medication Timing[1]	4	75%	47%	54%
Heart Failure Care				
ACE Inhibitor or ARB for LVSD	29	97%	96%	94%
Discharge Instructions	33	100%	91%	88%
Evaluation of LVS Function	54	100%	99%	98%
Smoking Cessation Advice[1]	4	75%	99%	98%
Pneumonia Care				
Appropriate Initial Antibiotic	67	93%	92%	92%
Blood Culture Timing	78	94%	96%	96%
Influenza Vaccine	54	98%	93%	91%
Initial Antibiotic Timing	80	100%	96%	95%
Pneumococcal Vaccine	74	96%	95%	93%
Smoking Cessation Advice[1]	17	88%	98%	97%
Surgical Care Improvement Project				
Appropriate VTP Within 24 Hours	50	92%	92%	92%
Appropriate Hair Removal	131	99%	100%	99%
Appropriate Beta Blocker Usage	28	93%	94%	93%
Controlled Postoperative Blood Glucose	0	-	94%	93%
Prophylactic Antibiotic Timing	96	91%	97%	97%
Prophylactic Antibiotic Timing (Outpatient)	35	71%	91%	92%
Prophylactic Antibiotic Selection	96	94%	98%	97%
Prophylactic Antibiotic Select. (Outpatient)	27	85%	94%	94%
Prophylactic Antibiotic Stopped	95	94%	95%	94%
Recommended VTP Ordered	50	92%	94%	94%
Urinary Catheter Removal	28	89%	91%	90%
Children's Asthma Care				
Received Systemic Corticosteroids	-	-	-	100%
Received Home Management Plan	-	-	-	71%
Received Reliever Medication	-	-	-	100%
Use of Medical Imaging				
Combination Abdominal CT Scan	254	0.142	0.164	0.191
Combination Chest CT Scan	154	0.013	0.038	0.054
Follow-up Mammogram/Ultrasound	435	14.0%	8.4%	8.4%
MRI for Low Back Pain	67	35.8%	30.2%	32.7%
Survey of Patients' Hospital Experiences				
Area Around Room 'Always' Quiet at Night	(a)	50%	-	58%
Doctors 'Always' Communicated Well	(a)	80%	-	80%
Home Recovery Information Given	(a)	82%	-	82%
Hospital Given 9 or 10 on 10 Point Scale	(a)	71%	-	67%
Meds 'Always' Explained Before Given	(a)	60%	-	60%
Nurses 'Always' Communicated Well	(a)	81%	-	76%
Pain 'Always' Well Controlled	(a)	73%	-	69%
Room and Bathroom 'Always' Clean	(a)	79%	-	71%
Timely Help 'Always' Received	(a)	75%	-	64%
Would Definitely Recommend Hospital	(a)	75%	-	69%

NOTE: Hospital profiles are in alphabetical order by state, then city, then hospital within the city; Rankings exclude hospitals with less than 25 cases except for patient surveys which excludes hospitals with less than 100 cases; (a) 100–299 cases; (1) The number of cases is too small to be sure how well a hospital is performing; (2) The hospital indicated that the data submitted for this measure were based on a sample of cases; (3) Data was collected during a shorter time period (fewer quarters) than the maximum possible time for this measure; (4) Suppressed for one or more quarters by CMS; (5) No data is available from the hospital for this measure; (6) Fewer than 100 patients completed the HCAHPS survey. Use these rates with caution, as the number of surveys may be too low to reliably assess hospital performance; (7) Survey results are based on less than 12 months of data; (8) Survey results are not available for this reporting period; (9) No or very few patients were eligible for the HCAHPS survey. The scores shown, if any, reflect a very small number of surveys; (10) A state average was not calculated because too few hospitals in the state submitted data; (11) There were discrepancies in the data collection process; Please refer to the User's Guide for a full explanation of data.

Doctors Hospital

5100 West Broad Street
Columbus, OH 43228
Type: Acute Care Hospitals
Ownership: Voluntary Non-Profit - Private

Phone: 614-544-1000
Fax: 614-544-1710
Emergency Services: Yes
Beds: 478

Key Personnel:

CEO/President	Kreg Gruber
Chief of Medical Staff	William Emlich, DO
Infection Control	Lee Chamberlin
Operating Room	Roberta Bannon, RN
Pediatric Ambulatory Care	Maureen Kollar, DO
Pediatric In-Patient Care	Maureen Kollar, DO
Quality Assurance	Kathy Kunkleman
Radiology	Thomas Anderson

Measure	Cases	This Hosp.	State Avg.	U.S. Avg.
Heart Attack Care				
ACE Inhibitor or ARB for LVSD	32	97%	97%	96%
Aspirin at Arrival	175	100%	99%	99%
Aspirin at Discharge	195	99%	99%	98%
Beta Blocker at Discharge	192	100%	99%	98%
Fibrinolytic Medication Timing	0	-	14%	55%
PCI Within 90 Minutes of Arrival	37	97%	92%	90%
Smoking Cessation Advice	98	100%	100%	99%
Chest Pain/Possible Heart Attack Care				
Aspirin at Arrival[1]	21	81%	96%	95%
Median Time to ECG (minutes)[1]	21	3	7	8
Median Time to Transfer (minutes)[5]	0	-	61	61
Fibrinolytic Medication Timing[3]	0	-	47%	54%
Heart Failure Care				
ACE Inhibitor or ARB for LVSD	89	97%	96%	94%
Discharge Instructions	180	98%	91%	88%
Evaluation of LVS Function	158	100%	99%	98%
Smoking Cessation Advice	44	100%	99%	98%
Pneumonia Care				
Appropriate Initial Antibiotic	182	97%	92%	92%
Blood Culture Timing	183	97%	96%	96%
Influenza Vaccine	176	90%	93%	91%
Initial Antibiotic Timing	277	98%	96%	95%
Pneumococcal Vaccine	177	97%	95%	93%
Smoking Cessation Advice	155	100%	98%	97%
Surgical Care Improvement Project				
Appropriate VTP Within 24 Hours[2]	137	99%	92%	92%
Appropriate Hair Removal[2]	523	100%	100%	99%
Appropriate Beta Blocker Usage[2]	146	97%	94%	93%
Controlled Postoperative Blood Glucose[2]	94	99%	94%	93%
Prophylactic Antibiotic Timing[2]	387	99%	97%	97%
Prophylactic Antibiotic Timing (Outpatient)	201	92%	91%	92%
Prophylactic Antibiotic Selection[2]	391	98%	98%	97%
Prophylactic Antibiotic Select. (Outpatient)	189	98%	94%	94%
Prophylactic Antibiotic Stopped[2]	375	99%	95%	94%
Recommended VTP Ordered[2]	137	99%	94%	94%
Urinary Catheter Removal[2]	122	98%	91%	90%
Children's Asthma Care				
Received Systemic Corticosteroids	-	-	-	100%
Received Home Management Plan	-	-	-	71%
Received Reliever Medication	-	-	-	100%
Use of Medical Imaging				
Combination Abdominal CT Scan	498	0.074	0.164	0.191
Combination Chest CT Scan	391	0.013	0.038	0.054
Follow-up Mammogram/Ultrasound	582	6.7%	8.4%	8.4%
MRI for Low Back Pain	96	17.7%	30.2%	32.7%
Survey of Patients' Hospital Experiences				
Area Around Room 'Always' Quiet at Night	300+	58%	-	58%
Doctors 'Always' Communicated Well	300+	79%	-	80%
Home Recovery Information Given	300+	82%	-	82%
Hospital Given 9 or 10 on 10 Point Scale	300+	72%	-	67%
Meds 'Always' Explained Before Given	300+	64%	-	60%
Nurses 'Always' Communicated Well	300+	81%	-	76%
Pain 'Always' Well Controlled	300+	69%	-	69%
Room and Bathroom 'Always' Clean	300+	68%	-	71%
Timely Help 'Always' Received	300+	69%	-	64%
Would Definitely Recommend Hospital	300+	73%	-	69%

Grant Medical Center

111 South Grant Avenue
Columbus, OH 43215
URL: www.ohiohealth.com
Type: Acute Care Hospitals
Ownership: Voluntary Non-Profit - Church

Phone: 614-566-9978
Fax: 614-566-8045

Emergency Services: Yes
Beds: 337

Key Personnel:

CEO/President	Karen Connors

Measure	Cases	This Hosp.	State Avg.	U.S. Avg.
Heart Attack Care				
ACE Inhibitor or ARB for LVSD	41	100%	97%	96%
Aspirin at Arrival	179	100%	99%	99%
Aspirin at Discharge	306	100%	99%	98%
Beta Blocker at Discharge	306	99%	99%	98%
Fibrinolytic Medication Timing	0	-	14%	55%
PCI Within 90 Minutes of Arrival	42	93%	92%	90%
Smoking Cessation Advice	138	100%	100%	99%
Chest Pain/Possible Heart Attack Care				
Aspirin at Arrival[1]	1	100%	96%	95%
Median Time to ECG (minutes)[1]	1	10	7	8
Median Time to Transfer (minutes)[5]	0	-	61	61
Fibrinolytic Medication Timing[5]	0	-	47%	54%
Heart Failure Care				
ACE Inhibitor or ARB for LVSD[2]	129	99%	96%	94%
Discharge Instructions[2]	266	100%	91%	88%
Evaluation of LVS Function[2]	306	100%	99%	98%
Smoking Cessation Advice[2]	76	100%	99%	98%
Pneumonia Care				
Appropriate Initial Antibiotic[2]	91	98%	92%	92%
Blood Culture Timing[2]	105	99%	96%	96%
Influenza Vaccine[2]	68	96%	93%	91%
Initial Antibiotic Timing[2]	151	97%	96%	95%
Pneumococcal Vaccine[2]	75	100%	95%	93%
Smoking Cessation Advice[2]	102	100%	98%	97%
Surgical Care Improvement Project				
Appropriate VTP Within 24 Hours[2]	188	98%	92%	92%
Appropriate Hair Removal[2]	886	100%	100%	99%
Appropriate Beta Blocker Usage[2]	265	100%	94%	93%
Controlled Postoperative Blood Glucose[2]	180	97%	94%	93%
Prophylactic Antibiotic Timing[2]	693	100%	97%	97%
Prophylactic Antibiotic Timing (Outpatient)	627	97%	91%	92%
Prophylactic Antibiotic Selection[2]	699	99%	98%	97%
Prophylactic Antibiotic Select. (Outpatient)	616	97%	94%	94%
Prophylactic Antibiotic Stopped[2]	676	99%	95%	94%
Recommended VTP Ordered[2]	188	100%	94%	94%
Urinary Catheter Removal[2]	218	98%	91%	90%
Children's Asthma Care				
Received Systemic Corticosteroids	-	-	-	100%
Received Home Management Plan	-	-	-	71%
Received Reliever Medication	-	-	-	100%
Use of Medical Imaging				
Combination Abdominal CT Scan	658	0.032	0.164	0.191
Combination Chest CT Scan	441	0.009	0.038	0.054
Follow-up Mammogram/Ultrasound	485	10.1%	8.4%	8.4%
MRI for Low Back Pain	122	23.0%	30.2%	32.7%
Survey of Patients' Hospital Experiences				
Area Around Room 'Always' Quiet at Night	300+	51%	-	58%
Doctors 'Always' Communicated Well	300+	79%	-	80%
Home Recovery Information Given	300+	87%	-	82%
Hospital Given 9 or 10 on 10 Point Scale	300+	68%	-	67%
Meds 'Always' Explained Before Given	300+	61%	-	60%
Nurses 'Always' Communicated Well	300+	78%	-	76%
Pain 'Always' Well Controlled	300+	70%	-	69%
Room and Bathroom 'Always' Clean	300+	70%	-	71%
Timely Help 'Always' Received	300+	62%	-	64%
Would Definitely Recommend Hospital	300+	74%	-	69%

Mount Carmel Health

793 West State Street
Columbus, OH 43222
URL: www.mountcarmelhealth.com
Type: Acute Care Hospitals
Ownership: Voluntary Non-Profit - Other

Phone: 614-546-4533
Fax: 614-234-0456

Emergency Services: Yes
Beds: 523

Key Personnel:

CEO/President	Jay Kasey
Chief of Medical Staff	Edward Brand, MD
Infection Control	Carol Elder
Operating Room	Vicki Carpenter
Pediatric Ambulatory Care	Craig Anderson, MD
Pediatric In-Patient Care	Craig Anderson, MD
Quality Assurance	Anita Morrison
Radiology	David Paull, MD

Measure	Cases	This Hosp.	State Avg.	U.S. Avg.
Heart Attack Care				
ACE Inhibitor or ARB for LVSD	133	100%	97%	96%
Aspirin at Arrival	688	100%	99%	99%
Aspirin at Discharge	855	100%	99%	98%
Beta Blocker at Discharge	819	100%	99%	98%
Fibrinolytic Medication Timing	0	-	14%	55%
PCI Within 90 Minutes of Arrival	170	96%	92%	90%
Smoking Cessation Advice	355	100%	100%	99%
Chest Pain/Possible Heart Attack Care				
Aspirin at Arrival[1]	5	100%	96%	95%
Median Time to ECG (minutes)[1]	6	0	7	8
Median Time to Transfer (minutes)[5]	0	-	61	61
Fibrinolytic Medication Timing[5]	0	-	47%	54%
Heart Failure Care				
ACE Inhibitor or ARB for LVSD	411	100%	96%	94%
Discharge Instructions	956	86%	91%	88%
Evaluation of LVS Function	1,208	100%	99%	98%
Smoking Cessation Advice	194	100%	99%	98%
Pneumonia Care				
Appropriate Initial Antibiotic[2]	240	95%	92%	92%
Blood Culture Timing[2]	383	96%	96%	96%
Influenza Vaccine[2]	218	85%	93%	91%
Initial Antibiotic Timing[2]	344	95%	96%	95%
Pneumococcal Vaccine[2]	306	89%	95%	93%
Smoking Cessation Advice[2]	150	99%	98%	97%
Surgical Care Improvement Project				
Appropriate VTP Within 24 Hours[2]	208	92%	92%	92%
Appropriate Hair Removal[2]	1,104	100%	100%	99%
Appropriate Beta Blocker Usage[2]	427	93%	94%	93%
Controlled Postoperative Blood Glucose[2]	206	96%	94%	93%
Prophylactic Antibiotic Timing[2]	839	98%	97%	97%
Prophylactic Antibiotic Timing (Outpatient)	758	97%	91%	92%
Prophylactic Antibiotic Selection[2]	851	98%	98%	97%
Prophylactic Antibiotic Select. (Outpatient)	746	93%	94%	94%
Prophylactic Antibiotic Stopped[2]	818	98%	95%	94%
Recommended VTP Ordered[2]	209	96%	94%	94%
Urinary Catheter Removal[2]	344	95%	91%	90%
Children's Asthma Care				
Received Systemic Corticosteroids	-	-	-	100%
Received Home Management Plan	-	-	-	71%
Received Reliever Medication	-	-	-	100%
Use of Medical Imaging				
Combination Abdominal CT Scan	2,279	0.050	0.164	0.191
Combination Chest CT Scan	1,181	0.018	0.038	0.054
Follow-up Mammogram/Ultrasound	3,959	6.4%	8.4%	8.4%
MRI for Low Back Pain	439	33.7%	30.2%	32.7%
Survey of Patients' Hospital Experiences				
Area Around Room 'Always' Quiet at Night	300+	50%	-	58%
Doctors 'Always' Communicated Well	300+	80%	-	80%
Home Recovery Information Given	300+	83%	-	82%
Hospital Given 9 or 10 on 10 Point Scale	300+	68%	-	67%
Meds 'Always' Explained Before Given	300+	57%	-	60%
Nurses 'Always' Communicated Well	300+	76%	-	76%
Pain 'Always' Well Controlled	300+	69%	-	69%
Room and Bathroom 'Always' Clean	300+	64%	-	71%
Timely Help 'Always' Received	300+	60%	-	64%
Would Definitely Recommend Hospital	300+	72%	-	69%

NOTE: Hospital profiles are in alphabetical order by state, then city, then hospital within the city; Rankings exclude hospitals with less than 25 cases except for patient surveys which excludes hospitals with less than 100 cases; (a) 100–299 cases; (1) The number of cases is too small to be sure how well a hospital is performing; (2) The hospital indicated that the data submitted for this measure were based on a sample of cases; (3) Data was collected during a shorter time period (fewer quarters) than the maximum possible time for this measure; (4) Suppressed for one or more quarters by CMS; (5) No data is available from the hospital for this measure; (6) Fewer than 100 patients completed the HCAHPS survey. Use these rates with caution, as the number of surveys may be too low to reliably assess hospital performance; (7) Survey results are based on less than 12 months of data; (8) Survey results are not available for this reporting period; (9) No or very few patients were eligible for the HCAHPS survey. The scores shown, if any, reflect a very small number of surveys; (10) A state average was not calculated because too few hospitals in the state submitted data; (11) There were discrepancies in the data collection process; Please refer to the User's Guide for a full explanation of data.

Ohio State University Hospitals

410 West 10th Avenue	Phone: 614-293-9700
Columbus, OH 43210	Fax: 614-293-3080
URL: www.jamesline.com
Type: Acute Care Hospitals	Emergency Services: Yes
Ownership: Government - State	Beds: 156

Key Personnel:
Chief of Medical Staff.......... William B Farrar
Radiology.................. David Bates

Measure	Cases	This Hosp.	State Avg.	U.S. Avg.
Heart Attack Care				
ACE Inhibitor or ARB for LVSD[2]	66	97%	97%	96%
Aspirin at Arrival[2]	120	99%	99%	99%
Aspirin at Discharge[2]	279	99%	99%	98%
Beta Blocker at Discharge[2]	284	100%	99%	98%
Fibrinolytic Medication Timing[2]	0	-	14%	55%
PCI Within 90 Minutes of Arrival[1,2]	12	83%	92%	90%
Smoking Cessation Advice[2]	110	100%	100%	99%
Chest Pain/Possible Heart Attack Care				
Aspirin at Arrival[5]	0	-	96%	95%
Median Time to ECG (minutes)[5]	0	-	7	8
Median Time to Transfer (minutes)[5]	0	-	61	61
Fibrinolytic Medication Timing[5]	0	-	47%	54%
Heart Failure Care				
ACE Inhibitor or ARB for LVSD[2]	139	99%	96%	94%
Discharge Instructions[2]	260	100%	91%	88%
Evaluation of LVS Function[2]	295	100%	99%	98%
Smoking Cessation Advice[2]	76	100%	99%	98%
Pneumonia Care				
Appropriate Initial Antibiotic[2]	51	96%	92%	92%
Blood Culture Timing[2]	95	94%	96%	96%
Influenza Vaccine[2]	42	90%	93%	91%
Initial Antibiotic Timing[2]	97	95%	96%	95%
Pneumococcal Vaccine[2]	56	93%	95%	93%
Smoking Cessation Advice[2]	86	100%	98%	97%
Surgical Care Improvement Project				
Appropriate VTP Within 24 Hours[2]	184	95%	92%	92%
Appropriate Hair Removal[2]	607	100%	100%	99%
Appropriate Beta Blocker Usage[2]	206	92%	94%	93%
Controlled Postoperative Blood Glucose[2]	129	98%	94%	93%
Prophylactic Antibiotic Timing[2]	385	99%	97%	97%
Prophylactic Antibiotic Timing (Outpatient)	377	97%	91%	92%
Prophylactic Antibiotic Selection[2]	396	98%	98%	97%
Prophylactic Antibiotic Select. (Outpatient)	370	97%	94%	94%
Prophylactic Antibiotic Stopped[2]	371	98%	95%	94%
Recommended VTP Ordered[2]	184	96%	94%	94%
Urinary Catheter Removal[2]	145	91%	91%	90%
Children's Asthma Care				
Received Systemic Corticosteroids	-	-	-	100%
Received Home Management Plan	-	-	-	71%
Received Reliever Medication	-	-	-	100%
Use of Medical Imaging				
Combination Abdominal CT Scan	1,351	0.028	0.164	0.191
Combination Chest CT Scan	1,010	0.048	0.038	0.054
Follow-up Mammogram/Ultrasound	382	7.6%	8.4%	8.4%
MRI for Low Back Pain	198	25.3%	30.2%	32.7%
Survey of Patients' Hospital Experiences				
Area Around Room 'Always' Quiet at Night	300+	53%	-	58%
Doctors 'Always' Communicated Well	300+	76%	-	80%
Home Recovery Information Given	300+	84%	-	82%
Hospital Given 9 or 10 on 10 Point Scale	300+	71%	-	67%
Meds 'Always' Explained Before Given	300+	59%	-	60%
Nurses 'Always' Communicated Well	300+	77%	-	76%
Pain 'Always' Well Controlled	300+	70%	-	69%
Room and Bathroom 'Always' Clean	300+	68%	-	71%
Timely Help 'Always' Received	300+	62%	-	64%
Would Definitely Recommend Hospital	300+	73%	-	69%

Riverside Methodist Hospital

3535 Olentangy River Rd	Phone: 614-566-5000
Columbus, OH 43214	Fax: 614-566-6760
URL: www.ohiohealth.com
Type: Acute Care Hospitals	Emergency Services: Yes
Ownership: Voluntary Non-Profit - Private	Beds: 1,049

Key Personnel:
CEO/President............... Bruce Hagen
Cardiac Laboratory............ Marty Yoder, RN
Chief of Medical Staff.......... Mark Montoney, MD
Coronary Care............... Linda Wagner
Operating Room.............. Mary Spyros
Pediatric Ambulatory Care...... Patrick Wall, MD
Pediatric In-Patient Care....... Patrick Wall, MD
Radiology................... Kyle Sharp

Measure	Cases	This Hosp.	State Avg.	U.S. Avg.
Heart Attack Care				
ACE Inhibitor or ARB for LVSD[2]	125	97%	97%	96%
Aspirin at Arrival[2]	296	98%	99%	99%
Aspirin at Discharge[2]	581	99%	99%	98%
Beta Blocker at Discharge[2]	572	98%	99%	98%
Fibrinolytic Medication Timing[2]	0	-	14%	55%
PCI Within 90 Minutes of Arrival[2]	87	98%	92%	90%
Smoking Cessation Advice[2]	209	100%	100%	99%
Chest Pain/Possible Heart Attack Care				
Aspirin at Arrival[1,3]	2	100%	96%	95%
Median Time to ECG (minutes)[1,3]	2	2	7	8
Median Time to Transfer (minutes)[5]	0	-	61	61
Fibrinolytic Medication Timing[5]	0	-	47%	54%
Heart Failure Care				
ACE Inhibitor or ARB for LVSD[2]	252	98%	96%	94%
Discharge Instructions[2]	487	100%	91%	88%
Evaluation of LVS Function[2]	648	100%	99%	98%
Smoking Cessation Advice[2]	100	100%	99%	98%
Pneumonia Care				
Appropriate Initial Antibiotic[2]	212	95%	92%	92%
Blood Culture Timing[2]	322	99%	96%	96%
Influenza Vaccine[2]	181	93%	93%	91%
Initial Antibiotic Timing[2]	288	97%	96%	95%
Pneumococcal Vaccine[2]	307	95%	95%	93%
Smoking Cessation Advice[2]	153	100%	98%	97%
Surgical Care Improvement Project				
Appropriate VTP Within 24 Hours[2]	880	98%	92%	92%
Appropriate Hair Removal[2]	3,209	100%	100%	99%
Appropriate Beta Blocker Usage[2]	1,072	97%	94%	93%
Controlled Postoperative Blood Glucose[2]	527	95%	94%	93%
Prophylactic Antibiotic Timing[2]	2,123	99%	97%	97%
Prophylactic Antibiotic Timing (Outpatient)	806	95%	91%	92%
Prophylactic Antibiotic Selection[2]	2,151	99%	98%	97%
Prophylactic Antibiotic Select. (Outpatient)	780	98%	94%	94%
Prophylactic Antibiotic Stopped[2]	2,064	97%	95%	94%
Recommended VTP Ordered[2]	881	99%	94%	94%
Urinary Catheter Removal	1,408	93%	91%	90%
Children's Asthma Care				
Received Systemic Corticosteroids	-	-	-	100%
Received Home Management Plan	-	-	-	71%
Received Reliever Medication	-	-	-	100%
Use of Medical Imaging				
Combination Abdominal CT Scan	2,908	0.113	0.164	0.191
Combination Chest CT Scan	2,735	0.056	0.038	0.054
Follow-up Mammogram/Ultrasound	5,816	8.5%	8.4%	8.4%
MRI for Low Back Pain	537	30.5%	30.2%	32.7%
Survey of Patients' Hospital Experiences				
Area Around Room 'Always' Quiet at Night	300+	48%	-	58%
Doctors 'Always' Communicated Well	300+	79%	-	80%
Home Recovery Information Given	300+	85%	-	82%
Hospital Given 9 or 10 on 10 Point Scale	300+	74%	-	67%
Meds 'Always' Explained Before Given	300+	62%	-	60%
Nurses 'Always' Communicated Well	300+	79%	-	76%
Pain 'Always' Well Controlled	300+	71%	-	69%
Room and Bathroom 'Always' Clean	300+	66%	-	71%
Timely Help 'Always' Received	300+	61%	-	64%
Would Definitely Recommend Hospital	300+	83%	-	69%

The Woods at Parkside

349 Olde Ridenour Road	Phone: 614-471-2552
Columbus, OH 43230	Fax: 614-471-0167
URL: www.thewoodsatparkside.com
Type: Acute Care Hospitals	Emergency Services: No
Ownership: Proprietary	Beds: 44

Key Personnel:
Chief of Medical Staff.......... Dr Harry Nguyen

Measure	Cases	This Hosp.	State Avg.	U.S. Avg.
Heart Attack Care				
ACE Inhibitor or ARB for LVSD[5]	0	-	97%	96%
Aspirin at Arrival[5]	0	-	99%	99%
Aspirin at Discharge[5]	0	-	99%	98%
Beta Blocker at Discharge[5]	0	-	99%	98%
Fibrinolytic Medication Timing[5]	0	-	14%	55%
PCI Within 90 Minutes of Arrival[5]	0	-	92%	90%
Smoking Cessation Advice[5]	0	-	100%	99%
Chest Pain/Possible Heart Attack Care				
Aspirin at Arrival[5]	0	-	96%	95%
Median Time to ECG (minutes)[5]	0	-	7	8
Median Time to Transfer (minutes)[5]	0	-	61	61
Fibrinolytic Medication Timing[5]	0	-	47%	54%
Heart Failure Care				
ACE Inhibitor or ARB for LVSD[5]	0	-	96%	94%
Discharge Instructions[5]	0	-	91%	88%
Evaluation of LVS Function[5]	0	-	99%	98%
Smoking Cessation Advice[5]	0	-	99%	98%
Pneumonia Care				
Appropriate Initial Antibiotic[5]	0	-	92%	92%
Blood Culture Timing[5]	0	-	96%	96%
Influenza Vaccine[5]	0	-	93%	91%
Initial Antibiotic Timing[5]	0	-	96%	95%
Pneumococcal Vaccine[5]	0	-	95%	93%
Smoking Cessation Advice[5]	0	-	98%	97%
Surgical Care Improvement Project				
Appropriate VTP Within 24 Hours[5]	0	-	92%	92%
Appropriate Hair Removal[5]	0	-	100%	99%
Appropriate Beta Blocker Usage[5]	0	-	94%	93%
Controlled Postoperative Blood Glucose[5]	0	-	94%	93%
Prophylactic Antibiotic Timing[5]	0	-	97%	97%
Prophylactic Antibiotic Timing (Outpatient)[5]	0	-	91%	92%
Prophylactic Antibiotic Selection[5]	0	-	98%	97%
Prophylactic Antibiotic Select. (Outpatient)[5]	0	-	94%	94%
Prophylactic Antibiotic Stopped[5]	0	-	95%	94%
Recommended VTP Ordered[5]	0	-	94%	94%
Urinary Catheter Removal[5]	0	-	91%	90%
Children's Asthma Care				
Received Systemic Corticosteroids	-	-	-	100%
Received Home Management Plan	-	-	-	71%
Received Reliever Medication	-	-	-	100%
Use of Medical Imaging				
Combination Abdominal CT Scan[5]	0	-	0.164	0.191
Combination Chest CT Scan[5]	0	-	0.038	0.054
Follow-up Mammogram/Ultrasound[5]	0	-	8.4%	8.4%
MRI for Low Back Pain[5]	0	-	30.2%	32.7%
Survey of Patients' Hospital Experiences				
Area Around Room 'Always' Quiet at Night[9]	-	-	-	58%
Doctors 'Always' Communicated Well[9]	-	-	-	80%
Home Recovery Information Given[9]	-	-	-	82%
Hospital Given 9 or 10 on 10 Point Scale[9]	-	-	-	67%
Meds 'Always' Explained Before Given[9]	-	-	-	60%
Nurses 'Always' Communicated Well[9]	-	-	-	76%
Pain 'Always' Well Controlled[9]	-	-	-	69%
Room and Bathroom 'Always' Clean[9]	-	-	-	71%
Timely Help 'Always' Received[9]	-	-	-	64%
Would Definitely Recommend Hospital[9]	-	-	-	69%

NOTE: Hospital profiles are in alphabetical order by state, then city, then hospital within the city; Rankings exclude hospitals with less than 25 cases except for patient surveys which excludes hospitals with less than 100 cases; (a) 100–299 cases; (1) The number of cases is too small to be sure how well a hospital is performing; (2) The hospital indicated that the data submitted for this measure were based on a sample of cases; (3) Data was collected during a shorter time period (fewer quarters) than the maximum possible time for this measure; (4) Suppressed for one or more quarters by CMS; (5) No data is available from the hospital for this measure; (6) Fewer than 100 patients completed the HCAHPS survey. Use these rates with caution, as the number of surveys may be too low to reliably assess hospital performance; (7) Survey results are based on less than 12 months of data; (8) Survey results are not available for this reporting period; (9) No or very few patients were eligible for the HCAHPS survey. The scores shown, if any, reflect a very small number of surveys; (10) A state average was not calculated because too few hospitals in the state submitted data; (11) There were discrepancies in the data collection process; Please refer to the User's Guide for a full explanation of data.

Lake Health

7590 Auburn Road Phone: 440-953-9600
Concord, OH 44077
Type: Acute Care Hospitals Emergency Services: Yes
Ownership: Voluntary Non-Profit - Private

Measure	Cases	This Hosp.	State Avg.	U.S. Avg.
Heart Attack Care				
ACE Inhibitor or ARB for LVSD[2]	51	100%	97%	96%
Aspirin at Arrival[2]	259	98%	99%	99%
Aspirin at Discharge[2]	271	99%	99%	98%
Beta Blocker at Discharge[2]	280	100%	99%	98%
Fibrinolytic Medication Timing[2]	0	-	14%	55%
PCI Within 90 Minutes of Arrival[2]	50	90%	92%	90%
Smoking Cessation Advice[2]	97	98%	100%	99%
Chest Pain/Possible Heart Attack Care				
Aspirin at Arrival	48	94%	96%	95%
Median Time to ECG (minutes)	49	6	7	8
Median Time to Transfer (minutes)[1,3]	2	79	61	61
Fibrinolytic Medication Timing[3]	0	-	47%	54%
Heart Failure Care				
ACE Inhibitor or ARB for LVSD[2]	119	91%	96%	94%
Discharge Instructions[2]	371	85%	91%	88%
Evaluation of LVS Function[2]	511	98%	99%	98%
Smoking Cessation Advice[2]	82	99%	99%	98%
Pneumonia Care				
Appropriate Initial Antibiotic[2]	284	88%	92%	92%
Blood Culture Timing[2]	333	91%	96%	96%
Influenza Vaccine	273	97%	93%	91%
Initial Antibiotic Timing[2]	394	92%	96%	95%
Pneumococcal Vaccine[2]	388	95%	95%	93%
Smoking Cessation Advice[2]	147	93%	98%	97%
Surgical Care Improvement Project				
Appropriate VTP Within 24 Hours[2]	146	68%	92%	92%
Appropriate Hair Removal[2]	530	99%	100%	99%
Appropriate Beta Blocker Usage[2]	201	81%	94%	93%
Controlled Postoperative Blood Glucose[2]	99	91%	94%	93%
Prophylactic Antibiotic Timing[2]	377	92%	97%	97%
Prophylactic Antibiotic Timing (Outpatient)	377	85%	91%	92%
Prophylactic Antibiotic Selection[2]	381	96%	98%	97%
Prophylactic Antibiotic Select. (Outpatient)	354	96%	94%	94%
Prophylactic Antibiotic Stopped[2]	355	82%	95%	94%
Recommended VTP Ordered[2]	146	72%	94%	94%
Urinary Catheter Removal[2]	97	76%	91%	90%
Children's Asthma Care				
Received Systemic Corticosteroids	-	-	-	100%
Received Home Management Plan	-	-	-	71%
Received Reliever Medication	-	-	-	100%
Use of Medical Imaging				
Combination Abdominal CT Scan	1,628	0.045	0.164	0.191
Combination Chest CT Scan	1,310	0.004	0.038	0.054
Follow-up Mammogram/Ultrasound	2,629	7.2%	8.4%	8.4%
MRI for Low Back Pain	171	38.0%	30.2%	32.7%
Survey of Patients' Hospital Experiences				
Area Around Room 'Always' Quiet at Night	300+	49%	-	58%
Doctors 'Always' Communicated Well	300+	74%	-	80%
Home Recovery Information Given	300+	84%	-	82%
Hospital Given 9 or 10 on 10 Point Scale	300+	63%	-	67%
Meds 'Always' Explained Before Given	300+	57%	-	60%
Nurses 'Always' Communicated Well	300+	73%	-	76%
Pain 'Always' Well Controlled	300+	66%	-	69%
Room and Bathroom 'Always' Clean	300+	70%	-	71%
Timely Help 'Always' Received	300+	58%	-	64%
Would Definitely Recommend Hospital	300+	67%	-	69%

University Hospitals Conneaut Medical Center

158 West Main Road Phone: 440-593-1131
Conneaut, OH 44030 Fax: 440-593-5050
Type: Critical Access Hospitals Emergency Services: Yes
Ownership: Voluntary Non-Profit - Other Beds: 86

Key Personnel:
CEO/President. . . . . William Lawrence

Measure	Cases	This Hosp.	State Avg.	U.S. Avg.
Heart Attack Care				
ACE Inhibitor or ARB for LVSD[3]	0	-	97%	96%
Aspirin at Arrival[1,3]	2	100%	99%	99%
Aspirin at Discharge[1,3]	1	100%	99%	98%
Beta Blocker at Discharge[1,3]	3	100%	99%	98%
Fibrinolytic Medication Timing[3]	0	-	14%	55%
PCI Within 90 Minutes of Arrival[3]	0	-	92%	90%
Smoking Cessation Advice[1,3]	1	100%	100%	99%
Chest Pain/Possible Heart Attack Care				
Aspirin at Arrival	56	100%	96%	95%
Median Time to ECG (minutes)	60	7	7	8
Median Time to Transfer (minutes)[1,3]	2	145	61	61
Fibrinolytic Medication Timing[1]	2	50%	47%	54%
Heart Failure Care				
ACE Inhibitor or ARB for LVSD[1]	6	100%	96%	94%
Discharge Instructions	25	100%	91%	88%
Evaluation of LVS Function	38	100%	99%	98%
Smoking Cessation Advice[1]	2	100%	99%	98%
Pneumonia Care				
Appropriate Initial Antibiotic	28	93%	92%	92%
Blood Culture Timing	31	100%	96%	96%
Influenza Vaccine[1]	20	100%	93%	91%
Initial Antibiotic Timing	30	100%	96%	95%
Pneumococcal Vaccine[1]	24	100%	95%	93%
Smoking Cessation Advice[1]	10	90%	98%	97%
Surgical Care Improvement Project				
Appropriate VTP Within 24 Hours[1,3]	5	100%	92%	92%
Appropriate Hair Removal[3]	92	99%	100%	99%
Appropriate Beta Blocker Usage[3]	26	100%	94%	93%
Controlled Postoperative Blood Glucose[3]	0	-	94%	93%
Prophylactic Antibiotic Timing[3]	76	99%	97%	97%
Prophylactic Antibiotic Timing (Outpatient)[1]	6	83%	91%	92%
Prophylactic Antibiotic Selection[3]	76	100%	98%	97%
Prophylactic Antibiotic Select. (Outpatient)[1]	5	100%	94%	94%
Prophylactic Antibiotic Stopped[3]	75	100%	95%	94%
Recommended VTP Ordered[1,3]	5	100%	94%	94%
Urinary Catheter Removal	74	100%	91%	90%
Children's Asthma Care				
Received Systemic Corticosteroids	-	-	-	100%
Received Home Management Plan	-	-	-	71%
Received Reliever Medication	-	-	-	100%
Use of Medical Imaging				
Combination Abdominal CT Scan	178	0.146	0.164	0.191
Combination Chest CT Scan	108	0.009	0.038	0.054
Follow-up Mammogram/Ultrasound	221	4.5%	8.4%	8.4%
MRI for Low Back Pain[1]	8	12.5%	30.2%	32.7%
Survey of Patients' Hospital Experiences				
Area Around Room 'Always' Quiet at Night[11]	(a)	64%	-	58%
Doctors 'Always' Communicated Well[11]	(a)	87%	-	80%
Home Recovery Information Given[11]	(a)	86%	-	82%
Hospital Given 9 or 10 on 10 Point Scale[11]	(a)	83%	-	67%
Meds 'Always' Explained Before Given[11]	(a)	74%	-	60%
Nurses 'Always' Communicated Well[11]	(a)	87%	-	76%
Pain 'Always' Well Controlled[11]	(a)	75%	-	69%
Room and Bathroom 'Always' Clean[11]	(a)	89%	-	71%
Timely Help 'Always' Received[11]	(a)	85%	-	64%
Would Definitely Recommend Hospital[11]	(a)	82%	-	69%

Coshocton County Memorial Hospital

1460 Orange Street Phone: 740-622-6411
Coshocton, OH 43812 Fax: 740-623-4095
Type: Acute Care Hospitals Emergency Services: No
Ownership: Voluntary Non-Profit - Private Beds: 61

Key Personnel:
Chief of Medical Staff . . . . Gary Carver
Infection Control. . . . . Marjorie Erman
Operating Room. . . . . Judi Shaffer, RN
Quality Assurance . . . . Kathy Bauman, RN
Radiology. . . . . Linda J Magness, MD
Emergency Room . . . . R Patel, MD
Intensive Care Unit. . . . . Gwen Miller, RN

Measure	Cases	This Hosp.	State Avg.	U.S. Avg.
Heart Attack Care				
ACE Inhibitor or ARB for LVSD	0	-	97%	96%
Aspirin at Arrival[1]	2	100%	99%	99%
Aspirin at Discharge[1]	2	100%	99%	98%
Beta Blocker at Discharge[1]	2	100%	99%	98%
Fibrinolytic Medication Timing	0	-	14%	55%
PCI Within 90 Minutes of Arrival	0	-	92%	90%
Smoking Cessation Advice	0	-	100%	99%
Chest Pain/Possible Heart Attack Care				
Aspirin at Arrival	228	94%	96%	95%
Median Time to ECG (minutes)	236	12	7	8
Median Time to Transfer (minutes)[1]	6	78	61	61
Fibrinolytic Medication Timing[1]	4	25%	47%	54%
Heart Failure Care				
ACE Inhibitor or ARB for LVSD[1]	9	67%	96%	94%
Discharge Instructions	36	75%	91%	88%
Evaluation of LVS Function	48	96%	99%	98%
Smoking Cessation Advice[1]	6	100%	99%	98%
Pneumonia Care				
Appropriate Initial Antibiotic	30	73%	92%	92%
Blood Culture Timing	37	92%	96%	96%
Influenza Vaccine	31	87%	93%	91%
Initial Antibiotic Timing	42	93%	96%	95%
Pneumococcal Vaccine	36	94%	95%	93%
Smoking Cessation Advice[1]	15	93%	98%	97%
Surgical Care Improvement Project				
Appropriate VTP Within 24 Hours	29	72%	92%	92%
Appropriate Hair Removal	74	99%	100%	99%
Appropriate Beta Blocker Usage[1]	16	94%	94%	93%
Controlled Postoperative Blood Glucose	0	-	94%	93%
Prophylactic Antibiotic Timing	43	98%	97%	97%
Prophylactic Antibiotic Timing (Outpatient)[1]	19	74%	91%	92%
Prophylactic Antibiotic Selection	43	93%	98%	97%
Prophylactic Antibiotic Select. (Outpatient)[1]	15	80%	94%	94%
Prophylactic Antibiotic Stopped	42	81%	95%	94%
Recommended VTP Ordered	31	81%	94%	94%
Urinary Catheter Removal[1]	4	75%	91%	90%
Children's Asthma Care				
Received Systemic Corticosteroids	-	-	-	100%
Received Home Management Plan	-	-	-	71%
Received Reliever Medication	-	-	-	100%
Use of Medical Imaging				
Combination Abdominal CT Scan	315	0.098	0.164	0.191
Combination Chest CT Scan	207	0.024	0.038	0.054
Follow-up Mammogram/Ultrasound	654	9.2%	8.4%	8.4%
MRI for Low Back Pain	68	27.9%	30.2%	32.7%
Survey of Patients' Hospital Experiences				
Area Around Room 'Always' Quiet at Night	300+	47%	-	58%
Doctors 'Always' Communicated Well	300+	76%	-	80%
Home Recovery Information Given	300+	80%	-	82%
Hospital Given 9 or 10 on 10 Point Scale	300+	58%	-	67%
Meds 'Always' Explained Before Given	300+	55%	-	60%
Nurses 'Always' Communicated Well	300+	74%	-	76%
Pain 'Always' Well Controlled	300+	65%	-	69%
Room and Bathroom 'Always' Clean	300+	72%	-	71%
Timely Help 'Always' Received	300+	65%	-	64%
Would Definitely Recommend Hospital	300+	51%	-	69%

NOTE: Hospital profiles are in alphabetical order by state, then city, then hospital within the city; Rankings exclude hospitals with less than 25 cases except for patient surveys which excludes hospitals with less than 100 cases; (a) 100–299 cases; (1) The number of cases is too small to be sure how well a hospital is performing; (2) The hospital indicated that the data submitted for this measure were based on a sample of cases; (3) Data was collected during a shorter time period (fewer quarters) than the maximum possible time for this measure; (4) Suppressed for one or more quarters by CMS; (5) No data is available from the hospital for this measure; (6) Fewer than 100 patients completed the HCAHPS survey. Use these rates with caution, as the number of surveys may be too low to reliably assess hospital performance; (7) Survey results are based on less than 12 months of data; (8) Survey results are not available for this reporting period; (9) No or very few patients were eligible for the HCAHPS survey. The scores shown, if any, reflect a very small number of surveys; (10) A state average was not calculated because too few hospitals in the state submitted data; (11) There were discrepancies in the data collection process; Please refer to the User's Guide for a full explanation of data.

Edwin Shaw Rehabilitation Institute

330 Broadway East
Cuyahoga Falls, OH 44221
URL: www.akrongeneral.org
Type: Acute Care Hospitals
Ownership: Government - Local

Phone: 330-436-0910

Emergency Services: No

Measure	Cases	This Hosp.	State Avg.	U.S. Avg.
Heart Attack Care				
ACE Inhibitor or ARB for LVSD[5]	0	-	97%	96%
Aspirin at Arrival[5]	0	-	99%	99%
Aspirin at Discharge[5]	0	-	99%	98%
Beta Blocker at Discharge[5]	0	-	99%	98%
Fibrinolytic Medication Timing[5]	0	-	14%	55%
PCI Within 90 Minutes of Arrival[5]	0	-	92%	90%
Smoking Cessation Advice[5]	0	-	100%	99%
Chest Pain/Possible Heart Attack Care				
Aspirin at Arrival	-	-	96%	95%
Median Time to ECG (minutes)	-	-	7	8
Median Time to Transfer (minutes)	-	-	61	61
Fibrinolytic Medication Timing	-	-	47%	54%
Heart Failure Care				
ACE Inhibitor or ARB for LVSD[5]	0	-	96%	94%
Discharge Instructions[5]	0	-	91%	88%
Evaluation of LVS Function[5]	0	-	99%	98%
Smoking Cessation Advice[5]	0	-	99%	98%
Pneumonia Care				
Appropriate Initial Antibiotic[5]	0	-	92%	92%
Blood Culture Timing[5]	0	-	96%	96%
Influenza Vaccine[5]	0	-	93%	91%
Initial Antibiotic Timing[5]	0	-	96%	95%
Pneumococcal Vaccine[5]	0	-	95%	93%
Smoking Cessation Advice[5]	0	-	98%	97%
Surgical Care Improvement Project				
Appropriate VTP Within 24 Hours[5]	0	-	92%	92%
Appropriate Hair Removal[5]	0	-	100%	99%
Appropriate Beta Blocker Usage[5]	0	-	94%	93%
Controlled Postoperative Blood Glucose[5]	0	-	94%	93%
Prophylactic Antibiotic Timing[5]	0	-	97%	97%
Prophylactic Antibiotic Timing (Outpatient)	-	-	91%	92%
Prophylactic Antibiotic Selection[5]	0	-	98%	97%
Prophylactic Antibiotic Select. (Outpatient)	-	-	94%	94%
Prophylactic Antibiotic Stopped[5]	0	-	95%	94%
Recommended VTP Ordered[5]	0	-	94%	94%
Urinary Catheter Removal[5]	0	-	91%	90%
Children's Asthma Care				
Received Systemic Corticosteroids	-	-	-	100%
Received Home Management Plan	-	-	-	71%
Received Reliever Medication	-	-	-	100%
Use of Medical Imaging				
Combination Abdominal CT Scan	-	-	0.164	0.191
Combination Chest CT Scan	-	-	0.038	0.054
Follow-up Mammogram/Ultrasound	-	-	8.4%	8.4%
MRI for Low Back Pain	-	-	30.2%	32.7%
Survey of Patients' Hospital Experiences				
Area Around Room 'Always' Quiet at Night[9]	-	-	-	58%
Doctors 'Always' Communicated Well[9]	-	-	-	80%
Home Recovery Information Given[9]	-	-	-	82%
Hospital Given 9 or 10 on 10 Point Scale[9]	-	-	-	67%
Meds 'Always' Explained Before Given[9]	-	-	-	60%
Nurses 'Always' Communicated Well[9]	-	-	-	76%
Pain 'Always' Well Controlled[9]	-	-	-	69%
Room and Bathroom 'Always' Clean[9]	-	-	-	71%
Timely Help 'Always' Received[9]	-	-	-	64%
Would Definitely Recommend Hospital[9]	-	-	-	69%

Summa Western Reserve Hospital

1900 23rd Street
Cuyahoga Falls, OH 44223
Type: Acute Care Hospitals
Ownership: Voluntary Non-Profit - Other

Phone: 330-971-7000
Fax: 330-971-7155
Emergency Services: Yes
Beds: 257

Key Personnel:
CEO/President . . . . Kathleen Rice
Chief of Medical Staff . . . . Leroy Refer
Quality Assurance . . . . Denise Haynes
Radiology . . . . GL Classen, DO

Measure	Cases	This Hosp.	State Avg.	U.S. Avg.
Heart Attack Care				
ACE Inhibitor or ARB for LVSD[1]	1	100%	97%	96%
Aspirin at Arrival[1]	15	100%	99%	99%
Aspirin at Discharge[1]	10	90%	99%	98%
Beta Blocker at Discharge[1]	7	100%	99%	98%
Fibrinolytic Medication Timing	0	-	14%	55%
PCI Within 90 Minutes of Arrival	0	-	92%	90%
Smoking Cessation Advice[1]	3	100%	100%	99%
Chest Pain/Possible Heart Attack Care				
Aspirin at Arrival	40	92%	96%	95%
Median Time to ECG (minutes)	43	11	7	8
Median Time to Transfer (minutes)[1]	11	48	61	61
Fibrinolytic Medication Timing	0	-	47%	54%
Heart Failure Care				
ACE Inhibitor or ARB for LVSD	27	100%	96%	94%
Discharge Instructions	80	84%	91%	88%
Evaluation of LVS Function	95	94%	99%	98%
Smoking Cessation Advice[1]	9	100%	99%	98%
Pneumonia Care				
Appropriate Initial Antibiotic	111	94%	92%	92%
Blood Culture Timing	128	95%	96%	96%
Influenza Vaccine	93	94%	93%	91%
Initial Antibiotic Timing	149	100%	96%	95%
Pneumococcal Vaccine	132	87%	95%	93%
Smoking Cessation Advice	40	100%	98%	97%
Surgical Care Improvement Project				
Appropriate VTP Within 24 Hours[2]	84	81%	92%	92%
Appropriate Hair Removal[2]	261	100%	100%	99%
Appropriate Beta Blocker Usage[2]	55	82%	94%	93%
Controlled Postoperative Blood Glucose[2]	0	-	94%	93%
Prophylactic Antibiotic Timing[2]	172	95%	97%	97%
Prophylactic Antibiotic Timing (Outpatient)	122	97%	91%	92%
Prophylactic Antibiotic Selection[2]	172	100%	98%	97%
Prophylactic Antibiotic Select. (Outpatient)	118	94%	94%	94%
Prophylactic Antibiotic Stopped[2]	165	93%	95%	94%
Recommended VTP Ordered[2]	84	88%	94%	94%
Urinary Catheter Removal[2]	53	89%	91%	90%
Children's Asthma Care				
Received Systemic Corticosteroids	-	-	-	100%
Received Home Management Plan	-	-	-	71%
Received Reliever Medication	-	-	-	100%
Use of Medical Imaging				
Combination Abdominal CT Scan	254	0.075	0.164	0.191
Combination Chest CT Scan	205	0.005	0.038	0.054
Follow-up Mammogram/Ultrasound[5]	0	-	8.4%	8.4%
MRI for Low Back Pain	128	29.7%	30.2%	32.7%
Survey of Patients' Hospital Experiences				
Area Around Room 'Always' Quiet at Night	300+	61%	-	58%
Doctors 'Always' Communicated Well	300+	77%	-	80%
Home Recovery Information Given	300+	81%	-	82%
Hospital Given 9 or 10 on 10 Point Scale	300+	70%	-	67%
Meds 'Always' Explained Before Given	300+	57%	-	60%
Nurses 'Always' Communicated Well	300+	75%	-	76%
Pain 'Always' Well Controlled	300+	66%	-	69%
Room and Bathroom 'Always' Clean	300+	69%	-	71%
Timely Help 'Always' Received	300+	63%	-	64%
Would Definitely Recommend Hospital	300+	75%	-	69%

Dayton VA Medical Center

4100 West Third Street
Dayton, OH 45428
URL: www.dayton.va.gov
Type: Acute Care-Veterans Administration
Ownership: Government - Federal

Phone: 937-268-6511
Fax: 937-262-2170

Emergency Services: No
Beds: 539

Key Personnel:
CEO/President . . . . Steven Cohen, MD
Chief of Medical Staff . . . . Edward Sperber, MD
Ambulatory Care . . . . Ronald Beaulied, ACOS

Measure	Cases	This Hosp.	State Avg.	U.S. Avg.
Heart Attack Care				
ACE Inhibitor or ARB for LVSD[1]	1	100%	97%	96%
Aspirin at Arrival[1]	21	100%	99%	99%
Aspirin at Discharge[1]	20	100%	99%	98%
Beta Blocker at Discharge[1]	19	100%	99%	98%
Fibrinolytic Medication Timing[5]	0	-	14%	55%
PCI Within 90 Minutes of Arrival[5]	0	-	92%	90%
Smoking Cessation Advice[1]	9	100%	100%	99%
Chest Pain/Possible Heart Attack Care				
Aspirin at Arrival	-	-	96%	95%
Median Time to ECG (minutes)	-	-	7	8
Median Time to Transfer (minutes)	-	-	61	61
Fibrinolytic Medication Timing	-	-	47%	54%
Heart Failure Care				
ACE Inhibitor or ARB for LVSD	70	96%	96%	94%
Discharge Instructions	150	89%	91%	88%
Evaluation of LVS Function	174	100%	99%	98%
Smoking Cessation Advice	49	94%	99%	98%
Pneumonia Care				
Appropriate Initial Antibiotic	79	91%	92%	92%
Blood Culture Timing	113	98%	96%	96%
Influenza Vaccine	92	95%	93%	91%
Initial Antibiotic Timing	119	91%	96%	95%
Pneumococcal Vaccine	93	98%	95%	93%
Smoking Cessation Advice	53	98%	98%	97%
Surgical Care Improvement Project				
Appropriate VTP Within 24 Hours[2]	40	95%	92%	92%
Appropriate Hair Removal[2]	156	100%	100%	99%
Appropriate Beta Blocker Usage[2]	64	98%	94%	93%
Controlled Postoperative Blood Glucose[2,5]	0	-	94%	93%
Prophylactic Antibiotic Timing	111	98%	97%	97%
Prophylactic Antibiotic Timing (Outpatient)	-	-	91%	92%
Prophylactic Antibiotic Selection	111	100%	98%	97%
Prophylactic Antibiotic Select. (Outpatient)	-	-	94%	94%
Prophylactic Antibiotic Stopped	109	99%	95%	94%
Recommended VTP Ordered[2]	40	95%	94%	94%
Urinary Catheter Removal[1,2]	17	94%	91%	90%
Children's Asthma Care				
Received Systemic Corticosteroids	-	-	-	100%
Received Home Management Plan	-	-	-	71%
Received Reliever Medication	-	-	-	100%
Use of Medical Imaging				
Combination Abdominal CT Scan	-	-	0.164	0.191
Combination Chest CT Scan	-	-	0.038	0.054
Follow-up Mammogram/Ultrasound	-	-	8.4%	8.4%
MRI for Low Back Pain	-	-	30.2%	32.7%
Survey of Patients' Hospital Experiences				
Area Around Room 'Always' Quiet at Night	-	-	-	58%
Doctors 'Always' Communicated Well	-	-	-	80%
Home Recovery Information Given	-	-	-	82%
Hospital Given 9 or 10 on 10 Point Scale	-	-	-	67%
Meds 'Always' Explained Before Given	-	-	-	60%
Nurses 'Always' Communicated Well	-	-	-	76%
Pain 'Always' Well Controlled	-	-	-	69%
Room and Bathroom 'Always' Clean	-	-	-	71%
Timely Help 'Always' Received	-	-	-	64%
Would Definitely Recommend Hospital	-	-	-	69%

NOTE: Hospital profiles are in alphabetical order by state, then city, then hospital within the city; Rankings exclude hospitals with less than 25 cases except for patient surveys which excludes hospitals with less than 100 cases; (a) 100–299 cases; (1) The number of cases is too small to be sure how well a hospital is performing; (2) The hospital indicated that the data submitted for this measure were based on a sample of cases; (3) Data was collected during a shorter time period (fewer quarters) than the maximum possible time for this measure; (4) Suppressed for one or more quarters by CMS; (5) No data is available from the hospital for this measure; (6) Fewer than 100 patients completed the HCAHPS survey. Use these rates with caution, as the number of surveys may be too low to reliably assess hospital performance; (7) Survey results are based on less than 12 months of data; (8) Survey results are not available for this reporting period; (9) No or very few patients were eligible for the HCAHPS survey. The scores shown, if any, reflect a very small number of surveys; (10) A state average was not calculated because too few hospitals in the state submitted data; (11) There were discrepancies in the data collection process; Please refer to the User's Guide for a full explanation of data.

Good Samaritan Hospital

2222 Philadelphia Drive — Phone: 937-278-2612
Dayton, OH 45406 — Fax: 937-276-8244
Type: Acute Care Hospitals — Emergency Services: Yes
Ownership: Voluntary Non-Profit - Church — Beds: 560

Key Personnel:
CEO/President. . . . . Mark S Shaker
Chief of Medical Staff . . . . Timothy B Sorg, MD
Infection Control. . . . . Sandy Iams
Pediatric Ambulatory Care . . . . . . G Youra, MD
Pediatric In-Patient Care . . . . . . G Youra, MD
Quality Assurance . . . . Mary Gutman
Radiology. . . . . Randall J Reilman, MD
Emergency Room . . . . Richard Garrison, MD

Measure	Cases	This Hosp.	State Avg.	U.S. Avg.
Heart Attack Care				
ACE Inhibitor or ARB for LVSD	74	95%	97%	96%
Aspirin at Arrival	324	100%	99%	99%
Aspirin at Discharge	493	98%	99%	98%
Beta Blocker at Discharge	474	99%	99%	98%
Fibrinolytic Medication Timing	0	-	14%	55%
PCI Within 90 Minutes of Arrival	66	91%	92%	90%
Smoking Cessation Advice	175	99%	100%	99%
Chest Pain/Possible Heart Attack Care				
Aspirin at Arrival[1]	6	100%	96%	95%
Median Time to ECG (minutes)[1]	7	9	7	8
Median Time to Transfer (minutes)[5]	0	-	61	61
Fibrinolytic Medication Timing[5]	0	-	47%	54%
Heart Failure Care				
ACE Inhibitor or ARB for LVSD[2]	100	92%	96%	94%
Discharge Instructions[2]	248	91%	91%	88%
Evaluation of LVS Function[2]	290	100%	99%	98%
Smoking Cessation Advice[2]	54	100%	99%	98%
Pneumonia Care				
Appropriate Initial Antibiotic[2]	78	99%	92%	92%
Blood Culture Timing[2]	131	85%	96%	96%
Influenza Vaccine[2]	59	93%	93%	91%
Initial Antibiotic Timing[2]	123	97%	96%	95%
Pneumococcal Vaccine[2]	100	92%	95%	93%
Smoking Cessation Advice[2]	63	98%	98%	97%
Surgical Care Improvement Project				
Appropriate VTP Within 24 Hours[2]	122	89%	92%	92%
Appropriate Hair Removal[2]	650	100%	100%	99%
Appropriate Beta Blocker Usage[2]	220	95%	94%	93%
Controlled Postoperative Blood Glucose[2]	162	95%	94%	93%
Prophylactic Antibiotic Timing[2]	488	96%	97%	97%
Prophylactic Antibiotic Timing (Outpatient)	609	85%	91%	92%
Prophylactic Antibiotic Selection[2]	500	98%	98%	97%
Prophylactic Antibiotic Select. (Outpatient)	593	97%	94%	94%
Prophylactic Antibiotic Stopped[2]	464	92%	95%	94%
Recommended VTP Ordered[2]	123	92%	94%	94%
Urinary Catheter Removal[2]	148	95%	91%	90%
Children's Asthma Care				
Received Systemic Corticosteroids	-	-	-	100%
Received Home Management Plan	-	-	-	71%
Received Reliever Medication	-	-	-	100%
Use of Medical Imaging				
Combination Abdominal CT Scan	1,102	0.047	0.164	0.191
Combination Chest CT Scan	1,070	0.011	0.038	0.054
Follow-up Mammogram/Ultrasound	2,531	9.7%	8.4%	8.4%
MRI for Low Back Pain	200	33.5%	30.2%	32.7%
Survey of Patients' Hospital Experiences				
Area Around Room 'Always' Quiet at Night	300+	50%	-	58%
Doctors 'Always' Communicated Well	300+	73%	-	80%
Home Recovery Information Given	300+	85%	-	82%
Hospital Given 9 or 10 on 10 Point Scale	300+	62%	-	67%
Meds 'Always' Explained Before Given	300+	54%	-	60%
Nurses 'Always' Communicated Well	300+	71%	-	76%
Pain 'Always' Well Controlled	300+	64%	-	69%
Room and Bathroom 'Always' Clean	300+	58%	-	71%
Timely Help 'Always' Received	300+	53%	-	64%
Would Definitely Recommend Hospital	300+	65%	-	69%

Grandview Hospital & Medical Center

405 Grand Avenue — Phone: 937-723-4988
Dayton, OH 45405 — Fax: 937-461-0020
URL: www.kmcnetwork.org
Type: Acute Care Hospitals — Emergency Services: Yes
Ownership: Voluntary Non-Profit - Other — Beds: 452

Key Personnel:
CEO/President. . . . . Francisco J Perez
Chief of Medical Staff . . . . Kevin Reid, DO
Operating Room. . . . . Rannie MD, RN
Pediatric In-Patient Care . . . . . . Robert Myers, DO
Quality Assurance . . . . Diane Setty
Radiology. . . . . David Volarich, DO
Anesthesiology. . . . . Wayne Anderson, DO
Emergency Room . . . . Charles K MacIntosh, DO

Measure	Cases	This Hosp.	State Avg.	U.S. Avg.
Heart Attack Care				
ACE Inhibitor or ARB for LVSD	28	100%	97%	96%
Aspirin at Arrival	132	98%	99%	99%
Aspirin at Discharge	177	99%	99%	98%
Beta Blocker at Discharge	175	99%	99%	98%
Fibrinolytic Medication Timing	0	-	14%	55%
PCI Within 90 Minutes of Arrival	34	85%	92%	90%
Smoking Cessation Advice	74	100%	100%	99%
Chest Pain/Possible Heart Attack Care				
Aspirin at Arrival[1]	8	75%	96%	95%
Median Time to ECG (minutes)[1]	8	4	7	8
Median Time to Transfer (minutes)[5]	0	-	61	61
Fibrinolytic Medication Timing[3]	0	-	47%	54%
Heart Failure Care				
ACE Inhibitor or ARB for LVSD	93	100%	96%	94%
Discharge Instructions	315	97%	91%	88%
Evaluation of LVS Function	410	100%	99%	98%
Smoking Cessation Advice	74	100%	99%	98%
Pneumonia Care				
Appropriate Initial Antibiotic	165	98%	92%	92%
Blood Culture Timing	280	99%	96%	96%
Influenza Vaccine	175	99%	93%	91%
Initial Antibiotic Timing	236	97%	96%	95%
Pneumococcal Vaccine	215	100%	95%	93%
Smoking Cessation Advice	115	100%	98%	97%
Surgical Care Improvement Project				
Appropriate VTP Within 24 Hours[2]	276	96%	92%	92%
Appropriate Hair Removal[2]	1,007	100%	100%	99%
Appropriate Beta Blocker Usage[2]	316	97%	94%	93%
Controlled Postoperative Blood Glucose[2]	126	89%	94%	93%
Prophylactic Antibiotic Timing[2]	780	99%	97%	97%
Prophylactic Antibiotic Timing (Outpatient)	559	95%	91%	92%
Prophylactic Antibiotic Selection[2]	786	97%	98%	97%
Prophylactic Antibiotic Select. (Outpatient)	547	96%	94%	94%
Prophylactic Antibiotic Stopped[2]	737	96%	95%	94%
Recommended VTP Ordered[2]	277	97%	94%	94%
Urinary Catheter Removal[2]	95	92%	91%	90%
Children's Asthma Care				
Received Systemic Corticosteroids	-	-	-	100%
Received Home Management Plan	-	-	-	71%
Received Reliever Medication	-	-	-	100%
Use of Medical Imaging				
Combination Abdominal CT Scan	1,413	0.263	0.164	0.191
Combination Chest CT Scan	643	0.171	0.038	0.054
Follow-up Mammogram/Ultrasound	942	5.9%	8.4%	8.4%
MRI for Low Back Pain	235	29.8%	30.2%	32.7%
Survey of Patients' Hospital Experiences				
Area Around Room 'Always' Quiet at Night	300+	51%	-	58%
Doctors 'Always' Communicated Well	300+	79%	-	80%
Home Recovery Information Given	300+	83%	-	82%
Hospital Given 9 or 10 on 10 Point Scale	300+	68%	-	67%
Meds 'Always' Explained Before Given	300+	55%	-	60%
Nurses 'Always' Communicated Well	300+	75%	-	76%
Pain 'Always' Well Controlled	300+	66%	-	69%
Room and Bathroom 'Always' Clean	300+	67%	-	71%
Timely Help 'Always' Received	300+	59%	-	64%
Would Definitely Recommend Hospital	300+	71%	-	69%

Medical Center at Elizabeth Place

One Elizabeth Place — Phone: 937-853-1053
Dayton, OH 45408
URL: www.mcep.us
Type: Acute Care Hospitals — Emergency Services: Yes
Ownership: Government - Federal — Beds: 26

Key Personnel:
CEO . . . . Alex Rintoul

Measure	Cases	This Hosp.	State Avg.	U.S. Avg.
Heart Attack Care				
ACE Inhibitor or ARB for LVSD[5]	0	-	97%	96%
Aspirin at Arrival[5]	0	-	99%	99%
Aspirin at Discharge[5]	0	-	99%	98%
Beta Blocker at Discharge[5]	0	-	99%	98%
Fibrinolytic Medication Timing[5]	0	-	14%	55%
PCI Within 90 Minutes of Arrival[5]	0	-	92%	90%
Smoking Cessation Advice[5]	0	-	100%	99%
Chest Pain/Possible Heart Attack Care				
Aspirin at Arrival[5]	0	-	96%	95%
Median Time to ECG (minutes)[5]	0	-	7	8
Median Time to Transfer (minutes)[5]	0	-	61	61
Fibrinolytic Medication Timing[5]	0	-	47%	54%
Heart Failure Care				
ACE Inhibitor or ARB for LVSD[1,3]	1	100%	96%	94%
Discharge Instructions[1,3]	3	67%	91%	88%
Evaluation of LVS Function[1,3]	4	75%	99%	98%
Smoking Cessation Advice[1,3]	1	0%	99%	98%
Pneumonia Care				
Appropriate Initial Antibiotic[3]	0	-	92%	92%
Blood Culture Timing[3]	0	-	96%	96%
Influenza Vaccine[1]	2	100%	93%	91%
Initial Antibiotic Timing[1,3]	1	100%	96%	95%
Pneumococcal Vaccine[3]	0	-	95%	93%
Smoking Cessation Advice[1,3]	1	100%	98%	97%
Surgical Care Improvement Project				
Appropriate VTP Within 24 Hours[1]	10	80%	92%	92%
Appropriate Hair Removal	160	100%	100%	99%
Appropriate Beta Blocker Usage	27	100%	94%	93%
Controlled Postoperative Blood Glucose	0	-	94%	93%
Prophylactic Antibiotic Timing	63	97%	97%	97%
Prophylactic Antibiotic Timing (Outpatient)	111	94%	91%	92%
Prophylactic Antibiotic Selection	65	85%	98%	97%
Prophylactic Antibiotic Select. (Outpatient)	109	84%	94%	94%
Prophylactic Antibiotic Stopped	63	92%	95%	94%
Recommended VTP Ordered[1]	10	80%	94%	94%
Urinary Catheter Removal[1]	5	100%	91%	90%
Children's Asthma Care				
Received Systemic Corticosteroids	-	-	-	100%
Received Home Management Plan	-	-	-	71%
Received Reliever Medication	-	-	-	100%
Use of Medical Imaging				
Combination Abdominal CT Scan	80	0.063	0.164	0.191
Combination Chest CT Scan	66	0.061	0.038	0.054
Follow-up Mammogram/Ultrasound[5]	0	-	8.4%	8.4%
MRI for Low Back Pain	110	20.9%	30.2%	32.7%
Survey of Patients' Hospital Experiences				
Area Around Room 'Always' Quiet at Night	(a)	78%	-	58%
Doctors 'Always' Communicated Well	(a)	79%	-	80%
Home Recovery Information Given	(a)	88%	-	82%
Hospital Given 9 or 10 on 10 Point Scale	(a)	79%	-	67%
Meds 'Always' Explained Before Given	(a)	63%	-	60%
Nurses 'Always' Communicated Well	(a)	85%	-	76%
Pain 'Always' Well Controlled	(a)	77%	-	69%
Room and Bathroom 'Always' Clean	(a)	75%	-	71%
Timely Help 'Always' Received	(a)	79%	-	64%
Would Definitely Recommend Hospital	(a)	76%	-	69%

NOTE: Hospital profiles are in alphabetical order by state, then city, then hospital within the city; Rankings exclude hospitals with less than 25 cases except for patient surveys which excludes hospitals with less than 100 cases; (a) 100–299 cases; (1) The number of cases is too small to be sure how well a hospital is performing; (2) The hospital indicated that the data submitted for this measure were based on a sample of cases; (3) Data was collected during a shorter time period (fewer quarters) than the maximum possible time for this measure; (4) Suppressed for one or more quarters by CMS; (5) No data is available from the hospital for this measure; (6) Fewer than 100 patients completed the HCAHPS survey. Use these rates with caution, as the number of surveys may be too low to reliably assess hospital performance; (7) Survey results are based on less than 12 months of data; (8) Survey results are not available for this reporting period; (9) No or very few patients were eligible for the HCAHPS survey. The scores shown, if any, reflect a very small number of surveys; (10) A state average was not calculated because too few hospitals in the state submitted data; (11) There were discrepancies in the data collection process; Please refer to the User's Guide for a full explanation of data.

Miami Valley Hospital

One Wyoming Street Phone: 937-208-8000
Dayton, OH 45409 Fax: 937-341-8611
URL: www.miamivalleyhospital.com
Type: Acute Care Hospitals Emergency Services: Yes
Ownership: Voluntary Non-Profit - Private Beds: 848

Key Personnel:

CEO/President. . . . . James R Pancoast
Chief of Medical Staff. . . . . Howard Wunderlich, MD
Infection Control . . . . Tim Collins
Operating Room. . . . . Randy Woods
Pediatric Ambulatory Care . . . . . . William Spohn, MD
Pediatric In-Patient Care . . . . William Spohn, MD
Quality Assurance . . . . Tim Collins
Radiology. . . . . Larry D Buchanan, MD

Measure	Cases	This Hosp.	State Avg.	U.S. Avg.
Heart Attack Care				
ACE Inhibitor or ARB for LVSD[2]	59	92%	97%	96%
Aspirin at Arrival[2]	263	100%	99%	99%
Aspirin at Discharge[2]	321	100%	99%	98%
Beta Blocker at Discharge[2]	318	99%	99%	98%
Fibrinolytic Medication Timing[2]	0	-	14%	55%
PCI Within 90 Minutes of Arrival[2]	60	92%	92%	90%
Smoking Cessation Advice[2]	149	100%	100%	99%
Chest Pain/Possible Heart Attack Care				
Aspirin at Arrival[1]	20	90%	96%	95%
Median Time to ECG (minutes)[1]	21	12	7	8
Median Time to Transfer (minutes)[5]	0	-	61	61
Fibrinolytic Medication Timing[3]	0	-	47%	54%
Heart Failure Care				
ACE Inhibitor or ARB for LVSD[2]	106	95%	96%	94%
Discharge Instructions[2]	253	85%	91%	88%
Evaluation of LVS Function[2]	317	100%	99%	98%
Smoking Cessation Advice[2]	84	100%	99%	98%
Pneumonia Care				
Appropriate Initial Antibiotic[2]	104	87%	92%	92%
Blood Culture Timing[2]	174	94%	96%	96%
Influenza Vaccine[2]	102	86%	93%	91%
Initial Antibiotic Timing[2]	159	96%	96%	95%
Pneumococcal Vaccine[2]	156	87%	95%	93%
Smoking Cessation Advice[2]	91	98%	98%	97%
Surgical Care Improvement Project				
Appropriate VTP Within 24 Hours[2]	206	87%	92%	92%
Appropriate Hair Removal[2]	729	100%	100%	99%
Appropriate Beta Blocker Usage[2]	239	90%	94%	93%
Controlled Postoperative Blood Glucose[2]	135	99%	94%	93%
Prophylactic Antibiotic Timing[2]	492	96%	97%	97%
Prophylactic Antibiotic Timing (Outpatient)	912	97%	91%	92%
Prophylactic Antibiotic Selection[2]	499	99%	98%	97%
Prophylactic Antibiotic Select. (Outpatient)	913	96%	94%	94%
Prophylactic Antibiotic Stopped[2]	465	90%	95%	94%
Recommended VTP Ordered[2]	206	92%	94%	94%
Urinary Catheter Removal[2]	137	89%	91%	90%
Children's Asthma Care				
Received Systemic Corticosteroids	-	-	-	100%
Received Home Management Plan	-	-	-	71%
Received Reliever Medication	-	-	-	100%
Use of Medical Imaging				
Combination Abdominal CT Scan	2,133	0.076	0.164	0.191
Combination Chest CT Scan	1,834	0.017	0.038	0.054
Follow-up Mammogram/Ultrasound	2,588	5.6%	8.4%	8.4%
MRI for Low Back Pain	350	29.4%	30.2%	32.7%
Survey of Patients' Hospital Experiences				
Area Around Room 'Always' Quiet at Night	300+	46%	-	58%
Doctors 'Always' Communicated Well	300+	74%	-	80%
Home Recovery Information Given	300+	88%	-	82%
Hospital Given 9 or 10 on 10 Point Scale	300+	66%	-	67%
Meds 'Always' Explained Before Given	300+	56%	-	60%
Nurses 'Always' Communicated Well	300+	74%	-	76%
Pain 'Always' Well Controlled	300+	68%	-	69%
Room and Bathroom 'Always' Clean	300+	61%	-	71%
Timely Help 'Always' Received	300+	55%	-	64%
Would Definitely Recommend Hospital	300+	72%	-	69%

Defiance Regional Medical Center

1200 Ralston Avenue Phone: 419-783-6955
Defiance, OH 43512 Fax: 419-783-6904
Type: Critical Access Hospitals Emergency Services: Yes
Ownership: Voluntary Non-Profit - Private Beds: 61

Key Personnel:

Cardiac Laboratory. . . . . Raza Hashmi, MD
Chief of Medical Staff. . . . . Robert Barnett, MD
Coronary Care . . . . Anne Minic, RN
Infection Control. . . . . Elizabeth Rettig
Operating Room. . . . . LouAnn Walton, RN
Quality Assurance . . . . Elizabeth Rettig, RN

Measure	Cases	This Hosp.	State Avg.	U.S. Avg.
Heart Attack Care				
ACE Inhibitor or ARB for LVSD[1]	4	25%	97%	96%
Aspirin at Arrival[1]	15	100%	99%	99%
Aspirin at Discharge[1]	12	100%	99%	98%
Beta Blocker at Discharge[1]	12	92%	99%	98%
Fibrinolytic Medication Timing	0	-	14%	55%
PCI Within 90 Minutes of Arrival	0	-	92%	90%
Smoking Cessation Advice[1]	3	67%	100%	99%
Chest Pain/Possible Heart Attack Care				
Aspirin at Arrival	-	-	96%	95%
Median Time to ECG (minutes)	-	-	7	8
Median Time to Transfer (minutes)	-	-	61	61
Fibrinolytic Medication Timing	-	-	47%	54%
Heart Failure Care				
ACE Inhibitor or ARB for LVSD[1]	7	100%	96%	94%
Discharge Instructions	27	96%	91%	88%
Evaluation of LVS Function	37	100%	99%	98%
Smoking Cessation Advice[1]	6	100%	99%	98%
Pneumonia Care				
Appropriate Initial Antibiotic	52	96%	92%	92%
Blood Culture Timing	68	97%	96%	96%
Influenza Vaccine	53	98%	93%	91%
Initial Antibiotic Timing	75	100%	96%	95%
Pneumococcal Vaccine	62	98%	95%	93%
Smoking Cessation Advice	37	97%	98%	97%
Surgical Care Improvement Project				
Appropriate VTP Within 24 Hours	48	88%	92%	92%
Appropriate Hair Removal	162	99%	100%	99%
Appropriate Beta Blocker Usage[5]	0	-	94%	93%
Controlled Postoperative Blood Glucose	0	-	94%	93%
Prophylactic Antibiotic Timing	125	98%	97%	97%
Prophylactic Antibiotic Timing (Outpatient)	-	-	91%	92%
Prophylactic Antibiotic Selection	126	96%	98%	97%
Prophylactic Antibiotic Select. (Outpatient)	-	-	94%	94%
Prophylactic Antibiotic Stopped	114	95%	95%	94%
Recommended VTP Ordered	48	94%	94%	94%
Urinary Catheter Removal[1]	18	89%	91%	90%
Children's Asthma Care				
Received Systemic Corticosteroids	-	-	-	100%
Received Home Management Plan	-	-	-	71%
Received Reliever Medication	-	-	-	100%
Use of Medical Imaging				
Combination Abdominal CT Scan	-	-	0.164	0.191
Combination Chest CT Scan	-	-	0.038	0.054
Follow-up Mammogram/Ultrasound	-	-	8.4%	8.4%
MRI for Low Back Pain	-	-	30.2%	32.7%
Survey of Patients' Hospital Experiences				
Area Around Room 'Always' Quiet at Night	300+	63%	-	58%
Doctors 'Always' Communicated Well	300+	77%	-	80%
Home Recovery Information Given	300+	85%	-	82%
Hospital Given 9 or 10 on 10 Point Scale	300+	75%	-	67%
Meds 'Always' Explained Before Given	300+	60%	-	60%
Nurses 'Always' Communicated Well	300+	77%	-	76%
Pain 'Always' Well Controlled	300+	68%	-	69%
Room and Bathroom 'Always' Clean	300+	76%	-	71%
Timely Help 'Always' Received	300+	69%	-	64%
Would Definitely Recommend Hospital	300+	77%	-	69%

Mercy Hospital of Defiance

1404 East Second Street Phone: 419-782-8444
Defiance, OH 43512
Type: Acute Care Hospitals Emergency Services: Yes
Ownership: Proprietary

Measure	Cases	This Hosp.	State Avg.	U.S. Avg.
Heart Attack Care				
ACE Inhibitor or ARB for LVSD[3]	0	-	97%	96%
Aspirin at Arrival[1,3]	2	100%	99%	99%
Aspirin at Discharge[1,3]	1	100%	99%	98%
Beta Blocker at Discharge[1,3]	1	100%	99%	98%
Fibrinolytic Medication Timing[3]	0	-	14%	55%
PCI Within 90 Minutes of Arrival[3]	0	-	92%	90%
Smoking Cessation Advice[3]	0	-	100%	99%
Chest Pain/Possible Heart Attack Care				
Aspirin at Arrival	62	98%	96%	95%
Median Time to ECG (minutes)	66	4	7	8
Median Time to Transfer (minutes)[1]	8	115	61	61
Fibrinolytic Medication Timing	0	-	47%	54%
Heart Failure Care				
ACE Inhibitor or ARB for LVSD[1]	10	100%	96%	94%
Discharge Instructions	26	96%	91%	88%
Evaluation of LVS Function	36	100%	99%	98%
Smoking Cessation Advice[1]	4	100%	99%	98%
Pneumonia Care				
Appropriate Initial Antibiotic	64	98%	92%	92%
Blood Culture Timing	83	99%	96%	96%
Influenza Vaccine	46	100%	93%	91%
Initial Antibiotic Timing	84	99%	96%	95%
Pneumococcal Vaccine	72	100%	95%	93%
Smoking Cessation Advice[1]	13	100%	98%	97%
Surgical Care Improvement Project				
Appropriate VTP Within 24 Hours	62	98%	92%	92%
Appropriate Hair Removal	113	100%	100%	99%
Appropriate Beta Blocker Usage	34	94%	94%	93%
Controlled Postoperative Blood Glucose	0	-	94%	93%
Prophylactic Antibiotic Timing	84	98%	97%	97%
Prophylactic Antibiotic Timing (Outpatient)[1]	12	100%	91%	92%
Prophylactic Antibiotic Selection	85	99%	98%	97%
Prophylactic Antibiotic Select. (Outpatient)[1]	12	83%	94%	94%
Prophylactic Antibiotic Stopped	83	96%	95%	94%
Recommended VTP Ordered	62	98%	94%	94%
Urinary Catheter Removal	35	100%	91%	90%
Children's Asthma Care				
Received Systemic Corticosteroids	-	-	-	100%
Received Home Management Plan	-	-	-	71%
Received Reliever Medication	-	-	-	100%
Use of Medical Imaging				
Combination Abdominal CT Scan	151	0.046	0.164	0.191
Combination Chest CT Scan	78	0.013	0.038	0.054
Follow-up Mammogram/Ultrasound[5]	0	-	8.4%	8.4%
MRI for Low Back Pain[5]	0	-	30.2%	32.7%
Survey of Patients' Hospital Experiences				
Area Around Room 'Always' Quiet at Night	300+	62%	-	58%
Doctors 'Always' Communicated Well	300+	84%	-	80%
Home Recovery Information Given	300+	88%	-	82%
Hospital Given 9 or 10 on 10 Point Scale	300+	77%	-	67%
Meds 'Always' Explained Before Given	300+	63%	-	60%
Nurses 'Always' Communicated Well	300+	83%	-	76%
Pain 'Always' Well Controlled	300+	80%	-	69%
Room and Bathroom 'Always' Clean	300+	84%	-	71%
Timely Help 'Always' Received	300+	78%	-	64%
Would Definitely Recommend Hospital	300+	78%	-	69%

NOTE: Hospital profiles are in alphabetical order by state, then city, then hospital within the city; Rankings exclude hospitals with less than 25 cases except for patient surveys which excludes hospitals with less than 100 cases; (a) 100–299 cases; (1) The number of cases is too small to be sure how well a hospital is performing; (2) The hospital indicated that the data submitted for this measure were based on a sample of cases; (3) Data was collected during a shorter time period (fewer quarters) than the maximum possible time for this measure; (4) Suppressed for one or more quarters by CMS; (5) No data is available from the hospital for this measure; (6) Fewer than 100 patients completed the HCAHPS survey. Use these rates with caution, as the number of surveys may be too low to reliably assess hospital performance; (7) Survey results are based on less than 12 months of data; (8) Survey results are not available for this reporting period; (9) No or very few patients were eligible for the HCAHPS survey. The scores shown, if any, reflect a very small number of surveys; (10) A state average was not calculated because too few hospitals in the state submitted data; (11) There were discrepancies in the data collection process; Please refer to the User's Guide for a full explanation of data.

Grady Memorial Hospital

561 West Central Avenue
Delaware, OH 43015
URL: www.gradyhospital.com
Type: Acute Care Hospitals
Ownership: Voluntary Non-Profit - Private

Phone: 740-368-5145
Fax: 740-368-5213

Emergency Services: Yes
Beds: 135

Key Personnel:
CEO/President. . . . . Everett P Weber Jr

Measure	Cases	This Hosp.	State Avg.	U.S. Avg.
Heart Attack Care				
ACE Inhibitor or ARB for LVSD[1]	1	100%	97%	96%
Aspirin at Arrival[1]	17	100%	99%	99%
Aspirin at Discharge[1]	5	100%	99%	98%
Beta Blocker at Discharge[1]	7	100%	99%	98%
Fibrinolytic Medication Timing	0	-	14%	55%
PCI Within 90 Minutes of Arrival	0	-	92%	90%
Smoking Cessation Advice	0	-	100%	99%
Chest Pain/Possible Heart Attack Care				
Aspirin at Arrival	123	99%	96%	95%
Median Time to ECG (minutes)	133	4	7	8
Median Time to Transfer (minutes)[1]	10	58	61	61
Fibrinolytic Medication Timing[1]	2	50%	47%	54%
Heart Failure Care				
ACE Inhibitor or ARB for LVSD	35	94%	96%	94%
Discharge Instructions	95	98%	91%	88%
Evaluation of LVS Function	115	98%	99%	98%
Smoking Cessation Advice[1]	15	100%	99%	98%
Pneumonia Care				
Appropriate Initial Antibiotic	77	88%	92%	92%
Blood Culture Timing	68	97%	96%	96%
Influenza Vaccine	62	98%	93%	91%
Initial Antibiotic Timing	104	100%	96%	95%
Pneumococcal Vaccine	85	98%	95%	93%
Smoking Cessation Advice	37	100%	98%	97%
Surgical Care Improvement Project				
Appropriate VTP Within 24 Hours	96	98%	92%	92%
Appropriate Hair Removal	221	100%	100%	99%
Appropriate Beta Blocker Usage	64	92%	94%	93%
Controlled Postoperative Blood Glucose	0	-	94%	93%
Prophylactic Antibiotic Timing	142	99%	97%	97%
Prophylactic Antibiotic Timing (Outpatient)	113	92%	91%	92%
Prophylactic Antibiotic Selection	142	100%	98%	97%
Prophylactic Antibiotic Select. (Outpatient)	110	94%	94%	94%
Prophylactic Antibiotic Stopped	137	99%	95%	94%
Recommended VTP Ordered	96	99%	94%	94%
Urinary Catheter Removal	60	93%	91%	90%
Children's Asthma Care				
Received Systemic Corticosteroids	-	-	-	100%
Received Home Management Plan	-	-	-	71%
Received Reliever Medication	-	-	-	100%
Use of Medical Imaging				
Combination Abdominal CT Scan	346	0.040	0.164	0.191
Combination Chest CT Scan	195	0.010	0.038	0.054
Follow-up Mammogram/Ultrasound	527	12.1%	8.4%	8.4%
MRI for Low Back Pain	64	23.4%	30.2%	32.7%
Survey of Patients' Hospital Experiences				
Area Around Room 'Always' Quiet at Night	300+	53%	-	58%
Doctors 'Always' Communicated Well	300+	81%	-	80%
Home Recovery Information Given	300+	83%	-	82%
Hospital Given 9 or 10 on 10 Point Scale	300+	67%	-	67%
Meds 'Always' Explained Before Given	300+	59%	-	60%
Nurses 'Always' Communicated Well	300+	76%	-	76%
Pain 'Always' Well Controlled	300+	69%	-	69%
Room and Bathroom 'Always' Clean	300+	72%	-	71%
Timely Help 'Always' Received	300+	60%	-	64%
Would Definitely Recommend Hospital	300+	68%	-	69%

Twin City Hospital

819 North First Street
Dennison, OH 44621
URL: www.twincityhospital.org
Type: Critical Access Hospitals
Ownership: Voluntary Non-Profit - Other

Phone: 740-922-2800
Fax: 740-922-6945

Emergency Services: Yes
Beds: 25

Key Personnel:
CEO/President. . . . . Frank Swinehart, CEO
Chief of Medical Staff . . . . Tim McKnight, MD
Infection Control . . . . Ruthann Belknap, RN
Operating Room . . . . Ruthann Belknap, RN
Anesthesiology. . . . . Laura Rollandini
Emergency Room . . . . Sue Walters, RN
Intensive Care Unit . . . . Tui Wanosik, RN
Patient Relations . . . . Cindy Unrue

Measure	Cases	This Hosp.	State Avg.	U.S. Avg.
Heart Attack Care				
ACE Inhibitor or ARB for LVSD[3]	0	-	97%	96%
Aspirin at Arrival[3]	0	-	99%	99%
Aspirin at Discharge[3]	0	-	99%	98%
Beta Blocker at Discharge[3]	0	-	99%	98%
Fibrinolytic Medication Timing[3]	0	-	14%	55%
PCI Within 90 Minutes of Arrival[5]	0	-	92%	90%
Smoking Cessation Advice[3]	0	-	100%	99%
Chest Pain/Possible Heart Attack Care				
Aspirin at Arrival	-	-	96%	95%
Median Time to ECG (minutes)	-	-	7	8
Median Time to Transfer (minutes)	-	-	61	61
Fibrinolytic Medication Timing	-	-	47%	54%
Heart Failure Care				
ACE Inhibitor or ARB for LVSD[1]	3	100%	96%	94%
Discharge Instructions[1]	14	21%	91%	88%
Evaluation of LVS Function[1]	15	93%	99%	98%
Smoking Cessation Advice[1]	2	50%	99%	98%
Pneumonia Care				
Appropriate Initial Antibiotic[1]	9	100%	92%	92%
Blood Culture Timing[1]	12	100%	96%	96%
Influenza Vaccine[1]	6	100%	93%	91%
Initial Antibiotic Timing[1]	12	100%	96%	95%
Pneumococcal Vaccine[1]	10	100%	95%	93%
Smoking Cessation Advice[1]	3	100%	98%	97%
Surgical Care Improvement Project				
Appropriate VTP Within 24 Hours[5]	0	-	92%	92%
Appropriate Hair Removal[5]	0	-	100%	99%
Appropriate Beta Blocker Usage[5]	0	-	94%	93%
Controlled Postoperative Blood Glucose[5]	0	-	94%	93%
Prophylactic Antibiotic Timing[5]	0	-	97%	97%
Prophylactic Antibiotic Timing (Outpatient)	-	-	91%	92%
Prophylactic Antibiotic Selection[5]	0	-	98%	97%
Prophylactic Antibiotic Select. (Outpatient)	-	-	94%	94%
Prophylactic Antibiotic Stopped[5]	0	-	95%	94%
Recommended VTP Ordered[5]	0	-	94%	94%
Urinary Catheter Removal[5]	0	-	91%	90%
Children's Asthma Care				
Received Systemic Corticosteroids	-	-	-	100%
Received Home Management Plan	-	-	-	71%
Received Reliever Medication	-	-	-	100%
Use of Medical Imaging				
Combination Abdominal CT Scan	-	-	0.164	0.191
Combination Chest CT Scan	-	-	0.038	0.054
Follow-up Mammogram/Ultrasound	-	-	8.4%	8.4%
MRI for Low Back Pain	-	-	30.2%	32.7%
Survey of Patients' Hospital Experiences				
Area Around Room 'Always' Quiet at Night[8]	-	-	-	58%
Doctors 'Always' Communicated Well[8]	-	-	-	80%
Home Recovery Information Given[8]	-	-	-	82%
Hospital Given 9 or 10 on 10 Point Scale[8]	-	-	-	67%
Meds 'Always' Explained Before Given[8]	-	-	-	60%
Nurses 'Always' Communicated Well[8]	-	-	-	76%
Pain 'Always' Well Controlled[8]	-	-	-	69%
Room and Bathroom 'Always' Clean[8]	-	-	-	71%
Timely Help 'Always' Received[8]	-	-	-	64%
Would Definitely Recommend Hospital[8]	-	-	-	69%

Union Hospital

659 Boulevard
Dover, OH 44622
URL: www.unionhospital.org
Type: Acute Care Hospitals
Ownership: Voluntary Non-Profit - Other

Phone: 330-343-3311
Fax: 330-364-0951

Emergency Services: Yes
Beds: 105

Key Personnel:
CEO/President. . . . . William Harding
Chief of Medical Staff . . . . Donald R Braden
Operating Room . . . . Miguel Bravo, RN
Pediatric Ambulatory Care . . . . . . Anita S Olmos, MD
Pediatric In-Patient Care . . . . Anita S Olmos, MD
Quality Assurance . . . . Cathy Corbett
Radiology. . . . . Robert L Basista, DO
Emergency Room . . . . Carma J Clarke, RN

Measure	Cases	This Hosp.	State Avg.	U.S. Avg.
Heart Attack Care				
ACE Inhibitor or ARB for LVSD[1]	7	100%	97%	96%
Aspirin at Arrival	63	100%	99%	99%
Aspirin at Discharge	42	100%	99%	98%
Beta Blocker at Discharge	44	98%	99%	98%
Fibrinolytic Medication Timing	0	-	14%	55%
PCI Within 90 Minutes of Arrival	0	-	92%	90%
Smoking Cessation Advice[1]	5	100%	100%	99%
Chest Pain/Possible Heart Attack Care				
Aspirin at Arrival	185	97%	96%	95%
Median Time to ECG (minutes)	195	11	7	8
Median Time to Transfer (minutes)	42	48	61	61
Fibrinolytic Medication Timing	0	-	47%	54%
Heart Failure Care				
ACE Inhibitor or ARB for LVSD	72	100%	96%	94%
Discharge Instructions	210	98%	91%	88%
Evaluation of LVS Function	301	100%	99%	98%
Smoking Cessation Advice	38	100%	99%	98%
Pneumonia Care				
Appropriate Initial Antibiotic	184	95%	92%	92%
Blood Culture Timing	231	97%	96%	96%
Influenza Vaccine	220	98%	93%	91%
Initial Antibiotic Timing	302	98%	96%	95%
Pneumococcal Vaccine	303	98%	95%	93%
Smoking Cessation Advice	98	97%	98%	97%
Surgical Care Improvement Project				
Appropriate VTP Within 24 Hours[2]	114	93%	92%	92%
Appropriate Hair Removal[2]	404	100%	100%	99%
Appropriate Beta Blocker Usage[2]	109	97%	94%	93%
Controlled Postoperative Blood Glucose[2]	0	-	94%	93%
Prophylactic Antibiotic Timing[2]	266	99%	97%	97%
Prophylactic Antibiotic Timing (Outpatient)	143	93%	91%	92%
Prophylactic Antibiotic Selection[2]	268	99%	98%	97%
Prophylactic Antibiotic Select. (Outpatient)	139	99%	94%	94%
Prophylactic Antibiotic Stopped[2]	254	99%	95%	94%
Recommended VTP Ordered[2]	114	99%	94%	94%
Urinary Catheter Removal	69	96%	91%	90%
Children's Asthma Care				
Received Systemic Corticosteroids	-	-	-	100%
Received Home Management Plan	-	-	-	71%
Received Reliever Medication	-	-	-	100%
Use of Medical Imaging				
Combination Abdominal CT Scan	759	0.101	0.164	0.191
Combination Chest CT Scan	610	0.005	0.038	0.054
Follow-up Mammogram/Ultrasound	776	6.6%	8.4%	8.4%
MRI for Low Back Pain	139	33.1%	30.2%	32.7%
Survey of Patients' Hospital Experiences				
Area Around Room 'Always' Quiet at Night	300+	46%	-	58%
Doctors 'Always' Communicated Well	300+	80%	-	80%
Home Recovery Information Given	300+	82%	-	82%
Hospital Given 9 or 10 on 10 Point Scale	300+	66%	-	67%
Meds 'Always' Explained Before Given	300+	57%	-	60%
Nurses 'Always' Communicated Well	300+	73%	-	76%
Pain 'Always' Well Controlled	300+	68%	-	69%
Room and Bathroom 'Always' Clean	300+	71%	-	71%
Timely Help 'Always' Received	300+	64%	-	64%
Would Definitely Recommend Hospital	300+	63%	-	69%

NOTE: Hospital profiles are in alphabetical order by state, then city, then hospital within the city; Rankings exclude hospitals with less than 25 cases except for patient surveys which excludes hospitals with less than 100 cases; (a) 100–299 cases; (1) The number of cases is too small to be sure how well a hospital is performing; (2) The hospital indicated that the data submitted for this measure were based on a sample of cases; (3) Data was collected during a shorter time period (fewer quarters) than the maximum possible time for this measure; (4) Suppressed for one or more quarters by CMS; (5) No data is available from the hospital for this measure; (6) Fewer than 100 patients completed the HCAHPS survey. Use these rates with caution, as the number of surveys may be too low to reliably assess hospital performance; (7) Survey results are based on less than 12 months of data; (8) Survey results are based on less than 12 months of data; (9) No or very few patients were eligible for the HCAHPS survey. The scores shown, if any, reflect a very small number of surveys; (10) A state average was not calculated because too few hospitals in the state submitted data; (11) There were discrepancies in the data collection process; Please refer to the User's Guide for a full explanation of data.

Dublin Methodist Hospital

7500 Hospital Avenue — Phone: 614-544-8000
Dublin, OH 43016
URL: www.ohiohealth.com
Type: Acute Care Hospitals — Emergency Services: Yes
Ownership: Voluntary Non-Profit - Church

Key Personnel:
President . . . . Bruce P Hagan

Measure	Cases	This Hosp.	State Avg.	U.S. Avg.
Heart Attack Care				
ACE Inhibitor or ARB for LVSD[1]	1	100%	97%	96%
Aspirin at Arrival[1]	4	100%	99%	99%
Aspirin at Discharge[1]	2	100%	99%	98%
Beta Blocker at Discharge[1]	2	100%	99%	98%
Fibrinolytic Medication Timing	0	-	14%	55%
PCI Within 90 Minutes of Arrival	0	-	92%	90%
Smoking Cessation Advice	0	-	100%	99%
Chest Pain/Possible Heart Attack Care				
Aspirin at Arrival	120	91%	96%	95%
Median Time to ECG (minutes)	123	9	7	8
Median Time to Transfer (minutes)[1]	18	80	61	61
Fibrinolytic Medication Timing	0	-	47%	54%
Heart Failure Care				
ACE Inhibitor or ARB for LVSD[1]	7	100%	96%	94%
Discharge Instructions	35	100%	91%	88%
Evaluation of LVS Function	46	98%	99%	98%
Smoking Cessation Advice[1]	6	100%	99%	98%
Pneumonia Care				
Appropriate Initial Antibiotic	87	95%	92%	92%
Blood Culture Timing	109	98%	96%	96%
Influenza Vaccine	56	89%	93%	91%
Initial Antibiotic Timing	110	100%	96%	95%
Pneumococcal Vaccine	67	96%	95%	93%
Smoking Cessation Advice	29	100%	98%	97%
Surgical Care Improvement Project				
Appropriate VTP Within 24 Hours	75	95%	92%	92%
Appropriate Hair Removal	166	100%	100%	99%
Appropriate Beta Blocker Usage	26	100%	94%	93%
Controlled Postoperative Blood Glucose	0	-	94%	93%
Prophylactic Antibiotic Timing	95	100%	97%	97%
Prophylactic Antibiotic Timing (Outpatient)	541	98%	91%	92%
Prophylactic Antibiotic Selection	95	93%	98%	97%
Prophylactic Antibiotic Select. (Outpatient)	536	100%	94%	94%
Prophylactic Antibiotic Stopped	94	98%	95%	94%
Recommended VTP Ordered	75	97%	94%	94%
Urinary Catheter Removal[1]	23	61%	91%	90%
Children's Asthma Care				
Received Systemic Corticosteroids	-	-	-	100%
Received Home Management Plan	-	-	-	71%
Received Reliever Medication	-	-	-	100%
Use of Medical Imaging				
Combination Abdominal CT Scan	142	0.035	0.164	0.191
Combination Chest CT Scan	85	0.035	0.038	0.054
Follow-up Mammogram/Ultrasound[1]	2	0.0%	8.4%	8.4%
MRI for Low Back Pain[1]	7	42.9%	30.2%	32.7%
Survey of Patients' Hospital Experiences				
Area Around Room 'Always' Quiet at Night	300+	78%	-	58%
Doctors 'Always' Communicated Well	300+	83%	-	80%
Home Recovery Information Given	300+	81%	-	82%
Hospital Given 9 or 10 on 10 Point Scale	300+	82%	-	67%
Meds 'Always' Explained Before Given	300+	65%	-	60%
Nurses 'Always' Communicated Well	300+	80%	-	76%
Pain 'Always' Well Controlled	300+	71%	-	69%
Room and Bathroom 'Always' Clean	300+	73%	-	71%
Timely Help 'Always' Received	300+	67%	-	64%
Would Definitely Recommend Hospital	300+	86%	-	69%

East Liverpool City Hospital

425 West 5th Street — Phone: 330-385-7200
East Liverpool, OH 43920
URL: www.elch.org
Type: Acute Care Hospitals — Emergency Services: Yes
Ownership: Voluntary Non-Profit - Private — Beds: 199

Key Personnel:
CEO/President. . . . . Melvin R Creeley
Chief of Medical Staff. . . . . Mark W Swift
Infection Control . . . . Pamela Fox
Operating Room. . . . . Joseph Lach
Pediatric Ambulatory Care . . . . . . Helouise Mapa MD
Pediatric In-Patient Care . . . . Helouise Mapa MD
Quality Assurance . . . . Michelle Miller
Radiology. . . . . Boris A Karaman

Measure	Cases	This Hosp.	State Avg.	U.S. Avg.
Heart Attack Care				
ACE Inhibitor or ARB for LVSD[1]	2	100%	97%	96%
Aspirin at Arrival[1]	13	85%	99%	99%
Aspirin at Discharge[1]	7	86%	99%	98%
Beta Blocker at Discharge[1]	7	86%	99%	98%
Fibrinolytic Medication Timing	0	-	14%	55%
PCI Within 90 Minutes of Arrival	0	-	92%	90%
Smoking Cessation Advice	0	-	100%	99%
Chest Pain/Possible Heart Attack Care				
Aspirin at Arrival	124	85%	96%	95%
Median Time to ECG (minutes)	126	20	7	8
Median Time to Transfer (minutes)	28	77	61	61
Fibrinolytic Medication Timing[1]	2	0%	47%	54%
Heart Failure Care				
ACE Inhibitor or ARB for LVSD	48	96%	96%	94%
Discharge Instructions	162	95%	91%	88%
Evaluation of LVS Function	193	95%	99%	98%
Smoking Cessation Advice	41	90%	99%	98%
Pneumonia Care				
Appropriate Initial Antibiotic[2]	114	72%	92%	92%
Blood Culture Timing[2]	103	88%	96%	96%
Influenza Vaccine[2]	78	65%	93%	91%
Initial Antibiotic Timing[2]	141	92%	96%	95%
Pneumococcal Vaccine[2]	90	96%	95%	93%
Smoking Cessation Advice[2]	66	92%	98%	97%
Surgical Care Improvement Project				
Appropriate VTP Within 24 Hours	53	77%	92%	92%
Appropriate Hair Removal	141	100%	100%	99%
Appropriate Beta Blocker Usage	42	60%	94%	93%
Controlled Postoperative Blood Glucose	0	-	94%	93%
Prophylactic Antibiotic Timing	94	87%	97%	97%
Prophylactic Antibiotic Timing (Outpatient)[1]	18	67%	91%	92%
Prophylactic Antibiotic Selection	94	93%	98%	97%
Prophylactic Antibiotic Select. (Outpatient)[1]	12	75%	94%	94%
Prophylactic Antibiotic Stopped	88	85%	95%	94%
Recommended VTP Ordered	53	83%	94%	94%
Urinary Catheter Removal[1]	14	79%	91%	90%
Children's Asthma Care				
Received Systemic Corticosteroids	-	-	-	100%
Received Home Management Plan	-	-	-	71%
Received Reliever Medication	-	-	-	100%
Use of Medical Imaging				
Combination Abdominal CT Scan	390	0.079	0.164	0.191
Combination Chest CT Scan	274	0.069	0.038	0.054
Follow-up Mammogram/Ultrasound	446	7.2%	8.4%	8.4%
MRI for Low Back Pain	98	32.7%	30.2%	32.7%
Survey of Patients' Hospital Experiences				
Area Around Room 'Always' Quiet at Night	300+	50%	-	58%
Doctors 'Always' Communicated Well	300+	78%	-	80%
Home Recovery Information Given	300+	76%	-	82%
Hospital Given 9 or 10 on 10 Point Scale	300+	55%	-	67%
Meds 'Always' Explained Before Given	300+	57%	-	60%
Nurses 'Always' Communicated Well	300+	70%	-	76%
Pain 'Always' Well Controlled	300+	63%	-	69%
Room and Bathroom 'Always' Clean	300+	69%	-	71%
Timely Help 'Always' Received	300+	60%	-	64%
Would Definitely Recommend Hospital	300+	50%	-	69%

Emh Regional Medical Center

630 East River Street — Phone: 440-329-7500
Elyria, OH 44035 — Fax: 440-329-7505
Type: Acute Care Hospitals — Emergency Services: Yes
Ownership: Voluntary Non-Profit - Private — Beds: 348

Key Personnel:
CEO/President. . . . . Kevin C Martin
Chief of Medical Staff . . . . Kenneth Bescak, MD
Infection Control. . . . . Peggy Gnizak
Quality Assurance . . . . Sue Ballard
Radiology. . . . . Eduardo Martinez
Emergency Room . . . . JoAnn Hozalski
Patient Relations . . . . Deb Jones

Measure	Cases	This Hosp.	State Avg.	U.S. Avg.
Heart Attack Care				
ACE Inhibitor or ARB for LVSD[2]	58	91%	97%	96%
Aspirin at Arrival[2]	244	97%	99%	99%
Aspirin at Discharge[2]	291	100%	99%	98%
Beta Blocker at Discharge[2]	292	99%	99%	98%
Fibrinolytic Medication Timing[2]	0	-	14%	55%
PCI Within 90 Minutes of Arrival[2]	40	98%	92%	90%
Smoking Cessation Advice[2]	106	100%	100%	99%
Chest Pain/Possible Heart Attack Care				
Aspirin at Arrival	110	85%	96%	95%
Median Time to ECG (minutes)	120	9	7	8
Median Time to Transfer (minutes)[3]	0	-	61	61
Fibrinolytic Medication Timing[3]	0	-	47%	54%
Heart Failure Care				
ACE Inhibitor or ARB for LVSD[2]	108	87%	96%	94%
Discharge Instructions[2]	229	72%	91%	88%
Evaluation of LVS Function[2]	287	98%	99%	98%
Smoking Cessation Advice[2]	49	96%	99%	98%
Pneumonia Care				
Appropriate Initial Antibiotic[2]	79	89%	92%	92%
Blood Culture Timing[2]	70	99%	96%	96%
Influenza Vaccine[2]	100	58%	93%	91%
Initial Antibiotic Timing[2]	116	91%	96%	95%
Pneumococcal Vaccine[2]	143	81%	95%	93%
Smoking Cessation Advice[2]	58	100%	98%	97%
Surgical Care Improvement Project				
Appropriate VTP Within 24 Hours[2]	193	94%	92%	92%
Appropriate Hair Removal[2]	620	100%	100%	99%
Appropriate Beta Blocker Usage[2]	249	90%	94%	93%
Controlled Postoperative Blood Glucose[2]	117	77%	94%	93%
Prophylactic Antibiotic Timing[2]	449	98%	97%	97%
Prophylactic Antibiotic Timing (Outpatient)	459	94%	91%	92%
Prophylactic Antibiotic Selection[2]	453	98%	98%	97%
Prophylactic Antibiotic Select. (Outpatient)	448	95%	94%	94%
Prophylactic Antibiotic Stopped[2]	442	79%	95%	94%
Recommended VTP Ordered[2]	199	93%	94%	94%
Urinary Catheter Removal[2]	142	76%	91%	90%
Children's Asthma Care				
Received Systemic Corticosteroids	-	-	-	100%
Received Home Management Plan	-	-	-	71%
Received Reliever Medication	-	-	-	100%
Use of Medical Imaging				
Combination Abdominal CT Scan	1,118	0.053	0.164	0.191
Combination Chest CT Scan	722	0.001	0.038	0.054
Follow-up Mammogram/Ultrasound	558	6.1%	8.4%	8.4%
MRI for Low Back Pain	117	28.2%	30.2%	32.7%
Survey of Patients' Hospital Experiences				
Area Around Room 'Always' Quiet at Night	300+	45%	-	58%
Doctors 'Always' Communicated Well	300+	71%	-	80%
Home Recovery Information Given	300+	79%	-	82%
Hospital Given 9 or 10 on 10 Point Scale	300+	60%	-	67%
Meds 'Always' Explained Before Given	300+	55%	-	60%
Nurses 'Always' Communicated Well	300+	71%	-	76%
Pain 'Always' Well Controlled	300+	64%	-	69%
Room and Bathroom 'Always' Clean	300+	62%	-	71%
Timely Help 'Always' Received	300+	60%	-	64%
Would Definitely Recommend Hospital	300+	62%	-	69%

NOTE: Hospital profiles are in alphabetical order by state, then city, then hospital within the city; Rankings exclude hospitals with less than 25 cases except for patient surveys which excludes hospitals with less than 100 cases; (a) 100–299 cases; (1) The number of cases is too small to be sure how well a hospital is performing; (2) The hospital indicated that the data submitted for this measure were based on a sample of cases; (3) Data was collected during a shorter time period (fewer quarters) than the maximum possible time for this measure; (4) Suppressed for one or more quarters by CMS; (5) No data is available from the hospital for this measure; (6) Fewer than 100 patients completed the HCAHPS survey. Use these rates with caution, as the number of surveys may be too low to reliably assess hospital performance; (7) Survey results are based on less than 12 months of data; (8) Survey results are not available for this reporting period; (9) No or very few patients were eligible for the HCAHPS survey. The scores shown, if any, reflect a very small number of surveys; (10) A state average was not calculated because too few hospitals in the state submitted data; (11) There were discrepancies in the data collection process; Please refer to the User's Guide for a full explanation of data.

Euclid Hospital

18901 Lake Shore Boulevard Phone: 216-531-9000
Euclid, OH 44119 Fax: 216-692-7473
URL: www.euclidhospital.org
Type: Acute Care Hospitals Emergency Services: Yes
Ownership: Voluntary Non-Profit - Other Beds: 371

Key Personnel:
CEO/President. . . . . Lauren Rock
Chief of Medical Staff. . . . . Tommas Anton
Operating Room. . . . . Mark Janzen, MD
Radiology. . . . . Ellen Park

Measure	Cases	This Hosp.	State Avg.	U.S. Avg.
Heart Attack Care				
ACE Inhibitor or ARB for LVSD[1]	2	100%	97%	96%
Aspirin at Arrival	29	97%	99%	99%
Aspirin at Discharge[1]	23	100%	99%	98%
Beta Blocker at Discharge[1]	21	100%	99%	98%
Fibrinolytic Medication Timing	0	-	14%	55%
PCI Within 90 Minutes of Arrival	0	-	92%	90%
Smoking Cessation Advice[1]	11	100%	100%	99%
Chest Pain/Possible Heart Attack Care				
Aspirin at Arrival	84	98%	96%	95%
Median Time to ECG (minutes)	91	5	7	8
Median Time to Transfer (minutes)[1]	11	55	61	61
Fibrinolytic Medication Timing	0	-	47%	54%
Heart Failure Care				
ACE Inhibitor or ARB for LVSD	84	98%	96%	94%
Discharge Instructions	222	91%	91%	88%
Evaluation of LVS Function	309	100%	99%	98%
Smoking Cessation Advice	84	100%	99%	98%
Pneumonia Care				
Appropriate Initial Antibiotic	73	99%	92%	92%
Blood Culture Timing	132	97%	96%	96%
Influenza Vaccine	76	93%	93%	91%
Initial Antibiotic Timing	144	98%	96%	95%
Pneumococcal Vaccine	125	93%	95%	93%
Smoking Cessation Advice	69	100%	98%	97%
Surgical Care Improvement Project				
Appropriate VTP Within 24 Hours[2]	214	97%	92%	92%
Appropriate Hair Removal[2]	948	100%	100%	99%
Appropriate Beta Blocker Usage[2]	264	94%	94%	93%
Controlled Postoperative Blood Glucose[2]	0	-	94%	93%
Prophylactic Antibiotic Timing[2]	765	96%	97%	97%
Prophylactic Antibiotic Timing (Outpatient)	90	92%	91%	92%
Prophylactic Antibiotic Selection[2]	768	100%	98%	97%
Prophylactic Antibiotic Select. (Outpatient)	86	98%	94%	94%
Prophylactic Antibiotic Stopped[2]	744	99%	95%	94%
Recommended VTP Ordered[2]	214	98%	94%	94%
Urinary Catheter Removal[2]	369	93%	91%	90%
Children's Asthma Care				
Received Systemic Corticosteroids	-	-	-	100%
Received Home Management Plan	-	-	-	71%
Received Reliever Medication	-	-	-	100%
Use of Medical Imaging				
Combination Abdominal CT Scan	291	0.065	0.164	0.191
Combination Chest CT Scan	248	0.000	0.038	0.054
Follow-up Mammogram/Ultrasound	422	9.7%	8.4%	8.4%
MRI for Low Back Pain[1]	47	17.0%	30.2%	32.7%
Survey of Patients' Hospital Experiences				
Area Around Room 'Always' Quiet at Night	300+	52%	-	58%
Doctors 'Always' Communicated Well	300+	76%	-	80%
Home Recovery Information Given	300+	84%	-	82%
Hospital Given 9 or 10 on 10 Point Scale	300+	63%	-	67%
Meds 'Always' Explained Before Given	300+	58%	-	60%
Nurses 'Always' Communicated Well	300+	75%	-	76%
Pain 'Always' Well Controlled	300+	67%	-	69%
Room and Bathroom 'Always' Clean	300+	63%	-	71%
Timely Help 'Always' Received	300+	56%	-	64%
Would Definitely Recommend Hospital	300+	68%	-	69%

Mercy Hospital Fairfield

3000 Mack Road Phone: 513-870-7197
Fairfield, OH 45014 Fax: 513-870-7065
Type: Acute Care Hospitals Emergency Services: Yes
Ownership: Voluntary Non-Profit - Church Beds: 167

Key Personnel:
CEO/President. . . . . Tom Urban
Emergency Room . . . . Marla Yost

Measure	Cases	This Hosp.	State Avg.	U.S. Avg.
Heart Attack Care				
ACE Inhibitor or ARB for LVSD	54	100%	97%	96%
Aspirin at Arrival	268	99%	99%	99%
Aspirin at Discharge	291	100%	99%	98%
Beta Blocker at Discharge	273	99%	99%	98%
Fibrinolytic Medication Timing	0	-	14%	55%
PCI Within 90 Minutes of Arrival	48	94%	92%	90%
Smoking Cessation Advice	110	100%	100%	99%
Chest Pain/Possible Heart Attack Care				
Aspirin at Arrival[1]	7	100%	96%	95%
Median Time to ECG (minutes)[1]	8	10	7	8
Median Time to Transfer (minutes)[5]	0	-	61	61
Fibrinolytic Medication Timing[5]	0	-	47%	54%
Heart Failure Care				
ACE Inhibitor or ARB for LVSD	138	99%	96%	94%
Discharge Instructions	347	96%	91%	88%
Evaluation of LVS Function	411	99%	99%	98%
Smoking Cessation Advice	68	100%	99%	98%
Pneumonia Care				
Appropriate Initial Antibiotic	237	92%	92%	92%
Blood Culture Timing	388	99%	96%	96%
Influenza Vaccine	210	99%	93%	91%
Initial Antibiotic Timing	340	98%	96%	95%
Pneumococcal Vaccine	255	98%	95%	93%
Smoking Cessation Advice	127	100%	98%	97%
Surgical Care Improvement Project				
Appropriate VTP Within 24 Hours[2]	260	91%	92%	92%
Appropriate Hair Removal[2]	963	100%	100%	99%
Appropriate Beta Blocker Usage[2]	268	92%	94%	93%
Controlled Postoperative Blood Glucose[2]	187	96%	94%	93%
Prophylactic Antibiotic Timing[2]	716	96%	97%	97%
Prophylactic Antibiotic Timing (Outpatient)	159	89%	91%	92%
Prophylactic Antibiotic Selection[2]	716	97%	98%	97%
Prophylactic Antibiotic Select. (Outpatient)	181	90%	94%	94%
Prophylactic Antibiotic Stopped[2]	691	95%	95%	94%
Recommended VTP Ordered[2]	260	94%	94%	94%
Urinary Catheter Removal[2]	249	91%	91%	90%
Children's Asthma Care				
Received Systemic Corticosteroids	-	-	-	100%
Received Home Management Plan	-	-	-	71%
Received Reliever Medication	-	-	-	100%
Use of Medical Imaging				
Combination Abdominal CT Scan	1,221	0.045	0.164	0.191
Combination Chest CT Scan	820	0.026	0.038	0.054
Follow-up Mammogram/Ultrasound	1,186	3.0%	8.4%	8.4%
MRI for Low Back Pain	215	25.1%	30.2%	32.7%
Survey of Patients' Hospital Experiences				
Area Around Room 'Always' Quiet at Night	300+	54%	-	58%
Doctors 'Always' Communicated Well	300+	76%	-	80%
Home Recovery Information Given	300+	80%	-	82%
Hospital Given 9 or 10 on 10 Point Scale	300+	70%	-	67%
Meds 'Always' Explained Before Given	300+	60%	-	60%
Nurses 'Always' Communicated Well	300+	77%	-	76%
Pain 'Always' Well Controlled	300+	71%	-	69%
Room and Bathroom 'Always' Clean	300+	68%	-	71%
Timely Help 'Always' Received	300+	65%	-	64%
Would Definitely Recommend Hospital	300+	75%	-	69%

Blanchard Valley Hospital

1900 South Main Street Phone: 419-423-4500
Findlay, OH 45840 Fax: 419-423-5358
URL: www.bvha.org
Type: Acute Care Hospitals Emergency Services: Yes
Ownership: Voluntary Non-Profit - Other Beds: 150

Key Personnel:
CEO/President. . . . . Marilyn Kerr
Chief of Medical Staff. . . . . Richard Polder
Coronary Care . . . . Sherri Winegardner
Operating Room. . . . . Eric Browning
Pediatric Ambulatory Care . . . . . . A Ritz, MD
Quality Assurance . . . . Sandy Shutt
Radiology. . . . . Edward Bok

Measure	Cases	This Hosp.	State Avg.	U.S. Avg.
Heart Attack Care				
ACE Inhibitor or ARB for LVSD[1]	19	100%	97%	96%
Aspirin at Arrival	124	100%	99%	99%
Aspirin at Discharge	128	100%	99%	98%
Beta Blocker at Discharge	117	100%	99%	98%
Fibrinolytic Medication Timing	0	-	14%	55%
PCI Within 90 Minutes of Arrival	50	94%	92%	90%
Smoking Cessation Advice	45	98%	100%	99%
Chest Pain/Possible Heart Attack Care				
Aspirin at Arrival[1,3]	3	100%	96%	95%
Median Time to ECG (minutes)[1,3]	4	8	7	8
Median Time to Transfer (minutes)[5]	0	-	61	61
Fibrinolytic Medication Timing[5]	0	-	47%	54%
Heart Failure Care				
ACE Inhibitor or ARB for LVSD	47	100%	96%	94%
Discharge Instructions	70	96%	91%	88%
Evaluation of LVS Function	105	100%	99%	98%
Smoking Cessation Advice[1]	14	100%	99%	98%
Pneumonia Care				
Appropriate Initial Antibiotic	95	89%	92%	92%
Blood Culture Timing	120	98%	96%	96%
Influenza Vaccine	90	99%	93%	91%
Initial Antibiotic Timing	118	97%	96%	95%
Pneumococcal Vaccine	127	100%	95%	93%
Smoking Cessation Advice	44	93%	98%	97%
Surgical Care Improvement Project				
Appropriate VTP Within 24 Hours[2]	183	86%	92%	92%
Appropriate Hair Removal[2]	754	100%	100%	99%
Appropriate Beta Blocker Usage[2]	216	87%	94%	93%
Controlled Postoperative Blood Glucose[2]	69	96%	94%	93%
Prophylactic Antibiotic Timing[2]	604	98%	97%	97%
Prophylactic Antibiotic Timing (Outpatient)	545	98%	91%	92%
Prophylactic Antibiotic Selection[2]	614	98%	98%	97%
Prophylactic Antibiotic Select. (Outpatient)	538	97%	94%	94%
Prophylactic Antibiotic Stopped[2]	585	97%	95%	94%
Recommended VTP Ordered[2]	184	88%	94%	94%
Urinary Catheter Removal[2]	131	82%	91%	90%
Children's Asthma Care				
Received Systemic Corticosteroids	-	-	-	100%
Received Home Management Plan	-	-	-	71%
Received Reliever Medication	-	-	-	100%
Use of Medical Imaging				
Combination Abdominal CT Scan	1,107	0.121	0.164	0.191
Combination Chest CT Scan	582	0.034	0.038	0.054
Follow-up Mammogram/Ultrasound	1,414	9.3%	8.4%	8.4%
MRI for Low Back Pain	339	27.1%	30.2%	32.7%
Survey of Patients' Hospital Experiences				
Area Around Room 'Always' Quiet at Night	300+	61%	-	58%
Doctors 'Always' Communicated Well	300+	83%	-	80%
Home Recovery Information Given	300+	83%	-	82%
Hospital Given 9 or 10 on 10 Point Scale	300+	72%	-	67%
Meds 'Always' Explained Before Given	300+	62%	-	60%
Nurses 'Always' Communicated Well	300+	76%	-	76%
Pain 'Always' Well Controlled	300+	71%	-	69%
Room and Bathroom 'Always' Clean	300+	82%	-	71%
Timely Help 'Always' Received	300+	67%	-	64%
Would Definitely Recommend Hospital	300+	72%	-	69%

NOTE: Hospital profiles are in alphabetical order by state, then city, then hospital within the city; Rankings exclude hospitals with less than 25 cases except for patient surveys which excludes hospitals with less than 100 cases; (a) 100–299 cases; (1) The number of cases is too small to be sure how well a hospital is performing; (2) The hospital indicated that the data submitted for this measure were based on a sample of cases; (3) Data was collected during a shorter time period (fewer quarters) than the maximum possible time for this measure; (4) Suppressed for one or more quarters by CMS; (5) No data is available from the hospital for this measure; (6) Fewer than 100 patients completed the HCAHPS survey. Use these rates with caution, as the number of surveys may be too low to reliably assess hospital performance; (7) Survey results are based on less than 12 months of data; (8) Survey results are not available for this reporting period; (9) No or very few patients were eligible for the HCAHPS survey. The scores shown, if any, reflect a very small number of surveys; (10) A state average was not calculated because too few hospitals in the state submitted data; (11) There were discrepancies in the data collection process; Please refer to the User's Guide for a full explanation of data.

Fostoria Community Hospital

501 Van Buren Street
Fostoria, OH 44830
Phone: 419-435-7734
Fax: 419-436-6602
Type: Critical Access Hospitals
Emergency Services: Yes
Ownership: Voluntary Non-Profit - Private
Beds: 66

Key Personnel:
CEO/President. . . . . Tim Jakacki
Chief of Medical Staff . . . . D Ross, MD
Emergency Room . . . . Amy Preble

Measure	Cases	This Hosp.	State Avg.	U.S. Avg.
Heart Attack Care				
ACE Inhibitor or ARB for LVSD[1]	1	100%	97%	96%
Aspirin at Arrival[1]	14	100%	99%	99%
Aspirin at Discharge[1]	6	100%	99%	98%
Beta Blocker at Discharge[1]	9	89%	99%	98%
Fibrinolytic Medication Timing	0	-	14%	55%
PCI Within 90 Minutes of Arrival	0	-	92%	90%
Smoking Cessation Advice	0	-	100%	99%
Chest Pain/Possible Heart Attack Care				
Aspirin at Arrival	-	-	96%	95%
Median Time to ECG (minutes)	-	-	7	8
Median Time to Transfer (minutes)	-	-	61	61
Fibrinolytic Medication Timing	-	-	47%	54%
Heart Failure Care				
ACE Inhibitor or ARB for LVSD[1]	8	100%	96%	94%
Discharge Instructions	29	97%	91%	88%
Evaluation of LVS Function	32	100%	99%	98%
Smoking Cessation Advice[1]	9	100%	99%	98%
Pneumonia Care				
Appropriate Initial Antibiotic	38	97%	92%	92%
Blood Culture Timing	36	100%	96%	96%
Influenza Vaccine	25	88%	93%	91%
Initial Antibiotic Timing	46	100%	96%	95%
Pneumococcal Vaccine	35	97%	95%	93%
Smoking Cessation Advice[1]	17	100%	98%	97%
Surgical Care Improvement Project				
Appropriate VTP Within 24 Hours[1]	12	100%	92%	92%
Appropriate Hair Removal	141	100%	100%	99%
Appropriate Beta Blocker Usage[5]	0	-	94%	93%
Controlled Postoperative Blood Glucose	0	-	94%	93%
Prophylactic Antibiotic Timing	135	100%	97%	97%
Prophylactic Antibiotic Timing (Outpatient)	-	-	91%	92%
Prophylactic Antibiotic Selection	135	99%	98%	97%
Prophylactic Antibiotic Select. (Outpatient)	-	-	94%	94%
Prophylactic Antibiotic Stopped	132	100%	95%	94%
Recommended VTP Ordered[1]	12	100%	94%	94%
Urinary Catheter Removal	0	-	91%	90%
Children's Asthma Care				
Received Systemic Corticosteroids	-	-	-	100%
Received Home Management Plan	-	-	-	71%
Received Reliever Medication	-	-	-	100%
Use of Medical Imaging				
Combination Abdominal CT Scan	-	-	0.164	0.191
Combination Chest CT Scan	-	-	0.038	0.054
Follow-up Mammogram/Ultrasound	-	-	8.4%	8.4%
MRI for Low Back Pain	-	-	30.2%	32.7%
Survey of Patients' Hospital Experiences				
Area Around Room 'Always' Quiet at Night	300+	59%	-	58%
Doctors 'Always' Communicated Well	300+	80%	-	80%
Home Recovery Information Given	300+	87%	-	82%
Hospital Given 9 or 10 on 10 Point Scale	300+	70%	-	67%
Meds 'Always' Explained Before Given	300+	61%	-	60%
Nurses 'Always' Communicated Well	300+	79%	-	76%
Pain 'Always' Well Controlled	300+	72%	-	69%
Room and Bathroom 'Always' Clean	300+	77%	-	71%
Timely Help 'Always' Received	300+	71%	-	64%
Would Definitely Recommend Hospital	300+	74%	-	69%

Atrium Medical Center

One Medical Center Drive
Franklin, OH 45005
Phone: 513-424-2111
URL: www.atriummedcenter.org
Type: Acute Care Hospitals
Emergency Services: Yes
Ownership: Voluntary Non-Profit - Private
Beds: 250

Key Personnel:
CEO/President. . . . . McNeill Doug
Pediatric Ambulatory Care . . . . . . Diana E Small MD
Radiology. . . . . Chris Chung MD

Measure	Cases	This Hosp.	State Avg.	U.S. Avg.
Heart Attack Care				
ACE Inhibitor or ARB for LVSD[2]	42	100%	97%	96%
Aspirin at Arrival[2]	280	100%	99%	99%
Aspirin at Discharge[2]	251	100%	99%	98%
Beta Blocker at Discharge[2]	240	100%	99%	98%
Fibrinolytic Medication Timing[2]	0	-	14%	55%
PCI Within 90 Minutes of Arrival[2]	54	85%	92%	90%
Smoking Cessation Advice[2]	98	100%	100%	99%
Chest Pain/Possible Heart Attack Care				
Aspirin at Arrival	31	100%	96%	95%
Median Time to ECG (minutes)	31	7	7	8
Median Time to Transfer (minutes)[1,3]	2	54	61	61
Fibrinolytic Medication Timing	0	-	47%	54%
Heart Failure Care				
ACE Inhibitor or ARB for LVSD	64	98%	96%	94%
Discharge Instructions	290	91%	91%	88%
Evaluation of LVS Function	358	100%	99%	98%
Smoking Cessation Advice	86	100%	99%	98%
Pneumonia Care				
Appropriate Initial Antibiotic	182	93%	92%	92%
Blood Culture Timing	286	97%	96%	96%
Influenza Vaccine	201	98%	93%	91%
Initial Antibiotic Timing	268	97%	96%	95%
Pneumococcal Vaccine	264	98%	95%	93%
Smoking Cessation Advice	181	100%	98%	97%
Surgical Care Improvement Project				
Appropriate VTP Within 24 Hours[2]	312	97%	92%	92%
Appropriate Hair Removal[2]	894	100%	100%	99%
Appropriate Beta Blocker Usage[2]	256	100%	94%	93%
Controlled Postoperative Blood Glucose[2]	97	96%	94%	93%
Prophylactic Antibiotic Timing[2]	508	99%	97%	97%
Prophylactic Antibiotic Timing (Outpatient)	255	91%	91%	92%
Prophylactic Antibiotic Selection[2]	512	99%	98%	97%
Prophylactic Antibiotic Select. (Outpatient)	238	95%	94%	94%
Prophylactic Antibiotic Stopped[2]	483	98%	95%	94%
Recommended VTP Ordered[2]	312	99%	94%	94%
Urinary Catheter Removal	167	98%	91%	90%
Children's Asthma Care				
Received Systemic Corticosteroids	-	-	-	100%
Received Home Management Plan	-	-	-	71%
Received Reliever Medication	-	-	-	100%
Use of Medical Imaging				
Combination Abdominal CT Scan	961	0.062	0.164	0.191
Combination Chest CT Scan	765	0.016	0.038	0.054
Follow-up Mammogram/Ultrasound	1,455	8.9%	8.4%	8.4%
MRI for Low Back Pain	147	29.9%	30.2%	32.7%
Survey of Patients' Hospital Experiences				
Area Around Room 'Always' Quiet at Night	300+	59%	-	58%
Doctors 'Always' Communicated Well	300+	76%	-	80%
Home Recovery Information Given	300+	82%	-	82%
Hospital Given 9 or 10 on 10 Point Scale	300+	64%	-	67%
Meds 'Always' Explained Before Given	300+	57%	-	60%
Nurses 'Always' Communicated Well	300+	73%	-	76%
Pain 'Always' Well Controlled	300+	68%	-	69%
Room and Bathroom 'Always' Clean	300+	73%	-	71%
Timely Help 'Always' Received	300+	55%	-	64%
Would Definitely Recommend Hospital	300+	65%	-	69%

Memorial Hospital

715 South Taft Avenue
Fremont, OH 43420
Phone: 419-334-6617
Fax: 419-332-5875
URL: www.freemontmemorial.org
Type: Acute Care Hospitals
Emergency Services: Yes
Ownership: Voluntary Non-Profit - Other
Beds: 186

Key Personnel:
Chief of Medical Staff . . . . Robert Marshall, MD
Infection Control. . . . . Tami Binger
Operating Room. . . . . Michael E Grillis
Quality Assurance . . . . Brenda McClain
Radiology. . . . . Bruce L Hammond
Emergency Room . . . . Dana Levy

Measure	Cases	This Hosp.	State Avg.	U.S. Avg.
Heart Attack Care				
ACE Inhibitor or ARB for LVSD[1]	1	100%	97%	96%
Aspirin at Arrival[1]	12	100%	99%	99%
Aspirin at Discharge[1]	8	88%	99%	98%
Beta Blocker at Discharge[1]	8	88%	99%	98%
Fibrinolytic Medication Timing[1]	1	0%	14%	55%
PCI Within 90 Minutes of Arrival	0	-	92%	90%
Smoking Cessation Advice	0	-	100%	99%
Chest Pain/Possible Heart Attack Care				
Aspirin at Arrival	98	89%	96%	95%
Median Time to ECG (minutes)	108	14	7	8
Median Time to Transfer (minutes)[1]	6	90	61	61
Fibrinolytic Medication Timing[1]	2	50%	47%	54%
Heart Failure Care				
ACE Inhibitor or ARB for LVSD[1]	14	93%	96%	94%
Discharge Instructions	34	79%	91%	88%
Evaluation of LVS Function	44	95%	99%	98%
Smoking Cessation Advice[1]	8	100%	99%	98%
Pneumonia Care				
Appropriate Initial Antibiotic	40	82%	92%	92%
Blood Culture Timing	73	93%	96%	96%
Influenza Vaccine	46	78%	93%	91%
Initial Antibiotic Timing	71	92%	96%	95%
Pneumococcal Vaccine	56	88%	95%	93%
Smoking Cessation Advice	28	89%	98%	97%
Surgical Care Improvement Project				
Appropriate VTP Within 24 Hours	62	81%	92%	92%
Appropriate Hair Removal	220	99%	100%	99%
Appropriate Beta Blocker Usage	62	85%	94%	93%
Controlled Postoperative Blood Glucose	0	-	94%	93%
Prophylactic Antibiotic Timing	173	83%	97%	97%
Prophylactic Antibiotic Timing (Outpatient)	79	65%	91%	92%
Prophylactic Antibiotic Selection	174	97%	98%	97%
Prophylactic Antibiotic Select. (Outpatient)	54	93%	94%	94%
Prophylactic Antibiotic Stopped	171	71%	95%	94%
Recommended VTP Ordered	64	80%	94%	94%
Urinary Catheter Removal	62	94%	91%	90%
Children's Asthma Care				
Received Systemic Corticosteroids	-	-	-	100%
Received Home Management Plan	-	-	-	71%
Received Reliever Medication	-	-	-	100%
Use of Medical Imaging				
Combination Abdominal CT Scan	468	0.639	0.164	0.191
Combination Chest CT Scan	392	0.227	0.038	0.054
Follow-up Mammogram/Ultrasound	807	6.9%	8.4%	8.4%
MRI for Low Back Pain	125	26.4%	30.2%	32.7%
Survey of Patients' Hospital Experiences				
Area Around Room 'Always' Quiet at Night	300+	55%	-	58%
Doctors 'Always' Communicated Well	300+	84%	-	80%
Home Recovery Information Given	300+	87%	-	82%
Hospital Given 9 or 10 on 10 Point Scale	300+	65%	-	67%
Meds 'Always' Explained Before Given	300+	61%	-	60%
Nurses 'Always' Communicated Well	300+	78%	-	76%
Pain 'Always' Well Controlled	300+	70%	-	69%
Room and Bathroom 'Always' Clean	300+	75%	-	71%
Timely Help 'Always' Received	300+	68%	-	64%
Would Definitely Recommend Hospital	300+	62%	-	69%

NOTE: Hospital profiles are in alphabetical order by state, then city, then hospital within the city; Rankings exclude hospitals with less than 25 cases except for patient surveys which excludes hospitals with less than 100 cases; (a) 100–299 cases; (1) The number of cases is too small to be sure how well a hospital is performing; (2) The hospital indicated that the data submitted for this measure were based on a sample of cases; (3) Data was collected during a shorter time period (fewer quarters) than the maximum possible time for this measure; (4) Suppressed for one or more quarters by CMS; (5) No data is available from the hospital for this measure; (6) Fewer than 100 patients completed the HCAHPS survey. Use these rates with caution, as the number of surveys may be too low to reliably assess hospital performance; (7) Survey results are based on less than 12 months of data; (8) Survey results are not available for this reporting period; (9) No or very few patients were eligible for the HCAHPS survey. The scores shown, if any, reflect a very small number of surveys; (10) A state average was not calculated because too few hospitals in the state submitted data; (11) There were discrepancies in the data collection process; Please refer to the User's Guide for a full explanation of data.

Physician's Choice Hospital - Fremont

2390 Enterprise Drive
Phone: 419-461-1057
Fremont, OH 43420
URL: www.physicianschoicehospital.com
Type: Acute Care Hospitals
Emergency Services: Yes
Ownership: Voluntary Non-Profit - Private

Measure	Cases	This Hosp.	State Avg.	U.S. Avg.
Heart Attack Care				
ACE Inhibitor or ARB for LVSD[2,3]	0	-	97%	96%
Aspirin at Arrival[1,2,3]	2	50%	99%	99%
Aspirin at Discharge[1,2,3]	1	100%	99%	98%
Beta Blocker at Discharge[1,2,3]	1	0%	99%	98%
Fibrinolytic Medication Timing[2,3]	0	-	14%	55%
PCI Within 90 Minutes of Arrival[2,3]	0	-	92%	90%
Smoking Cessation Advice[2,3]	0	-	100%	99%
Chest Pain/Possible Heart Attack Care				
Aspirin at Arrival	-	-	96%	95%
Median Time to ECG (minutes)	-	-	7	8
Median Time to Transfer (minutes)	-	-	61	61
Fibrinolytic Medication Timing	-	-	47%	54%
Heart Failure Care				
ACE Inhibitor or ARB for LVSD[1,2,3]	1	0%	96%	94%
Discharge Instructions[1,2,3]	3	0%	91%	88%
Evaluation of LVS Function[1,2,3]	3	67%	99%	98%
Smoking Cessation Advice[2,3]	0	-	99%	98%
Pneumonia Care				
Appropriate Initial Antibiotic[2,3]	0	-	92%	92%
Blood Culture Timing[1,2,3]	2	50%	96%	96%
Influenza Vaccine[2,3]	0	-	93%	91%
Initial Antibiotic Timing[1,2,3]	1	100%	96%	95%
Pneumococcal Vaccine[1,2,3]	1	100%	95%	93%
Smoking Cessation Advice[2,3]	0	-	98%	97%
Surgical Care Improvement Project				
Appropriate VTP Within 24 Hours[5]	0	-	92%	92%
Appropriate Hair Removal[5]	0	-	100%	99%
Appropriate Beta Blocker Usage[5]	0	-	94%	93%
Controlled Postoperative Blood Glucose[5]	0	-	94%	93%
Prophylactic Antibiotic Timing[5]	0	-	97%	97%
Prophylactic Antibiotic Timing (Outpatient)	-	-	91%	92%
Prophylactic Antibiotic Selection[5]	0	-	98%	97%
Prophylactic Antibiotic Select. (Outpatient)	-	-	94%	94%
Prophylactic Antibiotic Stopped[5]	0	-	95%	94%
Recommended VTP Ordered[5]	0	-	94%	94%
Urinary Catheter Removal[5]	0	-	91%	90%
Children's Asthma Care				
Received Systemic Corticosteroids	-	-	-	100%
Received Home Management Plan	-	-	-	71%
Received Reliever Medication	-	-	-	100%
Use of Medical Imaging				
Combination Abdominal CT Scan	-	-	0.164	0.191
Combination Chest CT Scan	-	-	0.038	0.054
Follow-up Mammogram/Ultrasound	-	-	8.4%	8.4%
MRI for Low Back Pain	-	-	30.2%	32.7%
Survey of Patients' Hospital Experiences				
Area Around Room 'Always' Quiet at Night[8]	-	-	-	58%
Doctors 'Always' Communicated Well[8]	-	-	-	80%
Home Recovery Information Given[8]	-	-	-	82%
Hospital Given 9 or 10 on 10 Point Scale[8]	-	-	-	67%
Meds 'Always' Explained Before Given[8]	-	-	-	60%
Nurses 'Always' Communicated Well[8]	-	-	-	76%
Pain 'Always' Well Controlled[8]	-	-	-	69%
Room and Bathroom 'Always' Clean[8]	-	-	-	71%
Timely Help 'Always' Received[8]	-	-	-	64%
Would Definitely Recommend Hospital[8]	-	-	-	69%

Galion Community Hospital

269 Portland Way South
Phone: 419-468-4841
Galion, OH 44833
Fax: 419-468-2381
URL: www.galionhospital.org
Type: Critical Access Hospitals
Emergency Services: Yes
Ownership: Voluntary Non-Profit - Church
Beds: 25

Key Personnel:
CEO/President. . . . . LaMar Wyse
Chief of Medical Staff . . . . Julie C Beard
Quality Assurance . . . . Helen Burdine
Radiology. . . . . James J Jerele
Emergency Room . . . . John Schoettmer
Intensive Care Unit. . . . . Shirley Fitz
Patient Relations . . . . Rebecca Miller

Measure	Cases	This Hosp.	State Avg.	U.S. Avg.
Heart Attack Care				
ACE Inhibitor or ARB for LVSD[3]	0	-	97%	96%
Aspirin at Arrival[1,3]	6	83%	99%	99%
Aspirin at Discharge[1,3]	4	50%	99%	98%
Beta Blocker at Discharge[1,3]	4	100%	99%	98%
Fibrinolytic Medication Timing[3]	0	-	14%	55%
PCI Within 90 Minutes of Arrival[3]	0	-	92%	90%
Smoking Cessation Advice[3]	0	-	100%	99%
Chest Pain/Possible Heart Attack Care				
Aspirin at Arrival	-	-	96%	95%
Median Time to ECG (minutes)	-	-	7	8
Median Time to Transfer (minutes)	-	-	61	61
Fibrinolytic Medication Timing	-	-	47%	54%
Heart Failure Care				
ACE Inhibitor or ARB for LVSD[1,3]	9	78%	96%	94%
Discharge Instructions[1,3]	13	92%	91%	88%
Evaluation of LVS Function[1,3]	21	95%	99%	98%
Smoking Cessation Advice[1,3]	4	75%	99%	98%
Pneumonia Care				
Appropriate Initial Antibiotic[1,3]	19	95%	92%	92%
Blood Culture Timing[1,3]	21	86%	96%	96%
Influenza Vaccine[1]	13	85%	93%	91%
Initial Antibiotic Timing[1,3]	23	100%	96%	95%
Pneumococcal Vaccine[1,3]	13	100%	95%	93%
Smoking Cessation Advice[1,3]	9	89%	98%	97%
Surgical Care Improvement Project				
Appropriate VTP Within 24 Hours[1,3]	24	96%	92%	92%
Appropriate Hair Removal[3]	123	100%	100%	99%
Appropriate Beta Blocker Usage[3]	40	80%	94%	93%
Controlled Postoperative Blood Glucose[3]	0	-	94%	93%
Prophylactic Antibiotic Timing[3]	112	94%	97%	97%
Prophylactic Antibiotic Timing (Outpatient)	-	-	91%	92%
Prophylactic Antibiotic Selection[3]	114	96%	98%	97%
Prophylactic Antibiotic Select. (Outpatient)	-	-	94%	94%
Prophylactic Antibiotic Stopped[3]	112	96%	95%	94%
Recommended VTP Ordered[1,3]	24	96%	94%	94%
Urinary Catheter Removal[1,3]	18	72%	91%	90%
Children's Asthma Care				
Received Systemic Corticosteroids	-	-	-	100%
Received Home Management Plan	-	-	-	71%
Received Reliever Medication	-	-	-	100%
Use of Medical Imaging				
Combination Abdominal CT Scan	-	-	0.164	0.191
Combination Chest CT Scan	-	-	0.038	0.054
Follow-up Mammogram/Ultrasound	-	-	8.4%	8.4%
MRI for Low Back Pain	-	-	30.2%	32.7%
Survey of Patients' Hospital Experiences				
Area Around Room 'Always' Quiet at Night	300+	55%	-	58%
Doctors 'Always' Communicated Well	300+	88%	-	80%
Home Recovery Information Given	300+	89%	-	82%
Hospital Given 9 or 10 on 10 Point Scale	300+	73%	-	67%
Meds 'Always' Explained Before Given	300+	69%	-	60%
Nurses 'Always' Communicated Well	300+	83%	-	76%
Pain 'Always' Well Controlled	300+	77%	-	69%
Room and Bathroom 'Always' Clean	300+	81%	-	71%
Timely Help 'Always' Received	300+	79%	-	64%
Would Definitely Recommend Hospital	300+	73%	-	69%

Holzer Medical Center

100 Jackson Pike
Phone: 740-446-5000
Gallipolis, OH 45631
Fax: 740-446-5522
URL: www.holzer.org
Type: Acute Care Hospitals
Emergency Services: Yes
Ownership: Voluntary Non-Profit - Private
Beds: 269

Key Personnel:
CEO/President. . . . . James Phillippe
Chief of Medical Staff . . . . Jamal Haddad
Coronary Care . . . . Glenda Skinner
Infection Control. . . . . Nancy Childs, RN
Pediatric Ambulatory Care . . . . . . Cindy Harrison
Pediatric In-Patient Care . . . . Cindy Harrison
Quality Assurance . . . . Thomas Judy
Radiology. . . . . Mike Roe

Measure	Cases	This Hosp.	State Avg.	U.S. Avg.
Heart Attack Care				
ACE Inhibitor or ARB for LVSD[1]	14	86%	97%	96%
Aspirin at Arrival	95	96%	99%	99%
Aspirin at Discharge	95	92%	99%	98%
Beta Blocker at Discharge	98	95%	99%	98%
Fibrinolytic Medication Timing	0	-	14%	55%
PCI Within 90 Minutes of Arrival[1]	11	73%	92%	90%
Smoking Cessation Advice	30	97%	100%	99%
Chest Pain/Possible Heart Attack Care				
Aspirin at Arrival	33	82%	96%	95%
Median Time to ECG (minutes)	31	5	7	8
Median Time to Transfer (minutes)[1,3]	1	125	61	61
Fibrinolytic Medication Timing[1]	1	0%	47%	54%
Heart Failure Care				
ACE Inhibitor or ARB for LVSD	84	86%	96%	94%
Discharge Instructions	253	85%	91%	88%
Evaluation of LVS Function	309	97%	99%	98%
Smoking Cessation Advice	43	93%	99%	98%
Pneumonia Care				
Appropriate Initial Antibiotic[2]	115	85%	92%	92%
Blood Culture Timing[2]	115	90%	96%	96%
Influenza Vaccine[2]	91	86%	93%	91%
Initial Antibiotic Timing[2]	136	95%	96%	95%
Pneumococcal Vaccine[2]	122	98%	95%	93%
Smoking Cessation Advice[2]	76	95%	98%	97%
Surgical Care Improvement Project				
Appropriate VTP Within 24 Hours	94	86%	92%	92%
Appropriate Hair Removal	302	99%	100%	99%
Appropriate Beta Blocker Usage	117	87%	94%	93%
Controlled Postoperative Blood Glucose	35	91%	94%	93%
Prophylactic Antibiotic Timing	179	97%	97%	97%
Prophylactic Antibiotic Timing (Outpatient)	59	90%	91%	92%
Prophylactic Antibiotic Selection	179	95%	98%	97%
Prophylactic Antibiotic Select. (Outpatient)	54	98%	94%	94%
Prophylactic Antibiotic Stopped	175	87%	95%	94%
Recommended VTP Ordered	98	86%	94%	94%
Urinary Catheter Removal	44	80%	91%	90%
Children's Asthma Care				
Received Systemic Corticosteroids	-	-	-	100%
Received Home Management Plan	-	-	-	71%
Received Reliever Medication	-	-	-	100%
Use of Medical Imaging				
Combination Abdominal CT Scan	294	0.061	0.164	0.191
Combination Chest CT Scan	110	0.009	0.038	0.054
Follow-up Mammogram/Ultrasound[5]	0	-	8.4%	8.4%
MRI for Low Back Pain[5]	0	-	30.2%	32.7%
Survey of Patients' Hospital Experiences				
Area Around Room 'Always' Quiet at Night	300+	57%	-	58%
Doctors 'Always' Communicated Well	300+	80%	-	80%
Home Recovery Information Given	300+	85%	-	82%
Hospital Given 9 or 10 on 10 Point Scale	300+	65%	-	67%
Meds 'Always' Explained Before Given	300+	61%	-	60%
Nurses 'Always' Communicated Well	300+	79%	-	76%
Pain 'Always' Well Controlled	300+	73%	-	69%
Room and Bathroom 'Always' Clean	300+	77%	-	71%
Timely Help 'Always' Received	300+	68%	-	64%
Would Definitely Recommend Hospital	300+	63%	-	69%

NOTE: Hospital profiles are in alphabetical order by state, then city, then hospital within the city; Rankings exclude hospitals with less than 25 cases except for patient surveys which excludes hospitals with less than 100 cases; (a) 100–299 cases; (1) The number of cases is too small to be sure how well a hospital is performing; (2) The hospital indicated that the data submitted for this measure were based on a sample of cases; (3) Data was collected during a shorter time period (fewer quarters) than the maximum possible time for this measure; (4) Suppressed for one or more quarters by CMS; (5) No data is available from the hospital for this measure; (6) Fewer than 100 patients completed the HCAHPS survey. Use these rates with caution, as the number of surveys may be too low to reliably assess hospital performance; (7) Survey results are based on less than 12 months of data; (8) Survey results are not available for this reporting period; (9) No or very few patients were eligible for the HCAHPS survey. The scores shown, if any, reflect a very small number of surveys; (10) A state average was not calculated because too few hospitals in the state submitted data; (11) There were discrepancies in the data collection process; Please refer to the User's Guide for a full explanation of data.

Marymount Hospital

12300 Mccracken Road
Garfield Heights, OH 44125
Phone: 216-581-0500
Fax: 216-587-8967
E-mail: marketing@marymount.org
URL: www.marymount.org
Type: Acute Care Hospitals
Emergency Services: Yes
Ownership: Voluntary Non-Profit - Church
Beds: 312

Key Personnel:
CEO/President. . . . . David J Kilarski
Chief of Medical Staff. . . . . Richard Ungvarsky, MD
Radiology. . . . . Indu Agarwal

Measure	Cases	This Hosp.	State Avg.	U.S. Avg.
Heart Attack Care				
ACE Inhibitor or ARB for LVSD[1]	5	100%	97%	96%
Aspirin at Arrival	62	100%	99%	99%
Aspirin at Discharge	37	100%	99%	98%
Beta Blocker at Discharge	38	100%	99%	98%
Fibrinolytic Medication Timing	0	-	14%	55%
PCI Within 90 Minutes of Arrival	0	-	92%	90%
Smoking Cessation Advice[1]	6	100%	100%	99%
Chest Pain/Possible Heart Attack Care				
Aspirin at Arrival	134	96%	96%	95%
Median Time to ECG (minutes)	137	7	7	8
Median Time to Transfer (minutes)	33	55	61	61
Fibrinolytic Medication Timing	0	-	47%	54%
Heart Failure Care				
ACE Inhibitor or ARB for LVSD	178	95%	96%	94%
Discharge Instructions	439	92%	91%	88%
Evaluation of LVS Function	623	99%	99%	98%
Smoking Cessation Advice	98	97%	99%	98%
Pneumonia Care				
Appropriate Initial Antibiotic	140	94%	92%	92%
Blood Culture Timing	293	97%	96%	96%
Influenza Vaccine	249	93%	93%	91%
Initial Antibiotic Timing	280	96%	96%	95%
Pneumococcal Vaccine	324	94%	95%	93%
Smoking Cessation Advice	125	100%	98%	97%
Surgical Care Improvement Project				
Appropriate VTP Within 24 Hours[2]	182	87%	92%	92%
Appropriate Hair Removal[2]	526	100%	100%	99%
Appropriate Beta Blocker Usage[2]	173	91%	94%	93%
Controlled Postoperative Blood Glucose[2]	0	-	94%	93%
Prophylactic Antibiotic Timing[2]	363	99%	97%	97%
Prophylactic Antibiotic Timing (Outpatient)	254	97%	91%	92%
Prophylactic Antibiotic Selection[2]	367	97%	98%	97%
Prophylactic Antibiotic Select. (Outpatient)	297	94%	94%	94%
Prophylactic Antibiotic Stopped[2]	351	97%	95%	94%
Recommended VTP Ordered[2]	182	87%	94%	94%
Urinary Catheter Removal[2]	139	89%	91%	90%
Children's Asthma Care				
Received Systemic Corticosteroids	-	-	-	100%
Received Home Management Plan	-	-	-	71%
Received Reliever Medication	-	-	-	100%
Use of Medical Imaging				
Combination Abdominal CT Scan	766	0.244	0.164	0.191
Combination Chest CT Scan	502	0.008	0.038	0.054
Follow-up Mammogram/Ultrasound	1,116	8.0%	8.4%	8.4%
MRI for Low Back Pain	151	37.1%	30.2%	32.7%
Survey of Patients' Hospital Experiences				
Area Around Room 'Always' Quiet at Night	300+	41%	-	58%
Doctors 'Always' Communicated Well	300+	72%	-	80%
Home Recovery Information Given	300+	83%	-	82%
Hospital Given 9 or 10 on 10 Point Scale	300+	55%	-	67%
Meds 'Always' Explained Before Given	300+	52%	-	60%
Nurses 'Always' Communicated Well	300+	69%	-	76%
Pain 'Always' Well Controlled	300+	62%	-	69%
Room and Bathroom 'Always' Clean	300+	65%	-	71%
Timely Help 'Always' Received	300+	55%	-	64%
Would Definitely Recommend Hospital	300+	57%	-	69%

UHHS Memorial Hospital of Geneva

870 West Main Street
Geneva, OH 44041
Phone: 440-466-1141
Fax: 440-466-0903
Type: Critical Access Hospitals
Emergency Services: Yes
Ownership: Voluntary Non-Profit - Private
Beds: 46

Key Personnel:
CEO/President. . . . . Thomas Zenty, III
Chief of Medical Staff. . . . . Emolyn Defensor, MD
Infection Control. . . . . Robert Malinowski, DO
Operating Room. . . . . Sue Hopkins, RN
Quality Assurance . . . . Laurie Lewis, ART
Emergency Room . . . . Sue Hopkins, RN
Intensive Care Unit. . . . . Debra Greiner, RN

Measure	Cases	This Hosp.	State Avg.	U.S. Avg.
Heart Attack Care				
ACE Inhibitor or ARB for LVSD	0	-	97%	96%
Aspirin at Arrival[1]	4	100%	99%	99%
Aspirin at Discharge[1]	1	100%	99%	98%
Beta Blocker at Discharge[1]	1	100%	99%	98%
Fibrinolytic Medication Timing	0	-	14%	55%
PCI Within 90 Minutes of Arrival	0	-	92%	90%
Smoking Cessation Advice	0	-	100%	99%
Chest Pain/Possible Heart Attack Care				
Aspirin at Arrival	222	100%	96%	95%
Median Time to ECG (minutes)	235	5	7	8
Median Time to Transfer (minutes)[1]	21	49	61	61
Fibrinolytic Medication Timing	0	-	47%	54%
Heart Failure Care				
ACE Inhibitor or ARB for LVSD[1]	19	100%	96%	94%
Discharge Instructions[1]	24	96%	91%	88%
Evaluation of LVS Function	44	100%	99%	98%
Smoking Cessation Advice[1]	15	100%	99%	98%
Pneumonia Care				
Appropriate Initial Antibiotic	49	94%	92%	92%
Blood Culture Timing	90	99%	96%	96%
Influenza Vaccine	41	93%	93%	91%
Initial Antibiotic Timing	69	100%	96%	95%
Pneumococcal Vaccine	48	100%	95%	93%
Smoking Cessation Advice	28	100%	98%	97%
Surgical Care Improvement Project				
Appropriate VTP Within 24 Hours[1]	5	100%	92%	92%
Appropriate Hair Removal	25	100%	100%	99%
Appropriate Beta Blocker Usage[1,3]	6	100%	94%	93%
Controlled Postoperative Blood Glucose	0	-	94%	93%
Prophylactic Antibiotic Timing[1]	19	100%	97%	97%
Prophylactic Antibiotic Timing (Outpatient)	51	100%	91%	92%
Prophylactic Antibiotic Selection[1]	19	100%	98%	97%
Prophylactic Antibiotic Select. (Outpatient)	51	100%	94%	94%
Prophylactic Antibiotic Stopped[1]	18	100%	95%	94%
Recommended VTP Ordered[1]	5	100%	94%	94%
Urinary Catheter Removal[1]	2	100%	91%	90%
Children's Asthma Care				
Received Systemic Corticosteroids	-	-	-	100%
Received Home Management Plan	-	-	-	71%
Received Reliever Medication	-	-	-	100%
Use of Medical Imaging				
Combination Abdominal CT Scan	431	0.142	0.164	0.191
Combination Chest CT Scan	508	0.004	0.038	0.054
Follow-up Mammogram/Ultrasound	258	11.2%	8.4%	8.4%
MRI for Low Back Pain	62	24.2%	30.2%	32.7%
Survey of Patients' Hospital Experiences				
Area Around Room 'Always' Quiet at Night[11]	300+	47%	-	58%
Doctors 'Always' Communicated Well[11]	300+	83%	-	80%
Home Recovery Information Given[11]	300+	83%	-	82%
Hospital Given 9 or 10 on 10 Point Scale[11]	300+	72%	-	67%
Meds 'Always' Explained Before Given[11]	300+	63%	-	60%
Nurses 'Always' Communicated Well[11]	300+	80%	-	76%
Pain 'Always' Well Controlled[11]	300+	70%	-	69%
Room and Bathroom 'Always' Clean[11]	300+	82%	-	71%
Timely Help 'Always' Received[11]	300+	73%	-	64%
Would Definitely Recommend Hospital[11]	300+	76%	-	69%

Brown County Hospital

425 Home Street
Georgetown, OH 45121
Phone: 513-378-7500
Fax: 937-378-7744
E-mail: c_beck@bcrhc.org
URL: www.browncountygeneralhospital.com
Type: Acute Care Hospitals
Emergency Services: Yes
Ownership: Government - Local
Beds: 127

Key Personnel:
CEO/President. . . . . Bruce A Bennett
Chief of Medical Staff. . . . . Todd Williams, MD
Infection Control. . . . . Mino Wright, RN
Operating Room. . . . . Lisa Michael
Radiology. . . . . Kevin A Aukerman, MD
Anesthesiology. . . . . Dr. Kirschner, MD
Emergency Room . . . . Scott Walden, MD
Intensive Care Unit. . . . . Cindy Edmister

Measure	Cases	This Hosp.	State Avg.	U.S. Avg.
Heart Attack Care				
ACE Inhibitor or ARB for LVSD	0	-	97%	96%
Aspirin at Arrival[1]	4	100%	99%	99%
Aspirin at Discharge[1]	2	100%	99%	98%
Beta Blocker at Discharge[1]	2	100%	99%	98%
Fibrinolytic Medication Timing	0	-	14%	55%
PCI Within 90 Minutes of Arrival	0	-	92%	90%
Smoking Cessation Advice[1]	1	0%	100%	99%
Chest Pain/Possible Heart Attack Care				
Aspirin at Arrival	87	99%	96%	95%
Median Time to ECG (minutes)	94	6	7	8
Median Time to Transfer (minutes)	0	-	61	61
Fibrinolytic Medication Timing	0	-	47%	54%
Heart Failure Care				
ACE Inhibitor or ARB for LVSD[1]	16	100%	96%	94%
Discharge Instructions	39	87%	91%	88%
Evaluation of LVS Function	62	100%	99%	98%
Smoking Cessation Advice[1]	12	92%	99%	98%
Pneumonia Care				
Appropriate Initial Antibiotic[2]	44	98%	92%	92%
Blood Culture Timing[2]	112	94%	96%	96%
Influenza Vaccine[2]	65	94%	93%	91%
Initial Antibiotic Timing[2]	107	99%	96%	95%
Pneumococcal Vaccine[2]	93	97%	95%	93%
Smoking Cessation Advice[2]	43	98%	98%	97%
Surgical Care Improvement Project				
Appropriate VTP Within 24 Hours[1,2]	10	100%	92%	92%
Appropriate Hair Removal[2]	39	100%	100%	99%
Appropriate Beta Blocker Usage[1,2]	8	100%	94%	93%
Controlled Postoperative Blood Glucose[2]	0	-	94%	93%
Prophylactic Antibiotic Timing[1,2]	19	79%	97%	97%
Prophylactic Antibiotic Timing (Outpatient)	38	84%	91%	92%
Prophylactic Antibiotic Selection[1,2]	21	86%	98%	97%
Prophylactic Antibiotic Select. (Outpatient)	36	92%	94%	94%
Prophylactic Antibiotic Stopped[1,2]	19	89%	95%	94%
Recommended VTP Ordered[1,2]	10	100%	94%	94%
Urinary Catheter Removal[1,2]	4	100%	91%	90%
Children's Asthma Care				
Received Systemic Corticosteroids	-	-	-	100%
Received Home Management Plan	-	-	-	71%
Received Reliever Medication	-	-	-	100%
Use of Medical Imaging				
Combination Abdominal CT Scan	241	0.041	0.164	0.191
Combination Chest CT Scan	132	0.053	0.038	0.054
Follow-up Mammogram/Ultrasound	299	9.4%	8.4%	8.4%
MRI for Low Back Pain	60	50.0%	30.2%	32.7%
Survey of Patients' Hospital Experiences				
Area Around Room 'Always' Quiet at Night	300+	49%	-	58%
Doctors 'Always' Communicated Well	300+	72%	-	80%
Home Recovery Information Given	300+	80%	-	82%
Hospital Given 9 or 10 on 10 Point Scale	300+	51%	-	67%
Meds 'Always' Explained Before Given	300+	51%	-	60%
Nurses 'Always' Communicated Well	300+	71%	-	76%
Pain 'Always' Well Controlled	300+	61%	-	69%
Room and Bathroom 'Always' Clean	300+	70%	-	71%
Timely Help 'Always' Received	300+	59%	-	64%
Would Definitely Recommend Hospital	300+	51%	-	69%

NOTE: Hospital profiles are in alphabetical order by state, then city, then hospital within the city; Rankings exclude hospitals with less than 25 cases except for patient surveys which excludes hospitals with less than 100 cases; (a) 100–299 cases; (1) The number of cases is too small to be sure how well a hospital is performing; (2) The hospital indicated that the data submitted for this measure were based on a sample of cases; (3) Data was collected during a shorter time period (fewer quarters) than the maximum possible time for this measure; (4) Suppressed for one or more quarters by CMS; (5) No data is available from the hospital for this measure; (6) Fewer than 100 patients completed the HCAHPS survey. Use these rates with caution, as the number of surveys may be too low to reliably assess hospital performance; (7) Survey results are based on less than 12 months of data; (8) Survey results are not available for this reporting period; (9) No or very few patients were eligible for the HCAHPS survey. The scores shown, if any, reflect a very small number of surveys; (10) A state average was not calculated because too few hospitals in the state submitted data; (11) There were discrepancies in the data collection process; Please refer to the User's Guide for a full explanation of data.

Greenfield Area Medical Center

550 Mirabeau Street Phone: 937-981-9400
Greenfield, OH 45123 Fax: 937-981-9499
URL: www.adena.org
Type: Critical Access Hospitals Emergency Services: Yes
Ownership: Voluntary Non-Profit - Private Beds: 46

Key Personnel:
CEO/President. . . . . Mark Shuter
Chief of Medical Staff. . . . . Wayne W Beam Jr
Radiology. . . . . Bryan I Borland
Emergency Room . . . . Kevin Dorothy

Measure	Cases	This Hosp.	State Avg.	U.S. Avg.
Heart Attack Care				
ACE Inhibitor or ARB for LVSD	-	-	97%	96%
Aspirin at Arrival	-	-	99%	99%
Aspirin at Discharge	-	-	99%	98%
Beta Blocker at Discharge	-	-	99%	98%
Fibrinolytic Medication Timing	-	-	14%	55%
PCI Within 90 Minutes of Arrival	-	-	92%	90%
Smoking Cessation Advice	-	-	100%	99%
Chest Pain/Possible Heart Attack Care				
Aspirin at Arrival[5]	0	-	96%	95%
Median Time to ECG (minutes)[5]	0	-	7	8
Median Time to Transfer (minutes)[5]	0	-	61	61
Fibrinolytic Medication Timing[5]	0	-	47%	54%
Heart Failure Care				
ACE Inhibitor or ARB for LVSD	-	-	96%	94%
Discharge Instructions	-	-	91%	88%
Evaluation of LVS Function	-	-	99%	98%
Smoking Cessation Advice	-	-	99%	98%
Pneumonia Care				
Appropriate Initial Antibiotic	-	-	92%	92%
Blood Culture Timing	-	-	96%	96%
Influenza Vaccine	-	-	93%	91%
Initial Antibiotic Timing	-	-	96%	95%
Pneumococcal Vaccine	-	-	95%	93%
Smoking Cessation Advice	-	-	98%	97%
Surgical Care Improvement Project				
Appropriate VTP Within 24 Hours	-	-	92%	92%
Appropriate Hair Removal	-	-	100%	99%
Appropriate Beta Blocker Usage	-	-	94%	93%
Controlled Postoperative Blood Glucose	-	-	94%	93%
Prophylactic Antibiotic Timing	-	-	97%	97%
Prophylactic Antibiotic Timing (Outpatient)[5]	0	-	91%	92%
Prophylactic Antibiotic Selection	-	-	98%	97%
Prophylactic Antibiotic Select. (Outpatient)[5]	0	-	94%	94%
Prophylactic Antibiotic Stopped	-	-	95%	94%
Recommended VTP Ordered	-	-	94%	94%
Urinary Catheter Removal	-	-	91%	90%
Children's Asthma Care				
Received Systemic Corticosteroids	-	-	-	100%
Received Home Management Plan	-	-	-	71%
Received Reliever Medication	-	-	-	100%
Use of Medical Imaging				
Combination Abdominal CT Scan	110	0.027	0.164	0.191
Combination Chest CT Scan[1]	63	0.111	0.038	0.054
Follow-up Mammogram/Ultrasound	112	8.9%	8.4%	8.4%
MRI for Low Back Pain[5]	0	-	30.2%	32.7%
Survey of Patients' Hospital Experiences				
Area Around Room 'Always' Quiet at Night	-	-	-	58%
Doctors 'Always' Communicated Well	-	-	-	80%
Home Recovery Information Given	-	-	-	82%
Hospital Given 9 or 10 on 10 Point Scale	-	-	-	67%
Meds 'Always' Explained Before Given	-	-	-	60%
Nurses 'Always' Communicated Well	-	-	-	76%
Pain 'Always' Well Controlled	-	-	-	69%
Room and Bathroom 'Always' Clean	-	-	-	71%
Timely Help 'Always' Received	-	-	-	64%
Would Definitely Recommend Hospital	-	-	-	69%

Wayne Hospital

835 Sweitzer Street Phone: 937-547-5926
Greenville, OH 45331 Fax: 937-547-5712
URL: www.waynehospital.com
Type: Acute Care Hospitals Emergency Services: Yes
Ownership: Voluntary Non-Profit - Private Beds: 92

Key Personnel:
Chief of Medical Staff . . . . James Appleman
Infection Control. . . . . Nancy Raffel
Operating Room. . . . . Holly Lemar, RN
Quality Assurance . . . . Susan Weisenberger
Emergency Room . . . . Robert Girmann, DO
Intensive Care Unit. . . . . Shirley Winger, RN

Measure	Cases	This Hosp.	State Avg.	U.S. Avg.
Heart Attack Care				
ACE Inhibitor or ARB for LVSD	0	-	97%	96%
Aspirin at Arrival[1]	6	83%	99%	99%
Aspirin at Discharge[1]	3	100%	99%	98%
Beta Blocker at Discharge[1]	3	100%	99%	98%
Fibrinolytic Medication Timing	0	-	14%	55%
PCI Within 90 Minutes of Arrival	0	-	92%	90%
Smoking Cessation Advice	0	-	100%	99%
Chest Pain/Possible Heart Attack Care				
Aspirin at Arrival	134	93%	96%	95%
Median Time to ECG (minutes)	150	22	7	8
Median Time to Transfer (minutes)[1,3]	9	85	61	61
Fibrinolytic Medication Timing[1]	3	67%	47%	54%
Heart Failure Care				
ACE Inhibitor or ARB for LVSD[1]	15	100%	96%	94%
Discharge Instructions	84	51%	91%	88%
Evaluation of LVS Function	120	86%	99%	98%
Smoking Cessation Advice[1]	18	83%	99%	98%
Pneumonia Care				
Appropriate Initial Antibiotic	62	81%	92%	92%
Blood Culture Timing	97	91%	96%	96%
Influenza Vaccine	67	96%	93%	91%
Initial Antibiotic Timing	91	98%	96%	95%
Pneumococcal Vaccine	86	92%	95%	93%
Smoking Cessation Advice	28	89%	98%	97%
Surgical Care Improvement Project				
Appropriate VTP Within 24 Hours	82	90%	92%	92%
Appropriate Hair Removal	207	96%	100%	99%
Appropriate Beta Blocker Usage	48	94%	94%	93%
Controlled Postoperative Blood Glucose	0	-	94%	93%
Prophylactic Antibiotic Timing	140	99%	97%	97%
Prophylactic Antibiotic Timing (Outpatient)[1]	21	62%	91%	92%
Prophylactic Antibiotic Selection	141	88%	98%	97%
Prophylactic Antibiotic Select. (Outpatient)	36	89%	94%	94%
Prophylactic Antibiotic Stopped	137	82%	95%	94%
Recommended VTP Ordered	82	96%	94%	94%
Urinary Catheter Removal	37	65%	91%	90%
Children's Asthma Care				
Received Systemic Corticosteroids	-	-	-	100%
Received Home Management Plan	-	-	-	71%
Received Reliever Medication	-	-	-	100%
Use of Medical Imaging				
Combination Abdominal CT Scan	458	0.024	0.164	0.191
Combination Chest CT Scan	308	0.000	0.038	0.054
Follow-up Mammogram/Ultrasound	846	9.0%	8.4%	8.4%
MRI for Low Back Pain	98	33.7%	30.2%	32.7%
Survey of Patients' Hospital Experiences				
Area Around Room 'Always' Quiet at Night	300+	53%	-	58%
Doctors 'Always' Communicated Well	300+	77%	-	80%
Home Recovery Information Given	300+	80%	-	82%
Hospital Given 9 or 10 on 10 Point Scale	300+	59%	-	67%
Meds 'Always' Explained Before Given	300+	59%	-	60%
Nurses 'Always' Communicated Well	300+	74%	-	76%
Pain 'Always' Well Controlled	300+	68%	-	69%
Room and Bathroom 'Always' Clean	300+	73%	-	71%
Timely Help 'Always' Received	300+	68%	-	64%
Would Definitely Recommend Hospital	300+	57%	-	69%

Butler County Medical Center

3125 Hamilton Mason Road Phone: 513-894-8888
Hamilton, OH 45011
Type: Acute Care Hospitals Emergency Services: No
Ownership: Proprietary

Measure	Cases	This Hosp.	State Avg.	U.S. Avg.
Heart Attack Care				
ACE Inhibitor or ARB for LVSD[5]	0	-	97%	96%
Aspirin at Arrival[5]	0	-	99%	99%
Aspirin at Discharge[5]	0	-	99%	98%
Beta Blocker at Discharge[5]	0	-	99%	98%
Fibrinolytic Medication Timing[5]	0	-	14%	55%
PCI Within 90 Minutes of Arrival[5]	0	-	92%	90%
Smoking Cessation Advice[5]	0	-	100%	99%
Chest Pain/Possible Heart Attack Care				
Aspirin at Arrival[5]	0	-	96%	95%
Median Time to ECG (minutes)[5]	0	-	7	8
Median Time to Transfer (minutes)[5]	0	-	61	61
Fibrinolytic Medication Timing[5]	0	-	47%	54%
Heart Failure Care				
ACE Inhibitor or ARB for LVSD[5]	0	-	96%	94%
Discharge Instructions[5]	0	-	91%	88%
Evaluation of LVS Function[5]	0	-	99%	98%
Smoking Cessation Advice[5]	0	-	99%	98%
Pneumonia Care				
Appropriate Initial Antibiotic[5]	0	-	92%	92%
Blood Culture Timing[5]	0	-	96%	96%
Influenza Vaccine[5]	0	-	93%	91%
Initial Antibiotic Timing[5]	0	-	96%	95%
Pneumococcal Vaccine[5]	0	-	95%	93%
Smoking Cessation Advice[5]	0	-	98%	97%
Surgical Care Improvement Project				
Appropriate VTP Within 24 Hours[1]	7	86%	92%	92%
Appropriate Hair Removal	209	100%	100%	99%
Appropriate Beta Blocker Usage	41	61%	94%	93%
Controlled Postoperative Blood Glucose	0	-	94%	93%
Prophylactic Antibiotic Timing	190	93%	97%	97%
Prophylactic Antibiotic Timing (Outpatient)	90	82%	91%	92%
Prophylactic Antibiotic Selection	186	95%	98%	97%
Prophylactic Antibiotic Select. (Outpatient)	75	93%	94%	94%
Prophylactic Antibiotic Stopped	180	95%	95%	94%
Recommended VTP Ordered[1]	7	86%	94%	94%
Urinary Catheter Removal[1]	14	86%	91%	90%
Children's Asthma Care				
Received Systemic Corticosteroids	-	-	-	100%
Received Home Management Plan	-	-	-	71%
Received Reliever Medication	-	-	-	100%
Use of Medical Imaging				
Combination Abdominal CT Scan	286	0.087	0.164	0.191
Combination Chest CT Scan	244	0.004	0.038	0.054
Follow-up Mammogram/Ultrasound	166	12.7%	8.4%	8.4%
MRI for Low Back Pain	168	30.4%	30.2%	32.7%
Survey of Patients' Hospital Experiences				
Area Around Room 'Always' Quiet at Night	(a)	80%	-	58%
Doctors 'Always' Communicated Well	(a)	97%	-	80%
Home Recovery Information Given	(a)	91%	-	82%
Hospital Given 9 or 10 on 10 Point Scale	(a)	93%	-	67%
Meds 'Always' Explained Before Given	(a)	77%	-	60%
Nurses 'Always' Communicated Well	(a)	92%	-	76%
Pain 'Always' Well Controlled	(a)	86%	-	69%
Room and Bathroom 'Always' Clean	(a)	88%	-	71%
Timely Help 'Always' Received	(a)	88%	-	64%
Would Definitely Recommend Hospital	(a)	90%	-	69%

NOTE: Hospital profiles are in alphabetical order by state, then city, then hospital within the city; Rankings exclude hospitals with less than 25 cases except for patient surveys which excludes hospitals with less than 100 cases; (a) 100–299 cases; (1) The number of cases is too small to be sure how well a hospital is performing; (2) The hospital indicated that the data submitted for this measure were based on a sample of cases; (3) Data was collected during a shorter time period (fewer quarters) than the maximum possible time for this measure; (4) Suppressed for one or more quarters by CMS; (5) No data is available from the hospital for this measure; (6) Fewer than 100 patients completed the HCAHPS survey. Use these rates with caution, as the number of surveys may be too low to reliably assess hospital performance; (7) Survey results are based on less than 12 months of data; (8) Survey results are not available for this reporting period; (9) No or very few patients were eligible for the HCAHPS survey. The scores shown, if any, reflect a very small number of surveys; (10) A state average was not calculated because too few hospitals in the state submitted data; (11) There were discrepancies in the data collection process; Please refer to the User's Guide for a full explanation of data.

Fort Hamilton Hughes Memorial Hospital

630 Eaton Avenue
Hamilton, OH 45013
URL: www.forthamiltonhospital.com
Type: Acute Care Hospitals
Ownership: Voluntary Non-Profit - Private

Phone: 513-867-2124
Fax: 513-867-2620

Emergency Services: Yes
Beds: 310

Key Personnel:
CEO/President. . . . . Lynn Oswald, FACHE
Chief of Medical Staff. . . . . H.S. Ramadas, MD
Operating Room . . . . Cheryl Creach
Pediatric In-Patient Care . . . . . . Marc Richardson, MD
Quality Assurance . . . . Nancy Cohen
Radiology. . . . . Karen Wilson
Emergency Room . . . . Pam Klaber

Measure	Cases	This Hosp.	State Avg.	U.S. Avg.
Heart Attack Care				
ACE Inhibitor or ARB for LVSD[1]	7	100%	97%	96%
Aspirin at Arrival	40	98%	99%	99%
Aspirin at Discharge	26	96%	99%	98%
Beta Blocker at Discharge	25	100%	99%	98%
Fibrinolytic Medication Timing	0	-	14%	55%
PCI Within 90 Minutes of Arrival[1]	1	100%	92%	90%
Smoking Cessation Advice[1]	7	100%	100%	99%
Chest Pain/Possible Heart Attack Care				
Aspirin at Arrival	36	100%	96%	95%
Median Time to ECG (minutes)	38	4	7	8
Median Time to Transfer (minutes)[1,3]	2	95	61	61
Fibrinolytic Medication Timing	0	-	47%	54%
Heart Failure Care				
ACE Inhibitor or ARB for LVSD	69	99%	96%	94%
Discharge Instructions	211	98%	91%	88%
Evaluation of LVS Function	269	100%	99%	98%
Smoking Cessation Advice	54	100%	99%	98%
Pneumonia Care				
Appropriate Initial Antibiotic[2]	73	96%	92%	92%
Blood Culture Timing[2]	113	97%	96%	96%
Influenza Vaccine[2]	97	99%	93%	91%
Initial Antibiotic Timing[2]	126	95%	96%	95%
Pneumococcal Vaccine[2]	134	100%	95%	93%
Smoking Cessation Advice[2]	72	100%	98%	97%
Surgical Care Improvement Project				
Appropriate VTP Within 24 Hours[2]	147	99%	92%	92%
Appropriate Hair Removal[2]	353	100%	100%	99%
Appropriate Beta Blocker Usage[2]	81	95%	94%	93%
Controlled Postoperative Blood Glucose[2]	0	-	94%	93%
Prophylactic Antibiotic Timing[2]	185	98%	97%	97%
Prophylactic Antibiotic Timing (Outpatient)	78	92%	91%	92%
Prophylactic Antibiotic Selection[2]	184	93%	98%	97%
Prophylactic Antibiotic Select. (Outpatient)	78	97%	94%	94%
Prophylactic Antibiotic Stopped[2]	155	96%	95%	94%
Recommended VTP Ordered[2]	147	99%	94%	94%
Urinary Catheter Removal	48	96%	91%	90%
Children's Asthma Care				
Received Systemic Corticosteroids	-	-	-	100%
Received Home Management Plan	-	-	-	71%
Received Reliever Medication	-	-	-	100%
Use of Medical Imaging				
Combination Abdominal CT Scan	645	0.057	0.164	0.191
Combination Chest CT Scan	441	0.002	0.038	0.054
Follow-up Mammogram/Ultrasound	983	9.3%	8.4%	8.4%
MRI for Low Back Pain	119	36.1%	30.2%	32.7%
Survey of Patients' Hospital Experiences				
Area Around Room 'Always' Quiet at Night	300+	49%	-	58%
Doctors 'Always' Communicated Well	300+	75%	-	80%
Home Recovery Information Given	300+	75%	-	82%
Hospital Given 9 or 10 on 10 Point Scale	300+	55%	-	67%
Meds 'Always' Explained Before Given	300+	54%	-	60%
Nurses 'Always' Communicated Well	300+	74%	-	76%
Pain 'Always' Well Controlled	300+	66%	-	69%
Room and Bathroom 'Always' Clean	300+	70%	-	71%
Timely Help 'Always' Received	300+	60%	-	64%
Would Definitely Recommend Hospital	300+	58%	-	69%

Highland District Hospital

1275 North High Street
Hillsboro, OH 45133
E-mail: hdhadm@bright.net
URL: www.hdh.org
Type: Critical Access Hospitals
Ownership: Govt - Hospital Dist/Auth

Phone: 937-393-6100
Fax: 937-393-6278

Emergency Services: Yes
Beds: 65

Key Personnel:
CEO/President. . . . . Paula Detterman
Chief of Medical Staff . . . . David Gunderman
Quality Assurance . . . . Bob Barger
Radiology. . . . . Jeffrey Cushman
Emergency Room . . . . Terri Balser

Measure	Cases	This Hosp.	State Avg.	U.S. Avg.
Heart Attack Care				
ACE Inhibitor or ARB for LVSD[3]	0	-	97%	96%
Aspirin at Arrival[1,3]	1	100%	99%	99%
Aspirin at Discharge[1,3]	1	100%	99%	98%
Beta Blocker at Discharge[1,3]	1	100%	99%	98%
Fibrinolytic Medication Timing[3]	0	-	14%	55%
PCI Within 90 Minutes of Arrival[3]	0	-	92%	90%
Smoking Cessation Advice[3]	0	-	100%	99%
Chest Pain/Possible Heart Attack Care				
Aspirin at Arrival[1,3]	19	100%	96%	95%
Median Time to ECG (minutes)[1,3]	20	6	7	8
Median Time to Transfer (minutes)[5]	0	-	61	61
Fibrinolytic Medication Timing[3]	0	-	47%	54%
Heart Failure Care				
ACE Inhibitor or ARB for LVSD[1]	21	86%	96%	94%
Discharge Instructions	53	66%	91%	88%
Evaluation of LVS Function	70	81%	99%	98%
Smoking Cessation Advice[1]	7	100%	99%	98%
Pneumonia Care				
Appropriate Initial Antibiotic	90	80%	92%	92%
Blood Culture Timing	98	83%	96%	96%
Influenza Vaccine	60	83%	93%	91%
Initial Antibiotic Timing	68	94%	96%	95%
Pneumococcal Vaccine	68	87%	95%	93%
Smoking Cessation Advice	26	92%	98%	97%
Surgical Care Improvement Project				
Appropriate VTP Within 24 Hours[5]	0	-	92%	92%
Appropriate Hair Removal[5]	0	-	100%	99%
Appropriate Beta Blocker Usage[5]	0	-	94%	93%
Controlled Postoperative Blood Glucose[5]	0	-	94%	93%
Prophylactic Antibiotic Timing	26	92%	97%	97%
Prophylactic Antibiotic Timing (Outpatient)[1,3]	19	58%	91%	92%
Prophylactic Antibiotic Selection	25	88%	98%	97%
Prophylactic Antibiotic Select. (Outpatient)[1,3]	11	91%	94%	94%
Prophylactic Antibiotic Stopped	25	100%	95%	94%
Recommended VTP Ordered[5]	0	-	94%	94%
Urinary Catheter Removal	0	-	91%	90%
Children's Asthma Care				
Received Systemic Corticosteroids	-	-	-	100%
Received Home Management Plan	-	-	-	71%
Received Reliever Medication	-	-	-	100%
Use of Medical Imaging				
Combination Abdominal CT Scan	507	0.613	0.164	0.191
Combination Chest CT Scan	330	0.333	0.038	0.054
Follow-up Mammogram/Ultrasound	461	11.9%	8.4%	8.4%
MRI for Low Back Pain	72	33.3%	30.2%	32.7%
Survey of Patients' Hospital Experiences				
Area Around Room 'Always' Quiet at Night[8]	-	-	-	58%
Doctors 'Always' Communicated Well[8]	-	-	-	80%
Home Recovery Information Given[8]	-	-	-	82%
Hospital Given 9 or 10 on 10 Point Scale[8]	-	-	-	67%
Meds 'Always' Explained Before Given[8]	-	-	-	60%
Nurses 'Always' Communicated Well[8]	-	-	-	76%
Pain 'Always' Well Controlled[8]	-	-	-	69%
Room and Bathroom 'Always' Clean[8]	-	-	-	71%
Timely Help 'Always' Received[8]	-	-	-	64%
Would Definitely Recommend Hospital[8]	-	-	-	69%

Holzer Medical Center Jackson

500 Burlington Road
Jackson, OH 45640
Type: Critical Access Hospitals
Ownership: Voluntary Non-Profit - Private

Phone: 740-395-8500

Emergency Services: Yes

Measure	Cases	This Hosp.	State Avg.	U.S. Avg.
Heart Attack Care				
ACE Inhibitor or ARB for LVSD	0	-	97%	96%
Aspirin at Arrival[1]	8	75%	99%	99%
Aspirin at Discharge[1]	4	75%	99%	98%
Beta Blocker at Discharge[1]	5	100%	99%	98%
Fibrinolytic Medication Timing	0	-	14%	55%
PCI Within 90 Minutes of Arrival	0	-	92%	90%
Smoking Cessation Advice	0	-	100%	99%
Chest Pain/Possible Heart Attack Care				
Aspirin at Arrival[5]	0	-	96%	95%
Median Time to ECG (minutes)[5]	0	-	7	8
Median Time to Transfer (minutes)[5]	0	-	61	61
Fibrinolytic Medication Timing[5]	0	-	47%	54%
Heart Failure Care				
ACE Inhibitor or ARB for LVSD[1]	19	84%	96%	94%
Discharge Instructions	74	80%	91%	88%
Evaluation of LVS Function	108	81%	99%	98%
Smoking Cessation Advice[1]	11	100%	99%	98%
Pneumonia Care				
Appropriate Initial Antibiotic	108	85%	92%	92%
Blood Culture Timing	117	93%	96%	96%
Influenza Vaccine	49	86%	93%	91%
Initial Antibiotic Timing	113	96%	96%	95%
Pneumococcal Vaccine	78	86%	95%	93%
Smoking Cessation Advice	38	100%	98%	97%
Surgical Care Improvement Project				
Appropriate VTP Within 24 Hours	34	79%	92%	92%
Appropriate Hair Removal	171	99%	100%	99%
Appropriate Beta Blocker Usage[5]	0	-	94%	93%
Controlled Postoperative Blood Glucose	0	-	94%	93%
Prophylactic Antibiotic Timing	158	84%	97%	97%
Prophylactic Antibiotic Timing (Outpatient)[5]	0	-	91%	92%
Prophylactic Antibiotic Selection	156	99%	98%	97%
Prophylactic Antibiotic Select. (Outpatient)[5]	0	-	94%	94%
Prophylactic Antibiotic Stopped	158	92%	95%	94%
Recommended VTP Ordered	34	79%	94%	94%
Urinary Catheter Removal	29	97%	91%	90%
Children's Asthma Care				
Received Systemic Corticosteroids	-	-	-	100%
Received Home Management Plan	-	-	-	71%
Received Reliever Medication	-	-	-	100%
Use of Medical Imaging				
Combination Abdominal CT Scan	416	0.041	0.164	0.191
Combination Chest CT Scan	107	0.000	0.038	0.054
Follow-up Mammogram/Ultrasound	70	4.3%	8.4%	8.4%
MRI for Low Back Pain[1]	34	26.5%	30.2%	32.7%
Survey of Patients' Hospital Experiences				
Area Around Room 'Always' Quiet at Night	300+	71%	-	58%
Doctors 'Always' Communicated Well	300+	80%	-	80%
Home Recovery Information Given	300+	85%	-	82%
Hospital Given 9 or 10 on 10 Point Scale	300+	70%	-	67%
Meds 'Always' Explained Before Given	300+	65%	-	60%
Nurses 'Always' Communicated Well	300+	84%	-	76%
Pain 'Always' Well Controlled	300+	75%	-	69%
Room and Bathroom 'Always' Clean	300+	81%	-	71%
Timely Help 'Always' Received	300+	77%	-	64%
Would Definitely Recommend Hospital	300+	70%	-	69%

NOTE: Hospital profiles are in alphabetical order by state, then city, then hospital within the city; Rankings exclude hospitals with less than 25 cases except for patient surveys which excludes hospitals with less than 100 cases; (a) 100–299 cases; (1) The number of cases is too small to be sure how well a hospital is performing; (2) The hospital indicated that the data submitted for this measure were based on a sample of cases; (3) Data was collected during a shorter time period (fewer quarters) than the maximum possible time for this measure; (4) Suppressed for one or more quarters by CMS; (5) No data is available from the hospital for this measure; (6) Fewer than 100 patients completed the HCAHPS survey. Use these rates with caution, as the number of surveys may be too low to reliably assess hospital performance; (7) Survey results are not available for this reporting period; (8) Survey results are based on less than 12 months of data; (9) No or very few patients were eligible for the HCAHPS survey. The scores shown, if any, reflect a very small number of surveys; (10) A state average was not calculated because too few hospitals in the state submitted data; (11) There were discrepancies in the data collection process; Please refer to the User's Guide for a full explanation of data.

Hardin Memorial Hospital

921 East Franklin Street
Kenton, OH 43326
Phone: 419-673-0761
Fax: 419-673-1097
E-mail: publicrelations@hardinmemorial.org
URL: www.hardinmemorial.org
Type: Critical Access Hospitals
Emergency Services: Yes
Ownership: Voluntary Non-Profit - Other
Beds: 103

Key Personnel:
Chief of Medical Staff. . . . . Katherine Johnson, MD
Infection Control. . . . . Cindy Althouse, RN
Operating Room. . . . . M Saadallah Abdulkarim, RN
Emergency Room . . . . Roxanne Tackett

Measure	Cases	This Hosp.	State Avg.	U.S. Avg.
Heart Attack Care				
ACE Inhibitor or ARB for LVSD[1]	1	100%	97%	96%
Aspirin at Arrival	0	-	99%	99%
Aspirin at Discharge	0	-	99%	98%
Beta Blocker at Discharge[1]	1	100%	99%	98%
Fibrinolytic Medication Timing	0	-	14%	55%
PCI Within 90 Minutes of Arrival	0	-	92%	90%
Smoking Cessation Advice	0	-	100%	99%
Chest Pain/Possible Heart Attack Care				
Aspirin at Arrival	-	-	96%	95%
Median Time to ECG (minutes)	-	-	7	8
Median Time to Transfer (minutes)	-	-	61	61
Fibrinolytic Medication Timing	-	-	47%	54%
Heart Failure Care				
ACE Inhibitor or ARB for LVSD[1]	8	88%	96%	94%
Discharge Instructions	29	100%	91%	88%
Evaluation of LVS Function	42	100%	99%	98%
Smoking Cessation Advice[1]	7	100%	99%	98%
Pneumonia Care				
Appropriate Initial Antibiotic	41	93%	92%	92%
Blood Culture Timing	41	93%	96%	96%
Influenza Vaccine[1]	21	100%	93%	91%
Initial Antibiotic Timing	39	95%	96%	95%
Pneumococcal Vaccine	25	96%	95%	93%
Smoking Cessation Advice[1]	19	100%	98%	97%
Surgical Care Improvement Project				
Appropriate VTP Within 24 Hours[5]	0	-	92%	92%
Appropriate Hair Removal[5]	0	-	100%	99%
Appropriate Beta Blocker Usage[5]	0	-	94%	93%
Controlled Postoperative Blood Glucose[5]	0	-	94%	93%
Prophylactic Antibiotic Timing[5]	0	-	97%	97%
Prophylactic Antibiotic Timing (Outpatient)	-	-	91%	92%
Prophylactic Antibiotic Selection[5]	0	-	98%	97%
Prophylactic Antibiotic Select. (Outpatient)	-	-	94%	94%
Prophylactic Antibiotic Stopped[5]	0	-	95%	94%
Recommended VTP Ordered[5]	0	-	94%	94%
Urinary Catheter Removal[5]	0	-	91%	90%
Children's Asthma Care				
Received Systemic Corticosteroids	-	-	-	100%
Received Home Management Plan	-	-	-	71%
Received Reliever Medication	-	-	-	100%
Use of Medical Imaging				
Combination Abdominal CT Scan	-	-	0.164	0.191
Combination Chest CT Scan	-	-	0.038	0.054
Follow-up Mammogram/Ultrasound	-	-	8.4%	8.4%
MRI for Low Back Pain	-	-	30.2%	32.7%
Survey of Patients' Hospital Experiences				
Area Around Room 'Always' Quiet at Night	(a)	61%	-	58%
Doctors 'Always' Communicated Well	(a)	78%	-	80%
Home Recovery Information Given	(a)	76%	-	82%
Hospital Given 9 or 10 on 10 Point Scale	(a)	67%	-	67%
Meds 'Always' Explained Before Given	(a)	62%	-	60%
Nurses 'Always' Communicated Well	(a)	78%	-	76%
Pain 'Always' Well Controlled	(a)	68%	-	69%
Room and Bathroom 'Always' Clean	(a)	79%	-	71%
Timely Help 'Always' Received	(a)	69%	-	64%
Would Definitely Recommend Hospital	(a)	59%	-	69%

Kettering Medical Center

3535 Southern Boulevard
Kettering, OH 45429
Phone: 937-395-8311
Fax: 937-395-8355
URL: www.khnetwork.org
Type: Acute Care Hospitals
Emergency Services: Yes
Ownership: Voluntary Non-Profit - Church
Beds: 522

Key Personnel:
CEO/President. . . . . Roy Chew
Chief of Medical Staff. . . . . R Gupta, MD
Infection Control. . . . . Sandy Shrader, MD
Operating Room. . . . . Kae Quinlan
Pediatric Ambulatory Care . . . . . . Thomas Sorauf, MD
Pediatric In-Patient Care . . . . Thomas Sorauf, MD
Quality Assurance . . . . Carolyn Peterson
Radiology. . . . . Theodore Miller, MD

Measure	Cases	This Hosp.	State Avg.	U.S. Avg.
Heart Attack Care				
ACE Inhibitor or ARB for LVSD	86	99%	97%	96%
Aspirin at Arrival	260	100%	99%	99%
Aspirin at Discharge	372	99%	99%	98%
Beta Blocker at Discharge	365	99%	99%	98%
Fibrinolytic Medication Timing	0	-	14%	55%
PCI Within 90 Minutes of Arrival	60	92%	92%	90%
Smoking Cessation Advice	100	100%	100%	99%
Chest Pain/Possible Heart Attack Care				
Aspirin at Arrival[1,3]	3	67%	96%	95%
Median Time to ECG (minutes)[1,3]	3	11	7	8
Median Time to Transfer (minutes)[5]	0	-	61	61
Fibrinolytic Medication Timing[5]	0	-	47%	54%
Heart Failure Care				
ACE Inhibitor or ARB for LVSD	195	99%	96%	94%
Discharge Instructions	387	95%	91%	88%
Evaluation of LVS Function	500	100%	99%	98%
Smoking Cessation Advice	61	100%	99%	98%
Pneumonia Care				
Appropriate Initial Antibiotic	189	97%	92%	92%
Blood Culture Timing	320	100%	96%	96%
Influenza Vaccine	231	96%	93%	91%
Initial Antibiotic Timing	287	99%	96%	95%
Pneumococcal Vaccine	260	99%	95%	93%
Smoking Cessation Advice	111	99%	98%	97%
Surgical Care Improvement Project				
Appropriate VTP Within 24 Hours[2]	617	100%	92%	92%
Appropriate Hair Removal[2]	2,599	100%	100%	99%
Appropriate Beta Blocker Usage[2]	892	98%	94%	93%
Controlled Postoperative Blood Glucose[2]	355	97%	94%	93%
Prophylactic Antibiotic Timing[2]	2,258	100%	97%	97%
Prophylactic Antibiotic Timing (Outpatient)	622	95%	91%	92%
Prophylactic Antibiotic Selection[2]	2,280	100%	98%	97%
Prophylactic Antibiotic Select. (Outpatient)	615	97%	94%	94%
Prophylactic Antibiotic Stopped[2]	2,191	99%	95%	94%
Recommended VTP Ordered[2]	617	100%	94%	94%
Urinary Catheter Removal[2]	683	99%	91%	90%
Children's Asthma Care				
Received Systemic Corticosteroids	-	-	-	100%
Received Home Management Plan	-	-	-	71%
Received Reliever Medication	-	-	-	100%
Use of Medical Imaging				
Combination Abdominal CT Scan	1,540	0.119	0.164	0.191
Combination Chest CT Scan	1,350	0.028	0.038	0.054
Follow-up Mammogram/Ultrasound[5]	0	-	8.4%	8.4%
MRI for Low Back Pain	172	32.0%	30.2%	32.7%
Survey of Patients' Hospital Experiences				
Area Around Room 'Always' Quiet at Night	300+	44%	-	58%
Doctors 'Always' Communicated Well	300+	77%	-	80%
Home Recovery Information Given	300+	86%	-	82%
Hospital Given 9 or 10 on 10 Point Scale	300+	68%	-	67%
Meds 'Always' Explained Before Given	300+	58%	-	60%
Nurses 'Always' Communicated Well	300+	75%	-	76%
Pain 'Always' Well Controlled	300+	67%	-	69%
Room and Bathroom 'Always' Clean	300+	64%	-	71%
Timely Help 'Always' Received	300+	56%	-	64%
Would Definitely Recommend Hospital	300+	75%	-	69%

Lakewood Hospital

14519 Detroit Avenue
Lakewood, OH 44107
Phone: 216-529-4200
Fax: 216-227-2621
URL: www.lakewoodhospital.org
Type: Acute Care Hospitals
Emergency Services: Yes
Ownership: Voluntary Non-Profit - Private
Beds: 400

Key Personnel:
CEO/President. . . . . Jack Gustin, MBA
Chief of Medical Staff. . . . . Marvin Shie III, MD

Measure	Cases	This Hosp.	State Avg.	U.S. Avg.
Heart Attack Care				
ACE Inhibitor or ARB for LVSD[1]	16	94%	97%	96%
Aspirin at Arrival	96	97%	99%	99%
Aspirin at Discharge	87	98%	99%	98%
Beta Blocker at Discharge	89	99%	99%	98%
Fibrinolytic Medication Timing	0	-	14%	55%
PCI Within 90 Minutes of Arrival	28	82%	92%	90%
Smoking Cessation Advice	38	100%	100%	99%
Chest Pain/Possible Heart Attack Care				
Aspirin at Arrival	29	93%	96%	95%
Median Time to ECG (minutes)	29	5	7	8
Median Time to Transfer (minutes)[5]	0	-	61	61
Fibrinolytic Medication Timing[5]	0	-	47%	54%
Heart Failure Care				
ACE Inhibitor or ARB for LVSD	67	99%	96%	94%
Discharge Instructions	187	98%	91%	88%
Evaluation of LVS Function	306	99%	99%	98%
Smoking Cessation Advice	68	100%	99%	98%
Pneumonia Care				
Appropriate Initial Antibiotic	89	89%	92%	92%
Blood Culture Timing	164	97%	96%	96%
Influenza Vaccine	88	97%	93%	91%
Initial Antibiotic Timing	158	95%	96%	95%
Pneumococcal Vaccine	110	99%	95%	93%
Smoking Cessation Advice	68	99%	98%	97%
Surgical Care Improvement Project				
Appropriate VTP Within 24 Hours	245	96%	92%	92%
Appropriate Hair Removal	564	100%	100%	99%
Appropriate Beta Blocker Usage	191	96%	94%	93%
Controlled Postoperative Blood Glucose	0	-	94%	93%
Prophylactic Antibiotic Timing	363	96%	97%	97%
Prophylactic Antibiotic Timing (Outpatient)	151	88%	91%	92%
Prophylactic Antibiotic Selection	364	99%	98%	97%
Prophylactic Antibiotic Select. (Outpatient)	138	94%	94%	94%
Prophylactic Antibiotic Stopped	342	99%	95%	94%
Recommended VTP Ordered	245	97%	94%	94%
Urinary Catheter Removal	175	99%	91%	90%
Children's Asthma Care				
Received Systemic Corticosteroids	-	-	-	100%
Received Home Management Plan	-	-	-	71%
Received Reliever Medication	-	-	-	100%
Use of Medical Imaging				
Combination Abdominal CT Scan	444	0.047	0.164	0.191
Combination Chest CT Scan	324	0.015	0.038	0.054
Follow-up Mammogram/Ultrasound	717	6.8%	8.4%	8.4%
MRI for Low Back Pain	76	35.5%	30.2%	32.7%
Survey of Patients' Hospital Experiences				
Area Around Room 'Always' Quiet at Night	300+	45%	-	58%
Doctors 'Always' Communicated Well	300+	73%	-	80%
Home Recovery Information Given	300+	79%	-	82%
Hospital Given 9 or 10 on 10 Point Scale	300+	59%	-	67%
Meds 'Always' Explained Before Given	300+	56%	-	60%
Nurses 'Always' Communicated Well	300+	74%	-	76%
Pain 'Always' Well Controlled	300+	66%	-	69%
Room and Bathroom 'Always' Clean	300+	68%	-	71%
Timely Help 'Always' Received	300+	57%	-	64%
Would Definitely Recommend Hospital	300+	66%	-	69%

NOTE: Hospital profiles are in alphabetical order by state, then city, then hospital within the city; Rankings exclude hospitals with less than 25 cases except for patient surveys which excludes hospitals with less than 100 cases; (a) 100–299 cases; (1) The number of cases is too small to be sure how well a hospital is performing; (2) The hospital indicated that the data submitted for this measure were based on a sample of cases; (3) Data was collected during a shorter time period (fewer quarters) than the maximum possible time for this measure; (4) Suppressed for one or more quarters by CMS; (5) No data is available from the hospital for this measure; (6) Fewer than 100 patients completed the HCAHPS survey. Use these rates with caution, as the number of surveys may be too low to reliably assess hospital performance; (7) Survey results are based on less than 12 months of data; (8) Survey results are not available for this reporting period; (9) No or very few patients were eligible for the HCAHPS survey. The scores shown, if any, reflect a very small number of surveys; (10) A state average was not calculated because too few hospitals in the state submitted data; (11) There were discrepancies in the data collection process; Please refer to the User's Guide for a full explanation of data.

Fairfield Medical Center

401 North Ewing Street Phone: 740-687-8009
Lancaster, OH 43130 Fax: 740-687-8115
URL: www.fmchealth.org
Type: Acute Care Hospitals Emergency Services: Yes
Ownership: Voluntary Non-Profit - Other Beds: 229

Key Personnel:
CEO/President. . . . . Mina Ubbing
Cardiac Laboratory. . . . . Misty Newsome
Chief of Medical Staff. . . . . Sarah Alley, MD
Coronary Care . . . . Anne Brown
Operating Room. . . . . Steven D Cox
Pediatric In-Patient Care . . . . Dora Metzger
Quality Assurance . . . . Roxanne Mathias
Radiology. . . . . Ricardo B Barboza

Measure	Cases	This Hosp.	State Avg.	U.S. Avg.
Heart Attack Care				
ACE Inhibitor or ARB for LVSD	53	98%	97%	96%
Aspirin at Arrival	243	99%	99%	99%
Aspirin at Discharge	252	97%	99%	98%
Beta Blocker at Discharge	240	100%	99%	98%
Fibrinolytic Medication Timing	0	-	14%	55%
PCI Within 90 Minutes of Arrival	52	81%	92%	90%
Smoking Cessation Advice	93	99%	100%	99%
Chest Pain/Possible Heart Attack Care				
Aspirin at Arrival	33	97%	96%	95%
Median Time to ECG (minutes)	37	11	7	8
Median Time to Transfer (minutes)[1,3]	1	86	61	61
Fibrinolytic Medication Timing[3]	0	-	47%	54%
Heart Failure Care				
ACE Inhibitor or ARB for LVSD	92	98%	96%	94%
Discharge Instructions	298	99%	91%	88%
Evaluation of LVS Function	362	100%	99%	98%
Smoking Cessation Advice	73	100%	99%	98%
Pneumonia Care				
Appropriate Initial Antibiotic	140	88%	92%	92%
Blood Culture Timing	289	95%	96%	96%
Influenza Vaccine	259	93%	93%	91%
Initial Antibiotic Timing	285	92%	96%	95%
Pneumococcal Vaccine	339	95%	95%	93%
Smoking Cessation Advice	155	100%	98%	97%
Surgical Care Improvement Project				
Appropriate VTP Within 24 Hours[2]	209	97%	92%	92%
Appropriate Hair Removal[2]	990	99%	100%	99%
Appropriate Beta Blocker Usage[2]	312	86%	94%	93%
Controlled Postoperative Blood Glucose[2]	154	78%	94%	93%
Prophylactic Antibiotic Timing[2]	761	94%	97%	97%
Prophylactic Antibiotic Timing (Outpatient)	427	87%	91%	92%
Prophylactic Antibiotic Selection[2]	769	98%	98%	97%
Prophylactic Antibiotic Select. (Outpatient)	388	92%	94%	94%
Prophylactic Antibiotic Stopped[2]	722	96%	95%	94%
Recommended VTP Ordered[2]	214	95%	94%	94%
Urinary Catheter Removal[2]	234	87%	91%	90%
Children's Asthma Care				
Received Systemic Corticosteroids	-	-	-	100%
Received Home Management Plan	-	-	-	71%
Received Reliever Medication	-	-	-	100%
Use of Medical Imaging				
Combination Abdominal CT Scan	853	0.081	0.164	0.191
Combination Chest CT Scan	550	0.002	0.038	0.054
Follow-up Mammogram/Ultrasound	655	9.6%	8.4%	8.4%
MRI for Low Back Pain	96	27.1%	30.2%	32.7%
Survey of Patients' Hospital Experiences				
Area Around Room 'Always' Quiet at Night	300+	42%	-	58%
Doctors 'Always' Communicated Well	300+	76%	-	80%
Home Recovery Information Given	300+	83%	-	82%
Hospital Given 9 or 10 on 10 Point Scale	300+	64%	-	67%
Meds 'Always' Explained Before Given	300+	56%	-	60%
Nurses 'Always' Communicated Well	300+	76%	-	76%
Pain 'Always' Well Controlled	300+	68%	-	69%
Room and Bathroom 'Always' Clean	300+	72%	-	71%
Timely Help 'Always' Received	300+	64%	-	64%
Would Definitely Recommend Hospital	300+	68%	-	69%

Institute for Orthopedic Surgery

801 Medical Drive, Suite B Phone: 419-224-7586
Lima, OH 45804
Type: Acute Care Hospitals Emergency Services: No
Ownership: Proprietary

Key Personnel:
CEO/President. . . . . Mark McDonald MD

Measure	Cases	This Hosp.	State Avg.	U.S. Avg.
Heart Attack Care				
ACE Inhibitor or ARB for LVSD[5]	0	-	97%	96%
Aspirin at Arrival[5]	0	-	99%	99%
Aspirin at Discharge[5]	0	-	99%	98%
Beta Blocker at Discharge[5]	0	-	99%	98%
Fibrinolytic Medication Timing[5]	0	-	14%	55%
PCI Within 90 Minutes of Arrival[5]	0	-	92%	90%
Smoking Cessation Advice[5]	0	-	100%	99%
Chest Pain/Possible Heart Attack Care				
Aspirin at Arrival[5]	0	-	96%	95%
Median Time to ECG (minutes)[5]	0	-	7	8
Median Time to Transfer (minutes)[5]	0	-	61	61
Fibrinolytic Medication Timing[5]	0	-	47%	54%
Heart Failure Care				
ACE Inhibitor or ARB for LVSD[5]	0	-	96%	94%
Discharge Instructions[5]	0	-	91%	88%
Evaluation of LVS Function[5]	0	-	99%	98%
Smoking Cessation Advice[5]	0	-	99%	98%
Pneumonia Care				
Appropriate Initial Antibiotic[5]	0	-	92%	92%
Blood Culture Timing[5]	0	-	96%	96%
Influenza Vaccine[5]	0	-	93%	91%
Initial Antibiotic Timing[5]	0	-	96%	95%
Pneumococcal Vaccine[5]	0	-	95%	93%
Smoking Cessation Advice[5]	0	-	98%	97%
Surgical Care Improvement Project				
Appropriate VTP Within 24 Hours[1,2]	9	100%	92%	92%
Appropriate Hair Removal[2]	214	99%	100%	99%
Appropriate Beta Blocker Usage[2]	64	97%	94%	93%
Controlled Postoperative Blood Glucose[2]	0	-	94%	93%
Prophylactic Antibiotic Timing[2]	191	100%	97%	97%
Prophylactic Antibiotic Timing (Outpatient)	83	100%	91%	92%
Prophylactic Antibiotic Selection[2]	191	100%	98%	97%
Prophylactic Antibiotic Select. (Outpatient)	83	98%	94%	94%
Prophylactic Antibiotic Stopped[2]	189	98%	95%	94%
Recommended VTP Ordered[1,2]	9	100%	94%	94%
Urinary Catheter Removal[1,2]	16	100%	91%	90%
Children's Asthma Care				
Received Systemic Corticosteroids	-	-	-	100%
Received Home Management Plan	-	-	-	71%
Received Reliever Medication	-	-	-	100%
Use of Medical Imaging				
Combination Abdominal CT Scan[5]	0	-	0.164	0.191
Combination Chest CT Scan[5]	0	-	0.038	0.054
Follow-up Mammogram/Ultrasound[5]	0	-	8.4%	8.4%
MRI for Low Back Pain[5]	0	-	30.2%	32.7%
Survey of Patients' Hospital Experiences				
Area Around Room 'Always' Quiet at Night	300+	78%	-	58%
Doctors 'Always' Communicated Well	300+	90%	-	80%
Home Recovery Information Given	300+	95%	-	82%
Hospital Given 9 or 10 on 10 Point Scale	300+	92%	-	67%
Meds 'Always' Explained Before Given	300+	78%	-	60%
Nurses 'Always' Communicated Well	300+	91%	-	76%
Pain 'Always' Well Controlled	300+	80%	-	69%
Room and Bathroom 'Always' Clean	300+	82%	-	71%
Timely Help 'Always' Received	300+	88%	-	64%
Would Definitely Recommend Hospital	300+	94%	-	69%

Lima Memorial Health System

1001 Bellefontaine Avenue Phone: 419-998-4731
Lima, OH 45804 Fax: 419-998-4509
URL: www.limamemorial.org
Type: Acute Care Hospitals Emergency Services: Yes
Ownership: Voluntary Non-Profit - Other Beds: 308

Key Personnel:
CEO/President. . . . . Mike Swick
Chief of Medical Staff . . . . Jean Johns
Operating Room. . . . . Jeff Collins
Pediatric Ambulatory Care . . . . . . J Liggett, MD
Quality Assurance . . . . Anita Good
Radiology. . . . . PK Malhotra, MD
Emergency Room . . . . Sue Fickel, RN, MS

Measure	Cases	This Hosp.	State Avg.	U.S. Avg.
Heart Attack Care				
ACE Inhibitor or ARB for LVSD	29	100%	97%	96%
Aspirin at Arrival	136	100%	99%	99%
Aspirin at Discharge	232	100%	99%	98%
Beta Blocker at Discharge	210	99%	99%	98%
Fibrinolytic Medication Timing[1]	3	0%	14%	55%
PCI Within 90 Minutes of Arrival[1]	14	100%	92%	90%
Smoking Cessation Advice	81	100%	100%	99%
Chest Pain/Possible Heart Attack Care				
Aspirin at Arrival[1,3]	3	67%	96%	95%
Median Time to ECG (minutes)[1,3]	4	4	7	8
Median Time to Transfer (minutes)[5]	0	-	61	61
Fibrinolytic Medication Timing[5]	0	-	47%	54%
Heart Failure Care				
ACE Inhibitor or ARB for LVSD	63	98%	96%	94%
Discharge Instructions	158	92%	91%	88%
Evaluation of LVS Function	191	100%	99%	98%
Smoking Cessation Advice	26	100%	99%	98%
Pneumonia Care				
Appropriate Initial Antibiotic	120	93%	92%	92%
Blood Culture Timing	160	99%	96%	96%
Influenza Vaccine	132	98%	93%	91%
Initial Antibiotic Timing	140	96%	96%	95%
Pneumococcal Vaccine	151	98%	95%	93%
Smoking Cessation Advice	66	100%	98%	97%
Surgical Care Improvement Project				
Appropriate VTP Within 24 Hours[2]	140	91%	92%	92%
Appropriate Hair Removal[2]	580	100%	100%	99%
Appropriate Beta Blocker Usage[2]	185	95%	94%	93%
Controlled Postoperative Blood Glucose[2]	240	96%	94%	93%
Prophylactic Antibiotic Timing[2]	406	95%	97%	97%
Prophylactic Antibiotic Timing (Outpatient)	370	87%	91%	92%
Prophylactic Antibiotic Selection[2]	410	99%	98%	97%
Prophylactic Antibiotic Select. (Outpatient)	359	99%	94%	94%
Prophylactic Antibiotic Stopped[2]	382	93%	95%	94%
Recommended VTP Ordered[2]	141	96%	94%	94%
Urinary Catheter Removal[2]	78	64%	91%	90%
Children's Asthma Care				
Received Systemic Corticosteroids	-	-	-	100%
Received Home Management Plan	-	-	-	71%
Received Reliever Medication	-	-	-	100%
Use of Medical Imaging				
Combination Abdominal CT Scan	694	0.046	0.164	0.191
Combination Chest CT Scan	582	0.005	0.038	0.054
Follow-up Mammogram/Ultrasound	1,360	12.1%	8.4%	8.4%
MRI for Low Back Pain	173	29.5%	30.2%	32.7%
Survey of Patients' Hospital Experiences				
Area Around Room 'Always' Quiet at Night	300+	57%	-	58%
Doctors 'Always' Communicated Well	300+	78%	-	80%
Home Recovery Information Given	300+	89%	-	82%
Hospital Given 9 or 10 on 10 Point Scale	300+	69%	-	67%
Meds 'Always' Explained Before Given	300+	57%	-	60%
Nurses 'Always' Communicated Well	300+	72%	-	76%
Pain 'Always' Well Controlled	300+	67%	-	69%
Room and Bathroom 'Always' Clean	300+	74%	-	71%
Timely Help 'Always' Received	300+	57%	-	64%
Would Definitely Recommend Hospital	300+	75%	-	69%

NOTE: Hospital profiles are in alphabetical order by state, then city, then hospital within the city; Rankings exclude hospitals with less than 25 cases except for patient surveys which excludes hospitals with less than 100 cases; (a) 100–299 cases; (1) The number of cases is too small to be sure how well a hospital is performing; (2) The hospital indicated that the data submitted for this measure were based on a sample of cases; (3) Data was collected during a shorter time period (fewer quarters) than the maximum possible time for this measure; (4) Suppressed for one or more quarters by CMS; (5) No data is available from the hospital for this measure; (6) Fewer than 100 patients completed the HCAHPS survey. Use these rates with caution, as the number of surveys may be too low to reliably assess hospital performance; (7) Survey results are based on less than 12 months of data; (8) Survey results are not available for this reporting period; (9) No or very few patients were eligible for the HCAHPS survey. The scores shown, if any, reflect a very small number of surveys; (10) A state average was not calculated because too few hospitals in the state submitted data; (11) There were discrepancies in the data collection process; Please refer to the User's Guide for a full explanation of data.

Saint Rita's Medical Center

730 West Market Street
Lima, OH 45801
Phone: 419-227-3361
Fax: 419-226-9718
URL: www.stritas.org
Type: Acute Care Hospitals
Emergency Services: Yes
Ownership: Voluntary Non-Profit - Church
Beds: 424

Key Personnel:
CEO/President. . . . . James P Reber
Chief of Medical Staff . . . . DL Imler, DO
Infection Control. . . . . KM Griffith, MD
Operating Room. . . . . Jo Shough
Pediatric Ambulatory Care . . . . . . JS Liggett, MD
Pediatric In-Patient Care . . . . JS Liggett, MD
Quality Assurance . . . . Cindy Mefferd
Radiology. . . . . EV Bostick, MD

Measure	Cases	This Hosp.	State Avg.	U.S. Avg.
Heart Attack Care				
ACE Inhibitor or ARB for LVSD	71	99%	97%	96%
Aspirin at Arrival	252	100%	99%	99%
Aspirin at Discharge	301	100%	99%	98%
Beta Blocker at Discharge	302	100%	99%	98%
Fibrinolytic Medication Timing	0	-	14%	55%
PCI Within 90 Minutes of Arrival	49	100%	92%	90%
Smoking Cessation Advice	121	100%	100%	99%
Chest Pain/Possible Heart Attack Care				
Aspirin at Arrival	58	100%	96%	95%
Median Time to ECG (minutes)	66	9	7	8
Median Time to Transfer (minutes)[1,3]	1	28	61	61
Fibrinolytic Medication Timing[3]	0	-	47%	54%
Heart Failure Care				
ACE Inhibitor or ARB for LVSD	152	97%	96%	94%
Discharge Instructions	267	97%	91%	88%
Evaluation of LVS Function	343	99%	99%	98%
Smoking Cessation Advice	62	100%	99%	98%
Pneumonia Care				
Appropriate Initial Antibiotic	157	98%	92%	92%
Blood Culture Timing	321	96%	96%	96%
Influenza Vaccine	133	100%	93%	91%
Initial Antibiotic Timing	217	98%	96%	95%
Pneumococcal Vaccine	229	99%	95%	93%
Smoking Cessation Advice	132	100%	98%	97%
Surgical Care Improvement Project				
Appropriate VTP Within 24 Hours	388	92%	92%	92%
Appropriate Hair Removal	1,164	99%	100%	99%
Appropriate Beta Blocker Usage	436	97%	94%	93%
Controlled Postoperative Blood Glucose	163	100%	94%	93%
Prophylactic Antibiotic Timing	693	98%	97%	97%
Prophylactic Antibiotic Timing (Outpatient)	275	91%	91%	92%
Prophylactic Antibiotic Selection	703	98%	98%	97%
Prophylactic Antibiotic Select. (Outpatient)	266	96%	94%	94%
Prophylactic Antibiotic Stopped	669	92%	95%	94%
Recommended VTP Ordered	388	95%	94%	94%
Urinary Catheter Removal	171	82%	91%	90%
Children's Asthma Care				
Received Systemic Corticosteroids	-	-	-	100%
Received Home Management Plan	-	-	-	71%
Received Reliever Medication	-	-	-	100%
Use of Medical Imaging				
Combination Abdominal CT Scan	1,586	0.091	0.164	0.191
Combination Chest CT Scan	952	0.015	0.038	0.054
Follow-up Mammogram/Ultrasound	2,427	8.2%	8.4%	8.4%
MRI for Low Back Pain	288	28.1%	30.2%	32.7%
Survey of Patients' Hospital Experiences				
Area Around Room 'Always' Quiet at Night	300+	55%	-	58%
Doctors 'Always' Communicated Well	300+	78%	-	80%
Home Recovery Information Given	300+	85%	-	82%
Hospital Given 9 or 10 on 10 Point Scale	300+	73%	-	67%
Meds 'Always' Explained Before Given	300+	60%	-	60%
Nurses 'Always' Communicated Well	300+	78%	-	76%
Pain 'Always' Well Controlled	300+	69%	-	69%
Room and Bathroom 'Always' Clean	300+	69%	-	71%
Timely Help 'Always' Received	300+	69%	-	64%
Would Definitely Recommend Hospital	300+	76%	-	69%

Lodi Community Hospital

225 Elyria Street
Lodi, OH 44254
Phone: 330-948-1222
Fax: 330-948-2614
URL: www.lodihospital.com
Type: Critical Access Hospitals
Emergency Services: Yes
Ownership: Voluntary Non-Profit - Private
Beds: 25

Key Personnel:
CEO/President. . . . . Thomas Whelan
Chief of Medical Staff . . . . Mary Hancock, MD
Operating Room. . . . . Molly Saal, RN
Emergency Room . . . . Christine Snow, RN
Patient Relations . . . . Dana Kocsis, RN

Measure	Cases	This Hosp.	State Avg.	U.S. Avg.
Heart Attack Care				
ACE Inhibitor or ARB for LVSD[5]	0	-	97%	96%
Aspirin at Arrival[5]	0	-	99%	99%
Aspirin at Discharge[5]	0	-	99%	98%
Beta Blocker at Discharge[5]	0	-	99%	98%
Fibrinolytic Medication Timing[5]	0	-	14%	55%
PCI Within 90 Minutes of Arrival[5]	0	-	92%	90%
Smoking Cessation Advice[5]	0	-	100%	99%
Chest Pain/Possible Heart Attack Care				
Aspirin at Arrival	134	99%	96%	95%
Median Time to ECG (minutes)	138	7	7	8
Median Time to Transfer (minutes)[1,3]	4	58	61	61
Fibrinolytic Medication Timing	0	-	47%	54%
Heart Failure Care				
ACE Inhibitor or ARB for LVSD[5]	0	-	96%	94%
Discharge Instructions[5]	0	-	91%	88%
Evaluation of LVS Function[5]	0	-	99%	98%
Smoking Cessation Advice[5]	0	-	99%	98%
Pneumonia Care				
Appropriate Initial Antibiotic[1]	15	100%	92%	92%
Blood Culture Timing[1]	15	100%	96%	96%
Influenza Vaccine[1]	5	100%	93%	91%
Initial Antibiotic Timing[1]	15	100%	96%	95%
Pneumococcal Vaccine[1]	8	100%	95%	93%
Smoking Cessation Advice[1]	5	80%	98%	97%
Surgical Care Improvement Project				
Appropriate VTP Within 24 Hours[5]	0	-	92%	92%
Appropriate Hair Removal[5]	0	-	100%	99%
Appropriate Beta Blocker Usage[5]	0	-	94%	93%
Controlled Postoperative Blood Glucose[5]	0	-	94%	93%
Prophylactic Antibiotic Timing[5]	0	-	97%	97%
Prophylactic Antibiotic Timing (Outpatient)[5]	0	-	91%	92%
Prophylactic Antibiotic Selection[5]	0	-	98%	97%
Prophylactic Antibiotic Select. (Outpatient)[5]	0	-	94%	94%
Prophylactic Antibiotic Stopped[5]	0	-	95%	94%
Recommended VTP Ordered[5]	0	-	94%	94%
Urinary Catheter Removal[5]	0	-	91%	90%
Children's Asthma Care				
Received Systemic Corticosteroids	-	-	-	100%
Received Home Management Plan	-	-	-	71%
Received Reliever Medication	-	-	-	100%
Use of Medical Imaging				
Combination Abdominal CT Scan	105	0.076	0.164	0.191
Combination Chest CT Scan[1]	44	0.045	0.038	0.054
Follow-up Mammogram/Ultrasound	134	16.4%	8.4%	8.4%
MRI for Low Back Pain[1]	6	83.3%	30.2%	32.7%
Survey of Patients' Hospital Experiences				
Area Around Room 'Always' Quiet at Night[11]	(a)	61%	-	58%
Doctors 'Always' Communicated Well[11]	(a)	79%	-	80%
Home Recovery Information Given[11]	(a)	90%	-	82%
Hospital Given 9 or 10 on 10 Point Scale[11]	(a)	84%	-	67%
Meds 'Always' Explained Before Given[11]	(a)	63%	-	60%
Nurses 'Always' Communicated Well[11]	(a)	87%	-	76%
Pain 'Always' Well Controlled[11]	(a)	75%	-	69%
Room and Bathroom 'Always' Clean[11]	(a)	84%	-	71%
Timely Help 'Always' Received[11]	(a)	74%	-	64%
Would Definitely Recommend Hospital[11]	(a)	86%	-	69%

Hocking Valley Community Hospital

State Route 664n
Logan, OH 43138
Phone: 740-380-8000
Fax: 740-385-9771
Type: Critical Access Hospitals
Emergency Services: Yes
Ownership: Voluntary Non-Profit - Other
Beds: 93

Key Personnel:
Chief of Medical Staff . . . . Prakash Kudlapur
Infection Control. . . . . Connie Gaib
Operating Room. . . . . Mary Rosier
Pediatric Ambulatory Care . . . . . . Rosario Labrador
Pediatric In-Patient Care . . . . Rosario Labrador
Quality Assurance . . . . Connie Gaib
Radiology. . . . . Robert Cox
Intensive Care Unit. . . . . Katy Daubenmeir

Measure	Cases	This Hosp.	State Avg.	U.S. Avg.
Heart Attack Care				
ACE Inhibitor or ARB for LVSD	0	-	97%	96%
Aspirin at Arrival	0	-	99%	99%
Aspirin at Discharge	0	-	99%	98%
Beta Blocker at Discharge	0	-	99%	98%
Fibrinolytic Medication Timing	0	-	14%	55%
PCI Within 90 Minutes of Arrival	0	-	92%	90%
Smoking Cessation Advice	0	-	100%	99%
Chest Pain/Possible Heart Attack Care				
Aspirin at Arrival	-	-	96%	95%
Median Time to ECG (minutes)	-	-	7	8
Median Time to Transfer (minutes)	-	-	61	61
Fibrinolytic Medication Timing	-	-	47%	54%
Heart Failure Care				
ACE Inhibitor or ARB for LVSD[1]	8	100%	96%	94%
Discharge Instructions[1]	16	38%	91%	88%
Evaluation of LVS Function[1]	21	86%	99%	98%
Smoking Cessation Advice[1]	4	50%	99%	98%
Pneumonia Care				
Appropriate Initial Antibiotic	58	83%	92%	92%
Blood Culture Timing	43	84%	96%	96%
Influenza Vaccine	28	93%	93%	91%
Initial Antibiotic Timing	52	96%	96%	95%
Pneumococcal Vaccine	31	97%	95%	93%
Smoking Cessation Advice[1]	18	56%	98%	97%
Surgical Care Improvement Project				
Appropriate VTP Within 24 Hours	25	96%	92%	92%
Appropriate Hair Removal	57	100%	100%	99%
Appropriate Beta Blocker Usage[5]	0	-	94%	93%
Controlled Postoperative Blood Glucose	0	-	94%	93%
Prophylactic Antibiotic Timing	51	94%	97%	97%
Prophylactic Antibiotic Timing (Outpatient)	-	-	91%	92%
Prophylactic Antibiotic Selection	51	96%	98%	97%
Prophylactic Antibiotic Select. (Outpatient)	-	-	94%	94%
Prophylactic Antibiotic Stopped	51	94%	95%	94%
Recommended VTP Ordered	25	96%	94%	94%
Urinary Catheter Removal[1]	18	100%	91%	90%
Children's Asthma Care				
Received Systemic Corticosteroids	-	-	-	100%
Received Home Management Plan	-	-	-	71%
Received Reliever Medication	-	-	-	100%
Use of Medical Imaging				
Combination Abdominal CT Scan	-	-	0.164	0.191
Combination Chest CT Scan	-	-	0.038	0.054
Follow-up Mammogram/Ultrasound	-	-	8.4%	8.4%
MRI for Low Back Pain	-	-	30.2%	32.7%
Survey of Patients' Hospital Experiences				
Area Around Room 'Always' Quiet at Night	300+	62%	-	58%
Doctors 'Always' Communicated Well	300+	83%	-	80%
Home Recovery Information Given	300+	88%	-	82%
Hospital Given 9 or 10 on 10 Point Scale	300+	76%	-	67%
Meds 'Always' Explained Before Given	300+	64%	-	60%
Nurses 'Always' Communicated Well	300+	81%	-	76%
Pain 'Always' Well Controlled	300+	76%	-	69%
Room and Bathroom 'Always' Clean	300+	73%	-	71%
Timely Help 'Always' Received	300+	71%	-	64%
Would Definitely Recommend Hospital	300+	66%	-	69%

NOTE: Hospital profiles are in alphabetical order by state, then city, then hospital within the city; Rankings exclude hospitals with less than 25 cases except for patient surveys which excludes hospitals with less than 100 cases; (a) 100–299 cases; (1) The number of cases is too small to be sure how well a hospital is performing; (2) The hospital indicated that the data submitted for this measure were based on a sample of cases; (3) Data was collected during a shorter time period (fewer quarters) than the maximum possible time for this measure; (4) Suppressed for one or more quarters by CMS; (5) No data is available from the hospital for this measure; (6) Fewer than 100 patients completed the HCAHPS survey. Use these rates with caution, as the number of surveys may be too low to reliably assess hospital performance; (7) Survey results are based on less than 12 months of data; (8) Survey results are not available for this reporting period; (9) No or very few patients were eligible for the HCAHPS survey. The scores shown, if any, reflect a very small number of surveys; (10) A state average was not calculated because too few hospitals in the state submitted data; (11) There were discrepancies in the data collection process; Please refer to the User's Guide for a full explanation of data.

Madison County Hospital

210 North Main Street
London, OH 43140
Phone: 740-845-7010
Fax: 740-852-3315
Type: Acute Care Hospitals
Emergency Services: Yes
Ownership: Voluntary Non-Profit - Other
Beds: 102

Key Personnel:
CEO/President. . . . . Fred L Kolb
Chief of Medical Staff. . . . . Michael Turner, MD
Infection Control. . . . . Millie Newman
Operating Room. . . . . AJ Beisler, RN
Pediatric Ambulatory Care . . . . . . Sooja Kim
Pediatric In-Patient Care . . . . Sooja Kim
Quality Assurance . . . . Darla Howland

Measure	Cases	This Hosp.	State Avg.	U.S. Avg.
Heart Attack Care				
ACE Inhibitor or ARB for LVSD[1,3]	1	0%	97%	96%
Aspirin at Arrival[1,3]	4	100%	99%	99%
Aspirin at Discharge[1,3]	1	100%	99%	98%
Beta Blocker at Discharge[1,3]	1	100%	99%	98%
Fibrinolytic Medication Timing[3]	0	-	14%	55%
PCI Within 90 Minutes of Arrival[3]	0	-	92%	90%
Smoking Cessation Advice[3]	0	-	100%	99%
Chest Pain/Possible Heart Attack Care				
Aspirin at Arrival	115	97%	96%	95%
Median Time to ECG (minutes)	117	4	7	8
Median Time to Transfer (minutes)[1,3]	2	187	61	61
Fibrinolytic Medication Timing[1]	5	20%	47%	54%
Heart Failure Care				
ACE Inhibitor or ARB for LVSD[1]	15	100%	96%	94%
Discharge Instructions	57	74%	91%	88%
Evaluation of LVS Function	67	85%	99%	98%
Smoking Cessation Advice[1]	15	93%	99%	98%
Pneumonia Care				
Appropriate Initial Antibiotic	60	93%	92%	92%
Blood Culture Timing	43	98%	96%	96%
Influenza Vaccine	43	88%	93%	91%
Initial Antibiotic Timing	62	95%	96%	95%
Pneumococcal Vaccine	50	90%	95%	93%
Smoking Cessation Advice[1]	20	100%	98%	97%
Surgical Care Improvement Project				
Appropriate VTP Within 24 Hours	31	84%	92%	92%
Appropriate Hair Removal	105	100%	100%	99%
Appropriate Beta Blocker Usage[1]	22	50%	94%	93%
Controlled Postoperative Blood Glucose	0	-	94%	93%
Prophylactic Antibiotic Timing	62	94%	97%	97%
Prophylactic Antibiotic Timing (Outpatient)	40	40%	91%	92%
Prophylactic Antibiotic Selection	62	98%	98%	97%
Prophylactic Antibiotic Select. (Outpatient)[1]	19	89%	94%	94%
Prophylactic Antibiotic Stopped	59	93%	95%	94%
Recommended VTP Ordered	32	84%	94%	94%
Urinary Catheter Removal[1]	22	95%	91%	90%
Children's Asthma Care				
Received Systemic Corticosteroids	-	-	-	100%
Received Home Management Plan	-	-	-	71%
Received Reliever Medication	-	-	-	100%
Use of Medical Imaging				
Combination Abdominal CT Scan	165	0.042	0.164	0.191
Combination Chest CT Scan	128	0.000	0.038	0.054
Follow-up Mammogram/Ultrasound	256	6.6%	8.4%	8.4%
MRI for Low Back Pain[1]	22	13.6%	30.2%	32.7%
Survey of Patients' Hospital Experiences				
Area Around Room 'Always' Quiet at Night	300+	56%	-	58%
Doctors 'Always' Communicated Well	300+	83%	-	80%
Home Recovery Information Given	300+	79%	-	82%
Hospital Given 9 or 10 on 10 Point Scale	300+	66%	-	67%
Meds 'Always' Explained Before Given	300+	60%	-	60%
Nurses 'Always' Communicated Well	300+	79%	-	76%
Pain 'Always' Well Controlled	300+	74%	-	69%
Room and Bathroom 'Always' Clean	300+	73%	-	71%
Timely Help 'Always' Received	300+	71%	-	64%
Would Definitely Recommend Hospital	300+	66%	-	69%

Community Regional Medical Center

3700 Kolbe Road
Lorain, OH 44053
Phone: 440-960-3295
Type: Acute Care Hospitals
Emergency Services: Yes
Ownership: Voluntary Non-Profit - Church

Measure	Cases	This Hosp.	State Avg.	U.S. Avg.
Heart Attack Care				
ACE Inhibitor or ARB for LVSD	43	100%	97%	96%
Aspirin at Arrival	228	100%	99%	99%
Aspirin at Discharge	228	100%	99%	98%
Beta Blocker at Discharge	228	100%	99%	98%
Fibrinolytic Medication Timing	0	-	14%	55%
PCI Within 90 Minutes of Arrival	50	88%	92%	90%
Smoking Cessation Advice	98	98%	100%	99%
Chest Pain/Possible Heart Attack Care				
Aspirin at Arrival[1]	11	100%	96%	95%
Median Time to ECG (minutes)[1]	13	6	7	8
Median Time to Transfer (minutes)[5]	0	-	61	61
Fibrinolytic Medication Timing[5]	0	-	47%	54%
Heart Failure Care				
ACE Inhibitor or ARB for LVSD	121	98%	96%	94%
Discharge Instructions	317	96%	91%	88%
Evaluation of LVS Function	402	100%	99%	98%
Smoking Cessation Advice	62	100%	99%	98%
Pneumonia Care				
Appropriate Initial Antibiotic	221	94%	92%	92%
Blood Culture Timing	386	98%	96%	96%
Influenza Vaccine	225	96%	93%	91%
Initial Antibiotic Timing	348	97%	96%	95%
Pneumococcal Vaccine	290	97%	95%	93%
Smoking Cessation Advice	152	99%	98%	97%
Surgical Care Improvement Project				
Appropriate VTP Within 24 Hours[2]	258	97%	92%	92%
Appropriate Hair Removal[2]	621	100%	100%	99%
Appropriate Beta Blocker Usage[2]	264	98%	94%	93%
Controlled Postoperative Blood Glucose[2]	42	95%	94%	93%
Prophylactic Antibiotic Timing[2]	481	100%	97%	97%
Prophylactic Antibiotic Timing (Outpatient)	307	98%	91%	92%
Prophylactic Antibiotic Selection[2]	485	97%	98%	97%
Prophylactic Antibiotic Select. (Outpatient)	307	94%	94%	94%
Prophylactic Antibiotic Stopped[2]	453	99%	95%	94%
Recommended VTP Ordered[2]	260	97%	94%	94%
Urinary Catheter Removal[2]	156	99%	91%	90%
Children's Asthma Care				
Received Systemic Corticosteroids	-	-	-	100%
Received Home Management Plan	-	-	-	71%
Received Reliever Medication	-	-	-	100%
Use of Medical Imaging				
Combination Abdominal CT Scan	995	0.051	0.164	0.191
Combination Chest CT Scan	759	0.269	0.038	0.054
Follow-up Mammogram/Ultrasound	2,206	7.4%	8.4%	8.4%
MRI for Low Back Pain	246	27.6%	30.2%	32.7%
Survey of Patients' Hospital Experiences				
Area Around Room 'Always' Quiet at Night	300+	52%	-	58%
Doctors 'Always' Communicated Well	300+	77%	-	80%
Home Recovery Information Given	300+	85%	-	82%
Hospital Given 9 or 10 on 10 Point Scale	300+	60%	-	67%
Meds 'Always' Explained Before Given	300+	58%	-	60%
Nurses 'Always' Communicated Well	300+	73%	-	76%
Pain 'Always' Well Controlled	300+	65%	-	69%
Room and Bathroom 'Always' Clean	300+	70%	-	71%
Timely Help 'Always' Received	300+	57%	-	64%
Would Definitely Recommend Hospital	300+	59%	-	69%

Medcentral Health System

335 Glessner Avenue
Mansfield, OH 44903
Phone: 419-526-8000
Fax: 419-521-7960
E-mail: medcentral@medcentral.org
URL: www.medcentral.org
Type: Acute Care Hospitals
Emergency Services: Yes
Ownership: Voluntary Non-Profit - Private
Beds: 398

Key Personnel:
CEO/President. . . . . James E Meyer
Chief of Medical Staff. . . . . Terry Weston MD
Coronary Care . . . . Patti Kastelic
Infection Control. . . . . Liz DeHaan
Operating Room. . . . . Linda Nelson
Pediatric In-Patient Care . . . . Susan Brown
Quality Assurance . . . . Janene Yeater
Radiology. . . . . Terry Baker

Measure	Cases	This Hosp.	State Avg.	U.S. Avg.
Heart Attack Care				
ACE Inhibitor or ARB for LVSD[2]	50	96%	97%	96%
Aspirin at Arrival[2]	266	98%	99%	99%
Aspirin at Discharge[2]	377	94%	99%	98%
Beta Blocker at Discharge[2]	397	97%	99%	98%
Fibrinolytic Medication Timing[2]	0	-	14%	55%
PCI Within 90 Minutes of Arrival[2]	39	79%	92%	90%
Smoking Cessation Advice[2]	165	100%	100%	99%
Chest Pain/Possible Heart Attack Care				
Aspirin at Arrival	55	91%	96%	95%
Median Time to ECG (minutes)	63	7	7	8
Median Time to Transfer (minutes)[1,3]	4	122	61	61
Fibrinolytic Medication Timing	0	-	47%	54%
Heart Failure Care				
ACE Inhibitor or ARB for LVSD[2]	86	92%	96%	94%
Discharge Instructions[2]	254	100%	91%	88%
Evaluation of LVS Function[2]	330	98%	99%	98%
Smoking Cessation Advice[2]	60	98%	99%	98%
Pneumonia Care				
Appropriate Initial Antibiotic[2]	195	91%	92%	92%
Blood Culture Timing[2]	328	94%	96%	96%
Influenza Vaccine	284	92%	93%	91%
Initial Antibiotic Timing[2]	371	91%	96%	95%
Pneumococcal Vaccine[2]	342	95%	95%	93%
Smoking Cessation Advice[2]	135	99%	98%	97%
Surgical Care Improvement Project				
Appropriate VTP Within 24 Hours[2]	288	88%	92%	92%
Appropriate Hair Removal[2]	930	97%	100%	99%
Appropriate Beta Blocker Usage[2]	380	96%	94%	93%
Controlled Postoperative Blood Glucose[2]	304	96%	94%	93%
Prophylactic Antibiotic Timing[2]	639	97%	97%	97%
Prophylactic Antibiotic Timing (Outpatient)	319	84%	91%	92%
Prophylactic Antibiotic Selection[2]	647	96%	98%	97%
Prophylactic Antibiotic Select. (Outpatient)	275	87%	94%	94%
Prophylactic Antibiotic Stopped[2]	624	92%	95%	94%
Recommended VTP Ordered[2]	289	90%	94%	94%
Urinary Catheter Removal[2]	213	74%	91%	90%
Children's Asthma Care				
Received Systemic Corticosteroids	-	-	-	100%
Received Home Management Plan	-	-	-	71%
Received Reliever Medication	-	-	-	100%
Use of Medical Imaging				
Combination Abdominal CT Scan	1,143	0.035	0.164	0.191
Combination Chest CT Scan	833	0.060	0.038	0.054
Follow-up Mammogram/Ultrasound	1,715	8.3%	8.4%	8.4%
MRI for Low Back Pain	198	25.8%	30.2%	32.7%
Survey of Patients' Hospital Experiences				
Area Around Room 'Always' Quiet at Night	300+	39%	-	58%
Doctors 'Always' Communicated Well	300+	71%	-	80%
Home Recovery Information Given	300+	83%	-	82%
Hospital Given 9 or 10 on 10 Point Scale	300+	62%	-	67%
Meds 'Always' Explained Before Given	300+	52%	-	60%
Nurses 'Always' Communicated Well	300+	72%	-	76%
Pain 'Always' Well Controlled	300+	64%	-	69%
Room and Bathroom 'Always' Clean	300+	68%	-	71%
Timely Help 'Always' Received	300+	62%	-	64%
Would Definitely Recommend Hospital	300+	61%	-	69%

NOTE: Hospital profiles are in alphabetical order by state, then city, then hospital within the city; Rankings exclude hospitals with less than 25 cases except for patient surveys which excludes hospitals with less than 100 cases; (a) 100–299 cases; (1) The number of cases is too small to be sure how well a hospital is performing; (2) The hospital indicated that the data submitted for this measure were based on a sample of cases; (3) Data was collected during a shorter time period (fewer quarters) than the maximum possible time for this measure; (4) Suppressed for one or more quarters by CMS; (5) No data is available from the hospital for this measure; (6) Fewer than 100 patients completed the HCAHPS survey. Use these rates with caution, as the number of surveys may be too low to reliably assess hospital performance; (7) Survey results are based on less than 12 months of data; (8) Survey results are not available for this reporting period; (9) No or very few patients were eligible for the HCAHPS survey. The scores shown, if any, reflect a very small number of surveys; (10) A state average was not calculated because too few hospitals in the state submitted data; (11) There were discrepancies in the data collection process; Please refer to the User's Guide for a full explanation of data.

Marietta Memorial Hospital

401 Matthew Street
Marietta, OH 45750
Phone: 740-374-1400
Fax: 740-376-5045
URL: www.mmhospital.org
Type: Acute Care Hospitals
Emergency Services: Yes
Ownership: Voluntary Non-Profit - Other
Beds: 204

Key Personnel:
CEO/President. . . . . Larry Unroe
Chief of Medical Staff . . . . Joseph Cooper, MD
Infection Control . . . . Suzanne Baker
Operating Room. . . . . Bradley Carman
Pediatric Ambulatory Care . . . . . William Jacoby, MD
Pediatric In-Patient Care . . . . . . William Jacoby, MD
Quality Assurance . . . . Bonnie Flannery
Radiology. . . . . Steve Boker, MD

Measure	Cases	This Hosp.	State Avg.	U.S. Avg.
Heart Attack Care				
ACE Inhibitor or ARB for LVSD[1]	24	100%	97%	96%
Aspirin at Arrival	95	99%	99%	99%
Aspirin at Discharge	81	100%	99%	98%
Beta Blocker at Discharge	88	100%	99%	98%
Fibrinolytic Medication Timing	0	-	14%	55%
PCI Within 90 Minutes of Arrival[1]	12	92%	92%	90%
Smoking Cessation Advice	27	100%	100%	99%
Chest Pain/Possible Heart Attack Care				
Aspirin at Arrival	50	94%	96%	95%
Median Time to ECG (minutes)	51	10	7	8
Median Time to Transfer (minutes)[1,3]	2	51	61	61
Fibrinolytic Medication Timing	0	-	47%	54%
Heart Failure Care				
ACE Inhibitor or ARB for LVSD	74	99%	96%	94%
Discharge Instructions	217	85%	91%	88%
Evaluation of LVS Function	278	100%	99%	98%
Smoking Cessation Advice	45	100%	99%	98%
Pneumonia Care				
Appropriate Initial Antibiotic[2]	40	92%	92%	92%
Blood Culture Timing[2]	81	100%	96%	96%
Influenza Vaccine[2]	58	98%	93%	91%
Initial Antibiotic Timing[2]	110	95%	96%	95%
Pneumococcal Vaccine[2]	100	95%	95%	93%
Smoking Cessation Advice[2]	41	100%	98%	97%
Surgical Care Improvement Project				
Appropriate VTP Within 24 Hours	214	96%	92%	92%
Appropriate Hair Removal	610	100%	100%	99%
Appropriate Beta Blocker Usage	188	90%	94%	93%
Controlled Postoperative Blood Glucose	0	-	94%	93%
Prophylactic Antibiotic Timing	473	92%	97%	97%
Prophylactic Antibiotic Timing (Outpatient)	162	71%	91%	92%
Prophylactic Antibiotic Selection	476	99%	98%	97%
Prophylactic Antibiotic Select. (Outpatient)	126	93%	94%	94%
Prophylactic Antibiotic Stopped	451	96%	95%	94%
Recommended VTP Ordered	215	97%	94%	94%
Urinary Catheter Removal	131	92%	91%	90%
Children's Asthma Care				
Received Systemic Corticosteroids	-	-	-	100%
Received Home Management Plan	-	-	-	71%
Received Reliever Medication	-	-	-	100%
Use of Medical Imaging				
Combination Abdominal CT Scan	783	0.755	0.164	0.191
Combination Chest CT Scan	942	0.137	0.038	0.054
Follow-up Mammogram/Ultrasound	1,015	4.9%	8.4%	8.4%
MRI for Low Back Pain	159	37.7%	30.2%	32.7%
Survey of Patients' Hospital Experiences				
Area Around Room 'Always' Quiet at Night	300+	40%	-	58%
Doctors 'Always' Communicated Well	300+	74%	-	80%
Home Recovery Information Given	300+	87%	-	82%
Hospital Given 9 or 10 on 10 Point Scale	300+	62%	-	67%
Meds 'Always' Explained Before Given	300+	54%	-	60%
Nurses 'Always' Communicated Well	300+	73%	-	76%
Pain 'Always' Well Controlled	300+	68%	-	69%
Room and Bathroom 'Always' Clean	300+	67%	-	71%
Timely Help 'Always' Received	300+	62%	-	64%
Would Definitely Recommend Hospital	300+	64%	-	69%

Selby General Hospital

1106 Colegate Drive
Marietta, OH 45750
Phone: 740-568-2000
Fax: 740-568-2089
E-mail: ceo@selbygeneralhospital.com
URL: www.selbygeneralhospital.con
Type: Critical Access Hospitals
Emergency Services: Yes
Ownership: Voluntary Non-Profit - Private
Beds: 80

Key Personnel:
CEO/President. . . . . Kevin P Calhoun
Chief of Medical Staff . . . . Charles Merrill
Operating Room. . . . . Nancy Chandler
Anesthesiology. . . . . Joseph Castle DO
Emergency Room . . . . James Conde
Intensive Care Unit. . . . . Angela Saffell RN

Measure	Cases	This Hosp.	State Avg.	U.S. Avg.
Heart Attack Care				
ACE Inhibitor or ARB for LVSD[3]	0	-	97%	96%
Aspirin at Arrival[1,3]	1	100%	99%	99%
Aspirin at Discharge[1,3]	1	100%	99%	98%
Beta Blocker at Discharge[1,3]	1	100%	99%	98%
Fibrinolytic Medication Timing[3]	0	-	14%	55%
PCI Within 90 Minutes of Arrival[3]	0	-	92%	90%
Smoking Cessation Advice[1,3]	1	100%	100%	99%
Chest Pain/Possible Heart Attack Care				
Aspirin at Arrival[5]	0	-	96%	95%
Median Time to ECG (minutes)[5]	0	-	7	8
Median Time to Transfer (minutes)[5]	0	-	61	61
Fibrinolytic Medication Timing[5]	0	-	47%	54%
Heart Failure Care				
ACE Inhibitor or ARB for LVSD[1]	4	75%	96%	94%
Discharge Instructions	25	60%	91%	88%
Evaluation of LVS Function	32	75%	99%	98%
Smoking Cessation Advice[1]	8	100%	99%	98%
Pneumonia Care				
Appropriate Initial Antibiotic[1]	19	53%	92%	92%
Blood Culture Timing[1]	6	83%	96%	96%
Influenza Vaccine[1]	15	87%	93%	91%
Initial Antibiotic Timing[1]	12	67%	96%	95%
Pneumococcal Vaccine[1]	8	100%	95%	93%
Smoking Cessation Advice[1]	15	93%	98%	97%
Surgical Care Improvement Project				
Appropriate VTP Within 24 Hours[3]	32	100%	92%	92%
Appropriate Hair Removal[3]	82	98%	100%	99%
Appropriate Beta Blocker Usage[5]	0	-	94%	93%
Controlled Postoperative Blood Glucose[3]	0	-	94%	93%
Prophylactic Antibiotic Timing[3]	70	89%	97%	97%
Prophylactic Antibiotic Timing (Outpatient)[5]	0	-	91%	92%
Prophylactic Antibiotic Selection[3]	69	96%	98%	97%
Prophylactic Antibiotic Select. (Outpatient)[5]	0	-	94%	94%
Prophylactic Antibiotic Stopped[3]	67	91%	95%	94%
Recommended VTP Ordered[3]	32	100%	94%	94%
Urinary Catheter Removal[1,3]	14	93%	91%	90%
Children's Asthma Care				
Received Systemic Corticosteroids	-	-	-	100%
Received Home Management Plan	-	-	-	71%
Received Reliever Medication	-	-	-	100%
Use of Medical Imaging				
Combination Abdominal CT Scan	143	0.727	0.164	0.191
Combination Chest CT Scan	91	0.000	0.038	0.054
Follow-up Mammogram/Ultrasound	135	5.9%	8.4%	8.4%
MRI for Low Back Pain[1]	8	62.5%	30.2%	32.7%
Survey of Patients' Hospital Experiences				
Area Around Room 'Always' Quiet at Night[8]	-	-	-	58%
Doctors 'Always' Communicated Well[8]	-	-	-	80%
Home Recovery Information Given[8]	-	-	-	82%
Hospital Given 9 or 10 on 10 Point Scale[8]	-	-	-	67%
Meds 'Always' Explained Before Given[8]	-	-	-	60%
Nurses 'Always' Communicated Well[8]	-	-	-	76%
Pain 'Always' Well Controlled[8]	-	-	-	69%
Room and Bathroom 'Always' Clean[8]	-	-	-	71%
Timely Help 'Always' Received[8]	-	-	-	64%
Would Definitely Recommend Hospital[8]	-	-	-	69%

Marion General Hospital

1000 Mckinley Park Drive
Marion, OH 43302
Phone: 740-383-8400
URL: www.mariongeneral.com
Type: Acute Care Hospitals
Emergency Services: Yes
Ownership: Voluntary Non-Profit - Private

Key Personnel:
Chief of Medical Staff . . . . Aaron M Fritz DO

Measure	Cases	This Hosp.	State Avg.	U.S. Avg.
Heart Attack Care				
ACE Inhibitor or ARB for LVSD	35	97%	97%	96%
Aspirin at Arrival	164	100%	99%	99%
Aspirin at Discharge	169	100%	99%	98%
Beta Blocker at Discharge	169	99%	99%	98%
Fibrinolytic Medication Timing	0	-	14%	55%
PCI Within 90 Minutes of Arrival	53	98%	92%	90%
Smoking Cessation Advice	72	100%	100%	99%
Chest Pain/Possible Heart Attack Care				
Aspirin at Arrival	134	99%	96%	95%
Median Time to ECG (minutes)	135	3	7	8
Median Time to Transfer (minutes)[5]	0	-	61	61
Fibrinolytic Medication Timing	0	-	47%	54%
Heart Failure Care				
ACE Inhibitor or ARB for LVSD	126	96%	96%	94%
Discharge Instructions	256	96%	91%	88%
Evaluation of LVS Function	339	99%	99%	98%
Smoking Cessation Advice	59	100%	99%	98%
Pneumonia Care				
Appropriate Initial Antibiotic	156	97%	92%	92%
Blood Culture Timing	200	98%	96%	96%
Influenza Vaccine	145	99%	93%	91%
Initial Antibiotic Timing	220	99%	96%	95%
Pneumococcal Vaccine	171	99%	95%	93%
Smoking Cessation Advice	87	100%	98%	97%
Surgical Care Improvement Project				
Appropriate VTP Within 24 Hours[2]	195	98%	92%	92%
Appropriate Hair Removal[2]	486	100%	100%	99%
Appropriate Beta Blocker Usage[2]	217	100%	94%	93%
Controlled Postoperative Blood Glucose[2]	59	100%	94%	93%
Prophylactic Antibiotic Timing[2]	406	99%	97%	97%
Prophylactic Antibiotic Timing (Outpatient)	198	97%	91%	92%
Prophylactic Antibiotic Selection[2]	409	98%	98%	97%
Prophylactic Antibiotic Select. (Outpatient)	197	99%	94%	94%
Prophylactic Antibiotic Stopped[2]	397	98%	95%	94%
Recommended VTP Ordered[2]	195	98%	94%	94%
Urinary Catheter Removal[2]	156	79%	91%	90%
Children's Asthma Care				
Received Systemic Corticosteroids	-	-	-	100%
Received Home Management Plan	-	-	-	71%
Received Reliever Medication	-	-	-	100%
Use of Medical Imaging				
Combination Abdominal CT Scan	221	0.027	0.164	0.191
Combination Chest CT Scan	52	0.019	0.038	0.054
Follow-up Mammogram/Ultrasound[5]	0	-	8.4%	8.4%
MRI for Low Back Pain[1]	6	50.0%	30.2%	32.7%
Survey of Patients' Hospital Experiences				
Area Around Room 'Always' Quiet at Night	300+	49%	-	58%
Doctors 'Always' Communicated Well	300+	81%	-	80%
Home Recovery Information Given	300+	87%	-	82%
Hospital Given 9 or 10 on 10 Point Scale	300+	68%	-	67%
Meds 'Always' Explained Before Given	300+	66%	-	60%
Nurses 'Always' Communicated Well	300+	80%	-	76%
Pain 'Always' Well Controlled	300+	71%	-	69%
Room and Bathroom 'Always' Clean	300+	75%	-	71%
Timely Help 'Always' Received	300+	70%	-	64%
Would Definitely Recommend Hospital	300+	69%	-	69%

NOTE: Hospital profiles are in alphabetical order by state, then city, then hospital within the city; Rankings exclude hospitals with less than 25 cases except for patient surveys which excludes hospitals with less than 100 cases; (a) 100–299 cases; (1) The number of cases is too small to be sure how well a hospital is performing; (2) The hospital indicated that the data submitted for this measure were based on a sample of cases; (3) Data was collected during a shorter time period (fewer quarters) than the maximum possible time for this measure; (4) Suppressed for one or more quarters by CMS; (5) No data is available from the hospital for this measure; (6) Fewer than 100 patients completed the HCAHPS survey. Use these rates with caution, as the number of surveys may be too low to reliably assess hospital performance; (7) Survey results are based on less than 12 months of data; (8) Survey results are not available for this reporting period; (9) No or very few patients were eligible for the HCAHPS survey. The scores shown, if any, reflect a very small number of surveys; (10) A state average was not calculated because too few hospitals in the state submitted data; (11) There were discrepancies in the data collection process; Please refer to the User's Guide for a full explanation of data.

East Ohio Regional Hospital

90 North Fourth Street
Martins Ferry, OH 43935
URL: www.eastohioregionalhospital.com
Type: Acute Care Hospitals
Ownership: Voluntary Non-Profit - Other
Phone: 740-633-4151
Fax: 740-633-4512
Emergency Services: Yes
Beds: 250

Measure	Cases	This Hosp.	State Avg.	U.S. Avg.
Heart Attack Care				
ACE Inhibitor or ARB for LVSD[1]	4	75%	97%	96%
Aspirin at Arrival	51	82%	99%	99%
Aspirin at Discharge[1]	20	95%	99%	98%
Beta Blocker at Discharge[1]	21	95%	99%	98%
Fibrinolytic Medication Timing	0	-	14%	55%
PCI Within 90 Minutes of Arrival	0	-	92%	90%
Smoking Cessation Advice[1]	1	100%	100%	99%
Chest Pain/Possible Heart Attack Care				
Aspirin at Arrival	47	94%	96%	95%
Median Time to ECG (minutes)	52	14	7	8
Median Time to Transfer (minutes)[1]	12	54	61	61
Fibrinolytic Medication Timing	0	-	47%	54%
Heart Failure Care				
ACE Inhibitor or ARB for LVSD	39	90%	96%	94%
Discharge Instructions	137	72%	91%	88%
Evaluation of LVS Function	204	100%	99%	98%
Smoking Cessation Advice[1]	23	100%	99%	98%
Pneumonia Care				
Appropriate Initial Antibiotic	110	87%	92%	92%
Blood Culture Timing	149	92%	96%	96%
Influenza Vaccine	78	64%	93%	91%
Initial Antibiotic Timing	167	95%	96%	95%
Pneumococcal Vaccine	104	81%	95%	93%
Smoking Cessation Advice	48	98%	98%	97%
Surgical Care Improvement Project				
Appropriate VTP Within 24 Hours	90	77%	92%	92%
Appropriate Hair Removal	353	100%	100%	99%
Appropriate Beta Blocker Usage	144	94%	94%	93%
Controlled Postoperative Blood Glucose	0	-	94%	93%
Prophylactic Antibiotic Timing	296	97%	97%	97%
Prophylactic Antibiotic Timing (Outpatient)	66	82%	91%	92%
Prophylactic Antibiotic Selection	297	99%	98%	97%
Prophylactic Antibiotic Select. (Outpatient)	58	95%	94%	94%
Prophylactic Antibiotic Stopped	293	94%	95%	94%
Recommended VTP Ordered	90	77%	94%	94%
Urinary Catheter Removal	113	90%	91%	90%
Children's Asthma Care				
Received Systemic Corticosteroids	-	-	-	100%
Received Home Management Plan	-	-	-	71%
Received Reliever Medication	-	-	-	100%
Use of Medical Imaging				
Combination Abdominal CT Scan	277	0.632	0.164	0.191
Combination Chest CT Scan	340	0.006	0.038	0.054
Follow-up Mammogram/Ultrasound	471	12.3%	8.4%	8.4%
MRI for Low Back Pain[1]	32	31.3%	30.2%	32.7%
Survey of Patients' Hospital Experiences				
Area Around Room 'Always' Quiet at Night	300+	37%	-	58%
Doctors 'Always' Communicated Well	300+	70%	-	80%
Home Recovery Information Given	300+	76%	-	82%
Hospital Given 9 or 10 on 10 Point Scale	300+	49%	-	67%
Meds 'Always' Explained Before Given	300+	51%	-	60%
Nurses 'Always' Communicated Well	300+	67%	-	76%
Pain 'Always' Well Controlled	300+	62%	-	69%
Room and Bathroom 'Always' Clean	300+	60%	-	71%
Timely Help 'Always' Received	300+	51%	-	64%
Would Definitely Recommend Hospital	300+	51%	-	69%

Memorial Hospital of Union County

500 London Avenue
Marysville, OH 43040
Type: Acute Care Hospitals
Ownership: Government - Local
Phone: 937-578-2289
Fax: 937-578-2806
Emergency Services: Yes
Beds: 82

Key Personnel:
CEO/President. . . . . Olas A Hubbs, III
Chief of Medical Staff . . . . David T Applegate, MD
Infection Control. . . . . Filiberto Cavazos, MD
Operating Room. . . . . Karen Hall, RN
Quality Assurance . . . . Laurie Whittington
Emergency Room . . . . Sharon Walls, RN
Intensive Care Unit. . . . . Sharon Walls, RN

Measure	Cases	This Hosp.	State Avg.	U.S. Avg.
Heart Attack Care				
ACE Inhibitor or ARB for LVSD[3]	0	-	97%	96%
Aspirin at Arrival[1,3]	5	100%	99%	99%
Aspirin at Discharge[1,3]	4	100%	99%	98%
Beta Blocker at Discharge[1,3]	4	100%	99%	98%
Fibrinolytic Medication Timing[1,3]	1	0%	14%	55%
PCI Within 90 Minutes of Arrival[3]	0	-	92%	90%
Smoking Cessation Advice[3]	0	-	100%	99%
Chest Pain/Possible Heart Attack Care				
Aspirin at Arrival	196	96%	96%	95%
Median Time to ECG (minutes)	205	4	7	8
Median Time to Transfer (minutes)[1]	12	47	61	61
Fibrinolytic Medication Timing[1]	3	33%	47%	54%
Heart Failure Care				
ACE Inhibitor or ARB for LVSD[1]	16	94%	96%	94%
Discharge Instructions	37	100%	91%	88%
Evaluation of LVS Function	51	100%	99%	98%
Smoking Cessation Advice[1]	8	100%	99%	98%
Pneumonia Care				
Appropriate Initial Antibiotic	64	89%	92%	92%
Blood Culture Timing	75	97%	96%	96%
Influenza Vaccine	51	96%	93%	91%
Initial Antibiotic Timing	84	95%	96%	95%
Pneumococcal Vaccine	62	98%	95%	93%
Smoking Cessation Advice	33	91%	98%	97%
Surgical Care Improvement Project				
Appropriate VTP Within 24 Hours	33	82%	92%	92%
Appropriate Hair Removal	122	99%	100%	99%
Appropriate Beta Blocker Usage	25	88%	94%	93%
Controlled Postoperative Blood Glucose	0	-	94%	93%
Prophylactic Antibiotic Timing	93	92%	97%	97%
Prophylactic Antibiotic Timing (Outpatient)	62	90%	91%	92%
Prophylactic Antibiotic Selection	93	98%	98%	97%
Prophylactic Antibiotic Select. (Outpatient)	61	95%	94%	94%
Prophylactic Antibiotic Stopped	90	93%	95%	94%
Recommended VTP Ordered	33	82%	94%	94%
Urinary Catheter Removal[1]	17	88%	91%	90%
Children's Asthma Care				
Received Systemic Corticosteroids	-	-	-	100%
Received Home Management Plan	-	-	-	71%
Received Reliever Medication	-	-	-	100%
Use of Medical Imaging				
Combination Abdominal CT Scan	306	0.088	0.164	0.191
Combination Chest CT Scan	222	0.018	0.038	0.054
Follow-up Mammogram/Ultrasound	435	10.1%	8.4%	8.4%
MRI for Low Back Pain	51	33.3%	30.2%	32.7%
Survey of Patients' Hospital Experiences				
Area Around Room 'Always' Quiet at Night	300+	62%	-	58%
Doctors 'Always' Communicated Well	300+	83%	-	80%
Home Recovery Information Given	300+	86%	-	82%
Hospital Given 9 or 10 on 10 Point Scale	300+	73%	-	67%
Meds 'Always' Explained Before Given	300+	67%	-	60%
Nurses 'Always' Communicated Well	300+	81%	-	76%
Pain 'Always' Well Controlled	300+	74%	-	69%
Room and Bathroom 'Always' Clean	300+	76%	-	71%
Timely Help 'Always' Received	300+	76%	-	64%
Would Definitely Recommend Hospital	300+	76%	-	69%

Affinity Medical Center

875 Eighth Street NE
Massillon, OH 44646
URL: www.affinitymedicalcenter.com
Type: Acute Care Hospitals
Ownership: Proprietary
Phone: 330-837-6863
Emergency Services: Yes
Beds: 451

Key Personnel:
CEO/President. . . . . Wendy Meighen

Measure	Cases	This Hosp.	State Avg.	U.S. Avg.
Heart Attack Care				
ACE Inhibitor or ARB for LVSD[1]	12	92%	97%	96%
Aspirin at Arrival	82	98%	99%	99%
Aspirin at Discharge	85	98%	99%	98%
Beta Blocker at Discharge	90	96%	99%	98%
Fibrinolytic Medication Timing	0	-	14%	55%
PCI Within 90 Minutes of Arrival	27	85%	92%	90%
Smoking Cessation Advice	35	100%	100%	99%
Chest Pain/Possible Heart Attack Care				
Aspirin at Arrival[1]	8	100%	96%	95%
Median Time to ECG (minutes)[1]	8	4	7	8
Median Time to Transfer (minutes)[5]	0	-	61	61
Fibrinolytic Medication Timing[5]	0	-	47%	54%
Heart Failure Care				
ACE Inhibitor or ARB for LVSD	50	94%	96%	94%
Discharge Instructions	119	87%	91%	88%
Evaluation of LVS Function	174	100%	99%	98%
Smoking Cessation Advice[1]	24	100%	99%	98%
Pneumonia Care				
Appropriate Initial Antibiotic	119	97%	92%	92%
Blood Culture Timing	198	93%	96%	96%
Influenza Vaccine	136	95%	93%	91%
Initial Antibiotic Timing	197	97%	96%	95%
Pneumococcal Vaccine	180	95%	95%	93%
Smoking Cessation Advice	80	100%	98%	97%
Surgical Care Improvement Project				
Appropriate VTP Within 24 Hours	134	99%	92%	92%
Appropriate Hair Removal	492	100%	100%	99%
Appropriate Beta Blocker Usage	177	94%	94%	93%
Controlled Postoperative Blood Glucose	88	93%	94%	93%
Prophylactic Antibiotic Timing	378	99%	97%	97%
Prophylactic Antibiotic Timing (Outpatient)	144	90%	91%	92%
Prophylactic Antibiotic Selection	384	100%	98%	97%
Prophylactic Antibiotic Select. (Outpatient)	140	89%	94%	94%
Prophylactic Antibiotic Stopped	355	97%	95%	94%
Recommended VTP Ordered	134	100%	94%	94%
Urinary Catheter Removal	147	99%	91%	90%
Children's Asthma Care				
Received Systemic Corticosteroids	-	-	-	100%
Received Home Management Plan	-	-	-	71%
Received Reliever Medication	-	-	-	100%
Use of Medical Imaging				
Combination Abdominal CT Scan	478	0.067	0.164	0.191
Combination Chest CT Scan	324	0.160	0.038	0.054
Follow-up Mammogram/Ultrasound	633	11.1%	8.4%	8.4%
MRI for Low Back Pain	66	25.8%	30.2%	32.7%
Survey of Patients' Hospital Experiences				
Area Around Room 'Always' Quiet at Night	300+	46%	-	58%
Doctors 'Always' Communicated Well	300+	77%	-	80%
Home Recovery Information Given	300+	85%	-	82%
Hospital Given 9 or 10 on 10 Point Scale	300+	64%	-	67%
Meds 'Always' Explained Before Given	300+	55%	-	60%
Nurses 'Always' Communicated Well	300+	72%	-	76%
Pain 'Always' Well Controlled	300+	69%	-	69%
Room and Bathroom 'Always' Clean	300+	67%	-	71%
Timely Help 'Always' Received	300+	57%	-	64%
Would Definitely Recommend Hospital	300+	65%	-	69%

NOTE: Hospital profiles are in alphabetical order by state, then city, then hospital within the city; Rankings exclude hospitals with less than 25 cases except for patient surveys which excludes hospitals with less than 100 cases; (a) 100–299 cases; (1) The number of cases is too small to be sure how well a hospital is performing; (2) The hospital indicated that the data submitted for this measure were based on a sample of cases; (3) Data was collected during a shorter time period (fewer quarters) than the maximum possible time for this measure; (4) Suppressed for one or more quarters by CMS; (5) No data is available from the hospital for this measure; (6) Fewer than 100 patients completed the HCAHPS survey. Use these rates with caution, as the number of surveys may be too low to reliably assess hospital performance; (7) Survey results are based on less than 12 months of data; (8) Survey results are not available for this reporting period; (9) No or very few patients were eligible for the HCAHPS survey. The scores shown, if any, reflect a very small number of surveys; (10) A state average was not calculated because too few hospitals in the state submitted data; (11) There were discrepancies in the data collection process; Please refer to the User's Guide for a full explanation of data.

Saint Luke's Hospital

5901 Monclova Road
Maumee, OH 43537
URL: www.stlukeshospital.com
Type: Acute Care Hospitals
Ownership: Voluntary Non-Profit - Other
Phone: 419-893-5900
Fax: 419-891-8079
Emergency Services: Yes
Beds: 314

Key Personnel:
CEO/President. . . . . Frank J Bartell, III
Chief of Medical Staff . . . . Stephen Bazelay, MD
Coronary Care . . . . Caroyln Gbur
Operating Room. . . . . Nadine Forton
Pediatric Ambulatory Care . . . . . . Ursula Xanthakos, MD
Pediatric In-Patient Care . . . . . . Ursula Xanthakos, MD
Quality Assurance . . . . Betsy Woodring
Emergency Room . . . . Cheryl Herr

Measure	Cases	This Hosp.	State Avg.	U.S. Avg.
Heart Attack Care				
ACE Inhibitor or ARB for LVSD	41	100%	97%	96%
Aspirin at Arrival	143	98%	99%	99%
Aspirin at Discharge	157	99%	99%	98%
Beta Blocker at Discharge	156	99%	99%	98%
Fibrinolytic Medication Timing	0	-	14%	55%
PCI Within 90 Minutes of Arrival	42	88%	92%	90%
Smoking Cessation Advice	55	98%	100%	99%
Chest Pain/Possible Heart Attack Care				
Aspirin at Arrival[1,3]	7	86%	96%	95%
Median Time to ECG (minutes)[1,3]	7	8	7	8
Median Time to Transfer (minutes)[5]	0	-	61	61
Fibrinolytic Medication Timing[5]	0	-	47%	54%
Heart Failure Care				
ACE Inhibitor or ARB for LVSD	97	98%	96%	94%
Discharge Instructions	254	96%	91%	88%
Evaluation of LVS Function	317	99%	99%	98%
Smoking Cessation Advice	32	94%	99%	98%
Pneumonia Care				
Appropriate Initial Antibiotic	137	94%	92%	92%
Blood Culture Timing	160	99%	96%	96%
Influenza Vaccine	128	94%	93%	91%
Initial Antibiotic Timing	182	97%	96%	95%
Pneumococcal Vaccine	155	95%	95%	93%
Smoking Cessation Advice	56	100%	98%	97%
Surgical Care Improvement Project				
Appropriate VTP Within 24 Hours	203	92%	92%	92%
Appropriate Hair Removal	893	99%	100%	99%
Appropriate Beta Blocker Usage	295	94%	94%	93%
Controlled Postoperative Blood Glucose	121	100%	94%	93%
Prophylactic Antibiotic Timing	632	98%	97%	97%
Prophylactic Antibiotic Timing (Outpatient)	262	95%	91%	92%
Prophylactic Antibiotic Selection	636	96%	98%	97%
Prophylactic Antibiotic Select. (Outpatient)	254	96%	94%	94%
Prophylactic Antibiotic Stopped	609	97%	95%	94%
Recommended VTP Ordered	203	97%	94%	94%
Urinary Catheter Removal	57	91%	91%	90%
Children's Asthma Care				
Received Systemic Corticosteroids	-	-	-	100%
Received Home Management Plan	-	-	-	71%
Received Reliever Medication	-	-	-	100%
Use of Medical Imaging				
Combination Abdominal CT Scan	826	0.088	0.164	0.191
Combination Chest CT Scan	420	0.102	0.038	0.054
Follow-up Mammogram/Ultrasound	482	4.8%	8.4%	8.4%
MRI for Low Back Pain	123	26.0%	30.2%	32.7%
Survey of Patients' Hospital Experiences				
Area Around Room 'Always' Quiet at Night	300+	52%	-	58%
Doctors 'Always' Communicated Well	300+	76%	-	80%
Home Recovery Information Given	300+	82%	-	82%
Hospital Given 9 or 10 on 10 Point Scale	300+	70%	-	67%
Meds 'Always' Explained Before Given	300+	61%	-	60%
Nurses 'Always' Communicated Well	300+	77%	-	76%
Pain 'Always' Well Controlled	300+	67%	-	69%
Room and Bathroom 'Always' Clean	300+	71%	-	71%
Timely Help 'Always' Received	300+	65%	-	64%
Would Definitely Recommend Hospital	300+	73%	-	69%

Hillcrest Hospital

6780 Mayfield Road
Mayfield Heights, OH 44124
URL: www.hillcresthospital.org
Type: Acute Care Hospitals
Ownership: Voluntary Non-Profit - Private
Phone: 440-312-4500
Fax: 440-312-6407
Emergency Services: Yes
Beds: 424

Key Personnel:
CEO/President. . . . . Glenn D Levy
Emergency Room . . . . Peg McDonald

Measure	Cases	This Hosp.	State Avg.	U.S. Avg.
Heart Attack Care				
ACE Inhibitor or ARB for LVSD	68	100%	97%	96%
Aspirin at Arrival	250	100%	99%	99%
Aspirin at Discharge	311	100%	99%	98%
Beta Blocker at Discharge	306	100%	99%	98%
Fibrinolytic Medication Timing	0	-	14%	55%
PCI Within 90 Minutes of Arrival	49	92%	92%	90%
Smoking Cessation Advice	81	100%	100%	99%
Chest Pain/Possible Heart Attack Care				
Aspirin at Arrival	48	92%	96%	95%
Median Time to ECG (minutes)	52	0	7	8
Median Time to Transfer (minutes)[5]	0	-	61	61
Fibrinolytic Medication Timing[3]	0	-	47%	54%
Heart Failure Care				
ACE Inhibitor or ARB for LVSD	167	99%	96%	94%
Discharge Instructions	398	86%	91%	88%
Evaluation of LVS Function	598	99%	99%	98%
Smoking Cessation Advice	51	100%	99%	98%
Pneumonia Care				
Appropriate Initial Antibiotic	204	94%	92%	92%
Blood Culture Timing	248	98%	96%	96%
Influenza Vaccine	208	96%	93%	91%
Initial Antibiotic Timing	316	94%	96%	95%
Pneumococcal Vaccine	368	92%	95%	93%
Smoking Cessation Advice	95	100%	98%	97%
Surgical Care Improvement Project				
Appropriate VTP Within 24 Hours[2]	307	95%	92%	92%
Appropriate Hair Removal[2]	837	100%	100%	99%
Appropriate Beta Blocker Usage[2]	297	93%	94%	93%
Controlled Postoperative Blood Glucose[2]	185	96%	94%	93%
Prophylactic Antibiotic Timing[2]	593	97%	97%	97%
Prophylactic Antibiotic Timing (Outpatient)	648	90%	91%	92%
Prophylactic Antibiotic Selection[2]	597	98%	98%	97%
Prophylactic Antibiotic Select. (Outpatient)	619	94%	94%	94%
Prophylactic Antibiotic Stopped[2]	580	92%	95%	94%
Recommended VTP Ordered[2]	307	96%	94%	94%
Urinary Catheter Removal[2]	160	79%	91%	90%
Children's Asthma Care				
Received Systemic Corticosteroids	-	-	-	100%
Received Home Management Plan	-	-	-	71%
Received Reliever Medication	-	-	-	100%
Use of Medical Imaging				
Combination Abdominal CT Scan	1,485	0.403	0.164	0.191
Combination Chest CT Scan	1,074	0.000	0.038	0.054
Follow-up Mammogram/Ultrasound	1,692	10.3%	8.4%	8.4%
MRI for Low Back Pain	214	27.6%	30.2%	32.7%
Survey of Patients' Hospital Experiences				
Area Around Room 'Always' Quiet at Night	300+	39%	-	58%
Doctors 'Always' Communicated Well	300+	73%	-	80%
Home Recovery Information Given	300+	76%	-	82%
Hospital Given 9 or 10 on 10 Point Scale	300+	59%	-	67%
Meds 'Always' Explained Before Given	300+	52%	-	60%
Nurses 'Always' Communicated Well	300+	68%	-	76%
Pain 'Always' Well Controlled	300+	63%	-	69%
Room and Bathroom 'Always' Clean	300+	63%	-	71%
Timely Help 'Always' Received	300+	56%	-	64%
Would Definitely Recommend Hospital	300+	65%	-	69%

Medina Hospital

1000 East Washington Street
Medina, OH 44256
Type: Acute Care Hospitals
Ownership: Voluntary Non-Profit - Private
Phone: 330-725-5600
Fax: 330-722-5812
Emergency Services: Yes
Beds: 118

Key Personnel:
CEO/President. . . . . Gary Hallman
Cardiac Laboratory. . . . . Sampath Ramanazartu
Chief of Medical Staff . . . . Patrick Sziraky
Radiology. . . . . Gregory L Arko
Emergency Room . . . . Kim Bowen

Measure	Cases	This Hosp.	State Avg.	U.S. Avg.
Heart Attack Care				
ACE Inhibitor or ARB for LVSD[1]	5	100%	97%	96%
Aspirin at Arrival	34	85%	99%	99%
Aspirin at Discharge[1]	19	74%	99%	98%
Beta Blocker at Discharge[1]	19	84%	99%	98%
Fibrinolytic Medication Timing	0	-	14%	55%
PCI Within 90 Minutes of Arrival	0	-	92%	90%
Smoking Cessation Advice[1]	4	100%	100%	99%
Chest Pain/Possible Heart Attack Care				
Aspirin at Arrival	123	91%	96%	95%
Median Time to ECG (minutes)	122	2	7	8
Median Time to Transfer (minutes)[3]	25	68	61	61
Fibrinolytic Medication Timing	0	-	47%	54%
Heart Failure Care				
ACE Inhibitor or ARB for LVSD	51	82%	96%	94%
Discharge Instructions	163	87%	91%	88%
Evaluation of LVS Function	225	99%	99%	98%
Smoking Cessation Advice[1]	22	91%	99%	98%
Pneumonia Care				
Appropriate Initial Antibiotic	176	84%	92%	92%
Blood Culture Timing	228	97%	96%	96%
Influenza Vaccine	173	91%	93%	91%
Initial Antibiotic Timing	238	92%	96%	95%
Pneumococcal Vaccine	222	96%	95%	93%
Smoking Cessation Advice	66	94%	98%	97%
Surgical Care Improvement Project				
Appropriate VTP Within 24 Hours[2]	152	88%	92%	92%
Appropriate Hair Removal[2]	426	100%	100%	99%
Appropriate Beta Blocker Usage[2]	127	90%	94%	93%
Controlled Postoperative Blood Glucose[2]	0	-	94%	93%
Prophylactic Antibiotic Timing[2]	303	99%	97%	97%
Prophylactic Antibiotic Timing (Outpatient)	214	90%	91%	92%
Prophylactic Antibiotic Selection[2]	305	100%	98%	97%
Prophylactic Antibiotic Select. (Outpatient)	203	93%	94%	94%
Prophylactic Antibiotic Stopped[2]	299	97%	95%	94%
Recommended VTP Ordered[2]	152	92%	94%	94%
Urinary Catheter Removal	123	79%	91%	90%
Children's Asthma Care				
Received Systemic Corticosteroids	-	-	-	100%
Received Home Management Plan	-	-	-	71%
Received Reliever Medication	-	-	-	100%
Use of Medical Imaging				
Combination Abdominal CT Scan	675	0.310	0.164	0.191
Combination Chest CT Scan	323	0.040	0.038	0.054
Follow-up Mammogram/Ultrasound	1,232	8.0%	8.4%	8.4%
MRI for Low Back Pain	114	28.9%	30.2%	32.7%
Survey of Patients' Hospital Experiences				
Area Around Room 'Always' Quiet at Night	300+	46%	-	58%
Doctors 'Always' Communicated Well	300+	78%	-	80%
Home Recovery Information Given	300+	78%	-	82%
Hospital Given 9 or 10 on 10 Point Scale	300+	60%	-	67%
Meds 'Always' Explained Before Given	300+	56%	-	60%
Nurses 'Always' Communicated Well	300+	72%	-	76%
Pain 'Always' Well Controlled	300+	66%	-	69%
Room and Bathroom 'Always' Clean	300+	66%	-	71%
Timely Help 'Always' Received	300+	59%	-	64%
Would Definitely Recommend Hospital	300+	62%	-	69%

NOTE: Hospital profiles are in alphabetical order by state, then city, then hospital within the city; Rankings exclude hospitals with less than 25 cases except for patient surveys which excludes hospitals with less than 100 cases; (a) 100–299 cases; (1) The number of cases is too small to be sure how well a hospital is performing; (2) The hospital indicated that the data submitted for this measure were based on a sample of cases; (3) Data was collected during a shorter time period (fewer quarters) than the maximum possible time for this measure; (4) Suppressed for one or more quarters by CMS; (5) No data is available from the hospital for this measure; (6) Fewer than 100 patients completed the HCAHPS survey. Use these rates with caution, as the number of surveys may be too low to reliably assess hospital performance; (7) Survey results are based on less than 12 months of data; (8) Survey results are not available for this reporting period; (9) No or very few patients were eligible for the HCAHPS survey. The scores shown, if any, reflect a very small number of surveys; (10) A state average was not calculated because too few hospitals in the state submitted data; (11) There were discrepancies in the data collection process; Please refer to the User's Guide for a full explanation of data.

Kettering Medical Center - Sycamore

4000 Miamisburg-Centerville Road   Phone: 937-384-8776
Miamisburg, OH 45342
URL: www.khnetwork.org/sycamore
Type: Acute Care Hospitals   Emergency Services: Yes
Ownership: Voluntary Non-Profit - Church   Beds: 181
Key Personnel:
CEO . . . . Frank Perez

Measure	Cases	This Hosp.	State Avg.	U.S. Avg.
Heart Attack Care				
ACE Inhibitor or ARB for LVSD[1]	2	100%	97%	96%
Aspirin at Arrival[1]	22	100%	99%	99%
Aspirin at Discharge[1]	15	100%	99%	98%
Beta Blocker at Discharge[1]	15	100%	99%	98%
Fibrinolytic Medication Timing	0	-	14%	55%
PCI Within 90 Minutes of Arrival	0	-	92%	90%
Smoking Cessation Advice[1]	4	100%	100%	99%
Chest Pain/Possible Heart Attack Care				
Aspirin at Arrival	97	99%	96%	95%
Median Time to ECG (minutes)	99	6	7	8
Median Time to Transfer (minutes)	25	44	61	61
Fibrinolytic Medication Timing	0	-	47%	54%
Heart Failure Care				
ACE Inhibitor or ARB for LVSD[1]	24	100%	96%	94%
Discharge Instructions	96	98%	91%	88%
Evaluation of LVS Function	127	100%	99%	98%
Smoking Cessation Advice[1]	15	100%	99%	98%
Pneumonia Care				
Appropriate Initial Antibiotic	114	99%	92%	92%
Blood Culture Timing	171	99%	96%	96%
Influenza Vaccine	143	99%	93%	91%
Initial Antibiotic Timing	165	100%	96%	95%
Pneumococcal Vaccine	173	99%	95%	93%
Smoking Cessation Advice	61	100%	98%	97%
Surgical Care Improvement Project				
Appropriate VTP Within 24 Hours[2]	215	99%	92%	92%
Appropriate Hair Removal[2]	447	100%	100%	99%
Appropriate Beta Blocker Usage[2]	164	99%	94%	93%
Controlled Postoperative Blood Glucose[2]	0	-	94%	93%
Prophylactic Antibiotic Timing[2]	304	99%	97%	97%
Prophylactic Antibiotic Timing (Outpatient)	145	92%	91%	92%
Prophylactic Antibiotic Selection[2]	305	100%	98%	97%
Prophylactic Antibiotic Select. (Outpatient)	169	99%	94%	94%
Prophylactic Antibiotic Stopped[2]	294	99%	95%	94%
Recommended VTP Ordered[2]	215	100%	94%	94%
Urinary Catheter Removal[2]	50	96%	91%	90%
Children's Asthma Care				
Received Systemic Corticosteroids	-	-	-	100%
Received Home Management Plan	-	-	-	71%
Received Reliever Medication	-	-	-	100%
Use of Medical Imaging				
Combination Abdominal CT Scan	922	0.088	0.164	0.191
Combination Chest CT Scan	507	0.014	0.038	0.054
Follow-up Mammogram/Ultrasound[5]	0	-	8.4%	8.4%
MRI for Low Back Pain	99	27.3%	30.2%	32.7%
Survey of Patients' Hospital Experiences				
Area Around Room 'Always' Quiet at Night	300+	48%	-	58%
Doctors 'Always' Communicated Well	300+	74%	-	80%
Home Recovery Information Given	300+	86%	-	82%
Hospital Given 9 or 10 on 10 Point Scale	300+	68%	-	67%
Meds 'Always' Explained Before Given	300+	53%	-	60%
Nurses 'Always' Communicated Well	300+	73%	-	76%
Pain 'Always' Well Controlled	300+	62%	-	69%
Room and Bathroom 'Always' Clean	300+	68%	-	71%
Timely Help 'Always' Received	300+	53%	-	64%
Would Definitely Recommend Hospital	300+	73%	-	69%

Southwest General Health Center

18697 Bagley Road   Phone: 440-816-8000
Middleburg Heights, OH 44130   Fax: 440-816-5299
URL: www.swgeneral.com
Type: Acute Care Hospitals   Emergency Services: Yes
Ownership: Voluntary Non-Profit - Private   Beds: 336
Key Personnel:
CEO/President . . . . Gary Rowe
Chief of Medical Staff . . . . Dr Kulbir Pannu
Coronary Care . . . . Robyn Szeles
Infection Control . . . . Debbie Winar
Pediatric Ambulatory Care . . . . . . Nancy Crow
Pediatric In-Patient Care . . . . Nancy Crow
Quality Assurance . . . . Sue Ferrante
Radiology . . . . Chris Blagojevic

Measure	Cases	This Hosp.	State Avg.	U.S. Avg.
Heart Attack Care				
ACE Inhibitor or ARB for LVSD	73	95%	97%	96%
Aspirin at Arrival	424	98%	99%	99%
Aspirin at Discharge	410	96%	99%	98%
Beta Blocker at Discharge	409	95%	99%	98%
Fibrinolytic Medication Timing	0	-	14%	55%
PCI Within 90 Minutes of Arrival	61	98%	92%	90%
Smoking Cessation Advice	105	98%	100%	99%
Chest Pain/Possible Heart Attack Care				
Aspirin at Arrival	84	89%	96%	95%
Median Time to ECG (minutes)	86	8	7	8
Median Time to Transfer (minutes)[5]	0	-	61	61
Fibrinolytic Medication Timing[3]	0	-	47%	54%
Heart Failure Care				
ACE Inhibitor or ARB for LVSD	141	100%	96%	94%
Discharge Instructions	374	98%	91%	88%
Evaluation of LVS Function	527	100%	99%	98%
Smoking Cessation Advice	52	96%	99%	98%
Pneumonia Care				
Appropriate Initial Antibiotic	255	92%	92%	92%
Blood Culture Timing	456	97%	96%	96%
Influenza Vaccine	236	83%	93%	91%
Initial Antibiotic Timing	427	96%	96%	95%
Pneumococcal Vaccine	358	85%	95%	93%
Smoking Cessation Advice	89	76%	98%	97%
Surgical Care Improvement Project				
Appropriate VTP Within 24 Hours[2]	160	86%	92%	92%
Appropriate Hair Removal[2]	1,092	100%	100%	99%
Appropriate Beta Blocker Usage[2]	429	95%	94%	93%
Controlled Postoperative Blood Glucose[2]	71	97%	94%	93%
Prophylactic Antibiotic Timing[2]	890	97%	97%	97%
Prophylactic Antibiotic Timing (Outpatient)	371	89%	91%	92%
Prophylactic Antibiotic Selection[2]	895	98%	98%	97%
Prophylactic Antibiotic Select. (Outpatient)	349	89%	94%	94%
Prophylactic Antibiotic Stopped[2]	879	95%	95%	94%
Recommended VTP Ordered[2]	160	91%	94%	94%
Urinary Catheter Removal[2]	317	90%	91%	90%
Children's Asthma Care				
Received Systemic Corticosteroids	-	-	-	100%
Received Home Management Plan	-	-	-	71%
Received Reliever Medication	-	-	-	100%
Use of Medical Imaging				
Combination Abdominal CT Scan	1,359	0.057	0.164	0.191
Combination Chest CT Scan	1,261	0.017	0.038	0.054
Follow-up Mammogram/Ultrasound	1,435	5.8%	8.4%	8.4%
MRI for Low Back Pain	110	32.7%	30.2%	32.7%
Survey of Patients' Hospital Experiences				
Area Around Room 'Always' Quiet at Night	300+	45%	-	58%
Doctors 'Always' Communicated Well	300+	78%	-	80%
Home Recovery Information Given	300+	80%	-	82%
Hospital Given 9 or 10 on 10 Point Scale	300+	68%	-	67%
Meds 'Always' Explained Before Given	300+	61%	-	60%
Nurses 'Always' Communicated Well	300+	79%	-	76%
Pain 'Always' Well Controlled	300+	70%	-	69%
Room and Bathroom 'Always' Clean	300+	66%	-	71%
Timely Help 'Always' Received	300+	65%	-	64%
Would Definitely Recommend Hospital	300+	71%	-	69%

Joel Pomerene Memorial Hospital

981 Wooster Road   Phone: 330-674-1015
Millersburg, OH 44654   Fax: 330-674-9707
Type: Acute Care Hospitals   Emergency Services: Yes
Ownership: Government - Local   Beds: 55
Key Personnel:
Chief of Medical Staff . . . . Roy Miller, MD
Operating Room . . . . Brian Black
Quality Assurance . . . . Sandy Cunningham
Radiology . . . . Claudia M Rozuk, MD
Anesthesiology . . . . Rick Koser, MD
Emergency Room . . . . Patrick Dunster, MD

Measure	Cases	This Hosp.	State Avg.	U.S. Avg.
Heart Attack Care				
ACE Inhibitor or ARB for LVSD	0	-	97%	96%
Aspirin at Arrival[1]	2	100%	99%	99%
Aspirin at Discharge[1]	1	100%	99%	98%
Beta Blocker at Discharge[1]	1	100%	99%	98%
Fibrinolytic Medication Timing	0	-	14%	55%
PCI Within 90 Minutes of Arrival	0	-	92%	90%
Smoking Cessation Advice	0	-	100%	99%
Chest Pain/Possible Heart Attack Care				
Aspirin at Arrival	140	96%	96%	95%
Median Time to ECG (minutes)	142	4	7	8
Median Time to Transfer (minutes)[1]	6	28	61	61
Fibrinolytic Medication Timing	0	-	47%	54%
Heart Failure Care				
ACE Inhibitor or ARB for LVSD[1]	9	100%	96%	94%
Discharge Instructions	38	97%	91%	88%
Evaluation of LVS Function	52	98%	99%	98%
Smoking Cessation Advice[1]	8	100%	99%	98%
Pneumonia Care				
Appropriate Initial Antibiotic	29	100%	92%	92%
Blood Culture Timing	78	100%	96%	96%
Influenza Vaccine	41	100%	93%	91%
Initial Antibiotic Timing	64	100%	96%	95%
Pneumococcal Vaccine	56	98%	95%	93%
Smoking Cessation Advice[1]	15	100%	98%	97%
Surgical Care Improvement Project				
Appropriate VTP Within 24 Hours	45	91%	92%	92%
Appropriate Hair Removal	113	100%	100%	99%
Appropriate Beta Blocker Usage	25	84%	94%	93%
Controlled Postoperative Blood Glucose	0	-	94%	93%
Prophylactic Antibiotic Timing	64	98%	97%	97%
Prophylactic Antibiotic Timing (Outpatient)[1]	23	91%	91%	92%
Prophylactic Antibiotic Selection	64	97%	98%	97%
Prophylactic Antibiotic Select. (Outpatient)[1]	22	77%	94%	94%
Prophylactic Antibiotic Stopped	61	93%	95%	94%
Recommended VTP Ordered	45	96%	94%	94%
Urinary Catheter Removal[1]	13	100%	91%	90%
Children's Asthma Care				
Received Systemic Corticosteroids	-	-	-	100%
Received Home Management Plan	-	-	-	71%
Received Reliever Medication	-	-	-	100%
Use of Medical Imaging				
Combination Abdominal CT Scan	109	0.101	0.164	0.191
Combination Chest CT Scan	99	0.000	0.038	0.054
Follow-up Mammogram/Ultrasound	233	8.2%	8.4%	8.4%
MRI for Low Back Pain[1]	25	24.0%	30.2%	32.7%
Survey of Patients' Hospital Experiences				
Area Around Room 'Always' Quiet at Night	300+	59%	-	58%
Doctors 'Always' Communicated Well	300+	80%	-	80%
Home Recovery Information Given	300+	83%	-	82%
Hospital Given 9 or 10 on 10 Point Scale	300+	67%	-	67%
Meds 'Always' Explained Before Given	300+	57%	-	60%
Nurses 'Always' Communicated Well	300+	76%	-	76%
Pain 'Always' Well Controlled	300+	65%	-	69%
Room and Bathroom 'Always' Clean	300+	78%	-	71%
Timely Help 'Always' Received	300+	62%	-	64%
Would Definitely Recommend Hospital	300+	60%	-	69%

Morrow County Hospital

651 West Marion Road
Mount Gilead, OH 43338
URL: www.morrowcountyhospital.com
Type: Critical Access Hospitals
Ownership: Government - Local
Phone: 419-949-3180
Fax: 419-949-3144
Emergency Services: Yes
Beds: 79

Key Personnel:
CEO/President. . . . . Diana D Fisher
Chief of Medical Staff. . . . . J Grant Galbraith, MD
Infection Control. . . . . Amy Bush
Operating Room. . . . . Amy Bush
Quality Assurance . . . . Carol McLaughlin
Radiology. . . . . Earnest Hetrick
Emergency Room . . . . Mark Davis
Intensive Care Unit. . . . . Laura Mahle

Measure	Cases	This Hosp.	State Avg.	U.S. Avg.
Heart Attack Care				
ACE Inhibitor or ARB for LVSD[3]	0	-	97%	96%
Aspirin at Arrival[3]	0	-	99%	99%
Aspirin at Discharge[3]	0	-	99%	98%
Beta Blocker at Discharge[3]	0	-	99%	98%
Fibrinolytic Medication Timing[3]	0	-	14%	55%
PCI Within 90 Minutes of Arrival[3]	0	-	92%	90%
Smoking Cessation Advice[3]	0	-	100%	99%
Chest Pain/Possible Heart Attack Care				
Aspirin at Arrival[3]	60	90%	96%	95%
Median Time to ECG (minutes)[3]	63	13	7	8
Median Time to Transfer (minutes)[1,3]	8	113	61	61
Fibrinolytic Medication Timing[1,3]	1	0%	47%	54%
Heart Failure Care				
ACE Inhibitor or ARB for LVSD[1,2]	7	86%	96%	94%
Discharge Instructions[1,2]	21	86%	91%	88%
Evaluation of LVS Function[2]	37	89%	99%	98%
Smoking Cessation Advice[1,2]	5	80%	99%	98%
Pneumonia Care				
Appropriate Initial Antibiotic	54	96%	92%	92%
Blood Culture Timing	75	96%	96%	96%
Influenza Vaccine	41	66%	93%	91%
Initial Antibiotic Timing	71	99%	96%	95%
Pneumococcal Vaccine	54	80%	95%	93%
Smoking Cessation Advice[1]	24	96%	98%	97%
Surgical Care Improvement Project				
Appropriate VTP Within 24 Hours[1,2]	6	50%	92%	92%
Appropriate Hair Removal[1,2]	19	100%	100%	99%
Appropriate Beta Blocker Usage[5]	0	-	94%	93%
Controlled Postoperative Blood Glucose[2]	0	-	94%	93%
Prophylactic Antibiotic Timing[1,2]	19	100%	97%	97%
Prophylactic Antibiotic Timing (Outpatient)[5]	0	-	91%	92%
Prophylactic Antibiotic Selection[1,2]	19	100%	98%	97%
Prophylactic Antibiotic Select. (Outpatient)[5]	0	-	94%	94%
Prophylactic Antibiotic Stopped[1,2]	19	95%	95%	94%
Recommended VTP Ordered[1,2]	6	50%	94%	94%
Urinary Catheter Removal[1]	8	88%	91%	90%
Children's Asthma Care				
Received Systemic Corticosteroids	-	-	-	100%
Received Home Management Plan	-	-	-	71%
Received Reliever Medication	-	-	-	100%
Use of Medical Imaging				
Combination Abdominal CT Scan	215	0.256	0.164	0.191
Combination Chest CT Scan	126	0.325	0.038	0.054
Follow-up Mammogram/Ultrasound	244	4.9%	8.4%	8.4%
MRI for Low Back Pain[1]	23	47.8%	30.2%	32.7%
Survey of Patients' Hospital Experiences				
Area Around Room 'Always' Quiet at Night	(a)	56%	-	58%
Doctors 'Always' Communicated Well	(a)	84%	-	80%
Home Recovery Information Given	(a)	91%	-	82%
Hospital Given 9 or 10 on 10 Point Scale	(a)	80%	-	67%
Meds 'Always' Explained Before Given	(a)	68%	-	60%
Nurses 'Always' Communicated Well	(a)	84%	-	76%
Pain 'Always' Well Controlled	(a)	65%	-	69%
Room and Bathroom 'Always' Clean	(a)	89%	-	71%
Timely Help 'Always' Received	(a)	77%	-	64%
Would Definitely Recommend Hospital	(a)	79%	-	69%

Knox Community Hospital

1330 Coshocton Road
Mount Vernon, OH 43050
Type: Acute Care Hospitals
Ownership: Voluntary Non-Profit - Other
Phone: 740-393-9000
Fax: 740-399-3130
Emergency Services: Yes
Beds: 115

Key Personnel:
CEO/President. . . . . Bruce White
Chief of Medical Staff. . . . . Judy Schwartz
Coronary Care . . . . Jaya Pala
Quality Assurance . . . . Peggy Penkhus
Radiology. . . . . Henry Windler
Emergency Room . . . . Lee Weiss

Measure	Cases	This Hosp.	State Avg.	U.S. Avg.
Heart Attack Care				
ACE Inhibitor or ARB for LVSD[1]	18	78%	97%	96%
Aspirin at Arrival	51	98%	99%	99%
Aspirin at Discharge	40	98%	99%	98%
Beta Blocker at Discharge	42	95%	99%	98%
Fibrinolytic Medication Timing	0	-	14%	55%
PCI Within 90 Minutes of Arrival	0	-	92%	90%
Smoking Cessation Advice[1]	4	75%	100%	99%
Chest Pain/Possible Heart Attack Care				
Aspirin at Arrival	48	94%	96%	95%
Median Time to ECG (minutes)	50	5	7	8
Median Time to Transfer (minutes)[1,3]	2	128	61	61
Fibrinolytic Medication Timing[3]	0	-	47%	54%
Heart Failure Care				
ACE Inhibitor or ARB for LVSD	55	98%	96%	94%
Discharge Instructions	132	71%	91%	88%
Evaluation of LVS Function	184	98%	99%	98%
Smoking Cessation Advice[1]	18	83%	99%	98%
Pneumonia Care				
Appropriate Initial Antibiotic	107	94%	92%	92%
Blood Culture Timing	153	84%	96%	96%
Influenza Vaccine	87	84%	93%	91%
Initial Antibiotic Timing	114	97%	96%	95%
Pneumococcal Vaccine	122	91%	95%	93%
Smoking Cessation Advice	41	85%	98%	97%
Surgical Care Improvement Project				
Appropriate VTP Within 24 Hours	86	87%	92%	92%
Appropriate Hair Removal	447	100%	100%	99%
Appropriate Beta Blocker Usage	117	89%	94%	93%
Controlled Postoperative Blood Glucose	0	-	94%	93%
Prophylactic Antibiotic Timing	382	98%	97%	97%
Prophylactic Antibiotic Timing (Outpatient)	85	76%	91%	92%
Prophylactic Antibiotic Selection	383	100%	98%	97%
Prophylactic Antibiotic Select. (Outpatient)	73	89%	94%	94%
Prophylactic Antibiotic Stopped	373	95%	95%	94%
Recommended VTP Ordered	86	93%	94%	94%
Urinary Catheter Removal	115	99%	91%	90%
Children's Asthma Care				
Received Systemic Corticosteroids	-	-	-	100%
Received Home Management Plan	-	-	-	71%
Received Reliever Medication	-	-	-	100%
Use of Medical Imaging				
Combination Abdominal CT Scan	611	0.540	0.164	0.191
Combination Chest CT Scan	337	0.101	0.038	0.054
Follow-up Mammogram/Ultrasound	736	5.4%	8.4%	8.4%
MRI for Low Back Pain	113	39.8%	30.2%	32.7%
Survey of Patients' Hospital Experiences				
Area Around Room 'Always' Quiet at Night	300+	53%	-	58%
Doctors 'Always' Communicated Well	300+	76%	-	80%
Home Recovery Information Given	300+	79%	-	82%
Hospital Given 9 or 10 on 10 Point Scale	300+	63%	-	67%
Meds 'Always' Explained Before Given	300+	57%	-	60%
Nurses 'Always' Communicated Well	300+	78%	-	76%
Pain 'Always' Well Controlled	300+	68%	-	69%
Room and Bathroom 'Always' Clean	300+	70%	-	71%
Timely Help 'Always' Received	300+	66%	-	64%
Would Definitely Recommend Hospital	300+	63%	-	69%

Henry County Hospital

1600 East Riverview Avenue
Napoleon, OH 43545
Type: Critical Access Hospitals
Ownership: Voluntary Non-Profit - Private
Phone: 419-592-4015
Fax: 419-592-4017
Emergency Services: Yes
Beds: 52

Key Personnel:
CEO/President. . . . . Kim Bordenkircher
Chief of Medical Staff. . . . . Stephen Knipe
Infection Control. . . . . Carol Borstelman
Quality Assurance . . . . Tara Frease
Radiology. . . . . Edmundo A Somoza
Emergency Room . . . . R Chesler, MD

Measure	Cases	This Hosp.	State Avg.	U.S. Avg.
Heart Attack Care				
ACE Inhibitor or ARB for LVSD[1,3]	1	100%	97%	96%
Aspirin at Arrival[1,3]	1	100%	99%	99%
Aspirin at Discharge[1,3]	1	100%	99%	98%
Beta Blocker at Discharge[1,3]	1	100%	99%	98%
Fibrinolytic Medication Timing[3]	0	-	14%	55%
PCI Within 90 Minutes of Arrival[3]	0	-	92%	90%
Smoking Cessation Advice[3]	0	-	100%	99%
Chest Pain/Possible Heart Attack Care				
Aspirin at Arrival	-	-	96%	95%
Median Time to ECG (minutes)	-	-	7	8
Median Time to Transfer (minutes)	-	-	61	61
Fibrinolytic Medication Timing	-	-	47%	54%
Heart Failure Care				
ACE Inhibitor or ARB for LVSD[1]	7	86%	96%	94%
Discharge Instructions	25	92%	91%	88%
Evaluation of LVS Function	39	92%	99%	98%
Smoking Cessation Advice[1]	2	100%	99%	98%
Pneumonia Care				
Appropriate Initial Antibiotic[1]	23	100%	92%	92%
Blood Culture Timing[1]	20	100%	96%	96%
Influenza Vaccine[1]	19	84%	93%	91%
Initial Antibiotic Timing	30	97%	96%	95%
Pneumococcal Vaccine[1]	24	96%	95%	93%
Smoking Cessation Advice[1]	9	100%	98%	97%
Surgical Care Improvement Project				
Appropriate VTP Within 24 Hours[1]	23	91%	92%	92%
Appropriate Hair Removal	48	100%	100%	99%
Appropriate Beta Blocker Usage[1]	12	83%	94%	93%
Controlled Postoperative Blood Glucose	0	-	94%	93%
Prophylactic Antibiotic Timing	39	97%	97%	97%
Prophylactic Antibiotic Timing (Outpatient)	-	-	91%	92%
Prophylactic Antibiotic Selection	39	97%	98%	97%
Prophylactic Antibiotic Select. (Outpatient)	-	-	94%	94%
Prophylactic Antibiotic Stopped	39	85%	95%	94%
Recommended VTP Ordered[1]	23	91%	94%	94%
Urinary Catheter Removal[1]	14	100%	91%	90%
Children's Asthma Care				
Received Systemic Corticosteroids	-	-	-	100%
Received Home Management Plan	-	-	-	71%
Received Reliever Medication	-	-	-	100%
Use of Medical Imaging				
Combination Abdominal CT Scan	-	-	0.164	0.191
Combination Chest CT Scan	-	-	0.038	0.054
Follow-up Mammogram/Ultrasound	-	-	8.4%	8.4%
MRI for Low Back Pain	-	-	30.2%	32.7%
Survey of Patients' Hospital Experiences				
Area Around Room 'Always' Quiet at Night	(a)	72%	-	58%
Doctors 'Always' Communicated Well	(a)	87%	-	80%
Home Recovery Information Given	(a)	90%	-	82%
Hospital Given 9 or 10 on 10 Point Scale	(a)	84%	-	67%
Meds 'Always' Explained Before Given	(a)	73%	-	60%
Nurses 'Always' Communicated Well	(a)	86%	-	76%
Pain 'Always' Well Controlled	(a)	81%	-	69%
Room and Bathroom 'Always' Clean	(a)	90%	-	71%
Timely Help 'Always' Received	(a)	84%	-	64%
Would Definitely Recommend Hospital	(a)	78%	-	69%

NOTE: Hospital profiles are in alphabetical order by state, then city, then hospital within the city; Rankings exclude hospitals with less than 25 cases except for patient surveys which excludes hospitals with less than 100 cases; (a) 100–299 cases; (1) The number of cases is too small to be sure how well a hospital is performing; (2) The hospital indicated that the data submitted for this measure were based on a sample of cases; (3) Data was collected during a shorter time period (fewer quarters) than the maximum possible time for this measure; (4) Suppressed for one or more quarters by CMS; (5) No data is available from the hospital for this measure; (6) Fewer than 100 patients completed the HCAHPS survey. Use these rates with caution, as the number of surveys may be too low to reliably assess hospital performance; (7) Survey results are based on less than 12 months of data; (8) Survey results are not available for this reporting period; (9) No or very few patients were eligible for the HCAHPS survey. The scores shown, if any, reflect a very small number of surveys; (10) A state average was not calculated because too few hospitals in the state submitted data; (11) There were discrepancies in the data collection process; Please refer to the User's Guide for a full explanation of data.

Doctors Hospital of Nelsonville

1950 Mount St Marys Drive Phone: 740-753-7302
Nelsonville, OH 45764 Fax: 740-753-2197
Type: Critical Access Hospitals Emergency Services: Yes
Ownership: Voluntary Non-Profit - Private Beds: 50

Key Personnel:
CEO/President.............. Steven Swart
Chief of Medical Staff.......... Patricia A Bacon
Coronary Care.............. Susan Bencley
Quality Assurance............ Robert Seamon
Radiology.................. Richard W Adams
Emergency Room............ Diane Viere

Measure	Cases	This Hosp.	State Avg.	U.S. Avg.
Heart Attack Care				
ACE Inhibitor or ARB for LVSD[3]	0	-	97%	96%
Aspirin at Arrival[3]	0	-	99%	99%
Aspirin at Discharge[3]	0	-	99%	98%
Beta Blocker at Discharge[3]	0	-	99%	98%
Fibrinolytic Medication Timing[3]	0	-	14%	55%
PCI Within 90 Minutes of Arrival[3]	0	-	92%	90%
Smoking Cessation Advice[3]	0	-	100%	99%
Chest Pain/Possible Heart Attack Care				
Aspirin at Arrival	-	-	96%	95%
Median Time to ECG (minutes)	-	-	7	8
Median Time to Transfer (minutes)	-	-	61	61
Fibrinolytic Medication Timing	-	-	47%	54%
Heart Failure Care				
ACE Inhibitor or ARB for LVSD[1]	5	100%	96%	94%
Discharge Instructions[1]	15	93%	91%	88%
Evaluation of LVS Function[1]	18	100%	99%	98%
Smoking Cessation Advice[1]	5	100%	99%	98%
Pneumonia Care				
Appropriate Initial Antibiotic	26	100%	92%	92%
Blood Culture Timing[1]	14	100%	96%	96%
Influenza Vaccine[1]	10	100%	93%	91%
Initial Antibiotic Timing	28	100%	96%	95%
Pneumococcal Vaccine[1]	16	100%	95%	93%
Smoking Cessation Advice[1]	11	91%	98%	97%
Surgical Care Improvement Project				
Appropriate VTP Within 24 Hours[1,3]	2	50%	92%	92%
Appropriate Hair Removal[1,3]	3	100%	100%	99%
Appropriate Beta Blocker Usage[1,3]	2	100%	94%	93%
Controlled Postoperative Blood Glucose[3]	0	-	94%	93%
Prophylactic Antibiotic Timing[3]	0	-	97%	97%
Prophylactic Antibiotic Timing (Outpatient)	-	-	91%	92%
Prophylactic Antibiotic Selection[3]	0	-	98%	97%
Prophylactic Antibiotic Select. (Outpatient)	-	-	94%	94%
Prophylactic Antibiotic Stopped[3]	0	-	95%	94%
Recommended VTP Ordered[1,3]	2	50%	94%	94%
Urinary Catheter Removal	0	-	91%	90%
Children's Asthma Care				
Received Systemic Corticosteroids	-	-	-	100%
Received Home Management Plan	-	-	-	71%
Received Reliever Medication	-	-	-	100%
Use of Medical Imaging				
Combination Abdominal CT Scan	-	-	0.164	0.191
Combination Chest CT Scan	-	-	0.038	0.054
Follow-up Mammogram/Ultrasound	-	-	8.4%	8.4%
MRI for Low Back Pain	-	-	30.2%	32.7%
Survey of Patients' Hospital Experiences				
Area Around Room 'Always' Quiet at Night[8]	-	-	-	58%
Doctors 'Always' Communicated Well[8]	-	-	-	80%
Home Recovery Information Given[8]	-	-	-	82%
Hospital Given 9 or 10 on 10 Point Scale[8]	-	-	-	67%
Meds 'Always' Explained Before Given[8]	-	-	-	60%
Nurses 'Always' Communicated Well[8]	-	-	-	76%
Pain 'Always' Well Controlled[8]	-	-	-	69%
Room and Bathroom 'Always' Clean[8]	-	-	-	71%
Timely Help 'Always' Received[8]	-	-	-	64%
Would Definitely Recommend Hospital[8]	-	-	-	69%

Mount Carmel New Albany Surgical Hospital

7333 Smith's Mill Road Phone: 614-546-4533
New Albany, OH 43054
Type: Acute Care Hospitals Emergency Services: No
Ownership: Proprietary

Measure	Cases	This Hosp.	State Avg.	U.S. Avg.
Heart Attack Care				
ACE Inhibitor or ARB for LVSD[5]	0	-	97%	96%
Aspirin at Arrival[5]	0	-	99%	99%
Aspirin at Discharge[5]	0	-	99%	98%
Beta Blocker at Discharge[5]	0	-	99%	98%
Fibrinolytic Medication Timing[5]	0	-	14%	55%
PCI Within 90 Minutes of Arrival[5]	0	-	92%	90%
Smoking Cessation Advice[5]	0	-	100%	99%
Chest Pain/Possible Heart Attack Care				
Aspirin at Arrival[5]	0	-	96%	95%
Median Time to ECG (minutes)[5]	0	-	7	8
Median Time to Transfer (minutes)[5]	0	-	61	61
Fibrinolytic Medication Timing[5]	0	-	47%	54%
Heart Failure Care				
ACE Inhibitor or ARB for LVSD[5]	0	-	96%	94%
Discharge Instructions[5]	0	-	91%	88%
Evaluation of LVS Function[5]	0	-	99%	98%
Smoking Cessation Advice[5]	0	-	99%	98%
Pneumonia Care				
Appropriate Initial Antibiotic[5]	0	-	92%	92%
Blood Culture Timing[5]	0	-	96%	96%
Influenza Vaccine[5]	0	-	93%	91%
Initial Antibiotic Timing[5]	0	-	96%	95%
Pneumococcal Vaccine[5]	0	-	95%	93%
Smoking Cessation Advice[5]	0	-	98%	97%
Surgical Care Improvement Project				
Appropriate VTP Within 24 Hours[2]	31	100%	92%	92%
Appropriate Hair Removal[2]	596	100%	100%	99%
Appropriate Beta Blocker Usage[2]	178	90%	94%	93%
Controlled Postoperative Blood Glucose[2]	0	-	94%	93%
Prophylactic Antibiotic Timing[2]	466	99%	97%	97%
Prophylactic Antibiotic Timing (Outpatient)	503	100%	91%	92%
Prophylactic Antibiotic Selection[2]	469	100%	98%	97%
Prophylactic Antibiotic Select. (Outpatient)	502	100%	94%	94%
Prophylactic Antibiotic Stopped[2]	462	99%	95%	94%
Recommended VTP Ordered[2]	31	100%	94%	94%
Urinary Catheter Removal[2]	183	100%	91%	90%
Children's Asthma Care				
Received Systemic Corticosteroids	-	-	-	100%
Received Home Management Plan	-	-	-	71%
Received Reliever Medication	-	-	-	100%
Use of Medical Imaging				
Combination Abdominal CT Scan[1]	11	0.182	0.164	0.191
Combination Chest CT Scan[1]	6	0.167	0.038	0.054
Follow-up Mammogram/Ultrasound[5]	0	-	8.4%	8.4%
MRI for Low Back Pain	63	22.2%	30.2%	32.7%
Survey of Patients' Hospital Experiences				
Area Around Room 'Always' Quiet at Night	300+	79%	-	58%
Doctors 'Always' Communicated Well	300+	85%	-	80%
Home Recovery Information Given	300+	90%	-	82%
Hospital Given 9 or 10 on 10 Point Scale	300+	86%	-	67%
Meds 'Always' Explained Before Given	300+	70%	-	60%
Nurses 'Always' Communicated Well	300+	84%	-	76%
Pain 'Always' Well Controlled	300+	76%	-	69%
Room and Bathroom 'Always' Clean	300+	81%	-	71%
Timely Help 'Always' Received	300+	72%	-	64%
Would Definitely Recommend Hospital	300+	89%	-	69%

Licking Memorial Hospital

1320 West Main Street Phone: 740-348-4000
Newark, OH 43055 Fax: 740-348-4055
Type: Acute Care Hospitals Emergency Services: Yes
Ownership: Voluntary Non-Profit - Private Beds: 195

Key Personnel:
CEO/President.............. Robert A Montagnese
Chief of Medical Staff.......... Craig Cairns
Operating Room.............. Deborah Young, RN
Quality Assurance............ Paula Alexander
Radiology.................. Subbarao Cherukuri, MD
Emergency Room............ Penny McCort

Measure	Cases	This Hosp.	State Avg.	U.S. Avg.
Heart Attack Care				
ACE Inhibitor or ARB for LVSD[1]	4	100%	97%	96%
Aspirin at Arrival	40	100%	99%	99%
Aspirin at Discharge	33	91%	99%	98%
Beta Blocker at Discharge	32	100%	99%	98%
Fibrinolytic Medication Timing	0	-	14%	55%
PCI Within 90 Minutes of Arrival	0	-	92%	90%
Smoking Cessation Advice[1]	10	100%	100%	99%
Chest Pain/Possible Heart Attack Care				
Aspirin at Arrival	64	95%	96%	95%
Median Time to ECG (minutes)	65	3	7	8
Median Time to Transfer (minutes)[1,3]	3	76	61	61
Fibrinolytic Medication Timing[1]	4	50%	47%	54%
Heart Failure Care				
ACE Inhibitor or ARB for LVSD	73	97%	96%	94%
Discharge Instructions	188	92%	91%	88%
Evaluation of LVS Function	239	99%	99%	98%
Smoking Cessation Advice	58	100%	99%	98%
Pneumonia Care				
Appropriate Initial Antibiotic[2]	166	85%	92%	92%
Blood Culture Timing[2]	207	98%	96%	96%
Influenza Vaccine[2]	174	95%	93%	91%
Initial Antibiotic Timing[2]	229	98%	96%	95%
Pneumococcal Vaccine[2]	180	98%	95%	93%
Smoking Cessation Advice[2]	136	99%	98%	97%
Surgical Care Improvement Project				
Appropriate VTP Within 24 Hours[2]	121	80%	92%	92%
Appropriate Hair Removal[2]	444	99%	100%	99%
Appropriate Beta Blocker Usage[2]	140	90%	94%	93%
Controlled Postoperative Blood Glucose[2]	0	-	94%	93%
Prophylactic Antibiotic Timing[2]	279	95%	97%	97%
Prophylactic Antibiotic Timing (Outpatient)	89	79%	91%	92%
Prophylactic Antibiotic Selection[2]	278	99%	98%	97%
Prophylactic Antibiotic Select. (Outpatient)	105	92%	94%	94%
Prophylactic Antibiotic Stopped[2]	266	97%	95%	94%
Recommended VTP Ordered[2]	121	87%	94%	94%
Urinary Catheter Removal	85	89%	91%	90%
Children's Asthma Care				
Received Systemic Corticosteroids	-	-	-	100%
Received Home Management Plan	-	-	-	71%
Received Reliever Medication	-	-	-	100%
Use of Medical Imaging				
Combination Abdominal CT Scan	1,257	0.019	0.164	0.191
Combination Chest CT Scan	666	0.000	0.038	0.054
Follow-up Mammogram/Ultrasound	2,142	2.4%	8.4%	8.4%
MRI for Low Back Pain	158	32.3%	30.2%	32.7%
Survey of Patients' Hospital Experiences				
Area Around Room 'Always' Quiet at Night	300+	58%	-	58%
Doctors 'Always' Communicated Well	300+	79%	-	80%
Home Recovery Information Given	300+	87%	-	82%
Hospital Given 9 or 10 on 10 Point Scale	300+	66%	-	67%
Meds 'Always' Explained Before Given	300+	59%	-	60%
Nurses 'Always' Communicated Well	300+	77%	-	76%
Pain 'Always' Well Controlled	300+	67%	-	69%
Room and Bathroom 'Always' Clean	300+	74%	-	71%
Timely Help 'Always' Received	300+	66%	-	64%
Would Definitely Recommend Hospital	300+	61%	-	69%

NOTE: Hospital profiles are in alphabetical order by state, then city, then hospital within the city; Rankings exclude hospitals with less than 25 cases except for patient surveys which excludes hospitals with less than 100 cases; (a) 100–299 cases; (1) The number of cases is too small to be sure how well a hospital is performing; (2) The hospital indicated that the data submitted for this measure were based on a sample of cases; (3) Data was collected during a shorter time period (fewer quarters) than the maximum possible time for this measure; (4) Suppressed for one or more quarters by CMS; (5) No data is available from the hospital for this measure; (6) Fewer than 100 patients completed the HCAHPS survey. Use these rates with caution, as the number of surveys may be too low to reliably assess hospital performance; (7) Survey results are based on less than 12 months of data; (8) Survey results are not available for this reporting period; (9) No or very few patients were eligible for the HCAHPS survey. The scores shown, if any, reflect a very small number of surveys; (10) A state average was not calculated because too few hospitals in the state submitted data; (11) There were discrepancies in the data collection process; Please refer to the User's Guide for a full explanation of data.

Medical Center of Newark

2000 Tamarack Road | Phone: 740-522-7800
Newark, OH 43055
URL: www.mcnohio.com
Type: Acute Care Hospitals | Emergency Services: No
Ownership: Voluntary Non-Profit - Private | Beds: 33

Key Personnel:
President . . . . Joe Murrell

Measure	Cases	This Hosp.	State Avg.	U.S. Avg.
Heart Attack Care				
ACE Inhibitor or ARB for LVSD[5]	0	-	97%	96%
Aspirin at Arrival[5]	0	-	99%	99%
Aspirin at Discharge[5]	0	-	99%	98%
Beta Blocker at Discharge[5]	0	-	99%	98%
Fibrinolytic Medication Timing[5]	0	-	14%	55%
PCI Within 90 Minutes of Arrival[5]	0	-	92%	90%
Smoking Cessation Advice[5]	0	-	100%	99%
Chest Pain/Possible Heart Attack Care				
Aspirin at Arrival[5]	0	-	96%	95%
Median Time to ECG (minutes)[5]	0	-	7	8
Median Time to Transfer (minutes)[5]	0	-	61	61
Fibrinolytic Medication Timing[5]	0	-	47%	54%
Heart Failure Care				
ACE Inhibitor or ARB for LVSD[1]	2	50%	96%	94%
Discharge Instructions[1]	8	12%	91%	88%
Evaluation of LVS Function[1]	13	38%	99%	98%
Smoking Cessation Advice[1]	1	0%	99%	98%
Pneumonia Care				
Appropriate Initial Antibiotic	26	81%	92%	92%
Blood Culture Timing	0	-	96%	96%
Influenza Vaccine[1]	11	9%	93%	91%
Initial Antibiotic Timing	27	89%	96%	95%
Pneumococcal Vaccine[1]	20	20%	95%	93%
Smoking Cessation Advice[1]	8	25%	98%	97%
Surgical Care Improvement Project				
Appropriate VTP Within 24 Hours	42	71%	92%	92%
Appropriate Hair Removal	104	98%	100%	99%
Appropriate Beta Blocker Usage[1]	23	61%	94%	93%
Controlled Postoperative Blood Glucose	0	-	94%	93%
Prophylactic Antibiotic Timing	72	90%	97%	97%
Prophylactic Antibiotic Timing (Outpatient)	43	63%	91%	92%
Prophylactic Antibiotic Selection	72	94%	98%	97%
Prophylactic Antibiotic Select. (Outpatient)	27	85%	94%	94%
Prophylactic Antibiotic Stopped	71	76%	95%	94%
Recommended VTP Ordered	43	70%	94%	94%
Urinary Catheter Removal	32	84%	91%	90%
Children's Asthma Care				
Received Systemic Corticosteroids	-	-	-	100%
Received Home Management Plan	-	-	-	71%
Received Reliever Medication	-	-	-	100%
Use of Medical Imaging				
Combination Abdominal CT Scan	276	0.145	0.164	0.191
Combination Chest CT Scan	165	0.000	0.038	0.054
Follow-up Mammogram/Ultrasound[5]	0	-	8.4%	8.4%
MRI for Low Back Pain	116	26.7%	30.2%	32.7%
Survey of Patients' Hospital Experiences				
Area Around Room 'Always' Quiet at Night	300+	73%	-	58%
Doctors 'Always' Communicated Well	300+	81%	-	80%
Home Recovery Information Given	300+	79%	-	82%
Hospital Given 9 or 10 on 10 Point Scale	300+	74%	-	67%
Meds 'Always' Explained Before Given	300+	60%	-	60%
Nurses 'Always' Communicated Well	300+	79%	-	76%
Pain 'Always' Well Controlled	300+	69%	-	69%
Room and Bathroom 'Always' Clean	300+	77%	-	71%
Timely Help 'Always' Received	300+	72%	-	64%
Would Definitely Recommend Hospital	300+	78%	-	69%

Fisher Titus Memorial Hospital

272 Benedict Avenue | Phone: 419-668-8101
Norwalk, OH 44857 | Fax: 419-663-6036
E-mail: jraboin@fimc.com
URL: www.fisher-titus.com
Type: Acute Care Hospitals | Emergency Services: Yes
Ownership: Voluntary Non-Profit - Private | Beds: 112

Key Personnel:
CEO/President. . . . . Patrick J Martin
Chief of Medical Staff . . . . William B Cornell, MD
Infection Control. . . . . Rae Colahan, RN
Operating Room. . . . . Souheil M Al-Jadda, RN
Pediatric Ambulatory Care . . . . . . Glenn Trippe
Pediatric In-Patient Care . . . . Glenn Trippe
Quality Assurance . . . . Cherlie Spragg, RN
Radiology. . . . . William L Ferber, DO

Measure	Cases	This Hosp.	State Avg.	U.S. Avg.
Heart Attack Care				
ACE Inhibitor or ARB for LVSD[1]	4	100%	97%	96%
Aspirin at Arrival[1]	12	100%	99%	99%
Aspirin at Discharge[1]	6	100%	99%	98%
Beta Blocker at Discharge[1]	8	100%	99%	98%
Fibrinolytic Medication Timing	0	-	14%	55%
PCI Within 90 Minutes of Arrival	0	-	92%	90%
Smoking Cessation Advice[1]	1	100%	100%	99%
Chest Pain/Possible Heart Attack Care				
Aspirin at Arrival	74	95%	96%	95%
Median Time to ECG (minutes)	76	6	7	8
Median Time to Transfer (minutes)	25	74	61	61
Fibrinolytic Medication Timing	0	-	47%	54%
Heart Failure Care				
ACE Inhibitor or ARB for LVSD	39	87%	96%	94%
Discharge Instructions	80	90%	91%	88%
Evaluation of LVS Function	109	99%	99%	98%
Smoking Cessation Advice[1]	13	100%	99%	98%
Pneumonia Care				
Appropriate Initial Antibiotic	110	95%	92%	92%
Blood Culture Timing	167	97%	96%	96%
Influenza Vaccine	101	90%	93%	91%
Initial Antibiotic Timing	158	99%	96%	95%
Pneumococcal Vaccine	147	97%	95%	93%
Smoking Cessation Advice	51	98%	98%	97%
Surgical Care Improvement Project				
Appropriate VTP Within 24 Hours	82	82%	92%	92%
Appropriate Hair Removal	298	100%	100%	99%
Appropriate Beta Blocker Usage	121	90%	94%	93%
Controlled Postoperative Blood Glucose	0	-	94%	93%
Prophylactic Antibiotic Timing	211	96%	97%	97%
Prophylactic Antibiotic Timing (Outpatient)	93	86%	91%	92%
Prophylactic Antibiotic Selection	210	98%	98%	97%
Prophylactic Antibiotic Select. (Outpatient)	88	91%	94%	94%
Prophylactic Antibiotic Stopped	200	92%	95%	94%
Recommended VTP Ordered	82	90%	94%	94%
Urinary Catheter Removal	113	95%	91%	90%
Children's Asthma Care				
Received Systemic Corticosteroids	-	-	-	100%
Received Home Management Plan	-	-	-	71%
Received Reliever Medication	-	-	-	100%
Use of Medical Imaging				
Combination Abdominal CT Scan	395	0.106	0.164	0.191
Combination Chest CT Scan	281	0.014	0.038	0.054
Follow-up Mammogram/Ultrasound	661	9.2%	8.4%	8.4%
MRI for Low Back Pain	85	30.6%	30.2%	32.7%
Survey of Patients' Hospital Experiences				
Area Around Room 'Always' Quiet at Night	300+	55%	-	58%
Doctors 'Always' Communicated Well	300+	74%	-	80%
Home Recovery Information Given	300+	86%	-	82%
Hospital Given 9 or 10 on 10 Point Scale	300+	71%	-	67%
Meds 'Always' Explained Before Given	300+	63%	-	60%
Nurses 'Always' Communicated Well	300+	74%	-	76%
Pain 'Always' Well Controlled	300+	68%	-	69%
Room and Bathroom 'Always' Clean	300+	79%	-	71%
Timely Help 'Always' Received	300+	61%	-	64%
Would Definitely Recommend Hospital	300+	74%	-	69%

Allen Community Hospital

200 West Lorain Street | Phone: 440-775-1211
Oberlin, OH 44074 | Fax: 440-775-9153
URL: www.ehealthconnection.com/lorain
Type: Critical Access Hospitals | Emergency Services: Yes
Ownership: Voluntary Non-Profit - Private | Beds: 25

Key Personnel:
CEO/President. . . . . Jerome Morasko
Cardiac Laboratory. . . . . Geeth Mohan, MD
Chief of Medical Staff . . . . Georgia Newman, MD
Infection Control. . . . . Denise Perry
Operating Room. . . . . Nancy Eastaugh
Quality Assurance . . . . Kathy Neptune
Radiology. . . . . Thomas Wu
Patient Relations . . . . Dale Greathouse

Measure	Cases	This Hosp.	State Avg.	U.S. Avg.
Heart Attack Care				
ACE Inhibitor or ARB for LVSD	0	-	97%	96%
Aspirin at Arrival	0	-	99%	99%
Aspirin at Discharge[1]	1	100%	99%	98%
Beta Blocker at Discharge	0	-	99%	98%
Fibrinolytic Medication Timing	0	-	14%	55%
PCI Within 90 Minutes of Arrival	0	-	92%	90%
Smoking Cessation Advice	0	-	100%	99%
Chest Pain/Possible Heart Attack Care				
Aspirin at Arrival	-	-	96%	95%
Median Time to ECG (minutes)	-	-	7	8
Median Time to Transfer (minutes)	-	-	61	61
Fibrinolytic Medication Timing	-	-	47%	54%
Heart Failure Care				
ACE Inhibitor or ARB for LVSD[1]	4	100%	96%	94%
Discharge Instructions[1]	16	100%	91%	88%
Evaluation of LVS Function[1]	18	100%	99%	98%
Smoking Cessation Advice[1]	4	100%	99%	98%
Pneumonia Care				
Appropriate Initial Antibiotic	35	91%	92%	92%
Blood Culture Timing	35	100%	96%	96%
Influenza Vaccine[1]	17	100%	93%	91%
Initial Antibiotic Timing	42	100%	96%	95%
Pneumococcal Vaccine	25	100%	95%	93%
Smoking Cessation Advice[1]	13	100%	98%	97%
Surgical Care Improvement Project				
Appropriate VTP Within 24 Hours[1]	16	100%	92%	92%
Appropriate Hair Removal	118	100%	100%	99%
Appropriate Beta Blocker Usage[5]	0	-	94%	93%
Controlled Postoperative Blood Glucose	0	-	94%	93%
Prophylactic Antibiotic Timing	99	100%	97%	97%
Prophylactic Antibiotic Timing (Outpatient)	-	-	91%	92%
Prophylactic Antibiotic Selection	101	99%	98%	97%
Prophylactic Antibiotic Select. (Outpatient)	-	-	94%	94%
Prophylactic Antibiotic Stopped	99	100%	95%	94%
Recommended VTP Ordered[1]	16	100%	94%	94%
Urinary Catheter Removal	49	100%	91%	90%
Children's Asthma Care				
Received Systemic Corticosteroids	-	-	-	100%
Received Home Management Plan	-	-	-	71%
Received Reliever Medication	-	-	-	100%
Use of Medical Imaging				
Combination Abdominal CT Scan	-	-	0.164	0.191
Combination Chest CT Scan	-	-	0.038	0.054
Follow-up Mammogram/Ultrasound	-	-	8.4%	8.4%
MRI for Low Back Pain	-	-	30.2%	32.7%
Survey of Patients' Hospital Experiences				
Area Around Room 'Always' Quiet at Night	300+	56%	-	58%
Doctors 'Always' Communicated Well	300+	84%	-	80%
Home Recovery Information Given	300+	83%	-	82%
Hospital Given 9 or 10 on 10 Point Scale	300+	75%	-	67%
Meds 'Always' Explained Before Given	300+	66%	-	60%
Nurses 'Always' Communicated Well	300+	82%	-	76%
Pain 'Always' Well Controlled	300+	76%	-	69%
Room and Bathroom 'Always' Clean	300+	79%	-	71%
Timely Help 'Always' Received	300+	71%	-	64%
Would Definitely Recommend Hospital	300+	75%	-	69%

NOTE: Hospital profiles are in alphabetical order by state, then city, then hospital within the city; Rankings exclude hospitals with less than 25 cases except for patient surveys which excludes hospitals with less than 100 cases; (a) 100–299 cases; (1) The number of cases is too small to be sure how well a hospital is performing; (2) The hospital indicated that the data submitted for this measure were based on a sample of cases; (3) Data was collected during a shorter time period (fewer quarters) than the maximum possible time for this measure; (4) Suppressed for one or more quarters by CMS; (5) No data is available from the hospital for this measure; (6) Fewer than 100 patients completed the HCAHPS survey. Use these rates with caution, as the number of surveys may be too low to reliably assess hospital performance; (7) Survey results are based on less than 12 months of data; (8) Survey results are not available for this reporting period; (9) No or very few patients were eligible for the HCAHPS survey. The scores shown, if any, reflect a very small number of surveys; (10) A state average was not calculated because too few hospitals in the state submitted data; (11) There were discrepancies in the data collection process; Please refer to the User's Guide for a full explanation of data.

Bay Park Community Hospital

2801 Bay Park Drive   Phone: 419-690-7700
Oregon, OH 43616   Fax: 419-690-7746
URL: www.promedica.org
Type: Acute Care Hospitals   Emergency Services: Yes
Ownership: Voluntary Non-Profit - Other   Beds: 70
Key Personnel:
CEO/President . . . . William M Mueller, FACHE
Chief of Medical Staff . . . . Bryan Badik

Measure	Cases	This Hosp.	State Avg.	U.S. Avg.
Heart Attack Care				
ACE Inhibitor or ARB for LVSD	0	-	97%	96%
Aspirin at Arrival[1]	20	100%	99%	99%
Aspirin at Discharge[1]	13	100%	99%	98%
Beta Blocker at Discharge[1]	14	100%	99%	98%
Fibrinolytic Medication Timing	0	-	14%	55%
PCI Within 90 Minutes of Arrival	0	-	92%	90%
Smoking Cessation Advice[1]	2	100%	100%	99%
Chest Pain/Possible Heart Attack Care				
Aspirin at Arrival	46	100%	96%	95%
Median Time to ECG (minutes)	46	4	7	8
Median Time to Transfer (minutes)[1,3]	4	70	61	61
Fibrinolytic Medication Timing	0	-	47%	54%
Heart Failure Care				
ACE Inhibitor or ARB for LVSD	25	100%	96%	94%
Discharge Instructions	100	100%	91%	88%
Evaluation of LVS Function	139	100%	99%	98%
Smoking Cessation Advice[1]	21	100%	99%	98%
Pneumonia Care				
Appropriate Initial Antibiotic	94	93%	92%	92%
Blood Culture Timing	121	98%	96%	96%
Influenza Vaccine	91	99%	93%	91%
Initial Antibiotic Timing	138	99%	96%	95%
Pneumococcal Vaccine	123	98%	95%	93%
Smoking Cessation Advice	46	100%	98%	97%
Surgical Care Improvement Project				
Appropriate VTP Within 24 Hours	114	92%	92%	92%
Appropriate Hair Removal	348	100%	100%	99%
Appropriate Beta Blocker Usage	121	94%	94%	93%
Controlled Postoperative Blood Glucose	0	-	94%	93%
Prophylactic Antibiotic Timing	263	97%	97%	97%
Prophylactic Antibiotic Timing (Outpatient)	78	92%	91%	92%
Prophylactic Antibiotic Selection	264	97%	98%	97%
Prophylactic Antibiotic Select. (Outpatient)	73	99%	94%	94%
Prophylactic Antibiotic Stopped	252	94%	95%	94%
Recommended VTP Ordered	114	97%	94%	94%
Urinary Catheter Removal	127	87%	91%	90%
Children's Asthma Care				
Received Systemic Corticosteroids	-	-	-	100%
Received Home Management Plan	-	-	-	71%
Received Reliever Medication	-	-	-	100%
Use of Medical Imaging				
Combination Abdominal CT Scan	246	0.045	0.164	0.191
Combination Chest CT Scan	254	0.004	0.038	0.054
Follow-up Mammogram/Ultrasound	484	8.9%	8.4%	8.4%
MRI for Low Back Pain	58	36.2%	30.2%	32.7%
Survey of Patients' Hospital Experiences				
Area Around Room 'Always' Quiet at Night	300+	60%	-	58%
Doctors 'Always' Communicated Well	300+	73%	-	80%
Home Recovery Information Given	300+	86%	-	82%
Hospital Given 9 or 10 on 10 Point Scale	300+	74%	-	67%
Meds 'Always' Explained Before Given	300+	61%	-	60%
Nurses 'Always' Communicated Well	300+	78%	-	76%
Pain 'Always' Well Controlled	300+	70%	-	69%
Room and Bathroom 'Always' Clean	300+	74%	-	71%
Timely Help 'Always' Received	300+	66%	-	64%
Would Definitely Recommend Hospital	300+	76%	-	69%

Mercy St Charles Hospital

2600 Navarre Avenue   Phone: 419-696-7200
Oregon, OH 43616
URL: www.mercyweb.org/st_charles
Type: Acute Care Hospitals   Emergency Services: Yes
Ownership: Voluntary Non-Profit - Church   Beds: 390
Key Personnel:
President/CEO . . . . Steven L Mickus

Measure	Cases	This Hosp.	State Avg.	U.S. Avg.
Heart Attack Care				
ACE Inhibitor or ARB for LVSD[1]	7	100%	97%	96%
Aspirin at Arrival	40	92%	99%	99%
Aspirin at Discharge[1]	22	91%	99%	98%
Beta Blocker at Discharge[1]	24	88%	99%	98%
Fibrinolytic Medication Timing	0	-	14%	55%
PCI Within 90 Minutes of Arrival	0	-	92%	90%
Smoking Cessation Advice[1]	5	100%	100%	99%
Chest Pain/Possible Heart Attack Care				
Aspirin at Arrival	83	100%	96%	95%
Median Time to ECG (minutes)	85	4	7	8
Median Time to Transfer (minutes)[1]	14	63	61	61
Fibrinolytic Medication Timing[1]	1	0%	47%	54%
Heart Failure Care				
ACE Inhibitor or ARB for LVSD	67	90%	96%	94%
Discharge Instructions	172	98%	91%	88%
Evaluation of LVS Function	217	100%	99%	98%
Smoking Cessation Advice	41	100%	99%	98%
Pneumonia Care				
Appropriate Initial Antibiotic	112	90%	92%	92%
Blood Culture Timing	174	99%	96%	96%
Influenza Vaccine	120	98%	93%	91%
Initial Antibiotic Timing	180	94%	96%	95%
Pneumococcal Vaccine	154	95%	95%	93%
Smoking Cessation Advice	96	99%	98%	97%
Surgical Care Improvement Project				
Appropriate VTP Within 24 Hours[2]	170	89%	92%	92%
Appropriate Hair Removal[2]	489	100%	100%	99%
Appropriate Beta Blocker Usage[2]	171	98%	94%	93%
Controlled Postoperative Blood Glucose[2]	0	-	94%	93%
Prophylactic Antibiotic Timing[2]	331	99%	97%	97%
Prophylactic Antibiotic Timing (Outpatient)	108	93%	91%	92%
Prophylactic Antibiotic Selection[2]	345	99%	98%	97%
Prophylactic Antibiotic Select. (Outpatient)	102	98%	94%	94%
Prophylactic Antibiotic Stopped[2]	322	97%	95%	94%
Recommended VTP Ordered[2]	170	92%	94%	94%
Urinary Catheter Removal[2]	142	98%	91%	90%
Children's Asthma Care				
Received Systemic Corticosteroids	-	-	-	100%
Received Home Management Plan	-	-	-	71%
Received Reliever Medication	-	-	-	100%
Use of Medical Imaging				
Combination Abdominal CT Scan	811	0.022	0.164	0.191
Combination Chest CT Scan	667	0.003	0.038	0.054
Follow-up Mammogram/Ultrasound	1,176	12.0%	8.4%	8.4%
MRI for Low Back Pain	167	28.7%	30.2%	32.7%
Survey of Patients' Hospital Experiences				
Area Around Room 'Always' Quiet at Night	300+	49%	-	58%
Doctors 'Always' Communicated Well	300+	72%	-	80%
Home Recovery Information Given	300+	81%	-	82%
Hospital Given 9 or 10 on 10 Point Scale	300+	71%	-	67%
Meds 'Always' Explained Before Given	300+	55%	-	60%
Nurses 'Always' Communicated Well	300+	78%	-	76%
Pain 'Always' Well Controlled	300+	69%	-	69%
Room and Bathroom 'Always' Clean	300+	80%	-	71%
Timely Help 'Always' Received	300+	67%	-	64%
Would Definitely Recommend Hospital	300+	73%	-	69%

Dunlap Memorial Hospital

832 South Main Street   Phone: 330-682-3010
Orrville, OH 44667   Fax: 330-683-2130
Type: Critical Access Hospitals   Emergency Services: Yes
Ownership: Voluntary Non-Profit - Private   Beds: 51
Key Personnel:
Chief of Medical Staff . . . . Robert H Hutson
Infection Control . . . . Jan Oberly, RN
Operating Room . . . . Laura Brelin
Radiology . . . . Karla Volke
Emergency Room . . . . Michael Corko

Measure	Cases	This Hosp.	State Avg.	U.S. Avg.
Heart Attack Care				
ACE Inhibitor or ARB for LVSD[5]	0	-	97%	96%
Aspirin at Arrival[5]	0	-	99%	99%
Aspirin at Discharge[5]	0	-	99%	98%
Beta Blocker at Discharge[5]	0	-	99%	98%
Fibrinolytic Medication Timing[5]	0	-	14%	55%
PCI Within 90 Minutes of Arrival[5]	0	-	92%	90%
Smoking Cessation Advice[5]	0	-	100%	99%
Chest Pain/Possible Heart Attack Care				
Aspirin at Arrival	-	-	96%	95%
Median Time to ECG (minutes)	-	-	7	8
Median Time to Transfer (minutes)	-	-	61	61
Fibrinolytic Medication Timing	-	-	47%	54%
Heart Failure Care				
ACE Inhibitor or ARB for LVSD[1,3]	4	100%	96%	94%
Discharge Instructions[1,3]	15	47%	91%	88%
Evaluation of LVS Function[1,3]	18	50%	99%	98%
Smoking Cessation Advice[1,3]	1	100%	99%	98%
Pneumonia Care				
Appropriate Initial Antibiotic[1,3]	14	93%	92%	92%
Blood Culture Timing[1,3]	11	100%	96%	96%
Influenza Vaccine[1,3]	10	100%	93%	91%
Initial Antibiotic Timing[1,3]	15	100%	96%	95%
Pneumococcal Vaccine[1,3]	18	94%	95%	93%
Smoking Cessation Advice[1,3]	4	75%	98%	97%
Surgical Care Improvement Project				
Appropriate VTP Within 24 Hours[1,3]	7	57%	92%	92%
Appropriate Hair Removal[1,3]	23	91%	100%	99%
Appropriate Beta Blocker Usage[5]	0	-	94%	93%
Controlled Postoperative Blood Glucose[3]	0	-	94%	93%
Prophylactic Antibiotic Timing[1,3]	10	80%	97%	97%
Prophylactic Antibiotic Timing (Outpatient)	-	-	91%	92%
Prophylactic Antibiotic Selection[1,3]	9	100%	98%	97%
Prophylactic Antibiotic Select. (Outpatient)	-	-	94%	94%
Prophylactic Antibiotic Stopped[1,3]	9	100%	95%	94%
Recommended VTP Ordered[1,3]	7	57%	94%	94%
Urinary Catheter Removal[1]	3	67%	91%	90%
Children's Asthma Care				
Received Systemic Corticosteroids	-	-	-	100%
Received Home Management Plan	-	-	-	71%
Received Reliever Medication	-	-	-	100%
Use of Medical Imaging				
Combination Abdominal CT Scan	-	-	0.164	0.191
Combination Chest CT Scan	-	-	0.038	0.054
Follow-up Mammogram/Ultrasound	-	-	8.4%	8.4%
MRI for Low Back Pain	-	-	30.2%	32.7%
Survey of Patients' Hospital Experiences				
Area Around Room 'Always' Quiet at Night[8]	-	-	-	58%
Doctors 'Always' Communicated Well[8]	-	-	-	80%
Home Recovery Information Given[8]	-	-	-	82%
Hospital Given 9 or 10 on 10 Point Scale[8]	-	-	-	67%
Meds 'Always' Explained Before Given[8]	-	-	-	60%
Nurses 'Always' Communicated Well[8]	-	-	-	76%
Pain 'Always' Well Controlled[8]	-	-	-	69%
Room and Bathroom 'Always' Clean[8]	-	-	-	71%
Timely Help 'Always' Received[8]	-	-	-	64%
Would Definitely Recommend Hospital[8]	-	-	-	69%

NOTE: Hospital profiles are in alphabetical order by state, then city, then hospital within the city; Rankings exclude hospitals with less than 25 cases except for patient surveys which excludes hospitals with less than 100 cases; (a) 100–299 cases; (1) The number of cases is too small to be sure how well a hospital is performing; (2) The hospital indicated that the data submitted for this measure were based on a sample of cases; (3) Data was collected during a shorter time period (fewer quarters) than the maximum possible time for this measure; (4) Suppressed for one or more quarters by CMS; (5) No data is available from the hospital for this measure; (6) Fewer than 100 patients completed the HCAHPS survey. Use these rates with caution, as the number of surveys may be too low to reliably assess hospital performance; (7) Survey results are based on less than 12 months of data; (8) Survey results are not available for this reporting period; (9) No or very few patients were eligible for the HCAHPS survey. The scores shown, if any, reflect a very small number of surveys; (10) A state average was not calculated because too few hospitals in the state submitted data; (11) There were discrepancies in the data collection process; Please refer to the User's Guide for a full explanation of data.

McCullough-Hyde Memorial Hospital

110 North Poplar Street   Phone: 513-523-2111
Oxford, OH 45056
URL: www.mhmh.org
Type: Acute Care Hospitals   Emergency Services: Yes
Ownership: Voluntary Non-Profit - Private   Beds: 60

Key Personnel:
CEO/President . . . . Bryan D Henemann FACHE
Chief of Medical Staff . . . . Bruce Gray MD
Radiology . . . . Lynn Brown

Measure	Cases	This Hosp.	State Avg.	U.S. Avg.
Heart Attack Care				
ACE Inhibitor or ARB for LVSD[1]	1	100%	97%	96%
Aspirin at Arrival[1]	10	100%	99%	99%
Aspirin at Discharge[1]	2	100%	99%	98%
Beta Blocker at Discharge[1]	2	50%	99%	98%
Fibrinolytic Medication Timing	0	-	14%	55%
PCI Within 90 Minutes of Arrival	0	-	92%	90%
Smoking Cessation Advice	0	-	100%	99%
Chest Pain/Possible Heart Attack Care				
Aspirin at Arrival	64	100%	96%	95%
Median Time to ECG (minutes)	65	3	7	8
Median Time to Transfer (minutes)[1]	7	82	61	61
Fibrinolytic Medication Timing[1]	2	100%	47%	54%
Heart Failure Care				
ACE Inhibitor or ARB for LVSD	34	94%	96%	94%
Discharge Instructions	70	99%	91%	88%
Evaluation of LVS Function	113	99%	99%	98%
Smoking Cessation Advice[1]	8	100%	99%	98%
Pneumonia Care				
Appropriate Initial Antibiotic	84	89%	92%	92%
Blood Culture Timing	98	96%	96%	96%
Influenza Vaccine	69	91%	93%	91%
Initial Antibiotic Timing	101	98%	96%	95%
Pneumococcal Vaccine	90	88%	95%	93%
Smoking Cessation Advice	48	96%	98%	97%
Surgical Care Improvement Project				
Appropriate VTP Within 24 Hours	120	97%	92%	92%
Appropriate Hair Removal	265	100%	100%	99%
Appropriate Beta Blocker Usage	54	93%	94%	93%
Controlled Postoperative Blood Glucose	0	-	94%	93%
Prophylactic Antibiotic Timing	207	96%	97%	97%
Prophylactic Antibiotic Timing (Outpatient)	42	95%	91%	92%
Prophylactic Antibiotic Selection	208	98%	98%	97%
Prophylactic Antibiotic Select. (Outpatient)	40	92%	94%	94%
Prophylactic Antibiotic Stopped	204	98%	95%	94%
Recommended VTP Ordered	121	96%	94%	94%
Urinary Catheter Removal	77	92%	91%	90%
Children's Asthma Care				
Received Systemic Corticosteroids	-	-	-	100%
Received Home Management Plan	-	-	-	71%
Received Reliever Medication	-	-	-	100%
Use of Medical Imaging				
Combination Abdominal CT Scan	358	0.059	0.164	0.191
Combination Chest CT Scan	273	0.000	0.038	0.054
Follow-up Mammogram/Ultrasound	421	14.7%	8.4%	8.4%
MRI for Low Back Pain	98	34.7%	30.2%	32.7%
Survey of Patients' Hospital Experiences				
Area Around Room 'Always' Quiet at Night	300+	60%	-	58%
Doctors 'Always' Communicated Well	300+	84%	-	80%
Home Recovery Information Given	300+	82%	-	82%
Hospital Given 9 or 10 on 10 Point Scale	300+	75%	-	67%
Meds 'Always' Explained Before Given	300+	65%	-	60%
Nurses 'Always' Communicated Well	300+	81%	-	76%
Pain 'Always' Well Controlled	300+	75%	-	69%
Room and Bathroom 'Always' Clean	300+	83%	-	71%
Timely Help 'Always' Received	300+	70%	-	64%
Would Definitely Recommend Hospital	300+	76%	-	69%

Parma Community General Hospital

7007 Powers Boulevard   Phone: 440-743-3000
Parma, OH 44129   Fax: 440-743-4092
E-mail: amatyas@parmahospital.org
URL: www.parmahospital.org
Type: Acute Care Hospitals   Emergency Services: Yes
Ownership: Voluntary Non-Profit - Private   Beds: 348

Key Personnel:
CEO/President . . . . Patricia A Ruflin
Chief of Medical Staff . . . . Tom Sidor, MD
Coronary Care . . . . Carolyn Holy, RN
Infection Control . . . . Sara Barwacz
Operating Room . . . . Dale Winsberg
Quality Assurance . . . . Barbara Wojtala, RN
Radiology . . . . Linda Nicklas

Measure	Cases	This Hosp.	State Avg.	U.S. Avg.
Heart Attack Care				
ACE Inhibitor or ARB for LVSD	72	93%	97%	96%
Aspirin at Arrival	303	98%	99%	99%
Aspirin at Discharge	313	99%	99%	98%
Beta Blocker at Discharge	305	96%	99%	98%
Fibrinolytic Medication Timing	0	-	14%	55%
PCI Within 90 Minutes of Arrival	61	93%	92%	90%
Smoking Cessation Advice	85	99%	100%	99%
Chest Pain/Possible Heart Attack Care				
Aspirin at Arrival	43	95%	96%	95%
Median Time to ECG (minutes)	43	2	7	8
Median Time to Transfer (minutes)[5]	0	-	61	61
Fibrinolytic Medication Timing[3]	0	-	47%	54%
Heart Failure Care				
ACE Inhibitor or ARB for LVSD	208	87%	96%	94%
Discharge Instructions	418	81%	91%	88%
Evaluation of LVS Function	625	99%	99%	98%
Smoking Cessation Advice	46	91%	99%	98%
Pneumonia Care				
Appropriate Initial Antibiotic	276	87%	92%	92%
Blood Culture Timing	409	99%	96%	96%
Influenza Vaccine	334	87%	93%	91%
Initial Antibiotic Timing	438	95%	96%	95%
Pneumococcal Vaccine	467	96%	95%	93%
Smoking Cessation Advice	114	99%	98%	97%
Surgical Care Improvement Project				
Appropriate VTP Within 24 Hours	320	92%	92%	92%
Appropriate Hair Removal	1,136	100%	100%	99%
Appropriate Beta Blocker Usage	423	94%	94%	93%
Controlled Postoperative Blood Glucose	97	92%	94%	93%
Prophylactic Antibiotic Timing	819	96%	97%	97%
Prophylactic Antibiotic Timing (Outpatient)	263	74%	91%	92%
Prophylactic Antibiotic Selection	822	99%	98%	97%
Prophylactic Antibiotic Select. (Outpatient)	211	70%	94%	94%
Prophylactic Antibiotic Stopped	790	98%	95%	94%
Recommended VTP Ordered	321	94%	94%	94%
Urinary Catheter Removal	325	97%	91%	90%
Children's Asthma Care				
Received Systemic Corticosteroids	-	-	-	100%
Received Home Management Plan	-	-	-	71%
Received Reliever Medication	-	-	-	100%
Use of Medical Imaging				
Combination Abdominal CT Scan	1,159	0.041	0.164	0.191
Combination Chest CT Scan	859	0.014	0.038	0.054
Follow-up Mammogram/Ultrasound	1,649	5.7%	8.4%	8.4%
MRI for Low Back Pain	115	33.9%	30.2%	32.7%
Survey of Patients' Hospital Experiences				
Area Around Room 'Always' Quiet at Night	300+	45%	-	58%
Doctors 'Always' Communicated Well	300+	77%	-	80%
Home Recovery Information Given	300+	83%	-	82%
Hospital Given 9 or 10 on 10 Point Scale	300+	60%	-	67%
Meds 'Always' Explained Before Given	300+	53%	-	60%
Nurses 'Always' Communicated Well	300+	72%	-	76%
Pain 'Always' Well Controlled	300+	67%	-	69%
Room and Bathroom 'Always' Clean	300+	65%	-	71%
Timely Help 'Always' Received	300+	58%	-	64%
Would Definitely Recommend Hospital	300+	62%	-	69%

Paulding County Hospital

1035 West Wayne St   Phone: 419-399-4080
Paulding, OH 45879   Fax: 419-399-5560
E-mail: pch@bright.net
URL: www.pauldingcountyhospital.com
Type: Critical Access Hospitals   Emergency Services: Yes
Ownership: Government - Local   Beds: 25

Key Personnel:
CEO/President . . . . Gary Adkins
Chief of Medical Staff . . . . Wendell Spangler, MD
Infection Control . . . . Sherry Wilhelm, RN
Operating Room . . . . Brent Savage, MD
Quality Assurance . . . . Mary Hohenberger, RN
Ambulatory Care . . . . Sherry Wilhelm, RN
Emergency Room . . . . Sherry Wilhelm, RN

Measure	Cases	This Hosp.	State Avg.	U.S. Avg.
Heart Attack Care				
ACE Inhibitor or ARB for LVSD[3]	0	-	97%	96%
Aspirin at Arrival[1,3]	2	100%	99%	99%
Aspirin at Discharge[1,3]	1	100%	99%	98%
Beta Blocker at Discharge[1,3]	1	100%	99%	98%
Fibrinolytic Medication Timing[3]	0	-	14%	55%
PCI Within 90 Minutes of Arrival[5]	0	-	92%	90%
Smoking Cessation Advice[3]	0	-	100%	99%
Chest Pain/Possible Heart Attack Care				
Aspirin at Arrival	-	-	96%	95%
Median Time to ECG (minutes)	-	-	7	8
Median Time to Transfer (minutes)	-	-	61	61
Fibrinolytic Medication Timing	-	-	47%	54%
Heart Failure Care				
ACE Inhibitor or ARB for LVSD[1,3]	1	100%	96%	94%
Discharge Instructions[1,3]	12	67%	91%	88%
Evaluation of LVS Function[1,3]	16	94%	99%	98%
Smoking Cessation Advice[1,3]	1	100%	99%	98%
Pneumonia Care				
Appropriate Initial Antibiotic[1,3]	21	95%	92%	92%
Blood Culture Timing[1,3]	14	100%	96%	96%
Influenza Vaccine[1,3]	8	50%	93%	91%
Initial Antibiotic Timing[1,3]	18	100%	96%	95%
Pneumococcal Vaccine[1,3]	16	88%	95%	93%
Smoking Cessation Advice[1,3]	5	100%	98%	97%
Surgical Care Improvement Project				
Appropriate VTP Within 24 Hours[1,2,3]	2	100%	92%	92%
Appropriate Hair Removal[1,2,3]	9	100%	100%	99%
Appropriate Beta Blocker Usage[5]	0	-	94%	93%
Controlled Postoperative Blood Glucose[5]	0	-	94%	93%
Prophylactic Antibiotic Timing[1,2,3]	9	44%	97%	97%
Prophylactic Antibiotic Timing (Outpatient)	-	-	91%	92%
Prophylactic Antibiotic Selection[1,2,3]	9	100%	98%	97%
Prophylactic Antibiotic Select. (Outpatient)	-	-	94%	94%
Prophylactic Antibiotic Stopped[1,2,3]	9	100%	95%	94%
Recommended VTP Ordered[1,2,3]	2	100%	94%	94%
Urinary Catheter Removal[1,2,3]	3	100%	91%	90%
Children's Asthma Care				
Received Systemic Corticosteroids	-	-	-	100%
Received Home Management Plan	-	-	-	71%
Received Reliever Medication	-	-	-	100%
Use of Medical Imaging				
Combination Abdominal CT Scan	-	-	0.164	0.191
Combination Chest CT Scan	-	-	0.038	0.054
Follow-up Mammogram/Ultrasound	-	-	8.4%	8.4%
MRI for Low Back Pain	-	-	30.2%	32.7%
Survey of Patients' Hospital Experiences				
Area Around Room 'Always' Quiet at Night[8]	-	-	-	58%
Doctors 'Always' Communicated Well[8]	-	-	-	80%
Home Recovery Information Given[8]	-	-	-	82%
Hospital Given 9 or 10 on 10 Point Scale[8]	-	-	-	67%
Meds 'Always' Explained Before Given[8]	-	-	-	60%
Nurses 'Always' Communicated Well[8]	-	-	-	76%
Pain 'Always' Well Controlled[8]	-	-	-	69%
Room and Bathroom 'Always' Clean[8]	-	-	-	71%
Timely Help 'Always' Received[8]	-	-	-	64%
Would Definitely Recommend Hospital[8]	-	-	-	69%

NOTE: Hospital profiles are in alphabetical order by state, then city, then hospital within the city; Rankings exclude hospitals with less than 25 cases except for patient surveys which excludes hospitals with less than 100 cases; (a) 100–299 cases; (1) The number of cases is too small to be sure how well a hospital is performing; (2) The hospital indicated that the data submitted for this measure were based on a sample of cases; (3) Data was collected during a shorter time period (fewer quarters) than the maximum possible time for this measure; (4) Suppressed for one or more quarters by CMS; (5) No data is available from the hospital for this measure; (6) Fewer than 100 patients completed the HCAHPS survey. Use these rates with caution, as the number of surveys may be too low to reliably assess hospital performance; (7) Survey results are based on less than 12 months of data; (8) Survey results are not available for this reporting period; (9) No or very few patients were eligible for the HCAHPS survey. The scores shown, if any, reflect a very small number of surveys; (10) A state average was not calculated because too few hospitals in the state submitted data; (11) There were discrepancies in the data collection process; Please refer to the User's Guide for a full explanation of data.

H B Magruder Memorial Hospital

615 Fulton St
Port Clinton, OH 43452
Type: Critical Access Hospitals
Ownership: Voluntary Non-Profit - Private

Phone: 419-734-3131
Fax: 419-734-8217
Emergency Services: Yes
Beds: 98

Key Personnel:
CEO/President . . . . David Norwine, FACHE
Chief of Medical Staff . . . . Barry Cover, MD
Quality Assurance . . . . Michael Long
Radiology . . . . Sina Hazneci
Emergency Room . . . . Julie Norway, RN

Measure	Cases	This Hosp.	State Avg.	U.S. Avg.
Heart Attack Care				
ACE Inhibitor or ARB for LVSD[5]	0	-	97%	96%
Aspirin at Arrival[5]	0	-	99%	99%
Aspirin at Discharge[5]	0	-	99%	98%
Beta Blocker at Discharge[5]	0	-	99%	98%
Fibrinolytic Medication Timing[5]	0	-	14%	55%
PCI Within 90 Minutes of Arrival[5]	0	-	92%	90%
Smoking Cessation Advice[5]	0	-	100%	99%
Chest Pain/Possible Heart Attack Care				
Aspirin at Arrival	-	-	96%	95%
Median Time to ECG (minutes)	-	-	7	8
Median Time to Transfer (minutes)	-	-	61	61
Fibrinolytic Medication Timing	-	-	47%	54%
Heart Failure Care				
ACE Inhibitor or ARB for LVSD[1]	16	88%	96%	94%
Discharge Instructions	26	69%	91%	88%
Evaluation of LVS Function	33	100%	99%	98%
Smoking Cessation Advice[1]	7	57%	99%	98%
Pneumonia Care				
Appropriate Initial Antibiotic	26	81%	92%	92%
Blood Culture Timing	40	92%	96%	96%
Influenza Vaccine	30	97%	93%	91%
Initial Antibiotic Timing	39	100%	96%	95%
Pneumococcal Vaccine	35	91%	95%	93%
Smoking Cessation Advice[1]	10	100%	98%	97%
Surgical Care Improvement Project				
Appropriate VTP Within 24 Hours[1]	24	79%	92%	92%
Appropriate Hair Removal	57	100%	100%	99%
Appropriate Beta Blocker Usage[5]	0	-	94%	93%
Controlled Postoperative Blood Glucose	0	-	94%	93%
Prophylactic Antibiotic Timing	41	98%	97%	97%
Prophylactic Antibiotic Timing (Outpatient)	-	-	91%	92%
Prophylactic Antibiotic Selection	41	100%	98%	97%
Prophylactic Antibiotic Select. (Outpatient)	-	-	94%	94%
Prophylactic Antibiotic Stopped	38	92%	95%	94%
Recommended VTP Ordered[1]	24	79%	94%	94%
Urinary Catheter Removal[1]	10	70%	91%	90%
Children's Asthma Care				
Received Systemic Corticosteroids	-	-	-	100%
Received Home Management Plan	-	-	-	71%
Received Reliever Medication	-	-	-	100%
Use of Medical Imaging				
Combination Abdominal CT Scan	-	-	0.164	0.191
Combination Chest CT Scan	-	-	0.038	0.054
Follow-up Mammogram/Ultrasound	-	-	8.4%	8.4%
MRI for Low Back Pain	-	-	30.2%	32.7%
Survey of Patients' Hospital Experiences				
Area Around Room 'Always' Quiet at Night	300+	66%	-	58%
Doctors 'Always' Communicated Well	300+	90%	-	80%
Home Recovery Information Given	300+	82%	-	82%
Hospital Given 9 or 10 on 10 Point Scale	300+	81%	-	67%
Meds 'Always' Explained Before Given	300+	71%	-	60%
Nurses 'Always' Communicated Well	300+	88%	-	76%
Pain 'Always' Well Controlled	300+	77%	-	69%
Room and Bathroom 'Always' Clean	300+	85%	-	71%
Timely Help 'Always' Received	300+	83%	-	64%
Would Definitely Recommend Hospital	300+	81%	-	69%

Southern Ohio Medical Center

1805 27th Street
Portsmouth, OH 45662
URL: www.somc.org
Type: Acute Care Hospitals
Ownership: Voluntary Non-Profit - Other

Phone: 740-354-5000
Fax: 740-353-5644
Emergency Services: Yes
Beds: 488

Key Personnel:
CEO/President . . . . Randal M Arnett
Chief of Medical Staff . . . . Kendall Stewart
Infection Control . . . . Randy Sosolik, MD
Operating Room . . . . Teresa Lute, RN
Pediatric Ambulatory Care . . . . . . Randy Sosolik, MD
Pediatric In-Patient Care . . . . Randy Sosolik, MD
Quality Assurance . . . . Rebecca Hall
Radiology . . . . George Johnson, MD

Measure	Cases	This Hosp.	State Avg.	U.S. Avg.
Heart Attack Care				
ACE Inhibitor or ARB for LVSD	39	97%	97%	96%
Aspirin at Arrival	203	100%	99%	99%
Aspirin at Discharge	181	100%	99%	98%
Beta Blocker at Discharge	189	100%	99%	98%
Fibrinolytic Medication Timing	0	-	14%	55%
PCI Within 90 Minutes of Arrival	46	98%	92%	90%
Smoking Cessation Advice	86	100%	100%	99%
Chest Pain/Possible Heart Attack Care				
Aspirin at Arrival	104	97%	96%	95%
Median Time to ECG (minutes)	113	5	7	8
Median Time to Transfer (minutes)[5]	0	-	61	61
Fibrinolytic Medication Timing	0	-	47%	54%
Heart Failure Care				
ACE Inhibitor or ARB for LVSD	123	99%	96%	94%
Discharge Instructions	334	100%	91%	88%
Evaluation of LVS Function	419	100%	99%	98%
Smoking Cessation Advice	71	100%	99%	98%
Pneumonia Care				
Appropriate Initial Antibiotic	252	87%	92%	92%
Blood Culture Timing	293	93%	96%	96%
Influenza Vaccine	103	94%	93%	91%
Initial Antibiotic Timing	311	96%	96%	95%
Pneumococcal Vaccine	262	97%	95%	93%
Smoking Cessation Advice	134	99%	98%	97%
Surgical Care Improvement Project				
Appropriate VTP Within 24 Hours	237	93%	92%	92%
Appropriate Hair Removal	867	100%	100%	99%
Appropriate Beta Blocker Usage	275	93%	94%	93%
Controlled Postoperative Blood Glucose	137	95%	94%	93%
Prophylactic Antibiotic Timing	600	96%	97%	97%
Prophylactic Antibiotic Timing (Outpatient)	161	94%	91%	92%
Prophylactic Antibiotic Selection	610	98%	98%	97%
Prophylactic Antibiotic Select. (Outpatient)	155	95%	94%	94%
Prophylactic Antibiotic Stopped	565	96%	95%	94%
Recommended VTP Ordered	238	92%	94%	94%
Urinary Catheter Removal	214	99%	91%	90%
Children's Asthma Care				
Received Systemic Corticosteroids	-	-	-	100%
Received Home Management Plan	-	-	-	71%
Received Reliever Medication	-	-	-	100%
Use of Medical Imaging				
Combination Abdominal CT Scan	1,527	0.547	0.164	0.191
Combination Chest CT Scan	1,359	0.110	0.038	0.054
Follow-up Mammogram/Ultrasound	1,356	5.7%	8.4%	8.4%
MRI for Low Back Pain	257	37.4%	30.2%	32.7%
Survey of Patients' Hospital Experiences				
Area Around Room 'Always' Quiet at Night	300+	65%	-	58%
Doctors 'Always' Communicated Well	300+	83%	-	80%
Home Recovery Information Given	300+	88%	-	82%
Hospital Given 9 or 10 on 10 Point Scale	300+	75%	-	67%
Meds 'Always' Explained Before Given	300+	64%	-	60%
Nurses 'Always' Communicated Well	300+	83%	-	76%
Pain 'Always' Well Controlled	300+	81%	-	69%
Room and Bathroom 'Always' Clean	300+	81%	-	71%
Timely Help 'Always' Received	300+	68%	-	64%
Would Definitely Recommend Hospital	300+	73%	-	69%

Three Gables Surgery Center

5897 Sr 7
Proctorville, OH 45669
URL: www.threegablessurgery.com
Type: Acute Care Hospitals
Ownership: Proprietary

Phone: 740-886-9911
Fax: 740-886-9922
Emergency Services: No

Key Personnel:
CEO/President . . . . John Stone

Measure	Cases	This Hosp.	State Avg.	U.S. Avg.
Heart Attack Care				
ACE Inhibitor or ARB for LVSD[5]	0	-	97%	96%
Aspirin at Arrival[5]	0	-	99%	99%
Aspirin at Discharge[5]	0	-	99%	98%
Beta Blocker at Discharge[5]	0	-	99%	98%
Fibrinolytic Medication Timing[5]	0	-	14%	55%
PCI Within 90 Minutes of Arrival[5]	0	-	92%	90%
Smoking Cessation Advice[5]	0	-	100%	99%
Chest Pain/Possible Heart Attack Care				
Aspirin at Arrival[5]	0	-	96%	95%
Median Time to ECG (minutes)[5]	0	-	7	8
Median Time to Transfer (minutes)[5]	0	-	61	61
Fibrinolytic Medication Timing[5]	0	-	47%	54%
Heart Failure Care				
ACE Inhibitor or ARB for LVSD[5]	0	-	96%	94%
Discharge Instructions[5]	0	-	91%	88%
Evaluation of LVS Function[5]	0	-	99%	98%
Smoking Cessation Advice[5]	0	-	99%	98%
Pneumonia Care				
Appropriate Initial Antibiotic[5]	0	-	92%	92%
Blood Culture Timing[5]	0	-	96%	96%
Influenza Vaccine[5]	0	-	93%	91%
Initial Antibiotic Timing[5]	0	-	96%	95%
Pneumococcal Vaccine[5]	0	-	95%	93%
Smoking Cessation Advice[5]	0	-	98%	97%
Surgical Care Improvement Project				
Appropriate VTP Within 24 Hours[5]	0	-	92%	92%
Appropriate Hair Removal[5]	0	-	100%	99%
Appropriate Beta Blocker Usage[5]	0	-	94%	93%
Controlled Postoperative Blood Glucose[5]	0	-	94%	93%
Prophylactic Antibiotic Timing[5]	0	-	97%	97%
Prophylactic Antibiotic Timing (Outpatient)	57	95%	91%	92%
Prophylactic Antibiotic Selection[5]	0	-	98%	97%
Prophylactic Antibiotic Select. (Outpatient)	54	22%	94%	94%
Prophylactic Antibiotic Stopped[5]	0	-	95%	94%
Recommended VTP Ordered[5]	0	-	94%	94%
Urinary Catheter Removal[5]	0	-	91%	90%
Children's Asthma Care				
Received Systemic Corticosteroids	-	-	-	100%
Received Home Management Plan	-	-	-	71%
Received Reliever Medication	-	-	-	100%
Use of Medical Imaging				
Combination Abdominal CT Scan[1]	1	1.000	0.164	0.191
Combination Chest CT Scan[1]	5	0.200	0.038	0.054
Follow-up Mammogram/Ultrasound[5]	0	-	8.4%	8.4%
MRI for Low Back Pain[1]	10	30.0%	30.2%	32.7%
Survey of Patients' Hospital Experiences				
Area Around Room 'Always' Quiet at Night[6]	<100	87%	-	58%
Doctors 'Always' Communicated Well[6]	<100	89%	-	80%
Home Recovery Information Given[6]	<100	83%	-	82%
Hospital Given 9 or 10 on 10 Point Scale[6]	<100	76%	-	67%
Meds 'Always' Explained Before Given[6]	<100	24%	-	60%
Nurses 'Always' Communicated Well[6]	<100	79%	-	76%
Pain 'Always' Well Controlled[6]	<100	65%	-	69%
Room and Bathroom 'Always' Clean[6]	<100	89%	-	71%
Timely Help 'Always' Received[6]	<100	80%	-	64%
Would Definitely Recommend Hospital[6]	<100	76%	-	69%

Robinson Memorial Hospital

6847 N Chestnut
Ravenna, OH 44266
Phone: 330-297-2300
Fax: 330-297-2949
URL: www.robinsonmemorial.org
Type: Acute Care Hospitals
Emergency Services: Yes
Ownership: Government - Local
Beds: 285

Key Personnel:
CEO/President. . . . . Stephen Colecchi

Measure	Cases	This Hosp.	State Avg.	U.S. Avg.
Heart Attack Care				
ACE Inhibitor or ARB for LVSD[1]	15	93%	97%	96%
Aspirin at Arrival	81	96%	99%	99%
Aspirin at Discharge	55	98%	99%	98%
Beta Blocker at Discharge	56	98%	99%	98%
Fibrinolytic Medication Timing	0	-	14%	55%
PCI Within 90 Minutes of Arrival	0	-	92%	90%
Smoking Cessation Advice[1]	14	100%	100%	99%
Chest Pain/Possible Heart Attack Care				
Aspirin at Arrival	115	98%	96%	95%
Median Time to ECG (minutes)	117	7	7	8
Median Time to Transfer (minutes)	40	50	61	61
Fibrinolytic Medication Timing	0	-	47%	54%
Heart Failure Care				
ACE Inhibitor or ARB for LVSD	78	94%	96%	94%
Discharge Instructions	267	100%	91%	88%
Evaluation of LVS Function	336	99%	99%	98%
Smoking Cessation Advice	52	100%	99%	98%
Pneumonia Care				
Appropriate Initial Antibiotic[2]	134	95%	92%	92%
Blood Culture Timing[2]	157	89%	96%	96%
Influenza Vaccine[2]	77	100%	93%	91%
Initial Antibiotic Timing[2]	193	97%	96%	95%
Pneumococcal Vaccine[2]	151	97%	95%	93%
Smoking Cessation Advice[2]	65	100%	98%	97%
Surgical Care Improvement Project				
Appropriate VTP Within 24 Hours[2]	175	86%	92%	92%
Appropriate Hair Removal[2]	451	100%	100%	99%
Appropriate Beta Blocker Usage[2]	139	96%	94%	93%
Controlled Postoperative Blood Glucose[2]	0	-	94%	93%
Prophylactic Antibiotic Timing[2]	296	99%	97%	97%
Prophylactic Antibiotic Timing (Outpatient)	264	94%	91%	92%
Prophylactic Antibiotic Selection[2]	297	96%	98%	97%
Prophylactic Antibiotic Select. (Outpatient)	273	95%	94%	94%
Prophylactic Antibiotic Stopped[2]	279	95%	95%	94%
Recommended VTP Ordered[2]	176	91%	94%	94%
Urinary Catheter Removal[2]	89	84%	91%	90%
Children's Asthma Care				
Received Systemic Corticosteroids	-	-	-	100%
Received Home Management Plan	-	-	-	71%
Received Reliever Medication	-	-	-	100%
Use of Medical Imaging				
Combination Abdominal CT Scan	751	0.148	0.164	0.191
Combination Chest CT Scan	437	0.000	0.038	0.054
Follow-up Mammogram/Ultrasound	1,328	7.6%	8.4%	8.4%
MRI for Low Back Pain	154	26.6%	30.2%	32.7%
Survey of Patients' Hospital Experiences				
Area Around Room 'Always' Quiet at Night	300+	46%	-	58%
Doctors 'Always' Communicated Well	300+	78%	-	80%
Home Recovery Information Given	300+	78%	-	82%
Hospital Given 9 or 10 on 10 Point Scale	300+	64%	-	67%
Meds 'Always' Explained Before Given	300+	56%	-	60%
Nurses 'Always' Communicated Well	300+	76%	-	76%
Pain 'Always' Well Controlled	300+	69%	-	69%
Room and Bathroom 'Always' Clean	300+	70%	-	71%
Timely Help 'Always' Received	300+	59%	-	64%
Would Definitely Recommend Hospital	300+	62%	-	69%

UHHS Richmond Heights Hospital

27100 Chardon Road
Richmond Heights, OH 44143
Phone: 440-585-6170
Fax: 440-585-6341
URL: www.uhhospitals.org
Type: Acute Care Hospitals
Emergency Services: No
Ownership: Proprietary
Beds: 250

Key Personnel:
CEO/President. . . . . William P Lawrence
Cardiac Laboratory. . . . . Larry Martin
Chief of Medical Staff . . . . David Rapkin, MD
Emergency Room . . . . Robin McCrone
Patient Relations . . . . Paul A Bailey

Measure	Cases	This Hosp.	State Avg.	U.S. Avg.
Heart Attack Care				
ACE Inhibitor or ARB for LVSD[1]	5	100%	97%	96%
Aspirin at Arrival	31	100%	99%	99%
Aspirin at Discharge[1]	22	100%	99%	98%
Beta Blocker at Discharge	25	100%	99%	98%
Fibrinolytic Medication Timing	0	-	14%	55%
PCI Within 90 Minutes of Arrival	0	-	92%	90%
Smoking Cessation Advice[1]	5	100%	100%	99%
Chest Pain/Possible Heart Attack Care				
Aspirin at Arrival	63	94%	96%	95%
Median Time to ECG (minutes)	68	6	7	8
Median Time to Transfer (minutes)[1]	12	45	61	61
Fibrinolytic Medication Timing	0	-	47%	54%
Heart Failure Care				
ACE Inhibitor or ARB for LVSD	63	92%	96%	94%
Discharge Instructions	148	93%	91%	88%
Evaluation of LVS Function	215	100%	99%	98%
Smoking Cessation Advice	26	100%	99%	98%
Pneumonia Care				
Appropriate Initial Antibiotic	46	96%	92%	92%
Blood Culture Timing	73	97%	96%	96%
Influenza Vaccine	60	95%	93%	91%
Initial Antibiotic Timing	89	96%	96%	95%
Pneumococcal Vaccine	79	95%	95%	93%
Smoking Cessation Advice[1]	24	100%	98%	97%
Surgical Care Improvement Project				
Appropriate VTP Within 24 Hours	75	93%	92%	92%
Appropriate Hair Removal	218	100%	100%	99%
Appropriate Beta Blocker Usage	67	97%	94%	93%
Controlled Postoperative Blood Glucose	0	-	94%	93%
Prophylactic Antibiotic Timing	146	98%	97%	97%
Prophylactic Antibiotic Timing (Outpatient)	87	90%	91%	92%
Prophylactic Antibiotic Selection	147	99%	98%	97%
Prophylactic Antibiotic Select. (Outpatient)	90	93%	94%	94%
Prophylactic Antibiotic Stopped	142	96%	95%	94%
Recommended VTP Ordered	75	97%	94%	94%
Urinary Catheter Removal	71	94%	91%	90%
Children's Asthma Care				
Received Systemic Corticosteroids	-	-	-	100%
Received Home Management Plan	-	-	-	71%
Received Reliever Medication	-	-	-	100%
Use of Medical Imaging				
Combination Abdominal CT Scan	272	0.294	0.164	0.191
Combination Chest CT Scan	195	0.087	0.038	0.054
Follow-up Mammogram/Ultrasound	395	3.5%	8.4%	8.4%
MRI for Low Back Pain	64	34.4%	30.2%	32.7%
Survey of Patients' Hospital Experiences				
Area Around Room 'Always' Quiet at Night[11]	300+	43%	-	58%
Doctors 'Always' Communicated Well[11]	300+	70%	-	80%
Home Recovery Information Given[11]	300+	74%	-	82%
Hospital Given 9 or 10 on 10 Point Scale[11]	300+	54%	-	67%
Meds 'Always' Explained Before Given[11]	300+	52%	-	60%
Nurses 'Always' Communicated Well[11]	300+	66%	-	76%
Pain 'Always' Well Controlled[11]	300+	62%	-	69%
Room and Bathroom 'Always' Clean[11]	300+	59%	-	71%
Timely Help 'Always' Received[11]	300+	48%	-	64%
Would Definitely Recommend Hospital[11]	300+	56%	-	69%

Glenbeigh

2863 State Route 45
Rock Creek, OH 44084
Phone: 440-563-3400
Fax: 440-563-9619
E-mail: helen@glenbeigh.com
URL: www.glenbeigh.com
Type: Acute Care Hospitals
Emergency Services: No
Ownership: Voluntary Non-Profit - Private
Beds: 80

Key Personnel:
CEO/President. . . . . Pat Weston-Hall, LISW
Chief of Medical Staff. . . . . Chester J Prusinski, DO
Infection Control. . . . . Renee Enstrom, RN
Quality Assurance . . . . Ruth Leslie, RN

Measure	Cases	This Hosp.	State Avg.	U.S. Avg.
Heart Attack Care				
ACE Inhibitor or ARB for LVSD[5]	0	-	97%	96%
Aspirin at Arrival[5]	0	-	99%	99%
Aspirin at Discharge[5]	0	-	99%	98%
Beta Blocker at Discharge[5]	0	-	99%	98%
Fibrinolytic Medication Timing[5]	0	-	14%	55%
PCI Within 90 Minutes of Arrival[5]	0	-	92%	90%
Smoking Cessation Advice[5]	0	-	100%	99%
Chest Pain/Possible Heart Attack Care				
Aspirin at Arrival[5]	0	-	96%	95%
Median Time to ECG (minutes)[5]	0	-	7	8
Median Time to Transfer (minutes)[5]	0	-	61	61
Fibrinolytic Medication Timing[5]	0	-	47%	54%
Heart Failure Care				
ACE Inhibitor or ARB for LVSD[5]	0	-	96%	94%
Discharge Instructions[5]	0	-	91%	88%
Evaluation of LVS Function[5]	0	-	99%	98%
Smoking Cessation Advice[5]	0	-	99%	98%
Pneumonia Care				
Appropriate Initial Antibiotic[5]	0	-	92%	92%
Blood Culture Timing[5]	0	-	96%	96%
Influenza Vaccine[5]	0	-	93%	91%
Initial Antibiotic Timing[5]	0	-	96%	95%
Pneumococcal Vaccine[5]	0	-	95%	93%
Smoking Cessation Advice[5]	0	-	98%	97%
Surgical Care Improvement Project				
Appropriate VTP Within 24 Hours[5]	0	-	92%	92%
Appropriate Hair Removal[5]	0	-	100%	99%
Appropriate Beta Blocker Usage[5]	0	-	94%	93%
Controlled Postoperative Blood Glucose[5]	0	-	94%	93%
Prophylactic Antibiotic Timing[5]	0	-	97%	97%
Prophylactic Antibiotic Timing (Outpatient)[5]	0	-	91%	92%
Prophylactic Antibiotic Selection[5]	0	-	98%	97%
Prophylactic Antibiotic Select. (Outpatient)[5]	0	-	94%	94%
Prophylactic Antibiotic Stopped[5]	0	-	95%	94%
Recommended VTP Ordered[5]	0	-	94%	94%
Urinary Catheter Removal[5]	0	-	91%	90%
Children's Asthma Care				
Received Systemic Corticosteroids	-	-	-	100%
Received Home Management Plan	-	-	-	71%
Received Reliever Medication	-	-	-	100%
Use of Medical Imaging				
Combination Abdominal CT Scan[5]	0	-	0.164	0.191
Combination Chest CT Scan[5]	0	-	0.038	0.054
Follow-up Mammogram/Ultrasound[5]	0	-	8.4%	8.4%
MRI for Low Back Pain[5]	0	-	30.2%	32.7%
Survey of Patients' Hospital Experiences				
Area Around Room 'Always' Quiet at Night[9]	-	-	-	58%
Doctors 'Always' Communicated Well[9]	-	-	-	80%
Home Recovery Information Given[9]	-	-	-	82%
Hospital Given 9 or 10 on 10 Point Scale[9]	-	-	-	67%
Meds 'Always' Explained Before Given[9]	-	-	-	60%
Nurses 'Always' Communicated Well[9]	-	-	-	76%
Pain 'Always' Well Controlled[9]	-	-	-	69%
Room and Bathroom 'Always' Clean[9]	-	-	-	71%
Timely Help 'Always' Received[9]	-	-	-	64%
Would Definitely Recommend Hospital[9]	-	-	-	69%

NOTE: Hospital profiles are in alphabetical order by state, then city, then hospital within the city; Rankings exclude hospitals with less than 25 cases except for patient surveys which excludes hospitals with less than 100 cases; (a) 100–299 cases; (1) The number of cases is too small to be sure how well a hospital is performing; (2) The hospital indicated that the data submitted for this measure were based on a sample of cases; (3) Data was collected during a shorter time period (fewer quarters) than the maximum possible time for this measure; (4) Suppressed for one or more quarters by CMS; (5) No data is available from the hospital for this measure; (6) Fewer than 100 patients completed the HCAHPS survey. Use these rates with caution, as the number of surveys may be too low to reliably assess hospital performance; (7) Survey results are based on less than 12 months of data; (8) Survey results are not available for this reporting period; (9) No or very few patients were eligible for the HCAHPS survey. The scores shown, if any, reflect a very small number of surveys; (10) A state average was not calculated because too few hospitals in the state submitted data; (11) There were discrepancies in the data collection process; Please refer to the User's Guide for a full explanation of data.

Joint Township District Memorial Hospital

200 Saint Clair Street Phone: 419-394-3335
Saint Marys, OH 45885 Fax: 419-394-8485
Type: Acute Care Hospitals Emergency Services: Yes
Ownership: Voluntary Non-Profit - Private Beds: 130

Key Personnel:
CEO/President. . . . . Kevin Harlan
Chief of Medical Staff . . . . Gregory Bergman
Radiology. . . . . Ashni K Behal

Measure	Cases	This Hosp.	State Avg.	U.S. Avg.
Heart Attack Care				
ACE Inhibitor or ARB for LVSD[1]	11	91%	97%	96%
Aspirin at Arrival[1]	24	96%	99%	99%
Aspirin at Discharge[1]	18	100%	99%	98%
Beta Blocker at Discharge[1]	20	100%	99%	98%
Fibrinolytic Medication Timing	0	-	14%	55%
PCI Within 90 Minutes of Arrival	0	-	92%	90%
Smoking Cessation Advice[1]	1	100%	100%	99%
Chest Pain/Possible Heart Attack Care				
Aspirin at Arrival	136	94%	96%	95%
Median Time to ECG (minutes)	150	7	7	8
Median Time to Transfer (minutes)[1,3]	5	53	61	61
Fibrinolytic Medication Timing	0	-	47%	54%
Heart Failure Care				
ACE Inhibitor or ARB for LVSD	48	94%	96%	94%
Discharge Instructions	99	79%	91%	88%
Evaluation of LVS Function	121	99%	99%	98%
Smoking Cessation Advice[1]	13	100%	99%	98%
Pneumonia Care				
Appropriate Initial Antibiotic	73	100%	92%	92%
Blood Culture Timing	67	96%	96%	96%
Influenza Vaccine	51	88%	93%	91%
Initial Antibiotic Timing	84	100%	96%	95%
Pneumococcal Vaccine	84	95%	95%	93%
Smoking Cessation Advice	25	100%	98%	97%
Surgical Care Improvement Project				
Appropriate VTP Within 24 Hours	68	88%	92%	92%
Appropriate Hair Removal	189	97%	100%	99%
Appropriate Beta Blocker Usage	60	80%	94%	93%
Controlled Postoperative Blood Glucose	0	-	94%	93%
Prophylactic Antibiotic Timing	146	92%	97%	97%
Prophylactic Antibiotic Timing (Outpatient)	31	87%	91%	92%
Prophylactic Antibiotic Selection	146	97%	98%	97%
Prophylactic Antibiotic Select. (Outpatient)	28	96%	94%	94%
Prophylactic Antibiotic Stopped	142	92%	95%	94%
Recommended VTP Ordered	70	89%	94%	94%
Urinary Catheter Removal	40	75%	91%	90%
Children's Asthma Care				
Received Systemic Corticosteroids	-	-	-	100%
Received Home Management Plan	-	-	-	71%
Received Reliever Medication	-	-	-	100%
Use of Medical Imaging				
Combination Abdominal CT Scan	354	0.582	0.164	0.191
Combination Chest CT Scan	257	0.074	0.038	0.054
Follow-up Mammogram/Ultrasound	553	5.4%	8.4%	8.4%
MRI for Low Back Pain	82	24.4%	30.2%	32.7%
Survey of Patients' Hospital Experiences				
Area Around Room 'Always' Quiet at Night	300+	59%	-	58%
Doctors 'Always' Communicated Well	300+	81%	-	80%
Home Recovery Information Given	300+	85%	-	82%
Hospital Given 9 or 10 on 10 Point Scale	300+	72%	-	67%
Meds 'Always' Explained Before Given	300+	68%	-	60%
Nurses 'Always' Communicated Well	300+	81%	-	76%
Pain 'Always' Well Controlled	300+	73%	-	69%
Room and Bathroom 'Always' Clean	300+	82%	-	71%
Timely Help 'Always' Received	300+	72%	-	64%
Would Definitely Recommend Hospital	300+	73%	-	69%

Salem Community Hospital

1995 East State Street Phone: 330-332-1551
Salem, OH 44460 Fax: 330-332-7691
E-mail: info@salemhosp.com
URL: www.salemhosp.com
Type: Acute Care Hospitals Emergency Services: Yes
Ownership: Voluntary Non-Profit - Private Beds: 183

Key Personnel:
CEO/President. . . . . Howard E Rohleder
Chief of Medical Staff . . . . Marc Ucchino
Radiology. . . . . Peter L Apicella
Emergency Room . . . . Lisa A Bennett

Measure	Cases	This Hosp.	State Avg.	U.S. Avg.
Heart Attack Care				
ACE Inhibitor or ARB for LVSD[1]	8	88%	97%	96%
Aspirin at Arrival	44	95%	99%	99%
Aspirin at Discharge[1]	21	86%	99%	98%
Beta Blocker at Discharge[1]	23	87%	99%	98%
Fibrinolytic Medication Timing	0	-	14%	55%
PCI Within 90 Minutes of Arrival	0	-	92%	90%
Smoking Cessation Advice[1]	4	75%	100%	99%
Chest Pain/Possible Heart Attack Care				
Aspirin at Arrival	75	93%	96%	95%
Median Time to ECG (minutes)	75	4	7	8
Median Time to Transfer (minutes)[1]	21	62	61	61
Fibrinolytic Medication Timing[1]	1	100%	47%	54%
Heart Failure Care				
ACE Inhibitor or ARB for LVSD	27	93%	96%	94%
Discharge Instructions	122	91%	91%	88%
Evaluation of LVS Function	165	99%	99%	98%
Smoking Cessation Advice[1]	15	93%	99%	98%
Pneumonia Care				
Appropriate Initial Antibiotic	123	93%	92%	92%
Blood Culture Timing	147	96%	96%	96%
Influenza Vaccine	119	92%	93%	91%
Initial Antibiotic Timing	188	95%	96%	95%
Pneumococcal Vaccine	164	89%	95%	93%
Smoking Cessation Advice	46	80%	98%	97%
Surgical Care Improvement Project				
Appropriate VTP Within 24 Hours[2]	135	76%	92%	92%
Appropriate Hair Removal[2]	351	100%	100%	99%
Appropriate Beta Blocker Usage[2]	100	95%	94%	93%
Controlled Postoperative Blood Glucose[2]	0	-	94%	93%
Prophylactic Antibiotic Timing[2]	228	96%	97%	97%
Prophylactic Antibiotic Timing (Outpatient)	98	83%	91%	92%
Prophylactic Antibiotic Selection[2]	228	95%	98%	97%
Prophylactic Antibiotic Select. (Outpatient)	82	94%	94%	94%
Prophylactic Antibiotic Stopped[2]	222	97%	95%	94%
Recommended VTP Ordered[2]	135	76%	94%	94%
Urinary Catheter Removal[2]	91	84%	91%	90%
Children's Asthma Care				
Received Systemic Corticosteroids	-	-	-	100%
Received Home Management Plan	-	-	-	71%
Received Reliever Medication	-	-	-	100%
Use of Medical Imaging				
Combination Abdominal CT Scan	811	0.102	0.164	0.191
Combination Chest CT Scan	710	0.001	0.038	0.054
Follow-up Mammogram/Ultrasound	1,087	7.9%	8.4%	8.4%
MRI for Low Back Pain	171	29.8%	30.2%	32.7%
Survey of Patients' Hospital Experiences				
Area Around Room 'Always' Quiet at Night	300+	35%	-	58%
Doctors 'Always' Communicated Well	300+	77%	-	80%
Home Recovery Information Given	300+	80%	-	82%
Hospital Given 9 or 10 on 10 Point Scale	300+	57%	-	67%
Meds 'Always' Explained Before Given	300+	53%	-	60%
Nurses 'Always' Communicated Well	300+	69%	-	76%
Pain 'Always' Well Controlled	300+	60%	-	69%
Room and Bathroom 'Always' Clean	300+	63%	-	71%
Timely Help 'Always' Received	300+	58%	-	64%
Would Definitely Recommend Hospital	300+	59%	-	69%

Firelands Regional Medical Center

1111 Hayes Avenue Phone: 419-557-7400
Sandusky, OH 44870 Fax: 419-557-6835
URL: www.firelands.com
Type: Acute Care Hospitals Emergency Services: Yes
Ownership: Voluntary Non-Profit - Private Beds: 325

Key Personnel:
CEO/President. . . . . Charles A Stark FACHE
Chief of Medical Staff . . . . Brenda Violette
Infection Control. . . . . Beth Frank
Operating Room. . . . . Ann Arnold RN
Pediatric Ambulatory Care . . . . . . Ann Arnold RN
Pediatric In-Patient Care . . . . Linda Ricci RN
Quality Assurance . . . . Amy Bohn-Green RN
Radiology. . . . . Mike Vickery

Measure	Cases	This Hosp.	State Avg.	U.S. Avg.
Heart Attack Care				
ACE Inhibitor or ARB for LVSD	28	100%	97%	96%
Aspirin at Arrival	89	100%	99%	99%
Aspirin at Discharge	129	100%	99%	98%
Beta Blocker at Discharge	125	98%	99%	98%
Fibrinolytic Medication Timing	0	-	14%	55%
PCI Within 90 Minutes of Arrival[1]	19	95%	92%	90%
Smoking Cessation Advice	45	100%	100%	99%
Chest Pain/Possible Heart Attack Care				
Aspirin at Arrival[1]	24	96%	96%	95%
Median Time to ECG (minutes)	25	5	7	8
Median Time to Transfer (minutes)[1,3]	9	62	61	61
Fibrinolytic Medication Timing[3]	0	-	47%	54%
Heart Failure Care				
ACE Inhibitor or ARB for LVSD	81	100%	96%	94%
Discharge Instructions	183	96%	91%	88%
Evaluation of LVS Function	255	98%	99%	98%
Smoking Cessation Advice	42	98%	99%	98%
Pneumonia Care				
Appropriate Initial Antibiotic	99	90%	92%	92%
Blood Culture Timing	152	97%	96%	96%
Influenza Vaccine	100	99%	93%	91%
Initial Antibiotic Timing	166	98%	96%	95%
Pneumococcal Vaccine	135	99%	95%	93%
Smoking Cessation Advice	53	98%	98%	97%
Surgical Care Improvement Project				
Appropriate VTP Within 24 Hours[2]	144	90%	92%	92%
Appropriate Hair Removal[2]	517	99%	100%	99%
Appropriate Beta Blocker Usage[2]	184	89%	94%	93%
Controlled Postoperative Blood Glucose[2]	31	90%	94%	93%
Prophylactic Antibiotic Timing[2]	353	95%	97%	97%
Prophylactic Antibiotic Timing (Outpatient)	281	88%	91%	92%
Prophylactic Antibiotic Selection[2]	352	91%	98%	97%
Prophylactic Antibiotic Select. (Outpatient)	254	90%	94%	94%
Prophylactic Antibiotic Stopped[2]	342	93%	95%	94%
Recommended VTP Ordered[2]	145	92%	94%	94%
Urinary Catheter Removal[2]	135	89%	91%	90%
Children's Asthma Care				
Received Systemic Corticosteroids	-	-	-	100%
Received Home Management Plan	-	-	-	71%
Received Reliever Medication	-	-	-	100%
Use of Medical Imaging				
Combination Abdominal CT Scan	851	0.150	0.164	0.191
Combination Chest CT Scan	527	0.032	0.038	0.054
Follow-up Mammogram/Ultrasound	1,373	4.4%	8.4%	8.4%
MRI for Low Back Pain	173	27.2%	30.2%	32.7%
Survey of Patients' Hospital Experiences				
Area Around Room 'Always' Quiet at Night	300+	54%	-	58%
Doctors 'Always' Communicated Well	300+	78%	-	80%
Home Recovery Information Given	300+	83%	-	82%
Hospital Given 9 or 10 on 10 Point Scale	300+	65%	-	67%
Meds 'Always' Explained Before Given	300+	59%	-	60%
Nurses 'Always' Communicated Well	300+	77%	-	76%
Pain 'Always' Well Controlled	300+	67%	-	69%
Room and Bathroom 'Always' Clean	300+	82%	-	71%
Timely Help 'Always' Received	300+	63%	-	64%
Would Definitely Recommend Hospital	300+	69%	-	69%

NOTE: Hospital profiles are in alphabetical order by state, then city, then hospital within the city; Rankings exclude hospitals with less than 25 cases except for patient surveys which excludes hospitals with less than 100 cases; (a) 100–299 cases; (1) The number of cases is too small to be sure how well a hospital is performing; (2) The hospital indicated that the data submitted for this measure were based on a sample of cases; (3) Data was collected during a shorter time period (fewer quarters) than the maximum possible time for this measure; (4) Suppressed for one or more quarters by CMS; (5) No data is available from the hospital for this measure; (6) Fewer than 100 patients completed the HCAHPS survey. Use these rates with caution, as the number of surveys may be too low to reliably assess hospital performance; (7) Survey results are based on less than 12 months of data; (8) Survey results are not available for this reporting period; (9) No or very few patients were eligible for the HCAHPS survey. The scores shown, if any, reflect a very small number of surveys; (10) A state average was not calculated because too few hospitals in the state submitted data; (11) There were discrepancies in the data collection process; Please refer to the User's Guide for a full explanation of data.

Adams County Regional Medical Center

230 Medical Center Drive
Seaman, OH 45679
Phone: 937-386-3400
URL: acrmc.com
Type: Critical Access Hospitals
Emergency Services: Yes
Ownership: Government - Local

Key Personnel:
Imaging . . . . Thomas Heffernan, MD
Surgery . . . . Tyler Campbell, MD
Emergency . . . . Olayinka Aina, MD

Measure	Cases	This Hosp.	State Avg.	U.S. Avg.
Heart Attack Care				
ACE Inhibitor or ARB for LVSD[1,3]	1	100%	97%	96%
Aspirin at Arrival[3]	0	-	99%	99%
Aspirin at Discharge[1,3]	1	100%	99%	98%
Beta Blocker at Discharge[1,3]	1	100%	99%	98%
Fibrinolytic Medication Timing[3]	0	-	14%	55%
PCI Within 90 Minutes of Arrival[3]	0	-	92%	90%
Smoking Cessation Advice[3]	0	-	100%	99%
Chest Pain/Possible Heart Attack Care				
Aspirin at Arrival	-	-	96%	95%
Median Time to ECG (minutes)	-	-	7	8
Median Time to Transfer (minutes)	-	-	61	61
Fibrinolytic Medication Timing	-	-	47%	54%
Heart Failure Care				
ACE Inhibitor or ARB for LVSD[1]	6	83%	96%	94%
Discharge Instructions[1]	19	53%	91%	88%
Evaluation of LVS Function	26	100%	99%	98%
Smoking Cessation Advice[1]	8	100%	99%	98%
Pneumonia Care				
Appropriate Initial Antibiotic	58	91%	92%	92%
Blood Culture Timing	74	96%	96%	96%
Influenza Vaccine	42	98%	93%	91%
Initial Antibiotic Timing	53	98%	96%	95%
Pneumococcal Vaccine	48	100%	95%	93%
Smoking Cessation Advice	33	100%	98%	97%
Surgical Care Improvement Project				
Appropriate VTP Within 24 Hours[1,3]	1	100%	92%	92%
Appropriate Hair Removal[1,3]	3	100%	100%	99%
Appropriate Beta Blocker Usage[5]	0	-	94%	93%
Controlled Postoperative Blood Glucose[3]	0	-	94%	93%
Prophylactic Antibiotic Timing[1,3]	3	67%	97%	97%
Prophylactic Antibiotic Timing (Outpatient)	-	-	91%	92%
Prophylactic Antibiotic Selection[1,3]	3	67%	98%	97%
Prophylactic Antibiotic Select. (Outpatient)	-	-	94%	94%
Prophylactic Antibiotic Stopped[1,3]	3	67%	95%	94%
Recommended VTP Ordered[1,3]	1	100%	94%	94%
Urinary Catheter Removal[5]	0	-	91%	90%
Children's Asthma Care				
Received Systemic Corticosteroids	-	-	-	100%
Received Home Management Plan	-	-	-	71%
Received Reliever Medication	-	-	-	100%
Use of Medical Imaging				
Combination Abdominal CT Scan	-	-	0.164	0.191
Combination Chest CT Scan	-	-	0.038	0.054
Follow-up Mammogram/Ultrasound	-	-	8.4%	8.4%
MRI for Low Back Pain	-	-	30.2%	32.7%
Survey of Patients' Hospital Experiences				
Area Around Room 'Always' Quiet at Night[8]	-	-	-	58%
Doctors 'Always' Communicated Well[8]	-	-	-	80%
Home Recovery Information Given[8]	-	-	-	82%
Hospital Given 9 or 10 on 10 Point Scale[8]	-	-	-	67%
Meds 'Always' Explained Before Given[8]	-	-	-	60%
Nurses 'Always' Communicated Well[8]	-	-	-	76%
Pain 'Always' Well Controlled[8]	-	-	-	69%
Room and Bathroom 'Always' Clean[8]	-	-	-	71%
Timely Help 'Always' Received[8]	-	-	-	64%
Would Definitely Recommend Hospital[8]	-	-	-	69%

Medcentral Health System Shelby Hospital

199 West Main Street
Shelby, OH 44875
Phone: 419-342-5015
Fax: 419-521-7960
Type: Critical Access Hospitals
Emergency Services: Yes
Ownership: Voluntary Non-Profit - Private
Beds: 68

Key Personnel:
CEO/President. . . . . Jim Meyer
Radiology. . . . . Paul Buehrer

Measure	Cases	This Hosp.	State Avg.	U.S. Avg.
Heart Attack Care				
ACE Inhibitor or ARB for LVSD[5]	0	-	97%	96%
Aspirin at Arrival[5]	0	-	99%	99%
Aspirin at Discharge[5]	0	-	99%	98%
Beta Blocker at Discharge[5]	0	-	99%	98%
Fibrinolytic Medication Timing[5]	0	-	14%	55%
PCI Within 90 Minutes of Arrival[5]	0	-	92%	90%
Smoking Cessation Advice[5]	0	-	100%	99%
Chest Pain/Possible Heart Attack Care				
Aspirin at Arrival	-	-	96%	95%
Median Time to ECG (minutes)	-	-	7	8
Median Time to Transfer (minutes)	-	-	61	61
Fibrinolytic Medication Timing	-	-	47%	54%
Heart Failure Care				
ACE Inhibitor or ARB for LVSD[5]	0	-	96%	94%
Discharge Instructions[5]	0	-	91%	88%
Evaluation of LVS Function[5]	0	-	99%	98%
Smoking Cessation Advice[5]	0	-	99%	98%
Pneumonia Care				
Appropriate Initial Antibiotic[5]	0	-	92%	92%
Blood Culture Timing[5]	0	-	96%	96%
Influenza Vaccine[5]	0	-	93%	91%
Initial Antibiotic Timing[5]	0	-	96%	95%
Pneumococcal Vaccine[5]	0	-	95%	93%
Smoking Cessation Advice[5]	0	-	98%	97%
Surgical Care Improvement Project				
Appropriate VTP Within 24 Hours[5]	0	-	92%	92%
Appropriate Hair Removal[5]	0	-	100%	99%
Appropriate Beta Blocker Usage[5]	0	-	94%	93%
Controlled Postoperative Blood Glucose[5]	0	-	94%	93%
Prophylactic Antibiotic Timing[5]	0	-	97%	97%
Prophylactic Antibiotic Timing (Outpatient)	-	-	91%	92%
Prophylactic Antibiotic Selection[5]	0	-	98%	97%
Prophylactic Antibiotic Select. (Outpatient)			94%	94%
Prophylactic Antibiotic Stopped[5]	0	-	95%	94%
Recommended VTP Ordered[5]	0	-	94%	94%
Urinary Catheter Removal[5]	0	-	91%	90%
Children's Asthma Care				
Received Systemic Corticosteroids	-	-	-	100%
Received Home Management Plan	-	-	-	71%
Received Reliever Medication	-	-	-	100%
Use of Medical Imaging				
Combination Abdominal CT Scan	-	-	0.164	0.191
Combination Chest CT Scan	-	-	0.038	0.054
Follow-up Mammogram/Ultrasound	-	-	8.4%	8.4%
MRI for Low Back Pain	-	-	30.2%	32.7%
Survey of Patients' Hospital Experiences				
Area Around Room 'Always' Quiet at Night	300+	53%	-	58%
Doctors 'Always' Communicated Well	300+	82%	-	80%
Home Recovery Information Given	300+	88%	-	82%
Hospital Given 9 or 10 on 10 Point Scale	300+	73%	-	67%
Meds 'Always' Explained Before Given	300+	64%	-	60%
Nurses 'Always' Communicated Well	300+	84%	-	76%
Pain 'Always' Well Controlled	300+	73%	-	69%
Room and Bathroom 'Always' Clean	300+	78%	-	71%
Timely Help 'Always' Received	300+	77%	-	64%
Would Definitely Recommend Hospital	300+	78%	-	69%

Wilson Memorial Hospital

915 West Michigan Street
Sidney, OH 45365
Phone: 937-498-5418
Fax: 937-497-8251
URL: www.wilsonhospital.com
Type: Acute Care Hospitals
Emergency Services: Yes
Ownership: Voluntary Non-Profit - Other
Beds: 112

Key Personnel:
CEO/President. . . . . Tom Boecker
Chief of Medical Staff. . . . . Robert McDevitt
Infection Control. . . . . Linda Smith, RN
Quality Assurance . . . . Elizabeth Custis
Radiology. . . . . C H Bahng
Emergency Room . . . . Fred Haussman
Intensive Care Unit. . . . . Linda Maurer
Patient Relations . . . . Connie Burgess

Measure	Cases	This Hosp.	State Avg.	U.S. Avg.
Heart Attack Care				
ACE Inhibitor or ARB for LVSD[1]	1	0%	97%	96%
Aspirin at Arrival[1]	7	100%	99%	99%
Aspirin at Discharge[1]	4	75%	99%	98%
Beta Blocker at Discharge[1]	4	75%	99%	98%
Fibrinolytic Medication Timing	0	-	14%	55%
PCI Within 90 Minutes of Arrival	0	-	92%	90%
Smoking Cessation Advice[1]	1	100%	100%	99%
Chest Pain/Possible Heart Attack Care				
Aspirin at Arrival	99	99%	96%	95%
Median Time to ECG (minutes)	100	12	7	8
Median Time to Transfer (minutes)[1,3]	4	90	61	61
Fibrinolytic Medication Timing[1]	13	46%	47%	54%
Heart Failure Care				
ACE Inhibitor or ARB for LVSD[1]	21	81%	96%	94%
Discharge Instructions	41	88%	91%	88%
Evaluation of LVS Function	73	95%	99%	98%
Smoking Cessation Advice[1]	7	100%	99%	98%
Pneumonia Care				
Appropriate Initial Antibiotic	78	82%	92%	92%
Blood Culture Timing	124	99%	96%	96%
Influenza Vaccine	79	94%	93%	91%
Initial Antibiotic Timing	93	97%	96%	95%
Pneumococcal Vaccine	108	96%	95%	93%
Smoking Cessation Advice[1]	22	77%	98%	97%
Surgical Care Improvement Project				
Appropriate VTP Within 24 Hours	54	96%	92%	92%
Appropriate Hair Removal	165	100%	100%	99%
Appropriate Beta Blocker Usage	47	89%	94%	93%
Controlled Postoperative Blood Glucose	0	-	94%	93%
Prophylactic Antibiotic Timing	110	95%	97%	97%
Prophylactic Antibiotic Timing (Outpatient)	115	91%	91%	92%
Prophylactic Antibiotic Selection	108	97%	98%	97%
Prophylactic Antibiotic Select. (Outpatient)	113	89%	94%	94%
Prophylactic Antibiotic Stopped	108	87%	95%	94%
Recommended VTP Ordered	54	98%	94%	94%
Urinary Catheter Removal	25	96%	91%	90%
Children's Asthma Care				
Received Systemic Corticosteroids	-	-	-	100%
Received Home Management Plan	-	-	-	71%
Received Reliever Medication	-	-	-	100%
Use of Medical Imaging				
Combination Abdominal CT Scan	364	0.236	0.164	0.191
Combination Chest CT Scan	298	0.158	0.038	0.054
Follow-up Mammogram/Ultrasound	645	13.5%	8.4%	8.4%
MRI for Low Back Pain	80	32.5%	30.2%	32.7%
Survey of Patients' Hospital Experiences				
Area Around Room 'Always' Quiet at Night	300+	60%	-	58%
Doctors 'Always' Communicated Well	300+	84%	-	80%
Home Recovery Information Given	300+	81%	-	82%
Hospital Given 9 or 10 on 10 Point Scale	300+	69%	-	67%
Meds 'Always' Explained Before Given	300+	62%	-	60%
Nurses 'Always' Communicated Well	300+	80%	-	76%
Pain 'Always' Well Controlled	300+	70%	-	69%
Room and Bathroom 'Always' Clean	300+	80%	-	71%
Timely Help 'Always' Received	300+	68%	-	64%
Would Definitely Recommend Hospital	300+	64%	-	69%

NOTE: Hospital profiles are in alphabetical order by state, then city, then hospital within the city; Rankings exclude hospitals with less than 25 cases except for patient surveys which excludes hospitals with less than 100 cases; (a) 100–299 cases; (1) The number of cases is too small to be sure how well a hospital is performing; (2) The hospital indicated that the data submitted for this measure were based on a sample of cases; (3) Data was collected during a shorter time period (fewer quarters) than the maximum possible time for this measure; (4) Suppressed for one or more quarters by CMS; (5) No data is available from the hospital for this measure; (6) Fewer than 100 patients completed the HCAHPS survey. Use these rates with caution, as the number of surveys may be too low to reliably assess hospital performance; (7) Survey results are based on less than 12 months of data; (8) Survey results are not available for this reporting period; (9) No or very few patients were eligible for the HCAHPS survey. The scores shown, if any, reflect a very small number of surveys; (10) A state average was not calculated because too few hospitals in the state submitted data; (11) There were discrepancies in the data collection process; Please refer to the User's Guide for a full explanation of data.

Ohio Valley Medical Center

100 West Main Street
Springfield, OH 45502   Phone: 937-521-3900
URL: www.ovmc-online.com
Type: Acute Care Hospitals   Emergency Services: No
Ownership: Voluntary Non-Profit - Private

Measure	Cases	This Hosp.	State Avg.	U.S. Avg.
Heart Attack Care				
ACE Inhibitor or ARB for LVSD[5]	0	-	97%	96%
Aspirin at Arrival[5]	0	-	99%	99%
Aspirin at Discharge[5]	0	-	99%	98%
Beta Blocker at Discharge[5]	0	-	99%	98%
Fibrinolytic Medication Timing[5]	0	-	14%	55%
PCI Within 90 Minutes of Arrival[5]	0	-	92%	90%
Smoking Cessation Advice[5]	0	-	100%	99%
Chest Pain/Possible Heart Attack Care				
Aspirin at Arrival[5]	0	-	96%	95%
Median Time to ECG (minutes)[5]	0	-	7	8
Median Time to Transfer (minutes)[5]	0	-	61	61
Fibrinolytic Medication Timing[5]	0	-	47%	54%
Heart Failure Care				
ACE Inhibitor or ARB for LVSD[5]	0	-	96%	94%
Discharge Instructions[5]	0	-	91%	88%
Evaluation of LVS Function[5]	0	-	99%	98%
Smoking Cessation Advice[5]	0	-	99%	98%
Pneumonia Care				
Appropriate Initial Antibiotic[5]	0	-	92%	92%
Blood Culture Timing[5]	0	-	96%	96%
Influenza Vaccine[5]	0	-	93%	91%
Initial Antibiotic Timing[5]	0	-	96%	95%
Pneumococcal Vaccine[5]	0	-	95%	93%
Smoking Cessation Advice[5]	0	-	98%	97%
Surgical Care Improvement Project				
Appropriate VTP Within 24 Hours[3]	26	100%	92%	92%
Appropriate Hair Removal[3]	230	100%	100%	99%
Appropriate Beta Blocker Usage[3]	43	81%	94%	93%
Controlled Postoperative Blood Glucose[3]	0	-	94%	93%
Prophylactic Antibiotic Timing[3]	202	100%	97%	97%
Prophylactic Antibiotic Timing (Outpatient)[3]	31	94%	91%	92%
Prophylactic Antibiotic Selection[3]	202	99%	98%	97%
Prophylactic Antibiotic Select. (Outpatient)[3]	31	97%	94%	94%
Prophylactic Antibiotic Stopped[3]	200	99%	95%	94%
Recommended VTP Ordered[3]	26	100%	94%	94%
Urinary Catheter Removal	68	91%	91%	90%
Children's Asthma Care				
Received Systemic Corticosteroids	-	-	-	100%
Received Home Management Plan	-	-	-	71%
Received Reliever Medication	-	-	-	100%
Use of Medical Imaging				
Combination Abdominal CT Scan[5]	0	-	0.164	0.191
Combination Chest CT Scan[5]	0	-	0.038	0.054
Follow-up Mammogram/Ultrasound[5]	0	-	8.4%	8.4%
MRI for Low Back Pain[5]	0	-	30.2%	32.7%
Survey of Patients' Hospital Experiences				
Area Around Room 'Always' Quiet at Night[8]	-	-	-	58%
Doctors 'Always' Communicated Well[8]	-	-	-	80%
Home Recovery Information Given[8]	-	-	-	82%
Hospital Given 9 or 10 on 10 Point Scale[8]	-	-	-	67%
Meds 'Always' Explained Before Given[8]	-	-	-	60%
Nurses 'Always' Communicated Well[8]	-	-	-	76%
Pain 'Always' Well Controlled[8]	-	-	-	69%
Room and Bathroom 'Always' Clean[8]	-	-	-	71%
Timely Help 'Always' Received[8]	-	-	-	64%
Would Definitely Recommend Hospital[8]	-	-	-	69%

Springfield Regional Medical Center

2615 East High Street
Springfield, OH 45505   Phone: 937-325-0531
   Fax: 937-328-8770
E-mail: comrel@communityhospital.com
URL: www.communityhospital.com
Type: Acute Care Hospitals   Emergency Services: Yes
Ownership: Voluntary Non-Profit - Church   Beds: 324
Key Personnel:
CEO/President . . . . Mark Wiener
Cardiac Laboratory . . . . Chris Fritts
Chief of Medical Staff . . . . Stephen Feagins, MD
Coronary Care . . . . Mary Ann Roberts
Operating Room . . . . Tedros Andom
Quality Assurance . . . . Nancy Shively
Radiology . . . . Jerry Tobler
Intensive Care Unit . . . . Penny Brubaker

Measure	Cases	This Hosp.	State Avg.	U.S. Avg.
Heart Attack Care				
ACE Inhibitor or ARB for LVSD	71	96%	97%	96%
Aspirin at Arrival	310	97%	99%	99%
Aspirin at Discharge	348	98%	99%	98%
Beta Blocker at Discharge	339	97%	99%	98%
Fibrinolytic Medication Timing	0	-	14%	55%
PCI Within 90 Minutes of Arrival	49	88%	92%	90%
Smoking Cessation Advice	126	100%	100%	99%
Chest Pain/Possible Heart Attack Care				
Aspirin at Arrival[1]	9	67%	96%	95%
Median Time to ECG (minutes)[1]	11	10	7	8
Median Time to Transfer (minutes)[5]	0	-	61	61
Fibrinolytic Medication Timing[5]	0	-	47%	54%
Heart Failure Care				
ACE Inhibitor or ARB for LVSD	180	97%	96%	94%
Discharge Instructions	368	92%	91%	88%
Evaluation of LVS Function	470	99%	99%	98%
Smoking Cessation Advice	88	99%	99%	98%
Pneumonia Care				
Appropriate Initial Antibiotic	304	95%	92%	92%
Blood Culture Timing	455	98%	96%	96%
Influenza Vaccine	277	98%	93%	91%
Initial Antibiotic Timing	469	95%	96%	95%
Pneumococcal Vaccine	344	98%	95%	93%
Smoking Cessation Advice	179	98%	98%	97%
Surgical Care Improvement Project				
Appropriate VTP Within 24 Hours	384	86%	92%	92%
Appropriate Hair Removal	1,068	100%	100%	99%
Appropriate Beta Blocker Usage	386	98%	94%	93%
Controlled Postoperative Blood Glucose	172	98%	94%	93%
Prophylactic Antibiotic Timing	635	98%	97%	97%
Prophylactic Antibiotic Timing (Outpatient)	197	87%	91%	92%
Prophylactic Antibiotic Selection	647	98%	98%	97%
Prophylactic Antibiotic Select. (Outpatient)	174	91%	94%	94%
Prophylactic Antibiotic Stopped	615	98%	95%	94%
Recommended VTP Ordered	386	91%	94%	94%
Urinary Catheter Removal	99	86%	91%	90%
Children's Asthma Care				
Received Systemic Corticosteroids	-	-	-	100%
Received Home Management Plan	-	-	-	71%
Received Reliever Medication	-	-	-	100%
Use of Medical Imaging				
Combination Abdominal CT Scan	1,085	0.083	0.164	0.191
Combination Chest CT Scan	803	0.035	0.038	0.054
Follow-up Mammogram/Ultrasound	1,449	5.9%	8.4%	8.4%
MRI for Low Back Pain	177	30.5%	30.2%	32.7%
Survey of Patients' Hospital Experiences				
Area Around Room 'Always' Quiet at Night	300+	40%	-	58%
Doctors 'Always' Communicated Well	300+	75%	-	80%
Home Recovery Information Given	300+	74%	-	82%
Hospital Given 9 or 10 on 10 Point Scale	300+	45%	-	67%
Meds 'Always' Explained Before Given	300+	54%	-	60%
Nurses 'Always' Communicated Well	300+	66%	-	76%
Pain 'Always' Well Controlled	300+	60%	-	69%
Room and Bathroom 'Always' Clean	300+	56%	-	71%
Timely Help 'Always' Received	300+	49%	-	64%
Would Definitely Recommend Hospital	300+	45%	-	69%

Trinity Medical Center East & Trinity Medical Center West

380 Summit Avenue
Steubenville, OH 43952   Phone: 740-264-7212
   Fax: 740-283-7104
URL: www.trinityhealth.com
Type: Acute Care Hospitals   Emergency Services: Yes
Ownership: Voluntary Non-Profit - Other   Beds: 401
Key Personnel:
Chief of Medical Staff . . . . A Reddy, MD
Operating Room . . . . Emily Milich-Franusic
Quality Assurance . . . . Susan McLamara
Radiology . . . . Frank Hamilton
Emergency Room . . . . David Sarcon

Measure	Cases	This Hosp.	State Avg.	U.S. Avg.
Heart Attack Care				
ACE Inhibitor or ARB for LVSD	89	93%	97%	96%
Aspirin at Arrival	251	96%	99%	99%
Aspirin at Discharge	317	98%	99%	98%
Beta Blocker at Discharge	324	97%	99%	98%
Fibrinolytic Medication Timing	0	-	14%	55%
PCI Within 90 Minutes of Arrival	33	73%	92%	90%
Smoking Cessation Advice	105	100%	100%	99%
Chest Pain/Possible Heart Attack Care				
Aspirin at Arrival[1,3]	3	100%	96%	95%
Median Time to ECG (minutes)[1,3]	4	12	7	8
Median Time to Transfer (minutes)[5]	0	-	61	61
Fibrinolytic Medication Timing[5]	0	-	47%	54%
Heart Failure Care				
ACE Inhibitor or ARB for LVSD	205	84%	96%	94%
Discharge Instructions	406	92%	91%	88%
Evaluation of LVS Function	579	99%	99%	98%
Smoking Cessation Advice	85	100%	99%	98%
Pneumonia Care				
Appropriate Initial Antibiotic	212	93%	92%	92%
Blood Culture Timing	309	97%	96%	96%
Influenza Vaccine	208	90%	93%	91%
Initial Antibiotic Timing	311	98%	96%	95%
Pneumococcal Vaccine	261	90%	95%	93%
Smoking Cessation Advice	111	100%	98%	97%
Surgical Care Improvement Project				
Appropriate VTP Within 24 Hours[2]	138	90%	92%	92%
Appropriate Hair Removal[2]	547	100%	100%	99%
Appropriate Beta Blocker Usage[2]	206	88%	94%	93%
Controlled Postoperative Blood Glucose[2]	109	90%	94%	93%
Prophylactic Antibiotic Timing[2]	410	97%	97%	97%
Prophylactic Antibiotic Timing (Outpatient)	270	93%	91%	92%
Prophylactic Antibiotic Selection[2]	415	98%	98%	97%
Prophylactic Antibiotic Select. (Outpatient)	262	95%	94%	94%
Prophylactic Antibiotic Stopped[2]	400	91%	95%	94%
Recommended VTP Ordered[2]	139	91%	94%	94%
Urinary Catheter Removal[2]	110	87%	91%	90%
Children's Asthma Care				
Received Systemic Corticosteroids	-	-	-	100%
Received Home Management Plan	-	-	-	71%
Received Reliever Medication	-	-	-	100%
Use of Medical Imaging				
Combination Abdominal CT Scan	543	0.659	0.164	0.191
Combination Chest CT Scan	411	0.708	0.038	0.054
Follow-up Mammogram/Ultrasound	982	8.5%	8.4%	8.4%
MRI for Low Back Pain	128	30.5%	30.2%	32.7%
Survey of Patients' Hospital Experiences				
Area Around Room 'Always' Quiet at Night	300+	51%	-	58%
Doctors 'Always' Communicated Well	300+	79%	-	80%
Home Recovery Information Given	300+	86%	-	82%
Hospital Given 9 or 10 on 10 Point Scale	300+	64%	-	67%
Meds 'Always' Explained Before Given	300+	60%	-	60%
Nurses 'Always' Communicated Well	300+	75%	-	76%
Pain 'Always' Well Controlled	300+	68%	-	69%
Room and Bathroom 'Always' Clean	300+	70%	-	71%
Timely Help 'Always' Received	300+	62%	-	64%
Would Definitely Recommend Hospital	300+	66%	-	69%

NOTE: Hospital profiles are in alphabetical order by state, then city, then hospital within the city; Rankings exclude hospitals with less than 25 cases except for patient surveys which excludes hospitals with less than 100 cases; (a) 100–299 cases; (1) The number of cases is too small to be sure how well a hospital is performing; (2) The hospital indicated that the data submitted for this measure were based on a sample of cases; (3) Data was collected during a shorter time period (fewer quarters) than the maximum possible time for this measure; (4) Suppressed for one or more quarters by CMS; (5) No data is available from the hospital for this measure; (6) Fewer than 100 patients completed the HCAHPS survey. Use these rates with caution, as the number of surveys may be too low to reliably assess hospital performance; (7) Survey results are based on less than 12 months of data; (8) Survey results are not available for this reporting period; (9) No or very few patients were eligible for the HCAHPS survey. The scores shown, if any, reflect a very small number of surveys; (10) A state average was not calculated because too few hospitals in the state submitted data; (11) There were discrepancies in the data collection process; Please refer to the User's Guide for a full explanation of data.

Flower Hospital

5200 Harroun Road Phone: 419-824-1444
Sylvania, OH 43560
URL: www.promedica.org
Type: Acute Care Hospitals Emergency Services: Yes
Ownership: Voluntary Non-Profit - Private Beds: 279

Measure	Cases	This Hosp.	State Avg.	U.S. Avg.
Heart Attack Care				
ACE Inhibitor or ARB for LVSD[1]	4	75%	97%	96%
Aspirin at Arrival	61	100%	99%	99%
Aspirin at Discharge	38	95%	99%	98%
Beta Blocker at Discharge	41	100%	99%	98%
Fibrinolytic Medication Timing	0	-	14%	55%
PCI Within 90 Minutes of Arrival	0	-	92%	90%
Smoking Cessation Advice[1]	7	100%	100%	99%
Chest Pain/Possible Heart Attack Care				
Aspirin at Arrival	53	96%	96%	95%
Median Time to ECG (minutes)	57	5	7	8
Median Time to Transfer (minutes)[1]	16	66	61	61
Fibrinolytic Medication Timing	0	-	47%	54%
Heart Failure Care				
ACE Inhibitor or ARB for LVSD	41	100%	96%	94%
Discharge Instructions	146	87%	91%	88%
Evaluation of LVS Function	210	97%	99%	98%
Smoking Cessation Advice[1]	21	100%	99%	98%
Pneumonia Care				
Appropriate Initial Antibiotic	120	93%	92%	92%
Blood Culture Timing	199	97%	96%	96%
Influenza Vaccine	146	92%	93%	91%
Initial Antibiotic Timing	188	98%	96%	95%
Pneumococcal Vaccine	181	94%	95%	93%
Smoking Cessation Advice	65	97%	98%	97%
Surgical Care Improvement Project				
Appropriate VTP Within 24 Hours[2]	202	93%	92%	92%
Appropriate Hair Removal[2]	473	99%	100%	99%
Appropriate Beta Blocker Usage[2]	152	96%	94%	93%
Controlled Postoperative Blood Glucose[2]	0	-	94%	93%
Prophylactic Antibiotic Timing[2]	314	97%	97%	97%
Prophylactic Antibiotic Timing (Outpatient)	179	89%	91%	92%
Prophylactic Antibiotic Selection[2]	316	98%	98%	97%
Prophylactic Antibiotic Select. (Outpatient)	174	94%	94%	94%
Prophylactic Antibiotic Stopped[2]	295	98%	95%	94%
Recommended VTP Ordered[2]	202	94%	94%	94%
Urinary Catheter Removal[2]	100	94%	91%	90%
Children's Asthma Care				
Received Systemic Corticosteroids	-	-	-	100%
Received Home Management Plan	-	-	-	71%
Received Reliever Medication	-	-	-	100%
Use of Medical Imaging				
Combination Abdominal CT Scan	458	0.022	0.164	0.191
Combination Chest CT Scan	378	0.016	0.038	0.054
Follow-up Mammogram/Ultrasound	661	8.5%	8.4%	8.4%
MRI for Low Back Pain	97	32.0%	30.2%	32.7%
Survey of Patients' Hospital Experiences				
Area Around Room 'Always' Quiet at Night	300+	50%	-	58%
Doctors 'Always' Communicated Well	300+	78%	-	80%
Home Recovery Information Given	300+	87%	-	82%
Hospital Given 9 or 10 on 10 Point Scale	300+	70%	-	67%
Meds 'Always' Explained Before Given	300+	57%	-	60%
Nurses 'Always' Communicated Well	300+	77%	-	76%
Pain 'Always' Well Controlled	300+	67%	-	69%
Room and Bathroom 'Always' Clean	300+	71%	-	71%
Timely Help 'Always' Received	300+	61%	-	64%
Would Definitely Recommend Hospital	300+	73%	-	69%

Mercy Tiffin Hospital

45 St Lawrence Drive Phone: 419-455-7000
Tiffin, OH 44883 Fax: 419-448-3181
Type: Acute Care Hospitals Emergency Services: Yes
Ownership: Voluntary Non-Profit - Private Beds: 105

Key Personnel:
CEO/President. . . . . Adam Dittman
Chief of Medical Staff . . . . James Anthony, MD, MRO
Infection Control. . . . . Susan Weithman
Operating Room. . . . . Linda Hayman, RN
Pediatric Ambulatory Care . . . . . . Prasad Kakaiala, MD
Pediatric In-Patient Care . . . . Prasad Kakaiala, MD
Quality Assurance . . . . Anne Zimmerman
Radiology. . . . . Jorge Cepeda

Measure	Cases	This Hosp.	State Avg.	U.S. Avg.
Heart Attack Care				
ACE Inhibitor or ARB for LVSD[1]	1	100%	97%	96%
Aspirin at Arrival[1]	14	100%	99%	99%
Aspirin at Discharge[1]	9	100%	99%	98%
Beta Blocker at Discharge[1]	8	100%	99%	98%
Fibrinolytic Medication Timing	0	-	14%	55%
PCI Within 90 Minutes of Arrival	0	-	92%	90%
Smoking Cessation Advice	0	-	100%	99%
Chest Pain/Possible Heart Attack Care				
Aspirin at Arrival	100	91%	96%	95%
Median Time to ECG (minutes)	105	6	7	8
Median Time to Transfer (minutes)[1]	14	110	61	61
Fibrinolytic Medication Timing[1]	3	0%	47%	54%
Heart Failure Care				
ACE Inhibitor or ARB for LVSD[1]	20	100%	96%	94%
Discharge Instructions	66	97%	91%	88%
Evaluation of LVS Function	103	99%	99%	98%
Smoking Cessation Advice[1]	8	100%	99%	98%
Pneumonia Care				
Appropriate Initial Antibiotic	62	94%	92%	92%
Blood Culture Timing	82	99%	96%	96%
Influenza Vaccine	65	94%	93%	91%
Initial Antibiotic Timing	84	100%	96%	95%
Pneumococcal Vaccine	88	93%	95%	93%
Smoking Cessation Advice	37	97%	98%	97%
Surgical Care Improvement Project				
Appropriate VTP Within 24 Hours	50	80%	92%	92%
Appropriate Hair Removal	166	100%	100%	99%
Appropriate Beta Blocker Usage	52	94%	94%	93%
Controlled Postoperative Blood Glucose	0	-	94%	93%
Prophylactic Antibiotic Timing	136	99%	97%	97%
Prophylactic Antibiotic Timing (Outpatient)	43	60%	91%	92%
Prophylactic Antibiotic Selection	136	98%	98%	97%
Prophylactic Antibiotic Select. (Outpatient)	62	69%	94%	94%
Prophylactic Antibiotic Stopped	134	98%	95%	94%
Recommended VTP Ordered	50	98%	94%	94%
Urinary Catheter Removal[1]	10	100%	91%	90%
Children's Asthma Care				
Received Systemic Corticosteroids	-	-	-	100%
Received Home Management Plan	-	-	-	71%
Received Reliever Medication	-	-	-	100%
Use of Medical Imaging				
Combination Abdominal CT Scan	431	0.691	0.164	0.191
Combination Chest CT Scan	241	0.079	0.038	0.054
Follow-up Mammogram/Ultrasound	600	6.0%	8.4%	8.4%
MRI for Low Back Pain	129	24.0%	30.2%	32.7%
Survey of Patients' Hospital Experiences				
Area Around Room 'Always' Quiet at Night	300+	62%	-	58%
Doctors 'Always' Communicated Well	300+	84%	-	80%
Home Recovery Information Given	300+	89%	-	82%
Hospital Given 9 or 10 on 10 Point Scale	300+	73%	-	67%
Meds 'Always' Explained Before Given	300+	67%	-	60%
Nurses 'Always' Communicated Well	300+	82%	-	76%
Pain 'Always' Well Controlled	300+	71%	-	69%
Room and Bathroom 'Always' Clean	300+	83%	-	71%
Timely Help 'Always' Received	300+	68%	-	64%
Would Definitely Recommend Hospital	300+	69%	-	69%

Mercy St Anne Hospital

3404 Sylvania Avenue Phone: 419-407-2663
Toledo, OH 43623 Fax: 419-251-2104
URL: www.mercyweb.org
Type: Acute Care Hospitals Emergency Services: Yes
Ownership: Voluntary Non-Profit - Church Beds: 88

Key Personnel:
CEO/President. . . . . Karen Connors
Chief of Medical Staff . . . . Steven Ariss, MD
Infection Control. . . . . Arlene Hustivick, RN
Operating Room. . . . . Sanjiv Bais, RN
Pediatric Ambulatory Care . . . . . . M Shaw
Pediatric In-Patient Care . . . . M Shaw
Quality Assurance . . . . Deb Nicotra
Radiology. . . . . David R Cervantes, MD

Measure	Cases	This Hosp.	State Avg.	U.S. Avg.
Heart Attack Care				
ACE Inhibitor or ARB for LVSD[1]	3	100%	97%	96%
Aspirin at Arrival	37	95%	99%	99%
Aspirin at Discharge[1]	23	96%	99%	98%
Beta Blocker at Discharge[1]	21	100%	99%	98%
Fibrinolytic Medication Timing	0	-	14%	55%
PCI Within 90 Minutes of Arrival	0	-	92%	90%
Smoking Cessation Advice[1]	5	100%	100%	99%
Chest Pain/Possible Heart Attack Care				
Aspirin at Arrival	71	100%	96%	95%
Median Time to ECG (minutes)	75	21	7	8
Median Time to Transfer (minutes)[1,3]	11	69	61	61
Fibrinolytic Medication Timing[3]	0	-	47%	54%
Heart Failure Care				
ACE Inhibitor or ARB for LVSD	47	91%	96%	94%
Discharge Instructions	157	97%	91%	88%
Evaluation of LVS Function	195	99%	99%	98%
Smoking Cessation Advice	43	98%	99%	98%
Pneumonia Care				
Appropriate Initial Antibiotic	107	95%	92%	92%
Blood Culture Timing	166	98%	96%	96%
Influenza Vaccine	80	96%	93%	91%
Initial Antibiotic Timing	140	99%	96%	95%
Pneumococcal Vaccine	94	97%	95%	93%
Smoking Cessation Advice	75	100%	98%	97%
Surgical Care Improvement Project				
Appropriate VTP Within 24 Hours[2]	170	96%	92%	92%
Appropriate Hair Removal[2]	412	100%	100%	99%
Appropriate Beta Blocker Usage[2]	143	98%	94%	93%
Controlled Postoperative Blood Glucose[2]	0	-	94%	93%
Prophylactic Antibiotic Timing[2]	284	95%	97%	97%
Prophylactic Antibiotic Timing (Outpatient)	101	97%	91%	92%
Prophylactic Antibiotic Selection[2]	285	98%	98%	97%
Prophylactic Antibiotic Select. (Outpatient)	99	97%	94%	94%
Prophylactic Antibiotic Stopped[2]	267	94%	95%	94%
Recommended VTP Ordered[2]	170	97%	94%	94%
Urinary Catheter Removal[2]	103	99%	91%	90%
Children's Asthma Care				
Received Systemic Corticosteroids	-	-	-	100%
Received Home Management Plan	-	-	-	71%
Received Reliever Medication	-	-	-	100%
Use of Medical Imaging				
Combination Abdominal CT Scan	473	0.021	0.164	0.191
Combination Chest CT Scan	315	0.000	0.038	0.054
Follow-up Mammogram/Ultrasound	1,406	6.8%	8.4%	8.4%
MRI for Low Back Pain	73	32.9%	30.2%	32.7%
Survey of Patients' Hospital Experiences				
Area Around Room 'Always' Quiet at Night	300+	64%	-	58%
Doctors 'Always' Communicated Well	300+	75%	-	80%
Home Recovery Information Given	300+	85%	-	82%
Hospital Given 9 or 10 on 10 Point Scale	300+	74%	-	67%
Meds 'Always' Explained Before Given	300+	59%	-	60%
Nurses 'Always' Communicated Well	300+	78%	-	76%
Pain 'Always' Well Controlled	300+	70%	-	69%
Room and Bathroom 'Always' Clean	300+	78%	-	71%
Timely Help 'Always' Received	300+	64%	-	64%
Would Definitely Recommend Hospital	300+	78%	-	69%

NOTE: Hospital profiles are in alphabetical order by state, then city, then hospital within the city; Rankings exclude hospitals with less than 25 cases except for patient surveys which excludes hospitals with less than 100 cases; (a) 100–299 cases; (1) The number of cases is too small to be sure how well a hospital is performing; (2) The hospital indicated that the data submitted for this measure were based on a sample of cases; (3) Data was collected during a shorter time period (fewer quarters) than the maximum possible time for this measure; (4) Suppressed for one or more quarters by CMS; (5) No data is available from the hospital for this measure; (6) Fewer than 100 patients completed the HCAHPS survey. Use these rates with caution, as the number of surveys may be too low to reliably assess hospital performance; (7) Survey results are based on less than 12 months of data; (8) Survey results are not available for this reporting period; (9) No or very few patients were eligible for the HCAHPS survey. The scores shown, if any, reflect a very small number of surveys; (10) A state average was not calculated because too few hospitals in the state submitted data; (11) There were discrepancies in the data collection process; Please refer to the User's Guide for a full explanation of data.

Mercy St Vincent Medical Center

2213 Cherry Street
Toledo, OH 43608
URL: www.mhsnr.org
Type: Acute Care Hospitals
Ownership: Voluntary Non-Profit - Church
Phone: 419-251-3232
Fax: 419-242-9806
Emergency Services: Yes
Beds: 588

Key Personnel:
CEO/President. . . . . Jeffrey Peterson
Chief of Medical Staff . . . . Robert Nawarre, MD

Measure	Cases	This Hosp.	State Avg.	U.S. Avg.
Heart Attack Care				
ACE Inhibitor or ARB for LVSD	149	97%	97%	96%
Aspirin at Arrival	331	99%	99%	99%
Aspirin at Discharge	645	100%	99%	98%
Beta Blocker at Discharge	632	100%	99%	98%
Fibrinolytic Medication Timing	0	-	14%	55%
PCI Within 90 Minutes of Arrival	82	93%	92%	90%
Smoking Cessation Advice	283	100%	100%	99%
Chest Pain/Possible Heart Attack Care				
Aspirin at Arrival[1]	13	85%	96%	95%
Median Time to ECG (minutes)[1]	13	5	7	8
Median Time to Transfer (minutes)[1,3]	1	173	61	61
Fibrinolytic Medication Timing[3]	0	-	47%	54%
Heart Failure Care				
ACE Inhibitor or ARB for LVSD	324	97%	96%	94%
Discharge Instructions	565	100%	91%	88%
Evaluation of LVS Function	657	100%	99%	98%
Smoking Cessation Advice	190	100%	99%	98%
Pneumonia Care				
Appropriate Initial Antibiotic	97	92%	92%	92%
Blood Culture Timing	212	95%	96%	96%
Influenza Vaccine	160	96%	93%	91%
Initial Antibiotic Timing	183	97%	96%	95%
Pneumococcal Vaccine	167	96%	95%	93%
Smoking Cessation Advice	154	100%	98%	97%
Surgical Care Improvement Project				
Appropriate VTP Within 24 Hours[2]	175	90%	92%	92%
Appropriate Hair Removal[2]	872	100%	100%	99%
Appropriate Beta Blocker Usage[2]	319	95%	94%	93%
Controlled Postoperative Blood Glucose[2]	314	100%	94%	93%
Prophylactic Antibiotic Timing[2]	672	98%	97%	97%
Prophylactic Antibiotic Timing (Outpatient)	474	97%	91%	92%
Prophylactic Antibiotic Selection[2]	681	99%	98%	97%
Prophylactic Antibiotic Select. (Outpatient)	474	90%	94%	94%
Prophylactic Antibiotic Stopped[2]	647	98%	95%	94%
Recommended VTP Ordered[2]	175	97%	94%	94%
Urinary Catheter Removal[2]	172	98%	91%	90%
Children's Asthma Care				
Received Systemic Corticosteroids	-	-	-	100%
Received Home Management Plan	-	-	-	71%
Received Reliever Medication	-	-	-	100%
Use of Medical Imaging				
Combination Abdominal CT Scan	436	0.023	0.164	0.191
Combination Chest CT Scan	410	0.002	0.038	0.054
Follow-up Mammogram/Ultrasound	471	8.5%	8.4%	8.4%
MRI for Low Back Pain	75	32.0%	30.2%	32.7%
Survey of Patients' Hospital Experiences				
Area Around Room 'Always' Quiet at Night	300+	55%	-	58%
Doctors 'Always' Communicated Well	300+	73%	-	80%
Home Recovery Information Given	300+	85%	-	82%
Hospital Given 9 or 10 on 10 Point Scale	300+	67%	-	67%
Meds 'Always' Explained Before Given	300+	57%	-	60%
Nurses 'Always' Communicated Well	300+	76%	-	76%
Pain 'Always' Well Controlled	300+	65%	-	69%
Room and Bathroom 'Always' Clean	300+	73%	-	71%
Timely Help 'Always' Received	300+	63%	-	64%
Would Definitely Recommend Hospital	300+	73%	-	69%

The Toledo Hospital

2142 North Cove Boulevard
Toledo, OH 43606
URL: www.promedica.org
Type: Acute Care Hospitals
Ownership: Voluntary Non-Profit - Private
Phone: 419-291-7463
Fax: 419-469-3791
Emergency Services: Yes
Beds: 794

Key Personnel:
CEO/President. . . . . Barbara Steele

Measure	Cases	This Hosp.	State Avg.	U.S. Avg.
Heart Attack Care				
ACE Inhibitor or ARB for LVSD[2]	60	97%	97%	96%
Aspirin at Arrival[2]	125	99%	99%	99%
Aspirin at Discharge[2]	300	99%	99%	98%
Beta Blocker at Discharge[2]	303	100%	99%	98%
Fibrinolytic Medication Timing[2]	0	-	14%	55%
PCI Within 90 Minutes of Arrival[1,2]	17	100%	92%	90%
Smoking Cessation Advice[2]	123	99%	100%	99%
Chest Pain/Possible Heart Attack Care				
Aspirin at Arrival[1,3]	1	100%	96%	95%
Median Time to ECG (minutes)[1,3]	2	8	7	8
Median Time to Transfer (minutes)[5]	0	-	61	61
Fibrinolytic Medication Timing[5]	0	-	47%	54%
Heart Failure Care				
ACE Inhibitor or ARB for LVSD[2]	75	95%	96%	94%
Discharge Instructions[2]	224	64%	91%	88%
Evaluation of LVS Function[2]	286	98%	99%	98%
Smoking Cessation Advice[2]	44	100%	99%	98%
Pneumonia Care				
Appropriate Initial Antibiotic[2]	65	86%	92%	92%
Blood Culture Timing[2]	106	96%	96%	96%
Influenza Vaccine[2]	73	90%	93%	91%
Initial Antibiotic Timing[2]	103	96%	96%	95%
Pneumococcal Vaccine[2]	97	91%	95%	93%
Smoking Cessation Advice[2]	49	90%	98%	97%
Surgical Care Improvement Project				
Appropriate VTP Within 24 Hours[2]	152	89%	92%	92%
Appropriate Hair Removal[2]	674	100%	100%	99%
Appropriate Beta Blocker Usage[2]	268	97%	94%	93%
Controlled Postoperative Blood Glucose[2]	151	90%	94%	93%
Prophylactic Antibiotic Timing[2]	486	96%	97%	97%
Prophylactic Antibiotic Timing (Outpatient)	588	97%	91%	92%
Prophylactic Antibiotic Selection[2]	495	97%	98%	97%
Prophylactic Antibiotic Select. (Outpatient)	581	93%	94%	94%
Prophylactic Antibiotic Stopped[2]	468	91%	95%	94%
Recommended VTP Ordered[2]	152	91%	94%	94%
Urinary Catheter Removal[2]	153	88%	91%	90%
Children's Asthma Care				
Received Systemic Corticosteroids	201	100%	-	100%
Received Home Management Plan	201	95%	-	71%
Received Reliever Medication	201	100%	-	100%
Use of Medical Imaging				
Combination Abdominal CT Scan	790	0.049	0.164	0.191
Combination Chest CT Scan	654	0.017	0.038	0.054
Follow-up Mammogram/Ultrasound	2,091	9.0%	8.4%	8.4%
MRI for Low Back Pain	193	22.8%	30.2%	32.7%
Survey of Patients' Hospital Experiences				
Area Around Room 'Always' Quiet at Night	300+	48%	-	58%
Doctors 'Always' Communicated Well	300+	70%	-	80%
Home Recovery Information Given	300+	85%	-	82%
Hospital Given 9 or 10 on 10 Point Scale	300+	63%	-	67%
Meds 'Always' Explained Before Given	300+	52%	-	60%
Nurses 'Always' Communicated Well	300+	68%	-	76%
Pain 'Always' Well Controlled	300+	65%	-	69%
Room and Bathroom 'Always' Clean	300+	68%	-	71%
Timely Help 'Always' Received	300+	56%	-	64%
Would Definitely Recommend Hospital	300+	66%	-	69%

University of Toledo Medical Center

3000 Arlington Avenue
Toledo, OH 43699
E-mail: utmc.webmaster@utoledo.edu
URL: utmc.utoledo.edu
Type: Acute Care Hospitals
Ownership: Government - State
Phone: 419-383-3413
Fax: 419-383-2800
Emergency Services: Yes
Beds: 319

Key Personnel:
CEO/President. . . . . Lloyd Jacobs
Chief of Medical Staff . . . . Daniel Morrissett, MD
Operating Room. . . . . Connie Ashbaugh, RN
Pediatric Ambulatory Care . . . . . . Mark Puczynski, MD
Pediatric In-Patient Care . . . . Mark Puczynski, MD
Quality Assurance . . . . Mary Shapiro
Radiology. . . . . Lee S Woldenberg, MD
Emergency Room . . . . Diane Ness

Measure	Cases	This Hosp.	State Avg.	U.S. Avg.
Heart Attack Care				
ACE Inhibitor or ARB for LVSD	32	100%	97%	96%
Aspirin at Arrival	100	99%	99%	99%
Aspirin at Discharge	178	99%	99%	98%
Beta Blocker at Discharge	172	100%	99%	98%
Fibrinolytic Medication Timing	0	-	14%	55%
PCI Within 90 Minutes of Arrival	25	92%	92%	90%
Smoking Cessation Advice	75	100%	100%	99%
Chest Pain/Possible Heart Attack Care				
Aspirin at Arrival[5]	0	-	96%	95%
Median Time to ECG (minutes)[5]	0	-	7	8
Median Time to Transfer (minutes)[5]	0	-	61	61
Fibrinolytic Medication Timing[5]	0	-	47%	54%
Heart Failure Care				
ACE Inhibitor or ARB for LVSD[2]	85	99%	96%	94%
Discharge Instructions[2]	212	93%	91%	88%
Evaluation of LVS Function[2]	244	100%	99%	98%
Smoking Cessation Advice[2]	43	100%	99%	98%
Pneumonia Care				
Appropriate Initial Antibiotic[2]	53	75%	92%	92%
Blood Culture Timing[2]	83	94%	96%	96%
Influenza Vaccine[2]	78	82%	93%	91%
Initial Antibiotic Timing[2]	76	96%	96%	95%
Pneumococcal Vaccine[2]	87	78%	95%	93%
Smoking Cessation Advice[2]	55	100%	98%	97%
Surgical Care Improvement Project				
Appropriate VTP Within 24 Hours[2]	152	96%	92%	92%
Appropriate Hair Removal[2]	477	100%	100%	99%
Appropriate Beta Blocker Usage[2]	200	96%	94%	93%
Controlled Postoperative Blood Glucose[2]	94	90%	94%	93%
Prophylactic Antibiotic Timing[2]	337	96%	97%	97%
Prophylactic Antibiotic Timing (Outpatient)	196	97%	91%	92%
Prophylactic Antibiotic Selection[2]	345	98%	98%	97%
Prophylactic Antibiotic Select. (Outpatient)	210	95%	94%	94%
Prophylactic Antibiotic Stopped[2]	295	97%	95%	94%
Recommended VTP Ordered[2]	152	100%	94%	94%
Urinary Catheter Removal[2]	102	98%	91%	90%
Children's Asthma Care				
Received Systemic Corticosteroids	-	-	-	100%
Received Home Management Plan	-	-	-	71%
Received Reliever Medication	-	-	-	100%
Use of Medical Imaging				
Combination Abdominal CT Scan	505	0.341	0.164	0.191
Combination Chest CT Scan	366	0.027	0.038	0.054
Follow-up Mammogram/Ultrasound	536	4.1%	8.4%	8.4%
MRI for Low Back Pain	181	27.1%	30.2%	32.7%
Survey of Patients' Hospital Experiences				
Area Around Room 'Always' Quiet at Night	300+	35%	-	58%
Doctors 'Always' Communicated Well	300+	66%	-	80%
Home Recovery Information Given	300+	80%	-	82%
Hospital Given 9 or 10 on 10 Point Scale	300+	52%	-	67%
Meds 'Always' Explained Before Given	300+	53%	-	60%
Nurses 'Always' Communicated Well	300+	63%	-	76%
Pain 'Always' Well Controlled	300+	60%	-	69%
Room and Bathroom 'Always' Clean	300+	52%	-	71%
Timely Help 'Always' Received	300+	51%	-	64%
Would Definitely Recommend Hospital	300+	53%	-	69%

NOTE: Hospital profiles are in alphabetical order by state, then city, then hospital within the city; Rankings exclude hospitals with less than 25 cases except for patient surveys which excludes hospitals with less than 100 cases; (a) 100–299 cases; (1) The number of cases is too small to be sure how well a hospital is performing; (2) The hospital indicated that the data submitted for this measure were based on a sample of cases; (3) Data was collected during a shorter time period (fewer quarters) than the maximum possible time for this measure; (4) Suppressed for one or more quarters by CMS; (5) No data is available from the hospital for this measure; (6) Fewer than 100 patients completed the HCAHPS survey. Use these rates with caution, as the number of surveys may be too low to reliably assess hospital performance; (7) Survey results are based on less than 12 months of data; (8) Survey results are not available for this reporting period; (9) No or very few patients were eligible for the HCAHPS survey. The scores shown, if any, reflect a very small number of surveys; (10) A state average was not calculated because too few hospitals in the state submitted data; (11) There were discrepancies in the data collection process; Please refer to the User's Guide for a full explanation of data.

Upper Valley Medical Center

3130 North County Road 25a
Troy, OH 45373
Phone: 937-440-7853
Fax: 937-440-7739
E-mail: bwilson@uvmc.com
URL: www.uvmc.com
Type: Acute Care Hospitals
Emergency Services: Yes
Ownership: Voluntary Non-Profit - Private
Beds: 128

Key Personnel:
CEO/President. . . . . David J Meckstroth
Chief of Medical Staff . . . . Sayed Ali
Quality Assurance . . . . Tony White
Radiology. . . . . Diane Anderson
Emergency Room . . . . Dee Mullen

Measure	Cases	This Hosp.	State Avg.	U.S. Avg.
Heart Attack Care				
ACE Inhibitor or ARB for LVSD[1]	13	100%	97%	96%
Aspirin at Arrival	85	99%	99%	99%
Aspirin at Discharge	59	98%	99%	98%
Beta Blocker at Discharge	58	98%	99%	98%
Fibrinolytic Medication Timing	0	-	14%	55%
PCI Within 90 Minutes of Arrival	0	-	92%	90%
Smoking Cessation Advice[1]	6	83%	100%	99%
Chest Pain/Possible Heart Attack Care				
Aspirin at Arrival	124	96%	96%	95%
Median Time to ECG (minutes)	126	8	7	8
Median Time to Transfer (minutes)	57	65	61	61
Fibrinolytic Medication Timing[1]	1	100%	47%	54%
Heart Failure Care				
ACE Inhibitor or ARB for LVSD	44	100%	96%	94%
Discharge Instructions	173	92%	91%	88%
Evaluation of LVS Function	221	100%	99%	98%
Smoking Cessation Advice[1]	15	100%	99%	98%
Pneumonia Care				
Appropriate Initial Antibiotic	188	94%	92%	92%
Blood Culture Timing	301	96%	96%	96%
Influenza Vaccine	141	91%	93%	91%
Initial Antibiotic Timing	263	99%	96%	95%
Pneumococcal Vaccine	246	93%	95%	93%
Smoking Cessation Advice	87	98%	98%	97%
Surgical Care Improvement Project				
Appropriate VTP Within 24 Hours	185	95%	92%	92%
Appropriate Hair Removal	420	100%	100%	99%
Appropriate Beta Blocker Usage	105	93%	94%	93%
Controlled Postoperative Blood Glucose	0	-	94%	93%
Prophylactic Antibiotic Timing	264	96%	97%	97%
Prophylactic Antibiotic Timing (Outpatient)	100	95%	91%	92%
Prophylactic Antibiotic Selection	266	96%	98%	97%
Prophylactic Antibiotic Select. (Outpatient)	96	91%	94%	94%
Prophylactic Antibiotic Stopped	250	90%	95%	94%
Recommended VTP Ordered	185	98%	94%	94%
Urinary Catheter Removal	34	94%	91%	90%
Children's Asthma Care				
Received Systemic Corticosteroids	-	-	-	100%
Received Home Management Plan	-	-	-	71%
Received Reliever Medication	-	-	-	100%
Use of Medical Imaging				
Combination Abdominal CT Scan	869	0.066	0.164	0.191
Combination Chest CT Scan	711	0.010	0.038	0.054
Follow-up Mammogram/Ultrasound	1,622	5.4%	8.4%	8.4%
MRI for Low Back Pain	116	22.4%	30.2%	32.7%
Survey of Patients' Hospital Experiences				
Area Around Room 'Always' Quiet at Night	300+	47%	-	58%
Doctors 'Always' Communicated Well	300+	76%	-	80%
Home Recovery Information Given	300+	82%	-	82%
Hospital Given 9 or 10 on 10 Point Scale	300+	59%	-	67%
Meds 'Always' Explained Before Given	300+	57%	-	60%
Nurses 'Always' Communicated Well	300+	74%	-	76%
Pain 'Always' Well Controlled	300+	66%	-	69%
Room and Bathroom 'Always' Clean	300+	67%	-	71%
Timely Help 'Always' Received	300+	63%	-	64%
Would Definitely Recommend Hospital	300+	60%	-	69%

Wyandot Memorial Hospital

885 North Sandusky Avenue
Upper Sandusky, OH 43351
Phone: 419-294-4991
Fax: 419-294-2233
URL: www.wyandotmemorial.com
Type: Critical Access Hospitals
Emergency Services: Yes
Ownership: Govt - Hospital Dist/Auth
Beds: 45

Key Personnel:
CEO/President. . . . . Joseph A D'Ettorre
Cardiac Laboratory. . . . . Russ Merrin
Chief of Medical Staff . . . . Mary Anne Schwenning, MD
Coronary Care . . . . Russ Merrin, BS CMT
Infection Control. . . . . Valerie Schalk, RN
Operating Room. . . . . LuAnn Montz, RN
Quality Assurance . . . . Vicki Underwood

Measure	Cases	This Hosp.	State Avg.	U.S. Avg.
Heart Attack Care				
ACE Inhibitor or ARB for LVSD	0	-	97%	96%
Aspirin at Arrival[1]	3	100%	99%	99%
Aspirin at Discharge	0	-	99%	98%
Beta Blocker at Discharge	0	-	99%	98%
Fibrinolytic Medication Timing	0	-	14%	55%
PCI Within 90 Minutes of Arrival	0	-	92%	90%
Smoking Cessation Advice	0	-	100%	99%
Chest Pain/Possible Heart Attack Care				
Aspirin at Arrival	-	-	96%	95%
Median Time to ECG (minutes)	-	-	7	8
Median Time to Transfer (minutes)	-	-	61	61
Fibrinolytic Medication Timing	-	-	47%	54%
Heart Failure Care				
ACE Inhibitor or ARB for LVSD[1]	6	100%	96%	94%
Discharge Instructions[1]	23	78%	91%	88%
Evaluation of LVS Function	26	96%	99%	98%
Smoking Cessation Advice[1]	1	100%	99%	98%
Pneumonia Care				
Appropriate Initial Antibiotic[1]	12	100%	92%	92%
Blood Culture Timing[1]	13	100%	96%	96%
Influenza Vaccine[1]	6	83%	93%	91%
Initial Antibiotic Timing[1]	15	87%	96%	95%
Pneumococcal Vaccine[1]	12	100%	95%	93%
Smoking Cessation Advice[1]	6	83%	98%	97%
Surgical Care Improvement Project				
Appropriate VTP Within 24 Hours[1]	14	100%	92%	92%
Appropriate Hair Removal	31	100%	100%	99%
Appropriate Beta Blocker Usage[5]	0	-	94%	93%
Controlled Postoperative Blood Glucose	0	-	94%	93%
Prophylactic Antibiotic Timing	29	79%	97%	97%
Prophylactic Antibiotic Timing (Outpatient)	-	-	91%	92%
Prophylactic Antibiotic Selection	29	97%	98%	97%
Prophylactic Antibiotic Select. (Outpatient)	-	-	94%	94%
Prophylactic Antibiotic Stopped	29	90%	95%	94%
Recommended VTP Ordered[1]	14	100%	94%	94%
Urinary Catheter Removal[1]	9	78%	91%	90%
Children's Asthma Care				
Received Systemic Corticosteroids	-	-	-	100%
Received Home Management Plan	-	-	-	71%
Received Reliever Medication	-	-	-	100%
Use of Medical Imaging				
Combination Abdominal CT Scan	-	-	0.164	0.191
Combination Chest CT Scan	-	-	0.038	0.054
Follow-up Mammogram/Ultrasound	-	-	8.4%	8.4%
MRI for Low Back Pain	-	-	30.2%	32.7%
Survey of Patients' Hospital Experiences				
Area Around Room 'Always' Quiet at Night[8]	-	-	-	58%
Doctors 'Always' Communicated Well[8]	-	-	-	80%
Home Recovery Information Given[8]	-	-	-	82%
Hospital Given 9 or 10 on 10 Point Scale[8]	-	-	-	67%
Meds 'Always' Explained Before Given[8]	-	-	-	60%
Nurses 'Always' Communicated Well[8]	-	-	-	76%
Pain 'Always' Well Controlled[8]	-	-	-	69%
Room and Bathroom 'Always' Clean[8]	-	-	-	71%
Timely Help 'Always' Received[8]	-	-	-	64%
Would Definitely Recommend Hospital[8]	-	-	-	69%

Mercy Memorial Hospital

904 Scioto Avenue
Urbana, OH 43078
Phone: 937-484-6147
Fax: 513-390-5554
Type: Critical Access Hospitals
Emergency Services: Yes
Ownership: Voluntary Non-Profit - Church
Beds: 73

Key Personnel:
Chief of Medical Staff . . . . Joseph Metz

Measure	Cases	This Hosp.	State Avg.	U.S. Avg.
Heart Attack Care				
ACE Inhibitor or ARB for LVSD[1]	1	100%	97%	96%
Aspirin at Arrival[1]	6	100%	99%	99%
Aspirin at Discharge[1]	4	100%	99%	98%
Beta Blocker at Discharge[1]	4	100%	99%	98%
Fibrinolytic Medication Timing	0	-	14%	55%
PCI Within 90 Minutes of Arrival	0	-	92%	90%
Smoking Cessation Advice[1]	2	100%	100%	99%
Chest Pain/Possible Heart Attack Care				
Aspirin at Arrival	-	-	96%	95%
Median Time to ECG (minutes)	-	-	7	8
Median Time to Transfer (minutes)	-	-	61	61
Fibrinolytic Medication Timing	-	-	47%	54%
Heart Failure Care				
ACE Inhibitor or ARB for LVSD[1]	23	91%	96%	94%
Discharge Instructions	52	100%	91%	88%
Evaluation of LVS Function	64	100%	99%	98%
Smoking Cessation Advice[1]	12	100%	99%	98%
Pneumonia Care				
Appropriate Initial Antibiotic	57	100%	92%	92%
Blood Culture Timing	83	99%	96%	96%
Influenza Vaccine	48	100%	93%	91%
Initial Antibiotic Timing	79	99%	96%	95%
Pneumococcal Vaccine	59	98%	95%	93%
Smoking Cessation Advice[1]	20	100%	98%	97%
Surgical Care Improvement Project				
Appropriate VTP Within 24 Hours[1]	16	100%	92%	92%
Appropriate Hair Removal[1]	20	100%	100%	99%
Appropriate Beta Blocker Usage[5]	0	-	94%	93%
Controlled Postoperative Blood Glucose	0	-	94%	93%
Prophylactic Antibiotic Timing[1]	8	88%	97%	97%
Prophylactic Antibiotic Timing (Outpatient)	-	-	91%	92%
Prophylactic Antibiotic Selection[1]	8	88%	98%	97%
Prophylactic Antibiotic Select. (Outpatient)	-	-	94%	94%
Prophylactic Antibiotic Stopped[1]	7	100%	95%	94%
Recommended VTP Ordered[1]	16	100%	94%	94%
Urinary Catheter Removal[1]	2	100%	91%	90%
Children's Asthma Care				
Received Systemic Corticosteroids	-	-	-	100%
Received Home Management Plan	-	-	-	71%
Received Reliever Medication	-	-	-	100%
Use of Medical Imaging				
Combination Abdominal CT Scan	-	-	0.164	0.191
Combination Chest CT Scan	-	-	0.038	0.054
Follow-up Mammogram/Ultrasound	-	-	8.4%	8.4%
MRI for Low Back Pain	-	-	30.2%	32.7%
Survey of Patients' Hospital Experiences				
Area Around Room 'Always' Quiet at Night	300+	44%	-	58%
Doctors 'Always' Communicated Well	300+	77%	-	80%
Home Recovery Information Given	300+	81%	-	82%
Hospital Given 9 or 10 on 10 Point Scale	300+	70%	-	67%
Meds 'Always' Explained Before Given	300+	62%	-	60%
Nurses 'Always' Communicated Well	300+	81%	-	76%
Pain 'Always' Well Controlled	300+	68%	-	69%
Room and Bathroom 'Always' Clean	300+	83%	-	71%
Timely Help 'Always' Received	300+	73%	-	64%
Would Definitely Recommend Hospital	300+	68%	-	69%

NOTE: Hospital profiles are in alphabetical order by state, then city, then hospital within the city; Rankings exclude hospitals with less than 25 cases except for patient surveys which excludes hospitals with less than 100 cases; (a) 100–299 cases; (1) The number of cases is too small to be sure how well a hospital is performing; (2) The hospital indicated that the data submitted for this measure were based on a sample of cases; (3) Data was collected during a shorter time period (fewer quarters) than the maximum possible time for this measure; (4) Suppressed for one or more quarters by CMS; (5) No data is available from the hospital for this measure; (6) Fewer than 100 patients completed the HCAHPS survey. Use these rates with caution, as the number of surveys may be too low to reliably assess hospital performance; (7) Survey results are based on less than 12 months of data; (8) Survey results are not available for this reporting period; (9) No or very few patients were eligible for the HCAHPS survey. The scores shown, if any, reflect a very small number of surveys; (10) A state average was not calculated because too few hospitals in the state submitted data; (11) There were discrepancies in the data collection process; Please refer to the User's Guide for a full explanation of data.

Van Wert County Hospital

1250 S Washington Street
Van Wert, OH 45891
URL: www.vanwerthospital.org
Type: Acute Care Hospitals
Ownership: Voluntary Non-Profit - Private
Phone: 419-238-8627
Fax: 419-238-2409

Emergency Services: Yes
Beds: 100

Key Personnel:
CEO/President . . . . Mark Minick
Chief of Medical Staff . . . . Eric Jelinger, MD
Infection Control . . . . Linner Kelly
Operating Room . . . . Brenda Wobler
Radiology . . . . Ashni Behal
Emergency Room . . . . Kathy Fischer

Measure	Cases	This Hosp.	State Avg.	U.S. Avg.
Heart Attack Care				
ACE Inhibitor or ARB for LVSD[1]	1	0%	97%	96%
Aspirin at Arrival[1]	10	100%	99%	99%
Aspirin at Discharge[1]	5	100%	99%	98%
Beta Blocker at Discharge[1]	6	100%	99%	98%
Fibrinolytic Medication Timing	0	-	14%	55%
PCI Within 90 Minutes of Arrival	0	-	92%	90%
Smoking Cessation Advice[1]	2	100%	100%	99%
Chest Pain/Possible Heart Attack Care				
Aspirin at Arrival	172	95%	96%	95%
Median Time to ECG (minutes)	176	13	7	8
Median Time to Transfer (minutes)[1,3]	5	85	61	61
Fibrinolytic Medication Timing[1]	7	29%	47%	54%
Heart Failure Care				
ACE Inhibitor or ARB for LVSD[1]	14	93%	96%	94%
Discharge Instructions	28	79%	91%	88%
Evaluation of LVS Function	53	98%	99%	98%
Smoking Cessation Advice[1]	7	86%	99%	98%
Pneumonia Care				
Appropriate Initial Antibiotic	65	92%	92%	92%
Blood Culture Timing	54	89%	96%	96%
Influenza Vaccine	32	88%	93%	91%
Initial Antibiotic Timing	64	98%	96%	95%
Pneumococcal Vaccine	52	87%	95%	93%
Smoking Cessation Advice[1]	13	92%	98%	97%
Surgical Care Improvement Project				
Appropriate VTP Within 24 Hours	62	81%	92%	92%
Appropriate Hair Removal	157	100%	100%	99%
Appropriate Beta Blocker Usage	56	100%	94%	93%
Controlled Postoperative Blood Glucose	0	-	94%	93%
Prophylactic Antibiotic Timing	113	93%	97%	97%
Prophylactic Antibiotic Timing (Outpatient)	88	97%	91%	92%
Prophylactic Antibiotic Selection	114	89%	98%	97%
Prophylactic Antibiotic Select. (Outpatient)	88	93%	94%	94%
Prophylactic Antibiotic Stopped	107	91%	95%	94%
Recommended VTP Ordered	62	81%	94%	94%
Urinary Catheter Removal[1]	17	94%	91%	90%
Children's Asthma Care				
Received Systemic Corticosteroids	-	-	-	100%
Received Home Management Plan	-	-	-	71%
Received Reliever Medication	-	-	-	100%
Use of Medical Imaging				
Combination Abdominal CT Scan	421	0.672	0.164	0.191
Combination Chest CT Scan	214	0.065	0.038	0.054
Follow-up Mammogram/Ultrasound	297	3.0%	8.4%	8.4%
MRI for Low Back Pain	70	27.1%	30.2%	32.7%
Survey of Patients' Hospital Experiences				
Area Around Room 'Always' Quiet at Night	300+	54%	-	58%
Doctors 'Always' Communicated Well	300+	81%	-	80%
Home Recovery Information Given	300+	87%	-	82%
Hospital Given 9 or 10 on 10 Point Scale	300+	68%	-	67%
Meds 'Always' Explained Before Given	300+	65%	-	60%
Nurses 'Always' Communicated Well	300+	78%	-	76%
Pain 'Always' Well Controlled	300+	73%	-	69%
Room and Bathroom 'Always' Clean	300+	79%	-	71%
Timely Help 'Always' Received	300+	68%	-	64%
Would Definitely Recommend Hospital	300+	65%	-	69%

Summa Wadsworth-Rittman Hospital

195 Wadsworth Road
Wadsworth, OH 44281
E-mail: prwrh@bright.net
URL: www.wrhospital.com
Type: Acute Care Hospitals
Ownership: Voluntary Non-Profit - Private
Phone: 330-334-1504
Fax: 330-336-0107

Emergency Services: Yes
Beds: 113

Key Personnel:
CEO/President . . . . James Pope
Chief of Medical Staff . . . . Jeffrey S Morris
Radiology . . . . Norman Crocker
Emergency Room . . . . Jay Carter

Measure	Cases	This Hosp.	State Avg.	U.S. Avg.
Heart Attack Care				
ACE Inhibitor or ARB for LVSD	0	-	97%	96%
Aspirin at Arrival[1]	9	100%	99%	99%
Aspirin at Discharge[1]	7	100%	99%	98%
Beta Blocker at Discharge[1]	5	100%	99%	98%
Fibrinolytic Medication Timing	0	-	14%	55%
PCI Within 90 Minutes of Arrival	0	-	92%	90%
Smoking Cessation Advice	0	-	100%	99%
Chest Pain/Possible Heart Attack Care				
Aspirin at Arrival	99	99%	96%	95%
Median Time to ECG (minutes)	102	4	7	8
Median Time to Transfer (minutes)[1]	16	44	61	61
Fibrinolytic Medication Timing	0	-	47%	54%
Heart Failure Care				
ACE Inhibitor or ARB for LVSD[1]	22	100%	96%	94%
Discharge Instructions	69	93%	91%	88%
Evaluation of LVS Function	87	99%	99%	98%
Smoking Cessation Advice[1]	5	100%	99%	98%
Pneumonia Care				
Appropriate Initial Antibiotic	103	93%	92%	92%
Blood Culture Timing	136	98%	96%	96%
Influenza Vaccine	70	96%	93%	91%
Initial Antibiotic Timing	118	97%	96%	95%
Pneumococcal Vaccine	87	98%	95%	93%
Smoking Cessation Advice	49	100%	98%	97%
Surgical Care Improvement Project				
Appropriate VTP Within 24 Hours	57	95%	92%	92%
Appropriate Hair Removal	172	100%	100%	99%
Appropriate Beta Blocker Usage	53	98%	94%	93%
Controlled Postoperative Blood Glucose	0	-	94%	93%
Prophylactic Antibiotic Timing	127	98%	97%	97%
Prophylactic Antibiotic Timing (Outpatient)	81	99%	91%	92%
Prophylactic Antibiotic Selection	127	99%	98%	97%
Prophylactic Antibiotic Select. (Outpatient)	80	99%	94%	94%
Prophylactic Antibiotic Stopped	124	96%	95%	94%
Recommended VTP Ordered	57	95%	94%	94%
Urinary Catheter Removal[1]	13	92%	91%	90%
Children's Asthma Care				
Received Systemic Corticosteroids	-	-	-	100%
Received Home Management Plan	-	-	-	71%
Received Reliever Medication	-	-	-	100%
Use of Medical Imaging				
Combination Abdominal CT Scan	415	0.101	0.164	0.191
Combination Chest CT Scan	276	0.025	0.038	0.054
Follow-up Mammogram/Ultrasound	639	2.8%	8.4%	8.4%
MRI for Low Back Pain	71	31.0%	30.2%	32.7%
Survey of Patients' Hospital Experiences				
Area Around Room 'Always' Quiet at Night	300+	40%	-	58%
Doctors 'Always' Communicated Well	300+	76%	-	80%
Home Recovery Information Given	300+	85%	-	82%
Hospital Given 9 or 10 on 10 Point Scale	300+	64%	-	67%
Meds 'Always' Explained Before Given	300+	54%	-	60%
Nurses 'Always' Communicated Well	300+	74%	-	76%
Pain 'Always' Well Controlled	300+	67%	-	69%
Room and Bathroom 'Always' Clean	300+	69%	-	71%
Timely Help 'Always' Received	300+	67%	-	64%
Would Definitely Recommend Hospital	300+	67%	-	69%

Saint Joseph Health Center

667 Eastland Ave SE
Warren, OH 44481
Type: Acute Care Hospitals
Ownership: Voluntary Non-Profit - Other
Phone: 330-841-4000

Emergency Services: Yes
Beds: 165

Key Personnel:
CEO/President . . . . Robert Shroder
Chief of Medical Staff . . . . Richard Weitzel, MD

Measure	Cases	This Hosp.	State Avg.	U.S. Avg.
Heart Attack Care				
ACE Inhibitor or ARB for LVSD[1]	5	100%	97%	96%
Aspirin at Arrival	46	100%	99%	99%
Aspirin at Discharge[1]	11	100%	99%	98%
Beta Blocker at Discharge[1]	15	100%	99%	98%
Fibrinolytic Medication Timing	0	-	14%	55%
PCI Within 90 Minutes of Arrival	0	-	92%	90%
Smoking Cessation Advice[1]	5	100%	100%	99%
Chest Pain/Possible Heart Attack Care				
Aspirin at Arrival	134	99%	96%	95%
Median Time to ECG (minutes)	139	5	7	8
Median Time to Transfer (minutes)	46	62	61	61
Fibrinolytic Medication Timing[1]	1	0%	47%	54%
Heart Failure Care				
ACE Inhibitor or ARB for LVSD[2]	71	97%	96%	94%
Discharge Instructions[2]	209	100%	91%	88%
Evaluation of LVS Function[2]	254	100%	99%	98%
Smoking Cessation Advice[2]	61	100%	99%	98%
Pneumonia Care				
Appropriate Initial Antibiotic[2]	90	94%	92%	92%
Blood Culture Timing[2]	80	99%	96%	96%
Influenza Vaccine[2]	83	95%	93%	91%
Initial Antibiotic Timing[2]	126	96%	96%	95%
Pneumococcal Vaccine[2]	103	96%	95%	93%
Smoking Cessation Advice[2]	67	100%	98%	97%
Surgical Care Improvement Project				
Appropriate VTP Within 24 Hours[2]	151	93%	92%	92%
Appropriate Hair Removal[2]	417	100%	100%	99%
Appropriate Beta Blocker Usage[2]	111	95%	94%	93%
Controlled Postoperative Blood Glucose[2]	0	-	94%	93%
Prophylactic Antibiotic Timing[2]	269	98%	97%	97%
Prophylactic Antibiotic Timing (Outpatient)	249	83%	91%	92%
Prophylactic Antibiotic Selection[2]	269	96%	98%	97%
Prophylactic Antibiotic Select. (Outpatient)	226	92%	94%	94%
Prophylactic Antibiotic Stopped[2]	253	98%	95%	94%
Recommended VTP Ordered[2]	151	95%	94%	94%
Urinary Catheter Removal[2]	63	97%	91%	90%
Children's Asthma Care				
Received Systemic Corticosteroids	-	-	-	100%
Received Home Management Plan	-	-	-	71%
Received Reliever Medication	-	-	-	100%
Use of Medical Imaging				
Combination Abdominal CT Scan	749	0.662	0.164	0.191
Combination Chest CT Scan	608	0.015	0.038	0.054
Follow-up Mammogram/Ultrasound	811	10.4%	8.4%	8.4%
MRI for Low Back Pain	153	24.2%	30.2%	32.7%
Survey of Patients' Hospital Experiences				
Area Around Room 'Always' Quiet at Night	300+	42%	-	58%
Doctors 'Always' Communicated Well	300+	78%	-	80%
Home Recovery Information Given	300+	82%	-	82%
Hospital Given 9 or 10 on 10 Point Scale	300+	68%	-	67%
Meds 'Always' Explained Before Given	300+	57%	-	60%
Nurses 'Always' Communicated Well	300+	72%	-	76%
Pain 'Always' Well Controlled	300+	64%	-	69%
Room and Bathroom 'Always' Clean	300+	64%	-	71%
Timely Help 'Always' Received	300+	57%	-	64%
Would Definitely Recommend Hospital	300+	73%	-	69%

Trumbull Memorial Hospital

1350 East Market Street Phone: 330-841-9820
Warren, OH 44482 Fax: 330-841-9281
URL: www.trumhosp.org
Type: Acute Care Hospitals Emergency Services: Yes
Ownership: Voluntary Non-Profit - Other Beds: 350

Key Personnel:
CEO/President. . . . . N Kristopher Hoce
Chief of Medical Staff. . . . . Yogesh Sheth, MD
Operating Room. . . . . Claudia Maksimoff, RN
Radiology. . . . . Thomas Groner, MD
Anesthesiology. . . . . Rickie Monroe, MD
Emergency Room . . . . JM Sudimack, MD
Intensive Care Unit. . . . . Martha Laurie, RN

Measure	Cases	This Hosp.	State Avg.	U.S. Avg.
Heart Attack Care				
ACE Inhibitor or ARB for LVSD	35	100%	97%	96%
Aspirin at Arrival	194	100%	99%	99%
Aspirin at Discharge	180	100%	99%	98%
Beta Blocker at Discharge	177	100%	99%	98%
Fibrinolytic Medication Timing[1]	1	0%	14%	55%
PCI Within 90 Minutes of Arrival	42	76%	92%	90%
Smoking Cessation Advice	61	100%	100%	99%
Chest Pain/Possible Heart Attack Care				
Aspirin at Arrival[1,3]	5	60%	96%	95%
Median Time to ECG (minutes)[1,3]	6	4	7	8
Median Time to Transfer (minutes)[5]	0	-	61	61
Fibrinolytic Medication Timing[3]	0	-	47%	54%
Heart Failure Care				
ACE Inhibitor or ARB for LVSD	117	100%	96%	94%
Discharge Instructions	408	74%	91%	88%
Evaluation of LVS Function	519	100%	99%	98%
Smoking Cessation Advice	84	100%	99%	98%
Pneumonia Care				
Appropriate Initial Antibiotic[2]	232	89%	92%	92%
Blood Culture Timing[2]	236	99%	96%	96%
Influenza Vaccine[2]	196	95%	93%	91%
Initial Antibiotic Timing[2]	280	91%	96%	95%
Pneumococcal Vaccine[2]	292	96%	95%	93%
Smoking Cessation Advice[2]	101	98%	98%	97%
Surgical Care Improvement Project				
Appropriate VTP Within 24 Hours[2]	196	85%	92%	92%
Appropriate Hair Removal[2]	699	99%	100%	99%
Appropriate Beta Blocker Usage[2]	201	89%	94%	93%
Controlled Postoperative Blood Glucose[2]	86	84%	94%	93%
Prophylactic Antibiotic Timing[2]	475	95%	97%	97%
Prophylactic Antibiotic Timing (Outpatient)	304	94%	91%	92%
Prophylactic Antibiotic Selection[2]	477	97%	98%	97%
Prophylactic Antibiotic Select. (Outpatient)	303	85%	94%	94%
Prophylactic Antibiotic Stopped[2]	463	97%	95%	94%
Recommended VTP Ordered[2]	197	89%	94%	94%
Urinary Catheter Removal[2]	57	79%	91%	90%
Children's Asthma Care				
Received Systemic Corticosteroids	-	-	-	100%
Received Home Management Plan	-	-	-	71%
Received Reliever Medication	-	-	-	100%
Use of Medical Imaging				
Combination Abdominal CT Scan	1,081	0.648	0.164	0.191
Combination Chest CT Scan	846	0.008	0.038	0.054
Follow-up Mammogram/Ultrasound	2,456	9.4%	8.4%	8.4%
MRI for Low Back Pain	218	26.6%	30.2%	32.7%
Survey of Patients' Hospital Experiences				
Area Around Room 'Always' Quiet at Night	300+	41%	-	58%
Doctors 'Always' Communicated Well	300+	77%	-	80%
Home Recovery Information Given	300+	80%	-	82%
Hospital Given 9 or 10 on 10 Point Scale	300+	54%	-	67%
Meds 'Always' Explained Before Given	300+	50%	-	60%
Nurses 'Always' Communicated Well	300+	67%	-	76%
Pain 'Always' Well Controlled	300+	59%	-	69%
Room and Bathroom 'Always' Clean	300+	56%	-	71%
Timely Help 'Always' Received	300+	55%	-	64%
Would Definitely Recommend Hospital	300+	57%	-	69%

South Pointe Hospital

20000 Harvard Road Phone: 216-491-6000
Warrensville Heights, OH 44122 Fax: 216-491-7260
URL: www.southpointehospital.org
Type: Acute Care Hospitals Emergency Services: Yes
Ownership: Voluntary Non-Profit - Other Beds: 232

Key Personnel:
CEO/President. . . . . Beverly Lozar
Cardiac Laboratory. . . . . Mark Pace
Chief of Medical Staff . . . . Charles Webb
Emergency Room . . . . Jonathan Klein

Measure	Cases	This Hosp.	State Avg.	U.S. Avg.
Heart Attack Care				
ACE Inhibitor or ARB for LVSD[1]	7	100%	97%	96%
Aspirin at Arrival	52	100%	99%	99%
Aspirin at Discharge	28	100%	99%	98%
Beta Blocker at Discharge	36	100%	99%	98%
Fibrinolytic Medication Timing	0	-	14%	55%
PCI Within 90 Minutes of Arrival	0	-	92%	90%
Smoking Cessation Advice[1]	7	100%	100%	99%
Chest Pain/Possible Heart Attack Care				
Aspirin at Arrival	398	98%	96%	95%
Median Time to ECG (minutes)	411	7	7	8
Median Time to Transfer (minutes)	29	60	61	61
Fibrinolytic Medication Timing	0	-	47%	54%
Heart Failure Care				
ACE Inhibitor or ARB for LVSD	137	99%	96%	94%
Discharge Instructions	301	99%	91%	88%
Evaluation of LVS Function	399	100%	99%	98%
Smoking Cessation Advice	98	100%	99%	98%
Pneumonia Care				
Appropriate Initial Antibiotic	118	95%	92%	92%
Blood Culture Timing	137	99%	96%	96%
Influenza Vaccine	146	97%	93%	91%
Initial Antibiotic Timing	244	98%	96%	95%
Pneumococcal Vaccine	200	98%	95%	93%
Smoking Cessation Advice	114	100%	98%	97%
Surgical Care Improvement Project				
Appropriate VTP Within 24 Hours	141	93%	92%	92%
Appropriate Hair Removal	305	100%	100%	99%
Appropriate Beta Blocker Usage	102	98%	94%	93%
Controlled Postoperative Blood Glucose	0	-	94%	93%
Prophylactic Antibiotic Timing	176	93%	97%	97%
Prophylactic Antibiotic Timing (Outpatient)	167	69%	91%	92%
Prophylactic Antibiotic Selection	176	95%	98%	97%
Prophylactic Antibiotic Select. (Outpatient)	134	82%	94%	94%
Prophylactic Antibiotic Stopped	169	96%	95%	94%
Recommended VTP Ordered	141	96%	94%	94%
Urinary Catheter Removal	76	84%	91%	90%
Children's Asthma Care				
Received Systemic Corticosteroids	-	-	-	100%
Received Home Management Plan	-	-	-	71%
Received Reliever Medication	-	-	-	100%
Use of Medical Imaging				
Combination Abdominal CT Scan	869	0.067	0.164	0.191
Combination Chest CT Scan	513	0.103	0.038	0.054
Follow-up Mammogram/Ultrasound	945	5.7%	8.4%	8.4%
MRI for Low Back Pain	141	31.9%	30.2%	32.7%
Survey of Patients' Hospital Experiences				
Area Around Room 'Always' Quiet at Night	300+	50%	-	58%
Doctors 'Always' Communicated Well	300+	74%	-	80%
Home Recovery Information Given	300+	80%	-	82%
Hospital Given 9 or 10 on 10 Point Scale	300+	60%	-	67%
Meds 'Always' Explained Before Given	300+	54%	-	60%
Nurses 'Always' Communicated Well	300+	70%	-	76%
Pain 'Always' Well Controlled	300+	66%	-	69%
Room and Bathroom 'Always' Clean	300+	63%	-	71%
Timely Help 'Always' Received	300+	60%	-	64%
Would Definitely Recommend Hospital	300+	59%	-	69%

Fayette County Memorial Hospital

1430 Columbus Avenue Phone: 740-333-1210
Washington Court House, OH 43160 Fax: 740-333-2998
E-mail: brenda_hughes@fcmh.org
Type: Critical Access Hospitals Emergency Services: Yes
Ownership: Government - Local Beds: 70

Key Personnel:
CEO/President. . . . . Lyndon Christman
Chief of Medical Staff . . . . Dale Reno, DO
Infection Control. . . . . Lin Glass, RN
Operating Room. . . . . Pam Melvin, RN
Quality Assurance . . . . Lin Glass, NR
Radiology. . . . . Steven R Mustric

Measure	Cases	This Hosp.	State Avg.	U.S. Avg.
Heart Attack Care				
ACE Inhibitor or ARB for LVSD[5]	0	-	97%	96%
Aspirin at Arrival[5]	0	-	99%	99%
Aspirin at Discharge[5]	0	-	99%	98%
Beta Blocker at Discharge[5]	0	-	99%	98%
Fibrinolytic Medication Timing[5]	0	-	14%	55%
PCI Within 90 Minutes of Arrival[5]	0	-	92%	90%
Smoking Cessation Advice[5]	0	-	100%	99%
Chest Pain/Possible Heart Attack Care				
Aspirin at Arrival	143	97%	96%	95%
Median Time to ECG (minutes)	153	6	7	8
Median Time to Transfer (minutes)[1]	8	58	61	61
Fibrinolytic Medication Timing[1]	4	25%	47%	54%
Heart Failure Care				
ACE Inhibitor or ARB for LVSD[1]	15	93%	96%	94%
Discharge Instructions	39	74%	91%	88%
Evaluation of LVS Function	45	93%	99%	98%
Smoking Cessation Advice[1]	10	100%	99%	98%
Pneumonia Care				
Appropriate Initial Antibiotic	37	92%	92%	92%
Blood Culture Timing	59	88%	96%	96%
Influenza Vaccine[1]	21	76%	93%	91%
Initial Antibiotic Timing	51	96%	96%	95%
Pneumococcal Vaccine	37	84%	95%	93%
Smoking Cessation Advice[1]	17	100%	98%	97%
Surgical Care Improvement Project				
Appropriate VTP Within 24 Hours[1,2]	12	100%	92%	92%
Appropriate Hair Removal[2]	28	100%	100%	99%
Appropriate Beta Blocker Usage[1,2]	10	90%	94%	93%
Controlled Postoperative Blood Glucose[2]	0	-	94%	93%
Prophylactic Antibiotic Timing[1,2]	15	100%	97%	97%
Prophylactic Antibiotic Timing (Outpatient)	61	92%	91%	92%
Prophylactic Antibiotic Selection[1,2]	15	100%	98%	97%
Prophylactic Antibiotic Select. (Outpatient)	58	98%	94%	94%
Prophylactic Antibiotic Stopped[1,2]	15	93%	95%	94%
Recommended VTP Ordered[1,2]	12	100%	94%	94%
Urinary Catheter Removal[1]	2	100%	91%	90%
Children's Asthma Care				
Received Systemic Corticosteroids	-	-	-	100%
Received Home Management Plan	-	-	-	71%
Received Reliever Medication	-	-	-	100%
Use of Medical Imaging				
Combination Abdominal CT Scan	343	0.044	0.164	0.191
Combination Chest CT Scan	176	0.006	0.038	0.054
Follow-up Mammogram/Ultrasound	344	10.8%	8.4%	8.4%
MRI for Low Back Pain[1]	32	37.5%	30.2%	32.7%
Survey of Patients' Hospital Experiences				
Area Around Room 'Always' Quiet at Night	(a)	53%	-	58%
Doctors 'Always' Communicated Well	(a)	75%	-	80%
Home Recovery Information Given	(a)	81%	-	82%
Hospital Given 9 or 10 on 10 Point Scale	(a)	59%	-	67%
Meds 'Always' Explained Before Given	(a)	61%	-	60%
Nurses 'Always' Communicated Well	(a)	76%	-	76%
Pain 'Always' Well Controlled	(a)	61%	-	69%
Room and Bathroom 'Always' Clean	(a)	74%	-	71%
Timely Help 'Always' Received	(a)	70%	-	64%
Would Definitely Recommend Hospital	(a)	54%	-	69%

NOTE: Hospital profiles are in alphabetical order by state, then city, then hospital within the city; Rankings exclude hospitals with less than 25 cases except for patient surveys which excludes hospitals with less than 100 cases; (a) 100–299 cases; (1) The number of cases is too small to be sure how well a hospital is performing; (2) The hospital indicated that the data submitted for this measure were based on a sample of cases; (3) Data was collected during a shorter time period (fewer quarters) than the maximum possible time for this measure; (4) Suppressed for one or more quarters by CMS; (5) No data is available from the hospital for this measure; (6) Fewer than 100 patients completed the HCAHPS survey. Use these rates with caution, as the number of surveys may be too low to reliably assess hospital performance; (7) Survey results are based on less than 12 months of data; (8) Survey results are not available for this reporting period; (9) No or very few patients were eligible for the HCAHPS survey. The scores shown, if any, reflect a very small number of surveys; (10) A state average was not calculated because too few hospitals in the state submitted data; (11) There were discrepancies in the data collection process; Please refer to the User's Guide for a full explanation of data.

Fulton County Health Center

725 South Shoop Avenue	Phone: 419-335-2015
Wauseon, OH 43567	Fax: 419-330-2602
Type: Critical Access Hospitals	Emergency Services: Yes
Ownership: Voluntary Non-Profit - Private	Beds: 119

Key Personnel:
CEO/President. . . . . Dean Beck, MD
Chief of Medical Staff . . . . Jana Bourn
Radiology. . . . . John Patrick Ewonus

Measure	Cases	This Hosp.	State Avg.	U.S. Avg.
Heart Attack Care				
ACE Inhibitor or ARB for LVSD[1,3]	1	100%	97%	96%
Aspirin at Arrival[1,3]	5	80%	99%	99%
Aspirin at Discharge[1,3]	4	100%	99%	98%
Beta Blocker at Discharge[1,3]	5	100%	99%	98%
Fibrinolytic Medication Timing[3]	0	-	14%	55%
PCI Within 90 Minutes of Arrival[3]	0	-	92%	90%
Smoking Cessation Advice[1,3]	1	100%	100%	99%
Chest Pain/Possible Heart Attack Care				
Aspirin at Arrival	107	74%	96%	95%
Median Time to ECG (minutes)	114	15	7	8
Median Time to Transfer (minutes)[1,3]	3	143	61	61
Fibrinolytic Medication Timing	0	-	47%	54%
Heart Failure Care				
ACE Inhibitor or ARB for LVSD[1]	14	79%	96%	94%
Discharge Instructions	26	69%	91%	88%
Evaluation of LVS Function	37	81%	99%	98%
Smoking Cessation Advice[1]	2	100%	99%	98%
Pneumonia Care				
Appropriate Initial Antibiotic	40	100%	92%	92%
Blood Culture Timing	39	85%	96%	96%
Influenza Vaccine	34	91%	93%	91%
Initial Antibiotic Timing	51	98%	96%	95%
Pneumococcal Vaccine	48	94%	95%	93%
Smoking Cessation Advice[1]	13	92%	98%	97%
Surgical Care Improvement Project				
Appropriate VTP Within 24 Hours	50	66%	92%	92%
Appropriate Hair Removal	263	100%	100%	99%
Appropriate Beta Blocker Usage	92	79%	94%	93%
Controlled Postoperative Blood Glucose	0	-	94%	93%
Prophylactic Antibiotic Timing	208	96%	97%	97%
Prophylactic Antibiotic Timing (Outpatient)	141	70%	91%	92%
Prophylactic Antibiotic Selection	208	98%	98%	97%
Prophylactic Antibiotic Select. (Outpatient)	121	74%	94%	94%
Prophylactic Antibiotic Stopped	206	98%	95%	94%
Recommended VTP Ordered	50	82%	94%	94%
Urinary Catheter Removal[1]	6	67%	91%	90%
Children's Asthma Care				
Received Systemic Corticosteroids	-	-	-	100%
Received Home Management Plan	-	-	-	71%
Received Reliever Medication	-	-	-	100%
Use of Medical Imaging				
Combination Abdominal CT Scan	387	0.173	0.164	0.191
Combination Chest CT Scan	217	0.041	0.038	0.054
Follow-up Mammogram/Ultrasound	512	3.9%	8.4%	8.4%
MRI for Low Back Pain[1]	55	25.5%	30.2%	32.7%
Survey of Patients' Hospital Experiences				
Area Around Room 'Always' Quiet at Night	300+	50%	-	58%
Doctors 'Always' Communicated Well	300+	80%	-	80%
Home Recovery Information Given	300+	85%	-	82%
Hospital Given 9 or 10 on 10 Point Scale	300+	73%	-	67%
Meds 'Always' Explained Before Given	300+	58%	-	60%
Nurses 'Always' Communicated Well	300+	74%	-	76%
Pain 'Always' Well Controlled	300+	72%	-	69%
Room and Bathroom 'Always' Clean	300+	84%	-	71%
Timely Help 'Always' Received	300+	68%	-	64%
Would Definitely Recommend Hospital	300+	72%	-	69%

Pike Community Hospital

100 Dawn Lane	Phone: 740-947-2186
Waverly, OH 45690	Fax: 740-947-6538
E-mail: pch1@bright.net
Type: Critical Access Hospitals	Emergency Services: Yes
Ownership: Voluntary Non-Profit - Private	Beds: 63

Key Personnel:
CEO/President. . . . . Richard E Sobota
Chief of Medical Staff . . . . David Roddy, MD
Infection Control . . . . Angela Pelphrey, RN
Operating Room. . . . . Pam Brown
Quality Assurance . . . . John Kovacic
Emergency Room . . . . Nikki McKee, RN

Measure	Cases	This Hosp.	State Avg.	U.S. Avg.
Heart Attack Care				
ACE Inhibitor or ARB for LVSD[5]	0	-	97%	96%
Aspirin at Arrival[5]	0	-	99%	99%
Aspirin at Discharge[5]	0	-	99%	98%
Beta Blocker at Discharge[5]	0	-	99%	98%
Fibrinolytic Medication Timing[5]	0	-	14%	55%
PCI Within 90 Minutes of Arrival[5]	0	-	92%	90%
Smoking Cessation Advice[5]	0	-	100%	99%
Chest Pain/Possible Heart Attack Care				
Aspirin at Arrival	-	-	96%	95%
Median Time to ECG (minutes)	-	-	7	8
Median Time to Transfer (minutes)	-	-	61	61
Fibrinolytic Medication Timing	-	-	47%	54%
Heart Failure Care				
ACE Inhibitor or ARB for LVSD[1]	11	82%	96%	94%
Discharge Instructions[1]	23	91%	91%	88%
Evaluation of LVS Function	39	44%	99%	98%
Smoking Cessation Advice[1]	1	100%	99%	98%
Pneumonia Care				
Appropriate Initial Antibiotic	40	85%	92%	92%
Blood Culture Timing	58	95%	96%	96%
Influenza Vaccine[1]	21	95%	93%	91%
Initial Antibiotic Timing	61	95%	96%	95%
Pneumococcal Vaccine	41	68%	95%	93%
Smoking Cessation Advice[1]	7	86%	98%	97%
Surgical Care Improvement Project				
Appropriate VTP Within 24 Hours[5]	0	-	92%	92%
Appropriate Hair Removal[5]	0	-	100%	99%
Appropriate Beta Blocker Usage[5]	0	-	94%	93%
Controlled Postoperative Blood Glucose[5]	0	-	94%	93%
Prophylactic Antibiotic Timing[5]	0	-	97%	97%
Prophylactic Antibiotic Timing (Outpatient)	-	-	91%	92%
Prophylactic Antibiotic Selection[5]	0	-	98%	97%
Prophylactic Antibiotic Select. (Outpatient)	-	-	94%	94%
Prophylactic Antibiotic Stopped[5]	0	-	95%	94%
Recommended VTP Ordered[5]	0	-	94%	94%
Urinary Catheter Removal[5]	0	-	91%	90%
Children's Asthma Care				
Received Systemic Corticosteroids	-	-	-	100%
Received Home Management Plan	-	-	-	71%
Received Reliever Medication	-	-	-	100%
Use of Medical Imaging				
Combination Abdominal CT Scan	-	-	0.164	0.191
Combination Chest CT Scan	-	-	0.038	0.054
Follow-up Mammogram/Ultrasound	-	-	8.4%	8.4%
MRI for Low Back Pain	-	-	30.2%	32.7%
Survey of Patients' Hospital Experiences				
Area Around Room 'Always' Quiet at Night[8]	-	-	-	58%
Doctors 'Always' Communicated Well[8]	-	-	-	80%
Home Recovery Information Given[8]	-	-	-	82%
Hospital Given 9 or 10 on 10 Point Scale[8]	-	-	-	67%
Meds 'Always' Explained Before Given[8]	-	-	-	60%
Nurses 'Always' Communicated Well[8]	-	-	-	76%
Pain 'Always' Well Controlled[8]	-	-	-	69%
Room and Bathroom 'Always' Clean[8]	-	-	-	71%
Timely Help 'Always' Received[8]	-	-	-	64%
Would Definitely Recommend Hospital[8]	-	-	-	69%

University Pointe Surgical Hospital

7750 University Court	Phone: 513-475-8300
West Chester, OH 45069	Fax: 513-475-8301
E-mail: upsh-info@uchealth.com
URL: www.uchealth.com/surgical hospital
Type: Acute Care Hospitals	Emergency Services: No
Ownership: Voluntary Non-Profit - Other	Beds: 8

Key Personnel:
Chief of Medical Staff . . . . Lesley Gilbertson

Measure	Cases	This Hosp.	State Avg.	U.S. Avg.
Heart Attack Care				
ACE Inhibitor or ARB for LVSD[5]	0	-	97%	96%
Aspirin at Arrival[5]	0	-	99%	99%
Aspirin at Discharge[5]	0	-	99%	98%
Beta Blocker at Discharge[5]	0	-	99%	98%
Fibrinolytic Medication Timing[5]	0	-	14%	55%
PCI Within 90 Minutes of Arrival[5]	0	-	92%	90%
Smoking Cessation Advice[5]	0	-	100%	99%
Chest Pain/Possible Heart Attack Care				
Aspirin at Arrival[5]	0	-	96%	95%
Median Time to ECG (minutes)[5]	0	-	7	8
Median Time to Transfer (minutes)[5]	0	-	61	61
Fibrinolytic Medication Timing[5]	0	-	47%	54%
Heart Failure Care				
ACE Inhibitor or ARB for LVSD[5]	0	-	96%	94%
Discharge Instructions[5]	0	-	91%	88%
Evaluation of LVS Function[5]	0	-	99%	98%
Smoking Cessation Advice[5]	0	-	99%	98%
Pneumonia Care				
Appropriate Initial Antibiotic[5]	0	-	92%	92%
Blood Culture Timing[5]	0	-	96%	96%
Influenza Vaccine[5]	0	-	93%	91%
Initial Antibiotic Timing[5]	0	-	96%	95%
Pneumococcal Vaccine[5]	0	-	95%	93%
Smoking Cessation Advice[5]	0	-	98%	97%
Surgical Care Improvement Project				
Appropriate VTP Within 24 Hours[2,3]	0	-	92%	92%
Appropriate Hair Removal[1,2,3]	5	100%	100%	99%
Appropriate Beta Blocker Usage[2,3]	0	-	94%	93%
Controlled Postoperative Blood Glucose[2,3]	0	-	94%	93%
Prophylactic Antibiotic Timing[1,2,3]	4	100%	97%	97%
Prophylactic Antibiotic Timing (Outpatient)[1,3]	8	100%	91%	92%
Prophylactic Antibiotic Selection[1,2,3]	4	25%	98%	97%
Prophylactic Antibiotic Select. (Outpatient)[1,3]	8	88%	94%	94%
Prophylactic Antibiotic Stopped[1,2,3]	4	100%	95%	94%
Recommended VTP Ordered[2,3]	0	-	94%	94%
Urinary Catheter Removal[3]	0	-	91%	90%
Children's Asthma Care				
Received Systemic Corticosteroids	-	-	-	100%
Received Home Management Plan	-	-	-	71%
Received Reliever Medication	-	-	-	100%
Use of Medical Imaging				
Combination Abdominal CT Scan	267	0.105	0.164	0.191
Combination Chest CT Scan	326	0.009	0.038	0.054
Follow-up Mammogram/Ultrasound	139	12.9%	8.4%	8.4%
MRI for Low Back Pain	56	42.9%	30.2%	32.7%
Survey of Patients' Hospital Experiences				
Area Around Room 'Always' Quiet at Night[6]	<100	93%	-	58%
Doctors 'Always' Communicated Well[6]	<100	93%	-	80%
Home Recovery Information Given[6]	<100	92%	-	82%
Hospital Given 9 or 10 on 10 Point Scale[6]	<100	93%	-	67%
Meds 'Always' Explained Before Given[6]	<100	70%	-	60%
Nurses 'Always' Communicated Well[6]	<100	95%	-	76%
Pain 'Always' Well Controlled[6]	<100	83%	-	69%
Room and Bathroom 'Always' Clean[6]	<100	92%	-	71%
Timely Help 'Always' Received[6]	<100	92%	-	64%
Would Definitely Recommend Hospital	<100	89%	-	69%

NOTE: Hospital profiles are in alphabetical order by state, then city, then hospital within the city; Rankings exclude hospitals with less than 25 cases except for patient surveys which excludes hospitals with less than 100 cases; (a) 100–299 cases; (1) The number of cases is too small to be sure how well a hospital is performing; (2) The hospital indicated that the data submitted for this measure were based on a sample of cases; (3) Data was collected during a shorter time period (fewer quarters) than the maximum possible time for this measure; (4) Suppressed for one or more quarters by CMS; (5) No data is available from the hospital for this measure; (6) Fewer than 100 patients completed the HCAHPS survey. Use these rates with caution, as the number of surveys may be too low to reliably assess hospital performance; (7) Survey results are based on less than 12 months of data; (8) Survey results are not available for this reporting period; (9) No or very few patients were eligible for the HCAHPS survey. The scores shown, if any, reflect a very small number of surveys; (10) A state average was not calculated because too few hospitals in the state submitted data; (11) There were discrepancies in the data collection process; Please refer to the User's Guide for a full explanation of data.

West Chester Medical Center

7700 University Drive Phone: 513-298-7700
West Chester, OH 45069
URL: westchesterhospital.uchealth.com
Type: Acute Care Hospitals Emergency Services: No
Ownership: Voluntary Non-Profit - Private

Key Personnel:

President/CEO.............. Kevin Joseph, MD
Cardiology.................. Mohamed Effat, MD
Radiology.................. Tom Brown, MD
Emergency.................. Elizabeth Leenellet, MD

Measure	Cases	This Hosp.	State Avg.	U.S. Avg.
Heart Attack Care				
ACE Inhibitor or ARB for LVSD[1]	2	100%	97%	96%
Aspirin at Arrival[1]	15	100%	99%	99%
Aspirin at Discharge[1]	10	100%	99%	98%
Beta Blocker at Discharge[1]	9	89%	99%	98%
Fibrinolytic Medication Timing[1]	1	100%	14%	55%
PCI Within 90 Minutes of Arrival	0	-	92%	90%
Smoking Cessation Advice[1]	3	100%	100%	99%
Chest Pain/Possible Heart Attack Care				
Aspirin at Arrival	46	98%	96%	95%
Median Time to ECG (minutes)	47	11	7	8
Median Time to Transfer (minutes)[1]	9	65	61	61
Fibrinolytic Medication Timing[1]	2	0%	47%	54%
Heart Failure Care				
ACE Inhibitor or ARB for LVSD	40	98%	96%	94%
Discharge Instructions	64	95%	91%	88%
Evaluation of LVS Function	102	99%	99%	98%
Smoking Cessation Advice[1]	10	100%	99%	98%
Pneumonia Care				
Appropriate Initial Antibiotic	77	86%	92%	92%
Blood Culture Timing	128	97%	96%	96%
Influenza Vaccine	60	93%	93%	91%
Initial Antibiotic Timing	85	94%	96%	95%
Pneumococcal Vaccine	96	94%	95%	93%
Smoking Cessation Advice	39	92%	98%	97%
Surgical Care Improvement Project				
Appropriate VTP Within 24 Hours	130	92%	92%	92%
Appropriate Hair Removal	402	100%	100%	99%
Appropriate Beta Blocker Usage	111	89%	94%	93%
Controlled Postoperative Blood Glucose	0	-	94%	93%
Prophylactic Antibiotic Timing	297	98%	97%	97%
Prophylactic Antibiotic Timing (Outpatient)	67	94%	91%	92%
Prophylactic Antibiotic Selection	300	98%	98%	97%
Prophylactic Antibiotic Select. (Outpatient)	65	100%	94%	94%
Prophylactic Antibiotic Stopped	288	98%	95%	94%
Recommended VTP Ordered	130	95%	94%	94%
Urinary Catheter Removal	145	97%	91%	90%
Children's Asthma Care				
Received Systemic Corticosteroids	-	-	-	100%
Received Home Management Plan	-	-	-	71%
Received Reliever Medication	-	-	-	100%
Use of Medical Imaging				
Combination Abdominal CT Scan[5]	0	-	0.164	0.191
Combination Chest CT Scan[5]	0	-	0.038	0.054
Follow-up Mammogram/Ultrasound[5]	0	-	8.4%	8.4%
MRI for Low Back Pain[5]	0	-	30.2%	32.7%
Survey of Patients' Hospital Experiences				
Area Around Room 'Always' Quiet at Night	300+	71%	-	58%
Doctors 'Always' Communicated Well	300+	79%	-	80%
Home Recovery Information Given	300+	85%	-	82%
Hospital Given 9 or 10 on 10 Point Scale	300+	80%	-	67%
Meds 'Always' Explained Before Given	300+	61%	-	60%
Nurses 'Always' Communicated Well	300+	81%	-	76%
Pain 'Always' Well Controlled	300+	74%	-	69%
Room and Bathroom 'Always' Clean	300+	73%	-	71%
Timely Help 'Always' Received	300+	65%	-	64%
Would Definitely Recommend Hospital	300+	85%	-	69%

Mount Carmel St Ann's Hospital

500 South Cleveland Avenue Phone: 614-546-4533
Westerville, OH 43081 Fax: 614-898-8668
URL: www.mchs.com
Type: Acute Care Hospitals Emergency Services: Yes
Ownership: Voluntary Non-Profit - Church Beds: 180

Key Personnel:

CEO/President.............. Joseph Calvaruso
Chief of Medical Staff.......... Frank Orth
Infection Control.............. Barbara Shaw
Operating Room.............. Pam Evans
Pediatric Ambulatory Care ...... Steve Lindner, MD
Pediatric In-Patient Care .... Steve Lindner, MD
Quality Assurance .... Judy Marshall
Radiology.................. Guillermo A Arbona

Measure	Cases	This Hosp.	State Avg.	U.S. Avg.
Heart Attack Care				
ACE Inhibitor or ARB for LVSD[1]	10	100%	97%	96%
Aspirin at Arrival	118	100%	99%	99%
Aspirin at Discharge	88	100%	99%	98%
Beta Blocker at Discharge	83	99%	99%	98%
Fibrinolytic Medication Timing	0	-	14%	55%
PCI Within 90 Minutes of Arrival	33	97%	92%	90%
Smoking Cessation Advice[1]	23	100%	100%	99%
Chest Pain/Possible Heart Attack Care				
Aspirin at Arrival	30	93%	96%	95%
Median Time to ECG (minutes)	30	4	7	8
Median Time to Transfer (minutes)[3]	0	-	61	61
Fibrinolytic Medication Timing[3]	0	-	47%	54%
Heart Failure Care				
ACE Inhibitor or ARB for LVSD	97	100%	96%	94%
Discharge Instructions	247	91%	91%	88%
Evaluation of LVS Function	337	100%	99%	98%
Smoking Cessation Advice	44	100%	99%	98%
Pneumonia Care				
Appropriate Initial Antibiotic[2]	173	96%	92%	92%
Blood Culture Timing[2]	243	97%	96%	96%
Influenza Vaccine[2]	111	81%	93%	91%
Initial Antibiotic Timing[2]	231	97%	96%	95%
Pneumococcal Vaccine[2]	160	89%	95%	93%
Smoking Cessation Advice[2]	96	99%	98%	97%
Surgical Care Improvement Project				
Appropriate VTP Within 24 Hours[2]	150	97%	92%	92%
Appropriate Hair Removal[2]	553	100%	100%	99%
Appropriate Beta Blocker Usage[2]	193	96%	94%	93%
Controlled Postoperative Blood Glucose[2]	0	-	94%	93%
Prophylactic Antibiotic Timing[2]	380	99%	97%	97%
Prophylactic Antibiotic Timing (Outpatient)	240	61%	91%	92%
Prophylactic Antibiotic Selection[2]	380	98%	98%	97%
Prophylactic Antibiotic Select. (Outpatient)	149	91%	94%	94%
Prophylactic Antibiotic Stopped[2]	364	96%	95%	94%
Recommended VTP Ordered[2]	150	99%	94%	94%
Urinary Catheter Removal[2]	104	92%	91%	90%
Children's Asthma Care				
Received Systemic Corticosteroids	-	-	-	100%
Received Home Management Plan	-	-	-	71%
Received Reliever Medication	-	-	-	100%
Use of Medical Imaging				
Combination Abdominal CT Scan	815	0.060	0.164	0.191
Combination Chest CT Scan	354	0.011	0.038	0.054
Follow-up Mammogram/Ultrasound	1,369	8.7%	8.4%	8.4%
MRI for Low Back Pain	122	33.6%	30.2%	32.7%
Survey of Patients' Hospital Experiences				
Area Around Room 'Always' Quiet at Night	300+	49%	-	58%
Doctors 'Always' Communicated Well	300+	78%	-	80%
Home Recovery Information Given	300+	83%	-	82%
Hospital Given 9 or 10 on 10 Point Scale	300+	68%	-	67%
Meds 'Always' Explained Before Given	300+	56%	-	60%
Nurses 'Always' Communicated Well	300+	74%	-	76%
Pain 'Always' Well Controlled	300+	68%	-	69%
Room and Bathroom 'Always' Clean	300+	63%	-	71%
Timely Help 'Always' Received	300+	61%	-	64%
Would Definitely Recommend Hospital	300+	71%	-	69%

Saint John Medical Center

29000 Center Ridge Road Phone: 440-835-8000
Westlake, OH 44145 Fax: 440-827-5283
URL: www.sjws.net
Type: Acute Care Hospitals Emergency Services: Yes
Ownership: Voluntary Non-Profit - Private Beds: 200

Key Personnel:

CEO/President.............. Cliff J Coker
Cardiac Laboratory............ Ken Nodes
Chief of Medical Staff.......... Philip Blitz, DO
Operating Room.............. Adnan Mourany
Pediatric Ambulatory Care ...... Ararind DePauly
Pediatric In-Patient Care .... Ararind DePauly
Radiology.................. Robert Konstan
Emergency Room .... Leslie Bush

Measure	Cases	This Hosp.	State Avg.	U.S. Avg.
Heart Attack Care				
ACE Inhibitor or ARB for LVSD[1,2]	20	100%	97%	96%
Aspirin at Arrival[2]	214	100%	99%	99%
Aspirin at Discharge[2]	190	100%	99%	98%
Beta Blocker at Discharge[2]	194	100%	99%	98%
Fibrinolytic Medication Timing[2]	0	-	14%	55%
PCI Within 90 Minutes of Arrival[2]	44	100%	92%	90%
Smoking Cessation Advice[2]	70	100%	100%	99%
Chest Pain/Possible Heart Attack Care				
Aspirin at Arrival	36	97%	96%	95%
Median Time to ECG (minutes)	38	5	7	8
Median Time to Transfer (minutes)[5]	0	-	61	61
Fibrinolytic Medication Timing[5]	0	-	47%	54%
Heart Failure Care				
ACE Inhibitor or ARB for LVSD[2]	40	90%	96%	94%
Discharge Instructions[2]	143	100%	91%	88%
Evaluation of LVS Function[2]	206	100%	99%	98%
Smoking Cessation Advice[1,2]	17	100%	99%	98%
Pneumonia Care				
Appropriate Initial Antibiotic[2]	98	96%	92%	92%
Blood Culture Timing[2]	137	96%	96%	96%
Influenza Vaccine[2]	62	95%	93%	91%
Initial Antibiotic Timing[2]	142	98%	96%	95%
Pneumococcal Vaccine[2]	110	98%	95%	93%
Smoking Cessation Advice[2]	41	100%	98%	97%
Surgical Care Improvement Project				
Appropriate VTP Within 24 Hours[2]	160	87%	92%	92%
Appropriate Hair Removal[2]	417	100%	100%	99%
Appropriate Beta Blocker Usage[2]	148	97%	94%	93%
Controlled Postoperative Blood Glucose[2]	51	96%	94%	93%
Prophylactic Antibiotic Timing[2]	285	95%	97%	97%
Prophylactic Antibiotic Timing (Outpatient)	276	96%	91%	92%
Prophylactic Antibiotic Selection[2]	289	99%	98%	97%
Prophylactic Antibiotic Select. (Outpatient)	269	88%	94%	94%
Prophylactic Antibiotic Stopped[2]	265	94%	95%	94%
Recommended VTP Ordered[2]	160	87%	94%	94%
Urinary Catheter Removal[2]	114	92%	91%	90%
Children's Asthma Care				
Received Systemic Corticosteroids[2]	28	100%	-	100%
Received Home Management Plan[1]	24	83%	-	71%
Received Reliever Medication[2]	28	100%	-	100%
Use of Medical Imaging				
Combination Abdominal CT Scan	526	0.057	0.164	0.191
Combination Chest CT Scan	519	0.000	0.038	0.054
Follow-up Mammogram/Ultrasound	648	10.2%	8.4%	8.4%
MRI for Low Back Pain	62	33.9%	30.2%	32.7%
Survey of Patients' Hospital Experiences				
Area Around Room 'Always' Quiet at Night	300+	56%	-	58%
Doctors 'Always' Communicated Well	300+	78%	-	80%
Home Recovery Information Given	300+	86%	-	82%
Hospital Given 9 or 10 on 10 Point Scale	300+	71%	-	67%
Meds 'Always' Explained Before Given	300+	56%	-	60%
Nurses 'Always' Communicated Well	300+	74%	-	76%
Pain 'Always' Well Controlled	300+	69%	-	69%
Room and Bathroom 'Always' Clean	300+	65%	-	71%
Timely Help 'Always' Received	300+	59%	-	64%
Would Definitely Recommend Hospital	300+	72%	-	69%

NOTE: Hospital profiles are in alphabetical order by state, then city, then hospital within the city; Rankings exclude hospitals with less than 25 cases except for patient surveys which excludes hospitals with less than 100 cases; (a) 100–299 cases; (1) The number of cases is too small to be sure how well a hospital is performing; (2) The hospital indicated that the data submitted for this measure were based on a sample of cases; (3) Data was collected during a shorter time period (fewer quarters) than the maximum possible time for this measure; (4) Suppressed for one or more quarters by CMS; (5) No data is available from the hospital for this measure; (6) Fewer than 100 patients completed the HCAHPS survey. Use these rates with caution, as the number of surveys may be too low to reliably assess hospital performance; (7) Survey results are based on less than 12 months of data; (8) Survey results are not available for this reporting period; (9) No or very few patients were eligible for the HCAHPS survey. The scores shown, if any, reflect a very small number of surveys; (10) A state average was not calculated because too few hospitals in the state submitted data; (11) There were discrepancies in the data collection process; Please refer to the User's Guide for a full explanation of data.

Mercy Hospital of Willard

110 E Howard St
Willard, OH 44890
Phone: 419-964-5000

Type: Critical Access Hospitals
Emergency Services: Yes
Ownership: Voluntary Non-Profit - Other
Beds: 25

Key Personnel:
CEO/President............... Lynn Detterman

Measure	Cases	This Hosp.	State Avg.	U.S. Avg.
Heart Attack Care				
ACE Inhibitor or ARB for LVSD[3]	0	-	97%	96%
Aspirin at Arrival[3]	0	-	99%	99%
Aspirin at Discharge[3]	0	-	99%	98%
Beta Blocker at Discharge[3]	0	-	99%	98%
Fibrinolytic Medication Timing[3]	0	-	14%	55%
PCI Within 90 Minutes of Arrival[3]	0	-	92%	90%
Smoking Cessation Advice[3]	0	-	100%	99%
Chest Pain/Possible Heart Attack Care				
Aspirin at Arrival[5]	0	-	96%	95%
Median Time to ECG (minutes)[5]	0	-	7	8
Median Time to Transfer (minutes)[5]	0	-	61	61
Fibrinolytic Medication Timing[5]	0	-	47%	54%
Heart Failure Care				
ACE Inhibitor or ARB for LVSD[1]	10	90%	96%	94%
Discharge Instructions[1]	20	100%	91%	88%
Evaluation of LVS Function[1]	23	100%	99%	98%
Smoking Cessation Advice[1]	6	100%	99%	98%
Pneumonia Care				
Appropriate Initial Antibiotic[1]	18	89%	92%	92%
Blood Culture Timing[1]	19	100%	96%	96%
Influenza Vaccine[1]	16	100%	93%	91%
Initial Antibiotic Timing[1]	20	100%	96%	95%
Pneumococcal Vaccine[1]	19	100%	95%	93%
Smoking Cessation Advice[1]	6	100%	98%	97%
Surgical Care Improvement Project				
Appropriate VTP Within 24 Hours[1]	12	92%	92%	92%
Appropriate Hair Removal	42	100%	100%	99%
Appropriate Beta Blocker Usage[5]	0	-	94%	93%
Controlled Postoperative Blood Glucose	0	-	94%	93%
Prophylactic Antibiotic Timing	35	94%	97%	97%
Prophylactic Antibiotic Timing (Outpatient)[5]	0	-	91%	92%
Prophylactic Antibiotic Selection	36	97%	98%	97%
Prophylactic Antibiotic Select. (Outpatient)[5]	0	-	94%	94%
Prophylactic Antibiotic Stopped	33	100%	95%	94%
Recommended VTP Ordered[1]	12	92%	94%	94%
Urinary Catheter Removal[1]	5	100%	91%	90%
Children's Asthma Care				
Received Systemic Corticosteroids	-	-	-	100%
Received Home Management Plan	-	-	-	71%
Received Reliever Medication	-	-	-	100%
Use of Medical Imaging				
Combination Abdominal CT Scan	139	0.281	0.164	0.191
Combination Chest CT Scan	72	0.056	0.038	0.054
Follow-up Mammogram/Ultrasound	261	5.7%	8.4%	8.4%
MRI for Low Back Pain[1]	21	33.3%	30.2%	32.7%
Survey of Patients' Hospital Experiences				
Area Around Room 'Always' Quiet at Night	(a)	57%	-	58%
Doctors 'Always' Communicated Well	(a)	93%	-	80%
Home Recovery Information Given	(a)	90%	-	82%
Hospital Given 9 or 10 on 10 Point Scale	(a)	85%	-	67%
Meds 'Always' Explained Before Given	(a)	73%	-	60%
Nurses 'Always' Communicated Well	(a)	87%	-	76%
Pain 'Always' Well Controlled	(a)	84%	-	69%
Room and Bathroom 'Always' Clean	(a)	85%	-	71%
Timely Help 'Always' Received	(a)	84%	-	64%
Would Definitely Recommend Hospital	(a)	84%	-	69%

CMH Regional Health System

610 West Main Street
Wilmington, OH 45177
Phone: 937-382-6611
Fax: 937-382-9278

E-mail: clintonmemorialhospital@in-touch.net
Type: Acute Care Hospitals
Emergency Services: Yes
Ownership: Government - Local
Beds: 150

Key Personnel:
CEO/President............... Tim Crowley
Chief of Medical Staff......... Phillip Aschi
Radiology................... Richard L Conti

Measure	Cases	This Hosp.	State Avg.	U.S. Avg.
Heart Attack Care				
ACE Inhibitor or ARB for LVSD[1]	4	100%	97%	96%
Aspirin at Arrival[1]	18	100%	99%	99%
Aspirin at Discharge[1]	12	100%	99%	98%
Beta Blocker at Discharge[1]	13	100%	99%	98%
Fibrinolytic Medication Timing	0	-	14%	55%
PCI Within 90 Minutes of Arrival	0	-	92%	90%
Smoking Cessation Advice[1]	1	100%	100%	99%
Chest Pain/Possible Heart Attack Care				
Aspirin at Arrival	97	98%	96%	95%
Median Time to ECG (minutes)	110	10	7	8
Median Time to Transfer (minutes)[1]	21	102	61	61
Fibrinolytic Medication Timing[1]	1	0%	47%	54%
Heart Failure Care				
ACE Inhibitor or ARB for LVSD	40	100%	96%	94%
Discharge Instructions	130	100%	91%	88%
Evaluation of LVS Function	160	99%	99%	98%
Smoking Cessation Advice	25	100%	99%	98%
Pneumonia Care				
Appropriate Initial Antibiotic	82	87%	92%	92%
Blood Culture Timing	130	97%	96%	96%
Influenza Vaccine	95	96%	93%	91%
Initial Antibiotic Timing	121	97%	96%	95%
Pneumococcal Vaccine	115	99%	95%	93%
Smoking Cessation Advice	26	96%	98%	97%
Surgical Care Improvement Project				
Appropriate VTP Within 24 Hours[2]	66	97%	92%	92%
Appropriate Hair Removal[2]	254	100%	100%	99%
Appropriate Beta Blocker Usage[2]	69	97%	94%	93%
Controlled Postoperative Blood Glucose[2]	0	-	94%	93%
Prophylactic Antibiotic Timing[2]	190	96%	97%	97%
Prophylactic Antibiotic Timing (Outpatient)	134	90%	91%	92%
Prophylactic Antibiotic Selection[2]	188	96%	98%	97%
Prophylactic Antibiotic Select. (Outpatient)	122	89%	94%	94%
Prophylactic Antibiotic Stopped[2]	187	97%	95%	94%
Recommended VTP Ordered[2]	66	97%	94%	94%
Urinary Catheter Removal[2]	76	100%	91%	90%
Children's Asthma Care				
Received Systemic Corticosteroids	-	-	-	100%
Received Home Management Plan	-	-	-	71%
Received Reliever Medication	-	-	-	100%
Use of Medical Imaging				
Combination Abdominal CT Scan	528	0.563	0.164	0.191
Combination Chest CT Scan	447	0.025	0.038	0.054
Follow-up Mammogram/Ultrasound	980	8.1%	8.4%	8.4%
MRI for Low Back Pain	113	30.1%	30.2%	32.7%
Survey of Patients' Hospital Experiences				
Area Around Room 'Always' Quiet at Night	300+	54%	-	58%
Doctors 'Always' Communicated Well	300+	77%	-	80%
Home Recovery Information Given	300+	87%	-	82%
Hospital Given 9 or 10 on 10 Point Scale	300+	69%	-	67%
Meds 'Always' Explained Before Given	300+	64%	-	60%
Nurses 'Always' Communicated Well	300+	78%	-	76%
Pain 'Always' Well Controlled	300+	66%	-	69%
Room and Bathroom 'Always' Clean	300+	83%	-	71%
Timely Help 'Always' Received	300+	69%	-	64%
Would Definitely Recommend Hospital	300+	67%	-	69%

Life Line Hospital

200 School Street
Wintersville, OH 43953
Phone: 740-346-2600

Type: Acute Care Hospitals
Emergency Services: No
Ownership: Voluntary Non-Profit - Private

Measure	Cases	This Hosp.	State Avg.	U.S. Avg.
Heart Attack Care				
ACE Inhibitor or ARB for LVSD[5]	0	-	97%	96%
Aspirin at Arrival[5]	0	-	99%	99%
Aspirin at Discharge[5]	0	-	99%	98%
Beta Blocker at Discharge[5]	0	-	99%	98%
Fibrinolytic Medication Timing[5]	0	-	14%	55%
PCI Within 90 Minutes of Arrival[5]	0	-	92%	90%
Smoking Cessation Advice[5]	0	-	100%	99%
Chest Pain/Possible Heart Attack Care				
Aspirin at Arrival	-	-	96%	95%
Median Time to ECG (minutes)	-	-	7	8
Median Time to Transfer (minutes)	-	-	61	61
Fibrinolytic Medication Timing	-	-	47%	54%
Heart Failure Care				
ACE Inhibitor or ARB for LVSD[5]	0	-	96%	94%
Discharge Instructions[5]	0	-	91%	88%
Evaluation of LVS Function[5]	0	-	99%	98%
Smoking Cessation Advice[5]	0	-	99%	98%
Pneumonia Care				
Appropriate Initial Antibiotic[5]	0	-	92%	92%
Blood Culture Timing[5]	0	-	96%	96%
Influenza Vaccine[5]	0	-	93%	91%
Initial Antibiotic Timing[5]	0	-	96%	95%
Pneumococcal Vaccine[5]	0	-	95%	93%
Smoking Cessation Advice[5]	0	-	98%	97%
Surgical Care Improvement Project				
Appropriate VTP Within 24 Hours[5]	0	-	92%	92%
Appropriate Hair Removal[5]	0	-	100%	99%
Appropriate Beta Blocker Usage[5]	0	-	94%	93%
Controlled Postoperative Blood Glucose[5]	0	-	94%	93%
Prophylactic Antibiotic Timing[5]	0	-	97%	97%
Prophylactic Antibiotic Timing (Outpatient)	-	-	91%	92%
Prophylactic Antibiotic Selection[5]	0	-	98%	97%
Prophylactic Antibiotic Select. (Outpatient)	-	-	94%	94%
Prophylactic Antibiotic Stopped[5]	0	-	95%	94%
Recommended VTP Ordered[5]	0	-	94%	94%
Urinary Catheter Removal[5]	0	-	91%	90%
Children's Asthma Care				
Received Systemic Corticosteroids	-	-	-	100%
Received Home Management Plan	-	-	-	71%
Received Reliever Medication	-	-	-	100%
Use of Medical Imaging				
Combination Abdominal CT Scan	-	-	0.164	0.191
Combination Chest CT Scan	-	-	0.038	0.054
Follow-up Mammogram/Ultrasound	-	-	8.4%	8.4%
MRI for Low Back Pain	-	-	30.2%	32.7%
Survey of Patients' Hospital Experiences				
Area Around Room 'Always' Quiet at Night[8]	-	-	-	58%
Doctors 'Always' Communicated Well[8]	-	-	-	80%
Home Recovery Information Given[8]	-	-	-	82%
Hospital Given 9 or 10 on 10 Point Scale[8]	-	-	-	67%
Meds 'Always' Explained Before Given[8]	-	-	-	60%
Nurses 'Always' Communicated Well[8]	-	-	-	76%
Pain 'Always' Well Controlled[8]	-	-	-	69%
Room and Bathroom 'Always' Clean[8]	-	-	-	71%
Timely Help 'Always' Received[8]	-	-	-	64%
Would Definitely Recommend Hospital[8]	-	-	-	69%

NOTE: Hospital profiles are in alphabetical order by state, then city, then hospital within the city; Rankings exclude hospitals with less than 25 cases except for patient surveys which excludes hospitals with less than 100 cases; (a) 100–299 cases; (1) The number of cases is too small to be sure how well a hospital is performing; (2) The hospital indicated that the data submitted for this measure were based on a sample of cases; (3) Data was collected during a shorter time period (fewer quarters) than the maximum possible time for this measure; (4) Suppressed for one or more quarters by CMS; (5) No data is available from the hospital for this measure; (6) Fewer than 100 patients completed the HCAHPS survey. Use these rates with caution, as the number of surveys may be too low to reliably assess hospital performance; (7) Survey results are based on less than 12 months of data; (8) Survey results are not available for this reporting period; (9) No or very few patients were eligible for the HCAHPS survey. The scores shown, if any, reflect a very small number of surveys; (10) A state average was not calculated because too few hospitals in the state submitted data; (11) There were discrepancies in the data collection process; Please refer to the User's Guide for a full explanation of data.

Wooster Community Hospital

1761 Beall Avenue Phone: 330-263-8100
Wooster, OH 44691 Fax: 330-263-8497
URL: www.woosterhospital.org
Type: Acute Care Hospitals Emergency Services: Yes
Ownership: Government - Local Beds: 130

Key Personnel:
CEO/President. . . . . Bill Sheron
Cardiac Laboratory. . . . . Joel Chupp
Chief of Medical Staff. . . . . Timothy Playl
Quality Assurance . . . . Kathy Sisseroim
Radiology. . . . . Brian A Aronson
Emergency Room . . . . William Elliott, MD

Measure	Cases	This Hosp.	State Avg.	U.S. Avg.
Heart Attack Care				
ACE Inhibitor or ARB for LVSD[1]	2	100%	97%	96%
Aspirin at Arrival	34	88%	99%	99%
Aspirin at Discharge[1]	20	95%	99%	98%
Beta Blocker at Discharge[1]	20	100%	99%	98%
Fibrinolytic Medication Timing	0	-	14%	55%
PCI Within 90 Minutes of Arrival	0	-	92%	90%
Smoking Cessation Advice	0	-	100%	99%
Chest Pain/Possible Heart Attack Care				
Aspirin at Arrival	218	98%	96%	95%
Median Time to ECG (minutes)	229	5	7	8
Median Time to Transfer (minutes)[1]	23	44	61	61
Fibrinolytic Medication Timing	0	-	47%	54%
Heart Failure Care				
ACE Inhibitor or ARB for LVSD	27	89%	96%	94%
Discharge Instructions	81	85%	91%	88%
Evaluation of LVS Function	104	92%	99%	98%
Smoking Cessation Advice[1]	15	93%	99%	98%
Pneumonia Care				
Appropriate Initial Antibiotic	120	90%	92%	92%
Blood Culture Timing	169	98%	96%	96%
Influenza Vaccine	154	98%	93%	91%
Initial Antibiotic Timing	212	97%	96%	95%
Pneumococcal Vaccine	216	99%	95%	93%
Smoking Cessation Advice	67	99%	98%	97%
Surgical Care Improvement Project				
Appropriate VTP Within 24 Hours	75	68%	92%	92%
Appropriate Hair Removal	465	99%	100%	99%
Appropriate Beta Blocker Usage	122	80%	94%	93%
Controlled Postoperative Blood Glucose	0	-	94%	93%
Prophylactic Antibiotic Timing	387	94%	97%	97%
Prophylactic Antibiotic Timing (Outpatient)	191	87%	91%	92%
Prophylactic Antibiotic Selection	387	95%	98%	97%
Prophylactic Antibiotic Select. (Outpatient)	170	95%	94%	94%
Prophylactic Antibiotic Stopped	385	95%	95%	94%
Recommended VTP Ordered	75	75%	94%	94%
Urinary Catheter Removal[1]	19	89%	91%	90%
Children's Asthma Care				
Received Systemic Corticosteroids	-	-	-	100%
Received Home Management Plan	-	-	-	71%
Received Reliever Medication	-	-	-	100%
Use of Medical Imaging				
Combination Abdominal CT Scan	507	0.124	0.164	0.191
Combination Chest CT Scan	496	0.131	0.038	0.054
Follow-up Mammogram/Ultrasound	602	18.1%	8.4%	8.4%
MRI for Low Back Pain	96	22.9%	30.2%	32.7%
Survey of Patients' Hospital Experiences				
Area Around Room 'Always' Quiet at Night	300+	53%	-	58%
Doctors 'Always' Communicated Well	300+	80%	-	80%
Home Recovery Information Given	300+	84%	-	82%
Hospital Given 9 or 10 on 10 Point Scale	300+	75%	-	67%
Meds 'Always' Explained Before Given	300+	60%	-	60%
Nurses 'Always' Communicated Well	300+	80%	-	76%
Pain 'Always' Well Controlled	300+	74%	-	69%
Room and Bathroom 'Always' Clean	300+	77%	-	71%
Timely Help 'Always' Received	300+	64%	-	64%
Would Definitely Recommend Hospital	300+	76%	-	69%

Greene Memorial Hospital

1141 North Monroe Drive Phone: 937-352-2000
Xenia, OH 45385 Fax: 937-376-6983
Type: Acute Care Hospitals Emergency Services: Yes
Ownership: Voluntary Non-Profit - Private Beds: 231

Key Personnel:
CEO/President. . . . . Michael R Stephens
Chief of Medical Staff . . . . Craig Hurak
Operating Room. . . . . Bonnie Hoagland, RN
Quality Assurance . . . . Sheila Harris
Radiology. . . . . David Brown MD
Emergency Room . . . . Shanda Zaharako

Measure	Cases	This Hosp.	State Avg.	U.S. Avg.
Heart Attack Care				
ACE Inhibitor or ARB for LVSD[1]	3	100%	97%	96%
Aspirin at Arrival	29	100%	99%	99%
Aspirin at Discharge[1]	16	94%	99%	98%
Beta Blocker at Discharge[1]	18	94%	99%	98%
Fibrinolytic Medication Timing	0	-	14%	55%
PCI Within 90 Minutes of Arrival	0	-	92%	90%
Smoking Cessation Advice[1]	1	100%	100%	99%
Chest Pain/Possible Heart Attack Care				
Aspirin at Arrival	56	98%	96%	95%
Median Time to ECG (minutes)	58	6	7	8
Median Time to Transfer (minutes)[1]	21	85	61	61
Fibrinolytic Medication Timing	0	-	47%	54%
Heart Failure Care				
ACE Inhibitor or ARB for LVSD	32	88%	96%	94%
Discharge Instructions	127	98%	91%	88%
Evaluation of LVS Function	157	100%	99%	98%
Smoking Cessation Advice	25	100%	99%	98%
Pneumonia Care				
Appropriate Initial Antibiotic	151	93%	92%	92%
Blood Culture Timing	239	98%	96%	96%
Influenza Vaccine	167	97%	93%	91%
Initial Antibiotic Timing	173	99%	96%	95%
Pneumococcal Vaccine	208	96%	95%	93%
Smoking Cessation Advice	83	100%	98%	97%
Surgical Care Improvement Project				
Appropriate VTP Within 24 Hours	83	89%	92%	92%
Appropriate Hair Removal	239	100%	100%	99%
Appropriate Beta Blocker Usage	74	95%	94%	93%
Controlled Postoperative Blood Glucose	0	-	94%	93%
Prophylactic Antibiotic Timing	155	99%	97%	97%
Prophylactic Antibiotic Timing (Outpatient)	72	93%	91%	92%
Prophylactic Antibiotic Selection	155	97%	98%	97%
Prophylactic Antibiotic Select. (Outpatient)	70	99%	94%	94%
Prophylactic Antibiotic Stopped	150	95%	95%	94%
Recommended VTP Ordered	83	96%	94%	94%
Urinary Catheter Removal	63	98%	91%	90%
Children's Asthma Care				
Received Systemic Corticosteroids	-	-	-	100%
Received Home Management Plan	-	-	-	71%
Received Reliever Medication	-	-	-	100%
Use of Medical Imaging				
Combination Abdominal CT Scan	467	0.107	0.164	0.191
Combination Chest CT Scan	287	0.188	0.038	0.054
Follow-up Mammogram/Ultrasound	704	11.1%	8.4%	8.4%
MRI for Low Back Pain	63	23.8%	30.2%	32.7%
Survey of Patients' Hospital Experiences				
Area Around Room 'Always' Quiet at Night	300+	46%	-	58%
Doctors 'Always' Communicated Well	300+	77%	-	80%
Home Recovery Information Given	300+	81%	-	82%
Hospital Given 9 or 10 on 10 Point Scale	300+	56%	-	67%
Meds 'Always' Explained Before Given	300+	57%	-	60%
Nurses 'Always' Communicated Well	300+	72%	-	76%
Pain 'Always' Well Controlled	300+	65%	-	69%
Room and Bathroom 'Always' Clean	300+	64%	-	71%
Timely Help 'Always' Received	300+	56%	-	64%
Would Definitely Recommend Hospital	300+	59%	-	69%

Northside Medical Center

500 Gypsy Lane Phone: 330-884-1000
Youngstown, OH 44501 Fax: 330-884-3740
Type: Acute Care Hospitals Emergency Services: Yes
Ownership: Voluntary Non-Profit - Private Beds: 830

Key Personnel:
CEO/President. . . . . Kris Hoce
Chief of Medical Staff . . . . Robert Sinsheimer, MD
Operating Room. . . . . Sandy Johnson-Prater
Quality Assurance . . . . Mike am Keating
Radiology. . . . . S Vibanker, MD
Anesthesiology. . . . . V Perni, MD
Emergency Room . . . . Craig Soltis, MD
Patient Relations . . . . Marta Cimino

Measure	Cases	This Hosp.	State Avg.	U.S. Avg.
Heart Attack Care				
ACE Inhibitor or ARB for LVSD[1]	21	100%	97%	96%
Aspirin at Arrival	101	100%	99%	99%
Aspirin at Discharge	153	100%	99%	98%
Beta Blocker at Discharge	154	100%	99%	98%
Fibrinolytic Medication Timing	0	-	14%	55%
PCI Within 90 Minutes of Arrival[1]	16	62%	92%	90%
Smoking Cessation Advice	51	100%	100%	99%
Chest Pain/Possible Heart Attack Care				
Aspirin at Arrival[5]	0	-	96%	95%
Median Time to ECG (minutes)[5]	0	-	7	8
Median Time to Transfer (minutes)[5]	0	-	61	61
Fibrinolytic Medication Timing[5]	0	-	47%	54%
Heart Failure Care				
ACE Inhibitor or ARB for LVSD	71	99%	96%	94%
Discharge Instructions	238	96%	91%	88%
Evaluation of LVS Function	293	99%	99%	98%
Smoking Cessation Advice	51	100%	99%	98%
Pneumonia Care				
Appropriate Initial Antibiotic	100	86%	92%	92%
Blood Culture Timing	189	92%	96%	96%
Influenza Vaccine	130	97%	93%	91%
Initial Antibiotic Timing	199	93%	96%	95%
Pneumococcal Vaccine	190	97%	95%	93%
Smoking Cessation Advice	77	96%	98%	97%
Surgical Care Improvement Project				
Appropriate VTP Within 24 Hours	269	94%	92%	92%
Appropriate Hair Removal	1,070	100%	100%	99%
Appropriate Beta Blocker Usage	352	95%	94%	93%
Controlled Postoperative Blood Glucose	98	92%	94%	93%
Prophylactic Antibiotic Timing	829	97%	97%	97%
Prophylactic Antibiotic Timing (Outpatient)	260	93%	91%	92%
Prophylactic Antibiotic Selection	836	98%	98%	97%
Prophylactic Antibiotic Select. (Outpatient)	252	94%	94%	94%
Prophylactic Antibiotic Stopped	816	94%	95%	94%
Recommended VTP Ordered	269	96%	94%	94%
Urinary Catheter Removal	177	92%	91%	90%
Children's Asthma Care				
Received Systemic Corticosteroids	-	-	-	100%
Received Home Management Plan	-	-	-	71%
Received Reliever Medication	-	-	-	100%
Use of Medical Imaging				
Combination Abdominal CT Scan	530	0.057	0.164	0.191
Combination Chest CT Scan	333	0.003	0.038	0.054
Follow-up Mammogram/Ultrasound	566	10.1%	8.4%	8.4%
MRI for Low Back Pain[1]	5	20.0%	30.2%	32.7%
Survey of Patients' Hospital Experiences				
Area Around Room 'Always' Quiet at Night	300+	40%	-	58%
Doctors 'Always' Communicated Well	300+	74%	-	80%
Home Recovery Information Given	300+	80%	-	82%
Hospital Given 9 or 10 on 10 Point Scale	300+	59%	-	67%
Meds 'Always' Explained Before Given	300+	53%	-	60%
Nurses 'Always' Communicated Well	300+	71%	-	76%
Pain 'Always' Well Controlled	300+	66%	-	69%
Room and Bathroom 'Always' Clean	300+	63%	-	71%
Timely Help 'Always' Received	300+	55%	-	64%
Would Definitely Recommend Hospital	300+	64%	-	69%

NOTE: Hospital profiles are in alphabetical order by state, then city, then hospital within the city; Rankings exclude hospitals with less than 25 cases except for patient surveys which excludes hospitals with less than 100 cases; (a) 100–299 cases; (1) The number of cases is too small to be sure how well a hospital is performing; (2) The hospital indicated that the data submitted for this measure were based on a sample of cases; (3) Data was collected during a shorter time period (fewer quarters) than the maximum possible time for this measure; (4) Suppressed for one or more quarters by CMS; (5) No data is available from the hospital for this measure; (6) Fewer than 100 patients completed the HCAHPS survey. Use these rates with caution, as the number of surveys may be too low to reliably assess hospital performance; (7) Survey results are based on less than 12 months of data; (8) Survey results are not available for this reporting period; (9) No or very few patients were eligible for the HCAHPS survey. The scores shown, if any, reflect a very small number of surveys; (10) A state average was not calculated because too few hospitals in the state submitted data; (11) There were discrepancies in the data collection process; Please refer to the User's Guide for a full explanation of data.

Saint Elizabeth Boardman Health Center

8401 Market Street   Phone: 330-729-2929
Youngstown, OH 44512
URL: www.ehealthconnection.com
Type: Acute Care Hospitals   Emergency Services: Yes
Ownership: Voluntary Non-Profit - Church
Key Personnel:
President/CEO . . . . Bob Shroder

Measure	Cases	This Hosp.	State Avg.	U.S. Avg.
Heart Attack Care				
ACE Inhibitor or ARB for LVSD[1]	9	100%	97%	96%
Aspirin at Arrival	42	100%	99%	99%
Aspirin at Discharge	25	100%	99%	98%
Beta Blocker at Discharge	30	100%	99%	98%
Fibrinolytic Medication Timing	0	-	14%	55%
PCI Within 90 Minutes of Arrival	0	-	92%	90%
Smoking Cessation Advice[1]	5	100%	100%	99%
Chest Pain/Possible Heart Attack Care				
Aspirin at Arrival	119	97%	96%	95%
Median Time to ECG (minutes)	125	6	7	8
Median Time to Transfer (minutes)	56	48	61	61
Fibrinolytic Medication Timing	0	-	47%	54%
Heart Failure Care				
ACE Inhibitor or ARB for LVSD[2]	58	93%	96%	94%
Discharge Instructions[2]	153	100%	91%	88%
Evaluation of LVS Function[2]	224	99%	99%	98%
Smoking Cessation Advice[2]	25	100%	99%	98%
Pneumonia Care				
Appropriate Initial Antibiotic[2]	76	93%	92%	92%
Blood Culture Timing[2]	98	100%	96%	96%
Influenza Vaccine[2]	82	100%	93%	91%
Initial Antibiotic Timing[2]	126	96%	96%	95%
Pneumococcal Vaccine[2]	126	99%	95%	93%
Smoking Cessation Advice[2]	33	100%	98%	97%
Surgical Care Improvement Project				
Appropriate VTP Within 24 Hours[2]	157	92%	92%	92%
Appropriate Hair Removal[2]	363	100%	100%	99%
Appropriate Beta Blocker Usage[2]	105	95%	94%	93%
Controlled Postoperative Blood Glucose[2]	0	-	94%	93%
Prophylactic Antibiotic Timing[2]	226	99%	97%	97%
Prophylactic Antibiotic Timing (Outpatient)	135	78%	91%	92%
Prophylactic Antibiotic Selection[2]	226	99%	98%	97%
Prophylactic Antibiotic Select. (Outpatient)	119	91%	94%	94%
Prophylactic Antibiotic Stopped[2]	219	98%	95%	94%
Recommended VTP Ordered[2]	157	94%	94%	94%
Urinary Catheter Removal[2]	103	98%	91%	90%
Children's Asthma Care				
Received Systemic Corticosteroids	-	-	-	100%
Received Home Management Plan	-	-	-	71%
Received Reliever Medication	-	-	-	100%
Use of Medical Imaging				
Combination Abdominal CT Scan	496	0.028	0.164	0.191
Combination Chest CT Scan	205	0.034	0.038	0.054
Follow-up Mammogram/Ultrasound	70	2.9%	8.4%	8.4%
MRI for Low Back Pain[1]	16	18.8%	30.2%	32.7%
Survey of Patients' Hospital Experiences				
Area Around Room 'Always' Quiet at Night	300+	56%	-	58%
Doctors 'Always' Communicated Well	300+	77%	-	80%
Home Recovery Information Given	300+	79%	-	82%
Hospital Given 9 or 10 on 10 Point Scale	300+	78%	-	67%
Meds 'Always' Explained Before Given	300+	60%	-	60%
Nurses 'Always' Communicated Well	300+	79%	-	76%
Pain 'Always' Well Controlled	300+	68%	-	69%
Room and Bathroom 'Always' Clean	300+	72%	-	71%
Timely Help 'Always' Received	300+	57%	-	64%
Would Definitely Recommend Hospital	300+	82%	-	69%

Saint Elizabeth Health Center

1044 Belmont Avenue   Phone: 330-746-7211
Youngstown, OH 44501   Fax: 330-480-2617
URL: www.hmhs.org
Type: Acute Care Hospitals   Emergency Services: Yes
Ownership: Voluntary Non-Profit - Church   Beds: 350
Key Personnel:
CEO/President . . . . Robert Shroder
Chief of Medical Staff . . . . Ken Heaps
Coronary Care . . . . Lisa Parish
Operating Room . . . . Pat Stedman
Pediatric Ambulatory Care . . . . . . Elenna Rossi, MD
Pediatric In-Patient Care . . . . Elenna Rossi, MD
Quality Assurance . . . . Mike Keating
Radiology . . . . Ken Lavin

Measure	Cases	This Hosp.	State Avg.	U.S. Avg.
Heart Attack Care				
ACE Inhibitor or ARB for LVSD	79	97%	97%	96%
Aspirin at Arrival	274	100%	99%	99%
Aspirin at Discharge	490	100%	99%	98%
Beta Blocker at Discharge	487	100%	99%	98%
Fibrinolytic Medication Timing	0	-	14%	55%
PCI Within 90 Minutes of Arrival	62	95%	92%	90%
Smoking Cessation Advice	190	100%	100%	99%
Chest Pain/Possible Heart Attack Care				
Aspirin at Arrival	63	97%	96%	95%
Median Time to ECG (minutes)	64	6	7	8
Median Time to Transfer (minutes)[5]	0	-	61	61
Fibrinolytic Medication Timing[3]	0	-	47%	54%
Heart Failure Care				
ACE Inhibitor or ARB for LVSD[2]	85	100%	96%	94%
Discharge Instructions[2]	221	100%	91%	88%
Evaluation of LVS Function[2]	301	100%	99%	98%
Smoking Cessation Advice[2]	55	100%	99%	98%
Pneumonia Care				
Appropriate Initial Antibiotic[2]	58	97%	92%	92%
Blood Culture Timing[2]	52	98%	96%	96%
Influenza Vaccine[2]	78	86%	93%	91%
Initial Antibiotic Timing[2]	90	91%	96%	95%
Pneumococcal Vaccine[2]	94	97%	95%	93%
Smoking Cessation Advice[2]	51	100%	98%	97%
Surgical Care Improvement Project				
Appropriate VTP Within 24 Hours[2]	174	97%	92%	92%
Appropriate Hair Removal[2]	660	100%	100%	99%
Appropriate Beta Blocker Usage[2]	249	97%	94%	93%
Controlled Postoperative Blood Glucose[2]	144	92%	94%	93%
Prophylactic Antibiotic Timing[2]	463	98%	97%	97%
Prophylactic Antibiotic Timing (Outpatient)	528	89%	91%	92%
Prophylactic Antibiotic Selection[2]	467	96%	98%	97%
Prophylactic Antibiotic Select. (Outpatient)	511	95%	94%	94%
Prophylactic Antibiotic Stopped[2]	445	97%	95%	94%
Recommended VTP Ordered[2]	175	97%	94%	94%
Urinary Catheter Removal[2]	143	99%	91%	90%
Children's Asthma Care				
Received Systemic Corticosteroids	-	-	-	100%
Received Home Management Plan	-	-	-	71%
Received Reliever Medication	-	-	-	100%
Use of Medical Imaging				
Combination Abdominal CT Scan	883	0.131	0.164	0.191
Combination Chest CT Scan	524	0.038	0.038	0.054
Follow-up Mammogram/Ultrasound	584	4.8%	8.4%	8.4%
MRI for Low Back Pain	71	36.6%	30.2%	32.7%
Survey of Patients' Hospital Experiences				
Area Around Room 'Always' Quiet at Night	300+	42%	-	58%
Doctors 'Always' Communicated Well	300+	77%	-	80%
Home Recovery Information Given	300+	78%	-	82%
Hospital Given 9 or 10 on 10 Point Scale	300+	59%	-	67%
Meds 'Always' Explained Before Given	300+	53%	-	60%
Nurses 'Always' Communicated Well	300+	69%	-	76%
Pain 'Always' Well Controlled	300+	61%	-	69%
Room and Bathroom 'Always' Clean	300+	61%	-	71%
Timely Help 'Always' Received	300+	53%	-	64%
Would Definitely Recommend Hospital	300+	61%	-	69%

Surgical Hospital at Southwoods

7630 Southern Blvd   Phone: 330-758-1954
Youngstown, OH 44512
URL: surgeryatsouthwoods.com
Type: Acute Care Hospitals   Emergency Services: No
Ownership: Voluntary Non-Profit - Private

Measure	Cases	This Hosp.	State Avg.	U.S. Avg.
Heart Attack Care				
ACE Inhibitor or ARB for LVSD[5]	0	-	97%	96%
Aspirin at Arrival[5]	0	-	99%	99%
Aspirin at Discharge[5]	0	-	99%	98%
Beta Blocker at Discharge[5]	0	-	99%	98%
Fibrinolytic Medication Timing[5]	0	-	14%	55%
PCI Within 90 Minutes of Arrival[5]	0	-	92%	90%
Smoking Cessation Advice[5]	0	-	100%	99%
Chest Pain/Possible Heart Attack Care				
Aspirin at Arrival[5]	0	-	96%	95%
Median Time to ECG (minutes)[5]	0	-	7	8
Median Time to Transfer (minutes)[5]	0	-	61	61
Fibrinolytic Medication Timing[5]	0	-	47%	54%
Heart Failure Care				
ACE Inhibitor or ARB for LVSD[5]	0	-	96%	94%
Discharge Instructions[5]	0	-	91%	88%
Evaluation of LVS Function[5]	0	-	99%	98%
Smoking Cessation Advice[5]	0	-	99%	98%
Pneumonia Care				
Appropriate Initial Antibiotic[5]	0	-	92%	92%
Blood Culture Timing[5]	0	-	96%	96%
Influenza Vaccine[5]	0	-	93%	91%
Initial Antibiotic Timing[5]	0	-	96%	95%
Pneumococcal Vaccine[5]	0	-	95%	93%
Smoking Cessation Advice[5]	0	-	98%	97%
Surgical Care Improvement Project				
Appropriate VTP Within 24 Hours[1,2]	21	95%	92%	92%
Appropriate Hair Removal[2]	289	100%	100%	99%
Appropriate Beta Blocker Usage[2]	47	98%	94%	93%
Controlled Postoperative Blood Glucose[2]	0	-	94%	93%
Prophylactic Antibiotic Timing[2]	267	91%	97%	97%
Prophylactic Antibiotic Timing (Outpatient)	218	66%	91%	92%
Prophylactic Antibiotic Selection[2]	269	94%	98%	97%
Prophylactic Antibiotic Select. (Outpatient)	182	87%	94%	94%
Prophylactic Antibiotic Stopped[2]	265	97%	95%	94%
Recommended VTP Ordered[1,2]	21	95%	94%	94%
Urinary Catheter Removal[2]	68	99%	91%	90%
Children's Asthma Care				
Received Systemic Corticosteroids	-	-	-	100%
Received Home Management Plan	-	-	-	71%
Received Reliever Medication	-	-	-	100%
Use of Medical Imaging				
Combination Abdominal CT Scan[5]	0	-	0.164	0.191
Combination Chest CT Scan[5]	0	-	0.038	0.054
Follow-up Mammogram/Ultrasound[5]	0	-	8.4%	8.4%
MRI for Low Back Pain[5]	0	-	30.2%	32.7%
Survey of Patients' Hospital Experiences				
Area Around Room 'Always' Quiet at Night	(a)	84%	-	58%
Doctors 'Always' Communicated Well	(a)	98%	-	80%
Home Recovery Information Given	(a)	93%	-	82%
Hospital Given 9 or 10 on 10 Point Scale	(a)	100%	-	67%
Meds 'Always' Explained Before Given	(a)	80%	-	60%
Nurses 'Always' Communicated Well	(a)	97%	-	76%
Pain 'Always' Well Controlled	(a)	90%	-	69%
Room and Bathroom 'Always' Clean	(a)	87%	-	71%
Timely Help 'Always' Received	(a)	92%	-	64%
Would Definitely Recommend Hospital	(a)	97%	-	69%

Genesis Healthcare System

2951 Maple Avenue   Phone: 740-454-5000
Zanesville, OH 43701   Fax: 740-454-4781
URL: www.genesishcs.org
Type: Acute Care Hospitals   Emergency Services: No
Ownership: Voluntary Non-Profit - Private   Beds: 352

Key Personnel:
CEO/President . . . . Matthew Perry
Chief of Medical Staff . . . . Theresa Millinger
Infection Control . . . . Kathy Blair
Operating Room . . . . Firas Eladoumikdachi
Quality Assurance . . . . Mike Greene
Radiology . . . . Shane Backu
Emergency Room . . . . Bradley Allen

Measure	Cases	This Hosp.	State Avg.	U.S. Avg.
Heart Attack Care				
ACE Inhibitor or ARB for LVSD	63	98%	97%	96%
Aspirin at Arrival	281	98%	99%	99%
Aspirin at Discharge	388	99%	99%	98%
Beta Blocker at Discharge	379	99%	99%	98%
Fibrinolytic Medication Timing	0	-	14%	55%
PCI Within 90 Minutes of Arrival	58	91%	92%	90%
Smoking Cessation Advice	149	99%	100%	99%
Chest Pain/Possible Heart Attack Care				
Aspirin at Arrival[1]	6	100%	96%	95%
Median Time to ECG (minutes)[1]	6	5	7	8
Median Time to Transfer (minutes)[5]	0	-	61	61
Fibrinolytic Medication Timing[3]	0	-	47%	54%
Heart Failure Care				
ACE Inhibitor or ARB for LVSD	100	90%	96%	94%
Discharge Instructions	331	96%	91%	88%
Evaluation of LVS Function	392	100%	99%	98%
Smoking Cessation Advice	64	100%	99%	98%
Pneumonia Care				
Appropriate Initial Antibiotic	261	97%	92%	92%
Blood Culture Timing	392	95%	96%	96%
Influenza Vaccine	282	87%	93%	91%
Initial Antibiotic Timing	396	96%	96%	95%
Pneumococcal Vaccine	343	87%	95%	93%
Smoking Cessation Advice	172	99%	98%	97%
Surgical Care Improvement Project				
Appropriate VTP Within 24 Hours[2]	107	94%	92%	92%
Appropriate Hair Removal[2]	518	100%	100%	99%
Appropriate Beta Blocker Usage[2]	193	97%	94%	93%
Controlled Postoperative Blood Glucose[2]	97	98%	94%	93%
Prophylactic Antibiotic Timing[2]	368	93%	97%	97%
Prophylactic Antibiotic Timing (Outpatient)	188	69%	91%	92%
Prophylactic Antibiotic Selection[2]	374	99%	98%	97%
Prophylactic Antibiotic Select. (Outpatient)	182	91%	94%	94%
Prophylactic Antibiotic Stopped[2]	359	97%	95%	94%
Recommended VTP Ordered[2]	108	94%	94%	94%
Urinary Catheter Removal[2]	52	60%	91%	90%
Children's Asthma Care				
Received Systemic Corticosteroids	-	-	-	100%
Received Home Management Plan	-	-	-	71%
Received Reliever Medication	-	-	-	100%
Use of Medical Imaging				
Combination Abdominal CT Scan	756	0.085	0.164	0.191
Combination Chest CT Scan	485	0.000	0.038	0.054
Follow-up Mammogram/Ultrasound	101	5.0%	8.4%	8.4%
MRI for Low Back Pain	38	42.1%	30.2%	32.7%
Survey of Patients' Hospital Experiences				
Area Around Room 'Always' Quiet at Night	300+	57%	-	58%
Doctors 'Always' Communicated Well	300+	78%	-	80%
Home Recovery Information Given	300+	82%	-	82%
Hospital Given 9 or 10 on 10 Point Scale	300+	69%	-	67%
Meds 'Always' Explained Before Given	300+	61%	-	60%
Nurses 'Always' Communicated Well	300+	79%	-	76%
Pain 'Always' Well Controlled	300+	72%	-	69%
Room and Bathroom 'Always' Clean	300+	72%	-	71%
Timely Help 'Always' Received	300+	71%	-	64%
Would Definitely Recommend Hospital	300+	70%	-	69%

NOTE: Hospital profiles are in alphabetical order by state, then city, then hospital within the city; Rankings exclude hospitals with less than 25 cases except for patient surveys which excludes hospitals with less than 100 cases; (a) 100–299 cases; (1) The number of cases is too small to be sure how well a hospital is performing; (2) The hospital indicated that the data submitted for this measure were based on a sample of cases; (3) Data was collected during a shorter time period (fewer quarters) than the maximum possible time for this measure; (4) Suppressed for one or more quarters by CMS; (5) No data is available from the hospital for this measure; (6) Fewer than 100 patients completed the HCAHPS survey. Use these rates with caution, as the number of surveys may be too low to reliably assess hospital performance; (7) Survey results are based on less than 12 months of data; (8) Survey results are not available for this reporting period; (9) No or very few patients were eligible for the HCAHPS survey. The scores shown, if any, reflect a very small number of surveys; (10) A state average was not calculated because too few hospitals in the state submitted data; (11) There were discrepancies in the data collection process; Please refer to the User's Guide for a full explanation of data.

Heart Attack Care

1. ACE Inhibitor or ARB for LVSD

Hospital Name	City	Rate	Cases
Allegheny General Hospital	Pittsburgh	100%	110
Aria Health	Philadelphia	100%	63
Butler Memorial Hospital	Butler	100%	62
Chester County Hospital	West Chester	100%	34
Doylestown Hospital[2]	Doylestown	100%	37
Dubois Regional Medical Center	Dubois	100%	66
Easton Hospital	Easton	100%	48
Good Samaritan Hospital	Lebanon	100%	36
Hahnemann University Hospital	Philadelphia	100%	43
Main Line Hospital Bryn Mawr Campus	Bryn Mawr	100%	27
Main Line Hospital Lankenau	Wynnewood	100%	52
Mercy Hospital Scranton[2]	Scranton	100%	59
Riddle Memorial Hospital	Media	100%	25
Saint Luke's Hospital Bethlehem	Bethlehem	100%	62
Saint Mary Medical Center	Langhorne	100%	51
Thomas Jefferson University Hospital	Philadelphia	100%	60
UPMC Presbyterian Shadyside	Pittsburgh	100%	189
Geisinger Medical Center	Danville	99%	102
Hamot Medical Center	Erie	99%	148
UPMC Mercy	Pittsburgh	99%	73
Crozer Chester Medical Center	Upland	98%	65
Heritage Valley Beaver	Beaver	98%	63
Holy Spirit Hospital	Camp Hill	98%	66
Hospital of Univ of Pennsylvania	Philadelphia	98%	40
Mercy Fitzgerald Hospital	Darby	98%	48
Reading Hospital Medical Center	Reading	98%	51
Saint Vincent Health Center	Erie	98%	80
UPMC Passavant	Pittsburgh	98%	61
The Washington Hospital	Washington	98%	65
Albert Einstein Medical Center	Philadelphia	97%	68
Jeanes Hospital	Philadelphia	97%	30
Lehigh Valley Hospital - Muhlenberg	Bethlehem	97%	33
Milton S Hershey Medical Center	Hershey	97%	35
Pinnacle Health Hospitals	Harrisburg	97%	149
Pocono Medical Center	E Stroudsburg	97%	66
Robert Packer Hospital	Sayre	97%	94
Temple University Hospital	Philadelphia	97%	90
Western Pennsylvania Hospital	Pittsburgh	97%	37
Abington Memorial Hospital	Abington	96%	73
Chambersburg Hospital	Chambersburg	96%	70
Community Medical Center	Scranton	96%	50
Lehigh Valley Hospital	Allentown	96%	149
Geisinger Wyoming Valley Medical Center	Wilkes-Barre	95%	40
Penn Presbyterian Medical Center	Philadelphia	95%	140
York Hospital	York	95%	125
Montgomery Hospital	Norristown	94%	32
Penn Hosp of the Univ of Penn Health Sys	Philadelphia	93%	45
Holy Redeemer Hospital and Medical Center	Meadowbrook	92%	26
Phoenixville Hospital	Phoenixville	92%	40
Lancaster General Hospital	Lancaster	91%	117
Western Penn Hosp-Forbes Reg Campus	Monroeville	91%	32
Williamsport Hospital & Medical Center	Williamsport	91%	43
Jefferson Regional Medical Center	Pittsburgh	90%	60
Wilkes-Barre General Hospital	Wilkes-Barre	89%	70
Altoona Regional Health System	Altoona	86%	141
Excela Health Westmoreland Reg Hosp	Greensburg	86%	79
Conemaugh Valley Memorial Hospital	Johnstown	81%	136
Hanover Hospital	Hanover	79%	29
Saint Clair Memorial Hospital	Pittsburgh	76%	34

2. Aspirin at Arrival

Hospital Name	City	Rate	Cases
Allegheny General Hospital	Pittsburgh	100%	310
Bradford Regional Medical Center	Bradford	100%	48
Butler Memorial Hospital	Butler	100%	201
Chester County Hospital	West Chester	100%	189
Chestnut Hill Hospital	Philadelphia	100%	40
Doylestown Hospital[2]	Doylestown	100%	240
Dubois Regional Medical Center	Dubois	100%	126
Gettysburg Hospital	Gettysburg	100%	43
Good Samaritan Hospital	Lebanon	100%	200
Hospital of Univ of Pennsylvania	Philadelphia	100%	112
Jennersville Regional Hospital	West Grove	100%	26
Lansdale Hospital	Lansdale	100%	60
Lehigh Valley Hospital	Allentown	100%	648
Lehigh Valley Hospital - Muhlenberg	Bethlehem	100%	288
Main Line Hospital Bryn Mawr Campus	Bryn Mawr	100%	206
Main Line Hospital Lankenau	Wynnewood	100%	216
Mercy Fitzgerald Hospital	Darby	100%	183
Mercy Suburban Hospital	Norristown	100%	35
Milton S Hershey Medical Center	Hershey	100%	234
Moses Taylor Hospital	Scranton	100%	42
Nazareth Hospital	Philadelphia	100%	109
Penn Presbyterian Medical Center	Philadelphia	100%	408
Penn Hosp of the Univ of Penn Health Sys	Philadelphia	100%	132
Pottstown Memorial Medical Center	Pottstown	100%	48
Saint Mary Medical Center	Langhorne	100%	416
Saint Vincent Health Center	Erie	100%	240
Sharon Regional Health System	Sharon	100%	157
UPMC Mckeesport	McKeesport	100%	108
UPMC Northwest	Seneca	100%	38
UPMC Passavant	Pittsburgh	100%	316
UPMC Presbyterian Shadyside	Pittsburgh	100%	456
VA Pittsburgh Healthcare System	Pittsburgh	100%	41
The Washington Hospital	Washington	100%	285
Western Penn Hosp-Forbes Reg Campus	Monroeville	100%	230
Abington Memorial Hospital	Abington	99%	358
Albert Einstein Medical Center	Philadelphia	99%	243
Aria Health	Philadelphia	99%	460
Community Medical Center	Scranton	99%	171
Crozer Chester Medical Center	Upland	99%	275
Easton Hospital	Easton	99%	171
Evangelical Community Hospital	Lewisburg	99%	149
Excela Health Westmoreland Reg Hosp	Greensburg	99%	328
Geisinger Medical Center	Danville	99%	260
Geisinger Wyoming Valley Medical Center	Wilkes-Barre	99%	182
Grand View Hospital	Sellersville	99%	69
Hamot Medical Center	Erie	99%	278
Jefferson Regional Medical Center	Pittsburgh	99%	271
Main Line Hospital Paoli	Paoli	99%	153
Mount Nittany Medical Center	State College	99%	139
Phoenixville Hospital	Phoenixville	99%	157
Pinnacle Health Hospitals	Harrisburg	99%	545
Reading Hospital Medical Center	Reading	99%	399
Robert Packer Hospital	Sayre	99%	161
Saint Joseph Medical Center	Reading	99%	144
Shamokin Area Community Hospital	Coal Township	99%	100
Somerset Hospital	Somerset	99%	76
Temple University Hospital	Philadelphia	99%	235
Thomas Jefferson University Hospital	Philadelphia	99%	184
Uniontown Hospital	Uniontown	99%	128
Western Pennsylvania Hospital	Pittsburgh	99%	110
Williamsport Hospital & Medical Center	Williamsport	99%	185
Alle Kiski Medical Center	Natrona	98%	167
Altoona Regional Health System	Altoona	98%	362
Brandywine Hospital	Coatesville	98%	137
Chambersburg Hospital	Chambersburg	98%	292
Conemaugh Valley Memorial Hospital	Johnstown	98%	452
Delaware County Memorial Hospital	Drexel Hill	98%	65
Ephrata Community Hospital	Ephrata	98%	49
Hahnemann University Hospital	Philadelphia	98%	103
Heritage Valley Sewickley	Sewickley	98%	43
Holy Spirit Hospital	Camp Hill	98%	308
Jeanes Hospital	Philadelphia	98%	164
Lancaster General Hospital	Lancaster	98%	717
Lancaster Regional Medical Center	Lancaster	98%	40
Lower Bucks Hospital	Bristol	98%	124
Memorial Hospital York	York	98%	62
Mercy Hospital Scranton[2]	Scranton	98%	204
Montgomery Hospital	Norristown	98%	128
Pocono Medical Center	E Stroudsburg	98%	297
Riddle Memorial Hospital	Media	98%	130
Saint Luke's Hospital Bethlehem	Bethlehem	98%	367
UPMC Horizon	Greenville	98%	61
UPMC Mercy	Pittsburgh	98%	259
York Hospital	York	98%	437
Excela Health Latrobe Hospital	Latrobe	97%	61
Hanover Hospital	Hanover	97%	174
Hazleton General Hospital	Hazleton	97%	61
Heritage Valley Beaver	Beaver	97%	336
Holy Redeemer Hospital and Medical Center	Meadowbrook	97%	176
Jameson Memorial Hospital	New Castle	97%	137
Lewistown Hospital	Lewistown	97%	123
Sacred Heart Hospital	Allentown	97%	31
Saint Clair Memorial Hospital	Pittsburgh	97%	269
Waynesboro Hospital	Waynesboro	97%	34
Wilkes-Barre General Hospital	Wilkes-Barre	97%	341
Berwick Hospital Center	Berwick	96%	27
Carlisle Regional Medical Center	Carlisle	96%	52
Monongahela Valley Hospital	Monongahela	96%	107
Schuylkill Med Ctr-S Jackson Street	Pottsville	96%	45
UPMC Saint Margaret	Pittsburgh	96%	102
Canonsburg General Hospital	Canonsburg	95%	41
Indiana Regional Medical Center	Indiana	95%	80
Roxborough Memorial Hospital	Phila	95%	41
Schuylkill Med Ctr-East Norwegian Street	Pottsville	95%	61
Wayne Memorial Hospital	Honesdale	93%	46
ACMH Hospital	Kittanning	91%	55
Windber Hospital	Windber	91%	33
Saint Joseph's Hospital	Philadelphia	89%	56
Excela Health Frick Hospital	Mount Pleasant	87%	30

3. Aspirin at Discharge

Hospital Name	City	Rate	Cases
Alle Kiski Medical Center	Natrona	100%	103
Allegheny General Hospital	Pittsburgh	100%	581
Aria Health	Philadelphia	100%	465
Butler Memorial Hospital	Butler	100%	261
Delaware County Memorial Hospital	Drexel Hill	100%	34
Doylestown Hospital[2]	Doylestown	100%	301
Geisinger Medical Center	Danville	100%	679
Good Samaritan Hospital	Lebanon	100%	192
Grand View Hospital	Sellersville	100%	49
Holy Spirit Hospital	Camp Hill	100%	334
Hospital of Univ of Pennsylvania	Philadelphia	100%	204
Jefferson Regional Medical Center	Pittsburgh	100%	309
Lancaster General Hospital	Lancaster	100%	749
Lancaster Regional Medical Center	Lancaster	100%	52
Lansdale Hospital	Lansdale	100%	33
Main Line Hospital Bryn Mawr Campus	Bryn Mawr	100%	232
Main Line Hospital Lankenau	Wynnewood	100%	298
Main Line Hospital Paoli	Paoli	100%	136
Memorial Hospital York	York	100%	38
Penn Presbyterian Medical Center	Philadelphia	100%	696
Phoenixville Hospital	Phoenixville	100%	217
Pottstown Memorial Medical Center	Pottstown	100%	26
Reading Hospital Medical Center	Reading	100%	397
Riddle Memorial Hospital	Media	100%	100
Saint Clair Memorial Hospital	Pittsburgh	100%	257
Saint Mary Medical Center	Langhorne	100%	407
Saint Vincent Health Center	Erie	100%	461
Sharon Regional Health System	Sharon	100%	145
Uniontown Hospital	Uniontown	100%	98
UPMC Horizon	Greenville	100%	42
UPMC Mckeesport	McKeesport	100%	78
UPMC Mercy	Pittsburgh	100%	374
UPMC Passavant	Pittsburgh	100%	449
UPMC Presbyterian Shadyside	Pittsburgh	100%	1034
UPMC Saint Margaret	Pittsburgh	100%	49
VA Pittsburgh Healthcare System	Pittsburgh	100%	46
Western Pennsylvania Hospital	Pittsburgh	100%	215
Williamsport Hospital & Medical Center	Williamsport	100%	265
Abington Memorial Hospital	Abington	99%	393
Albert Einstein Medical Center	Philadelphia	99%	301
Chester County Hospital	West Chester	99%	181
Community Medical Center	Scranton	99%	223
Conemaugh Valley Memorial Hospital	Johnstown	99%	590
Crozer Chester Medical Center	Upland	99%	354
Dubois Regional Medical Center	Dubois	99%	323
Easton Hospital	Easton	99%	202
Excela Health Westmoreland Reg Hosp	Greensburg	99%	451
Geisinger Wyoming Valley Medical Center	Wilkes-Barre	99%	189
Hahnemann University Hospital	Philadelphia	99%	195
Hamot Medical Center	Erie	99%	713
Jeanes Hospital	Philadelphia	99%	146
Lehigh Valley Hospital	Allentown	99%	976
Lehigh Valley Hospital - Muhlenberg	Bethlehem	99%	281
Mercy Fitzgerald Hospital	Darby	99%	179
Mercy Hospital Scranton[2]	Scranton	99%	287
Milton S Hershey Medical Center	Hershey	99%	349
Penn Hosp of the Univ of Penn Health Sys	Philadelphia	99%	186
Pinnacle Health Hospitals	Harrisburg	99%	637
Pocono Medical Center	E Stroudsburg	99%	283
Robert Packer Hospital	Sayre	99%	345
Saint Joseph Medical Center	Reading	99%	159
Saint Luke's Hospital Bethlehem	Bethlehem	99%	445
Temple University Hospital	Philadelphia	99%	297
Thomas Jefferson University Hospital	Philadelphia	99%	263
The Washington Hospital	Washington	99%	359
York Hospital	York	99%	531
Chambersburg Hospital	Chambersburg	98%	329
Heritage Valley Beaver	Beaver	98%	412
Montgomery Hospital	Norristown	98%	131
Mount Nittany Medical Center	State College	98%	120
Somerset Hospital	Somerset	98%	62
Altoona Regional Health System	Altoona	97%	522
Evangelical Community Hospital	Lewisburg	97%	122
Gettysburg Hospital	Gettysburg	97%	31
Hazleton General Hospital	Hazleton	97%	39
Holy Redeemer Hospital and Medical Center	Meadowbrook	97%	139
Indiana Regional Medical Center	Indiana	97%	59
Nazareth Hospital	Philadelphia	97%	60
Wilkes-Barre General Hospital	Wilkes-Barre	97%	329
Bradford Regional Medical Center	Bradford	96%	26
Jameson Memorial Hospital	New Castle	96%	98
Lower Bucks Hospital	Bristol	96%	114
Shamokin Area Community Hospital	Coal Township	96%	76
Western Penn Hosp-Forbes Reg Campus	Monroeville	96%	222
Schuylkill Med Ctr-East Norwegian Street	Pottsville	95%	38
Brandywine Hospital	Coatesville	93%	122
Lewistown Hospital	Lewistown	93%	76
Monongahela Valley Hospital	Monongahela	92%	63
Wayne Memorial Hospital	Honesdale	92%	25
Excela Health Latrobe Hospital	Latrobe	91%	35
Hanover Hospital	Hanover	88%	114
ACMH Hospital	Kittanning	81%	32

NOTE: Hospital profiles are in alphabetical order by state, then city, then hospital within the city; Rankings exclude hospitals with less than 25 cases except for patient surveys which excludes hospitals with less than 100 cases; (a) 100–299 cases; (1) The number of cases is too small to be sure how well a hospital is performing; (2) The hospital indicated that the data submitted for this measure were based on a sample of cases; (3) Data was collected during a shorter time period (fewer quarters) than the maximum possible time for this measure; (4) Suppressed for one or more quarters by CMS; (5) No data is available from the hospital for this measure; (6) Fewer than 100 patients completed the HCAHPS survey. Use these rates with caution, as the number of surveys may be too low to reliably assess hospital performance; (7) Survey results are based on less than 12 months of data; (8) Survey results are not available for this reporting period; (9) No or very few patients were eligible for the HCAHPS survey. The scores shown, if any, reflect a very small number of surveys; (10) A state average was not calculated because too few hospitals in the state submitted data; (11) There were discrepancies in the data collection process; Please refer to the User's Guide for a full explanation of data.

4. Beta Blocker at Discharge

Hospital Name	City	Rate	Cases
Alle Kiski Medical Center	Natrona	100%	104
Butler Memorial Hospital	Butler	100%	246
Carlisle Regional Medical Center	Carlisle	100%	25
Community Medical Center	Scranton	100%	230
Delaware County Memorial Hospital	Drexel Hill	100%	32
Doylestown Hospital[2]	Doylestown	100%	281
Dubois Regional Medical Center	Dubois	100%	321
Geisinger Medical Center	Danville	100%	660
Geisinger Wyoming Valley Medical Center	Wilkes-Barre	100%	186
Gettysburg Hospital	Gettysburg	100%	30
Good Samaritan Hospital	Lebanon	100%	193
Grand View Hospital	Sellersville	100%	46
Hahnemann University Hospital	Philadelphia	100%	192
Hazleton General Hospital	Hazleton	100%	48
Heritage Valley Beaver	Beaver	100%	367
Holy Spirit Hospital	Camp Hill	100%	324
Lancaster Regional Medical Center	Lancaster	100%	48
Lansdale Hospital	Lansdale	100%	33
Lehigh Valley Hospital - Muhlenberg	Bethlehem	100%	283
Main Line Hospital Bryn Mawr Campus	Bryn Mawr	100%	212
Main Line Hospital Lankenau	Wynnewood	100%	293
Mercy Hospital Scranton[2]	Scranton	100%	274
Moses Taylor Hospital	Scranton	100%	25
Phoenixville Hospital	Phoenixville	100%	215
Pottstown Memorial Medical Center	Pottstown	100%	25
Reading Hospital Medical Center	Reading	100%	392
Riddle Memorial Hospital	Media	100%	99
Saint Joseph Medical Center	Reading	100%	157
Saint Mary Medical Center	Langhorne	100%	383
Sharon Regional Health System	Sharon	100%	136
Somerset Hospital	Somerset	100%	62
Temple University Hospital	Philadelphia	100%	277
Thomas Jefferson University Hospital	Philadelphia	100%	250
UPMC Horizon	Greenville	100%	44
UPMC Mckeesport	McKeesport	100%	85
UPMC Mercy	Pittsburgh	100%	353
UPMC Passavant	Pittsburgh	100%	440
UPMC Presbyterian Shadyside	Pittsburgh	100%	998
UPMC Saint Margaret	Pittsburgh	100%	61
VA Pittsburgh Healthcare System	Pittsburgh	100%	47
Allegheny General Hospital	Pittsburgh	99%	523
Aria Health	Philadelphia	99%	451
Chester County Hospital	West Chester	99%	181
Crozer Chester Medical Center	Upland	99%	351
Easton Hospital	Easton	99%	204
Hamot Medical Center	Erie	99%	703
Jameson Memorial Hospital	New Castle	99%	95
Jefferson Regional Medical Center	Pittsburgh	99%	300
Lehigh Valley Hospital	Allentown	99%	951
Lewistown Hospital	Lewistown	99%	86
Main Line Hospital Paoli	Paoli	99%	131
Mercy Fitzgerald Hospital	Darby	99%	177
Milton S Hershey Medical Center	Hershey	99%	340
Penn Presbyterian Medical Center	Philadelphia	99%	692
Pinnacle Health Hospitals	Harrisburg	99%	633
Pocono Medical Center	E Stroudsburg	99%	258
Robert Packer Hospital	Sayre	99%	330
Saint Luke's Hospital Bethlehem	Bethlehem	99%	434
Saint Vincent Health Center	Erie	99%	457
The Washington Hospital	Washington	99%	349
Western Pennsylvania Hospital	Pittsburgh	99%	205
Western Penn Hosp-Forbes Reg Campus	Monroeville	99%	218
York Hospital	York	99%	538
Albert Einstein Medical Center	Philadelphia	98%	292
Evangelical Community Hospital	Lewisburg	98%	129
Holy Redeemer Hospital and Medical Center	Meadowbrook	98%	141
Hospital of Univ of Pennsylvania	Philadelphia	98%	198
Indiana Regional Medical Center	Indiana	98%	62
Jeanes Hospital	Philadelphia	98%	164
Lancaster General Hospital	Lancaster	98%	733
Montgomery Hospital	Norristown	98%	133
Mount Nittany Medical Center	State College	98%	121
Nazareth Hospital	Philadelphia	98%	63
Williamsport Hospital & Medical Center	Williamsport	98%	260
Abington Memorial Hospital	Abington	97%	393
Altoona Regional Health System	Altoona	97%	515
Chambersburg Hospital	Chambersburg	97%	338
Excela Health Latrobe Hospital	Latrobe	97%	36
Lower Bucks Hospital	Bristol	97%	119
Memorial Hospital York	York	97%	34
Penn Hosp of the Univ of Penn Health Sys	Philadelphia	97%	172
Saint Clair Memorial Hospital	Pittsburgh	97%	240
Schuylkill Med Ctr-S Jackson Street	Pottsville	97%	29
Shamokin Area Community Hospital	Coal Township	97%	91
Conemaugh Valley Memorial Hospital	Johnstown	96%	588
Excela Health Westmoreland Reg Hosp	Greensburg	96%	420
Monongahela Valley Hospital	Monongahela	96%	72
Wayne Memorial Hospital	Honesdale	96%	25
Wilkes-Barre General Hospital	Wilkes-Barre	96%	337
Brandywine Hospital	Coatesville	95%	121
Uniontown Hospital	Uniontown	94%	94
Bradford Regional Medical Center	Bradford	91%	35
Schuylkill Med Ctr-East Norwegian Street	Pottsville	91%	45
Hanover Hospital	Hanover	90%	112
ACMH Hospital	Kittanning	86%	37

6. PCI Within 90 Minutes of Arrival

Hospital Name	City	Rate	Cases
Easton Hospital	Easton	100%	40
Main Line Hospital Bryn Mawr Campus	Bryn Mawr	100%	30
Montgomery Hospital	Norristown	100%	25
Saint Joseph Medical Center	Reading	100%	43
Main Line Hospital Lankenau	Wynnewood	98%	42
Holy Spirit Hospital	Camp Hill	97%	68
Pinnacle Health Hospitals	Harrisburg	97%	90
UPMC Passavant	Pittsburgh	97%	30
Geisinger Medical Center	Danville	96%	52
Lehigh Valley Hospital	Allentown	96%	118
Pocono Medical Center	E Stroudsburg	96%	83
Albert Einstein Medical Center	Philadelphia	95%	42
Saint Mary Medical Center	Langhorne	95%	55
Crozer Chester Medical Center	Upland	94%	31
Doylestown Hospital[2]	Doylestown	94%	53
Saint Clair Memorial Hospital	Pittsburgh	94%	71
UPMC Presbyterian Shadyside	Pittsburgh	94%	85
The Washington Hospital	Washington	94%	50
Allegheny General Hospital	Pittsburgh	93%	55
Brandywine Hospital	Coatesville	93%	29
Butler Memorial Hospital	Butler	93%	30
Mercy Hospital Scranton[2]	Scranton	93%	45
Reading Hospital Medical Center	Reading	92%	112
Chester County Hospital	West Chester	91%	34
Hamot Medical Center	Erie	91%	64
Altoona Regional Health System	Altoona	90%	70
York Hospital	York	90%	102
Conemaugh Valley Memorial Hospital	Johnstown	89%	64
Lehigh Valley Hospital - Muhlenberg	Bethlehem	89%	71
Aria Health	Philadelphia	88%	52
Good Samaritan Hospital	Lebanon	88%	48
Main Line Hospital Paoli	Paoli	88%	25
Milton S Hershey Medical Center	Hershey	88%	41
Riddle Memorial Hospital	Media	88%	32
Uniontown Hospital	Uniontown	88%	25
Saint Luke's Hospital Bethlehem	Bethlehem	87%	46
Abington Memorial Hospital	Abington	86%	65
Chambersburg Hospital	Chambersburg	85%	46
Holy Redeemer Hospital and Medical Center	Meadowbrook	85%	33
Mount Nittany Medical Center	State College	85%	39
Community Medical Center	Scranton	84%	31
Williamsport Hospital & Medical Center	Williamsport	83%	42
Heritage Valley Beaver	Beaver	82%	66
Saint Vincent Health Center	Erie	82%	49
Excela Health Westmoreland Reg Hosp	Greensburg	81%	64
Jefferson Regional Medical Center	Pittsburgh	81%	64
UPMC Mercy	Pittsburgh	80%	45
Lancaster General Hospital	Lancaster	79%	122
Western Penn Hosp-Forbes Reg Campus	Monroeville	79%	42
Geisinger Wyoming Valley Medical Center	Wilkes-Barre	76%	42
Wilkes-Barre General Hospital	Wilkes-Barre	73%	41
Hospital of Univ of Pennsylvania	Philadelphia	72%	29

7. Smoking Cessation Advice

Hospital Name	City	Rate	Cases
Abington Memorial Hospital	Abington	100%	96
Albert Einstein Medical Center	Philadelphia	100%	114
Allegheny General Hospital	Pittsburgh	100%	193
Altoona Regional Health System	Altoona	100%	172
Aria Health	Philadelphia	100%	172
Butler Memorial Hospital	Butler	100%	99
Community Medical Center	Scranton	100%	83
Crozer Chester Medical Center	Upland	100%	114
Doylestown Hospital[2]	Doylestown	100%	62
Dubois Regional Medical Center	Dubois	100%	112
Easton Hospital	Easton	100%	80
Geisinger Medical Center	Danville	100%	226
Geisinger Wyoming Valley Medical Center	Wilkes-Barre	100%	61
Good Samaritan Hospital	Lebanon	100%	68
Hahnemann University Hospital	Philadelphia	100%	72
Hamot Medical Center	Erie	100%	275
Heritage Valley Beaver	Beaver	100%	135
Holy Redeemer Hospital and Medical Center	Meadowbrook	100%	30
Holy Spirit Hospital	Camp Hill	100%	100
Jameson Memorial Hospital	New Castle	100%	27
Jeanes Hospital	Philadelphia	100%	42
Lancaster General Hospital	Lancaster	100%	211
Lehigh Valley Hospital	Allentown	100%	247
Lehigh Valley Hospital - Muhlenberg	Bethlehem	100%	78
Main Line Hospital Bryn Mawr Campus	Bryn Mawr	100%	47
Main Line Hospital Lankenau	Wynnewood	100%	58
Mercy Fitzgerald Hospital	Darby	100%	65
Mercy Hospital Scranton[2]	Scranton	100%	110
Milton S Hershey Medical Center	Hershey	100%	89
Montgomery Hospital	Norristown	100%	44
Mount Nittany Medical Center	State College	100%	27
Penn Presbyterian Medical Center	Philadelphia	100%	208
Penn Hosp of the Univ of Penn Health Sys	Philadelphia	100%	79
Pinnacle Health Hospitals	Harrisburg	100%	183
Pocono Medical Center	E Stroudsburg	100%	112
Reading Hospital Medical Center	Reading	100%	115
Riddle Memorial Hospital	Media	100%	29
Robert Packer Hospital	Sayre	100%	112
Saint Clair Memorial Hospital	Pittsburgh	100%	68
Saint Luke's Hospital Bethlehem	Bethlehem	100%	128
Saint Mary Medical Center	Langhorne	100%	105
Saint Vincent Health Center	Erie	100%	173
Temple University Hospital	Philadelphia	100%	122
Thomas Jefferson University Hospital	Philadelphia	100%	88
UPMC Mercy	Pittsburgh	100%	149
UPMC Passavant	Pittsburgh	100%	123
UPMC Presbyterian Shadyside	Pittsburgh	100%	374
The Washington Hospital	Washington	100%	117
Western Pennsylvania Hospital	Pittsburgh	100%	72
Western Penn Hosp-Forbes Reg Campus	Monroeville	100%	64
Wilkes-Barre General Hospital	Wilkes-Barre	100%	104
Williamsport Hospital & Medical Center	Williamsport	100%	91
York Hospital	York	100%	200
Chambersburg Hospital	Chambersburg	99%	102
Excela Health Westmoreland Reg Hosp	Greensburg	99%	137
Hospital of Univ of Pennsylvania	Philadelphia	99%	70
Jefferson Regional Medical Center	Pittsburgh	99%	104
Brandywine Hospital	Coatesville	98%	56
Chester County Hospital	West Chester	98%	46
Conemaugh Valley Memorial Hospital	Johnstown	98%	170
Phoenixville Hospital	Phoenixville	98%	64
Saint Joseph Medical Center	Reading	98%	51
Sharon Regional Health System	Sharon	97%	35
Uniontown Hospital	Uniontown	97%	32
Lower Bucks Hospital	Bristol	92%	49

Chest Pain/Possible Heart Attack Care

8. Aspirin at Arrival

Hospital Name	City	Rate	Cases
Bradford Regional Medical Center	Bradford	100%	30
Jennersville Regional Hospital	West Grove	100%	29
Memorial Hospital York	York	100%	50
Troy Community Hospital[3]	Troy	100%	30
Canonsburg General Hospital	Canonsburg	99%	83
Excela Health Frick Hospital	Mount Pleasant	99%	106
Gettysburg Hospital	Gettysburg	99%	74
Grand View Hospital	Sellersville	99%	67
Monongahela Valley Hospital	Monongahela	99%	86
Pottstown Memorial Medical Center	Pottstown	99%	70
Soldiers and Sailors Memorial Hospital	Wellsboro	99%	84
UPMC Horizon	Greenville	99%	130
UPMC Northwest	Seneca	99%	141
Grove City Medical Center	Grove City	98%	158
Marian Community Hospital	Carbondale	98%	48
Meadville Medical Center	Meadville	98%	152
Ohio Valley General Hospital	Mckees Rocks	98%	47
Schuylkill Med Ctr-S Jackson Street	Pottsville	98%	85
Titusville Hospital	Titusville	98%	116
UPMC Passavant	Pittsburgh	98%	48
UPMC Saint Margaret	Pittsburgh	98%	132
Warren General Hospital	Warren	98%	167
Windber Hospital	Windber	98%	62
Carlisle Regional Medical Center	Carlisle	97%	116
Ellwood City Hospital	Ellwood City	97%	68
Excela Health Latrobe Hospital	Latrobe	97%	173
Indiana Regional Medical Center	Indiana	97%	212
Mercy Suburban Hospital	Norristown	97%	30
Moses Taylor Hospital	Scranton	97%	37
Nazareth Hospital	Philadelphia	97%	61
Uniontown Hospital	Uniontown	97%	68
UPMC Bedford	Everett	97%	118
UPMC Mckeesport	McKeesport	97%	30
Alle Kiski Medical Center	Natrona	96%	158
Berwick Hospital Center	Berwick	96%	51
Evangelical Community Hospital	Lewisburg	96%	150
Heritage Valley Sewickley	Sewickley	96%	70
Lewistown Hospital	Lewistown	96%	47
St Catherine Med Ctr Fountain Springs	Ashland	96%	46
Waynesboro Hospital	Waynesboro	96%	47
Clarion Hospital	Clarion	95%	63
Delaware County Memorial Hospital	Drexel Hill	95%	44
Ephrata Community Hospital	Ephrata	95%	38
Gnaden Huetten Memorial Hospital	Lehighton	95%	94
Shamokin Area Community Hospital	Coal Township	95%	88

NOTE: Hospital profiles are in alphabetical order by state, then city, then hospital within the city; Rankings exclude hospitals with less than 25 cases except for patient surveys which excludes hospitals with less than 100 cases; (a) 100–299 cases; (1) The number of cases is too small to be sure how well a hospital is performing; (2) The hospital indicated that the data submitted for this measure were based on a sample of cases; (3) Data was collected during a shorter time period (fewer quarters) than the maximum possible time for this measure; (4) Suppressed for one or more quarters by CMS; (5) No data is available from the hospital for this measure; (6) Fewer than 100 patients completed the HCAHPS survey. Use these rates with caution, as the number of surveys may be too low to reliably assess hospital performance; (7) Survey results are based on less than 12 months of data; (8) Survey results are not available for this reporting period; (9) No or very few patients were eligible for the HCAHPS survey. The scores shown, if any, reflect a very small number of surveys; (10) A state average was not calculated because too few hospitals in the state submitted data; (11) There were discrepancies in the data collection process; Please refer to the User's Guide for a full explanation of data.

UPMC Presbyterian Shadyside	Pittsburgh	95%	217
Wayne Memorial Hospital	Honesdale	95%	38
ACMH Hospital	Kittanning	94%	135
Lansdale Hospital	Lansdale	94%	48
Lock Haven Hospital	Lock Haven	94%	34
Nason Hospital	Roaring Spring	94%	34
Schuylkill Med Ctr-East Norwegian Street	Pottsville	94%	48
Southwest Regional Medical Center	Waynesburg	94%	107
Clearfield Hospital	Clearfield	93%	128
Elk Regional Health Center	Saint Marys	93%	90
Hanover Hospital	Hanover	93%	59
Memorial Hospital - Towanda	Towanda	93%	42
Bloomsburg Hospital	Bloomsburg	92%	101
Charles Cole Memorial Hospital	Coudersport	92%	39
Hazleton General Hospital	Hazleton	92%	321
Mercy Tyler Hospital	Tunkhannock	92%	60
Miners Medical Center	Hastings	92%	117
Chambersburg Hospital	Chambersburg	90%	31
Chestnut Hill Hospital	Philadelphia	90%	59
J C Blair Memorial Hospital	Huntingdon	90%	151
Palmerton Hospital	Palmerton	90%	40
Sunbury Community Hospital	Sunbury	90%	42
Western Penn Hosp-Forbes Reg Campus	Monroeville	86%	86
Excela Health Westmoreland Reg Hosp	Greensburg	81%	32
Highlands Hospital	Connellsville	81%	98

9. Median Time to ECG (minutes)

Hospital Name	City	Min.	Cases
Bloomsburg Hospital	Bloomsburg	0	106
Clearfield Hospital	Clearfield	2	138
Shamokin Area Community Hospital	Coal Township	2	92
Elk Regional Health Center	Saint Marys	4	91
Ephrata Community Hospital	Ephrata	4	39
Palmerton Hospital	Palmerton	4	42
Wayne Memorial Hospital	Honesdale	4	38
Waynesboro Hospital	Waynesboro	4	56
Carlisle Regional Medical Center	Carlisle	5	119
Grand View Hospital	Sellersville	5	67
Hanover Hospital	Hanover	5	63
UPMC Northwest	Seneca	5	148
ACMH Hospital	Kittanning	6	140
Berwick Hospital Center	Berwick	6	52
Charles Cole Memorial Hospital	Coudersport	6	42
Evangelical Community Hospital	Lewisburg	6	153
Excela Health Frick Hospital	Mount Pleasant	6	110
Gnaden Huetten Memorial Hospital	Lehighton	6	101
Grove City Medical Center	Grove City	6	164
Memorial Hospital - Towanda	Towanda	6	47
Schuylkill Med Ctr-S Jackson Street	Pottsville	6	87
Soldiers and Sailors Memorial Hospital	Wellsboro	6	85
Warren General Hospital	Warren	6	173
Bradford Regional Medical Center	Bradford	7	31
Jennersville Regional Hospital	West Grove	7	31
Lewistown Hospital	Lewistown	7	47
Memorial Hospital York	York	7	51
Nason Hospital	Roaring Spring	7	35
Troy Community Hospital[3]	Troy	7	32
Western Penn Hosp-Forbes Reg Campus	Monroeville	7	92
Delaware County Memorial Hospital	Drexel Hill	8	45
Marian Community Hospital	Carbondale	8	49
Schuylkill Med Ctr-East Norwegian Street	Pottsville	8	47
Titusville Hospital	Titusville	8	119
Gettysburg Hospital	Gettysburg	9	76
Lock Haven Hospital	Lock Haven	9	37
Meadville Medical Center	Meadville	9	156
Nazareth Hospital	Philadelphia	9	66
UPMC Bedford	Everett	9	126
UPMC Passavant	Pittsburgh	9	51
UPMC Presbyterian Shadyside	Pittsburgh	9	226
Alle Kiski Medical Center	Natrona	10	165
Monongahela Valley Hospital	Monongahela	10	91
Pottstown Memorial Medical Center	Pottstown	10	73
Southwest Regional Medical Center	Waynesburg	10	110
Excela Health Latrobe Hospital	Latrobe	11	176
Lansdale Hospital	Lansdale	11	50
Mercy Suburban Hospital	Norristown	11	30
Sunbury Community Hospital	Sunbury	11	46
Canonsburg General Hospital	Canonsburg	12	86
Chambersburg Hospital	Chambersburg	12	34
Heritage Valley Sewickley	Sewickley	12	72
Highlands Hospital	Connellsville	12	102
J C Blair Memorial Hospital	Huntingdon	12	158
Mercy Tyler Hospital	Tunkhannock	12	62
UPMC Horizon	Greenville	12	138
UPMC Mckeesport	McKeesport	12	32
UPMC Saint Margaret	Pittsburgh	12	138
Windber Hospital	Windber	12	66
Excela Health Westmoreland Reg Hosp	Greensburg	14	30
Hazleton General Hospital	Hazleton	14	333
Indiana Regional Medical Center	Indiana	14	217
Moses Taylor Hospital	Scranton	14	37
St Catherine Med Ctr Fountain Springs	Ashland	14	44
Ellwood City Hospital	Ellwood City	15	72
Chestnut Hill Hospital	Philadelphia	16	62
Miners Medical Center	Hastings	16	123
Clarion Hospital	Clarion	21	65
Ohio Valley General Hospital	Mckees Rocks	21	47
Uniontown Hospital	Uniontown	22	71

10. Median Time to Transfer (minutes)

Hospital Name	City	Min.	Cases
Hazleton General Hospital	Hazleton	52	44
ACMH Hospital	Kittanning	54	27
Alle Kiski Medical Center	Natrona	55	27
Chestnut Hill Hospital	Philadelphia	64	28
Bloomsburg Hospital	Bloomsburg	65	33
Excela Health Latrobe Hospital	Latrobe	70	35
Nazareth Hospital	Philadelphia	72	26
Indiana Regional Medical Center	Indiana	82	49
UPMC Saint Margaret	Pittsburgh	92	34

Heart Failure Care

12. ACE Inhibitor or ARB for LVSD

Hospital Name	City	Rate	Cases
Bradford Regional Medical Center	Bradford	100%	43
Geisinger Medical Center	Danville	100%	103
Grand View Hospital	Sellersville	100%	58
Heritage Valley Beaver	Beaver	100%	184
Heritage Valley Sewickley	Sewickley	100%	74
Lebanon VA Medical Center	Lebanon	100%	32
Lehigh Valley Hospital - Muhlenberg	Bethlehem	100%	106
Main Line Hospital Paoli	Paoli	100%	68
Mercy Hospital Scranton[2]	Scranton	100%	84
Mercy Suburban Hospital	Norristown	100%	62
Nazareth Hospital	Philadelphia	100%	50
Pinnacle Health Hospitals	Harrisburg	100%	256
Reading Hospital Medical Center	Reading	100%	193
Saint Joseph Medical Center	Reading	100%	109
Saint Mary Medical Center	Langhorne	100%	149
Soldiers and Sailors Memorial Hospital	Wellsboro	100%	28
UPMC Horizon	Greenville	100%	55
UPMC Mckeesport	McKeesport	100%	107
UPMC Northwest	Seneca	100%	49
UPMC Passavant	Pittsburgh	100%	144
UPMC Presbyterian Shadyside	Pittsburgh	100%	515
Wilkes-Barre VA Medical Center	Wilkes-Barre	100%	39
Allegheny General Hospital	Pittsburgh	99%	285
Butler Memorial Hospital	Butler	99%	121
Chestnut Hill Hospital	Philadelphia	99%	99
Good Samaritan Hospital	Lebanon	99%	67
Hahnemann University Hospital	Philadelphia	99%	389
Lehigh Valley Hospital	Allentown	99%	308
Main Line Hospital Bryn Mawr Campus	Bryn Mawr	99%	143
Main Line Hospital Lankenau	Wynnewood	99%	331
Mercy Fitzgerald Hospital	Darby	99%	487
Milton S Hershey Medical Center	Hershey	99%	113
Phoenixville Hospital	Phoenixville	99%	102
Thomas Jefferson University Hospital	Philadelphia	99%	412
UPMC Mercy	Pittsburgh	99%	168
VA Pittsburgh Healthcare System	Pittsburgh	99%	72
The Washington Hospital	Washington	99%	190
Abington Memorial Hospital	Abington	98%	335
Chester County Hospital	West Chester	98%	98
Doylestown Hospital	Doylestown	98%	133
Easton Hospital	Easton	98%	126
Ellwood City Hospital	Ellwood City	98%	42
Gettysburg Hospital	Gettysburg	98%	42
Hazleton General Hospital	Hazleton	98%	53
Holy Redeemer Hospital and Medical Center	Meadowbrook	98%	63
Hospital of Univ of Pennsylvania	Philadelphia	98%	402
Lancaster Regional Medical Center	Lancaster	98%	47
Penn Presbyterian Medical Center	Philadelphia	98%	350
Saint Luke's Hospital Bethlehem	Bethlehem	98%	247
Holy Spirit Hospital	Camp Hill	97%	117
Riddle Memorial Hospital	Media	97%	66
Somerset Hospital	Somerset	97%	38
Waynesboro Hospital	Waynesboro	97%	31
Williamsport Hospital & Medical Center	Williamsport	97%	89
Alle Kiski Medical Center	Natrona	96%	96
Aria Health	Philadelphia	96%	333
Temple University Hospital	Philadelphia	96%	692
UPMC Saint Margaret	Pittsburgh	96%	113
Wayne Memorial Hospital	Honesdale	96%	26
Western Penn Hosp-Forbes Reg Campus	Monroeville	96%	173
Delaware County Memorial Hospital	Drexel Hill	95%	87
Hamot Medical Center	Erie	95%	171
Lansdale Hospital	Lansdale	95%	61
Moses Taylor Hospital	Scranton	95%	41
Robert Packer Hospital	Sayre	95%	208
Chambersburg Hospital	Chambersburg	94%	95
Dubois Regional Medical Center	Dubois	94%	89
Meadville Medical Center	Meadville	94%	31
Western Pennsylvania Hospital	Pittsburgh	94%	141
Albert Einstein Medical Center[2]	Philadelphia	93%	142
Lancaster General Hospital	Lancaster	93%	284
Philadelphia VA Medical Center	Philadelphia	93%	135
Pocono Medical Center	E Stroudsburg	93%	136
Pottstown Memorial Medical Center	Pottstown	93%	104
Windber Hospital	Windber	93%	29
York Hospital	York	93%	203
Canonsburg General Hospital	Canonsburg	92%	40
Jeanes Hospital	Philadelphia	92%	115
Monongahela Valley Hospital	Monongahela	92%	96
Mount Nittany Medical Center	State College	92%	60
Penn Hosp of the Univ of Penn Health Sys	Philadelphia	92%	132
ACMH Hospital	Kittanning	91%	35
Ephrata Community Hospital	Ephrata	91%	46
Excela Health Frick Hospital	Mount Pleasant	91%	46
Excela Health Latrobe Hospital	Latrobe	91%	76
Carlisle Regional Medical Center	Carlisle	90%	61
Community Medical Center	Scranton	90%	110
Crozer Chester Medical Center	Upland	90%	345
Saint Vincent Health Center	Erie	90%	147
Sharon Regional Health System	Sharon	90%	48
Southwest Regional Medical Center	Waynesburg	90%	40
Clearfield Hospital	Clearfield	89%	37
Evangelical Community Hospital	Lewisburg	89%	27
Lower Bucks Hospital	Bristol	89%	88
Memorial Hospital York	York	89%	37
Altoona Regional Health System	Altoona	88%	165
Montgomery Hospital	Norristown	88%	69
Roxborough Memorial Hospital	Phila	87%	69
Uniontown Hospital	Uniontown	87%	100
Elk Regional Health Center	Saint Marys	86%	44
Excela Health Westmoreland Reg Hosp	Greensburg	86%	170
Bloomsburg Hospital	Bloomsburg	85%	26
Grove City Medical Center	Grove City	85%	27
Indiana Regional Medical Center	Indiana	85%	151
Jefferson Regional Medical Center	Pittsburgh	85%	217
Lewistown Hospital	Lewistown	85%	54
Saint Clair Memorial Hospital	Pittsburgh	84%	152
Schuylkill Med Ctr-East Norwegian Street	Pottsville	84%	63
Conemaugh Valley Memorial Hospital	Johnstown	83%	222
Geisinger Wyoming Valley Medical Center	Wilkes-Barre	83%	94
Jameson Memorial Hospital	New Castle	83%	94
Palmerton Hospital	Palmerton	83%	30
Brandywine Hospital	Coatesville	81%	70
Hanover Hospital	Hanover	81%	62
Warren General Hospital	Warren	81%	32
Ohio Valley General Hospital	Mckees Rocks	80%	70
Wilkes-Barre General Hospital	Wilkes-Barre	80%	135
Schuylkill Med Ctr-S Jackson Street	Pottsville	79%	39
Saint Joseph's Hospital	Philadelphia	76%	80
Clarion Hospital	Clarion	73%	30

13. Discharge Instructions

Hospital Name	City	Rate	Cases
Holy Redeemer Hospital and Medical Center	Meadowbrook	100%	232
Jennersville Regional Hospital	West Grove	100%	53
Jersey Shore Hospital	Jersey Shore	100%	72
Magee Womens Hosp of UPMC Health Sys	Pittsburgh	100%	59
Memorial Hospital - Towanda	Towanda	100%	42
Mercy Hospital Scranton[2]	Scranton	100%	202
Saint Luke's Miners Memorial Hospital	Coaldale	100%	55
Saint Mary Medical Center	Langhorne	100%	458
Gnaden Huetten Memorial Hospital	Lehighton	99%	99
Main Line Hospital Paoli	Paoli	99%	181
Nazareth Hospital	Philadelphia	99%	230
Somerset Hospital	Somerset	99%	92
UPMC Horizon	Greenville	99%	165
UPMC Mckeesport	McKeesport	99%	305
Wilkes-Barre VA Medical Center	Wilkes-Barre	99%	109
Ellwood City Hospital	Ellwood City	98%	99
Lebanon VA Medical Center	Lebanon	98%	57
Lehigh Valley Hospital - Muhlenberg	Bethlehem	98%	366
Main Line Hospital Bryn Mawr Campus	Bryn Mawr	98%	339
Mercy Fitzgerald Hospital	Darby	98%	842
Mercy Suburban Hospital	Norristown	98%	137
Reading Hospital Medical Center	Reading	98%	582
Thomas Jefferson University Hospital	Philadelphia	98%	853
UPMC Presbyterian Shadyside	Pittsburgh	98%	1113
Butler Memorial Hospital	Butler	97%	304
Chestnut Hill Hospital	Philadelphia	97%	171
Crozer Chester Medical Center	Upland	97%	801
Delaware County Memorial Hospital	Drexel Hill	97%	279
Excela Health Frick Hospital	Mount Pleasant	97%	197
Hahnemann University Hospital	Philadelphia	97%	642
James E. Van Zandt VA Med Ctr-Altoona	Altoona	97%	35
Lock Haven Hospital	Lock Haven	97%	60

NOTE: Hospital profiles are in alphabetical order by state, then city, then hospital within the city; Rankings exclude hospitals with less than 25 cases except for patient surveys which excludes hospitals with less than 100 cases; (a) 100–299 cases; (1) The number of cases is too small to be sure how well a hospital is performing; (2) The hospital indicated that the data submitted for this measure were based on a sample of cases; (3) Data was collected during a shorter time period (fewer quarters) than the maximum possible time for this measure; (4) Suppressed for one or more quarters by CMS; (5) No data is available from the hospital for this measure; (6) Fewer than 100 patients completed the HCAHPS survey. Use these rates with caution, as the number of surveys may be too low to reliably assess hospital performance; (7) Survey results are based on less than 12 months of data; (8) Survey results are not available for this reporting period; (9) No or very few patients were eligible for the HCAHPS survey. The scores shown, if any, reflect a very small number of surveys; (10) A state average was not calculated because too few hospitals in the state submitted data; (11) There were discrepancies in the data collection process; Please refer to the User's Guide for a full explanation of data.

Nason Hospital	Roaring Spring	97%	62
Penn Hosp of the Univ of Penn Health Sys	Philadelphia	97%	384
Soldiers and Sailors Memorial Hospital	Wellsboro	97%	77
UPMC Passavant	Pittsburgh	97%	347
Albert Einstein Medical Center[2]	Philadelphia	96%	221
Geisinger Medical Center	Danville	96%	304
Gettysburg Hospital	Gettysburg	96%	90
Holy Spirit Hospital	Camp Hill	96%	339
Memorial Hospital York	York	96%	114
Saint Joseph Medical Center	Reading	96%	301
Temple University Hospital	Philadelphia	96%	1216
VA Pittsburgh Healthcare System	Pittsburgh	96%	217
Allegheny General Hospital	Pittsburgh	95%	571
Corry Memorial Hospital	Corry	95%	58
Evangelical Community Hospital	Lewisburg	95%	106
Hazleton General Hospital	Hazleton	95%	183
Lancaster Regional Medical Center	Lancaster	95%	87
Lehigh Valley Hospital	Allentown	95%	879
Marian Community Hospital	Carbondale	95%	65
Phoenixville Hospital	Phoenixville	95%	207
Pottstown Memorial Medical Center	Pottstown	95%	183
Saint Vincent Health Center	Erie	95%	390
Aria Health	Philadelphia	94%	765
Brandywine Hospital	Coatesville	94%	157
Grove City Medical Center	Grove City	94%	51
Hanover Hospital	Hanover	94%	156
Jeanes Hospital	Philadelphia	94%	278
Main Line Hospital Lankenau	Wynnewood	94%	666
Sharon Regional Health System	Sharon	94%	153
Wayne Memorial Hospital	Honesdale	94%	83
Heritage Valley Beaver	Beaver	93%	638
Heritage Valley Sewickley	Sewickley	93%	241
Monongahela Valley Hospital	Monongahela	93%	354
Roxborough Memorial Hospital	Phila	93%	131
Saint Luke's Quakertown Hospital	Quakertown	93%	55
The Washington Hospital	Washington	93%	528
Doylestown Hospital	Doylestown	92%	357
Easton Hospital	Easton	92%	312
Good Samaritan Hospital	Lebanon	92%	160
St Catherine Med Ctr Fountain Springs	Ashland	92%	64
Saint Luke's Hospital Bethlehem	Bethlehem	92%	770
UPMC Northwest	Seneca	92%	138
Excela Health Latrobe Hospital	Latrobe	91%	223
Grand View Hospital	Sellersville	91%	245
Hamot Medical Center	Erie	91%	422
Jameson Memorial Hospital	New Castle	91%	285
Montgomery Hospital	Norristown	91%	191
UPMC Saint Margaret	Pittsburgh	91%	389
Community Medical Center	Scranton	90%	225
Excela Health Westmoreland Reg Hosp	Greensburg	90%	536
Jefferson Regional Medical Center	Pittsburgh	90%	605
Moses Taylor Hospital	Scranton	90%	125
Sacred Heart Hospital	Allentown	90%	93
Schuylkill Med Ctr-East Norwegian Street	Pottsville	90%	186
Western Pennsylvania Hospital	Pittsburgh	90%	288
Williamsport Hospital & Medical Center	Williamsport	90%	198
Altoona Regional Health System	Altoona	89%	402
Berwick Hospital Center	Berwick	89%	113
Carlisle Regional Medical Center	Carlisle	89%	165
Erie VA Medical Center	Erie	89%	28
Lewistown Hospital	Lewistown	89%	178
Milton S Hershey Medical Center	Hershey	89%	399
Palmerton Hospital	Palmerton	89%	90
Penn Presbyterian Medical Center	Philadelphia	89%	691
Pinnacle Health Hospitals	Harrisburg	89%	605
Titusville Hospital	Titusville	89%	46
Abington Memorial Hospital	Abington	88%	701
Chambersburg Hospital	Chambersburg	88%	314
Chester County Hospital	West Chester	88%	265
Hospital of Univ of Pennsylvania	Philadelphia	88%	708
Riddle Memorial Hospital	Media	88%	192
Schuylkill Med Ctr-S Jackson Street	Pottsville	88%	152
Wilkes-Barre General Hospital	Wilkes-Barre	88%	395
Windber Hospital	Windber	88%	92
ACMH Hospital	Kittanning	87%	111
Bloomsburg Hospital	Bloomsburg	87%	67
Bradford Regional Medical Center	Bradford	87%	62
Charles Cole Memorial Hospital	Coudersport	87%	47
Dubois Regional Medical Center	Dubois	87%	226
Robert Packer Hospital	Sayre	87%	303
UPMC Mercy	Pittsburgh	87%	366
Mount Nittany Medical Center	State College	86%	235
Highlands Hospital	Connellsville	85%	59
Indiana Regional Medical Center	Indiana	85%	260
Waynesboro Hospital	Waynesboro	85%	87
Western Penn Hosp-Forbes Reg Campus	Monroeville	85%	470
Alle Kiski Medical Center	Natrona	84%	370
Brookville Hospital	Brookville	83%	53
Geisinger Wyoming Valley Medical Center	Wilkes-Barre	83%	193
Southwest Regional Medical Center	Waynesburg	83%	156
Sunbury Community Hospital	Sunbury	83%	65
Ephrata Community Hospital	Ephrata	82%	131
York Hospital	York	82%	617
Philadelphia VA Medical Center	Philadelphia	81%	272
Millcreek Community Hospital	Erie	80%	46
UPMC Bedford	Everett	80%	45
J C Blair Memorial Hospital	Huntingdon	79%	57
Saint Clair Memorial Hospital	Pittsburgh	79%	454
Conemaugh Valley Memorial Hospital	Johnstown	78%	614
Lansdale Hospital	Lansdale	77%	146
Meadville Medical Center	Meadville	77%	91
Uniontown Hospital	Uniontown	76%	309
Punxsutawney Area Hospital	Punxsutawney	75%	48
Lancaster General Hospital	Lancaster	74%	794
Muncy Valley Hospital	Muncy	73%	26
Shamokin Area Community Hospital	Coal Township	72%	102
Lower Bucks Hospital	Bristol	71%	215
Pocono Medical Center	E Stroudsburg	68%	367
Clarion Hospital	Clarion	67%	86
Clearfield Hospital	Clearfield	67%	114
Ohio Valley General Hospital	Mckees Rocks	67%	151
Canonsburg General Hospital	Canonsburg	65%	105
Warren General Hospital	Warren	60%	78
Elk Regional Health Center	Saint Marys	58%	122
Miners Medical Center	Hastings	41%	27
Mercy Tyler Hospital	Tunkhannock	26%	39
Saint Joseph's Hospital	Philadelphia	23%	213
Kane Community Hospital	Kane	18%	74

14. Evaluation of LVS Function

Hospital Name	City	Rate	Cases
Abington Memorial Hospital	Abington	100%	923
ACMH Hospital	Kittanning	100%	151
Alle Kiski Medical Center	Natrona	100%	469
Allegheny General Hospital	Pittsburgh	100%	674
Aria Health	Philadelphia	100%	953
Brandywine Hospital	Coatesville	100%	231
Butler Memorial Hospital	Butler	100%	387
Chester County Hospital	West Chester	100%	351
Doylestown Hospital	Doylestown	100%	462
Dubois Regional Medical Center	Dubois	100%	263
Easton Hospital	Easton	100%	428
Ellwood City Hospital	Ellwood City	100%	130
Ephrata Community Hospital	Ephrata	100%	183
Erie VA Medical Center	Erie	100%	34
Excela Health Frick Hospital	Mount Pleasant	100%	223
Excela Health Latrobe Hospital	Latrobe	100%	293
Excela Health Westmoreland Reg Hosp	Greensburg	100%	758
Geisinger Medical Center	Danville	100%	402
Geisinger Wyoming Valley Medical Center	Wilkes-Barre	100%	255
Gettysburg Hospital	Gettysburg	100%	131
Grand View Hospital	Sellersville	100%	310
Hahnemann University Hospital	Philadelphia	100%	699
Hamot Medical Center	Erie	100%	538
Hazleton General Hospital	Hazleton	100%	282
Highlands Hospital	Connellsville	100%	61
Holy Spirit Hospital	Camp Hill	100%	468
Hospital of Univ of Pennsylvania	Philadelphia	100%	781
James E. Van Zandt VA Med Ctr-Altoona	Altoona	100%	37
Jennersville Regional Hospital	West Grove	100%	95
Jersey Shore Hospital	Jersey Shore	100%	86
Lancaster Regional Medical Center	Lancaster	100%	112
Lebanon VA Medical Center	Lebanon	100%	76
Lehigh Valley Hospital - Muhlenberg	Bethlehem	100%	466
Lewistown Hospital	Lewistown	100%	274
Magee Womens Hosp of UPMC Health Sys	Pittsburgh	100%	83
Main Line Hospital Bryn Mawr Campus	Bryn Mawr	100%	491
Main Line Hospital Lankenau	Wynnewood	100%	857
Main Line Hospital Paoli	Paoli	100%	246
Mercy Suburban Hospital	Norristown	100%	193
Mid-Valley Hospital[2,3]	Peckville	100%	33
Muncy Valley Hospital	Muncy	100%	35
Nason Hospital	Roaring Spring	100%	82
Nazareth Hospital	Philadelphia	100%	398
Ohio Valley General Hospital	Mckees Rocks	100%	212
Penn Hosp of the Univ of Penn Health Sys	Philadelphia	100%	433
Pinnacle Health Hospitals	Harrisburg	100%	769
Reading Hospital Medical Center	Reading	100%	789
Robert Packer Hospital	Sayre	100%	370
Saint Joseph Medical Center	Reading	100%	368
Saint Mary Medical Center	Langhorne	100%	598
Saint Vincent Health Center	Erie	100%	539
Somerset Hospital	Somerset	100%	114
UPMC Bedford	Everett	100%	63
UPMC Horizon	Greenville	100%	224
UPMC Mckeesport	McKeesport	100%	442
UPMC Mercy	Pittsburgh	100%	487
UPMC Northwest	Seneca	100%	201
UPMC Passavant	Pittsburgh	100%	508
UPMC Presbyterian Shadyside	Pittsburgh	100%	1383
UPMC Saint Margaret	Pittsburgh	100%	573
VA Pittsburgh Healthcare System	Pittsburgh	100%	237
The Washington Hospital	Washington	100%	666
Wilkes-Barre VA Medical Center	Wilkes-Barre	100%	129
Albert Einstein Medical Center[2]	Philadelphia	99%	305
Altoona Regional Health System	Altoona	99%	542
Berwick Hospital Center	Berwick	99%	160
Canonsburg General Hospital	Canonsburg	99%	152
Carlisle Regional Medical Center	Carlisle	99%	245
Clearfield Hospital	Clearfield	99%	159
Community Medical Center	Scranton	99%	304
Delaware County Memorial Hospital	Drexel Hill	99%	342
Evangelical Community Hospital	Lewisburg	99%	143
Gnaden Huetten Memorial Hospital	Lehighton	99%	127
Good Samaritan Hospital	Lebanon	99%	237
Heritage Valley Beaver	Beaver	99%	787
Heritage Valley Sewickley	Sewickley	99%	312
Holy Redeemer Hospital and Medical Center	Meadowbrook	99%	339
Jefferson Regional Medical Center	Pittsburgh	99%	744
Lancaster General Hospital	Lancaster	99%	1005
Lansdale Hospital	Lansdale	99%	222
Lehigh Valley Hospital	Allentown	99%	1112
Lock Haven Hospital	Lock Haven	99%	79
Memorial Hospital York	York	99%	144
Mercy Fitzgerald Hospital	Darby	99%	973
Mercy Hospital Scranton[2]	Scranton	99%	303
Milton S Hershey Medical Center	Hershey	99%	462
Monongahela Valley Hospital	Monongahela	99%	399
Montgomery Hospital	Norristown	99%	234
Moses Taylor Hospital	Scranton	99%	197
Mount Nittany Medical Center	State College	99%	298
Penn Presbyterian Medical Center	Philadelphia	99%	804
Philadelphia VA Medical Center	Philadelphia	99%	282
Pocono Medical Center	E Stroudsburg	99%	433
Pottstown Memorial Medical Center	Pottstown	99%	253
Riddle Memorial Hospital	Media	99%	286
Roxborough Memorial Hospital	Phila	99%	206
Saint Luke's Hospital Bethlehem	Bethlehem	99%	992
Saint Luke's Quakertown Hospital	Quakertown	99%	93
Shamokin Area Community Hospital	Coal Township	99%	174
Sharon Regional Health System	Sharon	99%	202
Temple University Hospital	Philadelphia	99%	1294
Thomas Jefferson University Hospital	Philadelphia	99%	985
Waynesboro Hospital	Waynesboro	99%	106
Western Pennsylvania Hospital	Pittsburgh	99%	334
Western Penn Hosp-Forbes Reg Campus	Monroeville	99%	667
Williamsport Hospital & Medical Center	Williamsport	99%	253
York Hospital	York	99%	756
Crozer Chester Medical Center	Upland	98%	927
Heart of Lancaster Regional Medical Center	Lititz	98%	46
Jeanes Hospital	Philadelphia	98%	355
Lower Bucks Hospital	Bristol	98%	262
Marian Community Hospital	Carbondale	98%	93
Millcreek Community Hospital	Erie	98%	80
Saint Clair Memorial Hospital	Pittsburgh	98%	614
Soldiers and Sailors Memorial Hospital	Wellsboro	98%	94
Sunbury Community Hospital	Sunbury	98%	106
Uniontown Hospital	Uniontown	98%	410
Wayne Memorial Hospital	Honesdale	98%	102
Windber Hospital	Windber	98%	118
Brookville Hospital	Brookville	97%	63
Chambersburg Hospital	Chambersburg	97%	394
Chestnut Hill Hospital	Philadelphia	97%	296
Grove City Medical Center	Grove City	97%	98
Indiana Regional Medical Center	Indiana	97%	333
Meadville Medical Center	Meadville	97%	129
Saint Luke's Miners Memorial Hospital	Coaldale	97%	74
Titusville Hospital	Titusville	97%	63
Conemaugh Valley Memorial Hospital	Johnstown	96%	803
Jameson Memorial Hospital	New Castle	96%	365
Phoenixville Hospital	Phoenixville	96%	257
Southwest Regional Medical Center	Waynesburg	96%	198
Bradford Regional Medical Center	Bradford	95%	86
Sacred Heart Hospital	Allentown	95%	130
Schuylkill Med Ctr-East Norwegian Street	Pottsville	95%	297
Mercy Tyler Hospital	Tunkhannock	94%	50
Palmerton Hospital	Palmerton	94%	115
Wilkes-Barre General Hospital	Wilkes-Barre	94%	579
Punxsutawney Area Hospital	Punxsutawney	93%	57
Warren General Hospital	Warren	93%	111
J C Blair Memorial Hospital	Huntingdon	92%	75
Memorial Hospital - Towanda	Towanda	92%	52
Elk Regional Health Center	Saint Marys	90%	178
Bloomsburg Hospital	Bloomsburg	89%	91
Clarion Hospital	Clarion	88%	112
Charles Cole Memorial Hospital	Coudersport	87%	70
Corry Memorial Hospital	Corry	86%	76
Miners Medical Center	Hastings	85%	34
St Catherine Med Ctr Fountain Springs	Ashland	84%	87
Kane Community Hospital	Kane	82%	95
Saint Joseph's Hospital	Philadelphia	79%	257
Schuylkill Med Ctr-S Jackson Street	Pottsville	79%	218

NOTE: Hospital profiles are in alphabetical order by state, then city, then hospital within the city; Rankings exclude hospitals with less than 25 cases except for patient surveys which excludes hospitals with less than 100 cases; (a) 100–299 cases; (1) The number of cases is too small to be sure how well a hospital is performing; (2) The hospital indicated that the data submitted for this measure were based on a sample of cases; (3) Data was collected during a shorter time period (fewer quarters) than the maximum possible time for this measure; (4) Suppressed for one or more quarters by CMS; (5) No data is available from the hospital for this measure; (6) Fewer than 100 patients completed the HCAHPS survey. Use these rates with caution, as the number of surveys may be too low to reliably assess hospital performance; (7) Survey results are based on less than 12 months of data; (8) Survey results are not available for this reporting period; (9) No or very few patients were eligible for the HCAHPS survey. The scores shown, if any, reflect a very small number of surveys; (10) A state average was not calculated because too few hospitals in the state submitted data; (11) There were discrepancies in the data collection process; Please refer to the User's Guide for a full explanation of data.

Hanover Hospital	Hanover	76%	197
Montrose General Hospital	Montrose	70%	27

15. Smoking Cessation Advice

Hospital Name	City	Rate	Cases
Abington Memorial Hospital	Abington	100%	91
Albert Einstein Medical Center[2]	Philadelphia	100%	96
Alle Kiski Medical Center	Natrona	100%	55
Allegheny General Hospital	Pittsburgh	100%	109
Altoona Regional Health System	Altoona	100%	57
Aria Health	Philadelphia	100%	201
Brandywine Hospital	Coatesville	100%	36
Butler Memorial Hospital	Butler	100%	49
Carlisle Regional Medical Center	Carlisle	100%	33
Chester County Hospital	West Chester	100%	55
Chestnut Hill Hospital	Philadelphia	100%	29
Community Medical Center	Scranton	100%	37
Conemaugh Valley Memorial Hospital	Johnstown	100%	94
Crozer Chester Medical Center	Upland	100%	203
Delaware County Memorial Hospital	Drexel Hill	100%	50
Dubois Regional Medical Center	Dubois	100%	36
Easton Hospital	Easton	100%	49
Excela Health Frick Hospital	Mount Pleasant	100%	37
Excela Health Latrobe Hospital	Latrobe	100%	26
Excela Health Westmoreland Reg Hosp	Greensburg	100%	54
Geisinger Medical Center	Danville	100%	68
Geisinger Wyoming Valley Medical Center	Wilkes-Barre	100%	34
Hamot Medical Center	Erie	100%	91
Hazleton General Hospital	Hazleton	100%	32
Heritage Valley Beaver	Beaver	100%	83
Holy Spirit Hospital	Camp Hill	100%	52
Jameson Memorial Hospital	New Castle	100%	35
Jeanes Hospital	Philadelphia	100%	39
Jefferson Regional Medical Center	Pittsburgh	100%	74
Lancaster General Hospital	Lancaster	100%	126
Lancaster Regional Medical Center	Lancaster	100%	31
Lehigh Valley Hospital	Allentown	100%	115
Lehigh Valley Hospital - Muhlenberg	Bethlehem	100%	41
Main Line Hospital Lankenau	Wynnewood	100%	139
Mercy Fitzgerald Hospital	Darby	100%	305
Mercy Hospital Scranton[2]	Scranton	100%	36
Mercy Suburban Hospital	Norristown	100%	25
Monongahela Valley Hospital	Monongahela	100%	47
Montgomery Hospital	Norristown	100%	39
Moses Taylor Hospital	Scranton	100%	34
Mount Nittany Medical Center	State College	100%	31
Nazareth Hospital	Philadelphia	100%	37
Penn Presbyterian Medical Center	Philadelphia	100%	160
Penn Hosp of the Univ of Penn Health Sys	Philadelphia	100%	66
Pinnacle Health Hospitals	Harrisburg	100%	113
Pottstown Memorial Medical Center	Pottstown	100%	27
Reading Hospital Medical Center	Reading	100%	87
Robert Packer Hospital	Sayre	100%	31
Roxborough Memorial Hospital	Phila	100%	51
Saint Clair Memorial Hospital	Pittsburgh	100%	54
Saint Mary Medical Center	Langhorne	100%	51
Saint Vincent Health Center	Erie	100%	58
Temple University Hospital	Philadelphia	100%	84
Thomas Jefferson University Hospital	Philadelphia	100%	229
UPMC Horizon	Greenville	100%	31
UPMC Mckeesport	McKeesport	100%	52
UPMC Mercy	Pittsburgh	100%	96
UPMC Northwest	Seneca	100%	28
UPMC Passavant	Pittsburgh	100%	37
UPMC Presbyterian Shadyside	Pittsburgh	100%	260
UPMC Saint Margaret	Pittsburgh	100%	60
VA Pittsburgh Healthcare System	Pittsburgh	100%	51
The Washington Hospital	Washington	100%	105
Western Pennsylvania Hospital	Pittsburgh	100%	64
Western Penn Hosp-Forbes Reg Campus	Monroeville	100%	77
Hospital of Univ of Pennsylvania	Philadelphia	99%	174
Philadelphia VA Medical Center	Philadelphia	99%	107
Saint Luke's Hospital Bethlehem	Bethlehem	99%	110
Hahnemann University Hospital	Philadelphia	98%	193
Heritage Valley Sewickley	Sewickley	98%	41
Milton S Hershey Medical Center	Hershey	98%	54
Pocono Medical Center	E Stroudsburg	98%	83
Saint Joseph Medical Center	Reading	98%	55
Wilkes-Barre General Hospital	Wilkes-Barre	98%	55
Chambersburg Hospital	Chambersburg	97%	61
Doylestown Hospital	Doylestown	97%	31
York Hospital	York	97%	126
Phoenixville Hospital	Phoenixville	96%	28
Indiana Regional Medical Center	Indiana	94%	35
Uniontown Hospital	Uniontown	94%	63
Williamsport Hospital & Medical Center	Williamsport	94%	35
Ohio Valley General Hospital	Mckees Rocks	92%	25
Southwest Regional Medical Center	Waynesburg	92%	37
Lower Bucks Hospital	Bristol	90%	39
Saint Joseph's Hospital	Philadelphia	61%	112

Pneumonia Care

16. Appropriate Initial Antibiotic

Hospital Name	City	Rate	Cases
Heart of Lancaster Regional Medical Center	Lititz	100%	28
UPMC Presbyterian Shadyside	Pittsburgh	100%	240
Wilkes-Barre VA Medical Center	Wilkes-Barre	100%	42
York Hospital	York	100%	223
Gettysburg Hospital	Gettysburg	99%	71
Grand View Hospital	Sellersville	99%	146
Holy Spirit Hospital	Camp Hill	99%	256
Main Line Hospital Bryn Mawr Campus	Bryn Mawr	99%	145
Waynesboro Hospital	Waynesboro	99%	71
Albert Einstein Medical Center	Philadelphia	98%	99
Charles Cole Memorial Hospital	Coudersport	98%	44
Grove City Medical Center	Grove City	98%	65
Jeanes Hospital	Philadelphia	98%	122
Roxborough Memorial Hospital	Phila	98%	43
Southwest Regional Medical Center	Waynesburg	98%	111
UPMC Mckeesport	McKeesport	98%	103
ACMH Hospital	Kittanning	97%	91
Aria Health	Philadelphia	97%	505
Butler Memorial Hospital	Butler	97%	188
Carlisle Regional Medical Center	Carlisle	97%	93
Community Medical Center	Scranton	97%	175
Geisinger Medical Center	Danville	97%	102
Hahnemann University Hospital	Philadelphia	97%	99
Main Line Hospital Lankenau	Wynnewood	97%	124
Main Line Hospital Paoli	Paoli	97%	127
Meadville Medical Center	Meadville	97%	92
Mercy Suburban Hospital	Norristown	97%	63
Nazareth Hospital	Philadelphia	97%	143
Pinnacle Health Hospitals	Harrisburg	97%	229
Pottstown Memorial Medical Center	Pottstown	97%	195
Saint Luke's Quakertown Hospital	Quakertown	97%	78
UPMC Bedford	Everett	97%	59
Abington Memorial Hospital	Abington	96%	249
Allegheny General Hospital	Pittsburgh	96%	109
Chestnut Hill Hospital	Philadelphia	96%	77
Excela Health Latrobe Hospital	Latrobe	96%	124
Geisinger Wyoming Valley Medical Center	Wilkes-Barre	96%	129
Lansdale Hospital	Lansdale	96%	78
Lehigh Valley Hospital - Muhlenberg	Bethlehem	96%	158
Lock Haven Hospital	Lock Haven	96%	50
Riddle Memorial Hospital	Media	96%	150
Robert Packer Hospital	Sayre	96%	95
Saint Clair Memorial Hospital	Pittsburgh	96%	360
Soldiers and Sailors Memorial Hospital	Wellsboro	96%	72
Troy Community Hospital	Troy	96%	26
Bloomsburg Hospital	Bloomsburg	95%	91
Crozer Chester Medical Center	Upland	95%	352
Delaware County Memorial Hospital	Drexel Hill	95%	111
Evangelical Community Hospital	Lewisburg	95%	117
Hamot Medical Center	Erie	95%	180
Lancaster General Hospital	Lancaster	95%	243
Mercy Fitzgerald Hospital	Darby	95%	186
Milton S Hershey Medical Center	Hershey	95%	129
Mount Nittany Medical Center	State College	95%	134
Muncy Valley Hospital	Muncy	95%	38
Punxsutawney Area Hospital	Punxsutawney	95%	61
Reading Hospital Medical Center	Reading	95%	331
Saint Luke's Hospital Bethlehem	Bethlehem	95%	300
Saint Mary Medical Center	Langhorne	95%	256
UPMC Horizon	Greenville	95%	147
UPMC Saint Margaret	Pittsburgh	95%	221
Brookville Hospital	Brookville	94%	31
Corry Memorial Hospital	Corry	94%	52
Jennersville Regional Hospital	West Grove	94%	151
Lancaster Regional Medical Center	Lancaster	94%	70
Lehigh Valley Hospital	Allentown	94%	257
Magee Womens Hosp of UPMC Health Sys	Pittsburgh	94%	34
Memorial Hospital York	York	94%	127
Monongahela Valley Hospital	Monongahela	94%	170
Nason Hospital	Roaring Spring	94%	63
Pocono Medical Center	E Stroudsburg	94%	207
Sunbury Community Hospital	Sunbury	94%	67
Temple University Hospital	Philadelphia	94%	218
UPMC Northwest	Seneca	94%	107
The Washington Hospital	Washington	94%	244
Western Penn Hosp-Forbes Reg Campus	Monroeville	94%	215
Williamsport Hospital & Medical Center	Williamsport	94%	149
Canonsburg General Hospital	Canonsburg	93%	72
Conemaugh Valley Memorial Hospital	Johnstown	93%	209
Hazleton General Hospital	Hazleton	93%	141
Heritage Valley Sewickley	Sewickley	93%	150
J C Blair Memorial Hospital	Huntingdon	93%	44
Jameson Memorial Hospital	New Castle	93%	162
Saint Vincent Health Center	Erie	93%	154
Western Pennsylvania Hospital	Pittsburgh	93%	104
Windber Hospital	Windber	93%	59
Bradford Regional Medical Center	Bradford	92%	59
Brandywine Hospital	Coatesville	92%	129
Clearfield Hospital	Clearfield	92%	118
Excela Health Westmoreland Reg Hosp	Greensburg	92%	185
Heritage Valley Beaver	Beaver	92%	211
Indiana Regional Medical Center	Indiana	92%	126
James E. Van Zandt VA Med Ctr-Altoona	Altoona	92%	36
Lewistown Hospital	Lewistown	92%	128
Schuylkill Med Ctr-East Norwegian Street	Pottsville	92%	64
Thomas Jefferson University Hospital	Philadelphia	92%	264
UPMC Mercy	Pittsburgh	92%	212
Wayne Memorial Hospital	Honesdale	92%	83
Alle Kiski Medical Center	Natrona	91%	148
Erie VA Medical Center	Erie	91%	33
Good Samaritan Hospital	Lebanon	91%	160
Holy Redeemer Hospital and Medical Center	Meadowbrook	91%	109
Penn Presbyterian Medical Center	Philadelphia	91%	76
Uniontown Hospital	Uniontown	91%	183
Wilkes-Barre General Hospital	Wilkes-Barre	91%	260
Altoona Regional Health System	Altoona	90%	198
Chester County Hospital	West Chester	90%	156
Ellwood City Hospital	Ellwood City	90%	42
Ephrata Community Hospital	Ephrata	90%	144
Excela Health Frick Hospital	Mount Pleasant	90%	73
Jefferson Regional Medical Center	Pittsburgh	90%	232
Marian Community Hospital	Carbondale	90%	108
Mercy Hospital Scranton[2]	Scranton	90%	71
Montgomery Hospital	Norristown	90%	82
Penn Hosp of the Univ of Penn Health Sys	Philadelphia	90%	99
Phoenixville Hospital	Phoenixville	90%	105
Saint Luke's Miners Memorial Hospital	Coaldale	90%	39
Chambersburg Hospital	Chambersburg	89%	152
Clarion Hospital	Clarion	89%	94
Dubois Regional Medical Center	Dubois	89%	70
Saint Joseph Medical Center	Reading	89%	124
Shamokin Area Community Hospital	Coal Township	89%	37
Somerset Hospital	Somerset	89%	76
VA Pittsburgh Healthcare System	Pittsburgh	89%	56
Hospital of Univ of Pennsylvania	Philadelphia	88%	96
Jersey Shore Hospital	Jersey Shore	88%	60
UPMC Passavant	Pittsburgh	88%	263
Berwick Hospital Center	Berwick	87%	53
Doylestown Hospital	Doylestown	87%	183
Sharon Regional Health System	Sharon	87%	94
Titusville Hospital	Titusville	87%	47
Warren General Hospital	Warren	87%	67
Philadelphia VA Medical Center	Philadelphia	86%	58
Elk Regional Health Center	Saint Marys	85%	111
Hanover Hospital	Hanover	85%	93
Moses Taylor Hospital	Scranton	85%	121
Schuylkill Med Ctr-S Jackson Street	Pottsville	85%	99
Easton Hospital	Easton	84%	123
Kane Community Hospital	Kane	84%	44
Lower Bucks Hospital	Bristol	84%	90
Ohio Valley General Hospital	Mckees Rocks	84%	98
Gnaden Huetten Memorial Hospital	Lehighton	83%	48
Highlands Hospital	Connellsville	82%	60
Mercy Tyler Hospital	Tunkhannock	82%	68
Sacred Heart Hospital	Allentown	80%	51
Miners Medical Center	Hastings	79%	43
St Catherine Med Ctr Fountain Springs	Ashland	78%	32
Palmerton Hospital	Palmerton	76%	41
Memorial Hospital - Towanda	Towanda	74%	61
Saint Joseph's Hospital	Philadelphia	68%	37

17. Blood Culture Timing

Hospital Name	City	Rate	Cases
Brookville Hospital	Brookville	100%	37
Butler Memorial Hospital	Butler	100%	217
Canonsburg General Hospital	Canonsburg	100%	143
Corry Memorial Hospital	Corry	100%	46
Excela Health Frick Hospital	Mount Pleasant	100%	97
Grove City Medical Center	Grove City	100%	80
Heart of Lancaster Regional Medical Center	Lititz	100%	50
Jameson Memorial Hospital	New Castle	100%	248
Lock Haven Hospital	Lock Haven	100%	59
Magee Womens Hosp of UPMC Health Sys	Pittsburgh	100%	32
Main Line Hospital Bryn Mawr Campus	Bryn Mawr	100%	271
Main Line Hospital Paoli	Paoli	100%	164
Moses Taylor Hospital	Scranton	100%	184
Nason Hospital	Roaring Spring	100%	76
Saint Luke's Miners Memorial Hospital	Coaldale	100%	57
Southwest Regional Medical Center	Waynesburg	100%	120
UPMC Mckeesport	McKeesport	100%	252
UPMC Presbyterian Shadyside	Pittsburgh	100%	447
The Washington Hospital	Washington	100%	301
Windber Hospital	Windber	100%	72
Alle Kiski Medical Center	Natrona	99%	69
Community Medical Center	Scranton	99%	211
Dubois Regional Medical Center	Dubois	99%	109
Excela Health Westmoreland Reg Hosp	Greensburg	99%	284

NOTE: Hospital profiles are in alphabetical order by state, then city, then hospital within the city; Rankings exclude hospitals with less than 25 cases except for patient surveys which excludes hospitals with less than 100 cases; (a) 100–299 cases; (1) The number of cases is too small to be sure how well a hospital is performing; (2) The hospital indicated that the data submitted for this measure were based on a sample of cases; (3) Data was collected during a shorter time period (fewer quarters) than the maximum possible time for this measure; (4) Suppressed for one or more quarters by CMS; (5) No data is available from the hospital for this measure; (6) Fewer than 100 patients completed the HCAHPS survey. Use these rates with caution, as the number of surveys may be too low to reliably assess hospital performance; (7) Survey results are based on less than 12 months of data; (8) Survey results are not available for this reporting period; (9) No or very few patients were eligible for the HCAHPS survey. The scores shown, if any, reflect a very small number of surveys; (10) A state average was not calculated because too few hospitals in the state submitted data; (11) There were discrepancies in the data collection process; Please refer to the User's Guide for a full explanation of data.

Grand View Hospital	Sellersville	99%	229
Heritage Valley Sewickley	Sewickley	99%	240
Holy Spirit Hospital	Camp Hill	99%	369
Lewistown Hospital	Lewistown	99%	224
Main Line Hospital Lankenau	Wynnewood	99%	278
Mercy Hospital Scranton[2]	Scranton	99%	99
Saint Mary Medical Center	Langhorne	99%	435
UPMC Horizon	Greenville	99%	179
UPMC Northwest	Seneca	99%	160
UPMC Saint Margaret	Pittsburgh	99%	259
VA Pittsburgh Healthcare System	Pittsburgh	99%	121
Wilkes-Barre VA Medical Center	Wilkes-Barre	99%	77
Aria Health	Philadelphia	98%	829
Chambersburg Hospital	Chambersburg	98%	223
Chestnut Hill Hospital	Philadelphia	98%	184
Conemaugh Valley Memorial Hospital	Johnstown	98%	343
Crozer Chester Medical Center	Upland	98%	466
Erie VA Medical Center	Erie	98%	55
Excela Health Latrobe Hospital	Latrobe	98%	200
Hahnemann University Hospital	Philadelphia	98%	200
Heritage Valley Beaver	Beaver	98%	361
Highlands Hospital	Connellsville	98%	61
Indiana Regional Medical Center	Indiana	98%	204
J C Blair Memorial Hospital	Huntingdon	98%	51
Lehigh Valley Hospital	Allentown	98%	489
Meadville Medical Center	Meadville	98%	129
Mercy Suburban Hospital	Norristown	98%	146
Monongahela Valley Hospital	Monongahela	98%	130
Nazareth Hospital	Philadelphia	98%	303
Pottstown Memorial Medical Center	Pottstown	98%	327
Saint Clair Memorial Hospital	Pittsburgh	98%	401
Saint Luke's Quakertown Hospital	Quakertown	98%	92
Sharon Regional Health System	Sharon	98%	126
UPMC Bedford	Everett	98%	87
UPMC Mercy	Pittsburgh	98%	242
UPMC Passavant	Pittsburgh	98%	387
Western Penn Hosp-Forbes Reg Campus	Monroeville	98%	180
Williamsport Hospital & Medical Center	Williamsport	98%	152
Altoona Regional Health System	Altoona	97%	323
Brandywine Hospital	Coatesville	97%	166
Evangelical Community Hospital	Lewisburg	97%	199
Hazleton General Hospital	Hazleton	97%	171
James E. Van Zandt VA Med Ctr-Altoona	Altoona	97%	38
Jeanes Hospital	Philadelphia	97%	188
Jefferson Regional Medical Center	Pittsburgh	97%	229
Jennersville Regional Hospital	West Grove	97%	233
Lancaster General Hospital	Lancaster	97%	356
Lehigh Valley Hospital - Muhlenberg	Bethlehem	97%	312
Lower Bucks Hospital	Bristol	97%	125
Memorial Hospital York	York	97%	197
Mercy Fitzgerald Hospital	Darby	97%	392
Montgomery Hospital	Norristown	97%	66
Philadelphia VA Medical Center	Philadelphia	97%	88
Saint Luke's Hospital Bethlehem	Bethlehem	97%	470
Sunbury Community Hospital	Sunbury	97%	128
Wayne Memorial Hospital	Honesdale	97%	102
ACMH Hospital	Kittanning	96%	109
Berwick Hospital Center	Berwick	96%	76
Chester County Hospital	West Chester	96%	251
Delaware County Memorial Hospital	Drexel Hill	96%	184
Ephrata Community Hospital	Ephrata	96%	196
Holy Redeemer Hospital and Medical Center	Meadowbrook	96%	228
Jersey Shore Hospital	Jersey Shore	96%	56
Marian Community Hospital	Carbondale	96%	160
Palmerton Hospital	Palmerton	96%	55
Penn Hosp of the Univ of Penn Health Sys	Philadelphia	96%	147
Pinnacle Health Hospitals	Harrisburg	96%	333
Robert Packer Hospital	Sayre	96%	147
Sacred Heart Hospital	Allentown	96%	67
Titusville Hospital	Titusville	96%	55
Uniontown Hospital	Uniontown	96%	115
Waynesboro Hospital	Waynesboro	96%	84
Western Pennsylvania Hospital	Pittsburgh	96%	134
Wilkes-Barre General Hospital	Wilkes-Barre	96%	394
Abington Memorial Hospital	Abington	95%	558
Allegheny General Hospital	Pittsburgh	95%	206
Carlisle Regional Medical Center	Carlisle	95%	175
Doylestown Hospital	Doylestown	95%	295
Easton Hospital	Easton	95%	201
Lancaster Regional Medical Center	Lancaster	95%	86
Millcreek Community Hospital	Erie	95%	40
Penn Presbyterian Medical Center	Philadelphia	95%	155
Reading Hospital Medical Center	Reading	95%	633
Temple University Hospital	Philadelphia	95%	298
Albert Einstein Medical Center	Philadelphia	94%	203
Bradford Regional Medical Center	Bradford	94%	88
Charles Cole Memorial Hospital	Coudersport	94%	71
Elk Regional Health Center	Saint Marys	94%	187
Gettysburg Hospital	Gettysburg	94%	158
Gnaden Huetten Memorial Hospital	Lehighton	94%	67
Hamot Medical Center	Erie	94%	288
Mount Nittany Medical Center	State College	94%	209
Muncy Valley Hospital	Muncy	94%	31
Saint Vincent Health Center	Erie	94%	224
Schuylkill Med Ctr-East Norwegian Street	Pottsville	94%	122
Shamokin Area Community Hospital	Coal Township	94%	86
Troy Community Hospital	Troy	94%	34
Warren General Hospital	Warren	94%	95
Good Samaritan Hospital	Lebanon	93%	202
Lebanon VA Medical Center	Lebanon	93%	29
Mercy Tyler Hospital	Tunkhannock	93%	72
Phoenixville Hospital	Phoenixville	93%	140
Riddle Memorial Hospital	Media	93%	204
St Catherine Med Ctr Fountain Springs	Ashland	93%	43
Saint Joseph Medical Center	Reading	93%	188
Soldiers and Sailors Memorial Hospital	Wellsboro	93%	98
Clearfield Hospital	Clearfield	92%	211
Ellwood City Hospital	Ellwood City	92%	38
Pocono Medical Center	E Stroudsburg	92%	253
Schuylkill Med Ctr-S Jackson Street	Pottsville	92%	170
Hanover Hospital	Hanover	91%	141
Memorial Hospital - Towanda	Towanda	91%	66
Clarion Hospital	Clarion	90%	125
Geisinger Wyoming Valley Medical Center	Wilkes-Barre	90%	194
Lansdale Hospital	Lansdale	90%	132
Mid-Valley Hospital[3]	Peckville	90%	31
Punxsutawney Area Hospital	Punxsutawney	90%	62
Roxborough Memorial Hospital	Phila	90%	92
Kane Community Hospital	Kane	89%	54
Milton S Hershey Medical Center	Hershey	89%	275
Geisinger Medical Center	Danville	88%	187
Ohio Valley General Hospital	Mckees Rocks	87%	93
Somerset Hospital	Somerset	87%	124
Thomas Jefferson University Hospital	Philadelphia	86%	435
Bloomsburg Hospital	Bloomsburg	85%	136
York Hospital	York	84%	608
Saint Joseph's Hospital	Philadelphia	81%	75
Miners Medical Center	Hastings	74%	35
Hospital of Univ of Pennsylvania	Philadelphia	66%	161

18. Influenza Vaccine

Hospital Name	City	Rate	Cases
Aria Health	Philadelphia	100%	465
Berwick Hospital Center	Berwick	100%	56
Heart of Lancaster Regional Medical Center	Lititz	100%	29
Heritage Valley Beaver	Beaver	100%	229
James E. Van Zandt VA Med Ctr-Altoona	Altoona	100%	35
Jennersville Regional Hospital	West Grove	100%	130
Lancaster Regional Medical Center	Lancaster	100%	35
Lebanon VA Medical Center	Lebanon	100%	25
Main Line Hospital Bryn Mawr Campus	Bryn Mawr	100%	177
Mercy Hospital Scranton[2]	Scranton	100%	81
Millcreek Community Hospital	Erie	100%	33
Nason Hospital	Roaring Spring	100%	53
Saint Luke's Miners Memorial Hospital	Coaldale	100%	39
Saint Mary Medical Center	Langhorne	100%	246
Shamokin Area Community Hospital	Coal Township	100%	103
UPMC Bedford	Everett	100%	45
Allegheny General Hospital	Pittsburgh	99%	201
Altoona Regional Health System	Altoona	99%	221
Excela Health Frick Hospital	Mount Pleasant	99%	81
Grand View Hospital	Sellersville	99%	159
Heritage Valley Sewickley	Sewickley	99%	148
Jeanes Hospital	Philadelphia	99%	97
Reading Hospital Medical Center	Reading	99%	420
UPMC Horizon	Greenville	99%	155
UPMC Northwest	Seneca	99%	120
UPMC Presbyterian Shadyside	Pittsburgh	99%	421
UPMC Saint Margaret	Pittsburgh	99%	207
Butler Memorial Hospital	Butler	98%	143
Carlisle Regional Medical Center	Carlisle	98%	106
Gettysburg Hospital	Gettysburg	98%	116
Hazleton General Hospital	Hazleton	98%	198
Holy Redeemer Hospital and Medical Center	Meadowbrook	98%	163
Lehigh Valley Hospital	Allentown	98%	353
Lehigh Valley Hospital - Muhlenberg	Bethlehem	98%	200
Mercy Suburban Hospital	Norristown	98%	64
Saint Joseph Medical Center	Reading	98%	145
Soldiers and Sailors Memorial Hospital	Wellsboro	98%	55
Somerset Hospital	Somerset	98%	62
UPMC Passavant	Pittsburgh	98%	288
The Washington Hospital	Washington	98%	274
Waynesboro Hospital	Waynesboro	98%	52
Wilkes-Barre VA Medical Center	Wilkes-Barre	98%	41
Easton Hospital	Easton	97%	153
Ephrata Community Hospital	Ephrata	97%	111
Erie VA Medical Center	Erie	97%	38
Lock Haven Hospital	Lock Haven	97%	31
Riddle Memorial Hospital	Media	97%	149
Robert Packer Hospital	Sayre	97%	141
Saint Luke's Quakertown Hospital	Quakertown	97%	65
UPMC Mckeesport	McKeesport	97%	199
York Hospital	York	97%	245
Chambersburg Hospital	Chambersburg	96%	139
Holy Spirit Hospital	Camp Hill	96%	258
Jefferson Regional Medical Center	Pittsburgh	96%	250
Lancaster General Hospital	Lancaster	96%	342
Main Line Hospital Paoli	Paoli	96%	132
Marian Community Hospital	Carbondale	96%	81
Alle Kiski Medical Center	Natrona	95%	191
Brandywine Hospital	Coatesville	95%	126
Corry Memorial Hospital	Corry	95%	42
Doylestown Hospital	Doylestown	95%	210
Dubois Regional Medical Center	Dubois	95%	73
Evangelical Community Hospital	Lewisburg	95%	123
Excela Health Westmoreland Reg Hosp	Greensburg	95%	220
Monongahela Valley Hospital	Monongahela	95%	162
Moses Taylor Hospital	Scranton	95%	129
Pottstown Memorial Medical Center	Pottstown	95%	193
Punxsutawney Area Hospital	Punxsutawney	95%	41
VA Pittsburgh Healthcare System	Pittsburgh	95%	61
Chestnut Hill Hospital	Philadelphia	94%	108
Crozer Chester Medical Center	Upland	94%	362
Gnaden Huetten Memorial Hospital	Lehighton	94%	48
Hahnemann University Hospital	Philadelphia	94%	117
Pinnacle Health Hospitals	Harrisburg	94%	321
Sunbury Community Hospital	Sunbury	94%	85
Wayne Memorial Hospital	Honesdale	94%	66
Clarion Hospital	Clarion	93%	72
Ellwood City Hospital	Ellwood City	93%	44
Hamot Medical Center	Erie	93%	235
J C Blair Memorial Hospital	Huntingdon	93%	42
Mercy Fitzgerald Hospital	Darby	93%	133
Mount Nittany Medical Center	State College	93%	179
Abington Memorial Hospital	Abington	92%	336
Brookville Hospital	Brookville	92%	38
Delaware County Memorial Hospital	Drexel Hill	92%	117
Lansdale Hospital	Lansdale	92%	80
Meadville Medical Center	Meadville	92%	85
Pocono Medical Center	E Stroudsburg	92%	207
Saint Luke's Hospital Bethlehem	Bethlehem	92%	313
Sharon Regional Health System	Sharon	92%	99
Temple University Hospital	Philadelphia	92%	240
ACMH Hospital	Kittanning	91%	104
Clearfield Hospital	Clearfield	91%	105
Excela Health Latrobe Hospital	Latrobe	91%	159
Magee Womens Hosp of UPMC Health Sys	Pittsburgh	91%	45
Main Line Hospital Lankenau	Wynnewood	91%	134
Montgomery Hospital	Norristown	91%	68
Saint Clair Memorial Hospital	Pittsburgh	91%	389
Bloomsburg Hospital	Bloomsburg	90%	84
Chester County Hospital	West Chester	90%	167
Conemaugh Valley Memorial Hospital	Johnstown	90%	346
Geisinger Medical Center	Danville	90%	207
Grove City Medical Center	Grove City	90%	49
Roxborough Memorial Hospital	Phila	90%	49
Thomas Jefferson University Hospital	Philadelphia	90%	241
UPMC Mercy	Pittsburgh	90%	205
Williamsport Hospital & Medical Center	Williamsport	90%	156
Hospital of Univ of Pennsylvania	Philadelphia	89%	84
Palmerton Hospital	Palmerton	89%	35
Saint Vincent Health Center	Erie	89%	189
Schuylkill Med Ctr-East Norwegian Street	Pottsville	89%	117
Jersey Shore Hospital	Jersey Shore	88%	42
Philadelphia VA Medical Center	Philadelphia	88%	58
Wilkes-Barre General Hospital	Wilkes-Barre	88%	290
Windber Hospital	Windber	88%	50
Geisinger Wyoming Valley Medical Center	Wilkes-Barre	87%	174
Memorial Hospital York	York	87%	99
Titusville Hospital	Titusville	87%	46
Charles Cole Memorial Hospital	Coudersport	86%	36
Lewistown Hospital	Lewistown	86%	139
Western Pennsylvania Hospital	Pittsburgh	86%	122
Western Penn Hosp-Forbes Reg Campus	Monroeville	86%	229
Bradford Regional Medical Center	Bradford	85%	78
Elk Regional Health Center	Saint Marys	85%	114
Indiana Regional Medical Center	Indiana	85%	134
Muncy Valley Hospital	Muncy	85%	27
Phoenixville Hospital	Phoenixville	85%	131
Schuylkill Med Ctr-S Jackson Street	Pottsville	85%	134
Warren General Hospital	Warren	85%	47
Community Medical Center	Scranton	84%	143
Jameson Memorial Hospital	New Castle	84%	210
Albert Einstein Medical Center	Philadelphia	83%	138
Uniontown Hospital	Uniontown	83%	163
Good Samaritan Hospital	Lebanon	82%	136
Nazareth Hospital	Philadelphia	82%	152
Hanover Hospital	Hanover	81%	113
Sacred Heart Hospital	Allentown	80%	54
Highlands Hospital	Connellsville	79%	33
Penn Hosp of the Univ of Penn Health Sys	Philadelphia	79%	66
St Catherine Med Ctr Fountain Springs	Ashland	79%	39

NOTE: Hospital profiles are in alphabetical order by state, then city, then hospital within the city; Rankings exclude hospitals with less than 25 cases except for patient surveys which excludes hospitals with less than 100 cases; (a) 100–299 cases; (1) The number of cases is too small to be sure how well a hospital is performing; (2) The hospital indicated that the data submitted for this measure were based on a sample of cases; (3) Data was collected during a shorter time period (fewer quarters) than the maximum possible time for this measure; (4) Suppressed for one or more quarters by CMS; (5) No data is available from the hospital for this measure; (6) Fewer than 100 patients completed the HCAHPS survey. Use these rates with caution, as the number of surveys may be too low to reliably assess hospital performance; (7) Survey results are based on less than 12 months of data; (8) Survey results are not available for this reporting period; (9) No or very few patients were eligible for the HCAHPS survey. The scores shown, if any, reflect a very small number of surveys; (10) A state average was not calculated because too few hospitals in the state submitted data; (11) There were discrepancies in the data collection process; Please refer to the User's Guide for a full explanation of data.

Milton S Hershey Medical Center	Hershey	78%	188
Ohio Valley General Hospital	Mckees Rocks	76%	75
Southwest Regional Medical Center	Waynesburg	73%	116
Canonsburg General Hospital	Canonsburg	69%	106
Memorial Hospital - Towanda	Towanda	68%	40
Mercy Tyler Hospital	Tunkhannock	67%	63
Penn Presbyterian Medical Center	Philadelphia	61%	95
Lower Bucks Hospital	Bristol	57%	51
Miners Medical Center	Hastings	38%	37
Saint Joseph's Hospital	Philadelphia	30%	37
Kane Community Hospital	Kane	27%	52

19. Initial Antibiotic Timing

Hospital Name	City	Rate	Cases
Heart of Lancaster Regional Medical Center	Lititz	100%	48
Magee Womens Hosp of UPMC Health Sys	Pittsburgh	100%	40
Saint Mary Medical Center	Langhorne	100%	437
Alle Kiski Medical Center	Natrona	99%	244
Clearfield Hospital	Clearfield	99%	203
Corry Memorial Hospital	Corry	99%	72
Excela Health Frick Hospital	Mount Pleasant	99%	109
Grand View Hospital	Sellersville	99%	211
Heritage Valley Beaver	Beaver	99%	327
Main Line Hospital Bryn Mawr Campus	Bryn Mawr	99%	224
Marian Community Hospital	Carbondale	99%	158
Mercy Tyler Hospital	Tunkhannock	99%	92
Nason Hospital	Roaring Spring	99%	77
Southwest Regional Medical Center	Waynesburg	99%	154
UPMC Bedford	Everett	99%	74
UPMC Northwest	Seneca	99%	164
UPMC Presbyterian Shadyside	Pittsburgh	99%	545
Windber Hospital	Windber	99%	87
ACMH Hospital	Kittanning	98%	129
Albert Einstein Medical Center	Philadelphia	98%	241
Allegheny General Hospital	Pittsburgh	98%	247
Bloomsburg Hospital	Bloomsburg	98%	137
Brookville Hospital	Brookville	98%	43
Butler Memorial Hospital	Butler	98%	233
Ellwood City Hospital	Ellwood City	98%	64
Erie VA Medical Center	Erie	98%	51
Geisinger Medical Center	Danville	98%	195
Gettysburg Hospital	Gettysburg	98%	131
Grove City Medical Center	Grove City	98%	88
Jameson Memorial Hospital	New Castle	98%	269
Lansdale Hospital	Lansdale	98%	123
Lehigh Valley Hospital - Muhlenberg	Bethlehem	98%	323
Lock Haven Hospital	Lock Haven	98%	59
Main Line Hospital Lankenau	Wynnewood	98%	240
Meadville Medical Center	Meadville	98%	139
Mercy Fitzgerald Hospital	Darby	98%	359
Mercy Hospital Scranton[2]	Scranton	98%	135
Moses Taylor Hospital	Scranton	98%	171
Pottstown Memorial Medical Center	Pottstown	98%	318
Riddle Memorial Hospital	Media	98%	261
Roxborough Memorial Hospital	Phila	98%	104
Saint Luke's Quakertown Hospital	Quakertown	98%	99
UPMC Horizon	Greenville	98%	188
UPMC Mckeesport	McKeesport	98%	251
Abington Memorial Hospital	Abington	97%	565
Clarion Hospital	Clarion	97%	144
Doylestown Hospital	Doylestown	97%	291
Dubois Regional Medical Center	Dubois	97%	114
Evangelical Community Hospital	Lewisburg	97%	183
Excela Health Westmoreland Reg Hosp	Greensburg	97%	319
Hahnemann University Hospital	Philadelphia	97%	192
Hazleton General Hospital	Hazleton	97%	257
Heritage Valley Sewickley	Sewickley	97%	234
Highlands Hospital	Connellsville	97%	67
Holy Redeemer Hospital and Medical Center	Meadowbrook	97%	236
J C Blair Memorial Hospital	Huntingdon	97%	59
James E. Van Zandt VA Med Ctr-Altoona	Altoona	97%	37
Jennersville Regional Hospital	West Grove	97%	222
Lewistown Hospital	Lewistown	97%	189
Montrose General Hospital	Montrose	97%	30
Nazareth Hospital	Philadelphia	97%	279
Penn Presbyterian Medical Center	Philadelphia	97%	139
Reading Hospital Medical Center	Reading	97%	555
Saint Luke's Miners Memorial Hospital	Coaldale	97%	58
Saint Vincent Health Center	Erie	97%	253
Shamokin Area Community Hospital	Coal Township	97%	135
Soldiers and Sailors Memorial Hospital	Wellsboro	97%	103
Warren General Hospital	Warren	97%	95
Williamsport Hospital & Medical Center	Williamsport	97%	193
Altoona Regional Health System	Altoona	96%	317
Berwick Hospital Center	Berwick	96%	78
Canonsburg General Hospital	Canonsburg	96%	128
Carlisle Regional Medical Center	Carlisle	96%	154
Chambersburg Hospital	Chambersburg	96%	221
Chestnut Hill Hospital	Philadelphia	96%	183
Community Medical Center	Scranton	96%	269
Delaware County Memorial Hospital	Drexel Hill	96%	192
Hanover Hospital	Hanover	96%	127
Holy Spirit Hospital	Camp Hill	96%	348
Indiana Regional Medical Center	Indiana	96%	190
Jefferson Regional Medical Center	Pittsburgh	96%	357
Lancaster Regional Medical Center	Lancaster	96%	92
Lower Bucks Hospital	Bristol	96%	113
Main Line Hospital Paoli	Paoli	96%	168
Millcreek Community Hospital	Erie	96%	47
Miners Medical Center	Hastings	96%	53
Pinnacle Health Hospitals	Harrisburg	96%	342
Pocono Medical Center	E Stroudsburg	96%	322
Punxsutawney Area Hospital	Punxsutawney	96%	74
Saint Clair Memorial Hospital	Pittsburgh	96%	540
Saint Luke's Hospital Bethlehem	Bethlehem	96%	493
Schuylkill Med Ctr-East Norwegian Street	Pottsville	96%	162
UPMC Mercy	Pittsburgh	96%	329
UPMC Saint Margaret	Pittsburgh	96%	327
The Washington Hospital	Washington	96%	360
Wayne Memorial Hospital	Honesdale	96%	104
Waynesboro Hospital	Waynesboro	96%	108
Wilkes-Barre VA Medical Center	Wilkes-Barre	96%	70
Aria Health	Philadelphia	95%	819
Bradford Regional Medical Center	Bradford	95%	111
Crozer Chester Medical Center	Upland	95%	588
Elk Regional Health Center	Saint Marys	95%	171
Excela Health Latrobe Hospital	Latrobe	95%	186
Hamot Medical Center	Erie	95%	347
Lancaster General Hospital	Lancaster	95%	384
Lehigh Valley Hospital	Allentown	95%	519
Mercy Suburban Hospital	Norristown	95%	133
Milton S Hershey Medical Center	Hershey	95%	237
Phoenixville Hospital	Phoenixville	95%	172
Sacred Heart Hospital	Allentown	95%	76
Schuylkill Med Ctr-S Jackson Street	Pottsville	95%	208
UPMC Passavant	Pittsburgh	95%	413
Charles Cole Memorial Hospital	Coudersport	94%	66
Conemaugh Valley Memorial Hospital	Johnstown	94%	453
Gnaden Huetten Memorial Hospital	Lehighton	94%	69
Jeanes Hospital	Philadelphia	94%	175
Memorial Hospital - Towanda	Towanda	94%	68
Memorial Hospital York	York	94%	177
Monongahela Valley Hospital	Monongahela	94%	249
Muncy Valley Hospital	Muncy	94%	34
Sharon Regional Health System	Sharon	94%	140
Somerset Hospital	Somerset	94%	114
Sunbury Community Hospital	Sunbury	94%	125
Western Pennsylvania Hospital	Pittsburgh	94%	152
Wilkes-Barre General Hospital	Wilkes-Barre	94%	432
Geisinger Wyoming Valley Medical Center	Wilkes-Barre	93%	193
Good Samaritan Hospital	Lebanon	93%	208
Jersey Shore Hospital	Jersey Shore	93%	76
Mid-Valley Hospital[3]	Peckville	93%	30
Montgomery Hospital	Norristown	93%	105
Saint Joseph Medical Center	Reading	93%	178
Uniontown Hospital	Uniontown	93%	231
VA Pittsburgh Healthcare System	Pittsburgh	93%	136
Brandywine Hospital	Coatesville	92%	197
Chester County Hospital	West Chester	92%	256
Fulton County Medical Center[3]	Mcconnellsburg	92%	25
Hospital of Univ of Pennsylvania	Philadelphia	92%	174
Kane Community Hospital	Kane	92%	74
Mount Nittany Medical Center	State College	92%	226
Western Penn Hosp-Forbes Reg Campus	Monroeville	92%	303
York Hospital	York	92%	559
Easton Hospital	Easton	91%	224
Ohio Valley General Hospital	Mckees Rocks	91%	134
Palmerton Hospital	Palmerton	91%	56
Penn Hosp of the Univ of Penn Health Sys	Philadelphia	90%	154
Temple University Hospital	Philadelphia	90%	360
Titusville Hospital	Titusville	90%	71
Robert Packer Hospital	Sayre	89%	144
St Catherine Med Ctr Fountain Springs	Ashland	89%	53
Thomas Jefferson University Hospital	Philadelphia	88%	400
Lebanon VA Medical Center	Lebanon	87%	31
Ephrata Community Hospital	Ephrata	86%	188
Philadelphia VA Medical Center	Philadelphia	85%	72
Saint Joseph's Hospital	Philadelphia	77%	79

20. Pneumococcal Vaccine

Hospital Name	City	Rate	Cases
Excela Health Frick Hospital	Mount Pleasant	100%	105
Heart of Lancaster Regional Medical Center	Lititz	100%	42
Heritage Valley Sewickley	Sewickley	100%	202
James E. Van Zandt VA Med Ctr-Altoona	Altoona	100%	32
Jennersville Regional Hospital	West Grove	100%	194
Mid-Valley Hospital[3]	Peckville	100%	32
Millcreek Community Hospital	Erie	100%	46
Nason Hospital	Roaring Spring	100%	72
Punxsutawney Area Hospital	Punxsutawney	100%	64
Reading Hospital Medical Center	Reading	100%	586
Saint Luke's Miners Memorial Hospital	Coaldale	100%	62
Saint Mary Medical Center	Langhorne	100%	328
Shamokin Area Community Hospital	Coal Township	100%	142
UPMC Horizon	Greenville	100%	201
UPMC Mckeesport	McKeesport	100%	253
UPMC Presbyterian Shadyside	Pittsburgh	100%	488
Wilkes-Barre VA Medical Center	Wilkes-Barre	100%	63
Aria Health	Philadelphia	99%	518
Carlisle Regional Medical Center	Carlisle	99%	145
Corry Memorial Hospital	Corry	99%	71
Ephrata Community Hospital	Ephrata	99%	183
Grand View Hospital	Sellersville	99%	234
Hazleton General Hospital	Hazleton	99%	276
Heritage Valley Beaver	Beaver	99%	281
Lancaster Regional Medical Center	Lancaster	99%	67
Lehigh Valley Hospital - Muhlenberg	Bethlehem	99%	308
Main Line Hospital Bryn Mawr Campus	Bryn Mawr	99%	273
Main Line Hospital Paoli	Paoli	99%	186
Marian Community Hospital	Carbondale	99%	125
Meadville Medical Center	Meadville	99%	114
Mercy Suburban Hospital	Norristown	99%	87
Riddle Memorial Hospital	Media	99%	242
Saint Luke's Quakertown Hospital	Quakertown	99%	92
UPMC Bedford	Everett	99%	72
UPMC Passavant	Pittsburgh	99%	408
VA Pittsburgh Healthcare System	Pittsburgh	99%	72
Waynesboro Hospital	Waynesboro	99%	107
Windber Hospital	Windber	99%	72
Allegheny General Hospital	Pittsburgh	98%	264
Altoona Regional Health System	Altoona	98%	326
Brandywine Hospital	Coatesville	98%	167
Butler Memorial Hospital	Butler	98%	232
Dubois Regional Medical Center	Dubois	98%	120
Easton Hospital	Easton	98%	252
Erie VA Medical Center	Erie	98%	53
Excela Health Westmoreland Reg Hosp	Greensburg	98%	336
Gnaden Huetten Memorial Hospital	Lehighton	98%	57
Holy Redeemer Hospital and Medical Center	Meadowbrook	98%	244
Mercy Hospital Scranton[2]	Scranton	98%	146
Moses Taylor Hospital	Scranton	98%	180
Mount Nittany Medical Center	State College	98%	251
Muncy Valley Hospital	Muncy	98%	44
Palmerton Hospital	Palmerton	98%	54
Philadelphia VA Medical Center	Philadelphia	98%	50
Pinnacle Health Hospitals	Harrisburg	98%	380
Sharon Regional Health System	Sharon	98%	129
Soldiers and Sailors Memorial Hospital	Wellsboro	98%	91
UPMC Northwest	Seneca	98%	184
UPMC Saint Margaret	Pittsburgh	98%	279
Alle Kiski Medical Center	Natrona	97%	292
Chambersburg Hospital	Chambersburg	97%	219
Ellwood City Hospital	Ellwood City	97%	62
Excela Health Latrobe Hospital	Latrobe	97%	238
Grove City Medical Center	Grove City	97%	69
Holy Spirit Hospital	Camp Hill	97%	348
Main Line Hospital Lankenau	Wynnewood	97%	209
Montrose General Hospital	Montrose	97%	37
Penn Presbyterian Medical Center	Philadelphia	97%	110
Robert Packer Hospital	Sayre	97%	223
Saint Joseph Medical Center	Reading	97%	193
The Washington Hospital	Washington	97%	364
Williamsport Hospital & Medical Center	Williamsport	97%	220
Abington Memorial Hospital	Abington	96%	487
Chestnut Hill Hospital	Philadelphia	96%	166
Elk Regional Health Center	Saint Marys	96%	155
Hamot Medical Center	Erie	96%	356
Lehigh Valley Hospital	Allentown	96%	499
Mercy Fitzgerald Hospital	Darby	96%	185
Pottstown Memorial Medical Center	Pottstown	96%	271
Saint Vincent Health Center	Erie	96%	268
Wayne Memorial Hospital	Honesdale	96%	97
York Hospital	York	96%	463
ACMH Hospital	Kittanning	95%	133
Chester County Hospital	West Chester	95%	245
Crozer Chester Medical Center	Upland	95%	444
Doylestown Hospital	Doylestown	95%	326
Evangelical Community Hospital	Lewisburg	95%	208
Geisinger Medical Center	Danville	95%	254
Gettysburg Hospital	Gettysburg	95%	143
Lancaster General Hospital	Lancaster	95%	434
Nazareth Hospital	Philadelphia	95%	202
Somerset Hospital	Somerset	95%	94
Berwick Hospital Center	Berwick	94%	71
Bradford Regional Medical Center	Bradford	94%	99
Brookville Hospital	Brookville	94%	50
Charles Cole Memorial Hospital	Coudersport	94%	70
Clearfield Hospital	Clearfield	94%	176
Geisinger Wyoming Valley Medical Center	Wilkes-Barre	94%	272
Hahnemann University Hospital	Philadelphia	94%	109
Highlands Hospital	Connellsville	94%	51

NOTE: Hospital profiles are in alphabetical order by state, then city, then hospital within the city; Rankings exclude hospitals with less than 25 cases except for patient surveys which excludes hospitals with less than 100 cases; (a) 100–299 cases; (1) The number of cases is too small to be sure how well a hospital is performing; (2) The hospital indicated that the data submitted for this measure were based on a sample of cases; (3) Data was collected during a shorter time period (fewer quarters) than the maximum possible time for this measure; (4) Suppressed for one or more quarters by CMS; (5) No data is available from the hospital for this measure; (6) Fewer than 100 patients completed the HCAHPS survey. Use these rates with caution, as the number of surveys may be too low to reliably assess hospital performance; (7) Survey results are based on less than 12 months of data; (8) Survey results are not available for this reporting period; (9) No or very few patients were eligible for the HCAHPS survey. The scores shown, if any, reflect a very small number of surveys; (10) A state average was not calculated because too few hospitals in the state submitted data; (11) There were discrepancies in the data collection process; Please refer to the User's Guide for a full explanation of data.

Jeanes Hospital	Philadelphia	94%	158
Jefferson Regional Medical Center	Pittsburgh	94%	323
Schuylkill Med Ctr-East Norwegian Street	Pottsville	94%	164
UPMC Mercy	Pittsburgh	94%	274
Conemaugh Valley Memorial Hospital	Johnstown	93%	475
Hanover Hospital	Hanover	93%	136
Mercy Tyler Hospital	Tunkhannock	93%	102
Monongahela Valley Hospital	Monongahela	93%	210
Saint Clair Memorial Hospital	Pittsburgh	93%	554
Saint Luke's Hospital Bethlehem	Bethlehem	93%	414
Thomas Jefferson University Hospital	Philadelphia	93%	289
Western Penn Hosp-Forbes Reg Campus	Monroeville	93%	311
Albert Einstein Medical Center	Philadelphia	92%	176
Delaware County Memorial Hospital	Drexel Hill	92%	144
Hospital of Univ of Pennsylvania	Philadelphia	92%	160
Lock Haven Hospital	Lock Haven	92%	40
Magee Womens Hosp of UPMC Health Sys	Pittsburgh	92%	51
Montgomery Hospital	Norristown	92%	90
Phoenixville Hospital	Phoenixville	92%	195
Indiana Regional Medical Center	Indiana	91%	185
J C Blair Memorial Hospital	Huntingdon	91%	55
Jersey Shore Hospital	Jersey Shore	91%	65
Lewistown Hospital	Lewistown	91%	188
Memorial Hospital York	York	91%	138
Penn Hosp of the Univ of Penn Health Sys	Philadelphia	91%	103
Roxborough Memorial Hospital	Phila	91%	98
Bloomsburg Hospital	Bloomsburg	90%	101
Community Medical Center	Scranton	90%	183
Sunbury Community Hospital	Sunbury	90%	109
Jameson Memorial Hospital	New Castle	89%	299
Pocono Medical Center	E Stroudsburg	89%	316
Warren General Hospital	Warren	89%	79
Canonsburg General Hospital	Canonsburg	88%	138
Schuylkill Med Ctr-S Jackson Street	Pottsville	88%	186
Wilkes-Barre General Hospital	Wilkes-Barre	88%	406
Good Samaritan Hospital	Lebanon	87%	186
Lansdale Hospital	Lansdale	86%	132
Ohio Valley General Hospital	Mckees Rocks	86%	106
Temple University Hospital	Philadelphia	86%	226
Uniontown Hospital	Uniontown	86%	212
Titusville Hospital	Titusville	83%	72
Milton S Hershey Medical Center	Hershey	82%	285
Clarion Hospital	Clarion	80%	112
St Catherine Med Ctr Fountain Springs	Ashland	80%	51
Western Pennsylvania Hospital	Pittsburgh	80%	127
Southwest Regional Medical Center	Waynesburg	79%	131
Sacred Heart Hospital	Allentown	78%	73
Troy Community Hospital	Troy	78%	27
Memorial Hospital - Towanda	Towanda	70%	50
Lower Bucks Hospital	Bristol	67%	70
Saint Joseph's Hospital	Philadelphia	52%	48
Miners Medical Center	Hastings	36%	50
Kane Community Hospital	Kane	22%	85

21. Smoking Cessation Advice

Hospital Name	City	Rate	Cases
Abington Memorial Hospital	Abington	100%	140
ACMH Hospital	Kittanning	100%	46
Albert Einstein Medical Center	Philadelphia	100%	155
Alle Kiski Medical Center	Natrona	100%	112
Altoona Regional Health System	Altoona	100%	127
Aria Health	Philadelphia	100%	367
Brandywine Hospital	Coatesville	100%	72
Canonsburg General Hospital	Canonsburg	100%	39
Carlisle Regional Medical Center	Carlisle	100%	40
Chester County Hospital	West Chester	100%	76
Chestnut Hill Hospital	Philadelphia	100%	46
Clearfield Hospital	Clearfield	100%	35
Crozer Chester Medical Center	Upland	100%	254
Delaware County Memorial Hospital	Drexel Hill	100%	62
Dubois Regional Medical Center	Dubois	100%	52
Easton Hospital	Easton	100%	56
Excela Health Frick Hospital	Mount Pleasant	100%	29
Geisinger Medical Center	Danville	100%	107
Geisinger Wyoming Valley Medical Center	Wilkes-Barre	100%	99
Gettysburg Hospital	Gettysburg	100%	40
Gnaden Huetten Memorial Hospital	Lehighton	100%	29
Grand View Hospital	Sellersville	100%	55
Hamot Medical Center	Erie	100%	178
Heritage Valley Beaver	Beaver	100%	132
Heritage Valley Sewickley	Sewickley	100%	65
Holy Spirit Hospital	Camp Hill	100%	88
Jameson Memorial Hospital	New Castle	100%	122
Jeanes Hospital	Philadelphia	100%	48
Jennersville Regional Hospital	West Grove	100%	72
Lancaster General Hospital	Lancaster	100%	145
Lancaster Regional Medical Center	Lancaster	100%	40
Lehigh Valley Hospital	Allentown	100%	149
Lehigh Valley Hospital - Muhlenberg	Bethlehem	100%	92
Magee Womens Hosp of UPMC Health Sys	Pittsburgh	100%	33
Main Line Hospital Bryn Mawr Campus	Bryn Mawr	100%	44
Main Line Hospital Lankenau	Wynnewood	100%	75
Main Line Hospital Paoli	Paoli	100%	34
Marian Community Hospital	Carbondale	100%	31
Meadville Medical Center	Meadville	100%	50
Memorial Hospital York	York	100%	47
Mercy Suburban Hospital	Norristown	100%	45
Montgomery Hospital	Norristown	100%	29
Moses Taylor Hospital	Scranton	100%	78
Mount Nittany Medical Center	State College	100%	62
Penn Presbyterian Medical Center	Philadelphia	100%	71
Penn Hosp of the Univ of Penn Health Sys	Philadelphia	100%	62
Philadelphia VA Medical Center	Philadelphia	100%	33
Pottstown Memorial Medical Center	Pottstown	100%	112
Reading Hospital Medical Center	Reading	100%	154
Robert Packer Hospital	Sayre	100%	68
Roxborough Memorial Hospital	Phila	100%	37
Saint Clair Memorial Hospital	Pittsburgh	100%	131
Saint Joseph Medical Center	Reading	100%	59
Saint Luke's Hospital Bethlehem	Bethlehem	100%	161
Saint Luke's Quakertown Hospital	Quakertown	100%	35
Saint Mary Medical Center	Langhorne	100%	116
Saint Vincent Health Center	Erie	100%	99
Schuylkill Med Ctr-East Norwegian Street	Pottsville	100%	31
Temple University Hospital	Philadelphia	100%	274
UPMC Horizon	Greenville	100%	59
UPMC Mckeesport	McKeesport	100%	96
UPMC Mercy	Pittsburgh	100%	197
UPMC Northwest	Seneca	100%	58
UPMC Presbyterian Shadyside	Pittsburgh	100%	326
UPMC Saint Margaret	Pittsburgh	100%	93
VA Pittsburgh Healthcare System	Pittsburgh	100%	36
Wayne Memorial Hospital	Honesdale	100%	36
Waynesboro Hospital	Waynesboro	100%	26
Western Pennsylvania Hospital	Pittsburgh	100%	87
Western Penn Hosp-Forbes Reg Campus	Monroeville	100%	97
York Hospital	York	100%	162
Butler Memorial Hospital	Butler	99%	107
Excela Health Latrobe Hospital	Latrobe	99%	70
Hazleton General Hospital	Hazleton	99%	90
Mercy Fitzgerald Hospital	Darby	99%	187
Milton S Hershey Medical Center	Hershey	99%	93
Pinnacle Health Hospitals	Harrisburg	99%	140
Thomas Jefferson University Hospital	Philadelphia	99%	177
UPMC Passavant	Pittsburgh	99%	111
The Washington Hospital	Washington	99%	134
Wilkes-Barre General Hospital	Wilkes-Barre	99%	146
Holy Redeemer Hospital and Medical Center	Meadowbrook	98%	42
Nazareth Hospital	Philadelphia	98%	66
Phoenixville Hospital	Phoenixville	98%	43
Schuylkill Med Ctr-S Jackson Street	Pottsville	98%	64
Williamsport Hospital & Medical Center	Williamsport	98%	89
Allegheny General Hospital	Pittsburgh	97%	160
Good Samaritan Hospital	Lebanon	97%	61
Lower Bucks Hospital	Bristol	97%	36
Pocono Medical Center	E Stroudsburg	97%	157
Community Medical Center	Scranton	96%	77
Conemaugh Valley Memorial Hospital	Johnstown	96%	170
Doylestown Hospital	Doylestown	96%	78
Hahnemann University Hospital	Philadelphia	96%	120
Hanover Hospital	Hanover	96%	27
Monongahela Valley Hospital	Monongahela	96%	91
Ohio Valley General Hospital	Mckees Rocks	96%	54
Sacred Heart Hospital	Allentown	96%	25
Warren General Hospital	Warren	96%	26
Hospital of Univ of Pennsylvania	Philadelphia	95%	96
Jefferson Regional Medical Center	Pittsburgh	95%	95
Riddle Memorial Hospital	Media	95%	64
Sharon Regional Health System	Sharon	95%	44
Bradford Regional Medical Center	Bradford	94%	31
Chambersburg Hospital	Chambersburg	94%	85
Elk Regional Health Center	Saint Marys	94%	52
Excela Health Westmoreland Reg Hosp	Greensburg	94%	105
Evangelical Community Hospital	Lewisburg	93%	44
Shamokin Area Community Hospital	Coal Township	93%	30
Southwest Regional Medical Center	Waynesburg	93%	59
Mercy Hospital Scranton[2]	Scranton	92%	37
Uniontown Hospital	Uniontown	91%	85
Indiana Regional Medical Center	Indiana	88%	56
Lewistown Hospital	Lewistown	88%	60
Punxsutawney Area Hospital	Punxsutawney	88%	25
Soldiers and Sailors Memorial Hospital	Wellsboro	88%	26
Bloomsburg Hospital	Bloomsburg	85%	34
Ephrata Community Hospital	Ephrata	85%	53
Titusville Hospital	Titusville	80%	30
Mercy Tyler Hospital	Tunkhannock	76%	29
Somerset Hospital	Somerset	72%	32
Clarion Hospital	Clarion	71%	45
Saint Joseph's Hospital	Philadelphia	40%	25

Surgical Care Improvement Project

22. Appropriate VTP Within 24 Hours

Hospital Name	City	Rate	Cases
Alle Kiski Medical Center	Natrona	100%	220
Brookville Hospital	Brookville	100%	29
Coordinated Health Orthopedic Hospital[2]	Bethlehem	100%	26
Delaware County Memorial Hospital[2]	Drexel Hill	100%	348
Jennersville Regional Hospital[2]	West Grove	100%	64
Main Line Hospital Bryn Mawr Campus[2]	Bryn Mawr	100%	224
Mercy Fitzgerald Hospital[2]	Darby	100%	272
Nason Hospital	Roaring Spring	100%	76
UPMC Bedford	Everett	100%	64
UPMC Mckeesport	McKeesport	100%	209
Western Pennsylvania Hospital[2]	Pittsburgh	100%	218
Albert Einstein Medical Center[2]	Philadelphia	99%	308
Grand View Hospital[2]	Sellersville	99%	165
Hospital of Univ of Pennsylvania[2]	Philadelphia	99%	384
Lancaster Regional Medical Center[2]	Lancaster	99%	177
Moses Taylor Hospital	Scranton	99%	254
Saint Joseph Medical Center[2]	Reading	99%	183
Sharon Regional Health System[2]	Sharon	99%	244
UPMC Presbyterian Shadyside	Pittsburgh	99%	3593
UPMC Saint Margaret	Pittsburgh	99%	849
Abington Memorial Hospital[2]	Abington	98%	138
Allegheny General Hospital[2]	Pittsburgh	98%	1416
Aria Health[2]	Philadelphia	98%	311
Ephrata Community Hospital	Ephrata	98%	239
Heart of Lancaster Regional Medical Center	Lititz	98%	83
Holy Redeemer Hospital and Medical Center	Meadowbrook	98%	254
Jeanes Hospital	Philadelphia	98%	235
Lehigh Valley Hospital	Allentown	98%	1432
Main Line Hospital Paoli[2]	Paoli	98%	234
Saint Luke's Miners Memorial Hospital	Coaldale	98%	58
Schuylkill Med Ctr-S Jackson Street	Pottsville	98%	146
Thomas Jefferson University Hospital[2]	Philadelphia	98%	814
UPMC Horizon	Greenville	98%	384
UPMC Mercy[2]	Pittsburgh	98%	227
UPMC Northwest	Seneca	98%	129
UPMC Passavant	Pittsburgh	98%	970
VA Pittsburgh Healthcare System[2]	Pittsburgh	98%	176
ACMH Hospital	Kittanning	97%	159
Butler Memorial Hospital	Butler	97%	271
Canonsburg General Hospital	Canonsburg	97%	152
Community Medical Center	Scranton	97%	381
Crozer Chester Medical Center[2]	Upland	97%	343
Easton Hospital[2]	Easton	97%	225
Excela Health Frick Hospital	Mount Pleasant	97%	64
Excela Health Westmoreland Reg Hosp	Greensburg	97%	507
Hamot Medical Center	Erie	97%	613
Magee Womens Hosp of UPMC Health Sys	Pittsburgh	97%	549
Main Line Hospital Lankenau[2]	Wynnewood	97%	300
Mercy Suburban Hospital	Norristown	97%	123
Nazareth Hospital	Philadelphia	97%	236
Reading Hospital Medical Center[2]	Reading	97%	521
Robert Packer Hospital	Sayre	97%	500
Temple University Hospital[2]	Philadelphia	97%	394
Western Penn Hosp-Forbes Reg Campus	Monroeville	97%	299
Williamsport Hospital & Medical Center[2]	Williamsport	97%	536
Chester County Hospital	West Chester	96%	371
Doylestown Hospital[2]	Doylestown	96%	315
Gettysburg Hospital	Gettysburg	96%	161
Gnaden Huetten Memorial Hospital	Lehighton	96%	72
Jameson Memorial Hospital	New Castle	96%	299
Lehigh Valley Hospital - Muhlenberg	Bethlehem	96%	352
Mercy Hospital Scranton[2]	Scranton	96%	147
Penn Hosp of the Univ of Penn Health Sys[2]	Philadelphia	96%	245
Philadelphia VA Medical Center[2]	Philadelphia	96%	67
Wayne Memorial Hospital[2]	Honesdale	96%	109
Chambersburg Hospital[2]	Chambersburg	95%	344
Charles Cole Memorial Hospital	Coudersport	95%	57
Conemaugh Valley Memorial Hospital	Johnstown	95%	584
Geisinger Medical Center[2]	Danville	95%	176
Jefferson Regional Medical Center	Pittsburgh	95%	700
Meadville Medical Center	Meadville	95%	182
Millcreek Community Hospital	Erie	95%	43
Milton S Hershey Medical Center[2]	Hershey	95%	426
Monongahela Valley Hospital	Monongahela	95%	333
Pinnacle Health Hospitals[2]	Harrisburg	95%	746
Roxborough Memorial Hospital	Phila	95%	81
Saint Vincent Health Center	Erie	95%	498
Schuylkill Med Ctr-East Norwegian Street	Pottsville	95%	159
Uniontown Hospital	Uniontown	95%	308
The Washington Hospital[2]	Washington	95%	218
Windber Hospital	Windber	95%	38
Altoona Regional Health System	Altoona	94%	488
Carlisle Regional Medical Center[2]	Carlisle	94%	187
Clearfield Hospital	Clearfield	94%	156
Dubois Regional Medical Center	Dubois	94%	112
Good Samaritan Hospital[2]	Lebanon	94%	170
Hazleton General Hospital	Hazleton	94%	153

NOTE: Hospital profiles are in alphabetical order by state, then city, then hospital within the city; Rankings exclude hospitals with less than 25 cases except for patient surveys which excludes hospitals with less than 100 cases; (a) 100–299 cases; (1) The number of cases is too small to be sure how well a hospital is performing; (2) The hospital indicated that the data submitted for this measure were based on a sample of cases; (3) Data was collected during a shorter time period (fewer quarters) than the maximum possible time for this measure; (4) Suppressed for one or more quarters by CMS; (5) No data is available from the hospital for this measure; (6) Fewer than 100 patients completed the HCAHPS survey. Use these rates with caution, as the number of surveys may be too low to reliably assess hospital performance; (7) Survey results are based on less than 12 months of data; (8) Survey results are not available for this reporting period; (9) No or very few patients were eligible for the HCAHPS survey. The scores shown, if any, reflect a very small number of surveys; (10) A state average was not calculated because too few hospitals in the state submitted data; (11) There were discrepancies in the data collection process; Please refer to the User's Guide for a full explanation of data.

J C Blair Memorial Hospital	Huntingdon	94%	33
Lancaster General Hospital[2]	Lancaster	94%	679
Lansdale Hospital[2]	Lansdale	94%	141
Marian Community Hospital	Carbondale	94%	33
Mount Nittany Medical Center	State College	94%	373
Penn Presbyterian Medical Center	Philadelphia	94%	576
Saint Luke's Hospital Bethlehem[2]	Bethlehem	94%	430
Somerset Hospital	Somerset	94%	97
Wilkes-Barre VA Medical Center[2]	Wilkes-Barre	94%	34
Ellwood City Hospital	Ellwood City	93%	56
Ohio Valley General Hospital	Mckees Rocks	93%	163
Phoenixville Hospital[2]	Phoenixville	93%	224
Saint Clair Memorial Hospital[2]	Pittsburgh	93%	569
Saint Luke's Quakertown Hospital	Quakertown	93%	45
York Hospital[2]	York	93%	611
Chestnut Hill Hospital[2]	Philadelphia	92%	133
Excela Health Latrobe Hospital	Latrobe	92%	276
Geisinger Wyoming Valley Medical Center[2]	Wilkes-Barre	92%	167
Riddle Memorial Hospital[2]	Media	92%	272
Cancer Treatment Centers of America	Philadelphia	91%	76
Heritage Valley Sewickley	Sewickley	91%	259
Indiana Regional Medical Center	Indiana	91%	159
Memorial Hospital York	York	91%	133
Punxsutawney Area Hospital	Punxsutawney	91%	58
Saint Mary Medical Center[2]	Langhorne	91%	158
Lebanon VA Medical Center[2]	Lebanon	90%	58
Pocono Medical Center	E Stroudsburg	90%	230
Soldiers and Sailors Memorial Hospital	Wellsboro	90%	77
Wilkes-Barre General Hospital[2]	Wilkes-Barre	90%	616
Bradford Regional Medical Center	Bradford	89%	57
Hahnemann University Hospital[2]	Philadelphia	89%	294
Holy Spirit Hospital[2]	Camp Hill	89%	279
Pottstown Memorial Medical Center[2]	Pottstown	89%	244
Southwest Regional Medical Center	Waynesburg	89%	47
Waynesboro Hospital	Waynesboro	89%	81
Palmerton Hospital	Palmerton	88%	58
Shamokin Area Community Hospital	Coal Township	88%	41
Hanover Hospital	Hanover	87%	163
Berwick Hospital Center[2]	Berwick	86%	42
Clarion Hospital	Clarion	86%	43
Evangelical Community Hospital[2]	Lewisburg	85%	131
Heritage Valley Beaver	Beaver	85%	358
Sacred Heart Hospital	Allentown	85%	155
Highlands Hospital[2]	Connellsville	84%	45
Saint Joseph's Hospital	Philadelphia	84%	38
Surgical Institute of Reading	Wyomissing	84%	49
Brandywine Hospital[2]	Coatesville	83%	106
Lewistown Hospital	Lewistown	81%	100
Bloomsburg Hospital	Bloomsburg	80%	60
Lower Bucks Hospital[2]	Bristol	80%	102
Sunbury Community Hospital[2]	Sunbury	80%	44
Mercy Tyler Hospital	Tunkhannock	79%	28
Elk Regional Health Center	Saint Marys	78%	76
Grove City Medical Center	Grove City	77%	35
Warren General Hospital	Warren	72%	50
Montgomery Hospital[2]	Norristown	68%	60
Titusville Hospital	Titusville	54%	37
Jersey Shore Hospital	Jersey Shore	45%	53

23. Appropriate Hair Removal

Hospital Name	City	Rate	Cases
ACMH Hospital	Kittanning	100%	480
Albert Einstein Medical Center[2]	Philadelphia	100%	738
Alle Kiski Medical Center	Natrona	100%	509
Allegheny General Hospital[2]	Pittsburgh	100%	2957
Altoona Regional Health System	Altoona	100%	2077
Aria Health[2]	Philadelphia	100%	710
Berwick Hospital Center[2]	Berwick	100%	169
Bloomsburg Hospital	Bloomsburg	100%	274
Brandywine Hospital[2]	Coatesville	100%	300
Brookville Hospital	Brookville	100%	54
Bucks County Specialty Hospital[2,3]	Bensalem	100%	99
Butler Memorial Hospital	Butler	100%	1315
Canonsburg General Hospital	Canonsburg	100%	479
Carlisle Regional Medical Center[2]	Carlisle	100%	561
Chambersburg Hospital[2]	Chambersburg	100%	921
Chester County Hospital	West Chester	100%	1081
Chestnut Hill Hospital[2]	Philadelphia	100%	309
Clarion Hospital	Clarion	100%	238
Community Medical Center	Scranton	100%	1141
Coordinated Health Orthopedic Hospital[2]	Bethlehem	100%	202
Crozer Chester Medical Center[2]	Upland	100%	1128
Delaware County Memorial Hospital[2]	Drexel Hill	100%	551
Doylestown Hospital[2]	Doylestown	100%	944
Easton Hospital[2]	Easton	100%	741
Edgewood Surgical Hospital	Transfer	100%	127
Elk Regional Health Center	Saint Marys	100%	248
Ephrata Community Hospital	Ephrata	100%	597
Erie VA Medical Center[2]	Erie	100%	45
Evangelical Community Hospital[2]	Lewisburg	100%	466
Excela Health Latrobe Hospital	Latrobe	100%	610
Geisinger Medical Center[2]	Danville	100%	767
Geisinger Wyoming Valley Medical Center[2]	Wilkes-Barre	100%	713
Gettysburg Hospital	Gettysburg	100%	409
Gnaden Huetten Memorial Hospital	Lehighton	100%	161
Good Samaritan Hospital[2]	Lebanon	100%	509
Grand View Hospital[2]	Sellersville	100%	454
Grove City Medical Center	Grove City	100%	152
Hamot Medical Center	Erie	100%	1832
Hanover Hospital	Hanover	100%	750
Hazleton General Hospital	Hazleton	100%	323
Heart of Lancaster Regional Medical Center	Lititz	100%	184
Heritage Valley Beaver	Beaver	100%	1303
Heritage Valley Sewickley	Sewickley	100%	1182
Holy Redeemer Hospital and Medical Center	Meadowbrook	100%	829
Holy Spirit Hospital[2]	Camp Hill	100%	1007
Hospital of Univ of Pennsylvania[2]	Philadelphia	100%	982
Indiana Regional Medical Center	Indiana	100%	394
J C Blair Memorial Hospital	Huntingdon	100%	58
Jameson Memorial Hospital	New Castle	100%	561
Jefferson Regional Medical Center	Pittsburgh	100%	1780
Jennersville Regional Hospital[2]	West Grove	100%	144
Jersey Shore Hospital	Jersey Shore	100%	84
Lancaster Regional Medical Center[2]	Lancaster	100%	498
Lansdale Hospital[2]	Lansdale	100%	213
Lebanon VA Medical Center[2]	Lebanon	100%	234
Lehigh Valley Hospital	Allentown	100%	4121
Lehigh Valley Hospital - Muhlenberg	Bethlehem	100%	802
Lewistown Hospital	Lewistown	100%	267
Lock Haven Hospital[2]	Lock Haven	100%	63
Lower Bucks Hospital[2]	Bristol	100%	293
Magee Womens Hosp of UPMC Health Sys	Pittsburgh	100%	2291
Main Line Hospital Bryn Mawr Campus[2]	Bryn Mawr	100%	1526
Main Line Hospital Lankenau[2]	Wynnewood	100%	1423
Main Line Hospital Paoli[2]	Paoli	100%	912
Marian Community Hospital	Carbondale	100%	108
Meadville Medical Center	Meadville	100%	824
Memorial Hospital - Towanda	Towanda	100%	26
Memorial Hospital York	York	100%	554
Mercy Fitzgerald Hospital[2]	Darby	100%	525
Mercy Hospital Scranton[2]	Scranton	100%	581
Mercy Suburban Hospital	Norristown	100%	316
Mercy Tyler Hospital	Tunkhannock	100%	40
Monongahela Valley Hospital	Monongahela	100%	665
Montgomery Hospital[2]	Norristown	100%	291
Moses Taylor Hospital	Scranton	100%	613
Nazareth Hospital	Philadelphia	100%	643
Ohio Valley General Hospital	Mckees Rocks	100%	307
Palmerton Hospital	Palmerton	100%	106
Penn Presbyterian Medical Center	Philadelphia	100%	2635
Penn Hosp of the Univ of Penn Health Sys[2]	Philadelphia	100%	689
Philadelphia VA Medical Center[2]	Philadelphia	100%	90
Phoenixville Hospital[2]	Phoenixville	100%	550
Pinnacle Health Hospitals[2]	Harrisburg	100%	3582
Pocono Medical Center	E Stroudsburg	100%	659
Pottstown Memorial Medical Center[2]	Pottstown	100%	491
Punxsutawney Area Hospital	Punxsutawney	100%	146
Reading Hospital Medical Center[2]	Reading	100%	1981
Robert Packer Hospital	Sayre	100%	1482
Roxborough Memorial Hospital	Phila	100%	144
St Catherine Med Ctr Fountain Springs	Ashland	100%	53
Saint Joseph Medical Center[2]	Reading	100%	613
Saint Luke's Hospital Bethlehem[2]	Bethlehem	100%	1622
Saint Luke's Miners Memorial Hospital	Coaldale	100%	188
Saint Luke's Quakertown Hospital	Quakertown	100%	106
Saint Mary Medical Center[2]	Langhorne	100%	701
Saint Vincent Health Center	Erie	100%	1898
Schuylkill Med Ctr-S Jackson Street	Pottsville	100%	413
Shamokin Area Community Hospital	Coal Township	100%	128
Sharon Regional Health System[2]	Sharon	100%	621
Somerset Hospital	Somerset	100%	293
Southwest Regional Medical Center	Waynesburg	100%	114
Sunbury Community Hospital[2]	Sunbury	100%	102
Surgical Specialty Ctr-Coordinated Health[2,3]	Allentown	100%	71
Temple University Hospital[2]	Philadelphia	100%	1112
Thomas Jefferson University Hospital[2]	Philadelphia	100%	3104
Uniontown Hospital	Uniontown	100%	910
UPMC Bedford	Everett	100%	157
UPMC Horizon	Greenville	100%	778
UPMC Mckeesport	McKeesport	100%	377
UPMC Mercy[2]	Pittsburgh	100%	617
UPMC Northwest	Seneca	100%	369
UPMC Passavant	Pittsburgh	100%	1951
UPMC Presbyterian Shadyside	Pittsburgh	100%	7812
UPMC Saint Margaret	Pittsburgh	100%	1600
VA Pittsburgh Healthcare System[2]	Pittsburgh	100%	457
Warren General Hospital	Warren	100%	231
The Washington Hospital[2]	Washington	100%	835
Wayne Memorial Hospital[2]	Honesdale	100%	255
Waynesboro Hospital	Waynesboro	100%	192
Western Pennsylvania Hospital[2]	Pittsburgh	100%	1030
Wilkes-Barre General Hospital[2]	Wilkes-Barre	100%	1668
Wilkes-Barre VA Medical Center[2]	Wilkes-Barre	100%	48
York Hospital[2]	York	100%	2258
Abington Memorial Hospital[2]	Abington	99%	651
Bradford Regional Medical Center	Bradford	99%	137
Clearfield Hospital	Clearfield	99%	273
Conemaugh Valley Memorial Hospital	Johnstown	99%	1837
Dubois Regional Medical Center	Dubois	99%	554
Ellwood City Hospital	Ellwood City	99%	96
Excela Health Frick Hospital	Mount Pleasant	99%	82
Excela Health Westmoreland Reg Hosp	Greensburg	99%	1561
Highlands Hospital[2]	Connellsville	99%	70
Millcreek Community Hospital	Erie	99%	126
Nason Hospital	Roaring Spring	99%	155
Riddle Memorial Hospital[2]	Media	99%	1284
Sacred Heart Hospital	Allentown	99%	397
Saint Clair Memorial Hospital[2]	Pittsburgh	99%	1508
Schuylkill Med Ctr-East Norwegian Street	Pottsville	99%	265
Soldiers and Sailors Memorial Hospital	Wellsboro	99%	195
Surgical Institute of Reading	Wyomissing	99%	418
Titusville Hospital	Titusville	99%	118
Western Penn Hosp-Forbes Reg Campus	Monroeville	99%	969
Williamsport Hospital & Medical Center[2]	Williamsport	99%	1184
Windber Hospital	Windber	99%	138
Charles Cole Memorial Hospital	Coudersport	98%	239
Hahnemann University Hospital[2]	Philadelphia	98%	686
Milton S Hershey Medical Center[2]	Hershey	98%	1642
Mount Nittany Medical Center	State College	98%	1632
Westfield Hospital	Allentown	97%	29
Lancaster General Hospital[2]	Lancaster	96%	2163
Jeanes Hospital	Philadelphia	95%	658
Saint Joseph's Hospital	Philadelphia	87%	63
Kane Community Hospital	Kane	69%	26
Cancer Treatment Centers of America	Philadelphia	43%	82

24. Appropriate Beta Blocker Usage

Hospital Name	City	Rate	Cases
Gnaden Huetten Memorial Hospital	Lehighton	100%	33
Lancaster Regional Medical Center[2]	Lancaster	100%	146
Nason Hospital	Roaring Spring	100%	43
Penn Presbyterian Medical Center	Philadelphia	100%	787
Roxborough Memorial Hospital	Phila	100%	40
Saint Joseph Medical Center[2]	Reading	100%	232
Gettysburg Hospital	Gettysburg	99%	110
Jeanes Hospital	Philadelphia	99%	196
Jefferson Regional Medical Center	Pittsburgh	99%	643
Lehigh Valley Hospital	Allentown	99%	1325
Main Line Hospital Paoli[2]	Paoli	99%	237
Mercy Hospital Scranton[2]	Scranton	99%	212
Phoenixville Hospital[2]	Phoenixville	99%	189
Sharon Regional Health System[2]	Sharon	99%	204
Somerset Hospital	Somerset	99%	82
UPMC Mckeesport	McKeesport	99%	114
UPMC Saint Margaret	Pittsburgh	99%	531
Western Pennsylvania Hospital[2]	Pittsburgh	99%	273
Albert Einstein Medical Center[2]	Philadelphia	98%	200
Evangelical Community Hospital[2]	Lewisburg	98%	131
Lansdale Hospital[2]	Lansdale	98%	60
Main Line Hospital Bryn Mawr Campus[2]	Bryn Mawr	98%	427
Memorial Hospital York	York	98%	111
Monongahela Valley Hospital	Monongahela	98%	162
Schuylkill Med Ctr-S Jackson Street	Pottsville	98%	113
Soldiers and Sailors Memorial Hospital	Wellsboro	98%	51
UPMC Mercy[2]	Pittsburgh	98%	197
UPMC Northwest	Seneca	98%	94
UPMC Passavant	Pittsburgh	98%	627
UPMC Presbyterian Shadyside	Pittsburgh	98%	2600
VA Pittsburgh Healthcare System[2]	Pittsburgh	98%	236
Western Penn Hosp-Forbes Reg Campus	Monroeville	98%	341
Grove City Medical Center	Grove City	97%	37
Heart of Lancaster Regional Medical Center	Lititz	97%	32
Indiana Regional Medical Center	Indiana	97%	117
Lebanon VA Medical Center[2]	Lebanon	97%	95
Main Line Hospital Lankenau[2]	Wynnewood	97%	505
Moses Taylor Hospital	Scranton	97%	161
Punxsutawney Area Hospital	Punxsutawney	97%	33
Saint Mary Medical Center[2]	Langhorne	97%	261
Williamsport Hospital & Medical Center[2]	Williamsport	97%	425
Ephrata Community Hospital	Ephrata	96%	161
Excela Health Westmoreland Reg Hosp	Greensburg	96%	490
Grand View Hospital[2]	Sellersville	96%	114
Hamot Medical Center	Erie	96%	688
Lehigh Valley Hospital - Muhlenberg	Bethlehem	96%	248
Meadville Medical Center	Meadville	96%	262
Mercy Suburban Hospital	Norristown	96%	89
Pocono Medical Center	E Stroudsburg	96%	214
Thomas Jefferson University Hospital[2]	Philadelphia	96%	763
UPMC Horizon	Greenville	96%	254
ACMH Hospital	Kittanning	95%	108
Allegheny General Hospital[2]	Pittsburgh	95%	875

NOTE: Hospital profiles are in alphabetical order by state, then city, then hospital within the city; Rankings exclude hospitals with less than 25 cases except for patient surveys which excludes hospitals with less than 100 cases; (a) 100–299 cases; (1) The number of cases is too small to be sure how well a hospital is performing; (2) The hospital indicated that the data submitted for this measure were based on a sample of cases; (3) Data was collected during a shorter time period (fewer quarters) than the maximum possible time for this measure; (4) Suppressed for one or more quarters by CMS; (5) No data is available from the hospital for this measure; (6) Fewer than 100 patients completed the HCAHPS survey. Use these rates with caution, as the number of surveys may be too low to reliably assess hospital performance; (7) Survey results are based on less than 12 months of data; (8) Survey results are not available for this reporting period; (9) No or very few patients were eligible for the HCAHPS survey. The scores shown, if any, reflect a very small number of surveys; (10) A state average was not calculated because too few hospitals in the state submitted data; (11) There were discrepancies in the data collection process; Please refer to the User's Guide for a full explanation of data.

Aria Health[2]	Philadelphia	95%	236
Chambersburg Hospital[2]	Chambersburg	95%	301
Chestnut Hill Hospital[2]	Philadelphia	95%	76
Community Medical Center	Scranton	95%	424
Crozer Chester Medical Center[2]	Upland	95%	302
Dubois Regional Medical Center	Dubois	95%	224
Excela Health Latrobe Hospital	Latrobe	95%	150
Hahnemann University Hospital[2]	Philadelphia	95%	214
Hanover Hospital	Hanover	95%	207
Magee Womens Hosp of UPMC Health Sys	Pittsburgh	95%	436
Nazareth Hospital	Philadelphia	95%	190
Saint Vincent Health Center	Erie	95%	621
Uniontown Hospital	Uniontown	95%	220
Berwick Hospital Center[2]	Berwick	94%	32
Chester County Hospital	West Chester	94%	328
Conemaugh Valley Memorial Hospital	Johnstown	94%	712
Hazleton General Hospital	Hazleton	94%	94
Jennersville Regional Hospital[2]	West Grove	94%	33
Lewistown Hospital	Lewistown	94%	78
Palmerton Hospital	Palmerton	94%	31
Pinnacle Health Hospitals[2]	Harrisburg	94%	1087
Reading Hospital Medical Center[2]	Reading	94%	730
Riddle Memorial Hospital[2]	Media	94%	308
The Washington Hospital[2]	Washington	94%	258
Windber Hospital	Windber	94%	34
Bucks County Specialty Hospital[2,3]	Bensalem	93%	27
Carlisle Regional Medical Center[2]	Carlisle	93%	179
Doylestown Hospital[2]	Doylestown	93%	302
Excela Health Frick Hospital	Mount Pleasant	93%	27
Waynesboro Hospital	Waynesboro	93%	43
Butler Memorial Hospital	Butler	92%	420
Good Samaritan Hospital[2]	Lebanon	92%	230
Jameson Memorial Hospital	New Castle	92%	146
Mercy Fitzgerald Hospital[2]	Darby	92%	142
Saint Clair Memorial Hospital[2]	Pittsburgh	92%	438
Saint Luke's Quakertown Hospital	Quakertown	92%	38
York Hospital[2]	York	92%	775
Delaware County Memorial Hospital[2]	Drexel Hill	91%	140
Easton Hospital[2]	Easton	91%	277
Sunbury Community Hospital[2]	Sunbury	91%	35
Titusville Hospital	Titusville	91%	33
UPMC Bedford	Everett	91%	44
Clearfield Hospital	Clearfield	90%	93
Geisinger Medical Center[2]	Danville	90%	322
Heritage Valley Sewickley	Sewickley	90%	331
Lower Bucks Hospital[2]	Bristol	90%	89
Wilkes-Barre General Hospital[2]	Wilkes-Barre	90%	600
Brandywine Hospital[2]	Coatesville	89%	114
Holy Redeemer Hospital and Medical Center	Meadowbrook	89%	228
Holy Spirit Hospital[2]	Camp Hill	89%	387
Lancaster General Hospital[2]	Lancaster	89%	764
Marian Community Hospital	Carbondale	89%	45
Mount Nittany Medical Center	State College	89%	482
Shamokin Area Community Hospital	Coal Township	88%	56
Surgical Institute of Reading	Wyomissing	88%	112
Altoona Regional Health System	Altoona	87%	634
Montgomery Hospital[2]	Norristown	87%	106
Penn Hosp of the Univ of Penn Health Sys[2]	Philadelphia	87%	218
Sacred Heart Hospital	Allentown	87%	99
Saint Luke's Hospital Bethlehem[2]	Bethlehem	87%	550
Schuylkill Med Ctr-East Norwegian Street	Pottsville	87%	101
Abington Memorial Hospital[2]	Abington	86%	217
Ellwood City Hospital	Ellwood City	86%	29
Milton S Hershey Medical Center[2]	Hershey	86%	534
Temple University Hospital[2]	Philadelphia	86%	289
Alle Kiski Medical Center	Natrona	84%	148
Robert Packer Hospital	Sayre	84%	529
Bradford Regional Medical Center	Bradford	83%	35
Canonsburg General Hospital	Canonsburg	83%	133
Geisinger Wyoming Valley Medical Center[2]	Wilkes-Barre	83%	314
Southwest Regional Medical Center	Waynesburg	82%	34
Ohio Valley General Hospital	Mckees Rocks	81%	78
Heritage Valley Beaver	Beaver	80%	363
Clarion Hospital	Clarion	79%	48
Elk Regional Health Center	Saint Marys	79%	70
Hospital of Univ of Pennsylvania[2]	Philadelphia	77%	293
Pottstown Memorial Medical Center[2]	Pottstown	76%	102
Wayne Memorial Hospital[2]	Honesdale	76%	54
Bloomsburg Hospital	Bloomsburg	75%	75
Millcreek Community Hospital	Erie	73%	30
Warren General Hospital	Warren	69%	61
Saint Luke's Miners Memorial Hospital	Coaldale	67%	52

25. Controlled Postoperative Blood Glucose

Hospital Name	City	Rate	Cases
Community Medical Center	Scranton	100%	226
Wilkes-Barre General Hospital[2]	Wilkes-Barre	100%	264
Williamsport Hospital & Medical Center[2]	Williamsport	100%	119
Butler Memorial Hospital	Butler	99%	326
Chester County Hospital	West Chester	99%	90
Doylestown Hospital[2]	Doylestown	99%	192
Dubois Regional Medical Center	Dubois	99%	148
Geisinger Medical Center[2]	Danville	99%	167
Holy Spirit Hospital[2]	Camp Hill	99%	272
Main Line Hospital Lankenau[2]	Wynnewood	99%	456
Pinnacle Health Hospitals[2]	Harrisburg	99%	497
Easton Hospital[2]	Easton	98%	121
Excela Health Westmoreland Reg Hosp	Greensburg	98%	348
Geisinger Wyoming Valley Medical Center[2]	Wilkes-Barre	98%	123
Hospital of Univ of Pennsylvania[2]	Philadelphia	98%	278
Jefferson Regional Medical Center	Pittsburgh	98%	363
Lehigh Valley Hospital	Allentown	98%	581
Main Line Hospital Bryn Mawr Campus[2]	Bryn Mawr	98%	89
Penn Presbyterian Medical Center	Philadelphia	98%	394
Reading Hospital Medical Center[2]	Reading	98%	213
The Washington Hospital[2]	Washington	98%	162
Western Pennsylvania Hospital[2]	Pittsburgh	98%	206
Aria Health[2]	Philadelphia	97%	88
Lehigh Valley Hospital - Muhlenberg	Bethlehem	97%	119
Saint Luke's Hospital Bethlehem[2]	Bethlehem	97%	227
Saint Mary Medical Center[2]	Langhorne	97%	155
Western Penn Hosp-Forbes Reg Campus	Monroeville	97%	180
Abington Memorial Hospital[2]	Abington	96%	150
Crozer Chester Medical Center[2]	Upland	96%	130
Lancaster General Hospital[2]	Lancaster	96%	278
Mercy Fitzgerald Hospital[2]	Darby	96%	72
Phoenixville Hospital[2]	Phoenixville	96%	99
Pocono Medical Center	E Stroudsburg	96%	165
Saint Clair Memorial Hospital[2]	Pittsburgh	96%	204
Saint Vincent Health Center	Erie	96%	423
UPMC Mercy[2]	Pittsburgh	96%	132
UPMC Presbyterian Shadyside	Pittsburgh	96%	894
Conemaugh Valley Memorial Hospital	Johnstown	95%	201
Good Samaritan Hospital[2]	Lebanon	95%	131
Heritage Valley Beaver	Beaver	95%	243
Main Line Hospital Paoli[2]	Paoli	95%	82
Robert Packer Hospital	Sayre	95%	187
UPMC Passavant	Pittsburgh	95%	392
Allegheny General Hospital[2]	Pittsburgh	94%	383
Altoona Regional Health System	Altoona	94%	256
Hahnemann University Hospital[2]	Philadelphia	94%	137
Jeanes Hospital	Philadelphia	94%	87
VA Pittsburgh Healthcare System[2]	Pittsburgh	94%	156
Albert Einstein Medical Center[2]	Philadelphia	93%	89
Lancaster Regional Medical Center[2]	Lancaster	93%	54
Saint Joseph Medical Center[2]	Reading	93%	121
Sharon Regional Health System[2]	Sharon	93%	84
Lower Bucks Hospital[2]	Bristol	92%	38
Mercy Hospital Scranton[2]	Scranton	92%	179
Milton S Hershey Medical Center[2]	Hershey	92%	333
Hamot Medical Center	Erie	91%	375
York Hospital[2]	York	90%	366
Temple University Hospital[2]	Philadelphia	87%	141
Thomas Jefferson University Hospital[2]	Philadelphia	87%	184
Penn Hosp of the Univ of Penn Health Sys[2]	Philadelphia	84%	106

26. Prophylactic Antibiotic Timing

Hospital Name	City	Rate	Cases
Brookville Hospital	Brookville	100%	34
Chestnut Hill Hospital[2]	Philadelphia	100%	203
Gettysburg Hospital	Gettysburg	100%	297
Gnaden Huetten Memorial Hospital	Lehighton	100%	96
Jennersville Regional Hospital[2]	West Grove	100%	91
Mercy Suburban Hospital	Norristown	100%	184
Nason Hospital	Roaring Spring	100%	91
Riddle Memorial Hospital[2]	Media	100%	996
Sunbury Community Hospital[2]	Sunbury	100%	71
UPMC Northwest	Seneca	100%	251
Western Pennsylvania Hospital[2]	Pittsburgh	100%	870
Western Penn Hosp-Forbes Reg Campus	Monroeville	100%	703
Allegheny General Hospital[2]	Pittsburgh	99%	1377
Butler Memorial Hospital	Butler	99%	990
Carlisle Regional Medical Center[2]	Carlisle	99%	394
Chester County Hospital	West Chester	99%	730
Community Medical Center	Scranton	99%	781
Conemaugh Valley Memorial Hospital	Johnstown	99%	1157
Edgewood Surgical Hospital	Transfer	99%	119
Excela Health Westmoreland Reg Hosp	Greensburg	99%	1095
Grand View Hospital[2]	Sellersville	99%	312
Grove City Medical Center	Grove City	99%	113
Heart of Lancaster Regional Medical Center	Lititz	99%	91
Holy Redeemer Hospital and Medical Center	Meadowbrook	99%	601
Hospital of Univ of Pennsylvania[2]	Philadelphia	99%	580
Jefferson Regional Medical Center	Pittsburgh	99%	1174
Lancaster Regional Medical Center[2]	Lancaster	99%	269
Lebanon VA Medical Center	Lebanon	99%	187
Main Line Hospital Bryn Mawr Campus[2]	Bryn Mawr	99%	1296
Main Line Hospital Lankenau[2]	Wynnewood	99%	1161
Main Line Hospital Paoli[2]	Paoli	99%	715
Marian Community Hospital	Carbondale	99%	93
Mercy Hospital Scranton[2]	Scranton	99%	423
Moses Taylor Hospital	Scranton	99%	400
Nazareth Hospital	Philadelphia	99%	479
Pinnacle Health Hospitals[2]	Harrisburg	99%	2975
Pocono Medical Center	E Stroudsburg	99%	379
Saint Luke's Hospital Bethlehem[2]	Bethlehem	99%	1242
Saint Luke's Miners Memorial Hospital	Coaldale	99%	158
Saint Luke's Quakertown Hospital	Quakertown	99%	68
Saint Mary Medical Center[2]	Langhorne	99%	517
Thomas Jefferson University Hospital[2]	Philadelphia	99%	2538
UPMC Mckeesport	McKeesport	99%	195
UPMC Presbyterian Shadyside	Pittsburgh	99%	2801
VA Pittsburgh Healthcare System	Pittsburgh	99%	366
The Washington Hospital[2]	Washington	99%	625
Albert Einstein Medical Center[2]	Philadelphia	98%	498
Berwick Hospital Center[2]	Berwick	98%	129
Chambersburg Hospital[2]	Chambersburg	98%	798
Coordinated Health Orthopedic Hospital[2]	Bethlehem	98%	180
Crozer Chester Medical Center[2]	Upland	98%	845
Erie VA Medical Center	Erie	98%	41
Excela Health Latrobe Hospital	Latrobe	98%	400
Hamot Medical Center	Erie	98%	1107
Heritage Valley Beaver	Beaver	98%	911
Heritage Valley Sewickley	Sewickley	98%	889
Indiana Regional Medical Center	Indiana	98%	287
Jameson Memorial Hospital	New Castle	98%	377
Jeanes Hospital	Philadelphia	98%	456
Lewistown Hospital	Lewistown	98%	176
Magee Womens Hosp of UPMC Health Sys	Pittsburgh	98%	1880
Meadville Medical Center	Meadville	98%	631
Mercy Fitzgerald Hospital[2]	Darby	98%	264
Penn Hosp of the Univ of Penn Health Sys[2]	Philadelphia	98%	483
Reading Hospital Medical Center[2]	Reading	98%	1568
Roxborough Memorial Hospital	Phila	98%	66
Saint Joseph Medical Center[2]	Reading	98%	456
Sharon Regional Health System[2]	Sharon	98%	472
UPMC Bedford	Everett	98%	114
Wilkes-Barre General Hospital[2]	Wilkes-Barre	98%	1114
ACMH Hospital	Kittanning	97%	378
Alle Kiski Medical Center	Natrona	97%	344
Altoona Regional Health System	Altoona	97%	1524
Bloomsburg Hospital	Bloomsburg	97%	213
Brandywine Hospital[2]	Coatesville	97%	169
Bucks County Specialty Hospital[2,3]	Bensalem	97%	99
Canonsburg General Hospital	Canonsburg	97%	339
Delaware County Memorial Hospital[2]	Drexel Hill	97%	379
Excela Health Frick Hospital	Mount Pleasant	97%	39
Geisinger Medical Center[2]	Danville	97%	471
Hanover Hospital	Hanover	97%	628
Hazleton General Hospital	Hazleton	97%	178
Holy Spirit Hospital[2]	Camp Hill	97%	842
Lehigh Valley Hospital	Allentown	97%	2490
Monongahela Valley Hospital	Monongahela	97%	425
Mount Nittany Medical Center	State College	97%	1229
Penn Presbyterian Medical Center	Philadelphia	97%	1482
Phoenixville Hospital[2]	Phoenixville	97%	325
Punxsutawney Area Hospital	Punxsutawney	97%	102
Saint Vincent Health Center	Erie	97%	1319
Surgical Specialty Ctr-Coordinated Health[2,3]	Allentown	97%	65
Temple University Hospital[2]	Philadelphia	97%	789
Uniontown Hospital	Uniontown	97%	640
UPMC Horizon	Greenville	97%	537
UPMC Passavant	Pittsburgh	97%	1232
Wayne Memorial Hospital[2]	Honesdale	97%	162
Wilkes-Barre VA Medical Center	Wilkes-Barre	97%	32
Abington Memorial Hospital[2]	Abington	96%	494
Aria Health[2]	Philadelphia	96%	353
Clarion Hospital	Clarion	96%	186
Dubois Regional Medical Center	Dubois	96%	443
Geisinger Wyoming Valley Medical Center[2]	Wilkes-Barre	96%	454
Hahnemann University Hospital[2]	Philadelphia	96%	468
Lansdale Hospital[2]	Lansdale	96%	112
Lehigh Valley Hospital - Muhlenberg	Bethlehem	96%	495
Lock Haven Hospital[2]	Lock Haven	96%	25
Lower Bucks Hospital[2]	Bristol	96%	190
Memorial Hospital York	York	96%	447
Robert Packer Hospital	Sayre	96%	878
Schuylkill Med Ctr-S Jackson Street	Pottsville	96%	302
UPMC Saint Margaret	Pittsburgh	96%	1095
Waynesboro Hospital	Waynesboro	96%	134
Williamsport Hospital & Medical Center[2]	Williamsport	96%	917
Windber Hospital	Windber	96%	94
York Hospital[2]	York	96%	1723
Evangelical Community Hospital[2]	Lewisburg	95%	321
Lancaster General Hospital[2]	Lancaster	95%	1457
Pottstown Memorial Medical Center[2]	Pottstown	95%	287
Shamokin Area Community Hospital	Coal Township	95%	92
Soldiers and Sailors Memorial Hospital	Wellsboro	95%	127
UPMC Mercy[2]	Pittsburgh	95%	425
Doylestown Hospital[2]	Doylestown	94%	644
Easton Hospital[2]	Easton	94%	858

NOTE: Hospital profiles are in alphabetical order by state, then city, then hospital within the city; Rankings exclude hospitals with less than 25 cases except for patient surveys which excludes hospitals with less than 100 cases; (a) 100–299 cases; (1) The number of cases is too small to be sure how well a hospital is performing; (2) The hospital indicated that the data submitted for this measure were based on a sample of cases; (3) Data was collected during a shorter time period (fewer quarters) than the maximum possible time for this measure; (4) Suppressed for one or more quarters by CMS; (5) No data is available from the hospital for this measure; (6) Fewer than 100 patients completed the HCAHPS survey. Use these rates with caution, as the number of surveys may be too low to reliably assess hospital performance; (7) Survey results are based on less than 12 months of data; (8) Survey results are not available for this reporting period; (9) No or very few patients were eligible for the HCAHPS survey. The scores shown, if any, reflect a very small number of surveys; (10) A state average was not calculated because too few hospitals in the state submitted data; (11) There were discrepancies in the data collection process; Please refer to the User's Guide for a full explanation of data.

Ellwood City Hospital	Ellwood City	94%	32
Ephrata Community Hospital	Ephrata	94%	431
Saint Clair Memorial Hospital[2]	Pittsburgh	94%	1086
Surgical Institute of Reading	Wyomissing	94%	395
Bradford Regional Medical Center	Bradford	93%	90
Millcreek Community Hospital	Erie	93%	85
Milton S Hershey Medical Center[2]	Hershey	93%	1275
Palmerton Hospital	Palmerton	93%	55
Sacred Heart Hospital	Allentown	93%	280
Schuylkill Med Ctr-East Norwegian Street	Pottsville	93%	149
Warren General Hospital	Warren	93%	228
Montgomery Hospital[2]	Norristown	92%	197
Ohio Valley General Hospital	Mckees Rocks	92%	210
St Catherine Med Ctr Fountain Springs	Ashland	92%	25
Somerset Hospital	Somerset	92%	212
Clearfield Hospital	Clearfield	91%	203
Good Samaritan Hospital[2]	Lebanon	91%	383
J C Blair Memorial Hospital	Huntingdon	88%	33
Philadelphia VA Medical Center	Philadelphia	88%	32
Southwest Regional Medical Center	Waynesburg	88%	64
Charles Cole Memorial Hospital	Coudersport	87%	195
Elk Regional Health Center	Saint Marys	87%	167
Titusville Hospital	Titusville	85%	85
Jersey Shore Hospital	Jersey Shore	78%	37
Highlands Hospital[2]	Connellsville	75%	32
Mercy Tyler Hospital	Tunkhannock	71%	31
Montrose General Hospital	Montrose	59%	97

27. Prophylactic Antibiotic Timing (Outpatient)

Hospital Name	City	Rate	Cases
Berwick Hospital Center	Berwick	100%	36
Coordinated Health Orthopedic Hospital[3]	Bethlehem	100%	33
Delaware County Memorial Hospital	Drexel Hill	100%	69
Lancaster Regional Medical Center	Lancaster	100%	305
Nazareth Hospital	Philadelphia	100%	73
Roxborough Memorial Hospital	Phila	100%	52
Heart of Lancaster Regional Medical Center	Lititz	99%	77
ACMH Hospital	Kittanning	98%	82
Crozer Chester Medical Center	Upland	98%	177
Jennersville Regional Hospital	West Grove	98%	47
Lansdale Hospital	Lansdale	98%	50
Lehigh Valley Hospital	Allentown	98%	1177
Mercy Suburban Hospital	Norristown	98%	58
Penn Hosp of the Univ of Penn Health Sys	Philadelphia	98%	572
Phoenixville Hospital	Phoenixville	98%	114
Sharon Regional Health System	Sharon	98%	157
Surgical Institute of Reading	Wyomissing	98%	204
Western Pennsylvania Hospital	Pittsburgh	98%	350
Abington Memorial Hospital	Abington	97%	412
Allegheny General Hospital	Pittsburgh	97%	541
Community Medical Center	Scranton	97%	461
Gettysburg Hospital	Gettysburg	97%	104
Memorial Hospital - Towanda	Towanda	97%	30
Millcreek Community Hospital	Erie	97%	30
Pocono Medical Center	E Stroudsburg	97%	192
Riddle Memorial Hospital	Media	97%	238
Saint Mary Medical Center	Langhorne	97%	273
Saint Vincent Health Center	Erie	97%	333
UPMC Mckeesport	McKeesport	97%	95
UPMC Presbyterian Shadyside	Pittsburgh	97%	970
Clearfield Hospital	Clearfield	96%	99
Hamot Medical Center	Erie	96%	421
Indiana Regional Medical Center	Indiana	96%	177
Lehigh Valley Hospital - Muhlenberg	Bethlehem	96%	277
Pinnacle Health Hospitals	Harrisburg	96%	1109
Punxsutawney Area Hospital	Punxsutawney	96%	70
UPMC Saint Margaret	Pittsburgh	96%	357
York Hospital	York	96%	832
Butler Memorial Hospital	Butler	95%	220
Dubois Regional Medical Center	Dubois	95%	319
Excela Health Frick Hospital	Mount Pleasant	95%	43
Grove City Medical Center	Grove City	95%	88
Hahnemann University Hospital	Philadelphia	95%	416
Lewistown Hospital	Lewistown	95%	119
Main Line Hospital Paoli	Paoli	95%	197
Monongahela Valley Hospital	Monongahela	95%	94
Montgomery Hospital	Norristown	95%	59
Moses Taylor Hospital	Scranton	95%	58
Mount Nittany Medical Center	State College	95%	221
Robert Packer Hospital	Sayre	95%	618
UPMC Northwest	Seneca	95%	139
Aria Health	Philadelphia	94%	293
Brandywine Hospital	Coatesville	94%	105
Grand View Hospital	Sellersville	94%	121
Holy Spirit Hospital	Camp Hill	94%	588
Jeanes Hospital	Philadelphia	94%	48
Jefferson Regional Medical Center	Pittsburgh	94%	268
Memorial Hospital York	York	94%	96
Somerset Hospital	Somerset	94%	77
Albert Einstein Medical Center	Philadelphia	93%	252
Chester County Hospital	West Chester	93%	248
Chestnut Hill Hospital	Philadelphia	93%	110
Evangelical Community Hospital	Lewisburg	93%	402
Geisinger Medical Center	Danville	93%	820
Main Line Hospital Bryn Mawr Campus	Bryn Mawr	93%	238
Main Line Hospital Lankenau	Wynnewood	93%	348
Meadville Medical Center	Meadville	93%	178
Milton S Hershey Medical Center	Hershey	93%	710
Temple University Hospital	Philadelphia	93%	402
UPMC Mercy	Pittsburgh	93%	441
UPMC Passavant	Pittsburgh	93%	519
Williamsport Hospital & Medical Center	Williamsport	93%	396
Chambersburg Hospital	Chambersburg	92%	71
Ephrata Community Hospital	Ephrata	92%	304
Excela Health Latrobe Hospital	Latrobe	92%	191
Geisinger Wyoming Valley Medical Center	Wilkes-Barre	92%	531
Hazleton General Hospital	Hazleton	92%	78
Saint Joseph Medical Center	Reading	92%	201
The Washington Hospital	Washington	92%	216
Elk Regional Health Center	Saint Marys	91%	141
Excela Health Westmoreland Reg Hosp	Greensburg	91%	245
Hanover Hospital	Hanover	91%	194
Lancaster General Hospital	Lancaster	91%	1616
Magee Womens Hosp of UPMC Health Sys	Pittsburgh	91%	330
Mercy Fitzgerald Hospital	Darby	91%	151
Nason Hospital	Roaring Spring	91%	58
Sacred Heart Hospital	Allentown	91%	85
UPMC Horizon	Greenville	91%	201
Wilkes-Barre General Hospital	Wilkes-Barre	91%	423
Windber Hospital	Windber	91%	44
Conemaugh Valley Memorial Hospital	Johnstown	90%	628
Easton Hospital	Easton	90%	84
Good Samaritan Hospital	Lebanon	90%	338
Penn Presbyterian Medical Center	Philadelphia	90%	343
Altoona Regional Health System	Altoona	89%	694
Ellwood City Hospital	Ellwood City	89%	35
Pottstown Memorial Medical Center	Pottstown	89%	146
Reading Hospital Medical Center	Reading	89%	747
Saint Luke's Hospital Bethlehem	Bethlehem	89%	700
Wayne Memorial Hospital	Honesdale	89%	47
Alle Kiski Medical Center	Natrona	88%	210
Bradford Regional Medical Center	Bradford	88%	42
Doylestown Hospital	Doylestown	88%	196
Jameson Memorial Hospital	New Castle	88%	77
Lower Bucks Hospital	Bristol	88%	83
Southwest Regional Medical Center	Waynesburg	88%	33
Carlisle Regional Medical Center	Carlisle	87%	137
Heritage Valley Beaver	Beaver	87%	196
Heritage Valley Sewickley	Sewickley	87%	119
Gnaden Huetten Memorial Hospital	Lehighton	86%	71
Saint Luke's Quakertown Hospital	Quakertown	86%	29
Thomas Jefferson University Hospital	Philadelphia	84%	487
Uniontown Hospital	Uniontown	84%	141
Clarion Hospital	Clarion	83%	30
Soldiers and Sailors Memorial Hospital	Wellsboro	83%	48
UPMC Bedford	Everett	83%	36
Western Penn Hosp-Forbes Reg Campus	Monroeville	83%	281
Mercy Hospital Scranton	Scranton	82%	281
Ohio Valley General Hospital	Mckees Rocks	80%	45
Waynesboro Hospital	Waynesboro	77%	26
Saint Clair Memorial Hospital	Pittsburgh	76%	336
Holy Redeemer Hospital and Medical Center	Meadowbrook	74%	58
Canonsburg General Hospital	Canonsburg	72%	36
Sunbury Community Hospital	Sunbury	72%	32
Charles Cole Memorial Hospital	Coudersport	71%	34
Warren General Hospital	Warren	71%	35
Palmerton Hospital	Palmerton	69%	78
Schuylkill Med Ctr-S Jackson Street	Pottsville	68%	122
Titusville Hospital	Titusville	58%	38
Hospital of Univ of Pennsylvania	Philadelphia	51%	690
Bloomsburg Hospital	Bloomsburg	45%	113

28. Prophylactic Antibiotic Selection

Hospital Name	City	Rate	Cases
Bucks County Specialty Hospital[2,3]	Bensalem	100%	99
Edgewood Surgical Hospital	Transfer	100%	119
Excela Health Frick Hospital	Mount Pleasant	100%	39
Grove City Medical Center	Grove City	100%	113
Heart of Lancaster Regional Medical Center	Lititz	100%	93
Montrose General Hospital	Montrose	100%	97
Punxsutawney Area Hospital	Punxsutawney	100%	103
Surgical Specialty Ctr-Coordinated Health[2,3]	Allentown	100%	65
UPMC Northwest	Seneca	100%	252
Abington Memorial Hospital[2]	Abington	99%	498
Allegheny General Hospital[2]	Pittsburgh	99%	1417
Bloomsburg Hospital	Bloomsburg	99%	215
Butler Memorial Hospital	Butler	99%	999
Chester County Hospital	West Chester	99%	734
Chestnut Hill Hospital[2]	Philadelphia	99%	206
Community Medical Center	Scranton	99%	795
Conemaugh Valley Memorial Hospital	Johnstown	99%	1164
Evangelical Community Hospital[2]	Lewisburg	99%	322
Excela Health Westmoreland Reg Hosp	Greensburg	99%	1109
Geisinger Medical Center[2]	Danville	99%	480
Hamot Medical Center	Erie	99%	1126
Heritage Valley Sewickley	Sewickley	99%	893
Indiana Regional Medical Center	Indiana	99%	287
Jefferson Regional Medical Center	Pittsburgh	99%	1197
Jennersville Regional Hospital[2]	West Grove	99%	90
Lebanon VA Medical Center	Lebanon	99%	190
Lehigh Valley Hospital	Allentown	99%	2523
Main Line Hospital Bryn Mawr Campus[2]	Bryn Mawr	99%	1307
Meadville Medical Center	Meadville	99%	633
Mercy Hospital Scranton[2]	Scranton	99%	436
Mount Nittany Medical Center	State College	99%	1232
Nason Hospital	Roaring Spring	99%	91
Nazareth Hospital	Philadelphia	99%	480
Robert Packer Hospital	Sayre	99%	887
Saint Luke's Miners Memorial Hospital	Coaldale	99%	159
Saint Luke's Quakertown Hospital	Quakertown	99%	68
Saint Mary Medical Center[2]	Langhorne	99%	523
Sharon Regional Health System[2]	Sharon	99%	477
Sunbury Community Hospital[2]	Sunbury	99%	71
UPMC Presbyterian Shadyside	Pittsburgh	99%	2889
UPMC Saint Margaret	Pittsburgh	99%	1100
VA Pittsburgh Healthcare System	Pittsburgh	99%	372
Waynesboro Hospital	Waynesboro	99%	132
ACMH Hospital	Kittanning	98%	378
Albert Einstein Medical Center[2]	Philadelphia	98%	511
Clarion Hospital	Clarion	98%	185
Coordinated Health Orthopedic Hospital[2]	Bethlehem	98%	180
Doylestown Hospital[2]	Doylestown	98%	648
Easton Hospital[2]	Easton	98%	462
Ephrata Community Hospital	Ephrata	98%	432
Excela Health Latrobe Hospital	Latrobe	98%	402
Grand View Hospital[2]	Sellersville	98%	313
Hanover Hospital	Hanover	98%	624
Hazleton General Hospital	Hazleton	98%	179
Holy Redeemer Hospital and Medical Center	Meadowbrook	98%	601
Holy Spirit Hospital[2]	Camp Hill	98%	854
Jeanes Hospital	Philadelphia	98%	459
Lancaster General Hospital[2]	Lancaster	98%	1477
Lansdale Hospital[2]	Lansdale	98%	113
Main Line Hospital Lankenau[2]	Wynnewood	98%	1183
Main Line Hospital Paoli[2]	Paoli	98%	720
Milton S Hershey Medical Center[2]	Hershey	98%	1287
Montgomery Hospital[2]	Norristown	98%	194
Palmerton Hospital	Palmerton	98%	55
Penn Presbyterian Medical Center	Philadelphia	98%	1485
Phoenixville Hospital[2]	Phoenixville	98%	328
Reading Hospital Medical Center[2]	Reading	98%	1580
Riddle Memorial Hospital[2]	Media	98%	1002
Saint Luke's Hospital Bethlehem[2]	Bethlehem	98%	1266
Shamokin Area Community Hospital	Coal Township	98%	92
Thomas Jefferson University Hospital[2]	Philadelphia	98%	2558
UPMC Bedford	Everett	98%	114
UPMC Mercy[2]	Pittsburgh	98%	436
UPMC Passavant	Pittsburgh	98%	1248
Western Penn Hosp-Forbes Reg Campus	Monroeville	98%	712
Williamsport Hospital & Medical Center[2]	Williamsport	98%	926
Alle Kiski Medical Center	Natrona	97%	344
Altoona Regional Health System	Altoona	97%	1559
Aria Health[2]	Philadelphia	97%	357
Carlisle Regional Medical Center[2]	Carlisle	97%	395
Chambersburg Hospital[2]	Chambersburg	97%	800
Charles Cole Memorial Hospital	Coudersport	97%	192
Delaware County Memorial Hospital[2]	Drexel Hill	97%	382
Geisinger Wyoming Valley Medical Center[2]	Wilkes-Barre	97%	465
Gettysburg Hospital	Gettysburg	97%	301
Good Samaritan Hospital[2]	Lebanon	97%	389
Hahnemann University Hospital[2]	Philadelphia	97%	473
Lancaster Regional Medical Center[2]	Lancaster	97%	275
Lehigh Valley Hospital - Muhlenberg	Bethlehem	97%	499
Magee Womens Hosp of UPMC Health Sys	Pittsburgh	97%	1878
Memorial Hospital York	York	97%	447
Mercy Fitzgerald Hospital[2]	Darby	97%	272
Mercy Suburban Hospital	Norristown	97%	185
Monongahela Valley Hospital	Monongahela	97%	425
Penn Hosp of the Univ of Penn Health Sys[2]	Philadelphia	97%	494
Pinnacle Health Hospitals[2]	Harrisburg	97%	3010
Pocono Medical Center	E Stroudsburg	97%	380
Saint Clair Memorial Hospital[2]	Pittsburgh	97%	1098
Saint Vincent Health Center	Erie	97%	1336
Schuylkill Med Ctr-East Norwegian Street	Pottsville	97%	148
UPMC Horizon	Greenville	97%	539
UPMC Mckeesport	McKeesport	97%	197
The Washington Hospital[2]	Washington	97%	630
Wilkes-Barre General Hospital[2]	Wilkes-Barre	97%	1127
Wilkes-Barre VA Medical Center	Wilkes-Barre	97%	32
Canonsburg General Hospital	Canonsburg	96%	340
Crozer Chester Medical Center[2]	Upland	96%	850

NOTE: Hospital profiles are in alphabetical order by state, then city, then hospital within the city; Rankings exclude hospitals with less than 25 cases except for patient surveys which excludes hospitals with less than 100 cases; (a) 100–299 cases; (1) The number of cases is too small to be sure how well a hospital is performing; (2) The hospital indicated that the data submitted for this measure were based on a sample of cases; (3) Data was collected during a shorter time period (fewer quarters) than the maximum possible time for this measure; (4) Suppressed for one or more quarters by CMS; (5) No data is available from the hospital for this measure; (6) Fewer than 100 patients completed the HCAHPS survey. Use these rates with caution, as the number of surveys may be too low to reliably assess hospital performance; (7) Survey results are based on less than 12 months of data; (8) Survey results are not available for this reporting period; (9) No or very few patients were eligible for the HCAHPS survey. The scores shown, if any, reflect a very small number of surveys; (10) A state average was not calculated because too few hospitals in the state submitted data; (11) There were discrepancies in the data collection process; Please refer to the User's Guide for a full explanation of data.

Dubois Regional Medical Center	Dubois	96%	449
Heritage Valley Beaver	Beaver	96%	924
Hospital of Univ of Pennsylvania[2]	Philadelphia	96%	598
Moses Taylor Hospital	Scranton	96%	400
Roxborough Memorial Hospital	Phila	96%	70
Saint Joseph Medical Center[2]	Reading	96%	468
Surgical Institute of Reading	Wyomissing	96%	395
Western Pennsylvania Hospital[2]	Pittsburgh	96%	886
Windber Hospital	Windber	96%	94
York Hospital[2]	York	96%	1760
Berwick Hospital Center[2]	Berwick	95%	131
Clearfield Hospital	Clearfield	95%	203
Erie VA Medical Center	Erie	95%	41
Gnaden Huetten Memorial Hospital	Lehighton	95%	96
Lewistown Hospital	Lewistown	95%	176
Millcreek Community Hospital	Erie	95%	87
Ohio Valley General Hospital	Mckees Rocks	95%	213
Southwest Regional Medical Center	Waynesburg	95%	64
Temple University Hospital[2]	Philadelphia	95%	804
Uniontown Hospital	Uniontown	95%	644
Wayne Memorial Hospital[2]	Honesdale	95%	162
Highlands Hospital[2]	Connellsville	94%	32
Jameson Memorial Hospital	New Castle	94%	379
Philadelphia VA Medical Center	Philadelphia	94%	31
Sacred Heart Hospital	Allentown	94%	280
Soldiers and Sailors Memorial Hospital	Wellsboro	94%	127
Warren General Hospital	Warren	94%	229
Brandywine Hospital[2]	Coatesville	93%	169
Marian Community Hospital	Carbondale	93%	95
Pottstown Memorial Medical Center[2]	Pottstown	93%	289
Elk Regional Health Center	Saint Marys	92%	167
Brookville Hospital	Brookville	91%	34
Lower Bucks Hospital[2]	Bristol	91%	189
Schuylkill Med Ctr-S Jackson Street	Pottsville	91%	301
Mercy Tyler Hospital	Tunkhannock	90%	30
Bradford Regional Medical Center	Bradford	89%	89
Somerset Hospital	Somerset	86%	214
J C Blair Memorial Hospital	Huntingdon	79%	33
Ellwood City Hospital	Ellwood City	78%	32
Titusville Hospital	Titusville	73%	84
St Catherine Med Ctr Fountain Springs	Ashland	72%	25
Jersey Shore Hospital	Jersey Shore	71%	35

29. Prophylactic Antibiotic Selection (Outpatient)

Hospital Name	City	Rate	Cases
Coordinated Health Orthopedic Hospital[3]	Bethlehem	100%	33
Lansdale Hospital	Lansdale	100%	50
Windber Hospital	Windber	100%	41
Gettysburg Hospital	Gettysburg	99%	101
Lancaster Regional Medical Center	Lancaster	99%	305
Soldiers and Sailors Memorial Hospital	Wellsboro	99%	109
Thomas Jefferson University Hospital	Philadelphia	99%	485
UPMC Northwest	Seneca	99%	242
UPMC Saint Margaret	Pittsburgh	99%	350
Williamsport Hospital & Medical Center	Williamsport	99%	386
Altoona Regional Health System	Altoona	98%	646
Aria Health	Philadelphia	98%	276
Bloomsburg Hospital	Bloomsburg	98%	51
Chestnut Hill Hospital	Philadelphia	98%	104
Community Medical Center	Scranton	98%	451
Evangelical Community Hospital	Lewisburg	98%	393
Grand View Hospital	Sellersville	98%	124
Jeanes Hospital	Philadelphia	98%	49
Jennersville Regional Hospital	West Grove	98%	98
Roxborough Memorial Hospital	Phila	98%	52
Sharon Regional Health System	Sharon	98%	155
Brandywine Hospital	Coatesville	97%	100
Canonsburg General Hospital	Canonsburg	97%	31
Clearfield Hospital	Clearfield	97%	97
Crozer Chester Medical Center	Upland	97%	174
Delaware County Memorial Hospital	Drexel Hill	97%	69
Dubois Regional Medical Center	Dubois	97%	409
Ephrata Community Hospital	Ephrata	97%	286
Geisinger Medical Center	Danville	97%	1064
Geisinger Wyoming Valley Medical Center	Wilkes-Barre	97%	596
Hahnemann University Hospital	Philadelphia	97%	419
Hamot Medical Center	Erie	97%	424
Heart of Lancaster Regional Medical Center	Lititz	97%	76
Indiana Regional Medical Center	Indiana	97%	213
Lancaster General Hospital	Lancaster	97%	1535
Lewistown Hospital	Lewistown	97%	117
Main Line Hospital Lankenau	Wynnewood	97%	341
Nazareth Hospital	Philadelphia	97%	73
Riddle Memorial Hospital	Media	97%	234
UPMC Presbyterian Shadyside	Pittsburgh	97%	973
Western Pennsylvania Hospital	Pittsburgh	97%	347
Abington Memorial Hospital	Abington	96%	411
Hanover Hospital	Hanover	96%	183
Lehigh Valley Hospital	Allentown	96%	1169
Lehigh Valley Hospital - Muhlenberg	Bethlehem	96%	270
Mercy Suburban Hospital	Norristown	96%	57
Mount Nittany Medical Center	State College	96%	215
Penn Hosp of the Univ of Penn Health Sys	Philadelphia	96%	571
Robert Packer Hospital	Sayre	96%	605
Saint Joseph Medical Center	Reading	96%	187
York Hospital	York	96%	831
Excela Health Westmoreland Reg Hosp	Greensburg	95%	240
Good Samaritan Hospital	Lebanon	95%	320
Holy Spirit Hospital	Camp Hill	95%	564
Pocono Medical Center	E Stroudsburg	95%	186
Punxsutawney Area Hospital	Punxsutawney	95%	98
Reading Hospital Medical Center	Reading	95%	724
Sunbury Community Hospital	Sunbury	95%	38
Surgical Institute of Reading	Wyomissing	95%	202
UPMC Mercy	Pittsburgh	95%	419
ACMH Hospital	Kittanning	94%	81
Alle Kiski Medical Center	Natrona	94%	217
Butler Memorial Hospital	Butler	94%	217
Chester County Hospital	West Chester	94%	237
Lock Haven Hospital	Lock Haven	94%	35
Magee Womens Hosp of UPMC Health Sys	Pittsburgh	94%	309
Milton S Hershey Medical Center	Hershey	94%	702
Conemaugh Valley Memorial Hospital	Johnstown	93%	586
Mercy Fitzgerald Hospital	Darby	93%	155
Mercy Hospital Scranton	Scranton	93%	250
Montgomery Hospital	Norristown	93%	58
Moses Taylor Hospital	Scranton	93%	56
Phoenixville Hospital	Phoenixville	93%	115
Saint Clair Memorial Hospital	Pittsburgh	93%	287
Saint Mary Medical Center	Langhorne	93%	264
Saint Vincent Health Center	Erie	93%	338
The Washington Hospital	Washington	93%	244
Albert Einstein Medical Center	Philadelphia	92%	240
Berwick Hospital Center	Berwick	92%	36
Charles Cole Memorial Hospital	Coudersport	92%	26
Easton Hospital	Easton	92%	83
Heritage Valley Beaver	Beaver	92%	186
Main Line Hospital Paoli	Paoli	92%	193
Saint Luke's Hospital Bethlehem	Bethlehem	92%	639
Carlisle Regional Medical Center	Carlisle	91%	120
Elk Regional Health Center	Saint Marys	91%	135
Excela Health Frick Hospital	Mount Pleasant	91%	43
Palmerton Hospital	Palmerton	91%	64
Penn Presbyterian Medical Center	Philadelphia	91%	313
Southwest Regional Medical Center	Waynesburg	91%	33
Temple University Hospital	Philadelphia	91%	394
UPMC Horizon	Greenville	91%	195
UPMC Passavant	Pittsburgh	91%	519
Wilkes-Barre General Hospital	Wilkes-Barre	91%	402
Excela Health Latrobe Hospital	Latrobe	90%	188
Lower Bucks Hospital	Bristol	90%	80
Memorial Hospital - Towanda	Towanda	90%	30
Pottstown Memorial Medical Center	Pottstown	90%	143
UPMC Mckeesport	McKeesport	90%	93
Grove City Medical Center	Grove City	89%	84
Heritage Valley Sewickley	Sewickley	89%	114
Monongahela Valley Hospital	Monongahela	89%	90
Bradford Regional Medical Center	Bradford	88%	40
Ellwood City Hospital	Ellwood City	88%	32
Main Line Hospital Bryn Mawr Campus	Bryn Mawr	88%	224
Sacred Heart Hospital	Allentown	88%	80
Saint Luke's Quakertown Hospital	Quakertown	88%	25
Uniontown Hospital	Uniontown	88%	128
Wayne Memorial Hospital	Honesdale	88%	49
Gnaden Huetten Memorial Hospital	Lehighton	87%	70
Pinnacle Health Hospitals	Harrisburg	87%	1086
Holy Redeemer Hospital and Medical Center	Meadowbrook	86%	44
Jameson Memorial Hospital	New Castle	86%	70
Millcreek Community Hospital	Erie	86%	29
Hazleton General Hospital	Hazleton	85%	75
Meadville Medical Center	Meadville	85%	219
Western Penn Hosp-Forbes Reg Campus	Monroeville	85%	242
Schuylkill Med Ctr-S Jackson Street	Pottsville	84%	90
Nason Hospital	Roaring Spring	82%	55
Ohio Valley General Hospital	Mckees Rocks	82%	38
Somerset Hospital	Somerset	82%	76
UPMC Bedford	Everett	82%	33
Memorial Hospital York	York	81%	94
Jefferson Regional Medical Center	Pittsburgh	80%	258
Hospital of Univ of Pennsylvania	Philadelphia	77%	538
Chambersburg Hospital	Chambersburg	74%	69
Clarion Hospital	Clarion	71%	28
Warren General Hospital	Warren	63%	27
Titusville Hospital	Titusville	61%	31
Allegheny General Hospital	Pittsburgh	60%	537
Doylestown Hospital	Doylestown	51%	190

30. Prophylactic Antibiotic Stopped

Hospital Name	City	Rate	Cases
Bucks County Specialty Hospital[2,3]	Bensalem	100%	99
Edgewood Surgical Hospital	Transfer	100%	119
Jennersville Regional Hospital[2]	West Grove	100%	90
Main Line Hospital Bryn Mawr Campus[2]	Bryn Mawr	100%	1262
Montgomery Hospital[2]	Norristown	100%	192
Surgical Institute of Reading	Wyomissing	100%	393
Surgical Specialty Ctr-Coordinated Health[2,3]	Allentown	100%	65
UPMC Mckeesport	McKeesport	100%	191
UPMC Northwest	Seneca	100%	240
Albert Einstein Medical Center[2]	Philadelphia	99%	481
Chestnut Hill Hospital[2]	Philadelphia	99%	189
Heart of Lancaster Regional Medical Center	Lititz	99%	88
Main Line Hospital Lankenau[2]	Wynnewood	99%	1116
Main Line Hospital Paoli[2]	Paoli	99%	660
Mount Nittany Medical Center	State College	99%	1201
Nazareth Hospital	Philadelphia	99%	465
Soldiers and Sailors Memorial Hospital	Wellsboro	99%	126
Temple University Hospital[2]	Philadelphia	99%	618
UPMC Presbyterian Shadyside	Pittsburgh	99%	2516
Dubois Regional Medical Center	Dubois	98%	409
Excela Health Latrobe Hospital	Latrobe	98%	377
Geisinger Medical Center[2]	Danville	98%	445
Grand View Hospital[2]	Sellersville	98%	296
Lebanon VA Medical Center	Lebanon	98%	186
Lehigh Valley Hospital	Allentown	98%	2407
Marian Community Hospital	Carbondale	98%	91
Nason Hospital	Roaring Spring	98%	89
Punxsutawney Area Hospital	Punxsutawney	98%	99
Thomas Jefferson University Hospital[2]	Philadelphia	98%	2489
UPMC Passavant	Pittsburgh	98%	1190
Waynesboro Hospital	Waynesboro	98%	129
Western Penn Hosp-Forbes Reg Campus	Monroeville	98%	682
ACMH Hospital	Kittanning	97%	369
Bloomsburg Hospital	Bloomsburg	97%	208
Canonsburg General Hospital	Canonsburg	97%	336
Carlisle Regional Medical Center[2]	Carlisle	97%	375
Community Medical Center	Scranton	97%	768
Conemaugh Valley Memorial Hospital	Johnstown	97%	1124
Crozer Chester Medical Center[2]	Upland	97%	814
Delaware County Memorial Hospital[2]	Drexel Hill	97%	354
Heritage Valley Sewickley	Sewickley	97%	836
Holy Redeemer Hospital and Medical Center	Meadowbrook	97%	577
Jameson Memorial Hospital	New Castle	97%	355
Lewistown Hospital	Lewistown	97%	166
Pocono Medical Center	E Stroudsburg	97%	355
Riddle Memorial Hospital[2]	Media	97%	980
Robert Packer Hospital	Sayre	97%	844
Saint Clair Memorial Hospital[2]	Pittsburgh	97%	1046
Saint Joseph Medical Center[2]	Reading	97%	445
Saint Luke's Hospital Bethlehem[2]	Bethlehem	97%	1203
UPMC Horizon	Greenville	97%	506
Western Pennsylvania Hospital[2]	Pittsburgh	97%	844
Aria Health[2]	Philadelphia	96%	308
Chester County Hospital	West Chester	96%	680
Easton Hospital[2]	Easton	96%	444
Excela Health Westmoreland Reg Hosp	Greensburg	96%	1039
Geisinger Wyoming Valley Medical Center[2]	Wilkes-Barre	96%	438
Gettysburg Hospital	Gettysburg	96%	291
Hamot Medical Center	Erie	96%	1076
Heritage Valley Beaver	Beaver	96%	879
Holy Spirit Hospital[2]	Camp Hill	96%	811
Lancaster General Hospital[2]	Lancaster	96%	1401
Lehigh Valley Hospital - Muhlenberg	Bethlehem	96%	475
Magee Womens Hosp of UPMC Health Sys	Pittsburgh	96%	1854
Meadville Medical Center	Meadville	96%	617
Mercy Hospital Scranton[2]	Scranton	96%	385
Mercy Suburban Hospital	Norristown	96%	179
Saint Luke's Quakertown Hospital	Quakertown	96%	57
Saint Mary Medical Center[2]	Langhorne	96%	483
Saint Vincent Health Center	Erie	96%	1297
Sharon Regional Health System[2]	Sharon	96%	467
UPMC Saint Margaret	Pittsburgh	96%	1056
The Washington Hospital[2]	Washington	96%	604
Wayne Memorial Hospital[2]	Honesdale	96%	158
Williamsport Hospital & Medical Center[2]	Williamsport	96%	902
Abington Memorial Hospital[2]	Abington	95%	478
Allegheny General Hospital[2]	Pittsburgh	95%	1265
Brandywine Hospital[2]	Coatesville	95%	152
Charles Cole Memorial Hospital	Coudersport	95%	186
Erie VA Medical Center	Erie	95%	39
Evangelical Community Hospital[2]	Lewisburg	95%	315
Grove City Medical Center	Grove City	95%	113
Hazleton General Hospital	Hazleton	95%	169
Lancaster Regional Medical Center[2]	Lancaster	95%	255
Pinnacle Health Hospitals[2]	Harrisburg	95%	2912
Saint Luke's Miners Memorial Hospital	Coaldale	95%	153
Uniontown Hospital	Uniontown	95%	620
Wilkes-Barre General Hospital[2]	Wilkes-Barre	95%	1079
York Hospital[2]	York	95%	1668
Alle Kiski Medical Center	Natrona	94%	327
Butler Memorial Hospital	Butler	94%	953
Chambersburg Hospital[2]	Chambersburg	94%	764

NOTE: Hospital profiles are in alphabetical order by state, then city, then hospital within the city; Rankings exclude hospitals with less than 25 cases except for patient surveys which excludes hospitals with less than 100 cases; (a) 100–299 cases; (1) The number of cases is too small to be sure how well a hospital is performing; (2) The hospital indicated that the data submitted for this measure were based on a sample of cases; (3) Data was collected during a shorter time period (fewer quarters) than the maximum possible time for this measure; (4) Suppressed for one or more quarters by CMS; (5) No data is available from the hospital for this measure; (6) Fewer than 100 patients completed the HCAHPS survey. Use these rates with caution, as the number of surveys may be too low to reliably assess hospital performance; (7) Survey results are based on less than 12 months of data; (8) Survey results are not available for this reporting period; (9) No or very few patients were eligible for the HCAHPS survey. The scores shown, if any, reflect a very small number of surveys; (10) A state average was not calculated because too few hospitals in the state submitted data; (11) There were discrepancies in the data collection process; Please refer to the User's Guide for a full explanation of data.

Indiana Regional Medical Center	Indiana	94%	271
Jeanes Hospital	Philadelphia	94%	441
Jefferson Regional Medical Center	Pittsburgh	94%	1150
Lansdale Hospital[2]	Lansdale	94%	111
Mercy Fitzgerald Hospital[2]	Darby	94%	248
Milton S Hershey Medical Center[2]	Hershey	94%	1205
Monongahela Valley Hospital	Monongahela	94%	398
Reading Hospital Medical Center[2]	Reading	94%	1462
UPMC Bedford	Everett	94%	109
UPMC Mercy[2]	Pittsburgh	94%	393
Altoona Regional Health System	Altoona	93%	1491
Brookville Hospital	Brookville	93%	30
Clarion Hospital	Clarion	93%	184
Coordinated Health Orthopedic Hospital[2]	Bethlehem	93%	180
Ephrata Community Hospital	Ephrata	93%	410
Moses Taylor Hospital	Scranton	93%	388
Doylestown Hospital[2]	Doylestown	92%	605
Hahnemann University Hospital[2]	Philadelphia	92%	455
Memorial Hospital York	York	92%	438
Phoenixville Hospital[2]	Phoenixville	92%	304
Southwest Regional Medical Center	Waynesburg	92%	61
Windber Hospital	Windber	92%	99
Clearfield Hospital	Clearfield	91%	195
Roxborough Memorial Hospital	Phila	91%	64
VA Pittsburgh Healthcare System	Pittsburgh	91%	358
Berwick Hospital Center[2]	Berwick	90%	126
Excela Health Frick Hospital	Mount Pleasant	90%	39
Warren General Hospital	Warren	90%	221
Gnaden Huetten Memorial Hospital	Lehighton	89%	90
Schuylkill Med Ctr-S Jackson Street	Pottsville	89%	290
Good Samaritan Hospital[2]	Lebanon	88%	364
Hanover Hospital	Hanover	88%	619
Bradford Regional Medical Center	Bradford	87%	85
Elk Regional Health Center	Saint Marys	87%	167
Ellwood City Hospital	Ellwood City	87%	31
Ohio Valley General Hospital	Mckees Rocks	87%	198
Palmerton Hospital	Palmerton	87%	54
Pottstown Memorial Medical Center[2]	Pottstown	87%	275
Lower Bucks Hospital[2]	Bristol	86%	186
Penn Presbyterian Medical Center	Philadelphia	86%	1440
Millcreek Community Hospital	Erie	85%	81
Shamokin Area Community Hospital	Coal Township	85%	89
Titusville Hospital	Titusville	85%	78
Highlands Hospital[2]	Connellsville	84%	31
Somerset Hospital	Somerset	84%	210
Mercy Tyler Hospital	Tunkhannock	83%	29
Sacred Heart Hospital	Allentown	82%	276
Wilkes-Barre VA Medical Center	Wilkes-Barre	82%	28
Sunbury Community Hospital[2]	Sunbury	80%	65
Penn Hosp of the Univ of Penn Health Sys[2]	Philadelphia	79%	464
Philadelphia VA Medical Center	Philadelphia	77%	26
Hospital of Univ of Pennsylvania[2]	Philadelphia	76%	557
Jersey Shore Hospital	Jersey Shore	71%	35
Schuylkill Med Ctr-East Norwegian Street	Pottsville	71%	140
J C Blair Memorial Hospital	Huntingdon	69%	29
Montrose General Hospital	Montrose	46%	97

31. Recommended VTP Ordered

Hospital Name	City	Rate	Cases
Alle Kiski Medical Center	Natrona	100%	220
Brookville Hospital	Brookville	100%	29
Coordinated Health Orthopedic Hospital[2]	Bethlehem	100%	26
Delaware County Memorial Hospital[2]	Drexel Hill	100%	349
Hospital of Univ of Pennsylvania[2]	Philadelphia	100%	384
Jennersville Regional Hospital[2]	West Grove	100%	64
Main Line Hospital Bryn Mawr Campus[2]	Bryn Mawr	100%	224
Mercy Fitzgerald Hospital[2]	Darby	100%	272
Nason Hospital	Roaring Spring	100%	76
Saint Joseph Medical Center[2]	Reading	100%	183
Saint Luke's Miners Memorial Hospital	Coaldale	100%	58
UPMC Bedford	Everett	100%	64
UPMC Mckeesport	McKeesport	100%	209
UPMC Saint Margaret	Pittsburgh	100%	849
Albert Einstein Medical Center[2]	Philadelphia	99%	308
Allegheny General Hospital[2]	Pittsburgh	99%	1416
Aria Health[2]	Philadelphia	99%	311
Butler Memorial Hospital	Butler	99%	271
Carlisle Regional Medical Center[2]	Carlisle	99%	187
Grand View Hospital[2]	Sellersville	99%	165
Lancaster Regional Medical Center[2]	Lancaster	99%	177
Lehigh Valley Hospital	Allentown	99%	1433
Main Line Hospital Lankenau[2]	Wynnewood	99%	300
Main Line Hospital Paoli[2]	Paoli	99%	235
Moses Taylor Hospital	Scranton	99%	254
Penn Presbyterian Medical Center	Philadelphia	99%	576
Pinnacle Health Hospitals[2]	Harrisburg	99%	746
Temple University Hospital[2]	Philadelphia	99%	394
Thomas Jefferson University Hospital[2]	Philadelphia	99%	816
UPMC Mercy[2]	Pittsburgh	99%	227
UPMC Passavant	Pittsburgh	99%	971
UPMC Presbyterian Shadyside	Pittsburgh	99%	3593
Abington Memorial Hospital[2]	Abington	98%	139
Canonsburg General Hospital	Canonsburg	98%	152
Chestnut Hill Hospital[2]	Philadelphia	98%	133
Crozer Chester Medical Center[2]	Upland	98%	343
Easton Hospital[2]	Easton	98%	225
Ephrata Community Hospital	Ephrata	98%	239
Excela Health Westmoreland Reg Hosp	Greensburg	98%	507
Gettysburg Hospital	Gettysburg	98%	161
Hamot Medical Center	Erie	98%	613
Heart of Lancaster Regional Medical Center	Lititz	98%	83
Holy Redeemer Hospital and Medical Center	Meadowbrook	98%	254
Magee Womens Hosp of UPMC Health Sys	Pittsburgh	98%	550
Mercy Suburban Hospital	Norristown	98%	123
Nazareth Hospital	Philadelphia	98%	236
Reading Hospital Medical Center[2]	Reading	98%	522
Robert Packer Hospital	Sayre	98%	502
Sharon Regional Health System[2]	Sharon	98%	247
Uniontown Hospital	Uniontown	98%	308
UPMC Horizon	Greenville	98%	384
UPMC Northwest	Seneca	98%	129
VA Pittsburgh Healthcare System[2]	Pittsburgh	98%	176
Western Pennsylvania Hospital[2]	Pittsburgh	98%	221
Western Penn Hosp-Forbes Reg Campus	Monroeville	98%	300
Williamsport Hospital & Medical Center[2]	Williamsport	98%	537
ACMH Hospital	Kittanning	97%	159
Cancer Treatment Centers of America	Philadelphia	97%	76
Chester County Hospital	West Chester	97%	371
Community Medical Center	Scranton	97%	383
Conemaugh Valley Memorial Hospital	Johnstown	97%	584
Doylestown Hospital[2]	Doylestown	97%	315
Excela Health Frick Hospital	Mount Pleasant	97%	64
Geisinger Medical Center[2]	Danville	97%	176
Hazleton General Hospital	Hazleton	97%	153
Jameson Memorial Hospital	New Castle	97%	301
Jeanes Hospital	Philadelphia	97%	239
Lehigh Valley Hospital - Muhlenberg	Bethlehem	97%	355
Marian Community Hospital	Carbondale	97%	33
Mercy Hospital Scranton[2]	Scranton	97%	147
Penn Hosp of the Univ of Penn Health Sys[2]	Philadelphia	97%	247
Philadelphia VA Medical Center[2]	Philadelphia	97%	67
Schuylkill Med Ctr-East Norwegian Street	Pottsville	97%	159
Schuylkill Med Ctr-S Jackson Street	Pottsville	97%	148
The Washington Hospital[2]	Washington	97%	218
Windber Hospital	Windber	97%	38
Chambersburg Hospital[2]	Chambersburg	96%	344
Dubois Regional Medical Center	Dubois	96%	112
Excela Health Latrobe Hospital	Latrobe	96%	276
Gnaden Huetten Memorial Hospital	Lehighton	96%	72
Jefferson Regional Medical Center	Pittsburgh	96%	703
Phoenixville Hospital[2]	Phoenixville	96%	224
Roxborough Memorial Hospital	Phila	96%	81
Saint Clair Memorial Hospital[2]	Pittsburgh	96%	569
Saint Luke's Quakertown Hospital	Quakertown	96%	45
Saint Vincent Health Center	Erie	96%	499
Wayne Memorial Hospital[2]	Honesdale	96%	109
York Hospital[2]	York	96%	617
Clearfield Hospital	Clearfield	95%	156
Lancaster General Hospital[2]	Lancaster	95%	681
Meadville Medical Center	Meadville	95%	186
Milton S Hershey Medical Center[2]	Hershey	95%	428
Monongahela Valley Hospital	Monongahela	95%	333
Mount Nittany Medical Center	State College	95%	373
Saint Luke's Hospital Bethlehem[2]	Bethlehem	95%	432
Geisinger Wyoming Valley Medical Center[2]	Wilkes-Barre	94%	167
Good Samaritan Hospital[2]	Lebanon	94%	171
Indiana Regional Medical Center	Indiana	94%	161
J C Blair Memorial Hospital	Huntingdon	94%	34
Lansdale Hospital[2]	Lansdale	94%	141
Ohio Valley General Hospital	Mckees Rocks	94%	164
Saint Mary Medical Center[2]	Langhorne	94%	158
Somerset Hospital	Somerset	94%	97
Wilkes-Barre VA Medical Center[2]	Wilkes-Barre	94%	34
Altoona Regional Health System	Altoona	93%	494
Bradford Regional Medical Center	Bradford	93%	57
Ellwood City Hospital	Ellwood City	93%	56
Millcreek Community Hospital	Erie	93%	44
Pottstown Memorial Medical Center[2]	Pottstown	93%	245
Riddle Memorial Hospital[2]	Media	93%	272
Charles Cole Memorial Hospital	Coudersport	92%	59
Heritage Valley Sewickley	Sewickley	92%	260
Holy Spirit Hospital[2]	Camp Hill	92%	279
Memorial Hospital York	York	92%	133
Punxsutawney Area Hospital	Punxsutawney	92%	59
Southwest Regional Medical Center	Waynesburg	92%	48
Lebanon VA Medical Center[2]	Lebanon	91%	58
Pocono Medical Center	E Stroudsburg	91%	234
Sacred Heart Hospital	Allentown	91%	162
Wilkes-Barre General Hospital[2]	Wilkes-Barre	91%	617
Shamokin Area Community Hospital	Coal Township	90%	41
Soldiers and Sailors Memorial Hospital	Wellsboro	90%	77
Hahnemann University Hospital[2]	Philadelphia	89%	295
Heritage Valley Beaver	Beaver	89%	359
Highlands Hospital[2]	Connellsville	89%	45
Waynesboro Hospital	Waynesboro	89%	81
Brandywine Hospital[2]	Coatesville	88%	107
Hanover Hospital	Hanover	88%	164
Palmerton Hospital	Palmerton	88%	58
Berwick Hospital Center[2]	Berwick	86%	43
Clarion Hospital	Clarion	86%	43
Evangelical Community Hospital[2]	Lewisburg	86%	131
Saint Joseph's Hospital	Philadelphia	85%	41
Surgical Institute of Reading	Wyomissing	84%	49
Lewistown Hospital	Lewistown	82%	102
Lower Bucks Hospital[2]	Bristol	82%	102
Bloomsburg Hospital	Bloomsburg	80%	60
Grove City Medical Center	Grove City	80%	35
Sunbury Community Hospital[2]	Sunbury	80%	44
Elk Regional Health Center	Saint Marys	79%	78
Mercy Tyler Hospital	Tunkhannock	79%	28
Montgomery Hospital[2]	Norristown	78%	60
Warren General Hospital	Warren	64%	58
Titusville Hospital	Titusville	62%	37
Jersey Shore Hospital	Jersey Shore	47%	53

32. Urinary Catheter Removal

Hospital Name	City	Rate	Cases
Coordinated Health Orthopedic Hospital[2]	Bethlehem	100%	72
Grand View Hospital[2]	Sellersville	100%	27
Hazleton General Hospital	Hazleton	100%	54
Holy Redeemer Hospital and Medical Center	Meadowbrook	100%	191
Magee Womens Hosp of UPMC Health Sys	Pittsburgh	100%	525
Main Line Hospital Bryn Mawr Campus[2]	Bryn Mawr	100%	134
Main Line Hospital Paoli[2]	Paoli	100%	241
Memorial Hospital York	York	100%	39
Saint Luke's Quakertown Hospital	Quakertown	100%	28
Surgical Specialty Ctr-Coordinated Health[2]	Allentown	100%	66
UPMC Northwest	Seneca	100%	40
Wilkes-Barre General Hospital	Wilkes-Barre	100%	404
Charles Cole Memorial Hospital	Coudersport	99%	81
Main Line Hospital Lankenau[2]	Wynnewood	99%	343
Penn Presbyterian Medical Center	Philadelphia	99%	734
Riddle Memorial Hospital[2]	Media	99%	460
Surgical Institute of Reading	Wyomissing	99%	189
Bloomsburg Hospital	Bloomsburg	98%	54
Carlisle Regional Medical Center	Carlisle	98%	59
Ephrata Community Hospital	Ephrata	98%	195
Geisinger Medical Center[2]	Danville	98%	131
Holy Spirit Hospital[2]	Camp Hill	98%	170
Lansdale Hospital[2]	Lansdale	98%	43
Mercy Hospital Scranton[2]	Scranton	98%	58
Pinnacle Health Hospitals[2]	Harrisburg	98%	624
Saint Luke's Hospital Bethlehem[2]	Bethlehem	98%	457
Saint Mary Medical Center[2]	Langhorne	98%	182
Shamokin Area Community Hospital	Coal Township	98%	50
Somerset Hospital	Somerset	98%	43
UPMC Horizon	Greenville	98%	43
Western Pennsylvania Hospital[2]	Pittsburgh	98%	207
Allegheny General Hospital[2]	Pittsburgh	97%	651
Aria Health[2]	Philadelphia	97%	147
Evangelical Community Hospital[2]	Lewisburg	97%	144
Hahnemann University Hospital[2]	Philadelphia	97%	143
Jefferson Regional Medical Center	Pittsburgh	97%	583
Lancaster Regional Medical Center[2]	Lancaster	97%	146
Lebanon VA Medical Center[2]	Lebanon	97%	87
Roxborough Memorial Hospital	Phila	97%	39
Thomas Jefferson University Hospital[2]	Philadelphia	97%	978
UPMC Mckeesport	McKeesport	97%	39
Western Penn Hosp-Forbes Reg Campus	Monroeville	97%	285
Williamsport Hospital & Medical Center[2]	Williamsport	97%	311
Abington Memorial Hospital[2]	Abington	96%	166
Doylestown Hospital[2]	Doylestown	96%	277
Dubois Regional Medical Center	Dubois	96%	133
Easton Hospital	Easton	96%	136
Geisinger Wyoming Valley Medical Center[2]	Wilkes-Barre	96%	188
Hamot Medical Center	Erie	96%	538
Reading Hospital Medical Center[2]	Reading	96%	433
Saint Joseph Medical Center[2]	Reading	96%	156
Uniontown Hospital	Uniontown	96%	109
UPMC Saint Margaret	Pittsburgh	96%	549
The Washington Hospital[2]	Washington	96%	121
Albert Einstein Medical Center[2]	Philadelphia	95%	222
Hanover Hospital	Hanover	95%	262
Lancaster General Hospital[2]	Lancaster	95%	591
Lehigh Valley Hospital	Allentown	95%	975
Sharon Regional Health System[2]	Sharon	95%	112
UPMC Presbyterian Shadyside	Pittsburgh	95%	1697
Alle Kiski Medical Center	Natrona	94%	141
Brandywine Hospital	Coatesville	94%	71
Butler Memorial Hospital	Butler	94%	227
Crozer Chester Medical Center[2]	Upland	94%	302

NOTE: Hospital profiles are in alphabetical order by state, then city, then hospital within the city; Rankings exclude hospitals with less than 25 cases except for patient surveys which excludes hospitals with less than 100 cases; (a) 100–299 cases; (1) The number of cases is too small to be sure how well a hospital is performing; (2) The hospital indicated that the data submitted for this measure were based on a sample of cases; (3) Data was collected during a shorter time period (fewer quarters) than the maximum possible time for this measure; (4) Suppressed for one or more quarters by CMS; (5) No data is available from the hospital for this measure; (6) Fewer than 100 patients completed the HCAHPS survey. Use these rates with caution, as the number of surveys may be too low to reliably assess hospital performance; (7) Survey results are based on less than 12 months of data; (8) Survey results are not available for this reporting period; (9) No or very few patients were eligible for the HCAHPS survey. The scores shown, if any, reflect a very small number of surveys; (10) A state average was not calculated because too few hospitals in the state submitted data; (11) There were discrepancies in the data collection process; Please refer to the User's Guide for a full explanation of data.

Gettysburg Hospital	Gettysburg	94%	32
Mercy Suburban Hospital	Norristown	94%	32
Mount Nittany Medical Center	State College	94%	228
Pottstown Memorial Medical Center	Pottstown	94%	129
Sunbury Community Hospital	Sunbury	94%	35
Conemaugh Valley Memorial Hospital	Johnstown	93%	292
Heritage Valley Beaver	Beaver	93%	279
Heritage Valley Sewickley	Sewickley	93%	374
Mercy Fitzgerald Hospital[2]	Darby	93%	84
Nazareth Hospital	Philadelphia	93%	213
Bucks County Specialty Hospital[2]	Bensalem	92%	39
Chestnut Hill Hospital	Philadelphia	92%	49
Delaware County Memorial Hospital[2]	Drexel Hill	92%	165
Good Samaritan Hospital[2]	Lebanon	92%	124
Indiana Regional Medical Center	Indiana	92%	109
Milton S Hershey Medical Center[2]	Hershey	92%	349
Penn Hosp of the Univ of Penn Health Sys[2]	Philadelphia	92%	199
Saint Clair Memorial Hospital[2]	Pittsburgh	92%	167
York Hospital[2]	York	92%	424
Chester County Hospital	West Chester	91%	220
Community Medical Center	Scranton	91%	203
Pocono Medical Center	E Stroudsburg	91%	156
Punxsutawney Area Hospital	Punxsutawney	91%	32
UPMC Mercy[2]	Pittsburgh	91%	118
ACMH Hospital	Kittanning	90%	78
Clarion Hospital	Clarion	90%	52
Elk Regional Health Center	Saint Marys	90%	50
Excela Health Westmoreland Reg Hosp	Greensburg	90%	353
Gnaden Huetten Memorial Hospital	Lehighton	90%	41
Phoenixville Hospital	Phoenixville	90%	126
Schuylkill Med Ctr-S Jackson Street	Pottsville	90%	29
UPMC Passavant	Pittsburgh	90%	397
Lehigh Valley Hospital - Muhlenberg	Bethlehem	89%	135
Saint Vincent Health Center	Erie	89%	476
Soldiers and Sailors Memorial Hospital	Wellsboro	89%	36
Excela Health Latrobe Hospital	Latrobe	88%	68
Palmerton Hospital	Palmerton	88%	25
Altoona Regional Health System	Altoona	87%	173
Hospital of Univ of Pennsylvania[2]	Philadelphia	87%	175
Meadville Medical Center	Meadville	87%	31
Lower Bucks Hospital[2]	Bristol	86%	42
VA Pittsburgh Healthcare System[2]	Pittsburgh	86%	220
Monongahela Valley Hospital	Monongahela	84%	64
Sacred Heart Hospital	Allentown	84%	45
Saint Luke's Miners Memorial Hospital	Coaldale	84%	74
Robert Packer Hospital	Sayre	83%	185
Chambersburg Hospital[2]	Chambersburg	82%	56
Jameson Memorial Hospital	New Castle	82%	65
Moses Taylor Hospital	Scranton	81%	125
Temple University Hospital[2]	Philadelphia	81%	159
Wayne Memorial Hospital[2]	Honesdale	79%	63
Schuylkill Med Ctr-East Norwegian Street	Pottsville	78%	41
Warren General Hospital	Warren	78%	55
Canonsburg General Hospital	Canonsburg	72%	29
Clearfield Hospital	Clearfield	61%	28
Philadelphia VA Medical Center[2]	Philadelphia	61%	33

Children's Asthma Care

33. Received Systemic Corticosteroids

Hospital Name	City	Rate	Cases
Children's Hospital of Philadelphia[2]	Philadelphia	100%	547
Children's Hospital of Pittsburgh of UPMC	Pittsburgh	100%	476
Saint Luke's Hospital Bethlehem	Bethlehem	100%	74

34. Received Home Management Plan of Care

Hospital Name	City	Rate	Cases
Saint Luke's Hospital Bethlehem	Bethlehem	64%	72
Children's Hospital of Pittsburgh of UPMC	Pittsburgh	57%	476
Children's Hospital of Philadelphia[2]	Philadelphia	47%	546

35. Received Reliever Medication

Hospital Name	City	Rate	Cases
Children's Hospital of Philadelphia[2]	Philadelphia	100%	548
Children's Hospital of Pittsburgh of UPMC	Pittsburgh	100%	478
Saint Luke's Hospital Bethlehem	Bethlehem	100%	74

Use of Medical Imaging

36. Combination Abdominal CT Scan

Hospital Name	City	Ratio	Cases
Excela Health Frick Hospital	Mount Pleasant	0.007	271
Windber Hospital	Windber	0.014	278
Hazleton General Hospital	Hazleton	0.017	579
Lehigh Valley Hospital	Allentown	0.017	779
UPMC Bedford	Everett	0.017	343
Conemaugh Valley Memorial Hospital	Johnstown	0.019	723
Excela Health Westmoreland Reg Hosp	Greensburg	0.021	653
J C Blair Memorial Hospital	Huntingdon	0.022	409
Troy Community Hospital	Troy	0.022	228
Miners Medical Center	Hastings	0.024	254
Charles Cole Memorial Hospital	Coudersport	0.025	237
Penn Presbyterian Medical Center	Philadelphia	0.025	324
Palmerton Hospital	Palmerton	0.026	347
Millcreek Community Hospital	Erie	0.030	100
Schuylkill Med Ctr-S Jackson Street	Pottsville	0.030	778
Aria Health	Philadelphia	0.034	1382
Abington Memorial Hospital	Abington	0.039	2284
Excela Health Latrobe Hospital	Latrobe	0.041	555
Holy Redeemer Hospital and Medical Center	Meadowbrook	0.045	622
Meadville Medical Center	Meadville	0.048	702
Nason Hospital	Roaring Spring	0.049	185
Hamot Medical Center	Erie	0.052	690
Grand View Hospital	Sellersville	0.059	901
Mercy Suburban Hospital	Norristown	0.059	410
Saint Mary Medical Center	Langhorne	0.059	1193
Westfield Hospital[1]	Allentown	0.061	49
Jameson Memorial Hospital	New Castle	0.063	458
Memorial Hospital - Towanda	Towanda	0.063	239
Schuylkill Med Ctr-East Norwegian Street	Pottsville	0.063	587
Evangelical Community Hospital	Lewisburg	0.064	1019
Reading Hospital Medical Center	Reading	0.067	2807
Gnaden Huetten Memorial Hospital	Lehighton	0.068	443
Jeanes Hospital	Philadelphia	0.068	559
Pocono Medical Center	E Stroudsburg	0.069	1120
Nazareth Hospital	Philadelphia	0.070	441
Moses Taylor Hospital	Scranton	0.071	538
Penn Hosp of the Univ of Penn Health Sys	Philadelphia	0.071	794
Mercy Fitzgerald Hospital	Darby	0.073	578
UPMC Northwest	Seneca	0.076	1032
Hahnemann University Hospital	Philadelphia	0.079	302
Jersey Shore Hospital	Jersey Shore	0.080	374
Saint Clair Memorial Hospital	Pittsburgh	0.080	981
Ellwood City Hospital	Ellwood City	0.081	124
Lehigh Valley Hospital - Muhlenberg	Bethlehem	0.082	1040
Ohio Valley General Hospital	Mckees Rocks	0.083	157
Western Penn Hosp-Forbes Reg Campus	Monroeville	0.083	483
Williamsport Hospital & Medical Center	Williamsport	0.083	1095
Lansdale Hospital	Lansdale	0.084	407
Lancaster Regional Medical Center	Lancaster	0.090	266
Bradford Regional Medical Center	Bradford	0.092	469
Hanover Hospital	Hanover	0.093	890
UPMC Mercy	Pittsburgh	0.093	301
Albert Einstein Medical Center	Philadelphia	0.094	838
Chester County Hospital	West Chester	0.094	981
Chestnut Hill Hospital	Philadelphia	0.094	459
Geisinger Medical Center	Danville	0.097	1575
Sunbury Community Hospital	Sunbury	0.099	192
UPMC Mckeesport	McKeesport	0.108	372
Community Medical Center	Scranton	0.109	588
Roxborough Memorial Hospital	Phila	0.110	146
Saint Vincent Health Center	Erie	0.111	946
Montgomery Hospital	Norristown	0.112	465
Heritage Valley Sewickley	Sewickley	0.113	337
Main Line Hospital Paoli	Paoli	0.113	1237
York Hospital	York	0.118	2450
Wayne Memorial Hospital	Honesdale	0.127	647
UPMC Horizon	Greenville	0.128	889
Mount Nittany Medical Center	State College	0.129	581
Saint Luke's Quakertown Hospital	Quakertown	0.130	354
Butler Memorial Hospital	Butler	0.131	677
Jefferson Regional Medical Center	Pittsburgh	0.134	625
Waynesboro Hospital	Waynesboro	0.135	446
Heritage Valley Beaver	Beaver	0.136	698
Robert Packer Hospital	Sayre	0.136	1657
Easton Hospital	Easton	0.137	818
Hospital of Univ of Pennsylvania	Philadelphia	0.141	1579
Main Line Hospital Lankenau	Wynnewood	0.142	1174
ACMH Hospital	Kittanning	0.147	184
Heart of Lancaster Regional Medical Center	Lititz	0.151	152
The Washington Hospital	Washington	0.153	393
Magee Womens Hosp of UPMC Health Sys	Pittsburgh	0.156	545
Western Pennsylvania Hospital	Pittsburgh	0.156	391
Jennersville Regional Hospital	West Grove	0.157	261
Mercy Hospital Scranton	Scranton	0.163	771
Titusville Hospital	Titusville	0.163	282
Temple University Hospital	Philadelphia	0.164	633
Brandywine Hospital	Coatesville	0.166	355
Carlisle Regional Medical Center	Carlisle	0.178	759
Doylestown Hospital	Doylestown	0.180	899
Sacred Heart Hospital	Allentown	0.182	472
Chambersburg Hospital	Chambersburg	0.190	1277
Pottstown Memorial Medical Center	Pottstown	0.190	823
Thomas Jefferson University Hospital	Philadelphia	0.195	1346
Crozer Chester Medical Center	Upland	0.196	1278
Milton S Hershey Medical Center	Hershey	0.206	1858
Grove City Medical Center	Grove City	0.211	237
Saint Luke's Miners Memorial Hospital	Coaldale	0.218	349
UPMC Saint Margaret	Pittsburgh	0.221	810
Main Line Hospital Bryn Mawr Campus	Bryn Mawr	0.228	1068
Saint Luke's Hospital Bethlehem	Bethlehem	0.254	2147
UPMC Presbyterian Shadyside	Pittsburgh	0.256	3464
Lower Bucks Hospital	Bristol	0.262	275
Pinnacle Health Hospitals	Harrisburg	0.272	993
Dubois Regional Medical Center	Dubois	0.278	1231
Lewistown Hospital	Lewistown	0.278	701
Wilkes-Barre General Hospital	Wilkes-Barre	0.311	1842
Altoona Regional Health System	Altoona	0.321	1317
Berwick Hospital Center	Berwick	0.335	185
Phoenixville Hospital	Phoenixville	0.338	470
Bloomsburg Hospital	Bloomsburg	0.340	206
Holy Spirit Hospital	Camp Hill	0.361	850
Mercy Tyler Hospital	Tunkhannock	0.364	187
Uniontown Hospital	Uniontown	0.381	833
Marian Community Hospital	Carbondale	0.394	297
Alle Kiski Medical Center	Natrona	0.397	536
Lancaster General Hospital	Lancaster	0.412	2670
Warren General Hospital	Warren	0.415	470
Lock Haven Hospital	Lock Haven	0.430	223
Delaware County Memorial Hospital	Drexel Hill	0.435	706
Sharon Regional Health System	Sharon	0.439	827
Allegheny General Hospital	Pittsburgh	0.472	1052
Good Samaritan Hospital	Lebanon	0.482	1288
Punxsutawney Area Hospital	Punxsutawney	0.484	283
Clarion Hospital	Clarion	0.491	379
Ephrata Community Hospital	Ephrata	0.496	811
Indiana Regional Medical Center	Indiana	0.512	385
Canonsburg General Hospital	Canonsburg	0.544	206
Somerset Hospital	Somerset	0.562	315
Soldiers and Sailors Memorial Hospital	Wellsboro	0.571	464
Kane Community Hospital	Kane	0.575	247
Southwest Regional Medical Center	Waynesburg	0.576	158
St Catherine Med Ctr Fountain Springs	Ashland	0.581	93
UPMC Passavant	Pittsburgh	0.593	958
Elk Regional Health Center	Saint Marys	0.611	707
Monongahela Valley Hospital	Monongahela	0.612	397
Riddle Memorial Hospital	Media	0.612	701
Geisinger Wyoming Valley Medical Center	Wilkes-Barre	0.624	901
Shamokin Area Community Hospital	Coal Township	0.626	321
Clearfield Hospital	Clearfield	0.663	854
Gettysburg Hospital	Gettysburg	0.664	658
Highlands Hospital	Connellsville	0.673	113
Saint Joseph Medical Center	Reading	0.700	543
Cancer Treatment Centers of America	Philadelphia	0.785	181

37. Combination Chest CT Scan

Hospital Name	City	Ratio	Cases
Evangelical Community Hospital	Lewisburg	0.000	434
Excela Health Westmoreland Reg Hosp	Greensburg	0.000	503
Hazleton General Hospital	Hazleton	0.000	410
Heritage Valley Sewickley	Sewickley	0.000	236
Holy Redeemer Hospital and Medical Center	Meadowbrook	0.000	563
Jennersville Regional Hospital	West Grove	0.000	223
Mercy Suburban Hospital	Norristown	0.000	217
Millcreek Community Hospital[1]	Erie	0.000	31
Monongahela Valley Hospital	Monongahela	0.000	185
Moses Taylor Hospital	Scranton	0.000	325
Ohio Valley General Hospital	Mckees Rocks	0.000	146
Punxsutawney Area Hospital	Punxsutawney	0.000	142
Saint Clair Memorial Hospital	Pittsburgh	0.000	672
Schuylkill Med Ctr-S Jackson Street	Pottsville	0.000	357
Titusville Hospital	Titusville	0.000	244
The Washington Hospital	Washington	0.000	380
Windber Hospital	Windber	0.000	231
Hospital of Univ of Pennsylvania	Philadelphia	0.001	2172
UPMC Saint Margaret	Pittsburgh	0.001	691
Conemaugh Valley Memorial Hospital	Johnstown	0.002	489
Doylestown Hospital	Doylestown	0.002	928
Heritage Valley Beaver	Beaver	0.002	487
Lewistown Hospital	Lewistown	0.002	536
Uniontown Hospital	Uniontown	0.002	471
UPMC Horizon	Greenville	0.002	553
Aria Health	Philadelphia	0.003	1164
Jameson Memorial Hospital	New Castle	0.003	359
Western Pennsylvania Hospital	Pittsburgh	0.003	363
Delaware County Memorial Hospital	Drexel Hill	0.004	539
Dubois Regional Medical Center	Dubois	0.004	728
Magee Womens Hosp of UPMC Health Sys	Pittsburgh	0.004	505
Palmerton Hospital	Palmerton	0.004	268
Saint Luke's Hospital Bethlehem	Bethlehem	0.004	1810
Warren General Hospital	Warren	0.004	282
Alle Kiski Medical Center	Natrona	0.005	412
Excela Health Frick Hospital	Mount Pleasant	0.005	188
J C Blair Memorial Hospital	Huntingdon	0.005	204
Nazareth Hospital	Philadelphia	0.005	380
Robert Packer Hospital	Sayre	0.005	1324
Saint Vincent Health Center	Erie	0.005	424
Grove City Medical Center	Grove City	0.006	161
Milton S Hershey Medical Center	Hershey	0.006	1991

NOTE: Hospital profiles are in alphabetical order by state, then city, then hospital within the city; Rankings exclude hospitals with less than 25 cases except for patient surveys which excludes hospitals with less than 100 cases; (a) 100–299 cases; (1) The number of cases is too small to be sure how well a hospital is performing; (2) The hospital indicated that the data submitted for this measure were based on a sample of cases; (3) Data was collected during a shorter time period (fewer quarters) than the maximum possible time for this measure; (4) Suppressed for one or more quarters by CMS; (5) No data is available from the hospital for this measure; (6) Fewer than 100 patients completed the HCAHPS survey. Use these rates with caution, as the number of surveys may be too low to reliably assess hospital performance; (7) Survey results are based on less than 12 months of data; (8) Survey results are not available for this reporting period; (9) No or very few patients were eligible for the HCAHPS survey. The scores shown, if any, reflect a very small number of surveys; (10) A state average was not calculated because too few hospitals in the state submitted data; (11) There were discrepancies in the data collection process; Please refer to the User's Guide for a full explanation of data.

Montgomery Hospital	Norristown	0.006	348
Schuylkill Med Ctr-East Norwegian Street	Pottsville	0.006	341
York Hospital	York	0.006	2749
Charles Cole Memorial Hospital	Coudersport	0.007	142
Grand View Hospital	Sellersville	0.007	842
Crozer Chester Medical Center	Upland	0.008	1085
Hahnemann University Hospital	Philadelphia	0.008	237
Hamot Medical Center	Erie	0.008	242
Indiana Regional Medical Center	Indiana	0.008	257
Meadville Medical Center	Meadville	0.008	514
Miners Medical Center	Hastings	0.008	130
Sharon Regional Health System	Sharon	0.008	712
Soldiers and Sailors Memorial Hospital	Wellsboro	0.008	242
Troy Community Hospital	Troy	0.008	129
UPMC Mercy	Pittsburgh	0.008	251
Wilkes-Barre General Hospital	Wilkes-Barre	0.008	1323
Cancer Treatment Centers of America	Philadelphia	0.009	220
Holy Spirit Hospital	Camp Hill	0.009	530
Ellwood City Hospital	Ellwood City	0.010	105
Brandywine Hospital	Coatesville	0.011	270
Excela Health Latrobe Hospital	Latrobe	0.011	448
Geisinger Medical Center	Danville	0.011	1407
Jersey Shore Hospital	Jersey Shore	0.011	180
Lower Bucks Hospital	Bristol	0.011	266
Memorial Hospital - Towanda	Towanda	0.011	93
Thomas Jefferson University Hospital	Philadelphia	0.011	1046
Abington Memorial Hospital	Abington	0.012	1943
Butler Memorial Hospital	Butler	0.012	500
Chester County Hospital	West Chester	0.012	864
UPMC Passavant	Pittsburgh	0.012	847
Canonsburg General Hospital	Canonsburg	0.013	149
Penn Hosp of the Univ of Penn Health Sys	Philadelphia	0.013	716
Saint Joseph Medical Center	Reading	0.014	499
UPMC Presbyterian Shadyside	Pittsburgh	0.014	3991
Jeanes Hospital	Philadelphia	0.015	272
Lansdale Hospital	Lansdale	0.016	244
Mount Nittany Medical Center	State College	0.017	539
Temple University Hospital	Philadelphia	0.017	827
Williamsport Hospital & Medical Center	Williamsport	0.017	535
Riddle Memorial Hospital	Media	0.018	507
Roxborough Memorial Hospital	Phila	0.018	112
Waynesboro Hospital	Waynesboro	0.018	271
Hanover Hospital	Hanover	0.019	697
Main Line Hospital Lankenau	Wynnewood	0.019	1079
Main Line Hospital Paoli	Paoli	0.019	1044
Nason Hospital	Roaring Spring	0.019	103
ACMH Hospital	Kittanning	0.020	147
Geisinger Wyoming Valley Medical Center	Wilkes-Barre	0.020	846
Good Samaritan Hospital	Lebanon	0.020	919
Lancaster Regional Medical Center	Lancaster	0.020	255
Saint Mary Medical Center	Langhorne	0.020	836
UPMC Northwest	Seneca	0.020	938
Western Penn Hosp-Forbes Reg Campus	Monroeville	0.020	345
Albert Einstein Medical Center	Philadelphia	0.021	533
St Catherine Med Ctr Fountain Springs	Ashland	0.022	45
Ephrata Community Hospital	Ephrata	0.023	740
Main Line Hospital Bryn Mawr Campus	Bryn Mawr	0.023	972
Marian Community Hospital	Carbondale	0.023	177
Mercy Hospital Scranton	Scranton	0.023	655
Chestnut Hill Hospital	Philadelphia	0.024	333
Penn Presbyterian Medical Center	Philadelphia	0.024	255
Mercy Fitzgerald Hospital	Darby	0.028	578
Mercy Tyler Hospital	Tunkhannock	0.029	103
Sacred Heart Hospital	Allentown	0.029	375
Easton Hospital	Easton	0.030	573
UPMC Bedford	Everett	0.030	165
Bradford Regional Medical Center	Bradford	0.031	325
Lancaster General Hospital	Lancaster	0.032	2583
Clearfield Hospital	Clearfield	0.033	303
Lehigh Valley Hospital - Muhlenberg	Bethlehem	0.033	932
Pocono Medical Center	E Stroudsburg	0.034	558
Altoona Regional Health System	Altoona	0.036	873
Lock Haven Hospital	Lock Haven	0.037	109
Pottstown Memorial Medical Center	Pottstown	0.038	478
Gnaden Huetten Memorial Hospital	Lehighton	0.042	312
Sunbury Community Hospital	Sunbury	0.042	143
Phoenixville Hospital	Phoenixville	0.045	424
Wayne Memorial Hospital	Honesdale	0.045	581
Chambersburg Hospital	Chambersburg	0.046	698
UPMC Mckeesport	McKeesport	0.051	293
Lehigh Valley Hospital	Allentown	0.058	514
Reading Hospital Medical Center	Reading	0.061	2818
Jefferson Regional Medical Center	Pittsburgh	0.063	432
Shamokin Area Community Hospital	Coal Township	0.064	264
Gettysburg Hospital	Gettysburg	0.082	379
Highlands Hospital[1]	Connellsville	0.083	60
Saint Luke's Miners Memorial Hospital	Coaldale	0.084	239
Heart of Lancaster Regional Medical Center	Lititz	0.085	94
Saint Luke's Quakertown Hospital	Quakertown	0.088	240
Allegheny General Hospital	Pittsburgh	0.100	872
Community Medical Center	Scranton	0.100	329
Berwick Hospital Center	Berwick	0.117	120
Southwest Regional Medical Center	Waynesburg	0.157	115
Pinnacle Health Hospitals	Harrisburg	0.158	608
Carlisle Regional Medical Center	Carlisle	0.164	549
Somerset Hospital	Somerset	0.325	163
Bloomsburg Hospital	Bloomsburg	0.484	64
Clarion Hospital	Clarion	0.512	207
Elk Regional Health Center	Saint Marys	0.567	305
Kane Community Hospital	Kane	0.750	124

38. Follow-up Mammogram/Ultrasound

Hospital Name	City	Rate	Cases
Millcreek Community Hospital	Erie	0.0%	56
Saint Joseph's Hospital[1]	Philadelphia	0.0%	41
Titusville Hospital	Titusville	0.4%	538
Warren General Hospital	Warren	2.0%	816
Sunbury Community Hospital	Sunbury	2.8%	435
UPMC Mckeesport	McKeesport	3.1%	260
Schuylkill Med Ctr-S Jackson Street	Pottsville	3.3%	1162
Meadville Medical Center	Meadville	3.5%	1434
Heart of Lancaster Regional Medical Center	Lititz	3.7%	188
Saint Luke's Miners Memorial Hospital	Coaldale	3.7%	406
Carlisle Regional Medical Center	Carlisle	3.9%	563
Good Samaritan Hospital	Lebanon	4.0%	2993
Clearfield Hospital	Clearfield	4.3%	769
Highlands Hospital	Connellsville	4.3%	184
Miners Medical Center	Hastings	4.4%	135
UPMC Bedford	Everett	4.5%	420
Jeanes Hospital	Philadelphia	4.6%	828
Lansdale Hospital	Lansdale	4.6%	673
Uniontown Hospital	Uniontown	4.6%	718
Saint Joseph Medical Center	Reading	4.7%	1549
Monongahela Valley Hospital	Monongahela	4.9%	536
Altoona Regional Health System	Altoona	5.0%	1148
Milton S Hershey Medical Center	Hershey	5.0%	1085
Conemaugh Valley Memorial Hospital	Johnstown	5.1%	950
Mercy Fitzgerald Hospital	Darby	5.1%	1236
Roxborough Memorial Hospital	Phila	5.2%	327
Albert Einstein Medical Center	Philadelphia	5.4%	2369
Chambersburg Hospital	Chambersburg	5.5%	2854
Delaware County Memorial Hospital	Drexel Hill	5.5%	566
Wayne Memorial Hospital	Honesdale	5.6%	1071
Temple University Hospital	Philadelphia	5.7%	888
Memorial Hospital - Towanda	Towanda	5.9%	337
Windber Hospital	Windber	5.9%	461
J C Blair Memorial Hospital	Huntingdon	6.0%	804
Jersey Shore Hospital	Jersey Shore	6.0%	399
Somerset Hospital	Somerset	6.1%	363
Hospital of Univ of Pennsylvania	Philadelphia	6.2%	1136
Community Medical Center	Scranton	6.3%	761
UPMC Saint Margaret	Pittsburgh	6.4%	561
Marian Community Hospital	Carbondale	6.5%	567
Reading Hospital Medical Center	Reading	6.5%	5143
Dubois Regional Medical Center	Dubois	6.7%	1688
Lehigh Valley Hospital	Allentown	6.7%	3682
Lehigh Valley Hospital - Muhlenberg	Bethlehem	6.7%	1557
Pottstown Memorial Medical Center	Pottstown	6.7%	1064
Saint Vincent Health Center	Erie	6.7%	1253
Evangelical Community Hospital	Lewisburg	6.8%	1761
Montgomery Hospital	Norristown	6.8%	725
Shamokin Area Community Hospital	Coal Township	6.8%	921
Main Line Hospital Bryn Mawr Campus	Bryn Mawr	6.9%	1404
Soldiers and Sailors Memorial Hospital	Wellsboro	6.9%	978
Mercy Tyler Hospital	Tunkhannock	7.1%	239
Chestnut Hill Hospital	Philadelphia	7.2%	1295
Main Line Hospital Paoli	Paoli	7.2%	1544
Punxsutawney Area Hospital	Punxsutawney	7.2%	375
Wilkes-Barre General Hospital	Wilkes-Barre	7.2%	2678
Mercy Hospital Scranton	Scranton	7.3%	731
The Washington Hospital	Washington	7.3%	959
Charles Cole Memorial Hospital	Coudersport	7.4%	488
Saint Mary Medical Center	Langhorne	7.4%	1535
UPMC Horizon	Greenville	7.4%	1168
Hazleton General Hospital	Hazleton	7.5%	345
UPMC Mercy	Pittsburgh	7.5%	292
UPMC Northwest	Seneca	7.5%	1769
St Catherine Med Ctr Fountain Springs	Ashland	7.6%	131
Waynesboro Hospital	Waynesboro	7.6%	1073
Holy Spirit Hospital	Camp Hill	7.7%	728
Indiana Regional Medical Center	Indiana	7.7%	674
Lower Bucks Hospital	Bristol	7.7%	671
Mercy Suburban Hospital	Norristown	7.7%	363
Pinnacle Health Hospitals	Harrisburg	7.7%	1189
Saint Luke's Quakertown Hospital	Quakertown	7.8%	486
Lancaster General Hospital	Lancaster	7.9%	5423
Grand View Hospital	Sellersville	8.1%	1568
Allegheny General Hospital	Pittsburgh	8.2%	833
Bloomsburg Hospital	Bloomsburg	8.2%	474
Main Line Hospital Lankenau	Wynnewood	8.2%	2031
Saint Luke's Hospital Bethlehem	Bethlehem	8.4%	3599
Magee Womens Hosp of UPMC Health Sys	Pittsburgh	8.5%	3186
Sharon Regional Health System	Sharon	8.5%	988
Aria Health	Philadelphia	8.6%	1126
Crozer Chester Medical Center	Upland	8.6%	1887
Excela Health Westmoreland Reg Hosp	Greensburg	8.7%	959
Holy Redeemer Hospital and Medical Center	Meadowbrook	8.8%	1264
Bradford Regional Medical Center	Bradford	8.9%	697
Pocono Medical Center	E Stroudsburg	9.0%	357
Thomas Jefferson University Hospital	Philadelphia	9.0%	3292
Phoenixville Hospital	Phoenixville	9.2%	841
York Hospital	York	9.5%	5709
Easton Hospital	Easton	9.7%	1525
Butler Memorial Hospital	Butler	9.9%	1060
Western Pennsylvania Hospital	Pittsburgh	9.9%	605
Grove City Medical Center	Grove City	10.0%	370
Excela Health Frick Hospital	Mount Pleasant	10.1%	237
Hahnemann University Hospital	Philadelphia	10.1%	435
Penn Presbyterian Medical Center	Philadelphia	10.1%	207
Mount Nittany Medical Center	State College	10.2%	1584
Abington Memorial Hospital	Abington	10.3%	2769
Nason Hospital	Roaring Spring	10.3%	377
Jameson Memorial Hospital	New Castle	10.4%	451
Lewistown Hospital	Lewistown	10.4%	895
Clarion Hospital	Clarion	10.5%	561
Nazareth Hospital	Philadelphia	10.5%	418
Schuylkill Med Ctr-East Norwegian Street	Pottsville	10.5%	740
Chester County Hospital	West Chester	10.6%	1780
Memorial Hospital York	York	10.6%	795
Excela Health Latrobe Hospital	Latrobe	10.7%	571
Doylestown Hospital	Doylestown	10.9%	2039
Geisinger Medical Center	Danville	11.0%	1366
UPMC Passavant	Pittsburgh	11.1%	587
Saint Clair Memorial Hospital	Pittsburgh	11.2%	699
Heritage Valley Beaver	Beaver	11.3%	1183
Heritage Valley Sewickley	Sewickley	11.3%	247
Berwick Hospital Center	Berwick	11.6%	372
Penn Hosp of the Univ of Penn Health Sys	Philadelphia	11.6%	946
Southwest Regional Medical Center	Waynesburg	11.8%	203
Elk Regional Health Center	Saint Marys	12.0%	897
Hanover Hospital	Hanover	12.0%	1172
Moses Taylor Hospital	Scranton	12.2%	699
Troy Community Hospital	Troy	12.3%	310
Ellwood City Hospital	Ellwood City	12.4%	226
Ohio Valley General Hospital	Mckees Rocks	12.4%	177
Gnaden Huetten Memorial Hospital	Lehighton	12.6%	625
Geisinger Wyoming Valley Medical Center	Wilkes-Barre	12.9%	735
Lock Haven Hospital	Lock Haven	12.9%	271
Canonsburg General Hospital	Canonsburg	13.0%	247
Robert Packer Hospital	Sayre	13.6%	1612
Jennersville Regional Hospital	West Grove	14.1%	377
Gettysburg Hospital	Gettysburg	14.8%	1343
ACMH Hospital	Kittanning	15.2%	356
Ephrata Community Hospital	Ephrata	15.4%	1492
Palmerton Hospital	Palmerton	15.4%	505
Brandywine Hospital	Coatesville	15.7%	623
Alle Kiski Medical Center	Natrona	17.4%	700
Western Penn Hosp-Forbes Reg Campus	Monroeville	17.6%	324
Jefferson Regional Medical Center	Pittsburgh	21.4%	248
Sacred Heart Hospital	Allentown	23.4%	824
Kane Community Hospital	Kane	43.6%	236

39. MRI for Low Back Pain

Hospital Name	City	Rate	Cases
Berwick Hospital Center[1]	Berwick	17.2%	58
Lansdale Hospital[1]	Lansdale	18.4%	49
Kane Community Hospital[1]	Kane	19.4%	36
Pocono Medical Center	E Stroudsburg	20.0%	70
Carlisle Regional Medical Center	Carlisle	20.8%	77
Montgomery Hospital	Norristown	22.1%	77
Grand View Hospital	Sellersville	24.0%	146
Hanover Hospital	Hanover	24.2%	236
Jeanes Hospital	Philadelphia	24.2%	91
Ephrata Community Hospital	Ephrata	25.3%	162
Gettysburg Hospital	Gettysburg	25.4%	209
Saint Mary Medical Center	Langhorne	25.7%	148
UPMC Mckeesport[1]	McKeesport	25.8%	31
Bloomsburg Hospital[1]	Bloomsburg	26.0%	50
Geisinger Medical Center	Danville	26.2%	221
Doylestown Hospital	Doylestown	26.5%	196
Milton S Hershey Medical Center	Hershey	26.6%	319
Hamot Medical Center	Erie	27.1%	133
Thomas Jefferson University Hospital	Philadelphia	27.4%	201
Marian Community Hospital[1]	Carbondale	27.5%	51
Nazareth Hospital	Philadelphia	27.8%	151
Memorial Hospital York	York	28.0%	82
Titusville Hospital	Titusville	28.3%	60
Evangelical Community Hospital	Lewisburg	28.4%	169
Main Line Hospital Lankenau	Wynnewood	28.9%	190
Reading Hospital Medical Center	Reading	28.9%	602
Saint Luke's Quakertown Hospital	Quakertown	29.2%	89

NOTE: Hospital profiles are in alphabetical order by state, then city, then hospital within the city; Rankings exclude hospitals with less than 25 cases except for patient surveys which excludes hospitals with less than 100 cases; (a) 100–299 cases; (1) The number of cases is too small to be sure how well a hospital is performing; (2) The hospital indicated that the data submitted for this measure were based on a sample of cases; (3) Data was collected during a shorter time period (fewer quarters) than the maximum possible time for this measure; (4) Suppressed for one or more quarters by CMS; (5) No data is available from the hospital for this measure; (6) Fewer than 100 patients completed the HCAHPS survey. Use these rates with caution, as the number of surveys may be too low to reliably assess hospital performance; (7) Survey results are based on less than 12 months of data; (8) Survey results are not available for this reporting period; (9) No or very few patients were eligible for the HCAHPS survey. The scores shown, if any, reflect a very small number of surveys; (10) A state average was not calculated because too few hospitals in the state submitted data; (11) There were discrepancies in the data collection process; Please refer to the User's Guide for a full explanation of data.

Geisinger Wyoming Valley Medical Center	Wilkes-Barre	29.3%	150
Heritage Valley Beaver	Beaver	29.3%	92
Mount Nittany Medical Center	State College	29.3%	82
Albert Einstein Medical Center	Philadelphia	29.4%	143
Jennersville Regional Hospital	West Grove	29.5%	78
Western Pennsylvania Hospital	Pittsburgh	29.6%	54
Abington Memorial Hospital	Abington	29.7%	370
Hahnemann University Hospital[1]	Philadelphia	30.0%	50
Chester County Hospital	West Chester	30.2%	126
Lehigh Valley Hospital - Muhlenberg	Bethlehem	30.3%	76
Schuylkill Med Ctr-East Norwegian Street	Pottsville	30.3%	142
Saint Luke's Miners Memorial Hospital	Coaldale	30.4%	69
Community Medical Center[1]	Scranton	30.6%	36
Meadville Medical Center	Meadville	31.0%	268
Punxsutawney Area Hospital[1]	Punxsutawney	31.0%	29
Hazleton General Hospital	Hazleton	31.2%	109
Saint Vincent Health Center	Erie	31.3%	291
Butler Memorial Hospital	Butler	31.4%	194
Brandywine Hospital	Coatesville	31.5%	92
Mercy Fitzgerald Hospital	Darby	31.6%	114
Altoona Regional Health System	Altoona	31.8%	148
Jersey Shore Hospital[1]	Jersey Shore	31.8%	44
Schuylkill Med Ctr-S Jackson Street	Pottsville	31.8%	148
Chambersburg Hospital	Chambersburg	31.9%	367
Pinnacle Health Hospitals	Harrisburg	32.2%	118
UPMC Horizon	Greenville	32.4%	188
Clarion Hospital	Clarion	32.6%	86
Sharon Regional Health System	Sharon	32.7%	147
Indiana Regional Medical Center	Indiana	32.8%	67
Soldiers and Sailors Memorial Hospital	Wellsboro	32.8%	122
Excela Health Latrobe Hospital	Latrobe	32.9%	85
Warren General Hospital	Warren	32.9%	164
Crozer Chester Medical Center	Upland	33.2%	292
Penn Presbyterian Medical Center[1]	Philadelphia	33.3%	36
UPMC Northwest	Seneca	33.3%	306
Hospital of Univ of Pennsylvania	Philadelphia	33.5%	212
Gnaden Huetten Memorial Hospital	Lehighton	33.7%	190
Chestnut Hill Hospital	Philadelphia	33.9%	62
Westfield Hospital	Allentown	33.9%	56
UPMC Passavant	Pittsburgh	34.0%	150
UPMC Presbyterian Shadyside	Pittsburgh	34.1%	270
Ohio Valley General Hospital[1]	Mckees Rocks	34.3%	35
Pottstown Memorial Medical Center	Pottstown	34.3%	210
Uniontown Hospital	Uniontown	34.3%	99
York Hospital	York	34.3%	207
Delaware County Memorial Hospital	Drexel Hill	34.4%	64
Robert Packer Hospital	Sayre	34.4%	195
Saint Joseph Medical Center	Reading	34.4%	151
Sacred Heart Hospital	Allentown	34.6%	52
Troy Community Hospital[1]	Troy	34.6%	26
UPMC Bedford[1]	Everett	34.6%	26
Elk Regional Health Center	Saint Marys	34.8%	164
Saint Luke's Hospital Bethlehem	Bethlehem	35.1%	239
Lock Haven Hospital[1]	Lock Haven	35.3%	34
Excela Health Westmoreland Reg Hosp	Greensburg	35.8%	95
Mercy Tyler Hospital	Tunkhannock	36.0%	50
Phoenixville Hospital	Phoenixville	36.1%	133
Mercy Suburban Hospital	Norristown	36.4%	55
Saint Clair Memorial Hospital	Pittsburgh	36.5%	156
Wilkes-Barre General Hospital	Wilkes-Barre	36.7%	139
Lewistown Hospital	Lewistown	36.9%	255
Memorial Hospital - Towanda	Towanda	37.1%	89
Somerset Hospital	Somerset	37.5%	64
Mercy Hospital Scranton	Scranton	37.8%	74
Southwest Regional Medical Center[1]	Waynesburg	38.2%	34
UPMC Saint Margaret	Pittsburgh	39.0%	159
Edgewood Surgical Hospital	Transfer	39.3%	117
Waynesboro Hospital	Waynesboro	39.5%	81
Allegheny General Hospital	Pittsburgh	39.6%	96
ACMH Hospital[1]	Kittanning	40.0%	35
Sunbury Community Hospital[1]	Sunbury	40.0%	30
Clearfield Hospital	Clearfield	40.3%	77
Holy Spirit Hospital	Camp Hill	40.3%	62
Shamokin Area Community Hospital	Coal Township	40.4%	94
Temple University Hospital	Philadelphia	40.5%	79
Grove City Medical Center	Grove City	40.8%	49
Windber Hospital	Windber	41.5%	53
Heritage Valley Sewickley	Sewickley	42.1%	57
Alle Kiski Medical Center	Natrona	42.7%	82
The Washington Hospital	Washington	43.1%	116
Easton Hospital	Easton	43.5%	46
Wayne Memorial Hospital	Honesdale	44.7%	94
Bradford Regional Medical Center	Bradford	45.2%	84
Canonsburg General Hospital[1]	Canonsburg	45.5%	33
UPMC Mercy	Pittsburgh	45.7%	35
Excela Health Frick Hospital	Mount Pleasant	45.9%	37
Jameson Memorial Hospital	New Castle	46.2%	52
J C Blair Memorial Hospital	Huntingdon	46.3%	41
Western Penn Hosp-Forbes Reg Campus	Monroeville	46.5%	43
Miners Medical Center	Hastings	47.7%	44
Charles Cole Memorial Hospital	Coudersport	48.2%	56
Moses Taylor Hospital	Scranton	48.6%	35
Monongahela Valley Hospital	Monongahela	50.5%	97

Survey of Patients' Hospital Experiences

40. Area Around Room 'Always' Quiet at Night

Hospital Name	City	Rate	Cases
Edgewood Surgical Hospital	Transfer	87%	(a)
Coordinated Health Orthopedic Hospital	Bethlehem	80%	300+
Surgical Institute of Reading	Wyomissing	74%	300+
Westfield Hospital	Allentown	68%	(a)
Miners Medical Center	Hastings	67%	(a)
Titusville Hospital	Titusville	66%	300+
Memorial Hospital - Towanda	Towanda	62%	300+
Cancer Treatment Centers of America	Philadelphia	61%	(a)
Charles Cole Memorial Hospital	Coudersport	60%	300+
Hahnemann University Hospital	Philadelphia	59%	300+
Muncy Valley Hospital	Muncy	59%	(a)
Ellwood City Hospital	Ellwood City	58%	300+
Lock Haven Hospital	Lock Haven	58%	300+
Sacred Heart Hospital	Allentown	58%	300+
Heart of Lancaster Regional Medical Center	Lititz	57%	300+
Lancaster Regional Medical Center	Lancaster	57%	300+
Monongahela Valley Hospital	Monongahela	57%	300+
Saint Joseph Medical Center	Reading	57%	300+
Chestnut Hill Hospital	Philadelphia	56%	300+
Nason Hospital	Roaring Spring	56%	300+
Ohio Valley General Hospital	Mckees Rocks	56%	300+
Windber Hospital	Windber	56%	300+
Berwick Hospital Center	Berwick	55%	300+
Community Medical Center	Scranton	54%	300+
Jeanes Hospital	Philadelphia	54%	300+
Main Line Hospital Paoli	Paoli	54%	300+
Nazareth Hospital	Philadelphia	54%	300+
Phoenixville Hospital	Phoenixville	54%	300+
Shamokin Area Community Hospital	Coal Township	54%	300+
Altoona Regional Health System	Altoona	53%	300+
Holy Redeemer Hospital and Medical Center	Meadowbrook	53%	300+
Jennersville Regional Hospital	West Grove	53%	300+
Kane Community Hospital	Kane	53%	(a)
Lansdale Hospital	Lansdale	53%	300+
Moses Taylor Hospital	Scranton	53%	300+
Penn Presbyterian Medical Center	Philadelphia	53%	300+
Punxsutawney Area Hospital	Punxsutawney	53%	300+
St Catherine Med Ctr Fountain Springs	Ashland	53%	(a)
Temple University Hospital	Philadelphia	53%	300+
UPMC Bedford	Everett	53%	300+
Western Pennsylvania Hospital	Pittsburgh	53%	300+
Canonsburg General Hospital	Canonsburg	52%	300+
Carlisle Regional Medical Center	Carlisle	52%	300+
Dubois Regional Medical Center	Dubois	52%	300+
Grand View Hospital	Sellersville	52%	300+
Grove City Medical Center	Grove City	52%	300+
Mercy Fitzgerald Hospital	Darby	52%	300+
Palmerton Hospital	Palmerton	52%	300+
Soldiers and Sailors Memorial Hospital	Wellsboro	52%	300+
Southwest Regional Medical Center	Waynesburg	52%	300+
Waynesboro Hospital	Waynesboro	52%	300+
Bloomsburg Hospital	Bloomsburg	51%	300+
Doylestown Hospital	Doylestown	51%	300+
Evangelical Community Hospital	Lewisburg	51%	300+
J C Blair Memorial Hospital	Huntingdon	51%	300+
Lehigh Valley Hospital - Muhlenberg	Bethlehem	51%	300+
Lower Bucks Hospital	Bristol	51%	300+
Meadville Medical Center	Meadville	51%	300+
Millcreek Community Hospital	Erie	51%	300+
Saint Clair Memorial Hospital	Pittsburgh	51%	300+
Saint Luke's Hospital Bethlehem	Bethlehem	51%	300+
Saint Luke's Miners Memorial Hospital	Coaldale	51%	300+
Saint Vincent Health Center	Erie	51%	300+
Uniontown Hospital	Uniontown	51%	300+
Albert Einstein Medical Center	Philadelphia	50%	300+
Clarion Hospital	Clarion	50%	300+
Delaware County Memorial Hospital	Drexel Hill	50%	300+
Heritage Valley Sewickley	Sewickley	50%	300+
Montgomery Hospital	Norristown	50%	300+
Penn Hosp of the Univ of Penn Health Sys	Philadelphia	50%	300+
Pocono Medical Center	E Stroudsburg	50%	300+
Robert Packer Hospital	Sayre	50%	300+
Saint Luke's Quakertown Hospital	Quakertown	50%	300+
Thomas Jefferson University Hospital	Philadelphia	50%	300+
UPMC Mckeesport	McKeesport	50%	300+
Aria Health	Philadelphia	49%	300+
Crozer Chester Medical Center	Upland	49%	300+
Easton Hospital	Easton	49%	300+
Excela Health Frick Hospital	Mount Pleasant	49%	300+
Geisinger Wyoming Valley Medical Center	Wilkes-Barre	49%	300+
Jefferson Regional Medical Center	Pittsburgh	49%	300+
Saint Joseph's Hospital	Philadelphia	49%	(a)
Butler Memorial Hospital	Butler	48%	300+
Hamot Medical Center	Erie	48%	300+
Lancaster General Hospital	Lancaster	48%	300+
Lehigh Valley Hospital	Allentown	48%	300+
Main Line Hospital Lankenau	Wynnewood	48%	300+
Sunbury Community Hospital	Sunbury	48%	300+
UPMC Mercy	Pittsburgh	48%	300+
UPMC Northwest	Seneca	48%	300+
Warren General Hospital	Warren	48%	300+
The Washington Hospital	Washington	48%	300+
Williamsport Hospital & Medical Center	Williamsport	48%	300+
Allegheny General Hospital	Pittsburgh	47%	300+
Chester County Hospital	West Chester	47%	300+
Conemaugh Valley Memorial Hospital	Johnstown	47%	300+
Gnaden Huetten Memorial Hospital	Lehighton	47%	300+
Mercy Hospital Scranton	Scranton	47%	300+
Reading Hospital Medical Center	Reading	47%	300+
Abington Memorial Hospital	Abington	46%	300+
Chambersburg Hospital	Chambersburg	46%	300+
Good Samaritan Hospital	Lebanon	46%	300+
Highlands Hospital	Connellsville	46%	300+
Hospital of Univ of Pennsylvania	Philadelphia	46%	300+
Indiana Regional Medical Center	Indiana	46%	300+
Pinnacle Health Hospitals	Harrisburg	46%	300+
Riddle Memorial Hospital	Media	46%	300+
Wayne Memorial Hospital	Honesdale	46%	300+
Excela Health Latrobe Hospital	Latrobe	45%	300+
Hanover Hospital	Hanover	45%	300+
Hazleton General Hospital	Hazleton	45%	300+
Main Line Hospital Bryn Mawr Campus	Bryn Mawr	45%	300+
Marian Community Hospital	Carbondale	45%	300+
Pottstown Memorial Medical Center	Pottstown	45%	300+
Schuylkill Med Ctr-S Jackson Street	Pottsville	45%	300+
Sharon Regional Health System	Sharon	45%	300+
UPMC Presbyterian Shadyside	Pittsburgh	45%	300+
UPMC Saint Margaret	Pittsburgh	45%	300+
Wilkes-Barre General Hospital	Wilkes-Barre	45%	300+
Brandywine Hospital	Coatesville	44%	300+
Clearfield Hospital	Clearfield	44%	300+
Elk Regional Health Center	Saint Marys	44%	300+
Excela Health Westmoreland Reg Hosp	Greensburg	44%	300+
Gettysburg Hospital	Gettysburg	44%	300+
Holy Spirit Hospital	Camp Hill	44%	300+
Jameson Memorial Hospital[11]	New Castle	44%	300+
Lewistown Hospital	Lewistown	44%	300+
Magee Womens Hosp of UPMC Health Sys	Pittsburgh	44%	300+
Somerset Hospital	Somerset	44%	300+
York Hospital	York	44%	300+
Bradford Regional Medical Center	Bradford	43%	300+
Ephrata Community Hospital	Ephrata	43%	300+
Geisinger Medical Center	Danville	43%	300+
Saint Mary Medical Center	Langhorne	43%	300+
UPMC Passavant	Pittsburgh	43%	300+
Memorial Hospital York	York	42%	300+
Milton S Hershey Medical Center	Hershey	42%	300+
UPMC Horizon	Greenville	42%	300+
Western Penn Hosp-Forbes Reg Campus	Monroeville	42%	300+
ACMH Hospital	Kittanning	41%	300+
Heritage Valley Beaver	Beaver	41%	300+
Mercy Tyler Hospital	Tunkhannock	41%	(a)
Mount Nittany Medical Center	State College	41%	300+
Roxborough Memorial Hospital	Phila	40%	300+
Alle Kiski Medical Center	Natrona	39%	300+
Schuylkill Med Ctr-East Norwegian Street	Pottsville	39%	300+
Corry Memorial Hospital	Corry	37%	(a)
Mercy Suburban Hospital	Norristown	37%	300+

41. Doctors 'Always' Communicated Well

Hospital Name	City	Rate	Cases
Surgical Institute of Reading	Wyomissing	94%	300+
Edgewood Surgical Hospital	Transfer	92%	(a)
Highlands Hospital	Connellsville	90%	300+
Miners Medical Center	Hastings	89%	(a)
Cancer Treatment Centers of America	Philadelphia	87%	(a)
Coordinated Health Orthopedic Hospital	Bethlehem	87%	300+
Titusville Hospital	Titusville	87%	300+
Windber Hospital	Windber	87%	300+
Muncy Valley Hospital	Muncy	86%	(a)
Shamokin Area Community Hospital	Coal Township	86%	300+
St Catherine Med Ctr Fountain Springs	Ashland	85%	(a)
Soldiers and Sailors Memorial Hospital	Wellsboro	85%	300+
Excela Health Frick Hospital	Mount Pleasant	84%	300+
Mercy Tyler Hospital	Tunkhannock	84%	(a)
Southwest Regional Medical Center	Waynesburg	84%	300+
ACMH Hospital	Kittanning	83%	300+
Berwick Hospital Center	Berwick	83%	300+
Charles Cole Memorial Hospital	Coudersport	83%	300+
Grove City Medical Center	Grove City	83%	300+
J C Blair Memorial Hospital	Huntingdon	83%	300+
Kane Community Hospital	Kane	83%	(a)
Memorial Hospital - Towanda	Towanda	83%	300+

NOTE: Hospital profiles are in alphabetical order by state, then city, then hospital within the city; Rankings exclude hospitals with less than 25 cases except for patient surveys which excludes hospitals with less than 100 cases; (a) 100–299 cases; (1) The number of cases is too small to be sure how well a hospital is performing; (2) The hospital indicated that the data submitted for this measure were based on a sample of cases; (3) Data was collected during a shorter time period (fewer quarters) than the maximum possible time for this measure; (4) Suppressed for one or more quarters by CMS; (5) No data is available from the hospital for this measure; (6) Fewer than 100 patients completed the HCAHPS survey. Use these rates with caution, as the number of surveys may be too low to reliably assess hospital performance; (7) Survey results are based on less than 12 months of data; (8) Survey results are not available for this reporting period; (9) No or very few patients were eligible for the HCAHPS survey. The scores shown, if any, reflect a very small number of surveys; (10) A state average was not calculated because too few hospitals in the state submitted data; (11) There were discrepancies in the data collection process; Please refer to the User's Guide for a full explanation of data.

Millcreek Community Hospital	Erie	83%	300+
Monongahela Valley Hospital	Monongahela	83%	300+
Nason Hospital	Roaring Spring	83%	300+
Williamsport Hospital & Medical Center	Williamsport	83%	300+
Altoona Regional Health System	Altoona	82%	300+
Doylestown Hospital	Doylestown	82%	300+
Hahnemann University Hospital	Philadelphia	82%	300+
Heritage Valley Sewickley	Sewickley	82%	300+
Indiana Regional Medical Center	Indiana	82%	300+
Meadville Medical Center	Meadville	82%	300+
Punxsutawney Area Hospital	Punxsutawney	82%	300+
Sharon Regional Health System	Sharon	82%	300+
Uniontown Hospital	Uniontown	82%	300+
The Washington Hospital	Washington	82%	300+
Corry Memorial Hospital	Corry	81%	(a)
Geisinger Wyoming Valley Medical Center	Wilkes-Barre	81%	300+
Jeanes Hospital	Philadelphia	81%	300+
Marian Community Hospital	Carbondale	81%	300+
Moses Taylor Hospital	Scranton	81%	300+
Mount Nittany Medical Center	State College	81%	300+
Sunbury Community Hospital	Sunbury	81%	300+
Canonsburg General Hospital	Canonsburg	80%	300+
Chester County Hospital	West Chester	80%	300+
Clearfield Hospital	Clearfield	80%	300+
Evangelical Community Hospital	Lewisburg	80%	300+
Excela Health Latrobe Hospital	Latrobe	80%	300+
Hazleton General Hospital	Hazleton	80%	300+
Holy Redeemer Hospital and Medical Center	Meadowbrook	80%	300+
Hospital of Univ of Pennsylvania	Philadelphia	80%	300+
Jefferson Regional Medical Center	Pittsburgh	80%	300+
Lancaster Regional Medical Center	Lancaster	80%	300+
Main Line Hospital Lankenau	Wynnewood	80%	300+
Penn Presbyterian Medical Center	Philadelphia	80%	300+
Saint Luke's Miners Memorial Hospital	Coaldale	80%	300+
UPMC Horizon	Greenville	80%	300+
Western Pennsylvania Hospital	Pittsburgh	80%	300+
Wilkes-Barre General Hospital	Wilkes-Barre	80%	300+
Community Medical Center	Scranton	79%	300+
Dubois Regional Medical Center	Dubois	79%	300+
Excela Health Westmoreland Reg Hosp	Greensburg	79%	300+
Geisinger Medical Center	Danville	79%	300+
Hanover Hospital	Hanover	79%	300+
Heritage Valley Beaver	Beaver	79%	300+
Jameson Memorial Hospital[11]	New Castle	79%	300+
Lehigh Valley Hospital	Allentown	79%	300+
Main Line Hospital Paoli	Paoli	79%	300+
UPMC Mckeesport	McKeesport	79%	300+
Waynesboro Hospital	Waynesboro	79%	300+
Westfield Hospital	Allentown	79%	(a)
Clarion Hospital	Clarion	78%	300+
Gettysburg Hospital	Gettysburg	78%	300+
Hamot Medical Center	Erie	78%	300+
Lehigh Valley Hospital - Muhlenberg	Bethlehem	78%	300+
Mercy Hospital Scranton	Scranton	78%	300+
Pocono Medical Center	E Stroudsburg	78%	300+
Robert Packer Hospital	Sayre	78%	300+
Saint Clair Memorial Hospital	Pittsburgh	78%	300+
Saint Luke's Hospital Bethlehem	Bethlehem	78%	300+
Saint Luke's Quakertown Hospital	Quakertown	78%	300+
UPMC Bedford	Everett	78%	300+
Wayne Memorial Hospital	Honesdale	78%	300+
Abington Memorial Hospital	Abington	77%	300+
Bloomsburg Hospital	Bloomsburg	77%	300+
Butler Memorial Hospital	Butler	77%	300+
Conemaugh Valley Memorial Hospital	Johnstown	77%	300+
Delaware County Memorial Hospital	Drexel Hill	77%	300+
Ellwood City Hospital	Ellwood City	77%	300+
Good Samaritan Hospital	Lebanon	77%	300+
Heart of Lancaster Regional Medical Center	Lititz	77%	300+
Lock Haven Hospital	Lock Haven	77%	300+
Ohio Valley General Hospital	Mckees Rocks	77%	300+
Riddle Memorial Hospital	Media	77%	300+
Saint Joseph Medical Center	Reading	77%	300+
Schuylkill Med Ctr-S Jackson Street	Pottsville	77%	300+
Temple University Hospital	Philadelphia	77%	300+
Thomas Jefferson University Hospital	Philadelphia	77%	300+
UPMC Saint Margaret	Pittsburgh	77%	300+
Warren General Hospital	Warren	77%	300+
Bradford Regional Medical Center	Bradford	76%	300+
Carlisle Regional Medical Center	Carlisle	76%	300+
Chambersburg Hospital	Chambersburg	76%	300+
Chestnut Hill Hospital	Philadelphia	76%	300+
Magee Womens Hosp of UPMC Health Sys	Pittsburgh	76%	300+
Main Line Hospital Bryn Mawr Campus	Bryn Mawr	76%	300+
Mercy Suburban Hospital	Norristown	76%	300+
Milton S Hershey Medical Center	Hershey	76%	300+
Montgomery Hospital	Norristown	76%	300+
Penn Hosp of the Univ of Penn Health Sys	Philadelphia	76%	300+
Reading Hospital Medical Center	Reading	76%	300+
Saint Vincent Health Center	Erie	76%	300+
York Hospital	York	76%	300+
Crozer Chester Medical Center	Upland	75%	300+
Easton Hospital	Easton	75%	300+
Elk Regional Health Center	Saint Marys	75%	300+
Ephrata Community Hospital	Ephrata	75%	300+
Gnaden Huetten Memorial Hospital	Lehighton	75%	300+
Grand View Hospital	Sellersville	75%	300+
Lansdale Hospital	Lansdale	75%	300+
Lewistown Hospital	Lewistown	75%	300+
Lower Bucks Hospital	Bristol	75%	300+
Palmerton Hospital	Palmerton	75%	300+
Sacred Heart Hospital	Allentown	75%	300+
Schuylkill Med Ctr-East Norwegian Street	Pottsville	75%	300+
Somerset Hospital	Somerset	75%	300+
UPMC Passavant	Pittsburgh	75%	300+
UPMC Presbyterian Shadyside	Pittsburgh	75%	300+
Brandywine Hospital	Coatesville	74%	300+
Lancaster General Hospital	Lancaster	74%	300+
Nazareth Hospital	Philadelphia	74%	300+
Pinnacle Health Hospitals	Harrisburg	74%	300+
Roxborough Memorial Hospital	Phila	74%	300+
Saint Mary Medical Center	Langhorne	74%	300+
UPMC Mercy	Pittsburgh	74%	300+
UPMC Northwest	Seneca	74%	300+
Western Penn Hosp-Forbes Reg Campus	Monroeville	74%	300+
Albert Einstein Medical Center	Philadelphia	73%	300+
Alle Kiski Medical Center	Natrona	73%	300+
Allegheny General Hospital	Pittsburgh	73%	300+
Mercy Fitzgerald Hospital	Darby	73%	300+
Phoenixville Hospital	Phoenixville	73%	300+
Aria Health	Philadelphia	72%	300+
Holy Spirit Hospital	Camp Hill	72%	300+
Jennersville Regional Hospital	West Grove	72%	300+
Memorial Hospital York	York	71%	300+
Pottstown Memorial Medical Center	Pottstown	71%	300+
Saint Joseph's Hospital	Philadelphia	70%	(a)

42. Home Recovery Information Given

Hospital Name	City	Rate	Cases
Surgical Institute of Reading	Wyomissing	94%	300+
Edgewood Surgical Hospital	Transfer	93%	(a)
Punxsutawney Area Hospital	Punxsutawney	92%	300+
Cancer Treatment Centers of America	Philadelphia	90%	(a)
Butler Memorial Hospital	Butler	89%	300+
Coordinated Health Orthopedic Hospital	Bethlehem	89%	300+
Milton S Hershey Medical Center	Hershey	89%	300+
Charles Cole Memorial Hospital	Coudersport	88%	300+
Geisinger Medical Center	Danville	88%	300+
Uniontown Hospital	Uniontown	88%	300+
Dubois Regional Medical Center	Dubois	87%	300+
Gettysburg Hospital	Gettysburg	87%	300+
Grove City Medical Center	Grove City	87%	300+
Hospital of Univ of Pennsylvania	Philadelphia	87%	300+
Indiana Regional Medical Center	Indiana	87%	300+
UPMC Saint Margaret	Pittsburgh	87%	300+
Windber Hospital	Windber	87%	300+
Doylestown Hospital	Doylestown	86%	300+
Grand View Hospital	Sellersville	86%	300+
Highlands Hospital	Connellsville	86%	300+
Lancaster General Hospital	Lancaster	86%	300+
St Catherine Med Ctr Fountain Springs	Ashland	86%	(a)
Wayne Memorial Hospital	Honesdale	86%	300+
Evangelical Community Hospital	Lewisburg	85%	300+
Jefferson Regional Medical Center	Pittsburgh	85%	300+
Lancaster Regional Medical Center	Lancaster	85%	300+
Lehigh Valley Hospital	Allentown	85%	300+
Lehigh Valley Hospital - Muhlenberg	Bethlehem	85%	300+
Mercy Suburban Hospital	Norristown	85%	300+
Mercy Tyler Hospital	Tunkhannock	85%	(a)
Reading Hospital Medical Center	Reading	85%	300+
Saint Joseph Medical Center	Reading	85%	300+
Soldiers and Sailors Memorial Hospital	Wellsboro	85%	300+
Titusville Hospital	Titusville	85%	300+
UPMC Presbyterian Shadyside	Pittsburgh	85%	300+
Waynesboro Hospital	Waynesboro	85%	300+
Williamsport Hospital & Medical Center	Williamsport	85%	300+
Altoona Regional Health System	Altoona	84%	300+
Clearfield Hospital	Clearfield	84%	300+
Conemaugh Valley Memorial Hospital	Johnstown	84%	300+
Excela Health Frick Hospital	Mount Pleasant	84%	300+
J C Blair Memorial Hospital	Huntingdon	84%	300+
Jameson Memorial Hospital[11]	New Castle	84%	300+
Kane Community Hospital	Kane	84%	(a)
Marian Community Hospital	Carbondale	84%	300+
Memorial Hospital - Towanda	Towanda	84%	300+
Mount Nittany Medical Center	State College	84%	300+
Muncy Valley Hospital	Muncy	84%	(a)
Penn Presbyterian Medical Center	Philadelphia	84%	300+
Pocono Medical Center	E Stroudsburg	84%	300+
Saint Vincent Health Center	Erie	84%	300+
Somerset Hospital	Somerset	84%	300+
Southwest Regional Medical Center	Waynesburg	84%	300+
Thomas Jefferson University Hospital	Philadelphia	84%	300+
UPMC Passavant	Pittsburgh	84%	300+
York Hospital	York	84%	300+
ACMH Hospital	Kittanning	83%	300+
Delaware County Memorial Hospital	Drexel Hill	83%	300+
Ephrata Community Hospital	Ephrata	83%	300+
Geisinger Wyoming Valley Medical Center	Wilkes-Barre	83%	300+
Gnaden Huetten Memorial Hospital	Lehighton	83%	300+
Good Samaritan Hospital	Lebanon	83%	300+
Hahnemann University Hospital	Philadelphia	83%	300+
Hamot Medical Center	Erie	83%	300+
Miners Medical Center	Hastings	83%	(a)
Nazareth Hospital	Philadelphia	83%	300+
Saint Luke's Quakertown Hospital	Quakertown	83%	300+
Shamokin Area Community Hospital	Coal Township	83%	300+
UPMC Bedford	Everett	83%	300+
The Washington Hospital	Washington	83%	300+
Carlisle Regional Medical Center	Carlisle	82%	300+
Community Medical Center	Scranton	82%	300+
Easton Hospital	Easton	82%	300+
Elk Regional Health Center	Saint Marys	82%	300+
Heritage Valley Sewickley	Sewickley	82%	300+
Jennersville Regional Hospital	West Grove	82%	300+
Lock Haven Hospital	Lock Haven	82%	300+
Main Line Hospital Bryn Mawr Campus	Bryn Mawr	82%	300+
Meadville Medical Center	Meadville	82%	300+
Palmerton Hospital	Palmerton	82%	300+
Pottstown Memorial Medical Center	Pottstown	82%	300+
Sacred Heart Hospital	Allentown	82%	300+
Saint Luke's Miners Memorial Hospital	Coaldale	82%	300+
Sunbury Community Hospital	Sunbury	82%	300+
Temple University Hospital	Philadelphia	82%	300+
UPMC Horizon	Greenville	82%	300+
Alle Kiski Medical Center	Natrona	81%	300+
Aria Health	Philadelphia	81%	300+
Chambersburg Hospital	Chambersburg	81%	300+
Clarion Hospital	Clarion	81%	300+
Corry Memorial Hospital	Corry	81%	(a)
Ellwood City Hospital	Ellwood City	81%	300+
Hanover Hospital	Hanover	81%	300+
Jeanes Hospital	Philadelphia	81%	300+
Mercy Fitzgerald Hospital	Darby	81%	300+
Moses Taylor Hospital	Scranton	81%	300+
Phoenixville Hospital	Phoenixville	81%	300+
Riddle Memorial Hospital	Media	81%	300+
Robert Packer Hospital	Sayre	81%	300+
Saint Clair Memorial Hospital	Pittsburgh	81%	300+
Western Pennsylvania Hospital	Pittsburgh	81%	300+
Abington Memorial Hospital	Abington	80%	300+
Allegheny General Hospital	Pittsburgh	80%	300+
Brandywine Hospital	Coatesville	80%	300+
Chestnut Hill Hospital	Philadelphia	80%	300+
Excela Health Latrobe Hospital	Latrobe	80%	300+
Heart of Lancaster Regional Medical Center	Lititz	80%	300+
Holy Redeemer Hospital and Medical Center	Meadowbrook	80%	300+
Lower Bucks Hospital	Bristol	80%	300+
Memorial Hospital York	York	80%	300+
Mercy Hospital Scranton	Scranton	80%	300+
Ohio Valley General Hospital	Mckees Rocks	80%	300+
Penn Hosp of the Univ of Penn Health Sys	Philadelphia	80%	300+
Sharon Regional Health System	Sharon	80%	300+
UPMC Mercy	Pittsburgh	80%	300+
Wilkes-Barre General Hospital	Wilkes-Barre	80%	300+
Excela Health Westmoreland Reg Hosp	Greensburg	79%	300+
Magee Womens Hosp of UPMC Health Sys	Pittsburgh	79%	300+
Main Line Hospital Lankenau	Wynnewood	79%	300+
Main Line Hospital Paoli	Paoli	79%	300+
Monongahela Valley Hospital	Monongahela	79%	300+
Montgomery Hospital	Norristown	79%	300+
Saint Mary Medical Center	Langhorne	79%	300+
UPMC Mckeesport	McKeesport	79%	300+
Western Penn Hosp-Forbes Reg Campus	Monroeville	79%	300+
Berwick Hospital Center	Berwick	78%	300+
Chester County Hospital	West Chester	78%	300+
Crozer Chester Medical Center	Upland	78%	300+
Lewistown Hospital	Lewistown	78%	300+
Pinnacle Health Hospitals	Harrisburg	78%	300+
Saint Luke's Hospital Bethlehem	Bethlehem	78%	300+
Westfield Hospital	Allentown	78%	(a)
Albert Einstein Medical Center	Philadelphia	77%	300+
Bloomsburg Hospital	Bloomsburg	77%	300+
Bradford Regional Medical Center	Bradford	77%	300+
Holy Spirit Hospital	Camp Hill	77%	300+
Nason Hospital	Roaring Spring	77%	300+
Schuylkill Med Ctr-East Norwegian Street	Pottsville	77%	300+
UPMC Northwest	Seneca	77%	300+
Canonsburg General Hospital	Canonsburg	76%	300+
Heritage Valley Beaver	Beaver	76%	300+
Roxborough Memorial Hospital	Phila	76%	300+
Warren General Hospital	Warren	75%	300+

NOTE: Hospital profiles are in alphabetical order by state, then city, then hospital within the city; Rankings exclude hospitals with less than 25 cases except for patient surveys which excludes hospitals with less than 100 cases; (a) 100–299 cases; (1) The number of cases is too small to be sure how well a hospital is performing; (2) The hospital indicated that the data submitted for this measure were based on a sample of cases; (3) Data was collected during a shorter time period (fewer quarters) than the maximum possible time for this measure; (4) Suppressed for one or more quarters by CMS; (5) No data is available from the hospital for this measure; (6) Fewer than 100 patients completed the HCAHPS survey. Use these rates with caution, as the number of surveys may be too low to reliably assess hospital performance; (7) Survey results are based on less than 12 months of data; (8) Survey results are not available for this reporting period; (9) No or very few patients were eligible for the HCAHPS survey. The scores shown, if any, reflect a very small number of surveys; (10) A state average was not calculated because too few hospitals in the state submitted data; (11) There were discrepancies in the data collection process; Please refer to the User's Guide for a full explanation of data.

Hazleton General Hospital	Hazleton	74%	300+
Lansdale Hospital	Lansdale	74%	300+
Millcreek Community Hospital	Erie	74%	300+
Schuylkill Med Ctr-S Jackson Street	Pottsville	73%	300+
Saint Joseph's Hospital	Philadelphia	64%	(a)

43. Hospital Given 9 or 10 on 10 Point Scale

Hospital Name	City	Rate	Cases
Surgical Institute of Reading	Wyomissing	93%	300+
Coordinated Health Orthopedic Hospital	Bethlehem	90%	300+
Cancer Treatment Centers of America	Philadelphia	88%	(a)
Edgewood Surgical Hospital	Transfer	87%	(a)
Shamokin Area Community Hospital	Coal Township	82%	300+
Main Line Hospital Paoli	Paoli	81%	300+
Doylestown Hospital	Doylestown	79%	300+
Westfield Hospital	Allentown	79%	(a)
Memorial Hospital - Towanda	Towanda	77%	300+
Miners Medical Center	Hastings	77%	(a)
Geisinger Medical Center	Danville	76%	300+
Lehigh Valley Hospital - Muhlenberg	Bethlehem	76%	300+
Nason Hospital	Roaring Spring	76%	300+
Saint Mary Medical Center	Langhorne	76%	300+
Titusville Hospital	Titusville	76%	300+
Windber Hospital	Windber	76%	300+
Main Line Hospital Lankenau	Wynnewood	75%	300+
Robert Packer Hospital	Sayre	75%	300+
Main Line Hospital Bryn Mawr Campus	Bryn Mawr	74%	300+
Muncy Valley Hospital	Muncy	74%	(a)
Grand View Hospital	Sellersville	73%	300+
Lehigh Valley Hospital	Allentown	73%	300+
Saint Luke's Hospital Bethlehem	Bethlehem	73%	300+
Soldiers and Sailors Memorial Hospital	Wellsboro	73%	300+
Waynesboro Hospital	Waynesboro	73%	300+
Holy Redeemer Hospital and Medical Center	Meadowbrook	72%	300+
Milton S Hershey Medical Center	Hershey	72%	300+
Saint Joseph Medical Center	Reading	72%	300+
Chester County Hospital	West Chester	71%	300+
Evangelical Community Hospital	Lewisburg	71%	300+
Excela Health Frick Hospital	Mount Pleasant	71%	300+
Hamot Medical Center	Erie	71%	300+
Highlands Hospital	Connellsville	71%	300+
Hospital of Univ of Pennsylvania	Philadelphia	71%	300+
Jefferson Regional Medical Center	Pittsburgh	71%	300+
Lancaster General Hospital	Lancaster	71%	300+
Saint Clair Memorial Hospital	Pittsburgh	71%	300+
Williamsport Hospital & Medical Center	Williamsport	71%	300+
Abington Memorial Hospital	Abington	70%	300+
Bloomsburg Hospital	Bloomsburg	70%	300+
Dubois Regional Medical Center	Dubois	70%	300+
Grove City Medical Center	Grove City	70%	300+
Lancaster Regional Medical Center	Lancaster	70%	300+
Monongahela Valley Hospital	Monongahela	70%	300+
Thomas Jefferson University Hospital	Philadelphia	70%	300+
Indiana Regional Medical Center	Indiana	69%	300+
Altoona Regional Health System	Altoona	68%	300+
Canonsburg General Hospital	Canonsburg	68%	300+
Charles Cole Memorial Hospital	Coudersport	68%	300+
Heritage Valley Sewickley	Sewickley	68%	300+
Jeanes Hospital	Philadelphia	68%	300+
Meadville Medical Center	Meadville	68%	300+
Penn Presbyterian Medical Center	Philadelphia	68%	300+
Saint Luke's Quakertown Hospital	Quakertown	68%	300+
Butler Memorial Hospital	Butler	67%	300+
York Hospital	York	67%	300+
Hahnemann University Hospital	Philadelphia	66%	300+
UPMC Saint Margaret	Pittsburgh	66%	300+
Aria Health	Philadelphia	65%	300+
Conemaugh Valley Memorial Hospital	Johnstown	65%	300+
Ellwood City Hospital	Ellwood City	65%	300+
Good Samaritan Hospital	Lebanon	65%	300+
Heart of Lancaster Regional Medical Center	Lititz	65%	300+
Kane Community Hospital	Kane	65%	(a)
Mount Nittany Medical Center	State College	65%	300+
Punxsutawney Area Hospital	Punxsutawney	65%	300+
Saint Vincent Health Center	Erie	65%	300+
Chambersburg Hospital	Chambersburg	64%	300+
Geisinger Wyoming Valley Medical Center	Wilkes-Barre	64%	300+
Hanover Hospital	Hanover	64%	300+
Holy Spirit Hospital	Camp Hill	64%	300+
Magee Womens Hosp of UPMC Health Sys	Pittsburgh	64%	300+
Memorial Hospital York	York	64%	300+
Mercy Hospital Scranton	Scranton	64%	300+
Mercy Tyler Hospital	Tunkhannock	64%	(a)
Moses Taylor Hospital	Scranton	64%	300+
Penn Hosp of the Univ of Penn Health Sys	Philadelphia	64%	300+
Phoenixville Hospital	Phoenixville	64%	300+
Reading Hospital Medical Center	Reading	64%	300+
The Washington Hospital	Washington	64%	300+
Western Pennsylvania Hospital	Pittsburgh	64%	300+
ACMH Hospital	Kittanning	63%	300+
Ephrata Community Hospital	Ephrata	63%	300+
Ohio Valley General Hospital	Mckees Rocks	63%	300+
Pocono Medical Center	E Stroudsburg	63%	300+
Riddle Memorial Hospital	Media	63%	300+
Sharon Regional Health System	Sharon	63%	300+
Uniontown Hospital	Uniontown	63%	300+
UPMC Presbyterian Shadyside	Pittsburgh	63%	300+
Warren General Hospital	Warren	63%	300+
Wayne Memorial Hospital	Honesdale	63%	300+
Chestnut Hill Hospital	Philadelphia	62%	300+
Community Medical Center	Scranton	62%	300+
Excela Health Latrobe Hospital	Latrobe	62%	300+
J C Blair Memorial Hospital	Huntingdon	62%	300+
Sunbury Community Hospital	Sunbury	62%	300+
Allegheny General Hospital	Pittsburgh	61%	300+
Clarion Hospital	Clarion	61%	300+
Delaware County Memorial Hospital	Drexel Hill	61%	300+
Marian Community Hospital	Carbondale	61%	300+
Millcreek Community Hospital	Erie	61%	300+
Palmerton Hospital	Palmerton	61%	300+
St Catherine Med Ctr Fountain Springs	Ashland	61%	(a)
Saint Luke's Miners Memorial Hospital	Coaldale	61%	300+
Southwest Regional Medical Center	Waynesburg	61%	300+
Gettysburg Hospital	Gettysburg	60%	300+
UPMC Bedford	Everett	60%	300+
UPMC Horizon	Greenville	60%	300+
UPMC Passavant	Pittsburgh	60%	300+
Berwick Hospital Center	Berwick	59%	300+
Heritage Valley Beaver	Beaver	59%	300+
Lock Haven Hospital	Lock Haven	59%	300+
Nazareth Hospital	Philadelphia	59%	300+
Pinnacle Health Hospitals	Harrisburg	59%	300+
Sacred Heart Hospital	Allentown	59%	300+
Temple University Hospital	Philadelphia	59%	300+
UPMC Mckeesport	McKeesport	59%	300+
Wilkes-Barre General Hospital	Wilkes-Barre	59%	300+
Alle Kiski Medical Center	Natrona	58%	300+
Carlisle Regional Medical Center	Carlisle	58%	300+
Crozer Chester Medical Center	Upland	58%	300+
Excela Health Westmoreland Reg Hosp	Greensburg	58%	300+
Brandywine Hospital	Coatesville	57%	300+
Gnaden Huetten Memorial Hospital	Lehighton	57%	300+
Jennersville Regional Hospital	West Grove	57%	300+
Mercy Suburban Hospital	Norristown	57%	300+
Schuylkill Med Ctr-East Norwegian Street	Pottsville	57%	300+
Western Penn Hosp-Forbes Reg Campus	Monroeville	57%	300+
Somerset Hospital	Somerset	56%	300+
Albert Einstein Medical Center	Philadelphia	55%	300+
Easton Hospital	Easton	55%	300+
Lansdale Hospital	Lansdale	55%	300+
Lewistown Hospital	Lewistown	55%	300+
Lower Bucks Hospital	Bristol	55%	300+
Mercy Fitzgerald Hospital	Darby	55%	300+
Pottstown Memorial Medical Center	Pottstown	55%	300+
Schuylkill Med Ctr-S Jackson Street	Pottsville	55%	300+
Bradford Regional Medical Center	Bradford	54%	300+
Clearfield Hospital	Clearfield	54%	300+
Jameson Memorial Hospital[11]	New Castle	53%	300+
UPMC Mercy	Pittsburgh	53%	300+
UPMC Northwest	Seneca	53%	300+
Montgomery Hospital	Norristown	52%	300+
Elk Regional Health Center	Saint Marys	51%	300+
Corry Memorial Hospital	Corry	50%	(a)
Roxborough Memorial Hospital	Phila	50%	300+
Hazleton General Hospital	Hazleton	49%	300+
Saint Joseph's Hospital	Philadelphia	40%	(a)

44. Meds 'Always' Explained Before Given

Hospital Name	City	Rate	Cases
Edgewood Surgical Hospital	Transfer	77%	(a)
Surgical Institute of Reading	Wyomissing	74%	300+
Coordinated Health Orthopedic Hospital	Bethlehem	73%	300+
Cancer Treatment Centers of America	Philadelphia	70%	(a)
Grove City Medical Center	Grove City	68%	300+
Soldiers and Sailors Memorial Hospital	Wellsboro	67%	300+
Waynesboro Hospital	Waynesboro	67%	300+
Charles Cole Memorial Hospital	Coudersport	66%	300+
Dubois Regional Medical Center	Dubois	66%	300+
Westfield Hospital	Allentown	66%	(a)
Grand View Hospital	Sellersville	65%	300+
Hahnemann University Hospital	Philadelphia	65%	300+
Highlands Hospital	Connellsville	65%	300+
Windber Hospital	Windber	65%	300+
Doylestown Hospital	Doylestown	64%	300+
Excela Health Frick Hospital	Mount Pleasant	64%	300+
Kane Community Hospital	Kane	64%	(a)
Mercy Tyler Hospital	Tunkhannock	64%	(a)
Muncy Valley Hospital	Muncy	64%	(a)
Hospital of Univ of Pennsylvania	Philadelphia	63%	300+
Memorial Hospital - Towanda	Towanda	63%	300+
Nason Hospital	Roaring Spring	63%	300+
Palmerton Hospital	Palmerton	63%	300+
Penn Presbyterian Medical Center	Philadelphia	63%	300+
Robert Packer Hospital	Sayre	63%	300+
Saint Luke's Hospital Bethlehem	Bethlehem	63%	300+
Saint Luke's Quakertown Hospital	Quakertown	63%	300+
Williamsport Hospital & Medical Center	Williamsport	63%	300+
Berwick Hospital Center	Berwick	62%	300+
Chester County Hospital	West Chester	62%	300+
Excela Health Westmoreland Reg Hosp	Greensburg	62%	300+
Geisinger Medical Center	Danville	62%	300+
Heritage Valley Sewickley	Sewickley	62%	300+
Indiana Regional Medical Center	Indiana	62%	300+
Miners Medical Center	Hastings	62%	(a)
Moses Taylor Hospital	Scranton	62%	300+
ACMH Hospital	Kittanning	61%	300+
Altoona Regional Health System	Altoona	61%	300+
Corry Memorial Hospital	Corry	61%	(a)
Delaware County Memorial Hospital	Drexel Hill	61%	300+
Gettysburg Hospital	Gettysburg	61%	300+
Good Samaritan Hospital	Lebanon	61%	300+
Hamot Medical Center	Erie	61%	300+
Lehigh Valley Hospital - Muhlenberg	Bethlehem	61%	300+
Main Line Hospital Paoli	Paoli	61%	300+
Mount Nittany Medical Center	State College	61%	300+
Pocono Medical Center	E Stroudsburg	61%	300+
Punxsutawney Area Hospital	Punxsutawney	61%	300+
St Catherine Med Ctr Fountain Springs	Ashland	61%	(a)
Shamokin Area Community Hospital	Coal Township	61%	300+
Sharon Regional Health System	Sharon	61%	300+
Thomas Jefferson University Hospital	Philadelphia	61%	300+
Titusville Hospital	Titusville	61%	300+
UPMC Bedford	Everett	61%	300+
Warren General Hospital	Warren	61%	300+
The Washington Hospital	Washington	61%	300+
Butler Memorial Hospital	Butler	60%	300+
Conemaugh Valley Memorial Hospital	Johnstown	60%	300+
Ellwood City Hospital	Ellwood City	60%	300+
Evangelical Community Hospital	Lewisburg	60%	300+
Excela Health Latrobe Hospital	Latrobe	60%	300+
Holy Redeemer Hospital and Medical Center	Meadowbrook	60%	300+
Lancaster Regional Medical Center	Lancaster	60%	300+
Lehigh Valley Hospital	Allentown	60%	300+
Main Line Hospital Bryn Mawr Campus	Bryn Mawr	60%	300+
Main Line Hospital Lankenau	Wynnewood	60%	300+
Marian Community Hospital	Carbondale	60%	300+
Monongahela Valley Hospital	Monongahela	60%	300+
Riddle Memorial Hospital	Media	60%	300+
Uniontown Hospital	Uniontown	60%	300+
Abington Memorial Hospital	Abington	59%	300+
Canonsburg General Hospital	Canonsburg	59%	300+
Chambersburg Hospital	Chambersburg	59%	300+
Clearfield Hospital	Clearfield	59%	300+
Crozer Chester Medical Center	Upland	59%	300+
Heart of Lancaster Regional Medical Center	Lititz	59%	300+
Jeanes Hospital	Philadelphia	59%	300+
Jennersville Regional Hospital	West Grove	59%	300+
Lansdale Hospital	Lansdale	59%	300+
Lower Bucks Hospital	Bristol	59%	300+
Meadville Medical Center	Meadville	59%	300+
Saint Mary Medical Center	Langhorne	59%	300+
UPMC Mckeesport	McKeesport	59%	300+
Wayne Memorial Hospital	Honesdale	59%	300+
York Hospital	York	59%	300+
Aria Health	Philadelphia	58%	300+
Elk Regional Health Center	Saint Marys	58%	300+
Gnaden Huetten Memorial Hospital	Lehighton	58%	300+
J C Blair Memorial Hospital	Huntingdon	58%	300+
Mercy Suburban Hospital	Norristown	58%	300+
Milton S Hershey Medical Center	Hershey	58%	300+
Penn Hosp of the Univ of Penn Health Sys	Philadelphia	58%	300+
Saint Luke's Miners Memorial Hospital	Coaldale	58%	300+
Western Pennsylvania Hospital	Pittsburgh	58%	300+
Bloomsburg Hospital	Bloomsburg	57%	300+
Ephrata Community Hospital	Ephrata	57%	300+
Jefferson Regional Medical Center	Pittsburgh	57%	300+
Lock Haven Hospital	Lock Haven	57%	300+
Millcreek Community Hospital	Erie	57%	300+
Montgomery Hospital	Norristown	57%	300+
Phoenixville Hospital	Phoenixville	57%	300+
Saint Clair Memorial Hospital	Pittsburgh	57%	300+
Southwest Regional Medical Center	Waynesburg	57%	300+
UPMC Saint Margaret	Pittsburgh	57%	300+
Albert Einstein Medical Center	Philadelphia	56%	300+
Community Medical Center	Scranton	56%	300+
Geisinger Wyoming Valley Medical Center	Wilkes-Barre	56%	300+
Jameson Memorial Hospital[11]	New Castle	56%	300+
Lancaster General Hospital	Lancaster	56%	300+
Memorial Hospital York	York	56%	300+
Nazareth Hospital	Philadelphia	56%	300+
Pinnacle Health Hospitals	Harrisburg	56%	300+

NOTE: Hospital profiles are in alphabetical order by state, then city, then hospital within the city; Rankings exclude hospitals with less than 25 cases except for patient surveys which excludes hospitals with less than 100 cases; (a) 100–299 cases; (1) The number of cases is too small to be sure how well a hospital is performing; (2) The hospital indicated that the data submitted for this measure were based on a sample of cases; (3) Data was collected during a shorter time period (fewer quarters) than the maximum possible time for this measure; (4) Suppressed for one or more quarters by CMS; (5) No data is available from the hospital for this measure; (6) Fewer than 100 patients completed the HCAHPS survey. Use these rates with caution, as the number of surveys may be too low to reliably assess hospital performance; (7) Survey results are based on less than 12 months of data; (8) Survey results are not available for this reporting period; (9) No or very few patients were eligible for the HCAHPS survey. The scores shown, if any, reflect a very small number of surveys; (10) A state average was not calculated because too few hospitals in the state submitted data; (11) There were discrepancies in the data collection process; Please refer to the User's Guide for a full explanation of data.

Sunbury Community Hospital	Sunbury	56%	300+
Temple University Hospital	Philadelphia	56%	300+
UPMC Horizon	Greenville	56%	300+
UPMC Presbyterian Shadyside	Pittsburgh	56%	300+
Wilkes-Barre General Hospital	Wilkes-Barre	56%	300+
Alle Kiski Medical Center	Natrona	55%	300+
Allegheny General Hospital	Pittsburgh	55%	300+
Holy Spirit Hospital	Camp Hill	55%	300+
Ohio Valley General Hospital	Mckees Rocks	55%	300+
Reading Hospital Medical Center	Reading	55%	300+
Saint Vincent Health Center	Erie	55%	300+
Schuylkill Med Ctr-East Norwegian Street	Pottsville	55%	300+
Somerset Hospital	Somerset	55%	300+
Western Penn Hosp-Forbes Reg Campus	Monroeville	55%	300+
Clarion Hospital	Clarion	54%	300+
Easton Hospital	Easton	54%	300+
Magee Womens Hosp of UPMC Health Sys	Pittsburgh	54%	300+
Mercy Hospital Scranton	Scranton	54%	300+
Pottstown Memorial Medical Center	Pottstown	54%	300+
Roxborough Memorial Hospital	Phila	54%	300+
Sacred Heart Hospital	Allentown	54%	300+
Saint Joseph Medical Center	Reading	54%	300+
Bradford Regional Medical Center	Bradford	53%	300+
Carlisle Regional Medical Center	Carlisle	53%	300+
Chestnut Hill Hospital	Philadelphia	53%	300+
Hazleton General Hospital	Hazleton	53%	300+
Heritage Valley Beaver	Beaver	53%	300+
Schuylkill Med Ctr-S Jackson Street	Pottsville	53%	300+
Hanover Hospital	Hanover	52%	300+
Mercy Fitzgerald Hospital	Darby	52%	300+
UPMC Northwest	Seneca	52%	300+
UPMC Passavant	Pittsburgh	52%	300+
Lewistown Hospital	Lewistown	51%	300+
UPMC Mercy	Pittsburgh	51%	300+
Brandywine Hospital	Coatesville	50%	300+
Saint Joseph's Hospital	Philadelphia	45%	(a)

45. Nurses 'Always' Communicated Well

Hospital Name	City	Rate	Cases
Coordinated Health Orthopedic Hospital	Bethlehem	92%	300+
Edgewood Surgical Hospital	Transfer	88%	(a)
Surgical Institute of Reading	Wyomissing	88%	300+
Miners Medical Center	Hastings	86%	(a)
Doylestown Hospital	Doylestown	84%	300+
Shamokin Area Community Hospital	Coal Township	83%	300+
Soldiers and Sailors Memorial Hospital	Wellsboro	83%	300+
Cancer Treatment Centers of America	Philadelphia	82%	(a)
Excela Health Frick Hospital	Mount Pleasant	82%	300+
Highlands Hospital	Connellsville	82%	300+
Muncy Valley Hospital	Muncy	82%	(a)
Saint Luke's Quakertown Hospital	Quakertown	82%	300+
Waynesboro Hospital	Waynesboro	82%	300+
Altoona Regional Health System	Altoona	81%	300+
Indiana Regional Medical Center	Indiana	81%	300+
Memorial Hospital - Towanda	Towanda	81%	300+
Titusville Hospital	Titusville	81%	300+
Westfield Hospital	Allentown	81%	(a)
Windber Hospital	Windber	81%	300+
Canonsburg General Hospital	Canonsburg	80%	300+
Charles Cole Memorial Hospital	Coudersport	80%	300+
Heritage Valley Sewickley	Sewickley	80%	300+
Jefferson Regional Medical Center	Pittsburgh	80%	300+
Main Line Hospital Paoli	Paoli	80%	300+
Monongahela Valley Hospital	Monongahela	80%	300+
Williamsport Hospital & Medical Center	Williamsport	80%	300+
Bloomsburg Hospital	Bloomsburg	79%	300+
Dubois Regional Medical Center	Dubois	79%	300+
Excela Health Latrobe Hospital	Latrobe	79%	300+
Geisinger Medical Center	Danville	79%	300+
Hamot Medical Center	Erie	79%	300+
Lehigh Valley Hospital	Allentown	79%	300+
Lehigh Valley Hospital - Muhlenberg	Bethlehem	79%	300+
Main Line Hospital Bryn Mawr Campus	Bryn Mawr	79%	300+
Nason Hospital	Roaring Spring	79%	300+
Robert Packer Hospital	Sayre	79%	300+
Saint Clair Memorial Hospital	Pittsburgh	79%	300+
The Washington Hospital	Washington	79%	300+
ACMH Hospital	Kittanning	78%	300+
Aria Health	Philadelphia	78%	300+
Chester County Hospital	West Chester	78%	300+
Evangelical Community Hospital	Lewisburg	78%	300+
Grand View Hospital	Sellersville	78%	300+
Hahnemann University Hospital	Philadelphia	78%	300+
Holy Redeemer Hospital and Medical Center	Meadowbrook	78%	300+
J C Blair Memorial Hospital	Huntingdon	78%	300+
Kane Community Hospital	Kane	78%	(a)
Punxsutawney Area Hospital	Punxsutawney	78%	300+
Saint Luke's Hospital Bethlehem	Bethlehem	78%	300+
Warren General Hospital	Warren	78%	300+
Abington Memorial Hospital	Abington	77%	300+
Berwick Hospital Center	Berwick	77%	300+
Butler Memorial Hospital	Butler	77%	300+
Chambersburg Hospital	Chambersburg	77%	300+
Conemaugh Valley Memorial Hospital	Johnstown	77%	300+
Ellwood City Hospital	Ellwood City	77%	300+
Ephrata Community Hospital	Ephrata	77%	300+
Good Samaritan Hospital	Lebanon	77%	300+
Grove City Medical Center	Grove City	77%	300+
Main Line Hospital Lankenau	Wynnewood	77%	300+
Meadville Medical Center	Meadville	77%	300+
Penn Presbyterian Medical Center	Philadelphia	77%	300+
Riddle Memorial Hospital	Media	77%	300+
Saint Luke's Miners Memorial Hospital	Coaldale	77%	300+
Saint Mary Medical Center	Langhorne	77%	300+
Southwest Regional Medical Center	Waynesburg	77%	300+
Thomas Jefferson University Hospital	Philadelphia	77%	300+
Wayne Memorial Hospital	Honesdale	77%	300+
Hospital of Univ of Pennsylvania	Philadelphia	76%	300+
Moses Taylor Hospital	Scranton	76%	300+
Mount Nittany Medical Center	State College	76%	300+
Pocono Medical Center	E Stroudsburg	76%	300+
St Catherine Med Ctr Fountain Springs	Ashland	76%	(a)
Sharon Regional Health System	Sharon	76%	300+
Uniontown Hospital	Uniontown	76%	300+
UPMC Bedford	Everett	76%	300+
Wilkes-Barre General Hospital	Wilkes-Barre	76%	300+
York Hospital	York	76%	300+
Community Medical Center	Scranton	75%	300+
Delaware County Memorial Hospital	Drexel Hill	75%	300+
Gettysburg Hospital	Gettysburg	75%	300+
Lancaster Regional Medical Center	Lancaster	75%	300+
Marian Community Hospital	Carbondale	75%	300+
Mercy Tyler Hospital	Tunkhannock	75%	(a)
Montgomery Hospital	Norristown	75%	300+
Saint Joseph Medical Center	Reading	75%	300+
Sunbury Community Hospital	Sunbury	75%	300+
Western Pennsylvania Hospital	Pittsburgh	75%	300+
Bradford Regional Medical Center	Bradford	74%	300+
Excela Health Westmoreland Reg Hosp	Greensburg	74%	300+
Geisinger Wyoming Valley Medical Center	Wilkes-Barre	74%	300+
Gnaden Huetten Memorial Hospital	Lehighton	74%	300+
Heritage Valley Beaver	Beaver	74%	300+
Jeanes Hospital	Philadelphia	74%	300+
Jennersville Regional Hospital	West Grove	74%	300+
Lancaster General Hospital	Lancaster	74%	300+
Lock Haven Hospital	Lock Haven	74%	300+
Lower Bucks Hospital	Bristol	74%	300+
Milton S Hershey Medical Center	Hershey	74%	300+
Palmerton Hospital	Palmerton	74%	300+
UPMC Mckeesport	McKeesport	74%	300+
UPMC Saint Margaret	Pittsburgh	74%	300+
Carlisle Regional Medical Center	Carlisle	73%	300+
Chestnut Hill Hospital	Philadelphia	73%	300+
Corry Memorial Hospital	Corry	73%	(a)
Crozer Chester Medical Center	Upland	73%	300+
Jameson Memorial Hospital[11]	New Castle	73%	300+
Lansdale Hospital	Lansdale	73%	300+
Ohio Valley General Hospital	Mckees Rocks	73%	300+
Phoenixville Hospital	Phoenixville	73%	300+
Reading Hospital Medical Center	Reading	73%	300+
Saint Vincent Health Center	Erie	73%	300+
Schuylkill Med Ctr-East Norwegian Street	Pottsville	73%	300+
UPMC Presbyterian Shadyside	Pittsburgh	73%	300+
Alle Kiski Medical Center	Natrona	72%	300+
Elk Regional Health Center	Saint Marys	72%	300+
Heart of Lancaster Regional Medical Center	Lititz	72%	300+
Holy Spirit Hospital	Camp Hill	72%	300+
Mercy Hospital Scranton	Scranton	72%	300+
Millcreek Community Hospital	Erie	72%	300+
Pinnacle Health Hospitals	Harrisburg	72%	300+
Somerset Hospital	Somerset	72%	300+
Allegheny General Hospital	Pittsburgh	71%	300+
Brandywine Hospital	Coatesville	71%	300+
Clarion Hospital	Clarion	71%	300+
Clearfield Hospital	Clearfield	71%	300+
Easton Hospital	Easton	71%	300+
Hanover Hospital	Hanover	71%	300+
Hazleton General Hospital	Hazleton	71%	300+
Mercy Suburban Hospital	Norristown	71%	300+
Nazareth Hospital	Philadelphia	71%	300+
Sacred Heart Hospital	Allentown	71%	300+
Schuylkill Med Ctr-S Jackson Street	Pottsville	71%	300+
UPMC Horizon	Greenville	71%	300+
Western Penn Hosp-Forbes Reg Campus	Monroeville	71%	300+
Lewistown Hospital	Lewistown	70%	300+
Magee Womens Hosp of UPMC Health Sys	Pittsburgh	70%	300+
Memorial Hospital York	York	70%	300+
Mercy Fitzgerald Hospital	Darby	70%	300+
Penn Hosp of the Univ of Penn Health Sys	Philadelphia	70%	300+
Pottstown Memorial Medical Center	Pottstown	70%	300+
Roxborough Memorial Hospital	Phila	70%	300+
Temple University Hospital	Philadelphia	69%	300+
UPMC Northwest	Seneca	69%	300+
UPMC Passavant	Pittsburgh	69%	300+
Albert Einstein Medical Center	Philadelphia	67%	300+
UPMC Mercy	Pittsburgh	64%	300+
Saint Joseph's Hospital	Philadelphia	56%	(a)

46. Pain 'Always' Well Controlled

Hospital Name	City	Rate	Cases
Cancer Treatment Centers of America	Philadelphia	80%	(a)
Coordinated Health Orthopedic Hospital	Bethlehem	80%	300+
Edgewood Surgical Hospital	Transfer	80%	(a)
Surgical Institute of Reading	Wyomissing	80%	300+
Miners Medical Center	Hastings	79%	(a)
Doylestown Hospital	Doylestown	78%	300+
Highlands Hospital	Connellsville	78%	300+
Meadville Medical Center	Meadville	75%	300+
Memorial Hospital - Towanda	Towanda	75%	300+
St Catherine Med Ctr Fountain Springs	Ashland	75%	(a)
Soldiers and Sailors Memorial Hospital	Wellsboro	75%	300+
Titusville Hospital	Titusville	75%	300+
Wayne Memorial Hospital	Honesdale	75%	300+
Nason Hospital	Roaring Spring	74%	300+
Waynesboro Hospital	Waynesboro	74%	300+
Dubois Regional Medical Center	Dubois	73%	300+
Heritage Valley Sewickley	Sewickley	73%	300+
Main Line Hospital Paoli	Paoli	73%	300+
Mount Nittany Medical Center	State College	73%	300+
Muncy Valley Hospital	Muncy	73%	(a)
Altoona Regional Health System	Altoona	72%	300+
Charles Cole Memorial Hospital	Coudersport	72%	300+
Excela Health Frick Hospital	Mount Pleasant	72%	300+
Grove City Medical Center	Grove City	72%	300+
Hahnemann University Hospital	Philadelphia	72%	300+
Hamot Medical Center	Erie	72%	300+
Jeanes Hospital	Philadelphia	72%	300+
Jefferson Regional Medical Center	Pittsburgh	72%	300+
Penn Presbyterian Medical Center	Philadelphia	72%	300+
Pocono Medical Center	E Stroudsburg	72%	300+
Robert Packer Hospital	Sayre	72%	300+
Saint Clair Memorial Hospital	Pittsburgh	72%	300+
Shamokin Area Community Hospital	Coal Township	72%	300+
Aria Health	Philadelphia	71%	300+
Chester County Hospital	West Chester	71%	300+
Ellwood City Hospital	Ellwood City	71%	300+
Evangelical Community Hospital	Lewisburg	71%	300+
J C Blair Memorial Hospital	Huntingdon	71%	300+
Lower Bucks Hospital	Bristol	71%	300+
Palmerton Hospital	Palmerton	71%	300+
Punxsutawney Area Hospital	Punxsutawney	71%	300+
Saint Luke's Hospital Bethlehem	Bethlehem	71%	300+
Saint Luke's Quakertown Hospital	Quakertown	71%	300+
Saint Mary Medical Center	Langhorne	71%	300+
Warren General Hospital	Warren	71%	300+
Williamsport Hospital & Medical Center	Williamsport	71%	300+
Windber Hospital	Windber	71%	300+
Bloomsburg Hospital	Bloomsburg	70%	300+
Butler Memorial Hospital	Butler	70%	300+
Good Samaritan Hospital	Lebanon	70%	300+
Hospital of Univ of Pennsylvania	Philadelphia	70%	300+
Lehigh Valley Hospital	Allentown	70%	300+
Main Line Hospital Bryn Mawr Campus	Bryn Mawr	70%	300+
Main Line Hospital Lankenau	Wynnewood	70%	300+
Sharon Regional Health System	Sharon	70%	300+
Southwest Regional Medical Center	Waynesburg	70%	300+
Thomas Jefferson University Hospital	Philadelphia	70%	300+
Uniontown Hospital	Uniontown	70%	300+
The Washington Hospital	Washington	70%	300+
Westfield Hospital	Allentown	70%	(a)
Bradford Regional Medical Center	Bradford	69%	300+
Canonsburg General Hospital	Canonsburg	69%	300+
Chambersburg Hospital	Chambersburg	69%	300+
Community Medical Center	Scranton	69%	300+
Conemaugh Valley Memorial Hospital	Johnstown	69%	300+
Excela Health Westmoreland Reg Hosp	Greensburg	69%	300+
Indiana Regional Medical Center	Indiana	69%	300+
Lancaster Regional Medical Center	Lancaster	69%	300+
Lock Haven Hospital	Lock Haven	69%	300+
Mercy Tyler Hospital	Tunkhannock	69%	(a)
Monongahela Valley Hospital	Monongahela	69%	300+
Riddle Memorial Hospital	Media	69%	300+
Saint Joseph Medical Center	Reading	69%	300+
ACMH Hospital	Kittanning	68%	300+
Berwick Hospital Center	Berwick	68%	300+
Excela Health Latrobe Hospital	Latrobe	68%	300+
Geisinger Medical Center	Danville	68%	300+
Grand View Hospital	Sellersville	68%	300+
Heritage Valley Beaver	Beaver	68%	300+
Holy Redeemer Hospital and Medical Center	Meadowbrook	68%	300+
Lehigh Valley Hospital - Muhlenberg	Bethlehem	68%	300+

NOTE: Hospital profiles are in alphabetical order by state, then city, then hospital within the city; Rankings exclude hospitals with less than 25 cases except for patient surveys which excludes hospitals with less than 100 cases; (a) 100–299 cases; (1) The number of cases is too small to be sure how well a hospital is performing; (2) The hospital indicated that the data submitted for this measure were based on a sample of cases; (3) Data was collected during a shorter time period (fewer quarters) than the maximum possible time for this measure; (4) Suppressed for one or more quarters by CMS; (5) No data is available from the hospital for this measure; (6) Fewer than 100 patients completed the HCAHPS survey. Use these rates with caution, as the number of surveys may be too low to reliably assess hospital performance; (7) Survey results are based on less than 12 months of data; (8) Survey results are not available for this reporting period; (9) No or very few patients were eligible for the HCAHPS survey. The scores shown, if any, reflect a very small number of surveys; (10) A state average was not calculated because too few hospitals in the state submitted data; (11) There were discrepancies in the data collection process; Please refer to the User's Guide for a full explanation of data.

Mercy Hospital Scranton	Scranton	68%	300+
Milton S Hershey Medical Center	Hershey	68%	300+
Wilkes-Barre General Hospital	Wilkes-Barre	68%	300+
York Hospital	York	68%	300+
Carlisle Regional Medical Center	Carlisle	67%	300+
Chestnut Hill Hospital	Philadelphia	67%	300+
Clarion Hospital	Clarion	67%	300+
Crozer Chester Medical Center	Upland	67%	300+
Easton Hospital	Easton	67%	300+
Elk Regional Health Center	Saint Marys	67%	300+
Gettysburg Hospital	Gettysburg	67%	300+
Gnaden Huetten Memorial Hospital	Lehighton	67%	300+
Hanover Hospital	Hanover	67%	300+
Jameson Memorial Hospital[11]	New Castle	67%	300+
Jennersville Regional Hospital	West Grove	67%	300+
Kane Community Hospital	Kane	67%	(a)
Montgomery Hospital	Norristown	67%	300+
Pinnacle Health Hospitals	Harrisburg	67%	300+
Reading Hospital Medical Center	Reading	67%	300+
Saint Luke's Miners Memorial Hospital	Coaldale	67%	300+
UPMC Bedford	Everett	67%	300+
UPMC Mckeesport	McKeesport	67%	300+
Western Pennsylvania Hospital	Pittsburgh	67%	300+
Abington Memorial Hospital	Abington	66%	300+
Ephrata Community Hospital	Ephrata	66%	300+
Hazleton General Hospital	Hazleton	66%	300+
Holy Spirit Hospital	Camp Hill	66%	300+
Lancaster General Hospital	Lancaster	66%	300+
Lansdale Hospital	Lansdale	66%	300+
Marian Community Hospital	Carbondale	66%	300+
Moses Taylor Hospital	Scranton	66%	300+
Nazareth Hospital	Philadelphia	66%	300+
Phoenixville Hospital	Phoenixville	66%	300+
Schuylkill Med Ctr-East Norwegian Street	Pottsville	66%	300+
Sunbury Community Hospital	Sunbury	66%	300+
UPMC Northwest	Seneca	66%	300+
UPMC Saint Margaret	Pittsburgh	66%	300+
Western Penn Hosp-Forbes Reg Campus	Monroeville	66%	300+
Delaware County Memorial Hospital	Drexel Hill	65%	300+
Geisinger Wyoming Valley Medical Center	Wilkes-Barre	65%	300+
Heart of Lancaster Regional Medical Center	Lititz	65%	300+
Mercy Suburban Hospital	Norristown	65%	300+
Penn Hosp of the Univ of Penn Health Sys	Philadelphia	65%	300+
Pottstown Memorial Medical Center	Pottstown	65%	300+
UPMC Passavant	Pittsburgh	65%	300+
UPMC Presbyterian Shadyside	Pittsburgh	65%	300+
Albert Einstein Medical Center	Philadelphia	64%	300+
Brandywine Hospital	Coatesville	64%	300+
Clearfield Hospital	Clearfield	64%	300+
Millcreek Community Hospital	Erie	64%	300+
Ohio Valley General Hospital	Mckees Rocks	64%	300+
Saint Vincent Health Center	Erie	64%	300+
Somerset Hospital	Somerset	64%	300+
UPMC Horizon	Greenville	64%	300+
Magee Womens Hosp of UPMC Health Sys	Pittsburgh	63%	300+
Memorial Hospital York	York	63%	300+
Schuylkill Med Ctr-S Jackson Street	Pottsville	63%	300+
Corry Memorial Hospital	Corry	62%	(a)
Sacred Heart Hospital	Allentown	62%	300+
Temple University Hospital	Philadelphia	62%	300+
Lewistown Hospital	Lewistown	61%	300+
Mercy Fitzgerald Hospital	Darby	61%	300+
Alle Kiski Medical Center	Natrona	60%	300+
Allegheny General Hospital	Pittsburgh	60%	300+
Roxborough Memorial Hospital	Phila	60%	300+
Saint Joseph's Hospital	Philadelphia	59%	(a)
UPMC Mercy	Pittsburgh	58%	300+

47. Room and Bathroom 'Always' Clean

Hospital Name	City	Rate	Cases
Shamokin Area Community Hospital	Coal Township	89%	300+
Soldiers and Sailors Memorial Hospital	Wellsboro	86%	300+
Coordinated Health Orthopedic Hospital	Bethlehem	85%	300+
Surgical Institute of Reading	Wyomissing	85%	300+
Memorial Hospital - Towanda	Towanda	84%	300+
Cancer Treatment Centers of America	Philadelphia	83%	(a)
St Catherine Med Ctr Fountain Springs	Ashland	83%	(a)
Titusville Hospital	Titusville	83%	300+
Grand View Hospital	Sellersville	82%	300+
Highlands Hospital	Connellsville	82%	300+
Windber Hospital	Windber	82%	300+
Edgewood Surgical Hospital	Transfer	81%	(a)
Muncy Valley Hospital	Muncy	81%	(a)
Nason Hospital	Roaring Spring	81%	300+
Westfield Hospital	Allentown	81%	(a)
Lancaster Regional Medical Center	Lancaster	80%	300+
Saint Luke's Miners Memorial Hospital	Coaldale	79%	300+
Grove City Medical Center	Grove City	78%	300+
Marian Community Hospital	Carbondale	78%	300+
UPMC Bedford	Everett	78%	300+
The Washington Hospital	Washington	78%	300+
Good Samaritan Hospital	Lebanon	77%	300+
J C Blair Memorial Hospital	Huntingdon	77%	300+
Kane Community Hospital	Kane	77%	(a)
Meadville Medical Center	Meadville	77%	300+
Miners Medical Center	Hastings	77%	(a)
Charles Cole Memorial Hospital	Coudersport	76%	300+
Ellwood City Hospital	Ellwood City	76%	300+
Excela Health Frick Hospital	Mount Pleasant	76%	300+
Mercy Tyler Hospital	Tunkhannock	76%	(a)
Monongahela Valley Hospital	Monongahela	76%	300+
Mount Nittany Medical Center	State College	76%	300+
Altoona Regional Health System	Altoona	75%	300+
Carlisle Regional Medical Center	Carlisle	75%	300+
Chambersburg Hospital	Chambersburg	75%	300+
Geisinger Medical Center	Danville	75%	300+
Hazleton General Hospital	Hazleton	75%	300+
Indiana Regional Medical Center	Indiana	75%	300+
Robert Packer Hospital	Sayre	75%	300+
Conemaugh Valley Memorial Hospital	Johnstown	74%	300+
Doylestown Hospital	Doylestown	74%	300+
Evangelical Community Hospital	Lewisburg	74%	300+
Hanover Hospital	Hanover	74%	300+
Lewistown Hospital	Lewistown	74%	300+
Palmerton Hospital	Palmerton	74%	300+
Alle Kiski Medical Center	Natrona	73%	300+
Gnaden Huetten Memorial Hospital	Lehighton	73%	300+
Jameson Memorial Hospital[11]	New Castle	73%	300+
Main Line Hospital Paoli	Paoli	73%	300+
Somerset Hospital	Somerset	73%	300+
Wayne Memorial Hospital	Honesdale	73%	300+
Waynesboro Hospital	Waynesboro	73%	300+
Elk Regional Health Center	Saint Marys	72%	300+
Heart of Lancaster Regional Medical Center	Lititz	72%	300+
Lehigh Valley Hospital - Muhlenberg	Bethlehem	72%	300+
Punxsutawney Area Hospital	Punxsutawney	72%	300+
Warren General Hospital	Warren	72%	300+
Berwick Hospital Center	Berwick	71%	300+
Bloomsburg Hospital	Bloomsburg	71%	300+
Corry Memorial Hospital	Corry	71%	(a)
Jefferson Regional Medical Center	Pittsburgh	71%	300+
Millcreek Community Hospital	Erie	71%	300+
Pocono Medical Center	E Stroudsburg	71%	300+
Saint Luke's Hospital Bethlehem	Bethlehem	71%	300+
Saint Mary Medical Center	Langhorne	71%	300+
Schuylkill Med Ctr-East Norwegian Street	Pottsville	71%	300+
Schuylkill Med Ctr-S Jackson Street	Pottsville	71%	300+
Uniontown Hospital	Uniontown	71%	300+
Williamsport Hospital & Medical Center	Williamsport	71%	300+
Aria Health	Philadelphia	70%	300+
Hamot Medical Center	Erie	70%	300+
Lancaster General Hospital	Lancaster	70%	300+
Moses Taylor Hospital	Scranton	70%	300+
Nazareth Hospital	Philadelphia	70%	300+
Saint Luke's Quakertown Hospital	Quakertown	70%	300+
UPMC Northwest	Seneca	70%	300+
Clearfield Hospital	Clearfield	69%	300+
Community Medical Center	Scranton	69%	300+
Ephrata Community Hospital	Ephrata	69%	300+
Saint Clair Memorial Hospital	Pittsburgh	69%	300+
Sharon Regional Health System	Sharon	69%	300+
UPMC Mckeesport	McKeesport	69%	300+
Hahnemann University Hospital	Philadelphia	68%	300+
Lock Haven Hospital	Lock Haven	68%	300+
Memorial Hospital York	York	68%	300+
Ohio Valley General Hospital	Mckees Rocks	68%	300+
Sunbury Community Hospital	Sunbury	68%	300+
UPMC Horizon	Greenville	68%	300+
Bradford Regional Medical Center	Bradford	67%	300+
Canonsburg General Hospital	Canonsburg	67%	300+
Chester County Hospital	West Chester	67%	300+
Dubois Regional Medical Center	Dubois	67%	300+
Geisinger Wyoming Valley Medical Center	Wilkes-Barre	67%	300+
Heritage Valley Sewickley	Sewickley	67%	300+
Jeanes Hospital	Philadelphia	67%	300+
Penn Presbyterian Medical Center	Philadelphia	67%	300+
Sacred Heart Hospital	Allentown	67%	300+
Saint Joseph Medical Center	Reading	67%	300+
Excela Health Westmoreland Reg Hosp	Greensburg	66%	300+
Gettysburg Hospital	Gettysburg	66%	300+
Heritage Valley Beaver	Beaver	66%	300+
Holy Redeemer Hospital and Medical Center	Meadowbrook	66%	300+
Holy Spirit Hospital	Camp Hill	66%	300+
Jennersville Regional Hospital	West Grove	66%	300+
Thomas Jefferson University Hospital	Philadelphia	66%	300+
Chestnut Hill Hospital	Philadelphia	65%	300+
Clarion Hospital	Clarion	65%	300+
Delaware County Memorial Hospital	Drexel Hill	65%	300+
Easton Hospital	Easton	65%	300+
Lower Bucks Hospital	Bristol	65%	300+
Main Line Hospital Bryn Mawr Campus	Bryn Mawr	65%	300+
Main Line Hospital Lankenau	Wynnewood	65%	300+
Milton S Hershey Medical Center	Hershey	65%	300+
ACMH Hospital	Kittanning	64%	300+
Butler Memorial Hospital	Butler	64%	300+
Crozer Chester Medical Center	Upland	64%	300+
Lansdale Hospital	Lansdale	64%	300+
Penn Hosp of the Univ of Penn Health Sys	Philadelphia	64%	300+
Southwest Regional Medical Center	Waynesburg	64%	300+
Temple University Hospital	Philadelphia	64%	300+
Western Pennsylvania Hospital	Pittsburgh	64%	300+
Wilkes-Barre General Hospital	Wilkes-Barre	64%	300+
Magee Womens Hosp of UPMC Health Sys	Pittsburgh	63%	300+
Lehigh Valley Hospital	Allentown	62%	300+
Mercy Fitzgerald Hospital	Darby	62%	300+
Phoenixville Hospital	Phoenixville	62%	300+
Reading Hospital Medical Center	Reading	62%	300+
Riddle Memorial Hospital	Media	62%	300+
Brandywine Hospital	Coatesville	61%	300+
Excela Health Latrobe Hospital	Latrobe	61%	300+
Saint Joseph's Hospital	Philadelphia	61%	(a)
UPMC Saint Margaret	Pittsburgh	61%	300+
Abington Memorial Hospital	Abington	60%	300+
Albert Einstein Medical Center	Philadelphia	60%	300+
Allegheny General Hospital	Pittsburgh	60%	300+
Montgomery Hospital	Norristown	60%	300+
Pinnacle Health Hospitals	Harrisburg	60%	300+
Pottstown Memorial Medical Center	Pottstown	60%	300+
Western Penn Hosp-Forbes Reg Campus	Monroeville	60%	300+
Mercy Hospital Scranton	Scranton	57%	300+
Mercy Suburban Hospital	Norristown	57%	300+
Saint Vincent Health Center	Erie	57%	300+
UPMC Presbyterian Shadyside	Pittsburgh	57%	300+
Roxborough Memorial Hospital	Phila	56%	300+
York Hospital	York	56%	300+
Hospital of Univ of Pennsylvania	Philadelphia	55%	300+
UPMC Mercy	Pittsburgh	55%	300+
UPMC Passavant	Pittsburgh	55%	300+

48. Timely Help 'Always' Received

Hospital Name	City	Rate	Cases
Coordinated Health Orthopedic Hospital	Bethlehem	90%	300+
Edgewood Surgical Hospital	Transfer	84%	(a)
Surgical Institute of Reading	Wyomissing	84%	300+
Miners Medical Center	Hastings	83%	(a)
Westfield Hospital	Allentown	82%	(a)
Soldiers and Sailors Memorial Hospital	Wellsboro	79%	300+
Shamokin Area Community Hospital	Coal Township	78%	300+
Waynesboro Hospital	Waynesboro	78%	300+
Memorial Hospital - Towanda	Towanda	77%	300+
Highlands Hospital	Connellsville	75%	300+
Doylestown Hospital	Doylestown	74%	300+
Muncy Valley Hospital	Muncy	74%	(a)
Titusville Hospital	Titusville	74%	300+
Charles Cole Memorial Hospital	Coudersport	73%	300+
Cancer Treatment Centers of America	Philadelphia	72%	(a)
Windber Hospital	Windber	72%	300+
Bradford Regional Medical Center	Bradford	70%	300+
Indiana Regional Medical Center	Indiana	70%	300+
J C Blair Memorial Hospital	Huntingdon	70%	300+
Lancaster Regional Medical Center	Lancaster	70%	300+
Nason Hospital	Roaring Spring	70%	300+
Punxsutawney Area Hospital	Punxsutawney	70%	300+
St Catherine Med Ctr Fountain Springs	Ashland	70%	(a)
Evangelical Community Hospital	Lewisburg	69%	300+
Excela Health Frick Hospital	Mount Pleasant	69%	300+
Excela Health Latrobe Hospital	Latrobe	69%	300+
Grand View Hospital	Sellersville	69%	300+
Mercy Tyler Hospital	Tunkhannock	69%	(a)
ACMH Hospital	Kittanning	68%	300+
Bloomsburg Hospital	Bloomsburg	68%	300+
Geisinger Medical Center	Danville	68%	300+
Grove City Medical Center	Grove City	68%	300+
Lock Haven Hospital	Lock Haven	68%	300+
Marian Community Hospital	Carbondale	68%	300+
Saint Mary Medical Center	Langhorne	68%	300+
Wayne Memorial Hospital	Honesdale	68%	300+
Altoona Regional Health System	Altoona	67%	300+
Aria Health	Philadelphia	67%	300+
Chester County Hospital	West Chester	67%	300+
Ellwood City Hospital	Ellwood City	67%	300+
Meadville Medical Center	Meadville	67%	300+
Monongahela Valley Hospital	Monongahela	67%	300+
Sharon Regional Health System	Sharon	67%	300+
Thomas Jefferson University Hospital	Philadelphia	67%	300+
Warren General Hospital	Warren	67%	300+
Williamsport Hospital & Medical Center	Williamsport	67%	300+
York Hospital	York	67%	300+
Dubois Regional Medical Center	Dubois	66%	300+
Hamot Medical Center	Erie	66%	300+
Heritage Valley Sewickley	Sewickley	66%	300+

NOTE: Hospital profiles are in alphabetical order by state, then city, then hospital within the city; Rankings exclude hospitals with less than 25 cases except for patient surveys which excludes hospitals with less than 100 cases; (a) 100–299 cases; (1) The number of cases is too small to be sure how well a hospital is performing; (2) The hospital indicated that the data submitted for this measure were based on a sample of cases; (3) Data was collected during a shorter time period (fewer quarters) than the maximum possible time for this measure; (4) Suppressed for one or more quarters by CMS; (5) No data is available from the hospital for this measure; (6) Fewer than 100 patients completed the HCAHPS survey. Use these rates with caution, as the number of surveys may be too low to reliably assess hospital performance; (7) Survey results are based on less than 12 months of data; (8) Survey results are not available for this reporting period; (9) No or very few patients were eligible for the HCAHPS survey. The scores shown, if any, reflect a very small number of surveys; (10) A state average was not calculated because too few hospitals in the state submitted data; (11) There were discrepancies in the data collection process; Please refer to the User's Guide for a full explanation of data.

Mount Nittany Medical Center	State College	66%	300+
Robert Packer Hospital	Sayre	66%	300+
Sunbury Community Hospital	Sunbury	66%	300+
Canonsburg General Hospital	Canonsburg	65%	300+
Chambersburg Hospital	Chambersburg	65%	300+
Clarion Hospital	Clarion	65%	300+
Kane Community Hospital	Kane	65%	(a)
Ohio Valley General Hospital	Mckees Rocks	65%	300+
Riddle Memorial Hospital	Media	65%	300+
Saint Luke's Quakertown Hospital	Quakertown	65%	300+
The Washington Hospital	Washington	65%	300+
Community Medical Center	Scranton	64%	300+
Excela Health Westmoreland Reg Hosp	Greensburg	64%	300+
Gettysburg Hospital	Gettysburg	64%	300+
Hahnemann University Hospital	Philadelphia	64%	300+
Montgomery Hospital	Norristown	64%	300+
Saint Clair Memorial Hospital	Pittsburgh	64%	300+
Saint Luke's Hospital Bethlehem	Bethlehem	64%	300+
Schuylkill Med Ctr-S Jackson Street	Pottsville	64%	300+
Southwest Regional Medical Center	Waynesburg	64%	300+
UPMC Bedford	Everett	64%	300+
Elk Regional Health Center	Saint Marys	63%	300+
Ephrata Community Hospital	Ephrata	63%	300+
Good Samaritan Hospital	Lebanon	63%	300+
Heart of Lancaster Regional Medical Center	Lititz	63%	300+
Holy Redeemer Hospital and Medical Center	Meadowbrook	63%	300+
Lower Bucks Hospital	Bristol	63%	300+
Main Line Hospital Paoli	Paoli	63%	300+
Millcreek Community Hospital	Erie	63%	300+
Pocono Medical Center	E Stroudsburg	63%	300+
Uniontown Hospital	Uniontown	63%	300+
Western Penn Hosp-Forbes Reg Campus	Monroeville	63%	300+
Abington Memorial Hospital	Abington	62%	300+
Butler Memorial Hospital	Butler	62%	300+
Carlisle Regional Medical Center	Carlisle	62%	300+
Conemaugh Valley Memorial Hospital	Johnstown	62%	300+
Gnaden Huetten Memorial Hospital	Lehighton	62%	300+
Hazleton General Hospital	Hazleton	62%	300+
Heritage Valley Beaver	Beaver	62%	300+
Main Line Hospital Bryn Mawr Campus	Bryn Mawr	62%	300+
Palmerton Hospital	Palmerton	62%	300+
Saint Joseph Medical Center	Reading	62%	300+
Geisinger Wyoming Valley Medical Center	Wilkes-Barre	61%	300+
Lehigh Valley Hospital	Allentown	61%	300+
Lehigh Valley Hospital - Muhlenberg	Bethlehem	61%	300+
Penn Presbyterian Medical Center	Philadelphia	61%	300+
Western Pennsylvania Hospital	Pittsburgh	61%	300+
Berwick Hospital Center	Berwick	60%	300+
Corry Memorial Hospital	Corry	60%	(a)
Hospital of Univ of Pennsylvania	Philadelphia	60%	300+
Jefferson Regional Medical Center	Pittsburgh	60%	300+
Lewistown Hospital	Lewistown	60%	300+
UPMC Mckeesport	McKeesport	60%	300+
UPMC Northwest	Seneca	60%	300+
Clearfield Hospital	Clearfield	59%	300+
Milton S Hershey Medical Center	Hershey	59%	300+
Moses Taylor Hospital	Scranton	59%	300+
Saint Vincent Health Center	Erie	59%	300+
Wilkes-Barre General Hospital	Wilkes-Barre	59%	300+
Alle Kiski Medical Center	Natrona	58%	300+
Jennersville Regional Hospital	West Grove	58%	300+
Lansdale Hospital	Lansdale	58%	300+
Reading Hospital Medical Center	Reading	58%	300+
Saint Luke's Miners Memorial Hospital	Coaldale	58%	300+
Crozer Chester Medical Center	Upland	57%	300+
Delaware County Memorial Hospital	Drexel Hill	57%	300+
Hanover Hospital	Hanover	57%	300+
Holy Spirit Hospital	Camp Hill	57%	300+
Main Line Hospital Lankenau	Wynnewood	57%	300+
Somerset Hospital	Somerset	57%	300+
UPMC Horizon	Greenville	57%	300+
Jeanes Hospital	Philadelphia	56%	300+
Lancaster General Hospital	Lancaster	56%	300+
Magee Womens Hosp of UPMC Health Sys	Pittsburgh	56%	300+
Nazareth Hospital	Philadelphia	56%	300+
Schuylkill Med Ctr-East Norwegian Street	Pottsville	56%	300+
UPMC Presbyterian Shadyside	Pittsburgh	56%	300+
UPMC Saint Margaret	Pittsburgh	56%	300+
Penn Hosp of the Univ of Penn Health Sys	Philadelphia	55%	300+
Sacred Heart Hospital	Allentown	55%	300+
Memorial Hospital York	York	54%	300+
Mercy Hospital Scranton	Scranton	54%	300+
Phoenixville Hospital	Phoenixville	54%	300+
Jameson Memorial Hospital[11]	New Castle	53%	300+
Pinnacle Health Hospitals	Harrisburg	53%	300+
Pottstown Memorial Medical Center	Pottstown	53%	300+
Allegheny General Hospital	Pittsburgh	52%	300+
Brandywine Hospital	Coatesville	52%	300+
Chestnut Hill Hospital	Philadelphia	52%	300+
UPMC Passavant	Pittsburgh	52%	300+
Albert Einstein Medical Center	Philadelphia	51%	300+
Mercy Suburban Hospital	Norristown	51%	300+
Roxborough Memorial Hospital	Phila	51%	300+
Temple University Hospital	Philadelphia	50%	300+
Easton Hospital	Easton	49%	300+
Mercy Fitzgerald Hospital	Darby	49%	300+
UPMC Mercy	Pittsburgh	45%	300+
Saint Joseph's Hospital	Philadelphia	43%	(a)

49. Would Definitely Recommend Hospital

Hospital Name	City	Rate	Cases
Cancer Treatment Centers of America	Philadelphia	95%	(a)
Surgical Institute of Reading	Wyomissing	94%	300+
Coordinated Health Orthopedic Hospital	Bethlehem	90%	300+
Edgewood Surgical Hospital	Transfer	87%	(a)
Main Line Hospital Paoli	Paoli	87%	300+
Doylestown Hospital	Doylestown	85%	300+
Shamokin Area Community Hospital	Coal Township	83%	300+
Grand View Hospital	Sellersville	82%	300+
Geisinger Medical Center	Danville	81%	300+
Hospital of Univ of Pennsylvania	Philadelphia	81%	300+
Lehigh Valley Hospital - Muhlenberg	Bethlehem	81%	300+
Evangelical Community Hospital	Lewisburg	80%	300+
Lancaster General Hospital	Lancaster	80%	300+
Main Line Hospital Bryn Mawr Campus	Bryn Mawr	80%	300+
Main Line Hospital Lankenau	Wynnewood	80%	300+
Saint Mary Medical Center	Langhorne	80%	300+
Dubois Regional Medical Center	Dubois	79%	300+
Lehigh Valley Hospital	Allentown	79%	300+
Windber Hospital	Windber	79%	300+
Milton S Hershey Medical Center	Hershey	78%	300+
Saint Luke's Hospital Bethlehem	Bethlehem	78%	300+
Westfield Hospital	Allentown	78%	(a)
Chester County Hospital	West Chester	77%	300+
Hamot Medical Center	Erie	77%	300+
Holy Redeemer Hospital and Medical Center	Meadowbrook	77%	300+
Nason Hospital	Roaring Spring	77%	300+
Robert Packer Hospital	Sayre	77%	300+
Abington Memorial Hospital	Abington	76%	300+
Jefferson Regional Medical Center	Pittsburgh	76%	300+
Saint Joseph Medical Center	Reading	76%	300+
Waynesboro Hospital	Waynesboro	76%	300+
Muncy Valley Hospital	Muncy	75%	(a)
Saint Clair Memorial Hospital	Pittsburgh	75%	300+
Thomas Jefferson University Hospital	Philadelphia	75%	300+
Miners Medical Center	Hastings	74%	(a)
Penn Presbyterian Medical Center	Philadelphia	74%	300+
Canonsburg General Hospital	Canonsburg	73%	300+
Titusville Hospital	Titusville	73%	300+
UPMC Saint Margaret	Pittsburgh	73%	300+
Altoona Regional Health System	Altoona	72%	300+
Bloomsburg Hospital	Bloomsburg	72%	300+
Excela Health Frick Hospital	Mount Pleasant	72%	300+
Heritage Valley Sewickley	Sewickley	72%	300+
Highlands Hospital	Connellsville	72%	300+
Magee Womens Hosp of UPMC Health Sys	Pittsburgh	72%	300+
Hahnemann University Hospital	Philadelphia	71%	300+
Lancaster Regional Medical Center	Lancaster	71%	300+
Memorial Hospital York	York	71%	300+
Penn Hosp of the Univ of Penn Health Sys	Philadelphia	71%	300+
Saint Luke's Quakertown Hospital	Quakertown	71%	300+
York Hospital	York	71%	300+
Geisinger Wyoming Valley Medical Center	Wilkes-Barre	70%	300+
Indiana Regional Medical Center	Indiana	70%	300+
Jeanes Hospital	Philadelphia	70%	300+
Memorial Hospital - Towanda	Towanda	70%	300+
Moses Taylor Hospital	Scranton	70%	300+
Saint Vincent Health Center	Erie	70%	300+
Soldiers and Sailors Memorial Hospital	Wellsboro	70%	300+
Ephrata Community Hospital	Ephrata	69%	300+
Ohio Valley General Hospital	Mckees Rocks	69%	300+
UPMC Presbyterian Shadyside	Pittsburgh	69%	300+
Williamsport Hospital & Medical Center	Williamsport	69%	300+
Butler Memorial Hospital	Butler	68%	300+
Ellwood City Hospital	Ellwood City	68%	300+
Heart of Lancaster Regional Medical Center	Lititz	68%	300+
Pinnacle Health Hospitals	Harrisburg	68%	300+
Riddle Memorial Hospital	Media	68%	300+
Aria Health	Philadelphia	67%	300+
Charles Cole Memorial Hospital	Coudersport	67%	300+
Conemaugh Valley Memorial Hospital	Johnstown	67%	300+
Delaware County Memorial Hospital	Drexel Hill	67%	300+
Mercy Hospital Scranton	Scranton	67%	300+
Monongahela Valley Hospital	Monongahela	67%	300+
Mount Nittany Medical Center	State College	67%	300+
Punxsutawney Area Hospital	Punxsutawney	67%	300+
Reading Hospital Medical Center	Reading	67%	300+
Western Pennsylvania Hospital	Pittsburgh	67%	300+
Community Medical Center	Scranton	66%	300+
Good Samaritan Hospital	Lebanon	66%	300+
Grove City Medical Center	Grove City	66%	300+
Holy Spirit Hospital	Camp Hill	66%	300+
Sharon Regional Health System	Sharon	66%	300+
The Washington Hospital	Washington	66%	300+
Allegheny General Hospital	Pittsburgh	65%	300+
Excela Health Latrobe Hospital	Latrobe	65%	300+
Hanover Hospital	Hanover	65%	300+
Kane Community Hospital	Kane	65%	(a)
Meadville Medical Center	Meadville	65%	300+
Pocono Medical Center	E Stroudsburg	65%	300+
ACMH Hospital	Kittanning	64%	300+
Mercy Tyler Hospital	Tunkhannock	64%	(a)
Phoenixville Hospital	Phoenixville	64%	300+
Saint Luke's Miners Memorial Hospital	Coaldale	64%	300+
UPMC Passavant	Pittsburgh	64%	300+
Chambersburg Hospital	Chambersburg	63%	300+
Excela Health Westmoreland Reg Hosp	Greensburg	63%	300+
Uniontown Hospital	Uniontown	63%	300+
Wayne Memorial Hospital	Honesdale	63%	300+
Chestnut Hill Hospital	Philadelphia	62%	300+
UPMC Horizon	Greenville	62%	300+
Warren General Hospital	Warren	62%	300+
Western Penn Hosp-Forbes Reg Campus	Monroeville	62%	300+
Gettysburg Hospital	Gettysburg	61%	300+
Heritage Valley Beaver	Beaver	61%	300+
Sunbury Community Hospital	Sunbury	61%	300+
Temple University Hospital	Philadelphia	61%	300+
Crozer Chester Medical Center	Upland	60%	300+
Millcreek Community Hospital	Erie	60%	300+
Southwest Regional Medical Center	Waynesburg	60%	300+
Wilkes-Barre General Hospital	Wilkes-Barre	60%	300+
Berwick Hospital Center	Berwick	59%	300+
Clarion Hospital	Clarion	59%	300+
Nazareth Hospital	Philadelphia	59%	300+
J C Blair Memorial Hospital	Huntingdon	58%	300+
Mercy Suburban Hospital	Norristown	58%	300+
Sacred Heart Hospital	Allentown	58%	300+
Carlisle Regional Medical Center	Carlisle	57%	300+
Gnaden Huetten Memorial Hospital	Lehighton	57%	300+
Lansdale Hospital	Lansdale	57%	300+
Marian Community Hospital	Carbondale	57%	300+
Schuylkill Med Ctr-East Norwegian Street	Pottsville	57%	300+
UPMC Mckeesport	McKeesport	57%	300+
UPMC Mercy	Pittsburgh	57%	300+
Palmerton Hospital	Palmerton	56%	300+
St Catherine Med Ctr Fountain Springs	Ashland	56%	(a)
UPMC Bedford	Everett	56%	300+
Albert Einstein Medical Center	Philadelphia	55%	300+
Brandywine Hospital	Coatesville	55%	300+
Jennersville Regional Hospital	West Grove	55%	300+
Lower Bucks Hospital	Bristol	55%	300+
Alle Kiski Medical Center	Natrona	54%	300+
Montgomery Hospital	Norristown	54%	300+
Schuylkill Med Ctr-S Jackson Street	Pottsville	54%	300+
Bradford Regional Medical Center	Bradford	53%	300+
Easton Hospital	Easton	53%	300+
Elk Regional Health Center	Saint Marys	53%	300+
Mercy Fitzgerald Hospital	Darby	53%	300+
Pottstown Memorial Medical Center	Pottstown	53%	300+
Somerset Hospital	Somerset	52%	300+
Clearfield Hospital	Clearfield	51%	300+
Lock Haven Hospital	Lock Haven	50%	300+
UPMC Northwest	Seneca	50%	300+
Jameson Memorial Hospital[11]	New Castle	47%	300+
Lewistown Hospital	Lewistown	47%	300+
Roxborough Memorial Hospital	Phila	47%	300+
Corry Memorial Hospital	Corry	45%	(a)
Hazleton General Hospital	Hazleton	44%	300+
Saint Joseph's Hospital	Philadelphia	35%	(a)

NOTE: Hospital profiles are in alphabetical order by state, then city, then hospital within the city; Rankings exclude hospitals with less than 25 cases except for patient surveys which excludes hospitals with less than 100 cases; (a) 100–299 cases; (1) The number of cases is too small to be sure how well a hospital is performing; (2) The hospital indicated that the data submitted for this measure were based on a sample of cases; (3) Data was collected during a shorter time period (fewer quarters) than the maximum possible time for this measure; (4) Suppressed for one or more quarters by CMS; (5) No data is available from the hospital for this measure; (6) Fewer than 100 patients completed the HCAHPS survey. Use these rates with caution, as the number of surveys may be too low to reliably assess hospital performance; (7) Survey results are based on less than 12 months of data; (8) Survey results are not available for this reporting period; (9) No or very few patients were eligible for the HCAHPS survey. The scores shown, if any, reflect a very small number of surveys; (10) A state average was not calculated because too few hospitals in the state submitted data; (11) There were discrepancies in the data collection process; Please refer to the User's Guide for a full explanation of data.

Abington Memorial Hospital

1200 Old York Road
Abington, PA 19001
Phone: 215-481-2000
Fax: 215-481-3619
URL: www.amh.org
Type: Acute Care Hospitals
Emergency Services: Yes
Ownership: Voluntary Non-Profit - Private
Beds: 508

Key Personnel:

CEO/President. . . . . Richard L Jones, JR
Chief of Medical Staff. . . . . Jack Kelly, MD
Infection Control. . . . . Beth Stunn
Operating Room. . . . . Teresa Howard
Pediatric Ambulatory Care . . . . . . Joseph Cirotti, MD
Pediatric In-Patient Care . . . . Joseph Cirotti, MD
Quality Assurance . . . . Tony Simek
Radiology. . . . . John Breckenridge, MD

Measure	Cases	This Hosp.	State Avg.	U.S. Avg.
Heart Attack Care				
ACE Inhibitor or ARB for LVSD	73	96%	95%	96%
Aspirin at Arrival	358	99%	99%	99%
Aspirin at Discharge	393	99%	99%	98%
Beta Blocker at Discharge	393	97%	99%	98%
Fibrinolytic Medication Timing	0	-	40%	55%
PCI Within 90 Minutes of Arrival	65	86%	88%	90%
Smoking Cessation Advice	96	100%	100%	99%
Chest Pain/Possible Heart Attack Care				
Aspirin at Arrival[5]	0	-	95%	95%
Median Time to ECG (minutes)[5]	0	-	8	8
Median Time to Transfer (minutes)[5]	0	-	68	61
Fibrinolytic Medication Timing[5]	0	-	48%	54%
Heart Failure Care				
ACE Inhibitor or ARB for LVSD	335	98%	95%	94%
Discharge Instructions	701	88%	90%	88%
Evaluation of LVS Function	923	100%	99%	98%
Smoking Cessation Advice	91	100%	98%	98%
Pneumonia Care				
Appropriate Initial Antibiotic	249	96%	93%	92%
Blood Culture Timing	558	95%	96%	96%
Influenza Vaccine	336	92%	92%	91%
Initial Antibiotic Timing	565	97%	96%	95%
Pneumococcal Vaccine	487	96%	95%	93%
Smoking Cessation Advice	140	100%	98%	97%
Surgical Care Improvement Project				
Appropriate VTP Within 24 Hours[2]	138	98%	95%	92%
Appropriate Hair Removal[2]	651	99%	100%	99%
Appropriate Beta Blocker Usage[2]	217	86%	94%	93%
Controlled Postoperative Blood Glucose[2]	150	96%	96%	93%
Prophylactic Antibiotic Timing[2]	494	96%	97%	97%
Prophylactic Antibiotic Timing (Outpatient)	412	97%	92%	92%
Prophylactic Antibiotic Selection[2]	498	99%	98%	97%
Prophylactic Antibiotic Select. (Outpatient)	411	96%	93%	94%
Prophylactic Antibiotic Stopped[2]	478	95%	95%	94%
Recommended VTP Ordered[2]	139	98%	97%	94%
Urinary Catheter Removal[2]	166	96%	95%	90%
Children's Asthma Care				
Received Systemic Corticosteroids	-	-	-	100%
Received Home Management Plan	-	-	-	71%
Received Reliever Medication	-	-	-	100%
Use of Medical Imaging				
Combination Abdominal CT Scan	2,284	0.039	0.203	0.191
Combination Chest CT Scan	1,943	0.012	0.026	0.054
Follow-up Mammogram/Ultrasound	2,769	10.3%	8.2%	8.4%
MRI for Low Back Pain	370	29.7%	32.4%	32.7%
Survey of Patients' Hospital Experiences				
Area Around Room 'Always' Quiet at Night	300+	46%	-	58%
Doctors 'Always' Communicated Well	300+	77%	-	80%
Home Recovery Information Given	300+	80%	-	82%
Hospital Given 9 or 10 on 10 Point Scale	300+	70%	-	67%
Meds 'Always' Explained Before Given	300+	59%	-	60%
Nurses 'Always' Communicated Well	300+	77%	-	76%
Pain 'Always' Well Controlled	300+	66%	-	69%
Room and Bathroom 'Always' Clean	300+	60%	-	71%
Timely Help 'Always' Received	300+	62%	-	64%
Would Definitely Recommend Hospital	300+	76%	-	69%

Lehigh Valley Hospital

PO Box 689
Allentown, PA 18105
Phone: 610-402-2273
Fax: 610-402-7523
URL: www.lvhhn.org
Type: Acute Care Hospitals
Emergency Services: Yes
Ownership: Voluntary Non-Profit - Other
Beds: 800

Key Personnel:

CEO/President. . . . . Elliot J Sussman, MD
Chief of Medical Staff . . . . Ronald W Swinfard, MD
Infection Control. . . . . Terry Lynn Burger
Operating Room. . . . . Brian Leader
Quality Assurance . . . . Georgene Saliba
Radiology. . . . . Sheila Sferrella

Measure	Cases	This Hosp.	State Avg.	U.S. Avg.
Heart Attack Care				
ACE Inhibitor or ARB for LVSD	149	96%	95%	96%
Aspirin at Arrival	648	100%	99%	99%
Aspirin at Discharge	976	99%	99%	98%
Beta Blocker at Discharge	951	99%	99%	98%
Fibrinolytic Medication Timing	0	-	40%	55%
PCI Within 90 Minutes of Arrival	118	96%	88%	90%
Smoking Cessation Advice	247	100%	100%	99%
Chest Pain/Possible Heart Attack Care				
Aspirin at Arrival[1,3]	4	75%	95%	95%
Median Time to ECG (minutes)[1,3]	5	12	8	8
Median Time to Transfer (minutes)[5]	0	-	68	61
Fibrinolytic Medication Timing[5]	0	-	48%	54%
Heart Failure Care				
ACE Inhibitor or ARB for LVSD	308	99%	95%	94%
Discharge Instructions	879	95%	90%	88%
Evaluation of LVS Function	1,112	99%	99%	98%
Smoking Cessation Advice	115	100%	98%	98%
Pneumonia Care				
Appropriate Initial Antibiotic	257	94%	93%	92%
Blood Culture Timing	489	98%	96%	96%
Influenza Vaccine	353	98%	92%	91%
Initial Antibiotic Timing	519	95%	96%	95%
Pneumococcal Vaccine	499	96%	95%	93%
Smoking Cessation Advice	149	100%	98%	97%
Surgical Care Improvement Project				
Appropriate VTP Within 24 Hours	1,432	98%	95%	92%
Appropriate Hair Removal	4,121	100%	100%	99%
Appropriate Beta Blocker Usage	1,325	99%	94%	93%
Controlled Postoperative Blood Glucose	581	98%	96%	93%
Prophylactic Antibiotic Timing	2,490	97%	97%	97%
Prophylactic Antibiotic Timing (Outpatient)	1,177	98%	92%	92%
Prophylactic Antibiotic Selection	2,523	99%	98%	97%
Prophylactic Antibiotic Select. (Outpatient)	1,169	96%	93%	94%
Prophylactic Antibiotic Stopped	2,407	98%	95%	94%
Recommended VTP Ordered	1,433	99%	97%	94%
Urinary Catheter Removal	975	95%	95%	90%
Children's Asthma Care				
Received Systemic Corticosteroids	-	-	-	100%
Received Home Management Plan	-	-	-	71%
Received Reliever Medication	-	-	-	100%
Use of Medical Imaging				
Combination Abdominal CT Scan	779	0.017	0.203	0.191
Combination Chest CT Scan	514	0.058	0.026	0.054
Follow-up Mammogram/Ultrasound	3,682	6.7%	8.2%	8.4%
MRI for Low Back Pain[1]	11	18.2%	32.4%	32.7%
Survey of Patients' Hospital Experiences				
Area Around Room 'Always' Quiet at Night	300+	48%	-	58%
Doctors 'Always' Communicated Well	300+	79%	-	80%
Home Recovery Information Given	300+	85%	-	82%
Hospital Given 9 or 10 on 10 Point Scale	300+	73%	-	67%
Meds 'Always' Explained Before Given	300+	60%	-	60%
Nurses 'Always' Communicated Well	300+	79%	-	76%
Pain 'Always' Well Controlled	300+	70%	-	69%
Room and Bathroom 'Always' Clean	300+	62%	-	71%
Timely Help 'Always' Received	300+	61%	-	64%
Would Definitely Recommend Hospital	300+	79%	-	69%

Sacred Heart Hospital

421 Chew Street
Allentown, PA 18102
Phone: 610-776-4900
Fax: 610-776-4559
E-mail: csodl@shh.org
URL: www.shh.org
Type: Acute Care Hospitals
Emergency Services: Yes
Ownership: Voluntary Non-Profit - Private
Beds: 243

Key Personnel:

CEO/President. . . . . Frank Sparandero
Cardiac Laboratory. . . . . Sarrokh Sader
Chief of Medical Staff. . . . . Mary Roth, MD
Infection Control. . . . . Mary Pavone
Operating Room. . . . . Ronald W Ambe, RN
Quality Assurance . . . . Lucia Williams
Radiology. . . . . Jeffrey Blinder

Measure	Cases	This Hosp.	State Avg.	U.S. Avg.
Heart Attack Care				
ACE Inhibitor or ARB for LVSD[1]	4	50%	95%	96%
Aspirin at Arrival	31	97%	99%	99%
Aspirin at Discharge[1]	21	100%	99%	98%
Beta Blocker at Discharge[1]	19	100%	99%	98%
Fibrinolytic Medication Timing	0	-	40%	55%
PCI Within 90 Minutes of Arrival	0	-	88%	90%
Smoking Cessation Advice[1]	3	100%	100%	99%
Chest Pain/Possible Heart Attack Care				
Aspirin at Arrival[1,3]	8	100%	95%	95%
Median Time to ECG (minutes)[1,3]	8	9	8	8
Median Time to Transfer (minutes)[1,3]	4	67	68	61
Fibrinolytic Medication Timing[3]	0	-	48%	54%
Heart Failure Care				
ACE Inhibitor or ARB for LVSD[1]	24	96%	95%	94%
Discharge Instructions	93	90%	90%	88%
Evaluation of LVS Function	130	95%	99%	98%
Smoking Cessation Advice[1]	15	93%	98%	98%
Pneumonia Care				
Appropriate Initial Antibiotic	51	80%	93%	92%
Blood Culture Timing	67	96%	96%	96%
Influenza Vaccine	54	80%	92%	91%
Initial Antibiotic Timing	76	95%	96%	95%
Pneumococcal Vaccine	73	78%	95%	93%
Smoking Cessation Advice	25	96%	98%	97%
Surgical Care Improvement Project				
Appropriate VTP Within 24 Hours	155	85%	95%	92%
Appropriate Hair Removal	397	99%	100%	99%
Appropriate Beta Blocker Usage	99	87%	94%	93%
Controlled Postoperative Blood Glucose[1]	1	0%	96%	93%
Prophylactic Antibiotic Timing	280	93%	97%	97%
Prophylactic Antibiotic Timing (Outpatient)	85	91%	92%	92%
Prophylactic Antibiotic Selection	280	94%	98%	97%
Prophylactic Antibiotic Select. (Outpatient)	80	88%	93%	94%
Prophylactic Antibiotic Stopped	276	82%	95%	94%
Recommended VTP Ordered	162	91%	97%	94%
Urinary Catheter Removal	45	84%	95%	90%
Children's Asthma Care				
Received Systemic Corticosteroids	-	-	-	100%
Received Home Management Plan	-	-	-	71%
Received Reliever Medication	-	-	-	100%
Use of Medical Imaging				
Combination Abdominal CT Scan	472	0.182	0.203	0.191
Combination Chest CT Scan	375	0.029	0.026	0.054
Follow-up Mammogram/Ultrasound	824	23.4%	8.2%	8.4%
MRI for Low Back Pain	52	34.6%	32.4%	32.7%
Survey of Patients' Hospital Experiences				
Area Around Room 'Always' Quiet at Night	300+	58%	-	58%
Doctors 'Always' Communicated Well	300+	75%	-	80%
Home Recovery Information Given	300+	82%	-	82%
Hospital Given 9 or 10 on 10 Point Scale	300+	59%	-	67%
Meds 'Always' Explained Before Given	300+	54%	-	60%
Nurses 'Always' Communicated Well	300+	71%	-	76%
Pain 'Always' Well Controlled	300+	62%	-	69%
Room and Bathroom 'Always' Clean	300+	67%	-	71%
Timely Help 'Always' Received	300+	55%	-	64%
Would Definitely Recommend Hospital	300+	58%	-	69%

NOTE: Hospital profiles are in alphabetical order by state, then city, then hospital within the city; Rankings exclude hospitals with less than 25 cases except for patient surveys which excludes hospitals with less than 100 cases; (a) 100–299 cases; (1) The number of cases is too small to be sure how well a hospital is performing; (2) The hospital indicated that the data submitted for this measure were based on a sample of cases; (3) Data was collected during a shorter time period (fewer quarters) than the maximum possible time for this measure; (4) Suppressed for one or more quarters by CMS; (5) No data is available from the hospital for this measure; (6) Fewer than 100 patients completed the HCAHPS survey. Use these rates with caution, as the number of surveys may be too low to reliably assess hospital performance; (7) Survey results are based on less than 12 months of data; (8) Survey results are not available for this reporting period; (9) No or very few patients were eligible for the HCAHPS survey. The scores shown, if any, reflect a very small number of surveys; (10) A state average was not calculated because too few hospitals in the state submitted data; (11) There were discrepancies in the data collection process; Please refer to the User's Guide for a full explanation of data.

Surgical Specialty Center at Coordinated Health

1503 Cedar Crest Boulevard Phone: 610-871-9110
Allentown, PA 18104
URL: www.coordinatedhealth.com
Type: Acute Care Hospitals Emergency Services: No
Ownership: Proprietary

Measure	Cases	This Hosp.	State Avg.	U.S. Avg.
Heart Attack Care				
ACE Inhibitor or ARB for LVSD[5]	0	-	95%	96%
Aspirin at Arrival[5]	0	-	99%	99%
Aspirin at Discharge[5]	0	-	99%	98%
Beta Blocker at Discharge[5]	0	-	99%	98%
Fibrinolytic Medication Timing[5]	0	-	40%	55%
PCI Within 90 Minutes of Arrival[5]	0	-	88%	90%
Smoking Cessation Advice[5]	0	-	100%	99%
Chest Pain/Possible Heart Attack Care				
Aspirin at Arrival[5]	0	-	95%	95%
Median Time to ECG (minutes)[5]	0	-	8	8
Median Time to Transfer (minutes)[5]	0	-	68	61
Fibrinolytic Medication Timing[5]	0	-	48%	54%
Heart Failure Care				
ACE Inhibitor or ARB for LVSD[5]	0	-	95%	94%
Discharge Instructions[5]	0	-	90%	88%
Evaluation of LVS Function[5]	0	-	99%	98%
Smoking Cessation Advice[5]	0	-	98%	98%
Pneumonia Care				
Appropriate Initial Antibiotic[5]	0	-	93%	92%
Blood Culture Timing[5]	0	-	96%	96%
Influenza Vaccine[5]	0	-	92%	91%
Initial Antibiotic Timing[5]	0	-	96%	95%
Pneumococcal Vaccine[5]	0	-	95%	93%
Smoking Cessation Advice[5]	0	-	98%	97%
Surgical Care Improvement Project				
Appropriate VTP Within 24 Hours[1,2,3]	4	100%	95%	92%
Appropriate Hair Removal[2,3]	71	100%	100%	99%
Appropriate Beta Blocker Usage[1,2,3]	7	29%	94%	93%
Controlled Postoperative Blood Glucose[2,3]	0	-	96%	93%
Prophylactic Antibiotic Timing[2,3]	65	97%	97%	97%
Prophylactic Antibiotic Timing (Outpatient)[5]	0	-	92%	92%
Prophylactic Antibiotic Selection[2,3]	65	100%	98%	97%
Prophylactic Antibiotic Select. (Outpatient)[5]	0	-	93%	94%
Prophylactic Antibiotic Stopped[2,3]	65	100%	95%	94%
Recommended VTP Ordered[1,2,3]	4	100%	97%	94%
Urinary Catheter Removal[2]	66	100%	95%	90%
Children's Asthma Care				
Received Systemic Corticosteroids	-	-	-	100%
Received Home Management Plan	-	-	-	71%
Received Reliever Medication	-	-	-	100%
Use of Medical Imaging				
Combination Abdominal CT Scan[5]	0	-	0.203	0.191
Combination Chest CT Scan[5]	0	-	0.026	0.054
Follow-up Mammogram/Ultrasound[5]	0	-	8.2%	8.4%
MRI for Low Back Pain[5]	0	-	32.4%	32.7%
Survey of Patients' Hospital Experiences				
Area Around Room 'Always' Quiet at Night[8]	-	-	-	58%
Doctors 'Always' Communicated Well[8]	-	-	-	80%
Home Recovery Information Given[8]	-	-	-	82%
Hospital Given 9 or 10 on 10 Point Scale[8]	-	-	-	67%
Meds 'Always' Explained Before Given[8]	-	-	-	60%
Nurses 'Always' Communicated Well[8]	-	-	-	76%
Pain 'Always' Well Controlled[8]	-	-	-	69%
Room and Bathroom 'Always' Clean[8]	-	-	-	71%
Timely Help 'Always' Received[8]	-	-	-	64%
Would Definitely Recommend Hospital[8]	-	-	-	69%

Westfield Hospital

4815 Tilghman Street Phone: 610-973-8400
Allentown, PA 18105
URL: www.westfieldhospital.com
Type: Acute Care Hospitals Emergency Services: Yes
Ownership: Proprietary
Key Personnel:
President . . . . Sherry Beers

Measure	Cases	This Hosp.	State Avg.	U.S. Avg.
Heart Attack Care				
ACE Inhibitor or ARB for LVSD[3]	0	-	95%	96%
Aspirin at Arrival[1,3]	1	0%	99%	99%
Aspirin at Discharge[3]	0	-	99%	98%
Beta Blocker at Discharge[3]	0	-	99%	98%
Fibrinolytic Medication Timing[3]	0	-	40%	55%
PCI Within 90 Minutes of Arrival[3]	0	-	88%	90%
Smoking Cessation Advice[3]	0	-	100%	99%
Chest Pain/Possible Heart Attack Care				
Aspirin at Arrival[5]	0	-	95%	95%
Median Time to ECG (minutes)[5]	0	-	8	8
Median Time to Transfer (minutes)[5]	0	-	68	61
Fibrinolytic Medication Timing[5]	0	-	48%	54%
Heart Failure Care				
ACE Inhibitor or ARB for LVSD	0	-	95%	94%
Discharge Instructions[1]	2	0%	90%	88%
Evaluation of LVS Function[1]	4	0%	99%	98%
Smoking Cessation Advice	0	-	98%	98%
Pneumonia Care				
Appropriate Initial Antibiotic[1]	12	92%	93%	92%
Blood Culture Timing[1]	8	75%	96%	96%
Influenza Vaccine[1]	4	75%	92%	91%
Initial Antibiotic Timing[1]	4	100%	96%	95%
Pneumococcal Vaccine[1]	7	43%	95%	93%
Smoking Cessation Advice[1]	3	67%	98%	97%
Surgical Care Improvement Project				
Appropriate VTP Within 24 Hours[1]	5	40%	95%	92%
Appropriate Hair Removal	29	97%	100%	99%
Appropriate Beta Blocker Usage[1]	4	25%	94%	93%
Controlled Postoperative Blood Glucose	0	-	96%	93%
Prophylactic Antibiotic Timing[1]	19	37%	97%	97%
Prophylactic Antibiotic Timing (Outpatient)[5]	0	-	92%	92%
Prophylactic Antibiotic Selection[1]	15	87%	98%	97%
Prophylactic Antibiotic Select. (Outpatient)[5]	0	-	93%	94%
Prophylactic Antibiotic Stopped[1]	15	87%	95%	94%
Recommended VTP Ordered[1]	5	40%	97%	94%
Urinary Catheter Removal[1]	1	100%	95%	90%
Children's Asthma Care				
Received Systemic Corticosteroids	-	-	-	100%
Received Home Management Plan	-	-	-	71%
Received Reliever Medication	-	-	-	100%
Use of Medical Imaging				
Combination Abdominal CT Scan[1]	49	0.061	0.203	0.191
Combination Chest CT Scan[1]	15	0.067	0.026	0.054
Follow-up Mammogram/Ultrasound[5]	0	-	8.2%	8.4%
MRI for Low Back Pain	56	33.9%	32.4%	32.7%
Survey of Patients' Hospital Experiences				
Area Around Room 'Always' Quiet at Night	(a)	68%	-	58%
Doctors 'Always' Communicated Well	(a)	79%	-	80%
Home Recovery Information Given	(a)	78%	-	82%
Hospital Given 9 or 10 on 10 Point Scale	(a)	79%	-	67%
Meds 'Always' Explained Before Given	(a)	66%	-	60%
Nurses 'Always' Communicated Well	(a)	81%	-	76%
Pain 'Always' Well Controlled	(a)	70%	-	69%
Room and Bathroom 'Always' Clean	(a)	81%	-	71%
Timely Help 'Always' Received	(a)	82%	-	64%
Would Definitely Recommend Hospital	(a)	78%	-	69%

Altoona Regional Health System

620 Howard Avenue Phone: 814-889-2011
Altoona, PA 16601 Fax: 814-949-3115
E-mail: info@altoonaregional.org
URL: www.altoonaregional.org
Type: Acute Care Hospitals Emergency Services: Yes
Ownership: Voluntary Non-Profit - Other Beds: 470
Key Personnel:
CEO/President. . . . . James W Barner
Chief of Medical Staff . . . . Anthony J Maniglia, MD
Infection Control. . . . . Margaret Adams
Operating Room. . . . . Jan Schachtner, RN
Pediatric Ambulatory Care . . . . . . Sharon Roscia, RN
Quality Assurance . . . . Kathy J Mecklen
Radiology. . . . . Michael Corso

Measure	Cases	This Hosp.	State Avg.	U.S. Avg.
Heart Attack Care				
ACE Inhibitor or ARB for LVSD	141	86%	95%	96%
Aspirin at Arrival	362	98%	99%	99%
Aspirin at Discharge	522	97%	99%	98%
Beta Blocker at Discharge	515	97%	99%	98%
Fibrinolytic Medication Timing	0	-	40%	55%
PCI Within 90 Minutes of Arrival	70	90%	88%	90%
Smoking Cessation Advice	172	100%	100%	99%
Chest Pain/Possible Heart Attack Care				
Aspirin at Arrival[5]	0	-	95%	95%
Median Time to ECG (minutes)[5]	0	-	8	8
Median Time to Transfer (minutes)[5]	0	-	68	61
Fibrinolytic Medication Timing[5]	0	-	48%	54%
Heart Failure Care				
ACE Inhibitor or ARB for LVSD	165	88%	95%	94%
Discharge Instructions	402	89%	90%	88%
Evaluation of LVS Function	542	99%	99%	98%
Smoking Cessation Advice	57	100%	98%	98%
Pneumonia Care				
Appropriate Initial Antibiotic	198	90%	93%	92%
Blood Culture Timing	323	97%	96%	96%
Influenza Vaccine	221	99%	92%	91%
Initial Antibiotic Timing	317	96%	96%	95%
Pneumococcal Vaccine	326	98%	95%	93%
Smoking Cessation Advice	127	100%	98%	97%
Surgical Care Improvement Project				
Appropriate VTP Within 24 Hours	488	94%	95%	92%
Appropriate Hair Removal	2,077	100%	100%	99%
Appropriate Beta Blocker Usage	634	87%	94%	93%
Controlled Postoperative Blood Glucose	256	94%	96%	93%
Prophylactic Antibiotic Timing	1,524	97%	97%	97%
Prophylactic Antibiotic Timing (Outpatient)	694	89%	92%	92%
Prophylactic Antibiotic Selection	1,559	97%	98%	97%
Prophylactic Antibiotic Select. (Outpatient)	646	98%	93%	94%
Prophylactic Antibiotic Stopped	1,491	93%	95%	94%
Recommended VTP Ordered	494	93%	97%	94%
Urinary Catheter Removal	173	87%	95%	90%
Children's Asthma Care				
Received Systemic Corticosteroids	-	-	-	100%
Received Home Management Plan	-	-	-	71%
Received Reliever Medication	-	-	-	100%
Use of Medical Imaging				
Combination Abdominal CT Scan	1,317	0.321	0.203	0.191
Combination Chest CT Scan	873	0.036	0.026	0.054
Follow-up Mammogram/Ultrasound	1,148	5.0%	8.2%	8.4%
MRI for Low Back Pain	148	31.8%	32.4%	32.7%
Survey of Patients' Hospital Experiences				
Area Around Room 'Always' Quiet at Night	300+	53%	-	58%
Doctors 'Always' Communicated Well	300+	82%	-	80%
Home Recovery Information Given	300+	84%	-	82%
Hospital Given 9 or 10 on 10 Point Scale	300+	68%	-	67%
Meds 'Always' Explained Before Given	300+	61%	-	60%
Nurses 'Always' Communicated Well	300+	81%	-	76%
Pain 'Always' Well Controlled	300+	72%	-	69%
Room and Bathroom 'Always' Clean	300+	75%	-	71%
Timely Help 'Always' Received	300+	67%	-	64%
Would Definitely Recommend Hospital	300+	72%	-	69%

NOTE: Hospital profiles are in alphabetical order by state, then city, then hospital within the city; Rankings exclude hospitals with less than 25 cases except for patient surveys which excludes hospitals with less than 100 cases; (a) 100–299 cases; (1) The number of cases is too small to be sure how well a hospital is performing; (2) The hospital indicated that the data submitted for this measure were based on a sample of cases; (3) Data was collected during a shorter time period (fewer quarters) than the maximum possible time for this measure; (4) Suppressed for one or more quarters by CMS; (5) No data is available from the hospital for this measure; (6) Fewer than 100 patients completed the HCAHPS survey. Use these rates with caution, as the number of surveys may be too low to reliably assess hospital performance; (7) Survey results are based on less than 12 months of data; (8) Survey results are not available for this reporting period; (9) No or very few patients were eligible for the HCAHPS survey. The scores shown, if any, reflect a very small number of surveys; (10) A state average was not calculated because too few hospitals in the state submitted data; (11) There were discrepancies in the data collection process; Please refer to the User's Guide for a full explanation of data.

James E. Van Zandt VA Medical Center - Altoona

2907 Pleasant Valley Boulevar
Altoona, PA 16602
Phone: 814-943-8164
Fax: 814-940-7898
URL: www.va.gov

Type: Acute Care-Veterans Administration
Ownership: Government - Federal
Emergency Services: No
Beds: 68

Key Personnel:

Chief of Medical Staff.......... Santha Kurian, MD
Infection Control.............. Jennifer Fouse

Measure	Cases	This Hosp.	State Avg.	U.S. Avg.
Heart Attack Care				
ACE Inhibitor or ARB for LVSD[1]	1	100%	95%	96%
Aspirin at Arrival[1]	11	100%	99%	99%
Aspirin at Discharge[1]	5	100%	99%	98%
Beta Blocker at Discharge[1]	5	100%	99%	98%
Fibrinolytic Medication Timing[5]	0	-	40%	55%
PCI Within 90 Minutes of Arrival[5]	0	-	88%	90%
Smoking Cessation Advice[1]	1	100%	100%	99%
Chest Pain/Possible Heart Attack Care				
Aspirin at Arrival	-	-	95%	95%
Median Time to ECG (minutes)	-	-	8	8
Median Time to Transfer (minutes)	-	-	68	61
Fibrinolytic Medication Timing	-	-	48%	54%
Heart Failure Care				
ACE Inhibitor or ARB for LVSD[1]	17	100%	95%	94%
Discharge Instructions	35	97%	90%	88%
Evaluation of LVS Function	37	100%	99%	98%
Smoking Cessation Advice[1]	3	100%	98%	98%
Pneumonia Care				
Appropriate Initial Antibiotic	36	92%	93%	92%
Blood Culture Timing	38	97%	96%	96%
Influenza Vaccine	35	100%	92%	91%
Initial Antibiotic Timing	37	97%	96%	95%
Pneumococcal Vaccine	32	100%	95%	93%
Smoking Cessation Advice[1]	17	100%	98%	97%
Surgical Care Improvement Project				
Appropriate VTP Within 24 Hours[2,5]	0	-	95%	92%
Appropriate Hair Removal[2,5]	0	-	100%	99%
Appropriate Beta Blocker Usage[2,5]	0	-	94%	93%
Controlled Postoperative Blood Glucose[2,5]	0	-	96%	93%
Prophylactic Antibiotic Timing[5]	0	-	97%	97%
Prophylactic Antibiotic Timing (Outpatient)	-	-	92%	92%
Prophylactic Antibiotic Selection[5]	0	-	98%	97%
Prophylactic Antibiotic Select. (Outpatient)	-	-	93%	94%
Prophylactic Antibiotic Stopped[5]	0	-	95%	94%
Recommended VTP Ordered[2,5]	0	-	97%	94%
Urinary Catheter Removal[2,5]	0	-	95%	90%
Children's Asthma Care				
Received Systemic Corticosteroids	-	-	-	100%
Received Home Management Plan	-	-	-	71%
Received Reliever Medication	-	-	-	100%
Use of Medical Imaging				
Combination Abdominal CT Scan	-	-	0.203	0.191
Combination Chest CT Scan	-	-	0.026	0.054
Follow-up Mammogram/Ultrasound	-	-	8.2%	8.4%
MRI for Low Back Pain	-	-	32.4%	32.7%
Survey of Patients' Hospital Experiences				
Area Around Room 'Always' Quiet at Night	-	-	-	58%
Doctors 'Always' Communicated Well	-	-	-	80%
Home Recovery Information Given	-	-	-	82%
Hospital Given 9 or 10 on 10 Point Scale	-	-	-	67%
Meds 'Always' Explained Before Given	-	-	-	60%
Nurses 'Always' Communicated Well	-	-	-	76%
Pain 'Always' Well Controlled	-	-	-	69%
Room and Bathroom 'Always' Clean	-	-	-	71%
Timely Help 'Always' Received	-	-	-	64%
Would Definitely Recommend Hospital	-	-	-	69%

Saint Catherine Medical Center Fountain Springs

101 Broad Street
Ashland, PA 17921
Phone: 570-875-2000
Fax: 570-875-6075
URL: www.stchc.com/scmcfs

Type: Acute Care Hospitals
Ownership: Voluntary Non-Profit - Private
Emergency Services: Yes
Beds: 141

Key Personnel:

CEO/President............... Daniel A. Colon
Cardiac Laboratory............ Charles Minehart, MD
Chief of Medical Staff.......... John Stefovic, MD
Radiology.................. Juan Peralta, MD
Anesthesiology.............. George Chalhoub, MD
Hemotology Center .... Ed Ashtar, MD

Measure	Cases	This Hosp.	State Avg.	U.S. Avg.
Heart Attack Care				
ACE Inhibitor or ARB for LVSD[1]	4	75%	95%	96%
Aspirin at Arrival[1]	12	100%	99%	99%
Aspirin at Discharge[1]	6	100%	99%	98%
Beta Blocker at Discharge[1]	8	88%	99%	98%
Fibrinolytic Medication Timing	0	-	40%	55%
PCI Within 90 Minutes of Arrival	0	-	88%	90%
Smoking Cessation Advice	0	-	100%	99%
Chest Pain/Possible Heart Attack Care				
Aspirin at Arrival	46	96%	95%	95%
Median Time to ECG (minutes)	44	14	8	8
Median Time to Transfer (minutes)[1]	8	69	68	61
Fibrinolytic Medication Timing[1]	1	0%	48%	54%
Heart Failure Care				
ACE Inhibitor or ARB for LVSD[1]	16	94%	95%	94%
Discharge Instructions	64	92%	90%	88%
Evaluation of LVS Function	87	84%	99%	98%
Smoking Cessation Advice[1]	18	100%	98%	98%
Pneumonia Care				
Appropriate Initial Antibiotic	32	78%	93%	92%
Blood Culture Timing	43	93%	96%	96%
Influenza Vaccine	39	79%	92%	91%
Initial Antibiotic Timing	53	89%	96%	95%
Pneumococcal Vaccine	51	80%	95%	93%
Smoking Cessation Advice[1]	20	100%	98%	97%
Surgical Care Improvement Project				
Appropriate VTP Within 24 Hours[1]	20	100%	95%	92%
Appropriate Hair Removal	53	100%	100%	99%
Appropriate Beta Blocker Usage[1]	10	100%	94%	93%
Controlled Postoperative Blood Glucose	0	-	96%	93%
Prophylactic Antibiotic Timing	25	92%	97%	97%
Prophylactic Antibiotic Timing (Outpatient)[1,3]	9	56%	92%	92%
Prophylactic Antibiotic Selection	25	72%	98%	97%
Prophylactic Antibiotic Select. (Outpatient)[1,3]	5	100%	93%	94%
Prophylactic Antibiotic Stopped[1]	24	79%	95%	94%
Recommended VTP Ordered[1]	21	95%	97%	94%
Urinary Catheter Removal[1]	7	71%	95%	90%
Children's Asthma Care				
Received Systemic Corticosteroids	-	-	-	100%
Received Home Management Plan	-	-	-	71%
Received Reliever Medication	-	-	-	100%
Use of Medical Imaging				
Combination Abdominal CT Scan	93	0.581	0.203	0.191
Combination Chest CT Scan	45	0.022	0.026	0.054
Follow-up Mammogram/Ultrasound	131	7.6%	8.2%	8.4%
MRI for Low Back Pain[1]	17	23.5%	32.4%	32.7%
Survey of Patients' Hospital Experiences				
Area Around Room 'Always' Quiet at Night	(a)	53%	-	58%
Doctors 'Always' Communicated Well	(a)	85%	-	80%
Home Recovery Information Given	(a)	86%	-	82%
Hospital Given 9 or 10 on 10 Point Scale	(a)	61%	-	67%
Meds 'Always' Explained Before Given	(a)	61%	-	60%
Nurses 'Always' Communicated Well	(a)	76%	-	76%
Pain 'Always' Well Controlled	(a)	75%	-	69%
Room and Bathroom 'Always' Clean	(a)	83%	-	71%
Timely Help 'Always' Received	(a)	70%	-	64%
Would Definitely Recommend Hospital	(a)	56%	-	69%

Heritage Valley Beaver

1000 Dutch Ridge Road
Beaver, PA 15009
Phone: 412-728-7000
Fax: 724-773-8210
URL: www.heritagevalley.org

Type: Acute Care Hospitals
Ownership: Voluntary Non-Profit - Private
Emergency Services: Yes
Beds: 358

Key Personnel:

CEO/President............... Larry A Crowell
Cardiac Laboratory............ Rhonda Beltz
Chief of Medical Staff.......... Fatish Dhagart, MD
Infection Control............. Bruce Chamovitz, MD
Pediatric Ambulatory Care ...... Krishana Kasi, MD
Pediatric In-Patient Care .... Krishana Kasi, MD
Quality Assurance .... Debbie Grady
Radiology.................. Roland McGraner

Measure	Cases	This Hosp.	State Avg.	U.S. Avg.
Heart Attack Care				
ACE Inhibitor or ARB for LVSD	63	98%	95%	96%
Aspirin at Arrival	336	97%	99%	99%
Aspirin at Discharge	412	98%	99%	98%
Beta Blocker at Discharge	367	100%	99%	98%
Fibrinolytic Medication Timing	0	-	40%	55%
PCI Within 90 Minutes of Arrival	66	82%	88%	90%
Smoking Cessation Advice	135	100%	100%	99%
Chest Pain/Possible Heart Attack Care				
Aspirin at Arrival[1]	9	100%	95%	95%
Median Time to ECG (minutes)[1]	10	12	8	8
Median Time to Transfer (minutes)[5]	0	-	68	61
Fibrinolytic Medication Timing[5]	0	-	48%	54%
Heart Failure Care				
ACE Inhibitor or ARB for LVSD	184	100%	95%	94%
Discharge Instructions	638	93%	90%	88%
Evaluation of LVS Function	787	99%	99%	98%
Smoking Cessation Advice	83	100%	98%	98%
Pneumonia Care				
Appropriate Initial Antibiotic	211	92%	93%	92%
Blood Culture Timing	361	98%	96%	96%
Influenza Vaccine	229	100%	92%	91%
Initial Antibiotic Timing	327	99%	96%	95%
Pneumococcal Vaccine	281	99%	95%	93%
Smoking Cessation Advice	132	100%	98%	97%
Surgical Care Improvement Project				
Appropriate VTP Within 24 Hours	358	85%	95%	92%
Appropriate Hair Removal	1,303	100%	100%	99%
Appropriate Beta Blocker Usage	363	80%	94%	93%
Controlled Postoperative Blood Glucose	243	95%	96%	93%
Prophylactic Antibiotic Timing	911	98%	97%	97%
Prophylactic Antibiotic Timing (Outpatient)	196	87%	92%	92%
Prophylactic Antibiotic Selection	924	96%	98%	97%
Prophylactic Antibiotic Select. (Outpatient)	186	92%	93%	94%
Prophylactic Antibiotic Stopped	879	96%	95%	94%
Recommended VTP Ordered	359	89%	97%	94%
Urinary Catheter Removal	279	93%	95%	90%
Children's Asthma Care				
Received Systemic Corticosteroids	-	-	-	100%
Received Home Management Plan	-	-	-	71%
Received Reliever Medication	-	-	-	100%
Use of Medical Imaging				
Combination Abdominal CT Scan	698	0.136	0.203	0.191
Combination Chest CT Scan	487	0.002	0.026	0.054
Follow-up Mammogram/Ultrasound	1,183	11.3%	8.2%	8.4%
MRI for Low Back Pain	92	29.3%	32.4%	32.7%
Survey of Patients' Hospital Experiences				
Area Around Room 'Always' Quiet at Night	300+	41%	-	58%
Doctors 'Always' Communicated Well	300+	79%	-	80%
Home Recovery Information Given	300+	76%	-	82%
Hospital Given 9 or 10 on 10 Point Scale	300+	59%	-	67%
Meds 'Always' Explained Before Given	300+	53%	-	60%
Nurses 'Always' Communicated Well	300+	74%	-	76%
Pain 'Always' Well Controlled	300+	68%	-	69%
Room and Bathroom 'Always' Clean	300+	66%	-	71%
Timely Help 'Always' Received	300+	62%	-	64%
Would Definitely Recommend Hospital	300+	61%	-	69%

NOTE: Hospital profiles are in alphabetical order by state, then city, then hospital within the city; Rankings exclude hospitals with less than 25 cases except for patient surveys which excludes hospitals with less than 100 cases; (a) 100–299 cases; (1) The number of cases is too small to be sure how well a hospital is performing; (2) The hospital indicated that the data submitted for this measure were based on a sample of cases; (3) Data was collected during a shorter time period (fewer quarters) than the maximum possible time for this measure; (4) Suppressed for one or more quarters by CMS; (5) No data is available from the hospital for this measure; (6) Fewer than 100 patients completed the HCAHPS survey. Use these rates with caution, as the number of surveys may be too low to reliably assess hospital performance; (7) Survey results are based on less than 12 months of data; (8) Survey results are not available for this reporting period; (9) No or very few patients were eligible for the HCAHPS survey. The scores shown, if any, reflect a very small number of surveys; (10) A state average was not calculated because too few hospitals in the state submitted data; (11) There were discrepancies in the data collection process; Please refer to the User's Guide for a full explanation of data.

Bucks County Specialty Hospital

3300 Tillman Drive
Bensalem, PA 19020 — Phone: 215-639-7513
URL: www.bcshospital.com
Type: Acute Care Hospitals — Emergency Services: No
Ownership: Proprietary

Measure	Cases	This Hosp.	State Avg.	U.S. Avg.
Heart Attack Care				
ACE Inhibitor or ARB for LVSD[5]	0	-	95%	96%
Aspirin at Arrival[5]	0	-	99%	99%
Aspirin at Discharge[5]	0	-	99%	98%
Beta Blocker at Discharge[5]	0	-	99%	98%
Fibrinolytic Medication Timing[5]	0	-	40%	55%
PCI Within 90 Minutes of Arrival[5]	0	-	88%	90%
Smoking Cessation Advice[5]	0	-	100%	99%
Chest Pain/Possible Heart Attack Care				
Aspirin at Arrival	-	-	95%	95%
Median Time to ECG (minutes)	-	-	8	8
Median Time to Transfer (minutes)	-	-	68	61
Fibrinolytic Medication Timing	-	-	48%	54%
Heart Failure Care				
ACE Inhibitor or ARB for LVSD[5]	0	-	95%	94%
Discharge Instructions[5]	0	-	90%	88%
Evaluation of LVS Function[5]	0	-	99%	98%
Smoking Cessation Advice[5]	0	-	98%	98%
Pneumonia Care				
Appropriate Initial Antibiotic[5]	0	-	93%	92%
Blood Culture Timing[5]	0	-	96%	96%
Influenza Vaccine[5]	0	-	92%	91%
Initial Antibiotic Timing[5]	0	-	96%	95%
Pneumococcal Vaccine[5]	0	-	95%	93%
Smoking Cessation Advice[5]	0	-	98%	97%
Surgical Care Improvement Project				
Appropriate VTP Within 24 Hours[2,3]	0	-	95%	92%
Appropriate Hair Removal[2,3]	99	100%	100%	99%
Appropriate Beta Blocker Usage[2,3]	27	93%	94%	93%
Controlled Postoperative Blood Glucose[2,3]	0	-	96%	93%
Prophylactic Antibiotic Timing[2,3]	99	97%	97%	97%
Prophylactic Antibiotic Timing (Outpatient)	-	-	92%	92%
Prophylactic Antibiotic Selection[2,3]	99	100%	98%	97%
Prophylactic Antibiotic Select. (Outpatient)	-	-	93%	94%
Prophylactic Antibiotic Stopped[2,3]	99	100%	95%	94%
Recommended VTP Ordered[2,3]	0	-	97%	94%
Urinary Catheter Removal[2]	39	92%	95%	90%
Children's Asthma Care				
Received Systemic Corticosteroids	-	-	-	100%
Received Home Management Plan	-	-	-	71%
Received Reliever Medication	-	-	-	100%
Use of Medical Imaging				
Combination Abdominal CT Scan	-	-	0.203	0.191
Combination Chest CT Scan	-	-	0.026	0.054
Follow-up Mammogram/Ultrasound	-	-	8.2%	8.4%
MRI for Low Back Pain	-	-	32.4%	32.7%
Survey of Patients' Hospital Experiences				
Area Around Room 'Always' Quiet at Night[8]	-	-	-	58%
Doctors 'Always' Communicated Well[8]	-	-	-	80%
Home Recovery Information Given[8]	-	-	-	82%
Hospital Given 9 or 10 on 10 Point Scale[8]	-	-	-	67%
Meds 'Always' Explained Before Given[8]	-	-	-	60%
Nurses 'Always' Communicated Well[8]	-	-	-	76%
Pain 'Always' Well Controlled[8]	-	-	-	69%
Room and Bathroom 'Always' Clean[8]	-	-	-	71%
Timely Help 'Always' Received[8]	-	-	-	64%
Would Definitely Recommend Hospital[8]	-	-	-	69%

Berwick Hospital Center

701 East 16th Street
Berwick, PA 18603 — Phone: 570-759-5000 / Fax: 570-759-3473
URL: www.berwick-hospital.com
Type: Acute Care Hospitals — Emergency Services: Yes
Ownership: Proprietary — Beds: 130

Key Personnel:
CEO/President . . . . Donald Henderson
Chief of Medical Staff . . . . Michael Kenny
Quality Assurance . . . . Megan Benson

Measure	Cases	This Hosp.	State Avg.	U.S. Avg.
Heart Attack Care				
ACE Inhibitor or ARB for LVSD[1]	2	100%	95%	96%
Aspirin at Arrival	27	96%	99%	99%
Aspirin at Discharge[1]	19	100%	99%	98%
Beta Blocker at Discharge[1]	24	100%	99%	98%
Fibrinolytic Medication Timing	0	-	40%	55%
PCI Within 90 Minutes of Arrival	0	-	88%	90%
Smoking Cessation Advice[1]	4	100%	100%	99%
Chest Pain/Possible Heart Attack Care				
Aspirin at Arrival	51	96%	95%	95%
Median Time to ECG (minutes)	52	6	8	8
Median Time to Transfer (minutes)[1]	18	46	68	61
Fibrinolytic Medication Timing	0	-	48%	54%
Heart Failure Care				
ACE Inhibitor or ARB for LVSD[1]	24	100%	95%	94%
Discharge Instructions	113	89%	90%	88%
Evaluation of LVS Function	160	99%	99%	98%
Smoking Cessation Advice[1]	21	100%	98%	98%
Pneumonia Care				
Appropriate Initial Antibiotic	53	87%	93%	92%
Blood Culture Timing	76	96%	96%	96%
Influenza Vaccine	56	100%	92%	91%
Initial Antibiotic Timing	78	96%	96%	95%
Pneumococcal Vaccine	71	94%	95%	93%
Smoking Cessation Advice[1]	22	100%	98%	97%
Surgical Care Improvement Project				
Appropriate VTP Within 24 Hours[2]	42	86%	95%	92%
Appropriate Hair Removal[2]	169	100%	100%	99%
Appropriate Beta Blocker Usage[2]	32	94%	94%	93%
Controlled Postoperative Blood Glucose[2]	0	-	96%	93%
Prophylactic Antibiotic Timing[2]	129	98%	97%	97%
Prophylactic Antibiotic Timing (Outpatient)	36	100%	92%	92%
Prophylactic Antibiotic Selection[2]	131	95%	98%	97%
Prophylactic Antibiotic Select. (Outpatient)	36	92%	93%	94%
Prophylactic Antibiotic Stopped[2]	126	90%	95%	94%
Recommended VTP Ordered[2]	43	86%	97%	94%
Urinary Catheter Removal[1]	6	83%	95%	90%
Children's Asthma Care				
Received Systemic Corticosteroids	-	-	-	100%
Received Home Management Plan	-	-	-	71%
Received Reliever Medication	-	-	-	100%
Use of Medical Imaging				
Combination Abdominal CT Scan	185	0.335	0.203	0.191
Combination Chest CT Scan	120	0.117	0.026	0.054
Follow-up Mammogram/Ultrasound	372	11.6%	8.2%	8.4%
MRI for Low Back Pain[1]	58	17.2%	32.4%	32.7%
Survey of Patients' Hospital Experiences				
Area Around Room 'Always' Quiet at Night	300+	55%	-	58%
Doctors 'Always' Communicated Well	300+	83%	-	80%
Home Recovery Information Given	300+	78%	-	82%
Hospital Given 9 or 10 on 10 Point Scale	300+	59%	-	67%
Meds 'Always' Explained Before Given	300+	62%	-	60%
Nurses 'Always' Communicated Well	300+	77%	-	76%
Pain 'Always' Well Controlled	300+	68%	-	69%
Room and Bathroom 'Always' Clean	300+	71%	-	71%
Timely Help 'Always' Received	300+	60%	-	64%
Would Definitely Recommend Hospital	300+	59%	-	69%

Coordinated Health Orthopedic Hospital

2310 Highland Avenue
Bethlehem, PA 18017 — Phone: 610-691-4300
Type: Acute Care Hospitals — Emergency Services: No
Ownership: Proprietary

Key Personnel:
CEO/President . . . . Emil J DiIorio MD

Measure	Cases	This Hosp.	State Avg.	U.S. Avg.
Heart Attack Care				
ACE Inhibitor or ARB for LVSD[5]	0	-	95%	96%
Aspirin at Arrival[5]	0	-	99%	99%
Aspirin at Discharge[5]	0	-	99%	98%
Beta Blocker at Discharge[5]	0	-	99%	98%
Fibrinolytic Medication Timing[5]	0	-	40%	55%
PCI Within 90 Minutes of Arrival[5]	0	-	88%	90%
Smoking Cessation Advice[5]	0	-	100%	99%
Chest Pain/Possible Heart Attack Care				
Aspirin at Arrival[5]	0	-	95%	95%
Median Time to ECG (minutes)[5]	0	-	8	8
Median Time to Transfer (minutes)[5]	0	-	68	61
Fibrinolytic Medication Timing[5]	0	-	48%	54%
Heart Failure Care				
ACE Inhibitor or ARB for LVSD[5]	0	-	95%	94%
Discharge Instructions[5]	0	-	90%	88%
Evaluation of LVS Function[5]	0	-	99%	98%
Smoking Cessation Advice[5]	0	-	98%	98%
Pneumonia Care				
Appropriate Initial Antibiotic[5]	0	-	93%	92%
Blood Culture Timing[5]	0	-	96%	96%
Influenza Vaccine[5]	0	-	92%	91%
Initial Antibiotic Timing[5]	0	-	96%	95%
Pneumococcal Vaccine[5]	0	-	95%	93%
Smoking Cessation Advice[5]	0	-	98%	97%
Surgical Care Improvement Project				
Appropriate VTP Within 24 Hours[2]	26	100%	95%	92%
Appropriate Hair Removal[2]	202	100%	100%	99%
Appropriate Beta Blocker Usage[1,2]	12	92%	94%	93%
Controlled Postoperative Blood Glucose[2]	0	-	96%	93%
Prophylactic Antibiotic Timing[2]	180	98%	97%	97%
Prophylactic Antibiotic Timing (Outpatient)[3]	33	100%	92%	92%
Prophylactic Antibiotic Selection[2]	180	98%	98%	97%
Prophylactic Antibiotic Select. (Outpatient)[3]	33	100%	93%	94%
Prophylactic Antibiotic Stopped[2]	180	93%	95%	94%
Recommended VTP Ordered[2]	26	100%	97%	94%
Urinary Catheter Removal[2]	72	100%	95%	90%
Children's Asthma Care				
Received Systemic Corticosteroids	-	-	-	100%
Received Home Management Plan	-	-	-	71%
Received Reliever Medication	-	-	-	100%
Use of Medical Imaging				
Combination Abdominal CT Scan[5]	0	-	0.203	0.191
Combination Chest CT Scan[5]	0	-	0.026	0.054
Follow-up Mammogram/Ultrasound[5]	0	-	8.2%	8.4%
MRI for Low Back Pain[5]	0	-	32.4%	32.7%
Survey of Patients' Hospital Experiences				
Area Around Room 'Always' Quiet at Night	300+	80%	-	58%
Doctors 'Always' Communicated Well	300+	87%	-	80%
Home Recovery Information Given	300+	89%	-	82%
Hospital Given 9 or 10 on 10 Point Scale	300+	90%	-	67%
Meds 'Always' Explained Before Given	300+	73%	-	60%
Nurses 'Always' Communicated Well	300+	92%	-	76%
Pain 'Always' Well Controlled	300+	80%	-	69%
Room and Bathroom 'Always' Clean	300+	85%	-	71%
Timely Help 'Always' Received	300+	90%	-	64%
Would Definitely Recommend Hospital	300+	90%	-	69%

Lehigh Valley Hospital - Muhlenberg

2545 Schoenersville Road — Phone: 610-402-2273
Bethlehem, PA 18017 — Fax: 610-402-7523
URL: www.lvhn.org
Type: Acute Care Hospitals — Emergency Services: Yes
Ownership: Voluntary Non-Profit - Other — Beds: 148

Key Personnel:
CEO/President. . . . . Elliot J Sussman
Chief of Medical Staff . . . . Linda L Lapos, MD
Infection Control. . . . . Terry Burger, RN
Operating Room. . . . . Thomas V Whalen
Pediatric Ambulatory Care . . . . . . John Van Brakle, MD
Pediatric In-Patient Care . . . . John Van Brakle, MD
Quality Assurance . . . . Sue Lawrence

Measure	Cases	This Hosp.	State Avg.	U.S. Avg.
Heart Attack Care				
ACE Inhibitor or ARB for LVSD	33	97%	95%	96%
Aspirin at Arrival	288	100%	99%	99%
Aspirin at Discharge	281	99%	99%	98%
Beta Blocker at Discharge	283	100%	99%	98%
Fibrinolytic Medication Timing	0	-	40%	55%
PCI Within 90 Minutes of Arrival	71	89%	88%	90%
Smoking Cessation Advice	78	100%	100%	99%
Chest Pain/Possible Heart Attack Care				
Aspirin at Arrival[1,3]	9	89%	95%	95%
Median Time to ECG (minutes)[1,3]	9	9	8	8
Median Time to Transfer (minutes)[5]	0	-	68	61
Fibrinolytic Medication Timing[3]	0	-	48%	54%
Heart Failure Care				
ACE Inhibitor or ARB for LVSD	106	100%	95%	94%
Discharge Instructions	366	98%	90%	88%
Evaluation of LVS Function	466	100%	99%	98%
Smoking Cessation Advice	41	100%	98%	98%
Pneumonia Care				
Appropriate Initial Antibiotic	158	96%	93%	92%
Blood Culture Timing	312	97%	96%	96%
Influenza Vaccine	200	98%	92%	91%
Initial Antibiotic Timing	323	98%	96%	95%
Pneumococcal Vaccine	308	99%	95%	93%
Smoking Cessation Advice	92	100%	98%	97%
Surgical Care Improvement Project				
Appropriate VTP Within 24 Hours	352	96%	95%	92%
Appropriate Hair Removal	802	100%	100%	99%
Appropriate Beta Blocker Usage	248	96%	94%	93%
Controlled Postoperative Blood Glucose	119	97%	96%	93%
Prophylactic Antibiotic Timing	495	96%	97%	97%
Prophylactic Antibiotic Timing (Outpatient)	277	96%	92%	92%
Prophylactic Antibiotic Selection	499	97%	98%	97%
Prophylactic Antibiotic Select. (Outpatient)	270	96%	93%	94%
Prophylactic Antibiotic Stopped	475	96%	95%	94%
Recommended VTP Ordered	355	97%	97%	94%
Urinary Catheter Removal	135	89%	95%	90%
Children's Asthma Care				
Received Systemic Corticosteroids	-	-	-	100%
Received Home Management Plan	-	-	-	71%
Received Reliever Medication	-	-	-	100%
Use of Medical Imaging				
Combination Abdominal CT Scan	1,040	0.082	0.203	0.191
Combination Chest CT Scan	932	0.033	0.026	0.054
Follow-up Mammogram/Ultrasound	1,557	6.7%	8.2%	8.4%
MRI for Low Back Pain	76	30.3%	32.4%	32.7%
Survey of Patients' Hospital Experiences				
Area Around Room 'Always' Quiet at Night	300+	51%	-	58%
Doctors 'Always' Communicated Well	300+	78%	-	80%
Home Recovery Information Given	300+	85%	-	82%
Hospital Given 9 or 10 on 10 Point Scale	300+	76%	-	67%
Meds 'Always' Explained Before Given	300+	61%	-	60%
Nurses 'Always' Communicated Well	300+	79%	-	76%
Pain 'Always' Well Controlled	300+	68%	-	69%
Room and Bathroom 'Always' Clean	300+	72%	-	71%
Timely Help 'Always' Received	300+	61%	-	64%
Would Definitely Recommend Hospital	300+	81%	-	69%

Saint Luke's Hospital Bethlehem

801 Ostrum Street — Phone: 610-954-4000
Bethlehem, PA 18015 — Fax: 610-954-4979
URL: www.slhn-lehighvalley.org
Type: Acute Care Hospitals — Emergency Services: Yes
Ownership: Voluntary Non-Profit - Other — Beds: 436

Key Personnel:
Chief of Medical Staff . . . . James A Cowan, MD
Infection Control. . . . . Jeffrey A Jahre, MD
Operating Room. . . . . Patricia A Krenn, RN
Pediatric Ambulatory Care . . . . . . Stanley Stein, MD
Pediatric In-Patient Care . . . . . . Stanley Stein, MD
Quality Assurance . . . . Janice Rader
Radiology. . . . . G Edward Streubert, MD

Measure	Cases	This Hosp.	State Avg.	U.S. Avg.
Heart Attack Care				
ACE Inhibitor or ARB for LVSD	62	100%	95%	96%
Aspirin at Arrival	367	98%	99%	99%
Aspirin at Discharge	445	99%	99%	98%
Beta Blocker at Discharge	434	99%	99%	98%
Fibrinolytic Medication Timing	0	-	40%	55%
PCI Within 90 Minutes of Arrival	46	87%	88%	90%
Smoking Cessation Advice	128	100%	100%	99%
Chest Pain/Possible Heart Attack Care				
Aspirin at Arrival[5]	0	-	95%	95%
Median Time to ECG (minutes)[5]	0	-	8	8
Median Time to Transfer (minutes)[5]	0	-	68	61
Fibrinolytic Medication Timing[5]	0	-	48%	54%
Heart Failure Care				
ACE Inhibitor or ARB for LVSD	247	98%	95%	94%
Discharge Instructions	770	92%	90%	88%
Evaluation of LVS Function	992	99%	99%	98%
Smoking Cessation Advice	110	99%	98%	98%
Pneumonia Care				
Appropriate Initial Antibiotic	300	95%	93%	92%
Blood Culture Timing	470	97%	96%	96%
Influenza Vaccine	313	92%	92%	91%
Initial Antibiotic Timing	493	96%	96%	95%
Pneumococcal Vaccine	414	93%	95%	93%
Smoking Cessation Advice	161	100%	98%	97%
Surgical Care Improvement Project				
Appropriate VTP Within 24 Hours[2]	430	94%	95%	92%
Appropriate Hair Removal[2]	1,622	100%	100%	99%
Appropriate Beta Blocker Usage[2]	550	87%	94%	93%
Controlled Postoperative Blood Glucose[2]	227	97%	96%	93%
Prophylactic Antibiotic Timing[2]	1,242	99%	97%	97%
Prophylactic Antibiotic Timing (Outpatient)	700	89%	92%	92%
Prophylactic Antibiotic Selection[2]	1,266	98%	98%	97%
Prophylactic Antibiotic Select. (Outpatient)	639	92%	93%	94%
Prophylactic Antibiotic Stopped[2]	1,203	97%	95%	94%
Recommended VTP Ordered[2]	432	95%	97%	94%
Urinary Catheter Removal[2]	457	98%	95%	90%
Children's Asthma Care				
Received Systemic Corticosteroids	74	100%	-	100%
Received Home Management Plan	72	64%	-	71%
Received Reliever Medication	74	100%	-	100%
Use of Medical Imaging				
Combination Abdominal CT Scan	2,147	0.254	0.203	0.191
Combination Chest CT Scan	1,810	0.004	0.026	0.054
Follow-up Mammogram/Ultrasound	3,599	8.4%	8.2%	8.4%
MRI for Low Back Pain	239	35.1%	32.4%	32.7%
Survey of Patients' Hospital Experiences				
Area Around Room 'Always' Quiet at Night	300+	51%	-	58%
Doctors 'Always' Communicated Well	300+	78%	-	80%
Home Recovery Information Given	300+	78%	-	82%
Hospital Given 9 or 10 on 10 Point Scale	300+	73%	-	67%
Meds 'Always' Explained Before Given	300+	63%	-	60%
Nurses 'Always' Communicated Well	300+	78%	-	76%
Pain 'Always' Well Controlled	300+	71%	-	69%
Room and Bathroom 'Always' Clean	300+	71%	-	71%
Timely Help 'Always' Received	300+	64%	-	64%
Would Definitely Recommend Hospital	300+	78%	-	69%

Bloomsburg Hospital

549 East Fair Street — Phone: 570-387-2100
Bloomsburg, PA 17815 — Fax: 570-387-2434
E-mail: tbhadmin@sunlink.net
URL: www.tbhonline.org
Type: Acute Care Hospitals — Emergency Services: Yes
Ownership: Voluntary Non-Profit - Private — Beds: 117

Key Personnel:
CEO/President. . . . . Regis PJ Cabonori
Chief of Medical Staff . . . . Paul A Saloky, DO

Measure	Cases	This Hosp.	State Avg.	U.S. Avg.
Heart Attack Care				
ACE Inhibitor or ARB for LVSD[1]	3	100%	95%	96%
Aspirin at Arrival[1]	16	100%	99%	99%
Aspirin at Discharge[1]	10	80%	99%	98%
Beta Blocker at Discharge[1]	10	80%	99%	98%
Fibrinolytic Medication Timing	0	-	40%	55%
PCI Within 90 Minutes of Arrival	0	-	88%	90%
Smoking Cessation Advice[1]	1	0%	100%	99%
Chest Pain/Possible Heart Attack Care				
Aspirin at Arrival	101	92%	95%	95%
Median Time to ECG (minutes)	106	0	8	8
Median Time to Transfer (minutes)	33	65	68	61
Fibrinolytic Medication Timing	0	-	48%	54%
Heart Failure Care				
ACE Inhibitor or ARB for LVSD	26	85%	95%	94%
Discharge Instructions	67	87%	90%	88%
Evaluation of LVS Function	91	89%	99%	98%
Smoking Cessation Advice[1]	8	75%	98%	98%
Pneumonia Care				
Appropriate Initial Antibiotic	91	95%	93%	92%
Blood Culture Timing	136	85%	96%	96%
Influenza Vaccine	84	90%	92%	91%
Initial Antibiotic Timing	137	98%	96%	95%
Pneumococcal Vaccine	101	90%	95%	93%
Smoking Cessation Advice	34	85%	98%	97%
Surgical Care Improvement Project				
Appropriate VTP Within 24 Hours	60	80%	95%	92%
Appropriate Hair Removal	274	100%	100%	99%
Appropriate Beta Blocker Usage	75	75%	94%	93%
Controlled Postoperative Blood Glucose	0	-	96%	93%
Prophylactic Antibiotic Timing	213	97%	97%	97%
Prophylactic Antibiotic Timing (Outpatient)	113	45%	92%	92%
Prophylactic Antibiotic Selection	215	99%	98%	97%
Prophylactic Antibiotic Select. (Outpatient)	51	98%	93%	94%
Prophylactic Antibiotic Stopped	208	97%	95%	94%
Recommended VTP Ordered	60	80%	97%	94%
Urinary Catheter Removal	54	98%	95%	90%
Children's Asthma Care				
Received Systemic Corticosteroids	-	-	-	100%
Received Home Management Plan	-	-	-	71%
Received Reliever Medication	-	-	-	100%
Use of Medical Imaging				
Combination Abdominal CT Scan	206	0.340	0.203	0.191
Combination Chest CT Scan	64	0.484	0.026	0.054
Follow-up Mammogram/Ultrasound	474	8.2%	8.2%	8.4%
MRI for Low Back Pain[1]	50	26.0%	32.4%	32.7%
Survey of Patients' Hospital Experiences				
Area Around Room 'Always' Quiet at Night	300+	51%	-	58%
Doctors 'Always' Communicated Well	300+	77%	-	80%
Home Recovery Information Given	300+	77%	-	82%
Hospital Given 9 or 10 on 10 Point Scale	300+	70%	-	67%
Meds 'Always' Explained Before Given	300+	57%	-	60%
Nurses 'Always' Communicated Well	300+	79%	-	76%
Pain 'Always' Well Controlled	300+	70%	-	69%
Room and Bathroom 'Always' Clean	300+	71%	-	71%
Timely Help 'Always' Received	300+	68%	-	64%
Would Definitely Recommend Hospital	300+	72%	-	69%

NOTE: Hospital profiles are in alphabetical order by state, then city, then hospital within the city; Rankings exclude hospitals with less than 25 cases except for patient surveys which excludes hospitals with less than 100 cases; (a) 100–299 cases; (1) The number of cases is too small to be sure how well a hospital is performing; (2) The hospital indicated that the data submitted for this measure were based on a sample of cases; (3) Data was collected during a shorter time period (fewer quarters) than the maximum possible time for this measure; (4) Suppressed for one or more quarters by CMS; (5) No data is available from the hospital for this measure; (6) Fewer than 100 patients completed the HCAHPS survey. Use these rates with caution, as the number of surveys may be too low to reliably assess hospital performance; (7) Survey results are based on less than 12 months of data; (8) Survey results are not available for this reporting period; (9) No or very few patients were eligible for the HCAHPS survey. The scores shown, if any, reflect a very small number of surveys; (10) A state average was not calculated because too few hospitals in the state submitted data; (11) There were discrepancies in the data collection process; Please refer to the User's Guide for a full explanation of data.

Bradford Regional Medical Center

116 Interstate Parkway — Phone: 814-368-4143
Bradford, PA 16701 — Fax: 814-368-5722
E-mail: webdirector@brmc.org
URL: www.bfdmed.org
Type: Acute Care Hospitals — Emergency Services: Yes
Ownership: Voluntary Non-Profit - Private — Beds: 127

Key Personnel:

CEO/President. . . . . George E Leonhardt
Chief of Medical Staff . . . . Peter Vaccaro, MD
Infection Control. . . . . Teri O'Brien, RN
Operating Room. . . . . Luis C Gonzalez, MD
Pediatric Ambulatory Care . . . . . . Anil Pradhan, MD
Pediatric In-Patient Care . . . . Anil Pradhan, MD
Quality Assurance . . . . Gayle Gronemeir, RN
Radiology. . . . . G Michael Maresca, MD

Measure	Cases	This Hosp.	State Avg.	U.S. Avg.
Heart Attack Care				
ACE Inhibitor or ARB for LVSD[1]	11	100%	95%	96%
Aspirin at Arrival	48	100%	99%	99%
Aspirin at Discharge	26	96%	99%	98%
Beta Blocker at Discharge	35	91%	99%	98%
Fibrinolytic Medication Timing	0	-	40%	55%
PCI Within 90 Minutes of Arrival	0	-	88%	90%
Smoking Cessation Advice[1]	7	86%	100%	99%
Chest Pain/Possible Heart Attack Care				
Aspirin at Arrival	30	100%	95%	95%
Median Time to ECG (minutes)	31	7	8	8
Median Time to Transfer (minutes)[1,3]	2	198	68	61
Fibrinolytic Medication Timing[1]	4	50%	48%	54%
Heart Failure Care				
ACE Inhibitor or ARB for LVSD	43	100%	95%	94%
Discharge Instructions	62	87%	90%	88%
Evaluation of LVS Function	86	95%	99%	98%
Smoking Cessation Advice[1]	5	80%	98%	98%
Pneumonia Care				
Appropriate Initial Antibiotic	59	92%	93%	92%
Blood Culture Timing	88	94%	96%	96%
Influenza Vaccine	78	85%	92%	91%
Initial Antibiotic Timing	111	95%	96%	95%
Pneumococcal Vaccine	99	94%	95%	93%
Smoking Cessation Advice	31	94%	98%	97%
Surgical Care Improvement Project				
Appropriate VTP Within 24 Hours	57	89%	95%	92%
Appropriate Hair Removal	137	99%	100%	99%
Appropriate Beta Blocker Usage	35	83%	94%	93%
Controlled Postoperative Blood Glucose	0	-	96%	93%
Prophylactic Antibiotic Timing	90	93%	97%	97%
Prophylactic Antibiotic Timing (Outpatient)	42	88%	92%	92%
Prophylactic Antibiotic Selection	89	89%	98%	97%
Prophylactic Antibiotic Select. (Outpatient)	40	88%	93%	94%
Prophylactic Antibiotic Stopped	85	87%	95%	94%
Recommended VTP Ordered	57	93%	97%	94%
Urinary Catheter Removal[1]	15	73%	95%	90%
Children's Asthma Care				
Received Systemic Corticosteroids	-	-	-	100%
Received Home Management Plan	-	-	-	71%
Received Reliever Medication	-	-	-	100%
Use of Medical Imaging				
Combination Abdominal CT Scan	469	0.092	0.203	0.191
Combination Chest CT Scan	325	0.031	0.026	0.054
Follow-up Mammogram/Ultrasound	697	8.9%	8.2%	8.4%
MRI for Low Back Pain	84	45.2%	32.4%	32.7%
Survey of Patients' Hospital Experiences				
Area Around Room 'Always' Quiet at Night	300+	43%	-	58%
Doctors 'Always' Communicated Well	300+	76%	-	80%
Home Recovery Information Given	300+	77%	-	82%
Hospital Given 9 or 10 on 10 Point Scale	300+	54%	-	67%
Meds 'Always' Explained Before Given	300+	53%	-	60%
Nurses 'Always' Communicated Well	300+	74%	-	76%
Pain 'Always' Well Controlled	300+	69%	-	69%
Room and Bathroom 'Always' Clean	300+	67%	-	71%
Timely Help 'Always' Received	300+	70%	-	64%
Would Definitely Recommend Hospital	300+	53%	-	69%

Lower Bucks Hospital

501 Bath Road — Phone: 215-785-9200
Bristol, PA 19007 — Fax: 215-785-9172
E-mail: LowerBucksHospital@LowerBucksHospital.org
URL: www.lowerbuckshospital.org
Type: Acute Care Hospitals — Emergency Services: No
Ownership: Voluntary Non-Profit - Private — Beds: 150

Key Personnel:

CEO/President. . . . . Nathan Bosk
Chief of Medical Staff . . . . Bruce Dershaw, MD
Pediatric In-Patient Care . . . . Gerry Green, DO
Quality Assurance . . . . Carol Evans
Radiology. . . . . Frederick Kraus, MD
Emergency Room . . . . Jennie Lutz, RN

Measure	Cases	This Hosp.	State Avg.	U.S. Avg.
Heart Attack Care				
ACE Inhibitor or ARB for LVSD[1]	15	87%	95%	96%
Aspirin at Arrival	124	98%	99%	99%
Aspirin at Discharge	114	96%	99%	98%
Beta Blocker at Discharge	119	97%	99%	98%
Fibrinolytic Medication Timing	0	-	40%	55%
PCI Within 90 Minutes of Arrival[1]	5	60%	88%	90%
Smoking Cessation Advice	49	92%	100%	99%
Chest Pain/Possible Heart Attack Care				
Aspirin at Arrival[5]	0	-	95%	95%
Median Time to ECG (minutes)[5]	0	-	8	8
Median Time to Transfer (minutes)[5]	0	-	68	61
Fibrinolytic Medication Timing[5]	0	-	48%	54%
Heart Failure Care				
ACE Inhibitor or ARB for LVSD	88	89%	95%	94%
Discharge Instructions	215	71%	90%	88%
Evaluation of LVS Function	262	98%	99%	98%
Smoking Cessation Advice	39	90%	98%	98%
Pneumonia Care				
Appropriate Initial Antibiotic	90	84%	93%	92%
Blood Culture Timing	125	97%	96%	96%
Influenza Vaccine	51	57%	92%	91%
Initial Antibiotic Timing	113	96%	96%	95%
Pneumococcal Vaccine	70	67%	95%	93%
Smoking Cessation Advice	36	97%	98%	97%
Surgical Care Improvement Project				
Appropriate VTP Within 24 Hours[2]	102	80%	95%	92%
Appropriate Hair Removal[2]	293	100%	100%	99%
Appropriate Beta Blocker Usage[2]	89	90%	94%	93%
Controlled Postoperative Blood Glucose[2]	38	92%	96%	93%
Prophylactic Antibiotic Timing[2]	190	96%	97%	97%
Prophylactic Antibiotic Timing (Outpatient)	83	88%	92%	92%
Prophylactic Antibiotic Selection[2]	189	91%	98%	97%
Prophylactic Antibiotic Select. (Outpatient)	80	90%	93%	94%
Prophylactic Antibiotic Stopped[2]	186	86%	95%	94%
Recommended VTP Ordered[2]	102	82%	97%	94%
Urinary Catheter Removal[2]	42	86%	95%	90%
Children's Asthma Care				
Received Systemic Corticosteroids	-	-	-	100%
Received Home Management Plan	-	-	-	71%
Received Reliever Medication	-	-	-	100%
Use of Medical Imaging				
Combination Abdominal CT Scan	275	0.262	0.203	0.191
Combination Chest CT Scan	266	0.011	0.026	0.054
Follow-up Mammogram/Ultrasound	671	7.7%	8.2%	8.4%
MRI for Low Back Pain[5]	0	-	32.4%	32.7%
Survey of Patients' Hospital Experiences				
Area Around Room 'Always' Quiet at Night	300+	51%	-	58%
Doctors 'Always' Communicated Well	300+	75%	-	80%
Home Recovery Information Given	300+	80%	-	82%
Hospital Given 9 or 10 on 10 Point Scale	300+	55%	-	67%
Meds 'Always' Explained Before Given	300+	59%	-	60%
Nurses 'Always' Communicated Well	300+	74%	-	76%
Pain 'Always' Well Controlled	300+	71%	-	69%
Room and Bathroom 'Always' Clean	300+	65%	-	71%
Timely Help 'Always' Received	300+	63%	-	64%
Would Definitely Recommend Hospital	300+	55%	-	69%

Brookville Hospital

100 Hospital Road — Phone: 814-849-2312
Brookville, PA 15825 — Fax: 814-849-4841
URL: www.brookvillehospital.org
Type: Critical Access Hospitals — Emergency Services: Yes
Ownership: Voluntary Non-Profit - Private — Beds: 63

Key Personnel:

CEO/President. . . . . John Sutika
Chief of Medical Staff . . . . Joseph Prusakowski, DO
Infection Control. . . . . Patricia Abell, RN
Operating Room. . . . . Richard Bucheit, RN
Quality Assurance . . . . Tere Byerly
Anesthesiology. . . . . Emerson Turnbull, CRNA
Emergency Room . . . . Paul E Harvey, MD
Intensive Care Unit. . . . . David Buchanan, RN

Measure	Cases	This Hosp.	State Avg.	U.S. Avg.
Heart Attack Care				
ACE Inhibitor or ARB for LVSD[1]	1	100%	95%	96%
Aspirin at Arrival[1]	7	86%	99%	99%
Aspirin at Discharge[1]	3	100%	99%	98%
Beta Blocker at Discharge[1]	7	86%	99%	98%
Fibrinolytic Medication Timing	0	-	40%	55%
PCI Within 90 Minutes of Arrival	0	-	88%	90%
Smoking Cessation Advice	0	-	100%	99%
Chest Pain/Possible Heart Attack Care				
Aspirin at Arrival	-	-	95%	95%
Median Time to ECG (minutes)	-	-	8	8
Median Time to Transfer (minutes)	-	-	68	61
Fibrinolytic Medication Timing	-	-	48%	54%
Heart Failure Care				
ACE Inhibitor or ARB for LVSD[1]	17	100%	95%	94%
Discharge Instructions	53	83%	90%	88%
Evaluation of LVS Function	63	97%	99%	98%
Smoking Cessation Advice[1]	6	100%	98%	98%
Pneumonia Care				
Appropriate Initial Antibiotic	31	94%	93%	92%
Blood Culture Timing	37	100%	96%	96%
Influenza Vaccine	38	92%	92%	91%
Initial Antibiotic Timing	43	98%	96%	95%
Pneumococcal Vaccine	50	94%	95%	93%
Smoking Cessation Advice[1]	21	95%	98%	97%
Surgical Care Improvement Project				
Appropriate VTP Within 24 Hours	29	100%	95%	92%
Appropriate Hair Removal	54	100%	100%	99%
Appropriate Beta Blocker Usage[5]	0	-	94%	93%
Controlled Postoperative Blood Glucose	0	-	96%	93%
Prophylactic Antibiotic Timing	34	100%	97%	97%
Prophylactic Antibiotic Timing (Outpatient)	-	-	92%	92%
Prophylactic Antibiotic Selection	34	91%	98%	97%
Prophylactic Antibiotic Select. (Outpatient)	-	-	93%	94%
Prophylactic Antibiotic Stopped	30	93%	95%	94%
Recommended VTP Ordered	29	100%	97%	94%
Urinary Catheter Removal[1]	12	100%	95%	90%
Children's Asthma Care				
Received Systemic Corticosteroids	-	-	-	100%
Received Home Management Plan	-	-	-	71%
Received Reliever Medication	-	-	-	100%
Use of Medical Imaging				
Combination Abdominal CT Scan	-	-	0.203	0.191
Combination Chest CT Scan	-	-	0.026	0.054
Follow-up Mammogram/Ultrasound	-	-	8.2%	8.4%
MRI for Low Back Pain	-	-	32.4%	32.7%
Survey of Patients' Hospital Experiences				
Area Around Room 'Always' Quiet at Night[8]	-	-	-	58%
Doctors 'Always' Communicated Well[8]	-	-	-	80%
Home Recovery Information Given[8]	-	-	-	82%
Hospital Given 9 or 10 on 10 Point Scale[8]	-	-	-	67%
Meds 'Always' Explained Before Given[8]	-	-	-	60%
Nurses 'Always' Communicated Well[8]	-	-	-	76%
Pain 'Always' Well Controlled[8]	-	-	-	69%
Room and Bathroom 'Always' Clean[8]	-	-	-	71%
Timely Help 'Always' Received[8]	-	-	-	64%
Would Definitely Recommend Hospital[8]	-	-	-	69%

NOTE: Hospital profiles are in alphabetical order by state, then city, then hospital within the city; Rankings exclude hospitals with less than 25 cases except for patient surveys which excludes hospitals with less than 100 cases; (a) 100–299 cases; (1) The number of cases is too small to be sure how well a hospital is performing; (2) The hospital indicated that the data submitted for this measure were based on a sample of cases; (3) Data was collected during a shorter time period (fewer quarters) than the maximum possible time for this measure; (4) Suppressed for one or more quarters by CMS; (5) No data is available from the hospital for this measure; (6) Fewer than 100 patients completed the HCAHPS survey. Use these rates with caution, as the number of surveys may be too low to reliably assess hospital performance; (7) Survey results are based on less than 12 months of data; (8) Survey results are not available for this reporting period; (9) No or very few patients were eligible for the HCAHPS survey. The scores shown, if any, reflect a very small number of surveys; (10) A state average was not calculated because too few hospitals in the state submitted data; (11) There were discrepancies in the data collection process; Please refer to the User's Guide for a full explanation of data.

Main Line Hospital Bryn Mawr Campus

130 South Bryn Mawr Ave Phone: 610-526-3000
Bryn Mawr, PA 19010 Fax: 610-526-3068
URL: www.mainlinehealth.org
Type: Acute Care Hospitals Emergency Services: Yes
Ownership: Voluntary Non-Profit - Private Beds: 307

Key Personnel:
CEO/President. . . . . Andrea Gilbert
Chief of Medical Staff . . . . James L McCabe, Jr, MD
Infection Control. . . . . Patti McBride, RN
Pediatric In-Patient Care . . . . Robert L Stavis, MD
Quality Assurance . . . . Lee Patrick
Radiology. . . . . Emma L Simpson, MD

Measure	Cases	This Hosp.	State Avg.	U.S. Avg.
Heart Attack Care				
ACE Inhibitor or ARB for LVSD	27	100%	95%	96%
Aspirin at Arrival	206	100%	99%	99%
Aspirin at Discharge	232	100%	99%	98%
Beta Blocker at Discharge	212	100%	99%	98%
Fibrinolytic Medication Timing	0	-	40%	55%
PCI Within 90 Minutes of Arrival	30	100%	88%	90%
Smoking Cessation Advice	47	100%	100%	99%
Chest Pain/Possible Heart Attack Care				
Aspirin at Arrival[1,3]	1	100%	95%	95%
Median Time to ECG (minutes)[1,3]	1	11	8	8
Median Time to Transfer (minutes)[5]	0	-	68	61
Fibrinolytic Medication Timing[5]	0	-	48%	54%
Heart Failure Care				
ACE Inhibitor or ARB for LVSD	143	99%	95%	94%
Discharge Instructions	339	98%	90%	88%
Evaluation of LVS Function	491	100%	99%	98%
Smoking Cessation Advice[1]	22	100%	98%	98%
Pneumonia Care				
Appropriate Initial Antibiotic	145	99%	93%	92%
Blood Culture Timing	271	100%	96%	96%
Influenza Vaccine	177	100%	92%	91%
Initial Antibiotic Timing	224	99%	96%	95%
Pneumococcal Vaccine	273	99%	95%	93%
Smoking Cessation Advice	44	100%	98%	97%
Surgical Care Improvement Project				
Appropriate VTP Within 24 Hours[2]	224	100%	95%	92%
Appropriate Hair Removal[2]	1,526	100%	100%	99%
Appropriate Beta Blocker Usage[2]	427	98%	94%	93%
Controlled Postoperative Blood Glucose[2]	89	98%	96%	93%
Prophylactic Antibiotic Timing[2]	1,296	99%	97%	97%
Prophylactic Antibiotic Timing (Outpatient)	238	93%	92%	92%
Prophylactic Antibiotic Selection[2]	1,307	99%	98%	97%
Prophylactic Antibiotic Select. (Outpatient)	224	88%	93%	94%
Prophylactic Antibiotic Stopped[2]	1,262	100%	95%	94%
Recommended VTP Ordered[2]	224	100%	97%	94%
Urinary Catheter Removal[2]	134	100%	95%	90%
Children's Asthma Care				
Received Systemic Corticosteroids	-	-	-	100%
Received Home Management Plan	-	-	-	71%
Received Reliever Medication	-	-	-	100%
Use of Medical Imaging				
Combination Abdominal CT Scan	1,068	0.228	0.203	0.191
Combination Chest CT Scan	972	0.023	0.026	0.054
Follow-up Mammogram/Ultrasound	1,404	6.9%	8.2%	8.4%
MRI for Low Back Pain[1]	2	0.0%	32.4%	32.7%
Survey of Patients' Hospital Experiences				
Area Around Room 'Always' Quiet at Night	300+	45%	-	58%
Doctors 'Always' Communicated Well	300+	76%	-	80%
Home Recovery Information Given	300+	82%	-	82%
Hospital Given 9 or 10 on 10 Point Scale	300+	74%	-	67%
Meds 'Always' Explained Before Given	300+	60%	-	60%
Nurses 'Always' Communicated Well	300+	79%	-	76%
Pain 'Always' Well Controlled	300+	70%	-	69%
Room and Bathroom 'Always' Clean	300+	65%	-	71%
Timely Help 'Always' Received	300+	62%	-	64%
Would Definitely Recommend Hospital	300+	80%	-	69%

Butler Memorial Hospital

One Hospital Way Phone: 724-283-6666
Butler, PA 16001 Fax: 724-477-3607
URL: www.butlerhealthsystem.org
Type: Acute Care Hospitals Emergency Services: Yes
Ownership: Voluntary Non-Profit - Other Beds: 268

Key Personnel:
CEO/President. . . . . Joseph Stewart
Cardiac Laboratory. . . . . Margie McLaughlin
Chief of Medical Staff . . . . A Thomas McGill, MD
Infection Control. . . . . Sharon Stephens
Pediatric In-Patient Care . . . . . . William Ashbaugh
Quality Assurance . . . . Mark Edwards
Radiology. . . . . James W Backstrom

Measure	Cases	This Hosp.	State Avg.	U.S. Avg.
Heart Attack Care				
ACE Inhibitor or ARB for LVSD	62	100%	95%	96%
Aspirin at Arrival	201	100%	99%	99%
Aspirin at Discharge	261	100%	99%	98%
Beta Blocker at Discharge	246	100%	99%	98%
Fibrinolytic Medication Timing	0	-	40%	55%
PCI Within 90 Minutes of Arrival	30	93%	88%	90%
Smoking Cessation Advice	99	100%	100%	99%
Chest Pain/Possible Heart Attack Care				
Aspirin at Arrival[5]	0	-	95%	95%
Median Time to ECG (minutes)[5]	0	-	8	8
Median Time to Transfer (minutes)[5]	0	-	68	61
Fibrinolytic Medication Timing[5]	0	-	48%	54%
Heart Failure Care				
ACE Inhibitor or ARB for LVSD	121	99%	95%	94%
Discharge Instructions	304	97%	90%	88%
Evaluation of LVS Function	387	100%	99%	98%
Smoking Cessation Advice	49	100%	98%	98%
Pneumonia Care				
Appropriate Initial Antibiotic	188	97%	93%	92%
Blood Culture Timing	217	100%	96%	96%
Influenza Vaccine	143	98%	92%	91%
Initial Antibiotic Timing	233	98%	96%	95%
Pneumococcal Vaccine	232	98%	95%	93%
Smoking Cessation Advice	107	99%	98%	97%
Surgical Care Improvement Project				
Appropriate VTP Within 24 Hours	271	97%	95%	92%
Appropriate Hair Removal	1,315	100%	100%	99%
Appropriate Beta Blocker Usage	420	92%	94%	93%
Controlled Postoperative Blood Glucose	326	99%	96%	93%
Prophylactic Antibiotic Timing	990	99%	97%	97%
Prophylactic Antibiotic Timing (Outpatient)	220	95%	92%	92%
Prophylactic Antibiotic Selection	999	99%	98%	97%
Prophylactic Antibiotic Select. (Outpatient)	217	94%	93%	94%
Prophylactic Antibiotic Stopped	953	94%	95%	94%
Recommended VTP Ordered	271	99%	97%	94%
Urinary Catheter Removal	227	94%	95%	90%
Children's Asthma Care				
Received Systemic Corticosteroids	-	-	-	100%
Received Home Management Plan	-	-	-	71%
Received Reliever Medication	-	-	-	100%
Use of Medical Imaging				
Combination Abdominal CT Scan	677	0.131	0.203	0.191
Combination Chest CT Scan	500	0.012	0.026	0.054
Follow-up Mammogram/Ultrasound	1,060	9.9%	8.2%	8.4%
MRI for Low Back Pain	194	31.4%	32.4%	32.7%
Survey of Patients' Hospital Experiences				
Area Around Room 'Always' Quiet at Night	300+	48%	-	58%
Doctors 'Always' Communicated Well	300+	77%	-	80%
Home Recovery Information Given	300+	89%	-	82%
Hospital Given 9 or 10 on 10 Point Scale	300+	67%	-	67%
Meds 'Always' Explained Before Given	300+	60%	-	60%
Nurses 'Always' Communicated Well	300+	77%	-	76%
Pain 'Always' Well Controlled	300+	70%	-	69%
Room and Bathroom 'Always' Clean	300+	64%	-	71%
Timely Help 'Always' Received	300+	62%	-	64%
Would Definitely Recommend Hospital	300+	68%	-	69%

Holy Spirit Hospital

503 North 21st Street Phone: 717-763-2100
Camp Hill, PA 17011 Fax: 717-763-2183
E-mail: info@hsh.org
URL: www.hsh.org
Type: Acute Care Hospitals Emergency Services: Yes
Ownership: Voluntary Non-Profit - Private Beds: 332

Key Personnel:
CEO/President. . . . . Romaine Niemeyer, SCC
Cardiac Laboratory. . . . . Chirstine Erdman
Chief of Medical Staff . . . . Joseph Torchia, MD
Infection Control. . . . . Joseph Torchia, MD
Quality Assurance . . . . Franchesca Charney, RN
Radiology. . . . . Ken Gable
Emergency Room . . . . Ramesh Arora, MD
Patient Relations . . . . Mary Buhrman

Measure	Cases	This Hosp.	State Avg.	U.S. Avg.
Heart Attack Care				
ACE Inhibitor or ARB for LVSD	66	98%	95%	96%
Aspirin at Arrival	308	98%	99%	99%
Aspirin at Discharge	334	100%	99%	98%
Beta Blocker at Discharge	324	100%	99%	98%
Fibrinolytic Medication Timing	0	-	40%	55%
PCI Within 90 Minutes of Arrival	68	97%	88%	90%
Smoking Cessation Advice	100	100%	100%	99%
Chest Pain/Possible Heart Attack Care				
Aspirin at Arrival[5]	0	-	95%	95%
Median Time to ECG (minutes)[5]	0	-	8	8
Median Time to Transfer (minutes)[5]	0	-	68	61
Fibrinolytic Medication Timing[5]	0	-	48%	54%
Heart Failure Care				
ACE Inhibitor or ARB for LVSD	117	97%	95%	94%
Discharge Instructions	339	96%	90%	88%
Evaluation of LVS Function	468	100%	99%	98%
Smoking Cessation Advice	52	100%	98%	98%
Pneumonia Care				
Appropriate Initial Antibiotic	256	99%	93%	92%
Blood Culture Timing	369	99%	96%	96%
Influenza Vaccine	258	96%	92%	91%
Initial Antibiotic Timing	348	96%	96%	95%
Pneumococcal Vaccine	348	97%	95%	93%
Smoking Cessation Advice	88	100%	98%	97%
Surgical Care Improvement Project				
Appropriate VTP Within 24 Hours[2]	279	89%	95%	92%
Appropriate Hair Removal[2]	1,007	100%	100%	99%
Appropriate Beta Blocker Usage[2]	387	89%	94%	93%
Controlled Postoperative Blood Glucose[2]	272	99%	96%	93%
Prophylactic Antibiotic Timing[2]	842	97%	97%	97%
Prophylactic Antibiotic Timing (Outpatient)	588	94%	92%	92%
Prophylactic Antibiotic Selection[2]	854	98%	98%	97%
Prophylactic Antibiotic Select. (Outpatient)	564	95%	93%	94%
Prophylactic Antibiotic Stopped[2]	811	96%	95%	94%
Recommended VTP Ordered[2]	279	92%	97%	94%
Urinary Catheter Removal[2]	170	98%	95%	90%
Children's Asthma Care				
Received Systemic Corticosteroids	-	-	-	100%
Received Home Management Plan	-	-	-	71%
Received Reliever Medication	-	-	-	100%
Use of Medical Imaging				
Combination Abdominal CT Scan	850	0.361	0.203	0.191
Combination Chest CT Scan	530	0.009	0.026	0.054
Follow-up Mammogram/Ultrasound	728	7.7%	8.2%	8.4%
MRI for Low Back Pain	62	40.3%	32.4%	32.7%
Survey of Patients' Hospital Experiences				
Area Around Room 'Always' Quiet at Night	300+	44%	-	58%
Doctors 'Always' Communicated Well	300+	72%	-	80%
Home Recovery Information Given	300+	77%	-	82%
Hospital Given 9 or 10 on 10 Point Scale	300+	64%	-	67%
Meds 'Always' Explained Before Given	300+	55%	-	60%
Nurses 'Always' Communicated Well	300+	72%	-	76%
Pain 'Always' Well Controlled	300+	66%	-	69%
Room and Bathroom 'Always' Clean	300+	66%	-	71%
Timely Help 'Always' Received	300+	57%	-	64%
Would Definitely Recommend Hospital	300+	66%	-	69%

NOTE: Hospital profiles are in alphabetical order by state, then city, then hospital within the city; Rankings exclude hospitals with less than 25 cases except for patient surveys which excludes hospitals with less than 100 cases; (a) 100–299 cases; (1) The number of cases is too small to be sure how well a hospital is performing; (2) The hospital indicated that the data submitted for this measure were based on a sample of cases; (3) Data was collected during a shorter time period (fewer quarters) than the maximum possible time for this measure; (4) Suppressed for one or more quarters by CMS; (5) No data is available from the hospital for this measure; (6) Fewer than 100 patients completed the HCAHPS survey. Use these rates with caution, as the number of surveys may be too low to reliably assess hospital performance; (7) Survey results are based on less than 12 months of data; (8) Survey results are not available for this reporting period; (9) No or very few patients were eligible for the HCAHPS survey. The scores shown, if any, reflect a very small number of surveys; (10) A state average was not calculated because too few hospitals in the state submitted data; (11) There were discrepancies in the data collection process; Please refer to the User's Guide for a full explanation of data.

Canonsburg General Hospital

100 Medical Boulevard Phone: 724-873-5892
Canonsburg, PA 15317 Fax: 724-873-5876
URL: www.wpahs.org/cgh
Type: Acute Care Hospitals Emergency Services: Yes
Ownership: Voluntary Non-Profit - Other Beds: 120

Key Personnel:
CEO/President. . . . . Kim Malinky
Chief of Medical Staff. . . . . Michael Catena
Quality Assurance . . . . Kathy Hayes
Emergency Room . . . . Jan Mandik

Measure	Cases	This Hosp.	State Avg.	U.S. Avg.
Heart Attack Care				
ACE Inhibitor or ARB for LVSD[1]	4	100%	95%	96%
Aspirin at Arrival	41	95%	99%	99%
Aspirin at Discharge[1]	15	93%	99%	98%
Beta Blocker at Discharge[1]	13	92%	99%	98%
Fibrinolytic Medication Timing	0	-	40%	55%
PCI Within 90 Minutes of Arrival	0	-	88%	90%
Smoking Cessation Advice[1]	2	100%	100%	99%
Chest Pain/Possible Heart Attack Care				
Aspirin at Arrival	83	99%	95%	95%
Median Time to ECG (minutes)	86	12	8	8
Median Time to Transfer (minutes)[1]	10	83	68	61
Fibrinolytic Medication Timing	0	-	48%	54%
Heart Failure Care				
ACE Inhibitor or ARB for LVSD	40	92%	95%	94%
Discharge Instructions	105	65%	90%	88%
Evaluation of LVS Function	152	99%	99%	98%
Smoking Cessation Advice[1]	15	100%	98%	98%
Pneumonia Care				
Appropriate Initial Antibiotic	72	93%	93%	92%
Blood Culture Timing	143	100%	96%	96%
Influenza Vaccine	106	69%	92%	91%
Initial Antibiotic Timing	128	96%	96%	95%
Pneumococcal Vaccine	138	88%	95%	93%
Smoking Cessation Advice	39	100%	98%	97%
Surgical Care Improvement Project				
Appropriate VTP Within 24 Hours	152	97%	95%	92%
Appropriate Hair Removal	479	100%	100%	99%
Appropriate Beta Blocker Usage	133	83%	94%	93%
Controlled Postoperative Blood Glucose	0	-	96%	93%
Prophylactic Antibiotic Timing	339	97%	97%	97%
Prophylactic Antibiotic Timing (Outpatient)	36	72%	92%	92%
Prophylactic Antibiotic Selection	340	96%	98%	97%
Prophylactic Antibiotic Select. (Outpatient)	31	97%	93%	94%
Prophylactic Antibiotic Stopped	336	97%	95%	94%
Recommended VTP Ordered	152	98%	97%	94%
Urinary Catheter Removal	29	72%	95%	90%
Children's Asthma Care				
Received Systemic Corticosteroids	-	-	-	100%
Received Home Management Plan	-	-	-	71%
Received Reliever Medication	-	-	-	100%
Use of Medical Imaging				
Combination Abdominal CT Scan	206	0.544	0.203	0.191
Combination Chest CT Scan	149	0.013	0.026	0.054
Follow-up Mammogram/Ultrasound	247	13.0%	8.2%	8.4%
MRI for Low Back Pain[1]	33	45.5%	32.4%	32.7%
Survey of Patients' Hospital Experiences				
Area Around Room 'Always' Quiet at Night	300+	52%	-	58%
Doctors 'Always' Communicated Well	300+	80%	-	80%
Home Recovery Information Given	300+	76%	-	82%
Hospital Given 9 or 10 on 10 Point Scale	300+	68%	-	67%
Meds 'Always' Explained Before Given	300+	59%	-	60%
Nurses 'Always' Communicated Well	300+	80%	-	76%
Pain 'Always' Well Controlled	300+	69%	-	69%
Room and Bathroom 'Always' Clean	300+	67%	-	71%
Timely Help 'Always' Received	300+	65%	-	64%
Would Definitely Recommend Hospital	300+	73%	-	69%

Marian Community Hospital

100 Lincoln Avenue Phone: 570-282-2100
Carbondale, PA 18407 Fax: 570-281-5390
E-mail: mariad@marianhospital.org
URL: www.marianhospital.org
Type: Acute Care Hospitals Emergency Services: Yes
Ownership: Voluntary Non-Profit - Church Beds: 104

Key Personnel:
CEO/President. . . . . Mary Theresa Vautrinot
Chief of Medical Staff. . . . . Jeffrey Mogerman, MD
Coronary Care . . . . Michelle Churney
Infection Control. . . . . Maria Noone
Operating Room. . . . . James Roche
Pediatric In-Patient Care . . . . Pat Cornell
Quality Assurance . . . . Jean Deecki
Radiology. . . . . Mark Alimoski

Measure	Cases	This Hosp.	State Avg.	U.S. Avg.
Heart Attack Care				
ACE Inhibitor or ARB for LVSD[1]	1	100%	95%	96%
Aspirin at Arrival[1]	16	100%	99%	99%
Aspirin at Discharge[1]	6	50%	99%	98%
Beta Blocker at Discharge[1]	5	100%	99%	98%
Fibrinolytic Medication Timing	0	-	40%	55%
PCI Within 90 Minutes of Arrival	0	-	88%	90%
Smoking Cessation Advice	0	-	100%	99%
Chest Pain/Possible Heart Attack Care				
Aspirin at Arrival	48	98%	95%	95%
Median Time to ECG (minutes)	49	8	8	8
Median Time to Transfer (minutes)[1]	11	43	68	61
Fibrinolytic Medication Timing	0	-	48%	54%
Heart Failure Care				
ACE Inhibitor or ARB for LVSD[1]	20	95%	95%	94%
Discharge Instructions	65	95%	90%	88%
Evaluation of LVS Function	93	98%	99%	98%
Smoking Cessation Advice[1]	5	100%	98%	98%
Pneumonia Care				
Appropriate Initial Antibiotic	108	90%	93%	92%
Blood Culture Timing	160	96%	96%	96%
Influenza Vaccine	81	96%	92%	91%
Initial Antibiotic Timing	158	99%	96%	95%
Pneumococcal Vaccine	125	99%	95%	93%
Smoking Cessation Advice	31	100%	98%	97%
Surgical Care Improvement Project				
Appropriate VTP Within 24 Hours	33	94%	95%	92%
Appropriate Hair Removal	108	100%	100%	99%
Appropriate Beta Blocker Usage	45	89%	94%	93%
Controlled Postoperative Blood Glucose	0	-	96%	93%
Prophylactic Antibiotic Timing	93	99%	97%	97%
Prophylactic Antibiotic Timing (Outpatient)[1,3]	19	84%	92%	92%
Prophylactic Antibiotic Selection	95	93%	98%	97%
Prophylactic Antibiotic Select. (Outpatient)[1,3]	17	94%	93%	94%
Prophylactic Antibiotic Stopped	91	98%	95%	94%
Recommended VTP Ordered	33	97%	97%	94%
Urinary Catheter Removal[1]	23	96%	95%	90%
Children's Asthma Care				
Received Systemic Corticosteroids	-	-	-	100%
Received Home Management Plan	-	-	-	71%
Received Reliever Medication	-	-	-	100%
Use of Medical Imaging				
Combination Abdominal CT Scan	297	0.394	0.203	0.191
Combination Chest CT Scan	177	0.023	0.026	0.054
Follow-up Mammogram/Ultrasound	567	6.5%	8.2%	8.4%
MRI for Low Back Pain[1]	51	27.5%	32.4%	32.7%
Survey of Patients' Hospital Experiences				
Area Around Room 'Always' Quiet at Night	300+	45%	-	58%
Doctors 'Always' Communicated Well	300+	81%	-	80%
Home Recovery Information Given	300+	84%	-	82%
Hospital Given 9 or 10 on 10 Point Scale	300+	61%	-	67%
Meds 'Always' Explained Before Given	300+	60%	-	60%
Nurses 'Always' Communicated Well	300+	75%	-	76%
Pain 'Always' Well Controlled	300+	66%	-	69%
Room and Bathroom 'Always' Clean	300+	78%	-	71%
Timely Help 'Always' Received	300+	68%	-	64%
Would Definitely Recommend Hospital	300+	57%	-	69%

Carlisle Regional Medical Center

361 Alexander Spring Road Phone: 717-249-1212
Carlisle, PA 17015 Fax: 717-960-3256
E-mail: livelifewell@crmcpa.hma-corp.com
URL: www.carlislermc.com
Type: Acute Care Hospitals Emergency Services: Yes
Ownership: Proprietary Beds: 200

Key Personnel:
CEO/President. . . . . Nathan Staggs
Chief of Medical Staff. . . . . Joseph T Acri
Operating Room. . . . . David Bryant
Pediatric In-Patient Care . . . . Deb Raubenstine
Quality Assurance . . . . Georgina Laughman
Radiology. . . . . Dennis M Burton

Measure	Cases	This Hosp.	State Avg.	U.S. Avg.
Heart Attack Care				
ACE Inhibitor or ARB for LVSD[1]	9	67%	95%	96%
Aspirin at Arrival	52	96%	99%	99%
Aspirin at Discharge[1]	22	91%	99%	98%
Beta Blocker at Discharge	25	100%	99%	98%
Fibrinolytic Medication Timing	0	-	40%	55%
PCI Within 90 Minutes of Arrival	0	-	88%	90%
Smoking Cessation Advice[1]	2	100%	100%	99%
Chest Pain/Possible Heart Attack Care				
Aspirin at Arrival	116	97%	95%	95%
Median Time to ECG (minutes)	119	5	8	8
Median Time to Transfer (minutes)[1]	14	51	68	61
Fibrinolytic Medication Timing	0	-	48%	54%
Heart Failure Care				
ACE Inhibitor or ARB for LVSD	61	90%	95%	94%
Discharge Instructions	165	89%	90%	88%
Evaluation of LVS Function	245	99%	99%	98%
Smoking Cessation Advice	33	100%	98%	98%
Pneumonia Care				
Appropriate Initial Antibiotic	93	97%	93%	92%
Blood Culture Timing	175	95%	96%	96%
Influenza Vaccine	106	98%	92%	91%
Initial Antibiotic Timing	154	96%	96%	95%
Pneumococcal Vaccine	145	99%	95%	93%
Smoking Cessation Advice	40	100%	98%	97%
Surgical Care Improvement Project				
Appropriate VTP Within 24 Hours[2]	187	94%	95%	92%
Appropriate Hair Removal[2]	561	100%	100%	99%
Appropriate Beta Blocker Usage[2]	179	93%	94%	93%
Controlled Postoperative Blood Glucose[2]	0	-	96%	93%
Prophylactic Antibiotic Timing[2]	394	99%	97%	97%
Prophylactic Antibiotic Timing (Outpatient)	137	87%	92%	92%
Prophylactic Antibiotic Selection[2]	395	97%	98%	97%
Prophylactic Antibiotic Select. (Outpatient)	120	91%	93%	94%
Prophylactic Antibiotic Stopped[2]	375	97%	95%	94%
Recommended VTP Ordered[2]	187	99%	97%	94%
Urinary Catheter Removal	59	98%	95%	90%
Children's Asthma Care				
Received Systemic Corticosteroids	-	-	-	100%
Received Home Management Plan	-	-	-	71%
Received Reliever Medication	-	-	-	100%
Use of Medical Imaging				
Combination Abdominal CT Scan	759	0.178	0.203	0.191
Combination Chest CT Scan	549	0.164	0.026	0.054
Follow-up Mammogram/Ultrasound	563	3.9%	8.2%	8.4%
MRI for Low Back Pain	77	20.8%	32.4%	32.7%
Survey of Patients' Hospital Experiences				
Area Around Room 'Always' Quiet at Night	300+	52%	-	58%
Doctors 'Always' Communicated Well	300+	76%	-	80%
Home Recovery Information Given	300+	82%	-	82%
Hospital Given 9 or 10 on 10 Point Scale	300+	58%	-	67%
Meds 'Always' Explained Before Given	300+	53%	-	60%
Nurses 'Always' Communicated Well	300+	73%	-	76%
Pain 'Always' Well Controlled	300+	67%	-	69%
Room and Bathroom 'Always' Clean	300+	75%	-	71%
Timely Help 'Always' Received	300+	62%	-	64%
Would Definitely Recommend Hospital	300+	57%	-	69%

NOTE: Hospital profiles are in alphabetical order by state, then city, then hospital within the city; Rankings exclude hospitals with less than 25 cases except for patient surveys which excludes hospitals with less than 100 cases; (a) 100–299 cases; (1) The number of cases is too small to be sure how well a hospital is performing; (2) The hospital indicated that the data submitted for this measure were based on a sample of cases; (3) Data was collected during a shorter time period (fewer quarters) than the maximum possible time for this measure; (4) Suppressed for one or more quarters by CMS; (5) No data is available from the hospital for this measure; (6) Fewer than 100 patients completed the HCAHPS survey. Use these rates with caution, as the number of surveys may be too low to reliably assess hospital performance; (7) Survey results are based on less than 12 months of data; (8) Survey results are not available for this reporting period; (9) No or very few patients were eligible for the HCAHPS survey. The scores shown, if any, reflect a very small number of surveys; (10) A state average was not calculated because too few hospitals in the state submitted data; (11) There were discrepancies in the data collection process; Please refer to the User's Guide for a full explanation of data.

Chambersburg Hospital

112 North Seventh Street
Chambersburg, PA 17201
URL: www.summithealth.org
Type: Acute Care Hospitals
Ownership: Voluntary Non-Profit - Other
Phone: 717-267-3000
Fax: 717-267-7920
Emergency Services: Yes
Beds: 248

Key Personnel:
Chief of Medical Staff . . . . Mark A Swatrz, MD
Operating Room. . . . . Stephen Lindsay Carter, RN
Pediatric Ambulatory Care . . . . . Carolyn Kent, RN
Quality Assurance . . . . Patricia Goulding, RN
Radiology. . . . . Amir R Batouli, MD
Emergency Room . . . . James Agnew, RN

Measure	Cases	This Hosp.	State Avg.	U.S. Avg.
Heart Attack Care				
ACE Inhibitor or ARB for LVSD	70	96%	95%	96%
Aspirin at Arrival	292	98%	99%	99%
Aspirin at Discharge	329	98%	99%	98%
Beta Blocker at Discharge	338	97%	99%	98%
Fibrinolytic Medication Timing	0	-	40%	55%
PCI Within 90 Minutes of Arrival	46	85%	88%	90%
Smoking Cessation Advice	102	99%	100%	99%
Chest Pain/Possible Heart Attack Care				
Aspirin at Arrival	31	90%	95%	95%
Median Time to ECG (minutes)	34	12	8	8
Median Time to Transfer (minutes)[5]	0	-	68	61
Fibrinolytic Medication Timing[3]	0	-	48%	54%
Heart Failure Care				
ACE Inhibitor or ARB for LVSD	95	94%	95%	94%
Discharge Instructions	314	88%	90%	88%
Evaluation of LVS Function	394	97%	99%	98%
Smoking Cessation Advice	61	97%	98%	98%
Pneumonia Care				
Appropriate Initial Antibiotic	152	89%	93%	92%
Blood Culture Timing	223	98%	96%	96%
Influenza Vaccine	139	96%	92%	91%
Initial Antibiotic Timing	221	96%	96%	95%
Pneumococcal Vaccine	219	97%	95%	93%
Smoking Cessation Advice	85	94%	98%	97%
Surgical Care Improvement Project				
Appropriate VTP Within 24 Hours[2]	344	95%	95%	92%
Appropriate Hair Removal[2]	921	100%	100%	99%
Appropriate Beta Blocker Usage[2]	301	95%	94%	93%
Controlled Postoperative Blood Glucose[2]	0	-	96%	93%
Prophylactic Antibiotic Timing[2]	798	98%	97%	97%
Prophylactic Antibiotic Timing (Outpatient)	71	92%	92%	92%
Prophylactic Antibiotic Selection[2]	800	97%	98%	97%
Prophylactic Antibiotic Select. (Outpatient)	69	74%	93%	94%
Prophylactic Antibiotic Stopped[2]	764	94%	95%	94%
Recommended VTP Ordered[2]	344	96%	97%	94%
Urinary Catheter Removal[2]	56	82%	95%	90%
Children's Asthma Care				
Received Systemic Corticosteroids	-	-	-	100%
Received Home Management Plan	-	-	-	71%
Received Reliever Medication	-	-	-	100%
Use of Medical Imaging				
Combination Abdominal CT Scan	1,277	0.190	0.203	0.191
Combination Chest CT Scan	698	0.046	0.026	0.054
Follow-up Mammogram/Ultrasound	2,854	5.5%	8.2%	8.4%
MRI for Low Back Pain	367	31.9%	32.4%	32.7%
Survey of Patients' Hospital Experiences				
Area Around Room 'Always' Quiet at Night	300+	46%	-	58%
Doctors 'Always' Communicated Well	300+	76%	-	80%
Home Recovery Information Given	300+	81%	-	82%
Hospital Given 9 or 10 on 10 Point Scale	300+	64%	-	67%
Meds 'Always' Explained Before Given	300+	59%	-	60%
Nurses 'Always' Communicated Well	300+	77%	-	76%
Pain 'Always' Well Controlled	300+	69%	-	69%
Room and Bathroom 'Always' Clean	300+	75%	-	71%
Timely Help 'Always' Received	300+	65%	-	64%
Would Definitely Recommend Hospital	300+	63%	-	69%

Clarion Hospital

One Hospital Drive
Clarion, PA 16214
URL: www.clarionhospital.org
Type: Acute Care Hospitals
Ownership: Voluntary Non-Profit - Other
Phone: 814-226-9500
Fax: 814-226-1224
Emergency Services: Yes
Beds: 96

Key Personnel:
Chief of Medical Staff . . . . John Meyers
Operating Room. . . . . Connie Aaron, RN
Quality Assurance . . . . Paul Edder
Anesthesiology. . . . . Ronald Buckley, D.O.
Emergency Room . . . . Arthur Dortort, DO

Measure	Cases	This Hosp.	State Avg.	U.S. Avg.
Heart Attack Care				
ACE Inhibitor or ARB for LVSD[1]	6	100%	95%	96%
Aspirin at Arrival[1]	20	90%	99%	99%
Aspirin at Discharge[1]	13	92%	99%	98%
Beta Blocker at Discharge[1]	13	100%	99%	98%
Fibrinolytic Medication Timing[1]	1	100%	40%	55%
PCI Within 90 Minutes of Arrival	0	-	88%	90%
Smoking Cessation Advice[1]	1	100%	100%	99%
Chest Pain/Possible Heart Attack Care				
Aspirin at Arrival	63	95%	95%	95%
Median Time to ECG (minutes)	65	21	8	8
Median Time to Transfer (minutes)[1,3]	4	71	68	61
Fibrinolytic Medication Timing[1]	3	0%	48%	54%
Heart Failure Care				
ACE Inhibitor or ARB for LVSD	30	73%	95%	94%
Discharge Instructions	86	67%	90%	88%
Evaluation of LVS Function	112	88%	99%	98%
Smoking Cessation Advice[1]	6	50%	98%	98%
Pneumonia Care				
Appropriate Initial Antibiotic	94	89%	93%	92%
Blood Culture Timing	125	90%	96%	96%
Influenza Vaccine	72	93%	92%	91%
Initial Antibiotic Timing	144	97%	96%	95%
Pneumococcal Vaccine	112	80%	95%	93%
Smoking Cessation Advice	45	71%	98%	97%
Surgical Care Improvement Project				
Appropriate VTP Within 24 Hours	43	86%	95%	92%
Appropriate Hair Removal	238	100%	100%	99%
Appropriate Beta Blocker Usage	48	79%	94%	93%
Controlled Postoperative Blood Glucose	0	-	96%	93%
Prophylactic Antibiotic Timing	186	96%	97%	97%
Prophylactic Antibiotic Timing (Outpatient)	30	83%	92%	92%
Prophylactic Antibiotic Selection	185	98%	98%	97%
Prophylactic Antibiotic Select. (Outpatient)	28	71%	93%	94%
Prophylactic Antibiotic Stopped	184	93%	95%	94%
Recommended VTP Ordered	43	86%	97%	94%
Urinary Catheter Removal	52	90%	95%	90%
Children's Asthma Care				
Received Systemic Corticosteroids	-	-	-	100%
Received Home Management Plan	-	-	-	71%
Received Reliever Medication	-	-	-	100%
Use of Medical Imaging				
Combination Abdominal CT Scan	379	0.491	0.203	0.191
Combination Chest CT Scan	207	0.512	0.026	0.054
Follow-up Mammogram/Ultrasound	561	10.5%	8.2%	8.4%
MRI for Low Back Pain	86	32.6%	32.4%	32.7%
Survey of Patients' Hospital Experiences				
Area Around Room 'Always' Quiet at Night	300+	50%	-	58%
Doctors 'Always' Communicated Well	300+	78%	-	80%
Home Recovery Information Given	300+	81%	-	82%
Hospital Given 9 or 10 on 10 Point Scale	300+	61%	-	67%
Meds 'Always' Explained Before Given	300+	54%	-	60%
Nurses 'Always' Communicated Well	300+	71%	-	76%
Pain 'Always' Well Controlled	300+	67%	-	69%
Room and Bathroom 'Always' Clean	300+	65%	-	71%
Timely Help 'Always' Received	300+	65%	-	64%
Would Definitely Recommend Hospital	300+	59%	-	69%

Clearfield Hospital

809 Turnpike Ave
Clearfield, PA 16830
E-mail: info@clearfieldhosp.org
URL: www.clearfieldhosp.org
Type: Acute Care Hospitals
Ownership: Voluntary Non-Profit - Other
Phone: 814-765-5341
Fax: 814-768-2445
Emergency Services: Yes
Beds: 83

Key Personnel:
CEO/President. . . . . David J McConnell
Chief of Medical Staff . . . . Gregory Sheffo
Radiology. . . . . Alfred B Coren
Anesthesiology. . . . . Richard C Bedger Jr

Measure	Cases	This Hosp.	State Avg.	U.S. Avg.
Heart Attack Care				
ACE Inhibitor or ARB for LVSD[1]	2	100%	95%	96%
Aspirin at Arrival[1]	17	100%	99%	99%
Aspirin at Discharge[1]	7	100%	99%	98%
Beta Blocker at Discharge[1]	7	86%	99%	98%
Fibrinolytic Medication Timing	0	-	40%	55%
PCI Within 90 Minutes of Arrival	0	-	88%	90%
Smoking Cessation Advice	0	-	100%	99%
Chest Pain/Possible Heart Attack Care				
Aspirin at Arrival	128	93%	95%	95%
Median Time to ECG (minutes)	138	2	8	8
Median Time to Transfer (minutes)[1]	8	58	68	61
Fibrinolytic Medication Timing[1]	4	25%	48%	54%
Heart Failure Care				
ACE Inhibitor or ARB for LVSD	37	89%	95%	94%
Discharge Instructions	114	67%	90%	88%
Evaluation of LVS Function	159	99%	99%	98%
Smoking Cessation Advice[1]	17	100%	98%	98%
Pneumonia Care				
Appropriate Initial Antibiotic	118	92%	93%	92%
Blood Culture Timing	211	92%	96%	96%
Influenza Vaccine	105	91%	92%	91%
Initial Antibiotic Timing	203	99%	96%	95%
Pneumococcal Vaccine	176	94%	95%	93%
Smoking Cessation Advice	35	100%	98%	97%
Surgical Care Improvement Project				
Appropriate VTP Within 24 Hours	156	94%	95%	92%
Appropriate Hair Removal	273	99%	100%	99%
Appropriate Beta Blocker Usage	93	90%	94%	93%
Controlled Postoperative Blood Glucose	0	-	96%	93%
Prophylactic Antibiotic Timing	203	91%	97%	97%
Prophylactic Antibiotic Timing (Outpatient)	99	96%	92%	92%
Prophylactic Antibiotic Selection	203	95%	98%	97%
Prophylactic Antibiotic Select. (Outpatient)	97	97%	93%	94%
Prophylactic Antibiotic Stopped	195	91%	95%	94%
Recommended VTP Ordered	156	95%	97%	94%
Urinary Catheter Removal	28	61%	95%	90%
Children's Asthma Care				
Received Systemic Corticosteroids	-	-	-	100%
Received Home Management Plan	-	-	-	71%
Received Reliever Medication	-	-	-	100%
Use of Medical Imaging				
Combination Abdominal CT Scan	854	0.663	0.203	0.191
Combination Chest CT Scan	303	0.033	0.026	0.054
Follow-up Mammogram/Ultrasound	769	4.3%	8.2%	8.4%
MRI for Low Back Pain	77	40.3%	32.4%	32.7%
Survey of Patients' Hospital Experiences				
Area Around Room 'Always' Quiet at Night	300+	44%	-	58%
Doctors 'Always' Communicated Well	300+	80%	-	80%
Home Recovery Information Given	300+	84%	-	82%
Hospital Given 9 or 10 on 10 Point Scale	300+	54%	-	67%
Meds 'Always' Explained Before Given	300+	59%	-	60%
Nurses 'Always' Communicated Well	300+	71%	-	76%
Pain 'Always' Well Controlled	300+	64%	-	69%
Room and Bathroom 'Always' Clean	300+	69%	-	71%
Timely Help 'Always' Received	300+	59%	-	64%
Would Definitely Recommend Hospital	300+	51%	-	69%

NOTE: Hospital profiles are in alphabetical order by state, then city, then hospital within the city; Rankings exclude hospitals with less than 25 cases except for patient surveys which excludes hospitals with less than 100 cases; (a) 100–299 cases; (1) The number of cases is too small to be sure how well a hospital is performing; (2) The hospital indicated that the data submitted for this measure were based on a sample of cases; (3) Data was collected during a shorter time period (fewer quarters) than the maximum possible time for this measure; (4) Suppressed for one or more quarters by CMS; (5) No data is available from the hospital for this measure; (6) Fewer than 100 patients completed the HCAHPS survey. Use these rates with caution, as the number of surveys may be too low to reliably assess hospital performance; (7) Survey results are based on less than 12 months of data; (8) Survey results are not available for this reporting period; (9) No or very few patients were eligible for the HCAHPS survey. The scores shown, if any, reflect a very small number of surveys; (10) A state average was not calculated because too few hospitals in the state submitted data; (11) There were discrepancies in the data collection process; Please refer to the User's Guide for a full explanation of data.

Shamokin Area Community Hospital

4200 Hospital Road Phone: 570-644-4200
Coal Township, PA 17866 Fax: 570-644-4351
E-mail: webmaster@shamokinhospital.org
URL: www.shamokinhospital.org
Type: Acute Care Hospitals Emergency Services: Yes
Ownership: Voluntary Non-Profit - Private Beds: 61

Key Personnel:
CEO/President. . . . . Thomas R Harlow
Cardiac Laboratory. . . . . Maryann Woytoich
Chief of Medical Staff . . . . Suzanne M Mace, MD
Radiology. . . . . Jinan O Bahia
Emergency Room . . . . Ann Marie Augustine

Measure	Cases	This Hosp.	State Avg.	U.S. Avg.
Heart Attack Care				
ACE Inhibitor or ARB for LVSD[1]	12	100%	95%	96%
Aspirin at Arrival	100	99%	99%	99%
Aspirin at Discharge	76	96%	99%	98%
Beta Blocker at Discharge	91	97%	99%	98%
Fibrinolytic Medication Timing	0	-	40%	55%
PCI Within 90 Minutes of Arrival	0	-	88%	90%
Smoking Cessation Advice[1]	17	94%	100%	99%
Chest Pain/Possible Heart Attack Care				
Aspirin at Arrival	88	95%	95%	95%
Median Time to ECG (minutes)	92	2	8	8
Median Time to Transfer (minutes)[1,3]	14	50	68	61
Fibrinolytic Medication Timing	0	-	48%	54%
Heart Failure Care				
ACE Inhibitor or ARB for LVSD[1]	16	100%	95%	94%
Discharge Instructions	102	72%	90%	88%
Evaluation of LVS Function	174	99%	99%	98%
Smoking Cessation Advice[1]	7	86%	98%	98%
Pneumonia Care				
Appropriate Initial Antibiotic	37	89%	93%	92%
Blood Culture Timing	86	94%	96%	96%
Influenza Vaccine	103	100%	92%	91%
Initial Antibiotic Timing	135	97%	96%	95%
Pneumococcal Vaccine	142	100%	95%	93%
Smoking Cessation Advice	30	93%	98%	97%
Surgical Care Improvement Project				
Appropriate VTP Within 24 Hours	41	88%	95%	92%
Appropriate Hair Removal	128	100%	100%	99%
Appropriate Beta Blocker Usage	56	88%	94%	93%
Controlled Postoperative Blood Glucose	0	-	96%	93%
Prophylactic Antibiotic Timing	92	95%	97%	97%
Prophylactic Antibiotic Timing (Outpatient)[1,3]	20	85%	92%	92%
Prophylactic Antibiotic Selection	92	98%	98%	97%
Prophylactic Antibiotic Select. (Outpatient)[1,3]	19	84%	93%	94%
Prophylactic Antibiotic Stopped	89	85%	95%	94%
Recommended VTP Ordered	41	90%	97%	94%
Urinary Catheter Removal	50	98%	95%	90%
Children's Asthma Care				
Received Systemic Corticosteroids	-	-	-	100%
Received Home Management Plan	-	-	-	71%
Received Reliever Medication	-	-	-	100%
Use of Medical Imaging				
Combination Abdominal CT Scan	321	0.626	0.203	0.191
Combination Chest CT Scan	264	0.064	0.026	0.054
Follow-up Mammogram/Ultrasound	921	6.8%	8.2%	8.4%
MRI for Low Back Pain	94	40.4%	32.4%	32.7%
Survey of Patients' Hospital Experiences				
Area Around Room 'Always' Quiet at Night	300+	54%	-	58%
Doctors 'Always' Communicated Well	300+	86%	-	80%
Home Recovery Information Given	300+	83%	-	82%
Hospital Given 9 or 10 on 10 Point Scale	300+	82%	-	67%
Meds 'Always' Explained Before Given	300+	61%	-	60%
Nurses 'Always' Communicated Well	300+	83%	-	76%
Pain 'Always' Well Controlled	300+	72%	-	69%
Room and Bathroom 'Always' Clean	300+	89%	-	71%
Timely Help 'Always' Received	300+	78%	-	64%
Would Definitely Recommend Hospital	300+	83%	-	69%

Saint Luke's Miners Memorial Hospital

360 W Ruddle Street Phone: 570-645-2131
Coaldale, PA 18218 Fax: 570-645-2121
URL: www.slhn-lehighvalley.org
Type: Acute Care Hospitals Emergency Services: Yes
Ownership: Voluntary Non-Profit - Private Beds: 61

Key Personnel:
CEO/President. . . . . William J Crossin
Chief of Medical Staff. . . . . Arthur Kennedy, MD
Infection Control. . . . . Kathy Matika, RN BSN
Operating Room. . . . . Atul K Amin, RN
Quality Assurance . . . . Gail Marek
Radiology. . . . . James D Bohri MD
Anesthesiology. . . . . Smita Mody, MD
Emergency Room . . . . Eric Rodish, MD

Measure	Cases	This Hosp.	State Avg.	U.S. Avg.
Heart Attack Care				
ACE Inhibitor or ARB for LVSD[1]	1	100%	95%	96%
Aspirin at Arrival[1]	20	80%	99%	99%
Aspirin at Discharge[1]	14	71%	99%	98%
Beta Blocker at Discharge[1]	13	92%	99%	98%
Fibrinolytic Medication Timing	0	-	40%	55%
PCI Within 90 Minutes of Arrival	0	-	88%	90%
Smoking Cessation Advice	0	-	100%	99%
Chest Pain/Possible Heart Attack Care				
Aspirin at Arrival[5]	0	-	95%	95%
Median Time to ECG (minutes)[5]	0	-	8	8
Median Time to Transfer (minutes)[5]	0	-	68	61
Fibrinolytic Medication Timing[5]	0	-	48%	54%
Heart Failure Care				
ACE Inhibitor or ARB for LVSD[1]	18	89%	95%	94%
Discharge Instructions	55	100%	90%	88%
Evaluation of LVS Function	74	97%	99%	98%
Smoking Cessation Advice[1]	7	100%	98%	98%
Pneumonia Care				
Appropriate Initial Antibiotic	39	90%	93%	92%
Blood Culture Timing	57	100%	96%	96%
Influenza Vaccine	39	100%	92%	91%
Initial Antibiotic Timing	58	97%	96%	95%
Pneumococcal Vaccine	62	100%	95%	93%
Smoking Cessation Advice[1]	16	100%	98%	97%
Surgical Care Improvement Project				
Appropriate VTP Within 24 Hours	58	98%	95%	92%
Appropriate Hair Removal	188	100%	100%	99%
Appropriate Beta Blocker Usage	52	67%	94%	93%
Controlled Postoperative Blood Glucose	0	-	96%	93%
Prophylactic Antibiotic Timing	158	99%	97%	97%
Prophylactic Antibiotic Timing (Outpatient)[1]	19	84%	92%	92%
Prophylactic Antibiotic Selection	159	99%	98%	97%
Prophylactic Antibiotic Select. (Outpatient)[1]	16	94%	93%	94%
Prophylactic Antibiotic Stopped	153	95%	95%	94%
Recommended VTP Ordered	58	100%	97%	94%
Urinary Catheter Removal	74	84%	95%	90%
Children's Asthma Care				
Received Systemic Corticosteroids	-	-	-	100%
Received Home Management Plan	-	-	-	71%
Received Reliever Medication	-	-	-	100%
Use of Medical Imaging				
Combination Abdominal CT Scan	349	0.218	0.203	0.191
Combination Chest CT Scan	239	0.084	0.026	0.054
Follow-up Mammogram/Ultrasound	406	3.7%	8.2%	8.4%
MRI for Low Back Pain	69	30.4%	32.4%	32.7%
Survey of Patients' Hospital Experiences				
Area Around Room 'Always' Quiet at Night	300+	51%	-	58%
Doctors 'Always' Communicated Well	300+	80%	-	80%
Home Recovery Information Given	300+	82%	-	82%
Hospital Given 9 or 10 on 10 Point Scale	300+	61%	-	67%
Meds 'Always' Explained Before Given	300+	58%	-	60%
Nurses 'Always' Communicated Well	300+	77%	-	76%
Pain 'Always' Well Controlled	300+	67%	-	69%
Room and Bathroom 'Always' Clean	300+	79%	-	71%
Timely Help 'Always' Received	300+	58%	-	64%
Would Definitely Recommend Hospital	300+	64%	-	69%

Brandywine Hospital

201 Reeseville Road Phone: 610-383-8000
Coatesville, PA 19320 Fax: 610-383-8233
URL: www.brandywinehospital.com
Type: Acute Care Hospitals Emergency Services: Yes
Ownership: Proprietary Beds: 168

Key Personnel:
CEO/President. . . . . Marion McGowan
Chief of Medical Staff. . . . . Robert Satriale, MD
Pediatric In-Patient Care . . . . F D'Urso, MD
Quality Assurance . . . . Kathy Zoph Herling
Radiology. . . . . Ronald Adelman, MD

Measure	Cases	This Hosp.	State Avg.	U.S. Avg.
Heart Attack Care				
ACE Inhibitor or ARB for LVSD[1]	10	90%	95%	96%
Aspirin at Arrival	137	98%	99%	99%
Aspirin at Discharge	122	93%	99%	98%
Beta Blocker at Discharge	121	95%	99%	98%
Fibrinolytic Medication Timing	0	-	40%	55%
PCI Within 90 Minutes of Arrival	29	93%	88%	90%
Smoking Cessation Advice	56	98%	100%	99%
Chest Pain/Possible Heart Attack Care				
Aspirin at Arrival[1]	5	100%	95%	95%
Median Time to ECG (minutes)[1]	5	4	8	8
Median Time to Transfer (minutes)[1,3]	1	50	68	61
Fibrinolytic Medication Timing[3]	0	-	48%	54%
Heart Failure Care				
ACE Inhibitor or ARB for LVSD	70	81%	95%	94%
Discharge Instructions	157	94%	90%	88%
Evaluation of LVS Function	231	100%	99%	98%
Smoking Cessation Advice	36	100%	98%	98%
Pneumonia Care				
Appropriate Initial Antibiotic	129	92%	93%	92%
Blood Culture Timing	166	97%	96%	96%
Influenza Vaccine	126	95%	92%	91%
Initial Antibiotic Timing	197	92%	96%	95%
Pneumococcal Vaccine	167	98%	95%	93%
Smoking Cessation Advice	72	100%	98%	97%
Surgical Care Improvement Project				
Appropriate VTP Within 24 Hours[2]	106	83%	95%	92%
Appropriate Hair Removal[2]	300	100%	100%	99%
Appropriate Beta Blocker Usage[2]	114	89%	94%	93%
Controlled Postoperative Blood Glucose[1,2]	21	95%	96%	93%
Prophylactic Antibiotic Timing[2]	169	97%	97%	97%
Prophylactic Antibiotic Timing (Outpatient)	105	94%	92%	92%
Prophylactic Antibiotic Selection[2]	169	93%	98%	97%
Prophylactic Antibiotic Select. (Outpatient)	100	97%	93%	94%
Prophylactic Antibiotic Stopped[2]	152	95%	95%	94%
Recommended VTP Ordered[2]	107	88%	97%	94%
Urinary Catheter Removal	71	94%	95%	90%
Children's Asthma Care				
Received Systemic Corticosteroids	-	-	-	100%
Received Home Management Plan	-	-	-	71%
Received Reliever Medication	-	-	-	100%
Use of Medical Imaging				
Combination Abdominal CT Scan	355	0.166	0.203	0.191
Combination Chest CT Scan	270	0.011	0.026	0.054
Follow-up Mammogram/Ultrasound	623	15.7%	8.2%	8.4%
MRI for Low Back Pain	92	31.5%	32.4%	32.7%
Survey of Patients' Hospital Experiences				
Area Around Room 'Always' Quiet at Night	300+	44%	-	58%
Doctors 'Always' Communicated Well	300+	74%	-	80%
Home Recovery Information Given	300+	80%	-	82%
Hospital Given 9 or 10 on 10 Point Scale	300+	57%	-	67%
Meds 'Always' Explained Before Given	300+	50%	-	60%
Nurses 'Always' Communicated Well	300+	71%	-	76%
Pain 'Always' Well Controlled	300+	64%	-	69%
Room and Bathroom 'Always' Clean	300+	61%	-	71%
Timely Help 'Always' Received	300+	52%	-	64%
Would Definitely Recommend Hospital	300+	55%	-	69%

NOTE: Hospital profiles are in alphabetical order by state, then city, then hospital within the city; Rankings exclude hospitals with less than 25 cases except for patient surveys which excludes hospitals with less than 100 cases; (a) 100–299 cases; (1) The number of cases is too small to be sure how well a hospital is performing; (2) The hospital indicated that the data submitted for this measure were based on a sample of cases; (3) Data was collected during a shorter time period (fewer quarters) than the maximum possible time for this measure; (4) Suppressed for one or more quarters by CMS; (5) No data is available from the hospital for this measure; (6) Fewer than 100 patients completed the HCAHPS survey. Use these rates with caution, as the number of surveys may be too low to reliably assess hospital performance; (7) Survey results are based on less than 12 months of data; (8) Survey results are not available for this reporting period; (9) No or very few patients were eligible for the HCAHPS survey. The scores shown, if any, reflect a very small number of surveys; (10) A state average was not calculated because too few hospitals in the state submitted data; (11) There were discrepancies in the data collection process; Please refer to the User's Guide for a full explanation of data.

Coatesville VA Medical Center

1400 Black Horse Hill Road   Phone: 610-384-7711
Coatesville, PA 19320   Fax: 610-383-0207
Type: Acute Care-Veterans Administration   Emergency Services: No
Ownership: Government - Federal
Key Personnel:
Quality Assurance . . . . JoAnn Reny, RN

Measure	Cases	This Hosp.	State Avg.	U.S. Avg.
Heart Attack Care				
ACE Inhibitor or ARB for LVSD[5]	0	-	95%	96%
Aspirin at Arrival[5]	0	-	99%	99%
Aspirin at Discharge[5]	0	-	99%	98%
Beta Blocker at Discharge[5]	0	-	99%	98%
Fibrinolytic Medication Timing[5]	0	-	40%	55%
PCI Within 90 Minutes of Arrival[5]	0	-	88%	90%
Smoking Cessation Advice[5]	0	-	100%	99%
Chest Pain/Possible Heart Attack Care				
Aspirin at Arrival	-	-	95%	95%
Median Time to ECG (minutes)	-	-	8	8
Median Time to Transfer (minutes)	-	-	68	61
Fibrinolytic Medication Timing	-	-	48%	54%
Heart Failure Care				
ACE Inhibitor or ARB for LVSD[5]	0	-	95%	94%
Discharge Instructions[5]	0	-	90%	88%
Evaluation of LVS Function[5]	0	-	99%	98%
Smoking Cessation Advice[5]	0	-	98%	98%
Pneumonia Care				
Appropriate Initial Antibiotic[1]	1	0%	93%	92%
Blood Culture Timing[1]	1	100%	96%	96%
Influenza Vaccine[1]	3	100%	92%	91%
Initial Antibiotic Timing[1]	2	100%	96%	95%
Pneumococcal Vaccine[1]	1	100%	95%	93%
Smoking Cessation Advice[1]	1	100%	98%	97%
Surgical Care Improvement Project				
Appropriate VTP Within 24 Hours[2,5]	0	-	95%	92%
Appropriate Hair Removal[2,5]	0	-	100%	99%
Appropriate Beta Blocker Usage[2,5]	0	-	94%	93%
Controlled Postoperative Blood Glucose[2,5]	0	-	96%	93%
Prophylactic Antibiotic Timing[5]	0	-	97%	97%
Prophylactic Antibiotic Timing (Outpatient)	-	-	92%	92%
Prophylactic Antibiotic Selection[5]	0	-	98%	97%
Prophylactic Antibiotic Select. (Outpatient)	-	-	93%	94%
Prophylactic Antibiotic Stopped[5]	0	-	95%	94%
Recommended VTP Ordered[2,5]	0	-	97%	94%
Urinary Catheter Removal[2,5]	0	-	95%	90%
Children's Asthma Care				
Received Systemic Corticosteroids	-	-	-	100%
Received Home Management Plan	-	-	-	71%
Received Reliever Medication	-	-	-	100%
Use of Medical Imaging				
Combination Abdominal CT Scan	-	-	0.203	0.191
Combination Chest CT Scan	-	-	0.026	0.054
Follow-up Mammogram/Ultrasound	-	-	8.2%	8.4%
MRI for Low Back Pain	-	-	32.4%	32.7%
Survey of Patients' Hospital Experiences				
Area Around Room 'Always' Quiet at Night	-	-	-	58%
Doctors 'Always' Communicated Well	-	-	-	80%
Home Recovery Information Given	-	-	-	82%
Hospital Given 9 or 10 on 10 Point Scale	-	-	-	67%
Meds 'Always' Explained Before Given	-	-	-	60%
Nurses 'Always' Communicated Well	-	-	-	76%
Pain 'Always' Well Controlled	-	-	-	69%
Room and Bathroom 'Always' Clean	-	-	-	71%
Timely Help 'Always' Received	-	-	-	64%
Would Definitely Recommend Hospital	-	-	-	69%

Highlands Hospital

401 East Murphy Avenue   Phone: 724-628-1500
Connellsville, PA 15425   Fax: 724-626-2334
E-mail: webmaster@highlandshospital.org
URL: www.highlandshospital.org
Type: Acute Care Hospitals   Emergency Services: Yes
Ownership: Voluntary Non-Profit - Private   Beds: 87
Key Personnel:
CEO/President . . . . Michelle Cuttingham
Chief of Medical Staff . . . . Albert Enany, MD
Quality Assurance . . . . Barbra Morrison
Emergency Room . . . . Peter Stevenson

Measure	Cases	This Hosp.	State Avg.	U.S. Avg.
Heart Attack Care				
ACE Inhibitor or ARB for LVSD[1,3]	1	0%	95%	96%
Aspirin at Arrival[1,3]	5	100%	99%	99%
Aspirin at Discharge[1,3]	4	100%	99%	98%
Beta Blocker at Discharge[1,3]	4	100%	99%	98%
Fibrinolytic Medication Timing[3]	0	-	40%	55%
PCI Within 90 Minutes of Arrival[3]	0	-	88%	90%
Smoking Cessation Advice[3]	0	-	100%	99%
Chest Pain/Possible Heart Attack Care				
Aspirin at Arrival	98	81%	95%	95%
Median Time to ECG (minutes)	102	12	8	8
Median Time to Transfer (minutes)[1]	15	75	68	61
Fibrinolytic Medication Timing	0	-	48%	54%
Heart Failure Care				
ACE Inhibitor or ARB for LVSD[1]	13	85%	95%	94%
Discharge Instructions	59	85%	90%	88%
Evaluation of LVS Function	61	100%	99%	98%
Smoking Cessation Advice[1]	3	100%	98%	98%
Pneumonia Care				
Appropriate Initial Antibiotic	60	82%	93%	92%
Blood Culture Timing	61	98%	96%	96%
Influenza Vaccine	33	79%	92%	91%
Initial Antibiotic Timing	67	97%	96%	95%
Pneumococcal Vaccine	51	94%	95%	93%
Smoking Cessation Advice[1]	24	100%	98%	97%
Surgical Care Improvement Project				
Appropriate VTP Within 24 Hours[2]	45	84%	95%	92%
Appropriate Hair Removal[2]	70	99%	100%	99%
Appropriate Beta Blocker Usage[2,1]	16	94%	94%	93%
Controlled Postoperative Blood Glucose[2]	0	-	96%	93%
Prophylactic Antibiotic Timing[2]	32	75%	97%	97%
Prophylactic Antibiotic Timing (Outpatient)[1,3]	8	62%	92%	92%
Prophylactic Antibiotic Selection[2]	32	94%	98%	97%
Prophylactic Antibiotic Select. (Outpatient)[1,3]	6	83%	93%	94%
Prophylactic Antibiotic Stopped[2]	31	84%	95%	94%
Recommended VTP Ordered[2]	45	89%	97%	94%
Urinary Catheter Removal[1]	20	80%	95%	90%
Children's Asthma Care				
Received Systemic Corticosteroids	-	-	-	100%
Received Home Management Plan	-	-	-	71%
Received Reliever Medication	-	-	-	100%
Use of Medical Imaging				
Combination Abdominal CT Scan	113	0.673	0.203	0.191
Combination Chest CT Scan[1]	60	0.083	0.026	0.054
Follow-up Mammogram/Ultrasound	184	4.3%	8.2%	8.4%
MRI for Low Back Pain[5]	0	-	32.4%	32.7%
Survey of Patients' Hospital Experiences				
Area Around Room 'Always' Quiet at Night	300+	46%	-	58%
Doctors 'Always' Communicated Well	300+	90%	-	80%
Home Recovery Information Given	300+	86%	-	82%
Hospital Given 9 or 10 on 10 Point Scale	300+	71%	-	67%
Meds 'Always' Explained Before Given	300+	65%	-	60%
Nurses 'Always' Communicated Well	300+	82%	-	76%
Pain 'Always' Well Controlled	300+	78%	-	69%
Room and Bathroom 'Always' Clean	300+	82%	-	71%
Timely Help 'Always' Received	300+	75%	-	64%
Would Definitely Recommend Hospital	300+	72%	-	69%

Corry Memorial Hospital

612 West Smith Street   Phone: 814-664-4641
Corry, PA 16407   Fax: 814-664-7967
E-mail: info@corryhospital.org
URL: www.corryhospital.org
Type: Critical Access Hospitals   Emergency Services: Yes
Ownership: Voluntary Non-Profit - Private   Beds: 55
Key Personnel:
CEO/President . . . . Barbara D Nichols
Chief of Medical Staff . . . . John E Balmer
Radiology . . . . Paul A McGeehan

Measure	Cases	This Hosp.	State Avg.	U.S. Avg.
Heart Attack Care				
ACE Inhibitor or ARB for LVSD[3]	0	-	95%	96%
Aspirin at Arrival[1,3]	1	100%	99%	99%
Aspirin at Discharge[3]	0	-	99%	98%
Beta Blocker at Discharge[3]	0	-	99%	98%
Fibrinolytic Medication Timing[3]	0	-	40%	55%
PCI Within 90 Minutes of Arrival[3]	0	-	88%	90%
Smoking Cessation Advice[3]	0	-	100%	99%
Chest Pain/Possible Heart Attack Care				
Aspirin at Arrival	-	-	95%	95%
Median Time to ECG (minutes)	-	-	8	8
Median Time to Transfer (minutes)	-	-	68	61
Fibrinolytic Medication Timing	-	-	48%	54%
Heart Failure Care				
ACE Inhibitor or ARB for LVSD[1]	15	87%	95%	94%
Discharge Instructions	58	95%	90%	88%
Evaluation of LVS Function	76	86%	99%	98%
Smoking Cessation Advice[1]	7	100%	98%	98%
Pneumonia Care				
Appropriate Initial Antibiotic	52	94%	93%	92%
Blood Culture Timing	46	100%	96%	96%
Influenza Vaccine	42	95%	92%	91%
Initial Antibiotic Timing	72	99%	96%	95%
Pneumococcal Vaccine	71	99%	95%	93%
Smoking Cessation Advice[1]	20	100%	98%	97%
Surgical Care Improvement Project				
Appropriate VTP Within 24 Hours[5]	0	-	95%	92%
Appropriate Hair Removal[5]	0	-	100%	99%
Appropriate Beta Blocker Usage[5]	0	-	94%	93%
Controlled Postoperative Blood Glucose[5]	0	-	96%	93%
Prophylactic Antibiotic Timing[5]	0	-	97%	97%
Prophylactic Antibiotic Timing (Outpatient)	-	-	92%	92%
Prophylactic Antibiotic Selection[5]	0	-	98%	97%
Prophylactic Antibiotic Select. (Outpatient)	-	-	93%	94%
Prophylactic Antibiotic Stopped[5]	0	-	95%	94%
Recommended VTP Ordered[5]	0	-	97%	94%
Urinary Catheter Removal[5]	0	-	95%	90%
Children's Asthma Care				
Received Systemic Corticosteroids	-	-	-	100%
Received Home Management Plan	-	-	-	71%
Received Reliever Medication	-	-	-	100%
Use of Medical Imaging				
Combination Abdominal CT Scan	-	-	0.203	0.191
Combination Chest CT Scan	-	-	0.026	0.054
Follow-up Mammogram/Ultrasound	-	-	8.2%	8.4%
MRI for Low Back Pain	-	-	32.4%	32.7%
Survey of Patients' Hospital Experiences				
Area Around Room 'Always' Quiet at Night	(a)	37%	-	58%
Doctors 'Always' Communicated Well	(a)	81%	-	80%
Home Recovery Information Given	(a)	81%	-	82%
Hospital Given 9 or 10 on 10 Point Scale	(a)	50%	-	67%
Meds 'Always' Explained Before Given	(a)	61%	-	60%
Nurses 'Always' Communicated Well	(a)	73%	-	76%
Pain 'Always' Well Controlled	(a)	62%	-	69%
Room and Bathroom 'Always' Clean	(a)	71%	-	71%
Timely Help 'Always' Received	(a)	60%	-	64%
Would Definitely Recommend Hospital	(a)	45%	-	69%

Charles Cole Memorial Hospital

1001 East Second Street
Coudersport, PA 16915
URL: www.charlescolehospital.com
Type: Critical Access Hospitals
Ownership: Voluntary Non-Profit - Other

Phone: 814-274-9301
Fax: 814-274-0884

Emergency Services: Yes
Beds: 140

Key Personnel:
CEO/President . . . . David Acker
Anesthesiology . . . . David Tonkin, MD
Emergency Room . . . . Michael Lettieri

Measure	Cases	This Hosp.	State Avg.	U.S. Avg.
Heart Attack Care				
ACE Inhibitor or ARB for LVSD[1]	2	100%	95%	96%
Aspirin at Arrival[1]	12	92%	99%	99%
Aspirin at Discharge[1]	10	100%	99%	98%
Beta Blocker at Discharge[1]	8	100%	99%	98%
Fibrinolytic Medication Timing	0	-	40%	55%
PCI Within 90 Minutes of Arrival	0	-	88%	90%
Smoking Cessation Advice[1]	2	100%	100%	99%
Chest Pain/Possible Heart Attack Care				
Aspirin at Arrival	39	92%	95%	95%
Median Time to ECG (minutes)	42	6	8	8
Median Time to Transfer (minutes)[1]	9	91	68	61
Fibrinolytic Medication Timing[1]	1	0%	48%	54%
Heart Failure Care				
ACE Inhibitor or ARB for LVSD[1]	12	100%	95%	94%
Discharge Instructions	47	87%	90%	88%
Evaluation of LVS Function	70	87%	99%	98%
Smoking Cessation Advice[1]	6	100%	98%	98%
Pneumonia Care				
Appropriate Initial Antibiotic	44	98%	93%	92%
Blood Culture Timing	71	94%	96%	96%
Influenza Vaccine	36	86%	92%	91%
Initial Antibiotic Timing	66	94%	96%	95%
Pneumococcal Vaccine	70	94%	95%	93%
Smoking Cessation Advice[1]	13	100%	98%	97%
Surgical Care Improvement Project				
Appropriate VTP Within 24 Hours	57	95%	95%	92%
Appropriate Hair Removal	239	98%	100%	99%
Appropriate Beta Blocker Usage[1,3]	19	100%	94%	93%
Controlled Postoperative Blood Glucose	0	-	96%	93%
Prophylactic Antibiotic Timing	195	87%	97%	97%
Prophylactic Antibiotic Timing (Outpatient)	34	71%	92%	92%
Prophylactic Antibiotic Selection	192	97%	98%	97%
Prophylactic Antibiotic Select. (Outpatient)	26	92%	93%	94%
Prophylactic Antibiotic Stopped	186	95%	95%	94%
Recommended VTP Ordered	59	92%	97%	94%
Urinary Catheter Removal	81	99%	95%	90%
Children's Asthma Care				
Received Systemic Corticosteroids	-	-	-	100%
Received Home Management Plan	-	-	-	71%
Received Reliever Medication	-	-	-	100%
Use of Medical Imaging				
Combination Abdominal CT Scan	237	0.025	0.203	0.191
Combination Chest CT Scan	142	0.007	0.026	0.054
Follow-up Mammogram/Ultrasound	488	7.4%	8.2%	8.4%
MRI for Low Back Pain	56	48.2%	32.4%	32.7%
Survey of Patients' Hospital Experiences				
Area Around Room 'Always' Quiet at Night	300+	60%	-	58%
Doctors 'Always' Communicated Well	300+	83%	-	80%
Home Recovery Information Given	300+	88%	-	82%
Hospital Given 9 or 10 on 10 Point Scale	300+	68%	-	67%
Meds 'Always' Explained Before Given	300+	66%	-	60%
Nurses 'Always' Communicated Well	300+	80%	-	76%
Pain 'Always' Well Controlled	300+	72%	-	69%
Room and Bathroom 'Always' Clean	300+	76%	-	71%
Timely Help 'Always' Received	300+	73%	-	64%
Would Definitely Recommend Hospital	300+	67%	-	69%

Geisinger Medical Center

100 North Academy Avenue
Danville, PA 17822
URL: www.geisinger.org
Type: Acute Care Hospitals
Ownership: Voluntary Non-Profit - Other

Phone: 570-271-6211
Fax: 570-271-5060

Emergency Services: Yes
Beds: 403

Key Personnel:
CEO/President . . . . Glenn Steele, Jr, MD PhD
Chief of Medical Staff . . . . Dennis Toretti
Infection Control . . . . James E Bross, MD
Operating Room . . . . Susan Sneider
Pediatric In-Patient Care . . . . . . Michael Ryan
Quality Assurance . . . . Chuck Miller
Radiology . . . . Joseph Rosen
Emergency Room . . . . John Skiendzielewski

Measure	Cases	This Hosp.	State Avg.	U.S. Avg.
Heart Attack Care				
ACE Inhibitor or ARB for LVSD	102	99%	95%	96%
Aspirin at Arrival	260	99%	99%	99%
Aspirin at Discharge	679	100%	99%	98%
Beta Blocker at Discharge	660	100%	99%	98%
Fibrinolytic Medication Timing	0	-	40%	55%
PCI Within 90 Minutes of Arrival	52	96%	88%	90%
Smoking Cessation Advice	226	100%	100%	99%
Chest Pain/Possible Heart Attack Care				
Aspirin at Arrival[5]	0	-	95%	95%
Median Time to ECG (minutes)[5]	0	-	8	8
Median Time to Transfer (minutes)[5]	0	-	68	61
Fibrinolytic Medication Timing[5]	0	-	48%	54%
Heart Failure Care				
ACE Inhibitor or ARB for LVSD	103	100%	95%	94%
Discharge Instructions	304	96%	90%	88%
Evaluation of LVS Function	402	100%	99%	98%
Smoking Cessation Advice	68	100%	98%	98%
Pneumonia Care				
Appropriate Initial Antibiotic	102	97%	93%	92%
Blood Culture Timing	187	88%	96%	96%
Influenza Vaccine	207	90%	92%	91%
Initial Antibiotic Timing	195	98%	96%	95%
Pneumococcal Vaccine	254	95%	95%	93%
Smoking Cessation Advice	107	100%	98%	97%
Surgical Care Improvement Project				
Appropriate VTP Within 24 Hours[2]	176	95%	95%	92%
Appropriate Hair Removal[2]	767	100%	100%	99%
Appropriate Beta Blocker Usage[2]	322	90%	94%	93%
Controlled Postoperative Blood Glucose[2]	167	99%	96%	93%
Prophylactic Antibiotic Timing[2]	471	97%	97%	97%
Prophylactic Antibiotic Timing (Outpatient)[2]	820	93%	92%	92%
Prophylactic Antibiotic Selection[2]	480	99%	98%	97%
Prophylactic Antibiotic Select. (Outpatient)[2]	1,064	97%	93%	94%
Prophylactic Antibiotic Stopped[2]	445	98%	95%	94%
Recommended VTP Ordered[2]	176	97%	97%	94%
Urinary Catheter Removal[2]	131	98%	95%	90%
Children's Asthma Care				
Received Systemic Corticosteroids	-	-	-	100%
Received Home Management Plan	-	-	-	71%
Received Reliever Medication	-	-	-	100%
Use of Medical Imaging				
Combination Abdominal CT Scan	1,575	0.097	0.203	0.191
Combination Chest CT Scan	1,407	0.011	0.026	0.054
Follow-up Mammogram/Ultrasound	1,366	11.0%	8.2%	8.4%
MRI for Low Back Pain	221	26.2%	32.4%	32.7%
Survey of Patients' Hospital Experiences				
Area Around Room 'Always' Quiet at Night	300+	43%	-	58%
Doctors 'Always' Communicated Well	300+	79%	-	80%
Home Recovery Information Given	300+	88%	-	82%
Hospital Given 9 or 10 on 10 Point Scale	300+	76%	-	67%
Meds 'Always' Explained Before Given	300+	62%	-	60%
Nurses 'Always' Communicated Well	300+	79%	-	76%
Pain 'Always' Well Controlled	300+	68%	-	69%
Room and Bathroom 'Always' Clean	300+	75%	-	71%
Timely Help 'Always' Received	300+	68%	-	64%
Would Definitely Recommend Hospital	300+	81%	-	69%

Mercy Fitzgerald Hospital

Lansdowne & Baily Rds
Darby, PA 19023
E-mail: info@mercyhealth.org
URL: www.mercyhealth.org
Type: Acute Care Hospitals
Ownership: Voluntary Non-Profit - Other

Phone: 215-237-4000
Fax: 610-237-4202

Emergency Services: Yes
Beds: 218

Key Personnel:
CEO/President . . . . Brian Finestein
Chief of Medical Staff . . . . Sharon Carney MD
Quality Assurance . . . . Mary Stein Esq.

Measure	Cases	This Hosp.	State Avg.	U.S. Avg.
Heart Attack Care				
ACE Inhibitor or ARB for LVSD	48	98%	95%	96%
Aspirin at Arrival	183	100%	99%	99%
Aspirin at Discharge	179	99%	99%	98%
Beta Blocker at Discharge	177	99%	99%	98%
Fibrinolytic Medication Timing	0	-	40%	55%
PCI Within 90 Minutes of Arrival[1]	21	86%	88%	90%
Smoking Cessation Advice	65	100%	100%	99%
Chest Pain/Possible Heart Attack Care				
Aspirin at Arrival[1]	8	88%	95%	95%
Median Time to ECG (minutes)[1]	8	16	8	8
Median Time to Transfer (minutes)[5]	0	-	68	61
Fibrinolytic Medication Timing[5]	0	-	48%	54%
Heart Failure Care				
ACE Inhibitor or ARB for LVSD	487	99%	95%	94%
Discharge Instructions	842	98%	90%	88%
Evaluation of LVS Function	973	99%	99%	98%
Smoking Cessation Advice	305	100%	98%	98%
Pneumonia Care				
Appropriate Initial Antibiotic	186	95%	93%	92%
Blood Culture Timing	392	97%	96%	96%
Influenza Vaccine	133	93%	92%	91%
Initial Antibiotic Timing	359	98%	96%	95%
Pneumococcal Vaccine	185	96%	95%	93%
Smoking Cessation Advice	187	99%	98%	97%
Surgical Care Improvement Project				
Appropriate VTP Within 24 Hours[2]	272	100%	95%	92%
Appropriate Hair Removal[2]	525	100%	100%	99%
Appropriate Beta Blocker Usage[2]	142	92%	94%	93%
Controlled Postoperative Blood Glucose[2]	72	96%	96%	93%
Prophylactic Antibiotic Timing[2]	264	98%	97%	97%
Prophylactic Antibiotic Timing (Outpatient)[2]	151	91%	92%	92%
Prophylactic Antibiotic Selection[2]	272	97%	98%	97%
Prophylactic Antibiotic Select. (Outpatient)[2]	155	93%	93%	94%
Prophylactic Antibiotic Stopped[2]	248	94%	95%	94%
Recommended VTP Ordered[2]	272	100%	97%	94%
Urinary Catheter Removal[2]	84	93%	95%	90%
Children's Asthma Care				
Received Systemic Corticosteroids	-	-	-	100%
Received Home Management Plan	-	-	-	71%
Received Reliever Medication	-	-	-	100%
Use of Medical Imaging				
Combination Abdominal CT Scan	578	0.073	0.203	0.191
Combination Chest CT Scan	578	0.028	0.026	0.054
Follow-up Mammogram/Ultrasound	1,236	5.1%	8.2%	8.4%
MRI for Low Back Pain	114	31.6%	32.4%	32.7%
Survey of Patients' Hospital Experiences				
Area Around Room 'Always' Quiet at Night	300+	52%	-	58%
Doctors 'Always' Communicated Well	300+	73%	-	80%
Home Recovery Information Given	300+	81%	-	82%
Hospital Given 9 or 10 on 10 Point Scale	300+	55%	-	67%
Meds 'Always' Explained Before Given	300+	52%	-	60%
Nurses 'Always' Communicated Well	300+	70%	-	76%
Pain 'Always' Well Controlled	300+	61%	-	69%
Room and Bathroom 'Always' Clean	300+	62%	-	71%
Timely Help 'Always' Received	300+	49%	-	64%
Would Definitely Recommend Hospital	300+	53%	-	69%

Doylestown Hospital

595 West State St
Doylestown, PA 18901
URL: www.dh.org
Type: Acute Care Hospitals
Ownership: Voluntary Non-Profit - Private
Phone: 215-345-2200
Fax: 215-345-2827
Emergency Services: Yes
Beds: 165

Key Personnel:
CEO/President. . . . . Richard A Reif
Cardiac Laboratory. . . . . Dave Martens
Chief of Medical Staff . . . . Scott S Levy
Radiology. . . . . Linda Barnhurst

Measure	Cases	This Hosp.	State Avg.	U.S. Avg.
Heart Attack Care				
ACE Inhibitor or ARB for LVSD[2]	37	100%	95%	96%
Aspirin at Arrival[2]	240	100%	99%	99%
Aspirin at Discharge[2]	301	100%	99%	98%
Beta Blocker at Discharge[2]	281	100%	99%	98%
Fibrinolytic Medication Timing[2]	0	-	40%	55%
PCI Within 90 Minutes of Arrival[2]	53	94%	88%	90%
Smoking Cessation Advice[2]	62	100%	100%	99%
Chest Pain/Possible Heart Attack Care				
Aspirin at Arrival[5]	0	-	95%	95%
Median Time to ECG (minutes)[5]	0	-	8	8
Median Time to Transfer (minutes)[5]	0	-	68	61
Fibrinolytic Medication Timing[5]	0	-	48%	54%
Heart Failure Care				
ACE Inhibitor or ARB for LVSD	133	98%	95%	94%
Discharge Instructions	357	92%	90%	88%
Evaluation of LVS Function	462	100%	99%	98%
Smoking Cessation Advice	31	97%	98%	98%
Pneumonia Care				
Appropriate Initial Antibiotic	183	87%	93%	92%
Blood Culture Timing	295	95%	96%	96%
Influenza Vaccine	210	95%	92%	91%
Initial Antibiotic Timing	291	97%	96%	95%
Pneumococcal Vaccine	326	95%	95%	93%
Smoking Cessation Advice	78	96%	98%	97%
Surgical Care Improvement Project				
Appropriate VTP Within 24 Hours[2]	315	96%	95%	92%
Appropriate Hair Removal[2]	944	100%	100%	99%
Appropriate Beta Blocker Usage[2]	302	93%	94%	93%
Controlled Postoperative Blood Glucose[2]	192	99%	96%	93%
Prophylactic Antibiotic Timing[2]	644	94%	97%	97%
Prophylactic Antibiotic Timing (Outpatient)	196	88%	92%	92%
Prophylactic Antibiotic Selection[2]	648	98%	98%	97%
Prophylactic Antibiotic Select. (Outpatient)	190	51%	93%	94%
Prophylactic Antibiotic Stopped[2]	605	92%	95%	94%
Recommended VTP Ordered[2]	315	97%	97%	94%
Urinary Catheter Removal[2]	277	96%	95%	90%
Children's Asthma Care				
Received Systemic Corticosteroids	-	-	-	100%
Received Home Management Plan	-	-	-	71%
Received Reliever Medication	-	-	-	100%
Use of Medical Imaging				
Combination Abdominal CT Scan	899	0.180	0.203	0.191
Combination Chest CT Scan	928	0.002	0.026	0.054
Follow-up Mammogram/Ultrasound	2,039	10.9%	8.2%	8.4%
MRI for Low Back Pain	196	26.5%	32.4%	32.7%
Survey of Patients' Hospital Experiences				
Area Around Room 'Always' Quiet at Night	300+	51%	-	58%
Doctors 'Always' Communicated Well	300+	82%	-	80%
Home Recovery Information Given	300+	86%	-	82%
Hospital Given 9 or 10 on 10 Point Scale	300+	79%	-	67%
Meds 'Always' Explained Before Given	300+	64%	-	60%
Nurses 'Always' Communicated Well	300+	84%	-	76%
Pain 'Always' Well Controlled	300+	78%	-	69%
Room and Bathroom 'Always' Clean	300+	74%	-	71%
Timely Help 'Always' Received	300+	74%	-	64%
Would Definitely Recommend Hospital	300+	85%	-	69%

Delaware County Memorial Hospital

501 North Lansdowne Ave
Drexel Hill, PA 19026
URL: www.crozer.org
Type: Acute Care Hospitals
Ownership: Voluntary Non-Profit - Private
Phone: 215-284-8100
Fax: 610-284-8993
Emergency Services: Yes
Beds: 247

Key Personnel:
CEO/President. . . . . Joan K Richards
Chief of Medical Staff . . . . Lawrence Mayer, MD
Operating Room. . . . . Seth A Malin, RN
Pediatric In-Patient Care . . . . David Pollack, MD
Quality Assurance . . . . Joan Meighan
Radiology. . . . . Thomas A DiLiberto, DO
Emergency Room . . . . John Reilley, MD

Measure	Cases	This Hosp.	State Avg.	U.S. Avg.
Heart Attack Care				
ACE Inhibitor or ARB for LVSD[1]	2	100%	95%	96%
Aspirin at Arrival	65	98%	99%	99%
Aspirin at Discharge	34	100%	99%	98%
Beta Blocker at Discharge	32	100%	99%	98%
Fibrinolytic Medication Timing	0	-	40%	55%
PCI Within 90 Minutes of Arrival	0	-	88%	90%
Smoking Cessation Advice[1]	8	100%	100%	99%
Chest Pain/Possible Heart Attack Care				
Aspirin at Arrival	44	95%	95%	95%
Median Time to ECG (minutes)	45	8	8	8
Median Time to Transfer (minutes)[1]	12	72	68	61
Fibrinolytic Medication Timing	0	-	48%	54%
Heart Failure Care				
ACE Inhibitor or ARB for LVSD	87	95%	95%	94%
Discharge Instructions	279	97%	90%	88%
Evaluation of LVS Function	342	99%	99%	98%
Smoking Cessation Advice	50	100%	98%	98%
Pneumonia Care				
Appropriate Initial Antibiotic	111	95%	93%	92%
Blood Culture Timing	184	96%	96%	96%
Influenza Vaccine	117	92%	92%	91%
Initial Antibiotic Timing	192	96%	96%	95%
Pneumococcal Vaccine	144	92%	95%	93%
Smoking Cessation Advice	62	100%	98%	97%
Surgical Care Improvement Project				
Appropriate VTP Within 24 Hours[2]	348	100%	95%	92%
Appropriate Hair Removal[2]	551	100%	100%	99%
Appropriate Beta Blocker Usage[2]	140	91%	94%	93%
Controlled Postoperative Blood Glucose[2]	0	-	96%	93%
Prophylactic Antibiotic Timing[2]	379	97%	97%	97%
Prophylactic Antibiotic Timing (Outpatient)	69	100%	92%	92%
Prophylactic Antibiotic Selection[2]	382	97%	98%	97%
Prophylactic Antibiotic Select. (Outpatient)	69	97%	93%	94%
Prophylactic Antibiotic Stopped[2]	354	97%	95%	94%
Recommended VTP Ordered[2]	349	100%	97%	94%
Urinary Catheter Removal[2]	165	92%	95%	90%
Children's Asthma Care				
Received Systemic Corticosteroids	-	-	-	100%
Received Home Management Plan	-	-	-	71%
Received Reliever Medication	-	-	-	100%
Use of Medical Imaging				
Combination Abdominal CT Scan	706	0.435	0.203	0.191
Combination Chest CT Scan	539	0.004	0.026	0.054
Follow-up Mammogram/Ultrasound	566	5.5%	8.2%	8.4%
MRI for Low Back Pain	64	34.4%	32.4%	32.7%
Survey of Patients' Hospital Experiences				
Area Around Room 'Always' Quiet at Night	300+	50%	-	58%
Doctors 'Always' Communicated Well	300+	77%	-	80%
Home Recovery Information Given	300+	83%	-	82%
Hospital Given 9 or 10 on 10 Point Scale	300+	61%	-	67%
Meds 'Always' Explained Before Given	300+	61%	-	60%
Nurses 'Always' Communicated Well	300+	75%	-	76%
Pain 'Always' Well Controlled	300+	65%	-	69%
Room and Bathroom 'Always' Clean	300+	65%	-	71%
Timely Help 'Always' Received	300+	57%	-	64%
Would Definitely Recommend Hospital	300+	67%	-	69%

Dubois Regional Medical Center

100 Hospital Avenue
Dubois, PA 15801
URL: www.drmc.org
Type: Acute Care Hospitals
Ownership: Voluntary Non-Profit - Other
Phone: 814-371-2200
Fax: 814-375-3342
Emergency Services: Yes
Beds: 214

Key Personnel:
CEO/President. . . . . Raymond Graeca
Infection Control. . . . . Carole Berger
Operating Room. . . . . Mary Ann Nicometo
Radiology. . . . . George M Kosco
Emergency Room . . . . Russell E Cameron
Hemotology Center . . . . Rose Campbell
Intensive Care Unit. . . . . Jean Matsko

Measure	Cases	This Hosp.	State Avg.	U.S. Avg.
Heart Attack Care				
ACE Inhibitor or ARB for LVSD	66	100%	95%	96%
Aspirin at Arrival	126	100%	99%	99%
Aspirin at Discharge	323	99%	99%	98%
Beta Blocker at Discharge	321	100%	99%	98%
Fibrinolytic Medication Timing	0	-	40%	55%
PCI Within 90 Minutes of Arrival[1]	23	87%	88%	90%
Smoking Cessation Advice	112	100%	100%	99%
Chest Pain/Possible Heart Attack Care				
Aspirin at Arrival[5]	0	-	95%	95%
Median Time to ECG (minutes)[5]	0	-	8	8
Median Time to Transfer (minutes)[5]	0	-	68	61
Fibrinolytic Medication Timing[5]	0	-	48%	54%
Heart Failure Care				
ACE Inhibitor or ARB for LVSD	89	94%	95%	94%
Discharge Instructions	226	87%	90%	88%
Evaluation of LVS Function	263	100%	99%	98%
Smoking Cessation Advice	36	100%	98%	98%
Pneumonia Care				
Appropriate Initial Antibiotic	70	89%	93%	92%
Blood Culture Timing	109	99%	96%	96%
Influenza Vaccine	73	95%	92%	91%
Initial Antibiotic Timing	114	97%	96%	95%
Pneumococcal Vaccine	120	98%	95%	93%
Smoking Cessation Advice	52	100%	98%	97%
Surgical Care Improvement Project				
Appropriate VTP Within 24 Hours	112	94%	95%	92%
Appropriate Hair Removal	554	99%	100%	99%
Appropriate Beta Blocker Usage	224	95%	94%	93%
Controlled Postoperative Blood Glucose	148	99%	96%	93%
Prophylactic Antibiotic Timing	443	96%	97%	97%
Prophylactic Antibiotic Timing (Outpatient)	319	95%	92%	92%
Prophylactic Antibiotic Selection	449	96%	98%	97%
Prophylactic Antibiotic Select. (Outpatient)	409	97%	93%	94%
Prophylactic Antibiotic Stopped	409	98%	95%	94%
Recommended VTP Ordered	112	96%	97%	94%
Urinary Catheter Removal	133	96%	95%	90%
Children's Asthma Care				
Received Systemic Corticosteroids	-	-	-	100%
Received Home Management Plan	-	-	-	71%
Received Reliever Medication	-	-	-	100%
Use of Medical Imaging				
Combination Abdominal CT Scan	1,231	0.278	0.203	0.191
Combination Chest CT Scan	728	0.004	0.026	0.054
Follow-up Mammogram/Ultrasound	1,688	6.7%	8.2%	8.4%
MRI for Low Back Pain[1]	1	0.0%	32.4%	32.7%
Survey of Patients' Hospital Experiences				
Area Around Room 'Always' Quiet at Night	300+	52%	-	58%
Doctors 'Always' Communicated Well	300+	79%	-	80%
Home Recovery Information Given	300+	87%	-	82%
Hospital Given 9 or 10 on 10 Point Scale	300+	70%	-	67%
Meds 'Always' Explained Before Given	300+	66%	-	60%
Nurses 'Always' Communicated Well	300+	79%	-	76%
Pain 'Always' Well Controlled	300+	73%	-	69%
Room and Bathroom 'Always' Clean	300+	67%	-	71%
Timely Help 'Always' Received	300+	66%	-	64%
Would Definitely Recommend Hospital	300+	79%	-	69%

NOTE: Hospital profiles are in alphabetical order by state, then city, then hospital within the city; Rankings exclude hospitals with less than 25 cases except for patient surveys which excludes hospitals with less than 100 cases; (a) 100–299 cases; (1) The number of cases is too small to be sure how well a hospital is performing; (2) The hospital indicated that the data submitted for this measure were based on a sample of cases; (3) Data was collected during a shorter time period (fewer quarters) than the maximum possible time for this measure; (4) Suppressed for one or more quarters by CMS; (5) No data is available from the hospital for this measure; (6) Fewer than 100 patients completed the HCAHPS survey. Use these rates with caution, as the number of surveys may be too low to reliably assess hospital performance; (7) Survey results are based on less than 12 months of data; (8) Survey results are not available for this reporting period; (9) No or very few patients were eligible for the HCAHPS survey. The scores shown, if any, reflect a very small number of surveys; (10) A state average was not calculated because too few hospitals in the state submitted data; (11) There were discrepancies in the data collection process; Please refer to the User's Guide for a full explanation of data.

Eagleville Hospital

100 Eagleville Rd
Eagleville, PA 19408
Phone: 215-539-6000
Fax: 610-539-8319
URL: www.eaglevillehospital.org
Type: Acute Care Hospitals
Emergency Services: Yes
Ownership: Voluntary Non-Profit - Other
Beds: 350
Key Personnel:
CEO/President. . . . . Maureen King Pollock

Measure	Cases	This Hosp.	State Avg.	U.S. Avg.
Heart Attack Care				
ACE Inhibitor or ARB for LVSD[5]	0	-	95%	96%
Aspirin at Arrival[5]	0	-	99%	99%
Aspirin at Discharge[5]	0	-	99%	98%
Beta Blocker at Discharge[5]	0	-	99%	98%
Fibrinolytic Medication Timing[5]	0	-	40%	55%
PCI Within 90 Minutes of Arrival[5]	0	-	88%	90%
Smoking Cessation Advice[5]	0	-	100%	99%
Chest Pain/Possible Heart Attack Care				
Aspirin at Arrival[5]	0	-	95%	95%
Median Time to ECG (minutes)[5]	0	-	8	8
Median Time to Transfer (minutes)[5]	0	-	68	61
Fibrinolytic Medication Timing[5]	0	-	48%	54%
Heart Failure Care				
ACE Inhibitor or ARB for LVSD[5]	0	-	95%	94%
Discharge Instructions[5]	0	-	90%	88%
Evaluation of LVS Function[5]	0	-	99%	98%
Smoking Cessation Advice[5]	0	-	98%	98%
Pneumonia Care				
Appropriate Initial Antibiotic[5]	0	-	93%	92%
Blood Culture Timing[5]	0	-	96%	96%
Influenza Vaccine[5]	0	-	92%	91%
Initial Antibiotic Timing[5]	0	-	96%	95%
Pneumococcal Vaccine[5]	0	-	95%	93%
Smoking Cessation Advice[5]	0	-	98%	97%
Surgical Care Improvement Project				
Appropriate VTP Within 24 Hours[5]	0	-	95%	92%
Appropriate Hair Removal[5]	0	-	100%	99%
Appropriate Beta Blocker Usage[5]	0	-	94%	93%
Controlled Postoperative Blood Glucose[5]	0	-	96%	93%
Prophylactic Antibiotic Timing[5]	0	-	97%	97%
Prophylactic Antibiotic Timing (Outpatient)[5]	0	-	92%	92%
Prophylactic Antibiotic Selection[5]	0	-	98%	97%
Prophylactic Antibiotic Select. (Outpatient)[5]	0	-	93%	94%
Prophylactic Antibiotic Stopped[5]	0	-	95%	94%
Recommended VTP Ordered[5]	0	-	97%	94%
Urinary Catheter Removal[5]	0	-	95%	90%
Children's Asthma Care				
Received Systemic Corticosteroids	-	-	-	100%
Received Home Management Plan	-	-	-	71%
Received Reliever Medication	-	-	-	100%
Use of Medical Imaging				
Combination Abdominal CT Scan[5]	0	-	0.203	0.191
Combination Chest CT Scan[5]	0	-	0.026	0.054
Follow-up Mammogram/Ultrasound[5]	0	-	8.2%	8.4%
MRI for Low Back Pain[5]	0	-	32.4%	32.7%
Survey of Patients' Hospital Experiences				
Area Around Room 'Always' Quiet at Night[9]	-	-	-	58%
Doctors 'Always' Communicated Well[9]	-	-	-	80%
Home Recovery Information Given[9]	-	-	-	82%
Hospital Given 9 or 10 on 10 Point Scale[9]	-	-	-	67%
Meds 'Always' Explained Before Given[9]	-	-	-	60%
Nurses 'Always' Communicated Well[9]	-	-	-	76%
Pain 'Always' Well Controlled[9]	-	-	-	69%
Room and Bathroom 'Always' Clean[9]	-	-	-	71%
Timely Help 'Always' Received[9]	-	-	-	64%
Would Definitely Recommend Hospital[9]	-	-	-	69%

Pocono Medical Center

206 East Brown Street
East Stroudsburg, PA 18301
Phone: 570-476-3348
Fax: 570-476-3604
E-mail: feedback@pmchealthsystem.org
URL: www.poconohealthsystem.org
Type: Acute Care Hospitals
Emergency Services: Yes
Ownership: Voluntary Non-Profit - Other
Beds: 192
Key Personnel:
CEO/President. . . . . Michael A Wilk
Cardiac Laboratory. . . . . Georganne DeGavany
Chief of Medical Staff. . . . . Howard Davis, MD
Operating Room. . . . . Thomas Gerold
Pediatric Ambulatory Care . . . . . . Arthur Dixon, MD
Pediatric In-Patient Care . . . . Arthur Dixon, MD
Quality Assurance . . . . Eileen Caden
Radiology. . . . . Dana Burke, MD

Measure	Cases	This Hosp.	State Avg.	U.S. Avg.
Heart Attack Care				
ACE Inhibitor or ARB for LVSD	66	97%	95%	96%
Aspirin at Arrival	297	98%	99%	99%
Aspirin at Discharge	283	99%	99%	98%
Beta Blocker at Discharge	258	99%	99%	98%
Fibrinolytic Medication Timing	0	-	40%	55%
PCI Within 90 Minutes of Arrival	83	96%	88%	90%
Smoking Cessation Advice	112	100%	100%	99%
Chest Pain/Possible Heart Attack Care				
Aspirin at Arrival[1,3]	3	100%	95%	95%
Median Time to ECG (minutes)[1,3]	4	6	8	8
Median Time to Transfer (minutes)[5]	0	-	68	61
Fibrinolytic Medication Timing[5]	0	-	48%	54%
Heart Failure Care				
ACE Inhibitor or ARB for LVSD	136	93%	95%	94%
Discharge Instructions	367	68%	90%	88%
Evaluation of LVS Function	433	99%	99%	98%
Smoking Cessation Advice	83	98%	98%	98%
Pneumonia Care				
Appropriate Initial Antibiotic	207	94%	93%	92%
Blood Culture Timing	253	92%	96%	96%
Influenza Vaccine	207	92%	92%	91%
Initial Antibiotic Timing	322	96%	96%	95%
Pneumococcal Vaccine	316	89%	95%	93%
Smoking Cessation Advice	157	97%	98%	97%
Surgical Care Improvement Project				
Appropriate VTP Within 24 Hours	230	90%	95%	92%
Appropriate Hair Removal	659	100%	100%	99%
Appropriate Beta Blocker Usage	214	96%	94%	93%
Controlled Postoperative Blood Glucose	165	96%	96%	93%
Prophylactic Antibiotic Timing	379	99%	97%	97%
Prophylactic Antibiotic Timing (Outpatient)	192	97%	92%	92%
Prophylactic Antibiotic Selection	380	97%	98%	97%
Prophylactic Antibiotic Select. (Outpatient)	186	95%	93%	94%
Prophylactic Antibiotic Stopped	355	97%	95%	94%
Recommended VTP Ordered	234	91%	97%	94%
Urinary Catheter Removal	156	91%	95%	90%
Children's Asthma Care				
Received Systemic Corticosteroids	-	-	-	100%
Received Home Management Plan	-	-	-	71%
Received Reliever Medication	-	-	-	100%
Use of Medical Imaging				
Combination Abdominal CT Scan	1,120	0.069	0.203	0.191
Combination Chest CT Scan	558	0.034	0.026	0.054
Follow-up Mammogram/Ultrasound	357	9.0%	8.2%	8.4%
MRI for Low Back Pain	70	20.0%	32.4%	32.7%
Survey of Patients' Hospital Experiences				
Area Around Room 'Always' Quiet at Night	300+	50%	-	58%
Doctors 'Always' Communicated Well	300+	78%	-	80%
Home Recovery Information Given	300+	84%	-	82%
Hospital Given 9 or 10 on 10 Point Scale	300+	63%	-	67%
Meds 'Always' Explained Before Given	300+	61%	-	60%
Nurses 'Always' Communicated Well	300+	76%	-	76%
Pain 'Always' Well Controlled	300+	72%	-	69%
Room and Bathroom 'Always' Clean	300+	71%	-	71%
Timely Help 'Always' Received	300+	63%	-	64%
Would Definitely Recommend Hospital	300+	65%	-	69%

Easton Hospital

250 South 21st Street
Easton, PA 18042
Phone: 610-250-4076
Fax: 610-250-4078
URL: www.easton-hospital.com
Type: Acute Care Hospitals
Emergency Services: Yes
Ownership: Proprietary
Beds: 233
Key Personnel:
CEO/President. . . . . Roy Boyd
Infection Control. . . . . Lisa Knaak
Operating Room. . . . . Dave Kasprzak
Pediatric In-Patient Care . . . . Prem K Marlapudi, MD
Quality Assurance . . . . Tara Reid
Radiology. . . . . Charmaine Wallaesa
Anesthesiology. . . . . Michael Feldman, MD
Emergency Room . . . . Robert N Slade, MD

Measure	Cases	This Hosp.	State Avg.	U.S. Avg.
Heart Attack Care				
ACE Inhibitor or ARB for LVSD	48	100%	95%	96%
Aspirin at Arrival	171	99%	99%	99%
Aspirin at Discharge	202	99%	99%	98%
Beta Blocker at Discharge	204	99%	99%	98%
Fibrinolytic Medication Timing	0	-	40%	55%
PCI Within 90 Minutes of Arrival	40	100%	88%	90%
Smoking Cessation Advice	80	100%	100%	99%
Chest Pain/Possible Heart Attack Care				
Aspirin at Arrival[1,3]	1	100%	95%	95%
Median Time to ECG (minutes)[1,3]	1	6	8	8
Median Time to Transfer (minutes)[5]	0	-	68	61
Fibrinolytic Medication Timing[5]	0	-	48%	54%
Heart Failure Care				
ACE Inhibitor or ARB for LVSD	126	98%	95%	94%
Discharge Instructions	312	92%	90%	88%
Evaluation of LVS Function	428	100%	99%	98%
Smoking Cessation Advice	49	100%	98%	98%
Pneumonia Care				
Appropriate Initial Antibiotic	123	84%	93%	92%
Blood Culture Timing	201	95%	96%	96%
Influenza Vaccine	153	97%	92%	91%
Initial Antibiotic Timing	224	91%	96%	95%
Pneumococcal Vaccine	252	98%	95%	93%
Smoking Cessation Advice	56	100%	98%	97%
Surgical Care Improvement Project				
Appropriate VTP Within 24 Hours[2]	225	97%	95%	92%
Appropriate Hair Removal[2]	741	100%	100%	99%
Appropriate Beta Blocker Usage[2]	277	91%	94%	93%
Controlled Postoperative Blood Glucose[2]	121	98%	96%	93%
Prophylactic Antibiotic Timing[2]	458	94%	97%	97%
Prophylactic Antibiotic Timing (Outpatient)	84	90%	92%	92%
Prophylactic Antibiotic Selection[2]	462	98%	98%	97%
Prophylactic Antibiotic Select. (Outpatient)	83	92%	93%	94%
Prophylactic Antibiotic Stopped[2]	444	96%	95%	94%
Recommended VTP Ordered[2]	225	98%	97%	94%
Urinary Catheter Removal	136	96%	95%	90%
Children's Asthma Care				
Received Systemic Corticosteroids	-	-	-	100%
Received Home Management Plan	-	-	-	71%
Received Reliever Medication	-	-	-	100%
Use of Medical Imaging				
Combination Abdominal CT Scan	818	0.137	0.203	0.191
Combination Chest CT Scan	573	0.030	0.026	0.054
Follow-up Mammogram/Ultrasound	1,525	9.7%	8.2%	8.4%
MRI for Low Back Pain	46	43.5%	32.4%	32.7%
Survey of Patients' Hospital Experiences				
Area Around Room 'Always' Quiet at Night	300+	49%	-	58%
Doctors 'Always' Communicated Well	300+	75%	-	80%
Home Recovery Information Given	300+	82%	-	82%
Hospital Given 9 or 10 on 10 Point Scale	300+	55%	-	67%
Meds 'Always' Explained Before Given	300+	54%	-	60%
Nurses 'Always' Communicated Well	300+	71%	-	76%
Pain 'Always' Well Controlled	300+	67%	-	69%
Room and Bathroom 'Always' Clean	300+	65%	-	71%
Timely Help 'Always' Received	300+	49%	-	64%
Would Definitely Recommend Hospital	300+	53%	-	69%

NOTE: Hospital profiles are in alphabetical order by state, then city, then hospital within the city; Rankings exclude hospitals with less than 25 cases except for patient surveys which excludes hospitals with less than 100 cases; (a) 100–299 cases; (1) The number of cases is too small to be sure how well a hospital is performing; (2) The hospital indicated that the data submitted for this measure were based on a sample of cases; (3) Data was collected during a shorter time period (fewer quarters) than the maximum possible time for this measure; (4) Suppressed for one or more quarters by CMS; (5) No data is available from the hospital for this measure; (6) Fewer than 100 patients completed the HCAHPS survey. Use these rates with caution, as the number of surveys may be too low to reliably assess hospital performance; (7) Survey results are based on less than 12 months of data; (8) Survey results are not available for this reporting period; (9) No or very few patients were eligible for the HCAHPS survey. The scores shown, if any, reflect a very small number of surveys; (10) A state average was not calculated because too few hospitals in the state submitted data; (11) There were discrepancies in the data collection process; Please refer to the User's Guide for a full explanation of data.

Ellwood City Hospital

724 Pershing Street
Ellwood City, PA 16117
URL: www.echospital.org
Type: Acute Care Hospitals
Ownership: Voluntary Non-Profit - Other

Phone: 724-752-0081
Fax: 724-752-0966

Emergency Services: Yes
Beds: 95

Key Personnel:
CEO/President . . . . Herbert S Skuba
Chief of Medical Staff . . . . Peter Volpe

Measure	Cases	This Hosp.	State Avg.	U.S. Avg.
Heart Attack Care				
ACE Inhibitor or ARB for LVSD[1]	1	100%	95%	96%
Aspirin at Arrival[1]	14	100%	99%	99%
Aspirin at Discharge[1]	6	100%	99%	98%
Beta Blocker at Discharge[1]	6	67%	99%	98%
Fibrinolytic Medication Timing	0	-	40%	55%
PCI Within 90 Minutes of Arrival	0	-	88%	90%
Smoking Cessation Advice	0	-	100%	99%
Chest Pain/Possible Heart Attack Care				
Aspirin at Arrival	68	97%	95%	95%
Median Time to ECG (minutes)	72	15	8	8
Median Time to Transfer (minutes)[1,3]	22	86	68	61
Fibrinolytic Medication Timing	0	-	48%	54%
Heart Failure Care				
ACE Inhibitor or ARB for LVSD	42	98%	95%	94%
Discharge Instructions	99	98%	90%	88%
Evaluation of LVS Function	130	100%	99%	98%
Smoking Cessation Advice[1]	14	100%	98%	98%
Pneumonia Care				
Appropriate Initial Antibiotic	42	90%	93%	92%
Blood Culture Timing	38	92%	96%	96%
Influenza Vaccine	44	93%	92%	91%
Initial Antibiotic Timing	64	98%	96%	95%
Pneumococcal Vaccine	62	97%	95%	93%
Smoking Cessation Advice[1]	20	95%	98%	97%
Surgical Care Improvement Project				
Appropriate VTP Within 24 Hours	56	93%	95%	92%
Appropriate Hair Removal	96	99%	100%	99%
Appropriate Beta Blocker Usage	29	86%	94%	93%
Controlled Postoperative Blood Glucose	0	-	96%	93%
Prophylactic Antibiotic Timing	32	94%	97%	97%
Prophylactic Antibiotic Timing (Outpatient)	35	89%	92%	92%
Prophylactic Antibiotic Selection	32	78%	98%	97%
Prophylactic Antibiotic Select. (Outpatient)	32	88%	93%	94%
Prophylactic Antibiotic Stopped	31	87%	95%	94%
Recommended VTP Ordered	56	93%	97%	94%
Urinary Catheter Removal[1]	6	33%	95%	90%
Children's Asthma Care				
Received Systemic Corticosteroids	-	-	-	100%
Received Home Management Plan	-	-	-	71%
Received Reliever Medication	-	-	-	100%
Use of Medical Imaging				
Combination Abdominal CT Scan	124	0.081	0.203	0.191
Combination Chest CT Scan	105	0.010	0.026	0.054
Follow-up Mammogram/Ultrasound	226	12.4%	8.2%	8.4%
MRI for Low Back Pain[1]	21	14.3%	32.4%	32.7%
Survey of Patients' Hospital Experiences				
Area Around Room 'Always' Quiet at Night	300+	58%	-	58%
Doctors 'Always' Communicated Well	300+	77%	-	80%
Home Recovery Information Given	300+	81%	-	82%
Hospital Given 9 or 10 on 10 Point Scale	300+	65%	-	67%
Meds 'Always' Explained Before Given	300+	60%	-	60%
Nurses 'Always' Communicated Well	300+	77%	-	76%
Pain 'Always' Well Controlled	300+	71%	-	69%
Room and Bathroom 'Always' Clean	300+	76%	-	71%
Timely Help 'Always' Received	300+	67%	-	64%
Would Definitely Recommend Hospital	300+	68%	-	69%

Ephrata Community Hospital

169 Martin Avenue
Ephrata, PA 17522
URL: www.ephratahospital.org
Type: Acute Care Hospitals
Ownership: Voluntary Non-Profit - Other

Phone: 717-733-0311
Fax: 717-733-0876

Emergency Services: Yes
Beds: 133

Key Personnel:
CEO/President . . . . John Porter
Chief of Medical Staff . . . . Christopher Hager

Measure	Cases	This Hosp.	State Avg.	U.S. Avg.
Heart Attack Care				
ACE Inhibitor or ARB for LVSD[1]	1	100%	95%	96%
Aspirin at Arrival	49	98%	99%	99%
Aspirin at Discharge[1]	21	95%	99%	98%
Beta Blocker at Discharge[1]	22	82%	99%	98%
Fibrinolytic Medication Timing	0	-	40%	55%
PCI Within 90 Minutes of Arrival	0	-	88%	90%
Smoking Cessation Advice[1]	6	83%	100%	99%
Chest Pain/Possible Heart Attack Care				
Aspirin at Arrival	38	95%	95%	95%
Median Time to ECG (minutes)	39	4	8	8
Median Time to Transfer (minutes)[1,3]	8	38	68	61
Fibrinolytic Medication Timing[3]	0	-	48%	54%
Heart Failure Care				
ACE Inhibitor or ARB for LVSD	46	91%	95%	94%
Discharge Instructions	131	82%	90%	88%
Evaluation of LVS Function	183	100%	99%	98%
Smoking Cessation Advice[1]	16	62%	98%	98%
Pneumonia Care				
Appropriate Initial Antibiotic	144	90%	93%	92%
Blood Culture Timing	196	96%	96%	96%
Influenza Vaccine	111	97%	92%	91%
Initial Antibiotic Timing	188	86%	96%	95%
Pneumococcal Vaccine	183	99%	95%	93%
Smoking Cessation Advice	53	85%	98%	97%
Surgical Care Improvement Project				
Appropriate VTP Within 24 Hours	239	98%	95%	92%
Appropriate Hair Removal	597	100%	100%	99%
Appropriate Beta Blocker Usage	161	96%	94%	93%
Controlled Postoperative Blood Glucose	0	-	96%	93%
Prophylactic Antibiotic Timing	431	94%	97%	97%
Prophylactic Antibiotic Timing (Outpatient)	304	92%	92%	92%
Prophylactic Antibiotic Selection	432	98%	98%	97%
Prophylactic Antibiotic Select. (Outpatient)	286	97%	93%	94%
Prophylactic Antibiotic Stopped	410	93%	95%	94%
Recommended VTP Ordered	239	98%	97%	94%
Urinary Catheter Removal	195	98%	95%	90%
Children's Asthma Care				
Received Systemic Corticosteroids	-	-	-	100%
Received Home Management Plan	-	-	-	71%
Received Reliever Medication	-	-	-	100%
Use of Medical Imaging				
Combination Abdominal CT Scan	811	0.496	0.203	0.191
Combination Chest CT Scan	740	0.023	0.026	0.054
Follow-up Mammogram/Ultrasound	1,492	15.4%	8.2%	8.4%
MRI for Low Back Pain	162	25.3%	32.4%	32.7%
Survey of Patients' Hospital Experiences				
Area Around Room 'Always' Quiet at Night	300+	43%	-	58%
Doctors 'Always' Communicated Well	300+	75%	-	80%
Home Recovery Information Given	300+	83%	-	82%
Hospital Given 9 or 10 on 10 Point Scale	300+	63%	-	67%
Meds 'Always' Explained Before Given	300+	57%	-	60%
Nurses 'Always' Communicated Well	300+	77%	-	76%
Pain 'Always' Well Controlled	300+	66%	-	69%
Room and Bathroom 'Always' Clean	300+	69%	-	71%
Timely Help 'Always' Received	300+	63%	-	64%
Would Definitely Recommend Hospital	300+	69%	-	69%

Erie VA Medical Center

135 East 38th Street
Erie, PA 16504
Type: Acute Care-Veterans Administration
Ownership: Government - Federal

Phone: 814-860-2576
Fax: 814-860-2135

Emergency Services: No
Beds: 81

Key Personnel:
Chief of Medical Staff . . . . Anthony Behm, DO
Operating Room. . . . . Prabhu Negi, MD
Quality Assurance . . . . Beth Thornton

Measure	Cases	This Hosp.	State Avg.	U.S. Avg.
Heart Attack Care				
ACE Inhibitor or ARB for LVSD[5]	0	-	95%	96%
Aspirin at Arrival[5]	0	-	99%	99%
Aspirin at Discharge[5]	0	-	99%	98%
Beta Blocker at Discharge[5]	0	-	99%	98%
Fibrinolytic Medication Timing[5]	0	-	40%	55%
PCI Within 90 Minutes of Arrival[5]	0	-	88%	90%
Smoking Cessation Advice[5]	0	-	100%	99%
Chest Pain/Possible Heart Attack Care				
Aspirin at Arrival	-	-	95%	95%
Median Time to ECG (minutes)	-	-	8	8
Median Time to Transfer (minutes)	-	-	68	61
Fibrinolytic Medication Timing	-	-	48%	54%
Heart Failure Care				
ACE Inhibitor or ARB for LVSD[1]	8	75%	95%	94%
Discharge Instructions	28	89%	90%	88%
Evaluation of LVS Function	34	100%	99%	98%
Smoking Cessation Advice[1]	7	86%	98%	98%
Pneumonia Care				
Appropriate Initial Antibiotic	33	91%	93%	92%
Blood Culture Timing	55	98%	96%	96%
Influenza Vaccine	38	97%	92%	91%
Initial Antibiotic Timing	51	98%	96%	95%
Pneumococcal Vaccine	53	98%	95%	93%
Smoking Cessation Advice[1]	21	81%	98%	97%
Surgical Care Improvement Project				
Appropriate VTP Within 24 Hours[1,2]	14	100%	95%	92%
Appropriate Hair Removal[2]	45	100%	100%	99%
Appropriate Beta Blocker Usage[1,2]	19	100%	94%	93%
Controlled Postoperative Blood Glucose[2,5]	0	-	96%	93%
Prophylactic Antibiotic Timing	41	98%	97%	97%
Prophylactic Antibiotic Timing (Outpatient)	-	-	92%	92%
Prophylactic Antibiotic Selection	41	95%	98%	97%
Prophylactic Antibiotic Select. (Outpatient)	-	-	93%	94%
Prophylactic Antibiotic Stopped	39	95%	95%	94%
Recommended VTP Ordered[1,2]	14	100%	97%	94%
Urinary Catheter Removal[1,2]	1	100%	95%	90%
Children's Asthma Care				
Received Systemic Corticosteroids	-	-	-	100%
Received Home Management Plan	-	-	-	71%
Received Reliever Medication	-	-	-	100%
Use of Medical Imaging				
Combination Abdominal CT Scan	-	-	0.203	0.191
Combination Chest CT Scan	-	-	0.026	0.054
Follow-up Mammogram/Ultrasound	-	-	8.2%	8.4%
MRI for Low Back Pain	-	-	32.4%	32.7%
Survey of Patients' Hospital Experiences				
Area Around Room 'Always' Quiet at Night	-	-	-	58%
Doctors 'Always' Communicated Well	-	-	-	80%
Home Recovery Information Given	-	-	-	82%
Hospital Given 9 or 10 on 10 Point Scale	-	-	-	67%
Meds 'Always' Explained Before Given	-	-	-	60%
Nurses 'Always' Communicated Well	-	-	-	76%
Pain 'Always' Well Controlled	-	-	-	69%
Room and Bathroom 'Always' Clean	-	-	-	71%
Timely Help 'Always' Received	-	-	-	64%
Would Definitely Recommend Hospital	-	-	-	69%

NOTE: Hospital profiles are in alphabetical order by state, then city, then hospital within the city; Rankings exclude hospitals with less than 25 cases except for patient surveys which excludes hospitals with less than 100 cases; (a) 100–299 cases; (1) The number of cases is too small to be sure how well a hospital is performing; (2) The hospital indicated that the data submitted for this measure were based on a sample of cases; (3) Data was collected during a shorter time period (fewer quarters) than the maximum possible time for this measure; (4) Suppressed for one or more quarters by CMS; (5) No data is available from the hospital for this measure; (6) Fewer than 100 patients completed the HCAHPS survey. Use these rates with caution, as the number of surveys may be too low to reliably assess hospital performance; (7) Survey results are based on less than 12 months of data; (8) Survey results are not available for this reporting period; (9) No or very few patients were eligible for the HCAHPS survey. The scores shown, if any, reflect a very small number of surveys; (10) A state average was not calculated because too few hospitals in the state submitted data; (11) There were discrepancies in the data collection process; Please refer to the User's Guide for a full explanation of data.

Hamot Medical Center

201 State Street
Erie, PA 16550
Phone: 814-877-6000
Fax: 814-877-7590
E-mail: info@hamot.org
URL: www.hamot.org
Type: Acute Care Hospitals
Emergency Services: Yes
Ownership: Voluntary Non-Profit - Private
Beds: 360

Key Personnel:
CEO/President. . . . . John Malone
Chief of Medical Staff. . . . . J David Albert II, MD
Infection Control. . . . . Lee P VanVoris, MD
Operating Room. . . . . Mary Ellen Stoddart
Pediatric Ambulatory Care . . . . . . Ronald F Zieziula, MD
Pediatric In-Patient Care . . . . Ronald F Zieziula, MD
Quality Assurance . . . . Paul Huckno
Radiology. . . . . Richard Willion

Measure	Cases	This Hosp.	State Avg.	U.S. Avg.
Heart Attack Care				
ACE Inhibitor or ARB for LVSD	148	99%	95%	96%
Aspirin at Arrival	278	99%	99%	99%
Aspirin at Discharge	713	99%	99%	98%
Beta Blocker at Discharge	703	99%	99%	98%
Fibrinolytic Medication Timing	0	-	40%	55%
PCI Within 90 Minutes of Arrival	64	91%	88%	90%
Smoking Cessation Advice	275	100%	100%	99%
Chest Pain/Possible Heart Attack Care				
Aspirin at Arrival[1,3]	1	100%	95%	95%
Median Time to ECG (minutes)[1,3]	1	5	8	8
Median Time to Transfer (minutes)[5]	0	-	68	61
Fibrinolytic Medication Timing[5]	0	-	48%	54%
Heart Failure Care				
ACE Inhibitor or ARB for LVSD	171	95%	95%	94%
Discharge Instructions	422	91%	90%	88%
Evaluation of LVS Function	538	100%	99%	98%
Smoking Cessation Advice	91	100%	98%	98%
Pneumonia Care				
Appropriate Initial Antibiotic	180	95%	93%	92%
Blood Culture Timing	288	94%	96%	96%
Influenza Vaccine	235	93%	92%	91%
Initial Antibiotic Timing	347	95%	96%	95%
Pneumococcal Vaccine	356	96%	95%	93%
Smoking Cessation Advice	178	100%	98%	97%
Surgical Care Improvement Project				
Appropriate VTP Within 24 Hours	613	97%	95%	92%
Appropriate Hair Removal	1,832	100%	100%	99%
Appropriate Beta Blocker Usage	688	96%	94%	93%
Controlled Postoperative Blood Glucose	375	91%	96%	93%
Prophylactic Antibiotic Timing	1,107	98%	97%	97%
Prophylactic Antibiotic Timing (Outpatient)	421	96%	92%	92%
Prophylactic Antibiotic Selection	1,126	99%	98%	97%
Prophylactic Antibiotic Select. (Outpatient)	424	97%	93%	94%
Prophylactic Antibiotic Stopped	1,076	96%	95%	94%
Recommended VTP Ordered	613	98%	97%	94%
Urinary Catheter Removal	538	96%	95%	90%
Children's Asthma Care				
Received Systemic Corticosteroids	-	-	-	100%
Received Home Management Plan	-	-	-	71%
Received Reliever Medication	-	-	-	100%
Use of Medical Imaging				
Combination Abdominal CT Scan	690	0.052	0.203	0.191
Combination Chest CT Scan	242	0.008	0.026	0.054
Follow-up Mammogram/Ultrasound[5]	0	-	8.2%	8.4%
MRI for Low Back Pain	133	27.1%	32.4%	32.7%
Survey of Patients' Hospital Experiences				
Area Around Room 'Always' Quiet at Night	300+	48%	-	58%
Doctors 'Always' Communicated Well	300+	78%	-	80%
Home Recovery Information Given	300+	83%	-	82%
Hospital Given 9 or 10 on 10 Point Scale	300+	71%	-	67%
Meds 'Always' Explained Before Given	300+	61%	-	60%
Nurses 'Always' Communicated Well	300+	79%	-	76%
Pain 'Always' Well Controlled	300+	72%	-	69%
Room and Bathroom 'Always' Clean	300+	70%	-	71%
Timely Help 'Always' Received	300+	66%	-	64%
Would Definitely Recommend Hospital	300+	77%	-	69%

Millcreek Community Hospital

5515 Peach Street
Erie, PA 16509
Phone: 814-864-4031
Fax: 814-868-8142
URL: www.millcreekcommunityhospital.com
Type: Acute Care Hospitals
Emergency Services: Yes
Ownership: Voluntary Non-Profit - Other
Beds: 200

Key Personnel:
CEO/President. . . . . Mary L Eckert
Cardiac Laboratory. . . . . William A Esper
Emergency Room . . . . Dennis Augustini

Measure	Cases	This Hosp.	State Avg.	U.S. Avg.
Heart Attack Care				
ACE Inhibitor or ARB for LVSD[1,3]	1	0%	95%	96%
Aspirin at Arrival[1,3]	3	100%	99%	99%
Aspirin at Discharge[1,3]	1	0%	99%	98%
Beta Blocker at Discharge[3]	0	-	99%	98%
Fibrinolytic Medication Timing[3]	0	-	40%	55%
PCI Within 90 Minutes of Arrival[3]	0	-	88%	90%
Smoking Cessation Advice[3]	0	-	100%	99%
Chest Pain/Possible Heart Attack Care				
Aspirin at Arrival[1,3]	12	100%	95%	95%
Median Time to ECG (minutes)[1,3]	12	18	8	8
Median Time to Transfer (minutes)[3]	0	-	68	61
Fibrinolytic Medication Timing[3]	0	-	48%	54%
Heart Failure Care				
ACE Inhibitor or ARB for LVSD[1]	20	90%	95%	94%
Discharge Instructions	46	80%	90%	88%
Evaluation of LVS Function	80	98%	99%	98%
Smoking Cessation Advice[1]	11	100%	98%	98%
Pneumonia Care				
Appropriate Initial Antibiotic[1]	24	83%	93%	92%
Blood Culture Timing	40	95%	96%	96%
Influenza Vaccine	33	100%	92%	91%
Initial Antibiotic Timing	47	96%	96%	95%
Pneumococcal Vaccine	46	100%	95%	93%
Smoking Cessation Advice[1]	22	100%	98%	97%
Surgical Care Improvement Project				
Appropriate VTP Within 24 Hours	43	95%	95%	92%
Appropriate Hair Removal	126	99%	100%	99%
Appropriate Beta Blocker Usage	30	73%	94%	93%
Controlled Postoperative Blood Glucose	0	-	96%	93%
Prophylactic Antibiotic Timing	85	93%	97%	97%
Prophylactic Antibiotic Timing (Outpatient)	30	97%	92%	92%
Prophylactic Antibiotic Selection	87	95%	98%	97%
Prophylactic Antibiotic Select. (Outpatient)	29	86%	93%	94%
Prophylactic Antibiotic Stopped	81	85%	95%	94%
Recommended VTP Ordered	44	93%	97%	94%
Urinary Catheter Removal[1]	18	83%	95%	90%
Children's Asthma Care				
Received Systemic Corticosteroids	-	-	-	100%
Received Home Management Plan	-	-	-	71%
Received Reliever Medication	-	-	-	100%
Use of Medical Imaging				
Combination Abdominal CT Scan	100	0.030	0.203	0.191
Combination Chest CT Scan[1]	31	0.000	0.026	0.054
Follow-up Mammogram/Ultrasound	56	0.0%	8.2%	8.4%
MRI for Low Back Pain[1]	24	33.3%	32.4%	32.7%
Survey of Patients' Hospital Experiences				
Area Around Room 'Always' Quiet at Night	300+	51%	-	58%
Doctors 'Always' Communicated Well	300+	83%	-	80%
Home Recovery Information Given	300+	74%	-	82%
Hospital Given 9 or 10 on 10 Point Scale	300+	61%	-	67%
Meds 'Always' Explained Before Given	300+	57%	-	60%
Nurses 'Always' Communicated Well	300+	72%	-	76%
Pain 'Always' Well Controlled	300+	64%	-	69%
Room and Bathroom 'Always' Clean	300+	71%	-	71%
Timely Help 'Always' Received	300+	63%	-	64%
Would Definitely Recommend Hospital	300+	60%	-	69%

Saint Vincent Health Center

232 West 25th Street
Erie, PA 16544
Phone: 814-452-5000
Fax: 814-455-1675
URL: www.svhs.org
Type: Acute Care Hospitals
Emergency Services: Yes
Ownership: Voluntary Non-Profit - Church
Beds: 490

Key Personnel:
CEO/President. . . . . Catherine Manning
Chief of Medical Staff. . . . . Howard Nodworny, MD
Infection Control. . . . . Nancy Weissfox
Operating Room. . . . . Veronica Maras, RN
Pediatric Ambulatory Care . . . . . . Cynthia Bowers
Pediatric In-Patient Care . . . . Cynthia Bowers
Quality Assurance . . . . Bonnie Baughman
Radiology. . . . . Richard S Kocan, MD

Measure	Cases	This Hosp.	State Avg.	U.S. Avg.
Heart Attack Care				
ACE Inhibitor or ARB for LVSD	80	98%	95%	96%
Aspirin at Arrival	240	100%	99%	99%
Aspirin at Discharge	461	100%	99%	98%
Beta Blocker at Discharge	457	99%	99%	98%
Fibrinolytic Medication Timing[1]	1	0%	40%	55%
PCI Within 90 Minutes of Arrival	49	82%	88%	90%
Smoking Cessation Advice	173	100%	100%	99%
Chest Pain/Possible Heart Attack Care				
Aspirin at Arrival[3]	0	-	95%	95%
Median Time to ECG (minutes)[3]	0	-	8	8
Median Time to Transfer (minutes)[5]	0	-	68	61
Fibrinolytic Medication Timing[5]	0	-	48%	54%
Heart Failure Care				
ACE Inhibitor or ARB for LVSD	147	90%	95%	94%
Discharge Instructions	390	95%	90%	88%
Evaluation of LVS Function	539	100%	99%	98%
Smoking Cessation Advice	58	100%	98%	98%
Pneumonia Care				
Appropriate Initial Antibiotic	154	93%	93%	92%
Blood Culture Timing	224	94%	96%	96%
Influenza Vaccine	189	89%	92%	91%
Initial Antibiotic Timing	253	97%	96%	95%
Pneumococcal Vaccine	268	96%	95%	93%
Smoking Cessation Advice	99	100%	98%	97%
Surgical Care Improvement Project				
Appropriate VTP Within 24 Hours	498	95%	95%	92%
Appropriate Hair Removal	1,898	100%	100%	99%
Appropriate Beta Blocker Usage	621	95%	94%	93%
Controlled Postoperative Blood Glucose	423	96%	96%	93%
Prophylactic Antibiotic Timing	1,319	97%	97%	97%
Prophylactic Antibiotic Timing (Outpatient)	333	97%	92%	92%
Prophylactic Antibiotic Selection	1,336	97%	98%	97%
Prophylactic Antibiotic Select. (Outpatient)	338	93%	93%	94%
Prophylactic Antibiotic Stopped	1,297	96%	95%	94%
Recommended VTP Ordered	499	96%	97%	94%
Urinary Catheter Removal	476	89%	95%	90%
Children's Asthma Care				
Received Systemic Corticosteroids	-	-	-	100%
Received Home Management Plan	-	-	-	71%
Received Reliever Medication	-	-	-	100%
Use of Medical Imaging				
Combination Abdominal CT Scan	946	0.111	0.203	0.191
Combination Chest CT Scan	424	0.005	0.026	0.054
Follow-up Mammogram/Ultrasound	1,253	6.7%	8.2%	8.4%
MRI for Low Back Pain	291	31.3%	32.4%	32.7%
Survey of Patients' Hospital Experiences				
Area Around Room 'Always' Quiet at Night	300+	51%	-	58%
Doctors 'Always' Communicated Well	300+	76%	-	80%
Home Recovery Information Given	300+	84%	-	82%
Hospital Given 9 or 10 on 10 Point Scale	300+	65%	-	67%
Meds 'Always' Explained Before Given	300+	55%	-	60%
Nurses 'Always' Communicated Well	300+	73%	-	76%
Pain 'Always' Well Controlled	300+	64%	-	69%
Room and Bathroom 'Always' Clean	300+	57%	-	71%
Timely Help 'Always' Received	300+	59%	-	64%
Would Definitely Recommend Hospital	300+	70%	-	69%

NOTE: Hospital profiles are in alphabetical order by state, then city, then hospital within the city; Rankings exclude hospitals with less than 25 cases except for patient surveys which excludes hospitals with less than 100 cases; (a) 100–299 cases; (1) The number of cases is too small to be sure how well a hospital is performing; (2) The hospital indicated that the data submitted for this measure were based on a sample of cases; (3) Data was collected during a shorter time period (fewer quarters) than the maximum possible time for this measure; (4) Suppressed for one or more quarters by CMS; (5) No data is available from the hospital for this measure; (6) Fewer than 100 patients completed the HCAHPS survey. Use these rates with caution, as the number of surveys may be too low to reliably assess hospital performance; (7) Survey results are based on less than 12 months of data; (8) Survey results are not available for this reporting period; (9) No or very few patients were eligible for the HCAHPS survey. The scores shown, if any, reflect a very small number of surveys; (10) A state average was not calculated because too few hospitals in the state submitted data; (11) There were discrepancies in the data collection process; Please refer to the User's Guide for a full explanation of data.

UPMC Bedford

10455 Lincoln Highway
Everett, PA 15537
Phone: 814-623-6161
Fax: 814-624-4313
Type: Acute Care Hospitals
Emergency Services: Yes
Ownership: Voluntary Non-Profit - Other
Beds: 49

Key Personnel:
CEO/President. . . . . Roger P Winn
Chief of Medical Staff. . . . . David Farber, MD
Coronary Care . . . . Kathleen Quinn
Infection Control. . . . . Beth Hullihen, RN
Operating Room. . . . . Anne Allendorfer
Pediatric In-Patient Care . . . . Barbara Antinora
Quality Assurance . . . . Sherrill Wylie, RN
Radiology. . . . . Thomas Anderson

Measure	Cases	This Hosp.	State Avg.	U.S. Avg.
Heart Attack Care				
ACE Inhibitor or ARB for LVSD[3]	0	-	95%	96%
Aspirin at Arrival[1,3]	4	100%	99%	99%
Aspirin at Discharge[1,3]	4	100%	99%	98%
Beta Blocker at Discharge[1,3]	5	100%	99%	98%
Fibrinolytic Medication Timing[3]	0	-	40%	55%
PCI Within 90 Minutes of Arrival[3]	0	-	88%	90%
Smoking Cessation Advice[3]	0	-	100%	99%
Chest Pain/Possible Heart Attack Care				
Aspirin at Arrival	118	97%	95%	95%
Median Time to ECG (minutes)	126	9	8	8
Median Time to Transfer (minutes)[1]	14	74	68	61
Fibrinolytic Medication Timing[1]	2	50%	48%	54%
Heart Failure Care				
ACE Inhibitor or ARB for LVSD[1]	21	81%	95%	94%
Discharge Instructions	45	80%	90%	88%
Evaluation of LVS Function	63	100%	99%	98%
Smoking Cessation Advice[1]	9	100%	98%	98%
Pneumonia Care				
Appropriate Initial Antibiotic	59	97%	93%	92%
Blood Culture Timing	87	98%	96%	96%
Influenza Vaccine	45	100%	92%	91%
Initial Antibiotic Timing	74	99%	96%	95%
Pneumococcal Vaccine	72	99%	95%	93%
Smoking Cessation Advice[1]	14	86%	98%	97%
Surgical Care Improvement Project				
Appropriate VTP Within 24 Hours	64	100%	95%	92%
Appropriate Hair Removal	157	100%	100%	99%
Appropriate Beta Blocker Usage	44	91%	94%	93%
Controlled Postoperative Blood Glucose	0	-	96%	93%
Prophylactic Antibiotic Timing	114	98%	97%	97%
Prophylactic Antibiotic Timing (Outpatient)	36	83%	92%	92%
Prophylactic Antibiotic Selection	114	98%	98%	97%
Prophylactic Antibiotic Select. (Outpatient)	33	82%	93%	94%
Prophylactic Antibiotic Stopped	109	94%	95%	94%
Recommended VTP Ordered	64	100%	97%	94%
Urinary Catheter Removal[1]	20	95%	95%	90%
Children's Asthma Care				
Received Systemic Corticosteroids	-	-	-	100%
Received Home Management Plan	-	-	-	71%
Received Reliever Medication	-	-	-	100%
Use of Medical Imaging				
Combination Abdominal CT Scan	343	0.017	0.203	0.191
Combination Chest CT Scan	165	0.030	0.026	0.054
Follow-up Mammogram/Ultrasound	420	4.5%	8.2%	8.4%
MRI for Low Back Pain[1]	26	34.6%	32.4%	32.7%
Survey of Patients' Hospital Experiences				
Area Around Room 'Always' Quiet at Night	300+	53%	-	58%
Doctors 'Always' Communicated Well	300+	78%	-	80%
Home Recovery Information Given	300+	83%	-	82%
Hospital Given 9 or 10 on 10 Point Scale	300+	60%	-	67%
Meds 'Always' Explained Before Given	300+	61%	-	60%
Nurses 'Always' Communicated Well	300+	76%	-	76%
Pain 'Always' Well Controlled	300+	67%	-	69%
Room and Bathroom 'Always' Clean	300+	78%	-	71%
Timely Help 'Always' Received	300+	64%	-	64%
Would Definitely Recommend Hospital	300+	56%	-	69%

Gettysburg Hospital

147 Gettys Street
Gettysburg, PA 17325
Phone: 717-334-2121
Fax: 717-337-4162
URL: www.wellspan.org
Type: Acute Care Hospitals
Emergency Services: Yes
Ownership: Voluntary Non-Profit - Private
Beds: 76

Key Personnel:
Quality Assurance . . . . Tom Lawler

Measure	Cases	This Hosp.	State Avg.	U.S. Avg.
Heart Attack Care				
ACE Inhibitor or ARB for LVSD[1]	6	83%	95%	96%
Aspirin at Arrival	43	100%	99%	99%
Aspirin at Discharge	31	97%	99%	98%
Beta Blocker at Discharge	30	100%	99%	98%
Fibrinolytic Medication Timing	0	-	40%	55%
PCI Within 90 Minutes of Arrival	0	-	88%	90%
Smoking Cessation Advice[1]	6	100%	100%	99%
Chest Pain/Possible Heart Attack Care				
Aspirin at Arrival	74	99%	95%	95%
Median Time to ECG (minutes)	76	9	8	8
Median Time to Transfer (minutes)[1,3]	11	74	68	61
Fibrinolytic Medication Timing[1]	3	67%	48%	54%
Heart Failure Care				
ACE Inhibitor or ARB for LVSD	42	98%	95%	94%
Discharge Instructions	90	96%	90%	88%
Evaluation of LVS Function	131	100%	99%	98%
Smoking Cessation Advice[1]	9	100%	98%	98%
Pneumonia Care				
Appropriate Initial Antibiotic	71	99%	93%	92%
Blood Culture Timing	158	94%	96%	96%
Influenza Vaccine	116	98%	92%	91%
Initial Antibiotic Timing	131	98%	96%	95%
Pneumococcal Vaccine	143	95%	95%	93%
Smoking Cessation Advice	40	100%	98%	97%
Surgical Care Improvement Project				
Appropriate VTP Within 24 Hours	161	96%	95%	92%
Appropriate Hair Removal	409	100%	100%	99%
Appropriate Beta Blocker Usage	110	99%	94%	93%
Controlled Postoperative Blood Glucose	0	-	96%	93%
Prophylactic Antibiotic Timing	297	100%	97%	97%
Prophylactic Antibiotic Timing (Outpatient)	104	97%	92%	92%
Prophylactic Antibiotic Selection	301	97%	98%	97%
Prophylactic Antibiotic Select. (Outpatient)	101	99%	93%	94%
Prophylactic Antibiotic Stopped	291	96%	95%	94%
Recommended VTP Ordered	161	98%	97%	94%
Urinary Catheter Removal	32	94%	95%	90%
Children's Asthma Care				
Received Systemic Corticosteroids	-	-	-	100%
Received Home Management Plan	-	-	-	71%
Received Reliever Medication	-	-	-	100%
Use of Medical Imaging				
Combination Abdominal CT Scan	658	0.664	0.203	0.191
Combination Chest CT Scan	379	0.082	0.026	0.054
Follow-up Mammogram/Ultrasound	1,343	14.8%	8.2%	8.4%
MRI for Low Back Pain	209	25.4%	32.4%	32.7%
Survey of Patients' Hospital Experiences				
Area Around Room 'Always' Quiet at Night	300+	44%	-	58%
Doctors 'Always' Communicated Well	300+	78%	-	80%
Home Recovery Information Given	300+	87%	-	82%
Hospital Given 9 or 10 on 10 Point Scale	300+	60%	-	67%
Meds 'Always' Explained Before Given	300+	61%	-	60%
Nurses 'Always' Communicated Well	300+	75%	-	76%
Pain 'Always' Well Controlled	300+	67%	-	69%
Room and Bathroom 'Always' Clean	300+	66%	-	71%
Timely Help 'Always' Received	300+	64%	-	64%
Would Definitely Recommend Hospital	300+	61%	-	69%

Excela Health Westmoreland Regional Hospital

532 West Pittsburgh Street
Greensburg, PA 15601
Phone: 412-832-5050
Fax: 724-832-4313
URL: www.westmoreland.org
Type: Acute Care Hospitals
Emergency Services: Yes
Ownership: Voluntary Non-Profit - Other
Beds: 302

Key Personnel:
Chief of Medical Staff. . . . . Donald Kettering, MD
Infection Control. . . . . Lisa D'Amilo, RN
Operating Room. . . . . Maryann Singley
Quality Assurance . . . . Al Rosatti
Radiology. . . . . Sam Raneri
Emergency Room . . . . Robert Whipkey, MD
Intensive Care Unit. . . . . Pam Donovan

Measure	Cases	This Hosp.	State Avg.	U.S. Avg.
Heart Attack Care				
ACE Inhibitor or ARB for LVSD	79	86%	95%	96%
Aspirin at Arrival	328	99%	99%	99%
Aspirin at Discharge	451	99%	99%	98%
Beta Blocker at Discharge	420	96%	99%	98%
Fibrinolytic Medication Timing	0	-	40%	55%
PCI Within 90 Minutes of Arrival	64	81%	88%	90%
Smoking Cessation Advice	137	99%	100%	99%
Chest Pain/Possible Heart Attack Care				
Aspirin at Arrival	32	81%	95%	95%
Median Time to ECG (minutes)	30	14	8	8
Median Time to Transfer (minutes)[1,3]	1	67	68	61
Fibrinolytic Medication Timing[3]	0	-	48%	54%
Heart Failure Care				
ACE Inhibitor or ARB for LVSD	170	86%	95%	94%
Discharge Instructions	536	90%	90%	88%
Evaluation of LVS Function	758	100%	99%	98%
Smoking Cessation Advice	54	100%	98%	98%
Pneumonia Care				
Appropriate Initial Antibiotic	185	92%	93%	92%
Blood Culture Timing	284	99%	96%	96%
Influenza Vaccine	220	95%	92%	91%
Initial Antibiotic Timing	319	97%	96%	95%
Pneumococcal Vaccine	336	98%	95%	93%
Smoking Cessation Advice	105	94%	98%	97%
Surgical Care Improvement Project				
Appropriate VTP Within 24 Hours	507	97%	95%	92%
Appropriate Hair Removal	1,561	99%	100%	99%
Appropriate Beta Blocker Usage	490	96%	94%	93%
Controlled Postoperative Blood Glucose	348	98%	96%	93%
Prophylactic Antibiotic Timing	1,095	99%	97%	97%
Prophylactic Antibiotic Timing (Outpatient)	245	91%	92%	92%
Prophylactic Antibiotic Selection	1,109	99%	98%	97%
Prophylactic Antibiotic Select. (Outpatient)	240	95%	93%	94%
Prophylactic Antibiotic Stopped	1,039	96%	95%	94%
Recommended VTP Ordered	507	98%	97%	94%
Urinary Catheter Removal	353	90%	95%	90%
Children's Asthma Care				
Received Systemic Corticosteroids	-	-	-	100%
Received Home Management Plan	-	-	-	71%
Received Reliever Medication	-	-	-	100%
Use of Medical Imaging				
Combination Abdominal CT Scan	653	0.021	0.203	0.191
Combination Chest CT Scan	503	0.000	0.026	0.054
Follow-up Mammogram/Ultrasound	959	8.7%	8.2%	8.4%
MRI for Low Back Pain	95	35.8%	32.4%	32.7%
Survey of Patients' Hospital Experiences				
Area Around Room 'Always' Quiet at Night	300+	44%	-	58%
Doctors 'Always' Communicated Well	300+	79%	-	80%
Home Recovery Information Given	300+	79%	-	82%
Hospital Given 9 or 10 on 10 Point Scale	300+	58%	-	67%
Meds 'Always' Explained Before Given	300+	62%	-	60%
Nurses 'Always' Communicated Well	300+	74%	-	76%
Pain 'Always' Well Controlled	300+	69%	-	69%
Room and Bathroom 'Always' Clean	300+	66%	-	71%
Timely Help 'Always' Received	300+	64%	-	64%
Would Definitely Recommend Hospital	300+	63%	-	69%

NOTE: Hospital profiles are in alphabetical order by state, then city, then hospital within the city; Rankings exclude hospitals with less than 25 cases except for patient surveys which excludes hospitals with less than 100 cases; (a) 100–299 cases; (1) The number of cases is too small to be sure how well a hospital is performing; (2) The hospital indicated that the data submitted for this measure were based on a sample of cases; (3) Data was collected during a shorter time period (fewer quarters) than the maximum possible time for this measure; (4) Suppressed for one or more quarters by CMS; (5) No data is available from the hospital for this measure; (6) Fewer than 100 patients completed the HCAHPS survey. Use these rates with caution, as the number of surveys may be too low to reliably assess hospital performance; (7) Survey results are based on less than 12 months of data; (8) Survey results are not available for this reporting period; (9) No or very few patients were eligible for the HCAHPS survey. The scores shown, if any, reflect a very small number of surveys; (10) A state average was not calculated because too few hospitals in the state submitted data; (11) There were discrepancies in the data collection process; Please refer to the User's Guide for a full explanation of data.

UPMC Horizon

110 North Main Street Phone: 724-588-2100
Greenville, PA 16125 Fax: 724-983-8877
URL: www.upmc.com
Type: Acute Care Hospitals Emergency Services: Yes
Ownership: Voluntary Non-Profit - Private Beds: 218

Key Personnel:
CEO/President. . . . . Jeffrey A Romoff
Chief of Medical Staff. . . . . Robert Cindberg
Infection Control. . . . . Donna Carl, RN
Operating Room. . . . . Debbie Schuster
Emergency Room . . . . Joseph Noga
Hemotology Center . . . . Sharon Larson
Intensive Care Unit. . . . . Elaine Owen, RN
Patient Relations . . . . Paula Cica

Measure	Cases	This Hosp.	State Avg.	U.S. Avg.
Heart Attack Care				
ACE Inhibitor or ARB for LVSD[1]	12	100%	95%	96%
Aspirin at Arrival	61	98%	99%	99%
Aspirin at Discharge	42	100%	99%	98%
Beta Blocker at Discharge	44	100%	99%	98%
Fibrinolytic Medication Timing	0	-	40%	55%
PCI Within 90 Minutes of Arrival	0	-	88%	90%
Smoking Cessation Advice[1]	5	100%	100%	99%
Chest Pain/Possible Heart Attack Care				
Aspirin at Arrival	130	99%	95%	95%
Median Time to ECG (minutes)	138	12	8	8
Median Time to Transfer (minutes)[1]	22	62	68	61
Fibrinolytic Medication Timing[1]	5	40%	48%	54%
Heart Failure Care				
ACE Inhibitor or ARB for LVSD	55	100%	95%	94%
Discharge Instructions	165	99%	90%	88%
Evaluation of LVS Function	224	100%	99%	98%
Smoking Cessation Advice	31	100%	98%	98%
Pneumonia Care				
Appropriate Initial Antibiotic	147	95%	93%	92%
Blood Culture Timing	179	99%	96%	96%
Influenza Vaccine	155	99%	92%	91%
Initial Antibiotic Timing	188	98%	96%	95%
Pneumococcal Vaccine	201	100%	95%	93%
Smoking Cessation Advice	59	100%	98%	97%
Surgical Care Improvement Project				
Appropriate VTP Within 24 Hours	384	98%	95%	92%
Appropriate Hair Removal	778	100%	100%	99%
Appropriate Beta Blocker Usage	254	96%	94%	93%
Controlled Postoperative Blood Glucose	0	-	96%	93%
Prophylactic Antibiotic Timing	537	97%	97%	97%
Prophylactic Antibiotic Timing (Outpatient)	201	91%	92%	92%
Prophylactic Antibiotic Selection	539	97%	98%	97%
Prophylactic Antibiotic Select. (Outpatient)	195	91%	93%	94%
Prophylactic Antibiotic Stopped	506	97%	95%	94%
Recommended VTP Ordered	384	98%	97%	94%
Urinary Catheter Removal	43	98%	95%	90%
Children's Asthma Care				
Received Systemic Corticosteroids	-	-	-	100%
Received Home Management Plan	-	-	-	71%
Received Reliever Medication	-	-	-	100%
Use of Medical Imaging				
Combination Abdominal CT Scan	889	0.128	0.203	0.191
Combination Chest CT Scan	553	0.002	0.026	0.054
Follow-up Mammogram/Ultrasound	1,168	7.4%	8.2%	8.4%
MRI for Low Back Pain	188	32.4%	32.4%	32.7%
Survey of Patients' Hospital Experiences				
Area Around Room 'Always' Quiet at Night	300+	42%	-	58%
Doctors 'Always' Communicated Well	300+	80%	-	80%
Home Recovery Information Given	300+	82%	-	82%
Hospital Given 9 or 10 on 10 Point Scale	300+	60%	-	67%
Meds 'Always' Explained Before Given	300+	56%	-	60%
Nurses 'Always' Communicated Well	300+	71%	-	76%
Pain 'Always' Well Controlled	300+	64%	-	69%
Room and Bathroom 'Always' Clean	300+	68%	-	71%
Timely Help 'Always' Received	300+	57%	-	64%
Would Definitely Recommend Hospital	300+	62%	-	69%

Grove City Medical Center

631 North Broad Street Ext. Phone: 724-450-7000
Grove City, PA 16127 Fax: 724-450-7179
E-mail: ushcommrelations@uchpa.org
URL: www.uchpa.org
Type: Acute Care Hospitals Emergency Services: Yes
Ownership: Voluntary Non-Profit - Other Beds: 95

Key Personnel:
CEO/President. . . . . Robert Jackson
Chief of Medical Staff. . . . . S Sawardekar
Infection Control. . . . . Donna Leffler
Quality Assurance . . . . Bev Jack
Radiology. . . . . Gilbert Lawrence MD
Emergency Room . . . . Tony Bono RN
Intensive Care Unit. . . . . Sue Lee
Patient Relations . . . . Rob Jackson

Measure	Cases	This Hosp.	State Avg.	U.S. Avg.
Heart Attack Care				
ACE Inhibitor or ARB for LVSD[1]	4	75%	95%	96%
Aspirin at Arrival[1]	13	92%	99%	99%
Aspirin at Discharge[1]	13	85%	99%	98%
Beta Blocker at Discharge[1]	11	91%	99%	98%
Fibrinolytic Medication Timing	0	-	40%	55%
PCI Within 90 Minutes of Arrival	0	-	88%	90%
Smoking Cessation Advice[1]	2	50%	100%	99%
Chest Pain/Possible Heart Attack Care				
Aspirin at Arrival	158	98%	95%	95%
Median Time to ECG (minutes)	164	6	8	8
Median Time to Transfer (minutes)[1]	15	60	68	61
Fibrinolytic Medication Timing	0	-	48%	54%
Heart Failure Care				
ACE Inhibitor or ARB for LVSD	27	85%	95%	94%
Discharge Instructions	51	94%	90%	88%
Evaluation of LVS Function	98	97%	99%	98%
Smoking Cessation Advice[1]	6	100%	98%	98%
Pneumonia Care				
Appropriate Initial Antibiotic	65	98%	93%	92%
Blood Culture Timing	80	100%	96%	96%
Influenza Vaccine	49	90%	92%	91%
Initial Antibiotic Timing	88	98%	96%	95%
Pneumococcal Vaccine	69	97%	95%	93%
Smoking Cessation Advice[1]	17	88%	98%	97%
Surgical Care Improvement Project				
Appropriate VTP Within 24 Hours	35	77%	95%	92%
Appropriate Hair Removal	152	100%	100%	99%
Appropriate Beta Blocker Usage	37	97%	94%	93%
Controlled Postoperative Blood Glucose	0	-	96%	93%
Prophylactic Antibiotic Timing	113	99%	97%	97%
Prophylactic Antibiotic Timing (Outpatient)	88	95%	92%	92%
Prophylactic Antibiotic Selection	113	100%	98%	97%
Prophylactic Antibiotic Select. (Outpatient)	84	89%	93%	94%
Prophylactic Antibiotic Stopped	113	95%	95%	94%
Recommended VTP Ordered	35	80%	97%	94%
Urinary Catheter Removal[1]	19	89%	95%	90%
Children's Asthma Care				
Received Systemic Corticosteroids	-	-	-	100%
Received Home Management Plan	-	-	-	71%
Received Reliever Medication	-	-	-	100%
Use of Medical Imaging				
Combination Abdominal CT Scan	237	0.211	0.203	0.191
Combination Chest CT Scan	161	0.006	0.026	0.054
Follow-up Mammogram/Ultrasound	370	10.0%	8.2%	8.4%
MRI for Low Back Pain	49	40.8%	32.4%	32.7%
Survey of Patients' Hospital Experiences				
Area Around Room 'Always' Quiet at Night	300+	52%	-	58%
Doctors 'Always' Communicated Well	300+	83%	-	80%
Home Recovery Information Given	300+	87%	-	82%
Hospital Given 9 or 10 on 10 Point Scale	300+	70%	-	67%
Meds 'Always' Explained Before Given	300+	68%	-	60%
Nurses 'Always' Communicated Well	300+	77%	-	76%
Pain 'Always' Well Controlled	300+	72%	-	69%
Room and Bathroom 'Always' Clean	300+	78%	-	71%
Timely Help 'Always' Received	300+	68%	-	64%
Would Definitely Recommend Hospital	300+	66%	-	69%

Hanover Hospital

300 Highland Ave Phone: 717-637-3711
Hanover, PA 17331 Fax: 717-633-2217
URL: www.hanoverhospital.org
Type: Acute Care Hospitals Emergency Services: Yes
Ownership: Voluntary Non-Profit - Private Beds: 117

Key Personnel:
CEO/President. . . . . George Kyriacou
Chief of Medical Staff. . . . . John Lunsford Jr, MD
Infection Control. . . . . Jennifer Laughman
Operating Room. . . . . Connie Robinson
Quality Assurance . . . . Gary Grant
Radiology. . . . . Alicia M Cartagena
Emergency Room . . . . Anthony Alvarez, MSN, RN
Patient Relations . . . . Laurie Wolf

Measure	Cases	This Hosp.	State Avg.	U.S. Avg.
Heart Attack Care				
ACE Inhibitor or ARB for LVSD	29	79%	95%	96%
Aspirin at Arrival	174	97%	99%	99%
Aspirin at Discharge	114	88%	99%	98%
Beta Blocker at Discharge	112	90%	99%	98%
Fibrinolytic Medication Timing[1]	5	20%	40%	55%
PCI Within 90 Minutes of Arrival	0	-	88%	90%
Smoking Cessation Advice[1]	16	94%	100%	99%
Chest Pain/Possible Heart Attack Care				
Aspirin at Arrival	59	93%	95%	95%
Median Time to ECG (minutes)	63	5	8	8
Median Time to Transfer (minutes)[1]	8	76	68	61
Fibrinolytic Medication Timing[1]	7	71%	48%	54%
Heart Failure Care				
ACE Inhibitor or ARB for LVSD	62	81%	95%	94%
Discharge Instructions	156	94%	90%	88%
Evaluation of LVS Function	197	76%	99%	98%
Smoking Cessation Advice[1]	23	100%	98%	98%
Pneumonia Care				
Appropriate Initial Antibiotic	93	85%	93%	92%
Blood Culture Timing	141	91%	96%	96%
Influenza Vaccine	113	81%	92%	91%
Initial Antibiotic Timing	127	96%	96%	95%
Pneumococcal Vaccine	136	93%	95%	93%
Smoking Cessation Advice	27	96%	98%	97%
Surgical Care Improvement Project				
Appropriate VTP Within 24 Hours	163	87%	95%	92%
Appropriate Hair Removal	750	100%	100%	99%
Appropriate Beta Blocker Usage	207	95%	94%	93%
Controlled Postoperative Blood Glucose	0	-	96%	93%
Prophylactic Antibiotic Timing	628	97%	97%	97%
Prophylactic Antibiotic Timing (Outpatient)	194	91%	92%	92%
Prophylactic Antibiotic Selection	624	98%	98%	97%
Prophylactic Antibiotic Select. (Outpatient)	183	96%	93%	94%
Prophylactic Antibiotic Stopped	619	88%	95%	94%
Recommended VTP Ordered	164	88%	97%	94%
Urinary Catheter Removal	262	95%	95%	90%
Children's Asthma Care				
Received Systemic Corticosteroids	-	-	-	100%
Received Home Management Plan	-	-	-	71%
Received Reliever Medication	-	-	-	100%
Use of Medical Imaging				
Combination Abdominal CT Scan	890	0.093	0.203	0.191
Combination Chest CT Scan	697	0.019	0.026	0.054
Follow-up Mammogram/Ultrasound	1,172	12.0%	8.2%	8.4%
MRI for Low Back Pain	236	24.2%	32.4%	32.7%
Survey of Patients' Hospital Experiences				
Area Around Room 'Always' Quiet at Night	300+	45%	-	58%
Doctors 'Always' Communicated Well	300+	79%	-	80%
Home Recovery Information Given	300+	81%	-	82%
Hospital Given 9 or 10 on 10 Point Scale	300+	64%	-	67%
Meds 'Always' Explained Before Given	300+	52%	-	60%
Nurses 'Always' Communicated Well	300+	71%	-	76%
Pain 'Always' Well Controlled	300+	67%	-	69%
Room and Bathroom 'Always' Clean	300+	74%	-	71%
Timely Help 'Always' Received	300+	57%	-	64%
Would Definitely Recommend Hospital	300+	65%	-	69%

NOTE: Hospital profiles are in alphabetical order by state, then city, then hospital within the city; Rankings exclude hospitals with less than 25 cases except for patient surveys which excludes hospitals with less than 100 cases; (a) 100–299 cases; (1) The number of cases is too small to be sure how well a hospital is performing; (2) The hospital indicated that the data submitted for this measure were based on a sample of cases; (3) Data was collected during a shorter time period (fewer quarters) than the maximum possible time for this measure; (4) Suppressed for one or more quarters by CMS; (5) No data is available from the hospital for this measure; (6) Fewer than 100 patients completed the HCAHPS survey. Use these rates with caution, as the number of surveys may be too low to reliably assess hospital performance; (7) Survey results are based on less than 12 months of data; (8) Survey results are not available for this reporting period; (9) No or very few patients were eligible for the HCAHPS survey. The scores shown, if any, reflect a very small number of surveys; (10) A state average was not calculated because too few hospitals in the state submitted data; (11) There were discrepancies in the data collection process; Please refer to the User's Guide for a full explanation of data.

Pinnacle Health Hospitals

409 South Second Street
Harrisburg, PA 17105
Phone: 717-782-5181
URL: www.pinnaclehealth.org
Type: Acute Care Hospitals
Emergency Services: Yes
Ownership: Voluntary Non-Profit - Other
Key Personnel:
CEO/President. . . . . Roger Longenderfer

Measure	Cases	This Hosp.	State Avg.	U.S. Avg.
Heart Attack Care				
ACE Inhibitor or ARB for LVSD	149	97%	95%	96%
Aspirin at Arrival	545	99%	99%	99%
Aspirin at Discharge	637	99%	99%	98%
Beta Blocker at Discharge	633	99%	99%	98%
Fibrinolytic Medication Timing	0	-	40%	55%
PCI Within 90 Minutes of Arrival	90	97%	88%	90%
Smoking Cessation Advice	183	100%	100%	99%
Chest Pain/Possible Heart Attack Care				
Aspirin at Arrival[1,3]	2	100%	95%	95%
Median Time to ECG (minutes)[1,3]	2	1	8	8
Median Time to Transfer (minutes)[5]	0	-	68	61
Fibrinolytic Medication Timing[5]	0	-	48%	54%
Heart Failure Care				
ACE Inhibitor or ARB for LVSD	256	100%	95%	94%
Discharge Instructions	605	89%	90%	88%
Evaluation of LVS Function	769	100%	99%	98%
Smoking Cessation Advice	113	100%	98%	98%
Pneumonia Care				
Appropriate Initial Antibiotic	229	97%	93%	92%
Blood Culture Timing	333	96%	96%	96%
Influenza Vaccine	321	94%	92%	91%
Initial Antibiotic Timing	342	96%	96%	95%
Pneumococcal Vaccine	380	98%	95%	93%
Smoking Cessation Advice	140	99%	98%	97%
Surgical Care Improvement Project				
Appropriate VTP Within 24 Hours[2]	746	95%	95%	92%
Appropriate Hair Removal[2]	3,582	100%	100%	99%
Appropriate Beta Blocker Usage[2]	1,087	94%	94%	93%
Controlled Postoperative Blood Glucose[2]	497	99%	96%	93%
Prophylactic Antibiotic Timing[2]	2,975	99%	97%	97%
Prophylactic Antibiotic Timing (Outpatient)	1,109	96%	92%	92%
Prophylactic Antibiotic Selection[2]	3,010	97%	98%	97%
Prophylactic Antibiotic Select. (Outpatient)	1,086	87%	93%	94%
Prophylactic Antibiotic Stopped[2]	2,912	95%	95%	94%
Recommended VTP Ordered[2]	746	99%	97%	94%
Urinary Catheter Removal[2]	624	98%	95%	90%
Children's Asthma Care				
Received Systemic Corticosteroids	-	-	-	100%
Received Home Management Plan	-	-	-	71%
Received Reliever Medication	-	-	-	100%
Use of Medical Imaging				
Combination Abdominal CT Scan	993	0.272	0.203	0.191
Combination Chest CT Scan	608	0.158	0.026	0.054
Follow-up Mammogram/Ultrasound	1,189	7.7%	8.2%	8.4%
MRI for Low Back Pain	118	32.2%	32.4%	32.7%
Survey of Patients' Hospital Experiences				
Area Around Room 'Always' Quiet at Night	300+	46%	-	58%
Doctors 'Always' Communicated Well	300+	74%	-	80%
Home Recovery Information Given	300+	78%	-	82%
Hospital Given 9 or 10 on 10 Point Scale	300+	59%	-	67%
Meds 'Always' Explained Before Given	300+	56%	-	60%
Nurses 'Always' Communicated Well	300+	72%	-	76%
Pain 'Always' Well Controlled	300+	67%	-	69%
Room and Bathroom 'Always' Clean	300+	60%	-	71%
Timely Help 'Always' Received	300+	53%	-	64%
Would Definitely Recommend Hospital	300+	68%	-	69%

Miners Medical Center

290 Haida Avenue
Hastings, PA 16646
Phone: 814-247-3100
Fax: 814-247-3119
URL: www.minershosp.org
Type: Acute Care Hospitals
Emergency Services: Yes
Ownership: Voluntary Non-Profit - Private
Beds: 30
Key Personnel:
CEO/President. . . . . Bill Crowe
Chief of Medical Staff . . . . John Crawford
Radiology. . . . . Vallabhaneni Babu

Measure	Cases	This Hosp.	State Avg.	U.S. Avg.
Heart Attack Care				
ACE Inhibitor or ARB for LVSD[1]	1	100%	95%	96%
Aspirin at Arrival[1]	12	100%	99%	99%
Aspirin at Discharge[1]	8	100%	99%	98%
Beta Blocker at Discharge[1]	7	86%	99%	98%
Fibrinolytic Medication Timing	0	-	40%	55%
PCI Within 90 Minutes of Arrival	0	-	88%	90%
Smoking Cessation Advice	0	-	100%	99%
Chest Pain/Possible Heart Attack Care				
Aspirin at Arrival	117	92%	95%	95%
Median Time to ECG (minutes)	123	16	8	8
Median Time to Transfer (minutes)[1]	8	62	68	61
Fibrinolytic Medication Timing	0	-	48%	54%
Heart Failure Care				
ACE Inhibitor or ARB for LVSD[1]	12	67%	95%	94%
Discharge Instructions	27	41%	90%	88%
Evaluation of LVS Function	34	85%	99%	98%
Smoking Cessation Advice[1]	6	83%	98%	98%
Pneumonia Care				
Appropriate Initial Antibiotic	43	79%	93%	92%
Blood Culture Timing	35	74%	96%	96%
Influenza Vaccine	37	38%	92%	91%
Initial Antibiotic Timing	53	96%	96%	95%
Pneumococcal Vaccine	50	36%	95%	93%
Smoking Cessation Advice[1]	21	62%	98%	97%
Surgical Care Improvement Project				
Appropriate VTP Within 24 Hours[1]	19	47%	95%	92%
Appropriate Hair Removal[1]	24	79%	100%	99%
Appropriate Beta Blocker Usage[1]	8	12%	94%	93%
Controlled Postoperative Blood Glucose	0	-	96%	93%
Prophylactic Antibiotic Timing[1]	14	79%	97%	97%
Prophylactic Antibiotic Timing (Outpatient)[1,3]	3	33%	92%	92%
Prophylactic Antibiotic Selection[1]	14	93%	98%	97%
Prophylactic Antibiotic Select. (Outpatient)[1,3]	2	50%	93%	94%
Prophylactic Antibiotic Stopped[1]	13	100%	95%	94%
Recommended VTP Ordered[1]	19	47%	97%	94%
Urinary Catheter Removal[1]	2	50%	95%	90%
Children's Asthma Care				
Received Systemic Corticosteroids	-	-	-	100%
Received Home Management Plan	-	-	-	71%
Received Reliever Medication	-	-	-	100%
Use of Medical Imaging				
Combination Abdominal CT Scan	254	0.024	0.203	0.191
Combination Chest CT Scan	130	0.008	0.026	0.054
Follow-up Mammogram/Ultrasound	135	4.4%	8.2%	8.4%
MRI for Low Back Pain	44	47.7%	32.4%	32.7%
Survey of Patients' Hospital Experiences				
Area Around Room 'Always' Quiet at Night	(a)	67%	-	58%
Doctors 'Always' Communicated Well	(a)	89%	-	80%
Home Recovery Information Given	(a)	83%	-	82%
Hospital Given 9 or 10 on 10 Point Scale	(a)	77%	-	67%
Meds 'Always' Explained Before Given	(a)	62%	-	60%
Nurses 'Always' Communicated Well	(a)	86%	-	76%
Pain 'Always' Well Controlled	(a)	79%	-	69%
Room and Bathroom 'Always' Clean	(a)	77%	-	71%
Timely Help 'Always' Received	(a)	83%	-	64%
Would Definitely Recommend Hospital	(a)	74%	-	69%

Hazleton General Hospital

700 East Broad Street
Hazleton, PA 18201
Phone: 570-501-4000
Fax: 570-501-6203
URL: www.ghha.org
Type: Acute Care Hospitals
Emergency Services: Yes
Ownership: Voluntary Non-Profit - Other
Beds: 160
Key Personnel:
CEO/President. . . . . James D Edwards
Chief of Medical Staff . . . . Anthony Valente, MD
Infection Control . . . . Edna Reis
Operating Room. . . . . Kathy Guida
Quality Assurance . . . . Andrea Andrews
Radiology. . . . . Orest B Boyko
Emergency Room . . . . Paul Tayoun, DO
Patient Relations . . . . Sue Farley

Measure	Cases	This Hosp.	State Avg.	U.S. Avg.
Heart Attack Care				
ACE Inhibitor or ARB for LVSD[1]	3	100%	95%	96%
Aspirin at Arrival	61	97%	99%	99%
Aspirin at Discharge	39	97%	99%	98%
Beta Blocker at Discharge	48	100%	99%	98%
Fibrinolytic Medication Timing	0	-	40%	55%
PCI Within 90 Minutes of Arrival	0	-	88%	90%
Smoking Cessation Advice[1]	5	100%	100%	99%
Chest Pain/Possible Heart Attack Care				
Aspirin at Arrival	321	92%	95%	95%
Median Time to ECG (minutes)	333	14	8	8
Median Time to Transfer (minutes)	44	52	68	61
Fibrinolytic Medication Timing	0	-	48%	54%
Heart Failure Care				
ACE Inhibitor or ARB for LVSD	53	98%	95%	94%
Discharge Instructions	183	95%	90%	88%
Evaluation of LVS Function	282	100%	99%	98%
Smoking Cessation Advice	32	100%	98%	98%
Pneumonia Care				
Appropriate Initial Antibiotic	141	93%	93%	92%
Blood Culture Timing	171	97%	96%	96%
Influenza Vaccine	198	98%	92%	91%
Initial Antibiotic Timing	257	97%	96%	95%
Pneumococcal Vaccine	276	99%	95%	93%
Smoking Cessation Advice	90	99%	98%	97%
Surgical Care Improvement Project				
Appropriate VTP Within 24 Hours	153	94%	95%	92%
Appropriate Hair Removal	323	100%	100%	99%
Appropriate Beta Blocker Usage	94	94%	94%	93%
Controlled Postoperative Blood Glucose	0	-	96%	93%
Prophylactic Antibiotic Timing	178	97%	97%	97%
Prophylactic Antibiotic Timing (Outpatient)	78	92%	92%	92%
Prophylactic Antibiotic Selection	179	98%	98%	97%
Prophylactic Antibiotic Select. (Outpatient)	75	85%	93%	94%
Prophylactic Antibiotic Stopped	169	95%	95%	94%
Recommended VTP Ordered	153	97%	97%	94%
Urinary Catheter Removal	54	100%	95%	90%
Children's Asthma Care				
Received Systemic Corticosteroids	-	-	-	100%
Received Home Management Plan	-	-	-	71%
Received Reliever Medication	-	-	-	100%
Use of Medical Imaging				
Combination Abdominal CT Scan	579	0.017	0.203	0.191
Combination Chest CT Scan	410	0.000	0.026	0.054
Follow-up Mammogram/Ultrasound	345	7.5%	8.2%	8.4%
MRI for Low Back Pain	109	31.2%	32.4%	32.7%
Survey of Patients' Hospital Experiences				
Area Around Room 'Always' Quiet at Night	300+	45%	-	58%
Doctors 'Always' Communicated Well	300+	80%	-	80%
Home Recovery Information Given	300+	74%	-	82%
Hospital Given 9 or 10 on 10 Point Scale	300+	49%	-	67%
Meds 'Always' Explained Before Given	300+	53%	-	60%
Nurses 'Always' Communicated Well	300+	71%	-	76%
Pain 'Always' Well Controlled	300+	66%	-	69%
Room and Bathroom 'Always' Clean	300+	75%	-	71%
Timely Help 'Always' Received	300+	62%	-	64%
Would Definitely Recommend Hospital	300+	44%	-	69%

NOTE: Hospital profiles are in alphabetical order by state, then city, then hospital within the city; Rankings exclude hospitals with less than 25 cases except for patient surveys which excludes hospitals with less than 100 cases; (a) 100–299 cases; (1) The number of cases is too small to be sure how well a hospital is performing; (2) The hospital indicated that the data submitted for this measure were based on a sample of cases; (3) Data was collected during a shorter time period (fewer quarters) than the maximum possible time for this measure; (4) Suppressed for one or more quarters by CMS; (5) No data is available from the hospital for this measure; (6) Fewer than 100 patients completed the HCAHPS survey. Use these rates with caution, as the number of surveys may be too low to reliably assess hospital performance; (7) Survey results are based on less than 12 months of data; (8) Survey results are not available for this reporting period; (9) No or very few patients were eligible for the HCAHPS survey. The scores shown, if any, reflect a very small number of surveys; (10) A state average was not calculated because too few hospitals in the state submitted data; (11) There were discrepancies in the data collection process; Please refer to the User's Guide for a full explanation of data.

Milton S Hershey Medical Center

500 University Drive Phone: 717-531-8521
Hershey, PA 17033 Fax: 717-531-4162
URL: www.hmc.psu.edu
Type: Acute Care Hospitals Emergency Services: Yes
Ownership: Voluntary Non-Profit - Other Beds: 504

Key Personnel:

CEO/President. . . . . Harold Paz, MD
Cardiac Laboratory. . . . . Gerald Neccareli
Chief of Medical Staff . . . . Michael Weitecamp, MD
Emergency Room . . . . Kym Salness, MD

Measure	Cases	This Hosp.	State Avg.	U.S. Avg.
Heart Attack Care				
ACE Inhibitor or ARB for LVSD	35	97%	95%	96%
Aspirin at Arrival	234	100%	99%	99%
Aspirin at Discharge	349	99%	99%	98%
Beta Blocker at Discharge	340	99%	99%	98%
Fibrinolytic Medication Timing[1]	1	100%	40%	55%
PCI Within 90 Minutes of Arrival	41	88%	88%	90%
Smoking Cessation Advice	89	100%	100%	99%
Chest Pain/Possible Heart Attack Care				
Aspirin at Arrival[5]	0	-	95%	95%
Median Time to ECG (minutes)[5]	0	-	8	8
Median Time to Transfer (minutes)[5]	0	-	68	61
Fibrinolytic Medication Timing[5]	0	-	48%	54%
Heart Failure Care				
ACE Inhibitor or ARB for LVSD	113	99%	95%	94%
Discharge Instructions	399	89%	90%	88%
Evaluation of LVS Function	462	99%	99%	98%
Smoking Cessation Advice	54	98%	98%	98%
Pneumonia Care				
Appropriate Initial Antibiotic	129	95%	93%	92%
Blood Culture Timing	275	89%	96%	96%
Influenza Vaccine	188	78%	92%	91%
Initial Antibiotic Timing	237	95%	96%	95%
Pneumococcal Vaccine	285	82%	95%	93%
Smoking Cessation Advice	93	99%	98%	97%
Surgical Care Improvement Project				
Appropriate VTP Within 24 Hours[2]	426	95%	95%	92%
Appropriate Hair Removal[2]	1,642	98%	100%	99%
Appropriate Beta Blocker Usage[2]	534	86%	94%	93%
Controlled Postoperative Blood Glucose[2]	333	92%	96%	93%
Prophylactic Antibiotic Timing[2]	1,275	93%	97%	97%
Prophylactic Antibiotic Timing (Outpatient)	710	93%	92%	92%
Prophylactic Antibiotic Selection[2]	1,287	98%	98%	97%
Prophylactic Antibiotic Select. (Outpatient)	702	94%	93%	94%
Prophylactic Antibiotic Stopped[2]	1,205	94%	95%	94%
Recommended VTP Ordered[2]	428	95%	97%	94%
Urinary Catheter Removal[2]	349	92%	95%	90%
Children's Asthma Care				
Received Systemic Corticosteroids	-	-	-	100%
Received Home Management Plan	-	-	-	71%
Received Reliever Medication	-	-	-	100%
Use of Medical Imaging				
Combination Abdominal CT Scan	1,858	0.206	0.203	0.191
Combination Chest CT Scan	1,991	0.006	0.026	0.054
Follow-up Mammogram/Ultrasound	1,085	5.0%	8.2%	8.4%
MRI for Low Back Pain	319	26.6%	32.4%	32.7%
Survey of Patients' Hospital Experiences				
Area Around Room 'Always' Quiet at Night	300+	42%	-	58%
Doctors 'Always' Communicated Well	300+	76%	-	80%
Home Recovery Information Given	300+	89%	-	82%
Hospital Given 9 or 10 on 10 Point Scale	300+	72%	-	67%
Meds 'Always' Explained Before Given	300+	58%	-	60%
Nurses 'Always' Communicated Well	300+	74%	-	76%
Pain 'Always' Well Controlled	300+	68%	-	69%
Room and Bathroom 'Always' Clean	300+	65%	-	71%
Timely Help 'Always' Received	300+	59%	-	64%
Would Definitely Recommend Hospital	300+	78%	-	69%

Wayne Memorial Hospital

601 Park Street Phone: 570-253-8100
Honesdale, PA 18431 Fax: 570-253-8397
URL: www.wmh.org
Type: Acute Care Hospitals Emergency Services: Yes
Ownership: Voluntary Non-Profit - Private Beds: 95

Key Personnel:

CEO/President. . . . . David Hoff
Chief of Medical Staff . . . . George Tietjen, MD
Infection Control. . . . . Cinda Tietjen
Quality Assurance . . . . Marilyn Swendsen
Anesthesiology. . . . . RA Achecar, MD
Emergency Room . . . . Donna Eget, MD
Intensive Care Unit. . . . . Lisa Kinzinger

Measure	Cases	This Hosp.	State Avg.	U.S. Avg.
Heart Attack Care				
ACE Inhibitor or ARB for LVSD[1]	5	100%	95%	96%
Aspirin at Arrival	46	93%	99%	99%
Aspirin at Discharge	25	92%	99%	98%
Beta Blocker at Discharge	25	96%	99%	98%
Fibrinolytic Medication Timing	0	-	40%	55%
PCI Within 90 Minutes of Arrival	0	-	88%	90%
Smoking Cessation Advice[1]	7	100%	100%	99%
Chest Pain/Possible Heart Attack Care				
Aspirin at Arrival	38	95%	95%	95%
Median Time to ECG (minutes)	38	4	8	8
Median Time to Transfer (minutes)[1]	9	53	68	61
Fibrinolytic Medication Timing	0	-	48%	54%
Heart Failure Care				
ACE Inhibitor or ARB for LVSD	26	96%	95%	94%
Discharge Instructions	83	94%	90%	88%
Evaluation of LVS Function	102	98%	99%	98%
Smoking Cessation Advice[1]	18	100%	98%	98%
Pneumonia Care				
Appropriate Initial Antibiotic	83	92%	93%	92%
Blood Culture Timing	102	97%	96%	96%
Influenza Vaccine	66	94%	92%	91%
Initial Antibiotic Timing	104	96%	96%	95%
Pneumococcal Vaccine	97	96%	95%	93%
Smoking Cessation Advice	36	100%	98%	97%
Surgical Care Improvement Project				
Appropriate VTP Within 24 Hours[2]	109	96%	95%	92%
Appropriate Hair Removal[2]	255	100%	100%	99%
Appropriate Beta Blocker Usage[2]	54	76%	94%	93%
Controlled Postoperative Blood Glucose[2]	0	-	96%	93%
Prophylactic Antibiotic Timing[2]	162	97%	97%	97%
Prophylactic Antibiotic Timing (Outpatient)	47	89%	92%	92%
Prophylactic Antibiotic Selection[2]	162	95%	98%	97%
Prophylactic Antibiotic Select. (Outpatient)	49	88%	93%	94%
Prophylactic Antibiotic Stopped[2]	158	96%	95%	94%
Recommended VTP Ordered[2]	109	96%	97%	94%
Urinary Catheter Removal[2]	63	79%	95%	90%
Children's Asthma Care				
Received Systemic Corticosteroids	-	-	-	100%
Received Home Management Plan	-	-	-	71%
Received Reliever Medication	-	-	-	100%
Use of Medical Imaging				
Combination Abdominal CT Scan	647	0.127	0.203	0.191
Combination Chest CT Scan	581	0.045	0.026	0.054
Follow-up Mammogram/Ultrasound	1,071	5.6%	8.2%	8.4%
MRI for Low Back Pain	94	44.7%	32.4%	32.7%
Survey of Patients' Hospital Experiences				
Area Around Room 'Always' Quiet at Night	300+	46%	-	58%
Doctors 'Always' Communicated Well	300+	78%	-	80%
Home Recovery Information Given	300+	86%	-	82%
Hospital Given 9 or 10 on 10 Point Scale	300+	63%	-	67%
Meds 'Always' Explained Before Given	300+	59%	-	60%
Nurses 'Always' Communicated Well	300+	77%	-	76%
Pain 'Always' Well Controlled	300+	75%	-	69%
Room and Bathroom 'Always' Clean	300+	73%	-	71%
Timely Help 'Always' Received	300+	68%	-	64%
Would Definitely Recommend Hospital	300+	63%	-	69%

J C Blair Memorial Hospital

1225 Warm Springs Ave Phone: 814-643-2290
Huntingdon, PA 16652 Fax: 814-643-8813
URL: www.jcblair.org
Type: Acute Care Hospitals Emergency Services: Yes
Ownership: Voluntary Non-Profit - Other Beds: 104

Key Personnel:

CEO/President. . . . . Leland E Farnell, ACHE
Chief of Medical Staff . . . . Christopher J Patitsas, MD
Coronary Care . . . . Don McCaulley
Infection Control. . . . . Bethany Brown
Operating Room. . . . . Leigh Bizak, RN
Pediatric Ambulatory Care . . . . . . Rita Notestine
Quality Assurance . . . . Marlene Pierce
Radiology. . . . . Larry Garman

Measure	Cases	This Hosp.	State Avg.	U.S. Avg.
Heart Attack Care				
ACE Inhibitor or ARB for LVSD[3]	0	-	95%	96%
Aspirin at Arrival[1,3]	6	83%	99%	99%
Aspirin at Discharge[1,3]	2	100%	99%	98%
Beta Blocker at Discharge[1,3]	2	100%	99%	98%
Fibrinolytic Medication Timing[3]	0	-	40%	55%
PCI Within 90 Minutes of Arrival[3]	0	-	88%	90%
Smoking Cessation Advice[3]	0	-	100%	99%
Chest Pain/Possible Heart Attack Care				
Aspirin at Arrival	151	90%	95%	95%
Median Time to ECG (minutes)	158	12	8	8
Median Time to Transfer (minutes)[1]	12	86	68	61
Fibrinolytic Medication Timing[1]	1	100%	48%	54%
Heart Failure Care				
ACE Inhibitor or ARB for LVSD[1]	17	88%	95%	94%
Discharge Instructions	57	79%	90%	88%
Evaluation of LVS Function	75	92%	99%	98%
Smoking Cessation Advice[1]	12	100%	98%	98%
Pneumonia Care				
Appropriate Initial Antibiotic	44	93%	93%	92%
Blood Culture Timing	51	98%	96%	96%
Influenza Vaccine	42	93%	92%	91%
Initial Antibiotic Timing	59	97%	96%	95%
Pneumococcal Vaccine	55	91%	95%	93%
Smoking Cessation Advice[1]	17	94%	98%	97%
Surgical Care Improvement Project				
Appropriate VTP Within 24 Hours	33	94%	95%	92%
Appropriate Hair Removal	58	100%	100%	99%
Appropriate Beta Blocker Usage[1]	9	78%	94%	93%
Controlled Postoperative Blood Glucose	0	-	96%	93%
Prophylactic Antibiotic Timing	33	88%	97%	97%
Prophylactic Antibiotic Timing (Outpatient)[1]	17	76%	92%	92%
Prophylactic Antibiotic Selection	33	79%	98%	97%
Prophylactic Antibiotic Select. (Outpatient)[1]	15	100%	93%	94%
Prophylactic Antibiotic Stopped	29	69%	95%	94%
Recommended VTP Ordered	34	94%	97%	94%
Urinary Catheter Removal[1]	7	0%	95%	90%
Children's Asthma Care				
Received Systemic Corticosteroids	-	-	-	100%
Received Home Management Plan	-	-	-	71%
Received Reliever Medication	-	-	-	100%
Use of Medical Imaging				
Combination Abdominal CT Scan	409	0.022	0.203	0.191
Combination Chest CT Scan	204	0.005	0.026	0.054
Follow-up Mammogram/Ultrasound	804	6.0%	8.2%	8.4%
MRI for Low Back Pain	41	46.3%	32.4%	32.7%
Survey of Patients' Hospital Experiences				
Area Around Room 'Always' Quiet at Night	300+	51%	-	58%
Doctors 'Always' Communicated Well	300+	83%	-	80%
Home Recovery Information Given	300+	84%	-	82%
Hospital Given 9 or 10 on 10 Point Scale	300+	62%	-	67%
Meds 'Always' Explained Before Given	300+	58%	-	60%
Nurses 'Always' Communicated Well	300+	78%	-	76%
Pain 'Always' Well Controlled	300+	71%	-	69%
Room and Bathroom 'Always' Clean	300+	77%	-	71%
Timely Help 'Always' Received	300+	70%	-	64%
Would Definitely Recommend Hospital	300+	58%	-	69%

NOTE: Hospital profiles are in alphabetical order by state, then city, then hospital within the city; Rankings exclude hospitals with less than 25 cases except for patient surveys which excludes hospitals with less than 100 cases; (a) 100–299 cases; (1) The number of cases is too small to be sure how well a hospital is performing; (2) The hospital indicated that the data submitted for this measure were based on a sample of cases; (3) Data was collected during a shorter time period (fewer quarters) than the maximum possible time for this measure; (4) Suppressed for one or more quarters by CMS; (5) No data is available from the hospital for this measure; (6) Fewer than 100 patients completed the HCAHPS survey. Use these rates with caution, as the number of surveys may be too low to reliably assess hospital performance; (7) Survey results are based on less than 12 months of data; (8) Survey results are not available for this reporting period; (9) No or very few patients were eligible for the HCAHPS survey. The scores shown, if any, reflect a very small number of surveys; (10) A state average was not calculated because too few hospitals in the state submitted data; (11) There were discrepancies in the data collection process; Please refer to the User's Guide for a full explanation of data.

Indiana Regional Medical Center

835 Hospital Road Phone: 724-357-7000
Indiana, PA 15701 Fax: 724-357-7449
E-mail: info@indianarmc.org
URL: www.indianarmc.org
Type: Acute Care Hospitals Emergency Services: Yes
Ownership: Voluntary Non-Profit - Private Beds: 162

Key Personnel:

CEO/President. . . . . Stephen A Wolfe
Cardiac Laboratory. . . . . Lancy Brunetto
Chief of Medical Staff . . . . Bruce A Bush, MD
Infection Control. . . . . David McDevitt, RN
Operating Room. . . . . Loraine George, RN
Pediatric In-Patient Care . . . . . . Deborah Mikolic, RN
Quality Assurance . . . . Virginia Hostetter
Radiology. . . . . Frank Simone, MD

Measure	Cases	This Hosp.	State Avg.	U.S. Avg.
Heart Attack Care				
ACE Inhibitor or ARB for LVSD[1]	16	81%	95%	96%
Aspirin at Arrival	80	95%	99%	99%
Aspirin at Discharge	59	97%	99%	98%
Beta Blocker at Discharge	62	98%	99%	98%
Fibrinolytic Medication Timing[1]	1	100%	40%	55%
PCI Within 90 Minutes of Arrival	0	-	88%	90%
Smoking Cessation Advice[1]	4	100%	100%	99%
Chest Pain/Possible Heart Attack Care				
Aspirin at Arrival	212	97%	95%	95%
Median Time to ECG (minutes)	217	14	8	8
Median Time to Transfer (minutes)	49	82	68	61
Fibrinolytic Medication Timing	0	-	48%	54%
Heart Failure Care				
ACE Inhibitor or ARB for LVSD	151	85%	95%	94%
Discharge Instructions	260	85%	90%	88%
Evaluation of LVS Function	333	97%	99%	98%
Smoking Cessation Advice	35	94%	98%	98%
Pneumonia Care				
Appropriate Initial Antibiotic	126	92%	93%	92%
Blood Culture Timing	204	98%	96%	96%
Influenza Vaccine	134	85%	92%	91%
Initial Antibiotic Timing	190	96%	96%	95%
Pneumococcal Vaccine	185	91%	95%	93%
Smoking Cessation Advice	56	88%	98%	97%
Surgical Care Improvement Project				
Appropriate VTP Within 24 Hours	159	91%	95%	92%
Appropriate Hair Removal	394	100%	100%	99%
Appropriate Beta Blocker Usage	117	97%	94%	93%
Controlled Postoperative Blood Glucose	0	-	96%	93%
Prophylactic Antibiotic Timing	287	98%	97%	97%
Prophylactic Antibiotic Timing (Outpatient)	177	96%	92%	92%
Prophylactic Antibiotic Selection	287	99%	98%	97%
Prophylactic Antibiotic Select. (Outpatient)	213	97%	93%	94%
Prophylactic Antibiotic Stopped	271	94%	95%	94%
Recommended VTP Ordered	161	94%	97%	94%
Urinary Catheter Removal	109	92%	95%	90%
Children's Asthma Care				
Received Systemic Corticosteroids	-	-	-	100%
Received Home Management Plan	-	-	-	71%
Received Reliever Medication	-	-	-	100%
Use of Medical Imaging				
Combination Abdominal CT Scan	385	0.512	0.203	0.191
Combination Chest CT Scan	257	0.008	0.026	0.054
Follow-up Mammogram/Ultrasound	674	7.7%	8.2%	8.4%
MRI for Low Back Pain	67	32.8%	32.4%	32.7%
Survey of Patients' Hospital Experiences				
Area Around Room 'Always' Quiet at Night	300+	46%	-	58%
Doctors 'Always' Communicated Well	300+	82%	-	80%
Home Recovery Information Given	300+	87%	-	82%
Hospital Given 9 or 10 on 10 Point Scale	300+	69%	-	67%
Meds 'Always' Explained Before Given	300+	62%	-	60%
Nurses 'Always' Communicated Well	300+	81%	-	76%
Pain 'Always' Well Controlled	300+	69%	-	69%
Room and Bathroom 'Always' Clean	300+	75%	-	71%
Timely Help 'Always' Received	300+	70%	-	64%
Would Definitely Recommend Hospital	300+	70%	-	69%

Jersey Shore Hospital

Thompson Street Phone: 570-398-0100
Jersey Shore, PA 17740 Fax: 570-398-4412
URL: www.jsh.org
Type: Critical Access Hospitals Emergency Services: Yes
Ownership: Voluntary Non-Profit - Other Beds: 49

Key Personnel:

CEO/President. . . . . Lou Ditzel Jr
Chief of Medical Staff . . . . John Hunter
Operating Room. . . . . Barbara Kozlowski, RN
Radiology. . . . . Ed Sowul, RT/RDMS
Emergency Room . . . . Barbara Kozlowski, RN

Measure	Cases	This Hosp.	State Avg.	U.S. Avg.
Heart Attack Care				
ACE Inhibitor or ARB for LVSD	0	-	95%	96%
Aspirin at Arrival[1]	5	100%	99%	99%
Aspirin at Discharge[1]	4	100%	99%	98%
Beta Blocker at Discharge[1]	7	71%	99%	98%
Fibrinolytic Medication Timing	0	-	40%	55%
PCI Within 90 Minutes of Arrival	0	-	88%	90%
Smoking Cessation Advice	0	-	100%	99%
Chest Pain/Possible Heart Attack Care				
Aspirin at Arrival[5]	0	-	95%	95%
Median Time to ECG (minutes)[5]	0	-	8	8
Median Time to Transfer (minutes)[5]	0	-	68	61
Fibrinolytic Medication Timing[5]	0	-	48%	54%
Heart Failure Care				
ACE Inhibitor or ARB for LVSD[1]	12	100%	95%	94%
Discharge Instructions	72	100%	90%	88%
Evaluation of LVS Function	86	100%	99%	98%
Smoking Cessation Advice[1]	4	100%	98%	98%
Pneumonia Care				
Appropriate Initial Antibiotic	60	88%	93%	92%
Blood Culture Timing	56	96%	96%	96%
Influenza Vaccine	42	88%	92%	91%
Initial Antibiotic Timing	76	93%	96%	95%
Pneumococcal Vaccine	65	91%	95%	93%
Smoking Cessation Advice[1]	15	100%	98%	97%
Surgical Care Improvement Project				
Appropriate VTP Within 24 Hours	53	45%	95%	92%
Appropriate Hair Removal	84	100%	100%	99%
Appropriate Beta Blocker Usage[5]	0	-	94%	93%
Controlled Postoperative Blood Glucose	0	-	96%	93%
Prophylactic Antibiotic Timing	37	78%	97%	97%
Prophylactic Antibiotic Timing (Outpatient)[5]	0	-	92%	92%
Prophylactic Antibiotic Selection	35	71%	98%	97%
Prophylactic Antibiotic Select. (Outpatient)[5]	0	-	93%	94%
Prophylactic Antibiotic Stopped	35	71%	95%	94%
Recommended VTP Ordered	53	47%	97%	94%
Urinary Catheter Removal[1]	21	95%	95%	90%
Children's Asthma Care				
Received Systemic Corticosteroids	-	-	-	100%
Received Home Management Plan	-	-	-	71%
Received Reliever Medication	-	-	-	100%
Use of Medical Imaging				
Combination Abdominal CT Scan	374	0.080	0.203	0.191
Combination Chest CT Scan	180	0.011	0.026	0.054
Follow-up Mammogram/Ultrasound	399	6.0%	8.2%	8.4%
MRI for Low Back Pain[1]	44	31.8%	32.4%	32.7%
Survey of Patients' Hospital Experiences				
Area Around Room 'Always' Quiet at Night[8]	-	-	-	58%
Doctors 'Always' Communicated Well[8]	-	-	-	80%
Home Recovery Information Given[8]	-	-	-	82%
Hospital Given 9 or 10 on 10 Point Scale[8]	-	-	-	67%
Meds 'Always' Explained Before Given[8]	-	-	-	60%
Nurses 'Always' Communicated Well[8]	-	-	-	76%
Pain 'Always' Well Controlled[8]	-	-	-	69%
Room and Bathroom 'Always' Clean[8]	-	-	-	71%
Timely Help 'Always' Received[8]	-	-	-	64%
Would Definitely Recommend Hospital[8]	-	-	-	69%

Conemaugh Valley Memorial Hospital

1086 Franklin Street Phone: 814-534-9000
Johnstown, PA 15905 Fax: 814-534-3486
URL: www.conemaugh.org
Type: Acute Care Hospitals Emergency Services: Yes
Ownership: Voluntary Non-Profit - Other Beds: 474

Key Personnel:

CEO/President. . . . . Steven E Tucker
Cardiac Laboratory. . . . . Samir A Hadeed, MD
Chief of Medical Staff . . . . Adib N Khouzami, MD
Infection Control. . . . . Louis A Schenfeld
Operating Room. . . . . Thomas S Helling, MD
Pediatric Ambulatory Care . . . . . Matthew Masiello, MD
Quality Assurance . . . . Karen Leoffler
Radiology. . . . . Jonathan Abrahms

Measure	Cases	This Hosp.	State Avg.	U.S. Avg.
Heart Attack Care				
ACE Inhibitor or ARB for LVSD	136	81%	95%	96%
Aspirin at Arrival	452	98%	99%	99%
Aspirin at Discharge	590	99%	99%	98%
Beta Blocker at Discharge	588	96%	99%	98%
Fibrinolytic Medication Timing	0	-	40%	55%
PCI Within 90 Minutes of Arrival	64	89%	88%	90%
Smoking Cessation Advice	170	98%	100%	99%
Chest Pain/Possible Heart Attack Care				
Aspirin at Arrival[1]	5	80%	95%	95%
Median Time to ECG (minutes)[1]	5	13	8	8
Median Time to Transfer (minutes)[5]	0	-	68	61
Fibrinolytic Medication Timing[3]	0	-	48%	54%
Heart Failure Care				
ACE Inhibitor or ARB for LVSD	222	83%	95%	94%
Discharge Instructions	614	78%	90%	88%
Evaluation of LVS Function	803	96%	99%	98%
Smoking Cessation Advice	94	100%	98%	98%
Pneumonia Care				
Appropriate Initial Antibiotic	209	93%	93%	92%
Blood Culture Timing	343	98%	96%	96%
Influenza Vaccine	346	90%	92%	91%
Initial Antibiotic Timing	453	94%	96%	95%
Pneumococcal Vaccine	475	93%	95%	93%
Smoking Cessation Advice	170	96%	98%	97%
Surgical Care Improvement Project				
Appropriate VTP Within 24 Hours	584	95%	95%	92%
Appropriate Hair Removal	1,837	99%	100%	99%
Appropriate Beta Blocker Usage	712	94%	94%	93%
Controlled Postoperative Blood Glucose	201	95%	96%	93%
Prophylactic Antibiotic Timing	1,157	99%	97%	97%
Prophylactic Antibiotic Timing (Outpatient)	628	90%	92%	92%
Prophylactic Antibiotic Selection	1,164	99%	98%	97%
Prophylactic Antibiotic Select. (Outpatient)	586	93%	93%	94%
Prophylactic Antibiotic Stopped	1,124	97%	95%	94%
Recommended VTP Ordered	584	97%	97%	94%
Urinary Catheter Removal	292	93%	95%	90%
Children's Asthma Care				
Received Systemic Corticosteroids	-	-	-	100%
Received Home Management Plan	-	-	-	71%
Received Reliever Medication	-	-	-	100%
Use of Medical Imaging				
Combination Abdominal CT Scan	723	0.019	0.203	0.191
Combination Chest CT Scan	489	0.002	0.026	0.054
Follow-up Mammogram/Ultrasound	950	5.1%	8.2%	8.4%
MRI for Low Back Pain[1]	9	22.2%	32.4%	32.7%
Survey of Patients' Hospital Experiences				
Area Around Room 'Always' Quiet at Night	300+	47%	-	58%
Doctors 'Always' Communicated Well	300+	77%	-	80%
Home Recovery Information Given	300+	84%	-	82%
Hospital Given 9 or 10 on 10 Point Scale	300+	65%	-	67%
Meds 'Always' Explained Before Given	300+	60%	-	60%
Nurses 'Always' Communicated Well	300+	77%	-	76%
Pain 'Always' Well Controlled	300+	69%	-	69%
Room and Bathroom 'Always' Clean	300+	74%	-	71%
Timely Help 'Always' Received	300+	62%	-	64%
Would Definitely Recommend Hospital	300+	67%	-	69%

NOTE: Hospital profiles are in alphabetical order by state, then city, then hospital within the city; Rankings exclude hospitals with less than 25 cases except for patient surveys which excludes hospitals with less than 100 cases; (a) 100–299 cases; (1) The number of cases is too small to be sure how well a hospital is performing; (2) The hospital indicated that the data submitted for this measure were based on a sample of cases; (3) Data was collected during a shorter time period (fewer quarters) than the maximum possible time for this measure; (4) Suppressed for one or more quarters by CMS; (5) No data is available from the hospital for this measure; (6) Fewer than 100 patients completed the HCAHPS survey. Use these rates with caution, as the number of surveys may be too low to reliably assess hospital performance; (7) Survey results are based on less than 12 months of data; (8) Survey results are not available for this reporting period; (9) No or very few patients were eligible for the HCAHPS survey. The scores shown, if any, reflect a very small number of surveys; (10) A state average was not calculated because too few hospitals in the state submitted data; (11) There were discrepancies in the data collection process; Please refer to the User's Guide for a full explanation of data.

Kane Community Hospital

4372 Route 6
Kane, PA 16735
E-mail: info@kanehosp.com
URL: www.kanehosp.com
Type: Acute Care Hospitals
Ownership: Voluntary Non-Profit - Other

Phone: 814-837-8585
Fax: 814-837-7992

Emergency Services: Yes
Beds: 38

Key Personnel:
CEO/President . . . . J Gary Rhodes
Chief of Medical Staff . . . . Linda Rettger, MD
Infection Control . . . . Pam Bray
Operating Room . . . . K Joseph
Radiology . . . . Jamil Sarfraz, MD

Measure	Cases	This Hosp.	State Avg.	U.S. Avg.
Heart Attack Care				
ACE Inhibitor or ARB for LVSD[1,3]	2	100%	95%	96%
Aspirin at Arrival[1,3]	4	75%	99%	99%
Aspirin at Discharge[1,3]	4	100%	99%	98%
Beta Blocker at Discharge[1,3]	3	67%	99%	98%
Fibrinolytic Medication Timing[3]	0	-	40%	55%
PCI Within 90 Minutes of Arrival[3]	0	-	88%	90%
Smoking Cessation Advice[3]	0	-	100%	99%
Chest Pain/Possible Heart Attack Care				
Aspirin at Arrival[1,3]	11	100%	95%	95%
Median Time to ECG (minutes)[1,3]	12	6	8	8
Median Time to Transfer (minutes)[1,3]	3	227	68	61
Fibrinolytic Medication Timing[1,3]	1	0%	48%	54%
Heart Failure Care				
ACE Inhibitor or ARB for LVSD[1]	17	100%	95%	94%
Discharge Instructions	74	18%	90%	88%
Evaluation of LVS Function	95	82%	99%	98%
Smoking Cessation Advice[1]	7	43%	98%	98%
Pneumonia Care				
Appropriate Initial Antibiotic	44	84%	93%	92%
Blood Culture Timing	54	89%	96%	96%
Influenza Vaccine	52	27%	92%	91%
Initial Antibiotic Timing	74	92%	96%	95%
Pneumococcal Vaccine	85	22%	95%	93%
Smoking Cessation Advice[1]	21	67%	98%	97%
Surgical Care Improvement Project				
Appropriate VTP Within 24 Hours[1]	16	69%	95%	92%
Appropriate Hair Removal	26	69%	100%	99%
Appropriate Beta Blocker Usage[1]	6	0%	94%	93%
Controlled Postoperative Blood Glucose	0	-	96%	93%
Prophylactic Antibiotic Timing[1]	9	67%	97%	97%
Prophylactic Antibiotic Timing (Outpatient)[1,3]	4	50%	92%	92%
Prophylactic Antibiotic Selection[1]	9	100%	98%	97%
Prophylactic Antibiotic Select. (Outpatient)[1,3]	2	100%	93%	94%
Prophylactic Antibiotic Stopped[1]	9	78%	95%	94%
Recommended VTP Ordered[1]	16	75%	97%	94%
Urinary Catheter Removal[1]	4	50%	95%	90%
Children's Asthma Care				
Received Systemic Corticosteroids	-	-	-	100%
Received Home Management Plan	-	-	-	71%
Received Reliever Medication	-	-	-	100%
Use of Medical Imaging				
Combination Abdominal CT Scan	247	0.575	0.203	0.191
Combination Chest CT Scan	124	0.750	0.026	0.054
Follow-up Mammogram/Ultrasound	236	43.6%	8.2%	8.4%
MRI for Low Back Pain[1]	36	19.4%	32.4%	32.7%
Survey of Patients' Hospital Experiences				
Area Around Room 'Always' Quiet at Night	(a)	53%	-	58%
Doctors 'Always' Communicated Well	(a)	83%	-	80%
Home Recovery Information Given	(a)	84%	-	82%
Hospital Given 9 or 10 on 10 Point Scale	(a)	65%	-	67%
Meds 'Always' Explained Before Given	(a)	64%	-	60%
Nurses 'Always' Communicated Well	(a)	78%	-	76%
Pain 'Always' Well Controlled	(a)	67%	-	69%
Room and Bathroom 'Always' Clean	(a)	77%	-	71%
Timely Help 'Always' Received	(a)	65%	-	64%
Would Definitely Recommend Hospital	(a)	65%	-	69%

ACMH Hospital

One Nolte Drive
Kittanning, PA 16201
E-mail: comrel@acmh.org
URL: www.acmh.org
Type: Acute Care Hospitals
Ownership: Voluntary Non-Profit - Private

Phone: 724-543-8404
Fax: 724-543-8704

Emergency Services: Yes
Beds: 177

Key Personnel:
CEO/President . . . . John Lewis
Chief of Medical Staff . . . . Harold Altman, MD
Radiology . . . . Donley Charles

Measure	Cases	This Hosp.	State Avg.	U.S. Avg.
Heart Attack Care				
ACE Inhibitor or ARB for LVSD[1]	7	100%	95%	96%
Aspirin at Arrival	55	91%	99%	99%
Aspirin at Discharge	32	81%	99%	98%
Beta Blocker at Discharge	37	86%	99%	98%
Fibrinolytic Medication Timing	0	-	40%	55%
PCI Within 90 Minutes of Arrival	0	-	88%	90%
Smoking Cessation Advice[1]	2	100%	100%	99%
Chest Pain/Possible Heart Attack Care				
Aspirin at Arrival	135	94%	95%	95%
Median Time to ECG (minutes)	140	6	8	8
Median Time to Transfer (minutes)	27	54	68	61
Fibrinolytic Medication Timing	0	-	48%	54%
Heart Failure Care				
ACE Inhibitor or ARB for LVSD	35	91%	95%	94%
Discharge Instructions	111	87%	90%	88%
Evaluation of LVS Function	151	100%	99%	98%
Smoking Cessation Advice[1]	17	100%	98%	98%
Pneumonia Care				
Appropriate Initial Antibiotic	91	97%	93%	92%
Blood Culture Timing	109	96%	96%	96%
Influenza Vaccine	104	91%	92%	91%
Initial Antibiotic Timing	129	98%	96%	95%
Pneumococcal Vaccine	133	95%	95%	93%
Smoking Cessation Advice[1]	46	100%	98%	97%
Surgical Care Improvement Project				
Appropriate VTP Within 24 Hours	159	97%	95%	92%
Appropriate Hair Removal	480	100%	100%	99%
Appropriate Beta Blocker Usage	108	95%	94%	93%
Controlled Postoperative Blood Glucose	0	-	96%	93%
Prophylactic Antibiotic Timing	378	97%	97%	97%
Prophylactic Antibiotic Timing (Outpatient)	82	98%	92%	92%
Prophylactic Antibiotic Selection	378	98%	98%	97%
Prophylactic Antibiotic Select. (Outpatient)	81	94%	93%	94%
Prophylactic Antibiotic Stopped	369	97%	95%	94%
Recommended VTP Ordered	159	97%	97%	94%
Urinary Catheter Removal	78	90%	95%	90%
Children's Asthma Care				
Received Systemic Corticosteroids	-	-	-	100%
Received Home Management Plan	-	-	-	71%
Received Reliever Medication	-	-	-	100%
Use of Medical Imaging				
Combination Abdominal CT Scan	184	0.147	0.203	0.191
Combination Chest CT Scan	147	0.020	0.026	0.054
Follow-up Mammogram/Ultrasound	356	15.2%	8.2%	8.4%
MRI for Low Back Pain[1]	35	40.0%	32.4%	32.7%
Survey of Patients' Hospital Experiences				
Area Around Room 'Always' Quiet at Night	300+	41%	-	58%
Doctors 'Always' Communicated Well	300+	83%	-	80%
Home Recovery Information Given	300+	83%	-	82%
Hospital Given 9 or 10 on 10 Point Scale	300+	63%	-	67%
Meds 'Always' Explained Before Given	300+	61%	-	60%
Nurses 'Always' Communicated Well	300+	78%	-	76%
Pain 'Always' Well Controlled	300+	68%	-	69%
Room and Bathroom 'Always' Clean	300+	64%	-	71%
Timely Help 'Always' Received	300+	68%	-	64%
Would Definitely Recommend Hospital	300+	64%	-	69%

Lancaster General Hospital

555 North Duke Street
Lancaster, PA 17604
E-mail: info@lancastergeneral.org
URL: www.lancastergeneral.org
Type: Acute Care Hospitals
Ownership: Voluntary Non-Profit - Other

Phone: 717-299-5511

Emergency Services: Yes
Beds: 640

Key Personnel:
CEO/President . . . . Thomas E Beeman
Ambulatory Care . . . . Andrś W Renna

Measure	Cases	This Hosp.	State Avg.	U.S. Avg.
Heart Attack Care				
ACE Inhibitor or ARB for LVSD	117	91%	95%	96%
Aspirin at Arrival	717	98%	99%	99%
Aspirin at Discharge	749	100%	99%	98%
Beta Blocker at Discharge	733	98%	99%	98%
Fibrinolytic Medication Timing	0	-	40%	55%
PCI Within 90 Minutes of Arrival	122	79%	88%	90%
Smoking Cessation Advice	211	100%	100%	99%
Chest Pain/Possible Heart Attack Care				
Aspirin at Arrival[1,3]	1	100%	95%	95%
Median Time to ECG (minutes)[1,3]	1	0	8	8
Median Time to Transfer (minutes)[5]	0	-	68	61
Fibrinolytic Medication Timing[5]	0	-	48%	54%
Heart Failure Care				
ACE Inhibitor or ARB for LVSD	284	93%	95%	94%
Discharge Instructions	794	74%	90%	88%
Evaluation of LVS Function	1,005	99%	99%	98%
Smoking Cessation Advice	126	100%	98%	98%
Pneumonia Care				
Appropriate Initial Antibiotic	243	95%	93%	92%
Blood Culture Timing	356	97%	96%	96%
Influenza Vaccine	342	96%	92%	91%
Initial Antibiotic Timing	384	95%	96%	95%
Pneumococcal Vaccine	434	95%	95%	93%
Smoking Cessation Advice	145	100%	98%	97%
Surgical Care Improvement Project				
Appropriate VTP Within 24 Hours[2]	679	94%	95%	92%
Appropriate Hair Removal[2]	2,163	96%	100%	99%
Appropriate Beta Blocker Usage[2]	764	89%	94%	93%
Controlled Postoperative Blood Glucose[2]	278	96%	96%	93%
Prophylactic Antibiotic Timing[2]	1,457	95%	97%	97%
Prophylactic Antibiotic Timing (Outpatient)[2]	1,616	91%	92%	92%
Prophylactic Antibiotic Selection[2]	1,477	98%	98%	97%
Prophylactic Antibiotic Select. (Outpatient)[2]	1,535	97%	93%	94%
Prophylactic Antibiotic Stopped[2]	1,401	96%	95%	94%
Recommended VTP Ordered[2]	681	95%	97%	94%
Urinary Catheter Removal[2]	591	95%	95%	90%
Children's Asthma Care				
Received Systemic Corticosteroids	-	-	-	100%
Received Home Management Plan	-	-	-	71%
Received Reliever Medication	-	-	-	100%
Use of Medical Imaging				
Combination Abdominal CT Scan	2,670	0.412	0.203	0.191
Combination Chest CT Scan	2,583	0.032	0.026	0.054
Follow-up Mammogram/Ultrasound	5,423	7.9%	8.2%	8.4%
MRI for Low Back Pain[1]	2	0.0%	32.4%	32.7%
Survey of Patients' Hospital Experiences				
Area Around Room 'Always' Quiet at Night	300+	48%	-	58%
Doctors 'Always' Communicated Well	300+	74%	-	80%
Home Recovery Information Given	300+	86%	-	82%
Hospital Given 9 or 10 on 10 Point Scale	300+	71%	-	67%
Meds 'Always' Explained Before Given	300+	56%	-	60%
Nurses 'Always' Communicated Well	300+	74%	-	76%
Pain 'Always' Well Controlled	300+	66%	-	69%
Room and Bathroom 'Always' Clean	300+	70%	-	71%
Timely Help 'Always' Received	300+	56%	-	64%
Would Definitely Recommend Hospital	300+	80%	-	69%

Lancaster Regional Medical Center

250 College Avenue — Phone: 717-291-8123
Lancaster, PA 17604
Type: Acute Care Hospitals — Emergency Services: Yes
Ownership: Proprietary

Key Personnel:
CEO/President. . . . . Steve Midkiff
Emergency Room . . . . Cindy Sapp

Measure	Cases	This Hosp.	State Avg.	U.S. Avg.
Heart Attack Care				
ACE Inhibitor or ARB for LVSD[1]	10	100%	95%	96%
Aspirin at Arrival	40	98%	99%	99%
Aspirin at Discharge	52	100%	99%	98%
Beta Blocker at Discharge	48	100%	99%	98%
Fibrinolytic Medication Timing	0	-	40%	55%
PCI Within 90 Minutes of Arrival[1]	7	86%	88%	90%
Smoking Cessation Advice[1]	17	100%	100%	99%
Chest Pain/Possible Heart Attack Care				
Aspirin at Arrival[1,3]	1	100%	95%	95%
Median Time to ECG (minutes)[1,3]	1	0	8	8
Median Time to Transfer (minutes)[5]	0	-	68	61
Fibrinolytic Medication Timing[5]	0	-	48%	54%
Heart Failure Care				
ACE Inhibitor or ARB for LVSD	47	98%	95%	94%
Discharge Instructions	87	95%	90%	88%
Evaluation of LVS Function	112	100%	99%	98%
Smoking Cessation Advice	31	100%	98%	98%
Pneumonia Care				
Appropriate Initial Antibiotic	70	94%	93%	92%
Blood Culture Timing	86	95%	96%	96%
Influenza Vaccine	35	100%	92%	91%
Initial Antibiotic Timing	92	96%	96%	95%
Pneumococcal Vaccine	67	99%	95%	93%
Smoking Cessation Advice	40	100%	98%	97%
Surgical Care Improvement Project				
Appropriate VTP Within 24 Hours[2]	177	99%	95%	92%
Appropriate Hair Removal[2]	498	100%	100%	99%
Appropriate Beta Blocker Usage[2]	146	100%	94%	93%
Controlled Postoperative Blood Glucose[2]	54	93%	96%	93%
Prophylactic Antibiotic Timing[2]	269	99%	97%	97%
Prophylactic Antibiotic Timing (Outpatient)	305	100%	92%	92%
Prophylactic Antibiotic Selection[2]	275	97%	98%	97%
Prophylactic Antibiotic Select. (Outpatient)	305	99%	93%	94%
Prophylactic Antibiotic Stopped[2]	255	95%	95%	94%
Recommended VTP Ordered[2]	177	99%	97%	94%
Urinary Catheter Removal[2]	146	97%	95%	90%
Children's Asthma Care				
Received Systemic Corticosteroids	-	-	-	100%
Received Home Management Plan	-	-	-	71%
Received Reliever Medication	-	-	-	100%
Use of Medical Imaging				
Combination Abdominal CT Scan	266	0.090	0.203	0.191
Combination Chest CT Scan	255	0.020	0.026	0.054
Follow-up Mammogram/Ultrasound[5]	0	-	8.2%	8.4%
MRI for Low Back Pain[1]	23	47.8%	32.4%	32.7%
Survey of Patients' Hospital Experiences				
Area Around Room 'Always' Quiet at Night	300+	57%	-	58%
Doctors 'Always' Communicated Well	300+	80%	-	80%
Home Recovery Information Given	300+	85%	-	82%
Hospital Given 9 or 10 on 10 Point Scale	300+	70%	-	67%
Meds 'Always' Explained Before Given	300+	60%	-	60%
Nurses 'Always' Communicated Well	300+	75%	-	76%
Pain 'Always' Well Controlled	300+	69%	-	69%
Room and Bathroom 'Always' Clean	300+	80%	-	71%
Timely Help 'Always' Received	300+	70%	-	64%
Would Definitely Recommend Hospital	300+	71%	-	69%

Saint Mary Medical Center

Langhorne-Newtown Rd — Phone: 215-750-2003
Langhorne, PA 19047 — Fax: 215-710-5190
URL: www.stmaryhealthcare.org
Type: Acute Care Hospitals — Emergency Services: Yes
Ownership: Voluntary Non-Profit - Church — Beds: 327

Key Personnel:
CEO/President. . . . . Gregory T Wozniak
Chief of Medical Staff. . . . . John Newson, MD
Operating Room. . . . . Teri Grisi, RN
Pediatric Ambulatory Care . . . . . . Prem Marlapudi
Pediatric In-Patient Care . . . . Prem Marlapudi
Quality Assurance . . . . Deb Taonne, RN
Radiology. . . . . Suzanne Monte, MD
Emergency Room . . . . Sid Vail, MD

Measure	Cases	This Hosp.	State Avg.	U.S. Avg.
Heart Attack Care				
ACE Inhibitor or ARB for LVSD	51	100%	95%	96%
Aspirin at Arrival	416	100%	99%	99%
Aspirin at Discharge	407	100%	99%	98%
Beta Blocker at Discharge	383	100%	99%	98%
Fibrinolytic Medication Timing	0	-	40%	55%
PCI Within 90 Minutes of Arrival	55	95%	88%	90%
Smoking Cessation Advice	105	100%	100%	99%
Chest Pain/Possible Heart Attack Care				
Aspirin at Arrival[1,3]	4	100%	95%	95%
Median Time to ECG (minutes)[1,3]	4	12	8	8
Median Time to Transfer (minutes)[5]	0	-	68	61
Fibrinolytic Medication Timing[5]	0	-	48%	54%
Heart Failure Care				
ACE Inhibitor or ARB for LVSD	149	100%	95%	94%
Discharge Instructions	458	100%	90%	88%
Evaluation of LVS Function	598	100%	99%	98%
Smoking Cessation Advice	51	100%	98%	98%
Pneumonia Care				
Appropriate Initial Antibiotic	256	95%	93%	92%
Blood Culture Timing	435	99%	96%	96%
Influenza Vaccine	246	100%	92%	91%
Initial Antibiotic Timing	437	100%	96%	95%
Pneumococcal Vaccine	328	100%	95%	93%
Smoking Cessation Advice	116	100%	98%	97%
Surgical Care Improvement Project				
Appropriate VTP Within 24 Hours[2]	158	91%	95%	92%
Appropriate Hair Removal[2]	701	100%	100%	99%
Appropriate Beta Blocker Usage[2]	261	97%	94%	93%
Controlled Postoperative Blood Glucose[2]	155	97%	96%	93%
Prophylactic Antibiotic Timing[2]	517	99%	97%	97%
Prophylactic Antibiotic Timing (Outpatient)	273	97%	92%	92%
Prophylactic Antibiotic Selection[2]	523	99%	98%	97%
Prophylactic Antibiotic Select. (Outpatient)	264	93%	93%	94%
Prophylactic Antibiotic Stopped[2]	483	96%	95%	94%
Recommended VTP Ordered[2]	158	94%	97%	94%
Urinary Catheter Removal[2]	182	98%	95%	90%
Children's Asthma Care				
Received Systemic Corticosteroids	-	-	-	100%
Received Home Management Plan	-	-	-	71%
Received Reliever Medication	-	-	-	100%
Use of Medical Imaging				
Combination Abdominal CT Scan	1,193	0.059	0.203	0.191
Combination Chest CT Scan	836	0.020	0.026	0.054
Follow-up Mammogram/Ultrasound	1,535	7.4%	8.2%	8.4%
MRI for Low Back Pain	148	25.7%	32.4%	32.7%
Survey of Patients' Hospital Experiences				
Area Around Room 'Always' Quiet at Night	300+	43%	-	58%
Doctors 'Always' Communicated Well	300+	74%	-	80%
Home Recovery Information Given	300+	79%	-	82%
Hospital Given 9 or 10 on 10 Point Scale	300+	76%	-	67%
Meds 'Always' Explained Before Given	300+	59%	-	60%
Nurses 'Always' Communicated Well	300+	77%	-	76%
Pain 'Always' Well Controlled	300+	71%	-	69%
Room and Bathroom 'Always' Clean	300+	71%	-	71%
Timely Help 'Always' Received	300+	68%	-	64%
Would Definitely Recommend Hospital	300+	80%	-	69%

Lansdale Hospital

100 Medical Campus Drive — Phone: 215-368-2100
Lansdale, PA 19446 — Fax: 215-361-4933
URL: www.cmmc-uhs.com
Type: Acute Care Hospitals — Emergency Services: Yes
Ownership: Voluntary Non-Profit - Other — Beds: 125

Key Personnel:
CEO/President. . . . . Gary Candia
Chief of Medical Staff. . . . . Colleen Christian, MD
Infection Control. . . . . Mary Doherty, RN
Quality Assurance . . . . Suzanne Lion
Radiology. . . . . Ronald Adelman
Anesthesiology. . . . . Jay Mergaman, MD

Measure	Cases	This Hosp.	State Avg.	U.S. Avg.
Heart Attack Care				
ACE Inhibitor or ARB for LVSD[1]	12	100%	95%	96%
Aspirin at Arrival	60	100%	99%	99%
Aspirin at Discharge	33	100%	99%	98%
Beta Blocker at Discharge	33	100%	99%	98%
Fibrinolytic Medication Timing[1]	1	0%	40%	55%
PCI Within 90 Minutes of Arrival	0	-	88%	90%
Smoking Cessation Advice[1]	2	100%	100%	99%
Chest Pain/Possible Heart Attack Care				
Aspirin at Arrival	48	94%	95%	95%
Median Time to ECG (minutes)	50	11	8	8
Median Time to Transfer (minutes)[1]	4	58	68	61
Fibrinolytic Medication Timing	0	-	48%	54%
Heart Failure Care				
ACE Inhibitor or ARB for LVSD	61	95%	95%	94%
Discharge Instructions	146	77%	90%	88%
Evaluation of LVS Function	222	99%	99%	98%
Smoking Cessation Advice[1]	22	100%	98%	98%
Pneumonia Care				
Appropriate Initial Antibiotic	78	96%	93%	92%
Blood Culture Timing	132	90%	96%	96%
Influenza Vaccine	80	92%	92%	91%
Initial Antibiotic Timing	123	98%	96%	95%
Pneumococcal Vaccine	132	86%	95%	93%
Smoking Cessation Advice[1]	17	100%	98%	97%
Surgical Care Improvement Project				
Appropriate VTP Within 24 Hours[2]	141	94%	95%	92%
Appropriate Hair Removal[2]	213	100%	100%	99%
Appropriate Beta Blocker Usage[2]	60	98%	94%	93%
Controlled Postoperative Blood Glucose[2]	0	-	96%	93%
Prophylactic Antibiotic Timing[2]	112	96%	97%	97%
Prophylactic Antibiotic Timing (Outpatient)	50	98%	92%	92%
Prophylactic Antibiotic Selection[2]	113	98%	98%	97%
Prophylactic Antibiotic Select. (Outpatient)	50	100%	93%	94%
Prophylactic Antibiotic Stopped[2]	111	94%	95%	94%
Recommended VTP Ordered[2]	141	94%	97%	94%
Urinary Catheter Removal[2]	43	98%	95%	90%
Children's Asthma Care				
Received Systemic Corticosteroids	-	-	-	100%
Received Home Management Plan	-	-	-	71%
Received Reliever Medication	-	-	-	100%
Use of Medical Imaging				
Combination Abdominal CT Scan	407	0.084	0.203	0.191
Combination Chest CT Scan	244	0.016	0.026	0.054
Follow-up Mammogram/Ultrasound	673	4.6%	8.2%	8.4%
MRI for Low Back Pain[1]	49	18.4%	32.4%	32.7%
Survey of Patients' Hospital Experiences				
Area Around Room 'Always' Quiet at Night	300+	53%	-	58%
Doctors 'Always' Communicated Well	300+	75%	-	80%
Home Recovery Information Given	300+	74%	-	82%
Hospital Given 9 or 10 on 10 Point Scale	300+	55%	-	67%
Meds 'Always' Explained Before Given	300+	59%	-	60%
Nurses 'Always' Communicated Well	300+	73%	-	76%
Pain 'Always' Well Controlled	300+	66%	-	69%
Room and Bathroom 'Always' Clean	300+	64%	-	71%
Timely Help 'Always' Received	300+	58%	-	64%
Would Definitely Recommend Hospital	300+	57%	-	69%

NOTE: Hospital profiles are in alphabetical order by state, then city, then hospital within the city; Rankings exclude hospitals with less than 25 cases except for patient surveys which excludes hospitals with less than 100 cases; (a) 100–299 cases; (1) The number of cases is too small to be sure how well a hospital is performing; (2) The hospital indicated that the data submitted for this measure were based on a sample of cases; (3) Data was collected during a shorter time period (fewer quarters) than the maximum possible time for this measure; (4) Suppressed for one or more quarters by CMS; (5) No data is available from the hospital for this measure; (6) Fewer than 100 patients completed the HCAHPS survey. Use these rates with caution, as the number of surveys may be too low to reliably assess hospital performance; (7) Survey results are based on less than 12 months of data; (8) Survey results are not available for this reporting period; (9) No or very few patients were eligible for the HCAHPS survey. The scores shown, if any, reflect a very small number of surveys; (10) A state average was not calculated because too few hospitals in the state submitted data; (11) There were discrepancies in the data collection process; Please refer to the User's Guide for a full explanation of data.

Excela Health Latrobe Hospital

One Mellon Way
Latrobe, PA 15650
Phone: 724-537-1000
Type: Acute Care Hospitals
Emergency Services: Yes
Ownership: Voluntary Non-Profit - Private

Measure	Cases	This Hosp.	State Avg.	U.S. Avg.
Heart Attack Care				
ACE Inhibitor or ARB for LVSD[1]	17	100%	95%	96%
Aspirin at Arrival	61	97%	99%	99%
Aspirin at Discharge	35	91%	99%	98%
Beta Blocker at Discharge	36	97%	99%	98%
Fibrinolytic Medication Timing	0	-	40%	55%
PCI Within 90 Minutes of Arrival	0	-	88%	90%
Smoking Cessation Advice[1]	5	100%	100%	99%
Chest Pain/Possible Heart Attack Care				
Aspirin at Arrival	173	97%	95%	95%
Median Time to ECG (minutes)	176	11	8	8
Median Time to Transfer (minutes)	35	70	68	61
Fibrinolytic Medication Timing	0	-	48%	54%
Heart Failure Care				
ACE Inhibitor or ARB for LVSD	76	91%	95%	94%
Discharge Instructions	223	91%	90%	88%
Evaluation of LVS Function	293	100%	99%	98%
Smoking Cessation Advice	26	100%	98%	98%
Pneumonia Care				
Appropriate Initial Antibiotic	124	96%	93%	92%
Blood Culture Timing	200	98%	96%	96%
Influenza Vaccine	159	91%	92%	91%
Initial Antibiotic Timing	186	95%	96%	95%
Pneumococcal Vaccine	238	97%	95%	93%
Smoking Cessation Advice	70	99%	98%	97%
Surgical Care Improvement Project				
Appropriate VTP Within 24 Hours	276	92%	95%	92%
Appropriate Hair Removal	610	100%	100%	99%
Appropriate Beta Blocker Usage	150	95%	94%	93%
Controlled Postoperative Blood Glucose	0	-	96%	93%
Prophylactic Antibiotic Timing	400	98%	97%	97%
Prophylactic Antibiotic Timing (Outpatient)	191	92%	92%	92%
Prophylactic Antibiotic Selection	402	98%	98%	97%
Prophylactic Antibiotic Select. (Outpatient)	188	90%	93%	94%
Prophylactic Antibiotic Stopped	377	98%	95%	94%
Recommended VTP Ordered	276	96%	97%	94%
Urinary Catheter Removal	68	88%	95%	90%
Children's Asthma Care				
Received Systemic Corticosteroids	-		-	100%
Received Home Management Plan	-		-	71%
Received Reliever Medication	-		-	100%
Use of Medical Imaging				
Combination Abdominal CT Scan	555	0.041	0.203	0.191
Combination Chest CT Scan	448	0.011	0.026	0.054
Follow-up Mammogram/Ultrasound	571	10.7%	8.2%	8.4%
MRI for Low Back Pain	85	32.9%	32.4%	32.7%
Survey of Patients' Hospital Experiences				
Area Around Room 'Always' Quiet at Night	300+	45%	-	58%
Doctors 'Always' Communicated Well	300+	80%	-	80%
Home Recovery Information Given	300+	80%	-	82%
Hospital Given 9 or 10 on 10 Point Scale	300+	62%	-	67%
Meds 'Always' Explained Before Given	300+	60%	-	60%
Nurses 'Always' Communicated Well	300+	79%	-	76%
Pain 'Always' Well Controlled	300+	68%	-	69%
Room and Bathroom 'Always' Clean	300+	61%	-	71%
Timely Help 'Always' Received	300+	69%	-	64%
Would Definitely Recommend Hospital	300+	65%	-	69%

Good Samaritan Hospital

Fourth and Walnut Streets
Lebanon, PA 17042
Phone: 717-270-7500
URL: www.gshleb.org
Type: Acute Care Hospitals
Emergency Services: Yes
Ownership: Voluntary Non-Profit - Other

Measure	Cases	This Hosp.	State Avg.	U.S. Avg.
Heart Attack Care				
ACE Inhibitor or ARB for LVSD	36	100%	95%	96%
Aspirin at Arrival	200	100%	99%	99%
Aspirin at Discharge	192	100%	99%	98%
Beta Blocker at Discharge	193	100%	99%	98%
Fibrinolytic Medication Timing	0	-	40%	55%
PCI Within 90 Minutes of Arrival	48	88%	88%	90%
Smoking Cessation Advice	68	100%	100%	99%
Chest Pain/Possible Heart Attack Care				
Aspirin at Arrival[1]	1	100%	95%	95%
Median Time to ECG (minutes)[1]	1	10	8	8
Median Time to Transfer (minutes)[5]	0	-	68	61
Fibrinolytic Medication Timing[5]	0	-	48%	54%
Heart Failure Care				
ACE Inhibitor or ARB for LVSD	67	99%	95%	94%
Discharge Instructions	160	92%	90%	88%
Evaluation of LVS Function	237	99%	99%	98%
Smoking Cessation Advice[1]	18	100%	98%	98%
Pneumonia Care				
Appropriate Initial Antibiotic	160	91%	93%	92%
Blood Culture Timing	202	93%	96%	96%
Influenza Vaccine	136	82%	92%	91%
Initial Antibiotic Timing	208	93%	96%	95%
Pneumococcal Vaccine	186	87%	95%	93%
Smoking Cessation Advice	61	97%	98%	97%
Surgical Care Improvement Project				
Appropriate VTP Within 24 Hours[2]	170	94%	95%	92%
Appropriate Hair Removal[2]	509	100%	100%	99%
Appropriate Beta Blocker Usage[2]	230	92%	94%	93%
Controlled Postoperative Blood Glucose[2]	131	95%	96%	93%
Prophylactic Antibiotic Timing[2]	383	91%	97%	97%
Prophylactic Antibiotic Timing (Outpatient)	338	90%	92%	92%
Prophylactic Antibiotic Selection[2]	389	97%	98%	97%
Prophylactic Antibiotic Select. (Outpatient)	320	95%	93%	94%
Prophylactic Antibiotic Stopped[2]	364	88%	95%	94%
Recommended VTP Ordered[2]	171	94%	97%	94%
Urinary Catheter Removal[2]	124	92%	95%	90%
Children's Asthma Care				
Received Systemic Corticosteroids	-		-	100%
Received Home Management Plan	-		-	71%
Received Reliever Medication	-		-	100%
Use of Medical Imaging				
Combination Abdominal CT Scan	1,288	0.482	0.203	0.191
Combination Chest CT Scan	919	0.020	0.026	0.054
Follow-up Mammogram/Ultrasound	2,993	4.0%	8.2%	8.4%
MRI for Low Back Pain[5]	0	-	32.4%	32.7%
Survey of Patients' Hospital Experiences				
Area Around Room 'Always' Quiet at Night	300+	46%	-	58%
Doctors 'Always' Communicated Well	300+	77%	-	80%
Home Recovery Information Given	300+	83%	-	82%
Hospital Given 9 or 10 on 10 Point Scale	300+	65%	-	67%
Meds 'Always' Explained Before Given	300+	61%	-	60%
Nurses 'Always' Communicated Well	300+	77%	-	76%
Pain 'Always' Well Controlled	300+	70%	-	69%
Room and Bathroom 'Always' Clean	300+	77%	-	71%
Timely Help 'Always' Received	300+	63%	-	64%
Would Definitely Recommend Hospital	300+	66%	-	69%

Lebanon VA Medical Center

1700 South Lincoln Avenue
Lebanon, PA 17042
Phone: 717-228-5901
URL: www.lebanon.va.gov
Type: Acute Care-Veterans Administration
Emergency Services: No
Ownership: Government - Federal
Beds: 248

Measure	Cases	This Hosp.	State Avg.	U.S. Avg.
Heart Attack Care				
ACE Inhibitor or ARB for LVSD[5]	0	-	95%	96%
Aspirin at Arrival[5]	0	-	99%	99%
Aspirin at Discharge[5]	0	-	99%	98%
Beta Blocker at Discharge[5]	0	-	99%	98%
Fibrinolytic Medication Timing[5]	0	-	40%	55%
PCI Within 90 Minutes of Arrival[5]	0	-	88%	90%
Smoking Cessation Advice[5]	0	-	100%	99%
Chest Pain/Possible Heart Attack Care				
Aspirin at Arrival	-		95%	95%
Median Time to ECG (minutes)	-		8	8
Median Time to Transfer (minutes)	-		68	61
Fibrinolytic Medication Timing	-		48%	54%
Heart Failure Care				
ACE Inhibitor or ARB for LVSD	32	100%	95%	94%
Discharge Instructions	57	98%	90%	88%
Evaluation of LVS Function	76	100%	99%	98%
Smoking Cessation Advice[1]	16	100%	98%	98%
Pneumonia Care				
Appropriate Initial Antibiotic[1]	23	87%	93%	92%
Blood Culture Timing	29	93%	96%	96%
Influenza Vaccine	25	100%	92%	91%
Initial Antibiotic Timing	31	87%	96%	95%
Pneumococcal Vaccine[1]	19	100%	95%	93%
Smoking Cessation Advice[1]	20	100%	98%	97%
Surgical Care Improvement Project				
Appropriate VTP Within 24 Hours[2]	58	90%	95%	92%
Appropriate Hair Removal[2]	234	100%	100%	99%
Appropriate Beta Blocker Usage[2]	95	97%	94%	93%
Controlled Postoperative Blood Glucose[5,2]	0	-	96%	93%
Prophylactic Antibiotic Timing	187	99%	97%	97%
Prophylactic Antibiotic Timing (Outpatient)	-		92%	92%
Prophylactic Antibiotic Selection	190	99%	98%	97%
Prophylactic Antibiotic Select. (Outpatient)	-		93%	94%
Prophylactic Antibiotic Stopped	186	98%	95%	94%
Recommended VTP Ordered[2]	58	91%	97%	94%
Urinary Catheter Removal[2]	87	97%	95%	90%
Children's Asthma Care				
Received Systemic Corticosteroids	-		-	100%
Received Home Management Plan	-		-	71%
Received Reliever Medication	-		-	100%
Use of Medical Imaging				
Combination Abdominal CT Scan	-		0.203	0.191
Combination Chest CT Scan	-		0.026	0.054
Follow-up Mammogram/Ultrasound	-		8.2%	8.4%
MRI for Low Back Pain	-		32.4%	32.7%
Survey of Patients' Hospital Experiences				
Area Around Room 'Always' Quiet at Night	-		-	58%
Doctors 'Always' Communicated Well	-		-	80%
Home Recovery Information Given	-		-	82%
Hospital Given 9 or 10 on 10 Point Scale	-		-	67%
Meds 'Always' Explained Before Given	-		-	60%
Nurses 'Always' Communicated Well	-		-	76%
Pain 'Always' Well Controlled	-		-	69%
Room and Bathroom 'Always' Clean	-		-	71%
Timely Help 'Always' Received	-		-	64%
Would Definitely Recommend Hospital	-		-	69%

NOTE: Hospital profiles are in alphabetical order by state, then city, then hospital within the city; Rankings exclude hospitals with less than 25 cases except for patient surveys which excludes hospitals with less than 100 cases; (a) 100–299 cases; (1) The number of cases is too small to be sure how well a hospital is performing; (2) The hospital indicated that the data submitted for this measure were based on a sample of cases; (3) Data was collected during a shorter time period (fewer quarters) than the maximum possible time for this measure; (4) Suppressed for one or more quarters by CMS; (5) No data is available from the hospital for this measure; (6) Fewer than 100 patients completed the HCAHPS survey. Use these rates with caution, as the number of surveys may be too low to reliably assess hospital performance; (7) Survey results are based on less than 12 months of data; (8) Survey results are not available for this reporting period; (9) No or very few patients were eligible for the HCAHPS survey. The scores shown, if any, reflect a very small number of surveys; (10) A state average was not calculated because too few hospitals in the state submitted data; (11) There were discrepancies in the data collection process; Please refer to the User's Guide for a full explanation of data.

Gnaden Huetten Memorial Hospital

211 North 12th Street — Phone: 607-377-1300
Lehighton, PA 18235 — Fax: 610-377-7920
URL: www.bluemountainhealthsystem.org/services.asp
Type: Acute Care Hospitals — Emergency Services: Yes
Ownership: Voluntary Non-Profit - Private — Beds: 202

Key Personnel:
CEO/President. . . . . Robert J Clark
Ambulatory Care . . . . Joseph Lendvay
Anesthesiology. . . . . George Chmiel

Measure	Cases	This Hosp.	State Avg.	U.S. Avg.
Heart Attack Care				
ACE Inhibitor or ARB for LVSD[1]	1	100%	95%	96%
Aspirin at Arrival[1]	13	85%	99%	99%
Aspirin at Discharge[1]	7	100%	99%	98%
Beta Blocker at Discharge[1]	8	100%	99%	98%
Fibrinolytic Medication Timing	0	-	40%	55%
PCI Within 90 Minutes of Arrival	0	-	88%	90%
Smoking Cessation Advice[1]	1	100%	100%	99%
Chest Pain/Possible Heart Attack Care				
Aspirin at Arrival	94	95%	95%	95%
Median Time to ECG (minutes)	101	6	8	8
Median Time to Transfer (minutes)[1]	24	60	68	61
Fibrinolytic Medication Timing	0	-	48%	54%
Heart Failure Care				
ACE Inhibitor or ARB for LVSD[1]	20	95%	95%	94%
Discharge Instructions	99	99%	90%	88%
Evaluation of LVS Function	127	99%	99%	98%
Smoking Cessation Advice[1]	15	80%	98%	98%
Pneumonia Care				
Appropriate Initial Antibiotic	48	83%	93%	92%
Blood Culture Timing	67	94%	96%	96%
Influenza Vaccine	48	94%	92%	91%
Initial Antibiotic Timing	69	94%	96%	95%
Pneumococcal Vaccine	57	98%	95%	93%
Smoking Cessation Advice	29	100%	98%	97%
Surgical Care Improvement Project				
Appropriate VTP Within 24 Hours	72	96%	95%	92%
Appropriate Hair Removal	161	100%	100%	99%
Appropriate Beta Blocker Usage	33	100%	94%	93%
Controlled Postoperative Blood Glucose	0	-	96%	93%
Prophylactic Antibiotic Timing	96	100%	97%	97%
Prophylactic Antibiotic Timing (Outpatient)	71	86%	92%	92%
Prophylactic Antibiotic Selection	96	95%	98%	97%
Prophylactic Antibiotic Select. (Outpatient)	70	87%	93%	94%
Prophylactic Antibiotic Stopped	90	89%	95%	94%
Recommended VTP Ordered	72	96%	97%	94%
Urinary Catheter Removal	41	90%	95%	90%
Children's Asthma Care				
Received Systemic Corticosteroids	-	-	-	100%
Received Home Management Plan	-	-	-	71%
Received Reliever Medication	-	-	-	100%
Use of Medical Imaging				
Combination Abdominal CT Scan	443	0.068	0.203	0.191
Combination Chest CT Scan	312	0.042	0.026	0.054
Follow-up Mammogram/Ultrasound	625	12.6%	8.2%	8.4%
MRI for Low Back Pain	190	33.7%	32.4%	32.7%
Survey of Patients' Hospital Experiences				
Area Around Room 'Always' Quiet at Night	300+	47%	-	58%
Doctors 'Always' Communicated Well	300+	75%	-	80%
Home Recovery Information Given	300+	83%	-	82%
Hospital Given 9 or 10 on 10 Point Scale	300+	57%	-	67%
Meds 'Always' Explained Before Given	300+	58%	-	60%
Nurses 'Always' Communicated Well	300+	74%	-	76%
Pain 'Always' Well Controlled	300+	67%	-	69%
Room and Bathroom 'Always' Clean	300+	73%	-	71%
Timely Help 'Always' Received	300+	62%	-	64%
Would Definitely Recommend Hospital	300+	57%	-	69%

Evangelical Community Hospital

One Hospital Drive — Phone: 570-522-2200
Lewisburg, PA 17837 — Fax: 570-522-2868
E-mail: information@evanhospital.com
URL: www.evanhospital.com
Type: Acute Care Hospitals — Emergency Services: No
Ownership: Voluntary Non-Profit - Other — Beds: 134

Key Personnel:
CEO/President. . . . . Michael N O'Keefe
Chief of Medical Staff. . . . . J Lawrence Ginsburg, MD
Infection Control. . . . . Tamara Persina, RN
Pediatric In-Patient Care . . . . Ruth Nolan
Quality Assurance . . . . Leigh Donecker
Radiology. . . . . Naval Kant
Emergency Room . . . . Darlene Rowe, RN
Patient Relations . . . . Angela Brouse

Measure	Cases	This Hosp.	State Avg.	U.S. Avg.
Heart Attack Care				
ACE Inhibitor or ARB for LVSD[1]	15	87%	95%	96%
Aspirin at Arrival	149	99%	99%	99%
Aspirin at Discharge	122	97%	99%	98%
Beta Blocker at Discharge	129	98%	99%	98%
Fibrinolytic Medication Timing	0	-	40%	55%
PCI Within 90 Minutes of Arrival	0	-	88%	90%
Smoking Cessation Advice[1]	9	89%	100%	99%
Chest Pain/Possible Heart Attack Care				
Aspirin at Arrival	150	96%	95%	95%
Median Time to ECG (minutes)	153	6	8	8
Median Time to Transfer (minutes)[1]	24	58	68	61
Fibrinolytic Medication Timing	0	-	48%	54%
Heart Failure Care				
ACE Inhibitor or ARB for LVSD	27	89%	95%	94%
Discharge Instructions	106	95%	90%	88%
Evaluation of LVS Function	143	99%	99%	98%
Smoking Cessation Advice[1]	8	100%	98%	98%
Pneumonia Care				
Appropriate Initial Antibiotic	117	95%	93%	92%
Blood Culture Timing	199	97%	96%	96%
Influenza Vaccine	123	95%	92%	91%
Initial Antibiotic Timing	183	97%	96%	95%
Pneumococcal Vaccine	208	95%	95%	93%
Smoking Cessation Advice	44	93%	98%	97%
Surgical Care Improvement Project				
Appropriate VTP Within 24 Hours[2]	131	85%	95%	92%
Appropriate Hair Removal[2]	466	100%	100%	99%
Appropriate Beta Blocker Usage[2]	131	98%	94%	93%
Controlled Postoperative Blood Glucose[2]	0	-	96%	93%
Prophylactic Antibiotic Timing[2]	321	95%	97%	97%
Prophylactic Antibiotic Timing (Outpatient)	402	93%	92%	92%
Prophylactic Antibiotic Selection[2]	322	99%	98%	97%
Prophylactic Antibiotic Select. (Outpatient)	393	98%	93%	94%
Prophylactic Antibiotic Stopped[2]	315	95%	95%	94%
Recommended VTP Ordered[2]	131	86%	97%	94%
Urinary Catheter Removal[2]	144	97%	95%	90%
Children's Asthma Care				
Received Systemic Corticosteroids	-	-	-	100%
Received Home Management Plan	-	-	-	71%
Received Reliever Medication	-	-	-	100%
Use of Medical Imaging				
Combination Abdominal CT Scan	1,019	0.064	0.203	0.191
Combination Chest CT Scan	434	0.000	0.026	0.054
Follow-up Mammogram/Ultrasound	1,761	6.8%	8.2%	8.4%
MRI for Low Back Pain	169	28.4%	32.4%	32.7%
Survey of Patients' Hospital Experiences				
Area Around Room 'Always' Quiet at Night	300+	51%	-	58%
Doctors 'Always' Communicated Well	300+	80%	-	80%
Home Recovery Information Given	300+	85%	-	82%
Hospital Given 9 or 10 on 10 Point Scale	300+	71%	-	67%
Meds 'Always' Explained Before Given	300+	60%	-	60%
Nurses 'Always' Communicated Well	300+	78%	-	76%
Pain 'Always' Well Controlled	300+	71%	-	69%
Room and Bathroom 'Always' Clean	300+	74%	-	71%
Timely Help 'Always' Received	300+	69%	-	64%
Would Definitely Recommend Hospital	300+	80%	-	69%

Lewistown Hospital

400 Highland Avenue — Phone: 717-248-5411
Lewistown, PA 17044 — Fax: 717-242-7245
URL: www.lewistownhospital.org
Type: Acute Care Hospitals — Emergency Services: Yes
Ownership: Voluntary Non-Profit - Other — Beds: 139

Key Personnel:
CEO/President. . . . . Kay A Hamilton, RN MS
Chief of Medical Staff. . . . . Gurpreet S Bhalla, MD
Coronary Care . . . . Pamela Benson
Infection Control. . . . . Linda Flanagan
Operating Room. . . . . G Scott Anderson
Pediatric Ambulatory Care . . . . . . Paul Brahmakulam, MD
Quality Assurance . . . . Judi Olnick
Radiology. . . . . Jerome Derdel, MD

Measure	Cases	This Hosp.	State Avg.	U.S. Avg.
Heart Attack Care				
ACE Inhibitor or ARB for LVSD[1]	22	86%	95%	96%
Aspirin at Arrival	123	97%	99%	99%
Aspirin at Discharge	76	93%	99%	98%
Beta Blocker at Discharge	86	99%	99%	98%
Fibrinolytic Medication Timing[1]	1	0%	40%	55%
PCI Within 90 Minutes of Arrival	0	-	88%	90%
Smoking Cessation Advice[1]	8	88%	100%	99%
Chest Pain/Possible Heart Attack Care				
Aspirin at Arrival	47	96%	95%	95%
Median Time to ECG (minutes)	47	7	8	8
Median Time to Transfer (minutes)[1]	5	45	68	61
Fibrinolytic Medication Timing[1]	1	100%	48%	54%
Heart Failure Care				
ACE Inhibitor or ARB for LVSD	54	85%	95%	94%
Discharge Instructions	178	89%	90%	88%
Evaluation of LVS Function	274	100%	99%	98%
Smoking Cessation Advice[1]	20	85%	98%	98%
Pneumonia Care				
Appropriate Initial Antibiotic	128	92%	93%	92%
Blood Culture Timing	224	99%	96%	96%
Influenza Vaccine	139	86%	92%	91%
Initial Antibiotic Timing	189	97%	96%	95%
Pneumococcal Vaccine	188	91%	95%	93%
Smoking Cessation Advice	60	88%	98%	97%
Surgical Care Improvement Project				
Appropriate VTP Within 24 Hours	100	81%	95%	92%
Appropriate Hair Removal	267	100%	100%	99%
Appropriate Beta Blocker Usage	78	94%	94%	93%
Controlled Postoperative Blood Glucose	0	-	96%	93%
Prophylactic Antibiotic Timing	176	98%	97%	97%
Prophylactic Antibiotic Timing (Outpatient)	119	95%	92%	92%
Prophylactic Antibiotic Selection	176	95%	98%	97%
Prophylactic Antibiotic Select. (Outpatient)	117	97%	93%	94%
Prophylactic Antibiotic Stopped	166	97%	95%	94%
Recommended VTP Ordered	102	82%	97%	94%
Urinary Catheter Removal[1]	11	100%	95%	90%
Children's Asthma Care				
Received Systemic Corticosteroids	-	-	-	100%
Received Home Management Plan	-	-	-	71%
Received Reliever Medication	-	-	-	100%
Use of Medical Imaging				
Combination Abdominal CT Scan	701	0.278	0.203	0.191
Combination Chest CT Scan	536	0.002	0.026	0.054
Follow-up Mammogram/Ultrasound	895	10.4%	8.2%	8.4%
MRI for Low Back Pain	255	36.9%	32.4%	32.7%
Survey of Patients' Hospital Experiences				
Area Around Room 'Always' Quiet at Night	300+	44%	-	58%
Doctors 'Always' Communicated Well	300+	75%	-	80%
Home Recovery Information Given	300+	78%	-	82%
Hospital Given 9 or 10 on 10 Point Scale	300+	55%	-	67%
Meds 'Always' Explained Before Given	300+	51%	-	60%
Nurses 'Always' Communicated Well	300+	70%	-	76%
Pain 'Always' Well Controlled	300+	61%	-	69%
Room and Bathroom 'Always' Clean	300+	74%	-	71%
Timely Help 'Always' Received	300+	60%	-	64%
Would Definitely Recommend Hospital	300+	47%	-	69%

NOTE: Hospital profiles are in alphabetical order by state, then city, then hospital within the city; Rankings exclude hospitals with less than 25 cases except for patient surveys which excludes hospitals with less than 100 cases; (a) 100–299 cases; (1) The number of cases is too small to be sure how well a hospital is performing; (2) The hospital indicated that the data submitted for this measure were based on a sample of cases; (3) Data was collected during a shorter time period (fewer quarters) than the maximum possible time for this measure; (4) Suppressed for one or more quarters by CMS; (5) No data is available from the hospital for this measure; (6) Fewer than 100 patients completed the HCAHPS survey. Use these rates with caution, as the number of surveys may be too low to reliably assess hospital performance; (7) Survey results are based on less than 12 months of data; (8) Survey results are not available for this reporting period; (9) No or very few patients were eligible for the HCAHPS survey. The scores shown, if any, reflect a very small number of surveys; (10) A state average was not calculated because too few hospitals in the state submitted data; (11) There were discrepancies in the data collection process; Please refer to the User's Guide for a full explanation of data.

Heart of Lancaster Regional Medical Center

1500 Highlands Drive | Phone: 717-625-5000
Lititz, PA 17543 | Fax: 717-625-5619
URL: www.heartoflancaster.com
Type: Acute Care Hospitals | Emergency Services: Yes
Ownership: Proprietary | Beds: 154

Key Personnel:
CEO/President. . . . . Lee Christenson
Chief of Medical Staff. . . . . Peter Pityk
Radiology. . . . . Alan R Alexander
Anesthesiology. . . . . Terry Prager, CRNA

Measure	Cases	This Hosp.	State Avg.	U.S. Avg.
Heart Attack Care				
ACE Inhibitor or ARB for LVSD	0	-	95%	96%
Aspirin at Arrival[1]	10	100%	99%	99%
Aspirin at Discharge[1]	5	100%	99%	98%
Beta Blocker at Discharge[1]	4	100%	99%	98%
Fibrinolytic Medication Timing	0	-	40%	55%
PCI Within 90 Minutes of Arrival	0	-	88%	90%
Smoking Cessation Advice	0	-	100%	99%
Chest Pain/Possible Heart Attack Care				
Aspirin at Arrival[1]	17	100%	95%	95%
Median Time to ECG (minutes)[1]	18	4	8	8
Median Time to Transfer (minutes)[1,3]	4	68	68	61
Fibrinolytic Medication Timing[3]	0	-	48%	54%
Heart Failure Care				
ACE Inhibitor or ARB for LVSD[1]	16	94%	95%	94%
Discharge Instructions[1]	24	96%	90%	88%
Evaluation of LVS Function	46	98%	99%	98%
Smoking Cessation Advice[1]	4	100%	98%	98%
Pneumonia Care				
Appropriate Initial Antibiotic	28	100%	93%	92%
Blood Culture Timing	50	100%	96%	96%
Influenza Vaccine	29	100%	92%	91%
Initial Antibiotic Timing	48	100%	96%	95%
Pneumococcal Vaccine	42	100%	95%	93%
Smoking Cessation Advice[1]	16	100%	98%	97%
Surgical Care Improvement Project				
Appropriate VTP Within 24 Hours	83	98%	95%	92%
Appropriate Hair Removal	184	100%	100%	99%
Appropriate Beta Blocker Usage	32	97%	94%	93%
Controlled Postoperative Blood Glucose	0	-	96%	93%
Prophylactic Antibiotic Timing	91	99%	97%	97%
Prophylactic Antibiotic Timing (Outpatient)	77	99%	92%	92%
Prophylactic Antibiotic Selection	93	100%	98%	97%
Prophylactic Antibiotic Select. (Outpatient)	76	97%	93%	94%
Prophylactic Antibiotic Stopped	88	99%	95%	94%
Recommended VTP Ordered	83	98%	97%	94%
Urinary Catheter Removal[1]	22	100%	95%	90%
Children's Asthma Care				
Received Systemic Corticosteroids[1]	11	100%	-	100%
Received Home Management Plan[1]	11	100%	-	71%
Received Reliever Medication[1]	11	100%	-	100%
Use of Medical Imaging				
Combination Abdominal CT Scan	152	0.151	0.203	0.191
Combination Chest CT Scan	94	0.085	0.026	0.054
Follow-up Mammogram/Ultrasound	188	3.7%	8.2%	8.4%
MRI for Low Back Pain[1]	21	23.8%	32.4%	32.7%
Survey of Patients' Hospital Experiences				
Area Around Room 'Always' Quiet at Night	300+	57%	-	58%
Doctors 'Always' Communicated Well	300+	77%	-	80%
Home Recovery Information Given	300+	80%	-	82%
Hospital Given 9 or 10 on 10 Point Scale	300+	65%	-	67%
Meds 'Always' Explained Before Given	300+	59%	-	60%
Nurses 'Always' Communicated Well	300+	72%	-	76%
Pain 'Always' Well Controlled	300+	65%	-	69%
Room and Bathroom 'Always' Clean	300+	72%	-	71%
Timely Help 'Always' Received	300+	63%	-	64%
Would Definitely Recommend Hospital	300+	68%	-	69%

Lock Haven Hospital

24 Cree Drive | Phone: 570-893-5000
Lock Haven, PA 17745 | Fax: 570-893-5172
URL: www.lockhavenhospital.com
Type: Acute Care Hospitals | Emergency Services: Yes
Ownership: Proprietary | Beds: 260

Key Personnel:
CEO/President. . . . . Gary Rhoads
Chief of Medical Staff . . . . Keith Adams, MD
Infection Control. . . . . Nancry Bolze
Operating Room. . . . . Sue Counsil
Pediatric Ambulatory Care . . . . . . P Bhatt, MD
Pediatric In-Patient Care . . . . . . P Bhatt, MD
Quality Assurance . . . . Michelle Polk
Radiology. . . . . Cyndy Bower

Measure	Cases	This Hosp.	State Avg.	U.S. Avg.
Heart Attack Care				
ACE Inhibitor or ARB for LVSD[1]	1	100%	95%	96%
Aspirin at Arrival[1]	9	89%	99%	99%
Aspirin at Discharge[1]	7	71%	99%	98%
Beta Blocker at Discharge[1]	7	100%	99%	98%
Fibrinolytic Medication Timing	0	-	40%	55%
PCI Within 90 Minutes of Arrival	0	-	88%	90%
Smoking Cessation Advice[1]	4	100%	100%	99%
Chest Pain/Possible Heart Attack Care				
Aspirin at Arrival	34	94%	95%	95%
Median Time to ECG (minutes)	37	9	8	8
Median Time to Transfer (minutes)[1]	3	44	68	61
Fibrinolytic Medication Timing	0	-	48%	54%
Heart Failure Care				
ACE Inhibitor or ARB for LVSD[1]	14	100%	95%	94%
Discharge Instructions	60	97%	90%	88%
Evaluation of LVS Function	79	99%	99%	98%
Smoking Cessation Advice[1]	14	100%	98%	98%
Pneumonia Care				
Appropriate Initial Antibiotic	50	96%	93%	92%
Blood Culture Timing	59	100%	96%	96%
Influenza Vaccine	31	97%	92%	91%
Initial Antibiotic Timing	59	98%	96%	95%
Pneumococcal Vaccine	40	92%	95%	93%
Smoking Cessation Advice[1]	13	100%	98%	97%
Surgical Care Improvement Project				
Appropriate VTP Within 24 Hours[1,2]	19	84%	95%	92%
Appropriate Hair Removal[2]	63	100%	100%	99%
Appropriate Beta Blocker Usage[1,2]	13	77%	94%	93%
Controlled Postoperative Blood Glucose[2]	0	-	96%	93%
Prophylactic Antibiotic Timing[2]	25	96%	97%	97%
Prophylactic Antibiotic Timing (Outpatient)[1]	9	89%	92%	92%
Prophylactic Antibiotic Selection[1,2]	24	92%	98%	97%
Prophylactic Antibiotic Select. (Outpatient)	35	94%	93%	94%
Prophylactic Antibiotic Stopped[1,2]	24	83%	95%	94%
Recommended VTP Ordered[1,2]	20	85%	97%	94%
Urinary Catheter Removal[1]	6	100%	95%	90%
Children's Asthma Care				
Received Systemic Corticosteroids	-	-	-	100%
Received Home Management Plan	-	-	-	71%
Received Reliever Medication	-	-	-	100%
Use of Medical Imaging				
Combination Abdominal CT Scan	223	0.430	0.203	0.191
Combination Chest CT Scan	109	0.037	0.026	0.054
Follow-up Mammogram/Ultrasound	271	12.9%	8.2%	8.4%
MRI for Low Back Pain[1]	34	35.3%	32.4%	32.7%
Survey of Patients' Hospital Experiences				
Area Around Room 'Always' Quiet at Night	300+	58%	-	58%
Doctors 'Always' Communicated Well	300+	77%	-	80%
Home Recovery Information Given	300+	82%	-	82%
Hospital Given 9 or 10 on 10 Point Scale	300+	59%	-	67%
Meds 'Always' Explained Before Given	300+	57%	-	60%
Nurses 'Always' Communicated Well	300+	74%	-	76%
Pain 'Always' Well Controlled	300+	69%	-	69%
Room and Bathroom 'Always' Clean	300+	68%	-	71%
Timely Help 'Always' Received	300+	68%	-	64%
Would Definitely Recommend Hospital	300+	50%	-	69%

Fulton County Medical Center

214 Peach Orchard Road | Phone: 717-485-3155
Mcconnellsburg, PA 17233 | Fax: 717-485-5605
E-mail: marketing@fcmc-pa.org
URL: www.fcmcpa.org
Type: Critical Access Hospitals | Emergency Services: Yes
Ownership: Voluntary Non-Profit - Private | Beds: 82

Key Personnel:
CEO/President. . . . . Jason Hawkins
Cardiac Laboratory. . . . . Kim Hsmish
Chief of Medical Staff . . . . Sharon Martin, MD
Coronary Care . . . . Sherri Fisher
Infection Control. . . . . Barbara Weller
Operating Room. . . . . Cherry Hale

Measure	Cases	This Hosp.	State Avg.	U.S. Avg.
Heart Attack Care				
ACE Inhibitor or ARB for LVSD[3]	0	-	95%	96%
Aspirin at Arrival[3]	0	-	99%	99%
Aspirin at Discharge[3]	0	-	99%	98%
Beta Blocker at Discharge[3]	0	-	99%	98%
Fibrinolytic Medication Timing[3]	0	-	40%	55%
PCI Within 90 Minutes of Arrival[3]	0	-	88%	90%
Smoking Cessation Advice[3]	0	-	100%	99%
Chest Pain/Possible Heart Attack Care				
Aspirin at Arrival	-	-	95%	95%
Median Time to ECG (minutes)	-	-	8	8
Median Time to Transfer (minutes)	-	-	68	61
Fibrinolytic Medication Timing	-	-	48%	54%
Heart Failure Care				
ACE Inhibitor or ARB for LVSD[1,3]	6	100%	95%	94%
Discharge Instructions[1,3]	14	71%	90%	88%
Evaluation of LVS Function[1,3]	20	90%	99%	98%
Smoking Cessation Advice[1,3]	1	0%	98%	98%
Pneumonia Care				
Appropriate Initial Antibiotic[1,3]	24	96%	93%	92%
Blood Culture Timing[1,3]	15	93%	96%	96%
Influenza Vaccine[1,3]	20	90%	92%	91%
Initial Antibiotic Timing[3]	25	92%	96%	95%
Pneumococcal Vaccine[1,3]	24	83%	95%	93%
Smoking Cessation Advice[1,3]	10	10%	98%	97%
Surgical Care Improvement Project				
Appropriate VTP Within 24 Hours[5]	0	-	95%	92%
Appropriate Hair Removal[5]	0	-	100%	99%
Appropriate Beta Blocker Usage[5]	0	-	94%	93%
Controlled Postoperative Blood Glucose[5]	0	-	96%	93%
Prophylactic Antibiotic Timing[5]	0	-	97%	97%
Prophylactic Antibiotic Timing (Outpatient)	-	-	92%	92%
Prophylactic Antibiotic Selection[5]	0	-	98%	97%
Prophylactic Antibiotic Select. (Outpatient)	-	-	93%	94%
Prophylactic Antibiotic Stopped[5]	0	-	95%	94%
Recommended VTP Ordered[5]	0	-	97%	94%
Urinary Catheter Removal[5]	0	-	95%	90%
Children's Asthma Care				
Received Systemic Corticosteroids	-	-	-	100%
Received Home Management Plan	-	-	-	71%
Received Reliever Medication	-	-	-	100%
Use of Medical Imaging				
Combination Abdominal CT Scan	-	-	0.203	0.191
Combination Chest CT Scan	-	-	0.026	0.054
Follow-up Mammogram/Ultrasound	-	-	8.2%	8.4%
MRI for Low Back Pain	-	-	32.4%	32.7%
Survey of Patients' Hospital Experiences				
Area Around Room 'Always' Quiet at Night[8]	-	-	-	58%
Doctors 'Always' Communicated Well[8]	-	-	-	80%
Home Recovery Information Given[8]	-	-	-	82%
Hospital Given 9 or 10 on 10 Point Scale[8]	-	-	-	67%
Meds 'Always' Explained Before Given[8]	-	-	-	60%
Nurses 'Always' Communicated Well[8]	-	-	-	76%
Pain 'Always' Well Controlled[8]	-	-	-	69%
Room and Bathroom 'Always' Clean[8]	-	-	-	71%
Timely Help 'Always' Received[8]	-	-	-	64%
Would Definitely Recommend Hospital[8]	-	-	-	69%

NOTE: Hospital profiles are in alphabetical order by state, then city, then hospital within the city; Rankings exclude hospitals with less than 25 cases except for patient surveys which excludes hospitals with less than 100 cases; (a) 100–299 cases; (1) The number of cases is too small to be sure how well a hospital is performing; (2) The hospital indicated that the data submitted for this measure were based on a sample of cases; (3) Data was collected during a shorter time period (fewer quarters) than the maximum possible time for this measure; (4) Suppressed for one or more quarters by CMS; (5) No data is available from the hospital for this measure; (6) Fewer than 100 patients completed the HCAHPS survey. Use these rates with caution, as the number of surveys may be too low to reliably assess hospital performance; (7) Survey results are based on less than 12 months of data; (8) Survey results are not available for this reporting period; (9) No or very few patients were eligible for the HCAHPS survey. The scores shown, if any, reflect a very small number of surveys; (10) A state average was not calculated because too few hospitals in the state submitted data; (11) There were discrepancies in the data collection process; Please refer to the User's Guide for a full explanation of data.

Ohio Valley General Hospital

25 Heckel Road
Mckees Rocks, PA 15136
Phone: 412-777-6161
Fax: 412-777-6189
URL: www.ohiovalleyhospital.org
Type: Acute Care Hospitals
Emergency Services: Yes
Ownership: Voluntary Non-Profit - Private
Beds: 119

Key Personnel:
CEO/President. . . . . William Provenzano
Chief of Medical Staff . . . . Roberta L Bashore
Emergency Room . . . . William Held

Measure	Cases	This Hosp.	State Avg.	U.S. Avg.
Heart Attack Care				
ACE Inhibitor or ARB for LVSD	0	-	95%	96%
Aspirin at Arrival[1]	18	100%	99%	99%
Aspirin at Discharge[1]	9	100%	99%	98%
Beta Blocker at Discharge[1]	10	100%	99%	98%
Fibrinolytic Medication Timing	0	-	40%	55%
PCI Within 90 Minutes of Arrival	0	-	88%	90%
Smoking Cessation Advice[1]	1	100%	100%	99%
Chest Pain/Possible Heart Attack Care				
Aspirin at Arrival	47	98%	95%	95%
Median Time to ECG (minutes)	47	21	8	8
Median Time to Transfer (minutes)[1]	12	75	68	61
Fibrinolytic Medication Timing	0	-	48%	54%
Heart Failure Care				
ACE Inhibitor or ARB for LVSD	70	80%	95%	94%
Discharge Instructions	151	67%	90%	88%
Evaluation of LVS Function	212	100%	99%	98%
Smoking Cessation Advice	25	92%	98%	98%
Pneumonia Care				
Appropriate Initial Antibiotic	98	84%	93%	92%
Blood Culture Timing	93	87%	96%	96%
Influenza Vaccine	75	76%	92%	91%
Initial Antibiotic Timing	134	91%	96%	95%
Pneumococcal Vaccine	106	86%	95%	93%
Smoking Cessation Advice	54	96%	98%	97%
Surgical Care Improvement Project				
Appropriate VTP Within 24 Hours	163	93%	95%	92%
Appropriate Hair Removal	307	100%	100%	99%
Appropriate Beta Blocker Usage	78	81%	94%	93%
Controlled Postoperative Blood Glucose	0	-	96%	93%
Prophylactic Antibiotic Timing	210	92%	97%	97%
Prophylactic Antibiotic Timing (Outpatient)	45	80%	92%	92%
Prophylactic Antibiotic Selection	213	95%	98%	97%
Prophylactic Antibiotic Select. (Outpatient)	38	82%	93%	94%
Prophylactic Antibiotic Stopped	198	87%	95%	94%
Recommended VTP Ordered	164	94%	97%	94%
Urinary Catheter Removal[1]	23	78%	95%	90%
Children's Asthma Care				
Received Systemic Corticosteroids	-	-	-	100%
Received Home Management Plan	-	-	-	71%
Received Reliever Medication	-	-	-	100%
Use of Medical Imaging				
Combination Abdominal CT Scan	157	0.083	0.203	0.191
Combination Chest CT Scan	146	0.000	0.026	0.054
Follow-up Mammogram/Ultrasound	177	12.4%	8.2%	8.4%
MRI for Low Back Pain[1]	35	34.3%	32.4%	32.7%
Survey of Patients' Hospital Experiences				
Area Around Room 'Always' Quiet at Night	300+	56%	-	58%
Doctors 'Always' Communicated Well	300+	77%	-	80%
Home Recovery Information Given	300+	80%	-	82%
Hospital Given 9 or 10 on 10 Point Scale	300+	63%	-	67%
Meds 'Always' Explained Before Given	300+	55%	-	60%
Nurses 'Always' Communicated Well	300+	73%	-	76%
Pain 'Always' Well Controlled	300+	64%	-	69%
Room and Bathroom 'Always' Clean	300+	68%	-	71%
Timely Help 'Always' Received	300+	65%	-	64%
Would Definitely Recommend Hospital	300+	69%	-	69%

UPMC Mckeesport

1500 Fifth Avenue
McKeesport, PA 15132
Phone: 412-664-2000
Fax: 412-664-2925
URL: www.selectmedicalcorp.com
Type: Acute Care Hospitals
Emergency Services: Yes
Ownership: Voluntary Non-Profit - Private
Beds: 30

Key Personnel:
CEO/President. . . . . Martin F Jackson
Chief of Medical Staff . . . . Mehboob K Chaudhry
Pediatric In-Patient Care . . . . LJ Silberman, MD
Quality Assurance . . . . Joseph Ferraro

Measure	Cases	This Hosp.	State Avg.	U.S. Avg.
Heart Attack Care				
ACE Inhibitor or ARB for LVSD[1]	19	100%	95%	96%
Aspirin at Arrival	108	100%	99%	99%
Aspirin at Discharge	78	100%	99%	98%
Beta Blocker at Discharge	85	100%	99%	98%
Fibrinolytic Medication Timing	0	-	40%	55%
PCI Within 90 Minutes of Arrival	0	-	88%	90%
Smoking Cessation Advice[1]	21	100%	100%	99%
Chest Pain/Possible Heart Attack Care				
Aspirin at Arrival	30	97%	95%	95%
Median Time to ECG (minutes)	32	12	8	8
Median Time to Transfer (minutes)[5]	0	-	68	61
Fibrinolytic Medication Timing[3]	0	-	48%	54%
Heart Failure Care				
ACE Inhibitor or ARB for LVSD	107	100%	95%	94%
Discharge Instructions	305	99%	90%	88%
Evaluation of LVS Function	442	100%	99%	98%
Smoking Cessation Advice	52	100%	98%	98%
Pneumonia Care				
Appropriate Initial Antibiotic	103	98%	93%	92%
Blood Culture Timing	252	100%	96%	96%
Influenza Vaccine	199	97%	92%	91%
Initial Antibiotic Timing	251	98%	96%	95%
Pneumococcal Vaccine	253	100%	95%	93%
Smoking Cessation Advice	96	100%	98%	97%
Surgical Care Improvement Project				
Appropriate VTP Within 24 Hours	209	100%	95%	92%
Appropriate Hair Removal	377	100%	100%	99%
Appropriate Beta Blocker Usage	114	99%	94%	93%
Controlled Postoperative Blood Glucose	0	-	96%	93%
Prophylactic Antibiotic Timing	195	99%	97%	97%
Prophylactic Antibiotic Timing (Outpatient)	95	97%	92%	92%
Prophylactic Antibiotic Selection	197	97%	98%	97%
Prophylactic Antibiotic Select. (Outpatient)	93	90%	93%	94%
Prophylactic Antibiotic Stopped	191	100%	95%	94%
Recommended VTP Ordered	209	100%	97%	94%
Urinary Catheter Removal	39	97%	95%	90%
Children's Asthma Care				
Received Systemic Corticosteroids	-	-	-	100%
Received Home Management Plan	-	-	-	71%
Received Reliever Medication	-	-	-	100%
Use of Medical Imaging				
Combination Abdominal CT Scan	372	0.108	0.203	0.191
Combination Chest CT Scan	293	0.051	0.026	0.054
Follow-up Mammogram/Ultrasound	260	3.1%	8.2%	8.4%
MRI for Low Back Pain[1]	31	25.8%	32.4%	32.7%
Survey of Patients' Hospital Experiences				
Area Around Room 'Always' Quiet at Night	300+	50%	-	58%
Doctors 'Always' Communicated Well	300+	79%	-	80%
Home Recovery Information Given	300+	79%	-	82%
Hospital Given 9 or 10 on 10 Point Scale	300+	59%	-	67%
Meds 'Always' Explained Before Given	300+	59%	-	60%
Nurses 'Always' Communicated Well	300+	74%	-	76%
Pain 'Always' Well Controlled	300+	67%	-	69%
Room and Bathroom 'Always' Clean	300+	69%	-	71%
Timely Help 'Always' Received	300+	60%	-	64%
Would Definitely Recommend Hospital	300+	57%	-	69%

Holy Redeemer Hospital and Medical Center

1648 Huntingdon Pike
Meadowbrook, PA 19046
Phone: 215-947-3000
Fax: 215-938-3232
E-mail: inforef@holyredeemer.com
URL: www.holyredeemer.com
Type: Acute Care Hospitals
Emergency Services: Yes
Ownership: Voluntary Non-Profit - Church
Beds: 249

Key Personnel:
CEO/President. . . . . Mark T Jones
Chief of Medical Staff . . . . William Gibbons, MD
Operating Room. . . . . Donna M Angotti, RN
Pediatric Ambulatory Care . . . . . . L Stewart Barbera, MD
Pediatric In-Patient Care . . . . L Stewart Barbera, MD
Quality Assurance . . . . Debra Shank

Measure	Cases	This Hosp.	State Avg.	U.S. Avg.
Heart Attack Care				
ACE Inhibitor or ARB for LVSD	26	92%	95%	96%
Aspirin at Arrival	176	97%	99%	99%
Aspirin at Discharge	139	97%	99%	98%
Beta Blocker at Discharge	141	98%	99%	98%
Fibrinolytic Medication Timing	0	-	40%	55%
PCI Within 90 Minutes of Arrival	33	85%	88%	90%
Smoking Cessation Advice	30	100%	100%	99%
Chest Pain/Possible Heart Attack Care				
Aspirin at Arrival[1,3]	1	100%	95%	95%
Median Time to ECG (minutes)[1,3]	1	308178	8	8
Median Time to Transfer (minutes)[5]	0	-	68	61
Fibrinolytic Medication Timing[5]	0	-	48%	54%
Heart Failure Care				
ACE Inhibitor or ARB for LVSD	63	98%	95%	94%
Discharge Instructions	232	100%	90%	88%
Evaluation of LVS Function	339	99%	99%	98%
Smoking Cessation Advice[1]	21	100%	98%	98%
Pneumonia Care				
Appropriate Initial Antibiotic	109	91%	93%	92%
Blood Culture Timing	228	96%	96%	96%
Influenza Vaccine	163	98%	92%	91%
Initial Antibiotic Timing	236	97%	96%	95%
Pneumococcal Vaccine	244	98%	95%	93%
Smoking Cessation Advice	42	98%	98%	97%
Surgical Care Improvement Project				
Appropriate VTP Within 24 Hours	254	98%	95%	92%
Appropriate Hair Removal	829	100%	100%	99%
Appropriate Beta Blocker Usage	228	89%	94%	93%
Controlled Postoperative Blood Glucose	0	-	96%	93%
Prophylactic Antibiotic Timing	601	99%	97%	97%
Prophylactic Antibiotic Timing (Outpatient)	58	74%	92%	92%
Prophylactic Antibiotic Selection	601	98%	98%	97%
Prophylactic Antibiotic Select. (Outpatient)	44	86%	93%	94%
Prophylactic Antibiotic Stopped	577	97%	95%	94%
Recommended VTP Ordered	254	98%	97%	94%
Urinary Catheter Removal	191	100%	95%	90%
Children's Asthma Care				
Received Systemic Corticosteroids	-	-	-	100%
Received Home Management Plan	-	-	-	71%
Received Reliever Medication	-	-	-	100%
Use of Medical Imaging				
Combination Abdominal CT Scan	622	0.045	0.203	0.191
Combination Chest CT Scan	563	0.000	0.026	0.054
Follow-up Mammogram/Ultrasound	1,264	8.8%	8.2%	8.4%
MRI for Low Back Pain[5]	0	-	32.4%	32.7%
Survey of Patients' Hospital Experiences				
Area Around Room 'Always' Quiet at Night	300+	53%	-	58%
Doctors 'Always' Communicated Well	300+	80%	-	80%
Home Recovery Information Given	300+	80%	-	82%
Hospital Given 9 or 10 on 10 Point Scale	300+	72%	-	67%
Meds 'Always' Explained Before Given	300+	60%	-	60%
Nurses 'Always' Communicated Well	300+	78%	-	76%
Pain 'Always' Well Controlled	300+	68%	-	69%
Room and Bathroom 'Always' Clean	300+	66%	-	71%
Timely Help 'Always' Received	300+	63%	-	64%
Would Definitely Recommend Hospital	300+	77%	-	69%

NOTE: Hospital profiles are in alphabetical order by state, then city, then hospital within the city; Rankings exclude hospitals with less than 25 cases except for patient surveys which excludes hospitals with less than 100 cases; (a) 100–299 cases; (1) The number of cases is too small to be sure how well a hospital is performing; (2) The hospital indicated that the data submitted for this measure were based on a sample of cases; (3) Data was collected during a shorter time period (fewer quarters) than the maximum possible time for this measure; (4) Suppressed for one or more quarters by CMS; (5) No data is available from the hospital for this measure; (6) Fewer than 100 patients completed the HCAHPS survey. Use these rates with caution, as the number of surveys may be too low to reliably assess hospital performance; (7) Survey results are based on less than 12 months of data; (8) Survey results are not available for this reporting period; (9) No or very few patients were eligible for the HCAHPS survey. The scores shown, if any, reflect a very small number of surveys; (10) A state average was not calculated because too few hospitals in the state submitted data; (11) There were discrepancies in the data collection process; Please refer to the User's Guide for a full explanation of data.

Meadville Medical Center

751 Liberty Street Phone: 814-333-5000
Meadville, PA 16335 Fax: 814-333-9456
URL: www.mmchs.org
Type: Acute Care Hospitals Emergency Services: Yes
Ownership: Voluntary Non-Profit - Other Beds: 277

Key Personnel:
CEO/President. . . . . Anthony De'Fail
Chief of Medical Staff. . . . . Richard Schoeschroecken, MD
Quality Assurance . . . . Connie Brady
Emergency Room . . . . Peter Lultschik, MD

Measure	Cases	This Hosp.	State Avg.	U.S. Avg.
Heart Attack Care				
ACE Inhibitor or ARB for LVSD[1]	1	100%	95%	96%
Aspirin at Arrival[1]	21	100%	99%	99%
Aspirin at Discharge[1]	9	78%	99%	98%
Beta Blocker at Discharge[1]	8	88%	99%	98%
Fibrinolytic Medication Timing	0	-	40%	55%
PCI Within 90 Minutes of Arrival	0	-	88%	90%
Smoking Cessation Advice[1]	2	50%	100%	99%
Chest Pain/Possible Heart Attack Care				
Aspirin at Arrival	152	98%	95%	95%
Median Time to ECG (minutes)	156	9	8	8
Median Time to Transfer (minutes)[1]	11	70	68	61
Fibrinolytic Medication Timing[1]	5	40%	48%	54%
Heart Failure Care				
ACE Inhibitor or ARB for LVSD	31	94%	95%	94%
Discharge Instructions	91	77%	90%	88%
Evaluation of LVS Function	129	97%	99%	98%
Smoking Cessation Advice[1]	14	100%	98%	98%
Pneumonia Care				
Appropriate Initial Antibiotic	92	97%	93%	92%
Blood Culture Timing	129	98%	96%	96%
Influenza Vaccine	85	92%	92%	91%
Initial Antibiotic Timing	139	98%	96%	95%
Pneumococcal Vaccine	114	99%	95%	93%
Smoking Cessation Advice	50	100%	98%	97%
Surgical Care Improvement Project				
Appropriate VTP Within 24 Hours	182	95%	95%	92%
Appropriate Hair Removal	824	100%	100%	99%
Appropriate Beta Blocker Usage	262	96%	94%	93%
Controlled Postoperative Blood Glucose	0	-	96%	93%
Prophylactic Antibiotic Timing	631	98%	97%	97%
Prophylactic Antibiotic Timing (Outpatient)	178	93%	92%	92%
Prophylactic Antibiotic Selection	633	99%	98%	97%
Prophylactic Antibiotic Select. (Outpatient)	219	85%	93%	94%
Prophylactic Antibiotic Stopped	617	96%	95%	94%
Recommended VTP Ordered	186	95%	97%	94%
Urinary Catheter Removal	31	87%	95%	90%
Children's Asthma Care				
Received Systemic Corticosteroids	-	-	-	100%
Received Home Management Plan	-	-	-	71%
Received Reliever Medication	-	-	-	100%
Use of Medical Imaging				
Combination Abdominal CT Scan	702	0.048	0.203	0.191
Combination Chest CT Scan	514	0.008	0.026	0.054
Follow-up Mammogram/Ultrasound	1,434	3.5%	8.2%	8.4%
MRI for Low Back Pain	268	31.0%	32.4%	32.7%
Survey of Patients' Hospital Experiences				
Area Around Room 'Always' Quiet at Night	300+	51%	-	58%
Doctors 'Always' Communicated Well	300+	82%	-	80%
Home Recovery Information Given	300+	82%	-	82%
Hospital Given 9 or 10 on 10 Point Scale	300+	68%	-	67%
Meds 'Always' Explained Before Given	300+	59%	-	60%
Nurses 'Always' Communicated Well	300+	77%	-	76%
Pain 'Always' Well Controlled	300+	75%	-	69%
Room and Bathroom 'Always' Clean	300+	77%	-	71%
Timely Help 'Always' Received	300+	67%	-	64%
Would Definitely Recommend Hospital	300+	65%	-	69%

Riddle Memorial Hospital

1068 West Baltimore Pike Phone: 610-566-9400
Media, PA 19063 Fax: 610-891-3592
URL: www.riddlehospital.org
Type: Acute Care Hospitals Emergency Services: Yes
Ownership: Voluntary Non-Profit - Private Beds: 248

Key Personnel:
CEO/President. . . . . Daniel E Kennedy
Chief of Medical Staff. . . . . George Lieb, MD
Infection Control. . . . . Carolyn Bingeman
Operating Room. . . . . William H Ayers, RN
Quality Assurance . . . . Janet Webb
Emergency Room . . . . Louise Hummel, RN
Intensive Care Unit. . . . . Marianne Schwalbe
Patient Relations . . . . Cathy Boyer

Measure	Cases	This Hosp.	State Avg.	U.S. Avg.
Heart Attack Care				
ACE Inhibitor or ARB for LVSD	25	100%	95%	96%
Aspirin at Arrival	130	98%	99%	99%
Aspirin at Discharge	100	100%	99%	98%
Beta Blocker at Discharge	99	100%	99%	98%
Fibrinolytic Medication Timing	0	-	40%	55%
PCI Within 90 Minutes of Arrival	32	88%	88%	90%
Smoking Cessation Advice	29	100%	100%	99%
Chest Pain/Possible Heart Attack Care				
Aspirin at Arrival[1,3]	1	100%	95%	95%
Median Time to ECG (minutes)[1,3]	1	68	8	8
Median Time to Transfer (minutes)[5]	0	-	68	61
Fibrinolytic Medication Timing[5]	0	-	48%	54%
Heart Failure Care				
ACE Inhibitor or ARB for LVSD	66	97%	95%	94%
Discharge Instructions	192	88%	90%	88%
Evaluation of LVS Function	286	99%	99%	98%
Smoking Cessation Advice[1]	23	96%	98%	98%
Pneumonia Care				
Appropriate Initial Antibiotic	150	96%	93%	92%
Blood Culture Timing	204	93%	96%	96%
Influenza Vaccine	149	97%	92%	91%
Initial Antibiotic Timing	261	98%	96%	95%
Pneumococcal Vaccine	242	99%	95%	93%
Smoking Cessation Advice	64	95%	98%	97%
Surgical Care Improvement Project				
Appropriate VTP Within 24 Hours[2]	272	92%	95%	92%
Appropriate Hair Removal[2]	1,284	99%	100%	99%
Appropriate Beta Blocker Usage[2]	308	94%	94%	93%
Controlled Postoperative Blood Glucose[2]	0	-	96%	93%
Prophylactic Antibiotic Timing[2]	996	100%	97%	97%
Prophylactic Antibiotic Timing (Outpatient)	238	97%	92%	92%
Prophylactic Antibiotic Selection[2]	1,002	98%	98%	97%
Prophylactic Antibiotic Select. (Outpatient)	234	97%	93%	94%
Prophylactic Antibiotic Stopped[2]	980	97%	95%	94%
Recommended VTP Ordered[2]	272	93%	97%	94%
Urinary Catheter Removal[2]	460	99%	95%	90%
Children's Asthma Care				
Received Systemic Corticosteroids	-	-	-	100%
Received Home Management Plan	-	-	-	71%
Received Reliever Medication	-	-	-	100%
Use of Medical Imaging				
Combination Abdominal CT Scan	701	0.612	0.203	0.191
Combination Chest CT Scan	507	0.018	0.026	0.054
Follow-up Mammogram/Ultrasound[1]	1	0.0%	8.2%	8.4%
MRI for Low Back Pain[1]	5	20.0%	32.4%	32.7%
Survey of Patients' Hospital Experiences				
Area Around Room 'Always' Quiet at Night	300+	46%	-	58%
Doctors 'Always' Communicated Well	300+	77%	-	80%
Home Recovery Information Given	300+	81%	-	82%
Hospital Given 9 or 10 on 10 Point Scale	300+	63%	-	67%
Meds 'Always' Explained Before Given	300+	60%	-	60%
Nurses 'Always' Communicated Well	300+	77%	-	76%
Pain 'Always' Well Controlled	300+	69%	-	69%
Room and Bathroom 'Always' Clean	300+	62%	-	71%
Timely Help 'Always' Received	300+	65%	-	64%
Would Definitely Recommend Hospital	300+	68%	-	69%

Monongahela Valley Hospital

1163 Country Club Road Phone: 724-258-1000
Monongahela, PA 15063 Fax: 724-258-1884
E-mail: mail@monvalleyhospital.com
URL: www.monvalleyhospital.com
Type: Acute Care Hospitals Emergency Services: Yes
Ownership: Voluntary Non-Profit - Other Beds: 226

Key Personnel:
CEO/President. . . . . Louis J Panza, Jr
Operating Room. . . . . Fernand N Parent, RN
Quality Assurance . . . . Diane Cooper, RN
Radiology. . . . . Douglas Wilson

Measure	Cases	This Hosp.	State Avg.	U.S. Avg.
Heart Attack Care				
ACE Inhibitor or ARB for LVSD[1]	8	100%	95%	96%
Aspirin at Arrival	107	96%	99%	99%
Aspirin at Discharge	63	92%	99%	98%
Beta Blocker at Discharge	72	96%	99%	98%
Fibrinolytic Medication Timing	0	-	40%	55%
PCI Within 90 Minutes of Arrival[1]	5	20%	88%	90%
Smoking Cessation Advice[1]	11	100%	100%	99%
Chest Pain/Possible Heart Attack Care				
Aspirin at Arrival	86	99%	95%	95%
Median Time to ECG (minutes)	91	10	8	8
Median Time to Transfer (minutes)[1]	14	86	68	61
Fibrinolytic Medication Timing	0	-	48%	54%
Heart Failure Care				
ACE Inhibitor or ARB for LVSD	96	92%	95%	94%
Discharge Instructions	354	93%	90%	88%
Evaluation of LVS Function	399	99%	99%	98%
Smoking Cessation Advice	47	100%	98%	98%
Pneumonia Care				
Appropriate Initial Antibiotic	170	94%	93%	92%
Blood Culture Timing	130	98%	96%	96%
Influenza Vaccine	162	95%	92%	91%
Initial Antibiotic Timing	249	94%	96%	95%
Pneumococcal Vaccine	210	93%	95%	93%
Smoking Cessation Advice	91	96%	98%	97%
Surgical Care Improvement Project				
Appropriate VTP Within 24 Hours	333	95%	95%	92%
Appropriate Hair Removal	665	100%	100%	99%
Appropriate Beta Blocker Usage	162	98%	94%	93%
Controlled Postoperative Blood Glucose	0	-	96%	93%
Prophylactic Antibiotic Timing	425	97%	97%	97%
Prophylactic Antibiotic Timing (Outpatient)	94	95%	92%	92%
Prophylactic Antibiotic Selection	425	97%	98%	97%
Prophylactic Antibiotic Select. (Outpatient)	90	89%	93%	94%
Prophylactic Antibiotic Stopped	398	94%	95%	94%
Recommended VTP Ordered	333	95%	97%	94%
Urinary Catheter Removal	64	84%	95%	90%
Children's Asthma Care				
Received Systemic Corticosteroids	-	-	-	100%
Received Home Management Plan	-	-	-	71%
Received Reliever Medication	-	-	-	100%
Use of Medical Imaging				
Combination Abdominal CT Scan	397	0.612	0.203	0.191
Combination Chest CT Scan	185	0.000	0.026	0.054
Follow-up Mammogram/Ultrasound	536	4.9%	8.2%	8.4%
MRI for Low Back Pain	97	50.5%	32.4%	32.7%
Survey of Patients' Hospital Experiences				
Area Around Room 'Always' Quiet at Night	300+	57%	-	58%
Doctors 'Always' Communicated Well	300+	83%	-	80%
Home Recovery Information Given	300+	79%	-	82%
Hospital Given 9 or 10 on 10 Point Scale	300+	70%	-	67%
Meds 'Always' Explained Before Given	300+	60%	-	60%
Nurses 'Always' Communicated Well	300+	80%	-	76%
Pain 'Always' Well Controlled	300+	69%	-	69%
Room and Bathroom 'Always' Clean	300+	76%	-	71%
Timely Help 'Always' Received	300+	67%	-	64%
Would Definitely Recommend Hospital	300+	67%	-	69%

NOTE: Hospital profiles are in alphabetical order by state, then city, then hospital within the city; Rankings exclude hospitals with less than 25 cases except for patient surveys which excludes hospitals with less than 100 cases; (a) 100–299 cases; (1) The number of cases is too small to be sure how well a hospital is performing; (2) The hospital indicated that the data submitted for this measure were based on a sample of cases; (3) Data was collected during a shorter time period (fewer quarters) than the maximum possible time for this measure; (4) Suppressed for one or more quarters by CMS; (5) No data is available from the hospital for this measure; (6) Fewer than 100 patients completed the HCAHPS survey. Use these rates with caution, as the number of surveys may be too low to reliably assess hospital performance; (7) Survey results are based on less than 12 months of data; (8) Survey results are not available for this reporting period; (9) No or very few patients were eligible for the HCAHPS survey. The scores shown, if any, reflect a very small number of surveys; (10) A state average was not calculated because too few hospitals in the state submitted data; (11) There were discrepancies in the data collection process; Please refer to the User's Guide for a full explanation of data.

Western Pennsylvania Hospital - Forbes Regional Campus

2570 Haymaker Rd
Monroeville, PA 15146
URL: www.wpahs.org
Phone: 412-858-2000
Fax: 412-858-2532
Type: Acute Care Hospitals
Emergency Services: Yes
Ownership: Voluntary Non-Profit - Other
Beds: 340

Key Personnel:
CEO/President . . . . Jim Collins
Quality Assurance . . . . Ann Mitchell
Emergency Room . . . . Angela Henzler
Patient Relations . . . . Jaye Faher

Measure	Cases	This Hosp.	State Avg.	U.S. Avg.
Heart Attack Care				
ACE Inhibitor or ARB for LVSD	32	91%	95%	96%
Aspirin at Arrival	230	100%	99%	99%
Aspirin at Discharge	222	96%	99%	98%
Beta Blocker at Discharge	218	99%	99%	98%
Fibrinolytic Medication Timing	0	-	40%	55%
PCI Within 90 Minutes of Arrival	42	79%	88%	90%
Smoking Cessation Advice	64	100%	100%	99%
Chest Pain/Possible Heart Attack Care				
Aspirin at Arrival	86	86%	95%	95%
Median Time to ECG (minutes)	92	7	8	8
Median Time to Transfer (minutes)[1,3]	1	75	68	61
Fibrinolytic Medication Timing[3]	0	-	48%	54%
Heart Failure Care				
ACE Inhibitor or ARB for LVSD	173	96%	95%	94%
Discharge Instructions	470	85%	90%	88%
Evaluation of LVS Function	667	99%	99%	98%
Smoking Cessation Advice	77	100%	98%	98%
Pneumonia Care				
Appropriate Initial Antibiotic	215	94%	93%	92%
Blood Culture Timing	180	98%	96%	96%
Influenza Vaccine	229	86%	92%	91%
Initial Antibiotic Timing	303	92%	96%	95%
Pneumococcal Vaccine	311	93%	95%	93%
Smoking Cessation Advice	97	100%	98%	97%
Surgical Care Improvement Project				
Appropriate VTP Within 24 Hours	299	97%	95%	92%
Appropriate Hair Removal	969	99%	100%	99%
Appropriate Beta Blocker Usage	341	98%	94%	93%
Controlled Postoperative Blood Glucose	180	97%	96%	93%
Prophylactic Antibiotic Timing	703	100%	97%	97%
Prophylactic Antibiotic Timing (Outpatient)	281	83%	92%	92%
Prophylactic Antibiotic Selection	712	98%	98%	97%
Prophylactic Antibiotic Select. (Outpatient)	242	85%	93%	94%
Prophylactic Antibiotic Stopped	682	98%	95%	94%
Recommended VTP Ordered	300	98%	97%	94%
Urinary Catheter Removal	285	97%	95%	90%
Children's Asthma Care				
Received Systemic Corticosteroids	-	-	-	100%
Received Home Management Plan	-	-	-	71%
Received Reliever Medication	-	-	-	100%
Use of Medical Imaging				
Combination Abdominal CT Scan	483	0.083	0.203	0.191
Combination Chest CT Scan	345	0.020	0.026	0.054
Follow-up Mammogram/Ultrasound	324	17.6%	8.2%	8.4%
MRI for Low Back Pain	43	46.5%	32.4%	32.7%
Survey of Patients' Hospital Experiences				
Area Around Room 'Always' Quiet at Night	300+	42%	-	58%
Doctors 'Always' Communicated Well	300+	74%	-	80%
Home Recovery Information Given	300+	79%	-	82%
Hospital Given 9 or 10 on 10 Point Scale	300+	57%	-	67%
Meds 'Always' Explained Before Given	300+	55%	-	60%
Nurses 'Always' Communicated Well	300+	71%	-	76%
Pain 'Always' Well Controlled	300+	66%	-	69%
Room and Bathroom 'Always' Clean	300+	60%	-	71%
Timely Help 'Always' Received	300+	63%	-	64%
Would Definitely Recommend Hospital	300+	62%	-	69%

Montrose General Hospital

25 Grow Avenue
Montrose, PA 18801
E-mail: emhsweb@hotmail.com
URL: www.endlesscare.org
Phone: 570-278-3801
Fax: 570-278-3648
Type: Critical Access Hospitals
Emergency Services: Yes
Ownership: Voluntary Non-Profit - Private
Beds: 22

Key Personnel:
CEO/President . . . . Rexford O Catlin
Chief of Medical Staff . . . . Joseph Speicher, DO
Infection Control . . . . Joseph Speicher, DO
Operating Room . . . . David J Bertsch, RN
Quality Assurance . . . . Rex Catlin
Radiology . . . . Paul Shaderowfs, MD
Emergency Room . . . . Ihab Dana, MD
Intensive Care Unit . . . . Ann Marie Baldwin

Measure	Cases	This Hosp.	State Avg.	U.S. Avg.
Heart Attack Care				
ACE Inhibitor or ARB for LVSD[1,3]	1	100%	95%	96%
Aspirin at Arrival[1,3]	3	100%	99%	99%
Aspirin at Discharge[1,3]	1	100%	99%	98%
Beta Blocker at Discharge[1,3]	2	100%	99%	98%
Fibrinolytic Medication Timing[1,3]	1	100%	40%	55%
PCI Within 90 Minutes of Arrival[3]	0	-	88%	90%
Smoking Cessation Advice[3]	0	-	100%	99%
Chest Pain/Possible Heart Attack Care				
Aspirin at Arrival	-	-	95%	95%
Median Time to ECG (minutes)	-	-	8	8
Median Time to Transfer (minutes)	-	-	68	61
Fibrinolytic Medication Timing	-	-	48%	54%
Heart Failure Care				
ACE Inhibitor or ARB for LVSD[1]	11	91%	95%	94%
Discharge Instructions[1]	20	70%	90%	88%
Evaluation of LVS Function	27	70%	99%	98%
Smoking Cessation Advice[1]	4	100%	98%	98%
Pneumonia Care				
Appropriate Initial Antibiotic[1]	21	57%	93%	92%
Blood Culture Timing[1]	5	80%	96%	96%
Influenza Vaccine[1]	14	93%	92%	91%
Initial Antibiotic Timing	30	97%	96%	95%
Pneumococcal Vaccine	37	97%	95%	93%
Smoking Cessation Advice[1]	6	83%	98%	97%
Surgical Care Improvement Project				
Appropriate VTP Within 24 Hours[5]	0	-	95%	92%
Appropriate Hair Removal[5]	0	-	100%	99%
Appropriate Beta Blocker Usage[5]	0	-	94%	93%
Controlled Postoperative Blood Glucose[5]	0	-	96%	93%
Prophylactic Antibiotic Timing	97	59%	97%	97%
Prophylactic Antibiotic Timing (Outpatient)	-	-	92%	92%
Prophylactic Antibiotic Selection	97	100%	98%	97%
Prophylactic Antibiotic Select. (Outpatient)	-	-	93%	94%
Prophylactic Antibiotic Stopped	97	46%	95%	94%
Recommended VTP Ordered[5]	0	-	97%	94%
Urinary Catheter Removal[5]	0	-	95%	90%
Children's Asthma Care				
Received Systemic Corticosteroids	-	-	-	100%
Received Home Management Plan	-	-	-	71%
Received Reliever Medication	-	-	-	100%
Use of Medical Imaging				
Combination Abdominal CT Scan	-	-	0.203	0.191
Combination Chest CT Scan	-	-	0.026	0.054
Follow-up Mammogram/Ultrasound	-	-	8.2%	8.4%
MRI for Low Back Pain	-	-	32.4%	32.7%
Survey of Patients' Hospital Experiences				
Area Around Room 'Always' Quiet at Night[8]	-	-	-	58%
Doctors 'Always' Communicated Well[8]	-	-	-	80%
Home Recovery Information Given[8]	-	-	-	82%
Hospital Given 9 or 10 on 10 Point Scale[8]	-	-	-	67%
Meds 'Always' Explained Before Given[8]	-	-	-	60%
Nurses 'Always' Communicated Well[8]	-	-	-	76%
Pain 'Always' Well Controlled[8]	-	-	-	69%
Room and Bathroom 'Always' Clean[8]	-	-	-	71%
Timely Help 'Always' Received[8]	-	-	-	64%
Would Definitely Recommend Hospital[8]	-	-	-	69%

Excela Health Frick Hospital

508 South Church Street
Mount Pleasant, PA 15666
URL: www.excelahealth.org
Phone: 724-547-1500
Fax: 724-547-1131
Type: Acute Care Hospitals
Emergency Services: Yes
Ownership: Voluntary Non-Profit - Other
Beds: 171

Key Personnel:
CEO/President . . . . Joseph Teluso
Chief of Medical Staff . . . . Bruce Teich, MD
Operating Room . . . . Melissa Kaufman
Quality Assurance . . . . Al Rosatti
Radiology . . . . Matthew Banks

Measure	Cases	This Hosp.	State Avg.	U.S. Avg.
Heart Attack Care				
ACE Inhibitor or ARB for LVSD[1]	1	0%	95%	96%
Aspirin at Arrival	30	87%	99%	99%
Aspirin at Discharge[1]	13	92%	99%	98%
Beta Blocker at Discharge[1]	14	93%	99%	98%
Fibrinolytic Medication Timing	0	-	40%	55%
PCI Within 90 Minutes of Arrival	0	-	88%	90%
Smoking Cessation Advice	0	-	100%	99%
Chest Pain/Possible Heart Attack Care				
Aspirin at Arrival	106	99%	95%	95%
Median Time to ECG (minutes)	110	6	8	8
Median Time to Transfer (minutes)[1]	20	56	68	61
Fibrinolytic Medication Timing	0	-	48%	54%
Heart Failure Care				
ACE Inhibitor or ARB for LVSD	46	91%	95%	94%
Discharge Instructions	197	97%	90%	88%
Evaluation of LVS Function	223	100%	99%	98%
Smoking Cessation Advice	37	100%	98%	98%
Pneumonia Care				
Appropriate Initial Antibiotic	73	90%	93%	92%
Blood Culture Timing	97	100%	96%	96%
Influenza Vaccine	81	99%	92%	91%
Initial Antibiotic Timing	109	99%	96%	95%
Pneumococcal Vaccine	105	100%	95%	93%
Smoking Cessation Advice	29	100%	98%	97%
Surgical Care Improvement Project				
Appropriate VTP Within 24 Hours	64	97%	95%	92%
Appropriate Hair Removal	82	99%	100%	99%
Appropriate Beta Blocker Usage	27	93%	94%	93%
Controlled Postoperative Blood Glucose	0	-	96%	93%
Prophylactic Antibiotic Timing	39	97%	97%	97%
Prophylactic Antibiotic Timing (Outpatient)	43	95%	92%	92%
Prophylactic Antibiotic Selection	39	100%	98%	97%
Prophylactic Antibiotic Select. (Outpatient)	43	91%	93%	94%
Prophylactic Antibiotic Stopped	39	90%	95%	94%
Recommended VTP Ordered	64	97%	97%	94%
Urinary Catheter Removal[1]	14	100%	95%	90%
Children's Asthma Care				
Received Systemic Corticosteroids	-	-	-	100%
Received Home Management Plan	-	-	-	71%
Received Reliever Medication	-	-	-	100%
Use of Medical Imaging				
Combination Abdominal CT Scan	271	0.007	0.203	0.191
Combination Chest CT Scan	188	0.005	0.026	0.054
Follow-up Mammogram/Ultrasound	237	10.1%	8.2%	8.4%
MRI for Low Back Pain	37	45.9%	32.4%	32.7%
Survey of Patients' Hospital Experiences				
Area Around Room 'Always' Quiet at Night	300+	49%	-	58%
Doctors 'Always' Communicated Well	300+	84%	-	80%
Home Recovery Information Given	300+	84%	-	82%
Hospital Given 9 or 10 on 10 Point Scale	300+	71%	-	67%
Meds 'Always' Explained Before Given	300+	64%	-	60%
Nurses 'Always' Communicated Well	300+	82%	-	76%
Pain 'Always' Well Controlled	300+	72%	-	69%
Room and Bathroom 'Always' Clean	300+	76%	-	71%
Timely Help 'Always' Received	300+	69%	-	64%
Would Definitely Recommend Hospital	300+	72%	-	69%

NOTE: Hospital profiles are in alphabetical order by state, then city, then hospital within the city; Rankings exclude hospitals with less than 25 cases except for patient surveys which excludes hospitals with less than 100 cases; (a) 100–299 cases; (1) The number of cases is too small to be sure how well a hospital is performing; (2) The hospital indicated that the data submitted for this measure were based on a sample of cases; (3) Data was collected during a shorter time period (fewer quarters) than the maximum possible time for this measure; (4) Suppressed for one or more quarters by CMS; (5) No data is available from the hospital for this measure; (6) Fewer than 100 patients completed the HCAHPS survey. Use these rates with caution, as the number of surveys may be too low to reliably assess hospital performance; (7) Survey results are based on less than 12 months of data; (8) Survey results are not available for this reporting period; (9) No or very few patients were eligible for the HCAHPS survey. The scores shown, if any, reflect a very small number of surveys; (10) A state average was not calculated because too few hospitals in the state submitted data; (11) There were discrepancies in the data collection process; Please refer to the User's Guide for a full explanation of data.

Muncy Valley Hospital

215 East Water Street | Phone: 570-546-8282
Muncy, PA 17756 | Fax: 570-546-8009
URL: www.shscares.org
Type: Critical Access Hospitals | Emergency Services: Yes
Ownership: Voluntary Non-Profit - Church | Beds: 139

Key Personnel:
CEO/President. . . . . Steven P Johnson
Chief of Medical Staff. . . . . Timothy A Mannello
Quality Assurance . . . . Robert C Wallace
Emergency Room . . . . Mark Beyer, MD

Measure	Cases	This Hosp.	State Avg.	U.S. Avg.
Heart Attack Care				
ACE Inhibitor or ARB for LVSD[3]	0	-	95%	96%
Aspirin at Arrival[1,3]	3	100%	99%	99%
Aspirin at Discharge[1,3]	3	100%	99%	98%
Beta Blocker at Discharge[1,3]	3	100%	99%	98%
Fibrinolytic Medication Timing[3]	0	-	40%	55%
PCI Within 90 Minutes of Arrival[3]	0	-	88%	90%
Smoking Cessation Advice[3]	0	-	100%	99%
Chest Pain/Possible Heart Attack Care				
Aspirin at Arrival	-	-	95%	95%
Median Time to ECG (minutes)	-	-	8	8
Median Time to Transfer (minutes)	-	-	68	61
Fibrinolytic Medication Timing	-	-	48%	54%
Heart Failure Care				
ACE Inhibitor or ARB for LVSD[1]	11	91%	95%	94%
Discharge Instructions	26	73%	90%	88%
Evaluation of LVS Function	35	100%	99%	98%
Smoking Cessation Advice[1]	4	100%	98%	98%
Pneumonia Care				
Appropriate Initial Antibiotic	38	95%	93%	92%
Blood Culture Timing	31	94%	96%	96%
Influenza Vaccine	27	85%	92%	91%
Initial Antibiotic Timing	34	94%	96%	95%
Pneumococcal Vaccine	44	98%	95%	93%
Smoking Cessation Advice[1]	6	100%	98%	97%
Surgical Care Improvement Project				
Appropriate VTP Within 24 Hours[1]	13	85%	95%	92%
Appropriate Hair Removal[1]	14	86%	100%	99%
Appropriate Beta Blocker Usage[1]	3	100%	94%	93%
Controlled Postoperative Blood Glucose	0	-	96%	93%
Prophylactic Antibiotic Timing[1]	8	62%	97%	97%
Prophylactic Antibiotic Timing (Outpatient)	-	-	92%	92%
Prophylactic Antibiotic Selection[1]	8	88%	98%	97%
Prophylactic Antibiotic Select. (Outpatient)	-	-	93%	94%
Prophylactic Antibiotic Stopped[1]	8	88%	95%	94%
Recommended VTP Ordered[1]	13	85%	97%	94%
Urinary Catheter Removal[1]	2	100%	95%	90%
Children's Asthma Care				
Received Systemic Corticosteroids	-	-	-	100%
Received Home Management Plan	-	-	-	71%
Received Reliever Medication	-	-	-	100%
Use of Medical Imaging				
Combination Abdominal CT Scan	-	-	0.203	0.191
Combination Chest CT Scan	-	-	0.026	0.054
Follow-up Mammogram/Ultrasound	-	-	8.2%	8.4%
MRI for Low Back Pain	-	-	32.4%	32.7%
Survey of Patients' Hospital Experiences				
Area Around Room 'Always' Quiet at Night	(a)	59%	-	58%
Doctors 'Always' Communicated Well	(a)	86%	-	80%
Home Recovery Information Given	(a)	84%	-	82%
Hospital Given 9 or 10 on 10 Point Scale	(a)	74%	-	67%
Meds 'Always' Explained Before Given	(a)	64%	-	60%
Nurses 'Always' Communicated Well	(a)	82%	-	76%
Pain 'Always' Well Controlled	(a)	73%	-	69%
Room and Bathroom 'Always' Clean	(a)	81%	-	71%
Timely Help 'Always' Received	(a)	74%	-	64%
Would Definitely Recommend Hospital	(a)	75%	-	69%

Alle Kiski Medical Center

1301 Carlisle St | Phone: 412-224-5100
Natrona, PA 15065 | Fax: 724-226-7490
URL: www.wpahs.org
Type: Acute Care Hospitals | Emergency Services: Yes
Ownership: Voluntary Non-Profit - Other | Beds: 260

Key Personnel:
CEO/President. . . . . Ned Laubacher
Chief of Medical Staff. . . . . Mohan M. Patel, MD
Ambulatory Care . . . . Jeff Polana
Anesthesiology. . . . . Fred Weniger

Measure	Cases	This Hosp.	State Avg.	U.S. Avg.
Heart Attack Care				
ACE Inhibitor or ARB for LVSD[1]	16	100%	95%	96%
Aspirin at Arrival	167	98%	99%	99%
Aspirin at Discharge	103	100%	99%	98%
Beta Blocker at Discharge	104	100%	99%	98%
Fibrinolytic Medication Timing	0	-	40%	55%
PCI Within 90 Minutes of Arrival	0	-	88%	90%
Smoking Cessation Advice[1]	11	100%	100%	99%
Chest Pain/Possible Heart Attack Care				
Aspirin at Arrival	158	96%	95%	95%
Median Time to ECG (minutes)	165	10	8	8
Median Time to Transfer (minutes)	27	55	68	61
Fibrinolytic Medication Timing	0	-	48%	54%
Heart Failure Care				
ACE Inhibitor or ARB for LVSD	96	96%	95%	94%
Discharge Instructions	370	84%	90%	88%
Evaluation of LVS Function	469	100%	99%	98%
Smoking Cessation Advice	55	100%	98%	98%
Pneumonia Care				
Appropriate Initial Antibiotic	148	91%	93%	92%
Blood Culture Timing	69	99%	96%	96%
Influenza Vaccine	191	95%	92%	91%
Initial Antibiotic Timing	244	99%	96%	95%
Pneumococcal Vaccine	292	97%	95%	93%
Smoking Cessation Advice	112	100%	98%	97%
Surgical Care Improvement Project				
Appropriate VTP Within 24 Hours	220	100%	95%	92%
Appropriate Hair Removal	509	100%	100%	99%
Appropriate Beta Blocker Usage	148	84%	94%	93%
Controlled Postoperative Blood Glucose	0	-	96%	93%
Prophylactic Antibiotic Timing	344	97%	97%	97%
Prophylactic Antibiotic Timing (Outpatient)	210	88%	92%	92%
Prophylactic Antibiotic Selection	344	97%	98%	97%
Prophylactic Antibiotic Select. (Outpatient)	217	94%	93%	94%
Prophylactic Antibiotic Stopped	327	94%	95%	94%
Recommended VTP Ordered	220	100%	97%	94%
Urinary Catheter Removal	141	94%	95%	90%
Children's Asthma Care				
Received Systemic Corticosteroids	-	-	-	100%
Received Home Management Plan	-	-	-	71%
Received Reliever Medication	-	-	-	100%
Use of Medical Imaging				
Combination Abdominal CT Scan	536	0.397	0.203	0.191
Combination Chest CT Scan	412	0.005	0.026	0.054
Follow-up Mammogram/Ultrasound	700	17.4%	8.2%	8.4%
MRI for Low Back Pain	82	42.7%	32.4%	32.7%
Survey of Patients' Hospital Experiences				
Area Around Room 'Always' Quiet at Night	300+	39%	-	58%
Doctors 'Always' Communicated Well	300+	73%	-	80%
Home Recovery Information Given	300+	81%	-	82%
Hospital Given 9 or 10 on 10 Point Scale	300+	58%	-	67%
Meds 'Always' Explained Before Given	300+	55%	-	60%
Nurses 'Always' Communicated Well	300+	72%	-	76%
Pain 'Always' Well Controlled	300+	60%	-	69%
Room and Bathroom 'Always' Clean	300+	73%	-	71%
Timely Help 'Always' Received	300+	58%	-	64%
Would Definitely Recommend Hospital	300+	54%	-	69%

Jameson Memorial Hospital

1211 Wilmington Avenue | Phone: 724-658-9001
New Castle, PA 16105 | Fax: 724-656-4142
Type: Acute Care Hospitals | Emergency Services: Yes
Ownership: Voluntary Non-Profit - Other | Beds: 230

Key Personnel:
CEO/President. . . . . Douglas Danko, MD
Quality Assurance . . . . Holly Hampe
Radiology. . . . . Julian Proctor
Emergency Room . . . . Richard Wadas

Measure	Cases	This Hosp.	State Avg.	U.S. Avg.
Heart Attack Care				
ACE Inhibitor or ARB for LVSD[1]	12	75%	95%	96%
Aspirin at Arrival	137	97%	99%	99%
Aspirin at Discharge	98	96%	99%	98%
Beta Blocker at Discharge	95	99%	99%	98%
Fibrinolytic Medication Timing	0	-	40%	55%
PCI Within 90 Minutes of Arrival[1]	7	43%	88%	90%
Smoking Cessation Advice	27	100%	100%	99%
Chest Pain/Possible Heart Attack Care				
Aspirin at Arrival[1,3]	23	100%	95%	95%
Median Time to ECG (minutes)[1,3]	24	9	8	8
Median Time to Transfer (minutes)[1,3]	8	68	68	61
Fibrinolytic Medication Timing[3]	0	-	48%	54%
Heart Failure Care				
ACE Inhibitor or ARB for LVSD	94	83%	95%	94%
Discharge Instructions	285	91%	90%	88%
Evaluation of LVS Function	365	96%	99%	98%
Smoking Cessation Advice	35	100%	98%	98%
Pneumonia Care				
Appropriate Initial Antibiotic	162	93%	93%	92%
Blood Culture Timing	248	100%	96%	96%
Influenza Vaccine	210	84%	92%	91%
Initial Antibiotic Timing	269	98%	96%	95%
Pneumococcal Vaccine	299	89%	95%	93%
Smoking Cessation Advice	122	100%	98%	97%
Surgical Care Improvement Project				
Appropriate VTP Within 24 Hours	299	96%	95%	92%
Appropriate Hair Removal	561	100%	100%	99%
Appropriate Beta Blocker Usage	146	92%	94%	93%
Controlled Postoperative Blood Glucose	0	-	96%	93%
Prophylactic Antibiotic Timing	377	98%	97%	97%
Prophylactic Antibiotic Timing (Outpatient)	77	88%	92%	92%
Prophylactic Antibiotic Selection	379	94%	98%	97%
Prophylactic Antibiotic Select. (Outpatient)	70	86%	93%	94%
Prophylactic Antibiotic Stopped	355	97%	95%	94%
Recommended VTP Ordered	301	97%	97%	94%
Urinary Catheter Removal	65	82%	95%	90%
Children's Asthma Care				
Received Systemic Corticosteroids	-	-	-	100%
Received Home Management Plan	-	-	-	71%
Received Reliever Medication	-	-	-	100%
Use of Medical Imaging				
Combination Abdominal CT Scan	458	0.063	0.203	0.191
Combination Chest CT Scan	359	0.003	0.026	0.054
Follow-up Mammogram/Ultrasound	451	10.4%	8.2%	8.4%
MRI for Low Back Pain	52	46.2%	32.4%	32.7%
Survey of Patients' Hospital Experiences				
Area Around Room 'Always' Quiet at Night[11]	300+	44%	-	58%
Doctors 'Always' Communicated Well[11]	300+	79%	-	80%
Home Recovery Information Given[11]	300+	84%	-	82%
Hospital Given 9 or 10 on 10 Point Scale[11]	300+	53%	-	67%
Meds 'Always' Explained Before Given[11]	300+	56%	-	60%
Nurses 'Always' Communicated Well[11]	300+	73%	-	76%
Pain 'Always' Well Controlled[11]	300+	67%	-	69%
Room and Bathroom 'Always' Clean[11]	300+	73%	-	71%
Timely Help 'Always' Received[11]	300+	53%	-	64%
Would Definitely Recommend Hospital[11]	300+	47%	-	69%

NOTE: Hospital profiles are in alphabetical order by state, then city, then hospital within the city; Rankings exclude hospitals with less than 25 cases except for patient surveys which excludes hospitals with less than 100 cases; (a) 100–299 cases; (1) The number of cases is too small to be sure how well a hospital is performing; (2) The hospital indicated that the data submitted for this measure were based on a sample of cases; (3) Data was collected during a shorter time period (fewer quarters) than the maximum possible time for this measure; (4) Suppressed for one or more quarters by CMS; (5) No data is available from the hospital for this measure; (6) Fewer than 100 patients completed the HCAHPS survey. Use these rates with caution, as the number of surveys may be too low to reliably assess hospital performance; (7) Survey results are based on less than 12 months of data; (8) Survey results are not available for this reporting period; (9) No or very few patients were eligible for the HCAHPS survey. The scores shown, if any, reflect a very small number of surveys; (10) A state average was not calculated because too few hospitals in the state submitted data; (11) There were discrepancies in the data collection process; Please refer to the User's Guide for a full explanation of data.

Mercy Suburban Hospital

2701 Dekalb Pike
Norristown, PA 19401
URL: www.mercyhealth.org
Phone: 215-278-2000
Fax: 610-272-4642
Type: Acute Care Hospitals
Emergency Services: Yes
Ownership: Voluntary Non-Profit - Church
Beds: 140

Key Personnel:
Chief of Medical Staff.......... Joseph Koehler, DO
Infection Control.............. Cyndy Darcy, RN
Operating Room.............. Marc Alpert, RN
Quality Assurance............ Susan Paparella, RN
Radiology.................. David M Bolden, DO
Emergency Room........... Patrick Moran

Measure	Cases	This Hosp.	State Avg.	U.S. Avg.
Heart Attack Care				
ACE Inhibitor or ARB for LVSD[1]	1	100%	95%	96%
Aspirin at Arrival	35	100%	99%	99%
Aspirin at Discharge[1]	16	94%	99%	98%
Beta Blocker at Discharge[1]	20	100%	99%	98%
Fibrinolytic Medication Timing	0	-	40%	55%
PCI Within 90 Minutes of Arrival	0	-	88%	90%
Smoking Cessation Advice[1]	1	100%	100%	99%
Chest Pain/Possible Heart Attack Care				
Aspirin at Arrival	30	97%	95%	95%
Median Time to ECG (minutes)	30	11	8	8
Median Time to Transfer (minutes)[5]	0	-	68	61
Fibrinolytic Medication Timing[5]	0	-	48%	54%
Heart Failure Care				
ACE Inhibitor or ARB for LVSD	62	100%	95%	94%
Discharge Instructions	137	98%	90%	88%
Evaluation of LVS Function	193	100%	99%	98%
Smoking Cessation Advice	25	100%	98%	98%
Pneumonia Care				
Appropriate Initial Antibiotic	63	97%	93%	92%
Blood Culture Timing	146	98%	96%	96%
Influenza Vaccine	64	98%	92%	91%
Initial Antibiotic Timing	133	95%	96%	95%
Pneumococcal Vaccine	87	99%	95%	93%
Smoking Cessation Advice	45	100%	98%	97%
Surgical Care Improvement Project				
Appropriate VTP Within 24 Hours	123	97%	95%	92%
Appropriate Hair Removal	316	100%	100%	99%
Appropriate Beta Blocker Usage	89	96%	94%	93%
Controlled Postoperative Blood Glucose	0	-	96%	93%
Prophylactic Antibiotic Timing	184	100%	97%	97%
Prophylactic Antibiotic Timing (Outpatient)	58	98%	92%	92%
Prophylactic Antibiotic Selection	185	97%	98%	97%
Prophylactic Antibiotic Select. (Outpatient)	57	96%	93%	94%
Prophylactic Antibiotic Stopped	179	96%	95%	94%
Recommended VTP Ordered	123	98%	97%	94%
Urinary Catheter Removal	32	94%	95%	90%
Children's Asthma Care				
Received Systemic Corticosteroids	-	-	-	100%
Received Home Management Plan	-	-	-	71%
Received Reliever Medication	-	-	-	100%
Use of Medical Imaging				
Combination Abdominal CT Scan	410	0.059	0.203	0.191
Combination Chest CT Scan	217	0.000	0.026	0.054
Follow-up Mammogram/Ultrasound	363	7.7%	8.2%	8.4%
MRI for Low Back Pain	55	36.4%	32.4%	32.7%
Survey of Patients' Hospital Experiences				
Area Around Room 'Always' Quiet at Night	300+	37%	-	58%
Doctors 'Always' Communicated Well	300+	76%	-	80%
Home Recovery Information Given	300+	85%	-	82%
Hospital Given 9 or 10 on 10 Point Scale	300+	57%	-	67%
Meds 'Always' Explained Before Given	300+	58%	-	60%
Nurses 'Always' Communicated Well	300+	71%	-	76%
Pain 'Always' Well Controlled	300+	65%	-	69%
Room and Bathroom 'Always' Clean	300+	57%	-	71%
Timely Help 'Always' Received	300+	51%	-	64%
Would Definitely Recommend Hospital	300+	58%	-	69%

Montgomery Hospital

Powell & Fornance Streets
Norristown, PA 19401
URL: www.montgomeryhospital.org
Phone: 610-270-2000
Fax: 610-270-2728
Type: Acute Care Hospitals
Emergency Services: Yes
Ownership: Voluntary Non-Profit - Private
Beds: 210

Key Personnel:
CEO/President............... Timothy M Casey
Chief of Medical Staff.......... James Obrien, MD
Operating Room.............. Cosme Manzarbeitia, RN
Pediatric In-Patient Care....... Mary Ann Gazdick, MD
Quality Assurance............ Linda Bieber
Radiology.................. John E Devenney
Emergency Room........... Linda West

Measure	Cases	This Hosp.	State Avg.	U.S. Avg.
Heart Attack Care				
ACE Inhibitor or ARB for LVSD	32	94%	95%	96%
Aspirin at Arrival	128	98%	99%	99%
Aspirin at Discharge	131	98%	99%	98%
Beta Blocker at Discharge	133	98%	99%	98%
Fibrinolytic Medication Timing	0	-	40%	55%
PCI Within 90 Minutes of Arrival	25	100%	88%	90%
Smoking Cessation Advice	44	100%	100%	99%
Chest Pain/Possible Heart Attack Care				
Aspirin at Arrival[5]	0	-	95%	95%
Median Time to ECG (minutes)[5]	0	-	8	8
Median Time to Transfer (minutes)[5]	0	-	68	61
Fibrinolytic Medication Timing[5]	0	-	48%	54%
Heart Failure Care				
ACE Inhibitor or ARB for LVSD	69	88%	95%	94%
Discharge Instructions	191	91%	90%	88%
Evaluation of LVS Function	234	99%	99%	98%
Smoking Cessation Advice	39	100%	98%	98%
Pneumonia Care				
Appropriate Initial Antibiotic	82	90%	93%	92%
Blood Culture Timing	66	97%	96%	96%
Influenza Vaccine	68	91%	92%	91%
Initial Antibiotic Timing	105	93%	96%	95%
Pneumococcal Vaccine	90	92%	95%	93%
Smoking Cessation Advice	29	100%	98%	97%
Surgical Care Improvement Project				
Appropriate VTP Within 24 Hours[2]	60	68%	95%	92%
Appropriate Hair Removal[2]	291	100%	100%	99%
Appropriate Beta Blocker Usage[2]	106	87%	94%	93%
Controlled Postoperative Blood Glucose[2]	0	-	96%	93%
Prophylactic Antibiotic Timing[2]	197	92%	97%	97%
Prophylactic Antibiotic Timing (Outpatient)	59	95%	92%	92%
Prophylactic Antibiotic Selection[2]	194	98%	98%	97%
Prophylactic Antibiotic Select. (Outpatient)	58	93%	93%	94%
Prophylactic Antibiotic Stopped[2]	192	100%	95%	94%
Recommended VTP Ordered[2]	60	78%	97%	94%
Urinary Catheter Removal[1,2]	19	84%	95%	90%
Children's Asthma Care				
Received Systemic Corticosteroids	-	-	-	100%
Received Home Management Plan	-	-	-	71%
Received Reliever Medication	-	-	-	100%
Use of Medical Imaging				
Combination Abdominal CT Scan	465	0.112	0.203	0.191
Combination Chest CT Scan	348	0.006	0.026	0.054
Follow-up Mammogram/Ultrasound	725	6.8%	8.2%	8.4%
MRI for Low Back Pain	77	22.1%	32.4%	32.7%
Survey of Patients' Hospital Experiences				
Area Around Room 'Always' Quiet at Night	300+	50%	-	58%
Doctors 'Always' Communicated Well	300+	76%	-	80%
Home Recovery Information Given	300+	79%	-	82%
Hospital Given 9 or 10 on 10 Point Scale	300+	52%	-	67%
Meds 'Always' Explained Before Given	300+	57%	-	60%
Nurses 'Always' Communicated Well	300+	75%	-	76%
Pain 'Always' Well Controlled	300+	67%	-	69%
Room and Bathroom 'Always' Clean	300+	60%	-	71%
Timely Help 'Always' Received	300+	64%	-	64%
Would Definitely Recommend Hospital	300+	54%	-	69%

Valley Forge Medical Center and Hospital

1033 W Germantown Pike
Norristown, PA 19401
E-mail: gslocum@vfmc.net
URL: www.vfmc.net
Phone: 215-539-8500
Fax: 610-539-0910
Type: Acute Care Hospitals
Emergency Services: No
Ownership: Proprietary
Beds: 78

Key Personnel:
CEO/President............... Marian Colcher, MSW
Chief of Medical Staff.......... Robert E Colcher, MD
Quality Assurance............ Frederick Jakes
Patient Relations............ Maureen King

Measure	Cases	This Hosp.	State Avg.	U.S. Avg.
Heart Attack Care				
ACE Inhibitor or ARB for LVSD[5]	0	-	95%	96%
Aspirin at Arrival[5]	0	-	99%	99%
Aspirin at Discharge[5]	0	-	99%	98%
Beta Blocker at Discharge[5]	0	-	99%	98%
Fibrinolytic Medication Timing[5]	0	-	40%	55%
PCI Within 90 Minutes of Arrival[5]	0	-	88%	90%
Smoking Cessation Advice[5]	0	-	100%	99%
Chest Pain/Possible Heart Attack Care				
Aspirin at Arrival	-	-	95%	95%
Median Time to ECG (minutes)	-	-	8	8
Median Time to Transfer (minutes)	-	-	68	61
Fibrinolytic Medication Timing	-	-	48%	54%
Heart Failure Care				
ACE Inhibitor or ARB for LVSD[5]	0	-	95%	94%
Discharge Instructions[5]	0	-	90%	88%
Evaluation of LVS Function[5]	0	-	99%	98%
Smoking Cessation Advice[5]	0	-	98%	98%
Pneumonia Care				
Appropriate Initial Antibiotic[5]	0	-	93%	92%
Blood Culture Timing[5]	0	-	96%	96%
Influenza Vaccine[5]	0	-	92%	91%
Initial Antibiotic Timing[5]	0	-	96%	95%
Pneumococcal Vaccine[5]	0	-	95%	93%
Smoking Cessation Advice[5]	0	-	98%	97%
Surgical Care Improvement Project				
Appropriate VTP Within 24 Hours[5]	0	-	95%	92%
Appropriate Hair Removal[5]	0	-	100%	99%
Appropriate Beta Blocker Usage[5]	0	-	94%	93%
Controlled Postoperative Blood Glucose[5]	0	-	96%	93%
Prophylactic Antibiotic Timing[5]	0	-	97%	97%
Prophylactic Antibiotic Timing (Outpatient)	-	-	92%	92%
Prophylactic Antibiotic Selection[5]	0	-	98%	97%
Prophylactic Antibiotic Select. (Outpatient)	-	-	93%	94%
Prophylactic Antibiotic Stopped[5]	0	-	95%	94%
Recommended VTP Ordered[5]	0	-	97%	94%
Urinary Catheter Removal[5]	0	-	95%	90%
Children's Asthma Care				
Received Systemic Corticosteroids	-	-	-	100%
Received Home Management Plan	-	-	-	71%
Received Reliever Medication	-	-	-	100%
Use of Medical Imaging				
Combination Abdominal CT Scan	-	-	0.203	0.191
Combination Chest CT Scan	-	-	0.026	0.054
Follow-up Mammogram/Ultrasound	-	-	8.2%	8.4%
MRI for Low Back Pain	-	-	32.4%	32.7%
Survey of Patients' Hospital Experiences				
Area Around Room 'Always' Quiet at Night[9]	-	-	-	58%
Doctors 'Always' Communicated Well[9]	-	-	-	80%
Home Recovery Information Given[9]	-	-	-	82%
Hospital Given 9 or 10 on 10 Point Scale[9]	-	-	-	67%
Meds 'Always' Explained Before Given[9]	-	-	-	60%
Nurses 'Always' Communicated Well[9]	-	-	-	76%
Pain 'Always' Well Controlled[9]	-	-	-	69%
Room and Bathroom 'Always' Clean[9]	-	-	-	71%
Timely Help 'Always' Received[9]	-	-	-	64%
Would Definitely Recommend Hospital[9]	-	-	-	69%

NOTE: Hospital profiles are in alphabetical order by state, then city, then hospital within the city; Rankings exclude hospitals with less than 25 cases except for patient surveys which excludes hospitals with less than 100 cases; (a) 100–299 cases; (1) The number of cases is too small to be sure how well a hospital is performing; (2) The hospital indicated that the data submitted for this measure were based on a sample of cases; (3) Data was collected during a shorter time period (fewer quarters) than the maximum possible time for this measure; (4) Suppressed for one or more quarters by CMS; (5) No data is available from the hospital for this measure; (6) Fewer than 100 patients completed the HCAHPS survey. Use these rates with caution, as the number of surveys may be too low to reliably assess hospital performance; (7) Survey results are based on less than 12 months of data; (8) Survey results are not available for this reporting period; (9) No or very few patients were eligible for the HCAHPS survey. The scores shown, if any, reflect a very small number of surveys; (10) A state average was not calculated because too few hospitals in the state submitted data; (11) There were discrepancies in the data collection process; Please refer to the User's Guide for a full explanation of data.

Palmerton Hospital

135 Lafayette Avenue Phone: 610-826-3141
Palmerton, PA 18071 Fax: 610-826-1282
URL: www.palmertonhospital.com
Type: Acute Care Hospitals Emergency Services: Yes
Ownership: Voluntary Non-Profit - Other Beds: 70

Key Personnel:
CEO/President. . . . . Richard Hager
Chief of Medical Staff. . . . . Thomas Tachousky, MD
Infection Control. . . . . Doreen Harleman, RN
Operating Room. . . . . Betty Ann Flyte, RN
Pediatric In-Patient Care . . . . . . Nancy Andreas, RN
Quality Assurance . . . . Susanne Garszczynski, PhD
Radiology. . . . . Edie Berger
Patient Relations . . . . Dana Beisel

Measure	Cases	This Hosp.	State Avg.	U.S. Avg.
Heart Attack Care				
ACE Inhibitor or ARB for LVSD[1]	2	50%	95%	96%
Aspirin at Arrival[1]	15	93%	99%	99%
Aspirin at Discharge[1]	9	100%	99%	98%
Beta Blocker at Discharge[1]	8	100%	99%	98%
Fibrinolytic Medication Timing	0	-	40%	55%
PCI Within 90 Minutes of Arrival	0	-	88%	90%
Smoking Cessation Advice[1]	2	100%	100%	99%
Chest Pain/Possible Heart Attack Care				
Aspirin at Arrival	40	90%	95%	95%
Median Time to ECG (minutes)	42	4	8	8
Median Time to Transfer (minutes)[1]	7	58	68	61
Fibrinolytic Medication Timing	0	-	48%	54%
Heart Failure Care				
ACE Inhibitor or ARB for LVSD	30	83%	95%	94%
Discharge Instructions	90	89%	90%	88%
Evaluation of LVS Function	115	94%	99%	98%
Smoking Cessation Advice[1]	7	86%	98%	98%
Pneumonia Care				
Appropriate Initial Antibiotic	41	76%	93%	92%
Blood Culture Timing	55	96%	96%	96%
Influenza Vaccine	35	89%	92%	91%
Initial Antibiotic Timing	56	91%	96%	95%
Pneumococcal Vaccine	54	98%	95%	93%
Smoking Cessation Advice[1]	15	93%	98%	97%
Surgical Care Improvement Project				
Appropriate VTP Within 24 Hours	58	88%	95%	92%
Appropriate Hair Removal	106	100%	100%	99%
Appropriate Beta Blocker Usage	31	94%	94%	93%
Controlled Postoperative Blood Glucose	0	-	96%	93%
Prophylactic Antibiotic Timing	55	93%	97%	97%
Prophylactic Antibiotic Timing (Outpatient)	78	69%	92%	92%
Prophylactic Antibiotic Selection	55	98%	98%	97%
Prophylactic Antibiotic Select. (Outpatient)	64	91%	93%	94%
Prophylactic Antibiotic Stopped	54	87%	95%	94%
Recommended VTP Ordered	58	88%	97%	94%
Urinary Catheter Removal	25	88%	95%	90%
Children's Asthma Care				
Received Systemic Corticosteroids	-	-	-	100%
Received Home Management Plan	-	-	-	71%
Received Reliever Medication	-	-	-	100%
Use of Medical Imaging				
Combination Abdominal CT Scan	347	0.026	0.203	0.191
Combination Chest CT Scan	268	0.004	0.026	0.054
Follow-up Mammogram/Ultrasound	505	15.4%	8.2%	8.4%
MRI for Low Back Pain[5]	0	-	32.4%	32.7%
Survey of Patients' Hospital Experiences				
Area Around Room 'Always' Quiet at Night	300+	52%	-	58%
Doctors 'Always' Communicated Well	300+	75%	-	80%
Home Recovery Information Given	300+	82%	-	82%
Hospital Given 9 or 10 on 10 Point Scale	300+	61%	-	67%
Meds 'Always' Explained Before Given	300+	63%	-	60%
Nurses 'Always' Communicated Well	300+	74%	-	76%
Pain 'Always' Well Controlled	300+	71%	-	69%
Room and Bathroom 'Always' Clean	300+	74%	-	71%
Timely Help 'Always' Received	300+	62%	-	64%
Would Definitely Recommend Hospital	300+	56%	-	69%

Main Line Hospital Paoli

255 West Lancaster Avenue Phone: 610-648-1000
Paoli, PA 19301 Fax: 610-526-4047
URL: www.mainlinehealth.org
Type: Acute Care Hospitals Emergency Services: Yes
Ownership: Voluntary Non-Profit - Private Beds: 208

Key Personnel:
CEO/President. . . . . Barbara Tachovsky, RN/MS
Infection Control. . . . . David Trevino, MD
Operating Room. . . . . William M Dellevigne
Emergency Room . . . . Donald J Armstrong, MD

Measure	Cases	This Hosp.	State Avg.	U.S. Avg.
Heart Attack Care				
ACE Inhibitor or ARB for LVSD[1]	10	100%	95%	96%
Aspirin at Arrival	153	99%	99%	99%
Aspirin at Discharge	136	100%	99%	98%
Beta Blocker at Discharge	131	99%	99%	98%
Fibrinolytic Medication Timing	0	-	40%	55%
PCI Within 90 Minutes of Arrival	25	88%	88%	90%
Smoking Cessation Advice[1]	19	100%	100%	99%
Chest Pain/Possible Heart Attack Care				
Aspirin at Arrival[1]	9	67%	95%	95%
Median Time to ECG (minutes)[1]	9	5	8	8
Median Time to Transfer (minutes)[5]	0	-	68	61
Fibrinolytic Medication Timing[5]	0	-	48%	54%
Heart Failure Care				
ACE Inhibitor or ARB for LVSD	68	100%	95%	94%
Discharge Instructions	181	99%	90%	88%
Evaluation of LVS Function	246	100%	99%	98%
Smoking Cessation Advice[1]	20	100%	98%	98%
Pneumonia Care				
Appropriate Initial Antibiotic	127	97%	93%	92%
Blood Culture Timing	164	100%	96%	96%
Influenza Vaccine	132	96%	92%	91%
Initial Antibiotic Timing	168	96%	96%	95%
Pneumococcal Vaccine	186	99%	95%	93%
Smoking Cessation Advice	34	100%	98%	97%
Surgical Care Improvement Project				
Appropriate VTP Within 24 Hours[2]	234	98%	95%	92%
Appropriate Hair Removal[2]	912	100%	100%	99%
Appropriate Beta Blocker Usage[2]	237	99%	94%	93%
Controlled Postoperative Blood Glucose[2]	82	95%	96%	93%
Prophylactic Antibiotic Timing[2]	715	99%	97%	97%
Prophylactic Antibiotic Timing (Outpatient)	197	95%	92%	92%
Prophylactic Antibiotic Selection[2]	720	98%	98%	97%
Prophylactic Antibiotic Select. (Outpatient)	193	92%	93%	94%
Prophylactic Antibiotic Stopped[2]	660	99%	95%	94%
Recommended VTP Ordered[2]	235	99%	97%	94%
Urinary Catheter Removal[2]	241	100%	95%	90%
Children's Asthma Care				
Received Systemic Corticosteroids	-	-	-	100%
Received Home Management Plan	-	-	-	71%
Received Reliever Medication	-	-	-	100%
Use of Medical Imaging				
Combination Abdominal CT Scan	1,237	0.113	0.203	0.191
Combination Chest CT Scan	1,044	0.019	0.026	0.054
Follow-up Mammogram/Ultrasound	1,544	7.2%	8.2%	8.4%
MRI for Low Back Pain[1]	2	50.0%	32.4%	32.7%
Survey of Patients' Hospital Experiences				
Area Around Room 'Always' Quiet at Night	300+	54%	-	58%
Doctors 'Always' Communicated Well	300+	79%	-	80%
Home Recovery Information Given	300+	79%	-	82%
Hospital Given 9 or 10 on 10 Point Scale	300+	81%	-	67%
Meds 'Always' Explained Before Given	300+	61%	-	60%
Nurses 'Always' Communicated Well	300+	80%	-	76%
Pain 'Always' Well Controlled	300+	73%	-	69%
Room and Bathroom 'Always' Clean	300+	73%	-	71%
Timely Help 'Always' Received	300+	63%	-	64%
Would Definitely Recommend Hospital	300+	87%	-	69%

Mid-Valley Hospital

1400 South Main Street Phone: 570-383-5500
Peckville, PA 18452 Fax: 570-383-5504
Type: Critical Access Hospitals Emergency Services: Yes
Ownership: Voluntary Non-Profit - Other Beds: 25

Key Personnel:
Cardiac Laboratory. . . . . W David Filvatatrick
Quality Assurance . . . . Katie Sunday
Emergency Room . . . . Frank Schell, MD

Measure	Cases	This Hosp.	State Avg.	U.S. Avg.
Heart Attack Care				
ACE Inhibitor or ARB for LVSD[1,3]	1	0%	95%	96%
Aspirin at Arrival[1,3]	6	83%	99%	99%
Aspirin at Discharge[1,3]	1	0%	99%	98%
Beta Blocker at Discharge[1,3]	2	100%	99%	98%
Fibrinolytic Medication Timing[3]	0	-	40%	55%
PCI Within 90 Minutes of Arrival[3]	0	-	88%	90%
Smoking Cessation Advice[3]	0	-	100%	99%
Chest Pain/Possible Heart Attack Care				
Aspirin at Arrival	-	-	95%	95%
Median Time to ECG (minutes)	-	-	8	8
Median Time to Transfer (minutes)	-	-	68	61
Fibrinolytic Medication Timing	-	-	48%	54%
Heart Failure Care				
ACE Inhibitor or ARB for LVSD[1,2,3]	7	100%	95%	94%
Discharge Instructions[1,2,3]	22	95%	90%	88%
Evaluation of LVS Function[2,3]	33	100%	99%	98%
Smoking Cessation Advice[1,2,3]	2	100%	98%	98%
Pneumonia Care				
Appropriate Initial Antibiotic[1,3]	19	95%	93%	92%
Blood Culture Timing[3]	31	90%	96%	96%
Influenza Vaccine[1,3]	14	100%	92%	91%
Initial Antibiotic Timing[3]	30	93%	96%	95%
Pneumococcal Vaccine[3]	32	100%	95%	93%
Smoking Cessation Advice[1,3]	5	100%	98%	97%
Surgical Care Improvement Project				
Appropriate VTP Within 24 Hours[5]	0	-	95%	92%
Appropriate Hair Removal[5]	0	-	100%	99%
Appropriate Beta Blocker Usage[5]	0	-	94%	93%
Controlled Postoperative Blood Glucose[5]	0	-	96%	93%
Prophylactic Antibiotic Timing[5]	0	-	97%	97%
Prophylactic Antibiotic Timing (Outpatient)	-	-	92%	92%
Prophylactic Antibiotic Selection[5]	0	-	98%	97%
Prophylactic Antibiotic Select. (Outpatient)	-	-	93%	94%
Prophylactic Antibiotic Stopped[5]	0	-	95%	94%
Recommended VTP Ordered[5]	0	-	97%	94%
Urinary Catheter Removal[5]	0	-	95%	90%
Children's Asthma Care				
Received Systemic Corticosteroids	-	-	-	100%
Received Home Management Plan	-	-	-	71%
Received Reliever Medication	-	-	-	100%
Use of Medical Imaging				
Combination Abdominal CT Scan	-	-	0.203	0.191
Combination Chest CT Scan	-	-	0.026	0.054
Follow-up Mammogram/Ultrasound	-	-	8.2%	8.4%
MRI for Low Back Pain	-	-	32.4%	32.7%
Survey of Patients' Hospital Experiences				
Area Around Room 'Always' Quiet at Night[8]	-	-	-	58%
Doctors 'Always' Communicated Well[8]	-	-	-	80%
Home Recovery Information Given[8]	-	-	-	82%
Hospital Given 9 or 10 on 10 Point Scale[8]	-	-	-	67%
Meds 'Always' Explained Before Given[8]	-	-	-	60%
Nurses 'Always' Communicated Well[8]	-	-	-	76%
Pain 'Always' Well Controlled[8]	-	-	-	69%
Room and Bathroom 'Always' Clean[8]	-	-	-	71%
Timely Help 'Always' Received[8]	-	-	-	64%
Would Definitely Recommend Hospital[8]	-	-	-	69%

NOTE: Hospital profiles are in alphabetical order by state, then city, then hospital within the city; Rankings exclude hospitals with less than 25 cases except for patient surveys which excludes hospitals with less than 100 cases; (a) 100–299 cases; (1) The number of cases is too small to be sure how well a hospital is performing; (2) The hospital indicated that the data submitted for this measure were based on a sample of cases; (3) Data was collected during a shorter time period (fewer quarters) than the maximum possible time for this measure; (4) Suppressed for one or more quarters by CMS; (5) No data is available from the hospital for this measure; (6) Fewer than 100 patients completed the HCAHPS survey. Use these rates with caution, as the number of surveys may be too low to reliably assess hospital performance; (7) Survey results are based on less than 12 months of data; (8) Survey results are not available for this reporting period; (9) No or very few patients were eligible for the HCAHPS survey. The scores shown, if any, reflect a very small number of surveys; (10) A state average was not calculated because too few hospitals in the state submitted data; (11) There were discrepancies in the data collection process; Please refer to the User's Guide for a full explanation of data.

Roxborough Memorial Hospital

5800 Ridge Ave — Phone: 215-483-9900
Phila, PA 19128 — Fax: 215-487-4221
URL: www.roxboroughmemorial.com
Type: Acute Care Hospitals — Emergency Services: No
Ownership: Proprietary — Beds: 165

Key Personnel:
CEO/President. . . . . John J Donnelly, Jr
Pediatric Ambulatory Care . . . . . . Charlene Brock, MD
Pediatric In-Patient Care . . . . Charlene Brock, MD
Quality Assurance . . . . Kathleen Phillips
Radiology. . . . . Laurie Gutstein, MD
Emergency Room . . . . Robert Cameron, MD

Measure	Cases	This Hosp.	State Avg.	U.S. Avg.
Heart Attack Care				
ACE Inhibitor or ARB for LVSD[1]	2	50%	95%	96%
Aspirin at Arrival	41	95%	99%	99%
Aspirin at Discharge[1]	21	90%	99%	98%
Beta Blocker at Discharge[1]	21	100%	99%	98%
Fibrinolytic Medication Timing	0	-	40%	55%
PCI Within 90 Minutes of Arrival	0	-	88%	90%
Smoking Cessation Advice[1]	6	100%	100%	99%
Chest Pain/Possible Heart Attack Care				
Aspirin at Arrival[5]	0	-	95%	95%
Median Time to ECG (minutes)[5]	0	-	8	8
Median Time to Transfer (minutes)[5]	0	-	68	61
Fibrinolytic Medication Timing[5]	0	-	48%	54%
Heart Failure Care				
ACE Inhibitor or ARB for LVSD	69	87%	95%	94%
Discharge Instructions	131	93%	90%	88%
Evaluation of LVS Function	206	99%	99%	98%
Smoking Cessation Advice	51	100%	98%	98%
Pneumonia Care				
Appropriate Initial Antibiotic	43	98%	93%	92%
Blood Culture Timing	92	90%	96%	96%
Influenza Vaccine	49	90%	92%	91%
Initial Antibiotic Timing	104	98%	96%	95%
Pneumococcal Vaccine	98	91%	95%	93%
Smoking Cessation Advice	37	100%	98%	97%
Surgical Care Improvement Project				
Appropriate VTP Within 24 Hours	81	95%	95%	92%
Appropriate Hair Removal	144	100%	100%	99%
Appropriate Beta Blocker Usage	40	100%	94%	93%
Controlled Postoperative Blood Glucose	0	-	96%	93%
Prophylactic Antibiotic Timing	66	98%	97%	97%
Prophylactic Antibiotic Timing (Outpatient)	52	100%	92%	92%
Prophylactic Antibiotic Selection	70	96%	98%	97%
Prophylactic Antibiotic Select. (Outpatient)	52	98%	93%	94%
Prophylactic Antibiotic Stopped	64	91%	95%	94%
Recommended VTP Ordered	81	96%	97%	94%
Urinary Catheter Removal	39	97%	95%	90%
Children's Asthma Care				
Received Systemic Corticosteroids	-	-	-	100%
Received Home Management Plan	-	-	-	71%
Received Reliever Medication	-	-	-	100%
Use of Medical Imaging				
Combination Abdominal CT Scan	146	0.110	0.203	0.191
Combination Chest CT Scan	112	0.018	0.026	0.054
Follow-up Mammogram/Ultrasound	327	5.2%	8.2%	8.4%
MRI for Low Back Pain[1]	9	44.4%	32.4%	32.7%
Survey of Patients' Hospital Experiences				
Area Around Room 'Always' Quiet at Night	300+	40%	-	58%
Doctors 'Always' Communicated Well	300+	74%	-	80%
Home Recovery Information Given	300+	76%	-	82%
Hospital Given 9 or 10 on 10 Point Scale	300+	50%	-	67%
Meds 'Always' Explained Before Given	300+	54%	-	60%
Nurses 'Always' Communicated Well	300+	70%	-	76%
Pain 'Always' Well Controlled	300+	60%	-	69%
Room and Bathroom 'Always' Clean	300+	56%	-	71%
Timely Help 'Always' Received	300+	51%	-	64%
Would Definitely Recommend Hospital	300+	47%	-	69%

Albert Einstein Medical Center

5501 Old York Road — Phone: 215-456-6090
Philadelphia, PA 19141 — Fax: 215-456-6242
URL: www.einstein.edu
Type: Acute Care Hospitals — Emergency Services: Yes
Ownership: Voluntary Non-Profit - Other — Beds: 987

Key Personnel:
CEO/President. . . . . Martin Goldsmith
Chief of Medical Staff . . . . Leonard Greenberg, MD
Infection Control. . . . . Robert Fisher, MD
Operating Room. . . . . Cathy Costello
Pediatric In-Patient Care . . . . Allan Arbeter, MD
Quality Assurance . . . . Sara Potter
Radiology. . . . . Henrietta Rosenburg, MD
Emergency Room . . . . Patty Lynch

Measure	Cases	This Hosp.	State Avg.	U.S. Avg.
Heart Attack Care				
ACE Inhibitor or ARB for LVSD	68	97%	95%	96%
Aspirin at Arrival	243	99%	99%	99%
Aspirin at Discharge	301	99%	99%	98%
Beta Blocker at Discharge	292	98%	99%	98%
Fibrinolytic Medication Timing[1]	1	100%	40%	55%
PCI Within 90 Minutes of Arrival	42	95%	88%	90%
Smoking Cessation Advice	114	100%	100%	99%
Chest Pain/Possible Heart Attack Care				
Aspirin at Arrival[1,3]	2	100%	95%	95%
Median Time to ECG (minutes)[1,3]	2	8	8	8
Median Time to Transfer (minutes)[5]	0	-	68	61
Fibrinolytic Medication Timing[5]	0	-	48%	54%
Heart Failure Care				
ACE Inhibitor or ARB for LVSD[2]	142	93%	95%	94%
Discharge Instructions[2]	221	96%	90%	88%
Evaluation of LVS Function[2]	305	99%	99%	98%
Smoking Cessation Advice[2]	96	100%	98%	98%
Pneumonia Care				
Appropriate Initial Antibiotic	99	98%	93%	92%
Blood Culture Timing	203	94%	96%	96%
Influenza Vaccine	138	83%	92%	91%
Initial Antibiotic Timing	241	98%	96%	95%
Pneumococcal Vaccine	176	92%	95%	93%
Smoking Cessation Advice	155	100%	98%	97%
Surgical Care Improvement Project				
Appropriate VTP Within 24 Hours[2]	308	99%	95%	92%
Appropriate Hair Removal[2]	738	100%	100%	99%
Appropriate Beta Blocker Usage[2]	200	98%	94%	93%
Controlled Postoperative Blood Glucose[2]	89	93%	96%	93%
Prophylactic Antibiotic Timing[2]	498	98%	97%	97%
Prophylactic Antibiotic Timing (Outpatient)	252	93%	92%	92%
Prophylactic Antibiotic Selection[2]	511	98%	98%	97%
Prophylactic Antibiotic Select. (Outpatient)	240	92%	93%	94%
Prophylactic Antibiotic Stopped[2]	481	99%	95%	94%
Recommended VTP Ordered[2]	308	99%	97%	94%
Urinary Catheter Removal[2]	222	95%	95%	90%
Children's Asthma Care				
Received Systemic Corticosteroids	-	-	-	100%
Received Home Management Plan	-	-	-	71%
Received Reliever Medication	-	-	-	100%
Use of Medical Imaging				
Combination Abdominal CT Scan	838	0.094	0.203	0.191
Combination Chest CT Scan	533	0.021	0.026	0.054
Follow-up Mammogram/Ultrasound	2,369	5.4%	8.2%	8.4%
MRI for Low Back Pain	143	29.4%	32.4%	32.7%
Survey of Patients' Hospital Experiences				
Area Around Room 'Always' Quiet at Night	300+	50%	-	58%
Doctors 'Always' Communicated Well	300+	73%	-	80%
Home Recovery Information Given	300+	77%	-	82%
Hospital Given 9 or 10 on 10 Point Scale	300+	55%	-	67%
Meds 'Always' Explained Before Given	300+	56%	-	60%
Nurses 'Always' Communicated Well	300+	67%	-	76%
Pain 'Always' Well Controlled	300+	64%	-	69%
Room and Bathroom 'Always' Clean	300+	60%	-	71%
Timely Help 'Always' Received	300+	51%	-	64%
Would Definitely Recommend Hospital	300+	55%	-	69%

Aria Health

10800 Knights Road — Phone: 215-612-4129
Philadelphia, PA 19114
URL: www.ariahealth.com
Type: Acute Care Hospitals — Emergency Services: Yes
Ownership: Voluntary Non-Profit - Private — Beds: 252

Key Personnel:
Cardiology . . . . Khalid Almuti, MD
Pediatrics. . . . . Barbara Gold, MD
Radiology. . . . . Ronald Adelman, MD
Emergency . . . . Jeffrey D Anderson, MD

Measure	Cases	This Hosp.	State Avg.	U.S. Avg.
Heart Attack Care				
ACE Inhibitor or ARB for LVSD	63	100%	95%	96%
Aspirin at Arrival	460	99%	99%	99%
Aspirin at Discharge	465	100%	99%	98%
Beta Blocker at Discharge	451	99%	99%	98%
Fibrinolytic Medication Timing[1]	1	0%	40%	55%
PCI Within 90 Minutes of Arrival	52	88%	88%	90%
Smoking Cessation Advice	172	100%	100%	99%
Chest Pain/Possible Heart Attack Care				
Aspirin at Arrival[1]	17	82%	95%	95%
Median Time to ECG (minutes)[1]	18	7	8	8
Median Time to Transfer (minutes)[5]	0	-	68	61
Fibrinolytic Medication Timing[3]	0	-	48%	54%
Heart Failure Care				
ACE Inhibitor or ARB for LVSD	333	96%	95%	94%
Discharge Instructions	765	94%	90%	88%
Evaluation of LVS Function	953	100%	99%	98%
Smoking Cessation Advice	201	100%	98%	98%
Pneumonia Care				
Appropriate Initial Antibiotic	505	97%	93%	92%
Blood Culture Timing	829	98%	96%	96%
Influenza Vaccine	465	100%	92%	91%
Initial Antibiotic Timing	819	95%	96%	95%
Pneumococcal Vaccine	518	99%	95%	93%
Smoking Cessation Advice	367	100%	98%	97%
Surgical Care Improvement Project				
Appropriate VTP Within 24 Hours[2]	311	98%	95%	92%
Appropriate Hair Removal[2]	710	100%	100%	99%
Appropriate Beta Blocker Usage[2]	236	95%	94%	93%
Controlled Postoperative Blood Glucose[2]	88	97%	96%	93%
Prophylactic Antibiotic Timing[2]	353	96%	97%	97%
Prophylactic Antibiotic Timing (Outpatient)	293	94%	92%	92%
Prophylactic Antibiotic Selection[2]	357	97%	98%	97%
Prophylactic Antibiotic Select. (Outpatient)	276	98%	93%	94%
Prophylactic Antibiotic Stopped[2]	308	96%	95%	94%
Recommended VTP Ordered[2]	311	99%	97%	94%
Urinary Catheter Removal[2]	147	97%	95%	90%
Children's Asthma Care				
Received Systemic Corticosteroids	-	-	-	100%
Received Home Management Plan	-	-	-	71%
Received Reliever Medication	-	-	-	100%
Use of Medical Imaging				
Combination Abdominal CT Scan	1,382	0.034	0.203	0.191
Combination Chest CT Scan	1,164	0.003	0.026	0.054
Follow-up Mammogram/Ultrasound	1,126	8.6%	8.2%	8.4%
MRI for Low Back Pain[5]	0	-	32.4%	32.7%
Survey of Patients' Hospital Experiences				
Area Around Room 'Always' Quiet at Night	300+	49%	-	58%
Doctors 'Always' Communicated Well	300+	72%	-	80%
Home Recovery Information Given	300+	81%	-	82%
Hospital Given 9 or 10 on 10 Point Scale	300+	65%	-	67%
Meds 'Always' Explained Before Given	300+	58%	-	60%
Nurses 'Always' Communicated Well	300+	78%	-	76%
Pain 'Always' Well Controlled	300+	71%	-	69%
Room and Bathroom 'Always' Clean	300+	70%	-	71%
Timely Help 'Always' Received	300+	67%	-	64%
Would Definitely Recommend Hospital	300+	67%	-	69%

NOTE: Hospital profiles are in alphabetical order by state, then city, then hospital within the city; Rankings exclude hospitals with less than 25 cases except for patient surveys which excludes hospitals with less than 100 cases; (a) 100–299 cases; (1) The number of cases is too small to be sure how well a hospital is performing; (2) The hospital indicated that the data submitted for this measure were based on a sample of cases; (3) Data was collected during a shorter time period (fewer quarters) than the maximum possible time for this measure; (4) Suppressed for one or more quarters by CMS; (5) No data is available from the hospital for this measure; (6) Fewer than 100 patients completed the HCAHPS survey. Use these rates with caution, as the number of surveys may be too low to reliably assess hospital performance; (7) Survey results are based on less than 12 months of data; (8) Survey results are not available for this reporting period; (9) No or very few patients were eligible for the HCAHPS survey. The scores shown, if any, reflect a very small number of surveys; (10) A state average was not calculated because too few hospitals in the state submitted data; (11) There were discrepancies in the data collection process; Please refer to the User's Guide for a full explanation of data.

Cancer Treatment Centers of America

1331 East Wyoming Avenue | Phone: 215-744-6728
Philadelphia, PA 19124 | Fax: 215-537-7899
URL: www.cancercenter.com
Type: Acute Care Hospitals | Emergency Services: No
Ownership: Voluntary Non-Profit - Private | Beds: 22

Key Personnel:
CEO/President.............. Robert Amon
Chief of Medical Staff.......... Holly Leppert, DO
Operating Room.............. Lynn Frechette, RN
Pediatric In-Patient Care .... Stewart Cooler, MD
Quality Assurance .... Sandra Sacks
Emergency Room .... Carol Behrle, RN

Measure	Cases	This Hosp.	State Avg.	U.S. Avg.
Heart Attack Care				
ACE Inhibitor or ARB for LVSD[3]	0	-	95%	96%
Aspirin at Arrival[1,3]	1	100%	99%	99%
Aspirin at Discharge[1,3]	1	100%	99%	98%
Beta Blocker at Discharge[1,3]	1	100%	99%	98%
Fibrinolytic Medication Timing[3]	0	-	40%	55%
PCI Within 90 Minutes of Arrival[3]	0	-	88%	90%
Smoking Cessation Advice[3]	0	-	100%	99%
Chest Pain/Possible Heart Attack Care				
Aspirin at Arrival[5]	0	-	95%	95%
Median Time to ECG (minutes)[5]	0	-	8	8
Median Time to Transfer (minutes)[5]	0	-	68	61
Fibrinolytic Medication Timing[5]	0	-	48%	54%
Heart Failure Care				
ACE Inhibitor or ARB for LVSD[1,3]	1	100%	95%	94%
Discharge Instructions[1,3]	1	100%	90%	88%
Evaluation of LVS Function[1,3]	1	100%	99%	98%
Smoking Cessation Advice[3]	0	-	98%	98%
Pneumonia Care				
Appropriate Initial Antibiotic	0	-	93%	92%
Blood Culture Timing	0	-	96%	96%
Influenza Vaccine[1]	4	25%	92%	91%
Initial Antibiotic Timing[1]	14	64%	96%	95%
Pneumococcal Vaccine[1]	1	0%	95%	93%
Smoking Cessation Advice[1]	1	0%	98%	97%
Surgical Care Improvement Project				
Appropriate VTP Within 24 Hours	76	91%	95%	92%
Appropriate Hair Removal	82	43%	100%	99%
Appropriate Beta Blocker Usage[1]	9	56%	94%	93%
Controlled Postoperative Blood Glucose	0	-	96%	93%
Prophylactic Antibiotic Timing[1]	21	81%	97%	97%
Prophylactic Antibiotic Timing (Outpatient)[1,3]	5	100%	92%	92%
Prophylactic Antibiotic Selection[1]	22	86%	98%	97%
Prophylactic Antibiotic Select. (Outpatient)[1,3]	5	100%	93%	94%
Prophylactic Antibiotic Stopped[1]	21	86%	95%	94%
Recommended VTP Ordered	76	97%	97%	94%
Urinary Catheter Removal[1]	10	70%	95%	90%
Children's Asthma Care				
Received Systemic Corticosteroids	-	-	-	100%
Received Home Management Plan	-	-	-	71%
Received Reliever Medication	-	-	-	100%
Use of Medical Imaging				
Combination Abdominal CT Scan	181	0.785	0.203	0.191
Combination Chest CT Scan	220	0.009	0.026	0.054
Follow-up Mammogram/Ultrasound[5]	0	-	8.2%	8.4%
MRI for Low Back Pain[5]	0	-	32.4%	32.7%
Survey of Patients' Hospital Experiences				
Area Around Room 'Always' Quiet at Night	(a)	61%	-	58%
Doctors 'Always' Communicated Well	(a)	87%	-	80%
Home Recovery Information Given	(a)	90%	-	82%
Hospital Given 9 or 10 on 10 Point Scale	(a)	88%	-	67%
Meds 'Always' Explained Before Given	(a)	70%	-	60%
Nurses 'Always' Communicated Well	(a)	82%	-	76%
Pain 'Always' Well Controlled	(a)	80%	-	69%
Room and Bathroom 'Always' Clean	(a)	83%	-	71%
Timely Help 'Always' Received	(a)	72%	-	64%
Would Definitely Recommend Hospital	(a)	95%	-	69%

Chestnut Hill Hospital

8835 Germantown Ave | Phone: 215-248-8200
Philadelphia, PA 19118 | Fax: 215-248-8053
URL: www.chh.org
Type: Acute Care Hospitals | Emergency Services: Yes
Ownership: Proprietary | Beds: 200

Key Personnel:
CEO/President.............. Brooks Turkel
Chief of Medical Staff.......... John Scanlon
Quality Assurance .... James Danihel
Radiology.................. Kevin Byrne
Emergency Room .... Ann Mary Pata

Measure	Cases	This Hosp.	State Avg.	U.S. Avg.
Heart Attack Care				
ACE Inhibitor or ARB for LVSD[1]	8	100%	95%	96%
Aspirin at Arrival	40	100%	99%	99%
Aspirin at Discharge[1]	23	91%	99%	98%
Beta Blocker at Discharge[1]	22	95%	99%	98%
Fibrinolytic Medication Timing	0	-	40%	55%
PCI Within 90 Minutes of Arrival	0	-	88%	90%
Smoking Cessation Advice[1]	3	100%	100%	99%
Chest Pain/Possible Heart Attack Care				
Aspirin at Arrival	59	90%	95%	95%
Median Time to ECG (minutes)	62	16	8	8
Median Time to Transfer (minutes)	28	64	68	61
Fibrinolytic Medication Timing[1]	1	100%	48%	54%
Heart Failure Care				
ACE Inhibitor or ARB for LVSD	99	99%	95%	94%
Discharge Instructions	171	97%	90%	88%
Evaluation of LVS Function	296	97%	99%	98%
Smoking Cessation Advice	29	100%	98%	98%
Pneumonia Care				
Appropriate Initial Antibiotic	77	96%	93%	92%
Blood Culture Timing	184	98%	96%	96%
Influenza Vaccine	108	94%	92%	91%
Initial Antibiotic Timing	183	96%	96%	95%
Pneumococcal Vaccine	166	96%	95%	93%
Smoking Cessation Advice	46	100%	98%	97%
Surgical Care Improvement Project				
Appropriate VTP Within 24 Hours[2]	133	92%	95%	92%
Appropriate Hair Removal[2]	309	100%	100%	99%
Appropriate Beta Blocker Usage[2]	76	95%	94%	93%
Controlled Postoperative Blood Glucose[2]	0	-	96%	93%
Prophylactic Antibiotic Timing[2]	203	100%	97%	97%
Prophylactic Antibiotic Timing (Outpatient)	110	93%	92%	92%
Prophylactic Antibiotic Selection[2]	206	99%	98%	97%
Prophylactic Antibiotic Select. (Outpatient)	104	98%	93%	94%
Prophylactic Antibiotic Stopped[2]	189	99%	95%	94%
Recommended VTP Ordered[2]	133	98%	97%	94%
Urinary Catheter Removal	49	92%	95%	90%
Children's Asthma Care				
Received Systemic Corticosteroids	-	-	-	100%
Received Home Management Plan	-	-	-	71%
Received Reliever Medication	-	-	-	100%
Use of Medical Imaging				
Combination Abdominal CT Scan	459	0.094	0.203	0.191
Combination Chest CT Scan	333	0.024	0.026	0.054
Follow-up Mammogram/Ultrasound	1,295	7.2%	8.2%	8.4%
MRI for Low Back Pain	62	33.9%	32.4%	32.7%
Survey of Patients' Hospital Experiences				
Area Around Room 'Always' Quiet at Night	300+	56%	-	58%
Doctors 'Always' Communicated Well	300+	76%	-	80%
Home Recovery Information Given	300+	80%	-	82%
Hospital Given 9 or 10 on 10 Point Scale	300+	62%	-	67%
Meds 'Always' Explained Before Given	300+	53%	-	60%
Nurses 'Always' Communicated Well	300+	73%	-	76%
Pain 'Always' Well Controlled	300+	67%	-	69%
Room and Bathroom 'Always' Clean	300+	65%	-	71%
Timely Help 'Always' Received	300+	52%	-	64%
Would Definitely Recommend Hospital	300+	62%	-	69%

Children's Hospital of Philadelphia

34th St & Civic Center Blvd | Phone: 215-590-3745
Philadelphia, PA 19104 | Fax: 215-860-4090
URL: www.chop.edu
Type: Childrens | Emergency Services: Yes
Ownership: Voluntary Non-Profit - Private | Beds: 430

Key Personnel:
CEO/President.............. Edmond Notebaert
Radiology.................. Kenneth E Fellows, Jr, DM

Measure	Cases	This Hosp.	State Avg.	U.S. Avg.
Heart Attack Care				
ACE Inhibitor or ARB for LVSD	-	-	95%	96%
Aspirin at Arrival	-	-	99%	99%
Aspirin at Discharge	-	-	99%	98%
Beta Blocker at Discharge	-	-	99%	98%
Fibrinolytic Medication Timing	-	-	40%	55%
PCI Within 90 Minutes of Arrival	-	-	88%	90%
Smoking Cessation Advice	-	-	100%	99%
Chest Pain/Possible Heart Attack Care				
Aspirin at Arrival	-	-	95%	95%
Median Time to ECG (minutes)	-	-	8	8
Median Time to Transfer (minutes)	-	-	68	61
Fibrinolytic Medication Timing	-	-	48%	54%
Heart Failure Care				
ACE Inhibitor or ARB for LVSD	-	-	95%	94%
Discharge Instructions	-	-	90%	88%
Evaluation of LVS Function	-	-	99%	98%
Smoking Cessation Advice	-	-	98%	98%
Pneumonia Care				
Appropriate Initial Antibiotic	-	-	93%	92%
Blood Culture Timing	-	-	96%	96%
Influenza Vaccine	-	-	92%	91%
Initial Antibiotic Timing	-	-	96%	95%
Pneumococcal Vaccine	-	-	95%	93%
Smoking Cessation Advice	-	-	98%	97%
Surgical Care Improvement Project				
Appropriate VTP Within 24 Hours	-	-	95%	92%
Appropriate Hair Removal	-	-	100%	99%
Appropriate Beta Blocker Usage	-	-	94%	93%
Controlled Postoperative Blood Glucose	-	-	96%	93%
Prophylactic Antibiotic Timing	-	-	97%	97%
Prophylactic Antibiotic Timing (Outpatient)	-	-	92%	92%
Prophylactic Antibiotic Selection	-	-	98%	97%
Prophylactic Antibiotic Select. (Outpatient)	-	-	93%	94%
Prophylactic Antibiotic Stopped	-	-	95%	94%
Recommended VTP Ordered	-	-	97%	94%
Urinary Catheter Removal	-	-	95%	90%
Children's Asthma Care				
Received Systemic Corticosteroids[2]	547	100%	-	100%
Received Home Management Plan[2]	546	47%	-	71%
Received Reliever Medication[2]	548	100%	-	100%
Use of Medical Imaging				
Combination Abdominal CT Scan	-	-	0.203	0.191
Combination Chest CT Scan	-	-	0.026	0.054
Follow-up Mammogram/Ultrasound	-	-	8.2%	8.4%
MRI for Low Back Pain	-	-	32.4%	32.7%
Survey of Patients' Hospital Experiences				
Area Around Room 'Always' Quiet at Night	-	-	-	58%
Doctors 'Always' Communicated Well	-	-	-	80%
Home Recovery Information Given	-	-	-	82%
Hospital Given 9 or 10 on 10 Point Scale	-	-	-	67%
Meds 'Always' Explained Before Given	-	-	-	60%
Nurses 'Always' Communicated Well	-	-	-	76%
Pain 'Always' Well Controlled	-	-	-	69%
Room and Bathroom 'Always' Clean	-	-	-	71%
Timely Help 'Always' Received	-	-	-	64%
Would Definitely Recommend Hospital	-	-	-	69%

NOTE: Hospital profiles are in alphabetical order by state, then city, then hospital within the city; Rankings exclude hospitals with less than 25 cases except for patient surveys which excludes hospitals with less than 100 cases; (a) 100–299 cases; (1) The number of cases is too small to be sure how well a hospital is performing; (2) The hospital indicated that the data submitted for this measure were based on a sample of cases; (3) Data was collected during a shorter time period (fewer quarters) than the maximum possible time for this measure; (4) Suppressed for one or more quarters by CMS; (5) No data is available from the hospital for this measure; (6) Fewer than 100 patients completed the HCAHPS survey. Use these rates with caution, as the number of surveys may be too low to reliably assess hospital performance; (7) Survey results are based on less than 12 months of data; (8) Survey results are not available for this reporting period; (9) No or very few patients were eligible for the HCAHPS survey. The scores shown, if any, reflect a very small number of surveys; (10) A state average was not calculated because too few hospitals in the state submitted data; (11) There were discrepancies in the data collection process; Please refer to the User's Guide for a full explanation of data.

Hahnemann University Hospital

230 North Broad Street Phone: 215-762-7000
Philadelphia, PA 19102 Fax: 215-762-8109
URL: www.hahnemannhospital.com
Type: Acute Care Hospitals Emergency Services: Yes
Ownership: Proprietary Beds: 540

Key Personnel:
CEO/President. . . . . Michael Halter, FACHE
Chief of Medical Staff . . . . Jeffrey Glassroth
Infection Control. . . . . Kathy Arias
Operating Room. . . . . Patty Robertson
Pediatric In-Patient Care . . . . James DeMarco
Quality Assurance . . . . Doug McCusker
Radiology. . . . . Charles Mulhern
Emergency Room . . . . Phillip Mead, MD

Measure	Cases	This Hosp.	State Avg.	U.S. Avg.
Heart Attack Care				
ACE Inhibitor or ARB for LVSD	43	100%	95%	96%
Aspirin at Arrival	103	98%	99%	99%
Aspirin at Discharge	195	99%	99%	98%
Beta Blocker at Discharge	192	100%	99%	98%
Fibrinolytic Medication Timing	0	-	40%	55%
PCI Within 90 Minutes of Arrival[1]	8	88%	88%	90%
Smoking Cessation Advice	72	100%	100%	99%
Chest Pain/Possible Heart Attack Care				
Aspirin at Arrival[1,3]	1	100%	95%	95%
Median Time to ECG (minutes)[1,3]	1	40	8	8
Median Time to Transfer (minutes)[5]	0	-	68	61
Fibrinolytic Medication Timing[5]	0	-	48%	54%
Heart Failure Care				
ACE Inhibitor or ARB for LVSD	389	99%	95%	94%
Discharge Instructions	642	97%	90%	88%
Evaluation of LVS Function	699	100%	99%	98%
Smoking Cessation Advice	193	98%	98%	98%
Pneumonia Care				
Appropriate Initial Antibiotic	99	97%	93%	92%
Blood Culture Timing	200	98%	96%	96%
Influenza Vaccine	117	94%	92%	91%
Initial Antibiotic Timing	192	97%	96%	95%
Pneumococcal Vaccine	109	94%	95%	93%
Smoking Cessation Advice	120	96%	98%	97%
Surgical Care Improvement Project				
Appropriate VTP Within 24 Hours[2]	294	89%	95%	92%
Appropriate Hair Removal[2]	686	98%	100%	99%
Appropriate Beta Blocker Usage[2]	214	95%	94%	93%
Controlled Postoperative Blood Glucose[2]	137	94%	96%	93%
Prophylactic Antibiotic Timing[2]	468	96%	97%	97%
Prophylactic Antibiotic Timing (Outpatient)	416	95%	92%	92%
Prophylactic Antibiotic Selection[2]	473	97%	98%	97%
Prophylactic Antibiotic Select. (Outpatient)	419	97%	93%	94%
Prophylactic Antibiotic Stopped[2]	455	92%	95%	94%
Recommended VTP Ordered[2]	295	89%	97%	94%
Urinary Catheter Removal[2]	143	97%	95%	90%
Children's Asthma Care				
Received Systemic Corticosteroids	-	-	-	100%
Received Home Management Plan	-	-	-	71%
Received Reliever Medication	-	-	-	100%
Use of Medical Imaging				
Combination Abdominal CT Scan	302	0.079	0.203	0.191
Combination Chest CT Scan	237	0.008	0.026	0.054
Follow-up Mammogram/Ultrasound	435	10.1%	8.2%	8.4%
MRI for Low Back Pain[1]	50	30.0%	32.4%	32.7%
Survey of Patients' Hospital Experiences				
Area Around Room 'Always' Quiet at Night	300+	59%	-	58%
Doctors 'Always' Communicated Well	300+	82%	-	80%
Home Recovery Information Given	300+	83%	-	82%
Hospital Given 9 or 10 on 10 Point Scale	300+	66%	-	67%
Meds 'Always' Explained Before Given	300+	65%	-	60%
Nurses 'Always' Communicated Well	300+	78%	-	76%
Pain 'Always' Well Controlled	300+	72%	-	69%
Room and Bathroom 'Always' Clean	300+	68%	-	71%
Timely Help 'Always' Received	300+	64%	-	64%
Would Definitely Recommend Hospital	300+	71%	-	69%

Hospital of Univ of Pennsylvania

34th & Spruce Sts Phone: 215-662-3227
Philadelphia, PA 19104 Fax: 215-349-5864
URL: www.upenn.edu
Type: Acute Care Hospitals Emergency Services: Yes
Ownership: Voluntary Non-Profit - Private Beds: 725

Key Personnel:
CEO/President. . . . . Robert D Marlin
Chief of Medical Staff . . . . Stanley Goldfarb, MD
Infection Control. . . . . Harvey Friedman, MD
Operating Room. . . . . Noreen McHugh, RN
Quality Assurance . . . . Mary Ellen Nepps
Radiology. . . . . R Nick Bryan, MD
Emergency Room . . . . William Baxt, MD

Measure	Cases	This Hosp.	State Avg.	U.S. Avg.
Heart Attack Care				
ACE Inhibitor or ARB for LVSD	40	98%	95%	96%
Aspirin at Arrival	112	100%	99%	99%
Aspirin at Discharge	204	100%	99%	98%
Beta Blocker at Discharge	198	98%	99%	98%
Fibrinolytic Medication Timing	0	-	40%	55%
PCI Within 90 Minutes of Arrival	29	72%	88%	90%
Smoking Cessation Advice	70	99%	100%	99%
Chest Pain/Possible Heart Attack Care				
Aspirin at Arrival[5]	0	-	95%	95%
Median Time to ECG (minutes)[5]	0	-	8	8
Median Time to Transfer (minutes)[5]	0	-	68	61
Fibrinolytic Medication Timing[5]	0	-	48%	54%
Heart Failure Care				
ACE Inhibitor or ARB for LVSD	402	98%	95%	94%
Discharge Instructions	708	88%	90%	88%
Evaluation of LVS Function	781	100%	99%	98%
Smoking Cessation Advice	174	99%	98%	98%
Pneumonia Care				
Appropriate Initial Antibiotic	96	88%	93%	92%
Blood Culture Timing	161	66%	96%	96%
Influenza Vaccine	84	89%	92%	91%
Initial Antibiotic Timing	174	92%	96%	95%
Pneumococcal Vaccine	160	92%	95%	93%
Smoking Cessation Advice	96	95%	98%	97%
Surgical Care Improvement Project				
Appropriate VTP Within 24 Hours[2]	384	99%	95%	92%
Appropriate Hair Removal[2]	982	100%	100%	99%
Appropriate Beta Blocker Usage[2]	293	77%	94%	93%
Controlled Postoperative Blood Glucose[2]	278	98%	96%	93%
Prophylactic Antibiotic Timing[2]	580	99%	97%	97%
Prophylactic Antibiotic Timing (Outpatient)	690	51%	92%	92%
Prophylactic Antibiotic Selection[2]	598	96%	98%	97%
Prophylactic Antibiotic Select. (Outpatient)	538	77%	93%	94%
Prophylactic Antibiotic Stopped[2]	557	76%	95%	94%
Recommended VTP Ordered[2]	384	100%	97%	94%
Urinary Catheter Removal[2]	175	87%	95%	90%
Children's Asthma Care				
Received Systemic Corticosteroids	-	-	-	100%
Received Home Management Plan	-	-	-	71%
Received Reliever Medication	-	-	-	100%
Use of Medical Imaging				
Combination Abdominal CT Scan	1,579	0.141	0.203	0.191
Combination Chest CT Scan	2,172	0.001	0.026	0.054
Follow-up Mammogram/Ultrasound	1,136	6.2%	8.2%	8.4%
MRI for Low Back Pain	212	33.5%	32.4%	32.7%
Survey of Patients' Hospital Experiences				
Area Around Room 'Always' Quiet at Night	300+	46%	-	58%
Doctors 'Always' Communicated Well	300+	80%	-	80%
Home Recovery Information Given	300+	87%	-	82%
Hospital Given 9 or 10 on 10 Point Scale	300+	71%	-	67%
Meds 'Always' Explained Before Given	300+	63%	-	60%
Nurses 'Always' Communicated Well	300+	76%	-	76%
Pain 'Always' Well Controlled	300+	70%	-	69%
Room and Bathroom 'Always' Clean	300+	55%	-	71%
Timely Help 'Always' Received	300+	60%	-	64%
Would Definitely Recommend Hospital	300+	81%	-	69%

Jeanes Hospital

7600 Central Ave Phone: 215-728-2000
Philadelphia, PA 19111 Fax: 215-728-3345
E-mail: information.jeanes@tuhs.temple.edu
URL: www.jeanes.com
Type: Acute Care Hospitals Emergency Services: Yes
Ownership: Voluntary Non-Profit - Private Beds: 197

Key Personnel:
CEO/President. . . . . Linda Grass
Chief of Medical Staff . . . . Joel Weissman
Infection Control. . . . . Simone Woodwell
Operating Room. . . . . Carole Campbell
Quality Assurance . . . . Deborah Dunaj
Anesthesiology. . . . . Subash Reddy, MD
Emergency Room . . . . Lawrence Albert
Patient Relations . . . . Sally Ziska

Measure	Cases	This Hosp.	State Avg.	U.S. Avg.
Heart Attack Care				
ACE Inhibitor or ARB for LVSD	30	97%	95%	96%
Aspirin at Arrival	164	98%	99%	99%
Aspirin at Discharge	146	99%	99%	98%
Beta Blocker at Discharge	164	98%	99%	98%
Fibrinolytic Medication Timing	0	-	40%	55%
PCI Within 90 Minutes of Arrival[1]	20	45%	88%	90%
Smoking Cessation Advice	42	100%	100%	99%
Chest Pain/Possible Heart Attack Care				
Aspirin at Arrival[1,3]	3	100%	95%	95%
Median Time to ECG (minutes)[1,3]	3	11	8	8
Median Time to Transfer (minutes)[5]	0	-	68	61
Fibrinolytic Medication Timing[3]	0	-	48%	54%
Heart Failure Care				
ACE Inhibitor or ARB for LVSD	115	92%	95%	94%
Discharge Instructions	278	94%	90%	88%
Evaluation of LVS Function	355	98%	99%	98%
Smoking Cessation Advice	39	100%	98%	98%
Pneumonia Care				
Appropriate Initial Antibiotic	122	98%	93%	92%
Blood Culture Timing	188	97%	96%	96%
Influenza Vaccine	97	99%	92%	91%
Initial Antibiotic Timing	175	94%	96%	95%
Pneumococcal Vaccine	158	94%	95%	93%
Smoking Cessation Advice	48	100%	98%	97%
Surgical Care Improvement Project				
Appropriate VTP Within 24 Hours	235	98%	95%	92%
Appropriate Hair Removal	658	95%	100%	99%
Appropriate Beta Blocker Usage	196	99%	94%	93%
Controlled Postoperative Blood Glucose	87	94%	96%	93%
Prophylactic Antibiotic Timing	456	98%	97%	97%
Prophylactic Antibiotic Timing (Outpatient)	48	94%	92%	92%
Prophylactic Antibiotic Selection	459	98%	98%	97%
Prophylactic Antibiotic Select. (Outpatient)	49	98%	93%	94%
Prophylactic Antibiotic Stopped	441	94%	95%	94%
Recommended VTP Ordered	239	97%	97%	94%
Urinary Catheter Removal[1]	1	100%	95%	90%
Children's Asthma Care				
Received Systemic Corticosteroids	-	-	-	100%
Received Home Management Plan	-	-	-	71%
Received Reliever Medication	-	-	-	100%
Use of Medical Imaging				
Combination Abdominal CT Scan	559	0.068	0.203	0.191
Combination Chest CT Scan	272	0.015	0.026	0.054
Follow-up Mammogram/Ultrasound	828	4.6%	8.2%	8.4%
MRI for Low Back Pain	91	24.2%	32.4%	32.7%
Survey of Patients' Hospital Experiences				
Area Around Room 'Always' Quiet at Night	300+	54%	-	58%
Doctors 'Always' Communicated Well	300+	81%	-	80%
Home Recovery Information Given	300+	81%	-	82%
Hospital Given 9 or 10 on 10 Point Scale	300+	68%	-	67%
Meds 'Always' Explained Before Given	300+	59%	-	60%
Nurses 'Always' Communicated Well	300+	74%	-	76%
Pain 'Always' Well Controlled	300+	72%	-	69%
Room and Bathroom 'Always' Clean	300+	67%	-	71%
Timely Help 'Always' Received	300+	56%	-	64%
Would Definitely Recommend Hospital	300+	70%	-	69%

NOTE: Hospital profiles are in alphabetical order by state, then city, then hospital within the city; Rankings exclude hospitals with less than 25 cases except for patient surveys which excludes hospitals with less than 100 cases; (a) 100–299 cases; (1) The number of cases is too small to be sure how well a hospital is performing; (2) The hospital indicated that the data submitted for this measure were based on a sample of cases; (3) Data was collected during a shorter time period (fewer quarters) than the maximum possible time for this measure; (4) Suppressed for one or more quarters by CMS; (5) No data is available from the hospital for this measure; (6) Fewer than 100 patients completed the HCAHPS survey. Use these rates with caution, as the number of surveys may be too low to reliably assess hospital performance; (7) Survey results are based on less than 12 months of data; (8) Survey results are not available for this reporting period; (9) No or very few patients were eligible for the HCAHPS survey. The scores shown, if any, reflect a very small number of surveys; (10) A state average was not calculated because too few hospitals in the state submitted data; (11) There were discrepancies in the data collection process; Please refer to the User's Guide for a full explanation of data.

Kensington Hospital

136 W Diamond Street   Phone: 215-426-8100
Philadelphia, PA 19122   Fax: 215-291-6030
Type: Acute Care Hospitals   Emergency Services: No
Ownership: Voluntary Non-Profit - Other   Beds: 45
Key Personnel:
Infection Control . . . . Judy Arentzen
Operating Room . . . . Bill Mihal

Measure	Cases	This Hosp.	State Avg.	U.S. Avg.
Heart Attack Care				
ACE Inhibitor or ARB for LVSD[5]	0	-	95%	96%
Aspirin at Arrival[5]	0	-	99%	99%
Aspirin at Discharge[5]	0	-	99%	98%
Beta Blocker at Discharge[5]	0	-	99%	98%
Fibrinolytic Medication Timing[5]	0	-	40%	55%
PCI Within 90 Minutes of Arrival[5]	0	-	88%	90%
Smoking Cessation Advice[5]	0	-	100%	99%
Chest Pain/Possible Heart Attack Care				
Aspirin at Arrival[5]	0	-	95%	95%
Median Time to ECG (minutes)[5]	0	-	8	8
Median Time to Transfer (minutes)[5]	0	-	68	61
Fibrinolytic Medication Timing[5]	0	-	48%	54%
Heart Failure Care				
ACE Inhibitor or ARB for LVSD[5]	0	-	95%	94%
Discharge Instructions[5]	0	-	90%	88%
Evaluation of LVS Function[5]	0	-	99%	98%
Smoking Cessation Advice[5]	0	-	98%	98%
Pneumonia Care				
Appropriate Initial Antibiotic[5]	0	-	93%	92%
Blood Culture Timing[5]	0	-	96%	96%
Influenza Vaccine[5]	0	-	92%	91%
Initial Antibiotic Timing[5]	0	-	96%	95%
Pneumococcal Vaccine[5]	0	-	95%	93%
Smoking Cessation Advice[5]	0	-	98%	97%
Surgical Care Improvement Project				
Appropriate VTP Within 24 Hours[5]	0	-	95%	92%
Appropriate Hair Removal[5]	0	-	100%	99%
Appropriate Beta Blocker Usage[5]	0	-	94%	93%
Controlled Postoperative Blood Glucose[5]	0	-	96%	93%
Prophylactic Antibiotic Timing[5]	0	-	97%	97%
Prophylactic Antibiotic Timing (Outpatient)[5]	0	-	92%	92%
Prophylactic Antibiotic Selection[5]	0	-	98%	97%
Prophylactic Antibiotic Select. (Outpatient)[5]	0	-	93%	94%
Prophylactic Antibiotic Stopped[5]	0	-	95%	94%
Recommended VTP Ordered[5]	0	-	97%	94%
Urinary Catheter Removal[5]	0	-	95%	90%
Children's Asthma Care				
Received Systemic Corticosteroids	-	-	-	100%
Received Home Management Plan	-	-	-	71%
Received Reliever Medication	-	-	-	100%
Use of Medical Imaging				
Combination Abdominal CT Scan[5]	0	-	0.203	0.191
Combination Chest CT Scan[5]	0	-	0.026	0.054
Follow-up Mammogram/Ultrasound[1]	18	0.0%	8.2%	8.4%
MRI for Low Back Pain[5]	0	-	32.4%	32.7%
Survey of Patients' Hospital Experiences				
Area Around Room 'Always' Quiet at Night[9,6]	<100	47%	-	58%
Doctors 'Always' Communicated Well[9,6]	<100	47%	-	80%
Home Recovery Information Given[9,6]	<100	-	-	82%
Hospital Given 9 or 10 on 10 Point Scale[9,6]	<100	-	-	67%
Meds 'Always' Explained Before Given[9,6]	<100	-	-	60%
Nurses 'Always' Communicated Well[9,6]	<100	46%	-	76%
Pain 'Always' Well Controlled[9,6]	<100	47%	-	69%
Room and Bathroom 'Always' Clean[9,6]	<100	100%	-	71%
Timely Help 'Always' Received[9,6]	<100	22%	-	64%
Would Definitely Recommend Hospital[9]	<100	-	-	69%

Nazareth Hospital

2601 Holme Ave   Phone: 215-335-6000
Philadelphia, PA 19152   Fax: 215-335-6668
E-mail: info@nazarethhospital.org
URL: www.nazarethhospital.org
Type: Acute Care Hospitals   Emergency Services: Yes
Ownership: Voluntary Non-Profit - Church   Beds: 347
Key Personnel:
CEO/President . . . . Pat DeAngelis
Chief of Medical Staff . . . . George Duber, MD
Operating Room . . . . Sandra Larson
Quality Assurance . . . . Nancy Anderson
Radiology . . . . Donald Ostrum, MD
Emergency Room . . . . Trisha Harbison

Measure	Cases	This Hosp.	State Avg.	U.S. Avg.
Heart Attack Care				
ACE Inhibitor or ARB for LVSD[1]	6	100%	95%	96%
Aspirin at Arrival	109	100%	99%	99%
Aspirin at Discharge	60	97%	99%	98%
Beta Blocker at Discharge	63	98%	99%	98%
Fibrinolytic Medication Timing	0	-	40%	55%
PCI Within 90 Minutes of Arrival	0	-	88%	90%
Smoking Cessation Advice[1]	3	100%	100%	99%
Chest Pain/Possible Heart Attack Care				
Aspirin at Arrival	61	97%	95%	95%
Median Time to ECG (minutes)	66	9	8	8
Median Time to Transfer (minutes)	26	72	68	61
Fibrinolytic Medication Timing[1]	2	0%	48%	54%
Heart Failure Care				
ACE Inhibitor or ARB for LVSD	50	100%	95%	94%
Discharge Instructions	230	99%	90%	88%
Evaluation of LVS Function	398	100%	99%	98%
Smoking Cessation Advice	37	100%	98%	98%
Pneumonia Care				
Appropriate Initial Antibiotic	143	97%	93%	92%
Blood Culture Timing	303	98%	96%	96%
Influenza Vaccine	152	82%	92%	91%
Initial Antibiotic Timing	279	97%	96%	95%
Pneumococcal Vaccine	202	95%	95%	93%
Smoking Cessation Advice	66	98%	98%	97%
Surgical Care Improvement Project				
Appropriate VTP Within 24 Hours	236	97%	95%	92%
Appropriate Hair Removal	643	100%	100%	99%
Appropriate Beta Blocker Usage	190	95%	94%	93%
Controlled Postoperative Blood Glucose	0	-	96%	93%
Prophylactic Antibiotic Timing	479	99%	97%	97%
Prophylactic Antibiotic Timing (Outpatient)	73	100%	92%	92%
Prophylactic Antibiotic Selection	480	99%	98%	97%
Prophylactic Antibiotic Select. (Outpatient)	73	97%	93%	94%
Prophylactic Antibiotic Stopped	465	99%	95%	94%
Recommended VTP Ordered	236	98%	97%	94%
Urinary Catheter Removal	213	93%	95%	90%
Children's Asthma Care				
Received Systemic Corticosteroids	-	-	-	100%
Received Home Management Plan	-	-	-	71%
Received Reliever Medication	-	-	-	100%
Use of Medical Imaging				
Combination Abdominal CT Scan	441	0.070	0.203	0.191
Combination Chest CT Scan	380	0.005	0.026	0.054
Follow-up Mammogram/Ultrasound	418	10.5%	8.2%	8.4%
MRI for Low Back Pain	151	27.8%	32.4%	32.7%
Survey of Patients' Hospital Experiences				
Area Around Room 'Always' Quiet at Night	300+	54%	-	58%
Doctors 'Always' Communicated Well	300+	74%	-	80%
Home Recovery Information Given	300+	83%	-	82%
Hospital Given 9 or 10 on 10 Point Scale	300+	59%	-	67%
Meds 'Always' Explained Before Given	300+	56%	-	60%
Nurses 'Always' Communicated Well	300+	71%	-	76%
Pain 'Always' Well Controlled	300+	66%	-	69%
Room and Bathroom 'Always' Clean	300+	70%	-	71%
Timely Help 'Always' Received	300+	56%	-	64%
Would Definitely Recommend Hospital	300+	59%	-	69%

Penn Presbyterian Medical Center

51 North 39th Street   Phone: 215-662-8000
Philadelphia, PA 19104   Fax: 215-662-8936
URL: www.pennhealth.com
Type: Acute Care Hospitals   Emergency Services: Yes
Ownership: Voluntary Non-Profit - Other   Beds: 344
Key Personnel:
CEO/President . . . . Michele Volpe
Chief of Medical Staff . . . . Lawrence Gavin, MD
Operating Room . . . . Barbara Schock
Quality Assurance . . . . Rhoda Vaflor
Radiology . . . . David Freiman, MD
Emergency Room . . . . Cheryl Ann Smaller

Measure	Cases	This Hosp.	State Avg.	U.S. Avg.
Heart Attack Care				
ACE Inhibitor or ARB for LVSD	140	95%	95%	96%
Aspirin at Arrival	408	100%	99%	99%
Aspirin at Discharge	696	100%	99%	98%
Beta Blocker at Discharge	692	99%	99%	98%
Fibrinolytic Medication Timing	0	-	40%	55%
PCI Within 90 Minutes of Arrival[1]	2	100%	88%	90%
Smoking Cessation Advice	208	100%	100%	99%
Chest Pain/Possible Heart Attack Care				
Aspirin at Arrival[5]	0	-	95%	95%
Median Time to ECG (minutes)[5]	0	-	8	8
Median Time to Transfer (minutes)[5]	0	-	68	61
Fibrinolytic Medication Timing[5]	0	-	48%	54%
Heart Failure Care				
ACE Inhibitor or ARB for LVSD	350	98%	95%	94%
Discharge Instructions	691	89%	90%	88%
Evaluation of LVS Function	804	99%	99%	98%
Smoking Cessation Advice	160	100%	98%	98%
Pneumonia Care				
Appropriate Initial Antibiotic	76	91%	93%	92%
Blood Culture Timing	155	95%	96%	96%
Influenza Vaccine	95	61%	92%	91%
Initial Antibiotic Timing	139	97%	96%	95%
Pneumococcal Vaccine	110	97%	95%	93%
Smoking Cessation Advice	71	100%	98%	97%
Surgical Care Improvement Project				
Appropriate VTP Within 24 Hours	576	94%	95%	92%
Appropriate Hair Removal	2,635	100%	100%	99%
Appropriate Beta Blocker Usage	787	100%	94%	93%
Controlled Postoperative Blood Glucose	394	98%	96%	93%
Prophylactic Antibiotic Timing	1,482	97%	97%	97%
Prophylactic Antibiotic Timing (Outpatient)	343	90%	92%	92%
Prophylactic Antibiotic Selection	1,485	98%	98%	97%
Prophylactic Antibiotic Select. (Outpatient)	313	91%	93%	94%
Prophylactic Antibiotic Stopped	1,440	86%	95%	94%
Recommended VTP Ordered	576	99%	97%	94%
Urinary Catheter Removal	734	99%	95%	90%
Children's Asthma Care				
Received Systemic Corticosteroids	-	-	-	100%
Received Home Management Plan	-	-	-	71%
Received Reliever Medication	-	-	-	100%
Use of Medical Imaging				
Combination Abdominal CT Scan	324	0.025	0.203	0.191
Combination Chest CT Scan	255	0.024	0.026	0.054
Follow-up Mammogram/Ultrasound	207	10.1%	8.2%	8.4%
MRI for Low Back Pain[1]	36	33.3%	32.4%	32.7%
Survey of Patients' Hospital Experiences				
Area Around Room 'Always' Quiet at Night	300+	53%	-	58%
Doctors 'Always' Communicated Well	300+	80%	-	80%
Home Recovery Information Given	300+	84%	-	82%
Hospital Given 9 or 10 on 10 Point Scale	300+	68%	-	67%
Meds 'Always' Explained Before Given	300+	63%	-	60%
Nurses 'Always' Communicated Well	300+	77%	-	76%
Pain 'Always' Well Controlled	300+	72%	-	69%
Room and Bathroom 'Always' Clean	300+	67%	-	71%
Timely Help 'Always' Received	300+	61%	-	64%
Would Definitely Recommend Hospital	300+	74%	-	69%

NOTE: Hospital profiles are in alphabetical order by state, then city, then hospital within the city; Rankings exclude hospitals with less than 25 cases except for patient surveys which excludes hospitals with less than 100 cases; (a) 100–299 cases; (1) The number of cases is too small to be sure how well a hospital is performing; (2) The hospital indicated that the data submitted for this measure were based on a sample of cases; (3) Data was collected during a shorter time period (fewer quarters) than the maximum possible time for this measure; (4) Suppressed for one or more quarters by CMS; (5) No data is available from the hospital for this measure; (6) Fewer than 100 patients completed the HCAHPS survey. Use these rates with caution, as the number of surveys may be too low to reliably assess hospital performance; (7) Survey results are based on less than 12 months of data; (8) Survey results are not available for this reporting period; (9) No or very few patients were eligible for the HCAHPS survey. The scores shown, if any, reflect a very small number of surveys; (10) A state average was not calculated because too few hospitals in the state submitted data; (11) There were discrepancies in the data collection process; Please refer to the User's Guide for a full explanation of data.

Pennsylvania Hospital of the Univ of Penn Health System

800 Spruce Street
Philadelphia, PA 19107
URL: www.pennmedicine.org/pahosp
Type: Acute Care Hospitals
Ownership: Voluntary Non-Profit - Private
Phone: 215-829-3000
Fax: 215-349-8312
Emergency Services: Yes
Beds: 515

Key Personnel:
Cardiac Laboratory. . . . . Howard C. Herman, MD
Chief of Medical Staff. . . . . Charles Wolf, MD
Infection Control. . . . . Jessica Bunson
Radiology. . . . . Harold I. Litt, MD, PhD
Anesthesiology. . . . . Jason Cwik, MD
Emergency Room . . . . Kathleen Nasci, MD
Hemotology Center . . . . David M Mintzer, MD
Intensive Care Unit. . . . . Francis Kempf, MD

Measure	Cases	This Hosp.	State Avg.	U.S. Avg.
Heart Attack Care				
ACE Inhibitor or ARB for LVSD	45	93%	95%	96%
Aspirin at Arrival	132	100%	99%	99%
Aspirin at Discharge	186	99%	99%	98%
Beta Blocker at Discharge	172	97%	99%	98%
Fibrinolytic Medication Timing[1]	1	100%	40%	55%
PCI Within 90 Minutes of Arrival[1]	23	48%	88%	90%
Smoking Cessation Advice	79	100%	100%	99%
Chest Pain/Possible Heart Attack Care				
Aspirin at Arrival[5]	0	-	95%	95%
Median Time to ECG (minutes)[5]	0	-	8	8
Median Time to Transfer (minutes)[5]	0	-	68	61
Fibrinolytic Medication Timing[5]	0	-	48%	54%
Heart Failure Care				
ACE Inhibitor or ARB for LVSD	132	92%	95%	94%
Discharge Instructions	384	97%	90%	88%
Evaluation of LVS Function	433	100%	99%	98%
Smoking Cessation Advice	66	100%	98%	98%
Pneumonia Care				
Appropriate Initial Antibiotic	99	90%	93%	92%
Blood Culture Timing	147	96%	96%	96%
Influenza Vaccine	66	79%	92%	91%
Initial Antibiotic Timing	154	90%	96%	95%
Pneumococcal Vaccine	103	91%	95%	93%
Smoking Cessation Advice	62	100%	98%	97%
Surgical Care Improvement Project				
Appropriate VTP Within 24 Hours[2]	245	96%	95%	92%
Appropriate Hair Removal[2]	689	100%	100%	99%
Appropriate Beta Blocker Usage[2]	218	87%	94%	93%
Controlled Postoperative Blood Glucose[2]	106	84%	96%	93%
Prophylactic Antibiotic Timing[2]	483	98%	97%	97%
Prophylactic Antibiotic Timing (Outpatient)	572	98%	92%	92%
Prophylactic Antibiotic Selection[2]	494	97%	98%	97%
Prophylactic Antibiotic Select. (Outpatient)	571	96%	93%	94%
Prophylactic Antibiotic Stopped[2]	464	79%	95%	94%
Recommended VTP Ordered[2]	247	97%	97%	94%
Urinary Catheter Removal[2]	199	92%	95%	90%
Children's Asthma Care				
Received Systemic Corticosteroids	-	-	-	100%
Received Home Management Plan	-	-	-	71%
Received Reliever Medication	-	-	-	100%
Use of Medical Imaging				
Combination Abdominal CT Scan	794	0.071	0.203	0.191
Combination Chest CT Scan	716	0.013	0.026	0.054
Follow-up Mammogram/Ultrasound	946	11.6%	8.2%	8.4%
MRI for Low Back Pain[1]	3	33.3%	32.4%	32.7%
Survey of Patients' Hospital Experiences				
Area Around Room 'Always' Quiet at Night	300+	50%	-	58%
Doctors 'Always' Communicated Well	300+	76%	-	80%
Home Recovery Information Given	300+	80%	-	82%
Hospital Given 9 or 10 on 10 Point Scale	300+	64%	-	67%
Meds 'Always' Explained Before Given	300+	58%	-	60%
Nurses 'Always' Communicated Well	300+	70%	-	76%
Pain 'Always' Well Controlled	300+	65%	-	69%
Room and Bathroom 'Always' Clean	300+	64%	-	71%
Timely Help 'Always' Received	300+	55%	-	64%
Would Definitely Recommend Hospital	300+	71%	-	69%

Philadelphia VA Medical Center

University and Woodland Avenue
Philadelphia, PA 19104
URL: www.philadelphia.va.gov
Type: Acute Care-Veterans Administration
Ownership: Government - Federal
Phone: 215-823-5857
Fax: 215-823-6054
Emergency Services: No
Beds: 675

Key Personnel:
CEO/President. . . . . Richard S Citron, FACHE
Chief of Medical Staff . . . . Peter R McCombs, MD
Quality Assurance . . . . Rosemary Campbell, RN
Radiology. . . . . M Scanlon, MD
Emergency Room . . . . J Abraham, MD

Measure	Cases	This Hosp.	State Avg.	U.S. Avg.
Heart Attack Care				
ACE Inhibitor or ARB for LVSD[5]	0	-	95%	96%
Aspirin at Arrival[5]	0	-	99%	99%
Aspirin at Discharge[5]	0	-	99%	98%
Beta Blocker at Discharge[5]	0	-	99%	98%
Fibrinolytic Medication Timing[5]	0	-	40%	55%
PCI Within 90 Minutes of Arrival[5]	0	-	88%	90%
Smoking Cessation Advice[5]	0	-	100%	99%
Chest Pain/Possible Heart Attack Care				
Aspirin at Arrival	-	-	95%	95%
Median Time to ECG (minutes)	-	-	8	8
Median Time to Transfer (minutes)	-	-	68	61
Fibrinolytic Medication Timing	-	-	48%	54%
Heart Failure Care				
ACE Inhibitor or ARB for LVSD	135	93%	95%	94%
Discharge Instructions	272	81%	90%	88%
Evaluation of LVS Function	282	99%	99%	98%
Smoking Cessation Advice	107	99%	98%	98%
Pneumonia Care				
Appropriate Initial Antibiotic	58	86%	93%	92%
Blood Culture Timing	88	97%	96%	96%
Influenza Vaccine	58	88%	92%	91%
Initial Antibiotic Timing	72	85%	96%	95%
Pneumococcal Vaccine	50	98%	95%	93%
Smoking Cessation Advice	33	100%	98%	97%
Surgical Care Improvement Project				
Appropriate VTP Within 24 Hours[2]	67	96%	95%	92%
Appropriate Hair Removal[2]	90	100%	100%	99%
Appropriate Beta Blocker Usage[1,2]	24	100%	94%	93%
Controlled Postoperative Blood Glucose[2,5]	0	-	96%	93%
Prophylactic Antibiotic Timing	32	88%	97%	97%
Prophylactic Antibiotic Timing (Outpatient)	-	-	92%	92%
Prophylactic Antibiotic Selection	31	94%	98%	97%
Prophylactic Antibiotic Select. (Outpatient)	-	-	93%	94%
Prophylactic Antibiotic Stopped	26	77%	95%	94%
Recommended VTP Ordered[2]	67	97%	97%	94%
Urinary Catheter Removal[2]	33	61%	95%	90%
Children's Asthma Care				
Received Systemic Corticosteroids	-	-	-	100%
Received Home Management Plan	-	-	-	71%
Received Reliever Medication	-	-	-	100%
Use of Medical Imaging				
Combination Abdominal CT Scan	-	-	0.203	0.191
Combination Chest CT Scan	-	-	0.026	0.054
Follow-up Mammogram/Ultrasound	-	-	8.2%	8.4%
MRI for Low Back Pain	-	-	32.4%	32.7%
Survey of Patients' Hospital Experiences				
Area Around Room 'Always' Quiet at Night	-	-	-	58%
Doctors 'Always' Communicated Well	-	-	-	80%
Home Recovery Information Given	-	-	-	82%
Hospital Given 9 or 10 on 10 Point Scale	-	-	-	67%
Meds 'Always' Explained Before Given	-	-	-	60%
Nurses 'Always' Communicated Well	-	-	-	76%
Pain 'Always' Well Controlled	-	-	-	69%
Room and Bathroom 'Always' Clean	-	-	-	71%
Timely Help 'Always' Received	-	-	-	64%
Would Definitely Recommend Hospital	-	-	-	69%

Saint Joseph's Hospital

1600 West Girard Avenue
Philadelphia, PA 19130
URL: www.nphs.com
Type: Acute Care Hospitals
Ownership: Voluntary Non-Profit - Private
Phone: 215-787-2000
Fax: 215-787-2195
Emergency Services: Yes
Beds: 168

Key Personnel:
CEO/President. . . . . George J Walmsley
Chief of Medical Staff. . . . . Shailendra Vaidya, MD
Operating Room. . . . . Jackie Dixon
Quality Assurance . . . . Wilda Seymour
Emergency Room . . . . H Greene

Measure	Cases	This Hosp.	State Avg.	U.S. Avg.
Heart Attack Care				
ACE Inhibitor or ARB for LVSD[1]	4	50%	95%	96%
Aspirin at Arrival	56	89%	99%	99%
Aspirin at Discharge[1]	17	82%	99%	98%
Beta Blocker at Discharge[1]	19	68%	99%	98%
Fibrinolytic Medication Timing[1]	1	0%	40%	55%
PCI Within 90 Minutes of Arrival	0	-	88%	90%
Smoking Cessation Advice[1]	5	60%	100%	99%
Chest Pain/Possible Heart Attack Care				
Aspirin at Arrival[1,3]	5	100%	95%	95%
Median Time to ECG (minutes)[1,3]	3	8	8	8
Median Time to Transfer (minutes)[5]	0	-	68	61
Fibrinolytic Medication Timing[3]	0	-	48%	54%
Heart Failure Care				
ACE Inhibitor or ARB for LVSD	80	76%	95%	94%
Discharge Instructions	213	23%	90%	88%
Evaluation of LVS Function	257	79%	99%	98%
Smoking Cessation Advice	112	61%	98%	98%
Pneumonia Care				
Appropriate Initial Antibiotic	37	68%	93%	92%
Blood Culture Timing	75	81%	96%	96%
Influenza Vaccine	37	30%	92%	91%
Initial Antibiotic Timing	79	77%	96%	95%
Pneumococcal Vaccine	48	52%	95%	93%
Smoking Cessation Advice	25	40%	98%	97%
Surgical Care Improvement Project				
Appropriate VTP Within 24 Hours	38	84%	95%	92%
Appropriate Hair Removal	63	87%	100%	99%
Appropriate Beta Blocker Usage[1]	10	70%	94%	93%
Controlled Postoperative Blood Glucose	0	-	96%	93%
Prophylactic Antibiotic Timing[1]	13	38%	97%	97%
Prophylactic Antibiotic Timing (Outpatient)[1,3]	16	62%	92%	92%
Prophylactic Antibiotic Selection[1]	13	69%	98%	97%
Prophylactic Antibiotic Select. (Outpatient)[1,3]	13	100%	93%	94%
Prophylactic Antibiotic Stopped[1]	13	38%	95%	94%
Recommended VTP Ordered	41	85%	97%	94%
Urinary Catheter Removal[1]	6	83%	95%	90%
Children's Asthma Care				
Received Systemic Corticosteroids	-	-	-	100%
Received Home Management Plan	-	-	-	71%
Received Reliever Medication	-	-	-	100%
Use of Medical Imaging				
Combination Abdominal CT Scan[1]	15	0.133	0.203	0.191
Combination Chest CT Scan[1]	6	0.000	0.026	0.054
Follow-up Mammogram/Ultrasound[1]	41	0.0%	8.2%	8.4%
MRI for Low Back Pain[5]	0	-	32.4%	32.7%
Survey of Patients' Hospital Experiences				
Area Around Room 'Always' Quiet at Night	(a)	49%	-	58%
Doctors 'Always' Communicated Well	(a)	70%	-	80%
Home Recovery Information Given	(a)	64%	-	82%
Hospital Given 9 or 10 on 10 Point Scale	(a)	40%	-	67%
Meds 'Always' Explained Before Given	(a)	45%	-	60%
Nurses 'Always' Communicated Well	(a)	56%	-	76%
Pain 'Always' Well Controlled	(a)	59%	-	69%
Room and Bathroom 'Always' Clean	(a)	61%	-	71%
Timely Help 'Always' Received	(a)	43%	-	64%
Would Definitely Recommend Hospital	(a)	35%	-	69%

NOTE: Hospital profiles are in alphabetical order by state, then city, then hospital within the city; Rankings exclude hospitals with less than 25 cases except for patient surveys which excludes hospitals with less than 100 cases; (a) 100–299 cases; (1) The number of cases is too small to be sure how well a hospital is performing; (2) The hospital indicated that the data submitted for this measure were based on a sample of cases; (3) Data was collected during a shorter time period (fewer quarters) than the maximum possible time for this measure; (4) Suppressed for one or more quarters by CMS; (5) No data is available from the hospital for this measure; (6) Fewer than 100 patients completed the HCAHPS survey. Use these rates with caution, as the number of surveys may be too low to reliably assess hospital performance; (7) Survey results are based on less than 12 months of data; (8) Survey results are not available for this reporting period; (9) No or very few patients were eligible for the HCAHPS survey. The scores shown, if any, reflect a very small number of surveys; (10) A state average was not calculated because too few hospitals in the state submitted data; (11) There were discrepancies in the data collection process; Please refer to the User's Guide for a full explanation of data.

Temple University Hospital

3401 North Broad Street Phone: 215-707-2000
Philadelphia, PA 19140 Fax: 215-707-8012
Type: Acute Care Hospitals Emergency Services: Yes
Ownership: Voluntary Non-Profit - Private Beds: 514

Key Personnel:
Chief of Medical Staff.......... Sidney Cohen
Infection Control.............. Keith St. John
Operating Room.............. Marsha Reddin, RN
Pediatric Ambulatory Care...... Stephen Aronoff
Pediatric In-Patient Care....... Stephen Aronoff
Quality Assurance............ Janet Leach
Radiology.................. Robert A Gatenby

Measure	Cases	This Hosp.	State Avg.	U.S. Avg.
Heart Attack Care				
ACE Inhibitor or ARB for LVSD	90	97%	95%	96%
Aspirin at Arrival	235	99%	99%	99%
Aspirin at Discharge	297	99%	99%	98%
Beta Blocker at Discharge	277	100%	99%	98%
Fibrinolytic Medication Timing	0	-	40%	55%
PCI Within 90 Minutes of Arrival[1]	23	74%	88%	90%
Smoking Cessation Advice	122	100%	100%	99%
Chest Pain/Possible Heart Attack Care				
Aspirin at Arrival[1,3]	9	100%	95%	95%
Median Time to ECG (minutes)[1,3]	10	14	8	8
Median Time to Transfer (minutes)[5]	0	-	68	61
Fibrinolytic Medication Timing[3]	0	-	48%	54%
Heart Failure Care				
ACE Inhibitor or ARB for LVSD	692	96%	95%	94%
Discharge Instructions	1,216	96%	90%	88%
Evaluation of LVS Function	1,294	99%	99%	98%
Smoking Cessation Advice	428	100%	98%	98%
Pneumonia Care				
Appropriate Initial Antibiotic	218	94%	93%	92%
Blood Culture Timing	298	95%	96%	96%
Influenza Vaccine	240	92%	92%	91%
Initial Antibiotic Timing	360	90%	96%	95%
Pneumococcal Vaccine	226	86%	95%	93%
Smoking Cessation Advice	274	100%	98%	97%
Surgical Care Improvement Project				
Appropriate VTP Within 24 Hours[2]	394	97%	95%	92%
Appropriate Hair Removal[2]	1,112	100%	100%	99%
Appropriate Beta Blocker Usage[2]	289	86%	94%	93%
Controlled Postoperative Blood Glucose[2]	141	87%	96%	93%
Prophylactic Antibiotic Timing[2]	789	97%	97%	97%
Prophylactic Antibiotic Timing (Outpatient)	402	93%	92%	92%
Prophylactic Antibiotic Selection[2]	804	95%	98%	97%
Prophylactic Antibiotic Select. (Outpatient)	394	91%	93%	94%
Prophylactic Antibiotic Stopped[2]	618	99%	95%	94%
Recommended VTP Ordered[2]	394	99%	97%	94%
Urinary Catheter Removal[2]	159	81%	95%	90%
Children's Asthma Care				
Received Systemic Corticosteroids	-	-	-	100%
Received Home Management Plan	-	-	-	71%
Received Reliever Medication	-	-	-	100%
Use of Medical Imaging				
Combination Abdominal CT Scan	633	0.164	0.203	0.191
Combination Chest CT Scan	827	0.017	0.026	0.054
Follow-up Mammogram/Ultrasound	888	5.7%	8.2%	8.4%
MRI for Low Back Pain	79	40.5%	32.4%	32.7%
Survey of Patients' Hospital Experiences				
Area Around Room 'Always' Quiet at Night	300+	53%	-	58%
Doctors 'Always' Communicated Well	300+	77%	-	80%
Home Recovery Information Given	300+	82%	-	82%
Hospital Given 9 or 10 on 10 Point Scale	300+	59%	-	67%
Meds 'Always' Explained Before Given	300+	56%	-	60%
Nurses 'Always' Communicated Well	300+	69%	-	76%
Pain 'Always' Well Controlled	300+	62%	-	69%
Room and Bathroom 'Always' Clean	300+	64%	-	71%
Timely Help 'Always' Received	300+	50%	-	64%
Would Definitely Recommend Hospital	300+	61%	-	69%

Thomas Jefferson University Hospital

111 South 11th Street Phone: 215-955-6000
Philadelphia, PA 19107 Fax: 215-955-2197
URL: www.jeffersonhospital.org
Type: Acute Care Hospitals Emergency Services: Yes
Ownership: Voluntary Non-Profit - Private Beds: 957

Key Personnel:
CEO/President.............. Thomas J Lewis
Chief of Medical Staff........ Geno Merli, MD, FACP

Measure	Cases	This Hosp.	State Avg.	U.S. Avg.
Heart Attack Care				
ACE Inhibitor or ARB for LVSD	60	100%	95%	96%
Aspirin at Arrival	184	99%	99%	99%
Aspirin at Discharge	263	99%	99%	98%
Beta Blocker at Discharge	250	100%	99%	98%
Fibrinolytic Medication Timing	0	-	40%	55%
PCI Within 90 Minutes of Arrival[1]	7	86%	88%	90%
Smoking Cessation Advice	88	100%	100%	99%
Chest Pain/Possible Heart Attack Care				
Aspirin at Arrival[5]	0	-	95%	95%
Median Time to ECG (minutes)[5]	0	-	8	8
Median Time to Transfer (minutes)[5]	0	-	68	61
Fibrinolytic Medication Timing[5]	0	-	48%	54%
Heart Failure Care				
ACE Inhibitor or ARB for LVSD	412	99%	95%	94%
Discharge Instructions	853	98%	90%	88%
Evaluation of LVS Function	985	99%	99%	98%
Smoking Cessation Advice	229	100%	98%	98%
Pneumonia Care				
Appropriate Initial Antibiotic	264	92%	93%	92%
Blood Culture Timing	435	86%	96%	96%
Influenza Vaccine	241	90%	92%	91%
Initial Antibiotic Timing	400	88%	96%	95%
Pneumococcal Vaccine	289	93%	95%	93%
Smoking Cessation Advice	177	99%	98%	97%
Surgical Care Improvement Project				
Appropriate VTP Within 24 Hours[2]	814	98%	95%	92%
Appropriate Hair Removal[2]	3,104	100%	100%	99%
Appropriate Beta Blocker Usage[2]	763	96%	94%	93%
Controlled Postoperative Blood Glucose[2]	184	87%	96%	93%
Prophylactic Antibiotic Timing[2]	2,538	99%	97%	97%
Prophylactic Antibiotic Timing (Outpatient)	487	84%	92%	92%
Prophylactic Antibiotic Selection[2]	2,558	98%	98%	97%
Prophylactic Antibiotic Select. (Outpatient)	485	99%	93%	94%
Prophylactic Antibiotic Stopped[2]	2,489	98%	95%	94%
Recommended VTP Ordered[2]	816	99%	97%	94%
Urinary Catheter Removal[2]	978	97%	95%	90%
Children's Asthma Care				
Received Systemic Corticosteroids	-	-	-	100%
Received Home Management Plan	-	-	-	71%
Received Reliever Medication	-	-	-	100%
Use of Medical Imaging				
Combination Abdominal CT Scan	1,346	0.195	0.203	0.191
Combination Chest CT Scan	1,046	0.011	0.026	0.054
Follow-up Mammogram/Ultrasound	3,292	9.0%	8.2%	8.4%
MRI for Low Back Pain	201	27.4%	32.4%	32.7%
Survey of Patients' Hospital Experiences				
Area Around Room 'Always' Quiet at Night	300+	50%	-	58%
Doctors 'Always' Communicated Well	300+	77%	-	80%
Home Recovery Information Given	300+	84%	-	82%
Hospital Given 9 or 10 on 10 Point Scale	300+	70%	-	67%
Meds 'Always' Explained Before Given	300+	61%	-	60%
Nurses 'Always' Communicated Well	300+	77%	-	76%
Pain 'Always' Well Controlled	300+	70%	-	69%
Room and Bathroom 'Always' Clean	300+	66%	-	71%
Timely Help 'Always' Received	300+	67%	-	64%
Would Definitely Recommend Hospital	300+	75%	-	69%

Phoenixville Hospital

140 Nutt Road Phone: 610-983-1000
Phoenixville, PA 19460 Fax: 610-983-1488
URL: www.pennhealth.com
Type: Acute Care Hospitals Emergency Services: Yes
Ownership: Proprietary Beds: 106

Key Personnel:
CEO/President.............. Mark B Real, MD
Chief of Medical Staff.......... Joel W Eisner, MD
Infection Control.............. Carolyn Peterson
Operating Room.............. Barbara Shaffer
Pediatric Ambulatory Care...... Maurice Rozwat, MD
Pediatric In-Patient Care....... Maurice Rozwat, MD
Quality Assurance............ Sue Detwiler, RN
Radiology.................. Geoffrey A Agrons, MD

Measure	Cases	This Hosp.	State Avg.	U.S. Avg.
Heart Attack Care				
ACE Inhibitor or ARB for LVSD	40	92%	95%	96%
Aspirin at Arrival	157	99%	99%	99%
Aspirin at Discharge	217	100%	99%	98%
Beta Blocker at Discharge	215	100%	99%	98%
Fibrinolytic Medication Timing	0	-	40%	55%
PCI Within 90 Minutes of Arrival[1]	22	86%	88%	90%
Smoking Cessation Advice	64	98%	100%	99%
Chest Pain/Possible Heart Attack Care				
Aspirin at Arrival[1,3]	3	100%	95%	95%
Median Time to ECG (minutes)[1,3]	3	5	8	8
Median Time to Transfer (minutes)[5]	0	-	68	61
Fibrinolytic Medication Timing[5]	0	-	48%	54%
Heart Failure Care				
ACE Inhibitor or ARB for LVSD	102	99%	95%	94%
Discharge Instructions	207	95%	90%	88%
Evaluation of LVS Function	257	96%	99%	98%
Smoking Cessation Advice	28	96%	98%	98%
Pneumonia Care				
Appropriate Initial Antibiotic	105	90%	93%	92%
Blood Culture Timing	140	93%	96%	96%
Influenza Vaccine	131	85%	92%	91%
Initial Antibiotic Timing	172	95%	96%	95%
Pneumococcal Vaccine	195	92%	95%	93%
Smoking Cessation Advice	43	98%	98%	97%
Surgical Care Improvement Project				
Appropriate VTP Within 24 Hours[2]	224	93%	95%	92%
Appropriate Hair Removal[2]	550	100%	100%	99%
Appropriate Beta Blocker Usage[2]	189	99%	94%	93%
Controlled Postoperative Blood Glucose[2]	99	96%	96%	93%
Prophylactic Antibiotic Timing[2]	325	97%	97%	97%
Prophylactic Antibiotic Timing (Outpatient)	114	98%	92%	92%
Prophylactic Antibiotic Selection[2]	328	98%	98%	97%
Prophylactic Antibiotic Select. (Outpatient)	115	93%	93%	94%
Prophylactic Antibiotic Stopped[2]	304	92%	95%	94%
Recommended VTP Ordered[2]	224	96%	97%	94%
Urinary Catheter Removal	126	90%	95%	90%
Children's Asthma Care				
Received Systemic Corticosteroids	-	-	-	100%
Received Home Management Plan	-	-	-	71%
Received Reliever Medication	-	-	-	100%
Use of Medical Imaging				
Combination Abdominal CT Scan	470	0.338	0.203	0.191
Combination Chest CT Scan	424	0.045	0.026	0.054
Follow-up Mammogram/Ultrasound	841	9.2%	8.2%	8.4%
MRI for Low Back Pain	133	36.1%	32.4%	32.7%
Survey of Patients' Hospital Experiences				
Area Around Room 'Always' Quiet at Night	300+	54%	-	58%
Doctors 'Always' Communicated Well	300+	73%	-	80%
Home Recovery Information Given	300+	81%	-	82%
Hospital Given 9 or 10 on 10 Point Scale	300+	64%	-	67%
Meds 'Always' Explained Before Given	300+	57%	-	60%
Nurses 'Always' Communicated Well	300+	73%	-	76%
Pain 'Always' Well Controlled	300+	66%	-	69%
Room and Bathroom 'Always' Clean	300+	62%	-	71%
Timely Help 'Always' Received	300+	54%	-	64%
Would Definitely Recommend Hospital	300+	64%	-	69%

NOTE: Hospital profiles are in alphabetical order by state, then city, then hospital within the city; Rankings exclude hospitals with less than 25 cases except for patient surveys which excludes hospitals with less than 100 cases; (a) 100–299 cases; (1) The number of cases is too small to be sure how well a hospital is performing; (2) The hospital indicated that the data submitted for this measure were based on a sample of cases; (3) Data was collected during a shorter time period (fewer quarters) than the maximum possible time for this measure; (4) Suppressed for one or more quarters by CMS; (5) No data is available from the hospital for this measure; (6) Fewer than 100 patients completed the HCAHPS survey. Use these rates with caution, as the number of surveys may be too low to reliably assess hospital performance; (7) Survey results are based on less than 12 months of data; (8) Survey results are not available for this reporting period; (9) No or very few patients were eligible for the HCAHPS survey. The scores shown, if any, reflect a very small number of surveys; (10) A state average was not calculated because too few hospitals in the state submitted data; (11) There were discrepancies in the data collection process; Please refer to the User's Guide for a full explanation of data.

Allegheny General Hospital

320 East North Avenue
Pittsburgh, PA 15212
URL: www.allhealth.edu
Phone: 412-359-3131
Fax: 412-359-3888
Type: Acute Care Hospitals
Ownership: Voluntary Non-Profit - Other
Emergency Services: Yes
Beds: 755

Key Personnel:
CEO/President. . . . . Connie M Cibrone
Chief of Medical Staff. . . . . Christopher Bonnet, MD
Infection Control. . . . . Cheryl Herbert
Operating Room. . . . . Vicky Butler, RN
Pediatric Ambulatory Care . . . . . . Mary Goessler, MD
Pediatric In-Patient Care . . . . Mary Goessler, MD
Quality Assurance . . . . Kathleen Engelmeier
Radiology. . . . . David Parda, MD

Measure	Cases	This Hosp.	State Avg.	U.S. Avg.
Heart Attack Care				
ACE Inhibitor or ARB for LVSD	110	100%	95%	96%
Aspirin at Arrival	310	100%	99%	99%
Aspirin at Discharge	581	100%	99%	98%
Beta Blocker at Discharge	523	99%	99%	98%
Fibrinolytic Medication Timing	0	-	40%	55%
PCI Within 90 Minutes of Arrival	55	93%	88%	90%
Smoking Cessation Advice	193	100%	100%	99%
Chest Pain/Possible Heart Attack Care				
Aspirin at Arrival[1]	23	96%	95%	95%
Median Time to ECG (minutes)[1]	22	14	8	8
Median Time to Transfer (minutes)[1,3]	2	68	68	61
Fibrinolytic Medication Timing[3]	0	-	48%	54%
Heart Failure Care				
ACE Inhibitor or ARB for LVSD	285	99%	95%	94%
Discharge Instructions	571	95%	90%	88%
Evaluation of LVS Function	674	100%	99%	98%
Smoking Cessation Advice	109	100%	98%	98%
Pneumonia Care				
Appropriate Initial Antibiotic	109	96%	93%	92%
Blood Culture Timing	206	95%	96%	96%
Influenza Vaccine	201	99%	92%	91%
Initial Antibiotic Timing	247	98%	96%	95%
Pneumococcal Vaccine	264	98%	95%	93%
Smoking Cessation Advice	160	97%	98%	97%
Surgical Care Improvement Project				
Appropriate VTP Within 24 Hours[2]	1,416	98%	95%	92%
Appropriate Hair Removal[2]	2,957	100%	100%	99%
Appropriate Beta Blocker Usage[2]	875	95%	94%	93%
Controlled Postoperative Blood Glucose[2]	383	94%	96%	93%
Prophylactic Antibiotic Timing[2]	1,377	99%	97%	97%
Prophylactic Antibiotic Timing (Outpatient)	541	97%	92%	92%
Prophylactic Antibiotic Selection[2]	1,417	99%	98%	97%
Prophylactic Antibiotic Select. (Outpatient)	537	60%	93%	94%
Prophylactic Antibiotic Stopped[2]	1,265	95%	95%	94%
Recommended VTP Ordered[2]	1,416	99%	97%	94%
Urinary Catheter Removal[2]	651	97%	95%	90%
Children's Asthma Care				
Received Systemic Corticosteroids	-	-	-	100%
Received Home Management Plan	-	-	-	71%
Received Reliever Medication	-	-	-	100%
Use of Medical Imaging				
Combination Abdominal CT Scan	1,052	0.472	0.203	0.191
Combination Chest CT Scan	872	0.100	0.026	0.054
Follow-up Mammogram/Ultrasound	833	8.2%	8.2%	8.4%
MRI for Low Back Pain	96	39.6%	32.4%	32.7%
Survey of Patients' Hospital Experiences				
Area Around Room 'Always' Quiet at Night	300+	47%	-	58%
Doctors 'Always' Communicated Well	300+	73%	-	80%
Home Recovery Information Given	300+	80%	-	82%
Hospital Given 9 or 10 on 10 Point Scale	300+	61%	-	67%
Meds 'Always' Explained Before Given	300+	55%	-	60%
Nurses 'Always' Communicated Well	300+	71%	-	76%
Pain 'Always' Well Controlled	300+	60%	-	69%
Room and Bathroom 'Always' Clean	300+	60%	-	71%
Timely Help 'Always' Received	300+	52%	-	64%
Would Definitely Recommend Hospital	300+	65%	-	69%

Children's Hospital of Pittsburgh of UPMC

4401 Penn Avenue
Pittsburgh, PA 15224
URL: www.chp.edu
Phone: 412-692-5325
Fax: 412-692-5800
Type: Childrens
Ownership: Voluntary Non-Profit - Other
Emergency Services: Yes
Beds: 260

Key Personnel:
CEO/President. . . . . Christopher A Gessner
Chief of Medical Staff. . . . . Steven G Docimo, MD
Infection Control. . . . . Adrian Farley, RN
Operating Room. . . . . Diane Hupp, RN
Pediatric Ambulatory Care . . . . . . David H Perlmutter, MD
Pediatric In-Patient Care . . . . George K Gittes, MD
Quality Assurance . . . . Karen Calhoon
Radiology. . . . . Charles Finz, MD

Measure	Cases	This Hosp.	State Avg.	U.S. Avg.
Heart Attack Care				
ACE Inhibitor or ARB for LVSD	-	-	95%	96%
Aspirin at Arrival	-	-	99%	99%
Aspirin at Discharge	-	-	99%	98%
Beta Blocker at Discharge	-	-	99%	98%
Fibrinolytic Medication Timing	-	-	40%	55%
PCI Within 90 Minutes of Arrival	-	-	88%	90%
Smoking Cessation Advice	-	-	100%	99%
Chest Pain/Possible Heart Attack Care				
Aspirin at Arrival	-	-	95%	95%
Median Time to ECG (minutes)	-	-	8	8
Median Time to Transfer (minutes)	-	-	68	61
Fibrinolytic Medication Timing	-	-	48%	54%
Heart Failure Care				
ACE Inhibitor or ARB for LVSD	-	-	95%	94%
Discharge Instructions	-	-	90%	88%
Evaluation of LVS Function	-	-	99%	98%
Smoking Cessation Advice	-	-	98%	98%
Pneumonia Care				
Appropriate Initial Antibiotic	-	-	93%	92%
Blood Culture Timing	-	-	96%	96%
Influenza Vaccine	-	-	92%	91%
Initial Antibiotic Timing	-	-	96%	95%
Pneumococcal Vaccine	-	-	95%	93%
Smoking Cessation Advice	-	-	98%	97%
Surgical Care Improvement Project				
Appropriate VTP Within 24 Hours	-	-	95%	92%
Appropriate Hair Removal	-	-	100%	99%
Appropriate Beta Blocker Usage	-	-	94%	93%
Controlled Postoperative Blood Glucose	-	-	96%	93%
Prophylactic Antibiotic Timing	-	-	97%	97%
Prophylactic Antibiotic Timing (Outpatient)	-	-	92%	92%
Prophylactic Antibiotic Selection	-	-	98%	97%
Prophylactic Antibiotic Select. (Outpatient)	-	-	93%	94%
Prophylactic Antibiotic Stopped	-	-	95%	94%
Recommended VTP Ordered	-	-	97%	94%
Urinary Catheter Removal	-	-	95%	90%
Children's Asthma Care				
Received Systemic Corticosteroids	476	100%	-	100%
Received Home Management Plan	476	57%	-	71%
Received Reliever Medication	478	100%	-	100%
Use of Medical Imaging				
Combination Abdominal CT Scan	-	-	0.203	0.191
Combination Chest CT Scan	-	-	0.026	0.054
Follow-up Mammogram/Ultrasound	-	-	8.2%	8.4%
MRI for Low Back Pain	-	-	32.4%	32.7%
Survey of Patients' Hospital Experiences				
Area Around Room 'Always' Quiet at Night	-	-	-	58%
Doctors 'Always' Communicated Well	-	-	-	80%
Home Recovery Information Given	-	-	-	82%
Hospital Given 9 or 10 on 10 Point Scale	-	-	-	67%
Meds 'Always' Explained Before Given	-	-	-	60%
Nurses 'Always' Communicated Well	-	-	-	76%
Pain 'Always' Well Controlled	-	-	-	69%
Room and Bathroom 'Always' Clean	-	-	-	71%
Timely Help 'Always' Received	-	-	-	64%
Would Definitely Recommend Hospital	-	-	-	69%

Jefferson Regional Medical Center

565 Coal Valley Rd
Pittsburgh, PA 15236
URL: www.jeffersonregional.com
Phone: 412-469-5000
Fax: 412-469-2495
Type: Acute Care Hospitals
Ownership: Voluntary Non-Profit - Other
Emergency Services: Yes
Beds: 390

Key Personnel:
CEO/President. . . . . Thomas P Timcho
Quality Assurance . . . . Edward Guzik
Radiology. . . . . Kate Labuskes
Intensive Care Unit. . . . . Jewell Coulter

Measure	Cases	This Hosp.	State Avg.	U.S. Avg.
Heart Attack Care				
ACE Inhibitor or ARB for LVSD	60	90%	95%	96%
Aspirin at Arrival	271	99%	99%	99%
Aspirin at Discharge	309	100%	99%	98%
Beta Blocker at Discharge	300	99%	99%	98%
Fibrinolytic Medication Timing	0	-	40%	55%
PCI Within 90 Minutes of Arrival	64	81%	88%	90%
Smoking Cessation Advice	104	99%	100%	99%
Chest Pain/Possible Heart Attack Care				
Aspirin at Arrival[1]	9	89%	95%	95%
Median Time to ECG (minutes)[1]	10	4	8	8
Median Time to Transfer (minutes)[5]	0	-	68	61
Fibrinolytic Medication Timing[3]	0	-	48%	54%
Heart Failure Care				
ACE Inhibitor or ARB for LVSD	217	85%	95%	94%
Discharge Instructions	605	90%	90%	88%
Evaluation of LVS Function	744	99%	99%	98%
Smoking Cessation Advice	74	100%	98%	98%
Pneumonia Care				
Appropriate Initial Antibiotic	232	90%	93%	92%
Blood Culture Timing	229	97%	96%	96%
Influenza Vaccine	250	96%	92%	91%
Initial Antibiotic Timing	357	96%	96%	95%
Pneumococcal Vaccine	323	94%	95%	93%
Smoking Cessation Advice	95	95%	98%	97%
Surgical Care Improvement Project				
Appropriate VTP Within 24 Hours	700	95%	95%	92%
Appropriate Hair Removal	1,780	100%	100%	99%
Appropriate Beta Blocker Usage	643	99%	94%	93%
Controlled Postoperative Blood Glucose	363	98%	96%	93%
Prophylactic Antibiotic Timing	1,174	99%	97%	97%
Prophylactic Antibiotic Timing (Outpatient)	268	94%	92%	92%
Prophylactic Antibiotic Selection	1,197	99%	98%	97%
Prophylactic Antibiotic Select. (Outpatient)	258	80%	93%	94%
Prophylactic Antibiotic Stopped	1,150	94%	95%	94%
Recommended VTP Ordered	703	96%	97%	94%
Urinary Catheter Removal	583	97%	95%	90%
Children's Asthma Care				
Received Systemic Corticosteroids	-	-	-	100%
Received Home Management Plan	-	-	-	71%
Received Reliever Medication	-	-	-	100%
Use of Medical Imaging				
Combination Abdominal CT Scan	625	0.134	0.203	0.191
Combination Chest CT Scan	432	0.063	0.026	0.054
Follow-up Mammogram/Ultrasound	248	21.4%	8.2%	8.4%
MRI for Low Back Pain[1]	14	57.1%	32.4%	32.7%
Survey of Patients' Hospital Experiences				
Area Around Room 'Always' Quiet at Night	300+	49%	-	58%
Doctors 'Always' Communicated Well	300+	80%	-	80%
Home Recovery Information Given	300+	85%	-	82%
Hospital Given 9 or 10 on 10 Point Scale	300+	71%	-	67%
Meds 'Always' Explained Before Given	300+	57%	-	60%
Nurses 'Always' Communicated Well	300+	80%	-	76%
Pain 'Always' Well Controlled	300+	72%	-	69%
Room and Bathroom 'Always' Clean	300+	71%	-	71%
Timely Help 'Always' Received	300+	60%	-	64%
Would Definitely Recommend Hospital	300+	76%	-	69%

NOTE: Hospital profiles are in alphabetical order by state, then city, then hospital within the city; Rankings exclude hospitals with less than 25 cases except for patient surveys which excludes hospitals with less than 100 cases; (a) 100–299 cases; (1) The number of cases is too small to be sure how well a hospital is performing; (2) The hospital indicated that the data submitted for this measure were based on a sample of cases; (3) Data was collected during a shorter time period (fewer quarters) than the maximum possible time for this measure; (4) Suppressed for one or more quarters by CMS; (5) No data is available from the hospital for this measure; (6) Fewer than 100 patients completed the HCAHPS survey. Use these rates with caution, as the number of surveys may be too low to reliably assess hospital performance; (7) Survey results are based on less than 12 months of data; (8) Survey results are not available for this reporting period; (9) No or very few patients were eligible for the HCAHPS survey. The scores shown, if any, reflect a very small number of surveys; (10) A state average was not calculated because too few hospitals in the state submitted data; (11) There were discrepancies in the data collection process; Please refer to the User's Guide for a full explanation of data.

Magee Womens Hospital of UPMC Health System

300 Halket Street
Pittsburgh, PA 15213
Phone: 412-641-4010
Fax: 412-641-4343
E-mail: upmcweb@upmc.edu
URL: www.magee.edu
Type: Acute Care Hospitals
Emergency Services: Yes
Ownership: Voluntary Non-Profit - Other
Beds: 287

Key Personnel:
Chief of Medical Staff.......... Jerome H Aarons, MD
Operating Room............. Linda Pechin
Pediatric In-Patient Care .... Sherin Devaskar, MD
Quality Assurance .... Sandra Read-Triebsch
Radiology.................. Jules J Sumkin, DO
Anesthesiology.............. Sivam Ramanathan, MD
Emergency Room .... Carol Simmons, MD
Intensive Care Unit............ Herbert Jacob, MD

Measure	Cases	This Hosp.	State Avg.	U.S. Avg.
Heart Attack Care				
ACE Inhibitor or ARB for LVSD[3]	0	-	95%	96%
Aspirin at Arrival[1,3]	3	100%	99%	99%
Aspirin at Discharge[1,3]	3	100%	99%	98%
Beta Blocker at Discharge[1,3]	3	100%	99%	98%
Fibrinolytic Medication Timing[3]	0	-	40%	55%
PCI Within 90 Minutes of Arrival[3]	0	-	88%	90%
Smoking Cessation Advice[3]	0	-	100%	99%
Chest Pain/Possible Heart Attack Care				
Aspirin at Arrival[5]	0	-	95%	95%
Median Time to ECG (minutes)[5]	0	-	8	8
Median Time to Transfer (minutes)[5]	0	-	68	61
Fibrinolytic Medication Timing[5]	0	-	48%	54%
Heart Failure Care				
ACE Inhibitor or ARB for LVSD[1]	21	100%	95%	94%
Discharge Instructions	59	100%	90%	88%
Evaluation of LVS Function	83	100%	99%	98%
Smoking Cessation Advice[1]	12	100%	98%	98%
Pneumonia Care				
Appropriate Initial Antibiotic	34	94%	93%	92%
Blood Culture Timing	32	100%	96%	96%
Influenza Vaccine	45	91%	92%	91%
Initial Antibiotic Timing	40	100%	96%	95%
Pneumococcal Vaccine	51	92%	95%	93%
Smoking Cessation Advice	33	100%	98%	97%
Surgical Care Improvement Project				
Appropriate VTP Within 24 Hours	549	97%	95%	92%
Appropriate Hair Removal	2,291	100%	100%	99%
Appropriate Beta Blocker Usage	436	95%	94%	93%
Controlled Postoperative Blood Glucose	0	-	96%	93%
Prophylactic Antibiotic Timing	1,880	98%	97%	97%
Prophylactic Antibiotic Timing (Outpatient)	330	91%	92%	92%
Prophylactic Antibiotic Selection	1,878	97%	98%	97%
Prophylactic Antibiotic Select. (Outpatient)	309	94%	93%	94%
Prophylactic Antibiotic Stopped	1,854	96%	95%	94%
Recommended VTP Ordered	550	98%	97%	94%
Urinary Catheter Removal	525	100%	95%	90%
Children's Asthma Care				
Received Systemic Corticosteroids	-	-	-	100%
Received Home Management Plan	-	-	-	71%
Received Reliever Medication	-	-	-	100%
Use of Medical Imaging				
Combination Abdominal CT Scan	545	0.156	0.203	0.191
Combination Chest CT Scan	505	0.004	0.026	0.054
Follow-up Mammogram/Ultrasound	3,186	8.5%	8.2%	8.4%
MRI for Low Back Pain[1]	10	30.0%	32.4%	32.7%
Survey of Patients' Hospital Experiences				
Area Around Room 'Always' Quiet at Night	300+	44%	-	58%
Doctors 'Always' Communicated Well	300+	76%	-	80%
Home Recovery Information Given	300+	79%	-	82%
Hospital Given 9 or 10 on 10 Point Scale	300+	64%	-	67%
Meds 'Always' Explained Before Given	300+	54%	-	60%
Nurses 'Always' Communicated Well	300+	70%	-	76%
Pain 'Always' Well Controlled	300+	63%	-	69%
Room and Bathroom 'Always' Clean	300+	63%	-	71%
Timely Help 'Always' Received	300+	56%	-	64%
Would Definitely Recommend Hospital	300+	72%	-	69%

Saint Clair Memorial Hospital

1000 Bower Hill Road
Pittsburgh, PA 15243
Phone: 412-561-4900
Fax: 412-572-6561
URL: www.stclair.org
Type: Acute Care Hospitals
Emergency Services: Yes
Ownership: Voluntary Non-Profit - Other
Beds: 314

Key Personnel:
Operating Room............. Barbara Mentzer
Pediatric Ambulatory Care ...... Charles Silverstein, MD
Pediatric In-Patient Care .... Charles Silverstein, MD
Quality Assurance .... Linda Lattner
Radiology.................. Donald P Orr, MD
Emergency Room .... Karen Klein, RN

Measure	Cases	This Hosp.	State Avg.	U.S. Avg.
Heart Attack Care				
ACE Inhibitor or ARB for LVSD	34	76%	95%	96%
Aspirin at Arrival	269	97%	99%	99%
Aspirin at Discharge	257	100%	99%	98%
Beta Blocker at Discharge	240	97%	99%	98%
Fibrinolytic Medication Timing	0	-	40%	55%
PCI Within 90 Minutes of Arrival	71	94%	88%	90%
Smoking Cessation Advice	68	100%	100%	99%
Chest Pain/Possible Heart Attack Care				
Aspirin at Arrival[1]	12	92%	95%	95%
Median Time to ECG (minutes)[1]	12	2	8	8
Median Time to Transfer (minutes)[3]	0	-	68	61
Fibrinolytic Medication Timing[3]	0	-	48%	54%
Heart Failure Care				
ACE Inhibitor or ARB for LVSD	152	84%	95%	94%
Discharge Instructions	454	79%	90%	88%
Evaluation of LVS Function	614	98%	99%	98%
Smoking Cessation Advice	54	100%	98%	98%
Pneumonia Care				
Appropriate Initial Antibiotic	360	96%	93%	92%
Blood Culture Timing	401	98%	96%	96%
Influenza Vaccine	389	91%	92%	91%
Initial Antibiotic Timing	540	96%	96%	95%
Pneumococcal Vaccine	554	93%	95%	93%
Smoking Cessation Advice	131	100%	98%	97%
Surgical Care Improvement Project				
Appropriate VTP Within 24 Hours[2]	569	93%	95%	92%
Appropriate Hair Removal[2]	1,508	99%	100%	99%
Appropriate Beta Blocker Usage[2]	438	92%	94%	93%
Controlled Postoperative Blood Glucose[2]	204	96%	96%	93%
Prophylactic Antibiotic Timing[2]	1,086	94%	97%	97%
Prophylactic Antibiotic Timing (Outpatient)	336	76%	92%	92%
Prophylactic Antibiotic Selection[2]	1,098	97%	98%	97%
Prophylactic Antibiotic Select. (Outpatient)	287	93%	93%	94%
Prophylactic Antibiotic Stopped[2]	1,046	97%	95%	94%
Recommended VTP Ordered[2]	569	96%	97%	94%
Urinary Catheter Removal[2]	167	92%	95%	90%
Children's Asthma Care				
Received Systemic Corticosteroids	-	-	-	100%
Received Home Management Plan	-	-	-	71%
Received Reliever Medication	-	-	-	100%
Use of Medical Imaging				
Combination Abdominal CT Scan	981	0.080	0.203	0.191
Combination Chest CT Scan	672	0.000	0.026	0.054
Follow-up Mammogram/Ultrasound	699	11.2%	8.2%	8.4%
MRI for Low Back Pain	156	36.5%	32.4%	32.7%
Survey of Patients' Hospital Experiences				
Area Around Room 'Always' Quiet at Night	300+	51%	-	58%
Doctors 'Always' Communicated Well	300+	78%	-	80%
Home Recovery Information Given	300+	81%	-	82%
Hospital Given 9 or 10 on 10 Point Scale	300+	71%	-	67%
Meds 'Always' Explained Before Given	300+	57%	-	60%
Nurses 'Always' Communicated Well	300+	79%	-	76%
Pain 'Always' Well Controlled	300+	72%	-	69%
Room and Bathroom 'Always' Clean	300+	69%	-	71%
Timely Help 'Always' Received	300+	64%	-	64%
Would Definitely Recommend Hospital	300+	75%	-	69%

UPMC Mercy

1400 Locust Street
Pittsburgh, PA 15219
Phone: 412-232-8111
Fax: 412-232-7408
URL: www.upmc.com/HospitalsFacilities/Mercy/Pages/default.aspx
Type: Acute Care Hospitals
Emergency Services: Yes
Ownership: Voluntary Non-Profit - Other
Beds: 416

Key Personnel:
CEO/President............... Kenneth A Eshak
Chief of Medical Staff.......... John Brungo, MD
Infection Control............. Sharon Krystofiak
Operating Room............. Claudia Osburn
Pediatric In-Patient Care .... Bradley J Bradford, MD
Quality Assurance .... Mary Menegazzi
Radiology.................. Sylvia Lesic

Measure	Cases	This Hosp.	State Avg.	U.S. Avg.
Heart Attack Care				
ACE Inhibitor or ARB for LVSD	73	99%	95%	96%
Aspirin at Arrival	259	98%	99%	99%
Aspirin at Discharge	374	100%	99%	98%
Beta Blocker at Discharge	353	100%	99%	98%
Fibrinolytic Medication Timing	0	-	40%	55%
PCI Within 90 Minutes of Arrival	45	80%	88%	90%
Smoking Cessation Advice	149	100%	100%	99%
Chest Pain/Possible Heart Attack Care				
Aspirin at Arrival[5]	0	-	95%	95%
Median Time to ECG (minutes)[5]	0	-	8	8
Median Time to Transfer (minutes)[5]	0	-	68	61
Fibrinolytic Medication Timing[5]	0	-	48%	54%
Heart Failure Care				
ACE Inhibitor or ARB for LVSD	168	99%	95%	94%
Discharge Instructions	366	87%	90%	88%
Evaluation of LVS Function	487	100%	99%	98%
Smoking Cessation Advice	96	100%	98%	98%
Pneumonia Care				
Appropriate Initial Antibiotic	212	92%	93%	92%
Blood Culture Timing	242	98%	96%	96%
Influenza Vaccine	205	90%	92%	91%
Initial Antibiotic Timing	329	96%	96%	95%
Pneumococcal Vaccine	274	94%	95%	93%
Smoking Cessation Advice	197	100%	98%	97%
Surgical Care Improvement Project				
Appropriate VTP Within 24 Hours[2]	227	98%	95%	92%
Appropriate Hair Removal[2]	617	100%	100%	99%
Appropriate Beta Blocker Usage[2]	197	98%	94%	93%
Controlled Postoperative Blood Glucose[2]	132	96%	96%	93%
Prophylactic Antibiotic Timing[2]	425	95%	97%	97%
Prophylactic Antibiotic Timing (Outpatient)	441	93%	92%	92%
Prophylactic Antibiotic Selection[2]	436	98%	98%	97%
Prophylactic Antibiotic Select. (Outpatient)	419	95%	93%	94%
Prophylactic Antibiotic Stopped[2]	393	94%	95%	94%
Recommended VTP Ordered[2]	227	99%	97%	94%
Urinary Catheter Removal[2]	118	91%	95%	90%
Children's Asthma Care				
Received Systemic Corticosteroids	-	-	-	100%
Received Home Management Plan	-	-	-	71%
Received Reliever Medication	-	-	-	100%
Use of Medical Imaging				
Combination Abdominal CT Scan	301	0.093	0.203	0.191
Combination Chest CT Scan	251	0.008	0.026	0.054
Follow-up Mammogram/Ultrasound	292	7.5%	8.2%	8.4%
MRI for Low Back Pain	35	45.7%	32.4%	32.7%
Survey of Patients' Hospital Experiences				
Area Around Room 'Always' Quiet at Night	300+	48%	-	58%
Doctors 'Always' Communicated Well	300+	74%	-	80%
Home Recovery Information Given	300+	80%	-	82%
Hospital Given 9 or 10 on 10 Point Scale	300+	53%	-	67%
Meds 'Always' Explained Before Given	300+	51%	-	60%
Nurses 'Always' Communicated Well	300+	64%	-	76%
Pain 'Always' Well Controlled	300+	58%	-	69%
Room and Bathroom 'Always' Clean	300+	55%	-	71%
Timely Help 'Always' Received	300+	45%	-	64%
Would Definitely Recommend Hospital	300+	57%	-	69%

NOTE: Hospital profiles are in alphabetical order by state, then city, then hospital within the city; Rankings exclude hospitals with less than 25 cases except for patient surveys which excludes hospitals with less than 100 cases; (a) 100–299 cases; (1) The number of cases is too small to be sure how well a hospital is performing; (2) The hospital indicated that the data submitted for this measure were based on a sample of cases; (3) Data was collected during a shorter time period (fewer quarters) than the maximum possible time for this measure; (4) Suppressed for one or more quarters by CMS; (5) No data is available from the hospital for this measure; (6) Fewer than 100 patients completed the HCAHPS survey. Use these rates with caution, as the number of surveys may be too low to reliably assess hospital performance; (7) Survey results are based on less than 12 months of data; (8) Survey results are not available for this reporting period; (9) No or very few patients were eligible for the HCAHPS survey. The scores shown, if any, reflect a very small number of surveys; (10) A state average was not calculated because too few hospitals in the state submitted data; (11) There were discrepancies in the data collection process; Please refer to the User's Guide for a full explanation of data.

UPMC Passavant

9100 Babcock Boulevard Phone: 412-367-6700
Pittsburgh, PA 15237 Fax: 412-367-6527
URL: passavant.upmc.com
Type: Acute Care Hospitals Emergency Services: Yes
Ownership: Voluntary Non-Profit - Private Beds: 272

Key Personnel:
CEO/President. . . . . Raymond Beck
Chief of Medical Staff. . . . . Thomas Shcauble, MD
Pediatric Ambulatory Care . . . . . . Howard K Scott
Pediatric In-Patient Care . . . . Howard K Scott
Quality Assurance . . . . Connie Susich
Radiology. . . . . Robert A Erbstein, MD
Emergency Room . . . . William Kristin, MD

Measure	Cases	This Hosp.	State Avg.	U.S. Avg.
Heart Attack Care				
ACE Inhibitor or ARB for LVSD	61	98%	95%	96%
Aspirin at Arrival	316	100%	99%	99%
Aspirin at Discharge	449	100%	99%	98%
Beta Blocker at Discharge	440	100%	99%	98%
Fibrinolytic Medication Timing	0	-	40%	55%
PCI Within 90 Minutes of Arrival	30	97%	88%	90%
Smoking Cessation Advice	123	100%	100%	99%
Chest Pain/Possible Heart Attack Care				
Aspirin at Arrival	48	98%	95%	95%
Median Time to ECG (minutes)	51	9	8	8
Median Time to Transfer (minutes)[1,3]	1	92	68	61
Fibrinolytic Medication Timing[3]	0	-	48%	54%
Heart Failure Care				
ACE Inhibitor or ARB for LVSD	144	100%	95%	94%
Discharge Instructions	347	97%	90%	88%
Evaluation of LVS Function	508	100%	99%	98%
Smoking Cessation Advice	37	100%	98%	98%
Pneumonia Care				
Appropriate Initial Antibiotic	263	88%	93%	92%
Blood Culture Timing	387	98%	96%	96%
Influenza Vaccine	288	98%	92%	91%
Initial Antibiotic Timing	413	95%	96%	95%
Pneumococcal Vaccine	408	99%	95%	93%
Smoking Cessation Advice	111	99%	98%	97%
Surgical Care Improvement Project				
Appropriate VTP Within 24 Hours	970	98%	95%	92%
Appropriate Hair Removal	1,951	100%	100%	99%
Appropriate Beta Blocker Usage	627	98%	94%	93%
Controlled Postoperative Blood Glucose	392	95%	96%	93%
Prophylactic Antibiotic Timing	1,232	97%	97%	97%
Prophylactic Antibiotic Timing (Outpatient)	519	93%	92%	92%
Prophylactic Antibiotic Selection	1,248	98%	98%	97%
Prophylactic Antibiotic Select. (Outpatient)	519	91%	93%	94%
Prophylactic Antibiotic Stopped	1,190	98%	95%	94%
Recommended VTP Ordered	971	99%	97%	94%
Urinary Catheter Removal	397	90%	95%	90%
Children's Asthma Care				
Received Systemic Corticosteroids	-	-	-	100%
Received Home Management Plan	-	-	-	71%
Received Reliever Medication	-	-	-	100%
Use of Medical Imaging				
Combination Abdominal CT Scan	958	0.593	0.203	0.191
Combination Chest CT Scan	847	0.012	0.026	0.054
Follow-up Mammogram/Ultrasound	587	11.1%	8.2%	8.4%
MRI for Low Back Pain	150	34.0%	32.4%	32.7%
Survey of Patients' Hospital Experiences				
Area Around Room 'Always' Quiet at Night	300+	43%	-	58%
Doctors 'Always' Communicated Well	300+	75%	-	80%
Home Recovery Information Given	300+	84%	-	82%
Hospital Given 9 or 10 on 10 Point Scale	300+	60%	-	67%
Meds 'Always' Explained Before Given	300+	52%	-	60%
Nurses 'Always' Communicated Well	300+	69%	-	76%
Pain 'Always' Well Controlled	300+	65%	-	69%
Room and Bathroom 'Always' Clean	300+	55%	-	71%
Timely Help 'Always' Received	300+	52%	-	64%
Would Definitely Recommend Hospital	300+	64%	-	69%

UPMC Presbyterian Shadyside

200 Lothrop Street Phone: 412-647-8788
Pittsburgh, PA 15213 Fax: 412-647-4881
URL: www.upmc.edu
Type: Acute Care Hospitals Emergency Services: Yes
Ownership: Voluntary Non-Profit - Private Beds: 1,227

Key Personnel:
CEO/President. . . . . Jeffrey Romoff
Chief of Medical Staff . . . . Edward Wing, MD
Quality Assurance . . . . April Lana Forf
Radiology. . . . . Jules H Sumkin, MD
Anesthesiology. . . . . Peter Winters, MD
Emergency Room . . . . Andrew B Peitzman, MD
Hemotology Center . . . . Ronald Herberman, MD
Intensive Care Unit. . . . . Jorge Rakela, MD

Measure	Cases	This Hosp.	State Avg.	U.S. Avg.
Heart Attack Care				
ACE Inhibitor or ARB for LVSD	189	100%	95%	96%
Aspirin at Arrival	456	100%	99%	99%
Aspirin at Discharge	1,034	100%	99%	98%
Beta Blocker at Discharge	998	100%	99%	98%
Fibrinolytic Medication Timing	0	-	40%	55%
PCI Within 90 Minutes of Arrival	85	94%	88%	90%
Smoking Cessation Advice	374	100%	100%	99%
Chest Pain/Possible Heart Attack Care				
Aspirin at Arrival	217	95%	95%	95%
Median Time to ECG (minutes)	226	9	8	8
Median Time to Transfer (minutes)[5]	0	-	68	61
Fibrinolytic Medication Timing[3]	0	-	48%	54%
Heart Failure Care				
ACE Inhibitor or ARB for LVSD	515	100%	95%	94%
Discharge Instructions	1,113	98%	90%	88%
Evaluation of LVS Function	1,383	100%	99%	98%
Smoking Cessation Advice	260	100%	98%	98%
Pneumonia Care				
Appropriate Initial Antibiotic	240	100%	93%	92%
Blood Culture Timing	447	100%	96%	96%
Influenza Vaccine	421	99%	92%	91%
Initial Antibiotic Timing	545	99%	96%	95%
Pneumococcal Vaccine	488	100%	95%	93%
Smoking Cessation Advice	326	100%	98%	97%
Surgical Care Improvement Project				
Appropriate VTP Within 24 Hours	3,593	99%	95%	92%
Appropriate Hair Removal	7,812	100%	100%	99%
Appropriate Beta Blocker Usage	2,600	98%	94%	93%
Controlled Postoperative Blood Glucose	894	96%	96%	93%
Prophylactic Antibiotic Timing	2,801	99%	97%	97%
Prophylactic Antibiotic Timing (Outpatient)	970	97%	92%	92%
Prophylactic Antibiotic Selection	2,889	99%	98%	97%
Prophylactic Antibiotic Select. (Outpatient)	973	97%	93%	94%
Prophylactic Antibiotic Stopped	2,516	99%	95%	94%
Recommended VTP Ordered	3,593	99%	97%	94%
Urinary Catheter Removal	1,697	95%	95%	90%
Children's Asthma Care				
Received Systemic Corticosteroids	-	-	-	100%
Received Home Management Plan	-	-	-	71%
Received Reliever Medication	-	-	-	100%
Use of Medical Imaging				
Combination Abdominal CT Scan	3,464	0.256	0.203	0.191
Combination Chest CT Scan	3,991	0.014	0.026	0.054
Follow-up Mammogram/Ultrasound[5]	0	-	8.2%	8.4%
MRI for Low Back Pain	270	34.1%	32.4%	32.7%
Survey of Patients' Hospital Experiences				
Area Around Room 'Always' Quiet at Night	300+	45%	-	58%
Doctors 'Always' Communicated Well	300+	75%	-	80%
Home Recovery Information Given	300+	85%	-	82%
Hospital Given 9 or 10 on 10 Point Scale	300+	63%	-	67%
Meds 'Always' Explained Before Given	300+	56%	-	60%
Nurses 'Always' Communicated Well	300+	73%	-	76%
Pain 'Always' Well Controlled	300+	65%	-	69%
Room and Bathroom 'Always' Clean	300+	57%	-	71%
Timely Help 'Always' Received	300+	56%	-	64%
Would Definitely Recommend Hospital	300+	69%	-	69%

UPMC Saint Margaret

815 Freeport Road Phone: 412-784-4000
Pittsburgh, PA 15215 Fax: 412-784-4788
URL: www.stmargaret.upmc.com
Type: Acute Care Hospitals Emergency Services: Yes
Ownership: Voluntary Non-Profit - Private Beds: 250

Key Personnel:
CEO/President. . . . . Richard E Sobehart
Cardiac Laboratory. . . . . Jean Culhane
Operating Room. . . . . M Cook, RN
Radiology. . . . . Bill Simmons

Measure	Cases	This Hosp.	State Avg.	U.S. Avg.
Heart Attack Care				
ACE Inhibitor or ARB for LVSD[1]	9	100%	95%	96%
Aspirin at Arrival	102	96%	99%	99%
Aspirin at Discharge	49	100%	99%	98%
Beta Blocker at Discharge	61	100%	99%	98%
Fibrinolytic Medication Timing	0	-	40%	55%
PCI Within 90 Minutes of Arrival	0	-	88%	90%
Smoking Cessation Advice[1]	4	100%	100%	99%
Chest Pain/Possible Heart Attack Care				
Aspirin at Arrival	132	98%	95%	95%
Median Time to ECG (minutes)	138	12	8	8
Median Time to Transfer (minutes)	34	92	68	61
Fibrinolytic Medication Timing[1]	1	0%	48%	54%
Heart Failure Care				
ACE Inhibitor or ARB for LVSD	113	96%	95%	94%
Discharge Instructions	389	91%	90%	88%
Evaluation of LVS Function	573	100%	99%	98%
Smoking Cessation Advice	60	100%	98%	98%
Pneumonia Care				
Appropriate Initial Antibiotic	221	95%	93%	92%
Blood Culture Timing	259	99%	96%	96%
Influenza Vaccine	207	99%	92%	91%
Initial Antibiotic Timing	327	96%	96%	95%
Pneumococcal Vaccine	279	98%	95%	93%
Smoking Cessation Advice	93	100%	98%	97%
Surgical Care Improvement Project				
Appropriate VTP Within 24 Hours	849	99%	95%	92%
Appropriate Hair Removal	1,600	100%	100%	99%
Appropriate Beta Blocker Usage	531	99%	94%	93%
Controlled Postoperative Blood Glucose[1]	1	100%	96%	93%
Prophylactic Antibiotic Timing	1,095	96%	97%	97%
Prophylactic Antibiotic Timing (Outpatient)	357	96%	92%	92%
Prophylactic Antibiotic Selection	1,100	99%	98%	97%
Prophylactic Antibiotic Select. (Outpatient)	350	99%	93%	94%
Prophylactic Antibiotic Stopped	1,056	96%	95%	94%
Recommended VTP Ordered	849	100%	97%	94%
Urinary Catheter Removal	549	96%	95%	90%
Children's Asthma Care				
Received Systemic Corticosteroids	-	-	-	100%
Received Home Management Plan	-	-	-	71%
Received Reliever Medication	-	-	-	100%
Use of Medical Imaging				
Combination Abdominal CT Scan	810	0.221	0.203	0.191
Combination Chest CT Scan	691	0.001	0.026	0.054
Follow-up Mammogram/Ultrasound	561	6.4%	8.2%	8.4%
MRI for Low Back Pain	159	39.0%	32.4%	32.7%
Survey of Patients' Hospital Experiences				
Area Around Room 'Always' Quiet at Night	300+	45%	-	58%
Doctors 'Always' Communicated Well	300+	77%	-	80%
Home Recovery Information Given	300+	87%	-	82%
Hospital Given 9 or 10 on 10 Point Scale	300+	66%	-	67%
Meds 'Always' Explained Before Given	300+	57%	-	60%
Nurses 'Always' Communicated Well	300+	74%	-	76%
Pain 'Always' Well Controlled	300+	66%	-	69%
Room and Bathroom 'Always' Clean	300+	61%	-	71%
Timely Help 'Always' Received	300+	56%	-	64%
Would Definitely Recommend Hospital	300+	73%	-	69%

NOTE: Hospital profiles are in alphabetical order by state, then city, then hospital within the city; Rankings exclude hospitals with less than 25 cases except for patient surveys which excludes hospitals with less than 100 cases; (a) 100–299 cases; (1) The number of cases is too small to be sure how well a hospital is performing; (2) The hospital indicated that the data submitted for this measure were based on a sample of cases; (3) Data was collected during a shorter time period (fewer quarters) than the maximum possible time for this measure; (4) Suppressed for one or more quarters by CMS; (5) No data is available from the hospital for this measure; (6) Fewer than 100 patients completed the HCAHPS survey. Use these rates with caution, as the number of surveys may be too low to reliably assess hospital performance; (7) Survey results are based on less than 12 months of data; (8) Survey results are not available for this reporting period; (9) No or very few patients were eligible for the HCAHPS survey. The scores shown, if any, reflect a very small number of surveys; (10) A state average was not calculated because too few hospitals in the state submitted data; (11) There were discrepancies in the data collection process; Please refer to the User's Guide for a full explanation of data.

VA Pittsburgh Healthcare System

University Drive C Phone: 412-688-6100
Pittsburgh, PA 15240 Fax: 412-688-6121
URL: www.pittsburg.va.gov
Type: Acute Care-Veterans Administration Emergency Services: No
Ownership: Government - Federal Beds: 146

Key Personnel:
CEO/President. . . . . Terry Gerick Wolf, FACHE
Chief of Medical Staff . . . . Rajiv Jain, MD
Infection Control . . . . Robert Muder
Operating Room. . . . . Mark Wilson, MD, PhD
Quality Assurance . . . . Barbara Reichbaum, RN
Radiology. . . . . B Kart, MD
Anesthesiology. . . . . Richard J Bjerke, MD
Intensive Care Unit. . . . . Paul Rogers, MD

Measure	Cases	This Hosp.	State Avg.	U.S. Avg.
Heart Attack Care				
ACE Inhibitor or ARB for LVSD[1]	3	100%	95%	96%
Aspirin at Arrival	41	100%	99%	99%
Aspirin at Discharge	46	100%	99%	98%
Beta Blocker at Discharge	47	100%	99%	98%
Fibrinolytic Medication Timing[5]	0	-	40%	55%
PCI Within 90 Minutes of Arrival[1]	11	73%	88%	90%
Smoking Cessation Advice[1]	16	100%	100%	99%
Chest Pain/Possible Heart Attack Care				
Aspirin at Arrival	-	-	95%	95%
Median Time to ECG (minutes)	-	-	8	8
Median Time to Transfer (minutes)	-	-	68	61
Fibrinolytic Medication Timing	-	-	48%	54%
Heart Failure Care				
ACE Inhibitor or ARB for LVSD	72	99%	95%	94%
Discharge Instructions	217	96%	90%	88%
Evaluation of LVS Function	237	100%	99%	98%
Smoking Cessation Advice	51	100%	98%	98%
Pneumonia Care				
Appropriate Initial Antibiotic	56	89%	93%	92%
Blood Culture Timing	121	99%	96%	96%
Influenza Vaccine	61	95%	92%	91%
Initial Antibiotic Timing	136	93%	96%	95%
Pneumococcal Vaccine	72	99%	95%	93%
Smoking Cessation Advice	36	100%	98%	97%
Surgical Care Improvement Project				
Appropriate VTP Within 24 Hours[2]	176	98%	95%	92%
Appropriate Hair Removal[2]	457	100%	100%	99%
Appropriate Beta Blocker Usage[2]	236	98%	94%	93%
Controlled Postoperative Blood Glucose[2]	156	94%	96%	93%
Prophylactic Antibiotic Timing	366	99%	97%	97%
Prophylactic Antibiotic Timing (Outpatient)	-	-	92%	92%
Prophylactic Antibiotic Selection	372	99%	98%	97%
Prophylactic Antibiotic Select. (Outpatient)	-	-	93%	94%
Prophylactic Antibiotic Stopped	358	91%	95%	94%
Recommended VTP Ordered[2]	176	98%	97%	94%
Urinary Catheter Removal[2]	220	86%	95%	90%
Children's Asthma Care				
Received Systemic Corticosteroids	-	-	-	100%
Received Home Management Plan	-	-	-	71%
Received Reliever Medication	-	-	-	100%
Use of Medical Imaging				
Combination Abdominal CT Scan	-	-	0.203	0.191
Combination Chest CT Scan	-	-	0.026	0.054
Follow-up Mammogram/Ultrasound	-	-	8.2%	8.4%
MRI for Low Back Pain	-	-	32.4%	32.7%
Survey of Patients' Hospital Experiences				
Area Around Room 'Always' Quiet at Night	-	-	-	58%
Doctors 'Always' Communicated Well	-	-	-	80%
Home Recovery Information Given	-	-	-	82%
Hospital Given 9 or 10 on 10 Point Scale	-	-	-	67%
Meds 'Always' Explained Before Given	-	-	-	60%
Nurses 'Always' Communicated Well	-	-	-	76%
Pain 'Always' Well Controlled	-	-	-	69%
Room and Bathroom 'Always' Clean	-	-	-	71%
Timely Help 'Always' Received	-	-	-	64%
Would Definitely Recommend Hospital	-	-	-	69%

Western Pennsylvania Hospital

4800 Friendship Avenue Phone: 412-578-5000
Pittsburgh, PA 15224 Fax: 412-578-1296
URL: www.wpahs.org/wph/contact/index.html
Type: Acute Care Hospitals Emergency Services: Yes
Ownership: Voluntary Non-Profit - Private Beds: 542

Key Personnel:
CEO/President. . . . . Dawn M Gideon
Cardiac Laboratory. . . . . Alan H Gradman, MD
Chief of Medical Staff . . . . Alan Lantzy, MD
Infection Control . . . . David L Weinbaum, MD
Operating Room. . . . . Philip F Caushaj, MD
Pediatric In-Patient Care . . . . Alan Lamtzy, MD
Radiology. . . . . Paul Kiproff, MD
Emergency Room . . . . Thomas Campbell, MD

Measure	Cases	This Hosp.	State Avg.	U.S. Avg.
Heart Attack Care				
ACE Inhibitor or ARB for LVSD	37	97%	95%	96%
Aspirin at Arrival	110	99%	99%	99%
Aspirin at Discharge	215	100%	99%	98%
Beta Blocker at Discharge	205	99%	99%	98%
Fibrinolytic Medication Timing	0	-	40%	55%
PCI Within 90 Minutes of Arrival[1]	15	87%	88%	90%
Smoking Cessation Advice	72	100%	100%	99%
Chest Pain/Possible Heart Attack Care				
Aspirin at Arrival[1,3]	1	100%	95%	95%
Median Time to ECG (minutes)[1,3]	1	12	8	8
Median Time to Transfer (minutes)[5]	0	-	68	61
Fibrinolytic Medication Timing[5]	0	-	48%	54%
Heart Failure Care				
ACE Inhibitor or ARB for LVSD	141	94%	95%	94%
Discharge Instructions	288	90%	90%	88%
Evaluation of LVS Function	334	99%	99%	98%
Smoking Cessation Advice	64	100%	98%	98%
Pneumonia Care				
Appropriate Initial Antibiotic	104	93%	93%	92%
Blood Culture Timing	134	96%	96%	96%
Influenza Vaccine	122	86%	92%	91%
Initial Antibiotic Timing	152	94%	96%	95%
Pneumococcal Vaccine	127	80%	95%	93%
Smoking Cessation Advice	87	100%	98%	97%
Surgical Care Improvement Project				
Appropriate VTP Within 24 Hours[2]	218	100%	95%	92%
Appropriate Hair Removal[2]	1,030	100%	100%	99%
Appropriate Beta Blocker Usage[2]	273	99%	94%	93%
Controlled Postoperative Blood Glucose[2]	206	98%	96%	93%
Prophylactic Antibiotic Timing[2]	870	100%	97%	97%
Prophylactic Antibiotic Timing (Outpatient)	350	98%	92%	92%
Prophylactic Antibiotic Selection[2]	886	96%	98%	97%
Prophylactic Antibiotic Select. (Outpatient)	347	97%	93%	94%
Prophylactic Antibiotic Stopped[2]	844	97%	95%	94%
Recommended VTP Ordered[2]	221	98%	97%	94%
Urinary Catheter Removal[2]	207	98%	95%	90%
Children's Asthma Care				
Received Systemic Corticosteroids	-	-	-	100%
Received Home Management Plan	-	-	-	71%
Received Reliever Medication	-	-	-	100%
Use of Medical Imaging				
Combination Abdominal CT Scan	391	0.156	0.203	0.191
Combination Chest CT Scan	363	0.003	0.026	0.054
Follow-up Mammogram/Ultrasound	605	9.9%	8.2%	8.4%
MRI for Low Back Pain	54	29.6%	32.4%	32.7%
Survey of Patients' Hospital Experiences				
Area Around Room 'Always' Quiet at Night	300+	53%	-	58%
Doctors 'Always' Communicated Well	300+	80%	-	80%
Home Recovery Information Given	300+	81%	-	82%
Hospital Given 9 or 10 on 10 Point Scale	300+	64%	-	67%
Meds 'Always' Explained Before Given	300+	58%	-	60%
Nurses 'Always' Communicated Well	300+	75%	-	76%
Pain 'Always' Well Controlled	300+	67%	-	69%
Room and Bathroom 'Always' Clean	300+	64%	-	71%
Timely Help 'Always' Received	300+	61%	-	64%
Would Definitely Recommend Hospital	300+	67%	-	69%

Pottstown Memorial Medical Center

1600 E High St and Armand Hammer Blvd Phone: 610-327-7000
Pottstown, PA 19464 Fax: 610-327-7432
URL: www.pmmctr.org
Type: Acute Care Hospitals Emergency Services: No
Ownership: Proprietary Beds: 299

Key Personnel:
CEO/President. . . . . John Kirby
Chief of Medical Staff . . . . Richard F Saylor, MD
Infection Control . . . . Elizabeth Jabbs
Operating Room. . . . . Cindy Iannelli
Quality Assurance . . . . Nancy Yocom
Radiology. . . . . Stephen Whitmoyer
Emergency Room . . . . Marvin Silverman, DO
Patient Relations . . . . Karen Reifsnyder

Measure	Cases	This Hosp.	State Avg.	U.S. Avg.
Heart Attack Care				
ACE Inhibitor or ARB for LVSD[1]	7	100%	95%	96%
Aspirin at Arrival	48	100%	99%	99%
Aspirin at Discharge	26	100%	99%	98%
Beta Blocker at Discharge	25	100%	99%	98%
Fibrinolytic Medication Timing	0	-	40%	55%
PCI Within 90 Minutes of Arrival	0	-	88%	90%
Smoking Cessation Advice[1]	3	100%	100%	99%
Chest Pain/Possible Heart Attack Care				
Aspirin at Arrival	70	99%	95%	95%
Median Time to ECG (minutes)	73	10	8	8
Median Time to Transfer (minutes)[1]	14	62	68	61
Fibrinolytic Medication Timing	0	-	48%	54%
Heart Failure Care				
ACE Inhibitor or ARB for LVSD	104	93%	95%	94%
Discharge Instructions	183	95%	90%	88%
Evaluation of LVS Function	253	99%	99%	98%
Smoking Cessation Advice	27	100%	98%	98%
Pneumonia Care				
Appropriate Initial Antibiotic	195	97%	93%	92%
Blood Culture Timing	327	98%	96%	96%
Influenza Vaccine	193	95%	92%	91%
Initial Antibiotic Timing	318	98%	96%	95%
Pneumococcal Vaccine	271	96%	95%	93%
Smoking Cessation Advice	112	100%	98%	97%
Surgical Care Improvement Project				
Appropriate VTP Within 24 Hours[2]	244	89%	95%	92%
Appropriate Hair Removal[2]	491	100%	100%	99%
Appropriate Beta Blocker Usage[2]	102	76%	94%	93%
Controlled Postoperative Blood Glucose[2]	0	-	96%	93%
Prophylactic Antibiotic Timing[2]	287	95%	97%	97%
Prophylactic Antibiotic Timing (Outpatient)	146	89%	92%	92%
Prophylactic Antibiotic Selection[2]	289	93%	98%	97%
Prophylactic Antibiotic Select. (Outpatient)	143	90%	93%	94%
Prophylactic Antibiotic Stopped[2]	275	87%	95%	94%
Recommended VTP Ordered[2]	245	93%	97%	94%
Urinary Catheter Removal	129	94%	95%	90%
Children's Asthma Care				
Received Systemic Corticosteroids	-	-	-	100%
Received Home Management Plan	-	-	-	71%
Received Reliever Medication	-	-	-	100%
Use of Medical Imaging				
Combination Abdominal CT Scan	823	0.190	0.203	0.191
Combination Chest CT Scan	478	0.038	0.026	0.054
Follow-up Mammogram/Ultrasound	1,064	6.7%	8.2%	8.4%
MRI for Low Back Pain	210	34.3%	32.4%	32.7%
Survey of Patients' Hospital Experiences				
Area Around Room 'Always' Quiet at Night	300+	45%	-	58%
Doctors 'Always' Communicated Well	300+	71%	-	80%
Home Recovery Information Given	300+	82%	-	82%
Hospital Given 9 or 10 on 10 Point Scale	300+	55%	-	67%
Meds 'Always' Explained Before Given	300+	54%	-	60%
Nurses 'Always' Communicated Well	300+	70%	-	76%
Pain 'Always' Well Controlled	300+	65%	-	69%
Room and Bathroom 'Always' Clean	300+	60%	-	71%
Timely Help 'Always' Received	300+	53%	-	64%
Would Definitely Recommend Hospital	300+	53%	-	69%

NOTE: Hospital profiles are in alphabetical order by state, then city, then hospital within the city; Rankings exclude hospitals with less than 25 cases except for patient surveys which excludes hospitals with less than 100 cases; (a) 100–299 cases; (1) The number of cases is too small to be sure how well a hospital is performing; (2) The hospital indicated that the data submitted for this measure were based on a sample of cases; (3) Data was collected during a shorter time period (fewer quarters) than the maximum possible time for this measure; (4) Suppressed for one or more quarters by CMS; (5) No data is available from the hospital for this measure; (6) Fewer than 100 patients completed the HCAHPS survey. Use these rates with caution, as the number of surveys may be too low to reliably assess hospital performance; (7) Survey results are based on less than 12 months of data; (8) Survey results are not available for this reporting period; (9) No or very few patients were eligible for the HCAHPS survey. The scores shown, if any, reflect a very small number of surveys; (10) A state average was not calculated because too few hospitals in the state submitted data; (11) There were discrepancies in the data collection process; Please refer to the User's Guide for a full explanation of data.

Schuylkill Medical Center - East Norwegian Street

700 East Norwegian Street Phone: 570-621-4000
Pottsville, PA 17901 Fax: 570-621-4775
URL: www.schuylkillhealth.com
Type: Acute Care Hospitals Emergency Services: Yes
Ownership: Voluntary Non-Profit - Church Beds: 221

Key Personnel:
CEO/President. . . . . Peter U Bergmann
Chief of Medical Staff. . . . . Thomas McLaughlin, MD
Coronary Care . . . . Cynthia Cappel
Infection Control. . . . . Susan Light
Operating Room. . . . . Rose Ann Mucci
Pediatric In-Patient Care . . . . . . Carol Rowan, RN
Quality Assurance . . . . Patricia Baldwin

Measure	Cases	This Hosp.	State Avg.	U.S. Avg.
Heart Attack Care				
ACE Inhibitor or ARB for LVSD[1]	3	33%	95%	96%
Aspirin at Arrival	61	95%	99%	99%
Aspirin at Discharge	38	95%	99%	98%
Beta Blocker at Discharge	45	91%	99%	98%
Fibrinolytic Medication Timing	0	-	40%	55%
PCI Within 90 Minutes of Arrival	0	-	88%	90%
Smoking Cessation Advice[1]	5	100%	100%	99%
Chest Pain/Possible Heart Attack Care				
Aspirin at Arrival	48	94%	95%	95%
Median Time to ECG (minutes)	47	8	8	8
Median Time to Transfer (minutes)[1]	7	55	68	61
Fibrinolytic Medication Timing[1]	1	0%	48%	54%
Heart Failure Care				
ACE Inhibitor or ARB for LVSD	63	84%	95%	94%
Discharge Instructions	186	90%	90%	88%
Evaluation of LVS Function	297	95%	99%	98%
Smoking Cessation Advice[1]	15	100%	98%	98%
Pneumonia Care				
Appropriate Initial Antibiotic	64	92%	93%	92%
Blood Culture Timing	122	94%	96%	96%
Influenza Vaccine	117	89%	92%	91%
Initial Antibiotic Timing	162	96%	96%	95%
Pneumococcal Vaccine	164	94%	95%	93%
Smoking Cessation Advice	31	100%	98%	97%
Surgical Care Improvement Project				
Appropriate VTP Within 24 Hours	159	95%	95%	92%
Appropriate Hair Removal	265	99%	100%	99%
Appropriate Beta Blocker Usage	101	87%	94%	93%
Controlled Postoperative Blood Glucose	0	-	96%	93%
Prophylactic Antibiotic Timing	149	93%	97%	97%
Prophylactic Antibiotic Timing (Outpatient)[1]	12	92%	92%	92%
Prophylactic Antibiotic Selection	148	97%	98%	97%
Prophylactic Antibiotic Select. (Outpatient)[1]	12	67%	93%	94%
Prophylactic Antibiotic Stopped	140	71%	95%	94%
Recommended VTP Ordered	159	97%	97%	94%
Urinary Catheter Removal	41	78%	95%	90%
Children's Asthma Care				
Received Systemic Corticosteroids	-	-	-	100%
Received Home Management Plan	-	-	-	71%
Received Reliever Medication	-	-	-	100%
Use of Medical Imaging				
Combination Abdominal CT Scan	587	0.063	0.203	0.191
Combination Chest CT Scan	341	0.006	0.026	0.054
Follow-up Mammogram/Ultrasound	740	10.5%	8.2%	8.4%
MRI for Low Back Pain	142	30.3%	32.4%	32.7%
Survey of Patients' Hospital Experiences				
Area Around Room 'Always' Quiet at Night	300+	39%	-	58%
Doctors 'Always' Communicated Well	300+	75%	-	80%
Home Recovery Information Given	300+	77%	-	82%
Hospital Given 9 or 10 on 10 Point Scale	300+	57%	-	67%
Meds 'Always' Explained Before Given	300+	55%	-	60%
Nurses 'Always' Communicated Well	300+	73%	-	76%
Pain 'Always' Well Controlled	300+	66%	-	69%
Room and Bathroom 'Always' Clean	300+	71%	-	71%
Timely Help 'Always' Received	300+	56%	-	64%
Would Definitely Recommend Hospital	300+	57%	-	69%

Schuylkill Medical Center - South Jackson Street

420 South Jackson Street Phone: 570-621-5000
Pottsville, PA 17901
URL: www.pottsvillehospital.com
Type: Acute Care Hospitals Emergency Services: Yes
Ownership: Voluntary Non-Profit - Private Beds: 200

Key Personnel:
CEO/President. . . . . John E. Simodejka

Measure	Cases	This Hosp.	State Avg.	U.S. Avg.
Heart Attack Care				
ACE Inhibitor or ARB for LVSD	7	100%	95%	96%
Aspirin at Arrival	45	96%	99%	99%
Aspirin at Discharge[1]	23	91%	99%	98%
Beta Blocker at Discharge	29	97%	99%	98%
Fibrinolytic Medication Timing	0	-	40%	55%
PCI Within 90 Minutes of Arrival	0	-	88%	90%
Smoking Cessation Advice[1]	4	100%	100%	99%
Chest Pain/Possible Heart Attack Care				
Aspirin at Arrival	85	98%	95%	95%
Median Time to ECG (minutes)	87	6	8	8
Median Time to Transfer (minutes)[1]	14	56	68	61
Fibrinolytic Medication Timing[1]	1	100%	48%	54%
Heart Failure Care				
ACE Inhibitor or ARB for LVSD	39	79%	95%	94%
Discharge Instructions	152	88%	90%	88%
Evaluation of LVS Function	218	79%	99%	98%
Smoking Cessation Advice[1]	23	96%	98%	98%
Pneumonia Care				
Appropriate Initial Antibiotic	99	85%	93%	92%
Blood Culture Timing	170	92%	96%	96%
Influenza Vaccine	134	85%	92%	91%
Initial Antibiotic Timing	208	95%	96%	95%
Pneumococcal Vaccine	186	88%	95%	93%
Smoking Cessation Advice	64	98%	98%	97%
Surgical Care Improvement Project				
Appropriate VTP Within 24 Hours	146	98%	95%	92%
Appropriate Hair Removal	413	100%	100%	99%
Appropriate Beta Blocker Usage	113	98%	94%	93%
Controlled Postoperative Blood Glucose	0	-	96%	93%
Prophylactic Antibiotic Timing	302	96%	97%	97%
Prophylactic Antibiotic Timing (Outpatient)	122	68%	92%	92%
Prophylactic Antibiotic Selection	301	91%	98%	97%
Prophylactic Antibiotic Select. (Outpatient)	90	84%	93%	94%
Prophylactic Antibiotic Stopped	290	89%	95%	94%
Recommended VTP Ordered	148	97%	97%	94%
Urinary Catheter Removal	29	90%	95%	90%
Children's Asthma Care				
Received Systemic Corticosteroids	-	-	-	100%
Received Home Management Plan	-	-	-	71%
Received Reliever Medication	-	-	-	100%
Use of Medical Imaging				
Combination Abdominal CT Scan	778	0.030	0.203	0.191
Combination Chest CT Scan	357	0.000	0.026	0.054
Follow-up Mammogram/Ultrasound	1,162	3.3%	8.2%	8.4%
MRI for Low Back Pain	148	31.8%	32.4%	32.7%
Survey of Patients' Hospital Experiences				
Area Around Room 'Always' Quiet at Night	300+	45%	-	58%
Doctors 'Always' Communicated Well	300+	77%	-	80%
Home Recovery Information Given	300+	73%	-	82%
Hospital Given 9 or 10 on 10 Point Scale	300+	55%	-	67%
Meds 'Always' Explained Before Given	300+	53%	-	60%
Nurses 'Always' Communicated Well	300+	71%	-	76%
Pain 'Always' Well Controlled	300+	63%	-	69%
Room and Bathroom 'Always' Clean	300+	71%	-	71%
Timely Help 'Always' Received	300+	64%	-	64%
Would Definitely Recommend Hospital	300+	54%	-	69%

Punxsutawney Area Hospital

81 Hillcrest Drive Phone: 814-938-1800
Punxsutawney, PA 15767 Fax: 814-938-1630
URL: www.pah.org
Type: Acute Care Hospitals Emergency Services: Yes
Ownership: Voluntary Non-Profit - Private Beds: 55

Key Personnel:
Chief of Medical Staff . . . . Nancy Meehan
Infection Control. . . . . Kathleen Crowell
Operating Room. . . . . Pat Parrish
Quality Assurance . . . . Kathleen Crowell
Radiology. . . . . Richard Foster, MD
Emergency Room . . . . Earl Morgan, MD
Intensive Care Unit. . . . . Shirley Brothers

Measure	Cases	This Hosp.	State Avg.	U.S. Avg.
Heart Attack Care				
ACE Inhibitor or ARB for LVSD[1]	2	100%	95%	96%
Aspirin at Arrival[1]	9	100%	99%	99%
Aspirin at Discharge[1]	3	100%	99%	98%
Beta Blocker at Discharge[1]	3	100%	99%	98%
Fibrinolytic Medication Timing	0	-	40%	55%
PCI Within 90 Minutes of Arrival	0	-	88%	90%
Smoking Cessation Advice	0	-	100%	99%
Chest Pain/Possible Heart Attack Care				
Aspirin at Arrival[1]	22	100%	95%	95%
Median Time to ECG (minutes)[1]	22	8	8	8
Median Time to Transfer (minutes)[1,3]	3	88	68	61
Fibrinolytic Medication Timing[3]	0	-	48%	54%
Heart Failure Care				
ACE Inhibitor or ARB for LVSD[1]	12	100%	95%	94%
Discharge Instructions	48	75%	90%	88%
Evaluation of LVS Function	57	93%	99%	98%
Smoking Cessation Advice[1]	7	100%	98%	98%
Pneumonia Care				
Appropriate Initial Antibiotic	61	95%	93%	92%
Blood Culture Timing	62	90%	96%	96%
Influenza Vaccine	41	95%	92%	91%
Initial Antibiotic Timing	74	96%	96%	95%
Pneumococcal Vaccine	64	100%	95%	93%
Smoking Cessation Advice	25	88%	98%	97%
Surgical Care Improvement Project				
Appropriate VTP Within 24 Hours	58	91%	95%	92%
Appropriate Hair Removal	146	100%	100%	99%
Appropriate Beta Blocker Usage	33	97%	94%	93%
Controlled Postoperative Blood Glucose	0	-	96%	93%
Prophylactic Antibiotic Timing	102	97%	97%	97%
Prophylactic Antibiotic Timing (Outpatient)	70	96%	92%	92%
Prophylactic Antibiotic Selection	103	100%	98%	97%
Prophylactic Antibiotic Select. (Outpatient)	98	95%	93%	94%
Prophylactic Antibiotic Stopped	99	98%	95%	94%
Recommended VTP Ordered	59	92%	97%	94%
Urinary Catheter Removal	32	91%	95%	90%
Children's Asthma Care				
Received Systemic Corticosteroids	-	-	-	100%
Received Home Management Plan	-	-	-	71%
Received Reliever Medication	-	-	-	100%
Use of Medical Imaging				
Combination Abdominal CT Scan	283	0.484	0.203	0.191
Combination Chest CT Scan	142	0.000	0.026	0.054
Follow-up Mammogram/Ultrasound	375	7.2%	8.2%	8.4%
MRI for Low Back Pain[1]	29	31.0%	32.4%	32.7%
Survey of Patients' Hospital Experiences				
Area Around Room 'Always' Quiet at Night	300+	53%	-	58%
Doctors 'Always' Communicated Well	300+	82%	-	80%
Home Recovery Information Given	300+	92%	-	82%
Hospital Given 9 or 10 on 10 Point Scale	300+	65%	-	67%
Meds 'Always' Explained Before Given	300+	61%	-	60%
Nurses 'Always' Communicated Well	300+	78%	-	76%
Pain 'Always' Well Controlled	300+	71%	-	69%
Room and Bathroom 'Always' Clean	300+	72%	-	71%
Timely Help 'Always' Received	300+	70%	-	64%
Would Definitely Recommend Hospital	300+	67%	-	69%

NOTE: Hospital profiles are in alphabetical order by state, then city, then hospital within the city; Rankings exclude hospitals with less than 25 cases except for patient surveys which excludes hospitals with less than 100 cases; (a) 100–299 cases; (1) The number of cases is too small to be sure how well a hospital is performing; (2) The hospital indicated that the data submitted for this measure were based on a sample of cases; (3) Data was collected during a shorter time period (fewer quarters) than the maximum possible time for this measure; (4) Suppressed for one or more quarters by CMS; (5) No data is available from the hospital for this measure; (6) Fewer than 100 patients completed the HCAHPS survey. Use these rates with caution, as the number of surveys may be too low to reliably assess hospital performance; (7) Survey results are based on less than 12 months of data; (8) Survey results are not available for this reporting period; (9) No or very few patients were eligible for the HCAHPS survey. The scores shown, if any, reflect a very small number of surveys; (10) A state average was not calculated because too few hospitals in the state submitted data; (11) There were discrepancies in the data collection process; Please refer to the User's Guide for a full explanation of data.

Saint Luke's Quakertown Hospital

1021 Park Avenue Phone: 215-538-4500
Quakertown, PA 18951 Fax: 215-529-5294
URL: www.slhn-lehighvalley.com
Type: Acute Care Hospitals Emergency Services: Yes
Ownership: Voluntary Non-Profit - Private Beds: 89

Key Personnel:
CEO/President. . . . . Edward Nawrocki
Chief of Medical Staff. . . . . Thomas Filipowitz, MD
Radiology. . . . . James D Bohri

Measure	Cases	This Hosp.	State Avg.	U.S. Avg.
Heart Attack Care				
ACE Inhibitor or ARB for LVSD[1]	3	100%	95%	96%
Aspirin at Arrival[1]	23	91%	99%	99%
Aspirin at Discharge[1]	13	92%	99%	98%
Beta Blocker at Discharge[1]	12	100%	99%	98%
Fibrinolytic Medication Timing	0	-	40%	55%
PCI Within 90 Minutes of Arrival	0	-	88%	90%
Smoking Cessation Advice	0	-	100%	99%
Chest Pain/Possible Heart Attack Care				
Aspirin at Arrival[5]	0	-	95%	95%
Median Time to ECG (minutes)[5]	0	-	8	8
Median Time to Transfer (minutes)[5]	0	-	68	61
Fibrinolytic Medication Timing[5]	0	-	48%	54%
Heart Failure Care				
ACE Inhibitor or ARB for LVSD[1]	23	100%	95%	94%
Discharge Instructions	55	93%	90%	88%
Evaluation of LVS Function	93	99%	99%	98%
Smoking Cessation Advice[1]	14	100%	98%	98%
Pneumonia Care				
Appropriate Initial Antibiotic	78	97%	93%	92%
Blood Culture Timing	92	98%	96%	96%
Influenza Vaccine	65	97%	92%	91%
Initial Antibiotic Timing	99	98%	96%	95%
Pneumococcal Vaccine	92	99%	95%	93%
Smoking Cessation Advice	35	100%	98%	97%
Surgical Care Improvement Project				
Appropriate VTP Within 24 Hours	45	93%	95%	92%
Appropriate Hair Removal	106	100%	100%	99%
Appropriate Beta Blocker Usage	38	92%	94%	93%
Controlled Postoperative Blood Glucose	0	-	96%	93%
Prophylactic Antibiotic Timing	68	99%	97%	97%
Prophylactic Antibiotic Timing (Outpatient)	29	86%	92%	92%
Prophylactic Antibiotic Selection	68	99%	98%	97%
Prophylactic Antibiotic Select. (Outpatient)	25	88%	93%	94%
Prophylactic Antibiotic Stopped	57	96%	95%	94%
Recommended VTP Ordered	45	96%	97%	94%
Urinary Catheter Removal	28	100%	95%	90%
Children's Asthma Care				
Received Systemic Corticosteroids	-	-	-	100%
Received Home Management Plan	-	-	-	71%
Received Reliever Medication	-	-	-	100%
Use of Medical Imaging				
Combination Abdominal CT Scan	354	0.130	0.203	0.191
Combination Chest CT Scan	240	0.088	0.026	0.054
Follow-up Mammogram/Ultrasound	486	7.8%	8.2%	8.4%
MRI for Low Back Pain	89	29.2%	32.4%	32.7%
Survey of Patients' Hospital Experiences				
Area Around Room 'Always' Quiet at Night	300+	50%	-	58%
Doctors 'Always' Communicated Well	300+	78%	-	80%
Home Recovery Information Given	300+	83%	-	82%
Hospital Given 9 or 10 on 10 Point Scale	300+	68%	-	67%
Meds 'Always' Explained Before Given	300+	63%	-	60%
Nurses 'Always' Communicated Well	300+	82%	-	76%
Pain 'Always' Well Controlled	300+	71%	-	69%
Room and Bathroom 'Always' Clean	300+	70%	-	71%
Timely Help 'Always' Received	300+	65%	-	64%
Would Definitely Recommend Hospital	300+	71%	-	69%

Reading Hospital Medical Center

Sixth Avenue and Spruce St Phone: 610-988-8000
Reading, PA 19603 Fax: 610-988-5192
E-mail: info@readinghospital.org
URL: www.readinghospital.org
Type: Acute Care Hospitals Emergency Services: Yes
Ownership: Voluntary Non-Profit - Other Beds: 804

Key Personnel:
CEO/President. . . . . Scott R Wolfe
Chief of Medical Staff. . . . . Gerald Malick, MD
Infection Control. . . . . Kenneth J DeBenedictis, MD
Quality Assurance . . . . Debra Levengood
Radiology. . . . . Albert Yuen
Anesthesiology. . . . . Francis Plucinsley, MD
Emergency Room . . . . Kristen Sandel

Measure	Cases	This Hosp.	State Avg.	U.S. Avg.
Heart Attack Care				
ACE Inhibitor or ARB for LVSD	51	98%	95%	96%
Aspirin at Arrival	399	99%	99%	99%
Aspirin at Discharge	397	100%	99%	98%
Beta Blocker at Discharge	392	100%	99%	98%
Fibrinolytic Medication Timing	0	-	40%	55%
PCI Within 90 Minutes of Arrival	112	92%	88%	90%
Smoking Cessation Advice	115	100%	100%	99%
Chest Pain/Possible Heart Attack Care				
Aspirin at Arrival[1,3]	1	100%	95%	95%
Median Time to ECG (minutes)[1,3]	4	8	8	8
Median Time to Transfer (minutes)[5]	0	-	68	61
Fibrinolytic Medication Timing[5]	0	-	48%	54%
Heart Failure Care				
ACE Inhibitor or ARB for LVSD	193	100%	95%	94%
Discharge Instructions	582	98%	90%	88%
Evaluation of LVS Function	789	100%	99%	98%
Smoking Cessation Advice	87	100%	98%	98%
Pneumonia Care				
Appropriate Initial Antibiotic	331	95%	93%	92%
Blood Culture Timing	633	95%	96%	96%
Influenza Vaccine	420	99%	92%	91%
Initial Antibiotic Timing	555	97%	96%	95%
Pneumococcal Vaccine	586	100%	95%	93%
Smoking Cessation Advice	154	100%	98%	97%
Surgical Care Improvement Project				
Appropriate VTP Within 24 Hours[2]	521	97%	95%	92%
Appropriate Hair Removal[2]	1,981	100%	100%	99%
Appropriate Beta Blocker Usage[2]	730	94%	94%	93%
Controlled Postoperative Blood Glucose[2]	213	98%	96%	93%
Prophylactic Antibiotic Timing[2]	1,568	98%	97%	97%
Prophylactic Antibiotic Timing (Outpatient)	747	89%	92%	92%
Prophylactic Antibiotic Selection[2]	1,580	98%	98%	97%
Prophylactic Antibiotic Select. (Outpatient)	724	95%	93%	94%
Prophylactic Antibiotic Stopped[2]	1,462	94%	95%	94%
Recommended VTP Ordered[2]	522	98%	97%	94%
Urinary Catheter Removal[2]	433	96%	95%	90%
Children's Asthma Care				
Received Systemic Corticosteroids	-	-	-	100%
Received Home Management Plan	-	-	-	71%
Received Reliever Medication	-	-	-	100%
Use of Medical Imaging				
Combination Abdominal CT Scan	2,807	0.067	0.203	0.191
Combination Chest CT Scan	2,818	0.061	0.026	0.054
Follow-up Mammogram/Ultrasound	5,143	6.5%	8.2%	8.4%
MRI for Low Back Pain	602	28.9%	32.4%	32.7%
Survey of Patients' Hospital Experiences				
Area Around Room 'Always' Quiet at Night	300+	47%	-	58%
Doctors 'Always' Communicated Well	300+	76%	-	80%
Home Recovery Information Given	300+	85%	-	82%
Hospital Given 9 or 10 on 10 Point Scale	300+	64%	-	67%
Meds 'Always' Explained Before Given	300+	55%	-	60%
Nurses 'Always' Communicated Well	300+	73%	-	76%
Pain 'Always' Well Controlled	300+	67%	-	69%
Room and Bathroom 'Always' Clean	300+	62%	-	71%
Timely Help 'Always' Received	300+	58%	-	64%
Would Definitely Recommend Hospital	300+	67%	-	69%

Saint Joseph Medical Center

2500 Bernville Road Phone: 610-378-2300
Reading, PA 19605 Fax: 610-378-2706
URL: www.sjmcberks.org
Type: Acute Care Hospitals Emergency Services: Yes
Ownership: Voluntary Non-Profit - Church Beds: 220

Key Personnel:
CEO/President. . . . . John Morahan
Chief of Medical Staff. . . . . Erwing Ehrlich, MD
Operating Room. . . . . Cyndie Miller, RN
Pediatric Ambulatory Care . . . . . . Mary Ann Mancano, MD
Pediatric In-Patient Care . . . . Mary Ann Mancano, MD
Quality Assurance . . . . Loretta Boyd, RN
Radiology. . . . . Steven R Chmielewski, MD
Emergency Room . . . . Ann Tranqualto, RN

Measure	Cases	This Hosp.	State Avg.	U.S. Avg.
Heart Attack Care				
ACE Inhibitor or ARB for LVSD[1]	21	100%	95%	96%
Aspirin at Arrival	144	99%	99%	99%
Aspirin at Discharge	159	99%	99%	98%
Beta Blocker at Discharge	157	100%	99%	98%
Fibrinolytic Medication Timing	0	-	40%	55%
PCI Within 90 Minutes of Arrival	43	100%	88%	90%
Smoking Cessation Advice	51	98%	100%	99%
Chest Pain/Possible Heart Attack Care				
Aspirin at Arrival[5]	0	-	95%	95%
Median Time to ECG (minutes)[5]	0	-	8	8
Median Time to Transfer (minutes)[5]	0	-	68	61
Fibrinolytic Medication Timing[5]	0	-	48%	54%
Heart Failure Care				
ACE Inhibitor or ARB for LVSD	109	100%	95%	94%
Discharge Instructions	301	96%	90%	88%
Evaluation of LVS Function	368	100%	99%	98%
Smoking Cessation Advice	55	98%	98%	98%
Pneumonia Care				
Appropriate Initial Antibiotic	124	89%	93%	92%
Blood Culture Timing	188	93%	96%	96%
Influenza Vaccine	145	98%	92%	91%
Initial Antibiotic Timing	178	93%	96%	95%
Pneumococcal Vaccine	193	97%	95%	93%
Smoking Cessation Advice	59	100%	98%	97%
Surgical Care Improvement Project				
Appropriate VTP Within 24 Hours[2]	183	99%	95%	92%
Appropriate Hair Removal[2]	613	100%	100%	99%
Appropriate Beta Blocker Usage[2]	232	100%	94%	93%
Controlled Postoperative Blood Glucose[2]	121	93%	96%	93%
Prophylactic Antibiotic Timing[2]	456	98%	97%	97%
Prophylactic Antibiotic Timing (Outpatient)	201	92%	92%	92%
Prophylactic Antibiotic Selection[2]	468	96%	98%	97%
Prophylactic Antibiotic Select. (Outpatient)	187	96%	93%	94%
Prophylactic Antibiotic Stopped[2]	445	97%	95%	94%
Recommended VTP Ordered[2]	183	100%	97%	94%
Urinary Catheter Removal[2]	156	96%	95%	90%
Children's Asthma Care				
Received Systemic Corticosteroids	-	-	-	100%
Received Home Management Plan	-	-	-	71%
Received Reliever Medication	-	-	-	100%
Use of Medical Imaging				
Combination Abdominal CT Scan	543	0.700	0.203	0.191
Combination Chest CT Scan	499	0.014	0.026	0.054
Follow-up Mammogram/Ultrasound	1,549	4.7%	8.2%	8.4%
MRI for Low Back Pain	151	34.4%	32.4%	32.7%
Survey of Patients' Hospital Experiences				
Area Around Room 'Always' Quiet at Night	300+	57%	-	58%
Doctors 'Always' Communicated Well	300+	77%	-	80%
Home Recovery Information Given	300+	85%	-	82%
Hospital Given 9 or 10 on 10 Point Scale	300+	72%	-	67%
Meds 'Always' Explained Before Given	300+	54%	-	60%
Nurses 'Always' Communicated Well	300+	75%	-	76%
Pain 'Always' Well Controlled	300+	69%	-	69%
Room and Bathroom 'Always' Clean	300+	67%	-	71%
Timely Help 'Always' Received	300+	62%	-	64%
Would Definitely Recommend Hospital	300+	76%	-	69%

NOTE: Hospital profiles are in alphabetical order by state, then city, then hospital within the city; Rankings exclude hospitals with less than 25 cases except for patient surveys which excludes hospitals with less than 100 cases; (a) 100–299 cases; (1) The number of cases is too small to be sure how well a hospital is performing; (2) The hospital indicated that the data submitted for this measure were based on a sample of cases; (3) Data was collected during a shorter time period (fewer quarters) than the maximum possible time for this measure; (4) Suppressed for one or more quarters by CMS; (5) No data is available from the hospital for this measure; (6) Fewer than 100 patients completed the HCAHPS survey. Use these rates with caution, as the number of surveys may be too low to reliably assess hospital performance; (7) Survey results are based on less than 12 months of data; (8) Survey results are not available for this reporting period; (9) No or very few patients were eligible for the HCAHPS survey. The scores shown, if any, reflect a very small number of surveys; (10) A state average was not calculated because too few hospitals in the state submitted data; (11) There were discrepancies in the data collection process; Please refer to the User's Guide for a full explanation of data.

Nason Hospital

105 Nason Drive
Roaring Spring, PA 16673
Phone: 814-224-2141
Fax: 814-224-6236
URL: www.nasonhospital.com
Type: Acute Care Hospitals
Emergency Services: Yes
Ownership: Voluntary Non-Profit - Private
Beds: 40

Key Personnel:

CEO/President. . . . . Garrett W Hoover, MA/MHA
Chief of Medical Staff . . . . Darron Locke, MD
Infection Control. . . . . Janice Kanode, RN
Operating Room. . . . . Howard M Black, RN
Pediatric Ambulatory Care . . . . . . Joseph Castel, MD
Pediatric In-Patient Care . . . . . . Joseph Castel, MD
Quality Assurance . . . . Faith Shea
Radiology. . . . . Francis X Pessolano

Measure	Cases	This Hosp.	State Avg.	U.S. Avg.
Heart Attack Care				
ACE Inhibitor or ARB for LVSD	0	-	95%	96%
Aspirin at Arrival[1]	22	100%	99%	99%
Aspirin at Discharge[1]	3	100%	99%	98%
Beta Blocker at Discharge[1]	3	100%	99%	98%
Fibrinolytic Medication Timing	0	-	40%	55%
PCI Within 90 Minutes of Arrival	0	-	88%	90%
Smoking Cessation Advice	0	-	100%	99%
Chest Pain/Possible Heart Attack Care				
Aspirin at Arrival	34	94%	95%	95%
Median Time to ECG (minutes)	35	7	8	8
Median Time to Transfer (minutes)[3]	0	-	68	61
Fibrinolytic Medication Timing[1]	4	100%	48%	54%
Heart Failure Care				
ACE Inhibitor or ARB for LVSD[1]	21	100%	95%	94%
Discharge Instructions	62	97%	90%	88%
Evaluation of LVS Function	82	100%	99%	98%
Smoking Cessation Advice[1]	4	100%	98%	98%
Pneumonia Care				
Appropriate Initial Antibiotic	63	94%	93%	92%
Blood Culture Timing	76	100%	96%	96%
Influenza Vaccine	53	100%	92%	91%
Initial Antibiotic Timing	77	99%	96%	95%
Pneumococcal Vaccine	72	100%	95%	93%
Smoking Cessation Advice[1]	18	94%	98%	97%
Surgical Care Improvement Project				
Appropriate VTP Within 24 Hours	76	100%	95%	92%
Appropriate Hair Removal	155	99%	100%	99%
Appropriate Beta Blocker Usage	43	100%	94%	93%
Controlled Postoperative Blood Glucose	0	-	96%	93%
Prophylactic Antibiotic Timing	91	100%	97%	97%
Prophylactic Antibiotic Timing (Outpatient)	58	91%	92%	92%
Prophylactic Antibiotic Selection	91	99%	98%	97%
Prophylactic Antibiotic Select. (Outpatient)	55	82%	93%	94%
Prophylactic Antibiotic Stopped	89	98%	95%	94%
Recommended VTP Ordered	76	100%	97%	94%
Urinary Catheter Removal[1]	19	79%	95%	90%
Children's Asthma Care				
Received Systemic Corticosteroids	-	-	-	100%
Received Home Management Plan	-	-	-	71%
Received Reliever Medication	-	-	-	100%
Use of Medical Imaging				
Combination Abdominal CT Scan	185	0.049	0.203	0.191
Combination Chest CT Scan	103	0.019	0.026	0.054
Follow-up Mammogram/Ultrasound	377	10.3%	8.2%	8.4%
MRI for Low Back Pain[1]	24	33.3%	32.4%	32.7%
Survey of Patients' Hospital Experiences				
Area Around Room 'Always' Quiet at Night	300+	56%	-	58%
Doctors 'Always' Communicated Well	300+	83%	-	80%
Home Recovery Information Given	300+	77%	-	82%
Hospital Given 9 or 10 on 10 Point Scale	300+	76%	-	67%
Meds 'Always' Explained Before Given	300+	63%	-	60%
Nurses 'Always' Communicated Well	300+	79%	-	76%
Pain 'Always' Well Controlled	300+	74%	-	69%
Room and Bathroom 'Always' Clean	300+	81%	-	71%
Timely Help 'Always' Received	300+	70%	-	64%
Would Definitely Recommend Hospital	300+	77%	-	69%

Elk Regional Health Center

763 Johnsonburg Road
Saint Marys, PA 15857
Phone: 814-788-8000
Fax: 814-788-8046
URL: www.elkregional.org
Type: Acute Care Hospitals
Emergency Services: Yes
Ownership: Voluntary Non-Profit - Other
Beds: 87

Key Personnel:

CEO/President. . . . . Greg Bauer, NHA/CHE
Chief of Medical Staff . . . . David Caruso
Operating Room. . . . . Kaye Schneider
Quality Assurance . . . . Kathy Wonderly, RN
Radiology. . . . . Richard Bolden
Emergency Room . . . . Jayant L Patankar, MD

Measure	Cases	This Hosp.	State Avg.	U.S. Avg.
Heart Attack Care				
ACE Inhibitor or ARB for LVSD[1]	3	67%	95%	96%
Aspirin at Arrival[1]	24	79%	99%	99%
Aspirin at Discharge[1]	12	50%	99%	98%
Beta Blocker at Discharge[1]	15	87%	99%	98%
Fibrinolytic Medication Timing	0	-	40%	55%
PCI Within 90 Minutes of Arrival	0	-	88%	90%
Smoking Cessation Advice[1]	2	100%	100%	99%
Chest Pain/Possible Heart Attack Care				
Aspirin at Arrival	90	93%	95%	95%
Median Time to ECG (minutes)	91	4	8	8
Median Time to Transfer (minutes)[1]	10	57	68	61
Fibrinolytic Medication Timing[1]	8	38%	48%	54%
Heart Failure Care				
ACE Inhibitor or ARB for LVSD	44	86%	95%	94%
Discharge Instructions	122	58%	90%	88%
Evaluation of LVS Function	178	90%	99%	98%
Smoking Cessation Advice[1]	17	100%	98%	98%
Pneumonia Care				
Appropriate Initial Antibiotic	111	85%	93%	92%
Blood Culture Timing	187	94%	96%	96%
Influenza Vaccine	114	85%	92%	91%
Initial Antibiotic Timing	171	95%	96%	95%
Pneumococcal Vaccine	155	96%	95%	93%
Smoking Cessation Advice	52	94%	98%	97%
Surgical Care Improvement Project				
Appropriate VTP Within 24 Hours	76	78%	95%	92%
Appropriate Hair Removal	248	100%	100%	99%
Appropriate Beta Blocker Usage	70	79%	94%	93%
Controlled Postoperative Blood Glucose	0	-	96%	93%
Prophylactic Antibiotic Timing	167	87%	97%	97%
Prophylactic Antibiotic Timing (Outpatient)	141	91%	92%	92%
Prophylactic Antibiotic Selection	167	92%	98%	97%
Prophylactic Antibiotic Select. (Outpatient)	135	91%	93%	94%
Prophylactic Antibiotic Stopped	167	87%	95%	94%
Recommended VTP Ordered	78	79%	97%	94%
Urinary Catheter Removal	50	90%	95%	90%
Children's Asthma Care				
Received Systemic Corticosteroids	-	-	-	100%
Received Home Management Plan	-	-	-	71%
Received Reliever Medication	-	-	-	100%
Use of Medical Imaging				
Combination Abdominal CT Scan	707	0.611	0.203	0.191
Combination Chest CT Scan	305	0.567	0.026	0.054
Follow-up Mammogram/Ultrasound	897	12.0%	8.2%	8.4%
MRI for Low Back Pain	164	34.8%	32.4%	32.7%
Survey of Patients' Hospital Experiences				
Area Around Room 'Always' Quiet at Night	300+	44%	-	58%
Doctors 'Always' Communicated Well	300+	75%	-	80%
Home Recovery Information Given	300+	82%	-	82%
Hospital Given 9 or 10 on 10 Point Scale	300+	51%	-	67%
Meds 'Always' Explained Before Given	300+	58%	-	60%
Nurses 'Always' Communicated Well	300+	72%	-	76%
Pain 'Always' Well Controlled	300+	67%	-	69%
Room and Bathroom 'Always' Clean	300+	72%	-	71%
Timely Help 'Always' Received	300+	63%	-	64%
Would Definitely Recommend Hospital	300+	53%	-	69%

Robert Packer Hospital

One Guthrie Square
Sayre, PA 18840
Phone: 570-888-6666
Fax: 570-882-5152
URL: www.guthrie.org
Type: Acute Care Hospitals
Emergency Services: Yes
Ownership: Voluntary Non-Profit - Other
Beds: 238

Key Personnel:

CEO/President. . . . . Marie Droege
Chief of Medical Staff . . . . Ferrol J Lee, MD
Infection Control. . . . . Allen Kilbourne
Pediatric In-Patient Care . . . . . . Gerry Terwilliger, MD
Quality Assurance . . . . Theresa Godrich
Emergency Room . . . . Edward Jones
Intensive Care Unit. . . . . Lisa Jarvis

Measure	Cases	This Hosp.	State Avg.	U.S. Avg.
Heart Attack Care				
ACE Inhibitor or ARB for LVSD	94	97%	95%	96%
Aspirin at Arrival	161	99%	99%	99%
Aspirin at Discharge	345	99%	99%	98%
Beta Blocker at Discharge	330	99%	99%	98%
Fibrinolytic Medication Timing	0	-	40%	55%
PCI Within 90 Minutes of Arrival[1]	23	78%	88%	90%
Smoking Cessation Advice	112	100%	100%	99%
Chest Pain/Possible Heart Attack Care				
Aspirin at Arrival[3]	0	-	95%	95%
Median Time to ECG (minutes)[3]	0	-	8	8
Median Time to Transfer (minutes)[5]	0	-	68	61
Fibrinolytic Medication Timing[5]	0	-	48%	54%
Heart Failure Care				
ACE Inhibitor or ARB for LVSD	208	95%	95%	94%
Discharge Instructions	303	87%	90%	88%
Evaluation of LVS Function	370	100%	99%	98%
Smoking Cessation Advice	31	100%	98%	98%
Pneumonia Care				
Appropriate Initial Antibiotic	95	96%	93%	92%
Blood Culture Timing	147	96%	96%	96%
Influenza Vaccine	141	97%	92%	91%
Initial Antibiotic Timing	144	89%	96%	95%
Pneumococcal Vaccine	223	97%	95%	93%
Smoking Cessation Advice	68	100%	98%	97%
Surgical Care Improvement Project				
Appropriate VTP Within 24 Hours	500	97%	95%	92%
Appropriate Hair Removal	1,482	100%	100%	99%
Appropriate Beta Blocker Usage	529	84%	94%	93%
Controlled Postoperative Blood Glucose	187	95%	96%	93%
Prophylactic Antibiotic Timing	878	96%	97%	97%
Prophylactic Antibiotic Timing (Outpatient)	618	95%	92%	92%
Prophylactic Antibiotic Selection	887	99%	98%	97%
Prophylactic Antibiotic Select. (Outpatient)	605	96%	93%	94%
Prophylactic Antibiotic Stopped	844	97%	95%	94%
Recommended VTP Ordered	502	98%	97%	94%
Urinary Catheter Removal	185	83%	95%	90%
Children's Asthma Care				
Received Systemic Corticosteroids	-	-	-	100%
Received Home Management Plan	-	-	-	71%
Received Reliever Medication	-	-	-	100%
Use of Medical Imaging				
Combination Abdominal CT Scan	1,657	0.136	0.203	0.191
Combination Chest CT Scan	1,324	0.005	0.026	0.054
Follow-up Mammogram/Ultrasound	1,612	13.6%	8.2%	8.4%
MRI for Low Back Pain	195	34.4%	32.4%	32.7%
Survey of Patients' Hospital Experiences				
Area Around Room 'Always' Quiet at Night	300+	50%	-	58%
Doctors 'Always' Communicated Well	300+	78%	-	80%
Home Recovery Information Given	300+	81%	-	82%
Hospital Given 9 or 10 on 10 Point Scale	300+	75%	-	67%
Meds 'Always' Explained Before Given	300+	63%	-	60%
Nurses 'Always' Communicated Well	300+	79%	-	76%
Pain 'Always' Well Controlled	300+	72%	-	69%
Room and Bathroom 'Always' Clean	300+	75%	-	71%
Timely Help 'Always' Received	300+	66%	-	64%
Would Definitely Recommend Hospital	300+	77%	-	69%

NOTE: Hospital profiles are in alphabetical order by state, then city, then hospital within the city; Rankings exclude hospitals with less than 25 cases except for patient surveys which excludes hospitals with less than 100 cases; (a) 100–299 cases; (1) The number of cases is too small to be sure how well a hospital is performing; (2) The hospital indicated that the data submitted for this measure were based on a sample of cases; (3) Data was collected during a shorter time period (fewer quarters) than the maximum possible time for this measure; (4) Suppressed for one or more quarters by CMS; (5) No data is available from the hospital for this measure; (6) Fewer than 100 patients completed the HCAHPS survey. Use these rates with caution, as the number of surveys may be too low to reliably assess hospital performance; (7) Survey results are based on less than 12 months of data; (8) Survey results are not available for this reporting period; (9) No or very few patients were eligible for the HCAHPS survey. The scores shown, if any, reflect a very small number of surveys; (10) A state average was not calculated because too few hospitals in the state submitted data; (11) There were discrepancies in the data collection process; Please refer to the User's Guide for a full explanation of data.

Community Medical Center

1822 Mulberry Street
Scranton, PA 18510
Phone: 570-969-8240
Fax: 570-969-7191
URL: www.cmchealthsys.org
Type: Acute Care Hospitals
Emergency Services: Yes
Ownership: Voluntary Non-Profit - Private
Beds: 299

Key Personnel:

CEO/President. . . . . C Richard Hartman, MD
Cardiac Laboratory. . . . . Chaufe Huang, MD
Chief of Medical Staff . . . . Vincent Ross, MD
Coronary Care . . . . Si Ramakrishna, MD
Infection Control. . . . . Trina Augustine
Operating Room. . . . . John Delmar
Quality Assurance . . . . Marge Gallagher, RN
Radiology. . . . . Burton Marks, DO

Measure	Cases	This Hosp.	State Avg.	U.S. Avg.
Heart Attack Care				
ACE Inhibitor or ARB for LVSD	50	96%	95%	96%
Aspirin at Arrival	171	99%	99%	99%
Aspirin at Discharge	223	99%	99%	98%
Beta Blocker at Discharge	230	100%	99%	98%
Fibrinolytic Medication Timing	0	-	40%	55%
PCI Within 90 Minutes of Arrival	31	84%	88%	90%
Smoking Cessation Advice	83	100%	100%	99%
Chest Pain/Possible Heart Attack Care				
Aspirin at Arrival[5]	0	-	95%	95%
Median Time to ECG (minutes)[5]	0	-	8	8
Median Time to Transfer (minutes)[5]	0	-	68	61
Fibrinolytic Medication Timing[5]	0	-	48%	54%
Heart Failure Care				
ACE Inhibitor or ARB for LVSD	110	90%	95%	94%
Discharge Instructions	225	90%	90%	88%
Evaluation of LVS Function	304	99%	99%	98%
Smoking Cessation Advice	37	100%	98%	98%
Pneumonia Care				
Appropriate Initial Antibiotic	175	97%	93%	92%
Blood Culture Timing	211	99%	96%	96%
Influenza Vaccine	143	84%	92%	91%
Initial Antibiotic Timing	269	96%	96%	95%
Pneumococcal Vaccine	183	90%	95%	93%
Smoking Cessation Advice	77	96%	98%	97%
Surgical Care Improvement Project				
Appropriate VTP Within 24 Hours	381	97%	95%	92%
Appropriate Hair Removal	1,141	100%	100%	99%
Appropriate Beta Blocker Usage	424	95%	94%	93%
Controlled Postoperative Blood Glucose	226	100%	96%	93%
Prophylactic Antibiotic Timing	781	99%	97%	97%
Prophylactic Antibiotic Timing (Outpatient)	461	97%	92%	92%
Prophylactic Antibiotic Selection	795	99%	98%	97%
Prophylactic Antibiotic Select. (Outpatient)	451	98%	93%	94%
Prophylactic Antibiotic Stopped	768	97%	95%	94%
Recommended VTP Ordered	383	97%	97%	94%
Urinary Catheter Removal	203	91%	95%	90%
Children's Asthma Care				
Received Systemic Corticosteroids	-	-	-	100%
Received Home Management Plan	-	-	-	71%
Received Reliever Medication	-	-	-	100%
Use of Medical Imaging				
Combination Abdominal CT Scan	588	0.109	0.203	0.191
Combination Chest CT Scan	329	0.100	0.026	0.054
Follow-up Mammogram/Ultrasound	761	6.3%	8.2%	8.4%
MRI for Low Back Pain[1]	36	30.6%	32.4%	32.7%
Survey of Patients' Hospital Experiences				
Area Around Room 'Always' Quiet at Night	300+	54%	-	58%
Doctors 'Always' Communicated Well	300+	79%	-	80%
Home Recovery Information Given	300+	82%	-	82%
Hospital Given 9 or 10 on 10 Point Scale	300+	62%	-	67%
Meds 'Always' Explained Before Given	300+	56%	-	60%
Nurses 'Always' Communicated Well	300+	75%	-	76%
Pain 'Always' Well Controlled	300+	69%	-	69%
Room and Bathroom 'Always' Clean	300+	69%	-	71%
Timely Help 'Always' Received	300+	64%	-	64%
Would Definitely Recommend Hospital	300+	66%	-	69%

Mercy Hospital Scranton

746 Jefferson Avenue
Scranton, PA 18501
Phone: 570-348-7100
Fax: 570-348-7639
URL: www.mercyhealthpartners.com
Type: Acute Care Hospitals
Emergency Services: Yes
Ownership: Voluntary Non-Profit - Church
Beds: 373

Key Personnel:

CEO/President. . . . . John Nespoli

Measure	Cases	This Hosp.	State Avg.	U.S. Avg.
Heart Attack Care				
ACE Inhibitor or ARB for LVSD[2]	59	100%	95%	96%
Aspirin at Arrival[2]	204	98%	99%	99%
Aspirin at Discharge[2]	287	99%	99%	98%
Beta Blocker at Discharge[2]	274	100%	99%	98%
Fibrinolytic Medication Timing[1,2]	1	0%	40%	55%
PCI Within 90 Minutes of Arrival[2]	45	93%	88%	90%
Smoking Cessation Advice[2]	110	100%	100%	99%
Chest Pain/Possible Heart Attack Care				
Aspirin at Arrival[5]	0	-	95%	95%
Median Time to ECG (minutes)[5]	0	-	8	8
Median Time to Transfer (minutes)[5]	0	-	68	61
Fibrinolytic Medication Timing[5]	0	-	48%	54%
Heart Failure Care				
ACE Inhibitor or ARB for LVSD[2]	84	100%	95%	94%
Discharge Instructions[2]	202	100%	90%	88%
Evaluation of LVS Function[2]	303	99%	99%	98%
Smoking Cessation Advice[2]	36	100%	98%	98%
Pneumonia Care				
Appropriate Initial Antibiotic[2]	71	90%	93%	92%
Blood Culture Timing[2]	99	99%	96%	96%
Influenza Vaccine[2]	81	100%	92%	91%
Initial Antibiotic Timing[2]	135	98%	96%	95%
Pneumococcal Vaccine[2]	146	98%	95%	93%
Smoking Cessation Advice[2]	37	92%	98%	97%
Surgical Care Improvement Project				
Appropriate VTP Within 24 Hours[2]	147	96%	95%	92%
Appropriate Hair Removal[2]	581	100%	100%	99%
Appropriate Beta Blocker Usage[2]	212	99%	94%	93%
Controlled Postoperative Blood Glucose[2]	179	92%	96%	93%
Prophylactic Antibiotic Timing[2]	423	99%	97%	97%
Prophylactic Antibiotic Timing (Outpatient)	281	82%	92%	92%
Prophylactic Antibiotic Selection[2]	436	99%	98%	97%
Prophylactic Antibiotic Select. (Outpatient)	250	93%	93%	94%
Prophylactic Antibiotic Stopped[2]	385	96%	95%	94%
Recommended VTP Ordered[2]	147	97%	97%	94%
Urinary Catheter Removal[2]	58	98%	95%	90%
Children's Asthma Care				
Received Systemic Corticosteroids	-	-	-	100%
Received Home Management Plan	-	-	-	71%
Received Reliever Medication	-	-	-	100%
Use of Medical Imaging				
Combination Abdominal CT Scan	771	0.163	0.203	0.191
Combination Chest CT Scan	655	0.023	0.026	0.054
Follow-up Mammogram/Ultrasound	731	7.3%	8.2%	8.4%
MRI for Low Back Pain	74	37.8%	32.4%	32.7%
Survey of Patients' Hospital Experiences				
Area Around Room 'Always' Quiet at Night	300+	47%	-	58%
Doctors 'Always' Communicated Well	300+	78%	-	80%
Home Recovery Information Given	300+	80%	-	82%
Hospital Given 9 or 10 on 10 Point Scale	300+	64%	-	67%
Meds 'Always' Explained Before Given	300+	54%	-	60%
Nurses 'Always' Communicated Well	300+	72%	-	76%
Pain 'Always' Well Controlled	300+	68%	-	69%
Room and Bathroom 'Always' Clean	300+	57%	-	71%
Timely Help 'Always' Received	300+	54%	-	64%
Would Definitely Recommend Hospital	300+	67%	-	69%

Moses Taylor Hospital

700 Quincy Avenue
Scranton, PA 18510
Phone: 570-340-2100
Fax: 570-969-2629
E-mail: mediaser@mth.org
URL: www.mth.org
Type: Acute Care Hospitals
Emergency Services: Yes
Ownership: Voluntary Non-Profit - Private
Beds: 224

Key Personnel:

CEO/President. . . . . Harold E Anderson
Chief of Medical Staff . . . . Carmen A Brutico Jr, MD
Infection Control. . . . . Alice McDonald, RN
Operating Room. . . . . Terence A Cochran, RN
Pediatric Ambulatory Care . . . . . . Stanley Blondek, MD
Pediatric In-Patient Care . . . . Stanley Blondek, MD
Quality Assurance . . . . Pam Maidlatesi, RN

Measure	Cases	This Hosp.	State Avg.	U.S. Avg.
Heart Attack Care				
ACE Inhibitor or ARB for LVSD[1]	6	83%	95%	96%
Aspirin at Arrival	42	100%	99%	99%
Aspirin at Discharge[1]	20	100%	99%	98%
Beta Blocker at Discharge	25	100%	99%	98%
Fibrinolytic Medication Timing	0	-	40%	55%
PCI Within 90 Minutes of Arrival	0	-	88%	90%
Smoking Cessation Advice[1]	3	100%	100%	99%
Chest Pain/Possible Heart Attack Care				
Aspirin at Arrival	37	97%	95%	95%
Median Time to ECG (minutes)	37	14	8	8
Median Time to Transfer (minutes)[1]	11	125	68	61
Fibrinolytic Medication Timing	0	-	48%	54%
Heart Failure Care				
ACE Inhibitor or ARB for LVSD	41	95%	95%	94%
Discharge Instructions	125	90%	90%	88%
Evaluation of LVS Function	197	99%	99%	98%
Smoking Cessation Advice	34	100%	98%	98%
Pneumonia Care				
Appropriate Initial Antibiotic	121	85%	93%	92%
Blood Culture Timing	184	100%	96%	96%
Influenza Vaccine	129	95%	92%	91%
Initial Antibiotic Timing	171	98%	96%	95%
Pneumococcal Vaccine	180	98%	95%	93%
Smoking Cessation Advice	78	100%	98%	97%
Surgical Care Improvement Project				
Appropriate VTP Within 24 Hours	254	99%	95%	92%
Appropriate Hair Removal	613	100%	100%	99%
Appropriate Beta Blocker Usage	161	97%	94%	93%
Controlled Postoperative Blood Glucose[1]	1	100%	96%	93%
Prophylactic Antibiotic Timing	400	99%	97%	97%
Prophylactic Antibiotic Timing (Outpatient)	58	95%	92%	92%
Prophylactic Antibiotic Selection	400	96%	98%	97%
Prophylactic Antibiotic Select. (Outpatient)	56	93%	93%	94%
Prophylactic Antibiotic Stopped	388	93%	95%	94%
Recommended VTP Ordered	254	99%	97%	94%
Urinary Catheter Removal	125	81%	95%	90%
Children's Asthma Care				
Received Systemic Corticosteroids	-	-	-	100%
Received Home Management Plan	-	-	-	71%
Received Reliever Medication	-	-	-	100%
Use of Medical Imaging				
Combination Abdominal CT Scan	538	0.071	0.203	0.191
Combination Chest CT Scan	325	0.000	0.026	0.054
Follow-up Mammogram/Ultrasound	699	12.2%	8.2%	8.4%
MRI for Low Back Pain	35	48.6%	32.4%	32.7%
Survey of Patients' Hospital Experiences				
Area Around Room 'Always' Quiet at Night	300+	53%	-	58%
Doctors 'Always' Communicated Well	300+	81%	-	80%
Home Recovery Information Given	300+	81%	-	82%
Hospital Given 9 or 10 on 10 Point Scale	300+	64%	-	67%
Meds 'Always' Explained Before Given	300+	62%	-	60%
Nurses 'Always' Communicated Well	300+	76%	-	76%
Pain 'Always' Well Controlled	300+	66%	-	69%
Room and Bathroom 'Always' Clean	300+	70%	-	71%
Timely Help 'Always' Received	300+	59%	-	64%
Would Definitely Recommend Hospital	300+	70%	-	69%

NOTE: Hospital profiles are in alphabetical order by state, then city, then hospital within the city; Rankings exclude hospitals with less than 25 cases except for patient surveys which excludes hospitals with less than 100 cases; (a) 100–299 cases; (1) The number of cases is too small to be sure how well a hospital is performing; (2) The hospital indicated that the data submitted for this measure were based on a sample of cases; (3) Data was collected during a shorter time period (fewer quarters) than the maximum possible time for this measure; (4) Suppressed for one or more quarters by CMS; (5) No data is available from the hospital for this measure; (6) Fewer than 100 patients completed the HCAHPS survey. Use these rates with caution, as the number of surveys may be too low to reliably assess hospital performance; (7) Survey results are based on less than 12 months of data; (8) Survey results are not available for this reporting period; (9) No or very few patients were eligible for the HCAHPS survey. The scores shown, if any, reflect a very small number of surveys; (10) A state average was not calculated because too few hospitals in the state submitted data; (11) There were discrepancies in the data collection process; Please refer to the User's Guide for a full explanation of data.

Grand View Hospital

700 Lawn Avenue
Sellersville, PA 18960
Phone: 215-453-4615
Fax: 215-453-9151
E-mail: info@gvh.org
URL: www.gvh.org
Type: Acute Care Hospitals
Emergency Services: Yes
Ownership: Voluntary Non-Profit - Other
Beds: 198

Key Personnel:
CEO/President. . . . . Stuart H Fine
Chief of Medical Staff. . . . . Anthony Foderaro, MD
Coronary Care . . . . Teresa Shoultes
Infection Control. . . . . Dean Miller
Pediatric Ambulatory Care . . . . . . Marie Clarke
Pediatric In-Patient Care . . . . Andrew Chu, MD
Quality Assurance . . . . Kathleen Slagel
Radiology. . . . . Anthony E Foderaro

Measure	Cases	This Hosp.	State Avg.	U.S. Avg.
Heart Attack Care				
ACE Inhibitor or ARB for LVSD[1]	10	100%	95%	96%
Aspirin at Arrival	69	99%	99%	99%
Aspirin at Discharge	49	100%	99%	98%
Beta Blocker at Discharge	46	100%	99%	98%
Fibrinolytic Medication Timing	0	-	40%	55%
PCI Within 90 Minutes of Arrival[1]	4	75%	88%	90%
Smoking Cessation Advice[1]	4	100%	100%	99%
Chest Pain/Possible Heart Attack Care				
Aspirin at Arrival	67	99%	95%	95%
Median Time to ECG (minutes)	67	5	8	8
Median Time to Transfer (minutes)[1]	23	38	68	61
Fibrinolytic Medication Timing	0	-	48%	54%
Heart Failure Care				
ACE Inhibitor or ARB for LVSD	58	100%	95%	94%
Discharge Instructions	245	91%	90%	88%
Evaluation of LVS Function	310	100%	99%	98%
Smoking Cessation Advice[1]	13	100%	98%	98%
Pneumonia Care				
Appropriate Initial Antibiotic	146	99%	93%	92%
Blood Culture Timing	229	99%	96%	96%
Influenza Vaccine	159	99%	92%	91%
Initial Antibiotic Timing	211	99%	96%	95%
Pneumococcal Vaccine	234	99%	95%	93%
Smoking Cessation Advice	55	100%	98%	97%
Surgical Care Improvement Project				
Appropriate VTP Within 24 Hours[2]	165	99%	95%	92%
Appropriate Hair Removal[2]	454	100%	100%	99%
Appropriate Beta Blocker Usage[2]	114	96%	94%	93%
Controlled Postoperative Blood Glucose[2]	0	-	96%	93%
Prophylactic Antibiotic Timing[2]	312	99%	97%	97%
Prophylactic Antibiotic Timing (Outpatient)	121	94%	92%	92%
Prophylactic Antibiotic Selection[2]	313	98%	98%	97%
Prophylactic Antibiotic Select. (Outpatient)	124	98%	93%	94%
Prophylactic Antibiotic Stopped[2]	296	98%	95%	94%
Recommended VTP Ordered[2]	165	99%	97%	94%
Urinary Catheter Removal[2]	27	100%	95%	90%
Children's Asthma Care				
Received Systemic Corticosteroids	-	-	-	100%
Received Home Management Plan	-	-	-	71%
Received Reliever Medication	-	-	-	100%
Use of Medical Imaging				
Combination Abdominal CT Scan	901	0.059	0.203	0.191
Combination Chest CT Scan	842	0.007	0.026	0.054
Follow-up Mammogram/Ultrasound	1,568	8.1%	8.2%	8.4%
MRI for Low Back Pain	146	24.0%	32.4%	32.7%
Survey of Patients' Hospital Experiences				
Area Around Room 'Always' Quiet at Night	300+	52%	-	58%
Doctors 'Always' Communicated Well	300+	75%	-	80%
Home Recovery Information Given	300+	86%	-	82%
Hospital Given 9 or 10 on 10 Point Scale	300+	73%	-	67%
Meds 'Always' Explained Before Given	300+	65%	-	60%
Nurses 'Always' Communicated Well	300+	78%	-	76%
Pain 'Always' Well Controlled	300+	68%	-	69%
Room and Bathroom 'Always' Clean	300+	82%	-	71%
Timely Help 'Always' Received	300+	69%	-	64%
Would Definitely Recommend Hospital	300+	82%	-	69%

UPMC Northwest

100 Fairfield Drive
Seneca, PA 16346
Phone: 814-676-7600
URL: northwest.upmc.com
Type: Acute Care Hospitals
Emergency Services: Yes
Ownership: Voluntary Non-Profit - Other

Key Personnel:
CEO/President. . . . . David P. Gibbons
Infection Control. . . . . Karen Latshaw

Measure	Cases	This Hosp.	State Avg.	U.S. Avg.
Heart Attack Care				
ACE Inhibitor or ARB for LVSD[1]	5	80%	95%	96%
Aspirin at Arrival	38	100%	99%	99%
Aspirin at Discharge[1]	20	100%	99%	98%
Beta Blocker at Discharge[1]	17	100%	99%	98%
Fibrinolytic Medication Timing	0	-	40%	55%
PCI Within 90 Minutes of Arrival	0	-	88%	90%
Smoking Cessation Advice[1]	3	100%	100%	99%
Chest Pain/Possible Heart Attack Care				
Aspirin at Arrival	141	99%	95%	95%
Median Time to ECG (minutes)	148	5	8	8
Median Time to Transfer (minutes)[1,3]	3	125	68	61
Fibrinolytic Medication Timing[1]	10	70%	48%	54%
Heart Failure Care				
ACE Inhibitor or ARB for LVSD	49	100%	95%	94%
Discharge Instructions	138	92%	90%	88%
Evaluation of LVS Function	201	100%	99%	98%
Smoking Cessation Advice	28	100%	98%	98%
Pneumonia Care				
Appropriate Initial Antibiotic	107	94%	93%	92%
Blood Culture Timing	160	99%	96%	96%
Influenza Vaccine	120	99%	92%	91%
Initial Antibiotic Timing	164	99%	96%	95%
Pneumococcal Vaccine	184	98%	95%	93%
Smoking Cessation Advice	58	100%	98%	97%
Surgical Care Improvement Project				
Appropriate VTP Within 24 Hours	129	98%	95%	92%
Appropriate Hair Removal	369	100%	100%	99%
Appropriate Beta Blocker Usage	94	98%	94%	93%
Controlled Postoperative Blood Glucose[1]	1	100%	96%	93%
Prophylactic Antibiotic Timing	251	100%	97%	97%
Prophylactic Antibiotic Timing (Outpatient)	139	95%	92%	92%
Prophylactic Antibiotic Selection	252	100%	98%	97%
Prophylactic Antibiotic Select. (Outpatient)	242	99%	93%	94%
Prophylactic Antibiotic Stopped	240	100%	95%	94%
Recommended VTP Ordered	129	98%	97%	94%
Urinary Catheter Removal	40	100%	95%	90%
Children's Asthma Care				
Received Systemic Corticosteroids	-	-	-	100%
Received Home Management Plan	-	-	-	71%
Received Reliever Medication	-	-	-	100%
Use of Medical Imaging				
Combination Abdominal CT Scan	1,032	0.076	0.203	0.191
Combination Chest CT Scan	938	0.020	0.026	0.054
Follow-up Mammogram/Ultrasound	1,769	7.5%	8.2%	8.4%
MRI for Low Back Pain	306	33.3%	32.4%	32.7%
Survey of Patients' Hospital Experiences				
Area Around Room 'Always' Quiet at Night	300+	48%	-	58%
Doctors 'Always' Communicated Well	300+	74%	-	80%
Home Recovery Information Given	300+	77%	-	82%
Hospital Given 9 or 10 on 10 Point Scale	300+	53%	-	67%
Meds 'Always' Explained Before Given	300+	52%	-	60%
Nurses 'Always' Communicated Well	300+	69%	-	76%
Pain 'Always' Well Controlled	300+	66%	-	69%
Room and Bathroom 'Always' Clean	300+	70%	-	71%
Timely Help 'Always' Received	300+	60%	-	64%
Would Definitely Recommend Hospital	300+	50%	-	69%

Heritage Valley Sewickley

720 Blackburn Road
Sewickley, PA 15143
Phone: 412-741-6600
Fax: 412-749-7400
Type: Acute Care Hospitals
Emergency Services: Yes
Ownership: Voluntary Non-Profit - Private
Beds: 221

Key Personnel:
CEO/President. . . . . Norman S Mitry
Chief of Medical Staff. . . . . Daniel Brooks
Operating Room. . . . . Michael D Felix
Pediatric Ambulatory Care . . . . . . Thom J Roberts
Pediatric In-Patient Care . . . . Thom J Roberts
Quality Assurance . . . . Catherine Williams
Emergency Room . . . . Lind Honyk

Measure	Cases	This Hosp.	State Avg.	U.S. Avg.
Heart Attack Care				
ACE Inhibitor or ARB for LVSD[1]	4	100%	95%	96%
Aspirin at Arrival	43	98%	99%	99%
Aspirin at Discharge[1]	21	90%	99%	98%
Beta Blocker at Discharge[1]	20	95%	99%	98%
Fibrinolytic Medication Timing	0	-	40%	55%
PCI Within 90 Minutes of Arrival	0	-	88%	90%
Smoking Cessation Advice[1]	1	100%	100%	99%
Chest Pain/Possible Heart Attack Care				
Aspirin at Arrival	70	96%	95%	95%
Median Time to ECG (minutes)	72	12	8	8
Median Time to Transfer (minutes)[5]	0	-	68	61
Fibrinolytic Medication Timing[5]	0	-	48%	54%
Heart Failure Care				
ACE Inhibitor or ARB for LVSD	74	100%	95%	94%
Discharge Instructions	241	93%	90%	88%
Evaluation of LVS Function	312	99%	99%	98%
Smoking Cessation Advice	41	98%	98%	98%
Pneumonia Care				
Appropriate Initial Antibiotic	150	93%	93%	92%
Blood Culture Timing	240	99%	96%	96%
Influenza Vaccine	148	99%	92%	91%
Initial Antibiotic Timing	234	97%	96%	95%
Pneumococcal Vaccine	202	100%	95%	93%
Smoking Cessation Advice	65	100%	98%	97%
Surgical Care Improvement Project				
Appropriate VTP Within 24 Hours	259	91%	95%	92%
Appropriate Hair Removal	1,182	100%	100%	99%
Appropriate Beta Blocker Usage	331	90%	94%	93%
Controlled Postoperative Blood Glucose	0	-	96%	93%
Prophylactic Antibiotic Timing	889	98%	97%	97%
Prophylactic Antibiotic Timing (Outpatient)	119	87%	92%	92%
Prophylactic Antibiotic Selection	893	99%	98%	97%
Prophylactic Antibiotic Select. (Outpatient)	114	89%	93%	94%
Prophylactic Antibiotic Stopped	836	97%	95%	94%
Recommended VTP Ordered	260	92%	97%	94%
Urinary Catheter Removal	374	93%	95%	90%
Children's Asthma Care				
Received Systemic Corticosteroids	-	-	-	100%
Received Home Management Plan	-	-	-	71%
Received Reliever Medication	-	-	-	100%
Use of Medical Imaging				
Combination Abdominal CT Scan	337	0.113	0.203	0.191
Combination Chest CT Scan	236	0.000	0.026	0.054
Follow-up Mammogram/Ultrasound	247	11.3%	8.2%	8.4%
MRI for Low Back Pain	57	42.1%	32.4%	32.7%
Survey of Patients' Hospital Experiences				
Area Around Room 'Always' Quiet at Night	300+	50%	-	58%
Doctors 'Always' Communicated Well	300+	82%	-	80%
Home Recovery Information Given	300+	82%	-	82%
Hospital Given 9 or 10 on 10 Point Scale	300+	68%	-	67%
Meds 'Always' Explained Before Given	300+	62%	-	60%
Nurses 'Always' Communicated Well	300+	80%	-	76%
Pain 'Always' Well Controlled	300+	73%	-	69%
Room and Bathroom 'Always' Clean	300+	67%	-	71%
Timely Help 'Always' Received	300+	66%	-	64%
Would Definitely Recommend Hospital	300+	72%	-	69%

NOTE: Hospital profiles are in alphabetical order by state, then city, then hospital within the city; Rankings exclude hospitals with less than 25 cases except for patient surveys which excludes hospitals with less than 100 cases; (a) 100–299 cases; (1) The number of cases is too small to be sure how well a hospital is performing; (2) The hospital indicated that the data submitted for this measure were based on a sample of cases; (3) Data was collected during a shorter time period (fewer quarters) than the maximum possible time for this measure; (4) Suppressed for one or more quarters by CMS; (5) No data is available from the hospital for this measure; (6) Fewer than 100 patients completed the HCAHPS survey. Use these rates with caution, as the number of surveys may be too low to reliably assess hospital performance; (7) Survey results are based on less than 12 months of data; (8) Survey results are not available for this reporting period; (9) No or very few patients were eligible for the HCAHPS survey. The scores shown, if any, reflect a very small number of surveys; (10) A state average was not calculated because too few hospitals in the state submitted data; (11) There were discrepancies in the data collection process; Please refer to the User's Guide for a full explanation of data.

Sharon Regional Health System

740 East State Street
Sharon, PA 16146
Phone: 724-983-3912
Fax: 724-983-3896
E-mail: info@srhs.org
URL: www.sharonregional.com
Type: Acute Care Hospitals
Emergency Services: Yes
Ownership: Voluntary Non-Profit - Other
Beds: 240

Key Personnel:
CEO/President.............. John A Zidansek
Chief of Medical Staff.......... Matthew D Crago
Coronary Care............... Mary Jane Altham RN
Infection Control.............. Sally Tice RN
Operating Room............... Michelle Aurin
Quality Assurance............ Ginny Catterson
Radiology.................... Arlene B Baratz

Measure	Cases	This Hosp.	State Avg.	U.S. Avg.
Heart Attack Care				
ACE Inhibitor or ARB for LVSD[1]	18	100%	95%	96%
Aspirin at Arrival	157	100%	99%	99%
Aspirin at Discharge	145	100%	99%	98%
Beta Blocker at Discharge	136	100%	99%	98%
Fibrinolytic Medication Timing	0	-	40%	55%
PCI Within 90 Minutes of Arrival[1]	22	100%	88%	90%
Smoking Cessation Advice	35	97%	100%	99%
Chest Pain/Possible Heart Attack Care				
Aspirin at Arrival[1]	9	67%	95%	95%
Median Time to ECG (minutes)[1]	9	12	8	8
Median Time to Transfer (minutes)[5]	0	-	68	61
Fibrinolytic Medication Timing[3]	0	-	48%	54%
Heart Failure Care				
ACE Inhibitor or ARB for LVSD	48	90%	95%	94%
Discharge Instructions	153	94%	90%	88%
Evaluation of LVS Function	202	99%	99%	98%
Smoking Cessation Advice[1]	23	87%	98%	98%
Pneumonia Care				
Appropriate Initial Antibiotic	94	87%	93%	92%
Blood Culture Timing	126	98%	96%	96%
Influenza Vaccine	99	92%	92%	91%
Initial Antibiotic Timing	140	94%	96%	95%
Pneumococcal Vaccine	129	98%	95%	93%
Smoking Cessation Advice	44	95%	98%	97%
Surgical Care Improvement Project				
Appropriate VTP Within 24 Hours[2]	244	99%	95%	92%
Appropriate Hair Removal[2]	621	100%	100%	99%
Appropriate Beta Blocker Usage[2]	204	99%	94%	93%
Controlled Postoperative Blood Glucose[2]	84	93%	96%	93%
Prophylactic Antibiotic Timing[2]	472	98%	97%	97%
Prophylactic Antibiotic Timing (Outpatient)	157	98%	92%	92%
Prophylactic Antibiotic Selection[2]	477	99%	98%	97%
Prophylactic Antibiotic Select. (Outpatient)	155	98%	93%	94%
Prophylactic Antibiotic Stopped[2]	467	96%	95%	94%
Recommended VTP Ordered[2]	247	98%	97%	94%
Urinary Catheter Removal[2]	112	95%	95%	90%
Children's Asthma Care				
Received Systemic Corticosteroids	-	-	-	100%
Received Home Management Plan	-	-	-	71%
Received Reliever Medication	-	-	-	100%
Use of Medical Imaging				
Combination Abdominal CT Scan	827	0.439	0.203	0.191
Combination Chest CT Scan	712	0.008	0.026	0.054
Follow-up Mammogram/Ultrasound	988	8.5%	8.2%	8.4%
MRI for Low Back Pain	147	32.7%	32.4%	32.7%
Survey of Patients' Hospital Experiences				
Area Around Room 'Always' Quiet at Night	300+	45%	-	58%
Doctors 'Always' Communicated Well	300+	82%	-	80%
Home Recovery Information Given	300+	80%	-	82%
Hospital Given 9 or 10 on 10 Point Scale	300+	63%	-	67%
Meds 'Always' Explained Before Given	300+	61%	-	60%
Nurses 'Always' Communicated Well	300+	76%	-	76%
Pain 'Always' Well Controlled	300+	70%	-	69%
Room and Bathroom 'Always' Clean	300+	69%	-	71%
Timely Help 'Always' Received	300+	67%	-	64%
Would Definitely Recommend Hospital	300+	66%	-	69%

Somerset Hospital

225 South Center Avenue
Somerset, PA 15501
Phone: 814-443-5000
Fax: 814-443-4937
E-mail: admin@schol.com
URL: www.somersethospital.com
Type: Acute Care Hospitals
Emergency Services: Yes
Ownership: Voluntary Non-Profit - Other
Beds: 167

Key Personnel:
CEO/President............... Michael J Farrell
Chief of Medical Staff.......... Wassim Abosamra
Infection Control.............. Erika Marker
Operating Room.............. Donna Zimmera
Quality Assurance........... Pam Ream
Radiology................... Thomas M Anderson, Jr
Emergency Room........... Shomendra K Moitra, MD
Intensive Care Unit........... M Boyce, RN

Measure	Cases	This Hosp.	State Avg.	U.S. Avg.
Heart Attack Care				
ACE Inhibitor or ARB for LVSD[1]	6	100%	95%	96%
Aspirin at Arrival	76	99%	99%	99%
Aspirin at Discharge	62	98%	99%	98%
Beta Blocker at Discharge	62	100%	99%	98%
Fibrinolytic Medication Timing	0	-	40%	55%
PCI Within 90 Minutes of Arrival[1]	12	58%	88%	90%
Smoking Cessation Advice[1]	12	92%	100%	99%
Chest Pain/Possible Heart Attack Care				
Aspirin at Arrival[1]	19	100%	95%	95%
Median Time to ECG (minutes)[1]	19	12	8	8
Median Time to Transfer (minutes)[1,3]	2	70	68	61
Fibrinolytic Medication Timing[3]	0	-	48%	54%
Heart Failure Care				
ACE Inhibitor or ARB for LVSD	38	97%	95%	94%
Discharge Instructions	92	99%	90%	88%
Evaluation of LVS Function	114	100%	99%	98%
Smoking Cessation Advice[1]	12	92%	98%	98%
Pneumonia Care				
Appropriate Initial Antibiotic	76	89%	93%	92%
Blood Culture Timing	124	87%	96%	96%
Influenza Vaccine	62	98%	92%	91%
Initial Antibiotic Timing	114	94%	96%	95%
Pneumococcal Vaccine	94	95%	95%	93%
Smoking Cessation Advice	32	72%	98%	97%
Surgical Care Improvement Project				
Appropriate VTP Within 24 Hours	97	94%	95%	92%
Appropriate Hair Removal	293	100%	100%	99%
Appropriate Beta Blocker Usage	82	99%	94%	93%
Controlled Postoperative Blood Glucose	0	-	96%	93%
Prophylactic Antibiotic Timing	212	92%	97%	97%
Prophylactic Antibiotic Timing (Outpatient)	77	94%	92%	92%
Prophylactic Antibiotic Selection	214	86%	98%	97%
Prophylactic Antibiotic Select. (Outpatient)	76	82%	93%	94%
Prophylactic Antibiotic Stopped	210	84%	95%	94%
Recommended VTP Ordered	97	94%	97%	94%
Urinary Catheter Removal	43	98%	95%	90%
Children's Asthma Care				
Received Systemic Corticosteroids	-	-	-	100%
Received Home Management Plan	-	-	-	71%
Received Reliever Medication	-	-	-	100%
Use of Medical Imaging				
Combination Abdominal CT Scan	315	0.562	0.203	0.191
Combination Chest CT Scan	163	0.325	0.026	0.054
Follow-up Mammogram/Ultrasound	363	6.1%	8.2%	8.4%
MRI for Low Back Pain	64	37.5%	32.4%	32.7%
Survey of Patients' Hospital Experiences				
Area Around Room 'Always' Quiet at Night	300+	44%	-	58%
Doctors 'Always' Communicated Well	300+	75%	-	80%
Home Recovery Information Given	300+	84%	-	82%
Hospital Given 9 or 10 on 10 Point Scale	300+	56%	-	67%
Meds 'Always' Explained Before Given	300+	55%	-	60%
Nurses 'Always' Communicated Well	300+	72%	-	76%
Pain 'Always' Well Controlled	300+	64%	-	69%
Room and Bathroom 'Always' Clean	300+	73%	-	71%
Timely Help 'Always' Received	300+	57%	-	64%
Would Definitely Recommend Hospital	300+	52%	-	69%

Mount Nittany Medical Center

1800 East Park Ave
State College, PA 16803
Phone: 814-231-7000
Fax: 814-234-6100
E-mail: info@mountnittany.org
URL: www.mountnittany.org
Type: Acute Care Hospitals
Emergency Services: Yes
Ownership: Voluntary Non-Profit - Other
Beds: 201

Key Personnel:
CEO/President............... Thomas J Murray, FACHE
Chief of Medical Staff.......... Jeffrey A Ratner, MD
Coronary Care............... Jeffrey Eaton, MD
Infection Control.............. Marlene Stetson, RN
Operating Room.............. James S Martin, MD
Pediatric In-Patient Care....... Tracy Trudel, MD
Quality Assurance............ Gail Miller
Radiology.................... Ari Geselowitz, MD

Measure	Cases	This Hosp.	State Avg.	U.S. Avg.
Heart Attack Care				
ACE Inhibitor or ARB for LVSD[1]	18	94%	95%	96%
Aspirin at Arrival	139	99%	99%	99%
Aspirin at Discharge	120	98%	99%	98%
Beta Blocker at Discharge	121	98%	99%	98%
Fibrinolytic Medication Timing	0	-	40%	55%
PCI Within 90 Minutes of Arrival	39	85%	88%	90%
Smoking Cessation Advice	27	100%	100%	99%
Chest Pain/Possible Heart Attack Care				
Aspirin at Arrival[1,3]	14	100%	95%	95%
Median Time to ECG (minutes)[1,3]	14	16	8	8
Median Time to Transfer (minutes)[1,3]	1	51	68	61
Fibrinolytic Medication Timing[3]	0	-	48%	54%
Heart Failure Care				
ACE Inhibitor or ARB for LVSD	60	92%	95%	94%
Discharge Instructions	235	86%	90%	88%
Evaluation of LVS Function	298	99%	99%	98%
Smoking Cessation Advice	31	100%	98%	98%
Pneumonia Care				
Appropriate Initial Antibiotic	134	95%	93%	92%
Blood Culture Timing	209	94%	96%	96%
Influenza Vaccine	179	93%	92%	91%
Initial Antibiotic Timing	226	92%	96%	95%
Pneumococcal Vaccine	251	98%	95%	93%
Smoking Cessation Advice	62	100%	98%	97%
Surgical Care Improvement Project				
Appropriate VTP Within 24 Hours	373	94%	95%	92%
Appropriate Hair Removal	1,632	98%	100%	99%
Appropriate Beta Blocker Usage	482	89%	94%	93%
Controlled Postoperative Blood Glucose	0	-	96%	93%
Prophylactic Antibiotic Timing	1,229	97%	97%	97%
Prophylactic Antibiotic Timing (Outpatient)	221	95%	92%	92%
Prophylactic Antibiotic Selection	1,232	99%	98%	97%
Prophylactic Antibiotic Select. (Outpatient)	215	96%	93%	94%
Prophylactic Antibiotic Stopped	1,201	99%	95%	94%
Recommended VTP Ordered	373	95%	97%	94%
Urinary Catheter Removal	228	94%	95%	90%
Children's Asthma Care				
Received Systemic Corticosteroids	-	-	-	100%
Received Home Management Plan	-	-	-	71%
Received Reliever Medication	-	-	-	100%
Use of Medical Imaging				
Combination Abdominal CT Scan	581	0.129	0.203	0.191
Combination Chest CT Scan	539	0.017	0.026	0.054
Follow-up Mammogram/Ultrasound	1,584	10.2%	8.2%	8.4%
MRI for Low Back Pain	82	29.3%	32.4%	32.7%
Survey of Patients' Hospital Experiences				
Area Around Room 'Always' Quiet at Night	300+	41%	-	58%
Doctors 'Always' Communicated Well	300+	81%	-	80%
Home Recovery Information Given	300+	84%	-	82%
Hospital Given 9 or 10 on 10 Point Scale	300+	65%	-	67%
Meds 'Always' Explained Before Given	300+	61%	-	60%
Nurses 'Always' Communicated Well	300+	76%	-	76%
Pain 'Always' Well Controlled	300+	73%	-	69%
Room and Bathroom 'Always' Clean	300+	76%	-	71%
Timely Help 'Always' Received	300+	66%	-	64%
Would Definitely Recommend Hospital	300+	67%	-	69%

NOTE: Hospital profiles are in alphabetical order by state, then city, then hospital within the city; Rankings exclude hospitals with less than 25 cases except for patient surveys which excludes hospitals with less than 100 cases; (a) 100–299 cases; (1) The number of cases is too small to be sure how well a hospital is performing; (2) The hospital indicated that the data submitted for this measure were based on a sample of cases; (3) Data was collected during a shorter time period (fewer quarters) than the maximum possible time for this measure; (4) Suppressed for one or more quarters by CMS; (5) No data is available from the hospital for this measure; (6) Fewer than 100 patients completed the HCAHPS survey. Use these rates with caution, as the number of surveys may be too low to reliably assess hospital performance; (7) Survey results are based on less than 12 months of data; (8) Survey results are not available for this reporting period; (9) No or very few patients were eligible for the HCAHPS survey. The scores shown, if any, reflect a very small number of surveys; (10) A state average was not calculated because too few hospitals in the state submitted data; (11) There were discrepancies in the data collection process; Please refer to the User's Guide for a full explanation of data.

Sunbury Community Hospital

350 North 11th Street
Sunbury, PA 17801
URL: www.schopc.org
Type: Acute Care Hospitals
Ownership: Proprietary
Phone: 570-286-3333
Fax: 570-286-3576
Emergency Services: Yes
Beds: 123

Key Personnel:
CEO/President. . . . . R Clifford Park
Chief of Medical Staff . . . . John C Ninos, MD
Operating Room. . . . . Brian A Batman, MD
Quality Assurance . . . . Liz Bendas, RN
Anesthesiology. . . . . Francisco A Furtado, MD
Emergency Room . . . . Frederick Burke, RN/BSN

Measure	Cases	This Hosp.	State Avg.	U.S. Avg.
Heart Attack Care				
ACE Inhibitor or ARB for LVSD[1]	3	67%	95%	96%
Aspirin at Arrival[1]	17	100%	99%	99%
Aspirin at Discharge[1]	6	100%	99%	98%
Beta Blocker at Discharge[1]	7	100%	99%	98%
Fibrinolytic Medication Timing	0	-	40%	55%
PCI Within 90 Minutes of Arrival	0	-	88%	90%
Smoking Cessation Advice[1]	1	100%	100%	99%
Chest Pain/Possible Heart Attack Care				
Aspirin at Arrival	42	90%	95%	95%
Median Time to ECG (minutes)	46	11	8	8
Median Time to Transfer (minutes)[1]	11	49	68	61
Fibrinolytic Medication Timing	0	-	48%	54%
Heart Failure Care				
ACE Inhibitor or ARB for LVSD[1]	16	81%	95%	94%
Discharge Instructions	65	83%	90%	88%
Evaluation of LVS Function	106	98%	99%	98%
Smoking Cessation Advice[1]	16	94%	98%	98%
Pneumonia Care				
Appropriate Initial Antibiotic	67	94%	93%	92%
Blood Culture Timing	128	97%	96%	96%
Influenza Vaccine	85	94%	92%	91%
Initial Antibiotic Timing	125	94%	96%	95%
Pneumococcal Vaccine	109	90%	95%	93%
Smoking Cessation Advice[1]	19	84%	98%	97%
Surgical Care Improvement Project				
Appropriate VTP Within 24 Hours[2]	44	80%	95%	92%
Appropriate Hair Removal[2]	102	100%	100%	99%
Appropriate Beta Blocker Usage[2]	35	91%	94%	93%
Controlled Postoperative Blood Glucose[2]	0	-	96%	93%
Prophylactic Antibiotic Timing[2]	71	100%	97%	97%
Prophylactic Antibiotic Timing (Outpatient)	32	72%	92%	92%
Prophylactic Antibiotic Selection[2]	71	99%	98%	97%
Prophylactic Antibiotic Select. (Outpatient)	38	95%	93%	94%
Prophylactic Antibiotic Stopped[2]	65	80%	95%	94%
Recommended VTP Ordered[2]	44	80%	97%	94%
Urinary Catheter Removal	35	94%	95%	90%
Children's Asthma Care				
Received Systemic Corticosteroids	-	-	-	100%
Received Home Management Plan	-	-	-	71%
Received Reliever Medication	-	-	-	100%
Use of Medical Imaging				
Combination Abdominal CT Scan	192	0.099	0.203	0.191
Combination Chest CT Scan	143	0.042	0.026	0.054
Follow-up Mammogram/Ultrasound	435	2.8%	8.2%	8.4%
MRI for Low Back Pain[1]	30	40.0%	32.4%	32.7%
Survey of Patients' Hospital Experiences				
Area Around Room 'Always' Quiet at Night	300+	48%	-	58%
Doctors 'Always' Communicated Well	300+	81%	-	80%
Home Recovery Information Given	300+	82%	-	82%
Hospital Given 9 or 10 on 10 Point Scale	300+	62%	-	67%
Meds 'Always' Explained Before Given	300+	56%	-	60%
Nurses 'Always' Communicated Well	300+	75%	-	76%
Pain 'Always' Well Controlled	300+	66%	-	69%
Room and Bathroom 'Always' Clean	300+	68%	-	71%
Timely Help 'Always' Received	300+	66%	-	64%
Would Definitely Recommend Hospital	300+	61%	-	69%

Titusville Hospital

406 West Oak Street
Titusville, PA 16354
URL: www.titusvillehospital.org
Type: Acute Care Hospitals
Ownership: Voluntary Non-Profit - Private
Phone: 814-827-1851
Fax: 814-827-3099
Emergency Services: Yes
Beds: 95

Key Personnel:
Chief of Medical Staff . . . . Terri See
Infection Control. . . . . Brenda Burnett
Operating Room. . . . . Anil Dutt, RN
Quality Assurance . . . . Linda Harris

Measure	Cases	This Hosp.	State Avg.	U.S. Avg.
Heart Attack Care				
ACE Inhibitor or ARB for LVSD[1]	1	100%	95%	96%
Aspirin at Arrival[1]	3	100%	99%	99%
Aspirin at Discharge[1]	4	100%	99%	98%
Beta Blocker at Discharge[1]	4	100%	99%	98%
Fibrinolytic Medication Timing	0	-	40%	55%
PCI Within 90 Minutes of Arrival	0	-	88%	90%
Smoking Cessation Advice	0	-	100%	99%
Chest Pain/Possible Heart Attack Care				
Aspirin at Arrival	116	98%	95%	95%
Median Time to ECG (minutes)	119	8	8	8
Median Time to Transfer (minutes)[1,3]	1	65	68	61
Fibrinolytic Medication Timing[1]	2	50%	48%	54%
Heart Failure Care				
ACE Inhibitor or ARB for LVSD[1]	17	76%	95%	94%
Discharge Instructions	46	89%	90%	88%
Evaluation of LVS Function	63	97%	99%	98%
Smoking Cessation Advice[1]	7	57%	98%	98%
Pneumonia Care				
Appropriate Initial Antibiotic	47	87%	93%	92%
Blood Culture Timing	55	96%	96%	96%
Influenza Vaccine	46	87%	92%	91%
Initial Antibiotic Timing	71	90%	96%	95%
Pneumococcal Vaccine	72	83%	95%	93%
Smoking Cessation Advice	30	80%	98%	97%
Surgical Care Improvement Project				
Appropriate VTP Within 24 Hours	37	54%	95%	92%
Appropriate Hair Removal	118	99%	100%	99%
Appropriate Beta Blocker Usage	33	91%	94%	93%
Controlled Postoperative Blood Glucose	0	-	96%	93%
Prophylactic Antibiotic Timing	85	85%	97%	97%
Prophylactic Antibiotic Timing (Outpatient)	38	58%	92%	92%
Prophylactic Antibiotic Selection	84	73%	98%	97%
Prophylactic Antibiotic Select. (Outpatient)	31	61%	93%	94%
Prophylactic Antibiotic Stopped	78	85%	95%	94%
Recommended VTP Ordered	37	62%	97%	94%
Urinary Catheter Removal[1]	3	33%	95%	90%
Children's Asthma Care				
Received Systemic Corticosteroids	-	-	-	100%
Received Home Management Plan	-	-	-	71%
Received Reliever Medication	-	-	-	100%
Use of Medical Imaging				
Combination Abdominal CT Scan	282	0.163	0.203	0.191
Combination Chest CT Scan	244	0.000	0.026	0.054
Follow-up Mammogram/Ultrasound	538	0.4%	8.2%	8.4%
MRI for Low Back Pain	60	28.3%	32.4%	32.7%
Survey of Patients' Hospital Experiences				
Area Around Room 'Always' Quiet at Night	300+	66%	-	58%
Doctors 'Always' Communicated Well	300+	87%	-	80%
Home Recovery Information Given	300+	85%	-	82%
Hospital Given 9 or 10 on 10 Point Scale	300+	76%	-	67%
Meds 'Always' Explained Before Given	300+	61%	-	60%
Nurses 'Always' Communicated Well	300+	81%	-	76%
Pain 'Always' Well Controlled	300+	75%	-	69%
Room and Bathroom 'Always' Clean	300+	83%	-	71%
Timely Help 'Always' Received	300+	74%	-	64%
Would Definitely Recommend Hospital	300+	73%	-	69%

Memorial Hospital - Towanda

91 Hospital Drive
Towanda, PA 18848
E-mail: memhosp@epix.net
URL: www.memorialhospital.org
Type: Acute Care Hospitals
Ownership: Voluntary Non-Profit - Other
Phone: 570-268-2270
Fax: 570-265-5763
Emergency Services: Yes
Beds: 94

Key Personnel:
CEO/President. . . . . Gary A Baker
Chief of Medical Staff . . . . Stephen Becker, MD
Operating Room. . . . . Caroline Brown, RN
Quality Assurance . . . . Anita Bennett
Radiology. . . . . Dave Sickler
Patient Relations . . . . Lynn Dibble

Measure	Cases	This Hosp.	State Avg.	U.S. Avg.
Heart Attack Care				
ACE Inhibitor or ARB for LVSD[1]	2	100%	95%	96%
Aspirin at Arrival[1]	6	100%	99%	99%
Aspirin at Discharge[1]	3	100%	99%	98%
Beta Blocker at Discharge[1]	3	100%	99%	98%
Fibrinolytic Medication Timing	0	-	40%	55%
PCI Within 90 Minutes of Arrival	0	-	88%	90%
Smoking Cessation Advice[1]	1	100%	100%	99%
Chest Pain/Possible Heart Attack Care				
Aspirin at Arrival	42	93%	95%	95%
Median Time to ECG (minutes)	47	6	8	8
Median Time to Transfer (minutes)[1]	5	92	68	61
Fibrinolytic Medication Timing	0	-	48%	54%
Heart Failure Care				
ACE Inhibitor or ARB for LVSD[1]	10	80%	95%	94%
Discharge Instructions	42	100%	90%	88%
Evaluation of LVS Function	52	92%	99%	98%
Smoking Cessation Advice[1]	5	100%	98%	98%
Pneumonia Care				
Appropriate Initial Antibiotic	61	74%	93%	92%
Blood Culture Timing	66	91%	96%	96%
Influenza Vaccine	40	68%	92%	91%
Initial Antibiotic Timing	68	94%	96%	95%
Pneumococcal Vaccine	50	70%	95%	93%
Smoking Cessation Advice[1]	22	100%	98%	97%
Surgical Care Improvement Project				
Appropriate VTP Within 24 Hours[1]	14	93%	95%	92%
Appropriate Hair Removal	26	100%	100%	99%
Appropriate Beta Blocker Usage[1]	4	75%	94%	93%
Controlled Postoperative Blood Glucose	0	-	96%	93%
Prophylactic Antibiotic Timing[1]	14	86%	97%	97%
Prophylactic Antibiotic Timing (Outpatient)	30	97%	92%	92%
Prophylactic Antibiotic Selection[1]	14	79%	98%	97%
Prophylactic Antibiotic Select. (Outpatient)	30	90%	93%	94%
Prophylactic Antibiotic Stopped[1]	13	77%	95%	94%
Recommended VTP Ordered[1]	14	93%	97%	94%
Urinary Catheter Removal[1]	2	100%	95%	90%
Children's Asthma Care				
Received Systemic Corticosteroids	-	-	-	100%
Received Home Management Plan	-	-	-	71%
Received Reliever Medication	-	-	-	100%
Use of Medical Imaging				
Combination Abdominal CT Scan	239	0.063	0.203	0.191
Combination Chest CT Scan	93	0.011	0.026	0.054
Follow-up Mammogram/Ultrasound	337	5.9%	8.2%	8.4%
MRI for Low Back Pain	89	37.1%	32.4%	32.7%
Survey of Patients' Hospital Experiences				
Area Around Room 'Always' Quiet at Night	300+	62%	-	58%
Doctors 'Always' Communicated Well	300+	83%	-	80%
Home Recovery Information Given	300+	84%	-	82%
Hospital Given 9 or 10 on 10 Point Scale	300+	77%	-	67%
Meds 'Always' Explained Before Given	300+	63%	-	60%
Nurses 'Always' Communicated Well	300+	81%	-	76%
Pain 'Always' Well Controlled	300+	75%	-	69%
Room and Bathroom 'Always' Clean	300+	84%	-	71%
Timely Help 'Always' Received	300+	77%	-	64%
Would Definitely Recommend Hospital	300+	70%	-	69%

NOTE: Hospital profiles are in alphabetical order by state, then city, then hospital within the city; Rankings exclude hospitals with less than 25 cases except for patient surveys which excludes hospitals with less than 100 cases; (a) 100–299 cases; (1) The number of cases is too small to be sure how well a hospital is performing; (2) The hospital indicated that the data submitted for this measure were based on a sample of cases; (3) Data was collected during a shorter time period (fewer quarters) than the maximum possible time for this measure; (4) Suppressed for one or more quarters by CMS; (5) No data is available from the hospital for this measure; (6) Fewer than 100 patients completed the HCAHPS survey. Use these rates with caution, as the number of surveys may be too low to reliably assess hospital performance; (7) Survey results are based on less than 12 months of data; (8) Survey results are not available for this reporting period; (9) No or very few patients were eligible for the HCAHPS survey. The scores shown, if any, reflect a very small number of surveys; (10) A state average was not calculated because too few hospitals in the state submitted data; (11) There were discrepancies in the data collection process; Please refer to the User's Guide for a full explanation of data.

Edgewood Surgical Hospital

239 Edgewood Drive Extension
Transfer, PA 16154
E-mail: mailbox@edgewoodsurgical.com
URL: www.edgewoodsurgical.com
Type: Acute Care Hospitals
Ownership: Proprietary

Phone: 724-646-0400
Fax: 724-646-0413

Emergency Services: Yes

Key Personnel:
CEO/President. . . . . Anthony J Puorro FACHE

Measure	Cases	This Hosp.	State Avg.	U.S. Avg.
Heart Attack Care				
ACE Inhibitor or ARB for LVSD[5]	0	-	95%	96%
Aspirin at Arrival[5]	0	-	99%	99%
Aspirin at Discharge[5]	0	-	99%	98%
Beta Blocker at Discharge[5]	0	-	99%	98%
Fibrinolytic Medication Timing[5]	0	-	40%	55%
PCI Within 90 Minutes of Arrival[5]	0	-	88%	90%
Smoking Cessation Advice[5]	0	-	100%	99%
Chest Pain/Possible Heart Attack Care				
Aspirin at Arrival[5]	0	-	95%	95%
Median Time to ECG (minutes)[5]	0	-	8	8
Median Time to Transfer (minutes)[5]	0	-	68	61
Fibrinolytic Medication Timing[5]	0	-	48%	54%
Heart Failure Care				
ACE Inhibitor or ARB for LVSD[5]	0	-	95%	94%
Discharge Instructions[5]	0	-	90%	88%
Evaluation of LVS Function[5]	0	-	99%	98%
Smoking Cessation Advice[5]	0	-	98%	98%
Pneumonia Care				
Appropriate Initial Antibiotic[5]	0	-	93%	92%
Blood Culture Timing[5]	0	-	96%	96%
Influenza Vaccine[5]	0	-	92%	91%
Initial Antibiotic Timing[5]	0	-	96%	95%
Pneumococcal Vaccine[5]	0	-	95%	93%
Smoking Cessation Advice[5]	0	-	98%	97%
Surgical Care Improvement Project				
Appropriate VTP Within 24 Hours[1]	7	100%	95%	92%
Appropriate Hair Removal	127	100%	100%	99%
Appropriate Beta Blocker Usage[1]	24	100%	94%	93%
Controlled Postoperative Blood Glucose	0	-	96%	93%
Prophylactic Antibiotic Timing	119	99%	97%	97%
Prophylactic Antibiotic Timing (Outpatient)[5]	0	-	92%	92%
Prophylactic Antibiotic Selection	119	100%	98%	97%
Prophylactic Antibiotic Select. (Outpatient)[5]	0	-	93%	94%
Prophylactic Antibiotic Stopped	119	100%	95%	94%
Recommended VTP Ordered[1]	7	100%	97%	94%
Urinary Catheter Removal[1]	15	100%	95%	90%
Children's Asthma Care				
Received Systemic Corticosteroids	-	-	-	100%
Received Home Management Plan	-	-	-	71%
Received Reliever Medication	-	-	-	100%
Use of Medical Imaging				
Combination Abdominal CT Scan[5]	0	-	0.203	0.191
Combination Chest CT Scan[5]	0	-	0.026	0.054
Follow-up Mammogram/Ultrasound[5]	0	-	8.2%	8.4%
MRI for Low Back Pain	117	39.3%	32.4%	32.7%
Survey of Patients' Hospital Experiences				
Area Around Room 'Always' Quiet at Night	(a)	87%	-	58%
Doctors 'Always' Communicated Well	(a)	92%	-	80%
Home Recovery Information Given	(a)	93%	-	82%
Hospital Given 9 or 10 on 10 Point Scale	(a)	87%	-	67%
Meds 'Always' Explained Before Given	(a)	77%	-	60%
Nurses 'Always' Communicated Well	(a)	88%	-	76%
Pain 'Always' Well Controlled	(a)	80%	-	69%
Room and Bathroom 'Always' Clean	(a)	81%	-	71%
Timely Help 'Always' Received	(a)	84%	-	64%
Would Definitely Recommend Hospital	(a)	87%	-	69%

Troy Community Hospital

101 Elmira Street
Troy, PA 16947
Type: Critical Access Hospitals
Ownership: Voluntary Non-Profit - Private

Phone: 570-297-2121
Fax: 570-297-3970
Emergency Services: Yes
Beds: 32

Key Personnel:
Chief of Medical Staff. . . . . Vance Good, MD
Infection Control. . . . . Sheila Angove, BSN
Operating Room. . . . . Mark O Connell, RN
Quality Assurance . . . . Joan Delovich
Emergency Room . . . . George P Abraham, MD
Patient Relations . . . . Beverly Jackson, RN

Measure	Cases	This Hosp.	State Avg.	U.S. Avg.
Heart Attack Care				
ACE Inhibitor or ARB for LVSD[3]	0	-	95%	96%
Aspirin at Arrival[1,3]	2	100%	99%	99%
Aspirin at Discharge[1,3]	1	100%	99%	98%
Beta Blocker at Discharge[1,3]	1	100%	99%	98%
Fibrinolytic Medication Timing[5]	0	-	40%	55%
PCI Within 90 Minutes of Arrival[5]	0	-	88%	90%
Smoking Cessation Advice[3]	0	-	100%	99%
Chest Pain/Possible Heart Attack Care				
Aspirin at Arrival[3]	30	100%	95%	95%
Median Time to ECG (minutes)[3]	32	7	8	8
Median Time to Transfer (minutes)[1,3]	11	155	68	61
Fibrinolytic Medication Timing[3]	0	-	48%	54%
Heart Failure Care				
ACE Inhibitor or ARB for LVSD[1]	9	78%	95%	94%
Discharge Instructions[1]	7	86%	90%	88%
Evaluation of LVS Function[1]	14	93%	99%	98%
Smoking Cessation Advice[1]	3	33%	98%	98%
Pneumonia Care				
Appropriate Initial Antibiotic	26	96%	93%	92%
Blood Culture Timing	34	94%	96%	96%
Influenza Vaccine[1]	17	94%	92%	91%
Initial Antibiotic Timing[1]	2	100%	96%	95%
Pneumococcal Vaccine	27	78%	95%	93%
Smoking Cessation Advice[1]	4	100%	98%	97%
Surgical Care Improvement Project				
Appropriate VTP Within 24 Hours[5]	0	-	95%	92%
Appropriate Hair Removal[5]	0	-	100%	99%
Appropriate Beta Blocker Usage[5]	0	-	94%	93%
Controlled Postoperative Blood Glucose[5]	0	-	96%	93%
Prophylactic Antibiotic Timing[5]	0	-	97%	97%
Prophylactic Antibiotic Timing (Outpatient)[5]	0	-	92%	92%
Prophylactic Antibiotic Selection[5]	0	-	98%	97%
Prophylactic Antibiotic Select. (Outpatient)[5]	0	-	93%	94%
Prophylactic Antibiotic Stopped[5]	0	-	95%	94%
Recommended VTP Ordered[5]	0	-	97%	94%
Urinary Catheter Removal[5]	0	-	95%	90%
Children's Asthma Care				
Received Systemic Corticosteroids	-	-	-	100%
Received Home Management Plan	-	-	-	71%
Received Reliever Medication	-	-	-	100%
Use of Medical Imaging				
Combination Abdominal CT Scan	228	0.022	0.203	0.191
Combination Chest CT Scan	129	0.008	0.026	0.054
Follow-up Mammogram/Ultrasound	310	12.3%	8.2%	8.4%
MRI for Low Back Pain[1]	26	34.6%	32.4%	32.7%
Survey of Patients' Hospital Experiences				
Area Around Room 'Always' Quiet at Night[8]	-	-	-	58%
Doctors 'Always' Communicated Well[8]	-	-	-	80%
Home Recovery Information Given[8]	-	-	-	82%
Hospital Given 9 or 10 on 10 Point Scale[8]	-	-	-	67%
Meds 'Always' Explained Before Given[8]	-	-	-	60%
Nurses 'Always' Communicated Well[8]	-	-	-	76%
Pain 'Always' Well Controlled[8]	-	-	-	69%
Room and Bathroom 'Always' Clean[8]	-	-	-	71%
Timely Help 'Always' Received[8]	-	-	-	64%
Would Definitely Recommend Hospital[8]	-	-	-	69%

Mercy Tyler Hospital

880 State Route 6 West
Tunkhannock, PA 18657
E-mail: mercytyler@health-partners.org
URL: www.tylerhospital.com
Type: Acute Care Hospitals
Ownership: Voluntary Non-Profit - Other

Phone: 570-836-2161
Fax: 570-836-7057

Emergency Services: Yes
Beds: 58

Key Personnel:
CEO/President. . . . . Denise Gieski
Cardiac Laboratory. . . . . Joyce Enders
Chief of Medical Staff . . . . Pamela A Shields, CPCS
Infection Control. . . . . Kathy Ritter
Operating Room. . . . . Robert Glicini
Quality Assurance . . . . Kathy Ritter
Radiology. . . . . Ian A Kellman, MD

Measure	Cases	This Hosp.	State Avg.	U.S. Avg.
Heart Attack Care				
ACE Inhibitor or ARB for LVSD[1,3]	1	0%	95%	96%
Aspirin at Arrival[1,3]	4	100%	99%	99%
Aspirin at Discharge[1,3]	1	100%	99%	98%
Beta Blocker at Discharge[1,3]	1	100%	99%	98%
Fibrinolytic Medication Timing[3]	0	-	40%	55%
PCI Within 90 Minutes of Arrival[3]	0	-	88%	90%
Smoking Cessation Advice[1,3]	1	0%	100%	99%
Chest Pain/Possible Heart Attack Care				
Aspirin at Arrival	60	92%	95%	95%
Median Time to ECG (minutes)	62	12	8	8
Median Time to Transfer (minutes)[1,3]	9	94	68	61
Fibrinolytic Medication Timing	0	-	48%	54%
Heart Failure Care				
ACE Inhibitor or ARB for LVSD[1]	10	70%	95%	94%
Discharge Instructions	39	26%	90%	88%
Evaluation of LVS Function	50	94%	99%	98%
Smoking Cessation Advice[1]	6	67%	98%	98%
Pneumonia Care				
Appropriate Initial Antibiotic	68	82%	93%	92%
Blood Culture Timing	72	93%	96%	96%
Influenza Vaccine	63	67%	92%	91%
Initial Antibiotic Timing	92	99%	96%	95%
Pneumococcal Vaccine	102	93%	95%	93%
Smoking Cessation Advice	29	76%	98%	97%
Surgical Care Improvement Project				
Appropriate VTP Within 24 Hours	28	79%	95%	92%
Appropriate Hair Removal	40	100%	100%	99%
Appropriate Beta Blocker Usage[1]	15	80%	94%	93%
Controlled Postoperative Blood Glucose	0	-	96%	93%
Prophylactic Antibiotic Timing	31	71%	97%	97%
Prophylactic Antibiotic Timing (Outpatient)[1]	16	69%	92%	92%
Prophylactic Antibiotic Selection	30	90%	98%	97%
Prophylactic Antibiotic Select. (Outpatient)[1]	15	80%	93%	94%
Prophylactic Antibiotic Stopped	29	83%	95%	94%
Recommended VTP Ordered	28	79%	97%	94%
Urinary Catheter Removal[1]	10	80%	95%	90%
Children's Asthma Care				
Received Systemic Corticosteroids	-	-	-	100%
Received Home Management Plan	-	-	-	71%
Received Reliever Medication	-	-	-	100%
Use of Medical Imaging				
Combination Abdominal CT Scan	187	0.364	0.203	0.191
Combination Chest CT Scan	103	0.029	0.026	0.054
Follow-up Mammogram/Ultrasound	239	7.1%	8.2%	8.4%
MRI for Low Back Pain	50	36.0%	32.4%	32.7%
Survey of Patients' Hospital Experiences				
Area Around Room 'Always' Quiet at Night	(a)	41%	-	58%
Doctors 'Always' Communicated Well	(a)	84%	-	80%
Home Recovery Information Given	(a)	85%	-	82%
Hospital Given 9 or 10 on 10 Point Scale	(a)	64%	-	67%
Meds 'Always' Explained Before Given	(a)	64%	-	60%
Nurses 'Always' Communicated Well	(a)	75%	-	76%
Pain 'Always' Well Controlled	(a)	69%	-	69%
Room and Bathroom 'Always' Clean	(a)	76%	-	71%
Timely Help 'Always' Received	(a)	69%	-	64%
Would Definitely Recommend Hospital	(a)	64%	-	69%

NOTE: Hospital profiles are in alphabetical order by state, then city, then hospital within the city; Rankings exclude hospitals with less than 25 cases except for patient surveys which excludes hospitals with less than 100 cases; (a) 100–299 cases; (1) The number of cases is too small to be sure how well a hospital is performing; (2) The hospital indicated that the data submitted for this measure were based on a sample of cases; (3) Data was collected during a shorter time period (fewer quarters) than the maximum possible time for this measure; (4) Suppressed for one or more quarters by CMS; (5) No data is available from the hospital for this measure; (6) Fewer than 100 patients completed the HCAHPS survey. Use these rates with caution, as the number of surveys may be too low to reliably assess hospital performance; (7) Survey results are not available for this reporting period; (9) No or very few patients were eligible for the HCAHPS survey. The scores shown, if any, reflect a very small number of surveys; (10) A state average was not calculated because too few hospitals in the state submitted data; (11) There were discrepancies in the data collection process; Please refer to the User's Guide for a full explanation of data.

Uniontown Hospital

500 West Berkeley Street
Uniontown, PA 15401
URL: www.uniontownhospital.com
Type: Acute Care Hospitals
Ownership: Voluntary Non-Profit - Other
Phone: 724-430-5000
Fax: 724-430-3342
Emergency Services: Yes
Beds: 209

Key Personnel:
Cardiac Laboratory. . . . . Kris Shiley
Chief of Medical Staff. . . . . Danette Minehart
Operating Room. . . . . Brandon M Ball
Pediatric In-Patient Care . . . . Mani Balu, MD
Quality Assurance . . . . Jan Curry
Radiology. . . . . Judith Taylor, MD
Emergency Room . . . . Cataldo Corrado

Measure	Cases	This Hosp.	State Avg.	U.S. Avg.
Heart Attack Care				
ACE Inhibitor or ARB for LVSD[1]	22	86%	95%	96%
Aspirin at Arrival	128	99%	99%	99%
Aspirin at Discharge	98	100%	99%	98%
Beta Blocker at Discharge	94	94%	99%	98%
Fibrinolytic Medication Timing	0	-	40%	55%
PCI Within 90 Minutes of Arrival	25	88%	88%	90%
Smoking Cessation Advice	32	97%	100%	99%
Chest Pain/Possible Heart Attack Care				
Aspirin at Arrival	68	97%	95%	95%
Median Time to ECG (minutes)	71	22	8	8
Median Time to Transfer (minutes)[1]	8	92	68	61
Fibrinolytic Medication Timing	0	-	48%	54%
Heart Failure Care				
ACE Inhibitor or ARB for LVSD	100	87%	95%	94%
Discharge Instructions	309	76%	90%	88%
Evaluation of LVS Function	410	98%	99%	98%
Smoking Cessation Advice	63	94%	98%	98%
Pneumonia Care				
Appropriate Initial Antibiotic	183	91%	93%	92%
Blood Culture Timing	115	96%	96%	96%
Influenza Vaccine	163	83%	92%	91%
Initial Antibiotic Timing	231	93%	96%	95%
Pneumococcal Vaccine	212	86%	95%	93%
Smoking Cessation Advice	85	91%	98%	97%
Surgical Care Improvement Project				
Appropriate VTP Within 24 Hours	308	95%	95%	92%
Appropriate Hair Removal	910	100%	100%	99%
Appropriate Beta Blocker Usage	220	95%	94%	93%
Controlled Postoperative Blood Glucose	0	-	96%	93%
Prophylactic Antibiotic Timing	640	97%	97%	97%
Prophylactic Antibiotic Timing (Outpatient)	141	84%	92%	92%
Prophylactic Antibiotic Selection	644	95%	98%	97%
Prophylactic Antibiotic Select. (Outpatient)	128	88%	93%	94%
Prophylactic Antibiotic Stopped	620	95%	95%	94%
Recommended VTP Ordered	308	98%	97%	94%
Urinary Catheter Removal	109	96%	95%	90%
Children's Asthma Care				
Received Systemic Corticosteroids	-	-	-	100%
Received Home Management Plan	-	-	-	71%
Received Reliever Medication	-	-	-	100%
Use of Medical Imaging				
Combination Abdominal CT Scan	833	0.381	0.203	0.191
Combination Chest CT Scan	471	0.002	0.026	0.054
Follow-up Mammogram/Ultrasound	718	4.6%	8.2%	8.4%
MRI for Low Back Pain	99	34.3%	32.4%	32.7%
Survey of Patients' Hospital Experiences				
Area Around Room 'Always' Quiet at Night	300+	51%	-	58%
Doctors 'Always' Communicated Well	300+	82%	-	80%
Home Recovery Information Given	300+	88%	-	82%
Hospital Given 9 or 10 on 10 Point Scale	300+	63%	-	67%
Meds 'Always' Explained Before Given	300+	60%	-	60%
Nurses 'Always' Communicated Well	300+	76%	-	76%
Pain 'Always' Well Controlled	300+	70%	-	69%
Room and Bathroom 'Always' Clean	300+	71%	-	71%
Timely Help 'Always' Received	300+	63%	-	64%
Would Definitely Recommend Hospital	300+	63%	-	69%

Crozer Chester Medical Center

One Medical Center Boulevard
Upland, PA 19013
URL: www.crozer.org
Type: Acute Care Hospitals
Ownership: Voluntary Non-Profit - Other
Phone: 610-447-2000
Fax: 610-447-2234
Emergency Services: Yes
Beds: 422

Key Personnel:
CEO/President. . . . . Joan Richards
Chief of Medical Staff . . . . Paul Woolf, MD
Infection Control . . . . Sally Ryan, RN
Operating Room. . . . . Diane Wolk, RN
Pediatric Ambulatory Care . . . . . . Gerald Kolsky, MD
Pediatric In-Patient Care . . . . Gerald Kolsky, MD
Quality Assurance . . . . Linda Ramsey
Radiology. . . . . Joseph R Stock, MD

Measure	Cases	This Hosp.	State Avg.	U.S. Avg.
Heart Attack Care				
ACE Inhibitor or ARB for LVSD	65	98%	95%	96%
Aspirin at Arrival	275	99%	99%	99%
Aspirin at Discharge	354	99%	99%	98%
Beta Blocker at Discharge	351	99%	99%	98%
Fibrinolytic Medication Timing[1]	2	0%	40%	55%
PCI Within 90 Minutes of Arrival	31	94%	88%	90%
Smoking Cessation Advice	114	100%	100%	99%
Chest Pain/Possible Heart Attack Care				
Aspirin at Arrival[1,3]	5	80%	95%	95%
Median Time to ECG (minutes)[1,3]	6	16	8	8
Median Time to Transfer (minutes)[1,3]	1	300	68	61
Fibrinolytic Medication Timing[3]	0	-	48%	54%
Heart Failure Care				
ACE Inhibitor or ARB for LVSD	345	90%	95%	94%
Discharge Instructions	801	97%	90%	88%
Evaluation of LVS Function	927	98%	99%	98%
Smoking Cessation Advice	203	100%	98%	98%
Pneumonia Care				
Appropriate Initial Antibiotic	352	95%	93%	92%
Blood Culture Timing	466	98%	96%	96%
Influenza Vaccine	362	94%	92%	91%
Initial Antibiotic Timing	588	95%	96%	95%
Pneumococcal Vaccine	444	95%	95%	93%
Smoking Cessation Advice	254	100%	98%	97%
Surgical Care Improvement Project				
Appropriate VTP Within 24 Hours[2]	343	97%	95%	92%
Appropriate Hair Removal[2]	1,128	100%	100%	99%
Appropriate Beta Blocker Usage[2]	302	95%	94%	93%
Controlled Postoperative Blood Glucose[2]	130	96%	96%	93%
Prophylactic Antibiotic Timing[2]	845	98%	97%	97%
Prophylactic Antibiotic Timing (Outpatient)	177	98%	92%	92%
Prophylactic Antibiotic Selection[2]	850	96%	98%	97%
Prophylactic Antibiotic Select. (Outpatient)	174	97%	93%	94%
Prophylactic Antibiotic Stopped[2]	814	97%	95%	94%
Recommended VTP Ordered[2]	343	98%	97%	94%
Urinary Catheter Removal[2]	302	94%	95%	90%
Children's Asthma Care				
Received Systemic Corticosteroids	-	-	-	100%
Received Home Management Plan	-	-	-	71%
Received Reliever Medication	-	-	-	100%
Use of Medical Imaging				
Combination Abdominal CT Scan	1,278	0.196	0.203	0.191
Combination Chest CT Scan	1,085	0.008	0.026	0.054
Follow-up Mammogram/Ultrasound	1,887	8.6%	8.2%	8.4%
MRI for Low Back Pain	292	33.2%	32.4%	32.7%
Survey of Patients' Hospital Experiences				
Area Around Room 'Always' Quiet at Night	300+	49%	-	58%
Doctors 'Always' Communicated Well	300+	75%	-	80%
Home Recovery Information Given	300+	78%	-	82%
Hospital Given 9 or 10 on 10 Point Scale	300+	58%	-	67%
Meds 'Always' Explained Before Given	300+	59%	-	60%
Nurses 'Always' Communicated Well	300+	73%	-	76%
Pain 'Always' Well Controlled	300+	67%	-	69%
Room and Bathroom 'Always' Clean	300+	64%	-	71%
Timely Help 'Always' Received	300+	57%	-	64%
Would Definitely Recommend Hospital	300+	60%	-	69%

Warren General Hospital

Two Crescent Park West
Warren, PA 16365
Type: Acute Care Hospitals
Ownership: Voluntary Non-Profit - Private
Phone: 814-723-3300
Fax: 814-723-2248
Emergency Services: Yes
Beds: 89

Key Personnel:
CEO/President. . . . . John P Papalia
Pediatric Ambulatory Care . . . . . . David McConnell, Jr, MD
Pediatric In-Patient Care . . . . David McConnell, Jr, MD
Radiology. . . . . Julius Berta, MD
Anesthesiology. . . . . Niaz Ahmed, MD

Measure	Cases	This Hosp.	State Avg.	U.S. Avg.
Heart Attack Care				
ACE Inhibitor or ARB for LVSD	0	-	95%	96%
Aspirin at Arrival[1]	12	83%	99%	99%
Aspirin at Discharge[1]	7	86%	99%	98%
Beta Blocker at Discharge[1]	10	80%	99%	98%
Fibrinolytic Medication Timing	0	-	40%	55%
PCI Within 90 Minutes of Arrival	0	-	88%	90%
Smoking Cessation Advice	0	-	100%	99%
Chest Pain/Possible Heart Attack Care				
Aspirin at Arrival	167	98%	95%	95%
Median Time to ECG (minutes)	173	6	8	8
Median Time to Transfer (minutes)[1,3]	5	218	68	61
Fibrinolytic Medication Timing[1]	5	40%	48%	54%
Heart Failure Care				
ACE Inhibitor or ARB for LVSD	32	81%	95%	94%
Discharge Instructions	78	60%	90%	88%
Evaluation of LVS Function	111	93%	99%	98%
Smoking Cessation Advice[1]	8	88%	98%	98%
Pneumonia Care				
Appropriate Initial Antibiotic	67	87%	93%	92%
Blood Culture Timing	95	94%	96%	96%
Influenza Vaccine	47	85%	92%	91%
Initial Antibiotic Timing	95	97%	96%	95%
Pneumococcal Vaccine	79	89%	95%	93%
Smoking Cessation Advice	26	96%	98%	97%
Surgical Care Improvement Project				
Appropriate VTP Within 24 Hours	50	72%	95%	92%
Appropriate Hair Removal	231	100%	100%	99%
Appropriate Beta Blocker Usage	61	69%	94%	93%
Controlled Postoperative Blood Glucose	0	-	96%	93%
Prophylactic Antibiotic Timing	228	93%	97%	97%
Prophylactic Antibiotic Timing (Outpatient)	35	71%	92%	92%
Prophylactic Antibiotic Selection	229	94%	98%	97%
Prophylactic Antibiotic Select. (Outpatient)	27	63%	93%	94%
Prophylactic Antibiotic Stopped	221	90%	95%	94%
Recommended VTP Ordered	58	64%	97%	94%
Urinary Catheter Removal	55	78%	95%	90%
Children's Asthma Care				
Received Systemic Corticosteroids	-	-	-	100%
Received Home Management Plan	-	-	-	71%
Received Reliever Medication	-	-	-	100%
Use of Medical Imaging				
Combination Abdominal CT Scan	470	0.415	0.203	0.191
Combination Chest CT Scan	282	0.004	0.026	0.054
Follow-up Mammogram/Ultrasound	816	2.0%	8.2%	8.4%
MRI for Low Back Pain	164	32.9%	32.4%	32.7%
Survey of Patients' Hospital Experiences				
Area Around Room 'Always' Quiet at Night	300+	48%	-	58%
Doctors 'Always' Communicated Well	300+	77%	-	80%
Home Recovery Information Given	300+	75%	-	82%
Hospital Given 9 or 10 on 10 Point Scale	300+	63%	-	67%
Meds 'Always' Explained Before Given	300+	61%	-	60%
Nurses 'Always' Communicated Well	300+	78%	-	76%
Pain 'Always' Well Controlled	300+	71%	-	69%
Room and Bathroom 'Always' Clean	300+	72%	-	71%
Timely Help 'Always' Received	300+	67%	-	64%
Would Definitely Recommend Hospital	300+	62%	-	69%

NOTE: Hospital profiles are in alphabetical order by state, then city, then hospital within the city; Rankings exclude hospitals with less than 25 cases except for patient surveys which excludes hospitals with less than 100 cases; (a) 100–299 cases; (1) The number of cases is too small to be sure how well a hospital is performing; (2) The hospital indicated that the data submitted for this measure were based on a sample of cases; (3) Data was collected during a shorter time period (fewer quarters) than the maximum possible time for this measure; (4) Suppressed for one or more quarters by CMS; (5) No data is available from the hospital for this measure; (6) Fewer than 100 patients completed the HCAHPS survey. Use these rates with caution, as the number of surveys may be too low to reliably assess hospital performance; (7) Survey results are based on less than 12 months of data; (8) Survey results are not available for this reporting period; (9) No or very few patients were eligible for the HCAHPS survey. The scores shown, if any, reflect a very small number of surveys; (10) A state average was not calculated because too few hospitals in the state submitted data; (11) There were discrepancies in the data collection process; Please refer to the User's Guide for a full explanation of data.

Advanced Surgical Hospital

100 Trich Drive
Washington, PA 15301
Phone: 724-884-0710
Type: Acute Care Hospitals
Emergency Services: No
Ownership: Proprietary
Beds: 14

Key Personnel:
CEO . . . . Lloyd Scarrow

Measure	Cases	This Hosp.	State Avg.	U.S. Avg.
Heart Attack Care				
ACE Inhibitor or ARB for LVSD[5]	0	-	95%	96%
Aspirin at Arrival[5]	0	-	99%	99%
Aspirin at Discharge[5]	0	-	99%	98%
Beta Blocker at Discharge[5]	0	-	99%	98%
Fibrinolytic Medication Timing[5]	0	-	40%	55%
PCI Within 90 Minutes of Arrival[5]	0	-	88%	90%
Smoking Cessation Advice[5]	0	-	100%	99%
Chest Pain/Possible Heart Attack Care				
Aspirin at Arrival	-	-	95%	95%
Median Time to ECG (minutes)	-	-	8	8
Median Time to Transfer (minutes)	-	-	68	61
Fibrinolytic Medication Timing	-	-	48%	54%
Heart Failure Care				
ACE Inhibitor or ARB for LVSD[5]	0	-	95%	94%
Discharge Instructions[5]	0	-	90%	88%
Evaluation of LVS Function[5]	0	-	99%	98%
Smoking Cessation Advice[5]	0	-	98%	98%
Pneumonia Care				
Appropriate Initial Antibiotic[5]	0	-	93%	92%
Blood Culture Timing[5]	0	-	96%	96%
Influenza Vaccine[5]	0	-	92%	91%
Initial Antibiotic Timing[5]	0	-	96%	95%
Pneumococcal Vaccine[5]	0	-	95%	93%
Smoking Cessation Advice[5]	0	-	98%	97%
Surgical Care Improvement Project				
Appropriate VTP Within 24 Hours[5]	0	-	95%	92%
Appropriate Hair Removal[5]	0	-	100%	99%
Appropriate Beta Blocker Usage[5]	0	-	94%	93%
Controlled Postoperative Blood Glucose[5]	0	-	96%	93%
Prophylactic Antibiotic Timing[5]	0	-	97%	97%
Prophylactic Antibiotic Timing (Outpatient)	-	-	92%	92%
Prophylactic Antibiotic Selection[5]	0	-	98%	97%
Prophylactic Antibiotic Select. (Outpatient)	-	-	93%	94%
Prophylactic Antibiotic Stopped[5]	0	-	95%	94%
Recommended VTP Ordered[5]	0	-	97%	94%
Urinary Catheter Removal[5]	0	-	95%	90%
Children's Asthma Care				
Received Systemic Corticosteroids	-	-	-	100%
Received Home Management Plan	-	-	-	71%
Received Reliever Medication	-	-	-	100%
Use of Medical Imaging				
Combination Abdominal CT Scan	-	-	0.203	0.191
Combination Chest CT Scan	-	-	0.026	0.054
Follow-up Mammogram/Ultrasound	-	-	8.2%	8.4%
MRI for Low Back Pain	-	-	32.4%	32.7%
Survey of Patients' Hospital Experiences				
Area Around Room 'Always' Quiet at Night[8]	-	-	-	58%
Doctors 'Always' Communicated Well[8]	-	-	-	80%
Home Recovery Information Given[8]	-	-	-	82%
Hospital Given 9 or 10 on 10 Point Scale[8]	-	-	-	67%
Meds 'Always' Explained Before Given[8]	-	-	-	60%
Nurses 'Always' Communicated Well[8]	-	-	-	76%
Pain 'Always' Well Controlled[8]	-	-	-	69%
Room and Bathroom 'Always' Clean[8]	-	-	-	71%
Timely Help 'Always' Received[8]	-	-	-	64%
Would Definitely Recommend Hospital[8]	-	-	-	69%

The Washington Hospital

155 Wilson Avenue
Washington, PA 15301
Phone: 724-225-7000
Fax: 724-223-3784
E-mail: info@washingtonhospital.org
URL: www.washingtonhospital.org
Type: Acute Care Hospitals
Emergency Services: Yes
Ownership: Government - Local
Beds: 239

Key Personnel:
CEO/President. . . . . Telford W Thomas
Chief of Medical Staff . . . . Dennis P Brown, MD
Operating Room. . . . . Kathy Hearn
Pediatric Ambulatory Care . . . . . . Paul M Wodlinger, MD
Pediatric In-Patient Care . . . . Paul M Wodlinger, MD
Quality Assurance . . . . Colleen C Allison
Radiology. . . . . Giovanna M Aracri

Measure	Cases	This Hosp.	State Avg.	U.S. Avg.
Heart Attack Care				
ACE Inhibitor or ARB for LVSD	65	98%	95%	96%
Aspirin at Arrival	285	100%	99%	99%
Aspirin at Discharge	359	99%	99%	98%
Beta Blocker at Discharge	349	99%	99%	98%
Fibrinolytic Medication Timing	0	-	40%	55%
PCI Within 90 Minutes of Arrival	50	94%	88%	90%
Smoking Cessation Advice	117	100%	100%	99%
Chest Pain/Possible Heart Attack Care				
Aspirin at Arrival[1]	9	100%	95%	95%
Median Time to ECG (minutes)[1]	10	13	8	8
Median Time to Transfer (minutes)[5]	0	-	68	61
Fibrinolytic Medication Timing[5]	0	-	48%	54%
Heart Failure Care				
ACE Inhibitor or ARB for LVSD	190	99%	95%	94%
Discharge Instructions	528	93%	90%	88%
Evaluation of LVS Function	666	100%	99%	98%
Smoking Cessation Advice	105	100%	98%	98%
Pneumonia Care				
Appropriate Initial Antibiotic	244	94%	93%	92%
Blood Culture Timing	301	100%	96%	96%
Influenza Vaccine	274	98%	92%	91%
Initial Antibiotic Timing	360	96%	96%	95%
Pneumococcal Vaccine	364	97%	95%	93%
Smoking Cessation Advice	134	99%	98%	97%
Surgical Care Improvement Project				
Appropriate VTP Within 24 Hours[2]	218	95%	95%	92%
Appropriate Hair Removal[2]	835	100%	100%	99%
Appropriate Beta Blocker Usage[2]	258	94%	94%	93%
Controlled Postoperative Blood Glucose[2]	162	98%	96%	93%
Prophylactic Antibiotic Timing[2]	625	99%	97%	97%
Prophylactic Antibiotic Timing (Outpatient)	216	92%	92%	92%
Prophylactic Antibiotic Selection[2]	630	97%	98%	97%
Prophylactic Antibiotic Select. (Outpatient)	244	93%	93%	94%
Prophylactic Antibiotic Stopped[2]	604	96%	95%	94%
Recommended VTP Ordered[2]	218	97%	97%	94%
Urinary Catheter Removal[2]	121	96%	95%	90%
Children's Asthma Care				
Received Systemic Corticosteroids	-	-	-	100%
Received Home Management Plan	-	-	-	71%
Received Reliever Medication	-	-	-	100%
Use of Medical Imaging				
Combination Abdominal CT Scan	393	0.153	0.203	0.191
Combination Chest CT Scan	380	0.000	0.026	0.054
Follow-up Mammogram/Ultrasound	959	7.3%	8.2%	8.4%
MRI for Low Back Pain	116	43.1%	32.4%	32.7%
Survey of Patients' Hospital Experiences				
Area Around Room 'Always' Quiet at Night	300+	48%	-	58%
Doctors 'Always' Communicated Well	300+	82%	-	80%
Home Recovery Information Given	300+	83%	-	82%
Hospital Given 9 or 10 on 10 Point Scale	300+	64%	-	67%
Meds 'Always' Explained Before Given	300+	61%	-	60%
Nurses 'Always' Communicated Well	300+	79%	-	76%
Pain 'Always' Well Controlled	300+	70%	-	69%
Room and Bathroom 'Always' Clean	300+	78%	-	71%
Timely Help 'Always' Received	300+	65%	-	64%
Would Definitely Recommend Hospital	300+	66%	-	69%

Waynesboro Hospital

501 East Main St
Waynesboro, PA 17268
Phone: 717-765-4000
Fax: 717-765-3431
URL: www.summithealth.org
Type: Acute Care Hospitals
Emergency Services: Yes
Ownership: Voluntary Non-Profit - Other
Beds: 64

Key Personnel:
CEO/President. . . . . Norman B Epstein
Chief of Medical Staff . . . . Shannsul M Hag, MD
Infection Control. . . . . Mary McDonald, RN
Operating Room. . . . . Christopher S Andrews
Quality Assurance . . . . Debra Davis, RN
Radiology. . . . . Amir R Batouli
Emergency Room . . . . Thomas E Anderson, DO
Intensive Care Unit. . . . . Karen Clark

Measure	Cases	This Hosp.	State Avg.	U.S. Avg.
Heart Attack Care				
ACE Inhibitor or ARB for LVSD[1]	6	100%	95%	96%
Aspirin at Arrival	34	97%	99%	99%
Aspirin at Discharge[1]	17	100%	99%	98%
Beta Blocker at Discharge[1]	22	95%	99%	98%
Fibrinolytic Medication Timing	0	-	40%	55%
PCI Within 90 Minutes of Arrival	0	-	88%	90%
Smoking Cessation Advice[1]	2	100%	100%	99%
Chest Pain/Possible Heart Attack Care				
Aspirin at Arrival	47	96%	95%	95%
Median Time to ECG (minutes)	56	4	8	8
Median Time to Transfer (minutes)[1]	11	48	68	61
Fibrinolytic Medication Timing	0	-	48%	54%
Heart Failure Care				
ACE Inhibitor or ARB for LVSD	31	97%	95%	94%
Discharge Instructions	87	85%	90%	88%
Evaluation of LVS Function	106	99%	99%	98%
Smoking Cessation Advice[1]	7	100%	98%	98%
Pneumonia Care				
Appropriate Initial Antibiotic	71	99%	93%	92%
Blood Culture Timing	84	96%	96%	96%
Influenza Vaccine	52	98%	92%	91%
Initial Antibiotic Timing	108	96%	96%	95%
Pneumococcal Vaccine	107	99%	95%	93%
Smoking Cessation Advice	26	100%	98%	97%
Surgical Care Improvement Project				
Appropriate VTP Within 24 Hours	81	89%	95%	92%
Appropriate Hair Removal	192	100%	100%	99%
Appropriate Beta Blocker Usage	43	93%	94%	93%
Controlled Postoperative Blood Glucose	0	-	96%	93%
Prophylactic Antibiotic Timing	134	96%	97%	97%
Prophylactic Antibiotic Timing (Outpatient)	26	77%	92%	92%
Prophylactic Antibiotic Selection	132	99%	98%	97%
Prophylactic Antibiotic Select. (Outpatient)[1]	22	86%	93%	94%
Prophylactic Antibiotic Stopped	129	98%	95%	94%
Recommended VTP Ordered	81	89%	97%	94%
Urinary Catheter Removal[1]	14	93%	95%	90%
Children's Asthma Care				
Received Systemic Corticosteroids	-	-	-	100%
Received Home Management Plan	-	-	-	71%
Received Reliever Medication	-	-	-	100%
Use of Medical Imaging				
Combination Abdominal CT Scan	446	0.135	0.203	0.191
Combination Chest CT Scan	271	0.018	0.026	0.054
Follow-up Mammogram/Ultrasound	1,073	7.6%	8.2%	8.4%
MRI for Low Back Pain	81	39.5%	32.4%	32.7%
Survey of Patients' Hospital Experiences				
Area Around Room 'Always' Quiet at Night	300+	52%	-	58%
Doctors 'Always' Communicated Well	300+	79%	-	80%
Home Recovery Information Given	300+	85%	-	82%
Hospital Given 9 or 10 on 10 Point Scale	300+	73%	-	67%
Meds 'Always' Explained Before Given	300+	67%	-	60%
Nurses 'Always' Communicated Well	300+	82%	-	76%
Pain 'Always' Well Controlled	300+	74%	-	69%
Room and Bathroom 'Always' Clean	300+	73%	-	71%
Timely Help 'Always' Received	300+	78%	-	64%
Would Definitely Recommend Hospital	300+	76%	-	69%

NOTE: Hospital profiles are in alphabetical order by state, then city, then hospital within the city; Rankings exclude hospitals with less than 25 cases except for patient surveys which excludes hospitals with less than 100 cases; (a) 100–299 cases; (1) The number of cases is too small to be sure how well a hospital is performing; (2) The hospital indicated that the data submitted for this measure were based on a sample of cases; (3) Data was collected during a shorter time period (fewer quarters) than the maximum possible time for this measure; (4) Suppressed for one or more quarters by CMS; (5) No data is available from the hospital for this measure; (6) Fewer than 100 patients completed the HCAHPS survey. Use these rates with caution, as the number of surveys may be too low to reliably assess hospital performance; (7) Survey results are based on less than 12 months of data; (8) Survey results are not available for this reporting period; (9) No or very few patients were eligible for the HCAHPS survey. The scores shown, if any, reflect a very small number of surveys; (10) A state average was not calculated because too few hospitals in the state submitted data; (11) There were discrepancies in the data collection process; Please refer to the User's Guide for a full explanation of data.

Southwest Regional Medical Center

350 Bonar Avenue Phone: 724-627-2602
Waynesburg, PA 15370 Fax: 724-627-7639
E-mail: jeggleston@gcmhcare.com
URL: www.gcmhcare.com
Type: Acute Care Hospitals Emergency Services: Yes
Ownership: Proprietary Beds: 54

Key Personnel:
CEO/President. . . . . Raoul M Walsh
Chief of Medical Staff. . . . . Bernard Imrich, MD
Coronary Care . . . . Barbara Walters
Infection Control. . . . . Mary Lee Headlee, RN
Operating Room. . . . . Billy Wood, RN
Pediatric Ambulatory Care . . . . . . Satish Kumar, MD
Pediatric In-Patient Care . . . . . . Daniel Church, MD
Quality Assurance . . . . Carroll Phillips, RN

Measure	Cases	This Hosp.	State Avg.	U.S. Avg.
Heart Attack Care				
ACE Inhibitor or ARB for LVSD	0	-	95%	96%
Aspirin at Arrival[1]	13	92%	99%	99%
Aspirin at Discharge[1]	11	73%	99%	98%
Beta Blocker at Discharge[1]	9	89%	99%	98%
Fibrinolytic Medication Timing	0	-	40%	55%
PCI Within 90 Minutes of Arrival	0	-	88%	90%
Smoking Cessation Advice	0	-	100%	99%
Chest Pain/Possible Heart Attack Care				
Aspirin at Arrival	107	94%	95%	95%
Median Time to ECG (minutes)	110	10	8	8
Median Time to Transfer (minutes)[1,3]	11	67	68	61
Fibrinolytic Medication Timing	0	-	48%	54%
Heart Failure Care				
ACE Inhibitor or ARB for LVSD	40	90%	95%	94%
Discharge Instructions	156	83%	90%	88%
Evaluation of LVS Function	198	96%	99%	98%
Smoking Cessation Advice	37	92%	98%	98%
Pneumonia Care				
Appropriate Initial Antibiotic	111	98%	93%	92%
Blood Culture Timing	120	100%	96%	96%
Influenza Vaccine	116	73%	92%	91%
Initial Antibiotic Timing	154	99%	96%	95%
Pneumococcal Vaccine	131	79%	95%	93%
Smoking Cessation Advice	59	93%	98%	97%
Surgical Care Improvement Project				
Appropriate VTP Within 24 Hours	47	89%	95%	92%
Appropriate Hair Removal	114	100%	100%	99%
Appropriate Beta Blocker Usage	34	82%	94%	93%
Controlled Postoperative Blood Glucose	0	-	96%	93%
Prophylactic Antibiotic Timing	64	88%	97%	97%
Prophylactic Antibiotic Timing (Outpatient)	33	88%	92%	92%
Prophylactic Antibiotic Selection	64	95%	98%	97%
Prophylactic Antibiotic Select. (Outpatient)	33	91%	93%	94%
Prophylactic Antibiotic Stopped	61	92%	95%	94%
Recommended VTP Ordered	48	92%	97%	94%
Urinary Catheter Removal[1]	16	94%	95%	90%
Children's Asthma Care				
Received Systemic Corticosteroids	-	-	-	100%
Received Home Management Plan	-	-	-	71%
Received Reliever Medication	-	-	-	100%
Use of Medical Imaging				
Combination Abdominal CT Scan	158	0.576	0.203	0.191
Combination Chest CT Scan	115	0.157	0.026	0.054
Follow-up Mammogram/Ultrasound	203	11.8%	8.2%	8.4%
MRI for Low Back Pain[1]	34	38.2%	32.4%	32.7%
Survey of Patients' Hospital Experiences				
Area Around Room 'Always' Quiet at Night	300+	52%	-	58%
Doctors 'Always' Communicated Well	300+	84%	-	80%
Home Recovery Information Given	300+	84%	-	82%
Hospital Given 9 or 10 on 10 Point Scale	300+	61%	-	67%
Meds 'Always' Explained Before Given	300+	57%	-	60%
Nurses 'Always' Communicated Well	300+	77%	-	76%
Pain 'Always' Well Controlled	300+	70%	-	69%
Room and Bathroom 'Always' Clean	300+	64%	-	71%
Timely Help 'Always' Received	300+	64%	-	64%
Would Definitely Recommend Hospital	300+	60%	-	69%

Soldiers and Sailors Memorial Hospital

32-36 Central Avenue Phone: 570-724-1631
Wellsboro, PA 16901 Fax: 570-724-7235
URL: www.laurelhs.org
Type: Acute Care Hospitals Emergency Services: Yes
Ownership: Voluntary Non-Profit - Other Beds: 103

Key Personnel:
CEO/President. . . . . Ronald Butler
Chief of Medical Staff . . . . Anthony Nespola, MD
Quality Assurance . . . . Judy Feil
Radiology. . . . . Enrico J Doganiero
Emergency Room . . . . Susan Held, Dir

Measure	Cases	This Hosp.	State Avg.	U.S. Avg.
Heart Attack Care				
ACE Inhibitor or ARB for LVSD[1]	2	100%	95%	96%
Aspirin at Arrival[1]	6	83%	99%	99%
Aspirin at Discharge[1]	4	100%	99%	98%
Beta Blocker at Discharge[1]	5	100%	99%	98%
Fibrinolytic Medication Timing	0	-	40%	55%
PCI Within 90 Minutes of Arrival	0	-	88%	90%
Smoking Cessation Advice[1]	2	100%	100%	99%
Chest Pain/Possible Heart Attack Care				
Aspirin at Arrival	84	99%	95%	95%
Median Time to ECG (minutes)	85	6	8	8
Median Time to Transfer (minutes)[1]	12	86	68	61
Fibrinolytic Medication Timing[1]	5	40%	48%	54%
Heart Failure Care				
ACE Inhibitor or ARB for LVSD	28	100%	95%	94%
Discharge Instructions	77	97%	90%	88%
Evaluation of LVS Function	94	98%	99%	98%
Smoking Cessation Advice[1]	11	100%	98%	98%
Pneumonia Care				
Appropriate Initial Antibiotic	72	96%	93%	92%
Blood Culture Timing	98	93%	96%	96%
Influenza Vaccine	55	98%	92%	91%
Initial Antibiotic Timing	103	97%	96%	95%
Pneumococcal Vaccine	91	98%	95%	93%
Smoking Cessation Advice	26	88%	98%	97%
Surgical Care Improvement Project				
Appropriate VTP Within 24 Hours	77	90%	95%	92%
Appropriate Hair Removal	195	99%	100%	99%
Appropriate Beta Blocker Usage	51	98%	94%	93%
Controlled Postoperative Blood Glucose	0	-	96%	93%
Prophylactic Antibiotic Timing	127	95%	97%	97%
Prophylactic Antibiotic Timing (Outpatient)	48	83%	92%	92%
Prophylactic Antibiotic Selection	127	94%	98%	97%
Prophylactic Antibiotic Select. (Outpatient)	109	99%	93%	94%
Prophylactic Antibiotic Stopped	126	99%	95%	94%
Recommended VTP Ordered	77	90%	97%	94%
Urinary Catheter Removal	36	89%	95%	90%
Children's Asthma Care				
Received Systemic Corticosteroids	-	-	-	100%
Received Home Management Plan	-	-	-	71%
Received Reliever Medication	-	-	-	100%
Use of Medical Imaging				
Combination Abdominal CT Scan	464	0.571	0.203	0.191
Combination Chest CT Scan	242	0.008	0.026	0.054
Follow-up Mammogram/Ultrasound	978	6.9%	8.2%	8.4%
MRI for Low Back Pain	122	32.8%	32.4%	32.7%
Survey of Patients' Hospital Experiences				
Area Around Room 'Always' Quiet at Night	300+	52%	-	58%
Doctors 'Always' Communicated Well	300+	85%	-	80%
Home Recovery Information Given	300+	85%	-	82%
Hospital Given 9 or 10 on 10 Point Scale	300+	73%	-	67%
Meds 'Always' Explained Before Given	300+	67%	-	60%
Nurses 'Always' Communicated Well	300+	83%	-	76%
Pain 'Always' Well Controlled	300+	75%	-	69%
Room and Bathroom 'Always' Clean	300+	86%	-	71%
Timely Help 'Always' Received	300+	79%	-	64%
Would Definitely Recommend Hospital	300+	70%	-	69%

Chester County Hospital

701 East Marshall St Phone: 610-431-5000
West Chester, PA 19380 Fax: 610-430-2956
URL: www.cchosp.com
Type: Acute Care Hospitals Emergency Services: Yes
Ownership: Voluntary Non-Profit - Private Beds: 261

Key Personnel:
CEO/President. . . . . HL Perry Pepper
Chief of Medical Staff . . . . Azam Husain, MD
Operating Room. . . . . Shirl Portwood
Pediatric Ambulatory Care . . . . . . Neil Pennington, MD
Pediatric In-Patient Care . . . . . . Neil Pennington, MD
Quality Assurance . . . . Virginia Handler
Radiology. . . . . William J Barry
Emergency Room . . . . Donna Froio

Measure	Cases	This Hosp.	State Avg.	U.S. Avg.
Heart Attack Care				
ACE Inhibitor or ARB for LVSD	34	100%	95%	96%
Aspirin at Arrival	189	100%	99%	99%
Aspirin at Discharge	181	99%	99%	98%
Beta Blocker at Discharge	181	99%	99%	98%
Fibrinolytic Medication Timing	0	-	40%	55%
PCI Within 90 Minutes of Arrival	34	91%	88%	90%
Smoking Cessation Advice	46	98%	100%	99%
Chest Pain/Possible Heart Attack Care				
Aspirin at Arrival[1,3]	7	100%	95%	95%
Median Time to ECG (minutes)[1,3]	7	10	8	8
Median Time to Transfer (minutes)[1,3]	1	44	68	61
Fibrinolytic Medication Timing[3]	0	-	48%	54%
Heart Failure Care				
ACE Inhibitor or ARB for LVSD	98	98%	95%	94%
Discharge Instructions	265	88%	90%	88%
Evaluation of LVS Function	351	100%	99%	98%
Smoking Cessation Advice	55	100%	98%	98%
Pneumonia Care				
Appropriate Initial Antibiotic	156	90%	93%	92%
Blood Culture Timing	251	96%	96%	96%
Influenza Vaccine	167	90%	92%	91%
Initial Antibiotic Timing	256	92%	96%	95%
Pneumococcal Vaccine	245	95%	95%	93%
Smoking Cessation Advice	76	100%	98%	97%
Surgical Care Improvement Project				
Appropriate VTP Within 24 Hours	371	96%	95%	92%
Appropriate Hair Removal	1,081	100%	100%	99%
Appropriate Beta Blocker Usage	328	94%	94%	93%
Controlled Postoperative Blood Glucose	90	99%	96%	93%
Prophylactic Antibiotic Timing	730	99%	97%	97%
Prophylactic Antibiotic Timing (Outpatient)	248	93%	92%	92%
Prophylactic Antibiotic Selection	734	99%	98%	97%
Prophylactic Antibiotic Select. (Outpatient)	237	94%	93%	94%
Prophylactic Antibiotic Stopped	680	96%	95%	94%
Recommended VTP Ordered	371	97%	97%	94%
Urinary Catheter Removal	220	91%	95%	90%
Children's Asthma Care				
Received Systemic Corticosteroids	-	-	-	100%
Received Home Management Plan	-	-	-	71%
Received Reliever Medication	-	-	-	100%
Use of Medical Imaging				
Combination Abdominal CT Scan	981	0.094	0.203	0.191
Combination Chest CT Scan	864	0.012	0.026	0.054
Follow-up Mammogram/Ultrasound	1,780	10.6%	8.2%	8.4%
MRI for Low Back Pain	126	30.2%	32.4%	32.7%
Survey of Patients' Hospital Experiences				
Area Around Room 'Always' Quiet at Night	300+	47%	-	58%
Doctors 'Always' Communicated Well	300+	80%	-	80%
Home Recovery Information Given	300+	78%	-	82%
Hospital Given 9 or 10 on 10 Point Scale	300+	71%	-	67%
Meds 'Always' Explained Before Given	300+	62%	-	60%
Nurses 'Always' Communicated Well	300+	78%	-	76%
Pain 'Always' Well Controlled	300+	71%	-	69%
Room and Bathroom 'Always' Clean	300+	67%	-	71%
Timely Help 'Always' Received	300+	67%	-	64%
Would Definitely Recommend Hospital	300+	77%	-	69%

NOTE: Hospital profiles are in alphabetical order by state, then city, then hospital within the city; Rankings exclude hospitals with less than 25 cases except for patient surveys which excludes hospitals with less than 100 cases; (a) 100–299 cases; (1) The number of cases is too small to be sure how well a hospital is performing; (2) The hospital indicated that the data submitted for this measure were based on a sample of cases; (3) Data was collected during a shorter time period (fewer quarters) than the maximum possible time for this measure; (4) Suppressed for one or more quarters by CMS; (5) No data is available from the hospital for this measure; (6) Fewer than 100 patients completed the HCAHPS survey. Use these rates with caution, as the number of surveys may be too low to reliably assess hospital performance; (7) Survey results are based on less than 12 months of data; (8) Survey results are not available for this reporting period; (9) No or very few patients were eligible for the HCAHPS survey. The scores shown, if any, reflect a very small number of surveys; (10) A state average was not calculated because too few hospitals in the state submitted data; (11) There were discrepancies in the data collection process; Please refer to the User's Guide for a full explanation of data.

Jennersville Regional Hospital

1015 West Baltimore Pike Phone: 610-869-1000
West Grove, PA 19390 Fax: 610-869-1362
URL: www.jennersville.com
Type: Acute Care Hospitals Emergency Services: Yes
Ownership: Proprietary Beds: 64
Key Personnel:
CEO/President. . . . . Scott Phillips
Operating Room. . . . . Elaine Cook

Measure	Cases	This Hosp.	State Avg.	U.S. Avg.
Heart Attack Care				
ACE Inhibitor or ARB for LVSD[1]	5	100%	95%	96%
Aspirin at Arrival	26	100%	99%	99%
Aspirin at Discharge[1]	14	100%	99%	98%
Beta Blocker at Discharge[1]	14	100%	99%	98%
Fibrinolytic Medication Timing	0	-	40%	55%
PCI Within 90 Minutes of Arrival	0	-	88%	90%
Smoking Cessation Advice[1]	3	100%	100%	99%
Chest Pain/Possible Heart Attack Care				
Aspirin at Arrival	29	100%	95%	95%
Median Time to ECG (minutes)	31	7	8	8
Median Time to Transfer (minutes)[1]	12	132	68	61
Fibrinolytic Medication Timing[1]	2	0%	48%	54%
Heart Failure Care				
ACE Inhibitor or ARB for LVSD[1]	11	100%	95%	94%
Discharge Instructions	53	100%	90%	88%
Evaluation of LVS Function	95	100%	99%	98%
Smoking Cessation Advice[1]	9	100%	98%	98%
Pneumonia Care				
Appropriate Initial Antibiotic	151	94%	93%	92%
Blood Culture Timing	233	97%	96%	96%
Influenza Vaccine	130	100%	92%	91%
Initial Antibiotic Timing	222	97%	96%	95%
Pneumococcal Vaccine	194	100%	95%	93%
Smoking Cessation Advice	72	100%	98%	97%
Surgical Care Improvement Project				
Appropriate VTP Within 24 Hours[2]	64	100%	95%	92%
Appropriate Hair Removal[2]	144	100%	100%	99%
Appropriate Beta Blocker Usage[2]	33	94%	94%	93%
Controlled Postoperative Blood Glucose[2]	0	-	96%	93%
Prophylactic Antibiotic Timing[2]	91	100%	97%	97%
Prophylactic Antibiotic Timing (Outpatient)	47	98%	92%	92%
Prophylactic Antibiotic Selection[2]	90	99%	98%	97%
Prophylactic Antibiotic Select. (Outpatient)	98	98%	93%	94%
Prophylactic Antibiotic Stopped[2]	90	100%	95%	94%
Recommended VTP Ordered[2]	64	100%	97%	94%
Urinary Catheter Removal[1]	18	100%	95%	90%
Children's Asthma Care				
Received Systemic Corticosteroids	-	-	-	100%
Received Home Management Plan	-	-	-	71%
Received Reliever Medication	-	-	-	100%
Use of Medical Imaging				
Combination Abdominal CT Scan	261	0.157	0.203	0.191
Combination Chest CT Scan	223	0.000	0.026	0.054
Follow-up Mammogram/Ultrasound	377	14.1%	8.2%	8.4%
MRI for Low Back Pain	78	29.5%	32.4%	32.7%
Survey of Patients' Hospital Experiences				
Area Around Room 'Always' Quiet at Night	300+	53%	-	58%
Doctors 'Always' Communicated Well	300+	72%	-	80%
Home Recovery Information Given	300+	82%	-	82%
Hospital Given 9 or 10 on 10 Point Scale	300+	57%	-	67%
Meds 'Always' Explained Before Given	300+	59%	-	60%
Nurses 'Always' Communicated Well	300+	74%	-	76%
Pain 'Always' Well Controlled	300+	67%	-	69%
Room and Bathroom 'Always' Clean	300+	66%	-	71%
Timely Help 'Always' Received	300+	58%	-	64%
Would Definitely Recommend Hospital	300+	55%	-	69%

Geisinger Wyoming Valley Medical Center

100o East Mountain Boulevard Phone: 570-826-7300
Wilkes-Barre, PA 18711 Fax: 570-819-5545
URL: www.geisinger.org
Type: Acute Care Hospitals Emergency Services: No
Ownership: Voluntary Non-Profit - Private Beds: 177
Key Personnel:
CEO/President. . . . . Glenn Steele Jr, MD
Chief of Medical Staff . . . . Howard R Grant
Operating Room. . . . . Rosalie King, RN
Pediatric In-Patient Care . . . . Janis Maksimak, MD
Quality Assurance . . . . Pat McCulloch, RN
Radiology. . . . . John Arthur Baxter, MD

Measure	Cases	This Hosp.	State Avg.	U.S. Avg.
Heart Attack Care				
ACE Inhibitor or ARB for LVSD	40	95%	95%	96%
Aspirin at Arrival	182	99%	99%	99%
Aspirin at Discharge	189	99%	99%	98%
Beta Blocker at Discharge	186	100%	99%	98%
Fibrinolytic Medication Timing	0	-	40%	55%
PCI Within 90 Minutes of Arrival	42	76%	88%	90%
Smoking Cessation Advice	61	100%	100%	99%
Chest Pain/Possible Heart Attack Care				
Aspirin at Arrival[1,3]	3	67%	95%	95%
Median Time to ECG (minutes)[1,3]	4	1	8	8
Median Time to Transfer (minutes)[5]	0	-	68	61
Fibrinolytic Medication Timing[3]	0	-	48%	54%
Heart Failure Care				
ACE Inhibitor or ARB for LVSD	94	83%	95%	94%
Discharge Instructions	193	83%	90%	88%
Evaluation of LVS Function	255	100%	99%	98%
Smoking Cessation Advice	34	100%	98%	98%
Pneumonia Care				
Appropriate Initial Antibiotic	129	96%	93%	92%
Blood Culture Timing	194	90%	96%	96%
Influenza Vaccine	174	87%	92%	91%
Initial Antibiotic Timing	193	93%	96%	95%
Pneumococcal Vaccine	272	94%	95%	93%
Smoking Cessation Advice	99	100%	98%	97%
Surgical Care Improvement Project				
Appropriate VTP Within 24 Hours[2]	167	92%	95%	92%
Appropriate Hair Removal[2]	713	100%	100%	99%
Appropriate Beta Blocker Usage[2]	314	83%	94%	93%
Controlled Postoperative Blood Glucose[2]	123	98%	96%	93%
Prophylactic Antibiotic Timing[2]	454	96%	97%	97%
Prophylactic Antibiotic Timing (Outpatient)	531	92%	92%	92%
Prophylactic Antibiotic Selection[2]	465	97%	98%	97%
Prophylactic Antibiotic Select. (Outpatient)	596	97%	93%	94%
Prophylactic Antibiotic Stopped[2]	438	96%	95%	94%
Recommended VTP Ordered[2]	167	94%	97%	94%
Urinary Catheter Removal[2]	188	96%	95%	90%
Children's Asthma Care				
Received Systemic Corticosteroids	-	-	-	100%
Received Home Management Plan	-	-	-	71%
Received Reliever Medication	-	-	-	100%
Use of Medical Imaging				
Combination Abdominal CT Scan	901	0.624	0.203	0.191
Combination Chest CT Scan	846	0.020	0.026	0.054
Follow-up Mammogram/Ultrasound	735	12.9%	8.2%	8.4%
MRI for Low Back Pain	150	29.3%	32.4%	32.7%
Survey of Patients' Hospital Experiences				
Area Around Room 'Always' Quiet at Night	300+	49%	-	58%
Doctors 'Always' Communicated Well	300+	81%	-	80%
Home Recovery Information Given	300+	83%	-	82%
Hospital Given 9 or 10 on 10 Point Scale	300+	64%	-	67%
Meds 'Always' Explained Before Given	300+	56%	-	60%
Nurses 'Always' Communicated Well	300+	74%	-	76%
Pain 'Always' Well Controlled	300+	65%	-	69%
Room and Bathroom 'Always' Clean	300+	67%	-	71%
Timely Help 'Always' Received	300+	61%	-	64%
Would Definitely Recommend Hospital	300+	70%	-	69%

Wilkes-Barre General Hospital

575 North River Street Phone: 570-829-8111
Wilkes-Barre, PA 18764 Fax: 570-552-7410
URL: www.wvhcs.org
Type: Acute Care Hospitals Emergency Services: Yes
Ownership: Voluntary Non-Profit - Private Beds: 519
Key Personnel:
CEO/President. . . . . Ron Stern
Chief of Medical Staff . . . . Robert Brown
Infection Control. . . . . Nancy Alonzo
Pediatric Ambulatory Care . . . . . . Michael Imbrogno, MD
Pediatric In-Patient Care . . . . Michael Imbrogno, MD
Quality Assurance . . . . Gwen Michaels
Radiology. . . . . N Shah, MD
Emergency Room . . . . Cynthia Liskof, MD

Measure	Cases	This Hosp.	State Avg.	U.S. Avg.
Heart Attack Care				
ACE Inhibitor or ARB for LVSD	70	89%	95%	96%
Aspirin at Arrival	341	97%	99%	99%
Aspirin at Discharge	329	97%	99%	98%
Beta Blocker at Discharge	337	96%	99%	98%
Fibrinolytic Medication Timing	0	-	40%	55%
PCI Within 90 Minutes of Arrival	41	73%	88%	90%
Smoking Cessation Advice	104	100%	100%	99%
Chest Pain/Possible Heart Attack Care				
Aspirin at Arrival[1]	7	100%	95%	95%
Median Time to ECG (minutes)[1]	8	8	8	8
Median Time to Transfer (minutes)[1,3]	1	18	68	61
Fibrinolytic Medication Timing[3]	0	-	48%	54%
Heart Failure Care				
ACE Inhibitor or ARB for LVSD	135	80%	95%	94%
Discharge Instructions	395	88%	90%	88%
Evaluation of LVS Function	579	94%	99%	98%
Smoking Cessation Advice	55	98%	98%	98%
Pneumonia Care				
Appropriate Initial Antibiotic	260	91%	93%	92%
Blood Culture Timing	394	96%	96%	96%
Influenza Vaccine	290	88%	92%	91%
Initial Antibiotic Timing	432	94%	96%	95%
Pneumococcal Vaccine	406	88%	95%	93%
Smoking Cessation Advice	146	99%	98%	97%
Surgical Care Improvement Project				
Appropriate VTP Within 24 Hours[2]	616	90%	95%	92%
Appropriate Hair Removal[2]	1,668	100%	100%	99%
Appropriate Beta Blocker Usage[2]	600	90%	94%	93%
Controlled Postoperative Blood Glucose[2]	264	100%	96%	93%
Prophylactic Antibiotic Timing[2]	1,114	98%	97%	97%
Prophylactic Antibiotic Timing (Outpatient)	423	91%	92%	92%
Prophylactic Antibiotic Selection[2]	1,127	97%	98%	97%
Prophylactic Antibiotic Select. (Outpatient)	402	91%	93%	94%
Prophylactic Antibiotic Stopped[2]	1,079	95%	95%	94%
Recommended VTP Ordered[2]	617	91%	97%	94%
Urinary Catheter Removal	404	100%	95%	90%
Children's Asthma Care				
Received Systemic Corticosteroids	-	-	-	100%
Received Home Management Plan	-	-	-	71%
Received Reliever Medication	-	-	-	100%
Use of Medical Imaging				
Combination Abdominal CT Scan	1,842	0.311	0.203	0.191
Combination Chest CT Scan	1,323	0.008	0.026	0.054
Follow-up Mammogram/Ultrasound	2,678	7.2%	8.2%	8.4%
MRI for Low Back Pain	139	36.7%	32.4%	32.7%
Survey of Patients' Hospital Experiences				
Area Around Room 'Always' Quiet at Night	300+	45%	-	58%
Doctors 'Always' Communicated Well	300+	80%	-	80%
Home Recovery Information Given	300+	80%	-	82%
Hospital Given 9 or 10 on 10 Point Scale	300+	59%	-	67%
Meds 'Always' Explained Before Given	300+	56%	-	60%
Nurses 'Always' Communicated Well	300+	76%	-	76%
Pain 'Always' Well Controlled	300+	68%	-	69%
Room and Bathroom 'Always' Clean	300+	64%	-	71%
Timely Help 'Always' Received	300+	59%	-	64%
Would Definitely Recommend Hospital	300+	60%	-	69%

NOTE: Hospital profiles are in alphabetical order by state, then city, then hospital within the city; Rankings exclude hospitals with less than 25 cases except for patient surveys which excludes hospitals with less than 100 cases; (a) 100–299 cases; (1) The number of cases is too small to be sure how well a hospital is performing; (2) The hospital indicated that the data submitted for this measure were based on a sample of cases; (3) Data was collected during a shorter time period (fewer quarters) than the maximum possible time for this measure; (4) Suppressed for one or more quarters by CMS; (5) No data is available from the hospital for this measure; (6) Fewer than 100 patients completed the HCAHPS survey. Use these rates with caution, as the number of surveys may be too low to reliably assess hospital performance; (7) Survey results are based on less than 12 months of data; (8) Survey results are not available for this reporting period; (9) No or very few patients were eligible for the HCAHPS survey. The scores shown, if any, reflect a very small number of surveys; (10) A state average was not calculated because too few hospitals in the state submitted data; (11) There were discrepancies in the data collection process; Please refer to the User's Guide for a full explanation of data.

Wilkes-Barre VA Medical Center

1111 East End Boulevard
Wilkes-Barre, PA 18711
Phone: 570-824-3521
Fax: 570-821-7264
URL: www.va.gov
Type: Acute Care-Veterans Administration
Emergency Services: No
Ownership: Government - Federal
Beds: 111

Key Personnel:
CEO/President. . . . . Roland E Moore
Chief of Medical Staff . . . . William K Grossman, MD
Infection Control. . . . . Patricia Baldwin, RN
Quality Assurance . . . . Yvonne Bohlander, RN
Anesthesiology. . . . . Mufti Basta, MD

Measure	Cases	This Hosp.	State Avg.	U.S. Avg.
Heart Attack Care				
ACE Inhibitor or ARB for LVSD[5]	0	-	95%	96%
Aspirin at Arrival[5]	0	-	99%	99%
Aspirin at Discharge[5]	0	-	99%	98%
Beta Blocker at Discharge[5]	0	-	99%	98%
Fibrinolytic Medication Timing[5]	0	-	40%	55%
PCI Within 90 Minutes of Arrival[5]	0	-	88%	90%
Smoking Cessation Advice[5]	0	-	100%	99%
Chest Pain/Possible Heart Attack Care				
Aspirin at Arrival	-	-	95%	95%
Median Time to ECG (minutes)	-	-	8	8
Median Time to Transfer (minutes)	-	-	68	61
Fibrinolytic Medication Timing	-	-	48%	54%
Heart Failure Care				
ACE Inhibitor or ARB for LVSD	39	100%	95%	94%
Discharge Instructions	109	99%	90%	88%
Evaluation of LVS Function	129	100%	99%	98%
Smoking Cessation Advice[1]	22	100%	98%	98%
Pneumonia Care				
Appropriate Initial Antibiotic	42	100%	93%	92%
Blood Culture Timing	77	99%	96%	96%
Influenza Vaccine	41	98%	92%	91%
Initial Antibiotic Timing	70	96%	96%	95%
Pneumococcal Vaccine	63	100%	95%	93%
Smoking Cessation Advice[1]	24	96%	98%	97%
Surgical Care Improvement Project				
Appropriate VTP Within 24 Hours[2]	34	94%	95%	92%
Appropriate Hair Removal[2]	48	100%	100%	99%
Appropriate Beta Blocker Usage[1,2]	18	83%	94%	93%
Controlled Postoperative Blood Glucose[2,5]	0	-	96%	93%
Prophylactic Antibiotic Timing	32	97%	97%	97%
Prophylactic Antibiotic Timing (Outpatient)	-	-	92%	92%
Prophylactic Antibiotic Selection	32	97%	98%	97%
Prophylactic Antibiotic Select. (Outpatient)	-	-	93%	94%
Prophylactic Antibiotic Stopped	28	82%	95%	94%
Recommended VTP Ordered[2]	34	94%	97%	94%
Urinary Catheter Removal[1,2]	22	86%	95%	90%
Children's Asthma Care				
Received Systemic Corticosteroids	-	-	-	100%
Received Home Management Plan	-	-	-	71%
Received Reliever Medication	-	-	-	100%
Use of Medical Imaging				
Combination Abdominal CT Scan	-	-	0.203	0.191
Combination Chest CT Scan	-	-	0.026	0.054
Follow-up Mammogram/Ultrasound	-	-	8.2%	8.4%
MRI for Low Back Pain	-	-	32.4%	32.7%
Survey of Patients' Hospital Experiences				
Area Around Room 'Always' Quiet at Night	-	-	-	58%
Doctors 'Always' Communicated Well	-	-	-	80%
Home Recovery Information Given	-	-	-	82%
Hospital Given 9 or 10 on 10 Point Scale	-	-	-	67%
Meds 'Always' Explained Before Given	-	-	-	60%
Nurses 'Always' Communicated Well	-	-	-	76%
Pain 'Always' Well Controlled	-	-	-	69%
Room and Bathroom 'Always' Clean	-	-	-	71%
Timely Help 'Always' Received	-	-	-	64%
Would Definitely Recommend Hospital	-	-	-	69%

Williamsport Hospital & Medical Center

777 Rural Ave
Williamsport, PA 17701
Phone: 570-321-1000
URL: www.susquehannahealth.org
Type: Acute Care Hospitals
Emergency Services: Yes
Ownership: Voluntary Non-Profit - Other

Key Personnel:
CEO/President. . . . . Steven P. Johnson

Measure	Cases	This Hosp.	State Avg.	U.S. Avg.
Heart Attack Care				
ACE Inhibitor or ARB for LVSD	43	91%	95%	96%
Aspirin at Arrival	185	99%	99%	99%
Aspirin at Discharge	265	100%	99%	98%
Beta Blocker at Discharge	260	98%	99%	98%
Fibrinolytic Medication Timing	0	-	40%	55%
PCI Within 90 Minutes of Arrival	42	83%	88%	90%
Smoking Cessation Advice	91	100%	100%	99%
Chest Pain/Possible Heart Attack Care				
Aspirin at Arrival[1]	8	88%	95%	95%
Median Time to ECG (minutes)[1]	8	7	8	8
Median Time to Transfer (minutes)[5]	0	-	68	61
Fibrinolytic Medication Timing[5]	0	-	48%	54%
Heart Failure Care				
ACE Inhibitor or ARB for LVSD	89	97%	95%	94%
Discharge Instructions	198	90%	90%	88%
Evaluation of LVS Function	253	99%	99%	98%
Smoking Cessation Advice	35	94%	98%	98%
Pneumonia Care				
Appropriate Initial Antibiotic	149	94%	93%	92%
Blood Culture Timing	152	98%	96%	96%
Influenza Vaccine	156	90%	92%	91%
Initial Antibiotic Timing	193	97%	96%	95%
Pneumococcal Vaccine	220	97%	95%	93%
Smoking Cessation Advice	89	98%	98%	97%
Surgical Care Improvement Project				
Appropriate VTP Within 24 Hours[2]	536	97%	95%	92%
Appropriate Hair Removal[2]	1,184	99%	100%	99%
Appropriate Beta Blocker Usage[2]	425	97%	94%	93%
Controlled Postoperative Blood Glucose[2]	119	100%	96%	93%
Prophylactic Antibiotic Timing[2]	917	96%	97%	97%
Prophylactic Antibiotic Timing (Outpatient)	396	93%	92%	92%
Prophylactic Antibiotic Selection[2]	926	98%	98%	97%
Prophylactic Antibiotic Select. (Outpatient)	386	99%	93%	94%
Prophylactic Antibiotic Stopped[2]	902	96%	95%	94%
Recommended VTP Ordered[2]	537	98%	97%	94%
Urinary Catheter Removal[2]	311	97%	95%	90%
Children's Asthma Care				
Received Systemic Corticosteroids	-	-	-	100%
Received Home Management Plan	-	-	-	71%
Received Reliever Medication	-	-	-	100%
Use of Medical Imaging				
Combination Abdominal CT Scan	1,095	0.083	0.203	0.191
Combination Chest CT Scan	535	0.017	0.026	0.054
Follow-up Mammogram/Ultrasound[5]	0	-	8.2%	8.4%
MRI for Low Back Pain[5]	0	-	32.4%	32.7%
Survey of Patients' Hospital Experiences				
Area Around Room 'Always' Quiet at Night	300+	48%	-	58%
Doctors 'Always' Communicated Well	300+	83%	-	80%
Home Recovery Information Given	300+	85%	-	82%
Hospital Given 9 or 10 on 10 Point Scale	300+	71%	-	67%
Meds 'Always' Explained Before Given	300+	63%	-	60%
Nurses 'Always' Communicated Well	300+	80%	-	76%
Pain 'Always' Well Controlled	300+	71%	-	69%
Room and Bathroom 'Always' Clean	300+	71%	-	71%
Timely Help 'Always' Received	300+	67%	-	64%
Would Definitely Recommend Hospital	300+	69%	-	69%

Windber Hospital

600 Somerset Avenue
Windber, PA 15963
Phone: 814-467-3000
Fax: 814-467-3451
E-mail: info@windbercare.com
URL: www.windbercare.com
Type: Acute Care Hospitals
Emergency Services: Yes
Ownership: Voluntary Non-Profit - Private
Beds: 82

Key Personnel:
Chief of Medical Staff . . . . Jerry L Gray, MD
Infection Control. . . . . Lynn Berger, RN
Operating Room. . . . . Darlene Falvo, RN
Pediatric In-Patient Care . . . . Masood Boroumand, MD
Quality Assurance . . . . Diane Pringle, RN
Radiology. . . . . Jonathan Abraha, MD
Emergency Room . . . . James Eckenrod, MD
Intensive Care Unit. . . . . Chris Spinos, RN

Measure	Cases	This Hosp.	State Avg.	U.S. Avg.
Heart Attack Care				
ACE Inhibitor or ARB for LVSD[1]	1	100%	95%	96%
Aspirin at Arrival	33	91%	99%	99%
Aspirin at Discharge[1]	18	94%	99%	98%
Beta Blocker at Discharge[1]	16	94%	99%	98%
Fibrinolytic Medication Timing	0	-	40%	55%
PCI Within 90 Minutes of Arrival	0	-	88%	90%
Smoking Cessation Advice	0	-	100%	99%
Chest Pain/Possible Heart Attack Care				
Aspirin at Arrival	62	98%	95%	95%
Median Time to ECG (minutes)	66	12	8	8
Median Time to Transfer (minutes)[1]	9	71	68	61
Fibrinolytic Medication Timing	0	-	48%	54%
Heart Failure Care				
ACE Inhibitor or ARB for LVSD	29	93%	95%	94%
Discharge Instructions	92	88%	90%	88%
Evaluation of LVS Function	118	98%	99%	98%
Smoking Cessation Advice[1]	9	89%	98%	98%
Pneumonia Care				
Appropriate Initial Antibiotic	59	93%	93%	92%
Blood Culture Timing	72	100%	96%	96%
Influenza Vaccine	50	88%	92%	91%
Initial Antibiotic Timing	87	99%	96%	95%
Pneumococcal Vaccine	72	99%	95%	93%
Smoking Cessation Advice[1]	12	75%	98%	97%
Surgical Care Improvement Project				
Appropriate VTP Within 24 Hours	38	95%	95%	92%
Appropriate Hair Removal	138	99%	100%	99%
Appropriate Beta Blocker Usage	34	94%	94%	93%
Controlled Postoperative Blood Glucose	0	-	96%	93%
Prophylactic Antibiotic Timing	94	96%	97%	97%
Prophylactic Antibiotic Timing (Outpatient)	44	91%	92%	92%
Prophylactic Antibiotic Selection	94	96%	98%	97%
Prophylactic Antibiotic Select. (Outpatient)	41	100%	93%	94%
Prophylactic Antibiotic Stopped	92	92%	95%	94%
Recommended VTP Ordered	38	97%	97%	94%
Urinary Catheter Removal[1]	23	91%	95%	90%
Children's Asthma Care				
Received Systemic Corticosteroids	-	-	-	100%
Received Home Management Plan	-	-	-	71%
Received Reliever Medication	-	-	-	100%
Use of Medical Imaging				
Combination Abdominal CT Scan	278	0.014	0.203	0.191
Combination Chest CT Scan	231	0.000	0.026	0.054
Follow-up Mammogram/Ultrasound	461	5.9%	8.2%	8.4%
MRI for Low Back Pain	53	41.5%	32.4%	32.7%
Survey of Patients' Hospital Experiences				
Area Around Room 'Always' Quiet at Night	300+	56%	-	58%
Doctors 'Always' Communicated Well	300+	87%	-	80%
Home Recovery Information Given	300+	87%	-	82%
Hospital Given 9 or 10 on 10 Point Scale	300+	76%	-	67%
Meds 'Always' Explained Before Given	300+	65%	-	60%
Nurses 'Always' Communicated Well	300+	81%	-	76%
Pain 'Always' Well Controlled	300+	71%	-	69%
Room and Bathroom 'Always' Clean	300+	82%	-	71%
Timely Help 'Always' Received	300+	72%	-	64%
Would Definitely Recommend Hospital	300+	79%	-	69%

NOTE: Hospital profiles are in alphabetical order by state, then city, then hospital within the city; Rankings exclude hospitals with less than 25 cases except for patient surveys which excludes hospitals with less than 100 cases; (a) 100–299 cases; (1) The number of cases is too small to be sure how well a hospital is performing; (2) The hospital indicated that the data submitted for this measure were based on a sample of cases; (3) Data was collected during a shorter time period (fewer quarters) than the maximum possible time for this measure; (4) Suppressed for one or more quarters by CMS; (5) No data is available from the hospital for this measure; (6) Fewer than 100 patients completed the HCAHPS survey. Use these rates with caution, as the number of surveys may be too low to reliably assess hospital performance; (7) Survey results are based on less than 12 months of data; (8) Survey results are not available for this reporting period; (9) No or very few patients were eligible for the HCAHPS survey. The scores shown, if any, reflect a very small number of surveys; (10) A state average was not calculated because too few hospitals in the state submitted data; (11) There were discrepancies in the data collection process; Please refer to the User's Guide for a full explanation of data.

Main Line Hospital Lankenau

100 Lancaster Ave   Phone: 610-645-2000
Wynnewood, PA 19096   Fax: 610-645-8007
URL: www.mainlinehealth.org/lh
Type: Acute Care Hospitals   Emergency Services: Yes
Ownership: Voluntary Non-Profit - Private   Beds: 341
Key Personnel:
CEO/President . . . . John Lynch
Quality Assurance . . . . Joan Anders

Measure	Cases	This Hosp.	State Avg.	U.S. Avg.
Heart Attack Care				
ACE Inhibitor or ARB for LVSD	52	100%	95%	96%
Aspirin at Arrival	216	100%	99%	99%
Aspirin at Discharge	298	100%	99%	98%
Beta Blocker at Discharge	293	100%	99%	98%
Fibrinolytic Medication Timing[1]	1	100%	40%	55%
PCI Within 90 Minutes of Arrival	42	98%	88%	90%
Smoking Cessation Advice	58	100%	100%	99%
Chest Pain/Possible Heart Attack Care				
Aspirin at Arrival[1,3]	3	67%	95%	95%
Median Time to ECG (minutes)[1,3]	3	20	8	8
Median Time to Transfer (minutes)[5]	0	-	68	61
Fibrinolytic Medication Timing[5]	0	-	48%	54%
Heart Failure Care				
ACE Inhibitor or ARB for LVSD	331	99%	95%	94%
Discharge Instructions	666	94%	90%	88%
Evaluation of LVS Function	857	100%	99%	98%
Smoking Cessation Advice	139	100%	98%	98%
Pneumonia Care				
Appropriate Initial Antibiotic	124	97%	93%	92%
Blood Culture Timing	278	99%	96%	96%
Influenza Vaccine	134	91%	92%	91%
Initial Antibiotic Timing	240	98%	96%	95%
Pneumococcal Vaccine	209	97%	95%	93%
Smoking Cessation Advice	75	100%	98%	97%
Surgical Care Improvement Project				
Appropriate VTP Within 24 Hours[2]	300	97%	95%	92%
Appropriate Hair Removal[2]	1,423	100%	100%	99%
Appropriate Beta Blocker Usage[2]	505	97%	94%	93%
Controlled Postoperative Blood Glucose[2]	456	99%	96%	93%
Prophylactic Antibiotic Timing[2]	1,161	99%	97%	97%
Prophylactic Antibiotic Timing (Outpatient)	348	93%	92%	92%
Prophylactic Antibiotic Selection[2]	1,183	98%	98%	97%
Prophylactic Antibiotic Select. (Outpatient)	341	97%	93%	94%
Prophylactic Antibiotic Stopped[2]	1,116	99%	95%	94%
Recommended VTP Ordered[2]	300	99%	97%	94%
Urinary Catheter Removal[2]	343	99%	95%	90%
Children's Asthma Care				
Received Systemic Corticosteroids	-	-	-	100%
Received Home Management Plan	-	-	-	71%
Received Reliever Medication	-	-	-	100%
Use of Medical Imaging				
Combination Abdominal CT Scan	1,174	0.142	0.203	0.191
Combination Chest CT Scan	1,079	0.019	0.026	0.054
Follow-up Mammogram/Ultrasound	2,031	8.2%	8.2%	8.4%
MRI for Low Back Pain	190	28.9%	32.4%	32.7%
Survey of Patients' Hospital Experiences				
Area Around Room 'Always' Quiet at Night	300+	48%	-	58%
Doctors 'Always' Communicated Well	300+	80%	-	80%
Home Recovery Information Given	300+	79%	-	82%
Hospital Given 9 or 10 on 10 Point Scale	300+	75%	-	67%
Meds 'Always' Explained Before Given	300+	60%	-	60%
Nurses 'Always' Communicated Well	300+	77%	-	76%
Pain 'Always' Well Controlled	300+	70%	-	69%
Room and Bathroom 'Always' Clean	300+	65%	-	71%
Timely Help 'Always' Received	300+	57%	-	64%
Would Definitely Recommend Hospital	300+	80%	-	69%

Surgical Institute of Reading

2752 Century Boulevard   Phone: 717-999-9999
Wyomissing, PA 19610
URL: www.sireading.com
Type: Acute Care Hospitals   Emergency Services: No
Ownership: Proprietary
Key Personnel:
Administrator . . . . Deborah Beissel

Measure	Cases	This Hosp.	State Avg.	U.S. Avg.
Heart Attack Care				
ACE Inhibitor or ARB for LVSD[5]	0	-	95%	96%
Aspirin at Arrival[5]	0	-	99%	99%
Aspirin at Discharge[5]	0	-	99%	98%
Beta Blocker at Discharge[5]	0	-	99%	98%
Fibrinolytic Medication Timing[5]	0	-	40%	55%
PCI Within 90 Minutes of Arrival[5]	0	-	88%	90%
Smoking Cessation Advice[5]	0	-	100%	99%
Chest Pain/Possible Heart Attack Care				
Aspirin at Arrival[5]	0	-	95%	95%
Median Time to ECG (minutes)[5]	0	-	8	8
Median Time to Transfer (minutes)[5]	0	-	68	61
Fibrinolytic Medication Timing[5]	0	-	48%	54%
Heart Failure Care				
ACE Inhibitor or ARB for LVSD[5]	0	-	95%	94%
Discharge Instructions[5]	0	-	90%	88%
Evaluation of LVS Function[5]	0	-	99%	98%
Smoking Cessation Advice[5]	0	-	98%	98%
Pneumonia Care				
Appropriate Initial Antibiotic[5]	0	-	93%	92%
Blood Culture Timing[5]	0	-	96%	96%
Influenza Vaccine[5]	0	-	92%	91%
Initial Antibiotic Timing[5]	0	-	96%	95%
Pneumococcal Vaccine[5]	0	-	95%	93%
Smoking Cessation Advice[5]	0	-	98%	97%
Surgical Care Improvement Project				
Appropriate VTP Within 24 Hours	49	84%	95%	92%
Appropriate Hair Removal	418	99%	100%	99%
Appropriate Beta Blocker Usage	112	88%	94%	93%
Controlled Postoperative Blood Glucose	0	-	96%	93%
Prophylactic Antibiotic Timing	395	94%	97%	97%
Prophylactic Antibiotic Timing (Outpatient)	204	98%	92%	92%
Prophylactic Antibiotic Selection	395	96%	98%	97%
Prophylactic Antibiotic Select. (Outpatient)	202	95%	93%	94%
Prophylactic Antibiotic Stopped	393	100%	95%	94%
Recommended VTP Ordered	49	84%	97%	94%
Urinary Catheter Removal	189	99%	95%	90%
Children's Asthma Care				
Received Systemic Corticosteroids	-	-	-	100%
Received Home Management Plan	-	-	-	71%
Received Reliever Medication	-	-	-	100%
Use of Medical Imaging				
Combination Abdominal CT Scan[1]	10	0.100	0.203	0.191
Combination Chest CT Scan[1]	12	0.000	0.026	0.054
Follow-up Mammogram/Ultrasound[5]	0	-	8.2%	8.4%
MRI for Low Back Pain[5]	0	-	32.4%	32.7%
Survey of Patients' Hospital Experiences				
Area Around Room 'Always' Quiet at Night	300+	74%	-	58%
Doctors 'Always' Communicated Well	300+	94%	-	80%
Home Recovery Information Given	300+	94%	-	82%
Hospital Given 9 or 10 on 10 Point Scale	300+	93%	-	67%
Meds 'Always' Explained Before Given	300+	74%	-	60%
Nurses 'Always' Communicated Well	300+	88%	-	76%
Pain 'Always' Well Controlled	300+	80%	-	69%
Room and Bathroom 'Always' Clean	300+	85%	-	71%
Timely Help 'Always' Received	300+	84%	-	64%
Would Definitely Recommend Hospital	300+	94%	-	69%

Memorial Hospital York

325 South Belmont Street   Phone: 717-843-8623
York, PA 17403   Fax: 717-849-5329
URL: www.mhyork.org
Type: Acute Care Hospitals   Emergency Services: Yes
Ownership: Voluntary Non-Profit - Private   Beds: 100
Key Personnel:
CEO/President . . . . Sally J Dixon
Cardiac Laboratory . . . . Jeanne Long
Chief of Medical Staff . . . . Hugh E Palmer, DO
Infection Control . . . . Carol Harvey, RN
Operating Room . . . . Sandy Kimbrell, RN
Pediatric Ambulatory Care . . . . . Philip Eppley, DO
Pediatric In-Patient Care . . . . . . Philip Eppley, DO
Quality Assurance . . . . Susan Nelson

Measure	Cases	This Hosp.	State Avg.	U.S. Avg.
Heart Attack Care				
ACE Inhibitor or ARB for LVSD[1]	6	100%	95%	96%
Aspirin at Arrival	62	98%	99%	99%
Aspirin at Discharge	38	100%	99%	98%
Beta Blocker at Discharge	34	97%	99%	98%
Fibrinolytic Medication Timing	0	-	40%	55%
PCI Within 90 Minutes of Arrival[1]	4	75%	88%	90%
Smoking Cessation Advice[1]	10	90%	100%	99%
Chest Pain/Possible Heart Attack Care				
Aspirin at Arrival	50	100%	95%	95%
Median Time to ECG (minutes)	51	7	8	8
Median Time to Transfer (minutes)[1]	18	81	68	61
Fibrinolytic Medication Timing	0	-	48%	54%
Heart Failure Care				
ACE Inhibitor or ARB for LVSD	37	89%	95%	94%
Discharge Instructions	114	96%	90%	88%
Evaluation of LVS Function	144	99%	99%	98%
Smoking Cessation Advice[1]	17	100%	98%	98%
Pneumonia Care				
Appropriate Initial Antibiotic	127	94%	93%	92%
Blood Culture Timing	197	97%	96%	96%
Influenza Vaccine	99	87%	92%	91%
Initial Antibiotic Timing	177	94%	96%	95%
Pneumococcal Vaccine	138	91%	95%	93%
Smoking Cessation Advice	47	100%	98%	97%
Surgical Care Improvement Project				
Appropriate VTP Within 24 Hours	133	91%	95%	92%
Appropriate Hair Removal	554	100%	100%	99%
Appropriate Beta Blocker Usage	111	98%	94%	93%
Controlled Postoperative Blood Glucose	0	-	96%	93%
Prophylactic Antibiotic Timing	447	96%	97%	97%
Prophylactic Antibiotic Timing (Outpatient)	96	94%	92%	92%
Prophylactic Antibiotic Selection	447	97%	98%	97%
Prophylactic Antibiotic Select. (Outpatient)	94	81%	93%	94%
Prophylactic Antibiotic Stopped	438	92%	95%	94%
Recommended VTP Ordered	133	92%	97%	94%
Urinary Catheter Removal	39	100%	95%	90%
Children's Asthma Care				
Received Systemic Corticosteroids	-	-	-	100%
Received Home Management Plan	-	-	-	71%
Received Reliever Medication	-	-	-	100%
Use of Medical Imaging				
Combination Abdominal CT Scan[1]	2	0.500	0.203	0.191
Combination Chest CT Scan[1]	2	0.000	0.026	0.054
Follow-up Mammogram/Ultrasound	795	10.6%	8.2%	8.4%
MRI for Low Back Pain	82	28.0%	32.4%	32.7%
Survey of Patients' Hospital Experiences				
Area Around Room 'Always' Quiet at Night	300+	42%	-	58%
Doctors 'Always' Communicated Well	300+	71%	-	80%
Home Recovery Information Given	300+	80%	-	82%
Hospital Given 9 or 10 on 10 Point Scale	300+	64%	-	67%
Meds 'Always' Explained Before Given	300+	56%	-	60%
Nurses 'Always' Communicated Well	300+	70%	-	76%
Pain 'Always' Well Controlled	300+	63%	-	69%
Room and Bathroom 'Always' Clean	300+	68%	-	71%
Timely Help 'Always' Received	300+	54%	-	64%
Would Definitely Recommend Hospital	300+	71%	-	69%

NOTE: Hospital profiles are in alphabetical order by state, then city, then hospital within the city; Rankings exclude hospitals with less than 25 cases except for patient surveys which excludes hospitals with less than 100 cases; (a) 100–299 cases; (1) The number of cases is too small to be sure how well a hospital is performing; (2) The hospital indicated that the data submitted for this measure were based on a sample of cases; (3) Data was collected during a shorter time period (fewer quarters) than the maximum possible time for this measure; (4) Suppressed for one or more quarters by CMS; (5) No data is available from the hospital for this measure; (6) Fewer than 100 patients completed the HCAHPS survey. Use these rates with caution, as the number of surveys may be too low to reliably assess hospital performance; (7) Survey results are based on less than 12 months of data; (8) Survey results are not available for this reporting period; (9) No or very few patients were eligible for the HCAHPS survey. The scores shown, if any, reflect a very small number of surveys; (10) A state average was not calculated because too few hospitals in the state submitted data; (11) There were discrepancies in the data collection process; Please refer to the User's Guide for a full explanation of data.

York Hospital
1001 South George Street
York, PA 17403
URL: www.wellspan.org
Type: Acute Care Hospitals
Ownership: Voluntary Non-Profit - Private

Phone: 717-851-2345
Fax: 717-851-3100

Emergency Services: Yes
Beds: 466

Key Personnel:
CEO/President . . . . Bruce M Bartels
Chief of Medical Staff . . . . John H McConville, MD
Infection Control . . . . John H McConville, MD
Operating Room . . . . Dawn E Noll, RN
Pediatric In-Patient Care . . . . David Turkewitz, MD

Measure	Cases	This Hosp.	State Avg.	U.S. Avg.
Heart Attack Care				
ACE Inhibitor or ARB for LVSD	125	95%	95%	96%
Aspirin at Arrival	437	98%	99%	99%
Aspirin at Discharge	531	99%	99%	98%
Beta Blocker at Discharge	538	99%	99%	98%
Fibrinolytic Medication Timing	0	-	40%	55%
PCI Within 90 Minutes of Arrival	102	90%	88%	90%
Smoking Cessation Advice	200	100%	100%	99%
Chest Pain/Possible Heart Attack Care				
Aspirin at Arrival[5]	0	-	95%	95%
Median Time to ECG (minutes)[5]	0	-	8	8
Median Time to Transfer (minutes)[5]	0	-	68	61
Fibrinolytic Medication Timing[5]	0	-	48%	54%
Heart Failure Care				
ACE Inhibitor or ARB for LVSD	203	93%	95%	94%
Discharge Instructions	617	82%	90%	88%
Evaluation of LVS Function	756	99%	99%	98%
Smoking Cessation Advice	126	97%	98%	98%
Pneumonia Care				
Appropriate Initial Antibiotic	223	100%	93%	92%
Blood Culture Timing	608	84%	96%	96%
Influenza Vaccine	245	97%	92%	91%
Initial Antibiotic Timing	559	92%	96%	95%
Pneumococcal Vaccine	463	96%	95%	93%
Smoking Cessation Advice	162	100%	98%	97%
Surgical Care Improvement Project				
Appropriate VTP Within 24 Hours[2]	611	93%	95%	92%
Appropriate Hair Removal[2]	2,258	100%	100%	99%
Appropriate Beta Blocker Usage[2]	775	92%	94%	93%
Controlled Postoperative Blood Glucose[2]	366	90%	96%	93%
Prophylactic Antibiotic Timing[2]	1,723	96%	97%	97%
Prophylactic Antibiotic Timing (Outpatient)	832	96%	92%	92%
Prophylactic Antibiotic Selection[2]	1,760	96%	98%	97%
Prophylactic Antibiotic Select. (Outpatient)	831	96%	93%	94%
Prophylactic Antibiotic Stopped[2]	1,668	95%	95%	94%
Recommended VTP Ordered[2]	617	96%	97%	94%
Urinary Catheter Removal[2]	424	92%	95%	90%
Children's Asthma Care				
Received Systemic Corticosteroids	-	-	-	100%
Received Home Management Plan	-	-	-	71%
Received Reliever Medication	-	-	-	100%
Use of Medical Imaging				
Combination Abdominal CT Scan	2,450	0.118	0.203	0.191
Combination Chest CT Scan	2,749	0.006	0.026	0.054
Follow-up Mammogram/Ultrasound	5,709	9.5%	8.2%	8.4%
MRI for Low Back Pain	207	34.3%	32.4%	32.7%
Survey of Patients' Hospital Experiences				
Area Around Room 'Always' Quiet at Night	300+	44%	-	58%
Doctors 'Always' Communicated Well	300+	76%	-	80%
Home Recovery Information Given	300+	84%	-	82%
Hospital Given 9 or 10 on 10 Point Scale	300+	67%	-	67%
Meds 'Always' Explained Before Given	300+	59%	-	60%
Nurses 'Always' Communicated Well	300+	76%	-	76%
Pain 'Always' Well Controlled	300+	68%	-	69%
Room and Bathroom 'Always' Clean	300+	56%	-	71%
Timely Help 'Always' Received	300+	67%	-	64%
Would Definitely Recommend Hospital	300+	71%	-	69%

NOTE: Hospital profiles are in alphabetical order by state, then city, then hospital within the city; Rankings exclude hospitals with less than 25 cases except for patient surveys which excludes hospitals with less than 100 cases; (a) 100–299 cases; (1) The number of cases is too small to be sure how well a hospital is performing; (2) The hospital indicated that the data submitted for this measure were based on a sample of cases; (3) Data was collected during a shorter time period (fewer quarters) than the maximum possible time for this measure; (4) Suppressed for one or more quarters by CMS; (5) No data is available from the hospital for this measure; (6) Fewer than 100 patients completed the HCAHPS survey. Use these rates with caution, as the number of surveys may be too low to reliably assess hospital performance; (7) Survey results are based on less than 12 months of data; (8) Survey results are not available for this reporting period; (9) No or very few patients were eligible for the HCAHPS survey. The scores shown, if any, reflect a very small number of surveys; (10) A state average was not calculated because too few hospitals in the state submitted data; (11) There were discrepancies in the data collection process; Please refer to the User's Guide for a full explanation of data.

Heart Attack Care

1. ACE Inhibitor or ARB for LVSD

Hospital Name	City	Rate	Cases
Rhode Island Hospital	Providence	99%	83
Miriam Hospital	Providence	98%	115

2. Aspirin at Arrival

Hospital Name	City	Rate	Cases
Rhode Island Hospital	Providence	100%	407
South County Hospital	Wakefield	100%	29
Landmark Medical Center	Woonsocket	99%	143
Miriam Hospital	Providence	99%	344
Roger Williams Medical Center	Providence	98%	66
Kent County Memorial Hospital	Warwick	97%	184
St Joseph Health Services of RI	N Providence	97%	60
Memorial Hospital of Rhode Island	Pawtucket	96%	51

3. Aspirin at Discharge

Hospital Name	City	Rate	Cases
Memorial Hospital of Rhode Island	Pawtucket	100%	25
Miriam Hospital	Providence	100%	629
Rhode Island Hospital	Providence	100%	643
Kent County Memorial Hospital	Warwick	98%	123
Landmark Medical Center	Woonsocket	98%	111
St Joseph Health Services of RI	N Providence	97%	37
Roger Williams Medical Center	Providence	92%	50

4. Beta Blocker at Discharge

Hospital Name	City	Rate	Cases
Memorial Hospital of Rhode Island	Pawtucket	100%	25
Rhode Island Hospital	Providence	100%	616
Roger Williams Medical Center	Providence	100%	50
Kent County Memorial Hospital	Warwick	99%	122
Miriam Hospital	Providence	99%	610
St Joseph Health Services of RI	N Providence	98%	41
Landmark Medical Center	Woonsocket	97%	112

6. PCI Within 90 Minutes of Arrival

Hospital Name	City	Rate	Cases
Rhode Island Hospital	Providence	94%	80
Miriam Hospital	Providence	85%	66

7. Smoking Cessation Advice

Hospital Name	City	Rate	Cases
Miriam Hospital	Providence	100%	187
Rhode Island Hospital	Providence	100%	212
Landmark Medical Center	Woonsocket	97%	31

Chest Pain/Possible Heart Attack Care

8. Aspirin at Arrival

Hospital Name	City	Rate	Cases
Westerly Hospital	Westerly	98%	51
Landmark Medical Center	Woonsocket	97%	30
Memorial Hospital of Rhode Island	Pawtucket	97%	39
Newport Hospital	Newport	97%	78
St Joseph Health Services of RI	N Providence	97%	32
Kent County Memorial Hospital	Warwick	95%	104
South County Hospital	Wakefield	94%	35
Women and Infants Hospital of Rhode Island	Providence	65%	43

9. Median Time to ECG (minutes)

Hospital Name	City	Min.	Cases
St Joseph Health Services of RI	N Providence	0	32
Landmark Medical Center	Woonsocket	4	31
Kent County Memorial Hospital	Warwick	5	109
Newport Hospital	Newport	8	76
South County Hospital	Wakefield	10	35
Westerly Hospital	Westerly	10	51
Women and Infants Hospital of Rhode Island	Providence	14	38
Memorial Hospital of Rhode Island	Pawtucket	18	39

10. Median Time to Transfer (minutes)

Hospital Name	City	Min.	Cases
Kent County Memorial Hospital	Warwick	57	43

Heart Failure Care

12. ACE Inhibitor or ARB for LVSD

Hospital Name	City	Rate	Cases
South County Hospital	Wakefield	100%	31
Landmark Medical Center	Woonsocket	99%	79
Providence VA Medical Center	Providence	96%	57
Miriam Hospital[2]	Providence	95%	165
Kent County Memorial Hospital	Warwick	94%	98
Newport Hospital	Newport	94%	51
Rhode Island Hospital[2]	Providence	94%	130
St Joseph Health Services of RI	N Providence	93%	44
Westerly Hospital	Westerly	92%	51
Memorial Hospital of Rhode Island	Pawtucket	85%	62
Roger Williams Medical Center	Providence	85%	34

13. Discharge Instructions

Hospital Name	City	Rate	Cases
Newport Hospital	Newport	97%	119
South County Hospital	Wakefield	97%	88
Memorial Hospital of Rhode Island	Pawtucket	93%	175
Landmark Medical Center	Woonsocket	92%	206
Providence VA Medical Center	Providence	92%	131
Miriam Hospital[2]	Providence	91%	421
Rhode Island Hospital[2]	Providence	87%	267
Kent County Memorial Hospital	Warwick	78%	348
St Joseph Health Services of RI	N Providence	72%	155
Westerly Hospital	Westerly	72%	122
Roger Williams Medical Center	Providence	67%	109

14. Evaluation of LVS Function

Hospital Name	City	Rate	Cases
South County Hospital	Wakefield	100%	111
Kent County Memorial Hospital	Warwick	99%	529
Landmark Medical Center	Woonsocket	99%	319
Miriam Hospital[2]	Providence	99%	541
Newport Hospital	Newport	99%	162
Providence VA Medical Center	Providence	99%	169
Rhode Island Hospital[2]	Providence	99%	346
Memorial Hospital of Rhode Island	Pawtucket	98%	242
St Joseph Health Services of RI	N Providence	97%	261
Roger Williams Medical Center	Providence	96%	162
Westerly Hospital	Westerly	96%	180

15. Smoking Cessation Advice

Hospital Name	City	Rate	Cases
Landmark Medical Center	Woonsocket	100%	50
Memorial Hospital of Rhode Island	Pawtucket	100%	37
Miriam Hospital[2]	Providence	100%	67
Rhode Island Hospital[2]	Providence	100%	54
Westerly Hospital	Westerly	96%	25
Kent County Memorial Hospital	Warwick	91%	67
Providence VA Medical Center	Providence	85%	27

Pneumonia Care

16. Appropriate Initial Antibiotic

Hospital Name	City	Rate	Cases
Newport Hospital[2]	Newport	97%	118
Rhode Island Hospital[2]	Providence	97%	59
Landmark Medical Center	Woonsocket	96%	116
Miriam Hospital[2]	Providence	96%	98
St Joseph Health Services of RI	N Providence	95%	108
Memorial Hospital of Rhode Island	Pawtucket	92%	92
Providence VA Medical Center	Providence	92%	25
South County Hospital	Wakefield	92%	99
Roger Williams Medical Center[2]	Providence	88%	78
Westerly Hospital	Westerly	88%	99
Kent County Memorial Hospital[2]	Warwick	86%	158

17. Blood Culture Timing

Hospital Name	City	Rate	Cases
Landmark Medical Center	Woonsocket	98%	168
Miriam Hospital[2]	Providence	98%	167
Newport Hospital[2]	Newport	98%	193
South County Hospital	Wakefield	98%	156
Westerly Hospital	Westerly	98%	91
Providence VA Medical Center	Providence	97%	73
Rhode Island Hospital[2]	Providence	97%	129
Memorial Hospital of Rhode Island	Pawtucket	96%	105
St Joseph Health Services of RI	N Providence	94%	195
Roger Williams Medical Center[2]	Providence	92%	109
Kent County Memorial Hospital[2]	Warwick	89%	273

18. Influenza Vaccine

Hospital Name	City	Rate	Cases
South County Hospital	Wakefield	100%	104
Miriam Hospital[2]	Providence	96%	105
Newport Hospital[2]	Newport	96%	85
Memorial Hospital of Rhode Island	Pawtucket	94%	100
Providence VA Medical Center	Providence	93%	40
Landmark Medical Center	Woonsocket	92%	133
Rhode Island Hospital[2]	Providence	82%	78
Westerly Hospital	Westerly	79%	77
St Joseph Health Services of RI	N Providence	75%	99
Roger Williams Medical Center	Providence	74%	69
Kent County Memorial Hospital[2]	Warwick	67%	150

19. Initial Antibiotic Timing

Hospital Name	City	Rate	Cases
Landmark Medical Center	Woonsocket	98%	199
St Joseph Health Services of RI	N Providence	98%	153
Miriam Hospital[2]	Providence	97%	176
Newport Hospital[2]	Newport	97%	185
South County Hospital	Wakefield	96%	156
Providence VA Medical Center	Providence	95%	76
Westerly Hospital	Westerly	95%	151
Kent County Memorial Hospital[2]	Warwick	94%	236
Rhode Island Hospital[2]	Providence	94%	138
Roger Williams Medical Center[2]	Providence	92%	146
Memorial Hospital of Rhode Island	Pawtucket	91%	172

20. Pneumococcal Vaccine

Hospital Name	City	Rate	Cases
Providence VA Medical Center	Providence	99%	74
South County Hospital	Wakefield	99%	148
Newport Hospital[2]	Newport	96%	148
Miriam Hospital[2]	Providence	91%	162
Memorial Hospital of Rhode Island	Pawtucket	88%	160
Landmark Medical Center	Woonsocket	87%	172
Kent County Memorial Hospital[2]	Warwick	85%	243
Rhode Island Hospital[2]	Providence	85%	115
St Joseph Health Services of RI	N Providence	85%	183
Roger Williams Medical Center[2]	Providence	72%	125
Westerly Hospital	Westerly	69%	139

21. Smoking Cessation Advice

Hospital Name	City	Rate	Cases
Miriam Hospital[2]	Providence	100%	46
Newport Hospital[2]	Newport	100%	33
Rhode Island Hospital[2]	Providence	100%	52
Roger Williams Medical Center[2]	Providence	100%	33
Memorial Hospital of Rhode Island	Pawtucket	99%	72
Landmark Medical Center	Woonsocket	97%	66
South County Hospital	Wakefield	97%	33
St Joseph Health Services of RI	N Providence	96%	49
Westerly Hospital	Westerly	96%	27
Kent County Memorial Hospital[2]	Warwick	93%	99

Surgical Care Improvement Project

22. Appropriate VTP Within 24 Hours

Hospital Name	City	Rate	Cases
Providence VA Medical Center[2]	Providence	99%	90
Rhode Island Hospital[2]	Providence	99%	221
Women and Infants Hospital of Rhode Island[2]	Providence	99%	86
Roger Williams Medical Center[2]	Providence	97%	181
Memorial Hospital of Rhode Island	Pawtucket	95%	149
Landmark Medical Center	Woonsocket	94%	137
South County Hospital[2]	Wakefield	94%	140
Kent County Memorial Hospital[2]	Warwick	93%	436
Miriam Hospital[2]	Providence	93%	442
Newport Hospital[2]	Newport	93%	186
St Joseph Health Services of RI[2]	N Providence	89%	206
Westerly Hospital	Westerly	85%	114

23. Appropriate Hair Removal

Hospital Name	City	Rate	Cases
Landmark Medical Center	Woonsocket	100%	283
Miriam Hospital[2]	Providence	100%	1111
Newport Hospital[2]	Newport	100%	287
Providence VA Medical Center[2]	Providence	100%	140
Rhode Island Hospital[2]	Providence	100%	687
Roger Williams Medical Center[2]	Providence	100%	377
St Joseph Health Services of RI[2]	N Providence	100%	467
South County Hospital[2]	Wakefield	100%	431
Kent County Memorial Hospital[2]	Warwick	99%	721
Westerly Hospital[2]	Westerly	99%	338
Women and Infants Hospital of Rhode Island[2]	Providence	99%	328
Memorial Hospital of Rhode Island	Pawtucket	98%	322

24. Appropriate Beta Blocker Usage

Hospital Name	City	Rate	Cases
St Joseph Health Services of RI[2]	N Providence	99%	163
Roger Williams Medical Center[2]	Providence	98%	112
Newport Hospital[2]	Newport	97%	77
Rhode Island Hospital[2]	Providence	97%	255
South County Hospital[2]	Wakefield	97%	110
Miriam Hospital[2]	Providence	96%	455
Women and Infants Hospital of Rhode Island[2]	Providence	96%	52
Providence VA Medical Center[2]	Providence	92%	53

NOTE: Hospital profiles are in alphabetical order by state, then city, then hospital within the city; Rankings exclude hospitals with less than 25 cases except for patient surveys which excludes hospitals with less than 100 cases; (a) 100–299 cases; (1) The number of cases is too small to be sure how well a hospital is performing; (2) The hospital indicated that the data submitted for this measure were based on a sample of cases; (3) Data was collected during a shorter time period (fewer quarters) than the maximum possible time for this measure; (4) Suppressed for one or more quarters by CMS; (5) No data is available from the hospital for this measure; (6) Fewer than 100 patients completed the HCAHPS survey. Use these rates with caution, as the number of surveys may be too low to reliably assess hospital performance; (7) Survey results are based on less than 12 months of data; (8) Survey results are not available for this reporting period; (9) No or very few patients were eligible for the HCAHPS survey. The scores shown, if any, reflect a very small number of surveys; (10) A state average was not calculated because too few hospitals in the state submitted data; (11) There were discrepancies in the data collection process; Please refer to the User's Guide for a full explanation of data.

Kent County Memorial Hospital[2]	Warwick	90%	230
Landmark Medical Center	Woonsocket	90%	86
Memorial Hospital of Rhode Island	Pawtucket	88%	81
Westerly Hospital	Westerly	83%	117

25. Controlled Postoperative Blood Glucose

Hospital Name	City	Rate	Cases
Miriam Hospital[2]	Providence	94%	195
Rhode Island Hospital[2]	Providence	94%	160

26. Prophylactic Antibiotic Timing

Hospital Name	City	Rate	Cases
Roger Williams Medical Center[2]	Providence	100%	255
Landmark Medical Center	Woonsocket	98%	179
Memorial Hospital of Rhode Island	Pawtucket	98%	187
Miriam Hospital[2]	Providence	98%	728
St Joseph Health Services of RI[2]	N Providence	98%	280
South County Hospital[2]	Wakefield	98%	285
Newport Hospital[2]	Newport	97%	180
Rhode Island Hospital[2]	Providence	97%	447
Westerly Hospital	Westerly	97%	232
Providence VA Medical Center	Providence	95%	74
Kent County Memorial Hospital[2]	Warwick	93%	460
Women and Infants Hospital of Rhode Island[2]	Providence	92%	237

27. Prophylactic Antibiotic Timing (Outpatient)

Hospital Name	City	Rate	Cases
Westerly Hospital	Westerly	99%	80
Memorial Hospital of Rhode Island	Pawtucket	98%	208
St Joseph Health Services of RI	N Providence	96%	476
Miriam Hospital	Providence	95%	289
Landmark Medical Center	Woonsocket	94%	155
South County Hospital	Wakefield	94%	109
Rhode Island Hospital	Providence	93%	479
Newport Hospital	Newport	92%	80
Kent County Memorial Hospital	Warwick	90%	262
Roger Williams Medical Center	Providence	90%	138
Women and Infants Hospital of Rhode Island	Providence	88%	189

28. Prophylactic Antibiotic Selection

Hospital Name	City	Rate	Cases
Miriam Hospital[2]	Providence	99%	729
Rhode Island Hospital[2]	Providence	99%	449
South County Hospital[2]	Wakefield	99%	288
Kent County Memorial Hospital[2]	Warwick	98%	464
St Joseph Health Services of RI[2]	N Providence	98%	280
Women and Infants Hospital of Rhode Island[2]	Providence	98%	234
Roger Williams Medical Center[2]	Providence	97%	256
Westerly Hospital	Westerly	97%	232
Landmark Medical Center	Woonsocket	96%	182
Memorial Hospital of Rhode Island	Pawtucket	96%	187
Newport Hospital[2]	Newport	96%	180
Providence VA Medical Center	Providence	96%	75

29. Prophylactic Antibiotic Selection (Outpatient)

Hospital Name	City	Rate	Cases
Westerly Hospital	Westerly	100%	80
Miriam Hospital	Providence	99%	280
Newport Hospital	Newport	99%	77
Roger Williams Medical Center	Providence	98%	130
South County Hospital	Wakefield	98%	106
Rhode Island Hospital	Providence	96%	531
St Joseph Health Services of RI	N Providence	96%	464
Kent County Memorial Hospital	Warwick	95%	255
Landmark Medical Center	Woonsocket	94%	153
Memorial Hospital of Rhode Island	Pawtucket	93%	207
Women and Infants Hospital of Rhode Island	Providence	91%	186

30. Prophylactic Antibiotic Stopped

Hospital Name	City	Rate	Cases
Memorial Hospital of Rhode Island	Pawtucket	99%	172
Rhode Island Hospital[2]	Providence	98%	408
Women and Infants Hospital of Rhode Island[2]	Providence	98%	231
Miriam Hospital[2]	Providence	97%	704
Roger Williams Medical Center[2]	Providence	97%	247
Landmark Medical Center	Woonsocket	96%	161
Westerly Hospital	Westerly	96%	227
Newport Hospital[2]	Newport	94%	171
South County Hospital[2]	Wakefield	94%	278
St Joseph Health Services of RI[2]	N Providence	93%	275
Kent County Memorial Hospital[2]	Warwick	92%	445
Providence VA Medical Center	Providence	90%	71

31. Recommended VTP Ordered

Hospital Name	City	Rate	Cases
Women and Infants Hospital of Rhode Island[2]	Providence	100%	86
Providence VA Medical Center[2]	Providence	99%	90
Rhode Island Hospital[2]	Providence	99%	221
Roger Williams Medical Center[2]	Providence	99%	181
Landmark Medical Center	Woonsocket	97%	138
Newport Hospital[2]	Newport	95%	186
Kent County Memorial Hospital[2]	Warwick	94%	437
Miriam Hospital[2]	Providence	94%	442
South County Hospital[2]	Wakefield	94%	140
Memorial Hospital of Rhode Island	Pawtucket	92%	156
St Joseph Health Services of RI[2]	N Providence	91%	206
Westerly Hospital	Westerly	91%	114

32. Urinary Catheter Removal

Hospital Name	City	Rate	Cases
Providence VA Medical Center[2]	Providence	96%	53
Westerly Hospital	Westerly	94%	93
Newport Hospital[2]	Newport	93%	28
South County Hospital[2]	Wakefield	93%	127
Memorial Hospital of Rhode Island	Pawtucket	90%	51
Rhode Island Hospital[2]	Providence	88%	164
Roger Williams Medical Center[2]	Providence	86%	140
Miriam Hospital[2]	Providence	85%	330
Kent County Memorial Hospital	Warwick	82%	184
St Joseph Health Services of RI[2]	N Providence	72%	79
Landmark Medical Center	Woonsocket	69%	32

Use of Medical Imaging

36. Combination Abdominal CT Scan

Hospital Name	City	Ratio	Cases
Women and Infants Hospital of Rhode Island	Providence	0.031	256
Newport Hospital	Newport	0.069	779
Landmark Medical Center	Woonsocket	0.071	491
Miriam Hospital	Providence	0.071	1293
Westerly Hospital	Westerly	0.079	684
Kent County Memorial Hospital	Warwick	0.082	655
Roger Williams Medical Center	Providence	0.085	399
Rhode Island Hospital	Providence	0.100	1687
St Joseph Health Services of RI	N Providence	0.124	565
Memorial Hospital of Rhode Island	Pawtucket	0.130	431
South County Hospital	Wakefield	0.160	470

37. Combination Chest CT Scan

Hospital Name	City	Ratio	Cases
Miriam Hospital	Providence	0.000	1071
St Joseph Health Services of RI	N Providence	0.000	291
Women and Infants Hospital of Rhode Island	Providence	0.000	244
Westerly Hospital	Westerly	0.004	566
Newport Hospital	Newport	0.005	432
Landmark Medical Center	Woonsocket	0.018	272
Roger Williams Medical Center	Providence	0.022	368
Memorial Hospital of Rhode Island	Pawtucket	0.025	324
South County Hospital	Wakefield	0.031	386
Kent County Memorial Hospital	Warwick	0.040	428
Rhode Island Hospital	Providence	0.062	1377

38. Follow-up Mammogram/Ultrasound

Hospital Name	City	Rate	Cases
Roger Williams Medical Center	Providence	4.9%	266
Landmark Medical Center	Woonsocket	5.1%	746
Newport Hospital	Newport	5.9%	1128
Rhode Island Hospital	Providence	6.7%	1163
Memorial Hospital of Rhode Island	Pawtucket	9.0%	525
Women and Infants Hospital of Rhode Island	Providence	9.1%	647
South County Hospital	Wakefield	10.6%	738
Kent County Memorial Hospital	Warwick	11.5%	1185
Miriam Hospital	Providence	12.1%	680
Westerly Hospital	Westerly	13.5%	1029
St Joseph Health Services of RI	N Providence	14.0%	414

39. MRI for Low Back Pain

Hospital Name	City	Rate	Cases
South County Hospital	Wakefield	26.0%	104
Kent County Memorial Hospital	Warwick	28.3%	106
Rhode Island Hospital	Providence	29.8%	94
Miriam Hospital	Providence	30.1%	73
Westerly Hospital	Westerly	31.2%	141
Newport Hospital	Newport	32.8%	189
St Joseph Health Services of RI[1]	N Providence	33.3%	30
Memorial Hospital of Rhode Island	Pawtucket	33.9%	56
Landmark Medical Center	Woonsocket	37.4%	91
Roger Williams Medical Center[1]	Providence	48.3%	29

Survey of Patients' Hospital Experiences

40. Area Around Room 'Always' Quiet at Night

Hospital Name	City	Rate	Cases
South County Hospital	Wakefield	60%	300+
Women and Infants Hospital of Rhode Island	Providence	59%	300+
Newport Hospital	Newport	58%	300+
Westerly Hospital	Westerly	54%	300+
Memorial Hospital of Rhode Island	Pawtucket	53%	300+
Miriam Hospital	Providence	49%	300+
Roger Williams Medical Center	Providence	48%	300+
Kent County Memorial Hospital	Warwick	46%	300+
Rhode Island Hospital	Providence	46%	300+
St Joseph Health Services of RI	N Providence	45%	300+
Landmark Medical Center	Woonsocket	41%	300+

41. Doctors 'Always' Communicated Well

Hospital Name	City	Rate	Cases
Women and Infants Hospital of Rhode Island	Providence	84%	300+
Miriam Hospital	Providence	82%	300+
South County Hospital	Wakefield	82%	300+
Westerly Hospital	Westerly	82%	300+
Memorial Hospital of Rhode Island	Pawtucket	81%	300+
Newport Hospital	Newport	78%	300+
Roger Williams Medical Center	Providence	78%	300+
Rhode Island Hospital	Providence	77%	300+
St Joseph Health Services of RI	N Providence	76%	300+
Kent County Memorial Hospital	Warwick	75%	300+
Landmark Medical Center	Woonsocket	75%	300+

42. Home Recovery Information Given

Hospital Name	City	Rate	Cases
Newport Hospital	Newport	86%	300+
Roger Williams Medical Center	Providence	85%	300+
Miriam Hospital	Providence	84%	300+
South County Hospital	Wakefield	84%	300+
Landmark Medical Center	Woonsocket	83%	300+
Women and Infants Hospital of Rhode Island	Providence	83%	300+
Memorial Hospital of Rhode Island	Pawtucket	82%	300+
Rhode Island Hospital	Providence	82%	300+
Kent County Memorial Hospital	Warwick	81%	300+
St Joseph Health Services of RI	N Providence	81%	300+
Westerly Hospital	Westerly	80%	300+

43. Hospital Given 9 or 10 on 10 Point Scale

Hospital Name	City	Rate	Cases
South County Hospital	Wakefield	77%	300+
Miriam Hospital	Providence	76%	300+
Women and Infants Hospital of Rhode Island	Providence	74%	300+
Newport Hospital	Newport	71%	300+
Westerly Hospital	Westerly	68%	300+
Memorial Hospital of Rhode Island	Pawtucket	65%	300+
Rhode Island Hospital	Providence	62%	300+
Kent County Memorial Hospital	Warwick	58%	300+
Roger Williams Medical Center	Providence	58%	300+
Landmark Medical Center	Woonsocket	52%	300+
St Joseph Health Services of RI	N Providence	49%	300+

44. Meds 'Always' Explained Before Given

Hospital Name	City	Rate	Cases
South County Hospital	Wakefield	65%	300+
Newport Hospital	Newport	63%	300+
Miriam Hospital	Providence	62%	300+
Women and Infants Hospital of Rhode Island	Providence	62%	300+
Westerly Hospital	Westerly	60%	300+
Memorial Hospital of Rhode Island	Pawtucket	58%	300+
Rhode Island Hospital	Providence	55%	300+
Roger Williams Medical Center	Providence	55%	300+
Landmark Medical Center	Woonsocket	54%	300+
Kent County Memorial Hospital	Warwick	53%	300+
St Joseph Health Services of RI	N Providence	52%	300+

45. Nurses 'Always' Communicated Well

Hospital Name	City	Rate	Cases
Miriam Hospital	Providence	81%	300+
South County Hospital	Wakefield	80%	300+
Women and Infants Hospital of Rhode Island	Providence	79%	300+
Newport Hospital	Newport	78%	300+
Westerly Hospital	Westerly	77%	300+
Memorial Hospital of Rhode Island	Pawtucket	76%	300+
Kent County Memorial Hospital	Warwick	74%	300+
Rhode Island Hospital	Providence	73%	300+
Roger Williams Medical Center	Providence	72%	300+
Landmark Medical Center	Woonsocket	69%	300+
St Joseph Health Services of RI	N Providence	67%	300+

46. Pain 'Always' Well Controlled

Hospital Name	City	Rate	Cases
Women and Infants Hospital of Rhode Island	Providence	78%	300+
Westerly Hospital	Westerly	76%	300+
South County Hospital	Wakefield	75%	300+
Miriam Hospital	Providence	73%	300+

NOTE: Hospital profiles are in alphabetical order by state, then city, then hospital within the city; Rankings exclude hospitals with less than 25 cases except for patient surveys which excludes hospitals with less than 100 cases; (a) 100–299 cases; (1) The number of cases is too small to be sure how well a hospital is performing; (2) The hospital indicated that the data submitted for this measure were based on a sample of cases; (3) Data was collected during a shorter time period (fewer quarters) than the maximum possible time for this measure; (4) Suppressed for one or more quarters by CMS; (5) No data is available from the hospital for this measure; (6) Fewer than 100 patients completed the HCAHPS survey. Use these rates with caution, as the number of surveys may be too low to reliably assess hospital performance; (7) Survey results are based on less than 12 months of data; (8) Survey results are not available for this reporting period; (9) No or very few patients were eligible for the HCAHPS survey. The scores shown, if any, reflect a very small number of surveys; (10) A state average was not calculated because too few hospitals in the state submitted data; (11) There were discrepancies in the data collection process; Please refer to the User's Guide for a full explanation of data.

Hospital Name	City	Rate	Cases
Memorial Hospital of Rhode Island	Pawtucket	70%	300+
Kent County Memorial Hospital	Warwick	69%	300+
Newport Hospital	Newport	69%	300+
Rhode Island Hospital	Providence	67%	300+
Landmark Medical Center	Woonsocket	65%	300+
Roger Williams Medical Center	Providence	65%	300+
St Joseph Health Services of RI	N Providence	63%	300+

47. Room and Bathroom 'Always' Clean

Hospital Name	City	Rate	Cases
Westerly Hospital	Westerly	83%	300+
Miriam Hospital	Providence	74%	300+
Newport Hospital	Newport	74%	300+
South County Hospital	Wakefield	74%	300+
Memorial Hospital of Rhode Island	Pawtucket	72%	300+
Women and Infants Hospital of Rhode Island	Providence	72%	300+
Rhode Island Hospital	Providence	70%	300+
Roger Williams Medical Center	Providence	69%	300+
Kent County Memorial Hospital	Warwick	66%	300+
Landmark Medical Center	Woonsocket	65%	300+
St Joseph Health Services of RI	N Providence	61%	300+

48. Timely Help 'Always' Received

Hospital Name	City	Rate	Cases
South County Hospital	Wakefield	72%	300+
Women and Infants Hospital of Rhode Island	Providence	68%	300+
Westerly Hospital	Westerly	66%	300+
Memorial Hospital of Rhode Island	Pawtucket	63%	300+
Kent County Memorial Hospital	Warwick	62%	300+
Miriam Hospital	Providence	62%	300+
Newport Hospital	Newport	62%	300+
Rhode Island Hospital	Providence	60%	300+
Roger Williams Medical Center	Providence	58%	300+
Landmark Medical Center	Woonsocket	57%	300+
St Joseph Health Services of RI	N Providence	50%	300+

49. Would Definitely Recommend Hospital

Hospital Name	City	Rate	Cases
Women and Infants Hospital of Rhode Island	Providence	85%	300+
Miriam Hospital	Providence	84%	300+
South County Hospital	Wakefield	80%	300+
Newport Hospital	Newport	74%	300+
Westerly Hospital	Westerly	73%	300+
Memorial Hospital of Rhode Island	Pawtucket	68%	300+
Rhode Island Hospital	Providence	67%	300+
Roger Williams Medical Center	Providence	62%	300+
Kent County Memorial Hospital	Warwick	60%	300+
Landmark Medical Center	Woonsocket	53%	300+
St Joseph Health Services of RI	N Providence	52%	300+

Newport Hospital

Friendship Street
Newport, RI 02840
URL: www.newporthospital.org
Type: Acute Care Hospitals
Ownership: Voluntary Non-Profit - Private

Phone: 401-846-6400
Fax: 401-845-1089
Emergency Services: Yes
Beds: 129

Key Personnel:
CEO/President. . . . . Arthur J Sampson
Operating Room. . . . . Mark A Billington
Pediatric In-Patient Care . . . . Keivan Ettefagh MD
Quality Assurance . . . . Ann Travis RN
Radiology. . . . . Donald B Fletcher
Emergency Room . . . . Benjamin Walker MD

Measure	Cases	This Hosp.	State Avg.	U.S. Avg.
Heart Attack Care				
ACE Inhibitor or ARB for LVSD[1]	4	100%	98%	96%
Aspirin at Arrival[1]	21	90%	99%	99%
Aspirin at Discharge[1]	13	100%	99%	98%
Beta Blocker at Discharge[1]	9	100%	99%	98%
Fibrinolytic Medication Timing	0	-	0%	55%
PCI Within 90 Minutes of Arrival	0	-	91%	90%
Smoking Cessation Advice[1]	1	100%	99%	99%
Chest Pain/Possible Heart Attack Care				
Aspirin at Arrival	78	97%	94%	95%
Median Time to ECG (minutes)	76	8	7	8
Median Time to Transfer (minutes)[1]	12	90	67	61
Fibrinolytic Medication Timing	0	-	88%	54%
Heart Failure Care				
ACE Inhibitor or ARB for LVSD	51	94%	94%	94%
Discharge Instructions	119	97%	85%	88%
Evaluation of LVS Function	162	99%	98%	98%
Smoking Cessation Advice[1]	9	100%	98%	98%
Pneumonia Care				
Appropriate Initial Antibiotic[2]	118	97%	92%	92%
Blood Culture Timing[2]	193	98%	95%	96%
Influenza Vaccine[2]	85	96%	85%	91%
Initial Antibiotic Timing[2]	185	97%	95%	95%
Pneumococcal Vaccine[2]	148	96%	86%	93%
Smoking Cessation Advice[2]	33	100%	97%	97%
Surgical Care Improvement Project				
Appropriate VTP Within 24 Hours[2]	186	93%	94%	92%
Appropriate Hair Removal[2]	287	100%	100%	99%
Appropriate Beta Blocker Usage[2]	77	97%	94%	93%
Controlled Postoperative Blood Glucose[2]	0	-	94%	93%
Prophylactic Antibiotic Timing[2]	180	97%	97%	97%
Prophylactic Antibiotic Timing (Outpatient)	80	92%	94%	92%
Prophylactic Antibiotic Selection[2]	180	96%	98%	97%
Prophylactic Antibiotic Select. (Outpatient)	77	99%	96%	94%
Prophylactic Antibiotic Stopped[2]	171	94%	96%	94%
Recommended VTP Ordered[2]	186	95%	95%	94%
Urinary Catheter Removal[2]	28	93%	86%	90%
Children's Asthma Care				
Received Systemic Corticosteroids	-	-	-	100%
Received Home Management Plan	-	-	-	71%
Received Reliever Medication	-	-	-	100%
Use of Medical Imaging				
Combination Abdominal CT Scan	779	0.069	0.091	0.191
Combination Chest CT Scan	432	0.005	0.024	0.054
Follow-up Mammogram/Ultrasound	1,128	5.9%	9.3%	8.4%
MRI for Low Back Pain	189	32.8%	31.8%	32.7%
Survey of Patients' Hospital Experiences				
Area Around Room 'Always' Quiet at Night	300+	58%	-	58%
Doctors 'Always' Communicated Well	300+	78%	-	80%
Home Recovery Information Given	300+	86%	-	82%
Hospital Given 9 or 10 on 10 Point Scale	300+	71%	-	67%
Meds 'Always' Explained Before Given	300+	63%	-	60%
Nurses 'Always' Communicated Well	300+	78%	-	76%
Pain 'Always' Well Controlled	300+	69%	-	69%
Room and Bathroom 'Always' Clean	300+	74%	-	71%
Timely Help 'Always' Received	300+	62%	-	64%
Would Definitely Recommend Hospital	300+	74%	-	69%

Saint Joseph Health Services of Rhode Island

200 High Service Avenue
North Providence, RI 02904
URL: www.fatimahospital.com
Type: Acute Care Hospitals
Ownership: Voluntary Non-Profit - Private

Phone: 401-456-3000
Fax: 401-456-3028
Emergency Services: Yes
Beds: 386

Key Personnel:
CEO/President. . . . . H John Keimig
Infection Control. . . . . Marlene Fishman
Operating Room. . . . . Kathy Squillante
Pediatric Ambulatory Care . . . . . . Alfred Toselli, MD
Pediatric In-Patient Care . . . . Alfred Toselli, MD
Quality Assurance . . . . Bruce Campbell
Radiology. . . . . Denise Driscoll

Measure	Cases	This Hosp.	State Avg.	U.S. Avg.
Heart Attack Care				
ACE Inhibitor or ARB for LVSD[1]	10	100%	98%	96%
Aspirin at Arrival	60	97%	99%	99%
Aspirin at Discharge	37	97%	99%	98%
Beta Blocker at Discharge	41	98%	99%	98%
Fibrinolytic Medication Timing	0	-	0%	55%
PCI Within 90 Minutes of Arrival	0	-	91%	90%
Smoking Cessation Advice[1]	3	67%	99%	99%
Chest Pain/Possible Heart Attack Care				
Aspirin at Arrival	32	97%	94%	95%
Median Time to ECG (minutes)	32	0	7	8
Median Time to Transfer (minutes)[1]	8	58	67	61
Fibrinolytic Medication Timing	0	-	88%	54%
Heart Failure Care				
ACE Inhibitor or ARB for LVSD	44	93%	94%	94%
Discharge Instructions	155	72%	85%	88%
Evaluation of LVS Function	261	97%	98%	98%
Smoking Cessation Advice[1]	23	96%	98%	98%
Pneumonia Care				
Appropriate Initial Antibiotic	108	95%	92%	92%
Blood Culture Timing	195	94%	95%	96%
Influenza Vaccine	99	75%	85%	91%
Initial Antibiotic Timing	153	98%	95%	95%
Pneumococcal Vaccine	183	85%	86%	93%
Smoking Cessation Advice	49	96%	97%	97%
Surgical Care Improvement Project				
Appropriate VTP Within 24 Hours[2]	206	89%	94%	92%
Appropriate Hair Removal[2]	467	100%	100%	99%
Appropriate Beta Blocker Usage[2]	163	99%	94%	93%
Controlled Postoperative Blood Glucose[2]	0	-	94%	93%
Prophylactic Antibiotic Timing[2]	280	98%	97%	97%
Prophylactic Antibiotic Timing (Outpatient)	476	96%	94%	92%
Prophylactic Antibiotic Selection[2]	280	98%	98%	97%
Prophylactic Antibiotic Select. (Outpatient)	464	96%	96%	94%
Prophylactic Antibiotic Stopped[2]	275	93%	96%	94%
Recommended VTP Ordered[2]	206	91%	95%	94%
Urinary Catheter Removal[2]	79	72%	86%	90%
Children's Asthma Care				
Received Systemic Corticosteroids	-	-	-	100%
Received Home Management Plan	-	-	-	71%
Received Reliever Medication	-	-	-	100%
Use of Medical Imaging				
Combination Abdominal CT Scan	565	0.124	0.091	0.191
Combination Chest CT Scan	291	0.000	0.024	0.054
Follow-up Mammogram/Ultrasound	414	14.0%	9.3%	8.4%
MRI for Low Back Pain[1]	30	33.3%	31.8%	32.7%
Survey of Patients' Hospital Experiences				
Area Around Room 'Always' Quiet at Night	300+	45%	-	58%
Doctors 'Always' Communicated Well	300+	76%	-	80%
Home Recovery Information Given	300+	81%	-	82%
Hospital Given 9 or 10 on 10 Point Scale	300+	49%	-	67%
Meds 'Always' Explained Before Given	300+	52%	-	60%
Nurses 'Always' Communicated Well	300+	67%	-	76%
Pain 'Always' Well Controlled	300+	63%	-	69%
Room and Bathroom 'Always' Clean	300+	61%	-	71%
Timely Help 'Always' Received	300+	50%	-	64%
Would Definitely Recommend Hospital	300+	52%	-	69%

Memorial Hospital of Rhode Island

111 Brewster Street
Pawtucket, RI 02860
URL: mhriweb.org
Type: Acute Care Hospitals
Ownership: Voluntary Non-Profit - Other

Phone: 401-729-2000
Fax: 401-729-3054
Emergency Services: Yes
Beds: 294

Key Personnel:
CEO/President. . . . . Francis R Dietz
Pediatric Ambulatory Care . . . . . . Louise Kiessling, MD
Pediatric In-Patient Care . . . . Louise Kiessling, MD

Measure	Cases	This Hosp.	State Avg.	U.S. Avg.
Heart Attack Care				
ACE Inhibitor or ARB for LVSD[1]	7	86%	98%	96%
Aspirin at Arrival	51	96%	99%	99%
Aspirin at Discharge	25	100%	99%	98%
Beta Blocker at Discharge	25	100%	99%	98%
Fibrinolytic Medication Timing	0	-	0%	55%
PCI Within 90 Minutes of Arrival	0	-	91%	90%
Smoking Cessation Advice[1]	7	100%	99%	99%
Chest Pain/Possible Heart Attack Care				
Aspirin at Arrival	39	97%	94%	95%
Median Time to ECG (minutes)	39	18	7	8
Median Time to Transfer (minutes)[1]	24	98	67	61
Fibrinolytic Medication Timing	0	-	88%	54%
Heart Failure Care				
ACE Inhibitor or ARB for LVSD	62	85%	94%	94%
Discharge Instructions	175	93%	85%	88%
Evaluation of LVS Function	242	98%	98%	98%
Smoking Cessation Advice	37	100%	98%	98%
Pneumonia Care				
Appropriate Initial Antibiotic	92	92%	92%	92%
Blood Culture Timing	105	96%	95%	96%
Influenza Vaccine	100	94%	85%	91%
Initial Antibiotic Timing	172	91%	95%	95%
Pneumococcal Vaccine	160	88%	86%	93%
Smoking Cessation Advice	72	99%	97%	97%
Surgical Care Improvement Project				
Appropriate VTP Within 24 Hours	149	95%	94%	92%
Appropriate Hair Removal	322	98%	100%	99%
Appropriate Beta Blocker Usage	81	88%	94%	93%
Controlled Postoperative Blood Glucose	0	-	94%	93%
Prophylactic Antibiotic Timing	187	98%	97%	97%
Prophylactic Antibiotic Timing (Outpatient)	208	98%	94%	92%
Prophylactic Antibiotic Selection	187	96%	98%	97%
Prophylactic Antibiotic Select. (Outpatient)	207	93%	96%	94%
Prophylactic Antibiotic Stopped	172	99%	96%	94%
Recommended VTP Ordered	156	92%	95%	94%
Urinary Catheter Removal	51	90%	86%	90%
Children's Asthma Care				
Received Systemic Corticosteroids	-	-	-	100%
Received Home Management Plan	-	-	-	71%
Received Reliever Medication	-	-	-	100%
Use of Medical Imaging				
Combination Abdominal CT Scan	431	0.130	0.091	0.191
Combination Chest CT Scan	324	0.025	0.024	0.054
Follow-up Mammogram/Ultrasound	525	9.0%	9.3%	8.4%
MRI for Low Back Pain	56	33.9%	31.8%	32.7%
Survey of Patients' Hospital Experiences				
Area Around Room 'Always' Quiet at Night	300+	53%	-	58%
Doctors 'Always' Communicated Well	300+	81%	-	80%
Home Recovery Information Given	300+	82%	-	82%
Hospital Given 9 or 10 on 10 Point Scale	300+	65%	-	67%
Meds 'Always' Explained Before Given	300+	58%	-	60%
Nurses 'Always' Communicated Well	300+	76%	-	76%
Pain 'Always' Well Controlled	300+	70%	-	69%
Room and Bathroom 'Always' Clean	300+	72%	-	71%
Timely Help 'Always' Received	300+	63%	-	64%
Would Definitely Recommend Hospital	300+	68%	-	69%

NOTE: Hospital profiles are in alphabetical order by state, then city, then hospital within the city; Rankings exclude hospitals with less than 25 cases except for patient surveys which excludes hospitals with less than 100 cases; (a) 100–299 cases; (1) The number of cases is too small to be sure how well a hospital is performing; (2) The hospital indicated that the data submitted for this measure were based on a sample of cases; (3) Data was collected during a shorter time period (fewer quarters) than the maximum possible time for this measure; (4) Suppressed for one or more quarters by CMS; (5) No data is available from the hospital for this measure; (6) Fewer than 100 patients completed the HCAHPS survey. Use these rates with caution, as the number of surveys may be too low to reliably assess hospital performance; (7) Survey results are based on less than 12 months of data; (8) Survey results are not available for this reporting period; (9) No or very few patients were eligible for the HCAHPS survey. The scores shown, if any, reflect a very small number of surveys; (10) A state average was not calculated because too few hospitals in the state submitted data; (11) There were discrepancies in the data collection process; Please refer to the User's Guide for a full explanation of data.

Miriam Hospital

164 Summit Avenue Phone: 401-793-2500
Providence, RI 02906 Fax: 401-793-2923
URL: www.lifespan.org/partners/tmh
Type: Acute Care Hospitals Emergency Services: Yes
Ownership: Voluntary Non-Profit - Private Beds: 247

Key Personnel:
CEO/President.............. Kathleen Hittner, MD
Chief of Medical Staff.......... William Corwin

Measure	Cases	This Hosp.	State Avg.	U.S. Avg.
Heart Attack Care				
ACE Inhibitor or ARB for LVSD	115	98%	98%	96%
Aspirin at Arrival	344	99%	99%	99%
Aspirin at Discharge	629	100%	99%	98%
Beta Blocker at Discharge	610	99%	99%	98%
Fibrinolytic Medication Timing	0	-	0%	55%
PCI Within 90 Minutes of Arrival	66	85%	91%	90%
Smoking Cessation Advice	187	100%	99%	99%
Chest Pain/Possible Heart Attack Care				
Aspirin at Arrival[1]	4	100%	94%	95%
Median Time to ECG (minutes)[1]	4	10	7	8
Median Time to Transfer (minutes)[5]	0	-	67	61
Fibrinolytic Medication Timing[5]	0	-	88%	54%
Heart Failure Care				
ACE Inhibitor or ARB for LVSD[2]	165	95%	94%	94%
Discharge Instructions[2]	421	91%	85%	88%
Evaluation of LVS Function[2]	541	99%	98%	98%
Smoking Cessation Advice[2]	67	100%	98%	98%
Pneumonia Care				
Appropriate Initial Antibiotic[2]	98	96%	92%	92%
Blood Culture Timing[2]	167	98%	95%	96%
Influenza Vaccine[2]	105	96%	85%	91%
Initial Antibiotic Timing[2]	176	97%	95%	95%
Pneumococcal Vaccine[2]	162	91%	86%	93%
Smoking Cessation Advice[2]	46	100%	97%	97%
Surgical Care Improvement Project				
Appropriate VTP Within 24 Hours[2]	442	93%	94%	92%
Appropriate Hair Removal[2]	1,111	100%	100%	99%
Appropriate Beta Blocker Usage[2]	455	96%	94%	93%
Controlled Postoperative Blood Glucose[2]	195	94%	94%	93%
Prophylactic Antibiotic Timing[2]	728	98%	97%	97%
Prophylactic Antibiotic Timing (Outpatient)	289	95%	94%	92%
Prophylactic Antibiotic Selection[2]	729	99%	98%	97%
Prophylactic Antibiotic Select. (Outpatient)	280	99%	96%	94%
Prophylactic Antibiotic Stopped[2]	704	97%	96%	94%
Recommended VTP Ordered[2]	442	94%	95%	94%
Urinary Catheter Removal[2]	330	85%	86%	90%
Children's Asthma Care				
Received Systemic Corticosteroids	-	-	-	100%
Received Home Management Plan	-	-	-	71%
Received Reliever Medication	-	-	-	100%
Use of Medical Imaging				
Combination Abdominal CT Scan	1,293	0.071	0.091	0.191
Combination Chest CT Scan	1,071	0.000	0.024	0.054
Follow-up Mammogram/Ultrasound	680	12.1%	9.3%	8.4%
MRI for Low Back Pain	73	30.1%	31.8%	32.7%
Survey of Patients' Hospital Experiences				
Area Around Room 'Always' Quiet at Night	300+	49%	-	58%
Doctors 'Always' Communicated Well	300+	82%	-	80%
Home Recovery Information Given	300+	84%	-	82%
Hospital Given 9 or 10 on 10 Point Scale	300+	76%	-	67%
Meds 'Always' Explained Before Given	300+	62%	-	60%
Nurses 'Always' Communicated Well	300+	81%	-	76%
Pain 'Always' Well Controlled	300+	73%	-	69%
Room and Bathroom 'Always' Clean	300+	74%	-	71%
Timely Help 'Always' Received	300+	62%	-	64%
Would Definitely Recommend Hospital	300+	84%	-	69%

Providence VA Medical Center

830 Chalkstone Avenue Phone: 401-457-3042
Providence, RI 02908 Fax: 401-457-3370
URL: www.visn1.med.va.gov/providence
Type: Acute Care-Veterans Administration Emergency Services: No
Ownership: Government - Federal Beds: 73

Key Personnel:
Chief of Medical Staff.......... Gregory M Gillette
Emergency Room.............. Satish Sharma, MD
Patient Relations.............. Deborah A Clickner, MEd RN

Measure	Cases	This Hosp.	State Avg.	U.S. Avg.
Heart Attack Care				
ACE Inhibitor or ARB for LVSD[5]	0	-	98%	96%
Aspirin at Arrival[5]	0	-	99%	99%
Aspirin at Discharge[5]	0	-	99%	98%
Beta Blocker at Discharge[5]	0	-	99%	98%
Fibrinolytic Medication Timing[5]	0	-	0%	55%
PCI Within 90 Minutes of Arrival[5]	0	-	91%	90%
Smoking Cessation Advice[5]	0	-	99%	99%
Chest Pain/Possible Heart Attack Care				
Aspirin at Arrival	-	-	94%	95%
Median Time to ECG (minutes)	-	-	7	8
Median Time to Transfer (minutes)	-	-	67	61
Fibrinolytic Medication Timing	-	-	88%	54%
Heart Failure Care				
ACE Inhibitor or ARB for LVSD	57	96%	94%	94%
Discharge Instructions	131	92%	85%	88%
Evaluation of LVS Function	169	99%	98%	98%
Smoking Cessation Advice	27	85%	98%	98%
Pneumonia Care				
Appropriate Initial Antibiotic	25	92%	92%	92%
Blood Culture Timing	73	97%	95%	96%
Influenza Vaccine	40	93%	85%	91%
Initial Antibiotic Timing	76	95%	95%	95%
Pneumococcal Vaccine	74	99%	86%	93%
Smoking Cessation Advice[1]	16	100%	97%	97%
Surgical Care Improvement Project				
Appropriate VTP Within 24 Hours[2]	90	99%	94%	92%
Appropriate Hair Removal[2]	140	100%	100%	99%
Appropriate Beta Blocker Usage[2]	53	92%	94%	93%
Controlled Postoperative Blood Glucose[2,5]	0	-	94%	93%
Prophylactic Antibiotic Timing	74	95%	97%	97%
Prophylactic Antibiotic Timing (Outpatient)	-	-	94%	92%
Prophylactic Antibiotic Selection	75	96%	98%	97%
Prophylactic Antibiotic Select. (Outpatient)	-	-	96%	94%
Prophylactic Antibiotic Stopped	71	90%	96%	94%
Recommended VTP Ordered[2]	90	99%	95%	94%
Urinary Catheter Removal[2]	53	96%	86%	90%
Children's Asthma Care				
Received Systemic Corticosteroids	-	-	-	100%
Received Home Management Plan	-	-	-	71%
Received Reliever Medication	-	-	-	100%
Use of Medical Imaging				
Combination Abdominal CT Scan	-	-	0.091	0.191
Combination Chest CT Scan	-	-	0.024	0.054
Follow-up Mammogram/Ultrasound	-	-	9.3%	8.4%
MRI for Low Back Pain	-	-	31.8%	32.7%
Survey of Patients' Hospital Experiences				
Area Around Room 'Always' Quiet at Night	-	-	-	58%
Doctors 'Always' Communicated Well	-	-	-	80%
Home Recovery Information Given	-	-	-	82%
Hospital Given 9 or 10 on 10 Point Scale	-	-	-	67%
Meds 'Always' Explained Before Given	-	-	-	60%
Nurses 'Always' Communicated Well	-	-	-	76%
Pain 'Always' Well Controlled	-	-	-	69%
Room and Bathroom 'Always' Clean	-	-	-	71%
Timely Help 'Always' Received	-	-	-	64%
Would Definitely Recommend Hospital	-	-	-	69%

Rhode Island Hospital

593 Eddy Street Phone: 401-444-4000
Providence, RI 02902 Fax: 401-444-4218
URL: www.rhodeislandhospital.org
Type: Acute Care Hospitals Emergency Services: Yes
Ownership: Voluntary Non-Profit - Private Beds: 719

Key Personnel:
CEO/President.............. Timothy J Babineau MD
Chief of Medical Staff.......... John B Murphy, MD
Coronary Care.............. George McKendall MD
Operating Room.............. Barbara Riley RN
Quality Assurance............ Joan Flynn
Radiology.................. John Cronan MD
Emergency Room............ Frantz Gibbs MD

Measure	Cases	This Hosp.	State Avg.	U.S. Avg.
Heart Attack Care				
ACE Inhibitor or ARB for LVSD	83	99%	98%	96%
Aspirin at Arrival	407	100%	99%	99%
Aspirin at Discharge	643	100%	99%	98%
Beta Blocker at Discharge	616	100%	99%	98%
Fibrinolytic Medication Timing[1]	1	0%	0%	55%
PCI Within 90 Minutes of Arrival	80	94%	91%	90%
Smoking Cessation Advice	212	100%	99%	99%
Chest Pain/Possible Heart Attack Care				
Aspirin at Arrival[1,3]	2	100%	94%	95%
Median Time to ECG (minutes)[1,3]	2	8	7	8
Median Time to Transfer (minutes)[5]	0	-	67	61
Fibrinolytic Medication Timing[3]	0	-	88%	54%
Heart Failure Care				
ACE Inhibitor or ARB for LVSD[2]	130	94%	94%	94%
Discharge Instructions[2]	267	87%	85%	88%
Evaluation of LVS Function[2]	346	99%	98%	98%
Smoking Cessation Advice[2]	54	100%	98%	98%
Pneumonia Care				
Appropriate Initial Antibiotic[2]	59	97%	92%	92%
Blood Culture Timing[2]	129	97%	95%	96%
Influenza Vaccine[2]	78	82%	85%	91%
Initial Antibiotic Timing[2]	138	94%	95%	95%
Pneumococcal Vaccine[2]	115	85%	86%	93%
Smoking Cessation Advice[2]	52	100%	97%	97%
Surgical Care Improvement Project				
Appropriate VTP Within 24 Hours[2]	221	99%	94%	92%
Appropriate Hair Removal[2]	687	100%	100%	99%
Appropriate Beta Blocker Usage[2]	255	97%	94%	93%
Controlled Postoperative Blood Glucose[2]	160	94%	94%	93%
Prophylactic Antibiotic Timing[2]	447	97%	97%	97%
Prophylactic Antibiotic Timing (Outpatient)	479	93%	94%	92%
Prophylactic Antibiotic Selection[2]	449	99%	98%	97%
Prophylactic Antibiotic Select. (Outpatient)	531	96%	96%	94%
Prophylactic Antibiotic Stopped[2]	408	98%	96%	94%
Recommended VTP Ordered[2]	221	99%	95%	94%
Urinary Catheter Removal[2]	164	88%	86%	90%
Children's Asthma Care				
Received Systemic Corticosteroids	-	-	-	100%
Received Home Management Plan	-	-	-	71%
Received Reliever Medication	-	-	-	100%
Use of Medical Imaging				
Combination Abdominal CT Scan	1,687	0.100	0.091	0.191
Combination Chest CT Scan	1,377	0.062	0.024	0.054
Follow-up Mammogram/Ultrasound	1,163	6.7%	9.3%	8.4%
MRI for Low Back Pain	94	29.8%	31.8%	32.7%
Survey of Patients' Hospital Experiences				
Area Around Room 'Always' Quiet at Night	300+	46%	-	58%
Doctors 'Always' Communicated Well	300+	77%	-	80%
Home Recovery Information Given	300+	82%	-	82%
Hospital Given 9 or 10 on 10 Point Scale	300+	62%	-	67%
Meds 'Always' Explained Before Given	300+	55%	-	60%
Nurses 'Always' Communicated Well	300+	73%	-	76%
Pain 'Always' Well Controlled	300+	67%	-	69%
Room and Bathroom 'Always' Clean	300+	70%	-	71%
Timely Help 'Always' Received	300+	60%	-	64%
Would Definitely Recommend Hospital	300+	67%	-	69%

NOTE: Hospital profiles are in alphabetical order by state, then city, then hospital within the city; Rankings exclude hospitals with less than 25 cases except for patient surveys which excludes hospitals with less than 100 cases; (a) 100–299 cases; (1) The number of cases is too small to be sure how well a hospital is performing; (2) The hospital indicated that the data submitted for this measure were based on a sample of cases; (3) Data was collected during a shorter time period (fewer quarters) than the maximum possible time for this measure; (4) Suppressed for one or more quarters by CMS; (5) No data is available from the hospital for this measure; (6) Fewer than 100 patients completed the HCAHPS survey. Use these rates with caution, as the number of surveys may be too low to reliably assess hospital performance; (7) Survey results are based on less than 12 months of data; (8) Survey results are not available for this reporting period; (9) No or very few patients were eligible for the HCAHPS survey. The scores shown, if any, reflect a very small number of surveys; (10) A state average was not calculated because too few hospitals in the state submitted data; (11) There were discrepancies in the data collection process; Please refer to the User's Guide for a full explanation of data.

Roger Williams Medical Center

825 Chalkstone Avenue · Phone: 401-456-2000
Providence, RI 02908 · Fax: 401-456-2029
URL: www.rwmc.com
Type: Acute Care Hospitals · Emergency Services: Yes
Ownership: Voluntary Non-Profit - Private · Beds: 238

Key Personnel:
CEO/President . . . . Robert A Urciuoli
Chief of Medical Staff . . . . Thomas Dennucci
Quality Assurance . . . . Joyce Hackley
Emergency Room . . . . Michael Bonitati

Measure	Cases	This Hosp.	State Avg.	U.S. Avg.
Heart Attack Care				
ACE Inhibitor or ARB for LVSD[1]	9	89%	98%	96%
Aspirin at Arrival	66	98%	99%	99%
Aspirin at Discharge	50	92%	99%	98%
Beta Blocker at Discharge	50	100%	99%	98%
Fibrinolytic Medication Timing	0	-	0%	55%
PCI Within 90 Minutes of Arrival	0	-	91%	90%
Smoking Cessation Advice[1]	7	100%	99%	99%
Chest Pain/Possible Heart Attack Care				
Aspirin at Arrival[1,3]	13	100%	94%	95%
Median Time to ECG (minutes)[1,3]	13	9	7	8
Median Time to Transfer (minutes)[1,3]	5	72	67	61
Fibrinolytic Medication Timing[3]	0	-	88%	54%
Heart Failure Care				
ACE Inhibitor or ARB for LVSD	34	85%	94%	94%
Discharge Instructions	109	67%	85%	88%
Evaluation of LVS Function	162	96%	98%	98%
Smoking Cessation Advice[1]	14	100%	98%	98%
Pneumonia Care				
Appropriate Initial Antibiotic[2]	78	88%	92%	92%
Blood Culture Timing[2]	109	92%	95%	96%
Influenza Vaccine	69	74%	85%	91%
Initial Antibiotic Timing[2]	146	92%	95%	95%
Pneumococcal Vaccine[2]	125	72%	86%	93%
Smoking Cessation Advice[2]	33	100%	97%	97%
Surgical Care Improvement Project				
Appropriate VTP Within 24 Hours[2]	181	97%	94%	92%
Appropriate Hair Removal[2]	377	100%	100%	99%
Appropriate Beta Blocker Usage[2]	112	98%	94%	93%
Controlled Postoperative Blood Glucose[1,2]	1	100%	94%	93%
Prophylactic Antibiotic Timing[2]	255	100%	97%	97%
Prophylactic Antibiotic Timing (Outpatient)	138	90%	94%	92%
Prophylactic Antibiotic Selection[2]	256	97%	98%	97%
Prophylactic Antibiotic Select. (Outpatient)	130	98%	96%	94%
Prophylactic Antibiotic Stopped[2]	247	97%	96%	94%
Recommended VTP Ordered[2]	181	99%	95%	94%
Urinary Catheter Removal[2]	140	86%	86%	90%
Children's Asthma Care				
Received Systemic Corticosteroids	-	-	-	100%
Received Home Management Plan	-	-	-	71%
Received Reliever Medication	-	-	-	100%
Use of Medical Imaging				
Combination Abdominal CT Scan	399	0.085	0.091	0.191
Combination Chest CT Scan	368	0.022	0.024	0.054
Follow-up Mammogram/Ultrasound	266	4.9%	9.3%	8.4%
MRI for Low Back Pain[1]	29	48.3%	31.8%	32.7%
Survey of Patients' Hospital Experiences				
Area Around Room 'Always' Quiet at Night	300+	48%	-	58%
Doctors 'Always' Communicated Well	300+	78%	-	80%
Home Recovery Information Given	300+	85%	-	82%
Hospital Given 9 or 10 on 10 Point Scale	300+	58%	-	67%
Meds 'Always' Explained Before Given	300+	55%	-	60%
Nurses 'Always' Communicated Well	300+	72%	-	76%
Pain 'Always' Well Controlled	300+	65%	-	69%
Room and Bathroom 'Always' Clean	300+	69%	-	71%
Timely Help 'Always' Received	300+	58%	-	64%
Would Definitely Recommend Hospital	300+	62%	-	69%

Women and Infants Hospital of Rhode Island

101 Dudley Street · Phone: 401-274-1100
Providence, RI 02905 · Fax: 401-453-7666
E-mail: mkernan@wihri.org
URL: www.womenandinfants.com
Type: Acute Care Hospitals · Emergency Services: No
Ownership: Voluntary Non-Profit - Other · Beds: 137

Key Personnel:
CEO/President . . . . Constance A Howes
Chief of Medical Staff . . . . Karen Rosene-Montell, MD
Infection Control . . . . Fatima Muriel
Pediatric In-Patient Care . . . . James Padbury, MD
Quality Assurance . . . . Deborah L Gard
Radiology . . . . Michael Atalay, MD
Anesthesiology . . . . Kue Choi, MD
Patient Relations . . . . Paula Gillette, RN

Measure	Cases	This Hosp.	State Avg.	U.S. Avg.
Heart Attack Care				
ACE Inhibitor or ARB for LVSD[5]	0	-	98%	96%
Aspirin at Arrival[5]	0	-	99%	99%
Aspirin at Discharge[5]	0	-	99%	98%
Beta Blocker at Discharge[5]	0	-	99%	98%
Fibrinolytic Medication Timing[5]	0	-	0%	55%
PCI Within 90 Minutes of Arrival[5]	0	-	91%	90%
Smoking Cessation Advice[5]	0	-	99%	99%
Chest Pain/Possible Heart Attack Care				
Aspirin at Arrival	43	65%	94%	95%
Median Time to ECG (minutes)	38	14	7	8
Median Time to Transfer (minutes)[5]	0	-	67	61
Fibrinolytic Medication Timing[5]	0	-	88%	54%
Heart Failure Care				
ACE Inhibitor or ARB for LVSD[3]	0	-	94%	94%
Discharge Instructions[1,3]	1	0%	85%	88%
Evaluation of LVS Function[1,3]	1	0%	98%	98%
Smoking Cessation Advice[3]	0	-	98%	98%
Pneumonia Care				
Appropriate Initial Antibiotic[1]	1	0%	92%	92%
Blood Culture Timing[1]	3	100%	95%	96%
Influenza Vaccine[1]	7	57%	85%	91%
Initial Antibiotic Timing[1]	10	80%	95%	95%
Pneumococcal Vaccine[1]	6	33%	86%	93%
Smoking Cessation Advice[1]	2	100%	97%	97%
Surgical Care Improvement Project				
Appropriate VTP Within 24 Hours[2]	86	99%	94%	92%
Appropriate Hair Removal[2]	328	99%	100%	99%
Appropriate Beta Blocker Usage[2]	52	96%	94%	93%
Controlled Postoperative Blood Glucose[2]	0	-	94%	93%
Prophylactic Antibiotic Timing[2]	237	92%	97%	97%
Prophylactic Antibiotic Timing (Outpatient)	189	88%	94%	92%
Prophylactic Antibiotic Selection[2]	234	98%	98%	97%
Prophylactic Antibiotic Select. (Outpatient)	186	91%	96%	94%
Prophylactic Antibiotic Stopped[2]	231	98%	96%	94%
Recommended VTP Ordered[2]	86	100%	95%	94%
Urinary Catheter Removal[1,2]	4	100%	86%	90%
Children's Asthma Care				
Received Systemic Corticosteroids	-	-	-	100%
Received Home Management Plan	-	-	-	71%
Received Reliever Medication	-	-	-	100%
Use of Medical Imaging				
Combination Abdominal CT Scan	256	0.031	0.091	0.191
Combination Chest CT Scan	244	0.000	0.024	0.054
Follow-up Mammogram/Ultrasound	647	9.1%	9.3%	8.4%
MRI for Low Back Pain[1]	3	33.3%	31.8%	32.7%
Survey of Patients' Hospital Experiences				
Area Around Room 'Always' Quiet at Night	300+	59%	-	58%
Doctors 'Always' Communicated Well	300+	84%	-	80%
Home Recovery Information Given	300+	83%	-	82%
Hospital Given 9 or 10 on 10 Point Scale	300+	74%	-	67%
Meds 'Always' Explained Before Given	300+	62%	-	60%
Nurses 'Always' Communicated Well	300+	79%	-	76%
Pain 'Always' Well Controlled	300+	78%	-	69%
Room and Bathroom 'Always' Clean	300+	72%	-	71%
Timely Help 'Always' Received	300+	68%	-	64%
Would Definitely Recommend Hospital	300+	85%	-	69%

South County Hospital

100 Kenyon Ave · Phone: 401-782-8000
Wakefield, RI 02879 · Fax: 401-783-6330
E-mail: info@schospital.com
URL: www.schospital.com
Type: Acute Care Hospitals · Emergency Services: Yes
Ownership: Voluntary Non-Profit - Private · Beds: 100

Key Personnel:
CEO/President . . . . Louis R Giancola
Cardiac Laboratory . . . . Sherri Zinno
Chief of Medical Staff . . . . Richard A Black, MD
Infection Control . . . . Lee Ann Buenn
Quality Assurance . . . . Debra Keaney
Radiology . . . . Jeffrey E Silverstein
Emergency Room . . . . Donna Fairchild
Patient Relations . . . . Barbara Seagrave

Measure	Cases	This Hosp.	State Avg.	U.S. Avg.
Heart Attack Care				
ACE Inhibitor or ARB for LVSD[1]	3	100%	98%	96%
Aspirin at Arrival	29	100%	99%	99%
Aspirin at Discharge[1]	15	100%	99%	98%
Beta Blocker at Discharge[1]	16	94%	99%	98%
Fibrinolytic Medication Timing	0	-	0%	55%
PCI Within 90 Minutes of Arrival	0	-	91%	90%
Smoking Cessation Advice[1]	1	100%	99%	99%
Chest Pain/Possible Heart Attack Care				
Aspirin at Arrival	35	94%	94%	95%
Median Time to ECG (minutes)	35	10	7	8
Median Time to Transfer (minutes)[1]	8	52	67	61
Fibrinolytic Medication Timing[1]	2	50%	88%	54%
Heart Failure Care				
ACE Inhibitor or ARB for LVSD	31	100%	94%	94%
Discharge Instructions	88	97%	85%	88%
Evaluation of LVS Function	111	100%	98%	98%
Smoking Cessation Advice[1]	8	100%	98%	98%
Pneumonia Care				
Appropriate Initial Antibiotic	99	92%	92%	92%
Blood Culture Timing	156	98%	95%	96%
Influenza Vaccine	104	100%	85%	91%
Initial Antibiotic Timing	156	96%	95%	95%
Pneumococcal Vaccine	148	99%	86%	93%
Smoking Cessation Advice	33	97%	97%	97%
Surgical Care Improvement Project				
Appropriate VTP Within 24 Hours[2]	140	94%	94%	92%
Appropriate Hair Removal[2]	431	100%	100%	99%
Appropriate Beta Blocker Usage[2]	110	97%	94%	93%
Controlled Postoperative Blood Glucose[2]	0	-	94%	93%
Prophylactic Antibiotic Timing[2]	285	98%	97%	97%
Prophylactic Antibiotic Timing (Outpatient)	109	94%	94%	92%
Prophylactic Antibiotic Selection[2]	288	99%	98%	97%
Prophylactic Antibiotic Select. (Outpatient)	106	98%	96%	94%
Prophylactic Antibiotic Stopped[2]	278	94%	96%	94%
Recommended VTP Ordered[2]	140	94%	95%	94%
Urinary Catheter Removal[2]	127	93%	86%	90%
Children's Asthma Care				
Received Systemic Corticosteroids	-	-	-	100%
Received Home Management Plan	-	-	-	71%
Received Reliever Medication	-	-	-	100%
Use of Medical Imaging				
Combination Abdominal CT Scan	470	0.160	0.091	0.191
Combination Chest CT Scan	386	0.031	0.024	0.054
Follow-up Mammogram/Ultrasound	738	10.6%	9.3%	8.4%
MRI for Low Back Pain	104	26.0%	31.8%	32.7%
Survey of Patients' Hospital Experiences				
Area Around Room 'Always' Quiet at Night	300+	60%	-	58%
Doctors 'Always' Communicated Well	300+	82%	-	80%
Home Recovery Information Given	300+	84%	-	82%
Hospital Given 9 or 10 on 10 Point Scale	300+	77%	-	67%
Meds 'Always' Explained Before Given	300+	65%	-	60%
Nurses 'Always' Communicated Well	300+	80%	-	76%
Pain 'Always' Well Controlled	300+	75%	-	69%
Room and Bathroom 'Always' Clean	300+	74%	-	71%
Timely Help 'Always' Received	300+	72%	-	64%
Would Definitely Recommend Hospital	300+	80%	-	69%

NOTE: Hospital profiles are in alphabetical order by state, then city, then hospital within the city; Rankings exclude hospitals with less than 25 cases except for patient surveys which excludes hospitals with less than 100 cases; (a) 100–299 cases; (1) The number of cases is too small to be sure how well a hospital is performing; (2) The hospital indicated that the data submitted for this measure were based on a sample of cases; (3) Data was collected during a shorter time period (fewer quarters) than the maximum possible time for this measure; (4) Suppressed for one or more quarters by CMS; (5) No data is available from the hospital for this measure; (6) Fewer than 100 patients completed the HCAHPS survey. Use these rates with caution, as the number of surveys may be too low to reliably assess hospital performance; (7) Survey results are based on less than 12 months of data; (8) Survey results are not available for this reporting period; (9) No or very few patients were eligible for the HCAHPS survey. The scores shown, if any, reflect a very small number of surveys; (10) A state average was not calculated because too few hospitals in the state submitted data; (11) There were discrepancies in the data collection process; Please refer to the User's Guide for a full explanation of data.

Kent County Memorial Hospital

455 Toll Gate Rd
Warwick, RI 02886
Phone: 401-737-7000
Fax: 401-736-1000
E-mail: info@kentri.org
URL: www.kentri.org
Type: Acute Care Hospitals
Emergency Services: Yes
Ownership: Voluntary Non-Profit - Other
Beds: 359

Key Personnel:
CEO/President. . . . . Sandra L. Coletta
Patient Relations . . . . Mary Ann Glynn, RN, MBA

Measure	Cases	This Hosp.	State Avg.	U.S. Avg.
Heart Attack Care				
ACE Inhibitor or ARB for LVSD[1]	11	100%	98%	96%
Aspirin at Arrival	184	97%	99%	99%
Aspirin at Discharge	123	98%	99%	98%
Beta Blocker at Discharge	122	99%	99%	98%
Fibrinolytic Medication Timing	0	-	0%	55%
PCI Within 90 Minutes of Arrival	0	-	91%	90%
Smoking Cessation Advice[1]	23	96%	99%	99%
Chest Pain/Possible Heart Attack Care				
Aspirin at Arrival	104	95%	94%	95%
Median Time to ECG (minutes)	109	5	7	8
Median Time to Transfer (minutes)	43	57	67	61
Fibrinolytic Medication Timing	0	-	88%	54%
Heart Failure Care				
ACE Inhibitor or ARB for LVSD	98	94%	94%	94%
Discharge Instructions	348	78%	85%	88%
Evaluation of LVS Function	529	99%	98%	98%
Smoking Cessation Advice	67	91%	98%	98%
Pneumonia Care				
Appropriate Initial Antibiotic[2]	158	86%	92%	92%
Blood Culture Timing[2]	273	89%	95%	96%
Influenza Vaccine[2]	150	67%	85%	91%
Initial Antibiotic Timing[2]	236	94%	95%	95%
Pneumococcal Vaccine[2]	243	85%	86%	93%
Smoking Cessation Advice[2]	99	93%	97%	97%
Surgical Care Improvement Project				
Appropriate VTP Within 24 Hours[2]	436	93%	94%	92%
Appropriate Hair Removal[2]	721	99%	100%	99%
Appropriate Beta Blocker Usage[2]	230	90%	94%	93%
Controlled Postoperative Blood Glucose[2]	0	-	94%	93%
Prophylactic Antibiotic Timing[2]	460	93%	97%	97%
Prophylactic Antibiotic Timing (Outpatient)	262	90%	94%	92%
Prophylactic Antibiotic Selection[2]	464	98%	98%	97%
Prophylactic Antibiotic Select. (Outpatient)	255	95%	96%	94%
Prophylactic Antibiotic Stopped[2]	445	92%	96%	94%
Recommended VTP Ordered[2]	437	94%	95%	94%
Urinary Catheter Removal	184	82%	86%	90%
Children's Asthma Care				
Received Systemic Corticosteroids	-	-	-	100%
Received Home Management Plan	-	-	-	71%
Received Reliever Medication	-	-	-	100%
Use of Medical Imaging				
Combination Abdominal CT Scan	655	0.082	0.091	0.191
Combination Chest CT Scan	428	0.040	0.024	0.054
Follow-up Mammogram/Ultrasound	1,185	11.5%	9.3%	8.4%
MRI for Low Back Pain	106	28.3%	31.8%	32.7%
Survey of Patients' Hospital Experiences				
Area Around Room 'Always' Quiet at Night	300+	46%	-	58%
Doctors 'Always' Communicated Well	300+	75%	-	80%
Home Recovery Information Given	300+	81%	-	82%
Hospital Given 9 or 10 on 10 Point Scale	300+	58%	-	67%
Meds 'Always' Explained Before Given	300+	53%	-	60%
Nurses 'Always' Communicated Well	300+	74%	-	76%
Pain 'Always' Well Controlled	300+	69%	-	69%
Room and Bathroom 'Always' Clean	300+	66%	-	71%
Timely Help 'Always' Received	300+	62%	-	64%
Would Definitely Recommend Hospital	300+	60%	-	69%

Westerly Hospital

25 Wells Street
Westerly, RI 02891
Phone: 401-596-6000
Fax: 401-348-3714
Type: Acute Care Hospitals
Emergency Services: Yes
Ownership: Voluntary Non-Profit - Private
Beds: 125

Key Personnel:
CEO/President. . . . . Charles S Kinney

Measure	Cases	This Hosp.	State Avg.	U.S. Avg.
Heart Attack Care				
ACE Inhibitor or ARB for LVSD[1]	2	100%	98%	96%
Aspirin at Arrival[1]	21	90%	99%	99%
Aspirin at Discharge[1]	15	93%	99%	98%
Beta Blocker at Discharge[1]	12	100%	99%	98%
Fibrinolytic Medication Timing	0	-	0%	55%
PCI Within 90 Minutes of Arrival	0	-	91%	90%
Smoking Cessation Advice[1]	6	83%	99%	99%
Chest Pain/Possible Heart Attack Care				
Aspirin at Arrival	51	98%	94%	95%
Median Time to ECG (minutes)	51	10	7	8
Median Time to Transfer (minutes)[1]	9	80	67	61
Fibrinolytic Medication Timing[1]	6	100%	88%	54%
Heart Failure Care				
ACE Inhibitor or ARB for LVSD	51	92%	94%	94%
Discharge Instructions	122	72%	85%	88%
Evaluation of LVS Function	180	96%	98%	98%
Smoking Cessation Advice	25	96%	98%	98%
Pneumonia Care				
Appropriate Initial Antibiotic	99	88%	92%	92%
Blood Culture Timing	91	98%	95%	96%
Influenza Vaccine	77	79%	85%	91%
Initial Antibiotic Timing	151	95%	95%	95%
Pneumococcal Vaccine	139	69%	86%	93%
Smoking Cessation Advice	27	96%	97%	97%
Surgical Care Improvement Project				
Appropriate VTP Within 24 Hours	114	85%	94%	92%
Appropriate Hair Removal	338	99%	100%	99%
Appropriate Beta Blocker Usage	117	83%	94%	93%
Controlled Postoperative Blood Glucose	0	-	94%	93%
Prophylactic Antibiotic Timing	232	97%	97%	97%
Prophylactic Antibiotic Timing (Outpatient)	80	99%	94%	92%
Prophylactic Antibiotic Selection	232	97%	98%	97%
Prophylactic Antibiotic Select. (Outpatient)	80	100%	96%	94%
Prophylactic Antibiotic Stopped	227	96%	96%	94%
Recommended VTP Ordered	114	91%	95%	94%
Urinary Catheter Removal	93	94%	86%	90%
Children's Asthma Care				
Received Systemic Corticosteroids	-	-	-	100%
Received Home Management Plan	-	-	-	71%
Received Reliever Medication	-	-	-	100%
Use of Medical Imaging				
Combination Abdominal CT Scan	684	0.079	0.091	0.191
Combination Chest CT Scan	566	0.004	0.024	0.054
Follow-up Mammogram/Ultrasound	1,029	13.5%	9.3%	8.4%
MRI for Low Back Pain	141	31.2%	31.8%	32.7%
Survey of Patients' Hospital Experiences				
Area Around Room 'Always' Quiet at Night	300+	54%	-	58%
Doctors 'Always' Communicated Well	300+	82%	-	80%
Home Recovery Information Given	300+	80%	-	82%
Hospital Given 9 or 10 on 10 Point Scale	300+	68%	-	67%
Meds 'Always' Explained Before Given	300+	60%	-	60%
Nurses 'Always' Communicated Well	300+	77%	-	76%
Pain 'Always' Well Controlled	300+	76%	-	69%
Room and Bathroom 'Always' Clean	300+	83%	-	71%
Timely Help 'Always' Received	300+	66%	-	64%
Would Definitely Recommend Hospital	300+	73%	-	69%

Landmark Medical Center

115 Cass Ave
Woonsocket, RI 02895
Phone: 401-769-4100
Fax: 401-767-1674
URL: www.landmarkmedical.org
Type: Acute Care Hospitals
Emergency Services: Yes
Ownership: Voluntary Non-Profit - Private
Beds: 233

Key Personnel:
CEO/President. . . . . Gary J Gaube
Chief of Medical Staff. . . . . Edward Anderson
Coronary Care . . . . Patricia Bibeault, RN
Infection Control. . . . . Isabelle Reis, RN
Pediatric Ambulatory Care . . . . . . Richard Smith, MD
Pediatric In-Patient Care . . . . Richard Smith, MD
Quality Assurance . . . . Linda Kissick
Radiology. . . . . Vincent A DeCesaris

Measure	Cases	This Hosp.	State Avg.	U.S. Avg.
Heart Attack Care				
ACE Inhibitor or ARB for LVSD[1]	20	100%	98%	96%
Aspirin at Arrival	143	99%	99%	99%
Aspirin at Discharge	111	98%	99%	98%
Beta Blocker at Discharge	112	97%	99%	98%
Fibrinolytic Medication Timing	0	-	0%	55%
PCI Within 90 Minutes of Arrival[1]	23	100%	91%	90%
Smoking Cessation Advice	31	97%	99%	99%
Chest Pain/Possible Heart Attack Care				
Aspirin at Arrival	30	97%	94%	95%
Median Time to ECG (minutes)	31	4	7	8
Median Time to Transfer (minutes)[1,3]	1	37	67	61
Fibrinolytic Medication Timing[3]	0	-	88%	54%
Heart Failure Care				
ACE Inhibitor or ARB for LVSD	79	99%	94%	94%
Discharge Instructions	206	92%	85%	88%
Evaluation of LVS Function	319	99%	98%	98%
Smoking Cessation Advice	50	100%	98%	98%
Pneumonia Care				
Appropriate Initial Antibiotic	116	96%	92%	92%
Blood Culture Timing	168	98%	95%	96%
Influenza Vaccine	133	92%	85%	91%
Initial Antibiotic Timing	199	98%	95%	95%
Pneumococcal Vaccine	172	87%	86%	93%
Smoking Cessation Advice	66	97%	97%	97%
Surgical Care Improvement Project				
Appropriate VTP Within 24 Hours	137	94%	94%	92%
Appropriate Hair Removal	283	100%	100%	99%
Appropriate Beta Blocker Usage	86	90%	94%	93%
Controlled Postoperative Blood Glucose	0	-	94%	93%
Prophylactic Antibiotic Timing	179	98%	97%	97%
Prophylactic Antibiotic Timing (Outpatient)	155	94%	94%	92%
Prophylactic Antibiotic Selection	182	96%	98%	97%
Prophylactic Antibiotic Select. (Outpatient)	153	94%	96%	94%
Prophylactic Antibiotic Stopped	161	96%	96%	94%
Recommended VTP Ordered	138	97%	95%	94%
Urinary Catheter Removal	32	69%	86%	90%
Children's Asthma Care				
Received Systemic Corticosteroids	-	-	-	100%
Received Home Management Plan	-	-	-	71%
Received Reliever Medication	-	-	-	100%
Use of Medical Imaging				
Combination Abdominal CT Scan	491	0.071	0.091	0.191
Combination Chest CT Scan	272	0.018	0.024	0.054
Follow-up Mammogram/Ultrasound	746	5.1%	9.3%	8.4%
MRI for Low Back Pain	91	37.4%	31.8%	32.7%
Survey of Patients' Hospital Experiences				
Area Around Room 'Always' Quiet at Night	300+	41%	-	58%
Doctors 'Always' Communicated Well	300+	75%	-	80%
Home Recovery Information Given	300+	83%	-	82%
Hospital Given 9 or 10 on 10 Point Scale	300+	52%	-	67%
Meds 'Always' Explained Before Given	300+	54%	-	60%
Nurses 'Always' Communicated Well	300+	69%	-	76%
Pain 'Always' Well Controlled	300+	65%	-	69%
Room and Bathroom 'Always' Clean	300+	65%	-	71%
Timely Help 'Always' Received	300+	57%	-	64%
Would Definitely Recommend Hospital	300+	53%	-	69%

NOTE: Hospital profiles are in alphabetical order by state, then city, then hospital within the city; Rankings exclude hospitals with less than 25 cases except for patient surveys which excludes hospitals with less than 100 cases; (a) 100–299 cases; (1) The number of cases is too small to be sure how well a hospital is performing; (2) The hospital indicated that the data submitted for this measure were based on a sample of cases; (3) Data was collected during a shorter time period (fewer quarters) than the maximum possible time for this measure; (4) Suppressed for one or more quarters by CMS; (5) No data is available from the hospital for this measure; (6) Fewer than 100 patients completed the HCAHPS survey. Use these rates with caution, as the number of surveys may be too low to reliably assess hospital performance; (7) Survey results are based on less than 12 months of data; (8) Survey results are not available for this reporting period; (9) No or very few patients were eligible for the HCAHPS survey. The scores shown, if any, reflect a very small number of surveys; (10) A state average was not calculated because too few hospitals in the state submitted data; (11) There were discrepancies in the data collection process; Please refer to the User's Guide for a full explanation of data.

Heart Attack Care

1. ACE Inhibitor or ARB for LVSD

Hospital Name	City	Rate	Cases
Centennial Medical Center	Nashville	100%	104
Erlanger Medical Center	Chattanooga	100%	52
Fort Sanders Regional Medical Center	Knoxville	100%	53
Memorial Healthcare System	Chattanooga	100%	122
Methodist Medical Center of Oak Ridge	Oak Ridge	100%	64
Saint Francis Hospital	Memphis	100%	39
VA Middle Tennessee Healthcare System	Nashville	100%	40
Vanderbilt University Hospital[2]	Nashville	100%	53
Baptist Memorial Hospital	Memphis	99%	117
Methodist Healthcare Memphis Hospitals	Memphis	99%	182
University of Tennessee Memorial Hospital[2]	Knoxville	98%	62
Wellmont Holston Valley Medical Center[2]	Kingsport	98%	60
Regional Hospital of Jackson	Jackson	97%	34
Baptist Hospital	Nashville	96%	51
Cookeville Regional Medical Center	Cookeville	96%	143
Gateway Medical Center	Clarksville	95%	37
Mercy Medical Center	Knoxville	95%	111
Parkwest Medical Center	Knoxville	95%	84
Saint Thomas Hospital	Nashville	95%	283
Blount Memorial Hospital[2]	Maryville	94%	32
Middle Tennessee Medical Center	Murfreesboro	94%	34
Maury Regional Hospital	Columbia	93%	88
Johnson City Medical Center[2]	Johnson City	92%	51
Wellmont Bristol Regional Medical Center[2]	Bristol	92%	49
Jackson-Madison County General Hospital[2]	Jackson	91%	194

2. Aspirin at Arrival

Hospital Name	City	Rate	Cases
Centennial Medical Center	Nashville	100%	141
Fort Sanders Regional Medical Center	Knoxville	100%	166
Harton Regional Medical Center	Tullahoma	100%	59
Hendersonville Medical Center	Hendersonville	100%	42
Indian Path Medical Center[2]	Kingsport	100%	46
Memphis VA Medical Center	Memphis	100%	68
Methodist Healthcare Memphis Hospitals	Memphis	100%	741
Mountain Home VA Medical Center	Mountain Home	100%	79
Northcrest Medical Center	Springfield	100%	56
Parkridge Medical Center	Chattanooga	100%	111
Saint Francis Bartlett Medical Center	Bartlett	100%	26
Skyline Medical Center	Nashville	100%	152
Stonecrest Medical Center	Smyrna	100%	27
Summit Medical Center	Hermitage	100%	112
University of Tennessee Memorial Hospital[2]	Knoxville	100%	212
Baptist Hospital	Nashville	99%	199
Blount Memorial Hospital[2]	Maryville	99%	191
Cookeville Regional Medical Center	Cookeville	99%	320
Erlanger Medical Center	Chattanooga	99%	234
Gateway Medical Center	Clarksville	99%	180
Memorial Healthcare System	Chattanooga	99%	530
Mercy Medical Center	Knoxville	99%	337
Methodist Medical Center of Oak Ridge	Oak Ridge	99%	191
Morristown Hamblen Hospital Association	Morristown	99%	195
Parkwest Medical Center	Knoxville	99%	333
Saint Thomas Hospital	Nashville	99%	423
Southern Hills Medical Center	Nashville	99%	78
VA Middle Tennessee Healthcare System	Nashville	99%	142
Vanderbilt University Hospital[2]	Nashville	99%	148
Baptist Memorial Hospital	Memphis	98%	519
Horizon Medical Center	Dickson	98%	48
Johnson City Medical Center[2]	Johnson City	98%	140
Maury Regional Hospital	Columbia	98%	199
Saint Francis Hospital	Memphis	98%	248
Skyridge Medical Center	Cleveland	98%	94
Sumner Regional Medical Center	Gallatin	98%	111
Wellmont Bristol Regional Medical Center[2]	Bristol	98%	183
Wellmont Holston Valley Medical Center[2]	Kingsport	98%	124
Williamson Medical Center	Franklin	98%	137
Middle Tennessee Medical Center	Murfreesboro	97%	212
University Medical Center	Lebanon	97%	37
Regional Hospital of Jackson	Jackson	96%	52
Cumberland Medical Center	Crossville	95%	40
Jackson-Madison County General Hospital[2]	Jackson	95%	553
Metro Nashville General Hospital[2]	Nashville	93%	90
Regional Medical Center at Memphis	Memphis	91%	46
Southern Tennessee Medical Center	Winchester	89%	28

3. Aspirin at Discharge

Hospital Name	City	Rate	Cases
Centennial Medical Center	Nashville	100%	555
Cumberland Medical Center	Crossville	100%	30
Erlanger Medical Center	Chattanooga	100%	391
Fort Sanders Regional Medical Center	Knoxville	100%	302
Harton Regional Medical Center	Tullahoma	100%	52
Hendersonville Medical Center	Hendersonville	100%	48
Horizon Medical Center	Dickson	100%	37
Indian Path Medical Center[2]	Kingsport	100%	42
Memorial Healthcare System	Chattanooga	100%	746
Memphis VA Medical Center	Memphis	100%	65
Methodist Healthcare Memphis Hospitals	Memphis	100%	950
Mountain Home VA Medical Center	Mountain Home	100%	62
Northcrest Medical Center	Springfield	100%	42
Parkridge Medical Center	Chattanooga	100%	230
Parkwest Medical Center	Knoxville	100%	506
Skyridge Medical Center	Cleveland	100%	47
Summit Medical Center	Hermitage	100%	95
Vanderbilt University Hospital[2]	Nashville	100%	359
Wellmont Bristol Regional Medical Center[2]	Bristol	100%	267
Wellmont Holston Valley Medical Center[2]	Kingsport	100%	259
Baptist Hospital	Nashville	99%	235
Blount Memorial Hospital[2]	Maryville	99%	177
Cookeville Regional Medical Center	Cookeville	99%	522
Johnson City Medical Center[2]	Johnson City	99%	284
Maury Regional Hospital	Columbia	99%	267
Mercy Medical Center	Knoxville	99%	559
Middle Tennessee Medical Center	Murfreesboro	99%	190
Saint Thomas Hospital	Nashville	99%	1322
Skyline Medical Center	Nashville	99%	127
University of Tennessee Memorial Hospital[2]	Knoxville	99%	316
VA Middle Tennessee Healthcare System	Nashville	99%	136
Baptist Memorial Hospital	Memphis	98%	692
Methodist Medical Center of Oak Ridge	Oak Ridge	98%	281
Morristown Hamblen Hospital Association	Morristown	98%	202
Regional Medical Center at Memphis	Memphis	98%	43
Saint Francis Hospital	Memphis	98%	292
Williamson Medical Center	Franklin	98%	133
Jackson-Madison County General Hospital[2]	Jackson	96%	994
Metro Nashville General Hospital[2]	Nashville	95%	87
Regional Hospital of Jackson	Jackson	95%	164
Southern Hills Medical Center	Nashville	95%	58
Gateway Medical Center	Clarksville	94%	188
Sumner Regional Medical Center	Gallatin	94%	101

4. Beta Blocker at Discharge

Hospital Name	City	Rate	Cases
Baptist Hospital	Nashville	100%	237
Blount Memorial Hospital[2]	Maryville	100%	170
Centennial Medical Center	Nashville	100%	528
Erlanger Medical Center	Chattanooga	100%	354
Fort Sanders Regional Medical Center	Knoxville	100%	287
Harton Regional Medical Center	Tullahoma	100%	51
Hendersonville Medical Center	Hendersonville	100%	47
Horizon Medical Center	Dickson	100%	34
Indian Path Medical Center[2]	Kingsport	100%	45
Memorial Healthcare System	Chattanooga	100%	705
Memphis VA Medical Center	Memphis	100%	61
Methodist Healthcare Memphis Hospitals	Memphis	100%	941
Mountain Home VA Medical Center	Mountain Home	100%	61
Northcrest Medical Center	Springfield	100%	43
Parkridge Medical Center	Chattanooga	100%	218
Saint Francis Hospital	Memphis	100%	289
Skyline Medical Center	Nashville	100%	124
VA Middle Tennessee Healthcare System	Nashville	100%	139
Wellmont Bristol Regional Medical Center[2]	Bristol	100%	262
Wellmont Holston Valley Medical Center[2]	Kingsport	100%	257
Cookeville Regional Medical Center	Cookeville	99%	514
Mercy Medical Center	Knoxville	99%	554
Methodist Medical Center of Oak Ridge	Oak Ridge	99%	269
Metro Nashville General Hospital[2]	Nashville	99%	82
Parkwest Medical Center	Knoxville	99%	505
University of Tennessee Memorial Hospital[2]	Knoxville	99%	321
Vanderbilt University Hospital[2]	Nashville	99%	349
Williamson Medical Center	Franklin	99%	128
Baptist Memorial Hospital	Memphis	98%	654
Maury Regional Hospital	Columbia	98%	254
Middle Tennessee Medical Center	Murfreesboro	98%	178
Saint Thomas Hospital	Nashville	98%	1283
Skyridge Medical Center	Cleveland	98%	52
Summit Medical Center	Hermitage	98%	97
Cumberland Medical Center	Crossville	97%	31
Johnson City Medical Center[2]	Johnson City	97%	280
Morristown Hamblen Hospital Association	Morristown	97%	209
Regional Hospital of Jackson	Jackson	96%	152
Southern Hills Medical Center	Nashville	96%	69
Jackson-Madison County General Hospital[2]	Jackson	95%	967
Regional Medical Center at Memphis	Memphis	95%	40
Sumner Regional Medical Center	Gallatin	95%	99
Gateway Medical Center	Clarksville	94%	194

6. PCI Within 90 Minutes of Arrival

Hospital Name	City	Rate	Cases
Baptist Hospital	Nashville	100%	25
Methodist Medical Center of Oak Ridge	Oak Ridge	100%	51
Skyline Medical Center	Nashville	100%	33
Summit Medical Center	Hermitage	100%	25
Wellmont Bristol Regional Medical Center[2]	Bristol	100%	26
Methodist Healthcare Memphis Hospitals	Memphis	99%	155
Fort Sanders Regional Medical Center	Knoxville	98%	57
Saint Thomas Hospital	Nashville	98%	65
Morristown Hamblen Hospital Association	Morristown	96%	51
Maury Regional Hospital	Columbia	94%	36
Blount Memorial Hospital[2]	Maryville	93%	43
Erlanger Medical Center	Chattanooga	92%	72
Parkwest Medical Center	Knoxville	92%	78
Cookeville Regional Medical Center	Cookeville	89%	82
Johnson City Medical Center[2]	Johnson City	89%	27
University of Tennessee Memorial Hospital[2]	Knoxville	89%	61
Saint Francis Hospital	Memphis	86%	44
Williamson Medical Center	Franklin	86%	44
Jackson-Madison County General Hospital[2]	Jackson	85%	72
Memorial Healthcare System	Chattanooga	85%	104
Middle Tennessee Medical Center	Murfreesboro	82%	49
Mercy Medical Center	Knoxville	81%	48
Baptist Memorial Hospital	Memphis	80%	44
Gateway Medical Center	Clarksville	76%	45

7. Smoking Cessation Advice

Hospital Name	City	Rate	Cases
Baptist Hospital	Nashville	100%	87
Baptist Memorial Hospital	Memphis	100%	214
Blount Memorial Hospital[2]	Maryville	100%	62
Centennial Medical Center	Nashville	100%	250
Cookeville Regional Medical Center	Cookeville	100%	219
Erlanger Medical Center	Chattanooga	100%	208
Fort Sanders Regional Medical Center	Knoxville	100%	120
Gateway Medical Center	Clarksville	100%	104
Johnson City Medical Center[2]	Johnson City	100%	112
Maury Regional Hospital	Columbia	100%	124
Memorial Healthcare System	Chattanooga	100%	240
Memphis VA Medical Center	Memphis	100%	28
Mercy Medical Center	Knoxville	100%	255
Methodist Healthcare Memphis Hospitals	Memphis	100%	435
Methodist Medical Center of Oak Ridge	Oak Ridge	100%	118
Metro Nashville General Hospital[2]	Nashville	100%	48
Middle Tennessee Medical Center	Murfreesboro	100%	90
Parkridge Medical Center	Chattanooga	100%	117
Parkwest Medical Center	Knoxville	100%	212
Regional Hospital of Jackson	Jackson	100%	76
Regional Medical Center at Memphis	Memphis	100%	32
Saint Francis Hospital	Memphis	100%	96
Saint Thomas Hospital	Nashville	100%	472
Skyline Medical Center	Nashville	100%	52
Southern Hills Medical Center	Nashville	100%	36
Summit Medical Center	Hermitage	100%	32
Sumner Regional Medical Center	Gallatin	100%	48
University of Tennessee Memorial Hospital[2]	Knoxville	100%	156
VA Middle Tennessee Healthcare System	Nashville	100%	57
Vanderbilt University Hospital[2]	Nashville	100%	144
Wellmont Bristol Regional Medical Center[2]	Bristol	100%	117
Wellmont Holston Valley Medical Center[2]	Kingsport	100%	104
Williamson Medical Center	Franklin	100%	47
Jackson-Madison County General Hospital[2]	Jackson	99%	436
Morristown Hamblen Hospital Association	Morristown	99%	95

Chest Pain/Possible Heart Attack Care

8. Aspirin at Arrival

Hospital Name	City	Rate	Cases
Centennial Medical Center of Ashland City	Ashland City	100%	107
Dyersburg Regional Medical Center	Dyersburg	100%	207
Fort Loudoun Medical Center	Lenoir City	100%	56
Henderson County Community Hospital	Lexington	100%	116
Hendersonville Medical Center	Hendersonville	100%	40
Jamestown Regional Medical Center	Jamestown	100%	92
Livingston Regional Hospital	Livingston	100%	69
Saint Francis Bartlett Medical Center	Bartlett	100%	60
Scott County Hospital	Oneida	100%	120
Southern Hills Medical Center	Nashville	100%	31
Summit Medical Center	Hermitage	100%	70
Athens Regional Medical Center	Athens	99%	203
Cumberland Medical Center	Crossville	99%	123
McKenzie Regional Hospital	McKenzie	99%	142
Skyline Medical Center	Nashville	99%	72
Stonecrest Medical Center	Smyrna	99%	109
Unicoi County Memorial Hospital	Erwin	99%	153
Baptist Memorial Hospital Union City	Union City	98%	157
Crockett Hospital	Lawrenceburg	98%	240
Gateway Medical Center	Clarksville	98%	124
Leconte Medical Center	Sevierville	98%	194
Parkridge Medical Center	Chattanooga	98%	65
Riverview Regional Medical Center North	Carthage	98%	125
Skyridge Medical Center	Cleveland	98%	91
Takoma Regional Hospital	Greeneville	98%	65
Woods Memorial Hospital	Etowah	98%	43
Bolivar General Hospital	Bolivar	97%	86
Decatur County General Hospital	Parsons	97%	124

NOTE: Hospital profiles are in alphabetical order by state, then city, then hospital within the city; Rankings exclude hospitals with less than 25 cases except for patient surveys which excludes hospitals with less than 100 cases; (a) 100–299 cases; (1) The number of cases is too small to be sure how well a hospital is performing; (2) The hospital indicated that the data submitted for this measure were based on a sample of cases; (3) Data was collected during a shorter time period (fewer quarters) than the maximum possible time for this measure; (4) Suppressed for one or more quarters by CMS; (5) No data is available from the hospital for this measure; (6) Fewer than 100 patients completed the HCAHPS survey. Use these rates with caution, as the number of surveys may be too low to reliably assess hospital performance; (7) Survey results are based on less than 12 months of data; (8) Survey results are not available for this reporting period; (9) No or very few patients were eligible for the HCAHPS survey. The scores shown, if any, reflect a very small number of surveys; (10) A state average was not calculated because too few hospitals in the state submitted data; (11) There were discrepancies in the data collection process; Please refer to the User's Guide for a full explanation of data.

Grandview Medical Center	Jasper	97%	210
Hardin Medical Center	Savannah	97%	324
Heritage Medical Center	Shelbyville	97%	155
Horizon Medical Center	Dickson	97%	159
Laughlin Memorial Hospital	Greeneville	97%	299
McNairy Regional Hospital	Selmer	97%	140
Methodist Healthcare Fayette Hospital	Somerville	97%	97
Saint Mary's Jefferson Memorial Hospital	Jefferson City	97%	191
Southern Tennessee Medical Center	Winchester	97%	213
Sweetwater Hospital Association	Sweetwater	97%	144
Volunteer Community Hospital	Martin	97%	276
Williamson Medical Center	Franklin	97%	33
Baptist Hospital of Cocke County	Newport	96%	315
Cookeville Regional Medical Center	Cookeville	96%	27
Haywood Park Community Hospital	Brownsville	96%	105
Henry County Medical Center	Paris	96%	219
Lincoln Medical Center	Fayetteville	96%	322
Roane Medical Center	Harriman	96%	180
Sumner Regional Medical Center	Gallatin	96%	48
University Medical Center	Lebanon	96%	95
White County Community Hospital	Sparta	96%	47
River Park Hospital	McMinnville	95%	163
St Mary's Med Ctr of Campbell County	La Follette	95%	136
Gibson General Hospital	Trenton	94%	70
Harton Regional Medical Center	Tullahoma	94%	65
Hillside Hospital	Pulaski	94%	281
Indian Path Medical Center	Kingsport	94%	34
Johnson County Community Hospital	Mountain City	94%	138
Lauderdale Community Hospital[3]	Ripley	94%	81
Memorial Healthcare System	Chattanooga	94%	33
Stones River Hosp & Dekalb Comm Hosp	Woodbury	94%	48
Stones River Hosp/Dekalb Comm Hosp	Smithville	94%	99
Macon County General Hospital	Lafayette	93%	71
Milan General Hospital	Milan	93%	123
Baptist Memorial Hospital Huntingdon	Huntingdon	92%	104
Jellico Community Hospital	Jellico	92%	71
Maury Regional Hospital	Columbia	92%	48
Northcrest Medical Center	Springfield	91%	34
Wayne Medical Center	Waynesboro	91%	53
Wellmont Hawkins County Memorial Hospital	Rogersville	91%	121
Baptist Memorial Hospital Tipton	Covington	90%	185
Claiborne County Hospital	Tazewell	90%	130
Franklin Woods Community Hospital	Johnson City	87%	135
Sycamore Shoals Hospital	Elizabethton	87%	157
Humboldt General Hospital	Humboldt	86%	90
Rhea Medical Center	Dayton	86%	159
Perry Community Hospital	Linden	85%	41
Medical Center of Manchester	Manchester	84%	81
Middle Tennessee Medical Center	Murfreesboro	84%	75
Copper Basin Medical Center	Copperhill	83%	75
United Regional Medical Center	Manchester	55%	51

9. Median Time to ECG (minutes)

Hospital Name	City	Min.	Cases
Methodist Healthcare Fayette Hospital	Somerville	0	100
Dyersburg Regional Medical Center	Dyersburg	1	218
Henderson County Community Hospital	Lexington	2	130
Memorial Healthcare System	Chattanooga	2	31
Baptist Memorial Hospital Union City	Union City	4	164
Franklin Woods Community Hospital	Johnson City	4	145
Gateway Medical Center	Clarksville	4	129
Haywood Park Community Hospital	Brownsville	4	108
Heritage Medical Center	Shelbyville	4	162
Indian Path Medical Center	Kingsport	4	35
Livingston Regional Hospital	Livingston	4	81
River Park Hospital	McMinnville	4	173
Skyline Medical Center	Nashville	4	73
Summit Medical Center	Hermitage	4	72
Sumner Regional Medical Center	Gallatin	4	52
Athens Regional Medical Center	Athens	5	210
Cookeville Regional Medical Center	Cookeville	5	25
Crockett Hospital	Lawrenceburg	5	250
Hendersonville Medical Center	Hendersonville	5	45
Hillside Hospital	Pulaski	5	292
Jamestown Regional Medical Center	Jamestown	5	99
Lincoln Medical Center	Fayetteville	5	334
Maury Regional Hospital	Columbia	5	53
Stonecrest Medical Center	Smyrna	5	119
Decatur County General Hospital	Parsons	6	137
Harton Regional Medical Center	Tullahoma	6	66
Henry County Medical Center	Paris	6	217
Horizon Medical Center	Dickson	6	170
McNairy Regional Hospital	Selmer	6	150
Parkridge Medical Center	Chattanooga	6	71
St Mary's Med Ctr of Campbell County	La Follette	6	152
Scott County Hospital	Oneida	6	131
Sweetwater Hospital Association	Sweetwater	6	152
Williamson Medical Center	Franklin	6	36
Baptist Memorial Hospital Huntingdon	Huntingdon	7	113
Northcrest Medical Center	Springfield	7	36
Rhea Medical Center	Dayton	7	167
Roane Medical Center	Harriman	7	190
Southern Hills Medical Center	Nashville	7	33
Southern Tennessee Medical Center	Winchester	7	225
Stones River Hosp & Dekalb Comm Hosp	Woodbury	7	51
University Medical Center	Lebanon	7	99
Centennial Medical Center of Ashland City	Ashland City	8	120
Fort Loudoun Medical Center	Lenoir City	8	58
McKenzie Regional Hospital	McKenzie	8	154
Riverview Regional Medical Center North	Carthage	8	138
Stones River Hosp/Dekalb Comm Hosp	Smithville	8	105
Unicoi County Memorial Hospital	Erwin	8	165
Hardin Medical Center	Savannah	9	345
Lauderdale Community Hospital[3]	Ripley	9	81
Leconte Medical Center	Sevierville	9	198
Perry Community Hospital	Linden	9	55
Claiborne County Hospital	Tazewell	10	137
Jellico Community Hospital	Jellico	10	73
Laughlin Memorial Hospital	Greeneville	10	316
Macon County General Hospital	Lafayette	10	72
Middle Tennessee Medical Center	Murfreesboro	10	60
Skyridge Medical Center	Cleveland	10	95
Takoma Regional Hospital	Greeneville	10	71
White County Community Hospital	Sparta	10	47
Morristown Hamblen Hospital Association	Morristown	11	25
Woods Memorial Hospital	Etowah	11	45
Grandview Medical Center	Jasper	12	229
Milan General Hospital	Milan	12	138
Volunteer Community Hospital	Martin	12	294
Wellmont Hawkins County Memorial Hospital	Rogersville	12	122
Cumberland Medical Center	Crossville	13	122
Johnson County Community Hospital	Mountain City	13	149
Wayne Medical Center	Waynesboro	13	57
Medical Center of Manchester	Manchester	14	84
Saint Francis Bartlett Medical Center	Bartlett	14	63
Saint Mary's Jefferson Memorial Hospital	Jefferson City	14	195
Bolivar General Hospital	Bolivar	15	102
Baptist Hospital of Cocke County	Newport	17	334
Baptist Memorial Hospital Tipton	Covington	20	198
Copper Basin Medical Center	Copperhill	21	77
Gibson General Hospital	Trenton	21	73
Sycamore Shoals Hospital	Elizabethton	21	165
United Regional Medical Center	Manchester	22	52
Humboldt General Hospital	Humboldt	33	93

10. Median Time to Transfer (minutes)

Hospital Name	City	Min.	Cases
Stonecrest Medical Center	Smyrna	42	28
Laughlin Memorial Hospital	Greeneville	54	25
Leconte Medical Center	Sevierville	55	31
Skyridge Medical Center	Cleveland	73	54

Heart Failure Care

12. ACE Inhibitor or ARB for LVSD

Hospital Name	City	Rate	Cases
Fort Sanders Regional Medical Center	Knoxville	100%	123
Harton Regional Medical Center	Tullahoma	100%	51
Hendersonville Medical Center	Hendersonville	100%	32
Henry County Medical Center	Paris	100%	38
Indian Path Medical Center[2]	Kingsport	100%	37
Laughlin Memorial Hospital	Greeneville	100%	34
Metro Nashville General Hospital[2]	Nashville	100%	91
Regional Medical Center at Memphis	Memphis	100%	151
Saint Francis Bartlett Medical Center	Bartlett	100%	45
Southern Hills Medical Center	Nashville	100%	32
Summit Medical Center	Hermitage	100%	64
Blount Memorial Hospital[2]	Maryville	99%	78
Mercy Medical Center	Knoxville	99%	171
Methodist Healthcare Memphis Hospitals[2]	Memphis	99%	531
Parkridge Medical Center	Chattanooga	99%	98
Skyline Medical Center	Nashville	99%	94
Dyersburg Regional Medical Center	Dyersburg	98%	51
Memorial Healthcare System	Chattanooga	98%	249
Memphis VA Medical Center	Memphis	98%	126
Methodist Medical Center of Oak Ridge	Oak Ridge	98%	93
Morristown Hamblen Hospital Association	Morristown	98%	63
Mountain Home VA Medical Center	Mountain Home	98%	53
Northcrest Medical Center	Springfield	98%	53
Saint Francis Hospital	Memphis	98%	293
Wellmont Holston Valley Medical Center[2]	Kingsport	98%	109
Williamson Medical Center	Franklin	98%	58
Erlanger Medical Center	Chattanooga	97%	133
Sycamore Shoals Hospital[2]	Elizabethton	97%	31
Baptist Memorial Hospital	Memphis	96%	448
Gateway Medical Center	Clarksville	96%	108
Horizon Medical Center	Dickson	96%	45
Leconte Medical Center	Sevierville	96%	25
University Medical Center	Lebanon	96%	25
Wellmont Hawkins County Memorial Hospital	Rogersville	96%	25
Baptist Hospital	Nashville	95%	193
Centennial Medical Center	Nashville	95%	221
Maury Regional Hospital	Columbia	95%	174
Regional Hospital of Jackson	Jackson	95%	60
Skyridge Medical Center	Cleveland	95%	61
Southern Tennessee Medical Center	Winchester	95%	38
Parkwest Medical Center	Knoxville	94%	86
Saint Thomas Hospital	Nashville	94%	399
Baptist Hospital of Cocke County	Newport	93%	27
River Park Hospital	McMinnville	93%	29
VA Middle Tennessee Healthcare System	Nashville	93%	160
Vanderbilt University Hospital[2]	Nashville	93%	150
Woods Memorial Hospital	Etowah	93%	44
Saint Mary's Jefferson Memorial Hospital	Jefferson City	92%	51
Delta Medical Center	Memphis	91%	56
Sumner Regional Medical Center	Gallatin	91%	55
Jackson-Madison County General Hospital[2]	Jackson	90%	369
Wellmont Bristol Regional Medical Center[2]	Bristol	90%	83
University of Tennessee Memorial Hospital[2]	Knoxville	89%	115
Middle Tennessee Medical Center	Murfreesboro	88%	137
Johnson City Medical Center[2]	Johnson City	87%	109
Cookeville Regional Medical Center	Cookeville	86%	138
Heritage Medical Center	Shelbyville	86%	29
Cumberland Medical Center	Crossville	82%	60
Athens Regional Medical Center	Athens	81%	32

13. Discharge Instructions

Hospital Name	City	Rate	Cases
Haywood Park Community Hospital	Brownsville	100%	35
Henderson County Community Hospital	Lexington	100%	46
Laughlin Memorial Hospital	Greeneville	100%	113
Livingston Regional Hospital	Livingston	100%	67
Mountain Home VA Medical Center	Mountain Home	100%	156
Saint Francis Bartlett Medical Center	Bartlett	100%	138
Skyline Medical Center	Nashville	100%	246
Summit Medical Center	Hermitage	100%	171
Hendersonville Medical Center	Hendersonville	99%	97
Jamestown Regional Medical Center	Jamestown	99%	83
Memphis VA Medical Center	Memphis	99%	246
Southern Hills Medical Center	Nashville	99%	109
Wellmont Holston Valley Medical Center[2]	Kingsport	99%	231
Baptist Memorial Hospital Huntingdon	Huntingdon	98%	40
Fort Sanders Regional Medical Center	Knoxville	98%	353
Jellico Community Hospital	Jellico	98%	48
St Mary's Med Ctr of Campbell County	La Follette	98%	129
Stonecrest Medical Center	Smyrna	98%	66
VA Middle Tennessee Healthcare System	Nashville	98%	347
Parkridge Medical Center	Chattanooga	97%	258
Riverview Regional Medical Center North	Carthage	97%	36
Trousdale Medical Center	Hartsville	97%	33
Copper Basin Medical Center[2]	Copperhill	96%	27
Cumberland River Hospital	Celina	96%	25
Fort Loudoun Medical Center	Lenoir City	96%	81
Gateway Medical Center	Clarksville	96%	286
Humboldt General Hospital	Humboldt	96%	25
Lakeway Regional Hospital	Morristown	96%	57
Middle Tennessee Medical Center	Murfreesboro	96%	308
Northcrest Medical Center	Springfield	96%	117
Woods Memorial Hospital	Etowah	96%	48
Dyersburg Regional Medical Center	Dyersburg	95%	197
Harton Regional Medical Center	Tullahoma	95%	164
Saint Francis Hospital	Memphis	95%	660
Centennial Medical Center	Nashville	94%	482
Delta Medical Center	Memphis	94%	149
Leconte Medical Center	Sevierville	94%	121
Methodist Healthcare Memphis Hospitals[2]	Memphis	94%	1084
Methodist Medical Center of Oak Ridge	Oak Ridge	94%	287
Takoma Regional Hospital	Greeneville	94%	49
Wellmont Bristol Regional Medical Center[2]	Bristol	94%	229
Athens Regional Medical Center	Athens	93%	82
Baptist Memorial Hospital Union City	Union City	93%	61
Hardin Medical Center	Savannah	93%	43
Maury Regional Hospital	Columbia	93%	333
McNairy Regional Hospital	Selmer	93%	44
Parkwest Medical Center	Knoxville	93%	318
Scott County Hospital	Oneida	93%	70
Southern Tennessee Medical Center	Winchester	93%	125
Sycamore Shoals Hospital[2]	Elizabethton	93%	56
Skyridge Medical Center	Cleveland	92%	205
Vanderbilt University Hospital[2]	Nashville	92%	333
Crockett Hospital	Lawrenceburg	91%	58
Horizon Medical Center	Dickson	90%	140
Regional Hospital of Jackson	Jackson	90%	162
University Medical Center	Lebanon	90%	122
White County Community Hospital	Sparta	89%	36
Blount Memorial Hospital[2]	Maryville	88%	205
Cumberland Medical Center	Crossville	88%	258
Erlanger Medical Center	Chattanooga	88%	304
Morristown Hamblen Hospital Association	Morristown	88%	245
Claiborne County Hospital[2]	Tazewell	87%	135

NOTE: Hospital profiles are in alphabetical order by state, then city, then hospital within the city; Rankings exclude hospitals with less than 25 cases except for patient surveys which excludes hospitals with less than 100 cases; (a) 100–299 cases; (1) The number of cases is too small to be sure how well a hospital is performing; (2) The hospital indicated that the data submitted for this measure were based on a sample of cases; (3) Data was collected during a shorter time period (fewer quarters) than the maximum possible time for this measure; (4) Suppressed for one or more quarters by CMS; (5) No data is available from the hospital for this measure; (6) Fewer than 100 patients completed the HCAHPS survey. Use these rates with caution, as the number of surveys may be too low to reliably assess hospital performance; (7) Survey results are based on less than 12 months of data; (8) Survey results are not available for this reporting period; (9) No or very few patients were eligible for the HCAHPS survey. The scores shown, if any, reflect a very small number of surveys; (10) A state average was not calculated because too few hospitals in the state submitted data; (11) There were discrepancies in the data collection process; Please refer to the User's Guide for a full explanation of data.

Mercy Medical Center	Knoxville	87%	487
Roane Medical Center	Harriman	87%	67
Saint Mary's Jefferson Memorial Hospital	Jefferson City	87%	109
Sumner Regional Medical Center	Gallatin	87%	154
Williamson Medical Center	Franklin	87%	167
Saint Thomas Hospital	Nashville	86%	925
University of Tennessee Memorial Hospital[2]	Knoxville	86%	276
Baptist Hospital	Nashville	85%	503
Indian Path Medical Center[2]	Kingsport	85%	130
Volunteer Community Hospital	Martin	85%	33
Baptist Memorial Hospital	Memphis	84%	1171
Memorial Healthcare System	Chattanooga	84%	663
River Park Hospital	McMinnville	83%	127
Wellmont Hawkins County Memorial Hospital	Rogersville	83%	84
Baptist Memorial Hospital Tipton	Covington	80%	45
Heritage Medical Center	Shelbyville	79%	67
Johnson City Medical Center[2]	Johnson City	79%	231
Regional Medical Center at Memphis	Memphis	79%	241
Henry County Medical Center	Paris	78%	76
Metro Nashville General Hospital[2]	Nashville	77%	174
Lincoln Medical Center	Fayetteville	74%	42
Cookeville Regional Medical Center	Cookeville	71%	300
Baptist Hospital of Cocke County	Newport	69%	59
Wayne Medical Center	Waynesboro	69%	26
Bolivar General Hospital	Bolivar	68%	25
Grandview Medical Center	Jasper	64%	28
Jackson-Madison County General Hospital[2]	Jackson	62%	720
Stones River Hosp/Dekalb Comm Hosp	Smithville	61%	51
Unicoi County Memorial Hospital	Erwin	58%	26
Sweetwater Hospital Association	Sweetwater	53%	73
Lauderdale Community Hospital	Ripley	46%	28
Perry Community Hospital[2]	Linden	10%	39
United Regional Medical Center	Manchester	3%	33

14. Evaluation of LVS Function

Hospital Name	City	Rate	Cases
Baptist Memorial Hospital	Memphis	100%	1294
Baptist Memorial Hospital Union City	Union City	100%	84
Centennial Medical Center	Nashville	100%	537
Dyersburg Regional Medical Center	Dyersburg	100%	252
Fort Loudoun Medical Center	Lenoir City	100%	92
Fort Sanders Regional Medical Center	Knoxville	100%	424
Franklin Woods Community Hospital[2]	Johnson City	100%	26
Grandview Medical Center	Jasper	100%	33
Harton Regional Medical Center	Tullahoma	100%	194
Haywood Park Community Hospital	Brownsville	100%	44
Henderson County Community Hospital	Lexington	100%	64
Hendersonville Medical Center	Hendersonville	100%	121
Hillside Hospital	Pulaski	100%	25
Horizon Medical Center	Dickson	100%	178
Jamestown Regional Medical Center	Jamestown	100%	96
Jellico Community Hospital	Jellico	100%	54
Leconte Medical Center	Sevierville	100%	133
Livingston Regional Hospital	Livingston	100%	103
Maury Regional Hospital	Columbia	100%	422
Mercy Medical Center	Knoxville	100%	589
Methodist Healthcare Memphis Hospitals[2]	Memphis	100%	1215
Metro Nashville General Hospital[2]	Nashville	100%	172
Mountain Home VA Medical Center	Mountain Home	100%	172
Parkridge Medical Center	Chattanooga	100%	323
Regional Medical Center at Memphis	Memphis	100%	254
Saint Francis Hospital	Memphis	100%	763
Stones River Hosp/Dekalb Comm Hosp	Smithville	100%	74
Sycamore Shoals Hospital[2]	Elizabethton	100%	78
Takoma Regional Hospital	Greeneville	100%	64
University of Tennessee Memorial Hospital[2]	Knoxville	100%	323
Williamson Medical Center	Franklin	100%	213
Athens Regional Medical Center	Athens	99%	101
Baptist Hospital of Cocke County	Newport	99%	69
Blount Memorial Hospital[2]	Maryville	99%	267
Erlanger Medical Center	Chattanooga	99%	341
Henry County Medical Center	Paris	99%	97
Indian Path Medical Center[2]	Kingsport	99%	164
Johnson City Medical Center[2]	Johnson City	99%	298
Laughlin Memorial Hospital	Greeneville	99%	163
Memorial Healthcare System	Chattanooga	99%	785
Memphis VA Medical Center	Memphis	99%	255
Methodist Medical Center of Oak Ridge	Oak Ridge	99%	344
Middle Tennessee Medical Center	Murfreesboro	99%	397
Morristown Hamblen Hospital Association	Morristown	99%	270
Northcrest Medical Center	Springfield	99%	140
Parkwest Medical Center	Knoxville	99%	396
Regional Hospital of Jackson	Jackson	99%	181
River Park Hospital	McMinnville	99%	161
Roane Medical Center	Harriman	99%	88
Saint Francis Bartlett Medical Center	Bartlett	99%	162
St Mary's Med Ctr of Campbell County	La Follette	99%	163
Saint Thomas Hospital	Nashville	99%	1049
Skyline Medical Center[2]	Nashville	99%	285
Skyridge Medical Center	Cleveland	99%	241

University Medical Center	Lebanon	99%	144
VA Middle Tennessee Healthcare System	Nashville	99%	361
Vanderbilt University Hospital[2]	Nashville	99%	367
Wellmont Hawkins County Memorial Hospital	Rogersville	99%	94
Baptist Hospital	Nashville	98%	574
Baptist Memorial Hospital Huntingdon	Huntingdon	98%	58
Cookeville Regional Medical Center	Cookeville	98%	350
Hardin Medical Center	Savannah	98%	64
Heritage Medical Center	Shelbyville	98%	86
Jackson-Madison County General Hospital[2]	Jackson	98%	882
Lakeway Regional Hospital	Morristown	98%	66
McNairy Regional Hospital	Selmer	98%	63
Southern Hills Medical Center	Nashville	98%	122
Stonecrest Medical Center	Smyrna	98%	84
Summit Medical Center	Hermitage	98%	212
Copper Basin Medical Center[2]	Copperhill	97%	29
Cumberland Medical Center	Crossville	97%	293
Decatur County General Hospital	Parsons	97%	31
Saint Mary's Jefferson Memorial Hospital	Jefferson City	97%	137
Southern Tennessee Medical Center	Winchester	97%	154
Wellmont Bristol Regional Medical Center[2]	Bristol	97%	274
Wellmont Holston Valley Medical Center[2]	Kingsport	97%	272
Crockett Hospital	Lawrenceburg	96%	77
Delta Medical Center	Memphis	96%	161
Rhea Medical Center	Dayton	96%	27
Volunteer Community Hospital	Martin	96%	67
Baptist Memorial Hospital Tipton	Covington	95%	62
Sumner Regional Medical Center	Gallatin	93%	194
Humboldt General Hospital	Humboldt	91%	33
Lincoln Medical Center	Fayetteville	91%	58
Scott County Hospital	Oneida	91%	69
White County Community Hospital	Sparta	91%	45
Riverview Regional Medical Center North	Carthage	90%	50
Sweetwater Hospital Association	Sweetwater	89%	91
Gateway Medical Center	Clarksville	88%	322
Lauderdale Community Hospital	Ripley	88%	40
Woods Memorial Hospital	Etowah	87%	55
Cumberland River Hospital	Celina	86%	36
Wayne Medical Center	Waynesboro	85%	34
Gibson General Hospital	Trenton	81%	27
Unicoi County Memorial Hospital	Erwin	80%	35
Trousdale Medical Center	Hartsville	77%	61
Patients' Choice Medical Center of Erin	Erin	62%	50
Bolivar General Hospital	Bolivar	59%	29
United Regional Medical Center	Manchester	42%	40
Claiborne County Hospital[2]	Tazewell	37%	175
Medical Center of Manchester	Manchester	14%	29
Perry Community Hospital[2]	Linden	2%	85

15. Smoking Cessation Advice

Hospital Name	City	Rate	Cases
Baptist Hospital	Nashville	100%	109
Baptist Memorial Hospital	Memphis	100%	229
Blount Memorial Hospital[2]	Maryville	100%	30
Centennial Medical Center	Nashville	100%	123
Claiborne County Hospital[2]	Tazewell	100%	39
Cumberland Medical Center	Crossville	100%	54
Dyersburg Regional Medical Center	Dyersburg	100%	46
Erlanger Medical Center	Chattanooga	100%	117
Fort Sanders Regional Medical Center	Knoxville	100%	73
Harton Regional Medical Center	Tullahoma	100%	34
Hendersonville Medical Center	Hendersonville	100%	25
Indian Path Medical Center[2]	Kingsport	100%	34
Jackson-Madison County General Hospital[2]	Jackson	100%	201
Johnson City Medical Center[2]	Johnson City	100%	53
Maury Regional Hospital	Columbia	100%	105
Memphis VA Medical Center	Memphis	100%	79
Methodist Healthcare Memphis Hospitals[2]	Memphis	100%	268
Methodist Medical Center of Oak Ridge	Oak Ridge	100%	57
Metro Nashville General Hospital[2]	Nashville	100%	92
Middle Tennessee Medical Center	Murfreesboro	100%	71
Mountain Home VA Medical Center	Mountain Home	100%	37
Northcrest Medical Center	Springfield	100%	30
Parkridge Medical Center	Chattanooga	100%	85
Parkwest Medical Center	Knoxville	100%	71
Regional Hospital of Jackson	Jackson	100%	39
Regional Medical Center at Memphis	Memphis	100%	118
Saint Francis Bartlett Medical Center	Bartlett	100%	27
Saint Francis Hospital	Memphis	100%	117
St Mary's Med Ctr of Campbell County	La Follette	100%	31
Saint Thomas Hospital	Nashville	100%	149
Skyline Medical Center[2]	Nashville	100%	79
Skyridge Medical Center	Cleveland	100%	53
Southern Hills Medical Center	Nashville	100%	32
Summit Medical Center	Hermitage	100%	35
University of Tennessee Memorial Hospital[2]	Knoxville	100%	64
Vanderbilt University Hospital[2]	Nashville	100%	70
Wellmont Bristol Regional Medical Center[2]	Bristol	100%	46
Gateway Medical Center	Clarksville	99%	79
Mercy Medical Center	Knoxville	99%	128

VA Middle Tennessee Healthcare System	Nashville	99%	96
Cookeville Regional Medical Center	Cookeville	98%	61
Memorial Healthcare System	Chattanooga	98%	129
River Park Hospital	McMinnville	98%	42
Wellmont Holston Valley Medical Center[2]	Kingsport	98%	57
Horizon Medical Center	Dickson	97%	33
Morristown Hamblen Hospital Association	Morristown	97%	69
Sumner Regional Medical Center	Gallatin	97%	32
Delta Medical Center	Memphis	96%	46
Trousdale Medical Center	Hartsville	93%	27

Pneumonia Care

16. Appropriate Initial Antibiotic

Hospital Name	City	Rate	Cases
Baptist Memorial Hospital Union City	Union City	100%	56
Cumberland River Hospital	Celina	100%	26
Henderson County Community Hospital	Lexington	100%	26
McKenzie Regional Hospital	McKenzie	100%	40
Memorial Healthcare System	Chattanooga	100%	411
Riverview Regional Medical Center North	Carthage	100%	58
Trousdale Medical Center	Hartsville	100%	25
Memphis VA Medical Center	Memphis	99%	99
Athens Regional Medical Center	Athens	98%	126
Delta Medical Center	Memphis	98%	40
Lakeway Regional Hospital	Morristown	98%	51
Methodist Medical Center of Oak Ridge	Oak Ridge	98%	276
Regional Medical Center at Memphis	Memphis	98%	46
Grandview Medical Center	Jasper	97%	117
Methodist Healthcare Fayette Hospital	Somerville	97%	29
Mountain Home VA Medical Center	Mountain Home	97%	91
Northcrest Medical Center	Springfield	97%	149
Parkridge Medical Center	Chattanooga	97%	171
Saint Francis Bartlett Medical Center	Bartlett	97%	206
Southern Hills Medical Center	Nashville	97%	118
Vanderbilt University Hospital[2]	Nashville	97%	39
Jamestown Regional Medical Center	Jamestown	96%	68
Leconte Medical Center	Sevierville	96%	137
Roane Medical Center	Harriman	96%	133
Sycamore Shoals Hospital[2]	Elizabethton	96%	73
Centennial Medical Center	Nashville	95%	88
Crockett Hospital	Lawrenceburg	95%	115
Hendersonville Medical Center	Hendersonville	95%	60
Henry County Medical Center	Paris	95%	111
Horizon Medical Center	Dickson	95%	133
Stones River Hosp & Dekalb Comm Hosp	Woodbury	95%	39
Takoma Regional Hospital	Greeneville	95%	96
Blount Memorial Hospital[2]	Maryville	94%	79
Fort Sanders Regional Medical Center	Knoxville	94%	198
Gateway Medical Center	Clarksville	94%	204
Heritage Medical Center	Shelbyville	94%	101
Jackson-Madison County General Hospital[2]	Jackson	94%	80
Livingston Regional Hospital	Livingston	94%	98
Saint Mary's Jefferson Memorial Hospital	Jefferson City	94%	123
St Mary's Med Ctr of Campbell County	La Follette	94%	185
Skyline Medical Center[2]	Nashville	94%	102
Stones River Hosp/Dekalb Comm Hosp	Smithville	94%	121
Williamson Medical Center	Franklin	94%	111
Fort Loudoun Medical Center[2]	Lenoir City	93%	86
Hardin Medical Center	Savannah	93%	87
Hillside Hospital	Pulaski	93%	60
Indian Path Medical Center[2]	Kingsport	93%	76
Mercy Medical Center	Knoxville	93%	469
Methodist Healthcare Memphis Hospitals[2]	Memphis	93%	289
Metro Nashville General Hospital[2]	Nashville	93%	54
Summit Medical Center	Hermitage	93%	233
Sweetwater Hospital Association	Sweetwater	93%	88
University of Tennessee Memorial Hospital[2]	Knoxville	93%	69
Baptist Memorial Hospital	Memphis	92%	451
Dyersburg Regional Medical Center	Dyersburg	92%	75
Franklin Woods Community Hospital[2]	Johnson City	92%	83
Johnson City Medical Center[2]	Johnson City	92%	72
Lincoln Medical Center	Fayetteville	92%	80
Parkwest Medical Center	Knoxville	92%	298
Regional Hospital of Jackson	Jackson	92%	62
Stonecrest Medical Center	Smyrna	92%	111
VA Middle Tennessee Healthcare System	Nashville	92%	118
Wellmont Bristol Regional Medical Center[2]	Bristol	92%	61
White County Community Hospital	Sparta	92%	73
Woods Memorial Hospital	Etowah	92%	37
Baptist Hospital	Nashville	91%	159
Baptist Memorial Hospital Tipton	Covington	91%	47
Erlanger Medical Center	Chattanooga	91%	113
Harton Regional Medical Center	Tullahoma	91%	94
Middle Tennessee Medical Center	Murfreesboro	91%	254
Saint Thomas Hospital	Nashville	91%	206
Southern Tennessee Medical Center	Winchester	91%	97
Wayne Medical Center	Waynesboro	91%	34
Rhea Medical Center	Dayton	90%	107
University Medical Center	Lebanon	90%	137

NOTE: Hospital profiles are in alphabetical order by state, then city, then hospital within the city; Rankings exclude hospitals with less than 25 cases except for patient surveys which excludes hospitals with less than 100 cases; (a) 100–299 cases; (1) The number of cases is too small to be sure how well a hospital is performing; (2) The hospital indicated that the data submitted for this measure were based on a sample of cases; (3) Data was collected during a shorter time period (fewer quarters) than the maximum possible time for this measure; (4) Suppressed for one or more quarters by CMS; (5) No data is available from the hospital for this measure; (6) Fewer than 100 patients completed the HCAHPS survey. Use these rates with caution, as the number of surveys may be too low to reliably assess hospital performance; (7) Survey results are based on less than 12 months of data; (8) Survey results are not available for this reporting period; (9) No or very few patients were eligible for the HCAHPS survey. The scores shown, if any, reflect a very small number of surveys; (10) A state average was not calculated because too few hospitals in the state submitted data; (11) There were discrepancies in the data collection process; Please refer to the User's Guide for a full explanation of data.

Wellmont Hawkins County Memorial Hospital	Rogersville	90%	129
Baptist Hospital of Cocke County	Newport	89%	142
Claiborne County Hospital[2]	Tazewell	89%	28
Decatur County General Hospital	Parsons	89%	44
Jellico Community Hospital	Jellico	89%	73
Laughlin Memorial Hospital	Greeneville	89%	161
McNairy Regional Hospital	Selmer	89%	38
Skyridge Medical Center	Cleveland	89%	253
Sumner Regional Medical Center	Gallatin	89%	135
Unicoi County Memorial Hospital	Erwin	89%	57
Volunteer Community Hospital	Martin	89%	53
Patients' Choice Medical Center of Erin	Erin	88%	33
River Park Hospital	McMinnville	88%	149
Saint Francis Hospital	Memphis	88%	108
Wellmont Holston Valley Medical Center[2]	Kingsport	88%	57
Morristown Hamblen Hospital Association	Morristown	87%	203
Baptist Memorial Hospital Huntingdon	Huntingdon	86%	28
Scott County Hospital[2]	Oneida	86%	102
Cookeville Regional Medical Center	Cookeville	85%	243
Maury Regional Hospital[2]	Columbia	85%	66
Cumberland Medical Center	Crossville	82%	272
Lauderdale Community Hospital	Ripley	81%	32
United Regional Medical Center	Manchester	77%	115
Perry Community Hospital[2]	Linden	35%	48

17. Blood Culture Timing

Hospital Name	City	Rate	Cases
Athens Regional Medical Center	Athens	100%	116
Baptist Hospital	Nashville	100%	247
Baptist Memorial Hospital Union City	Union City	100%	55
Cumberland River Hospital	Celina	100%	44
Fort Loudoun Medical Center[2]	Lenoir City	100%	127
Henderson County Community Hospital	Lexington	100%	28
Hillside Hospital	Pulaski	100%	54
Jamestown Regional Medical Center	Jamestown	100%	73
Lakeway Regional Hospital	Morristown	100%	58
Livingston Regional Hospital	Livingston	100%	128
McKenzie Regional Hospital	McKenzie	100%	49
Methodist Healthcare Fayette Hospital	Somerville	100%	33
Regional Hospital of Jackson	Jackson	100%	89
Southern Hills Medical Center	Nashville	100%	172
Volunteer Community Hospital	Martin	100%	60
Fort Sanders Regional Medical Center	Knoxville	99%	357
Hendersonville Medical Center	Hendersonville	99%	79
Horizon Medical Center	Dickson	99%	179
Memorial Healthcare System	Chattanooga	99%	724
Memphis VA Medical Center	Memphis	99%	154
Morristown Hamblen Hospital Association	Morristown	99%	288
Parkridge Medical Center	Chattanooga	99%	171
Riverview Regional Medical Center North	Carthage	99%	86
Saint Francis Bartlett Medical Center	Bartlett	99%	308
Saint Mary's Jefferson Memorial Hospital	Jefferson City	99%	153
Stonecrest Medical Center	Smyrna	99%	163
VA Middle Tennessee Healthcare System	Nashville	99%	190
White County Community Hospital	Sparta	99%	101
Baptist Memorial Hospital	Memphis	98%	530
Baptist Memorial Hospital Huntingdon	Huntingdon	98%	41
Centennial Medical Center	Nashville	98%	105
Dyersburg Regional Medical Center	Dyersburg	98%	100
Franklin Woods Community Hospital[2]	Johnson City	98%	93
Harton Regional Medical Center	Tullahoma	98%	127
Heritage Medical Center	Shelbyville	98%	93
Methodist Healthcare Memphis Hospitals[2]	Memphis	98%	453
Methodist Medical Center of Oak Ridge	Oak Ridge	98%	525
Middle Tennessee Medical Center	Murfreesboro	98%	376
Mountain Home VA Medical Center	Mountain Home	98%	143
Northcrest Medical Center	Springfield	98%	270
St Mary's Med Ctr of Campbell County	La Follette	98%	291
Scott County Hospital[2]	Oneida	98%	98
Skyline Medical Center[2]	Nashville	98%	201
Skyridge Medical Center	Cleveland	98%	280
Summit Medical Center	Hermitage	98%	290
Wellmont Bristol Regional Medical Center[2]	Bristol	98%	46
Williamson Medical Center	Franklin	98%	156
Baptist Hospital of Cocke County	Newport	97%	195
Baptist Memorial Hospital Tipton	Covington	97%	66
Claiborne County Hospital[2]	Tazewell	97%	73
Delta Medical Center	Memphis	97%	59
Grandview Medical Center	Jasper	97%	99
Laughlin Memorial Hospital	Greeneville	97%	233
Roane Medical Center	Harriman	97%	160
Sycamore Shoals Hospital[2]	Elizabethton	97%	89
Takoma Regional Hospital	Greeneville	97%	169
Cookeville Regional Medical Center	Cookeville	96%	314
Cumberland Medical Center	Crossville	96%	289
Indian Path Medical Center[2]	Kingsport	96%	110
Jellico Community Hospital	Jellico	96%	113
Lauderdale Community Hospital	Ripley	96%	28
Maury Regional Hospital[2]	Columbia	96%	112
Mercy Medical Center	Knoxville	96%	649
Parkwest Medical Center	Knoxville	96%	413
Rhea Medical Center	Dayton	96%	106
Saint Thomas Hospital	Nashville	96%	348
Southern Tennessee Medical Center	Winchester	96%	102
University Medical Center	Lebanon	96%	166
Wellmont Hancock County Hospital	Sneedville	96%	26
Blount Memorial Hospital[2]	Maryville	95%	161
Erlanger Medical Center	Chattanooga	95%	175
Gateway Medical Center	Clarksville	95%	327
Henry County Medical Center	Paris	95%	88
Lincoln Medical Center	Fayetteville	95%	106
River Park Hospital	McMinnville	95%	210
Saint Francis Hospital	Memphis	95%	172
Sumner Regional Medical Center	Gallatin	95%	187
University of Tennessee Memorial Hospital[2]	Knoxville	95%	136
Woods Memorial Hospital	Etowah	95%	92
Decatur County General Hospital	Parsons	94%	50
Leconte Medical Center	Sevierville	94%	199
Stones River Hosp/Dekalb Comm Hosp	Smithville	94%	84
Sweetwater Hospital Association	Sweetwater	94%	131
Hardin Medical Center	Savannah	93%	100
Stones River Hosp & Dekalb Comm Hosp	Woodbury	93%	27
Crockett Hospital	Lawrenceburg	92%	108
Metro Nashville General Hospital[2]	Nashville	92%	80
Vanderbilt University Hospital[2]	Nashville	92%	100
Wellmont Hawkins County Memorial Hospital	Rogersville	92%	114
Jackson-Madison County General Hospital[2]	Jackson	91%	87
Wellmont Holston Valley Medical Center[2]	Kingsport	91%	94
Unicoi County Memorial Hospital	Erwin	89%	66
Johnson City Medical Center[2]	Johnson City	87%	99
Regional Medical Center at Memphis	Memphis	86%	73
Marshall Medical Center	Lewisburg	83%	29
Bolivar General Hospital	Bolivar	81%	26
United Regional Medical Center	Manchester	75%	28

18. Influenza Vaccine

Hospital Name	City	Rate	Cases
Athens Regional Medical Center	Athens	100%	89
Fort Sanders Regional Medical Center	Knoxville	100%	244
Grandview Medical Center	Jasper	100%	90
Henderson County Community Hospital	Lexington	100%	27
Horizon Medical Center	Dickson	100%	106
Jamestown Regional Medical Center	Jamestown	100%	67
Livingston Regional Hospital	Livingston	100%	94
McNairy Regional Hospital	Selmer	100%	33
Methodist Healthcare Memphis Hospitals[2]	Memphis	100%	219
Middle Tennessee Medical Center	Murfreesboro	100%	309
Parkridge Medical Center	Chattanooga	100%	153
Sycamore Shoals Hospital[2]	Elizabethton	100%	71
Takoma Regional Hospital	Greeneville	100%	90
Trousdale Medical Center	Hartsville	100%	30
Baptist Hospital of Cocke County	Newport	99%	121
Centennial Medical Center	Nashville	99%	207
Fort Loudoun Medical Center[2]	Lenoir City	99%	69
Harton Regional Medical Center	Tullahoma	99%	109
Hendersonville Medical Center	Hendersonville	99%	85
Memorial Healthcare System	Chattanooga	99%	488
Morristown Hamblen Hospital Association	Morristown	99%	162
Saint Francis Bartlett Medical Center	Bartlett	99%	152
Southern Hills Medical Center	Nashville	99%	78
Summit Medical Center	Hermitage	99%	212
Wellmont Bristol Regional Medical Center[2]	Bristol	99%	70
Baptist Hospital	Nashville	98%	211
Dyersburg Regional Medical Center	Dyersburg	98%	62
McKenzie Regional Hospital	McKenzie	98%	51
Mercy Medical Center	Knoxville	98%	474
Saint Thomas Hospital	Nashville	98%	301
Skyline Medical Center[2]	Nashville	98%	102
VA Middle Tennessee Healthcare System	Nashville	98%	177
Blount Memorial Hospital[2]	Maryville	97%	102
Crockett Hospital	Lawrenceburg	97%	79
Franklin Woods Community Hospital[2]	Johnson City	97%	62
Mountain Home VA Medical Center	Mountain Home	97%	115
Saint Mary's Jefferson Memorial Hospital	Jefferson City	97%	88
University Medical Center	Lebanon	97%	115
Wellmont Hawkins County Memorial Hospital	Rogersville	97%	98
Baptist Memorial Hospital	Memphis	96%	480
Baptist Memorial Hospital Union City	Union City	96%	50
Decatur County General Hospital	Parsons	96%	45
Erlanger Medical Center	Chattanooga	96%	163
Leconte Medical Center	Sevierville	96%	77
Methodist Medical Center of Oak Ridge	Oak Ridge	96%	382
Northcrest Medical Center	Springfield	96%	166
St Mary's Med Ctr of Campbell County	La Follette	96%	190
Stonecrest Medical Center	Smyrna	96%	78
Williamson Medical Center	Franklin	96%	108
Baptist Memorial Hospital Tipton	Covington	95%	41
Claiborne County Hospital[2]	Tazewell	95%	57
Indian Path Medical Center[2]	Kingsport	95%	85
Maury Regional Hospital[2]	Columbia	95%	97
River Park Hospital	McMinnville	95%	154
Roane Medical Center	Harriman	95%	100
Saint Francis Hospital	Memphis	95%	142
Skyridge Medical Center	Cleveland	95%	249
Volunteer Community Hospital	Martin	95%	75
Gateway Medical Center	Clarksville	94%	218
Regional Hospital of Jackson	Jackson	94%	98
Scott County Hospital[2]	Oneida	94%	51
Hillside Hospital	Pulaski	93%	57
Jellico Community Hospital	Jellico	93%	73
Lincoln Medical Center	Fayetteville	93%	58
Parkwest Medical Center	Knoxville	93%	280
University of Tennessee Memorial Hospital[2]	Knoxville	92%	83
Heritage Medical Center	Shelbyville	91%	88
Laughlin Memorial Hospital	Greeneville	91%	170
Rhea Medical Center	Dayton	90%	72
Johnson City Medical Center[2]	Johnson City	89%	106
Riverview Regional Medical Center North	Carthage	89%	56
Sweetwater Hospital Association	Sweetwater	89%	117
White County Community Hospital	Sparta	88%	66
Hardin Medical Center	Savannah	87%	61
Jackson-Madison County General Hospital[2]	Jackson	86%	170
Southern Tennessee Medical Center	Winchester	86%	113
Henry County Medical Center	Paris	85%	95
Lakeway Regional Hospital	Morristown	85%	41
Memphis VA Medical Center	Memphis	85%	108
Vanderbilt University Hospital[2]	Nashville	84%	81
Wellmont Holston Valley Medical Center[2]	Kingsport	83%	76
Cumberland River Hospital	Celina	80%	44
Cookeville Regional Medical Center	Cookeville	78%	250
Sumner Regional Medical Center	Gallatin	78%	153
Stones River Hosp & Dekalb Comm Hosp	Woodbury	70%	27
Woods Memorial Hospital	Etowah	69%	74
Patients' Choice Medical Center of Erin	Erin	68%	31
Stones River Hosp/Dekalb Comm Hosp	Smithville	68%	94
Cumberland Medical Center	Crossville	61%	221
United Regional Medical Center	Manchester	59%	107
Unicoi County Memorial Hospital	Erwin	55%	44
Wayne Medical Center	Waynesboro	49%	35
Perry Community Hospital[2]	Linden	0%	50

19. Initial Antibiotic Timing

Hospital Name	City	Rate	Cases
Baptist Memorial Hospital Union City	Union City	100%	76
Henderson County Community Hospital	Lexington	100%	36
Laughlin Memorial Hospital	Greeneville	100%	254
Marshall Medical Center	Lewisburg	100%	28
McKenzie Regional Hospital	McKenzie	100%	64
McNairy Regional Hospital	Selmer	100%	58
Parkridge Medical Center	Chattanooga	100%	226
Patients' Choice Medical Center of Erin	Erin	100%	45
Riverview Regional Medical Center North	Carthage	100%	92
Saint Francis Bartlett Medical Center	Bartlett	100%	270
Stones River Hosp & Dekalb Comm Hosp	Woodbury	100%	34
Takoma Regional Hospital	Greeneville	100%	152
Wayne Medical Center	Waynesboro	100%	66
Athens Regional Medical Center	Athens	99%	162
Baptist Hospital of Cocke County	Newport	99%	182
Centennial Medical Center	Nashville	99%	155
Dyersburg Regional Medical Center	Dyersburg	99%	113
Fort Sanders Regional Medical Center	Knoxville	99%	329
Franklin Woods Community Hospital[2]	Johnson City	99%	96
Horizon Medical Center	Dickson	99%	176
Livingston Regional Hospital	Livingston	99%	164
St Mary's Med Ctr of Campbell County	La Follette	99%	300
Scott County Hospital[2]	Oneida	99%	103
Skyline Medical Center[2]	Nashville	99%	163
Southern Hills Medical Center	Nashville	99%	165
Stonecrest Medical Center	Smyrna	99%	140
White County Community Hospital	Sparta	99%	104
Fort Loudoun Medical Center[2]	Lenoir City	98%	116
Grandview Medical Center	Jasper	98%	157
Heritage Medical Center	Shelbyville	98%	120
Hillside Hospital	Pulaski	98%	84
Lakeway Regional Hospital	Morristown	98%	90
Lincoln Medical Center	Fayetteville	98%	111
Methodist Healthcare Memphis Hospitals[2]	Memphis	98%	424
Methodist Medical Center of Oak Ridge	Oak Ridge	98%	444
Morristown Hamblen Hospital Association	Morristown	98%	300
Regional Hospital of Jackson	Jackson	98%	95
Sumner Regional Medical Center	Gallatin	98%	164
Woods Memorial Hospital	Etowah	98%	108
Cookeville Regional Medical Center	Cookeville	97%	356
Decatur County General Hospital	Parsons	97%	68
Harton Regional Medical Center	Tullahoma	97%	123
Jamestown Regional Medical Center	Jamestown	97%	129
Jellico Community Hospital	Jellico	97%	112
Northcrest Medical Center	Springfield	97%	225
Skyridge Medical Center	Cleveland	97%	349
Unicoi County Memorial Hospital	Erwin	97%	92

NOTE: Hospital profiles are in alphabetical order by state, then city, then hospital within the city; Rankings exclude hospitals with less than 25 cases except for patient surveys which excludes hospitals with less than 100 cases; (a) 100–299 cases; (1) The number of cases is too small to be sure how well a hospital is performing; (2) The hospital indicated that the data submitted for this measure were based on a sample of cases; (3) Data was collected during a shorter time period (fewer quarters) than the maximum possible time for this measure; (4) Suppressed for one or more quarters by CMS; (5) No data is available from the hospital for this measure; (6) Fewer than 100 patients completed the HCAHPS survey. Use these rates with caution, as the number of surveys may be too low to reliably assess hospital performance; (7) Survey results are based on less than 12 months of data; (8) Survey results are not available for this reporting period; (9) No or very few patients were eligible for the HCAHPS survey. The scores shown, if any, reflect a very small number of surveys; (10) A state average was not calculated because too few hospitals in the state submitted data; (11) There were discrepancies in the data collection process; Please refer to the User's Guide for a full explanation of data.

University Medical Center	Lebanon	97%	180
University of Tennessee Memorial Hospital[2]	Knoxville	97%	143
Baptist Memorial Hospital	Memphis	96%	617
Erlanger Medical Center	Chattanooga	96%	195
Gateway Medical Center	Clarksville	96%	315
Hendersonville Medical Center	Hendersonville	96%	83
Leconte Medical Center	Sevierville	96%	185
Maury Regional Hospital[2]	Columbia	96%	106
Memorial Healthcare System	Chattanooga	96%	815
Middle Tennessee Medical Center	Murfreesboro	96%	477
Parkwest Medical Center	Knoxville	96%	400
Rhea Medical Center	Dayton	96%	135
Southern Tennessee Medical Center	Winchester	96%	159
Summit Medical Center	Hermitage	96%	291
VA Middle Tennessee Healthcare System	Nashville	96%	179
Volunteer Community Hospital	Martin	96%	84
Wellmont Hawkins County Memorial Hospital	Rogersville	96%	163
Blount Memorial Hospital[2]	Maryville	95%	140
Crockett Hospital	Lawrenceburg	95%	132
Cumberland Medical Center	Crossville	95%	343
Hardin Medical Center	Savannah	95%	103
Indian Path Medical Center[2]	Kingsport	95%	109
Mercy Medical Center	Knoxville	95%	628
Methodist Healthcare Fayette Hospital	Somerville	95%	42
Mountain Home VA Medical Center	Mountain Home	95%	150
Roane Medical Center	Harriman	95%	164
Wellmont Bristol Regional Medical Center[2]	Bristol	95%	109
Williamson Medical Center	Franklin	95%	164
Baptist Hospital	Nashville	94%	254
Baptist Memorial Hospital Huntingdon	Huntingdon	94%	32
Claiborne County Hospital[2]	Tazewell	94%	114
Cumberland River Hospital	Celina	94%	72
Henry County Medical Center	Paris	94%	125
Memphis VA Medical Center	Memphis	94%	146
Saint Thomas Hospital	Nashville	94%	320
Stones River Hosp/Dekalb Comm Hosp	Smithville	94%	149
Vanderbilt University Hospital[2]	Nashville	94%	106
Bolivar General Hospital	Bolivar	93%	27
Wellmont Holston Valley Medical Center[2]	Kingsport	93%	88
Jackson-Madison County General Hospital[2]	Jackson	92%	149
Perry Community Hospital[2]	Linden	92%	75
Saint Francis Hospital	Memphis	92%	209
Saint Mary's Jefferson Memorial Hospital	Jefferson City	92%	171
Sycamore Shoals Hospital[2]	Elizabethton	92%	115
Baptist Memorial Hospital Tipton	Covington	91%	53
River Park Hospital	McMinnville	91%	229
Sweetwater Hospital Association	Sweetwater	91%	174
Trousdale Medical Center	Hartsville	91%	35
Delta Medical Center	Memphis	90%	52
Johnson City Medical Center[2]	Johnson City	90%	123
Lauderdale Community Hospital	Ripley	89%	46
Metro Nashville General Hospital[2]	Nashville	88%	78
United Regional Medical Center	Manchester	84%	170
Regional Medical Center at Memphis	Memphis	82%	80

20. Pneumococcal Vaccine

Hospital Name	City	Rate	Cases
Baptist Memorial Hospital Huntingdon	Huntingdon	100%	29
Centennial Medical Center	Nashville	100%	246
Fort Sanders Regional Medical Center	Knoxville	100%	346
Franklin Woods Community Hospital[2]	Johnson City	100%	69
Grandview Medical Center	Jasper	100%	121
Henderson County Community Hospital	Lexington	100%	35
Hendersonville Medical Center	Hendersonville	100%	97
McKenzie Regional Hospital	McKenzie	100%	57
McNairy Regional Hospital	Selmer	100%	63
Methodist Healthcare Fayette Hospital	Somerville	100%	36
Methodist Healthcare Memphis Hospitals[2]	Memphis	100%	294
Mountain Home VA Medical Center	Mountain Home	100%	136
Parkridge Medical Center	Chattanooga	100%	183
Saint Francis Bartlett Medical Center	Bartlett	100%	168
Skyline Medical Center[2]	Nashville	100%	144
Southern Hills Medical Center	Nashville	100%	90
Summit Medical Center	Hermitage	100%	263
Sycamore Shoals Hospital[2]	Elizabethton	100%	114
Trousdale Medical Center	Hartsville	100%	32
Baptist Hospital of Cocke County	Newport	99%	143
Blount Memorial Hospital[2]	Maryville	99%	146
Decatur County General Hospital	Parsons	99%	74
Harton Regional Medical Center	Tullahoma	99%	136
Hillside Hospital	Pulaski	99%	71
Horizon Medical Center	Dickson	99%	153
Jamestown Regional Medical Center	Jamestown	99%	78
Memorial Healthcare System	Chattanooga	99%	706
Middle Tennessee Medical Center	Murfreesboro	99%	377
Northcrest Medical Center	Springfield	99%	195
Takoma Regional Hospital	Greeneville	99%	111
University Medical Center	Lebanon	99%	140
VA Middle Tennessee Healthcare System	Nashville	99%	183
Athens Regional Medical Center	Athens	98%	130
Baptist Memorial Hospital Tipton	Covington	98%	41
Dyersburg Regional Medical Center	Dyersburg	98%	80
Erlanger Medical Center	Chattanooga	98%	164
Fort Loudoun Medical Center[2]	Lenoir City	98%	95
Jellico Community Hospital	Jellico	98%	98
Leconte Medical Center	Sevierville	98%	115
Livingston Regional Hospital	Livingston	98%	144
Mercy Medical Center	Knoxville	98%	595
Riverview Regional Medical Center North	Carthage	98%	58
Roane Medical Center	Harriman	98%	115
Skyridge Medical Center	Cleveland	98%	320
Wellmont Bristol Regional Medical Center[2]	Bristol	98%	105
Wellmont Hawkins County Memorial Hospital	Rogersville	98%	129
Laughlin Memorial Hospital	Greeneville	97%	233
Methodist Medical Center of Oak Ridge	Oak Ridge	97%	510
Parkwest Medical Center	Knoxville	97%	368
Saint Francis Hospital	Memphis	97%	192
Saint Mary's Jefferson Memorial Hospital	Jefferson City	97%	141
Saint Thomas Hospital	Nashville	97%	410
Stonecrest Medical Center	Smyrna	97%	113
Baptist Hospital	Nashville	96%	269
Baptist Memorial Hospital	Memphis	96%	584
Gateway Medical Center	Clarksville	96%	252
Indian Path Medical Center[2]	Kingsport	96%	140
Lincoln Medical Center	Fayetteville	96%	92
Scott County Hospital[2]	Oneida	96%	76
Southern Tennessee Medical Center	Winchester	96%	142
Crockett Hospital	Lawrenceburg	95%	116
Henry County Medical Center	Paris	95%	124
Johnson City Medical Center[2]	Johnson City	95%	119
Morristown Hamblen Hospital Association	Morristown	95%	216
St Mary's Med Ctr of Campbell County	La Follette	95%	251
Sweetwater Hospital Association	Sweetwater	95%	163
Volunteer Community Hospital	Martin	95%	97
Williamson Medical Center	Franklin	95%	153
Baptist Memorial Hospital Union City	Union City	94%	52
Hardin Medical Center	Savannah	94%	90
Heritage Medical Center	Shelbyville	94%	89
Memphis VA Medical Center	Memphis	94%	107
Wayne Medical Center	Waynesboro	94%	67
Maury Regional Hospital[2]	Columbia	93%	140
Regional Hospital of Jackson	Jackson	93%	105
University of Tennessee Memorial Hospital[2]	Knoxville	93%	100
River Park Hospital	McMinnville	92%	194
Claiborne County Hospital[2]	Tazewell	90%	89
Cumberland Medical Center	Crossville	89%	316
White County Community Hospital	Sparta	89%	91
Cookeville Regional Medical Center	Cookeville	87%	330
Wellmont Holston Valley Medical Center[2]	Kingsport	87%	109
Stones River Hosp/Dekalb Comm Hosp	Smithville	86%	132
Sumner Regional Medical Center	Gallatin	86%	185
Lakeway Regional Hospital	Morristown	85%	52
Rhea Medical Center	Dayton	84%	90
Jackson-Madison County General Hospital[2]	Jackson	83%	194
Vanderbilt University Hospital[2]	Nashville	83%	87
Stones River Hosp & Dekalb Comm Hosp	Woodbury	81%	36
Lauderdale Community Hospital	Ripley	79%	28
Woods Memorial Hospital	Etowah	76%	113
Patients' Choice Medical Center of Erin	Erin	72%	40
Cumberland River Hospital	Celina	69%	61
Unicoi County Memorial Hospital	Erwin	68%	73
Bolivar General Hospital	Bolivar	65%	26
United Regional Medical Center	Manchester	54%	148
Hickman Community Health Services	Centerville	16%	25
Perry Community Hospital[2]	Linden	1%	72

21. Smoking Cessation Advice

Hospital Name	City	Rate	Cases
Baptist Hospital	Nashville	100%	141
Baptist Hospital of Cocke County	Newport	100%	84
Baptist Memorial Hospital	Memphis	100%	226
Baptist Memorial Hospital Union City	Union City	100%	30
Claiborne County Hospital[2]	Tazewell	100%	38
Crockett Hospital	Lawrenceburg	100%	48
Dyersburg Regional Medical Center	Dyersburg	100%	50
Fort Loudoun Medical Center[2]	Lenoir City	100%	44
Fort Sanders Regional Medical Center	Knoxville	100%	239
Franklin Woods Community Hospital[2]	Johnson City	100%	62
Gateway Medical Center	Clarksville	100%	116
Harton Regional Medical Center	Tullahoma	100%	55
Hendersonville Medical Center	Hendersonville	100%	65
Henry County Medical Center	Paris	100%	50
Heritage Medical Center	Shelbyville	100%	57
Indian Path Medical Center[2]	Kingsport	100%	68
Jamestown Regional Medical Center	Jamestown	100%	55
Johnson City Medical Center[2]	Johnson City	100%	71
Lakeway Regional Hospital	Morristown	100%	42
Laughlin Memorial Hospital	Greeneville	100%	77
Leconte Medical Center	Sevierville	100%	63
Livingston Regional Hospital	Livingston	100%	66
Maury Regional Hospital[2]	Columbia	100%	66
McKenzie Regional Hospital	McKenzie	100%	26
Memorial Healthcare System	Chattanooga	100%	231
Memphis VA Medical Center	Memphis	100%	62
Mercy Medical Center	Knoxville	100%	403
Methodist Healthcare Memphis Hospitals[2]	Memphis	100%	235
Methodist Medical Center of Oak Ridge	Oak Ridge	100%	252
Metro Nashville General Hospital[2]	Nashville	100%	58
Middle Tennessee Medical Center	Murfreesboro	100%	196
Morristown Hamblen Hospital Association	Morristown	100%	139
Mountain Home VA Medical Center	Mountain Home	100%	67
Northcrest Medical Center	Springfield	100%	98
Parkridge Medical Center	Chattanooga	100%	149
Parkwest Medical Center	Knoxville	100%	141
Regional Medical Center at Memphis	Memphis	100%	67
Rhea Medical Center	Dayton	100%	54
River Park Hospital	McMinnville	100%	127
Saint Francis Bartlett Medical Center	Bartlett	100%	81
Saint Francis Hospital	Memphis	100%	79
St Mary's Med Ctr of Campbell County	La Follette	100%	143
Scott County Hospital[2]	Oneida	100%	35
Skyline Medical Center[2]	Nashville	100%	84
Skyridge Medical Center	Cleveland	100%	186
Southern Hills Medical Center	Nashville	100%	79
Southern Tennessee Medical Center	Winchester	100%	70
Stonecrest Medical Center	Smyrna	100%	64
Summit Medical Center	Hermitage	100%	121
Sycamore Shoals Hospital[2]	Elizabethton	100%	74
Takoma Regional Hospital	Greeneville	100%	82
University Medical Center	Lebanon	100%	110
University of Tennessee Memorial Hospital[2]	Knoxville	100%	90
VA Middle Tennessee Healthcare System	Nashville	100%	107
Vanderbilt University Hospital[2]	Nashville	100%	66
Volunteer Community Hospital	Martin	100%	35
Wellmont Bristol Regional Medical Center[2]	Bristol	100%	68
Wellmont Hawkins County Memorial Hospital	Rogersville	100%	99
White County Community Hospital	Sparta	100%	41
Athens Regional Medical Center	Athens	99%	74
Blount Memorial Hospital[2]	Maryville	99%	74
Centennial Medical Center	Nashville	99%	181
Cumberland Medical Center	Crossville	99%	140
Erlanger Medical Center	Chattanooga	99%	179
Grandview Medical Center	Jasper	99%	104
Jackson-Madison County General Hospital[2]	Jackson	99%	122
Jellico Community Hospital	Jellico	99%	88
Regional Hospital of Jackson	Jackson	99%	95
Roane Medical Center	Harriman	99%	76
Saint Thomas Hospital	Nashville	99%	196
Cookeville Regional Medical Center	Cookeville	98%	205
Horizon Medical Center	Dickson	98%	102
Lincoln Medical Center	Fayetteville	98%	40
Riverview Regional Medical Center North	Carthage	98%	48
Wellmont Holston Valley Medical Center[2]	Kingsport	98%	51
Delta Medical Center	Memphis	97%	35
Hillside Hospital	Pulaski	97%	35
Saint Mary's Jefferson Memorial Hospital	Jefferson City	97%	65
Unicoi County Memorial Hospital	Erwin	97%	29
Williamson Medical Center	Franklin	96%	55
Woods Memorial Hospital	Etowah	96%	54
Stones River Hosp/Dekalb Comm Hosp	Smithville	95%	63
Sumner Regional Medical Center	Gallatin	95%	97
Hardin Medical Center	Savannah	94%	32
Sweetwater Hospital Association	Sweetwater	94%	86
United Regional Medical Center	Manchester	79%	97

Surgical Care Improvement Project

22. Appropriate VTP Within 24 Hours

Hospital Name	City	Rate	Cases
Methodist Medical Center of Oak Ridge[2]	Oak Ridge	99%	224
Saint Thomas Hospital[2]	Nashville	99%	187
University of Tennessee Memorial Hospital[2]	Knoxville	99%	207
Vanderbilt University Hospital[2]	Nashville	99%	198
Centennial Medical Center[2]	Nashville	98%	276
Heritage Medical Center[2]	Shelbyville	98%	43
Northcrest Medical Center	Springfield	98%	85
Skyridge Medical Center[2]	Cleveland	98%	242
Southern Hills Medical Center	Nashville	98%	118
VA Middle Tennessee Healthcare System[2]	Nashville	98%	81
Erlanger Medical Center[2]	Chattanooga	97%	156
Indian Path Medical Center[2]	Kingsport	97%	185
Roane Medical Center	Harriman	97%	34
Wellmont Holston Valley Medical Center[2]	Kingsport	97%	151
Parkridge Medical Center[2]	Chattanooga	96%	198
Regional Hospital of Jackson[2]	Jackson	96%	197
River Park Hospital	McMinnville	96%	57
Southern Tennessee Medical Center	Winchester	96%	103
Stonecrest Medical Center	Smyrna	96%	116
Summit Medical Center[2]	Hermitage	96%	224
Laughlin Memorial Hospital	Greeneville	95%	139

NOTE: Hospital profiles are in alphabetical order by state, then city, then hospital within the city; Rankings exclude hospitals with less than 25 cases except for patient surveys which excludes hospitals with less than 100 cases; (a) 100–299 cases; (1) The number of cases is too small to be sure how well a hospital is performing; (2) The hospital indicated that the data submitted for this measure were based on a sample of cases; (3) Data was collected during a shorter time period (fewer quarters) than the maximum possible time for this measure; (4) Suppressed for one or more quarters by CMS; (5) No data is available from the hospital for this measure; (6) Fewer than 100 patients completed the HCAHPS survey. Use these rates with caution, as the number of surveys may be too low to reliably assess hospital performance; (7) Survey results are based on less than 12 months of data; (8) Survey results are not available for this reporting period; (9) No or very few patients were eligible for the HCAHPS survey. The scores shown, if any, reflect a very small number of surveys; (10) A state average was not calculated because too few hospitals in the state submitted data; (11) There were discrepancies in the data collection process; Please refer to the User's Guide for a full explanation of data.

Methodist Healthcare Memphis Hospitals[2]	Memphis	95%	1309
University Medical Center	Lebanon	95%	240
Fort Sanders Regional Medical Center[2]	Knoxville	94%	310
Hendersonville Medical Center	Hendersonville	94%	125
Henry County Medical Center	Paris	94%	199
Jackson-Madison County General Hospital[2]	Jackson	93%	635
Morristown Hamblen Hospital Association	Morristown	93%	130
Regional Medical Center at Memphis	Memphis	93%	318
Athens Regional Medical Center	Athens	92%	98
Blount Memorial Hospital[2]	Maryville	92%	178
Gateway Medical Center	Clarksville	92%	279
Parkwest Medical Center[2]	Knoxville	92%	408
Skyline Medical Center[2]	Nashville	92%	208
Volunteer Community Hospital[2]	Martin	92%	52
Dyersburg Regional Medical Center[2]	Dyersburg	91%	68
Mercy Medical Center[2]	Knoxville	91%	611
Saint Francis Bartlett Medical Center[2]	Bartlett	91%	114
Sycamore Shoals Hospital[2]	Elizabethton	91%	80
Williamson Medical Center[2]	Franklin	91%	154
Baptist Hospital[2]	Nashville	90%	211
Baptist Memorial Hospital[2]	Memphis	90%	362
Fort Loudoun Medical Center	Lenoir City	90%	30
Horizon Medical Center	Dickson	90%	103
Memorial Healthcare System[2]	Chattanooga	90%	657
Middle Tennessee Medical Center[2]	Murfreesboro	90%	215
Unicoi County Memorial Hospital	Erwin	90%	40
Cookeville Regional Medical Center	Cookeville	89%	377
Leconte Medical Center[2]	Sevierville	89%	83
Harton Regional Medical Center	Tullahoma	88%	86
Saint Francis Hospital[2]	Memphis	88%	236
Maury Regional Hospital[2]	Columbia	87%	162
Delta Medical Center	Memphis	85%	40
Livingston Regional Hospital	Livingston	85%	39
Baptist Memorial Hospital Union City[2]	Union City	84%	57
Metro Nashville General Hospital[2]	Nashville	84%	135
Sumner Regional Medical Center	Gallatin	84%	115
Takoma Regional Hospital	Greeneville	83%	36
Woods Memorial Hospital	Etowah	83%	35
Lakeway Regional Hospital[2]	Morristown	82%	51
Saint Mary's Jefferson Memorial Hospital	Jefferson City	82%	28
Sweetwater Hospital Association	Sweetwater	81%	59
Johnson City Medical Center[2]	Johnson City	78%	172
Cumberland Medical Center[2]	Crossville	73%	125
Wellmont Bristol Regional Medical Center[2]	Bristol	71%	144
Claiborne County Hospital[2]	Tazewell	69%	32

23. Appropriate Hair Removal

Hospital Name	City	Rate	Cases
Athens Regional Medical Center	Athens	100%	149
Baptist Hospital[2]	Nashville	100%	749
Baptist Memorial Hospital[2]	Memphis	100%	1112
Baptist Memorial Hospital Huntingdon	Huntingdon	100%	37
Baptist Memorial Hospital Union City[2]	Union City	100%	149
Blount Memorial Hospital[2]	Maryville	100%	454
Centennial Medical Center[2]	Nashville	100%	924
Claiborne County Hospital[2]	Tazewell	100%	42
Cookeville Regional Medical Center	Cookeville	100%	1288
Crockett Hospital	Lawrenceburg	100%	41
Delta Medical Center	Memphis	100%	131
Dyersburg Regional Medical Center[2]	Dyersburg	100%	114
Erlanger Medical Center[2]	Chattanooga	100%	518
Fort Loudoun Medical Center	Lenoir City	100%	38
Fort Sanders Regional Medical Center[2]	Knoxville	100%	1004
Hardin Medical Center	Savannah	100%	64
Harton Regional Medical Center	Tullahoma	100%	272
Hendersonville Medical Center	Hendersonville	100%	314
Henry County Medical Center	Paris	100%	524
Horizon Medical Center	Dickson	100%	156
Jellico Community Hospital	Jellico	100%	56
Johnson City Medical Center[2]	Johnson City	100%	634
Johnson City Specialty Hospital[2]	Johnson City	100%	33
Laughlin Memorial Hospital	Greeneville	100%	302
Leconte Medical Center[2]	Sevierville	100%	249
Livingston Regional Hospital	Livingston	100%	78
Maury Regional Hospital[2]	Columbia	100%	655
Memorial Healthcare System[2]	Chattanooga	100%	2756
Mercy Medical Center[2]	Knoxville	100%	2647
Methodist Healthcare Memphis Hospitals[2]	Memphis	100%	3589
Methodist Medical Center of Oak Ridge[2]	Oak Ridge	100%	1253
Middle Tennessee Medical Center[2]	Murfreesboro	100%	888
Morristown Hamblen Hospital Association	Morristown	100%	387
Northcrest Medical Center	Springfield	100%	196
Parkridge Medical Center[2]	Chattanooga	100%	696
Parkwest Medical Center[2]	Knoxville	100%	1918
Regional Hospital of Jackson[2]	Jackson	100%	359
Regional Medical Center at Memphis	Memphis	100%	486
River Park Hospital	McMinnville	100%	86
Roane Medical Center	Harriman	100%	55
Saint Francis Bartlett Medical Center[2]	Bartlett	100%	290
Saint Mary's Jefferson Memorial Hospital	Jefferson City	100%	61
Saint Thomas Hospital[2]	Nashville	100%	806
Skyline Medical Center[2]	Nashville	100%	481
Southern Hills Medical Center	Nashville	100%	293
Southern Tennessee Medical Center	Winchester	100%	271
Stonecrest Medical Center	Smyrna	100%	316
Stones River Hosp & Dekalb Comm Hosp[2]	Woodbury	100%	44
Stones River Hosp/Dekalb Comm Hosp	Smithville	100%	68
Summit Medical Center[2]	Hermitage	100%	440
Sumner Regional Medical Center	Gallatin	100%	385
Sycamore Shoals Hospital[2]	Elizabethton	100%	183
Takoma Regional Hospital	Greeneville	100%	83
University Medical Center	Lebanon	100%	456
University of Tennessee Memorial Hospital[2]	Knoxville	100%	658
VA Middle Tennessee Healthcare System[2]	Nashville	100%	222
Volunteer Community Hospital[2]	Martin	100%	74
Wellmont Holston Valley Medical Center[2]	Kingsport	100%	557
Williamson Medical Center[2]	Franklin	100%	373
Woods Memorial Hospital	Etowah	100%	75
Cumberland Medical Center[2]	Crossville	99%	200
Hillside Hospital	Pulaski	99%	72
Jackson-Madison County General Hospital[2]	Jackson	99%	1625
Lakeway Regional Hospital[2]	Morristown	99%	149
Metro Nashville General Hospital[2]	Nashville	99%	233
Saint Francis Hospital[2]	Memphis	99%	599
Skyridge Medical Center[2]	Cleveland	99%	427
Sweetwater Hospital Association	Sweetwater	99%	97
Unicoi County Memorial Hospital	Erwin	99%	91
Vanderbilt University Hospital[2]	Nashville	99%	682
Heritage Medical Center[2]	Shelbyville	98%	82
Indian Path Medical Center[2]	Kingsport	98%	394
Wellmont Bristol Regional Medical Center[2]	Bristol	98%	493
McKenzie Regional Hospital[2]	McKenzie	97%	59
White County Community Hospital[2]	Sparta	97%	66
Lincoln Medical Center	Fayetteville	96%	27
Gateway Medical Center	Clarksville	95%	767
Baptist Memorial Hospital Tipton	Covington	94%	31

24. Appropriate Beta Blocker Usage

Hospital Name	City	Rate	Cases
Baptist Memorial Hospital Union City[2]	Union City	100%	29
Blount Memorial Hospital[2]	Maryville	100%	130
Cumberland Medical Center[2]	Crossville	100%	71
Harton Regional Medical Center	Tullahoma	100%	64
Hendersonville Medical Center	Hendersonville	100%	78
Horizon Medical Center	Dickson	100%	40
Northcrest Medical Center	Springfield	100%	46
Southern Hills Medical Center	Nashville	100%	68
Summit Medical Center[2]	Hermitage	100%	99
University of Tennessee Memorial Hospital[2]	Knoxville	100%	225
Laughlin Memorial Hospital	Greeneville	99%	98
Leconte Medical Center[2]	Sevierville	99%	69
Regional Hospital of Jackson[2]	Jackson	99%	70
Southern Tennessee Medical Center	Winchester	99%	68
Centennial Medical Center[2]	Nashville	98%	346
Fort Sanders Regional Medical Center[2]	Knoxville	98%	201
Parkridge Medical Center[2]	Chattanooga	98%	212
Stonecrest Medical Center	Smyrna	98%	58
University Medical Center	Lebanon	98%	126
Gateway Medical Center	Clarksville	97%	215
Henry County Medical Center	Paris	97%	138
Johnson City Medical Center[2]	Johnson City	96%	239
Methodist Medical Center of Oak Ridge[2]	Oak Ridge	96%	193
Parkwest Medical Center[2]	Knoxville	96%	570
Williamson Medical Center[2]	Franklin	96%	106
Mercy Medical Center[2]	Knoxville	95%	867
Methodist Healthcare Memphis Hospitals[2]	Memphis	95%	988
Saint Thomas Hospital[2]	Nashville	95%	258
Indian Path Medical Center[2]	Kingsport	94%	103
Maury Regional Hospital[2]	Columbia	94%	170
Athens Regional Medical Center	Athens	93%	43
Baptist Hospital[2]	Nashville	93%	206
Lakeway Regional Hospital[2]	Morristown	93%	45
Skyline Medical Center[2]	Nashville	93%	136
Sumner Regional Medical Center	Gallatin	93%	104
Middle Tennessee Medical Center[2]	Murfreesboro	92%	207
VA Middle Tennessee Healthcare System[2]	Nashville	92%	104
Erlanger Medical Center[2]	Chattanooga	91%	140
Memorial Healthcare System[2]	Chattanooga	91%	888
Metro Nashville General Hospital[2]	Nashville	91%	32
Morristown Hamblen Hospital Association	Morristown	91%	122
Saint Francis Hospital[2]	Memphis	91%	208
Vanderbilt University Hospital[2]	Nashville	91%	186
Wellmont Holston Valley Medical Center[2]	Kingsport	91%	225
Baptist Memorial Hospital[2]	Memphis	89%	338
Cookeville Regional Medical Center	Cookeville	88%	508
Sycamore Shoals Hospital[2]	Elizabethton	88%	32
Skyridge Medical Center[2]	Cleveland	87%	92
Regional Medical Center at Memphis	Memphis	84%	50
Saint Francis Bartlett Medical Center[2]	Bartlett	84%	51
Jackson-Madison County General Hospital[2]	Jackson	79%	497
Wellmont Bristol Regional Medical Center[2]	Bristol	66%	164

25. Controlled Postoperative Blood Glucose

Hospital Name	City	Rate	Cases
Baptist Hospital[2]	Nashville	99%	118
Maury Regional Hospital[2]	Columbia	99%	74
Wellmont Holston Valley Medical Center[2]	Kingsport	98%	130
Fort Sanders Regional Medical Center[2]	Knoxville	97%	153
Methodist Healthcare Memphis Hospitals[2]	Memphis	97%	478
Methodist Medical Center of Oak Ridge[2]	Oak Ridge	97%	184
Gateway Medical Center	Clarksville	96%	80
Saint Francis Hospital[2]	Memphis	96%	166
VA Middle Tennessee Healthcare System[2]	Nashville	96%	105
Parkridge Medical Center[2]	Chattanooga	95%	157
University of Tennessee Memorial Hospital[2]	Knoxville	95%	150
Cookeville Regional Medical Center	Cookeville	94%	216
Mercy Medical Center[2]	Knoxville	94%	388
Jackson-Madison County General Hospital[2]	Jackson	93%	372
Saint Thomas Hospital[2]	Nashville	93%	174
Centennial Medical Center[2]	Nashville	92%	224
Vanderbilt University Hospital[2]	Nashville	92%	109
Erlanger Medical Center[2]	Chattanooga	91%	102
Memorial Healthcare System[2]	Chattanooga	89%	702
Parkwest Medical Center[2]	Knoxville	89%	341
Johnson City Medical Center[2]	Johnson City	88%	139
Baptist Memorial Hospital[2]	Memphis	86%	149
Wellmont Bristol Regional Medical Center[2]	Bristol	80%	88

26. Prophylactic Antibiotic Timing

Hospital Name	City	Rate	Cases
Crockett Hospital	Lawrenceburg	100%	26
Indian Path Medical Center[2]	Kingsport	100%	273
Johnson City Specialty Hospital[2]	Johnson City	100%	26
Livingston Regional Hospital	Livingston	100%	52
Southern Hills Medical Center	Nashville	100%	169
Stones River Hosp & Dekalb Comm Hosp[2]	Woodbury	100%	41
Takoma Regional Hospital	Greeneville	100%	49
Unicoi County Memorial Hospital	Erwin	100%	70
Centennial Medical Center[2]	Nashville	99%	622
Harton Regional Medical Center	Tullahoma	99%	170
Henry County Medical Center	Paris	99%	395
Horizon Medical Center	Dickson	99%	91
Leconte Medical Center[2]	Sevierville	99%	196
Mercy Medical Center[2]	Knoxville	99%	2001
Methodist Healthcare Memphis Hospitals[2]	Memphis	99%	2254
Methodist Medical Center of Oak Ridge[2]	Oak Ridge	99%	1019
Middle Tennessee Medical Center[2]	Murfreesboro	99%	671
Northcrest Medical Center	Springfield	99%	110
Parkridge Medical Center[2]	Chattanooga	99%	460
Parkwest Medical Center[2]	Knoxville	99%	1671
Saint Francis Bartlett Medical Center[2]	Bartlett	99%	189
Saint Thomas Hospital[2]	Nashville	99%	542
University Medical Center	Lebanon	99%	318
Vanderbilt University Hospital[2]	Nashville	99%	421
Williamson Medical Center[2]	Franklin	99%	257
Baptist Hospital[2]	Nashville	98%	514
Baptist Memorial Hospital Union City[2]	Union City	98%	99
Fort Sanders Regional Medical Center[2]	Knoxville	98%	772
Gateway Medical Center	Clarksville	98%	535
Heritage Medical Center[2]	Shelbyville	98%	50
Johnson City Medical Center[2]	Johnson City	98%	443
Lakeway Regional Hospital[2]	Morristown	98%	123
Maury Regional Hospital[2]	Columbia	98%	474
McKenzie Regional Hospital[2]	McKenzie	98%	57
Skyline Medical Center[2]	Nashville	98%	277
Southern Tennessee Medical Center	Winchester	98%	186
Stonecrest Medical Center	Smyrna	98%	202
Stones River Hosp/Dekalb Comm Hosp	Smithville	98%	50
Sycamore Shoals Hospital[2]	Elizabethton	98%	124
Volunteer Community Hospital[2]	Martin	98%	47
Wellmont Bristol Regional Medical Center[2]	Bristol	98%	317
Wellmont Holston Valley Medical Center[2]	Kingsport	98%	400
Erlanger Medical Center[2]	Chattanooga	97%	339
Hardin Medical Center	Savannah	97%	39
Laughlin Memorial Hospital	Greeneville	97%	207
Memorial Healthcare System[2]	Chattanooga	97%	2048
Morristown Hamblen Hospital Association	Morristown	97%	274
Regional Hospital of Jackson[2]	Jackson	97%	218
River Park Hospital	McMinnville	97%	61
Saint Mary's Jefferson Memorial Hospital	Jefferson City	97%	63
Summit Medical Center[2]	Hermitage	97%	241
Sumner Regional Medical Center	Gallatin	97%	280
Baptist Memorial Hospital[2]	Memphis	96%	701
Delta Medical Center	Memphis	96%	77
Dyersburg Regional Medical Center[2]	Dyersburg	96%	53
Hillside Hospital	Pulaski	96%	56
University of Tennessee Memorial Hospital[2]	Knoxville	96%	469
Cookeville Regional Medical Center	Cookeville	95%	870
Hendersonville Medical Center	Hendersonville	95%	189
Saint Francis Hospital[2]	Memphis	95%	418

NOTE: Hospital profiles are in alphabetical order by state, then city, then hospital within the city; Rankings exclude hospitals with less than 25 cases except for patient surveys which excludes hospitals with less than 100 cases; (a) 100–299 cases; (1) The number of cases is too small to be sure how well a hospital is performing; (2) The hospital indicated that the data submitted for this measure were based on a sample of cases; (3) Data was collected during a shorter time period (fewer quarters) than the maximum possible time for this measure; (4) Suppressed for one or more quarters by CMS; (5) No data is available from the hospital for this measure; (6) Fewer than 100 patients completed the HCAHPS survey. Use these rates with caution, as the number of surveys may be too low to reliably assess hospital performance; (7) Survey results are based on less than 12 months of data; (8) Survey results are not available for this reporting period; (9) No or very few patients were eligible for the HCAHPS survey. The scores shown, if any, reflect a very small number of surveys; (10) A state average was not calculated because too few hospitals in the state submitted data; (11) There were discrepancies in the data collection process; Please refer to the User's Guide for a full explanation of data.

Blount Memorial Hospital[2]	Maryville	94%	294
Regional Medical Center at Memphis	Memphis	93%	119
VA Middle Tennessee Healthcare System	Nashville	93%	138
Skyridge Medical Center[2]	Cleveland	90%	241
Sweetwater Hospital Association	Sweetwater	90%	42
White County Community Hospital[2]	Sparta	90%	42
Athens Regional Medical Center	Athens	89%	90
Jellico Community Hospital	Jellico	89%	37
Woods Memorial Hospital	Etowah	88%	52
Jackson-Madison County General Hospital[2]	Jackson	87%	1267
Cumberland Medical Center[2]	Crossville	77%	112
Metro Nashville General Hospital[2]	Nashville	71%	139

27. Prophylactic Antibiotic Timing (Outpatient)

Hospital Name	City	Rate	Cases
Baptist Memorial Hospital Union City	Union City	100%	98
The Center for Spinal Surgery	Nashville	100%	913
Harton Regional Medical Center	Tullahoma	99%	433
Johnson City Specialty Hospital	Johnson City	99%	280
Parkridge Medical Center	Chattanooga	99%	695
Southern Hills Medical Center	Nashville	99%	113
Summit Medical Center	Hermitage	99%	493
Williamson Medical Center	Franklin	99%	353
Centennial Medical Center	Nashville	98%	788
Leconte Medical Center	Sevierville	98%	117
Methodist Medical Center of Oak Ridge	Oak Ridge	98%	502
Middle Tennessee Medical Center	Murfreesboro	98%	505
Stonecrest Medical Center	Smyrna	98%	204
Volunteer Community Hospital	Martin	98%	111
Baptist Hospital	Nashville	97%	697
Cookeville Regional Medical Center	Cookeville	97%	714
Horizon Medical Center	Dickson	97%	76
Laughlin Memorial Hospital	Greeneville	97%	133
Livingston Regional Hospital	Livingston	97%	30
Saint Thomas Hospital	Nashville	97%	526
Skyline Medical Center	Nashville	97%	302
Stones River Hosp/Dekalb Comm Hosp	Smithville	97%	30
University Medical Center	Lebanon	97%	218
Athens Regional Medical Center	Athens	96%	104
Methodist Healthcare Memphis Hospitals	Memphis	96%	1189
Regional Hospital of Jackson	Jackson	96%	79
Regional Medical Center at Memphis	Memphis	96%	45
Saint Francis Bartlett Medical Center	Bartlett	96%	92
Wellmont Bristol Regional Medical Center	Bristol	96%	363
Dyersburg Regional Medical Center	Dyersburg	95%	109
Fort Loudoun Medical Center	Lenoir City	95%	44
Fort Sanders Regional Medical Center	Knoxville	95%	719
Lakeway Regional Hospital	Morristown	95%	168
Memorial Healthcare System	Chattanooga	95%	522
Parkwest Medical Center	Knoxville	95%	1443
Wellmont Holston Valley Medical Center	Kingsport	95%	561
Baptist Memorial Hospital	Memphis	94%	1372
Erlanger Medical Center	Chattanooga	94%	539
Gateway Medical Center	Clarksville	94%	174
Hendersonville Medical Center	Hendersonville	94%	178
Mercy Medical Center	Knoxville	94%	1180
Takoma Regional Hospital	Greeneville	94%	62
University of Tennessee Memorial Hospital	Knoxville	94%	852
Vanderbilt University Hospital	Nashville	94%	779
Saint Francis Hospital	Memphis	93%	461
Indian Path Medical Center	Kingsport	92%	225
Southern Tennessee Medical Center	Winchester	92%	140
Maury Regional Hospital	Columbia	91%	453
Grandview Medical Center	Jasper	90%	29
Lincoln Medical Center	Fayetteville	90%	31
Northcrest Medical Center	Springfield	90%	100
Morristown Hamblen Hospital Association	Morristown	88%	271
Sycamore Shoals Hospital	Elizabethton	88%	66
River Park Hospital	McMinnville	86%	183
Skyridge Medical Center	Cleveland	84%	316
Jackson-Madison County General Hospital	Jackson	83%	1600
Johnson City Medical Center	Johnson City	83%	681
Sumner Regional Medical Center	Gallatin	83%	115
Blount Memorial Hospital	Maryville	82%	278
St Mary's Med Ctr of Campbell County	La Follette	82%	28
Saint Mary's Jefferson Memorial Hospital	Jefferson City	81%	27
Hardin Medical Center	Savannah	79%	28
Henry County Medical Center	Paris	78%	46
Sweetwater Hospital Association	Sweetwater	77%	48
Cumberland Medical Center	Crossville	71%	194
Metro Nashville General Hospital	Nashville	58%	88
Claiborne County Hospital	Tazewell	50%	34

28. Prophylactic Antibiotic Selection

Hospital Name	City	Rate	Cases
Baptist Memorial Hospital Huntingdon	Huntingdon	100%	25
Baptist Memorial Hospital Union City[2]	Union City	100%	99
Crockett Hospital	Lawrenceburg	100%	26
Dyersburg Regional Medical Center[2]	Dyersburg	100%	53
Hardin Medical Center	Savannah	100%	39
Memorial Healthcare System[2]	Chattanooga	100%	2064
Parkwest Medical Center[2]	Knoxville	100%	1686
Regional Hospital of Jackson[2]	Jackson	100%	218
Stones River Hosp & Dekalb Comm Hosp[2]	Woodbury	100%	41
Sumner Regional Medical Center	Gallatin	100%	276
Unicoi County Memorial Hospital	Erwin	100%	70
Baptist Hospital[2]	Nashville	99%	525
Centennial Medical Center[2]	Nashville	99%	634
Delta Medical Center	Memphis	99%	79
Fort Sanders Regional Medical Center[2]	Knoxville	99%	773
Harton Regional Medical Center	Tullahoma	99%	172
Henry County Medical Center	Paris	99%	403
Indian Path Medical Center[2]	Kingsport	99%	275
Johnson City Medical Center[2]	Johnson City	99%	452
Lakeway Regional Hospital[2]	Morristown	99%	126
Leconte Medical Center[2]	Sevierville	99%	198
Mercy Medical Center[2]	Knoxville	99%	2023
Morristown Hamblen Hospital Association	Morristown	99%	278
Saint Thomas Hospital[2]	Nashville	99%	552
Skyline Medical Center[2]	Nashville	99%	278
Summit Medical Center[2]	Hermitage	99%	242
VA Middle Tennessee Healthcare System	Nashville	99%	139
Athens Regional Medical Center	Athens	98%	91
Blount Memorial Hospital[2]	Maryville	98%	296
Erlanger Medical Center[2]	Chattanooga	98%	351
Gateway Medical Center	Clarksville	98%	542
Hendersonville Medical Center	Hendersonville	98%	190
Heritage Medical Center[2]	Shelbyville	98%	50
Hillside Hospital	Pulaski	98%	56
Laughlin Memorial Hospital	Greeneville	98%	208
Methodist Medical Center of Oak Ridge[2]	Oak Ridge	98%	1017
Parkridge Medical Center[2]	Chattanooga	98%	470
Saint Mary's Jefferson Memorial Hospital	Jefferson City	98%	63
Southern Tennessee Medical Center	Winchester	98%	187
Stonecrest Medical Center	Smyrna	98%	204
University Medical Center	Lebanon	98%	321
Vanderbilt University Hospital[2]	Nashville	98%	434
Wellmont Holston Valley Medical Center[2]	Kingsport	98%	401
Woods Memorial Hospital	Etowah	98%	52
Baptist Memorial Hospital[2]	Memphis	97%	707
Horizon Medical Center	Dickson	97%	91
Jellico Community Hospital	Jellico	97%	33
Methodist Healthcare Memphis Hospitals[2]	Memphis	97%	2277
Middle Tennessee Medical Center[2]	Murfreesboro	97%	675
River Park Hospital	McMinnville	97%	63
Southern Hills Medical Center	Nashville	97%	172
University of Tennessee Memorial Hospital[2]	Knoxville	97%	479
Wellmont Bristol Regional Medical Center[2]	Bristol	97%	323
Cookeville Regional Medical Center	Cookeville	96%	877
Maury Regional Hospital[2]	Columbia	96%	483
Stones River Hosp/Dekalb Comm Hosp	Smithville	96%	50
Sycamore Shoals Hospital[2]	Elizabethton	96%	128
Northcrest Medical Center	Springfield	95%	110
Regional Medical Center at Memphis	Memphis	95%	123
Saint Francis Hospital[2]	Memphis	95%	425
Livingston Regional Hospital	Livingston	94%	52
Skyridge Medical Center[2]	Cleveland	94%	240
Takoma Regional Hospital	Greeneville	94%	50
Volunteer Community Hospital[2]	Martin	94%	47
Williamson Medical Center[2]	Franklin	94%	262
Jackson-Madison County General Hospital[2]	Jackson	93%	1272
McKenzie Regional Hospital[2]	McKenzie	93%	57
Metro Nashville General Hospital[2]	Nashville	90%	127
Johnson City Specialty Hospital[2]	Johnson City	88%	26
White County Community Hospital[2]	Sparta	84%	43
Saint Francis Bartlett Medical Center[2]	Bartlett	83%	191
Sweetwater Hospital Association	Sweetwater	77%	43
Cumberland Medical Center[2]	Crossville	76%	112

29. Prophylactic Antibiotic Selection (Outpatient)

Hospital Name	City	Rate	Cases
The Center for Spinal Surgery	Nashville	100%	913
Memorial Healthcare System	Chattanooga	99%	545
Centennial Medical Center	Nashville	98%	782
Fort Loudoun Medical Center	Lenoir City	98%	43
Harton Regional Medical Center	Tullahoma	98%	435
Hendersonville Medical Center	Hendersonville	98%	177
Middle Tennessee Medical Center	Murfreesboro	98%	502
Parkridge Medical Center	Chattanooga	98%	693
Skyline Medical Center	Nashville	98%	299
Stonecrest Medical Center	Smyrna	98%	212
Takoma Regional Hospital	Greeneville	98%	59
Fort Sanders Regional Medical Center	Knoxville	97%	708
Gateway Medical Center	Clarksville	97%	173
Horizon Medical Center	Dickson	97%	75
Leconte Medical Center	Sevierville	97%	116
Livingston Regional Hospital	Livingston	97%	29
Parkwest Medical Center	Knoxville	97%	1424
Regional Hospital of Jackson	Jackson	97%	79
Skyridge Medical Center	Cleveland	97%	294
Southern Hills Medical Center	Nashville	97%	112
Summit Medical Center	Hermitage	97%	489
Williamson Medical Center	Franklin	97%	353
Methodist Medical Center of Oak Ridge	Oak Ridge	96%	503
Vanderbilt University Hospital	Nashville	96%	911
Wellmont Bristol Regional Medical Center	Bristol	96%	362
Baptist Hospital	Nashville	95%	693
Baptist Memorial Hospital	Memphis	95%	1359
Erlanger Medical Center	Chattanooga	95%	525
Methodist Healthcare Memphis Hospitals	Memphis	95%	1177
Regional Medical Center at Memphis	Memphis	95%	44
Southern Tennessee Medical Center	Winchester	95%	132
Sweetwater Hospital Association	Sweetwater	95%	39
Sycamore Shoals Hospital	Elizabethton	95%	62
Volunteer Community Hospital	Martin	95%	110
Blount Memorial Hospital	Maryville	94%	255
Cookeville Regional Medical Center	Cookeville	94%	710
Dyersburg Regional Medical Center	Dyersburg	94%	126
Johnson City Specialty Hospital	Johnson City	94%	280
Maury Regional Hospital	Columbia	94%	424
Stones River Hosp/Dekalb Comm Hosp	Smithville	94%	31
University of Tennessee Memorial Hospital	Knoxville	94%	832
Laughlin Memorial Hospital	Greeneville	93%	132
University Medical Center	Lebanon	93%	215
Athens Regional Medical Center	Athens	92%	108
Henry County Medical Center	Paris	92%	37
Mercy Medical Center	Knoxville	92%	1164
River Park Hospital	McMinnville	92%	192
Saint Thomas Hospital	Nashville	92%	525
Indian Path Medical Center	Kingsport	91%	239
Morristown Hamblen Hospital Association	Morristown	91%	252
Saint Francis Hospital	Memphis	91%	449
Baptist Memorial Hospital Union City	Union City	90%	99
Cumberland Medical Center	Crossville	90%	181
Lakeway Regional Hospital	Morristown	90%	166
Lincoln Medical Center	Fayetteville	90%	30
Saint Francis Bartlett Medical Center	Bartlett	90%	89
Sumner Regional Medical Center	Gallatin	90%	107
Northcrest Medical Center	Springfield	89%	98
Saint Mary's Jefferson Memorial Hospital	Jefferson City	88%	25
Wellmont Holston Valley Medical Center	Kingsport	88%	561
Jackson-Madison County General Hospital	Jackson	87%	1551
Johnson City Medical Center	Johnson City	86%	674
Grandview Medical Center	Jasper	85%	27
Metro Nashville General Hospital	Nashville	59%	86

30. Prophylactic Antibiotic Stopped

Hospital Name	City	Rate	Cases
Crockett Hospital	Lawrenceburg	100%	26
McKenzie Regional Hospital[2]	McKenzie	100%	57
Stones River Hosp & Dekalb Comm Hosp[2]	Woodbury	100%	40
Fort Sanders Regional Medical Center[2]	Knoxville	99%	742
Hendersonville Medical Center	Hendersonville	99%	177
Saint Francis Bartlett Medical Center[2]	Bartlett	99%	188
Harton Regional Medical Center	Tullahoma	98%	134
Mercy Medical Center[2]	Knoxville	98%	1934
Methodist Medical Center of Oak Ridge[2]	Oak Ridge	98%	963
Parkwest Medical Center[2]	Knoxville	98%	1610
Southern Hills Medical Center	Nashville	98%	154
Henry County Medical Center	Paris	97%	369
Leconte Medical Center[2]	Sevierville	97%	192
Memorial Healthcare System[2]	Chattanooga	97%	2005
Parkridge Medical Center[2]	Chattanooga	97%	419
Saint Mary's Jefferson Memorial Hospital	Jefferson City	97%	61
Sumner Regional Medical Center	Gallatin	97%	271
Sycamore Shoals Hospital[2]	Elizabethton	97%	120
Vanderbilt University Hospital[2]	Nashville	97%	401
Wellmont Holston Valley Medical Center[2]	Kingsport	97%	377
Dyersburg Regional Medical Center[2]	Dyersburg	96%	49
Hillside Hospital	Pulaski	96%	54
Indian Path Medical Center[2]	Kingsport	96%	256
Livingston Regional Hospital	Livingston	96%	48
Regional Hospital of Jackson[2]	Jackson	96%	199
Skyline Medical Center[2]	Nashville	96%	244
Stonecrest Medical Center	Smyrna	96%	184
Summit Medical Center[2]	Hermitage	96%	223
Takoma Regional Hospital	Greeneville	96%	46
Blount Memorial Hospital[2]	Maryville	95%	279
Centennial Medical Center[2]	Nashville	95%	557
Laughlin Memorial Hospital	Greeneville	95%	190
Maury Regional Hospital[2]	Columbia	95%	446
Methodist Healthcare Memphis Hospitals[2]	Memphis	95%	2142
Morristown Hamblen Hospital Association	Morristown	95%	262
Northcrest Medical Center	Springfield	95%	104
Baptist Memorial Hospital Union City[2]	Union City	94%	93
Horizon Medical Center	Dickson	94%	88
Saint Thomas Hospital[2]	Nashville	94%	525
Southern Tennessee Medical Center	Winchester	94%	174
Baptist Hospital[2]	Nashville	93%	490
Cookeville Regional Medical Center	Cookeville	93%	831

NOTE: Hospital profiles are in alphabetical order by state, then city, then hospital within the city; Rankings exclude hospitals with less than 25 cases except for patient surveys which excludes hospitals with less than 100 cases; (a) 100–299 cases; (1) The number of cases is too small to be sure how well a hospital is performing; (2) The hospital indicated that the data submitted for this measure were based on a sample of cases; (3) Data was collected during a shorter time period (fewer quarters) than the maximum possible time for this measure; (4) Suppressed for one or more quarters by CMS; (5) No data is available from the hospital for this measure; (6) Fewer than 100 patients completed the HCAHPS survey. Use these rates with caution, as the number of surveys may be too low to reliably assess hospital performance; (7) Survey results are based on less than 12 months of data; (8) Survey results are not available for this reporting period; (9) No or very few patients were eligible for the HCAHPS survey. The scores shown, if any, reflect a very small number of surveys; (10) A state average was not calculated because too few hospitals in the state submitted data; (11) There were discrepancies in the data collection process; Please refer to the User's Guide for a full explanation of data.

Erlanger Medical Center[2]	Chattanooga	93%	321
Lakeway Regional Hospital[2]	Morristown	93%	122
Regional Medical Center at Memphis	Memphis	93%	116
River Park Hospital	McMinnville	93%	55
Unicoi County Memorial Hospital	Erwin	93%	68
University Medical Center	Lebanon	93%	296
Volunteer Community Hospital[2]	Martin	93%	45
Wellmont Bristol Regional Medical Center[2]	Bristol	93%	309
Delta Medical Center	Memphis	92%	73
Saint Francis Hospital[2]	Memphis	92%	396
University of Tennessee Memorial Hospital[2]	Knoxville	92%	441
Athens Regional Medical Center	Athens	91%	80
Middle Tennessee Medical Center[2]	Murfreesboro	91%	649
Skyridge Medical Center[2]	Cleveland	91%	220
VA Middle Tennessee Healthcare System	Nashville	91%	126
Baptist Memorial Hospital[2]	Memphis	90%	659
Gateway Medical Center	Clarksville	90%	512
Jellico Community Hospital	Jellico	90%	30
Hardin Medical Center	Savannah	89%	36
Williamson Medical Center[2]	Franklin	89%	241
Metro Nashville General Hospital[2]	Nashville	88%	117
Woods Memorial Hospital	Etowah	88%	50
Stones River Hosp/Dekalb Comm Hosp	Smithville	87%	46
Cumberland Medical Center[2]	Crossville	85%	110
Heritage Medical Center[2]	Shelbyville	85%	48
Jackson-Madison County General Hospital[2]	Jackson	84%	1197
Johnson City Specialty Hospital[2]	Johnson City	84%	25
Sweetwater Hospital Association	Sweetwater	83%	35
Johnson City Medical Center[2]	Johnson City	81%	421
White County Community Hospital[2]	Sparta	73%	41

31. Recommended VTP Ordered

Hospital Name	City	Rate	Cases
Heritage Medical Center[2]	Shelbyville	100%	43
Centennial Medical Center[2]	Nashville	99%	276
Erlanger Medical Center[2]	Chattanooga	99%	156
Methodist Medical Center of Oak Ridge[2]	Oak Ridge	99%	224
Saint Thomas Hospital[2]	Nashville	99%	187
Southern Tennessee Medical Center	Winchester	99%	103
University of Tennessee Memorial Hospital[2]	Knoxville	99%	207
Vanderbilt University Hospital[2]	Nashville	99%	198
Wellmont Holston Valley Medical Center[2]	Kingsport	99%	151
Indian Path Medical Center[2]	Kingsport	98%	186
Northcrest Medical Center	Springfield	98%	85
Regional Hospital of Jackson[2]	Jackson	98%	199
Skyridge Medical Center[2]	Cleveland	98%	243
Southern Hills Medical Center	Nashville	98%	118
Summit Medical Center[2]	Hermitage	98%	224
Hendersonville Medical Center	Hendersonville	97%	125
Jackson-Madison County General Hospital[2]	Jackson	97%	635
Morristown Hamblen Hospital Association	Morristown	97%	130
Parkridge Medical Center[2]	Chattanooga	97%	198
Roane Medical Center	Harriman	97%	34
Skyline Medical Center[2]	Nashville	97%	209
Stonecrest Medical Center	Smyrna	97%	116
Dyersburg Regional Medical Center[2]	Dyersburg	96%	68
Gateway Medical Center	Clarksville	96%	279
Methodist Healthcare Memphis Hospitals[2]	Memphis	96%	1318
Regional Medical Center at Memphis	Memphis	96%	318
River Park Hospital	McMinnville	96%	57
University Medical Center	Lebanon	96%	241
VA Middle Tennessee Healthcare System[2]	Nashville	96%	82
Athens Regional Medical Center	Athens	95%	98
Fort Sanders Regional Medical Center[2]	Knoxville	95%	311
Henry County Medical Center	Paris	95%	199
Laughlin Memorial Hospital	Greeneville	95%	139
Unicoi County Memorial Hospital	Erwin	95%	40
Baptist Hospital[2]	Nashville	94%	211
Leconte Medical Center[2]	Sevierville	94%	83
Baptist Memorial Hospital[2]	Memphis	93%	366
Blount Memorial Hospital[2]	Maryville	93%	178
Fort Loudoun Medical Center	Lenoir City	93%	30
Memorial Healthcare System[2]	Chattanooga	93%	658
Middle Tennessee Medical Center[2]	Murfreesboro	93%	215
Parkwest Medical Center[2]	Knoxville	93%	410
Saint Francis Bartlett Medical Center[2]	Bartlett	93%	115
Sumner Regional Medical Center	Gallatin	93%	115
Harton Regional Medical Center	Tullahoma	92%	87
Horizon Medical Center	Dickson	92%	103
Livingston Regional Hospital	Livingston	92%	39
Mercy Medical Center[2]	Knoxville	92%	613
Saint Francis Hospital[2]	Memphis	92%	236
Sycamore Shoals Hospital[2]	Elizabethton	92%	80
Volunteer Community Hospital[2]	Martin	92%	52
Maury Regional Hospital[2]	Columbia	91%	162
Cookeville Regional Medical Center	Cookeville	90%	377
Sweetwater Hospital Association	Sweetwater	90%	61
Williamson Medical Center[2]	Franklin	90%	155
Baptist Memorial Hospital Union City[2]	Union City	86%	57
Takoma Regional Hospital	Greeneville	86%	36
Lakeway Regional Hospital[2]	Morristown	85%	52
Johnson City Medical Center[2]	Johnson City	83%	173
Metro Nashville General Hospital[2]	Nashville	83%	138
Woods Memorial Hospital	Etowah	83%	35
Saint Mary's Jefferson Memorial Hospital	Jefferson City	82%	28
Delta Medical Center	Memphis	74%	46
Wellmont Bristol Regional Medical Center[2]	Bristol	74%	145
Cumberland Medical Center[2]	Crossville	72%	129
Claiborne County Hospital[2]	Tazewell	65%	34

32. Urinary Catheter Removal

Hospital Name	City	Rate	Cases
Hendersonville Medical Center	Hendersonville	100%	65
Unicoi County Memorial Hospital	Erwin	100%	25
Skyline Medical Center[2]	Nashville	99%	94
Summit Medical Center[2]	Hermitage	99%	87
Southern Hills Medical Center	Nashville	98%	61
Laughlin Memorial Hospital	Greeneville	97%	79
Mercy Medical Center	Knoxville	97%	870
Saint Mary's Jefferson Memorial Hospital	Jefferson City	97%	36
Stonecrest Medical Center	Smyrna	97%	58
University of Tennessee Memorial Hospital[2]	Knoxville	97%	174
Harton Regional Medical Center	Tullahoma	96%	28
Morristown Hamblen Hospital Association	Morristown	96%	102
Southern Tennessee Medical Center	Winchester	96%	84
Vanderbilt University Hospital[2]	Nashville	96%	151
Fort Sanders Regional Medical Center[2]	Knoxville	95%	205
Northcrest Medical Center	Springfield	95%	44
Centennial Medical Center[2]	Nashville	94%	218
Indian Path Medical Center[2]	Kingsport	94%	35
Sumner Regional Medical Center	Gallatin	93%	106
Williamson Medical Center[2]	Franklin	92%	89
University Medical Center	Lebanon	91%	85
Maury Regional Hospital[2]	Columbia	90%	119
Memorial Healthcare System[2]	Chattanooga	90%	754
Methodist Healthcare Memphis Hospitals[2]	Memphis	90%	452
Parkridge Medical Center[2]	Chattanooga	90%	109
Regional Hospital of Jackson	Jackson	90%	78
Baptist Hospital[2]	Nashville	89%	183
Gateway Medical Center	Clarksville	89%	185
Johnson City Medical Center[2]	Johnson City	89%	158
Lakeway Regional Hospital	Morristown	89%	44
Methodist Medical Center of Oak Ridge[2]	Oak Ridge	89%	217
Parkwest Medical Center[2]	Knoxville	89%	466
Saint Thomas Hospital[2]	Nashville	89%	179
Henry County Medical Center	Paris	88%	67
Horizon Medical Center	Dickson	88%	43
Middle Tennessee Medical Center[2]	Murfreesboro	88%	111
Sycamore Shoals Hospital[2]	Elizabethton	86%	29
Baptist Memorial Hospital[2]	Memphis	85%	128
Wellmont Holston Valley Medical Center[2]	Kingsport	85%	130
Cookeville Regional Medical Center	Cookeville	84%	347
VA Middle Tennessee Healthcare System[2]	Nashville	84%	44
Metro Nashville General Hospital[2]	Nashville	83%	52
Jackson-Madison County General Hospital[2]	Jackson	82%	419
Athens Regional Medical Center	Athens	80%	30
Blount Memorial Hospital[2]	Maryville	80%	99
Erlanger Medical Center[2]	Chattanooga	80%	64
Saint Francis Hospital[2]	Memphis	80%	101
Wellmont Bristol Regional Medical Center[2]	Bristol	77%	97
Regional Medical Center at Memphis	Memphis	73%	41
Skyridge Medical Center	Cleveland	73%	55
Cumberland Medical Center[2]	Crossville	72%	36

Children's Asthma Care

33. Received Systemic Corticosteroids

Hospital Name	City	Rate	Cases
Erlanger Medical Center	Chattanooga	100%	39
Johnson City Medical Center[2]	Johnson City	97%	66

34. Received Home Management Plan of Care

Hospital Name	City	Rate	Cases
Erlanger Medical Center	Chattanooga	82%	39
Johnson City Medical Center[2]	Johnson City	9%	66

35. Received Reliever Medication

Hospital Name	City	Rate	Cases
Erlanger Medical Center	Chattanooga	100%	39
Johnson City Medical Center[2]	Johnson City	100%	66

Use of Medical Imaging

36. Combination Abdominal CT Scan

Hospital Name	City	Ratio	Cases
Milan General Hospital	Milan	0.000	166
Stones River Hosp & Dekalb Comm Hosp[1]	Woodbury	0.000	43
Gibson General Hospital	Trenton	0.011	89
Bolivar General Hospital	Bolivar	0.013	153
Dyersburg Regional Medical Center	Dyersburg	0.013	454
Regional Hospital of Jackson	Jackson	0.013	228
River Park Hospital	McMinnville	0.023	385
Claiborne County Hospital	Tazewell	0.024	376
Baptist Memorial Hospital Tipton	Covington	0.025	323
Hardin Medical Center	Savannah	0.034	466
Methodist Healthcare Fayette Hospital	Somerville	0.038	184
Jackson-Madison County General Hospital	Jackson	0.039	1630
Gateway Medical Center	Clarksville	0.042	954
Saint Mary's Jefferson Memorial Hospital	Jefferson City	0.049	531
Lauderdale Community Hospital	Ripley	0.050	140
McNairy Regional Hospital	Selmer	0.050	161
Baptist Memorial Hospital	Memphis	0.051	1699
Baptist Memorial Hospital Union City	Union City	0.052	480
Saint Thomas Hospital	Nashville	0.055	902
Cookeville Regional Medical Center	Cookeville	0.057	888
Metro Nashville General Hospital	Nashville	0.057	70
Perry Community Hospital	Linden	0.058	104
Methodist Medical Center of Oak Ridge	Oak Ridge	0.059	1105
Southern Tennessee Medical Center	Winchester	0.061	396
Stonecrest Medical Center	Smyrna	0.064	346
Mercy Medical Center	Knoxville	0.066	1189
Haywood Park Community Hospital	Brownsville	0.069	102
Humboldt General Hospital	Humboldt	0.070	86
Northcrest Medical Center	Springfield	0.073	381
Centennial Medical Center of Ashland City	Ashland City	0.076	66
Jamestown Regional Medical Center	Jamestown	0.079	165
University of Tennessee Memorial Hospital	Knoxville	0.080	2016
Baptist Hospital of Cocke County	Newport	0.088	362
Sweetwater Hospital Association	Sweetwater	0.092	392
Rhea Medical Center	Dayton	0.096	384
United Regional Medical Center	Manchester	0.106	94
Centennial Medical Center	Nashville	0.107	863
Cumberland Medical Center	Crossville	0.110	970
Morristown Hamblen Hospital Association	Morristown	0.118	619
Southern Hills Medical Center	Nashville	0.122	395
Laughlin Memorial Hospital	Greeneville	0.128	897
Maury Regional Hospital	Columbia	0.128	1324
Blount Memorial Hospital	Maryville	0.129	1077
Horizon Medical Center	Dickson	0.136	440
Baptist Hospital	Nashville	0.139	894
Fort Sanders Regional Medical Center	Knoxville	0.141	740
Leconte Medical Center	Sevierville	0.141	802
Heritage Medical Center	Shelbyville	0.146	219
Volunteer Community Hospital	Martin	0.147	238
Unicoi County Memorial Hospital	Erwin	0.148	209
Parkwest Medical Center	Knoxville	0.155	885
Hillside Hospital	Pulaski	0.156	282
Roane Medical Center	Harriman	0.162	359
Parkridge Medical Center	Chattanooga	0.173	819
Wellmont Hawkins County Memorial Hospital	Rogersville	0.173	197
Hendersonville Medical Center	Hendersonville	0.174	522
University Medical Center	Lebanon	0.180	510
Skyridge Medical Center	Cleveland	0.195	967
Crockett Hospital	Lawrenceburg	0.210	405
Vanderbilt University Hospital	Nashville	0.212	2684
Middle Tennessee Medical Center	Murfreesboro	0.215	608
Copper Basin Medical Center	Copperhill	0.229	166
Methodist Healthcare Memphis Hospitals	Memphis	0.245	3067
Wellmont Holston Valley Medical Center	Kingsport	0.256	540
Williamson Medical Center	Franklin	0.256	632
Johnson County Community Hospital	Mountain City	0.272	162
Skyline Medical Center	Nashville	0.277	822
Grandview Medical Center	Jasper	0.283	311
Fort Loudoun Medical Center	Lenoir City	0.293	256
Erlanger Medical Center	Chattanooga	0.296	1071
Woods Memorial Hospital	Etowah	0.317	319
Stones River Hosp/Dekalb Comm Hosp	Smithville	0.327	226
Harton Regional Medical Center	Tullahoma	0.330	518
Franklin Woods Community Hospital	Johnson City	0.333	420
Medical Center of Manchester	Manchester	0.333	150
Summit Medical Center	Hermitage	0.341	722
St Mary's Med Ctr of Campbell County	La Follette	0.344	256
Johnson City Medical Center	Johnson City	0.349	1194
Athens Regional Medical Center	Athens	0.353	481
White County Community Hospital	Sparta	0.356	160
Henderson County Community Hospital	Lexington	0.363	91
Regional Medical Center at Memphis	Memphis	0.377	273
Sycamore Shoals Hospital	Elizabethton	0.386	541
Memorial Healthcare System	Chattanooga	0.390	2724
Riverview Regional Medical Center North	Carthage	0.403	191
Decatur County General Hospital	Parsons	0.410	173
McKenzie Regional Hospital	McKenzie	0.417	60
Takoma Regional Hospital	Greeneville	0.457	313
Sumner Regional Medical Center	Gallatin	0.552	600
Henry County Medical Center	Paris	0.563	710
Indian Path Medical Center	Kingsport	0.565	391
Macon County General Hospital	Lafayette	0.581	105
Lakeway Regional Hospital	Morristown	0.582	220
Jellico Community Hospital	Jellico	0.588	216

NOTE: Hospital profiles are in alphabetical order by state, then city, then hospital within the city; Rankings exclude hospitals with less than 25 cases except for patient surveys which excludes hospitals with less than 100 cases; (a) 100–299 cases; (1) The number of cases is too small to be sure how well a hospital is performing; (2) The hospital indicated that the data submitted for this measure were based on a sample of cases; (3) Data was collected during a shorter time period (fewer quarters) than the maximum possible time for this measure; (4) Suppressed for one or more quarters by CMS; (5) No data is available from the hospital for this measure; (6) Fewer than 100 patients completed the HCAHPS survey. Use these rates with caution, as the number of surveys may be too low to reliably assess hospital performance; (7) Survey results are based on less than 12 months of data; (8) Survey results are not available for this reporting period; (9) No or very few patients were eligible for the HCAHPS survey. The scores shown, if any, reflect a very small number of surveys; (10) A state average was not calculated because too few hospitals in the state submitted data; (11) There were discrepancies in the data collection process; Please refer to the User's Guide for a full explanation of data.

Delta Medical Center	Memphis	0.596	47
Wayne Medical Center	Waynesboro	0.615	91
Livingston Regional Hospital	Livingston	0.622	246
Lincoln Medical Center	Fayetteville	0.635	249
Baptist Memorial Hospital Huntingdon	Huntingdon	0.639	155
Cumberland River Hospital[1]	Celina	0.674	43
Saint Francis Bartlett Medical Center	Bartlett	0.694	369
Wellmont Bristol Regional Medical Center	Bristol	0.696	1463
Saint Francis Hospital	Memphis	0.747	770

37. Combination Chest CT Scan

Hospital Name	City	Ratio	Cases
Claiborne County Hospital	Tazewell	0.000	288
Henry County Medical Center	Paris	0.000	436
Humboldt General Hospital	Humboldt	0.000	49
Milan General Hospital	Milan	0.000	71
Stones River Hosp & Dekalb Comm Hosp	Woodbury	0.000	52
Methodist Medical Center of Oak Ridge	Oak Ridge	0.003	738
Skyline Medical Center	Nashville	0.003	629
Saint Francis Hospital	Memphis	0.004	525
Baptist Memorial Hospital Tipton	Covington	0.005	213
Gateway Medical Center	Clarksville	0.005	768
Regional Hospital of Jackson	Jackson	0.005	197
Hillside Hospital	Pulaski	0.006	159
Northcrest Medical Center	Springfield	0.006	316
Jackson-Madison County General Hospital	Jackson	0.008	1313
Lauderdale Community Hospital	Ripley	0.009	115
Saint Francis Bartlett Medical Center	Bartlett	0.010	208
Dyersburg Regional Medical Center	Dyersburg	0.011	280
Hardin Medical Center	Savannah	0.011	261
Horizon Medical Center	Dickson	0.012	163
Southern Tennessee Medical Center	Winchester	0.012	167
Skyridge Medical Center	Cleveland	0.014	702
Hendersonville Medical Center	Hendersonville	0.017	346
Saint Thomas Hospital	Nashville	0.017	896
Haywood Park Community Hospital	Brownsville	0.018	56
Middle Tennessee Medical Center	Murfreesboro	0.018	111
University of Tennessee Memorial Hospital	Knoxville	0.018	2392
Vanderbilt University Hospital	Nashville	0.018	2521
Bolivar General Hospital	Bolivar	0.020	50
Mercy Medical Center	Knoxville	0.020	841
Methodist Healthcare Fayette Hospital	Somerville	0.020	101
Southern Hills Medical Center	Nashville	0.020	246
Jamestown Regional Medical Center	Jamestown	0.022	89
Saint Mary's Jefferson Memorial Hospital	Jefferson City	0.022	320
Crockett Hospital	Lawrenceburg	0.023	393
White County Community Hospital	Sparta	0.023	132
Wellmont Holston Valley Medical Center	Kingsport	0.024	289
Athens Regional Medical Center	Athens	0.026	190
Centennial Medical Center of Ashland City[1]	Ashland City	0.029	35
Metro Nashville General Hospital[1]	Nashville	0.030	33
Wellmont Hawkins County Memorial Hospital	Rogersville	0.030	167
Stonecrest Medical Center	Smyrna	0.032	155
Baptist Memorial Hospital Union City	Union City	0.038	316
Centennial Medical Center	Nashville	0.040	606
Perry Community Hospital	Linden	0.040	75
Sweetwater Hospital Association	Sweetwater	0.041	295
Woods Memorial Hospital	Etowah	0.041	145
Memorial Healthcare System	Chattanooga	0.045	1359
McNairy Regional Hospital	Selmer	0.049	81
Decatur County General Hospital	Parsons	0.051	98
Stones River Hosp/Dekalb Comm Hosp	Smithville	0.057	175
Maury Regional Hospital	Columbia	0.059	1232
Baptist Memorial Hospital	Memphis	0.060	1306
Delta Medical Center[1]	Memphis	0.060	50
Blount Memorial Hospital	Maryville	0.064	643
Leconte Medical Center	Sevierville	0.066	711
Summit Medical Center	Hermitage	0.069	421
Parkwest Medical Center	Knoxville	0.076	682
Gibson General Hospital[1]	Trenton	0.077	26
Cookeville Regional Medical Center	Cookeville	0.078	694
Volunteer Community Hospital	Martin	0.085	164
Baptist Hospital of Cocke County	Newport	0.090	266
Fort Sanders Regional Medical Center	Knoxville	0.103	692
Laughlin Memorial Hospital	Greeneville	0.105	459
Rhea Medical Center	Dayton	0.110	200
Parkridge Medical Center	Chattanooga	0.119	311
Regional Medical Center at Memphis	Memphis	0.119	260
United Regional Medical Center	Manchester	0.122	82
Cumberland Medical Center	Crossville	0.129	1038
Unicoi County Memorial Hospital	Erwin	0.129	139
Baptist Hospital	Nashville	0.132	768
Methodist Healthcare Memphis Hospitals	Memphis	0.150	2231
University Medical Center	Lebanon	0.150	367
Erlanger Medical Center	Chattanooga	0.153	940
Morristown Hamblen Hospital Association	Morristown	0.159	389
Roane Medical Center	Harriman	0.164	323
Fort Loudoun Medical Center	Lenoir City	0.166	290
Wellmont Bristol Regional Medical Center	Bristol	0.167	927
Williamson Medical Center	Franklin	0.172	344
St Mary's Med Ctr of Campbell County	La Follette	0.180	206
Copper Basin Medical Center	Copperhill	0.189	90
Grandview Medical Center	Jasper	0.234	124
River Park Hospital	McMinnville	0.252	393
Harton Regional Medical Center	Tullahoma	0.301	309
Sycamore Shoals Hospital	Elizabethton	0.321	293
Riverview Regional Medical Center North	Carthage	0.361	119
Takoma Regional Hospital	Greeneville	0.367	221
Heritage Medical Center	Shelbyville	0.413	138
Johnson City Medical Center	Johnson City	0.418	813
Sumner Regional Medical Center	Gallatin	0.422	597
Lincoln Medical Center	Fayetteville	0.434	175
Franklin Woods Community Hospital	Johnson City	0.455	200
Johnson County Community Hospital	Mountain City	0.458	83
Medical Center of Manchester	Manchester	0.469	49
Macon County General Hospital	Lafayette	0.494	85
Indian Path Medical Center	Kingsport	0.520	177
Lakeway Regional Hospital	Morristown	0.610	82
Baptist Memorial Hospital Huntingdon	Huntingdon	0.649	94
Wayne Medical Center	Waynesboro	0.731	67
Jellico Community Hospital	Jellico	0.754	199
McKenzie Regional Hospital[1]	McKenzie	0.833	30
Livingston Regional Hospital	Livingston	0.874	111

38. Follow-up Mammogram/Ultrasound

Hospital Name	City	Rate	Cases
Humboldt General Hospital	Humboldt	2.2%	268
St Mary's Med Ctr of Campbell County	La Follette	2.8%	320
Copper Basin Medical Center	Copperhill	2.9%	238
Livingston Regional Hospital	Livingston	3.0%	337
Metro Nashville General Hospital	Nashville	3.2%	124
Jamestown Regional Medical Center	Jamestown	3.7%	376
Williamson Medical Center	Franklin	3.8%	996
Bolivar General Hospital	Bolivar	4.0%	149
Wellmont Holston Valley Medical Center	Kingsport	4.0%	1696
Lauderdale Community Hospital	Ripley	4.1%	318
Roane Medical Center	Harriman	4.1%	534
Volunteer Community Hospital	Martin	4.2%	120
Centennial Medical Center of Ashland City	Ashland City	4.3%	46
Memorial Healthcare System	Chattanooga	4.6%	4438
McNairy Regional Hospital	Selmer	4.8%	294
River Park Hospital	McMinnville	4.8%	744
Erlanger Medical Center	Chattanooga	5.1%	2058
Skyridge Medical Center	Cleveland	5.1%	1145
Southern Tennessee Medical Center	Winchester	5.1%	891
Horizon Medical Center	Dickson	5.2%	650
Cumberland Medical Center	Crossville	5.3%	2102
Cumberland River Hospital	Celina	5.3%	94
Henry County Medical Center	Paris	5.3%	836
Heritage Medical Center	Shelbyville	5.4%	444
Southern Hills Medical Center	Nashville	5.9%	656
Haywood Park Community Hospital	Brownsville	6.0%	348
Grandview Medical Center	Jasper	6.2%	355
Fort Sanders Regional Medical Center	Knoxville	6.4%	593
Parkwest Medical Center	Knoxville	6.4%	779
Gateway Medical Center	Clarksville	6.5%	1261
Gibson General Hospital	Trenton	6.6%	228
University of Tennessee Memorial Hospital	Knoxville	6.6%	1935
Baptist Memorial Hospital Union City	Union City	6.7%	360
Wayne Medical Center	Waynesboro	6.8%	162
Takoma Regional Hospital	Greeneville	6.9%	420
Cookeville Regional Medical Center	Cookeville	7.0%	1003
Dyersburg Regional Medical Center	Dyersburg	7.0%	672
Saint Francis Bartlett Medical Center	Bartlett	7.0%	314
Jackson-Madison County General Hospital	Jackson	7.2%	1994
Lincoln Medical Center	Fayetteville	7.2%	429
Centennial Medical Center	Nashville	7.3%	1051
Saint Francis Hospital	Memphis	7.3%	1212
Regional Medical Center at Memphis	Memphis	7.4%	257
United Regional Medical Center	Manchester	7.4%	256
Leconte Medical Center	Sevierville	7.5%	933
Baptist Memorial Hospital Tipton	Covington	7.6%	331
Delta Medical Center	Memphis	7.6%	119
Johnson City Medical Center	Johnson City	7.6%	2602
Middle Tennessee Medical Center	Murfreesboro	7.8%	729
Morristown Hamblen Hospital Association	Morristown	7.8%	541
Saint Thomas Hospital	Nashville	7.8%	1619
Stones River Hosp & Dekalb Comm Hosp	Woodbury	7.8%	77
Sweetwater Hospital Association	Sweetwater	7.8%	257
Johnson City Specialty Hospital	Johnson City	7.9%	114
Skyline Medical Center	Nashville	7.9%	1095
Henderson County Community Hospital	Lexington	8.2%	255
Indian Path Medical Center	Kingsport	8.4%	598
Methodist Healthcare Fayette Hospital	Somerville	8.4%	202
Stones River Hosp/Dekalb Comm Hosp	Smithville	8.4%	323
Johnson County Community Hospital	Mountain City	8.5%	176
Unicoi County Memorial Hospital	Erwin	8.5%	342
Wellmont Bristol Regional Medical Center	Bristol	8.5%	1183
Laughlin Memorial Hospital	Greeneville	8.7%	969
Regional Hospital of Jackson	Jackson	8.7%	161
Methodist Medical Center of Oak Ridge	Oak Ridge	8.8%	2390
Lakeway Regional Hospital	Morristown	8.9%	157
Claiborne County Hospital	Tazewell	9.0%	299
Stonecrest Medical Center	Smyrna	9.0%	480
Milan General Hospital	Milan	9.2%	271
Hillside Hospital	Pulaski	9.4%	499
White County Community Hospital	Sparta	9.5%	338
Sycamore Shoals Hospital	Elizabethton	9.9%	708
Baptist Memorial Hospital	Memphis	10.0%	3419
Methodist Healthcare Memphis Hospitals	Memphis	10.0%	4237
Baptist Hospital	Nashville	10.1%	1712
Crockett Hospital	Lawrenceburg	10.1%	662
Saint Mary's Jefferson Memorial Hospital	Jefferson City	10.1%	596
Blount Memorial Hospital	Maryville	10.2%	1525
Summit Medical Center	Hermitage	10.2%	1258
University Medical Center	Lebanon	10.4%	595
Maury Regional Hospital	Columbia	10.7%	1690
Mercy Medical Center	Knoxville	10.8%	742
Harton Regional Medical Center	Tullahoma	11.2%	1036
Hendersonville Medical Center	Hendersonville	11.2%	721
Athens Regional Medical Center	Athens	11.3%	961
Vanderbilt University Hospital	Nashville	11.3%	990
Rhea Medical Center	Dayton	11.6%	380
Baptist Hospital of Cocke County	Newport	11.9%	506
Parkridge Medical Center	Chattanooga	12.3%	625
Sumner Regional Medical Center	Gallatin	12.5%	615
Baptist Memorial Hospital Huntingdon	Huntingdon	12.8%	243
Fort Loudoun Medical Center	Lenoir City	12.8%	337
Woods Memorial Hospital	Etowah	12.8%	345
Wellmont Hawkins County Memorial Hospital	Rogersville	13.0%	223
Northcrest Medical Center	Springfield	13.1%	672
McKenzie Regional Hospital	McKenzie	13.3%	264
Jellico Community Hospital	Jellico	15.9%	308
Decatur County General Hospital	Parsons	17.4%	281
Hardin Medical Center	Savannah	19.0%	399
Macon County General Hospital	Lafayette	23.2%	155

39. MRI for Low Back Pain

Hospital Name	City	Rate	Cases
Jamestown Regional Medical Center[1]	Jamestown	14.0%	43
River Park Hospital	McMinnville	17.8%	157
Morristown Hamblen Hospital Association	Morristown	19.6%	189
Riverview Regional Medical Center North[1]	Carthage	20.0%	55
Franklin Woods Community Hospital	Johnson City	20.5%	127
Henderson County Community Hospital	Lexington	21.0%	62
Baptist Memorial Hospital Tipton	Covington	22.6%	62
Hillside Hospital[1]	Pulaski	22.8%	57
United Regional Medical Center	Manchester	22.8%	215
University of Tennessee Memorial Hospital	Knoxville	23.2%	323
Hendersonville Medical Center	Hendersonville	23.6%	178
Parkwest Medical Center	Knoxville	24.4%	176
University Medical Center	Lebanon	24.4%	82
Methodist Medical Center of Oak Ridge	Oak Ridge	24.6%	357
Lakeway Regional Hospital	Morristown	25.2%	107
Cookeville Regional Medical Center	Cookeville	25.4%	331
Sumner Regional Medical Center	Gallatin	25.5%	141
Summit Medical Center	Hermitage	25.7%	257
Grandview Medical Center	Jasper	25.8%	66
Southern Hills Medical Center	Nashville	25.8%	62
Takoma Regional Hospital	Greeneville	26.3%	76
Harton Regional Medical Center	Tullahoma	26.4%	178
Dyersburg Regional Medical Center	Dyersburg	26.8%	142
Regional Hospital of Jackson	Jackson	26.8%	56
Stones River Hosp & Dekalb Comm Hosp[1]	Woodbury	26.8%	41
Medical Center of Manchester[1]	Manchester	26.9%	26
Johnson City Medical Center	Johnson City	27.3%	414
Macon County General Hospital[1]	Lafayette	27.8%	36
Maury Regional Hospital	Columbia	27.8%	230
White County Community Hospital[1]	Sparta	28.3%	53
Gateway Medical Center	Clarksville	28.4%	268
Saint Thomas Hospital	Nashville	28.6%	147
Horizon Medical Center	Dickson	28.7%	178
Vanderbilt University Hospital	Nashville	28.7%	101
Wellmont Holston Valley Medical Center[1]	Kingsport	28.9%	45
Mercy Medical Center	Knoxville	29.0%	383
Henry County Medical Center	Paris	29.8%	181
Livingston Regional Hospital	Livingston	29.8%	84
Volunteer Community Hospital	Martin	30.0%	60
Jackson-Madison County General Hospital	Jackson	30.4%	678
Indian Path Medical Center	Kingsport	30.5%	105
Baptist Memorial Hospital Huntingdon	Huntingdon	31.2%	93
Cumberland Medical Center	Crossville	31.3%	415
Saint Francis Hospital	Memphis	31.4%	210
Skyridge Medical Center	Cleveland	31.5%	317
Blount Memorial Hospital	Maryville	31.6%	282
Skyline Medical Center	Nashville	31.6%	244
Rhea Medical Center	Dayton	32.1%	53
Claiborne County Hospital	Tazewell	32.6%	86
Heritage Medical Center	Shelbyville	32.8%	64
Unicoi County Memorial Hospital	Erwin	32.8%	58

NOTE: Hospital profiles are in alphabetical order by state, then city, then hospital within the city; Rankings exclude hospitals with less than 25 cases except for patient surveys which excludes hospitals with less than 100 cases; (a) 100–299 cases; (1) The number of cases is too small to be sure how well a hospital is performing; (2) The hospital indicated that the data submitted for this measure were based on a sample of cases; (3) Data was collected during a shorter time period (fewer quarters) than the maximum possible time for this measure; (4) Suppressed for one or more quarters by CMS; (5) No data is available from the hospital for this measure; (6) Fewer than 100 patients completed the HCAHPS survey. Use these rates with caution, as the number of surveys may be too low to reliably assess hospital performance; (7) Survey results are based on less than 12 months of data; (8) Survey results are not available for this reporting period; (9) No or very few patients were eligible for the HCAHPS survey. The scores shown, if any, reflect a very small number of surveys; (10) A state average was not calculated because too few hospitals in the state submitted data; (11) There were discrepancies in the data collection process; Please refer to the User's Guide for a full explanation of data.

Fort Sanders Regional Medical Center	Knoxville	33.1%	248
Southern Tennessee Medical Center	Winchester	33.1%	142
Centennial Medical Center	Nashville	33.3%	180
Memorial Healthcare System	Chattanooga	33.3%	568
Roane Medical Center	Harriman	33.3%	66
Methodist Healthcare Memphis Hospitals	Memphis	33.5%	505
Laughlin Memorial Hospital	Greeneville	33.6%	214
Northcrest Medical Center	Springfield	33.7%	95
Stonecrest Medical Center	Smyrna	33.8%	65
Parkridge Medical Center	Chattanooga	33.9%	118
Fort Loudoun Medical Center	Lenoir City	34.2%	79
Baptist Memorial Hospital Union City	Union City	35.1%	111
Lincoln Medical Center	Fayetteville	35.1%	57
Saint Mary's Jefferson Memorial Hospital	Jefferson City	35.1%	114
Saint Francis Bartlett Medical Center	Bartlett	35.3%	68
Woods Memorial Hospital	Etowah	35.4%	79
Athens Regional Medical Center	Athens	35.5%	138
Stones River Hosp/Dekalb Comm Hosp	Smithville	35.5%	62
Baptist Memorial Hospital	Memphis	35.8%	268
Wellmont Bristol Regional Medical Center	Bristol	35.8%	439
Crockett Hospital	Lawrenceburg	36.0%	136
Wayne Medical Center	Waynesboro	36.2%	47
Erlanger Medical Center	Chattanooga	36.6%	164
Williamson Medical Center	Franklin	36.8%	68
Sycamore Shoals Hospital	Elizabethton	37.1%	210
McNairy Regional Hospital	Selmer	37.5%	48
Middle Tennessee Medical Center[1]	Murfreesboro	38.9%	36
Wellmont Hawkins County Memorial Hospital	Rogersville	39.2%	74
Baptist Hospital	Nashville	39.6%	144
Hardin Medical Center	Savannah	39.6%	106
Leconte Medical Center	Sevierville	40.1%	172
Sweetwater Hospital Association	Sweetwater	43.3%	90
Baptist Hospital of Cocke County	Newport	44.2%	104
St Mary's Med Ctr of Campbell County	La Follette	47.1%	119
Jellico Community Hospital	Jellico	67.9%	56

Survey of Patients' Hospital Experiences

40. Area Around Room 'Always' Quiet at Night

Hospital Name	City	Rate	Cases
The Center for Spinal Surgery	Nashville	91%	300+
Methodist Healthcare Fayette Hospital	Somerville	87%	(a)
Haywood Park Community Hospital	Brownsville	79%	(a)
Baptist Memorial Hospital Huntingdon	Huntingdon	76%	(a)
Delta Medical Center	Memphis	76%	300+
United Regional Medical Center	Manchester	76%	300+
Gibson General Hospital	Trenton	75%	(a)
Johnson City Specialty Hospital	Johnson City	75%	300+
Wellmont Hawkins County Memorial Hospital	Rogersville	75%	300+
Hardin Medical Center	Savannah	74%	300+
McNairy Regional Hospital	Selmer	74%	(a)
Humboldt General Hospital	Humboldt	73%	(a)
Saint Francis Bartlett Medical Center	Bartlett	72%	300+
White County Community Hospital	Sparta	72%	300+
Fort Loudoun Medical Center	Lenoir City	71%	300+
Henderson County Community Hospital	Lexington	71%	(a)
Roane Medical Center	Harriman	71%	300+
McKenzie Regional Hospital	McKenzie	70%	300+
Riverview Regional Medical Center North	Carthage	70%	(a)
Stonecrest Medical Center	Smyrna	70%	300+
Sycamore Shoals Hospital	Elizabethton	70%	300+
Woods Memorial Hospital	Etowah	70%	300+
Parkwest Medical Center	Knoxville	69%	300+
Baptist Memorial Hospital Union City	Union City	68%	300+
Henry County Medical Center	Paris	68%	300+
Memorial Healthcare System	Chattanooga	68%	300+
Athens Regional Medical Center	Athens	67%	300+
Centennial Medical Center	Nashville	67%	300+
Jackson-Madison County General Hospital	Jackson	67%	300+
Regional Hospital of Jackson	Jackson	67%	300+
Saint Francis Hospital	Memphis	67%	300+
Stones River Hosp/Dekalb Comm Hosp	Smithville	67%	300+
Trousdale Medical Center	Hartsville	67%	(a)
Stones River Hosp & Dekalb Comm Hosp	Woodbury	66%	(a)
Williamson Medical Center	Franklin	66%	300+
Dyersburg Regional Medical Center	Dyersburg	65%	300+
Fort Sanders Regional Medical Center	Knoxville	65%	300+
Grandview Medical Center	Jasper	65%	(a)
Jellico Community Hospital	Jellico	65%	(a)
Lakeway Regional Hospital	Morristown	65%	300+
Leconte Medical Center	Sevierville	65%	300+
Mercy Medical Center	Knoxville	65%	300+
Methodist Medical Center of Oak Ridge	Oak Ridge	65%	300+
Parkridge Medical Center	Chattanooga	65%	300+
Scott County Hospital	Oneida	65%	(a)
Skyline Medical Center	Nashville	65%	300+
Southern Hills Medical Center	Nashville	65%	300+
Baptist Memorial Hospital Tipton	Covington	64%	(a)
Crockett Hospital	Lawrenceburg	64%	300+
Southern Tennessee Medical Center	Winchester	64%	300+
Baptist Memorial Hospital	Memphis	63%	300+
Hillside Hospital	Pulaski	63%	(a)
Jamestown Regional Medical Center	Jamestown	63%	300+
Lincoln Medical Center	Fayetteville	63%	300+
Maury Regional Hospital	Columbia	63%	300+
Methodist Healthcare Memphis Hospitals	Memphis	63%	300+
River Park Hospital	McMinnville	63%	300+
Summit Medical Center	Hermitage	63%	300+
Takoma Regional Hospital	Greeneville	63%	(a)
University of Tennessee Memorial Hospital	Knoxville	63%	300+
Wayne Medical Center	Waynesboro	63%	(a)
Baptist Hospital	Nashville	62%	300+
Erlanger Medical Center	Chattanooga	62%	300+
Metro Nashville General Hospital	Nashville	62%	300+
Sweetwater Hospital Association	Sweetwater	62%	(a)
Volunteer Community Hospital	Martin	62%	300+
Hendersonville Medical Center	Hendersonville	61%	300+
Heritage Medical Center	Shelbyville	61%	300+
Rhea Medical Center	Dayton	61%	300+
University Medical Center	Lebanon	61%	300+
Horizon Medical Center	Dickson	60%	300+
Skyridge Medical Center	Cleveland	60%	300+
Sumner Regional Medical Center	Gallatin	60%	300+
Baptist Hospital of Cocke County	Newport	59%	300+
Cookeville Regional Medical Center	Cookeville	59%	300+
Decatur County General Hospital	Parsons	59%	(a)
Franklin Woods Community Hospital	Johnson City	59%	(a)
Livingston Regional Hospital	Livingston	59%	300+
Northcrest Medical Center	Springfield	59%	300+
Gateway Medical Center	Clarksville	58%	300+
Regional Medical Center at Memphis	Memphis	58%	300+
Wellmont Bristol Regional Medical Center	Bristol	58%	300+
Cumberland Medical Center	Crossville	57%	300+
Harton Regional Medical Center	Tullahoma	57%	300+
Indian Path Medical Center	Kingsport	57%	300+
Middle Tennessee Medical Center	Murfreesboro	57%	300+
St Mary's Med Ctr of Campbell County	La Follette	57%	300+
Unicoi County Memorial Hospital	Erwin	57%	300+
Cumberland River Hospital	Celina	56%	(a)
Laughlin Memorial Hospital	Greeneville	56%	300+
Saint Mary's Jefferson Memorial Hospital	Jefferson City	56%	300+
Vanderbilt University Hospital	Nashville	55%	300+
Wellmont Holston Valley Medical Center	Kingsport	55%	300+
Johnson City Medical Center	Johnson City	54%	300+
Morristown Hamblen Hospital Association	Morristown	54%	300+
Claiborne County Hospital	Tazewell	53%	(a)
Saint Thomas Hospital	Nashville	51%	300+
Blount Memorial Hospital	Maryville	48%	300+

41. Doctors 'Always' Communicated Well

Hospital Name	City	Rate	Cases
Methodist Healthcare Fayette Hospital	Somerville	95%	(a)
The Center for Spinal Surgery	Nashville	93%	300+
Humboldt General Hospital	Humboldt	93%	(a)
Johnson City Specialty Hospital	Johnson City	92%	300+
United Regional Medical Center	Manchester	91%	300+
Gibson General Hospital	Trenton	90%	(a)
Hardin Medical Center	Savannah	90%	300+
Stones River Hosp/Dekalb Comm Hosp	Smithville	90%	300+
Trousdale Medical Center	Hartsville	89%	(a)
Athens Regional Medical Center	Athens	88%	300+
Baptist Memorial Hospital Huntingdon	Huntingdon	88%	(a)
Rhea Medical Center	Dayton	88%	300+
Wellmont Hawkins County Memorial Hospital	Rogersville	88%	300+
Haywood Park Community Hospital	Brownsville	87%	(a)
Sweetwater Hospital Association	Sweetwater	87%	(a)
Unicoi County Memorial Hospital	Erwin	87%	300+
Woods Memorial Hospital	Etowah	87%	300+
Claiborne County Hospital	Tazewell	86%	(a)
Jellico Community Hospital	Jellico	86%	(a)
Leconte Medical Center	Sevierville	86%	300+
Livingston Regional Hospital	Livingston	86%	300+
Centennial Medical Center	Nashville	85%	300+
Hillside Hospital	Pulaski	85%	(a)
McNairy Regional Hospital	Selmer	85%	(a)
Parkwest Medical Center	Knoxville	85%	300+
Scott County Hospital	Oneida	85%	(a)
Stones River Hosp & Dekalb Comm Hosp	Woodbury	85%	(a)
White County Community Hospital	Sparta	85%	300+
Baptist Hospital	Nashville	84%	300+
Cumberland River Hospital	Celina	84%	(a)
Fort Loudoun Medical Center	Lenoir City	84%	300+
Henry County Medical Center	Paris	84%	300+
Heritage Medical Center	Shelbyville	84%	300+
Laughlin Memorial Hospital	Greeneville	84%	300+
Maury Regional Hospital	Columbia	84%	300+
Memorial Healthcare System	Chattanooga	84%	300+
Middle Tennessee Medical Center	Murfreesboro	84%	300+
Riverview Regional Medical Center North	Carthage	84%	(a)
Saint Mary's Jefferson Memorial Hospital	Jefferson City	84%	300+
Sycamore Shoals Hospital	Elizabethton	84%	300+
Williamson Medical Center	Franklin	84%	300+
Baptist Memorial Hospital Union City	Union City	83%	300+
Fort Sanders Regional Medical Center	Knoxville	83%	300+
Horizon Medical Center	Dickson	83%	300+
Jamestown Regional Medical Center	Jamestown	83%	300+
Parkridge Medical Center	Chattanooga	83%	300+
Saint Francis Bartlett Medical Center	Bartlett	83%	300+
Saint Francis Hospital	Memphis	83%	300+
St Mary's Med Ctr of Campbell County	La Follette	83%	300+
Saint Thomas Hospital	Nashville	83%	300+
University of Tennessee Memorial Hospital	Knoxville	83%	300+
Vanderbilt University Hospital	Nashville	83%	300+
Wellmont Holston Valley Medical Center	Kingsport	83%	300+
Baptist Hospital of Cocke County	Newport	82%	300+
Baptist Memorial Hospital Tipton	Covington	82%	(a)
Crockett Hospital	Lawrenceburg	82%	300+
Hendersonville Medical Center	Hendersonville	82%	300+
Mercy Medical Center	Knoxville	82%	300+
Methodist Medical Center of Oak Ridge	Oak Ridge	82%	300+
Metro Nashville General Hospital	Nashville	82%	300+
Northcrest Medical Center	Springfield	82%	300+
Southern Hills Medical Center	Nashville	82%	300+
Southern Tennessee Medical Center	Winchester	82%	300+
Stonecrest Medical Center	Smyrna	82%	300+
Summit Medical Center	Hermitage	82%	300+
Volunteer Community Hospital	Martin	82%	300+
Baptist Memorial Hospital	Memphis	81%	300+
Cumberland Medical Center	Crossville	81%	300+
Decatur County General Hospital	Parsons	81%	(a)
Erlanger Medical Center	Chattanooga	81%	300+
Indian Path Medical Center	Kingsport	81%	300+
McKenzie Regional Hospital	McKenzie	81%	300+
Morristown Hamblen Hospital Association	Morristown	81%	300+
Regional Hospital of Jackson	Jackson	81%	300+
Roane Medical Center	Harriman	81%	300+
Sumner Regional Medical Center	Gallatin	81%	300+
Cookeville Regional Medical Center	Cookeville	80%	300+
Henderson County Community Hospital	Lexington	80%	(a)
Skyline Medical Center	Nashville	80%	300+
University Medical Center	Lebanon	80%	300+
Dyersburg Regional Medical Center	Dyersburg	79%	300+
Gateway Medical Center	Clarksville	79%	300+
Grandview Medical Center	Jasper	79%	(a)
Jackson-Madison County General Hospital	Jackson	79%	300+
Regional Medical Center at Memphis	Memphis	79%	300+
Wayne Medical Center	Waynesboro	79%	(a)
Blount Memorial Hospital	Maryville	78%	300+
Harton Regional Medical Center	Tullahoma	78%	300+
Lakeway Regional Hospital	Morristown	78%	300+
Lincoln Medical Center	Fayetteville	78%	300+
Skyridge Medical Center	Cleveland	78%	300+
Takoma Regional Hospital	Greeneville	78%	(a)
Wellmont Bristol Regional Medical Center	Bristol	78%	300+
Methodist Healthcare Memphis Hospitals	Memphis	77%	300+
River Park Hospital	McMinnville	77%	300+
Johnson City Medical Center	Johnson City	76%	300+
Delta Medical Center	Memphis	73%	300+
Franklin Woods Community Hospital	Johnson City	73%	(a)

42. Home Recovery Information Given

Hospital Name	City	Rate	Cases
The Center for Spinal Surgery	Nashville	90%	300+
Johnson City Specialty Hospital	Johnson City	90%	300+
Leconte Medical Center	Sevierville	89%	300+
Morristown Hamblen Hospital Association	Morristown	88%	300+
Summit Medical Center	Hermitage	88%	300+
Centennial Medical Center	Nashville	87%	300+
Horizon Medical Center	Dickson	87%	300+
Stonecrest Medical Center	Smyrna	87%	300+
Hardin Medical Center	Savannah	86%	300+
Northcrest Medical Center	Springfield	86%	300+
Parkwest Medical Center	Knoxville	86%	300+
Takoma Regional Hospital	Greeneville	86%	(a)
Fort Loudoun Medical Center	Lenoir City	85%	300+
Franklin Woods Community Hospital	Johnson City	85%	(a)
Memorial Healthcare System	Chattanooga	85%	300+
Southern Hills Medical Center	Nashville	85%	300+
Trousdale Medical Center	Hartsville	85%	(a)
United Regional Medical Center	Manchester	85%	300+
Vanderbilt University Hospital	Nashville	85%	300+
Baptist Hospital	Nashville	84%	300+
Blount Memorial Hospital	Maryville	84%	300+
Hendersonville Medical Center	Hendersonville	84%	300+
Methodist Healthcare Fayette Hospital	Somerville	84%	(a)
Middle Tennessee Medical Center	Murfreesboro	84%	300+
Saint Thomas Hospital	Nashville	84%	300+
Skyline Medical Center	Nashville	84%	300+
Stones River Hosp/Dekalb Comm Hosp	Smithville	84%	300+
White County Community Hospital	Sparta	84%	300+

NOTE: Hospital profiles are in alphabetical order by state, then city, then hospital within the city; Rankings exclude hospitals with less than 25 cases except for patient surveys which excludes hospitals with less than 100 cases; (a) 100–299 cases; (1) The number of cases is too small to be sure how well a hospital is performing; (2) The hospital indicated that the data submitted for this measure were based on a sample of cases; (3) Data was collected during a shorter time period (fewer quarters) than the maximum possible time for this measure; (4) Suppressed for one or more quarters by CMS; (5) No data is available from the hospital for this measure; (6) Fewer than 100 patients completed the HCAHPS survey. Use these rates with caution, as the number of surveys may be too low to reliably assess hospital performance; (7) Survey results are based on less than 12 months of data; (8) Survey results are not available for this reporting period; (9) No or very few patients were eligible for the HCAHPS survey. The scores shown, if any, reflect a very small number of surveys; (10) A state average was not calculated because too few hospitals in the state submitted data; (11) There were discrepancies in the data collection process; Please refer to the User's Guide for a full explanation of data.

Williamson Medical Center	Franklin	84%	300+
Athens Regional Medical Center	Athens	83%	300+
Baptist Memorial Hospital Union City	Union City	83%	300+
Fort Sanders Regional Medical Center	Knoxville	83%	300+
Indian Path Medical Center	Kingsport	83%	300+
Maury Regional Hospital	Columbia	83%	300+
Mercy Medical Center	Knoxville	83%	300+
Methodist Medical Center of Oak Ridge	Oak Ridge	83%	300+
Parkridge Medical Center	Chattanooga	83%	300+
Saint Francis Bartlett Medical Center	Bartlett	83%	300+
Sweetwater Hospital Association	Sweetwater	83%	(a)
Wellmont Hawkins County Memorial Hospital	Rogersville	83%	300+
Woods Memorial Hospital	Etowah	83%	300+
Baptist Memorial Hospital Huntingdon	Huntingdon	82%	(a)
Cumberland River Hospital	Celina	82%	(a)
Henry County Medical Center	Paris	82%	300+
Jellico Community Hospital	Jellico	82%	(a)
Roane Medical Center	Harriman	82%	300+
Stones River Hosp & Dekalb Comm Hosp	Woodbury	82%	(a)
University of Tennessee Memorial Hospital	Knoxville	82%	300+
Cookeville Regional Medical Center	Cookeville	81%	300+
Heritage Medical Center	Shelbyville	81%	300+
Hillside Hospital	Pulaski	81%	(a)
Jackson-Madison County General Hospital	Jackson	81%	300+
Johnson City Medical Center	Johnson City	81%	300+
Lakeway Regional Hospital	Morristown	81%	300+
Metro Nashville General Hospital	Nashville	81%	300+
Regional Medical Center at Memphis	Memphis	81%	300+
River Park Hospital	McMinnville	81%	300+
Saint Mary's Jefferson Memorial Hospital	Jefferson City	81%	300+
Sycamore Shoals Hospital	Elizabethton	81%	300+
Erlanger Medical Center	Chattanooga	80%	300+
Harton Regional Medical Center	Tullahoma	80%	300+
Henderson County Community Hospital	Lexington	80%	(a)
McKenzie Regional Hospital	McKenzie	80%	300+
Saint Francis Hospital	Memphis	80%	300+
Scott County Hospital	Oneida	80%	(a)
Southern Tennessee Medical Center	Winchester	80%	300+
University Medical Center	Lebanon	80%	300+
Baptist Hospital of Cocke County	Newport	79%	300+
Baptist Memorial Hospital	Memphis	79%	300+
Claiborne County Hospital	Tazewell	79%	(a)
Methodist Healthcare Memphis Hospitals	Memphis	79%	300+
St Mary's Med Ctr of Campbell County	La Follette	79%	300+
Volunteer Community Hospital	Martin	79%	300+
Wellmont Bristol Regional Medical Center	Bristol	79%	300+
Wellmont Holston Valley Medical Center	Kingsport	79%	300+
Dyersburg Regional Medical Center	Dyersburg	78%	300+
Grandview Medical Center	Jasper	78%	(a)
McNairy Regional Hospital	Selmer	78%	(a)
Regional Hospital of Jackson	Jackson	78%	300+
Riverview Regional Medical Center North	Carthage	78%	(a)
Skyridge Medical Center	Cleveland	78%	300+
Decatur County General Hospital	Parsons	77%	(a)
Gateway Medical Center	Clarksville	77%	300+
Gibson General Hospital	Trenton	77%	(a)
Haywood Park Community Hospital	Brownsville	77%	(a)
Rhea Medical Center	Dayton	77%	300+
Unicoi County Memorial Hospital	Erwin	77%	300+
Cumberland Medical Center	Crossville	76%	300+
Sumner Regional Medical Center	Gallatin	76%	300+
Baptist Memorial Hospital Tipton	Covington	75%	(a)
Jamestown Regional Medical Center	Jamestown	75%	300+
Livingston Regional Hospital	Livingston	75%	300+
Crockett Hospital	Lawrenceburg	74%	300+
Laughlin Memorial Hospital	Greeneville	74%	300+
Lincoln Medical Center	Fayetteville	74%	300+
Wayne Medical Center	Waynesboro	73%	(a)
Delta Medical Center	Memphis	72%	300+
Humboldt General Hospital	Humboldt	67%	(a)

43. Hospital Given 9 or 10 on 10 Point Scale

Hospital Name	City	Rate	Cases
The Center for Spinal Surgery	Nashville	93%	300+
Johnson City Specialty Hospital	Johnson City	90%	300+
Parkwest Medical Center	Knoxville	82%	300+
Saint Thomas Hospital	Nashville	81%	300+
Centennial Medical Center	Nashville	79%	300+
Memorial Healthcare System	Chattanooga	78%	300+
University of Tennessee Memorial Hospital	Knoxville	76%	300+
Fort Sanders Regional Medical Center	Knoxville	75%	300+
Maury Regional Hospital	Columbia	75%	300+
Methodist Healthcare Fayette Hospital	Somerville	75%	(a)
Baptist Memorial Hospital Huntingdon	Huntingdon	74%	(a)
Leconte Medical Center	Sevierville	74%	300+
Sycamore Shoals Hospital	Elizabethton	74%	300+
Vanderbilt University Hospital	Nashville	74%	300+
Williamson Medical Center	Franklin	74%	300+
Fort Loudoun Medical Center	Lenoir City	73%	300+
Parkridge Medical Center	Chattanooga	73%	300+
Wellmont Hawkins County Memorial Hospital	Rogersville	73%	300+
Woods Memorial Hospital	Etowah	73%	300+
Baptist Memorial Hospital	Memphis	72%	300+
Humboldt General Hospital	Humboldt	72%	(a)
Mercy Medical Center	Knoxville	72%	300+
Saint Francis Bartlett Medical Center	Bartlett	72%	300+
Summit Medical Center	Hermitage	72%	300+
Unicoi County Memorial Hospital	Erwin	72%	300+
Baptist Hospital	Nashville	71%	300+
Baptist Memorial Hospital Union City	Union City	71%	300+
Hardin Medical Center	Savannah	71%	300+
Indian Path Medical Center	Kingsport	71%	300+
Regional Hospital of Jackson	Jackson	71%	300+
Stonecrest Medical Center	Smyrna	71%	300+
Stones River Hosp/Dekalb Comm Hosp	Smithville	71%	300+
Cookeville Regional Medical Center	Cookeville	70%	300+
Northcrest Medical Center	Springfield	70%	300+
Trousdale Medical Center	Hartsville	70%	(a)
Franklin Woods Community Hospital	Johnson City	69%	(a)
Henry County Medical Center	Paris	69%	300+
Sweetwater Hospital Association	Sweetwater	69%	(a)
Athens Regional Medical Center	Athens	68%	300+
Cumberland River Hospital	Celina	68%	(a)
Gibson General Hospital	Trenton	68%	(a)
Jellico Community Hospital	Jellico	68%	(a)
Johnson City Medical Center	Johnson City	68%	300+
Methodist Healthcare Memphis Hospitals	Memphis	68%	300+
Roane Medical Center	Harriman	68%	300+
Takoma Regional Hospital	Greeneville	68%	(a)
White County Community Hospital	Sparta	68%	300+
Horizon Medical Center	Dickson	67%	300+
Laughlin Memorial Hospital	Greeneville	67%	300+
Rhea Medical Center	Dayton	67%	300+
Saint Mary's Jefferson Memorial Hospital	Jefferson City	67%	300+
Southern Hills Medical Center	Nashville	67%	300+
Wellmont Bristol Regional Medical Center	Bristol	67%	300+
Erlanger Medical Center	Chattanooga	66%	300+
Heritage Medical Center	Shelbyville	66%	300+
Jackson-Madison County General Hospital	Jackson	66%	300+
Methodist Medical Center of Oak Ridge	Oak Ridge	66%	300+
Riverview Regional Medical Center North	Carthage	66%	(a)
Skyline Medical Center	Nashville	66%	300+
Volunteer Community Hospital	Martin	66%	300+
Haywood Park Community Hospital	Brownsville	65%	(a)
Hendersonville Medical Center	Hendersonville	65%	300+
Hillside Hospital	Pulaski	65%	(a)
Lakeway Regional Hospital	Morristown	65%	300+
McKenzie Regional Hospital	McKenzie	65%	300+
McNairy Regional Hospital	Selmer	65%	(a)
Metro Nashville General Hospital	Nashville	65%	300+
Morristown Hamblen Hospital Association	Morristown	65%	300+
Saint Francis Hospital	Memphis	65%	300+
Baptist Hospital of Cocke County	Newport	64%	300+
Sumner Regional Medical Center	Gallatin	64%	300+
Wellmont Holston Valley Medical Center	Kingsport	64%	300+
Claiborne County Hospital	Tazewell	63%	(a)
Crockett Hospital	Lawrenceburg	63%	300+
Cumberland Medical Center	Crossville	63%	300+
Decatur County General Hospital	Parsons	63%	(a)
Grandview Medical Center	Jasper	63%	(a)
Livingston Regional Hospital	Livingston	62%	300+
United Regional Medical Center	Manchester	62%	300+
Henderson County Community Hospital	Lexington	61%	(a)
Southern Tennessee Medical Center	Winchester	61%	300+
Wayne Medical Center	Waynesboro	61%	(a)
Blount Memorial Hospital	Maryville	60%	300+
Delta Medical Center	Memphis	60%	300+
Gateway Medical Center	Clarksville	60%	300+
Scott County Hospital	Oneida	60%	(a)
Baptist Memorial Hospital Tipton	Covington	59%	(a)
River Park Hospital	McMinnville	59%	300+
University Medical Center	Lebanon	59%	300+
Harton Regional Medical Center	Tullahoma	58%	300+
St Mary's Med Ctr of Campbell County	La Follette	58%	300+
Skyridge Medical Center	Cleveland	58%	300+
Stones River Hosp & Dekalb Comm Hosp	Woodbury	58%	(a)
Dyersburg Regional Medical Center	Dyersburg	57%	300+
Middle Tennessee Medical Center	Murfreesboro	57%	300+
Jamestown Regional Medical Center	Jamestown	55%	300+
Regional Medical Center at Memphis	Memphis	55%	300+
Lincoln Medical Center	Fayetteville	53%	300+

44. Meds 'Always' Explained Before Given

Hospital Name	City	Rate	Cases
Methodist Healthcare Fayette Hospital	Somerville	79%	(a)
The Center for Spinal Surgery	Nashville	78%	300+
Johnson City Specialty Hospital	Johnson City	74%	300+
Haywood Park Community Hospital	Brownsville	72%	(a)
Trousdale Medical Center	Hartsville	72%	(a)
Hardin Medical Center	Savannah	71%	300+
Maury Regional Hospital	Columbia	69%	300+
Wellmont Hawkins County Memorial Hospital	Rogersville	69%	300+
Baptist Memorial Hospital Huntingdon	Huntingdon	68%	(a)
Sweetwater Hospital Association	Sweetwater	68%	(a)
Sycamore Shoals Hospital	Elizabethton	68%	300+
Centennial Medical Center	Nashville	67%	300+
Cumberland River Hospital	Celina	66%	(a)
Fort Loudoun Medical Center	Lenoir City	66%	300+
Gibson General Hospital	Trenton	66%	(a)
Leconte Medical Center	Sevierville	66%	300+
Parkwest Medical Center	Knoxville	66%	300+
Athens Regional Medical Center	Athens	65%	300+
Baptist Memorial Hospital Tipton	Covington	65%	(a)
Henry County Medical Center	Paris	65%	300+
Jellico Community Hospital	Jellico	65%	(a)
Scott County Hospital	Oneida	65%	(a)
Unicoi County Memorial Hospital	Erwin	65%	300+
White County Community Hospital	Sparta	65%	300+
Baptist Memorial Hospital Union City	Union City	64%	300+
McNairy Regional Hospital	Selmer	64%	(a)
Northcrest Medical Center	Springfield	64%	300+
Baptist Hospital	Nashville	63%	300+
Claiborne County Hospital	Tazewell	63%	(a)
Humboldt General Hospital	Humboldt	63%	(a)
Jamestown Regional Medical Center	Jamestown	63%	300+
Memorial Healthcare System	Chattanooga	63%	300+
Methodist Medical Center of Oak Ridge	Oak Ridge	63%	300+
Saint Francis Hospital	Memphis	63%	300+
Takoma Regional Hospital	Greeneville	63%	(a)
United Regional Medical Center	Manchester	63%	300+
Williamson Medical Center	Franklin	63%	300+
Dyersburg Regional Medical Center	Dyersburg	62%	300+
Johnson City Medical Center	Johnson City	62%	300+
McKenzie Regional Hospital	McKenzie	62%	300+
Metro Nashville General Hospital	Nashville	62%	300+
Roane Medical Center	Harriman	62%	300+
Saint Francis Bartlett Medical Center	Bartlett	62%	300+
St Mary's Med Ctr of Campbell County	La Follette	62%	300+
Baptist Hospital of Cocke County	Newport	61%	300+
Baptist Memorial Hospital	Memphis	61%	300+
Erlanger Medical Center	Chattanooga	61%	300+
Franklin Woods Community Hospital	Johnson City	61%	(a)
Henderson County Community Hospital	Lexington	61%	(a)
Hillside Hospital	Pulaski	61%	(a)
Lincoln Medical Center	Fayetteville	61%	300+
Morristown Hamblen Hospital Association	Morristown	61%	300+
Parkridge Medical Center	Chattanooga	61%	300+
Riverview Regional Medical Center North	Carthage	61%	(a)
Saint Thomas Hospital	Nashville	61%	300+
Stonecrest Medical Center	Smyrna	61%	300+
University of Tennessee Memorial Hospital	Knoxville	61%	300+
Heritage Medical Center	Shelbyville	60%	300+
Horizon Medical Center	Dickson	60%	300+
Middle Tennessee Medical Center	Murfreesboro	60%	300+
Saint Mary's Jefferson Memorial Hospital	Jefferson City	60%	300+
Southern Tennessee Medical Center	Winchester	60%	300+
Vanderbilt University Hospital	Nashville	60%	300+
Fort Sanders Regional Medical Center	Knoxville	59%	300+
Indian Path Medical Center	Kingsport	59%	300+
Lakeway Regional Hospital	Morristown	59%	300+
Mercy Medical Center	Knoxville	59%	300+
Methodist Healthcare Memphis Hospitals	Memphis	59%	300+
Skyline Medical Center	Nashville	59%	300+
Southern Hills Medical Center	Nashville	59%	300+
Summit Medical Center	Hermitage	59%	300+
Wellmont Holston Valley Medical Center	Kingsport	59%	300+
Cumberland Medical Center	Crossville	58%	300+
Decatur County General Hospital	Parsons	58%	(a)
Hendersonville Medical Center	Hendersonville	58%	300+
Laughlin Memorial Hospital	Greeneville	58%	300+
Regional Hospital of Jackson	Jackson	58%	300+
Rhea Medical Center	Dayton	58%	300+
Stones River Hosp/Dekalb Comm Hosp	Smithville	58%	300+
Cookeville Regional Medical Center	Cookeville	57%	300+
Regional Medical Center at Memphis	Memphis	57%	300+
River Park Hospital	McMinnville	57%	300+
Sumner Regional Medical Center	Gallatin	57%	300+
Woods Memorial Hospital	Etowah	57%	300+
Crockett Hospital	Lawrenceburg	56%	300+
Gateway Medical Center	Clarksville	56%	300+
Jackson-Madison County General Hospital	Jackson	56%	300+
Livingston Regional Hospital	Livingston	56%	300+
Volunteer Community Hospital	Martin	56%	300+
Wayne Medical Center	Waynesboro	56%	(a)
Wellmont Bristol Regional Medical Center	Bristol	56%	300+
Delta Medical Center	Memphis	55%	300+
Harton Regional Medical Center	Tullahoma	55%	300+
Stones River Hosp & Dekalb Comm Hosp	Woodbury	55%	(a)
Blount Memorial Hospital	Maryville	54%	300+
University Medical Center	Lebanon	54%	300+
Grandview Medical Center	Jasper	53%	(a)

NOTE: Hospital profiles are in alphabetical order by state, then city, then hospital within the city; Rankings exclude hospitals with less than 25 cases except for patient surveys which excludes hospitals with less than 100 cases; (a) 100–299 cases; (1) The number of cases is too small to be sure how well a hospital is performing; (2) The hospital indicated that the data submitted for this measure were based on a sample of cases; (3) Data was collected during a shorter time period (fewer quarters) than the maximum possible time for this measure; (4) Suppressed for one or more quarters by CMS; (5) No data is available from the hospital for this measure; (6) Fewer than 100 patients completed the HCAHPS survey. Use these rates with caution, as the number of surveys may be too low to reliably assess hospital performance; (7) Survey results are based on less than 12 months of data; (8) Survey results are not available for this reporting period; (9) No or very few patients were eligible for the HCAHPS survey. The scores shown, if any, reflect a very small number of surveys; (10) A state average was not calculated because too few hospitals in the state submitted data; (11) There were discrepancies in the data collection process; Please refer to the User's Guide for a full explanation of data.

Skyridge Medical Center	Cleveland	53%	300+

45. Nurses 'Always' Communicated Well

Hospital Name	City	Rate	Cases
The Center for Spinal Surgery	Nashville	92%	300+
Johnson City Specialty Hospital	Johnson City	89%	300+
Methodist Healthcare Fayette Hospital	Somerville	89%	(a)
Baptist Memorial Hospital Huntingdon	Huntingdon	87%	(a)
Hardin Medical Center	Savannah	85%	300+
Humboldt General Hospital	Humboldt	85%	(a)
Trousdale Medical Center	Hartsville	85%	(a)
Gibson General Hospital	Trenton	84%	(a)
United Regional Medical Center	Manchester	84%	300+
Maury Regional Hospital	Columbia	83%	300+
Stones River Hosp/Dekalb Comm Hosp	Smithville	83%	300+
Wellmont Hawkins County Memorial Hospital	Rogersville	83%	300+
Decatur County General Hospital	Parsons	82%	(a)
Memorial Healthcare System	Chattanooga	82%	300+
Sycamore Shoals Hospital	Elizabethton	82%	300+
Baptist Hospital of Cocke County	Newport	81%	300+
Centennial Medical Center	Nashville	81%	300+
Cumberland River Hospital	Celina	81%	(a)
University of Tennessee Memorial Hospital	Knoxville	81%	300+
Baptist Memorial Hospital Union City	Union City	80%	300+
Fort Loudoun Medical Center	Lenoir City	80%	300+
Fort Sanders Regional Medical Center	Knoxville	80%	300+
Woods Memorial Hospital	Etowah	80%	300+
Franklin Woods Community Hospital	Johnson City	79%	(a)
Henderson County Community Hospital	Lexington	79%	(a)
Horizon Medical Center	Dickson	79%	300+
Leconte Medical Center	Sevierville	79%	300+
Morristown Hamblen Hospital Association	Morristown	79%	300+
Parkwest Medical Center	Knoxville	79%	300+
Saint Thomas Hospital	Nashville	79%	300+
Baptist Hospital	Nashville	78%	300+
Indian Path Medical Center	Kingsport	78%	300+
Jamestown Regional Medical Center	Jamestown	78%	300+
Jellico Community Hospital	Jellico	78%	(a)
McNairy Regional Hospital	Selmer	78%	(a)
Northcrest Medical Center	Springfield	78%	300+
Parkridge Medical Center	Chattanooga	78%	300+
Regional Hospital of Jackson	Jackson	78%	300+
Rhea Medical Center	Dayton	78%	300+
Roane Medical Center	Harriman	78%	300+
Saint Francis Bartlett Medical Center	Bartlett	78%	300+
Scott County Hospital	Oneida	78%	(a)
Vanderbilt University Hospital	Nashville	78%	300+
Wayne Medical Center	Waynesboro	78%	(a)
Williamson Medical Center	Franklin	78%	300+
Athens Regional Medical Center	Athens	77%	300+
Baptist Memorial Hospital Tipton	Covington	77%	(a)
Claiborne County Hospital	Tazewell	77%	(a)
Cookeville Regional Medical Center	Cookeville	77%	300+
Cumberland Medical Center	Crossville	77%	300+
Haywood Park Community Hospital	Brownsville	77%	(a)
Johnson City Medical Center	Johnson City	77%	300+
Mercy Medical Center	Knoxville	77%	300+
Riverview Regional Medical Center North	Carthage	77%	(a)
St Mary's Med Ctr of Campbell County	La Follette	77%	300+
Stonecrest Medical Center	Smyrna	77%	300+
Volunteer Community Hospital	Martin	77%	300+
Wellmont Bristol Regional Medical Center	Bristol	77%	300+
Baptist Memorial Hospital	Memphis	76%	300+
Erlanger Medical Center	Chattanooga	76%	300+
Henry County Medical Center	Paris	76%	300+
Hillside Hospital	Pulaski	76%	(a)
Lincoln Medical Center	Fayetteville	76%	300+
Methodist Medical Center of Oak Ridge	Oak Ridge	76%	300+
Stones River Hosp & Dekalb Comm Hosp	Woodbury	76%	(a)
Summit Medical Center	Hermitage	76%	300+
Sweetwater Hospital Association	Sweetwater	76%	(a)
Wellmont Holston Valley Medical Center	Kingsport	76%	300+
White County Community Hospital	Sparta	76%	300+
Crockett Hospital	Lawrenceburg	75%	300+
Dyersburg Regional Medical Center	Dyersburg	75%	300+
Grandview Medical Center	Jasper	75%	(a)
Hendersonville Medical Center	Hendersonville	75%	300+
Jackson-Madison County General Hospital	Jackson	75%	300+
Livingston Regional Hospital	Livingston	75%	300+
Saint Francis Hospital	Memphis	75%	300+
Saint Mary's Jefferson Memorial Hospital	Jefferson City	75%	300+
Skyline Medical Center	Nashville	75%	300+
Southern Hills Medical Center	Nashville	75%	300+
Southern Tennessee Medical Center	Winchester	75%	300+
Sumner Regional Medical Center	Gallatin	75%	300+
Takoma Regional Hospital	Greeneville	75%	(a)
Unicoi County Memorial Hospital	Erwin	75%	300+
Heritage Medical Center	Shelbyville	74%	300+
Lakeway Regional Hospital	Morristown	74%	300+
Laughlin Memorial Hospital	Greeneville	74%	300+
Methodist Healthcare Memphis Hospitals	Memphis	74%	300+
Middle Tennessee Medical Center	Murfreesboro	74%	300+
Blount Memorial Hospital	Maryville	73%	300+
Gateway Medical Center	Clarksville	73%	300+
McKenzie Regional Hospital	McKenzie	73%	300+
Metro Nashville General Hospital	Nashville	73%	300+
Skyridge Medical Center	Cleveland	73%	300+
River Park Hospital	McMinnville	72%	300+
University Medical Center	Lebanon	72%	300+
Delta Medical Center	Memphis	71%	300+
Harton Regional Medical Center	Tullahoma	71%	300+
Regional Medical Center at Memphis	Memphis	69%	300+

46. Pain 'Always' Well Controlled

Hospital Name	City	Rate	Cases
Methodist Healthcare Fayette Hospital	Somerville	87%	(a)
Gibson General Hospital	Trenton	86%	(a)
Johnson City Specialty Hospital	Johnson City	85%	300+
The Center for Spinal Surgery	Nashville	84%	300+
Hardin Medical Center	Savannah	82%	300+
Humboldt General Hospital	Humboldt	80%	(a)
United Regional Medical Center	Manchester	79%	300+
Baptist Memorial Hospital Huntingdon	Huntingdon	78%	(a)
Stones River Hosp/Dekalb Comm Hosp	Smithville	77%	300+
Sycamore Shoals Hospital	Elizabethton	77%	300+
Maury Regional Hospital	Columbia	76%	300+
Trousdale Medical Center	Hartsville	76%	(a)
Wellmont Hawkins County Memorial Hospital	Rogersville	76%	300+
Athens Regional Medical Center	Athens	75%	300+
Centennial Medical Center	Nashville	75%	300+
Franklin Woods Community Hospital	Johnson City	75%	(a)
Scott County Hospital	Oneida	75%	(a)
Fort Loudoun Medical Center	Lenoir City	74%	300+
McNairy Regional Hospital	Selmer	74%	(a)
Memorial Healthcare System	Chattanooga	74%	300+
Parkwest Medical Center	Knoxville	74%	300+
Woods Memorial Hospital	Etowah	74%	300+
Parkridge Medical Center	Chattanooga	73%	300+
Saint Francis Bartlett Medical Center	Bartlett	73%	300+
Saint Thomas Hospital	Nashville	73%	300+
Stonecrest Medical Center	Smyrna	73%	300+
Baptist Hospital	Nashville	72%	300+
Baptist Hospital of Cocke County	Newport	72%	300+
Baptist Memorial Hospital Tipton	Covington	72%	(a)
Decatur County General Hospital	Parsons	72%	(a)
Horizon Medical Center	Dickson	72%	300+
Leconte Medical Center	Sevierville	72%	300+
University of Tennessee Memorial Hospital	Knoxville	72%	300+
Volunteer Community Hospital	Martin	72%	300+
White County Community Hospital	Sparta	72%	300+
Baptist Memorial Hospital Union City	Union City	71%	300+
Dyersburg Regional Medical Center	Dyersburg	71%	300+
Indian Path Medical Center	Kingsport	71%	300+
Mercy Medical Center	Knoxville	71%	300+
Northcrest Medical Center	Springfield	71%	300+
Regional Hospital of Jackson	Jackson	71%	300+
St Mary's Med Ctr of Campbell County	La Follette	71%	300+
Southern Tennessee Medical Center	Winchester	71%	300+
Baptist Memorial Hospital	Memphis	70%	300+
Cumberland River Hospital	Celina	70%	(a)
Gateway Medical Center	Clarksville	70%	300+
Haywood Park Community Hospital	Brownsville	70%	(a)
Henry County Medical Center	Paris	70%	300+
Jellico Community Hospital	Jellico	70%	(a)
Summit Medical Center	Hermitage	70%	300+
Vanderbilt University Hospital	Nashville	70%	300+
Cookeville Regional Medical Center	Cookeville	69%	300+
Cumberland Medical Center	Crossville	69%	300+
Erlanger Medical Center	Chattanooga	69%	300+
Fort Sanders Regional Medical Center	Knoxville	69%	300+
Hendersonville Medical Center	Hendersonville	69%	300+
Hillside Hospital	Pulaski	69%	(a)
Livingston Regional Hospital	Livingston	69%	300+
Middle Tennessee Medical Center	Murfreesboro	69%	300+
Saint Francis Hospital	Memphis	69%	300+
Skyline Medical Center	Nashville	69%	300+
Southern Hills Medical Center	Nashville	69%	300+
Stones River Hosp & Dekalb Comm Hosp	Woodbury	69%	(a)
Sumner Regional Medical Center	Gallatin	69%	300+
Sweetwater Hospital Association	Sweetwater	69%	(a)
Wellmont Holston Valley Medical Center	Kingsport	69%	300+
Williamson Medical Center	Franklin	69%	300+
Crockett Hospital	Lawrenceburg	68%	300+
Heritage Medical Center	Shelbyville	68%	300+
Methodist Healthcare Memphis Hospitals	Memphis	68%	300+
Skyridge Medical Center	Cleveland	68%	300+
Blount Memorial Hospital	Maryville	67%	300+
Morristown Hamblen Hospital Association	Morristown	67%	300+
Riverview Regional Medical Center North	Carthage	67%	(a)
Takoma Regional Hospital	Greeneville	67%	(a)
Claiborne County Hospital	Tazewell	66%	(a)
Jackson-Madison County General Hospital	Jackson	66%	300+
Johnson City Medical Center	Johnson City	66%	300+
Laughlin Memorial Hospital	Greeneville	66%	300+
McKenzie Regional Hospital	McKenzie	66%	300+
Methodist Medical Center of Oak Ridge	Oak Ridge	66%	300+
Metro Nashville General Hospital	Nashville	66%	300+
Rhea Medical Center	Dayton	66%	300+
Roane Medical Center	Harriman	66%	300+
Grandview Medical Center	Jasper	65%	(a)
Henderson County Community Hospital	Lexington	65%	(a)
Jamestown Regional Medical Center	Jamestown	65%	300+
Lakeway Regional Hospital	Morristown	65%	300+
River Park Hospital	McMinnville	65%	300+
Unicoi County Memorial Hospital	Erwin	65%	300+
University Medical Center	Lebanon	65%	300+
Lincoln Medical Center	Fayetteville	64%	300+
Wellmont Bristol Regional Medical Center	Bristol	64%	300+
Delta Medical Center	Memphis	63%	300+
Saint Mary's Jefferson Memorial Hospital	Jefferson City	63%	300+
Wayne Medical Center	Waynesboro	63%	(a)
Harton Regional Medical Center	Tullahoma	61%	300+
Regional Medical Center at Memphis	Memphis	60%	300+

47. Room and Bathroom 'Always' Clean

Hospital Name	City	Rate	Cases
Trousdale Medical Center	Hartsville	92%	(a)
Johnson City Specialty Hospital	Johnson City	85%	300+
The Center for Spinal Surgery	Nashville	83%	300+
Methodist Healthcare Fayette Hospital	Somerville	83%	(a)
Cumberland River Hospital	Celina	82%	(a)
Riverview Regional Medical Center North	Carthage	82%	(a)
Wellmont Hawkins County Memorial Hospital	Rogersville	82%	300+
Scott County Hospital	Oneida	81%	(a)
United Regional Medical Center	Manchester	80%	300+
Baptist Memorial Hospital Union City	Union City	78%	300+
Decatur County General Hospital	Parsons	77%	(a)
Maury Regional Hospital	Columbia	77%	300+
Morristown Hamblen Hospital Association	Morristown	77%	300+
White County Community Hospital	Sparta	77%	300+
Humboldt General Hospital	Humboldt	76%	(a)
Leconte Medical Center	Sevierville	76%	300+
Sumner Regional Medical Center	Gallatin	76%	300+
Sycamore Shoals Hospital	Elizabethton	76%	300+
Unicoi County Memorial Hospital	Erwin	76%	300+
Wayne Medical Center	Waynesboro	76%	(a)
Baptist Memorial Hospital Huntingdon	Huntingdon	75%	(a)
Cookeville Regional Medical Center	Cookeville	75%	300+
Cumberland Medical Center	Crossville	75%	300+
Hardin Medical Center	Savannah	75%	300+
Jellico Community Hospital	Jellico	75%	(a)
Roane Medical Center	Harriman	75%	300+
Stones River Hosp/Dekalb Comm Hosp	Smithville	75%	300+
University of Tennessee Memorial Hospital	Knoxville	75%	300+
Baptist Memorial Hospital Tipton	Covington	74%	(a)
Centennial Medical Center	Nashville	74%	300+
Delta Medical Center	Memphis	74%	300+
Fort Loudoun Medical Center	Lenoir City	74%	300+
Methodist Medical Center of Oak Ridge	Oak Ridge	74%	300+
Stonecrest Medical Center	Smyrna	74%	300+
Sweetwater Hospital Association	Sweetwater	74%	(a)
Heritage Medical Center	Shelbyville	73%	300+
Parkridge Medical Center	Chattanooga	73%	300+
Saint Mary's Jefferson Memorial Hospital	Jefferson City	73%	300+
Takoma Regional Hospital	Greeneville	73%	(a)
Baptist Hospital of Cocke County	Newport	72%	300+
Baptist Memorial Hospital	Memphis	72%	300+
Northcrest Medical Center	Springfield	72%	300+
Parkwest Medical Center	Knoxville	72%	300+
Franklin Woods Community Hospital	Johnson City	71%	(a)
Grandview Medical Center	Jasper	71%	(a)
Horizon Medical Center	Dickson	71%	300+
Jamestown Regional Medical Center	Jamestown	71%	300+
Memorial Healthcare System	Chattanooga	71%	300+
Mercy Medical Center	Knoxville	71%	300+
Stones River Hosp & Dekalb Comm Hosp	Woodbury	71%	(a)
Summit Medical Center	Hermitage	71%	300+
Volunteer Community Hospital	Martin	71%	300+
Woods Memorial Hospital	Etowah	71%	300+
Claiborne County Hospital	Tazewell	70%	(a)
Indian Path Medical Center	Kingsport	70%	300+
McNairy Regional Hospital	Selmer	70%	(a)
Southern Hills Medical Center	Nashville	70%	300+
University Medical Center	Lebanon	70%	300+
Williamson Medical Center	Franklin	70%	300+
Fort Sanders Regional Medical Center	Knoxville	69%	300+
Gibson General Hospital	Trenton	69%	(a)
Laughlin Memorial Hospital	Greeneville	69%	300+
St Mary's Med Ctr of Campbell County	La Follette	69%	300+
Wellmont Holston Valley Medical Center	Kingsport	69%	300+

NOTE: Hospital profiles are in alphabetical order by state, then city, then hospital within the city; Rankings exclude hospitals with less than 25 cases except for patient surveys which excludes hospitals with less than 100 cases; (a) 100–299 cases; (1) The number of cases is too small to be sure how well a hospital is performing; (2) The hospital indicated that the data submitted for this measure were based on a sample of cases; (3) Data was collected during a shorter time period (fewer quarters) than the maximum possible time for this measure; (4) Suppressed for one or more quarters by CMS; (5) No data is available from the hospital for this measure; (6) Fewer than 100 patients completed the HCAHPS survey. Use these rates with caution, as the number of surveys may be too low to reliably assess hospital performance; (7) Survey results are based on less than 12 months of data; (8) Survey results are not available for this reporting period; (9) No or very few patients were eligible for the HCAHPS survey. The scores shown, if any, reflect a very small number of surveys; (10) A state average was not calculated because too few hospitals in the state submitted data; (11) There were discrepancies in the data collection process; Please refer to the User's Guide for a full explanation of data.

Harton Regional Medical Center	Tullahoma	68%	300+
Henry County Medical Center	Paris	68%	300+
Lincoln Medical Center	Fayetteville	68%	300+
Livingston Regional Hospital	Livingston	68%	300+
McKenzie Regional Hospital	McKenzie	68%	300+
Metro Nashville General Hospital	Nashville	68%	300+
Saint Francis Bartlett Medical Center	Bartlett	68%	300+
Athens Regional Medical Center	Athens	67%	300+
Blount Memorial Hospital	Maryville	67%	300+
Crockett Hospital	Lawrenceburg	67%	300+
Hendersonville Medical Center	Hendersonville	66%	300+
Regional Hospital of Jackson	Jackson	66%	300+
Skyline Medical Center	Nashville	66%	300+
Southern Tennessee Medical Center	Winchester	66%	300+
Gateway Medical Center	Clarksville	65%	300+
Henderson County Community Hospital	Lexington	65%	(a)
Jackson-Madison County General Hospital	Jackson	65%	300+
Lakeway Regional Hospital	Morristown	65%	300+
Rhea Medical Center	Dayton	65%	300+
Saint Thomas Hospital	Nashville	65%	300+
Baptist Hospital	Nashville	64%	300+
Dyersburg Regional Medical Center	Dyersburg	64%	300+
Hillside Hospital	Pulaski	64%	(a)
Johnson City Medical Center	Johnson City	64%	300+
Methodist Healthcare Memphis Hospitals	Memphis	64%	300+
River Park Hospital	McMinnville	64%	300+
Vanderbilt University Hospital	Nashville	64%	300+
Wellmont Bristol Regional Medical Center	Bristol	64%	300+
Saint Francis Hospital	Memphis	63%	300+
Skyridge Medical Center	Cleveland	63%	300+
Erlanger Medical Center	Chattanooga	62%	300+
Haywood Park Community Hospital	Brownsville	60%	(a)
Regional Medical Center at Memphis	Memphis	59%	300+
Middle Tennessee Medical Center	Murfreesboro	58%	300+

48. Timely Help 'Always' Received

Hospital Name	City	Rate	Cases
The Center for Spinal Surgery	Nashville	85%	300+
Johnson City Specialty Hospital	Johnson City	81%	300+
Gibson General Hospital	Trenton	79%	(a)
Hardin Medical Center	Savannah	79%	300+
Humboldt General Hospital	Humboldt	79%	(a)
Methodist Healthcare Fayette Hospital	Somerville	79%	(a)
Cumberland River Hospital	Celina	77%	(a)
Roane Medical Center	Harriman	75%	300+
United Regional Medical Center	Manchester	75%	300+
Baptist Memorial Hospital Huntingdon	Huntingdon	74%	(a)
Maury Regional Hospital	Columbia	74%	300+
Wellmont Hawkins County Memorial Hospital	Rogersville	73%	300+
Decatur County General Hospital	Parsons	72%	(a)
Sycamore Shoals Hospital	Elizabethton	72%	300+
Woods Memorial Hospital	Etowah	72%	300+
Baptist Memorial Hospital Union City	Union City	71%	300+
Centennial Medical Center	Nashville	71%	300+
Scott County Hospital	Oneida	71%	(a)
Riverview Regional Medical Center North	Carthage	70%	(a)
Baptist Hospital of Cocke County	Newport	69%	300+
Fort Loudoun Medical Center	Lenoir City	69%	300+
Memorial Healthcare System	Chattanooga	69%	300+
Horizon Medical Center	Dickson	68%	300+
St Mary's Med Ctr of Campbell County	La Follette	68%	300+
Stones River Hosp/Dekalb Comm Hosp	Smithville	68%	300+
Sweetwater Hospital Association	Sweetwater	68%	(a)
White County Community Hospital	Sparta	68%	300+
Cookeville Regional Medical Center	Cookeville	67%	300+
Haywood Park Community Hospital	Brownsville	67%	(a)
Henderson County Community Hospital	Lexington	67%	(a)
McNairy Regional Hospital	Selmer	67%	(a)
Northcrest Medical Center	Springfield	67%	300+
Trousdale Medical Center	Hartsville	67%	(a)
Baptist Hospital	Nashville	66%	300+
Jamestown Regional Medical Center	Jamestown	66%	300+
Leconte Medical Center	Sevierville	66%	300+
Morristown Hamblen Hospital Association	Morristown	66%	300+
Parkwest Medical Center	Knoxville	66%	300+
Saint Francis Bartlett Medical Center	Bartlett	66%	300+
Stones River Hosp & Dekalb Comm Hosp	Woodbury	66%	(a)
Summit Medical Center	Hermitage	66%	300+
Takoma Regional Hospital	Greeneville	66%	(a)
Athens Regional Medical Center	Athens	65%	300+
Baptist Memorial Hospital Tipton	Covington	65%	(a)
Dyersburg Regional Medical Center	Dyersburg	65%	300+
Franklin Woods Community Hospital	Johnson City	65%	(a)
Hillside Hospital	Pulaski	65%	(a)
Indian Path Medical Center	Kingsport	65%	300+
Mercy Medical Center	Knoxville	65%	300+
Parkridge Medical Center	Chattanooga	65%	300+
Regional Hospital of Jackson	Jackson	65%	300+
Unicoi County Memorial Hospital	Erwin	65%	300+
Williamson Medical Center	Franklin	65%	300+
Claiborne County Hospital	Tazewell	64%	(a)
Cumberland Medical Center	Crossville	64%	300+
Fort Sanders Regional Medical Center	Knoxville	64%	300+
Johnson City Medical Center	Johnson City	64%	300+
Laughlin Memorial Hospital	Greeneville	64%	300+
Livingston Regional Hospital	Livingston	64%	300+
Stonecrest Medical Center	Smyrna	64%	300+
Rhea Medical Center	Dayton	63%	300+
University of Tennessee Memorial Hospital	Knoxville	63%	300+
Volunteer Community Hospital	Martin	63%	300+
Baptist Memorial Hospital	Memphis	62%	300+
Skyline Medical Center	Nashville	62%	300+
Sumner Regional Medical Center	Gallatin	62%	300+
Vanderbilt University Hospital	Nashville	62%	300+
Wayne Medical Center	Waynesboro	62%	(a)
Wellmont Holston Valley Medical Center	Kingsport	62%	300+
Crockett Hospital	Lawrenceburg	61%	300+
Erlanger Medical Center	Chattanooga	61%	300+
Gateway Medical Center	Clarksville	61%	300+
Hendersonville Medical Center	Hendersonville	61%	300+
Henry County Medical Center	Paris	61%	300+
Jackson-Madison County General Hospital	Jackson	61%	300+
Jellico Community Hospital	Jellico	61%	(a)
Lincoln Medical Center	Fayetteville	61%	300+
McKenzie Regional Hospital	McKenzie	61%	300+
Methodist Medical Center of Oak Ridge	Oak Ridge	61%	300+
Saint Thomas Hospital	Nashville	61%	300+
Grandview Medical Center	Jasper	60%	(a)
Heritage Medical Center	Shelbyville	60%	300+
River Park Hospital	McMinnville	60%	300+
Southern Hills Medical Center	Nashville	60%	300+
Blount Memorial Hospital	Maryville	59%	300+
Lakeway Regional Hospital	Morristown	59%	300+
Southern Tennessee Medical Center	Winchester	59%	300+
Saint Mary's Jefferson Memorial Hospital	Jefferson City	58%	300+
Skyridge Medical Center	Cleveland	58%	300+
Methodist Healthcare Memphis Hospitals	Memphis	57%	300+
Metro Nashville General Hospital	Nashville	57%	300+
Middle Tennessee Medical Center	Murfreesboro	57%	300+
Saint Francis Hospital	Memphis	57%	300+
Wellmont Bristol Regional Medical Center	Bristol	57%	300+
Harton Regional Medical Center	Tullahoma	56%	300+
University Medical Center	Lebanon	55%	300+
Delta Medical Center	Memphis	51%	300+
Regional Medical Center at Memphis	Memphis	51%	300+

49. Would Definitely Recommend Hospital

Hospital Name	City	Rate	Cases
The Center for Spinal Surgery	Nashville	95%	300+
Johnson City Specialty Hospital	Johnson City	94%	300+
Saint Thomas Hospital	Nashville	87%	300+
Methodist Healthcare Fayette Hospital	Somerville	86%	(a)
Parkwest Medical Center	Knoxville	86%	300+
Memorial Healthcare System	Chattanooga	84%	300+
University of Tennessee Memorial Hospital	Knoxville	82%	300+
Centennial Medical Center	Nashville	81%	300+
Unicoi County Memorial Hospital	Erwin	81%	300+
Vanderbilt University Hospital	Nashville	81%	300+
Williamson Medical Center	Franklin	78%	300+
Baptist Hospital	Nashville	77%	300+
Baptist Memorial Hospital Huntingdon	Huntingdon	77%	(a)
Saint Francis Bartlett Medical Center	Bartlett	77%	300+
Stonecrest Medical Center	Smyrna	77%	300+
United Regional Medical Center	Manchester	77%	300+
Baptist Memorial Hospital	Memphis	76%	300+
Cookeville Regional Medical Center	Cookeville	76%	300+
Fort Loudoun Medical Center	Lenoir City	76%	300+
Fort Sanders Regional Medical Center	Knoxville	76%	300+
Humboldt General Hospital	Humboldt	76%	(a)
Maury Regional Hospital	Columbia	76%	300+
Mercy Medical Center	Knoxville	76%	300+
Methodist Medical Center of Oak Ridge	Oak Ridge	76%	300+
Parkridge Medical Center	Chattanooga	76%	300+
Woods Memorial Hospital	Etowah	76%	300+
Summit Medical Center	Hermitage	75%	300+
Sycamore Shoals Hospital	Elizabethton	75%	300+
Wellmont Hawkins County Memorial Hospital	Rogersville	75%	300+
Erlanger Medical Center	Chattanooga	74%	300+
Indian Path Medical Center	Kingsport	74%	300+
Regional Hospital of Jackson	Jackson	74%	300+
Stones River Hosp/Dekalb Comm Hosp	Smithville	73%	300+
Wellmont Holston Valley Medical Center	Kingsport	73%	300+
Cumberland River Hospital	Celina	72%	(a)
Franklin Woods Community Hospital	Johnson City	72%	(a)
Leconte Medical Center	Sevierville	72%	300+
Methodist Healthcare Memphis Hospitals	Memphis	72%	300+
Hardin Medical Center	Savannah	71%	300+
Henry County Medical Center	Paris	71%	300+
Morristown Hamblen Hospital Association	Morristown	71%	300+
Saint Mary's Jefferson Memorial Hospital	Jefferson City	71%	300+
Takoma Regional Hospital	Greeneville	71%	(a)
Trousdale Medical Center	Hartsville	71%	(a)
Jackson-Madison County General Hospital	Jackson	70%	300+
Johnson City Medical Center	Johnson City	70%	300+
Laughlin Memorial Hospital	Greeneville	70%	300+
Skyline Medical Center	Nashville	70%	300+
Saint Francis Hospital	Memphis	69%	300+
Athens Regional Medical Center	Athens	68%	300+
Baptist Memorial Hospital Union City	Union City	68%	300+
Northcrest Medical Center	Springfield	68%	300+
Rhea Medical Center	Dayton	68%	300+
Claiborne County Hospital	Tazewell	67%	(a)
Hendersonville Medical Center	Hendersonville	67%	300+
Sumner Regional Medical Center	Gallatin	67%	300+
Wellmont Bristol Regional Medical Center	Bristol	67%	300+
Cumberland Medical Center	Crossville	66%	300+
Horizon Medical Center	Dickson	66%	300+
Jellico Community Hospital	Jellico	66%	(a)
Lakeway Regional Hospital	Morristown	66%	300+
McNairy Regional Hospital	Selmer	66%	(a)
Baptist Hospital of Cocke County	Newport	65%	300+
McKenzie Regional Hospital	McKenzie	65%	300+
Southern Hills Medical Center	Nashville	65%	300+
Livingston Regional Hospital	Livingston	64%	300+
Metro Nashville General Hospital	Nashville	64%	300+
Sweetwater Hospital Association	Sweetwater	64%	(a)
Volunteer Community Hospital	Martin	64%	300+
Heritage Medical Center	Shelbyville	63%	300+
Regional Medical Center at Memphis	Memphis	63%	300+
Scott County Hospital	Oneida	63%	(a)
Southern Tennessee Medical Center	Winchester	63%	300+
White County Community Hospital	Sparta	63%	300+
Blount Memorial Hospital	Maryville	62%	300+
Middle Tennessee Medical Center	Murfreesboro	62%	300+
Roane Medical Center	Harriman	62%	300+
Wayne Medical Center	Waynesboro	62%	(a)
Hillside Hospital	Pulaski	61%	(a)
Baptist Memorial Hospital Tipton	Covington	60%	(a)
Crockett Hospital	Lawrenceburg	60%	300+
Gateway Medical Center	Clarksville	60%	300+
Gibson General Hospital	Trenton	60%	(a)
Harton Regional Medical Center	Tullahoma	60%	300+
Riverview Regional Medical Center North	Carthage	60%	(a)
Henderson County Community Hospital	Lexington	59%	(a)
Stones River Hosp & Dekalb Comm Hosp	Woodbury	59%	(a)
Decatur County General Hospital	Parsons	58%	(a)
St Mary's Med Ctr of Campbell County	La Follette	58%	300+
University Medical Center	Lebanon	58%	300+
Delta Medical Center	Memphis	57%	300+
Grandview Medical Center	Jasper	57%	(a)
River Park Hospital	McMinnville	57%	300+
Skyridge Medical Center	Cleveland	56%	300+
Dyersburg Regional Medical Center	Dyersburg	54%	300+
Haywood Park Community Hospital	Brownsville	53%	(a)
Jamestown Regional Medical Center	Jamestown	52%	300+
Lincoln Medical Center	Fayetteville	50%	300+

NOTE: Hospital profiles are in alphabetical order by state, then city, then hospital within the city; Rankings exclude hospitals with less than 25 cases except for patient surveys which excludes hospitals with less than 100 cases; (a) 100–299 cases; (1) The number of cases is too small to be sure how well a hospital is performing; (2) The hospital indicated that the data submitted for this measure were based on a sample of cases; (3) Data was collected during a shorter time period (fewer quarters) than the maximum possible time for this measure; (4) Suppressed for one or more quarters by CMS; (5) No data is available from the hospital for this measure; (6) Fewer than 100 patients completed the HCAHPS survey. Use these rates with caution, as the number of surveys may be too low to reliably assess hospital performance; (7) Survey results are based on less than 12 months of data; (8) Survey results are not available for this reporting period; (9) No or very few patients were eligible for the HCAHPS survey. The scores shown, if any, reflect a very small number of surveys; (10) A state average was not calculated because too few hospitals in the state submitted data; (11) There were discrepancies in the data collection process; Please refer to the User's Guide for a full explanation of data.

Centennial Medical Center of Ashland City

313 North Main St
Ashland City, TN 37015
Phone: 615-792-3030
URL: www.centennialashlandcity.com
Type: Critical Access Hospitals
Emergency Services: Yes
Ownership: Proprietary
Beds: 12

Key Personnel:

Administrator . . . . Darrell White, RN

Measure	Cases	This Hosp.	State Avg.	U.S. Avg.
Heart Attack Care				
ACE Inhibitor or ARB for LVSD[5]	0	-	96%	96%
Aspirin at Arrival[5]	0	-	98%	99%
Aspirin at Discharge[5]	0	-	99%	98%
Beta Blocker at Discharge[5]	0	-	98%	98%
Fibrinolytic Medication Timing[5]	0	-	67%	55%
PCI Within 90 Minutes of Arrival[5]	0	-	91%	90%
Smoking Cessation Advice[5]	0	-	100%	99%
Chest Pain/Possible Heart Attack Care				
Aspirin at Arrival	107	100%	95%	95%
Median Time to ECG (minutes)	120	8	8	8
Median Time to Transfer (minutes)[1,3]	10	40	65	61
Fibrinolytic Medication Timing[1,3]	2	50%	49%	54%
Heart Failure Care				
ACE Inhibitor or ARB for LVSD[5]	0	-	95%	94%
Discharge Instructions[5]	0	-	88%	88%
Evaluation of LVS Function[5]	0	-	97%	98%
Smoking Cessation Advice[5]	0	-	99%	98%
Pneumonia Care				
Appropriate Initial Antibiotic[1,3]	2	100%	92%	92%
Blood Culture Timing[3]	0	-	97%	96%
Influenza Vaccine[1]	3	100%	93%	91%
Initial Antibiotic Timing[1,3]	1	100%	96%	95%
Pneumococcal Vaccine[1,3]	2	100%	95%	93%
Smoking Cessation Advice[1,3]	2	100%	99%	97%
Surgical Care Improvement Project				
Appropriate VTP Within 24 Hours[5]	0	-	92%	92%
Appropriate Hair Removal[5]	0	-	100%	99%
Appropriate Beta Blocker Usage[5]	0	-	93%	93%
Controlled Postoperative Blood Glucose[5]	0	-	93%	93%
Prophylactic Antibiotic Timing[5]	0	-	97%	97%
Prophylactic Antibiotic Timing (Outpatient)[5]	0	-	94%	92%
Prophylactic Antibiotic Selection[5]	0	-	97%	97%
Prophylactic Antibiotic Select. (Outpatient)[5]	0	-	94%	94%
Prophylactic Antibiotic Stopped[5]	0	-	94%	94%
Recommended VTP Ordered[5]	0	-	94%	94%
Urinary Catheter Removal[5]	0	-	90%	90%
Children's Asthma Care				
Received Systemic Corticosteroids	-	-	-	100%
Received Home Management Plan	-	-	-	71%
Received Reliever Medication	-	-	-	100%
Use of Medical Imaging				
Combination Abdominal CT Scan	66	0.076	0.219	0.191
Combination Chest CT Scan[1]	35	0.029	0.102	0.054
Follow-up Mammogram/Ultrasound	46	4.3%	8%	8.4%
MRI for Low Back Pain[1]	15	33.3%	30.7%	32.7%
Survey of Patients' Hospital Experiences				
Area Around Room 'Always' Quiet at Night[6]	<100	80%	-	58%
Doctors 'Always' Communicated Well[6]	<100	92%	-	80%
Home Recovery Information Given[6]	<100	76%	-	82%
Hospital Given 9 or 10 on 10 Point Scale[6]	<100	87%	-	67%
Meds 'Always' Explained Before Given[6]	<100	67%	-	60%
Nurses 'Always' Communicated Well[6]	<100	82%	-	76%
Pain 'Always' Well Controlled[6]	<100	71%	-	69%
Room and Bathroom 'Always' Clean[6]	<100	74%	-	71%
Timely Help 'Always' Received[6]	<100	69%	-	64%
Would Definitely Recommend Hospital	<100	95%	-	69%

Athens Regional Medical Center

1114 W Madison Ave
Athens, TN 37371
Phone: 423-745-1411
Fax: 423-745-8630
URL: www.athensrmc.com
Type: Acute Care Hospitals
Emergency Services: Yes
Ownership: Proprietary
Beds: 118

Key Personnel:

CEO/President. . . . . John Workman
Cardiac Laboratory. . . . . Judy Parham
Chief of Medical Staff . . . . Michael Hahn
Radiology. . . . . Douglas S Hayes, RT
Emergency Room . . . . Brett Atchley, MD

Measure	Cases	This Hosp.	State Avg.	U.S. Avg.
Heart Attack Care				
ACE Inhibitor or ARB for LVSD	0	-	96%	96%
Aspirin at Arrival[1]	4	100%	98%	99%
Aspirin at Discharge[1]	2	100%	99%	98%
Beta Blocker at Discharge[1]	2	100%	98%	98%
Fibrinolytic Medication Timing	0	-	67%	55%
PCI Within 90 Minutes of Arrival	0	-	91%	90%
Smoking Cessation Advice	0	-	100%	99%
Chest Pain/Possible Heart Attack Care				
Aspirin at Arrival	203	99%	95%	95%
Median Time to ECG (minutes)	210	5	8	8
Median Time to Transfer (minutes)[1]	17	59	65	61
Fibrinolytic Medication Timing[1]	5	40%	49%	54%
Heart Failure Care				
ACE Inhibitor or ARB for LVSD	32	81%	95%	94%
Discharge Instructions	82	93%	88%	88%
Evaluation of LVS Function	101	99%	97%	98%
Smoking Cessation Advice[1]	23	100%	99%	98%
Pneumonia Care				
Appropriate Initial Antibiotic	126	98%	92%	92%
Blood Culture Timing	116	100%	97%	96%
Influenza Vaccine	89	100%	93%	91%
Initial Antibiotic Timing	162	99%	96%	95%
Pneumococcal Vaccine	130	98%	95%	93%
Smoking Cessation Advice	74	99%	99%	97%
Surgical Care Improvement Project				
Appropriate VTP Within 24 Hours	98	92%	92%	92%
Appropriate Hair Removal	149	100%	100%	99%
Appropriate Beta Blocker Usage	43	93%	93%	93%
Controlled Postoperative Blood Glucose	0	-	93%	93%
Prophylactic Antibiotic Timing	90	89%	97%	97%
Prophylactic Antibiotic Timing (Outpatient)	104	96%	94%	92%
Prophylactic Antibiotic Selection	91	98%	97%	97%
Prophylactic Antibiotic Select. (Outpatient)	108	92%	94%	94%
Prophylactic Antibiotic Stopped	80	91%	94%	94%
Recommended VTP Ordered	98	95%	94%	94%
Urinary Catheter Removal	30	80%	90%	90%
Children's Asthma Care				
Received Systemic Corticosteroids	-	-	-	100%
Received Home Management Plan	-	-	-	71%
Received Reliever Medication	-	-	-	100%
Use of Medical Imaging				
Combination Abdominal CT Scan	481	0.353	0.219	0.191
Combination Chest CT Scan	190	0.026	0.102	0.054
Follow-up Mammogram/Ultrasound	961	11.3%	8%	8.4%
MRI for Low Back Pain	138	35.5%	30.7%	32.7%
Survey of Patients' Hospital Experiences				
Area Around Room 'Always' Quiet at Night	300+	67%	-	58%
Doctors 'Always' Communicated Well	300+	88%	-	80%
Home Recovery Information Given	300+	83%	-	82%
Hospital Given 9 or 10 on 10 Point Scale	300+	68%	-	67%
Meds 'Always' Explained Before Given	300+	65%	-	60%
Nurses 'Always' Communicated Well	300+	77%	-	76%
Pain 'Always' Well Controlled	300+	75%	-	69%
Room and Bathroom 'Always' Clean	300+	67%	-	71%
Timely Help 'Always' Received	300+	65%	-	64%
Would Definitely Recommend Hospital	300+	68%	-	69%

Saint Francis Bartlett Medical Center

2986 Kate Bond Rd
Bartlett, TN 38133
Phone: 901-820-7050
Fax: 901-820-7051
URL: www.saintfrancisbartlett.com
Type: Acute Care Hospitals
Emergency Services: Yes
Ownership: Proprietary
Beds: 100

Key Personnel:

CEO/President. . . . . Kem Mullins
Chief of Medical Staff . . . . Peter Lindy, MD
Emergency Room . . . . Clinton Price

Measure	Cases	This Hosp.	State Avg.	U.S. Avg.
Heart Attack Care				
ACE Inhibitor or ARB for LVSD[1]	3	100%	96%	96%
Aspirin at Arrival	26	100%	98%	99%
Aspirin at Discharge[1]	15	100%	99%	98%
Beta Blocker at Discharge[1]	19	95%	98%	98%
Fibrinolytic Medication Timing	0	-	67%	55%
PCI Within 90 Minutes of Arrival	0	-	91%	90%
Smoking Cessation Advice[1]	6	100%	100%	99%
Chest Pain/Possible Heart Attack Care				
Aspirin at Arrival	60	100%	95%	95%
Median Time to ECG (minutes)	63	14	8	8
Median Time to Transfer (minutes)[1,3]	5	63	65	61
Fibrinolytic Medication Timing[1]	1	100%	49%	54%
Heart Failure Care				
ACE Inhibitor or ARB for LVSD	45	100%	95%	94%
Discharge Instructions	138	100%	88%	88%
Evaluation of LVS Function	162	99%	97%	98%
Smoking Cessation Advice	27	100%	99%	98%
Pneumonia Care				
Appropriate Initial Antibiotic	206	97%	92%	92%
Blood Culture Timing	308	99%	97%	96%
Influenza Vaccine	152	99%	93%	91%
Initial Antibiotic Timing	270	100%	96%	95%
Pneumococcal Vaccine	168	100%	95%	93%
Smoking Cessation Advice	81	100%	99%	97%
Surgical Care Improvement Project				
Appropriate VTP Within 24 Hours[2]	114	91%	92%	92%
Appropriate Hair Removal[2]	290	100%	100%	99%
Appropriate Beta Blocker Usage[2]	51	84%	93%	93%
Controlled Postoperative Blood Glucose[2]	0	-	93%	93%
Prophylactic Antibiotic Timing[2]	189	99%	97%	97%
Prophylactic Antibiotic Timing (Outpatient)	92	96%	94%	92%
Prophylactic Antibiotic Selection[2]	191	83%	97%	97%
Prophylactic Antibiotic Select. (Outpatient)	89	90%	94%	94%
Prophylactic Antibiotic Stopped[2]	188	99%	94%	94%
Recommended VTP Ordered[2]	115	93%	94%	94%
Urinary Catheter Removal[1,2]	22	86%	90%	90%
Children's Asthma Care				
Received Systemic Corticosteroids	-	-	-	100%
Received Home Management Plan	-	-	-	71%
Received Reliever Medication	-	-	-	100%
Use of Medical Imaging				
Combination Abdominal CT Scan	369	0.694	0.219	0.191
Combination Chest CT Scan	208	0.010	0.102	0.054
Follow-up Mammogram/Ultrasound	314	7.0%	8%	8.4%
MRI for Low Back Pain	68	35.3%	30.7%	32.7%
Survey of Patients' Hospital Experiences				
Area Around Room 'Always' Quiet at Night	300+	72%	-	58%
Doctors 'Always' Communicated Well	300+	83%	-	80%
Home Recovery Information Given	300+	83%	-	82%
Hospital Given 9 or 10 on 10 Point Scale	300+	72%	-	67%
Meds 'Always' Explained Before Given	300+	62%	-	60%
Nurses 'Always' Communicated Well	300+	78%	-	76%
Pain 'Always' Well Controlled	300+	73%	-	69%
Room and Bathroom 'Always' Clean	300+	68%	-	71%
Timely Help 'Always' Received	300+	66%	-	64%
Would Definitely Recommend Hospital	300+	77%	-	69%

NOTE: Hospital profiles are in alphabetical order by state, then city, then hospital within the city; Rankings exclude hospitals with less than 25 cases except for patient surveys which excludes hospitals with less than 100 cases; (a) 100–299 cases; (1) The number of cases is too small to be sure how well a hospital is performing; (2) The hospital indicated that the data submitted for this measure were based on a sample of cases; (3) Data was collected during a shorter time period (fewer quarters) than the maximum possible time for this measure; (4) Suppressed for one or more quarters by CMS; (5) No data is available from the hospital for this measure; (6) Fewer than 100 patients completed the HCAHPS survey. Use these rates with caution, as the number of surveys may be too low to reliably assess hospital performance; (7) Survey results are based on less than 12 months of data; (8) Survey results are not available for this reporting period; (9) No or very few patients were eligible for the HCAHPS survey. The scores shown, if any, reflect a very small number of surveys; (10) A state average was not calculated because too few hospitals in the state submitted data; (11) There were discrepancies in the data collection process; Please refer to the User's Guide for a full explanation of data.

Bolivar General Hospital

650 Nuckolls Road
Bolivar, TN 38008
URL: www.wth.net
Type: Acute Care Hospitals
Ownership: Govt - Hospital Dist/Auth
Phone: 731-658-3100
Fax: 731-658-2843
Emergency Services: No
Beds: 61

Key Personnel:
CEO/President. . . . . Ruby Kirby
Chief of Medical Staff. . . . . Charles Frost
Radiology. . . . . Gregory Bruno

Measure	Cases	This Hosp.	State Avg.	U.S. Avg.
Heart Attack Care				
ACE Inhibitor or ARB for LVSD[3]	0	-	96%	96%
Aspirin at Arrival[3]	0	-	98%	99%
Aspirin at Discharge[3]	0	-	99%	98%
Beta Blocker at Discharge[3]	0	-	98%	98%
Fibrinolytic Medication Timing[3]	0	-	67%	55%
PCI Within 90 Minutes of Arrival[3]	0	-	91%	90%
Smoking Cessation Advice[3]	0	-	100%	99%
Chest Pain/Possible Heart Attack Care				
Aspirin at Arrival	86	97%	95%	95%
Median Time to ECG (minutes)	102	15	8	8
Median Time to Transfer (minutes)[1,3]	4	453	65	61
Fibrinolytic Medication Timing[1]	2	0%	49%	54%
Heart Failure Care				
ACE Inhibitor or ARB for LVSD[1]	8	100%	95%	94%
Discharge Instructions	25	68%	88%	88%
Evaluation of LVS Function	29	59%	97%	98%
Smoking Cessation Advice[1]	5	100%	99%	98%
Pneumonia Care				
Appropriate Initial Antibiotic[1]	17	76%	92%	92%
Blood Culture Timing	26	81%	97%	96%
Influenza Vaccine[1]	18	61%	93%	91%
Initial Antibiotic Timing	27	93%	96%	95%
Pneumococcal Vaccine	26	65%	95%	93%
Smoking Cessation Advice[1]	9	89%	99%	97%
Surgical Care Improvement Project				
Appropriate VTP Within 24 Hours[5]	0	-	92%	92%
Appropriate Hair Removal[5]	0	-	100%	99%
Appropriate Beta Blocker Usage[5]	0	-	93%	93%
Controlled Postoperative Blood Glucose[5]	0	-	93%	93%
Prophylactic Antibiotic Timing[5]	0	-	97%	97%
Prophylactic Antibiotic Timing (Outpatient)[1,3]	5	0%	94%	92%
Prophylactic Antibiotic Selection[5]	0	-	97%	97%
Prophylactic Antibiotic Select. (Outpatient)[3]	0	-	94%	94%
Prophylactic Antibiotic Stopped[5]	0	-	94%	94%
Recommended VTP Ordered[5]	0	-	94%	94%
Urinary Catheter Removal[5]	0	-	90%	90%
Children's Asthma Care				
Received Systemic Corticosteroids	-	-	-	100%
Received Home Management Plan	-	-	-	71%
Received Reliever Medication	-	-	-	100%
Use of Medical Imaging				
Combination Abdominal CT Scan	153	0.013	0.219	0.191
Combination Chest CT Scan	50	0.020	0.102	0.054
Follow-up Mammogram/Ultrasound	149	4.0%	8%	8.4%
MRI for Low Back Pain[5]	0	-	30.7%	32.7%
Survey of Patients' Hospital Experiences				
Area Around Room 'Always' Quiet at Night[6]	<100	78%	-	58%
Doctors 'Always' Communicated Well[6]	<100	79%	-	80%
Home Recovery Information Given[6]	<100	54%	-	82%
Hospital Given 9 or 10 on 10 Point Scale[6]	<100	59%	-	67%
Meds 'Always' Explained Before Given[6]	<100	63%	-	60%
Nurses 'Always' Communicated Well[6]	<100	80%	-	76%
Pain 'Always' Well Controlled[6]	<100	62%	-	69%
Room and Bathroom 'Always' Clean[6]	<100	88%	-	71%
Timely Help 'Always' Received[6]	<100	67%	-	64%
Would Definitely Recommend Hospital	<100	47%	-	69%

Wellmont Bristol Regional Medical Center

One Medical Park Blvd
Bristol, TN 37620
URL: www.wellmont.org
Type: Acute Care Hospitals
Ownership: Govt - Hospital Dist/Auth
Phone: 423-844-1121
Fax: 423-844-4202
Emergency Services: No
Beds: 348

Key Personnel:
CEO/President. . . . . Bart Hove
Chief of Medical Staff. . . . . Gail Stanley, MD
Anesthesiology. . . . . Dennis Aguirre, MD

Measure	Cases	This Hosp.	State Avg.	U.S. Avg.
Heart Attack Care				
ACE Inhibitor or ARB for LVSD[2]	49	92%	96%	96%
Aspirin at Arrival[2]	183	98%	98%	99%
Aspirin at Discharge[2]	267	100%	99%	98%
Beta Blocker at Discharge[2]	262	100%	98%	98%
Fibrinolytic Medication Timing[2]	0	-	67%	55%
PCI Within 90 Minutes of Arrival[2]	26	100%	91%	90%
Smoking Cessation Advice[2]	117	100%	100%	99%
Chest Pain/Possible Heart Attack Care				
Aspirin at Arrival[1]	4	75%	95%	95%
Median Time to ECG (minutes)[1]	4	4	8	8
Median Time to Transfer (minutes)[5]	0	-	65	61
Fibrinolytic Medication Timing[5]	0	-	49%	54%
Heart Failure Care				
ACE Inhibitor or ARB for LVSD[2]	83	90%	95%	94%
Discharge Instructions[2]	229	94%	88%	88%
Evaluation of LVS Function[2]	274	97%	97%	98%
Smoking Cessation Advice[2]	46	100%	99%	98%
Pneumonia Care				
Appropriate Initial Antibiotic[2]	61	92%	92%	92%
Blood Culture Timing[2]	46	98%	97%	96%
Influenza Vaccine[2]	70	99%	93%	91%
Initial Antibiotic Timing[2]	109	95%	96%	95%
Pneumococcal Vaccine[2]	105	98%	95%	93%
Smoking Cessation Advice[2]	68	100%	99%	97%
Surgical Care Improvement Project				
Appropriate VTP Within 24 Hours[2]	144	71%	92%	92%
Appropriate Hair Removal[2]	493	98%	100%	99%
Appropriate Beta Blocker Usage[2]	164	66%	93%	93%
Controlled Postoperative Blood Glucose[2]	88	80%	93%	93%
Prophylactic Antibiotic Timing[2]	317	98%	97%	97%
Prophylactic Antibiotic Timing (Outpatient)	363	96%	94%	92%
Prophylactic Antibiotic Selection[2]	323	97%	97%	97%
Prophylactic Antibiotic Select. (Outpatient)	362	96%	94%	94%
Prophylactic Antibiotic Stopped[2]	309	93%	94%	94%
Recommended VTP Ordered[2]	145	74%	94%	94%
Urinary Catheter Removal[2]	97	77%	90%	90%
Children's Asthma Care				
Received Systemic Corticosteroids	-	-	-	100%
Received Home Management Plan	-	-	-	71%
Received Reliever Medication	-	-	-	100%
Use of Medical Imaging				
Combination Abdominal CT Scan	1,463	0.696	0.219	0.191
Combination Chest CT Scan	927	0.167	0.102	0.054
Follow-up Mammogram/Ultrasound	1,183	8.5%	8%	8.4%
MRI for Low Back Pain	439	35.8%	30.7%	32.7%
Survey of Patients' Hospital Experiences				
Area Around Room 'Always' Quiet at Night	300+	58%	-	58%
Doctors 'Always' Communicated Well	300+	78%	-	80%
Home Recovery Information Given	300+	79%	-	82%
Hospital Given 9 or 10 on 10 Point Scale	300+	67%	-	67%
Meds 'Always' Explained Before Given	300+	56%	-	60%
Nurses 'Always' Communicated Well	300+	77%	-	76%
Pain 'Always' Well Controlled	300+	64%	-	69%
Room and Bathroom 'Always' Clean	300+	64%	-	71%
Timely Help 'Always' Received	300+	57%	-	64%
Would Definitely Recommend Hospital	300+	67%	-	69%

Haywood Park Community Hospital

2545 N Washington Ave
Brownsville, TN 38012
Type: Acute Care Hospitals
Ownership: Proprietary
Phone: 731-772-4110
Fax: 731-772-9428
Emergency Services: Yes
Beds: 62

Key Personnel:
CEO/President. . . . . Kim Anthony
Infection Control. . . . . Hannah Vickers, RN
Operating Room. . . . . Dr Percival
Radiology. . . . . Ann Tran

Measure	Cases	This Hosp.	State Avg.	U.S. Avg.
Heart Attack Care				
ACE Inhibitor or ARB for LVSD	0	-	96%	96%
Aspirin at Arrival[1]	1	100%	98%	99%
Aspirin at Discharge	0	-	99%	98%
Beta Blocker at Discharge	0	-	98%	98%
Fibrinolytic Medication Timing	0	-	67%	55%
PCI Within 90 Minutes of Arrival	0	-	91%	90%
Smoking Cessation Advice	0	-	100%	99%
Chest Pain/Possible Heart Attack Care				
Aspirin at Arrival	105	96%	95%	95%
Median Time to ECG (minutes)	108	4	8	8
Median Time to Transfer (minutes)[3]	0	-	65	61
Fibrinolytic Medication Timing[1]	2	50%	49%	54%
Heart Failure Care				
ACE Inhibitor or ARB for LVSD[1]	10	80%	95%	94%
Discharge Instructions	35	100%	88%	88%
Evaluation of LVS Function	44	100%	97%	98%
Smoking Cessation Advice[1]	7	100%	99%	98%
Pneumonia Care				
Appropriate Initial Antibiotic[1]	16	100%	92%	92%
Blood Culture Timing[1]	8	100%	97%	96%
Influenza Vaccine[1]	17	88%	93%	91%
Initial Antibiotic Timing[1]	22	100%	96%	95%
Pneumococcal Vaccine[1]	16	100%	95%	93%
Smoking Cessation Advice[1]	10	100%	99%	97%
Surgical Care Improvement Project				
Appropriate VTP Within 24 Hours[5]	0	-	92%	92%
Appropriate Hair Removal[5]	0	-	100%	99%
Appropriate Beta Blocker Usage[5]	0	-	93%	93%
Controlled Postoperative Blood Glucose[5]	0	-	93%	93%
Prophylactic Antibiotic Timing[5]	0	-	97%	97%
Prophylactic Antibiotic Timing (Outpatient)[1,3]	2	50%	94%	92%
Prophylactic Antibiotic Selection[5]	0	-	97%	97%
Prophylactic Antibiotic Select. (Outpatient)[1,3]	1	100%	94%	94%
Prophylactic Antibiotic Stopped[5]	0	-	94%	94%
Recommended VTP Ordered[5]	0	-	94%	94%
Urinary Catheter Removal[5]	0	-	90%	90%
Children's Asthma Care				
Received Systemic Corticosteroids	-	-	-	100%
Received Home Management Plan	-	-	-	71%
Received Reliever Medication	-	-	-	100%
Use of Medical Imaging				
Combination Abdominal CT Scan	102	0.069	0.219	0.191
Combination Chest CT Scan	56	0.018	0.102	0.054
Follow-up Mammogram/Ultrasound	348	6.0%	8%	8.4%
MRI for Low Back Pain[5]	0	-	30.7%	32.7%
Survey of Patients' Hospital Experiences				
Area Around Room 'Always' Quiet at Night	(a)	79%	-	58%
Doctors 'Always' Communicated Well	(a)	87%	-	80%
Home Recovery Information Given	(a)	77%	-	82%
Hospital Given 9 or 10 on 10 Point Scale	(a)	65%	-	67%
Meds 'Always' Explained Before Given	(a)	72%	-	60%
Nurses 'Always' Communicated Well	(a)	77%	-	76%
Pain 'Always' Well Controlled	(a)	70%	-	69%
Room and Bathroom 'Always' Clean	(a)	60%	-	71%
Timely Help 'Always' Received	(a)	67%	-	64%
Would Definitely Recommend Hospital	(a)	53%	-	69%

NOTE: Hospital profiles are in alphabetical order by state, then city, then hospital within the city; Rankings exclude hospitals with less than 25 cases except for patient surveys which excludes hospitals with less than 100 cases; (a) 100–299 cases; (1) The number of cases is too small to be sure how well a hospital is performing; (2) The hospital indicated that the data submitted for this measure were based on a sample of cases; (3) Data was collected during a shorter time period (fewer quarters) than the maximum possible time for this measure; (4) Suppressed for one or more quarters by CMS; (5) No data is available from the hospital for this measure; (6) Fewer than 100 patients completed the HCAHPS survey. Use these rates with caution, as the number of surveys may be too low to reliably assess hospital performance; (7) Survey results are based on less than 12 months of data; (8) Survey results are not available for this reporting period; (9) No or very few patients were eligible for the HCAHPS survey. The scores shown, if any, reflect a very small number of surveys; (10) A state average was not calculated because too few hospitals in the state submitted data; (11) There were discrepancies in the data collection process; Please refer to the User's Guide for a full explanation of data.

Camden General Hospital

175 Hospital Drive
Camden, TN 38320
Phone: 731-584-6135
Fax: 731-584-0124
URL: www.wth.net
Type: Critical Access Hospitals
Emergency Services: Yes
Ownership: Govt - Hospital Dist/Auth
Beds: 83

Key Personnel:

CEO/President. . . . . Jim Moss
Chief of Medical Staff . . . . Jon R Winter, DO
Emergency Room . . . . Jim Craig

Measure	Cases	This Hosp.	State Avg.	U.S. Avg.
Heart Attack Care				
ACE Inhibitor or ARB for LVSD[5]	0	-	96%	96%
Aspirin at Arrival[5]	0	-	98%	99%
Aspirin at Discharge[5]	0	-	99%	98%
Beta Blocker at Discharge[5]	0	-	98%	98%
Fibrinolytic Medication Timing[5]	0	-	67%	55%
PCI Within 90 Minutes of Arrival[5]	0	-	91%	90%
Smoking Cessation Advice[5]	0	-	100%	99%
Chest Pain/Possible Heart Attack Care				
Aspirin at Arrival	-	-	95%	95%
Median Time to ECG (minutes)	-	-	8	8
Median Time to Transfer (minutes)	-	-	65	61
Fibrinolytic Medication Timing	-	-	49%	54%
Heart Failure Care				
ACE Inhibitor or ARB for LVSD[5]	0	-	95%	94%
Discharge Instructions[5]	0	-	88%	88%
Evaluation of LVS Function[5]	0	-	97%	98%
Smoking Cessation Advice[5]	0	-	99%	98%
Pneumonia Care				
Appropriate Initial Antibiotic[1]	4	100%	92%	92%
Blood Culture Timing[1]	6	100%	97%	96%
Influenza Vaccine[1]	1	100%	93%	91%
Initial Antibiotic Timing[1]	7	100%	96%	95%
Pneumococcal Vaccine[1]	1	100%	95%	93%
Smoking Cessation Advice[1]	2	100%	99%	97%
Surgical Care Improvement Project				
Appropriate VTP Within 24 Hours[5]	0	-	92%	92%
Appropriate Hair Removal[5]	0	-	100%	99%
Appropriate Beta Blocker Usage[5]	0	-	93%	93%
Controlled Postoperative Blood Glucose[5]	0	-	93%	93%
Prophylactic Antibiotic Timing[5]	0	-	97%	97%
Prophylactic Antibiotic Timing (Outpatient)	-	-	94%	92%
Prophylactic Antibiotic Selection[5]	0	-	97%	97%
Prophylactic Antibiotic Select. (Outpatient)	-	-	94%	94%
Prophylactic Antibiotic Stopped[5]	0	-	94%	94%
Recommended VTP Ordered[5]	0	-	94%	94%
Urinary Catheter Removal[5]	0	-	90%	90%
Children's Asthma Care				
Received Systemic Corticosteroids	-	-	-	100%
Received Home Management Plan	-	-	-	71%
Received Reliever Medication	-	-	-	100%
Use of Medical Imaging				
Combination Abdominal CT Scan	-	-	0.219	0.191
Combination Chest CT Scan	-	-	0.102	0.054
Follow-up Mammogram/Ultrasound	-	-	8%	8.4%
MRI for Low Back Pain	-	-	30.7%	32.7%
Survey of Patients' Hospital Experiences				
Area Around Room 'Always' Quiet at Night[6]	<100	63%	-	58%
Doctors 'Always' Communicated Well[6]	<100	79%	-	80%
Home Recovery Information Given[6]	<100	78%	-	82%
Hospital Given 9 or 10 on 10 Point Scale[6]	<100	59%	-	67%
Meds 'Always' Explained Before Given[6]	<100	45%	-	60%
Nurses 'Always' Communicated Well[6]	<100	76%	-	76%
Pain 'Always' Well Controlled[6]	<100	76%	-	69%
Room and Bathroom 'Always' Clean[6]	<100	74%	-	71%
Timely Help 'Always' Received[6]	<100	77%	-	64%
Would Definitely Recommend Hospital	<100	57%	-	69%

Riverview Regional Medical Center North

158 Hospital Drive
Carthage, TN 37030
Phone: 615-735-1560
Fax: 615-735-5118
URL: www.sumner.org
Type: Acute Care Hospitals
Emergency Services: Yes
Ownership: Government - Local
Beds: 63

Key Personnel:

CEO/President. . . . . Ed Chip Sanford
Chief of Medical Staff . . . . Richard Rutherford
Infection Control. . . . . Brenda Allison
Operating Room. . . . . Shirley Hailey, RN
Quality Assurance . . . . Patty Anderson
Radiology. . . . . Paul Dedick
Anesthesiology. . . . . Wayne Winfree
Emergency Room . . . . Lori Nixon, MD

Measure	Cases	This Hosp.	State Avg.	U.S. Avg.
Heart Attack Care				
ACE Inhibitor or ARB for LVSD[3]	0	-	96%	96%
Aspirin at Arrival[1,3]	1	100%	98%	99%
Aspirin at Discharge[1,3]	1	100%	99%	98%
Beta Blocker at Discharge[1,3]	1	100%	98%	98%
Fibrinolytic Medication Timing[3]	0	-	67%	55%
PCI Within 90 Minutes of Arrival[3]	0	-	91%	90%
Smoking Cessation Advice[3]	0	-	100%	99%
Chest Pain/Possible Heart Attack Care				
Aspirin at Arrival	125	98%	95%	95%
Median Time to ECG (minutes)	138	8	8	8
Median Time to Transfer (minutes)[1,3]	1	165	65	61
Fibrinolytic Medication Timing[1]	2	50%	49%	54%
Heart Failure Care				
ACE Inhibitor or ARB for LVSD[1]	7	86%	95%	94%
Discharge Instructions	36	97%	88%	88%
Evaluation of LVS Function	50	90%	97%	98%
Smoking Cessation Advice[1]	8	100%	99%	98%
Pneumonia Care				
Appropriate Initial Antibiotic	58	100%	92%	92%
Blood Culture Timing	86	99%	97%	96%
Influenza Vaccine	56	89%	93%	91%
Initial Antibiotic Timing	92	100%	96%	95%
Pneumococcal Vaccine	58	98%	95%	93%
Smoking Cessation Advice	48	98%	99%	97%
Surgical Care Improvement Project				
Appropriate VTP Within 24 Hours[1]	11	91%	92%	92%
Appropriate Hair Removal[1]	21	100%	100%	99%
Appropriate Beta Blocker Usage[1]	3	100%	93%	93%
Controlled Postoperative Blood Glucose	0	-	93%	93%
Prophylactic Antibiotic Timing[1]	12	75%	97%	97%
Prophylactic Antibiotic Timing (Outpatient)[1,3]	3	67%	94%	92%
Prophylactic Antibiotic Selection[1]	12	92%	97%	97%
Prophylactic Antibiotic Select. (Outpatient)[1,3]	2	100%	94%	94%
Prophylactic Antibiotic Stopped[1]	11	91%	94%	94%
Recommended VTP Ordered[1]	11	100%	94%	94%
Urinary Catheter Removal[1]	5	80%	90%	90%
Children's Asthma Care				
Received Systemic Corticosteroids	-	-	-	100%
Received Home Management Plan	-	-	-	71%
Received Reliever Medication	-	-	-	100%
Use of Medical Imaging				
Combination Abdominal CT Scan	191	0.403	0.219	0.191
Combination Chest CT Scan	119	0.361	0.102	0.054
Follow-up Mammogram/Ultrasound[5]	0	-	8%	8.4%
MRI for Low Back Pain[1]	55	20.0%	30.7%	32.7%
Survey of Patients' Hospital Experiences				
Area Around Room 'Always' Quiet at Night	(a)	70%	-	58%
Doctors 'Always' Communicated Well	(a)	84%	-	80%
Home Recovery Information Given	(a)	78%	-	82%
Hospital Given 9 or 10 on 10 Point Scale	(a)	66%	-	67%
Meds 'Always' Explained Before Given	(a)	61%	-	60%
Nurses 'Always' Communicated Well	(a)	77%	-	76%
Pain 'Always' Well Controlled	(a)	67%	-	69%
Room and Bathroom 'Always' Clean	(a)	82%	-	71%
Timely Help 'Always' Received	(a)	70%	-	64%
Would Definitely Recommend Hospital	(a)	60%	-	69%

Riverview Regional Medical Center South

130 Lebanon Highway
Carthage, TN 37030
Phone: 615-735-9815
URL: www.sumner.org
Type: Critical Access Hospitals
Emergency Services: Yes
Ownership: Proprietary
Beds: 25

Key Personnel:

CEO/President. . . . . Ed Chip Sanford
Chief of Medical Staff . . . . Glenn Nabors
Operating Room. . . . . Susie Dennis
Quality Assurance . . . . Marcie Mofield, RN
Anesthesiology. . . . . Wayne Winfree, CRNA
Emergency Room . . . . Holly Bush, RN

Measure	Cases	This Hosp.	State Avg.	U.S. Avg.
Heart Attack Care				
ACE Inhibitor or ARB for LVSD[5]	0	-	96%	96%
Aspirin at Arrival[5]	0	-	98%	99%
Aspirin at Discharge[5]	0	-	99%	98%
Beta Blocker at Discharge[5]	0	-	98%	98%
Fibrinolytic Medication Timing[5]	0	-	67%	55%
PCI Within 90 Minutes of Arrival[5]	0	-	91%	90%
Smoking Cessation Advice[5]	0	-	100%	99%
Chest Pain/Possible Heart Attack Care				
Aspirin at Arrival	-	-	95%	95%
Median Time to ECG (minutes)	-	-	8	8
Median Time to Transfer (minutes)	-	-	65	61
Fibrinolytic Medication Timing	-	-	49%	54%
Heart Failure Care				
ACE Inhibitor or ARB for LVSD[5]	0	-	95%	94%
Discharge Instructions[5]	0	-	88%	88%
Evaluation of LVS Function[5]	0	-	97%	98%
Smoking Cessation Advice[5]	0	-	99%	98%
Pneumonia Care				
Appropriate Initial Antibiotic[5]	0	-	92%	92%
Blood Culture Timing[5]	0	-	97%	96%
Influenza Vaccine[5]	0	-	93%	91%
Initial Antibiotic Timing[5]	0	-	96%	95%
Pneumococcal Vaccine[5]	0	-	95%	93%
Smoking Cessation Advice[5]	0	-	99%	97%
Surgical Care Improvement Project				
Appropriate VTP Within 24 Hours[5]	0	-	92%	92%
Appropriate Hair Removal[5]	0	-	100%	99%
Appropriate Beta Blocker Usage[5]	0	-	93%	93%
Controlled Postoperative Blood Glucose[5]	0	-	93%	93%
Prophylactic Antibiotic Timing[5]	0	-	97%	97%
Prophylactic Antibiotic Timing (Outpatient)	-	-	94%	92%
Prophylactic Antibiotic Selection[5]	0	-	97%	97%
Prophylactic Antibiotic Select. (Outpatient)	-	-	94%	94%
Prophylactic Antibiotic Stopped[5]	0	-	94%	94%
Recommended VTP Ordered[5]	0	-	94%	94%
Urinary Catheter Removal[5]	0	-	90%	90%
Children's Asthma Care				
Received Systemic Corticosteroids	-	-	-	100%
Received Home Management Plan	-	-	-	71%
Received Reliever Medication	-	-	-	100%
Use of Medical Imaging				
Combination Abdominal CT Scan	-	-	0.219	0.191
Combination Chest CT Scan	-	-	0.102	0.054
Follow-up Mammogram/Ultrasound	-	-	8%	8.4%
MRI for Low Back Pain	-	-	30.7%	32.7%
Survey of Patients' Hospital Experiences				
Area Around Room 'Always' Quiet at Night[8]	-	-	-	58%
Doctors 'Always' Communicated Well[8]	-	-	-	80%
Home Recovery Information Given[8]	-	-	-	82%
Hospital Given 9 or 10 on 10 Point Scale[8]	-	-	-	67%
Meds 'Always' Explained Before Given[8]	-	-	-	60%
Nurses 'Always' Communicated Well[8]	-	-	-	76%
Pain 'Always' Well Controlled[8]	-	-	-	69%
Room and Bathroom 'Always' Clean[8]	-	-	-	71%
Timely Help 'Always' Received[8]	-	-	-	64%
Would Definitely Recommend Hospital[8]	-	-	-	69%

NOTE: Hospital profiles are in alphabetical order by state, then city, then hospital within the city; Rankings exclude hospitals with less than 25 cases except for patient surveys which excludes hospitals with less than 100 cases; (a) 100–299 cases; (1) The number of cases is too small to be sure how well a hospital is performing; (2) The hospital indicated that the data submitted for this measure were based on a sample of cases; (3) Data was collected during a shorter time period (fewer quarters) than the maximum possible time for this measure; (4) Suppressed for one or more quarters by CMS; (5) No data is available from the hospital for this measure; (6) Fewer than 100 patients completed the HCAHPS survey. Use these rates with caution, as the number of surveys may be too low to reliably assess hospital performance; (7) Survey results are based on less than 12 months of data; (8) Survey results are not available for this reporting period; (9) No or very few patients were eligible for the HCAHPS survey. The scores shown, if any, reflect a very small number of surveys; (10) A state average was not calculated because too few hospitals in the state submitted data; (11) There were discrepancies in the data collection process; Please refer to the User's Guide for a full explanation of data.

Cumberland River Hospital

100 Old Jefferson St
Celina, TN 38551
Phone: 931-243-3581
Fax: 931-243-5263
Type: Acute Care Hospitals
Emergency Services: Yes
Ownership: Proprietary
Beds: 26

Key Personnel:
CEO/President. . . . . Andrea McLerran
Chief of Medical Staff. . . . . Kenneth Beaty
Radiology. . . . . Jim Hayes

Measure	Cases	This Hosp.	State Avg.	U.S. Avg.
Heart Attack Care				
ACE Inhibitor or ARB for LVSD[3]	0	-	96%	96%
Aspirin at Arrival[1,3]	2	100%	98%	99%
Aspirin at Discharge[1,3]	1	100%	99%	98%
Beta Blocker at Discharge[1,3]	1	100%	98%	98%
Fibrinolytic Medication Timing[3]	0	-	67%	55%
PCI Within 90 Minutes of Arrival[3]	0	-	91%	90%
Smoking Cessation Advice[3]	0	-	100%	99%
Chest Pain/Possible Heart Attack Care				
Aspirin at Arrival[1]	11	64%	95%	95%
Median Time to ECG (minutes)[1]	12	16	8	8
Median Time to Transfer (minutes)[1,3]	1	200	65	61
Fibrinolytic Medication Timing[1,3]	1	0%	49%	54%
Heart Failure Care				
ACE Inhibitor or ARB for LVSD[1]	12	100%	95%	94%
Discharge Instructions	25	96%	88%	88%
Evaluation of LVS Function	36	86%	97%	98%
Smoking Cessation Advice[1]	4	100%	99%	98%
Pneumonia Care				
Appropriate Initial Antibiotic	26	100%	92%	92%
Blood Culture Timing	44	100%	97%	96%
Influenza Vaccine	44	80%	93%	91%
Initial Antibiotic Timing	72	94%	96%	95%
Pneumococcal Vaccine	61	69%	95%	93%
Smoking Cessation Advice[1]	23	100%	99%	97%
Surgical Care Improvement Project				
Appropriate VTP Within 24 Hours[5]	0	-	92%	92%
Appropriate Hair Removal[5]	0	-	100%	99%
Appropriate Beta Blocker Usage[5]	0	-	93%	93%
Controlled Postoperative Blood Glucose[5]	0	-	93%	93%
Prophylactic Antibiotic Timing[5]	0	-	97%	97%
Prophylactic Antibiotic Timing (Outpatient)[5]	0	-	94%	92%
Prophylactic Antibiotic Selection[5]	0	-	97%	97%
Prophylactic Antibiotic Select. (Outpatient)[5]	0	-	94%	94%
Prophylactic Antibiotic Stopped[5]	0	-	94%	94%
Recommended VTP Ordered[5]	0	-	94%	94%
Urinary Catheter Removal[5]	0	-	90%	90%
Children's Asthma Care				
Received Systemic Corticosteroids	-	-	-	100%
Received Home Management Plan	-	-	-	71%
Received Reliever Medication	-	-	-	100%
Use of Medical Imaging				
Combination Abdominal CT Scan[1]	43	0.674	0.219	0.191
Combination Chest CT Scan[1]	23	0.739	0.102	0.054
Follow-up Mammogram/Ultrasound	94	5.3%	8%	8.4%
MRI for Low Back Pain[5]	0	-	30.7%	32.7%
Survey of Patients' Hospital Experiences				
Area Around Room 'Always' Quiet at Night	(a)	56%	-	58%
Doctors 'Always' Communicated Well	(a)	84%	-	80%
Home Recovery Information Given	(a)	82%	-	82%
Hospital Given 9 or 10 on 10 Point Scale	(a)	68%	-	67%
Meds 'Always' Explained Before Given	(a)	66%	-	60%
Nurses 'Always' Communicated Well	(a)	81%	-	76%
Pain 'Always' Well Controlled	(a)	70%	-	69%
Room and Bathroom 'Always' Clean	(a)	82%	-	71%
Timely Help 'Always' Received	(a)	77%	-	64%
Would Definitely Recommend Hospital	(a)	72%	-	69%

Hickman Community Health Services

135 East Swan Street
Centerville, TN 37033
Phone: 931-729-4271
Fax: 931-729-4612
Type: Critical Access Hospitals
Emergency Services: Yes
Ownership: Voluntary Non-Profit - Other
Beds: 25

Key Personnel:
CEO/President. . . . . Donna Bourdon
Chief of Medical Staff. . . . . Sai Oh
Emergency Room . . . . Darlene Swart, RN

Measure	Cases	This Hosp.	State Avg.	U.S. Avg.
Heart Attack Care				
ACE Inhibitor or ARB for LVSD[5]	0	-	96%	96%
Aspirin at Arrival[5]	0	-	98%	99%
Aspirin at Discharge[5]	0	-	99%	98%
Beta Blocker at Discharge[5]	0	-	98%	98%
Fibrinolytic Medication Timing[5]	0	-	67%	55%
PCI Within 90 Minutes of Arrival[5]	0	-	91%	90%
Smoking Cessation Advice[5]	0	-	100%	99%
Chest Pain/Possible Heart Attack Care				
Aspirin at Arrival	-	-	95%	95%
Median Time to ECG (minutes)	-	-	8	8
Median Time to Transfer (minutes)	-	-	65	61
Fibrinolytic Medication Timing	-	-	49%	54%
Heart Failure Care				
ACE Inhibitor or ARB for LVSD[5]	0	-	95%	94%
Discharge Instructions[5]	0	-	88%	88%
Evaluation of LVS Function[5]	0	-	97%	98%
Smoking Cessation Advice[5]	0	-	99%	98%
Pneumonia Care				
Appropriate Initial Antibiotic[1]	16	81%	92%	92%
Blood Culture Timing[1]	20	95%	97%	96%
Influenza Vaccine[1]	21	14%	93%	91%
Initial Antibiotic Timing[1]	16	88%	96%	95%
Pneumococcal Vaccine	25	16%	95%	93%
Smoking Cessation Advice[1]	2	100%	99%	97%
Surgical Care Improvement Project				
Appropriate VTP Within 24 Hours[5]	0	-	92%	92%
Appropriate Hair Removal[5]	0	-	100%	99%
Appropriate Beta Blocker Usage[5]	0	-	93%	93%
Controlled Postoperative Blood Glucose[5]	0	-	93%	93%
Prophylactic Antibiotic Timing[5]	0	-	97%	97%
Prophylactic Antibiotic Timing (Outpatient)	-	-	94%	92%
Prophylactic Antibiotic Selection[5]	0	-	97%	97%
Prophylactic Antibiotic Select. (Outpatient)	-	-	94%	94%
Prophylactic Antibiotic Stopped[5]	0	-	94%	94%
Recommended VTP Ordered[5]	0	-	94%	94%
Urinary Catheter Removal[5]	0	-	90%	90%
Children's Asthma Care				
Received Systemic Corticosteroids	-	-	-	100%
Received Home Management Plan	-	-	-	71%
Received Reliever Medication	-	-	-	100%
Use of Medical Imaging				
Combination Abdominal CT Scan	-	-	0.219	0.191
Combination Chest CT Scan	-	-	0.102	0.054
Follow-up Mammogram/Ultrasound	-	-	8%	8.4%
MRI for Low Back Pain	-	-	30.7%	32.7%
Survey of Patients' Hospital Experiences				
Area Around Room 'Always' Quiet at Night[8]	-	-	-	58%
Doctors 'Always' Communicated Well[8]	-	-	-	80%
Home Recovery Information Given[8]	-	-	-	82%
Hospital Given 9 or 10 on 10 Point Scale[8]	-	-	-	67%
Meds 'Always' Explained Before Given[8]	-	-	-	60%
Nurses 'Always' Communicated Well[8]	-	-	-	76%
Pain 'Always' Well Controlled[8]	-	-	-	69%
Room and Bathroom 'Always' Clean[8]	-	-	-	71%
Timely Help 'Always' Received[8]	-	-	-	64%
Would Definitely Recommend Hospital[8]	-	-	-	69%

Erlanger Medical Center

975 E 3rd St
Chattanooga, TN 37403
Phone: 423-778-7000
Fax: 423-778-7454
URL: www.erlanger.org
Type: Acute Care Hospitals
Emergency Services: Yes
Ownership: Govt - Hospital Dist/Auth
Beds: 819

Key Personnel:
CEO/President. . . . . Jim Brexler
Chief of Medical Staff . . . . Woods Blake, MD
Infection Control. . . . . Steve Hawkins, MD
Pediatric Ambulatory Care . . . . . . Nita Shumaker, MD
Pediatric In-Patient Care . . . . Nita Shumaker, MD
Quality Assurance . . . . Mike Bettinger
Radiology. . . . . Robert Phlegar, MD

Measure	Cases	This Hosp.	State Avg.	U.S. Avg.
Heart Attack Care				
ACE Inhibitor or ARB for LVSD	52	100%	96%	96%
Aspirin at Arrival	234	99%	98%	99%
Aspirin at Discharge	391	100%	99%	98%
Beta Blocker at Discharge	354	100%	98%	98%
Fibrinolytic Medication Timing	0	-	67%	55%
PCI Within 90 Minutes of Arrival	72	92%	91%	90%
Smoking Cessation Advice	208	100%	100%	99%
Chest Pain/Possible Heart Attack Care				
Aspirin at Arrival[1]	23	91%	95%	95%
Median Time to ECG (minutes)[1]	24	12	8	8
Median Time to Transfer (minutes)[1,3]	3	58	65	61
Fibrinolytic Medication Timing[3]	0	-	49%	54%
Heart Failure Care				
ACE Inhibitor or ARB for LVSD	133	97%	95%	94%
Discharge Instructions	304	88%	88%	88%
Evaluation of LVS Function	341	99%	97%	98%
Smoking Cessation Advice	117	100%	99%	98%
Pneumonia Care				
Appropriate Initial Antibiotic	113	91%	92%	92%
Blood Culture Timing	175	95%	97%	96%
Influenza Vaccine	163	96%	93%	91%
Initial Antibiotic Timing	195	96%	96%	95%
Pneumococcal Vaccine	164	98%	95%	93%
Smoking Cessation Advice	179	99%	99%	97%
Surgical Care Improvement Project				
Appropriate VTP Within 24 Hours[2]	156	97%	92%	92%
Appropriate Hair Removal[2]	518	100%	100%	99%
Appropriate Beta Blocker Usage[2]	140	91%	93%	93%
Controlled Postoperative Blood Glucose[2]	102	91%	93%	93%
Prophylactic Antibiotic Timing[2]	339	97%	97%	97%
Prophylactic Antibiotic Timing (Outpatient)	539	94%	94%	92%
Prophylactic Antibiotic Selection[2]	351	98%	97%	97%
Prophylactic Antibiotic Select. (Outpatient)	525	95%	94%	94%
Prophylactic Antibiotic Stopped[2]	321	93%	94%	94%
Recommended VTP Ordered[2]	156	99%	94%	94%
Urinary Catheter Removal[2]	64	80%	90%	90%
Children's Asthma Care				
Received Systemic Corticosteroids	39	100%	-	100%
Received Home Management Plan	39	82%	-	71%
Received Reliever Medication	39	100%	-	100%
Use of Medical Imaging				
Combination Abdominal CT Scan	1,071	0.296	0.219	0.191
Combination Chest CT Scan	940	0.153	0.102	0.054
Follow-up Mammogram/Ultrasound	2,058	5.1%	8%	8.4%
MRI for Low Back Pain	164	36.6%	30.7%	32.7%
Survey of Patients' Hospital Experiences				
Area Around Room 'Always' Quiet at Night	300+	62%	-	58%
Doctors 'Always' Communicated Well	300+	81%	-	80%
Home Recovery Information Given	300+	80%	-	82%
Hospital Given 9 or 10 on 10 Point Scale	300+	66%	-	67%
Meds 'Always' Explained Before Given	300+	61%	-	60%
Nurses 'Always' Communicated Well	300+	76%	-	76%
Pain 'Always' Well Controlled	300+	69%	-	69%
Room and Bathroom 'Always' Clean	300+	62%	-	71%
Timely Help 'Always' Received	300+	61%	-	64%
Would Definitely Recommend Hospital	300+	74%	-	69%

NOTE: Hospital profiles are in alphabetical order by state, then city, then hospital within the city; Rankings exclude hospitals with less than 25 cases except for patient surveys which excludes hospitals with less than 100 cases; (a) 100–299 cases; (1) The number of cases is too small to be sure how well a hospital is performing; (2) The hospital indicated that the data submitted for this measure were based on a sample of cases; (3) Data was collected during a shorter time period (fewer quarters) than the maximum possible time for this measure; (4) Suppressed for one or more quarters by CMS; (5) No data is available from the hospital for this measure; (6) Fewer than 100 patients completed the HCAHPS survey. Use these rates with caution, as the number of surveys may be too low to reliably assess hospital performance; (7) Survey results are based on less than 12 months of data; (8) Survey results are not available for this reporting period; (9) No or very few patients were eligible for the HCAHPS survey. The scores shown, if any, reflect a very small number of surveys; (10) A state average was not calculated because too few hospitals in the state submitted data; (11) There were discrepancies in the data collection process; Please refer to the User's Guide for a full explanation of data.

Healthsouth Chattanooga Rehab Hospital

2412 Mccallie Ave Phone: 423-698-0221
Chattanooga, TN 37404 Fax: 423-697-9295
URL: www.healthsouth.com
Type: Acute Care Hospitals Emergency Services: No
Ownership: Government - State Beds: 80

Key Personnel:
CEO/President. . . . . Karen G Davis
Chief of Medical Staff. . . . . Sai Oh
Quality Assurance . . . . Denise Smith
Intensive Care Unit. . . . . Mark J Tarr

Measure	Cases	This Hosp.	State Avg.	U.S. Avg.
Heart Attack Care				
ACE Inhibitor or ARB for LVSD[5]	0	-	96%	96%
Aspirin at Arrival[5]	0	-	98%	99%
Aspirin at Discharge[5]	0	-	99%	98%
Beta Blocker at Discharge[5]	0	-	98%	98%
Fibrinolytic Medication Timing[5]	0	-	67%	55%
PCI Within 90 Minutes of Arrival[5]	0	-	91%	90%
Smoking Cessation Advice[5]	0	-	100%	99%
Chest Pain/Possible Heart Attack Care				
Aspirin at Arrival	-	-	95%	95%
Median Time to ECG (minutes)	-	-	8	8
Median Time to Transfer (minutes)	-	-	65	61
Fibrinolytic Medication Timing	-	-	49%	54%
Heart Failure Care				
ACE Inhibitor or ARB for LVSD[5]	0	-	95%	94%
Discharge Instructions[5]	0	-	88%	88%
Evaluation of LVS Function[5]	0	-	97%	98%
Smoking Cessation Advice[5]	0	-	99%	98%
Pneumonia Care				
Appropriate Initial Antibiotic[5]	0	-	92%	92%
Blood Culture Timing[5]	0	-	97%	96%
Influenza Vaccine[5]	0	-	93%	91%
Initial Antibiotic Timing[5]	0	-	96%	95%
Pneumococcal Vaccine[5]	0	-	95%	93%
Smoking Cessation Advice[5]	0	-	99%	97%
Surgical Care Improvement Project				
Appropriate VTP Within 24 Hours[5]	0	-	92%	92%
Appropriate Hair Removal[5]	0	-	100%	99%
Appropriate Beta Blocker Usage[5]	0	-	93%	93%
Controlled Postoperative Blood Glucose[5]	0	-	93%	93%
Prophylactic Antibiotic Timing[5]	0	-	97%	97%
Prophylactic Antibiotic Timing (Outpatient)	-	-	94%	92%
Prophylactic Antibiotic Selection[5]	0	-	97%	97%
Prophylactic Antibiotic Select. (Outpatient)	-	-	94%	94%
Prophylactic Antibiotic Stopped[5]	0	-	94%	94%
Recommended VTP Ordered[5]	0	-	94%	94%
Urinary Catheter Removal[5]	0	-	90%	90%
Children's Asthma Care				
Received Systemic Corticosteroids	-	-	-	100%
Received Home Management Plan	-	-	-	71%
Received Reliever Medication	-	-	-	100%
Use of Medical Imaging				
Combination Abdominal CT Scan	-	-	0.219	0.191
Combination Chest CT Scan	-	-	0.102	0.054
Follow-up Mammogram/Ultrasound	-	-	8%	8.4%
MRI for Low Back Pain	-	-	30.7%	32.7%
Survey of Patients' Hospital Experiences				
Area Around Room 'Always' Quiet at Night[9]	-	-	-	58%
Doctors 'Always' Communicated Well[9]	-	-	-	80%
Home Recovery Information Given[9]	-	-	-	82%
Hospital Given 9 or 10 on 10 Point Scale[9]	-	-	-	67%
Meds 'Always' Explained Before Given[9]	-	-	-	60%
Nurses 'Always' Communicated Well[9]	-	-	-	76%
Pain 'Always' Well Controlled[9]	-	-	-	69%
Room and Bathroom 'Always' Clean[9]	-	-	-	71%
Timely Help 'Always' Received[9]	-	-	-	64%
Would Definitely Recommend Hospital[9]	-	-	-	69%

Memorial Healthcare System

2525 Desales Ave Phone: 423-495-2525
Chattanooga, TN 37404 Fax: 423-495-6722
URL: www.memorial.org
Type: Acute Care Hospitals Emergency Services: Yes
Ownership: Voluntary Non-Profit - Church Beds: 322

Key Personnel:
CEO/President. . . . . Dan L Bowers
Cardiac Laboratory. . . . . Laura Hartman, RN
Infection Control. . . . . Gwen Davis
Quality Assurance . . . . Beverly Gordon
Radiology. . . . . Stan Casteel
Emergency Room . . . . Runay Valentine

Measure	Cases	This Hosp.	State Avg.	U.S. Avg.
Heart Attack Care				
ACE Inhibitor or ARB for LVSD	122	100%	96%	96%
Aspirin at Arrival	530	99%	98%	99%
Aspirin at Discharge	746	100%	99%	98%
Beta Blocker at Discharge	705	100%	98%	98%
Fibrinolytic Medication Timing	0	-	67%	55%
PCI Within 90 Minutes of Arrival	104	85%	91%	90%
Smoking Cessation Advice	240	100%	100%	99%
Chest Pain/Possible Heart Attack Care				
Aspirin at Arrival	33	94%	95%	95%
Median Time to ECG (minutes)	31	2	8	8
Median Time to Transfer (minutes)[1]	11	57	65	61
Fibrinolytic Medication Timing	0	-	49%	54%
Heart Failure Care				
ACE Inhibitor or ARB for LVSD	249	98%	95%	94%
Discharge Instructions	663	84%	88%	88%
Evaluation of LVS Function	785	99%	97%	98%
Smoking Cessation Advice	129	98%	99%	98%
Pneumonia Care				
Appropriate Initial Antibiotic	411	100%	92%	92%
Blood Culture Timing	724	99%	97%	96%
Influenza Vaccine	488	99%	93%	91%
Initial Antibiotic Timing	815	96%	96%	95%
Pneumococcal Vaccine	706	99%	95%	93%
Smoking Cessation Advice	231	100%	99%	97%
Surgical Care Improvement Project				
Appropriate VTP Within 24 Hours[2]	657	90%	92%	92%
Appropriate Hair Removal[2]	2,756	100%	100%	99%
Appropriate Beta Blocker Usage[2]	888	91%	93%	93%
Controlled Postoperative Blood Glucose[2]	702	89%	93%	93%
Prophylactic Antibiotic Timing[2]	2,048	97%	97%	97%
Prophylactic Antibiotic Timing (Outpatient)	522	95%	94%	92%
Prophylactic Antibiotic Selection[2]	2,064	100%	97%	97%
Prophylactic Antibiotic Select. (Outpatient)	545	99%	94%	94%
Prophylactic Antibiotic Stopped[2]	2,005	97%	94%	94%
Recommended VTP Ordered[2]	658	93%	94%	94%
Urinary Catheter Removal[2]	754	90%	90%	90%
Children's Asthma Care				
Received Systemic Corticosteroids	-	-	-	100%
Received Home Management Plan	-	-	-	71%
Received Reliever Medication	-	-	-	100%
Use of Medical Imaging				
Combination Abdominal CT Scan	2,724	0.390	0.219	0.191
Combination Chest CT Scan	1,359	0.045	0.102	0.054
Follow-up Mammogram/Ultrasound	4,438	4.6%	8%	8.4%
MRI for Low Back Pain	568	33.3%	30.7%	32.7%
Survey of Patients' Hospital Experiences				
Area Around Room 'Always' Quiet at Night	300+	68%	-	58%
Doctors 'Always' Communicated Well	300+	84%	-	80%
Home Recovery Information Given	300+	85%	-	82%
Hospital Given 9 or 10 on 10 Point Scale	300+	78%	-	67%
Meds 'Always' Explained Before Given	300+	63%	-	60%
Nurses 'Always' Communicated Well	300+	82%	-	76%
Pain 'Always' Well Controlled	300+	74%	-	69%
Room and Bathroom 'Always' Clean	300+	71%	-	71%
Timely Help 'Always' Received	300+	69%	-	64%
Would Definitely Recommend Hospital	300+	84%	-	69%

Parkridge Medical Center

2333 Mccallie Ave Phone: 423-894-4220
Chattanooga, TN 37404 Fax: 423-493-1208
URL: www.TriStarHealth.com
Type: Acute Care Hospitals Emergency Services: Yes
Ownership: Proprietary Beds: 296

Key Personnel:
CEO/President. . . . . Darrell Moore
Chief of Medical Staff . . . . Kirk Brody, MD
Infection Control. . . . . Susan Schnell
Operating Room. . . . . Adam Royer
Pediatric In-Patient Care . . . . Teresa C Walker
Quality Assurance . . . . Judy Ketchersid
Radiology. . . . . Sharon Hobbs
Patient Relations . . . . Sherry Maxwell

Measure	Cases	This Hosp.	State Avg.	U.S. Avg.
Heart Attack Care				
ACE Inhibitor or ARB for LVSD[1]	24	100%	96%	96%
Aspirin at Arrival	111	100%	98%	99%
Aspirin at Discharge	230	100%	99%	98%
Beta Blocker at Discharge	218	100%	98%	98%
Fibrinolytic Medication Timing[1]	2	100%	67%	55%
PCI Within 90 Minutes of Arrival[1]	14	100%	91%	90%
Smoking Cessation Advice	117	100%	100%	99%
Chest Pain/Possible Heart Attack Care				
Aspirin at Arrival	65	98%	95%	95%
Median Time to ECG (minutes)	71	6	8	8
Median Time to Transfer (minutes)[1]	8	28	65	61
Fibrinolytic Medication Timing	0	-	49%	54%
Heart Failure Care				
ACE Inhibitor or ARB for LVSD	98	99%	95%	94%
Discharge Instructions	258	97%	88%	88%
Evaluation of LVS Function	323	100%	97%	98%
Smoking Cessation Advice	85	100%	99%	98%
Pneumonia Care				
Appropriate Initial Antibiotic	171	97%	92%	92%
Blood Culture Timing	171	99%	97%	96%
Influenza Vaccine	153	100%	93%	91%
Initial Antibiotic Timing	226	100%	96%	95%
Pneumococcal Vaccine	183	100%	95%	93%
Smoking Cessation Advice	149	100%	99%	97%
Surgical Care Improvement Project				
Appropriate VTP Within 24 Hours[2]	198	96%	92%	92%
Appropriate Hair Removal[2]	696	100%	100%	99%
Appropriate Beta Blocker Usage[2]	212	98%	93%	93%
Controlled Postoperative Blood Glucose[2]	157	95%	93%	93%
Prophylactic Antibiotic Timing[2]	460	99%	97%	97%
Prophylactic Antibiotic Timing (Outpatient)	695	99%	94%	92%
Prophylactic Antibiotic Selection[2]	470	98%	97%	97%
Prophylactic Antibiotic Select. (Outpatient)	693	98%	94%	94%
Prophylactic Antibiotic Stopped[2]	419	97%	94%	94%
Recommended VTP Ordered[2]	198	97%	94%	94%
Urinary Catheter Removal[2]	109	90%	90%	90%
Children's Asthma Care				
Received Systemic Corticosteroids	-	-	-	100%
Received Home Management Plan	-	-	-	71%
Received Reliever Medication	-	-	-	100%
Use of Medical Imaging				
Combination Abdominal CT Scan	819	0.173	0.219	0.191
Combination Chest CT Scan	311	0.119	0.102	0.054
Follow-up Mammogram/Ultrasound	625	12.3%	8%	8.4%
MRI for Low Back Pain	118	33.9%	30.7%	32.7%
Survey of Patients' Hospital Experiences				
Area Around Room 'Always' Quiet at Night	300+	65%	-	58%
Doctors 'Always' Communicated Well	300+	83%	-	80%
Home Recovery Information Given	300+	83%	-	82%
Hospital Given 9 or 10 on 10 Point Scale	300+	73%	-	67%
Meds 'Always' Explained Before Given	300+	61%	-	60%
Nurses 'Always' Communicated Well	300+	78%	-	76%
Pain 'Always' Well Controlled	300+	73%	-	69%
Room and Bathroom 'Always' Clean	300+	73%	-	71%
Timely Help 'Always' Received	300+	65%	-	64%
Would Definitely Recommend Hospital	300+	76%	-	69%

NOTE: Hospital profiles are in alphabetical order by state, then city, then hospital within the city; Rankings exclude hospitals with less than 25 cases except for patient surveys which excludes hospitals with less than 100 cases; (a) 100–299 cases; (1) The number of cases is too small to be sure how well a hospital is performing; (2) The hospital indicated that the data submitted for this measure were based on a sample of cases; (3) Data was collected during a shorter time period (fewer quarters) than the maximum possible time for this measure; (4) Suppressed for one or more quarters by CMS; (5) No data is available from the hospital for this measure; (6) Fewer than 100 patients completed the HCAHPS survey. Use these rates with caution, as the number of surveys may be too low to reliably assess hospital performance; (7) Survey results are based on less than 12 months of data; (8) Survey results are not available for this reporting period; (9) No or very few patients were eligible for the HCAHPS survey. The scores shown, if any, reflect a very small number of surveys; (10) A state average was not calculated because too few hospitals in the state submitted data; (11) There were discrepancies in the data collection process; Please refer to the User's Guide for a full explanation of data.

Gateway Medical Center

651 Dunlop Lane
Clarksville, TN 37040
Phone: 931-502-1000
URL: www.todaysgateway.com
Type: Acute Care Hospitals
Emergency Services: Yes
Ownership: Govt - Hospital Dist/Auth
Beds: 270

Key Personnel:

CEO . . . . Tim Puthoff
President . . . . Angie Allen
Radiology. . . . . Dan Starnes
Emergency . . . . Randy Likes

Measure	Cases	This Hosp.	State Avg.	U.S. Avg.
Heart Attack Care				
ACE Inhibitor or ARB for LVSD	37	95%	96%	96%
Aspirin at Arrival	180	99%	98%	99%
Aspirin at Discharge	188	94%	99%	98%
Beta Blocker at Discharge	194	94%	98%	98%
Fibrinolytic Medication Timing	0	-	67%	55%
PCI Within 90 Minutes of Arrival	45	76%	91%	90%
Smoking Cessation Advice	104	100%	100%	99%
Chest Pain/Possible Heart Attack Care				
Aspirin at Arrival	124	98%	95%	95%
Median Time to ECG (minutes)	129	4	8	8
Median Time to Transfer (minutes)[1,3]	5	53	65	61
Fibrinolytic Medication Timing[1]	1	0%	49%	54%
Heart Failure Care				
ACE Inhibitor or ARB for LVSD	108	96%	95%	94%
Discharge Instructions	286	96%	88%	88%
Evaluation of LVS Function	322	88%	97%	98%
Smoking Cessation Advice	79	99%	99%	98%
Pneumonia Care				
Appropriate Initial Antibiotic	204	94%	92%	92%
Blood Culture Timing	327	95%	97%	96%
Influenza Vaccine	218	94%	93%	91%
Initial Antibiotic Timing	315	96%	96%	95%
Pneumococcal Vaccine	252	96%	95%	93%
Smoking Cessation Advice	116	100%	99%	97%
Surgical Care Improvement Project				
Appropriate VTP Within 24 Hours	279	92%	92%	92%
Appropriate Hair Removal	767	95%	100%	99%
Appropriate Beta Blocker Usage	215	97%	93%	93%
Controlled Postoperative Blood Glucose	80	96%	93%	93%
Prophylactic Antibiotic Timing	535	98%	97%	97%
Prophylactic Antibiotic Timing (Outpatient)	174	94%	94%	92%
Prophylactic Antibiotic Selection	542	98%	97%	97%
Prophylactic Antibiotic Select. (Outpatient)	173	97%	94%	94%
Prophylactic Antibiotic Stopped	512	90%	94%	94%
Recommended VTP Ordered	279	96%	94%	94%
Urinary Catheter Removal	185	89%	90%	90%
Children's Asthma Care				
Received Systemic Corticosteroids	-	-	-	100%
Received Home Management Plan	-	-	-	71%
Received Reliever Medication	-	-	-	100%
Use of Medical Imaging				
Combination Abdominal CT Scan	954	0.042	0.219	0.191
Combination Chest CT Scan	768	0.005	0.102	0.054
Follow-up Mammogram/Ultrasound	1,261	6.5%	8%	8.4%
MRI for Low Back Pain	268	28.4%	30.7%	32.7%
Survey of Patients' Hospital Experiences				
Area Around Room 'Always' Quiet at Night	300+	58%	-	58%
Doctors 'Always' Communicated Well	300+	79%	-	80%
Home Recovery Information Given	300+	77%	-	82%
Hospital Given 9 or 10 on 10 Point Scale	300+	60%	-	67%
Meds 'Always' Explained Before Given	300+	56%	-	60%
Nurses 'Always' Communicated Well	300+	73%	-	76%
Pain 'Always' Well Controlled	300+	70%	-	69%
Room and Bathroom 'Always' Clean	300+	65%	-	71%
Timely Help 'Always' Received	300+	61%	-	64%
Would Definitely Recommend Hospital	300+	60%	-	69%

Skyridge Medical Center

2305 Chambliss Ave NW
Cleveland, TN 37311
Phone: 423-339-4132
URL: www.skyridgemedcenter.com
Type: Acute Care Hospitals
Emergency Services: Yes
Ownership: Proprietary

Key Personnel:

President/CEO. . . . . Maureen Tarrant
Emergency . . . . Stephen Heinz, MD

Measure	Cases	This Hosp.	State Avg.	U.S. Avg.
Heart Attack Care				
ACE Inhibitor or ARB for LVSD[1]	12	92%	96%	96%
Aspirin at Arrival	94	98%	98%	99%
Aspirin at Discharge	47	100%	99%	98%
Beta Blocker at Discharge	52	98%	98%	98%
Fibrinolytic Medication Timing	0	-	67%	55%
PCI Within 90 Minutes of Arrival	0	-	91%	90%
Smoking Cessation Advice[1]	14	100%	100%	99%
Chest Pain/Possible Heart Attack Care				
Aspirin at Arrival	91	98%	95%	95%
Median Time to ECG (minutes)	95	10	8	8
Median Time to Transfer (minutes)	54	73	65	61
Fibrinolytic Medication Timing	0	-	49%	54%
Heart Failure Care				
ACE Inhibitor or ARB for LVSD	61	95%	95%	94%
Discharge Instructions	205	92%	88%	88%
Evaluation of LVS Function	241	99%	97%	98%
Smoking Cessation Advice	53	100%	99%	98%
Pneumonia Care				
Appropriate Initial Antibiotic	253	89%	92%	92%
Blood Culture Timing	280	98%	97%	96%
Influenza Vaccine	249	95%	93%	91%
Initial Antibiotic Timing	349	97%	96%	95%
Pneumococcal Vaccine	320	98%	95%	93%
Smoking Cessation Advice	186	100%	99%	97%
Surgical Care Improvement Project				
Appropriate VTP Within 24 Hours[2]	242	98%	92%	92%
Appropriate Hair Removal[2]	427	99%	100%	99%
Appropriate Beta Blocker Usage[2]	92	87%	93%	93%
Controlled Postoperative Blood Glucose[2]	0	-	93%	93%
Prophylactic Antibiotic Timing[2]	241	90%	97%	97%
Prophylactic Antibiotic Timing (Outpatient)	316	84%	94%	92%
Prophylactic Antibiotic Selection[2]	240	94%	97%	97%
Prophylactic Antibiotic Select. (Outpatient)	294	97%	94%	94%
Prophylactic Antibiotic Stopped[2]	220	91%	94%	94%
Recommended VTP Ordered[2]	243	98%	94%	94%
Urinary Catheter Removal	55	73%	90%	90%
Children's Asthma Care				
Received Systemic Corticosteroids	-	-	-	100%
Received Home Management Plan	-	-	-	71%
Received Reliever Medication	-	-	-	100%
Use of Medical Imaging				
Combination Abdominal CT Scan	967	0.195	0.219	0.191
Combination Chest CT Scan	702	0.014	0.102	0.054
Follow-up Mammogram/Ultrasound	1,145	5.1%	8%	8.4%
MRI for Low Back Pain	317	31.5%	30.7%	32.7%
Survey of Patients' Hospital Experiences				
Area Around Room 'Always' Quiet at Night	300+	60%	-	58%
Doctors 'Always' Communicated Well	300+	78%	-	80%
Home Recovery Information Given	300+	78%	-	82%
Hospital Given 9 or 10 on 10 Point Scale	300+	58%	-	67%
Meds 'Always' Explained Before Given	300+	53%	-	60%
Nurses 'Always' Communicated Well	300+	73%	-	76%
Pain 'Always' Well Controlled	300+	68%	-	69%
Room and Bathroom 'Always' Clean	300+	63%	-	71%
Timely Help 'Always' Received	300+	58%	-	64%
Would Definitely Recommend Hospital	300+	56%	-	69%

Maury Regional Hospital

1224 Trotwood Ave
Columbia, TN 38401
Phone: 931-381-1111
Fax: 931-380-4016
URL: www.maurgregional.com
Type: Acute Care Hospitals
Emergency Services: Yes
Ownership: Government - Local
Beds: 255

Key Personnel:

CEO/President. . . . . Robert Otwell
Chief of Medical Staff . . . . Anthony D. Khim
Infection Control. . . . . Roger Anderson
Operating Room. . . . . Stephen Noe
Quality Assurance . . . . Sue Parsons
Radiology. . . . . Terrie Stinson
Anesthesiology. . . . . Jeff Kirkpatrick, MD
Patient Relations . . . . Cindy Fox

Measure	Cases	This Hosp.	State Avg.	U.S. Avg.
Heart Attack Care				
ACE Inhibitor or ARB for LVSD	88	93%	96%	96%
Aspirin at Arrival	199	98%	98%	99%
Aspirin at Discharge	267	99%	99%	98%
Beta Blocker at Discharge	254	98%	98%	98%
Fibrinolytic Medication Timing	0	-	67%	55%
PCI Within 90 Minutes of Arrival	36	94%	91%	90%
Smoking Cessation Advice	124	100%	100%	99%
Chest Pain/Possible Heart Attack Care				
Aspirin at Arrival	48	92%	95%	95%
Median Time to ECG (minutes)	53	5	8	8
Median Time to Transfer (minutes)[5]	0	-	65	61
Fibrinolytic Medication Timing[3]	0	-	49%	54%
Heart Failure Care				
ACE Inhibitor or ARB for LVSD	174	95%	95%	94%
Discharge Instructions	333	93%	88%	88%
Evaluation of LVS Function	422	100%	97%	98%
Smoking Cessation Advice	105	100%	99%	98%
Pneumonia Care				
Appropriate Initial Antibiotic[2]	66	85%	92%	92%
Blood Culture Timing[2]	112	96%	97%	96%
Influenza Vaccine[2]	97	95%	93%	91%
Initial Antibiotic Timing[2]	106	96%	96%	95%
Pneumococcal Vaccine[2]	140	93%	95%	93%
Smoking Cessation Advice[2]	66	100%	99%	97%
Surgical Care Improvement Project				
Appropriate VTP Within 24 Hours[2]	162	87%	92%	92%
Appropriate Hair Removal[2]	655	100%	100%	99%
Appropriate Beta Blocker Usage[2]	170	94%	93%	93%
Controlled Postoperative Blood Glucose[2]	74	99%	93%	93%
Prophylactic Antibiotic Timing[2]	474	98%	97%	97%
Prophylactic Antibiotic Timing (Outpatient)	453	91%	94%	92%
Prophylactic Antibiotic Selection[2]	483	96%	97%	97%
Prophylactic Antibiotic Select. (Outpatient)	424	94%	94%	94%
Prophylactic Antibiotic Stopped[2]	446	95%	94%	94%
Recommended VTP Ordered[2]	162	91%	94%	94%
Urinary Catheter Removal[2]	119	90%	90%	90%
Children's Asthma Care				
Received Systemic Corticosteroids	-	-	-	100%
Received Home Management Plan	-	-	-	71%
Received Reliever Medication	-	-	-	100%
Use of Medical Imaging				
Combination Abdominal CT Scan	1,324	0.128	0.219	0.191
Combination Chest CT Scan	1,232	0.059	0.102	0.054
Follow-up Mammogram/Ultrasound	1,690	10.7%	8%	8.4%
MRI for Low Back Pain	230	27.8%	30.7%	32.7%
Survey of Patients' Hospital Experiences				
Area Around Room 'Always' Quiet at Night	300+	63%	-	58%
Doctors 'Always' Communicated Well	300+	84%	-	80%
Home Recovery Information Given	300+	83%	-	82%
Hospital Given 9 or 10 on 10 Point Scale	300+	75%	-	67%
Meds 'Always' Explained Before Given	300+	69%	-	60%
Nurses 'Always' Communicated Well	300+	83%	-	76%
Pain 'Always' Well Controlled	300+	76%	-	69%
Room and Bathroom 'Always' Clean	300+	77%	-	71%
Timely Help 'Always' Received	300+	74%	-	64%
Would Definitely Recommend Hospital	300+	76%	-	69%

NOTE: Hospital profiles are in alphabetical order by state, then city, then hospital within the city; Rankings exclude hospitals with less than 25 cases except for patient surveys which excludes hospitals with less than 100 cases; (a) 100–299 cases; (1) The number of cases is too small to be sure how well a hospital is performing; (2) The hospital indicated that the data submitted for this measure were based on a sample of cases; (3) Data was collected during a shorter time period (fewer quarters) than the maximum possible time for this measure; (4) Suppressed for one or more quarters by CMS; (5) No data is available from the hospital for this measure; (6) Fewer than 100 patients completed the HCAHPS survey. Use these rates with caution, as the number of surveys may be too low to reliably assess hospital performance; (7) Survey results are based on less than 12 months of data; (8) Survey results are not available for this reporting period; (9) No or very few patients were eligible for the HCAHPS survey. The scores shown, if any, reflect a very small number of surveys; (10) A state average was not calculated because too few hospitals in the state submitted data; (11) There were discrepancies in the data collection process; Please refer to the User's Guide for a full explanation of data.

Cookeville Regional Medical Center

1 Medical Center Boulevard — Phone: 931-646-2000
Cookeville, TN 38501 — Fax: 931-646-2635
URL: www.crmchealth.org
Type: Acute Care Hospitals — Emergency Services: Yes
Ownership: Government - Local — Beds: 247

Key Personnel:
CEO/President. . . . . Bernard L Mattingly
Chief of Medical Staff . . . . Tim R Collins
Radiology. . . . . Ginny Charnock, MD
Anesthesiology. . . . . Blake Butler, MD

Measure	Cases	This Hosp.	State Avg.	U.S. Avg.
Heart Attack Care				
ACE Inhibitor or ARB for LVSD	143	96%	96%	96%
Aspirin at Arrival	320	99%	98%	99%
Aspirin at Discharge	522	99%	99%	98%
Beta Blocker at Discharge	514	99%	98%	98%
Fibrinolytic Medication Timing	0	-	67%	55%
PCI Within 90 Minutes of Arrival	82	89%	91%	90%
Smoking Cessation Advice	219	100%	100%	99%
Chest Pain/Possible Heart Attack Care				
Aspirin at Arrival	27	96%	95%	95%
Median Time to ECG (minutes)	25	5	8	8
Median Time to Transfer (minutes)[5]	0	-	65	61
Fibrinolytic Medication Timing[5]	0	-	49%	54%
Heart Failure Care				
ACE Inhibitor or ARB for LVSD	138	86%	95%	94%
Discharge Instructions	300	71%	88%	88%
Evaluation of LVS Function	350	98%	97%	98%
Smoking Cessation Advice	61	98%	99%	98%
Pneumonia Care				
Appropriate Initial Antibiotic	243	85%	92%	92%
Blood Culture Timing	314	96%	97%	96%
Influenza Vaccine	250	78%	93%	91%
Initial Antibiotic Timing	356	97%	96%	95%
Pneumococcal Vaccine	330	87%	95%	93%
Smoking Cessation Advice	205	98%	99%	97%
Surgical Care Improvement Project				
Appropriate VTP Within 24 Hours	377	89%	92%	92%
Appropriate Hair Removal	1,288	100%	100%	99%
Appropriate Beta Blocker Usage	508	88%	93%	93%
Controlled Postoperative Blood Glucose	216	94%	93%	93%
Prophylactic Antibiotic Timing	870	95%	97%	97%
Prophylactic Antibiotic Timing (Outpatient)	714	97%	94%	92%
Prophylactic Antibiotic Selection	877	96%	97%	97%
Prophylactic Antibiotic Select. (Outpatient)	710	94%	94%	94%
Prophylactic Antibiotic Stopped	831	93%	94%	94%
Recommended VTP Ordered	377	90%	94%	94%
Urinary Catheter Removal	347	84%	90%	90%
Children's Asthma Care				
Received Systemic Corticosteroids	-	-	-	100%
Received Home Management Plan	-	-	-	71%
Received Reliever Medication	-	-	-	100%
Use of Medical Imaging				
Combination Abdominal CT Scan	888	0.057	0.219	0.191
Combination Chest CT Scan	694	0.078	0.102	0.054
Follow-up Mammogram/Ultrasound	1,003	7.0%	8%	8.4%
MRI for Low Back Pain	331	25.4%	30.7%	32.7%
Survey of Patients' Hospital Experiences				
Area Around Room 'Always' Quiet at Night	300+	59%	-	58%
Doctors 'Always' Communicated Well	300+	80%	-	80%
Home Recovery Information Given	300+	81%	-	82%
Hospital Given 9 or 10 on 10 Point Scale	300+	70%	-	67%
Meds 'Always' Explained Before Given	300+	57%	-	60%
Nurses 'Always' Communicated Well	300+	77%	-	76%
Pain 'Always' Well Controlled	300+	69%	-	69%
Room and Bathroom 'Always' Clean	300+	75%	-	71%
Timely Help 'Always' Received	300+	67%	-	64%
Would Definitely Recommend Hospital	300+	76%	-	69%

Copper Basin Medical Center

Highway 68 — Phone: 423-496-5511
Copperhill, TN 37317 — Fax: 423-496-8171
Type: Critical Access Hospitals — Emergency Services: Yes
Ownership: Voluntary Non-Profit - Other — Beds: 44

Key Personnel:
CEO/President. . . . . David W Hyatt
Chief of Medical Staff . . . . Allen S Uhlik, MD
Infection Control. . . . . Nancy Gessling
Emergency Room . . . . Tonya Niz
Patient Relations . . . . Chris Cook

Measure	Cases	This Hosp.	State Avg.	U.S. Avg.
Heart Attack Care				
ACE Inhibitor or ARB for LVSD[1,2,3]	1	0%	96%	96%
Aspirin at Arrival[1,2,3]	1	100%	98%	99%
Aspirin at Discharge[1,2,3]	1	100%	99%	98%
Beta Blocker at Discharge[1,2,3]	2	50%	98%	98%
Fibrinolytic Medication Timing[2,3]	0	-	67%	55%
PCI Within 90 Minutes of Arrival[2,3]	0	-	91%	90%
Smoking Cessation Advice[2,3]	0	-	100%	99%
Chest Pain/Possible Heart Attack Care				
Aspirin at Arrival	75	83%	95%	95%
Median Time to ECG (minutes)	77	21	8	8
Median Time to Transfer (minutes)[1]	3	170	65	61
Fibrinolytic Medication Timing[1]	3	0%	49%	54%
Heart Failure Care				
ACE Inhibitor or ARB for LVSD[1,2]	9	89%	95%	94%
Discharge Instructions[2]	27	96%	88%	88%
Evaluation of LVS Function[2]	29	97%	97%	98%
Smoking Cessation Advice[1,2]	4	75%	99%	98%
Pneumonia Care				
Appropriate Initial Antibiotic[1,2]	13	92%	92%	92%
Blood Culture Timing[1,2]	7	71%	97%	96%
Influenza Vaccine[1,2]	10	80%	93%	91%
Initial Antibiotic Timing[1,2]	2	100%	96%	95%
Pneumococcal Vaccine[1,2]	16	88%	95%	93%
Smoking Cessation Advice[1,2]	5	80%	99%	97%
Surgical Care Improvement Project				
Appropriate VTP Within 24 Hours[5]	0	-	92%	92%
Appropriate Hair Removal[5]	0	-	100%	99%
Appropriate Beta Blocker Usage[5]	0	-	93%	93%
Controlled Postoperative Blood Glucose[5]	0	-	93%	93%
Prophylactic Antibiotic Timing[5]	0	-	97%	97%
Prophylactic Antibiotic Timing (Outpatient)[5]	0	-	94%	92%
Prophylactic Antibiotic Selection[5]	0	-	97%	97%
Prophylactic Antibiotic Select. (Outpatient)[5]	0	-	94%	94%
Prophylactic Antibiotic Stopped[5]	0	-	94%	94%
Recommended VTP Ordered[5]	0	-	94%	94%
Urinary Catheter Removal[5]	0	-	90%	90%
Children's Asthma Care				
Received Systemic Corticosteroids	-	-	-	100%
Received Home Management Plan	-	-	-	71%
Received Reliever Medication	-	-	-	100%
Use of Medical Imaging				
Combination Abdominal CT Scan	166	0.229	0.219	0.191
Combination Chest CT Scan	90	0.189	0.102	0.054
Follow-up Mammogram/Ultrasound	238	2.9%	8%	8.4%
MRI for Low Back Pain[1]	5	60.0%	30.7%	32.7%
Survey of Patients' Hospital Experiences				
Area Around Room 'Always' Quiet at Night[8]	-	-	-	58%
Doctors 'Always' Communicated Well[8]	-	-	-	80%
Home Recovery Information Given[8]	-	-	-	82%
Hospital Given 9 or 10 on 10 Point Scale[8]	-	-	-	67%
Meds 'Always' Explained Before Given[8]	-	-	-	60%
Nurses 'Always' Communicated Well[8]	-	-	-	76%
Pain 'Always' Well Controlled[8]	-	-	-	69%
Room and Bathroom 'Always' Clean[8]	-	-	-	71%
Timely Help 'Always' Received[8]	-	-	-	64%
Would Definitely Recommend Hospital[8]	-	-	-	69%

Baptist Memorial Hospital Tipton

1995 Highway 51 S — Phone: 901-476-2621
Covington, TN 38019 — Fax: 901-475-5504
URL: www.bmhcc.org
Type: Acute Care Hospitals — Emergency Services: Yes
Ownership: Voluntary Non-Profit - Church — Beds: 70

Key Personnel:
CEO/President. . . . . Stephen C Reynolds
Radiology. . . . . James D Acker

Measure	Cases	This Hosp.	State Avg.	U.S. Avg.
Heart Attack Care				
ACE Inhibitor or ARB for LVSD[3]	0	-	96%	96%
Aspirin at Arrival[1,3]	4	75%	98%	99%
Aspirin at Discharge[1,3]	2	50%	99%	98%
Beta Blocker at Discharge[1,3]	1	100%	98%	98%
Fibrinolytic Medication Timing[3]	0	-	67%	55%
PCI Within 90 Minutes of Arrival[3]	0	-	91%	90%
Smoking Cessation Advice[3]	0	-	100%	99%
Chest Pain/Possible Heart Attack Care				
Aspirin at Arrival	185	90%	95%	95%
Median Time to ECG (minutes)	198	20	8	8
Median Time to Transfer (minutes)[1]	12	170	65	61
Fibrinolytic Medication Timing[1]	5	20%	49%	54%
Heart Failure Care				
ACE Inhibitor or ARB for LVSD[1]	17	88%	95%	94%
Discharge Instructions	45	80%	88%	88%
Evaluation of LVS Function	62	95%	97%	98%
Smoking Cessation Advice[1]	10	100%	99%	98%
Pneumonia Care				
Appropriate Initial Antibiotic	47	91%	92%	92%
Blood Culture Timing	66	97%	97%	96%
Influenza Vaccine	41	95%	93%	91%
Initial Antibiotic Timing	53	91%	96%	95%
Pneumococcal Vaccine	41	98%	95%	93%
Smoking Cessation Advice[1]	24	96%	99%	97%
Surgical Care Improvement Project				
Appropriate VTP Within 24 Hours[1]	7	57%	92%	92%
Appropriate Hair Removal	31	94%	100%	99%
Appropriate Beta Blocker Usage[1]	1	0%	93%	93%
Controlled Postoperative Blood Glucose	0	-	93%	93%
Prophylactic Antibiotic Timing[1]	20	95%	97%	97%
Prophylactic Antibiotic Timing (Outpatient)[1]	13	85%	94%	92%
Prophylactic Antibiotic Selection[1]	21	95%	97%	97%
Prophylactic Antibiotic Select. (Outpatient)[1]	12	92%	94%	94%
Prophylactic Antibiotic Stopped[1]	20	90%	94%	94%
Recommended VTP Ordered[1]	7	57%	94%	94%
Urinary Catheter Removal	0	-	90%	90%
Children's Asthma Care				
Received Systemic Corticosteroids	-	-	-	100%
Received Home Management Plan	-	-	-	71%
Received Reliever Medication	-	-	-	100%
Use of Medical Imaging				
Combination Abdominal CT Scan	323	0.025	0.219	0.191
Combination Chest CT Scan	213	0.005	0.102	0.054
Follow-up Mammogram/Ultrasound	331	7.6%	8%	8.4%
MRI for Low Back Pain	62	22.6%	30.7%	32.7%
Survey of Patients' Hospital Experiences				
Area Around Room 'Always' Quiet at Night	(a)	64%	-	58%
Doctors 'Always' Communicated Well	(a)	82%	-	80%
Home Recovery Information Given	(a)	75%	-	82%
Hospital Given 9 or 10 on 10 Point Scale	(a)	59%	-	67%
Meds 'Always' Explained Before Given	(a)	65%	-	60%
Nurses 'Always' Communicated Well	(a)	77%	-	76%
Pain 'Always' Well Controlled	(a)	72%	-	69%
Room and Bathroom 'Always' Clean	(a)	74%	-	71%
Timely Help 'Always' Received	(a)	65%	-	64%
Would Definitely Recommend Hospital	(a)	60%	-	69%

NOTE: Hospital profiles are in alphabetical order by state, then city, then hospital within the city; Rankings exclude hospitals with less than 25 cases except for patient surveys which excludes hospitals with less than 100 cases; (a) 100–299 cases; (1) The number of cases is too small to be sure how well a hospital is performing; (2) The hospital indicated that the data submitted for this measure were based on a sample of cases; (3) Data was collected during a shorter time period (fewer quarters) than the maximum possible time for this measure; (4) Suppressed for one or more quarters by CMS; (5) No data is available from the hospital for this measure; (6) Fewer than 100 patients completed the HCAHPS survey. Use these rates with caution, as the number of surveys may be too low to reliably assess hospital performance; (7) Survey results are based on less than 12 months of data; (8) Survey results are not available for this reporting period; (9) No or very few patients were eligible for the HCAHPS survey. The scores shown, if any, reflect a very small number of surveys; (10) A state average was not calculated because too few hospitals in the state submitted data; (11) There were discrepancies in the data collection process; Please refer to the User's Guide for a full explanation of data.

Cumberland Medical Center

421 S Main St
Crossville, TN 38555
Phone: 931-484-9511
Fax: 931-707-8150
E-mail: jmartin@cmchealthcare.org
URL: www.cmchealthcare.org
Type: Acute Care Hospitals
Emergency Services: Yes
Ownership: Voluntary Non-Profit - Private
Beds: 202

Key Personnel:
CEO/President. . . . . Donna Franklin
Cardiac Laboratory. . . . . Dian Jones
Chief of Medical Staff . . . . Timothy Spitler
Pediatric Ambulatory Care . . . . . . MH Koucheki, MD
Radiology. . . . . Richard L Bilbrey, MD
Anesthesiology. . . . . Thomas LaSalle, DO
Emergency Room . . . . David McKinney

Measure	Cases	This Hosp.	State Avg.	U.S. Avg.
Heart Attack Care				
ACE Inhibitor or ARB for LVSD[1]	8	88%	96%	96%
Aspirin at Arrival	40	95%	98%	99%
Aspirin at Discharge	30	100%	99%	98%
Beta Blocker at Discharge	31	97%	98%	98%
Fibrinolytic Medication Timing	0	-	67%	55%
PCI Within 90 Minutes of Arrival	0	-	91%	90%
Smoking Cessation Advice[1]	5	100%	100%	99%
Chest Pain/Possible Heart Attack Care				
Aspirin at Arrival	123	99%	95%	95%
Median Time to ECG (minutes)	122	13	8	8
Median Time to Transfer (minutes)[3]	0	-	65	61
Fibrinolytic Medication Timing[1]	19	53%	49%	54%
Heart Failure Care				
ACE Inhibitor or ARB for LVSD	60	82%	95%	94%
Discharge Instructions	258	88%	88%	88%
Evaluation of LVS Function	293	97%	97%	98%
Smoking Cessation Advice	54	100%	99%	98%
Pneumonia Care				
Appropriate Initial Antibiotic	272	82%	92%	92%
Blood Culture Timing	289	96%	97%	96%
Influenza Vaccine	221	61%	93%	91%
Initial Antibiotic Timing	343	95%	96%	95%
Pneumococcal Vaccine	316	89%	95%	93%
Smoking Cessation Advice	140	99%	99%	97%
Surgical Care Improvement Project				
Appropriate VTP Within 24 Hours[2]	125	73%	92%	92%
Appropriate Hair Removal[2]	200	99%	100%	99%
Appropriate Beta Blocker Usage[2]	71	100%	93%	93%
Controlled Postoperative Blood Glucose[2]	0	-	93%	93%
Prophylactic Antibiotic Timing[2]	112	77%	97%	97%
Prophylactic Antibiotic Timing (Outpatient)	194	71%	94%	92%
Prophylactic Antibiotic Selection[2]	112	76%	97%	97%
Prophylactic Antibiotic Select. (Outpatient)	181	90%	94%	94%
Prophylactic Antibiotic Stopped[2]	110	85%	94%	94%
Recommended VTP Ordered[2]	129	72%	94%	94%
Urinary Catheter Removal[2]	36	72%	90%	90%
Children's Asthma Care				
Received Systemic Corticosteroids	-	-	-	100%
Received Home Management Plan	-	-	-	71%
Received Reliever Medication	-	-	-	100%
Use of Medical Imaging				
Combination Abdominal CT Scan	970	0.110	0.219	0.191
Combination Chest CT Scan	1,038	0.129	0.102	0.054
Follow-up Mammogram/Ultrasound	2,102	5.3%	8%	8.4%
MRI for Low Back Pain	415	31.3%	30.7%	32.7%
Survey of Patients' Hospital Experiences				
Area Around Room 'Always' Quiet at Night	300+	57%	-	58%
Doctors 'Always' Communicated Well	300+	81%	-	80%
Home Recovery Information Given	300+	76%	-	82%
Hospital Given 9 or 10 on 10 Point Scale	300+	63%	-	67%
Meds 'Always' Explained Before Given	300+	58%	-	60%
Nurses 'Always' Communicated Well	300+	77%	-	76%
Pain 'Always' Well Controlled	300+	69%	-	69%
Room and Bathroom 'Always' Clean	300+	75%	-	71%
Timely Help 'Always' Received	300+	64%	-	64%
Would Definitely Recommend Hospital	300+	66%	-	69%

Rhea Medical Center

9400 Rhea County Highway
Dayton, TN 37321
Phone: 423-775-1121
Fax: 423-775-6621
Type: Critical Access Hospitals
Emergency Services: Yes
Ownership: Proprietary
Beds: 131

Key Personnel:
CEO/President. . . . . Kennedy Croom
Radiology. . . . . Roger Miller
Emergency Room . . . . John Staley, MD

Measure	Cases	This Hosp.	State Avg.	U.S. Avg.
Heart Attack Care				
ACE Inhibitor or ARB for LVSD[3]	0	-	96%	96%
Aspirin at Arrival[1,3]	3	100%	98%	99%
Aspirin at Discharge[1,3]	2	100%	99%	98%
Beta Blocker at Discharge[1,3]	2	100%	98%	98%
Fibrinolytic Medication Timing[3]	0	-	67%	55%
PCI Within 90 Minutes of Arrival[3]	0	-	91%	90%
Smoking Cessation Advice[1,3]	1	100%	100%	99%
Chest Pain/Possible Heart Attack Care				
Aspirin at Arrival	159	86%	95%	95%
Median Time to ECG (minutes)	167	7	8	8
Median Time to Transfer (minutes)[1]	6	72	65	61
Fibrinolytic Medication Timing[1]	8	25%	49%	54%
Heart Failure Care				
ACE Inhibitor or ARB for LVSD[1]	6	100%	95%	94%
Discharge Instructions[1]	19	53%	88%	88%
Evaluation of LVS Function	27	96%	97%	98%
Smoking Cessation Advice[1]	5	80%	99%	98%
Pneumonia Care				
Appropriate Initial Antibiotic	107	90%	92%	92%
Blood Culture Timing	106	96%	97%	96%
Influenza Vaccine	72	90%	93%	91%
Initial Antibiotic Timing	135	96%	96%	95%
Pneumococcal Vaccine	90	84%	95%	93%
Smoking Cessation Advice	54	100%	99%	97%
Surgical Care Improvement Project				
Appropriate VTP Within 24 Hours[1]	5	100%	92%	92%
Appropriate Hair Removal[1]	9	100%	100%	99%
Appropriate Beta Blocker Usage[1]	3	100%	93%	93%
Controlled Postoperative Blood Glucose	0	-	93%	93%
Prophylactic Antibiotic Timing[1]	3	100%	97%	97%
Prophylactic Antibiotic Timing (Outpatient)[1,3]	1	100%	94%	92%
Prophylactic Antibiotic Selection[1]	3	67%	97%	97%
Prophylactic Antibiotic Select. (Outpatient)[1,3]	1	100%	94%	94%
Prophylactic Antibiotic Stopped[1]	2	100%	94%	94%
Recommended VTP Ordered[1]	5	100%	94%	94%
Urinary Catheter Removal[1]	2	100%	90%	90%
Children's Asthma Care				
Received Systemic Corticosteroids	-	-	-	100%
Received Home Management Plan	-	-	-	71%
Received Reliever Medication	-	-	-	100%
Use of Medical Imaging				
Combination Abdominal CT Scan	384	0.096	0.219	0.191
Combination Chest CT Scan	200	0.110	0.102	0.054
Follow-up Mammogram/Ultrasound	380	11.6%	8%	8.4%
MRI for Low Back Pain	53	32.1%	30.7%	32.7%
Survey of Patients' Hospital Experiences				
Area Around Room 'Always' Quiet at Night	300+	61%	-	58%
Doctors 'Always' Communicated Well	300+	88%	-	80%
Home Recovery Information Given	300+	77%	-	82%
Hospital Given 9 or 10 on 10 Point Scale	300+	67%	-	67%
Meds 'Always' Explained Before Given	300+	58%	-	60%
Nurses 'Always' Communicated Well	300+	78%	-	76%
Pain 'Always' Well Controlled	300+	66%	-	69%
Room and Bathroom 'Always' Clean	300+	65%	-	71%
Timely Help 'Always' Received	300+	63%	-	64%
Would Definitely Recommend Hospital	300+	68%	-	69%

Horizon Medical Center

111 Highway 70 East
Dickson, TN 37055
Phone: 615-446-0446
Fax: 615-441-2514
Type: Acute Care Hospitals
Emergency Services: Yes
Ownership: Proprietary
Beds: 150

Key Personnel:
CEO/President. . . . . John Marshall
Chief of Medical Staff . . . . Van Mills
Infection Control. . . . . Donna Clark
Operating Room. . . . . Megan Weiss
Quality Assurance . . . . Tori Howk
Radiology. . . . . John J Alarcon
Anesthesiology. . . . . Barry Brasfield, MD
Emergency Room . . . . Gina Bullington, RN

Measure	Cases	This Hosp.	State Avg.	U.S. Avg.
Heart Attack Care				
ACE Inhibitor or ARB for LVSD[1]	8	100%	96%	96%
Aspirin at Arrival	48	98%	98%	99%
Aspirin at Discharge	37	100%	99%	98%
Beta Blocker at Discharge	34	100%	98%	98%
Fibrinolytic Medication Timing	0	-	67%	55%
PCI Within 90 Minutes of Arrival[1]	4	100%	91%	90%
Smoking Cessation Advice[1]	14	100%	100%	99%
Chest Pain/Possible Heart Attack Care				
Aspirin at Arrival	159	97%	95%	95%
Median Time to ECG (minutes)	170	6	8	8
Median Time to Transfer (minutes)[1]	20	34	65	61
Fibrinolytic Medication Timing[1]	1	100%	49%	54%
Heart Failure Care				
ACE Inhibitor or ARB for LVSD	45	96%	95%	94%
Discharge Instructions	140	90%	88%	88%
Evaluation of LVS Function	178	100%	97%	98%
Smoking Cessation Advice	33	97%	99%	98%
Pneumonia Care				
Appropriate Initial Antibiotic	133	95%	92%	92%
Blood Culture Timing	179	99%	97%	96%
Influenza Vaccine	106	100%	93%	91%
Initial Antibiotic Timing	176	99%	96%	95%
Pneumococcal Vaccine	153	99%	95%	93%
Smoking Cessation Advice	102	98%	99%	97%
Surgical Care Improvement Project				
Appropriate VTP Within 24 Hours	103	90%	92%	92%
Appropriate Hair Removal	156	100%	100%	99%
Appropriate Beta Blocker Usage	40	100%	93%	93%
Controlled Postoperative Blood Glucose	0	-	93%	93%
Prophylactic Antibiotic Timing	91	99%	97%	97%
Prophylactic Antibiotic Timing (Outpatient)	76	97%	94%	92%
Prophylactic Antibiotic Selection	91	97%	97%	97%
Prophylactic Antibiotic Select. (Outpatient)	75	97%	94%	94%
Prophylactic Antibiotic Stopped	88	94%	94%	94%
Recommended VTP Ordered	103	92%	94%	94%
Urinary Catheter Removal	43	88%	90%	90%
Children's Asthma Care				
Received Systemic Corticosteroids	-	-	-	100%
Received Home Management Plan	-	-	-	71%
Received Reliever Medication	-	-	-	100%
Use of Medical Imaging				
Combination Abdominal CT Scan	440	0.136	0.219	0.191
Combination Chest CT Scan	163	0.012	0.102	0.054
Follow-up Mammogram/Ultrasound	650	5.2%	8%	8.4%
MRI for Low Back Pain	178	28.7%	30.7%	32.7%
Survey of Patients' Hospital Experiences				
Area Around Room 'Always' Quiet at Night	300+	60%	-	58%
Doctors 'Always' Communicated Well	300+	83%	-	80%
Home Recovery Information Given	300+	87%	-	82%
Hospital Given 9 or 10 on 10 Point Scale	300+	67%	-	67%
Meds 'Always' Explained Before Given	300+	60%	-	60%
Nurses 'Always' Communicated Well	300+	79%	-	76%
Pain 'Always' Well Controlled	300+	72%	-	69%
Room and Bathroom 'Always' Clean	300+	71%	-	71%
Timely Help 'Always' Received	300+	68%	-	64%
Would Definitely Recommend Hospital	300+	66%	-	69%

NOTE: Hospital profiles are in alphabetical order by state, then city, then hospital within the city; Rankings exclude hospitals with less than 25 cases except for patient surveys which excludes hospitals with less than 100 cases; (a) 100–299 cases; (1) The number of cases is too small to be sure how well a hospital is performing; (2) The hospital indicated that the data submitted for this measure were based on a sample of cases; (3) Data was collected during a shorter time period (fewer quarters) than the maximum possible time for this measure; (4) Suppressed for one or more quarters by CMS; (5) No data is available from the hospital for this measure; (6) Fewer than 100 patients completed the HCAHPS survey. Use these rates with caution, as the number of surveys may be too low to reliably assess hospital performance; (7) Survey results are based on less than 12 months of data; (8) Survey results are not available for this reporting period; (9) No or very few patients were eligible for the HCAHPS survey. The scores shown, if any, reflect a very small number of surveys; (10) A state average was not calculated because too few hospitals in the state submitted data; (11) There were discrepancies in the data collection process; Please refer to the User's Guide for a full explanation of data.

Dyersburg Regional Medical Center

400 Tickle St
Dyersburg, TN 38024
Type: Acute Care Hospitals
Ownership: Proprietary

Phone: 731-285-2410

Emergency Services: Yes

Measure	Cases	This Hosp.	State Avg.	U.S. Avg.
Heart Attack Care				
ACE Inhibitor or ARB for LVSD[1]	4	100%	96%	96%
Aspirin at Arrival[1]	22	91%	98%	99%
Aspirin at Discharge[1]	14	86%	99%	98%
Beta Blocker at Discharge[1]	14	100%	98%	98%
Fibrinolytic Medication Timing	0	-	67%	55%
PCI Within 90 Minutes of Arrival	0	-	91%	90%
Smoking Cessation Advice[1]	1	100%	100%	99%
Chest Pain/Possible Heart Attack Care				
Aspirin at Arrival	207	100%	95%	95%
Median Time to ECG (minutes)	218	1	8	8
Median Time to Transfer (minutes)[5]	0		65	61
Fibrinolytic Medication Timing[1]	12	83%	49%	54%
Heart Failure Care				
ACE Inhibitor or ARB for LVSD	51	98%	95%	94%
Discharge Instructions	197	95%	88%	88%
Evaluation of LVS Function	252	100%	97%	98%
Smoking Cessation Advice	46	100%	99%	98%
Pneumonia Care				
Appropriate Initial Antibiotic	75	92%	92%	92%
Blood Culture Timing	100	98%	97%	96%
Influenza Vaccine	62	98%	93%	91%
Initial Antibiotic Timing	113	99%	96%	95%
Pneumococcal Vaccine	80	98%	95%	93%
Smoking Cessation Advice	50	100%	99%	97%
Surgical Care Improvement Project				
Appropriate VTP Within 24 Hours[2]	68	91%	92%	92%
Appropriate Hair Removal[2]	114	100%	100%	99%
Appropriate Beta Blocker Usage[1,2]	17	100%	93%	93%
Controlled Postoperative Blood Glucose[2]	0	-	93%	93%
Prophylactic Antibiotic Timing[2]	53	96%	97%	97%
Prophylactic Antibiotic Timing (Outpatient)	109	95%	94%	92%
Prophylactic Antibiotic Selection[2]	53	100%	97%	97%
Prophylactic Antibiotic Select. (Outpatient)	126	94%	94%	94%
Prophylactic Antibiotic Stopped[2]	49	96%	94%	94%
Recommended VTP Ordered[2]	68	96%	94%	94%
Urinary Catheter Removal[1]	17	94%	90%	90%
Children's Asthma Care				
Received Systemic Corticosteroids	-	-	-	100%
Received Home Management Plan	-	-	-	71%
Received Reliever Medication	-	-	-	100%
Use of Medical Imaging				
Combination Abdominal CT Scan	454	0.013	0.219	0.191
Combination Chest CT Scan	280	0.011	0.102	0.054
Follow-up Mammogram/Ultrasound	672	7.0%	8%	8.4%
MRI for Low Back Pain	142	26.8%	30.7%	32.7%
Survey of Patients' Hospital Experiences				
Area Around Room 'Always' Quiet at Night	300+	65%	-	58%
Doctors 'Always' Communicated Well	300+	79%	-	80%
Home Recovery Information Given	300+	78%	-	82%
Hospital Given 9 or 10 on 10 Point Scale	300+	57%	-	67%
Meds 'Always' Explained Before Given	300+	62%	-	60%
Nurses 'Always' Communicated Well	300+	75%	-	76%
Pain 'Always' Well Controlled	300+	71%	-	69%
Room and Bathroom 'Always' Clean	300+	64%	-	71%
Timely Help 'Always' Received	300+	65%	-	64%
Would Definitely Recommend Hospital	300+	54%	-	69%

Sycamore Shoals Hospital

1501 West Elk Avenue
Elizabethton, TN 37643
URL: www.msha.com
Type: Acute Care Hospitals
Ownership: Voluntary Non-Profit - Private

Phone: 423-542-1300
Fax: 423-542-1439

Emergency Services: Yes
Beds: 121

Key Personnel:
CEO/President . . . . Scott Williams
Chief of Medical Staff . . . . Elizabeth Clemens
Radiology. . . . . Vincent Becker

Measure	Cases	This Hosp.	State Avg.	U.S. Avg.
Heart Attack Care				
ACE Inhibitor or ARB for LVSD[1,2,3]	1	100%	96%	96%
Aspirin at Arrival[1,2,3]	7	86%	98%	99%
Aspirin at Discharge[1,2,3]	5	80%	99%	98%
Beta Blocker at Discharge[1,2,3]	4	100%	98%	98%
Fibrinolytic Medication Timing[2,3]	0	-	67%	55%
PCI Within 90 Minutes of Arrival[2,3]	0	-	91%	90%
Smoking Cessation Advice[1,2,3]	1	100%	100%	99%
Chest Pain/Possible Heart Attack Care				
Aspirin at Arrival	157	87%	95%	95%
Median Time to ECG (minutes)	165	21	8	8
Median Time to Transfer (minutes)[1]	7	55	65	61
Fibrinolytic Medication Timing	0	-	49%	54%
Heart Failure Care				
ACE Inhibitor or ARB for LVSD[2]	31	97%	95%	94%
Discharge Instructions[2]	56	93%	88%	88%
Evaluation of LVS Function[2]	78	100%	97%	98%
Smoking Cessation Advice[1,2]	17	100%	99%	98%
Pneumonia Care				
Appropriate Initial Antibiotic[2]	73	96%	92%	92%
Blood Culture Timing[2]	89	97%	97%	96%
Influenza Vaccine[2]	71	100%	93%	91%
Initial Antibiotic Timing[2]	115	92%	96%	95%
Pneumococcal Vaccine[2]	114	100%	95%	93%
Smoking Cessation Advice[2]	74	100%	99%	97%
Surgical Care Improvement Project				
Appropriate VTP Within 24 Hours[2]	80	91%	92%	92%
Appropriate Hair Removal[2]	183	100%	100%	99%
Appropriate Beta Blocker Usage[2]	32	88%	93%	93%
Controlled Postoperative Blood Glucose[2]	0	-	93%	93%
Prophylactic Antibiotic Timing[2]	124	98%	97%	97%
Prophylactic Antibiotic Timing (Outpatient)	66	88%	94%	92%
Prophylactic Antibiotic Selection[2]	128	96%	97%	97%
Prophylactic Antibiotic Select. (Outpatient)	62	95%	94%	94%
Prophylactic Antibiotic Stopped[2]	120	97%	94%	94%
Recommended VTP Ordered[2]	80	92%	94%	94%
Urinary Catheter Removal[2]	29	86%	90%	90%
Children's Asthma Care				
Received Systemic Corticosteroids	-	-	-	100%
Received Home Management Plan	-	-	-	71%
Received Reliever Medication	-	-	-	100%
Use of Medical Imaging				
Combination Abdominal CT Scan	541	0.386	0.219	0.191
Combination Chest CT Scan	293	0.321	0.102	0.054
Follow-up Mammogram/Ultrasound	708	9.9%	8%	8.4%
MRI for Low Back Pain	210	37.1%	30.7%	32.7%
Survey of Patients' Hospital Experiences				
Area Around Room 'Always' Quiet at Night	300+	70%	-	58%
Doctors 'Always' Communicated Well	300+	84%	-	80%
Home Recovery Information Given	300+	81%	-	82%
Hospital Given 9 or 10 on 10 Point Scale	300+	74%	-	67%
Meds 'Always' Explained Before Given	300+	68%	-	60%
Nurses 'Always' Communicated Well	300+	82%	-	76%
Pain 'Always' Well Controlled	300+	77%	-	69%
Room and Bathroom 'Always' Clean	300+	76%	-	71%
Timely Help 'Always' Received	300+	72%	-	64%
Would Definitely Recommend Hospital	300+	75%	-	69%

Patients' Choice Medical Center of Erin

302 East Main Street
Erin, TN 37061
Type: Critical Access Hospitals
Ownership: Proprietary

Phone: 931-289-4211

Emergency Services: Yes

Measure	Cases	This Hosp.	State Avg.	U.S. Avg.
Heart Attack Care				
ACE Inhibitor or ARB for LVSD[3]	0	-	96%	96%
Aspirin at Arrival[3]	0	-	98%	99%
Aspirin at Discharge[3]	0	-	99%	98%
Beta Blocker at Discharge[1,3]	1	100%	98%	98%
Fibrinolytic Medication Timing[3]	0	-	67%	55%
PCI Within 90 Minutes of Arrival[3]	0	-	91%	90%
Smoking Cessation Advice[3]	0	-	100%	99%
Chest Pain/Possible Heart Attack Care				
Aspirin at Arrival	-		95%	95%
Median Time to ECG (minutes)	-		8	8
Median Time to Transfer (minutes)	-		65	61
Fibrinolytic Medication Timing	-		49%	54%
Heart Failure Care				
ACE Inhibitor or ARB for LVSD[1]	3	100%	95%	94%
Discharge Instructions[1]	15	73%	88%	88%
Evaluation of LVS Function	50	62%	97%	98%
Smoking Cessation Advice[1]	6	67%	99%	98%
Pneumonia Care				
Appropriate Initial Antibiotic	33	88%	92%	92%
Blood Culture Timing[1]	21	90%	97%	96%
Influenza Vaccine	31	68%	93%	91%
Initial Antibiotic Timing	45	100%	96%	95%
Pneumococcal Vaccine	40	72%	95%	93%
Smoking Cessation Advice[1]	11	64%	99%	97%
Surgical Care Improvement Project				
Appropriate VTP Within 24 Hours[5]	0	-	92%	92%
Appropriate Hair Removal[5]	0	-	100%	99%
Appropriate Beta Blocker Usage[5]	0	-	93%	93%
Controlled Postoperative Blood Glucose[5]	0	-	93%	93%
Prophylactic Antibiotic Timing[5]	0	-	97%	97%
Prophylactic Antibiotic Timing (Outpatient)	0	-	94%	92%
Prophylactic Antibiotic Selection[5]	0	-	97%	97%
Prophylactic Antibiotic Select. (Outpatient)	0	-	94%	94%
Prophylactic Antibiotic Stopped[5]	0	-	94%	94%
Recommended VTP Ordered[5]	0	-	94%	94%
Urinary Catheter Removal[5]	0	-	90%	90%
Children's Asthma Care				
Received Systemic Corticosteroids	-	-	-	100%
Received Home Management Plan	-	-	-	71%
Received Reliever Medication	-	-	-	100%
Use of Medical Imaging				
Combination Abdominal CT Scan	-	-	0.219	0.191
Combination Chest CT Scan	-	-	0.102	0.054
Follow-up Mammogram/Ultrasound	-	-	8%	8.4%
MRI for Low Back Pain	-	-	30.7%	32.7%
Survey of Patients' Hospital Experiences				
Area Around Room 'Always' Quiet at Night[8]	-	-	-	58%
Doctors 'Always' Communicated Well[8]	-	-	-	80%
Home Recovery Information Given[8]	-	-	-	82%
Hospital Given 9 or 10 on 10 Point Scale[8]	-	-	-	67%
Meds 'Always' Explained Before Given[8]	-	-	-	60%
Nurses 'Always' Communicated Well[8]	-	-	-	76%
Pain 'Always' Well Controlled[8]	-	-	-	69%
Room and Bathroom 'Always' Clean[8]	-	-	-	71%
Timely Help 'Always' Received[8]	-	-	-	64%
Would Definitely Recommend Hospital[8]	-	-	-	69%

NOTE: Hospital profiles are in alphabetical order by state, then city, then hospital within the city; Rankings exclude hospitals with less than 25 cases except for patient surveys which excludes hospitals with less than 100 cases; (a) 100–299 cases; (1) The number of cases is too small to be sure how well a hospital is performing; (2) The hospital indicated that the data submitted for this measure were based on a sample of cases; (3) Data was collected during a shorter time period (fewer quarters) than the maximum possible time for this measure; (4) Suppressed for one or more quarters by CMS; (5) No data is available from the hospital for this measure; (6) Fewer than 100 patients completed the HCAHPS survey. Use these rates with caution, as the number of surveys may be too low to reliably assess hospital performance; (7) Survey results are based on less than 12 months of data; (8) Survey results are not available for this reporting period; (9) No or very few patients were eligible for the HCAHPS survey. The scores shown, if any, reflect a very small number of surveys; (10) A state average was not calculated because too few hospitals in the state submitted data; (11) There were discrepancies in the data collection process; Please refer to the User's Guide for a full explanation of data.

Unicoi County Memorial Hospital

Greenway Circle · Phone: 423-743-3141
Erwin, TN 37650 · Fax: 423-743-2807
Type: Acute Care Hospitals · Emergency Services: Yes
Ownership: Voluntary Non-Profit - Other · Beds: 46

Key Personnel:
CEO/President. . . . . Jim Pate
Chief of Medical Staff. . . . . Joseph Beiberly
Radiology. . . . . Michael Slemp

Measure	Cases	This Hosp.	State Avg.	U.S. Avg.
Heart Attack Care				
ACE Inhibitor or ARB for LVSD[3]	0	-	96%	96%
Aspirin at Arrival[1,3]	1	0%	98%	99%
Aspirin at Discharge[1,3]	1	100%	99%	98%
Beta Blocker at Discharge[1,3]	1	100%	98%	98%
Fibrinolytic Medication Timing[3]	0	-	67%	55%
PCI Within 90 Minutes of Arrival[3]	0	-	91%	90%
Smoking Cessation Advice[3]	0	-	100%	99%
Chest Pain/Possible Heart Attack Care				
Aspirin at Arrival	153	99%	95%	95%
Median Time to ECG (minutes)	165	8	8	8
Median Time to Transfer (minutes)[1,3]	1	53	65	61
Fibrinolytic Medication Timing[3]	0	-	49%	54%
Heart Failure Care				
ACE Inhibitor or ARB for LVSD[1]	6	67%	95%	94%
Discharge Instructions	26	58%	88%	88%
Evaluation of LVS Function	35	80%	97%	98%
Smoking Cessation Advice[1]	4	100%	99%	98%
Pneumonia Care				
Appropriate Initial Antibiotic	57	89%	92%	92%
Blood Culture Timing	66	89%	97%	96%
Influenza Vaccine	44	55%	93%	91%
Initial Antibiotic Timing	92	97%	96%	95%
Pneumococcal Vaccine	73	68%	95%	93%
Smoking Cessation Advice	29	97%	99%	97%
Surgical Care Improvement Project				
Appropriate VTP Within 24 Hours	40	90%	92%	92%
Appropriate Hair Removal	91	99%	100%	99%
Appropriate Beta Blocker Usage[1]	23	96%	93%	93%
Controlled Postoperative Blood Glucose	0	-	93%	93%
Prophylactic Antibiotic Timing	70	100%	97%	97%
Prophylactic Antibiotic Timing (Outpatient)[1]	12	92%	94%	92%
Prophylactic Antibiotic Selection	70	100%	97%	97%
Prophylactic Antibiotic Select. (Outpatient)[1]	12	83%	94%	94%
Prophylactic Antibiotic Stopped	68	93%	94%	94%
Recommended VTP Ordered	40	95%	94%	94%
Urinary Catheter Removal	25	100%	90%	90%
Children's Asthma Care				
Received Systemic Corticosteroids	-	-	-	100%
Received Home Management Plan	-	-	-	71%
Received Reliever Medication	-	-	-	100%
Use of Medical Imaging				
Combination Abdominal CT Scan	209	0.148	0.219	0.191
Combination Chest CT Scan	139	0.129	0.102	0.054
Follow-up Mammogram/Ultrasound	342	8.5%	8%	8.4%
MRI for Low Back Pain	58	32.8%	30.7%	32.7%
Survey of Patients' Hospital Experiences				
Area Around Room 'Always' Quiet at Night	300+	57%	-	58%
Doctors 'Always' Communicated Well	300+	87%	-	80%
Home Recovery Information Given	300+	77%	-	82%
Hospital Given 9 or 10 on 10 Point Scale	300+	72%	-	67%
Meds 'Always' Explained Before Given	300+	65%	-	60%
Nurses 'Always' Communicated Well	300+	75%	-	76%
Pain 'Always' Well Controlled	300+	65%	-	69%
Room and Bathroom 'Always' Clean	300+	76%	-	71%
Timely Help 'Always' Received	300+	65%	-	64%
Would Definitely Recommend Hospital	300+	81%	-	69%

Woods Memorial Hospital

886 Highway 411 North · Phone: 423-263-3600
Etowah, TN 37331 · Fax: 423-263-3793
Type: Acute Care Hospitals · Emergency Services: No
Ownership: Govt - Hospital Dist/Auth · Beds: 160

Key Personnel:
CEO/President. . . . . Steve Clapp
Radiology. . . . . Stephen Lemings, MD
Emergency Room . . . . Rick Popp, MD
Hemotology Center . . . . Robert D Shumaker, MD

Measure	Cases	This Hosp.	State Avg.	U.S. Avg.
Heart Attack Care				
ACE Inhibitor or ARB for LVSD[1]	2	100%	96%	96%
Aspirin at Arrival[1]	5	100%	98%	99%
Aspirin at Discharge[1]	3	100%	99%	98%
Beta Blocker at Discharge[1]	2	100%	98%	98%
Fibrinolytic Medication Timing	0	-	67%	55%
PCI Within 90 Minutes of Arrival	0	-	91%	90%
Smoking Cessation Advice[1]	1	100%	100%	99%
Chest Pain/Possible Heart Attack Care				
Aspirin at Arrival	43	98%	95%	95%
Median Time to ECG (minutes)	45	11	8	8
Median Time to Transfer (minutes)[1]	8	94	65	61
Fibrinolytic Medication Timing	0	-	49%	54%
Heart Failure Care				
ACE Inhibitor or ARB for LVSD	44	93%	95%	94%
Discharge Instructions	48	96%	88%	88%
Evaluation of LVS Function	55	87%	97%	98%
Smoking Cessation Advice[1]	12	100%	99%	98%
Pneumonia Care				
Appropriate Initial Antibiotic	37	92%	92%	92%
Blood Culture Timing	92	95%	97%	96%
Influenza Vaccine	74	69%	93%	91%
Initial Antibiotic Timing	108	98%	96%	95%
Pneumococcal Vaccine	113	76%	95%	93%
Smoking Cessation Advice	54	96%	99%	97%
Surgical Care Improvement Project				
Appropriate VTP Within 24 Hours	35	83%	92%	92%
Appropriate Hair Removal	75	100%	100%	99%
Appropriate Beta Blocker Usage[1]	23	70%	93%	93%
Controlled Postoperative Blood Glucose	0	-	93%	93%
Prophylactic Antibiotic Timing	52	88%	97%	97%
Prophylactic Antibiotic Timing (Outpatient)[1]	16	100%	94%	92%
Prophylactic Antibiotic Selection	52	98%	97%	97%
Prophylactic Antibiotic Select. (Outpatient)[1]	16	94%	94%	94%
Prophylactic Antibiotic Stopped	50	88%	94%	94%
Recommended VTP Ordered	35	83%	94%	94%
Urinary Catheter Removal[1]	20	95%	90%	90%
Children's Asthma Care				
Received Systemic Corticosteroids	-	-	-	100%
Received Home Management Plan	-	-	-	71%
Received Reliever Medication	-	-	-	100%
Use of Medical Imaging				
Combination Abdominal CT Scan	319	0.317	0.219	0.191
Combination Chest CT Scan	145	0.041	0.102	0.054
Follow-up Mammogram/Ultrasound	345	12.8%	8%	8.4%
MRI for Low Back Pain	79	35.4%	30.7%	32.7%
Survey of Patients' Hospital Experiences				
Area Around Room 'Always' Quiet at Night	300+	70%	-	58%
Doctors 'Always' Communicated Well	300+	87%	-	80%
Home Recovery Information Given	300+	83%	-	82%
Hospital Given 9 or 10 on 10 Point Scale	300+	73%	-	67%
Meds 'Always' Explained Before Given	300+	57%	-	60%
Nurses 'Always' Communicated Well	300+	80%	-	76%
Pain 'Always' Well Controlled	300+	74%	-	69%
Room and Bathroom 'Always' Clean	300+	71%	-	71%
Timely Help 'Always' Received	300+	72%	-	64%
Would Definitely Recommend Hospital	300+	76%	-	69%

Lincoln Medical Center

106 Medical Center Blvd · Phone: 931-438-1100
Fayetteville, TN 37334 · Fax: 931-438-7456
URL: www.lchealthsystems.com
Type: Acute Care Hospitals · Emergency Services: Yes
Ownership: Government - Local · Beds: 49

Key Personnel:
CEO/President. . . . . Gary Kendrick

Measure	Cases	This Hosp.	State Avg.	U.S. Avg.
Heart Attack Care				
ACE Inhibitor or ARB for LVSD[3]	0	-	96%	96%
Aspirin at Arrival[1,3]	2	100%	98%	99%
Aspirin at Discharge[1,3]	2	100%	99%	98%
Beta Blocker at Discharge[1,3]	2	100%	98%	98%
Fibrinolytic Medication Timing[3]	0	-	67%	55%
PCI Within 90 Minutes of Arrival[3]	0	-	91%	90%
Smoking Cessation Advice[3]	0	-	100%	99%
Chest Pain/Possible Heart Attack Care				
Aspirin at Arrival	322	96%	95%	95%
Median Time to ECG (minutes)	334	5	8	8
Median Time to Transfer (minutes)[1,3]	1	66	65	61
Fibrinolytic Medication Timing[1]	8	38%	49%	54%
Heart Failure Care				
ACE Inhibitor or ARB for LVSD[1]	18	78%	95%	94%
Discharge Instructions	42	74%	88%	88%
Evaluation of LVS Function	58	91%	97%	98%
Smoking Cessation Advice[1]	4	100%	99%	98%
Pneumonia Care				
Appropriate Initial Antibiotic	80	92%	92%	92%
Blood Culture Timing	106	95%	97%	96%
Influenza Vaccine	58	93%	93%	91%
Initial Antibiotic Timing	111	98%	96%	95%
Pneumococcal Vaccine	92	96%	95%	93%
Smoking Cessation Advice	40	98%	99%	97%
Surgical Care Improvement Project				
Appropriate VTP Within 24 Hours[1]	13	69%	92%	92%
Appropriate Hair Removal	27	96%	100%	99%
Appropriate Beta Blocker Usage[1]	6	83%	93%	93%
Controlled Postoperative Blood Glucose	0	-	93%	93%
Prophylactic Antibiotic Timing[1]	17	94%	97%	97%
Prophylactic Antibiotic Timing (Outpatient)	31	90%	94%	92%
Prophylactic Antibiotic Selection[1]	17	100%	97%	97%
Prophylactic Antibiotic Select. (Outpatient)	30	90%	94%	94%
Prophylactic Antibiotic Stopped[1]	16	94%	94%	94%
Recommended VTP Ordered[1]	13	85%	94%	94%
Urinary Catheter Removal[1]	2	0%	90%	90%
Children's Asthma Care				
Received Systemic Corticosteroids	-	-	-	100%
Received Home Management Plan	-	-	-	71%
Received Reliever Medication	-	-	-	100%
Use of Medical Imaging				
Combination Abdominal CT Scan	249	0.635	0.219	0.191
Combination Chest CT Scan	175	0.434	0.102	0.054
Follow-up Mammogram/Ultrasound	429	7.2%	8%	8.4%
MRI for Low Back Pain	57	35.1%	30.7%	32.7%
Survey of Patients' Hospital Experiences				
Area Around Room 'Always' Quiet at Night	300+	63%	-	58%
Doctors 'Always' Communicated Well	300+	78%	-	80%
Home Recovery Information Given	300+	74%	-	82%
Hospital Given 9 or 10 on 10 Point Scale	300+	53%	-	67%
Meds 'Always' Explained Before Given	300+	61%	-	60%
Nurses 'Always' Communicated Well	300+	76%	-	76%
Pain 'Always' Well Controlled	300+	64%	-	69%
Room and Bathroom 'Always' Clean	300+	68%	-	71%
Timely Help 'Always' Received	300+	61%	-	64%
Would Definitely Recommend Hospital	300+	50%	-	69%

NOTE: Hospital profiles are in alphabetical order by state, then city, then hospital within the city; Rankings exclude hospitals with less than 25 cases except for patient surveys which excludes hospitals with less than 100 cases; (a) 100–299 cases; (1) The number of cases is too small to be sure how well a hospital is performing; (2) The hospital indicated that the data submitted for this measure were based on a sample of cases; (3) Data was collected during a shorter time period (fewer quarters) than the maximum possible time for this measure; (4) Suppressed for one or more quarters by CMS; (5) No data is available from the hospital for this measure; (6) Fewer than 100 patients completed the HCAHPS survey. Use these rates with caution, as the number of surveys may be too low to reliably assess hospital performance; (7) Survey results are based on less than 12 months of data; (8) Survey results are not available for this reporting period; (9) No or very few patients were eligible for the HCAHPS survey. The scores shown, if any, reflect a very small number of surveys; (10) A state average was not calculated because too few hospitals in the state submitted data; (11) There were discrepancies in the data collection process; Please refer to the User's Guide for a full explanation of data.

Williamson Medical Center

4321 Carothers Parkway Phone: 615-435-5000
Franklin, TN 37067 Fax: 615-435-5576
E-mail: information@wmed.org
URL: www.williamsonmedicalcenter.org
Type: Acute Care Hospitals Emergency Services: Yes
Ownership: Govt - Hospital Dist/Auth Beds: 185

Key Personnel:
CEO/President. . . . . Dennis Miller, FACHE
Chief of Medical Staff. . . . . Starling C Evins, MD
Radiology. . . . . John Alarcon

Measure	Cases	This Hosp.	State Avg.	U.S. Avg.
Heart Attack Care				
ACE Inhibitor or ARB for LVSD[1]	18	100%	96%	96%
Aspirin at Arrival	137	98%	98%	99%
Aspirin at Discharge	133	98%	99%	98%
Beta Blocker at Discharge	128	99%	98%	98%
Fibrinolytic Medication Timing	0	-	67%	55%
PCI Within 90 Minutes of Arrival	44	86%	91%	90%
Smoking Cessation Advice	47	100%	100%	99%
Chest Pain/Possible Heart Attack Care				
Aspirin at Arrival	33	97%	95%	95%
Median Time to ECG (minutes)	36	6	8	8
Median Time to Transfer (minutes)[1,3]	3	44	65	61
Fibrinolytic Medication Timing	0	-	49%	54%
Heart Failure Care				
ACE Inhibitor or ARB for LVSD	58	98%	95%	94%
Discharge Instructions	167	87%	88%	88%
Evaluation of LVS Function	213	100%	97%	98%
Smoking Cessation Advice[1]	21	100%	99%	98%
Pneumonia Care				
Appropriate Initial Antibiotic	111	94%	92%	92%
Blood Culture Timing	156	98%	97%	96%
Influenza Vaccine	108	96%	93%	91%
Initial Antibiotic Timing	164	95%	96%	95%
Pneumococcal Vaccine	153	95%	95%	93%
Smoking Cessation Advice	55	96%	99%	97%
Surgical Care Improvement Project				
Appropriate VTP Within 24 Hours[2]	154	91%	92%	92%
Appropriate Hair Removal[2]	373	100%	100%	99%
Appropriate Beta Blocker Usage[2]	106	96%	93%	93%
Controlled Postoperative Blood Glucose[2]	0	-	93%	93%
Prophylactic Antibiotic Timing[2]	257	99%	97%	97%
Prophylactic Antibiotic Timing (Outpatient)	353	99%	94%	92%
Prophylactic Antibiotic Selection[2]	262	94%	97%	97%
Prophylactic Antibiotic Select. (Outpatient)	353	97%	94%	94%
Prophylactic Antibiotic Stopped[2]	241	89%	94%	94%
Recommended VTP Ordered[2]	155	90%	94%	94%
Urinary Catheter Removal[2]	89	92%	90%	90%
Children's Asthma Care				
Received Systemic Corticosteroids	-	-	-	100%
Received Home Management Plan	-	-	-	71%
Received Reliever Medication	-	-	-	100%
Use of Medical Imaging				
Combination Abdominal CT Scan	632	0.256	0.219	0.191
Combination Chest CT Scan	344	0.172	0.102	0.054
Follow-up Mammogram/Ultrasound	996	3.8%	8%	8.4%
MRI for Low Back Pain	68	36.8%	30.7%	32.7%
Survey of Patients' Hospital Experiences				
Area Around Room 'Always' Quiet at Night	300+	66%	-	58%
Doctors 'Always' Communicated Well	300+	84%	-	80%
Home Recovery Information Given	300+	84%	-	82%
Hospital Given 9 or 10 on 10 Point Scale	300+	74%	-	67%
Meds 'Always' Explained Before Given	300+	63%	-	60%
Nurses 'Always' Communicated Well	300+	78%	-	76%
Pain 'Always' Well Controlled	300+	69%	-	69%
Room and Bathroom 'Always' Clean	300+	70%	-	71%
Timely Help 'Always' Received	300+	65%	-	64%
Would Definitely Recommend Hospital	300+	78%	-	69%

Sumner Regional Medical Center

555 Hartsville Pike Phone: 615-452-4210
Gallatin, TN 37066 Fax: 615-451-6145
Type: Acute Care Hospitals Emergency Services: Yes
Ownership: Proprietary Beds: 155

Key Personnel:
CEO/President. . . . . William T Sugg
Anesthesiology. . . . . Mark Carter, MD
Emergency Room . . . . James Robert Gill, MD

Measure	Cases	This Hosp.	State Avg.	U.S. Avg.
Heart Attack Care				
ACE Inhibitor or ARB for LVSD[1]	19	89%	96%	96%
Aspirin at Arrival	111	98%	98%	99%
Aspirin at Discharge	101	94%	99%	98%
Beta Blocker at Discharge	99	95%	98%	98%
Fibrinolytic Medication Timing	0	-	67%	55%
PCI Within 90 Minutes of Arrival[1]	11	82%	91%	90%
Smoking Cessation Advice	48	100%	100%	99%
Chest Pain/Possible Heart Attack Care				
Aspirin at Arrival	48	96%	95%	95%
Median Time to ECG (minutes)	52	4	8	8
Median Time to Transfer (minutes)[5]	0	-	65	61
Fibrinolytic Medication Timing	0	-	49%	54%
Heart Failure Care				
ACE Inhibitor or ARB for LVSD	55	91%	95%	94%
Discharge Instructions	154	87%	88%	88%
Evaluation of LVS Function	194	93%	97%	98%
Smoking Cessation Advice	32	97%	99%	98%
Pneumonia Care				
Appropriate Initial Antibiotic	135	89%	92%	92%
Blood Culture Timing	187	95%	97%	96%
Influenza Vaccine	153	78%	93%	91%
Initial Antibiotic Timing	164	98%	96%	95%
Pneumococcal Vaccine	185	86%	95%	93%
Smoking Cessation Advice	97	95%	99%	97%
Surgical Care Improvement Project				
Appropriate VTP Within 24 Hours	115	84%	92%	92%
Appropriate Hair Removal	385	100%	100%	99%
Appropriate Beta Blocker Usage	104	93%	93%	93%
Controlled Postoperative Blood Glucose[1]	1	0%	93%	93%
Prophylactic Antibiotic Timing	280	97%	97%	97%
Prophylactic Antibiotic Timing (Outpatient)	115	83%	94%	92%
Prophylactic Antibiotic Selection	276	100%	97%	97%
Prophylactic Antibiotic Select. (Outpatient)	107	90%	94%	94%
Prophylactic Antibiotic Stopped	271	97%	94%	94%
Recommended VTP Ordered	115	93%	94%	94%
Urinary Catheter Removal	106	93%	90%	90%
Children's Asthma Care				
Received Systemic Corticosteroids	-	-	-	100%
Received Home Management Plan	-	-	-	71%
Received Reliever Medication	-	-	-	100%
Use of Medical Imaging				
Combination Abdominal CT Scan	600	0.552	0.219	0.191
Combination Chest CT Scan	597	0.422	0.102	0.054
Follow-up Mammogram/Ultrasound	615	12.5%	8%	8.4%
MRI for Low Back Pain	141	25.5%	30.7%	32.7%
Survey of Patients' Hospital Experiences				
Area Around Room 'Always' Quiet at Night	300+	60%	-	58%
Doctors 'Always' Communicated Well	300+	81%	-	80%
Home Recovery Information Given	300+	76%	-	82%
Hospital Given 9 or 10 on 10 Point Scale	300+	64%	-	67%
Meds 'Always' Explained Before Given	300+	57%	-	60%
Nurses 'Always' Communicated Well	300+	75%	-	76%
Pain 'Always' Well Controlled	300+	69%	-	69%
Room and Bathroom 'Always' Clean	300+	76%	-	71%
Timely Help 'Always' Received	300+	62%	-	64%
Would Definitely Recommend Hospital	300+	67%	-	69%

Baptist Rehabilitation Germantown

2100 Exeter Road Phone: 901-757-1350
Germantown, TN 38138 Fax: 901-226-4519
URL: www.bmhcc.org
Type: Acute Care Hospitals Emergency Services: No
Ownership: Voluntary Non-Profit - Private Beds: 60

Key Personnel:
Radiology. . . . . James D Acker

Measure	Cases	This Hosp.	State Avg.	U.S. Avg.
Heart Attack Care				
ACE Inhibitor or ARB for LVSD[5]	0	-	96%	96%
Aspirin at Arrival[5]	0	-	98%	99%
Aspirin at Discharge[5]	0	-	99%	98%
Beta Blocker at Discharge[5]	0	-	98%	98%
Fibrinolytic Medication Timing[5]	0	-	67%	55%
PCI Within 90 Minutes of Arrival[5]	0	-	91%	90%
Smoking Cessation Advice[5]	0	-	100%	99%
Chest Pain/Possible Heart Attack Care				
Aspirin at Arrival	-	-	95%	95%
Median Time to ECG (minutes)	-	-	8	8
Median Time to Transfer (minutes)	-	-	65	61
Fibrinolytic Medication Timing	-	-	49%	54%
Heart Failure Care				
ACE Inhibitor or ARB for LVSD[5]	0	-	95%	94%
Discharge Instructions[5]	0	-	88%	88%
Evaluation of LVS Function[5]	0	-	97%	98%
Smoking Cessation Advice[5]	0	-	99%	98%
Pneumonia Care				
Appropriate Initial Antibiotic[5]	0	-	92%	92%
Blood Culture Timing[5]	0	-	97%	96%
Influenza Vaccine[5]	0	-	93%	91%
Initial Antibiotic Timing[5]	0	-	96%	95%
Pneumococcal Vaccine[5]	0	-	95%	93%
Smoking Cessation Advice[5]	0	-	99%	97%
Surgical Care Improvement Project				
Appropriate VTP Within 24 Hours[5]	0	-	92%	92%
Appropriate Hair Removal[5]	0	-	100%	99%
Appropriate Beta Blocker Usage[5]	0	-	93%	93%
Controlled Postoperative Blood Glucose[5]	0	-	93%	93%
Prophylactic Antibiotic Timing[5]	0	-	97%	97%
Prophylactic Antibiotic Timing (Outpatient)	-	-	94%	92%
Prophylactic Antibiotic Selection[5]	0	-	97%	97%
Prophylactic Antibiotic Select. (Outpatient)	-	-	94%	94%
Prophylactic Antibiotic Stopped[5]	0	-	94%	94%
Recommended VTP Ordered[5]	0	-	94%	94%
Urinary Catheter Removal[5]	0	-	90%	90%
Children's Asthma Care				
Received Systemic Corticosteroids	-	-	-	100%
Received Home Management Plan	-	-	-	71%
Received Reliever Medication	-	-	-	100%
Use of Medical Imaging				
Combination Abdominal CT Scan	-	-	0.219	0.191
Combination Chest CT Scan	-	-	0.102	0.054
Follow-up Mammogram/Ultrasound	-	-	8%	8.4%
MRI for Low Back Pain	-	-	30.7%	32.7%
Survey of Patients' Hospital Experiences				
Area Around Room 'Always' Quiet at Night[9]	-	-	-	58%
Doctors 'Always' Communicated Well[9]	-	-	-	80%
Home Recovery Information Given[9]	-	-	-	82%
Hospital Given 9 or 10 on 10 Point Scale[9]	-	-	-	67%
Meds 'Always' Explained Before Given[9]	-	-	-	60%
Nurses 'Always' Communicated Well[9]	-	-	-	76%
Pain 'Always' Well Controlled[9]	-	-	-	69%
Room and Bathroom 'Always' Clean[9]	-	-	-	71%
Timely Help 'Always' Received[9]	-	-	-	64%
Would Definitely Recommend Hospital[9]	-	-	-	69%

NOTE: Hospital profiles are in alphabetical order by state, then city, then hospital within the city; Rankings exclude hospitals with less than 25 cases except for patient surveys which excludes hospitals with less than 100 cases; (a) 100–299 cases; (1) The number of cases is too small to be sure how well a hospital is performing; (2) The hospital indicated that the data submitted for this measure were based on a sample of cases; (3) Data was collected during a shorter time period (fewer quarters) than the maximum possible time for this measure; (4) Suppressed for one or more quarters by CMS; (5) No data is available from the hospital for this measure; (6) Fewer than 100 patients completed the HCAHPS survey. Use these rates with caution, as the number of surveys may be too low to reliably assess hospital performance; (7) Survey results are based on less than 12 months of data; (8) Survey results are not available for this reporting period; (9) No or very few patients were eligible for the HCAHPS survey. The scores shown, if any, reflect a very small number of surveys; (10) A state average was not calculated because too few hospitals in the state submitted data; (11) There were discrepancies in the data collection process; Please refer to the User's Guide for a full explanation of data.

Laughlin Memorial Hospital

1420 Tusculum Blvd
Greeneville, TN 37745
Phone: 423-787-5000
Fax: 423-787-5083
Type: Acute Care Hospitals
Emergency Services: Yes
Ownership: Voluntary Non-Profit - Private
Beds: 230

Key Personnel:
CEO/President. . . . . Charles H Whitefield
Radiology. . . . . Phillip Marino

Measure	Cases	This Hosp.	State Avg.	U.S. Avg.
Heart Attack Care				
ACE Inhibitor or ARB for LVSD[1]	1	100%	96%	96%
Aspirin at Arrival[1]	9	100%	98%	99%
Aspirin at Discharge[1]	6	100%	99%	98%
Beta Blocker at Discharge[1]	5	100%	98%	98%
Fibrinolytic Medication Timing	0	-	67%	55%
PCI Within 90 Minutes of Arrival	0	-	91%	90%
Smoking Cessation Advice	0	-	100%	99%
Chest Pain/Possible Heart Attack Care				
Aspirin at Arrival	299	97%	95%	95%
Median Time to ECG (minutes)	316	10	8	8
Median Time to Transfer (minutes)	25	54	65	61
Fibrinolytic Medication Timing[1]	2	50%	49%	54%
Heart Failure Care				
ACE Inhibitor or ARB for LVSD	34	100%	95%	94%
Discharge Instructions	113	100%	88%	88%
Evaluation of LVS Function	163	99%	97%	98%
Smoking Cessation Advice[1]	18	100%	99%	98%
Pneumonia Care				
Appropriate Initial Antibiotic	161	89%	92%	92%
Blood Culture Timing	233	97%	97%	96%
Influenza Vaccine	170	91%	93%	91%
Initial Antibiotic Timing	254	100%	96%	95%
Pneumococcal Vaccine	233	97%	95%	93%
Smoking Cessation Advice	77	100%	99%	97%
Surgical Care Improvement Project				
Appropriate VTP Within 24 Hours	139	95%	92%	92%
Appropriate Hair Removal	302	100%	100%	99%
Appropriate Beta Blocker Usage	98	99%	93%	93%
Controlled Postoperative Blood Glucose	0	-	93%	93%
Prophylactic Antibiotic Timing	207	97%	97%	97%
Prophylactic Antibiotic Timing (Outpatient)	133	97%	94%	92%
Prophylactic Antibiotic Selection	208	98%	97%	97%
Prophylactic Antibiotic Select. (Outpatient)	132	93%	94%	94%
Prophylactic Antibiotic Stopped	190	95%	94%	94%
Recommended VTP Ordered	139	95%	94%	94%
Urinary Catheter Removal	79	97%	90%	90%
Children's Asthma Care				
Received Systemic Corticosteroids	-	-	-	100%
Received Home Management Plan	-	-	-	71%
Received Reliever Medication	-	-	-	100%
Use of Medical Imaging				
Combination Abdominal CT Scan	897	0.128	0.219	0.191
Combination Chest CT Scan	459	0.105	0.102	0.054
Follow-up Mammogram/Ultrasound	969	8.7%	8%	8.4%
MRI for Low Back Pain	214	33.6%	30.7%	32.7%
Survey of Patients' Hospital Experiences				
Area Around Room 'Always' Quiet at Night	300+	56%	-	58%
Doctors 'Always' Communicated Well	300+	84%	-	80%
Home Recovery Information Given	300+	74%	-	82%
Hospital Given 9 or 10 on 10 Point Scale	300+	67%	-	67%
Meds 'Always' Explained Before Given	300+	58%	-	60%
Nurses 'Always' Communicated Well	300+	74%	-	76%
Pain 'Always' Well Controlled	300+	66%	-	69%
Room and Bathroom 'Always' Clean	300+	69%	-	71%
Timely Help 'Always' Received	300+	64%	-	64%
Would Definitely Recommend Hospital	300+	70%	-	69%

Takoma Regional Hospital

401 Takoma Ave
Greeneville, TN 37743
Phone: 423-639-3151
Fax: 423-636-2374
URL: www.takoma.org
Type: Acute Care Hospitals
Emergency Services: Yes
Ownership: Voluntary Non-Profit - Church
Beds: 115

Key Personnel:
CEO/President. . . . . Carlyle Walton
Chief of Medical Staff . . . . Raymond Kohne, MD
Coronary Care . . . . Dwayne Covington
Infection Control. . . . . Peggy McCoy
Operating Room. . . . . William Bridges
Pediatric Ambulatory Care . . . . . . Yvonne Waddell
Quality Assurance . . . . Karen Tilson
Radiology. . . . . Raymond E Kohne

Measure	Cases	This Hosp.	State Avg.	U.S. Avg.
Heart Attack Care				
ACE Inhibitor or ARB for LVSD[1]	2	100%	96%	96%
Aspirin at Arrival[1]	8	100%	98%	99%
Aspirin at Discharge[1]	5	100%	99%	98%
Beta Blocker at Discharge[1]	7	100%	98%	98%
Fibrinolytic Medication Timing	0	-	67%	55%
PCI Within 90 Minutes of Arrival	0	-	91%	90%
Smoking Cessation Advice	0	-	100%	99%
Chest Pain/Possible Heart Attack Care				
Aspirin at Arrival	65	98%	95%	95%
Median Time to ECG (minutes)	71	10	8	8
Median Time to Transfer (minutes)[1,3]	1	158	65	61
Fibrinolytic Medication Timing[1]	5	80%	49%	54%
Heart Failure Care				
ACE Inhibitor or ARB for LVSD[1]	23	96%	95%	94%
Discharge Instructions	49	94%	88%	88%
Evaluation of LVS Function	64	100%	97%	98%
Smoking Cessation Advice[1]	5	100%	99%	98%
Pneumonia Care				
Appropriate Initial Antibiotic	96	95%	92%	92%
Blood Culture Timing	169	97%	97%	96%
Influenza Vaccine	90	100%	93%	91%
Initial Antibiotic Timing	152	100%	96%	95%
Pneumococcal Vaccine	111	99%	95%	93%
Smoking Cessation Advice	82	100%	99%	97%
Surgical Care Improvement Project				
Appropriate VTP Within 24 Hours	36	83%	92%	92%
Appropriate Hair Removal	83	100%	100%	99%
Appropriate Beta Blocker Usage[1]	14	79%	93%	93%
Controlled Postoperative Blood Glucose	0	-	93%	93%
Prophylactic Antibiotic Timing	49	100%	97%	97%
Prophylactic Antibiotic Timing (Outpatient)	62	94%	94%	92%
Prophylactic Antibiotic Selection	50	94%	97%	97%
Prophylactic Antibiotic Select. (Outpatient)	59	98%	94%	94%
Prophylactic Antibiotic Stopped	46	96%	94%	94%
Recommended VTP Ordered	36	86%	94%	94%
Urinary Catheter Removal[1]	13	100%	90%	90%
Children's Asthma Care				
Received Systemic Corticosteroids	-	-	-	100%
Received Home Management Plan	-	-	-	71%
Received Reliever Medication	-	-	-	100%
Use of Medical Imaging				
Combination Abdominal CT Scan	313	0.457	0.219	0.191
Combination Chest CT Scan	221	0.367	0.102	0.054
Follow-up Mammogram/Ultrasound	420	6.9%	8%	8.4%
MRI for Low Back Pain	76	26.3%	30.7%	32.7%
Survey of Patients' Hospital Experiences				
Area Around Room 'Always' Quiet at Night	(a)	63%	-	58%
Doctors 'Always' Communicated Well	(a)	78%	-	80%
Home Recovery Information Given	(a)	86%	-	82%
Hospital Given 9 or 10 on 10 Point Scale	(a)	68%	-	67%
Meds 'Always' Explained Before Given	(a)	63%	-	60%
Nurses 'Always' Communicated Well	(a)	75%	-	76%
Pain 'Always' Well Controlled	(a)	67%	-	69%
Room and Bathroom 'Always' Clean	(a)	73%	-	71%
Timely Help 'Always' Received	(a)	66%	-	64%
Would Definitely Recommend Hospital	(a)	71%	-	69%

Roane Medical Center

412 Devonia St
Harriman, TN 37748
Phone: 865-882-1323
Fax: 865-882-4484
URL: www.roanemedical.com
Type: Acute Care Hospitals
Emergency Services: Yes
Ownership: Govt - Hospital Dist/Auth
Beds: 85

Key Personnel:
CEO/President. . . . . Jim Gann
Radiology. . . . . Steven Addonizio

Measure	Cases	This Hosp.	State Avg.	U.S. Avg.
Heart Attack Care				
ACE Inhibitor or ARB for LVSD[1]	1	100%	96%	96%
Aspirin at Arrival[1]	10	100%	98%	99%
Aspirin at Discharge[1]	3	100%	99%	98%
Beta Blocker at Discharge[1]	2	100%	98%	98%
Fibrinolytic Medication Timing	0	-	67%	55%
PCI Within 90 Minutes of Arrival	0	-	91%	90%
Smoking Cessation Advice[1]	1	100%	100%	99%
Chest Pain/Possible Heart Attack Care				
Aspirin at Arrival	180	96%	95%	95%
Median Time to ECG (minutes)	190	7	8	8
Median Time to Transfer (minutes)[1,3]	8	125	65	61
Fibrinolytic Medication Timing[1]	6	50%	49%	54%
Heart Failure Care				
ACE Inhibitor or ARB for LVSD[1]	22	91%	95%	94%
Discharge Instructions	67	87%	88%	88%
Evaluation of LVS Function	88	99%	97%	98%
Smoking Cessation Advice[1]	17	94%	99%	98%
Pneumonia Care				
Appropriate Initial Antibiotic	133	96%	92%	92%
Blood Culture Timing	160	97%	97%	96%
Influenza Vaccine	100	95%	93%	91%
Initial Antibiotic Timing	164	95%	96%	95%
Pneumococcal Vaccine	115	98%	95%	93%
Smoking Cessation Advice	76	99%	99%	97%
Surgical Care Improvement Project				
Appropriate VTP Within 24 Hours	34	97%	92%	92%
Appropriate Hair Removal	55	100%	100%	99%
Appropriate Beta Blocker Usage[1]	6	100%	93%	93%
Controlled Postoperative Blood Glucose	0	-	93%	93%
Prophylactic Antibiotic Timing[1]	20	100%	97%	97%
Prophylactic Antibiotic Timing (Outpatient)[1,3]	3	100%	94%	92%
Prophylactic Antibiotic Selection[1]	20	95%	97%	97%
Prophylactic Antibiotic Select. (Outpatient)[1,3]	3	67%	94%	94%
Prophylactic Antibiotic Stopped[1]	16	100%	94%	94%
Recommended VTP Ordered	34	97%	94%	94%
Urinary Catheter Removal[1]	8	75%	90%	90%
Children's Asthma Care				
Received Systemic Corticosteroids	-	-	-	100%
Received Home Management Plan	-	-	-	71%
Received Reliever Medication	-	-	-	100%
Use of Medical Imaging				
Combination Abdominal CT Scan	359	0.162	0.219	0.191
Combination Chest CT Scan	323	0.164	0.102	0.054
Follow-up Mammogram/Ultrasound	534	4.1%	8%	8.4%
MRI for Low Back Pain	66	33.3%	30.7%	32.7%
Survey of Patients' Hospital Experiences				
Area Around Room 'Always' Quiet at Night	300+	71%	-	58%
Doctors 'Always' Communicated Well	300+	81%	-	80%
Home Recovery Information Given	300+	82%	-	82%
Hospital Given 9 or 10 on 10 Point Scale	300+	68%	-	67%
Meds 'Always' Explained Before Given	300+	62%	-	60%
Nurses 'Always' Communicated Well	300+	78%	-	76%
Pain 'Always' Well Controlled	300+	66%	-	69%
Room and Bathroom 'Always' Clean	300+	75%	-	71%
Timely Help 'Always' Received	300+	75%	-	64%
Would Definitely Recommend Hospital	300+	62%	-	69%

NOTE: Hospital profiles are in alphabetical order by state, then city, then hospital within the city; Rankings exclude hospitals with less than 25 cases except for patient surveys which excludes hospitals with less than 100 cases; (a) 100–299 cases; (1) The number of cases is too small to be sure how well a hospital is performing; (2) The hospital indicated that the data submitted for this measure were based on a sample of cases; (3) Data was collected during a shorter time period (fewer quarters) than the maximum possible time for this measure; (4) Suppressed for one or more quarters by CMS; (5) No data is available from the hospital for this measure; (6) Fewer than 100 patients completed the HCAHPS survey. Use these rates with caution, as the number of surveys may be too low to reliably assess hospital performance; (7) Survey results are based on less than 12 months of data; (8) Survey results are not available for this reporting period; (9) No or very few patients were eligible for the HCAHPS survey. The scores shown, if any, reflect a very small number of surveys; (10) A state average was not calculated because too few hospitals in the state submitted data; (11) There were discrepancies in the data collection process; Please refer to the User's Guide for a full explanation of data.

Trousdale Medical Center

500 Church Street Phone: 615-374-2221
Hartsville, TN 37074 Fax: 615-374-2928
Type: Critical Access Hospitals Emergency Services: Yes
Ownership: Voluntary Non-Profit - Other Beds: 25
Key Personnel:
Chief of Medical Staff. . . . . B T Samson
Infection Control. . . . . Kim Kichy
Quality Assurance . . . . Martha Stack
Radiology. . . . . Brent Frisbie
Emergency Room . . . . Floyd Reid

Measure	Cases	This Hosp.	State Avg.	U.S. Avg.
Heart Attack Care				
ACE Inhibitor or ARB for LVSD[3]	0	-	96%	96%
Aspirin at Arrival[3]	0	-	98%	99%
Aspirin at Discharge[3]	0	-	99%	98%
Beta Blocker at Discharge[3]	0	-	98%	98%
Fibrinolytic Medication Timing[3]	0	-	67%	55%
PCI Within 90 Minutes of Arrival[3]	0	-	91%	90%
Smoking Cessation Advice[3]	0	-	100%	99%
Chest Pain/Possible Heart Attack Care				
Aspirin at Arrival	-	-	95%	95%
Median Time to ECG (minutes)	-	-	8	8
Median Time to Transfer (minutes)	-	-	65	61
Fibrinolytic Medication Timing	-	-	49%	54%
Heart Failure Care				
ACE Inhibitor or ARB for LVSD[1]	9	78%	95%	94%
Discharge Instructions	33	97%	88%	88%
Evaluation of LVS Function	61	77%	97%	98%
Smoking Cessation Advice	27	93%	99%	98%
Pneumonia Care				
Appropriate Initial Antibiotic	25	100%	92%	92%
Blood Culture Timing[1]	12	92%	97%	96%
Influenza Vaccine	30	100%	93%	91%
Initial Antibiotic Timing	35	91%	96%	95%
Pneumococcal Vaccine	32	100%	95%	93%
Smoking Cessation Advice[1]	14	100%	99%	97%
Surgical Care Improvement Project				
Appropriate VTP Within 24 Hours[5]	0	-	92%	92%
Appropriate Hair Removal[5]	0	-	100%	99%
Appropriate Beta Blocker Usage[5]	0	-	93%	93%
Controlled Postoperative Blood Glucose[5]	0	-	93%	93%
Prophylactic Antibiotic Timing[5]	0	-	97%	97%
Prophylactic Antibiotic Timing (Outpatient)	-	-	94%	92%
Prophylactic Antibiotic Selection[5]	0	-	97%	97%
Prophylactic Antibiotic Select. (Outpatient)	-	-	94%	94%
Prophylactic Antibiotic Stopped[5]	0	-	94%	94%
Recommended VTP Ordered[5]	0	-	94%	94%
Urinary Catheter Removal[5]	0	-	90%	90%
Children's Asthma Care				
Received Systemic Corticosteroids	-	-	-	100%
Received Home Management Plan	-	-	-	71%
Received Reliever Medication	-	-	-	100%
Use of Medical Imaging				
Combination Abdominal CT Scan	-	-	0.219	0.191
Combination Chest CT Scan	-	-	0.102	0.054
Follow-up Mammogram/Ultrasound	-	-	8%	8.4%
MRI for Low Back Pain	-	-	30.7%	32.7%
Survey of Patients' Hospital Experiences				
Area Around Room 'Always' Quiet at Night	(a)	67%	-	58%
Doctors 'Always' Communicated Well	(a)	89%	-	80%
Home Recovery Information Given	(a)	85%	-	82%
Hospital Given 9 or 10 on 10 Point Scale	(a)	70%	-	67%
Meds 'Always' Explained Before Given	(a)	72%	-	60%
Nurses 'Always' Communicated Well	(a)	85%	-	76%
Pain 'Always' Well Controlled	(a)	76%	-	69%
Room and Bathroom 'Always' Clean	(a)	92%	-	71%
Timely Help 'Always' Received	(a)	67%	-	64%
Would Definitely Recommend Hospital	(a)	71%	-	69%

Hendersonville Medical Center

355 New Shackle Island Rd Phone: 615-338-1000
Hendersonville, TN 37075 Fax: 615-338-1101
URL: www.hendersonvillemedicalcenter.com
Type: Acute Care Hospitals Emergency Services: Yes
Ownership: Voluntary Non-Profit - Other Beds: 110
Key Personnel:
CEO/President. . . . . Regina Bartlett
Cardiac Laboratory. . . . . Jim Oliver
Chief of Medical Staff . . . . Tracy Callista, MD
Infection Control. . . . . Debbie Smith
Operating Room. . . . . John Andrew Boskind
Quality Assurance . . . . Karen Stanley
Radiology. . . . . John J Alarcon

Measure	Cases	This Hosp.	State Avg.	U.S. Avg.
Heart Attack Care				
ACE Inhibitor or ARB for LVSD[1]	10	100%	96%	96%
Aspirin at Arrival	42	100%	98%	99%
Aspirin at Discharge	48	100%	99%	98%
Beta Blocker at Discharge	47	100%	98%	98%
Fibrinolytic Medication Timing	0	-	67%	55%
PCI Within 90 Minutes of Arrival[1]	10	100%	91%	90%
Smoking Cessation Advice[1]	22	100%	100%	99%
Chest Pain/Possible Heart Attack Care				
Aspirin at Arrival	40	100%	95%	95%
Median Time to ECG (minutes)	45	5	8	8
Median Time to Transfer (minutes)[5]	0	-	65	61
Fibrinolytic Medication Timing	0	-	49%	54%
Heart Failure Care				
ACE Inhibitor or ARB for LVSD	32	100%	95%	94%
Discharge Instructions	97	99%	88%	88%
Evaluation of LVS Function	121	100%	97%	98%
Smoking Cessation Advice	25	100%	99%	98%
Pneumonia Care				
Appropriate Initial Antibiotic	60	95%	92%	92%
Blood Culture Timing	79	99%	97%	96%
Influenza Vaccine	85	99%	93%	91%
Initial Antibiotic Timing	83	96%	96%	95%
Pneumococcal Vaccine	97	100%	95%	93%
Smoking Cessation Advice	65	100%	99%	97%
Surgical Care Improvement Project				
Appropriate VTP Within 24 Hours	125	94%	92%	92%
Appropriate Hair Removal	314	100%	100%	99%
Appropriate Beta Blocker Usage	78	100%	93%	93%
Controlled Postoperative Blood Glucose	0	-	93%	93%
Prophylactic Antibiotic Timing	189	95%	97%	97%
Prophylactic Antibiotic Timing (Outpatient)	178	94%	94%	92%
Prophylactic Antibiotic Selection	190	98%	97%	97%
Prophylactic Antibiotic Select. (Outpatient)	177	98%	94%	94%
Prophylactic Antibiotic Stopped	177	99%	94%	94%
Recommended VTP Ordered	125	97%	94%	94%
Urinary Catheter Removal	65	100%	90%	90%
Children's Asthma Care				
Received Systemic Corticosteroids	-	-	-	100%
Received Home Management Plan	-	-	-	71%
Received Reliever Medication	-	-	-	100%
Use of Medical Imaging				
Combination Abdominal CT Scan	522	0.174	0.219	0.191
Combination Chest CT Scan	346	0.017	0.102	0.054
Follow-up Mammogram/Ultrasound	721	11.2%	8%	8.4%
MRI for Low Back Pain	178	23.6%	30.7%	32.7%
Survey of Patients' Hospital Experiences				
Area Around Room 'Always' Quiet at Night	300+	61%	-	58%
Doctors 'Always' Communicated Well	300+	82%	-	80%
Home Recovery Information Given	300+	84%	-	82%
Hospital Given 9 or 10 on 10 Point Scale	300+	65%	-	67%
Meds 'Always' Explained Before Given	300+	58%	-	60%
Nurses 'Always' Communicated Well	300+	75%	-	76%
Pain 'Always' Well Controlled	300+	69%	-	69%
Room and Bathroom 'Always' Clean	300+	66%	-	71%
Timely Help 'Always' Received	300+	61%	-	64%
Would Definitely Recommend Hospital	300+	67%	-	69%

Summit Medical Center

5655 Frist Blvd Phone: 615-316-3000
Hermitage, TN 37076 Fax: 615-316-3557
URL: www.summitmedctr.com
Type: Acute Care Hospitals Emergency Services: Yes
Ownership: Proprietary Beds: 204
Key Personnel:
CEO/President. . . . . Jeff Whitehorn
Chief of Medical Staff . . . . Wendy Brandon
Operating Room. . . . . Stephanie Davis
Quality Assurance . . . . Patsy Parrell
Radiology. . . . . Lisa A Altieri, MD
Emergency Room . . . . Randy Farrar

Measure	Cases	This Hosp.	State Avg.	U.S. Avg.
Heart Attack Care				
ACE Inhibitor or ARB for LVSD[1]	12	100%	96%	96%
Aspirin at Arrival	112	100%	98%	99%
Aspirin at Discharge	95	100%	99%	98%
Beta Blocker at Discharge	97	98%	98%	98%
Fibrinolytic Medication Timing[1]	1	100%	67%	55%
PCI Within 90 Minutes of Arrival	25	100%	91%	90%
Smoking Cessation Advice	32	100%	100%	99%
Chest Pain/Possible Heart Attack Care				
Aspirin at Arrival	70	100%	95%	95%
Median Time to ECG (minutes)	72	4	8	8
Median Time to Transfer (minutes)[1]	23	51	65	61
Fibrinolytic Medication Timing	0	-	49%	54%
Heart Failure Care				
ACE Inhibitor or ARB for LVSD	64	100%	95%	94%
Discharge Instructions	171	100%	88%	88%
Evaluation of LVS Function	212	98%	97%	98%
Smoking Cessation Advice	35	100%	99%	98%
Pneumonia Care				
Appropriate Initial Antibiotic	233	93%	92%	92%
Blood Culture Timing	290	98%	97%	96%
Influenza Vaccine	212	99%	93%	91%
Initial Antibiotic Timing	291	96%	96%	95%
Pneumococcal Vaccine	263	100%	95%	93%
Smoking Cessation Advice	121	100%	99%	97%
Surgical Care Improvement Project				
Appropriate VTP Within 24 Hours[2]	224	96%	92%	92%
Appropriate Hair Removal[2]	440	100%	100%	99%
Appropriate Beta Blocker Usage[2]	99	100%	93%	93%
Controlled Postoperative Blood Glucose[2]	0	-	93%	93%
Prophylactic Antibiotic Timing[2]	241	97%	97%	97%
Prophylactic Antibiotic Timing (Outpatient)	493	99%	94%	92%
Prophylactic Antibiotic Selection[2]	242	99%	97%	97%
Prophylactic Antibiotic Select. (Outpatient)	489	97%	94%	94%
Prophylactic Antibiotic Stopped[2]	223	96%	94%	94%
Recommended VTP Ordered[2]	224	98%	94%	94%
Urinary Catheter Removal[2]	87	99%	90%	90%
Children's Asthma Care				
Received Systemic Corticosteroids	-	-	-	100%
Received Home Management Plan	-	-	-	71%
Received Reliever Medication	-	-	-	100%
Use of Medical Imaging				
Combination Abdominal CT Scan	722	0.341	0.219	0.191
Combination Chest CT Scan	421	0.069	0.102	0.054
Follow-up Mammogram/Ultrasound	1,258	10.2%	8%	8.4%
MRI for Low Back Pain	257	25.7%	30.7%	32.7%
Survey of Patients' Hospital Experiences				
Area Around Room 'Always' Quiet at Night	300+	63%	-	58%
Doctors 'Always' Communicated Well	300+	82%	-	80%
Home Recovery Information Given	300+	88%	-	82%
Hospital Given 9 or 10 on 10 Point Scale	300+	72%	-	67%
Meds 'Always' Explained Before Given	300+	59%	-	60%
Nurses 'Always' Communicated Well	300+	76%	-	76%
Pain 'Always' Well Controlled	300+	70%	-	69%
Room and Bathroom 'Always' Clean	300+	71%	-	71%
Timely Help 'Always' Received	300+	66%	-	64%
Would Definitely Recommend Hospital	300+	75%	-	69%

NOTE: Hospital profiles are in alphabetical order by state, then city, then hospital within the city; Rankings exclude hospitals with less than 25 cases except for patient surveys which excludes hospitals with less than 100 cases; (a) 100–299 cases; (1) The number of cases is too small to be sure how well a hospital is performing; (2) The hospital indicated that the data submitted for this measure were based on a sample of cases; (3) Data was collected during a shorter time period (fewer quarters) than the maximum possible time for this measure; (4) Suppressed for one or more quarters by CMS; (5) No data is available from the hospital for this measure; (6) Fewer than 100 patients completed the HCAHPS survey. Use these rates with caution, as the number of surveys may be too low to reliably assess hospital performance; (7) Survey results are based on less than 12 months of data; (8) Survey results are not available for this reporting period; (9) No or very few patients were eligible for the HCAHPS survey. The scores shown, if any, reflect a very small number of surveys; (10) A state average was not calculated because too few hospitals in the state submitted data; (11) There were discrepancies in the data collection process; Please refer to the User's Guide for a full explanation of data.

Humboldt General Hospital

3525 Chere Carol Rd Phone: 731-784-2321
Humboldt, TN 38343 Fax: 731-824-5569
Type: Acute Care Hospitals Emergency Services: Yes
Ownership: Govt - Hospital Dist/Auth Beds: 62
Key Personnel:
CEO/President. . . . . Bill Kail
Chief of Medical Staff . . . . Jennifer Utley
Infection Control. . . . . Della Yarbrough
Operating Room. . . . . Linda Elmore
Radiology. . . . . Keith Garner
Emergency Room . . . . Renoda Crone

Measure	Cases	This Hosp.	State Avg.	U.S. Avg.
Heart Attack Care				
ACE Inhibitor or ARB for LVSD[3]	0	-	96%	96%
Aspirin at Arrival[1,3]	2	100%	98%	99%
Aspirin at Discharge[1,3]	2	50%	99%	98%
Beta Blocker at Discharge[1,3]	2	50%	98%	98%
Fibrinolytic Medication Timing[3]	0	-	67%	55%
PCI Within 90 Minutes of Arrival[3]	0	-	91%	90%
Smoking Cessation Advice[3]	0	-	100%	99%
Chest Pain/Possible Heart Attack Care				
Aspirin at Arrival	90	86%	95%	95%
Median Time to ECG (minutes)	93	33	8	8
Median Time to Transfer (minutes)[1,3]	3	135	65	61
Fibrinolytic Medication Timing[1]	3	0%	49%	54%
Heart Failure Care				
ACE Inhibitor or ARB for LVSD[1]	13	85%	95%	94%
Discharge Instructions	25	96%	88%	88%
Evaluation of LVS Function	33	91%	97%	98%
Smoking Cessation Advice[1]	9	100%	99%	98%
Pneumonia Care				
Appropriate Initial Antibiotic[1]	19	84%	92%	92%
Blood Culture Timing[1]	15	93%	97%	96%
Influenza Vaccine[1]	11	100%	93%	91%
Initial Antibiotic Timing[1]	24	92%	96%	95%
Pneumococcal Vaccine[1]	22	77%	95%	93%
Smoking Cessation Advice[1]	8	100%	99%	97%
Surgical Care Improvement Project				
Appropriate VTP Within 24 Hours[5]	0	-	92%	92%
Appropriate Hair Removal[5]	0	-	100%	99%
Appropriate Beta Blocker Usage[5]	0	-	93%	93%
Controlled Postoperative Blood Glucose[5]	0	-	93%	93%
Prophylactic Antibiotic Timing[5]	0	-	97%	97%
Prophylactic Antibiotic Timing (Outpatient)[1,3]	3	0%	94%	92%
Prophylactic Antibiotic Selection[5]	0	-	97%	97%
Prophylactic Antibiotic Select. (Outpatient)[3]	0	-	94%	94%
Prophylactic Antibiotic Stopped[5]	0	-	94%	94%
Recommended VTP Ordered[5]	0	-	94%	94%
Urinary Catheter Removal[5]	0	-	90%	90%
Children's Asthma Care				
Received Systemic Corticosteroids	-	-	-	100%
Received Home Management Plan	-	-	-	71%
Received Reliever Medication	-	-	-	100%
Use of Medical Imaging				
Combination Abdominal CT Scan	86	0.070	0.219	0.191
Combination Chest CT Scan	49	0.000	0.102	0.054
Follow-up Mammogram/Ultrasound	268	2.2%	8%	8.4%
MRI for Low Back Pain[5]	0	-	30.7%	32.7%
Survey of Patients' Hospital Experiences				
Area Around Room 'Always' Quiet at Night	(a)	73%	-	58%
Doctors 'Always' Communicated Well	(a)	93%	-	80%
Home Recovery Information Given	(a)	67%	-	82%
Hospital Given 9 or 10 on 10 Point Scale	(a)	72%	-	67%
Meds 'Always' Explained Before Given	(a)	63%	-	60%
Nurses 'Always' Communicated Well	(a)	85%	-	76%
Pain 'Always' Well Controlled	(a)	80%	-	69%
Room and Bathroom 'Always' Clean	(a)	76%	-	71%
Timely Help 'Always' Received	(a)	79%	-	64%
Would Definitely Recommend Hospital	(a)	76%	-	69%

Baptist Memorial Hospital Huntingdon

631 Rb Wilson Dr Phone: 731-986-4461
Huntingdon, TN 38344 Fax: 731-986-7288
URL: www.bmhcc.org
Type: Acute Care Hospitals Emergency Services: Yes
Ownership: Voluntary Non-Profit - Church Beds: 72
Key Personnel:
CEO/President. . . . . Susan M Breeden
Radiology. . . . . Jacob Abraham

Measure	Cases	This Hosp.	State Avg.	U.S. Avg.
Heart Attack Care				
ACE Inhibitor or ARB for LVSD	0	-	96%	96%
Aspirin at Arrival[1]	3	100%	98%	99%
Aspirin at Discharge[1]	1	100%	99%	98%
Beta Blocker at Discharge[1]	1	100%	98%	98%
Fibrinolytic Medication Timing	0	-	67%	55%
PCI Within 90 Minutes of Arrival	0	-	91%	90%
Smoking Cessation Advice	0	-	100%	99%
Chest Pain/Possible Heart Attack Care				
Aspirin at Arrival	104	92%	95%	95%
Median Time to ECG (minutes)	113	7	8	8
Median Time to Transfer (minutes)[1,3]	2	258	65	61
Fibrinolytic Medication Timing[1]	4	0%	49%	54%
Heart Failure Care				
ACE Inhibitor or ARB for LVSD[1]	13	100%	95%	94%
Discharge Instructions	40	98%	88%	88%
Evaluation of LVS Function	58	98%	97%	98%
Smoking Cessation Advice[1]	15	100%	99%	98%
Pneumonia Care				
Appropriate Initial Antibiotic	28	86%	92%	92%
Blood Culture Timing	41	98%	97%	96%
Influenza Vaccine[1]	18	100%	93%	91%
Initial Antibiotic Timing	32	94%	96%	95%
Pneumococcal Vaccine	29	100%	95%	93%
Smoking Cessation Advice[1]	17	100%	99%	97%
Surgical Care Improvement Project				
Appropriate VTP Within 24 Hours[1]	21	100%	92%	92%
Appropriate Hair Removal	37	100%	100%	99%
Appropriate Beta Blocker Usage[1]	6	100%	93%	93%
Controlled Postoperative Blood Glucose	0	-	93%	93%
Prophylactic Antibiotic Timing[1]	24	92%	97%	97%
Prophylactic Antibiotic Timing (Outpatient)[1,3]	7	86%	94%	92%
Prophylactic Antibiotic Selection	25	100%	97%	97%
Prophylactic Antibiotic Select. (Outpatient)[1,3]	6	100%	94%	94%
Prophylactic Antibiotic Stopped[1]	22	86%	94%	94%
Recommended VTP Ordered[1]	21	100%	94%	94%
Urinary Catheter Removal[1]	5	40%	90%	90%
Children's Asthma Care				
Received Systemic Corticosteroids	-	-	-	100%
Received Home Management Plan	-	-	-	71%
Received Reliever Medication	-	-	-	100%
Use of Medical Imaging				
Combination Abdominal CT Scan	155	0.639	0.219	0.191
Combination Chest CT Scan	94	0.649	0.102	0.054
Follow-up Mammogram/Ultrasound	243	12.8%	8%	8.4%
MRI for Low Back Pain	93	31.2%	30.7%	32.7%
Survey of Patients' Hospital Experiences				
Area Around Room 'Always' Quiet at Night	(a)	76%	-	58%
Doctors 'Always' Communicated Well	(a)	88%	-	80%
Home Recovery Information Given	(a)	82%	-	82%
Hospital Given 9 or 10 on 10 Point Scale	(a)	74%	-	67%
Meds 'Always' Explained Before Given	(a)	68%	-	60%
Nurses 'Always' Communicated Well	(a)	87%	-	76%
Pain 'Always' Well Controlled	(a)	78%	-	69%
Room and Bathroom 'Always' Clean	(a)	75%	-	71%
Timely Help 'Always' Received	(a)	74%	-	64%
Would Definitely Recommend Hospital	(a)	77%	-	69%

Jackson-Madison County General Hospital

620 Skyline Drive Phone: 731-541-5000
Jackson, TN 38301
Type: Acute Care Hospitals Emergency Services: Yes
Ownership: Voluntary Non-Profit - Other
Key Personnel:
CEO/President. . . . . Jim Moss
Infection Control. . . . . Ellena Henderson
Radiology. . . . . Kelly Yenawine
Hemotology Center . . . . Gina Myracle

Measure	Cases	This Hosp.	State Avg.	U.S. Avg.
Heart Attack Care				
ACE Inhibitor or ARB for LVSD[2]	194	91%	96%	96%
Aspirin at Arrival[2]	553	95%	98%	99%
Aspirin at Discharge[2]	994	96%	99%	98%
Beta Blocker at Discharge[2]	967	95%	98%	98%
Fibrinolytic Medication Timing[1,2]	1	0%	67%	55%
PCI Within 90 Minutes of Arrival[2]	72	85%	91%	90%
Smoking Cessation Advice[2]	436	99%	100%	99%
Chest Pain/Possible Heart Attack Care				
Aspirin at Arrival[1]	4	50%	95%	95%
Median Time to ECG (minutes)[1]	5	18	8	8
Median Time to Transfer (minutes)[5]	0	-	65	61
Fibrinolytic Medication Timing[3]	0	-	49%	54%
Heart Failure Care				
ACE Inhibitor or ARB for LVSD[2]	369	90%	95%	94%
Discharge Instructions[2]	720	62%	88%	88%
Evaluation of LVS Function[2]	882	98%	97%	98%
Smoking Cessation Advice[2]	201	100%	99%	98%
Pneumonia Care				
Appropriate Initial Antibiotic[2]	80	94%	92%	92%
Blood Culture Timing[2]	87	91%	97%	96%
Influenza Vaccine[2]	170	86%	93%	91%
Initial Antibiotic Timing[2]	149	92%	96%	95%
Pneumococcal Vaccine[2]	194	83%	95%	93%
Smoking Cessation Advice[2]	122	99%	99%	97%
Surgical Care Improvement Project				
Appropriate VTP Within 24 Hours[2]	635	93%	92%	92%
Appropriate Hair Removal[2]	1,625	99%	100%	99%
Appropriate Beta Blocker Usage[2]	497	79%	93%	93%
Controlled Postoperative Blood Glucose[2]	372	93%	93%	93%
Prophylactic Antibiotic Timing[2]	1,267	87%	97%	97%
Prophylactic Antibiotic Timing (Outpatient)	1,600	83%	94%	92%
Prophylactic Antibiotic Selection[2]	1,272	93%	97%	97%
Prophylactic Antibiotic Select. (Outpatient)	1,551	87%	94%	94%
Prophylactic Antibiotic Stopped[2]	1,197	84%	94%	94%
Recommended VTP Ordered[2]	635	97%	94%	94%
Urinary Catheter Removal[2]	419	82%	90%	90%
Children's Asthma Care				
Received Systemic Corticosteroids	-	-	-	100%
Received Home Management Plan	-	-	-	71%
Received Reliever Medication	-	-	-	100%
Use of Medical Imaging				
Combination Abdominal CT Scan	1,630	0.039	0.219	0.191
Combination Chest CT Scan	1,313	0.008	0.102	0.054
Follow-up Mammogram/Ultrasound	1,994	7.2%	8%	8.4%
MRI for Low Back Pain	678	30.4%	30.7%	32.7%
Survey of Patients' Hospital Experiences				
Area Around Room 'Always' Quiet at Night	300+	67%	-	58%
Doctors 'Always' Communicated Well	300+	79%	-	80%
Home Recovery Information Given	300+	81%	-	82%
Hospital Given 9 or 10 on 10 Point Scale	300+	66%	-	67%
Meds 'Always' Explained Before Given	300+	56%	-	60%
Nurses 'Always' Communicated Well	300+	75%	-	76%
Pain 'Always' Well Controlled	300+	66%	-	69%
Room and Bathroom 'Always' Clean	300+	65%	-	71%
Timely Help 'Always' Received	300+	61%	-	64%
Would Definitely Recommend Hospital	300+	70%	-	69%

NOTE: Hospital profiles are in alphabetical order by state, then city, then hospital within the city; Rankings exclude hospitals with less than 25 cases except for patient surveys which excludes hospitals with less than 100 cases; (a) 100–299 cases; (1) The number of cases is too small to be sure how well a hospital is performing; (2) The hospital indicated that the data submitted for this measure were based on a sample of cases; (3) Data was collected during a shorter time period (fewer quarters) than the maximum possible time for this measure; (4) Suppressed for one or more quarters by CMS; (5) No data is available from the hospital for this measure; (6) Fewer than 100 patients completed the HCAHPS survey. Use these rates with caution, as the number of surveys may be too low to reliably assess hospital performance; (7) Survey results are based on less than 12 months of data; (8) Survey results are not available for this reporting period; (9) No or very few patients were eligible for the HCAHPS survey. The scores shown, if any, reflect a very small number of surveys; (10) A state average was not calculated because too few hospitals in the state submitted data; (11) There were discrepancies in the data collection process; Please refer to the User's Guide for a full explanation of data.

Regional Hospital of Jackson

367 Hospital Blvd Phone: 731-661-2000
Jackson, TN 38305 Fax: 731-661-2257
URL: www.regionalhospitaljackson.com
Type: Acute Care Hospitals Emergency Services: Yes
Ownership: Proprietary Beds: 98

Key Personnel:
CEO/President. . . . . Tim Puthoff
Cardiac Laboratory. . . . . Jorge Delgado
Chief of Medical Staff. . . . . Laurence Martin, MD
Infection Control. . . . . Jill Kilby
Operating Room. . . . . Teresa Ayers
Radiology. . . . . Gary Weiss

Measure	Cases	This Hosp.	State Avg.	U.S. Avg.
Heart Attack Care				
ACE Inhibitor or ARB for LVSD	34	97%	96%	96%
Aspirin at Arrival	52	96%	98%	99%
Aspirin at Discharge	164	95%	99%	98%
Beta Blocker at Discharge	152	96%	98%	98%
Fibrinolytic Medication Timing	0	-	67%	55%
PCI Within 90 Minutes of Arrival[1]	7	57%	91%	90%
Smoking Cessation Advice	76	100%	100%	99%
Chest Pain/Possible Heart Attack Care				
Aspirin at Arrival[1,3]	9	100%	95%	95%
Median Time to ECG (minutes)[1,3]	10	6	8	8
Median Time to Transfer (minutes)[5]	0	-	65	61
Fibrinolytic Medication Timing[3]	0	-	49%	54%
Heart Failure Care				
ACE Inhibitor or ARB for LVSD	60	95%	95%	94%
Discharge Instructions	162	90%	88%	88%
Evaluation of LVS Function	181	99%	97%	98%
Smoking Cessation Advice	39	100%	99%	98%
Pneumonia Care				
Appropriate Initial Antibiotic	62	92%	92%	92%
Blood Culture Timing	89	100%	97%	96%
Influenza Vaccine	98	94%	93%	91%
Initial Antibiotic Timing	95	98%	96%	95%
Pneumococcal Vaccine	105	93%	95%	93%
Smoking Cessation Advice	95	99%	99%	97%
Surgical Care Improvement Project				
Appropriate VTP Within 24 Hours[2]	197	96%	92%	92%
Appropriate Hair Removal[2]	359	100%	100%	99%
Appropriate Beta Blocker Usage[2]	70	99%	93%	93%
Controlled Postoperative Blood Glucose[2]	0	-	93%	93%
Prophylactic Antibiotic Timing[2]	218	97%	97%	97%
Prophylactic Antibiotic Timing (Outpatient)	79	96%	94%	92%
Prophylactic Antibiotic Selection[2]	218	100%	97%	97%
Prophylactic Antibiotic Select. (Outpatient)	79	97%	94%	94%
Prophylactic Antibiotic Stopped[2]	199	96%	94%	94%
Recommended VTP Ordered[2]	199	98%	94%	94%
Urinary Catheter Removal	78	90%	90%	90%
Children's Asthma Care				
Received Systemic Corticosteroids	-	-	-	100%
Received Home Management Plan	-	-	-	71%
Received Reliever Medication	-	-	-	100%
Use of Medical Imaging				
Combination Abdominal CT Scan	228	0.013	0.219	0.191
Combination Chest CT Scan	197	0.005	0.102	0.054
Follow-up Mammogram/Ultrasound	161	8.7%	8%	8.4%
MRI for Low Back Pain	56	26.8%	30.7%	32.7%
Survey of Patients' Hospital Experiences				
Area Around Room 'Always' Quiet at Night	300+	67%	-	58%
Doctors 'Always' Communicated Well	300+	81%	-	80%
Home Recovery Information Given	300+	78%	-	82%
Hospital Given 9 or 10 on 10 Point Scale	300+	71%	-	67%
Meds 'Always' Explained Before Given	300+	58%	-	60%
Nurses 'Always' Communicated Well	300+	78%	-	76%
Pain 'Always' Well Controlled	300+	71%	-	69%
Room and Bathroom 'Always' Clean	300+	66%	-	71%
Timely Help 'Always' Received	300+	65%	-	64%
Would Definitely Recommend Hospital	300+	74%	-	69%

Jamestown Regional Medical Center

436 Central Avenue West Phone: 931-879-3352
Jamestown, TN 38556 Fax: 931-879-4896
URL: www.jamestownregional.org
Type: Acute Care Hospitals Emergency Services: Yes
Ownership: Proprietary Beds: 85

Key Personnel:
CEO/President. . . . . Kimberly Anthony
Chief of Medical Staff. . . . . Rockey Talley, MD
Infection Control. . . . . Machelle Lee, RN
Operating Room. . . . . Sue McDonald
Quality Assurance . . . . Jill Jones, RN
Radiology. . . . . Pat Gunter
Emergency Room . . . . Linda L Jackson, RN
Patient Relations . . . . Rhonda Tate

Measure	Cases	This Hosp.	State Avg.	U.S. Avg.
Heart Attack Care				
ACE Inhibitor or ARB for LVSD	0	-	96%	96%
Aspirin at Arrival[1]	5	100%	98%	99%
Aspirin at Discharge[1]	2	100%	99%	98%
Beta Blocker at Discharge[1]	4	100%	98%	98%
Fibrinolytic Medication Timing	0	-	67%	55%
PCI Within 90 Minutes of Arrival	0	-	91%	90%
Smoking Cessation Advice[1]	1	100%	100%	99%
Chest Pain/Possible Heart Attack Care				
Aspirin at Arrival	92	100%	95%	95%
Median Time to ECG (minutes)	99	5	8	8
Median Time to Transfer (minutes)[3]	0	-	65	61
Fibrinolytic Medication Timing[1]	1	100%	49%	54%
Heart Failure Care				
ACE Inhibitor or ARB for LVSD[1]	24	100%	95%	94%
Discharge Instructions	83	99%	88%	88%
Evaluation of LVS Function	96	100%	97%	98%
Smoking Cessation Advice[1]	23	100%	99%	98%
Pneumonia Care				
Appropriate Initial Antibiotic	68	96%	92%	92%
Blood Culture Timing	73	100%	97%	96%
Influenza Vaccine	67	100%	93%	91%
Initial Antibiotic Timing	129	97%	96%	95%
Pneumococcal Vaccine	78	99%	95%	93%
Smoking Cessation Advice	55	100%	99%	97%
Surgical Care Improvement Project				
Appropriate VTP Within 24 Hours[1,3]	5	60%	92%	92%
Appropriate Hair Removal[1,3]	19	100%	100%	99%
Appropriate Beta Blocker Usage[1,3]	2	100%	93%	93%
Controlled Postoperative Blood Glucose[3]	0	-	93%	93%
Prophylactic Antibiotic Timing[1,3]	15	100%	97%	97%
Prophylactic Antibiotic Timing (Outpatient)[1,3]	2	0%	94%	92%
Prophylactic Antibiotic Selection[1,3]	13	85%	97%	97%
Prophylactic Antibiotic Select. (Outpatient)[3]	0	-	94%	94%
Prophylactic Antibiotic Stopped[1,3]	11	91%	94%	94%
Recommended VTP Ordered[1,3]	5	60%	94%	94%
Urinary Catheter Removal[1]	3	100%	90%	90%
Children's Asthma Care				
Received Systemic Corticosteroids[1]	10	90%	-	100%
Received Home Management Plan[1]	10	80%	-	71%
Received Reliever Medication[1]	10	100%	-	100%
Use of Medical Imaging				
Combination Abdominal CT Scan	165	0.079	0.219	0.191
Combination Chest CT Scan	89	0.022	0.102	0.054
Follow-up Mammogram/Ultrasound	376	3.7%	8%	8.4%
MRI for Low Back Pain[1]	43	14.0%	30.7%	32.7%
Survey of Patients' Hospital Experiences				
Area Around Room 'Always' Quiet at Night	300+	63%	-	58%
Doctors 'Always' Communicated Well	300+	83%	-	80%
Home Recovery Information Given	300+	75%	-	82%
Hospital Given 9 or 10 on 10 Point Scale	300+	55%	-	67%
Meds 'Always' Explained Before Given	300+	63%	-	60%
Nurses 'Always' Communicated Well	300+	78%	-	76%
Pain 'Always' Well Controlled	300+	65%	-	69%
Room and Bathroom 'Always' Clean	300+	71%	-	71%
Timely Help 'Always' Received	300+	66%	-	64%
Would Definitely Recommend Hospital	300+	52%	-	69%

Grandview Medical Center

1000 Highway 28 Phone: 423-837-9500
Jasper, TN 37347 Fax: 423-837-9406
URL: www.grandviewhospital.com
Type: Acute Care Hospitals Emergency Services: Yes
Ownership: Voluntary Non-Profit - Private Beds: 100

Key Personnel:
CEO/President. . . . . Dan Aranda
Chief of Medical Staff. . . . . Charles Adcock
Infection Control. . . . . Sue Headrick
Operating Room. . . . . Conrad Manayan
Quality Assurance . . . . Holly Stewart
Emergency Room . . . . Helen McGowan

Measure	Cases	This Hosp.	State Avg.	U.S. Avg.
Heart Attack Care				
ACE Inhibitor or ARB for LVSD[1]	2	100%	96%	96%
Aspirin at Arrival[1]	3	100%	98%	99%
Aspirin at Discharge[1]	3	100%	99%	98%
Beta Blocker at Discharge[1]	3	100%	98%	98%
Fibrinolytic Medication Timing	0	-	67%	55%
PCI Within 90 Minutes of Arrival	0	-	91%	90%
Smoking Cessation Advice	0	-	100%	99%
Chest Pain/Possible Heart Attack Care				
Aspirin at Arrival	210	97%	95%	95%
Median Time to ECG (minutes)	229	12	8	8
Median Time to Transfer (minutes)[1]	13	54	65	61
Fibrinolytic Medication Timing[1]	5	60%	49%	54%
Heart Failure Care				
ACE Inhibitor or ARB for LVSD[1]	11	91%	95%	94%
Discharge Instructions	28	64%	88%	88%
Evaluation of LVS Function	33	100%	97%	98%
Smoking Cessation Advice[1]	11	91%	99%	98%
Pneumonia Care				
Appropriate Initial Antibiotic	117	97%	92%	92%
Blood Culture Timing	99	97%	97%	96%
Influenza Vaccine	90	100%	93%	91%
Initial Antibiotic Timing	157	98%	96%	95%
Pneumococcal Vaccine	121	100%	95%	93%
Smoking Cessation Advice	104	99%	99%	97%
Surgical Care Improvement Project				
Appropriate VTP Within 24 Hours[1]	20	80%	92%	92%
Appropriate Hair Removal[1]	24	100%	100%	99%
Appropriate Beta Blocker Usage[1]	5	80%	93%	93%
Controlled Postoperative Blood Glucose	0	-	93%	93%
Prophylactic Antibiotic Timing[1]	6	100%	97%	97%
Prophylactic Antibiotic Timing (Outpatient)	29	90%	94%	92%
Prophylactic Antibiotic Selection[1]	7	100%	97%	97%
Prophylactic Antibiotic Select. (Outpatient)	27	85%	94%	94%
Prophylactic Antibiotic Stopped[1]	6	100%	94%	94%
Recommended VTP Ordered[1]	20	90%	94%	94%
Urinary Catheter Removal[1]	4	100%	90%	90%
Children's Asthma Care				
Received Systemic Corticosteroids	-	-	-	100%
Received Home Management Plan	-	-	-	71%
Received Reliever Medication	-	-	-	100%
Use of Medical Imaging				
Combination Abdominal CT Scan	311	0.283	0.219	0.191
Combination Chest CT Scan	124	0.234	0.102	0.054
Follow-up Mammogram/Ultrasound	355	6.2%	8%	8.4%
MRI for Low Back Pain	66	25.8%	30.7%	32.7%
Survey of Patients' Hospital Experiences				
Area Around Room 'Always' Quiet at Night	(a)	65%	-	58%
Doctors 'Always' Communicated Well	(a)	79%	-	80%
Home Recovery Information Given	(a)	78%	-	82%
Hospital Given 9 or 10 on 10 Point Scale	(a)	63%	-	67%
Meds 'Always' Explained Before Given	(a)	53%	-	60%
Nurses 'Always' Communicated Well	(a)	75%	-	76%
Pain 'Always' Well Controlled	(a)	65%	-	69%
Room and Bathroom 'Always' Clean	(a)	71%	-	71%
Timely Help 'Always' Received	(a)	60%	-	64%
Would Definitely Recommend Hospital	(a)	57%	-	69%

NOTE: Hospital profiles are in alphabetical order by state, then city, then hospital within the city; Rankings exclude hospitals with less than 25 cases except for patient surveys which excludes hospitals with less than 100 cases; (a) 100–299 cases; (1) The number of cases is too small to be sure how well a hospital is performing; (2) The hospital indicated that the data submitted for this measure were based on a sample of cases; (3) Data was collected during a shorter time period (fewer quarters) than the maximum possible time for this measure; (4) Suppressed for one or more quarters by CMS; (5) No data is available from the hospital for this measure; (6) Fewer than 100 patients completed the HCAHPS survey. Use these rates with caution, as the number of surveys may be too low to reliably assess hospital performance; (7) Survey results are based on less than 12 months of data; (8) Survey results are not available for this reporting period; (9) No or very few patients were eligible for the HCAHPS survey. The scores shown, if any, reflect a very small number of surveys; (10) A state average was not calculated because too few hospitals in the state submitted data; (11) There were discrepancies in the data collection process; Please refer to the User's Guide for a full explanation of data.

Saint Mary's Jefferson Memorial Hospital

110 Hospital Drive
Jefferson City, TN 37760
URL: www.stmaryshealth.com
Type: Acute Care Hospitals
Ownership: Voluntary Non-Profit - Private

Phone: 865-471-2500
Fax: 865-471-2450

Emergency Services: Yes
Beds: 58

Key Personnel:
CEO/President . . . . Debra K London
Chief of Medical Staff . . . . Leann Byrd, MD
Radiology . . . . Christopher Aikens

Measure	Cases	This Hosp.	State Avg.	U.S. Avg.
Heart Attack Care				
ACE Inhibitor or ARB for LVSD[1]	6	100%	96%	96%
Aspirin at Arrival[1]	14	100%	98%	99%
Aspirin at Discharge[1]	11	100%	99%	98%
Beta Blocker at Discharge[1]	12	100%	98%	98%
Fibrinolytic Medication Timing	0	-	67%	55%
PCI Within 90 Minutes of Arrival	0	-	91%	90%
Smoking Cessation Advice	0	-	100%	99%
Chest Pain/Possible Heart Attack Care				
Aspirin at Arrival	191	97%	95%	95%
Median Time to ECG (minutes)	195	14	8	8
Median Time to Transfer (minutes)[1,3]	4	81	65	61
Fibrinolytic Medication Timing[1]	1	0%	49%	54%
Heart Failure Care				
ACE Inhibitor or ARB for LVSD	51	92%	95%	94%
Discharge Instructions	109	87%	88%	88%
Evaluation of LVS Function	137	97%	97%	98%
Smoking Cessation Advice[1]	22	100%	99%	98%
Pneumonia Care				
Appropriate Initial Antibiotic	123	94%	92%	92%
Blood Culture Timing	153	99%	97%	96%
Influenza Vaccine	88	97%	93%	91%
Initial Antibiotic Timing	171	92%	96%	95%
Pneumococcal Vaccine	141	97%	95%	93%
Smoking Cessation Advice	65	99%	99%	97%
Surgical Care Improvement Project				
Appropriate VTP Within 24 Hours	28	82%	92%	92%
Appropriate Hair Removal	61	100%	100%	99%
Appropriate Beta Blocker Usage[1]	21	90%	93%	93%
Controlled Postoperative Blood Glucose	0	-	93%	93%
Prophylactic Antibiotic Timing	63	97%	97%	97%
Prophylactic Antibiotic Timing (Outpatient)	27	81%	94%	92%
Prophylactic Antibiotic Selection	63	98%	97%	97%
Prophylactic Antibiotic Select. (Outpatient)	25	88%	94%	94%
Prophylactic Antibiotic Stopped	61	97%	94%	94%
Recommended VTP Ordered	28	82%	94%	94%
Urinary Catheter Removal	36	97%	90%	90%
Children's Asthma Care				
Received Systemic Corticosteroids	-	-	-	100%
Received Home Management Plan	-	-	-	71%
Received Reliever Medication	-	-	-	100%
Use of Medical Imaging				
Combination Abdominal CT Scan	531	0.049	0.219	0.191
Combination Chest CT Scan	320	0.022	0.102	0.054
Follow-up Mammogram/Ultrasound	596	10.1%	8%	8.4%
MRI for Low Back Pain	114	35.1%	30.7%	32.7%
Survey of Patients' Hospital Experiences				
Area Around Room 'Always' Quiet at Night	300+	56%	-	58%
Doctors 'Always' Communicated Well	300+	84%	-	80%
Home Recovery Information Given	300+	81%	-	82%
Hospital Given 9 or 10 on 10 Point Scale	300+	67%	-	67%
Meds 'Always' Explained Before Given	300+	60%	-	60%
Nurses 'Always' Communicated Well	300+	75%	-	76%
Pain 'Always' Well Controlled	300+	63%	-	69%
Room and Bathroom 'Always' Clean	300+	73%	-	71%
Timely Help 'Always' Received	300+	58%	-	64%
Would Definitely Recommend Hospital	300+	71%	-	69%

Jellico Community Hospital

188 Hospital Lane
Jellico, TN 37762
URL: www.jellicohospital.com
Type: Acute Care Hospitals
Ownership: Voluntary Non-Profit - Church

Phone: 423-784-7252
Fax: 423-784-1136

Emergency Services: Yes
Beds: 54

Key Personnel:
CEO/President . . . . David A Butler
Chief of Medical Staff . . . . David Bosscher, MD
Infection Control . . . . Judy McKiddy, RN
Operating Room . . . . Wilma Morgan
Quality Assurance . . . . Pam Hodge
Radiology . . . . Robert Anderson
Intensive Care Unit . . . . Joyee Reese, RN
Patient Relations . . . . Sharon Lewis

Measure	Cases	This Hosp.	State Avg.	U.S. Avg.
Heart Attack Care				
ACE Inhibitor or ARB for LVSD	0	-	96%	96%
Aspirin at Arrival	9	100%	98%	99%
Aspirin at Discharge[1]	1	100%	99%	98%
Beta Blocker at Discharge[1]	2	100%	98%	98%
Fibrinolytic Medication Timing	0	-	67%	55%
PCI Within 90 Minutes of Arrival	0	-	91%	90%
Smoking Cessation Advice	0	-	100%	99%
Chest Pain/Possible Heart Attack Care				
Aspirin at Arrival	71	92%	95%	95%
Median Time to ECG (minutes)	73	10	8	8
Median Time to Transfer (minutes)[1,3]	7	93	65	61
Fibrinolytic Medication Timing[1]	3	33%	49%	54%
Heart Failure Care				
ACE Inhibitor or ARB for LVSD[1]	13	92%	95%	94%
Discharge Instructions	48	98%	88%	88%
Evaluation of LVS Function	54	100%	97%	98%
Smoking Cessation Advice[1]	16	100%	99%	98%
Pneumonia Care				
Appropriate Initial Antibiotic	73	89%	92%	92%
Blood Culture Timing	113	96%	97%	96%
Influenza Vaccine	73	93%	93%	91%
Initial Antibiotic Timing	112	97%	96%	95%
Pneumococcal Vaccine	98	98%	95%	93%
Smoking Cessation Advice	88	99%	99%	97%
Surgical Care Improvement Project				
Appropriate VTP Within 24 Hours[1]	15	67%	92%	92%
Appropriate Hair Removal	56	100%	100%	99%
Appropriate Beta Blocker Usage[1]	13	100%	93%	93%
Controlled Postoperative Blood Glucose	0	-	93%	93%
Prophylactic Antibiotic Timing	37	89%	97%	97%
Prophylactic Antibiotic Timing (Outpatient)[1]	24	79%	94%	92%
Prophylactic Antibiotic Selection	33	97%	97%	97%
Prophylactic Antibiotic Select. (Outpatient)[1]	21	100%	94%	94%
Prophylactic Antibiotic Stopped	30	90%	94%	94%
Recommended VTP Ordered[1]	15	67%	94%	94%
Urinary Catheter Removal[1]	2	50%	90%	90%
Children's Asthma Care				
Received Systemic Corticosteroids	-	-	-	100%
Received Home Management Plan	-	-	-	71%
Received Reliever Medication	-	-	-	100%
Use of Medical Imaging				
Combination Abdominal CT Scan	216	0.588	0.219	0.191
Combination Chest CT Scan	199	0.754	0.102	0.054
Follow-up Mammogram/Ultrasound	308	15.9%	8%	8.4%
MRI for Low Back Pain	56	67.9%	30.7%	32.7%
Survey of Patients' Hospital Experiences				
Area Around Room 'Always' Quiet at Night	(a)	65%	-	58%
Doctors 'Always' Communicated Well	(a)	86%	-	80%
Home Recovery Information Given	(a)	82%	-	82%
Hospital Given 9 or 10 on 10 Point Scale	(a)	68%	-	67%
Meds 'Always' Explained Before Given	(a)	65%	-	60%
Nurses 'Always' Communicated Well	(a)	78%	-	76%
Pain 'Always' Well Controlled	(a)	70%	-	69%
Room and Bathroom 'Always' Clean	(a)	75%	-	71%
Timely Help 'Always' Received	(a)	61%	-	64%
Would Definitely Recommend Hospital	(a)	66%	-	69%

Franklin Woods Community Hospital

401 Princeton Rd
Johnson City, TN 37601
Type: Acute Care Hospitals
Ownership: Voluntary Non-Profit - Private

Phone: 423-854-5600
Fax: 423-854-5748

Emergency Services: Yes
Beds: 39

Key Personnel:
CEO/President . . . . John Melton
Chief of Medical Staff . . . . T Hopson
Emergency Room . . . . Atif Atyia

Measure	Cases	This Hosp.	State Avg.	U.S. Avg.
Heart Attack Care				
ACE Inhibitor or ARB for LVSD[5]	0	-	96%	96%
Aspirin at Arrival[5]	0	-	98%	99%
Aspirin at Discharge[5]	0	-	99%	98%
Beta Blocker at Discharge[5]	0	-	98%	98%
Fibrinolytic Medication Timing[5]	0	-	67%	55%
PCI Within 90 Minutes of Arrival[5]	0	-	91%	90%
Smoking Cessation Advice[5]	0	-	100%	99%
Chest Pain/Possible Heart Attack Care				
Aspirin at Arrival	135	87%	95%	95%
Median Time to ECG (minutes)	145	4	8	8
Median Time to Transfer (minutes)[1,3]	3	52	65	61
Fibrinolytic Medication Timing	0	-	49%	54%
Heart Failure Care				
ACE Inhibitor or ARB for LVSD[1,2]	4	100%	95%	94%
Discharge Instructions[1,2]	19	84%	88%	88%
Evaluation of LVS Function[2]	26	100%	97%	98%
Smoking Cessation Advice[1,2]	6	100%	99%	98%
Pneumonia Care				
Appropriate Initial Antibiotic[2]	83	92%	92%	92%
Blood Culture Timing[2]	93	98%	97%	96%
Influenza Vaccine[2]	62	97%	93%	91%
Initial Antibiotic Timing[2]	96	99%	96%	95%
Pneumococcal Vaccine[2]	69	100%	95%	93%
Smoking Cessation Advice[2]	62	100%	99%	97%
Surgical Care Improvement Project				
Appropriate VTP Within 24 Hours[5]	0	-	92%	92%
Appropriate Hair Removal[5]	0	-	100%	99%
Appropriate Beta Blocker Usage[5]	0	-	93%	93%
Controlled Postoperative Blood Glucose[5]	0	-	93%	93%
Prophylactic Antibiotic Timing[5]	0	-	97%	97%
Prophylactic Antibiotic Timing (Outpatient)[5]	0	-	94%	92%
Prophylactic Antibiotic Selection[5]	0	-	97%	97%
Prophylactic Antibiotic Select. (Outpatient)[5]	0	-	94%	94%
Prophylactic Antibiotic Stopped[5]	0	-	94%	94%
Recommended VTP Ordered[5]	0	-	94%	94%
Urinary Catheter Removal[5]	0	-	90%	90%
Children's Asthma Care				
Received Systemic Corticosteroids	-	-	-	100%
Received Home Management Plan	-	-	-	71%
Received Reliever Medication	-	-	-	100%
Use of Medical Imaging				
Combination Abdominal CT Scan	420	0.333	0.219	0.191
Combination Chest CT Scan	200	0.455	0.102	0.054
Follow-up Mammogram/Ultrasound[5]	0	-	8%	8.4%
MRI for Low Back Pain	127	20.5%	30.7%	32.7%
Survey of Patients' Hospital Experiences				
Area Around Room 'Always' Quiet at Night	(a)	59%	-	58%
Doctors 'Always' Communicated Well	(a)	73%	-	80%
Home Recovery Information Given	(a)	85%	-	82%
Hospital Given 9 or 10 on 10 Point Scale	(a)	69%	-	67%
Meds 'Always' Explained Before Given	(a)	61%	-	60%
Nurses 'Always' Communicated Well	(a)	79%	-	76%
Pain 'Always' Well Controlled	(a)	75%	-	69%
Room and Bathroom 'Always' Clean	(a)	71%	-	71%
Timely Help 'Always' Received	(a)	65%	-	64%
Would Definitely Recommend Hospital	(a)	72%	-	69%

Johnson City Medical Center

400 N State of Franklin Rd | Phone: 423-431-6111
Johnson City, TN 37604 | Fax: 423-431-2910
URL: www.msha.com
Type: Acute Care Hospitals | Emergency Services: Yes
Ownership: Voluntary Non-Profit - Private | Beds: 488

Key Personnel:
CEO/President. . . . . Dennis Vonderfecht
Cardiac Laboratory. . . . . Sindy Salyer
Chief of Medical Staff . . . . Kenneth Marshall, MD
Operating Room. . . . . Chris York
Radiology. . . . . George Spence, MD
Emergency Room . . . . Candace Jennings
Intensive Care Unit. . . . . Gayle Broyles
Patient Relations . . . . Tom Tull

Measure	Cases	This Hosp.	State Avg.	U.S. Avg.
Heart Attack Care				
ACE Inhibitor or ARB for LVSD[2]	51	92%	96%	96%
Aspirin at Arrival[2]	140	98%	98%	99%
Aspirin at Discharge[2]	284	99%	99%	98%
Beta Blocker at Discharge[2]	280	97%	98%	98%
Fibrinolytic Medication Timing[2]	0	-	67%	55%
PCI Within 90 Minutes of Arrival[2]	27	89%	91%	90%
Smoking Cessation Advice[2]	112	100%	100%	99%
Chest Pain/Possible Heart Attack Care				
Aspirin at Arrival[1,3]	5	80%	95%	95%
Median Time to ECG (minutes)[1,3]	5	3	8	8
Median Time to Transfer (minutes)[5]	0	-	65	61
Fibrinolytic Medication Timing[3]	0	-	49%	54%
Heart Failure Care				
ACE Inhibitor or ARB for LVSD[2]	109	87%	95%	94%
Discharge Instructions[2]	231	79%	88%	88%
Evaluation of LVS Function[2]	298	99%	97%	98%
Smoking Cessation Advice[2]	53	100%	99%	98%
Pneumonia Care				
Appropriate Initial Antibiotic[2]	72	92%	92%	92%
Blood Culture Timing[2]	99	87%	97%	96%
Influenza Vaccine[2]	106	89%	93%	91%
Initial Antibiotic Timing[2]	123	90%	96%	95%
Pneumococcal Vaccine[2]	119	95%	95%	93%
Smoking Cessation Advice[2]	71	100%	99%	97%
Surgical Care Improvement Project				
Appropriate VTP Within 24 Hours[2]	172	78%	92%	92%
Appropriate Hair Removal[2]	634	100%	100%	99%
Appropriate Beta Blocker Usage[2]	239	96%	93%	93%
Controlled Postoperative Blood Glucose[2]	139	88%	93%	93%
Prophylactic Antibiotic Timing[2]	443	98%	97%	97%
Prophylactic Antibiotic Timing (Outpatient)	681	83%	94%	92%
Prophylactic Antibiotic Selection[2]	452	99%	97%	97%
Prophylactic Antibiotic Select. (Outpatient)	674	86%	94%	94%
Prophylactic Antibiotic Stopped[2]	421	81%	94%	94%
Recommended VTP Ordered[2]	173	83%	94%	94%
Urinary Catheter Removal[2]	158	89%	90%	90%
Children's Asthma Care				
Received Systemic Corticosteroids[2]	66	97%	-	100%
Received Home Management Plan[2]	66	9%	-	71%
Received Reliever Medication[2]	66	100%	-	100%
Use of Medical Imaging				
Combination Abdominal CT Scan	1,194	0.349	0.219	0.191
Combination Chest CT Scan	813	0.418	0.102	0.054
Follow-up Mammogram/Ultrasound	2,602	7.6%	8%	8.4%
MRI for Low Back Pain	414	27.3%	30.7%	32.7%
Survey of Patients' Hospital Experiences				
Area Around Room 'Always' Quiet at Night	300+	54%	-	58%
Doctors 'Always' Communicated Well	300+	76%	-	80%
Home Recovery Information Given	300+	81%	-	82%
Hospital Given 9 or 10 on 10 Point Scale	300+	68%	-	67%
Meds 'Always' Explained Before Given	300+	62%	-	60%
Nurses 'Always' Communicated Well	300+	77%	-	76%
Pain 'Always' Well Controlled	300+	66%	-	69%
Room and Bathroom 'Always' Clean	300+	64%	-	71%
Timely Help 'Always' Received	300+	64%	-	64%
Would Definitely Recommend Hospital	300+	70%	-	69%

Johnson City Specialty Hospital

203 E Watauga Ave | Phone: 423-434-1400
Johnson City, TN 37601 | Fax: 423-979-6163
Type: Acute Care Hospitals | Emergency Services: No
Ownership: Voluntary Non-Profit - Private | Beds: 49

Key Personnel:
CEO/President. . . . . Dennis Vonderfecht

Measure	Cases	This Hosp.	State Avg.	U.S. Avg.
Heart Attack Care				
ACE Inhibitor or ARB for LVSD[5]	0	-	96%	96%
Aspirin at Arrival[5]	0	-	98%	99%
Aspirin at Discharge[5]	0	-	99%	98%
Beta Blocker at Discharge[5]	0	-	98%	98%
Fibrinolytic Medication Timing[5]	0	-	67%	55%
PCI Within 90 Minutes of Arrival[5]	0	-	91%	90%
Smoking Cessation Advice[5]	0	-	100%	99%
Chest Pain/Possible Heart Attack Care				
Aspirin at Arrival[5]	0	-	95%	95%
Median Time to ECG (minutes)[5]	0	-	8	8
Median Time to Transfer (minutes)[5]	0	-	65	61
Fibrinolytic Medication Timing[5]	0	-	49%	54%
Heart Failure Care				
ACE Inhibitor or ARB for LVSD[5]	0	-	95%	94%
Discharge Instructions[5]	0	-	88%	88%
Evaluation of LVS Function[5]	0	-	97%	98%
Smoking Cessation Advice[5]	0	-	99%	98%
Pneumonia Care				
Appropriate Initial Antibiotic[5]	0	-	92%	92%
Blood Culture Timing[5]	0	-	97%	96%
Influenza Vaccine[5]	0	-	93%	91%
Initial Antibiotic Timing[5]	0	-	96%	95%
Pneumococcal Vaccine[5]	0	-	95%	93%
Smoking Cessation Advice[5]	0	-	99%	97%
Surgical Care Improvement Project				
Appropriate VTP Within 24 Hours[1,2]	3	100%	92%	92%
Appropriate Hair Removal[2]	33	100%	100%	99%
Appropriate Beta Blocker Usage[1,2]	5	80%	93%	93%
Controlled Postoperative Blood Glucose[2]	0	-	93%	93%
Prophylactic Antibiotic Timing[2]	26	100%	97%	97%
Prophylactic Antibiotic Timing (Outpatient)	280	99%	94%	92%
Prophylactic Antibiotic Selection[2]	26	88%	97%	97%
Prophylactic Antibiotic Select. (Outpatient)	280	94%	94%	94%
Prophylactic Antibiotic Stopped[2]	25	84%	94%	94%
Recommended VTP Ordered[1,2]	3	100%	94%	94%
Urinary Catheter Removal[2]	0	-	90%	90%
Children's Asthma Care				
Received Systemic Corticosteroids	-	-	-	100%
Received Home Management Plan	-	-	-	71%
Received Reliever Medication	-	-	-	100%
Use of Medical Imaging				
Combination Abdominal CT Scan[5]	0	-	0.219	0.191
Combination Chest CT Scan[5]	0	-	0.102	0.054
Follow-up Mammogram/Ultrasound	114	7.9%	8%	8.4%
MRI for Low Back Pain[5]	0	-	30.7%	32.7%
Survey of Patients' Hospital Experiences				
Area Around Room 'Always' Quiet at Night	300+	75%	-	58%
Doctors 'Always' Communicated Well	300+	92%	-	80%
Home Recovery Information Given	300+	90%	-	82%
Hospital Given 9 or 10 on 10 Point Scale	300+	90%	-	67%
Meds 'Always' Explained Before Given	300+	74%	-	60%
Nurses 'Always' Communicated Well	300+	89%	-	76%
Pain 'Always' Well Controlled	300+	85%	-	69%
Room and Bathroom 'Always' Clean	300+	85%	-	71%
Timely Help 'Always' Received	300+	81%	-	64%
Would Definitely Recommend Hospital	300+	94%	-	69%

Indian Path Medical Center

2000 Brookside Dr | Phone: 423-431-1941
Kingsport, TN 37660
URL: www.msha.com
Type: Acute Care Hospitals | Emergency Services: Yes
Ownership: Voluntary Non-Profit - Private | Beds: 261

Key Personnel:
CEO/President. . . . . Monty McLauren
Emergency Room . . . . EC Goulding, MD
Hemotology Center . . . . Kyle Colvett MD

Measure	Cases	This Hosp.	State Avg.	U.S. Avg.
Heart Attack Care				
ACE Inhibitor or ARB for LVSD[1,2]	14	93%	96%	96%
Aspirin at Arrival[2]	46	100%	98%	99%
Aspirin at Discharge[2]	42	100%	99%	98%
Beta Blocker at Discharge[2]	45	100%	98%	98%
Fibrinolytic Medication Timing[2]	0	-	67%	55%
PCI Within 90 Minutes of Arrival[1,2]	3	100%	91%	90%
Smoking Cessation Advice[1,2]	13	100%	100%	99%
Chest Pain/Possible Heart Attack Care				
Aspirin at Arrival	34	94%	95%	95%
Median Time to ECG (minutes)	35	4	8	8
Median Time to Transfer (minutes)[1,3]	8	48	65	61
Fibrinolytic Medication Timing	0	-	49%	54%
Heart Failure Care				
ACE Inhibitor or ARB for LVSD[2]	37	100%	95%	94%
Discharge Instructions[2]	130	85%	88%	88%
Evaluation of LVS Function[2]	164	99%	97%	98%
Smoking Cessation Advice[2]	34	100%	99%	98%
Pneumonia Care				
Appropriate Initial Antibiotic[2]	76	93%	92%	92%
Blood Culture Timing[2]	110	96%	97%	96%
Influenza Vaccine[2]	85	95%	93%	91%
Initial Antibiotic Timing[2]	109	95%	96%	95%
Pneumococcal Vaccine[2]	140	96%	95%	93%
Smoking Cessation Advice[2]	68	100%	99%	97%
Surgical Care Improvement Project				
Appropriate VTP Within 24 Hours[2]	185	97%	92%	92%
Appropriate Hair Removal[2]	394	98%	100%	99%
Appropriate Beta Blocker Usage[2]	103	94%	93%	93%
Controlled Postoperative Blood Glucose[2]	0	-	93%	93%
Prophylactic Antibiotic Timing[2]	273	100%	97%	97%
Prophylactic Antibiotic Timing (Outpatient)	225	92%	94%	92%
Prophylactic Antibiotic Selection[2]	275	99%	97%	97%
Prophylactic Antibiotic Select. (Outpatient)	239	91%	94%	94%
Prophylactic Antibiotic Stopped[2]	256	96%	94%	94%
Recommended VTP Ordered[2]	186	98%	94%	94%
Urinary Catheter Removal[2]	35	94%	90%	90%
Children's Asthma Care				
Received Systemic Corticosteroids	-	-	-	100%
Received Home Management Plan	-	-	-	71%
Received Reliever Medication	-	-	-	100%
Use of Medical Imaging				
Combination Abdominal CT Scan	391	0.565	0.219	0.191
Combination Chest CT Scan	177	0.520	0.102	0.054
Follow-up Mammogram/Ultrasound	598	8.4%	8%	8.4%
MRI for Low Back Pain	105	30.5%	30.7%	32.7%
Survey of Patients' Hospital Experiences				
Area Around Room 'Always' Quiet at Night	300+	57%	-	58%
Doctors 'Always' Communicated Well	300+	81%	-	80%
Home Recovery Information Given	300+	83%	-	82%
Hospital Given 9 or 10 on 10 Point Scale	300+	71%	-	67%
Meds 'Always' Explained Before Given	300+	59%	-	60%
Nurses 'Always' Communicated Well	300+	78%	-	76%
Pain 'Always' Well Controlled	300+	71%	-	69%
Room and Bathroom 'Always' Clean	300+	70%	-	71%
Timely Help 'Always' Received	300+	65%	-	64%
Would Definitely Recommend Hospital	300+	74%	-	69%

NOTE: Hospital profiles are in alphabetical order by state, then city, then hospital within the city; Rankings exclude hospitals with less than 25 cases except for patient surveys which excludes hospitals with less than 100 cases; (a) 100–299 cases; (1) The number of cases is too small to be sure how well a hospital is performing; (2) The hospital indicated that the data submitted for this measure were based on a sample of cases; (3) Data was collected during a shorter time period (fewer quarters) than the maximum possible time for this measure; (4) Suppressed for one or more quarters by CMS; (5) No data is available from the hospital for this measure; (6) Fewer than 100 patients completed the HCAHPS survey. Use these rates with caution, as the number of surveys may be too low to reliably assess hospital performance; (7) Survey results are based on less than 12 months of data; (8) Survey results are not available for this reporting period; (9) No or very few patients were eligible for the HCAHPS survey. The scores shown, if any, reflect a very small number of surveys; (10) A state average was not calculated because too few hospitals in the state submitted data; (11) There were discrepancies in the data collection process; Please refer to the User's Guide for a full explanation of data.

Wellmont Holston Valley Medical Center

130 West Ravine Road
Kingsport, TN 37662
URL: www.wellmont.org
Phone: 423-224-4000
Fax: 423-224-6419
Type: Acute Care Hospitals
Emergency Services: Yes
Ownership: Voluntary Non-Profit - Private
Beds: 540

Key Personnel:
CEO/President. . . . . Virginia Frank
Chief of Medical Staff. . . . . Bruce S. Grover, MD
Infection Control. . . . . Eleanor Duncan
Operating Room. . . . . Ilene Hess, RN
Pediatric Ambulatory Care . . . . . . Art Garrett, MD
Pediatric In-Patient Care . . . . Art Garrett, MD
Quality Assurance . . . . Justine Hill
Radiology. . . . . Larry Westerfield, MD

Measure	Cases	This Hosp.	State Avg.	U.S. Avg.
Heart Attack Care				
ACE Inhibitor or ARB for LVSD[2]	60	98%	96%	96%
Aspirin at Arrival[2]	124	98%	98%	99%
Aspirin at Discharge[2]	259	100%	99%	98%
Beta Blocker at Discharge[2]	257	100%	98%	98%
Fibrinolytic Medication Timing[1,2]	1	0%	67%	55%
PCI Within 90 Minutes of Arrival[1,2]	24	96%	91%	90%
Smoking Cessation Advice[2]	104	100%	100%	99%
Chest Pain/Possible Heart Attack Care				
Aspirin at Arrival[1,3]	4	75%	95%	95%
Median Time to ECG (minutes)[1,3]	4	8	8	8
Median Time to Transfer (minutes)[5]	0	-	65	61
Fibrinolytic Medication Timing[3]	0	-	49%	54%
Heart Failure Care				
ACE Inhibitor or ARB for LVSD[2]	109	98%	95%	94%
Discharge Instructions[2]	231	99%	88%	88%
Evaluation of LVS Function[2]	272	97%	97%	98%
Smoking Cessation Advice[2]	57	98%	99%	98%
Pneumonia Care				
Appropriate Initial Antibiotic[2]	57	88%	92%	92%
Blood Culture Timing[2]	94	91%	97%	96%
Influenza Vaccine[2]	76	83%	93%	91%
Initial Antibiotic Timing[2]	88	93%	96%	95%
Pneumococcal Vaccine[2]	109	87%	95%	93%
Smoking Cessation Advice[2]	51	98%	99%	97%
Surgical Care Improvement Project				
Appropriate VTP Within 24 Hours[2]	151	97%	92%	92%
Appropriate Hair Removal[2]	557	100%	100%	99%
Appropriate Beta Blocker Usage[2]	225	91%	93%	93%
Controlled Postoperative Blood Glucose[2]	130	98%	93%	93%
Prophylactic Antibiotic Timing[2]	400	98%	97%	97%
Prophylactic Antibiotic Timing (Outpatient)	561	95%	94%	92%
Prophylactic Antibiotic Selection[2]	401	98%	97%	97%
Prophylactic Antibiotic Select. (Outpatient)	561	88%	94%	94%
Prophylactic Antibiotic Stopped[2]	377	97%	94%	94%
Recommended VTP Ordered[2]	151	99%	94%	94%
Urinary Catheter Removal[2]	130	85%	90%	90%
Children's Asthma Care				
Received Systemic Corticosteroids	-	-	-	100%
Received Home Management Plan	-	-	-	71%
Received Reliever Medication	-	-	-	100%
Use of Medical Imaging				
Combination Abdominal CT Scan	540	0.256	0.219	0.191
Combination Chest CT Scan	289	0.024	0.102	0.054
Follow-up Mammogram/Ultrasound	1,696	4.0%	8%	8.4%
MRI for Low Back Pain[1]	45	28.9%	30.7%	32.7%
Survey of Patients' Hospital Experiences				
Area Around Room 'Always' Quiet at Night	300+	55%	-	58%
Doctors 'Always' Communicated Well	300+	83%	-	80%
Home Recovery Information Given	300+	79%	-	82%
Hospital Given 9 or 10 on 10 Point Scale	300+	64%	-	67%
Meds 'Always' Explained Before Given	300+	59%	-	60%
Nurses 'Always' Communicated Well	300+	76%	-	76%
Pain 'Always' Well Controlled	300+	69%	-	69%
Room and Bathroom 'Always' Clean	300+	69%	-	71%
Timely Help 'Always' Received	300+	62%	-	64%
Would Definitely Recommend Hospital	300+	73%	-	69%

Baptist Hospital West

10820 Parkside Drive
Knoxville, TN 37934
Phone: 865-218-7090
Type: Acute Care Hospitals
Emergency Services: Yes
Ownership: Voluntary Non-Profit - Private

Measure	Cases	This Hosp.	State Avg.	U.S. Avg.
Heart Attack Care				
ACE Inhibitor or ARB for LVSD	-	-	96%	96%
Aspirin at Arrival	-	-	98%	99%
Aspirin at Discharge	-	-	99%	98%
Beta Blocker at Discharge	-	-	98%	98%
Fibrinolytic Medication Timing	-	-	67%	55%
PCI Within 90 Minutes of Arrival	-	-	91%	90%
Smoking Cessation Advice	-	-	100%	99%
Chest Pain/Possible Heart Attack Care				
Aspirin at Arrival	-	-	95%	95%
Median Time to ECG (minutes)	-	-	8	8
Median Time to Transfer (minutes)	-	-	65	61
Fibrinolytic Medication Timing	-	-	49%	54%
Heart Failure Care				
ACE Inhibitor or ARB for LVSD	-	-	95%	94%
Discharge Instructions	-	-	88%	88%
Evaluation of LVS Function	-	-	97%	98%
Smoking Cessation Advice	-	-	99%	98%
Pneumonia Care				
Appropriate Initial Antibiotic	-	-	92%	92%
Blood Culture Timing	-	-	97%	96%
Influenza Vaccine	-	-	93%	91%
Initial Antibiotic Timing	-	-	96%	95%
Pneumococcal Vaccine	-	-	95%	93%
Smoking Cessation Advice	-	-	99%	97%
Surgical Care Improvement Project				
Appropriate VTP Within 24 Hours	-	-	92%	92%
Appropriate Hair Removal	-	-	100%	99%
Appropriate Beta Blocker Usage	-	-	93%	93%
Controlled Postoperative Blood Glucose	-	-	93%	93%
Prophylactic Antibiotic Timing	-	-	97%	97%
Prophylactic Antibiotic Timing (Outpatient)	-	-	94%	92%
Prophylactic Antibiotic Selection	-	-	97%	97%
Prophylactic Antibiotic Select. (Outpatient)	-	-	94%	94%
Prophylactic Antibiotic Stopped	-	-	94%	94%
Recommended VTP Ordered	-	-	94%	94%
Urinary Catheter Removal	-	-	90%	90%
Children's Asthma Care				
Received Systemic Corticosteroids	-	-	-	100%
Received Home Management Plan	-	-	-	71%
Received Reliever Medication	-	-	-	100%
Use of Medical Imaging				
Combination Abdominal CT Scan	-	-	0.219	0.191
Combination Chest CT Scan	-	-	0.102	0.054
Follow-up Mammogram/Ultrasound	-	-	8%	8.4%
MRI for Low Back Pain	-	-	30.7%	32.7%
Survey of Patients' Hospital Experiences				
Area Around Room 'Always' Quiet at Night	-	-	-	58%
Doctors 'Always' Communicated Well	-	-	-	80%
Home Recovery Information Given	-	-	-	82%
Hospital Given 9 or 10 on 10 Point Scale	-	-	-	67%
Meds 'Always' Explained Before Given	-	-	-	60%
Nurses 'Always' Communicated Well	-	-	-	76%
Pain 'Always' Well Controlled	-	-	-	69%
Room and Bathroom 'Always' Clean	-	-	-	71%
Timely Help 'Always' Received	-	-	-	64%
Would Definitely Recommend Hospital	-	-	-	69%

Fort Sanders Regional Medical Center

1901 W Clinch Ave
Knoxville, TN 37916
URL: www.fsregional.com
Phone: 865-541-1101
Fax: 865-541-2840
Type: Acute Care Hospitals
Emergency Services: Yes
Ownership: Voluntary Non-Profit - Private
Beds: 541

Key Personnel:
CEO/President. . . . . Keith Altshuler
Chief of Medical Staff. . . . . David Ayers
Infection Control. . . . . John Adams, MD
Radiology. . . . . Steven J Addonizio
Anesthesiology. . . . . Wilson Beamer, MD
Emergency Room . . . . Charles Adams, MD

Measure	Cases	This Hosp.	State Avg.	U.S. Avg.
Heart Attack Care				
ACE Inhibitor or ARB for LVSD	53	100%	96%	96%
Aspirin at Arrival	166	100%	98%	99%
Aspirin at Discharge	302	100%	99%	98%
Beta Blocker at Discharge	287	100%	98%	98%
Fibrinolytic Medication Timing	0	-	67%	55%
PCI Within 90 Minutes of Arrival	57	98%	91%	90%
Smoking Cessation Advice	120	100%	100%	99%
Chest Pain/Possible Heart Attack Care				
Aspirin at Arrival[1,3]	1	0%	95%	95%
Median Time to ECG (minutes)[1,3]	1	0	8	8
Median Time to Transfer (minutes)[5]	0	-	65	61
Fibrinolytic Medication Timing[5]	0	-	49%	54%
Heart Failure Care				
ACE Inhibitor or ARB for LVSD	123	100%	95%	94%
Discharge Instructions	353	98%	88%	88%
Evaluation of LVS Function	424	100%	97%	98%
Smoking Cessation Advice	73	100%	99%	98%
Pneumonia Care				
Appropriate Initial Antibiotic	198	94%	92%	92%
Blood Culture Timing	357	99%	97%	96%
Influenza Vaccine	244	100%	93%	91%
Initial Antibiotic Timing	329	99%	96%	95%
Pneumococcal Vaccine	346	100%	95%	93%
Smoking Cessation Advice	239	100%	99%	97%
Surgical Care Improvement Project				
Appropriate VTP Within 24 Hours[2]	310	94%	92%	92%
Appropriate Hair Removal[2]	1,004	100%	100%	99%
Appropriate Beta Blocker Usage[2]	201	98%	93%	93%
Controlled Postoperative Blood Glucose[2]	153	97%	93%	93%
Prophylactic Antibiotic Timing[2]	772	98%	97%	97%
Prophylactic Antibiotic Timing (Outpatient)	719	95%	94%	92%
Prophylactic Antibiotic Selection[2]	773	99%	97%	97%
Prophylactic Antibiotic Select. (Outpatient)	708	97%	94%	94%
Prophylactic Antibiotic Stopped[2]	742	99%	94%	94%
Recommended VTP Ordered[2]	311	95%	94%	94%
Urinary Catheter Removal[2]	205	95%	90%	90%
Children's Asthma Care				
Received Systemic Corticosteroids	-	-	-	100%
Received Home Management Plan	-	-	-	71%
Received Reliever Medication	-	-	-	100%
Use of Medical Imaging				
Combination Abdominal CT Scan	740	0.141	0.219	0.191
Combination Chest CT Scan	692	0.103	0.102	0.054
Follow-up Mammogram/Ultrasound	593	6.4%	8%	8.4%
MRI for Low Back Pain	248	33.1%	30.7%	32.7%
Survey of Patients' Hospital Experiences				
Area Around Room 'Always' Quiet at Night	300+	65%	-	58%
Doctors 'Always' Communicated Well	300+	83%	-	80%
Home Recovery Information Given	300+	83%	-	82%
Hospital Given 9 or 10 on 10 Point Scale	300+	75%	-	67%
Meds 'Always' Explained Before Given	300+	59%	-	60%
Nurses 'Always' Communicated Well	300+	80%	-	76%
Pain 'Always' Well Controlled	300+	69%	-	69%
Room and Bathroom 'Always' Clean	300+	69%	-	71%
Timely Help 'Always' Received	300+	64%	-	64%
Would Definitely Recommend Hospital	300+	76%	-	69%

NOTE: Hospital profiles are in alphabetical order by state, then city, then hospital within the city; Rankings exclude hospitals with less than 25 cases except for patient surveys which excludes hospitals with less than 100 cases; (a) 100–299 cases; (1) The number of cases is too small to be sure how well a hospital is performing; (2) The hospital indicated that the data submitted for this measure were based on a sample of cases; (3) Data was collected during a shorter time period (fewer quarters) than the maximum possible time for this measure; (4) Suppressed for one or more quarters by CMS; (5) No data is available from the hospital for this measure; (6) Fewer than 100 patients completed the HCAHPS survey. Use these rates with caution, as the number of surveys may be too low to reliably assess hospital performance; (7) Survey results are based on less than 12 months of data; (8) Survey results are not available for this reporting period; (9) No or very few patients were eligible for the HCAHPS survey. The scores shown, if any, reflect a very small number of surveys; (10) A state average was not calculated because too few hospitals in the state submitted data; (11) There were discrepancies in the data collection process; Please refer to the User's Guide for a full explanation of data.

Mercy Medical Center

900 East Oak Hill Avenue
Knoxville, TN 37917
URL: www.stmaryshealth.com
Type: Acute Care Hospitals
Ownership: Voluntary Non-Profit - Church
Phone: 865-545-8000
Fax: 865-545-6732
Emergency Services: Yes
Beds: 506

Key Personnel:
Chief of Medical Staff . . . . Joseph Minardo
Infection Control . . . . Stephanie Brooks
Operating Room . . . . Kathy Romero
Quality Assurance . . . . Carol Kortz
Radiology . . . . William McKissick
Anesthesiology . . . . Paul Baker
Intensive Care Unit . . . . Doug Clark

Measure	Cases	This Hosp.	State Avg.	U.S. Avg.
Heart Attack Care				
ACE Inhibitor or ARB for LVSD	111	95%	96%	96%
Aspirin at Arrival	337	99%	98%	99%
Aspirin at Discharge	559	99%	99%	98%
Beta Blocker at Discharge	554	99%	98%	98%
Fibrinolytic Medication Timing	0	-	67%	55%
PCI Within 90 Minutes of Arrival	48	81%	91%	90%
Smoking Cessation Advice	255	100%	100%	99%
Chest Pain/Possible Heart Attack Care				
Aspirin at Arrival[1]	19	74%	95%	95%
Median Time to ECG (minutes)[1]	17	11	8	8
Median Time to Transfer (minutes)[1,3]	2	262876	65	61
Fibrinolytic Medication Timing	0	-	49%	54%
Heart Failure Care				
ACE Inhibitor or ARB for LVSD	171	99%	95%	94%
Discharge Instructions	487	87%	88%	88%
Evaluation of LVS Function	589	100%	97%	98%
Smoking Cessation Advice	128	99%	99%	98%
Pneumonia Care				
Appropriate Initial Antibiotic	469	93%	92%	92%
Blood Culture Timing	649	96%	97%	96%
Influenza Vaccine	474	98%	93%	91%
Initial Antibiotic Timing	628	95%	96%	95%
Pneumococcal Vaccine	595	98%	95%	93%
Smoking Cessation Advice	403	100%	99%	97%
Surgical Care Improvement Project				
Appropriate VTP Within 24 Hours[2]	611	91%	92%	92%
Appropriate Hair Removal[2]	2,647	100%	100%	99%
Appropriate Beta Blocker Usage[2]	867	95%	93%	93%
Controlled Postoperative Blood Glucose[2]	388	94%	93%	93%
Prophylactic Antibiotic Timing[2]	2,001	99%	97%	97%
Prophylactic Antibiotic Timing (Outpatient)	1,180	94%	94%	92%
Prophylactic Antibiotic Selection[2]	2,023	99%	97%	97%
Prophylactic Antibiotic Select. (Outpatient)	1,164	92%	94%	94%
Prophylactic Antibiotic Stopped[2]	1,934	98%	94%	94%
Recommended VTP Ordered[2]	613	92%	94%	94%
Urinary Catheter Removal	870	97%	90%	90%
Children's Asthma Care				
Received Systemic Corticosteroids	-	-	-	100%
Received Home Management Plan	-	-	-	71%
Received Reliever Medication	-	-	-	100%
Use of Medical Imaging				
Combination Abdominal CT Scan	1,189	0.066	0.219	0.191
Combination Chest CT Scan	841	0.020	0.102	0.054
Follow-up Mammogram/Ultrasound	742	10.8%	8%	8.4%
MRI for Low Back Pain	383	29.0%	30.7%	32.7%
Survey of Patients' Hospital Experiences				
Area Around Room 'Always' Quiet at Night	300+	65%	-	58%
Doctors 'Always' Communicated Well	300+	82%	-	80%
Home Recovery Information Given	300+	83%	-	82%
Hospital Given 9 or 10 on 10 Point Scale	300+	72%	-	67%
Meds 'Always' Explained Before Given	300+	59%	-	60%
Nurses 'Always' Communicated Well	300+	77%	-	76%
Pain 'Always' Well Controlled	300+	71%	-	69%
Room and Bathroom 'Always' Clean	300+	71%	-	71%
Timely Help 'Always' Received	300+	65%	-	64%
Would Definitely Recommend Hospital	300+	76%	-	69%

Parkwest Medical Center

9352 Park West Blvd
Knoxville, TN 37923
URL: www.yesparkwest.com
Type: Acute Care Hospitals
Ownership: Voluntary Non-Profit - Private
Phone: 865-373-1000
Fax: 865-373-1012
Emergency Services: Yes
Beds: 414

Key Personnel:
CEO/President . . . . Rick Lassiter
Cardiac Laboratory . . . . Laura Zeletnac
Chief of Medical Staff . . . . Mitchell Dickson, MD
Infection Control . . . . Margaret Chambers, RN
Operating Room . . . . Brenda Ginn, RN
Quality Assurance . . . . Linda Tillman, RN
Radiology . . . . Jeffrey Roesch, MD

Measure	Cases	This Hosp.	State Avg.	U.S. Avg.
Heart Attack Care				
ACE Inhibitor or ARB for LVSD	84	95%	96%	96%
Aspirin at Arrival	333	99%	98%	99%
Aspirin at Discharge	506	100%	99%	98%
Beta Blocker at Discharge	505	99%	98%	98%
Fibrinolytic Medication Timing	0	-	67%	55%
PCI Within 90 Minutes of Arrival	78	92%	91%	90%
Smoking Cessation Advice	212	100%	100%	99%
Chest Pain/Possible Heart Attack Care				
Aspirin at Arrival[1]	18	72%	95%	95%
Median Time to ECG (minutes)[1]	19	10	8	8
Median Time to Transfer (minutes)[5]	0	-	65	61
Fibrinolytic Medication Timing[3]	0	-	49%	54%
Heart Failure Care				
ACE Inhibitor or ARB for LVSD	86	94%	95%	94%
Discharge Instructions	318	93%	88%	88%
Evaluation of LVS Function	396	99%	97%	98%
Smoking Cessation Advice	71	100%	99%	98%
Pneumonia Care				
Appropriate Initial Antibiotic	298	92%	92%	92%
Blood Culture Timing	413	96%	97%	96%
Influenza Vaccine	280	93%	93%	91%
Initial Antibiotic Timing	400	96%	96%	95%
Pneumococcal Vaccine	368	97%	95%	93%
Smoking Cessation Advice	141	100%	99%	97%
Surgical Care Improvement Project				
Appropriate VTP Within 24 Hours[2]	408	92%	92%	92%
Appropriate Hair Removal[2]	1,918	100%	100%	99%
Appropriate Beta Blocker Usage[2]	570	96%	93%	93%
Controlled Postoperative Blood Glucose[2]	341	89%	93%	93%
Prophylactic Antibiotic Timing[2]	1,671	99%	97%	97%
Prophylactic Antibiotic Timing (Outpatient)	1,443	95%	94%	92%
Prophylactic Antibiotic Selection[2]	1,686	100%	97%	97%
Prophylactic Antibiotic Select. (Outpatient)	1,424	97%	94%	94%
Prophylactic Antibiotic Stopped[2]	1,610	98%	94%	94%
Recommended VTP Ordered[2]	410	93%	94%	94%
Urinary Catheter Removal[2]	466	89%	90%	90%
Children's Asthma Care				
Received Systemic Corticosteroids	-	-	-	100%
Received Home Management Plan	-	-	-	71%
Received Reliever Medication	-	-	-	100%
Use of Medical Imaging				
Combination Abdominal CT Scan	885	0.155	0.219	0.191
Combination Chest CT Scan	682	0.076	0.102	0.054
Follow-up Mammogram/Ultrasound	779	6.4%	8%	8.4%
MRI for Low Back Pain	176	24.4%	30.7%	32.7%
Survey of Patients' Hospital Experiences				
Area Around Room 'Always' Quiet at Night	300+	69%	-	58%
Doctors 'Always' Communicated Well	300+	85%	-	80%
Home Recovery Information Given	300+	86%	-	82%
Hospital Given 9 or 10 on 10 Point Scale	300+	82%	-	67%
Meds 'Always' Explained Before Given	300+	66%	-	60%
Nurses 'Always' Communicated Well	300+	79%	-	76%
Pain 'Always' Well Controlled	300+	74%	-	69%
Room and Bathroom 'Always' Clean	300+	72%	-	71%
Timely Help 'Always' Received	300+	66%	-	64%
Would Definitely Recommend Hospital	300+	86%	-	69%

University of Tennessee Memorial Hospital

1924 Alcoa Highway
Knoxville, TN 37920
URL: www.utmedicalcenter.org
Type: Acute Care Hospitals
Ownership: Voluntary Non-Profit - Private
Phone: 865-544-9000
Fax: 865-670-6112
Emergency Services: Yes
Beds: 602

Key Personnel:
CEO/President . . . . Joseph Landsman
Chief of Medical Staff . . . . Raymond Dideter
Infection Control . . . . Eva Harris, RN
Operating Room . . . . Gregory J Mancini, RN
Pediatric Ambulatory Care . . . . . . Eddie Moore, MD
Pediatric In-Patient Care . . . . Eddie Moore, MD
Quality Assurance . . . . Frances Wiesener
Radiology . . . . James W Boyd

Measure	Cases	This Hosp.	State Avg.	U.S. Avg.
Heart Attack Care				
ACE Inhibitor or ARB for LVSD[2]	62	98%	96%	96%
Aspirin at Arrival[2]	212	100%	98%	99%
Aspirin at Discharge[2]	316	99%	99%	98%
Beta Blocker at Discharge[2]	321	99%	98%	98%
Fibrinolytic Medication Timing[2]	0	-	67%	55%
PCI Within 90 Minutes of Arrival[2]	61	89%	91%	90%
Smoking Cessation Advice[2]	156	100%	100%	99%
Chest Pain/Possible Heart Attack Care				
Aspirin at Arrival[1,3]	1	100%	95%	95%
Median Time to ECG (minutes)[1,3]	1	23	8	8
Median Time to Transfer (minutes)[5]	0	-	65	61
Fibrinolytic Medication Timing[5]	0	-	49%	54%
Heart Failure Care				
ACE Inhibitor or ARB for LVSD[2]	115	89%	95%	94%
Discharge Instructions[2]	276	86%	88%	88%
Evaluation of LVS Function[2]	323	100%	97%	98%
Smoking Cessation Advice[2]	64	100%	99%	98%
Pneumonia Care				
Appropriate Initial Antibiotic[2]	69	93%	92%	92%
Blood Culture Timing[2]	136	95%	97%	96%
Influenza Vaccine[2]	83	92%	93%	91%
Initial Antibiotic Timing[2]	143	97%	96%	95%
Pneumococcal Vaccine[2]	100	93%	95%	93%
Smoking Cessation Advice[2]	90	100%	99%	97%
Surgical Care Improvement Project				
Appropriate VTP Within 24 Hours[2]	207	99%	92%	92%
Appropriate Hair Removal[2]	658	100%	100%	99%
Appropriate Beta Blocker Usage[2]	225	100%	93%	93%
Controlled Postoperative Blood Glucose[2]	150	95%	93%	93%
Prophylactic Antibiotic Timing[2]	469	96%	97%	97%
Prophylactic Antibiotic Timing (Outpatient)	852	94%	94%	92%
Prophylactic Antibiotic Selection[2]	479	97%	97%	97%
Prophylactic Antibiotic Select. (Outpatient)	832	94%	94%	94%
Prophylactic Antibiotic Stopped[2]	441	92%	94%	94%
Recommended VTP Ordered[2]	207	99%	94%	94%
Urinary Catheter Removal[2]	174	97%	90%	90%
Children's Asthma Care				
Received Systemic Corticosteroids	-	-	-	100%
Received Home Management Plan	-	-	-	71%
Received Reliever Medication	-	-	-	100%
Use of Medical Imaging				
Combination Abdominal CT Scan	2,016	0.080	0.219	0.191
Combination Chest CT Scan	2,392	0.018	0.102	0.054
Follow-up Mammogram/Ultrasound	1,935	6.6%	8%	8.4%
MRI for Low Back Pain	323	23.2%	30.7%	32.7%
Survey of Patients' Hospital Experiences				
Area Around Room 'Always' Quiet at Night	300+	63%	-	58%
Doctors 'Always' Communicated Well	300+	83%	-	80%
Home Recovery Information Given	300+	82%	-	82%
Hospital Given 9 or 10 on 10 Point Scale	300+	76%	-	67%
Meds 'Always' Explained Before Given	300+	61%	-	60%
Nurses 'Always' Communicated Well	300+	81%	-	76%
Pain 'Always' Well Controlled	300+	72%	-	69%
Room and Bathroom 'Always' Clean	300+	75%	-	71%
Timely Help 'Always' Received	300+	63%	-	64%
Would Definitely Recommend Hospital	300+	82%	-	69%

NOTE: Hospital profiles are in alphabetical order by state, then city, then hospital within the city; Rankings exclude hospitals with less than 25 cases except for patient surveys which excludes hospitals with less than 100 cases; (a) 100–299 cases; (1) The number of cases is too small to be sure how well a hospital is performing; (2) The hospital indicated that the data submitted for this measure were based on a sample of cases; (3) Data was collected during a shorter time period (fewer quarters) than the maximum possible time for this measure; (4) Suppressed for one or more quarters by CMS; (5) No data is available from the hospital for this measure; (6) Fewer than 100 patients completed the HCAHPS survey. Use these rates with caution, as the number of surveys may be too low to reliably assess hospital performance; (7) Survey results are based on less than 12 months of data; (8) Survey results are not available for this reporting period; (9) No or very few patients were eligible for the HCAHPS survey. The scores shown, if any, reflect a very small number of surveys; (10) A state average was not calculated because too few hospitals in the state submitted data; (11) There were discrepancies in the data collection process; Please refer to the User's Guide for a full explanation of data.

Saint Mary's Medical Center of Campbell County

923 East Central Avenue Phone: 423-907-1200
La Follette, TN 37766 Fax: 423-907-1164
URL: www.stmaryshealth.com
Type: Acute Care Hospitals Emergency Services: Yes
Ownership: Voluntary Non-Profit - Church Beds: 164

Key Personnel:
Chief of Medical Staff.......... Errol Britto
Radiology.................. Thomas Cohen

Measure	Cases	This Hosp.	State Avg.	U.S. Avg.
Heart Attack Care				
ACE Inhibitor or ARB for LVSD[1]	2	100%	96%	96%
Aspirin at Arrival[1]	18	100%	98%	99%
Aspirin at Discharge[1]	13	100%	99%	98%
Beta Blocker at Discharge[1]	16	100%	98%	98%
Fibrinolytic Medication Timing	0	-	67%	55%
PCI Within 90 Minutes of Arrival	0	-	91%	90%
Smoking Cessation Advice[1]	4	100%	100%	99%
Chest Pain/Possible Heart Attack Care				
Aspirin at Arrival	136	95%	95%	95%
Median Time to ECG (minutes)	152	6	8	8
Median Time to Transfer (minutes)[1]	13	100	65	61
Fibrinolytic Medication Timing[1]	3	67%	49%	54%
Heart Failure Care				
ACE Inhibitor or ARB for LVSD[1]	19	100%	95%	94%
Discharge Instructions	129	98%	88%	88%
Evaluation of LVS Function	163	99%	97%	98%
Smoking Cessation Advice	31	100%	99%	98%
Pneumonia Care				
Appropriate Initial Antibiotic	185	94%	92%	92%
Blood Culture Timing	291	98%	97%	96%
Influenza Vaccine	190	96%	93%	91%
Initial Antibiotic Timing	300	99%	96%	95%
Pneumococcal Vaccine	251	95%	95%	93%
Smoking Cessation Advice	143	100%	99%	97%
Surgical Care Improvement Project				
Appropriate VTP Within 24 Hours[1]	6	67%	92%	92%
Appropriate Hair Removal[1]	9	100%	100%	99%
Appropriate Beta Blocker Usage[1]	4	75%	93%	93%
Controlled Postoperative Blood Glucose	0	-	93%	93%
Prophylactic Antibiotic Timing[1]	2	100%	97%	97%
Prophylactic Antibiotic Timing (Outpatient)	28	82%	94%	92%
Prophylactic Antibiotic Selection[1]	3	100%	97%	97%
Prophylactic Antibiotic Select. (Outpatient)[1]	23	96%	94%	94%
Prophylactic Antibiotic Stopped[1]	2	100%	94%	94%
Recommended VTP Ordered[1]	7	57%	94%	94%
Urinary Catheter Removal[1]	1	100%	90%	90%
Children's Asthma Care				
Received Systemic Corticosteroids	-	-	-	100%
Received Home Management Plan	-	-	-	71%
Received Reliever Medication	-	-	-	100%
Use of Medical Imaging				
Combination Abdominal CT Scan	256	0.344	0.219	0.191
Combination Chest CT Scan	206	0.180	0.102	0.054
Follow-up Mammogram/Ultrasound	320	2.8%	8%	8.4%
MRI for Low Back Pain	119	47.1%	30.7%	32.7%
Survey of Patients' Hospital Experiences				
Area Around Room 'Always' Quiet at Night	300+	57%	-	58%
Doctors 'Always' Communicated Well	300+	83%	-	80%
Home Recovery Information Given	300+	79%	-	82%
Hospital Given 9 or 10 on 10 Point Scale	300+	58%	-	67%
Meds 'Always' Explained Before Given	300+	62%	-	60%
Nurses 'Always' Communicated Well	300+	77%	-	76%
Pain 'Always' Well Controlled	300+	71%	-	69%
Room and Bathroom 'Always' Clean	300+	69%	-	71%
Timely Help 'Always' Received	300+	68%	-	64%
Would Definitely Recommend Hospital	300+	58%	-	69%

Macon County General Hospital

204 Medical Drive Phone: 615-666-2147
Lafayette, TN 37083 Fax: 615-666-7002
URL: www.mcgh.net
Type: Critical Access Hospitals Emergency Services: Yes
Ownership: Voluntary Non-Profit - Private Beds: 43

Key Personnel:
CEO/President............... Dennis A Wolford
Infection Control.............. Dixie Wooten, LPN
Emergency Room .... Hanna C Ilia, MD

Measure	Cases	This Hosp.	State Avg.	U.S. Avg.
Heart Attack Care				
ACE Inhibitor or ARB for LVSD	-	-	96%	96%
Aspirin at Arrival	-	-	98%	99%
Aspirin at Discharge	-	-	99%	98%
Beta Blocker at Discharge	-	-	98%	98%
Fibrinolytic Medication Timing	-	-	67%	55%
PCI Within 90 Minutes of Arrival	-	-	91%	90%
Smoking Cessation Advice	-	-	100%	99%
Chest Pain/Possible Heart Attack Care				
Aspirin at Arrival	71	93%	95%	95%
Median Time to ECG (minutes)	72	10	8	8
Median Time to Transfer (minutes)[3]	0	-	65	61
Fibrinolytic Medication Timing[1]	1	0%	49%	54%
Heart Failure Care				
ACE Inhibitor or ARB for LVSD	-	-	95%	94%
Discharge Instructions	-	-	88%	88%
Evaluation of LVS Function	-	-	97%	98%
Smoking Cessation Advice	-	-	99%	98%
Pneumonia Care				
Appropriate Initial Antibiotic	-	-	92%	92%
Blood Culture Timing	-	-	97%	96%
Influenza Vaccine	-	-	93%	91%
Initial Antibiotic Timing	-	-	96%	95%
Pneumococcal Vaccine	-	-	95%	93%
Smoking Cessation Advice	-	-	99%	97%
Surgical Care Improvement Project				
Appropriate VTP Within 24 Hours	-	-	92%	92%
Appropriate Hair Removal	-	-	100%	99%
Appropriate Beta Blocker Usage	-	-	93%	93%
Controlled Postoperative Blood Glucose	-	-	93%	93%
Prophylactic Antibiotic Timing	-	-	97%	97%
Prophylactic Antibiotic Timing (Outpatient)[5]	0	-	94%	92%
Prophylactic Antibiotic Selection	-	-	97%	97%
Prophylactic Antibiotic Select. (Outpatient)[5]	0	-	94%	94%
Prophylactic Antibiotic Stopped	-	-	94%	94%
Recommended VTP Ordered	-	-	94%	94%
Urinary Catheter Removal	-	-	90%	90%
Children's Asthma Care				
Received Systemic Corticosteroids	-	-	-	100%
Received Home Management Plan	-	-	-	71%
Received Reliever Medication	-	-	-	100%
Use of Medical Imaging				
Combination Abdominal CT Scan	105	0.581	0.219	0.191
Combination Chest CT Scan	85	0.494	0.102	0.054
Follow-up Mammogram/Ultrasound	155	23.2%	8%	8.4%
MRI for Low Back Pain[1]	36	27.8%	30.7%	32.7%
Survey of Patients' Hospital Experiences				
Area Around Room 'Always' Quiet at Night	-	-	-	58%
Doctors 'Always' Communicated Well	-	-	-	80%
Home Recovery Information Given	-	-	-	82%
Hospital Given 9 or 10 on 10 Point Scale	-	-	-	67%
Meds 'Always' Explained Before Given	-	-	-	60%
Nurses 'Always' Communicated Well	-	-	-	76%
Pain 'Always' Well Controlled	-	-	-	69%
Room and Bathroom 'Always' Clean	-	-	-	71%
Timely Help 'Always' Received	-	-	-	64%
Would Definitely Recommend Hospital	-	-	-	69%

Crockett Hospital

Hwy 43 S Box 847 Phone: 931-762-6571
Lawrenceburg, TN 38464 Fax: 931-766-3248
E-mail: robert.augustin@lifepointhospitals.com
URL: www.crocketthospital.com
Type: Acute Care Hospitals Emergency Services: Yes
Ownership: Proprietary Beds: 107

Key Personnel:
CEO/President............... Jack Buck
Chief of Medical Staff.......... Kimberly Goodemote
Radiology.................. William Wesley Brewer

Measure	Cases	This Hosp.	State Avg.	U.S. Avg.
Heart Attack Care				
ACE Inhibitor or ARB for LVSD[3]	0	-	96%	96%
Aspirin at Arrival[1,3]	2	100%	98%	99%
Aspirin at Discharge[1,3]	1	100%	99%	98%
Beta Blocker at Discharge[1,3]	1	100%	98%	98%
Fibrinolytic Medication Timing[3]	0	-	67%	55%
PCI Within 90 Minutes of Arrival[3]	0	-	91%	90%
Smoking Cessation Advice[3]	0	-	100%	99%
Chest Pain/Possible Heart Attack Care				
Aspirin at Arrival	240	98%	95%	95%
Median Time to ECG (minutes)	250	5	8	8
Median Time to Transfer (minutes)[1]	13	122	65	61
Fibrinolytic Medication Timing[1]	10	60%	49%	54%
Heart Failure Care				
ACE Inhibitor or ARB for LVSD[1]	17	94%	95%	94%
Discharge Instructions	58	91%	88%	88%
Evaluation of LVS Function	77	96%	97%	98%
Smoking Cessation Advice[1]	6	100%	99%	98%
Pneumonia Care				
Appropriate Initial Antibiotic	115	95%	92%	92%
Blood Culture Timing	108	92%	97%	96%
Influenza Vaccine	79	97%	93%	91%
Initial Antibiotic Timing	132	95%	96%	95%
Pneumococcal Vaccine	116	95%	95%	93%
Smoking Cessation Advice	48	100%	99%	97%
Surgical Care Improvement Project				
Appropriate VTP Within 24 Hours[1]	17	94%	92%	92%
Appropriate Hair Removal	41	100%	100%	99%
Appropriate Beta Blocker Usage[1]	10	100%	93%	93%
Controlled Postoperative Blood Glucose	0	-	93%	93%
Prophylactic Antibiotic Timing	26	100%	97%	97%
Prophylactic Antibiotic Timing (Outpatient)[1]	19	79%	94%	92%
Prophylactic Antibiotic Selection	26	100%	97%	97%
Prophylactic Antibiotic Select. (Outpatient)[1]	17	94%	94%	94%
Prophylactic Antibiotic Stopped	26	100%	94%	94%
Recommended VTP Ordered[1]	17	100%	94%	94%
Urinary Catheter Removal[1]	3	100%	90%	90%
Children's Asthma Care				
Received Systemic Corticosteroids	-	-	-	100%
Received Home Management Plan	-	-	-	71%
Received Reliever Medication	-	-	-	100%
Use of Medical Imaging				
Combination Abdominal CT Scan	405	0.210	0.219	0.191
Combination Chest CT Scan	393	0.023	0.102	0.054
Follow-up Mammogram/Ultrasound	662	10.1%	8%	8.4%
MRI for Low Back Pain	136	36.0%	30.7%	32.7%
Survey of Patients' Hospital Experiences				
Area Around Room 'Always' Quiet at Night	300+	64%	-	58%
Doctors 'Always' Communicated Well	300+	82%	-	80%
Home Recovery Information Given	300+	74%	-	82%
Hospital Given 9 or 10 on 10 Point Scale	300+	63%	-	67%
Meds 'Always' Explained Before Given	300+	56%	-	60%
Nurses 'Always' Communicated Well	300+	75%	-	76%
Pain 'Always' Well Controlled	300+	68%	-	69%
Room and Bathroom 'Always' Clean	300+	67%	-	71%
Timely Help 'Always' Received	300+	61%	-	64%
Would Definitely Recommend Hospital	300+	60%	-	69%

NOTE: Hospital profiles are in alphabetical order by state, then city, then hospital within the city; Rankings exclude hospitals with less than 25 cases except for patient surveys which excludes hospitals with less than 100 cases; (a) 100–299 cases; (1) The number of cases is too small to be sure how well a hospital is performing; (2) The hospital indicated that the data submitted for this measure were based on a sample of cases; (3) Data was collected during a shorter time period (fewer quarters) than the maximum possible time for this measure; (4) Suppressed for one or more quarters by CMS; (5) No data is available from the hospital for this measure; (6) Fewer than 100 patients completed the HCAHPS survey. Use these rates with caution, as the number of surveys may be too low to reliably assess hospital performance; (7) Survey results are based on less than 12 months of data; (8) Survey results are not available for this reporting period; (9) No or very few patients were eligible for the HCAHPS survey. The scores shown, if any, reflect a very small number of surveys; (10) A state average was not calculated because too few hospitals in the state submitted data; (11) There were discrepancies in the data collection process; Please refer to the User's Guide for a full explanation of data.

University Medical Center

1411 Baddour Parkway
Lebanon, TN 37087
URL: www.universitymedicalcenter.com
Type: Acute Care Hospitals
Ownership: Voluntary Non-Profit - Private
Phone: 615-444-8262
Fax: 615-443-2553
Emergency Services: Yes
Beds: 257

Key Personnel:
CEO/President. . . . . Mark Craford
Emergency Room . . . . Scott Giles, MD

Measure	Cases	This Hosp.	State Avg.	U.S. Avg.
Heart Attack Care				
ACE Inhibitor or ARB for LVSD[1]	7	100%	96%	96%
Aspirin at Arrival	37	97%	98%	99%
Aspirin at Discharge[1]	16	100%	99%	98%
Beta Blocker at Discharge[1]	18	94%	98%	98%
Fibrinolytic Medication Timing	0	-	67%	55%
PCI Within 90 Minutes of Arrival	0	-	91%	90%
Smoking Cessation Advice[1]	7	100%	100%	99%
Chest Pain/Possible Heart Attack Care				
Aspirin at Arrival	95	96%	95%	95%
Median Time to ECG (minutes)	99	7	8	8
Median Time to Transfer (minutes)[1]	22	62	65	61
Fibrinolytic Medication Timing[1]	7	43%	49%	54%
Heart Failure Care				
ACE Inhibitor or ARB for LVSD	25	96%	95%	94%
Discharge Instructions	122	90%	88%	88%
Evaluation of LVS Function	144	99%	97%	98%
Smoking Cessation Advice[1]	24	100%	99%	98%
Pneumonia Care				
Appropriate Initial Antibiotic	137	90%	92%	92%
Blood Culture Timing	166	96%	97%	96%
Influenza Vaccine	115	97%	93%	91%
Initial Antibiotic Timing	180	97%	96%	95%
Pneumococcal Vaccine	140	99%	95%	93%
Smoking Cessation Advice	110	100%	99%	97%
Surgical Care Improvement Project				
Appropriate VTP Within 24 Hours	240	95%	92%	92%
Appropriate Hair Removal	456	100%	100%	99%
Appropriate Beta Blocker Usage	126	98%	93%	93%
Controlled Postoperative Blood Glucose	0	-	93%	93%
Prophylactic Antibiotic Timing	318	99%	97%	97%
Prophylactic Antibiotic Timing (Outpatient)	218	97%	94%	92%
Prophylactic Antibiotic Selection	321	98%	97%	97%
Prophylactic Antibiotic Select. (Outpatient)	215	93%	94%	94%
Prophylactic Antibiotic Stopped	296	93%	94%	94%
Recommended VTP Ordered	241	96%	94%	94%
Urinary Catheter Removal	85	91%	90%	90%
Children's Asthma Care				
Received Systemic Corticosteroids[1]	7	100%	-	100%
Received Home Management Plan[1]	7	71%	-	71%
Received Reliever Medication[1]	7	100%	-	100%
Use of Medical Imaging				
Combination Abdominal CT Scan	510	0.180	0.219	0.191
Combination Chest CT Scan	367	0.150	0.102	0.054
Follow-up Mammogram/Ultrasound	595	10.4%	8%	8.4%
MRI for Low Back Pain	82	24.4%	30.7%	32.7%
Survey of Patients' Hospital Experiences				
Area Around Room 'Always' Quiet at Night	300+	61%	-	58%
Doctors 'Always' Communicated Well	300+	80%	-	80%
Home Recovery Information Given	300+	80%	-	82%
Hospital Given 9 or 10 on 10 Point Scale	300+	59%	-	67%
Meds 'Always' Explained Before Given	300+	54%	-	60%
Nurses 'Always' Communicated Well	300+	72%	-	76%
Pain 'Always' Well Controlled	300+	65%	-	69%
Room and Bathroom 'Always' Clean	300+	70%	-	71%
Timely Help 'Always' Received	300+	55%	-	64%
Would Definitely Recommend Hospital	300+	58%	-	69%

Fort Loudoun Medical Center

550 Fort Loudoun Medical Center Dr
Lenoir City, TN 37772
URL: www.fsloudon.com
Type: Acute Care Hospitals
Ownership: Voluntary Non-Profit - Other
Phone: 865-271-6000
Fax: 865-271-6514
Emergency Services: Yes
Beds: 50

Key Personnel:
CEO/President. . . . . Jeffrey Feike
Chief of Medical Staff. . . . . Steven Knight, MD
Infection Control. . . . . Connie Moore
Operating Room. . . . . John Eason
Quality Assurance . . . . Connie Moore, RN
Radiology. . . . . Steven J Addonizio

Measure	Cases	This Hosp.	State Avg.	U.S. Avg.
Heart Attack Care				
ACE Inhibitor or ARB for LVSD[1]	4	100%	96%	96%
Aspirin at Arrival[1]	17	100%	98%	99%
Aspirin at Discharge[1]	10	100%	99%	98%
Beta Blocker at Discharge[1]	11	100%	98%	98%
Fibrinolytic Medication Timing	0	-	67%	55%
PCI Within 90 Minutes of Arrival	0	-	91%	90%
Smoking Cessation Advice[1]	1	100%	100%	99%
Chest Pain/Possible Heart Attack Care				
Aspirin at Arrival	56	100%	95%	95%
Median Time to ECG (minutes)	58	8	8	8
Median Time to Transfer (minutes)[1]	8	56	65	61
Fibrinolytic Medication Timing	0	-	49%	54%
Heart Failure Care				
ACE Inhibitor or ARB for LVSD[1]	18	100%	95%	94%
Discharge Instructions	81	96%	88%	88%
Evaluation of LVS Function	92	100%	97%	98%
Smoking Cessation Advice[1]	12	100%	99%	98%
Pneumonia Care				
Appropriate Initial Antibiotic[2]	86	93%	92%	92%
Blood Culture Timing[2]	127	100%	97%	96%
Influenza Vaccine[2]	69	99%	93%	91%
Initial Antibiotic Timing[2]	116	98%	96%	95%
Pneumococcal Vaccine[2]	95	98%	95%	93%
Smoking Cessation Advice[2]	44	100%	99%	97%
Surgical Care Improvement Project				
Appropriate VTP Within 24 Hours	30	90%	92%	92%
Appropriate Hair Removal	38	100%	100%	99%
Appropriate Beta Blocker Usage[1]	14	71%	93%	93%
Controlled Postoperative Blood Glucose	0	-	93%	93%
Prophylactic Antibiotic Timing[1]	10	90%	97%	97%
Prophylactic Antibiotic Timing (Outpatient)	44	95%	94%	92%
Prophylactic Antibiotic Selection[1]	10	80%	97%	97%
Prophylactic Antibiotic Select. (Outpatient)	43	98%	94%	94%
Prophylactic Antibiotic Stopped[1]	9	100%	94%	94%
Recommended VTP Ordered	30	93%	94%	94%
Urinary Catheter Removal[1]	6	67%	90%	90%
Children's Asthma Care				
Received Systemic Corticosteroids	-	-	-	100%
Received Home Management Plan	-	-	-	71%
Received Reliever Medication	-	-	-	100%
Use of Medical Imaging				
Combination Abdominal CT Scan	256	0.293	0.219	0.191
Combination Chest CT Scan	290	0.166	0.102	0.054
Follow-up Mammogram/Ultrasound	337	12.8%	8%	8.4%
MRI for Low Back Pain	79	34.2%	30.7%	32.7%
Survey of Patients' Hospital Experiences				
Area Around Room 'Always' Quiet at Night	300+	71%	-	58%
Doctors 'Always' Communicated Well	300+	84%	-	80%
Home Recovery Information Given	300+	85%	-	82%
Hospital Given 9 or 10 on 10 Point Scale	300+	73%	-	67%
Meds 'Always' Explained Before Given	300+	66%	-	60%
Nurses 'Always' Communicated Well	300+	80%	-	76%
Pain 'Always' Well Controlled	300+	74%	-	69%
Room and Bathroom 'Always' Clean	300+	74%	-	71%
Timely Help 'Always' Received	300+	69%	-	64%
Would Definitely Recommend Hospital	300+	76%	-	69%

Marshall Medical Center

1080 North Ellington Parkway
Lewisburg, TN 37091
Type: Critical Access Hospitals
Ownership: Govt - Hospital Dist/Auth
Phone: 931-359-6276
Fax: 931-359-9522
Emergency Services: Yes
Beds: 119

Key Personnel:
CEO/President. . . . . Phyllis Brown
Chief of Medical Staff . . . . Jerry Arnold, MD
Radiology. . . . . Robert J Mahoney

Measure	Cases	This Hosp.	State Avg.	U.S. Avg.
Heart Attack Care				
ACE Inhibitor or ARB for LVSD[5]	0	-	96%	96%
Aspirin at Arrival[5]	0	-	98%	99%
Aspirin at Discharge[5]	0	-	99%	98%
Beta Blocker at Discharge[5]	0	-	98%	98%
Fibrinolytic Medication Timing[5]	0	-	67%	55%
PCI Within 90 Minutes of Arrival[5]	0	-	91%	90%
Smoking Cessation Advice[5]	0	-	100%	99%
Chest Pain/Possible Heart Attack Care				
Aspirin at Arrival	-	-	95%	95%
Median Time to ECG (minutes)	-	-	8	8
Median Time to Transfer (minutes)	-	-	65	61
Fibrinolytic Medication Timing	-	-	49%	54%
Heart Failure Care				
ACE Inhibitor or ARB for LVSD[1]	5	80%	95%	94%
Discharge Instructions[1]	20	100%	88%	88%
Evaluation of LVS Function[1]	23	87%	97%	98%
Smoking Cessation Advice[1]	7	100%	99%	98%
Pneumonia Care				
Appropriate Initial Antibiotic[1]	21	95%	92%	92%
Blood Culture Timing	29	83%	97%	96%
Influenza Vaccine[1]	19	68%	93%	91%
Initial Antibiotic Timing	28	100%	96%	95%
Pneumococcal Vaccine[1]	21	95%	95%	93%
Smoking Cessation Advice[1]	16	100%	99%	97%
Surgical Care Improvement Project				
Appropriate VTP Within 24 Hours[5]	0	-	92%	92%
Appropriate Hair Removal[5]	0	-	100%	99%
Appropriate Beta Blocker Usage[5]	0	-	93%	93%
Controlled Postoperative Blood Glucose[5]	0	-	93%	93%
Prophylactic Antibiotic Timing[5]	0	-	97%	97%
Prophylactic Antibiotic Timing (Outpatient)	-	-	94%	92%
Prophylactic Antibiotic Selection[5]	0	-	97%	97%
Prophylactic Antibiotic Select. (Outpatient)	-	-	94%	94%
Prophylactic Antibiotic Stopped[5]	0	-	94%	94%
Recommended VTP Ordered[5]	0	-	94%	94%
Urinary Catheter Removal[5]	0	-	90%	90%
Children's Asthma Care				
Received Systemic Corticosteroids	-	-	-	100%
Received Home Management Plan	-	-	-	71%
Received Reliever Medication	-	-	-	100%
Use of Medical Imaging				
Combination Abdominal CT Scan	-	-	0.219	0.191
Combination Chest CT Scan	-	-	0.102	0.054
Follow-up Mammogram/Ultrasound	-	-	8%	8.4%
MRI for Low Back Pain	-	-	30.7%	32.7%
Survey of Patients' Hospital Experiences				
Area Around Room 'Always' Quiet at Night[8]	-	-	-	58%
Doctors 'Always' Communicated Well[8]	-	-	-	80%
Home Recovery Information Given[8]	-	-	-	82%
Hospital Given 9 or 10 on 10 Point Scale[8]	-	-	-	67%
Meds 'Always' Explained Before Given[8]	-	-	-	60%
Nurses 'Always' Communicated Well[8]	-	-	-	76%
Pain 'Always' Well Controlled[8]	-	-	-	69%
Room and Bathroom 'Always' Clean[8]	-	-	-	71%
Timely Help 'Always' Received[8]	-	-	-	64%
Would Definitely Recommend Hospital[8]	-	-	-	69%

NOTE: Hospital profiles are in alphabetical order by state, then city, then hospital within the city; Rankings exclude hospitals with less than 25 cases except for patient surveys which excludes hospitals with less than 100 cases; (a) 100–299 cases; (1) The number of cases is too small to be sure how well a hospital is performing; (2) The hospital indicated that the data submitted for this measure were based on a sample of cases; (3) Data was collected during a shorter time period (fewer quarters) than the maximum possible time for this measure; (4) Suppressed for one or more quarters by CMS; (5) No data is available from the hospital for this measure; (6) Fewer than 100 patients completed the HCAHPS survey. Use these rates with caution, as the number of surveys may be too low to reliably assess hospital performance; (7) Survey results are based on less than 12 months of data; (8) Survey results are not available for this reporting period; (9) No or very few patients were eligible for the HCAHPS survey. The scores shown, if any, reflect a very small number of surveys; (10) A state average was not calculated because too few hospitals in the state submitted data; (11) There were discrepancies in the data collection process; Please refer to the User's Guide for a full explanation of data.

Henderson County Community Hospital

200 W Church St
Lexington, TN 38351
Phone: 731-968-1801
Fax: 731-968-8113
Type: Acute Care Hospitals
Emergency Services: Yes
Ownership: Proprietary
Beds: 36

Key Personnel:
CEO/President. . . . . Holly Fowler
Chief of Medical Staff. . . . . Charles White Jr
Emergency Room . . . . Joe Wilhite, MD

Measure	Cases	This Hosp.	State Avg.	U.S. Avg.
Heart Attack Care				
ACE Inhibitor or ARB for LVSD[1]	1	100%	96%	96%
Aspirin at Arrival[1]	5	100%	98%	99%
Aspirin at Discharge[1]	4	100%	99%	98%
Beta Blocker at Discharge[1]	4	100%	98%	98%
Fibrinolytic Medication Timing	0	-	67%	55%
PCI Within 90 Minutes of Arrival	0	-	91%	90%
Smoking Cessation Advice[1]	1	100%	100%	99%
Chest Pain/Possible Heart Attack Care				
Aspirin at Arrival	116	100%	95%	95%
Median Time to ECG (minutes)	130	2	8	8
Median Time to Transfer (minutes)	0	-	65	61
Fibrinolytic Medication Timing[1]	3	100%	49%	54%
Heart Failure Care				
ACE Inhibitor or ARB for LVSD[1]	12	100%	95%	94%
Discharge Instructions	46	100%	88%	88%
Evaluation of LVS Function	64	100%	97%	98%
Smoking Cessation Advice[1]	16	100%	99%	98%
Pneumonia Care				
Appropriate Initial Antibiotic	26	100%	92%	92%
Blood Culture Timing	28	100%	97%	96%
Influenza Vaccine	27	100%	93%	91%
Initial Antibiotic Timing	36	100%	96%	95%
Pneumococcal Vaccine	35	100%	95%	93%
Smoking Cessation Advice[1]	17	100%	99%	97%
Surgical Care Improvement Project				
Appropriate VTP Within 24 Hours[1,2]	5	100%	92%	92%
Appropriate Hair Removal[1,2]	9	100%	100%	99%
Appropriate Beta Blocker Usage[1,2]	3	100%	93%	93%
Controlled Postoperative Blood Glucose[2]	0	-	93%	93%
Prophylactic Antibiotic Timing[1,2]	1	100%	97%	97%
Prophylactic Antibiotic Timing (Outpatient)[1,3]	2	100%	94%	92%
Prophylactic Antibiotic Selection[1,2]	1	100%	97%	97%
Prophylactic Antibiotic Select. (Outpatient)[1,3]	2	100%	94%	94%
Prophylactic Antibiotic Stopped[1,2]	1	100%	94%	94%
Recommended VTP Ordered[1,2]	5	100%	94%	94%
Urinary Catheter Removal	0	-	90%	90%
Children's Asthma Care				
Received Systemic Corticosteroids	-	-	-	100%
Received Home Management Plan	-	-	-	71%
Received Reliever Medication	-	-	-	100%
Use of Medical Imaging				
Combination Abdominal CT Scan	91	0.363	0.219	0.191
Combination Chest CT Scan[1]	21	0.476	0.102	0.054
Follow-up Mammogram/Ultrasound	255	8.2%	8%	8.4%
MRI for Low Back Pain	62	21.0%	30.7%	32.7%
Survey of Patients' Hospital Experiences				
Area Around Room 'Always' Quiet at Night	(a)	71%	-	58%
Doctors 'Always' Communicated Well	(a)	80%	-	80%
Home Recovery Information Given	(a)	80%	-	82%
Hospital Given 9 or 10 on 10 Point Scale	(a)	61%	-	67%
Meds 'Always' Explained Before Given	(a)	61%	-	60%
Nurses 'Always' Communicated Well	(a)	79%	-	76%
Pain 'Always' Well Controlled	(a)	65%	-	69%
Room and Bathroom 'Always' Clean	(a)	65%	-	71%
Timely Help 'Always' Received	(a)	67%	-	64%
Would Definitely Recommend Hospital	(a)	59%	-	69%

Perry Community Hospital

2718 Squirrel Hollow Drive
Linden, TN 37096
Phone: 931-589-2121
Fax: 931-589-3331
E-mail: pdbosp@mtcase.net
Type: Acute Care Hospitals
Emergency Services: Yes
Ownership: Proprietary
Beds: 53

Key Personnel:
Chief of Medical Staff . . . . Andrew Averett, MD
Quality Assurance . . . . Brenda Storn
Emergency Room . . . . Leah Watkins, RN

Measure	Cases	This Hosp.	State Avg.	U.S. Avg.
Heart Attack Care				
ACE Inhibitor or ARB for LVSD[2,3]	0	-	96%	96%
Aspirin at Arrival[1,2,3]	1	100%	98%	99%
Aspirin at Discharge[1,2,3]	1	100%	99%	98%
Beta Blocker at Discharge[1,2,3]	2	100%	98%	98%
Fibrinolytic Medication Timing[2,3]	0	-	67%	55%
PCI Within 90 Minutes of Arrival[2,3]	0	-	91%	90%
Smoking Cessation Advice[2,3]	0	-	100%	99%
Chest Pain/Possible Heart Attack Care				
Aspirin at Arrival	41	85%	95%	95%
Median Time to ECG (minutes)	55	9	8	8
Median Time to Transfer (minutes)[1,3]	2	96	65	61
Fibrinolytic Medication Timing[1,3]	4	50%	49%	54%
Heart Failure Care				
ACE Inhibitor or ARB for LVSD[1,2]	1	100%	95%	94%
Discharge Instructions[2]	39	10%	88%	88%
Evaluation of LVS Function[2]	85	2%	97%	98%
Smoking Cessation Advice[1,2]	10	30%	99%	98%
Pneumonia Care				
Appropriate Initial Antibiotic[2]	48	35%	92%	92%
Blood Culture Timing[1,2]	5	80%	97%	96%
Influenza Vaccine[2]	50	0%	93%	91%
Initial Antibiotic Timing[2]	75	92%	96%	95%
Pneumococcal Vaccine[2]	72	1%	95%	93%
Smoking Cessation Advice[1,2]	19	21%	99%	97%
Surgical Care Improvement Project				
Appropriate VTP Within 24 Hours[5]	0	-	92%	92%
Appropriate Hair Removal[5]	0	-	100%	99%
Appropriate Beta Blocker Usage[5]	0	-	93%	93%
Controlled Postoperative Blood Glucose[5]	0	-	93%	93%
Prophylactic Antibiotic Timing[5]	0	-	97%	97%
Prophylactic Antibiotic Timing (Outpatient)[5]	0	-	94%	92%
Prophylactic Antibiotic Selection[5]	0	-	97%	97%
Prophylactic Antibiotic Select. (Outpatient)[5]	0	-	94%	94%
Prophylactic Antibiotic Stopped[5]	0	-	94%	94%
Recommended VTP Ordered[5]	0	-	94%	94%
Urinary Catheter Removal[5]	0	-	90%	90%
Children's Asthma Care				
Received Systemic Corticosteroids	-	-	-	100%
Received Home Management Plan	-	-	-	71%
Received Reliever Medication	-	-	-	100%
Use of Medical Imaging				
Combination Abdominal CT Scan	104	0.058	0.219	0.191
Combination Chest CT Scan	75	0.040	0.102	0.054
Follow-up Mammogram/Ultrasound[5]	0	-	8%	8.4%
MRI for Low Back Pain[5]	0	-	30.7%	32.7%
Survey of Patients' Hospital Experiences				
Area Around Room 'Always' Quiet at Night[6]	<100	53%	-	58%
Doctors 'Always' Communicated Well[6]	<100	64%	-	80%
Home Recovery Information Given[6]	<100	45%	-	82%
Hospital Given 9 or 10 on 10 Point Scale[6]	<100	33%	-	67%
Meds 'Always' Explained Before Given[6]	<100	8%	-	60%
Nurses 'Always' Communicated Well[6]	<100	57%	-	76%
Pain 'Always' Well Controlled[6]	<100	37%	-	69%
Room and Bathroom 'Always' Clean[6]	<100	74%	-	71%
Timely Help 'Always' Received[6]	<100	39%	-	64%
Would Definitely Recommend Hospital	<100	6%	-	69%

Livingston Regional Hospital

315 Oak St Box 550
Livingston, TN 38570
Phone: 931-823-5611
Fax: 931-403-2334
URL: www.livingstonregionalhospital.com
Type: Acute Care Hospitals
Emergency Services: Yes
Ownership: Voluntary Non-Profit - Other
Beds: 114

Key Personnel:
CEO/President. . . . . Timothy W McGill
Chief of Medical Staff. . . . . John Clough, MD
Pediatric Ambulatory Care . . . . . . Jessie Lee Copeland, MD
Radiology. . . . . Donald Huff, MD
Emergency Room . . . . Richard Fields, MD

Measure	Cases	This Hosp.	State Avg.	U.S. Avg.
Heart Attack Care				
ACE Inhibitor or ARB for LVSD[1]	1	100%	96%	96%
Aspirin at Arrival[1]	8	88%	98%	99%
Aspirin at Discharge[1]	4	100%	99%	98%
Beta Blocker at Discharge[1]	4	100%	98%	98%
Fibrinolytic Medication Timing	0	-	67%	55%
PCI Within 90 Minutes of Arrival	0	-	91%	90%
Smoking Cessation Advice[1]	3	100%	100%	99%
Chest Pain/Possible Heart Attack Care				
Aspirin at Arrival	69	100%	95%	95%
Median Time to ECG (minutes)	81	4	8	8
Median Time to Transfer (minutes)[1]	7	70	65	61
Fibrinolytic Medication Timing[1]	1	0%	49%	54%
Heart Failure Care				
ACE Inhibitor or ARB for LVSD[1]	18	89%	95%	94%
Discharge Instructions	67	100%	88%	88%
Evaluation of LVS Function	103	100%	97%	98%
Smoking Cessation Advice[1]	22	100%	99%	98%
Pneumonia Care				
Appropriate Initial Antibiotic	98	94%	92%	92%
Blood Culture Timing	128	100%	97%	96%
Influenza Vaccine	94	100%	93%	91%
Initial Antibiotic Timing	164	99%	96%	95%
Pneumococcal Vaccine	144	98%	95%	93%
Smoking Cessation Advice	66	100%	99%	97%
Surgical Care Improvement Project				
Appropriate VTP Within 24 Hours	39	85%	92%	92%
Appropriate Hair Removal	78	100%	100%	99%
Appropriate Beta Blocker Usage[1]	18	83%	93%	93%
Controlled Postoperative Blood Glucose	0	-	93%	93%
Prophylactic Antibiotic Timing	52	100%	97%	97%
Prophylactic Antibiotic Timing (Outpatient)	30	97%	94%	92%
Prophylactic Antibiotic Selection	52	94%	97%	97%
Prophylactic Antibiotic Select. (Outpatient)	29	97%	94%	94%
Prophylactic Antibiotic Stopped	48	96%	94%	94%
Recommended VTP Ordered	39	92%	94%	94%
Urinary Catheter Removal[1]	16	94%	90%	90%
Children's Asthma Care				
Received Systemic Corticosteroids	-	-	-	100%
Received Home Management Plan	-	-	-	71%
Received Reliever Medication	-	-	-	100%
Use of Medical Imaging				
Combination Abdominal CT Scan	246	0.622	0.219	0.191
Combination Chest CT Scan	111	0.874	0.102	0.054
Follow-up Mammogram/Ultrasound	337	3.0%	8%	8.4%
MRI for Low Back Pain	84	29.8%	30.7%	32.7%
Survey of Patients' Hospital Experiences				
Area Around Room 'Always' Quiet at Night	300+	59%	-	58%
Doctors 'Always' Communicated Well	300+	86%	-	80%
Home Recovery Information Given	300+	75%	-	82%
Hospital Given 9 or 10 on 10 Point Scale	300+	62%	-	67%
Meds 'Always' Explained Before Given	300+	56%	-	60%
Nurses 'Always' Communicated Well	300+	75%	-	76%
Pain 'Always' Well Controlled	300+	69%	-	69%
Room and Bathroom 'Always' Clean	300+	68%	-	71%
Timely Help 'Always' Received	300+	64%	-	64%
Would Definitely Recommend Hospital	300+	64%	-	69%

NOTE: Hospital profiles are in alphabetical order by state, then city, then hospital within the city; Rankings exclude hospitals with less than 25 cases except for patient surveys which excludes hospitals with less than 100 cases; (a) 100–299 cases; (1) The number of cases is too small to be sure how well a hospital is performing; (2) The hospital indicated that the data submitted for this measure were based on a sample of cases; (3) Data was collected during a shorter time period (fewer quarters) than the maximum possible time for this measure; (4) Suppressed for one or more quarters by CMS; (5) No data is available from the hospital for this measure; (6) Fewer than 100 patients completed the HCAHPS survey. Use these rates with caution, as the number of surveys may be too low to reliably assess hospital performance; (7) Survey results are based on less than 12 months of data; (8) Survey results are not available for this reporting period; (9) No or very few patients were eligible for the HCAHPS survey. The scores shown, if any, reflect a very small number of surveys; (10) A state average was not calculated because too few hospitals in the state submitted data; (11) There were discrepancies in the data collection process; Please refer to the User's Guide for a full explanation of data.

Medical Center of Manchester

481 Interstate Drive
Manchester, TN 37355
Phone: 931-728-6354
Fax: 931-728-5420
Type: Critical Access Hospitals
Emergency Services: Yes
Ownership: Proprietary
Beds: 49

Key Personnel:
CEO/President. . . . . Robert J Couch
Chief of Medical Staff. . . . . AR Brandon, DO
Infection Control. . . . . Suzanne Knox, LPN
Operating Room. . . . . Lisa Winkler
Emergency Room . . . . Gina Brennan, RN
Intensive Care Unit. . . . . Brenda Ballard, RN

Measure	Cases	This Hosp.	State Avg.	U.S. Avg.
Heart Attack Care				
ACE Inhibitor or ARB for LVSD[5]	0	-	96%	96%
Aspirin at Arrival[5]	0	-	98%	99%
Aspirin at Discharge[5]	0	-	99%	98%
Beta Blocker at Discharge[5]	0	-	98%	98%
Fibrinolytic Medication Timing[5]	0	-	67%	55%
PCI Within 90 Minutes of Arrival[5]	0	-	91%	90%
Smoking Cessation Advice[5]	0	-	100%	99%
Chest Pain/Possible Heart Attack Care				
Aspirin at Arrival	81	84%	95%	95%
Median Time to ECG (minutes)	84	14	8	8
Median Time to Transfer (minutes)[1]	6	82	65	61
Fibrinolytic Medication Timing[1]	2	50%	49%	54%
Heart Failure Care				
ACE Inhibitor or ARB for LVSD[1]	4	100%	95%	94%
Discharge Instructions[1]	18	67%	88%	88%
Evaluation of LVS Function	29	14%	97%	98%
Smoking Cessation Advice[1]	5	0%	99%	98%
Pneumonia Care				
Appropriate Initial Antibiotic[1]	18	94%	92%	92%
Blood Culture Timing[1]	7	71%	97%	96%
Influenza Vaccine[1]	14	71%	93%	91%
Initial Antibiotic Timing[1]	15	80%	96%	95%
Pneumococcal Vaccine[1]	17	82%	95%	93%
Smoking Cessation Advice[1]	9	22%	99%	97%
Surgical Care Improvement Project				
Appropriate VTP Within 24 Hours[5]	0	-	92%	92%
Appropriate Hair Removal[5]	0	-	100%	99%
Appropriate Beta Blocker Usage[5]	0	-	93%	93%
Controlled Postoperative Blood Glucose[5]	0	-	93%	93%
Prophylactic Antibiotic Timing[5]	0	-	97%	97%
Prophylactic Antibiotic Timing (Outpatient)[5]	0	-	94%	92%
Prophylactic Antibiotic Selection[5]	0	-	97%	97%
Prophylactic Antibiotic Select. (Outpatient)[5]	0	-	94%	94%
Prophylactic Antibiotic Stopped[5]	0	-	94%	94%
Recommended VTP Ordered[5]	0	-	94%	94%
Urinary Catheter Removal[5]	0	-	90%	90%
Children's Asthma Care				
Received Systemic Corticosteroids	-	-	-	100%
Received Home Management Plan	-	-	-	71%
Received Reliever Medication	-	-	-	100%
Use of Medical Imaging				
Combination Abdominal CT Scan	150	0.333	0.219	0.191
Combination Chest CT Scan	49	0.469	0.102	0.054
Follow-up Mammogram/Ultrasound[5]	0	-	8%	8.4%
MRI for Low Back Pain[1]	26	26.9%	30.7%	32.7%
Survey of Patients' Hospital Experiences				
Area Around Room 'Always' Quiet at Night[8]	-	-	-	58%
Doctors 'Always' Communicated Well[8]	-	-	-	80%
Home Recovery Information Given[8]	-	-	-	82%
Hospital Given 9 or 10 on 10 Point Scale[8]	-	-	-	67%
Meds 'Always' Explained Before Given[8]	-	-	-	60%
Nurses 'Always' Communicated Well[8]	-	-	-	76%
Pain 'Always' Well Controlled[8]	-	-	-	69%
Room and Bathroom 'Always' Clean[8]	-	-	-	71%
Timely Help 'Always' Received[8]	-	-	-	64%
Would Definitely Recommend Hospital[8]	-	-	-	69%

United Regional Medical Center

1001 Mcarthur St
Manchester, TN 37355
Phone: 931-728-3586
Fax: 931-728-6877
Type: Acute Care Hospitals
Emergency Services: Yes
Ownership: Proprietary
Beds: 126

Key Personnel:
CEO/President. . . . . Robert George
Chief of Medical Staff. . . . . Glenn Davis
Infection Control. . . . . Virginia Smith RN
Operating Room. . . . . Councill C Rudolph
Quality Assurance . . . . Pam Adderson RN
Radiology. . . . . Wendell McAbee
Emergency Room . . . . Richie Lupo

Measure	Cases	This Hosp.	State Avg.	U.S. Avg.
Heart Attack Care				
ACE Inhibitor or ARB for LVSD[1,3]	1	100%	96%	96%
Aspirin at Arrival[1,3]	18	83%	98%	99%
Aspirin at Discharge[1,3]	17	53%	99%	98%
Beta Blocker at Discharge[1,3]	17	41%	98%	98%
Fibrinolytic Medication Timing[3]	0	-	67%	55%
PCI Within 90 Minutes of Arrival[3]	0	-	91%	90%
Smoking Cessation Advice[1,3]	6	50%	100%	99%
Chest Pain/Possible Heart Attack Care				
Aspirin at Arrival	51	55%	95%	95%
Median Time to ECG (minutes)	52	22	8	8
Median Time to Transfer (minutes)[1,3]	3	96	65	61
Fibrinolytic Medication Timing[1]	1	0%	49%	54%
Heart Failure Care				
ACE Inhibitor or ARB for LVSD[1]	4	100%	95%	94%
Discharge Instructions	33	3%	88%	88%
Evaluation of LVS Function	40	42%	97%	98%
Smoking Cessation Advice[1]	5	60%	99%	98%
Pneumonia Care				
Appropriate Initial Antibiotic	115	77%	92%	92%
Blood Culture Timing	28	75%	97%	96%
Influenza Vaccine	107	59%	93%	91%
Initial Antibiotic Timing	170	84%	96%	95%
Pneumococcal Vaccine	148	54%	95%	93%
Smoking Cessation Advice	97	79%	99%	97%
Surgical Care Improvement Project				
Appropriate VTP Within 24 Hours[5]	0	-	92%	92%
Appropriate Hair Removal[5]	0	-	100%	99%
Appropriate Beta Blocker Usage[5]	0	-	93%	93%
Controlled Postoperative Blood Glucose[5]	0	-	93%	93%
Prophylactic Antibiotic Timing[5]	0	-	97%	97%
Prophylactic Antibiotic Timing (Outpatient)[5]	0	-	94%	92%
Prophylactic Antibiotic Selection[5]	0	-	97%	97%
Prophylactic Antibiotic Select. (Outpatient)[5]	0	-	94%	94%
Prophylactic Antibiotic Stopped[5]	0	-	94%	94%
Recommended VTP Ordered[5]	0	-	94%	94%
Urinary Catheter Removal[5]	0	-	90%	90%
Children's Asthma Care				
Received Systemic Corticosteroids	-	-	-	100%
Received Home Management Plan	-	-	-	71%
Received Reliever Medication	-	-	-	100%
Use of Medical Imaging				
Combination Abdominal CT Scan	94	0.106	0.219	0.191
Combination Chest CT Scan	82	0.122	0.102	0.054
Follow-up Mammogram/Ultrasound	256	7.4%	8%	8.4%
MRI for Low Back Pain	215	22.8%	30.7%	32.7%
Survey of Patients' Hospital Experiences				
Area Around Room 'Always' Quiet at Night	300+	76%	-	58%
Doctors 'Always' Communicated Well	300+	91%	-	80%
Home Recovery Information Given	300+	85%	-	82%
Hospital Given 9 or 10 on 10 Point Scale	300+	62%	-	67%
Meds 'Always' Explained Before Given	300+	63%	-	60%
Nurses 'Always' Communicated Well	300+	84%	-	76%
Pain 'Always' Well Controlled	300+	79%	-	69%
Room and Bathroom 'Always' Clean	300+	80%	-	71%
Timely Help 'Always' Received	300+	75%	-	64%
Would Definitely Recommend Hospital	300+	77%	-	69%

Volunteer Community Hospital

161 Mount Pelia Rd
Martin, TN 38237
Phone: 731-587-4261
Fax: 731-587-6142
URL: www.chs.net
Type: Acute Care Hospitals
Emergency Services: Yes
Ownership: Proprietary
Beds: 65

Key Personnel:
CEO/President. . . . . Steve Westenhofer
Chief of Medical Staff. . . . . Cynthia Phillips
Infection Control. . . . . Betty Wilson
Operating Room. . . . . Michael Saridakis
Quality Assurance . . . . Lori Brown
Radiology. . . . . Michelle Melotti, MD
Emergency Room . . . . James A Whitlock, DO
Intensive Care Unit. . . . . Lois Shanks, RN

Measure	Cases	This Hosp.	State Avg.	U.S. Avg.
Heart Attack Care				
ACE Inhibitor or ARB for LVSD	0	-	96%	96%
Aspirin at Arrival[1]	3	100%	98%	99%
Aspirin at Discharge[1]	2	100%	99%	98%
Beta Blocker at Discharge[1]	4	100%	98%	98%
Fibrinolytic Medication Timing	0	-	67%	55%
PCI Within 90 Minutes of Arrival	0	-	91%	90%
Smoking Cessation Advice	0	-	100%	99%
Chest Pain/Possible Heart Attack Care				
Aspirin at Arrival	276	97%	95%	95%
Median Time to ECG (minutes)	294	12	8	8
Median Time to Transfer (minutes)[5]	0	-	65	61
Fibrinolytic Medication Timing[1]	1	0%	49%	54%
Heart Failure Care				
ACE Inhibitor or ARB for LVSD[1]	23	87%	95%	94%
Discharge Instructions	33	85%	88%	88%
Evaluation of LVS Function	67	96%	97%	98%
Smoking Cessation Advice[1]	6	100%	99%	98%
Pneumonia Care				
Appropriate Initial Antibiotic	53	89%	92%	92%
Blood Culture Timing	60	100%	97%	96%
Influenza Vaccine	75	95%	93%	91%
Initial Antibiotic Timing	84	96%	96%	95%
Pneumococcal Vaccine	97	95%	95%	93%
Smoking Cessation Advice	35	100%	99%	97%
Surgical Care Improvement Project				
Appropriate VTP Within 24 Hours[2]	52	92%	92%	92%
Appropriate Hair Removal[2]	74	100%	100%	99%
Appropriate Beta Blocker Usage[1,2]	21	81%	93%	93%
Controlled Postoperative Blood Glucose[2]	0	-	93%	93%
Prophylactic Antibiotic Timing[2]	47	98%	97%	97%
Prophylactic Antibiotic Timing (Outpatient)	111	98%	94%	92%
Prophylactic Antibiotic Selection[2]	47	94%	97%	97%
Prophylactic Antibiotic Select. (Outpatient)	110	95%	94%	94%
Prophylactic Antibiotic Stopped[2]	45	93%	94%	94%
Recommended VTP Ordered[2]	52	92%	94%	94%
Urinary Catheter Removal[1]	7	86%	90%	90%
Children's Asthma Care				
Received Systemic Corticosteroids	-	-	-	100%
Received Home Management Plan	-	-	-	71%
Received Reliever Medication	-	-	-	100%
Use of Medical Imaging				
Combination Abdominal CT Scan	238	0.147	0.219	0.191
Combination Chest CT Scan	164	0.085	0.102	0.054
Follow-up Mammogram/Ultrasound	120	4.2%	8%	8.4%
MRI for Low Back Pain	60	30.0%	30.7%	32.7%
Survey of Patients' Hospital Experiences				
Area Around Room 'Always' Quiet at Night	300+	62%	-	58%
Doctors 'Always' Communicated Well	300+	82%	-	80%
Home Recovery Information Given	300+	79%	-	82%
Hospital Given 9 or 10 on 10 Point Scale	300+	66%	-	67%
Meds 'Always' Explained Before Given	300+	56%	-	60%
Nurses 'Always' Communicated Well	300+	77%	-	76%
Pain 'Always' Well Controlled	300+	72%	-	69%
Room and Bathroom 'Always' Clean	300+	71%	-	71%
Timely Help 'Always' Received	300+	63%	-	64%
Would Definitely Recommend Hospital	300+	64%	-	69%

NOTE: Hospital profiles are in alphabetical order by state, then city, then hospital within the city; Rankings exclude hospitals with less than 25 cases except for patient surveys which excludes hospitals with less than 100 cases; (a) 100–299 cases; (1) The number of cases is too small to be sure how well a hospital is performing; (2) The hospital indicated that the data submitted for this measure were based on a sample of cases; (3) Data was collected during a shorter time period (fewer quarters) than the maximum possible time for this measure; (4) Suppressed for one or more quarters by CMS; (5) No data is available from the hospital for this measure; (6) Fewer than 100 patients completed the HCAHPS survey. Use these rates with caution, as the number of surveys may be too low to assess hospital performance; (7) Survey results are based on less than 12 months of data; (8) Survey results are not available for this reporting period; (9) No or very few patients were eligible for the HCAHPS survey. The scores shown, if any, reflect a very small number of surveys; (10) A state average was not calculated because too few hospitals in the state submitted data; (11) There were discrepancies in the data collection process; Please refer to the User's Guide for a full explanation of data.

Blount Memorial Hospital

907 E Lamar Alexander Parkway
Maryville, TN 37804
Phone: 865-983-7211
Fax: 865-977-5550
URL: www.blountmemorial.org
Type: Acute Care Hospitals
Emergency Services: Yes
Ownership: Government - Local
Beds: 272

Key Personnel:
CEO/President. . . . . Robert P Redwine
Chief of Medical Staff . . . . Marvin Beard, MD
Operating Room. . . . . Carolyn Phillips
Radiology. . . . . Daniel Cotton, MD
Emergency Room . . . . Shirley Hutton

Measure	Cases	This Hosp.	State Avg.	U.S. Avg.
Heart Attack Care				
ACE Inhibitor or ARB for LVSD[2]	32	94%	96%	96%
Aspirin at Arrival[2]	191	99%	98%	99%
Aspirin at Discharge[2]	177	99%	99%	98%
Beta Blocker at Discharge[2]	170	100%	98%	98%
Fibrinolytic Medication Timing[2]	0	-	67%	55%
PCI Within 90 Minutes of Arrival[2]	43	93%	91%	90%
Smoking Cessation Advice[2]	62	100%	100%	99%
Chest Pain/Possible Heart Attack Care				
Aspirin at Arrival[1]	11	82%	95%	95%
Median Time to ECG (minutes)[1]	12	8	8	8
Median Time to Transfer (minutes)[5]	0	-	65	61
Fibrinolytic Medication Timing[3]	0	-	49%	54%
Heart Failure Care				
ACE Inhibitor or ARB for LVSD[2]	78	99%	95%	94%
Discharge Instructions[2]	205	88%	88%	88%
Evaluation of LVS Function[2]	267	99%	97%	98%
Smoking Cessation Advice[2]	30	100%	99%	98%
Pneumonia Care				
Appropriate Initial Antibiotic[2]	79	94%	92%	92%
Blood Culture Timing[2]	161	95%	97%	96%
Influenza Vaccine[2]	102	97%	93%	91%
Initial Antibiotic Timing[2]	140	95%	96%	95%
Pneumococcal Vaccine[2]	146	99%	95%	93%
Smoking Cessation Advice[2]	74	99%	99%	97%
Surgical Care Improvement Project				
Appropriate VTP Within 24 Hours[2]	178	92%	92%	92%
Appropriate Hair Removal[2]	454	100%	100%	99%
Appropriate Beta Blocker Usage[2]	130	100%	93%	93%
Controlled Postoperative Blood Glucose[2]	0	-	93%	93%
Prophylactic Antibiotic Timing[2]	294	94%	97%	97%
Prophylactic Antibiotic Timing (Outpatient)	278	82%	94%	92%
Prophylactic Antibiotic Selection[2]	296	98%	97%	97%
Prophylactic Antibiotic Select. (Outpatient)	255	94%	94%	94%
Prophylactic Antibiotic Stopped[2]	279	95%	94%	94%
Recommended VTP Ordered[2]	178	93%	94%	94%
Urinary Catheter Removal[2]	99	80%	90%	90%
Children's Asthma Care				
Received Systemic Corticosteroids	-	-	-	100%
Received Home Management Plan	-	-	-	71%
Received Reliever Medication	-	-	-	100%
Use of Medical Imaging				
Combination Abdominal CT Scan	1,077	0.129	0.219	0.191
Combination Chest CT Scan	643	0.064	0.102	0.054
Follow-up Mammogram/Ultrasound	1,525	10.2%	8%	8.4%
MRI for Low Back Pain	282	31.6%	30.7%	32.7%
Survey of Patients' Hospital Experiences				
Area Around Room 'Always' Quiet at Night	300+	48%	-	58%
Doctors 'Always' Communicated Well	300+	78%	-	80%
Home Recovery Information Given	300+	84%	-	82%
Hospital Given 9 or 10 on 10 Point Scale	300+	60%	-	67%
Meds 'Always' Explained Before Given	300+	54%	-	60%
Nurses 'Always' Communicated Well	300+	73%	-	76%
Pain 'Always' Well Controlled	300+	67%	-	69%
Room and Bathroom 'Always' Clean	300+	67%	-	71%
Timely Help 'Always' Received	300+	59%	-	64%
Would Definitely Recommend Hospital	300+	62%	-	69%

McKenzie Regional Hospital

161 Hospital Drive
McKenzie, TN 38201
Phone: 731-352-5344
Fax: 731-352-2733
URL: www.mckenzieregionalhospital.com
Type: Acute Care Hospitals
Emergency Services: Yes
Ownership: Proprietary
Beds: 45

Key Personnel:
CEO/President. . . . . Darrell Blaylock
Chief of Medical Staff . . . . Terry Colotta, MD
Operating Room. . . . . Regina Lockaby
Radiology. . . . . Ricky Scott
Emergency Room . . . . Denna Jackson
Patient Relations . . . . Kim Ladd

Measure	Cases	This Hosp.	State Avg.	U.S. Avg.
Heart Attack Care				
ACE Inhibitor or ARB for LVSD	0	-	96%	96%
Aspirin at Arrival[1]	2	100%	98%	99%
Aspirin at Discharge[1]	1	100%	99%	98%
Beta Blocker at Discharge[1]	1	100%	98%	98%
Fibrinolytic Medication Timing	0	-	67%	55%
PCI Within 90 Minutes of Arrival	0	-	91%	90%
Smoking Cessation Advice	0	-	100%	99%
Chest Pain/Possible Heart Attack Care				
Aspirin at Arrival	142	99%	95%	95%
Median Time to ECG (minutes)	154	8	8	8
Median Time to Transfer (minutes)[5]	0	-	65	61
Fibrinolytic Medication Timing[1]	6	67%	49%	54%
Heart Failure Care				
ACE Inhibitor or ARB for LVSD[1]	2	100%	95%	94%
Discharge Instructions[1]	16	100%	88%	88%
Evaluation of LVS Function[1]	23	100%	97%	98%
Smoking Cessation Advice[1]	2	100%	99%	98%
Pneumonia Care				
Appropriate Initial Antibiotic	40	100%	92%	92%
Blood Culture Timing	49	100%	97%	96%
Influenza Vaccine	51	98%	93%	91%
Initial Antibiotic Timing	64	100%	96%	95%
Pneumococcal Vaccine	57	100%	95%	93%
Smoking Cessation Advice	26	100%	99%	97%
Surgical Care Improvement Project				
Appropriate VTP Within 24 Hours[1,2]	3	100%	92%	92%
Appropriate Hair Removal[2]	59	97%	100%	99%
Appropriate Beta Blocker Usage[1,2]	7	100%	93%	93%
Controlled Postoperative Blood Glucose[2]	0	-	93%	93%
Prophylactic Antibiotic Timing[2]	57	98%	97%	97%
Prophylactic Antibiotic Timing (Outpatient)[1,3]	2	100%	94%	92%
Prophylactic Antibiotic Selection[2]	57	93%	97%	97%
Prophylactic Antibiotic Select. (Outpatient)[1,3]	2	100%	94%	94%
Prophylactic Antibiotic Stopped[2]	57	100%	94%	94%
Recommended VTP Ordered[1,2]	3	100%	94%	94%
Urinary Catheter Removal[1]	2	100%	90%	90%
Children's Asthma Care				
Received Systemic Corticosteroids	-	-	-	100%
Received Home Management Plan	-	-	-	71%
Received Reliever Medication	-	-	-	100%
Use of Medical Imaging				
Combination Abdominal CT Scan	60	0.417	0.219	0.191
Combination Chest CT Scan[1]	30	0.833	0.102	0.054
Follow-up Mammogram/Ultrasound	264	13.3%	8%	8.4%
MRI for Low Back Pain[1]	6	33.3%	30.7%	32.7%
Survey of Patients' Hospital Experiences				
Area Around Room 'Always' Quiet at Night	300+	70%	-	58%
Doctors 'Always' Communicated Well	300+	81%	-	80%
Home Recovery Information Given	300+	80%	-	82%
Hospital Given 9 or 10 on 10 Point Scale	300+	65%	-	67%
Meds 'Always' Explained Before Given	300+	62%	-	60%
Nurses 'Always' Communicated Well	300+	73%	-	76%
Pain 'Always' Well Controlled	300+	66%	-	69%
Room and Bathroom 'Always' Clean	300+	68%	-	71%
Timely Help 'Always' Received	300+	61%	-	64%
Would Definitely Recommend Hospital	300+	65%	-	69%

River Park Hospital

1559 Sparta Street
McMinnville, TN 37110
Phone: 931-815-4101
Fax: 931-815-4638
URL: www.riverparkhospital.com
Type: Acute Care Hospitals
Emergency Services: Yes
Ownership: Proprietary
Beds: 127

Key Personnel:
CEO/President. . . . . John R McLain
Chief of Medical Staff . . . . Timothy M Fisher, DO
Operating Room. . . . . William Bradfor Brock
Pediatric Ambulatory Care . . . . . . Jeffrey K McVey, DO
Radiology. . . . . Wendell V McAbee, MD
Patient Relations . . . . Elaine Neal

Measure	Cases	This Hosp.	State Avg.	U.S. Avg.
Heart Attack Care				
ACE Inhibitor or ARB for LVSD[1]	4	100%	96%	96%
Aspirin at Arrival[1]	14	93%	98%	99%
Aspirin at Discharge[1]	10	100%	99%	98%
Beta Blocker at Discharge[1]	12	83%	98%	98%
Fibrinolytic Medication Timing	0	-	67%	55%
PCI Within 90 Minutes of Arrival	0	-	91%	90%
Smoking Cessation Advice[1]	4	100%	100%	99%
Chest Pain/Possible Heart Attack Care				
Aspirin at Arrival	163	95%	95%	95%
Median Time to ECG (minutes)	173	4	8	8
Median Time to Transfer (minutes)[1,3]	4	140	65	61
Fibrinolytic Medication Timing[1]	21	43%	49%	54%
Heart Failure Care				
ACE Inhibitor or ARB for LVSD	29	93%	95%	94%
Discharge Instructions	127	83%	88%	88%
Evaluation of LVS Function	161	99%	97%	98%
Smoking Cessation Advice	42	98%	99%	98%
Pneumonia Care				
Appropriate Initial Antibiotic	149	88%	92%	92%
Blood Culture Timing	210	95%	97%	96%
Influenza Vaccine	154	95%	93%	91%
Initial Antibiotic Timing	229	91%	96%	95%
Pneumococcal Vaccine	194	92%	95%	93%
Smoking Cessation Advice	127	100%	99%	97%
Surgical Care Improvement Project				
Appropriate VTP Within 24 Hours	57	96%	92%	92%
Appropriate Hair Removal	86	100%	100%	99%
Appropriate Beta Blocker Usage[1]	22	95%	93%	93%
Controlled Postoperative Blood Glucose	0	-	93%	93%
Prophylactic Antibiotic Timing	61	97%	97%	97%
Prophylactic Antibiotic Timing (Outpatient)	183	86%	94%	92%
Prophylactic Antibiotic Selection	63	97%	97%	97%
Prophylactic Antibiotic Select. (Outpatient)	192	92%	94%	94%
Prophylactic Antibiotic Stopped	55	93%	94%	94%
Recommended VTP Ordered	57	96%	94%	94%
Urinary Catheter Removal[1]	24	83%	90%	90%
Children's Asthma Care				
Received Systemic Corticosteroids	-	-	-	100%
Received Home Management Plan	-	-	-	71%
Received Reliever Medication	-	-	-	100%
Use of Medical Imaging				
Combination Abdominal CT Scan	385	0.023	0.219	0.191
Combination Chest CT Scan	393	0.252	0.102	0.054
Follow-up Mammogram/Ultrasound	744	4.8%	8%	8.4%
MRI for Low Back Pain	157	17.8%	30.7%	32.7%
Survey of Patients' Hospital Experiences				
Area Around Room 'Always' Quiet at Night	300+	63%	-	58%
Doctors 'Always' Communicated Well	300+	77%	-	80%
Home Recovery Information Given	300+	81%	-	82%
Hospital Given 9 or 10 on 10 Point Scale	300+	59%	-	67%
Meds 'Always' Explained Before Given	300+	57%	-	60%
Nurses 'Always' Communicated Well	300+	72%	-	76%
Pain 'Always' Well Controlled	300+	65%	-	69%
Room and Bathroom 'Always' Clean	300+	64%	-	71%
Timely Help 'Always' Received	300+	60%	-	64%
Would Definitely Recommend Hospital	300+	57%	-	69%

NOTE: Hospital profiles are in alphabetical order by state, then city, then hospital within the city; Rankings exclude hospitals with less than 25 cases except for patient surveys which excludes hospitals with less than 100 cases; (a) 100–299 cases; (1) The number of cases is too small to be sure how well a hospital is performing; (2) The hospital indicated that the data submitted for this measure were based on a sample of cases; (3) Data was collected during a shorter time period (fewer quarters) than the maximum possible time for this measure; (4) Suppressed for one or more quarters by CMS; (5) No data is available from the hospital for this measure; (6) Fewer than 100 patients completed the HCAHPS survey. Use these rates with caution, as the number of surveys may be too low to reliably assess hospital performance; (7) Survey results are based on less than 12 months of data; (8) Survey results are not available for this reporting period; (9) No or very few patients were eligible for the HCAHPS survey. The scores shown, if any, reflect a very small number of surveys; (10) A state average was not calculated because too few hospitals in the state submitted data; (11) There were discrepancies in the data collection process; Please refer to the User's Guide for a full explanation of data.

Baptist Memorial Hospital

6019 Walnut Grove Road Phone: 901-226-5000
Memphis, TN 38120 Fax: 901-227-6149
E-mail: info.memphis@bmhcc.org
URL: www.bmhcc.org
Type: Acute Care Hospitals Emergency Services: Yes
Ownership: Voluntary Non-Profit - Private Beds: 706

Key Personnel:
CEO/President. . . . . Zach Chandler
Infection Control. . . . . Katie Morrissette
Operating Room. . . . . Martha Ullrich
Radiology. . . . . Johnny Stanford
Emergency Room . . . . William Falvey, MD
Hemotology Center . . . . Ric Ransom

Measure	Cases	This Hosp.	State Avg.	U.S. Avg.
Heart Attack Care				
ACE Inhibitor or ARB for LVSD	117	99%	96%	96%
Aspirin at Arrival	519	98%	98%	99%
Aspirin at Discharge	692	98%	99%	98%
Beta Blocker at Discharge	654	98%	98%	98%
Fibrinolytic Medication Timing	0	-	67%	55%
PCI Within 90 Minutes of Arrival	44	80%	91%	90%
Smoking Cessation Advice	214	100%	100%	99%
Chest Pain/Possible Heart Attack Care				
Aspirin at Arrival[1]	22	91%	95%	95%
Median Time to ECG (minutes)[1]	21	23	8	8
Median Time to Transfer (minutes)[5]	0	-	65	61
Fibrinolytic Medication Timing[3]	0	-	49%	54%
Heart Failure Care				
ACE Inhibitor or ARB for LVSD	448	96%	95%	94%
Discharge Instructions	1,171	84%	88%	88%
Evaluation of LVS Function	1,294	100%	97%	98%
Smoking Cessation Advice	229	100%	99%	98%
Pneumonia Care				
Appropriate Initial Antibiotic	451	92%	92%	92%
Blood Culture Timing	530	98%	97%	96%
Influenza Vaccine	480	96%	93%	91%
Initial Antibiotic Timing	617	96%	96%	95%
Pneumococcal Vaccine	584	96%	95%	93%
Smoking Cessation Advice	226	100%	99%	97%
Surgical Care Improvement Project				
Appropriate VTP Within 24 Hours[2]	362	90%	92%	92%
Appropriate Hair Removal[2]	1,112	100%	100%	99%
Appropriate Beta Blocker Usage[2]	338	89%	93%	93%
Controlled Postoperative Blood Glucose[2]	149	86%	93%	93%
Prophylactic Antibiotic Timing[2]	701	96%	97%	97%
Prophylactic Antibiotic Timing (Outpatient)	1,372	94%	94%	92%
Prophylactic Antibiotic Selection[2]	707	97%	97%	97%
Prophylactic Antibiotic Select. (Outpatient)	1,359	95%	94%	94%
Prophylactic Antibiotic Stopped[2]	659	90%	94%	94%
Recommended VTP Ordered[2]	366	93%	94%	94%
Urinary Catheter Removal[2]	128	85%	90%	90%
Children's Asthma Care				
Received Systemic Corticosteroids	-	-	-	100%
Received Home Management Plan	-	-	-	71%
Received Reliever Medication	-	-	-	100%
Use of Medical Imaging				
Combination Abdominal CT Scan	1,699	0.051	0.219	0.191
Combination Chest CT Scan	1,306	0.060	0.102	0.054
Follow-up Mammogram/Ultrasound	3,419	10.0%	8%	8.4%
MRI for Low Back Pain	268	35.8%	30.7%	32.7%
Survey of Patients' Hospital Experiences				
Area Around Room 'Always' Quiet at Night	300+	63%	-	58%
Doctors 'Always' Communicated Well	300+	81%	-	80%
Home Recovery Information Given	300+	79%	-	82%
Hospital Given 9 or 10 on 10 Point Scale	300+	72%	-	67%
Meds 'Always' Explained Before Given	300+	61%	-	60%
Nurses 'Always' Communicated Well	300+	76%	-	76%
Pain 'Always' Well Controlled	300+	70%	-	69%
Room and Bathroom 'Always' Clean	300+	72%	-	71%
Timely Help 'Always' Received	300+	62%	-	64%
Would Definitely Recommend Hospital	300+	76%	-	69%

Delta Medical Center

3000 Getwell Rd Phone: 901-369-8100
Memphis, TN 38118 Fax: 901-369-8503
URL: www.deltamedcenter.com
Type: Acute Care Hospitals Emergency Services: Yes
Ownership: Proprietary Beds: 243

Key Personnel:
CEO/President. . . . . J Gene Faile
Chief of Medical Staff . . . . Gregory Vandevan
Coronary Care . . . . Mary Hammons
Infection Control. . . . . Debbie Braddock
Operating Room. . . . . Hazel Collins
Quality Assurance . . . . Shayne Racheals
Anesthesiology. . . . . Salwa Moustafa, MD
Emergency Room . . . . Rita Garner

Measure	Cases	This Hosp.	State Avg.	U.S. Avg.
Heart Attack Care				
ACE Inhibitor or ARB for LVSD[1]	1	100%	96%	96%
Aspirin at Arrival[1]	11	100%	98%	99%
Aspirin at Discharge[1]	5	80%	99%	98%
Beta Blocker at Discharge[1]	5	80%	98%	98%
Fibrinolytic Medication Timing	0	-	67%	55%
PCI Within 90 Minutes of Arrival	0	-	91%	90%
Smoking Cessation Advice[1]	3	100%	100%	99%
Chest Pain/Possible Heart Attack Care				
Aspirin at Arrival[5]	0	-	95%	95%
Median Time to ECG (minutes)[5]	0	-	8	8
Median Time to Transfer (minutes)[5]	0	-	65	61
Fibrinolytic Medication Timing[5]	0	-	49%	54%
Heart Failure Care				
ACE Inhibitor or ARB for LVSD	56	91%	95%	94%
Discharge Instructions	149	94%	88%	88%
Evaluation of LVS Function	161	96%	97%	98%
Smoking Cessation Advice	46	96%	99%	98%
Pneumonia Care				
Appropriate Initial Antibiotic	40	98%	92%	92%
Blood Culture Timing	59	97%	97%	96%
Influenza Vaccine[1]	23	87%	93%	91%
Initial Antibiotic Timing	52	90%	96%	95%
Pneumococcal Vaccine[1]	15	100%	95%	93%
Smoking Cessation Advice	35	97%	99%	97%
Surgical Care Improvement Project				
Appropriate VTP Within 24 Hours	40	85%	92%	92%
Appropriate Hair Removal	131	100%	100%	99%
Appropriate Beta Blocker Usage[1]	17	82%	93%	93%
Controlled Postoperative Blood Glucose	0	-	93%	93%
Prophylactic Antibiotic Timing	77	96%	97%	97%
Prophylactic Antibiotic Timing (Outpatient)[1]	9	89%	94%	92%
Prophylactic Antibiotic Selection	79	99%	97%	97%
Prophylactic Antibiotic Select. (Outpatient)[1]	9	100%	94%	94%
Prophylactic Antibiotic Stopped	73	92%	94%	94%
Recommended VTP Ordered	46	74%	94%	94%
Urinary Catheter Removal[1]	10	70%	90%	90%
Children's Asthma Care				
Received Systemic Corticosteroids	-	-	-	100%
Received Home Management Plan	-	-	-	71%
Received Reliever Medication	-	-	-	100%
Use of Medical Imaging				
Combination Abdominal CT Scan	47	0.596	0.219	0.191
Combination Chest CT Scan[1]	50	0.060	0.102	0.054
Follow-up Mammogram/Ultrasound	119	7.6%	8%	8.4%
MRI for Low Back Pain[1]	14	71.4%	30.7%	32.7%
Survey of Patients' Hospital Experiences				
Area Around Room 'Always' Quiet at Night	300+	76%	-	58%
Doctors 'Always' Communicated Well	300+	73%	-	80%
Home Recovery Information Given	300+	72%	-	82%
Hospital Given 9 or 10 on 10 Point Scale	300+	60%	-	67%
Meds 'Always' Explained Before Given	300+	55%	-	60%
Nurses 'Always' Communicated Well	300+	71%	-	76%
Pain 'Always' Well Controlled	300+	63%	-	69%
Room and Bathroom 'Always' Clean	300+	74%	-	71%
Timely Help 'Always' Received	300+	51%	-	64%
Would Definitely Recommend Hospital	300+	57%	-	69%

Memphis VA Medical Center

1030 Jefferson Avenue Phone: 901-577-7200
Memphis, TN 38104 Fax: 901-577-7251
URL: www.va.gov/sta/guide/home.asp
Type: Acute Care-Veterans Administration Emergency Services: No
Ownership: Government - Federal Beds: 263

Key Personnel:
CEO/President. . . . . James L Robinson, III
Cardiac Laboratory. . . . . K Ramanathan, MD
Chief of Medical Staff . . . . Margarette Hagemann, MD
Infection Control. . . . . Ellen W Whitnack, MD
Quality Assurance . . . . Melinda Kincade
Radiology. . . . . John R Ware, MD

Measure	Cases	This Hosp.	State Avg.	U.S. Avg.
Heart Attack Care				
ACE Inhibitor or ARB for LVSD[1]	17	94%	96%	96%
Aspirin at Arrival	68	100%	98%	99%
Aspirin at Discharge	65	100%	99%	98%
Beta Blocker at Discharge	61	100%	98%	98%
Fibrinolytic Medication Timing[5]	0	-	67%	55%
PCI Within 90 Minutes of Arrival[1]	5	100%	91%	90%
Smoking Cessation Advice	28	100%	100%	99%
Chest Pain/Possible Heart Attack Care				
Aspirin at Arrival	-	-	95%	95%
Median Time to ECG (minutes)	-	-	8	8
Median Time to Transfer (minutes)	-	-	65	61
Fibrinolytic Medication Timing	-	-	49%	54%
Heart Failure Care				
ACE Inhibitor or ARB for LVSD	126	98%	95%	94%
Discharge Instructions	246	99%	88%	88%
Evaluation of LVS Function	255	99%	97%	98%
Smoking Cessation Advice	79	100%	99%	98%
Pneumonia Care				
Appropriate Initial Antibiotic	99	99%	92%	92%
Blood Culture Timing	154	99%	97%	96%
Influenza Vaccine	108	85%	93%	91%
Initial Antibiotic Timing	146	94%	96%	95%
Pneumococcal Vaccine	107	94%	95%	93%
Smoking Cessation Advice	62	100%	99%	97%
Surgical Care Improvement Project				
Appropriate VTP Within 24 Hours[2,5]	0	-	92%	92%
Appropriate Hair Removal[2,5]	0	-	100%	99%
Appropriate Beta Blocker Usage[2,5]	0	-	93%	93%
Controlled Postoperative Blood Glucose[2,5]	0	-	93%	93%
Prophylactic Antibiotic Timing[5]	0	-	97%	97%
Prophylactic Antibiotic Timing (Outpatient)	-	-	94%	92%
Prophylactic Antibiotic Selection[5]	0	-	97%	97%
Prophylactic Antibiotic Select. (Outpatient)	-	-	94%	94%
Prophylactic Antibiotic Stopped[5]	0	-	94%	94%
Recommended VTP Ordered[2,5]	0	-	94%	94%
Urinary Catheter Removal[2,5]	0	-	90%	90%
Children's Asthma Care				
Received Systemic Corticosteroids	-	-	-	100%
Received Home Management Plan	-	-	-	71%
Received Reliever Medication	-	-	-	100%
Use of Medical Imaging				
Combination Abdominal CT Scan	-	-	0.219	0.191
Combination Chest CT Scan	-	-	0.102	0.054
Follow-up Mammogram/Ultrasound	-	-	8%	8.4%
MRI for Low Back Pain	-	-	30.7%	32.7%
Survey of Patients' Hospital Experiences				
Area Around Room 'Always' Quiet at Night	-	-	-	58%
Doctors 'Always' Communicated Well	-	-	-	80%
Home Recovery Information Given	-	-	-	82%
Hospital Given 9 or 10 on 10 Point Scale	-	-	-	67%
Meds 'Always' Explained Before Given	-	-	-	60%
Nurses 'Always' Communicated Well	-	-	-	76%
Pain 'Always' Well Controlled	-	-	-	69%
Room and Bathroom 'Always' Clean	-	-	-	71%
Timely Help 'Always' Received	-	-	-	64%
Would Definitely Recommend Hospital	-	-	-	69%

NOTE: Hospital profiles are in alphabetical order by state, then city, then hospital within the city; Rankings exclude hospitals with less than 25 cases except for patient surveys which excludes hospitals with less than 100 cases; (a) 100–299 cases; (1) The number of cases is too small to be sure how well a hospital is performing; (2) The hospital indicated that the data submitted for this measure were based on a sample of cases; (3) Data was collected during a shorter time period (fewer quarters) than the maximum possible time for this measure; (4) Suppressed for one or more quarters by CMS; (5) No data is available from the hospital for this measure; (6) Fewer than 100 patients completed the HCAHPS survey. Use these rates with caution, as the number of surveys may be too low to reliably assess hospital performance; (7) Survey results are based on less than 12 months of data; (8) Survey results are not available for this reporting period; (9) No or very few patients were eligible for the HCAHPS survey. The scores shown, if any, reflect a very small number of surveys; (10) A state average was not calculated because too few hospitals in the state submitted data; (11) There were discrepancies in the data collection process; Please refer to the User's Guide for a full explanation of data.

Methodist Healthcare Memphis Hospitals

1265 Union Ave Suite 700
Memphis, TN 38104
Phone: 901-516-8274
Fax: 901-516-0528
URL: www.methodisthealth.org
Type: Acute Care Hospitals
Emergency Services: Yes
Ownership: Voluntary Non-Profit - Church
Beds: 693

Key Personnel:

CEO/President. . . . . Gary Shorb
Infection Control. . . . . Bryan Simmons, MD
Operating Room. . . . . Bonnie Williams
Quality Assurance . . . . Carl Cross
Radiology. . . . . Davis Moser, MD
Emergency Room . . . . Ferrell Varner, Jr, DM
Hemotology Center . . . . Irving Fleming
Intensive Care Unit. . . . . Donna Brown

Measure	Cases	This Hosp.	State Avg.	U.S. Avg.
Heart Attack Care				
ACE Inhibitor or ARB for LVSD	182	99%	96%	96%
Aspirin at Arrival	741	100%	98%	99%
Aspirin at Discharge	950	100%	99%	98%
Beta Blocker at Discharge	941	100%	98%	98%
Fibrinolytic Medication Timing	0	-	67%	55%
PCI Within 90 Minutes of Arrival	155	99%	91%	90%
Smoking Cessation Advice	435	100%	100%	99%
Chest Pain/Possible Heart Attack Care				
Aspirin at Arrival[1]	20	80%	95%	95%
Median Time to ECG (minutes)[1]	23	8	8	8
Median Time to Transfer (minutes)[5]	0	-	65	61
Fibrinolytic Medication Timing[3]	0	-	49%	54%
Heart Failure Care				
ACE Inhibitor or ARB for LVSD[2]	531	99%	95%	94%
Discharge Instructions[2]	1,084	94%	88%	88%
Evaluation of LVS Function[2]	1,215	100%	97%	98%
Smoking Cessation Advice[2]	268	100%	99%	98%
Pneumonia Care				
Appropriate Initial Antibiotic[2]	289	93%	92%	92%
Blood Culture Timing[2]	453	98%	97%	96%
Influenza Vaccine[2]	219	100%	93%	91%
Initial Antibiotic Timing[2]	424	98%	96%	95%
Pneumococcal Vaccine[2]	294	100%	95%	93%
Smoking Cessation Advice[2]	235	100%	99%	97%
Surgical Care Improvement Project				
Appropriate VTP Within 24 Hours[2]	1,309	95%	92%	92%
Appropriate Hair Removal[2]	3,589	100%	100%	99%
Appropriate Beta Blocker Usage[2]	988	95%	93%	93%
Controlled Postoperative Blood Glucose[2]	478	97%	93%	93%
Prophylactic Antibiotic Timing[2]	2,254	99%	97%	97%
Prophylactic Antibiotic Timing (Outpatient)	1,189	96%	94%	92%
Prophylactic Antibiotic Selection[2]	2,277	97%	97%	97%
Prophylactic Antibiotic Select. (Outpatient)	1,177	95%	94%	94%
Prophylactic Antibiotic Stopped[2]	2,142	95%	94%	94%
Recommended VTP Ordered[2]	1,318	96%	94%	94%
Urinary Catheter Removal[2]	452	90%	90%	90%
Children's Asthma Care				
Received Systemic Corticosteroids	-	-	-	100%
Received Home Management Plan	-	-	-	71%
Received Reliever Medication	-	-	-	100%
Use of Medical Imaging				
Combination Abdominal CT Scan	3,067	0.245	0.219	0.191
Combination Chest CT Scan	2,231	0.150	0.102	0.054
Follow-up Mammogram/Ultrasound	4,237	10.0%	8%	8.4%
MRI for Low Back Pain	505	33.5%	30.7%	32.7%
Survey of Patients' Hospital Experiences				
Area Around Room 'Always' Quiet at Night	300+	63%	-	58%
Doctors 'Always' Communicated Well	300+	77%	-	80%
Home Recovery Information Given	300+	79%	-	82%
Hospital Given 9 or 10 on 10 Point Scale	300+	68%	-	67%
Meds 'Always' Explained Before Given	300+	59%	-	60%
Nurses 'Always' Communicated Well	300+	74%	-	76%
Pain 'Always' Well Controlled	300+	68%	-	69%
Room and Bathroom 'Always' Clean	300+	64%	-	71%
Timely Help 'Always' Received	300+	57%	-	64%
Would Definitely Recommend Hospital	300+	72%	-	69%

Regional Medical Center at Memphis

877 Jefferson Avenue
Memphis, TN 38103
Phone: 901-545-7928
Fax: 901-545-8649
E-mail: ssnell@the-med.org
URL: www.the-med.org
Type: Acute Care Hospitals
Emergency Services: Yes
Ownership: Govt - Hospital Dist/Auth
Beds: 631

Key Personnel:

CEO/President. . . . . Claude Watts, JR
Cardiac Laboratory. . . . . Brenda Theus
Chief of Medical Staff . . . . Stuart Polly MD
Infection Control. . . . . Stuart Polly MD
Operating Room. . . . . Linda Duncan
Quality Assurance . . . . Terri Adams
Radiology. . . . . Judy Perkins

Measure	Cases	This Hosp.	State Avg.	U.S. Avg.
Heart Attack Care				
ACE Inhibitor or ARB for LVSD[1]	9	100%	96%	96%
Aspirin at Arrival	46	91%	98%	99%
Aspirin at Discharge	43	98%	99%	98%
Beta Blocker at Discharge	40	95%	98%	98%
Fibrinolytic Medication Timing[1]	2	0%	67%	55%
PCI Within 90 Minutes of Arrival[1]	5	20%	91%	90%
Smoking Cessation Advice	32	100%	100%	99%
Chest Pain/Possible Heart Attack Care				
Aspirin at Arrival[5]	0	-	95%	95%
Median Time to ECG (minutes)[5]	0	-	8	8
Median Time to Transfer (minutes)[5]	0	-	65	61
Fibrinolytic Medication Timing[5]	0	-	49%	54%
Heart Failure Care				
ACE Inhibitor or ARB for LVSD	151	100%	95%	94%
Discharge Instructions	241	79%	88%	88%
Evaluation of LVS Function	254	100%	97%	98%
Smoking Cessation Advice	118	100%	99%	98%
Pneumonia Care				
Appropriate Initial Antibiotic	46	98%	92%	92%
Blood Culture Timing	73	86%	97%	96%
Influenza Vaccine[1]	12	92%	93%	91%
Initial Antibiotic Timing	80	82%	96%	95%
Pneumococcal Vaccine[1]	18	100%	95%	93%
Smoking Cessation Advice	67	100%	99%	97%
Surgical Care Improvement Project				
Appropriate VTP Within 24 Hours	318	93%	92%	92%
Appropriate Hair Removal	486	100%	100%	99%
Appropriate Beta Blocker Usage	50	84%	93%	93%
Controlled Postoperative Blood Glucose[1]	4	100%	93%	93%
Prophylactic Antibiotic Timing	119	93%	97%	97%
Prophylactic Antibiotic Timing (Outpatient)	45	96%	94%	92%
Prophylactic Antibiotic Selection	123	95%	97%	97%
Prophylactic Antibiotic Select. (Outpatient)	44	95%	94%	94%
Prophylactic Antibiotic Stopped	116	93%	94%	94%
Recommended VTP Ordered	318	96%	94%	94%
Urinary Catheter Removal	41	73%	90%	90%
Children's Asthma Care				
Received Systemic Corticosteroids	-	-	-	100%
Received Home Management Plan	-	-	-	71%
Received Reliever Medication	-	-	-	100%
Use of Medical Imaging				
Combination Abdominal CT Scan	273	0.377	0.219	0.191
Combination Chest CT Scan	260	0.119	0.102	0.054
Follow-up Mammogram/Ultrasound	257	7.4%	8%	8.4%
MRI for Low Back Pain[1]	24	37.5%	30.7%	32.7%
Survey of Patients' Hospital Experiences				
Area Around Room 'Always' Quiet at Night	300+	58%	-	58%
Doctors 'Always' Communicated Well	300+	79%	-	80%
Home Recovery Information Given	300+	81%	-	82%
Hospital Given 9 or 10 on 10 Point Scale	300+	55%	-	67%
Meds 'Always' Explained Before Given	300+	57%	-	60%
Nurses 'Always' Communicated Well	300+	69%	-	76%
Pain 'Always' Well Controlled	300+	60%	-	69%
Room and Bathroom 'Always' Clean	300+	59%	-	71%
Timely Help 'Always' Received	300+	51%	-	64%
Would Definitely Recommend Hospital	300+	63%	-	69%

Saint Francis Hospital

5959 Park Ave
Memphis, TN 38119
Phone: 901-765-1000
Fax: 901-765-1799
Type: Acute Care Hospitals
Emergency Services: No
Ownership: Proprietary
Beds: 651

Key Personnel:

Chief of Medical Staff. . . . . Robert Kraus, MD
Infection Control. . . . . Mike Todai
Pediatric In-Patient Care . . . . . . Isaac John, MD
Quality Assurance . . . . Tricia Caughley
Radiology. . . . . R Steven Roney, MD
Anesthesiology. . . . . Kays Nawaf, MD
Emergency Room . . . . Jack Bandura, MD

Measure	Cases	This Hosp.	State Avg.	U.S. Avg.
Heart Attack Care				
ACE Inhibitor or ARB for LVSD	39	100%	96%	96%
Aspirin at Arrival	248	98%	98%	99%
Aspirin at Discharge	292	98%	99%	98%
Beta Blocker at Discharge	289	100%	98%	98%
Fibrinolytic Medication Timing	0	-	67%	55%
PCI Within 90 Minutes of Arrival	44	86%	91%	90%
Smoking Cessation Advice	96	100%	100%	99%
Chest Pain/Possible Heart Attack Care				
Aspirin at Arrival[5]	0	-	95%	95%
Median Time to ECG (minutes)[5]	0	-	8	8
Median Time to Transfer (minutes)[5]	0	-	65	61
Fibrinolytic Medication Timing[5]	0	-	49%	54%
Heart Failure Care				
ACE Inhibitor or ARB for LVSD	293	98%	95%	94%
Discharge Instructions	660	95%	88%	88%
Evaluation of LVS Function	763	100%	97%	98%
Smoking Cessation Advice	117	100%	99%	98%
Pneumonia Care				
Appropriate Initial Antibiotic	108	88%	92%	92%
Blood Culture Timing	172	95%	97%	96%
Influenza Vaccine	142	95%	93%	91%
Initial Antibiotic Timing	209	92%	96%	95%
Pneumococcal Vaccine	192	97%	95%	93%
Smoking Cessation Advice	79	100%	99%	97%
Surgical Care Improvement Project				
Appropriate VTP Within 24 Hours[2]	236	88%	92%	92%
Appropriate Hair Removal[2]	599	99%	100%	99%
Appropriate Beta Blocker Usage[2]	208	91%	93%	93%
Controlled Postoperative Blood Glucose[2]	166	96%	93%	93%
Prophylactic Antibiotic Timing[2]	418	95%	97%	97%
Prophylactic Antibiotic Timing (Outpatient)	461	93%	94%	92%
Prophylactic Antibiotic Selection[2]	425	95%	97%	97%
Prophylactic Antibiotic Select. (Outpatient)	449	91%	94%	94%
Prophylactic Antibiotic Stopped[2]	396	92%	94%	94%
Recommended VTP Ordered[2]	236	92%	94%	94%
Urinary Catheter Removal[2]	101	80%	90%	90%
Children's Asthma Care				
Received Systemic Corticosteroids	-	-	-	100%
Received Home Management Plan	-	-	-	71%
Received Reliever Medication	-	-	-	100%
Use of Medical Imaging				
Combination Abdominal CT Scan	770	0.747	0.219	0.191
Combination Chest CT Scan	525	0.004	0.102	0.054
Follow-up Mammogram/Ultrasound	1,212	7.3%	8%	8.4%
MRI for Low Back Pain	210	31.4%	30.7%	32.7%
Survey of Patients' Hospital Experiences				
Area Around Room 'Always' Quiet at Night	300+	67%	-	58%
Doctors 'Always' Communicated Well	300+	83%	-	80%
Home Recovery Information Given	300+	80%	-	82%
Hospital Given 9 or 10 on 10 Point Scale	300+	65%	-	67%
Meds 'Always' Explained Before Given	300+	63%	-	60%
Nurses 'Always' Communicated Well	300+	75%	-	76%
Pain 'Always' Well Controlled	300+	69%	-	69%
Room and Bathroom 'Always' Clean	300+	63%	-	71%
Timely Help 'Always' Received	300+	57%	-	64%
Would Definitely Recommend Hospital	300+	69%	-	69%

NOTE: Hospital profiles are in alphabetical order by state, then city, then hospital within the city; Rankings exclude hospitals with less than 25 cases except for patient surveys which excludes hospitals with less than 100 cases; (a) 100–299 cases; (1) The number of cases is too small to be sure how well a hospital is performing; (2) The hospital indicated that the data submitted for this measure were based on a sample of cases; (3) Data was collected during a shorter time period (fewer quarters) than the maximum possible time for this measure; (4) Suppressed for one or more quarters by CMS; (5) No data is available from the hospital for this measure; (6) Fewer than 100 patients completed the HCAHPS survey. Use these rates with caution, as the number of surveys may be too low to reliably assess hospital performance; (7) Survey results are based on less than 12 months of data; (8) Survey results are not available for this reporting period; (9) No or very few patients were eligible for the HCAHPS survey. The scores shown, if any, reflect a very small number of surveys; (10) A state average was not calculated because too few hospitals in the state submitted data; (11) There were discrepancies in the data collection process; Please refer to the User's Guide for a full explanation of data.

Milan General Hospital

4039 Highland St
Milan, TN 38358
Phone: 731-686-1591
Fax: 731-686-5129
Type: Acute Care Hospitals
Emergency Services: Yes
Ownership: Government - Local
Beds: 72

Key Personnel:

Chief of Medical Staff.......... Kim Tozer, MD
Infection Control.............. Sandra Isbell
Operating Room............. June Bolton
Quality Assurance .... Jerry Barker

Measure	Cases	This Hosp.	State Avg.	U.S. Avg.
Heart Attack Care				
ACE Inhibitor or ARB for LVSD[3]	0	-	96%	96%
Aspirin at Arrival[3]	0	-	98%	99%
Aspirin at Discharge[3]	0	-	99%	98%
Beta Blocker at Discharge[3]	0	-	98%	98%
Fibrinolytic Medication Timing[3]	0	-	67%	55%
PCI Within 90 Minutes of Arrival[3]	0	-	91%	90%
Smoking Cessation Advice[3]	0	-	100%	99%
Chest Pain/Possible Heart Attack Care				
Aspirin at Arrival	123	93%	95%	95%
Median Time to ECG (minutes)	138	12	8	8
Median Time to Transfer (minutes)[5]	0	-	65	61
Fibrinolytic Medication Timing[1]	12	58%	49%	54%
Heart Failure Care				
ACE Inhibitor or ARB for LVSD[1]	2	100%	95%	94%
Discharge Instructions[1]	4	100%	88%	88%
Evaluation of LVS Function[1]	6	100%	97%	98%
Smoking Cessation Advice	0	-	99%	98%
Pneumonia Care				
Appropriate Initial Antibiotic[1]	16	75%	92%	92%
Blood Culture Timing[1]	16	100%	97%	96%
Influenza Vaccine[1]	7	100%	93%	91%
Initial Antibiotic Timing[1]	16	94%	96%	95%
Pneumococcal Vaccine[1]	12	100%	95%	93%
Smoking Cessation Advice[1]	4	100%	99%	97%
Surgical Care Improvement Project				
Appropriate VTP Within 24 Hours[1]	11	100%	92%	92%
Appropriate Hair Removal[1]	21	100%	100%	99%
Appropriate Beta Blocker Usage[1]	3	100%	93%	93%
Controlled Postoperative Blood Glucose	0	-	93%	93%
Prophylactic Antibiotic Timing[1]	4	100%	97%	97%
Prophylactic Antibiotic Timing (Outpatient)[1]	12	67%	94%	92%
Prophylactic Antibiotic Selection[1]	4	75%	97%	97%
Prophylactic Antibiotic Select. (Outpatient)[1]	8	62%	94%	94%
Prophylactic Antibiotic Stopped[1]	4	75%	94%	94%
Recommended VTP Ordered[1]	11	100%	94%	94%
Urinary Catheter Removal[1]	1	100%	90%	90%
Children's Asthma Care				
Received Systemic Corticosteroids	-	-	-	100%
Received Home Management Plan	-	-	-	71%
Received Reliever Medication	-	-	-	100%
Use of Medical Imaging				
Combination Abdominal CT Scan	166	0.000	0.219	0.191
Combination Chest CT Scan	71	0.000	0.102	0.054
Follow-up Mammogram/Ultrasound	271	9.2%	8%	8.4%
MRI for Low Back Pain[5]	0	-	30.7%	32.7%
Survey of Patients' Hospital Experiences				
Area Around Room 'Always' Quiet at Night[6]	<100	81%	-	58%
Doctors 'Always' Communicated Well[6]	<100	94%	-	80%
Home Recovery Information Given[6]	<100	84%	-	82%
Hospital Given 9 or 10 on 10 Point Scale[6]	<100	79%	-	67%
Meds 'Always' Explained Before Given[6]	<100	74%	-	60%
Nurses 'Always' Communicated Well[6]	<100	91%	-	76%
Pain 'Always' Well Controlled[6]	<100	88%	-	69%
Room and Bathroom 'Always' Clean[6]	<100	84%	-	71%
Timely Help 'Always' Received[6]	<100	82%	-	64%
Would Definitely Recommend Hospital	<100	79%	-	69%

Lakeway Regional Hospital

726 Mcfarland St
Morristown, TN 37814
Phone: 423-522-6000
Fax: 423-587-8548
Type: Acute Care Hospitals
Emergency Services: Yes
Ownership: Proprietary
Beds: 135

Key Personnel:

CEO/President................ Priscilla Mills
Chief of Medical Staff.......... Paul Cardall, MD
Infection Control............. Eva Stinson, RN
Operating Room.............. Pat Freeman
Quality Assurance .... Kristen Kilgore, RN
Radiology.................. Michael Adler
Emergency Room .... Debbie Boyd
Intensive Care Unit........... Anne Johnson, RN

Measure	Cases	This Hosp.	State Avg.	U.S. Avg.
Heart Attack Care				
ACE Inhibitor or ARB for LVSD[1]	3	67%	96%	96%
Aspirin at Arrival[1]	12	75%	98%	99%
Aspirin at Discharge[1]	14	79%	99%	98%
Beta Blocker at Discharge[1]	13	92%	98%	98%
Fibrinolytic Medication Timing	0	-	67%	55%
PCI Within 90 Minutes of Arrival	0	-	91%	90%
Smoking Cessation Advice[1]	3	100%	100%	99%
Chest Pain/Possible Heart Attack Care				
Aspirin at Arrival[1]	18	94%	95%	95%
Median Time to ECG (minutes)[1]	18	6	8	8
Median Time to Transfer (minutes)[1,3]	3	79	65	61
Fibrinolytic Medication Timing	0	-	49%	54%
Heart Failure Care				
ACE Inhibitor or ARB for LVSD[1]	8	100%	95%	94%
Discharge Instructions	57	96%	88%	88%
Evaluation of LVS Function	66	98%	97%	98%
Smoking Cessation Advice[1]	11	100%	99%	98%
Pneumonia Care				
Appropriate Initial Antibiotic	51	98%	92%	92%
Blood Culture Timing	58	100%	97%	96%
Influenza Vaccine	41	85%	93%	91%
Initial Antibiotic Timing	90	98%	96%	95%
Pneumococcal Vaccine	52	85%	95%	93%
Smoking Cessation Advice	42	100%	99%	97%
Surgical Care Improvement Project				
Appropriate VTP Within 24 Hours[2]	51	82%	92%	92%
Appropriate Hair Removal[2]	149	99%	100%	99%
Appropriate Beta Blocker Usage[2]	45	93%	93%	93%
Controlled Postoperative Blood Glucose[2]	0	-	93%	93%
Prophylactic Antibiotic Timing[2]	123	98%	97%	97%
Prophylactic Antibiotic Timing (Outpatient)	168	95%	94%	92%
Prophylactic Antibiotic Selection[2]	126	99%	97%	97%
Prophylactic Antibiotic Select. (Outpatient)	166	90%	94%	94%
Prophylactic Antibiotic Stopped[2]	122	93%	94%	94%
Recommended VTP Ordered[2]	52	85%	94%	94%
Urinary Catheter Removal	44	89%	90%	90%
Children's Asthma Care				
Received Systemic Corticosteroids	-	-	-	100%
Received Home Management Plan	-	-	-	71%
Received Reliever Medication	-	-	-	100%
Use of Medical Imaging				
Combination Abdominal CT Scan	220	0.582	0.219	0.191
Combination Chest CT Scan	82	0.610	0.102	0.054
Follow-up Mammogram/Ultrasound	157	8.9%	8%	8.4%
MRI for Low Back Pain	107	25.2%	30.7%	32.7%
Survey of Patients' Hospital Experiences				
Area Around Room 'Always' Quiet at Night	300+	65%	-	58%
Doctors 'Always' Communicated Well	300+	78%	-	80%
Home Recovery Information Given	300+	81%	-	82%
Hospital Given 9 or 10 on 10 Point Scale	300+	65%	-	67%
Meds 'Always' Explained Before Given	300+	59%	-	60%
Nurses 'Always' Communicated Well	300+	74%	-	76%
Pain 'Always' Well Controlled	300+	65%	-	69%
Room and Bathroom 'Always' Clean	300+	65%	-	71%
Timely Help 'Always' Received	300+	59%	-	64%
Would Definitely Recommend Hospital	300+	66%	-	69%

Morristown Hamblen Hospital Association

908 W 4th North St
Morristown, TN 37814
Phone: 423-586-4231
Fax: 423-585-1271
URL: www.mhhs1.org
Type: Acute Care Hospitals
Emergency Services: No
Ownership: Government - Local
Beds: 155

Key Personnel:

CEO/President.............. Richard L Clark
Chief of Medical Staff.......... Sunil Ramaprasad, MD
Infection Control............. Tarry Samsel
Operating Room.............. David Crawford
Quality Assurance .... Rita Bunch
Radiology.................. Stephen J Brown
Anesthesiology............... Mark Davenport, MD
Emergency Room .... Cynthia Thompson, RN

Measure	Cases	This Hosp.	State Avg.	U.S. Avg.
Heart Attack Care				
ACE Inhibitor or ARB for LVSD[1]	14	93%	96%	96%
Aspirin at Arrival	195	99%	98%	99%
Aspirin at Discharge	202	98%	99%	98%
Beta Blocker at Discharge	209	97%	98%	98%
Fibrinolytic Medication Timing	0	-	67%	55%
PCI Within 90 Minutes of Arrival	51	96%	91%	90%
Smoking Cessation Advice	95	99%	100%	99%
Chest Pain/Possible Heart Attack Care				
Aspirin at Arrival[1]	20	95%	95%	95%
Median Time to ECG (minutes)	25	11	8	8
Median Time to Transfer (minutes)[5]	0	-	65	61
Fibrinolytic Medication Timing[5]	0	-	49%	54%
Heart Failure Care				
ACE Inhibitor or ARB for LVSD	63	98%	95%	94%
Discharge Instructions	245	88%	88%	88%
Evaluation of LVS Function	270	99%	97%	98%
Smoking Cessation Advice	69	97%	99%	98%
Pneumonia Care				
Appropriate Initial Antibiotic	203	87%	92%	92%
Blood Culture Timing	288	99%	97%	96%
Influenza Vaccine	162	99%	93%	91%
Initial Antibiotic Timing	300	98%	96%	95%
Pneumococcal Vaccine	216	95%	95%	93%
Smoking Cessation Advice	139	100%	99%	97%
Surgical Care Improvement Project				
Appropriate VTP Within 24 Hours	130	93%	92%	92%
Appropriate Hair Removal	387	100%	100%	99%
Appropriate Beta Blocker Usage	122	91%	93%	93%
Controlled Postoperative Blood Glucose	0	-	93%	93%
Prophylactic Antibiotic Timing	274	97%	97%	97%
Prophylactic Antibiotic Timing (Outpatient)	271	88%	94%	92%
Prophylactic Antibiotic Selection	278	99%	97%	97%
Prophylactic Antibiotic Select. (Outpatient)	252	91%	94%	94%
Prophylactic Antibiotic Stopped	262	95%	94%	94%
Recommended VTP Ordered	130	97%	94%	94%
Urinary Catheter Removal	102	96%	90%	90%
Children's Asthma Care				
Received Systemic Corticosteroids	-	-	-	100%
Received Home Management Plan	-	-	-	71%
Received Reliever Medication	-	-	-	100%
Use of Medical Imaging				
Combination Abdominal CT Scan	619	0.118	0.219	0.191
Combination Chest CT Scan	389	0.159	0.102	0.054
Follow-up Mammogram/Ultrasound	541	7.8%	8%	8.4%
MRI for Low Back Pain	189	19.6%	30.7%	32.7%
Survey of Patients' Hospital Experiences				
Area Around Room 'Always' Quiet at Night	300+	54%	-	58%
Doctors 'Always' Communicated Well	300+	81%	-	80%
Home Recovery Information Given	300+	88%	-	82%
Hospital Given 9 or 10 on 10 Point Scale	300+	65%	-	67%
Meds 'Always' Explained Before Given	300+	61%	-	60%
Nurses 'Always' Communicated Well	300+	79%	-	76%
Pain 'Always' Well Controlled	300+	67%	-	69%
Room and Bathroom 'Always' Clean	300+	77%	-	71%
Timely Help 'Always' Received	300+	66%	-	64%
Would Definitely Recommend Hospital	300+	71%	-	69%

NOTE: Hospital profiles are in alphabetical order by state, then city, then hospital within the city; Rankings exclude hospitals with less than 25 cases except for patient surveys which excludes hospitals with less than 100 cases; (a) 100–299 cases; (1) The number of cases is too small to be sure how well a hospital is performing; (2) The hospital indicated that the data submitted for this measure were based on a sample of cases; (3) Data was collected during a shorter time period (fewer quarters) than the maximum possible time for this measure; (4) Suppressed for one or more quarters by CMS; (5) No data is available from the hospital for this measure; (6) Fewer than 100 patients completed the HCAHPS survey. Use these rates with caution, as the number of surveys may be too low to reliably assess hospital performance; (7) Survey results are based on less than 12 months of data; (8) Survey results are not available for this reporting period; (9) No or very few patients were eligible for the HCAHPS survey. The scores shown, if any, reflect a very small number of surveys; (10) A state average was not calculated because too few hospitals in the state submitted data; (11) There were discrepancies in the data collection process; Please refer to the User's Guide for a full explanation of data.

Johnson County Community Hospital

1901 S Shady St
Mountain City, TN 37683
URL: www.msha.com
Type: Critical Access Hospitals
Ownership: Voluntary Non-Profit - Other

Phone: 423-727-1110
Fax: 423-727-1105
Emergency Services: Yes
Beds: 2

Measure	Cases	This Hosp.	State Avg.	U.S. Avg.
Heart Attack Care				
ACE Inhibitor or ARB for LVSD	-	-	96%	96%
Aspirin at Arrival	-	-	98%	99%
Aspirin at Discharge	-	-	99%	98%
Beta Blocker at Discharge	-	-	98%	98%
Fibrinolytic Medication Timing	-	-	67%	55%
PCI Within 90 Minutes of Arrival	-	-	91%	90%
Smoking Cessation Advice	-	-	100%	99%
Chest Pain/Possible Heart Attack Care				
Aspirin at Arrival	138	94%	95%	95%
Median Time to ECG (minutes)	149	13	8	8
Median Time to Transfer (minutes)[5]	0	-	65	61
Fibrinolytic Medication Timing[5]	0	-	49%	54%
Heart Failure Care				
ACE Inhibitor or ARB for LVSD	-	-	95%	94%
Discharge Instructions	-	-	88%	88%
Evaluation of LVS Function	-	-	97%	98%
Smoking Cessation Advice	-	-	99%	98%
Pneumonia Care				
Appropriate Initial Antibiotic	-	-	92%	92%
Blood Culture Timing	-	-	97%	96%
Influenza Vaccine	-	-	93%	91%
Initial Antibiotic Timing	-	-	96%	95%
Pneumococcal Vaccine	-	-	95%	93%
Smoking Cessation Advice	-	-	99%	97%
Surgical Care Improvement Project				
Appropriate VTP Within 24 Hours	-	-	92%	92%
Appropriate Hair Removal	-	-	100%	99%
Appropriate Beta Blocker Usage	-	-	93%	93%
Controlled Postoperative Blood Glucose	-	-	93%	93%
Prophylactic Antibiotic Timing	-	-	97%	97%
Prophylactic Antibiotic Timing (Outpatient)[5]	0	-	94%	92%
Prophylactic Antibiotic Selection	-	-	97%	97%
Prophylactic Antibiotic Select. (Outpatient)[5]	0	-	94%	94%
Prophylactic Antibiotic Stopped	-	-	94%	94%
Recommended VTP Ordered	-	-	94%	94%
Urinary Catheter Removal	-	-	90%	90%
Children's Asthma Care				
Received Systemic Corticosteroids	-	-	-	100%
Received Home Management Plan	-	-	-	71%
Received Reliever Medication	-	-	-	100%
Use of Medical Imaging				
Combination Abdominal CT Scan	162	0.272	0.219	0.191
Combination Chest CT Scan	83	0.458	0.102	0.054
Follow-up Mammogram/Ultrasound	176	8.5%	8%	8.4%
MRI for Low Back Pain[5]	0	-	30.7%	32.7%
Survey of Patients' Hospital Experiences				
Area Around Room 'Always' Quiet at Night	-	-	-	58%
Doctors 'Always' Communicated Well	-	-	-	80%
Home Recovery Information Given	-	-	-	82%
Hospital Given 9 or 10 on 10 Point Scale	-	-	-	67%
Meds 'Always' Explained Before Given	-	-	-	60%
Nurses 'Always' Communicated Well	-	-	-	76%
Pain 'Always' Well Controlled	-	-	-	69%
Room and Bathroom 'Always' Clean	-	-	-	71%
Timely Help 'Always' Received	-	-	-	64%
Would Definitely Recommend Hospital	-	-	-	69%

Mountain Home VA Medical Center

Sidney & Lamont Streets
Mountain Home, TN 37684
Type: Acute Care-Veterans Administration
Ownership: Government - Federal

Phone: 423-926-1171
Fax: 423-979-3572
Emergency Services: No
Beds: 199

Key Personnel:
CEO/President. . . . . Carl J Gerber, MD
Chief of Medical Staff. . . . . Richard M Jordan, MD
Operating Room. . . . . Lori Hagen, RN
Quality Assurance . . . . Norma Swanson
Radiology. . . . . Pradeep Kumar, MD

Measure	Cases	This Hosp.	State Avg.	U.S. Avg.
Heart Attack Care				
ACE Inhibitor or ARB for LVSD[1]	14	100%	96%	96%
Aspirin at Arrival	79	100%	98%	99%
Aspirin at Discharge	62	100%	99%	98%
Beta Blocker at Discharge	61	100%	98%	98%
Fibrinolytic Medication Timing[5]	0	-	67%	55%
PCI Within 90 Minutes of Arrival[1]	13	31%	91%	90%
Smoking Cessation Advice[1]	24	100%	100%	99%
Chest Pain/Possible Heart Attack Care				
Aspirin at Arrival	-	-	95%	95%
Median Time to ECG (minutes)	-	-	8	8
Median Time to Transfer (minutes)	-	-	65	61
Fibrinolytic Medication Timing	-	-	49%	54%
Heart Failure Care				
ACE Inhibitor or ARB for LVSD	53	98%	95%	94%
Discharge Instructions	156	100%	88%	88%
Evaluation of LVS Function	172	100%	97%	98%
Smoking Cessation Advice	37	100%	99%	98%
Pneumonia Care				
Appropriate Initial Antibiotic	91	97%	92%	92%
Blood Culture Timing	143	98%	97%	96%
Influenza Vaccine	115	97%	93%	91%
Initial Antibiotic Timing	150	95%	96%	95%
Pneumococcal Vaccine	136	100%	95%	93%
Smoking Cessation Advice	67	100%	99%	97%
Surgical Care Improvement Project				
Appropriate VTP Within 24 Hours[2,5]	0	-	92%	92%
Appropriate Hair Removal[2,5]	0	-	100%	99%
Appropriate Beta Blocker Usage[2,5]	0	-	93%	93%
Controlled Postoperative Blood Glucose[2,5]	0	-	93%	93%
Prophylactic Antibiotic Timing[5]	0	-	97%	97%
Prophylactic Antibiotic Timing (Outpatient)	-	-	94%	92%
Prophylactic Antibiotic Selection[5]	0	-	97%	97%
Prophylactic Antibiotic Select. (Outpatient)	-	-	94%	94%
Prophylactic Antibiotic Stopped[5]	0	-	94%	94%
Recommended VTP Ordered[2,5]	0	-	94%	94%
Urinary Catheter Removal[2,5]	0	-	90%	90%
Children's Asthma Care				
Received Systemic Corticosteroids	-	-	-	100%
Received Home Management Plan	-	-	-	71%
Received Reliever Medication	-	-	-	100%
Use of Medical Imaging				
Combination Abdominal CT Scan	-	-	0.219	0.191
Combination Chest CT Scan	-	-	0.102	0.054
Follow-up Mammogram/Ultrasound	-	-	8%	8.4%
MRI for Low Back Pain	-	-	30.7%	32.7%
Survey of Patients' Hospital Experiences				
Area Around Room 'Always' Quiet at Night	-	-	-	58%
Doctors 'Always' Communicated Well	-	-	-	80%
Home Recovery Information Given	-	-	-	82%
Hospital Given 9 or 10 on 10 Point Scale	-	-	-	67%
Meds 'Always' Explained Before Given	-	-	-	60%
Nurses 'Always' Communicated Well	-	-	-	76%
Pain 'Always' Well Controlled	-	-	-	69%
Room and Bathroom 'Always' Clean	-	-	-	71%
Timely Help 'Always' Received	-	-	-	64%
Would Definitely Recommend Hospital	-	-	-	69%

Middle Tennessee Medical Center

1700 Medical Center Parkway
Murfreesboro, TN 37129
URL: www.mtmc.org
Type: Acute Care Hospitals
Ownership: Voluntary Non-Profit - Church

Phone: 615-396-4100
Fax: 615-396-4659
Emergency Services: Yes
Beds: 288

Key Personnel:
CEO/President. . . . . Gordon B Ferguson
Chief of Medical Staff . . . . Andy Brown, MD
Operating Room. . . . . Bennie Porter, RN
Quality Assurance . . . . Retta Fann
Radiology. . . . . Eric Dame
Emergency Room . . . . Patty Dixon

Measure	Cases	This Hosp.	State Avg.	U.S. Avg.
Heart Attack Care				
ACE Inhibitor or ARB for LVSD	34	94%	96%	96%
Aspirin at Arrival	212	97%	98%	99%
Aspirin at Discharge	190	99%	99%	98%
Beta Blocker at Discharge	178	98%	98%	98%
Fibrinolytic Medication Timing	0	-	67%	55%
PCI Within 90 Minutes of Arrival	49	82%	91%	90%
Smoking Cessation Advice	90	100%	100%	99%
Chest Pain/Possible Heart Attack Care				
Aspirin at Arrival	75	84%	95%	95%
Median Time to ECG (minutes)	60	10	8	8
Median Time to Transfer (minutes)[1,3]	6	298	65	61
Fibrinolytic Medication Timing	0	-	49%	54%
Heart Failure Care				
ACE Inhibitor or ARB for LVSD	137	88%	95%	94%
Discharge Instructions	308	96%	88%	88%
Evaluation of LVS Function	397	99%	97%	98%
Smoking Cessation Advice	71	100%	99%	98%
Pneumonia Care				
Appropriate Initial Antibiotic	254	91%	92%	92%
Blood Culture Timing	376	98%	97%	96%
Influenza Vaccine	309	100%	93%	91%
Initial Antibiotic Timing	477	96%	96%	95%
Pneumococcal Vaccine	377	99%	95%	93%
Smoking Cessation Advice	196	100%	99%	97%
Surgical Care Improvement Project				
Appropriate VTP Within 24 Hours[2]	215	90%	92%	92%
Appropriate Hair Removal[2]	888	100%	100%	99%
Appropriate Beta Blocker Usage[2]	207	92%	93%	93%
Controlled Postoperative Blood Glucose[2]	0	-	93%	93%
Prophylactic Antibiotic Timing[2]	671	99%	97%	97%
Prophylactic Antibiotic Timing (Outpatient)	505	98%	94%	92%
Prophylactic Antibiotic Selection[2]	675	97%	97%	97%
Prophylactic Antibiotic Select. (Outpatient)	502	98%	94%	94%
Prophylactic Antibiotic Stopped[2]	649	91%	94%	94%
Recommended VTP Ordered[2]	215	93%	94%	94%
Urinary Catheter Removal[2]	111	88%	90%	90%
Children's Asthma Care				
Received Systemic Corticosteroids	-	-	-	100%
Received Home Management Plan	-	-	-	71%
Received Reliever Medication	-	-	-	100%
Use of Medical Imaging				
Combination Abdominal CT Scan	608	0.215	0.219	0.191
Combination Chest CT Scan	111	0.018	0.102	0.054
Follow-up Mammogram/Ultrasound	729	7.8%	8%	8.4%
MRI for Low Back Pain[1]	36	38.9%	30.7%	32.7%
Survey of Patients' Hospital Experiences				
Area Around Room 'Always' Quiet at Night	300+	57%	-	58%
Doctors 'Always' Communicated Well	300+	84%	-	80%
Home Recovery Information Given	300+	84%	-	82%
Hospital Given 9 or 10 on 10 Point Scale	300+	57%	-	67%
Meds 'Always' Explained Before Given	300+	60%	-	60%
Nurses 'Always' Communicated Well	300+	74%	-	76%
Pain 'Always' Well Controlled	300+	69%	-	69%
Room and Bathroom 'Always' Clean	300+	58%	-	71%
Timely Help 'Always' Received	300+	57%	-	64%
Would Definitely Recommend Hospital	300+	62%	-	69%

NOTE: Hospital profiles are in alphabetical order by state, then city, then hospital within the city; Rankings exclude hospitals with less than 25 cases except for patient surveys which excludes hospitals with less than 100 cases; (a) 100–299 cases; (1) The number of cases is too small to be sure how well a hospital is performing; (2) The hospital indicated that the data submitted for this measure were based on a sample of cases; (3) Data was collected during a shorter time period (fewer quarters) than the maximum possible time for this measure; (4) Suppressed for one or more quarters by CMS; (5) No data is available from the hospital for this measure; (6) Fewer than 100 patients completed the HCAHPS survey. Use these rates with caution, as the number of surveys may be too low to reliably assess hospital performance; (7) Survey results are based on less than 12 months of data; (8) Survey results are not available for this reporting period; (9) No or very few patients were eligible for the HCAHPS survey. The scores shown, if any, reflect a very small number of surveys; (10) A state average was not calculated because too few hospitals in the state submitted data; (11) There were discrepancies in the data collection process; Please refer to the User's Guide for a full explanation of data.

Baptist Hospital

2000 Church St
Nashville, TN 37236
URL: www.baptisthospital.com
Type: Acute Care Hospitals
Ownership: Voluntary Non-Profit - Private
Phone: 615-284-5555
Fax: 615-284-8686
Emergency Services: Yes
Beds: 723

Key Personnel:
Chief of Medical Staff. . . . . Frank W Gluck Jr, MD
Infection Control. . . . . Virginia Tankersly, RN
Operating Room. . . . . Perri Lynn White
Pediatric Ambulatory Care . . . . . . Ralph Greenbaum, MD
Pediatric In-Patient Care . . . . . . Ralph Greenbaum, MD
Quality Assurance . . . . Sue Carter, RN
Radiology. . . . . Michael Seshul, MD

Measure	Cases	This Hosp.	State Avg.	U.S. Avg.
Heart Attack Care				
ACE Inhibitor or ARB for LVSD	51	96%	96%	96%
Aspirin at Arrival	199	99%	98%	99%
Aspirin at Discharge	235	99%	99%	98%
Beta Blocker at Discharge	237	100%	98%	98%
Fibrinolytic Medication Timing	0	-	67%	55%
PCI Within 90 Minutes of Arrival	25	100%	91%	90%
Smoking Cessation Advice	87	100%	100%	99%
Chest Pain/Possible Heart Attack Care				
Aspirin at Arrival[1,3]	2	100%	95%	95%
Median Time to ECG (minutes)[1,3]	2	9	8	8
Median Time to Transfer (minutes)[5]	0	-	65	61
Fibrinolytic Medication Timing[3]	0	-	49%	54%
Heart Failure Care				
ACE Inhibitor or ARB for LVSD	193	95%	95%	94%
Discharge Instructions	503	85%	88%	88%
Evaluation of LVS Function	574	98%	97%	98%
Smoking Cessation Advice	109	100%	99%	98%
Pneumonia Care				
Appropriate Initial Antibiotic	159	91%	92%	92%
Blood Culture Timing	247	100%	97%	96%
Influenza Vaccine	211	98%	93%	91%
Initial Antibiotic Timing	254	94%	96%	95%
Pneumococcal Vaccine	269	96%	95%	93%
Smoking Cessation Advice	141	100%	99%	97%
Surgical Care Improvement Project				
Appropriate VTP Within 24 Hours[2]	211	90%	92%	92%
Appropriate Hair Removal[2]	749	100%	100%	99%
Appropriate Beta Blocker Usage[2]	206	93%	93%	93%
Controlled Postoperative Blood Glucose[2]	118	99%	93%	93%
Prophylactic Antibiotic Timing[2]	514	98%	97%	97%
Prophylactic Antibiotic Timing (Outpatient)	697	97%	94%	92%
Prophylactic Antibiotic Selection[2]	525	99%	97%	97%
Prophylactic Antibiotic Select. (Outpatient)	693	95%	94%	94%
Prophylactic Antibiotic Stopped[2]	490	93%	94%	94%
Recommended VTP Ordered[2]	211	94%	94%	94%
Urinary Catheter Removal[2]	183	89%	90%	90%
Children's Asthma Care				
Received Systemic Corticosteroids	-	-	-	100%
Received Home Management Plan	-	-	-	71%
Received Reliever Medication	-	-	-	100%
Use of Medical Imaging				
Combination Abdominal CT Scan	894	0.139	0.219	0.191
Combination Chest CT Scan	768	0.132	0.102	0.054
Follow-up Mammogram/Ultrasound	1,712	10.1%	8%	8.4%
MRI for Low Back Pain	144	39.6%	30.7%	32.7%
Survey of Patients' Hospital Experiences				
Area Around Room 'Always' Quiet at Night	300+	62%	-	58%
Doctors 'Always' Communicated Well	300+	84%	-	80%
Home Recovery Information Given	300+	84%	-	82%
Hospital Given 9 or 10 on 10 Point Scale	300+	71%	-	67%
Meds 'Always' Explained Before Given	300+	63%	-	60%
Nurses 'Always' Communicated Well	300+	78%	-	76%
Pain 'Always' Well Controlled	300+	72%	-	69%
Room and Bathroom 'Always' Clean	300+	64%	-	71%
Timely Help 'Always' Received	300+	66%	-	64%
Would Definitely Recommend Hospital	300+	77%	-	69%

Centennial Medical Center

2300 Patterson Street
Nashville, TN 37203
Type: Acute Care Hospitals
Ownership: Proprietary
Phone: 615-342-1000
Emergency Services: Yes

Key Personnel:
CEO/President. . . . . Thomas L Herron FACHE

Measure	Cases	This Hosp.	State Avg.	U.S. Avg.
Heart Attack Care				
ACE Inhibitor or ARB for LVSD	104	100%	96%	96%
Aspirin at Arrival	141	100%	98%	99%
Aspirin at Discharge	555	100%	99%	98%
Beta Blocker at Discharge	528	100%	98%	98%
Fibrinolytic Medication Timing	0	-	67%	55%
PCI Within 90 Minutes of Arrival[1]	18	100%	91%	90%
Smoking Cessation Advice	250	100%	100%	99%
Chest Pain/Possible Heart Attack Care				
Aspirin at Arrival[1,3]	5	100%	95%	95%
Median Time to ECG (minutes)[1,3]	5	9	8	8
Median Time to Transfer (minutes)[5]	0	-	65	61
Fibrinolytic Medication Timing[5]	0	-	49%	54%
Heart Failure Care				
ACE Inhibitor or ARB for LVSD	221	95%	95%	94%
Discharge Instructions	482	94%	88%	88%
Evaluation of LVS Function	537	100%	97%	98%
Smoking Cessation Advice	123	100%	99%	98%
Pneumonia Care				
Appropriate Initial Antibiotic	88	95%	92%	92%
Blood Culture Timing	105	98%	97%	96%
Influenza Vaccine	207	99%	93%	91%
Initial Antibiotic Timing	155	99%	96%	95%
Pneumococcal Vaccine	246	100%	95%	93%
Smoking Cessation Advice	181	99%	99%	97%
Surgical Care Improvement Project				
Appropriate VTP Within 24 Hours[2]	276	98%	92%	92%
Appropriate Hair Removal[2]	924	100%	100%	99%
Appropriate Beta Blocker Usage[2]	346	98%	93%	93%
Controlled Postoperative Blood Glucose[2]	224	92%	93%	93%
Prophylactic Antibiotic Timing[2]	622	99%	97%	97%
Prophylactic Antibiotic Timing (Outpatient)	788	98%	94%	92%
Prophylactic Antibiotic Selection[2]	634	99%	97%	97%
Prophylactic Antibiotic Select. (Outpatient)	782	98%	94%	94%
Prophylactic Antibiotic Stopped[2]	557	95%	94%	94%
Recommended VTP Ordered[2]	276	99%	94%	94%
Urinary Catheter Removal[2]	218	94%	90%	90%
Children's Asthma Care				
Received Systemic Corticosteroids	-	-	-	100%
Received Home Management Plan	-	-	-	71%
Received Reliever Medication	-	-	-	100%
Use of Medical Imaging				
Combination Abdominal CT Scan	863	0.107	0.219	0.191
Combination Chest CT Scan	606	0.040	0.102	0.054
Follow-up Mammogram/Ultrasound	1,051	7.3%	8%	8.4%
MRI for Low Back Pain	180	33.3%	30.7%	32.7%
Survey of Patients' Hospital Experiences				
Area Around Room 'Always' Quiet at Night	300+	67%	-	58%
Doctors 'Always' Communicated Well	300+	85%	-	80%
Home Recovery Information Given	300+	87%	-	82%
Hospital Given 9 or 10 on 10 Point Scale	300+	79%	-	67%
Meds 'Always' Explained Before Given	300+	67%	-	60%
Nurses 'Always' Communicated Well	300+	81%	-	76%
Pain 'Always' Well Controlled	300+	75%	-	69%
Room and Bathroom 'Always' Clean	300+	74%	-	71%
Timely Help 'Always' Received	300+	71%	-	64%
Would Definitely Recommend Hospital	300+	81%	-	69%

The Center for Spinal Surgery

2011 Murphy Avenue
Nashville, TN 37203
Type: Acute Care Hospitals
Ownership: Proprietary
Phone: 615-515-8200
Emergency Services: No
Beds: 18

Key Personnel:
CEO/President. . . . . Elissa Christiansen

Measure	Cases	This Hosp.	State Avg.	U.S. Avg.
Heart Attack Care				
ACE Inhibitor or ARB for LVSD[5]	0	-	96%	96%
Aspirin at Arrival[5]	0	-	98%	99%
Aspirin at Discharge[5]	0	-	99%	98%
Beta Blocker at Discharge[5]	0	-	98%	98%
Fibrinolytic Medication Timing[5]	0	-	67%	55%
PCI Within 90 Minutes of Arrival[5]	0	-	91%	90%
Smoking Cessation Advice[5]	0	-	100%	99%
Chest Pain/Possible Heart Attack Care				
Aspirin at Arrival[5]	0	-	95%	95%
Median Time to ECG (minutes)[5]	0	-	8	8
Median Time to Transfer (minutes)[5]	0	-	65	61
Fibrinolytic Medication Timing[5]	0	-	49%	54%
Heart Failure Care				
ACE Inhibitor or ARB for LVSD[5]	0	-	95%	94%
Discharge Instructions[5]	0	-	88%	88%
Evaluation of LVS Function[5]	0	-	97%	98%
Smoking Cessation Advice[5]	0	-	99%	98%
Pneumonia Care				
Appropriate Initial Antibiotic[5]	0	-	92%	92%
Blood Culture Timing[5]	0	-	97%	96%
Influenza Vaccine[5]	0	-	93%	91%
Initial Antibiotic Timing[5]	0	-	96%	95%
Pneumococcal Vaccine[5]	0	-	95%	93%
Smoking Cessation Advice[5]	0	-	99%	97%
Surgical Care Improvement Project				
Appropriate VTP Within 24 Hours[5]	0	-	92%	92%
Appropriate Hair Removal[5]	0	-	100%	99%
Appropriate Beta Blocker Usage[5]	0	-	93%	93%
Controlled Postoperative Blood Glucose[5]	0	-	93%	93%
Prophylactic Antibiotic Timing[5]	0	-	97%	97%
Prophylactic Antibiotic Timing (Outpatient)	913	100%	94%	92%
Prophylactic Antibiotic Selection[5]	0	-	97%	97%
Prophylactic Antibiotic Select. (Outpatient)	913	100%	94%	94%
Prophylactic Antibiotic Stopped[5]	0	-	94%	94%
Recommended VTP Ordered[5]	0	-	94%	94%
Urinary Catheter Removal[5]	0	-	90%	90%
Children's Asthma Care				
Received Systemic Corticosteroids	-	-	-	100%
Received Home Management Plan	-	-	-	71%
Received Reliever Medication	-	-	-	100%
Use of Medical Imaging				
Combination Abdominal CT Scan[5]	0	-	0.219	0.191
Combination Chest CT Scan[5]	0	-	0.102	0.054
Follow-up Mammogram/Ultrasound[5]	0	-	8%	8.4%
MRI for Low Back Pain[5]	0	-	30.7%	32.7%
Survey of Patients' Hospital Experiences				
Area Around Room 'Always' Quiet at Night	300+	91%	-	58%
Doctors 'Always' Communicated Well	300+	93%	-	80%
Home Recovery Information Given	300+	90%	-	82%
Hospital Given 9 or 10 on 10 Point Scale	300+	93%	-	67%
Meds 'Always' Explained Before Given	300+	74%	-	60%
Nurses 'Always' Communicated Well	300+	92%	-	76%
Pain 'Always' Well Controlled	300+	84%	-	69%
Room and Bathroom 'Always' Clean	300+	83%	-	71%
Timely Help 'Always' Received	300+	85%	-	64%
Would Definitely Recommend Hospital	300+	95%	-	69%

NOTE: Hospital profiles are in alphabetical order by state, then city, then hospital within the city; Rankings exclude hospitals with less than 25 cases except for patient surveys which excludes hospitals with less than 100 cases; (a) 100–299 cases; (1) The number of cases is too small to be sure how well a hospital is performing; (2) The hospital indicated that the data submitted for this measure were based on a sample of cases; (3) Data was collected during a shorter time period (fewer quarters) than the maximum possible time for this measure; (4) Suppressed for one or more quarters by CMS; (5) No data is available from the hospital for this measure; (6) Fewer than 100 patients completed the HCAHPS survey. Use these rates with caution, as the number of surveys may be too low to reliably assess hospital performance; (7) Survey results are based on less than 12 months of data; (8) Survey results are not available for this reporting period; (9) No or very few patients were eligible for the HCAHPS survey. The scores shown, if any, reflect a very small number of surveys; (10) A state average was not calculated because too few hospitals in the state submitted data; (11) There were discrepancies in the data collection process; Please refer to the User's Guide for a full explanation of data.

Metro Nashville General Hospital

1818 Albion Street
Nashville, TN 37208
Type: Acute Care Hospitals
Ownership: Govt - Hospital Dist/Auth

Phone: 615-341-4490
Fax: 615-341-4493
Emergency Services: Yes
Beds: 150

Key Personnel:
CEO/President . . . . Roxane Spitzer, PHD
Chief of Medical Staff . . . . Reginald Coopwood, MD

Measure	Cases	This Hosp.	State Avg.	U.S. Avg.
Heart Attack Care				
ACE Inhibitor or ARB for LVSD[1,2]	20	100%	96%	96%
Aspirin at Arrival[2]	90	93%	98%	99%
Aspirin at Discharge[2]	87	95%	99%	98%
Beta Blocker at Discharge[2]	82	99%	98%	98%
Fibrinolytic Medication Timing[2]	0	-	67%	55%
PCI Within 90 Minutes of Arrival[1,2]	3	67%	91%	90%
Smoking Cessation Advice[2]	48	100%	100%	99%
Chest Pain/Possible Heart Attack Care				
Aspirin at Arrival[1]	8	100%	95%	95%
Median Time to ECG (minutes)[1]	9	24	8	8
Median Time to Transfer (minutes)[1,3]	4	281	65	61
Fibrinolytic Medication Timing[3]	0	-	49%	54%
Heart Failure Care				
ACE Inhibitor or ARB for LVSD[2]	91	100%	95%	94%
Discharge Instructions[2]	174	77%	88%	88%
Evaluation of LVS Function[2]	172	100%	97%	98%
Smoking Cessation Advice[2]	92	100%	99%	98%
Pneumonia Care				
Appropriate Initial Antibiotic[2]	54	93%	92%	92%
Blood Culture Timing[2]	80	92%	97%	96%
Influenza Vaccine[1,2]	19	100%	93%	91%
Initial Antibiotic Timing[2]	78	88%	96%	95%
Pneumococcal Vaccine[1,2]	19	63%	95%	93%
Smoking Cessation Advice[2]	58	100%	99%	97%
Surgical Care Improvement Project				
Appropriate VTP Within 24 Hours[2]	135	84%	92%	92%
Appropriate Hair Removal[2]	233	99%	100%	99%
Appropriate Beta Blocker Usage[2]	32	91%	93%	93%
Controlled Postoperative Blood Glucose[2]	0	-	93%	93%
Prophylactic Antibiotic Timing[2]	139	71%	97%	97%
Prophylactic Antibiotic Timing (Outpatient)	88	58%	94%	92%
Prophylactic Antibiotic Selection[2]	127	90%	97%	97%
Prophylactic Antibiotic Select. (Outpatient)	86	59%	94%	94%
Prophylactic Antibiotic Stopped[2]	117	88%	94%	94%
Recommended VTP Ordered[2]	138	83%	94%	94%
Urinary Catheter Removal[2]	52	83%	90%	90%
Children's Asthma Care				
Received Systemic Corticosteroids	-	-	-	100%
Received Home Management Plan	-	-	-	71%
Received Reliever Medication	-	-	-	100%
Use of Medical Imaging				
Combination Abdominal CT Scan	70	0.057	0.219	0.191
Combination Chest CT Scan[1]	33	0.030	0.102	0.054
Follow-up Mammogram/Ultrasound	124	3.2%	8%	8.4%
MRI for Low Back Pain[1]	7	57.1%	30.7%	32.7%
Survey of Patients' Hospital Experiences				
Area Around Room 'Always' Quiet at Night	300+	62%	-	58%
Doctors 'Always' Communicated Well	300+	82%	-	80%
Home Recovery Information Given	300+	81%	-	82%
Hospital Given 9 or 10 on 10 Point Scale	300+	65%	-	67%
Meds 'Always' Explained Before Given	300+	62%	-	60%
Nurses 'Always' Communicated Well	300+	73%	-	76%
Pain 'Always' Well Controlled	300+	66%	-	69%
Room and Bathroom 'Always' Clean	300+	68%	-	71%
Timely Help 'Always' Received	300+	57%	-	64%
Would Definitely Recommend Hospital	300+	64%	-	69%

Saint Thomas Hospital

4220 Harding Rd
Nashville, TN 37205
URL: www.stthomas.org
Type: Acute Care Hospitals
Ownership: Voluntary Non-Profit - Church

Phone: 615-222-2111
Fax: 615-222-4482

Emergency Services: Yes
Beds: 541

Key Personnel:
CEO/President . . . . Thomas E Beeman
Chief of Medical Staff . . . . John Johnson
Infection Control . . . . Deanie Lancaster
Quality Assurance . . . . Linda Poteete
Radiology. . . . . K James Schumacher, MD
Emergency Room . . . . Kevin Bonner, MD
Hemotology Center . . . . Paul Rosenblatt, MD
Intensive Care Unit. . . . . CS Thomas, Jr, MD

Measure	Cases	This Hosp.	State Avg.	U.S. Avg.
Heart Attack Care				
ACE Inhibitor or ARB for LVSD	283	95%	96%	96%
Aspirin at Arrival	423	99%	98%	99%
Aspirin at Discharge	1,322	99%	99%	98%
Beta Blocker at Discharge	1,283	98%	98%	98%
Fibrinolytic Medication Timing	0	-	67%	55%
PCI Within 90 Minutes of Arrival	65	98%	91%	90%
Smoking Cessation Advice	472	100%	100%	99%
Chest Pain/Possible Heart Attack Care				
Aspirin at Arrival[1,3]	3	100%	95%	95%
Median Time to ECG (minutes)[1,3]	4	4	8	8
Median Time to Transfer (minutes)[5]	0	-	65	61
Fibrinolytic Medication Timing[3]	0	-	49%	54%
Heart Failure Care				
ACE Inhibitor or ARB for LVSD	399	94%	95%	94%
Discharge Instructions	925	86%	88%	88%
Evaluation of LVS Function	1,049	99%	97%	98%
Smoking Cessation Advice	149	100%	99%	98%
Pneumonia Care				
Appropriate Initial Antibiotic	206	91%	92%	92%
Blood Culture Timing	348	96%	97%	96%
Influenza Vaccine	301	98%	93%	91%
Initial Antibiotic Timing	320	94%	96%	95%
Pneumococcal Vaccine	410	97%	95%	93%
Smoking Cessation Advice	196	99%	99%	97%
Surgical Care Improvement Project				
Appropriate VTP Within 24 Hours[2]	187	99%	92%	92%
Appropriate Hair Removal[2]	806	100%	100%	99%
Appropriate Beta Blocker Usage[2]	258	95%	93%	93%
Controlled Postoperative Blood Glucose[2]	174	93%	93%	93%
Prophylactic Antibiotic Timing[2]	542	99%	97%	97%
Prophylactic Antibiotic Timing (Outpatient)	526	97%	94%	92%
Prophylactic Antibiotic Selection[2]	552	99%	97%	97%
Prophylactic Antibiotic Select. (Outpatient)	525	92%	94%	94%
Prophylactic Antibiotic Stopped[2]	525	94%	94%	94%
Recommended VTP Ordered[2]	187	99%	94%	94%
Urinary Catheter Removal[2]	179	89%	90%	90%
Children's Asthma Care				
Received Systemic Corticosteroids	-	-	-	100%
Received Home Management Plan	-	-	-	71%
Received Reliever Medication	-	-	-	100%
Use of Medical Imaging				
Combination Abdominal CT Scan	902	0.055	0.219	0.191
Combination Chest CT Scan	896	0.017	0.102	0.054
Follow-up Mammogram/Ultrasound	1,619	7.8%	8%	8.4%
MRI for Low Back Pain	147	28.6%	30.7%	32.7%
Survey of Patients' Hospital Experiences				
Area Around Room 'Always' Quiet at Night	300+	51%	-	58%
Doctors 'Always' Communicated Well	300+	83%	-	80%
Home Recovery Information Given	300+	84%	-	82%
Hospital Given 9 or 10 on 10 Point Scale	300+	81%	-	67%
Meds 'Always' Explained Before Given	300+	61%	-	60%
Nurses 'Always' Communicated Well	300+	79%	-	76%
Pain 'Always' Well Controlled	300+	73%	-	69%
Room and Bathroom 'Always' Clean	300+	65%	-	71%
Timely Help 'Always' Received	300+	61%	-	64%
Would Definitely Recommend Hospital	300+	87%	-	69%

Skyline Medical Center

3441 Dickerson Pike
Nashville, TN 37207
URL: www.skylinemedicalcenter.com
Type: Acute Care Hospitals
Ownership: Voluntary Non-Profit - Private

Phone: 615-769-2000
Fax: 615-769-2211

Emergency Services: Yes
Beds: 196

Key Personnel:
CEO/President . . . . Mike Garfield
Radiology. . . . . Rick Phillips, CRA

Measure	Cases	This Hosp.	State Avg.	U.S. Avg.
Heart Attack Care				
ACE Inhibitor or ARB for LVSD[1]	13	100%	96%	96%
Aspirin at Arrival	152	100%	98%	99%
Aspirin at Discharge	127	99%	99%	98%
Beta Blocker at Discharge	124	100%	98%	98%
Fibrinolytic Medication Timing	0	-	67%	55%
PCI Within 90 Minutes of Arrival	33	100%	91%	90%
Smoking Cessation Advice	52	100%	100%	99%
Chest Pain/Possible Heart Attack Care				
Aspirin at Arrival	72	99%	95%	95%
Median Time to ECG (minutes)	73	4	8	8
Median Time to Transfer (minutes)[3]	0	-	65	61
Fibrinolytic Medication Timing[3]	0	-	49%	54%
Heart Failure Care				
ACE Inhibitor or ARB for LVSD	94	99%	95%	94%
Discharge Instructions	246	100%	88%	88%
Evaluation of LVS Function	285	99%	97%	98%
Smoking Cessation Advice	79	100%	99%	98%
Pneumonia Care				
Appropriate Initial Antibiotic[2]	102	94%	92%	92%
Blood Culture Timing[2]	201	98%	97%	96%
Influenza Vaccine[2]	102	98%	93%	91%
Initial Antibiotic Timing[2]	163	99%	96%	95%
Pneumococcal Vaccine[2]	144	100%	95%	93%
Smoking Cessation Advice[2]	84	100%	99%	97%
Surgical Care Improvement Project				
Appropriate VTP Within 24 Hours[2]	208	92%	92%	92%
Appropriate Hair Removal[2]	481	100%	100%	99%
Appropriate Beta Blocker Usage[2]	136	93%	93%	93%
Controlled Postoperative Blood Glucose[2]	0	-	93%	93%
Prophylactic Antibiotic Timing[2]	277	98%	97%	97%
Prophylactic Antibiotic Timing (Outpatient)	302	97%	94%	92%
Prophylactic Antibiotic Selection[2]	278	99%	97%	97%
Prophylactic Antibiotic Select. (Outpatient)	299	98%	94%	94%
Prophylactic Antibiotic Stopped[2]	244	96%	94%	94%
Recommended VTP Ordered[2]	209	97%	94%	94%
Urinary Catheter Removal[2]	94	99%	90%	90%
Children's Asthma Care				
Received Systemic Corticosteroids	-	-	-	100%
Received Home Management Plan	-	-	-	71%
Received Reliever Medication	-	-	-	100%
Use of Medical Imaging				
Combination Abdominal CT Scan	822	0.277	0.219	0.191
Combination Chest CT Scan	629	0.003	0.102	0.054
Follow-up Mammogram/Ultrasound	1,095	7.9%	8%	8.4%
MRI for Low Back Pain	244	31.6%	30.7%	32.7%
Survey of Patients' Hospital Experiences				
Area Around Room 'Always' Quiet at Night	300+	65%	-	58%
Doctors 'Always' Communicated Well	300+	80%	-	80%
Home Recovery Information Given	300+	84%	-	82%
Hospital Given 9 or 10 on 10 Point Scale	300+	66%	-	67%
Meds 'Always' Explained Before Given	300+	59%	-	60%
Nurses 'Always' Communicated Well	300+	75%	-	76%
Pain 'Always' Well Controlled	300+	69%	-	69%
Room and Bathroom 'Always' Clean	300+	66%	-	71%
Timely Help 'Always' Received	300+	62%	-	64%
Would Definitely Recommend Hospital	300+	70%	-	69%

NOTE: Hospital profiles are in alphabetical order by state, then city, then hospital within the city; Rankings exclude hospitals with less than 25 cases except for patient surveys which excludes hospitals with less than 100 cases; (a) 100–299 cases; (1) The number of cases is too small to be sure how well a hospital is performing; (2) The hospital indicated that the data submitted for this measure were based on a sample of cases; (3) Data was collected during a shorter time period (fewer quarters) than the maximum possible time for this measure; (4) Suppressed for one or more quarters by CMS; (5) No data is available from the hospital for this measure; (6) Fewer than 100 patients completed the HCAHPS survey. Use these rates with caution, as the number of surveys may be too low to reliably assess hospital performance; (7) Survey results are based on less than 12 months of data; (8) Survey results are not available for this reporting period; (9) No or very few patients were eligible for the HCAHPS survey. The scores shown, if any, reflect a very small number of surveys; (10) A state average was not calculated because too few hospitals in the state submitted data; (11) There were discrepancies in the data collection process; Please refer to the User's Guide for a full explanation of data.

Southern Hills Medical Center

391 Wallace Rd
Nashville, TN 37211
URL: www.southernhills.com
Type: Acute Care Hospitals
Ownership: Proprietary

Phone: 615-781-4000
Fax: 615-781-4113

Emergency Services: Yes
Beds: 160

Key Personnel:
CEO/President . . . . Thomas H Ozburn
Chief of Medical Staff . . . . Robert Bishop, MD
Infection Control . . . . Jane Harris
Operating Room. . . . . Suhail H Allos
Radiology. . . . . Christopher J Bodin
Emergency Room . . . . Eric Morris, MD
Intensive Care Unit. . . . . Darlene Cantrell

Measure	Cases	This Hosp.	State Avg.	U.S. Avg.
Heart Attack Care				
ACE Inhibitor or ARB for LVSD[1]	9	89%	96%	96%
Aspirin at Arrival	78	99%	98%	99%
Aspirin at Discharge	58	95%	99%	98%
Beta Blocker at Discharge	69	96%	98%	98%
Fibrinolytic Medication Timing[1]	3	100%	67%	55%
PCI Within 90 Minutes of Arrival[1]	23	100%	91%	90%
Smoking Cessation Advice	36	100%	100%	99%
Chest Pain/Possible Heart Attack Care				
Aspirin at Arrival	31	100%	95%	95%
Median Time to ECG (minutes)	33	7	8	8
Median Time to Transfer (minutes)[5]	0	-	65	61
Fibrinolytic Medication Timing[3]	0	-	49%	54%
Heart Failure Care				
ACE Inhibitor or ARB for LVSD	32	100%	95%	94%
Discharge Instructions	109	99%	88%	88%
Evaluation of LVS Function	122	98%	97%	98%
Smoking Cessation Advice	32	100%	99%	98%
Pneumonia Care				
Appropriate Initial Antibiotic	118	97%	92%	92%
Blood Culture Timing	172	100%	97%	96%
Influenza Vaccine	78	99%	93%	91%
Initial Antibiotic Timing	165	99%	96%	95%
Pneumococcal Vaccine	90	100%	95%	93%
Smoking Cessation Advice	79	100%	99%	97%
Surgical Care Improvement Project				
Appropriate VTP Within 24 Hours	118	98%	92%	92%
Appropriate Hair Removal	293	100%	100%	99%
Appropriate Beta Blocker Usage	68	100%	93%	93%
Controlled Postoperative Blood Glucose	0	-	93%	93%
Prophylactic Antibiotic Timing	169	100%	97%	97%
Prophylactic Antibiotic Timing (Outpatient)	113	99%	94%	92%
Prophylactic Antibiotic Selection	172	97%	97%	97%
Prophylactic Antibiotic Select. (Outpatient)	112	97%	94%	94%
Prophylactic Antibiotic Stopped	154	98%	94%	94%
Recommended VTP Ordered	118	98%	94%	94%
Urinary Catheter Removal	61	98%	90%	90%
Children's Asthma Care				
Received Systemic Corticosteroids	-	-	-	100%
Received Home Management Plan	-	-	-	71%
Received Reliever Medication	-	-	-	100%
Use of Medical Imaging				
Combination Abdominal CT Scan	395	0.122	0.219	0.191
Combination Chest CT Scan	246	0.020	0.102	0.054
Follow-up Mammogram/Ultrasound	656	5.9%	8%	8.4%
MRI for Low Back Pain	62	25.8%	30.7%	32.7%
Survey of Patients' Hospital Experiences				
Area Around Room 'Always' Quiet at Night	300+	65%	-	58%
Doctors 'Always' Communicated Well	300+	82%	-	80%
Home Recovery Information Given	300+	85%	-	82%
Hospital Given 9 or 10 on 10 Point Scale	300+	67%	-	67%
Meds 'Always' Explained Before Given	300+	59%	-	60%
Nurses 'Always' Communicated Well	300+	75%	-	76%
Pain 'Always' Well Controlled	300+	69%	-	69%
Room and Bathroom 'Always' Clean	300+	70%	-	71%
Timely Help 'Always' Received	300+	60%	-	64%
Would Definitely Recommend Hospital	300+	65%	-	69%

VA Middle Tennessee Healthcare System

1310 24th Avenue South
Nashville, TN 37212
Type: Acute Care-Veterans Administration
Ownership: Government - Federal

Phone: 615-327-5332
Fax: 615-321-6350
Emergency Services: No
Beds: 238

Key Personnel:
CEO/President . . . . David N Pannington
Chief of Medical Staff . . . . John H Newman, MD
Quality Assurance . . . . Dolores Kaplan, RN

Measure	Cases	This Hosp.	State Avg.	U.S. Avg.
Heart Attack Care				
ACE Inhibitor or ARB for LVSD	40	100%	96%	96%
Aspirin at Arrival	142	99%	98%	99%
Aspirin at Discharge	136	99%	99%	98%
Beta Blocker at Discharge	139	100%	98%	98%
Fibrinolytic Medication Timing[5]	0	-	67%	55%
PCI Within 90 Minutes of Arrival[1]	23	39%	91%	90%
Smoking Cessation Advice	57	100%	100%	99%
Chest Pain/Possible Heart Attack Care				
Aspirin at Arrival	-	-	95%	95%
Median Time to ECG (minutes)	-	-	8	8
Median Time to Transfer (minutes)	-	-	65	61
Fibrinolytic Medication Timing	-	-	49%	54%
Heart Failure Care				
ACE Inhibitor or ARB for LVSD	160	93%	95%	94%
Discharge Instructions	347	98%	88%	88%
Evaluation of LVS Function	361	99%	97%	98%
Smoking Cessation Advice	96	99%	99%	98%
Pneumonia Care				
Appropriate Initial Antibiotic	118	92%	92%	92%
Blood Culture Timing	190	99%	97%	96%
Influenza Vaccine	177	98%	93%	91%
Initial Antibiotic Timing	179	96%	96%	95%
Pneumococcal Vaccine	183	99%	95%	93%
Smoking Cessation Advice	107	100%	99%	97%
Surgical Care Improvement Project				
Appropriate VTP Within 24 Hours[2]	81	98%	92%	92%
Appropriate Hair Removal[2]	222	100%	100%	99%
Appropriate Beta Blocker Usage[2]	104	92%	93%	93%
Controlled Postoperative Blood Glucose[2]	105	96%	93%	93%
Prophylactic Antibiotic Timing	138	93%	97%	97%
Prophylactic Antibiotic Timing (Outpatient)	-	-	94%	92%
Prophylactic Antibiotic Selection	139	99%	97%	97%
Prophylactic Antibiotic Select. (Outpatient)	-	-	94%	94%
Prophylactic Antibiotic Stopped	126	91%	94%	94%
Recommended VTP Ordered[2]	82	96%	94%	94%
Urinary Catheter Removal[2]	44	84%	90%	90%
Children's Asthma Care				
Received Systemic Corticosteroids	-	-	-	100%
Received Home Management Plan	-	-	-	71%
Received Reliever Medication	-	-	-	100%
Use of Medical Imaging				
Combination Abdominal CT Scan	-	-	0.219	0.191
Combination Chest CT Scan	-	-	0.102	0.054
Follow-up Mammogram/Ultrasound	-	-	8%	8.4%
MRI for Low Back Pain	-	-	30.7%	32.7%
Survey of Patients' Hospital Experiences				
Area Around Room 'Always' Quiet at Night	-	-	-	58%
Doctors 'Always' Communicated Well	-	-	-	80%
Home Recovery Information Given	-	-	-	82%
Hospital Given 9 or 10 on 10 Point Scale	-	-	-	67%
Meds 'Always' Explained Before Given	-	-	-	60%
Nurses 'Always' Communicated Well	-	-	-	76%
Pain 'Always' Well Controlled	-	-	-	69%
Room and Bathroom 'Always' Clean	-	-	-	71%
Timely Help 'Always' Received	-	-	-	64%
Would Definitely Recommend Hospital	-	-	-	69%

Vanderbilt University Hospital

1161 21st Avenue South
Nashville, TN 37232
URL: www.mc.vanderbilt.edu
Type: Acute Care Hospitals
Ownership: Voluntary Non-Profit - Private

Phone: 615-322-3454
Fax: 615-343-7317

Emergency Services: Yes
Beds: 705

Key Personnel:
CEO/President . . . . Norman Burmy
Chief of Medical Staff . . . . Allen B Kaiser, MD
Infection Control. . . . . William Schaffner, MD
Operating Room. . . . . Nancy Feistrizer
Pediatric Ambulatory Care . . . . . . Thomas Graham, MD
Pediatric In-Patient Care . . . . Terrell Smith
Quality Assurance . . . . Paul Miles, MD
Radiology. . . . . Dennis Halahan, MD

Measure	Cases	This Hosp.	State Avg.	U.S. Avg.
Heart Attack Care				
ACE Inhibitor or ARB for LVSD[2]	53	100%	96%	96%
Aspirin at Arrival[2]	148	99%	98%	99%
Aspirin at Discharge[2]	359	100%	99%	98%
Beta Blocker at Discharge[2]	349	99%	98%	98%
Fibrinolytic Medication Timing[2]	0	-	67%	55%
PCI Within 90 Minutes of Arrival[1,2]	24	96%	91%	90%
Smoking Cessation Advice[2]	144	100%	100%	99%
Chest Pain/Possible Heart Attack Care				
Aspirin at Arrival[1,3]	2	100%	95%	95%
Median Time to ECG (minutes)[1,3]	2	8	8	8
Median Time to Transfer (minutes)[5]	0	-	65	61
Fibrinolytic Medication Timing[5]	0	-	49%	54%
Heart Failure Care				
ACE Inhibitor or ARB for LVSD[2]	150	93%	95%	94%
Discharge Instructions[2]	333	92%	88%	88%
Evaluation of LVS Function[2]	367	99%	97%	98%
Smoking Cessation Advice[2]	70	100%	99%	98%
Pneumonia Care				
Appropriate Initial Antibiotic[2]	39	97%	92%	92%
Blood Culture Timing[2]	100	92%	97%	96%
Influenza Vaccine[2]	81	84%	93%	91%
Initial Antibiotic Timing[2]	106	94%	96%	95%
Pneumococcal Vaccine[2]	87	83%	95%	93%
Smoking Cessation Advice[2]	66	100%	99%	97%
Surgical Care Improvement Project				
Appropriate VTP Within 24 Hours[2]	198	99%	92%	92%
Appropriate Hair Removal[2]	682	99%	100%	99%
Appropriate Beta Blocker Usage[2]	186	91%	93%	93%
Controlled Postoperative Blood Glucose[2]	109	92%	93%	93%
Prophylactic Antibiotic Timing[2]	421	99%	97%	97%
Prophylactic Antibiotic Timing (Outpatient)	779	94%	94%	92%
Prophylactic Antibiotic Selection[2]	434	98%	97%	97%
Prophylactic Antibiotic Select. (Outpatient)	911	96%	94%	94%
Prophylactic Antibiotic Stopped[2]	401	97%	94%	94%
Recommended VTP Ordered[2]	198	99%	94%	94%
Urinary Catheter Removal[2]	151	96%	90%	90%
Children's Asthma Care				
Received Systemic Corticosteroids	-	-	-	100%
Received Home Management Plan	-	-	-	71%
Received Reliever Medication	-	-	-	100%
Use of Medical Imaging				
Combination Abdominal CT Scan	2,684	0.212	0.219	0.191
Combination Chest CT Scan	2,521	0.018	0.102	0.054
Follow-up Mammogram/Ultrasound	990	11.3%	8%	8.4%
MRI for Low Back Pain	101	28.7%	30.7%	32.7%
Survey of Patients' Hospital Experiences				
Area Around Room 'Always' Quiet at Night	300+	55%	-	58%
Doctors 'Always' Communicated Well	300+	83%	-	80%
Home Recovery Information Given	300+	85%	-	82%
Hospital Given 9 or 10 on 10 Point Scale	300+	74%	-	67%
Meds 'Always' Explained Before Given	300+	60%	-	60%
Nurses 'Always' Communicated Well	300+	78%	-	76%
Pain 'Always' Well Controlled	300+	70%	-	69%
Room and Bathroom 'Always' Clean	300+	64%	-	71%
Timely Help 'Always' Received	300+	62%	-	64%
Would Definitely Recommend Hospital	300+	81%	-	69%

NOTE: Hospital profiles are in alphabetical order by state, then city, then hospital within the city; Rankings exclude hospitals with less than 25 cases except for patient surveys which excludes hospitals with less than 100 cases; (a) 100–299 cases; (1) The number of cases is too small to be sure how well a hospital is performing; (2) The hospital indicated that the data submitted for this measure were based on a sample of cases; (3) Data was collected during a shorter time period (fewer quarters) than the maximum possible time for this measure; (4) Suppressed for one or more quarters by CMS; (5) No data is available from the hospital for this measure; (6) Fewer than 100 patients completed the HCAHPS survey. Use these rates with caution, as the number of surveys may be too low to reliably assess hospital performance; (7) Survey results are based on less than 12 months of data; (8) Survey results are not available for this reporting period; (9) No or very few patients were eligible for the HCAHPS survey. The scores shown, if any, reflect a very small number of surveys; (10) A state average was not calculated because too few hospitals in the state submitted data; (11) There were discrepancies in the data collection process; Please refer to the User's Guide for a full explanation of data.

Baptist Hospital of Cocke County

435 2nd St
Newport, TN 37821
Phone: 423-625-2200
Fax: 423-625-2215
URL: www.baptistoneword.org
Type: Acute Care Hospitals
Emergency Services: Yes
Ownership: Voluntary Non-Profit - Church
Beds: 103

Key Personnel:
CEO/President. . . . . James Becker
Chief of Medical Staff . . . . Tish Perkins
Infection Control. . . . . Deanna Hill, RN
Operating Room. . . . . Sue Monroe, RN
Quality Assurance . . . . Sherry Rolen, RN
Radiology. . . . . John Stallworth
Emergency Room . . . . Kenneth Tazil, MD
Intensive Care Unit. . . . . Judy Henry, RN

Measure	Cases	This Hosp.	State Avg.	U.S. Avg.
Heart Attack Care				
ACE Inhibitor or ARB for LVSD	0	-	96%	96%
Aspirin at Arrival[1]	8	100%	98%	99%
Aspirin at Discharge[1]	4	100%	99%	98%
Beta Blocker at Discharge[1]	6	100%	98%	98%
Fibrinolytic Medication Timing	0	-	67%	55%
PCI Within 90 Minutes of Arrival	0	-	91%	90%
Smoking Cessation Advice	0	-	100%	99%
Chest Pain/Possible Heart Attack Care				
Aspirin at Arrival	315	96%	95%	95%
Median Time to ECG (minutes)	334	17	8	8
Median Time to Transfer (minutes)[1,3]	5	95	65	61
Fibrinolytic Medication Timing[1]	2	0%	49%	54%
Heart Failure Care				
ACE Inhibitor or ARB for LVSD	27	93%	95%	94%
Discharge Instructions	59	69%	88%	88%
Evaluation of LVS Function	69	99%	97%	98%
Smoking Cessation Advice[1]	22	95%	99%	98%
Pneumonia Care				
Appropriate Initial Antibiotic	142	89%	92%	92%
Blood Culture Timing	195	97%	97%	96%
Influenza Vaccine	121	99%	93%	91%
Initial Antibiotic Timing	182	99%	96%	95%
Pneumococcal Vaccine	143	99%	95%	93%
Smoking Cessation Advice	84	100%	99%	97%
Surgical Care Improvement Project				
Appropriate VTP Within 24 Hours[1,3]	6	33%	92%	92%
Appropriate Hair Removal[1,3]	6	100%	100%	99%
Appropriate Beta Blocker Usage[1,3]	1	100%	93%	93%
Controlled Postoperative Blood Glucose[3]	0	-	93%	93%
Prophylactic Antibiotic Timing[1,3]	4	50%	97%	97%
Prophylactic Antibiotic Timing (Outpatient)[1,3]	1	0%	94%	92%
Prophylactic Antibiotic Selection[1,3]	4	100%	97%	97%
Prophylactic Antibiotic Select. (Outpatient)[3]	0	-	94%	94%
Prophylactic Antibiotic Stopped[1,3]	3	100%	94%	94%
Recommended VTP Ordered[1,3]	6	33%	94%	94%
Urinary Catheter Removal[3]	0	-	90%	90%
Children's Asthma Care				
Received Systemic Corticosteroids	-	-	-	100%
Received Home Management Plan	-	-	-	71%
Received Reliever Medication	-	-	-	100%
Use of Medical Imaging				
Combination Abdominal CT Scan	362	0.088	0.219	0.191
Combination Chest CT Scan	266	0.090	0.102	0.054
Follow-up Mammogram/Ultrasound	506	11.9%	8%	8.4%
MRI for Low Back Pain	104	44.2%	30.7%	32.7%
Survey of Patients' Hospital Experiences				
Area Around Room 'Always' Quiet at Night	300+	59%	-	58%
Doctors 'Always' Communicated Well	300+	82%	-	80%
Home Recovery Information Given	300+	79%	-	82%
Hospital Given 9 or 10 on 10 Point Scale	300+	64%	-	67%
Meds 'Always' Explained Before Given	300+	61%	-	60%
Nurses 'Always' Communicated Well	300+	81%	-	76%
Pain 'Always' Well Controlled	300+	72%	-	69%
Room and Bathroom 'Always' Clean	300+	72%	-	71%
Timely Help 'Always' Received	300+	69%	-	64%
Would Definitely Recommend Hospital	300+	65%	-	69%

Methodist Medical Center of Oak Ridge

990 Oak Ridge Turnpike Box 529
Oak Ridge, TN 37830
Phone: 865-835-1000
Fax: 865-835-1795
URL: www.mmcoakridge.com
Type: Acute Care Hospitals
Emergency Services: Yes
Ownership: Voluntary Non-Profit - Private
Beds: 301

Key Personnel:
CEO/President. . . . . George Mathews
Cardiac Laboratory. . . . . Sue Harris, RN
Chief of Medical Staff . . . . Bill Molony, MD
Operating Room. . . . . Earlene Brewer
Quality Assurance . . . . Lee Young
Radiology. . . . . William Prater, MD

Measure	Cases	This Hosp.	State Avg.	U.S. Avg.
Heart Attack Care				
ACE Inhibitor or ARB for LVSD	64	100%	96%	96%
Aspirin at Arrival	191	99%	98%	99%
Aspirin at Discharge	281	98%	99%	98%
Beta Blocker at Discharge	269	99%	98%	98%
Fibrinolytic Medication Timing[1]	1	0%	67%	55%
PCI Within 90 Minutes of Arrival	51	100%	91%	90%
Smoking Cessation Advice	118	100%	100%	99%
Chest Pain/Possible Heart Attack Care				
Aspirin at Arrival[1]	10	90%	95%	95%
Median Time to ECG (minutes)[1]	12	8	8	8
Median Time to Transfer (minutes)[5]	0	-	65	61
Fibrinolytic Medication Timing[3]	0	-	49%	54%
Heart Failure Care				
ACE Inhibitor or ARB for LVSD	93	98%	95%	94%
Discharge Instructions	287	94%	88%	88%
Evaluation of LVS Function	344	99%	97%	98%
Smoking Cessation Advice	57	100%	99%	98%
Pneumonia Care				
Appropriate Initial Antibiotic	276	98%	92%	92%
Blood Culture Timing	525	98%	97%	96%
Influenza Vaccine	382	96%	93%	91%
Initial Antibiotic Timing	444	98%	96%	95%
Pneumococcal Vaccine	510	97%	95%	93%
Smoking Cessation Advice	252	100%	99%	97%
Surgical Care Improvement Project				
Appropriate VTP Within 24 Hours[2]	224	99%	92%	92%
Appropriate Hair Removal[2]	1,253	100%	100%	99%
Appropriate Beta Blocker Usage[2]	193	96%	93%	93%
Controlled Postoperative Blood Glucose[2]	184	97%	93%	93%
Prophylactic Antibiotic Timing[2]	1,019	99%	97%	97%
Prophylactic Antibiotic Timing (Outpatient)	502	98%	94%	92%
Prophylactic Antibiotic Selection[2]	1,017	98%	97%	97%
Prophylactic Antibiotic Select. (Outpatient)	503	96%	94%	94%
Prophylactic Antibiotic Stopped[2]	963	98%	94%	94%
Recommended VTP Ordered[2]	224	99%	94%	94%
Urinary Catheter Removal[2]	217	89%	90%	90%
Children's Asthma Care				
Received Systemic Corticosteroids	-	-	-	100%
Received Home Management Plan	-	-	-	71%
Received Reliever Medication	-	-	-	100%
Use of Medical Imaging				
Combination Abdominal CT Scan	1,105	0.059	0.219	0.191
Combination Chest CT Scan	738	0.003	0.102	0.054
Follow-up Mammogram/Ultrasound	2,390	8.8%	8%	8.4%
MRI for Low Back Pain	357	24.6%	30.7%	32.7%
Survey of Patients' Hospital Experiences				
Area Around Room 'Always' Quiet at Night	300+	65%	-	58%
Doctors 'Always' Communicated Well	300+	82%	-	80%
Home Recovery Information Given	300+	83%	-	82%
Hospital Given 9 or 10 on 10 Point Scale	300+	66%	-	67%
Meds 'Always' Explained Before Given	300+	63%	-	60%
Nurses 'Always' Communicated Well	300+	76%	-	76%
Pain 'Always' Well Controlled	300+	66%	-	69%
Room and Bathroom 'Always' Clean	300+	74%	-	71%
Timely Help 'Always' Received	300+	61%	-	64%
Would Definitely Recommend Hospital	300+	76%	-	69%

Scott County Hospital

18797 Alberta Avenue
Oneida, TN 37841
Phone: 423-569-8521
Fax: 423-569-5460
URL: www.scottcountyhostpital.com
Type: Critical Access Hospitals
Emergency Services: Yes
Ownership: Government - Local
Beds: 99

Key Personnel:
CEO/President. . . . . Larry Jater
Chief of Medical Staff . . . . Jan Robbins
Infection Control. . . . . Cheryl Jeffers
Operating Room. . . . . Pat Vanover
Quality Assurance . . . . Bob Rettig
Emergency Room . . . . Larry Turpin
Intensive Care Unit. . . . . Georgia Werley
Patient Relations . . . . Sonia Smithers

Measure	Cases	This Hosp.	State Avg.	U.S. Avg.
Heart Attack Care				
ACE Inhibitor or ARB for LVSD[1]	1	100%	96%	96%
Aspirin at Arrival[1]	3	100%	98%	99%
Aspirin at Discharge[1]	4	100%	99%	98%
Beta Blocker at Discharge[1]	5	100%	98%	98%
Fibrinolytic Medication Timing	0	-	67%	55%
PCI Within 90 Minutes of Arrival	0	-	91%	90%
Smoking Cessation Advice[1]	2	100%	100%	99%
Chest Pain/Possible Heart Attack Care				
Aspirin at Arrival	120	100%	95%	95%
Median Time to ECG (minutes)	131	6	8	8
Median Time to Transfer (minutes)[1]	2	48	65	61
Fibrinolytic Medication Timing[1]	6	50%	49%	54%
Heart Failure Care				
ACE Inhibitor or ARB for LVSD[1]	21	95%	95%	94%
Discharge Instructions	70	93%	88%	88%
Evaluation of LVS Function	69	91%	97%	98%
Smoking Cessation Advice[1]	12	100%	99%	98%
Pneumonia Care				
Appropriate Initial Antibiotic[2]	102	86%	92%	92%
Blood Culture Timing[2]	98	98%	97%	96%
Influenza Vaccine[2]	51	94%	93%	91%
Initial Antibiotic Timing[2]	103	99%	96%	95%
Pneumococcal Vaccine[2]	76	96%	95%	93%
Smoking Cessation Advice[2]	35	100%	99%	97%
Surgical Care Improvement Project				
Appropriate VTP Within 24 Hours[1]	6	0%	92%	92%
Appropriate Hair Removal[1]	9	100%	100%	99%
Appropriate Beta Blocker Usage[1]	2	100%	93%	93%
Controlled Postoperative Blood Glucose	0	-	93%	93%
Prophylactic Antibiotic Timing[1]	4	75%	97%	97%
Prophylactic Antibiotic Timing (Outpatient)[1,3]	1	100%	94%	92%
Prophylactic Antibiotic Selection[1]	4	25%	97%	97%
Prophylactic Antibiotic Select. (Outpatient)[1,3]	1	100%	94%	94%
Prophylactic Antibiotic Stopped[1]	4	100%	94%	94%
Recommended VTP Ordered[1]	6	0%	94%	94%
Urinary Catheter Removal	0	-	90%	90%
Children's Asthma Care				
Received Systemic Corticosteroids	-	-	-	100%
Received Home Management Plan	-	-	-	71%
Received Reliever Medication	-	-	-	100%
Use of Medical Imaging				
Combination Abdominal CT Scan[5]	0	-	0.219	0.191
Combination Chest CT Scan[5]	0	-	0.102	0.054
Follow-up Mammogram/Ultrasound[5]	0	-	8%	8.4%
MRI for Low Back Pain[5]	0	-	30.7%	32.7%
Survey of Patients' Hospital Experiences				
Area Around Room 'Always' Quiet at Night	(a)	65%	-	58%
Doctors 'Always' Communicated Well	(a)	85%	-	80%
Home Recovery Information Given	(a)	80%	-	82%
Hospital Given 9 or 10 on 10 Point Scale	(a)	60%	-	67%
Meds 'Always' Explained Before Given	(a)	65%	-	60%
Nurses 'Always' Communicated Well	(a)	78%	-	76%
Pain 'Always' Well Controlled	(a)	75%	-	69%
Room and Bathroom 'Always' Clean	(a)	81%	-	71%
Timely Help 'Always' Received	(a)	71%	-	64%
Would Definitely Recommend Hospital	(a)	63%	-	69%

NOTE: Hospital profiles are in alphabetical order by state, then city, then hospital within the city; Rankings exclude hospitals with less than 25 cases except for patient surveys which excludes hospitals with less than 100 cases; (a) 100–299 cases; (1) The number of cases is too small to be sure how well a hospital is performing; (2) The hospital indicated that the data submitted for this measure were based on a sample of cases; (3) Data was collected during a shorter time period (fewer quarters) than the maximum possible time for this measure; (4) Suppressed for one or more quarters by CMS; (5) No data is available from the hospital for this measure; (6) Fewer than 100 patients completed the HCAHPS survey. Use these rates with caution, as the number of surveys may be too low to reliably assess hospital performance; (7) Survey results are based on less than 12 months of data; (8) Survey results are not available for this reporting period; (9) No or very few patients were eligible for the HCAHPS survey. The scores shown, if any, reflect a very small number of surveys; (10) A state average was not calculated because too few hospitals in the state submitted data; (11) There were discrepancies in the data collection process; Please refer to the User's Guide for a full explanation of data.

Henry County Medical Center

301 Tyson Av
Paris, TN 38242
E-mail: hcmc@aeneas.net
URL: www.hcmc-tn.org
Type: Acute Care Hospitals
Ownership: Govt - Hospital Dist/Auth
Phone: 731-642-1220
Fax: 731-642-9588
Emergency Services: Yes
Beds: 142

Key Personnel:
CEO/President. . . . . Thomas H Gee
Chief of Medical Staff. . . . . Philip Nanney
Radiology. . . . . Robb Mitchell

Measure	Cases	This Hosp.	State Avg.	U.S. Avg.
Heart Attack Care				
ACE Inhibitor or ARB for LVSD[1]	4	100%	96%	96%
Aspirin at Arrival[1]	24	96%	98%	99%
Aspirin at Discharge[1]	17	88%	99%	98%
Beta Blocker at Discharge[1]	15	100%	98%	98%
Fibrinolytic Medication Timing	0	-	67%	55%
PCI Within 90 Minutes of Arrival	0	-	91%	90%
Smoking Cessation Advice[1]	3	100%	100%	99%
Chest Pain/Possible Heart Attack Care				
Aspirin at Arrival	219	96%	95%	95%
Median Time to ECG (minutes)	217	6	8	8
Median Time to Transfer (minutes)[1,3]	1	67	65	61
Fibrinolytic Medication Timing[1]	17	59%	49%	54%
Heart Failure Care				
ACE Inhibitor or ARB for LVSD	38	100%	95%	94%
Discharge Instructions	76	78%	88%	88%
Evaluation of LVS Function	97	99%	97%	98%
Smoking Cessation Advice[1]	19	100%	99%	98%
Pneumonia Care				
Appropriate Initial Antibiotic	111	95%	92%	92%
Blood Culture Timing	88	95%	97%	96%
Influenza Vaccine	95	85%	93%	91%
Initial Antibiotic Timing	125	94%	96%	95%
Pneumococcal Vaccine	124	95%	95%	93%
Smoking Cessation Advice	50	100%	99%	97%
Surgical Care Improvement Project				
Appropriate VTP Within 24 Hours	199	94%	92%	92%
Appropriate Hair Removal	524	100%	100%	99%
Appropriate Beta Blocker Usage	138	97%	93%	93%
Controlled Postoperative Blood Glucose	0	-	93%	93%
Prophylactic Antibiotic Timing	395	99%	97%	97%
Prophylactic Antibiotic Timing (Outpatient)	46	78%	94%	92%
Prophylactic Antibiotic Selection	403	99%	97%	97%
Prophylactic Antibiotic Select. (Outpatient)	37	92%	94%	94%
Prophylactic Antibiotic Stopped	369	97%	94%	94%
Recommended VTP Ordered	199	95%	94%	94%
Urinary Catheter Removal	67	88%	90%	90%
Children's Asthma Care				
Received Systemic Corticosteroids	-	-	-	100%
Received Home Management Plan	-	-	-	71%
Received Reliever Medication	-	-	-	100%
Use of Medical Imaging				
Combination Abdominal CT Scan	710	0.563	0.219	0.191
Combination Chest CT Scan	436	0.000	0.102	0.054
Follow-up Mammogram/Ultrasound	836	5.3%	8%	8.4%
MRI for Low Back Pain	181	29.8%	30.7%	32.7%
Survey of Patients' Hospital Experiences				
Area Around Room 'Always' Quiet at Night	300+	68%	-	58%
Doctors 'Always' Communicated Well	300+	84%	-	80%
Home Recovery Information Given	300+	82%	-	82%
Hospital Given 9 or 10 on 10 Point Scale	300+	69%	-	67%
Meds 'Always' Explained Before Given	300+	65%	-	60%
Nurses 'Always' Communicated Well	300+	76%	-	76%
Pain 'Always' Well Controlled	300+	70%	-	69%
Room and Bathroom 'Always' Clean	300+	68%	-	71%
Timely Help 'Always' Received	300+	61%	-	64%
Would Definitely Recommend Hospital	300+	71%	-	69%

Decatur County General Hospital

969 Tennessee Ave S
Parsons, TN 38363
E-mail: info@DCGH.org
URL: www.dcgh.org
Type: Acute Care Hospitals
Ownership: Government - Local
Phone: 731-847-3031
Fax: 731-847-1122
Emergency Services: Yes
Beds: 40

Key Personnel:
Chief of Medical Staff . . . . Thomas Hamilton
Infection Control. . . . . Linda Quinn
Operating Room. . . . . Charles Alderson
Quality Assurance . . . . Sue Ringger, RN
Radiology. . . . . Patrick Murphy, MD
Emergency Room . . . . Thomas Hamilton, MD
Intensive Care Unit. . . . . Wanda Hamm

Measure	Cases	This Hosp.	State Avg.	U.S. Avg.
Heart Attack Care				
ACE Inhibitor or ARB for LVSD[3]	0	-	96%	96%
Aspirin at Arrival[1,3]	3	100%	98%	99%
Aspirin at Discharge[1,3]	2	100%	99%	98%
Beta Blocker at Discharge[1,3]	2	100%	98%	98%
Fibrinolytic Medication Timing[3]	0	-	67%	55%
PCI Within 90 Minutes of Arrival[3]	0	-	91%	90%
Smoking Cessation Advice[3]	0	-	100%	99%
Chest Pain/Possible Heart Attack Care				
Aspirin at Arrival	124	97%	95%	95%
Median Time to ECG (minutes)	137	6	8	8
Median Time to Transfer (minutes)[1,3]	3	117	65	61
Fibrinolytic Medication Timing[1,3]	5	40%	49%	54%
Heart Failure Care				
ACE Inhibitor or ARB for LVSD[1]	3	67%	95%	94%
Discharge Instructions[1]	21	95%	88%	88%
Evaluation of LVS Function	31	97%	97%	98%
Smoking Cessation Advice[1]	2	100%	99%	98%
Pneumonia Care				
Appropriate Initial Antibiotic	44	89%	92%	92%
Blood Culture Timing	50	94%	97%	96%
Influenza Vaccine	45	96%	93%	91%
Initial Antibiotic Timing	68	97%	96%	95%
Pneumococcal Vaccine	74	99%	95%	93%
Smoking Cessation Advice[1]	11	100%	99%	97%
Surgical Care Improvement Project				
Appropriate VTP Within 24 Hours[5]	0	-	92%	92%
Appropriate Hair Removal[5]	0	-	100%	99%
Appropriate Beta Blocker Usage[5]	0	-	93%	93%
Controlled Postoperative Blood Glucose[5]	0	-	93%	93%
Prophylactic Antibiotic Timing[5]	0	-	97%	97%
Prophylactic Antibiotic Timing (Outpatient)[3]	0	-	94%	92%
Prophylactic Antibiotic Selection[5]	0	-	97%	97%
Prophylactic Antibiotic Select. (Outpatient)[3]	0	-	94%	94%
Prophylactic Antibiotic Stopped[5]	0	-	94%	94%
Recommended VTP Ordered[5]	0	-	94%	94%
Urinary Catheter Removal[5]	0	-	90%	90%
Children's Asthma Care				
Received Systemic Corticosteroids	-	-	-	100%
Received Home Management Plan	-	-	-	71%
Received Reliever Medication	-	-	-	100%
Use of Medical Imaging				
Combination Abdominal CT Scan	173	0.410	0.219	0.191
Combination Chest CT Scan	98	0.051	0.102	0.054
Follow-up Mammogram/Ultrasound	281	17.4%	8%	8.4%
MRI for Low Back Pain[1]	9	55.6%	30.7%	32.7%
Survey of Patients' Hospital Experiences				
Area Around Room 'Always' Quiet at Night	(a)	59%	-	58%
Doctors 'Always' Communicated Well	(a)	81%	-	80%
Home Recovery Information Given	(a)	77%	-	82%
Hospital Given 9 or 10 on 10 Point Scale	(a)	63%	-	67%
Meds 'Always' Explained Before Given	(a)	58%	-	60%
Nurses 'Always' Communicated Well	(a)	82%	-	76%
Pain 'Always' Well Controlled	(a)	72%	-	69%
Room and Bathroom 'Always' Clean	(a)	77%	-	71%
Timely Help 'Always' Received	(a)	72%	-	64%
Would Definitely Recommend Hospital	(a)	58%	-	69%

Hillside Hospital

1265 E College St
Pulaski, TN 38478
URL: www.hillsidehospital.com
Type: Acute Care Hospitals
Ownership: Proprietary
Phone: 931-363-7531
Fax: 931-424-7520
Emergency Services: Yes
Beds: 95

Key Personnel:
CEO/President. . . . . Donald Gavin
Chief of Medical Staff. . . . . Gigi Alejandrino, MD
Infection Control. . . . . Debbie Weaver
Operating Room. . . . . Denida Cox
Quality Assurance . . . . Penni Patterson
Radiology. . . . . Richard Stults
Emergency Room . . . . Miranda Danley

Measure	Cases	This Hosp.	State Avg.	U.S. Avg.
Heart Attack Care				
ACE Inhibitor or ARB for LVSD[3]	0	-	96%	96%
Aspirin at Arrival[1,3]	1	100%	98%	99%
Aspirin at Discharge[1,3]	1	0%	99%	98%
Beta Blocker at Discharge[1,3]	1	100%	98%	98%
Fibrinolytic Medication Timing[3]	0	-	67%	55%
PCI Within 90 Minutes of Arrival[3]	0	-	91%	90%
Smoking Cessation Advice[3]	0	-	100%	99%
Chest Pain/Possible Heart Attack Care				
Aspirin at Arrival	281	94%	95%	95%
Median Time to ECG (minutes)	292	5	8	8
Median Time to Transfer (minutes)[1]	3	79	65	61
Fibrinolytic Medication Timing[1]	4	50%	49%	54%
Heart Failure Care				
ACE Inhibitor or ARB for LVSD[1]	6	67%	95%	94%
Discharge Instructions[1]	19	95%	88%	88%
Evaluation of LVS Function	25	100%	97%	98%
Smoking Cessation Advice[1]	7	100%	99%	98%
Pneumonia Care				
Appropriate Initial Antibiotic	60	93%	92%	92%
Blood Culture Timing	54	100%	97%	96%
Influenza Vaccine	57	93%	93%	91%
Initial Antibiotic Timing	84	98%	96%	95%
Pneumococcal Vaccine	71	99%	95%	93%
Smoking Cessation Advice	35	97%	99%	97%
Surgical Care Improvement Project				
Appropriate VTP Within 24 Hours[1]	21	100%	92%	92%
Appropriate Hair Removal	72	99%	100%	99%
Appropriate Beta Blocker Usage[1]	14	79%	93%	93%
Controlled Postoperative Blood Glucose	0	-	93%	93%
Prophylactic Antibiotic Timing	56	96%	97%	97%
Prophylactic Antibiotic Timing (Outpatient)[1,3]	11	82%	94%	92%
Prophylactic Antibiotic Selection	56	98%	97%	97%
Prophylactic Antibiotic Select. (Outpatient)[1,3]	10	60%	94%	94%
Prophylactic Antibiotic Stopped	54	96%	94%	94%
Recommended VTP Ordered[1]	21	100%	94%	94%
Urinary Catheter Removal[1]	11	91%	90%	90%
Children's Asthma Care				
Received Systemic Corticosteroids	-	-	-	100%
Received Home Management Plan	-	-	-	71%
Received Reliever Medication	-	-	-	100%
Use of Medical Imaging				
Combination Abdominal CT Scan	282	0.156	0.219	0.191
Combination Chest CT Scan	159	0.006	0.102	0.054
Follow-up Mammogram/Ultrasound	499	9.4%	8%	8.4%
MRI for Low Back Pain[1]	57	22.8%	30.7%	32.7%
Survey of Patients' Hospital Experiences				
Area Around Room 'Always' Quiet at Night	(a)	63%	-	58%
Doctors 'Always' Communicated Well	(a)	85%	-	80%
Home Recovery Information Given	(a)	81%	-	82%
Hospital Given 9 or 10 on 10 Point Scale	(a)	65%	-	67%
Meds 'Always' Explained Before Given	(a)	61%	-	60%
Nurses 'Always' Communicated Well	(a)	76%	-	76%
Pain 'Always' Well Controlled	(a)	69%	-	69%
Room and Bathroom 'Always' Clean	(a)	64%	-	71%
Timely Help 'Always' Received	(a)	65%	-	64%
Would Definitely Recommend Hospital	(a)	61%	-	69%

NOTE: Hospital profiles are in alphabetical order by state, then city, then hospital within the city; Rankings exclude hospitals with less than 25 cases except for patient surveys which excludes hospitals with less than 100 cases; (a) 100–299 cases; (1) The number of cases is too small to be sure how well a hospital is performing; (2) The hospital indicated that the data submitted for this measure were based on a sample of cases; (3) Data was collected during a shorter time period (fewer quarters) than the maximum possible time for this measure; (4) Suppressed for one or more quarters by CMS; (5) No data is available from the hospital for this measure; (6) Fewer than 100 patients completed the HCAHPS survey. Use these rates with caution, as the number of surveys may be too low to reliably assess hospital performance; (7) Survey results are based on less than 12 months of data; (8) Survey results are not available for this reporting period; (9) No or very few patients were eligible for the HCAHPS survey. The scores shown, if any, reflect a very small number of surveys; (10) A state average was not calculated because too few hospitals in the state submitted data; (11) There were discrepancies in the data collection process; Please refer to the User's Guide for a full explanation of data.

Lauderdale Community Hospital

326 Asbury Avenue
Ripley, TN 38063
URL: www.lauderdalehospital.com
Type: Critical Access Hospitals
Ownership: Proprietary
Phone: 731-221-2200
Fax: 731-221-2499
Emergency Services: Yes
Beds: 25

Key Personnel:
CEO/President. . . . . Scott Tongate, CEO
Chief of Medical Staff. . . . . Syed A. Zaidi, MD
Infection Control. . . . . Cynthia Kidd, RN
Operating Room. . . . . Denise Blankenship, RN
Quality Assurance . . . . Cheryl Manns
Radiology. . . . . Billinda Baggett

Measure	Cases	This Hosp.	State Avg.	U.S. Avg.
Heart Attack Care				
ACE Inhibitor or ARB for LVSD[3]	0	-	96%	96%
Aspirin at Arrival[1,3]	1	100%	98%	99%
Aspirin at Discharge[1,3]	1	0%	99%	98%
Beta Blocker at Discharge[1,3]	3	100%	98%	98%
Fibrinolytic Medication Timing[3]	0	-	67%	55%
PCI Within 90 Minutes of Arrival[5]	0	-	91%	90%
Smoking Cessation Advice[3]	0	-	100%	99%
Chest Pain/Possible Heart Attack Care				
Aspirin at Arrival[3]	81	94%	95%	95%
Median Time to ECG (minutes)[3]	81	9	8	8
Median Time to Transfer (minutes)[5]	0	-	65	61
Fibrinolytic Medication Timing[1,3]	3	33%	49%	54%
Heart Failure Care				
ACE Inhibitor or ARB for LVSD[1]	10	100%	95%	94%
Discharge Instructions	28	46%	88%	88%
Evaluation of LVS Function	40	88%	97%	98%
Smoking Cessation Advice[1]	2	100%	99%	98%
Pneumonia Care				
Appropriate Initial Antibiotic	32	81%	92%	92%
Blood Culture Timing	28	96%	97%	96%
Influenza Vaccine[1]	20	100%	93%	91%
Initial Antibiotic Timing	46	89%	96%	95%
Pneumococcal Vaccine	28	79%	95%	93%
Smoking Cessation Advice[1]	17	100%	99%	97%
Surgical Care Improvement Project				
Appropriate VTP Within 24 Hours[5]	0	-	92%	92%
Appropriate Hair Removal[5]	0	-	100%	99%
Appropriate Beta Blocker Usage[5]	0	-	93%	93%
Controlled Postoperative Blood Glucose[5]	0	-	93%	93%
Prophylactic Antibiotic Timing[5]	0	-	97%	97%
Prophylactic Antibiotic Timing (Outpatient)[5]	0	-	94%	92%
Prophylactic Antibiotic Selection[5]	0	-	97%	97%
Prophylactic Antibiotic Select. (Outpatient)[5]	0	-	94%	94%
Prophylactic Antibiotic Stopped[5]	0	-	94%	94%
Recommended VTP Ordered[5]	0	-	94%	94%
Urinary Catheter Removal[5]	0	-	90%	90%
Children's Asthma Care				
Received Systemic Corticosteroids	-	-	-	100%
Received Home Management Plan	-	-	-	71%
Received Reliever Medication	-	-	-	100%
Use of Medical Imaging				
Combination Abdominal CT Scan	140	0.050	0.219	0.191
Combination Chest CT Scan	115	0.009	0.102	0.054
Follow-up Mammogram/Ultrasound	318	4.1%	8%	8.4%
MRI for Low Back Pain[1]	19	26.3%	30.7%	32.7%
Survey of Patients' Hospital Experiences				
Area Around Room 'Always' Quiet at Night[8]	-	-	-	58%
Doctors 'Always' Communicated Well[8]	-	-	-	80%
Home Recovery Information Given[8]	-	-	-	82%
Hospital Given 9 or 10 on 10 Point Scale[8]	-	-	-	67%
Meds 'Always' Explained Before Given[8]	-	-	-	60%
Nurses 'Always' Communicated Well[8]	-	-	-	76%
Pain 'Always' Well Controlled[8]	-	-	-	69%
Room and Bathroom 'Always' Clean[8]	-	-	-	71%
Timely Help 'Always' Received[8]	-	-	-	64%
Would Definitely Recommend Hospital[8]	-	-	-	69%

Wellmont Hawkins County Memorial Hospital

851 Locust Street
Rogersville, TN 37857
Type: Acute Care Hospitals
Ownership: Voluntary Non-Profit - Private
Phone: 423-921-7000
Fax: 423-921-7022
Emergency Services: Yes
Beds: 50

Key Personnel:
Chief of Medical Staff. . . . . Stephen Baumrucker, MD
Infection Control. . . . . Cathy Sandidge, RN
Operating Room. . . . . Charlene Presley, RN
Quality Assurance . . . . Mary Jo Fleenor
Radiology. . . . . Anton Allen

Measure	Cases	This Hosp.	State Avg.	U.S. Avg.
Heart Attack Care				
ACE Inhibitor or ARB for LVSD[1]	1	100%	96%	96%
Aspirin at Arrival[1]	10	90%	98%	99%
Aspirin at Discharge[1]	5	100%	99%	98%
Beta Blocker at Discharge[1]	6	100%	98%	98%
Fibrinolytic Medication Timing	0	-	67%	55%
PCI Within 90 Minutes of Arrival	0	-	91%	90%
Smoking Cessation Advice[1]	1	100%	100%	99%
Chest Pain/Possible Heart Attack Care				
Aspirin at Arrival	121	91%	95%	95%
Median Time to ECG (minutes)	122	12	8	8
Median Time to Transfer (minutes)[1]	8	180	65	61
Fibrinolytic Medication Timing[1]	1	0%	49%	54%
Heart Failure Care				
ACE Inhibitor or ARB for LVSD	25	96%	95%	94%
Discharge Instructions	84	83%	88%	88%
Evaluation of LVS Function	94	99%	97%	98%
Smoking Cessation Advice[1]	19	100%	99%	98%
Pneumonia Care				
Appropriate Initial Antibiotic	129	90%	92%	92%
Blood Culture Timing	114	92%	97%	96%
Influenza Vaccine	98	97%	93%	91%
Initial Antibiotic Timing	163	96%	96%	95%
Pneumococcal Vaccine	129	98%	95%	93%
Smoking Cessation Advice	99	100%	99%	97%
Surgical Care Improvement Project				
Appropriate VTP Within 24 Hours[1,2]	16	75%	92%	92%
Appropriate Hair Removal[1,2]	22	100%	100%	99%
Appropriate Beta Blocker Usage[1,2]	6	67%	93%	93%
Controlled Postoperative Blood Glucose[2]	0	-	93%	93%
Prophylactic Antibiotic Timing[1,2]	5	80%	97%	97%
Prophylactic Antibiotic Timing (Outpatient)[1,3]	5	100%	94%	92%
Prophylactic Antibiotic Selection[1,2]	5	100%	97%	97%
Prophylactic Antibiotic Select. (Outpatient)[1,3]	5	80%	94%	94%
Prophylactic Antibiotic Stopped[1,2]	4	75%	94%	94%
Recommended VTP Ordered[1,2]	16	75%	94%	94%
Urinary Catheter Removal[1,2]	2	100%	90%	90%
Children's Asthma Care				
Received Systemic Corticosteroids	-	-	-	100%
Received Home Management Plan	-	-	-	71%
Received Reliever Medication	-	-	-	100%
Use of Medical Imaging				
Combination Abdominal CT Scan	197	0.173	0.219	0.191
Combination Chest CT Scan	167	0.030	0.102	0.054
Follow-up Mammogram/Ultrasound	223	13.0%	8%	8.4%
MRI for Low Back Pain	74	39.2%	30.7%	32.7%
Survey of Patients' Hospital Experiences				
Area Around Room 'Always' Quiet at Night	300+	75%	-	58%
Doctors 'Always' Communicated Well	300+	88%	-	80%
Home Recovery Information Given	300+	83%	-	82%
Hospital Given 9 or 10 on 10 Point Scale	300+	73%	-	67%
Meds 'Always' Explained Before Given	300+	69%	-	60%
Nurses 'Always' Communicated Well	300+	83%	-	76%
Pain 'Always' Well Controlled	300+	76%	-	69%
Room and Bathroom 'Always' Clean	300+	82%	-	71%
Timely Help 'Always' Received	300+	73%	-	64%
Would Definitely Recommend Hospital	300+	75%	-	69%

Hardin Medical Center

935 Wayne Road
Savannah, TN 38372
Type: Acute Care Hospitals
Ownership: Government - Local
Phone: 731-926-8121
Fax: 731-926-8080
Emergency Services: Yes
Beds: 58

Key Personnel:
CEO/President. . . . . Charlotte Burns, CEO
Chief of Medical Staff. . . . . Gilbert Triger, MD
Infection Control. . . . . Diane DeBerry
Operating Room. . . . . Cindy Coleman
Quality Assurance . . . . Diane DeBerry
Emergency Room . . . . Suzanne Stricklin, RN
Hemotology Center . . . . Connie Hurt
Intensive Care Unit. . . . . Carolyn Carpenter

Measure	Cases	This Hosp.	State Avg.	U.S. Avg.
Heart Attack Care				
ACE Inhibitor or ARB for LVSD[3]	0	-	96%	96%
Aspirin at Arrival[1,3]	3	100%	98%	99%
Aspirin at Discharge[1,3]	3	67%	99%	98%
Beta Blocker at Discharge[1,3]	2	50%	98%	98%
Fibrinolytic Medication Timing[3]	0	-	67%	55%
PCI Within 90 Minutes of Arrival[3]	0	-	91%	90%
Smoking Cessation Advice[3]	0	-	100%	99%
Chest Pain/Possible Heart Attack Care				
Aspirin at Arrival	324	97%	95%	95%
Median Time to ECG (minutes)	345	9	8	8
Median Time to Transfer (minutes)[5]	0	-	65	61
Fibrinolytic Medication Timing[1]	16	62%	49%	54%
Heart Failure Care				
ACE Inhibitor or ARB for LVSD[1]	17	94%	95%	94%
Discharge Instructions	43	93%	88%	88%
Evaluation of LVS Function	64	98%	97%	98%
Smoking Cessation Advice[1]	13	100%	99%	98%
Pneumonia Care				
Appropriate Initial Antibiotic	87	93%	92%	92%
Blood Culture Timing	100	93%	97%	96%
Influenza Vaccine	61	87%	93%	91%
Initial Antibiotic Timing	103	95%	96%	95%
Pneumococcal Vaccine	90	94%	95%	93%
Smoking Cessation Advice	32	94%	99%	97%
Surgical Care Improvement Project				
Appropriate VTP Within 24 Hours[1]	23	87%	92%	92%
Appropriate Hair Removal	64	100%	100%	99%
Appropriate Beta Blocker Usage[1]	11	82%	93%	93%
Controlled Postoperative Blood Glucose	0	-	93%	93%
Prophylactic Antibiotic Timing	39	97%	97%	97%
Prophylactic Antibiotic Timing (Outpatient)	28	79%	94%	92%
Prophylactic Antibiotic Selection	39	100%	97%	97%
Prophylactic Antibiotic Select. (Outpatient)[1]	23	96%	94%	94%
Prophylactic Antibiotic Stopped	36	89%	94%	94%
Recommended VTP Ordered[1]	23	91%	94%	94%
Urinary Catheter Removal[1]	9	89%	90%	90%
Children's Asthma Care				
Received Systemic Corticosteroids	-	-	-	100%
Received Home Management Plan	-	-	-	71%
Received Reliever Medication	-	-	-	100%
Use of Medical Imaging				
Combination Abdominal CT Scan	466	0.034	0.219	0.191
Combination Chest CT Scan	261	0.011	0.102	0.054
Follow-up Mammogram/Ultrasound	399	19.0%	8%	8.4%
MRI for Low Back Pain	106	39.6%	30.7%	32.7%
Survey of Patients' Hospital Experiences				
Area Around Room 'Always' Quiet at Night	300+	74%	-	58%
Doctors 'Always' Communicated Well	300+	90%	-	80%
Home Recovery Information Given	300+	86%	-	82%
Hospital Given 9 or 10 on 10 Point Scale	300+	71%	-	67%
Meds 'Always' Explained Before Given	300+	71%	-	60%
Nurses 'Always' Communicated Well	300+	85%	-	76%
Pain 'Always' Well Controlled	300+	82%	-	69%
Room and Bathroom 'Always' Clean	300+	75%	-	71%
Timely Help 'Always' Received	300+	79%	-	64%
Would Definitely Recommend Hospital	300+	71%	-	69%

NOTE: Hospital profiles are in alphabetical order by state, then city, then hospital within the city; Rankings exclude hospitals with less than 25 cases except for patient surveys which excludes hospitals with less than 100 cases; (a) 100–299 cases; (1) The number of cases is too small to be sure how well a hospital is performing; (2) The hospital indicated that the data submitted for this measure were based on a sample of cases; (3) Data was collected during a shorter time period (fewer quarters) than the maximum possible time for this measure; (4) Suppressed for one or more quarters by CMS; (5) No data is available from the hospital for this measure; (6) Fewer than 100 patients completed the HCAHPS survey. Use these rates with caution, as the number of surveys may be too low to reliably assess hospital performance; (7) Survey results are based on less than 12 months of data; (8) Survey results are not available for this reporting period; (9) No or very few patients were eligible for the HCAHPS survey. The scores shown, if any, reflect a very small number of surveys; (10) A state average was not calculated because too few hospitals in the state submitted data; (11) There were discrepancies in the data collection process; Please refer to the User's Guide for a full explanation of data.

McNairy Regional Hospital

705 E Poplar Ave
Selmer, TN 38375
URL: www.mcnairyregionalhospital.com
Type: Acute Care Hospitals
Ownership: Proprietary

Phone: 731-645-3221

Emergency Services: Yes
Beds: 45

Key Personnel:
Radiology. . . . . Bonnie Lancaster
Anesthesiology. . . . . Jay Turner

Measure	Cases	This Hosp.	State Avg.	U.S. Avg.
Heart Attack Care				
ACE Inhibitor or ARB for LVSD[1]	3	67%	96%	96%
Aspirin at Arrival[1]	11	100%	98%	99%
Aspirin at Discharge[1]	7	86%	99%	98%
Beta Blocker at Discharge[1]	9	100%	98%	98%
Fibrinolytic Medication Timing	0	-	67%	55%
PCI Within 90 Minutes of Arrival	0	-	91%	90%
Smoking Cessation Advice	0	-	100%	99%
Chest Pain/Possible Heart Attack Care				
Aspirin at Arrival	140	97%	95%	95%
Median Time to ECG (minutes)	150	6	8	8
Median Time to Transfer (minutes)[5]	0	-	65	61
Fibrinolytic Medication Timing[1]	1	0%	49%	54%
Heart Failure Care				
ACE Inhibitor or ARB for LVSD[1]	15	80%	95%	94%
Discharge Instructions	44	93%	88%	88%
Evaluation of LVS Function	63	98%	97%	98%
Smoking Cessation Advice[1]	10	100%	99%	98%
Pneumonia Care				
Appropriate Initial Antibiotic	38	89%	92%	92%
Blood Culture Timing[1]	23	100%	97%	96%
Influenza Vaccine	33	100%	93%	91%
Initial Antibiotic Timing	58	100%	96%	95%
Pneumococcal Vaccine	40	100%	95%	93%
Smoking Cessation Advice[1]	19	100%	99%	97%
Surgical Care Improvement Project				
Appropriate VTP Within 24 Hours[1,2]	1	100%	92%	92%
Appropriate Hair Removal[1,2]	14	100%	100%	99%
Appropriate Beta Blocker Usage[1,2]	3	100%	93%	93%
Controlled Postoperative Blood Glucose[2]	0	-	93%	93%
Prophylactic Antibiotic Timing[1,2]	13	92%	97%	97%
Prophylactic Antibiotic Timing (Outpatient)[1,3]	16	94%	94%	92%
Prophylactic Antibiotic Selection[1,2]	13	92%	97%	97%
Prophylactic Antibiotic Select. (Outpatient)[1,3]	16	100%	94%	94%
Prophylactic Antibiotic Stopped[1,2]	13	100%	94%	94%
Recommended VTP Ordered[1,2]	1	100%	94%	94%
Urinary Catheter Removal	0	-	90%	90%
Children's Asthma Care				
Received Systemic Corticosteroids	-	-	-	100%
Received Home Management Plan	-	-	-	71%
Received Reliever Medication	-	-	-	100%
Use of Medical Imaging				
Combination Abdominal CT Scan	161	0.050	0.219	0.191
Combination Chest CT Scan	81	0.049	0.102	0.054
Follow-up Mammogram/Ultrasound	294	4.8%	8%	8.4%
MRI for Low Back Pain	48	37.5%	30.7%	32.7%
Survey of Patients' Hospital Experiences				
Area Around Room 'Always' Quiet at Night	(a)	74%	-	58%
Doctors 'Always' Communicated Well	(a)	85%	-	80%
Home Recovery Information Given	(a)	78%	-	82%
Hospital Given 9 or 10 on 10 Point Scale	(a)	65%	-	67%
Meds 'Always' Explained Before Given	(a)	64%	-	60%
Nurses 'Always' Communicated Well	(a)	78%	-	76%
Pain 'Always' Well Controlled	(a)	74%	-	69%
Room and Bathroom 'Always' Clean	(a)	70%	-	71%
Timely Help 'Always' Received	(a)	67%	-	64%
Would Definitely Recommend Hospital	(a)	66%	-	69%

Leconte Medical Center

742 Middlecreek Road
Sevierville, TN 37862
URL: www.lecontemedicalcenter.com
Type: Acute Care Hospitals
Ownership: Voluntary Non-Profit - Other

Phone: 865-429-6618

Emergency Services: Yes

Key Personnel:
President . . . . Ellen Wilhoit

Measure	Cases	This Hosp.	State Avg.	U.S. Avg.
Heart Attack Care				
ACE Inhibitor or ARB for LVSD[1]	3	100%	96%	96%
Aspirin at Arrival[1]	23	100%	98%	99%
Aspirin at Discharge[1]	19	95%	99%	98%
Beta Blocker at Discharge[1]	20	100%	98%	98%
Fibrinolytic Medication Timing	0	-	67%	55%
PCI Within 90 Minutes of Arrival	0	-	91%	90%
Smoking Cessation Advice[1]	4	100%	100%	99%
Chest Pain/Possible Heart Attack Care				
Aspirin at Arrival	194	98%	95%	95%
Median Time to ECG (minutes)	198	9	8	8
Median Time to Transfer (minutes)	31	55	65	61
Fibrinolytic Medication Timing	0	-	49%	54%
Heart Failure Care				
ACE Inhibitor or ARB for LVSD	25	96%	95%	94%
Discharge Instructions	121	94%	88%	88%
Evaluation of LVS Function	133	100%	97%	98%
Smoking Cessation Advice[1]	19	100%	99%	98%
Pneumonia Care				
Appropriate Initial Antibiotic	137	96%	92%	92%
Blood Culture Timing	199	94%	97%	96%
Influenza Vaccine	77	96%	93%	91%
Initial Antibiotic Timing	185	96%	96%	95%
Pneumococcal Vaccine	115	98%	95%	93%
Smoking Cessation Advice	63	100%	99%	97%
Surgical Care Improvement Project				
Appropriate VTP Within 24 Hours[2]	83	89%	92%	92%
Appropriate Hair Removal[2]	249	100%	100%	99%
Appropriate Beta Blocker Usage[2]	69	99%	93%	93%
Controlled Postoperative Blood Glucose[2]	0	-	93%	93%
Prophylactic Antibiotic Timing[2]	196	99%	97%	97%
Prophylactic Antibiotic Timing (Outpatient)	117	98%	94%	92%
Prophylactic Antibiotic Selection[2]	198	99%	97%	97%
Prophylactic Antibiotic Select. (Outpatient)	116	97%	94%	94%
Prophylactic Antibiotic Stopped[2]	192	97%	94%	94%
Recommended VTP Ordered[2]	83	94%	94%	94%
Urinary Catheter Removal[1,2]	4	100%	90%	90%
Children's Asthma Care				
Received Systemic Corticosteroids	-	-	-	100%
Received Home Management Plan	-	-	-	71%
Received Reliever Medication	-	-	-	100%
Use of Medical Imaging				
Combination Abdominal CT Scan	802	0.141	0.219	0.191
Combination Chest CT Scan	711	0.066	0.102	0.054
Follow-up Mammogram/Ultrasound	933	7.5%	8%	8.4%
MRI for Low Back Pain	172	40.1%	30.7%	32.7%
Survey of Patients' Hospital Experiences				
Area Around Room 'Always' Quiet at Night	300+	65%	-	58%
Doctors 'Always' Communicated Well	300+	86%	-	80%
Home Recovery Information Given	300+	89%	-	82%
Hospital Given 9 or 10 on 10 Point Scale	300+	74%	-	67%
Meds 'Always' Explained Before Given	300+	66%	-	60%
Nurses 'Always' Communicated Well	300+	79%	-	76%
Pain 'Always' Well Controlled	300+	72%	-	69%
Room and Bathroom 'Always' Clean	300+	76%	-	71%
Timely Help 'Always' Received	300+	66%	-	64%
Would Definitely Recommend Hospital	300+	72%	-	69%

Heritage Medical Center

2835 Hwy 231 N
Shelbyville, TN 37160
Type: Acute Care Hospitals
Ownership: Proprietary

Phone: 931-685-5433

Emergency Services: Yes

Measure	Cases	This Hosp.	State Avg.	U.S. Avg.
Heart Attack Care				
ACE Inhibitor or ARB for LVSD[1]	3	100%	96%	96%
Aspirin at Arrival[1]	13	100%	98%	99%
Aspirin at Discharge[1]	5	80%	99%	98%
Beta Blocker at Discharge[1]	5	100%	98%	98%
Fibrinolytic Medication Timing	0	-	67%	55%
PCI Within 90 Minutes of Arrival	0	-	91%	90%
Smoking Cessation Advice	0	-	100%	99%
Chest Pain/Possible Heart Attack Care				
Aspirin at Arrival	155	97%	95%	95%
Median Time to ECG (minutes)	162	4	8	8
Median Time to Transfer (minutes)[1]	5	42	65	61
Fibrinolytic Medication Timing[1]	2	50%	49%	54%
Heart Failure Care				
ACE Inhibitor or ARB for LVSD	29	86%	95%	94%
Discharge Instructions	67	79%	88%	88%
Evaluation of LVS Function	86	98%	97%	98%
Smoking Cessation Advice[1]	16	100%	99%	98%
Pneumonia Care				
Appropriate Initial Antibiotic	101	94%	92%	92%
Blood Culture Timing	93	98%	97%	96%
Influenza Vaccine	88	91%	93%	91%
Initial Antibiotic Timing	120	98%	96%	95%
Pneumococcal Vaccine	89	94%	95%	93%
Smoking Cessation Advice	57	100%	99%	97%
Surgical Care Improvement Project				
Appropriate VTP Within 24 Hours[2]	43	98%	92%	92%
Appropriate Hair Removal[2]	82	98%	100%	99%
Appropriate Beta Blocker Usage[1,2]	15	93%	93%	93%
Controlled Postoperative Blood Glucose[2]	0	-	93%	93%
Prophylactic Antibiotic Timing[2]	50	98%	97%	97%
Prophylactic Antibiotic Timing (Outpatient)[1]	8	100%	94%	92%
Prophylactic Antibiotic Selection[2]	50	98%	97%	97%
Prophylactic Antibiotic Select. (Outpatient)[1]	8	88%	94%	94%
Prophylactic Antibiotic Stopped[2]	48	85%	94%	94%
Recommended VTP Ordered[2]	43	100%	94%	94%
Urinary Catheter Removal[1]	19	84%	90%	90%
Children's Asthma Care				
Received Systemic Corticosteroids	-	-	-	100%
Received Home Management Plan	-	-	-	71%
Received Reliever Medication	-	-	-	100%
Use of Medical Imaging				
Combination Abdominal CT Scan	219	0.146	0.219	0.191
Combination Chest CT Scan	138	0.413	0.102	0.054
Follow-up Mammogram/Ultrasound	444	5.4%	8%	8.4%
MRI for Low Back Pain	64	32.8%	30.7%	32.7%
Survey of Patients' Hospital Experiences				
Area Around Room 'Always' Quiet at Night	300+	61%	-	58%
Doctors 'Always' Communicated Well	300+	84%	-	80%
Home Recovery Information Given	300+	81%	-	82%
Hospital Given 9 or 10 on 10 Point Scale	300+	66%	-	67%
Meds 'Always' Explained Before Given	300+	60%	-	60%
Nurses 'Always' Communicated Well	300+	74%	-	76%
Pain 'Always' Well Controlled	300+	68%	-	69%
Room and Bathroom 'Always' Clean	300+	73%	-	71%
Timely Help 'Always' Received	300+	60%	-	64%
Would Definitely Recommend Hospital	300+	63%	-	69%

NOTE: Hospital profiles are in alphabetical order by state, then city, then hospital within the city; Rankings exclude hospitals with less than 25 cases except for patient surveys which excludes hospitals with less than 100 cases; (a) 100–299 cases; (1) The number of cases is too small to be sure how well a hospital is performing; (2) The hospital indicated that the data submitted for this measure were based on a sample of cases; (3) Data was collected during a shorter time period (fewer quarters) than the maximum possible time for this measure; (4) Suppressed for one or more quarters by CMS; (5) No data is available from the hospital for this measure; (6) Fewer than 100 patients completed the HCAHPS survey. Use these rates with caution, as the number of surveys may be too low to reliably assess hospital performance; (7) The scores shown, if any, reflect a very small number of surveys; (8) Survey results are not available for this reporting period; (9) No or very few patients were eligible for the HCAHPS survey. The scores shown, if any, reflect a very small number of surveys; (10) A state average was not calculated because too few hospitals in the state submitted data; (11) There were discrepancies in the data collection process; Please refer to the User's Guide for a full explanation of data.

Stones River Hospital and Dekalb Community Hospital

520 W Main St
Smithville, TN 37166
Phone: 615-215-5000
Fax: 615-215-5604
URL: www.dekalb-hospital.com
Type: Acute Care Hospitals
Emergency Services: Yes
Ownership: Voluntary Non-Profit - Church
Beds: 71

Key Personnel:
CEO/President. . . . . Dennis Smock

Measure	Cases	This Hosp.	State Avg.	U.S. Avg.
Heart Attack Care				
ACE Inhibitor or ARB for LVSD	0	-	96%	96%
Aspirin at Arrival[1]	4	100%	98%	99%
Aspirin at Discharge[1]	2	100%	99%	98%
Beta Blocker at Discharge[1]	4	100%	98%	98%
Fibrinolytic Medication Timing	0	-	67%	55%
PCI Within 90 Minutes of Arrival	0	-	91%	90%
Smoking Cessation Advice	0	-	100%	99%
Chest Pain/Possible Heart Attack Care				
Aspirin at Arrival	99	94%	95%	95%
Median Time to ECG (minutes)	105	8	8	8
Median Time to Transfer (minutes)[5]	0	-	65	61
Fibrinolytic Medication Timing[1]	4	0%	49%	54%
Heart Failure Care				
ACE Inhibitor or ARB for LVSD[1]	10	100%	95%	94%
Discharge Instructions	51	61%	88%	88%
Evaluation of LVS Function	74	100%	97%	98%
Smoking Cessation Advice[1]	6	100%	99%	98%
Pneumonia Care				
Appropriate Initial Antibiotic	121	94%	92%	92%
Blood Culture Timing	84	94%	97%	96%
Influenza Vaccine	94	68%	93%	91%
Initial Antibiotic Timing	149	94%	96%	95%
Pneumococcal Vaccine	132	86%	95%	93%
Smoking Cessation Advice	63	95%	99%	97%
Surgical Care Improvement Project				
Appropriate VTP Within 24 Hours[1]	24	88%	92%	92%
Appropriate Hair Removal	68	100%	100%	99%
Appropriate Beta Blocker Usage[1]	22	100%	93%	93%
Controlled Postoperative Blood Glucose	0	-	93%	93%
Prophylactic Antibiotic Timing	50	98%	97%	97%
Prophylactic Antibiotic Timing (Outpatient)	30	97%	94%	92%
Prophylactic Antibiotic Selection	50	96%	97%	97%
Prophylactic Antibiotic Select. (Outpatient)	31	94%	94%	94%
Prophylactic Antibiotic Stopped	46	87%	94%	94%
Recommended VTP Ordered[1]	24	88%	94%	94%
Urinary Catheter Removal[1]	16	88%	90%	90%
Children's Asthma Care				
Received Systemic Corticosteroids	-	-	-	100%
Received Home Management Plan	-	-	-	71%
Received Reliever Medication	-	-	-	100%
Use of Medical Imaging				
Combination Abdominal CT Scan	226	0.327	0.219	0.191
Combination Chest CT Scan	175	0.057	0.102	0.054
Follow-up Mammogram/Ultrasound	323	8.4%	8%	8.4%
MRI for Low Back Pain	62	35.5%	30.7%	32.7%
Survey of Patients' Hospital Experiences				
Area Around Room 'Always' Quiet at Night	300+	67%	-	58%
Doctors 'Always' Communicated Well	300+	90%	-	80%
Home Recovery Information Given	300+	84%	-	82%
Hospital Given 9 or 10 on 10 Point Scale	300+	71%	-	67%
Meds 'Always' Explained Before Given	300+	58%	-	60%
Nurses 'Always' Communicated Well	300+	83%	-	76%
Pain 'Always' Well Controlled	300+	77%	-	69%
Room and Bathroom 'Always' Clean	300+	75%	-	71%
Timely Help 'Always' Received	300+	68%	-	64%
Would Definitely Recommend Hospital	300+	73%	-	69%

Stonecrest Medical Center

200 Stonecrest Boulevard
Smyrna, TN 37167
Phone: 615-768-2000
Fax: 615-768-2203
URL: www.stonecrestmedical.com
Type: Acute Care Hospitals
Emergency Services: Yes
Ownership: Proprietary
Beds: 75

Key Personnel:
CEO/President. . . . . Neil A Heatherly, CHE
Chief of Medical Staff. . . . . Anita Dhar
Radiology. . . . . Christopher J Bodin

Measure	Cases	This Hosp.	State Avg.	U.S. Avg.
Heart Attack Care				
ACE Inhibitor or ARB for LVSD[1]	3	100%	96%	96%
Aspirin at Arrival	27	100%	98%	99%
Aspirin at Discharge[1]	16	94%	99%	98%
Beta Blocker at Discharge[1]	20	100%	98%	98%
Fibrinolytic Medication Timing	0	-	67%	55%
PCI Within 90 Minutes of Arrival	0	-	91%	90%
Smoking Cessation Advice[1]	12	100%	100%	99%
Chest Pain/Possible Heart Attack Care				
Aspirin at Arrival	109	99%	95%	95%
Median Time to ECG (minutes)	119	5	8	8
Median Time to Transfer (minutes)	28	42	65	61
Fibrinolytic Medication Timing	0	-	49%	54%
Heart Failure Care				
ACE Inhibitor or ARB for LVSD[1]	20	100%	95%	94%
Discharge Instructions	66	98%	88%	88%
Evaluation of LVS Function	84	98%	97%	98%
Smoking Cessation Advice[1]	21	100%	99%	98%
Pneumonia Care				
Appropriate Initial Antibiotic	111	92%	92%	92%
Blood Culture Timing	163	99%	97%	96%
Influenza Vaccine	78	96%	93%	91%
Initial Antibiotic Timing	140	99%	96%	95%
Pneumococcal Vaccine	113	97%	95%	93%
Smoking Cessation Advice	64	100%	99%	97%
Surgical Care Improvement Project				
Appropriate VTP Within 24 Hours	116	96%	92%	92%
Appropriate Hair Removal	316	100%	100%	99%
Appropriate Beta Blocker Usage	58	98%	93%	93%
Controlled Postoperative Blood Glucose	0	-	93%	93%
Prophylactic Antibiotic Timing	202	98%	97%	97%
Prophylactic Antibiotic Timing (Outpatient)	204	98%	94%	92%
Prophylactic Antibiotic Selection	204	98%	97%	97%
Prophylactic Antibiotic Select. (Outpatient)	212	98%	94%	94%
Prophylactic Antibiotic Stopped	184	96%	94%	94%
Recommended VTP Ordered	116	97%	94%	94%
Urinary Catheter Removal	58	97%	90%	90%
Children's Asthma Care				
Received Systemic Corticosteroids	-	-	-	100%
Received Home Management Plan	-	-	-	71%
Received Reliever Medication	-	-	-	100%
Use of Medical Imaging				
Combination Abdominal CT Scan	346	0.064	0.219	0.191
Combination Chest CT Scan	155	0.032	0.102	0.054
Follow-up Mammogram/Ultrasound	480	9.0%	8%	8.4%
MRI for Low Back Pain	65	33.8%	30.7%	32.7%
Survey of Patients' Hospital Experiences				
Area Around Room 'Always' Quiet at Night	300+	70%	-	58%
Doctors 'Always' Communicated Well	300+	82%	-	80%
Home Recovery Information Given	300+	87%	-	82%
Hospital Given 9 or 10 on 10 Point Scale	300+	71%	-	67%
Meds 'Always' Explained Before Given	300+	61%	-	60%
Nurses 'Always' Communicated Well	300+	77%	-	76%
Pain 'Always' Well Controlled	300+	73%	-	69%
Room and Bathroom 'Always' Clean	300+	74%	-	71%
Timely Help 'Always' Received	300+	64%	-	64%
Would Definitely Recommend Hospital	300+	77%	-	69%

Wellmont Hancock County Hospital

1517 Main Street Hwy 33
Sneedville, TN 37869
Phone: 423-733-5001
URL: www.wellmont.org
Type: Critical Access Hospitals
Emergency Services: Yes
Ownership: Voluntary Non-Profit - Private

Key Personnel:
CEO/President. . . . . Fred Pelle
Chief of Medical Staff. . . . . John Short

Measure	Cases	This Hosp.	State Avg.	U.S. Avg.
Heart Attack Care				
ACE Inhibitor or ARB for LVSD[3]	0	-	96%	96%
Aspirin at Arrival[1,3]	1	100%	98%	99%
Aspirin at Discharge[1,3]	1	100%	99%	98%
Beta Blocker at Discharge[1,3]	1	100%	98%	98%
Fibrinolytic Medication Timing[3]	0	-	67%	55%
PCI Within 90 Minutes of Arrival[3]	0	-	91%	90%
Smoking Cessation Advice[1,3]	1	100%	100%	99%
Chest Pain/Possible Heart Attack Care				
Aspirin at Arrival	-	-	95%	95%
Median Time to ECG (minutes)	-	-	8	8
Median Time to Transfer (minutes)	-	-	65	61
Fibrinolytic Medication Timing	-	-	49%	54%
Heart Failure Care				
ACE Inhibitor or ARB for LVSD[1]	3	100%	95%	94%
Discharge Instructions[1]	16	100%	88%	88%
Evaluation of LVS Function[1]	18	89%	97%	98%
Smoking Cessation Advice[1]	5	100%	99%	98%
Pneumonia Care				
Appropriate Initial Antibiotic[1]	19	95%	92%	92%
Blood Culture Timing	26	96%	97%	96%
Influenza Vaccine[1]	13	100%	93%	91%
Initial Antibiotic Timing[1]	24	100%	96%	95%
Pneumococcal Vaccine[1]	20	100%	95%	93%
Smoking Cessation Advice[1]	11	100%	99%	97%
Surgical Care Improvement Project				
Appropriate VTP Within 24 Hours[5]	0	-	92%	92%
Appropriate Hair Removal[5]	0	-	100%	99%
Appropriate Beta Blocker Usage[5]	0	-	93%	93%
Controlled Postoperative Blood Glucose[5]	0	-	93%	93%
Prophylactic Antibiotic Timing[5]	0	-	97%	97%
Prophylactic Antibiotic Timing (Outpatient)	-	-	94%	92%
Prophylactic Antibiotic Selection[5]	0	-	97%	97%
Prophylactic Antibiotic Select. (Outpatient)	-	-	94%	94%
Prophylactic Antibiotic Stopped[5]	0	-	94%	94%
Recommended VTP Ordered[5]	0	-	94%	94%
Urinary Catheter Removal[5]	0	-	90%	90%
Children's Asthma Care				
Received Systemic Corticosteroids	-	-	-	100%
Received Home Management Plan	-	-	-	71%
Received Reliever Medication	-	-	-	100%
Use of Medical Imaging				
Combination Abdominal CT Scan	-	-	0.219	0.191
Combination Chest CT Scan	-	-	0.102	0.054
Follow-up Mammogram/Ultrasound	-	-	8%	8.4%
MRI for Low Back Pain	-	-	30.7%	32.7%
Survey of Patients' Hospital Experiences				
Area Around Room 'Always' Quiet at Night[8]	-	-	-	58%
Doctors 'Always' Communicated Well[8]	-	-	-	80%
Home Recovery Information Given[8]	-	-	-	82%
Hospital Given 9 or 10 on 10 Point Scale[8]	-	-	-	67%
Meds 'Always' Explained Before Given[8]	-	-	-	60%
Nurses 'Always' Communicated Well[8]	-	-	-	76%
Pain 'Always' Well Controlled[8]	-	-	-	69%
Room and Bathroom 'Always' Clean[8]	-	-	-	71%
Timely Help 'Always' Received[8]	-	-	-	64%
Would Definitely Recommend Hospital[8]	-	-	-	69%

NOTE: Hospital profiles are in alphabetical order by state, then city, then hospital within the city; Rankings exclude hospitals with less than 25 cases except for patient surveys which excludes hospitals with less than 100 cases; (a) 100–299 cases; (1) The number of cases is too small to be sure how well a hospital is performing; (2) The hospital indicated that the data submitted for this measure were based on a sample of cases; (3) Data was collected during a shorter time period (fewer quarters) than the maximum possible time for this measure; (4) Suppressed for one or more quarters by CMS; (5) No data is available from the hospital for this measure; (6) Fewer than 100 patients completed the HCAHPS survey. Use these rates with caution, as the number of surveys may be too low to reliably assess hospital performance; (7) Survey results are based on less than 12 months of data; (8) Survey results are not available for this reporting period; (9) No or very few patients were eligible for the HCAHPS survey. The scores shown, if any, reflect a very small number of surveys; (10) A state average was not calculated because too few hospitals in the state submitted data; (11) There were discrepancies in the data collection process; Please refer to the User's Guide for a full explanation of data.

Methodist Healthcare Fayette Hospital

214 Lakeview Rd
Somerville, TN 38068
Phone: 901-516-4014
Type: Acute Care Hospitals
Emergency Services: Yes
Ownership: Voluntary Non-Profit - Church

Key Personnel:
CEO/President. . . . . David Crislip

Measure	Cases	This Hosp.	State Avg.	U.S. Avg.
Heart Attack Care				
ACE Inhibitor or ARB for LVSD[5]	0	-	96%	96%
Aspirin at Arrival[5]	0	-	98%	99%
Aspirin at Discharge[5]	0	-	99%	98%
Beta Blocker at Discharge[5]	0	-	98%	98%
Fibrinolytic Medication Timing[5]	0	-	67%	55%
PCI Within 90 Minutes of Arrival[5]	0	-	91%	90%
Smoking Cessation Advice[5]	0	-	100%	99%
Chest Pain/Possible Heart Attack Care				
Aspirin at Arrival	97	97%	95%	95%
Median Time to ECG (minutes)	100	0	8	8
Median Time to Transfer (minutes)[1,3]	1	103	65	61
Fibrinolytic Medication Timing[1]	2	100%	49%	54%
Heart Failure Care				
ACE Inhibitor or ARB for LVSD[1,3]	4	100%	95%	94%
Discharge Instructions[1,3]	13	92%	88%	88%
Evaluation of LVS Function[1,3]	17	100%	97%	98%
Smoking Cessation Advice[1,3]	4	100%	99%	98%
Pneumonia Care				
Appropriate Initial Antibiotic	29	97%	92%	92%
Blood Culture Timing	33	100%	97%	96%
Influenza Vaccine[1]	23	91%	93%	91%
Initial Antibiotic Timing	42	95%	96%	95%
Pneumococcal Vaccine	36	100%	95%	93%
Smoking Cessation Advice[1]	13	92%	99%	97%
Surgical Care Improvement Project				
Appropriate VTP Within 24 Hours[1,3]	4	100%	92%	92%
Appropriate Hair Removal[1,3]	4	100%	100%	99%
Appropriate Beta Blocker Usage[1,3]	1	100%	93%	93%
Controlled Postoperative Blood Glucose[3]	0	-	93%	93%
Prophylactic Antibiotic Timing[1,3]	1	100%	97%	97%
Prophylactic Antibiotic Timing (Outpatient)[3]	0	-	94%	92%
Prophylactic Antibiotic Selection[1,3]	1	100%	97%	97%
Prophylactic Antibiotic Select. (Outpatient)[1,3]	1	0%	94%	94%
Prophylactic Antibiotic Stopped[1,3]	1	100%	94%	94%
Recommended VTP Ordered[1,3]	4	100%	94%	94%
Urinary Catheter Removal[5]	0	-	90%	90%
Children's Asthma Care				
Received Systemic Corticosteroids	-	-	-	100%
Received Home Management Plan	-	-	-	71%
Received Reliever Medication	-	-	-	100%
Use of Medical Imaging				
Combination Abdominal CT Scan	184	0.038	0.219	0.191
Combination Chest CT Scan	101	0.020	0.102	0.054
Follow-up Mammogram/Ultrasound	202	8.4%	8%	8.4%
MRI for Low Back Pain[1]	20	45.0%	30.7%	32.7%
Survey of Patients' Hospital Experiences				
Area Around Room 'Always' Quiet at Night	(a)	87%	-	58%
Doctors 'Always' Communicated Well	(a)	95%	-	80%
Home Recovery Information Given	(a)	84%	-	82%
Hospital Given 9 or 10 on 10 Point Scale	(a)	75%	-	67%
Meds 'Always' Explained Before Given	(a)	79%	-	60%
Nurses 'Always' Communicated Well	(a)	89%	-	76%
Pain 'Always' Well Controlled	(a)	87%	-	69%
Room and Bathroom 'Always' Clean	(a)	83%	-	71%
Timely Help 'Always' Received	(a)	79%	-	64%
Would Definitely Recommend Hospital	(a)	86%	-	69%

White County Community Hospital

401 Sewell Dr
Sparta, TN 38583
Phone: 931-738-9211
Fax: 931-837-4133
URL: www.whitecountyhospital.com
Type: Acute Care Hospitals
Emergency Services: Yes
Ownership: Proprietary
Beds: 60

Key Personnel:
CEO/President. . . . . Wayne Smith
Cardiac Laboratory. . . . . Greg Williams
Chief of Medical Staff. . . . . John Langloif
Emergency Room . . . . Herbert Smith, RN

Measure	Cases	This Hosp.	State Avg.	U.S. Avg.
Heart Attack Care				
ACE Inhibitor or ARB for LVSD	0	-	96%	96%
Aspirin at Arrival[1]	15	100%	98%	99%
Aspirin at Discharge[1]	9	100%	99%	98%
Beta Blocker at Discharge[1]	10	90%	98%	98%
Fibrinolytic Medication Timing	0	-	67%	55%
PCI Within 90 Minutes of Arrival	0	-	91%	90%
Smoking Cessation Advice[1]	1	100%	100%	99%
Chest Pain/Possible Heart Attack Care				
Aspirin at Arrival	47	96%	95%	95%
Median Time to ECG (minutes)	47	10	8	8
Median Time to Transfer (minutes)[1,3]	6	223	65	61
Fibrinolytic Medication Timing[1]	1	100%	49%	54%
Heart Failure Care				
ACE Inhibitor or ARB for LVSD[1]	7	100%	95%	94%
Discharge Instructions	36	89%	88%	88%
Evaluation of LVS Function	45	91%	97%	98%
Smoking Cessation Advice[1]	6	100%	99%	98%
Pneumonia Care				
Appropriate Initial Antibiotic	73	92%	92%	92%
Blood Culture Timing	101	99%	97%	96%
Influenza Vaccine	66	88%	93%	91%
Initial Antibiotic Timing	104	99%	96%	95%
Pneumococcal Vaccine	91	89%	95%	93%
Smoking Cessation Advice	41	100%	99%	97%
Surgical Care Improvement Project				
Appropriate VTP Within 24 Hours[1,2]	12	75%	92%	92%
Appropriate Hair Removal[2]	66	97%	100%	99%
Appropriate Beta Blocker Usage[1,2]	14	100%	93%	93%
Controlled Postoperative Blood Glucose[2]	0	-	93%	93%
Prophylactic Antibiotic Timing[2]	42	90%	97%	97%
Prophylactic Antibiotic Timing (Outpatient)[1]	24	79%	94%	92%
Prophylactic Antibiotic Selection[2]	43	84%	97%	97%
Prophylactic Antibiotic Select. (Outpatient)[1]	19	100%	94%	94%
Prophylactic Antibiotic Stopped[2]	41	73%	94%	94%
Recommended VTP Ordered[1,2]	13	69%	94%	94%
Urinary Catheter Removal[1,2]	3	67%	90%	90%
Children's Asthma Care				
Received Systemic Corticosteroids	-	-	-	100%
Received Home Management Plan	-	-	-	71%
Received Reliever Medication	-	-	-	100%
Use of Medical Imaging				
Combination Abdominal CT Scan	160	0.356	0.219	0.191
Combination Chest CT Scan	132	0.023	0.102	0.054
Follow-up Mammogram/Ultrasound	338	9.5%	8%	8.4%
MRI for Low Back Pain[1]	53	28.3%	30.7%	32.7%
Survey of Patients' Hospital Experiences				
Area Around Room 'Always' Quiet at Night	300+	72%	-	58%
Doctors 'Always' Communicated Well	300+	85%	-	80%
Home Recovery Information Given	300+	84%	-	82%
Hospital Given 9 or 10 on 10 Point Scale	300+	68%	-	67%
Meds 'Always' Explained Before Given	300+	65%	-	60%
Nurses 'Always' Communicated Well	300+	76%	-	76%
Pain 'Always' Well Controlled	300+	72%	-	69%
Room and Bathroom 'Always' Clean	300+	77%	-	71%
Timely Help 'Always' Received	300+	68%	-	64%
Would Definitely Recommend Hospital	300+	63%	-	69%

Northcrest Medical Center

100 Northcrest Drive
Springfield, TN 37172
Phone: 615-384-2411
Fax: 615-384-1509
URL: www.northcrest.com
Type: Acute Care Hospitals
Emergency Services: Yes
Ownership: Voluntary Non-Profit - Other
Beds: 109

Key Personnel:
Chief of Medical Staff . . . . Jeff Fosnes, MD
Infection Control. . . . . Marylin Worsham, RN
Operating Room. . . . . Daniel Davis, RN
Quality Assurance . . . . Carol Harrison
Radiology. . . . . Robert Stanton Amonette
Anesthesiology. . . . . Carol Cobb
Emergency Room . . . . Laura Zervas
Intensive Care Unit. . . . . Karen String, RN

Measure	Cases	This Hosp.	State Avg.	U.S. Avg.
Heart Attack Care				
ACE Inhibitor or ARB for LVSD[1]	4	100%	96%	96%
Aspirin at Arrival	56	100%	98%	99%
Aspirin at Discharge	42	100%	99%	98%
Beta Blocker at Discharge	43	100%	98%	98%
Fibrinolytic Medication Timing	0	-	67%	55%
PCI Within 90 Minutes of Arrival[1]	11	27%	91%	90%
Smoking Cessation Advice[1]	20	100%	100%	99%
Chest Pain/Possible Heart Attack Care				
Aspirin at Arrival	34	91%	95%	95%
Median Time to ECG (minutes)	36	7	8	8
Median Time to Transfer (minutes)[1,3]	1	114	65	61
Fibrinolytic Medication Timing[1]	1	0%	49%	54%
Heart Failure Care				
ACE Inhibitor or ARB for LVSD	53	98%	95%	94%
Discharge Instructions	117	96%	88%	88%
Evaluation of LVS Function	140	99%	97%	98%
Smoking Cessation Advice	30	100%	99%	98%
Pneumonia Care				
Appropriate Initial Antibiotic	149	97%	92%	92%
Blood Culture Timing	270	98%	97%	96%
Influenza Vaccine	166	96%	93%	91%
Initial Antibiotic Timing	225	97%	96%	95%
Pneumococcal Vaccine	195	99%	95%	93%
Smoking Cessation Advice	98	100%	99%	97%
Surgical Care Improvement Project				
Appropriate VTP Within 24 Hours	85	98%	92%	92%
Appropriate Hair Removal	196	100%	100%	99%
Appropriate Beta Blocker Usage	46	100%	93%	93%
Controlled Postoperative Blood Glucose	0	-	93%	93%
Prophylactic Antibiotic Timing	110	99%	97%	97%
Prophylactic Antibiotic Timing (Outpatient)	100	90%	94%	92%
Prophylactic Antibiotic Selection	110	95%	97%	97%
Prophylactic Antibiotic Select. (Outpatient)	98	89%	94%	94%
Prophylactic Antibiotic Stopped	104	95%	94%	94%
Recommended VTP Ordered	85	98%	94%	94%
Urinary Catheter Removal	44	95%	90%	90%
Children's Asthma Care				
Received Systemic Corticosteroids	-	-	-	100%
Received Home Management Plan	-	-	-	71%
Received Reliever Medication	-	-	-	100%
Use of Medical Imaging				
Combination Abdominal CT Scan	381	0.073	0.219	0.191
Combination Chest CT Scan	316	0.006	0.102	0.054
Follow-up Mammogram/Ultrasound	672	13.1%	8%	8.4%
MRI for Low Back Pain	95	33.7%	30.7%	32.7%
Survey of Patients' Hospital Experiences				
Area Around Room 'Always' Quiet at Night	300+	59%	-	58%
Doctors 'Always' Communicated Well	300+	82%	-	80%
Home Recovery Information Given	300+	86%	-	82%
Hospital Given 9 or 10 on 10 Point Scale	300+	70%	-	67%
Meds 'Always' Explained Before Given	300+	64%	-	60%
Nurses 'Always' Communicated Well	300+	78%	-	76%
Pain 'Always' Well Controlled	300+	71%	-	69%
Room and Bathroom 'Always' Clean	300+	72%	-	71%
Timely Help 'Always' Received	300+	67%	-	64%
Would Definitely Recommend Hospital	300+	68%	-	69%

NOTE: Hospital profiles are in alphabetical order by state, then city, then hospital within the city; Rankings exclude hospitals with less than 25 cases except for patient surveys which excludes hospitals with less than 100 cases; (a) 100–299 cases; (1) The number of cases is too small to be sure how well a hospital is performing; (2) The hospital indicated that the data submitted for this measure were based on a sample of cases; (3) Data was collected during a shorter time period (fewer quarters) than the maximum possible time for this measure; (4) Suppressed for one or more quarters by CMS; (5) No data is available from the hospital for this measure; (6) Fewer than 100 patients completed the HCAHPS survey. Use these rates with caution, as the number of surveys may be too low to reliably assess hospital performance; (7) Survey results are based on less than 12 months of data; (8) Survey results are not available for this reporting period; (9) No or very few patients were eligible for the HCAHPS survey. The scores shown, if any, reflect a very small number of surveys; (10) A state average was not calculated because too few hospitals in the state submitted data; (11) There were discrepancies in the data collection process; Please refer to the User's Guide for a full explanation of data.

Sweetwater Hospital Association

304 Wright St
Sweetwater, TN 37874
URL: www.sweetwaterhospital.org
Type: Acute Care Hospitals
Ownership: Voluntary Non-Profit - Other

Phone: 865-213-8200

Emergency Services: Yes
Beds: 59

Key Personnel:
CEO/President . . . . Scott Bowman
Radiology . . . . Bob Wilkins

Measure	Cases	This Hosp.	State Avg.	U.S. Avg.
Heart Attack Care				
ACE Inhibitor or ARB for LVSD	0	-	96%	96%
Aspirin at Arrival[1]	18	78%	98%	99%
Aspirin at Discharge[1]	11	82%	99%	98%
Beta Blocker at Discharge[1]	11	64%	98%	98%
Fibrinolytic Medication Timing	0	-	67%	55%
PCI Within 90 Minutes of Arrival	0	-	91%	90%
Smoking Cessation Advice[1]	5	100%	100%	99%
Chest Pain/Possible Heart Attack Care				
Aspirin at Arrival	144	97%	95%	95%
Median Time to ECG (minutes)	152	6	8	8
Median Time to Transfer (minutes)[1,3]	5	41	65	61
Fibrinolytic Medication Timing[1]	2	50%	49%	54%
Heart Failure Care				
ACE Inhibitor or ARB for LVSD[1]	17	88%	95%	94%
Discharge Instructions	73	53%	88%	88%
Evaluation of LVS Function	91	89%	97%	98%
Smoking Cessation Advice[1]	21	86%	99%	98%
Pneumonia Care				
Appropriate Initial Antibiotic	88	93%	92%	92%
Blood Culture Timing	131	94%	97%	96%
Influenza Vaccine	117	89%	93%	91%
Initial Antibiotic Timing	174	91%	96%	95%
Pneumococcal Vaccine	163	95%	95%	93%
Smoking Cessation Advice	86	94%	99%	97%
Surgical Care Improvement Project				
Appropriate VTP Within 24 Hours	59	81%	92%	92%
Appropriate Hair Removal	97	99%	100%	99%
Appropriate Beta Blocker Usage[1]	20	75%	93%	93%
Controlled Postoperative Blood Glucose	0	-	93%	93%
Prophylactic Antibiotic Timing	42	90%	97%	97%
Prophylactic Antibiotic Timing (Outpatient)	48	77%	94%	92%
Prophylactic Antibiotic Selection	43	77%	97%	97%
Prophylactic Antibiotic Select. (Outpatient)	39	95%	94%	94%
Prophylactic Antibiotic Stopped	35	83%	94%	94%
Recommended VTP Ordered	61	90%	94%	94%
Urinary Catheter Removal[1]	6	83%	90%	90%
Children's Asthma Care				
Received Systemic Corticosteroids	-	-	-	100%
Received Home Management Plan	-	-	-	71%
Received Reliever Medication	-	-	-	100%
Use of Medical Imaging				
Combination Abdominal CT Scan	392	0.092	0.219	0.191
Combination Chest CT Scan	295	0.041	0.102	0.054
Follow-up Mammogram/Ultrasound	257	7.8%	8%	8.4%
MRI for Low Back Pain	90	43.3%	30.7%	32.7%
Survey of Patients' Hospital Experiences				
Area Around Room 'Always' Quiet at Night	(a)	62%	-	58%
Doctors 'Always' Communicated Well	(a)	87%	-	80%
Home Recovery Information Given	(a)	83%	-	82%
Hospital Given 9 or 10 on 10 Point Scale	(a)	69%	-	67%
Meds 'Always' Explained Before Given	(a)	68%	-	60%
Nurses 'Always' Communicated Well	(a)	76%	-	76%
Pain 'Always' Well Controlled	(a)	69%	-	69%
Room and Bathroom 'Always' Clean	(a)	74%	-	71%
Timely Help 'Always' Received	(a)	68%	-	64%
Would Definitely Recommend Hospital	(a)	64%	-	69%

Claiborne County Hospital

1850 Old Knoxville Highway
Tazewell, TN 37879
URL: www.claibornehospital.org
Type: Acute Care Hospitals
Ownership: Government - Local

Phone: 423-626-4211
Fax: 423-626-9926

Emergency Services: Yes
Beds: 85

Key Personnel:
CEO/President . . . . Michael Hutchins
Chief of Medical Staff . . . . Richard Clark
Infection Control . . . . Mary Moore, RN
Operating Room . . . . Nancy Steadman
Quality Assurance . . . . Linda Vanlandingham
Emergency Room . . . . Tim Runions
Intensive Care Unit . . . . Jackie Carpenter

Measure	Cases	This Hosp.	State Avg.	U.S. Avg.
Heart Attack Care				
ACE Inhibitor or ARB for LVSD[1,2]	1	100%	96%	96%
Aspirin at Arrival[1,2]	10	80%	98%	99%
Aspirin at Discharge[1,2]	8	75%	99%	98%
Beta Blocker at Discharge[1,2]	10	60%	98%	98%
Fibrinolytic Medication Timing[2]	0	-	67%	55%
PCI Within 90 Minutes of Arrival[2]	0	-	91%	90%
Smoking Cessation Advice[1,2]	1	100%	100%	99%
Chest Pain/Possible Heart Attack Care				
Aspirin at Arrival	130	90%	95%	95%
Median Time to ECG (minutes)	137	10	8	8
Median Time to Transfer (minutes)[1,3]	13	65	65	61
Fibrinolytic Medication Timing[1]	2	0%	49%	54%
Heart Failure Care				
ACE Inhibitor or ARB for LVSD[1,2]	15	47%	95%	94%
Discharge Instructions[2]	135	87%	88%	88%
Evaluation of LVS Function[2]	175	37%	97%	98%
Smoking Cessation Advice[2]	39	100%	99%	98%
Pneumonia Care				
Appropriate Initial Antibiotic[2]	28	89%	92%	92%
Blood Culture Timing[2]	73	97%	97%	96%
Influenza Vaccine[2]	57	95%	93%	91%
Initial Antibiotic Timing[2]	114	94%	96%	95%
Pneumococcal Vaccine[2]	89	90%	95%	93%
Smoking Cessation Advice[2]	38	100%	99%	97%
Surgical Care Improvement Project				
Appropriate VTP Within 24 Hours[2]	32	69%	92%	92%
Appropriate Hair Removal[2]	42	100%	100%	99%
Appropriate Beta Blocker Usage[1,2]	8	75%	93%	93%
Controlled Postoperative Blood Glucose[2]	0	-	93%	93%
Prophylactic Antibiotic Timing[1,2]	19	74%	97%	97%
Prophylactic Antibiotic Timing (Outpatient)	34	50%	94%	92%
Prophylactic Antibiotic Selection[1,2]	20	85%	97%	97%
Prophylactic Antibiotic Select. (Outpatient)[1]	19	84%	94%	94%
Prophylactic Antibiotic Stopped[1,2]	18	67%	94%	94%
Recommended VTP Ordered[2]	34	65%	94%	94%
Urinary Catheter Removal[1,2]	11	45%	90%	90%
Children's Asthma Care				
Received Systemic Corticosteroids	-	-	-	100%
Received Home Management Plan	-	-	-	71%
Received Reliever Medication	-	-	-	100%
Use of Medical Imaging				
Combination Abdominal CT Scan	376	0.024	0.219	0.191
Combination Chest CT Scan	288	0.000	0.102	0.054
Follow-up Mammogram/Ultrasound	299	9.0%	8%	8.4%
MRI for Low Back Pain	86	32.6%	30.7%	32.7%
Survey of Patients' Hospital Experiences				
Area Around Room 'Always' Quiet at Night	(a)	53%	-	58%
Doctors 'Always' Communicated Well	(a)	86%	-	80%
Home Recovery Information Given	(a)	79%	-	82%
Hospital Given 9 or 10 on 10 Point Scale	(a)	63%	-	67%
Meds 'Always' Explained Before Given	(a)	63%	-	60%
Nurses 'Always' Communicated Well	(a)	77%	-	76%
Pain 'Always' Well Controlled	(a)	66%	-	69%
Room and Bathroom 'Always' Clean	(a)	70%	-	71%
Timely Help 'Always' Received	(a)	64%	-	64%
Would Definitely Recommend Hospital	(a)	67%	-	69%

Gibson General Hospital

200 Hospital Dr
Trenton, TN 38382
URL: www.wth.net
Type: Acute Care Hospitals
Ownership: Voluntary Non-Profit - Other

Phone: 731-855-7900
Fax: 731-855-7570

Emergency Services: Yes
Beds: 100

Key Personnel:
CEO/President . . . . Sherry Scruggs
Chief of Medical Staff . . . . Ezekiel O Adetunji
Radiology . . . . Gregory C Bruno

Measure	Cases	This Hosp.	State Avg.	U.S. Avg.
Heart Attack Care				
ACE Inhibitor or ARB for LVSD[1,3]	1	100%	96%	96%
Aspirin at Arrival[1,3]	3	100%	98%	99%
Aspirin at Discharge[1,3]	3	100%	99%	98%
Beta Blocker at Discharge[1,3]	3	67%	98%	98%
Fibrinolytic Medication Timing[3]	0	-	67%	55%
PCI Within 90 Minutes of Arrival[3]	0	-	91%	90%
Smoking Cessation Advice[1,3]	1	0%	100%	99%
Chest Pain/Possible Heart Attack Care				
Aspirin at Arrival	70	94%	95%	95%
Median Time to ECG (minutes)	73	21	8	8
Median Time to Transfer (minutes)[1,3]	1	685	65	61
Fibrinolytic Medication Timing[1]	5	20%	49%	54%
Heart Failure Care				
ACE Inhibitor or ARB for LVSD[1]	10	70%	95%	94%
Discharge Instructions[1]	12	67%	88%	88%
Evaluation of LVS Function	27	81%	97%	98%
Smoking Cessation Advice[1]	2	50%	99%	98%
Pneumonia Care				
Appropriate Initial Antibiotic[1]	12	75%	92%	92%
Blood Culture Timing[1]	21	95%	97%	96%
Influenza Vaccine[1]	7	86%	93%	91%
Initial Antibiotic Timing[1]	22	100%	96%	95%
Pneumococcal Vaccine[1]	17	71%	95%	93%
Smoking Cessation Advice[1]	4	100%	99%	97%
Surgical Care Improvement Project				
Appropriate VTP Within 24 Hours[1]	5	80%	92%	92%
Appropriate Hair Removal[1]	6	83%	100%	99%
Appropriate Beta Blocker Usage[1]	2	50%	93%	93%
Controlled Postoperative Blood Glucose	0	-	93%	93%
Prophylactic Antibiotic Timing[1]	6	67%	97%	97%
Prophylactic Antibiotic Timing (Outpatient)[1,3]	8	38%	94%	92%
Prophylactic Antibiotic Selection[1]	5	0%	97%	97%
Prophylactic Antibiotic Select. (Outpatient)[1,3]	3	100%	94%	94%
Prophylactic Antibiotic Stopped[1]	6	33%	94%	94%
Recommended VTP Ordered[1]	5	80%	94%	94%
Urinary Catheter Removal	0	-	90%	90%
Children's Asthma Care				
Received Systemic Corticosteroids	-	-	-	100%
Received Home Management Plan	-	-	-	71%
Received Reliever Medication	-	-	-	100%
Use of Medical Imaging				
Combination Abdominal CT Scan	89	0.011	0.219	0.191
Combination Chest CT Scan[1]	26	0.077	0.102	0.054
Follow-up Mammogram/Ultrasound	228	6.6%	8%	8.4%
MRI for Low Back Pain[5]	0	-	30.7%	32.7%
Survey of Patients' Hospital Experiences				
Area Around Room 'Always' Quiet at Night	(a)	75%	-	58%
Doctors 'Always' Communicated Well	(a)	90%	-	80%
Home Recovery Information Given	(a)	77%	-	82%
Hospital Given 9 or 10 on 10 Point Scale	(a)	68%	-	67%
Meds 'Always' Explained Before Given	(a)	66%	-	60%
Nurses 'Always' Communicated Well	(a)	84%	-	76%
Pain 'Always' Well Controlled	(a)	86%	-	69%
Room and Bathroom 'Always' Clean	(a)	69%	-	71%
Timely Help 'Always' Received	(a)	79%	-	64%
Would Definitely Recommend Hospital	(a)	60%	-	69%

Harton Regional Medical Center

1801 N Jackson St Box 460
Tullahoma, TN 37388
Phone: 931-393-3000
Fax: 931-455-4220
URL: www.hartonmedicalcenter.com
Type: Acute Care Hospitals
Emergency Services: Yes
Ownership: Voluntary Non-Profit - Other
Beds: 137

Key Personnel:

CEO/President. . . . . Dwayne Blaylock
Chief of Medical Staff. . . . . J Denny Crabtree, MD
Operating Room. . . . . Mark Blair
Quality Assurance . . . . Cindy Nadeau
Radiology. . . . . Joel S Birdwell

Measure	Cases	This Hosp.	State Avg.	U.S. Avg.
Heart Attack Care				
ACE Inhibitor or ARB for LVSD[1]	4	100%	96%	96%
Aspirin at Arrival	59	100%	98%	99%
Aspirin at Discharge	52	100%	99%	98%
Beta Blocker at Discharge	51	100%	98%	98%
Fibrinolytic Medication Timing[1]	3	100%	67%	55%
PCI Within 90 Minutes of Arrival[1]	11	91%	91%	90%
Smoking Cessation Advice[1]	23	100%	100%	99%
Chest Pain/Possible Heart Attack Care				
Aspirin at Arrival	65	94%	95%	95%
Median Time to ECG (minutes)	66	6	8	8
Median Time to Transfer (minutes)[1,3]	4	52	65	61
Fibrinolytic Medication Timing[1]	6	67%	49%	54%
Heart Failure Care				
ACE Inhibitor or ARB for LVSD	51	100%	95%	94%
Discharge Instructions	164	95%	88%	88%
Evaluation of LVS Function	194	100%	97%	98%
Smoking Cessation Advice	34	100%	99%	98%
Pneumonia Care				
Appropriate Initial Antibiotic	94	91%	92%	92%
Blood Culture Timing	127	98%	97%	96%
Influenza Vaccine	109	99%	93%	91%
Initial Antibiotic Timing	123	97%	96%	95%
Pneumococcal Vaccine	136	99%	95%	93%
Smoking Cessation Advice	55	100%	99%	97%
Surgical Care Improvement Project				
Appropriate VTP Within 24 Hours	86	88%	92%	92%
Appropriate Hair Removal	272	100%	100%	99%
Appropriate Beta Blocker Usage	64	100%	93%	93%
Controlled Postoperative Blood Glucose	0	-	93%	93%
Prophylactic Antibiotic Timing	170	99%	97%	97%
Prophylactic Antibiotic Timing (Outpatient)	433	99%	94%	92%
Prophylactic Antibiotic Selection	172	99%	97%	97%
Prophylactic Antibiotic Select. (Outpatient)	435	98%	94%	94%
Prophylactic Antibiotic Stopped	134	98%	94%	94%
Recommended VTP Ordered	87	92%	94%	94%
Urinary Catheter Removal	28	96%	90%	90%
Children's Asthma Care				
Received Systemic Corticosteroids[1]	20	95%	-	100%
Received Home Management Plan[1]	20	100%	-	71%
Received Reliever Medication[1]	20	100%	-	100%
Use of Medical Imaging				
Combination Abdominal CT Scan	518	0.330	0.219	0.191
Combination Chest CT Scan	309	0.301	0.102	0.054
Follow-up Mammogram/Ultrasound	1,036	11.2%	8%	8.4%
MRI for Low Back Pain	178	26.4%	30.7%	32.7%
Survey of Patients' Hospital Experiences				
Area Around Room 'Always' Quiet at Night	300+	57%	-	58%
Doctors 'Always' Communicated Well	300+	78%	-	80%
Home Recovery Information Given	300+	80%	-	82%
Hospital Given 9 or 10 on 10 Point Scale	300+	58%	-	67%
Meds 'Always' Explained Before Given	300+	55%	-	60%
Nurses 'Always' Communicated Well	300+	71%	-	76%
Pain 'Always' Well Controlled	300+	61%	-	69%
Room and Bathroom 'Always' Clean	300+	68%	-	71%
Timely Help 'Always' Received	300+	56%	-	64%
Would Definitely Recommend Hospital	300+	60%	-	69%

Baptist Memorial Hospital Union City

1201 Bishop Street
Union City, TN 38261
Phone: 731-885-2410
Fax: 731-884-8603
E-mail: info.unioncity@bmhcc.org
URL: www.bmhcc.org
Type: Acute Care Hospitals
Emergency Services: Yes
Ownership: Proprietary
Beds: 173

Key Personnel:

CEO/President. . . . . Mike Perryman
Cardiac Laboratory. . . . . James Hall, MD
Chief of Medical Staff. . . . . David StClair, MD

Measure	Cases	This Hosp.	State Avg.	U.S. Avg.
Heart Attack Care				
ACE Inhibitor or ARB for LVSD[1]	1	100%	96%	96%
Aspirin at Arrival[1]	12	100%	98%	99%
Aspirin at Discharge[1]	7	100%	99%	98%
Beta Blocker at Discharge[1]	8	100%	98%	98%
Fibrinolytic Medication Timing	0	-	67%	55%
PCI Within 90 Minutes of Arrival	0	-	91%	90%
Smoking Cessation Advice[1]	2	100%	100%	99%
Chest Pain/Possible Heart Attack Care				
Aspirin at Arrival	157	98%	95%	95%
Median Time to ECG (minutes)	164	4	8	8
Median Time to Transfer (minutes)[3,1]	3	118	65	61
Fibrinolytic Medication Timing[1]	10	60%	49%	54%
Heart Failure Care				
ACE Inhibitor or ARB for LVSD[1]	20	100%	95%	94%
Discharge Instructions	61	93%	88%	88%
Evaluation of LVS Function	84	100%	97%	98%
Smoking Cessation Advice[1]	15	100%	99%	98%
Pneumonia Care				
Appropriate Initial Antibiotic	56	100%	92%	92%
Blood Culture Timing	55	100%	97%	96%
Influenza Vaccine	50	96%	93%	91%
Initial Antibiotic Timing	76	100%	96%	95%
Pneumococcal Vaccine	52	94%	95%	93%
Smoking Cessation Advice	30	100%	99%	97%
Surgical Care Improvement Project				
Appropriate VTP Within 24 Hours[2]	57	84%	92%	92%
Appropriate Hair Removal[2]	149	100%	100%	99%
Appropriate Beta Blocker Usage[2]	29	100%	93%	93%
Controlled Postoperative Blood Glucose[2]	0	-	93%	93%
Prophylactic Antibiotic Timing[2]	99	98%	97%	97%
Prophylactic Antibiotic Timing (Outpatient)	98	100%	94%	92%
Prophylactic Antibiotic Selection[2]	99	100%	97%	97%
Prophylactic Antibiotic Select. (Outpatient)	99	90%	94%	94%
Prophylactic Antibiotic Stopped[2]	93	94%	94%	94%
Recommended VTP Ordered[2]	57	86%	94%	94%
Urinary Catheter Removal[1,2]	14	93%	90%	90%
Children's Asthma Care				
Received Systemic Corticosteroids	-	-	-	100%
Received Home Management Plan	-	-	-	71%
Received Reliever Medication	-	-	-	100%
Use of Medical Imaging				
Combination Abdominal CT Scan	480	0.052	0.219	0.191
Combination Chest CT Scan	316	0.038	0.102	0.054
Follow-up Mammogram/Ultrasound	360	6.7%	8%	8.4%
MRI for Low Back Pain	111	35.1%	30.7%	32.7%
Survey of Patients' Hospital Experiences				
Area Around Room 'Always' Quiet at Night	300+	68%	-	58%
Doctors 'Always' Communicated Well	300+	83%	-	80%
Home Recovery Information Given	300+	83%	-	82%
Hospital Given 9 or 10 on 10 Point Scale	300+	71%	-	67%
Meds 'Always' Explained Before Given	300+	64%	-	60%
Nurses 'Always' Communicated Well	300+	80%	-	76%
Pain 'Always' Well Controlled	300+	71%	-	69%
Room and Bathroom 'Always' Clean	300+	78%	-	71%
Timely Help 'Always' Received	300+	71%	-	64%
Would Definitely Recommend Hospital	300+	68%	-	69%

Wayne Medical Center

103 J V Mangubat Dr
Waynesboro, TN 38485
Phone: 931-722-5411
Fax: 931-722-7170
Type: Acute Care Hospitals
Emergency Services: Yes
Ownership: Voluntary Non-Profit - Other
Beds: 80

Key Personnel:

CEO/President. . . . . Mike Sears
Cardiac Laboratory. . . . . Dr Jaques Heibig
Chief of Medical Staff. . . . . Dr David Magas
Infection Control. . . . . Dr John Olson
Operating Room. . . . . Tammy Howell, RN
Quality Assurance . . . . Paula Petty, RN
Radiology. . . . . Hubert Langley, MD

Measure	Cases	This Hosp.	State Avg.	U.S. Avg.
Heart Attack Care				
ACE Inhibitor or ARB for LVSD[5]	0	-	96%	96%
Aspirin at Arrival[5]	0	-	98%	99%
Aspirin at Discharge[5]	0	-	99%	98%
Beta Blocker at Discharge[5]	0	-	98%	98%
Fibrinolytic Medication Timing[5]	0	-	67%	55%
PCI Within 90 Minutes of Arrival[5]	0	-	91%	90%
Smoking Cessation Advice[5]	0	-	100%	99%
Chest Pain/Possible Heart Attack Care				
Aspirin at Arrival	53	91%	95%	95%
Median Time to ECG (minutes)	57	13	8	8
Median Time to Transfer (minutes)[5]	0	-	65	61
Fibrinolytic Medication Timing[1]	1	100%	49%	54%
Heart Failure Care				
ACE Inhibitor or ARB for LVSD[1]	10	100%	95%	94%
Discharge Instructions	26	69%	88%	88%
Evaluation of LVS Function	34	85%	97%	98%
Smoking Cessation Advice[1]	3	100%	99%	98%
Pneumonia Care				
Appropriate Initial Antibiotic	34	91%	92%	92%
Blood Culture Timing[1]	21	100%	97%	96%
Influenza Vaccine	35	49%	93%	91%
Initial Antibiotic Timing	66	100%	96%	95%
Pneumococcal Vaccine	67	94%	95%	93%
Smoking Cessation Advice[1]	15	53%	99%	97%
Surgical Care Improvement Project				
Appropriate VTP Within 24 Hours[5]	0	-	92%	92%
Appropriate Hair Removal[5]	0	-	100%	99%
Appropriate Beta Blocker Usage[5]	0	-	93%	93%
Controlled Postoperative Blood Glucose[5]	0	-	93%	93%
Prophylactic Antibiotic Timing[5]	0	-	97%	97%
Prophylactic Antibiotic Timing (Outpatient)[5]	0	-	94%	92%
Prophylactic Antibiotic Selection[5]	0	-	97%	97%
Prophylactic Antibiotic Select. (Outpatient)[5]	0	-	94%	94%
Prophylactic Antibiotic Stopped[5]	0	-	94%	94%
Recommended VTP Ordered[5]	0	-	94%	94%
Urinary Catheter Removal[5]	0	-	90%	90%
Children's Asthma Care				
Received Systemic Corticosteroids	-	-	-	100%
Received Home Management Plan	-	-	-	71%
Received Reliever Medication	-	-	-	100%
Use of Medical Imaging				
Combination Abdominal CT Scan	91	0.615	0.219	0.191
Combination Chest CT Scan	67	0.731	0.102	0.054
Follow-up Mammogram/Ultrasound	162	6.8%	8%	8.4%
MRI for Low Back Pain	47	36.2%	30.7%	32.7%
Survey of Patients' Hospital Experiences				
Area Around Room 'Always' Quiet at Night	(a)	63%	-	58%
Doctors 'Always' Communicated Well	(a)	79%	-	80%
Home Recovery Information Given	(a)	73%	-	82%
Hospital Given 9 or 10 on 10 Point Scale	(a)	61%	-	67%
Meds 'Always' Explained Before Given	(a)	56%	-	60%
Nurses 'Always' Communicated Well	(a)	78%	-	76%
Pain 'Always' Well Controlled	(a)	63%	-	69%
Room and Bathroom 'Always' Clean	(a)	76%	-	71%
Timely Help 'Always' Received	(a)	62%	-	64%
Would Definitely Recommend Hospital	(a)	62%	-	69%

NOTE: Hospital profiles are in alphabetical order by state, then city, then hospital within the city; Rankings exclude hospitals with less than 25 cases except for patient surveys which excludes hospitals with less than 100 cases; (a) 100–299 cases; (1) The number of cases is too small to be sure how well a hospital is performing; (2) The hospital indicated that the data submitted for this measure were based on a sample of cases; (3) Data was collected during a shorter time period (fewer quarters) than the maximum possible time for this measure; (4) Suppressed for one or more quarters by CMS; (5) No data is available from the hospital for this measure; (6) Fewer than 100 patients completed the HCAHPS survey. Use these rates with caution, as the number of surveys may be too low to reliably assess hospital performance; (7) Survey results are based on less than 12 months of data; (8) Survey results are not available for this reporting period; (9) No or very few patients were eligible for the HCAHPS survey. The scores shown, if any, reflect a very small number of surveys; (10) A state average was not calculated because too few hospitals in the state submitted data; (11) There were discrepancies in the data collection process; Please refer to the User's Guide for a full explanation of data.

Southern Tennessee Medical Center

185 Hospital Road
Winchester, TN 37398
URL: www.southerntennessee.com
Type: Acute Care Hospitals
Ownership: Proprietary

Phone: 931-967-8295
Fax: 931-967-4464

Emergency Services: Yes
Beds: 131

Key Personnel:

CEO/President	Lenae King
Chief of Medical Staff	Lia C Boyanton
Radiology	Paul Ellis, MD
Anesthesiology	Esme H Brown, MD
Hemotology Center	Henry J Goolsby III, MD

Measure	Cases	This Hosp.	State Avg.	U.S. Avg.
Heart Attack Care				
ACE Inhibitor or ARB for LVSD[1]	8	100%	96%	96%
Aspirin at Arrival	28	89%	98%	99%
Aspirin at Discharge[1]	18	72%	99%	98%
Beta Blocker at Discharge[1]	22	82%	98%	98%
Fibrinolytic Medication Timing[1]	1	100%	67%	55%
PCI Within 90 Minutes of Arrival	0	-	91%	90%
Smoking Cessation Advice[1]	3	100%	100%	99%
Chest Pain/Possible Heart Attack Care				
Aspirin at Arrival	213	97%	95%	95%
Median Time to ECG (minutes)	225	7	8	8
Median Time to Transfer (minutes)[1,3]	1	36	65	61
Fibrinolytic Medication Timing[1]	8	88%	49%	54%
Heart Failure Care				
ACE Inhibitor or ARB for LVSD	38	95%	95%	94%
Discharge Instructions	125	93%	88%	88%
Evaluation of LVS Function	154	97%	97%	98%
Smoking Cessation Advice[1]	19	100%	99%	98%
Pneumonia Care				
Appropriate Initial Antibiotic	97	91%	92%	92%
Blood Culture Timing	102	96%	97%	96%
Influenza Vaccine	113	86%	93%	91%
Initial Antibiotic Timing	159	96%	96%	95%
Pneumococcal Vaccine	142	96%	95%	93%
Smoking Cessation Advice	70	100%	99%	97%
Surgical Care Improvement Project				
Appropriate VTP Within 24 Hours	103	96%	92%	92%
Appropriate Hair Removal	271	100%	100%	99%
Appropriate Beta Blocker Usage	68	99%	93%	93%
Controlled Postoperative Blood Glucose	0	-	93%	93%
Prophylactic Antibiotic Timing	186	98%	97%	97%
Prophylactic Antibiotic Timing (Outpatient)	140	92%	94%	92%
Prophylactic Antibiotic Selection	187	98%	97%	97%
Prophylactic Antibiotic Select. (Outpatient)	132	95%	94%	94%
Prophylactic Antibiotic Stopped	174	94%	94%	94%
Recommended VTP Ordered	103	99%	94%	94%
Urinary Catheter Removal	84	96%	90%	90%
Children's Asthma Care				
Received Systemic Corticosteroids	-	-	-	100%
Received Home Management Plan	-	-	-	71%
Received Reliever Medication	-	-	-	100%
Use of Medical Imaging				
Combination Abdominal CT Scan	396	0.061	0.219	0.191
Combination Chest CT Scan	167	0.012	0.102	0.054
Follow-up Mammogram/Ultrasound	891	5.1%	8%	8.4%
MRI for Low Back Pain	142	33.1%	30.7%	32.7%
Survey of Patients' Hospital Experiences				
Area Around Room 'Always' Quiet at Night	300+	64%	-	58%
Doctors 'Always' Communicated Well	300+	82%	-	80%
Home Recovery Information Given	300+	80%	-	82%
Hospital Given 9 or 10 on 10 Point Scale	300+	61%	-	67%
Meds 'Always' Explained Before Given	300+	60%	-	60%
Nurses 'Always' Communicated Well	300+	75%	-	76%
Pain 'Always' Well Controlled	300+	71%	-	69%
Room and Bathroom 'Always' Clean	300+	66%	-	71%
Timely Help 'Always' Received	300+	59%	-	64%
Would Definitely Recommend Hospital	300+	63%	-	69%

Stones River Hospital & Dekalb Community Hospital

324 Doolittle Road
Woodbury, TN 37190
E-mail: info@srhtn.com
URL: www.stonesriverhospital.com
Type: Acute Care Hospitals
Ownership: Proprietary

Phone: 615-563-4001
Fax: 615-563-7314

Emergency Services: Yes
Beds: 55

Key Personnel:

CEO/President	Don Downey
Chief of Medical Staff	Jeff Todd
Infection Control	Vida King, RN
Operating Room	Jim Fedusenko
Quality Assurance	Pamela Anderson
Radiology	Eric A Dam
Anesthesiology	Lloyd Trivett
Emergency Room	Gary Brynt, MD

Measure	Cases	This Hosp.	State Avg.	U.S. Avg.
Heart Attack Care				
ACE Inhibitor or ARB for LVSD[3]	0	-	96%	96%
Aspirin at Arrival[1,3]	3	100%	98%	99%
Aspirin at Discharge[1,3]	2	100%	99%	98%
Beta Blocker at Discharge[1,3]	2	100%	98%	98%
Fibrinolytic Medication Timing[3]	0	-	67%	55%
PCI Within 90 Minutes of Arrival[3]	0	-	91%	90%
Smoking Cessation Advice[1,3]	1	100%	100%	99%
Chest Pain/Possible Heart Attack Care				
Aspirin at Arrival	48	94%	95%	95%
Median Time to ECG (minutes)	51	7	8	8
Median Time to Transfer (minutes)[3]	0	-	65	61
Fibrinolytic Medication Timing[1]	2	0%	49%	54%
Heart Failure Care				
ACE Inhibitor or ARB for LVSD[1]	3	100%	95%	94%
Discharge Instructions[1]	12	92%	88%	88%
Evaluation of LVS Function[1]	16	100%	97%	98%
Smoking Cessation Advice	0	-	99%	98%
Pneumonia Care				
Appropriate Initial Antibiotic	39	95%	92%	92%
Blood Culture Timing	27	93%	97%	96%
Influenza Vaccine	27	70%	93%	91%
Initial Antibiotic Timing	34	100%	96%	95%
Pneumococcal Vaccine	36	81%	95%	93%
Smoking Cessation Advice[1]	24	100%	99%	97%
Surgical Care Improvement Project				
Appropriate VTP Within 24 Hours[1,2]	12	100%	92%	92%
Appropriate Hair Removal[2]	44	100%	100%	99%
Appropriate Beta Blocker Usage[1,2]	13	100%	93%	93%
Controlled Postoperative Blood Glucose[2]	0	-	93%	93%
Prophylactic Antibiotic Timing[2]	41	100%	97%	97%
Prophylactic Antibiotic Timing (Outpatient)[1]	5	100%	94%	92%
Prophylactic Antibiotic Selection[2]	41	100%	97%	97%
Prophylactic Antibiotic Select. (Outpatient)[1]	5	100%	94%	94%
Prophylactic Antibiotic Stopped[2]	40	100%	94%	94%
Recommended VTP Ordered[1,2]	12	100%	94%	94%
Urinary Catheter Removal[1,2]	17	100%	90%	90%
Children's Asthma Care				
Received Systemic Corticosteroids	-	-	-	100%
Received Home Management Plan	-	-	-	71%
Received Reliever Medication	-	-	-	100%
Use of Medical Imaging				
Combination Abdominal CT Scan[1]	43	0.000	0.219	0.191
Combination Chest CT Scan	52	0.000	0.102	0.054
Follow-up Mammogram/Ultrasound	77	7.8%	8%	8.4%
MRI for Low Back Pain[1]	41	26.8%	30.7%	32.7%
Survey of Patients' Hospital Experiences				
Area Around Room 'Always' Quiet at Night	(a)	66%	-	58%
Doctors 'Always' Communicated Well	(a)	85%	-	80%
Home Recovery Information Given	(a)	82%	-	82%
Hospital Given 9 or 10 on 10 Point Scale	(a)	58%	-	67%
Meds 'Always' Explained Before Given	(a)	55%	-	60%
Nurses 'Always' Communicated Well	(a)	76%	-	76%
Pain 'Always' Well Controlled	(a)	69%	-	69%
Room and Bathroom 'Always' Clean	(a)	71%	-	71%
Timely Help 'Always' Received	(a)	66%	-	64%
Would Definitely Recommend Hospital	(a)	59%	-	69%

NOTE: Hospital profiles are in alphabetical order by state, then city, then hospital within the city; Rankings exclude hospitals with less than 25 cases except for patient surveys which excludes hospitals with less than 100 cases; (a) 100–299 cases; (1) The number of cases is too small to be sure how well a hospital is performing; (2) The hospital indicated that the data submitted for this measure were based on a sample of cases; (3) Data was collected during a shorter time period (fewer quarters) than the maximum possible time for this measure; (4) Suppressed for one or more quarters by CMS; (5) No data is available from the hospital for this measure; (6) Fewer than 100 patients completed the HCAHPS survey. Use these rates with caution, as the number of surveys may be too low to reliably assess hospital performance; (7) Survey results are based on less than 12 months of data; (8) Survey results are not available for this reporting period; (9) No or very few patients were eligible for the HCAHPS survey. The scores shown, if any, reflect a very small number of surveys; (10) A state average was not calculated because too few hospitals in the state submitted data; (11) There were discrepancies in the data collection process; Please refer to the User's Guide for a full explanation of data.

Heart Attack Care

1. ACE Inhibitor or ARB for LVSD

Hospital Name	City	Rate	Cases
Fletcher Allen Hospital of Vermont	Burlington	97%	116

2. Aspirin at Arrival

Hospital Name	City	Rate	Cases
Fletcher Allen Hospital of Vermont	Burlington	100%	242
Southwestern Vermont Medical Center	Bennington	100%	36
Rutland Regional Medical Center	Rutland	97%	61

3. Aspirin at Discharge

Hospital Name	City	Rate	Cases
Fletcher Allen Hospital of Vermont	Burlington	99%	631
Rutland Regional Medical Center	Rutland	96%	45

4. Beta Blocker at Discharge

Hospital Name	City	Rate	Cases
Rutland Regional Medical Center	Rutland	100%	44
Southwestern Vermont Medical Center	Bennington	100%	25
Fletcher Allen Hospital of Vermont	Burlington	99%	627

7. Smoking Cessation Advice

Hospital Name	City	Rate	Cases
Fletcher Allen Hospital of Vermont	Burlington	100%	212

Chest Pain/Possible Heart Attack Care

8. Aspirin at Arrival

Hospital Name	City	Rate	Cases
Central Vermont Medical Center	Barre	99%	156
Northwestern Medical Center	Saint Albans	99%	127
Southwestern Vermont Medical Center	Bennington	99%	110
Rutland Regional Medical Center	Rutland	98%	96

9. Median Time to ECG (minutes)

Hospital Name	City	Min.	Cases
Northwestern Medical Center	Saint Albans	4	133
Central Vermont Medical Center	Barre	6	159
Rutland Regional Medical Center	Rutland	6	98
Southwestern Vermont Medical Center	Bennington	7	120

Heart Failure Care

12. ACE Inhibitor or ARB for LVSD

Hospital Name	City	Rate	Cases
Southwestern Vermont Medical Center	Bennington	100%	26
White River Junction VA Medical Center	White River Jct	100%	29
Fletcher Allen Hospital of Vermont	Burlington	94%	117
Rutland Regional Medical Center	Rutland	87%	38

13. Discharge Instructions

Hospital Name	City	Rate	Cases
Gifford Medical Center	Randolph	100%	44
Springfield Hospital	Springfield	100%	45
White River Junction VA Medical Center	White River Jct	100%	81
Fletcher Allen Hospital of Vermont	Burlington	91%	247
North Country Hospital and Health Center	Newport	91%	35
Southwestern Vermont Medical Center	Bennington	89%	89
Rutland Regional Medical Center	Rutland	83%	109
Central Vermont Medical Center	Barre	82%	51
Northwestern Medical Center	Saint Albans	78%	32
Northeastern Vermont Regional Hospital	Saint Johnsbury	52%	33

14. Evaluation of LVS Function

Hospital Name	City	Rate	Cases
Brattleboro Memorial Hospital	Brattleboro	100%	31
North Country Hospital and Health Center	Newport	100%	53
Northeastern Vermont Regional Hospital	Saint Johnsbury	100%	41
Northwestern Medical Center	Saint Albans	100%	39
Rutland Regional Medical Center	Rutland	100%	144
Springfield Hospital	Springfield	100%	62
White River Junction VA Medical Center	White River Jct	100%	88
Southwestern Vermont Medical Center	Bennington	99%	130
Fletcher Allen Hospital of Vermont	Burlington	98%	316
Central Vermont Medical Center	Barre	97%	65
Copley Hospital	Morrisville	96%	28
Porter Hospital	Middlebury	89%	27
Gifford Medical Center	Randolph	84%	56

15. Smoking Cessation Advice

Hospital Name	City	Rate	Cases
Fletcher Allen Hospital of Vermont	Burlington	100%	55

Pneumonia Care

16. Appropriate Initial Antibiotic

Hospital Name	City	Rate	Cases
Mount Ascutney Hospital	Windsor	100%	27
Central Vermont Medical Center	Barre	99%	84
Fletcher Allen Hospital of Vermont	Burlington	97%	138
Gifford Medical Center	Randolph	97%	36
Copley Hospital	Morrisville	96%	49
Northwestern Medical Center	Saint Albans	96%	85
Southwestern Vermont Medical Center	Bennington	96%	101
Springfield Hospital	Springfield	96%	112
Porter Hospital	Middlebury	95%	76
Brattleboro Memorial Hospital	Brattleboro	93%	42
Rutland Regional Medical Center	Rutland	92%	123
White River Junction VA Medical Center	White River Jct	89%	37
Northeastern Vermont Regional Hospital	Saint Johnsbury	87%	53

17. Blood Culture Timing

Hospital Name	City	Rate	Cases
Gifford Medical Center	Randolph	100%	42
Mount Ascutney Hospital	Windsor	100%	29
Springfield Hospital	Springfield	100%	150
Brattleboro Memorial Hospital	Brattleboro	98%	58
Northwestern Medical Center	Saint Albans	98%	115
Porter Hospital	Middlebury	97%	63
Southwestern Vermont Medical Center	Bennington	97%	193
White River Junction VA Medical Center	White River Jct	96%	52
Northeastern Vermont Regional Hospital	Saint Johnsbury	95%	62
Rutland Regional Medical Center	Rutland	94%	194
Central Vermont Medical Center	Barre	92%	52
Fletcher Allen Hospital of Vermont	Burlington	92%	227
Copley Hospital	Morrisville	81%	37

18. Influenza Vaccine

Hospital Name	City	Rate	Cases
Northeastern Vermont Regional Hospital	Saint Johnsbury	100%	36
Springfield Hospital	Springfield	100%	91
Central Vermont Medical Center	Barre	99%	88
White River Junction VA Medical Center	White River Jct	97%	38
Northwestern Medical Center	Saint Albans	96%	67
Brattleboro Memorial Hospital	Brattleboro	94%	36
Porter Hospital	Middlebury	94%	54
Fletcher Allen Hospital of Vermont	Burlington	92%	174
Southwestern Vermont Medical Center	Bennington	92%	118
Rutland Regional Medical Center	Rutland	89%	112
Gifford Medical Center	Randolph	84%	38
Copley Hospital	Morrisville	81%	32

19. Initial Antibiotic Timing

Hospital Name	City	Rate	Cases
Northwestern Medical Center	Saint Albans	100%	109
Springfield Hospital	Springfield	100%	145
Central Vermont Medical Center	Barre	99%	129
Porter Hospital	Middlebury	99%	108
Gifford Medical Center	Randolph	98%	58
Southwestern Vermont Medical Center	Bennington	98%	178
Brattleboro Memorial Hospital	Brattleboro	97%	66
Northeastern Vermont Regional Hospital	Saint Johnsbury	97%	70
Copley Hospital	Morrisville	96%	55
Fletcher Allen Hospital of Vermont	Burlington	96%	229
Mount Ascutney Hospital	Windsor	94%	33
Rutland Regional Medical Center	Rutland	94%	203
White River Junction VA Medical Center	White River Jct	92%	25

20. Pneumococcal Vaccine

Hospital Name	City	Rate	Cases
Central Vermont Medical Center	Barre	100%	126
North Country Hospital and Health Center	Newport	100%	26
Northeastern Vermont Regional Hospital	Saint Johnsbury	100%	59
Springfield Hospital	Springfield	100%	124
White River Junction VA Medical Center	White River Jct	100%	60
Porter Hospital	Middlebury	99%	102
Northwestern Medical Center	Saint Albans	97%	98
Fletcher Allen Hospital of Vermont	Burlington	94%	265
Rutland Regional Medical Center	Rutland	94%	201
Gifford Medical Center	Randolph	92%	52
Mount Ascutney Hospital	Windsor	92%	39
Southwestern Vermont Medical Center	Bennington	92%	195
Brattleboro Memorial Hospital	Brattleboro	91%	57
Copley Hospital	Morrisville	91%	56

21. Smoking Cessation Advice

Hospital Name	City	Rate	Cases
Central Vermont Medical Center	Barre	100%	45
Fletcher Allen Hospital of Vermont	Burlington	100%	131
Springfield Hospital	Springfield	100%	41
Southwestern Vermont Medical Center	Bennington	98%	48
Northwestern Medical Center	Saint Albans	93%	27
Rutland Regional Medical Center	Rutland	93%	71

Surgical Care Improvement Project

22. Appropriate VTP Within 24 Hours

Hospital Name	City	Rate	Cases
North Country Hospital and Health Center	Newport	100%	30
Porter Hospital[2]	Middlebury	100%	41
Springfield Hospital[2]	Springfield	100%	35
White River Junction VA Medical Center[2]	White River Jct	100%	91
Southwestern Vermont Medical Center[2]	Bennington	99%	136
Copley Hospital[2]	Morrisville	98%	44
Fletcher Allen Hospital of Vermont[2]	Burlington	97%	148
Brattleboro Memorial Hospital	Brattleboro	95%	99
Central Vermont Medical Center	Barre	94%	70
Rutland Regional Medical Center[2]	Rutland	94%	161
Northwestern Medical Center	Saint Albans	92%	38
Northeastern Vermont Regional Hospital[2]	Saint Johnsbury	86%	103

23. Appropriate Hair Removal

Hospital Name	City	Rate	Cases
Brattleboro Memorial Hospital	Brattleboro	100%	251
Central Vermont Medical Center	Barre	100%	186
Copley Hospital[2]	Morrisville	100%	140
Fletcher Allen Hospital of Vermont[2]	Burlington	100%	469
Gifford Medical Center	Randolph	100%	80
Mount Ascutney Hospital	Windsor	100%	32
North Country Hospital and Health Center	Newport	100%	59
Northeastern Vermont Regional Hospital[2]	Saint Johnsbury	100%	126
Northwestern Medical Center	Saint Albans	100%	183
Porter Hospital[2]	Middlebury	100%	168
Rutland Regional Medical Center[2]	Rutland	100%	601
Southwestern Vermont Medical Center[2]	Bennington	100%	273
Springfield Hospital[2]	Springfield	100%	100
White River Junction VA Medical Center[2]	White River Jct	100%	127

24. Appropriate Beta Blocker Usage

Hospital Name	City	Rate	Cases
Springfield Hospital[2]	Springfield	100%	38
White River Junction VA Medical Center[2]	White River Jct	97%	66
Northwestern Medical Center	Saint Albans	96%	46
Brattleboro Memorial Hospital	Brattleboro	95%	82
Fletcher Allen Hospital of Vermont[2]	Burlington	95%	193
Porter Hospital[2]	Middlebury	95%	40
Southwestern Vermont Medical Center[2]	Bennington	94%	79
Northeastern Vermont Regional Hospital[2]	Saint Johnsbury	91%	33
Central Vermont Medical Center	Barre	90%	51
Rutland Regional Medical Center[2]	Rutland	81%	202

25. Controlled Postoperative Blood Glucose

Hospital Name	City	Rate	Cases
Fletcher Allen Hospital of Vermont[2]	Burlington	90%	127

26. Prophylactic Antibiotic Timing

Hospital Name	City	Rate	Cases
North Country Hospital and Health Center	Newport	100%	55
Northeastern Vermont Regional Hospital[2]	Saint Johnsbury	100%	97
Southwestern Vermont Medical Center[2]	Bennington	100%	167
White River Junction VA Medical Center	White River Jct	100%	63
Northwestern Medical Center	Saint Albans	99%	144
Porter Hospital[2]	Middlebury	99%	135
Springfield Hospital[2]	Springfield	99%	73
Brattleboro Memorial Hospital	Brattleboro	98%	183
Rutland Regional Medical Center[2]	Rutland	98%	449
Central Vermont Medical Center	Barre	97%	123
Mount Ascutney Hospital	Windsor	97%	29
Fletcher Allen Hospital of Vermont[2]	Burlington	95%	432
Gifford Medical Center	Randolph	91%	77
Copley Hospital[2]	Morrisville	90%	115

27. Prophylactic Antibiotic Timing (Outpatient)

Hospital Name	City	Rate	Cases
Southwestern Vermont Medical Center	Bennington	99%	161
Brattleboro Memorial Hospital	Brattleboro	96%	73
Northwestern Medical Center	Saint Albans	96%	144
Fletcher Allen Hospital of Vermont	Burlington	95%	863
Rutland Regional Medical Center	Rutland	91%	169
Central Vermont Medical Center	Barre	78%	101

28. Prophylactic Antibiotic Selection

Hospital Name	City	Rate	Cases
Copley Hospital[2]	Morrisville	100%	115
Gifford Medical Center	Randolph	100%	77
Porter Hospital[2]	Middlebury	100%	135
Springfield Hospital[2]	Springfield	100%	73

NOTE: Hospital profiles are in alphabetical order by state, then city, then hospital within the city; Rankings exclude hospitals with less than 25 cases except for patient surveys which excludes hospitals with less than 100 cases; (a) 100–299 cases; (1) The number of cases is too small to be sure how well a hospital is performing; (2) The hospital indicated that the data submitted for this measure were based on a sample of cases; (3) Data was collected during a shorter time period (fewer quarters) than the maximum possible time for this measure; (4) Suppressed for one or more quarters by CMS; (5) No data is available from the hospital for this measure; (6) Fewer than 100 patients completed the HCAHPS survey. Use these rates with caution, as the number of surveys may be too low to reliably assess hospital performance; (7) Survey results are based on less than 12 months of data; (8) Survey results are not available for this reporting period; (9) No or very few patients were eligible for the HCAHPS survey. The scores shown, if any, reflect a very small number of surveys; (10) A state average was not calculated because too few hospitals in the state submitted data; (11) There were discrepancies in the data collection process; Please refer to the User's Guide for a full explanation of data.

Brattleboro Memorial Hospital	Brattleboro	99%	183
Central Vermont Medical Center	Barre	99%	122
Northeastern Vermont Regional Hospital[2]	Saint Johnsbury	99%	97
Northwestern Medical Center	Saint Albans	99%	144
Rutland Regional Medical Center[2]	Rutland	99%	450
Southwestern Vermont Medical Center[2]	Bennington	99%	168
Fletcher Allen Hospital of Vermont[2]	Burlington	97%	439
Mount Ascutney Hospital	Windsor	97%	29
North Country Hospital and Health Center	Newport	95%	55
White River Junction VA Medical Center	White River Jct	94%	64

29. Prophylactic Antibiotic Selection (Outpatient)

Hospital Name	City	Rate	Cases
Southwestern Vermont Medical Center	Bennington	99%	161
Rutland Regional Medical Center	Rutland	98%	161
Fletcher Allen Hospital of Vermont	Burlington	97%	844
Central Vermont Medical Center	Barre	96%	98
Northwestern Medical Center	Saint Albans	96%	138
Brattleboro Memorial Hospital	Brattleboro	93%	72

30. Prophylactic Antibiotic Stopped

Hospital Name	City	Rate	Cases
Southwestern Vermont Medical Center[2]	Bennington	100%	163
Springfield Hospital[2]	Springfield	100%	73
Fletcher Allen Hospital of Vermont[2]	Burlington	99%	418
Porter Hospital[2]	Middlebury	99%	134
Brattleboro Memorial Hospital	Brattleboro	98%	181
Northeastern Vermont Regional Hospital[2]	Saint Johnsbury	98%	97
White River Junction VA Medical Center	White River Jct	98%	60
Central Vermont Medical Center	Barre	97%	117
Rutland Regional Medical Center[2]	Rutland	97%	439
Gifford Medical Center	Randolph	96%	75
Mount Ascutney Hospital	Windsor	96%	28
Northwestern Medical Center	Saint Albans	96%	140
Copley Hospital[2]	Morrisville	91%	114
North Country Hospital and Health Center	Newport	74%	54

31. Recommended VTP Ordered

Hospital Name	City	Rate	Cases
North Country Hospital and Health Center	Newport	100%	30
Porter Hospital[2]	Middlebury	100%	41
Springfield Hospital[2]	Springfield	100%	35
White River Junction VA Medical Center[2]	White River Jct	100%	91
Brattleboro Memorial Hospital	Brattleboro	99%	99
Southwestern Vermont Medical Center[2]	Bennington	99%	136
Copley Hospital[2]	Morrisville	98%	44
Fletcher Allen Hospital of Vermont[2]	Burlington	97%	148
Central Vermont Medical Center	Barre	96%	70
Rutland Regional Medical Center[2]	Rutland	95%	161
Northwestern Medical Center	Saint Albans	90%	39
Northeastern Vermont Regional Hospital[2]	Saint Johnsbury	88%	103

32. Urinary Catheter Removal

Hospital Name	City	Rate	Cases
Copley Hospital[2]	Morrisville	100%	49
Fletcher Allen Hospital of Vermont[2]	Burlington	100%	135
Gifford Medical Center	Randolph	100%	31
Northwestern Medical Center	Saint Albans	100%	32
Springfield Hospital[2]	Springfield	100%	38
Brattleboro Memorial Hospital	Brattleboro	99%	76
Porter Hospital[2]	Middlebury	98%	60
Southwestern Vermont Medical Center[2]	Bennington	98%	62
White River Junction VA Medical Center[2]	White River Jct	98%	48
Northeastern Vermont Regional Hospital[2]	Saint Johnsbury	97%	39
Central Vermont Medical Center	Barre	94%	49
Rutland Regional Medical Center[2]	Rutland	90%	111

Use of Medical Imaging

36. Combination Abdominal CT Scan

Hospital Name	City	Ratio	Cases
Rutland Regional Medical Center	Rutland	0.046	677
Brattleboro Memorial Hospital	Brattleboro	0.099	312
Central Vermont Medical Center	Barre	0.103	650
Fletcher Allen Hospital of Vermont	Burlington	0.106	1844
Southwestern Vermont Medical Center	Bennington	0.107	758
Northwestern Medical Center	Saint Albans	0.110	538

37. Combination Chest CT Scan

Hospital Name	City	Ratio	Cases
Central Vermont Medical Center	Barre	0.000	386
Fletcher Allen Hospital of Vermont	Burlington	0.002	1878
Southwestern Vermont Medical Center	Bennington	0.016	575
Northwestern Medical Center	Saint Albans	0.017	346
Rutland Regional Medical Center	Rutland	0.042	501
Brattleboro Memorial Hospital	Brattleboro	0.062	162

38. Follow-up Mammogram/Ultrasound

Hospital Name	City	Rate	Cases
Rutland Regional Medical Center	Rutland	3.8%	1798
Brattleboro Memorial Hospital	Brattleboro	7.2%	1058
Southwestern Vermont Medical Center	Bennington	8.0%	1331
Fletcher Allen Hospital of Vermont	Burlington	8.9%	4637
Northwestern Medical Center	Saint Albans	11.7%	920
Central Vermont Medical Center	Barre	12.0%	1746

39. MRI for Low Back Pain

Hospital Name	City	Rate	Cases
Fletcher Allen Hospital of Vermont	Burlington	19.2%	411
Southwestern Vermont Medical Center	Bennington	23.1%	134
Brattleboro Memorial Hospital	Brattleboro	25.0%	92
Rutland Regional Medical Center	Rutland	29.5%	264
Central Vermont Medical Center	Barre	30.6%	85
Northwestern Medical Center	Saint Albans	36.5%	63

Survey of Patients' Hospital Experiences

40. Area Around Room 'Always' Quiet at Night

Hospital Name	City	Rate	Cases
Copley Hospital	Morrisville	61%	300+
Gifford Medical Center	Randolph	61%	300+
Northwestern Medical Center	Saint Albans	61%	300+
North Country Hospital and Health Center	Newport	60%	300+
Northeastern Vermont Regional Hospital	Saint Johnsbury	57%	300+
Porter Hospital	Middlebury	55%	300+
Central Vermont Medical Center	Barre	54%	300+
Southwestern Vermont Medical Center	Bennington	53%	300+
Brattleboro Memorial Hospital	Brattleboro	52%	300+
Springfield Hospital	Springfield	52%	300+
Mount Ascutney Hospital	Windsor	50%	(a)
Rutland Regional Medical Center	Rutland	49%	300+
Fletcher Allen Hospital of Vermont	Burlington	43%	300+

41. Doctors 'Always' Communicated Well

Hospital Name	City	Rate	Cases
North Country Hospital and Health Center	Newport	88%	300+
Copley Hospital	Morrisville	87%	300+
Mount Ascutney Hospital	Windsor	85%	(a)
Northeastern Vermont Regional Hospital	Saint Johnsbury	85%	300+
Porter Hospital	Middlebury	85%	300+
Southwestern Vermont Medical Center	Bennington	85%	300+
Springfield Hospital	Springfield	83%	300+
Northwestern Medical Center	Saint Albans	82%	300+
Brattleboro Memorial Hospital	Brattleboro	81%	300+
Gifford Medical Center	Randolph	80%	300+
Fletcher Allen Hospital of Vermont	Burlington	79%	300+
Rutland Regional Medical Center	Rutland	79%	300+
Central Vermont Medical Center	Barre	76%	300+

42. Home Recovery Information Given

Hospital Name	City	Rate	Cases
North Country Hospital and Health Center	Newport	90%	300+
Copley Hospital	Morrisville	88%	300+
Mount Ascutney Hospital	Windsor	88%	(a)
Northwestern Medical Center	Saint Albans	88%	300+
Porter Hospital	Middlebury	88%	300+
Central Vermont Medical Center	Barre	87%	300+
Fletcher Allen Hospital of Vermont	Burlington	87%	300+
Gifford Medical Center	Randolph	87%	300+
Northeastern Vermont Regional Hospital	Saint Johnsbury	87%	300+
Rutland Regional Medical Center	Rutland	86%	300+
Southwestern Vermont Medical Center	Bennington	86%	300+
Springfield Hospital	Springfield	84%	300+
Brattleboro Memorial Hospital	Brattleboro	82%	300+

43. Hospital Given 9 or 10 on 10 Point Scale

Hospital Name	City	Rate	Cases
Southwestern Vermont Medical Center	Bennington	76%	300+
Gifford Medical Center	Randolph	75%	300+
Copley Hospital	Morrisville	74%	300+
Northwestern Medical Center	Saint Albans	74%	300+
Mount Ascutney Hospital	Windsor	73%	(a)
Fletcher Allen Hospital of Vermont	Burlington	71%	300+
North Country Hospital and Health Center	Newport	71%	300+
Northeastern Vermont Regional Hospital	Saint Johnsbury	69%	300+
Porter Hospital	Middlebury	69%	300+
Brattleboro Memorial Hospital	Brattleboro	67%	300+
Springfield Hospital	Springfield	65%	300+
Rutland Regional Medical Center	Rutland	64%	300+
Central Vermont Medical Center	Barre	62%	300+

44. Meds 'Always' Explained Before Given

Hospital Name	City	Rate	Cases
Copley Hospital	Morrisville	68%	300+
Porter Hospital	Middlebury	68%	300+
Mount Ascutney Hospital	Windsor	67%	(a)
Northeastern Vermont Regional Hospital	Saint Johnsbury	67%	300+
Springfield Hospital	Springfield	67%	300+
Gifford Medical Center	Randolph	66%	300+
North Country Hospital and Health Center	Newport	66%	300+
Northwestern Medical Center	Saint Albans	66%	300+
Southwestern Vermont Medical Center	Bennington	66%	300+
Brattleboro Memorial Hospital	Brattleboro	64%	300+
Fletcher Allen Hospital of Vermont	Burlington	61%	300+
Central Vermont Medical Center	Barre	59%	300+
Rutland Regional Medical Center	Rutland	59%	300+

45. Nurses 'Always' Communicated Well

Hospital Name	City	Rate	Cases
North Country Hospital and Health Center	Newport	82%	300+
Northwestern Medical Center	Saint Albans	82%	300+
Southwestern Vermont Medical Center	Bennington	82%	300+
Springfield Hospital	Springfield	82%	300+
Copley Hospital	Morrisville	81%	300+
Porter Hospital	Middlebury	81%	300+
Brattleboro Memorial Hospital	Brattleboro	80%	300+
Gifford Medical Center	Randolph	79%	300+
Mount Ascutney Hospital	Windsor	79%	(a)
Northeastern Vermont Regional Hospital	Saint Johnsbury	79%	300+
Fletcher Allen Hospital of Vermont	Burlington	77%	300+
Rutland Regional Medical Center	Rutland	76%	300+
Central Vermont Medical Center	Barre	74%	300+

46. Pain 'Always' Well Controlled

Hospital Name	City	Rate	Cases
Copley Hospital	Morrisville	78%	300+
Mount Ascutney Hospital	Windsor	78%	(a)
Southwestern Vermont Medical Center	Bennington	76%	300+
Northwestern Medical Center	Saint Albans	74%	300+
Rutland Regional Medical Center	Rutland	74%	300+
Porter Hospital	Middlebury	73%	300+
Gifford Medical Center	Randolph	72%	300+
North Country Hospital and Health Center	Newport	72%	300+
Northeastern Vermont Regional Hospital	Saint Johnsbury	72%	300+
Springfield Hospital	Springfield	72%	300+
Brattleboro Memorial Hospital	Brattleboro	71%	300+
Fletcher Allen Hospital of Vermont	Burlington	69%	300+
Central Vermont Medical Center	Barre	64%	300+

47. Room and Bathroom 'Always' Clean

Hospital Name	City	Rate	Cases
Northeastern Vermont Regional Hospital	Saint Johnsbury	83%	300+
Northwestern Medical Center	Saint Albans	83%	300+
North Country Hospital and Health Center	Newport	82%	300+
Mount Ascutney Hospital	Windsor	81%	(a)
Southwestern Vermont Medical Center	Bennington	81%	300+
Brattleboro Memorial Hospital	Brattleboro	79%	300+
Central Vermont Medical Center	Barre	79%	300+
Springfield Hospital	Springfield	79%	300+
Fletcher Allen Hospital of Vermont	Burlington	77%	300+
Copley Hospital	Morrisville	76%	300+
Porter Hospital	Middlebury	74%	300+
Gifford Medical Center	Randolph	72%	300+
Rutland Regional Medical Center	Rutland	71%	300+

48. Timely Help 'Always' Received

Hospital Name	City	Rate	Cases
Copley Hospital	Morrisville	76%	300+
North Country Hospital and Health Center	Newport	75%	300+
Springfield Hospital	Springfield	75%	300+
Brattleboro Memorial Hospital	Brattleboro	72%	300+
Northeastern Vermont Regional Hospital	Saint Johnsbury	72%	300+
Southwestern Vermont Medical Center	Bennington	71%	300+
Gifford Medical Center	Randolph	70%	300+
Northwestern Medical Center	Saint Albans	70%	300+
Mount Ascutney Hospital	Windsor	69%	(a)
Rutland Regional Medical Center	Rutland	69%	300+
Porter Hospital	Middlebury	68%	300+
Central Vermont Medical Center	Barre	66%	300+
Fletcher Allen Hospital of Vermont	Burlington	65%	300+

49. Would Definitely Recommend Hospital

Hospital Name	City	Rate	Cases
Mount Ascutney Hospital	Windsor	81%	(a)
Southwestern Vermont Medical Center	Bennington	80%	300+
Northwestern Medical Center	Saint Albans	79%	300+
Copley Hospital	Morrisville	77%	300+
Fletcher Allen Hospital of Vermont	Burlington	77%	300+

NOTE: Hospital profiles are in alphabetical order by state, then city, then hospital within the city; Rankings exclude hospitals with less than 25 cases except for patient surveys which excludes hospitals with less than 100 cases; (a) 100–299 cases; (1) The number of cases is too small to be sure how well a hospital is performing; (2) The hospital indicated that the data submitted for this measure were based on a sample of cases; (3) Data was collected during a shorter time period (fewer quarters) than the maximum possible time for this measure; (4) Suppressed for one or more quarters by CMS; (5) No data is available from the hospital for this measure; (6) Fewer than 100 patients completed the HCAHPS survey. Use these rates with caution, as the number of surveys may be too low to reliably assess hospital performance; (7) Survey results are based on less than 12 months of data; (8) Survey results are not available for this reporting period; (9) No or very few patients were eligible for the HCAHPS survey. The scores shown, if any, reflect a very small number of surveys; (10) A state average was not calculated because too few hospitals in the state submitted data; (11) There were discrepancies in the data collection process; Please refer to the User's Guide for a full explanation of data.

Gifford Medical Center	Randolph	76%	300+
Porter Hospital	Middlebury	74%	300+
Brattleboro Memorial Hospital	Brattleboro	73%	300+
Northeastern Vermont Regional Hospital	Saint Johnsbury	73%	300+
North Country Hospital and Health Center	Newport	70%	300+
Springfield Hospital	Springfield	65%	300+
Rutland Regional Medical Center	Rutland	63%	300+
Central Vermont Medical Center	Barre	62%	300+

NOTE: Hospital profiles are in alphabetical order by state, then city, then hospital within the city; Rankings exclude hospitals with less than 25 cases except for patient surveys which excludes hospitals with less than 100 cases; (a) 100–299 cases; (1) The number of cases is too small to be sure how well a hospital is performing; (2) The hospital indicated that the data submitted for this measure were based on a sample of cases; (3) Data was collected during a shorter time period (fewer quarters) than the maximum possible time for this measure; (4) Suppressed for one or more quarters by CMS; (5) No data is available from the hospital for this measure; (6) Fewer than 100 patients completed the HCAHPS survey. Use these rates with caution, as the number of surveys may be too low to reliably assess hospital performance; (7) Survey results are based on less than 12 months of data; (8) Survey results are not available for this reporting period; (9) No or very few patients were eligible for the HCAHPS survey. The scores shown, if any, reflect a very small number of surveys; (10) A state average was not calculated because too few hospitals in the state submitted data; (11) There were discrepancies in the data collection process; Please refer to the User's Guide for a full explanation of data.

Central Vermont Medical Center

130 Fisher Road
Barre, VT 05641
Phone: 802-371-4100
Fax: 802-371-4401
URL: www.cvmc.hitchcock.org
Type: Acute Care Hospitals
Emergency Services: No
Ownership: Voluntary Non-Profit - Private
Beds: 210

Key Personnel:

CEO/President. . . . . Judy Tarr
Chief of Medical Staff . . . . Russle Davignon, DO
Infection Control. . . . . Jane Barranco
Operating Room. . . . . Karin Morrow
Pediatric Ambulatory Care . . . . . . William Gaidys, MD
Pediatric In-Patient Care . . . . William Gaidys, MD
Quality Assurance . . . . Russell Davignon, MD
Radiology. . . . . Robert D Johnson, MD

Measure	Cases	This Hosp.	State Avg.	U.S. Avg.
Heart Attack Care				
ACE Inhibitor or ARB for LVSD[1]	2	100%	97%	96%
Aspirin at Arrival[1]	7	100%	99%	99%
Aspirin at Discharge[1]	3	100%	99%	98%
Beta Blocker at Discharge[1]	5	100%	99%	98%
Fibrinolytic Medication Timing	0	-	0%	55%
PCI Within 90 Minutes of Arrival	0	-	-	90%
Smoking Cessation Advice	0	-	100%	99%
Chest Pain/Possible Heart Attack Care				
Aspirin at Arrival	156	99%	99%	95%
Median Time to ECG (minutes)	159	6	6	8
Median Time to Transfer (minutes)[1]	17	31	34	61
Fibrinolytic Medication Timing[1]	1	100%	71%	54%
Heart Failure Care				
ACE Inhibitor or ARB for LVSD[1]	15	93%	94%	94%
Discharge Instructions	51	82%	87%	88%
Evaluation of LVS Function	65	97%	98%	98%
Smoking Cessation Advice[1]	11	100%	99%	98%
Pneumonia Care				
Appropriate Initial Antibiotic	84	99%	95%	92%
Blood Culture Timing	52	92%	96%	96%
Influenza Vaccine	88	99%	93%	91%
Initial Antibiotic Timing	129	99%	97%	95%
Pneumococcal Vaccine	126	100%	95%	93%
Smoking Cessation Advice	45	100%	97%	97%
Surgical Care Improvement Project				
Appropriate VTP Within 24 Hours	70	94%	96%	92%
Appropriate Hair Removal	186	100%	100%	99%
Appropriate Beta Blocker Usage	51	90%	91%	93%
Controlled Postoperative Blood Glucose	0	-	90%	93%
Prophylactic Antibiotic Timing	123	97%	97%	97%
Prophylactic Antibiotic Timing (Outpatient)	101	78%	94%	92%
Prophylactic Antibiotic Selection	122	99%	99%	97%
Prophylactic Antibiotic Select. (Outpatient)	98	96%	97%	94%
Prophylactic Antibiotic Stopped	117	97%	97%	94%
Recommended VTP Ordered	70	96%	96%	94%
Urinary Catheter Removal	49	94%	97%	90%
Children's Asthma Care				
Received Systemic Corticosteroids	-	-	-	100%
Received Home Management Plan	-	-	-	71%
Received Reliever Medication	-	-	-	100%
Use of Medical Imaging				
Combination Abdominal CT Scan	650	0.103	0.086	0.191
Combination Chest CT Scan	386	0.000	0.015	0.054
Follow-up Mammogram/Ultrasound	1,746	12.0%	8.7%	8.4%
MRI for Low Back Pain	85	30.6%	27.1%	32.7%
Survey of Patients' Hospital Experiences				
Area Around Room 'Always' Quiet at Night	300+	54%	-	58%
Doctors 'Always' Communicated Well	300+	76%	-	80%
Home Recovery Information Given	300+	87%	-	82%
Hospital Given 9 or 10 on 10 Point Scale	300+	62%	-	67%
Meds 'Always' Explained Before Given	300+	59%	-	60%
Nurses 'Always' Communicated Well	300+	74%	-	76%
Pain 'Always' Well Controlled	300+	64%	-	69%
Room and Bathroom 'Always' Clean	300+	79%	-	71%
Timely Help 'Always' Received	300+	66%	-	64%
Would Definitely Recommend Hospital	300+	62%	-	69%

Southwestern Vermont Medical Center

100 Hospital Drive
Bennington, VT 05201
Phone: 802-442-6361
Fax: 802-442-8331
URL: www.svhealthcare.org
Type: Acute Care Hospitals
Emergency Services: Yes
Ownership: Voluntary Non-Profit - Private
Beds: 99

Key Personnel:

CEO/President. . . . . Harvey Yorke
Chief of Medical Staff . . . . Robert Pezzulich, MD
Quality Assurance . . . . Patricia Hebert
Radiology. . . . . Terrell L Coffield
Emergency Room . . . . Christopher Barsotti

Measure	Cases	This Hosp.	State Avg.	U.S. Avg.
Heart Attack Care				
ACE Inhibitor or ARB for LVSD[1]	3	100%	97%	96%
Aspirin at Arrival	36	100%	99%	99%
Aspirin at Discharge[1]	23	100%	99%	98%
Beta Blocker at Discharge	25	100%	99%	98%
Fibrinolytic Medication Timing	0	-	0%	55%
PCI Within 90 Minutes of Arrival	0	-	-	90%
Smoking Cessation Advice[1]	7	100%	100%	99%
Chest Pain/Possible Heart Attack Care				
Aspirin at Arrival	110	99%	99%	95%
Median Time to ECG (minutes)	120	7	6	8
Median Time to Transfer (minutes)[1]	4	96	34	61
Fibrinolytic Medication Timing[1]	4	50%	71%	54%
Heart Failure Care				
ACE Inhibitor or ARB for LVSD	26	100%	94%	94%
Discharge Instructions	89	89%	87%	88%
Evaluation of LVS Function	130	99%	98%	98%
Smoking Cessation Advice[1]	10	100%	99%	98%
Pneumonia Care				
Appropriate Initial Antibiotic	101	96%	95%	92%
Blood Culture Timing	193	97%	96%	96%
Influenza Vaccine	118	92%	93%	91%
Initial Antibiotic Timing	178	98%	97%	95%
Pneumococcal Vaccine	195	92%	95%	93%
Smoking Cessation Advice	48	98%	97%	97%
Surgical Care Improvement Project				
Appropriate VTP Within 24 Hours[2]	136	99%	96%	92%
Appropriate Hair Removal[2]	273	100%	100%	99%
Appropriate Beta Blocker Usage[2]	79	94%	91%	93%
Controlled Postoperative Blood Glucose[2]	0	-	90%	93%
Prophylactic Antibiotic Timing[2]	167	100%	97%	97%
Prophylactic Antibiotic Timing (Outpatient)	161	99%	94%	92%
Prophylactic Antibiotic Selection[2]	168	99%	99%	97%
Prophylactic Antibiotic Select. (Outpatient)	161	99%	97%	94%
Prophylactic Antibiotic Stopped[2]	163	100%	97%	94%
Recommended VTP Ordered[2]	136	99%	96%	94%
Urinary Catheter Removal[2]	62	98%	97%	90%
Children's Asthma Care				
Received Systemic Corticosteroids	-	-	-	100%
Received Home Management Plan	-	-	-	71%
Received Reliever Medication	-	-	-	100%
Use of Medical Imaging				
Combination Abdominal CT Scan	758	0.107	0.086	0.191
Combination Chest CT Scan	575	0.016	0.015	0.054
Follow-up Mammogram/Ultrasound	1,331	8.0%	8.7%	8.4%
MRI for Low Back Pain	134	23.1%	27.1%	32.7%
Survey of Patients' Hospital Experiences				
Area Around Room 'Always' Quiet at Night	300+	53%	-	58%
Doctors 'Always' Communicated Well	300+	85%	-	80%
Home Recovery Information Given	300+	86%	-	82%
Hospital Given 9 or 10 on 10 Point Scale	300+	76%	-	67%
Meds 'Always' Explained Before Given	300+	66%	-	60%
Nurses 'Always' Communicated Well	300+	82%	-	76%
Pain 'Always' Well Controlled	300+	76%	-	69%
Room and Bathroom 'Always' Clean	300+	81%	-	71%
Timely Help 'Always' Received	300+	71%	-	64%
Would Definitely Recommend Hospital	300+	80%	-	69%

Brattleboro Memorial Hospital

17 Belmont Ave
Brattleboro, VT 05301
Phone: 802-257-0341
Fax: 802-257-8822
E-mail: info@bmhvt.org
URL: www.bmhvt.org
Type: Acute Care Hospitals
Emergency Services: Yes
Ownership: Voluntary Non-Profit - Other
Beds: 47

Key Personnel:

CEO/President. . . . . Michael O Rogers
Chief of Medical Staff . . . . David Albright, MD
Quality Assurance . . . . Corinne Bristol, RN
Radiology. . . . . Edward F Elliott Jr

Measure	Cases	This Hosp.	State Avg.	U.S. Avg.
Heart Attack Care				
ACE Inhibitor or ARB for LVSD[1]	3	100%	97%	96%
Aspirin at Arrival[1]	13	100%	99%	99%
Aspirin at Discharge[1]	9	100%	99%	98%
Beta Blocker at Discharge[1]	10	100%	99%	98%
Fibrinolytic Medication Timing	0	-	0%	55%
PCI Within 90 Minutes of Arrival	0	-	-	90%
Smoking Cessation Advice[1]	1	100%	100%	99%
Chest Pain/Possible Heart Attack Care				
Aspirin at Arrival[1,3]	7	86%	99%	95%
Median Time to ECG (minutes)[1,3]	7	4	6	8
Median Time to Transfer (minutes)[1,3]	2	328	34	61
Fibrinolytic Medication Timing[3]	0	-	71%	54%
Heart Failure Care				
ACE Inhibitor or ARB for LVSD[1]	8	88%	94%	94%
Discharge Instructions[1]	23	96%	87%	88%
Evaluation of LVS Function	31	100%	98%	98%
Smoking Cessation Advice[1]	3	100%	99%	98%
Pneumonia Care				
Appropriate Initial Antibiotic	42	93%	95%	92%
Blood Culture Timing	58	98%	96%	96%
Influenza Vaccine	36	94%	93%	91%
Initial Antibiotic Timing	66	97%	97%	95%
Pneumococcal Vaccine	57	91%	95%	93%
Smoking Cessation Advice[1]	15	100%	97%	97%
Surgical Care Improvement Project				
Appropriate VTP Within 24 Hours	99	95%	96%	92%
Appropriate Hair Removal	251	100%	100%	99%
Appropriate Beta Blocker Usage	82	95%	91%	93%
Controlled Postoperative Blood Glucose	0	-	90%	93%
Prophylactic Antibiotic Timing	183	98%	97%	97%
Prophylactic Antibiotic Timing (Outpatient)	73	96%	94%	92%
Prophylactic Antibiotic Selection	183	99%	99%	97%
Prophylactic Antibiotic Select. (Outpatient)	72	93%	97%	94%
Prophylactic Antibiotic Stopped	181	98%	97%	94%
Recommended VTP Ordered	99	99%	96%	94%
Urinary Catheter Removal	76	99%	97%	90%
Children's Asthma Care				
Received Systemic Corticosteroids	-	-	-	100%
Received Home Management Plan	-	-	-	71%
Received Reliever Medication	-	-	-	100%
Use of Medical Imaging				
Combination Abdominal CT Scan	312	0.099	0.086	0.191
Combination Chest CT Scan	162	0.062	0.015	0.054
Follow-up Mammogram/Ultrasound	1,058	7.2%	8.7%	8.4%
MRI for Low Back Pain	92	25.0%	27.1%	32.7%
Survey of Patients' Hospital Experiences				
Area Around Room 'Always' Quiet at Night	300+	52%	-	58%
Doctors 'Always' Communicated Well	300+	81%	-	80%
Home Recovery Information Given	300+	82%	-	82%
Hospital Given 9 or 10 on 10 Point Scale	300+	67%	-	67%
Meds 'Always' Explained Before Given	300+	64%	-	60%
Nurses 'Always' Communicated Well	300+	80%	-	76%
Pain 'Always' Well Controlled	300+	71%	-	69%
Room and Bathroom 'Always' Clean	300+	79%	-	71%
Timely Help 'Always' Received	300+	72%	-	64%
Would Definitely Recommend Hospital	300+	73%	-	69%

NOTE: Hospital profiles are in alphabetical order by state, then city, then hospital within the city; Rankings exclude hospitals with less than 25 cases except for patient surveys which excludes hospitals with less than 100 cases; (a) 100–299 cases; (1) The number of cases is too small to be sure how well a hospital is performing; (2) The hospital indicated that the data submitted for this measure were based on a sample of cases; (3) Data was collected during a shorter time period (fewer quarters) than the maximum possible time for this measure; (4) Suppressed for one or more quarters by CMS; (5) No data is available from the hospital for this measure; (6) Fewer than 100 patients completed the HCAHPS survey. Use these rates with caution, as the number of surveys may be too low to reliably assess hospital performance; (7) Survey results are based on less than 12 months of data; (8) Survey results are not available for this reporting period; (9) No or very few patients were eligible for the HCAHPS survey. The scores shown, if any, reflect a very small number of surveys; (10) A state average was not calculated because too few hospitals in the state submitted data; (11) There were discrepancies in the data collection process; Please refer to the User's Guide for a full explanation of data.

Fletcher Allen Hospital of Vermont

111 Colchester Ave — Phone: 802-847-0000
Burlington, VT 05401 — Fax: 802-847-5540
URL: www.fletcherallen.org
Type: Acute Care Hospitals — Emergency Services: Yes
Ownership: Voluntary Non-Profit - Other — Beds: 562

Key Personnel:
Operating Room. . . . . Stephen Shackford, MD
Quality Assurance . . . . John Brumsted, MD
Radiology. . . . . Steve Braff
Emergency Room . . . . Ramsey Herrington, MD

Measure	Cases	This Hosp.	State Avg.	U.S. Avg.
Heart Attack Care				
ACE Inhibitor or ARB for LVSD	116	97%	97%	96%
Aspirin at Arrival	242	100%	99%	99%
Aspirin at Discharge	631	99%	99%	98%
Beta Blocker at Discharge	627	99%	99%	98%
Fibrinolytic Medication Timing	0	-	0%	55%
PCI Within 90 Minutes of Arrival	0	-	-	90%
Smoking Cessation Advice	212	100%	100%	99%
Chest Pain/Possible Heart Attack Care				
Aspirin at Arrival[5]	0	-	99%	95%
Median Time to ECG (minutes)[5]	0	-	6	8
Median Time to Transfer (minutes)[5]	0	-	34	61
Fibrinolytic Medication Timing[5]	0	-	71%	54%
Heart Failure Care				
ACE Inhibitor or ARB for LVSD	117	94%	94%	94%
Discharge Instructions	247	91%	87%	88%
Evaluation of LVS Function	316	98%	98%	98%
Smoking Cessation Advice	55	100%	99%	98%
Pneumonia Care				
Appropriate Initial Antibiotic	138	97%	95%	92%
Blood Culture Timing	227	92%	96%	96%
Influenza Vaccine	174	92%	93%	91%
Initial Antibiotic Timing	229	96%	97%	95%
Pneumococcal Vaccine	265	94%	95%	93%
Smoking Cessation Advice	131	100%	97%	97%
Surgical Care Improvement Project				
Appropriate VTP Within 24 Hours[2]	148	97%	96%	92%
Appropriate Hair Removal[2]	469	100%	100%	99%
Appropriate Beta Blocker Usage[2]	193	95%	91%	93%
Controlled Postoperative Blood Glucose[2]	127	90%	90%	93%
Prophylactic Antibiotic Timing[2]	432	95%	97%	97%
Prophylactic Antibiotic Timing (Outpatient)	863	95%	94%	92%
Prophylactic Antibiotic Selection[2]	439	97%	99%	97%
Prophylactic Antibiotic Select. (Outpatient)	844	97%	97%	94%
Prophylactic Antibiotic Stopped[2]	418	99%	97%	94%
Recommended VTP Ordered[2]	148	97%	96%	94%
Urinary Catheter Removal[2]	135	100%	97%	90%
Children's Asthma Care				
Received Systemic Corticosteroids	-	-	-	100%
Received Home Management Plan	-	-	-	71%
Received Reliever Medication	-	-	-	100%
Use of Medical Imaging				
Combination Abdominal CT Scan	1,844	0.106	0.086	0.191
Combination Chest CT Scan	1,878	0.002	0.015	0.054
Follow-up Mammogram/Ultrasound	4,637	8.9%	8.7%	8.4%
MRI for Low Back Pain	411	19.2%	27.1%	32.7%
Survey of Patients' Hospital Experiences				
Area Around Room 'Always' Quiet at Night	300+	43%	-	58%
Doctors 'Always' Communicated Well	300+	79%	-	80%
Home Recovery Information Given	300+	87%	-	82%
Hospital Given 9 or 10 on 10 Point Scale	300+	71%	-	67%
Meds 'Always' Explained Before Given	300+	61%	-	60%
Nurses 'Always' Communicated Well	300+	77%	-	76%
Pain 'Always' Well Controlled	300+	69%	-	69%
Room and Bathroom 'Always' Clean	300+	77%	-	71%
Timely Help 'Always' Received	300+	65%	-	64%
Would Definitely Recommend Hospital	300+	77%	-	69%

Porter Hospital

115 Porter Drive — Phone: 802-388-4701
Middlebury, VT 05753 — Fax: 802-388-8859
URL: www.portermedical.org
Type: Critical Access Hospitals — Emergency Services: Yes
Ownership: Voluntary Non-Profit - Private — Beds: 45

Key Personnel:
Chief of Medical Staff. . . . . Rebecca Adams, MD
Infection Control. . . . . Sheila Boise
Pediatric Ambulatory Care . . . . . . Johana Brakeley, MD
Pediatric In-Patient Care . . . . Johana Brakeley, MD
Quality Assurance . . . . Lyn Farr
Radiology. . . . . C Wade Cobb

Measure	Cases	This Hosp.	State Avg.	U.S. Avg.
Heart Attack Care				
ACE Inhibitor or ARB for LVSD[3]	0	-	97%	96%
Aspirin at Arrival[1,3]	3	67%	99%	99%
Aspirin at Discharge[1,3]	2	50%	99%	98%
Beta Blocker at Discharge[1,3]	2	100%	99%	98%
Fibrinolytic Medication Timing[3]	0	-	0%	55%
PCI Within 90 Minutes of Arrival[3]	0	-	-	90%
Smoking Cessation Advice[3]	0	-	100%	99%
Chest Pain/Possible Heart Attack Care				
Aspirin at Arrival	-	-	99%	95%
Median Time to ECG (minutes)	-	-	6	8
Median Time to Transfer (minutes)	-	-	34	61
Fibrinolytic Medication Timing	-	-	71%	54%
Heart Failure Care				
ACE Inhibitor or ARB for LVSD[1]	6	100%	94%	94%
Discharge Instructions[1]	23	83%	87%	88%
Evaluation of LVS Function	27	89%	98%	98%
Smoking Cessation Advice[1]	4	100%	99%	98%
Pneumonia Care				
Appropriate Initial Antibiotic	76	95%	95%	92%
Blood Culture Timing	63	97%	96%	96%
Influenza Vaccine	54	94%	93%	91%
Initial Antibiotic Timing	108	99%	97%	95%
Pneumococcal Vaccine	102	99%	95%	93%
Smoking Cessation Advice[1]	21	95%	97%	97%
Surgical Care Improvement Project				
Appropriate VTP Within 24 Hours[2]	41	100%	96%	92%
Appropriate Hair Removal[2]	168	100%	100%	99%
Appropriate Beta Blocker Usage[2]	40	95%	91%	93%
Controlled Postoperative Blood Glucose[2]	0	-	90%	93%
Prophylactic Antibiotic Timing[2]	135	99%	97%	97%
Prophylactic Antibiotic Timing (Outpatient)	-	-	94%	92%
Prophylactic Antibiotic Selection[2]	135	100%	99%	97%
Prophylactic Antibiotic Select. (Outpatient)	-	-	97%	94%
Prophylactic Antibiotic Stopped[2]	134	99%	97%	94%
Recommended VTP Ordered[2]	41	100%	96%	94%
Urinary Catheter Removal[2]	60	98%	97%	90%
Children's Asthma Care				
Received Systemic Corticosteroids	-	-	-	100%
Received Home Management Plan	-	-	-	71%
Received Reliever Medication	-	-	-	100%
Use of Medical Imaging				
Combination Abdominal CT Scan	-	-	0.086	0.191
Combination Chest CT Scan	-	-	0.015	0.054
Follow-up Mammogram/Ultrasound	-	-	8.7%	8.4%
MRI for Low Back Pain	-	-	27.1%	32.7%
Survey of Patients' Hospital Experiences				
Area Around Room 'Always' Quiet at Night	300+	55%	-	58%
Doctors 'Always' Communicated Well	300+	85%	-	80%
Home Recovery Information Given	300+	88%	-	82%
Hospital Given 9 or 10 on 10 Point Scale	300+	69%	-	67%
Meds 'Always' Explained Before Given	300+	68%	-	60%
Nurses 'Always' Communicated Well	300+	81%	-	76%
Pain 'Always' Well Controlled	300+	73%	-	69%
Room and Bathroom 'Always' Clean	300+	74%	-	71%
Timely Help 'Always' Received	300+	68%	-	64%
Would Definitely Recommend Hospital	300+	74%	-	69%

Copley Hospital

528 Washington Highway — Phone: 802-888-4231
Morrisville, VT 05661 — Fax: 802-888-8223
E-mail: pwright@chsi.org
URL: www.copleyvt.org
Type: Critical Access Hospitals — Emergency Services: Yes
Ownership: Government - Federal — Beds: 53

Key Personnel:
CEO/President. . . . . Melvyn Patashnick
Chief of Medical Staff. . . . . Brendan Buckley, MD
Infection Control. . . . . Carol Wood-Koob, RN
Operating Room. . . . . Patricia Jaqua
Quality Assurance . . . . Joseph Falworth
Radiology. . . . . Richard Bennum

Measure	Cases	This Hosp.	State Avg.	U.S. Avg.
Heart Attack Care				
ACE Inhibitor or ARB for LVSD[1]	3	100%	97%	96%
Aspirin at Arrival[1]	7	100%	99%	99%
Aspirin at Discharge[1]	6	100%	99%	98%
Beta Blocker at Discharge[1]	3	100%	99%	98%
Fibrinolytic Medication Timing	0	-	0%	55%
PCI Within 90 Minutes of Arrival	0	-	-	90%
Smoking Cessation Advice[1]	1	100%	100%	99%
Chest Pain/Possible Heart Attack Care				
Aspirin at Arrival	-	-	99%	95%
Median Time to ECG (minutes)	-	-	6	8
Median Time to Transfer (minutes)	-	-	34	61
Fibrinolytic Medication Timing	-	-	71%	54%
Heart Failure Care				
ACE Inhibitor or ARB for LVSD[1]	2	100%	94%	94%
Discharge Instructions[1]	22	95%	87%	88%
Evaluation of LVS Function	28	96%	98%	98%
Smoking Cessation Advice[1]	1	100%	99%	98%
Pneumonia Care				
Appropriate Initial Antibiotic	49	96%	95%	92%
Blood Culture Timing	37	81%	96%	96%
Influenza Vaccine	32	81%	93%	91%
Initial Antibiotic Timing	55	96%	97%	95%
Pneumococcal Vaccine	56	91%	95%	93%
Smoking Cessation Advice[1]	14	100%	97%	97%
Surgical Care Improvement Project				
Appropriate VTP Within 24 Hours[2]	44	98%	96%	92%
Appropriate Hair Removal[2]	140	100%	100%	99%
Appropriate Beta Blocker Usage[1,2]	23	100%	91%	93%
Controlled Postoperative Blood Glucose[2]	0	-	90%	93%
Prophylactic Antibiotic Timing[2]	115	90%	97%	97%
Prophylactic Antibiotic Timing (Outpatient)	-	-	94%	92%
Prophylactic Antibiotic Selection[2]	115	100%	99%	97%
Prophylactic Antibiotic Select. (Outpatient)	-	-	97%	94%
Prophylactic Antibiotic Stopped[2]	114	91%	97%	94%
Recommended VTP Ordered[2]	44	98%	96%	94%
Urinary Catheter Removal[2]	49	100%	97%	90%
Children's Asthma Care				
Received Systemic Corticosteroids	-	-	-	100%
Received Home Management Plan	-	-	-	71%
Received Reliever Medication	-	-	-	100%
Use of Medical Imaging				
Combination Abdominal CT Scan	-	-	0.086	0.191
Combination Chest CT Scan	-	-	0.015	0.054
Follow-up Mammogram/Ultrasound	-	-	8.7%	8.4%
MRI for Low Back Pain	-	-	27.1%	32.7%
Survey of Patients' Hospital Experiences				
Area Around Room 'Always' Quiet at Night	300+	61%	-	58%
Doctors 'Always' Communicated Well	300+	87%	-	80%
Home Recovery Information Given	300+	88%	-	82%
Hospital Given 9 or 10 on 10 Point Scale	300+	74%	-	67%
Meds 'Always' Explained Before Given	300+	68%	-	60%
Nurses 'Always' Communicated Well	300+	81%	-	76%
Pain 'Always' Well Controlled	300+	78%	-	69%
Room and Bathroom 'Always' Clean	300+	76%	-	71%
Timely Help 'Always' Received	300+	76%	-	64%
Would Definitely Recommend Hospital	300+	77%	-	69%

NOTE: Hospital profiles are in alphabetical order by state, then city, then hospital within the city; Rankings exclude hospitals with less than 25 cases except for patient surveys which excludes hospitals with less than 100 cases; (a) 100–299 cases; (1) The number of cases is too small to be sure how well a hospital is performing; (2) The hospital indicated that the data submitted for this measure were based on a sample of cases; (3) Data was collected during a shorter time period (fewer quarters) than the maximum possible time for this measure; (4) Suppressed for one or more quarters by CMS; (5) No data is available from the hospital for this measure; (6) Fewer than 100 patients completed the HCAHPS survey. Use these rates with caution, as the number of surveys may be too low to reliably assess hospital performance; (7) Survey results are based on less than 12 months of data; (8) Survey results are not available for this reporting period; (9) No or very few patients were eligible for the HCAHPS survey. The scores shown, if any, reflect a very small number of surveys; (10) A state average was not calculated because too few hospitals in the state submitted data; (11) There were discrepancies in the data collection process; Please refer to the User's Guide for a full explanation of data.

North Country Hospital and Health Center

189 Prouty Drive
Newport, VT 05855
Phone: 802-334-7331
Fax: 802-334-4510
URL: www.nchsi.org
Type: Critical Access Hospitals
Emergency Services: Yes
Ownership: Voluntary Non-Profit - Private
Beds: 25

Key Personnel:

CEO/President. . . . . Karen A Weller
Chief of Medical Staff. . . . . R Ron Holland, MD
Infection Control. . . . . Jean Holcomb
Pediatric In-Patient Care . . . . Kathy Fabian, RN
Quality Assurance . . . . Stephen Halikas
Radiology. . . . . Steven Perlin
Intensive Care Unit. . . . . Chris Convard
Patient Relations . . . . Carol Loux

Measure	Cases	This Hosp.	State Avg.	U.S. Avg.
Heart Attack Care				
ACE Inhibitor or ARB for LVSD	0	-	97%	96%
Aspirin at Arrival[1]	9	100%	99%	99%
Aspirin at Discharge[1]	7	100%	99%	98%
Beta Blocker at Discharge[1]	6	100%	99%	98%
Fibrinolytic Medication Timing	0	-	0%	55%
PCI Within 90 Minutes of Arrival	0	-	-	90%
Smoking Cessation Advice[1]	1	100%	100%	99%
Chest Pain/Possible Heart Attack Care				
Aspirin at Arrival	-	-	99%	95%
Median Time to ECG (minutes)	-	-	6	8
Median Time to Transfer (minutes)	-	-	34	61
Fibrinolytic Medication Timing	-	-	71%	54%
Heart Failure Care				
ACE Inhibitor or ARB for LVSD[1]	13	100%	94%	94%
Discharge Instructions	35	91%	87%	88%
Evaluation of LVS Function	53	100%	98%	98%
Smoking Cessation Advice[1]	4	100%	99%	98%
Pneumonia Care				
Appropriate Initial Antibiotic[1]	23	96%	95%	92%
Blood Culture Timing[1]	19	95%	96%	96%
Influenza Vaccine[1]	19	89%	93%	91%
Initial Antibiotic Timing[1]	24	100%	97%	95%
Pneumococcal Vaccine	26	100%	95%	93%
Smoking Cessation Advice[1]	7	100%	97%	97%
Surgical Care Improvement Project				
Appropriate VTP Within 24 Hours	30	100%	96%	92%
Appropriate Hair Removal	59	100%	100%	99%
Appropriate Beta Blocker Usage[1]	18	94%	91%	93%
Controlled Postoperative Blood Glucose	0	-	90%	93%
Prophylactic Antibiotic Timing	55	100%	97%	97%
Prophylactic Antibiotic Timing (Outpatient)	-	-	94%	92%
Prophylactic Antibiotic Selection	55	95%	99%	97%
Prophylactic Antibiotic Select. (Outpatient)	-	-	97%	94%
Prophylactic Antibiotic Stopped	54	74%	97%	94%
Recommended VTP Ordered	30	100%	96%	94%
Urinary Catheter Removal[1]	22	91%	97%	90%
Children's Asthma Care				
Received Systemic Corticosteroids	-	-	-	100%
Received Home Management Plan	-	-	-	71%
Received Reliever Medication	-	-	-	100%
Use of Medical Imaging				
Combination Abdominal CT Scan	-	-	0.086	0.191
Combination Chest CT Scan	-	-	0.015	0.054
Follow-up Mammogram/Ultrasound	-	-	8.7%	8.4%
MRI for Low Back Pain	-	-	27.1%	32.7%
Survey of Patients' Hospital Experiences				
Area Around Room 'Always' Quiet at Night	300+	60%	-	58%
Doctors 'Always' Communicated Well	300+	88%	-	80%
Home Recovery Information Given	300+	90%	-	82%
Hospital Given 9 or 10 on 10 Point Scale	300+	71%	-	67%
Meds 'Always' Explained Before Given	300+	66%	-	60%
Nurses 'Always' Communicated Well	300+	82%	-	76%
Pain 'Always' Well Controlled	300+	72%	-	69%
Room and Bathroom 'Always' Clean	300+	82%	-	71%
Timely Help 'Always' Received	300+	75%	-	64%
Would Definitely Recommend Hospital	300+	70%	-	69%

Gifford Medical Center

44 South Main Street
Randolph, VT 05060
Phone: 802-728-4441
Fax: 802-728-4245
E-mail: info@giffordmed.org
URL: www.giffordmed.org
Type: Critical Access Hospitals
Emergency Services: Yes
Ownership: Voluntary Non-Profit - Other
Beds: 55

Key Personnel:

CEO/President. . . . . Joseph Woodin
Chief of Medical Staff . . . . Louis DiNicola, MD
Infection Control. . . . . D Simpson, RN
Radiology. . . . . Erin M Tsai
Emergency Room . . . . Larry Ermold

Measure	Cases	This Hosp.	State Avg.	U.S. Avg.
Heart Attack Care				
ACE Inhibitor or ARB for LVSD[1]	2	100%	97%	96%
Aspirin at Arrival[1]	7	100%	99%	99%
Aspirin at Discharge[1]	6	100%	99%	98%
Beta Blocker at Discharge[1]	5	100%	99%	98%
Fibrinolytic Medication Timing[3]	0	-	0%	55%
PCI Within 90 Minutes of Arrival[3]	0	-	-	90%
Smoking Cessation Advice[1]	2	100%	100%	99%
Chest Pain/Possible Heart Attack Care				
Aspirin at Arrival	-	-	99%	95%
Median Time to ECG (minutes)	-	-	6	8
Median Time to Transfer (minutes)	-	-	34	61
Fibrinolytic Medication Timing	-	-	71%	54%
Heart Failure Care				
ACE Inhibitor or ARB for LVSD[1]	5	100%	94%	94%
Discharge Instructions	44	100%	87%	88%
Evaluation of LVS Function	56	84%	98%	98%
Smoking Cessation Advice[1]	4	100%	99%	98%
Pneumonia Care				
Appropriate Initial Antibiotic	36	97%	95%	92%
Blood Culture Timing	42	100%	96%	96%
Influenza Vaccine	38	84%	93%	91%
Initial Antibiotic Timing	58	98%	97%	95%
Pneumococcal Vaccine	52	92%	95%	93%
Smoking Cessation Advice[1]	13	100%	97%	97%
Surgical Care Improvement Project				
Appropriate VTP Within 24 Hours[1]	20	100%	96%	92%
Appropriate Hair Removal	80	100%	100%	99%
Appropriate Beta Blocker Usage[1,3]	5	100%	91%	93%
Controlled Postoperative Blood Glucose	0	-	90%	93%
Prophylactic Antibiotic Timing	77	91%	97%	97%
Prophylactic Antibiotic Timing (Outpatient)	-	-	94%	92%
Prophylactic Antibiotic Selection	77	100%	99%	97%
Prophylactic Antibiotic Select. (Outpatient)	-	-	97%	94%
Prophylactic Antibiotic Stopped	75	96%	97%	94%
Recommended VTP Ordered[1]	20	100%	96%	94%
Urinary Catheter Removal	31	100%	97%	90%
Children's Asthma Care				
Received Systemic Corticosteroids	-	-	-	100%
Received Home Management Plan	-	-	-	71%
Received Reliever Medication	-	-	-	100%
Use of Medical Imaging				
Combination Abdominal CT Scan	-	-	0.086	0.191
Combination Chest CT Scan	-	-	0.015	0.054
Follow-up Mammogram/Ultrasound	-	-	8.7%	8.4%
MRI for Low Back Pain	-	-	27.1%	32.7%
Survey of Patients' Hospital Experiences				
Area Around Room 'Always' Quiet at Night	300+	61%	-	58%
Doctors 'Always' Communicated Well	300+	80%	-	80%
Home Recovery Information Given	300+	87%	-	82%
Hospital Given 9 or 10 on 10 Point Scale	300+	75%	-	67%
Meds 'Always' Explained Before Given	300+	66%	-	60%
Nurses 'Always' Communicated Well	300+	79%	-	76%
Pain 'Always' Well Controlled	300+	72%	-	69%
Room and Bathroom 'Always' Clean	300+	72%	-	71%
Timely Help 'Always' Received	300+	70%	-	64%
Would Definitely Recommend Hospital	300+	76%	-	69%

Rutland Regional Medical Center

160 Allen St
Rutland, VT 05701
Phone: 802-775-7111
Fax: 802-747-6207
URL: www.rrmc.org
Type: Acute Care Hospitals
Emergency Services: Yes
Ownership: Voluntary Non-Profit - Private
Beds: 188

Key Personnel:

CEO/President. . . . . Thomas W Huebner
Chief of Medical Staff . . . . Richard D Lovett, MD
Operating Room. . . . . Carol Welsh, RN
Pediatric Ambulatory Care . . . . . . David Schneider, DO
Pediatric In-Patient Care . . . . David Schneider, DO
Quality Assurance . . . . Linda McElhinney
Radiology. . . . . Jean-Christophe Bieb, MD

Measure	Cases	This Hosp.	State Avg.	U.S. Avg.
Heart Attack Care				
ACE Inhibitor or ARB for LVSD[1]	7	100%	97%	96%
Aspirin at Arrival	61	97%	99%	99%
Aspirin at Discharge	45	96%	99%	98%
Beta Blocker at Discharge	44	100%	99%	98%
Fibrinolytic Medication Timing[1]	2	0%	0%	55%
PCI Within 90 Minutes of Arrival	0	-	-	90%
Smoking Cessation Advice[1]	9	100%	100%	99%
Chest Pain/Possible Heart Attack Care				
Aspirin at Arrival	96	98%	99%	95%
Median Time to ECG (minutes)	98	6	6	8
Median Time to Transfer (minutes)[1,3]	3	193	34	61
Fibrinolytic Medication Timing[1]	19	74%	71%	54%
Heart Failure Care				
ACE Inhibitor or ARB for LVSD	38	87%	94%	94%
Discharge Instructions	109	83%	87%	88%
Evaluation of LVS Function	144	100%	98%	98%
Smoking Cessation Advice[1]	13	92%	99%	98%
Pneumonia Care				
Appropriate Initial Antibiotic	123	92%	95%	92%
Blood Culture Timing	194	94%	96%	96%
Influenza Vaccine	112	89%	93%	91%
Initial Antibiotic Timing	203	94%	97%	95%
Pneumococcal Vaccine	201	94%	95%	93%
Smoking Cessation Advice	71	93%	97%	97%
Surgical Care Improvement Project				
Appropriate VTP Within 24 Hours[2]	161	94%	96%	92%
Appropriate Hair Removal[2]	601	100%	100%	99%
Appropriate Beta Blocker Usage[2]	202	81%	91%	93%
Controlled Postoperative Blood Glucose[2]	0	-	90%	93%
Prophylactic Antibiotic Timing[2]	449	98%	97%	97%
Prophylactic Antibiotic Timing (Outpatient)	169	91%	94%	92%
Prophylactic Antibiotic Selection[2]	450	99%	99%	97%
Prophylactic Antibiotic Select. (Outpatient)	161	98%	97%	94%
Prophylactic Antibiotic Stopped[2]	439	97%	97%	94%
Recommended VTP Ordered[2]	161	95%	96%	94%
Urinary Catheter Removal[2]	111	90%	97%	90%
Children's Asthma Care				
Received Systemic Corticosteroids	-	-	-	100%
Received Home Management Plan	-	-	-	71%
Received Reliever Medication	-	-	-	100%
Use of Medical Imaging				
Combination Abdominal CT Scan	677	0.046	0.086	0.191
Combination Chest CT Scan	501	0.042	0.015	0.054
Follow-up Mammogram/Ultrasound	1,798	3.8%	8.7%	8.4%
MRI for Low Back Pain	264	29.5%	27.1%	32.7%
Survey of Patients' Hospital Experiences				
Area Around Room 'Always' Quiet at Night	300+	49%	-	58%
Doctors 'Always' Communicated Well	300+	79%	-	80%
Home Recovery Information Given	300+	86%	-	82%
Hospital Given 9 or 10 on 10 Point Scale	300+	64%	-	67%
Meds 'Always' Explained Before Given	300+	59%	-	60%
Nurses 'Always' Communicated Well	300+	76%	-	76%
Pain 'Always' Well Controlled	300+	74%	-	69%
Room and Bathroom 'Always' Clean	300+	71%	-	71%
Timely Help 'Always' Received	300+	69%	-	64%
Would Definitely Recommend Hospital	300+	63%	-	69%

NOTE: Hospital profiles are in alphabetical order by state, then city, then hospital within the city; Rankings exclude hospitals with less than 25 cases except for patient surveys which excludes hospitals with less than 100 cases; (a) 100–299 cases; (1) The number of cases is too small to be sure how well a hospital is performing; (2) The hospital indicated that the data submitted for this measure were based on a sample of cases; (3) Data was collected during a shorter time period (fewer quarters) than the maximum possible time for this measure; (4) Suppressed for one or more quarters by CMS; (5) No data is available from the hospital for this measure; (6) Fewer than 100 patients completed the HCAHPS survey. Use these rates with caution, as the number of surveys may be too low to reliably assess hospital performance; (7) Survey results are based on less than 12 months of data; (8) Survey results are not available for this reporting period; (9) No or very few patients were eligible for the HCAHPS survey. The scores shown, if any, reflect a very small number of surveys; (10) A state average was not calculated because too few hospitals in the state submitted data; (11) There were discrepancies in the data collection process; Please refer to the User's Guide for a full explanation of data.

Northwestern Medical Center

133 Fairfield Street
Saint Albans, VT 05478
E-mail: insights@nmcinc.org
URL: www.northwesternmedicalcenter.org
Type: Acute Care Hospitals
Ownership: Voluntary Non-Profit - Other

Phone: 802-524-1231
Fax: 802-524-1238

Emergency Services: Yes
Beds: 70

Key Personnel:
CEO/President . . . . Peter Hofstetter
Chief of Medical Staff . . . . James Duncan
Quality Assurance . . . . Jane Catton
Radiology. . . . . Luis Gonzalez
Emergency Room . . . . Ed Haak, MD

Measure	Cases	This Hosp.	State Avg.	U.S. Avg.
Heart Attack Care				
ACE Inhibitor or ARB for LVSD[1]	5	100%	97%	96%
Aspirin at Arrival[1]	22	100%	99%	99%
Aspirin at Discharge[1]	17	94%	99%	98%
Beta Blocker at Discharge[1]	19	100%	99%	98%
Fibrinolytic Medication Timing	0	-	0%	55%
PCI Within 90 Minutes of Arrival	0	-	-	90%
Smoking Cessation Advice[1]	1	100%	100%	99%
Chest Pain/Possible Heart Attack Care				
Aspirin at Arrival	127	99%	99%	95%
Median Time to ECG (minutes)	133	4	6	8
Median Time to Transfer (minutes)[1]	17	31	34	61
Fibrinolytic Medication Timing	0	-	71%	54%
Heart Failure Care				
ACE Inhibitor or ARB for LVSD[1]	3	100%	94%	94%
Discharge Instructions	32	78%	87%	88%
Evaluation of LVS Function	39	100%	98%	98%
Smoking Cessation Advice[1]	12	100%	99%	98%
Pneumonia Care				
Appropriate Initial Antibiotic	85	96%	95%	92%
Blood Culture Timing	115	98%	96%	96%
Influenza Vaccine	67	96%	93%	91%
Initial Antibiotic Timing	109	100%	97%	95%
Pneumococcal Vaccine	98	97%	95%	93%
Smoking Cessation Advice	27	93%	97%	97%
Surgical Care Improvement Project				
Appropriate VTP Within 24 Hours	38	92%	96%	92%
Appropriate Hair Removal	183	100%	100%	99%
Appropriate Beta Blocker Usage	46	96%	91%	93%
Controlled Postoperative Blood Glucose	0	-	90%	93%
Prophylactic Antibiotic Timing	144	99%	97%	97%
Prophylactic Antibiotic Timing (Outpatient)	144	96%	94%	92%
Prophylactic Antibiotic Selection	144	99%	99%	97%
Prophylactic Antibiotic Select. (Outpatient)	138	96%	97%	94%
Prophylactic Antibiotic Stopped	140	96%	97%	94%
Recommended VTP Ordered	39	90%	96%	94%
Urinary Catheter Removal	32	100%	97%	90%
Children's Asthma Care				
Received Systemic Corticosteroids	-	-	-	100%
Received Home Management Plan	-	-	-	71%
Received Reliever Medication	-	-	-	100%
Use of Medical Imaging				
Combination Abdominal CT Scan	538	0.110	0.086	0.191
Combination Chest CT Scan	346	0.017	0.015	0.054
Follow-up Mammogram/Ultrasound	920	11.7%	8.7%	8.4%
MRI for Low Back Pain	63	36.5%	27.1%	32.7%
Survey of Patients' Hospital Experiences				
Area Around Room 'Always' Quiet at Night	300+	61%	-	58%
Doctors 'Always' Communicated Well	300+	82%	-	80%
Home Recovery Information Given	300+	88%	-	82%
Hospital Given 9 or 10 on 10 Point Scale	300+	74%	-	67%
Meds 'Always' Explained Before Given	300+	66%	-	60%
Nurses 'Always' Communicated Well	300+	82%	-	76%
Pain 'Always' Well Controlled	300+	74%	-	69%
Room and Bathroom 'Always' Clean	300+	83%	-	71%
Timely Help 'Always' Received	300+	70%	-	64%
Would Definitely Recommend Hospital	300+	79%	-	69%

Northeastern Vermont Regional Hospital

1315 Hospital Drive
Saint Johnsbury, VT 05819
URL: www.nvrh.org
Type: Critical Access Hospitals
Ownership: Voluntary Non-Profit - Private

Phone: 802-748-7400
Fax: 802-748-7398

Emergency Services: Yes
Beds: 100

Key Personnel:
CEO/President . . . . Paul Bengtson
Cardiac Laboratory. . . . . Mark Heipzman
Chief of Medical Staff . . . . Craig Schein, MD
Infection Control. . . . . Colleen Sinon
Operating Room. . . . . Dolores Vieua
Quality Assurance . . . . Colleen Sinon
Radiology. . . . . Richard Bennum
Emergency Room . . . . Stanley Baker

Measure	Cases	This Hosp.	State Avg.	U.S. Avg.
Heart Attack Care				
ACE Inhibitor or ARB for LVSD[1]	2	50%	97%	96%
Aspirin at Arrival[1]	12	100%	99%	99%
Aspirin at Discharge[1]	10	90%	99%	98%
Beta Blocker at Discharge[1]	11	100%	99%	98%
Fibrinolytic Medication Timing	0	-	0%	55%
PCI Within 90 Minutes of Arrival	0	-	-	90%
Smoking Cessation Advice	0	-	100%	99%
Chest Pain/Possible Heart Attack Care				
Aspirin at Arrival	-	-	99%	95%
Median Time to ECG (minutes)	-	-	6	8
Median Time to Transfer (minutes)	-	-	34	61
Fibrinolytic Medication Timing	-	-	71%	54%
Heart Failure Care				
ACE Inhibitor or ARB for LVSD[1]	13	100%	94%	94%
Discharge Instructions	33	52%	87%	88%
Evaluation of LVS Function	41	100%	98%	98%
Smoking Cessation Advice[1]	2	100%	99%	98%
Pneumonia Care				
Appropriate Initial Antibiotic	53	87%	95%	92%
Blood Culture Timing	62	95%	96%	96%
Influenza Vaccine	36	100%	93%	91%
Initial Antibiotic Timing	70	97%	97%	95%
Pneumococcal Vaccine	59	100%	95%	93%
Smoking Cessation Advice[1]	14	93%	97%	97%
Surgical Care Improvement Project				
Appropriate VTP Within 24 Hours[2]	103	86%	96%	92%
Appropriate Hair Removal[2]	126	100%	100%	99%
Appropriate Beta Blocker Usage[2]	33	91%	91%	93%
Controlled Postoperative Blood Glucose[2]	0	-	90%	93%
Prophylactic Antibiotic Timing[2]	97	100%	97%	97%
Prophylactic Antibiotic Timing (Outpatient)	-	-	94%	92%
Prophylactic Antibiotic Selection[2]	97	99%	99%	97%
Prophylactic Antibiotic Select. (Outpatient)	-	-	97%	94%
Prophylactic Antibiotic Stopped[2]	97	98%	97%	94%
Recommended VTP Ordered[2]	103	88%	96%	94%
Urinary Catheter Removal[2]	39	97%	97%	90%
Children's Asthma Care				
Received Systemic Corticosteroids	-	-	-	100%
Received Home Management Plan	-	-	-	71%
Received Reliever Medication	-	-	-	100%
Use of Medical Imaging				
Combination Abdominal CT Scan	-	-	0.086	0.191
Combination Chest CT Scan	-	-	0.015	0.054
Follow-up Mammogram/Ultrasound	-	-	8.7%	8.4%
MRI for Low Back Pain	-	-	27.1%	32.7%
Survey of Patients' Hospital Experiences				
Area Around Room 'Always' Quiet at Night	300+	57%	-	58%
Doctors 'Always' Communicated Well	300+	85%	-	80%
Home Recovery Information Given	300+	87%	-	82%
Hospital Given 9 or 10 on 10 Point Scale	300+	69%	-	67%
Meds 'Always' Explained Before Given	300+	67%	-	60%
Nurses 'Always' Communicated Well	300+	79%	-	76%
Pain 'Always' Well Controlled	300+	72%	-	69%
Room and Bathroom 'Always' Clean	300+	83%	-	71%
Timely Help 'Always' Received	300+	72%	-	64%
Would Definitely Recommend Hospital	300+	73%	-	69%

Springfield Hospital

PO Box 2003
Springfield, VT 05156
Type: Critical Access Hospitals
Ownership: Voluntary Non-Profit - Private

Phone: 802-885-2151
Fax: 802-885-3959

Emergency Services: Yes
Beds: 69

Key Personnel:
CEO/President . . . . Thomas Crawford
Chief of Medical Staff . . . . Karen Clay, MD
Infection Control. . . . . Becky Howe
Operating Room. . . . . Eric Warren, BSN
Quality Assurance . . . . Pam Brown
Radiology. . . . . Thomas E Brennan

Measure	Cases	This Hosp.	State Avg.	U.S. Avg.
Heart Attack Care				
ACE Inhibitor or ARB for LVSD[1]	1	100%	97%	96%
Aspirin at Arrival[1]	11	100%	99%	99%
Aspirin at Discharge[1]	9	100%	99%	98%
Beta Blocker at Discharge[1]	8	100%	99%	98%
Fibrinolytic Medication Timing	0	-	0%	55%
PCI Within 90 Minutes of Arrival	0	-	-	90%
Smoking Cessation Advice	0	-	100%	99%
Chest Pain/Possible Heart Attack Care				
Aspirin at Arrival	-	-	99%	95%
Median Time to ECG (minutes)	-	-	6	8
Median Time to Transfer (minutes)	-	-	34	61
Fibrinolytic Medication Timing	-	-	71%	54%
Heart Failure Care				
ACE Inhibitor or ARB for LVSD[1]	18	94%	94%	94%
Discharge Instructions	45	100%	87%	88%
Evaluation of LVS Function	62	100%	98%	98%
Smoking Cessation Advice[1]	2	100%	99%	98%
Pneumonia Care				
Appropriate Initial Antibiotic	112	96%	95%	92%
Blood Culture Timing	150	100%	96%	96%
Influenza Vaccine	91	100%	93%	91%
Initial Antibiotic Timing	145	100%	97%	95%
Pneumococcal Vaccine	124	100%	95%	93%
Smoking Cessation Advice	41	100%	97%	97%
Surgical Care Improvement Project				
Appropriate VTP Within 24 Hours[2]	35	100%	96%	92%
Appropriate Hair Removal[2]	100	100%	100%	99%
Appropriate Beta Blocker Usage[2]	38	100%	91%	93%
Controlled Postoperative Blood Glucose[2]	0	-	90%	93%
Prophylactic Antibiotic Timing[2]	73	99%	97%	97%
Prophylactic Antibiotic Timing (Outpatient)	-	-	94%	92%
Prophylactic Antibiotic Selection[2]	73	100%	99%	97%
Prophylactic Antibiotic Select. (Outpatient)	-	-	97%	94%
Prophylactic Antibiotic Stopped[2]	73	100%	97%	94%
Recommended VTP Ordered[2]	35	100%	96%	94%
Urinary Catheter Removal[2]	38	100%	97%	90%
Children's Asthma Care				
Received Systemic Corticosteroids	-	-	-	100%
Received Home Management Plan	-	-	-	71%
Received Reliever Medication	-	-	-	100%
Use of Medical Imaging				
Combination Abdominal CT Scan	-	-	0.086	0.191
Combination Chest CT Scan	-	-	0.015	0.054
Follow-up Mammogram/Ultrasound	-	-	8.7%	8.4%
MRI for Low Back Pain	-	-	27.1%	32.7%
Survey of Patients' Hospital Experiences				
Area Around Room 'Always' Quiet at Night	300+	52%	-	58%
Doctors 'Always' Communicated Well	300+	83%	-	80%
Home Recovery Information Given	300+	84%	-	82%
Hospital Given 9 or 10 on 10 Point Scale	300+	65%	-	67%
Meds 'Always' Explained Before Given	300+	67%	-	60%
Nurses 'Always' Communicated Well	300+	82%	-	76%
Pain 'Always' Well Controlled	300+	72%	-	69%
Room and Bathroom 'Always' Clean	300+	79%	-	71%
Timely Help 'Always' Received	300+	75%	-	64%
Would Definitely Recommend Hospital	300+	65%	-	69%

NOTE: Hospital profiles are in alphabetical order by state, then city, then hospital within the city; Rankings exclude hospitals with less than 25 cases except for patient surveys which excludes hospitals with less than 100 cases; (a) 100–299 cases; (1) The number of cases is too small to be sure how well a hospital is performing; (2) The hospital indicated that the data submitted for this measure were based on a sample of cases; (3) Data was collected during a shorter time period (fewer quarters) than the maximum possible time for this measure; (4) Suppressed for one or more quarters by CMS; (5) No data is available from the hospital for this measure; (6) Fewer than 100 patients completed the HCAHPS survey. Use these rates with caution, as the number of surveys may be too low to reliably assess hospital performance; (7) Survey results are based on less than 12 months of data; (8) Survey results are not available for this reporting period; (9) No or very few patients were eligible for the HCAHPS survey. The scores shown, if any, reflect a very small number of surveys; (10) A state average was not calculated because too few hospitals in the state submitted data; (11) There were discrepancies in the data collection process; Please refer to the User's Guide for a full explanation of data.

Grace Cottage Hospital

PO Box 216
Townshend, VT 05353
Phone: 802-365-7920
Fax: 802-365-7031
E-mail: info@gracecottage.org
URL: www.gracecottage.org
Type: Critical Access Hospitals
Emergency Services: Yes
Ownership: Proprietary
Beds: 19

Key Personnel:
CEO/President. . . . . Michael Brant
Chief of Medical Staff. . . . . Timothy Shafer
Quality Assurance . . . . Mary Morgan
Radiology. . . . . Edward Elliott

Measure	Cases	This Hosp.	State Avg.	U.S. Avg.
Heart Attack Care				
ACE Inhibitor or ARB for LVSD[5]	0	-	97%	96%
Aspirin at Arrival[5]	0	-	99%	99%
Aspirin at Discharge[5]	0	-	99%	98%
Beta Blocker at Discharge[5]	0	-	99%	98%
Fibrinolytic Medication Timing[5]	0	-	0%	55%
PCI Within 90 Minutes of Arrival[5]	0	-	-	90%
Smoking Cessation Advice[5]	0	-	100%	99%
Chest Pain/Possible Heart Attack Care				
Aspirin at Arrival	-	-	99%	95%
Median Time to ECG (minutes)	-	-	6	8
Median Time to Transfer (minutes)	-	-	34	61
Fibrinolytic Medication Timing	-	-	71%	54%
Heart Failure Care				
ACE Inhibitor or ARB for LVSD[1]	1	100%	94%	94%
Discharge Instructions[1]	4	75%	87%	88%
Evaluation of LVS Function[1]	5	80%	98%	98%
Smoking Cessation Advice[1]	1	100%	99%	98%
Pneumonia Care				
Appropriate Initial Antibiotic[1]	15	93%	95%	92%
Blood Culture Timing[1]	7	100%	96%	96%
Influenza Vaccine[1]	14	100%	93%	91%
Initial Antibiotic Timing[1]	17	88%	97%	95%
Pneumococcal Vaccine[1]	20	100%	95%	93%
Smoking Cessation Advice[1]	4	100%	97%	97%
Surgical Care Improvement Project				
Appropriate VTP Within 24 Hours[5]	0	-	96%	92%
Appropriate Hair Removal[5]	0	-	100%	99%
Appropriate Beta Blocker Usage[5]	0	-	91%	93%
Controlled Postoperative Blood Glucose[5]	0	-	90%	93%
Prophylactic Antibiotic Timing[5]	0	-	97%	97%
Prophylactic Antibiotic Timing (Outpatient)	-	-	94%	92%
Prophylactic Antibiotic Selection[5]	0	-	99%	97%
Prophylactic Antibiotic Select. (Outpatient)	-	-	97%	94%
Prophylactic Antibiotic Stopped[5]	0	-	97%	94%
Recommended VTP Ordered[5]	0	-	96%	94%
Urinary Catheter Removal[5]	0	-	97%	90%
Children's Asthma Care				
Received Systemic Corticosteroids	-	-	-	100%
Received Home Management Plan	-	-	-	71%
Received Reliever Medication	-	-	-	100%
Use of Medical Imaging				
Combination Abdominal CT Scan	-	-	0.086	0.191
Combination Chest CT Scan	-	-	0.015	0.054
Follow-up Mammogram/Ultrasound	-	-	8.7%	8.4%
MRI for Low Back Pain	-	-	27.1%	32.7%
Survey of Patients' Hospital Experiences				
Area Around Room 'Always' Quiet at Night[6]	<100	61%	-	58%
Doctors 'Always' Communicated Well[6]	<100	88%	-	80%
Home Recovery Information Given[6]	<100	85%	-	82%
Hospital Given 9 or 10 on 10 Point Scale[6]	<100	83%	-	67%
Meds 'Always' Explained Before Given[6]	<100	66%	-	60%
Nurses 'Always' Communicated Well[6]	<100	83%	-	76%
Pain 'Always' Well Controlled[6]	<100	73%	-	69%
Room and Bathroom 'Always' Clean[6]	<100	91%	-	71%
Timely Help 'Always' Received[6]	<100	75%	-	64%
Would Definitely Recommend Hospital	<100	93%	-	69%

White River Junction VA Medical Center

215 N. Main St.
White River Junction, VT 05009
Phone: 802-295-9363
Fax: 802-296-6354
E-mail: vhawrjwww@med.va.gov
URL: www.visn1.med.va.gov/wrj
Type: Acute Care-Veterans Administration
Emergency Services: No
Ownership: Government - Federal
Beds: 60

Key Personnel:
Chief of Medical Staff . . . . Thomas Parrino, MD
Infection Control. . . . . Laura Smith, RN
Operating Room. . . . . Frank Pindyck, MD
Quality Assurance . . . . Joanne B Puckett, RN MeD
Anesthesiology. . . . . Frederick Perkins, MD
Intensive Care Unit. . . . . James Geiling, MD

Measure	Cases	This Hosp.	State Avg.	U.S. Avg.
Heart Attack Care				
ACE Inhibitor or ARB for LVSD[1]	2	100%	97%	96%
Aspirin at Arrival[1]	6	100%	99%	99%
Aspirin at Discharge[1]	4	100%	99%	98%
Beta Blocker at Discharge[1]	4	100%	99%	98%
Fibrinolytic Medication Timing[5]	0	-	0%	55%
PCI Within 90 Minutes of Arrival[5]	0	-	-	90%
Smoking Cessation Advice[5]	0	-	100%	99%
Chest Pain/Possible Heart Attack Care				
Aspirin at Arrival	-	-	99%	95%
Median Time to ECG (minutes)	-	-	6	8
Median Time to Transfer (minutes)	-	-	34	61
Fibrinolytic Medication Timing	-	-	71%	54%
Heart Failure Care				
ACE Inhibitor or ARB for LVSD	29	100%	94%	94%
Discharge Instructions	81	100%	87%	88%
Evaluation of LVS Function	88	100%	98%	98%
Smoking Cessation Advice[1]	17	100%	99%	98%
Pneumonia Care				
Appropriate Initial Antibiotic	37	89%	95%	92%
Blood Culture Timing	52	96%	96%	96%
Influenza Vaccine	38	97%	93%	91%
Initial Antibiotic Timing	25	92%	97%	95%
Pneumococcal Vaccine	60	100%	95%	93%
Smoking Cessation Advice[1]	14	100%	97%	97%
Surgical Care Improvement Project				
Appropriate VTP Within 24 Hours[2]	91	100%	96%	92%
Appropriate Hair Removal[2]	127	100%	100%	99%
Appropriate Beta Blocker Usage[2]	66	97%	91%	93%
Controlled Postoperative Blood Glucose[2,5]	0	-	90%	93%
Prophylactic Antibiotic Timing	63	100%	97%	97%
Prophylactic Antibiotic Timing (Outpatient)	-	-	94%	92%
Prophylactic Antibiotic Selection	64	94%	99%	97%
Prophylactic Antibiotic Select. (Outpatient)	-	-	97%	94%
Prophylactic Antibiotic Stopped	60	98%	97%	94%
Recommended VTP Ordered[2]	91	100%	96%	94%
Urinary Catheter Removal[2]	48	98%	97%	90%
Children's Asthma Care				
Received Systemic Corticosteroids	-	-	-	100%
Received Home Management Plan	-	-	-	71%
Received Reliever Medication	-	-	-	100%
Use of Medical Imaging				
Combination Abdominal CT Scan	-	-	0.086	0.191
Combination Chest CT Scan	-	-	0.015	0.054
Follow-up Mammogram/Ultrasound	-	-	8.7%	8.4%
MRI for Low Back Pain	-	-	27.1%	32.7%
Survey of Patients' Hospital Experiences				
Area Around Room 'Always' Quiet at Night	-	-	-	58%
Doctors 'Always' Communicated Well	-	-	-	80%
Home Recovery Information Given	-	-	-	82%
Hospital Given 9 or 10 on 10 Point Scale	-	-	-	67%
Meds 'Always' Explained Before Given	-	-	-	60%
Nurses 'Always' Communicated Well	-	-	-	76%
Pain 'Always' Well Controlled	-	-	-	69%
Room and Bathroom 'Always' Clean	-	-	-	71%
Timely Help 'Always' Received	-	-	-	64%
Would Definitely Recommend Hospital	-	-	-	69%

Mount Ascutney Hospital

289 County Road
Windsor, VT 05089
Phone: 802-674-6711
Fax: 802-674-7155
URL: www.mtascutneyhospital.org
Type: Critical Access Hospitals
Emergency Services: Yes
Ownership: Voluntary Non-Profit - Private
Beds: 91

Key Personnel:
CEO/President. . . . . Richard Slusky
Cardiac Laboratory. . . . . J Jones
Chief of Medical Staff. . . . . David Russo
Infection Control. . . . . Mary Lou Campbell
Operating Room. . . . . Julie Weld, RN
Quality Assurance . . . . Cheryl Briere
Radiology. . . . . Robert M Friedlander, MD
Intensive Care Unit. . . . . William Palmer

Measure	Cases	This Hosp.	State Avg.	U.S. Avg.
Heart Attack Care				
ACE Inhibitor or ARB for LVSD[3]	0	-	97%	96%
Aspirin at Arrival[1,3]	1	100%	99%	99%
Aspirin at Discharge[3]	0	-	99%	98%
Beta Blocker at Discharge[3]	0	-	99%	98%
Fibrinolytic Medication Timing[3]	0	-	0%	55%
PCI Within 90 Minutes of Arrival[3]	0	-	-	90%
Smoking Cessation Advice[3]	0	-	100%	99%
Chest Pain/Possible Heart Attack Care				
Aspirin at Arrival	-	-	99%	95%
Median Time to ECG (minutes)	-	-	6	8
Median Time to Transfer (minutes)	-	-	34	61
Fibrinolytic Medication Timing	-	-	71%	54%
Heart Failure Care				
ACE Inhibitor or ARB for LVSD[1]	4	75%	94%	94%
Discharge Instructions[1]	12	75%	87%	88%
Evaluation of LVS Function[1]	24	100%	98%	98%
Smoking Cessation Advice[1]	1	100%	99%	98%
Pneumonia Care				
Appropriate Initial Antibiotic	27	100%	95%	92%
Blood Culture Timing	29	100%	96%	96%
Influenza Vaccine[1]	16	88%	93%	91%
Initial Antibiotic Timing	33	94%	97%	95%
Pneumococcal Vaccine	39	92%	95%	93%
Smoking Cessation Advice[1]	5	40%	97%	97%
Surgical Care Improvement Project				
Appropriate VTP Within 24 Hours[1]	21	95%	96%	92%
Appropriate Hair Removal	32	100%	100%	99%
Appropriate Beta Blocker Usage[1]	14	71%	91%	93%
Controlled Postoperative Blood Glucose	0	-	90%	93%
Prophylactic Antibiotic Timing	29	97%	97%	97%
Prophylactic Antibiotic Timing (Outpatient)	-	-	94%	92%
Prophylactic Antibiotic Selection	29	97%	99%	97%
Prophylactic Antibiotic Select. (Outpatient)	-	-	97%	94%
Prophylactic Antibiotic Stopped	28	96%	97%	94%
Recommended VTP Ordered[1]	21	95%	96%	94%
Urinary Catheter Removal[1]	10	100%	97%	90%
Children's Asthma Care				
Received Systemic Corticosteroids	-	-	-	100%
Received Home Management Plan	-	-	-	71%
Received Reliever Medication	-	-	-	100%
Use of Medical Imaging				
Combination Abdominal CT Scan	-	-	0.086	0.191
Combination Chest CT Scan	-	-	0.015	0.054
Follow-up Mammogram/Ultrasound	-	-	8.7%	8.4%
MRI for Low Back Pain	-	-	27.1%	32.7%
Survey of Patients' Hospital Experiences				
Area Around Room 'Always' Quiet at Night	(a)	50%	-	58%
Doctors 'Always' Communicated Well	(a)	85%	-	80%
Home Recovery Information Given	(a)	88%	-	82%
Hospital Given 9 or 10 on 10 Point Scale	(a)	73%	-	67%
Meds 'Always' Explained Before Given	(a)	67%	-	60%
Nurses 'Always' Communicated Well	(a)	79%	-	76%
Pain 'Always' Well Controlled	(a)	78%	-	69%
Room and Bathroom 'Always' Clean	(a)	81%	-	71%
Timely Help 'Always' Received	(a)	69%	-	64%
Would Definitely Recommend Hospital	(a)	81%	-	69%

NOTE: Hospital profiles are in alphabetical order by state, then city, then hospital within the city; Rankings exclude hospitals with less than 25 cases except for patient surveys which excludes hospitals with less than 100 cases; (a) 100–299 cases; (1) The number of cases is too small to be sure how well a hospital is performing; (2) The hospital indicated that the data submitted for this measure were based on a sample of cases; (3) Data was collected during a shorter time period (fewer quarters) than the maximum possible time for this measure; (4) Suppressed for one or more quarters by CMS; (5) No data is available from the hospital for this measure; (6) Fewer than 100 patients completed the HCAHPS survey. Use these rates with caution, as the number of surveys may be too low to reliably assess hospital performance; (7) Survey results are based on less than 12 months of data; (8) Survey results are not available for this reporting period; (9) No or very few patients were eligible for the HCAHPS survey. The scores shown, if any, reflect a very small number of surveys; (10) A state average was not calculated because too few hospitals in the state submitted data; (11) There were discrepancies in the data collection process; Please refer to the User's Guide for a full explanation of data.

Heart Attack Care

1. ACE Inhibitor or ARB for LVSD

Hospital Name	City	Rate	Cases
Bon Secours - Maryview Medical Center	Portsmouth	100%	43
Bon Secours - Memorial Regional Medical[2]	Mechanicsville	100%	88
Bon Secours - St Francis Medical Center	Midlothian	100%	29
Bon Secours - St Marys Hospital of Richmond	Richmond	100%	58
Chesapeake General Hospital	Chesapeake	100%	46
CJW Medical Center	Richmond	100%	93
Henrico Doctors' Hospital	Richmond	100%	53
Inova Fairfax Hospital[2]	Falls Church	100%	31
Lewis-Gale Medical Center	Salem	100%	55
Martha Jefferson Hospital	Charlottesville	100%	36
Riverside Regional Medical Center	Newport News	100%	52
Sentara Virginia Beach General Hospital	Virginia Beach	100%	63
Winchester Medical Center[2]	Winchester	100%	67
Mary Washington Hospital	Fredericksburg	99%	75
Sentara Norfolk General Hospital	Norfolk	99%	87
Rockingham Memorial Hospital	Harrisonburg	98%	44
University of Virginia Medical Center[2]	Charlottesville	98%	65
Centra Health	Lynchburg	97%	72
Virginia Hospital Center - Arlington	Arlington	96%	28
Carilion Medical Center	Roanoke	95%	228
Southside Regional Medical Center	Petersburg	95%	42
Inova Alexandria Hospital	Alexandria	94%	34
Virginia Commonwealth Univ Health Sys	Richmond	90%	93

2. Aspirin at Arrival

Hospital Name	City	Rate	Cases
Augusta Health	Fishersville	100%	129
Bon Secours - Maryview Medical Center	Portsmouth	100%	207
Bon Secours - Memorial Regional Medical[2]	Mechanicsville	100%	323
Centra Health	Lynchburg	100%	479
CJW Medical Center	Richmond	100%	376
Clinch Valley Medical Center	Richlands	100%	33
Community Memorial Healthcenter	South Hill	100%	54
The Fauquier Hospital	Warrenton	100%	28
Halifax Regional Hospital	Halifax	100%	58
Henrico Doctors' Hospital	Richmond	100%	180
Inova Fairfax Hospital[2]	Falls Church	100%	150
Inova Loudoun Hospital	Leesburg	100%	95
Inova Mount Vernon Hospital	Alexandria	100%	44
John Randolph Medical Center	Hopewell	100%	43
Lewis-Gale Medical Center	Salem	100%	203
Mary Immaculate Hospital	Newport News	100%	93
Mary Washington Hospital	Fredericksburg	100%	473
Montgomery Regional Hospital	Blacksburg	100%	61
Pulaski Community Hospital	Pulaski	100%	53
Reston Hospital Center	Reston	100%	103
Riverside Regional Medical Center	Newport News	100%	241
Salem VA Medical Center	Salem	100%	43
Sentara Bayside Hospital	Virginia Beach	100%	80
Sentara Careplex Hospital	Hampton	100%	150
Sentara Norfolk General Hospital	Norfolk	100%	133
Sentara Virginia Beach General Hospital	Virginia Beach	100%	196
Sentara Williamsburg Regional Med Ctr	Williamsburg	100%	120
Virginia Hospital Center - Arlington	Arlington	100%	185
Winchester Medical Center[2]	Winchester	100%	157
Bon Secours - St Francis Medical Center	Midlothian	99%	116
Bon Secours - St Marys Hospital of Richmond	Richmond	99%	195
Carilion Medical Center	Roanoke	99%	560
Danville Regional Medical Center	Danville	99%	166
Potomac Hospital	Woodbridge	99%	108
Rockingham Memorial Hospital	Harrisonburg	99%	349
Sentara Leigh Hospital	Norfolk	99%	110
University of Virginia Medical Center[2]	Charlottesville	99%	161
Virginia Commonwealth Univ Health Sys	Richmond	99%	255
Chesapeake General Hospital	Chesapeake	98%	267
Martha Jefferson Hospital	Charlottesville	98%	164
Richmond VA Medical Center	Richmond	98%	50
Sentara Obici Hospital	Suffolk	98%	125
Southside Regional Medical Center	Petersburg	98%	213
Bon Secours - Depaul Medical Center	Norfolk	97%	143
Inova Alexandria Hospital	Alexandria	97%	204
Inova Fair Oaks Hospital	Fairfax	97%	31
Riverside Walter Reed Hospital	Gloucester	97%	39
Mem Hosp of Martinsville & Henry County	Martinsville	96%	68
Prince William Hospital	Manassas	96%	84
Southern Virginia Regional Medical Center	Emporia	96%	51
Johnston Memorial Hospital[2]	Abingdon	93%	55
Wellmont Lonesome Pine Hospital	Big Stone Gap	93%	44

3. Aspirin at Discharge

Hospital Name	City	Rate	Cases
Bon Secours - Maryview Medical Center	Portsmouth	100%	227
Bon Secours - Memorial Regional Medical[2]	Mechanicsville	100%	319
Bon Secours - St Francis Medical Center	Midlothian	100%	98
Bon Secours - St Marys Hospital of Richmond	Richmond	100%	225
Centra Health	Lynchburg	100%	572
Chesapeake General Hospital	Chesapeake	100%	229
CJW Medical Center	Richmond	100%	435
Community Memorial Healthcenter	South Hill	100%	42
Halifax Regional Hospital	Halifax	100%	41
Henrico Doctors' Hospital	Richmond	100%	276
John Randolph Medical Center	Hopewell	100%	27
Lewis-Gale Medical Center	Salem	100%	355
Mem Hosp of Martinsville & Henry County	Martinsville	100%	50
Montgomery Regional Hospital	Blacksburg	100%	42
Prince William Hospital	Manassas	100%	29
Pulaski Community Hospital	Pulaski	100%	37
Reston Hospital Center	Reston	100%	79
Riverside Regional Medical Center	Newport News	100%	350
Salem VA Medical Center	Salem	100%	32
Sentara Bayside Hospital	Virginia Beach	100%	70
Sentara Careplex Hospital	Hampton	100%	125
Sentara Virginia Beach General Hospital	Virginia Beach	100%	241
Sentara Williamsburg Regional Med Ctr	Williamsburg	100%	101
Southern Virginia Regional Medical Center	Emporia	100%	26
Virginia Hospital Center - Arlington	Arlington	100%	202
Carilion Medical Center	Roanoke	99%	1249
Inova Alexandria Hospital	Alexandria	99%	228
Inova Fairfax Hospital[2]	Falls Church	99%	280
Martha Jefferson Hospital	Charlottesville	99%	155
Rockingham Memorial Hospital	Harrisonburg	99%	344
Sentara Leigh Hospital	Norfolk	99%	83
Sentara Norfolk General Hospital	Norfolk	99%	458
University of Virginia Medical Center[2]	Charlottesville	99%	322
Winchester Medical Center[2]	Winchester	99%	333
Bon Secours - Depaul Medical Center	Norfolk	98%	127
Danville Regional Medical Center	Danville	98%	132
Inova Loudoun Hospital	Leesburg	98%	85
Mary Immaculate Hospital	Newport News	98%	85
Mary Washington Hospital	Fredericksburg	98%	515
Richmond VA Medical Center	Richmond	98%	54
Sentara Obici Hospital	Suffolk	98%	88
Virginia Commonwealth Univ Health Sys	Richmond	98%	358
Potomac Hospital	Woodbridge	96%	55
Augusta Health	Fishersville	94%	115
Southside Regional Medical Center	Petersburg	94%	200
Johnston Memorial Hospital[2]	Abingdon	91%	33
Wellmont Lonesome Pine Hospital	Big Stone Gap	88%	32

4. Beta Blocker at Discharge

Hospital Name	City	Rate	Cases
Bon Secours - Maryview Medical Center	Portsmouth	100%	220
Bon Secours - Memorial Regional Medical[2]	Mechanicsville	100%	308
Bon Secours - St Marys Hospital of Richmond	Richmond	100%	220
Chesapeake General Hospital	Chesapeake	100%	227
CJW Medical Center	Richmond	100%	401
Clinch Valley Medical Center	Richlands	100%	28
Community Memorial Healthcenter	South Hill	100%	44
Halifax Regional Hospital	Halifax	100%	39
Henrico Doctors' Hospital	Richmond	100%	259
Inova Loudoun Hospital	Leesburg	100%	86
John Randolph Medical Center	Hopewell	100%	28
Lewis-Gale Medical Center	Salem	100%	356
Montgomery Regional Hospital	Blacksburg	100%	40
Prince William Hospital	Manassas	100%	33
Pulaski Community Hospital	Pulaski	100%	45
Reston Hospital Center	Reston	100%	77
Riverside Regional Medical Center	Newport News	100%	342
Salem VA Medical Center	Salem	100%	32
Sentara Bayside Hospital	Virginia Beach	100%	70
Sentara Leigh Hospital	Norfolk	100%	80
Sentara Virginia Beach General Hospital	Virginia Beach	100%	252
Southern Virginia Regional Medical Center	Emporia	100%	28
Centra Health	Lynchburg	99%	563
Danville Regional Medical Center	Danville	99%	132
Inova Alexandria Hospital	Alexandria	99%	222
Inova Fairfax Hospital[2]	Falls Church	99%	228
Martha Jefferson Hospital	Charlottesville	99%	142
Mary Washington Hospital	Fredericksburg	99%	495
Rockingham Memorial Hospital	Harrisonburg	99%	341
Sentara Careplex Hospital	Hampton	99%	119
Sentara Norfolk General Hospital	Norfolk	99%	448
Sentara Williamsburg Regional Med Ctr	Williamsburg	99%	108
Virginia Commonwealth Univ Health Sys	Richmond	99%	328
Virginia Hospital Center - Arlington	Arlington	99%	199
Winchester Medical Center[2]	Winchester	99%	316
Carilion Medical Center	Roanoke	98%	1264
Mary Immaculate Hospital	Newport News	98%	81
Mem Hosp of Martinsville & Henry County	Martinsville	98%	52
University of Virginia Medical Center[2]	Charlottesville	98%	289
Augusta Health	Fishersville	97%	105
Bon Secours - St Francis Medical Center	Midlothian	97%	94
Potomac Hospital	Woodbridge	96%	47
Richmond VA Medical Center	Richmond	96%	51
Sentara Obici Hospital	Suffolk	96%	82
Southside Regional Medical Center	Petersburg	96%	199
Johnston Memorial Hospital[2]	Abingdon	92%	36
Wellmont Lonesome Pine Hospital	Big Stone Gap	92%	37
Bon Secours - Depaul Medical Center	Norfolk	89%	129

6. PCI Within 90 Minutes of Arrival

Hospital Name	City	Rate	Cases
Bon Secours - St Marys Hospital of Richmond	Richmond	100%	46
Henrico Doctors' Hospital	Richmond	100%	34
Inova Fairfax Hospital[2]	Falls Church	100%	33
Rockingham Memorial Hospital	Harrisonburg	100%	59
Sentara Virginia Beach General Hospital	Virginia Beach	100%	42
CJW Medical Center	Richmond	98%	62
Lewis-Gale Medical Center	Salem	98%	41
Virginia Commonwealth Univ Health Sys	Richmond	98%	57
Centra Health	Lynchburg	97%	79
Sentara Careplex Hospital	Hampton	97%	33
Sentara Williamsburg Regional Med Ctr	Williamsburg	97%	30
Mary Washington Hospital	Fredericksburg	96%	55
Bon Secours - Memorial Regional Medical[2]	Mechanicsville	95%	60
Inova Alexandria Hospital	Alexandria	94%	32
Sentara Leigh Hospital	Norfolk	94%	33
Southside Regional Medical Center	Petersburg	94%	48
Winchester Medical Center[2]	Winchester	93%	30
Riverside Regional Medical Center	Newport News	92%	36
Martha Jefferson Hospital	Charlottesville	91%	43
Bon Secours - Maryview Medical Center	Portsmouth	90%	30
Carilion Medical Center	Roanoke	88%	104
Reston Hospital Center	Reston	88%	25
Sentara Obici Hospital	Suffolk	88%	26
Chesapeake General Hospital	Chesapeake	85%	52
Virginia Hospital Center - Arlington	Arlington	83%	41
Bon Secours - Depaul Medical Center	Norfolk	82%	28
University of Virginia Medical Center[2]	Charlottesville	80%	30

7. Smoking Cessation Advice

Hospital Name	City	Rate	Cases
Augusta Health	Fishersville	100%	37
Bon Secours - Depaul Medical Center	Norfolk	100%	51
Bon Secours - Maryview Medical Center	Portsmouth	100%	81
Bon Secours - Memorial Regional Medical[2]	Mechanicsville	100%	96
Bon Secours - St Francis Medical Center	Midlothian	100%	30
Bon Secours - St Marys Hospital of Richmond	Richmond	100%	71
Carilion Medical Center	Roanoke	100%	509
Centra Health	Lynchburg	100%	222
Chesapeake General Hospital	Chesapeake	100%	88
CJW Medical Center	Richmond	100%	166
Danville Regional Medical Center	Danville	100%	55
Henrico Doctors' Hospital	Richmond	100%	114
Inova Fairfax Hospital[2]	Falls Church	100%	63
Inova Loudoun Hospital	Leesburg	100%	27
Lewis-Gale Medical Center	Salem	100%	139
Martha Jefferson Hospital	Charlottesville	100%	32
Mary Immaculate Hospital	Newport News	100%	29
Mary Washington Hospital	Fredericksburg	100%	197
Riverside Regional Medical Center	Newport News	100%	129
Rockingham Memorial Hospital	Harrisonburg	100%	105
Sentara Careplex Hospital	Hampton	100%	49
Sentara Leigh Hospital	Norfolk	100%	29
Sentara Norfolk General Hospital	Norfolk	100%	165
Sentara Obici Hospital	Suffolk	100%	35
University of Virginia Medical Center[2]	Charlottesville	100%	126
Virginia Commonwealth Univ Health Sys	Richmond	100%	160
Virginia Hospital Center - Arlington	Arlington	100%	43
Winchester Medical Center[2]	Winchester	100%	137
Southside Regional Medical Center	Petersburg	99%	92
Sentara Virginia Beach General Hospital	Virginia Beach	98%	93
Inova Alexandria Hospital	Alexandria	97%	61

Chest Pain/Possible Heart Attack Care

8. Aspirin at Arrival

Hospital Name	City	Rate	Cases
Alleghany Regional Hospital	Low Moor	100%	74
Buchanan General Hospital	Grundy	100%	61
Carilion Giles Memorial Hospital[3]	Pearisburg	100%	48
Culpeper Regional Hospital	Culpeper	100%	64
John Randolph Medical Center	Hopewell	100%	26
Mary Washington Hospital	Fredericksburg	100%	39
Pulaski Community Hospital	Pulaski	100%	59
Sentara Careplex Hospital	Hampton	100%	39
Warren Memorial Hospital	Front Royal	100%	33
Wythe County Community Hospital	Wytheville	100%	159
Augusta Health	Fishersville	99%	108
Potomac Hospital	Woodbridge	99%	157
Stafford Hospital Center	Stafford	99%	67
The Fauquier Hospital	Warrenton	98%	83
Southern Virginia Regional Medical Center	Emporia	98%	44
Twin County Regional Hospital	Galax	98%	104

NOTE: Hospital profiles are in alphabetical order by state, then city, then hospital within the city; Rankings exclude hospitals with less than 25 cases except for patient surveys which excludes hospitals with less than 100 cases; (a) 100–299 cases; (1) The number of cases is too small to be sure how well a hospital is performing; (2) The hospital indicated that the data submitted for this measure were based on a sample of cases; (3) Data was collected during a shorter time period (fewer quarters) than the maximum possible time for this measure; (4) Suppressed for one or more quarters by CMS; (5) No data is available from the hospital for this measure; (6) Fewer than 100 patients completed the HCAHPS survey. Use these rates with caution, as the number of surveys may be too low to reliably assess hospital performance; (7) Survey results are based on less than 12 months of data; (8) Survey results are not available for this reporting period; (9) No or very few patients were eligible for the HCAHPS survey. The scores shown, if any, reflect a very small number of surveys; (10) A state average was not calculated because too few hospitals in the state submitted data; (11) There were discrepancies in the data collection process; Please refer to the User's Guide for a full explanation of data.

Clinch Valley Medical Center	Richlands	97%	63
Danville Regional Medical Center	Danville	97%	35
Johnston Memorial Hospital	Abingdon	97%	206
Lee Regional Medical Center	Pennington Gap	97%	29
Rappahannock General Hospital	Kilmarnock	97%	92
Sentara Bayside Hospital	Virginia Beach	97%	226
Sentara Obici Hospital	Suffolk	97%	78
Inova Mount Vernon Hospital	Alexandria	96%	48
Prince William Hospital	Manassas	96%	153
Riverside Tappahannock Hospital	Tappahannock	96%	46
Carilion New River Valley Medical Center	Christiansburg	95%	39
Dickenson Community Hospital	Clintwood	95%	111
Mem Hosp of Martinsville & Henry County	Martinsville	95%	174
Smyth County Community Hospital	Marion	95%	39
Southampton Memorial Hospital	Franklin	95%	55
Carilion Franklin Memorial Hospital	Rocky Mount	94%	204
Community Memorial Healthcenter	South Hill	94%	97
Inova Fairfax Hospital	Falls Church	94%	207
Riverside Walter Reed Hospital	Gloucester	94%	48
Norton Community Hospital	Norton	93%	140
Wellmont Lonesome Pine Hospital	Big Stone Gap	92%	63
Halifax Regional Hospital	Halifax	91%	34
Inova Fair Oaks Hospital	Fairfax	91%	123
Inova Loudoun Hospital	Leesburg	90%	91
Southside Community Hospital	Farmville	89%	93
Riverside Shore Memorial Hospital	Nassawadox	86%	36
Bedford Memorial Hospital	Bedford	83%	64
Russell County Medical Center	Lebanon	78%	59

9. Median Time to ECG (minutes)

Hospital Name	City	Min.	Cases
Riverside Walter Reed Hospital	Gloucester	0	51
Pulaski Community Hospital	Pulaski	1	66
Riverside Tappahannock Hospital	Tappahannock	2	45
Southampton Memorial Hospital	Franklin	3	55
Halifax Regional Hospital	Halifax	4	35
Johnston Memorial Hospital	Abingdon	4	212
Prince William Hospital	Manassas	5	161
Russell County Medical Center	Lebanon	5	58
Sentara Obici Hospital	Suffolk	5	78
Southern Virginia Regional Medical Center	Emporia	5	47
Alleghany Regional Hospital	Low Moor	6	76
Dickenson Community Hospital	Clintwood	6	117
Inova Fairfax Hospital	Falls Church	6	213
Sentara Careplex Hospital	Hampton	6	47
Southside Community Hospital	Farmville	6	96
Wythe County Community Hospital	Wytheville	6	165
Buchanan General Hospital	Grundy	7	62
Inova Loudoun Hospital	Leesburg	7	98
Inova Mount Vernon Hospital	Alexandria	7	47
Augusta Health	Fishersville	8	109
Community Memorial Healthcenter	South Hill	8	95
The Fauquier Hospital	Warrenton	8	87
John Randolph Medical Center	Hopewell	8	27
Rappahannock General Hospital	Kilmarnock	8	96
Sentara Bayside Hospital	Virginia Beach	8	225
Danville Regional Medical Center	Danville	9	37
Potomac Hospital	Woodbridge	9	164
Reston Hospital Center	Reston	9	25
Twin County Regional Hospital	Galax	9	117
Bedford Memorial Hospital	Bedford	10	66
Inova Fair Oaks Hospital	Fairfax	10	133
Lee Regional Medical Center	Pennington Gap	10	34
Warren Memorial Hospital	Front Royal	10	33
Mem Hosp of Martinsville & Henry County	Martinsville	11	179
Clinch Valley Medical Center	Richlands	12	70
Mary Washington Hospital	Fredericksburg	12	40
Stafford Hospital Center	Stafford	12	68
Norton Community Hospital	Norton	14	151
Riverside Shore Memorial Hospital	Nassawadox	15	36
Culpeper Regional Hospital	Culpeper	16	68
Wellmont Lonesome Pine Hospital	Big Stone Gap	17	66
Carilion Giles Memorial Hospital[3]	Pearisburg	18	53
Smyth County Community Hospital	Marion	21	41
Carilion New River Valley Medical Center	Christiansburg	25	27
Carilion Franklin Memorial Hospital	Rocky Mount	31	221

10. Median Time to Transfer (minutes)

Hospital Name	City	Min.	Cases
Johnston Memorial Hospital	Abingdon	35	34
Prince William Hospital	Manassas	43	33
Augusta Health	Fishersville	74	33

Heart Failure Care

12. ACE Inhibitor or ARB for LVSD

Hospital Name	City	Rate	Cases
Bon Secours - Maryview Medical Center	Portsmouth	100%	144
Bon Secours - Memorial Regional Medical[2]	Mechanicsville	100%	120
Bon Secours - St Francis Medical Center	Midlothian	100%	58
CJW Medical Center	Richmond	100%	224
Clinch Valley Medical Center	Richlands	100%	32
Community Memorial Healthcenter	South Hill	100%	51
The Fauquier Hospital	Warrenton	100%	55
Henrico Doctors' Hospital[2]	Richmond	100%	144
John Randolph Medical Center	Hopewell	100%	81
Lewis-Gale Medical Center	Salem	100%	121
Mary Washington Hospital[2]	Fredericksburg	100%	176
Montgomery Regional Hospital	Blacksburg	100%	25
Potomac Hospital[2]	Woodbridge	100%	65
Reston Hospital Center	Reston	100%	27
Riverside Regional Medical Center	Newport News	100%	166
Riverside Shore Memorial Hospital	Nassawadox	100%	53
Riverside Tappahannock Hospital	Tappahannock	100%	33
Salem VA Medical Center	Salem	100%	66
Sentara Bayside Hospital	Virginia Beach	100%	66
Sentara Careplex Hospital	Hampton	100%	113
Sentara Norfolk General Hospital	Norfolk	100%	345
Southern Virginia Regional Medical Center	Emporia	100%	62
Twin County Regional Hospital	Galax	100%	37
Mary Immaculate Hospital	Newport News	99%	74
Virginia Hospital Center - Arlington	Arlington	99%	93
Winchester Medical Center	Winchester	99%	208
Halifax Regional Hospital	Halifax	98%	57
Inova Alexandria Hospital[2]	Alexandria	98%	112
Inova Loudoun Hospital	Leesburg	98%	51
Inova Mount Vernon Hospital	Alexandria	98%	49
Sentara Virginia Beach General Hospital	Virginia Beach	98%	118
Southampton Memorial Hospital	Franklin	98%	61
University of Virginia Medical Center[2]	Charlottesville	98%	131
Culpeper Regional Hospital	Culpeper	97%	29
Inova Fair Oaks Hospital	Fairfax	97%	33
Mem Hosp of Martinsville & Henry County	Martinsville	97%	93
Richmond VA Medical Center	Richmond	97%	137
Rockingham Memorial Hospital[2]	Harrisonburg	97%	101
Sentara Williamsburg Regional Med Ctr	Williamsburg	97%	77
Southside Community Hospital	Farmville	97%	58
Augusta Health	Fishersville	96%	112
Bon Secours - Depaul Medical Center	Norfolk	96%	70
Centra Health[2]	Lynchburg	96%	219
Danville Regional Medical Center[2]	Danville	96%	130
Sentara Obici Hospital	Suffolk	96%	145
Wellmont Lonesome Pine Hospital	Big Stone Gap	96%	28
Bon Secours - St Marys Hospital of Richmond	Richmond	95%	107
Riverside Walter Reed Hospital	Gloucester	95%	41
Sentara Leigh Hospital	Norfolk	95%	147
Virginia Commonwealth Univ Health Sys	Richmond	95%	338
Chesapeake General Hospital	Chesapeake	94%	220
Prince William Hospital	Manassas	94%	48
Martha Jefferson Hospital	Charlottesville	93%	129
Inova Fairfax Hospital[2]	Falls Church	92%	95
Southside Regional Medical Center	Petersburg	92%	203
Carilion New River Valley Medical Center	Christiansburg	88%	34
Carilion Medical Center	Roanoke	87%	300
Johnston Memorial Hospital[2]	Abingdon	68%	31

13. Discharge Instructions

Hospital Name	City	Rate	Cases
Alleghany Regional Hospital	Low Moor	100%	94
Bon Secours - Memorial Regional Medical[2]	Mechanicsville	100%	293
Bon Secours - St Francis Medical Center	Midlothian	100%	176
Centra Health[2]	Lynchburg	100%	616
Community Memorial Healthcenter	South Hill	100%	158
Hampton VA Medical Center	Hampton	100%	78
Mountain View Regional Medical Center	Norton	100%	84
Pulaski Community Hospital	Pulaski	100%	65
Rappahannock General Hospital	Kilmarnock	100%	43
Reston Hospital Center	Reston	100%	144
CJW Medical Center	Richmond	99%	596
Clinch Valley Medical Center	Richlands	99%	150
Riverside Tappahannock Hospital	Tappahannock	99%	76
Sentara Leigh Hospital	Norfolk	99%	345
Bedford Memorial Hospital	Bedford	98%	55
Bon Secours - Maryview Medical Center	Portsmouth	98%	374
Bon Secours - St Marys Hospital of Richmond	Richmond	98%	324
Lewis-Gale Medical Center	Salem	98%	284
Montgomery Regional Hospital	Blacksburg	98%	56
Sentara Bayside Hospital	Virginia Beach	98%	186
John Randolph Medical Center	Hopewell	97%	153
Sentara Careplex Hospital	Hampton	97%	338
Southside Regional Medical Center	Petersburg	97%	376
Twin County Regional Hospital	Galax	97%	88
Virginia Commonwealth Univ Health Sys	Richmond	97%	659
Buchanan General Hospital	Grundy	96%	76
Riverside Walter Reed Hospital	Gloucester	96%	91
Southern Virginia Regional Medical Center	Emporia	96%	197
Bon Secours - Depaul Medical Center	Norfolk	95%	190
Inova Loudoun Hospital	Leesburg	95%	173
Richmond VA Medical Center	Richmond	95%	262
Riverside Shore Memorial Hospital	Nassawadox	95%	112
Sentara Norfolk General Hospital	Norfolk	95%	788
Halifax Regional Hospital	Halifax	94%	178
Mary Immaculate Hospital	Newport News	94%	142
Norton Community Hospital[2]	Norton	94%	84
Riverside Regional Medical Center	Newport News	94%	361
Sentara Williamsburg Regional Med Ctr	Williamsburg	94%	225
The Fauquier Hospital	Warrenton	93%	146
Henrico Doctors' Hospital[2]	Richmond	93%	330
Carilion Medical Center	Roanoke	92%	636
Sentara Virginia Beach General Hospital	Virginia Beach	92%	360
Augusta Health	Fishersville	91%	260
Carilion Franklin Memorial Hospital	Rocky Mount	91%	53
Chesapeake General Hospital	Chesapeake	91%	475
Inova Mount Vernon Hospital	Alexandria	91%	172
Rockingham Memorial Hospital[2]	Harrisonburg	91%	304
Wythe County Community Hospital	Wytheville	91%	75
Carilion Stonewall Jackson Hospital	Lexington	90%	49
Winchester Medical Center	Winchester	90%	573
Inova Fair Oaks Hospital	Fairfax	89%	160
Mary Washington Hospital[2]	Fredericksburg	89%	560
Page Memorial Hospital	Luray	89%	27
Carilion New River Valley Medical Center	Christiansburg	88%	100
Inova Fairfax Hospital[2]	Falls Church	88%	238
Southampton Memorial Hospital	Franklin	88%	108
Salem VA Medical Center	Salem	87%	121
Sentara Obici Hospital	Suffolk	86%	331
Carilion Giles Memorial Hospital	Pearisburg	85%	53
Russell County Medical Center[2]	Lebanon	84%	79
Potomac Hospital[2]	Woodbridge	83%	240
Stafford Hospital Center	Stafford	83%	88
Warren Memorial Hospital	Front Royal	83%	47
Culpeper Regional Hospital	Culpeper	82%	84
Johnston Memorial Hospital[2]	Abingdon	82%	125
Prince William Hospital	Manassas	80%	112
University of Virginia Medical Center[2]	Charlottesville	80%	240
Virginia Hospital Center - Arlington	Arlington	79%	225
Mem Hosp of Martinsville & Henry County	Martinsville	78%	195
Smyth County Community Hospital[2]	Marion	78%	50
Carilion Tazewell Community Hospital	Tazewell	77%	44
Danville Regional Medical Center[2]	Danville	76%	264
Bon Secours - Richmond Community Hospital	Richmond	75%	51
Martha Jefferson Hospital	Charlottesville	75%	273
Wellmont Lonesome Pine Hospital	Big Stone Gap	72%	86
Shenandoah Memorial Hospital	Woodstock	68%	31
Inova Alexandria Hospital[2]	Alexandria	67%	231
Southside Community Hospital	Farmville	66%	118
Lee Regional Medical Center	Pennington Gap	38%	80

14. Evaluation of LVS Function

Hospital Name	City	Rate	Cases
Alleghany Regional Hospital	Low Moor	100%	120
Augusta Health	Fishersville	100%	332
Bon Secours - Memorial Regional Medical[2]	Mechanicsville	100%	353
Bon Secours - St Marys Hospital of Richmond	Richmond	100%	423
Buchanan General Hospital	Grundy	100%	84
Carilion Stonewall Jackson Hospital	Lexington	100%	61
Chesapeake General Hospital	Chesapeake	100%	548
CJW Medical Center	Richmond	100%	734
Community Memorial Healthcenter	South Hill	100%	190
The Fauquier Hospital	Warrenton	100%	174
Halifax Regional Hospital	Halifax	100%	205
Hampton VA Medical Center	Hampton	100%	79
Henrico Doctors' Hospital[2]	Richmond	100%	432
John Randolph Medical Center	Hopewell	100%	190
Lewis-Gale Medical Center	Salem	100%	393
Martha Jefferson Hospital	Charlottesville	100%	321
Mary Washington Hospital[2]	Fredericksburg	100%	669
Mem Hosp of Martinsville & Henry County	Martinsville	100%	253
Montgomery Regional Hospital	Blacksburg	100%	79
Mountain View Regional Medical Center	Norton	100%	101
Page Memorial Hospital	Luray	100%	50
Pulaski Community Hospital	Pulaski	100%	88
Richmond VA Medical Center	Richmond	100%	273
Riverside Regional Medical Center	Newport News	100%	442
Riverside Shore Memorial Hospital	Nassawadox	100%	134
Riverside Tappahannock Hospital	Tappahannock	100%	93
Riverside Walter Reed Hospital	Gloucester	100%	128
Rockingham Memorial Hospital[2]	Harrisonburg	100%	388
Salem VA Medical Center	Salem	100%	143
Sentara Bayside Hospital	Virginia Beach	100%	219
Sentara Careplex Hospital	Hampton	100%	392
Sentara Leigh Hospital	Norfolk	100%	425
Sentara Norfolk General Hospital	Norfolk	100%	886
Sentara Obici Hospital	Suffolk	100%	416
Sentara Virginia Beach General Hospital	Virginia Beach	100%	453
Sentara Williamsburg Regional Med Ctr	Williamsburg	100%	275
Shenandoah Memorial Hospital	Woodstock	100%	41
Southern Virginia Regional Medical Center	Emporia	100%	219
Stafford Hospital Center	Stafford	100%	99

NOTE: Hospital profiles are in alphabetical order by state, then city, then hospital within the city; Rankings exclude hospitals with less than 25 cases except for patient surveys which excludes hospitals with less than 100 cases; (a) 100–299 cases; (1) The number of cases is too small to be sure how well a hospital is performing; (2) The hospital indicated that the data submitted for this measure were based on a sample of cases; (3) Data was collected during a shorter time period (fewer quarters) than the maximum possible time for this measure; (4) Suppressed for one or more quarters by CMS; (5) No data is available from the hospital for this measure; (6) Fewer than 100 patients completed the HCAHPS survey. Use these rates with caution, as the number of surveys may be too low to reliably assess hospital performance; (7) Survey results are based on less than 12 months of data; (8) Survey results are not available for this reporting period; (9) No or very few patients were eligible for the HCAHPS survey. The scores shown, if any, reflect a very small number of surveys; (10) A state average was not calculated because too few hospitals in the state submitted data; (11) There were discrepancies in the data collection process; Please refer to the User's Guide for a full explanation of data.

Twin County Regional Hospital	Galax	100%	122
Virginia Commonwealth Univ Health Sys	Richmond	100%	709
Warren Memorial Hospital	Front Royal	100%	55
Winchester Medical Center	Winchester	100%	660
Wythe County Community Hospital	Wytheville	100%	99
Bon Secours - Depaul Medical Center	Norfolk	99%	252
Bon Secours - Maryview Medical Center	Portsmouth	99%	429
Bon Secours - St Francis Medical Center	Midlothian	99%	211
Carilion New River Valley Medical Center	Christiansburg	99%	123
Centra Health[2]	Lynchburg	99%	818
Clinch Valley Medical Center	Richlands	99%	165
Inova Fairfax Hospital[2]	Falls Church	99%	290
Inova Loudoun Hospital	Leesburg	99%	209
Inova Mount Vernon Hospital	Alexandria	99%	216
Mary Immaculate Hospital	Newport News	99%	173
Prince William Hospital	Manassas	99%	133
Reston Hospital Center	Reston	99%	172
Smyth County Community Hospital[2]	Marion	99%	68
Southampton Memorial Hospital	Franklin	99%	133
Southside Regional Medical Center	Petersburg	99%	468
University of Virginia Medical Center[2]	Charlottesville	99%	282
Wellmont Lonesome Pine Hospital	Big Stone Gap	99%	108
Bon Secours - Richmond Community Hospital	Richmond	98%	57
Inova Fair Oaks Hospital	Fairfax	98%	187
Norton Community Hospital[2]	Norton	98%	94
Rappahannock General Hospital	Kilmarnock	98%	51
Danville Regional Medical Center[2]	Danville	97%	343
Southside Community Hospital	Farmville	97%	149
Carilion Franklin Memorial Hospital	Rocky Mount	96%	76
Carilion Medical Center	Roanoke	96%	780
Virginia Hospital Center - Arlington	Arlington	96%	292
Inova Alexandria Hospital[2]	Alexandria	95%	283
Culpeper Regional Hospital	Culpeper	94%	107
Johnston Memorial Hospital[2]	Abingdon	94%	155
Bedford Memorial Hospital	Bedford	93%	67
Potomac Hospital[2]	Woodbridge	93%	260
Russell County Medical Center[2]	Lebanon	90%	89
Carilion Tazewell Community Hospital	Tazewell	87%	55
Carilion Giles Memorial Hospital	Pearisburg	86%	65
Lee Regional Medical Center	Pennington Gap	71%	91

15. Smoking Cessation Advice

Hospital Name	City	Rate	Cases
Augusta Health	Fishersville	100%	53
Bon Secours - Maryview Medical Center	Portsmouth	100%	89
Bon Secours - Memorial Regional Medical[2]	Mechanicsville	100%	54
Bon Secours - Richmond Community Hospital	Richmond	100%	25
Bon Secours - St Francis Medical Center	Midlothian	100%	26
Bon Secours - St Marys Hospital of Richmond	Richmond	100%	56
Centra Health[2]	Lynchburg	100%	168
Chesapeake General Hospital	Chesapeake	100%	112
CJW Medical Center	Richmond	100%	141
Clinch Valley Medical Center	Richlands	100%	28
Community Memorial Healthcenter	South Hill	100%	37
Danville Regional Medical Center[2]	Danville	100%	86
The Fauquier Hospital	Warrenton	100%	34
Henrico Doctors' Hospital[2]	Richmond	100%	52
Inova Fairfax Hospital[2]	Falls Church	100%	27
Inova Loudoun Hospital	Leesburg	100%	25
Inova Mount Vernon Hospital	Alexandria	100%	25
John Randolph Medical Center	Hopewell	100%	52
Lewis-Gale Medical Center	Salem	100%	48
Mary Immaculate Hospital	Newport News	100%	27
Mary Washington Hospital[2]	Fredericksburg	100%	126
Mem Hosp of Martinsville & Henry County	Martinsville	100%	56
Norton Community Hospital[2]	Norton	100%	25
Prince William Hospital	Manassas	100%	25
Riverside Regional Medical Center	Newport News	100%	89
Riverside Shore Memorial Hospital	Nassawadox	100%	26
Rockingham Memorial Hospital[2]	Harrisonburg	100%	59
Salem VA Medical Center	Salem	100%	35
Sentara Bayside Hospital	Virginia Beach	100%	36
Sentara Careplex Hospital	Hampton	100%	96
Sentara Norfolk General Hospital	Norfolk	100%	193
Sentara Virginia Beach General Hospital	Virginia Beach	100%	75
Sentara Williamsburg Regional Med Ctr	Williamsburg	100%	62
Southampton Memorial Hospital	Franklin	100%	28
Southern Virginia Regional Medical Center	Emporia	100%	43
Southside Community Hospital	Farmville	100%	32
Southside Regional Medical Center	Petersburg	100%	110
Virginia Commonwealth Univ Health Sys	Richmond	100%	219
Virginia Hospital Center - Arlington	Arlington	100%	29
Winchester Medical Center	Winchester	100%	129
Sentara Leigh Hospital	Norfolk	99%	75
University of Virginia Medical Center[2]	Charlottesville	99%	74
Bon Secours - Depaul Medical Center	Norfolk	98%	56
Carilion Medical Center	Roanoke	98%	200
Halifax Regional Hospital	Halifax	98%	42
Potomac Hospital[2]	Woodbridge	98%	46
Sentara Obici Hospital	Suffolk	98%	80
Richmond VA Medical Center	Richmond	97%	58
Inova Alexandria Hospital[2]	Alexandria	95%	56
Martha Jefferson Hospital	Charlottesville	95%	55

Pneumonia Care

16. Appropriate Initial Antibiotic

Hospital Name	City	Rate	Cases
Bon Secours - Memorial Regional Medical[2]	Mechanicsville	100%	162
Virginia Hospital Center - Arlington[2]	Arlington	100%	74
Sentara Careplex Hospital	Hampton	99%	151
Twin County Regional Hospital	Galax	99%	118
Lewis-Gale Medical Center	Salem	98%	248
Sentara Norfolk General Hospital	Norfolk	98%	107
Sentara Williamsburg Regional Med Ctr	Williamsburg	98%	124
Wythe County Community Hospital	Wytheville	98%	103
Bon Secours - St Marys Hospital of Richmond	Richmond	97%	126
The Fauquier Hospital	Warrenton	97%	108
Halifax Regional Hospital	Halifax	97%	69
Inova Alexandria Hospital[2]	Alexandria	97%	90
Riverside Walter Reed Hospital	Gloucester	97%	121
Rockingham Memorial Hospital[2]	Harrisonburg	97%	123
Southern Virginia Regional Medical Center	Emporia	97%	115
CJW Medical Center	Richmond	96%	200
Danville Regional Medical Center[2]	Danville	96%	78
Hampton VA Medical Center	Hampton	96%	28
John Randolph Medical Center	Hopewell	96%	73
Reston Hospital Center	Reston	96%	111
Riverside Tappahannock Hospital	Tappahannock	96%	49
Sentara Leigh Hospital	Norfolk	96%	141
Stafford Hospital Center	Stafford	96%	72
Alleghany Regional Hospital	Low Moor	95%	106
Clinch Valley Medical Center	Richlands	95%	77
Community Memorial Healthcenter	South Hill	95%	65
Inova Mount Vernon Hospital	Alexandria	95%	63
Mary Washington Hospital[2]	Fredericksburg	95%	275
Montgomery Regional Hospital	Blacksburg	95%	78
Pulaski Community Hospital	Pulaski	95%	73
Riverside Regional Medical Center	Newport News	95%	119
Riverside Shore Memorial Hospital	Nassawadox	95%	59
Salem VA Medical Center	Salem	95%	62
Augusta Health	Fishersville	94%	204
Bon Secours - Maryview Medical Center	Portsmouth	94%	85
Buchanan General Hospital	Grundy	94%	63
Mem Hosp of Martinsville & Henry County	Martinsville	94%	109
Sentara Virginia Beach General Hospital	Virginia Beach	94%	173
Warren Memorial Hospital	Front Royal	94%	49
Carilion Franklin Memorial Hospital	Rocky Mount	93%	68
Chesapeake General Hospital	Chesapeake	93%	227
Inova Loudoun Hospital[2]	Leesburg	93%	111
Richmond VA Medical Center	Richmond	93%	85
Sentara Bayside Hospital	Virginia Beach	93%	96
Southside Regional Medical Center	Petersburg	93%	139
University of Virginia Medical Center[2]	Charlottesville	93%	54
Bon Secours - St Francis Medical Center	Midlothian	92%	129
Culpeper Regional Hospital	Culpeper	92%	77
Henrico Doctors' Hospital[2]	Richmond	92%	119
Inova Fair Oaks Hospital[2]	Fairfax	92%	84
Norton Community Hospital[2]	Norton	92%	89
Prince William Hospital	Manassas	92%	130
Sentara Obici Hospital	Suffolk	92%	119
Winchester Medical Center[2]	Winchester	92%	158
Johnston Memorial Hospital[2]	Abingdon	91%	111
Lee Regional Medical Center	Pennington Gap	91%	127
Martha Jefferson Hospital[2]	Charlottesville	91%	85
Potomac Hospital[2]	Woodbridge	91%	98
Smyth County Community Hospital[2]	Marion	91%	81
Southside Community Hospital	Farmville	91%	91
Mary Immaculate Hospital	Newport News	90%	84
Russell County Medical Center[2]	Lebanon	90%	103
Virginia Commonwealth Univ Health Sys	Richmond	90%	86
Carilion Giles Memorial Hospital	Pearisburg	89%	36
Inova Fairfax Hospital[2]	Falls Church	89%	57
Rappahannock General Hospital	Kilmarnock	89%	44
Centra Health[2]	Lynchburg	88%	209
Page Memorial Hospital	Luray	88%	25
Carilion Stonewall Jackson Hospital	Lexington	87%	31
Bon Secours - Depaul Medical Center	Norfolk	86%	78
Mountain View Regional Medical Center	Norton	86%	51
Carilion New River Valley Medical Center	Christiansburg	85%	132
Shenandoah Memorial Hospital	Woodstock	85%	61
Carilion Medical Center	Roanoke	84%	288
Southampton Memorial Hospital	Franklin	84%	56
Wellmont Lonesome Pine Hospital	Big Stone Gap	84%	73
Bon Secours - Richmond Community Hospital	Richmond	79%	47
Bedford Memorial Hospital	Bedford	75%	61
Carilion Tazewell Community Hospital	Tazewell	74%	38

17. Blood Culture Timing

Hospital Name	City	Rate	Cases
Alleghany Regional Hospital	Low Moor	100%	131
Bon Secours - Richmond Community Hospital	Richmond	100%	57
CJW Medical Center	Richmond	100%	400
John Randolph Medical Center	Hopewell	100%	120
Mountain View Regional Medical Center	Norton	100%	73
Rappahannock General Hospital	Kilmarnock	100%	68
Russell County Medical Center[2]	Lebanon	100%	98
Twin County Regional Hospital	Galax	100%	221
Buchanan General Hospital	Grundy	99%	86
Chesapeake General Hospital	Chesapeake	99%	364
Community Memorial Healthcenter	South Hill	99%	82
Inova Alexandria Hospital[2]	Alexandria	99%	143
Inova Fairfax Hospital[2]	Falls Church	99%	90
Lewis-Gale Medical Center	Salem	99%	370
Pulaski Community Hospital	Pulaski	99%	104
Reston Hospital Center	Reston	99%	179
Richmond VA Medical Center	Richmond	99%	150
Riverside Shore Memorial Hospital	Nassawadox	99%	119
Riverside Walter Reed Hospital	Gloucester	99%	195
Rockingham Memorial Hospital[2]	Harrisonburg	99%	170
Sentara Bayside Hospital	Virginia Beach	99%	161
Smyth County Community Hospital[2]	Marion	99%	76
Southern Virginia Regional Medical Center	Emporia	99%	76
Virginia Hospital Center - Arlington[2]	Arlington	99%	125
Wythe County Community Hospital	Wytheville	99%	107
Bon Secours - Depaul Medical Center	Norfolk	98%	129
Bon Secours - Maryview Medical Center	Portsmouth	98%	171
Bon Secours - Memorial Regional Medical[2]	Mechanicsville	98%	244
Hampton VA Medical Center	Hampton	98%	46
Inova Mount Vernon Hospital	Alexandria	98%	90
Lee Regional Medical Center	Pennington Gap	98%	150
Mary Immaculate Hospital	Newport News	98%	160
Montgomery Regional Hospital	Blacksburg	98%	119
Riverside Tappahannock Hospital	Tappahannock	98%	49
Salem VA Medical Center	Salem	98%	96
Sentara Leigh Hospital	Norfolk	98%	284
Sentara Williamsburg Regional Med Ctr	Williamsburg	98%	169
Bedford Memorial Hospital	Bedford	97%	96
Bon Secours - St Marys Hospital of Richmond	Richmond	97%	249
Clinch Valley Medical Center	Richlands	97%	109
Halifax Regional Hospital	Halifax	97%	89
Johnston Memorial Hospital[2]	Abingdon	97%	156
Prince William Hospital	Manassas	97%	223
Riverside Regional Medical Center	Newport News	97%	231
Sentara Careplex Hospital	Hampton	97%	294
Sentara Norfolk General Hospital	Norfolk	97%	211
Sentara Obici Hospital	Suffolk	97%	174
Southside Regional Medical Center	Petersburg	97%	175
Augusta Health	Fishersville	96%	329
Carilion Franklin Memorial Hospital	Rocky Mount	96%	120
Culpeper Regional Hospital	Culpeper	96%	156
Danville Regional Medical Center[2]	Danville	96%	123
The Fauquier Hospital	Warrenton	96%	202
Henrico Doctors' Hospital[2]	Richmond	96%	153
Inova Fair Oaks Hospital[2]	Fairfax	96%	135
Mary Washington Hospital[2]	Fredericksburg	96%	401
Mem Hosp of Martinsville & Henry County	Martinsville	96%	184
Page Memorial Hospital	Luray	96%	27
Sentara Virginia Beach General Hospital	Virginia Beach	96%	290
Southampton Memorial Hospital	Franklin	96%	83
Southside Community Hospital	Farmville	96%	123
Bon Secours - St Francis Medical Center	Midlothian	95%	183
Carilion Giles Memorial Hospital	Pearisburg	95%	57
Carilion Stonewall Jackson Hospital	Lexington	95%	41
Centra Health[2]	Lynchburg	95%	318
Shenandoah Memorial Hospital	Woodstock	95%	83
Stafford Hospital Center	Stafford	95%	80
University of Virginia Medical Center[2]	Charlottesville	95%	81
Warren Memorial Hospital	Front Royal	95%	63
Wellmont Lonesome Pine Hospital	Big Stone Gap	95%	92
Winchester Medical Center[2]	Winchester	95%	187
Carilion New River Valley Medical Center	Christiansburg	93%	163
Martha Jefferson Hospital[2]	Charlottesville	93%	103
Norton Community Hospital[2]	Norton	93%	153
Inova Loudoun Hospital[2]	Leesburg	92%	141
Potomac Hospital[2]	Woodbridge	89%	143
Carilion Medical Center	Roanoke	88%	398
Virginia Commonwealth Univ Health Sys	Richmond	86%	206
Carilion Tazewell Community Hospital	Tazewell	81%	58

18. Influenza Vaccine

Hospital Name	City	Rate	Cases
Alleghany Regional Hospital	Low Moor	100%	91
Bon Secours - Depaul Medical Center	Norfolk	100%	85
Community Memorial Healthcenter	South Hill	100%	50
John Randolph Medical Center	Hopewell	100%	62
Lewis-Gale Medical Center	Salem	100%	252
Montgomery Regional Hospital	Blacksburg	100%	92

NOTE: Hospital profiles are in alphabetical order by state, then city, then hospital within the city; Rankings exclude hospitals with less than 25 cases except for patient surveys which excludes hospitals with less than 100 cases; (a) 100–299 cases; (1) The number of cases is too small to be sure how well a hospital is performing; (2) The hospital indicated that the data submitted for this measure were based on a sample of cases; (3) Data was collected during a shorter time period (fewer quarters) than the maximum possible time for this measure; (4) Suppressed for one or more quarters by CMS; (5) No data is available from the hospital for this measure; (6) Fewer than 100 patients completed the HCAHPS survey. Use these rates with caution, as the number of surveys may be too low to reliably assess hospital performance; (7) Survey results are based on less than 12 months of data; (8) Survey results are not available for this reporting period; (9) No or very few patients were eligible for the HCAHPS survey. The scores shown, if any, reflect a very small number of surveys; (10) A state average was not calculated because too few hospitals in the state submitted data; (11) There were discrepancies in the data collection process; Please refer to the User's Guide for a full explanation of data.

Reston Hospital Center	Reston	100%	111
Riverside Tappahannock Hospital	Tappahannock	100%	32
Riverside Walter Reed Hospital	Gloucester	100%	108
Smyth County Community Hospital[2]	Marion	100%	73
Twin County Regional Hospital	Galax	100%	125
Warren Memorial Hospital	Front Royal	100%	35
Wythe County Community Hospital	Wytheville	100%	121
Mary Immaculate Hospital	Newport News	99%	79
Mem Hosp of Martinsville & Henry County	Martinsville	99%	111
Pulaski Community Hospital	Pulaski	99%	88
Russell County Medical Center[2]	Lebanon	99%	94
Sentara Virginia Beach General Hospital	Virginia Beach	99%	239
CJW Medical Center	Richmond	98%	246
Mountain View Regional Medical Center	Norton	98%	54
Riverside Regional Medical Center	Newport News	98%	135
Sentara Careplex Hospital	Hampton	98%	176
Sentara Williamsburg Regional Med Ctr	Williamsburg	98%	112
Bon Secours - St Marys Hospital of Richmond	Richmond	97%	198
Buchanan General Hospital	Grundy	97%	61
Carilion Giles Memorial Hospital	Pearisburg	97%	33
Clinch Valley Medical Center	Richlands	97%	60
Henrico Doctors' Hospital[2]	Richmond	97%	147
Norton Community Hospital[2]	Norton	97%	86
Salem VA Medical Center	Salem	97%	78
Sentara Norfolk General Hospital	Norfolk	97%	151
Sentara Obici Hospital	Suffolk	97%	137
Southern Virginia Regional Medical Center	Emporia	97%	86
Wellmont Lonesome Pine Hospital	Big Stone Gap	97%	76
Bon Secours - Memorial Regional Medical[2]	Mechanicsville	96%	118
Chesapeake General Hospital	Chesapeake	96%	251
The Fauquier Hospital	Warrenton	96%	102
Inova Fair Oaks Hospital[2]	Fairfax	96%	73
Sentara Bayside Hospital	Virginia Beach	96%	136
Carilion Tazewell Community Hospital	Tazewell	95%	39
Centra Health[2]	Lynchburg	95%	220
Riverside Shore Memorial Hospital	Nassawadox	95%	75
Augusta Health	Fishersville	94%	203
Carilion New River Valley Medical Center	Christiansburg	94%	94
Carilion Stonewall Jackson Hospital	Lexington	94%	35
Inova Alexandria Hospital[2]	Alexandria	94%	69
Inova Loudoun Hospital	Leesburg	94%	127
Richmond VA Medical Center	Richmond	94%	110
Southampton Memorial Hospital	Franklin	94%	49
Bon Secours - St Francis Medical Center	Midlothian	93%	76
Sentara Leigh Hospital	Norfolk	93%	205
Southside Community Hospital	Farmville	93%	69
Southside Regional Medical Center	Petersburg	93%	130
Virginia Hospital Center - Arlington[2]	Arlington	93%	126
Carilion Franklin Memorial Hospital	Rocky Mount	92%	63
Winchester Medical Center[2]	Winchester	92%	157
Inova Mount Vernon Hospital	Alexandria	91%	58
Mary Washington Hospital[2]	Fredericksburg	90%	211
Rockingham Memorial Hospital[2]	Harrisonburg	90%	140
Bon Secours - Maryview Medical Center	Portsmouth	89%	132
Carilion Medical Center	Roanoke	89%	270
Johnston Memorial Hospital[2]	Abingdon	89%	88
Prince William Hospital	Manassas	89%	122
University of Virginia Medical Center[2]	Charlottesville	88%	67
Bedford Memorial Hospital	Bedford	87%	31
Inova Fairfax Hospital[2]	Falls Church	87%	79
Shenandoah Memorial Hospital	Woodstock	84%	50
Virginia Commonwealth Univ Health Sys	Richmond	84%	146
Culpeper Regional Hospital	Culpeper	82%	89
Stafford Hospital Center	Stafford	80%	55
Potomac Hospital[2]	Woodbridge	79%	73
Martha Jefferson Hospital[2]	Charlottesville	78%	96
Danville Regional Medical Center[2]	Danville	76%	89
Lee Regional Medical Center	Pennington Gap	76%	102
Halifax Regional Hospital	Halifax	69%	112
Hampton VA Medical Center	Hampton	68%	31

19. Initial Antibiotic Timing

Hospital Name	City	Rate	Cases
Bon Secours - Memorial Regional Medical[2]	Mechanicsville	100%	230
Inova Mount Vernon Hospital	Alexandria	100%	86
Montgomery Regional Hospital	Blacksburg	100%	118
Rappahannock General Hospital	Kilmarnock	100%	70
Inova Alexandria Hospital[2]	Alexandria	99%	139
Inova Fair Oaks Hospital[2]	Fairfax	99%	130
Inova Fairfax Hospital[2]	Falls Church	99%	90
Reston Hospital Center	Reston	99%	137
Russell County Medical Center[2]	Lebanon	99%	143
Sentara Bayside Hospital	Virginia Beach	99%	165
Sentara Careplex Hospital	Hampton	99%	271
Southern Virginia Regional Medical Center	Emporia	99%	150
Twin County Regional Hospital	Galax	99%	190
Virginia Hospital Center - Arlington[2]	Arlington	99%	108
Wythe County Community Hospital	Wytheville	99%	147
Bon Secours - St Francis Medical Center	Midlothian	98%	163
Buchanan General Hospital	Grundy	98%	100
CJW Medical Center	Richmond	98%	338
John Randolph Medical Center	Hopewell	98%	103
Lee Regional Medical Center	Pennington Gap	98%	166
Lewis-Gale Medical Center	Salem	98%	354
Prince William Hospital	Manassas	98%	187
Riverside Walter Reed Hospital	Gloucester	98%	179
Sentara Norfolk General Hospital	Norfolk	98%	241
Smyth County Community Hospital[2]	Marion	98%	116
Stafford Hospital Center	Stafford	98%	64
Bon Secours - Depaul Medical Center	Norfolk	97%	131
Bon Secours - Richmond Community Hospital	Richmond	97%	61
Carilion Franklin Memorial Hospital	Rocky Mount	97%	108
Clinch Valley Medical Center	Richlands	97%	116
Community Memorial Healthcenter	South Hill	97%	93
Culpeper Regional Hospital	Culpeper	97%	134
Inova Loudoun Hospital[2]	Leesburg	97%	143
Johnston Memorial Hospital[2]	Abingdon	97%	150
Mary Washington Hospital[2]	Fredericksburg	97%	372
Pulaski Community Hospital	Pulaski	97%	59
Richmond VA Medical Center	Richmond	97%	157
Rockingham Memorial Hospital[2]	Harrisonburg	97%	175
Sentara Obici Hospital	Suffolk	97%	196
Sentara Williamsburg Regional Med Ctr	Williamsburg	97%	191
Shenandoah Memorial Hospital	Woodstock	97%	75
Alleghany Regional Hospital	Low Moor	96%	114
Augusta Health	Fishersville	96%	314
Bon Secours - St Marys Hospital of Richmond	Richmond	96%	227
Mary Immaculate Hospital	Newport News	96%	163
Mem Hosp of Martinsville & Henry County	Martinsville	96%	158
Mountain View Regional Medical Center	Norton	96%	75
Sentara Leigh Hospital	Norfolk	96%	272
Southampton Memorial Hospital	Franklin	96%	84
Bon Secours - Maryview Medical Center	Portsmouth	95%	157
Carilion Giles Memorial Hospital	Pearisburg	95%	55
Centra Health[2]	Lynchburg	95%	382
The Fauquier Hospital	Warrenton	95%	169
Hampton VA Medical Center	Hampton	95%	40
Henrico Doctors' Hospital[2]	Richmond	95%	208
Riverside Regional Medical Center	Newport News	95%	209
Riverside Shore Memorial Hospital	Nassawadox	95%	125
Salem VA Medical Center	Salem	95%	83
Southside Community Hospital	Farmville	95%	127
Southside Regional Medical Center	Petersburg	95%	213
Warren Memorial Hospital	Front Royal	95%	63
Wellmont Lonesome Pine Hospital	Big Stone Gap	95%	106
Winchester Medical Center[2]	Winchester	95%	222
Martha Jefferson Hospital[2]	Charlottesville	94%	129
Norton Community Hospital[2]	Norton	94%	142
Page Memorial Hospital	Luray	94%	33
Sentara Virginia Beach General Hospital	Virginia Beach	94%	299
Chesapeake General Hospital	Chesapeake	93%	352
Potomac Hospital[2]	Woodbridge	91%	132
Riverside Tappahannock Hospital	Tappahannock	91%	34
Virginia Commonwealth Univ Health Sys	Richmond	91%	226
Carilion New River Valley Medical Center	Christiansburg	90%	154
Bedford Memorial Hospital	Bedford	88%	26
Carilion Stonewall Jackson Hospital	Lexington	88%	43
Danville Regional Medical Center[2]	Danville	88%	132
Halifax Regional Hospital	Halifax	88%	126
Carilion Medical Center	Roanoke	87%	485
University of Virginia Medical Center[2]	Charlottesville	87%	93
Carilion Tazewell Community Hospital	Tazewell	79%	73

20. Pneumococcal Vaccine

Hospital Name	City	Rate	Cases
Alleghany Regional Hospital	Low Moor	100%	111
Buchanan General Hospital	Grundy	100%	74
CJW Medical Center	Richmond	100%	296
John Randolph Medical Center	Hopewell	100%	78
Lewis-Gale Medical Center	Salem	100%	378
Montgomery Regional Hospital	Blacksburg	100%	110
Mountain View Regional Medical Center	Norton	100%	74
Reston Hospital Center	Reston	100%	144
Riverside Tappahannock Hospital	Tappahannock	100%	42
Russell County Medical Center[2]	Lebanon	100%	122
Smyth County Community Hospital[2]	Marion	100%	89
Southern Virginia Regional Medical Center	Emporia	100%	89
Wythe County Community Hospital	Wytheville	100%	125
The Fauquier Hospital	Warrenton	99%	142
Mem Hosp of Martinsville & Henry County	Martinsville	99%	164
Pulaski Community Hospital	Pulaski	99%	109
Richmond VA Medical Center	Richmond	99%	105
Riverside Regional Medical Center	Newport News	99%	185
Riverside Walter Reed Hospital	Gloucester	99%	148
Sentara Bayside Hospital	Virginia Beach	99%	162
Twin County Regional Hospital	Galax	99%	198
Bon Secours - Memorial Regional Medical[2]	Mechanicsville	98%	178
Carilion Stonewall Jackson Hospital	Lexington	98%	40
Centra Health[2]	Lynchburg	98%	337
Henrico Doctors' Hospital[2]	Richmond	98%	235
Inova Fair Oaks Hospital[2]	Fairfax	98%	117
Inova Loudoun Hospital[2]	Leesburg	98%	158
Mary Immaculate Hospital	Newport News	98%	103
Salem VA Medical Center	Salem	98%	90
Sentara Careplex Hospital	Hampton	98%	228
Sentara Williamsburg Regional Med Ctr	Williamsburg	98%	165
Bon Secours - Depaul Medical Center	Norfolk	97%	111
Bon Secours - St Francis Medical Center	Midlothian	97%	118
Bon Secours - St Marys Hospital of Richmond	Richmond	97%	243
Clinch Valley Medical Center	Richlands	97%	75
Augusta Health	Fishersville	96%	299
Carilion Giles Memorial Hospital	Pearisburg	96%	57
Carilion New River Valley Medical Center	Christiansburg	96%	120
Community Memorial Healthcenter	South Hill	96%	76
Norton Community Hospital[2]	Norton	96%	119
Page Memorial Hospital	Luray	96%	28
Prince William Hospital	Manassas	96%	167
Sentara Virginia Beach General Hospital	Virginia Beach	96%	361
Shenandoah Memorial Hospital	Woodstock	96%	78
Southampton Memorial Hospital	Franklin	96%	98
Warren Memorial Hospital	Front Royal	96%	52
Wellmont Lonesome Pine Hospital	Big Stone Gap	96%	84
Sentara Leigh Hospital	Norfolk	95%	247
Sentara Norfolk General Hospital	Norfolk	95%	175
Sentara Obici Hospital	Suffolk	95%	177
Virginia Hospital Center - Arlington[2]	Arlington	95%	184
Carilion Franklin Memorial Hospital	Rocky Mount	94%	93
Chesapeake General Hospital	Chesapeake	94%	357
Mary Washington Hospital[2]	Fredericksburg	94%	325
Rappahannock General Hospital	Kilmarnock	94%	62
Riverside Shore Memorial Hospital	Nassawadox	94%	97
Southside Regional Medical Center	Petersburg	94%	167
Johnston Memorial Hospital[2]	Abingdon	93%	128
Carilion Medical Center	Roanoke	92%	366
Inova Fairfax Hospital[2]	Falls Church	92%	102
Inova Mount Vernon Hospital	Alexandria	92%	84
Winchester Medical Center[2]	Winchester	92%	218
Bon Secours - Maryview Medical Center	Portsmouth	91%	175
Inova Alexandria Hospital[2]	Alexandria	91%	105
Rockingham Memorial Hospital[2]	Harrisonburg	91%	204
Southside Community Hospital	Farmville	91%	103
University of Virginia Medical Center[2]	Charlottesville	91%	92
Carilion Tazewell Community Hospital	Tazewell	87%	53
Culpeper Regional Hospital	Culpeper	86%	126
Danville Regional Medical Center[2]	Danville	86%	139
Stafford Hospital Center	Stafford	86%	56
Halifax Regional Hospital	Halifax	83%	140
Virginia Commonwealth Univ Health Sys	Richmond	83%	113
Lee Regional Medical Center	Pennington Gap	81%	124
Martha Jefferson Hospital[2]	Charlottesville	77%	149
Potomac Hospital[2]	Woodbridge	77%	84
Bedford Memorial Hospital	Bedford	75%	61

21. Smoking Cessation Advice

Hospital Name	City	Rate	Cases
Alleghany Regional Hospital	Low Moor	100%	48
Bon Secours - Depaul Medical Center	Norfolk	100%	49
Bon Secours - Maryview Medical Center	Portsmouth	100%	73
Bon Secours - Memorial Regional Medical[2]	Mechanicsville	100%	72
Bon Secours - Richmond Community Hospital	Richmond	100%	35
Bon Secours - St Francis Medical Center	Midlothian	100%	38
Bon Secours - St Marys Hospital of Richmond	Richmond	100%	57
Buchanan General Hospital	Grundy	100%	41
Carilion Franklin Memorial Hospital	Rocky Mount	100%	38
Carilion New River Valley Medical Center	Christiansburg	100%	57
Chesapeake General Hospital	Chesapeake	100%	122
CJW Medical Center	Richmond	100%	135
Clinch Valley Medical Center	Richlands	100%	43
Community Memorial Healthcenter	South Hill	100%	31
Danville Regional Medical Center[2]	Danville	100%	72
Inova Alexandria Hospital[2]	Alexandria	100%	27
John Randolph Medical Center	Hopewell	100%	43
Mary Immaculate Hospital	Newport News	100%	30
Mary Washington Hospital[2]	Fredericksburg	100%	150
Mem Hosp of Martinsville & Henry County	Martinsville	100%	93
Montgomery Regional Hospital	Blacksburg	100%	53
Mountain View Regional Medical Center	Norton	100%	36
Pulaski Community Hospital	Pulaski	100%	41
Reston Hospital Center	Reston	100%	32
Riverside Regional Medical Center	Newport News	100%	80
Riverside Shore Memorial Hospital	Nassawadox	100%	33
Riverside Walter Reed Hospital	Gloucester	100%	52
Rockingham Memorial Hospital[2]	Harrisonburg	100%	76
Sentara Bayside Hospital	Virginia Beach	100%	81
Sentara Careplex Hospital	Hampton	100%	99
Sentara Williamsburg Regional Med Ctr	Williamsburg	100%	50
Southampton Memorial Hospital	Franklin	100%	34
Southern Virginia Regional Medical Center	Emporia	100%	50
Southside Community Hospital	Farmville	100%	39
Southside Regional Medical Center	Petersburg	100%	93

NOTE: Hospital profiles are in alphabetical order by state, then city, then hospital within the city; Rankings exclude hospitals with less than 25 cases except for patient surveys which excludes hospitals with less than 100 cases; (a) 100–299 cases; (1) The number of cases is too small to be sure how well a hospital is performing; (2) The hospital indicated that the data submitted for this measure were based on a sample of cases; (3) Data was collected during a shorter time period (fewer quarters) than the maximum possible time for this measure; (4) Suppressed for one or more quarters by CMS; (5) No data is available from the hospital for this measure; (6) Fewer than 100 patients completed the HCAHPS survey. Use these rates with caution, as the number of surveys may be too low to reliably assess hospital performance; (7) Survey results are based on less than 12 months of data; (8) Survey results are not available for this reporting period; (9) No or very few patients were eligible for the HCAHPS survey. The scores shown, if any, reflect a very small number of surveys; (10) A state average was not calculated because too few hospitals in the state submitted data; (11) There were discrepancies in the data collection process; Please refer to the User's Guide for a full explanation of data.

Stafford Hospital Center	Stafford	100%	25
Twin County Regional Hospital	Galax	100%	61
Virginia Hospital Center - Arlington[2]	Arlington	100%	37
Wellmont Lonesome Pine Hospital	Big Stone Gap	100%	58
Winchester Medical Center[2]	Winchester	100%	119
Wythe County Community Hospital	Wytheville	100%	63
Augusta Health	Fishersville	99%	105
Carilion Medical Center	Roanoke	99%	232
Centra Health[2]	Lynchburg	99%	177
Henrico Doctors' Hospital[2]	Richmond	99%	72
Lewis-Gale Medical Center	Salem	99%	115
Sentara Leigh Hospital	Norfolk	99%	105
Sentara Norfolk General Hospital	Norfolk	99%	121
Sentara Obici Hospital	Suffolk	99%	85
Virginia Commonwealth Univ Health Sys	Richmond	99%	183
Inova Loudoun Hospital[2]	Leesburg	98%	60
Richmond VA Medical Center	Richmond	98%	57
Sentara Virginia Beach General Hospital	Virginia Beach	98%	125
University of Virginia Medical Center[2]	Charlottesville	98%	56
Martha Jefferson Hospital[2]	Charlottesville	97%	31
Norton Community Hospital[2]	Norton	97%	67
The Fauquier Hospital	Warrenton	96%	57
Inova Fairfax Hospital[2]	Falls Church	96%	27
Russell County Medical Center[2]	Lebanon	96%	70
Halifax Regional Hospital	Halifax	94%	64
Salem VA Medical Center	Salem	94%	36
Culpeper Regional Hospital	Culpeper	92%	36
Smyth County Community Hospital[2]	Marion	92%	48
Prince William Hospital	Manassas	90%	70
Carilion Tazewell Community Hospital	Tazewell	89%	27
Johnston Memorial Hospital[2]	Abingdon	84%	62
Inova Fair Oaks Hospital[2]	Fairfax	81%	27
Potomac Hospital[2]	Woodbridge	80%	50
Lee Regional Medical Center	Pennington Gap	65%	68

Surgical Care Improvement Project

22. Appropriate VTP Within 24 Hours

Hospital Name	City	Rate	Cases
John Randolph Medical Center	Hopewell	100%	66
Pulaski Community Hospital	Pulaski	100%	43
Salem VA Medical Center[2]	Salem	100%	114
Bon Secours - St Marys Hospital of Richmond[2]	Richmond	99%	524
Montgomery Regional Hospital	Blacksburg	99%	108
Sentara Bayside Hospital	Virginia Beach	99%	104
Sentara Leigh Hospital[2]	Norfolk	99%	818
Bon Secours - Maryview Medical Center[2]	Portsmouth	98%	192
Centra Health[2]	Lynchburg	98%	408
The Fauquier Hospital	Warrenton	98%	168
Inova Fairfax Hospital[2]	Falls Church	98%	184
Lewis-Gale Medical Center[2]	Salem	98%	219
Richmond VA Medical Center[2]	Richmond	98%	163
Rockingham Memorial Hospital[2]	Harrisonburg	98%	181
Sentara Careplex Hospital[2]	Hampton	98%	126
Sentara Virginia Beach General Hospital[2]	Virginia Beach	98%	365
Twin County Regional Hospital	Galax	98%	90
Alleghany Regional Hospital[2]	Low Moor	97%	109
Bon Secours - Memorial Regional Medical[2]	Mechanicsville	97%	308
CJW Medical Center[2]	Richmond	97%	270
Potomac Hospital[2]	Woodbridge	97%	101
Riverside Walter Reed Hospital	Gloucester	97%	78
Sentara Norfolk General Hospital[2]	Norfolk	97%	187
Sentara Williamsburg Regional Med Ctr[2]	Williamsburg	97%	172
Shenandoah Memorial Hospital	Woodstock	97%	88
Southern Virginia Regional Medical Center[2]	Emporia	97%	32
Virginia Commonwealth Univ Health Sys[2]	Richmond	97%	259
Virginia Hospital Center - Arlington[2]	Arlington	97%	210
Winchester Medical Center[2]	Winchester	97%	274
Bon Secours - St Francis Medical Center	Midlothian	96%	288
Carilion Medical Center[2]	Roanoke	96%	447
Inova Fair Oaks Hospital[2]	Fairfax	96%	76
Riverside Tappahannock Hospital	Tappahannock	96%	77
Warren Memorial Hospital	Front Royal	96%	46
Chesapeake General Hospital[2]	Chesapeake	95%	177
Henrico Doctors' Hospital[2]	Richmond	95%	208
Inova Mount Vernon Hospital[2]	Alexandria	95%	94
Norton Community Hospital[2]	Norton	95%	37
Southside Community Hospital	Farmville	95%	66
Bon Secours - Depaul Medical Center[2]	Norfolk	94%	152
Reston Hospital Center[2]	Reston	94%	157
Riverside Regional Medical Center[2]	Newport News	94%	189
Sentara Obici Hospital[2]	Suffolk	94%	215
Carilion New River Valley Medical Center	Christiansburg	92%	124
Rappahannock General Hospital	Kilmarnock	92%	80
Carilion Stonewall Jackson Hospital	Lexington	91%	32
Martha Jefferson Hospital[2]	Charlottesville	91%	127
Danville Regional Medical Center[2]	Danville	90%	176
Inova Alexandria Hospital[2]	Alexandria	90%	146
Mary Washington Hospital[2]	Fredericksburg	90%	249
Southside Regional Medical Center[2]	Petersburg	90%	177
University of Virginia Medical Center[2]	Charlottesville	90%	193
Augusta Health[2]	Fishersville	89%	227
Culpeper Regional Hospital	Culpeper	89%	108
Mary Immaculate Hospital[2]	Newport News	89%	159
Southampton Memorial Hospital[2]	Franklin	89%	36
Smyth County Community Hospital[2]	Marion	88%	66
Johnston Memorial Hospital[2]	Abingdon	87%	132
Prince William Hospital[2]	Manassas	87%	117
Inova Loudoun Hospital[2]	Leesburg	86%	156
Riverside Shore Memorial Hospital	Nassawadox	83%	30
Clinch Valley Medical Center	Richlands	82%	33
Wythe County Community Hospital	Wytheville	82%	33
Mem Hosp of Martinsville & Henry County	Martinsville	81%	124
Stafford Hospital Center	Stafford	79%	52
Community Memorial Healthcenter[2]	South Hill	71%	49
Halifax Regional Hospital	Halifax	71%	120

23. Appropriate Hair Removal

Hospital Name	City	Rate	Cases
Alleghany Regional Hospital[2]	Low Moor	100%	233
Augusta Health[2]	Fishersville	100%	867
Bedford Memorial Hospital	Bedford	100%	29
Bon Secours - Depaul Medical Center[2]	Norfolk	100%	406
Bon Secours - Maryview Medical Center[2]	Portsmouth	100%	828
Bon Secours - Memorial Regional Medical[2]	Mechanicsville	100%	1049
Bon Secours - St Francis Medical Center	Midlothian	100%	1020
Bon Secours - St Marys Hospital of Richmond[2]	Richmond	100%	2049
Buchanan General Hospital	Grundy	100%	34
Carilion Franklin Memorial Hospital	Rocky Mount	100%	59
Carilion Medical Center[2]	Roanoke	100%	2675
Carilion Stonewall Jackson Hospital	Lexington	100%	64
Centra Health[2]	Lynchburg	100%	1548
Clinch Valley Medical Center	Richlands	100%	155
Community Memorial Healthcenter[2]	South Hill	100%	85
Culpeper Regional Hospital	Culpeper	100%	322
Danville Regional Medical Center[2]	Danville	100%	452
The Fauquier Hospital	Warrenton	100%	342
Hampton VA Medical Center[2]	Hampton	100%	71
Inova Alexandria Hospital[2]	Alexandria	100%	467
Inova Fair Oaks Hospital[2]	Fairfax	100%	337
Inova Fairfax Hospital[2]	Falls Church	100%	620
Inova Loudoun Hospital[2]	Leesburg	100%	449
Inova Mount Vernon Hospital[2]	Alexandria	100%	329
John Randolph Medical Center	Hopewell	100%	93
Johnston Memorial Hospital[2]	Abingdon	100%	429
Lee Regional Medical Center	Pennington Gap	100%	30
Lewis-Gale Medical Center[2]	Salem	100%	724
Martha Jefferson Hospital[2]	Charlottesville	100%	473
Mary Immaculate Hospital[2]	Newport News	100%	1451
Mary Washington Hospital[2]	Fredericksburg	100%	1000
Mem Hosp of Martinsville & Henry County	Martinsville	100%	299
Montgomery Regional Hospital	Blacksburg	100%	416
Norton Community Hospital[2]	Norton	100%	74
Potomac Hospital[2]	Woodbridge	100%	320
Prince William Hospital[2]	Manassas	100%	536
Pulaski Community Hospital	Pulaski	100%	82
Rappahannock General Hospital	Kilmarnock	100%	127
Reston Hospital Center[2]	Reston	100%	477
Richmond VA Medical Center[2]	Richmond	100%	351
Riverside Regional Medical Center[2]	Newport News	100%	577
Riverside Shore Memorial Hospital	Nassawadox	100%	85
Riverside Tappahannock Hospital	Tappahannock	100%	112
Riverside Walter Reed Hospital	Gloucester	100%	187
Rockingham Memorial Hospital[2]	Harrisonburg	100%	563
Salem VA Medical Center[2]	Salem	100%	214
Sentara Bayside Hospital	Virginia Beach	100%	226
Sentara Careplex Hospital[2]	Hampton	100%	540
Sentara Obici Hospital[2]	Suffolk	100%	746
Sentara Virginia Beach General Hospital[2]	Virginia Beach	100%	947
Sentara Williamsburg Regional Med Ctr[2]	Williamsburg	100%	445
Shenandoah Memorial Hospital	Woodstock	100%	261
Smyth County Community Hospital[2]	Marion	100%	175
Southampton Memorial Hospital[2]	Franklin	100%	126
Southern Virginia Regional Medical Center[2]	Emporia	100%	48
Southside Regional Medical Center[2]	Petersburg	100%	520
Stafford Hospital Center	Stafford	100%	142
Twin County Regional Hospital	Galax	100%	173
Virginia Hospital Center - Arlington[2]	Arlington	100%	632
Wellmont Lonesome Pine Hospital[2]	Big Stone Gap	100%	64
Winchester Medical Center[2]	Winchester	100%	952
Wythe County Community Hospital	Wytheville	100%	247
Carilion New River Valley Medical Center	Christiansburg	99%	347
Chesapeake General Hospital[2]	Chesapeake	99%	395
CJW Medical Center[2]	Richmond	99%	843
Henrico Doctors' Hospital[2]	Richmond	99%	875
Mountain View Regional Medical Center	Norton	99%	73
Sentara Leigh Hospital[2]	Norfolk	99%	1879
Sentara Norfolk General Hospital[2]	Norfolk	99%	1401
Southside Community Hospital	Farmville	99%	142
Warren Memorial Hospital	Front Royal	99%	92
Virginia Commonwealth Univ Health Sys[2]	Richmond	98%	741
Halifax Regional Hospital	Halifax	97%	275
University of Virginia Medical Center[2]	Charlottesville	96%	636

24. Appropriate Beta Blocker Usage

Hospital Name	City	Rate	Cases
Alleghany Regional Hospital[2]	Low Moor	100%	35
Bon Secours - Memorial Regional Medical[2]	Mechanicsville	100%	326
Centra Health[2]	Lynchburg	100%	528
Pulaski Community Hospital	Pulaski	100%	26
Richmond VA Medical Center[2]	Richmond	100%	150
Sentara Bayside Hospital	Virginia Beach	100%	45
Sentara Careplex Hospital[2]	Hampton	100%	145
Sentara Williamsburg Regional Med Ctr[2]	Williamsburg	100%	111
Southampton Memorial Hospital[2]	Franklin	100%	27
Twin County Regional Hospital	Galax	100%	34
Bon Secours - Maryview Medical Center[2]	Portsmouth	99%	229
The Fauquier Hospital	Warrenton	99%	68
Inova Fair Oaks Hospital[2]	Fairfax	99%	89
Lewis-Gale Medical Center[2]	Salem	99%	278
Mary Immaculate Hospital[2]	Newport News	99%	332
Mem Hosp of Martinsville & Henry County	Martinsville	99%	78
Montgomery Regional Hospital	Blacksburg	99%	115
Bon Secours - St Marys Hospital of Richmond[2]	Richmond	98%	514
CJW Medical Center[2]	Richmond	98%	281
Henrico Doctors' Hospital[2]	Richmond	98%	261
Inova Alexandria Hospital[2]	Alexandria	98%	128
Salem VA Medical Center[2]	Salem	98%	66
Riverside Tappahannock Hospital	Tappahannock	97%	31
Smyth County Community Hospital[2]	Marion	97%	33
Bon Secours - St Francis Medical Center	Midlothian	96%	228
Halifax Regional Hospital	Halifax	96%	96
Inova Fairfax Hospital[2]	Falls Church	96%	114
Inova Mount Vernon Hospital[2]	Alexandria	96%	92
Potomac Hospital[2]	Woodbridge	96%	55
Reston Hospital Center[2]	Reston	96%	105
Southside Regional Medical Center[2]	Petersburg	96%	114
Virginia Hospital Center - Arlington[2]	Arlington	96%	171
Inova Loudoun Hospital[2]	Leesburg	95%	102
Prince William Hospital[2]	Manassas	95%	118
Riverside Regional Medical Center[2]	Newport News	95%	175
Rockingham Memorial Hospital[2]	Harrisonburg	95%	190
Sentara Obici Hospital[2]	Suffolk	95%	207
Winchester Medical Center[2]	Winchester	95%	331
Sentara Norfolk General Hospital[2]	Norfolk	94%	645
Chesapeake General Hospital[2]	Chesapeake	93%	107
Clinch Valley Medical Center	Richlands	93%	27
Virginia Commonwealth Univ Health Sys[2]	Richmond	93%	211
Bon Secours - Depaul Medical Center[2]	Norfolk	92%	87
Culpeper Regional Hospital	Culpeper	92%	76
Mary Washington Hospital[2]	Fredericksburg	92%	318
Wythe County Community Hospital	Wytheville	92%	61
Augusta Health[2]	Fishersville	91%	247
Sentara Leigh Hospital[2]	Norfolk	91%	452
Sentara Virginia Beach General Hospital[2]	Virginia Beach	91%	233
Rappahannock General Hospital	Kilmarnock	90%	41
Riverside Walter Reed Hospital	Gloucester	89%	55
Shenandoah Memorial Hospital	Woodstock	89%	89
Carilion Medical Center[2]	Roanoke	88%	815
Johnston Memorial Hospital[2]	Abingdon	88%	129
Martha Jefferson Hospital[2]	Charlottesville	88%	126
Danville Regional Medical Center[2]	Danville	86%	154
University of Virginia Medical Center[2]	Charlottesville	86%	218
Carilion New River Valley Medical Center	Christiansburg	80%	111
Southside Community Hospital	Farmville	70%	37

25. Controlled Postoperative Blood Glucose

Hospital Name	City	Rate	Cases
Bon Secours - St Marys Hospital of Richmond[2]	Richmond	100%	257
Centra Health[2]	Lynchburg	100%	289
CJW Medical Center[2]	Richmond	99%	155
Danville Regional Medical Center[2]	Danville	99%	68
Lewis-Gale Medical Center[2]	Salem	99%	139
Bon Secours - Memorial Regional Medical[2]	Mechanicsville	98%	177
Henrico Doctors' Hospital[2]	Richmond	98%	172
Inova Alexandria Hospital[2]	Alexandria	98%	87
Inova Fairfax Hospital[2]	Falls Church	98%	114
Rockingham Memorial Hospital[2]	Harrisonburg	98%	85
Riverside Regional Medical Center[2]	Newport News	97%	97
Bon Secours - Maryview Medical Center[2]	Portsmouth	96%	124
Carilion Medical Center[2]	Roanoke	96%	570
Richmond VA Medical Center[2]	Richmond	96%	95
Sentara Norfolk General Hospital[2]	Norfolk	96%	781
Virginia Commonwealth Univ Health Sys[2]	Richmond	93%	140
Virginia Hospital Center - Arlington[2]	Arlington	93%	110
Mary Washington Hospital[2]	Fredericksburg	91%	188
Sentara Virginia Beach General Hospital[2]	Virginia Beach	88%	101
Winchester Medical Center[2]	Winchester	86%	194
University of Virginia Medical Center[2]	Charlottesville	85%	120

NOTE: Hospital profiles are in alphabetical order by state, then city, then hospital within the city; Rankings exclude hospitals with less than 25 cases except for patient surveys which excludes hospitals with less than 100 cases; (a) 100–299 cases; (1) The number of cases is too small to be sure how well a hospital is performing; (2) The hospital indicated that the data submitted for this measure were based on a sample of cases; (3) Data was collected during a shorter time period (fewer quarters) than the maximum possible time for this measure; (4) Suppressed for one or more quarters by CMS; (5) No data is available from the hospital for this measure; (6) Fewer than 100 patients completed the HCAHPS survey. Use these rates with caution, as the number of surveys may be too low to reliably assess hospital performance; (7) Survey results are based on less than 12 months of data; (8) Survey results are not available for this reporting period; (9) No or very few patients were eligible for the HCAHPS survey. The scores shown, if any, reflect a very small number of surveys; (10) A state average was not calculated because too few hospitals in the state submitted data; (11) There were discrepancies in the data collection process; Please refer to the User's Guide for a full explanation of data.

26. Prophylactic Antibiotic Timing

Hospital Name	City	Rate	Cases
Alleghany Regional Hospital[2]	Low Moor	100%	198
Carilion Stonewall Jackson Hospital	Lexington	100%	51
Centra Health[2]	Lynchburg	100%	1075
CJW Medical Center[2]	Richmond	100%	531
Hampton VA Medical Center	Hampton	100%	56
Inova Fair Oaks Hospital[2]	Fairfax	100%	226
John Randolph Medical Center	Hopewell	100%	41
Montgomery Regional Hospital	Blacksburg	100%	312
Pulaski Community Hospital	Pulaski	100%	38
Southampton Memorial Hospital[2]	Franklin	100%	101
Southern Virginia Regional Medical Center[2]	Emporia	100%	27
Twin County Regional Hospital	Galax	100%	100
Virginia Hospital Center - Arlington[2]	Arlington	100%	465
Warren Memorial Hospital	Front Royal	100%	55
Bon Secours - Depaul Medical Center[2]	Norfolk	99%	280
Bon Secours - Memorial Regional Medical[2]	Mechanicsville	99%	764
Bon Secours - St Marys Hospital of Richmond[2]	Richmond	99%	1769
Inova Mount Vernon Hospital[2]	Alexandria	99%	214
Lewis-Gale Medical Center[2]	Salem	99%	538
Riverside Regional Medical Center[2]	Newport News	99%	405
Riverside Tappahannock Hospital	Tappahannock	99%	87
Riverside Walter Reed Hospital	Gloucester	99%	134
Sentara Careplex Hospital[2]	Hampton	99%	384
Sentara Virginia Beach General Hospital[2]	Virginia Beach	99%	721
Southside Regional Medical Center[2]	Petersburg	99%	374
Wythe County Community Hospital	Wytheville	99%	204
Augusta Health[2]	Fishersville	98%	696
Henrico Doctors' Hospital[2]	Richmond	98%	599
Inova Alexandria Hospital[2]	Alexandria	98%	325
Prince William Hospital[2]	Manassas	98%	373
Reston Hospital Center[2]	Reston	98%	312
Sentara Bayside Hospital	Virginia Beach	98%	129
Sentara Leigh Hospital[2]	Norfolk	98%	1673
Sentara Norfolk General Hospital[2]	Norfolk	98%	1043
Sentara Obici Hospital[2]	Suffolk	98%	586
Smyth County Community Hospital[2]	Marion	98%	126
Bon Secours - St Francis Medical Center	Midlothian	97%	721
Carilion New River Valley Medical Center	Christiansburg	97%	238
Clinch Valley Medical Center	Richlands	97%	110
Community Memorial Healthcenter[2]	South Hill	97%	33
Martha Jefferson Hospital[2]	Charlottesville	97%	325
Rappahannock General Hospital	Kilmarnock	97%	79
Salem VA Medical Center	Salem	97%	141
Sentara Williamsburg Regional Med Ctr[2]	Williamsburg	97%	302
Chesapeake General Hospital[2]	Chesapeake	96%	265
Culpeper Regional Hospital	Culpeper	96%	246
Danville Regional Medical Center[2]	Danville	96%	309
Mary Immaculate Hospital[2]	Newport News	96%	1292
Mountain View Regional Medical Center	Norton	96%	56
Potomac Hospital[2]	Woodbridge	96%	194
Richmond VA Medical Center	Richmond	96%	253
University of Virginia Medical Center[2]	Charlottesville	96%	402
Carilion Medical Center[2]	Roanoke	95%	2261
The Fauquier Hospital	Warrenton	95%	240
Inova Fairfax Hospital[2]	Falls Church	95%	415
Inova Loudoun Hospital[2]	Leesburg	95%	270
Johnston Memorial Hospital[2]	Abingdon	95%	293
Norton Community Hospital[2]	Norton	95%	41
Winchester Medical Center[2]	Winchester	95%	639
Bon Secours - Maryview Medical Center[2]	Portsmouth	94%	654
Mary Washington Hospital[2]	Fredericksburg	94%	664
Mem Hosp of Martinsville & Henry County	Martinsville	94%	179
Virginia Commonwealth Univ Health Sys[2]	Richmond	93%	445
Stafford Hospital Center	Stafford	92%	88
Riverside Shore Memorial Hospital	Nassawadox	91%	57
Halifax Regional Hospital	Halifax	90%	186
Rockingham Memorial Hospital[2]	Harrisonburg	90%	385
Shenandoah Memorial Hospital	Woodstock	90%	178
Wellmont Lonesome Pine Hospital[2]	Big Stone Gap	90%	49
Southside Community Hospital	Farmville	89%	79
Carilion Franklin Memorial Hospital	Rocky Mount	86%	36

27. Prophylactic Antibiotic Timing (Outpatient)

Hospital Name	City	Rate	Cases
Pulaski Community Hospital	Pulaski	100%	39
Inova Fair Oaks Hospital	Fairfax	99%	656
Lewis-Gale Medical Center	Salem	99%	618
Montgomery Regional Hospital	Blacksburg	99%	92
John Randolph Medical Center	Hopewell	98%	58
Potomac Hospital	Woodbridge	98%	214
Reston Hospital Center	Reston	98%	948
Riverside Regional Medical Center	Newport News	98%	588
Alleghany Regional Hospital	Low Moor	97%	34
Bon Secours - Depaul Medical Center	Norfolk	97%	358
Henrico Doctors' Hospital	Richmond	97%	662
Sentara Leigh Hospital	Norfolk	97%	363
Bon Secours - St Marys Hospital of Richmond	Richmond	96%	606
Chesapeake General Hospital	Chesapeake	96%	464
Inova Loudoun Hospital	Leesburg	96%	342
Mary Washington Hospital	Fredericksburg	96%	588
Riverside Tappahannock Hospital	Tappahannock	96%	25
Sentara Obici Hospital	Suffolk	96%	141
Bon Secours - Maryview Medical Center	Portsmouth	95%	279
Clinch Valley Medical Center	Richlands	95%	62
Rappahannock General Hospital	Kilmarnock	95%	44
University of Virginia Medical Center	Charlottesville	95%	367
Virginia Hospital Center - Arlington	Arlington	95%	439
Bon Secours - Memorial Regional Medical	Mechanicsville	94%	460
Bon Secours - St Francis Medical Center	Midlothian	94%	392
CJW Medical Center	Richmond	94%	690
Culpeper Regional Hospital	Culpeper	94%	65
Halifax Regional Hospital	Halifax	94%	93
Inova Fairfax Hospital	Falls Church	94%	984
Sentara Virginia Beach General Hospital	Virginia Beach	94%	490
Wythe County Community Hospital	Wytheville	94%	51
Inova Alexandria Hospital	Alexandria	93%	309
Inova Mount Vernon Hospital	Alexandria	93%	70
Mem Hosp of Martinsville & Henry County	Martinsville	93%	175
Prince William Hospital	Manassas	93%	439
Rockingham Memorial Hospital	Harrisonburg	93%	257
Sentara Careplex Hospital	Hampton	93%	307
Centra Health	Lynchburg	92%	444
The Fauquier Hospital	Warrenton	92%	88
Martha Jefferson Hospital	Charlottesville	92%	204
Southside Regional Medical Center	Petersburg	92%	181
Augusta Health	Fishersville	91%	216
Carilion Medical Center	Roanoke	91%	598
Carilion New River Valley Medical Center	Christiansburg	90%	203
Riverside Shore Memorial Hospital	Nassawadox	90%	31
Sentara Williamsburg Regional Med Ctr	Williamsburg	90%	266
Sentara Norfolk General Hospital	Norfolk	89%	655
Warren Memorial Hospital	Front Royal	89%	35
Stafford Hospital Center	Stafford	86%	88
Virginia Commonwealth Univ Health Sys	Richmond	86%	866
Mary Immaculate Hospital	Newport News	85%	283
Norton Community Hospital	Norton	85%	27
Sentara Bayside Hospital	Virginia Beach	85%	147
Danville Regional Medical Center	Danville	83%	119
Riverside Walter Reed Hospital	Gloucester	83%	35
Smyth County Community Hospital	Marion	82%	49
Winchester Medical Center	Winchester	81%	642
Johnston Memorial Hospital	Abingdon	76%	125
Community Memorial Healthcenter	South Hill	74%	50
Mountain View Regional Medical Center	Norton	67%	54
Southampton Memorial Hospital	Franklin	65%	43
Bon Secours - Richmond Community Hospital	Richmond	63%	27

28. Prophylactic Antibiotic Selection

Hospital Name	City	Rate	Cases
Carilion Stonewall Jackson Hospital	Lexington	100%	52
John Randolph Medical Center	Hopewell	100%	41
Shenandoah Memorial Hospital	Woodstock	100%	179
Southern Virginia Regional Medical Center[2]	Emporia	100%	27
Wythe County Community Hospital	Wytheville	100%	204
Augusta Health[2]	Fishersville	99%	697
Bon Secours - Memorial Regional Medical[2]	Mechanicsville	99%	763
Bon Secours - St Marys Hospital of Richmond[2]	Richmond	99%	1777
Carilion New River Valley Medical Center	Christiansburg	99%	240
Culpeper Regional Hospital	Culpeper	99%	243
Inova Fair Oaks Hospital[2]	Fairfax	99%	229
Inova Mount Vernon Hospital[2]	Alexandria	99%	214
Lewis-Gale Medical Center[2]	Salem	99%	545
Mary Immaculate Hospital[2]	Newport News	99%	1295
Mary Washington Hospital[2]	Fredericksburg	99%	673
Montgomery Regional Hospital	Blacksburg	99%	317
Reston Hospital Center[2]	Reston	99%	321
Riverside Regional Medical Center[2]	Newport News	99%	409
Riverside Walter Reed Hospital	Gloucester	99%	134
Salem VA Medical Center	Salem	99%	144
Sentara Careplex Hospital[2]	Hampton	99%	385
Sentara Norfolk General Hospital[2]	Norfolk	99%	1087
Sentara Virginia Beach General Hospital[2]	Virginia Beach	99%	730
Sentara Williamsburg Regional Med Ctr[2]	Williamsburg	99%	304
Smyth County Community Hospital[2]	Marion	99%	126
Stafford Hospital Center	Stafford	99%	88
Winchester Medical Center[2]	Winchester	99%	647
Alleghany Regional Hospital[2]	Low Moor	98%	198
Bon Secours - St Francis Medical Center	Midlothian	98%	722
Carilion Medical Center[2]	Roanoke	98%	2269
Centra Health[2]	Lynchburg	98%	1090
CJW Medical Center[2]	Richmond	98%	543
The Fauquier Hospital	Warrenton	98%	240
Hampton VA Medical Center	Hampton	98%	57
Inova Alexandria Hospital[2]	Alexandria	98%	331
Johnston Memorial Hospital[2]	Abingdon	98%	293
Mountain View Regional Medical Center	Norton	98%	55
Potomac Hospital[2]	Woodbridge	98%	196
Prince William Hospital[2]	Manassas	98%	376
Rappahannock General Hospital	Kilmarnock	98%	80
Richmond VA Medical Center	Richmond	98%	257
Sentara Bayside Hospital	Virginia Beach	98%	130
Sentara Obici Hospital[2]	Suffolk	98%	589
Twin County Regional Hospital	Galax	98%	105
Wellmont Lonesome Pine Hospital[2]	Big Stone Gap	98%	49
Chesapeake General Hospital[2]	Chesapeake	97%	265
Community Memorial Healthcenter[2]	South Hill	97%	35
Danville Regional Medical Center[2]	Danville	97%	310
Henrico Doctors' Hospital[2]	Richmond	97%	606
Inova Fairfax Hospital[2]	Falls Church	97%	422
Inova Loudoun Hospital[2]	Leesburg	97%	272
Martha Jefferson Hospital[2]	Charlottesville	97%	326
Pulaski Community Hospital	Pulaski	97%	39
Riverside Tappahannock Hospital	Tappahannock	97%	87
Sentara Leigh Hospital[2]	Norfolk	97%	1674
Southampton Memorial Hospital[2]	Franklin	97%	101
Southside Community Hospital	Farmville	97%	79
Southside Regional Medical Center[2]	Petersburg	97%	375
University of Virginia Medical Center[2]	Charlottesville	97%	409
Virginia Commonwealth Univ Health Sys[2]	Richmond	97%	456
Virginia Hospital Center - Arlington[2]	Arlington	97%	469
Bon Secours - Depaul Medical Center[2]	Norfolk	96%	280
Halifax Regional Hospital	Halifax	96%	181
Mem Hosp of Martinsville & Henry County	Martinsville	96%	182
Warren Memorial Hospital	Front Royal	96%	56
Bon Secours - Maryview Medical Center[2]	Portsmouth	95%	657
Norton Community Hospital[2]	Norton	95%	41
Rockingham Memorial Hospital[2]	Harrisonburg	95%	386
Carilion Franklin Memorial Hospital	Rocky Mount	92%	36
Riverside Shore Memorial Hospital	Nassawadox	90%	59
Clinch Valley Medical Center	Richlands	88%	112

29. Prophylactic Antibiotic Selection (Outpatient)

Hospital Name	City	Rate	Cases
Alleghany Regional Hospital	Low Moor	100%	33
Halifax Regional Hospital	Halifax	99%	89
Lewis-Gale Medical Center	Salem	99%	620
Reston Hospital Center	Reston	99%	945
Riverside Tappahannock Hospital	Tappahannock	99%	75
Bon Secours - Depaul Medical Center	Norfolk	98%	353
Centra Health	Lynchburg	98%	432
Clinch Valley Medical Center	Richlands	98%	95
The Fauquier Hospital	Warrenton	98%	86
Henrico Doctors' Hospital	Richmond	98%	649
Montgomery Regional Hospital	Blacksburg	98%	98
Mountain View Regional Medical Center	Norton	98%	42
Pulaski Community Hospital	Pulaski	98%	40
Rappahannock General Hospital	Kilmarnock	98%	43
Virginia Hospital Center - Arlington	Arlington	98%	435
Bon Secours - Memorial Regional Medical	Mechanicsville	97%	455
Bon Secours - St Francis Medical Center	Midlothian	97%	385
Bon Secours - St Marys Hospital of Richmond	Richmond	97%	593
CJW Medical Center	Richmond	97%	680
Inova Mount Vernon Hospital	Alexandria	97%	70
John Randolph Medical Center	Hopewell	97%	58
Mary Washington Hospital	Fredericksburg	97%	583
Mem Hosp of Martinsville & Henry County	Martinsville	97%	168
Prince William Hospital	Manassas	97%	421
Riverside Regional Medical Center	Newport News	97%	583
Riverside Walter Reed Hospital	Gloucester	97%	33
Rockingham Memorial Hospital	Harrisonburg	97%	249
Sentara Norfolk General Hospital	Norfolk	97%	621
Southampton Memorial Hospital	Franklin	97%	59
Southside Regional Medical Center	Petersburg	97%	177
University of Virginia Medical Center	Charlottesville	97%	362
Winchester Medical Center	Winchester	97%	631
Augusta Health	Fishersville	96%	205
Carilion Medical Center	Roanoke	96%	575
Chesapeake General Hospital	Chesapeake	96%	450
Inova Alexandria Hospital	Alexandria	96%	300
Inova Fair Oaks Hospital	Fairfax	96%	655
Martha Jefferson Hospital	Charlottesville	96%	201
Sentara Careplex Hospital	Hampton	96%	508
Sentara Virginia Beach General Hospital	Virginia Beach	96%	480
Wythe County Community Hospital	Wytheville	96%	49
Norton Community Hospital	Norton	95%	41
Sentara Leigh Hospital	Norfolk	95%	354
Smyth County Community Hospital	Marion	95%	40
Stafford Hospital Center	Stafford	95%	80
Inova Fairfax Hospital	Falls Church	94%	937
Riverside Shore Memorial Hospital	Nassawadox	94%	62
Sentara Obici Hospital	Suffolk	94%	140
Warren Memorial Hospital	Front Royal	94%	35
Bon Secours - Maryview Medical Center	Portsmouth	93%	276
Mary Immaculate Hospital	Newport News	93%	273
Virginia Commonwealth Univ Health Sys	Richmond	93%	839
Johnston Memorial Hospital	Abingdon	92%	111
Sentara Bayside Hospital	Virginia Beach	92%	256
Inova Loudoun Hospital	Leesburg	91%	348

NOTE: Hospital profiles are in alphabetical order by state, then city, then hospital within the city; Rankings exclude hospitals with less than 25 cases except for patient surveys which excludes hospitals with less than 100 cases; (a) 100–299 cases; (1) The number of cases is too small to be sure how well a hospital is performing; (2) The hospital indicated that the data submitted for this measure were based on a sample of cases; (3) Data was collected during a shorter time period (fewer quarters) than the maximum possible time for this measure; (4) Suppressed for one or more quarters by CMS; (5) No data is available from the hospital for this measure; (6) Fewer than 100 patients completed the HCAHPS survey. Use these rates with caution, as the number of surveys may be too low to reliably assess hospital performance; (7) Survey results are based on less than 12 months of data; (8) Survey results are not available for this reporting period; (9) No or very few patients were eligible for the HCAHPS survey. The scores shown, if any, reflect a very small number of surveys; (10) A state average was not calculated because too few hospitals in the state submitted data; (11) There were discrepancies in the data collection process; Please refer to the User's Guide for a full explanation of data.

Potomac Hospital	Woodbridge	91%	220
Culpeper Regional Hospital	Culpeper	89%	65
Sentara Williamsburg Regional Med Ctr	Williamsburg	88%	286
Danville Regional Medical Center	Danville	84%	113
Carilion New River Valley Medical Center	Christiansburg	83%	212
Community Memorial Healthcenter	South Hill	73%	37

30. Prophylactic Antibiotic Stopped

Hospital Name	City	Rate	Cases
Centra Health[2]	Lynchburg	100%	1016
John Randolph Medical Center	Hopewell	100%	35
Pulaski Community Hospital	Pulaski	100%	33
Riverside Shore Memorial Hospital	Nassawadox	100%	56
Southern Virginia Regional Medical Center[2]	Emporia	100%	26
Clinch Valley Medical Center	Richlands	99%	107
Lewis-Gale Medical Center[2]	Salem	99%	521
Montgomery Regional Hospital	Blacksburg	99%	298
Riverside Tappahannock Hospital	Tappahannock	99%	85
Salem VA Medical Center	Salem	99%	140
Alleghany Regional Hospital[2]	Low Moor	98%	196
Augusta Health[2]	Fishersville	98%	684
Bon Secours - Memorial Regional Medical[2]	Mechanicsville	98%	733
Bon Secours - St Marys Hospital of Richmond[2]	Richmond	98%	1725
Carilion Stonewall Jackson Hospital	Lexington	98%	51
Danville Regional Medical Center[2]	Danville	98%	298
Martha Jefferson Hospital[2]	Charlottesville	98%	314
Riverside Walter Reed Hospital	Gloucester	98%	125
Sentara Careplex Hospital[2]	Hampton	98%	378
Sentara Leigh Hospital[2]	Norfolk	98%	1655
Southampton Memorial Hospital[2]	Franklin	98%	95
Twin County Regional Hospital	Galax	98%	86
Warren Memorial Hospital	Front Royal	98%	49
Bon Secours - St Francis Medical Center	Midlothian	97%	699
Carilion Franklin Memorial Hospital	Rocky Mount	97%	35
Community Memorial Healthcenter[2]	South Hill	97%	32
Riverside Regional Medical Center[2]	Newport News	97%	392
Sentara Williamsburg Regional Med Ctr[2]	Williamsburg	97%	289
Virginia Hospital Center - Arlington[2]	Arlington	97%	434
Wythe County Community Hospital	Wytheville	97%	203
The Fauquier Hospital	Warrenton	96%	226
Inova Fair Oaks Hospital[2]	Fairfax	96%	219
Inova Mount Vernon Hospital[2]	Alexandria	96%	207
Johnston Memorial Hospital[2]	Abingdon	96%	263
Mary Immaculate Hospital[2]	Newport News	96%	1263
Prince William Hospital[2]	Manassas	96%	367
Sentara Virginia Beach General Hospital[2]	Virginia Beach	96%	692
Bon Secours - Depaul Medical Center[2]	Norfolk	95%	265
Bon Secours - Maryview Medical Center[2]	Portsmouth	95%	641
Carilion Medical Center[2]	Roanoke	95%	2203
Carilion New River Valley Medical Center	Christiansburg	95%	231
CJW Medical Center[2]	Richmond	95%	491
Henrico Doctors' Hospital[2]	Richmond	95%	574
Mary Washington Hospital[2]	Fredericksburg	95%	630
Mem Hosp of Martinsville & Henry County	Martinsville	95%	160
Norton Community Hospital[2]	Norton	95%	39
Sentara Norfolk General Hospital[2]	Norfolk	95%	974
Sentara Obici Hospital[2]	Suffolk	95%	554
Shenandoah Memorial Hospital	Woodstock	95%	170
Winchester Medical Center[2]	Winchester	95%	603
Chesapeake General Hospital[2]	Chesapeake	94%	250
Inova Fairfax Hospital[2]	Falls Church	94%	407
Richmond VA Medical Center	Richmond	94%	232
Rockingham Memorial Hospital[2]	Harrisonburg	94%	351
Sentara Bayside Hospital	Virginia Beach	94%	124
Smyth County Community Hospital[2]	Marion	94%	123
Southside Regional Medical Center[2]	Petersburg	94%	361
Rappahannock General Hospital	Kilmarnock	93%	75
Reston Hospital Center[2]	Reston	93%	296
University of Virginia Medical Center[2]	Charlottesville	93%	387
Stafford Hospital Center	Stafford	92%	85
Hampton VA Medical Center	Hampton	91%	56
Southside Community Hospital	Farmville	90%	71
Halifax Regional Hospital	Halifax	89%	171
Inova Alexandria Hospital[2]	Alexandria	89%	316
Inova Loudoun Hospital[2]	Leesburg	89%	260
Wellmont Lonesome Pine Hospital[2]	Big Stone Gap	89%	45
Culpeper Regional Hospital	Culpeper	88%	239
Virginia Commonwealth Univ Health Sys[2]	Richmond	87%	423
Potomac Hospital[2]	Woodbridge	86%	186
Mountain View Regional Medical Center	Norton	81%	53

31. Recommended VTP Ordered

Hospital Name	City	Rate	Cases
John Randolph Medical Center	Hopewell	100%	66
Pulaski Community Hospital	Pulaski	100%	43
Salem VA Medical Center[2]	Salem	100%	114
Southern Virginia Regional Medical Center[2]	Emporia	100%	32
Bon Secours - St Marys Hospital of Richmond[2]	Richmond	99%	524
Centra Health[2]	Lynchburg	99%	408
The Fauquier Hospital	Warrenton	99%	168
Montgomery Regional Hospital	Blacksburg	99%	108
Rockingham Memorial Hospital[2]	Harrisonburg	99%	182
Sentara Bayside Hospital	Virginia Beach	99%	104
Sentara Careplex Hospital[2]	Hampton	99%	126
Sentara Leigh Hospital[2]	Norfolk	99%	820
Sentara Virginia Beach General Hospital[2]	Virginia Beach	99%	365
Twin County Regional Hospital	Galax	99%	90
Bon Secours - Maryview Medical Center[2]	Portsmouth	98%	192
Bon Secours - Memorial Regional Medical[2]	Mechanicsville	98%	308
Inova Fairfax Hospital[2]	Falls Church	98%	184
Lewis-Gale Medical Center[2]	Salem	98%	219
Richmond VA Medical Center[2]	Richmond	98%	163
Virginia Commonwealth Univ Health Sys[2]	Richmond	98%	259
Warren Memorial Hospital	Front Royal	98%	46
Alleghany Regional Hospital[2]	Low Moor	97%	109
Bon Secours - St Francis Medical Center	Midlothian	97%	288
Carilion New River Valley Medical Center	Christiansburg	97%	124
Carilion Stonewall Jackson Hospital	Lexington	97%	32
Chesapeake General Hospital[2]	Chesapeake	97%	177
CJW Medical Center[2]	Richmond	97%	271
Culpeper Regional Hospital	Culpeper	97%	108
Potomac Hospital[2]	Woodbridge	97%	101
Riverside Walter Reed Hospital	Gloucester	97%	79
Sentara Williamsburg Regional Med Ctr[2]	Williamsburg	97%	172
Shenandoah Memorial Hospital	Woodstock	97%	88
Southampton Memorial Hospital[2]	Franklin	97%	36
Virginia Hospital Center - Arlington[2]	Arlington	97%	210
Winchester Medical Center[2]	Winchester	97%	274
Carilion Medical Center[2]	Roanoke	96%	448
Henrico Doctors' Hospital[2]	Richmond	96%	208
Inova Fair Oaks Hospital[2]	Fairfax	96%	76
Inova Mount Vernon Hospital[2]	Alexandria	96%	95
Riverside Tappahannock Hospital	Tappahannock	96%	77
Sentara Norfolk General Hospital[2]	Norfolk	96%	188
Southside Community Hospital	Farmville	96%	67
Bon Secours - Depaul Medical Center[2]	Norfolk	95%	153
Mary Washington Hospital[2]	Fredericksburg	95%	249
Norton Community Hospital[2]	Norton	95%	37
Rappahannock General Hospital	Kilmarnock	95%	80
Reston Hospital Center[2]	Reston	95%	157
Sentara Obici Hospital[2]	Suffolk	95%	216
Inova Alexandria Hospital[2]	Alexandria	94%	146
Riverside Regional Medical Center[2]	Newport News	94%	189
University of Virginia Medical Center[2]	Charlottesville	94%	193
Danville Regional Medical Center[2]	Danville	93%	178
Martha Jefferson Hospital[2]	Charlottesville	93%	127
Southside Regional Medical Center[2]	Petersburg	93%	178
Augusta Health[2]	Fishersville	92%	227
Prince William Hospital[2]	Manassas	92%	118
Clinch Valley Medical Center	Richlands	91%	33
Inova Loudoun Hospital[2]	Leesburg	91%	156
Mary Immaculate Hospital[2]	Newport News	91%	159
Wythe County Community Hospital	Wytheville	91%	33
Smyth County Community Hospital[2]	Marion	88%	66
Johnston Memorial Hospital[2]	Abingdon	87%	133
Riverside Shore Memorial Hospital	Nassawadox	83%	30
Stafford Hospital Center	Stafford	81%	52
Community Memorial Healthcenter[2]	South Hill	80%	49
Mem Hosp of Martinsville & Henry County	Martinsville	80%	130
Halifax Regional Hospital	Halifax	75%	124

32. Urinary Catheter Removal

Hospital Name	City	Rate	Cases
Inova Fair Oaks Hospital[2]	Fairfax	100%	61
Mary Immaculate Hospital[2]	Newport News	100%	57
Potomac Hospital[2]	Woodbridge	100%	61
Riverside Walter Reed Hospital	Gloucester	100%	69
Sentara Bayside Hospital	Virginia Beach	100%	37
Sentara Careplex Hospital[2]	Hampton	100%	100
Montgomery Regional Hospital	Blacksburg	99%	79
Prince William Hospital[2]	Manassas	99%	123
Bon Secours - Maryview Medical Center[2]	Portsmouth	98%	258
Sentara Leigh Hospital[2]	Norfolk	98%	674
Stafford Hospital Center	Stafford	98%	40
Bon Secours - Memorial Regional Medical[2]	Mechanicsville	97%	347
Bon Secours - St Marys Hospital of Richmond[2]	Richmond	97%	651
Centra Health[2]	Lynchburg	97%	135
Riverside Regional Medical Center[2]	Newport News	97%	118
Sentara Virginia Beach General Hospital[2]	Virginia Beach	97%	220
Wythe County Community Hospital	Wytheville	97%	69
Carilion New River Valley Medical Center	Christiansburg	95%	73
CJW Medical Center[2]	Richmond	95%	195
Richmond VA Medical Center[2]	Richmond	95%	131
Sentara Williamsburg Regional Med Ctr[2]	Williamsburg	95%	112
Virginia Hospital Center - Arlington[2]	Arlington	95%	106
Carilion Medical Center[2]	Roanoke	94%	325
The Fauquier Hospital	Warrenton	94%	100
Inova Mount Vernon Hospital[2]	Alexandria	94%	133
Reston Hospital Center[2]	Reston	94%	130
Culpeper Regional Hospital	Culpeper	93%	107
Inova Alexandria Hospital[2]	Alexandria	93%	114
Inova Fairfax Hospital[2]	Falls Church	93%	163
Rockingham Memorial Hospital[2]	Harrisonburg	93%	108
Salem VA Medical Center[2]	Salem	93%	85
Mary Washington Hospital[2]	Fredericksburg	92%	185
Sentara Norfolk General Hospital[2]	Norfolk	92%	331
Mem Hosp of Martinsville & Henry County	Martinsville	91%	44
Bon Secours - Depaul Medical Center[2]	Norfolk	90%	39
Martha Jefferson Hospital[2]	Charlottesville	89%	66
Sentara Obici Hospital[2]	Suffolk	89%	135
Augusta Health[2]	Fishersville	88%	42
Henrico Doctors' Hospital[2]	Richmond	88%	195
Inova Loudoun Hospital[2]	Leesburg	88%	48
Lewis-Gale Medical Center[2]	Salem	88%	100
Rappahannock General Hospital	Kilmarnock	88%	33
Johnston Memorial Hospital[2]	Abingdon	86%	92
Bon Secours - St Francis Medical Center	Midlothian	85%	52
Shenandoah Memorial Hospital	Woodstock	85%	48
Southside Regional Medical Center	Petersburg	85%	81
Virginia Commonwealth Univ Health Sys[2]	Richmond	85%	161
Chesapeake General Hospital[2]	Chesapeake	79%	91
Winchester Medical Center[2]	Winchester	79%	141
Danville Regional Medical Center[2]	Danville	60%	43
University of Virginia Medical Center[2]	Charlottesville	59%	121
Halifax Regional Hospital	Halifax	55%	38
Southside Community Hospital	Farmville	50%	26

Children's Asthma Care

33. Received Systemic Corticosteroids

Hospital Name	City	Rate	Cases
Centra Health	Lynchburg	100%	74
Inova Fairfax Hospital[2]	Falls Church	100%	309
Mary Washington Hospital	Fredericksburg	100%	47
University of Virginia Medical Center[2]	Charlottesville	97%	38

34. Received Home Management Plan of Care

Hospital Name	City	Rate	Cases
Centra Health	Lynchburg	94%	70
Inova Fairfax Hospital[2]	Falls Church	78%	310
Mary Washington Hospital	Fredericksburg	76%	45
University of Virginia Medical Center[2]	Charlottesville	61%	38

35. Received Reliever Medication

Hospital Name	City	Rate	Cases
Centra Health	Lynchburg	100%	75
Inova Fairfax Hospital[2]	Falls Church	100%	310
Mary Washington Hospital	Fredericksburg	100%	47
University of Virginia Medical Center[2]	Charlottesville	100%	38

Use of Medical Imaging

36. Combination Abdominal CT Scan

Hospital Name	City	Ratio	Cases
Warren Memorial Hospital	Front Royal	0.010	290
Mary Washington Hospital	Fredericksburg	0.013	602
Inova Fairfax Hospital	Falls Church	0.026	1485
Carilion Medical Center	Roanoke	0.027	1721
Russell County Medical Center	Lebanon	0.027	148
Pulaski Community Hospital	Pulaski	0.031	359
Carilion Franklin Memorial Hospital	Rocky Mount	0.032	408
Wythe County Community Hospital	Wytheville	0.042	384
Riverside Tappahannock Hospital	Tappahannock	0.050	459
Rockingham Memorial Hospital	Harrisonburg	0.053	1312
Inova Fair Oaks Hospital	Fairfax	0.054	607
University of Virginia Medical Center	Charlottesville	0.056	589
Lewis-Gale Medical Center	Salem	0.057	1458
Mary Immaculate Hospital	Newport News	0.060	366
Alleghany Regional Hospital	Low Moor	0.061	443
The Fauquier Hospital	Warrenton	0.061	656
Sentara Williamsburg Regional Med Ctr	Williamsburg	0.065	1052
Inova Loudoun Hospital	Leesburg	0.066	797
Carilion Tazewell Community Hospital	Tazewell	0.067	135
Potomac Hospital	Woodbridge	0.070	660
Virginia Hospital Center - Arlington	Arlington	0.072	1478
Culpeper Regional Hospital	Culpeper	0.074	537
Prince William Hospital	Manassas	0.074	914
Montgomery Regional Hospital	Blacksburg	0.075	518
Mem Hosp of Martinsville & Henry County	Martinsville	0.076	719
Riverside Shore Memorial Hospital	Nassawadox	0.076	447
Reston Hospital Center	Reston	0.080	638
Carilion New River Valley Medical Center	Christiansburg	0.086	850
Riverside Walter Reed Hospital	Gloucester	0.086	570
Sentara Virginia Beach General Hospital	Virginia Beach	0.087	1523
Southside Community Hospital	Farmville	0.093	399
Inova Mount Vernon Hospital	Alexandria	0.095	613
Buchanan General Hospital	Grundy	0.097	278
Centra Health	Lynchburg	0.097	1628

NOTE: Hospital profiles are in alphabetical order by state, then city, then hospital within the city; Rankings exclude hospitals with less than 25 cases except for patient surveys which excludes hospitals with less than 100 cases; (a) 100–299 cases; (1) The number of cases is too small to be sure how well a hospital is performing; (2) The hospital indicated that the data submitted for this measure were based on a sample of cases; (3) Data was collected during a shorter time period (fewer quarters) than the maximum possible time for this measure; (4) Suppressed for one or more quarters by CMS; (5) No data is available from the hospital for this measure; (6) Fewer than 100 patients completed the HCAHPS survey. Use these rates with caution, as the number of surveys may be too low to reliably assess hospital performance; (7) Survey results are based on less than 12 months of data; (8) Survey results are not available for this reporting period; (9) No or very few patients were eligible for the HCAHPS survey. The scores shown, if any, reflect a very small number of surveys; (10) A state average was not calculated because too few hospitals in the state submitted data; (11) There were discrepancies in the data collection process; Please refer to the User's Guide for a full explanation of data.

Carilion Giles Memorial Hospital	Pearisburg	0.104	317
Rappahannock General Hospital	Kilmarnock	0.110	474
Winchester Medical Center	Winchester	0.111	1393
Bon Secours - Maryview Medical Center	Portsmouth	0.116	1505
Riverside Regional Medical Center	Newport News	0.117	1839
Sentara Bayside Hospital	Virginia Beach	0.119	1363
Sentara Norfolk General Hospital	Norfolk	0.120	1338
Inova Alexandria Hospital	Alexandria	0.123	819
Southern Virginia Regional Medical Center	Emporia	0.123	243
Virginia Commonwealth Univ Health Sys	Richmond	0.124	1225
Johnston Memorial Hospital	Abingdon	0.125	1032
Martha Jefferson Hospital	Charlottesville	0.125	1435
Sentara Leigh Hospital	Norfolk	0.126	1835
Sentara Careplex Hospital	Hampton	0.137	2040
Bon Secours - St Marys Hospital of Richmond	Richmond	0.138	1040
Bon Secours - Memorial Regional Medical	Mechanicsville	0.139	1472
Henrico Doctors' Hospital	Richmond	0.141	1202
Bon Secours - Depaul Medical Center	Norfolk	0.149	793
Augusta Health	Fishersville	0.163	1673
Sentara Obici Hospital	Suffolk	0.184	898
Danville Regional Medical Center	Danville	0.187	327
Southside Regional Medical Center	Petersburg	0.205	929
Bedford Memorial Hospital	Bedford	0.230	257
Bon Secours - Richmond Community Hospital	Richmond	0.233	103
Bon Secours - St Francis Medical Center	Midlothian	0.267	647
Mountain View Regional Medical Center	Norton	0.322	208
CJW Medical Center	Richmond	0.324	1776
Clinch Valley Medical Center	Richlands	0.333	708
Southampton Memorial Hospital	Franklin	0.352	347
Halifax Regional Hospital	Halifax	0.371	574
John Randolph Medical Center	Hopewell	0.384	631
Chesapeake General Hospital	Chesapeake	0.395	1313
Dickenson Community Hospital	Clintwood	0.402	102
Community Memorial Healthcenter	South Hill	0.409	545
Twin County Regional Hospital	Galax	0.530	776
Norton Community Hospital	Norton	0.543	468
Smyth County Community Hospital	Marion	0.560	377
Lee Regional Medical Center	Pennington Gap	0.614	197
Wellmont Lonesome Pine Hospital	Big Stone Gap	0.641	370

37. Combination Chest CT Scan

Hospital Name	City	Ratio	Cases
Alleghany Regional Hospital	Low Moor	0.000	346
Bedford Memorial Hospital	Bedford	0.000	170
Danville Regional Medical Center	Danville	0.000	301
The Fauquier Hospital	Warrenton	0.000	384
Martha Jefferson Hospital	Charlottesville	0.000	1024
Sentara Obici Hospital	Suffolk	0.000	514
Wythe County Community Hospital	Wytheville	0.000	240
Augusta Health	Fishersville	0.001	1236
Sentara Careplex Hospital	Hampton	0.002	1253
Virginia Hospital Center - Arlington	Arlington	0.002	1170
Bon Secours - Depaul Medical Center	Norfolk	0.003	718
Rockingham Memorial Hospital	Harrisonburg	0.003	745
University of Virginia Medical Center	Charlottesville	0.003	357
Riverside Walter Reed Hospital	Gloucester	0.004	454
Sentara Virginia Beach General Hospital	Virginia Beach	0.004	1375
Smyth County Community Hospital	Marion	0.004	229
Sentara Williamsburg Regional Med Ctr	Williamsburg	0.005	737
Bon Secours - Memorial Regional Medical	Mechanicsville	0.006	843
Southside Regional Medical Center	Petersburg	0.006	694
Chesapeake General Hospital	Chesapeake	0.007	1249
Culpeper Regional Hospital	Culpeper	0.007	304
John Randolph Medical Center	Hopewell	0.007	428
Sentara Leigh Hospital	Norfolk	0.007	1671
Lewis-Gale Medical Center	Salem	0.008	992
Sentara Norfolk General Hospital	Norfolk	0.008	1183
Warren Memorial Hospital	Front Royal	0.008	250
Mary Washington Hospital	Fredericksburg	0.009	109
Riverside Shore Memorial Hospital	Nassawadox	0.009	322
Inova Loudoun Hospital	Leesburg	0.010	775
Pulaski Community Hospital	Pulaski	0.010	202
Winchester Medical Center	Winchester	0.010	1384
Halifax Regional Hospital	Halifax	0.011	374
Inova Fairfax Hospital	Falls Church	0.011	1218
Bon Secours - St Marys Hospital of Richmond	Richmond	0.012	499
Henrico Doctors' Hospital	Richmond	0.012	890
Inova Alexandria Hospital	Alexandria	0.014	655
Prince William Hospital	Manassas	0.014	591
Centra Health	Lynchburg	0.016	1074
Inova Fair Oaks Hospital	Fairfax	0.019	540
Twin County Regional Hospital	Galax	0.020	244
Riverside Tappahannock Hospital	Tappahannock	0.021	375
Bon Secours - Richmond Community Hospital	Richmond	0.022	45
Bon Secours - St Francis Medical Center	Midlothian	0.022	369
Potomac Hospital	Woodbridge	0.022	631
Inova Mount Vernon Hospital	Alexandria	0.023	559
Riverside Regional Medical Center	Newport News	0.023	1627
Bon Secours - Maryview Medical Center	Portsmouth	0.028	1172
Montgomery Regional Hospital	Blacksburg	0.030	296
Mem Hosp of Martinsville & Henry County	Martinsville	0.032	440
Reston Hospital Center	Reston	0.032	501
Carilion Medical Center	Roanoke	0.038	1131
Southern Virginia Regional Medical Center	Emporia	0.039	129
Virginia Commonwealth Univ Health Sys	Richmond	0.040	1549
Carilion New River Valley Medical Center	Christiansburg	0.041	680
Mary Immaculate Hospital	Newport News	0.048	165
Sentara Bayside Hospital	Virginia Beach	0.048	986
CJW Medical Center	Richmond	0.052	897
Rappahannock General Hospital	Kilmarnock	0.053	320
Community Memorial Healthcenter	South Hill	0.059	321
Carilion Franklin Memorial Hospital	Rocky Mount	0.067	163
Johnston Memorial Hospital	Abingdon	0.095	761
Southampton Memorial Hospital	Franklin	0.098	183
Carilion Tazewell Community Hospital	Tazewell	0.114	79
Clinch Valley Medical Center	Richlands	0.122	615
Buchanan General Hospital	Grundy	0.155	181
Russell County Medical Center	Lebanon	0.240	125
Wellmont Lonesome Pine Hospital	Big Stone Gap	0.243	235
Carilion Giles Memorial Hospital	Pearisburg	0.287	129
Southside Community Hospital	Farmville	0.288	191
Mountain View Regional Medical Center	Norton	0.324	182
Dickenson Community Hospital	Clintwood	0.338	80
Norton Community Hospital	Norton	0.361	410
Lee Regional Medical Center	Pennington Gap	0.584	77

38. Follow-up Mammogram/Ultrasound

Hospital Name	City	Rate	Cases
Mem Hosp of Martinsville & Henry County	Martinsville	3.1%	2087
Southern Virginia Regional Medical Center	Emporia	3.4%	470
Riverside Shore Memorial Hospital	Nassawadox	3.6%	1034
Johnston Memorial Hospital	Abingdon	3.8%	1565
Pulaski Community Hospital	Pulaski	3.8%	420
Virginia Commonwealth Univ Health Sys	Richmond	3.9%	1917
Twin County Regional Hospital	Galax	4.0%	1485
Rappahannock General Hospital	Kilmarnock	4.2%	891
Carilion Medical Center	Roanoke	4.3%	4239
Carilion Franklin Memorial Hospital	Rocky Mount	4.4%	681
John Randolph Medical Center	Hopewell	4.5%	731
Community Memorial Healthcenter	South Hill	4.6%	1230
Carilion Giles Memorial Hospital	Pearisburg	4.7%	548
Carilion Tazewell Community Hospital	Tazewell	4.9%	223
Southampton Memorial Hospital	Franklin	4.9%	427
Riverside Walter Reed Hospital	Gloucester	5.3%	1037
CJW Medical Center	Richmond	5.6%	2755
Inova Fair Oaks Hospital	Fairfax	5.6%	356
Mountain View Regional Medical Center	Norton	5.6%	341
Bon Secours - Depaul Medical Center	Norfolk	5.7%	1458
Southside Community Hospital	Farmville	5.7%	663
Riverside Tappahannock Hospital	Tappahannock	6.0%	651
Virginia Hospital Center - Arlington	Arlington	6.0%	2248
Winchester Medical Center	Winchester	6.1%	2748
Rockingham Memorial Hospital	Harrisonburg	6.2%	2521
Sentara Virginia Beach General Hospital	Virginia Beach	6.3%	2093
Inova Alexandria Hospital	Alexandria	6.5%	417
Sentara Obici Hospital	Suffolk	7.0%	1260
Bon Secours - Maryview Medical Center	Portsmouth	7.3%	2111
Bon Secours - Memorial Regional Medical	Mechanicsville	7.4%	2636
Clinch Valley Medical Center	Richlands	7.4%	135
Danville Regional Medical Center	Danville	7.7%	117
Martha Jefferson Hospital	Charlottesville	7.8%	3457
Sentara Bayside Hospital	Virginia Beach	7.8%	1504
Bon Secours - St Marys Hospital of Richmond	Richmond	7.9%	3046
Sentara Leigh Hospital	Norfolk	7.9%	2507
Wythe County Community Hospital	Wytheville	7.9%	471
Henrico Doctors' Hospital	Richmond	8.0%	1467
Riverside Regional Medical Center	Newport News	8.1%	2204
Mary Immaculate Hospital	Newport News	8.2%	476
Sentara Norfolk General Hospital	Norfolk	8.4%	1752
Bedford Memorial Hospital	Bedford	8.5%	648
Southside Regional Medical Center	Petersburg	8.5%	1383
Carilion New River Valley Medical Center	Christiansburg	8.6%	1497
Inova Fairfax Hospital	Falls Church	8.6%	487
Inova Mount Vernon Hospital	Alexandria	8.7%	756
Lewis-Gale Medical Center	Salem	8.7%	2523
Wellmont Lonesome Pine Hospital	Big Stone Gap	8.7%	355
Sentara Williamsburg Regional Med Ctr	Williamsburg	8.9%	2860
Reston Hospital Center	Reston	9.5%	455
University of Virginia Medical Center	Charlottesville	9.6%	3221
Chesapeake General Hospital	Chesapeake	10.0%	1989
Alleghany Regional Hospital	Low Moor	10.1%	833
Lee Regional Medical Center	Pennington Gap	10.2%	305
The Fauquier Hospital	Warrenton	10.3%	769
Inova Loudoun Hospital	Leesburg	10.3%	544
Prince William Hospital	Manassas	10.3%	1023
Bon Secours - Richmond Community Hospital	Richmond	10.4%	202
Halifax Regional Hospital	Halifax	10.4%	1288
Culpeper Regional Hospital	Culpeper	10.8%	702
Sentara Careplex Hospital	Hampton	10.8%	2681
Montgomery Regional Hospital	Blacksburg	10.9%	827
Augusta Health	Fishersville	12.5%	2916
Warren Memorial Hospital	Front Royal	12.5%	407
Bon Secours - St Francis Medical Center	Midlothian	12.9%	457
Potomac Hospital	Woodbridge	13.8%	385
Russell County Medical Center	Lebanon	15.3%	163
Mary Washington Hospital	Fredericksburg	15.4%	228
Norton Community Hospital	Norton	16.6%	500
Smyth County Community Hospital	Marion	17.1%	578
Buchanan General Hospital	Grundy	17.9%	246

39. MRI for Low Back Pain

Hospital Name	City	Rate	Cases
Warren Memorial Hospital[1]	Front Royal	15.8%	38
Lee Regional Medical Center[1]	Pennington Gap	20.5%	39
Bon Secours - Maryview Medical Center	Portsmouth	21.8%	404
Sentara Virginia Beach General Hospital	Virginia Beach	21.9%	187
Potomac Hospital	Woodbridge	22.3%	157
Bon Secours - St Francis Medical Center[1]	Midlothian	23.5%	51
Southside Community Hospital	Farmville	23.8%	63
Mary Immaculate Hospital	Newport News	24.3%	70
Culpeper Regional Hospital	Culpeper	25.0%	128
Riverside Shore Memorial Hospital[1]	Nassawadox	25.0%	32
Riverside Regional Medical Center	Newport News	26.4%	277
Riverside Tappahannock Hospital[1]	Tappahannock	26.5%	34
Henrico Doctors' Hospital	Richmond	26.6%	214
Inova Loudoun Hospital	Leesburg	26.6%	124
Rappahannock General Hospital	Kilmarnock	26.7%	161
Sentara Bayside Hospital	Virginia Beach	26.7%	247
Sentara Leigh Hospital	Norfolk	27.1%	221
Pulaski Community Hospital	Pulaski	27.5%	80
Sentara Williamsburg Regional Med Ctr	Williamsburg	27.8%	237
Lewis-Gale Medical Center	Salem	28.0%	275
Sentara Norfolk General Hospital	Norfolk	28.0%	125
Bon Secours - Depaul Medical Center	Norfolk	28.4%	169
Centra Health	Lynchburg	28.5%	267
Sentara Obici Hospital	Suffolk	28.6%	220
Bon Secours - Memorial Regional Medical	Mechanicsville	28.7%	362
Virginia Commonwealth Univ Health Sys	Richmond	28.8%	226
Bon Secours - St Marys Hospital of Richmond	Richmond	29.6%	422
Inova Fair Oaks Hospital	Fairfax	29.6%	270
Winchester Medical Center	Winchester	30.3%	501
Southside Regional Medical Center	Petersburg	30.4%	181
Halifax Regional Hospital	Halifax	30.5%	128
Rockingham Memorial Hospital	Harrisonburg	30.7%	358
CJW Medical Center	Richmond	30.9%	282
Prince William Hospital	Manassas	31.3%	195
Martha Jefferson Hospital	Charlottesville	31.8%	330
Sentara Careplex Hospital	Hampton	31.9%	232
Virginia Hospital Center - Arlington	Arlington	31.9%	329
Inova Alexandria Hospital	Alexandria	32.2%	295
Danville Regional Medical Center[1]	Danville	32.4%	37
Chesapeake General Hospital	Chesapeake	32.6%	227
Carilion Medical Center	Roanoke	32.7%	459
Carilion Giles Memorial Hospital	Pearisburg	33.3%	57
Mary Washington Hospital[1]	Fredericksburg	33.3%	30
The Fauquier Hospital	Warrenton	33.6%	125
Alleghany Regional Hospital	Low Moor	33.7%	92
Norton Community Hospital	Norton	33.8%	65
Riverside Walter Reed Hospital	Gloucester	33.8%	145
Inova Fairfax Hospital	Falls Church	34.0%	147
Inova Mount Vernon Hospital	Alexandria	34.2%	190
Augusta Health	Fishersville	34.6%	503
Montgomery Regional Hospital	Blacksburg	35.0%	214
Carilion Franklin Memorial Hospital	Rocky Mount	38.2%	89
Wythe County Community Hospital	Wytheville	39.5%	86
John Randolph Medical Center	Hopewell	40.0%	115
Johnston Memorial Hospital	Abingdon	40.1%	324
Bedford Memorial Hospital	Bedford	41.3%	46
Buchanan General Hospital	Grundy	41.8%	79
Carilion New River Valley Medical Center	Christiansburg	42.0%	200
Mem Hosp of Martinsville & Henry County	Martinsville	42.9%	161
Smyth County Community Hospital	Marion	43.0%	79
Clinch Valley Medical Center	Richlands	43.2%	111
Twin County Regional Hospital	Galax	43.5%	147
Community Memorial Healthcenter	South Hill	47.1%	70
Wellmont Lonesome Pine Hospital	Big Stone Gap	47.5%	61
Carilion Tazewell Community Hospital[1]	Tazewell	48.0%	25
Mountain View Regional Medical Center	Norton	50.0%	66
Southampton Memorial Hospital[1]	Franklin	55.2%	29

Survey of Patients' Hospital Experiences

40. Area Around Room 'Always' Quiet at Night

Hospital Name	City	Rate	Cases
Bon Secours - Richmond Community Hospital	Richmond	77%	(a)
Carilion Tazewell Community Hospital	Tazewell	69%	(a)
Potomac Hospital	Woodbridge	67%	300+
Bon Secours - St Francis Medical Center	Midlothian	66%	300+
Southern Virginia Regional Medical Center	Emporia	66%	300+
Bon Secours - Maryview Medical Center	Portsmouth	65%	300+

NOTE: Hospital profiles are in alphabetical order by state, then city, then hospital within the city; Rankings exclude hospitals with less than 25 cases except for patient surveys which excludes hospitals with less than 100 cases; (a) 100–299 cases; (1) The number of cases is too small to be sure how well a hospital is performing; (2) The hospital indicated that the data submitted for this measure were based on a sample of cases; (3) Data was collected during a shorter time period (fewer quarters) than the maximum possible time for this measure; (4) Suppressed for one or more quarters by CMS; (5) No data is available from the hospital for this measure; (6) Fewer than 100 patients completed the HCAHPS survey. Use these rates with caution, as the number of surveys may be too low to reliably assess hospital performance; (7) Survey results are based on less than 12 months of data; (8) Survey results are not available for this reporting period; (9) No or very few patients were eligible for the HCAHPS survey. The scores shown, if any, reflect a very small number of surveys; (10) A state average was not calculated because too few hospitals in the state submitted data; (11) There were discrepancies in the data collection process; Please refer to the User's Guide for a full explanation of data.

Halifax Regional Hospital	Halifax	65%	300+
Southampton Memorial Hospital	Franklin	65%	300+
Bon Secours - St Marys Hospital of Richmond	Richmond	64%	300+
Danville Regional Medical Center	Danville	64%	300+
Mary Immaculate Hospital	Newport News	64%	300+
Montgomery Regional Hospital	Blacksburg	63%	300+
Carilion Giles Memorial Hospital	Pearisburg	62%	(a)
Reston Hospital Center	Reston	62%	300+
Bon Secours - Depaul Medical Center	Norfolk	61%	300+
Buchanan General Hospital	Grundy	61%	300+
Carilion Stonewall Jackson Hospital	Lexington	61%	300+
Clinch Valley Medical Center	Richlands	61%	300+
The Fauquier Hospital	Warrenton	61%	300+
Henrico Doctors' Hospital	Richmond	61%	300+
John Randolph Medical Center	Hopewell	61%	300+
Pulaski Community Hospital	Pulaski	61%	300+
Shenandoah Memorial Hospital	Woodstock	61%	300+
Alleghany Regional Hospital	Low Moor	60%	300+
Carilion Medical Center	Roanoke	60%	300+
Centra Health	Lynchburg	60%	300+
Community Memorial Healthcenter	South Hill	60%	300+
Sentara Careplex Hospital	Hampton	60%	300+
Wythe County Community Hospital	Wytheville	60%	300+
Carilion Franklin Memorial Hospital	Rocky Mount	59%	300+
Twin County Regional Hospital	Galax	59%	300+
Virginia Commonwealth Univ Health Sys	Richmond	59%	300+
Wellmont Lonesome Pine Hospital	Big Stone Gap	59%	300+
Bedford Memorial Hospital	Bedford	58%	300+
Carilion New River Valley Medical Center	Christiansburg	58%	300+
CJW Medical Center	Richmond	58%	300+
Sentara Williamsburg Regional Med Ctr	Williamsburg	58%	300+
Southside Community Hospital[11]	Farmville	58%	300+
Virginia Hospital Center - Arlington	Arlington	58%	300+
Bon Secours - Memorial Regional Medical	Mechanicsville	57%	300+
Culpeper Regional Hospital	Culpeper	56%	300+
Inova Mount Vernon Hospital	Alexandria	56%	300+
Southside Regional Medical Center	Petersburg	56%	300+
Chesapeake General Hospital	Chesapeake	55%	300+
Lewis-Gale Medical Center	Salem	55%	300+
Russell County Medical Center	Lebanon	55%	300+
Warren Memorial Hospital	Front Royal	55%	300+
Lee Regional Medical Center	Pennington Gap	54%	300+
Page Memorial Hospital	Luray	54%	(a)
Riverside Walter Reed Hospital	Gloucester	54%	300+
Sentara Bayside Hospital	Virginia Beach	54%	300+
Sentara Norfolk General Hospital	Norfolk	54%	300+
Sentara Obici Hospital	Suffolk	54%	300+
Smyth County Community Hospital	Marion	54%	300+
Stafford Hospital Center	Stafford	54%	300+
Martha Jefferson Hospital	Charlottesville	53%	300+
Mem Hosp of Martinsville & Henry County	Martinsville	53%	300+
Winchester Medical Center	Winchester	53%	(a)
Inova Alexandria Hospital	Alexandria	52%	300+
Johnston Memorial Hospital	Abingdon	52%	300+
Prince William Hospital	Manassas	52%	300+
Riverside Shore Memorial Hospital	Nassawadox	52%	300+
Rockingham Memorial Hospital	Harrisonburg	52%	300+
Sentara Virginia Beach General Hospital	Virginia Beach	52%	300+
Augusta Health	Fishersville	51%	300+
Mary Washington Hospital	Fredericksburg	51%	300+
Inova Fair Oaks Hospital	Fairfax	50%	300+
Mountain View Regional Medical Center	Norton	50%	(a)
Riverside Tappahannock Hospital	Tappahannock	50%	300+
Inova Fairfax Hospital	Falls Church	49%	300+
Rappahannock General Hospital	Kilmarnock	49%	300+
Norton Community Hospital	Norton	47%	300+
Inova Loudoun Hospital	Leesburg	45%	300+
Riverside Regional Medical Center	Newport News	45%	300+
Sentara Leigh Hospital	Norfolk	45%	300+
University of Virginia Medical Center	Charlottesville	42%	300+

41. Doctors 'Always' Communicated Well

Hospital Name	City	Rate	Cases
Bon Secours - Richmond Community Hospital	Richmond	88%	(a)
Martha Jefferson Hospital	Charlottesville	88%	300+
Bedford Memorial Hospital	Bedford	86%	300+
Buchanan General Hospital	Grundy	86%	300+
Carilion Giles Memorial Hospital	Pearisburg	86%	(a)
Carilion Stonewall Jackson Hospital	Lexington	86%	300+
Pulaski Community Hospital	Pulaski	86%	300+
Halifax Regional Hospital	Halifax	85%	300+
Riverside Shore Memorial Hospital	Nassawadox	85%	300+
Southern Virginia Regional Medical Center	Emporia	85%	300+
Wythe County Community Hospital	Wytheville	85%	300+
Bon Secours - Memorial Regional Medical	Mechanicsville	84%	300+
Clinch Valley Medical Center	Richlands	84%	300+
Johnston Memorial Hospital	Abingdon	84%	300+
Montgomery Regional Hospital	Blacksburg	84%	300+
Carilion Franklin Memorial Hospital	Rocky Mount	83%	300+
Centra Health	Lynchburg	83%	300+
Alleghany Regional Hospital	Low Moor	82%	300+
Community Memorial Healthcenter	South Hill	82%	300+
Henrico Doctors' Hospital	Richmond	82%	300+
Lewis-Gale Medical Center	Salem	82%	300+
Rappahannock General Hospital	Kilmarnock	82%	300+
Russell County Medical Center	Lebanon	82%	300+
Southampton Memorial Hospital	Franklin	82%	300+
Twin County Regional Hospital	Galax	82%	300+
Augusta Health	Fishersville	81%	300+
Bon Secours - Maryview Medical Center	Portsmouth	81%	300+
Bon Secours - St Marys Hospital of Richmond	Richmond	81%	300+
Carilion Tazewell Community Hospital	Tazewell	81%	(a)
Inova Mount Vernon Hospital	Alexandria	81%	300+
Mem Hosp of Martinsville & Henry County	Martinsville	81%	300+
Mountain View Regional Medical Center	Norton	81%	(a)
Riverside Walter Reed Hospital	Gloucester	81%	300+
Carilion New River Valley Medical Center	Christiansburg	80%	300+
CJW Medical Center	Richmond	80%	300+
The Fauquier Hospital	Warrenton	80%	300+
Inova Loudoun Hospital	Leesburg	80%	300+
Lee Regional Medical Center	Pennington Gap	80%	300+
Norton Community Hospital	Norton	80%	300+
Shenandoah Memorial Hospital	Woodstock	80%	300+
Virginia Commonwealth Univ Health Sys	Richmond	80%	300+
Winchester Medical Center	Winchester	80%	(a)
Mary Immaculate Hospital	Newport News	79%	300+
Prince William Hospital	Manassas	79%	300+
Reston Hospital Center	Reston	79%	300+
Sentara Norfolk General Hospital	Norfolk	79%	300+
Southside Community Hospital[11]	Farmville	79%	300+
Southside Regional Medical Center	Petersburg	79%	300+
Bon Secours - Depaul Medical Center	Norfolk	79%	300+
Carilion Medical Center	Roanoke	78%	300+
Inova Fair Oaks Hospital	Fairfax	78%	300+
Riverside Tappahannock Hospital	Tappahannock	78%	300+
Virginia Hospital Center - Arlington	Arlington	78%	300+
Bon Secours - St Francis Medical Center	Midlothian	77%	300+
Chesapeake General Hospital	Chesapeake	77%	300+
John Randolph Medical Center	Hopewell	77%	300+
Rockingham Memorial Hospital	Harrisonburg	77%	300+
Warren Memorial Hospital	Front Royal	77%	300+
Danville Regional Medical Center	Danville	76%	300+
Inova Fairfax Hospital	Falls Church	76%	300+
Potomac Hospital	Woodbridge	76%	300+
Riverside Regional Medical Center	Newport News	76%	300+
University of Virginia Medical Center	Charlottesville	76%	300+
Sentara Bayside Hospital	Virginia Beach	75%	300+
Sentara Careplex Hospital	Hampton	75%	300+
Sentara Williamsburg Regional Med Ctr	Williamsburg	75%	300+
Smyth County Community Hospital	Marion	75%	300+
Stafford Hospital Center	Stafford	75%	300+
Wellmont Lonesome Pine Hospital	Big Stone Gap	75%	300+
Inova Alexandria Hospital	Alexandria	74%	300+
Mary Washington Hospital	Fredericksburg	74%	300+
Page Memorial Hospital	Luray	74%	(a)
Sentara Virginia Beach General Hospital	Virginia Beach	74%	300+
Sentara Leigh Hospital	Norfolk	73%	300+
Sentara Obici Hospital	Suffolk	72%	300+
Culpeper Regional Hospital	Culpeper	68%	300+

42. Home Recovery Information Given

Hospital Name	City	Rate	Cases
Page Memorial Hospital	Luray	91%	(a)
Montgomery Regional Hospital	Blacksburg	88%	300+
Wythe County Community Hospital	Wytheville	88%	300+
Carilion New River Valley Medical Center	Christiansburg	87%	300+
Inova Loudoun Hospital	Leesburg	87%	300+
Lewis-Gale Medical Center	Salem	87%	300+
Shenandoah Memorial Hospital	Woodstock	87%	300+
Bon Secours - Memorial Regional Medical	Mechanicsville	86%	300+
Bon Secours - Richmond Community Hospital	Richmond	86%	(a)
Bon Secours - St Francis Medical Center	Midlothian	86%	300+
Pulaski Community Hospital	Pulaski	86%	300+
University of Virginia Medical Center	Charlottesville	86%	300+
Virginia Commonwealth Univ Health Sys	Richmond	86%	300+
Augusta Health	Fishersville	85%	300+
Bon Secours - Depaul Medical Center	Norfolk	85%	300+
Bon Secours - Maryview Medical Center	Portsmouth	85%	300+
Halifax Regional Hospital	Halifax	85%	300+
Martha Jefferson Hospital	Charlottesville	85%	300+
Carilion Medical Center	Roanoke	84%	300+
CJW Medical Center	Richmond	84%	300+
The Fauquier Hospital	Warrenton	84%	300+
Henrico Doctors' Hospital	Richmond	84%	300+
Mary Immaculate Hospital	Newport News	84%	300+
Prince William Hospital	Manassas	84%	300+
Sentara Leigh Hospital	Norfolk	84%	300+
Sentara Norfolk General Hospital	Norfolk	84%	300+
Sentara Obici Hospital	Suffolk	84%	300+
Sentara Virginia Beach General Hospital	Virginia Beach	84%	300+
Southampton Memorial Hospital	Franklin	84%	300+
Alleghany Regional Hospital	Low Moor	83%	300+
Bon Secours - St Marys Hospital of Richmond	Richmond	83%	300+
Carilion Franklin Memorial Hospital	Rocky Mount	83%	300+
Centra Health	Lynchburg	83%	300+
Clinch Valley Medical Center	Richlands	83%	300+
Community Memorial Healthcenter	South Hill	83%	300+
Inova Fairfax Hospital	Falls Church	83%	300+
Mem Hosp of Martinsville & Henry County	Martinsville	83%	300+
Sentara Bayside Hospital	Virginia Beach	83%	300+
Sentara Williamsburg Regional Med Ctr	Williamsburg	83%	300+
Carilion Giles Memorial Hospital	Pearisburg	82%	(a)
Carilion Stonewall Jackson Hospital	Lexington	82%	300+
Chesapeake General Hospital	Chesapeake	82%	300+
Inova Alexandria Hospital	Alexandria	82%	300+
Inova Fair Oaks Hospital	Fairfax	82%	300+
Inova Mount Vernon Hospital	Alexandria	82%	300+
Mountain View Regional Medical Center	Norton	82%	(a)
Southern Virginia Regional Medical Center	Emporia	82%	300+
Warren Memorial Hospital	Front Royal	82%	300+
Winchester Medical Center	Winchester	82%	(a)
John Randolph Medical Center	Hopewell	81%	300+
Reston Hospital Center	Reston	81%	300+
Riverside Regional Medical Center	Newport News	81%	300+
Riverside Shore Memorial Hospital	Nassawadox	81%	300+
Rockingham Memorial Hospital	Harrisonburg	81%	300+
Russell County Medical Center	Lebanon	81%	300+
Carilion Tazewell Community Hospital	Tazewell	80%	(a)
Johnston Memorial Hospital	Abingdon	80%	300+
Rappahannock General Hospital	Kilmarnock	80%	300+
Riverside Walter Reed Hospital	Gloucester	80%	300+
Southside Community Hospital[11]	Farmville	80%	300+
Twin County Regional Hospital	Galax	80%	300+
Bedford Memorial Hospital	Bedford	79%	300+
Culpeper Regional Hospital	Culpeper	79%	300+
Mary Washington Hospital	Fredericksburg	79%	300+
Potomac Hospital	Woodbridge	79%	300+
Riverside Tappahannock Hospital	Tappahannock	79%	300+
Smyth County Community Hospital	Marion	79%	300+
Southside Regional Medical Center	Petersburg	79%	300+
Stafford Hospital Center	Stafford	79%	300+
Sentara Careplex Hospital	Hampton	78%	300+
Buchanan General Hospital	Grundy	76%	300+
Danville Regional Medical Center	Danville	76%	300+
Norton Community Hospital	Norton	76%	300+
Virginia Hospital Center - Arlington	Arlington	76%	300+
Lee Regional Medical Center	Pennington Gap	74%	300+
Wellmont Lonesome Pine Hospital	Big Stone Gap	73%	300+

43. Hospital Given 9 or 10 on 10 Point Scale

Hospital Name	City	Rate	Cases
Bon Secours - St Francis Medical Center	Midlothian	75%	300+
Martha Jefferson Hospital	Charlottesville	75%	300+
Bon Secours - Memorial Regional Medical	Mechanicsville	74%	300+
Centra Health	Lynchburg	74%	300+
Virginia Hospital Center - Arlington	Arlington	74%	300+
Winchester Medical Center	Winchester	74%	(a)
Bon Secours - St Marys Hospital of Richmond	Richmond	72%	300+
Carilion Giles Memorial Hospital	Pearisburg	72%	(a)
Inova Loudoun Hospital	Leesburg	72%	300+
Lewis-Gale Medical Center	Salem	72%	300+
Carilion Franklin Memorial Hospital	Rocky Mount	71%	300+
Carilion Medical Center	Roanoke	71%	300+
Henrico Doctors' Hospital	Richmond	71%	300+
Inova Fair Oaks Hospital	Fairfax	71%	300+
Montgomery Regional Hospital	Blacksburg	71%	300+
Stafford Hospital Center	Stafford	71%	300+
The Fauquier Hospital	Warrenton	70%	300+
Pulaski Community Hospital	Pulaski	70%	300+
Sentara Norfolk General Hospital	Norfolk	70%	300+
Carilion New River Valley Medical Center	Christiansburg	69%	300+
Inova Fairfax Hospital	Falls Church	68%	300+
Rappahannock General Hospital	Kilmarnock	68%	300+
Shenandoah Memorial Hospital	Woodstock	68%	300+
Virginia Commonwealth Univ Health Sys	Richmond	68%	300+
Wythe County Community Hospital	Wytheville	68%	300+
Bon Secours - Richmond Community Hospital	Richmond	67%	(a)
Carilion Tazewell Community Hospital	Tazewell	67%	(a)
CJW Medical Center	Richmond	67%	300+
Halifax Regional Hospital	Halifax	67%	300+
Twin County Regional Hospital	Galax	67%	300+
Inova Mount Vernon Hospital	Alexandria	66%	300+
Sentara Virginia Beach General Hospital	Virginia Beach	66%	300+
Carilion Stonewall Jackson Hospital	Lexington	65%	300+
Inova Alexandria Hospital	Alexandria	65%	300+
Prince William Hospital	Manassas	65%	300+
Sentara Leigh Hospital	Norfolk	65%	300+
Southampton Memorial Hospital	Franklin	65%	300+
University of Virginia Medical Center	Charlottesville	65%	300+
Alleghany Regional Hospital	Low Moor	64%	300+

NOTE: Hospital profiles are in alphabetical order by state, then city, then hospital within the city; Rankings exclude hospitals with less than 25 cases except for patient surveys which excludes hospitals with less than 100 cases; (a) 100–299 cases; (1) The number of cases is too small to be sure how well a hospital is performing; (2) The hospital indicated that the data submitted for this measure were based on a sample of cases; (3) Data was collected during a shorter time period (fewer quarters) than the maximum possible time for this measure; (4) Suppressed for one or more quarters by CMS; (5) No data is available from the hospital for this measure; (6) Fewer than 100 patients completed the HCAHPS survey. Use these rates with caution, as the number of surveys may be too low to reliably assess hospital performance; (7) Survey results are based on less than 12 months of data; (8) Survey results are not available for this reporting period; (9) No or very few patients were eligible for the HCAHPS survey. The scores shown, if any, reflect a very small number of surveys; (10) A state average was not calculated because too few hospitals in the state submitted data; (11) There were discrepancies in the data collection process; Please refer to the User's Guide for a full explanation of data.

Bedford Memorial Hospital	Bedford	64%	300+
Buchanan General Hospital	Grundy	64%	300+
Augusta Health	Fishersville	63%	300+
Bon Secours - Depaul Medical Center	Norfolk	63%	300+
Chesapeake General Hospital	Chesapeake	63%	300+
Clinch Valley Medical Center	Richlands	63%	300+
Community Memorial Healthcenter	South Hill	63%	300+
Johnston Memorial Hospital	Abingdon	63%	300+
Reston Hospital Center	Reston	63%	300+
Rockingham Memorial Hospital	Harrisonburg	63%	300+
Sentara Williamsburg Regional Med Ctr	Williamsburg	63%	300+
Southside Regional Medical Center	Petersburg	63%	300+
Bon Secours - Maryview Medical Center	Portsmouth	62%	300+
Sentara Careplex Hospital	Hampton	62%	300+
Southern Virginia Regional Medical Center	Emporia	62%	300+
Culpeper Regional Hospital	Culpeper	61%	300+
Riverside Shore Memorial Hospital	Nassawadox	61%	300+
Sentara Bayside Hospital	Virginia Beach	61%	300+
Riverside Regional Medical Center	Newport News	60%	300+
John Randolph Medical Center	Hopewell	59%	300+
Mary Immaculate Hospital	Newport News	59%	300+
Norton Community Hospital	Norton	59%	300+
Potomac Hospital	Woodbridge	59%	300+
Riverside Tappahannock Hospital	Tappahannock	59%	300+
Riverside Walter Reed Hospital	Gloucester	59%	300+
Russell County Medical Center	Lebanon	59%	300+
Lee Regional Medical Center	Pennington Gap	58%	300+
Mary Washington Hospital	Fredericksburg	58%	300+
Mem Hosp of Martinsville & Henry County	Martinsville	58%	300+
Page Memorial Hospital	Luray	58%	(a)
Wellmont Lonesome Pine Hospital	Big Stone Gap	58%	300+
Southside Community Hospital[11]	Farmville	57%	300+
Mountain View Regional Medical Center	Norton	56%	(a)
Sentara Obici Hospital	Suffolk	56%	300+
Smyth County Community Hospital	Marion	56%	300+
Warren Memorial Hospital	Front Royal	55%	300+
Danville Regional Medical Center	Danville	51%	300+

44. Meds 'Always' Explained Before Given

Hospital Name	City	Rate	Cases
Bon Secours - Richmond Community Hospital	Richmond	69%	(a)
Carilion Stonewall Jackson Hospital	Lexington	68%	300+
Carilion Franklin Memorial Hospital	Rocky Mount	67%	300+
Carilion Medical Center	Roanoke	67%	300+
Community Memorial Healthcenter	South Hill	66%	300+
Martha Jefferson Hospital	Charlottesville	65%	300+
Carilion Giles Memorial Hospital	Pearisburg	64%	(a)
Pulaski Community Hospital	Pulaski	64%	300+
Buchanan General Hospital	Grundy	63%	300+
Carilion Tazewell Community Hospital	Tazewell	63%	(a)
Centra Health	Lynchburg	63%	300+
The Fauquier Hospital	Warrenton	63%	300+
Alleghany Regional Hospital	Low Moor	62%	300+
Rappahannock General Hospital	Kilmarnock	62%	300+
Smyth County Community Hospital	Marion	62%	300+
Augusta Health	Fishersville	61%	300+
Bedford Memorial Hospital	Bedford	61%	300+
Clinch Valley Medical Center	Richlands	61%	300+
Inova Fair Oaks Hospital	Fairfax	61%	300+
Russell County Medical Center	Lebanon	61%	300+
Southern Virginia Regional Medical Center	Emporia	61%	300+
Southside Community Hospital[11]	Farmville	61%	300+
Virginia Commonwealth Univ Health Sys	Richmond	61%	300+
Winchester Medical Center	Winchester	61%	(a)
Carilion New River Valley Medical Center	Christiansburg	60%	300+
Inova Loudoun Hospital	Leesburg	60%	300+
Inova Mount Vernon Hospital	Alexandria	60%	300+
Johnston Memorial Hospital	Abingdon	60%	300+
Montgomery Regional Hospital	Blacksburg	60%	300+
Norton Community Hospital	Norton	60%	300+
Riverside Shore Memorial Hospital	Nassawadox	60%	300+
Riverside Tappahannock Hospital	Tappahannock	60%	300+
Sentara Bayside Hospital	Virginia Beach	60%	300+
Shenandoah Memorial Hospital	Woodstock	60%	300+
Southampton Memorial Hospital	Franklin	60%	300+
Wythe County Community Hospital	Wytheville	60%	300+
Bon Secours - Memorial Regional Medical	Mechanicsville	59%	300+
Bon Secours - St Francis Medical Center	Midlothian	59%	300+
Henrico Doctors' Hospital	Richmond	59%	300+
Potomac Hospital	Woodbridge	59%	300+
Twin County Regional Hospital	Galax	59%	300+
Bon Secours - St Marys Hospital of Richmond	Richmond	58%	300+
Inova Fairfax Hospital	Falls Church	58%	300+
Lee Regional Medical Center	Pennington Gap	58%	300+
Lewis-Gale Medical Center	Salem	58%	300+
Virginia Hospital Center - Arlington	Arlington	58%	300+
Wellmont Lonesome Pine Hospital	Big Stone Gap	58%	300+
Bon Secours - Depaul Medical Center	Norfolk	57%	300+
Halifax Regional Hospital	Halifax	57%	300+
Reston Hospital Center	Reston	57%	300+
Stafford Hospital Center	Stafford	57%	300+
CJW Medical Center	Richmond	56%	300+
Culpeper Regional Hospital	Culpeper	56%	300+
John Randolph Medical Center	Hopewell	56%	300+
Mary Immaculate Hospital	Newport News	56%	300+
Rockingham Memorial Hospital	Harrisonburg	56%	300+
Sentara Leigh Hospital	Norfolk	56%	300+
Sentara Norfolk General Hospital	Norfolk	56%	300+
University of Virginia Medical Center	Charlottesville	56%	300+
Chesapeake General Hospital	Chesapeake	55%	300+
Mountain View Regional Medical Center	Norton	55%	(a)
Sentara Obici Hospital	Suffolk	55%	300+
Sentara Williamsburg Regional Med Ctr	Williamsburg	55%	300+
Southside Regional Medical Center	Petersburg	55%	300+
Bon Secours - Maryview Medical Center	Portsmouth	54%	300+
Danville Regional Medical Center	Danville	54%	300+
Inova Alexandria Hospital	Alexandria	54%	300+
Mary Washington Hospital	Fredericksburg	54%	300+
Mem Hosp of Martinsville & Henry County	Martinsville	54%	300+
Riverside Regional Medical Center	Newport News	54%	300+
Riverside Walter Reed Hospital	Gloucester	54%	300+
Sentara Virginia Beach General Hospital	Virginia Beach	54%	300+
Warren Memorial Hospital	Front Royal	54%	300+
Prince William Hospital	Manassas	53%	300+
Sentara Careplex Hospital	Hampton	51%	300+
Page Memorial Hospital	Luray	44%	(a)

45. Nurses 'Always' Communicated Well

Hospital Name	City	Rate	Cases
Carilion Giles Memorial Hospital	Pearisburg	83%	(a)
Carilion Franklin Memorial Hospital	Rocky Mount	82%	300+
Bedford Memorial Hospital	Bedford	81%	300+
Carilion Stonewall Jackson Hospital	Lexington	81%	300+
Centra Health	Lynchburg	81%	300+
Pulaski Community Hospital	Pulaski	81%	300+
Rappahannock General Hospital	Kilmarnock	81%	300+
Wythe County Community Hospital	Wytheville	81%	300+
Bon Secours - Memorial Regional Medical	Mechanicsville	80%	300+
Martha Jefferson Hospital	Charlottesville	80%	300+
Montgomery Regional Hospital	Blacksburg	80%	300+
Carilion Tazewell Community Hospital	Tazewell	79%	(a)
Russell County Medical Center	Lebanon	79%	300+
Shenandoah Memorial Hospital	Woodstock	79%	300+
Twin County Regional Hospital	Galax	79%	300+
Alleghany Regional Hospital	Low Moor	78%	300+
Bon Secours - Richmond Community Hospital	Richmond	78%	(a)
Buchanan General Hospital	Grundy	78%	300+
Carilion New River Valley Medical Center	Christiansburg	78%	300+
Halifax Regional Hospital	Halifax	78%	300+
Lee Regional Medical Center	Pennington Gap	78%	300+
Southampton Memorial Hospital	Franklin	78%	300+
Carilion Medical Center	Roanoke	77%	300+
Lewis-Gale Medical Center	Salem	77%	300+
Bon Secours - St Francis Medical Center	Midlothian	76%	300+
Bon Secours - St Marys Hospital of Richmond	Richmond	76%	300+
Clinch Valley Medical Center	Richlands	76%	300+
Community Memorial Healthcenter	South Hill	76%	300+
The Fauquier Hospital	Warrenton	76%	300+
Henrico Doctors' Hospital	Richmond	76%	300+
Inova Loudoun Hospital	Leesburg	76%	300+
Johnston Memorial Hospital	Abingdon	76%	300+
Norton Community Hospital	Norton	76%	300+
Smyth County Community Hospital	Marion	76%	300+
Southside Community Hospital[11]	Farmville	76%	300+
Inova Fair Oaks Hospital	Fairfax	75%	300+
Riverside Tappahannock Hospital	Tappahannock	75%	300+
Sentara Norfolk General Hospital	Norfolk	75%	300+
Virginia Commonwealth Univ Health Sys	Richmond	75%	300+
Wellmont Lonesome Pine Hospital	Big Stone Gap	75%	300+
Winchester Medical Center	Winchester	75%	(a)
Augusta Health	Fishersville	74%	300+
CJW Medical Center	Richmond	74%	300+
Mountain View Regional Medical Center	Norton	74%	(a)
Prince William Hospital	Manassas	74%	300+
Riverside Shore Memorial Hospital	Nassawadox	74%	300+
Riverside Walter Reed Hospital	Gloucester	74%	300+
Sentara Bayside Hospital	Virginia Beach	74%	300+
University of Virginia Medical Center	Charlottesville	74%	300+
Virginia Hospital Center - Arlington	Arlington	74%	300+
Bon Secours - Maryview Medical Center	Portsmouth	73%	300+
Inova Fairfax Hospital	Falls Church	73%	300+
John Randolph Medical Center	Hopewell	73%	300+
Rockingham Memorial Hospital	Harrisonburg	73%	300+
Southern Virginia Regional Medical Center	Emporia	73%	300+
Southside Regional Medical Center	Petersburg	73%	300+
Stafford Hospital Center	Stafford	73%	300+
Culpeper Regional Hospital	Culpeper	72%	300+
Page Memorial Hospital	Luray	72%	(a)
Warren Memorial Hospital	Front Royal	72%	300+
Inova Alexandria Hospital	Alexandria	71%	300+
Inova Mount Vernon Hospital	Alexandria	71%	300+
Mem Hosp of Martinsville & Henry County	Martinsville	71%	300+
Sentara Virginia Beach General Hospital	Virginia Beach	71%	300+
Bon Secours - Depaul Medical Center	Norfolk	70%	300+
Danville Regional Medical Center	Danville	70%	300+
Mary Washington Hospital	Fredericksburg	70%	300+
Potomac Hospital	Woodbridge	70%	300+
Sentara Obici Hospital	Suffolk	70%	300+
Sentara Williamsburg Regional Med Ctr	Williamsburg	70%	300+
Chesapeake General Hospital	Chesapeake	69%	300+
Mary Immaculate Hospital	Newport News	69%	300+
Reston Hospital Center	Reston	69%	300+
Riverside Regional Medical Center	Newport News	69%	300+
Sentara Leigh Hospital	Norfolk	68%	300+
Sentara Careplex Hospital	Hampton	67%	300+

46. Pain 'Always' Well Controlled

Hospital Name	City	Rate	Cases
Carilion Giles Memorial Hospital	Pearisburg	76%	(a)
Carilion Franklin Memorial Hospital	Rocky Mount	75%	300+
Bon Secours - Memorial Regional Medical	Mechanicsville	74%	300+
Bon Secours - Richmond Community Hospital	Richmond	74%	(a)
Carilion Stonewall Jackson Hospital	Lexington	74%	300+
Montgomery Regional Hospital	Blacksburg	74%	300+
Pulaski Community Hospital	Pulaski	74%	300+
Bedford Memorial Hospital	Bedford	73%	300+
Henrico Doctors' Hospital	Richmond	73%	300+
Martha Jefferson Hospital	Charlottesville	73%	300+
Twin County Regional Hospital	Galax	73%	300+
Alleghany Regional Hospital	Low Moor	72%	300+
Centra Health	Lynchburg	72%	300+
Bon Secours - St Marys Hospital of Richmond	Richmond	71%	300+
Carilion Tazewell Community Hospital	Tazewell	71%	(a)
The Fauquier Hospital	Warrenton	71%	300+
Johnston Memorial Hospital	Abingdon	71%	300+
Lewis-Gale Medical Center	Salem	71%	300+
Shenandoah Memorial Hospital	Woodstock	71%	300+
Wythe County Community Hospital	Wytheville	71%	300+
Halifax Regional Hospital	Halifax	70%	300+
John Randolph Medical Center	Hopewell	70%	300+
Prince William Hospital	Manassas	70%	300+
Rappahannock General Hospital	Kilmarnock	70%	300+
Riverside Shore Memorial Hospital	Nassawadox	70%	300+
Southampton Memorial Hospital	Franklin	70%	300+
Winchester Medical Center	Winchester	70%	(a)
Augusta Health	Fishersville	69%	300+
Bon Secours - Maryview Medical Center	Portsmouth	69%	300+
Bon Secours - St Francis Medical Center	Midlothian	69%	300+
Carilion Medical Center	Roanoke	69%	300+
CJW Medical Center	Richmond	69%	300+
Inova Alexandria Hospital	Alexandria	69%	300+
Riverside Tappahannock Hospital	Tappahannock	69%	300+
Sentara Bayside Hospital	Virginia Beach	69%	300+
Sentara Norfolk General Hospital	Norfolk	69%	300+
Virginia Commonwealth Univ Health Sys	Richmond	69%	300+
Bon Secours - Depaul Medical Center	Norfolk	68%	300+
Buchanan General Hospital	Grundy	68%	300+
Carilion New River Valley Medical Center	Christiansburg	68%	300+
Community Memorial Healthcenter	South Hill	68%	300+
Inova Fair Oaks Hospital	Fairfax	68%	300+
Inova Mount Vernon Hospital	Alexandria	68%	300+
Russell County Medical Center	Lebanon	68%	300+
Southern Virginia Regional Medical Center	Emporia	68%	300+
Southside Community Hospital[11]	Farmville	68%	300+
Southside Regional Medical Center	Petersburg	68%	300+
Virginia Hospital Center - Arlington	Arlington	68%	300+
Chesapeake General Hospital	Chesapeake	67%	300+
Clinch Valley Medical Center	Richlands	67%	300+
Inova Fairfax Hospital	Falls Church	67%	300+
Inova Loudoun Hospital	Leesburg	67%	300+
Mary Immaculate Hospital	Newport News	66%	300+
Norton Community Hospital	Norton	66%	300+
Riverside Regional Medical Center	Newport News	66%	300+
Riverside Walter Reed Hospital	Gloucester	66%	300+
Smyth County Community Hospital	Marion	66%	300+
Wellmont Lonesome Pine Hospital	Big Stone Gap	66%	300+
Danville Regional Medical Center	Danville	65%	300+
Mary Washington Hospital	Fredericksburg	65%	300+
Mem Hosp of Martinsville & Henry County	Martinsville	65%	300+
Page Memorial Hospital	Luray	65%	(a)
Potomac Hospital	Woodbridge	65%	300+
Reston Hospital Center	Reston	65%	300+
Rockingham Memorial Hospital	Harrisonburg	65%	300+
University of Virginia Medical Center	Charlottesville	65%	300+
Sentara Virginia Beach General Hospital	Virginia Beach	64%	300+
Stafford Hospital Center	Stafford	64%	300+
Sentara Leigh Hospital	Norfolk	63%	300+
Warren Memorial Hospital	Front Royal	63%	300+
Culpeper Regional Hospital	Culpeper	62%	300+
Lee Regional Medical Center	Pennington Gap	62%	300+

NOTE: Hospital profiles are in alphabetical order by state, then city, then hospital within the city; Rankings exclude hospitals with less than 25 cases except for patient surveys which excludes hospitals with less than 100 cases; (a) 100–299 cases; (1) The number of cases is too small to be sure how well a hospital is performing; (2) The hospital indicated that the data submitted for this measure were based on a sample of cases; (3) Data was collected during a shorter time period (fewer quarters) than the maximum possible time for this measure; (4) Suppressed for one or more quarters by CMS; (5) No data is available from the hospital for this measure; (6) Fewer than 100 patients completed the HCAHPS survey. Use these rates with caution, as the number of surveys may be too low to reliably assess hospital performance; (7) Survey results are based on less than 12 months of data; (8) Survey results are not available for this reporting period; (9) No or very few patients were eligible for the HCAHPS survey. The scores shown, if any, reflect a very small number of surveys; (10) A state average was not calculated because too few hospitals in the state submitted data; (11) There were discrepancies in the data collection process; Please refer to the User's Guide for a full explanation of data.

Sentara Obici Hospital	Suffolk	62%	300+
Sentara Williamsburg Regional Med Ctr	Williamsburg	62%	300+
Mountain View Regional Medical Center	Norton	61%	(a)
Sentara Careplex Hospital	Hampton	60%	300+

47. Room and Bathroom 'Always' Clean

Hospital Name	City	Rate	Cases
Twin County Regional Hospital	Galax	82%	300+
Shenandoah Memorial Hospital	Woodstock	80%	300+
Rappahannock General Hospital	Kilmarnock	79%	300+
Carilion Franklin Memorial Hospital	Rocky Mount	77%	300+
Centra Health	Lynchburg	77%	300+
Mountain View Regional Medical Center	Norton	77%	(a)
Montgomery Regional Hospital	Blacksburg	76%	300+
Potomac Hospital	Woodbridge	76%	300+
Carilion Giles Memorial Hospital	Pearisburg	75%	(a)
Carilion Stonewall Jackson Hospital	Lexington	75%	300+
Wellmont Lonesome Pine Hospital	Big Stone Gap	75%	300+
The Fauquier Hospital	Warrenton	74%	300+
Russell County Medical Center	Lebanon	74%	300+
Southampton Memorial Hospital	Franklin	74%	300+
Virginia Hospital Center - Arlington	Arlington	74%	300+
Augusta Health	Fishersville	73%	300+
Bon Secours - Richmond Community Hospital	Richmond	73%	(a)
Riverside Walter Reed Hospital	Gloucester	73%	300+
Southside Community Hospital[11]	Farmville	73%	300+
Bon Secours - St Francis Medical Center	Midlothian	72%	300+
Buchanan General Hospital	Grundy	72%	300+
Carilion Tazewell Community Hospital	Tazewell	72%	(a)
Culpeper Regional Hospital	Culpeper	72%	300+
Prince William Hospital	Manassas	72%	300+
Smyth County Community Hospital	Marion	72%	300+
Stafford Hospital Center	Stafford	72%	300+
Winchester Medical Center	Winchester	72%	(a)
Carilion New River Valley Medical Center	Christiansburg	71%	300+
Clinch Valley Medical Center	Richlands	71%	300+
Bedford Memorial Hospital	Bedford	70%	300+
Community Memorial Healthcenter	South Hill	70%	300+
Inova Fair Oaks Hospital	Fairfax	70%	300+
John Randolph Medical Center	Hopewell	70%	300+
Page Memorial Hospital	Luray	70%	(a)
Wythe County Community Hospital	Wytheville	70%	300+
Bon Secours - St Marys Hospital of Richmond	Richmond	69%	300+
Lee Regional Medical Center	Pennington Gap	69%	300+
Pulaski Community Hospital	Pulaski	69%	300+
Bon Secours - Depaul Medical Center	Norfolk	68%	300+
Bon Secours - Maryview Medical Center	Portsmouth	68%	300+
Halifax Regional Hospital	Halifax	68%	300+
Rockingham Memorial Hospital	Harrisonburg	68%	300+
Alleghany Regional Hospital	Low Moor	67%	300+
Lewis-Gale Medical Center	Salem	67%	300+
Sentara Obici Hospital	Suffolk	67%	300+
Bon Secours - Memorial Regional Medical	Mechanicsville	66%	300+
CJW Medical Center	Richmond	66%	300+
Danville Regional Medical Center	Danville	66%	300+
Henrico Doctors' Hospital	Richmond	66%	300+
Martha Jefferson Hospital	Charlottesville	66%	300+
Riverside Shore Memorial Hospital	Nassawadox	66%	300+
Sentara Williamsburg Regional Med Ctr	Williamsburg	66%	300+
Warren Memorial Hospital	Front Royal	66%	300+
Johnston Memorial Hospital	Abingdon	65%	300+
Mem Hosp of Martinsville & Henry County	Martinsville	65%	300+
Virginia Commonwealth Univ Health Sys	Richmond	65%	300+
Inova Loudoun Hospital	Leesburg	64%	300+
Reston Hospital Center	Reston	64%	300+
Sentara Bayside Hospital	Virginia Beach	64%	300+
Riverside Tappahannock Hospital	Tappahannock	63%	300+
Sentara Virginia Beach General Hospital	Virginia Beach	63%	300+
Southern Virginia Regional Medical Center	Emporia	63%	300+
Inova Alexandria Hospital	Alexandria	62%	300+
Inova Mount Vernon Hospital	Alexandria	62%	300+
Sentara Careplex Hospital	Hampton	62%	300+
Southside Regional Medical Center	Petersburg	62%	300+
University of Virginia Medical Center	Charlottesville	62%	300+
Norton Community Hospital	Norton	61%	300+
Riverside Regional Medical Center	Newport News	61%	300+
Carilion Medical Center	Roanoke	60%	300+
Inova Fairfax Hospital	Falls Church	60%	300+
Mary Washington Hospital	Fredericksburg	60%	300+
Sentara Norfolk General Hospital	Norfolk	60%	300+
Sentara Leigh Hospital	Norfolk	59%	300+
Chesapeake General Hospital	Chesapeake	56%	300+
Mary Immaculate Hospital	Newport News	56%	300+

48. Timely Help 'Always' Received

Hospital Name	City	Rate	Cases
Carilion Tazewell Community Hospital	Tazewell	76%	(a)
Carilion Stonewall Jackson Hospital	Lexington	75%	300+
Carilion Giles Memorial Hospital	Pearisburg	74%	(a)
Carilion New River Valley Medical Center	Christiansburg	74%	300+
Rappahannock General Hospital	Kilmarnock	74%	300+
Twin County Regional Hospital	Galax	73%	300+
Wythe County Community Hospital	Wytheville	73%	300+
Bedford Memorial Hospital	Bedford	72%	300+
Carilion Franklin Memorial Hospital	Rocky Mount	71%	300+
Bon Secours - Memorial Regional Medical	Mechanicsville	69%	300+
Lee Regional Medical Center	Pennington Gap	69%	300+
Pulaski Community Hospital	Pulaski	68%	300+
Buchanan General Hospital	Grundy	67%	300+
Halifax Regional Hospital	Halifax	67%	300+
Russell County Medical Center	Lebanon	67%	300+
Shenandoah Memorial Hospital	Woodstock	67%	300+
Augusta Health	Fishersville	66%	300+
Centra Health	Lynchburg	66%	300+
Johnston Memorial Hospital	Abingdon	66%	300+
Montgomery Regional Hospital	Blacksburg	66%	300+
Smyth County Community Hospital	Marion	66%	300+
Carilion Medical Center	Roanoke	65%	300+
The Fauquier Hospital	Warrenton	65%	300+
Henrico Doctors' Hospital	Richmond	65%	300+
Norton Community Hospital	Norton	65%	300+
Riverside Walter Reed Hospital	Gloucester	65%	300+
Martha Jefferson Hospital	Charlottesville	64%	300+
Sentara Norfolk General Hospital	Norfolk	64%	300+
Southside Community Hospital[11]	Farmville	64%	300+
Winchester Medical Center	Winchester	64%	(a)
Clinch Valley Medical Center	Richlands	63%	300+
Inova Loudoun Hospital	Leesburg	63%	300+
Southampton Memorial Hospital	Franklin	63%	300+
Bon Secours - Richmond Community Hospital	Richmond	62%	(a)
Bon Secours - St Marys Hospital of Richmond	Richmond	62%	300+
Mem Hosp of Martinsville & Henry County	Martinsville	62%	300+
Stafford Hospital Center	Stafford	62%	300+
Alleghany Regional Hospital	Low Moor	61%	300+
Bon Secours - Depaul Medical Center	Norfolk	61%	300+
Lewis-Gale Medical Center	Salem	61%	300+
Riverside Shore Memorial Hospital	Nassawadox	61%	300+
Virginia Hospital Center - Arlington	Arlington	61%	300+
Bon Secours - Maryview Medical Center	Portsmouth	60%	300+
Community Memorial Healthcenter	South Hill	60%	300+
Virginia Commonwealth Univ Health Sys	Richmond	60%	300+
CJW Medical Center	Richmond	59%	300+
Inova Alexandria Hospital	Alexandria	59%	300+
Inova Fairfax Hospital	Falls Church	59%	300+
Prince William Hospital	Manassas	59%	300+
Riverside Tappahannock Hospital	Tappahannock	59%	300+
Southern Virginia Regional Medical Center	Emporia	59%	300+
Warren Memorial Hospital	Front Royal	59%	300+
Bon Secours - St Francis Medical Center	Midlothian	58%	300+
Culpeper Regional Hospital	Culpeper	58%	300+
Rockingham Memorial Hospital	Harrisonburg	58%	300+
Chesapeake General Hospital	Chesapeake	57%	300+
Inova Fair Oaks Hospital	Fairfax	57%	300+
Inova Mount Vernon Hospital	Alexandria	57%	300+
John Randolph Medical Center	Hopewell	57%	300+
Wellmont Lonesome Pine Hospital	Big Stone Gap	57%	300+
Page Memorial Hospital	Luray	56%	(a)
Sentara Leigh Hospital	Norfolk	56%	300+
Sentara Obici Hospital	Suffolk	56%	300+
Mary Washington Hospital	Fredericksburg	55%	300+
Sentara Bayside Hospital	Virginia Beach	55%	300+
Mountain View Regional Medical Center	Norton	54%	(a)
Sentara Careplex Hospital	Hampton	54%	300+
Sentara Virginia Beach General Hospital	Virginia Beach	54%	300+
Potomac Hospital	Woodbridge	53%	300+
Southside Regional Medical Center	Petersburg	53%	300+
University of Virginia Medical Center	Charlottesville	53%	300+
Danville Regional Medical Center	Danville	52%	300+
Reston Hospital Center	Reston	52%	300+
Riverside Regional Medical Center	Newport News	52%	300+
Mary Immaculate Hospital	Newport News	51%	300+
Sentara Williamsburg Regional Med Ctr	Williamsburg	50%	300+

49. Would Definitely Recommend Hospital

Hospital Name	City	Rate	Cases
Martha Jefferson Hospital	Charlottesville	83%	300+
Winchester Medical Center	Winchester	82%	(a)
Centra Health	Lynchburg	81%	300+
Virginia Hospital Center - Arlington	Arlington	80%	300+
Bon Secours - Memorial Regional Medical	Mechanicsville	78%	300+
Bon Secours - St Francis Medical Center	Midlothian	78%	300+
Inova Fair Oaks Hospital	Fairfax	78%	300+
Bon Secours - St Marys Hospital of Richmond	Richmond	77%	300+
Carilion New River Valley Medical Center	Christiansburg	77%	300+
Lewis-Gale Medical Center	Salem	77%	300+
The Fauquier Hospital	Warrenton	76%	300+
Henrico Doctors' Hospital	Richmond	76%	300+
Sentara Norfolk General Hospital	Norfolk	76%	300+
Stafford Hospital Center	Stafford	76%	300+
Inova Fairfax Hospital	Falls Church	75%	300+
Carilion Medical Center	Roanoke	74%	300+
Inova Loudoun Hospital	Leesburg	74%	300+
Montgomery Regional Hospital	Blacksburg	74%	300+
University of Virginia Medical Center	Charlottesville	74%	300+
Inova Mount Vernon Hospital	Alexandria	72%	300+
Rappahannock General Hospital	Kilmarnock	72%	300+
Augusta Health	Fishersville	71%	300+
Pulaski Community Hospital	Pulaski	71%	300+
Shenandoah Memorial Hospital	Woodstock	71%	300+
Virginia Commonwealth Univ Health Sys	Richmond	71%	300+
Carilion Franklin Memorial Hospital	Rocky Mount	70%	300+
CJW Medical Center	Richmond	70%	300+
Sentara Leigh Hospital	Norfolk	70%	300+
Reston Hospital Center	Reston	69%	300+
Sentara Virginia Beach General Hospital	Virginia Beach	69%	300+
Bedford Memorial Hospital	Bedford	68%	300+
Carilion Giles Memorial Hospital	Pearisburg	68%	(a)
Chesapeake General Hospital	Chesapeake	68%	300+
Prince William Hospital	Manassas	68%	300+
Sentara Williamsburg Regional Med Ctr	Williamsburg	68%	300+
Carilion Tazewell Community Hospital	Tazewell	67%	(a)
Inova Alexandria Hospital	Alexandria	67%	300+
Rockingham Memorial Hospital	Harrisonburg	67%	300+
Alleghany Regional Hospital	Low Moor	66%	300+
Bon Secours - Depaul Medical Center	Norfolk	66%	300+
Johnston Memorial Hospital	Abingdon	66%	300+
Twin County Regional Hospital	Galax	66%	300+
Mary Immaculate Hospital	Newport News	65%	300+
Sentara Bayside Hospital	Virginia Beach	65%	300+
Wythe County Community Hospital	Wytheville	65%	300+
Buchanan General Hospital	Grundy	64%	300+
Clinch Valley Medical Center	Richlands	64%	300+
Culpeper Regional Hospital	Culpeper	64%	300+
Halifax Regional Hospital	Halifax	64%	300+
Sentara Careplex Hospital	Hampton	64%	300+
Carilion Stonewall Jackson Hospital	Lexington	63%	300+
Community Memorial Healthcenter	South Hill	63%	300+
Riverside Regional Medical Center	Newport News	63%	300+
Sentara Obici Hospital	Suffolk	63%	300+
Norton Community Hospital	Norton	62%	300+
Potomac Hospital	Woodbridge	62%	300+
Mary Washington Hospital	Fredericksburg	61%	300+
Riverside Tappahannock Hospital	Tappahannock	61%	300+
Southside Regional Medical Center	Petersburg	61%	300+
Bon Secours - Richmond Community Hospital	Richmond	60%	(a)
Mountain View Regional Medical Center	Norton	60%	(a)
Riverside Walter Reed Hospital	Gloucester	60%	300+
Wellmont Lonesome Pine Hospital	Big Stone Gap	59%	300+
Bon Secours - Maryview Medical Center	Portsmouth	58%	300+
John Randolph Medical Center	Hopewell	58%	300+
Page Memorial Hospital	Luray	58%	(a)
Russell County Medical Center	Lebanon	58%	300+
Southern Virginia Regional Medical Center	Emporia	58%	300+
Southampton Memorial Hospital	Franklin	57%	300+
Warren Memorial Hospital	Front Royal	57%	300+
Lee Regional Medical Center	Pennington Gap	54%	300+
Riverside Shore Memorial Hospital	Nassawadox	54%	300+
Southside Community Hospital[11]	Farmville	54%	300+
Mem Hosp of Martinsville & Henry County	Martinsville	53%	300+
Smyth County Community Hospital	Marion	53%	300+
Danville Regional Medical Center	Danville	44%	300+

NOTE: Hospital profiles are in alphabetical order by state, then city, then hospital within the city; Rankings exclude hospitals with less than 25 cases except for patient surveys which excludes hospitals with less than 100 cases; (a) 100–299 cases; (1) The number of cases is too small to be sure how well a hospital is performing; (2) The hospital indicated that the data submitted for this measure were based on a sample of cases; (3) Data was collected during a shorter time period (fewer quarters) than the maximum possible time for this measure; (4) Suppressed for one or more quarters by CMS; (5) No data is available from the hospital for this measure; (6) Fewer than 100 patients completed the HCAHPS survey. Use these rates with caution, as the number of surveys may be too low to reliably assess hospital performance; (7) Survey results are based on less than 12 months of data; (8) Survey results are not available for this reporting period; (9) No or very few patients were eligible for the HCAHPS survey. The scores shown, if any, reflect a very small number of surveys; (10) A state average was not calculated because too few hospitals in the state submitted data; (11) There were discrepancies in the data collection process; Please refer to the User's Guide for a full explanation of data.

Johnston Memorial Hospital

351 Court Street, NE
Abingdon, VA 24210
E-mail: info@jmh.org
URL: www.jmh.org
Type: Acute Care Hospitals
Ownership: Voluntary Non-Profit - Private
Phone: 276-676-7000
Fax: 276-676-2631
Emergency Services: Yes
Beds: 135

Key Personnel:
CEO/President. . . . . Sean S McMurray
Chief of Medical Staff . . . . Richard Buddington
Infection Control . . . . Sue Greco
Operating Room. . . . . Eleanor E Hess
Pediatric Ambulatory Care . . . . . . Donna Hudgens, MD
Pediatric In-Patient Care . . . . Donna Hudgens, MD
Quality Assurance . . . . Teresa Tignor, RN
Radiology. . . . . Matthew Cobb

Measure	Cases	This Hosp.	State Avg.	U.S. Avg.
Heart Attack Care				
ACE Inhibitor or ARB for LVSD[1,2]	4	75%	97%	96%
Aspirin at Arrival[2]	55	93%	99%	99%
Aspirin at Discharge[2]	33	91%	99%	98%
Beta Blocker at Discharge[2]	36	92%	99%	98%
Fibrinolytic Medication Timing[1,2]	1	100%	75%	55%
PCI Within 90 Minutes of Arrival[2]	0	-	93%	90%
Smoking Cessation Advice[1,2]	6	83%	100%	99%
Chest Pain/Possible Heart Attack Care				
Aspirin at Arrival	206	97%	95%	95%
Median Time to ECG (minutes)	212	4	8	8
Median Time to Transfer (minutes)	34	35	60	61
Fibrinolytic Medication Timing[1]	1	100%	59%	54%
Heart Failure Care				
ACE Inhibitor or ARB for LVSD[2]	31	68%	97%	94%
Discharge Instructions[2]	125	82%	92%	88%
Evaluation of LVS Function[2]	155	94%	99%	98%
Smoking Cessation Advice[1,2]	24	62%	99%	98%
Pneumonia Care				
Appropriate Initial Antibiotic[2]	111	91%	93%	92%
Blood Culture Timing[2]	156	97%	97%	96%
Influenza Vaccine[2]	88	89%	94%	91%
Initial Antibiotic Timing[2]	150	97%	96%	95%
Pneumococcal Vaccine[2]	128	93%	95%	93%
Smoking Cessation Advice[2]	62	84%	98%	97%
Surgical Care Improvement Project				
Appropriate VTP Within 24 Hours[2]	132	87%	94%	92%
Appropriate Hair Removal[2]	429	100%	100%	99%
Appropriate Beta Blocker Usage[2]	129	88%	94%	93%
Controlled Postoperative Blood Glucose[2]	0	-	96%	93%
Prophylactic Antibiotic Timing[2]	293	95%	97%	97%
Prophylactic Antibiotic Timing (Outpatient)	125	76%	93%	92%
Prophylactic Antibiotic Selection[2]	293	98%	98%	97%
Prophylactic Antibiotic Select. (Outpatient)	111	92%	96%	94%
Prophylactic Antibiotic Stopped[2]	263	96%	96%	94%
Recommended VTP Ordered[2]	133	87%	96%	94%
Urinary Catheter Removal[2]	92	86%	93%	90%
Children's Asthma Care				
Received Systemic Corticosteroids	-	-	-	100%
Received Home Management Plan	-	-	-	71%
Received Reliever Medication	-	-	-	100%
Use of Medical Imaging				
Combination Abdominal CT Scan	1,032	0.125	0.144	0.191
Combination Chest CT Scan	761	0.095	0.030	0.054
Follow-up Mammogram/Ultrasound	1,565	3.8%	7.5%	8.4%
MRI for Low Back Pain	324	40.1%	31.5%	32.7%
Survey of Patients' Hospital Experiences				
Area Around Room 'Always' Quiet at Night	300+	52%	-	58%
Doctors 'Always' Communicated Well	300+	84%	-	80%
Home Recovery Information Given	300+	80%	-	82%
Hospital Given 9 or 10 on 10 Point Scale	300+	63%	-	67%
Meds 'Always' Explained Before Given	300+	60%	-	60%
Nurses 'Always' Communicated Well	300+	76%	-	76%
Pain 'Always' Well Controlled	300+	71%	-	69%
Room and Bathroom 'Always' Clean	300+	65%	-	71%
Timely Help 'Always' Received	300+	66%	-	64%
Would Definitely Recommend Hospital	300+	66%	-	69%

Inova Alexandria Hospital

4320 Seminary Rd
Alexandria, VA 22304
Phone: 703-504-3000
Fax: 703-504-3700
URL: www.inova.com/inovapublic.srt/iah/index.jsp
Type: Acute Care Hospitals
Emergency Services: Yes
Ownership: Voluntary Non-Profit - Private
Beds: 320

Key Personnel:
CEO/President. . . . . Christine Candio
Chief of Medical Staff . . . . Stephen Rosenfeld, MD
Operating Room. . . . . Carol Webb
Pediatric In-Patient Care . . . . Jon Farber, MD
Quality Assurance . . . . Pam Baker
Radiology. . . . . Frank Schert

Measure	Cases	This Hosp.	State Avg.	U.S. Avg.
Heart Attack Care				
ACE Inhibitor or ARB for LVSD	34	94%	97%	96%
Aspirin at Arrival	204	97%	99%	99%
Aspirin at Discharge	228	99%	99%	98%
Beta Blocker at Discharge	222	99%	99%	98%
Fibrinolytic Medication Timing	0	-	75%	55%
PCI Within 90 Minutes of Arrival	32	94%	93%	90%
Smoking Cessation Advice	61	97%	100%	99%
Chest Pain/Possible Heart Attack Care				
Aspirin at Arrival[1,3]	9	89%	95%	95%
Median Time to ECG (minutes)[1,3]	10	0	8	8
Median Time to Transfer (minutes)[5]	0	-	60	61
Fibrinolytic Medication Timing[5]	0	-	59%	54%
Heart Failure Care				
ACE Inhibitor or ARB for LVSD[2]	112	98%	97%	94%
Discharge Instructions[2]	231	67%	92%	88%
Evaluation of LVS Function[2]	283	95%	99%	98%
Smoking Cessation Advice[2]	56	95%	99%	98%
Pneumonia Care				
Appropriate Initial Antibiotic[2]	90	97%	93%	92%
Blood Culture Timing[2]	143	99%	97%	96%
Influenza Vaccine[2]	69	94%	94%	91%
Initial Antibiotic Timing[2]	139	99%	96%	95%
Pneumococcal Vaccine[2]	105	91%	95%	93%
Smoking Cessation Advice[2]	27	100%	98%	97%
Surgical Care Improvement Project				
Appropriate VTP Within 24 Hours[2]	146	90%	94%	92%
Appropriate Hair Removal[2]	467	100%	100%	99%
Appropriate Beta Blocker Usage[2]	128	98%	94%	93%
Controlled Postoperative Blood Glucose[2]	87	98%	96%	93%
Prophylactic Antibiotic Timing[2]	325	98%	97%	97%
Prophylactic Antibiotic Timing (Outpatient)	309	93%	93%	92%
Prophylactic Antibiotic Selection[2]	331	98%	98%	97%
Prophylactic Antibiotic Select. (Outpatient)	300	96%	96%	94%
Prophylactic Antibiotic Stopped[2]	316	89%	96%	94%
Recommended VTP Ordered[2]	146	94%	96%	94%
Urinary Catheter Removal[2]	114	93%	93%	90%
Children's Asthma Care				
Received Systemic Corticosteroids	-	-	-	100%
Received Home Management Plan	-	-	-	71%
Received Reliever Medication	-	-	-	100%
Use of Medical Imaging				
Combination Abdominal CT Scan	819	0.123	0.144	0.191
Combination Chest CT Scan	655	0.014	0.030	0.054
Follow-up Mammogram/Ultrasound	417	6.5%	7.5%	8.4%
MRI for Low Back Pain	295	32.2%	31.5%	32.7%
Survey of Patients' Hospital Experiences				
Area Around Room 'Always' Quiet at Night	300+	52%	-	58%
Doctors 'Always' Communicated Well	300+	74%	-	80%
Home Recovery Information Given	300+	82%	-	82%
Hospital Given 9 or 10 on 10 Point Scale	300+	65%	-	67%
Meds 'Always' Explained Before Given	300+	54%	-	60%
Nurses 'Always' Communicated Well	300+	71%	-	76%
Pain 'Always' Well Controlled	300+	69%	-	69%
Room and Bathroom 'Always' Clean	300+	62%	-	71%
Timely Help 'Always' Received	300+	59%	-	64%
Would Definitely Recommend Hospital	300+	67%	-	69%

Inova Mount Vernon Hospital

2501 Parkers Lane
Alexandria, VA 22306
Phone: 703-664-7000
Fax: 703-664-7304
URL: www.inova.com/inovapublic.srt/imvh/index.jsp
Type: Acute Care Hospitals
Emergency Services: Yes
Ownership: Voluntary Non-Profit - Other
Beds: 232

Key Personnel:
CEO/President. . . . . Barbara Doyle
Chief of Medical Staff . . . . David M Abbot
Operating Room. . . . . Ann Vandervort
Pediatric In-Patient Care . . . . Nancy J Leykan, MD
Quality Assurance . . . . Judy Perry
Radiology. . . . . Maria C Alvano, MD

Measure	Cases	This Hosp.	State Avg.	U.S. Avg.
Heart Attack Care				
ACE Inhibitor or ARB for LVSD[1]	5	80%	97%	96%
Aspirin at Arrival	44	100%	99%	99%
Aspirin at Discharge[1]	18	94%	99%	98%
Beta Blocker at Discharge[1]	19	100%	99%	98%
Fibrinolytic Medication Timing	0	-	75%	55%
PCI Within 90 Minutes of Arrival	0	-	93%	90%
Smoking Cessation Advice[1]	2	100%	100%	99%
Chest Pain/Possible Heart Attack Care				
Aspirin at Arrival	48	96%	95%	95%
Median Time to ECG (minutes)	47	7	8	8
Median Time to Transfer (minutes)[1,3]	6	76	60	61
Fibrinolytic Medication Timing[3]	0	-	59%	54%
Heart Failure Care				
ACE Inhibitor or ARB for LVSD	49	98%	97%	94%
Discharge Instructions	172	91%	92%	88%
Evaluation of LVS Function	216	99%	99%	98%
Smoking Cessation Advice	25	100%	99%	98%
Pneumonia Care				
Appropriate Initial Antibiotic	63	95%	93%	92%
Blood Culture Timing	90	98%	97%	96%
Influenza Vaccine	58	91%	94%	91%
Initial Antibiotic Timing	86	100%	96%	95%
Pneumococcal Vaccine	84	92%	95%	93%
Smoking Cessation Advice[1]	24	100%	98%	97%
Surgical Care Improvement Project				
Appropriate VTP Within 24 Hours[2]	94	95%	94%	92%
Appropriate Hair Removal[2]	329	100%	100%	99%
Appropriate Beta Blocker Usage[2]	92	96%	94%	93%
Controlled Postoperative Blood Glucose[2]	0	-	96%	93%
Prophylactic Antibiotic Timing[2]	214	99%	97%	97%
Prophylactic Antibiotic Timing (Outpatient)	70	93%	93%	92%
Prophylactic Antibiotic Selection[2]	214	99%	98%	97%
Prophylactic Antibiotic Select. (Outpatient)	70	97%	96%	94%
Prophylactic Antibiotic Stopped[2]	207	96%	96%	94%
Recommended VTP Ordered[2]	95	96%	96%	94%
Urinary Catheter Removal[2]	133	94%	93%	90%
Children's Asthma Care				
Received Systemic Corticosteroids	-	-	-	100%
Received Home Management Plan	-	-	-	71%
Received Reliever Medication	-	-	-	100%
Use of Medical Imaging				
Combination Abdominal CT Scan	613	0.095	0.144	0.191
Combination Chest CT Scan	559	0.023	0.030	0.054
Follow-up Mammogram/Ultrasound	756	8.7%	7.5%	8.4%
MRI for Low Back Pain	190	34.2%	31.5%	32.7%
Survey of Patients' Hospital Experiences				
Area Around Room 'Always' Quiet at Night	300+	56%	-	58%
Doctors 'Always' Communicated Well	300+	81%	-	80%
Home Recovery Information Given	300+	82%	-	82%
Hospital Given 9 or 10 on 10 Point Scale	300+	66%	-	67%
Meds 'Always' Explained Before Given	300+	60%	-	60%
Nurses 'Always' Communicated Well	300+	71%	-	76%
Pain 'Always' Well Controlled	300+	68%	-	69%
Room and Bathroom 'Always' Clean	300+	62%	-	71%
Timely Help 'Always' Received	300+	57%	-	64%
Would Definitely Recommend Hospital	300+	72%	-	69%

NOTE: Hospital profiles are in alphabetical order by state, then city, then hospital within the city; Rankings exclude hospitals with less than 25 cases except for patient surveys which excludes hospitals with less than 100 cases; (a) 100–299 cases; (1) The number of cases is too small to be sure how well a hospital is performing; (2) The hospital indicated that the data submitted for this measure were based on a sample of cases; (3) Data was collected during a shorter time period (fewer quarters) than the maximum possible time for this measure; (4) Suppressed for one or more quarters by CMS; (5) No data is available from the hospital for this measure; (6) Fewer than 100 patients completed the HCAHPS survey. Use these rates with caution, as the number of surveys may be too low to reliably assess hospital performance; (7) Survey results are based on less than 12 months of data; (8) Survey results are not available for this reporting period; (9) No or very few patients were eligible for the HCAHPS survey. The scores shown, if any, reflect a very small number of surveys; (10) A state average was not calculated because too few hospitals in the state submitted data; (11) There were discrepancies in the data collection process; Please refer to the User's Guide for a full explanation of data.

Virginia Hospital Center - Arlington

1701 North George Mason Drive   Phone: 703-558-5000
Arlington, VA 22205   Fax: 703-558-6553
URL: www.virginiahospitalcenter.com
Type: Acute Care Hospitals   Emergency Services: Yes
Ownership: Voluntary Non-Profit - Private   Beds: 334

Key Personnel:
CEO/President . . . . James B Cole
Cardiac Laboratory . . . . Antonio Parente, MD
Operating Room . . . . Thomas Butler, MD
Pediatric Ambulatory Care . . . . . David Reese, MD
Radiology . . . . Russell McWey, MD
Anesthesiology . . . . Michael Chaikind, MD
Emergency Room . . . . Yorke Allen, MD
Patient Relations . . . . Carolyn McCosh

Measure	Cases	This Hosp.	State Avg.	U.S. Avg.
Heart Attack Care				
ACE Inhibitor or ARB for LVSD	28	96%	97%	96%
Aspirin at Arrival	185	100%	99%	99%
Aspirin at Discharge	202	100%	99%	98%
Beta Blocker at Discharge	199	99%	99%	98%
Fibrinolytic Medication Timing	0	-	75%	55%
PCI Within 90 Minutes of Arrival	41	83%	93%	90%
Smoking Cessation Advice	43	100%	100%	99%
Chest Pain/Possible Heart Attack Care				
Aspirin at Arrival[1,3]	3	100%	95%	95%
Median Time to ECG (minutes)[1,3]	4	0	8	8
Median Time to Transfer (minutes)[5]	0	-	60	61
Fibrinolytic Medication Timing[5]	0	-	59%	54%
Heart Failure Care				
ACE Inhibitor or ARB for LVSD	93	99%	97%	94%
Discharge Instructions	225	79%	92%	88%
Evaluation of LVS Function	292	96%	99%	98%
Smoking Cessation Advice	29	100%	99%	98%
Pneumonia Care				
Appropriate Initial Antibiotic[2]	74	100%	93%	92%
Blood Culture Timing[2]	125	99%	97%	96%
Influenza Vaccine[2]	126	93%	94%	91%
Initial Antibiotic Timing[2]	108	99%	96%	95%
Pneumococcal Vaccine[2]	184	95%	95%	93%
Smoking Cessation Advice[2]	37	100%	98%	97%
Surgical Care Improvement Project				
Appropriate VTP Within 24 Hours[2]	210	97%	94%	92%
Appropriate Hair Removal[2]	632	100%	100%	99%
Appropriate Beta Blocker Usage[2]	171	96%	94%	93%
Controlled Postoperative Blood Glucose[2]	110	93%	96%	93%
Prophylactic Antibiotic Timing[2]	465	100%	97%	97%
Prophylactic Antibiotic Timing (Outpatient)	439	95%	93%	92%
Prophylactic Antibiotic Selection[2]	469	97%	98%	97%
Prophylactic Antibiotic Select. (Outpatient)	435	98%	96%	94%
Prophylactic Antibiotic Stopped[2]	434	97%	96%	94%
Recommended VTP Ordered[2]	210	97%	96%	94%
Urinary Catheter Removal[2]	106	95%	93%	90%
Children's Asthma Care				
Received Systemic Corticosteroids	-	-	-	100%
Received Home Management Plan	-	-	-	71%
Received Reliever Medication	-	-	-	100%
Use of Medical Imaging				
Combination Abdominal CT Scan	1,478	0.072	0.144	0.191
Combination Chest CT Scan	1,170	0.002	0.030	0.054
Follow-up Mammogram/Ultrasound	2,248	6.0%	7.5%	8.4%
MRI for Low Back Pain	329	31.9%	31.5%	32.7%
Survey of Patients' Hospital Experiences				
Area Around Room 'Always' Quiet at Night	300+	58%	-	58%
Doctors 'Always' Communicated Well	300+	78%	-	80%
Home Recovery Information Given	300+	76%	-	82%
Hospital Given 9 or 10 on 10 Point Scale	300+	74%	-	67%
Meds 'Always' Explained Before Given	300+	58%	-	60%
Nurses 'Always' Communicated Well	300+	74%	-	76%
Pain 'Always' Well Controlled	300+	68%	-	69%
Room and Bathroom 'Always' Clean	300+	74%	-	71%
Timely Help 'Always' Received	300+	61%	-	64%
Would Definitely Recommend Hospital	300+	80%	-	69%

Bedford Memorial Hospital

1613 Oakwood Street   Phone: 540-586-2441
Bedford, VA 24523   Fax: 540-586-4342
URL: www.bmhva.com
Type: Acute Care Hospitals   Emergency Services: Yes
Ownership: Voluntary Non-Profit - Private   Beds: 161

Key Personnel:
CEO/President . . . . William Flattery
Chief of Medical Staff . . . . Linda S Beahm, MD
Infection Control . . . . Melisa Hobbs
Operating Room . . . . Eugene W Lowe
Quality Assurance . . . . Karen McBrite
Anesthesiology . . . . Martin Dittler
Emergency Room . . . . Darrell Vanness

Measure	Cases	This Hosp.	State Avg.	U.S. Avg.
Heart Attack Care				
ACE Inhibitor or ARB for LVSD[1]	3	100%	97%	96%
Aspirin at Arrival[1]	14	93%	99%	99%
Aspirin at Discharge[1]	10	100%	99%	98%
Beta Blocker at Discharge[1]	11	100%	99%	98%
Fibrinolytic Medication Timing	0	-	75%	55%
PCI Within 90 Minutes of Arrival	0	-	93%	90%
Smoking Cessation Advice[1]	3	100%	100%	99%
Chest Pain/Possible Heart Attack Care				
Aspirin at Arrival	64	83%	95%	95%
Median Time to ECG (minutes)	66	10	8	8
Median Time to Transfer (minutes)[1]	16	40	60	61
Fibrinolytic Medication Timing	0	-	59%	54%
Heart Failure Care				
ACE Inhibitor or ARB for LVSD[1]	19	95%	97%	94%
Discharge Instructions	55	98%	92%	88%
Evaluation of LVS Function	67	93%	99%	98%
Smoking Cessation Advice[1]	16	100%	99%	98%
Pneumonia Care				
Appropriate Initial Antibiotic	61	75%	93%	92%
Blood Culture Timing	96	97%	97%	96%
Influenza Vaccine	31	87%	94%	91%
Initial Antibiotic Timing	26	88%	96%	95%
Pneumococcal Vaccine	61	75%	95%	93%
Smoking Cessation Advice[1]	21	100%	98%	97%
Surgical Care Improvement Project				
Appropriate VTP Within 24 Hours[1]	13	62%	94%	92%
Appropriate Hair Removal	29	100%	100%	99%
Appropriate Beta Blocker Usage[1]	5	60%	94%	93%
Controlled Postoperative Blood Glucose	0	-	96%	93%
Prophylactic Antibiotic Timing[1]	18	100%	97%	97%
Prophylactic Antibiotic Timing (Outpatient)[1,3]	5	60%	93%	92%
Prophylactic Antibiotic Selection[1]	19	95%	98%	97%
Prophylactic Antibiotic Select. (Outpatient)[1,3]	3	100%	96%	94%
Prophylactic Antibiotic Stopped[1]	18	100%	96%	94%
Recommended VTP Ordered[1]	13	69%	96%	94%
Urinary Catheter Removal[1]	4	75%	93%	90%
Children's Asthma Care				
Received Systemic Corticosteroids	-	-	-	100%
Received Home Management Plan	-	-	-	71%
Received Reliever Medication	-	-	-	100%
Use of Medical Imaging				
Combination Abdominal CT Scan	257	0.230	0.144	0.191
Combination Chest CT Scan	170	0.000	0.030	0.054
Follow-up Mammogram/Ultrasound	648	8.5%	7.5%	8.4%
MRI for Low Back Pain	46	41.3%	31.5%	32.7%
Survey of Patients' Hospital Experiences				
Area Around Room 'Always' Quiet at Night	300+	58%	-	58%
Doctors 'Always' Communicated Well	300+	86%	-	80%
Home Recovery Information Given	300+	79%	-	82%
Hospital Given 9 or 10 on 10 Point Scale	300+	64%	-	67%
Meds 'Always' Explained Before Given	300+	61%	-	60%
Nurses 'Always' Communicated Well	300+	81%	-	76%
Pain 'Always' Well Controlled	300+	73%	-	69%
Room and Bathroom 'Always' Clean	300+	70%	-	71%
Timely Help 'Always' Received	300+	72%	-	64%
Would Definitely Recommend Hospital	300+	68%	-	69%

Wellmont Lonesome Pine Hospital

1990 Holton Avenue East   Phone: 703-523-3111
Big Stone Gap, VA 24219   Fax: 423-230-8224
URL: www.wellmont.org
Type: Acute Care Hospitals   Emergency Services: Yes
Ownership: Voluntary Non-Profit - Other   Beds: 60

Key Personnel:
CEO/President . . . . David Brash
Quality Assurance . . . . Paul Trammell
Emergency Room . . . . Jelly Carter

Measure	Cases	This Hosp.	State Avg.	U.S. Avg.
Heart Attack Care				
ACE Inhibitor or ARB for LVSD[1]	7	86%	97%	96%
Aspirin at Arrival	44	93%	99%	99%
Aspirin at Discharge	32	88%	99%	98%
Beta Blocker at Discharge	37	92%	99%	98%
Fibrinolytic Medication Timing	0	-	75%	55%
PCI Within 90 Minutes of Arrival	0	-	93%	90%
Smoking Cessation Advice[1]	8	100%	100%	99%
Chest Pain/Possible Heart Attack Care				
Aspirin at Arrival	63	92%	95%	95%
Median Time to ECG (minutes)	66	17	8	8
Median Time to Transfer (minutes)[1,3]	1	65	60	61
Fibrinolytic Medication Timing[1]	6	0%	59%	54%
Heart Failure Care				
ACE Inhibitor or ARB for LVSD	28	96%	97%	94%
Discharge Instructions	86	72%	92%	88%
Evaluation of LVS Function	108	99%	99%	98%
Smoking Cessation Advice[1]	22	100%	99%	98%
Pneumonia Care				
Appropriate Initial Antibiotic	73	84%	93%	92%
Blood Culture Timing	92	95%	97%	96%
Influenza Vaccine	76	97%	94%	91%
Initial Antibiotic Timing	106	95%	96%	95%
Pneumococcal Vaccine	84	96%	95%	93%
Smoking Cessation Advice	58	100%	98%	97%
Surgical Care Improvement Project				
Appropriate VTP Within 24 Hours[1,2]	22	82%	94%	92%
Appropriate Hair Removal[2]	64	100%	100%	99%
Appropriate Beta Blocker Usage[1,2]	13	69%	94%	93%
Controlled Postoperative Blood Glucose[2]	0	-	96%	93%
Prophylactic Antibiotic Timing[2]	49	90%	97%	97%
Prophylactic Antibiotic Timing (Outpatient)[1]	15	40%	93%	92%
Prophylactic Antibiotic Selection[2]	49	98%	98%	97%
Prophylactic Antibiotic Select. (Outpatient)[1]	6	50%	96%	94%
Prophylactic Antibiotic Stopped[2]	45	89%	96%	94%
Recommended VTP Ordered[1,2]	22	95%	96%	94%
Urinary Catheter Removal[1,2]	16	88%	93%	90%
Children's Asthma Care				
Received Systemic Corticosteroids	-	-	-	100%
Received Home Management Plan	-	-	-	71%
Received Reliever Medication	-	-	-	100%
Use of Medical Imaging				
Combination Abdominal CT Scan	370	0.641	0.144	0.191
Combination Chest CT Scan	235	0.243	0.030	0.054
Follow-up Mammogram/Ultrasound	355	8.7%	7.5%	8.4%
MRI for Low Back Pain	61	47.5%	31.5%	32.7%
Survey of Patients' Hospital Experiences				
Area Around Room 'Always' Quiet at Night	300+	59%	-	58%
Doctors 'Always' Communicated Well	300+	75%	-	80%
Home Recovery Information Given	300+	73%	-	82%
Hospital Given 9 or 10 on 10 Point Scale	300+	58%	-	67%
Meds 'Always' Explained Before Given	300+	58%	-	60%
Nurses 'Always' Communicated Well	300+	75%	-	76%
Pain 'Always' Well Controlled	300+	66%	-	69%
Room and Bathroom 'Always' Clean	300+	75%	-	71%
Timely Help 'Always' Received	300+	57%	-	64%
Would Definitely Recommend Hospital	300+	59%	-	69%

NOTE: Hospital profiles are in alphabetical order by state, then city, then hospital within the city; Rankings exclude hospitals with less than 25 cases except for patient surveys which excludes hospitals with less than 100 cases; (a) 100–299 cases; (1) The number of cases is too small to be sure how well a hospital is performing; (2) The hospital indicated that the data submitted for this measure were based on a sample of cases; (3) Data was collected during a shorter time period (fewer quarters) than the maximum possible time for this measure; (4) Suppressed for one or more quarters by CMS; (5) No data is available from the hospital for this measure; (6) Fewer than 100 patients completed the HCAHPS survey. Use these rates with caution, as the number of surveys may be too low to reliably assess hospital performance; (7) Survey results are based on less than 12 months of data; (8) Survey results are not available for this reporting period; (9) No or very few patients were eligible for the HCAHPS survey. The scores shown, if any, reflect a very small number of surveys; (10) A state average was not calculated because too few hospitals in the state submitted data; (11) There were discrepancies in the data collection process; Please refer to the User's Guide for a full explanation of data.

Montgomery Regional Hospital

3700 South Main Street
Blacksburg, VA 24060
Phone: 540-951-1111
Fax: 540-953-5295
URL: www.mrhospital.com
Type: Acute Care Hospitals
Emergency Services: No
Ownership: Proprietary
Beds: 146

Key Personnel:

CEO/President. . . . . David Darden
Chief of Medical Staff. . . . . Hing - Har Lo, MD
Infection Control. . . . . Jennifer Brumfield
Operating Room. . . . . Jolene B Henshaw
Pediatric Ambulatory Care . . . . . . Martha Wunsch, MD
Quality Assurance . . . . Lori Rakes
Radiology. . . . . Michael Aronson, MD
Intensive Care Unit. . . . . MJ Bean

Measure	Cases	This Hosp.	State Avg.	U.S. Avg.
Heart Attack Care				
ACE Inhibitor or ARB for LVSD[1]	6	100%	97%	96%
Aspirin at Arrival	61	100%	99%	99%
Aspirin at Discharge	42	100%	99%	98%
Beta Blocker at Discharge	40	100%	99%	98%
Fibrinolytic Medication Timing	0	-	75%	55%
PCI Within 90 Minutes of Arrival[1]	18	100%	93%	90%
Smoking Cessation Advice[1]	22	100%	100%	99%
Chest Pain/Possible Heart Attack Care				
Aspirin at Arrival[1]	22	100%	95%	95%
Median Time to ECG (minutes)[1]	22	10	8	8
Median Time to Transfer (minutes)[5]	0	-	60	61
Fibrinolytic Medication Timing[3]	0	-	59%	54%
Heart Failure Care				
ACE Inhibitor or ARB for LVSD	25	100%	97%	94%
Discharge Instructions	56	98%	92%	88%
Evaluation of LVS Function	79	100%	99%	98%
Smoking Cessation Advice[1]	8	100%	99%	98%
Pneumonia Care				
Appropriate Initial Antibiotic	78	95%	93%	92%
Blood Culture Timing	119	98%	97%	96%
Influenza Vaccine	92	100%	94%	91%
Initial Antibiotic Timing	118	100%	96%	95%
Pneumococcal Vaccine	110	100%	95%	93%
Smoking Cessation Advice	53	100%	98%	97%
Surgical Care Improvement Project				
Appropriate VTP Within 24 Hours	108	99%	94%	92%
Appropriate Hair Removal	416	100%	100%	99%
Appropriate Beta Blocker Usage	115	99%	94%	93%
Controlled Postoperative Blood Glucose	0	-	96%	93%
Prophylactic Antibiotic Timing	312	100%	97%	97%
Prophylactic Antibiotic Timing (Outpatient)	92	99%	93%	92%
Prophylactic Antibiotic Selection	317	99%	98%	97%
Prophylactic Antibiotic Select. (Outpatient)	98	98%	96%	94%
Prophylactic Antibiotic Stopped	298	99%	96%	94%
Recommended VTP Ordered	108	99%	96%	94%
Urinary Catheter Removal	79	99%	93%	90%
Children's Asthma Care				
Received Systemic Corticosteroids	-	-	-	100%
Received Home Management Plan	-	-	-	71%
Received Reliever Medication	-	-	-	100%
Use of Medical Imaging				
Combination Abdominal CT Scan	518	0.075	0.144	0.191
Combination Chest CT Scan	296	0.030	0.030	0.054
Follow-up Mammogram/Ultrasound	827	10.9%	7.5%	8.4%
MRI for Low Back Pain	214	35.0%	31.5%	32.7%
Survey of Patients' Hospital Experiences				
Area Around Room 'Always' Quiet at Night	300+	63%	-	58%
Doctors 'Always' Communicated Well	300+	84%	-	80%
Home Recovery Information Given	300+	88%	-	82%
Hospital Given 9 or 10 on 10 Point Scale	300+	71%	-	67%
Meds 'Always' Explained Before Given	300+	60%	-	60%
Nurses 'Always' Communicated Well	300+	80%	-	76%
Pain 'Always' Well Controlled	300+	74%	-	69%
Room and Bathroom 'Always' Clean	300+	76%	-	71%
Timely Help 'Always' Received	300+	66%	-	64%
Would Definitely Recommend Hospital	300+	74%	-	69%

Piedmont Geriatric Hospital

Highway 360 and 460
Burkeville, VA 23922
Phone: 804-767-4401
Fax: 434-767-4500
E-mail: mike.wimsatt@pgh.dmhmrsas.virginia.gov
URL: www.pgh.dmhmrsas.virginia.gov
Type: Acute Care Hospitals
Emergency Services: No
Ownership: Government - State
Beds: 150

Key Personnel:

CEO/President. . . . . WR Pirece, Jr
Chief of Medical Staff . . . . Hugo Falcon
Quality Assurance . . . . H Eugene Overton
Patient Relations . . . . Anne Stiles

Measure	Cases	This Hosp.	State Avg.	U.S. Avg.
Heart Attack Care				
ACE Inhibitor or ARB for LVSD[5]	0	-	97%	96%
Aspirin at Arrival[5]	0	-	99%	99%
Aspirin at Discharge[5]	0	-	99%	98%
Beta Blocker at Discharge[5]	0	-	99%	98%
Fibrinolytic Medication Timing[5]	0	-	75%	55%
PCI Within 90 Minutes of Arrival[5]	0	-	93%	90%
Smoking Cessation Advice[5]	0	-	100%	99%
Chest Pain/Possible Heart Attack Care				
Aspirin at Arrival	-	-	95%	95%
Median Time to ECG (minutes)	-	-	8	8
Median Time to Transfer (minutes)	-	-	60	61
Fibrinolytic Medication Timing	-	-	59%	54%
Heart Failure Care				
ACE Inhibitor or ARB for LVSD[5]	0	-	97%	94%
Discharge Instructions[5]	0	-	92%	88%
Evaluation of LVS Function[5]	0	-	99%	98%
Smoking Cessation Advice[5]	0	-	99%	98%
Pneumonia Care				
Appropriate Initial Antibiotic[5]	0	-	93%	92%
Blood Culture Timing[5]	0	-	97%	96%
Influenza Vaccine[5]	0	-	94%	91%
Initial Antibiotic Timing[5]	0	-	96%	95%
Pneumococcal Vaccine[5]	0	-	95%	93%
Smoking Cessation Advice[5]	0	-	98%	97%
Surgical Care Improvement Project				
Appropriate VTP Within 24 Hours[5]	0	-	94%	92%
Appropriate Hair Removal[5]	0	-	100%	99%
Appropriate Beta Blocker Usage[5]	0	-	94%	93%
Controlled Postoperative Blood Glucose[5]	0	-	96%	93%
Prophylactic Antibiotic Timing[5]	0	-	97%	97%
Prophylactic Antibiotic Timing (Outpatient)	-	-	93%	92%
Prophylactic Antibiotic Selection[5]	0	-	98%	97%
Prophylactic Antibiotic Select. (Outpatient)	-	-	96%	94%
Prophylactic Antibiotic Stopped[5]	0	-	96%	94%
Recommended VTP Ordered[5]	0	-	96%	94%
Urinary Catheter Removal[5]	0	-	93%	90%
Children's Asthma Care				
Received Systemic Corticosteroids	-	-	-	100%
Received Home Management Plan	-	-	-	71%
Received Reliever Medication	-	-	-	100%
Use of Medical Imaging				
Combination Abdominal CT Scan	-	-	0.144	0.191
Combination Chest CT Scan	-	-	0.030	0.054
Follow-up Mammogram/Ultrasound	-	-	7.5%	8.4%
MRI for Low Back Pain	-	-	31.5%	32.7%
Survey of Patients' Hospital Experiences				
Area Around Room 'Always' Quiet at Night[8]	-	-	-	58%
Doctors 'Always' Communicated Well[8]	-	-	-	80%
Home Recovery Information Given[8]	-	-	-	82%
Hospital Given 9 or 10 on 10 Point Scale[8]	-	-	-	67%
Meds 'Always' Explained Before Given[8]	-	-	-	60%
Nurses 'Always' Communicated Well[8]	-	-	-	76%
Pain 'Always' Well Controlled[8]	-	-	-	69%
Room and Bathroom 'Always' Clean[8]	-	-	-	71%
Timely Help 'Always' Received[8]	-	-	-	64%
Would Definitely Recommend Hospital[8]	-	-	-	69%

Martha Jefferson Hospital

459 Locust Ave
Charlottesville, VA 22902
Phone: 434-654-7326
Fax: 434-982-7759
URL: www.marthajefferson.org
Type: Acute Care Hospitals
Emergency Services: Yes
Ownership: Voluntary Non-Profit - Private
Beds: 176

Key Personnel:

CEO/President. . . . . James E Haden
Chief of Medical Staff. . . . . K Asao-Ragosta
Operating Room. . . . . Andrew A Bailey
Pediatric In-Patient Care . . . . Katherine D Mika, MD
Quality Assurance . . . . DD Sandridge
Emergency Room . . . . Sarah White

Measure	Cases	This Hosp.	State Avg.	U.S. Avg.
Heart Attack Care				
ACE Inhibitor or ARB for LVSD	36	100%	97%	96%
Aspirin at Arrival	164	98%	99%	99%
Aspirin at Discharge	155	99%	99%	98%
Beta Blocker at Discharge	142	99%	99%	98%
Fibrinolytic Medication Timing	0	-	75%	55%
PCI Within 90 Minutes of Arrival	43	91%	93%	90%
Smoking Cessation Advice	32	100%	100%	99%
Chest Pain/Possible Heart Attack Care				
Aspirin at Arrival[1,3]	3	100%	95%	95%
Median Time to ECG (minutes)[1,3]	3	11	8	8
Median Time to Transfer (minutes)[5]	0	-	60	61
Fibrinolytic Medication Timing[3]	0	-	59%	54%
Heart Failure Care				
ACE Inhibitor or ARB for LVSD	129	93%	97%	94%
Discharge Instructions	273	75%	92%	88%
Evaluation of LVS Function	321	100%	99%	98%
Smoking Cessation Advice	55	95%	99%	98%
Pneumonia Care				
Appropriate Initial Antibiotic[2]	85	91%	93%	92%
Blood Culture Timing[2]	103	93%	97%	96%
Influenza Vaccine[2]	96	78%	94%	91%
Initial Antibiotic Timing[2]	129	94%	96%	95%
Pneumococcal Vaccine[2]	149	77%	95%	93%
Smoking Cessation Advice[2]	31	97%	98%	97%
Surgical Care Improvement Project				
Appropriate VTP Within 24 Hours[2]	127	91%	94%	92%
Appropriate Hair Removal[2]	473	100%	100%	99%
Appropriate Beta Blocker Usage[2]	126	88%	94%	93%
Controlled Postoperative Blood Glucose[2]	0	-	96%	93%
Prophylactic Antibiotic Timing[2]	325	97%	97%	97%
Prophylactic Antibiotic Timing (Outpatient)	204	92%	93%	92%
Prophylactic Antibiotic Selection[2]	326	97%	98%	97%
Prophylactic Antibiotic Select. (Outpatient)	201	96%	96%	94%
Prophylactic Antibiotic Stopped[2]	314	98%	96%	94%
Recommended VTP Ordered[2]	127	93%	96%	94%
Urinary Catheter Removal[2]	66	89%	93%	90%
Children's Asthma Care				
Received Systemic Corticosteroids	-	-	-	100%
Received Home Management Plan	-	-	-	71%
Received Reliever Medication	-	-	-	100%
Use of Medical Imaging				
Combination Abdominal CT Scan	1,435	0.125	0.144	0.191
Combination Chest CT Scan	1,024	0.000	0.030	0.054
Follow-up Mammogram/Ultrasound	3,457	7.8%	7.5%	8.4%
MRI for Low Back Pain	330	31.8%	31.5%	32.7%
Survey of Patients' Hospital Experiences				
Area Around Room 'Always' Quiet at Night	300+	53%	-	58%
Doctors 'Always' Communicated Well	300+	88%	-	80%
Home Recovery Information Given	300+	85%	-	82%
Hospital Given 9 or 10 on 10 Point Scale	300+	75%	-	67%
Meds 'Always' Explained Before Given	300+	65%	-	60%
Nurses 'Always' Communicated Well	300+	80%	-	76%
Pain 'Always' Well Controlled	300+	73%	-	69%
Room and Bathroom 'Always' Clean	300+	66%	-	71%
Timely Help 'Always' Received	300+	64%	-	64%
Would Definitely Recommend Hospital	300+	83%	-	69%

NOTE: Hospital profiles are in alphabetical order by state, then city, then hospital within the city; Rankings exclude hospitals with less than 25 cases except for patient surveys which excludes hospitals with less than 100 cases; (a) 100–299 cases; (1) The number of cases is too small to be sure how well a hospital is performing; (2) The hospital indicated that the data submitted for this measure were based on a sample of cases; (3) Data was collected during a shorter time period (fewer quarters) than the maximum possible time for this measure; (4) Suppressed for one or more quarters by CMS; (5) No data is available from the hospital for this measure; (6) Fewer than 100 patients completed the HCAHPS survey. Use these rates with caution, as the number of surveys may be too low to reliably assess hospital performance; (7) Survey results are based on less than 12 months of data; (8) Survey results are not available for this reporting period; (9) No or very few patients were eligible for the HCAHPS survey. The scores shown, if any, reflect a very small number of surveys; (10) A state average was not calculated because too few hospitals in the state submitted data; (11) There were discrepancies in the data collection process; Please refer to the User's Guide for a full explanation of data.

University of Virginia Medical Center

Jefferson Park Ave
Charlottesville, VA 22908
Phone: 800-251-3627
URL: uvahealth.com
Type: Acute Care Hospitals
Ownership: Government - State
Emergency Services: Yes
Beds: 619

Key Personnel:
CEO/President. . . . . R.Edward Howell
Chief of Medical Staff. . . . . Jonathon D Truwit, MD MBA
Coronary Care . . . . Marian Lawson, RN
Infection Control . . . . Eve Giannetta
Pediatric Ambulatory Care . . . . . . Sheila Smith
Pediatric In-Patient Care . . . . Sheila Smith
Quality Assurance . . . . Abraham Segres
Radiology. . . . . James Cames

Measure	Cases	This Hosp.	State Avg.	U.S. Avg.
Heart Attack Care				
ACE Inhibitor or ARB for LVSD[2]	65	98%	97%	96%
Aspirin at Arrival[2]	161	99%	99%	99%
Aspirin at Discharge[2]	322	99%	99%	98%
Beta Blocker at Discharge[2]	289	98%	99%	98%
Fibrinolytic Medication Timing[1,2]	1	100%	75%	55%
PCI Within 90 Minutes of Arrival[2]	30	80%	93%	90%
Smoking Cessation Advice[2]	126	100%	100%	99%
Chest Pain/Possible Heart Attack Care				
Aspirin at Arrival[5]	0	-	95%	95%
Median Time to ECG (minutes)[5]	0	-	8	8
Median Time to Transfer (minutes)[5]	0	-	60	61
Fibrinolytic Medication Timing[5]	0	-	59%	54%
Heart Failure Care				
ACE Inhibitor or ARB for LVSD[2]	131	98%	97%	94%
Discharge Instructions[2]	240	80%	92%	88%
Evaluation of LVS Function[2]	282	99%	99%	98%
Smoking Cessation Advice[2]	74	99%	99%	98%
Pneumonia Care				
Appropriate Initial Antibiotic[2]	54	93%	93%	92%
Blood Culture Timing[2]	81	95%	97%	96%
Influenza Vaccine[2]	67	88%	94%	91%
Initial Antibiotic Timing[2]	93	87%	96%	95%
Pneumococcal Vaccine[2]	92	91%	95%	93%
Smoking Cessation Advice[2]	56	98%	98%	97%
Surgical Care Improvement Project				
Appropriate VTP Within 24 Hours[2]	193	90%	94%	92%
Appropriate Hair Removal[2]	636	96%	100%	99%
Appropriate Beta Blocker Usage[2]	218	86%	94%	93%
Controlled Postoperative Blood Glucose[2]	120	85%	96%	93%
Prophylactic Antibiotic Timing[2]	402	96%	97%	97%
Prophylactic Antibiotic Timing (Outpatient)	367	95%	93%	92%
Prophylactic Antibiotic Selection[2]	409	97%	98%	97%
Prophylactic Antibiotic Select. (Outpatient)	362	97%	96%	94%
Prophylactic Antibiotic Stopped[2]	387	93%	96%	94%
Recommended VTP Ordered[2]	193	94%	96%	94%
Urinary Catheter Removal[2]	121	59%	93%	90%
Children's Asthma Care				
Received Systemic Corticosteroids[2]	38	97%	-	100%
Received Home Management Plan[2]	38	61%	-	71%
Received Reliever Medication[2]	38	100%	-	100%
Use of Medical Imaging				
Combination Abdominal CT Scan	589	0.056	0.144	0.191
Combination Chest CT Scan	357	0.003	0.030	0.054
Follow-up Mammogram/Ultrasound	3,221	9.6%	7.5%	8.4%
MRI for Low Back Pain[1]	17	23.5%	31.5%	32.7%
Survey of Patients' Hospital Experiences				
Area Around Room 'Always' Quiet at Night	300+	42%	-	58%
Doctors 'Always' Communicated Well	300+	76%	-	80%
Home Recovery Information Given	300+	86%	-	82%
Hospital Given 9 or 10 on 10 Point Scale	300+	65%	-	67%
Meds 'Always' Explained Before Given	300+	56%	-	60%
Nurses 'Always' Communicated Well	300+	74%	-	76%
Pain 'Always' Well Controlled	300+	65%	-	69%
Room and Bathroom 'Always' Clean	300+	62%	-	71%
Timely Help 'Always' Received	300+	53%	-	64%
Would Definitely Recommend Hospital	300+	74%	-	69%

Chesapeake General Hospital

736 Battlefield Blvd North
Chesapeake, VA 23320
Phone: 757-312-8121
Fax: 757-312-6184
E-mail: info@chealth.org,
URL: www.chesapeakehealth.com
Type: Acute Care Hospitals
Ownership: Govt - Hospital Dist/Auth
Emergency Services: Yes
Beds: 260

Key Personnel:
CEO/President. . . . . Christopher Mosley
Chief of Medical Staff. . . . . Francis Watson, MD
Operating Room. . . . . Merle Wilson, RN
Pediatric Ambulatory Care . . . . . . Vernita Peeples, MD
Pediatric In-Patient Care . . . . Vernita Peeples, MD
Quality Assurance . . . . Sandra Chellew, RN
Radiology. . . . . James J Rinaldi, MD

Measure	Cases	This Hosp.	State Avg.	U.S. Avg.
Heart Attack Care				
ACE Inhibitor or ARB for LVSD	46	100%	97%	96%
Aspirin at Arrival	267	98%	99%	99%
Aspirin at Discharge	229	100%	99%	98%
Beta Blocker at Discharge	227	100%	99%	98%
Fibrinolytic Medication Timing	0	-	75%	55%
PCI Within 90 Minutes of Arrival	52	85%	93%	90%
Smoking Cessation Advice	88	100%	100%	99%
Chest Pain/Possible Heart Attack Care				
Aspirin at Arrival[5]	0	-	95%	95%
Median Time to ECG (minutes)[5]	0	-	8	8
Median Time to Transfer (minutes)[5]	0	-	60	61
Fibrinolytic Medication Timing[5]	0	-	59%	54%
Heart Failure Care				
ACE Inhibitor or ARB for LVSD	220	94%	97%	94%
Discharge Instructions	475	91%	92%	88%
Evaluation of LVS Function	548	100%	99%	98%
Smoking Cessation Advice	112	100%	99%	98%
Pneumonia Care				
Appropriate Initial Antibiotic	227	93%	93%	92%
Blood Culture Timing	364	99%	97%	96%
Influenza Vaccine	251	96%	94%	91%
Initial Antibiotic Timing	352	93%	96%	95%
Pneumococcal Vaccine	357	94%	95%	93%
Smoking Cessation Advice	122	100%	98%	97%
Surgical Care Improvement Project				
Appropriate VTP Within 24 Hours[2]	177	95%	94%	92%
Appropriate Hair Removal[2]	395	99%	100%	99%
Appropriate Beta Blocker Usage[2]	107	93%	94%	93%
Controlled Postoperative Blood Glucose[2]	0	-	96%	93%
Prophylactic Antibiotic Timing[2]	265	96%	97%	97%
Prophylactic Antibiotic Timing (Outpatient)	464	96%	93%	92%
Prophylactic Antibiotic Selection[2]	265	97%	98%	97%
Prophylactic Antibiotic Select. (Outpatient)	450	96%	96%	94%
Prophylactic Antibiotic Stopped[2]	250	94%	96%	94%
Recommended VTP Ordered[2]	177	97%	96%	94%
Urinary Catheter Removal[2]	91	79%	93%	90%
Children's Asthma Care				
Received Systemic Corticosteroids	-	-	-	100%
Received Home Management Plan	-	-	-	71%
Received Reliever Medication	-	-	-	100%
Use of Medical Imaging				
Combination Abdominal CT Scan	1,313	0.395	0.144	0.191
Combination Chest CT Scan	1,249	0.007	0.030	0.054
Follow-up Mammogram/Ultrasound	1,989	10.0%	7.5%	8.4%
MRI for Low Back Pain	227	32.6%	31.5%	32.7%
Survey of Patients' Hospital Experiences				
Area Around Room 'Always' Quiet at Night	300+	55%	-	58%
Doctors 'Always' Communicated Well	300+	77%	-	80%
Home Recovery Information Given	300+	82%	-	82%
Hospital Given 9 or 10 on 10 Point Scale	300+	63%	-	67%
Meds 'Always' Explained Before Given	300+	55%	-	60%
Nurses 'Always' Communicated Well	300+	69%	-	76%
Pain 'Always' Well Controlled	300+	67%	-	69%
Room and Bathroom 'Always' Clean	300+	56%	-	71%
Timely Help 'Always' Received	300+	57%	-	64%
Would Definitely Recommend Hospital	300+	68%	-	69%

Carilion New River Valley Medical Center

2900 Lamb Circle
Christiansburg, VA 24073
Phone: 540-731-2000
Fax: 540-731-2850
URL: www.carilion.com
Type: Acute Care Hospitals
Ownership: Voluntary Non-Profit - Other
Emergency Services: Yes
Beds: 97

Key Personnel:
CEO/President. . . . . Janet Crawford
Cardiac Laboratory. . . . . Carlos Fernandez
Pediatric Ambulatory Care . . . . . . Joyce Yearout
Emergency Room . . . . Gary S Abel

Measure	Cases	This Hosp.	State Avg.	U.S. Avg.
Heart Attack Care				
ACE Inhibitor or ARB for LVSD[1]	2	100%	97%	96%
Aspirin at Arrival[1]	23	100%	99%	99%
Aspirin at Discharge[1]	11	100%	99%	98%
Beta Blocker at Discharge[1]	11	100%	99%	98%
Fibrinolytic Medication Timing	0	-	75%	55%
PCI Within 90 Minutes of Arrival	0	-	93%	90%
Smoking Cessation Advice[1]	2	100%	100%	99%
Chest Pain/Possible Heart Attack Care				
Aspirin at Arrival	39	95%	95%	95%
Median Time to ECG (minutes)	27	25	8	8
Median Time to Transfer (minutes)[1,3]	4	50	60	61
Fibrinolytic Medication Timing[3]	0	-	59%	54%
Heart Failure Care				
ACE Inhibitor or ARB for LVSD	34	88%	97%	94%
Discharge Instructions	100	88%	92%	88%
Evaluation of LVS Function	123	99%	99%	98%
Smoking Cessation Advice[1]	22	100%	99%	98%
Pneumonia Care				
Appropriate Initial Antibiotic	132	85%	93%	92%
Blood Culture Timing	163	93%	97%	96%
Influenza Vaccine	94	94%	94%	91%
Initial Antibiotic Timing	154	90%	96%	95%
Pneumococcal Vaccine	120	96%	95%	93%
Smoking Cessation Advice	57	100%	98%	97%
Surgical Care Improvement Project				
Appropriate VTP Within 24 Hours	124	92%	94%	92%
Appropriate Hair Removal	347	99%	100%	99%
Appropriate Beta Blocker Usage	111	80%	94%	93%
Controlled Postoperative Blood Glucose	0	-	96%	93%
Prophylactic Antibiotic Timing	238	97%	97%	97%
Prophylactic Antibiotic Timing (Outpatient)	203	90%	93%	92%
Prophylactic Antibiotic Selection	240	99%	98%	97%
Prophylactic Antibiotic Select. (Outpatient)	212	83%	96%	94%
Prophylactic Antibiotic Stopped	231	95%	96%	94%
Recommended VTP Ordered	124	97%	96%	94%
Urinary Catheter Removal	73	95%	93%	90%
Children's Asthma Care				
Received Systemic Corticosteroids	-	-	-	100%
Received Home Management Plan	-	-	-	71%
Received Reliever Medication	-	-	-	100%
Use of Medical Imaging				
Combination Abdominal CT Scan	850	0.086	0.144	0.191
Combination Chest CT Scan	680	0.041	0.030	0.054
Follow-up Mammogram/Ultrasound	1,497	8.6%	7.5%	8.4%
MRI for Low Back Pain	200	42.0%	31.5%	32.7%
Survey of Patients' Hospital Experiences				
Area Around Room 'Always' Quiet at Night	300+	58%	-	58%
Doctors 'Always' Communicated Well	300+	80%	-	80%
Home Recovery Information Given	300+	87%	-	82%
Hospital Given 9 or 10 on 10 Point Scale	300+	69%	-	67%
Meds 'Always' Explained Before Given	300+	60%	-	60%
Nurses 'Always' Communicated Well	300+	78%	-	76%
Pain 'Always' Well Controlled	300+	68%	-	69%
Room and Bathroom 'Always' Clean	300+	71%	-	71%
Timely Help 'Always' Received	300+	74%	-	64%
Would Definitely Recommend Hospital	300+	77%	-	69%

NOTE: Hospital profiles are in alphabetical order by state, then city, then hospital within the city; Rankings exclude hospitals with less than 25 cases except for patient surveys which excludes hospitals with less than 100 cases; (a) 100–299 cases; (1) The number of cases is too small to be sure how well a hospital is performing; (2) The hospital indicated that the data submitted for this measure were based on a sample of cases; (3) Data was collected during a shorter time period (fewer quarters) than the maximum possible time for this measure; (4) Suppressed for one or more quarters by CMS; (5) No data is available from the hospital for this measure; (6) Fewer than 100 patients completed the HCAHPS survey. Use these rates with caution, as the number of surveys may be too low to reliably assess hospital performance; (7) Survey results are based on less than 12 months of data; (8) Survey results are not available for this reporting period; (9) No or very few patients were eligible for the HCAHPS survey. The scores shown, if any, reflect a very small number of surveys; (10) A state average was not calculated because too few hospitals in the state submitted data; (11) There were discrepancies in the data collection process; Please refer to the User's Guide for a full explanation of data.

Dickenson Community Hospital

312 Hospital Drive
Clintwood, VA 24228
Phone: 276-926-0300
Fax: 276-926-0329
URL: www.dchosp.com

Type: Critical Access Hospitals
Emergency Services: Yes
Ownership: Voluntary Non-Profit - Private
Beds: 15

Key Personnel:

CEO/President. . . . . Lee Turner
Operating Room. . . . . Carman Banks, RN
Quality Assurance . . . . Joan Curry
Radiology. . . . . Mark Blair, RT(R)

Measure	Cases	This Hosp.	State Avg.	U.S. Avg.
Heart Attack Care				
ACE Inhibitor or ARB for LVSD[5]	0	-	97%	96%
Aspirin at Arrival[5]	0	-	99%	99%
Aspirin at Discharge[5]	0	-	99%	98%
Beta Blocker at Discharge[5]	0	-	99%	98%
Fibrinolytic Medication Timing[5]	0	-	75%	55%
PCI Within 90 Minutes of Arrival[5]	0	-	93%	90%
Smoking Cessation Advice[5]	0	-	100%	99%
Chest Pain/Possible Heart Attack Care				
Aspirin at Arrival	111	95%	95%	95%
Median Time to ECG (minutes)	117	6	8	8
Median Time to Transfer (minutes)[3]	0	-	60	61
Fibrinolytic Medication Timing[1]	4	25%	59%	54%
Heart Failure Care				
ACE Inhibitor or ARB for LVSD[5]	0	-	97%	94%
Discharge Instructions[5]	0	-	92%	88%
Evaluation of LVS Function[5]	0	-	99%	98%
Smoking Cessation Advice[5]	0	-	99%	98%
Pneumonia Care				
Appropriate Initial Antibiotic[5]	0	-	93%	92%
Blood Culture Timing[5]	0	-	97%	96%
Influenza Vaccine[5]	0	-	94%	91%
Initial Antibiotic Timing[5]	0	-	96%	95%
Pneumococcal Vaccine[5]	0	-	95%	93%
Smoking Cessation Advice[5]	0	-	98%	97%
Surgical Care Improvement Project				
Appropriate VTP Within 24 Hours[5]	0	-	94%	92%
Appropriate Hair Removal[5]	0	-	100%	99%
Appropriate Beta Blocker Usage[5]	0	-	94%	93%
Controlled Postoperative Blood Glucose[5]	0	-	96%	93%
Prophylactic Antibiotic Timing[5]	0	-	97%	97%
Prophylactic Antibiotic Timing (Outpatient)[5]	0	-	93%	92%
Prophylactic Antibiotic Selection[5]	0	-	98%	97%
Prophylactic Antibiotic Select. (Outpatient)[5]	0	-	96%	94%
Prophylactic Antibiotic Stopped[5]	0	-	96%	94%
Recommended VTP Ordered[5]	0	-	96%	94%
Urinary Catheter Removal[5]	0	-	93%	90%
Children's Asthma Care				
Received Systemic Corticosteroids	-	-	-	100%
Received Home Management Plan	-	-	-	71%
Received Reliever Medication	-	-	-	100%
Use of Medical Imaging				
Combination Abdominal CT Scan	102	0.402	0.144	0.191
Combination Chest CT Scan	80	0.338	0.030	0.054
Follow-up Mammogram/Ultrasound[5]	0	-	7.5%	8.4%
MRI for Low Back Pain[5]	0	-	31.5%	32.7%
Survey of Patients' Hospital Experiences				
Area Around Room 'Always' Quiet at Night[8]	-	-	-	58%
Doctors 'Always' Communicated Well[8]	-	-	-	80%
Home Recovery Information Given[8]	-	-	-	82%
Hospital Given 9 or 10 on 10 Point Scale[8]	-	-	-	67%
Meds 'Always' Explained Before Given[8]	-	-	-	60%
Nurses 'Always' Communicated Well[8]	-	-	-	76%
Pain 'Always' Well Controlled[8]	-	-	-	69%
Room and Bathroom 'Always' Clean[8]	-	-	-	71%
Timely Help 'Always' Received[8]	-	-	-	64%
Would Definitely Recommend Hospital[8]	-	-	-	69%

Culpeper Regional Hospital

501 Sunset Lane
Culpeper, VA 22701
Phone: 540-829-4100
Fax: 540-829-4353
E-mail: webmaster@culpeperhospital.com
URL: www.culpeperhospital.com

Type: Acute Care Hospitals
Emergency Services: Yes
Ownership: Voluntary Non-Profit - Other
Beds: 70

Key Personnel:

CEO/President. . . . . Larry Fitzgerald
Chief of Medical Staff . . . . Sok Yi, MD
Infection Control. . . . . Lisa Richardson, RN
Operating Room. . . . . Tama Auville
Quality Assurance . . . . Patricia Mullins, RN
Emergency Room . . . . Michael Bost, MD
Hemotology Center . . . . Vicki Krohn, RN
Intensive Care Unit. . . . . Janice Beahm, RN

Measure	Cases	This Hosp.	State Avg.	U.S. Avg.
Heart Attack Care				
ACE Inhibitor or ARB for LVSD[1]	3	100%	97%	96%
Aspirin at Arrival[1]	15	100%	99%	99%
Aspirin at Discharge[1]	14	100%	99%	98%
Beta Blocker at Discharge[1]	14	100%	99%	98%
Fibrinolytic Medication Timing	0	-	75%	55%
PCI Within 90 Minutes of Arrival	0	-	93%	90%
Smoking Cessation Advice[1]	3	100%	100%	99%
Chest Pain/Possible Heart Attack Care				
Aspirin at Arrival	64	100%	95%	95%
Median Time to ECG (minutes)	68	16	8	8
Median Time to Transfer (minutes)[1]	9	60	60	61
Fibrinolytic Medication Timing	0	-	59%	54%
Heart Failure Care				
ACE Inhibitor or ARB for LVSD	29	97%	97%	94%
Discharge Instructions	84	82%	92%	88%
Evaluation of LVS Function	107	94%	99%	98%
Smoking Cessation Advice[1]	12	100%	99%	98%
Pneumonia Care				
Appropriate Initial Antibiotic	77	92%	93%	92%
Blood Culture Timing	156	96%	97%	96%
Influenza Vaccine	89	82%	94%	91%
Initial Antibiotic Timing	134	97%	96%	95%
Pneumococcal Vaccine	126	86%	95%	93%
Smoking Cessation Advice	36	92%	98%	97%
Surgical Care Improvement Project				
Appropriate VTP Within 24 Hours	108	89%	94%	92%
Appropriate Hair Removal	322	100%	100%	99%
Appropriate Beta Blocker Usage	76	92%	94%	93%
Controlled Postoperative Blood Glucose	0	-	96%	93%
Prophylactic Antibiotic Timing	246	96%	97%	97%
Prophylactic Antibiotic Timing (Outpatient)	65	94%	93%	92%
Prophylactic Antibiotic Selection	243	99%	98%	97%
Prophylactic Antibiotic Select. (Outpatient)	65	89%	96%	94%
Prophylactic Antibiotic Stopped	239	88%	96%	94%
Recommended VTP Ordered	108	97%	96%	94%
Urinary Catheter Removal	107	93%	93%	90%
Children's Asthma Care				
Received Systemic Corticosteroids	-	-	-	100%
Received Home Management Plan	-	-	-	71%
Received Reliever Medication	-	-	-	100%
Use of Medical Imaging				
Combination Abdominal CT Scan	537	0.074	0.144	0.191
Combination Chest CT Scan	304	0.007	0.030	0.054
Follow-up Mammogram/Ultrasound	702	10.8%	7.5%	8.4%
MRI for Low Back Pain	128	25.0%	31.5%	32.7%
Survey of Patients' Hospital Experiences				
Area Around Room 'Always' Quiet at Night	300+	56%	-	58%
Doctors 'Always' Communicated Well	300+	68%	-	80%
Home Recovery Information Given	300+	79%	-	82%
Hospital Given 9 or 10 on 10 Point Scale	300+	61%	-	67%
Meds 'Always' Explained Before Given	300+	56%	-	60%
Nurses 'Always' Communicated Well	300+	72%	-	76%
Pain 'Always' Well Controlled	300+	62%	-	69%
Room and Bathroom 'Always' Clean	300+	72%	-	71%
Timely Help 'Always' Received	300+	58%	-	64%
Would Definitely Recommend Hospital	300+	64%	-	69%

Danville Regional Medical Center

142 South Main Street
Danville, VA 24541
Phone: 434-799-2100
Fax: 434-799-4449
URL: www.danvilleregional.org

Type: Acute Care Hospitals
Emergency Services: Yes
Ownership: Proprietary
Beds: 350

Key Personnel:

CEO/President. . . . . Ruth Brinkley
Chief of Medical Staff . . . . Gary P Miller, MD
Operating Room. . . . . Kathy Dalton
Quality Assurance . . . . Kim Gibson
Radiology. . . . . Gerald Johnson, MD
Anesthesiology. . . . . Richard Pagano, MD
Emergency Room . . . . Mark Brande
Intensive Care Unit. . . . . Tari Wyatt

Measure	Cases	This Hosp.	State Avg.	U.S. Avg.
Heart Attack Care				
ACE Inhibitor or ARB for LVSD[1]	19	95%	97%	96%
Aspirin at Arrival	166	99%	99%	99%
Aspirin at Discharge	132	98%	99%	98%
Beta Blocker at Discharge	132	99%	99%	98%
Fibrinolytic Medication Timing[1]	8	88%	75%	55%
PCI Within 90 Minutes of Arrival[1]	17	94%	93%	90%
Smoking Cessation Advice	55	100%	100%	99%
Chest Pain/Possible Heart Attack Care				
Aspirin at Arrival	35	97%	95%	95%
Median Time to ECG (minutes)	37	9	8	8
Median Time to Transfer (minutes)[3]	0	-	60	61
Fibrinolytic Medication Timing[1]	7	86%	59%	54%
Heart Failure Care				
ACE Inhibitor or ARB for LVSD[2]	130	96%	97%	94%
Discharge Instructions[2]	264	76%	92%	88%
Evaluation of LVS Function[2]	343	97%	99%	98%
Smoking Cessation Advice[2]	86	100%	99%	98%
Pneumonia Care				
Appropriate Initial Antibiotic[2]	78	96%	93%	92%
Blood Culture Timing[2]	123	96%	97%	96%
Influenza Vaccine[2]	89	76%	94%	91%
Initial Antibiotic Timing[2]	132	88%	96%	95%
Pneumococcal Vaccine[2]	139	86%	95%	93%
Smoking Cessation Advice[2]	72	100%	98%	97%
Surgical Care Improvement Project				
Appropriate VTP Within 24 Hours[2]	176	90%	94%	92%
Appropriate Hair Removal[2]	452	100%	100%	99%
Appropriate Beta Blocker Usage[2]	154	86%	94%	93%
Controlled Postoperative Blood Glucose[2]	68	99%	96%	93%
Prophylactic Antibiotic Timing[2]	309	96%	97%	97%
Prophylactic Antibiotic Timing (Outpatient)	119	83%	93%	92%
Prophylactic Antibiotic Selection[2]	310	97%	98%	97%
Prophylactic Antibiotic Select. (Outpatient)	113	84%	96%	94%
Prophylactic Antibiotic Stopped[2]	298	98%	96%	94%
Recommended VTP Ordered[2]	178	93%	96%	94%
Urinary Catheter Removal[2]	43	60%	93%	90%
Children's Asthma Care				
Received Systemic Corticosteroids	-	-	-	100%
Received Home Management Plan	-	-	-	71%
Received Reliever Medication	-	-	-	100%
Use of Medical Imaging				
Combination Abdominal CT Scan	327	0.187	0.144	0.191
Combination Chest CT Scan	301	0.000	0.030	0.054
Follow-up Mammogram/Ultrasound	117	7.7%	7.5%	8.4%
MRI for Low Back Pain[1]	37	32.4%	31.5%	32.7%
Survey of Patients' Hospital Experiences				
Area Around Room 'Always' Quiet at Night	300+	64%	-	58%
Doctors 'Always' Communicated Well	300+	76%	-	80%
Home Recovery Information Given	300+	76%	-	82%
Hospital Given 9 or 10 on 10 Point Scale	300+	51%	-	67%
Meds 'Always' Explained Before Given	300+	54%	-	60%
Nurses 'Always' Communicated Well	300+	70%	-	76%
Pain 'Always' Well Controlled	300+	65%	-	69%
Room and Bathroom 'Always' Clean	300+	66%	-	71%
Timely Help 'Always' Received	300+	52%	-	64%
Would Definitely Recommend Hospital	300+	44%	-	69%

NOTE: Hospital profiles are in alphabetical order by state, then city, then hospital within the city; Rankings exclude hospitals with less than 25 cases except for patient surveys which excludes hospitals with less than 100 cases; (a) 100–299 cases; (1) The number of cases is too small to be sure how well a hospital is performing; (2) The hospital indicated that the data submitted for this measure were based on a sample of cases; (3) Data was collected during a shorter time period (fewer quarters) than the maximum possible time for this measure; (4) Suppressed for one or more quarters by CMS; (5) No data is available from the hospital for this measure; (6) Fewer than 100 patients completed the HCAHPS survey. Use these rates with caution, as the number of surveys may be too low to reliably assess hospital performance; (7) Survey results are based on less than 12 months of data; (8) Survey results are not available for this reporting period; (9) No or very few patients were eligible for the HCAHPS survey. The scores shown, if any, reflect a very small number of surveys; (10) A state average was not calculated because too few hospitals in the state submitted data; (11) There were discrepancies in the data collection process; Please refer to the User's Guide for a full explanation of data.

Southern Virginia Regional Medical Center

727 North Main Street Phone: 434-348-4400
Emporia, VA 23847 Fax: 434-348-4982
URL: www.svrmc.com
Type: Acute Care Hospitals Emergency Services: Yes
Ownership: Proprietary Beds: 80

Key Personnel:
CEO/President. . . . . Robert D Towler
Chief of Medical Staff. . . . . Michael Anderson
Anesthesiology. . . . . Manhal Saleeby, MD
Emergency Room . . . . Iqbal Singh, MD
Hemotology Center . . . . Mary Hackney, MD

Measure	Cases	This Hosp.	State Avg.	U.S. Avg.
Heart Attack Care				
ACE Inhibitor or ARB for LVSD[1]	8	100%	97%	96%
Aspirin at Arrival	51	96%	99%	99%
Aspirin at Discharge	26	100%	99%	98%
Beta Blocker at Discharge	28	100%	99%	98%
Fibrinolytic Medication Timing	0	-	75%	55%
PCI Within 90 Minutes of Arrival	0	-	93%	90%
Smoking Cessation Advice[1]	7	100%	100%	99%
Chest Pain/Possible Heart Attack Care				
Aspirin at Arrival	44	98%	95%	95%
Median Time to ECG (minutes)	47	5	8	8
Median Time to Transfer (minutes)[1]	7	57	60	61
Fibrinolytic Medication Timing	0	-	59%	54%
Heart Failure Care				
ACE Inhibitor or ARB for LVSD	62	100%	97%	94%
Discharge Instructions	197	96%	92%	88%
Evaluation of LVS Function	219	100%	99%	98%
Smoking Cessation Advice	43	100%	99%	98%
Pneumonia Care				
Appropriate Initial Antibiotic	115	97%	93%	92%
Blood Culture Timing	76	99%	97%	96%
Influenza Vaccine	86	97%	94%	91%
Initial Antibiotic Timing	150	99%	96%	95%
Pneumococcal Vaccine	89	100%	95%	93%
Smoking Cessation Advice	50	100%	98%	97%
Surgical Care Improvement Project				
Appropriate VTP Within 24 Hours[2]	32	97%	94%	92%
Appropriate Hair Removal[2]	48	100%	100%	99%
Appropriate Beta Blocker Usage[1,2]	10	90%	94%	93%
Controlled Postoperative Blood Glucose[2]	0	-	96%	93%
Prophylactic Antibiotic Timing[2]	27	100%	97%	97%
Prophylactic Antibiotic Timing (Outpatient)[1]	7	71%	93%	92%
Prophylactic Antibiotic Selection[2]	27	100%	98%	97%
Prophylactic Antibiotic Select. (Outpatient)[1]	20	100%	96%	94%
Prophylactic Antibiotic Stopped[2]	26	100%	96%	94%
Recommended VTP Ordered[2]	32	100%	96%	94%
Urinary Catheter Removal[1]	15	87%	93%	90%
Children's Asthma Care				
Received Systemic Corticosteroids	-	-	-	100%
Received Home Management Plan	-	-	-	71%
Received Reliever Medication	-	-	-	100%
Use of Medical Imaging				
Combination Abdominal CT Scan	243	0.123	0.144	0.191
Combination Chest CT Scan	129	0.039	0.030	0.054
Follow-up Mammogram/Ultrasound	470	3.4%	7.5%	8.4%
MRI for Low Back Pain[1]	13	30.8%	31.5%	32.7%
Survey of Patients' Hospital Experiences				
Area Around Room 'Always' Quiet at Night	300+	66%	-	58%
Doctors 'Always' Communicated Well	300+	85%	-	80%
Home Recovery Information Given	300+	82%	-	82%
Hospital Given 9 or 10 on 10 Point Scale	300+	62%	-	67%
Meds 'Always' Explained Before Given	300+	61%	-	60%
Nurses 'Always' Communicated Well	300+	73%	-	76%
Pain 'Always' Well Controlled	300+	68%	-	69%
Room and Bathroom 'Always' Clean	300+	63%	-	71%
Timely Help 'Always' Received	300+	59%	-	64%
Would Definitely Recommend Hospital	300+	58%	-	69%

Inova Fair Oaks Hospital

3600 Joseph Siewick Drive Phone: 703-391-3600
Fairfax, VA 22033 Fax: 703-391-3273
URL: www.inova.org/inovapublic.srt/ifoh/index.jsp
Type: Acute Care Hospitals Emergency Services: Yes
Ownership: Voluntary Non-Profit - Other Beds: 160

Key Personnel:
Chief of Medical Staff. . . . . Jay Tyroller, MD
Pediatric Ambulatory Care . . . . . . Alan E Silk, MD
Pediatric In-Patient Care . . . . Alan E Silk, MD
Quality Assurance . . . . Robbin Bixler
Anesthesiology. . . . . Ricky Lee Ramsey, MD
Emergency Room . . . . Ellen Ruja
Intensive Care Unit. . . . . Megan Winegarden

Measure	Cases	This Hosp.	State Avg.	U.S. Avg.
Heart Attack Care				
ACE Inhibitor or ARB for LVSD[1]	5	100%	97%	96%
Aspirin at Arrival	31	97%	99%	99%
Aspirin at Discharge[1]	19	89%	99%	98%
Beta Blocker at Discharge[1]	19	95%	99%	98%
Fibrinolytic Medication Timing	0	-	75%	55%
PCI Within 90 Minutes of Arrival	0	-	93%	90%
Smoking Cessation Advice[1]	3	100%	100%	99%
Chest Pain/Possible Heart Attack Care				
Aspirin at Arrival	123	91%	95%	95%
Median Time to ECG (minutes)	133	10	8	8
Median Time to Transfer (minutes)[1]	20	60	60	61
Fibrinolytic Medication Timing	0	-	59%	54%
Heart Failure Care				
ACE Inhibitor or ARB for LVSD	33	97%	97%	94%
Discharge Instructions	160	89%	92%	88%
Evaluation of LVS Function	187	98%	99%	98%
Smoking Cessation Advice[1]	16	94%	99%	98%
Pneumonia Care				
Appropriate Initial Antibiotic[2]	84	92%	93%	92%
Blood Culture Timing[2]	135	96%	97%	96%
Influenza Vaccine[2]	73	96%	94%	91%
Initial Antibiotic Timing[2]	130	99%	96%	95%
Pneumococcal Vaccine[2]	117	98%	95%	93%
Smoking Cessation Advice[2]	27	81%	98%	97%
Surgical Care Improvement Project				
Appropriate VTP Within 24 Hours[2]	76	96%	94%	92%
Appropriate Hair Removal[2]	337	100%	100%	99%
Appropriate Beta Blocker Usage[2]	89	99%	94%	93%
Controlled Postoperative Blood Glucose[2]	0	-	96%	93%
Prophylactic Antibiotic Timing[2]	226	100%	97%	97%
Prophylactic Antibiotic Timing (Outpatient)	656	99%	93%	92%
Prophylactic Antibiotic Selection[2]	229	99%	98%	97%
Prophylactic Antibiotic Select. (Outpatient)	655	96%	96%	94%
Prophylactic Antibiotic Stopped[2]	219	96%	96%	94%
Recommended VTP Ordered[2]	76	96%	96%	94%
Urinary Catheter Removal[2]	61	100%	93%	90%
Children's Asthma Care				
Received Systemic Corticosteroids	-	-	-	100%
Received Home Management Plan	-	-	-	71%
Received Reliever Medication	-	-	-	100%
Use of Medical Imaging				
Combination Abdominal CT Scan	607	0.054	0.144	0.191
Combination Chest CT Scan	540	0.019	0.030	0.054
Follow-up Mammogram/Ultrasound	356	5.6%	7.5%	8.4%
MRI for Low Back Pain	270	29.6%	31.5%	32.7%
Survey of Patients' Hospital Experiences				
Area Around Room 'Always' Quiet at Night	300+	50%	-	58%
Doctors 'Always' Communicated Well	300+	78%	-	80%
Home Recovery Information Given	300+	82%	-	82%
Hospital Given 9 or 10 on 10 Point Scale	300+	71%	-	67%
Meds 'Always' Explained Before Given	300+	61%	-	60%
Nurses 'Always' Communicated Well	300+	75%	-	76%
Pain 'Always' Well Controlled	300+	68%	-	69%
Room and Bathroom 'Always' Clean	300+	70%	-	71%
Timely Help 'Always' Received	300+	57%	-	64%
Would Definitely Recommend Hospital	300+	78%	-	69%

Inova Fairfax Hospital

3300 Gallows Rd Phone: 703-776-3332
Falls Church, VA 22042 Fax: 703-776-3623
URL: www.inova.org
Type: Acute Care Hospitals Emergency Services: Yes
Ownership: Voluntary Non-Profit - Other Beds: 833

Key Personnel:
CEO/President. . . . . L Reuven Pasternak
Chief of Medical Staff. . . . . F Joseph Hallal
Infection Control. . . . . Allan J Morrison, MD
Quality Assurance . . . . Betty Ann Wilkins
Emergency Room . . . . Robert Cates, MD

Measure	Cases	This Hosp.	State Avg.	U.S. Avg.
Heart Attack Care				
ACE Inhibitor or ARB for LVSD[2]	31	100%	97%	96%
Aspirin at Arrival[2]	150	100%	99%	99%
Aspirin at Discharge[2]	280	99%	99%	98%
Beta Blocker at Discharge[2]	228	99%	99%	98%
Fibrinolytic Medication Timing[2]	0	-	75%	55%
PCI Within 90 Minutes of Arrival[2]	33	100%	93%	90%
Smoking Cessation Advice[2]	63	100%	100%	99%
Chest Pain/Possible Heart Attack Care				
Aspirin at Arrival	207	94%	95%	95%
Median Time to ECG (minutes)	213	6	8	8
Median Time to Transfer (minutes)[1,3]	6	36	60	61
Fibrinolytic Medication Timing	0	-	59%	54%
Heart Failure Care				
ACE Inhibitor or ARB for LVSD[2]	95	92%	97%	94%
Discharge Instructions[2]	238	88%	92%	88%
Evaluation of LVS Function[2]	290	99%	99%	98%
Smoking Cessation Advice[2]	27	100%	99%	98%
Pneumonia Care				
Appropriate Initial Antibiotic[2]	57	89%	93%	92%
Blood Culture Timing[2]	90	99%	97%	96%
Influenza Vaccine[2]	79	87%	94%	91%
Initial Antibiotic Timing[2]	90	99%	96%	95%
Pneumococcal Vaccine[2]	102	92%	95%	93%
Smoking Cessation Advice[2]	27	96%	98%	97%
Surgical Care Improvement Project				
Appropriate VTP Within 24 Hours[2]	184	98%	94%	92%
Appropriate Hair Removal[2]	620	100%	100%	99%
Appropriate Beta Blocker Usage[2]	114	96%	94%	93%
Controlled Postoperative Blood Glucose[2]	114	98%	96%	93%
Prophylactic Antibiotic Timing[2]	415	95%	97%	97%
Prophylactic Antibiotic Timing (Outpatient)	984	94%	93%	92%
Prophylactic Antibiotic Selection[2]	422	97%	98%	97%
Prophylactic Antibiotic Select. (Outpatient)	937	94%	96%	94%
Prophylactic Antibiotic Stopped[2]	407	94%	96%	94%
Recommended VTP Ordered[2]	184	98%	96%	94%
Urinary Catheter Removal[2]	163	93%	93%	90%
Children's Asthma Care				
Received Systemic Corticosteroids[2]	309	100%	-	100%
Received Home Management Plan[2]	310	78%	-	71%
Received Reliever Medication[2]	310	100%	-	100%
Use of Medical Imaging				
Combination Abdominal CT Scan	1,485	0.026	0.144	0.191
Combination Chest CT Scan	1,218	0.011	0.030	0.054
Follow-up Mammogram/Ultrasound	487	8.6%	7.5%	8.4%
MRI for Low Back Pain	147	34.0%	31.5%	32.7%
Survey of Patients' Hospital Experiences				
Area Around Room 'Always' Quiet at Night	300+	49%	-	58%
Doctors 'Always' Communicated Well	300+	76%	-	80%
Home Recovery Information Given	300+	83%	-	82%
Hospital Given 9 or 10 on 10 Point Scale	300+	68%	-	67%
Meds 'Always' Explained Before Given	300+	58%	-	60%
Nurses 'Always' Communicated Well	300+	73%	-	76%
Pain 'Always' Well Controlled	300+	67%	-	69%
Room and Bathroom 'Always' Clean	300+	60%	-	71%
Timely Help 'Always' Received	300+	59%	-	64%
Would Definitely Recommend Hospital	300+	75%	-	69%

NOTE: Hospital profiles are in alphabetical order by state, then city, then hospital within the city; Rankings exclude hospitals with less than 25 cases except for patient surveys which excludes hospitals with less than 100 cases; (a) 100–299 cases; (1) The number of cases is too small to be sure how well a hospital is performing; (2) The hospital indicated that the data submitted for this measure were based on a sample of cases; (3) Data was collected during a shorter time period (fewer quarters) than the maximum possible time for this measure; (4) Suppressed for one or more quarters by CMS; (5) No data is available from the hospital for this measure; (6) Fewer than 100 patients completed the HCAHPS survey. Use these rates with caution, as the number of surveys may be too low to reliably assess hospital performance; (7) Survey results are based on less than 12 months of data; (8) Survey results are not available for this reporting period; (9) No or very few patients were eligible for the HCAHPS survey. The scores shown, if any, reflect a very small number of surveys; (10) A state average was not calculated because too few hospitals in the state submitted data; (11) There were discrepancies in the data collection process; Please refer to the User's Guide for a full explanation of data.

Southside Community Hospital

800 Oak Street
Farmville, VA 23901
E-mail: info@sch-farmville.org
URL: www.sch-farmville.org
Type: Acute Care Hospitals
Ownership: Voluntary Non-Profit - Private

Phone: 434-392-8811
Fax: 434-315-2581

Emergency Services: Yes
Beds: 116

Key Personnel:
CEO/President . . . . Gwen Eddleman, EdD
Chief of Medical Staff . . . . Dr. Charles Anderson
Quality Assurance . . . . Judy Neller
Emergency Room . . . . Kathleen Manis

Measure	Cases	This Hosp.	State Avg.	U.S. Avg.
Heart Attack Care				
ACE Inhibitor or ARB for LVSD[1]	2	100%	97%	96%
Aspirin at Arrival[1]	10	100%	99%	99%
Aspirin at Discharge[1]	7	100%	99%	98%
Beta Blocker at Discharge[1]	8	100%	99%	98%
Fibrinolytic Medication Timing	0	-	75%	55%
PCI Within 90 Minutes of Arrival	0	-	93%	90%
Smoking Cessation Advice[1]	1	100%	100%	99%
Chest Pain/Possible Heart Attack Care				
Aspirin at Arrival	93	89%	95%	95%
Median Time to ECG (minutes)	96	6	8	8
Median Time to Transfer (minutes)[1,3]	3	42	60	61
Fibrinolytic Medication Timing[1]	1	100%	59%	54%
Heart Failure Care				
ACE Inhibitor or ARB for LVSD	58	97%	97%	94%
Discharge Instructions	118	66%	92%	88%
Evaluation of LVS Function	149	97%	99%	98%
Smoking Cessation Advice	32	100%	99%	98%
Pneumonia Care				
Appropriate Initial Antibiotic	91	91%	93%	92%
Blood Culture Timing	123	96%	97%	96%
Influenza Vaccine	69	93%	94%	91%
Initial Antibiotic Timing	127	95%	96%	95%
Pneumococcal Vaccine	103	91%	95%	93%
Smoking Cessation Advice	39	100%	98%	97%
Surgical Care Improvement Project				
Appropriate VTP Within 24 Hours	66	95%	94%	92%
Appropriate Hair Removal	142	99%	100%	99%
Appropriate Beta Blocker Usage	37	70%	94%	93%
Controlled Postoperative Blood Glucose	0	-	96%	93%
Prophylactic Antibiotic Timing	79	89%	97%	97%
Prophylactic Antibiotic Timing (Outpatient)[1]	17	41%	93%	92%
Prophylactic Antibiotic Selection	79	97%	98%	97%
Prophylactic Antibiotic Select. (Outpatient)[1]	7	100%	96%	94%
Prophylactic Antibiotic Stopped	71	90%	96%	94%
Recommended VTP Ordered	67	96%	96%	94%
Urinary Catheter Removal	26	50%	93%	90%
Children's Asthma Care				
Received Systemic Corticosteroids	-	-	-	100%
Received Home Management Plan	-	-	-	71%
Received Reliever Medication	-	-	-	100%
Use of Medical Imaging				
Combination Abdominal CT Scan	399	0.093	0.144	0.191
Combination Chest CT Scan	191	0.288	0.030	0.054
Follow-up Mammogram/Ultrasound	663	5.7%	7.5%	8.4%
MRI for Low Back Pain	63	23.8%	31.5%	32.7%
Survey of Patients' Hospital Experiences				
Area Around Room 'Always' Quiet at Night[11]	300+	58%	-	58%
Doctors 'Always' Communicated Well[11]	300+	79%	-	80%
Home Recovery Information Given[11]	300+	80%	-	82%
Hospital Given 9 or 10 on 10 Point Scale[11]	300+	57%	-	67%
Meds 'Always' Explained Before Given[11]	300+	61%	-	60%
Nurses 'Always' Communicated Well[11]	300+	76%	-	76%
Pain 'Always' Well Controlled[11]	300+	68%	-	69%
Room and Bathroom 'Always' Clean[11]	300+	73%	-	71%
Timely Help 'Always' Received[11]	300+	64%	-	64%
Would Definitely Recommend Hospital[11]	300+	54%	-	69%

Augusta Health

78 Medical Center Drive
Fishersville, VA 22939
URL: www.augustamed.com
Type: Acute Care Hospitals
Ownership: Voluntary Non-Profit - Other

Phone: 540-932-4000
Fax: 540-332-4809

Emergency Services: Yes
Beds: 255

Key Personnel:
CEO/President . . . . Richard Graham
Chief of Medical Staff . . . . Joseph Ranzini
Infection Control . . . . Carolyn Palmer, RN
Pediatric Ambulatory Care . . . . . . Robert Gunther, MD
Pediatric In-Patient Care . . . . Robert Gunther, MD
Radiology . . . . David Tempkin, MD
Anesthesiology . . . . Louis Chaldars, MD
Emergency Room . . . . Sally Tucker, MD

Measure	Cases	This Hosp.	State Avg.	U.S. Avg.
Heart Attack Care				
ACE Inhibitor or ARB for LVSD[1]	21	95%	97%	96%
Aspirin at Arrival	129	100%	99%	99%
Aspirin at Discharge	115	94%	99%	98%
Beta Blocker at Discharge	105	97%	99%	98%
Fibrinolytic Medication Timing	0	-	75%	55%
PCI Within 90 Minutes of Arrival[1]	10	100%	93%	90%
Smoking Cessation Advice	37	100%	100%	99%
Chest Pain/Possible Heart Attack Care				
Aspirin at Arrival	108	99%	95%	95%
Median Time to ECG (minutes)	109	8	8	8
Median Time to Transfer (minutes)	33	74	60	61
Fibrinolytic Medication Timing[1]	3	67%	59%	54%
Heart Failure Care				
ACE Inhibitor or ARB for LVSD	112	96%	97%	94%
Discharge Instructions	260	91%	92%	88%
Evaluation of LVS Function	332	100%	99%	98%
Smoking Cessation Advice	53	100%	99%	98%
Pneumonia Care				
Appropriate Initial Antibiotic	204	94%	93%	92%
Blood Culture Timing	329	96%	97%	96%
Influenza Vaccine	203	94%	94%	91%
Initial Antibiotic Timing	314	96%	96%	95%
Pneumococcal Vaccine	299	96%	95%	93%
Smoking Cessation Advice	105	99%	98%	97%
Surgical Care Improvement Project				
Appropriate VTP Within 24 Hours[2]	227	89%	94%	92%
Appropriate Hair Removal[2]	867	100%	100%	99%
Appropriate Beta Blocker Usage[2]	247	91%	94%	93%
Controlled Postoperative Blood Glucose[2]	0	-	96%	93%
Prophylactic Antibiotic Timing[2]	696	98%	97%	97%
Prophylactic Antibiotic Timing (Outpatient)	216	91%	93%	92%
Prophylactic Antibiotic Selection[2]	697	99%	98%	97%
Prophylactic Antibiotic Select. (Outpatient)	205	96%	96%	94%
Prophylactic Antibiotic Stopped[2]	684	98%	96%	94%
Recommended VTP Ordered[2]	227	92%	96%	94%
Urinary Catheter Removal[2]	42	88%	93%	90%
Children's Asthma Care				
Received Systemic Corticosteroids	-	-	-	100%
Received Home Management Plan	-	-	-	71%
Received Reliever Medication	-	-	-	100%
Use of Medical Imaging				
Combination Abdominal CT Scan	1,673	0.163	0.144	0.191
Combination Chest CT Scan	1,236	0.001	0.030	0.054
Follow-up Mammogram/Ultrasound	2,916	12.5%	7.5%	8.4%
MRI for Low Back Pain	503	34.6%	31.5%	32.7%
Survey of Patients' Hospital Experiences				
Area Around Room 'Always' Quiet at Night	300+	51%	-	58%
Doctors 'Always' Communicated Well	300+	81%	-	80%
Home Recovery Information Given	300+	85%	-	82%
Hospital Given 9 or 10 on 10 Point Scale	300+	63%	-	67%
Meds 'Always' Explained Before Given	300+	61%	-	60%
Nurses 'Always' Communicated Well	300+	74%	-	76%
Pain 'Always' Well Controlled	300+	69%	-	69%
Room and Bathroom 'Always' Clean	300+	73%	-	71%
Timely Help 'Always' Received	300+	66%	-	64%
Would Definitely Recommend Hospital	300+	71%	-	69%

Southampton Memorial Hospital

100 Fairview Drive
Franklin, VA 23851
URL: www.smhfranklin.com
Type: Acute Care Hospitals
Ownership: Proprietary

Phone: 757-569-6100
Fax: 757-569-6390

Emergency Services: Yes
Beds: 221

Key Personnel:
CEO/President . . . . Gwen Eddleman
Chief of Medical Staff . . . . Rich Holm, MD
Operating Room . . . . Gregory Johnson
Pediatric Ambulatory Care . . . . . . Mike Cicero
Pediatric In-Patient Care . . . . Mike Cicero
Quality Assurance . . . . Margie Wilson
Emergency Room . . . . David Sields, RN

Measure	Cases	This Hosp.	State Avg.	U.S. Avg.
Heart Attack Care				
ACE Inhibitor or ARB for LVSD[1]	5	80%	97%	96%
Aspirin at Arrival[1]	12	100%	99%	99%
Aspirin at Discharge[1]	7	86%	99%	98%
Beta Blocker at Discharge[1]	7	100%	99%	98%
Fibrinolytic Medication Timing	0	-	75%	55%
PCI Within 90 Minutes of Arrival	0	-	93%	90%
Smoking Cessation Advice[1]	1	100%	100%	99%
Chest Pain/Possible Heart Attack Care				
Aspirin at Arrival	55	95%	95%	95%
Median Time to ECG (minutes)	55	3	8	8
Median Time to Transfer (minutes)[1,3]	8	155	60	61
Fibrinolytic Medication Timing	0	-	59%	54%
Heart Failure Care				
ACE Inhibitor or ARB for LVSD	61	98%	97%	94%
Discharge Instructions	108	88%	92%	88%
Evaluation of LVS Function	133	99%	99%	98%
Smoking Cessation Advice	28	100%	99%	98%
Pneumonia Care				
Appropriate Initial Antibiotic	56	84%	93%	92%
Blood Culture Timing	83	96%	97%	96%
Influenza Vaccine	63	94%	94%	91%
Initial Antibiotic Timing	84	96%	96%	95%
Pneumococcal Vaccine	98	96%	95%	93%
Smoking Cessation Advice	34	100%	98%	97%
Surgical Care Improvement Project				
Appropriate VTP Within 24 Hours[2]	36	89%	94%	92%
Appropriate Hair Removal[2]	126	100%	100%	99%
Appropriate Beta Blocker Usage[2]	27	100%	94%	93%
Controlled Postoperative Blood Glucose[2]	0	-	96%	93%
Prophylactic Antibiotic Timing[2]	101	100%	97%	97%
Prophylactic Antibiotic Timing (Outpatient)	43	65%	93%	92%
Prophylactic Antibiotic Selection[2]	101	97%	98%	97%
Prophylactic Antibiotic Select. (Outpatient)	59	97%	96%	94%
Prophylactic Antibiotic Stopped[2]	95	98%	96%	94%
Recommended VTP Ordered[2]	36	97%	96%	94%
Urinary Catheter Removal[1]	7	100%	93%	90%
Children's Asthma Care				
Received Systemic Corticosteroids	-	-	-	100%
Received Home Management Plan	-	-	-	71%
Received Reliever Medication	-	-	-	100%
Use of Medical Imaging				
Combination Abdominal CT Scan	347	0.352	0.144	0.191
Combination Chest CT Scan	183	0.098	0.030	0.054
Follow-up Mammogram/Ultrasound	427	4.9%	7.5%	8.4%
MRI for Low Back Pain[1]	29	55.2%	31.5%	32.7%
Survey of Patients' Hospital Experiences				
Area Around Room 'Always' Quiet at Night	300+	65%	-	58%
Doctors 'Always' Communicated Well	300+	82%	-	80%
Home Recovery Information Given	300+	84%	-	82%
Hospital Given 9 or 10 on 10 Point Scale	300+	65%	-	67%
Meds 'Always' Explained Before Given	300+	60%	-	60%
Nurses 'Always' Communicated Well	300+	78%	-	76%
Pain 'Always' Well Controlled	300+	70%	-	69%
Room and Bathroom 'Always' Clean	300+	74%	-	71%
Timely Help 'Always' Received	300+	63%	-	64%
Would Definitely Recommend Hospital	300+	57%	-	69%

NOTE: Hospital profiles are in alphabetical order by state, then city, then hospital within the city; Rankings exclude hospitals with less than 25 cases except for patient surveys which excludes hospitals with less than 100 cases; (a) 100–299 cases; (1) The number of cases is too small to be sure how well a hospital is performing; (2) The hospital indicated that the data submitted for this measure were based on a sample of cases; (3) Data was collected during a shorter time period (fewer quarters) than the maximum possible time for this measure; (4) Suppressed for one or more quarters by CMS; (5) No data is available from the hospital for this measure; (6) Fewer than 100 patients completed the HCAHPS survey. Use these rates with caution, as the number of surveys may be too low to reliably assess hospital performance; (7) Survey results are based on less than 12 months of data; (8) Survey results are not available for this reporting period; (9) No or very few patients were eligible for the HCAHPS survey. The scores shown, if any, reflect a very small number of surveys; (10) A state average was not calculated because too few hospitals in the state submitted data; (11) There were discrepancies in the data collection process; Please refer to the User's Guide for a full explanation of data.

Mary Washington Hospital

1001 Sam Perry Boulevard
Fredericksburg, VA 22401
URL: www.medicorp.org
Type: Acute Care Hospitals
Ownership: Voluntary Non-Profit - Private

Phone: 540-741-1100
Fax: 540-741-2571

Emergency Services: Yes
Beds: 412

Key Personnel:

CEO/President	Fred Rankin
Chief of Medical Staff	Daniel Hoffman, MD
Infection Control	Norman Bernstein, MD
Operating Room	Elyse Dorman
Pediatric Ambulatory Care	Claudia Sussdorf
Pediatric In-Patient Care	Claudia Sussdorf
Quality Assurance	Linda Wallace
Radiology	Michael Hewitt

Measure	Cases	This Hosp.	State Avg.	U.S. Avg.
Heart Attack Care				
ACE Inhibitor or ARB for LVSD	75	99%	97%	96%
Aspirin at Arrival	473	100%	99%	99%
Aspirin at Discharge	515	98%	99%	98%
Beta Blocker at Discharge	495	99%	99%	98%
Fibrinolytic Medication Timing	0	-	75%	55%
PCI Within 90 Minutes of Arrival	55	96%	93%	90%
Smoking Cessation Advice	197	100%	100%	99%
Chest Pain/Possible Heart Attack Care				
Aspirin at Arrival	39	100%	95%	95%
Median Time to ECG (minutes)	40	12	8	8
Median Time to Transfer (minutes)[5]	0	-	60	61
Fibrinolytic Medication Timing[5]	0	-	59%	54%
Heart Failure Care				
ACE Inhibitor or ARB for LVSD[2]	176	100%	97%	94%
Discharge Instructions[2]	560	89%	92%	88%
Evaluation of LVS Function[2]	669	100%	99%	98%
Smoking Cessation Advice[2]	126	100%	99%	98%
Pneumonia Care				
Appropriate Initial Antibiotic[2]	275	95%	93%	92%
Blood Culture Timing[2]	401	96%	97%	96%
Influenza Vaccine[2]	211	90%	94%	91%
Initial Antibiotic Timing[2]	372	97%	96%	95%
Pneumococcal Vaccine[2]	325	94%	95%	93%
Smoking Cessation Advice[2]	150	100%	98%	97%
Surgical Care Improvement Project				
Appropriate VTP Within 24 Hours[2]	249	90%	94%	92%
Appropriate Hair Removal[2]	1,000	100%	100%	99%
Appropriate Beta Blocker Usage[2]	318	92%	94%	93%
Controlled Postoperative Blood Glucose[2]	188	91%	96%	93%
Prophylactic Antibiotic Timing[2]	664	94%	97%	97%
Prophylactic Antibiotic Timing (Outpatient)	588	96%	93%	92%
Prophylactic Antibiotic Selection[2]	673	99%	98%	97%
Prophylactic Antibiotic Select. (Outpatient)	583	97%	96%	94%
Prophylactic Antibiotic Stopped[2]	630	95%	96%	94%
Recommended VTP Ordered[2]	249	95%	96%	94%
Urinary Catheter Removal[2]	185	92%	93%	90%
Children's Asthma Care				
Received Systemic Corticosteroids	47	100%	-	100%
Received Home Management Plan	45	76%	-	71%
Received Reliever Medication	47	100%	-	100%
Use of Medical Imaging				
Combination Abdominal CT Scan	602	0.013	0.144	0.191
Combination Chest CT Scan	109	0.009	0.030	0.054
Follow-up Mammogram/Ultrasound	228	15.4%	7.5%	8.4%
MRI for Low Back Pain[1]	30	33.3%	31.5%	32.7%
Survey of Patients' Hospital Experiences				
Area Around Room 'Always' Quiet at Night	300+	51%	-	58%
Doctors 'Always' Communicated Well	300+	74%	-	80%
Home Recovery Information Given	300+	79%	-	82%
Hospital Given 9 or 10 on 10 Point Scale	300+	58%	-	67%
Meds 'Always' Explained Before Given	300+	54%	-	60%
Nurses 'Always' Communicated Well	300+	70%	-	76%
Pain 'Always' Well Controlled	300+	65%	-	69%
Room and Bathroom 'Always' Clean	300+	60%	-	71%
Timely Help 'Always' Received	300+	55%	-	64%
Would Definitely Recommend Hospital	300+	61%	-	69%

Spotsylvania Regional Medical Center

4600 Spotsylvania Parkway
Fredericksburg, VA 22408
URL: www.spotsrmc.com
Type: Acute Care Hospitals
Ownership: Proprietary

Phone: 540-834-1500

Emergency Services: No

Key Personnel:

CEO	Tim Tobin

Measure	Cases	This Hosp.	State Avg.	U.S. Avg.
Heart Attack Care				
ACE Inhibitor or ARB for LVSD[5]	0	-	97%	96%
Aspirin at Arrival[5]	0	-	99%	99%
Aspirin at Discharge[5]	0	-	99%	98%
Beta Blocker at Discharge[5]	0	-	99%	98%
Fibrinolytic Medication Timing[5]	0	-	75%	55%
PCI Within 90 Minutes of Arrival[5]	0	-	93%	90%
Smoking Cessation Advice[5]	0	-	100%	99%
Chest Pain/Possible Heart Attack Care				
Aspirin at Arrival	0	-	95%	95%
Median Time to ECG (minutes)	0	-	8	8
Median Time to Transfer (minutes)	0	-	60	61
Fibrinolytic Medication Timing	0	-	59%	54%
Heart Failure Care				
ACE Inhibitor or ARB for LVSD[5]	0	-	97%	94%
Discharge Instructions[5]	0	-	92%	88%
Evaluation of LVS Function[5]	0	-	99%	98%
Smoking Cessation Advice[5]	0	-	99%	98%
Pneumonia Care				
Appropriate Initial Antibiotic[5]	0	-	93%	92%
Blood Culture Timing[5]	0	-	97%	96%
Influenza Vaccine[5]	0	-	94%	91%
Initial Antibiotic Timing[5]	0	-	96%	95%
Pneumococcal Vaccine[5]	0	-	95%	93%
Smoking Cessation Advice[5]	0	-	98%	97%
Surgical Care Improvement Project				
Appropriate VTP Within 24 Hours[5]	0	-	94%	92%
Appropriate Hair Removal[5]	0	-	100%	99%
Appropriate Beta Blocker Usage[5]	0	-	94%	93%
Controlled Postoperative Blood Glucose[5]	0	-	96%	93%
Prophylactic Antibiotic Timing[5]	0	-	97%	97%
Prophylactic Antibiotic Timing (Outpatient)	-	-	93%	92%
Prophylactic Antibiotic Selection[5]	0	-	98%	97%
Prophylactic Antibiotic Select. (Outpatient)	-	-	96%	94%
Prophylactic Antibiotic Stopped[5]	0	-	96%	94%
Recommended VTP Ordered[5]	0	-	96%	94%
Urinary Catheter Removal[5]	0	-	93%	90%
Children's Asthma Care				
Received Systemic Corticosteroids	-	-	-	100%
Received Home Management Plan	-	-	-	71%
Received Reliever Medication	-	-	-	100%
Use of Medical Imaging				
Combination Abdominal CT Scan	-	-	0.144	0.191
Combination Chest CT Scan	-	-	0.030	0.054
Follow-up Mammogram/Ultrasound	-	-	7.5%	8.4%
MRI for Low Back Pain	-	-	31.5%	32.7%
Survey of Patients' Hospital Experiences				
Area Around Room 'Always' Quiet at Night[8]	-	-	-	58%
Doctors 'Always' Communicated Well[8]	-	-	-	80%
Home Recovery Information Given[8]	-	-	-	82%
Hospital Given 9 or 10 on 10 Point Scale[8]	-	-	-	67%
Meds 'Always' Explained Before Given[8]	-	-	-	60%
Nurses 'Always' Communicated Well[8]	-	-	-	76%
Pain 'Always' Well Controlled[8]	-	-	-	69%
Room and Bathroom 'Always' Clean[8]	-	-	-	71%
Timely Help 'Always' Received[8]	-	-	-	64%
Would Definitely Recommend Hospital[8]	-	-	-	69%

Warren Memorial Hospital

1000 North Shenandoah Ave
Front Royal, VA 22630
URL: www.valleyhealthlink.com
Type: Acute Care Hospitals
Ownership: Voluntary Non-Profit - Other

Phone: 703-636-0300
Fax: 540-636-0258

Emergency Services: Yes
Beds: 196

Key Personnel:

CEO/President	Patrick B Nolan
Chief of Medical Staff	Floyd Bradd, III, MD
Infection Control	Trudi Riley, RN
Operating Room	Ronnie Duckworth, RN
Quality Assurance	Heather Silvious
Radiology	Namik Erdag
Intensive Care Unit	Susan Hawkins, RN
Patient Relations	Phyllis Himelright

Measure	Cases	This Hosp.	State Avg.	U.S. Avg.
Heart Attack Care				
ACE Inhibitor or ARB for LVSD	0	-	97%	96%
Aspirin at Arrival[1]	8	100%	99%	99%
Aspirin at Discharge[1]	4	75%	99%	98%
Beta Blocker at Discharge[1]	5	100%	99%	98%
Fibrinolytic Medication Timing	0	-	75%	55%
PCI Within 90 Minutes of Arrival	0	-	93%	90%
Smoking Cessation Advice[1]	1	100%	100%	99%
Chest Pain/Possible Heart Attack Care				
Aspirin at Arrival	33	100%	95%	95%
Median Time to ECG (minutes)	33	10	8	8
Median Time to Transfer (minutes)[5]	0	-	60	61
Fibrinolytic Medication Timing	0	-	59%	54%
Heart Failure Care				
ACE Inhibitor or ARB for LVSD[1]	23	91%	97%	94%
Discharge Instructions	47	83%	92%	88%
Evaluation of LVS Function	55	100%	99%	98%
Smoking Cessation Advice[1]	8	100%	99%	98%
Pneumonia Care				
Appropriate Initial Antibiotic	49	94%	93%	92%
Blood Culture Timing	63	95%	97%	96%
Influenza Vaccine	35	100%	94%	91%
Initial Antibiotic Timing	63	95%	96%	95%
Pneumococcal Vaccine	52	96%	95%	93%
Smoking Cessation Advice[1]	24	100%	98%	97%
Surgical Care Improvement Project				
Appropriate VTP Within 24 Hours	46	96%	94%	92%
Appropriate Hair Removal	92	99%	100%	99%
Appropriate Beta Blocker Usage[1]	21	100%	94%	93%
Controlled Postoperative Blood Glucose	0	-	96%	93%
Prophylactic Antibiotic Timing	55	100%	97%	97%
Prophylactic Antibiotic Timing (Outpatient)	35	89%	93%	92%
Prophylactic Antibiotic Selection	56	96%	98%	97%
Prophylactic Antibiotic Select. (Outpatient)	35	94%	96%	94%
Prophylactic Antibiotic Stopped	49	98%	96%	94%
Recommended VTP Ordered	46	98%	96%	94%
Urinary Catheter Removal[1]	5	100%	93%	90%
Children's Asthma Care				
Received Systemic Corticosteroids	-	-	-	100%
Received Home Management Plan	-	-	-	71%
Received Reliever Medication	-	-	-	100%
Use of Medical Imaging				
Combination Abdominal CT Scan	290	0.010	0.144	0.191
Combination Chest CT Scan	250	0.008	0.030	0.054
Follow-up Mammogram/Ultrasound	407	12.5%	7.5%	8.4%
MRI for Low Back Pain[1]	38	15.8%	31.5%	32.7%
Survey of Patients' Hospital Experiences				
Area Around Room 'Always' Quiet at Night	300+	55%	-	58%
Doctors 'Always' Communicated Well	300+	77%	-	80%
Home Recovery Information Given	300+	82%	-	82%
Hospital Given 9 or 10 on 10 Point Scale	300+	55%	-	67%
Meds 'Always' Explained Before Given	300+	54%	-	60%
Nurses 'Always' Communicated Well	300+	72%	-	76%
Pain 'Always' Well Controlled	300+	63%	-	69%
Room and Bathroom 'Always' Clean	300+	66%	-	71%
Timely Help 'Always' Received	300+	59%	-	64%
Would Definitely Recommend Hospital	300+	57%	-	69%

NOTE: Hospital profiles are in alphabetical order by state, then city, then hospital within the city; Rankings exclude hospitals with less than 25 cases except for patient surveys which excludes hospitals with less than 100 cases; (a) 100–299 cases; (1) The number of cases is too small to be sure how well a hospital is performing; (2) The hospital indicated that the data submitted for this measure were based on a sample of cases; (3) Data was collected during a shorter time period (fewer quarters) than the maximum possible time for this measure; (4) Suppressed for one or more quarters by CMS; (5) No data is available from the hospital for this measure; (6) Fewer than 100 patients completed the HCAHPS survey. Use these results with caution, as the number of surveys may be too low to reliably assess hospital performance; (7) Survey results are based on less than 12 months of data; (8) Survey results are not available for this reporting period; (9) No or very few patients were eligible for the HCAHPS survey. The scores shown, if any, reflect a very small number of surveys; (10) A state average was not calculated because too few hospitals in the state submitted data; (11) There were discrepancies in the data collection process; Please refer to the User's Guide for a full explanation of data.

Twin County Regional Hospital

200 Hospital Drive
Galax, VA 24333
Phone: 276-236-8181
Fax: 276-236-1718
E-mail: ppeterson@tcrh.hbocvan.com
URL: www.tcrh.org
Type: Acute Care Hospitals
Emergency Services: No
Ownership: Voluntary Non-Profit - Private
Beds: 141

Key Personnel:
CEO/President. . . . . Marcus Kuhn
Chief of Medical Staff. . . . . Julie Williams
Infection Control. . . . . Julia Banks
Operating Room. . . . . Shelby Luper, RN
Quality Assurance . . . . Michele Bobbitt
Radiology. . . . . John W Bolen Jr, MD
Anesthesiology. . . . . James Griffeth, MD
Emergency Room . . . . Scott Wright, MD

Measure	Cases	This Hosp.	State Avg.	U.S. Avg.
Heart Attack Care				
ACE Inhibitor or ARB for LVSD	0	-	97%	96%
Aspirin at Arrival[1]	14	93%	99%	99%
Aspirin at Discharge[1]	7	100%	99%	98%
Beta Blocker at Discharge[1]	10	100%	99%	98%
Fibrinolytic Medication Timing	0	-	75%	55%
PCI Within 90 Minutes of Arrival	0	-	93%	90%
Smoking Cessation Advice[1]	1	100%	100%	99%
Chest Pain/Possible Heart Attack Care				
Aspirin at Arrival	104	98%	95%	95%
Median Time to ECG (minutes)	117	9	8	8
Median Time to Transfer (minutes)[1]	4	190	60	61
Fibrinolytic Medication Timing[1]	14	64%	59%	54%
Heart Failure Care				
ACE Inhibitor or ARB for LVSD	37	100%	97%	94%
Discharge Instructions	88	97%	92%	88%
Evaluation of LVS Function	122	100%	99%	98%
Smoking Cessation Advice[1]	15	100%	99%	98%
Pneumonia Care				
Appropriate Initial Antibiotic	118	99%	93%	92%
Blood Culture Timing	221	100%	97%	96%
Influenza Vaccine	125	100%	94%	91%
Initial Antibiotic Timing	190	99%	96%	95%
Pneumococcal Vaccine	198	99%	95%	93%
Smoking Cessation Advice	61	100%	98%	97%
Surgical Care Improvement Project				
Appropriate VTP Within 24 Hours	90	98%	94%	92%
Appropriate Hair Removal	173	100%	100%	99%
Appropriate Beta Blocker Usage	34	100%	94%	93%
Controlled Postoperative Blood Glucose	0	-	96%	93%
Prophylactic Antibiotic Timing	100	100%	97%	97%
Prophylactic Antibiotic Timing (Outpatient)[1]	20	90%	93%	92%
Prophylactic Antibiotic Selection	105	98%	98%	97%
Prophylactic Antibiotic Select. (Outpatient)[1]	18	100%	96%	94%
Prophylactic Antibiotic Stopped	86	98%	96%	94%
Recommended VTP Ordered	90	99%	96%	94%
Urinary Catheter Removal[1]	24	100%	93%	90%
Children's Asthma Care				
Received Systemic Corticosteroids	-	-	-	100%
Received Home Management Plan	-	-	-	71%
Received Reliever Medication	-	-	-	100%
Use of Medical Imaging				
Combination Abdominal CT Scan	776	0.530	0.144	0.191
Combination Chest CT Scan	244	0.020	0.030	0.054
Follow-up Mammogram/Ultrasound	1,485	4.0%	7.5%	8.4%
MRI for Low Back Pain	147	43.5%	31.5%	32.7%
Survey of Patients' Hospital Experiences				
Area Around Room 'Always' Quiet at Night	300+	59%	-	58%
Doctors 'Always' Communicated Well	300+	82%	-	80%
Home Recovery Information Given	300+	80%	-	82%
Hospital Given 9 or 10 on 10 Point Scale	300+	67%	-	67%
Meds 'Always' Explained Before Given	300+	59%	-	60%
Nurses 'Always' Communicated Well	300+	79%	-	76%
Pain 'Always' Well Controlled	300+	73%	-	69%
Room and Bathroom 'Always' Clean	300+	82%	-	71%
Timely Help 'Always' Received	300+	73%	-	64%
Would Definitely Recommend Hospital	300+	66%	-	69%

Riverside Walter Reed Hospital

7519 Hospital Road
Gloucester, VA 23061
Phone: 804-693-8800
Fax: 804-693-8812
URL: www.riverside-online.com
Type: Acute Care Hospitals
Emergency Services: Yes
Ownership: Voluntary Non-Profit - Private
Beds: 67

Key Personnel:
CEO/President. . . . . Richard Pearce
Chief of Medical Staff . . . . Robert Cross, MD
Quality Assurance . . . . David Tate
Emergency Room . . . . Susan Frishkorn, RN

Measure	Cases	This Hosp.	State Avg.	U.S. Avg.
Heart Attack Care				
ACE Inhibitor or ARB for LVSD[1]	3	100%	97%	96%
Aspirin at Arrival	39	97%	99%	99%
Aspirin at Discharge[1]	14	93%	99%	98%
Beta Blocker at Discharge[1]	16	88%	99%	98%
Fibrinolytic Medication Timing	0	-	75%	55%
PCI Within 90 Minutes of Arrival	0	-	93%	90%
Smoking Cessation Advice[1]	2	100%	100%	99%
Chest Pain/Possible Heart Attack Care				
Aspirin at Arrival	48	94%	95%	95%
Median Time to ECG (minutes)	51	0	8	8
Median Time to Transfer (minutes)[1,3]	13	92	60	61
Fibrinolytic Medication Timing	0	-	59%	54%
Heart Failure Care				
ACE Inhibitor or ARB for LVSD	41	95%	97%	94%
Discharge Instructions	91	96%	92%	88%
Evaluation of LVS Function	128	100%	99%	98%
Smoking Cessation Advice[1]	15	100%	99%	98%
Pneumonia Care				
Appropriate Initial Antibiotic	121	97%	93%	92%
Blood Culture Timing	195	99%	97%	96%
Influenza Vaccine	108	100%	94%	91%
Initial Antibiotic Timing	179	98%	96%	95%
Pneumococcal Vaccine	148	99%	95%	93%
Smoking Cessation Advice	52	100%	98%	97%
Surgical Care Improvement Project				
Appropriate VTP Within 24 Hours	78	97%	94%	92%
Appropriate Hair Removal	187	100%	100%	99%
Appropriate Beta Blocker Usage	55	89%	94%	93%
Controlled Postoperative Blood Glucose	0	-	96%	93%
Prophylactic Antibiotic Timing	134	99%	97%	97%
Prophylactic Antibiotic Timing (Outpatient)	35	83%	93%	92%
Prophylactic Antibiotic Selection	134	99%	98%	97%
Prophylactic Antibiotic Select. (Outpatient)	33	97%	96%	94%
Prophylactic Antibiotic Stopped	125	98%	96%	94%
Recommended VTP Ordered	79	97%	96%	94%
Urinary Catheter Removal	69	100%	93%	90%
Children's Asthma Care				
Received Systemic Corticosteroids	-	-	-	100%
Received Home Management Plan	-	-	-	71%
Received Reliever Medication	-	-	-	100%
Use of Medical Imaging				
Combination Abdominal CT Scan	570	0.086	0.144	0.191
Combination Chest CT Scan	454	0.004	0.030	0.054
Follow-up Mammogram/Ultrasound	1,037	5.3%	7.5%	8.4%
MRI for Low Back Pain	145	33.8%	31.5%	32.7%
Survey of Patients' Hospital Experiences				
Area Around Room 'Always' Quiet at Night	300+	54%	-	58%
Doctors 'Always' Communicated Well	300+	81%	-	80%
Home Recovery Information Given	300+	80%	-	82%
Hospital Given 9 or 10 on 10 Point Scale	300+	59%	-	67%
Meds 'Always' Explained Before Given	300+	54%	-	60%
Nurses 'Always' Communicated Well	300+	74%	-	76%
Pain 'Always' Well Controlled	300+	66%	-	69%
Room and Bathroom 'Always' Clean	300+	73%	-	71%
Timely Help 'Always' Received	300+	65%	-	64%
Would Definitely Recommend Hospital	300+	60%	-	69%

Buchanan General Hospital

1535 Slate Creek Road
Grundy, VA 24614
Phone: 276-935-1000
Fax: 276-935-1469
E-mail: roger.cooper@bgh.org
URL: www.bgh.org
Type: Acute Care Hospitals
Emergency Services: Yes
Ownership: Voluntary Non-Profit - Other
Beds: 134

Key Personnel:
CEO/President. . . . . Roger Cooper
Chief of Medical Staff. . . . . JG Patel
Radiology. . . . . Dilip R Patel
Emergency Room . . . . Dwight Bagano

Measure	Cases	This Hosp.	State Avg.	U.S. Avg.
Heart Attack Care				
ACE Inhibitor or ARB for LVSD	0	-	97%	96%
Aspirin at Arrival[1]	17	94%	99%	99%
Aspirin at Discharge[1]	11	91%	99%	98%
Beta Blocker at Discharge[1]	11	91%	99%	98%
Fibrinolytic Medication Timing	0	-	75%	55%
PCI Within 90 Minutes of Arrival	0	-	93%	90%
Smoking Cessation Advice[1]	1	100%	100%	99%
Chest Pain/Possible Heart Attack Care				
Aspirin at Arrival	61	100%	95%	95%
Median Time to ECG (minutes)	62	7	8	8
Median Time to Transfer (minutes)[5]	0	-	60	61
Fibrinolytic Medication Timing[1]	1	100%	59%	54%
Heart Failure Care				
ACE Inhibitor or ARB for LVSD[1]	20	90%	97%	94%
Discharge Instructions	76	96%	92%	88%
Evaluation of LVS Function	84	100%	99%	98%
Smoking Cessation Advice[1]	5	100%	99%	98%
Pneumonia Care				
Appropriate Initial Antibiotic	63	94%	93%	92%
Blood Culture Timing	86	99%	97%	96%
Influenza Vaccine	61	97%	94%	91%
Initial Antibiotic Timing	100	98%	96%	95%
Pneumococcal Vaccine	74	100%	95%	93%
Smoking Cessation Advice	41	100%	98%	97%
Surgical Care Improvement Project				
Appropriate VTP Within 24 Hours[1]	24	54%	94%	92%
Appropriate Hair Removal	34	100%	100%	99%
Appropriate Beta Blocker Usage[1]	6	83%	94%	93%
Controlled Postoperative Blood Glucose	0	-	96%	93%
Prophylactic Antibiotic Timing[1]	8	100%	97%	97%
Prophylactic Antibiotic Timing (Outpatient)[5]	0	-	93%	92%
Prophylactic Antibiotic Selection[1]	8	100%	98%	97%
Prophylactic Antibiotic Select. (Outpatient)[5]	0	-	96%	94%
Prophylactic Antibiotic Stopped[1]	7	71%	96%	94%
Recommended VTP Ordered[1]	24	54%	96%	94%
Urinary Catheter Removal[1]	7	100%	93%	90%
Children's Asthma Care				
Received Systemic Corticosteroids	-	-	-	100%
Received Home Management Plan	-	-	-	71%
Received Reliever Medication	-	-	-	100%
Use of Medical Imaging				
Combination Abdominal CT Scan	278	0.097	0.144	0.191
Combination Chest CT Scan	181	0.155	0.030	0.054
Follow-up Mammogram/Ultrasound	246	17.9%	7.5%	8.4%
MRI for Low Back Pain	79	41.8%	31.5%	32.7%
Survey of Patients' Hospital Experiences				
Area Around Room 'Always' Quiet at Night	300+	61%	-	58%
Doctors 'Always' Communicated Well	300+	86%	-	80%
Home Recovery Information Given	300+	76%	-	82%
Hospital Given 9 or 10 on 10 Point Scale	300+	64%	-	67%
Meds 'Always' Explained Before Given	300+	63%	-	60%
Nurses 'Always' Communicated Well	300+	78%	-	76%
Pain 'Always' Well Controlled	300+	68%	-	69%
Room and Bathroom 'Always' Clean	300+	72%	-	71%
Timely Help 'Always' Received	300+	67%	-	64%
Would Definitely Recommend Hospital	300+	64%	-	69%

NOTE: Hospital profiles are in alphabetical order by state, then city, then hospital within the city; Rankings exclude hospitals with less than 25 cases except for patient surveys which excludes hospitals with less than 100 cases; (a) 100–299 cases; (1) The number of cases is too small to be sure how well a hospital is performing; (2) The hospital indicated that the data submitted for this measure were based on a sample of cases; (3) Data was collected during a shorter time period (fewer quarters) than the maximum possible time for this measure; (4) Suppressed for one or more quarters by CMS; (5) No data is available from the hospital for this measure; (6) Fewer than 100 patients completed the HCAHPS survey. Use these rates with caution, as the number of surveys may be too low to reliably assess hospital performance; (7) Survey results are based on less than 12 months of data; (8) Survey results are not available for this reporting period; (9) No or very few patients were eligible for the HCAHPS survey. The scores shown, if any, reflect a very small number of surveys; (10) A state average was not calculated because too few hospitals in the state submitted data; (11) There were discrepancies in the data collection process; Please refer to the User's Guide for a full explanation of data.

Halifax Regional Hospital

2204 Wilborn Avenue Phone: 434-517-3100
Halifax, VA 24558
Type: Acute Care Hospitals Emergency Services: Yes
Ownership: Voluntary Non-Profit - Other

Measure	Cases	This Hosp.	State Avg.	U.S. Avg.
Heart Attack Care				
ACE Inhibitor or ARB for LVSD[1]	7	100%	97%	96%
Aspirin at Arrival	58	100%	99%	99%
Aspirin at Discharge	41	100%	99%	98%
Beta Blocker at Discharge	39	100%	99%	98%
Fibrinolytic Medication Timing	0	-	75%	55%
PCI Within 90 Minutes of Arrival	0	-	93%	90%
Smoking Cessation Advice[1]	11	100%	100%	99%
Chest Pain/Possible Heart Attack Care				
Aspirin at Arrival	34	91%	95%	95%
Median Time to ECG (minutes)	35	4	8	8
Median Time to Transfer (minutes)[1,3]	1	69	60	61
Fibrinolytic Medication Timing[1]	6	100%	59%	54%
Heart Failure Care				
ACE Inhibitor or ARB for LVSD	57	98%	97%	94%
Discharge Instructions	178	94%	92%	88%
Evaluation of LVS Function	205	100%	99%	98%
Smoking Cessation Advice	42	98%	99%	98%
Pneumonia Care				
Appropriate Initial Antibiotic	69	97%	93%	92%
Blood Culture Timing	89	97%	97%	96%
Influenza Vaccine	112	69%	94%	91%
Initial Antibiotic Timing	126	88%	96%	95%
Pneumococcal Vaccine	140	83%	95%	93%
Smoking Cessation Advice	64	94%	98%	97%
Surgical Care Improvement Project				
Appropriate VTP Within 24 Hours	120	71%	94%	92%
Appropriate Hair Removal	275	97%	100%	99%
Appropriate Beta Blocker Usage	96	96%	94%	93%
Controlled Postoperative Blood Glucose	0	-	96%	93%
Prophylactic Antibiotic Timing	186	90%	97%	97%
Prophylactic Antibiotic Timing (Outpatient)	93	94%	93%	92%
Prophylactic Antibiotic Selection	181	96%	98%	97%
Prophylactic Antibiotic Select. (Outpatient)	89	99%	96%	94%
Prophylactic Antibiotic Stopped	171	89%	96%	94%
Recommended VTP Ordered	124	75%	96%	94%
Urinary Catheter Removal	38	55%	93%	90%
Children's Asthma Care				
Received Systemic Corticosteroids	-	-	-	100%
Received Home Management Plan	-	-	-	71%
Received Reliever Medication	-	-	-	100%
Use of Medical Imaging				
Combination Abdominal CT Scan	574	0.371	0.144	0.191
Combination Chest CT Scan	374	0.011	0.030	0.054
Follow-up Mammogram/Ultrasound	1,288	10.4%	7.5%	8.4%
MRI for Low Back Pain	128	30.5%	31.5%	32.7%
Survey of Patients' Hospital Experiences				
Area Around Room 'Always' Quiet at Night	300+	65%	-	58%
Doctors 'Always' Communicated Well	300+	85%	-	80%
Home Recovery Information Given	300+	85%	-	82%
Hospital Given 9 or 10 on 10 Point Scale	300+	67%	-	67%
Meds 'Always' Explained Before Given	300+	57%	-	60%
Nurses 'Always' Communicated Well	300+	78%	-	76%
Pain 'Always' Well Controlled	300+	70%	-	69%
Room and Bathroom 'Always' Clean	300+	68%	-	71%
Timely Help 'Always' Received	300+	67%	-	64%
Would Definitely Recommend Hospital	300+	64%	-	69%

Hampton VA Medical Center

100 Emancipation Drive Phone: 757-722-9961
Hampton, VA 23667 Fax: 757-728-7000
E-mail: Sheila.Bailey@va.gov
URL: www.va.gov
Type: Acute Care-Veterans Administration Emergency Services: No
Ownership: Government - Federal Beds: 516

Key Personnel:
CEO/President. . . . . Wanda Mims, MBA
Chief of Medical Staff. . . . . Gnamani Arul, MD
Infection Control. . . . . Debra Kerr, RN
Operating Room. . . . . Ida Robinson, RN
Quality Assurance . . . . Sharon Steinkamp, RN
Radiology. . . . . Haywood Davis, MD

Measure	Cases	This Hosp.	State Avg.	U.S. Avg.
Heart Attack Care				
ACE Inhibitor or ARB for LVSD[5]	0	-	97%	96%
Aspirin at Arrival[5]	0	-	99%	99%
Aspirin at Discharge[5]	0	-	99%	98%
Beta Blocker at Discharge[5]	0	-	99%	98%
Fibrinolytic Medication Timing[5]	0	-	75%	55%
PCI Within 90 Minutes of Arrival[5]	0	-	93%	90%
Smoking Cessation Advice[5]	0	-	100%	99%
Chest Pain/Possible Heart Attack Care				
Aspirin at Arrival	-	-	95%	95%
Median Time to ECG (minutes)	-	-	8	8
Median Time to Transfer (minutes)	-	-	60	61
Fibrinolytic Medication Timing	-	-	59%	54%
Heart Failure Care				
ACE Inhibitor or ARB for LVSD[1]	22	95%	97%	94%
Discharge Instructions	78	100%	92%	88%
Evaluation of LVS Function	79	100%	99%	98%
Smoking Cessation Advice[1]	22	100%	99%	98%
Pneumonia Care				
Appropriate Initial Antibiotic	28	96%	93%	92%
Blood Culture Timing	46	98%	97%	96%
Influenza Vaccine	31	68%	94%	91%
Initial Antibiotic Timing	40	95%	96%	95%
Pneumococcal Vaccine[1]	18	94%	95%	93%
Smoking Cessation Advice[1]	21	100%	98%	97%
Surgical Care Improvement Project				
Appropriate VTP Within 24 Hours[1,2]	18	100%	94%	92%
Appropriate Hair Removal[2]	71	100%	100%	99%
Appropriate Beta Blocker Usage[1,2]	17	100%	94%	93%
Controlled Postoperative Blood Glucose[2,5]	0	-	96%	93%
Prophylactic Antibiotic Timing	56	100%	97%	97%
Prophylactic Antibiotic Timing (Outpatient)	-	-	93%	92%
Prophylactic Antibiotic Selection	57	98%	98%	97%
Prophylactic Antibiotic Select. (Outpatient)	-	-	96%	94%
Prophylactic Antibiotic Stopped	56	91%	96%	94%
Recommended VTP Ordered[1,2]	18	100%	96%	94%
Urinary Catheter Removal[1,2]	4	100%	93%	90%
Children's Asthma Care				
Received Systemic Corticosteroids	-	-	-	100%
Received Home Management Plan	-	-	-	71%
Received Reliever Medication	-	-	-	100%
Use of Medical Imaging				
Combination Abdominal CT Scan	-	-	0.144	0.191
Combination Chest CT Scan	-	-	0.030	0.054
Follow-up Mammogram/Ultrasound	-	-	7.5%	8.4%
MRI for Low Back Pain	-	-	31.5%	32.7%
Survey of Patients' Hospital Experiences				
Area Around Room 'Always' Quiet at Night	-	-	-	58%
Doctors 'Always' Communicated Well	-	-	-	80%
Home Recovery Information Given	-	-	-	82%
Hospital Given 9 or 10 on 10 Point Scale	-	-	-	67%
Meds 'Always' Explained Before Given	-	-	-	60%
Nurses 'Always' Communicated Well	-	-	-	76%
Pain 'Always' Well Controlled	-	-	-	69%
Room and Bathroom 'Always' Clean	-	-	-	71%
Timely Help 'Always' Received	-	-	-	64%
Would Definitely Recommend Hospital	-	-	-	69%

Sentara Careplex Hospital

3000 Coliseum Drive Phone: 757-736-1000
Hampton, VA 23666
URL: www.sentara.com
Type: Acute Care Hospitals Emergency Services: No
Ownership: Voluntary Non-Profit - Private Beds: 224

Measure	Cases	This Hosp.	State Avg.	U.S. Avg.
Heart Attack Care				
ACE Inhibitor or ARB for LVSD[1]	13	100%	97%	96%
Aspirin at Arrival	150	100%	99%	99%
Aspirin at Discharge	125	100%	99%	98%
Beta Blocker at Discharge	119	99%	99%	98%
Fibrinolytic Medication Timing	0	-	75%	55%
PCI Within 90 Minutes of Arrival	33	97%	93%	90%
Smoking Cessation Advice	49	100%	100%	99%
Chest Pain/Possible Heart Attack Care				
Aspirin at Arrival	39	100%	95%	95%
Median Time to ECG (minutes)	47	6	8	8
Median Time to Transfer (minutes)[1]	5	53	60	61
Fibrinolytic Medication Timing	0	-	59%	54%
Heart Failure Care				
ACE Inhibitor or ARB for LVSD	113	100%	97%	94%
Discharge Instructions	338	97%	92%	88%
Evaluation of LVS Function	392	100%	99%	98%
Smoking Cessation Advice	96	100%	99%	98%
Pneumonia Care				
Appropriate Initial Antibiotic	151	99%	93%	92%
Blood Culture Timing	294	97%	97%	96%
Influenza Vaccine	176	98%	94%	91%
Initial Antibiotic Timing	271	99%	96%	95%
Pneumococcal Vaccine	228	98%	95%	93%
Smoking Cessation Advice	99	100%	98%	97%
Surgical Care Improvement Project				
Appropriate VTP Within 24 Hours[2]	126	98%	94%	92%
Appropriate Hair Removal[2]	540	100%	100%	99%
Appropriate Beta Blocker Usage[2]	145	100%	94%	93%
Controlled Postoperative Blood Glucose[2]	0	-	96%	93%
Prophylactic Antibiotic Timing[2]	384	99%	97%	97%
Prophylactic Antibiotic Timing (Outpatient)	307	93%	93%	92%
Prophylactic Antibiotic Selection[2]	385	99%	98%	97%
Prophylactic Antibiotic Select. (Outpatient)	508	96%	96%	94%
Prophylactic Antibiotic Stopped[2]	378	98%	96%	94%
Recommended VTP Ordered[2]	126	99%	96%	94%
Urinary Catheter Removal[2]	100	100%	93%	90%
Children's Asthma Care				
Received Systemic Corticosteroids	-	-	-	100%
Received Home Management Plan	-	-	-	71%
Received Reliever Medication	-	-	-	100%
Use of Medical Imaging				
Combination Abdominal CT Scan	2,040	0.137	0.144	0.191
Combination Chest CT Scan	1,253	0.002	0.030	0.054
Follow-up Mammogram/Ultrasound	2,681	10.8%	7.5%	8.4%
MRI for Low Back Pain	232	31.9%	31.5%	32.7%
Survey of Patients' Hospital Experiences				
Area Around Room 'Always' Quiet at Night	300+	60%	-	58%
Doctors 'Always' Communicated Well	300+	75%	-	80%
Home Recovery Information Given	300+	78%	-	82%
Hospital Given 9 or 10 on 10 Point Scale	300+	62%	-	67%
Meds 'Always' Explained Before Given	300+	51%	-	60%
Nurses 'Always' Communicated Well	300+	67%	-	76%
Pain 'Always' Well Controlled	300+	60%	-	69%
Room and Bathroom 'Always' Clean	300+	62%	-	71%
Timely Help 'Always' Received	300+	54%	-	64%
Would Definitely Recommend Hospital	300+	64%	-	69%

NOTE: Hospital profiles are in alphabetical order by state, then city, then hospital within the city; Rankings exclude hospitals with less than 25 cases except for patient surveys which excludes hospitals with less than 100 cases; (a) 100–299 cases; (1) The number of cases is too small to be sure how well a hospital is performing; (2) The hospital indicated that the data submitted for this measure were based on a sample of cases; (3) Data was collected during a shorter time period (fewer quarters) than the maximum possible time for this measure; (4) Suppressed for one or more quarters by CMS; (5) No data is available from the hospital for this measure; (6) Fewer than 100 patients completed the HCAHPS survey. Use these rates with caution, as the number of surveys may be too low to reliably assess hospital performance; (7) Survey results are based on less than 12 months of data; (8) Survey results are not available for this reporting period; (9) No or very few patients were eligible for the HCAHPS survey. The scores shown, if any, reflect a very small number of surveys; (10) A state average was not calculated because too few hospitals in the state submitted data; (11) There were discrepancies in the data collection process; Please refer to the User's Guide for a full explanation of data.

Rockingham Memorial Hospital

2010 Health Campus Drive
Harrisonburg, VA 22801
URL: www.rmhonline.com
Type: Acute Care Hospitals
Ownership: Voluntary Non-Profit - Private

Phone: 540-433-4100
Fax: 540-433-4576

Emergency Services: No
Beds: 270

Key Personnel:
CEO/President . . . . James Krauss
Operating Room . . . . Joan Ridley, RN
Quality Assurance . . . . Helen Youngs
Radiology . . . . Judy Budd
Emergency Room . . . . Mary Anne Nolan

Measure	Cases	This Hosp.	State Avg.	U.S. Avg.
Heart Attack Care				
ACE Inhibitor or ARB for LVSD	44	98%	97%	96%
Aspirin at Arrival	349	99%	99%	99%
Aspirin at Discharge	344	99%	99%	98%
Beta Blocker at Discharge	341	99%	99%	98%
Fibrinolytic Medication Timing	0	-	75%	55%
PCI Within 90 Minutes of Arrival	59	100%	93%	90%
Smoking Cessation Advice	105	100%	100%	99%
Chest Pain/Possible Heart Attack Care				
Aspirin at Arrival[1,3]	7	100%	95%	95%
Median Time to ECG (minutes)[1,3]	7	12	8	8
Median Time to Transfer (minutes)[5]	0	-	60	61
Fibrinolytic Medication Timing[3]	0	-	59%	54%
Heart Failure Care				
ACE Inhibitor or ARB for LVSD[2]	101	97%	97%	94%
Discharge Instructions[2]	304	91%	92%	88%
Evaluation of LVS Function[2]	388	100%	99%	98%
Smoking Cessation Advice[2]	59	100%	99%	98%
Pneumonia Care				
Appropriate Initial Antibiotic[2]	123	97%	93%	92%
Blood Culture Timing[2]	170	99%	97%	96%
Influenza Vaccine[2]	140	90%	94%	91%
Initial Antibiotic Timing[2]	175	97%	96%	95%
Pneumococcal Vaccine[2]	204	91%	95%	93%
Smoking Cessation Advice[2]	76	100%	98%	97%
Surgical Care Improvement Project				
Appropriate VTP Within 24 Hours[2]	181	98%	94%	92%
Appropriate Hair Removal[2]	563	100%	100%	99%
Appropriate Beta Blocker Usage[2]	190	95%	94%	93%
Controlled Postoperative Blood Glucose[2]	85	98%	96%	93%
Prophylactic Antibiotic Timing[2]	385	90%	97%	97%
Prophylactic Antibiotic Timing (Outpatient)	257	93%	93%	92%
Prophylactic Antibiotic Selection[2]	386	95%	98%	97%
Prophylactic Antibiotic Select. (Outpatient)	249	97%	96%	94%
Prophylactic Antibiotic Stopped[2]	351	94%	96%	94%
Recommended VTP Ordered[2]	182	99%	96%	94%
Urinary Catheter Removal[2]	108	93%	93%	90%
Children's Asthma Care				
Received Systemic Corticosteroids	-	-	-	100%
Received Home Management Plan	-	-	-	71%
Received Reliever Medication	-	-	-	100%
Use of Medical Imaging				
Combination Abdominal CT Scan	1,312	0.053	0.144	0.191
Combination Chest CT Scan	745	0.003	0.030	0.054
Follow-up Mammogram/Ultrasound	2,521	6.2%	7.5%	8.4%
MRI for Low Back Pain	358	30.7%	31.5%	32.7%
Survey of Patients' Hospital Experiences				
Area Around Room 'Always' Quiet at Night	300+	52%	-	58%
Doctors 'Always' Communicated Well	300+	77%	-	80%
Home Recovery Information Given	300+	81%	-	82%
Hospital Given 9 or 10 on 10 Point Scale	300+	63%	-	67%
Meds 'Always' Explained Before Given	300+	56%	-	60%
Nurses 'Always' Communicated Well	300+	73%	-	76%
Pain 'Always' Well Controlled	300+	65%	-	69%
Room and Bathroom 'Always' Clean	300+	68%	-	71%
Timely Help 'Always' Received	300+	58%	-	64%
Would Definitely Recommend Hospital	300+	67%	-	69%

John Randolph Medical Center

411 West Randolph Road
Hopewell, VA 23860
URL: www.johnrandolphmed.com
Type: Acute Care Hospitals
Ownership: Proprietary

Phone: 804-541-1600
Fax: 804-452-3699

Emergency Services: Yes
Beds: 257

Key Personnel:
CEO/President . . . . E Bernard Boone, III
Chief of Medical Staff . . . . Dr Mohammad Mojeebuddin
Coronary Care . . . . Debbie Young
Operating Room . . . . Joan Hirsch
Pediatric In-Patient Care . . . . . . Nancy Lasken, RN
Quality Assurance . . . . Jeanne Poindexter
Radiology . . . . Rhonda Munson

Measure	Cases	This Hosp.	State Avg.	U.S. Avg.
Heart Attack Care				
ACE Inhibitor or ARB for LVSD[1]	10	100%	97%	96%
Aspirin at Arrival	43	100%	99%	99%
Aspirin at Discharge	27	100%	99%	98%
Beta Blocker at Discharge	28	100%	99%	98%
Fibrinolytic Medication Timing	0	-	75%	55%
PCI Within 90 Minutes of Arrival	0	-	93%	90%
Smoking Cessation Advice[1]	8	100%	100%	99%
Chest Pain/Possible Heart Attack Care				
Aspirin at Arrival	26	100%	95%	95%
Median Time to ECG (minutes)	27	8	8	8
Median Time to Transfer (minutes)[1]	11	49	60	61
Fibrinolytic Medication Timing	0	-	59%	54%
Heart Failure Care				
ACE Inhibitor or ARB for LVSD	81	100%	97%	94%
Discharge Instructions	153	97%	92%	88%
Evaluation of LVS Function	190	100%	99%	98%
Smoking Cessation Advice	52	100%	99%	98%
Pneumonia Care				
Appropriate Initial Antibiotic	73	96%	93%	92%
Blood Culture Timing	120	100%	97%	96%
Influenza Vaccine	62	100%	94%	91%
Initial Antibiotic Timing	103	98%	96%	95%
Pneumococcal Vaccine	78	100%	95%	93%
Smoking Cessation Advice	43	100%	98%	97%
Surgical Care Improvement Project				
Appropriate VTP Within 24 Hours	66	100%	94%	92%
Appropriate Hair Removal	93	100%	100%	99%
Appropriate Beta Blocker Usage[1]	18	100%	94%	93%
Controlled Postoperative Blood Glucose	0	-	96%	93%
Prophylactic Antibiotic Timing	41	100%	97%	97%
Prophylactic Antibiotic Timing (Outpatient)	58	98%	93%	92%
Prophylactic Antibiotic Selection	41	100%	98%	97%
Prophylactic Antibiotic Select. (Outpatient)	58	97%	96%	94%
Prophylactic Antibiotic Stopped	35	100%	96%	94%
Recommended VTP Ordered	66	100%	96%	94%
Urinary Catheter Removal[1]	12	100%	93%	90%
Children's Asthma Care				
Received Systemic Corticosteroids	-	-	-	100%
Received Home Management Plan	-	-	-	71%
Received Reliever Medication	-	-	-	100%
Use of Medical Imaging				
Combination Abdominal CT Scan	631	0.384	0.144	0.191
Combination Chest CT Scan	428	0.007	0.030	0.054
Follow-up Mammogram/Ultrasound	731	4.5%	7.5%	8.4%
MRI for Low Back Pain	115	40.0%	31.5%	32.7%
Survey of Patients' Hospital Experiences				
Area Around Room 'Always' Quiet at Night	300+	61%	-	58%
Doctors 'Always' Communicated Well	300+	77%	-	80%
Home Recovery Information Given	300+	81%	-	82%
Hospital Given 9 or 10 on 10 Point Scale	300+	59%	-	67%
Meds 'Always' Explained Before Given	300+	56%	-	60%
Nurses 'Always' Communicated Well	300+	73%	-	76%
Pain 'Always' Well Controlled	300+	70%	-	69%
Room and Bathroom 'Always' Clean	300+	70%	-	71%
Timely Help 'Always' Received	300+	57%	-	64%
Would Definitely Recommend Hospital	300+	58%	-	69%

Bath County Community Hospital

106 Park Drive
Hot Springs, VA 24445
E-mail: dlipes@bcchospital.org
URL: www.bcchospital.org
Type: Critical Access Hospitals
Ownership: Voluntary Non-Profit - Other

Phone: 540-839-7000
Fax: 540-839-7060

Emergency Services: Yes
Beds: 25

Key Personnel:
CEO/President . . . . Deborah R Lipes
Chief of Medical Staff . . . . James Redington, MD
Infection Control . . . . Becky Armstrong
Operating Room . . . . Mary Ayers
Quality Assurance . . . . Amanda Thornsbury
Radiology . . . . Jo Lamb, MD
Emergency Room . . . . James Redington, MD

Measure	Cases	This Hosp.	State Avg.	U.S. Avg.
Heart Attack Care				
ACE Inhibitor or ARB for LVSD[5]	0	-	97%	96%
Aspirin at Arrival[5]	0	-	99%	99%
Aspirin at Discharge[5]	0	-	99%	98%
Beta Blocker at Discharge[5]	0	-	99%	98%
Fibrinolytic Medication Timing[5]	0	-	75%	55%
PCI Within 90 Minutes of Arrival[5]	0	-	93%	90%
Smoking Cessation Advice[5]	0	-	100%	99%
Chest Pain/Possible Heart Attack Care				
Aspirin at Arrival	-	-	95%	95%
Median Time to ECG (minutes)	-	-	8	8
Median Time to Transfer (minutes)	-	-	60	61
Fibrinolytic Medication Timing	-	-	59%	54%
Heart Failure Care				
ACE Inhibitor or ARB for LVSD[1]	6	100%	97%	94%
Discharge Instructions[1]	13	62%	92%	88%
Evaluation of LVS Function[1]	16	94%	99%	98%
Smoking Cessation Advice[1]	4	75%	99%	98%
Pneumonia Care				
Appropriate Initial Antibiotic[1]	15	80%	93%	92%
Blood Culture Timing[1]	13	92%	97%	96%
Influenza Vaccine[1]	12	75%	94%	91%
Initial Antibiotic Timing[1]	22	95%	96%	95%
Pneumococcal Vaccine[1]	19	68%	95%	93%
Smoking Cessation Advice[1]	6	83%	98%	97%
Surgical Care Improvement Project				
Appropriate VTP Within 24 Hours[5]	0	-	94%	92%
Appropriate Hair Removal[5]	0	-	100%	99%
Appropriate Beta Blocker Usage[5]	0	-	94%	93%
Controlled Postoperative Blood Glucose[5]	0	-	96%	93%
Prophylactic Antibiotic Timing[5]	0	-	97%	97%
Prophylactic Antibiotic Timing (Outpatient)	-	-	93%	92%
Prophylactic Antibiotic Selection[5]	0	-	98%	97%
Prophylactic Antibiotic Select. (Outpatient)	-	-	96%	94%
Prophylactic Antibiotic Stopped[5]	0	-	96%	94%
Recommended VTP Ordered[5]	0	-	96%	94%
Urinary Catheter Removal[5]	0	-	93%	90%
Children's Asthma Care				
Received Systemic Corticosteroids	-	-	-	100%
Received Home Management Plan	-	-	-	71%
Received Reliever Medication	-	-	-	100%
Use of Medical Imaging				
Combination Abdominal CT Scan	-	-	0.144	0.191
Combination Chest CT Scan	-	-	0.030	0.054
Follow-up Mammogram/Ultrasound	-	-	7.5%	8.4%
MRI for Low Back Pain	-	-	31.5%	32.7%
Survey of Patients' Hospital Experiences				
Area Around Room 'Always' Quiet at Night[8]	-	-	-	58%
Doctors 'Always' Communicated Well[8]	-	-	-	80%
Home Recovery Information Given[8]	-	-	-	82%
Hospital Given 9 or 10 on 10 Point Scale[8]	-	-	-	67%
Meds 'Always' Explained Before Given[8]	-	-	-	60%
Nurses 'Always' Communicated Well[8]	-	-	-	76%
Pain 'Always' Well Controlled[8]	-	-	-	69%
Room and Bathroom 'Always' Clean[8]	-	-	-	71%
Timely Help 'Always' Received[8]	-	-	-	64%
Would Definitely Recommend Hospital[8]	-	-	-	69%

NOTE: Hospital profiles are in alphabetical order by state, then city, then hospital within the city; Rankings exclude hospitals with less than 25 cases except for patient surveys which excludes hospitals with less than 100 cases; (a) 100–299 cases; (1) The number of cases is too small to be sure how well a hospital is performing; (2) The hospital indicated that the data submitted for this measure were based on a sample of cases; (3) Data was collected during a shorter time period (fewer quarters) than the maximum possible time for this measure; (4) Suppressed for one or more quarters by CMS; (5) No data is available from the hospital for this measure; (6) Fewer than 100 patients completed the HCAHPS survey. Use these rates with caution, as the number of surveys may be too low to reliably assess hospital performance; (7) Survey results are not available for this reporting period; (8) Survey results are based on less than 12 months of data; (8) Survey results, if any, reflect a very small number of surveys; (10) A state average was not calculated because too few hospitals in the state submitted data; (11) There were discrepancies in the data collection process; Please refer to the User's Guide for a full explanation of data.

Rappahannock General Hospital

101 Harris Road
Kilmarnock, VA 22482
Phone: 804-435-8000
Fax: 804-435-8543
E-mail: egravatt@hotmail.com
URL: www.RGH-Hospital.com
Type: Acute Care Hospitals
Emergency Services: Yes
Ownership: Voluntary Non-Profit - Private
Beds: 76

Key Personnel:

CEO/President. . . . . James M Holmes, Jr
Operating Room. . . . . Karen Farris, RN
Radiology. . . . . William B Olson
Emergency Room . . . . Virginia W Gale
Intensive Care Unit. . . . . Ann Gumina, RN
Patient Relations . . . . Betty Bryant

Measure	Cases	This Hosp.	State Avg.	U.S. Avg.
Heart Attack Care				
ACE Inhibitor or ARB for LVSD	0	-	97%	96%
Aspirin at Arrival[1]	8	100%	99%	99%
Aspirin at Discharge[1]	4	100%	99%	98%
Beta Blocker at Discharge[1]	2	100%	99%	98%
Fibrinolytic Medication Timing	0	-	75%	55%
PCI Within 90 Minutes of Arrival	0	-	93%	90%
Smoking Cessation Advice[1]	1	100%	100%	99%
Chest Pain/Possible Heart Attack Care				
Aspirin at Arrival	92	97%	95%	95%
Median Time to ECG (minutes)	96	8	8	8
Median Time to Transfer (minutes)[1]	7	63	60	61
Fibrinolytic Medication Timing[1]	9	33%	59%	54%
Heart Failure Care				
ACE Inhibitor or ARB for LVSD[1]	16	100%	97%	94%
Discharge Instructions	43	100%	92%	88%
Evaluation of LVS Function	51	98%	99%	98%
Smoking Cessation Advice[1]	8	100%	99%	98%
Pneumonia Care				
Appropriate Initial Antibiotic	44	89%	93%	92%
Blood Culture Timing	68	100%	97%	96%
Influenza Vaccine[1]	17	94%	94%	91%
Initial Antibiotic Timing	70	100%	96%	95%
Pneumococcal Vaccine	62	94%	95%	93%
Smoking Cessation Advice[1]	15	87%	98%	97%
Surgical Care Improvement Project				
Appropriate VTP Within 24 Hours	80	92%	94%	92%
Appropriate Hair Removal	127	100%	100%	99%
Appropriate Beta Blocker Usage	41	90%	94%	93%
Controlled Postoperative Blood Glucose	0	-	96%	93%
Prophylactic Antibiotic Timing	79	97%	97%	97%
Prophylactic Antibiotic Timing (Outpatient)	44	95%	93%	92%
Prophylactic Antibiotic Selection	80	98%	98%	97%
Prophylactic Antibiotic Select. (Outpatient)	43	98%	96%	94%
Prophylactic Antibiotic Stopped	75	93%	96%	94%
Recommended VTP Ordered	80	95%	96%	94%
Urinary Catheter Removal	33	88%	93%	90%
Children's Asthma Care				
Received Systemic Corticosteroids	-	-	-	100%
Received Home Management Plan	-	-	-	71%
Received Reliever Medication	-	-	-	100%
Use of Medical Imaging				
Combination Abdominal CT Scan	474	0.110	0.144	0.191
Combination Chest CT Scan	320	0.053	0.030	0.054
Follow-up Mammogram/Ultrasound	891	4.2%	7.5%	8.4%
MRI for Low Back Pain	161	26.7%	31.5%	32.7%
Survey of Patients' Hospital Experiences				
Area Around Room 'Always' Quiet at Night	300+	49%	-	58%
Doctors 'Always' Communicated Well	300+	82%	-	80%
Home Recovery Information Given	300+	80%	-	82%
Hospital Given 9 or 10 on 10 Point Scale	300+	68%	-	67%
Meds 'Always' Explained Before Given	300+	62%	-	60%
Nurses 'Always' Communicated Well	300+	81%	-	76%
Pain 'Always' Well Controlled	300+	70%	-	69%
Room and Bathroom 'Always' Clean	300+	79%	-	71%
Timely Help 'Always' Received	300+	74%	-	64%
Would Definitely Recommend Hospital	300+	72%	-	69%

Russell County Medical Center

58 Carroll Street
Lebanon, VA 24266
Phone: 276-883-8000
Fax: 276-883-8111
Type: Acute Care Hospitals
Emergency Services: Yes
Ownership: Proprietary
Beds: 78

Key Personnel:

CEO/President. . . . . David Parsh
Chief of Medical Staff . . . . Samuel Milton
Infection Control . . . . William Taylor, RN
Operating Room. . . . . Debbie Garrett, RN
Quality Assurance . . . . Brenda Banner
Anesthesiology. . . . . Jennifer Burton, D.O.
Emergency Room . . . . Norman Rexrode Jr, MD
Intensive Care Unit. . . . . Karen Chaney, RN

Measure	Cases	This Hosp.	State Avg.	U.S. Avg.
Heart Attack Care				
ACE Inhibitor or ARB for LVSD[2,3]	0	-	97%	96%
Aspirin at Arrival[1,2,3]	10	100%	99%	99%
Aspirin at Discharge[1,2,3]	5	80%	99%	98%
Beta Blocker at Discharge[1,2,3]	3	100%	99%	98%
Fibrinolytic Medication Timing[2,3]	0	-	75%	55%
PCI Within 90 Minutes of Arrival[2,3]	0	-	93%	90%
Smoking Cessation Advice[1,2,3]	1	100%	100%	99%
Chest Pain/Possible Heart Attack Care				
Aspirin at Arrival	59	78%	95%	95%
Median Time to ECG (minutes)	58	5	8	8
Median Time to Transfer (minutes)[5]	0	-	60	61
Fibrinolytic Medication Timing[1]	2	100%	59%	54%
Heart Failure Care				
ACE Inhibitor or ARB for LVSD[1,2]	20	95%	97%	94%
Discharge Instructions[2]	79	84%	92%	88%
Evaluation of LVS Function[2]	89	90%	99%	98%
Smoking Cessation Advice[1,2]	20	100%	99%	98%
Pneumonia Care				
Appropriate Initial Antibiotic[2]	103	90%	93%	92%
Blood Culture Timing[2]	98	100%	97%	96%
Influenza Vaccine[2]	94	99%	94%	91%
Initial Antibiotic Timing[2]	143	99%	96%	95%
Pneumococcal Vaccine[2]	122	100%	95%	93%
Smoking Cessation Advice[2]	70	96%	98%	97%
Surgical Care Improvement Project				
Appropriate VTP Within 24 Hours[5]	0	-	94%	92%
Appropriate Hair Removal[5]	0	-	100%	99%
Appropriate Beta Blocker Usage[5]	0	-	94%	93%
Controlled Postoperative Blood Glucose[5]	0	-	96%	93%
Prophylactic Antibiotic Timing[5]	0	-	97%	97%
Prophylactic Antibiotic Timing (Outpatient)[1,3]	1	100%	93%	92%
Prophylactic Antibiotic Selection[5]	0	-	98%	97%
Prophylactic Antibiotic Select. (Outpatient)[1,3]	1	0%	96%	94%
Prophylactic Antibiotic Stopped[5]	0	-	96%	94%
Recommended VTP Ordered[5]	0	-	96%	94%
Urinary Catheter Removal[5]	0	-	93%	90%
Children's Asthma Care				
Received Systemic Corticosteroids	-	-	-	100%
Received Home Management Plan	-	-	-	71%
Received Reliever Medication	-	-	-	100%
Use of Medical Imaging				
Combination Abdominal CT Scan	148	0.027	0.144	0.191
Combination Chest CT Scan	125	0.240	0.030	0.054
Follow-up Mammogram/Ultrasound	163	15.3%	7.5%	8.4%
MRI for Low Back Pain[1]	19	47.4%	31.5%	32.7%
Survey of Patients' Hospital Experiences				
Area Around Room 'Always' Quiet at Night	300+	55%	-	58%
Doctors 'Always' Communicated Well	300+	82%	-	80%
Home Recovery Information Given	300+	81%	-	82%
Hospital Given 9 or 10 on 10 Point Scale	300+	59%	-	67%
Meds 'Always' Explained Before Given	300+	61%	-	60%
Nurses 'Always' Communicated Well	300+	79%	-	76%
Pain 'Always' Well Controlled	300+	68%	-	69%
Room and Bathroom 'Always' Clean	300+	74%	-	71%
Timely Help 'Always' Received	300+	67%	-	64%
Would Definitely Recommend Hospital	300+	58%	-	69%

Inova Loudoun Hospital

44045 Riverside Parkway
Leesburg, VA 20176
Phone: 703-858-6600
Fax: 703-858-6610
URL: loudounhealthcare.org
Type: Acute Care Hospitals
Emergency Services: Yes
Ownership: Proprietary
Beds: 155

Key Personnel:

CEO/President. . . . . Randall Kelley
Cardiac Laboratory. . . . . Deidre Cahill
Chief of Medical Staff. . . . . Kevin O'Connor
Infection Control. . . . . Linda Belomonte
Operating Room. . . . . Barb McDonnell
Quality Assurance . . . . Diane Wilhite
Emergency Room . . . . Lisa Dugan

Measure	Cases	This Hosp.	State Avg.	U.S. Avg.
Heart Attack Care				
ACE Inhibitor or ARB for LVSD[1]	8	88%	97%	96%
Aspirin at Arrival	95	100%	99%	99%
Aspirin at Discharge	85	98%	99%	98%
Beta Blocker at Discharge	86	100%	99%	98%
Fibrinolytic Medication Timing	0	-	75%	55%
PCI Within 90 Minutes of Arrival[1]	24	83%	93%	90%
Smoking Cessation Advice	27	100%	100%	99%
Chest Pain/Possible Heart Attack Care				
Aspirin at Arrival	91	90%	95%	95%
Median Time to ECG (minutes)	98	7	8	8
Median Time to Transfer (minutes)[1,3]	20	72	60	61
Fibrinolytic Medication Timing[3]	0	-	59%	54%
Heart Failure Care				
ACE Inhibitor or ARB for LVSD	51	98%	97%	94%
Discharge Instructions	173	95%	92%	88%
Evaluation of LVS Function	209	99%	99%	98%
Smoking Cessation Advice	25	100%	99%	98%
Pneumonia Care				
Appropriate Initial Antibiotic[2]	111	93%	93%	92%
Blood Culture Timing[2]	141	92%	97%	96%
Influenza Vaccine	127	94%	94%	91%
Initial Antibiotic Timing[2]	143	97%	96%	95%
Pneumococcal Vaccine[2]	158	98%	95%	93%
Smoking Cessation Advice[2]	60	98%	98%	97%
Surgical Care Improvement Project				
Appropriate VTP Within 24 Hours[2]	156	86%	94%	92%
Appropriate Hair Removal[2]	449	100%	100%	99%
Appropriate Beta Blocker Usage[2]	102	95%	94%	93%
Controlled Postoperative Blood Glucose[2]	0	-	96%	93%
Prophylactic Antibiotic Timing[2]	270	95%	97%	97%
Prophylactic Antibiotic Timing (Outpatient)	342	96%	93%	92%
Prophylactic Antibiotic Selection[2]	272	97%	98%	97%
Prophylactic Antibiotic Select. (Outpatient)	348	91%	96%	94%
Prophylactic Antibiotic Stopped[2]	260	89%	96%	94%
Recommended VTP Ordered[2]	156	91%	96%	94%
Urinary Catheter Removal[2]	48	88%	93%	90%
Children's Asthma Care				
Received Systemic Corticosteroids	-	-	-	100%
Received Home Management Plan	-	-	-	71%
Received Reliever Medication	-	-	-	100%
Use of Medical Imaging				
Combination Abdominal CT Scan	797	0.066	0.144	0.191
Combination Chest CT Scan	775	0.010	0.030	0.054
Follow-up Mammogram/Ultrasound	544	10.3%	7.5%	8.4%
MRI for Low Back Pain	124	26.6%	31.5%	32.7%
Survey of Patients' Hospital Experiences				
Area Around Room 'Always' Quiet at Night	300+	45%	-	58%
Doctors 'Always' Communicated Well	300+	80%	-	80%
Home Recovery Information Given	300+	87%	-	82%
Hospital Given 9 or 10 on 10 Point Scale	300+	72%	-	67%
Meds 'Always' Explained Before Given	300+	60%	-	60%
Nurses 'Always' Communicated Well	300+	76%	-	76%
Pain 'Always' Well Controlled	300+	67%	-	69%
Room and Bathroom 'Always' Clean	300+	64%	-	71%
Timely Help 'Always' Received	300+	63%	-	64%
Would Definitely Recommend Hospital	300+	74%	-	69%

NOTE: Hospital profiles are in alphabetical order by state, then city, then hospital within the city; Rankings exclude hospitals with less than 25 cases except for patient surveys which excludes hospitals with less than 100 cases; (a) 100–299 cases; (1) The number of cases is too small to be sure how well a hospital is performing; (2) The hospital indicated that the data submitted for this measure were based on a sample of cases; (3) Data was collected during a shorter time period (fewer quarters) than the maximum possible time for this measure; (4) Suppressed for one or more quarters by CMS; (5) No data is available from the hospital for this measure; (6) Fewer than 100 patients completed the HCAHPS survey. Use these rates with caution, as the number of surveys may be too low to reliably assess hospital performance; (7) Survey results are based on less than 12 months of data; (8) Survey results are not available for this reporting period; (9) No or very few patients were eligible for the HCAHPS survey. The scores shown, if any, reflect a very small number of surveys; (10) A state average was not calculated because too few hospitals in the state submitted data; (11) There were discrepancies in the data collection process; Please refer to the User's Guide for a full explanation of data.

Carilion Stonewall Jackson Hospital

1 Health Circle
Lexington, VA 24450
E-mail: crassist@sjhospital.com
URL: www.sjhospital.com
Type: Critical Access Hospitals
Ownership: Voluntary Non-Profit - Private

Phone: 540-458-3503
Fax: 540-458-3545

Emergency Services: Yes
Beds: 130

Key Personnel:
CEO/President . . . . Thomas McNamara
Radiology . . . . Michael Clague

Measure	Cases	This Hosp.	State Avg.	U.S. Avg.
Heart Attack Care				
ACE Inhibitor or ARB for LVSD[1]	5	100%	97%	96%
Aspirin at Arrival[1]	20	95%	99%	99%
Aspirin at Discharge[1]	14	100%	99%	98%
Beta Blocker at Discharge[1]	14	100%	99%	98%
Fibrinolytic Medication Timing	0	-	75%	55%
PCI Within 90 Minutes of Arrival	0	-	93%	90%
Smoking Cessation Advice[1]	2	100%	100%	99%
Chest Pain/Possible Heart Attack Care				
Aspirin at Arrival	-	-	95%	95%
Median Time to ECG (minutes)	-	-	8	8
Median Time to Transfer (minutes)	-	-	60	61
Fibrinolytic Medication Timing	-	-	59%	54%
Heart Failure Care				
ACE Inhibitor or ARB for LVSD[1]	19	95%	97%	94%
Discharge Instructions	49	90%	92%	88%
Evaluation of LVS Function	61	100%	99%	98%
Smoking Cessation Advice[1]	7	100%	99%	98%
Pneumonia Care				
Appropriate Initial Antibiotic	31	87%	93%	92%
Blood Culture Timing	41	95%	97%	96%
Influenza Vaccine	35	94%	94%	91%
Initial Antibiotic Timing	43	88%	96%	95%
Pneumococcal Vaccine	40	98%	95%	93%
Smoking Cessation Advice[1]	12	100%	98%	97%
Surgical Care Improvement Project				
Appropriate VTP Within 24 Hours	32	91%	94%	92%
Appropriate Hair Removal	64	100%	100%	99%
Appropriate Beta Blocker Usage[1]	19	74%	94%	93%
Controlled Postoperative Blood Glucose[3]	0	-	96%	93%
Prophylactic Antibiotic Timing	51	100%	97%	97%
Prophylactic Antibiotic Timing (Outpatient)	-	-	93%	92%
Prophylactic Antibiotic Selection	52	100%	98%	97%
Prophylactic Antibiotic Select. (Outpatient)	-	-	96%	94%
Prophylactic Antibiotic Stopped	51	98%	96%	94%
Recommended VTP Ordered	32	97%	96%	94%
Urinary Catheter Removal[1]	19	95%	93%	90%
Children's Asthma Care				
Received Systemic Corticosteroids	-	-	-	100%
Received Home Management Plan	-	-	-	71%
Received Reliever Medication	-	-	-	100%
Use of Medical Imaging				
Combination Abdominal CT Scan	-	-	0.144	0.191
Combination Chest CT Scan	-	-	0.030	0.054
Follow-up Mammogram/Ultrasound	-	-	7.5%	8.4%
MRI for Low Back Pain	-	-	31.5%	32.7%
Survey of Patients' Hospital Experiences				
Area Around Room 'Always' Quiet at Night	300+	61%	-	58%
Doctors 'Always' Communicated Well	300+	86%	-	80%
Home Recovery Information Given	300+	82%	-	82%
Hospital Given 9 on 10 on 10 Point Scale	300+	65%	-	67%
Meds 'Always' Explained Before Given	300+	68%	-	60%
Nurses 'Always' Communicated Well	300+	81%	-	76%
Pain 'Always' Well Controlled	300+	74%	-	69%
Room and Bathroom 'Always' Clean	300+	75%	-	71%
Timely Help 'Always' Received	300+	75%	-	64%
Would Definitely Recommend Hospital	300+	63%	-	69%

Alleghany Regional Hospital

One Arh Lane
Low Moor, VA 24457
URL: www.alleghanyregional.com
Type: Acute Care Hospitals
Ownership: Proprietary

Phone: 540-862-6011
Fax: 540-862-6472

Emergency Services: Yes
Beds: 156

Key Personnel:
CEO/President . . . . Greg Madsen
Chief of Medical Staff . . . . James A McCoig
Operating Room . . . . Gayle Minson, RN
Quality Assurance . . . . Debbie Clark, RN
Radiology . . . . Bruce C Banning, MD

Measure	Cases	This Hosp.	State Avg.	U.S. Avg.
Heart Attack Care				
ACE Inhibitor or ARB for LVSD[1]	2	100%	97%	96%
Aspirin at Arrival[1]	14	93%	99%	99%
Aspirin at Discharge[1]	8	100%	99%	98%
Beta Blocker at Discharge[1]	10	100%	99%	98%
Fibrinolytic Medication Timing	0	-	75%	55%
PCI Within 90 Minutes of Arrival	0	-	93%	90%
Smoking Cessation Advice[1]	2	100%	100%	99%
Chest Pain/Possible Heart Attack Care				
Aspirin at Arrival	74	100%	95%	95%
Median Time to ECG (minutes)	76	6	8	8
Median Time to Transfer (minutes)	0	-	60	61
Fibrinolytic Medication Timing[1]	6	100%	59%	54%
Heart Failure Care				
ACE Inhibitor or ARB for LVSD[1]	21	95%	97%	94%
Discharge Instructions	94	100%	92%	88%
Evaluation of LVS Function	120	100%	99%	98%
Smoking Cessation Advice[1]	19	100%	99%	98%
Pneumonia Care				
Appropriate Initial Antibiotic	106	95%	93%	92%
Blood Culture Timing	131	100%	97%	96%
Influenza Vaccine	91	100%	94%	91%
Initial Antibiotic Timing	114	96%	96%	95%
Pneumococcal Vaccine	111	100%	95%	93%
Smoking Cessation Advice	48	100%	98%	97%
Surgical Care Improvement Project				
Appropriate VTP Within 24 Hours[2]	109	97%	94%	92%
Appropriate Hair Removal[2]	233	100%	100%	99%
Appropriate Beta Blocker Usage[2]	35	100%	94%	93%
Controlled Postoperative Blood Glucose[2]	0	-	96%	93%
Prophylactic Antibiotic Timing[2]	198	100%	97%	97%
Prophylactic Antibiotic Timing (Outpatient)	34	97%	93%	92%
Prophylactic Antibiotic Selection[2]	198	98%	98%	97%
Prophylactic Antibiotic Select. (Outpatient)	33	97%	96%	94%
Prophylactic Antibiotic Stopped[2]	196	98%	96%	94%
Recommended VTP Ordered[2]	109	97%	96%	94%
Urinary Catheter Removal[1,2]	12	83%	93%	90%
Children's Asthma Care				
Received Systemic Corticosteroids	-	-	-	100%
Received Home Management Plan	-	-	-	71%
Received Reliever Medication	-	-	-	100%
Use of Medical Imaging				
Combination Abdominal CT Scan	443	0.061	0.144	0.191
Combination Chest CT Scan	346	0.000	0.030	0.054
Follow-up Mammogram/Ultrasound	833	10.1%	7.5%	8.4%
MRI for Low Back Pain	92	33.7%	31.5%	32.7%
Survey of Patients' Hospital Experiences				
Area Around Room 'Always' Quiet at Night	300+	60%	-	58%
Doctors 'Always' Communicated Well	300+	82%	-	80%
Home Recovery Information Given	300+	83%	-	82%
Hospital Given 9 or 10 on 10 Point Scale	300+	64%	-	67%
Meds 'Always' Explained Before Given	300+	62%	-	60%
Nurses 'Always' Communicated Well	300+	78%	-	76%
Pain 'Always' Well Controlled	300+	72%	-	69%
Room and Bathroom 'Always' Clean	300+	67%	-	71%
Timely Help 'Always' Received	300+	61%	-	64%
Would Definitely Recommend Hospital	300+	66%	-	69%

Page Memorial Hospital

200 Memorial Drive
Luray, VA 22835
E-mail: pmh@shentel.net
URL: www.pagememorialhospital.org
Type: Critical Access Hospitals
Ownership: Voluntary Non-Profit - Private

Phone: 540-743-4561
Fax: 540-743-9560

Emergency Services: Yes
Beds: 54

Key Personnel:
CEO/President . . . . John Barrett
Infection Control . . . . John Vollmer
Quality Assurance . . . . Clara Layman
Radiology . . . . Donna M Sefczek
Emergency Room . . . . Erin Noser

Measure	Cases	This Hosp.	State Avg.	U.S. Avg.
Heart Attack Care				
ACE Inhibitor or ARB for LVSD	0	-	97%	96%
Aspirin at Arrival[1]	8	100%	99%	99%
Aspirin at Discharge[1]	6	100%	99%	98%
Beta Blocker at Discharge[1]	7	100%	99%	98%
Fibrinolytic Medication Timing	0	-	75%	55%
PCI Within 90 Minutes of Arrival	0	-	93%	90%
Smoking Cessation Advice	0	-	100%	99%
Chest Pain/Possible Heart Attack Care				
Aspirin at Arrival	-	-	95%	95%
Median Time to ECG (minutes)	-	-	8	8
Median Time to Transfer (minutes)	-	-	60	61
Fibrinolytic Medication Timing	-	-	59%	54%
Heart Failure Care				
ACE Inhibitor or ARB for LVSD[1]	22	77%	97%	94%
Discharge Instructions	27	89%	92%	88%
Evaluation of LVS Function	50	100%	99%	98%
Smoking Cessation Advice[1]	1	100%	99%	98%
Pneumonia Care				
Appropriate Initial Antibiotic	25	88%	93%	92%
Blood Culture Timing	27	96%	97%	96%
Influenza Vaccine[1]	19	89%	94%	91%
Initial Antibiotic Timing	33	94%	96%	95%
Pneumococcal Vaccine	28	96%	95%	93%
Smoking Cessation Advice[1]	9	89%	98%	97%
Surgical Care Improvement Project				
Appropriate VTP Within 24 Hours[5]	0	-	94%	92%
Appropriate Hair Removal[5]	0	-	100%	99%
Appropriate Beta Blocker Usage[5]	0	-	94%	93%
Controlled Postoperative Blood Glucose[5]	0	-	96%	93%
Prophylactic Antibiotic Timing[5]	0	-	97%	97%
Prophylactic Antibiotic Timing (Outpatient)	-	-	93%	92%
Prophylactic Antibiotic Selection[5]	0	-	98%	97%
Prophylactic Antibiotic Select. (Outpatient)	-	-	96%	94%
Prophylactic Antibiotic Stopped[5]	0	-	96%	94%
Recommended VTP Ordered[5]	0	-	96%	94%
Urinary Catheter Removal[5]	0	-	93%	90%
Children's Asthma Care				
Received Systemic Corticosteroids	-	-	-	100%
Received Home Management Plan	-	-	-	71%
Received Reliever Medication	-	-	-	100%
Use of Medical Imaging				
Combination Abdominal CT Scan	-	-	0.144	0.191
Combination Chest CT Scan	-	-	0.030	0.054
Follow-up Mammogram/Ultrasound	-	-	7.5%	8.4%
MRI for Low Back Pain	-	-	31.5%	32.7%
Survey of Patients' Hospital Experiences				
Area Around Room 'Always' Quiet at Night	(a)	54%	-	58%
Doctors 'Always' Communicated Well	(a)	74%	-	80%
Home Recovery Information Given	(a)	91%	-	82%
Hospital Given 9 or 10 on 10 Point Scale	(a)	58%	-	67%
Meds 'Always' Explained Before Given	(a)	44%	-	60%
Nurses 'Always' Communicated Well	(a)	72%	-	76%
Pain 'Always' Well Controlled	(a)	65%	-	69%
Room and Bathroom 'Always' Clean	(a)	70%	-	71%
Timely Help 'Always' Received	(a)	56%	-	64%
Would Definitely Recommend Hospital	(a)	58%	-	69%

Centra Health

1920 Atherholt Road
Lynchburg, VA 24501
URL: www.centrahealth.com
Type: Acute Care Hospitals
Ownership: Voluntary Non-Profit - Private

Phone: 434-947-4705

Emergency Services: Yes

Key Personnel:
President/CEO . . . . W Michael Bryant

Measure	Cases	This Hosp.	State Avg.	U.S. Avg.
Heart Attack Care				
ACE Inhibitor or ARB for LVSD	72	97%	97%	96%
Aspirin at Arrival	479	100%	99%	99%
Aspirin at Discharge	572	100%	99%	98%
Beta Blocker at Discharge	563	99%	99%	98%
Fibrinolytic Medication Timing	0	-	75%	55%
PCI Within 90 Minutes of Arrival	79	97%	93%	90%
Smoking Cessation Advice	222	100%	100%	99%
Chest Pain/Possible Heart Attack Care				
Aspirin at Arrival[1,3]	1	100%	95%	95%
Median Time to ECG (minutes)[1,3]	1	61	8	8
Median Time to Transfer (minutes)[5]	0	-	60	61
Fibrinolytic Medication Timing[5]	0	-	59%	54%
Heart Failure Care				
ACE Inhibitor or ARB for LVSD[2]	219	96%	97%	94%
Discharge Instructions[2]	616	100%	92%	88%
Evaluation of LVS Function[2]	818	99%	99%	98%
Smoking Cessation Advice[2]	168	100%	99%	98%
Pneumonia Care				
Appropriate Initial Antibiotic[2]	209	88%	93%	92%
Blood Culture Timing[2]	318	95%	97%	96%
Influenza Vaccine[2]	220	95%	94%	91%
Initial Antibiotic Timing[2]	382	95%	96%	95%
Pneumococcal Vaccine[2]	337	98%	95%	93%
Smoking Cessation Advice[2]	177	99%	98%	97%
Surgical Care Improvement Project				
Appropriate VTP Within 24 Hours[2]	408	98%	94%	92%
Appropriate Hair Removal[2]	1,548	100%	100%	99%
Appropriate Beta Blocker Usage[2]	528	100%	94%	93%
Controlled Postoperative Blood Glucose[2]	289	100%	96%	93%
Prophylactic Antibiotic Timing[2]	1,075	100%	97%	97%
Prophylactic Antibiotic Timing (Outpatient)	444	92%	93%	92%
Prophylactic Antibiotic Selection[2]	1,090	98%	98%	97%
Prophylactic Antibiotic Select. (Outpatient)	432	98%	96%	94%
Prophylactic Antibiotic Stopped[2]	1,016	100%	96%	94%
Recommended VTP Ordered[2]	408	99%	96%	94%
Urinary Catheter Removal[2]	135	97%	93%	90%
Children's Asthma Care				
Received Systemic Corticosteroids	74	100%	-	100%
Received Home Management Plan	70	94%	-	71%
Received Reliever Medication	75	100%	-	100%
Use of Medical Imaging				
Combination Abdominal CT Scan	1,628	0.097	0.144	0.191
Combination Chest CT Scan	1,074	0.016	0.030	0.054
Follow-up Mammogram/Ultrasound[1]	6	33.3%	7.5%	8.4%
MRI for Low Back Pain	267	28.5%	31.5%	32.7%
Survey of Patients' Hospital Experiences				
Area Around Room 'Always' Quiet at Night	300+	60%	-	58%
Doctors 'Always' Communicated Well	300+	83%	-	80%
Home Recovery Information Given	300+	83%	-	82%
Hospital Given 9 or 10 on 10 Point Scale	300+	74%	-	67%
Meds 'Always' Explained Before Given	300+	63%	-	60%
Nurses 'Always' Communicated Well	300+	81%	-	76%
Pain 'Always' Well Controlled	300+	72%	-	69%
Room and Bathroom 'Always' Clean	300+	77%	-	71%
Timely Help 'Always' Received	300+	66%	-	64%
Would Definitely Recommend Hospital	300+	81%	-	69%

Prince William Hospital

8700 Sudley Rd
Manassas, VA 20110
URL: www.pwhs.org
Type: Acute Care Hospitals
Ownership: Voluntary Non-Profit - Other

Phone: 703-369-8000
Fax: 703-369-8010

Emergency Services: Yes
Beds: 170

Key Personnel:
CEO/President . . . . Michael J Schwartz, MD
Chief of Medical Staff . . . . Vikram Khot, MD
Operating Room . . . . Beatrice Holt, RN
Pediatric Ambulatory Care . . . . . Marc Krenytzky
Quality Assurance . . . . Ginny Blairk
Radiology . . . . Namik Erdag
Emergency Room . . . . Ayan H Ahmed, MD
Patient Relations . . . . Sandy Rigsbee

Measure	Cases	This Hosp.	State Avg.	U.S. Avg.
Heart Attack Care				
ACE Inhibitor or ARB for LVSD[1]	11	91%	97%	96%
Aspirin at Arrival	84	96%	99%	99%
Aspirin at Discharge	29	100%	99%	98%
Beta Blocker at Discharge	33	100%	99%	98%
Fibrinolytic Medication Timing[1]	1	0%	75%	55%
PCI Within 90 Minutes of Arrival	0	-	93%	90%
Smoking Cessation Advice[1]	10	90%	100%	99%
Chest Pain/Possible Heart Attack Care				
Aspirin at Arrival	153	96%	95%	95%
Median Time to ECG (minutes)	161	5	8	8
Median Time to Transfer (minutes)	33	43	60	61
Fibrinolytic Medication Timing[1]	1	100%	59%	54%
Heart Failure Care				
ACE Inhibitor or ARB for LVSD	48	94%	97%	94%
Discharge Instructions	112	80%	92%	88%
Evaluation of LVS Function	133	99%	99%	98%
Smoking Cessation Advice	25	100%	99%	98%
Pneumonia Care				
Appropriate Initial Antibiotic	130	92%	93%	92%
Blood Culture Timing	223	97%	97%	96%
Influenza Vaccine	122	89%	94%	91%
Initial Antibiotic Timing	187	98%	96%	95%
Pneumococcal Vaccine	167	96%	95%	93%
Smoking Cessation Advice	70	90%	98%	97%
Surgical Care Improvement Project				
Appropriate VTP Within 24 Hours[2]	117	87%	94%	92%
Appropriate Hair Removal[2]	536	100%	100%	99%
Appropriate Beta Blocker Usage[2]	118	95%	94%	93%
Controlled Postoperative Blood Glucose[2]	0	-	96%	93%
Prophylactic Antibiotic Timing[2]	373	98%	97%	97%
Prophylactic Antibiotic Timing (Outpatient)	439	93%	93%	92%
Prophylactic Antibiotic Selection[2]	376	98%	98%	97%
Prophylactic Antibiotic Select. (Outpatient)	421	97%	96%	94%
Prophylactic Antibiotic Stopped[2]	367	96%	96%	94%
Recommended VTP Ordered[2]	118	92%	96%	94%
Urinary Catheter Removal[2]	123	99%	93%	90%
Children's Asthma Care				
Received Systemic Corticosteroids	-	-	-	100%
Received Home Management Plan	-	-	-	71%
Received Reliever Medication	-	-	-	100%
Use of Medical Imaging				
Combination Abdominal CT Scan	914	0.074	0.144	0.191
Combination Chest CT Scan	591	0.014	0.030	0.054
Follow-up Mammogram/Ultrasound	1,023	10.3%	7.5%	8.4%
MRI for Low Back Pain	195	31.3%	31.5%	32.7%
Survey of Patients' Hospital Experiences				
Area Around Room 'Always' Quiet at Night	300+	52%	-	58%
Doctors 'Always' Communicated Well	300+	79%	-	80%
Home Recovery Information Given	300+	84%	-	82%
Hospital Given 9 or 10 on 10 Point Scale	300+	65%	-	67%
Meds 'Always' Explained Before Given	300+	53%	-	60%
Nurses 'Always' Communicated Well	300+	74%	-	76%
Pain 'Always' Well Controlled	300+	70%	-	69%
Room and Bathroom 'Always' Clean	300+	72%	-	71%
Timely Help 'Always' Received	300+	59%	-	64%
Would Definitely Recommend Hospital	300+	68%	-	69%

Smyth County Community Hospital

565 Radio Hill Road
Marion, VA 24354
URL: www.scchosp.org
Type: Acute Care Hospitals
Ownership: Voluntary Non-Profit - Other

Phone: 276-782-1234
Fax: 276-782-1436

Emergency Services: Yes
Beds: 50

Key Personnel:
CEO/President . . . . Houston Bell
Quality Assurance . . . . Tim Anderson
Radiology . . . . Wesley L Asbury Jr
Emergency Room . . . . James Paterson

Measure	Cases	This Hosp.	State Avg.	U.S. Avg.
Heart Attack Care				
ACE Inhibitor or ARB for LVSD[1,2,3]	6	83%	97%	96%
Aspirin at Arrival[1,2,3]	15	100%	99%	99%
Aspirin at Discharge[1,2,3]	10	100%	99%	98%
Beta Blocker at Discharge[1,2,3]	11	100%	99%	98%
Fibrinolytic Medication Timing[2,3]	0	-	75%	55%
PCI Within 90 Minutes of Arrival[2,3]	0	-	93%	90%
Smoking Cessation Advice[1,2,3]	1	100%	100%	99%
Chest Pain/Possible Heart Attack Care				
Aspirin at Arrival	39	95%	95%	95%
Median Time to ECG (minutes)	41	21	8	8
Median Time to Transfer (minutes)[5]	0	-	60	61
Fibrinolytic Medication Timing[1]	5	20%	59%	54%
Heart Failure Care				
ACE Inhibitor or ARB for LVSD[1,2]	20	90%	97%	94%
Discharge Instructions[2]	50	78%	92%	88%
Evaluation of LVS Function[2]	68	99%	99%	98%
Smoking Cessation Advice[1,2]	11	82%	99%	98%
Pneumonia Care				
Appropriate Initial Antibiotic[2]	81	91%	93%	92%
Blood Culture Timing[2]	76	99%	97%	96%
Influenza Vaccine[2]	73	100%	94%	91%
Initial Antibiotic Timing[2]	116	98%	96%	95%
Pneumococcal Vaccine[2]	89	100%	95%	93%
Smoking Cessation Advice[2]	48	92%	98%	97%
Surgical Care Improvement Project				
Appropriate VTP Within 24 Hours[2]	66	88%	94%	92%
Appropriate Hair Removal[2]	175	100%	100%	99%
Appropriate Beta Blocker Usage[2]	33	97%	94%	93%
Controlled Postoperative Blood Glucose[2]	0	-	96%	93%
Prophylactic Antibiotic Timing[2]	126	98%	97%	97%
Prophylactic Antibiotic Timing (Outpatient)	49	82%	93%	92%
Prophylactic Antibiotic Selection[2]	126	99%	98%	97%
Prophylactic Antibiotic Select. (Outpatient)	40	95%	96%	94%
Prophylactic Antibiotic Stopped[2]	123	94%	96%	94%
Recommended VTP Ordered[2]	66	88%	96%	94%
Urinary Catheter Removal[1,2]	22	95%	93%	90%
Children's Asthma Care				
Received Systemic Corticosteroids	-	-	-	100%
Received Home Management Plan	-	-	-	71%
Received Reliever Medication	-	-	-	100%
Use of Medical Imaging				
Combination Abdominal CT Scan	377	0.560	0.144	0.191
Combination Chest CT Scan	229	0.004	0.030	0.054
Follow-up Mammogram/Ultrasound	578	17.1%	7.5%	8.4%
MRI for Low Back Pain	79	43.0%	31.5%	32.7%
Survey of Patients' Hospital Experiences				
Area Around Room 'Always' Quiet at Night	300+	54%	-	58%
Doctors 'Always' Communicated Well	300+	75%	-	80%
Home Recovery Information Given	300+	79%	-	82%
Hospital Given 9 or 10 on 10 Point Scale	300+	56%	-	67%
Meds 'Always' Explained Before Given	300+	62%	-	60%
Nurses 'Always' Communicated Well	300+	76%	-	76%
Pain 'Always' Well Controlled	300+	66%	-	69%
Room and Bathroom 'Always' Clean	300+	72%	-	71%
Timely Help 'Always' Received	300+	66%	-	64%
Would Definitely Recommend Hospital	300+	53%	-	69%

NOTE: Hospital profiles are in alphabetical order by state, then city, then hospital within the city; Rankings exclude hospitals with less than 25 cases except for patient surveys which excludes hospitals with less than 100 cases; (a) 100-299 cases; (1) The number of cases is too small to be sure how well a hospital is performing; (2) The hospital indicated that the data submitted for this measure were based on a sample of cases; (3) Data was collected during a shorter time period (fewer quarters) than the maximum possible time for this measure; (4) Suppressed for one or more quarters by CMS; (5) No data is available from the hospital for this measure; (6) Fewer than 100 patients completed the HCAHPS survey. Use these rates with caution, as the number of surveys may be too low to reliably assess hospital performance; (7) Survey results are based on less than 12 months of data; (8) Survey results are not available for this reporting period; (9) No or very few patients were eligible for the HCAHPS survey. The scores shown, if any, reflect a very small number of surveys; (10) A state average was not calculated because too few hospitals in the state submitted data; (11) There were discrepancies in the data collection process; Please refer to the User's Guide for a full explanation of data.

Southwestern Virginia Mental Health Institute

340 Bagley Circle Phone: 276-783-1217
Marion, VA 24354 Fax: 276-783-9712
URL: www.swvmhi.state.va.us
Type: Acute Care Hospitals Emergency Services: Yes
Ownership: Government - State Beds: 176

Key Personnel:
CEO/President.............. Cynthia McLure
Chief of Medical Staff.......... Donna Rigolrvo
Infection Control.............. Pam Rolen, RN
Quality Assurance .... Philip Jones

Measure	Cases	This Hosp.	State Avg.	U.S. Avg.
Heart Attack Care				
ACE Inhibitor or ARB for LVSD[5]	0	-	97%	96%
Aspirin at Arrival[5]	0	-	99%	99%
Aspirin at Discharge[5]	0	-	99%	98%
Beta Blocker at Discharge[5]	0	-	99%	98%
Fibrinolytic Medication Timing[5]	0	-	75%	55%
PCI Within 90 Minutes of Arrival[5]	0	-	93%	90%
Smoking Cessation Advice[5]	0	-	100%	99%
Chest Pain/Possible Heart Attack Care				
Aspirin at Arrival	-	-	95%	95%
Median Time to ECG (minutes)	-	-	8	8
Median Time to Transfer (minutes)	-	-	60	61
Fibrinolytic Medication Timing	-	-	59%	54%
Heart Failure Care				
ACE Inhibitor or ARB for LVSD[5]	0	-	97%	94%
Discharge Instructions[5]	0	-	92%	88%
Evaluation of LVS Function[5]	0	-	99%	98%
Smoking Cessation Advice[5]	0	-	99%	98%
Pneumonia Care				
Appropriate Initial Antibiotic[5]	0	-	93%	92%
Blood Culture Timing[5]	0	-	97%	96%
Influenza Vaccine[5]	0	-	94%	91%
Initial Antibiotic Timing[5]	0	-	96%	95%
Pneumococcal Vaccine[5]	0	-	95%	93%
Smoking Cessation Advice[5]	0	-	98%	97%
Surgical Care Improvement Project				
Appropriate VTP Within 24 Hours[5]	0	-	94%	92%
Appropriate Hair Removal[5]	0	-	100%	99%
Appropriate Beta Blocker Usage[5]	0	-	94%	93%
Controlled Postoperative Blood Glucose[5]	0	-	96%	93%
Prophylactic Antibiotic Timing[5]	0	-	97%	97%
Prophylactic Antibiotic Timing (Outpatient)	-	-	93%	92%
Prophylactic Antibiotic Selection[5]	0	-	98%	97%
Prophylactic Antibiotic Select. (Outpatient)	-	-	96%	94%
Prophylactic Antibiotic Stopped[5]	0	-	96%	94%
Recommended VTP Ordered[5]	0	-	96%	94%
Urinary Catheter Removal[5]	0	-	93%	90%
Children's Asthma Care				
Received Systemic Corticosteroids	-	-	-	100%
Received Home Management Plan	-	-	-	71%
Received Reliever Medication	-	-	-	100%
Use of Medical Imaging				
Combination Abdominal CT Scan	-	-	0.144	0.191
Combination Chest CT Scan	-	-	0.030	0.054
Follow-up Mammogram/Ultrasound	-	-	7.5%	8.4%
MRI for Low Back Pain	-	-	31.5%	32.7%
Survey of Patients' Hospital Experiences				
Area Around Room 'Always' Quiet at Night[8]	-	-	-	58%
Doctors 'Always' Communicated Well[8]	-	-	-	80%
Home Recovery Information Given[8]	-	-	-	82%
Hospital Given 9 or 10 on 10 Point Scale[8]	-	-	-	67%
Meds 'Always' Explained Before Given[8]	-	-	-	60%
Nurses 'Always' Communicated Well[8]	-	-	-	76%
Pain 'Always' Well Controlled[8]	-	-	-	69%
Room and Bathroom 'Always' Clean[8]	-	-	-	71%
Timely Help 'Always' Received[8]	-	-	-	64%
Would Definitely Recommend Hospital[8]	-	-	-	69%

Memorial Hospital of Martinsville & Henry County

320 Hospital Drive Phone: 276-666-7200
Martinsville, VA 24115 Fax: 276-666-7600
E-mail: info@mhmhc.com
URL: www.martinsvillehospital.com
Type: Acute Care Hospitals Emergency Services: No
Ownership: Proprietary Beds: 220

Key Personnel:
CEO/President.............. Joseph Roach
Chief of Medical Staff.......... LS Poirer, MD
Coronary Care.............. Martha Holland, RN BSN
Infection Control............ Faye Sedwick, RN MSN
Operating Room............ Thomas K Berry, RN
Quality Assurance .... Peggy Tunnell, RN
Radiology.................. Leonard S Poirier

Measure	Cases	This Hosp.	State Avg.	U.S. Avg.
Heart Attack Care				
ACE Inhibitor or ARB for LVSD[1]	8	100%	97%	96%
Aspirin at Arrival	68	96%	99%	99%
Aspirin at Discharge	50	100%	99%	98%
Beta Blocker at Discharge	52	98%	99%	98%
Fibrinolytic Medication Timing	0	-	75%	55%
PCI Within 90 Minutes of Arrival[1]	10	80%	93%	90%
Smoking Cessation Advice[1]	22	100%	100%	99%
Chest Pain/Possible Heart Attack Care				
Aspirin at Arrival	174	95%	95%	95%
Median Time to ECG (minutes)	179	11	8	8
Median Time to Transfer (minutes)[1]	13	158	60	61
Fibrinolytic Medication Timing[1]	11	36%	59%	54%
Heart Failure Care				
ACE Inhibitor or ARB for LVSD	93	97%	97%	94%
Discharge Instructions	195	78%	92%	88%
Evaluation of LVS Function	253	100%	99%	98%
Smoking Cessation Advice	56	100%	99%	98%
Pneumonia Care				
Appropriate Initial Antibiotic	109	94%	93%	92%
Blood Culture Timing	184	96%	97%	96%
Influenza Vaccine	111	99%	94%	91%
Initial Antibiotic Timing	158	96%	96%	95%
Pneumococcal Vaccine	164	99%	95%	93%
Smoking Cessation Advice	93	100%	98%	97%
Surgical Care Improvement Project				
Appropriate VTP Within 24 Hours	124	81%	94%	92%
Appropriate Hair Removal	299	100%	100%	99%
Appropriate Beta Blocker Usage	78	99%	94%	93%
Controlled Postoperative Blood Glucose	0	-	96%	93%
Prophylactic Antibiotic Timing	179	94%	97%	97%
Prophylactic Antibiotic Timing (Outpatient)	175	93%	93%	92%
Prophylactic Antibiotic Selection	182	96%	98%	97%
Prophylactic Antibiotic Select. (Outpatient)	168	97%	96%	94%
Prophylactic Antibiotic Stopped	160	95%	96%	94%
Recommended VTP Ordered	130	80%	96%	94%
Urinary Catheter Removal	44	91%	93%	90%
Children's Asthma Care				
Received Systemic Corticosteroids	-	-	-	100%
Received Home Management Plan	-	-	-	71%
Received Reliever Medication	-	-	-	100%
Use of Medical Imaging				
Combination Abdominal CT Scan	719	0.076	0.144	0.191
Combination Chest CT Scan	440	0.032	0.030	0.054
Follow-up Mammogram/Ultrasound	2,087	3.1%	7.5%	8.4%
MRI for Low Back Pain	161	42.9%	31.5%	32.7%
Survey of Patients' Hospital Experiences				
Area Around Room 'Always' Quiet at Night	300+	53%	-	58%
Doctors 'Always' Communicated Well	300+	81%	-	80%
Home Recovery Information Given	300+	83%	-	82%
Hospital Given 9 or 10 on 10 Point Scale	300+	58%	-	67%
Meds 'Always' Explained Before Given	300+	54%	-	60%
Nurses 'Always' Communicated Well	300+	71%	-	76%
Pain 'Always' Well Controlled	300+	65%	-	69%
Room and Bathroom 'Always' Clean	300+	65%	-	71%
Timely Help 'Always' Received	300+	62%	-	64%
Would Definitely Recommend Hospital	300+	53%	-	69%

Bon Secours - Memorial Regional Medical

8260 Atlee Road Phone: 804-764-6000
Mechanicsville, VA 23116 Fax: 804-764-6420
URL: www.bonsecours.com
Type: Acute Care Hospitals Emergency Services: No
Ownership: Voluntary Non-Profit - Church Beds: 225

Key Personnel:
CEO/President................ Michael Robinson
Cardiac Laboratory............ Timothy W Hagemann, MD
Chief of Medical Staff.......... John Bowman
Radiology.................... Todd B Baird
Emergency Room .... William Azzie

Measure	Cases	This Hosp.	State Avg.	U.S. Avg.
Heart Attack Care				
ACE Inhibitor or ARB for LVSD[2]	88	100%	97%	96%
Aspirin at Arrival[2]	323	100%	99%	99%
Aspirin at Discharge[2]	319	100%	99%	98%
Beta Blocker at Discharge[2]	308	100%	99%	98%
Fibrinolytic Medication Timing[2]	0	-	75%	55%
PCI Within 90 Minutes of Arrival[2]	60	95%	93%	90%
Smoking Cessation Advice[2]	96	100%	100%	99%
Chest Pain/Possible Heart Attack Care				
Aspirin at Arrival[1]	4	100%	95%	95%
Median Time to ECG (minutes)[1]	4	4	8	8
Median Time to Transfer (minutes)[5]	0	-	60	61
Fibrinolytic Medication Timing[5]	0	-	59%	54%
Heart Failure Care				
ACE Inhibitor or ARB for LVSD[2]	120	100%	97%	94%
Discharge Instructions[2]	293	100%	92%	88%
Evaluation of LVS Function[2]	353	100%	99%	98%
Smoking Cessation Advice[2]	54	100%	99%	98%
Pneumonia Care				
Appropriate Initial Antibiotic[2]	162	100%	93%	92%
Blood Culture Timing[2]	244	98%	97%	96%
Influenza Vaccine[2]	118	96%	94%	91%
Initial Antibiotic Timing[2]	230	100%	96%	95%
Pneumococcal Vaccine[2]	178	98%	95%	93%
Smoking Cessation Advice[2]	72	100%	98%	97%
Surgical Care Improvement Project				
Appropriate VTP Within 24 Hours[2]	308	97%	94%	92%
Appropriate Hair Removal[2]	1,049	100%	100%	99%
Appropriate Beta Blocker Usage[2]	326	100%	94%	93%
Controlled Postoperative Blood Glucose[2]	177	98%	96%	93%
Prophylactic Antibiotic Timing[2]	764	99%	97%	97%
Prophylactic Antibiotic Timing (Outpatient)	460	94%	93%	92%
Prophylactic Antibiotic Selection[2]	763	99%	98%	97%
Prophylactic Antibiotic Select. (Outpatient)	455	97%	96%	94%
Prophylactic Antibiotic Stopped[2]	733	98%	96%	94%
Recommended VTP Ordered[2]	308	98%	96%	94%
Urinary Catheter Removal[2]	347	97%	93%	90%
Children's Asthma Care				
Received Systemic Corticosteroids	-	-	-	100%
Received Home Management Plan	-	-	-	71%
Received Reliever Medication	-	-	-	100%
Use of Medical Imaging				
Combination Abdominal CT Scan	1,472	0.139	0.144	0.191
Combination Chest CT Scan	843	0.006	0.030	0.054
Follow-up Mammogram/Ultrasound	2,636	7.4%	7.5%	8.4%
MRI for Low Back Pain	362	28.7%	31.5%	32.7%
Survey of Patients' Hospital Experiences				
Area Around Room 'Always' Quiet at Night	300+	57%	-	58%
Doctors 'Always' Communicated Well	300+	84%	-	80%
Home Recovery Information Given	300+	86%	-	82%
Hospital Given 9 or 10 on 10 Point Scale	300+	74%	-	67%
Meds 'Always' Explained Before Given	300+	59%	-	60%
Nurses 'Always' Communicated Well	300+	80%	-	76%
Pain 'Always' Well Controlled	300+	74%	-	69%
Room and Bathroom 'Always' Clean	300+	66%	-	71%
Timely Help 'Always' Received	300+	69%	-	64%
Would Definitely Recommend Hospital	300+	78%	-	69%

NOTE: Hospital profiles are in alphabetical order by state, then city, then hospital within the city; Rankings exclude hospitals with less than 25 cases except for patient surveys which excludes hospitals with less than 100 cases; (a) 100–299 cases; (1) The number of cases is too small to be sure how well a hospital is performing; (2) The hospital indicated that the data submitted for this measure were based on a sample of cases; (3) Data was collected during a shorter time period (fewer quarters) than the maximum possible time for this measure; (4) Suppressed for one or more quarters by CMS; (5) No data is available from the hospital for this measure; (6) Fewer than 100 patients completed the HCAHPS survey. Use these rates with caution, as the number of surveys may be too low to reliably assess hospital performance; (7) Survey results are based on less than 12 months of data; (8) Survey results are not available for this reporting period; (9) No or very few patients were eligible for the HCAHPS survey. The scores shown, if any, reflect a very small number of surveys; (10) A state average was not calculated because too few hospitals in the state submitted data; (11) There were discrepancies in the data collection process; Please refer to the User's Guide for a full explanation of data.

Bon Secours - St Francis Medical Center

13700 Stfrancis Blvd Suite 100 Phone: 804-594-7400
Midlothian, VA 23114
Type: Acute Care Hospitals Emergency Services: Yes
Ownership: Voluntary Non-Profit - Church
Key Personnel:
CEO/President. . . . . Peter Gallagher

Measure	Cases	This Hosp.	State Avg.	U.S. Avg.
Heart Attack Care				
ACE Inhibitor or ARB for LVSD	29	100%	97%	96%
Aspirin at Arrival	116	99%	99%	99%
Aspirin at Discharge	98	100%	99%	98%
Beta Blocker at Discharge	94	97%	99%	98%
Fibrinolytic Medication Timing	0	-	75%	55%
PCI Within 90 Minutes of Arrival[1]	22	86%	93%	90%
Smoking Cessation Advice	30	100%	100%	99%
Chest Pain/Possible Heart Attack Care				
Aspirin at Arrival[1]	9	89%	95%	95%
Median Time to ECG (minutes)[1]	9	9	8	8
Median Time to Transfer (minutes)[5]	0	-	60	61
Fibrinolytic Medication Timing[3]	0	-	59%	54%
Heart Failure Care				
ACE Inhibitor or ARB for LVSD	58	100%	97%	94%
Discharge Instructions	176	100%	92%	88%
Evaluation of LVS Function	211	99%	99%	98%
Smoking Cessation Advice	26	100%	99%	98%
Pneumonia Care				
Appropriate Initial Antibiotic	129	92%	93%	92%
Blood Culture Timing	183	95%	97%	96%
Influenza Vaccine	76	93%	94%	91%
Initial Antibiotic Timing	163	98%	96%	95%
Pneumococcal Vaccine	118	97%	95%	93%
Smoking Cessation Advice	38	100%	98%	97%
Surgical Care Improvement Project				
Appropriate VTP Within 24 Hours	288	96%	94%	92%
Appropriate Hair Removal	1,020	100%	100%	99%
Appropriate Beta Blocker Usage	228	96%	94%	93%
Controlled Postoperative Blood Glucose	0	-	96%	93%
Prophylactic Antibiotic Timing	721	97%	97%	97%
Prophylactic Antibiotic Timing (Outpatient)	392	94%	93%	92%
Prophylactic Antibiotic Selection	722	98%	98%	97%
Prophylactic Antibiotic Select. (Outpatient)	385	97%	96%	94%
Prophylactic Antibiotic Stopped	699	97%	96%	94%
Recommended VTP Ordered	288	97%	96%	94%
Urinary Catheter Removal	52	85%	93%	90%
Children's Asthma Care				
Received Systemic Corticosteroids	-	-	-	100%
Received Home Management Plan	-	-	-	71%
Received Reliever Medication	-	-	-	100%
Use of Medical Imaging				
Combination Abdominal CT Scan	647	0.267	0.144	0.191
Combination Chest CT Scan	369	0.022	0.030	0.054
Follow-up Mammogram/Ultrasound	457	12.9%	7.5%	8.4%
MRI for Low Back Pain[1]	51	23.5%	31.5%	32.7%
Survey of Patients' Hospital Experiences				
Area Around Room 'Always' Quiet at Night	300+	66%	-	58%
Doctors 'Always' Communicated Well	300+	77%	-	80%
Home Recovery Information Given	300+	86%	-	82%
Hospital Given 9 or 10 on 10 Point Scale	300+	75%	-	67%
Meds 'Always' Explained Before Given	300+	59%	-	60%
Nurses 'Always' Communicated Well	300+	76%	-	76%
Pain 'Always' Well Controlled	300+	69%	-	69%
Room and Bathroom 'Always' Clean	300+	72%	-	71%
Timely Help 'Always' Received	300+	58%	-	64%
Would Definitely Recommend Hospital	300+	78%	-	69%

Riverside Shore Memorial Hospital

9507 Hospital Avenue Phone: 757-414-8000
Nassawadox, VA 23413 Fax: 757-414-8633
E-mail: shorehealth@esva.net
URL: www.shorehealthservices.org
Type: Acute Care Hospitals Emergency Services: Yes
Ownership: Voluntary Non-Profit - Private Beds: 143
Key Personnel:
CEO/President. . . . . Alan Markowitz
Chief of Medical Staff . . . . James L McDaniel, MD
Infection Control. . . . . Sharon Angle
Operating Room. . . . . Otis W Doss, MD
Pediatric Ambulatory Care . . . . . . Cathy Riopel, MD
Pediatric In-Patient Care . . . . Cathy Riopel, MD
Quality Assurance . . . . Sharon Angle
Radiology. . . . . Michael J Bigg, MD

Measure	Cases	This Hosp.	State Avg.	U.S. Avg.
Heart Attack Care				
ACE Inhibitor or ARB for LVSD[1]	3	100%	97%	96%
Aspirin at Arrival[1]	23	100%	99%	99%
Aspirin at Discharge[1]	12	100%	99%	98%
Beta Blocker at Discharge[1]	14	100%	99%	98%
Fibrinolytic Medication Timing	0	-	75%	55%
PCI Within 90 Minutes of Arrival	0	-	93%	90%
Smoking Cessation Advice[1]	2	100%	100%	99%
Chest Pain/Possible Heart Attack Care				
Aspirin at Arrival	36	86%	95%	95%
Median Time to ECG (minutes)	36	15	8	8
Median Time to Transfer (minutes)[1,3]	1	206	60	61
Fibrinolytic Medication Timing	0	-	59%	54%
Heart Failure Care				
ACE Inhibitor or ARB for LVSD	53	100%	97%	94%
Discharge Instructions	112	95%	92%	88%
Evaluation of LVS Function	134	100%	99%	98%
Smoking Cessation Advice	26	100%	99%	98%
Pneumonia Care				
Appropriate Initial Antibiotic	59	95%	93%	92%
Blood Culture Timing	119	99%	97%	96%
Influenza Vaccine	75	95%	94%	91%
Initial Antibiotic Timing	125	95%	96%	95%
Pneumococcal Vaccine	97	94%	95%	93%
Smoking Cessation Advice	33	100%	98%	97%
Surgical Care Improvement Project				
Appropriate VTP Within 24 Hours	30	83%	94%	92%
Appropriate Hair Removal	85	100%	100%	99%
Appropriate Beta Blocker Usage[1]	20	100%	94%	93%
Controlled Postoperative Blood Glucose	0	-	96%	93%
Prophylactic Antibiotic Timing	57	91%	97%	97%
Prophylactic Antibiotic Timing (Outpatient)	31	90%	93%	92%
Prophylactic Antibiotic Selection	59	90%	98%	97%
Prophylactic Antibiotic Select. (Outpatient)	62	94%	96%	94%
Prophylactic Antibiotic Stopped	56	100%	96%	94%
Recommended VTP Ordered	30	83%	96%	94%
Urinary Catheter Removal[1]	15	60%	93%	90%
Children's Asthma Care				
Received Systemic Corticosteroids	-	-	-	100%
Received Home Management Plan	-	-	-	71%
Received Reliever Medication	-	-	-	100%
Use of Medical Imaging				
Combination Abdominal CT Scan	447	0.076	0.144	0.191
Combination Chest CT Scan	322	0.009	0.030	0.054
Follow-up Mammogram/Ultrasound	1,034	3.6%	7.5%	8.4%
MRI for Low Back Pain[1]	32	25.0%	31.5%	32.7%
Survey of Patients' Hospital Experiences				
Area Around Room 'Always' Quiet at Night	300+	52%	-	58%
Doctors 'Always' Communicated Well	300+	85%	-	80%
Home Recovery Information Given	300+	81%	-	82%
Hospital Given 9 or 10 on 10 Point Scale	300+	61%	-	67%
Meds 'Always' Explained Before Given	300+	60%	-	60%
Nurses 'Always' Communicated Well	300+	74%	-	76%
Pain 'Always' Well Controlled	300+	70%	-	69%
Room and Bathroom 'Always' Clean	300+	66%	-	71%
Timely Help 'Always' Received	300+	61%	-	64%
Would Definitely Recommend Hospital	300+	54%	-	69%

Mary Immaculate Hospital

2 Bernardine Drive Phone: 757-886-6768
Newport News, VA 23602 Fax: 757-886-6605
URL: www.bonsecourshamptonroad.com
Type: Acute Care Hospitals Emergency Services: Yes
Ownership: Voluntary Non-Profit - Church Beds: 120
Key Personnel:
CEO/President. . . . . Pat L Robertson
Radiology. . . . . Harry III

Measure	Cases	This Hosp.	State Avg.	U.S. Avg.
Heart Attack Care				
ACE Inhibitor or ARB for LVSD[1]	21	90%	97%	96%
Aspirin at Arrival	93	100%	99%	99%
Aspirin at Discharge	85	98%	99%	98%
Beta Blocker at Discharge	81	98%	99%	98%
Fibrinolytic Medication Timing	0	-	75%	55%
PCI Within 90 Minutes of Arrival[1]	17	94%	93%	90%
Smoking Cessation Advice	29	100%	100%	99%
Chest Pain/Possible Heart Attack Care				
Aspirin at Arrival[1]	6	83%	95%	95%
Median Time to ECG (minutes)[1]	6	46	8	8
Median Time to Transfer (minutes)[3]	0	-	60	61
Fibrinolytic Medication Timing[3]	0	-	59%	54%
Heart Failure Care				
ACE Inhibitor or ARB for LVSD	74	99%	97%	94%
Discharge Instructions	142	94%	92%	88%
Evaluation of LVS Function	173	99%	99%	98%
Smoking Cessation Advice	27	100%	99%	98%
Pneumonia Care				
Appropriate Initial Antibiotic	84	90%	93%	92%
Blood Culture Timing	160	98%	97%	96%
Influenza Vaccine	79	99%	94%	91%
Initial Antibiotic Timing	163	96%	96%	95%
Pneumococcal Vaccine	103	98%	95%	93%
Smoking Cessation Advice	30	100%	98%	97%
Surgical Care Improvement Project				
Appropriate VTP Within 24 Hours[2]	159	89%	94%	92%
Appropriate Hair Removal[2]	1,451	100%	100%	99%
Appropriate Beta Blocker Usage[2]	332	99%	94%	93%
Controlled Postoperative Blood Glucose[2]	0	-	96%	93%
Prophylactic Antibiotic Timing[2]	1,292	96%	97%	97%
Prophylactic Antibiotic Timing (Outpatient)	283	85%	93%	92%
Prophylactic Antibiotic Selection[2]	1,295	99%	98%	97%
Prophylactic Antibiotic Select. (Outpatient)	273	93%	96%	94%
Prophylactic Antibiotic Stopped[2]	1,263	96%	96%	94%
Recommended VTP Ordered[2]	159	91%	96%	94%
Urinary Catheter Removal[2]	57	100%	93%	90%
Children's Asthma Care				
Received Systemic Corticosteroids	-	-	-	100%
Received Home Management Plan	-	-	-	71%
Received Reliever Medication	-	-	-	100%
Use of Medical Imaging				
Combination Abdominal CT Scan	366	0.060	0.144	0.191
Combination Chest CT Scan	165	0.048	0.030	0.054
Follow-up Mammogram/Ultrasound	476	8.2%	7.5%	8.4%
MRI for Low Back Pain	70	24.3%	31.5%	32.7%
Survey of Patients' Hospital Experiences				
Area Around Room 'Always' Quiet at Night	300+	64%	-	58%
Doctors 'Always' Communicated Well	300+	79%	-	80%
Home Recovery Information Given	300+	84%	-	82%
Hospital Given 9 or 10 on 10 Point Scale	300+	59%	-	67%
Meds 'Always' Explained Before Given	300+	56%	-	60%
Nurses 'Always' Communicated Well	300+	69%	-	76%
Pain 'Always' Well Controlled	300+	66%	-	69%
Room and Bathroom 'Always' Clean	300+	56%	-	71%
Timely Help 'Always' Received	300+	51%	-	64%
Would Definitely Recommend Hospital	300+	65%	-	69%

NOTE: Hospital profiles are in alphabetical order by state, then city, then hospital within the city; Rankings exclude hospitals with less than 25 cases except for patient surveys which excludes hospitals with less than 100 cases; (a) 100–299 cases; (1) The number of cases is too small to be sure how well a hospital is performing; (2) The hospital indicated that the data submitted for this measure were based on a sample of cases; (3) Data was collected during a shorter time period (fewer quarters) than the maximum possible time for this measure; (4) Suppressed for one or more quarters by CMS; (5) No data is available from the hospital for this measure; (6) Fewer than 100 patients completed the HCAHPS survey. Use these rates with caution, as the number of surveys may be too low to reliably assess hospital performance; (7) Survey results are based on less than 12 months of data; (8) Survey results are not available for this reporting period; (9) No or very few patients were eligible for the HCAHPS survey. The scores shown, if any, reflect a very small number of surveys; (10) A state average was not calculated because too few hospitals in the state submitted data; (11) There were discrepancies in the data collection process; Please refer to the User's Guide for a full explanation of data.

Riverside Regional Medical Center

500 J Clyde Morris Blvd
Newport News, VA 23601
URL: www.riversideonline.com
Type: Acute Care Hospitals
Ownership: Voluntary Non-Profit - Private
Phone: 757-594-2000
Fax: 757-594-3864
Emergency Services: No
Beds: 576

Key Personnel:
CEO/President. . . . . Richard J Pearce
Chief of Medical Staff. . . . . Dr Barry Gross
Coronary Care . . . . Donna Haughinberry
Operating Room. . . . . Sheila Rilee
Quality Assurance . . . . Jody Friend
Radiology. . . . . Paula Burcher
Intensive Care Unit. . . . . Donna Haughinberry
Patient Relations . . . . Medford Ramey

Measure	Cases	This Hosp.	State Avg.	U.S. Avg.
Heart Attack Care				
ACE Inhibitor or ARB for LVSD	52	100%	97%	96%
Aspirin at Arrival	241	100%	99%	99%
Aspirin at Discharge	350	100%	99%	98%
Beta Blocker at Discharge	342	100%	99%	98%
Fibrinolytic Medication Timing	0	-	75%	55%
PCI Within 90 Minutes of Arrival	36	92%	93%	90%
Smoking Cessation Advice	129	100%	100%	99%
Chest Pain/Possible Heart Attack Care				
Aspirin at Arrival[1,3]	2	100%	95%	95%
Median Time to ECG (minutes)[1,3]	2	5	8	8
Median Time to Transfer (minutes)[5]	0	-	60	61
Fibrinolytic Medication Timing[5]	0	-	59%	54%
Heart Failure Care				
ACE Inhibitor or ARB for LVSD	166	100%	97%	94%
Discharge Instructions	361	94%	92%	88%
Evaluation of LVS Function	442	100%	99%	98%
Smoking Cessation Advice	89	100%	99%	98%
Pneumonia Care				
Appropriate Initial Antibiotic	119	95%	93%	92%
Blood Culture Timing	231	97%	97%	96%
Influenza Vaccine	135	98%	94%	91%
Initial Antibiotic Timing	209	95%	96%	95%
Pneumococcal Vaccine	185	99%	95%	93%
Smoking Cessation Advice	80	100%	98%	97%
Surgical Care Improvement Project				
Appropriate VTP Within 24 Hours[2]	189	94%	94%	92%
Appropriate Hair Removal[2]	577	100%	100%	99%
Appropriate Beta Blocker Usage[2]	175	95%	94%	93%
Controlled Postoperative Blood Glucose[2]	97	97%	96%	93%
Prophylactic Antibiotic Timing[2]	405	99%	97%	97%
Prophylactic Antibiotic Timing (Outpatient)	588	98%	93%	92%
Prophylactic Antibiotic Selection[2]	409	99%	98%	97%
Prophylactic Antibiotic Select. (Outpatient)	583	97%	96%	94%
Prophylactic Antibiotic Stopped[2]	392	97%	96%	94%
Recommended VTP Ordered[2]	189	94%	96%	94%
Urinary Catheter Removal[2]	118	97%	93%	90%
Children's Asthma Care				
Received Systemic Corticosteroids	-	-	-	100%
Received Home Management Plan	-	-	-	71%
Received Reliever Medication	-	-	-	100%
Use of Medical Imaging				
Combination Abdominal CT Scan	1,839	0.117	0.144	0.191
Combination Chest CT Scan	1,627	0.023	0.030	0.054
Follow-up Mammogram/Ultrasound	2,204	8.1%	7.5%	8.4%
MRI for Low Back Pain	277	26.4%	31.5%	32.7%
Survey of Patients' Hospital Experiences				
Area Around Room 'Always' Quiet at Night	300+	45%	-	58%
Doctors 'Always' Communicated Well	300+	76%	-	80%
Home Recovery Information Given	300+	81%	-	82%
Hospital Given 9 or 10 on 10 Point Scale	300+	60%	-	67%
Meds 'Always' Explained Before Given	300+	54%	-	60%
Nurses 'Always' Communicated Well	300+	69%	-	76%
Pain 'Always' Well Controlled	300+	66%	-	69%
Room and Bathroom 'Always' Clean	300+	61%	-	71%
Timely Help 'Always' Received	300+	52%	-	64%
Would Definitely Recommend Hospital	300+	63%	-	69%

Bon Secours - Depaul Medical Center

150 Kingsley Lane
Norfolk, VA 23505
URL: www.bonsecourshamptonroads.com
Type: Acute Care Hospitals
Ownership: Voluntary Non-Profit - Church
Phone: 757-889-5000
Fax: 757-489-3450
Emergency Services: Yes
Beds: 189

Key Personnel:
CEO/President. . . . . Susan Erickson
Chief of Medical Staff . . . . Judy Meekins-James
Infection Control. . . . . Jessica Davis
Operating Room. . . . . L D Britt
Quality Assurance . . . . Amy Derion
Radiology. . . . . Harry A Allen, III
Emergency Room . . . . Jane Carty

Measure	Cases	This Hosp.	State Avg.	U.S. Avg.
Heart Attack Care				
ACE Inhibitor or ARB for LVSD[1]	16	94%	97%	96%
Aspirin at Arrival	143	97%	99%	99%
Aspirin at Discharge	127	98%	99%	98%
Beta Blocker at Discharge	129	89%	99%	98%
Fibrinolytic Medication Timing	0	-	75%	55%
PCI Within 90 Minutes of Arrival	28	82%	93%	90%
Smoking Cessation Advice	51	100%	100%	99%
Chest Pain/Possible Heart Attack Care				
Aspirin at Arrival[1]	14	86%	95%	95%
Median Time to ECG (minutes)[1]	15	0	8	8
Median Time to Transfer (minutes)[5]	0	-	60	61
Fibrinolytic Medication Timing[3]	0	-	59%	54%
Heart Failure Care				
ACE Inhibitor or ARB for LVSD	70	96%	97%	94%
Discharge Instructions	190	95%	92%	88%
Evaluation of LVS Function	252	99%	99%	98%
Smoking Cessation Advice	56	98%	99%	98%
Pneumonia Care				
Appropriate Initial Antibiotic	78	86%	93%	92%
Blood Culture Timing	129	98%	97%	96%
Influenza Vaccine	85	100%	94%	91%
Initial Antibiotic Timing	131	97%	96%	95%
Pneumococcal Vaccine	111	97%	95%	93%
Smoking Cessation Advice	49	100%	98%	97%
Surgical Care Improvement Project				
Appropriate VTP Within 24 Hours[2]	152	94%	94%	92%
Appropriate Hair Removal[2]	406	100%	100%	99%
Appropriate Beta Blocker Usage[2]	87	92%	94%	93%
Controlled Postoperative Blood Glucose[2]	0	-	96%	93%
Prophylactic Antibiotic Timing[2]	280	99%	97%	97%
Prophylactic Antibiotic Timing (Outpatient)	358	97%	93%	92%
Prophylactic Antibiotic Selection[2]	280	96%	98%	97%
Prophylactic Antibiotic Select. (Outpatient)	353	98%	96%	94%
Prophylactic Antibiotic Stopped[2]	265	95%	96%	94%
Recommended VTP Ordered[2]	153	95%	96%	94%
Urinary Catheter Removal[2]	39	90%	93%	90%
Children's Asthma Care				
Received Systemic Corticosteroids	-	-	-	100%
Received Home Management Plan	-	-	-	71%
Received Reliever Medication	-	-	-	100%
Use of Medical Imaging				
Combination Abdominal CT Scan	793	0.149	0.144	0.191
Combination Chest CT Scan	718	0.003	0.030	0.054
Follow-up Mammogram/Ultrasound	1,458	5.7%	7.5%	8.4%
MRI for Low Back Pain	169	28.4%	31.5%	32.7%
Survey of Patients' Hospital Experiences				
Area Around Room 'Always' Quiet at Night	300+	61%	-	58%
Doctors 'Always' Communicated Well	300+	78%	-	80%
Home Recovery Information Given	300+	85%	-	82%
Hospital Given 9 or 10 on 10 Point Scale	300+	63%	-	67%
Meds 'Always' Explained Before Given	300+	57%	-	60%
Nurses 'Always' Communicated Well	300+	70%	-	76%
Pain 'Always' Well Controlled	300+	68%	-	69%
Room and Bathroom 'Always' Clean	300+	68%	-	71%
Timely Help 'Always' Received	300+	61%	-	64%
Would Definitely Recommend Hospital	300+	66%	-	69%

Sentara Leigh Hospital

830 Kempsville Road
Norfolk, VA 23502
URL: www.sentara.com
Type: Acute Care Hospitals
Ownership: Voluntary Non-Profit - Other
Phone: 757-261-6601
Fax: 757-455-7164
Emergency Services: Yes
Beds: 250

Key Personnel:
CEO/President. . . . . Darlene Anderson
Chief of Medical Staff . . . . John Hurre, MD
Operating Room. . . . . Lisa Rogers
Quality Assurance . . . . Sam Byrd

Measure	Cases	This Hosp.	State Avg.	U.S. Avg.
Heart Attack Care				
ACE Inhibitor or ARB for LVSD[1]	16	88%	97%	96%
Aspirin at Arrival	110	99%	99%	99%
Aspirin at Discharge	83	99%	99%	98%
Beta Blocker at Discharge	80	100%	99%	98%
Fibrinolytic Medication Timing	0	-	75%	55%
PCI Within 90 Minutes of Arrival	33	94%	93%	90%
Smoking Cessation Advice	29	100%	100%	99%
Chest Pain/Possible Heart Attack Care				
Aspirin at Arrival[1]	16	100%	95%	95%
Median Time to ECG (minutes)[1]	16	10	8	8
Median Time to Transfer (minutes)[5]	0	-	60	61
Fibrinolytic Medication Timing	0	-	59%	54%
Heart Failure Care				
ACE Inhibitor or ARB for LVSD	147	95%	97%	94%
Discharge Instructions	345	99%	92%	88%
Evaluation of LVS Function	425	100%	99%	98%
Smoking Cessation Advice	75	99%	99%	98%
Pneumonia Care				
Appropriate Initial Antibiotic	141	96%	93%	92%
Blood Culture Timing	284	98%	97%	96%
Influenza Vaccine	205	93%	94%	91%
Initial Antibiotic Timing	272	96%	96%	95%
Pneumococcal Vaccine	247	95%	95%	93%
Smoking Cessation Advice	105	99%	98%	97%
Surgical Care Improvement Project				
Appropriate VTP Within 24 Hours[2]	818	99%	94%	92%
Appropriate Hair Removal[2]	1,879	99%	100%	99%
Appropriate Beta Blocker Usage[2]	452	91%	94%	93%
Controlled Postoperative Blood Glucose[2]	0	-	96%	93%
Prophylactic Antibiotic Timing[2]	1,673	98%	97%	97%
Prophylactic Antibiotic Timing (Outpatient)	363	97%	93%	92%
Prophylactic Antibiotic Selection[2]	1,674	97%	98%	97%
Prophylactic Antibiotic Select. (Outpatient)	354	95%	96%	94%
Prophylactic Antibiotic Stopped[2]	1,655	98%	96%	94%
Recommended VTP Ordered[2]	820	99%	96%	94%
Urinary Catheter Removal[2]	674	98%	93%	90%
Children's Asthma Care				
Received Systemic Corticosteroids	-	-	-	100%
Received Home Management Plan	-	-	-	71%
Received Reliever Medication	-	-	-	100%
Use of Medical Imaging				
Combination Abdominal CT Scan	1,835	0.126	0.144	0.191
Combination Chest CT Scan	1,671	0.007	0.030	0.054
Follow-up Mammogram/Ultrasound	2,507	7.9%	7.5%	8.4%
MRI for Low Back Pain	221	27.1%	31.5%	32.7%
Survey of Patients' Hospital Experiences				
Area Around Room 'Always' Quiet at Night	300+	45%	-	58%
Doctors 'Always' Communicated Well	300+	73%	-	80%
Home Recovery Information Given	300+	84%	-	82%
Hospital Given 9 or 10 on 10 Point Scale	300+	65%	-	67%
Meds 'Always' Explained Before Given	300+	56%	-	60%
Nurses 'Always' Communicated Well	300+	68%	-	76%
Pain 'Always' Well Controlled	300+	63%	-	69%
Room and Bathroom 'Always' Clean	300+	59%	-	71%
Timely Help 'Always' Received	300+	56%	-	64%
Would Definitely Recommend Hospital	300+	70%	-	69%

NOTE: Hospital profiles are in alphabetical order by state, then city, then hospital within the city; Rankings exclude hospitals with less than 25 cases except for patient surveys which excludes hospitals with less than 100 cases; (a) 100–299 cases; (1) The number of cases is too small to be sure how well a hospital is performing; (2) The hospital indicated that the data submitted for this measure were based on a sample of cases; (3) Data was collected during a shorter time period (fewer quarters) than the maximum possible time for this measure; (4) Suppressed for one or more quarters by CMS; (5) No data is available from the hospital for this measure; (6) Fewer than 100 patients completed the HCAHPS survey. Use these rates with caution, as the number of surveys may be too low to reliably assess hospital performance; (7) Survey results are based on less than 12 months of data; (8) Survey results are not available for this reporting period; (9) No or very few patients were eligible for the HCAHPS survey. The scores shown, if any, reflect a very small number of surveys; (10) A state average was not calculated because too few hospitals in the state submitted data; (11) There were discrepancies in the data collection process; Please refer to the User's Guide for a full explanation of data.

Sentara Norfolk General Hospital

600 Gresham Dr Phone: 757-388-3000
Norfolk, VA 23507 Fax: 757-455-7555
URL: www.sentara.com
Type: Acute Care Hospitals Emergency Services: Yes
Ownership: Voluntary Non-Profit - Other Beds: 569

Key Personnel:
CEO/President.............. Howard Kern
Cardiac Laboratory............ Matt Rheins
Chief of Medical Staff.......... Leonard Weineter, MD
Infection Control.............. Jackie Butler, RN
Operating Room.............. Pam Robertson
Pediatric Ambulatory Care...... Glen Green, MD
Quality Assurance............ Jaeque Mitchell
Radiology................... Brock Cutchins

Measure	Cases	This Hosp.	State Avg.	U.S. Avg.
Heart Attack Care				
ACE Inhibitor or ARB for LVSD	87	99%	97%	96%
Aspirin at Arrival	133	100%	99%	99%
Aspirin at Discharge	458	99%	99%	98%
Beta Blocker at Discharge	448	99%	99%	98%
Fibrinolytic Medication Timing	0	-	75%	55%
PCI Within 90 Minutes of Arrival[1]	23	87%	93%	90%
Smoking Cessation Advice	165	100%	100%	99%
Chest Pain/Possible Heart Attack Care				
Aspirin at Arrival[1,3]	1	100%	95%	95%
Median Time to ECG (minutes)[1,3]	1	20	8	8
Median Time to Transfer (minutes)[5]	0	-	60	61
Fibrinolytic Medication Timing[5]	0	-	59%	54%
Heart Failure Care				
ACE Inhibitor or ARB for LVSD	345	100%	97%	94%
Discharge Instructions	788	95%	92%	88%
Evaluation of LVS Function	886	100%	99%	98%
Smoking Cessation Advice	193	100%	99%	98%
Pneumonia Care				
Appropriate Initial Antibiotic	107	98%	93%	92%
Blood Culture Timing	211	97%	97%	96%
Influenza Vaccine	151	97%	94%	91%
Initial Antibiotic Timing	241	98%	96%	95%
Pneumococcal Vaccine	175	95%	95%	93%
Smoking Cessation Advice	121	99%	98%	97%
Surgical Care Improvement Project				
Appropriate VTP Within 24 Hours[2]	187	97%	94%	92%
Appropriate Hair Removal[2]	1,401	99%	100%	99%
Appropriate Beta Blocker Usage[2]	645	94%	94%	93%
Controlled Postoperative Blood Glucose[2]	781	96%	96%	93%
Prophylactic Antibiotic Timing[2]	1,043	98%	97%	97%
Prophylactic Antibiotic Timing (Outpatient)	655	89%	93%	92%
Prophylactic Antibiotic Selection[2]	1,087	99%	98%	97%
Prophylactic Antibiotic Select. (Outpatient)	621	97%	96%	94%
Prophylactic Antibiotic Stopped[2]	974	95%	96%	94%
Recommended VTP Ordered[2]	188	96%	96%	94%
Urinary Catheter Removal[2]	331	92%	93%	90%
Children's Asthma Care				
Received Systemic Corticosteroids	-	-	-	100%
Received Home Management Plan	-	-	-	71%
Received Reliever Medication	-	-	-	100%
Use of Medical Imaging				
Combination Abdominal CT Scan	1,338	0.120	0.144	0.191
Combination Chest CT Scan	1,183	0.008	0.030	0.054
Follow-up Mammogram/Ultrasound	1,752	8.4%	7.5%	8.4%
MRI for Low Back Pain	125	28.0%	31.5%	32.7%
Survey of Patients' Hospital Experiences				
Area Around Room 'Always' Quiet at Night	300+	54%	-	58%
Doctors 'Always' Communicated Well	300+	79%	-	80%
Home Recovery Information Given	300+	84%	-	82%
Hospital Given 9 or 10 on 10 Point Scale	300+	70%	-	67%
Meds 'Always' Explained Before Given	300+	56%	-	60%
Nurses 'Always' Communicated Well	300+	75%	-	76%
Pain 'Always' Well Controlled	300+	69%	-	69%
Room and Bathroom 'Always' Clean	300+	60%	-	71%
Timely Help 'Always' Received	300+	64%	-	64%
Would Definitely Recommend Hospital	300+	76%	-	69%

Mountain View Regional Medical Center

310 Third Street NE Phone: 276-679-9174
Norton, VA 24273 Fax: 276-679-1926
URL: www.smhnorton.org
Type: Acute Care Hospitals Emergency Services: Yes
Ownership: Voluntary Non-Profit - Private Beds: 133

Key Personnel:
CEO/President.............. Jamie W Guin Jr
Chief of Medical Staff.......... P Paul Barongan, MD
Infection Control.............. Peggy Yanez, LPN
Quality Assurance............ Shelby Collins, RN
Radiology.................. Kathleen DePont
Anesthesiology.............. Mina Guzman, MD
Emergency Room............ Happy Smith, MD
Intensive Care Unit............ Bonita Stair, RN

Measure	Cases	This Hosp.	State Avg.	U.S. Avg.
Heart Attack Care				
ACE Inhibitor or ARB for LVSD[1]	3	100%	97%	96%
Aspirin at Arrival[1]	17	100%	99%	99%
Aspirin at Discharge[1]	10	100%	99%	98%
Beta Blocker at Discharge[1]	12	100%	99%	98%
Fibrinolytic Medication Timing	0	-	75%	55%
PCI Within 90 Minutes of Arrival	0	-	93%	90%
Smoking Cessation Advice[1]	1	100%	100%	99%
Chest Pain/Possible Heart Attack Care				
Aspirin at Arrival[1]	21	86%	95%	95%
Median Time to ECG (minutes)[1]	24	2	8	8
Median Time to Transfer (minutes)[5]	0	-	60	61
Fibrinolytic Medication Timing[1]	8	38%	59%	54%
Heart Failure Care				
ACE Inhibitor or ARB for LVSD[1]	24	100%	97%	94%
Discharge Instructions	84	100%	92%	88%
Evaluation of LVS Function	101	100%	99%	98%
Smoking Cessation Advice[1]	15	100%	99%	98%
Pneumonia Care				
Appropriate Initial Antibiotic	51	86%	93%	92%
Blood Culture Timing	73	100%	97%	96%
Influenza Vaccine	54	98%	94%	91%
Initial Antibiotic Timing	75	96%	96%	95%
Pneumococcal Vaccine	74	100%	95%	93%
Smoking Cessation Advice	36	100%	98%	97%
Surgical Care Improvement Project				
Appropriate VTP Within 24 Hours[1]	23	91%	94%	92%
Appropriate Hair Removal	73	99%	100%	99%
Appropriate Beta Blocker Usage[1]	19	89%	94%	93%
Controlled Postoperative Blood Glucose	0	-	96%	93%
Prophylactic Antibiotic Timing	56	96%	97%	97%
Prophylactic Antibiotic Timing (Outpatient)	54	67%	93%	92%
Prophylactic Antibiotic Selection	55	98%	98%	97%
Prophylactic Antibiotic Select. (Outpatient)	42	98%	96%	94%
Prophylactic Antibiotic Stopped	53	81%	96%	94%
Recommended VTP Ordered[1]	23	96%	96%	94%
Urinary Catheter Removal[1]	16	81%	93%	90%
Children's Asthma Care				
Received Systemic Corticosteroids	-	-	-	100%
Received Home Management Plan	-	-	-	71%
Received Reliever Medication	-	-	-	100%
Use of Medical Imaging				
Combination Abdominal CT Scan	208	0.322	0.144	0.191
Combination Chest CT Scan	182	0.324	0.030	0.054
Follow-up Mammogram/Ultrasound	341	5.6%	7.5%	8.4%
MRI for Low Back Pain	66	50.0%	31.5%	32.7%
Survey of Patients' Hospital Experiences				
Area Around Room 'Always' Quiet at Night	(a)	50%	-	58%
Doctors 'Always' Communicated Well	(a)	81%	-	80%
Home Recovery Information Given	(a)	82%	-	82%
Hospital Given 9 or 10 on 10 Point Scale	(a)	56%	-	67%
Meds 'Always' Explained Before Given	(a)	55%	-	60%
Nurses 'Always' Communicated Well	(a)	74%	-	76%
Pain 'Always' Well Controlled	(a)	61%	-	69%
Room and Bathroom 'Always' Clean	(a)	77%	-	71%
Timely Help 'Always' Received	(a)	54%	-	64%
Would Definitely Recommend Hospital	(a)	60%	-	69%

Norton Community Hospital

100 15th St NW Phone: 703-679-9600
Norton, VA 24273 Fax: 276-679-9003
URL: www.nchosp.org
Type: Acute Care Hospitals Emergency Services: Yes
Ownership: Voluntary Non-Profit - Other Beds: 129

Key Personnel:
CEO/President.............. David Fuqua
Chief of Medical Staff.......... Nicanor Concepcion, MD
Infection Control.............. Barbara Mullins, RN
Operating Room.............. Mitch Kennedy, RN
Pediatric Ambulatory Care...... Nancy Woodward
Quality Assurance............ Madonna Baker
Radiology................... Bryan Mullins

Measure	Cases	This Hosp.	State Avg.	U.S. Avg.
Heart Attack Care				
ACE Inhibitor or ARB for LVSD[2,3]	0	-	97%	96%
Aspirin at Arrival[1,2,3]	3	100%	99%	99%
Aspirin at Discharge[1,2,3]	3	100%	99%	98%
Beta Blocker at Discharge[1,2,3]	3	100%	99%	98%
Fibrinolytic Medication Timing[2,3]	0	-	75%	55%
PCI Within 90 Minutes of Arrival[2,3]	0	-	93%	90%
Smoking Cessation Advice[2,3]	0	-	100%	99%
Chest Pain/Possible Heart Attack Care				
Aspirin at Arrival	140	93%	95%	95%
Median Time to ECG (minutes)	151	14	8	8
Median Time to Transfer (minutes)[3]	0	-	60	61
Fibrinolytic Medication Timing[1]	3	0%	59%	54%
Heart Failure Care				
ACE Inhibitor or ARB for LVSD[1,2]	15	100%	97%	94%
Discharge Instructions[2]	84	94%	92%	88%
Evaluation of LVS Function[2]	94	98%	99%	98%
Smoking Cessation Advice[2]	25	100%	99%	98%
Pneumonia Care				
Appropriate Initial Antibiotic[2]	89	92%	93%	92%
Blood Culture Timing[2]	153	93%	97%	96%
Influenza Vaccine[2]	86	97%	94%	91%
Initial Antibiotic Timing[2]	142	94%	96%	95%
Pneumococcal Vaccine[2]	119	96%	95%	93%
Smoking Cessation Advice[2]	67	97%	98%	97%
Surgical Care Improvement Project				
Appropriate VTP Within 24 Hours[2]	37	95%	94%	92%
Appropriate Hair Removal[2]	74	100%	100%	99%
Appropriate Beta Blocker Usage[1,2]	13	85%	94%	93%
Controlled Postoperative Blood Glucose[2]	0	-	96%	93%
Prophylactic Antibiotic Timing[2]	41	95%	97%	97%
Prophylactic Antibiotic Timing (Outpatient)	27	85%	93%	92%
Prophylactic Antibiotic Selection[2]	41	95%	98%	97%
Prophylactic Antibiotic Select. (Outpatient)	41	95%	96%	94%
Prophylactic Antibiotic Stopped[2]	39	95%	96%	94%
Recommended VTP Ordered[2]	37	95%	96%	94%
Urinary Catheter Removal[1,2]	7	86%	93%	90%
Children's Asthma Care				
Received Systemic Corticosteroids	-	-	-	100%
Received Home Management Plan	-	-	-	71%
Received Reliever Medication	-	-	-	100%
Use of Medical Imaging				
Combination Abdominal CT Scan	468	0.543	0.144	0.191
Combination Chest CT Scan	410	0.361	0.030	0.054
Follow-up Mammogram/Ultrasound	500	16.6%	7.5%	8.4%
MRI for Low Back Pain	65	33.8%	31.5%	32.7%
Survey of Patients' Hospital Experiences				
Area Around Room 'Always' Quiet at Night	300+	47%	-	58%
Doctors 'Always' Communicated Well	300+	80%	-	80%
Home Recovery Information Given	300+	76%	-	82%
Hospital Given 9 or 10 on 10 Point Scale	300+	59%	-	67%
Meds 'Always' Explained Before Given	300+	60%	-	60%
Nurses 'Always' Communicated Well	300+	76%	-	76%
Pain 'Always' Well Controlled	300+	66%	-	69%
Room and Bathroom 'Always' Clean	300+	61%	-	71%
Timely Help 'Always' Received	300+	65%	-	64%
Would Definitely Recommend Hospital	300+	62%	-	69%

NOTE: Hospital profiles are in alphabetical order by state, then city, then hospital within the city; Rankings exclude hospitals with less than 25 cases except for patient surveys which excludes hospitals with less than 100 cases; (a) 100–299 cases; (1) The number of cases is too small to be sure how well a hospital is performing; (2) The hospital indicated that the data submitted for this measure were based on a sample of cases; (3) Data was collected during a shorter time period (fewer quarters) than the maximum possible time for this measure; (4) Suppressed for one or more quarters by CMS; (5) No data is available from the hospital for this measure; (6) Fewer than 100 patients completed the HCAHPS survey. Use these rates with caution, as the number of surveys may be too low to reliably assess hospital performance; (7) Survey results are based on less than 12 months of data; (8) Survey results are not available for this reporting period; (9) No or very few patients were eligible for the HCAHPS survey. The scores shown, if any, reflect a very small number of surveys; (10) A state average was not calculated because too few hospitals in the state submitted data; (11) There were discrepancies in the data collection process; Please refer to the User's Guide for a full explanation of data.

Carilion Giles Memorial Hospital

159 Hartley Way
Pearisburg, VA 24134
URL: www.carilion.com/cgmh
Type: Critical Access Hospitals
Ownership: Voluntary Non-Profit - Private

Phone: 540-921-6035
Fax: 540-921-6858

Emergency Services: Yes
Beds: 65

Key Personnel:
CEO/President . . . . Morris Reese
Operating Room . . . . Beverly Rice
Radiology . . . . John L Tamminen

Measure	Cases	This Hosp.	State Avg.	U.S. Avg.
Heart Attack Care				
ACE Inhibitor or ARB for LVSD[1]	2	100%	97%	96%
Aspirin at Arrival[1]	17	100%	99%	99%
Aspirin at Discharge[1]	13	100%	99%	98%
Beta Blocker at Discharge[1]	12	100%	99%	98%
Fibrinolytic Medication Timing	0	-	75%	55%
PCI Within 90 Minutes of Arrival	0	-	93%	90%
Smoking Cessation Advice[1]	3	100%	100%	99%
Chest Pain/Possible Heart Attack Care				
Aspirin at Arrival[3]	48	100%	95%	95%
Median Time to ECG (minutes)[3]	53	18	8	8
Median Time to Transfer (minutes)[1,3]	1	60	60	61
Fibrinolytic Medication Timing[1,3]	1	0%	59%	54%
Heart Failure Care				
ACE Inhibitor or ARB for LVSD[1]	11	91%	97%	94%
Discharge Instructions	53	85%	92%	88%
Evaluation of LVS Function	65	86%	99%	98%
Smoking Cessation Advice[1]	11	100%	99%	98%
Pneumonia Care				
Appropriate Initial Antibiotic	36	89%	93%	92%
Blood Culture Timing	57	95%	97%	96%
Influenza Vaccine	33	97%	94%	91%
Initial Antibiotic Timing	55	95%	96%	95%
Pneumococcal Vaccine	57	96%	95%	93%
Smoking Cessation Advice[1]	17	94%	98%	97%
Surgical Care Improvement Project				
Appropriate VTP Within 24 Hours[1,3]	2	0%	94%	92%
Appropriate Hair Removal[1,3]	2	100%	100%	99%
Appropriate Beta Blocker Usage[1,3]	1	100%	94%	93%
Controlled Postoperative Blood Glucose[3]	0	-	96%	93%
Prophylactic Antibiotic Timing[1,3]	1	100%	97%	97%
Prophylactic Antibiotic Timing (Outpatient)[1,3]	1	0%	93%	92%
Prophylactic Antibiotic Selection[1,3]	1	100%	98%	97%
Prophylactic Antibiotic Select. (Outpatient)[3]	0	-	96%	94%
Prophylactic Antibiotic Stopped[1,3]	1	100%	96%	94%
Recommended VTP Ordered[1,3]	2	0%	96%	94%
Urinary Catheter Removal[5]	0	-	93%	90%
Children's Asthma Care				
Received Systemic Corticosteroids	-	-	-	100%
Received Home Management Plan	-	-	-	71%
Received Reliever Medication	-	-	-	100%
Use of Medical Imaging				
Combination Abdominal CT Scan	317	0.104	0.144	0.191
Combination Chest CT Scan	129	0.287	0.030	0.054
Follow-up Mammogram/Ultrasound	548	4.7%	7.5%	8.4%
MRI for Low Back Pain	57	33.3%	31.5%	32.7%
Survey of Patients' Hospital Experiences				
Area Around Room 'Always' Quiet at Night	(a)	62%	-	58%
Doctors 'Always' Communicated Well	(a)	86%	-	80%
Home Recovery Information Given	(a)	82%	-	82%
Hospital Given 9 or 10 on 10 Point Scale	(a)	72%	-	67%
Meds 'Always' Explained Before Given	(a)	64%	-	60%
Nurses 'Always' Communicated Well	(a)	83%	-	76%
Pain 'Always' Well Controlled	(a)	76%	-	69%
Room and Bathroom 'Always' Clean	(a)	75%	-	71%
Timely Help 'Always' Received	(a)	74%	-	64%
Would Definitely Recommend Hospital	(a)	68%	-	69%

Lee Regional Medical Center

1800 Combs Road
Pennington Gap, VA 24277
E-mail: info@LeeRegional.com
URL: www.leeregional.com
Type: Acute Care Hospitals
Ownership: Voluntary Non-Profit - Other

Phone: 276-546-1440
Fax: 276-546-5594

Emergency Services: Yes
Beds: 80

Key Personnel:
CEO/President . . . . David Brash
Chief of Medical Staff . . . . Marissa Vitocruz
Radiology . . . . Kathleen DePonte

Measure	Cases	This Hosp.	State Avg.	U.S. Avg.
Heart Attack Care				
ACE Inhibitor or ARB for LVSD	0	-	97%	96%
Aspirin at Arrival	23	91%	99%	99%
Aspirin at Discharge[1]	14	86%	99%	98%
Beta Blocker at Discharge[1]	12	100%	99%	98%
Fibrinolytic Medication Timing	0	-	75%	55%
PCI Within 90 Minutes of Arrival	0	-	93%	90%
Smoking Cessation Advice[1]	1	100%	100%	99%
Chest Pain/Possible Heart Attack Care				
Aspirin at Arrival	29	97%	95%	95%
Median Time to ECG (minutes)	34	10	8	8
Median Time to Transfer (minutes)[5]	0	-	60	61
Fibrinolytic Medication Timing[1]	3	67%	59%	54%
Heart Failure Care				
ACE Inhibitor or ARB for LVSD[1]	22	91%	97%	94%
Discharge Instructions	80	38%	92%	88%
Evaluation of LVS Function	91	71%	99%	98%
Smoking Cessation Advice[1]	13	77%	99%	98%
Pneumonia Care				
Appropriate Initial Antibiotic	127	91%	93%	92%
Blood Culture Timing	150	98%	97%	96%
Influenza Vaccine	102	76%	94%	91%
Initial Antibiotic Timing	166	98%	96%	95%
Pneumococcal Vaccine	124	81%	95%	93%
Smoking Cessation Advice	68	65%	98%	97%
Surgical Care Improvement Project				
Appropriate VTP Within 24 Hours[1]	24	54%	94%	92%
Appropriate Hair Removal	30	100%	100%	99%
Appropriate Beta Blocker Usage[1]	9	78%	94%	93%
Controlled Postoperative Blood Glucose	0	-	96%	93%
Prophylactic Antibiotic Timing[1]	7	57%	97%	97%
Prophylactic Antibiotic Timing (Outpatient)[1,3]	3	33%	93%	92%
Prophylactic Antibiotic Selection[1]	7	43%	98%	97%
Prophylactic Antibiotic Select. (Outpatient)[1,3]	1	0%	96%	94%
Prophylactic Antibiotic Stopped[1]	7	57%	96%	94%
Recommended VTP Ordered[1]	24	54%	96%	94%
Urinary Catheter Removal[1]	3	67%	93%	90%
Children's Asthma Care				
Received Systemic Corticosteroids	-	-	-	100%
Received Home Management Plan	-	-	-	71%
Received Reliever Medication	-	-	-	100%
Use of Medical Imaging				
Combination Abdominal CT Scan	197	0.614	0.144	0.191
Combination Chest CT Scan	77	0.584	0.030	0.054
Follow-up Mammogram/Ultrasound	305	10.2%	7.5%	8.4%
MRI for Low Back Pain[1]	39	20.5%	31.5%	32.7%
Survey of Patients' Hospital Experiences				
Area Around Room 'Always' Quiet at Night	300+	54%	-	58%
Doctors 'Always' Communicated Well	300+	80%	-	80%
Home Recovery Information Given	300+	74%	-	82%
Hospital Given 9 or 10 on 10 Point Scale	300+	58%	-	67%
Meds 'Always' Explained Before Given	300+	58%	-	60%
Nurses 'Always' Communicated Well	300+	78%	-	76%
Pain 'Always' Well Controlled	300+	62%	-	69%
Room and Bathroom 'Always' Clean	300+	69%	-	71%
Timely Help 'Always' Received	300+	69%	-	64%
Would Definitely Recommend Hospital	300+	54%	-	69%

Southside Regional Medical Center

200 Medical Park Boulevard
Petersburg, VA 23805
URL: www.srmconline.com
Type: Acute Care Hospitals
Ownership: Proprietary

Phone: 804-765-5000
Fax: 804-957-6000

Emergency Services: Yes
Beds: 408

Key Personnel:
CEO/President . . . . David Fikse
Cardiac Laboratory . . . . Lynn Sule
Coronary Care . . . . Margaret Greene, RN
Infection Control . . . . Linda Atkinson
Operating Room . . . . Sherry Wilkinson
Pediatric In-Patient Care . . . . Peggy Benton
Radiology . . . . Rita Baldwin

Measure	Cases	This Hosp.	State Avg.	U.S. Avg.
Heart Attack Care				
ACE Inhibitor or ARB for LVSD	42	95%	97%	96%
Aspirin at Arrival	213	98%	99%	99%
Aspirin at Discharge	200	94%	99%	98%
Beta Blocker at Discharge	199	96%	99%	98%
Fibrinolytic Medication Timing[1]	1	100%	75%	55%
PCI Within 90 Minutes of Arrival	48	94%	93%	90%
Smoking Cessation Advice	92	99%	100%	99%
Chest Pain/Possible Heart Attack Care				
Aspirin at Arrival	15	93%	95%	95%
Median Time to ECG (minutes)[1]	15	1	8	8
Median Time to Transfer (minutes)[1,3]	1	154	60	61
Fibrinolytic Medication Timing[3]	0	-	59%	54%
Heart Failure Care				
ACE Inhibitor or ARB for LVSD	203	92%	97%	94%
Discharge Instructions	376	97%	92%	88%
Evaluation of LVS Function	468	99%	99%	98%
Smoking Cessation Advice	110	100%	99%	98%
Pneumonia Care				
Appropriate Initial Antibiotic	139	93%	93%	92%
Blood Culture Timing	175	97%	97%	96%
Influenza Vaccine	130	93%	94%	91%
Initial Antibiotic Timing	213	95%	96%	95%
Pneumococcal Vaccine	167	94%	95%	93%
Smoking Cessation Advice	93	100%	98%	97%
Surgical Care Improvement Project				
Appropriate VTP Within 24 Hours[2]	177	90%	94%	92%
Appropriate Hair Removal[2]	520	100%	100%	99%
Appropriate Beta Blocker Usage[2]	114	96%	94%	93%
Controlled Postoperative Blood Glucose[1,2]	1	100%	96%	93%
Prophylactic Antibiotic Timing[2]	374	98%	97%	97%
Prophylactic Antibiotic Timing (Outpatient)	181	92%	93%	92%
Prophylactic Antibiotic Selection[2]	375	97%	98%	97%
Prophylactic Antibiotic Select. (Outpatient)	177	97%	96%	94%
Prophylactic Antibiotic Stopped[2]	361	94%	96%	94%
Recommended VTP Ordered[2]	178	93%	96%	94%
Urinary Catheter Removal	81	85%	93%	90%
Children's Asthma Care				
Received Systemic Corticosteroids	-	-	-	100%
Received Home Management Plan	-	-	-	71%
Received Reliever Medication	-	-	-	100%
Use of Medical Imaging				
Combination Abdominal CT Scan	929	0.205	0.144	0.191
Combination Chest CT Scan	694	0.006	0.030	0.054
Follow-up Mammogram/Ultrasound	1,383	8.5%	7.5%	8.4%
MRI for Low Back Pain	181	30.4%	31.5%	32.7%
Survey of Patients' Hospital Experiences				
Area Around Room 'Always' Quiet at Night	300+	56%	-	58%
Doctors 'Always' Communicated Well	300+	79%	-	80%
Home Recovery Information Given	300+	79%	-	82%
Hospital Given 9 or 10 on 10 Point Scale	300+	63%	-	67%
Meds 'Always' Explained Before Given	300+	55%	-	60%
Nurses 'Always' Communicated Well	300+	73%	-	76%
Pain 'Always' Well Controlled	300+	68%	-	69%
Room and Bathroom 'Always' Clean	300+	62%	-	71%
Timely Help 'Always' Received	300+	53%	-	64%
Would Definitely Recommend Hospital	300+	61%	-	69%

Bon Secours - Maryview Medical Center

3636 High Street Phone: 757-398-2200
Portsmouth, VA 23707 Fax: 757-398-4982
URL: www.bonsecourshamptonroads.com
Type: Acute Care Hospitals Emergency Services: Yes
Ownership: Voluntary Non-Profit - Church Beds: 346

Key Personnel:
CEO/President. . . . . Dominick Calgi
Operating Room. . . . . John Jacobs
Pediatric In-Patient Care . . . . Sandra Baucom
Quality Assurance . . . . Emma Truitt
Radiology. . . . . N Devanath

Measure	Cases	This Hosp.	State Avg.	U.S. Avg.
Heart Attack Care				
ACE Inhibitor or ARB for LVSD	43	100%	97%	96%
Aspirin at Arrival	207	100%	99%	99%
Aspirin at Discharge	227	100%	99%	98%
Beta Blocker at Discharge	220	100%	99%	98%
Fibrinolytic Medication Timing	0	-	75%	55%
PCI Within 90 Minutes of Arrival	30	90%	93%	90%
Smoking Cessation Advice	81	100%	100%	99%
Chest Pain/Possible Heart Attack Care				
Aspirin at Arrival[1]	21	95%	95%	95%
Median Time to ECG (minutes)[1]	22	11	8	8
Median Time to Transfer (minutes)[1,3]	3	57	60	61
Fibrinolytic Medication Timing[3]	0	-	59%	54%
Heart Failure Care				
ACE Inhibitor or ARB for LVSD	144	100%	97%	94%
Discharge Instructions	374	98%	92%	88%
Evaluation of LVS Function	429	99%	99%	98%
Smoking Cessation Advice	89	100%	99%	98%
Pneumonia Care				
Appropriate Initial Antibiotic	85	94%	93%	92%
Blood Culture Timing	171	98%	97%	96%
Influenza Vaccine	132	89%	94%	91%
Initial Antibiotic Timing	157	95%	96%	95%
Pneumococcal Vaccine	175	91%	95%	93%
Smoking Cessation Advice	73	100%	98%	97%
Surgical Care Improvement Project				
Appropriate VTP Within 24 Hours[2]	192	98%	94%	92%
Appropriate Hair Removal[2]	828	100%	100%	99%
Appropriate Beta Blocker Usage[2]	229	99%	94%	93%
Controlled Postoperative Blood Glucose[2]	124	96%	96%	93%
Prophylactic Antibiotic Timing[2]	654	94%	97%	97%
Prophylactic Antibiotic Timing (Outpatient)	279	95%	93%	92%
Prophylactic Antibiotic Selection[2]	657	95%	98%	97%
Prophylactic Antibiotic Select. (Outpatient)	276	93%	96%	94%
Prophylactic Antibiotic Stopped[2]	641	95%	96%	94%
Recommended VTP Ordered[2]	192	98%	96%	94%
Urinary Catheter Removal[2]	258	98%	93%	90%
Children's Asthma Care				
Received Systemic Corticosteroids	-	-	-	100%
Received Home Management Plan	-	-	-	71%
Received Reliever Medication	-	-	-	100%
Use of Medical Imaging				
Combination Abdominal CT Scan	1,505	0.116	0.144	0.191
Combination Chest CT Scan	1,172	0.028	0.030	0.054
Follow-up Mammogram/Ultrasound	2,111	7.3%	7.5%	8.4%
MRI for Low Back Pain	404	21.8%	31.5%	32.7%
Survey of Patients' Hospital Experiences				
Area Around Room 'Always' Quiet at Night	300+	65%	-	58%
Doctors 'Always' Communicated Well	300+	81%	-	80%
Home Recovery Information Given	300+	85%	-	82%
Hospital Given 9 or 10 on 10 Point Scale	300+	62%	-	67%
Meds 'Always' Explained Before Given	300+	54%	-	60%
Nurses 'Always' Communicated Well	300+	73%	-	76%
Pain 'Always' Well Controlled	300+	69%	-	69%
Room and Bathroom 'Always' Clean	300+	68%	-	71%
Timely Help 'Always' Received	300+	60%	-	64%
Would Definitely Recommend Hospital	300+	58%	-	69%

Pulaski Community Hospital

2400 Lee Highway Phone: 540-994-8100
Pulaski, VA 24301 Fax: 540-994-8333
URL: www.pch-va.com or www.PulaskiCommunityHospital.com
Type: Acute Care Hospitals Emergency Services: No
Ownership: Proprietary Beds: 147

Key Personnel:
CEO/President. . . . . W. Mark Rader
Cardiac Laboratory. . . . . Barbara Farris
Chief of Medical Staff. . . . . Dr. Paul D'Amico
Infection Control. . . . . Lee Cox
Operating Room. . . . . Yung C Chan
Pediatric In-Patient Care . . . . . . Greg Angle
Quality Assurance . . . . Bob Suddarth
Radiology. . . . . Allen Knull

Measure	Cases	This Hosp.	State Avg.	U.S. Avg.
Heart Attack Care				
ACE Inhibitor or ARB for LVSD[1]	21	100%	97%	96%
Aspirin at Arrival	53	100%	99%	99%
Aspirin at Discharge	37	100%	99%	98%
Beta Blocker at Discharge	45	100%	99%	98%
Fibrinolytic Medication Timing	0	-	75%	55%
PCI Within 90 Minutes of Arrival	0	-	93%	90%
Smoking Cessation Advice[1]	8	100%	100%	99%
Chest Pain/Possible Heart Attack Care				
Aspirin at Arrival	59	100%	95%	95%
Median Time to ECG (minutes)	66	1	8	8
Median Time to Transfer (minutes)[1,3]	5	59	60	61
Fibrinolytic Medication Timing	0	-	59%	54%
Heart Failure Care				
ACE Inhibitor or ARB for LVSD[1]	23	100%	97%	94%
Discharge Instructions	65	100%	92%	88%
Evaluation of LVS Function	88	100%	99%	98%
Smoking Cessation Advice[1]	5	100%	99%	98%
Pneumonia Care				
Appropriate Initial Antibiotic	73	95%	93%	92%
Blood Culture Timing	104	99%	97%	96%
Influenza Vaccine	88	99%	94%	91%
Initial Antibiotic Timing	59	97%	96%	95%
Pneumococcal Vaccine	109	99%	95%	93%
Smoking Cessation Advice	41	100%	98%	97%
Surgical Care Improvement Project				
Appropriate VTP Within 24 Hours	43	100%	94%	92%
Appropriate Hair Removal	82	100%	100%	99%
Appropriate Beta Blocker Usage	26	100%	94%	93%
Controlled Postoperative Blood Glucose	0	-	96%	93%
Prophylactic Antibiotic Timing	38	100%	97%	97%
Prophylactic Antibiotic Timing (Outpatient)	39	100%	93%	92%
Prophylactic Antibiotic Selection	39	97%	98%	97%
Prophylactic Antibiotic Select. (Outpatient)	40	98%	96%	94%
Prophylactic Antibiotic Stopped	33	100%	96%	94%
Recommended VTP Ordered	43	100%	96%	94%
Urinary Catheter Removal[1]	10	90%	93%	90%
Children's Asthma Care				
Received Systemic Corticosteroids	-	-	-	100%
Received Home Management Plan	-	-	-	71%
Received Reliever Medication	-	-	-	100%
Use of Medical Imaging				
Combination Abdominal CT Scan	359	0.031	0.144	0.191
Combination Chest CT Scan	202	0.010	0.030	0.054
Follow-up Mammogram/Ultrasound	420	3.8%	7.5%	8.4%
MRI for Low Back Pain	80	27.5%	31.5%	32.7%
Survey of Patients' Hospital Experiences				
Area Around Room 'Always' Quiet at Night	300+	61%	-	58%
Doctors 'Always' Communicated Well	300+	86%	-	80%
Home Recovery Information Given	300+	86%	-	82%
Hospital Given 9 or 10 on 10 Point Scale	300+	70%	-	67%
Meds 'Always' Explained Before Given	300+	64%	-	60%
Nurses 'Always' Communicated Well	300+	81%	-	76%
Pain 'Always' Well Controlled	300+	74%	-	69%
Room and Bathroom 'Always' Clean	300+	69%	-	71%
Timely Help 'Always' Received	300+	68%	-	64%
Would Definitely Recommend Hospital	300+	71%	-	69%

Reston Hospital Center

1850 Town Center Parkway Phone: 703-689-9018
Reston, VA 20190 Fax: 703-689-0840
E-mail: denise.dancy@hcahealthcare.com
URL: www.restonhospital.com
Type: Acute Care Hospitals Emergency Services: Yes
Ownership: Proprietary Beds: 160

Key Personnel:
CEO/President. . . . . William Adams
Cardiac Laboratory. . . . . Kim Elliotts
Operating Room. . . . . Jim Cliett, RN
Pediatric In-Patient Care . . . . Carrie Sutara, RN
Quality Assurance . . . . Judy Riggins
Radiology. . . . . David Dubois MD
Emergency Room . . . . Darren Lisse, MD

Measure	Cases	This Hosp.	State Avg.	U.S. Avg.
Heart Attack Care				
ACE Inhibitor or ARB for LVSD[1]	13	100%	97%	96%
Aspirin at Arrival	103	100%	99%	99%
Aspirin at Discharge	79	100%	99%	98%
Beta Blocker at Discharge	77	100%	99%	98%
Fibrinolytic Medication Timing	0	-	75%	55%
PCI Within 90 Minutes of Arrival	25	88%	93%	90%
Smoking Cessation Advice[1]	20	100%	100%	99%
Chest Pain/Possible Heart Attack Care				
Aspirin at Arrival[1]	24	100%	95%	95%
Median Time to ECG (minutes)	25	9	8	8
Median Time to Transfer (minutes)[5]	0	-	60	61
Fibrinolytic Medication Timing	0	-	59%	54%
Heart Failure Care				
ACE Inhibitor or ARB for LVSD	29	100%	97%	94%
Discharge Instructions	144	100%	92%	88%
Evaluation of LVS Function	172	99%	99%	98%
Smoking Cessation Advice[1]	12	100%	99%	98%
Pneumonia Care				
Appropriate Initial Antibiotic	111	96%	93%	92%
Blood Culture Timing	179	99%	97%	96%
Influenza Vaccine	111	100%	94%	91%
Initial Antibiotic Timing	137	99%	96%	95%
Pneumococcal Vaccine	144	100%	95%	93%
Smoking Cessation Advice	32	100%	98%	97%
Surgical Care Improvement Project				
Appropriate VTP Within 24 Hours[2]	157	94%	94%	92%
Appropriate Hair Removal[2]	477	100%	100%	99%
Appropriate Beta Blocker Usage[2]	105	96%	94%	93%
Controlled Postoperative Blood Glucose[2]	0	-	96%	93%
Prophylactic Antibiotic Timing[2]	312	98%	97%	97%
Prophylactic Antibiotic Timing (Outpatient)	948	98%	93%	92%
Prophylactic Antibiotic Selection[2]	321	99%	98%	97%
Prophylactic Antibiotic Select. (Outpatient)	945	99%	96%	94%
Prophylactic Antibiotic Stopped[2]	296	93%	96%	94%
Recommended VTP Ordered[2]	157	95%	96%	94%
Urinary Catheter Removal[2]	130	94%	93%	90%
Children's Asthma Care				
Received Systemic Corticosteroids	-	-	-	100%
Received Home Management Plan	-	-	-	71%
Received Reliever Medication	-	-	-	100%
Use of Medical Imaging				
Combination Abdominal CT Scan	638	0.080	0.144	0.191
Combination Chest CT Scan	501	0.032	0.030	0.054
Follow-up Mammogram/Ultrasound	455	9.5%	7.5%	8.4%
MRI for Low Back Pain[1]	5	60.0%	31.5%	32.7%
Survey of Patients' Hospital Experiences				
Area Around Room 'Always' Quiet at Night	300+	62%	-	58%
Doctors 'Always' Communicated Well	300+	79%	-	80%
Home Recovery Information Given	300+	81%	-	82%
Hospital Given 9 or 10 on 10 Point Scale	300+	63%	-	67%
Meds 'Always' Explained Before Given	300+	57%	-	60%
Nurses 'Always' Communicated Well	300+	69%	-	76%
Pain 'Always' Well Controlled	300+	65%	-	69%
Room and Bathroom 'Always' Clean	300+	64%	-	71%
Timely Help 'Always' Received	300+	52%	-	64%
Would Definitely Recommend Hospital	300+	69%	-	69%

NOTE: Hospital profiles are in alphabetical order by state, then city, then hospital within the city; Rankings exclude hospitals with less than 25 cases except for patient surveys which excludes hospitals with less than 100 cases; (a) 100–299 cases; (1) The number of cases is too small to be sure how well a hospital is performing; (2) The hospital indicated that the data submitted for this measure were based on a sample of cases; (3) Data was collected during a shorter time period (fewer quarters) than the maximum possible time for this measure; (4) Suppressed for one or more quarters by CMS; (5) No data is available from the hospital for this measure; (6) Fewer than 100 patients completed the HCAHPS survey. Use these rates with caution, as the number of surveys may be too low to reliably assess hospital performance; (7) Survey results are based on less than 12 months of data; (8) Survey results are not available for this reporting period; (9) No or very few patients were eligible for the HCAHPS survey. The scores shown, if any, reflect a very small number of surveys; (10) A state average was not calculated because too few hospitals in the state submitted data; (11) There were discrepancies in the data collection process; Please refer to the User's Guide for a full explanation of data.

Clinch Valley Medical Center

6801 Gov G C Peery Hwy
Richlands, VA 24641
Phone: 276-596-6000
Fax: 276-596-6009
E-mail: karel.fulton@lpnt.net
URL: clinchvalleymedicalcenter.com
Type: Acute Care Hospitals
Emergency Services: Yes
Ownership: Proprietary
Beds: 200

Key Personnel:
CEO/President. . . . . David Darden
Chief of Medical Staff . . . . Glenn Harrison, DDS
Infection Control . . . . Debi Riffe
Operating Room. . . . . Joseph C Claustro
Quality Assurance . . . . Jeanna Lambert
Radiology. . . . . Edson L Knapp
Intensive Care Unit. . . . . Rusty Osborne
Patient Relations . . . . Tracie Rinehardt

Measure	Cases	This Hosp.	State Avg.	U.S. Avg.
Heart Attack Care				
ACE Inhibitor or ARB for LVSD[1]	5	100%	97%	96%
Aspirin at Arrival	33	100%	99%	99%
Aspirin at Discharge[1]	22	100%	99%	98%
Beta Blocker at Discharge	28	100%	99%	98%
Fibrinolytic Medication Timing	0	-	75%	55%
PCI Within 90 Minutes of Arrival	0	-	93%	90%
Smoking Cessation Advice[1]	5	100%	100%	99%
Chest Pain/Possible Heart Attack Care				
Aspirin at Arrival	63	97%	95%	95%
Median Time to ECG (minutes)	70	12	8	8
Median Time to Transfer (minutes)[1,3]	1	86	60	61
Fibrinolytic Medication Timing[1]	22	82%	59%	54%
Heart Failure Care				
ACE Inhibitor or ARB for LVSD	32	100%	97%	94%
Discharge Instructions	150	99%	92%	88%
Evaluation of LVS Function	165	99%	99%	98%
Smoking Cessation Advice	28	100%	99%	98%
Pneumonia Care				
Appropriate Initial Antibiotic	77	95%	93%	92%
Blood Culture Timing	109	97%	97%	96%
Influenza Vaccine	60	97%	94%	91%
Initial Antibiotic Timing	116	97%	96%	95%
Pneumococcal Vaccine	75	97%	95%	93%
Smoking Cessation Advice	43	100%	98%	97%
Surgical Care Improvement Project				
Appropriate VTP Within 24 Hours	33	82%	94%	92%
Appropriate Hair Removal	155	100%	100%	99%
Appropriate Beta Blocker Usage	27	93%	94%	93%
Controlled Postoperative Blood Glucose	0	-	96%	93%
Prophylactic Antibiotic Timing	110	97%	97%	97%
Prophylactic Antibiotic Timing (Outpatient)	62	95%	93%	92%
Prophylactic Antibiotic Selection	112	88%	98%	97%
Prophylactic Antibiotic Select. (Outpatient)	95	98%	96%	94%
Prophylactic Antibiotic Stopped	107	99%	96%	94%
Recommended VTP Ordered	33	91%	96%	94%
Urinary Catheter Removal[1]	2	100%	93%	90%
Children's Asthma Care				
Received Systemic Corticosteroids	-	-	-	100%
Received Home Management Plan	-	-	-	71%
Received Reliever Medication	-	-	-	100%
Use of Medical Imaging				
Combination Abdominal CT Scan	708	0.333	0.144	0.191
Combination Chest CT Scan	615	0.122	0.030	0.054
Follow-up Mammogram/Ultrasound	135	7.4%	7.5%	8.4%
MRI for Low Back Pain	111	43.2%	31.5%	32.7%
Survey of Patients' Hospital Experiences				
Area Around Room 'Always' Quiet at Night	300+	61%	-	58%
Doctors 'Always' Communicated Well	300+	84%	-	80%
Home Recovery Information Given	300+	83%	-	82%
Hospital Given 9 or 10 on 10 Point Scale	300+	63%	-	67%
Meds 'Always' Explained Before Given	300+	61%	-	60%
Nurses 'Always' Communicated Well	300+	76%	-	76%
Pain 'Always' Well Controlled	300+	67%	-	69%
Room and Bathroom 'Always' Clean	300+	71%	-	71%
Timely Help 'Always' Received	300+	63%	-	64%
Would Definitely Recommend Hospital	300+	64%	-	69%

Bon Secours - Richmond Community Hospital

1500 N. 28th Street
Richmond, VA 23223
Phone: 804-225-1700
Fax: 804-627-5029
E-mail: webmaster@bshsi.org
URL: www.bonsecours.com
Type: Acute Care Hospitals
Emergency Services: Yes
Ownership: Voluntary Non-Profit - Private
Beds: 104

Key Personnel:
CEO/President. . . . . Paula R Autry
Infection Control . . . . Connie Jones
Operating Room. . . . . Jacqueline Manning
Quality Assurance . . . . Marlene McAnich
Radiology. . . . . Todd B Baird
Anesthesiology. . . . . Mark Kirshner
Emergency Room . . . . Dean Williams

Measure	Cases	This Hosp.	State Avg.	U.S. Avg.
Heart Attack Care				
ACE Inhibitor or ARB for LVSD[3]	0	-	97%	96%
Aspirin at Arrival[1,3]	5	100%	99%	99%
Aspirin at Discharge[1,3]	1	100%	99%	98%
Beta Blocker at Discharge[1,3]	1	100%	99%	98%
Fibrinolytic Medication Timing[3]	0	-	75%	55%
PCI Within 90 Minutes of Arrival[3]	0	-	93%	90%
Smoking Cessation Advice[3]	0	-	100%	99%
Chest Pain/Possible Heart Attack Care				
Aspirin at Arrival[1]	15	100%	95%	95%
Median Time to ECG (minutes)[1]	15	13	8	8
Median Time to Transfer (minutes)[1,3]	2	58	60	61
Fibrinolytic Medication Timing	0	-	59%	54%
Heart Failure Care				
ACE Inhibitor or ARB for LVSD[1]	15	100%	97%	94%
Discharge Instructions	51	75%	92%	88%
Evaluation of LVS Function	57	98%	99%	98%
Smoking Cessation Advice	25	100%	99%	98%
Pneumonia Care				
Appropriate Initial Antibiotic	47	79%	93%	92%
Blood Culture Timing	57	100%	97%	96%
Influenza Vaccine[1]	14	100%	94%	91%
Initial Antibiotic Timing	61	97%	96%	95%
Pneumococcal Vaccine[1]	18	94%	95%	93%
Smoking Cessation Advice	35	100%	98%	97%
Surgical Care Improvement Project				
Appropriate VTP Within 24 Hours[1]	10	80%	94%	92%
Appropriate Hair Removal[1]	13	100%	100%	99%
Appropriate Beta Blocker Usage[1]	2	50%	94%	93%
Controlled Postoperative Blood Glucose	0	-	96%	93%
Prophylactic Antibiotic Timing[1]	6	67%	97%	97%
Prophylactic Antibiotic Timing (Outpatient)	27	63%	93%	92%
Prophylactic Antibiotic Selection[1]	6	83%	98%	97%
Prophylactic Antibiotic Select. (Outpatient)[1]	22	95%	96%	94%
Prophylactic Antibiotic Stopped[1]	6	83%	96%	94%
Recommended VTP Ordered[1]	11	82%	96%	94%
Urinary Catheter Removal[1]	5	80%	93%	90%
Children's Asthma Care				
Received Systemic Corticosteroids	-	-	-	100%
Received Home Management Plan	-	-	-	71%
Received Reliever Medication	-	-	-	100%
Use of Medical Imaging				
Combination Abdominal CT Scan	103	0.233	0.144	0.191
Combination Chest CT Scan	45	0.022	0.030	0.054
Follow-up Mammogram/Ultrasound	202	10.4%	7.5%	8.4%
MRI for Low Back Pain[1]	18	44.4%	31.5%	32.7%
Survey of Patients' Hospital Experiences				
Area Around Room 'Always' Quiet at Night	(a)	77%	-	58%
Doctors 'Always' Communicated Well	(a)	88%	-	80%
Home Recovery Information Given	(a)	86%	-	82%
Hospital Given 9 or 10 on 10 Point Scale	(a)	67%	-	67%
Meds 'Always' Explained Before Given	(a)	69%	-	60%
Nurses 'Always' Communicated Well	(a)	78%	-	76%
Pain 'Always' Well Controlled	(a)	74%	-	69%
Room and Bathroom 'Always' Clean	(a)	73%	-	71%
Timely Help 'Always' Received	(a)	62%	-	64%
Would Definitely Recommend Hospital	(a)	60%	-	69%

Bon Secours - St Marys Hospital of Richmond

5801 Bremo Rd
Richmond, VA 23226
Phone: 804-285-2011
Fax: 804-285-1338
URL: www.bonsecours.com
Type: Acute Care Hospitals
Emergency Services: Yes
Ownership: Voluntary Non-Profit - Church
Beds: 391

Key Personnel:
CEO/President. . . . . Christopher M Carney
Chief of Medical Staff . . . . Thomas Davis, MD
Infection Control. . . . . Michael Mandel, MD
Operating Room. . . . . Khaki Kostetter, RN
Pediatric Ambulatory Care . . . . . . Grover Robinson, MD
Pediatric In-Patient Care . . . . Grover Robinson, MD
Quality Assurance . . . . Marie Kerns
Radiology. . . . . David Ekey, MD

Measure	Cases	This Hosp.	State Avg.	U.S. Avg.
Heart Attack Care				
ACE Inhibitor or ARB for LVSD	58	100%	97%	96%
Aspirin at Arrival	195	99%	99%	99%
Aspirin at Discharge	225	100%	99%	98%
Beta Blocker at Discharge	220	100%	99%	98%
Fibrinolytic Medication Timing	0	-	75%	55%
PCI Within 90 Minutes of Arrival	46	100%	93%	90%
Smoking Cessation Advice	71	100%	100%	99%
Chest Pain/Possible Heart Attack Care				
Aspirin at Arrival[1]	3	67%	95%	95%
Median Time to ECG (minutes)[1]	3	230	8	8
Median Time to Transfer (minutes)[5]	0	-	60	61
Fibrinolytic Medication Timing[5]	0	-	59%	54%
Heart Failure Care				
ACE Inhibitor or ARB for LVSD	107	95%	97%	94%
Discharge Instructions	324	98%	92%	88%
Evaluation of LVS Function	423	100%	99%	98%
Smoking Cessation Advice	56	100%	99%	98%
Pneumonia Care				
Appropriate Initial Antibiotic	126	97%	93%	92%
Blood Culture Timing	249	97%	97%	96%
Influenza Vaccine	198	97%	94%	91%
Initial Antibiotic Timing	227	96%	96%	95%
Pneumococcal Vaccine	243	97%	95%	93%
Smoking Cessation Advice	57	100%	98%	97%
Surgical Care Improvement Project				
Appropriate VTP Within 24 Hours[2]	524	99%	94%	92%
Appropriate Hair Removal[2]	2,049	100%	100%	99%
Appropriate Beta Blocker Usage[2]	514	98%	94%	93%
Controlled Postoperative Blood Glucose[2]	257	100%	96%	93%
Prophylactic Antibiotic Timing[2]	1,769	99%	97%	97%
Prophylactic Antibiotic Timing (Outpatient)	606	96%	93%	92%
Prophylactic Antibiotic Selection[2]	1,777	99%	98%	97%
Prophylactic Antibiotic Select. (Outpatient)	593	97%	96%	94%
Prophylactic Antibiotic Stopped[2]	1,725	96%	96%	94%
Recommended VTP Ordered[2]	524	99%	96%	94%
Urinary Catheter Removal[2]	651	97%	93%	90%
Children's Asthma Care				
Received Systemic Corticosteroids	-	-	-	100%
Received Home Management Plan	-	-	-	71%
Received Reliever Medication	-	-	-	100%
Use of Medical Imaging				
Combination Abdominal CT Scan	1,040	0.138	0.144	0.191
Combination Chest CT Scan	499	0.012	0.030	0.054
Follow-up Mammogram/Ultrasound	3,046	7.9%	7.5%	8.4%
MRI for Low Back Pain	422	29.6%	31.5%	32.7%
Survey of Patients' Hospital Experiences				
Area Around Room 'Always' Quiet at Night	300+	64%	-	58%
Doctors 'Always' Communicated Well	300+	81%	-	80%
Home Recovery Information Given	300+	83%	-	82%
Hospital Given 9 or 10 on 10 Point Scale	300+	72%	-	67%
Meds 'Always' Explained Before Given	300+	58%	-	60%
Nurses 'Always' Communicated Well	300+	76%	-	76%
Pain 'Always' Well Controlled	300+	71%	-	69%
Room and Bathroom 'Always' Clean	300+	69%	-	71%
Timely Help 'Always' Received	300+	62%	-	64%
Would Definitely Recommend Hospital	300+	77%	-	69%

NOTE: Hospital profiles are in alphabetical order by state, then city, then hospital within the city; Rankings exclude hospitals with less than 25 cases except for patient surveys which excludes hospitals with less than 100 cases; (a) 100–299 cases; (1) The number of cases is too small to be sure how well a hospital is performing; (2) The hospital indicated that the data submitted for this measure were based on a sample of cases; (3) Data was collected during a shorter time period (fewer quarters) than the maximum possible time for this measure; (4) Suppressed for one or more quarters by CMS; (5) No data is available from the hospital for this measure; (6) Fewer than 100 patients completed the HCAHPS survey. Use these rates with caution, as the number of surveys may be too low to reliably assess hospital performance; (7) Survey results are based on less than 12 months of data; (8) Survey results are not available for this reporting period; (9) No or very few patients were eligible for the HCAHPS survey. The scores shown, if any, reflect a very small number of surveys; (10) A state average was not calculated because too few hospitals in the state submitted data; (11) There were discrepancies in the data collection process; Please refer to the User's Guide for a full explanation of data.

CJW Medical Center

1401 Johnston Willis Drive — Phone: 804-330-2001
Richmond, VA 23235
Type: Acute Care Hospitals — Emergency Services: No
Ownership: Proprietary
Key Personnel:
CEO/President. . . . . Peter Marmerstrin

Measure	Cases	This Hosp.	State Avg.	U.S. Avg.
Heart Attack Care				
ACE Inhibitor or ARB for LVSD	93	100%	97%	96%
Aspirin at Arrival	376	100%	99%	99%
Aspirin at Discharge	435	100%	99%	98%
Beta Blocker at Discharge	401	100%	99%	98%
Fibrinolytic Medication Timing	0	-	75%	55%
PCI Within 90 Minutes of Arrival	62	98%	93%	90%
Smoking Cessation Advice	166	100%	100%	99%
Chest Pain/Possible Heart Attack Care				
Aspirin at Arrival[1,3]	4	100%	95%	95%
Median Time to ECG (minutes)[1,3]	4	4	8	8
Median Time to Transfer (minutes)[5]	0	-	60	61
Fibrinolytic Medication Timing[5]	0	-	59%	54%
Heart Failure Care				
ACE Inhibitor or ARB for LVSD	224	100%	97%	94%
Discharge Instructions	596	99%	92%	88%
Evaluation of LVS Function	734	100%	99%	98%
Smoking Cessation Advice	141	100%	99%	98%
Pneumonia Care				
Appropriate Initial Antibiotic	200	96%	93%	92%
Blood Culture Timing	400	100%	97%	96%
Influenza Vaccine	246	98%	94%	91%
Initial Antibiotic Timing	338	98%	96%	95%
Pneumococcal Vaccine	296	100%	95%	93%
Smoking Cessation Advice	135	100%	98%	97%
Surgical Care Improvement Project				
Appropriate VTP Within 24 Hours[2]	270	97%	94%	92%
Appropriate Hair Removal[2]	843	99%	100%	99%
Appropriate Beta Blocker Usage[2]	281	98%	94%	93%
Controlled Postoperative Blood Glucose[2]	155	99%	96%	93%
Prophylactic Antibiotic Timing[2]	531	100%	97%	97%
Prophylactic Antibiotic Timing (Outpatient)	690	94%	93%	92%
Prophylactic Antibiotic Selection[2]	543	98%	98%	97%
Prophylactic Antibiotic Select. (Outpatient)	680	97%	96%	94%
Prophylactic Antibiotic Stopped[2]	491	95%	96%	94%
Recommended VTP Ordered[2]	271	97%	96%	94%
Urinary Catheter Removal[2]	195	95%	93%	90%
Children's Asthma Care				
Received Systemic Corticosteroids	-	-	-	100%
Received Home Management Plan	-	-	-	71%
Received Reliever Medication	-	-	-	100%
Use of Medical Imaging				
Combination Abdominal CT Scan	1,776	0.324	0.144	0.191
Combination Chest CT Scan	897	0.052	0.030	0.054
Follow-up Mammogram/Ultrasound	2,755	5.6%	7.5%	8.4%
MRI for Low Back Pain	282	30.9%	31.5%	32.7%
Survey of Patients' Hospital Experiences				
Area Around Room 'Always' Quiet at Night	300+	58%	-	58%
Doctors 'Always' Communicated Well	300+	80%	-	80%
Home Recovery Information Given	300+	84%	-	82%
Hospital Given 9 or 10 on 10 Point Scale	300+	67%	-	67%
Meds 'Always' Explained Before Given	300+	56%	-	60%
Nurses 'Always' Communicated Well	300+	74%	-	76%
Pain 'Always' Well Controlled	300+	69%	-	69%
Room and Bathroom 'Always' Clean	300+	66%	-	71%
Timely Help 'Always' Received	300+	59%	-	64%
Would Definitely Recommend Hospital	300+	70%	-	69%

Henrico Doctors' Hospital

1602 Skipwith Road — Phone: 804-289-4500
Richmond, VA 23229 — Fax: 804-287-4358
URL: www.henricodoctors.com
Type: Acute Care Hospitals — Emergency Services: Yes
Ownership: Proprietary — Beds: 760
Key Personnel:
CEO/President. . . . . David Russell Williams
Chief of Medical Staff. . . . . Dr Richard Hamrick
Coronary Care. . . . . Steve Tarkington
Infection Control. . . . . Jeanette Daniel
Pediatric Ambulatory Care . . . . . . Judy Mathews
Pediatric In-Patient Care . . . . Judy Mathews
Quality Assurance . . . . Nancy Kindervater
Radiology. . . . . Bob Longley

Measure	Cases	This Hosp.	State Avg.	U.S. Avg.
Heart Attack Care				
ACE Inhibitor or ARB for LVSD	53	100%	97%	96%
Aspirin at Arrival	180	100%	99%	99%
Aspirin at Discharge	276	100%	99%	98%
Beta Blocker at Discharge	259	100%	99%	98%
Fibrinolytic Medication Timing	0	-	75%	55%
PCI Within 90 Minutes of Arrival	34	100%	93%	90%
Smoking Cessation Advice	114	100%	100%	99%
Chest Pain/Possible Heart Attack Care				
Aspirin at Arrival[1]	5	100%	95%	95%
Median Time to ECG (minutes)[1]	6	8	8	8
Median Time to Transfer (minutes)[1,3]	1	47	60	61
Fibrinolytic Medication Timing[3]	0	-	59%	54%
Heart Failure Care				
ACE Inhibitor or ARB for LVSD[2]	144	100%	97%	94%
Discharge Instructions[2]	330	93%	92%	88%
Evaluation of LVS Function[2]	432	100%	99%	98%
Smoking Cessation Advice[2]	52	100%	99%	98%
Pneumonia Care				
Appropriate Initial Antibiotic[2]	119	92%	93%	92%
Blood Culture Timing[2]	153	96%	97%	96%
Influenza Vaccine[2]	147	97%	94%	91%
Initial Antibiotic Timing[2]	208	95%	96%	95%
Pneumococcal Vaccine[2]	235	98%	95%	93%
Smoking Cessation Advice[2]	72	99%	98%	97%
Surgical Care Improvement Project				
Appropriate VTP Within 24 Hours[2]	208	95%	94%	92%
Appropriate Hair Removal[2]	875	99%	100%	99%
Appropriate Beta Blocker Usage[2]	261	98%	94%	93%
Controlled Postoperative Blood Glucose[2]	172	98%	96%	93%
Prophylactic Antibiotic Timing[2]	599	98%	97%	97%
Prophylactic Antibiotic Timing (Outpatient)	662	97%	93%	92%
Prophylactic Antibiotic Selection[2]	606	97%	98%	97%
Prophylactic Antibiotic Select. (Outpatient)	649	98%	96%	94%
Prophylactic Antibiotic Stopped[2]	574	95%	96%	94%
Recommended VTP Ordered[2]	208	96%	96%	94%
Urinary Catheter Removal[2]	195	88%	93%	90%
Children's Asthma Care				
Received Systemic Corticosteroids	-	-	-	100%
Received Home Management Plan	-	-	-	71%
Received Reliever Medication	-	-	-	100%
Use of Medical Imaging				
Combination Abdominal CT Scan	1,202	0.141	0.144	0.191
Combination Chest CT Scan	890	0.012	0.030	0.054
Follow-up Mammogram/Ultrasound	1,467	8.0%	7.5%	8.4%
MRI for Low Back Pain	214	26.6%	31.5%	32.7%
Survey of Patients' Hospital Experiences				
Area Around Room 'Always' Quiet at Night	300+	61%	-	58%
Doctors 'Always' Communicated Well	300+	82%	-	80%
Home Recovery Information Given	300+	84%	-	82%
Hospital Given 9 or 10 on 10 Point Scale	300+	71%	-	67%
Meds 'Always' Explained Before Given	300+	59%	-	60%
Nurses 'Always' Communicated Well	300+	76%	-	76%
Pain 'Always' Well Controlled	300+	73%	-	69%
Room and Bathroom 'Always' Clean	300+	66%	-	71%
Timely Help 'Always' Received	300+	65%	-	64%
Would Definitely Recommend Hospital	300+	76%	-	69%

Richmond VA Medical Center

1201 Broad Rock Boulevard — Phone: 804-675-5000
Richmond, VA 23249 — Fax: 804-675-5585
URL: www.med.va.gov
Type: Acute Care-Veterans Administration — Emergency Services: No
Ownership: Government - Federal — Beds: 427
Key Personnel:
Chief of Medical Staff. . . . . Julie Beals, MD
Infection Control. . . . . Edward Wong, MD
Operating Room. . . . . Bobbie C Branch, RN
Quality Assurance . . . . Margaret Supensky, RN
Radiology. . . . . Peter Quagliano, MD
Anesthesiology. . . . . Robert Litwack, MD
Emergency Room . . . . Charles Stuckey, MD
Intensive Care Unit. . . . . Mablene Bailey, RN

Measure	Cases	This Hosp.	State Avg.	U.S. Avg.
Heart Attack Care				
ACE Inhibitor or ARB for LVSD[1]	13	85%	97%	96%
Aspirin at Arrival	50	98%	99%	99%
Aspirin at Discharge	54	98%	99%	98%
Beta Blocker at Discharge	51	96%	99%	98%
Fibrinolytic Medication Timing[5]	0	-	75%	55%
PCI Within 90 Minutes of Arrival[1]	2	50%	93%	90%
Smoking Cessation Advice[1]	15	100%	100%	99%
Chest Pain/Possible Heart Attack Care				
Aspirin at Arrival	-	-	95%	95%
Median Time to ECG (minutes)	-	-	8	8
Median Time to Transfer (minutes)	-	-	60	61
Fibrinolytic Medication Timing	-	-	59%	54%
Heart Failure Care				
ACE Inhibitor or ARB for LVSD	137	97%	97%	94%
Discharge Instructions	262	95%	92%	88%
Evaluation of LVS Function	273	100%	99%	98%
Smoking Cessation Advice	58	97%	99%	98%
Pneumonia Care				
Appropriate Initial Antibiotic	85	93%	93%	92%
Blood Culture Timing	150	99%	97%	96%
Influenza Vaccine	110	94%	94%	91%
Initial Antibiotic Timing	157	97%	96%	95%
Pneumococcal Vaccine	105	99%	95%	93%
Smoking Cessation Advice	57	98%	98%	97%
Surgical Care Improvement Project				
Appropriate VTP Within 24 Hours[2]	163	98%	94%	92%
Appropriate Hair Removal[2]	351	100%	100%	99%
Appropriate Beta Blocker Usage[2]	150	100%	94%	93%
Controlled Postoperative Blood Glucose[2]	95	96%	96%	93%
Prophylactic Antibiotic Timing	253	96%	97%	97%
Prophylactic Antibiotic Timing (Outpatient)	-	-	93%	92%
Prophylactic Antibiotic Selection	257	98%	98%	97%
Prophylactic Antibiotic Select. (Outpatient)	-	-	96%	94%
Prophylactic Antibiotic Stopped	232	94%	96%	94%
Recommended VTP Ordered[2]	163	98%	96%	94%
Urinary Catheter Removal[2]	131	95%	93%	90%
Children's Asthma Care				
Received Systemic Corticosteroids	-	-	-	100%
Received Home Management Plan	-	-	-	71%
Received Reliever Medication	-	-	-	100%
Use of Medical Imaging				
Combination Abdominal CT Scan	-	-	0.144	0.191
Combination Chest CT Scan	-	-	0.030	0.054
Follow-up Mammogram/Ultrasound	-	-	7.5%	8.4%
MRI for Low Back Pain	-	-	31.5%	32.7%
Survey of Patients' Hospital Experiences				
Area Around Room 'Always' Quiet at Night	-	-	-	58%
Doctors 'Always' Communicated Well	-	-	-	80%
Home Recovery Information Given	-	-	-	82%
Hospital Given 9 or 10 on 10 Point Scale	-	-	-	67%
Meds 'Always' Explained Before Given	-	-	-	60%
Nurses 'Always' Communicated Well	-	-	-	76%
Pain 'Always' Well Controlled	-	-	-	69%
Room and Bathroom 'Always' Clean	-	-	-	71%
Timely Help 'Always' Received	-	-	-	64%
Would Definitely Recommend Hospital	-	-	-	69%

NOTE: Hospital profiles are in alphabetical order by state, then city, then hospital within the city; Rankings exclude hospitals with less than 25 cases except for patient surveys which excludes hospitals with less than 100 cases; (a) 100–299 cases; (1) The number of cases is too small to be sure how well a hospital is performing; (2) The hospital indicated that the data submitted for this measure were based on a sample of cases; (3) Data was collected during a shorter time period (fewer quarters) than the maximum possible time for this measure; (4) Suppressed for one or more quarters by CMS; (5) No data is available from the hospital for this measure; (6) Fewer than 100 patients completed the HCAHPS survey. Use these rates with caution, as the number of surveys may be too low to reliably assess hospital performance; (7) Survey results are based on less than 12 months of data; (8) Survey results are not available for this reporting period; (9) No or very few patients were eligible for the HCAHPS survey. The scores shown, if any, reflect a very small number of surveys; (10) A state average was not calculated because too few hospitals in the state submitted data; (11) There were discrepancies in the data collection process; Please refer to the User's Guide for a full explanation of data.

Virginia Commonwealth University Health System

1250 East Marshall Street
Richmond, VA 23298
Phone: 804-828-0938
Fax: 804-828-1657
E-mail: lcoles@mcvh-vcu.edu
URL: www.vcuhealth.org
Type: Acute Care Hospitals
Emergency Services: No
Ownership: Govt - Hospital Dist/Auth
Beds: 779

Key Personnel:

CEO/President. . . . . John Duval
Chief of Medical Staff. . . . . Ralph R Clark, MD
Coronary Care. . . . . Wanda Miller
Infection Control. . . . . Michael Edmond, MD MPH
Pediatric Ambulatory Care . . . . . . Joseph Laver
Pediatric In-Patient Care . . . . Lauren Goodloe
Quality Assurance . . . . Jennifer Adkins
Radiology. . . . . Ron Miller

Measure	Cases	This Hosp.	State Avg.	U.S. Avg.
Heart Attack Care				
ACE Inhibitor or ARB for LVSD	93	90%	97%	96%
Aspirin at Arrival	255	99%	99%	99%
Aspirin at Discharge	358	98%	99%	98%
Beta Blocker at Discharge	328	99%	99%	98%
Fibrinolytic Medication Timing	0	-	75%	55%
PCI Within 90 Minutes of Arrival	57	98%	93%	90%
Smoking Cessation Advice	160	100%	100%	99%
Chest Pain/Possible Heart Attack Care				
Aspirin at Arrival[5]	0	-	95%	95%
Median Time to ECG (minutes)[5]	0	-	8	8
Median Time to Transfer (minutes)[5]	0	-	60	61
Fibrinolytic Medication Timing[5]	0	-	59%	54%
Heart Failure Care				
ACE Inhibitor or ARB for LVSD	338	95%	97%	94%
Discharge Instructions	659	97%	92%	88%
Evaluation of LVS Function	709	100%	99%	98%
Smoking Cessation Advice	219	100%	99%	98%
Pneumonia Care				
Appropriate Initial Antibiotic	86	90%	93%	92%
Blood Culture Timing	206	86%	97%	96%
Influenza Vaccine	146	84%	94%	91%
Initial Antibiotic Timing	226	91%	96%	95%
Pneumococcal Vaccine	113	83%	95%	93%
Smoking Cessation Advice	183	99%	98%	97%
Surgical Care Improvement Project				
Appropriate VTP Within 24 Hours[2]	259	97%	94%	92%
Appropriate Hair Removal[2]	741	98%	100%	99%
Appropriate Beta Blocker Usage[2]	211	93%	94%	93%
Controlled Postoperative Blood Glucose[2]	140	93%	96%	93%
Prophylactic Antibiotic Timing[2]	445	93%	97%	97%
Prophylactic Antibiotic Timing (Outpatient)	866	86%	93%	92%
Prophylactic Antibiotic Selection[2]	456	97%	98%	97%
Prophylactic Antibiotic Select. (Outpatient)	839	93%	96%	94%
Prophylactic Antibiotic Stopped[2]	423	87%	96%	94%
Recommended VTP Ordered[2]	259	98%	96%	94%
Urinary Catheter Removal[2]	161	85%	93%	90%
Children's Asthma Care				
Received Systemic Corticosteroids	-	-	-	100%
Received Home Management Plan	-	-	-	71%
Received Reliever Medication	-	-	-	100%
Use of Medical Imaging				
Combination Abdominal CT Scan	1,225	0.124	0.144	0.191
Combination Chest CT Scan	1,549	0.040	0.030	0.054
Follow-up Mammogram/Ultrasound	1,917	3.9%	7.5%	8.4%
MRI for Low Back Pain	226	28.8%	31.5%	32.7%
Survey of Patients' Hospital Experiences				
Area Around Room 'Always' Quiet at Night	300+	59%	-	58%
Doctors 'Always' Communicated Well	300+	80%	-	80%
Home Recovery Information Given	300+	86%	-	82%
Hospital Given 9 or 10 on 10 Point Scale	300+	68%	-	67%
Meds 'Always' Explained Before Given	300+	61%	-	60%
Nurses 'Always' Communicated Well	300+	75%	-	76%
Pain 'Always' Well Controlled	300+	69%	-	69%
Room and Bathroom 'Always' Clean	300+	65%	-	71%
Timely Help 'Always' Received	300+	60%	-	64%
Would Definitely Recommend Hospital	300+	71%	-	69%

Carilion Medical Center

1906 Belleview Avenue
Roanoke, VA 24033
Phone: 540-981-7000
Fax: 540-983-1190
URL: www.carilion.com/crmh
Type: Acute Care Hospitals
Emergency Services: Yes
Ownership: Voluntary Non-Profit - Private
Beds: 520

Key Personnel:

CEO/President. . . . . Lucas A Snipes
Chief of Medical Staff. . . . . Jim Gooding
Infection Control . . . . Debora Demicco, MD
Operating Room. . . . . Jeannette Capella
Quality Assurance . . . . Judy Wilson
Radiology. . . . . Dana B Fathy, MD
Emergency Room . . . . Evelyn Menetta
Intensive Care Unit. . . . . Cindy Smith

Measure	Cases	This Hosp.	State Avg.	U.S. Avg.
Heart Attack Care				
ACE Inhibitor or ARB for LVSD	228	95%	97%	96%
Aspirin at Arrival	560	99%	99%	99%
Aspirin at Discharge	1,249	99%	99%	98%
Beta Blocker at Discharge	1,264	98%	99%	98%
Fibrinolytic Medication Timing	0	-	75%	55%
PCI Within 90 Minutes of Arrival	104	88%	93%	90%
Smoking Cessation Advice	509	100%	100%	99%
Chest Pain/Possible Heart Attack Care				
Aspirin at Arrival[3]	0	-	95%	95%
Median Time to ECG (minutes)[1,3]	1	91	8	8
Median Time to Transfer (minutes)[5]	0	-	60	61
Fibrinolytic Medication Timing[5]	0	-	59%	54%
Heart Failure Care				
ACE Inhibitor or ARB for LVSD	300	87%	97%	94%
Discharge Instructions	636	92%	92%	88%
Evaluation of LVS Function	780	96%	99%	98%
Smoking Cessation Advice	200	98%	99%	98%
Pneumonia Care				
Appropriate Initial Antibiotic	288	84%	93%	92%
Blood Culture Timing	398	88%	97%	96%
Influenza Vaccine	270	89%	94%	91%
Initial Antibiotic Timing	485	87%	96%	95%
Pneumococcal Vaccine	366	92%	95%	93%
Smoking Cessation Advice	232	99%	98%	97%
Surgical Care Improvement Project				
Appropriate VTP Within 24 Hours[2]	447	96%	94%	92%
Appropriate Hair Removal[2]	2,675	100%	100%	99%
Appropriate Beta Blocker Usage[2]	815	88%	94%	93%
Controlled Postoperative Blood Glucose[2]	570	96%	96%	93%
Prophylactic Antibiotic Timing[2]	2,261	95%	97%	97%
Prophylactic Antibiotic Timing (Outpatient)	598	91%	93%	92%
Prophylactic Antibiotic Selection[2]	2,269	98%	98%	97%
Prophylactic Antibiotic Select. (Outpatient)	575	96%	96%	94%
Prophylactic Antibiotic Stopped[2]	2,203	95%	96%	94%
Recommended VTP Ordered[2]	448	96%	96%	94%
Urinary Catheter Removal[2]	325	94%	93%	90%
Children's Asthma Care				
Received Systemic Corticosteroids	-	-	-	100%
Received Home Management Plan	-	-	-	71%
Received Reliever Medication	-	-	-	100%
Use of Medical Imaging				
Combination Abdominal CT Scan	1,721	0.027	0.144	0.191
Combination Chest CT Scan	1,131	0.038	0.030	0.054
Follow-up Mammogram/Ultrasound	4,239	4.3%	7.5%	8.4%
MRI for Low Back Pain	459	32.7%	31.5%	32.7%
Survey of Patients' Hospital Experiences				
Area Around Room 'Always' Quiet at Night	300+	60%	-	58%
Doctors 'Always' Communicated Well	300+	78%	-	80%
Home Recovery Information Given	300+	84%	-	82%
Hospital Given 9 or 10 on 10 Point Scale	300+	71%	-	67%
Meds 'Always' Explained Before Given	300+	67%	-	60%
Nurses 'Always' Communicated Well	300+	77%	-	76%
Pain 'Always' Well Controlled	300+	69%	-	69%
Room and Bathroom 'Always' Clean	300+	60%	-	71%
Timely Help 'Always' Received	300+	65%	-	64%
Would Definitely Recommend Hospital	300+	74%	-	69%

Carilion Franklin Memorial Hospital

180 Floyd Avenue
Rocky Mount, VA 24151
Phone: 540-483-5277
Fax: 540-489-6442
URL: www.carilion.com/cfmh
Type: Acute Care Hospitals
Emergency Services: Yes
Ownership: Voluntary Non-Profit - Other
Beds: 37

Key Personnel:

Chief of Medical Staff. . . . . Mark J Werner
Infection Control. . . . . Virginia Crouch
Operating Room. . . . . Charles A Harris
Quality Assurance . . . . Carol Melvin
Emergency Room . . . . Darrell Van Ness

Measure	Cases	This Hosp.	State Avg.	U.S. Avg.
Heart Attack Care				
ACE Inhibitor or ARB for LVSD[1]	2	100%	97%	96%
Aspirin at Arrival[1]	11	100%	99%	99%
Aspirin at Discharge[1]	8	100%	99%	98%
Beta Blocker at Discharge[1]	6	100%	99%	98%
Fibrinolytic Medication Timing	0	-	75%	55%
PCI Within 90 Minutes of Arrival	0	-	93%	90%
Smoking Cessation Advice	0	-	100%	99%
Chest Pain/Possible Heart Attack Care				
Aspirin at Arrival	204	94%	95%	95%
Median Time to ECG (minutes)	221	31	8	8
Median Time to Transfer (minutes)[1,3]	4	86	60	61
Fibrinolytic Medication Timing	0	-	59%	54%
Heart Failure Care				
ACE Inhibitor or ARB for LVSD[1]	9	100%	97%	94%
Discharge Instructions	53	91%	92%	88%
Evaluation of LVS Function	76	96%	99%	98%
Smoking Cessation Advice[1]	11	100%	99%	98%
Pneumonia Care				
Appropriate Initial Antibiotic	68	93%	93%	92%
Blood Culture Timing	120	96%	97%	96%
Influenza Vaccine	63	92%	94%	91%
Initial Antibiotic Timing	108	97%	96%	95%
Pneumococcal Vaccine	93	94%	95%	93%
Smoking Cessation Advice	38	100%	98%	97%
Surgical Care Improvement Project				
Appropriate VTP Within 24 Hours[1]	16	94%	94%	92%
Appropriate Hair Removal	59	100%	100%	99%
Appropriate Beta Blocker Usage[1]	8	62%	94%	93%
Controlled Postoperative Blood Glucose	0	-	96%	93%
Prophylactic Antibiotic Timing	36	86%	97%	97%
Prophylactic Antibiotic Timing (Outpatient)[1]	16	56%	93%	92%
Prophylactic Antibiotic Selection	36	92%	98%	97%
Prophylactic Antibiotic Select. (Outpatient)[1]	10	100%	96%	94%
Prophylactic Antibiotic Stopped	35	97%	96%	94%
Recommended VTP Ordered[1]	16	94%	96%	94%
Urinary Catheter Removal[1]	5	100%	93%	90%
Children's Asthma Care				
Received Systemic Corticosteroids	-	-	-	100%
Received Home Management Plan	-	-	-	71%
Received Reliever Medication	-	-	-	100%
Use of Medical Imaging				
Combination Abdominal CT Scan	408	0.032	0.144	0.191
Combination Chest CT Scan	163	0.067	0.030	0.054
Follow-up Mammogram/Ultrasound	681	4.4%	7.5%	8.4%
MRI for Low Back Pain	89	38.2%	31.5%	32.7%
Survey of Patients' Hospital Experiences				
Area Around Room 'Always' Quiet at Night	300+	59%	-	58%
Doctors 'Always' Communicated Well	300+	83%	-	80%
Home Recovery Information Given	300+	83%	-	82%
Hospital Given 9 or 10 on 10 Point Scale	300+	71%	-	67%
Meds 'Always' Explained Before Given	300+	67%	-	60%
Nurses 'Always' Communicated Well	300+	82%	-	76%
Pain 'Always' Well Controlled	300+	75%	-	69%
Room and Bathroom 'Always' Clean	300+	77%	-	71%
Timely Help 'Always' Received	300+	71%	-	64%
Would Definitely Recommend Hospital	300+	70%	-	69%

NOTE: Hospital profiles are in alphabetical order by state, then city, then hospital within the city; Rankings exclude hospitals with less than 25 cases except for patient surveys which excludes hospitals with less than 100 cases; (a) 100–299 cases; (1) The number of cases is too small to be sure how well a hospital is performing; (2) The hospital indicated that the data submitted for this measure were based on a sample of cases; (3) Data was collected during a shorter time period (fewer quarters) than the maximum possible time for this measure; (4) Suppressed for one or more quarters by CMS; (5) No data is available from the hospital for this measure; (6) Fewer than 100 patients completed the HCAHPS survey. Use these rates with caution, as the number of surveys may be too low to reliably assess hospital performance; (7) Survey results are based on less than 12 months of data; (8) Survey results are not available for this reporting period; (9) No or very few patients were eligible for the HCAHPS survey. The scores shown, if any, reflect a very small number of surveys; (10) A state average was not calculated because too few hospitals in the state submitted data; (11) There were discrepancies in the data collection process; Please refer to the User's Guide for a full explanation of data.

Lewis-Gale Medical Center

1900 Electric Road
Salem, VA 24153
Phone: 540-776-4100
Fax: 540-772-6411
E-mail: james.thweatt@hcahealthcare.com
URL: www.lewis-gale.com
Type: Acute Care Hospitals
Emergency Services: Yes
Ownership: Proprietary
Beds: 521

Key Personnel:

CEO/President.............. James W Thweatt, Jr
Chief of Medical Staff.......... Rajeev Sharma, MD
Infection Control.............. Teresa Stowasser, RN
Operating Room.............. Nancy Boyer, RN
Pediatric In-Patient Care .... Luther A Beazley, MD
Quality Assurance .... Charlotte Tyson
Radiology.................. John M Mathis, MD

Measure	Cases	This Hosp.	State Avg.	U.S. Avg.
Heart Attack Care				
ACE Inhibitor or ARB for LVSD	55	100%	97%	96%
Aspirin at Arrival	203	100%	99%	99%
Aspirin at Discharge	355	100%	99%	98%
Beta Blocker at Discharge	356	100%	99%	98%
Fibrinolytic Medication Timing	0	-	75%	55%
PCI Within 90 Minutes of Arrival	41	98%	93%	90%
Smoking Cessation Advice	139	100%	100%	99%
Chest Pain/Possible Heart Attack Care				
Aspirin at Arrival[1,3]	4	100%	95%	95%
Median Time to ECG (minutes)[1,3]	3	9	8	8
Median Time to Transfer (minutes)[5]	0	-	60	61
Fibrinolytic Medication Timing[3]	0	-	59%	54%
Heart Failure Care				
ACE Inhibitor or ARB for LVSD	121	100%	97%	94%
Discharge Instructions	284	98%	92%	88%
Evaluation of LVS Function	393	100%	99%	98%
Smoking Cessation Advice	48	100%	99%	98%
Pneumonia Care				
Appropriate Initial Antibiotic	248	98%	93%	92%
Blood Culture Timing	370	99%	97%	96%
Influenza Vaccine	252	100%	94%	91%
Initial Antibiotic Timing	354	98%	96%	95%
Pneumococcal Vaccine	378	100%	95%	93%
Smoking Cessation Advice	115	99%	98%	97%
Surgical Care Improvement Project				
Appropriate VTP Within 24 Hours[2]	219	98%	94%	92%
Appropriate Hair Removal[2]	724	100%	100%	99%
Appropriate Beta Blocker Usage[2]	278	99%	94%	93%
Controlled Postoperative Blood Glucose[2]	139	99%	96%	93%
Prophylactic Antibiotic Timing[2]	538	99%	97%	97%
Prophylactic Antibiotic Timing (Outpatient)	618	99%	93%	92%
Prophylactic Antibiotic Selection[2]	545	99%	98%	97%
Prophylactic Antibiotic Select. (Outpatient)	620	99%	96%	94%
Prophylactic Antibiotic Stopped[2]	521	99%	96%	94%
Recommended VTP Ordered[2]	219	98%	96%	94%
Urinary Catheter Removal[2]	100	88%	93%	90%
Children's Asthma Care				
Received Systemic Corticosteroids	-	-	-	100%
Received Home Management Plan	-	-	-	71%
Received Reliever Medication	-	-	-	100%
Use of Medical Imaging				
Combination Abdominal CT Scan	1,458	0.057	0.144	0.191
Combination Chest CT Scan	992	0.008	0.030	0.054
Follow-up Mammogram/Ultrasound	2,523	8.7%	7.5%	8.4%
MRI for Low Back Pain	275	28.0%	31.5%	32.7%
Survey of Patients' Hospital Experiences				
Area Around Room 'Always' Quiet at Night	300+	55%	-	58%
Doctors 'Always' Communicated Well	300+	82%	-	80%
Home Recovery Information Given	300+	87%	-	82%
Hospital Given 9 or 10 on 10 Point Scale	300+	72%	-	67%
Meds 'Always' Explained Before Given	300+	58%	-	60%
Nurses 'Always' Communicated Well	300+	77%	-	76%
Pain 'Always' Well Controlled	300+	71%	-	69%
Room and Bathroom 'Always' Clean	300+	67%	-	71%
Timely Help 'Always' Received	300+	61%	-	64%
Would Definitely Recommend Hospital	300+	77%	-	69%

Salem VA Medical Center

1970 Boulevard
Salem, VA 24153
Phone: 540-982-2463
Fax: 540-983-1096
URL: www.med.va.gov
Type: Acute Care-Veterans Administration
Emergency Services: No
Ownership: Government - Federal
Beds: 282

Key Personnel:

Cardiac Laboratory............ Nelson Bernardo, MD
Chief of Medical Staff.......... Maureen McCarthy, MD
Infection Control.............. Charlene McCadden
Operating Room.............. Wayne H Wilson
Quality Assurance .... Carol Carlson, RN
Radiology.................. Narain Srinivas, MD
Emergency Room .... Matthew T Barnette, RN
Patient Relations .... Debra Burgess

Measure	Cases	This Hosp.	State Avg.	U.S. Avg.
Heart Attack Care				
ACE Inhibitor or ARB for LVSD[1]	5	80%	97%	96%
Aspirin at Arrival	43	100%	99%	99%
Aspirin at Discharge	32	100%	99%	98%
Beta Blocker at Discharge	32	100%	99%	98%
Fibrinolytic Medication Timing[5]	0	-	75%	55%
PCI Within 90 Minutes of Arrival[1]	3	67%	93%	90%
Smoking Cessation Advice[1]	10	90%	100%	99%
Chest Pain/Possible Heart Attack Care				
Aspirin at Arrival	-	-	95%	95%
Median Time to ECG (minutes)	-	-	8	8
Median Time to Transfer (minutes)	-	-	60	61
Fibrinolytic Medication Timing	-	-	59%	54%
Heart Failure Care				
ACE Inhibitor or ARB for LVSD	66	100%	97%	94%
Discharge Instructions	121	87%	92%	88%
Evaluation of LVS Function	143	100%	99%	98%
Smoking Cessation Advice	35	100%	99%	98%
Pneumonia Care				
Appropriate Initial Antibiotic	62	95%	93%	92%
Blood Culture Timing	96	98%	97%	96%
Influenza Vaccine	78	97%	94%	91%
Initial Antibiotic Timing	83	95%	96%	95%
Pneumococcal Vaccine	90	98%	95%	93%
Smoking Cessation Advice	36	94%	98%	97%
Surgical Care Improvement Project				
Appropriate VTP Within 24 Hours[2]	114	100%	94%	92%
Appropriate Hair Removal[2]	214	100%	100%	99%
Appropriate Beta Blocker Usage[2]	66	98%	94%	93%
Controlled Postoperative Blood Glucose[2,5]	0	-	96%	93%
Prophylactic Antibiotic Timing	141	97%	97%	97%
Prophylactic Antibiotic Timing (Outpatient)	-	-	93%	92%
Prophylactic Antibiotic Selection	144	99%	98%	97%
Prophylactic Antibiotic Select. (Outpatient)	-	-	96%	94%
Prophylactic Antibiotic Stopped	140	99%	96%	94%
Recommended VTP Ordered[2]	114	100%	96%	94%
Urinary Catheter Removal[2]	85	93%	93%	90%
Children's Asthma Care				
Received Systemic Corticosteroids	-	-	-	100%
Received Home Management Plan	-	-	-	71%
Received Reliever Medication	-	-	-	100%
Use of Medical Imaging				
Combination Abdominal CT Scan	-	-	0.144	0.191
Combination Chest CT Scan	-	-	0.030	0.054
Follow-up Mammogram/Ultrasound	-	-	7.5%	8.4%
MRI for Low Back Pain	-	-	31.5%	32.7%
Survey of Patients' Hospital Experiences				
Area Around Room 'Always' Quiet at Night	-	-	-	58%
Doctors 'Always' Communicated Well	-	-	-	80%
Home Recovery Information Given	-	-	-	82%
Hospital Given 9 or 10 on 10 Point Scale	-	-	-	67%
Meds 'Always' Explained Before Given	-	-	-	60%
Nurses 'Always' Communicated Well	-	-	-	76%
Pain 'Always' Well Controlled	-	-	-	69%
Room and Bathroom 'Always' Clean	-	-	-	71%
Timely Help 'Always' Received	-	-	-	64%
Would Definitely Recommend Hospital	-	-	-	69%

Community Memorial Healthcenter

125 Buena Vista Circle
South Hill, VA 23970
Phone: 434-447-3151
Fax: 434-774-2485
E-mail: ethompson@cmh-sh.org
URL: www.cmh-sh.org
Type: Acute Care Hospitals
Emergency Services: Yes
Ownership: Voluntary Non-Profit - Private
Beds: 144

Key Personnel:

CEO/President.............. Scott W Burnette
Chief of Medical Staff.......... David Powers
Infection Control.............. Gayle Sutton, RN
Operating Room.............. Joanne Paynter, TN
Quality Assurance .... Edward Brandenburg
Radiology.................. Nirpendra Devanath
Emergency Room .... Wallace Horne
Patient Relations .... Ursula Butts

Measure	Cases	This Hosp.	State Avg.	U.S. Avg.
Heart Attack Care				
ACE Inhibitor or ARB for LVSD[1]	11	100%	97%	96%
Aspirin at Arrival	54	100%	99%	99%
Aspirin at Discharge	42	100%	99%	98%
Beta Blocker at Discharge	44	100%	99%	98%
Fibrinolytic Medication Timing[1]	3	67%	75%	55%
PCI Within 90 Minutes of Arrival	0	-	93%	90%
Smoking Cessation Advice[1]	6	100%	100%	99%
Chest Pain/Possible Heart Attack Care				
Aspirin at Arrival	97	94%	95%	95%
Median Time to ECG (minutes)	95	8	8	8
Median Time to Transfer (minutes)[5]	0	-	60	61
Fibrinolytic Medication Timing[1]	4	50%	59%	54%
Heart Failure Care				
ACE Inhibitor or ARB for LVSD	51	100%	97%	94%
Discharge Instructions	158	100%	92%	88%
Evaluation of LVS Function	190	100%	99%	98%
Smoking Cessation Advice	37	100%	99%	98%
Pneumonia Care				
Appropriate Initial Antibiotic	65	95%	93%	92%
Blood Culture Timing	82	99%	97%	96%
Influenza Vaccine	50	100%	94%	91%
Initial Antibiotic Timing	93	97%	96%	95%
Pneumococcal Vaccine	76	96%	95%	93%
Smoking Cessation Advice	31	100%	98%	97%
Surgical Care Improvement Project				
Appropriate VTP Within 24 Hours[2]	49	71%	94%	92%
Appropriate Hair Removal[2]	85	100%	100%	99%
Appropriate Beta Blocker Usage[1,2]	20	80%	94%	93%
Controlled Postoperative Blood Glucose[2]	0	-	96%	93%
Prophylactic Antibiotic Timing[2]	33	97%	97%	97%
Prophylactic Antibiotic Timing (Outpatient)	50	74%	93%	92%
Prophylactic Antibiotic Selection[2]	35	97%	98%	97%
Prophylactic Antibiotic Select. (Outpatient)	37	73%	96%	94%
Prophylactic Antibiotic Stopped[2]	32	97%	96%	94%
Recommended VTP Ordered[2]	49	80%	96%	94%
Urinary Catheter Removal[1,2]	8	100%	93%	90%
Children's Asthma Care				
Received Systemic Corticosteroids[1]	12	100%	-	100%
Received Home Management Plan[1]	12	100%	-	71%
Received Reliever Medication[1]	12	100%	-	100%
Use of Medical Imaging				
Combination Abdominal CT Scan	545	0.409	0.144	0.191
Combination Chest CT Scan	321	0.059	0.030	0.054
Follow-up Mammogram/Ultrasound	1,230	4.6%	7.5%	8.4%
MRI for Low Back Pain	70	47.1%	31.5%	32.7%
Survey of Patients' Hospital Experiences				
Area Around Room 'Always' Quiet at Night	300+	60%	-	58%
Doctors 'Always' Communicated Well	300+	82%	-	80%
Home Recovery Information Given	300+	83%	-	82%
Hospital Given 9 or 10 on 10 Point Scale	300+	63%	-	67%
Meds 'Always' Explained Before Given	300+	66%	-	60%
Nurses 'Always' Communicated Well	300+	76%	-	76%
Pain 'Always' Well Controlled	300+	68%	-	69%
Room and Bathroom 'Always' Clean	300+	70%	-	71%
Timely Help 'Always' Received	300+	60%	-	64%
Would Definitely Recommend Hospital	300+	63%	-	69%

NOTE: Hospital profiles are in alphabetical order by state, then city, then hospital within the city; Rankings exclude hospitals with less than 25 cases except for patient surveys which excludes hospitals with less than 100 cases; (a) 100–299 cases; (1) The number of cases is too small to be sure how well a hospital is performing; (2) The hospital indicated that the data submitted for this measure were based on a sample of cases; (3) Data was collected during a shorter time period (fewer quarters) than the maximum possible time for this measure; (4) Suppressed for one or more quarters by CMS; (5) No data is available from the hospital for this measure; (6) Fewer than 100 patients completed the HCAHPS survey. Use these rates with caution, as the number of surveys may be too low to reliably assess hospital performance; (7) Survey results are based on less than 12 months of data; (8) Survey results are not available for this reporting period; (9) No or very few patients were eligible for the HCAHPS survey. The scores shown, if any, reflect a very small number of surveys; (10) A state average was not calculated because too few hospitals in the state submitted data; (11) There were discrepancies in the data collection process; Please refer to the User's Guide for a full explanation of data.

Stafford Hospital Center

101 Hospital Center Blvd, Suite 307　Phone: 540-741-9033
Stafford, VA 22554
URL: www.marywashingtonhealthcare.com
Type: Acute Care Hospitals　Emergency Services: Yes
Ownership: Voluntary Non-Profit - Private　Beds: 100
Key Personnel:
Administrator . . . . Cathy Yablonski

Measure	Cases	This Hosp.	State Avg.	U.S. Avg.
Heart Attack Care				
ACE Inhibitor or ARB for LVSD	0	-	97%	96%
Aspirin at Arrival[1]	23	100%	99%	99%
Aspirin at Discharge[1]	12	92%	99%	98%
Beta Blocker at Discharge[1]	11	91%	99%	98%
Fibrinolytic Medication Timing	0	-	75%	55%
PCI Within 90 Minutes of Arrival	0	-	93%	90%
Smoking Cessation Advice	0	-	100%	99%
Chest Pain/Possible Heart Attack Care				
Aspirin at Arrival	67	99%	95%	95%
Median Time to ECG (minutes)	68	12	8	8
Median Time to Transfer (minutes)[1]	5	58	60	61
Fibrinolytic Medication Timing	0	-	59%	54%
Heart Failure Care				
ACE Inhibitor or ARB for LVSD[1]	15	100%	97%	94%
Discharge Instructions	88	83%	92%	88%
Evaluation of LVS Function	99	100%	99%	98%
Smoking Cessation Advice[1]	19	100%	99%	98%
Pneumonia Care				
Appropriate Initial Antibiotic	72	96%	93%	92%
Blood Culture Timing	80	95%	97%	96%
Influenza Vaccine	55	80%	94%	91%
Initial Antibiotic Timing	64	98%	96%	95%
Pneumococcal Vaccine	56	86%	95%	93%
Smoking Cessation Advice	25	100%	98%	97%
Surgical Care Improvement Project				
Appropriate VTP Within 24 Hours	52	79%	94%	92%
Appropriate Hair Removal	142	100%	100%	99%
Appropriate Beta Blocker Usage[1]	20	95%	94%	93%
Controlled Postoperative Blood Glucose	0	-	96%	93%
Prophylactic Antibiotic Timing	88	92%	97%	97%
Prophylactic Antibiotic Timing (Outpatient)	88	86%	93%	92%
Prophylactic Antibiotic Selection	88	99%	98%	97%
Prophylactic Antibiotic Select. (Outpatient)	80	95%	96%	94%
Prophylactic Antibiotic Stopped	85	92%	96%	94%
Recommended VTP Ordered	52	81%	96%	94%
Urinary Catheter Removal	40	98%	93%	90%
Children's Asthma Care				
Received Systemic Corticosteroids	-	-	-	100%
Received Home Management Plan	-	-	-	71%
Received Reliever Medication	-	-	-	100%
Use of Medical Imaging				
Combination Abdominal CT Scan[5]	0	-	0.144	0.191
Combination Chest CT Scan[5]	0	-	0.030	0.054
Follow-up Mammogram/Ultrasound[5]	0	-	7.5%	8.4%
MRI for Low Back Pain[5]	0	-	31.5%	32.7%
Survey of Patients' Hospital Experiences				
Area Around Room 'Always' Quiet at Night	300+	54%	-	58%
Doctors 'Always' Communicated Well	300+	75%	-	80%
Home Recovery Information Given	300+	79%	-	82%
Hospital Given 9 or 10 on 10 Point Scale	300+	71%	-	67%
Meds 'Always' Explained Before Given	300+	57%	-	60%
Nurses 'Always' Communicated Well	300+	73%	-	76%
Pain 'Always' Well Controlled	300+	64%	-	69%
Room and Bathroom 'Always' Clean	300+	72%	-	71%
Timely Help 'Always' Received	300+	62%	-	64%
Would Definitely Recommend Hospital	300+	76%	-	69%

Western State Hospital

1301 Richmond Avenue　Phone: 703-332-8000
Staunton, VA 24402　Fax: 540-332-8197
Type: Acute Care Hospitals　Emergency Services: Yes
Ownership: Government - State　Beds: 517
Key Personnel:
Chief of Medical Staff . . . . Marie Claire Smith
Infection Control . . . . Nancy Davis, RN
Quality Assurance . . . . Kathy Belcher
Radiology . . . . Lucy Hanger

Measure	Cases	This Hosp.	State Avg.	U.S. Avg.
Heart Attack Care				
ACE Inhibitor or ARB for LVSD[5]	0	-	97%	96%
Aspirin at Arrival[5]	0	-	99%	99%
Aspirin at Discharge[5]	0	-	99%	98%
Beta Blocker at Discharge[5]	0	-	99%	98%
Fibrinolytic Medication Timing[5]	0	-	75%	55%
PCI Within 90 Minutes of Arrival[5]	0	-	93%	90%
Smoking Cessation Advice[5]	0	-	100%	99%
Chest Pain/Possible Heart Attack Care				
Aspirin at Arrival[5]	0	-	95%	95%
Median Time to ECG (minutes)[5]	0	-	8	8
Median Time to Transfer (minutes)[5]	0	-	60	61
Fibrinolytic Medication Timing[5]	0	-	59%	54%
Heart Failure Care				
ACE Inhibitor or ARB for LVSD[5]	0	-	97%	94%
Discharge Instructions[5]	0	-	92%	88%
Evaluation of LVS Function[5]	0	-	99%	98%
Smoking Cessation Advice[5]	0	-	99%	98%
Pneumonia Care				
Appropriate Initial Antibiotic[5]	0	-	93%	92%
Blood Culture Timing[5]	0	-	97%	96%
Influenza Vaccine[5]	0	-	94%	91%
Initial Antibiotic Timing[5]	0	-	96%	95%
Pneumococcal Vaccine[5]	0	-	95%	93%
Smoking Cessation Advice[5]	0	-	98%	97%
Surgical Care Improvement Project				
Appropriate VTP Within 24 Hours[5]	0	-	94%	92%
Appropriate Hair Removal[5]	0	-	100%	99%
Appropriate Beta Blocker Usage[5]	0	-	94%	93%
Controlled Postoperative Blood Glucose[5]	0	-	96%	93%
Prophylactic Antibiotic Timing[5]	0	-	97%	97%
Prophylactic Antibiotic Timing (Outpatient)[5]	0	-	93%	92%
Prophylactic Antibiotic Selection[5]	0	-	98%	97%
Prophylactic Antibiotic Select. (Outpatient)[5]	0	-	96%	94%
Prophylactic Antibiotic Stopped[5]	0	-	96%	94%
Recommended VTP Ordered[5]	0	-	96%	94%
Urinary Catheter Removal[5]	0	-	93%	90%
Children's Asthma Care				
Received Systemic Corticosteroids	-	-	-	100%
Received Home Management Plan	-	-	-	71%
Received Reliever Medication	-	-	-	100%
Use of Medical Imaging				
Combination Abdominal CT Scan[5]	0	-	0.144	0.191
Combination Chest CT Scan[5]	0	-	0.030	0.054
Follow-up Mammogram/Ultrasound[5]	0	-	7.5%	8.4%
MRI for Low Back Pain[5]	0	-	31.5%	32.7%
Survey of Patients' Hospital Experiences				
Area Around Room 'Always' Quiet at Night[9]	-	-	-	58%
Doctors 'Always' Communicated Well[9]	-	-	-	80%
Home Recovery Information Given[9]	-	-	-	82%
Hospital Given 9 or 10 on 10 Point Scale[9]	-	-	-	67%
Meds 'Always' Explained Before Given[9]	-	-	-	60%
Nurses 'Always' Communicated Well[9]	-	-	-	76%
Pain 'Always' Well Controlled[9]	-	-	-	69%
Room and Bathroom 'Always' Clean[9]	-	-	-	71%
Timely Help 'Always' Received[9]	-	-	-	64%
Would Definitely Recommend Hospital[9]	-	-	-	69%

Pioneer Health Services of Patrick County

18688 Jeb Stuart Highway　Phone: 276-694-8678
Stuart, VA 24171　Fax: 276-694-8655
URL: www.rjrhospital.com
Type: Critical Access Hospitals　Emergency Services: Yes
Ownership: Proprietary　Beds: 50
Key Personnel:
CEO/President . . . . Janice Wilkins, RN/BSN
Chief of Medical Staff . . . . Richard Cole
Operating Room . . . . Sandy Rhodes
Emergency Room . . . . Cindy Fain

Measure	Cases	This Hosp.	State Avg.	U.S. Avg.
Heart Attack Care				
ACE Inhibitor or ARB for LVSD[5]	0	-	97%	96%
Aspirin at Arrival[5]	0	-	99%	99%
Aspirin at Discharge[5]	0	-	99%	98%
Beta Blocker at Discharge[5]	0	-	99%	98%
Fibrinolytic Medication Timing[5]	0	-	75%	55%
PCI Within 90 Minutes of Arrival[5]	0	-	93%	90%
Smoking Cessation Advice[5]	0	-	100%	99%
Chest Pain/Possible Heart Attack Care				
Aspirin at Arrival	-	-	95%	95%
Median Time to ECG (minutes)	-	-	8	8
Median Time to Transfer (minutes)	-	-	60	61
Fibrinolytic Medication Timing	-	-	59%	54%
Heart Failure Care				
ACE Inhibitor or ARB for LVSD[5]	0	-	97%	94%
Discharge Instructions[5]	0	-	92%	88%
Evaluation of LVS Function[5]	0	-	99%	98%
Smoking Cessation Advice[5]	0	-	99%	98%
Pneumonia Care				
Appropriate Initial Antibiotic[5]	0	-	93%	92%
Blood Culture Timing[5]	0	-	97%	96%
Influenza Vaccine[5]	0	-	94%	91%
Initial Antibiotic Timing[5]	0	-	96%	95%
Pneumococcal Vaccine[5]	0	-	95%	93%
Smoking Cessation Advice[5]	0	-	98%	97%
Surgical Care Improvement Project				
Appropriate VTP Within 24 Hours[5]	0	-	94%	92%
Appropriate Hair Removal[5]	0	-	100%	99%
Appropriate Beta Blocker Usage[5]	0	-	94%	93%
Controlled Postoperative Blood Glucose[5]	0	-	96%	93%
Prophylactic Antibiotic Timing[5]	0	-	97%	97%
Prophylactic Antibiotic Timing (Outpatient)	-	-	93%	92%
Prophylactic Antibiotic Selection[5]	0	-	98%	97%
Prophylactic Antibiotic Select. (Outpatient)	-	-	96%	94%
Prophylactic Antibiotic Stopped[5]	0	-	96%	94%
Recommended VTP Ordered[5]	0	-	96%	94%
Urinary Catheter Removal[5]	0	-	93%	90%
Children's Asthma Care				
Received Systemic Corticosteroids	-	-	-	100%
Received Home Management Plan	-	-	-	71%
Received Reliever Medication	-	-	-	100%
Use of Medical Imaging				
Combination Abdominal CT Scan	-	-	0.144	0.191
Combination Chest CT Scan	-	-	0.030	0.054
Follow-up Mammogram/Ultrasound	-	-	7.5%	8.4%
MRI for Low Back Pain	-	-	31.5%	32.7%
Survey of Patients' Hospital Experiences				
Area Around Room 'Always' Quiet at Night[8]	-	-	-	58%
Doctors 'Always' Communicated Well[8]	-	-	-	80%
Home Recovery Information Given[8]	-	-	-	82%
Hospital Given 9 or 10 on 10 Point Scale[8]	-	-	-	67%
Meds 'Always' Explained Before Given[8]	-	-	-	60%
Nurses 'Always' Communicated Well[8]	-	-	-	76%
Pain 'Always' Well Controlled[8]	-	-	-	69%
Room and Bathroom 'Always' Clean[8]	-	-	-	71%
Timely Help 'Always' Received[8]	-	-	-	64%
Would Definitely Recommend Hospital[8]	-	-	-	69%

NOTE: Hospital profiles are in alphabetical order by state, then city, then hospital within the city; Rankings exclude hospitals with less than 25 cases except for patient surveys which excludes hospitals with less than 100 cases; (a) 100–299 cases; (1) The number of cases is too small to be sure how well a hospital is performing; (2) The hospital indicated that the data submitted for this measure were based on a sample of cases; (3) Data was collected during a shorter time period (fewer quarters) than the maximum possible time for this measure; (4) Suppressed for one or more quarters by CMS; (5) No data is available from the hospital for this measure; (6) Fewer than 100 patients completed the HCAHPS survey. Use these rates with caution, as the number of surveys may be too low to reliably assess hospital performance; (7) Survey results are based on less than 12 months of data; (8) Survey results are not available for this reporting period; (9) No or very few patients were eligible for the HCAHPS survey. The scores shown, if any, reflect a very small number of surveys; (10) A state average was not calculated because too few hospitals in the state submitted data; (11) There were discrepancies in the data collection process; Please refer to the User's Guide for a full explanation of data.

Sentara Obici Hospital

2800 Godwin Boulevard
Suffolk, VA 23439
URL: www.sentara.com
Type: Acute Care Hospitals
Ownership: Voluntary Non-Profit - Other
Phone: 757-934-4000
Fax: 757-455-7155
Emergency Services: Yes
Beds: 150

Key Personnel:
CEO/President. . . . . Howard P Kern
Chief of Medical Staff. . . . . Gary R Yates, MD
Coronary Care . . . . Theresa Godfrey
Infection Control. . . . . Tammy Irving
Pediatric Ambulatory Care . . . . . . K Sankaran
Pediatric In-Patient Care . . . . K Sankaran
Quality Assurance . . . . Amanda Goodwin
Radiology. . . . . Gail Byrd

Measure	Cases	This Hosp.	State Avg.	U.S. Avg.
Heart Attack Care				
ACE Inhibitor or ARB for LVSD[1]	14	86%	97%	96%
Aspirin at Arrival	125	98%	99%	99%
Aspirin at Discharge	88	98%	99%	98%
Beta Blocker at Discharge	82	96%	99%	98%
Fibrinolytic Medication Timing	0	-	75%	55%
PCI Within 90 Minutes of Arrival	26	88%	93%	90%
Smoking Cessation Advice	35	100%	100%	99%
Chest Pain/Possible Heart Attack Care				
Aspirin at Arrival	78	97%	95%	95%
Median Time to ECG (minutes)	78	5	8	8
Median Time to Transfer (minutes)[1]	13	70	60	61
Fibrinolytic Medication Timing	0	-	59%	54%
Heart Failure Care				
ACE Inhibitor or ARB for LVSD	145	96%	97%	94%
Discharge Instructions	331	86%	92%	88%
Evaluation of LVS Function	416	100%	99%	98%
Smoking Cessation Advice	80	98%	99%	98%
Pneumonia Care				
Appropriate Initial Antibiotic	119	92%	93%	92%
Blood Culture Timing	174	97%	97%	96%
Influenza Vaccine	137	97%	94%	91%
Initial Antibiotic Timing	196	97%	96%	95%
Pneumococcal Vaccine	177	95%	95%	93%
Smoking Cessation Advice	85	99%	98%	97%
Surgical Care Improvement Project				
Appropriate VTP Within 24 Hours[2]	215	94%	94%	92%
Appropriate Hair Removal[2]	746	100%	100%	99%
Appropriate Beta Blocker Usage[2]	207	95%	94%	93%
Controlled Postoperative Blood Glucose[2]	0	-	96%	93%
Prophylactic Antibiotic Timing[2]	586	98%	97%	97%
Prophylactic Antibiotic Timing (Outpatient)	141	96%	93%	92%
Prophylactic Antibiotic Selection[2]	589	98%	98%	97%
Prophylactic Antibiotic Select. (Outpatient)	140	94%	96%	94%
Prophylactic Antibiotic Stopped[2]	554	95%	96%	94%
Recommended VTP Ordered[2]	216	95%	96%	94%
Urinary Catheter Removal[2]	135	89%	93%	90%
Children's Asthma Care				
Received Systemic Corticosteroids	-	-	-	100%
Received Home Management Plan	-	-	-	71%
Received Reliever Medication	-	-	-	100%
Use of Medical Imaging				
Combination Abdominal CT Scan	898	0.184	0.144	0.191
Combination Chest CT Scan	514	0.000	0.030	0.054
Follow-up Mammogram/Ultrasound	1,260	7.0%	7.5%	8.4%
MRI for Low Back Pain	220	28.6%	31.5%	32.7%
Survey of Patients' Hospital Experiences				
Area Around Room 'Always' Quiet at Night	300+	54%	-	58%
Doctors 'Always' Communicated Well	300+	72%	-	80%
Home Recovery Information Given	300+	84%	-	82%
Hospital Given 9 or 10 on 10 Point Scale	300+	56%	-	67%
Meds 'Always' Explained Before Given	300+	55%	-	60%
Nurses 'Always' Communicated Well	300+	70%	-	76%
Pain 'Always' Well Controlled	300+	62%	-	69%
Room and Bathroom 'Always' Clean	300+	67%	-	71%
Timely Help 'Always' Received	300+	56%	-	64%
Would Definitely Recommend Hospital	300+	63%	-	69%

Riverside Tappahannock Hospital

618 Hospital Road
Tappahannock, VA 22560
Type: Acute Care Hospitals
Ownership: Voluntary Non-Profit - Private
Phone: 804-443-3311
Fax: 804-443-6004
Emergency Services: Yes
Beds: 92

Key Personnel:
CEO/President. . . . . Elizabeth J Martin
Chief of Medical Staff. . . . . James R Dudley, MD
Infection Control. . . . . Donna Tigor
Operating Room. . . . . Terri Willaford
Quality Assurance . . . . Jodi Friend
Radiology. . . . . Elizabeth L Abell
Emergency Room . . . . Shafqat H Ashai, ENP

Measure	Cases	This Hosp.	State Avg.	U.S. Avg.
Heart Attack Care				
ACE Inhibitor or ARB for LVSD[1]	4	75%	97%	96%
Aspirin at Arrival[1]	24	100%	99%	99%
Aspirin at Discharge[1]	13	100%	99%	98%
Beta Blocker at Discharge[1]	14	100%	99%	98%
Fibrinolytic Medication Timing	0	-	75%	55%
PCI Within 90 Minutes of Arrival	0	-	93%	90%
Smoking Cessation Advice[1]	5	100%	100%	99%
Chest Pain/Possible Heart Attack Care				
Aspirin at Arrival	46	96%	95%	95%
Median Time to ECG (minutes)	45	2	8	8
Median Time to Transfer (minutes)[1]	5	89	60	61
Fibrinolytic Medication Timing[1]	1	0%	59%	54%
Heart Failure Care				
ACE Inhibitor or ARB for LVSD	33	100%	97%	94%
Discharge Instructions	76	99%	92%	88%
Evaluation of LVS Function	93	100%	99%	98%
Smoking Cessation Advice[1]	15	100%	99%	98%
Pneumonia Care				
Appropriate Initial Antibiotic	49	96%	93%	92%
Blood Culture Timing	49	98%	97%	96%
Influenza Vaccine	32	100%	94%	91%
Initial Antibiotic Timing	34	91%	96%	95%
Pneumococcal Vaccine	42	100%	95%	93%
Smoking Cessation Advice[1]	15	100%	98%	97%
Surgical Care Improvement Project				
Appropriate VTP Within 24 Hours	77	96%	94%	92%
Appropriate Hair Removal	112	100%	100%	99%
Appropriate Beta Blocker Usage	31	97%	94%	93%
Controlled Postoperative Blood Glucose	0	-	96%	93%
Prophylactic Antibiotic Timing	87	99%	97%	97%
Prophylactic Antibiotic Timing (Outpatient)	25	96%	93%	92%
Prophylactic Antibiotic Selection	87	97%	98%	97%
Prophylactic Antibiotic Select. (Outpatient)	75	99%	96%	94%
Prophylactic Antibiotic Stopped	85	99%	96%	94%
Recommended VTP Ordered	77	96%	96%	94%
Urinary Catheter Removal[1]	7	100%	93%	90%
Children's Asthma Care				
Received Systemic Corticosteroids	-	-	-	100%
Received Home Management Plan	-	-	-	71%
Received Reliever Medication	-	-	-	100%
Use of Medical Imaging				
Combination Abdominal CT Scan	459	0.050	0.144	0.191
Combination Chest CT Scan	375	0.021	0.030	0.054
Follow-up Mammogram/Ultrasound	651	6.0%	7.5%	8.4%
MRI for Low Back Pain[1]	34	26.5%	31.5%	32.7%
Survey of Patients' Hospital Experiences				
Area Around Room 'Always' Quiet at Night	300+	50%	-	58%
Doctors 'Always' Communicated Well	300+	78%	-	80%
Home Recovery Information Given	300+	79%	-	82%
Hospital Given 9 or 10 on 10 Point Scale	300+	59%	-	67%
Meds 'Always' Explained Before Given	300+	60%	-	60%
Nurses 'Always' Communicated Well	300+	75%	-	76%
Pain 'Always' Well Controlled	300+	69%	-	69%
Room and Bathroom 'Always' Clean	300+	63%	-	71%
Timely Help 'Always' Received	300+	59%	-	64%
Would Definitely Recommend Hospital	300+	61%	-	69%

Carilion Tazewell Community Hospital

141 Ben Bolt Avenue
Tazewell, VA 24651
URL: www.tazecommhospital.org
Type: Acute Care Hospitals
Ownership: Voluntary Non-Profit - Other
Phone: 276-988-8700
Fax: 276-988-8782
Emergency Services: Yes
Beds: 56

Key Personnel:
CEO/President. . . . . Chris Wearmouth
Anesthesiology. . . . . Alex Fernandez
Intensive Care Unit. . . . . Tanya Hess

Measure	Cases	This Hosp.	State Avg.	U.S. Avg.
Heart Attack Care				
ACE Inhibitor or ARB for LVSD[1]	1	100%	97%	96%
Aspirin at Arrival[1]	10	90%	99%	99%
Aspirin at Discharge[1]	8	100%	99%	98%
Beta Blocker at Discharge[1]	8	100%	99%	98%
Fibrinolytic Medication Timing	0	-	75%	55%
PCI Within 90 Minutes of Arrival	0	-	93%	90%
Smoking Cessation Advice[1]	2	100%	100%	99%
Chest Pain/Possible Heart Attack Care				
Aspirin at Arrival[1,3]	23	91%	95%	95%
Median Time to ECG (minutes)[1,3]	24	27	8	8
Median Time to Transfer (minutes)[1,3]	1	204	60	61
Fibrinolytic Medication Timing[1,3]	1	0%	59%	54%
Heart Failure Care				
ACE Inhibitor or ARB for LVSD[1]	15	80%	97%	94%
Discharge Instructions	44	77%	92%	88%
Evaluation of LVS Function	55	87%	99%	98%
Smoking Cessation Advice[1]	21	100%	99%	98%
Pneumonia Care				
Appropriate Initial Antibiotic	38	74%	93%	92%
Blood Culture Timing	58	81%	97%	96%
Influenza Vaccine	39	95%	94%	91%
Initial Antibiotic Timing	73	79%	96%	95%
Pneumococcal Vaccine	53	87%	95%	93%
Smoking Cessation Advice	27	89%	98%	97%
Surgical Care Improvement Project				
Appropriate VTP Within 24 Hours[1,3]	4	25%	94%	92%
Appropriate Hair Removal[1,3]	6	83%	100%	99%
Appropriate Beta Blocker Usage[1,3]	1	0%	94%	93%
Controlled Postoperative Blood Glucose[3]	0	-	96%	93%
Prophylactic Antibiotic Timing[1,3]	4	75%	97%	97%
Prophylactic Antibiotic Timing (Outpatient)[1]	7	71%	93%	92%
Prophylactic Antibiotic Selection[1,3]	4	100%	98%	97%
Prophylactic Antibiotic Select. (Outpatient)[1]	5	100%	96%	94%
Prophylactic Antibiotic Stopped[1,3]	4	100%	96%	94%
Recommended VTP Ordered[1,3]	5	20%	96%	94%
Urinary Catheter Removal[1,3]	3	0%	93%	90%
Children's Asthma Care				
Received Systemic Corticosteroids	-	-	-	100%
Received Home Management Plan	-	-	-	71%
Received Reliever Medication	-	-	-	100%
Use of Medical Imaging				
Combination Abdominal CT Scan	135	0.067	0.144	0.191
Combination Chest CT Scan	79	0.114	0.030	0.054
Follow-up Mammogram/Ultrasound	223	4.9%	7.5%	8.4%
MRI for Low Back Pain[1]	25	48.0%	31.5%	32.7%
Survey of Patients' Hospital Experiences				
Area Around Room 'Always' Quiet at Night	(a)	69%	-	58%
Doctors 'Always' Communicated Well	(a)	81%	-	80%
Home Recovery Information Given	(a)	80%	-	82%
Hospital Given 9 or 10 on 10 Point Scale	(a)	67%	-	67%
Meds 'Always' Explained Before Given	(a)	63%	-	60%
Nurses 'Always' Communicated Well	(a)	79%	-	76%
Pain 'Always' Well Controlled	(a)	71%	-	69%
Room and Bathroom 'Always' Clean	(a)	72%	-	71%
Timely Help 'Always' Received	(a)	76%	-	64%
Would Definitely Recommend Hospital	(a)	67%	-	69%

NOTE: Hospital profiles are in alphabetical order by state, then city, then hospital within the city; Rankings exclude hospitals with less than 25 cases except for patient surveys which excludes hospitals with less than 100 cases; (a) 100–299 cases; (1) The number of cases is too small to be sure how well a hospital is performing; (2) The hospital indicated that the data submitted for this measure were based on a sample of cases; (3) Data was collected during a shorter time period (fewer quarters) than the maximum possible time for this measure; (4) Suppressed for one or more quarters by CMS; (5) No data is available from the hospital for this measure; (6) Fewer than 100 patients completed the HCAHPS survey. Use these rates with caution, as the number of surveys may be too low to reliably assess hospital performance; (7) Survey results are based on less than 12 months of data; (8) Survey results are not available for this reporting period; (9) No or very few patients were eligible for the HCAHPS survey. The scores shown, if any, reflect a very small number of surveys; (10) A state average was not calculated because too few hospitals in the state submitted data; (11) There were discrepancies in the data collection process; Please refer to the User's Guide for a full explanation of data.

Sentara Bayside Hospital

800 Independence Blvd
Virginia Beach, VA 23455
URL: www.sentara.com
Type: Acute Care Hospitals
Ownership: Voluntary Non-Profit - Other
Phone: 757-363-6196
Fax: 757-363-6650
Emergency Services: Yes
Beds: 158

Key Personnel:
CEO/President. . . . . Mark Gaven
Operating Room. . . . . Thomas G Clifford Jr
Quality Assurance . . . . Sam Byrd
Emergency Room . . . . Su Harvell

Measure	Cases	This Hosp.	State Avg.	U.S. Avg.
Heart Attack Care				
ACE Inhibitor or ARB for LVSD[1]	9	89%	97%	96%
Aspirin at Arrival	80	100%	99%	99%
Aspirin at Discharge	70	100%	99%	98%
Beta Blocker at Discharge	70	100%	99%	98%
Fibrinolytic Medication Timing[1]	1	0%	75%	55%
PCI Within 90 Minutes of Arrival[1]	14	93%	93%	90%
Smoking Cessation Advice[1]	22	100%	100%	99%
Chest Pain/Possible Heart Attack Care				
Aspirin at Arrival	226	97%	95%	95%
Median Time to ECG (minutes)	225	8	8	8
Median Time to Transfer (minutes)[1]	13	54	60	61
Fibrinolytic Medication Timing	0	-	59%	54%
Heart Failure Care				
ACE Inhibitor or ARB for LVSD	66	100%	97%	94%
Discharge Instructions	186	98%	92%	88%
Evaluation of LVS Function	219	100%	99%	98%
Smoking Cessation Advice	36	100%	99%	98%
Pneumonia Care				
Appropriate Initial Antibiotic	96	93%	93%	92%
Blood Culture Timing	161	99%	97%	96%
Influenza Vaccine	136	96%	94%	91%
Initial Antibiotic Timing	165	99%	96%	95%
Pneumococcal Vaccine	162	99%	95%	93%
Smoking Cessation Advice	81	100%	98%	97%
Surgical Care Improvement Project				
Appropriate VTP Within 24 Hours	104	99%	94%	92%
Appropriate Hair Removal	226	100%	100%	99%
Appropriate Beta Blocker Usage	45	100%	94%	93%
Controlled Postoperative Blood Glucose	0	-	96%	93%
Prophylactic Antibiotic Timing	129	98%	97%	97%
Prophylactic Antibiotic Timing (Outpatient)	147	85%	93%	92%
Prophylactic Antibiotic Selection	130	98%	98%	97%
Prophylactic Antibiotic Select. (Outpatient)	256	92%	96%	94%
Prophylactic Antibiotic Stopped	124	94%	96%	94%
Recommended VTP Ordered	104	99%	96%	94%
Urinary Catheter Removal	37	100%	93%	90%
Children's Asthma Care				
Received Systemic Corticosteroids	-	-	-	100%
Received Home Management Plan	-	-	-	71%
Received Reliever Medication	-	-	-	100%
Use of Medical Imaging				
Combination Abdominal CT Scan	1,363	0.119	0.144	0.191
Combination Chest CT Scan	986	0.048	0.030	0.054
Follow-up Mammogram/Ultrasound	1,504	7.8%	7.5%	8.4%
MRI for Low Back Pain	247	26.7%	31.5%	32.7%
Survey of Patients' Hospital Experiences				
Area Around Room 'Always' Quiet at Night	300+	54%	-	58%
Doctors 'Always' Communicated Well	300+	75%	-	80%
Home Recovery Information Given	300+	83%	-	82%
Hospital Given 9 or 10 on 10 Point Scale	300+	61%	-	67%
Meds 'Always' Explained Before Given	300+	60%	-	60%
Nurses 'Always' Communicated Well	300+	74%	-	76%
Pain 'Always' Well Controlled	300+	69%	-	69%
Room and Bathroom 'Always' Clean	300+	64%	-	71%
Timely Help 'Always' Received	300+	55%	-	64%
Would Definitely Recommend Hospital	300+	65%	-	69%

Sentara Virginia Beach General Hospital

1060 First Colonial Road
Virginia Beach, VA 23454
URL: www.sentara.com
Type: Acute Care Hospitals
Ownership: Voluntary Non-Profit - Other
Phone: 757-395-8000
Fax: 757-455-7964
Emergency Services: Yes
Beds: 274

Key Personnel:
CEO/President. . . . . Robert Graves
Chief of Medical Staff . . . . HC Harrison
Operating Room. . . . . R William Hoefer
Pediatric Ambulatory Care . . . . . . Glenn Snyders, MD
Pediatric In-Patient Care . . . . Glenn Snyders, MD
Quality Assurance . . . . Deborah Pelech
Radiology. . . . . John Arvny, MD
Emergency Room . . . . Linda Baker

Measure	Cases	This Hosp.	State Avg.	U.S. Avg.
Heart Attack Care				
ACE Inhibitor or ARB for LVSD	63	100%	97%	96%
Aspirin at Arrival	196	100%	99%	99%
Aspirin at Discharge	241	100%	99%	98%
Beta Blocker at Discharge	252	100%	99%	98%
Fibrinolytic Medication Timing	0	-	75%	55%
PCI Within 90 Minutes of Arrival	42	100%	93%	90%
Smoking Cessation Advice	93	98%	100%	99%
Chest Pain/Possible Heart Attack Care				
Aspirin at Arrival[1]	7	100%	95%	95%
Median Time to ECG (minutes)[1]	7	11	8	8
Median Time to Transfer (minutes)[5]	0	-	60	61
Fibrinolytic Medication Timing[5]	0	-	59%	54%
Heart Failure Care				
ACE Inhibitor or ARB for LVSD	118	98%	97%	94%
Discharge Instructions	360	92%	92%	88%
Evaluation of LVS Function	453	100%	99%	98%
Smoking Cessation Advice	75	100%	99%	98%
Pneumonia Care				
Appropriate Initial Antibiotic	173	94%	93%	92%
Blood Culture Timing	290	96%	97%	96%
Influenza Vaccine	239	99%	94%	91%
Initial Antibiotic Timing	299	94%	96%	95%
Pneumococcal Vaccine	361	96%	95%	93%
Smoking Cessation Advice	125	98%	98%	97%
Surgical Care Improvement Project				
Appropriate VTP Within 24 Hours[2]	365	98%	94%	92%
Appropriate Hair Removal[2]	947	100%	100%	99%
Appropriate Beta Blocker Usage[2]	233	91%	94%	93%
Controlled Postoperative Blood Glucose[2]	101	88%	96%	93%
Prophylactic Antibiotic Timing[2]	721	99%	97%	97%
Prophylactic Antibiotic Timing (Outpatient)	490	94%	93%	92%
Prophylactic Antibiotic Selection[2]	730	99%	98%	97%
Prophylactic Antibiotic Select. (Outpatient)	480	96%	96%	94%
Prophylactic Antibiotic Stopped[2]	692	96%	96%	94%
Recommended VTP Ordered[2]	365	99%	96%	94%
Urinary Catheter Removal[2]	220	97%	93%	90%
Children's Asthma Care				
Received Systemic Corticosteroids	-	-	-	100%
Received Home Management Plan	-	-	-	71%
Received Reliever Medication	-	-	-	100%
Use of Medical Imaging				
Combination Abdominal CT Scan	1,523	0.087	0.144	0.191
Combination Chest CT Scan	1,375	0.004	0.030	0.054
Follow-up Mammogram/Ultrasound	2,093	6.3%	7.5%	8.4%
MRI for Low Back Pain	187	21.9%	31.5%	32.7%
Survey of Patients' Hospital Experiences				
Area Around Room 'Always' Quiet at Night	300+	52%	-	58%
Doctors 'Always' Communicated Well	300+	74%	-	80%
Home Recovery Information Given	300+	84%	-	82%
Hospital Given 9 or 10 on 10 Point Scale	300+	66%	-	67%
Meds 'Always' Explained Before Given	300+	54%	-	60%
Nurses 'Always' Communicated Well	300+	71%	-	76%
Pain 'Always' Well Controlled	300+	64%	-	69%
Room and Bathroom 'Always' Clean	300+	63%	-	71%
Timely Help 'Always' Received	300+	54%	-	64%
Would Definitely Recommend Hospital	300+	69%	-	69%

The Fauquier Hospital

500 Hospital Drive
Warrenton, VA 20186
E-mail: referral@fauquierhospital.org
URL: www.fauquierhospital.org
Type: Acute Care Hospitals
Ownership: Voluntary Non-Profit - Private
Phone: 540-316-5000
Fax: 540-341-0823
Emergency Services: Yes
Beds: 86

Key Personnel:
CEO/President. . . . . Rodger H Baker
Chief of Medical Staff . . . . Dr Thomas Sherman
Infection Control. . . . . Dorothy Siebert, RN
Operating Room. . . . . Angela Schob
Quality Assurance . . . . Lee Laughter
Radiology. . . . . Susan Bruns, MD
Emergency Room . . . . Joseph Serviedo, MD

Measure	Cases	This Hosp.	State Avg.	U.S. Avg.
Heart Attack Care				
ACE Inhibitor or ARB for LVSD[1]	5	100%	97%	96%
Aspirin at Arrival	28	100%	99%	99%
Aspirin at Discharge[1]	11	100%	99%	98%
Beta Blocker at Discharge[1]	11	100%	99%	98%
Fibrinolytic Medication Timing	0	-	75%	55%
PCI Within 90 Minutes of Arrival	0	-	93%	90%
Smoking Cessation Advice[1]	1	100%	100%	99%
Chest Pain/Possible Heart Attack Care				
Aspirin at Arrival	83	98%	95%	95%
Median Time to ECG (minutes)	87	8	8	8
Median Time to Transfer (minutes)[1]	19	79	60	61
Fibrinolytic Medication Timing[1]	2	50%	59%	54%
Heart Failure Care				
ACE Inhibitor or ARB for LVSD	55	100%	97%	94%
Discharge Instructions	146	93%	92%	88%
Evaluation of LVS Function	174	100%	99%	98%
Smoking Cessation Advice	34	100%	99%	98%
Pneumonia Care				
Appropriate Initial Antibiotic	108	97%	93%	92%
Blood Culture Timing	202	96%	97%	96%
Influenza Vaccine	102	96%	94%	91%
Initial Antibiotic Timing	169	95%	96%	95%
Pneumococcal Vaccine	142	99%	95%	93%
Smoking Cessation Advice	57	96%	98%	97%
Surgical Care Improvement Project				
Appropriate VTP Within 24 Hours	168	98%	94%	92%
Appropriate Hair Removal	342	100%	100%	99%
Appropriate Beta Blocker Usage	68	99%	94%	93%
Controlled Postoperative Blood Glucose	0	-	96%	93%
Prophylactic Antibiotic Timing	240	95%	97%	97%
Prophylactic Antibiotic Timing (Outpatient)	88	92%	93%	92%
Prophylactic Antibiotic Selection	240	98%	98%	97%
Prophylactic Antibiotic Select. (Outpatient)	86	98%	96%	94%
Prophylactic Antibiotic Stopped	226	96%	96%	94%
Recommended VTP Ordered	168	99%	96%	94%
Urinary Catheter Removal	100	94%	93%	90%
Children's Asthma Care				
Received Systemic Corticosteroids	-	-	-	100%
Received Home Management Plan	-	-	-	71%
Received Reliever Medication	-	-	-	100%
Use of Medical Imaging				
Combination Abdominal CT Scan	656	0.061	0.144	0.191
Combination Chest CT Scan	384	0.000	0.030	0.054
Follow-up Mammogram/Ultrasound	769	10.3%	7.5%	8.4%
MRI for Low Back Pain	125	33.6%	31.5%	32.7%
Survey of Patients' Hospital Experiences				
Area Around Room 'Always' Quiet at Night	300+	61%	-	58%
Doctors 'Always' Communicated Well	300+	80%	-	80%
Home Recovery Information Given	300+	84%	-	82%
Hospital Given 9 or 10 on 10 Point Scale	300+	70%	-	67%
Meds 'Always' Explained Before Given	300+	63%	-	60%
Nurses 'Always' Communicated Well	300+	76%	-	76%
Pain 'Always' Well Controlled	300+	71%	-	69%
Room and Bathroom 'Always' Clean	300+	74%	-	71%
Timely Help 'Always' Received	300+	65%	-	64%
Would Definitely Recommend Hospital	300+	76%	-	69%

NOTE: Hospital profiles are in alphabetical order by state, then city, then hospital within the city; Rankings exclude hospitals with less than 25 cases except for patient surveys which excludes hospitals with less than 100 cases; (a) 100–299 cases; (1) The number of cases is too small to be sure how well a hospital is performing; (2) The hospital indicated that the data submitted for this measure were based on a sample of cases; (3) Data was collected during a shorter time period (fewer quarters) than the maximum possible time for this measure; (4) Suppressed for one or more quarters by CMS; (5) No data is available from the hospital for this measure; (6) Fewer than 100 patients completed the HCAHPS survey. Use these rates with caution, as the number of surveys may be too low to reliably assess hospital performance; (7) Survey results are based on less than 12 months of data; (8) Survey results are not available for this reporting period; (9) No or very few patients were eligible for the HCAHPS survey. The scores shown, if any, reflect a very small number of surveys; (10) A state average was not calculated because too few hospitals in the state submitted data; (11) There were discrepancies in the data collection process; Please refer to the User's Guide for a full explanation of data.

Eastern State Hospital

4601 Ironbound Road
Williamsburg, VA 23188
Phone: 757-253-5161
Fax: 757-253-5065
URL: www.ehs.dmhmrsas.virginia.gov
Type: Acute Care Hospitals
Emergency Services: No
Ownership: Government - State
Beds: 362

Key Personnel:

CEO/President. . . . . John M Favret NHA
Chief of Medical Staff . . . . Guillermo Schrader MD, MD
Infection Control. . . . . Karol Curtis RN
Quality Assurance . . . . Barbara Lambert RN
Radiology. . . . . Mary Wilson, MT
Patient Relations . . . . Willie Barnes

Measure	Cases	This Hosp.	State Avg.	U.S. Avg.
Heart Attack Care				
ACE Inhibitor or ARB for LVSD[5]	0	-	97%	96%
Aspirin at Arrival[5]	0	-	99%	99%
Aspirin at Discharge[5]	0	-	99%	98%
Beta Blocker at Discharge[5]	0	-	99%	98%
Fibrinolytic Medication Timing[5]	0	-	75%	55%
PCI Within 90 Minutes of Arrival[5]	0	-	93%	90%
Smoking Cessation Advice[5]	0	-	100%	99%
Chest Pain/Possible Heart Attack Care				
Aspirin at Arrival[5]	0	-	95%	95%
Median Time to ECG (minutes)[5]	0	-	8	8
Median Time to Transfer (minutes)[5]	0	-	60	61
Fibrinolytic Medication Timing[5]	0	-	59%	54%
Heart Failure Care				
ACE Inhibitor or ARB for LVSD[5]	0	-	97%	94%
Discharge Instructions[5]	0	-	92%	88%
Evaluation of LVS Function[5]	0	-	99%	98%
Smoking Cessation Advice[5]	0	-	99%	98%
Pneumonia Care				
Appropriate Initial Antibiotic[2,3]	0	-	93%	92%
Blood Culture Timing[2,3]	0	-	97%	96%
Influenza Vaccine[1,2]	6	100%	94%	91%
Initial Antibiotic Timing[1,2,3]	9	100%	96%	95%
Pneumococcal Vaccine[1,2,3]	1	100%	95%	93%
Smoking Cessation Advice[2,3]	0	-	98%	97%
Surgical Care Improvement Project				
Appropriate VTP Within 24 Hours[5]	0	-	94%	92%
Appropriate Hair Removal[5]	0	-	100%	99%
Appropriate Beta Blocker Usage[5]	0	-	94%	93%
Controlled Postoperative Blood Glucose[5]	0	-	96%	93%
Prophylactic Antibiotic Timing[5]	0	-	97%	97%
Prophylactic Antibiotic Timing (Outpatient)[5]	0	-	93%	92%
Prophylactic Antibiotic Selection[5]	0	-	98%	97%
Prophylactic Antibiotic Select. (Outpatient)[5]	0	-	96%	94%
Prophylactic Antibiotic Stopped[5]	0	-	96%	94%
Recommended VTP Ordered[5]	0	-	96%	94%
Urinary Catheter Removal[5]	0	-	93%	90%
Children's Asthma Care				
Received Systemic Corticosteroids	-	-	-	100%
Received Home Management Plan	-	-	-	71%
Received Reliever Medication	-	-	-	100%
Use of Medical Imaging				
Combination Abdominal CT Scan[5]	0	-	0.144	0.191
Combination Chest CT Scan[5]	0	-	0.030	0.054
Follow-up Mammogram/Ultrasound[5]	0	-	7.5%	8.4%
MRI for Low Back Pain[5]	0	-	31.5%	32.7%
Survey of Patients' Hospital Experiences				
Area Around Room 'Always' Quiet at Night[9]	-	-	-	58%
Doctors 'Always' Communicated Well[9]	-	-	-	80%
Home Recovery Information Given[9]	-	-	-	82%
Hospital Given 9 or 10 on 10 Point Scale[9]	-	-	-	67%
Meds 'Always' Explained Before Given[9]	-	-	-	60%
Nurses 'Always' Communicated Well[9]	-	-	-	76%
Pain 'Always' Well Controlled[9]	-	-	-	69%
Room and Bathroom 'Always' Clean[9]	-	-	-	71%
Timely Help 'Always' Received[9]	-	-	-	64%
Would Definitely Recommend Hospital[9]	-	-	-	69%

Sentara Williamsburg Regional Medical Center

100 Sentara Circle
Williamsburg, VA 23188
Phone: 757-984-6000
Fax: 757-984-7421
Type: Acute Care Hospitals
Emergency Services: Yes
Ownership: Voluntary Non-Profit - Private
Beds: 139

Key Personnel:

Operating Room. . . . . Linda Silver

Measure	Cases	This Hosp.	State Avg.	U.S. Avg.
Heart Attack Care				
ACE Inhibitor or ARB for LVSD[1]	22	100%	97%	96%
Aspirin at Arrival	120	100%	99%	99%
Aspirin at Discharge	101	100%	99%	98%
Beta Blocker at Discharge	108	99%	99%	98%
Fibrinolytic Medication Timing	0	-	75%	55%
PCI Within 90 Minutes of Arrival	30	97%	93%	90%
Smoking Cessation Advice[1]	20	100%	100%	99%
Chest Pain/Possible Heart Attack Care				
Aspirin at Arrival[1]	11	91%	95%	95%
Median Time to ECG (minutes)[1]	12	7	8	8
Median Time to Transfer (minutes)[1,3]	1	44800	60	61
Fibrinolytic Medication Timing[3]	0	-	59%	54%
Heart Failure Care				
ACE Inhibitor or ARB for LVSD	77	97%	97%	94%
Discharge Instructions	225	94%	92%	88%
Evaluation of LVS Function	275	100%	99%	98%
Smoking Cessation Advice	62	100%	99%	98%
Pneumonia Care				
Appropriate Initial Antibiotic	124	98%	93%	92%
Blood Culture Timing	169	98%	97%	96%
Influenza Vaccine	112	98%	94%	91%
Initial Antibiotic Timing	191	97%	96%	95%
Pneumococcal Vaccine	165	98%	95%	93%
Smoking Cessation Advice	50	100%	98%	97%
Surgical Care Improvement Project				
Appropriate VTP Within 24 Hours[2]	172	97%	94%	92%
Appropriate Hair Removal[2]	445	100%	100%	99%
Appropriate Beta Blocker Usage[2]	111	100%	94%	93%
Controlled Postoperative Blood Glucose[2]	0	-	96%	93%
Prophylactic Antibiotic Timing[2]	302	97%	97%	97%
Prophylactic Antibiotic Timing (Outpatient)	266	90%	93%	92%
Prophylactic Antibiotic Selection[2]	304	99%	98%	97%
Prophylactic Antibiotic Select. (Outpatient)	286	88%	96%	94%
Prophylactic Antibiotic Stopped[2]	289	97%	96%	94%
Recommended VTP Ordered[2]	172	97%	96%	94%
Urinary Catheter Removal[2]	112	95%	93%	90%
Children's Asthma Care				
Received Systemic Corticosteroids	-	-	-	100%
Received Home Management Plan	-	-	-	71%
Received Reliever Medication	-	-	-	100%
Use of Medical Imaging				
Combination Abdominal CT Scan	1,052	0.065	0.144	0.191
Combination Chest CT Scan	737	0.005	0.030	0.054
Follow-up Mammogram/Ultrasound	2,860	8.9%	7.5%	8.4%
MRI for Low Back Pain	237	27.8%	31.5%	32.7%
Survey of Patients' Hospital Experiences				
Area Around Room 'Always' Quiet at Night	300+	58%	-	58%
Doctors 'Always' Communicated Well	300+	75%	-	80%
Home Recovery Information Given	300+	83%	-	82%
Hospital Given 9 or 10 on 10 Point Scale	300+	63%	-	67%
Meds 'Always' Explained Before Given	300+	55%	-	60%
Nurses 'Always' Communicated Well	300+	70%	-	76%
Pain 'Always' Well Controlled	300+	62%	-	69%
Room and Bathroom 'Always' Clean	300+	66%	-	71%
Timely Help 'Always' Received	300+	50%	-	64%
Would Definitely Recommend Hospital	300+	68%	-	69%

Winchester Medical Center

220 Campus Blvd Suite 210
Winchester, VA 22601
Phone: 540-536-7654
Fax: 540-536-8606
URL: www.valleyhealthlink.com
Type: Acute Care Hospitals
Emergency Services: Yes
Ownership: Voluntary Non-Profit - Private
Beds: 411

Key Personnel:

CEO/President. . . . . Al Pilong
Cardiac Laboratory. . . . . James Warner, MD
Chief of Medical Staff . . . . Robert Tucker, MD
Infection Control. . . . . Jack Armstrong, MD
Operating Room. . . . . Kathleen Johnson
Radiology. . . . . Namik Erdag
Emergency Room . . . . Ahmad Baray

Measure	Cases	This Hosp.	State Avg.	U.S. Avg.
Heart Attack Care				
ACE Inhibitor or ARB for LVSD[2]	67	100%	97%	96%
Aspirin at Arrival[2]	157	100%	99%	99%
Aspirin at Discharge[2]	333	99%	99%	98%
Beta Blocker at Discharge[2]	316	99%	99%	98%
Fibrinolytic Medication Timing[2]	0	-	75%	55%
PCI Within 90 Minutes of Arrival[2]	30	93%	93%	90%
Smoking Cessation Advice[2]	137	100%	100%	99%
Chest Pain/Possible Heart Attack Care				
Aspirin at Arrival[5]	0	-	95%	95%
Median Time to ECG (minutes)[5]	0	-	8	8
Median Time to Transfer (minutes)[5]	0	-	60	61
Fibrinolytic Medication Timing[5]	0	-	59%	54%
Heart Failure Care				
ACE Inhibitor or ARB for LVSD	208	99%	97%	94%
Discharge Instructions	573	90%	92%	88%
Evaluation of LVS Function	660	100%	99%	98%
Smoking Cessation Advice	129	100%	99%	98%
Pneumonia Care				
Appropriate Initial Antibiotic[2]	158	92%	93%	92%
Blood Culture Timing[2]	187	95%	97%	96%
Influenza Vaccine[2]	157	92%	94%	91%
Initial Antibiotic Timing[2]	222	95%	96%	95%
Pneumococcal Vaccine[2]	218	92%	95%	93%
Smoking Cessation Advice[2]	119	100%	98%	97%
Surgical Care Improvement Project				
Appropriate VTP Within 24 Hours[2]	274	97%	94%	92%
Appropriate Hair Removal[2]	952	100%	100%	99%
Appropriate Beta Blocker Usage[2]	331	95%	94%	93%
Controlled Postoperative Blood Glucose[2]	194	86%	96%	93%
Prophylactic Antibiotic Timing[2]	639	95%	97%	97%
Prophylactic Antibiotic Timing (Outpatient)	642	81%	93%	92%
Prophylactic Antibiotic Selection[2]	647	99%	98%	97%
Prophylactic Antibiotic Select. (Outpatient)	631	97%	96%	94%
Prophylactic Antibiotic Stopped[2]	603	95%	96%	94%
Recommended VTP Ordered[2]	274	97%	96%	94%
Urinary Catheter Removal[2]	141	79%	93%	90%
Children's Asthma Care				
Received Systemic Corticosteroids	-	-	-	100%
Received Home Management Plan	-	-	-	71%
Received Reliever Medication	-	-	-	100%
Use of Medical Imaging				
Combination Abdominal CT Scan	1,393	0.111	0.144	0.191
Combination Chest CT Scan	1,384	0.010	0.030	0.054
Follow-up Mammogram/Ultrasound	2,748	6.1%	7.5%	8.4%
MRI for Low Back Pain	501	30.3%	31.5%	32.7%
Survey of Patients' Hospital Experiences				
Area Around Room 'Always' Quiet at Night	(a)	53%	-	58%
Doctors 'Always' Communicated Well	(a)	80%	-	80%
Home Recovery Information Given	(a)	82%	-	82%
Hospital Given 9 or 10 on 10 Point Scale	(a)	74%	-	67%
Meds 'Always' Explained Before Given	(a)	61%	-	60%
Nurses 'Always' Communicated Well	(a)	75%	-	76%
Pain 'Always' Well Controlled	(a)	70%	-	69%
Room and Bathroom 'Always' Clean	(a)	72%	-	71%
Timely Help 'Always' Received	(a)	64%	-	64%
Would Definitely Recommend Hospital	(a)	82%	-	69%

NOTE: Hospital profiles are in alphabetical order by state, then city, then hospital within the city; Rankings exclude hospitals with less than 25 cases except for patient surveys which excludes hospitals with less than 100 cases; (a) 100–299 cases; (1) The number of cases is too small to be sure how well a hospital is performing; (2) The hospital indicated that the data submitted for this measure were based on a sample of cases; (3) Data was collected during a shorter time period (fewer quarters) than the maximum possible time for this measure; (4) Suppressed for one or more quarters by CMS; (5) No data is available from the hospital for this measure; (6) Fewer than 100 patients completed the HCAHPS survey. Use these rates with caution, as the number of surveys may be too low to reliably assess hospital performance; (7) Survey results are based on less than 12 months of data; (8) Survey results are not available for this reporting period; (9) No or very few patients were eligible for the HCAHPS survey. The scores shown, if any, reflect a very small number of surveys; (10) A state average was not calculated because too few hospitals in the state submitted data; (11) There were discrepancies in the data collection process; Please refer to the User's Guide for a full explanation of data.

Potomac Hospital

2300 Opitz Boulevard
Woodbridge, VA 22191
Phone: 703-670-1313
Fax: 703-670-7643
E-mail: email@potomachospital.com
URL: www.potomachospital.com

Type: Acute Care Hospitals — Emergency Services: Yes
Ownership: Voluntary Non-Profit - Other — Beds: 153

Key Personnel:

- CEO/President . . . . William M Moss
- Chief of Medical Staff . . . . Bill Reha
- Infection Control . . . . Suzanne Davis
- Operating Room . . . . Todd Henderson
- Pediatric Ambulatory Care . . . . . . William Carr, MD
- Pediatric In-Patient Care . . . . William Carr, MD
- Quality Assurance . . . . Valerie Keane
- Radiology . . . . Norbertina Bans, MD

Measure	Cases	This Hosp.	State Avg.	U.S. Avg.
Heart Attack Care				
ACE Inhibitor or ARB for LVSD[1]	23	96%	97%	96%
Aspirin at Arrival	108	99%	99%	99%
Aspirin at Discharge	55	96%	99%	98%
Beta Blocker at Discharge	47	96%	99%	98%
Fibrinolytic Medication Timing	0	-	75%	55%
PCI Within 90 Minutes of Arrival	0	-	93%	90%
Smoking Cessation Advice[1]	9	100%	100%	99%
Chest Pain/Possible Heart Attack Care				
Aspirin at Arrival	157	99%	95%	95%
Median Time to ECG (minutes)	164	9	8	8
Median Time to Transfer (minutes)[1]	4	77	60	61
Fibrinolytic Medication Timing	0	-	59%	54%
Heart Failure Care				
ACE Inhibitor or ARB for LVSD[2]	65	100%	97%	94%
Discharge Instructions[2]	240	83%	92%	88%
Evaluation of LVS Function[2]	260	93%	99%	98%
Smoking Cessation Advice[2]	46	98%	99%	98%
Pneumonia Care				
Appropriate Initial Antibiotic[2]	98	91%	93%	92%
Blood Culture Timing[2]	143	89%	97%	96%
Influenza Vaccine[2]	73	79%	94%	91%
Initial Antibiotic Timing[2]	132	91%	96%	95%
Pneumococcal Vaccine[2]	84	77%	95%	93%
Smoking Cessation Advice[2]	50	80%	98%	97%
Surgical Care Improvement Project				
Appropriate VTP Within 24 Hours[2]	101	97%	94%	92%
Appropriate Hair Removal[2]	320	100%	100%	99%
Appropriate Beta Blocker Usage[2]	55	96%	94%	93%
Controlled Postoperative Blood Glucose[2]	0	-	96%	93%
Prophylactic Antibiotic Timing[2]	194	96%	97%	97%
Prophylactic Antibiotic Timing (Outpatient)	214	98%	93%	92%
Prophylactic Antibiotic Selection[2]	196	98%	98%	97%
Prophylactic Antibiotic Select. (Outpatient)	220	91%	96%	94%
Prophylactic Antibiotic Stopped[2]	186	86%	96%	94%
Recommended VTP Ordered[2]	101	97%	96%	94%
Urinary Catheter Removal[2]	61	100%	93%	90%
Children's Asthma Care				
Received Systemic Corticosteroids	-	-	-	100%
Received Home Management Plan	-	-	-	71%
Received Reliever Medication	-	-	-	100%
Use of Medical Imaging				
Combination Abdominal CT Scan	660	0.070	0.144	0.191
Combination Chest CT Scan	631	0.022	0.030	0.054
Follow-up Mammogram/Ultrasound	385	13.8%	7.5%	8.4%
MRI for Low Back Pain	157	22.3%	31.5%	32.7%
Survey of Patients' Hospital Experiences				
Area Around Room 'Always' Quiet at Night	300+	67%	-	58%
Doctors 'Always' Communicated Well	300+	76%	-	80%
Home Recovery Information Given	300+	79%	-	82%
Hospital Given 9 or 10 on 10 Point Scale	300+	59%	-	67%
Meds 'Always' Explained Before Given	300+	59%	-	60%
Nurses 'Always' Communicated Well	300+	70%	-	76%
Pain 'Always' Well Controlled	300+	65%	-	69%
Room and Bathroom 'Always' Clean	300+	76%	-	71%
Timely Help 'Always' Received	300+	53%	-	64%
Would Definitely Recommend Hospital	300+	62%	-	69%

Shenandoah Memorial Hospital

759 South Main Street
Woodstock, VA 22664
Phone: 540-459-1100
Fax: 540-459-1136
E-mail: marketingmail@valleyhealthlink.com
URL: www.valleyhealthlink.com

Type: Critical Access Hospitals — Emergency Services: Yes
Ownership: Voluntary Non-Profit - Private — Beds: 25

Key Personnel:

- CEO/President . . . . Floyd Heater

Measure	Cases	This Hosp.	State Avg.	U.S. Avg.
Heart Attack Care				
ACE Inhibitor or ARB for LVSD[3]	0	-	97%	96%
Aspirin at Arrival[1,3]	6	100%	99%	99%
Aspirin at Discharge[1,3]	2	100%	99%	98%
Beta Blocker at Discharge[1,3]	2	50%	99%	98%
Fibrinolytic Medication Timing[3]	0	-	75%	55%
PCI Within 90 Minutes of Arrival[3]	0	-	93%	90%
Smoking Cessation Advice[1,3]	1	100%	100%	99%
Chest Pain/Possible Heart Attack Care				
Aspirin at Arrival	-	-	95%	95%
Median Time to ECG (minutes)	-	-	8	8
Median Time to Transfer (minutes)	-	-	60	61
Fibrinolytic Medication Timing	-	-	59%	54%
Heart Failure Care				
ACE Inhibitor or ARB for LVSD[1]	8	100%	97%	94%
Discharge Instructions	31	68%	92%	88%
Evaluation of LVS Function	41	100%	99%	98%
Smoking Cessation Advice[1]	4	100%	99%	98%
Pneumonia Care				
Appropriate Initial Antibiotic	61	85%	93%	92%
Blood Culture Timing	83	95%	97%	96%
Influenza Vaccine	50	84%	94%	91%
Initial Antibiotic Timing	75	97%	96%	95%
Pneumococcal Vaccine	78	96%	95%	93%
Smoking Cessation Advice[1]	23	96%	98%	97%
Surgical Care Improvement Project				
Appropriate VTP Within 24 Hours	88	97%	94%	92%
Appropriate Hair Removal	261	100%	100%	99%
Appropriate Beta Blocker Usage	89	89%	94%	93%
Controlled Postoperative Blood Glucose	0	-	96%	93%
Prophylactic Antibiotic Timing	178	90%	97%	97%
Prophylactic Antibiotic Timing (Outpatient)	-	-	93%	92%
Prophylactic Antibiotic Selection	179	100%	98%	97%
Prophylactic Antibiotic Select. (Outpatient)	-	-	96%	94%
Prophylactic Antibiotic Stopped	170	95%	96%	94%
Recommended VTP Ordered	88	97%	96%	94%
Urinary Catheter Removal	48	85%	93%	90%
Children's Asthma Care				
Received Systemic Corticosteroids	-	-	-	100%
Received Home Management Plan	-	-	-	71%
Received Reliever Medication	-	-	-	100%
Use of Medical Imaging				
Combination Abdominal CT Scan	-	-	0.144	0.191
Combination Chest CT Scan	-	-	0.030	0.054
Follow-up Mammogram/Ultrasound	-	-	7.5%	8.4%
MRI for Low Back Pain	-	-	31.5%	32.7%
Survey of Patients' Hospital Experiences				
Area Around Room 'Always' Quiet at Night	300+	61%	-	58%
Doctors 'Always' Communicated Well	300+	80%	-	80%
Home Recovery Information Given	300+	87%	-	82%
Hospital Given 9 or 10 on 10 Point Scale	300+	68%	-	67%
Meds 'Always' Explained Before Given	300+	60%	-	60%
Nurses 'Always' Communicated Well	300+	79%	-	76%
Pain 'Always' Well Controlled	300+	71%	-	69%
Room and Bathroom 'Always' Clean	300+	80%	-	71%
Timely Help 'Always' Received	300+	67%	-	64%
Would Definitely Recommend Hospital	300+	71%	-	69%

Wythe County Community Hospital

600 West Ridge Road
Wytheville, VA 24382
Phone: 276-228-0200
Fax: 276-228-0397
URL: www.wcch.org

Type: Acute Care Hospitals — Emergency Services: Yes
Ownership: Voluntary Non-Profit - Private — Beds: 104

Key Personnel:

- CEO/President . . . . B Eric Deaton
- Chief of Medical Staff . . . . Michael Stoker, MD
- Coronary Care . . . . Marsha Jones
- Infection Control . . . . Becky McDonald, RN
- Operating Room . . . . Paul Morin
- Quality Assurance . . . . Carolyn Rudzinski
- Radiology . . . . Karl Ritch

Measure	Cases	This Hosp.	State Avg.	U.S. Avg.
Heart Attack Care				
ACE Inhibitor or ARB for LVSD[1]	1	100%	97%	96%
Aspirin at Arrival[1]	21	100%	99%	99%
Aspirin at Discharge[1]	18	94%	99%	98%
Beta Blocker at Discharge[1]	17	100%	99%	98%
Fibrinolytic Medication Timing	0	-	75%	55%
PCI Within 90 Minutes of Arrival	0	-	93%	90%
Smoking Cessation Advice[1]	1	100%	100%	99%
Chest Pain/Possible Heart Attack Care				
Aspirin at Arrival	159	100%	95%	95%
Median Time to ECG (minutes)	165	6	8	8
Median Time to Transfer (minutes)[1,3]	3	51	60	61
Fibrinolytic Medication Timing[1]	15	73%	59%	54%
Heart Failure Care				
ACE Inhibitor or ARB for LVSD[1]	24	100%	97%	94%
Discharge Instructions	75	91%	92%	88%
Evaluation of LVS Function	99	100%	99%	98%
Smoking Cessation Advice[1]	11	100%	99%	98%
Pneumonia Care				
Appropriate Initial Antibiotic	103	98%	93%	92%
Blood Culture Timing	107	99%	97%	96%
Influenza Vaccine	121	100%	94%	91%
Initial Antibiotic Timing	147	99%	96%	95%
Pneumococcal Vaccine	125	100%	95%	93%
Smoking Cessation Advice	63	100%	98%	97%
Surgical Care Improvement Project				
Appropriate VTP Within 24 Hours	33	82%	94%	92%
Appropriate Hair Removal	247	100%	100%	99%
Appropriate Beta Blocker Usage	61	92%	94%	93%
Controlled Postoperative Blood Glucose	0	-	96%	93%
Prophylactic Antibiotic Timing	204	99%	97%	97%
Prophylactic Antibiotic Timing (Outpatient)	51	94%	93%	92%
Prophylactic Antibiotic Selection	204	100%	98%	97%
Prophylactic Antibiotic Select. (Outpatient)	49	96%	96%	94%
Prophylactic Antibiotic Stopped	203	97%	96%	94%
Recommended VTP Ordered	33	91%	96%	94%
Urinary Catheter Removal	69	97%	93%	90%
Children's Asthma Care				
Received Systemic Corticosteroids	-	-	-	100%
Received Home Management Plan	-	-	-	71%
Received Reliever Medication	-	-	-	100%
Use of Medical Imaging				
Combination Abdominal CT Scan	384	0.042	0.144	0.191
Combination Chest CT Scan	240	0.000	0.030	0.054
Follow-up Mammogram/Ultrasound	471	7.9%	7.5%	8.4%
MRI for Low Back Pain	86	39.5%	31.5%	32.7%
Survey of Patients' Hospital Experiences				
Area Around Room 'Always' Quiet at Night	300+	60%	-	58%
Doctors 'Always' Communicated Well	300+	85%	-	80%
Home Recovery Information Given	300+	88%	-	82%
Hospital Given 9 or 10 on 10 Point Scale	300+	68%	-	67%
Meds 'Always' Explained Before Given	300+	60%	-	60%
Nurses 'Always' Communicated Well	300+	81%	-	76%
Pain 'Always' Well Controlled	300+	71%	-	69%
Room and Bathroom 'Always' Clean	300+	70%	-	71%
Timely Help 'Always' Received	300+	73%	-	64%
Would Definitely Recommend Hospital	300+	65%	-	69%

NOTE: Hospital profiles are in alphabetical order by state, then city, then hospital within the city; Rankings exclude hospitals with less than 25 cases except for patient surveys which excludes hospitals with less than 100 cases; (a) 100–299 cases; (1) The number of cases is too small to be sure how well a hospital is performing; (2) The hospital indicated that the data submitted for this measure were based on a sample of cases; (3) Data was collected during a shorter time period (fewer quarters) than the maximum possible time for this measure; (4) Suppressed for one or more quarters by CMS; (5) No data is available from the hospital for this measure; (6) Fewer than 100 patients completed the HCAHPS survey. Use these rates with caution, as the number of surveys may be too low to reliably assess hospital performance; (7) Survey results are based on less than 12 months of data; (8) Survey results are not available for this reporting period; (9) No or very few patients were eligible for the HCAHPS survey. The scores shown, if any, reflect a very small number of surveys; (10) A state average was not calculated because too few hospitals in the state submitted data; (11) There were discrepancies in the data collection process; Please refer to the User's Guide for a full explanation of data.

Heart Attack Care

1. ACE Inhibitor or ARB for LVSD

Hospital Name	City	Rate	Cases
Monongalia County General Hospital	Morgantown	100%	71
Raleigh General Hospital	Beckley	100%	26
United Hospital Center	Bridgeport	100%	54
West Virginia University Hospitals	Morgantown	96%	85
Wheeling Hospital	Wheeling	95%	91
Charleston Area Medical Center[2]	Charleston	94%	218
Saint Mary's Medical Center	Huntington	94%	77
Saint Josephs Healthcare System	Parkersburg	92%	36

2. Aspirin at Arrival

Hospital Name	City	Rate	Cases
City Hospital	Martinsburg	100%	108
Clarksburg VA Medical Center	Clarksburg	100%	26
Raleigh General Hospital	Beckley	100%	159
United Hospital Center	Bridgeport	100%	192
West Virginia University Hospitals	Morgantown	100%	196
Monongalia County General Hospital	Morgantown	99%	138
Camden Clark Memorial Hospital	Parkersburg	98%	172
Charleston Area Medical Center[2]	Charleston	98%	469
Fairmont General Hospital	Fairmont	98%	61
Saint Mary's Medical Center	Huntington	98%	357
Wheeling Hospital	Wheeling	98%	245
Cabell-Huntington Hospital	Huntington	97%	32
Saint Francis Hospital	Charleston	97%	37
Saint Josephs Healthcare System	Parkersburg	96%	151
Bluefield Regional Medical Center	Bluefield	95%	42
Ohio Valley Medical Center	Wheeling	95%	66
Weirton Medical Center	Weirton	94%	68
Princeton Community Hospital	Princeton	93%	60
Wetzel County Hospital	New Martinsville	92%	25
Davis Memorial Hospital	Elkins	90%	30
Thomas Memorial Hospital[2]	S Charleston	90%	114
Reynolds Memorial Hospital	Glen Dale	86%	37
Beckley Arh Hospital	Beckley	81%	27

3. Aspirin at Discharge

Hospital Name	City	Rate	Cases
Fairmont General Hospital	Fairmont	100%	40
Monongalia County General Hospital	Morgantown	100%	264
Ohio Valley Medical Center	Wheeling	100%	38
Saint Mary's Medical Center	Huntington	100%	576
United Hospital Center	Bridgeport	100%	195
West Virginia University Hospitals	Morgantown	100%	461
Charleston Area Medical Center[2]	Charleston	99%	997
Camden Clark Memorial Hospital	Parkersburg	98%	108
Saint Josephs Healthcare System	Parkersburg	98%	234
Wheeling Hospital	Wheeling	98%	402
Raleigh General Hospital	Beckley	96%	185
Thomas Memorial Hospital[2]	S Charleston	94%	80
Saint Francis Hospital	Charleston	93%	60
Bluefield Regional Medical Center	Bluefield	88%	25
Princeton Community Hospital	Princeton	87%	38
Weirton Medical Center	Weirton	82%	57
City Hospital	Martinsburg	80%	54

4. Beta Blocker at Discharge

Hospital Name	City	Rate	Cases
Fairmont General Hospital	Fairmont	100%	44
Princeton Community Hospital	Princeton	100%	36
United Hospital Center	Bridgeport	100%	189
Camden Clark Memorial Hospital	Parkersburg	99%	104
Charleston Area Medical Center[2]	Charleston	99%	996
Monongalia County General Hospital	Morgantown	99%	266
Saint Josephs Healthcare System	Parkersburg	99%	230
Saint Mary's Medical Center	Huntington	99%	560
West Virginia University Hospitals	Morgantown	99%	453
Wheeling Hospital	Wheeling	99%	404
Ohio Valley Medical Center	Wheeling	98%	41
Saint Francis Hospital	Charleston	97%	60
Raleigh General Hospital	Beckley	96%	171
Bluefield Regional Medical Center	Bluefield	94%	31
Thomas Memorial Hospital[2]	S Charleston	91%	82
Weirton Medical Center	Weirton	90%	58
City Hospital	Martinsburg	81%	52

6. PCI Within 90 Minutes of Arrival

Hospital Name	City	Rate	Cases
United Hospital Center	Bridgeport	100%	33
Wheeling Hospital	Wheeling	98%	60
Saint Mary's Medical Center	Huntington	97%	64
West Virginia University Hospitals	Morgantown	97%	31
Monongalia County General Hospital	Morgantown	91%	35
Saint Josephs Healthcare System	Parkersburg	90%	30
Charleston Area Medical Center[2]	Charleston	67%	73
Raleigh General Hospital	Beckley	62%	29

7. Smoking Cessation Advice

Hospital Name	City	Rate	Cases
Charleston Area Medical Center[2]	Charleston	100%	410
Monongalia County General Hospital	Morgantown	100%	90
Raleigh General Hospital	Beckley	100%	78
Saint Francis Hospital	Charleston	100%	29
Saint Josephs Healthcare System	Parkersburg	100%	80
Saint Mary's Medical Center	Huntington	100%	257
Thomas Memorial Hospital[2]	S Charleston	100%	30
United Hospital Center	Bridgeport	100%	91
Wheeling Hospital	Wheeling	100%	164
West Virginia University Hospitals	Morgantown	97%	173

Chest Pain/Possible Heart Attack Care

8. Aspirin at Arrival

Hospital Name	City	Rate	Cases
Raleigh General Hospital	Beckley	100%	88
Saint Joseph Hospital	Buckhannon	100%	40
Fairmont General Hospital	Fairmont	98%	156
Logan Regional Medical Center	Logan	98%	239
Plateau Medical Center	Oak Hill	98%	131
Williamson Memorial Hospital	Williamson	98%	46
Cabell-Huntington Hospital	Huntington	97%	34
Davis Memorial Hospital	Elkins	97%	216
Greenbrier Valley Medical Center	Ronceverte	97%	76
Jackson General Hospital	Ripley	97%	104
Roane General Hospital	Spencer	97%	38
United Hospital Center	Bridgeport	97%	33
Stonewall Jackson Memorial Hospital	Weston	96%	45
Preston Memorial Hospital	Kingwood	95%	55
Princeton Community Hospital	Princeton	95%	187
Summersville Regional Medical Center	Summersville	94%	81
Bluefield Regional Medical Center	Bluefield	93%	121
City Hospital	Martinsburg	93%	110
Wetzel County Hospital	New Martinsville	92%	72
Camden Clark Memorial Hospital	Parkersburg	91%	56
Beckley Arh Hospital	Beckley	90%	48
Welch Community Hospital	Welch	90%	140
Pleasant Valley Hospital	Point Pleasant	89%	76
Ohio Valley Medical Center	Wheeling	88%	33

9. Median Time to ECG (minutes)

Hospital Name	City	Min.	Cases
Roane General Hospital	Spencer	0	40
Greenbrier Valley Medical Center	Ronceverte	3	83
City Hospital	Martinsburg	6	108
Davis Memorial Hospital	Elkins	7	229
Stonewall Jackson Memorial Hospital	Weston	7	48
Williamson Memorial Hospital	Williamson	7	59
Ohio Valley Medical Center	Wheeling	8	34
Fairmont General Hospital	Fairmont	9	160
Princeton Community Hospital	Princeton	9	201
Jackson General Hospital	Ripley	10	107
Pleasant Valley Hospital	Point Pleasant	10	78
Beckley Arh Hospital	Beckley	11	51
Cabell-Huntington Hospital	Huntington	11	36
Plateau Medical Center	Oak Hill	12	139
United Hospital Center	Bridgeport	13	31
Wetzel County Hospital	New Martinsville	13	83
Camden Clark Memorial Hospital	Parkersburg	14	55
Summersville Regional Medical Center	Summersville	14	86
Bluefield Regional Medical Center	Bluefield	16	123
Saint Joseph Hospital	Buckhannon	16	44
Logan Regional Medical Center	Logan	18	253
Raleigh General Hospital	Beckley	20	94
Preston Memorial Hospital	Kingwood	23	55
Camc Teays Valley Hospital	Hurricane	30	26
Welch Community Hospital	Welch	41	142

Heart Failure Care

12. ACE Inhibitor or ARB for LVSD

Hospital Name	City	Rate	Cases
Davis Memorial Hospital	Elkins	100%	45
Logan Regional Medical Center	Logan	100%	40
Saint Francis Hospital	Charleston	100%	52
Stonewall Jackson Memorial Hospital	Weston	100%	25
United Hospital Center	Bridgeport	100%	126
Camden Clark Memorial Hospital	Parkersburg	99%	76
Fairmont General Hospital	Fairmont	98%	45
West Virginia University Hospitals	Morgantown	98%	111
Princeton Community Hospital	Princeton	97%	68
Raleigh General Hospital	Beckley	97%	79
Weirton Medical Center	Weirton	97%	63
Cabell-Huntington Hospital	Huntington	96%	45
Clarksburg VA Medical Center	Clarksburg	96%	25
Huntington VA Medical Center	Huntington	94%	66
Martinsburg VA Medical Center	Martinsburg	93%	46
Beckley VA Medical Center	Beckley	92%	25
Charleston Area Medical Center[2]	Charleston	92%	259
Saint Mary's Medical Center	Huntington	92%	136
Wheeling Hospital	Wheeling	92%	123
Ohio Valley Medical Center	Wheeling	90%	49
Thomas Memorial Hospital[2]	S Charleston	90%	52
Camc Teays Valley Hospital	Hurricane	89%	36
Monongalia County General Hospital	Morgantown	83%	92
Bluefield Regional Medical Center	Bluefield	82%	62
Greenbrier Valley Medical Center	Ronceverte	79%	48
Saint Josephs Healthcare System	Parkersburg	78%	85
City Hospital	Martinsburg	77%	43
Reynolds Memorial Hospital	Glen Dale	72%	43
Beckley Arh Hospital	Beckley	64%	33
Pleasant Valley Hospital	Point Pleasant	58%	36

13. Discharge Instructions

Hospital Name	City	Rate	Cases
Beckley VA Medical Center	Beckley	100%	49
Clarksburg VA Medical Center	Clarksburg	100%	88
Huntington VA Medical Center	Huntington	100%	157
Stonewall Jackson Memorial Hospital	Weston	100%	69
Williamson Memorial Hospital	Williamson	100%	83
Logan Regional Medical Center	Logan	98%	178
Princeton Community Hospital	Princeton	98%	248
Saint Francis Hospital	Charleston	98%	88
West Virginia University Hospitals	Morgantown	97%	266
Ohio Valley Medical Center	Wheeling	96%	127
United Hospital Center	Bridgeport	95%	212
Wheeling Hospital	Wheeling	95%	239
Davis Memorial Hospital	Elkins	94%	126
Summers County ARH Hospital	Hinton	93%	29
Pleasant Valley Hospital	Point Pleasant	92%	87
Reynolds Memorial Hospital	Glen Dale	92%	87
Saint Mary's Medical Center	Huntington	90%	451
Camden Clark Memorial Hospital	Parkersburg	89%	255
Greenbrier Valley Medical Center	Ronceverte	89%	114
Cabell-Huntington Hospital	Huntington	87%	121
Fairmont General Hospital	Fairmont	87%	161
Monongalia County General Hospital	Morgantown	87%	229
Raleigh General Hospital	Beckley	86%	311
Weirton Medical Center	Weirton	86%	171
Thomas Memorial Hospital[2]	S Charleston	85%	163
Plateau Medical Center	Oak Hill	83%	54
Wetzel County Hospital	New Martinsville	80%	40
Montgomery General Hospital	Montgomery	79%	29
Jackson General Hospital	Ripley	78%	83
Grant Memorial Hospital	Petersburg	77%	35
Potomac Valley Hospital	Keyser	76%	34
Saint Josephs Healthcare System	Parkersburg	73%	268
Beckley Arh Hospital	Beckley	72%	124
Bluefield Regional Medical Center	Bluefield	72%	178
Martinsburg VA Medical Center	Martinsburg	72%	78
City Hospital	Martinsburg	71%	142
Camc Teays Valley Hospital	Hurricane	70%	47
Charleston Area Medical Center[2]	Charleston	67%	610
Braxton County Memorial Hospital	Gassaway	55%	31
Summersville Regional Medical Center[2]	Summersville	37%	35

14. Evaluation of LVS Function

Hospital Name	City	Rate	Cases
Beckley VA Medical Center	Beckley	100%	56
Camc Teays Valley Hospital	Hurricane	100%	60
Camden Clark Memorial Hospital	Parkersburg	100%	362
Davis Memorial Hospital	Elkins	100%	138
Fairmont General Hospital	Fairmont	100%	213
Huntington VA Medical Center	Huntington	100%	168
Jefferson Memorial Hospital	Ranson	100%	28
Logan Regional Medical Center	Logan	100%	213
Martinsburg VA Medical Center	Martinsburg	100%	97
Raleigh General Hospital	Beckley	100%	365
Saint Francis Hospital	Charleston	100%	100
Saint Mary's Medical Center	Huntington	100%	525
Stonewall Jackson Memorial Hospital	Weston	100%	76
Summers County ARH Hospital	Hinton	100%	43
United Hospital Center	Bridgeport	100%	258
Cabell-Huntington Hospital	Huntington	99%	150
Charleston Area Medical Center[2]	Charleston	99%	684
Greenbrier Valley Medical Center	Ronceverte	99%	139
Jackson General Hospital	Ripley	99%	103
Plateau Medical Center	Oak Hill	99%	78
Weirton Medical Center	Weirton	99%	212
West Virginia University Hospitals	Morgantown	99%	315
Wheeling Hospital	Wheeling	99%	312
Bluefield Regional Medical Center	Bluefield	98%	193
Clarksburg VA Medical Center	Clarksburg	98%	91
Monongalia County General Hospital	Morgantown	98%	276

NOTE: Hospital profiles are in alphabetical order by state, then city, then hospital within the city; Rankings exclude hospitals with less than 25 cases except for patient surveys which excludes hospitals with less than 100 cases; (a) 100–299 cases; (1) The number of cases is too small to be sure how well a hospital is performing; (2) The hospital indicated that the data submitted for this measure were based on a sample of cases; (3) Data was collected during a shorter time period (fewer quarters) than the maximum possible time for this measure; (4) Suppressed for one or more quarters by CMS; (5) No data is available from the hospital for this measure; (6) Fewer than 100 patients completed the HCAHPS survey. Use these rates with caution, as the number of surveys may be too low to reliably assess hospital performance; (7) Survey results are based on less than 12 months of data; (8) Survey results are not available for this reporting period; (9) No or very few patients were eligible for the HCAHPS survey. The scores shown, if any, reflect a very small number of surveys; (10) A state average was not calculated because too few hospitals in the state submitted data; (11) There were discrepancies in the data collection process; Please refer to the User's Guide for a full explanation of data.

Ohio Valley Medical Center	Wheeling	98%	177
Pleasant Valley Hospital	Point Pleasant	98%	116
Williamson Memorial Hospital	Williamson	97%	92
Princeton Community Hospital	Princeton	96%	282
Saint Josephs Healthcare System	Parkersburg	95%	323
Thomas Memorial Hospital[2]	S Charleston	95%	207
Reynolds Memorial Hospital	Glen Dale	94%	130
Summersville Regional Medical Center[2]	Summersville	94%	53
Potomac Valley Hospital	Keyser	92%	38
Beckley Arh Hospital	Beckley	91%	152
City Hospital	Martinsburg	89%	157
Wetzel County Hospital	New Martinsville	88%	58
Grant Memorial Hospital	Petersburg	81%	68
Montgomery General Hospital	Montgomery	78%	37
Braxton County Memorial Hospital	Gassaway	71%	35

15. Smoking Cessation Advice

Hospital Name	City	Rate	Cases
Cabell-Huntington Hospital	Huntington	100%	36
Camden Clark Memorial Hospital	Parkersburg	100%	42
Huntington VA Medical Center	Huntington	100%	43
Logan Regional Medical Center	Logan	100%	30
Martinsburg VA Medical Center	Martinsburg	100%	29
Monongalia County General Hospital	Morgantown	100%	39
Ohio Valley Medical Center	Wheeling	100%	27
Princeton Community Hospital	Princeton	100%	35
Raleigh General Hospital	Beckley	100%	86
Saint Francis Hospital	Charleston	100%	28
Saint Josephs Healthcare System	Parkersburg	100%	48
Saint Mary's Medical Center	Huntington	100%	102
United Hospital Center	Bridgeport	100%	46
Weirton Medical Center	Weirton	100%	35
Wheeling Hospital	Wheeling	100%	35
West Virginia University Hospitals	Morgantown	99%	69
Charleston Area Medical Center[2]	Charleston	98%	133
Beckley Arh Hospital	Beckley	97%	34
Thomas Memorial Hospital[2]	S Charleston	96%	27
City Hospital	Martinsburg	84%	25
Bluefield Regional Medical Center	Bluefield	76%	33

Pneumonia Care

16. Appropriate Initial Antibiotic

Hospital Name	City	Rate	Cases
Potomac Valley Hospital[2]	Keyser	100%	30
Cabell-Huntington Hospital	Huntington	98%	61
United Hospital Center	Bridgeport	98%	205
Williamson Memorial Hospital	Williamson	98%	57
Raleigh General Hospital	Beckley	97%	213
West Virginia University Hospitals	Morgantown	97%	99
Huntington VA Medical Center	Huntington	96%	77
Fairmont General Hospital	Fairmont	95%	105
Saint Mary's Medical Center	Huntington	95%	317
Martinsburg VA Medical Center	Martinsburg	94%	67
Saint Josephs Healthcare System	Parkersburg	94%	104
Summers County ARH Hospital	Hinton	94%	32
Beckley VA Medical Center	Beckley	93%	107
Braxton County Memorial Hospital	Gassaway	93%	30
Saint Francis Hospital	Charleston	93%	61
Welch Community Hospital	Welch	93%	45
Greenbrier Valley Medical Center	Ronceverte	92%	120
Jackson General Hospital	Ripley	92%	49
Weirton Medical Center	Weirton	92%	232
Camden Clark Memorial Hospital	Parkersburg	91%	199
City Hospital	Martinsburg	91%	176
Summersville Regional Medical Center	Summersville	91%	43
Clarksburg VA Medical Center	Clarksburg	90%	59
Saint Joseph Hospital	Buckhannon	90%	29
Camc Teays Valley Hospital	Hurricane	89%	70
Davis Memorial Hospital	Elkins	89%	92
Logan Regional Medical Center	Logan	88%	227
Monongalia County General Hospital	Morgantown	88%	103
Montgomery General Hospital	Montgomery	88%	75
Thomas Memorial Hospital[2]	S Charleston	88%	189
Wheeling Hospital[2]	Wheeling	88%	107
Stonewall Jackson Memorial Hospital	Weston	87%	93
Jefferson Memorial Hospital	Ranson	86%	28
Wetzel County Hospital	New Martinsville	86%	70
Charleston Area Medical Center[2]	Charleston	85%	340
Beckley Arh Hospital	Beckley	84%	64
Grant Memorial Hospital	Petersburg	84%	38
Plateau Medical Center	Oak Hill	83%	64
Reynolds Memorial Hospital	Glen Dale	83%	64
Ohio Valley Medical Center	Wheeling	82%	88
Pleasant Valley Hospital	Point Pleasant	81%	64
Princeton Community Hospital	Princeton	80%	210
Bluefield Regional Medical Center	Bluefield	75%	121
Boone Memorial Hospital	Madison	69%	29

17. Blood Culture Timing

Hospital Name	City	Rate	Cases
Camden Clark Memorial Hospital	Parkersburg	99%	294
Clarksburg VA Medical Center	Clarksburg	99%	93
Davis Memorial Hospital	Elkins	99%	118
Huntington VA Medical Center	Huntington	99%	178
Stonewall Jackson Memorial Hospital	Weston	99%	82
United Hospital Center	Bridgeport	99%	255
Weirton Medical Center	Weirton	99%	321
Jackson General Hospital	Ripley	98%	97
Monongalia County General Hospital	Morgantown	98%	125
Montgomery General Hospital	Montgomery	98%	82
Cabell-Huntington Hospital	Huntington	97%	193
Ohio Valley Medical Center	Wheeling	97%	133
Princeton Community Hospital	Princeton	97%	224
Saint Mary's Medical Center	Huntington	97%	590
Summers County ARH Hospital	Hinton	97%	34
Williamson Memorial Hospital	Williamson	97%	71
Beckley VA Medical Center	Beckley	96%	158
Fairmont General Hospital	Fairmont	96%	121
Martinsburg VA Medical Center	Martinsburg	96%	82
Potomac Valley Hospital[2]	Keyser	96%	28
Saint Josephs Healthcare System	Parkersburg	96%	173
Logan Regional Medical Center	Logan	95%	323
Plateau Medical Center	Oak Hill	95%	88
Wheeling Hospital[2]	Wheeling	95%	155
Charleston Area Medical Center[2]	Charleston	94%	541
Greenbrier Valley Medical Center	Ronceverte	94%	196
Pleasant Valley Hospital	Point Pleasant	94%	66
Thomas Memorial Hospital[2]	S Charleston	94%	282
West Virginia University Hospitals	Morgantown	94%	199
Bluefield Regional Medical Center	Bluefield	93%	169
Saint Francis Hospital	Charleston	93%	88
Wetzel County Hospital	New Martinsville	93%	55
Raleigh General Hospital	Beckley	92%	323
Camc Teays Valley Hospital	Hurricane	91%	95
City Hospital	Martinsburg	90%	208
Saint Joseph Hospital	Buckhannon	89%	36
Jefferson Memorial Hospital	Ranson	88%	52
Reynolds Memorial Hospital	Glen Dale	88%	48
Beckley Arh Hospital	Beckley	86%	105
Boone Memorial Hospital	Madison	86%	49
Preston Memorial Hospital[2]	Kingwood	80%	25
Summersville Regional Medical Center	Summersville	78%	101
Braxton County Memorial Hospital	Gassaway	72%	39

18. Influenza Vaccine

Hospital Name	City	Rate	Cases
Beckley VA Medical Center	Beckley	100%	104
Logan Regional Medical Center	Logan	100%	232
Williamson Memorial Hospital	Williamson	100%	42
Clarksburg VA Medical Center	Clarksburg	99%	68
Fairmont General Hospital	Fairmont	98%	116
Jackson General Hospital	Ripley	98%	56
Plateau Medical Center	Oak Hill	98%	60
Camden Clark Memorial Hospital	Parkersburg	97%	233
Martinsburg VA Medical Center	Martinsburg	97%	67
Princeton Community Hospital	Princeton	97%	218
Weirton Medical Center	Weirton	97%	210
Greenbrier Valley Medical Center	Ronceverte	96%	164
United Hospital Center	Bridgeport	96%	257
Huntington VA Medical Center	Huntington	95%	119
Monongalia County General Hospital	Morgantown	95%	96
West Virginia University Hospitals	Morgantown	94%	189
Cabell-Huntington Hospital	Huntington	93%	128
Pleasant Valley Hospital	Point Pleasant	93%	60
Wetzel County Hospital	New Martinsville	93%	58
Stonewall Jackson Memorial Hospital	Weston	92%	92
Davis Memorial Hospital	Elkins	91%	81
Saint Josephs Healthcare System	Parkersburg	91%	117
Raleigh General Hospital	Beckley	90%	218
Reynolds Memorial Hospital	Glen Dale	90%	61
Summers County ARH Hospital	Hinton	90%	29
Saint Francis Hospital	Charleston	89%	61
City Hospital	Martinsburg	88%	113
Montgomery General Hospital	Montgomery	88%	42
Saint Mary's Medical Center	Huntington	88%	285
Wheeling Hospital[2]	Wheeling	87%	140
Charleston Area Medical Center[2]	Charleston	85%	378
Camc Teays Valley Hospital	Hurricane	82%	68
Ohio Valley Medical Center	Wheeling	81%	109
Bluefield Regional Medical Center	Bluefield	80%	90
Summersville Regional Medical Center	Summersville	80%	59
Beckley Arh Hospital	Beckley	75%	69
Grant Memorial Hospital	Petersburg	72%	29
Thomas Memorial Hospital	S Charleston	72%	198
Braxton County Memorial Hospital	Gassaway	43%	35
Welch Community Hospital	Welch	34%	29

19. Initial Antibiotic Timing

Hospital Name	City	Rate	Cases
Montgomery General Hospital	Montgomery	100%	93
Summers County ARH Hospital	Hinton	100%	41
Fairmont General Hospital	Fairmont	99%	138
Huntington VA Medical Center	Huntington	99%	113
Beckley VA Medical Center	Beckley	98%	160
Raleigh General Hospital	Beckley	98%	319
Saint Joseph Hospital	Buckhannon	98%	42
Weirton Medical Center	Weirton	98%	313
Camden Clark Memorial Hospital	Parkersburg	97%	325
City Hospital	Martinsburg	97%	210
Clarksburg VA Medical Center	Clarksburg	97%	103
Davis Memorial Hospital	Elkins	97%	107
Greenbrier Valley Medical Center	Ronceverte	97%	198
Monongalia County General Hospital	Morgantown	97%	115
Stonewall Jackson Memorial Hospital	Weston	97%	149
United Hospital Center	Bridgeport	97%	116
Jackson General Hospital	Ripley	96%	103
Cabell-Huntington Hospital	Huntington	95%	192
Plateau Medical Center	Oak Hill	95%	94
Summersville Regional Medical Center	Summersville	95%	120
Wetzel County Hospital	New Martinsville	95%	82
Ohio Valley Medical Center	Wheeling	94%	167
Pleasant Valley Hospital	Point Pleasant	94%	105
Wheeling Hospital[2]	Wheeling	94%	182
Logan Regional Medical Center	Logan	93%	348
Martinsburg VA Medical Center	Martinsburg	93%	95
Reynolds Memorial Hospital	Glen Dale	93%	84
Saint Mary's Medical Center	Huntington	93%	580
Beckley Arh Hospital	Beckley	92%	107
Camc Teays Valley Hospital	Hurricane	92%	88
Roane General Hospital	Spencer	92%	25
Thomas Memorial Hospital[2]	S Charleston	92%	288
Saint Josephs Healthcare System	Parkersburg	91%	165
Grant Memorial Hospital	Petersburg	90%	48
Potomac Valley Hospital[2]	Keyser	90%	31
Saint Francis Hospital	Charleston	90%	93
West Virginia University Hospitals	Morgantown	90%	225
Braxton County Memorial Hospital	Gassaway	89%	44
Charleston Area Medical Center[2]	Charleston	89%	494
Princeton Community Hospital	Princeton	89%	332
Welch Community Hospital	Welch	89%	45
Bluefield Regional Medical Center	Bluefield	88%	172
Grafton City Hospital	Grafton	88%	25
Jefferson Memorial Hospital	Ranson	87%	54

20. Pneumococcal Vaccine

Hospital Name	City	Rate	Cases
Logan Regional Medical Center	Logan	100%	235
Martinsburg VA Medical Center	Martinsburg	100%	86
Williamson Memorial Hospital	Williamson	100%	37
Beckley VA Medical Center	Beckley	99%	162
Camden Clark Memorial Hospital	Parkersburg	99%	349
Clarksburg VA Medical Center	Clarksburg	99%	93
Fairmont General Hospital	Fairmont	99%	161
Greenbrier Valley Medical Center	Ronceverte	99%	205
Huntington VA Medical Center	Huntington	98%	168
Monongalia County General Hospital	Morgantown	98%	121
Pleasant Valley Hospital	Point Pleasant	98%	80
Cabell-Huntington Hospital	Huntington	97%	142
Jackson General Hospital	Ripley	97%	94
Raleigh General Hospital	Beckley	97%	249
United Hospital Center	Bridgeport	97%	319
Princeton Community Hospital	Princeton	96%	275
West Virginia University Hospitals	Morgantown	96%	199
Reynolds Memorial Hospital	Glen Dale	95%	87
Weirton Medical Center	Weirton	95%	286
Davis Memorial Hospital	Elkins	94%	102
Plateau Medical Center	Oak Hill	94%	71
Roane General Hospital	Spencer	93%	30
Stonewall Jackson Memorial Hospital	Weston	93%	127
Charleston Area Medical Center[2]	Charleston	92%	487
City Hospital	Martinsburg	92%	149
Ohio Valley Medical Center	Wheeling	92%	130
Saint Josephs Healthcare System	Parkersburg	92%	167
Saint Mary's Medical Center	Huntington	91%	445
Saint Joseph Hospital	Buckhannon	88%	26
Wheeling Hospital[2]	Wheeling	87%	206
Camc Teays Valley Hospital	Hurricane	86%	83
Summers County ARH Hospital	Hinton	86%	37
Bluefield Regional Medical Center	Bluefield	84%	136
Montgomery General Hospital	Montgomery	84%	69
Beckley Arh Hospital	Beckley	83%	81
Boone Memorial Hospital	Madison	82%	28
Summersville Regional Medical Center	Summersville	79%	86
Wetzel County Hospital	New Martinsville	79%	90
Saint Francis Hospital	Charleston	78%	76
Jefferson Memorial Hospital	Ranson	71%	34
Thomas Memorial Hospital[2]	S Charleston	70%	242

NOTE: Hospital profiles are in alphabetical order by state, then city, then hospital within the city; Rankings exclude hospitals with less than 25 cases except for patient surveys which excludes hospitals with less than 100 cases; (a) 100–299 cases; (1) The number of cases is too small to be sure how well a hospital is performing; (2) The hospital indicated that the data submitted for this measure were based on a sample of cases; (3) Data was collected during a shorter time period (fewer quarters) than the maximum possible time for this measure; (4) Suppressed for one or more quarters by CMS; (5) No data is available from the hospital for this measure; (6) Fewer than 100 patients completed the HCAHPS survey. Use these rates with caution, as the number of surveys may be too low to reliably assess hospital performance; (7) Survey results are based on less than 12 months of data; (8) Survey results are not available for this reporting period; (9) No or very few patients were eligible for the HCAHPS survey. The scores shown, if any, reflect a very small number of surveys; (10) A state average was not calculated because too few hospitals in the state submitted data; (11) There were discrepancies in the data collection process; Please refer to the User's Guide for a full explanation of data.

Grant Memorial Hospital	Petersburg	67%	42
Welch Community Hospital	Welch	50%	34
Braxton County Memorial Hospital	Gassaway	34%	41

21. Smoking Cessation Advice

Hospital Name	City	Rate	Cases
Beckley VA Medical Center	Beckley	100%	64
Cabell-Huntington Hospital	Huntington	100%	155
Clarksburg VA Medical Center	Clarksburg	100%	29
Davis Memorial Hospital	Elkins	100%	38
Fairmont General Hospital	Fairmont	100%	79
Huntington VA Medical Center	Huntington	100%	88
Ohio Valley Medical Center	Wheeling	100%	65
Princeton Community Hospital	Princeton	100%	143
Raleigh General Hospital	Beckley	100%	171
Saint Josephs Healthcare System	Parkersburg	100%	65
Stonewall Jackson Memorial Hospital	Weston	100%	53
United Hospital Center	Bridgeport	100%	149
Weirton Medical Center	Weirton	100%	139
Williamson Memorial Hospital	Williamson	100%	32
Logan Regional Medical Center	Logan	99%	162
Saint Mary's Medical Center	Huntington	99%	260
Camc Teays Valley Hospital	Hurricane	98%	43
Martinsburg VA Medical Center	Martinsburg	98%	47
Pleasant Valley Hospital	Point Pleasant	98%	48
Thomas Memorial Hospital[2]	S Charleston	98%	114
Charleston Area Medical Center[2]	Charleston	97%	375
Greenbrier Valley Medical Center	Ronceverte	97%	116
Montgomery General Hospital	Montgomery	97%	29
Reynolds Memorial Hospital	Glen Dale	97%	33
West Virginia University Hospitals	Morgantown	97%	131
Wetzel County Hospital	New Martinsville	97%	34
Plateau Medical Center	Oak Hill	96%	28
Beckley Arh Hospital	Beckley	95%	59
Bluefield Regional Medical Center	Bluefield	95%	62
Camden Clark Memorial Hospital	Parkersburg	95%	113
Monongalia County General Hospital	Morgantown	93%	46
Saint Francis Hospital	Charleston	89%	53
Wheeling Hospital[2]	Wheeling	88%	66
City Hospital	Martinsburg	84%	96
Welch Community Hospital	Welch	68%	25
Summersville Regional Medical Center	Summersville	67%	30

Surgical Care Improvement Project

22. Appropriate VTP Within 24 Hours

Hospital Name	City	Rate	Cases
Fairmont General Hospital	Fairmont	99%	117
West Virginia University Hospitals[2]	Morgantown	99%	287
Greenbrier Valley Medical Center	Ronceverte	98%	93
Huntington VA Medical Center[2]	Huntington	98%	94
Cabell-Huntington Hospital[2]	Huntington	97%	141
Monongalia County General Hospital[2]	Morgantown	97%	388
United Hospital Center[2]	Bridgeport	97%	254
Wheeling Hospital	Wheeling	97%	243
City Hospital	Martinsburg	96%	252
Charleston Area Medical Center[2]	Charleston	95%	465
Logan Regional Medical Center	Logan	95%	132
Summersville Regional Medical Center[2]	Summersville	95%	64
Davis Memorial Hospital	Elkins	94%	120
Plateau Medical Center[2]	Oak Hill	94%	48
Raleigh General Hospital	Beckley	94%	159
Princeton Community Hospital	Princeton	93%	179
Camden Clark Memorial Hospital[2]	Parkersburg	90%	233
Grant Memorial Hospital	Petersburg	88%	25
Saint Mary's Medical Center[2]	Huntington	88%	237
Saint Josephs Healthcare System[2]	Parkersburg	87%	157
Stonewall Jackson Memorial Hospital	Weston	87%	62
Weirton Medical Center[2]	Weirton	86%	118
Ohio Valley Medical Center	Wheeling	85%	146
Jefferson Memorial Hospital	Ranson	82%	34
Reynolds Memorial Hospital	Glen Dale	82%	44
Saint Francis Hospital	Charleston	81%	140
Camc Teays Valley Hospital	Hurricane	80%	70
Bluefield Regional Medical Center	Bluefield	76%	79
Beckley Arh Hospital	Beckley	75%	80
Pleasant Valley Hospital	Point Pleasant	71%	70
Thomas Memorial Hospital[2]	S Charleston	71%	235
Saint Joseph Hospital	Buckhannon	60%	25

23. Appropriate Hair Removal

Hospital Name	City	Rate	Cases
Cabell-Huntington Hospital[2]	Huntington	100%	441
Camden Clark Memorial Hospital[2]	Parkersburg	100%	756
Charleston Area Medical Center[2]	Charleston	100%	2464
City Hospital	Martinsburg	100%	573
Davis Memorial Hospital	Elkins	100%	322
Fairmont General Hospital	Fairmont	100%	216
Grant Memorial Hospital	Petersburg	100%	124
Greenbrier Valley Medical Center	Ronceverte	100%	199
Jefferson Memorial Hospital	Ranson	100%	55
Logan Regional Medical Center	Logan	100%	268
Monongalia County General Hospital[2]	Morgantown	100%	1210
Plateau Medical Center[2]	Oak Hill	100%	186
Princeton Community Hospital	Princeton	100%	618
Raleigh General Hospital	Beckley	100%	496
Reynolds Memorial Hospital	Glen Dale	100%	95
Saint Joseph Hospital	Buckhannon	100%	66
Saint Mary's Medical Center[2]	Huntington	100%	1204
Stonewall Jackson Memorial Hospital	Weston	100%	148
Summersville Regional Medical Center[2]	Summersville	100%	101
United Hospital Center[2]	Bridgeport	100%	739
West Virginia University Hospitals[2]	Morgantown	100%	1153
Williamson Memorial Hospital	Williamson	100%	27
Beckley Arh Hospital	Beckley	99%	152
Bluefield Regional Medical Center	Bluefield	99%	285
Camc Teays Valley Hospital	Hurricane	99%	155
Huntington VA Medical Center[2]	Huntington	99%	182
Saint Francis Hospital	Charleston	99%	598
Saint Josephs Healthcare System[2]	Parkersburg	99%	551
Pleasant Valley Hospital	Point Pleasant	98%	109
Weirton Medical Center[2]	Weirton	98%	329
Wheeling Hospital	Wheeling	98%	1191
Ohio Valley Medical Center	Wheeling	97%	363
Thomas Memorial Hospital[2]	S Charleston	96%	683
Welch Community Hospital	Welch	85%	26

24. Appropriate Beta Blocker Usage

Hospital Name	City	Rate	Cases
City Hospital	Martinsburg	100%	145
Huntington VA Medical Center[2]	Huntington	100%	75
Summersville Regional Medical Center[2]	Summersville	100%	32
United Hospital Center[2]	Bridgeport	100%	214
West Virginia University Hospitals[2]	Morgantown	100%	362
Camden Clark Memorial Hospital[2]	Parkersburg	97%	198
Fairmont General Hospital	Fairmont	97%	67
Plateau Medical Center[2]	Oak Hill	97%	61
Raleigh General Hospital	Beckley	97%	92
Saint Josephs Healthcare System[2]	Parkersburg	97%	181
Weirton Medical Center[2]	Weirton	97%	79
Charleston Area Medical Center[2]	Charleston	96%	928
Saint Mary's Medical Center[2]	Huntington	96%	453
Cabell-Huntington Hospital[2]	Huntington	94%	120
Logan Regional Medical Center	Logan	94%	64
Princeton Community Hospital	Princeton	94%	168
Greenbrier Valley Medical Center	Ronceverte	93%	60
Davis Memorial Hospital	Elkins	92%	85
Wheeling Hospital	Wheeling	92%	412
Monongalia County General Hospital[2]	Morgantown	90%	426
Reynolds Memorial Hospital	Glen Dale	90%	29
Stonewall Jackson Memorial Hospital	Weston	89%	28
Bluefield Regional Medical Center	Bluefield	86%	90
Camc Teays Valley Hospital	Hurricane	85%	52
Grant Memorial Hospital	Petersburg	85%	27
Thomas Memorial Hospital[2]	S Charleston	84%	215
Beckley Arh Hospital	Beckley	83%	41
Saint Francis Hospital	Charleston	82%	174
Ohio Valley Medical Center	Wheeling	76%	109
Pleasant Valley Hospital	Point Pleasant	76%	29

25. Controlled Postoperative Blood Glucose

Hospital Name	City	Rate	Cases
Saint Mary's Medical Center[2]	Huntington	98%	312
Saint Josephs Healthcare System[2]	Parkersburg	97%	72
Monongalia County General Hospital[2]	Morgantown	93%	211
Charleston Area Medical Center[2]	Charleston	91%	960
West Virginia University Hospitals[2]	Morgantown	86%	313
Wheeling Hospital	Wheeling	82%	243

26. Prophylactic Antibiotic Timing

Hospital Name	City	Rate	Cases
Stonewall Jackson Memorial Hospital	Weston	100%	95
Charleston Area Medical Center[2]	Charleston	99%	1885
Fairmont General Hospital	Fairmont	99%	139
Huntington VA Medical Center	Huntington	99%	121
Saint Josephs Healthcare System[2]	Parkersburg	99%	349
United Hospital Center[2]	Bridgeport	99%	552
West Virginia University Hospitals[2]	Morgantown	99%	926
Greenbrier Valley Medical Center	Ronceverte	98%	127
Princeton Community Hospital	Princeton	98%	498
Raleigh General Hospital	Beckley	98%	309
Saint Mary's Medical Center[2]	Huntington	98%	965
Bluefield Regional Medical Center	Bluefield	97%	260
Camden Clark Memorial Hospital[2]	Parkersburg	97%	532
Grant Memorial Hospital	Petersburg	97%	114
Logan Regional Medical Center	Logan	97%	165
Monongalia County General Hospital[2]	Morgantown	97%	1020
Plateau Medical Center[2]	Oak Hill	97%	130
Thomas Memorial Hospital[2]	S Charleston	97%	454
Weirton Medical Center[2]	Weirton	97%	245
Cabell-Huntington Hospital[2]	Huntington	96%	295
Reynolds Memorial Hospital	Glen Dale	96%	72
Saint Francis Hospital	Charleston	96%	482
Wheeling Hospital	Wheeling	96%	910
Davis Memorial Hospital	Elkins	95%	230
Ohio Valley Medical Center	Wheeling	95%	239
City Hospital	Martinsburg	94%	214
Summersville Regional Medical Center[2]	Summersville	93%	58
Camc Teays Valley Hospital	Hurricane	91%	85
Saint Joseph Hospital	Buckhannon	91%	44
Pleasant Valley Hospital	Point Pleasant	90%	73
Beckley Arh Hospital	Beckley	88%	42

27. Prophylactic Antibiotic Timing (Outpatient)

Hospital Name	City	Rate	Cases
Fairmont General Hospital	Fairmont	98%	89
Charleston Area Medical Center	Charleston	97%	903
Greenbrier Valley Medical Center	Ronceverte	97%	127
Raleigh General Hospital	Beckley	97%	179
Camc Teays Valley Hospital[3]	Hurricane	96%	48
Williamson Memorial Hospital	Williamson	96%	46
United Hospital Center	Bridgeport	95%	109
Reynolds Memorial Hospital	Glen Dale	94%	31
West Virginia University Hospitals	Morgantown	94%	285
Davis Memorial Hospital	Elkins	93%	170
Stonewall Jackson Memorial Hospital	Weston	92%	53
Saint Mary's Medical Center	Huntington	91%	448
City Hospital	Martinsburg	90%	112
Thomas Memorial Hospital	S Charleston	90%	156
Wheeling Hospital	Wheeling	90%	207
Bluefield Regional Medical Center	Bluefield	88%	133
Logan Regional Medical Center	Logan	87%	61
Monongalia County General Hospital	Morgantown	85%	361
Cabell-Huntington Hospital	Huntington	84%	186
Ohio Valley Medical Center	Wheeling	84%	80
Saint Francis Hospital	Charleston	84%	213
Princeton Community Hospital	Princeton	83%	147
Saint Josephs Healthcare System	Parkersburg	82%	155
Camden Clark Memorial Hospital	Parkersburg	80%	175
Summersville Regional Medical Center	Summersville	80%	56
Weirton Medical Center	Weirton	80%	85
Pleasant Valley Hospital	Point Pleasant	63%	54
Beckley Arh Hospital	Beckley	54%	84

28. Prophylactic Antibiotic Selection

Hospital Name	City	Rate	Cases
Fairmont General Hospital	Fairmont	100%	139
Huntington VA Medical Center	Huntington	100%	122
United Hospital Center[2]	Bridgeport	100%	561
Charleston Area Medical Center[2]	Charleston	99%	1943
Greenbrier Valley Medical Center	Ronceverte	99%	130
West Virginia University Hospitals[2]	Morgantown	99%	945
Monongalia County General Hospital[2]	Morgantown	98%	1030
Plateau Medical Center[2]	Oak Hill	98%	150
Saint Joseph Hospital	Buckhannon	98%	45
Saint Josephs Healthcare System[2]	Parkersburg	98%	351
Saint Mary's Medical Center[2]	Huntington	98%	981
Wheeling Hospital	Wheeling	98%	934
Camden Clark Memorial Hospital[2]	Parkersburg	97%	536
Davis Memorial Hospital	Elkins	97%	230
Grant Memorial Hospital	Petersburg	97%	114
Thomas Memorial Hospital[2]	S Charleston	97%	456
Ohio Valley Medical Center	Wheeling	96%	238
Princeton Community Hospital	Princeton	96%	499
Raleigh General Hospital	Beckley	96%	311
Stonewall Jackson Memorial Hospital	Weston	96%	96
Cabell-Huntington Hospital[2]	Huntington	95%	297
Camc Teays Valley Hospital	Hurricane	95%	88
City Hospital	Martinsburg	95%	220
Logan Regional Medical Center	Logan	95%	166
Weirton Medical Center[2]	Weirton	95%	245
Bluefield Regional Medical Center	Bluefield	93%	259
Reynolds Memorial Hospital	Glen Dale	93%	73
Pleasant Valley Hospital	Point Pleasant	92%	73
Saint Francis Hospital	Charleston	92%	483
Summersville Regional Medical Center[2]	Summersville	82%	57
Beckley Arh Hospital	Beckley	79%	43

29. Prophylactic Antibiotic Selection (Outpatient)

Hospital Name	City	Rate	Cases
Ohio Valley Medical Center	Wheeling	100%	70
Reynolds Memorial Hospital	Glen Dale	100%	29
Williamson Memorial Hospital	Williamson	100%	44
Saint Josephs Healthcare System	Parkersburg	99%	136
Stonewall Jackson Memorial Hospital	Weston	99%	72
Davis Memorial Hospital	Elkins	98%	162
Greenbrier Valley Medical Center	Ronceverte	98%	124

NOTE: Hospital profiles are in alphabetical order by state, then city, then hospital within the city; Rankings exclude hospitals with less than 25 cases except for patient surveys which excludes hospitals with less than 100 cases; (a) 100–299 cases; (1) The number of cases is too small to be sure how well a hospital is performing; (2) The hospital indicated that the data submitted for this measure were based on a sample of cases; (3) Data was collected during a shorter time period (fewer quarters) than the maximum possible time for this measure; (4) Suppressed for one or more quarters by CMS; (5) No data is available from the hospital for this measure; (6) Fewer than 100 patients completed the HCAHPS survey. Use these rates with caution, as the number of surveys may be too low to reliably assess hospital performance; (7) Survey results are based on less than 12 months of data; (8) Survey results are not available for this reporting period; (9) No or very few patients were eligible for the HCAHPS survey. The scores shown, if any, reflect a very small number of surveys; (10) A state average was not calculated because too few hospitals in the state submitted data; (11) There were discrepancies in the data collection process; Please refer to the User's Guide for a full explanation of data.

Monongalia County General Hospital	Morgantown	98%	316
Raleigh General Hospital	Beckley	98%	176
Cabell-Huntington Hospital	Huntington	96%	255
Thomas Memorial Hospital	S Charleston	96%	144
Bluefield Regional Medical Center	Bluefield	94%	121
Fairmont General Hospital	Fairmont	94%	87
United Hospital Center	Bridgeport	94%	107
West Virginia University Hospitals	Morgantown	94%	279
Beckley Arh Hospital	Beckley	91%	53
Charleston Area Medical Center	Charleston	91%	892
Saint Mary's Medical Center	Huntington	89%	422
City Hospital	Martinsburg	88%	104
Wheeling Hospital	Wheeling	88%	217
Logan Regional Medical Center	Logan	84%	57
Camc Teays Valley Hospital[3]	Hurricane	83%	47
Princeton Community Hospital	Princeton	83%	145
Camden Clark Memorial Hospital	Parkersburg	81%	144
Summersville Regional Medical Center	Summersville	78%	45
Saint Francis Hospital	Charleston	77%	197
Pleasant Valley Hospital	Point Pleasant	75%	53
Weirton Medical Center	Weirton	68%	82

30. Prophylactic Antibiotic Stopped

Hospital Name	City	Rate	Cases
Fairmont General Hospital	Fairmont	100%	124
Huntington VA Medical Center	Huntington	100%	116
Plateau Medical Center[2]	Oak Hill	98%	129
West Virginia University Hospitals[2]	Morgantown	98%	900
Camden Clark Memorial Hospital[2]	Parkersburg	97%	492
Monongalia County General Hospital[2]	Morgantown	97%	1003
United Hospital Center[2]	Bridgeport	97%	519
City Hospital	Martinsburg	96%	190
Davis Memorial Hospital	Elkins	96%	222
Princeton Community Hospital	Princeton	96%	471
Saint Mary's Medical Center[2]	Huntington	96%	904
Charleston Area Medical Center[2]	Charleston	95%	1639
Raleigh General Hospital	Beckley	95%	301
Reynolds Memorial Hospital	Glen Dale	95%	65
Cabell-Huntington Hospital[2]	Huntington	93%	283
Grant Memorial Hospital	Petersburg	93%	112
Greenbrier Valley Medical Center	Ronceverte	93%	121
Logan Regional Medical Center	Logan	93%	94
Ohio Valley Medical Center	Wheeling	93%	235
Wheeling Hospital	Wheeling	93%	850
Saint Josephs Healthcare System[2]	Parkersburg	92%	333
Saint Francis Hospital	Charleston	91%	482
Beckley Arh Hospital	Beckley	90%	40
Bluefield Regional Medical Center	Bluefield	90%	257
Camc Teays Valley Hospital	Hurricane	90%	83
Stonewall Jackson Memorial Hospital	Weston	90%	93
Weirton Medical Center[2]	Weirton	89%	236
Thomas Memorial Hospital[2]	S Charleston	87%	433
Pleasant Valley Hospital	Point Pleasant	83%	71
Saint Joseph Hospital	Buckhannon	81%	42
Summersville Regional Medical Center[2]	Summersville	80%	55

31. Recommended VTP Ordered

Hospital Name	City	Rate	Cases
Cabell-Huntington Hospital[2]	Huntington	99%	141
Fairmont General Hospital	Fairmont	99%	117
Huntington VA Medical Center[2]	Huntington	99%	94
West Virginia University Hospitals[2]	Morgantown	99%	287
Greenbrier Valley Medical Center	Ronceverte	98%	93
Raleigh General Hospital	Beckley	98%	160
United Hospital Center[2]	Bridgeport	98%	254
Monongalia County General Hospital[2]	Morgantown	97%	392
Summersville Regional Medical Center[2]	Summersville	97%	64
Wheeling Hospital	Wheeling	97%	244
City Hospital	Martinsburg	96%	252
Charleston Area Medical Center[2]	Charleston	95%	470
Davis Memorial Hospital	Elkins	95%	120
Logan Regional Medical Center	Logan	95%	132
Plateau Medical Center[2]	Oak Hill	94%	48
Princeton Community Hospital	Princeton	94%	181
Saint Mary's Medical Center[2]	Huntington	94%	237
Camden Clark Memorial Hospital[2]	Parkersburg	92%	234
Bluefield Regional Medical Center	Bluefield	89%	83
Camc Teays Valley Hospital	Hurricane	89%	70
Stonewall Jackson Memorial Hospital	Weston	89%	64
Weirton Medical Center[2]	Weirton	89%	118
Grant Memorial Hospital	Petersburg	88%	25
Saint Josephs Healthcare System[2]	Parkersburg	88%	161
Ohio Valley Medical Center	Wheeling	87%	149
Jefferson Memorial Hospital	Ranson	82%	34
Reynolds Memorial Hospital	Glen Dale	82%	44
Saint Francis Hospital	Charleston	80%	147
Thomas Memorial Hospital[2]	S Charleston	78%	237
Pleasant Valley Hospital	Point Pleasant	74%	70
Beckley Arh Hospital	Beckley	72%	85
Saint Joseph Hospital	Buckhannon	62%	26

32. Urinary Catheter Removal

Hospital Name	City	Rate	Cases
Huntington VA Medical Center[2]	Huntington	100%	103
West Virginia University Hospitals[2]	Morgantown	100%	284
United Hospital Center[2]	Bridgeport	99%	186
City Hospital	Martinsburg	98%	138
Plateau Medical Center	Oak Hill	98%	57
Fairmont General Hospital	Fairmont	97%	32
Raleigh General Hospital	Beckley	96%	50
Saint Mary's Medical Center[2]	Huntington	95%	383
Camc Teays Valley Hospital	Hurricane	94%	47
Charleston Area Medical Center[2]	Charleston	93%	418
Saint Josephs Healthcare System[2]	Parkersburg	93%	190
Davis Memorial Hospital	Elkins	90%	50
Saint Francis Hospital	Charleston	90%	205
Cabell-Huntington Hospital[2]	Huntington	89%	36
Camden Clark Memorial Hospital[2]	Parkersburg	89%	83
Thomas Memorial Hospital	S Charleston	85%	78
Princeton Community Hospital	Princeton	83%	35
Monongalia County General Hospital[2]	Morgantown	80%	103
Greenbrier Valley Medical Center	Ronceverte	79%	38
Logan Regional Medical Center	Logan	79%	28
Wheeling Hospital	Wheeling	73%	141
Weirton Medical Center	Weirton	70%	88
Ohio Valley Medical Center	Wheeling	53%	78

Children's Asthma Care

33. Received Systemic Corticosteroids

Hospital Name	City	Rate	Cases
Raleigh General Hospital	Beckley	100%	30
Williamson Memorial Hospital	Williamson	97%	34

34. Received Home Management Plan of Care

Hospital Name	City	Rate	Cases
Williamson Memorial Hospital	Williamson	100%	33
Raleigh General Hospital	Beckley	90%	30

35. Received Reliever Medication

Hospital Name	City	Rate	Cases
Raleigh General Hospital	Beckley	100%	31
Williamson Memorial Hospital	Williamson	100%	34

Use of Medical Imaging

36. Combination Abdominal CT Scan

Hospital Name	City	Ratio	Cases
Logan Regional Medical Center	Logan	0.005	571
Saint Josephs Healthcare System	Parkersburg	0.011	738
Saint Francis Hospital	Charleston	0.017	241
Thomas Memorial Hospital	S Charleston	0.030	876
City Hospital	Martinsburg	0.035	1129
Pleasant Valley Hospital	Point Pleasant	0.041	362
Cabell-Huntington Hospital	Huntington	0.046	988
Summersville Regional Medical Center	Summersville	0.046	502
Camc Teays Valley Hospital	Hurricane	0.055	417
Charleston Area Medical Center	Charleston	0.058	1752
Saint Mary's Medical Center	Huntington	0.083	1399
Williamson Memorial Hospital	Williamson	0.088	249
Plateau Medical Center	Oak Hill	0.132	182
Greenbrier Valley Medical Center	Ronceverte	0.145	757
Preston Memorial Hospital	Kingwood	0.146	89
Weirton Medical Center	Weirton	0.149	524
Jackson General Hospital	Ripley	0.150	314
Wheeling Hospital	Wheeling	0.165	752
West Virginia University Hospitals	Morgantown	0.189	824
Welch Community Hospital	Welch	0.258	62
Davis Memorial Hospital	Elkins	0.373	702
Reynolds Memorial Hospital	Glen Dale	0.423	163
Broaddus Hospital Association	Philippi	0.482	114
Wetzel County Hospital	New Martinsville	0.495	204
Saint Joseph Hospital	Buckhannon	0.498	217
Bluefield Regional Medical Center	Bluefield	0.500	688
Roane General Hospital	Spencer	0.523	132
Camden Clark Memorial Hospital	Parkersburg	0.595	1643
Beckley Arh Hospital	Beckley	0.615	356
Monongalia County General Hospital	Morgantown	0.638	939
Ohio Valley Medical Center	Wheeling	0.640	344
Stonewall Jackson Memorial Hospital	Weston	0.648	213
Fairmont General Hospital	Fairmont	0.673	710
Princeton Community Hospital	Princeton	0.720	1159
United Hospital Center	Bridgeport	0.750	1314
Raleigh General Hospital	Beckley	0.838	588

37. Combination Chest CT Scan

Hospital Name	City	Ratio	Cases
Jackson General Hospital	Ripley	0.000	189
Logan Regional Medical Center	Logan	0.000	547
Ohio Valley Medical Center	Wheeling	0.000	374
Reynolds Memorial Hospital	Glen Dale	0.000	129
Roane General Hospital	Spencer	0.000	83
Saint Francis Hospital	Charleston	0.000	111
Saint Joseph Hospital	Buckhannon	0.000	128
Saint Josephs Healthcare System	Parkersburg	0.000	572
Stonewall Jackson Memorial Hospital	Weston	0.000	103
Thomas Memorial Hospital	S Charleston	0.000	580
Wetzel County Hospital	New Martinsville	0.000	170
Saint Mary's Medical Center	Huntington	0.001	720
United Hospital Center	Bridgeport	0.001	886
Fairmont General Hospital	Fairmont	0.002	407
Greenbrier Valley Medical Center	Ronceverte	0.002	561
Camc Teays Valley Hospital	Hurricane	0.004	278
Monongalia County General Hospital	Morgantown	0.004	737
Charleston Area Medical Center	Charleston	0.006	1689
City Hospital	Martinsburg	0.011	463
Wheeling Hospital	Wheeling	0.013	894
Princeton Community Hospital	Princeton	0.019	745
Cabell-Huntington Hospital	Huntington	0.024	581
Camden Clark Memorial Hospital	Parkersburg	0.031	1071
Pleasant Valley Hospital	Point Pleasant	0.033	209
Weirton Medical Center	Weirton	0.037	352
Summersville Regional Medical Center	Summersville	0.050	261
Davis Memorial Hospital	Elkins	0.063	302
Preston Memorial Hospital	Kingwood	0.071	70
Williamson Memorial Hospital	Williamson	0.090	78
West Virginia University Hospitals	Morgantown	0.120	947
Plateau Medical Center	Oak Hill	0.219	105
Beckley Arh Hospital	Beckley	0.308	224
Bluefield Regional Medical Center	Bluefield	0.321	380
Broaddus Hospital Association	Philippi	0.642	67
Raleigh General Hospital	Beckley	0.716	535

38. Follow-up Mammogram/Ultrasound

Hospital Name	City	Rate	Cases
City Hospital	Martinsburg	2.0%	1091
Fairmont General Hospital	Fairmont	4.2%	648
Saint Josephs Healthcare System	Parkersburg	4.7%	1021
Welch Community Hospital	Welch	4.7%	106
Broaddus Hospital Association	Philippi	4.9%	162
Princeton Community Hospital	Princeton	5.1%	1076
Davis Memorial Hospital	Elkins	5.8%	824
Jackson General Hospital	Ripley	6.1%	410
Saint Francis Hospital	Charleston	6.4%	1003
United Hospital Center	Bridgeport	6.4%	1853
Beckley Arh Hospital	Beckley	6.6%	332
Camden Clark Memorial Hospital	Parkersburg	7.0%	2174
Williamson Memorial Hospital	Williamson	7.1%	98
Thomas Memorial Hospital	S Charleston	7.4%	1121
West Virginia University Hospitals	Morgantown	7.7%	1132
Saint Joseph Hospital	Buckhannon	8.3%	412
Wetzel County Hospital	New Martinsville	8.7%	343
Weirton Medical Center	Weirton	9.4%	552
Pleasant Valley Hospital	Point Pleasant	9.6%	334
Saint Mary's Medical Center	Huntington	9.7%	967
Summersville Regional Medical Center	Summersville	9.7%	236
Bluefield Regional Medical Center	Bluefield	9.8%	712
Charleston Area Medical Center	Charleston	9.8%	2401
Preston Memorial Hospital	Kingwood	9.8%	215
Monongalia County General Hospital	Morgantown	10.1%	835
Stonewall Jackson Memorial Hospital	Weston	10.1%	288
Camc Teays Valley Hospital	Hurricane	10.6%	339
Raleigh General Hospital	Beckley	10.9%	128
Reynolds Memorial Hospital	Glen Dale	11.0%	255
Plateau Medical Center	Oak Hill	11.3%	106
Cabell-Huntington Hospital	Huntington	11.4%	1749
Greenbrier Valley Medical Center	Ronceverte	12.7%	488
Ohio Valley Medical Center	Wheeling	13.3%	474
Wheeling Hospital	Wheeling	13.4%	1056
Logan Regional Medical Center	Logan	19.3%	420
Roane General Hospital	Spencer	23.0%	235

39. MRI for Low Back Pain

Hospital Name	City	Rate	Cases
Reynolds Memorial Hospital[1]	Glen Dale	28.9%	38
Saint Josephs Healthcare System	Parkersburg	29.9%	204
Ohio Valley Medical Center	Wheeling	31.1%	90
Weirton Medical Center	Weirton	31.7%	142
City Hospital	Martinsburg	31.9%	163
Davis Memorial Hospital	Elkins	33.3%	102
Camden Clark Memorial Hospital	Parkersburg	34.4%	355
Wheeling Hospital	Wheeling	34.4%	131
Greenbrier Valley Medical Center	Ronceverte	35.1%	202
Thomas Memorial Hospital	S Charleston	35.7%	406
Cabell-Huntington Hospital	Huntington	35.8%	134
Pleasant Valley Hospital	Point Pleasant	36.3%	113
Summersville Regional Medical Center	Summersville	37.2%	113
Beckley Arh Hospital	Beckley	37.3%	110

NOTE: Hospital profiles are in alphabetical order by state, then city, then hospital within the city; Rankings exclude hospitals with less than 25 cases except for patient surveys which excludes hospitals with less than 100 cases; (a) 100–299 cases; (1) The number of cases is too small to be sure how well a hospital is performing; (2) The hospital indicated that the data submitted for this measure were based on a sample of cases; (3) Data was collected during a shorter time period (fewer quarters) than the maximum possible time for this measure; (4) Suppressed for one or more quarters by CMS; (5) No data is available from the hospital for this measure; (6) Fewer than 100 patients completed the HCAHPS survey. Use these rates with caution, as the number of surveys may be too low to reliably assess hospital performance; (7) Survey results are based on less than 12 months of data; (8) Survey results are not available for this reporting period; (9) No or very few patients were eligible for the HCAHPS survey. The scores shown, if any, reflect a very small number of surveys; (10) A state average was not calculated because too few hospitals in the state submitted data; (11) There were discrepancies in the data collection process; Please refer to the User's Guide for a full explanation of data.

Saint Mary's Medical Center	Huntington	37.3%	75
Wetzel County Hospital	New Martinsville	37.3%	59
Monongalia County General Hospital	Morgantown	37.5%	104
Saint Francis Hospital	Charleston	38.6%	145
United Hospital Center	Bridgeport	39.3%	323
Camc Teays Valley Hospital	Hurricane	40.0%	95
Jackson General Hospital	Ripley	41.0%	105
Fairmont General Hospital	Fairmont	41.3%	143
Charleston Area Medical Center	Charleston	42.3%	333
Raleigh General Hospital	Beckley	44.2%	396
Bluefield Regional Medical Center	Bluefield	44.3%	88
Logan Regional Medical Center	Logan	45.5%	99
Princeton Community Hospital	Princeton	48.2%	251
Plateau Medical Center	Oak Hill	52.9%	34

Bluefield Regional Medical Center	Bluefield	79%	300+
Charleston Area Medical Center	Charleston	79%	300+
City Hospital	Martinsburg	79%	300+
Grant Memorial Hospital	Petersburg	79%	300+
Saint Mary's Medical Center	Huntington	79%	300+
Thomas Memorial Hospital	S Charleston	79%	300+
United Hospital Center	Bridgeport	79%	300+
Camc Teays Valley Hospital	Hurricane	78%	300+
Wheeling Hospital	Wheeling	78%	300+
Raleigh General Hospital	Beckley	77%	300+
Beckley Arh Hospital	Beckley	76%	300+
Camden Clark Memorial Hospital	Parkersburg	76%	300+
Ohio Valley Medical Center	Wheeling	76%	300+
Morgan County War Memorial	Berkeley Springs	74%	(a)
West Virginia University Hospitals	Morgantown	74%	300+
Weirton Medical Center	Weirton	73%	300+

Princeton Community Hospital	Princeton	62%	300+
Williamson Memorial Hospital	Williamson	62%	300+
Morgan County War Memorial	Berkeley Springs	61%	(a)
Camden Clark Memorial Hospital	Parkersburg	60%	300+
Greenbrier Valley Medical Center	Ronceverte	60%	300+
Summersville Regional Medical Center	Summersville	60%	300+
Thomas Memorial Hospital	S Charleston	60%	300+
Beckley Arh Hospital	Beckley	59%	300+
Camc Teays Valley Hospital	Hurricane	59%	300+
Grant Memorial Hospital	Petersburg	59%	300+
Jefferson Memorial Hospital	Ranson	59%	(a)
Bluefield Regional Medical Center	Bluefield	56%	300+
Logan Regional Medical Center	Logan	55%	300+
City Hospital	Martinsburg	53%	300+
United Hospital Center	Bridgeport	51%	300+
Weirton Medical Center	Weirton	44%	300+

Survey of Patients' Hospital Experiences

40. Area Around Room 'Always' Quiet at Night

Hospital Name	City	Rate	Cases
Welch Community Hospital	Welch	72%	(a)
Cabell-Huntington Hospital	Huntington	68%	300+
Saint Francis Hospital	Charleston	64%	300+
Summers County ARH Hospital	Hinton	63%	(a)
Boone Memorial Hospital	Madison	62%	(a)
Monongalia County General Hospital	Morgantown	61%	300+
Montgomery General Hospital	Montgomery	61%	(a)
Plateau Medical Center	Oak Hill	57%	300+
Pleasant Valley Hospital	Point Pleasant	57%	300+
Braxton County Memorial Hospital	Gassaway	56%	(a)
Fairmont General Hospital	Fairmont	56%	300+
Ohio Valley Medical Center	Wheeling	56%	300+
Roane General Hospital	Spencer	56%	(a)
Saint Joseph Hospital	Buckhannon	56%	(a)
Jefferson Memorial Hospital	Ranson	55%	(a)
Bluefield Regional Medical Center	Bluefield	54%	300+
Morgan County War Memorial	Berkeley Springs	54%	(a)
Saint Mary's Medical Center	Huntington	54%	300+
Wetzel County Hospital	New Martinsville	53%	300+
Williamson Memorial Hospital	Williamson	53%	300+
Beckley Arh Hospital	Beckley	52%	300+
Davis Memorial Hospital	Elkins	52%	300+
Logan Regional Medical Center	Logan	52%	300+
Princeton Community Hospital	Princeton	52%	300+
Stonewall Jackson Memorial Hospital	Weston	52%	300+
Greenbrier Valley Medical Center	Ronceverte	51%	300+
Raleigh General Hospital	Beckley	51%	300+
Reynolds Memorial Hospital	Glen Dale	51%	300+
Jackson General Hospital	Ripley	50%	300+
Wheeling Hospital	Wheeling	49%	300+
Grant Memorial Hospital	Petersburg	47%	300+
Preston Memorial Hospital	Kingwood	47%	(a)
West Virginia University Hospitals	Morgantown	47%	300+
Charleston Area Medical Center	Charleston	45%	300+
Saint Josephs Healthcare System	Parkersburg	44%	300+
Summersville Regional Medical Center	Summersville	44%	300+
Thomas Memorial Hospital	S Charleston	43%	300+
United Hospital Center	Bridgeport	43%	300+
City Hospital	Martinsburg	41%	300+
Camden Clark Memorial Hospital	Parkersburg	40%	300+
Weirton Medical Center	Weirton	36%	300+
Camc Teays Valley Hospital	Hurricane	35%	300+

41. Doctors 'Always' Communicated Well

Hospital Name	City	Rate	Cases
Summers County ARH Hospital	Hinton	92%	(a)
Braxton County Memorial Hospital	Gassaway	89%	(a)
Boone Memorial Hospital	Madison	88%	(a)
Jackson General Hospital	Ripley	86%	300+
Jefferson Memorial Hospital	Ranson	85%	(a)
Monongalia County General Hospital	Morgantown	85%	300+
Preston Memorial Hospital	Kingwood	85%	(a)
Saint Joseph Hospital	Buckhannon	85%	(a)
Welch Community Hospital	Welch	85%	(a)
Plateau Medical Center	Oak Hill	84%	300+
Roane General Hospital	Spencer	84%	(a)
Summersville Regional Medical Center	Summersville	84%	300+
Fairmont General Hospital	Fairmont	83%	300+
Stonewall Jackson Memorial Hospital	Weston	83%	300+
Williamson Memorial Hospital	Williamson	83%	300+
Logan Regional Medical Center	Logan	82%	300+
Princeton Community Hospital	Princeton	82%	300+
Wetzel County Hospital	New Martinsville	82%	300+
Greenbrier Valley Medical Center	Ronceverte	81%	300+
Pleasant Valley Hospital	Point Pleasant	81%	300+
Saint Francis Hospital	Charleston	81%	300+
Saint Josephs Healthcare System	Parkersburg	81%	300+
Cabell-Huntington Hospital	Huntington	80%	300+
Davis Memorial Hospital	Elkins	80%	300+
Montgomery General Hospital	Montgomery	80%	(a)
Reynolds Memorial Hospital	Glen Dale	80%	300+

42. Home Recovery Information Given

Hospital Name	City	Rate	Cases
Grant Memorial Hospital	Petersburg	88%	300+
Boone Memorial Hospital	Madison	87%	(a)
Jackson General Hospital	Ripley	87%	300+
Pleasant Valley Hospital	Point Pleasant	87%	300+
Reynolds Memorial Hospital	Glen Dale	87%	300+
Davis Memorial Hospital	Elkins	86%	300+
Wheeling Hospital	Wheeling	86%	300+
Princeton Community Hospital	Princeton	85%	300+
Roane General Hospital	Spencer	85%	(a)
Saint Joseph Hospital	Buckhannon	85%	(a)
Fairmont General Hospital	Fairmont	84%	300+
Saint Josephs Healthcare System	Parkersburg	84%	300+
Braxton County Memorial Hospital	Gassaway	83%	(a)
Cabell-Huntington Hospital	Huntington	83%	300+
Jefferson Memorial Hospital	Ranson	83%	(a)
Morgan County War Memorial	Berkeley Springs	83%	(a)
Saint Mary's Medical Center	Huntington	82%	300+
Thomas Memorial Hospital	S Charleston	82%	300+
Welch Community Hospital	Welch	82%	(a)
Bluefield Regional Medical Center	Bluefield	81%	300+
Saint Francis Hospital	Charleston	81%	300+
Summers County ARH Hospital	Hinton	81%	(a)
West Virginia University Hospitals	Morgantown	81%	300+
Greenbrier Valley Medical Center	Ronceverte	80%	300+
Raleigh General Hospital	Beckley	80%	300+
United Hospital Center	Bridgeport	80%	300+
Camden Clark Memorial Hospital	Parkersburg	79%	300+
Plateau Medical Center	Oak Hill	79%	300+
Preston Memorial Hospital	Kingwood	79%	(a)
Camc Teays Valley Hospital	Hurricane	78%	300+
Charleston Area Medical Center	Charleston	78%	300+
City Hospital	Martinsburg	78%	300+
Logan Regional Medical Center	Logan	78%	300+
Monongalia County General Hospital	Morgantown	78%	300+
Williamson Memorial Hospital	Williamson	77%	300+
Beckley Arh Hospital	Beckley	76%	300+
Ohio Valley Medical Center	Wheeling	76%	300+
Weirton Medical Center	Weirton	76%	300+
Summersville Regional Medical Center	Summersville	75%	300+
Stonewall Jackson Memorial Hospital	Weston	74%	300+
Wetzel County Hospital	New Martinsville	74%	300+
Montgomery General Hospital	Montgomery	72%	(a)

43. Hospital Given 9 or 10 on 10 Point Scale

Hospital Name	City	Rate	Cases
Summers County ARH Hospital	Hinton	81%	(a)
Roane General Hospital	Spencer	77%	(a)
Braxton County Memorial Hospital	Gassaway	76%	(a)
Monongalia County General Hospital	Morgantown	76%	300+
Cabell-Huntington Hospital	Huntington	75%	300+
Saint Francis Hospital	Charleston	75%	300+
Saint Joseph Hospital	Buckhannon	75%	(a)
Saint Mary's Medical Center	Huntington	74%	300+
Welch Community Hospital	Welch	74%	(a)
Montgomery General Hospital	Montgomery	72%	(a)
Boone Memorial Hospital	Madison	70%	(a)
Plateau Medical Center	Oak Hill	70%	300+
Jackson General Hospital	Ripley	67%	300+
Stonewall Jackson Memorial Hospital	Weston	67%	300+
Wheeling Hospital	Wheeling	67%	300+
Charleston Area Medical Center	Charleston	66%	300+
Pleasant Valley Hospital	Point Pleasant	66%	300+
Reynolds Memorial Hospital	Glen Dale	66%	300+
Wetzel County Hospital	New Martinsville	65%	300+
Raleigh General Hospital	Beckley	64%	300+
Saint Josephs Healthcare System	Parkersburg	64%	300+
West Virginia University Hospitals	Morgantown	64%	300+
Davis Memorial Hospital	Elkins	63%	300+
Fairmont General Hospital	Fairmont	63%	300+
Ohio Valley Medical Center	Wheeling	63%	300+
Preston Memorial Hospital	Kingwood	62%	(a)

44. Meds 'Always' Explained Before Given

Hospital Name	City	Rate	Cases
Boone Memorial Hospital	Madison	74%	(a)
Summers County ARH Hospital	Hinton	71%	(a)
Welch Community Hospital	Welch	69%	(a)
Grant Memorial Hospital	Petersburg	66%	300+
Fairmont General Hospital	Fairmont	65%	300+
Preston Memorial Hospital	Kingwood	65%	(a)
Saint Joseph Hospital	Buckhannon	65%	(a)
Braxton County Memorial Hospital	Gassaway	64%	(a)
Princeton Community Hospital	Princeton	64%	300+
Reynolds Memorial Hospital	Glen Dale	64%	300+
Wetzel County Hospital	New Martinsville	64%	300+
Stonewall Jackson Memorial Hospital	Weston	63%	300+
Cabell-Huntington Hospital	Huntington	62%	300+
Jefferson Memorial Hospital	Ranson	62%	(a)
Monongalia County General Hospital	Morgantown	62%	300+
Summersville Regional Medical Center	Summersville	62%	300+
Davis Memorial Hospital	Elkins	61%	300+
Jackson General Hospital	Ripley	61%	300+
West Virginia University Hospitals	Morgantown	61%	300+
Bluefield Regional Medical Center	Bluefield	60%	300+
Pleasant Valley Hospital	Point Pleasant	60%	300+
Roane General Hospital	Spencer	60%	(a)
Saint Mary's Medical Center	Huntington	60%	300+
Camc Teays Valley Hospital	Hurricane	59%	300+
City Hospital	Martinsburg	59%	300+
Montgomery General Hospital	Montgomery	59%	(a)
Williamson Memorial Hospital	Williamson	59%	300+
Plateau Medical Center	Oak Hill	58%	300+
Saint Francis Hospital	Charleston	58%	300+
Wheeling Hospital	Wheeling	58%	300+
Charleston Area Medical Center	Charleston	57%	300+
Morgan County War Memorial	Berkeley Springs	57%	(a)
Ohio Valley Medical Center	Wheeling	57%	300+
Raleigh General Hospital	Beckley	57%	300+
Greenbrier Valley Medical Center	Ronceverte	55%	300+
Beckley Arh Hospital	Beckley	54%	300+
Saint Josephs Healthcare System	Parkersburg	54%	300+
United Hospital Center	Bridgeport	54%	300+
Thomas Memorial Hospital	S Charleston	52%	300+
Camden Clark Memorial Hospital	Parkersburg	51%	300+
Logan Regional Medical Center	Logan	51%	300+
Weirton Medical Center	Weirton	51%	300+

45. Nurses 'Always' Communicated Well

Hospital Name	City	Rate	Cases
Summers County ARH Hospital	Hinton	86%	(a)
Welch Community Hospital	Welch	86%	(a)
Braxton County Memorial Hospital	Gassaway	85%	(a)
Boone Memorial Hospital	Madison	84%	(a)
Saint Joseph Hospital	Buckhannon	81%	(a)
Wetzel County Hospital	New Martinsville	81%	300+
Grant Memorial Hospital	Petersburg	80%	300+
Monongalia County General Hospital	Morgantown	80%	300+
Montgomery General Hospital	Montgomery	80%	(a)
Saint Mary's Medical Center	Huntington	80%	300+
Plateau Medical Center	Oak Hill	79%	300+
Preston Memorial Hospital	Kingwood	79%	(a)
Princeton Community Hospital	Princeton	79%	300+
Roane General Hospital	Spencer	79%	(a)
Saint Francis Hospital	Charleston	79%	300+
Stonewall Jackson Memorial Hospital	Weston	79%	300+
Davis Memorial Hospital	Elkins	78%	300+
Fairmont General Hospital	Fairmont	78%	300+
Williamson Memorial Hospital	Williamson	78%	300+
Cabell-Huntington Hospital	Huntington	77%	300+
Jackson General Hospital	Ripley	77%	300+
Reynolds Memorial Hospital	Glen Dale	76%	300+
West Virginia University Hospitals	Morgantown	76%	300+
Bluefield Regional Medical Center	Bluefield	75%	300+
Pleasant Valley Hospital	Point Pleasant	75%	300+
Jefferson Memorial Hospital	Ranson	74%	(a)

NOTE: Hospital profiles are in alphabetical order by state, then city, then hospital within the city; Rankings exclude hospitals with less than 25 cases except for patient surveys which excludes hospitals with less than 100 cases; (a) 100–299 cases; (1) The number of cases is too small to be sure how well a hospital is performing; (2) The hospital indicated that the data submitted for this measure were based on a sample of cases; (3) Data was collected during a shorter time period (fewer quarters) than the maximum possible time for this measure; (4) Suppressed for one or more quarters by CMS; (5) No data is available from the hospital for this measure; (6) Fewer than 100 patients completed the HCAHPS survey. Use these rates with caution, as the number of surveys may be too low to reliably assess hospital performance; (7) Survey results are based on less than 12 months of data; (8) Survey results are not available for this reporting period; (9) No or very few patients were eligible for the HCAHPS survey. The scores shown, if any, reflect a very small number of surveys; (10) A state average was not calculated because too few hospitals in the state submitted data; (11) There were discrepancies in the data collection process; Please refer to the User's Guide for a full explanation of data.

Summersville Regional Medical Center	Summersville	74%	300+
Wheeling Hospital	Wheeling	74%	300+
City Hospital	Martinsburg	73%	300+
Greenbrier Valley Medical Center	Ronceverte	73%	300+
Ohio Valley Medical Center	Wheeling	73%	300+
Raleigh General Hospital	Beckley	73%	300+
Charleston Area Medical Center	Charleston	72%	300+
Saint Josephs Healthcare System	Parkersburg	72%	300+
Beckley Arh Hospital	Beckley	71%	300+
Thomas Memorial Hospital	S Charleston	71%	300+
United Hospital Center	Bridgeport	70%	300+
Camden Clark Memorial Hospital	Parkersburg	69%	300+
Logan Regional Medical Center	Logan	69%	300+
Morgan County War Memorial	Berkeley Springs	69%	(a)
Camc Teays Valley Hospital	Hurricane	68%	300+
Weirton Medical Center	Weirton	62%	300+

46. Pain 'Always' Well Controlled

Hospital Name	City	Rate	Cases
Boone Memorial Hospital	Madison	83%	(a)
Summers County ARH Hospital	Hinton	81%	(a)
Saint Francis Hospital	Charleston	75%	300+
Welch Community Hospital	Welch	75%	(a)
Fairmont General Hospital	Fairmont	74%	300+
Saint Joseph Hospital	Buckhannon	74%	(a)
Braxton County Memorial Hospital	Gassaway	73%	(a)
Wetzel County Hospital	New Martinsville	73%	300+
Cabell-Huntington Hospital	Huntington	72%	300+
Jackson General Hospital	Ripley	72%	300+
Preston Memorial Hospital	Kingwood	71%	(a)
Roane General Hospital	Spencer	71%	(a)
Davis Memorial Hospital	Elkins	70%	300+
Princeton Community Hospital	Princeton	70%	300+
Raleigh General Hospital	Beckley	70%	300+
Saint Mary's Medical Center	Huntington	70%	300+
Stonewall Jackson Memorial Hospital	Weston	70%	300+
City Hospital	Martinsburg	69%	300+
Jefferson Memorial Hospital	Ranson	69%	(a)
Summersville Regional Medical Center	Summersville	69%	300+
Wheeling Hospital	Wheeling	69%	300+
Grant Memorial Hospital	Petersburg	68%	300+
Greenbrier Valley Medical Center	Ronceverte	68%	300+
Monongalia County General Hospital	Morgantown	68%	300+
Plateau Medical Center	Oak Hill	68%	300+
Pleasant Valley Hospital	Point Pleasant	68%	300+
Charleston Area Medical Center	Charleston	67%	300+
Ohio Valley Medical Center	Wheeling	67%	300+
Beckley Arh Hospital	Beckley	66%	300+
Bluefield Regional Medical Center	Bluefield	66%	300+
Montgomery General Hospital	Montgomery	66%	(a)
Reynolds Memorial Hospital	Glen Dale	66%	300+
Saint Josephs Healthcare System	Parkersburg	65%	300+
Thomas Memorial Hospital	S Charleston	65%	300+
West Virginia University Hospitals	Morgantown	65%	300+
Camc Teays Valley Hospital	Hurricane	64%	300+
Logan Regional Medical Center	Logan	63%	300+
Williamson Memorial Hospital	Williamson	63%	300+
Camden Clark Memorial Hospital	Parkersburg	61%	300+
Morgan County War Memorial	Berkeley Springs	61%	(a)
United Hospital Center	Bridgeport	61%	300+
Weirton Medical Center	Weirton	61%	300+

47. Room and Bathroom 'Always' Clean

Hospital Name	City	Rate	Cases
Grant Memorial Hospital	Petersburg	83%	300+
Jefferson Memorial Hospital	Ranson	83%	(a)
Summers County ARH Hospital	Hinton	83%	(a)
Boone Memorial Hospital	Madison	82%	(a)
Preston Memorial Hospital	Kingwood	82%	(a)
Welch Community Hospital	Welch	82%	(a)
Wetzel County Hospital	New Martinsville	81%	300+
Saint Mary's Medical Center	Huntington	80%	300+
Morgan County War Memorial	Berkeley Springs	79%	(a)
Jackson General Hospital	Ripley	78%	300+
Monongalia County General Hospital	Morgantown	78%	300+
Pleasant Valley Hospital	Point Pleasant	78%	300+
Roane General Hospital	Spencer	78%	(a)
Braxton County Memorial Hospital	Gassaway	77%	(a)
Stonewall Jackson Memorial Hospital	Weston	77%	300+
Davis Memorial Hospital	Elkins	76%	300+
Montgomery General Hospital	Montgomery	76%	(a)
Cabell-Huntington Hospital	Huntington	74%	300+
Fairmont General Hospital	Fairmont	74%	300+
Ohio Valley Medical Center	Wheeling	73%	300+
Williamson Memorial Hospital	Williamson	73%	300+
City Hospital	Martinsburg	71%	300+
Plateau Medical Center	Oak Hill	70%	300+
Reynolds Memorial Hospital	Glen Dale	70%	300+
Saint Joseph Hospital	Buckhannon	70%	(a)
Wheeling Hospital	Wheeling	70%	300+

Bluefield Regional Medical Center	Bluefield	69%	300+
Saint Francis Hospital	Charleston	69%	300+
Summersville Regional Medical Center	Summersville	69%	300+
Camc Teays Valley Hospital	Hurricane	65%	300+
Princeton Community Hospital	Princeton	65%	300+
Camden Clark Memorial Hospital	Parkersburg	64%	300+
Charleston Area Medical Center	Charleston	64%	300+
Raleigh General Hospital	Beckley	64%	300+
West Virginia University Hospitals	Morgantown	64%	300+
Greenbrier Valley Medical Center	Ronceverte	62%	300+
Saint Josephs Healthcare System	Parkersburg	62%	300+
United Hospital Center	Bridgeport	62%	300+
Logan Regional Medical Center	Logan	61%	300+
Thomas Memorial Hospital	S Charleston	60%	300+
Beckley Arh Hospital	Beckley	59%	300+
Weirton Medical Center	Weirton	51%	300+

48. Timely Help 'Always' Received

Hospital Name	City	Rate	Cases
Welch Community Hospital	Welch	78%	(a)
Boone Memorial Hospital	Madison	77%	(a)
Saint Joseph Hospital	Buckhannon	76%	(a)
Summers County ARH Hospital	Hinton	76%	(a)
Braxton County Memorial Hospital	Gassaway	74%	(a)
Roane General Hospital	Spencer	74%	(a)
Wetzel County Hospital	New Martinsville	72%	300+
Grant Memorial Hospital	Petersburg	71%	300+
Plateau Medical Center	Oak Hill	71%	300+
Reynolds Memorial Hospital	Glen Dale	71%	300+
Saint Francis Hospital	Charleston	69%	300+
Jackson General Hospital	Ripley	68%	300+
Cabell-Huntington Hospital	Huntington	67%	300+
Monongalia County General Hospital	Morgantown	67%	300+
Montgomery General Hospital	Montgomery	67%	(a)
Stonewall Jackson Memorial Hospital	Weston	67%	300+
City Hospital	Martinsburg	65%	300+
Davis Memorial Hospital	Elkins	65%	300+
Fairmont General Hospital	Fairmont	65%	300+
Pleasant Valley Hospital	Point Pleasant	65%	300+
Preston Memorial Hospital	Kingwood	65%	(a)
Morgan County War Memorial	Berkeley Springs	64%	(a)
Jefferson Memorial Hospital	Ranson	63%	(a)
Saint Mary's Medical Center	Huntington	63%	300+
Williamson Memorial Hospital	Williamson	62%	300+
Summersville Regional Medical Center	Summersville	61%	300+
Bluefield Regional Medical Center	Bluefield	60%	300+
Wheeling Hospital	Wheeling	60%	300+
Charleston Area Medical Center	Charleston	59%	300+
Princeton Community Hospital	Princeton	59%	300+
Thomas Memorial Hospital	S Charleston	58%	300+
West Virginia University Hospitals	Morgantown	58%	300+
Greenbrier Valley Medical Center	Ronceverte	57%	300+
Saint Josephs Healthcare System	Parkersburg	56%	300+
Camden Clark Memorial Hospital	Parkersburg	55%	300+
Logan Regional Medical Center	Logan	55%	300+
Ohio Valley Medical Center	Wheeling	55%	300+
United Hospital Center	Bridgeport	54%	300+
Beckley Arh Hospital	Beckley	53%	300+
Raleigh General Hospital	Beckley	53%	300+
Camc Teays Valley Hospital	Hurricane	50%	300+
Weirton Medical Center	Weirton	40%	300+

49. Would Definitely Recommend Hospital

Hospital Name	City	Rate	Cases
Monongalia County General Hospital	Morgantown	83%	300+
Summers County ARH Hospital	Hinton	81%	(a)
Saint Mary's Medical Center	Huntington	80%	300+
Saint Francis Hospital	Charleston	77%	300+
Cabell-Huntington Hospital	Huntington	76%	300+
Charleston Area Medical Center	Charleston	73%	300+
Saint Joseph Hospital	Buckhannon	73%	(a)
Braxton County Memorial Hospital	Gassaway	72%	(a)
Ohio Valley Medical Center	Wheeling	70%	300+
Wheeling Hospital	Wheeling	70%	300+
Plateau Medical Center	Oak Hill	69%	300+
Pleasant Valley Hospital	Point Pleasant	69%	300+
West Virginia University Hospitals	Morgantown	69%	300+
Stonewall Jackson Memorial Hospital	Weston	68%	300+
Jackson General Hospital	Ripley	67%	300+
Princeton Community Hospital	Princeton	67%	300+
Reynolds Memorial Hospital	Glen Dale	67%	300+
Camden Clark Memorial Hospital	Parkersburg	66%	300+
Saint Josephs Healthcare System	Parkersburg	66%	300+
Welch Community Hospital	Welch	66%	(a)
Wetzel County Hospital	New Martinsville	66%	300+
Beckley Arh Hospital	Beckley	65%	300+
Roane General Hospital	Spencer	65%	(a)
Williamson Memorial Hospital	Williamson	65%	300+
Summersville Regional Medical Center	Summersville	64%	300+
Preston Memorial Hospital	Kingwood	63%	(a)

Thomas Memorial Hospital	S Charleston	63%	300+
Davis Memorial Hospital	Elkins	62%	300+
Fairmont General Hospital	Fairmont	62%	300+
Morgan County War Memorial	Berkeley Springs	62%	(a)
Raleigh General Hospital	Beckley	62%	300+
Boone Memorial Hospital	Madison	61%	(a)
Montgomery General Hospital	Montgomery	61%	(a)
Camc Teays Valley Hospital	Hurricane	59%	300+
Grant Memorial Hospital	Petersburg	59%	300+
Greenbrier Valley Medical Center	Ronceverte	59%	300+
Jefferson Memorial Hospital	Ranson	59%	(a)
Bluefield Regional Medical Center	Bluefield	57%	300+
City Hospital	Martinsburg	55%	300+
United Hospital Center	Bridgeport	54%	300+
Logan Regional Medical Center	Logan	53%	300+
Weirton Medical Center	Weirton	41%	300+

NOTE: Hospital profiles are in alphabetical order by state, then city, then hospital within the city; Rankings exclude hospitals with less than 25 cases except for patient surveys which excludes hospitals with less than 100 cases; (a) 100–299 cases; (1) The number of cases is too small to be sure how well a hospital is performing; (2) The hospital indicated that the data submitted for this measure were based on a sample of cases; (3) Data was collected during a shorter time period (fewer quarters) than the maximum possible time for this measure; (4) Suppressed for one or more quarters by CMS; (5) No data is available from the hospital for this measure; (6) Fewer than 100 patients completed the HCAHPS survey. Use these rates with caution, as the number of surveys may be too low to reliably assess hospital performance; (7) Survey results are based on less than 12 months of data; (8) Survey results are not available for this reporting period; (9) No or very few patients were eligible for the HCAHPS survey. The scores shown, if any, reflect a very small number of surveys; (10) A state average was not calculated because too few hospitals in the state submitted data; (11) There were discrepancies in the data collection process; Please refer to the User's Guide for a full explanation of data.

Beckley Arh Hospital

306 Stanaford Road
Beckley, WV 25801
E-mail: beckleyArh@arh.org
URL: www.arh.org/beckley
Type: Acute Care Hospitals
Ownership: Voluntary Non-Profit - Private

Phone: 304-255-3456
Fax: 304-255-3544

Emergency Services: No
Beds: 173

Key Personnel:

CEO/President . . . . Stephen C Hanson
Chief of Medical Staff . . . . Syed Siddigi, MD
Infection Control . . . . Kathy Martin
Operating Room . . . . Elias Isaac
Quality Assurance . . . . Robert Wayne
Radiology . . . . Daniel D Maxwell
Emergency Room . . . . Rob Williams, MD
Intensive Care Unit . . . . Brenda Ward

Measure	Cases	This Hosp.	State Avg.	U.S. Avg.
Heart Attack Care				
ACE Inhibitor or ARB for LVSD[1]	2	50%	94%	96%
Aspirin at Arrival	27	81%	97%	99%
Aspirin at Discharge[1]	8	88%	98%	98%
Beta Blocker at Discharge[1]	8	100%	98%	98%
Fibrinolytic Medication Timing	0	-	29%	55%
PCI Within 90 Minutes of Arrival	0	-	85%	90%
Smoking Cessation Advice[1]	1	100%	99%	99%
Chest Pain/Possible Heart Attack Care				
Aspirin at Arrival	48	90%	95%	95%
Median Time to ECG (minutes)	51	11	12	8
Median Time to Transfer (minutes)[1,3]	3	55	77	61
Fibrinolytic Medication Timing[1]	10	60%	56%	54%
Heart Failure Care				
ACE Inhibitor or ARB for LVSD	33	64%	90%	94%
Discharge Instructions	124	72%	85%	88%
Evaluation of LVS Function	152	91%	97%	98%
Smoking Cessation Advice	34	97%	97%	98%
Pneumonia Care				
Appropriate Initial Antibiotic	64	84%	89%	92%
Blood Culture Timing	105	86%	95%	96%
Influenza Vaccine	69	75%	90%	91%
Initial Antibiotic Timing	107	92%	94%	95%
Pneumococcal Vaccine	81	83%	91%	93%
Smoking Cessation Advice	59	95%	96%	97%
Surgical Care Improvement Project				
Appropriate VTP Within 24 Hours	80	75%	91%	92%
Appropriate Hair Removal	152	99%	99%	99%
Appropriate Beta Blocker Usage	41	83%	93%	93%
Controlled Postoperative Blood Glucose	0	-	91%	93%
Prophylactic Antibiotic Timing	42	88%	97%	97%
Prophylactic Antibiotic Timing (Outpatient)	84	54%	90%	92%
Prophylactic Antibiotic Selection	43	79%	97%	97%
Prophylactic Antibiotic Select. (Outpatient)	53	91%	91%	94%
Prophylactic Antibiotic Stopped	40	90%	94%	94%
Recommended VTP Ordered	85	72%	92%	94%
Urinary Catheter Removal[1]	16	75%	90%	90%
Children's Asthma Care				
Received Systemic Corticosteroids	-	-	-	100%
Received Home Management Plan	-	-	-	71%
Received Reliever Medication	-	-	-	100%
Use of Medical Imaging				
Combination Abdominal CT Scan	356	0.615	0.304	0.191
Combination Chest CT Scan	224	0.308	0.063	0.054
Follow-up Mammogram/Ultrasound	332	6.6%	8.8%	8.4%
MRI for Low Back Pain	110	37.3%	38.5%	32.7%
Survey of Patients' Hospital Experiences				
Area Around Room 'Always' Quiet at Night	300+	52%	-	58%
Doctors 'Always' Communicated Well	300+	76%	-	80%
Home Recovery Information Given	300+	76%	-	82%
Hospital Given 9 or 10 on 10 Point Scale	300+	59%	-	67%
Meds 'Always' Explained Before Given	300+	54%	-	60%
Nurses 'Always' Communicated Well	300+	71%	-	76%
Pain 'Always' Well Controlled	300+	66%	-	69%
Room and Bathroom 'Always' Clean	300+	59%	-	71%
Timely Help 'Always' Received	300+	53%	-	64%
Would Definitely Recommend Hospital	300+	65%	-	69%

Beckley VA Medical Center

200 Veterans Avenue
Beckley, WV 25801
Type: Acute Care-Veterans Administration
Ownership: Government - Federal

Phone: 304-255-2121
Fax: 304-255-2431
Emergency Services: No
Beds: 111

Key Personnel:

Chief of Medical Staff . . . . Edward Shooler
Quality Assurance . . . . Sandra Mane
Emergency Room . . . . James Pawell

Measure	Cases	This Hosp.	State Avg.	U.S. Avg.
Heart Attack Care				
ACE Inhibitor or ARB for LVSD[1]	1	100%	94%	96%
Aspirin at Arrival[1]	4	100%	97%	99%
Aspirin at Discharge[1]	1	100%	98%	98%
Beta Blocker at Discharge[1]	1	100%	98%	98%
Fibrinolytic Medication Timing[5]	0	-	29%	55%
PCI Within 90 Minutes of Arrival[5]	0	-	85%	90%
Smoking Cessation Advice[5]	0	-	99%	99%
Chest Pain/Possible Heart Attack Care				
Aspirin at Arrival	-	-	95%	95%
Median Time to ECG (minutes)	-	-	12	8
Median Time to Transfer (minutes)	-	-	77	61
Fibrinolytic Medication Timing	-	-	56%	54%
Heart Failure Care				
ACE Inhibitor or ARB for LVSD	25	92%	90%	94%
Discharge Instructions	49	100%	85%	88%
Evaluation of LVS Function	56	100%	97%	98%
Smoking Cessation Advice[1]	10	100%	97%	98%
Pneumonia Care				
Appropriate Initial Antibiotic	107	93%	89%	92%
Blood Culture Timing	158	96%	95%	96%
Influenza Vaccine	104	100%	90%	91%
Initial Antibiotic Timing	160	98%	94%	95%
Pneumococcal Vaccine	162	99%	91%	93%
Smoking Cessation Advice	64	100%	96%	97%
Surgical Care Improvement Project				
Appropriate VTP Within 24 Hours[2,5]	0	-	91%	92%
Appropriate Hair Removal[2,5]	0	-	99%	99%
Appropriate Beta Blocker Usage[2,5]	0	-	93%	93%
Controlled Postoperative Blood Glucose[2,5]	0	-	91%	93%
Prophylactic Antibiotic Timing[5]	0	-	97%	97%
Prophylactic Antibiotic Timing (Outpatient)	-	-	90%	92%
Prophylactic Antibiotic Selection[5]	0	-	97%	97%
Prophylactic Antibiotic Select. (Outpatient)	-	-	91%	94%
Prophylactic Antibiotic Stopped[5]	0	-	94%	94%
Recommended VTP Ordered[2,5]	0	-	92%	94%
Urinary Catheter Removal[2,5]	0	-	90%	90%
Children's Asthma Care				
Received Systemic Corticosteroids	-	-	-	100%
Received Home Management Plan	-	-	-	71%
Received Reliever Medication	-	-	-	100%
Use of Medical Imaging				
Combination Abdominal CT Scan	-	-	0.304	0.191
Combination Chest CT Scan	-	-	0.063	0.054
Follow-up Mammogram/Ultrasound	-	-	8.8%	8.4%
MRI for Low Back Pain	-	-	38.5%	32.7%
Survey of Patients' Hospital Experiences				
Area Around Room 'Always' Quiet at Night	-	-	-	58%
Doctors 'Always' Communicated Well	-	-	-	80%
Home Recovery Information Given	-	-	-	82%
Hospital Given 9 or 10 on 10 Point Scale	-	-	-	67%
Meds 'Always' Explained Before Given	-	-	-	60%
Nurses 'Always' Communicated Well	-	-	-	76%
Pain 'Always' Well Controlled	-	-	-	69%
Room and Bathroom 'Always' Clean	-	-	-	71%
Timely Help 'Always' Received	-	-	-	64%
Would Definitely Recommend Hospital	-	-	-	69%

Raleigh General Hospital

1710 Harper Road
Beckley, WV 25801
Type: Acute Care Hospitals
Ownership: Voluntary Non-Profit - Private

Phone: 304-256-4100
Fax: 304-256-4009
Emergency Services: Yes
Beds: 392

Key Personnel:

CEO/President . . . . Karen Bowling
Chief of Medical Staff . . . . Anthony Dinh
Infection Control . . . . Nancy Ward
Operating Room . . . . Doug Wyandt
Pediatric Ambulatory Care . . . . . . Ted Solari, MD
Pediatric In-Patient Care . . . . Ted Solari, MD
Quality Assurance . . . . Shievonna Shamblin

Measure	Cases	This Hosp.	State Avg.	U.S. Avg.
Heart Attack Care				
ACE Inhibitor or ARB for LVSD	26	100%	94%	96%
Aspirin at Arrival	159	100%	97%	99%
Aspirin at Discharge	185	96%	98%	98%
Beta Blocker at Discharge	171	96%	98%	98%
Fibrinolytic Medication Timing[1]	1	0%	29%	55%
PCI Within 90 Minutes of Arrival	29	62%	85%	90%
Smoking Cessation Advice	78	100%	99%	99%
Chest Pain/Possible Heart Attack Care				
Aspirin at Arrival	88	100%	95%	95%
Median Time to ECG (minutes)	94	20	12	8
Median Time to Transfer (minutes)[1,3]	2	131	77	61
Fibrinolytic Medication Timing[1,3]	12	33%	56%	54%
Heart Failure Care				
ACE Inhibitor or ARB for LVSD	79	97%	90%	94%
Discharge Instructions	311	86%	85%	88%
Evaluation of LVS Function	365	100%	97%	98%
Smoking Cessation Advice	86	100%	97%	98%
Pneumonia Care				
Appropriate Initial Antibiotic	213	97%	89%	92%
Blood Culture Timing	323	92%	95%	96%
Influenza Vaccine	218	90%	90%	91%
Initial Antibiotic Timing	319	98%	94%	95%
Pneumococcal Vaccine	249	97%	91%	93%
Smoking Cessation Advice	171	100%	96%	97%
Surgical Care Improvement Project				
Appropriate VTP Within 24 Hours	159	94%	91%	92%
Appropriate Hair Removal	496	100%	99%	99%
Appropriate Beta Blocker Usage	92	97%	93%	93%
Controlled Postoperative Blood Glucose	0	-	91%	93%
Prophylactic Antibiotic Timing	309	98%	97%	97%
Prophylactic Antibiotic Timing (Outpatient)	179	97%	90%	92%
Prophylactic Antibiotic Selection	311	96%	97%	97%
Prophylactic Antibiotic Select. (Outpatient)	176	98%	91%	94%
Prophylactic Antibiotic Stopped	301	95%	94%	94%
Recommended VTP Ordered	160	98%	92%	94%
Urinary Catheter Removal	50	96%	90%	90%
Children's Asthma Care				
Received Systemic Corticosteroids	30	100%	-	100%
Received Home Management Plan	30	90%	-	71%
Received Reliever Medication	31	100%	-	100%
Use of Medical Imaging				
Combination Abdominal CT Scan	588	0.838	0.304	0.191
Combination Chest CT Scan	535	0.716	0.063	0.054
Follow-up Mammogram/Ultrasound	128	10.9%	8.8%	8.4%
MRI for Low Back Pain	396	44.2%	38.5%	32.7%
Survey of Patients' Hospital Experiences				
Area Around Room 'Always' Quiet at Night	300+	51%	-	58%
Doctors 'Always' Communicated Well	300+	77%	-	80%
Home Recovery Information Given	300+	80%	-	82%
Hospital Given 9 or 10 on 10 Point Scale	300+	64%	-	67%
Meds 'Always' Explained Before Given	300+	57%	-	60%
Nurses 'Always' Communicated Well	300+	73%	-	76%
Pain 'Always' Well Controlled	300+	70%	-	69%
Room and Bathroom 'Always' Clean	300+	64%	-	71%
Timely Help 'Always' Received	300+	53%	-	64%
Would Definitely Recommend Hospital	300+	62%	-	69%

NOTE: Hospital profiles are in alphabetical order by state, then city, then hospital within the city; Rankings exclude hospitals with less than 25 cases except for patient surveys which excludes hospitals with less than 100 cases; (a) 100–299 cases; (1) The number of cases is too small to be sure how well a hospital is performing; (2) The hospital indicated that the data submitted for this measure were based on a sample of cases; (3) Data was collected during a shorter time period (fewer quarters) than the maximum possible time for this measure; (4) Suppressed for one or more quarters by CMS; (5) No data is available from the hospital for this measure; (6) Fewer than 100 patients completed the HCAHPS survey. Use these rates with caution, as the number of surveys may be too low to reliably assess hospital performance; (7) Survey results are based on less than 12 months of data; (8) Survey results are not available for this reporting period; (9) No or very few patients were eligible for the HCAHPS survey. The scores shown, if any, reflect a very small number of surveys; (10) A state average was not calculated because too few hospitals in the state submitted data; (11) There were discrepancies in the data collection process; Please refer to the User's Guide for a full explanation of data.

Morgan County War Memorial

109 War Memorial
Berkeley Springs, WV 25411
Phone: 304-258-1234
Fax: 304-258-5618
Type: Critical Access Hospitals
Emergency Services: Yes
Ownership: Voluntary Non-Profit - Other
Beds: 60

Key Personnel:

CEO/President. . . . . David Applewood
Chief of Medical Staff. . . . . Joseph Hashem
Quality Assurance . . . . Evelyn Clonch, RN
Radiology. . . . . Stephen B Eigles

Measure	Cases	This Hosp.	State Avg.	U.S. Avg.
Heart Attack Care				
ACE Inhibitor or ARB for LVSD[3]	0	-	94%	96%
Aspirin at Arrival[3]	0	-	97%	99%
Aspirin at Discharge[3]	0	-	98%	98%
Beta Blocker at Discharge[3]	0	-	98%	98%
Fibrinolytic Medication Timing[1,3]	1	0%	29%	55%
PCI Within 90 Minutes of Arrival[5]	0	-	85%	90%
Smoking Cessation Advice[3]	0	-	99%	99%
Chest Pain/Possible Heart Attack Care				
Aspirin at Arrival	-	-	95%	95%
Median Time to ECG (minutes)	-	-	12	8
Median Time to Transfer (minutes)	-	-	77	61
Fibrinolytic Medication Timing	-	-	56%	54%
Heart Failure Care				
ACE Inhibitor or ARB for LVSD[1,3]	4	50%	90%	94%
Discharge Instructions[1,3]	8	62%	85%	88%
Evaluation of LVS Function[1,3]	15	80%	97%	98%
Smoking Cessation Advice[1,3]	1	0%	97%	98%
Pneumonia Care				
Appropriate Initial Antibiotic[1,3]	9	89%	89%	92%
Blood Culture Timing[1,3]	12	75%	95%	96%
Influenza Vaccine[1,3]	4	100%	90%	91%
Initial Antibiotic Timing[1,3]	14	93%	94%	95%
Pneumococcal Vaccine[1,3]	10	90%	91%	93%
Smoking Cessation Advice[1,3]	4	75%	96%	97%
Surgical Care Improvement Project				
Appropriate VTP Within 24 Hours[5]	0	-	91%	92%
Appropriate Hair Removal[5]	0	-	99%	99%
Appropriate Beta Blocker Usage[5]	0	-	93%	93%
Controlled Postoperative Blood Glucose[5]	0	-	91%	93%
Prophylactic Antibiotic Timing[5]	0	-	97%	97%
Prophylactic Antibiotic Timing (Outpatient)	-	-	90%	92%
Prophylactic Antibiotic Selection[5]	0	-	97%	97%
Prophylactic Antibiotic Select. (Outpatient)	-	-	91%	94%
Prophylactic Antibiotic Stopped[5]	0	-	94%	94%
Recommended VTP Ordered[5]	0	-	92%	94%
Urinary Catheter Removal[5]	0	-	90%	90%
Children's Asthma Care				
Received Systemic Corticosteroids	-	-	-	100%
Received Home Management Plan	-	-	-	71%
Received Reliever Medication	-	-	-	100%
Use of Medical Imaging				
Combination Abdominal CT Scan	-	-	0.304	0.191
Combination Chest CT Scan	-	-	0.063	0.054
Follow-up Mammogram/Ultrasound	-	-	8.8%	8.4%
MRI for Low Back Pain	-	-	38.5%	32.7%
Survey of Patients' Hospital Experiences				
Area Around Room 'Always' Quiet at Night	(a)	54%	-	58%
Doctors 'Always' Communicated Well	(a)	74%	-	80%
Home Recovery Information Given	(a)	83%	-	82%
Hospital Given 9 or 10 on 10 Point Scale	(a)	61%	-	67%
Meds 'Always' Explained Before Given	(a)	57%	-	60%
Nurses 'Always' Communicated Well	(a)	69%	-	76%
Pain 'Always' Well Controlled	(a)	61%	-	69%
Room and Bathroom 'Always' Clean	(a)	79%	-	71%
Timely Help 'Always' Received	(a)	64%	-	64%
Would Definitely Recommend Hospital	(a)	62%	-	69%

Bluefield Regional Medical Center

500 Cherry St
Bluefield, WV 24701
Phone: 304-327-1100
Fax: 304-327-1896
URL: www.bluefield.org
Type: Acute Care Hospitals
Emergency Services: Yes
Ownership: Voluntary Non-Profit - Other
Beds: 210

Key Personnel:

CEO/President. . . . . Leland Farnell
Chief of Medical Staff. . . . . Donald Asbury, MD
Operating Room. . . . . Martha Plant
Pediatric Ambulatory Care . . . . . . Thomas E Richardon, MD
Pediatric In-Patient Care . . . . Kathy Glover
Radiology. . . . . Kay Cooper
Emergency Room . . . . Gary Butt
Intensive Care Unit. . . . . Gary Butt

Measure	Cases	This Hosp.	State Avg.	U.S. Avg.
Heart Attack Care				
ACE Inhibitor or ARB for LVSD[1]	3	100%	94%	96%
Aspirin at Arrival	42	95%	97%	99%
Aspirin at Discharge	25	88%	98%	98%
Beta Blocker at Discharge	31	94%	98%	98%
Fibrinolytic Medication Timing[1]	1	0%	29%	55%
PCI Within 90 Minutes of Arrival	0	-	85%	90%
Smoking Cessation Advice[1]	6	100%	99%	99%
Chest Pain/Possible Heart Attack Care				
Aspirin at Arrival	121	93%	95%	95%
Median Time to ECG (minutes)	123	16	12	8
Median Time to Transfer (minutes)[1,3]	4	155	77	61
Fibrinolytic Medication Timing[1]	17	29%	56%	54%
Heart Failure Care				
ACE Inhibitor or ARB for LVSD	62	82%	90%	94%
Discharge Instructions	178	72%	85%	88%
Evaluation of LVS Function	193	98%	97%	98%
Smoking Cessation Advice	33	76%	97%	98%
Pneumonia Care				
Appropriate Initial Antibiotic	121	75%	89%	92%
Blood Culture Timing	169	93%	95%	96%
Influenza Vaccine	90	80%	90%	91%
Initial Antibiotic Timing	172	88%	94%	95%
Pneumococcal Vaccine	136	84%	91%	93%
Smoking Cessation Advice	62	95%	96%	97%
Surgical Care Improvement Project				
Appropriate VTP Within 24 Hours	79	76%	91%	92%
Appropriate Hair Removal	285	99%	99%	99%
Appropriate Beta Blocker Usage	90	86%	93%	93%
Controlled Postoperative Blood Glucose	0	-	91%	93%
Prophylactic Antibiotic Timing	260	97%	97%	97%
Prophylactic Antibiotic Timing (Outpatient)	133	88%	90%	92%
Prophylactic Antibiotic Selection	259	93%	97%	97%
Prophylactic Antibiotic Select. (Outpatient)	121	94%	91%	94%
Prophylactic Antibiotic Stopped	257	90%	94%	94%
Recommended VTP Ordered	83	89%	92%	94%
Urinary Catheter Removal[1]	16	62%	90%	90%
Children's Asthma Care				
Received Systemic Corticosteroids	-	-	-	100%
Received Home Management Plan	-	-	-	71%
Received Reliever Medication	-	-	-	100%
Use of Medical Imaging				
Combination Abdominal CT Scan	688	0.500	0.304	0.191
Combination Chest CT Scan	380	0.321	0.063	0.054
Follow-up Mammogram/Ultrasound	712	9.8%	8.8%	8.4%
MRI for Low Back Pain	88	44.3%	38.5%	32.7%
Survey of Patients' Hospital Experiences				
Area Around Room 'Always' Quiet at Night	300+	54%	-	58%
Doctors 'Always' Communicated Well	300+	79%	-	80%
Home Recovery Information Given	300+	81%	-	82%
Hospital Given 9 or 10 on 10 Point Scale	300+	56%	-	67%
Meds 'Always' Explained Before Given	300+	60%	-	60%
Nurses 'Always' Communicated Well	300+	75%	-	76%
Pain 'Always' Well Controlled	300+	66%	-	69%
Room and Bathroom 'Always' Clean	300+	69%	-	71%
Timely Help 'Always' Received	300+	60%	-	64%
Would Definitely Recommend Hospital	300+	57%	-	69%

United Hospital Center

327 Medical Park Drive
Bridgeport, WV 26330
Phone: 681-342-1000
URL: www.uhcwv.org
Type: Acute Care Hospitals
Emergency Services: Yes
Ownership: Voluntary Non-Profit - Private
Beds: 292

Key Personnel:

Radiology. . . . . Parke Thrush

Measure	Cases	This Hosp.	State Avg.	U.S. Avg.
Heart Attack Care				
ACE Inhibitor or ARB for LVSD	54	100%	94%	96%
Aspirin at Arrival	192	100%	97%	99%
Aspirin at Discharge	195	100%	98%	98%
Beta Blocker at Discharge	189	100%	98%	98%
Fibrinolytic Medication Timing	0	-	29%	55%
PCI Within 90 Minutes of Arrival	33	100%	85%	90%
Smoking Cessation Advice	91	100%	99%	99%
Chest Pain/Possible Heart Attack Care				
Aspirin at Arrival	33	97%	95%	95%
Median Time to ECG (minutes)	31	13	12	8
Median Time to Transfer (minutes)[3]	0	-	77	61
Fibrinolytic Medication Timing[3]	0	-	56%	54%
Heart Failure Care				
ACE Inhibitor or ARB for LVSD	126	100%	90%	94%
Discharge Instructions	212	95%	85%	88%
Evaluation of LVS Function	258	100%	97%	98%
Smoking Cessation Advice	46	100%	97%	98%
Pneumonia Care				
Appropriate Initial Antibiotic	205	98%	89%	92%
Blood Culture Timing	255	99%	95%	96%
Influenza Vaccine	257	96%	90%	91%
Initial Antibiotic Timing	116	97%	94%	95%
Pneumococcal Vaccine	319	97%	91%	93%
Smoking Cessation Advice	149	100%	96%	97%
Surgical Care Improvement Project				
Appropriate VTP Within 24 Hours[2]	254	97%	91%	92%
Appropriate Hair Removal[2]	739	100%	99%	99%
Appropriate Beta Blocker Usage[2]	214	100%	93%	93%
Controlled Postoperative Blood Glucose[2]	0	-	91%	93%
Prophylactic Antibiotic Timing[2]	552	99%	97%	97%
Prophylactic Antibiotic Timing (Outpatient)	109	95%	90%	92%
Prophylactic Antibiotic Selection[2]	561	100%	97%	97%
Prophylactic Antibiotic Select. (Outpatient)	107	94%	91%	94%
Prophylactic Antibiotic Stopped[2]	519	97%	94%	94%
Recommended VTP Ordered[2]	254	98%	92%	94%
Urinary Catheter Removal[2]	186	99%	90%	90%
Children's Asthma Care				
Received Systemic Corticosteroids	-	-	-	100%
Received Home Management Plan	-	-	-	71%
Received Reliever Medication	-	-	-	100%
Use of Medical Imaging				
Combination Abdominal CT Scan	1,314	0.750	0.304	0.191
Combination Chest CT Scan	886	0.001	0.063	0.054
Follow-up Mammogram/Ultrasound	1,853	6.4%	8.8%	8.4%
MRI for Low Back Pain	323	39.3%	38.5%	32.7%
Survey of Patients' Hospital Experiences				
Area Around Room 'Always' Quiet at Night	300+	43%	-	58%
Doctors 'Always' Communicated Well	300+	79%	-	80%
Home Recovery Information Given	300+	80%	-	82%
Hospital Given 9 or 10 on 10 Point Scale	300+	51%	-	67%
Meds 'Always' Explained Before Given	300+	54%	-	60%
Nurses 'Always' Communicated Well	300+	70%	-	76%
Pain 'Always' Well Controlled	300+	61%	-	69%
Room and Bathroom 'Always' Clean	300+	62%	-	71%
Timely Help 'Always' Received	300+	54%	-	64%
Would Definitely Recommend Hospital	300+	54%	-	69%

NOTE: Hospital profiles are in alphabetical order by state, then city, then hospital within the city; Rankings exclude hospitals with less than 25 cases except for patient surveys which excludes hospitals with less than 100 cases; (a) 100–299 cases; (1) The number of cases is too small to be sure how well a hospital is performing; (2) The hospital indicated that the data submitted for this measure were based on a sample of cases; (3) Data was collected during a shorter time period (fewer quarters) than the maximum possible time for this measure; (4) Suppressed for one or more quarters by CMS; (5) No data is available from the hospital for this measure; (6) Fewer than 100 patients completed the HCAHPS survey. Use these rates with caution, as the number of surveys may be too low to reliably assess hospital performance; (7) Survey results are based on less than 12 months of data; (8) Survey results are not available for this reporting period; (9) No or very few patients were eligible for the HCAHPS survey. The scores shown, if any, reflect a very small number of surveys; (10) A state average was not calculated because too few hospitals in the state submitted data; (11) There were discrepancies in the data collection process; Please refer to the User's Guide for a full explanation of data.

Pocahontas Memorial Hospital

Rr Box 52 West
Buckeye, WV 24924
Phone: 304-799-7400
Fax: 304-799-6636
Type: Critical Access Hospitals
Emergency Services: Yes
Ownership: Voluntary Non-Profit - Other
Beds: 27

Key Personnel:
Chief of Medical Staff.......... Luis Soriano
Quality Assurance .... Amy Wade
Emergency Room .... Dr. Luis Soriano

Measure	Cases	This Hosp.	State Avg.	U.S. Avg.
Heart Attack Care				
ACE Inhibitor or ARB for LVSD[5]	0	-	94%	96%
Aspirin at Arrival[5]	0	-	97%	99%
Aspirin at Discharge[5]	0	-	98%	98%
Beta Blocker at Discharge[5]	0	-	98%	98%
Fibrinolytic Medication Timing[5]	0	-	29%	55%
PCI Within 90 Minutes of Arrival[5]	0	-	85%	90%
Smoking Cessation Advice[5]	0	-	99%	99%
Chest Pain/Possible Heart Attack Care				
Aspirin at Arrival			95%	95%
Median Time to ECG (minutes)	-	-	12	8
Median Time to Transfer (minutes)	-	-	77	61
Fibrinolytic Medication Timing	-	-	56%	54%
Heart Failure Care				
ACE Inhibitor or ARB for LVSD[5]	0	-	90%	94%
Discharge Instructions[5]	0	-	85%	88%
Evaluation of LVS Function[5]	0	-	97%	98%
Smoking Cessation Advice[5]	0	-	97%	98%
Pneumonia Care				
Appropriate Initial Antibiotic[5]	0	-	89%	92%
Blood Culture Timing[5]	0	-	95%	96%
Influenza Vaccine[5]	0	-	90%	91%
Initial Antibiotic Timing[5]	0	-	94%	95%
Pneumococcal Vaccine[5]	0	-	91%	93%
Smoking Cessation Advice[5]	0	-	96%	97%
Surgical Care Improvement Project				
Appropriate VTP Within 24 Hours[5]	0	-	91%	92%
Appropriate Hair Removal[5]	0	-	99%	99%
Appropriate Beta Blocker Usage[5]	0	-	93%	93%
Controlled Postoperative Blood Glucose[5]	0	-	91%	93%
Prophylactic Antibiotic Timing[5]	0	-	97%	97%
Prophylactic Antibiotic Timing (Outpatient)		-	90%	92%
Prophylactic Antibiotic Selection[5]	0	-	97%	97%
Prophylactic Antibiotic Select. (Outpatient)		-	91%	94%
Prophylactic Antibiotic Stopped[5]	0	-	94%	94%
Recommended VTP Ordered[5]	0	-	92%	94%
Urinary Catheter Removal[5]	0	-	90%	90%
Children's Asthma Care				
Received Systemic Corticosteroids	-	-	-	100%
Received Home Management Plan	-	-	-	71%
Received Reliever Medication	-	-	-	100%
Use of Medical Imaging				
Combination Abdominal CT Scan		-	0.304	0.191
Combination Chest CT Scan		-	0.063	0.054
Follow-up Mammogram/Ultrasound		-	8.8%	8.4%
MRI for Low Back Pain		-	38.5%	32.7%
Survey of Patients' Hospital Experiences				
Area Around Room 'Always' Quiet at Night[8]	-	-	-	58%
Doctors 'Always' Communicated Well[8]	-	-	-	80%
Home Recovery Information Given[8]	-	-	-	82%
Hospital Given 9 or 10 on 10 Point Scale[8]	-	-	-	67%
Meds 'Always' Explained Before Given[8]	-	-	-	60%
Nurses 'Always' Communicated Well[8]	-	-	-	76%
Pain 'Always' Well Controlled[8]	-	-	-	69%
Room and Bathroom 'Always' Clean[8]	-	-	-	71%
Timely Help 'Always' Received[8]	-	-	-	64%
Would Definitely Recommend Hospital[8]	-	-	-	69%

Saint Joseph Hospital

1 Amalia Drive
Buckhannon, WV 26201
Phone: 304-472-2000
Fax: 304-472-6620
E-mail: webmaster@stj.net
URL: www.stj.net
Type: Acute Care Hospitals
Emergency Services: Yes
Ownership: Voluntary Non-Profit - Church
Beds: 95

Key Personnel:
CEO/President................. Wayne B Griffith
Quality Assurance .... Elly Mick
Emergency Room .... John Freed, MD

Measure	Cases	This Hosp.	State Avg.	U.S. Avg.
Heart Attack Care				
ACE Inhibitor or ARB for LVSD[1]	1	0%	94%	96%
Aspirin at Arrival[1]	7	100%	97%	99%
Aspirin at Discharge[1]	4	100%	98%	98%
Beta Blocker at Discharge[1]	5	100%	98%	98%
Fibrinolytic Medication Timing	0	-	29%	55%
PCI Within 90 Minutes of Arrival	0	-	85%	90%
Smoking Cessation Advice[1]	2	50%	99%	99%
Chest Pain/Possible Heart Attack Care				
Aspirin at Arrival	40	100%	95%	95%
Median Time to ECG (minutes)	44	16	12	8
Median Time to Transfer (minutes)[1,3]	1	218	77	61
Fibrinolytic Medication Timing[1]	3	100%	56%	54%
Heart Failure Care				
ACE Inhibitor or ARB for LVSD[1]	6	83%	90%	94%
Discharge Instructions[1]	20	75%	85%	88%
Evaluation of LVS Function[1]	23	91%	97%	98%
Smoking Cessation Advice[1]	5	60%	97%	98%
Pneumonia Care				
Appropriate Initial Antibiotic	29	90%	89%	92%
Blood Culture Timing	36	89%	95%	96%
Influenza Vaccine[1]	18	94%	90%	91%
Initial Antibiotic Timing	42	98%	94%	95%
Pneumococcal Vaccine	26	88%	91%	93%
Smoking Cessation Advice[1]	18	83%	96%	97%
Surgical Care Improvement Project				
Appropriate VTP Within 24 Hours	25	60%	91%	92%
Appropriate Hair Removal	66	100%	99%	99%
Appropriate Beta Blocker Usage[1]	12	100%	93%	93%
Controlled Postoperative Blood Glucose	0	-	91%	93%
Prophylactic Antibiotic Timing	44	91%	97%	97%
Prophylactic Antibiotic Timing (Outpatient)[1]	16	94%	90%	92%
Prophylactic Antibiotic Selection	45	98%	97%	97%
Prophylactic Antibiotic Select. (Outpatient)[1]	15	100%	91%	94%
Prophylactic Antibiotic Stopped	42	81%	94%	94%
Recommended VTP Ordered	26	62%	92%	94%
Urinary Catheter Removal[1]	13	92%	90%	90%
Children's Asthma Care				
Received Systemic Corticosteroids	-	-	-	100%
Received Home Management Plan	-	-	-	71%
Received Reliever Medication	-	-	-	100%
Use of Medical Imaging				
Combination Abdominal CT Scan	217	0.498	0.304	0.191
Combination Chest CT Scan	128	0.000	0.063	0.054
Follow-up Mammogram/Ultrasound	412	8.3%	8.8%	8.4%
MRI for Low Back Pain[1]	24	33.3%	38.5%	32.7%
Survey of Patients' Hospital Experiences				
Area Around Room 'Always' Quiet at Night	(a)	56%	-	58%
Doctors 'Always' Communicated Well	(a)	85%	-	80%
Home Recovery Information Given	(a)	85%	-	82%
Hospital Given 9 or 10 on 10 Point Scale	(a)	75%	-	67%
Meds 'Always' Explained Before Given	(a)	65%	-	60%
Nurses 'Always' Communicated Well	(a)	81%	-	76%
Pain 'Always' Well Controlled	(a)	74%	-	69%
Room and Bathroom 'Always' Clean	(a)	70%	-	71%
Timely Help 'Always' Received	(a)	76%	-	64%
Would Definitely Recommend Hospital	(a)	73%	-	69%

Charleston Area Medical Center

501 Morris Street
Charleston, WV 25301
Phone: 304-388-6203
Fax: 304-388-6314
URL: www.camc.org
Type: Acute Care Hospitals
Emergency Services: No
Ownership: Voluntary Non-Profit - Private
Beds: 400

Key Personnel:
CEO/President................. David Ramsey
Cardiac Laboratory............. Jamal Kahken
Infection Control............... Terrie Lee
Operating Room................ Susan Taber, RN
Pediatric Ambulatory Care ...... Stefan Maxwell, MD
Quality Assurance .... Jean Morgan
Radiology...................... Joseph Skeens, MD
Emergency Room .... David Seidler, MD

Measure	Cases	This Hosp.	State Avg.	U.S. Avg.
Heart Attack Care				
ACE Inhibitor or ARB for LVSD[2]	218	94%	94%	96%
Aspirin at Arrival[2]	469	98%	97%	99%
Aspirin at Discharge[2]	997	99%	98%	98%
Beta Blocker at Discharge[2]	996	99%	98%	98%
Fibrinolytic Medication Timing[1,2]	1	0%	29%	55%
PCI Within 90 Minutes of Arrival[2]	73	67%	85%	90%
Smoking Cessation Advice[2]	410	100%	99%	99%
Chest Pain/Possible Heart Attack Care				
Aspirin at Arrival[1,3]	1	100%	95%	95%
Median Time to ECG (minutes)[1,3]	1	53	12	8
Median Time to Transfer (minutes)[5]	0	-	77	61
Fibrinolytic Medication Timing[5]	0	-	56%	54%
Heart Failure Care				
ACE Inhibitor or ARB for LVSD[2]	259	92%	90%	94%
Discharge Instructions[2]	610	67%	85%	88%
Evaluation of LVS Function[2]	684	99%	97%	98%
Smoking Cessation Advice[2]	133	98%	97%	98%
Pneumonia Care				
Appropriate Initial Antibiotic[2]	340	85%	89%	92%
Blood Culture Timing[2]	541	94%	95%	96%
Influenza Vaccine[2]	378	85%	90%	91%
Initial Antibiotic Timing[2]	494	89%	94%	95%
Pneumococcal Vaccine[2]	487	92%	91%	93%
Smoking Cessation Advice[2]	375	97%	96%	97%
Surgical Care Improvement Project				
Appropriate VTP Within 24 Hours[2]	465	95%	91%	92%
Appropriate Hair Removal[2]	2,464	100%	99%	99%
Appropriate Beta Blocker Usage[2]	928	96%	93%	93%
Controlled Postoperative Blood Glucose[2]	960	91%	91%	93%
Prophylactic Antibiotic Timing[2]	1,885	99%	97%	97%
Prophylactic Antibiotic Timing (Outpatient)	903	97%	90%	92%
Prophylactic Antibiotic Selection[2]	1,943	99%	97%	97%
Prophylactic Antibiotic Select. (Outpatient)	892	91%	91%	94%
Prophylactic Antibiotic Stopped[2]	1,639	95%	94%	94%
Recommended VTP Ordered[2]	470	95%	92%	94%
Urinary Catheter Removal[2]	418	93%	90%	90%
Children's Asthma Care				
Received Systemic Corticosteroids	-	-	-	100%
Received Home Management Plan	-	-	-	71%
Received Reliever Medication	-	-	-	100%
Use of Medical Imaging				
Combination Abdominal CT Scan	1,752	0.058	0.304	0.191
Combination Chest CT Scan	1,689	0.006	0.063	0.054
Follow-up Mammogram/Ultrasound	2,401	9.8%	8.8%	8.4%
MRI for Low Back Pain	333	42.3%	38.5%	32.7%
Survey of Patients' Hospital Experiences				
Area Around Room 'Always' Quiet at Night	300+	45%	-	58%
Doctors 'Always' Communicated Well	300+	79%	-	80%
Home Recovery Information Given	300+	78%	-	82%
Hospital Given 9 or 10 on 10 Point Scale	300+	66%	-	67%
Meds 'Always' Explained Before Given	300+	57%	-	60%
Nurses 'Always' Communicated Well	300+	72%	-	76%
Pain 'Always' Well Controlled	300+	67%	-	69%
Room and Bathroom 'Always' Clean	300+	64%	-	71%
Timely Help 'Always' Received	300+	59%	-	64%
Would Definitely Recommend Hospital	300+	73%	-	69%

NOTE: Hospital profiles are in alphabetical order by state, then city, then hospital within the city; Rankings exclude hospitals with less than 25 cases except for patient surveys which excludes hospitals with less than 100 cases; (a) 100–299 cases; (1) The number of cases is too small to be sure how well a hospital is performing; (2) The hospital indicated that the data submitted for this measure were based on a sample of cases; (3) Data was collected during a shorter time period (fewer quarters) than the maximum possible time for this measure; (4) Suppressed for one or more quarters by CMS; (5) No data is available from the hospital for this measure; (6) Fewer than 100 patients completed the HCAHPS survey. Use these rates with caution, as the number of surveys may be too low to reliably assess hospital performance; (7) Survey results are based on less than 12 months of data; (8) Survey results are not available for this reporting period; (9) No or very few patients were eligible for the HCAHPS survey. The scores shown, if any, reflect a very small number of surveys; (10) A state average was not calculated because too few hospitals in the state submitted data; (11) There were discrepancies in the data collection process; Please refer to the User's Guide for a full explanation of data.

Charleston Surgical Hospital

1306 Kanawha Bl E
Charleston, WV 25301
E-mail: ashelton@citynet.net
URL: www.eyeandearclinicwv.com
Type: Acute Care Hospitals
Ownership: Proprietary
Phone: 304-343-4371
Fax: 304-353-0215
Emergency Services: No
Beds: 35

Key Personnel:
CEO/President. . . . . W Allen Shelton
Chief of Medical Staff . . . . Robert E Pollard, MD
Operating Room. . . . . Carmen Palmer, RN
Anesthesiology. . . . . Phillip Casingal, MD

Measure	Cases	This Hosp.	State Avg.	U.S. Avg.
Heart Attack Care				
ACE Inhibitor or ARB for LVSD[5]	0	-	94%	96%
Aspirin at Arrival[5]	0	-	97%	99%
Aspirin at Discharge[5]	0	-	98%	98%
Beta Blocker at Discharge[5]	0	-	98%	98%
Fibrinolytic Medication Timing[5]	0	-	29%	55%
PCI Within 90 Minutes of Arrival[5]	0	-	85%	90%
Smoking Cessation Advice[5]	0	-	99%	99%
Chest Pain/Possible Heart Attack Care				
Aspirin at Arrival[5]	0	-	95%	95%
Median Time to ECG (minutes)[5]	0	-	12	8
Median Time to Transfer (minutes)[5]	0	-	77	61
Fibrinolytic Medication Timing[5]	0	-	56%	54%
Heart Failure Care				
ACE Inhibitor or ARB for LVSD[5]	0	-	90%	94%
Discharge Instructions[5]	0	-	85%	88%
Evaluation of LVS Function[5]	0	-	97%	98%
Smoking Cessation Advice[5]	0	-	97%	98%
Pneumonia Care				
Appropriate Initial Antibiotic[5]	0	-	89%	92%
Blood Culture Timing[5]	0	-	95%	96%
Influenza Vaccine[5]	0	-	90%	91%
Initial Antibiotic Timing[5]	0	-	94%	95%
Pneumococcal Vaccine[5]	0	-	91%	93%
Smoking Cessation Advice[5]	0	-	96%	97%
Surgical Care Improvement Project				
Appropriate VTP Within 24 Hours[5]	0	-	91%	92%
Appropriate Hair Removal[5]	0	-	99%	99%
Appropriate Beta Blocker Usage[5]	0	-	93%	93%
Controlled Postoperative Blood Glucose[5]	0	-	91%	93%
Prophylactic Antibiotic Timing[5]	0	-	97%	97%
Prophylactic Antibiotic Timing (Outpatient)[1,3]	4	100%	90%	92%
Prophylactic Antibiotic Selection[5]	0	-	97%	97%
Prophylactic Antibiotic Select. (Outpatient)[1,3]	4	100%	91%	94%
Prophylactic Antibiotic Stopped[5]	0	-	94%	94%
Recommended VTP Ordered[5]	0	-	92%	94%
Urinary Catheter Removal[5]	0	-	90%	90%
Children's Asthma Care				
Received Systemic Corticosteroids	-	-	-	100%
Received Home Management Plan	-	-	-	71%
Received Reliever Medication	-	-	-	100%
Use of Medical Imaging				
Combination Abdominal CT Scan[5]	0	-	0.304	0.191
Combination Chest CT Scan[5]	0	-	0.063	0.054
Follow-up Mammogram/Ultrasound[5]	0	-	8.8%	8.4%
MRI for Low Back Pain[5]	0	-	38.5%	32.7%
Survey of Patients' Hospital Experiences				
Area Around Room 'Always' Quiet at Night[9]	-	-	-	58%
Doctors 'Always' Communicated Well[9]	-	-	-	80%
Home Recovery Information Given[9]	-	-	-	82%
Hospital Given 9 or 10 on 10 Point Scale[9]	-	-	-	67%
Meds 'Always' Explained Before Given[9]	-	-	-	60%
Nurses 'Always' Communicated Well[9]	-	-	-	76%
Pain 'Always' Well Controlled[9]	-	-	-	69%
Room and Bathroom 'Always' Clean[9]	-	-	-	71%
Timely Help 'Always' Received[9]	-	-	-	64%
Would Definitely Recommend Hospital[9]	-	-	-	69%

Saint Francis Hospital

333 Laidley St
Charleston, WV 25301
Type: Acute Care Hospitals
Ownership: Proprietary
Phone: 304-347-6500
Fax: 304-347-6885
Emergency Services: Yes
Beds: 155

Key Personnel:
CEO/President. . . . . Dan Lauffer
Cardiac Laboratory. . . . . Brian Lilly
Chief of Medical Staff . . . . Mallinath Kay, MD
Operating Room. . . . . Cindy Kranz
Quality Assurance . . . . Patty Skaff
Emergency Room . . . . Ed Bowdifh

Measure	Cases	This Hosp.	State Avg.	U.S. Avg.
Heart Attack Care				
ACE Inhibitor or ARB for LVSD[1]	15	100%	94%	96%
Aspirin at Arrival	37	97%	97%	99%
Aspirin at Discharge	60	93%	98%	98%
Beta Blocker at Discharge	60	97%	98%	98%
Fibrinolytic Medication Timing	0	-	29%	55%
PCI Within 90 Minutes of Arrival[1]	5	60%	85%	90%
Smoking Cessation Advice	29	100%	99%	99%
Chest Pain/Possible Heart Attack Care				
Aspirin at Arrival[5]	0	-	95%	95%
Median Time to ECG (minutes)[5]	0	-	12	8
Median Time to Transfer (minutes)[5]	0	-	77	61
Fibrinolytic Medication Timing[5]	0	-	56%	54%
Heart Failure Care				
ACE Inhibitor or ARB for LVSD	52	100%	90%	94%
Discharge Instructions	88	98%	85%	88%
Evaluation of LVS Function	100	100%	97%	98%
Smoking Cessation Advice	28	100%	97%	98%
Pneumonia Care				
Appropriate Initial Antibiotic	61	93%	89%	92%
Blood Culture Timing	88	93%	95%	96%
Influenza Vaccine	61	89%	90%	91%
Initial Antibiotic Timing	93	90%	94%	95%
Pneumococcal Vaccine	76	78%	91%	93%
Smoking Cessation Advice	53	89%	96%	97%
Surgical Care Improvement Project				
Appropriate VTP Within 24 Hours	140	81%	91%	92%
Appropriate Hair Removal	598	99%	99%	99%
Appropriate Beta Blocker Usage	174	82%	93%	93%
Controlled Postoperative Blood Glucose	0	-	91%	93%
Prophylactic Antibiotic Timing	482	96%	97%	97%
Prophylactic Antibiotic Timing (Outpatient)	213	84%	90%	92%
Prophylactic Antibiotic Selection	483	92%	97%	97%
Prophylactic Antibiotic Select. (Outpatient)	197	77%	91%	94%
Prophylactic Antibiotic Stopped	482	91%	94%	94%
Recommended VTP Ordered	147	80%	92%	94%
Urinary Catheter Removal	205	90%	90%	90%
Children's Asthma Care				
Received Systemic Corticosteroids	-	-	-	100%
Received Home Management Plan	-	-	-	71%
Received Reliever Medication	-	-	-	100%
Use of Medical Imaging				
Combination Abdominal CT Scan	241	0.017	0.304	0.191
Combination Chest CT Scan	111	0.000	0.063	0.054
Follow-up Mammogram/Ultrasound	1,003	6.4%	8.8%	8.4%
MRI for Low Back Pain	145	38.6%	38.5%	32.7%
Survey of Patients' Hospital Experiences				
Area Around Room 'Always' Quiet at Night	300+	64%	-	58%
Doctors 'Always' Communicated Well	300+	81%	-	80%
Home Recovery Information Given	300+	81%	-	82%
Hospital Given 9 or 10 on 10 Point Scale	300+	75%	-	67%
Meds 'Always' Explained Before Given	300+	58%	-	60%
Nurses 'Always' Communicated Well	300+	79%	-	76%
Pain 'Always' Well Controlled	300+	75%	-	69%
Room and Bathroom 'Always' Clean	300+	69%	-	71%
Timely Help 'Always' Received	300+	69%	-	64%
Would Definitely Recommend Hospital	300+	77%	-	69%

Clarksburg VA Medical Center

1 Medical Center Drive
Clarksburg, WV 26301
URL: www.clarksburg.va.gov
Type: Acute Care-Veterans Administration
Ownership: Government - Federal
Phone: 304-623-3461
Emergency Services: No

Measure	Cases	This Hosp.	State Avg.	U.S. Avg.
Heart Attack Care				
ACE Inhibitor or ARB for LVSD[1]	2	100%	94%	96%
Aspirin at Arrival	26	100%	97%	99%
Aspirin at Discharge[1]	15	93%	98%	98%
Beta Blocker at Discharge[1]	16	100%	98%	98%
Fibrinolytic Medication Timing[5]	0	-	29%	55%
PCI Within 90 Minutes of Arrival[5]	0	-	85%	90%
Smoking Cessation Advice[1]	1	100%	99%	99%
Chest Pain/Possible Heart Attack Care				
Aspirin at Arrival	-	-	95%	95%
Median Time to ECG (minutes)	-	-	12	8
Median Time to Transfer (minutes)	-	-	77	61
Fibrinolytic Medication Timing	-	-	56%	54%
Heart Failure Care				
ACE Inhibitor or ARB for LVSD	25	96%	90%	94%
Discharge Instructions	88	100%	85%	88%
Evaluation of LVS Function	91	98%	97%	98%
Smoking Cessation Advice[1]	15	100%	97%	98%
Pneumonia Care				
Appropriate Initial Antibiotic	59	90%	89%	92%
Blood Culture Timing	93	99%	95%	96%
Influenza Vaccine	68	99%	90%	91%
Initial Antibiotic Timing	103	97%	94%	95%
Pneumococcal Vaccine	93	99%	91%	93%
Smoking Cessation Advice	29	100%	96%	97%
Surgical Care Improvement Project				
Appropriate VTP Within 24 Hours[2,5]	0	-	91%	92%
Appropriate Hair Removal[2,5]	0	-	99%	99%
Appropriate Beta Blocker Usage[2,5]	0	-	93%	93%
Controlled Postoperative Blood Glucose[2,5]	0	-	91%	93%
Prophylactic Antibiotic Timing[5]	0	-	97%	97%
Prophylactic Antibiotic Timing (Outpatient)	-	-	90%	92%
Prophylactic Antibiotic Selection[5]	0	-	97%	97%
Prophylactic Antibiotic Select. (Outpatient)	-	-	91%	94%
Prophylactic Antibiotic Stopped[5]	0	-	94%	94%
Recommended VTP Ordered[2,5]	0	-	92%	94%
Urinary Catheter Removal[2,5]	0	-	90%	90%
Children's Asthma Care				
Received Systemic Corticosteroids	-	-	-	100%
Received Home Management Plan	-	-	-	71%
Received Reliever Medication	-	-	-	100%
Use of Medical Imaging				
Combination Abdominal CT Scan	-	-	0.304	0.191
Combination Chest CT Scan	-	-	0.063	0.054
Follow-up Mammogram/Ultrasound	-	-	8.8%	8.4%
MRI for Low Back Pain	-	-	38.5%	32.7%
Survey of Patients' Hospital Experiences				
Area Around Room 'Always' Quiet at Night	-	-	-	58%
Doctors 'Always' Communicated Well	-	-	-	80%
Home Recovery Information Given	-	-	-	82%
Hospital Given 9 or 10 on 10 Point Scale	-	-	-	67%
Meds 'Always' Explained Before Given	-	-	-	60%
Nurses 'Always' Communicated Well	-	-	-	76%
Pain 'Always' Well Controlled	-	-	-	69%
Room and Bathroom 'Always' Clean	-	-	-	71%
Timely Help 'Always' Received	-	-	-	64%
Would Definitely Recommend Hospital	-	-	-	69%

NOTE: Hospital profiles are in alphabetical order by state, then city, then hospital within the city; Rankings exclude hospitals with less than 25 cases except for patient surveys which excludes hospitals with less than 100 cases; (a) 100–299 cases; (1) The number of cases is too small to be sure how well a hospital is performing; (2) The hospital indicated that the data submitted for this measure were based on a sample of cases; (3) Data was collected during a shorter time period (fewer quarters) than the maximum possible time for this measure; (4) Suppressed for one or more quarters by CMS; (5) No data is available from the hospital for this measure; (6) Fewer than 100 patients completed the HCAHPS survey. Use these rates with caution, as the number of surveys may be too low to reliably assess hospital performance; (7) Survey results are based on less than 12 months of data; (8) Survey results are not available for this reporting period; (9) No or very few patients were eligible for the HCAHPS survey. The scores shown, if any, reflect a very small number of surveys; (10) A state average was not calculated because too few hospitals in the state submitted data; (11) There were discrepancies in the data collection process; Please refer to the User's Guide for a full explanation of data.

Davis Memorial Hospital

PO Box 1484 Phone: 304-636-3300
Elkins, WV 26241 Fax: 304-637-3384
URL: davishealthcare.org
Type: Acute Care Hospitals Emergency Services: Yes
Ownership: Voluntary Non-Profit - Other Beds: 90

Key Personnel:
CEO/President. . . . . Mark Doak
Infection Control. . . . . Margaret Emma, RN
Quality Assurance . . . . Sandra Phillips
Radiology. . . . . Steven M Barnett
Emergency Room . . . . Susan E Bobes, MD

Measure	Cases	This Hosp.	State Avg.	U.S. Avg.
Heart Attack Care				
ACE Inhibitor or ARB for LVSD[1]	7	100%	94%	96%
Aspirin at Arrival	30	90%	97%	99%
Aspirin at Discharge[1]	18	100%	98%	98%
Beta Blocker at Discharge[1]	20	95%	98%	98%
Fibrinolytic Medication Timing	0	-	29%	55%
PCI Within 90 Minutes of Arrival	0	-	85%	90%
Smoking Cessation Advice[1]	5	100%	99%	99%
Chest Pain/Possible Heart Attack Care				
Aspirin at Arrival	216	97%	95%	95%
Median Time to ECG (minutes)	229	7	12	8
Median Time to Transfer (minutes)[1]	7	200	77	61
Fibrinolytic Medication Timing[1]	12	75%	56%	54%
Heart Failure Care				
ACE Inhibitor or ARB for LVSD	45	100%	90%	94%
Discharge Instructions	126	94%	85%	88%
Evaluation of LVS Function	138	100%	97%	98%
Smoking Cessation Advice[1]	21	100%	97%	98%
Pneumonia Care				
Appropriate Initial Antibiotic	92	89%	89%	92%
Blood Culture Timing	118	99%	95%	96%
Influenza Vaccine	81	91%	90%	91%
Initial Antibiotic Timing	107	97%	94%	95%
Pneumococcal Vaccine	102	94%	91%	93%
Smoking Cessation Advice	38	100%	96%	97%
Surgical Care Improvement Project				
Appropriate VTP Within 24 Hours	120	94%	91%	92%
Appropriate Hair Removal	322	100%	99%	99%
Appropriate Beta Blocker Usage	85	92%	93%	93%
Controlled Postoperative Blood Glucose	0	-	91%	93%
Prophylactic Antibiotic Timing	230	95%	97%	97%
Prophylactic Antibiotic Timing (Outpatient)	170	93%	90%	92%
Prophylactic Antibiotic Selection	230	97%	97%	97%
Prophylactic Antibiotic Select. (Outpatient)	162	98%	91%	94%
Prophylactic Antibiotic Stopped	222	96%	94%	94%
Recommended VTP Ordered	120	95%	92%	94%
Urinary Catheter Removal	50	90%	90%	90%
Children's Asthma Care				
Received Systemic Corticosteroids	-	-	-	100%
Received Home Management Plan	-	-	-	71%
Received Reliever Medication	-	-	-	100%
Use of Medical Imaging				
Combination Abdominal CT Scan	702	0.373	0.304	0.191
Combination Chest CT Scan	302	0.063	0.063	0.054
Follow-up Mammogram/Ultrasound	824	5.8%	8.8%	8.4%
MRI for Low Back Pain	102	33.3%	38.5%	32.7%
Survey of Patients' Hospital Experiences				
Area Around Room 'Always' Quiet at Night	300+	52%	-	58%
Doctors 'Always' Communicated Well	300+	80%	-	80%
Home Recovery Information Given	300+	86%	-	82%
Hospital Given 9 or 10 on 10 Point Scale	300+	63%	-	67%
Meds 'Always' Explained Before Given	300+	61%	-	60%
Nurses 'Always' Communicated Well	300+	78%	-	76%
Pain 'Always' Well Controlled	300+	70%	-	69%
Room and Bathroom 'Always' Clean	300+	76%	-	71%
Timely Help 'Always' Received	300+	65%	-	64%
Would Definitely Recommend Hospital	300+	62%	-	69%

Fairmont General Hospital

1325 Locust Avenue Phone: 304-367-7100
Fairmont, WV 26554 Fax: 304-367-7167
E-mail: info@fghi.com
URL: www.fghi.com
Type: Acute Care Hospitals Emergency Services: Yes
Ownership: Voluntary Non-Profit - Private Beds: 268

Key Personnel:
CEO/President. . . . . Albert Pilkerson, III
Cardiac Laboratory. . . . . Paul Alappha
Chief of Medical Staff. . . . . Joedy Daristotle, MD
Infection Control. . . . . Janet Crigler
Emergency Room . . . . Tina Straight

Measure	Cases	This Hosp.	State Avg.	U.S. Avg.
Heart Attack Care				
ACE Inhibitor or ARB for LVSD[1]	10	100%	94%	96%
Aspirin at Arrival	61	98%	97%	99%
Aspirin at Discharge	40	100%	98%	98%
Beta Blocker at Discharge	44	100%	98%	98%
Fibrinolytic Medication Timing	0	-	29%	55%
PCI Within 90 Minutes of Arrival	0	-	85%	90%
Smoking Cessation Advice[1]	10	100%	99%	99%
Chest Pain/Possible Heart Attack Care				
Aspirin at Arrival	156	98%	95%	95%
Median Time to ECG (minutes)	160	9	12	8
Median Time to Transfer (minutes)[1]	6	48	77	61
Fibrinolytic Medication Timing[1]	9	67%	56%	54%
Heart Failure Care				
ACE Inhibitor or ARB for LVSD	45	98%	90%	94%
Discharge Instructions	161	87%	85%	88%
Evaluation of LVS Function	213	100%	97%	98%
Smoking Cessation Advice[1]	23	100%	97%	98%
Pneumonia Care				
Appropriate Initial Antibiotic	105	95%	89%	92%
Blood Culture Timing	121	96%	95%	96%
Influenza Vaccine	116	98%	90%	91%
Initial Antibiotic Timing	138	99%	94%	95%
Pneumococcal Vaccine	161	99%	91%	93%
Smoking Cessation Advice	79	100%	96%	97%
Surgical Care Improvement Project				
Appropriate VTP Within 24 Hours	117	99%	91%	92%
Appropriate Hair Removal	216	100%	99%	99%
Appropriate Beta Blocker Usage	67	97%	93%	93%
Controlled Postoperative Blood Glucose	0	-	91%	93%
Prophylactic Antibiotic Timing	139	99%	97%	97%
Prophylactic Antibiotic Timing (Outpatient)	89	98%	90%	92%
Prophylactic Antibiotic Selection	139	100%	97%	97%
Prophylactic Antibiotic Select. (Outpatient)	87	94%	91%	94%
Prophylactic Antibiotic Stopped	124	100%	94%	94%
Recommended VTP Ordered	117	99%	92%	94%
Urinary Catheter Removal	32	97%	90%	90%
Children's Asthma Care				
Received Systemic Corticosteroids	-	-	-	100%
Received Home Management Plan	-	-	-	71%
Received Reliever Medication	-	-	-	100%
Use of Medical Imaging				
Combination Abdominal CT Scan	710	0.673	0.304	0.191
Combination Chest CT Scan	407	0.002	0.063	0.054
Follow-up Mammogram/Ultrasound	648	4.2%	8.8%	8.4%
MRI for Low Back Pain	143	41.3%	38.5%	32.7%
Survey of Patients' Hospital Experiences				
Area Around Room 'Always' Quiet at Night	300+	56%	-	58%
Doctors 'Always' Communicated Well	300+	83%	-	80%
Home Recovery Information Given	300+	84%	-	82%
Hospital Given 9 or 10 on 10 Point Scale	300+	63%	-	67%
Meds 'Always' Explained Before Given	300+	65%	-	60%
Nurses 'Always' Communicated Well	300+	78%	-	76%
Pain 'Always' Well Controlled	300+	74%	-	69%
Room and Bathroom 'Always' Clean	300+	74%	-	71%
Timely Help 'Always' Received	300+	65%	-	64%
Would Definitely Recommend Hospital	300+	62%	-	69%

Braxton County Memorial Hospital

100 Hoylman Drive Phone: 304-364-5156
Gassaway, WV 26624 Fax: 304-364-1154
URL: www.braxtonmemorial.org
Type: Critical Access Hospitals Emergency Services: Yes
Ownership: Voluntary Non-Profit - Private Beds: 25

Key Personnel:
CEO/President. . . . . Barbara Adams
Chief of Medical Staff. . . . . Russell Stewart, MD
Infection Control. . . . . Sharon Gaston, RN
Operating Room. . . . . Pam Bender, RN
Quality Assurance . . . . Sharon Gaston, RN
Anesthesiology. . . . . Pam Bender, RN
Emergency Room . . . . Jill Cotrill, RN

Measure	Cases	This Hosp.	State Avg.	U.S. Avg.
Heart Attack Care				
ACE Inhibitor or ARB for LVSD[5]	0	-	94%	96%
Aspirin at Arrival[5]	0	-	97%	99%
Aspirin at Discharge[5]	0	-	98%	98%
Beta Blocker at Discharge[5]	0	-	98%	98%
Fibrinolytic Medication Timing[5]	0	-	29%	55%
PCI Within 90 Minutes of Arrival[5]	0	-	85%	90%
Smoking Cessation Advice[5]	0	-	99%	99%
Chest Pain/Possible Heart Attack Care				
Aspirin at Arrival	-	-	95%	95%
Median Time to ECG (minutes)	-	-	12	8
Median Time to Transfer (minutes)	-	-	77	61
Fibrinolytic Medication Timing	-	-	56%	54%
Heart Failure Care				
ACE Inhibitor or ARB for LVSD[1]	17	47%	90%	94%
Discharge Instructions	31	55%	85%	88%
Evaluation of LVS Function	35	71%	97%	98%
Smoking Cessation Advice[1]	3	100%	97%	98%
Pneumonia Care				
Appropriate Initial Antibiotic	30	93%	89%	92%
Blood Culture Timing	39	72%	95%	96%
Influenza Vaccine	35	43%	90%	91%
Initial Antibiotic Timing	44	89%	94%	95%
Pneumococcal Vaccine	41	34%	91%	93%
Smoking Cessation Advice[1]	8	75%	96%	97%
Surgical Care Improvement Project				
Appropriate VTP Within 24 Hours[5]	0	-	91%	92%
Appropriate Hair Removal[5]	0	-	99%	99%
Appropriate Beta Blocker Usage[5]	0	-	93%	93%
Controlled Postoperative Blood Glucose[5]	0	-	91%	93%
Prophylactic Antibiotic Timing[5]	0	-	97%	97%
Prophylactic Antibiotic Timing (Outpatient)	-	-	90%	92%
Prophylactic Antibiotic Selection[5]	0	-	97%	97%
Prophylactic Antibiotic Select. (Outpatient)	-	-	91%	94%
Prophylactic Antibiotic Stopped[5]	0	-	94%	94%
Recommended VTP Ordered[5]	0	-	92%	94%
Urinary Catheter Removal[5]	0	-	90%	90%
Children's Asthma Care				
Received Systemic Corticosteroids	-	-	-	100%
Received Home Management Plan	-	-	-	71%
Received Reliever Medication	-	-	-	100%
Use of Medical Imaging				
Combination Abdominal CT Scan	-	-	0.304	0.191
Combination Chest CT Scan	-	-	0.063	0.054
Follow-up Mammogram/Ultrasound	-	-	8.8%	8.4%
MRI for Low Back Pain	-	-	38.5%	32.7%
Survey of Patients' Hospital Experiences				
Area Around Room 'Always' Quiet at Night	(a)	56%	-	58%
Doctors 'Always' Communicated Well	(a)	89%	-	80%
Home Recovery Information Given	(a)	83%	-	82%
Hospital Given 9 or 10 on 10 Point Scale	(a)	76%	-	67%
Meds 'Always' Explained Before Given	(a)	64%	-	60%
Nurses 'Always' Communicated Well	(a)	85%	-	76%
Pain 'Always' Well Controlled	(a)	73%	-	69%
Room and Bathroom 'Always' Clean	(a)	77%	-	71%
Timely Help 'Always' Received	(a)	74%	-	64%
Would Definitely Recommend Hospital	(a)	72%	-	69%

NOTE: Hospital profiles are in alphabetical order by state, then city, then hospital within the city; Rankings exclude hospitals with less than 25 cases except for patient surveys which excludes hospitals with less than 100 cases; (a) 100–299 cases; (1) The number of cases is too small to be sure how well a hospital is performing; (2) The hospital indicated that the data submitted for this measure were based on a sample of cases; (3) Data was collected during a shorter time period (fewer quarters) than the maximum possible time for this measure; (4) Suppressed for one or more quarters by CMS; (5) No data is available from the hospital for this measure; (6) Fewer than 100 patients completed the HCAHPS survey. Use these rates with caution, as the number of surveys may be too low to reliably assess hospital performance; (7) Survey results are based on less than 12 months of data; (8) Survey results are not available for this reporting period; (9) No or very few patients were eligible for the HCAHPS survey. The scores shown, if any, reflect a very small number of surveys; (10) A state average was not calculated because too few hospitals in the state submitted data; (11) There were discrepancies in the data collection process; Please refer to the User's Guide for a full explanation of data.

Reynolds Memorial Hospital

800 Wheeling Ave
Glen Dale, WV 26038
Phone: 304-843-3230
Fax: 304-843-3202
URL: www.reynoldsmemorial.com
Type: Acute Care Hospitals
Emergency Services: Yes
Ownership: Voluntary Non-Profit - Private
Beds: 233

Key Personnel:

CEO/President. . . . . John A Sicurella
Chief of Medical Staff. . . . . Robert B Wade, MD
Coronary Care . . . . Patti Kimple, RN
Infection Control. . . . . Patti Kimpel, RN
Quality Assurance . . . . Patricia Downey
Radiology. . . . . Frank D Diettinger
Emergency Room . . . . Debra L Henry, MD

Measure	Cases	This Hosp.	State Avg.	U.S. Avg.
Heart Attack Care				
ACE Inhibitor or ARB for LVSD[1]	6	50%	94%	96%
Aspirin at Arrival	37	86%	97%	99%
Aspirin at Discharge[1]	20	90%	98%	98%
Beta Blocker at Discharge[1]	22	86%	98%	98%
Fibrinolytic Medication Timing	0	-	29%	55%
PCI Within 90 Minutes of Arrival	0	-	85%	90%
Smoking Cessation Advice[1]	3	100%	99%	99%
Chest Pain/Possible Heart Attack Care				
Aspirin at Arrival[1]	12	100%	95%	95%
Median Time to ECG (minutes)[1]	12	8	12	8
Median Time to Transfer (minutes)[1,3]	6	33	77	61
Fibrinolytic Medication Timing[1,3]	1	100%	56%	54%
Heart Failure Care				
ACE Inhibitor or ARB for LVSD	43	72%	90%	94%
Discharge Instructions	87	92%	85%	88%
Evaluation of LVS Function	130	94%	97%	98%
Smoking Cessation Advice[1]	23	100%	97%	98%
Pneumonia Care				
Appropriate Initial Antibiotic	64	83%	89%	92%
Blood Culture Timing	48	88%	95%	96%
Influenza Vaccine	61	90%	90%	91%
Initial Antibiotic Timing	84	93%	94%	95%
Pneumococcal Vaccine	87	95%	91%	93%
Smoking Cessation Advice	33	97%	96%	97%
Surgical Care Improvement Project				
Appropriate VTP Within 24 Hours	44	82%	91%	92%
Appropriate Hair Removal	95	100%	99%	99%
Appropriate Beta Blocker Usage	29	90%	93%	93%
Controlled Postoperative Blood Glucose	0	-	91%	93%
Prophylactic Antibiotic Timing	72	96%	97%	97%
Prophylactic Antibiotic Timing (Outpatient)	31	94%	90%	92%
Prophylactic Antibiotic Selection	73	93%	97%	97%
Prophylactic Antibiotic Select. (Outpatient)	29	100%	91%	94%
Prophylactic Antibiotic Stopped	65	95%	94%	94%
Recommended VTP Ordered	44	82%	92%	94%
Urinary Catheter Removal[1]	19	95%	90%	90%
Children's Asthma Care				
Received Systemic Corticosteroids	-	-	-	100%
Received Home Management Plan	-	-	-	71%
Received Reliever Medication	-	-	-	100%
Use of Medical Imaging				
Combination Abdominal CT Scan	163	0.423	0.304	0.191
Combination Chest CT Scan	129	0.000	0.063	0.054
Follow-up Mammogram/Ultrasound	255	11.0%	8.8%	8.4%
MRI for Low Back Pain[1]	38	28.9%	38.5%	32.7%
Survey of Patients' Hospital Experiences				
Area Around Room 'Always' Quiet at Night	300+	51%	-	58%
Doctors 'Always' Communicated Well	300+	80%	-	80%
Home Recovery Information Given	300+	87%	-	82%
Hospital Given 9 or 10 on 10 Point Scale	300+	66%	-	67%
Meds 'Always' Explained Before Given	300+	64%	-	60%
Nurses 'Always' Communicated Well	300+	76%	-	76%
Pain 'Always' Well Controlled	300+	66%	-	69%
Room and Bathroom 'Always' Clean	300+	70%	-	71%
Timely Help 'Always' Received	300+	71%	-	64%
Would Definitely Recommend Hospital	300+	67%	-	69%

Grafton City Hospital

500 Market Street
Grafton, WV 26354
Phone: 304-265-0400
Fax: 304-265-3926
URL: www.graftonhospital.com
Type: Critical Access Hospitals
Emergency Services: Yes
Ownership: Government - Local
Beds: 136

Key Personnel:

CEO/President. . . . . Jeff Lilley
Chief of Medical Staff . . . . Christopher Z Villaraza II, II
Infection Control. . . . . Diana Knight
Operating Room. . . . . Debbie Lemasters
Quality Assurance . . . . Dan Swiger
Anesthesiology. . . . . Mona Grandstaff CRNA
Emergency Room . . . . Thomas Lauderman
Patient Relations . . . . Kathy Matheney

Measure	Cases	This Hosp.	State Avg.	U.S. Avg.
Heart Attack Care				
ACE Inhibitor or ARB for LVSD[5]	0	-	94%	96%
Aspirin at Arrival[5]	0	-	97%	99%
Aspirin at Discharge[5]	0	-	98%	98%
Beta Blocker at Discharge[5]	0	-	98%	98%
Fibrinolytic Medication Timing[5]	0	-	29%	55%
PCI Within 90 Minutes of Arrival[5]	0	-	85%	90%
Smoking Cessation Advice[5]	0	-	99%	99%
Chest Pain/Possible Heart Attack Care				
Aspirin at Arrival	-	-	95%	95%
Median Time to ECG (minutes)	-	-	12	8
Median Time to Transfer (minutes)	-	-	77	61
Fibrinolytic Medication Timing	-	-	56%	54%
Heart Failure Care				
ACE Inhibitor or ARB for LVSD[1]	5	100%	90%	94%
Discharge Instructions[1]	14	100%	85%	88%
Evaluation of LVS Function[1]	18	100%	97%	98%
Smoking Cessation Advice[1]	2	100%	97%	98%
Pneumonia Care				
Appropriate Initial Antibiotic[1]	12	50%	89%	92%
Blood Culture Timing[1]	12	92%	95%	96%
Influenza Vaccine[1]	16	94%	90%	91%
Initial Antibiotic Timing	25	88%	94%	95%
Pneumococcal Vaccine[1]	20	85%	91%	93%
Smoking Cessation Advice[1]	9	33%	96%	97%
Surgical Care Improvement Project				
Appropriate VTP Within 24 Hours[5]	0	-	91%	92%
Appropriate Hair Removal[5]	0	-	99%	99%
Appropriate Beta Blocker Usage[5]	0	-	93%	93%
Controlled Postoperative Blood Glucose[5]	0	-	91%	93%
Prophylactic Antibiotic Timing[5]	0	-	97%	97%
Prophylactic Antibiotic Timing (Outpatient)	-	-	90%	92%
Prophylactic Antibiotic Selection[5]	0	-	97%	97%
Prophylactic Antibiotic Select. (Outpatient)	-	-	91%	94%
Prophylactic Antibiotic Stopped[5]	0	-	94%	94%
Recommended VTP Ordered[5]	0	-	92%	94%
Urinary Catheter Removal[5]	0	-	90%	90%
Children's Asthma Care				
Received Systemic Corticosteroids	-	-	-	100%
Received Home Management Plan	-	-	-	71%
Received Reliever Medication	-	-	-	100%
Use of Medical Imaging				
Combination Abdominal CT Scan	-	-	0.304	0.191
Combination Chest CT Scan	-	-	0.063	0.054
Follow-up Mammogram/Ultrasound	-	-	8.8%	8.4%
MRI for Low Back Pain	-	-	38.5%	32.7%
Survey of Patients' Hospital Experiences				
Area Around Room 'Always' Quiet at Night[8]	-	-	-	58%
Doctors 'Always' Communicated Well[8]	-	-	-	80%
Home Recovery Information Given[8]	-	-	-	82%
Hospital Given 9 or 10 on 10 Point Scale[8]	-	-	-	67%
Meds 'Always' Explained Before Given[8]	-	-	-	60%
Nurses 'Always' Communicated Well[8]	-	-	-	76%
Pain 'Always' Well Controlled[8]	-	-	-	69%
Room and Bathroom 'Always' Clean[8]	-	-	-	71%
Timely Help 'Always' Received[8]	-	-	-	64%
Would Definitely Recommend Hospital[8]	-	-	-	69%

Minnie Hamilton Health Care Center

186 Hospital Drive
Grantsville, WV 26147
Phone: 304-354-9244
Type: Critical Access Hospitals
Emergency Services: Yes
Ownership: Voluntary Non-Profit - Private

Key Personnel:

CEO/President. . . . . Barbara Lay
Chief of Medical Staff . . . . Vishwanath Hande MD
Quality Assurance . . . . Sandra Ellis
Radiology. . . . . Cheryl Balisciano
Emergency Room . . . . Trudy Anderson RN

Measure	Cases	This Hosp.	State Avg.	U.S. Avg.
Heart Attack Care				
ACE Inhibitor or ARB for LVSD[5]	0	-	94%	96%
Aspirin at Arrival[5]	0	-	97%	99%
Aspirin at Discharge[5]	0	-	98%	98%
Beta Blocker at Discharge[5]	0	-	98%	98%
Fibrinolytic Medication Timing[5]	0	-	29%	55%
PCI Within 90 Minutes of Arrival[5]	0	-	85%	90%
Smoking Cessation Advice[5]	0	-	99%	99%
Chest Pain/Possible Heart Attack Care				
Aspirin at Arrival	-	-	95%	95%
Median Time to ECG (minutes)	-	-	12	8
Median Time to Transfer (minutes)	-	-	77	61
Fibrinolytic Medication Timing	-	-	56%	54%
Heart Failure Care				
ACE Inhibitor or ARB for LVSD[5]	0	-	90%	94%
Discharge Instructions[5]	0	-	85%	88%
Evaluation of LVS Function[5]	0	-	97%	98%
Smoking Cessation Advice[5]	0	-	97%	98%
Pneumonia Care				
Appropriate Initial Antibiotic[5]	0	-	89%	92%
Blood Culture Timing[5]	0	-	95%	96%
Influenza Vaccine[5]	0	-	90%	91%
Initial Antibiotic Timing[5]	0	-	94%	95%
Pneumococcal Vaccine[5]	0	-	91%	93%
Smoking Cessation Advice[5]	0	-	96%	97%
Surgical Care Improvement Project				
Appropriate VTP Within 24 Hours[5]	0	-	91%	92%
Appropriate Hair Removal[5]	0	-	99%	99%
Appropriate Beta Blocker Usage[5]	0	-	93%	93%
Controlled Postoperative Blood Glucose[5]	0	-	91%	93%
Prophylactic Antibiotic Timing[5]	0	-	97%	97%
Prophylactic Antibiotic Timing (Outpatient)	-	-	90%	92%
Prophylactic Antibiotic Selection[5]	0	-	97%	97%
Prophylactic Antibiotic Select. (Outpatient)	-	-	91%	94%
Prophylactic Antibiotic Stopped[5]	0	-	94%	94%
Recommended VTP Ordered[5]	0	-	92%	94%
Urinary Catheter Removal[5]	0	-	90%	90%
Children's Asthma Care				
Received Systemic Corticosteroids	-	-	-	100%
Received Home Management Plan	-	-	-	71%
Received Reliever Medication	-	-	-	100%
Use of Medical Imaging				
Combination Abdominal CT Scan	-	-	0.304	0.191
Combination Chest CT Scan	-	-	0.063	0.054
Follow-up Mammogram/Ultrasound	-	-	8.8%	8.4%
MRI for Low Back Pain	-	-	38.5%	32.7%
Survey of Patients' Hospital Experiences				
Area Around Room 'Always' Quiet at Night[8]	-	-	-	58%
Doctors 'Always' Communicated Well[8]	-	-	-	80%
Home Recovery Information Given[8]	-	-	-	82%
Hospital Given 9 or 10 on 10 Point Scale[8]	-	-	-	67%
Meds 'Always' Explained Before Given[8]	-	-	-	60%
Nurses 'Always' Communicated Well[8]	-	-	-	76%
Pain 'Always' Well Controlled[8]	-	-	-	69%
Room and Bathroom 'Always' Clean[8]	-	-	-	71%
Timely Help 'Always' Received[8]	-	-	-	64%
Would Definitely Recommend Hospital[8]	-	-	-	69%

NOTE: Hospital profiles are in alphabetical order by state, then city, then hospital within the city; Rankings exclude hospitals with less than 25 cases except for patient surveys which excludes hospitals with less than 100 cases; (a) 100–299 cases; (1) The number of cases is too small to be sure how well a hospital is performing; (2) The hospital indicated that the data submitted for this measure were based on a sample of cases; (3) Data was collected during a shorter time period (fewer quarters) than the maximum possible time for this measure; (4) Suppressed for one or more quarters by CMS; (5) No data is available from the hospital for this measure; (6) Fewer than 100 patients completed the HCAHPS survey. Use these rates with caution, as the number of surveys may be too low to reliably assess hospital performance; (7) Survey results are based on less than 12 months of data; (8) Survey results are not available for this reporting period; (9) No or very few patients were eligible for the HCAHPS survey. The scores shown, if any, reflect a very small number of surveys; (10) A state average was not calculated because too few hospitals in the state submitted data; (11) There were discrepancies in the data collection process; Please refer to the User's Guide for a full explanation of data.

Summers County ARH Hospital

1500 Terrace Street Phone: 304-466-1000
Hinton, WV 25951 Fax: 304-466-1690
E-mail: nwhitleck@arh.org
URL: www.arh.org/summers%20county
Type: Critical Access Hospitals Emergency Services: Yes
Ownership: Voluntary Non-Profit - Private Beds: 89

Key Personnel:

CEO/President.............. Chris Vaught
Cardiac Laboratory............ Ajay Anand, MD
Radiology.................... Daniel D Maxwell
Emergency Room .... Amarinder S Chhabra, MD

Measure	Cases	This Hosp.	State Avg.	U.S. Avg.
Heart Attack Care				
ACE Inhibitor or ARB for LVSD	0	-	94%	96%
Aspirin at Arrival[1]	2	100%	97%	99%
Aspirin at Discharge	0	-	98%	98%
Beta Blocker at Discharge	0	-	98%	98%
Fibrinolytic Medication Timing	0	-	29%	55%
PCI Within 90 Minutes of Arrival	0	-	85%	90%
Smoking Cessation Advice	0	-	99%	99%
Chest Pain/Possible Heart Attack Care				
Aspirin at Arrival	-	-	95%	95%
Median Time to ECG (minutes)	-	-	12	8
Median Time to Transfer (minutes)	-	-	77	61
Fibrinolytic Medication Timing	-	-	56%	54%
Heart Failure Care				
ACE Inhibitor or ARB for LVSD[1]	13	92%	90%	94%
Discharge Instructions	29	93%	85%	88%
Evaluation of LVS Function	43	100%	97%	98%
Smoking Cessation Advice[1]	10	90%	97%	98%
Pneumonia Care				
Appropriate Initial Antibiotic	32	94%	89%	92%
Blood Culture Timing	34	97%	95%	96%
Influenza Vaccine	29	90%	90%	91%
Initial Antibiotic Timing	41	100%	94%	95%
Pneumococcal Vaccine	37	86%	91%	93%
Smoking Cessation Advice[1]	20	100%	96%	97%
Surgical Care Improvement Project				
Appropriate VTP Within 24 Hours[5]	0	-	91%	92%
Appropriate Hair Removal[5]	0	-	99%	99%
Appropriate Beta Blocker Usage[5]	0	-	93%	93%
Controlled Postoperative Blood Glucose[5]	0	-	91%	93%
Prophylactic Antibiotic Timing[5]	0	-	97%	97%
Prophylactic Antibiotic Timing (Outpatient)	-	-	90%	92%
Prophylactic Antibiotic Selection[5]	0	-	97%	97%
Prophylactic Antibiotic Select. (Outpatient)	-	-	91%	94%
Prophylactic Antibiotic Stopped[5]	0	-	94%	94%
Recommended VTP Ordered[5]	0	-	92%	94%
Urinary Catheter Removal[5]	0	-	90%	90%
Children's Asthma Care				
Received Systemic Corticosteroids	-	-	-	100%
Received Home Management Plan	-	-	-	71%
Received Reliever Medication	-	-	-	100%
Use of Medical Imaging				
Combination Abdominal CT Scan	-	-	0.304	0.191
Combination Chest CT Scan	-	-	0.063	0.054
Follow-up Mammogram/Ultrasound	-	-	8.8%	8.4%
MRI for Low Back Pain	-	-	38.5%	32.7%
Survey of Patients' Hospital Experiences				
Area Around Room 'Always' Quiet at Night	(a)	63%	-	58%
Doctors 'Always' Communicated Well	(a)	92%	-	80%
Home Recovery Information Given	(a)	81%	-	82%
Hospital Given 9 or 10 on 10 Point Scale	(a)	81%	-	67%
Meds 'Always' Explained Before Given	(a)	71%	-	60%
Nurses 'Always' Communicated Well	(a)	86%	-	76%
Pain 'Always' Well Controlled	(a)	81%	-	69%
Room and Bathroom 'Always' Clean	(a)	83%	-	71%
Timely Help 'Always' Received	(a)	76%	-	64%
Would Definitely Recommend Hospital	(a)	81%	-	69%

Cabell-Huntington Hospital

1340 Hal Greer Boulevard Phone: 304-526-2000
Huntington, WV 25701 Fax: 304-526-6077
E-mail: info@cabellhuntington.org
URL: www.cabellhuntington.org
Type: Acute Care Hospitals Emergency Services: Yes
Ownership: Voluntary Non-Profit - Private Beds: 280

Key Personnel:

CEO/President............... Brent A Marsteller
Chief of Medical Staff.......... Hoyt Burdick
Operating Room.............. Debbie Ball, RN
Pediatric In-Patient Care .... Gilbert Ratcliff
Quality Assurance .... Deanna Parsons
Radiology..................... John Duncan

Measure	Cases	This Hosp.	State Avg.	U.S. Avg.
Heart Attack Care				
ACE Inhibitor or ARB for LVSD[1]	7	100%	94%	96%
Aspirin at Arrival	32	97%	97%	99%
Aspirin at Discharge[1]	18	100%	98%	98%
Beta Blocker at Discharge[1]	19	95%	98%	98%
Fibrinolytic Medication Timing	0	-	29%	55%
PCI Within 90 Minutes of Arrival	0	-	85%	90%
Smoking Cessation Advice[1]	3	100%	99%	99%
Chest Pain/Possible Heart Attack Care				
Aspirin at Arrival	34	97%	95%	95%
Median Time to ECG (minutes)	36	11	12	8
Median Time to Transfer (minutes)[1,3]	13	112	77	61
Fibrinolytic Medication Timing[3]	0	-	56%	54%
Heart Failure Care				
ACE Inhibitor or ARB for LVSD	45	96%	90%	94%
Discharge Instructions	121	87%	85%	88%
Evaluation of LVS Function	150	99%	97%	98%
Smoking Cessation Advice	36	100%	97%	98%
Pneumonia Care				
Appropriate Initial Antibiotic	61	98%	89%	92%
Blood Culture Timing	193	97%	95%	96%
Influenza Vaccine	128	93%	90%	91%
Initial Antibiotic Timing	192	95%	94%	95%
Pneumococcal Vaccine	142	97%	91%	93%
Smoking Cessation Advice	155	100%	96%	97%
Surgical Care Improvement Project				
Appropriate VTP Within 24 Hours[2]	141	97%	91%	92%
Appropriate Hair Removal[2]	441	100%	99%	99%
Appropriate Beta Blocker Usage[2]	120	94%	93%	93%
Controlled Postoperative Blood Glucose[2]	0	-	91%	93%
Prophylactic Antibiotic Timing[2]	295	96%	97%	97%
Prophylactic Antibiotic Timing (Outpatient)	186	84%	90%	92%
Prophylactic Antibiotic Selection[2]	297	95%	97%	97%
Prophylactic Antibiotic Select. (Outpatient)	255	96%	91%	94%
Prophylactic Antibiotic Stopped[2]	283	93%	94%	94%
Recommended VTP Ordered[2]	141	99%	92%	94%
Urinary Catheter Removal[2]	36	89%	90%	90%
Children's Asthma Care				
Received Systemic Corticosteroids	-	-	-	100%
Received Home Management Plan	-	-	-	71%
Received Reliever Medication	-	-	-	100%
Use of Medical Imaging				
Combination Abdominal CT Scan	988	0.046	0.304	0.191
Combination Chest CT Scan	581	0.024	0.063	0.054
Follow-up Mammogram/Ultrasound	1,749	11.4%	8.8%	8.4%
MRI for Low Back Pain	134	35.8%	38.5%	32.7%
Survey of Patients' Hospital Experiences				
Area Around Room 'Always' Quiet at Night	300+	68%	-	58%
Doctors 'Always' Communicated Well	300+	80%	-	80%
Home Recovery Information Given	300+	83%	-	82%
Hospital Given 9 or 10 on 10 Point Scale	300+	75%	-	67%
Meds 'Always' Explained Before Given	300+	62%	-	60%
Nurses 'Always' Communicated Well	300+	77%	-	76%
Pain 'Always' Well Controlled	300+	72%	-	69%
Room and Bathroom 'Always' Clean	300+	74%	-	71%
Timely Help 'Always' Received	300+	67%	-	64%
Would Definitely Recommend Hospital	300+	76%	-	69%

Huntington VA Medical Center

1540 Spring Valley Road Phone: 304-429-0241
Huntington, WV 25704 Fax: 304-429-6713
E-mail: jerrishaffer@med.va.gov
URL: www.huntington.med.gov
Type: Acute Care-Veterans Administration Emergency Services: No
Ownership: Government - Federal Beds: 80

Key Personnel:

CEO/President.............. Gale Beamen
Cardiac Laboratory............ Richard Stevenson, MD
Chief of Medical Staff.......... Joseph A Pellecchia, MD
Infection Control.............. Roberta Messner, RN
Operating Room.............. Nancy Hutchinson, RN
Quality Assurance .... Carole Bachtel, RN

Measure	Cases	This Hosp.	State Avg.	U.S. Avg.
Heart Attack Care				
ACE Inhibitor or ARB for LVSD[1]	3	100%	94%	96%
Aspirin at Arrival[1]	23	100%	97%	99%
Aspirin at Discharge[1]	12	100%	98%	98%
Beta Blocker at Discharge[1]	12	100%	98%	98%
Fibrinolytic Medication Timing[5]	0	-	29%	55%
PCI Within 90 Minutes of Arrival[5]	0	-	85%	90%
Smoking Cessation Advice[1]	6	100%	99%	99%
Chest Pain/Possible Heart Attack Care				
Aspirin at Arrival	-	-	95%	95%
Median Time to ECG (minutes)	-	-	12	8
Median Time to Transfer (minutes)	-	-	77	61
Fibrinolytic Medication Timing	-	-	56%	54%
Heart Failure Care				
ACE Inhibitor or ARB for LVSD	66	94%	90%	94%
Discharge Instructions	157	100%	85%	88%
Evaluation of LVS Function	168	100%	97%	98%
Smoking Cessation Advice	43	100%	97%	98%
Pneumonia Care				
Appropriate Initial Antibiotic	77	96%	89%	92%
Blood Culture Timing	178	99%	95%	96%
Influenza Vaccine	119	95%	90%	91%
Initial Antibiotic Timing	113	99%	94%	95%
Pneumococcal Vaccine	168	98%	91%	93%
Smoking Cessation Advice	88	100%	96%	97%
Surgical Care Improvement Project				
Appropriate VTP Within 24 Hours[2]	94	98%	91%	92%
Appropriate Hair Removal[2]	182	99%	99%	99%
Appropriate Beta Blocker Usage[2]	75	100%	93%	93%
Controlled Postoperative Blood Glucose[2,5]	0	-	91%	93%
Prophylactic Antibiotic Timing	121	99%	97%	97%
Prophylactic Antibiotic Timing (Outpatient)	-	-	90%	92%
Prophylactic Antibiotic Selection	122	100%	97%	97%
Prophylactic Antibiotic Select. (Outpatient)	-	-	91%	94%
Prophylactic Antibiotic Stopped	116	100%	94%	94%
Recommended VTP Ordered[2]	94	99%	92%	94%
Urinary Catheter Removal[2]	103	100%	90%	90%
Children's Asthma Care				
Received Systemic Corticosteroids	-	-	-	100%
Received Home Management Plan	-	-	-	71%
Received Reliever Medication	-	-	-	100%
Use of Medical Imaging				
Combination Abdominal CT Scan	-	-	0.304	0.191
Combination Chest CT Scan	-	-	0.063	0.054
Follow-up Mammogram/Ultrasound	-	-	8.8%	8.4%
MRI for Low Back Pain	-	-	38.5%	32.7%
Survey of Patients' Hospital Experiences				
Area Around Room 'Always' Quiet at Night	-	-	-	58%
Doctors 'Always' Communicated Well	-	-	-	80%
Home Recovery Information Given	-	-	-	82%
Hospital Given 9 or 10 on 10 Point Scale	-	-	-	67%
Meds 'Always' Explained Before Given	-	-	-	60%
Nurses 'Always' Communicated Well	-	-	-	76%
Pain 'Always' Well Controlled	-	-	-	69%
Room and Bathroom 'Always' Clean	-	-	-	71%
Timely Help 'Always' Received	-	-	-	64%
Would Definitely Recommend Hospital	-	-	-	69%

NOTE: Hospital profiles are in alphabetical order by state, then city, then hospital within the city; Rankings exclude hospitals with less than 25 cases except for patient surveys which excludes hospitals with less than 100 cases; (a) 100–299 cases; (1) The number of cases is too small to be sure how well a hospital is performing; (2) The hospital indicated that the data submitted for this measure were based on a sample of cases; (3) Data was collected during a shorter time period (fewer quarters) than the maximum possible time for this measure; (4) Suppressed for one or more quarters by CMS; (5) No data is available from the hospital for this measure; (6) Fewer than 100 patients completed the HCAHPS survey. Use these rates with caution, as the number of surveys may be too low to reliably assess hospital performance; (7) Survey results are based on less than 12 months of data; (8) Survey results are not available for this reporting period; (9) No or very few patients were eligible for the HCAHPS survey. The scores shown, if any, reflect a very small number of surveys; (10) A state average was not calculated because too few hospitals in the state submitted data; (11) There were discrepancies in the data collection process; Please refer to the User's Guide for a full explanation of data.

Saint Mary's Medical Center

2900 1st Avenue
Huntington, WV 25701
URL: www.st-marys.org
Type: Acute Care Hospitals
Ownership: Voluntary Non-Profit - Church

Phone: 304-526-1234
Fax: 304-526-8996
Emergency Services: No
Beds: 393

Key Personnel:
CEO/President . . . . Michael G Selleards
Chief of Medical Staff . . . . James Goetz
Infection Control . . . . Anita Fahirety
Operating Room . . . . Tammy Nimmo
Pediatric Ambulatory Care . . . . . . James Lewis
Pediatric In-Patient Care . . . . James Lewis
Quality Assurance . . . . Pat Stultz
Radiology . . . . Paul Akers

Measure	Cases	This Hosp.	State Avg.	U.S. Avg.
Heart Attack Care				
ACE Inhibitor or ARB for LVSD	77	94%	94%	96%
Aspirin at Arrival	357	98%	97%	99%
Aspirin at Discharge	576	100%	98%	98%
Beta Blocker at Discharge	560	99%	98%	98%
Fibrinolytic Medication Timing	0	-	29%	55%
PCI Within 90 Minutes of Arrival	64	97%	85%	90%
Smoking Cessation Advice	257	100%	99%	99%
Chest Pain/Possible Heart Attack Care				
Aspirin at Arrival[5]	0	-	95%	95%
Median Time to ECG (minutes)[5]	0	-	12	8
Median Time to Transfer (minutes)[5]	0	-	77	61
Fibrinolytic Medication Timing[5]	0	-	56%	54%
Heart Failure Care				
ACE Inhibitor or ARB for LVSD	136	92%	90%	94%
Discharge Instructions	451	90%	85%	88%
Evaluation of LVS Function	525	100%	97%	98%
Smoking Cessation Advice	102	100%	97%	98%
Pneumonia Care				
Appropriate Initial Antibiotic	317	95%	89%	92%
Blood Culture Timing	590	97%	95%	96%
Influenza Vaccine	285	88%	90%	91%
Initial Antibiotic Timing	580	93%	94%	95%
Pneumococcal Vaccine	445	91%	91%	93%
Smoking Cessation Advice	260	99%	96%	97%
Surgical Care Improvement Project				
Appropriate VTP Within 24 Hours[2]	237	88%	91%	92%
Appropriate Hair Removal[2]	1,204	100%	99%	99%
Appropriate Beta Blocker Usage[2]	453	96%	93%	93%
Controlled Postoperative Blood Glucose[2]	312	98%	91%	93%
Prophylactic Antibiotic Timing[2]	965	98%	97%	97%
Prophylactic Antibiotic Timing (Outpatient)	448	91%	90%	92%
Prophylactic Antibiotic Selection[2]	981	98%	97%	97%
Prophylactic Antibiotic Select. (Outpatient)	422	89%	91%	94%
Prophylactic Antibiotic Stopped[2]	904	96%	94%	94%
Recommended VTP Ordered[2]	237	94%	92%	94%
Urinary Catheter Removal[2]	383	95%	90%	90%
Children's Asthma Care				
Received Systemic Corticosteroids	-	-	-	100%
Received Home Management Plan	-	-	-	71%
Received Reliever Medication	-	-	-	100%
Use of Medical Imaging				
Combination Abdominal CT Scan	1,399	0.083	0.304	0.191
Combination Chest CT Scan	720	0.001	0.063	0.054
Follow-up Mammogram/Ultrasound	967	9.7%	8.8%	8.4%
MRI for Low Back Pain	75	37.3%	38.5%	32.7%
Survey of Patients' Hospital Experiences				
Area Around Room 'Always' Quiet at Night	300+	54%	-	58%
Doctors 'Always' Communicated Well	300+	79%	-	80%
Home Recovery Information Given	300+	82%	-	82%
Hospital Given 9 or 10 on 10 Point Scale	300+	74%	-	67%
Meds 'Always' Explained Before Given	300+	60%	-	60%
Nurses 'Always' Communicated Well	300+	80%	-	76%
Pain 'Always' Well Controlled	300+	70%	-	69%
Room and Bathroom 'Always' Clean	300+	80%	-	71%
Timely Help 'Always' Received	300+	63%	-	64%
Would Definitely Recommend Hospital	300+	80%	-	69%

Camc Teays Valley Hospital

1400 Hospital Drive
Hurricane, WV 25526
Type: Acute Care Hospitals
Ownership: Voluntary Non-Profit - Private

Phone: 304-757-1700
Fax: 304-757-1732
Emergency Services: No
Beds: 68

Key Personnel:
CEO/President . . . . Patsy Hardy
Chief of Medical Staff . . . . Rick Houdersheldt, DO
Infection Control . . . . Sue Ellis, RN
Operating Room . . . . Jeff Fleck, RN
Quality Assurance . . . . Sue Ellis
Anesthesiology . . . . David Maxson, MD
Emergency Room . . . . Gregory Kelly, DO
Intensive Care Unit . . . . Tammie Hiles, RN

Measure	Cases	This Hosp.	State Avg.	U.S. Avg.
Heart Attack Care				
ACE Inhibitor or ARB for LVSD[1]	1	0%	94%	96%
Aspirin at Arrival[1]	15	87%	97%	99%
Aspirin at Discharge[1]	6	100%	98%	98%
Beta Blocker at Discharge[1]	6	100%	98%	98%
Fibrinolytic Medication Timing	0	-	29%	55%
PCI Within 90 Minutes of Arrival	0	-	85%	90%
Smoking Cessation Advice[1]	1	100%	99%	99%
Chest Pain/Possible Heart Attack Care				
Aspirin at Arrival[1]	24	83%	95%	95%
Median Time to ECG (minutes)	26	30	12	8
Median Time to Transfer (minutes)[5]	0	-	77	61
Fibrinolytic Medication Timing[3]	0	-	56%	54%
Heart Failure Care				
ACE Inhibitor or ARB for LVSD	36	89%	90%	94%
Discharge Instructions	47	70%	85%	88%
Evaluation of LVS Function	60	100%	97%	98%
Smoking Cessation Advice[1]	8	100%	97%	98%
Pneumonia Care				
Appropriate Initial Antibiotic	70	89%	89%	92%
Blood Culture Timing	95	91%	95%	96%
Influenza Vaccine	68	82%	90%	91%
Initial Antibiotic Timing	88	92%	94%	95%
Pneumococcal Vaccine	83	86%	91%	93%
Smoking Cessation Advice	43	98%	96%	97%
Surgical Care Improvement Project				
Appropriate VTP Within 24 Hours	70	80%	91%	92%
Appropriate Hair Removal	155	99%	99%	99%
Appropriate Beta Blocker Usage	52	85%	93%	93%
Controlled Postoperative Blood Glucose	0	-	91%	93%
Prophylactic Antibiotic Timing	85	91%	97%	97%
Prophylactic Antibiotic Timing (Outpatient)[3]	48	96%	90%	92%
Prophylactic Antibiotic Selection	88	95%	97%	97%
Prophylactic Antibiotic Select. (Outpatient)[3]	47	83%	91%	94%
Prophylactic Antibiotic Stopped	83	90%	94%	94%
Recommended VTP Ordered	70	89%	92%	94%
Urinary Catheter Removal	47	94%	90%	90%
Children's Asthma Care				
Received Systemic Corticosteroids	-	-	-	100%
Received Home Management Plan	-	-	-	71%
Received Reliever Medication	-	-	-	100%
Use of Medical Imaging				
Combination Abdominal CT Scan	417	0.055	0.304	0.191
Combination Chest CT Scan	278	0.004	0.063	0.054
Follow-up Mammogram/Ultrasound	339	10.6%	8.8%	8.4%
MRI for Low Back Pain	95	40.0%	38.5%	32.7%
Survey of Patients' Hospital Experiences				
Area Around Room 'Always' Quiet at Night	300+	35%	-	58%
Doctors 'Always' Communicated Well	300+	78%	-	80%
Home Recovery Information Given	300+	78%	-	82%
Hospital Given 9 or 10 on 10 Point Scale	300+	59%	-	67%
Meds 'Always' Explained Before Given	300+	59%	-	60%
Nurses 'Always' Communicated Well	300+	68%	-	76%
Pain 'Always' Well Controlled	300+	64%	-	69%
Room and Bathroom 'Always' Clean	300+	65%	-	71%
Timely Help 'Always' Received	300+	50%	-	64%
Would Definitely Recommend Hospital	300+	59%	-	69%

Potomac Valley Hospital

100 Pin Oak Lane
Keyser, WV 26726
Type: Critical Access Hospitals
Ownership: Voluntary Non-Profit - Private

Phone: 304-597-3500
Fax: 304-597-1118
Emergency Services: Yes
Beds: 25

Key Personnel:
CEO/President . . . . Michael Makosky

Measure	Cases	This Hosp.	State Avg.	U.S. Avg.
Heart Attack Care				
ACE Inhibitor or ARB for LVSD[1,3]	1	100%	94%	96%
Aspirin at Arrival[1,3]	7	86%	97%	99%
Aspirin at Discharge[1,3]	5	80%	98%	98%
Beta Blocker at Discharge[1,3]	5	100%	98%	98%
Fibrinolytic Medication Timing[3]	0	-	29%	55%
PCI Within 90 Minutes of Arrival[3]	0	-	85%	90%
Smoking Cessation Advice[3]	0	-	99%	99%
Chest Pain/Possible Heart Attack Care				
Aspirin at Arrival	-	-	95%	95%
Median Time to ECG (minutes)	-	-	12	8
Median Time to Transfer (minutes)	-	-	77	61
Fibrinolytic Medication Timing	-	-	56%	54%
Heart Failure Care				
ACE Inhibitor or ARB for LVSD[1]	11	91%	90%	94%
Discharge Instructions	34	76%	85%	88%
Evaluation of LVS Function	38	92%	97%	98%
Smoking Cessation Advice[1]	4	75%	97%	98%
Pneumonia Care				
Appropriate Initial Antibiotic[2]	30	100%	89%	92%
Blood Culture Timing[2]	28	96%	95%	96%
Influenza Vaccine[1,2]	19	68%	90%	91%
Initial Antibiotic Timing[2]	31	90%	94%	95%
Pneumococcal Vaccine[1,2]	21	86%	91%	93%
Smoking Cessation Advice[1,2]	9	100%	96%	97%
Surgical Care Improvement Project				
Appropriate VTP Within 24 Hours[1,3]	5	80%	91%	92%
Appropriate Hair Removal[1,3]	16	100%	99%	99%
Appropriate Beta Blocker Usage[5]	0	-	93%	93%
Controlled Postoperative Blood Glucose[3]	0	-	91%	93%
Prophylactic Antibiotic Timing[1,3]	13	77%	97%	97%
Prophylactic Antibiotic Timing (Outpatient)	-	-	90%	92%
Prophylactic Antibiotic Selection[1,3]	13	85%	97%	97%
Prophylactic Antibiotic Select. (Outpatient)	-	-	91%	94%
Prophylactic Antibiotic Stopped[1,3]	13	85%	94%	94%
Recommended VTP Ordered[1,3]	5	80%	92%	94%
Urinary Catheter Removal[1]	9	89%	90%	90%
Children's Asthma Care				
Received Systemic Corticosteroids	-	-	-	100%
Received Home Management Plan	-	-	-	71%
Received Reliever Medication	-	-	-	100%
Use of Medical Imaging				
Combination Abdominal CT Scan	-	-	0.304	0.191
Combination Chest CT Scan	-	-	0.063	0.054
Follow-up Mammogram/Ultrasound	-	-	8.8%	8.4%
MRI for Low Back Pain	-	-	38.5%	32.7%
Survey of Patients' Hospital Experiences				
Area Around Room 'Always' Quiet at Night[8]	-	-	-	58%
Doctors 'Always' Communicated Well[8]	-	-	-	80%
Home Recovery Information Given[8]	-	-	-	82%
Hospital Given 9 or 10 on 10 Point Scale[8]	-	-	-	67%
Meds 'Always' Explained Before Given[8]	-	-	-	60%
Nurses 'Always' Communicated Well[8]	-	-	-	76%
Pain 'Always' Well Controlled[8]	-	-	-	69%
Room and Bathroom 'Always' Clean[8]	-	-	-	71%
Timely Help 'Always' Received[8]	-	-	-	64%
Would Definitely Recommend Hospital[8]	-	-	-	69%

NOTE: Hospital profiles are in alphabetical order by state, then city, then hospital within the city; Rankings exclude hospitals with less than 25 cases except for patient surveys which excludes hospitals with less than 100 cases; (a) 100–299 cases; (1) The number of cases is too small to be sure how well a hospital is performing; (2) The hospital indicated that the data submitted for this measure were based on a sample of cases; (3) Data was collected during a shorter time period (fewer quarters) than the maximum possible time for this measure; (4) Suppressed for one or more quarters by CMS; (5) No data is available from the hospital for this measure; (6) Fewer than 100 patients completed the HCAHPS survey. Use these rates with caution, as the number of surveys may be too low to reliably assess hospital performance; (7) Survey results are based on less than 12 months of data; (8) Survey results are not available for this reporting period; (9) No or very few patients were eligible for the HCAHPS survey. The scores shown, if any, reflect a very small number of surveys; (10) A state average was not calculated because too few hospitals in the state submitted data; (11) There were discrepancies in the data collection process; Please refer to the User's Guide for a full explanation of data.

Preston Memorial Hospital

300 S Price Street
Kingwood, WV 26537
Phone: 304-329-1400
Fax: 304-329-1175
URL: www.prestonmemorial.com
Type: Critical Access Hospitals
Emergency Services: Yes
Ownership: Voluntary Non-Profit - Private
Beds: 76

Key Personnel:

CEO/President. . . . . Michael Thompson
Chief of Medical Staff. . . . . Frederick A. Conley
Operating Room. . . . . Susan Krause
Quality Assurance . . . . Kathy Wilson
Radiology. . . . . Leisa Stalnaker
Emergency Room . . . . Fred Conley, MD

Measure	Cases	This Hosp.	State Avg.	U.S. Avg.
Heart Attack Care				
ACE Inhibitor or ARB for LVSD[1,3]	1	0%	94%	96%
Aspirin at Arrival[1,3]	2	100%	97%	99%
Aspirin at Discharge[1,3]	2	100%	98%	98%
Beta Blocker at Discharge[1,3]	2	100%	98%	98%
Fibrinolytic Medication Timing[3]	0	-	29%	55%
PCI Within 90 Minutes of Arrival[3]	0	-	85%	90%
Smoking Cessation Advice[3]	0	-	99%	99%
Chest Pain/Possible Heart Attack Care				
Aspirin at Arrival	55	95%	95%	95%
Median Time to ECG (minutes)	55	23	12	8
Median Time to Transfer (minutes)[1,3]	1	112	77	61
Fibrinolytic Medication Timing[1]	1	0%	56%	54%
Heart Failure Care				
ACE Inhibitor or ARB for LVSD[1]	9	67%	90%	94%
Discharge Instructions[1]	21	76%	85%	88%
Evaluation of LVS Function[1]	23	83%	97%	98%
Smoking Cessation Advice[1]	1	0%	97%	98%
Pneumonia Care				
Appropriate Initial Antibiotic[1,2]	8	75%	89%	92%
Blood Culture Timing[2]	25	80%	95%	96%
Influenza Vaccine[1,2]	18	72%	90%	91%
Initial Antibiotic Timing[1,2]	20	85%	94%	95%
Pneumococcal Vaccine[1,2]	24	83%	91%	93%
Smoking Cessation Advice[1,2]	8	50%	96%	97%
Surgical Care Improvement Project				
Appropriate VTP Within 24 Hours[5]	0	-	91%	92%
Appropriate Hair Removal[5]	0	-	99%	99%
Appropriate Beta Blocker Usage[5]	0	-	93%	93%
Controlled Postoperative Blood Glucose[5]	0	-	91%	93%
Prophylactic Antibiotic Timing[5]	0	-	97%	97%
Prophylactic Antibiotic Timing (Outpatient)[5]	0	-	90%	92%
Prophylactic Antibiotic Selection[5]	0	-	97%	97%
Prophylactic Antibiotic Select. (Outpatient)[5]	0	-	91%	94%
Prophylactic Antibiotic Stopped[5]	0	-	94%	94%
Recommended VTP Ordered[5]	0	-	92%	94%
Urinary Catheter Removal[1]	3	100%	90%	90%
Children's Asthma Care				
Received Systemic Corticosteroids	-	-	-	100%
Received Home Management Plan	-	-	-	71%
Received Reliever Medication	-	-	-	100%
Use of Medical Imaging				
Combination Abdominal CT Scan	89	0.146	0.304	0.191
Combination Chest CT Scan	70	0.071	0.063	0.054
Follow-up Mammogram/Ultrasound	215	9.8%	8.8%	8.4%
MRI for Low Back Pain[1]	13	38.5%	38.5%	32.7%
Survey of Patients' Hospital Experiences				
Area Around Room 'Always' Quiet at Night	(a)	47%	-	58%
Doctors 'Always' Communicated Well	(a)	85%	-	80%
Home Recovery Information Given	(a)	79%	-	82%
Hospital Given 9 or 10 on 10 Point Scale	(a)	62%	-	67%
Meds 'Always' Explained Before Given	(a)	65%	-	60%
Nurses 'Always' Communicated Well	(a)	79%	-	76%
Pain 'Always' Well Controlled	(a)	71%	-	69%
Room and Bathroom 'Always' Clean	(a)	82%	-	71%
Timely Help 'Always' Received	(a)	65%	-	64%
Would Definitely Recommend Hospital	(a)	63%	-	69%

Logan Regional Medical Center

20 Hospital Drive
Logan, WV 25601
Phone: 304-831-1350
Fax: 304-831-1871
Type: Acute Care Hospitals
Emergency Services: Yes
Ownership: Voluntary Non-Profit - Other
Beds: 140

Key Personnel:

CEO/President. . . . . Kevin Fowler
Chief of Medical Staff . . . . S Chevy, MD
Operating Room. . . . . Richard Skibo
Quality Assurance . . . . Alisa Bently
Anesthesiology. . . . . Billy Mullen, DO
Intensive Care Unit. . . . . Jenny Baxter

Measure	Cases	This Hosp.	State Avg.	U.S. Avg.
Heart Attack Care				
ACE Inhibitor or ARB for LVSD	0	-	94%	96%
Aspirin at Arrival[1]	15	93%	97%	99%
Aspirin at Discharge[1]	5	100%	98%	98%
Beta Blocker at Discharge[1]	5	100%	98%	98%
Fibrinolytic Medication Timing	0	-	29%	55%
PCI Within 90 Minutes of Arrival	0	-	85%	90%
Smoking Cessation Advice[1]	2	100%	99%	99%
Chest Pain/Possible Heart Attack Care				
Aspirin at Arrival	239	98%	95%	95%
Median Time to ECG (minutes)	253	18	12	8
Median Time to Transfer (minutes)[1]	6	104	77	61
Fibrinolytic Medication Timing[1]	11	45%	56%	54%
Heart Failure Care				
ACE Inhibitor or ARB for LVSD	40	100%	90%	94%
Discharge Instructions	178	98%	85%	88%
Evaluation of LVS Function	213	100%	97%	98%
Smoking Cessation Advice	30	100%	97%	98%
Pneumonia Care				
Appropriate Initial Antibiotic	227	88%	89%	92%
Blood Culture Timing	323	95%	95%	96%
Influenza Vaccine	232	100%	90%	91%
Initial Antibiotic Timing	348	93%	94%	95%
Pneumococcal Vaccine	235	100%	91%	93%
Smoking Cessation Advice	162	99%	96%	97%
Surgical Care Improvement Project				
Appropriate VTP Within 24 Hours	132	95%	91%	92%
Appropriate Hair Removal	268	100%	99%	99%
Appropriate Beta Blocker Usage	64	94%	93%	93%
Controlled Postoperative Blood Glucose	0	-	91%	93%
Prophylactic Antibiotic Timing	165	97%	97%	97%
Prophylactic Antibiotic Timing (Outpatient)	61	87%	90%	92%
Prophylactic Antibiotic Selection	166	95%	97%	97%
Prophylactic Antibiotic Select. (Outpatient)	57	84%	91%	94%
Prophylactic Antibiotic Stopped	94	93%	94%	94%
Recommended VTP Ordered	132	95%	92%	94%
Urinary Catheter Removal	28	79%	90%	90%
Children's Asthma Care				
Received Systemic Corticosteroids	-	-	-	100%
Received Home Management Plan	-	-	-	71%
Received Reliever Medication	-	-	-	100%
Use of Medical Imaging				
Combination Abdominal CT Scan	571	0.005	0.304	0.191
Combination Chest CT Scan	547	0.000	0.063	0.054
Follow-up Mammogram/Ultrasound	420	19.3%	8.8%	8.4%
MRI for Low Back Pain	99	45.5%	38.5%	32.7%
Survey of Patients' Hospital Experiences				
Area Around Room 'Always' Quiet at Night	300+	52%	-	58%
Doctors 'Always' Communicated Well	300+	82%	-	80%
Home Recovery Information Given	300+	78%	-	82%
Hospital Given 9 or 10 on 10 Point Scale	300+	55%	-	67%
Meds 'Always' Explained Before Given	300+	51%	-	60%
Nurses 'Always' Communicated Well	300+	69%	-	76%
Pain 'Always' Well Controlled	300+	63%	-	69%
Room and Bathroom 'Always' Clean	300+	61%	-	71%
Timely Help 'Always' Received	300+	55%	-	64%
Would Definitely Recommend Hospital	300+	53%	-	69%

Boone Memorial Hospital

701 Madison Avenue
Madison, WV 25130
Phone: 304-369-1230
Fax: 304-369-1525
E-mail: mlinville@bmh.org
URL: www.bmh.org
Type: Critical Access Hospitals
Emergency Services: Yes
Ownership: Voluntary Non-Profit - Other
Beds: 25

Key Personnel:

CEO/President. . . . . Tommy H Mullins
Cardiac Laboratory. . . . . Matt Downey
Chief of Medical Staff . . . . Robert B Atkins
Infection Control. . . . . Teresa Meade
Radiology. . . . . Greg Zornes

Measure	Cases	This Hosp.	State Avg.	U.S. Avg.
Heart Attack Care				
ACE Inhibitor or ARB for LVSD[5]	0	-	94%	96%
Aspirin at Arrival[5]	0	-	97%	99%
Aspirin at Discharge[5]	0	-	98%	98%
Beta Blocker at Discharge[5]	0	-	98%	98%
Fibrinolytic Medication Timing[5]	0	-	29%	55%
PCI Within 90 Minutes of Arrival[5]	0	-	85%	90%
Smoking Cessation Advice[5]	0	-	99%	99%
Chest Pain/Possible Heart Attack Care				
Aspirin at Arrival	-	-	95%	95%
Median Time to ECG (minutes)	-	-	12	8
Median Time to Transfer (minutes)	-	-	77	61
Fibrinolytic Medication Timing	-	-	56%	54%
Heart Failure Care				
ACE Inhibitor or ARB for LVSD[1]	2	100%	90%	94%
Discharge Instructions[1]	13	69%	85%	88%
Evaluation of LVS Function[1]	13	46%	97%	98%
Smoking Cessation Advice[1]	1	0%	97%	98%
Pneumonia Care				
Appropriate Initial Antibiotic	29	69%	89%	92%
Blood Culture Timing	49	86%	95%	96%
Influenza Vaccine[1]	24	79%	90%	91%
Initial Antibiotic Timing[1]	11	91%	94%	95%
Pneumococcal Vaccine	28	82%	91%	93%
Smoking Cessation Advice[1]	18	83%	96%	97%
Surgical Care Improvement Project				
Appropriate VTP Within 24 Hours[5]	0	-	91%	92%
Appropriate Hair Removal[5]	0	-	99%	99%
Appropriate Beta Blocker Usage[5]	0	-	93%	93%
Controlled Postoperative Blood Glucose[5]	0	-	91%	93%
Prophylactic Antibiotic Timing[5]	0	-	97%	97%
Prophylactic Antibiotic Timing (Outpatient)	-	-	90%	92%
Prophylactic Antibiotic Selection[5]	0	-	97%	97%
Prophylactic Antibiotic Select. (Outpatient)	-	-	91%	94%
Prophylactic Antibiotic Stopped[5]	0	-	94%	94%
Recommended VTP Ordered[5]	0	-	92%	94%
Urinary Catheter Removal[5]	0	-	90%	90%
Children's Asthma Care				
Received Systemic Corticosteroids	-	-	-	100%
Received Home Management Plan	-	-	-	71%
Received Reliever Medication	-	-	-	100%
Use of Medical Imaging				
Combination Abdominal CT Scan	-	-	0.304	0.191
Combination Chest CT Scan	-	-	0.063	0.054
Follow-up Mammogram/Ultrasound	-	-	8.8%	8.4%
MRI for Low Back Pain	-	-	38.5%	32.7%
Survey of Patients' Hospital Experiences				
Area Around Room 'Always' Quiet at Night	(a)	62%	-	58%
Doctors 'Always' Communicated Well	(a)	88%	-	80%
Home Recovery Information Given	(a)	87%	-	82%
Hospital Given 9 or 10 on 10 Point Scale	(a)	70%	-	67%
Meds 'Always' Explained Before Given	(a)	74%	-	60%
Nurses 'Always' Communicated Well	(a)	84%	-	76%
Pain 'Always' Well Controlled	(a)	83%	-	69%
Room and Bathroom 'Always' Clean	(a)	82%	-	71%
Timely Help 'Always' Received	(a)	77%	-	64%
Would Definitely Recommend Hospital	(a)	61%	-	69%

NOTE: Hospital profiles are in alphabetical order by state, then city, then hospital within the city; Rankings exclude hospitals with less than 25 cases except for patient surveys which excludes hospitals with less than 100 cases; (a) 100–299 cases; (1) The number of cases is too small to be sure how well a hospital is performing; (2) The hospital indicated that the data submitted for this measure were based on a sample of cases; (3) Data was collected during a shorter time period (fewer quarters) than the maximum possible time for this measure; (4) Suppressed for one or more quarters by CMS; (5) No data is available from the hospital for this measure; (6) Fewer than 100 patients completed the HCAHPS survey. Use these rates with caution, as the number of surveys may be too low to reliably assess hospital performance; (7) Survey results are based on less than 12 months of data; (8) Survey results are not available for this reporting period; (9) No or very few patients were eligible for the HCAHPS survey. The scores shown, if any, reflect a very small number of surveys; (10) A state average was not calculated because too few hospitals in the state submitted data; (11) There were discrepancies in the data collection process; Please refer to the User's Guide for a full explanation of data.

City Hospital

2500 Hospital Drive
Martinsburg, WV 25401
URL: www.cityhospital.org
Type: Acute Care Hospitals
Ownership: Voluntary Non-Profit - Other
Phone: 304-264-1000
Fax: 304-264-1255
Emergency Services: Yes
Beds: 144

Key Personnel:
CEO/President. . . . . Jon Applebaum
Chief of Medical Staff. . . . . C Joseph Cincinnati, DO
Infection Control. . . . . Paula Donahue, RN
Pediatric In-Patient Care . . . . Mary Jo Ostrowski, RN
Quality Assurance . . . . Barbara Sherman
Radiology. . . . . Frederick Ammer
Hemotology Center . . . . Bernie Raney, RN
Intensive Care Unit. . . . . Mary Ellen Clark, RN

Measure	Cases	This Hosp.	State Avg.	U.S. Avg.
Heart Attack Care				
ACE Inhibitor or ARB for LVSD[1]	6	100%	94%	96%
Aspirin at Arrival	108	100%	97%	99%
Aspirin at Discharge	54	80%	98%	98%
Beta Blocker at Discharge	52	81%	98%	98%
Fibrinolytic Medication Timing[1]	2	100%	29%	55%
PCI Within 90 Minutes of Arrival	0	-	85%	90%
Smoking Cessation Advice[1]	14	93%	99%	99%
Chest Pain/Possible Heart Attack Care				
Aspirin at Arrival	110	93%	95%	95%
Median Time to ECG (minutes)	108	6	12	8
Median Time to Transfer (minutes)[1]	3	254	77	61
Fibrinolytic Medication Timing[1]	21	43%	56%	54%
Heart Failure Care				
ACE Inhibitor or ARB for LVSD	43	77%	90%	94%
Discharge Instructions	142	71%	85%	88%
Evaluation of LVS Function	157	89%	97%	98%
Smoking Cessation Advice	25	84%	97%	98%
Pneumonia Care				
Appropriate Initial Antibiotic	176	91%	89%	92%
Blood Culture Timing	208	90%	95%	96%
Influenza Vaccine	113	88%	90%	91%
Initial Antibiotic Timing	210	97%	94%	95%
Pneumococcal Vaccine	149	92%	91%	93%
Smoking Cessation Advice	96	84%	96%	97%
Surgical Care Improvement Project				
Appropriate VTP Within 24 Hours	252	96%	91%	92%
Appropriate Hair Removal	573	100%	99%	99%
Appropriate Beta Blocker Usage	145	100%	93%	93%
Controlled Postoperative Blood Glucose	0	-	91%	93%
Prophylactic Antibiotic Timing	214	94%	97%	97%
Prophylactic Antibiotic Timing (Outpatient)	112	90%	90%	92%
Prophylactic Antibiotic Selection	220	95%	97%	97%
Prophylactic Antibiotic Select. (Outpatient)	104	88%	91%	94%
Prophylactic Antibiotic Stopped	190	96%	94%	94%
Recommended VTP Ordered	252	96%	92%	94%
Urinary Catheter Removal	138	98%	90%	90%
Children's Asthma Care				
Received Systemic Corticosteroids	-	-	-	100%
Received Home Management Plan	-	-	-	71%
Received Reliever Medication	-	-	-	100%
Use of Medical Imaging				
Combination Abdominal CT Scan	1,129	0.035	0.304	0.191
Combination Chest CT Scan	463	0.011	0.063	0.054
Follow-up Mammogram/Ultrasound	1,091	2.0%	8.8%	8.4%
MRI for Low Back Pain	163	31.9%	38.5%	32.7%
Survey of Patients' Hospital Experiences				
Area Around Room 'Always' Quiet at Night	300+	41%	-	58%
Doctors 'Always' Communicated Well	300+	79%	-	80%
Home Recovery Information Given	300+	78%	-	82%
Hospital Given 9 or 10 on 10 Point Scale	300+	53%	-	67%
Meds 'Always' Explained Before Given	300+	59%	-	60%
Nurses 'Always' Communicated Well	300+	73%	-	76%
Pain 'Always' Well Controlled	300+	69%	-	69%
Room and Bathroom 'Always' Clean	300+	71%	-	71%
Timely Help 'Always' Received	300+	65%	-	64%
Would Definitely Recommend Hospital	300+	55%	-	69%

Martinsburg VA Medical Center

510 Butler Ave.
Martinsburg, WV 25401
URL: www.martinsburg.va.gov
Type: Acute Care-Veterans Administration
Ownership: Government - Federal
Phone: 304-263-0811
Fax: 304-262-7433
Emergency Services: No
Beds: 566

Key Personnel:
CEO/President. . . . . Fernando O. Rivera
Chief of Medical Staff . . . . Linda J Morris, MD
Coronary Care . . . . Sonya Racey, RN
Infection Control. . . . . Linda Coffman, RN
Operating Room. . . . . Kati Jo Brown, RN
Quality Assurance . . . . Debra Rogers
Radiology. Satinder Gill, MD

Measure	Cases	This Hosp.	State Avg.	U.S. Avg.
Heart Attack Care				
ACE Inhibitor or ARB for LVSD[1]	3	100%	94%	96%
Aspirin at Arrival[1]	13	100%	97%	99%
Aspirin at Discharge[1]	8	100%	98%	98%
Beta Blocker at Discharge[1]	10	100%	98%	98%
Fibrinolytic Medication Timing[5]	0	-	29%	55%
PCI Within 90 Minutes of Arrival[5]	0	-	85%	90%
Smoking Cessation Advice[1]	5	100%	99%	99%
Chest Pain/Possible Heart Attack Care				
Aspirin at Arrival	-	-	95%	95%
Median Time to ECG (minutes)	-	-	12	8
Median Time to Transfer (minutes)	-	-	77	61
Fibrinolytic Medication Timing	-	-	56%	54%
Heart Failure Care				
ACE Inhibitor or ARB for LVSD	46	93%	90%	94%
Discharge Instructions	78	72%	85%	88%
Evaluation of LVS Function	97	100%	97%	98%
Smoking Cessation Advice	29	100%	97%	98%
Pneumonia Care				
Appropriate Initial Antibiotic	67	94%	89%	92%
Blood Culture Timing	82	96%	95%	96%
Influenza Vaccine	67	97%	90%	91%
Initial Antibiotic Timing	95	93%	94%	95%
Pneumococcal Vaccine	86	100%	91%	93%
Smoking Cessation Advice	47	98%	96%	97%
Surgical Care Improvement Project				
Appropriate VTP Within 24 Hours[2,5]	0	-	91%	92%
Appropriate Hair Removal[2,5]	0	-	99%	99%
Appropriate Beta Blocker Usage[2,5]	0	-	93%	93%
Controlled Postoperative Blood Glucose[2,5]	0	-	91%	93%
Prophylactic Antibiotic Timing[5]	0	-	97%	97%
Prophylactic Antibiotic Timing (Outpatient)	-	-	90%	92%
Prophylactic Antibiotic Selection[5]	0	-	97%	97%
Prophylactic Antibiotic Select. (Outpatient)	-	-	91%	94%
Prophylactic Antibiotic Stopped[5]	0	-	94%	94%
Recommended VTP Ordered[2,5]	0	-	92%	94%
Urinary Catheter Removal[2,5]	0	-	90%	90%
Children's Asthma Care				
Received Systemic Corticosteroids	-	-	-	100%
Received Home Management Plan	-	-	-	71%
Received Reliever Medication	-	-	-	100%
Use of Medical Imaging				
Combination Abdominal CT Scan	-	-	0.304	0.191
Combination Chest CT Scan	-	-	0.063	0.054
Follow-up Mammogram/Ultrasound	-	-	8.8%	8.4%
MRI for Low Back Pain	-	-	38.5%	32.7%
Survey of Patients' Hospital Experiences				
Area Around Room 'Always' Quiet at Night	-	-	-	58%
Doctors 'Always' Communicated Well	-	-	-	80%
Home Recovery Information Given	-	-	-	82%
Hospital Given 9 or 10 on 10 Point Scale	-	-	-	67%
Meds 'Always' Explained Before Given	-	-	-	60%
Nurses 'Always' Communicated Well	-	-	-	76%
Pain 'Always' Well Controlled	-	-	-	69%
Room and Bathroom 'Always' Clean	-	-	-	71%
Timely Help 'Always' Received	-	-	-	64%
Would Definitely Recommend Hospital	-	-	-	69%

Montgomery General Hospital

401 Sixth Avenue, Fayette County
Montgomery, WV 25136
URL: www.montgomerygeneral.com
Type: Critical Access Hospitals
Ownership: Government - Local
Phone: 304-442-5151
Fax: 304-442-7494
Emergency Services: Yes
Beds: 191

Key Personnel:
CEO/President. . . . . Peter W Monge
Chief of Medical Staff . . . . John D Maylath
Patient Relations . . . . Marylou Watson, MS RN

Measure	Cases	This Hosp.	State Avg.	U.S. Avg.
Heart Attack Care				
ACE Inhibitor or ARB for LVSD[1]	1	0%	94%	96%
Aspirin at Arrival[1]	13	92%	97%	99%
Aspirin at Discharge[1]	11	73%	98%	98%
Beta Blocker at Discharge[1]	10	100%	98%	98%
Fibrinolytic Medication Timing	0	-	29%	55%
PCI Within 90 Minutes of Arrival	0	-	85%	90%
Smoking Cessation Advice	0	-	99%	99%
Chest Pain/Possible Heart Attack Care				
Aspirin at Arrival	-	-	95%	95%
Median Time to ECG (minutes)	-	-	12	8
Median Time to Transfer (minutes)	-	-	77	61
Fibrinolytic Medication Timing	-	-	56%	54%
Heart Failure Care				
ACE Inhibitor or ARB for LVSD[1]	13	54%	90%	94%
Discharge Instructions	29	79%	85%	88%
Evaluation of LVS Function	37	78%	97%	98%
Smoking Cessation Advice[1]	3	100%	97%	98%
Pneumonia Care				
Appropriate Initial Antibiotic	75	88%	89%	92%
Blood Culture Timing	82	98%	95%	96%
Influenza Vaccine	42	88%	90%	91%
Initial Antibiotic Timing	93	100%	94%	95%
Pneumococcal Vaccine	69	84%	91%	93%
Smoking Cessation Advice	29	97%	96%	97%
Surgical Care Improvement Project				
Appropriate VTP Within 24 Hours[5]	0	-	91%	92%
Appropriate Hair Removal[5]	0	-	99%	99%
Appropriate Beta Blocker Usage[5]	0	-	93%	93%
Controlled Postoperative Blood Glucose[5]	0	-	91%	93%
Prophylactic Antibiotic Timing[5]	0	-	97%	97%
Prophylactic Antibiotic Timing (Outpatient)	-	-	90%	92%
Prophylactic Antibiotic Selection[5]	0	-	97%	97%
Prophylactic Antibiotic Select. (Outpatient)	-	-	91%	94%
Prophylactic Antibiotic Stopped[5]	0	-	94%	94%
Recommended VTP Ordered[5]	0	-	92%	94%
Urinary Catheter Removal[5]	0	-	90%	90%
Children's Asthma Care				
Received Systemic Corticosteroids	-	-	-	100%
Received Home Management Plan	-	-	-	71%
Received Reliever Medication	-	-	-	100%
Use of Medical Imaging				
Combination Abdominal CT Scan	-	-	0.304	0.191
Combination Chest CT Scan	-	-	0.063	0.054
Follow-up Mammogram/Ultrasound	-	-	8.8%	8.4%
MRI for Low Back Pain	-	-	38.5%	32.7%
Survey of Patients' Hospital Experiences				
Area Around Room 'Always' Quiet at Night	(a)	61%	-	58%
Doctors 'Always' Communicated Well	(a)	80%	-	80%
Home Recovery Information Given	(a)	72%	-	82%
Hospital Given 9 or 10 on 10 Point Scale	(a)	72%	-	67%
Meds 'Always' Explained Before Given	(a)	59%	-	60%
Nurses 'Always' Communicated Well	(a)	80%	-	76%
Pain 'Always' Well Controlled	(a)	66%	-	69%
Room and Bathroom 'Always' Clean	(a)	76%	-	71%
Timely Help 'Always' Received	(a)	67%	-	64%
Would Definitely Recommend Hospital	(a)	61%	-	69%

NOTE: Hospital profiles are in alphabetical order by state, then city, then hospital within the city; Rankings exclude hospitals with less than 25 cases except for patient surveys which excludes hospitals with less than 100 cases; (a) 100–299 cases; (1) The number of cases is too small to be sure how well a hospital is performing; (2) The hospital indicated that the data submitted for this measure were based on a sample of cases; (3) Data was collected during a shorter time period (fewer quarters) than the maximum possible time for this measure; (4) Suppressed for one or more quarters by CMS; (5) No data is available from the hospital for this measure; (6) Fewer than 100 patients completed the HCAHPS survey. Use these rates with caution, as the number of surveys may be too low to reliably assess hospital performance; (7) Survey results are based on less than 12 months of data; (8) Survey results are not available for this reporting period; (9) No or very few patients were eligible for the HCAHPS survey. The scores shown, if any, reflect a very small number of surveys; (10) A state average was not calculated because too few hospitals in the state submitted data; (11) There were discrepancies in the data collection process; Please refer to the User's Guide for a full explanation of data.

Monongalia County General Hospital

1200 Jd Anderson Dr Phone: 304-598-1200
Morgantown, WV 26505 Fax: 304-599-8382
URL: www.mongeneral.com
Type: Acute Care Hospitals Emergency Services: Yes
Ownership: Voluntary Non-Profit - Private Beds: 199

Key Personnel:
CEO/President. . . . . Dave Robertson
Chief of Medical Staff . . . . Todd Tallman, MD
Operating Room. . . . . Roberto H Burns, RN
Radiology. . . . . Surendra V Pawar
Emergency Room . . . . Jo Anne Liptock

Measure	Cases	This Hosp.	State Avg.	U.S. Avg.
Heart Attack Care				
ACE Inhibitor or ARB for LVSD	71	100%	94%	96%
Aspirin at Arrival	138	99%	97%	99%
Aspirin at Discharge	264	100%	98%	98%
Beta Blocker at Discharge	266	99%	98%	98%
Fibrinolytic Medication Timing	0	-	29%	55%
PCI Within 90 Minutes of Arrival	35	91%	85%	90%
Smoking Cessation Advice	90	100%	99%	99%
Chest Pain/Possible Heart Attack Care				
Aspirin at Arrival[1,3]	2	100%	95%	95%
Median Time to ECG (minutes)[1,3]	2	7	12	8
Median Time to Transfer (minutes)[5]	0	-	77	61
Fibrinolytic Medication Timing[5]	0	-	56%	54%
Heart Failure Care				
ACE Inhibitor or ARB for LVSD	92	83%	90%	94%
Discharge Instructions	229	87%	85%	88%
Evaluation of LVS Function	276	98%	97%	98%
Smoking Cessation Advice	39	100%	97%	98%
Pneumonia Care				
Appropriate Initial Antibiotic	103	88%	89%	92%
Blood Culture Timing	125	98%	95%	96%
Influenza Vaccine	96	95%	90%	91%
Initial Antibiotic Timing	115	97%	94%	95%
Pneumococcal Vaccine	121	98%	91%	93%
Smoking Cessation Advice	46	93%	96%	97%
Surgical Care Improvement Project				
Appropriate VTP Within 24 Hours[2]	388	97%	91%	92%
Appropriate Hair Removal[2]	1,210	100%	99%	99%
Appropriate Beta Blocker Usage[2]	426	90%	93%	93%
Controlled Postoperative Blood Glucose[2]	211	93%	91%	93%
Prophylactic Antibiotic Timing[2]	1,020	97%	97%	97%
Prophylactic Antibiotic Timing (Outpatient)	361	85%	90%	92%
Prophylactic Antibiotic Selection[2]	1,030	98%	97%	97%
Prophylactic Antibiotic Select. (Outpatient)	316	98%	91%	94%
Prophylactic Antibiotic Stopped[2]	1,003	97%	94%	94%
Recommended VTP Ordered[2]	392	97%	92%	94%
Urinary Catheter Removal[2]	103	80%	90%	90%
Children's Asthma Care				
Received Systemic Corticosteroids	-	-	-	100%
Received Home Management Plan	-	-	-	71%
Received Reliever Medication	-	-	-	100%
Use of Medical Imaging				
Combination Abdominal CT Scan	939	0.638	0.304	0.191
Combination Chest CT Scan	737	0.004	0.063	0.054
Follow-up Mammogram/Ultrasound	835	10.1%	8.8%	8.4%
MRI for Low Back Pain	104	37.5%	38.5%	32.7%
Survey of Patients' Hospital Experiences				
Area Around Room 'Always' Quiet at Night	300+	61%	-	58%
Doctors 'Always' Communicated Well	300+	85%	-	80%
Home Recovery Information Given	300+	78%	-	82%
Hospital Given 9 or 10 on 10 Point Scale	300+	76%	-	67%
Meds 'Always' Explained Before Given	300+	62%	-	60%
Nurses 'Always' Communicated Well	300+	80%	-	76%
Pain 'Always' Well Controlled	300+	68%	-	69%
Room and Bathroom 'Always' Clean	300+	78%	-	71%
Timely Help 'Always' Received	300+	67%	-	64%
Would Definitely Recommend Hospital	300+	83%	-	69%

West Virginia University Hospitals

Medical Center Drive Phone: 304-598-4000
Morgantown, WV 26506 Fax: 304-598-4124
URL: www.wvuh.com
Type: Acute Care Hospitals Emergency Services: Yes
Ownership: Voluntary Non-Profit - Private Beds: 440

Key Personnel:
CEO/President. . . . . Bruce McClymounds
Chief of Medical Staff . . . . Kevin Halbritter
Infection Control. . . . . Rashida Khakoo, MD
Operating Room. . . . . Ehab Akkary
Radiology. . . . . Mary Cannon, MD
Anesthesiology. . . . . Robert Johnstone, MD
Emergency Room . . . . Ann Chinnis, MD

Measure	Cases	This Hosp.	State Avg.	U.S. Avg.
Heart Attack Care				
ACE Inhibitor or ARB for LVSD	85	96%	94%	96%
Aspirin at Arrival	196	100%	97%	99%
Aspirin at Discharge	461	100%	98%	98%
Beta Blocker at Discharge	453	99%	98%	98%
Fibrinolytic Medication Timing	0	-	29%	55%
PCI Within 90 Minutes of Arrival	31	97%	85%	90%
Smoking Cessation Advice	173	97%	99%	99%
Chest Pain/Possible Heart Attack Care				
Aspirin at Arrival[1,3]	2	100%	95%	95%
Median Time to ECG (minutes)[1,3]	2	46	12	8
Median Time to Transfer (minutes)[5]	0	-	77	61
Fibrinolytic Medication Timing[5]	0	-	56%	54%
Heart Failure Care				
ACE Inhibitor or ARB for LVSD	111	98%	90%	94%
Discharge Instructions	266	97%	85%	88%
Evaluation of LVS Function	315	99%	97%	98%
Smoking Cessation Advice	69	99%	97%	98%
Pneumonia Care				
Appropriate Initial Antibiotic	99	97%	89%	92%
Blood Culture Timing	199	94%	95%	96%
Influenza Vaccine	189	94%	90%	91%
Initial Antibiotic Timing	225	90%	94%	95%
Pneumococcal Vaccine	199	96%	91%	93%
Smoking Cessation Advice	131	97%	96%	97%
Surgical Care Improvement Project				
Appropriate VTP Within 24 Hours[2]	287	99%	91%	92%
Appropriate Hair Removal[2]	1,153	100%	99%	99%
Appropriate Beta Blocker Usage[2]	362	100%	93%	93%
Controlled Postoperative Blood Glucose[2]	313	86%	91%	93%
Prophylactic Antibiotic Timing[2]	926	99%	97%	97%
Prophylactic Antibiotic Timing (Outpatient)	285	94%	90%	92%
Prophylactic Antibiotic Selection[2]	945	99%	97%	97%
Prophylactic Antibiotic Select. (Outpatient)	279	94%	91%	94%
Prophylactic Antibiotic Stopped[2]	900	98%	94%	94%
Recommended VTP Ordered[2]	287	99%	92%	94%
Urinary Catheter Removal[2]	284	100%	90%	90%
Children's Asthma Care				
Received Systemic Corticosteroids	-	-	-	100%
Received Home Management Plan	-	-	-	71%
Received Reliever Medication	-	-	-	100%
Use of Medical Imaging				
Combination Abdominal CT Scan	824	0.189	0.304	0.191
Combination Chest CT Scan	947	0.120	0.063	0.054
Follow-up Mammogram/Ultrasound	1,132	7.7%	8.8%	8.4%
MRI for Low Back Pain[5]	0	-	38.5%	32.7%
Survey of Patients' Hospital Experiences				
Area Around Room 'Always' Quiet at Night	300+	47%	-	58%
Doctors 'Always' Communicated Well	300+	74%	-	80%
Home Recovery Information Given	300+	81%	-	82%
Hospital Given 9 or 10 on 10 Point Scale	300+	64%	-	67%
Meds 'Always' Explained Before Given	300+	61%	-	60%
Nurses 'Always' Communicated Well	300+	76%	-	76%
Pain 'Always' Well Controlled	300+	65%	-	69%
Room and Bathroom 'Always' Clean	300+	64%	-	71%
Timely Help 'Always' Received	300+	58%	-	64%
Would Definitely Recommend Hospital	300+	69%	-	69%

Wetzel County Hospital

#3 East Benjamin Drive Phone: 304-455-8000
New Martinsville, WV 26155 Fax: 304-455-4259
Type: Acute Care Hospitals Emergency Services: Yes
Ownership: Government - Local Beds: 68

Key Personnel:
CEO/President. . . . . George Couch
Cardiac Laboratory. . . . . Bradley Miller
Chief of Medical Staff . . . . Donald Blum
Infection Control. . . . . Jenny Abbott, RN
Operating Room. . . . . Debbie Starchen, RN
Quality Assurance . . . . Jane Flor, RN
Anesthesiology. . . . . Santwara Souani, MD
Emergency Room . . . . John King, MD

Measure	Cases	This Hosp.	State Avg.	U.S. Avg.
Heart Attack Care				
ACE Inhibitor or ARB for LVSD[1]	2	100%	94%	96%
Aspirin at Arrival	25	92%	97%	99%
Aspirin at Discharge[1]	14	64%	98%	98%
Beta Blocker at Discharge[1]	15	80%	98%	98%
Fibrinolytic Medication Timing	0	-	29%	55%
PCI Within 90 Minutes of Arrival	0	-	85%	90%
Smoking Cessation Advice[1]	1	100%	99%	99%
Chest Pain/Possible Heart Attack Care				
Aspirin at Arrival	72	92%	95%	95%
Median Time to ECG (minutes)	83	13	12	8
Median Time to Transfer (minutes)[1]	8	59	77	61
Fibrinolytic Medication Timing[1]	4	100%	56%	54%
Heart Failure Care				
ACE Inhibitor or ARB for LVSD[1]	18	72%	90%	94%
Discharge Instructions	40	80%	85%	88%
Evaluation of LVS Function	58	88%	97%	98%
Smoking Cessation Advice[1]	3	100%	97%	98%
Pneumonia Care				
Appropriate Initial Antibiotic	70	86%	89%	92%
Blood Culture Timing	55	93%	95%	96%
Influenza Vaccine	58	93%	90%	91%
Initial Antibiotic Timing	82	95%	94%	95%
Pneumococcal Vaccine	90	79%	91%	93%
Smoking Cessation Advice	34	97%	96%	97%
Surgical Care Improvement Project				
Appropriate VTP Within 24 Hours[1]	11	91%	91%	92%
Appropriate Hair Removal[1]	15	93%	99%	99%
Appropriate Beta Blocker Usage[1]	4	75%	93%	93%
Controlled Postoperative Blood Glucose	0	-	91%	93%
Prophylactic Antibiotic Timing[1]	7	86%	97%	97%
Prophylactic Antibiotic Timing (Outpatient)[1,3]	6	67%	90%	92%
Prophylactic Antibiotic Selection[1]	7	86%	97%	97%
Prophylactic Antibiotic Select. (Outpatient)[1,3]	5	100%	91%	94%
Prophylactic Antibiotic Stopped[1]	7	100%	94%	94%
Recommended VTP Ordered[1]	11	91%	92%	94%
Urinary Catheter Removal[1]	4	75%	90%	90%
Children's Asthma Care				
Received Systemic Corticosteroids	-	-	-	100%
Received Home Management Plan	-	-	-	71%
Received Reliever Medication	-	-	-	100%
Use of Medical Imaging				
Combination Abdominal CT Scan	204	0.495	0.304	0.191
Combination Chest CT Scan	170	0.000	0.063	0.054
Follow-up Mammogram/Ultrasound	343	8.7%	8.8%	8.4%
MRI for Low Back Pain	59	37.3%	38.5%	32.7%
Survey of Patients' Hospital Experiences				
Area Around Room 'Always' Quiet at Night	300+	53%	-	58%
Doctors 'Always' Communicated Well	300+	82%	-	80%
Home Recovery Information Given	300+	74%	-	82%
Hospital Given 9 or 10 on 10 Point Scale	300+	65%	-	67%
Meds 'Always' Explained Before Given	300+	64%	-	60%
Nurses 'Always' Communicated Well	300+	81%	-	76%
Pain 'Always' Well Controlled	300+	73%	-	69%
Room and Bathroom 'Always' Clean	300+	81%	-	71%
Timely Help 'Always' Received	300+	72%	-	64%
Would Definitely Recommend Hospital	300+	66%	-	69%

NOTE: Hospital profiles are in alphabetical order by state, then city, then hospital within the city; Rankings exclude hospitals with less than 25 cases except for patient surveys which excludes hospitals with less than 100 cases; (a) 100–299 cases; (1) The number of cases is too small to be sure how well a hospital is performing; (2) The hospital indicated that the data submitted for this measure were based on a sample of cases; (3) Data was collected during a shorter time period (fewer quarters) than the maximum possible time for this measure; (4) Suppressed for one or more quarters by CMS; (5) No data is available from the hospital for this measure; (6) Fewer than 100 patients completed the HCAHPS survey. Use these rates with caution, as the number of surveys may be too low to reliably assess hospital performance; (7) Survey results are based on less than 12 months of data; (8) Survey results are not available for this reporting period; (9) No or very few patients were eligible for the HCAHPS survey. The scores shown, if any, reflect a very small number of surveys; (10) A state average was not calculated because too few hospitals in the state submitted data; (11) There were discrepancies in the data collection process; Please refer to the User's Guide for a full explanation of data.

Plateau Medical Center

430 Main Street
Oak Hill, WV 25901
Phone: 304-469-8600
Fax: 304-469-8605
Type: Critical Access Hospitals
Emergency Services: Yes
Ownership: Proprietary
Beds: 90

Key Personnel:
CEO/President. . . . . David Bunch
Chief of Medical Staff. . . . . Clint Curtis
Infection Control. . . . . Linda Roach
Operating Room. . . . . Joyce Stover, RN
Quality Assurance . . . . Lynn Legg
Anesthesiology. . . . . Jessie Loot, MD
Emergency Room . . . . Burnon Stanly
Intensive Care Unit. . . . . Linda DeBord

Measure	Cases	This Hosp.	State Avg.	U.S. Avg.
Heart Attack Care				
ACE Inhibitor or ARB for LVSD[1]	1	100%	94%	96%
Aspirin at Arrival[1]	12	100%	97%	99%
Aspirin at Discharge[1]	9	100%	98%	98%
Beta Blocker at Discharge[1]	7	86%	98%	98%
Fibrinolytic Medication Timing	0	-	29%	55%
PCI Within 90 Minutes of Arrival	0	-	85%	90%
Smoking Cessation Advice[1]	2	100%	99%	99%
Chest Pain/Possible Heart Attack Care				
Aspirin at Arrival	131	98%	95%	95%
Median Time to ECG (minutes)	139	12	12	8
Median Time to Transfer (minutes)[1]	10	50	77	61
Fibrinolytic Medication Timing[1]	5	40%	56%	54%
Heart Failure Care				
ACE Inhibitor or ARB for LVSD[1]	13	85%	90%	94%
Discharge Instructions	54	83%	85%	88%
Evaluation of LVS Function	78	99%	97%	98%
Smoking Cessation Advice[1]	14	100%	97%	98%
Pneumonia Care				
Appropriate Initial Antibiotic	64	83%	89%	92%
Blood Culture Timing	88	95%	95%	96%
Influenza Vaccine	60	98%	90%	91%
Initial Antibiotic Timing	94	95%	94%	95%
Pneumococcal Vaccine	71	94%	91%	93%
Smoking Cessation Advice	28	96%	96%	97%
Surgical Care Improvement Project				
Appropriate VTP Within 24 Hours[2]	48	94%	91%	92%
Appropriate Hair Removal[2]	186	100%	99%	99%
Appropriate Beta Blocker Usage[2]	61	97%	93%	93%
Controlled Postoperative Blood Glucose[2]	0	-	91%	93%
Prophylactic Antibiotic Timing[2]	130	97%	97%	97%
Prophylactic Antibiotic Timing (Outpatient)[1]	12	75%	90%	92%
Prophylactic Antibiotic Selection[2]	150	98%	97%	97%
Prophylactic Antibiotic Select. (Outpatient)[1]	12	92%	91%	94%
Prophylactic Antibiotic Stopped[2]	129	98%	94%	94%
Recommended VTP Ordered[2]	48	94%	92%	94%
Urinary Catheter Removal	57	98%	90%	90%
Children's Asthma Care				
Received Systemic Corticosteroids	-	-	-	100%
Received Home Management Plan	-	-	-	71%
Received Reliever Medication	-	-	-	100%
Use of Medical Imaging				
Combination Abdominal CT Scan	182	0.132	0.304	0.191
Combination Chest CT Scan	105	0.219	0.063	0.054
Follow-up Mammogram/Ultrasound	106	11.3%	8.8%	8.4%
MRI for Low Back Pain	34	52.9%	38.5%	32.7%
Survey of Patients' Hospital Experiences				
Area Around Room 'Always' Quiet at Night	300+	57%	-	58%
Doctors 'Always' Communicated Well	300+	84%	-	80%
Home Recovery Information Given	300+	79%	-	82%
Hospital Given 9 or 10 on 10 Point Scale	300+	70%	-	67%
Meds 'Always' Explained Before Given	300+	58%	-	60%
Nurses 'Always' Communicated Well	300+	79%	-	76%
Pain 'Always' Well Controlled	300+	68%	-	69%
Room and Bathroom 'Always' Clean	300+	70%	-	71%
Timely Help 'Always' Received	300+	71%	-	64%
Would Definitely Recommend Hospital	300+	69%	-	69%

Camden Clark Memorial Hospital

800 Garfield Ave
Parkersburg, WV 26101
Phone: 304-424-2111
Fax: 304-424-2688
E-mail: prccmh@ccmh.org
URL: www.ccmh.org
Type: Acute Care Hospitals
Emergency Services: Yes
Ownership: Proprietary
Beds: 269

Key Personnel:
CEO/President. . . . . Thomas Corder
Chief of Medical Staff. . . . . Judy Kemp, MD
Infection Control. . . . . Susan Dearman
Quality Assurance . . . . Sherry Johnston
Radiology. . . . . Robert Al-Aly, MD
Emergency Room . . . . Dominic Bagnoli, MD
Intensive Care Unit. . . . . Patty Blanchard
Patient Relations . . . . Nancy Brooks

Measure	Cases	This Hosp.	State Avg.	U.S. Avg.
Heart Attack Care				
ACE Inhibitor or ARB for LVSD[1]	15	100%	94%	96%
Aspirin at Arrival	172	98%	97%	99%
Aspirin at Discharge	108	98%	98%	98%
Beta Blocker at Discharge	104	99%	98%	98%
Fibrinolytic Medication Timing	0	-	29%	55%
PCI Within 90 Minutes of Arrival[1]	2	50%	85%	90%
Smoking Cessation Advice[1]	24	100%	99%	99%
Chest Pain/Possible Heart Attack Care				
Aspirin at Arrival	56	91%	95%	95%
Median Time to ECG (minutes)	55	14	12	8
Median Time to Transfer (minutes)[1,3]	13	69	77	61
Fibrinolytic Medication Timing	0	-	56%	54%
Heart Failure Care				
ACE Inhibitor or ARB for LVSD	76	99%	90%	94%
Discharge Instructions	255	89%	85%	88%
Evaluation of LVS Function	362	100%	97%	98%
Smoking Cessation Advice	42	100%	97%	98%
Pneumonia Care				
Appropriate Initial Antibiotic	199	91%	89%	92%
Blood Culture Timing	294	99%	95%	96%
Influenza Vaccine	233	97%	90%	91%
Initial Antibiotic Timing	325	97%	94%	95%
Pneumococcal Vaccine	349	99%	91%	93%
Smoking Cessation Advice	113	95%	96%	97%
Surgical Care Improvement Project				
Appropriate VTP Within 24 Hours[2]	233	90%	91%	92%
Appropriate Hair Removal[2]	756	100%	99%	99%
Appropriate Beta Blocker Usage[2]	198	97%	93%	93%
Controlled Postoperative Blood Glucose[2]	0	-	91%	93%
Prophylactic Antibiotic Timing[2]	532	97%	97%	97%
Prophylactic Antibiotic Timing (Outpatient)	175	80%	90%	92%
Prophylactic Antibiotic Selection[2]	536	97%	97%	97%
Prophylactic Antibiotic Select. (Outpatient)	144	81%	91%	94%
Prophylactic Antibiotic Stopped[2]	492	97%	94%	94%
Recommended VTP Ordered[2]	234	92%	92%	94%
Urinary Catheter Removal[2]	83	89%	90%	90%
Children's Asthma Care				
Received Systemic Corticosteroids	-	-	-	100%
Received Home Management Plan	-	-	-	71%
Received Reliever Medication	-	-	-	100%
Use of Medical Imaging				
Combination Abdominal CT Scan	1,643	0.595	0.304	0.191
Combination Chest CT Scan	1,071	0.031	0.063	0.054
Follow-up Mammogram/Ultrasound	2,174	7.0%	8.8%	8.4%
MRI for Low Back Pain	355	34.4%	38.5%	32.7%
Survey of Patients' Hospital Experiences				
Area Around Room 'Always' Quiet at Night	300+	40%	-	58%
Doctors 'Always' Communicated Well	300+	76%	-	80%
Home Recovery Information Given	300+	79%	-	82%
Hospital Given 9 or 10 on 10 Point Scale	300+	60%	-	67%
Meds 'Always' Explained Before Given	300+	51%	-	60%
Nurses 'Always' Communicated Well	300+	69%	-	76%
Pain 'Always' Well Controlled	300+	61%	-	69%
Room and Bathroom 'Always' Clean	300+	64%	-	71%
Timely Help 'Always' Received	300+	55%	-	64%
Would Definitely Recommend Hospital	300+	66%	-	69%

Saint Josephs Healthcare System

1824 Murdoch Avenue
Parkersburg, WV 26102
Phone: 304-424-4382
Fax: 304-424-4807
URL: www.stjosephs-hospital.com
Type: Acute Care Hospitals
Emergency Services: Yes
Ownership: Voluntary Non-Profit - Other
Beds: 325

Key Personnel:
CEO/President. . . . . John D Julius
Cardiac Laboratory. . . . . H R Lockhart
Infection Control. . . . . Judy Miller RN
Operating Room. . . . . Beverly Reger RN
Quality Assurance . . . . Brenda Thompson
Radiology. . . . . Terri Allman
Intensive Care Unit. . . . . Angela Perkins RN
Patient Relations . . . . Jill Parsons

Measure	Cases	This Hosp.	State Avg.	U.S. Avg.
Heart Attack Care				
ACE Inhibitor or ARB for LVSD	36	92%	94%	96%
Aspirin at Arrival	151	96%	97%	99%
Aspirin at Discharge	234	98%	98%	98%
Beta Blocker at Discharge	230	99%	98%	98%
Fibrinolytic Medication Timing	0	-	29%	55%
PCI Within 90 Minutes of Arrival	30	90%	85%	90%
Smoking Cessation Advice	80	100%	99%	99%
Chest Pain/Possible Heart Attack Care				
Aspirin at Arrival[1]	6	83%	95%	95%
Median Time to ECG (minutes)[1]	7	15	12	8
Median Time to Transfer (minutes)[5]	0	-	77	61
Fibrinolytic Medication Timing[5]	0	-	56%	54%
Heart Failure Care				
ACE Inhibitor or ARB for LVSD	85	78%	90%	94%
Discharge Instructions	268	73%	85%	88%
Evaluation of LVS Function	323	95%	97%	98%
Smoking Cessation Advice	48	100%	97%	98%
Pneumonia Care				
Appropriate Initial Antibiotic	104	94%	89%	92%
Blood Culture Timing	173	96%	95%	96%
Influenza Vaccine	117	91%	90%	91%
Initial Antibiotic Timing	165	91%	94%	95%
Pneumococcal Vaccine	167	92%	91%	93%
Smoking Cessation Advice	65	100%	96%	97%
Surgical Care Improvement Project				
Appropriate VTP Within 24 Hours[2]	157	87%	91%	92%
Appropriate Hair Removal[2]	551	99%	99%	99%
Appropriate Beta Blocker Usage[2]	181	97%	93%	93%
Controlled Postoperative Blood Glucose[2]	72	97%	91%	93%
Prophylactic Antibiotic Timing[2]	349	99%	97%	97%
Prophylactic Antibiotic Timing (Outpatient)	155	82%	90%	92%
Prophylactic Antibiotic Selection[2]	351	98%	97%	97%
Prophylactic Antibiotic Select. (Outpatient)	136	99%	91%	94%
Prophylactic Antibiotic Stopped[2]	333	92%	94%	94%
Recommended VTP Ordered[2]	161	88%	92%	94%
Urinary Catheter Removal[2]	190	93%	90%	90%
Children's Asthma Care				
Received Systemic Corticosteroids	-	-	-	100%
Received Home Management Plan	-	-	-	71%
Received Reliever Medication	-	-	-	100%
Use of Medical Imaging				
Combination Abdominal CT Scan	738	0.011	0.304	0.191
Combination Chest CT Scan	572	0.000	0.063	0.054
Follow-up Mammogram/Ultrasound	1,021	4.7%	8.8%	8.4%
MRI for Low Back Pain	204	29.9%	38.5%	32.7%
Survey of Patients' Hospital Experiences				
Area Around Room 'Always' Quiet at Night	300+	44%	-	58%
Doctors 'Always' Communicated Well	300+	81%	-	80%
Home Recovery Information Given	300+	84%	-	82%
Hospital Given 9 or 10 on 10 Point Scale	300+	64%	-	67%
Meds 'Always' Explained Before Given	300+	54%	-	60%
Nurses 'Always' Communicated Well	300+	72%	-	76%
Pain 'Always' Well Controlled	300+	65%	-	69%
Room and Bathroom 'Always' Clean	300+	62%	-	71%
Timely Help 'Always' Received	300+	56%	-	64%
Would Definitely Recommend Hospital	300+	66%	-	69%

NOTE: Hospital profiles are in alphabetical order by state, then city, then hospital within the city; Rankings exclude hospitals with less than 25 cases except for patient surveys which excludes hospitals with less than 100 cases; (a) 100–299 cases; (1) The number of cases is too small to be sure how well a hospital is performing; (2) The hospital indicated that the data submitted for this measure were based on a sample of cases; (3) Data was collected during a shorter time period (fewer quarters) than the maximum possible time for this measure; (4) Suppressed for one or more quarters by CMS; (5) No data is available from the hospital for this measure; (6) Fewer than 100 patients completed the HCAHPS survey. Use these rates with caution, as the number of surveys may be too low to reliably assess hospital performance; (7) Survey results are based on less than 12 months of data; (8) Survey results are not available for this reporting period; (9) No or very few patients were eligible for the HCAHPS survey. The scores shown, if any, reflect a very small number of surveys; (10) A state average was not calculated because too few hospitals in the state submitted data; (11) There were discrepancies in the data collection process; Please refer to the User's Guide for a full explanation of data.

Grant Memorial Hospital

1 Hospital Drive
Petersburg, WV 26847
Type: Critical Access Hospitals
Ownership: Voluntary Non-Profit - Other

Phone: 304-257-1026
Fax: 304-257-2537
Emergency Services: Yes
Beds: 61

Key Personnel:
CEO/President . . . . Robert Harman
Emergency Room . . . . Randall L Turner

Measure	Cases	This Hosp.	State Avg.	U.S. Avg.
Heart Attack Care				
ACE Inhibitor or ARB for LVSD[3]	0	-	94%	96%
Aspirin at Arrival[1,3]	4	75%	97%	99%
Aspirin at Discharge[1,3]	4	100%	98%	98%
Beta Blocker at Discharge[1,3]	4	75%	98%	98%
Fibrinolytic Medication Timing[3]	0	-	29%	55%
PCI Within 90 Minutes of Arrival[3]	0	-	85%	90%
Smoking Cessation Advice[3]	0	-	99%	99%
Chest Pain/Possible Heart Attack Care				
Aspirin at Arrival	-	-	95%	95%
Median Time to ECG (minutes)	-	-	12	8
Median Time to Transfer (minutes)	-	-	77	61
Fibrinolytic Medication Timing	-	-	56%	54%
Heart Failure Care				
ACE Inhibitor or ARB for LVSD[1]	18	83%	90%	94%
Discharge Instructions	35	77%	85%	88%
Evaluation of LVS Function	68	81%	97%	98%
Smoking Cessation Advice[1]	3	67%	97%	98%
Pneumonia Care				
Appropriate Initial Antibiotic	38	84%	89%	92%
Blood Culture Timing[1]	20	95%	95%	96%
Influenza Vaccine	29	72%	90%	91%
Initial Antibiotic Timing	48	90%	94%	95%
Pneumococcal Vaccine	42	67%	91%	93%
Smoking Cessation Advice[1]	13	77%	96%	97%
Surgical Care Improvement Project				
Appropriate VTP Within 24 Hours	25	88%	91%	92%
Appropriate Hair Removal	124	100%	99%	99%
Appropriate Beta Blocker Usage	27	85%	93%	93%
Controlled Postoperative Blood Glucose	0	-	91%	93%
Prophylactic Antibiotic Timing	114	97%	97%	97%
Prophylactic Antibiotic Timing (Outpatient)	-	-	90%	92%
Prophylactic Antibiotic Selection	114	97%	97%	97%
Prophylactic Antibiotic Select. (Outpatient)	-	-	91%	94%
Prophylactic Antibiotic Stopped	112	93%	94%	94%
Recommended VTP Ordered	25	88%	92%	94%
Urinary Catheter Removal[1]	21	90%	90%	90%
Children's Asthma Care				
Received Systemic Corticosteroids	-	-	-	100%
Received Home Management Plan	-	-	-	71%
Received Reliever Medication	-	-	-	100%
Use of Medical Imaging				
Combination Abdominal CT Scan	-	-	0.304	0.191
Combination Chest CT Scan	-	-	0.063	0.054
Follow-up Mammogram/Ultrasound	-	-	8.8%	8.4%
MRI for Low Back Pain	-	-	38.5%	32.7%
Survey of Patients' Hospital Experiences				
Area Around Room 'Always' Quiet at Night	300+	47%	-	58%
Doctors 'Always' Communicated Well	300+	79%	-	80%
Home Recovery Information Given	300+	88%	-	82%
Hospital Given 9 or 10 on 10 Point Scale	300+	59%	-	67%
Meds 'Always' Explained Before Given	300+	66%	-	60%
Nurses 'Always' Communicated Well	300+	80%	-	76%
Pain 'Always' Well Controlled	300+	68%	-	69%
Room and Bathroom 'Always' Clean	300+	83%	-	71%
Timely Help 'Always' Received	300+	71%	-	64%
Would Definitely Recommend Hospital	300+	59%	-	69%

Broaddus Hospital Association

Mansfield Hill, PO Box 930
Philippi, WV 26416
E-mail: higginss@davishealthsystem.org
URL: www.davishealthcare.com
Type: Critical Access Hospitals
Ownership: Voluntary Non-Profit - Other

Phone: 304-457-1760
Fax: 304-457-1516

Emergency Services: Yes
Beds: 72

Key Personnel:
CEO/President . . . . Jeff Powpofon
Chief of Medical Staff . . . . Pecel Hollbert
Radiology . . . . Steven M Barnett
Emergency Room . . . . Sharon Mots, RN

Measure	Cases	This Hosp.	State Avg.	U.S. Avg.
Heart Attack Care				
ACE Inhibitor or ARB for LVSD[5]	0	-	94%	96%
Aspirin at Arrival[5]	0	-	97%	99%
Aspirin at Discharge[5]	0	-	98%	98%
Beta Blocker at Discharge[5]	0	-	98%	98%
Fibrinolytic Medication Timing[5]	0	-	29%	55%
PCI Within 90 Minutes of Arrival[5]	0	-	85%	90%
Smoking Cessation Advice[5]	0	-	99%	99%
Chest Pain/Possible Heart Attack Care				
Aspirin at Arrival[5]	0	-	95%	95%
Median Time to ECG (minutes)[5]	0	-	12	8
Median Time to Transfer (minutes)[5]	0	-	77	61
Fibrinolytic Medication Timing[5]	0	-	56%	54%
Heart Failure Care				
ACE Inhibitor or ARB for LVSD[3]	0	-	90%	94%
Discharge Instructions[1,3]	8	62%	85%	88%
Evaluation of LVS Function[1,3]	9	100%	97%	98%
Smoking Cessation Advice[3]	0	-	97%	98%
Pneumonia Care				
Appropriate Initial Antibiotic[1,3]	3	0%	89%	92%
Blood Culture Timing[1,3]	3	100%	95%	96%
Influenza Vaccine[1,3]	3	67%	90%	91%
Initial Antibiotic Timing[1,3]	5	80%	94%	95%
Pneumococcal Vaccine[1,3]	4	50%	91%	93%
Smoking Cessation Advice[3]	0	-	96%	97%
Surgical Care Improvement Project				
Appropriate VTP Within 24 Hours[5]	0	-	91%	92%
Appropriate Hair Removal[5]	0	-	99%	99%
Appropriate Beta Blocker Usage[5]	0	-	93%	93%
Controlled Postoperative Blood Glucose[5]	0	-	91%	93%
Prophylactic Antibiotic Timing[5]	0	-	97%	97%
Prophylactic Antibiotic Timing (Outpatient)[5]	0	-	90%	92%
Prophylactic Antibiotic Selection[5]	0	-	97%	97%
Prophylactic Antibiotic Select. (Outpatient)[5]	0	-	91%	94%
Prophylactic Antibiotic Stopped[5]	0	-	94%	94%
Recommended VTP Ordered[5]	0	-	92%	94%
Urinary Catheter Removal[5]	0	-	90%	90%
Children's Asthma Care				
Received Systemic Corticosteroids	-	-	-	100%
Received Home Management Plan	-	-	-	71%
Received Reliever Medication	-	-	-	100%
Use of Medical Imaging				
Combination Abdominal CT Scan	114	0.482	0.304	0.191
Combination Chest CT Scan	67	0.642	0.063	0.054
Follow-up Mammogram/Ultrasound	162	4.9%	8.8%	8.4%
MRI for Low Back Pain[1]	22	63.6%	38.5%	32.7%
Survey of Patients' Hospital Experiences				
Area Around Room 'Always' Quiet at Night[6]	<100	64%	-	58%
Doctors 'Always' Communicated Well[6]	<100	85%	-	80%
Home Recovery Information Given[6]	<100	89%	-	82%
Hospital Given 9 or 10 on 10 Point Scale[6]	<100	70%	-	67%
Meds 'Always' Explained Before Given[6]	<100	70%	-	60%
Nurses 'Always' Communicated Well[6]	<100	87%	-	76%
Pain 'Always' Well Controlled[6]	<100	76%	-	69%
Room and Bathroom 'Always' Clean[6]	<100	89%	-	71%
Timely Help 'Always' Received[6]	<100	78%	-	64%
Would Definitely Recommend Hospital	<100	73%	-	69%

Pleasant Valley Hospital

2520 Valley Drive
Point Pleasant, WV 25550
E-mail: ssprouse@pvalley.org
Type: Acute Care Hospitals
Ownership: Government - Local

Phone: 304-675-4340
Fax: 304-675-5243

Emergency Services: Yes
Beds: 201

Key Personnel:
CEO/President . . . . Alvin R Lawson, JD
Cardiac Laboratory . . . . Israel Jamora
Chief of Medical Staff . . . . Shrikant Vaidya, MD
Infection Control . . . . Susan Garten
Operating Room . . . . Doug Eades
Radiology . . . . Suresh K Agrawal
Intensive Care Unit . . . . Doug Eades
Patient Relations . . . . Sue Hussel

Measure	Cases	This Hosp.	State Avg.	U.S. Avg.
Heart Attack Care				
ACE Inhibitor or ARB for LVSD[1]	2	100%	94%	96%
Aspirin at Arrival[1]	22	91%	97%	99%
Aspirin at Discharge[1]	13	69%	98%	98%
Beta Blocker at Discharge[1]	13	77%	98%	98%
Fibrinolytic Medication Timing	0	-	29%	55%
PCI Within 90 Minutes of Arrival	0	-	85%	90%
Smoking Cessation Advice[1]	1	100%	99%	99%
Chest Pain/Possible Heart Attack Care				
Aspirin at Arrival	76	89%	95%	95%
Median Time to ECG (minutes)	78	10	12	8
Median Time to Transfer (minutes)[1,3]	10	66	77	61
Fibrinolytic Medication Timing[1]	1	100%	56%	54%
Heart Failure Care				
ACE Inhibitor or ARB for LVSD	36	58%	90%	94%
Discharge Instructions	87	92%	85%	88%
Evaluation of LVS Function	116	98%	97%	98%
Smoking Cessation Advice[1]	16	94%	97%	98%
Pneumonia Care				
Appropriate Initial Antibiotic	64	81%	89%	92%
Blood Culture Timing	66	94%	95%	96%
Influenza Vaccine	60	93%	90%	91%
Initial Antibiotic Timing	105	94%	94%	95%
Pneumococcal Vaccine	80	98%	91%	93%
Smoking Cessation Advice	48	98%	96%	97%
Surgical Care Improvement Project				
Appropriate VTP Within 24 Hours	70	71%	91%	92%
Appropriate Hair Removal	109	98%	99%	99%
Appropriate Beta Blocker Usage	29	76%	93%	93%
Controlled Postoperative Blood Glucose	0	-	91%	93%
Prophylactic Antibiotic Timing	73	90%	97%	97%
Prophylactic Antibiotic Timing (Outpatient)	54	63%	90%	92%
Prophylactic Antibiotic Selection	73	92%	97%	97%
Prophylactic Antibiotic Select. (Outpatient)	53	75%	91%	94%
Prophylactic Antibiotic Stopped	71	83%	94%	94%
Recommended VTP Ordered	70	74%	92%	94%
Urinary Catheter Removal[1]	7	43%	90%	90%
Children's Asthma Care				
Received Systemic Corticosteroids	-	-	-	100%
Received Home Management Plan	-	-	-	71%
Received Reliever Medication	-	-	-	100%
Use of Medical Imaging				
Combination Abdominal CT Scan	362	0.041	0.304	0.191
Combination Chest CT Scan	209	0.033	0.063	0.054
Follow-up Mammogram/Ultrasound	334	9.6%	8.8%	8.4%
MRI for Low Back Pain	113	36.3%	38.5%	32.7%
Survey of Patients' Hospital Experiences				
Area Around Room 'Always' Quiet at Night	300+	57%	-	58%
Doctors 'Always' Communicated Well	300+	81%	-	80%
Home Recovery Information Given	300+	87%	-	82%
Hospital Given 9 or 10 on 10 Point Scale	300+	66%	-	67%
Meds 'Always' Explained Before Given	300+	60%	-	60%
Nurses 'Always' Communicated Well	300+	75%	-	76%
Pain 'Always' Well Controlled	300+	68%	-	69%
Room and Bathroom 'Always' Clean	300+	78%	-	71%
Timely Help 'Always' Received	300+	65%	-	64%
Would Definitely Recommend Hospital	300+	69%	-	69%

NOTE: Hospital profiles are in alphabetical order by state, then city, then hospital within the city; Rankings exclude hospitals with less than 25 cases except for patient surveys which excludes hospitals with less than 100 cases; (a) 100–299 cases; (1) The number of cases is too small to be sure how well a hospital is performing; (2) The hospital indicated that the data submitted for this measure were based on a sample of cases; (3) Data was collected during a shorter time period (fewer quarters) than the maximum possible time for this measure; (4) Suppressed for one or more quarters by CMS; (5) No data is available from the hospital for this measure; (6) Fewer than 100 patients completed the HCAHPS survey. Use these rates with caution, as the number of surveys may be too low to reliably assess hospital performance; (7) Survey results are based on less than 12 months of data; (8) Survey results are not available for this reporting period; (9) No or very few patients were eligible for the HCAHPS survey. The scores shown, if any, reflect a very small number of surveys; (10) A state average was not calculated because too few hospitals in the state submitted data; (11) There were discrepancies in the data collection process; Please refer to the User's Guide for a full explanation of data.

Princeton Community Hospital

122 12th Street Phone: 304-487-7260
Princeton, WV 24740 Fax: 304-487-2161
URL: www.pchonline.org
Type: Acute Care Hospitals Emergency Services: Yes
Ownership: Government - Local Beds: 267

Key Personnel:
CEO/President. . . . . Wayne Griffith
Chief of Medical Staff. . . . . Philip Branson, MD
Infection Control. . . . . Cindy Belcher
Operating Room. . . . . Larry Perdue
Quality Assurance . . . . Rick Puckett

Measure	Cases	This Hosp.	State Avg.	U.S. Avg.
Heart Attack Care				
ACE Inhibitor or ARB for LVSD[1]	8	88%	94%	96%
Aspirin at Arrival	60	93%	97%	99%
Aspirin at Discharge	38	87%	98%	98%
Beta Blocker at Discharge	36	100%	98%	98%
Fibrinolytic Medication Timing	0	-	29%	55%
PCI Within 90 Minutes of Arrival	0	-	85%	90%
Smoking Cessation Advice[1]	3	100%	99%	99%
Chest Pain/Possible Heart Attack Care				
Aspirin at Arrival	187	95%	95%	95%
Median Time to ECG (minutes)	201	9	12	8
Median Time to Transfer (minutes)[1,3]	4	244	77	61
Fibrinolytic Medication Timing[1]	17	71%	56%	54%
Heart Failure Care				
ACE Inhibitor or ARB for LVSD	68	97%	90%	94%
Discharge Instructions	248	98%	85%	88%
Evaluation of LVS Function	282	96%	97%	98%
Smoking Cessation Advice	35	100%	97%	98%
Pneumonia Care				
Appropriate Initial Antibiotic	210	80%	89%	92%
Blood Culture Timing	224	97%	95%	96%
Influenza Vaccine	218	97%	90%	91%
Initial Antibiotic Timing	332	89%	94%	95%
Pneumococcal Vaccine	275	96%	91%	93%
Smoking Cessation Advice	143	100%	96%	97%
Surgical Care Improvement Project				
Appropriate VTP Within 24 Hours	179	93%	91%	92%
Appropriate Hair Removal	618	100%	99%	99%
Appropriate Beta Blocker Usage	168	94%	93%	93%
Controlled Postoperative Blood Glucose	0	-	91%	93%
Prophylactic Antibiotic Timing	498	98%	97%	97%
Prophylactic Antibiotic Timing (Outpatient)	147	83%	90%	92%
Prophylactic Antibiotic Selection	499	96%	97%	97%
Prophylactic Antibiotic Select. (Outpatient)	145	83%	91%	94%
Prophylactic Antibiotic Stopped	471	96%	94%	94%
Recommended VTP Ordered	181	94%	92%	94%
Urinary Catheter Removal	35	83%	90%	90%
Children's Asthma Care				
Received Systemic Corticosteroids	-	-	-	100%
Received Home Management Plan	-	-	-	71%
Received Reliever Medication	-	-	-	100%
Use of Medical Imaging				
Combination Abdominal CT Scan	1,159	0.720	0.304	0.191
Combination Chest CT Scan	745	0.019	0.063	0.054
Follow-up Mammogram/Ultrasound	1,076	5.1%	8.8%	8.4%
MRI for Low Back Pain	251	48.2%	38.5%	32.7%
Survey of Patients' Hospital Experiences				
Area Around Room 'Always' Quiet at Night	300+	52%	-	58%
Doctors 'Always' Communicated Well	300+	82%	-	80%
Home Recovery Information Given	300+	85%	-	82%
Hospital Given 9 or 10 on 10 Point Scale	300+	62%	-	67%
Meds 'Always' Explained Before Given	300+	64%	-	60%
Nurses 'Always' Communicated Well	300+	79%	-	76%
Pain 'Always' Well Controlled	300+	70%	-	69%
Room and Bathroom 'Always' Clean	300+	65%	-	71%
Timely Help 'Always' Received	300+	59%	-	64%
Would Definitely Recommend Hospital	300+	67%	-	69%

Jefferson Memorial Hospital

300 South Preston Street Phone: 304-728-1600
Ranson, WV 25438 Fax: 304-725-9492
E-mail: tstover@jeffmem.com
URL: www.jeffmem.com
Type: Critical Access Hospitals Emergency Services: Yes
Ownership: Voluntary Non-Profit - Private Beds: 114

Key Personnel:
CEO/President. . . . . John M Sherwood
Chief of Medical Staff. . . . . Vikram Dayal, MD
Infection Control. . . . . Robin Akin, RN
Pediatric Ambulatory Care . . . . . . Sarah Moerschel, MD
Pediatric In-Patient Care . . . . Linda Blanc
Quality Assurance . . . . Sarah Johnson
Intensive Care Unit. . . . . Tammy Fitch
Patient Relations . . . . Suzanne Shackelford

Measure	Cases	This Hosp.	State Avg.	U.S. Avg.
Heart Attack Care				
ACE Inhibitor or ARB for LVSD	0	-	94%	96%
Aspirin at Arrival[1]	3	67%	97%	99%
Aspirin at Discharge	0	-	98%	98%
Beta Blocker at Discharge	0	-	98%	98%
Fibrinolytic Medication Timing	0	-	29%	55%
PCI Within 90 Minutes of Arrival[5]	0	-	85%	90%
Smoking Cessation Advice	0	-	99%	99%
Chest Pain/Possible Heart Attack Care				
Aspirin at Arrival	-	-	95%	95%
Median Time to ECG (minutes)	-	-	12	8
Median Time to Transfer (minutes)	-	-	77	61
Fibrinolytic Medication Timing	-	-	56%	54%
Heart Failure Care				
ACE Inhibitor or ARB for LVSD[1]	5	100%	90%	94%
Discharge Instructions[1]	19	84%	85%	88%
Evaluation of LVS Function	28	100%	97%	98%
Smoking Cessation Advice[1]	4	100%	97%	98%
Pneumonia Care				
Appropriate Initial Antibiotic	28	86%	89%	92%
Blood Culture Timing	52	88%	95%	96%
Influenza Vaccine[1]	10	90%	90%	91%
Initial Antibiotic Timing	54	87%	94%	95%
Pneumococcal Vaccine	34	71%	91%	93%
Smoking Cessation Advice[1]	14	100%	96%	97%
Surgical Care Improvement Project				
Appropriate VTP Within 24 Hours	34	82%	91%	92%
Appropriate Hair Removal	55	100%	99%	99%
Appropriate Beta Blocker Usage[1]	6	100%	93%	93%
Controlled Postoperative Blood Glucose	0	-	91%	93%
Prophylactic Antibiotic Timing[1]	24	71%	97%	97%
Prophylactic Antibiotic Timing (Outpatient)	-	-	90%	92%
Prophylactic Antibiotic Selection[1]	24	83%	97%	97%
Prophylactic Antibiotic Select. (Outpatient)	-	-	91%	94%
Prophylactic Antibiotic Stopped[1]	18	61%	94%	94%
Recommended VTP Ordered	34	82%	92%	94%
Urinary Catheter Removal[1]	6	100%	90%	90%
Children's Asthma Care				
Received Systemic Corticosteroids	-	-	-	100%
Received Home Management Plan	-	-	-	71%
Received Reliever Medication	-	-	-	100%
Use of Medical Imaging				
Combination Abdominal CT Scan	-	-	0.304	0.191
Combination Chest CT Scan	-	-	0.063	0.054
Follow-up Mammogram/Ultrasound	-	-	8.8%	8.4%
MRI for Low Back Pain	-	-	38.5%	32.7%
Survey of Patients' Hospital Experiences				
Area Around Room 'Always' Quiet at Night	(a)	55%	-	58%
Doctors 'Always' Communicated Well	(a)	85%	-	80%
Home Recovery Information Given	(a)	83%	-	82%
Hospital Given 9 or 10 on 10 Point Scale	(a)	59%	-	67%
Meds 'Always' Explained Before Given	(a)	62%	-	60%
Nurses 'Always' Communicated Well	(a)	74%	-	76%
Pain 'Always' Well Controlled	(a)	69%	-	69%
Room and Bathroom 'Always' Clean	(a)	83%	-	71%
Timely Help 'Always' Received	(a)	63%	-	64%
Would Definitely Recommend Hospital	(a)	59%	-	69%

Jackson General Hospital

122 Pinnell St Phone: 304-372-2731
Ripley, WV 25271 Fax: 304-372-2749
E-mail: selza@jacksongeneral.com
URL: www.jacksongeneral.com
Type: Acute Care Hospitals Emergency Services: Yes
Ownership: Voluntary Non-Profit - Other Beds: 82

Key Personnel:
CEO/President. . . . . Sandra J Elza
Chief of Medical Staff. . . . . Brandon A Cestaric
Infection Control. . . . . Karen Hoschar
Operating Room. . . . . Karen Hoscar
Quality Assurance . . . . James Payne
Radiology. . . . . Glen Dean McKnight
Emergency Room . . . . Barbara LeGue
Intensive Care Unit. . . . . Sherry Quick RN

Measure	Cases	This Hosp.	State Avg.	U.S. Avg.
Heart Attack Care				
ACE Inhibitor or ARB for LVSD[1]	1	0%	94%	96%
Aspirin at Arrival[1]	11	91%	97%	99%
Aspirin at Discharge[1]	4	75%	98%	98%
Beta Blocker at Discharge[1]	4	100%	98%	98%
Fibrinolytic Medication Timing	0	-	29%	55%
PCI Within 90 Minutes of Arrival	0	-	85%	90%
Smoking Cessation Advice	0	-	99%	99%
Chest Pain/Possible Heart Attack Care				
Aspirin at Arrival	104	97%	95%	95%
Median Time to ECG (minutes)	107	10	12	8
Median Time to Transfer (minutes)[3]	0	-	77	61
Fibrinolytic Medication Timing[1]	16	81%	56%	54%
Heart Failure Care				
ACE Inhibitor or ARB for LVSD[1]	20	100%	90%	94%
Discharge Instructions	83	78%	85%	88%
Evaluation of LVS Function	103	99%	97%	98%
Smoking Cessation Advice[1]	12	100%	97%	98%
Pneumonia Care				
Appropriate Initial Antibiotic	49	92%	89%	92%
Blood Culture Timing	97	98%	95%	96%
Influenza Vaccine	56	98%	90%	91%
Initial Antibiotic Timing	103	96%	94%	95%
Pneumococcal Vaccine	94	97%	91%	93%
Smoking Cessation Advice[1]	22	95%	96%	97%
Surgical Care Improvement Project				
Appropriate VTP Within 24 Hours[1]	12	83%	91%	92%
Appropriate Hair Removal[1]	18	100%	99%	99%
Appropriate Beta Blocker Usage[1]	5	20%	93%	93%
Controlled Postoperative Blood Glucose	0	-	91%	93%
Prophylactic Antibiotic Timing[1]	2	100%	97%	97%
Prophylactic Antibiotic Timing (Outpatient)[1]	5	100%	90%	92%
Prophylactic Antibiotic Selection[1]	2	100%	97%	97%
Prophylactic Antibiotic Select. (Outpatient)[1]	5	100%	91%	94%
Prophylactic Antibiotic Stopped[1]	2	100%	94%	94%
Recommended VTP Ordered[1]	12	92%	92%	94%
Urinary Catheter Removal[1]	3	67%	90%	90%
Children's Asthma Care				
Received Systemic Corticosteroids	-	-	-	100%
Received Home Management Plan	-	-	-	71%
Received Reliever Medication	-	-	-	100%
Use of Medical Imaging				
Combination Abdominal CT Scan	314	0.150	0.304	0.191
Combination Chest CT Scan	189	0.000	0.063	0.054
Follow-up Mammogram/Ultrasound	410	6.1%	8.8%	8.4%
MRI for Low Back Pain	105	41.0%	38.5%	32.7%
Survey of Patients' Hospital Experiences				
Area Around Room 'Always' Quiet at Night	300+	50%	-	58%
Doctors 'Always' Communicated Well	300+	86%	-	80%
Home Recovery Information Given	300+	87%	-	82%
Hospital Given 9 or 10 on 10 Point Scale	300+	67%	-	67%
Meds 'Always' Explained Before Given	300+	61%	-	60%
Nurses 'Always' Communicated Well	300+	77%	-	76%
Pain 'Always' Well Controlled	300+	72%	-	69%
Room and Bathroom 'Always' Clean	300+	78%	-	71%
Timely Help 'Always' Received	300+	68%	-	64%
Would Definitely Recommend Hospital	300+	67%	-	69%

NOTE: Hospital profiles are in alphabetical order by state, then city, then hospital within the city; Rankings exclude hospitals with less than 25 cases except for patient surveys which excludes hospitals with less than 100 cases; (a) 100–299 cases; (1) The number of cases is too small to be sure how well a hospital is performing; (2) The hospital indicated that the data submitted for this measure were based on a sample of cases; (3) Data was collected during a shorter time period (fewer quarters) than the maximum possible time for this measure; (4) Suppressed for one or more quarters by CMS; (5) No data is available from the hospital for this measure; (6) Fewer than 100 patients completed the HCAHPS survey. Use these rates with caution, as the number of surveys may be too low to reliably assess hospital performance; (7) Survey results are based on less than 12 months of data; (8) Survey results are not available for this reporting period; (9) No or very few patients were eligible for the HCAHPS survey. The scores shown, if any, reflect a very small number of surveys; (10) A state average was not calculated because too few hospitals in the state submitted data; (11) There were discrepancies in the data collection process; Please refer to the User's Guide for a full explanation of data.

Hampshire Memorial Hospital

549 Center Avenue Phone: 304-822-4561
Romney, WV 26757 Fax: 304-822-7809
E-mail: hmhi@access.mountain.net
Type: Critical Access Hospitals Emergency Services: Yes
Ownership: Voluntary Non-Profit - Private Beds: 47

Key Personnel:
CEO/President. . . . . Harold A McBee, Sr
Chief of Medical Staff. . . . . Vijay K Chowdhary, MD
Infection Control. . . . . Jonathan R Walburn, MD
Operating Room. . . . . Carlotte Staudt
Quality Assurance . . . . Julia A Sites, RN
Emergency Room . . . . Anthony K Haywood, DO

Measure	Cases	This Hosp.	State Avg.	U.S. Avg.
Heart Attack Care				
ACE Inhibitor or ARB for LVSD[5]	0	-	94%	96%
Aspirin at Arrival[5]	0	-	97%	99%
Aspirin at Discharge[5]	0	-	98%	98%
Beta Blocker at Discharge[5]	0	-	98%	98%
Fibrinolytic Medication Timing[5]	0	-	29%	55%
PCI Within 90 Minutes of Arrival[5]	0	-	85%	90%
Smoking Cessation Advice[5]	0	-	99%	99%
Chest Pain/Possible Heart Attack Care				
Aspirin at Arrival	-	-	95%	95%
Median Time to ECG (minutes)	-	-	12	8
Median Time to Transfer (minutes)	-	-	77	61
Fibrinolytic Medication Timing	-	-	56%	54%
Heart Failure Care				
ACE Inhibitor or ARB for LVSD[5]	0	-	90%	94%
Discharge Instructions[5]	0	-	85%	88%
Evaluation of LVS Function[5]	0	-	97%	98%
Smoking Cessation Advice[5]	0	-	97%	98%
Pneumonia Care				
Appropriate Initial Antibiotic[5]	0	-	89%	92%
Blood Culture Timing[5]	0	-	95%	96%
Influenza Vaccine[5]	0	-	90%	91%
Initial Antibiotic Timing[5]	0	-	94%	95%
Pneumococcal Vaccine[5]	0	-	91%	93%
Smoking Cessation Advice[5]	0	-	96%	97%
Surgical Care Improvement Project				
Appropriate VTP Within 24 Hours[5]	0	-	91%	92%
Appropriate Hair Removal[5]	0	-	99%	99%
Appropriate Beta Blocker Usage[5]	0	-	93%	93%
Controlled Postoperative Blood Glucose[5]	0	-	91%	93%
Prophylactic Antibiotic Timing[5]	0	-	97%	97%
Prophylactic Antibiotic Timing (Outpatient)	-	-	90%	92%
Prophylactic Antibiotic Selection[5]	0	-	97%	97%
Prophylactic Antibiotic Select. (Outpatient)	-	-	91%	94%
Prophylactic Antibiotic Stopped[5]	0	-	94%	94%
Recommended VTP Ordered[5]	0	-	92%	94%
Urinary Catheter Removal[5]	0	-	90%	90%
Children's Asthma Care				
Received Systemic Corticosteroids	-	-	-	100%
Received Home Management Plan	-	-	-	71%
Received Reliever Medication	-	-	-	100%
Use of Medical Imaging				
Combination Abdominal CT Scan	-	-	0.304	0.191
Combination Chest CT Scan	-	-	0.063	0.054
Follow-up Mammogram/Ultrasound	-	-	8.8%	8.4%
MRI for Low Back Pain	-	-	38.5%	32.7%
Survey of Patients' Hospital Experiences				
Area Around Room 'Always' Quiet at Night[6]	<100	49%	-	58%
Doctors 'Always' Communicated Well[6]	<100	88%	-	80%
Home Recovery Information Given[6]	<100	80%	-	82%
Hospital Given 9 or 10 on 10 Point Scale[6]	<100	48%	-	67%
Meds 'Always' Explained Before Given[6]	<100	64%	-	60%
Nurses 'Always' Communicated Well[6]	<100	79%	-	76%
Pain 'Always' Well Controlled[6]	<100	60%	-	69%
Room and Bathroom 'Always' Clean[6]	<100	80%	-	71%
Timely Help 'Always' Received[6]	<100	81%	-	64%
Would Definitely Recommend Hospital	<100	60%	-	69%

Greenbrier Valley Medical Center

202 Maplewood Avenue Phone: 304-647-4411
Ronceverte, WV 24970 Fax: 304-647-6010
Type: Acute Care Hospitals Emergency Services: Yes
Ownership: Voluntary Non-Profit - Other Beds: 122

Key Personnel:
CEO/President. . . . . Mark Nosacka
Chief of Medical Staff. . . . . Oshfaq Ohsannidin, MD
Infection Control. . . . . Barbara Walker
Operating Room. . . . . Paula Bishop, RN
Radiology. . . . . David Maki
Anesthesiology. . . . . Colin Rose, MD
Emergency Room . . . . Jon Stout, DO
Intensive Care Unit. . . . . Tammy Murphy

Measure	Cases	This Hosp.	State Avg.	U.S. Avg.
Heart Attack Care				
ACE Inhibitor or ARB for LVSD[1]	1	100%	94%	96%
Aspirin at Arrival[1]	19	100%	97%	99%
Aspirin at Discharge[1]	8	100%	98%	98%
Beta Blocker at Discharge[1]	7	86%	98%	98%
Fibrinolytic Medication Timing	0	-	29%	55%
PCI Within 90 Minutes of Arrival	0	-	85%	90%
Smoking Cessation Advice[1]	2	100%	99%	99%
Chest Pain/Possible Heart Attack Care				
Aspirin at Arrival	76	97%	95%	95%
Median Time to ECG (minutes)	83	3	12	8
Median Time to Transfer (minutes)[1,3]	2	130	77	61
Fibrinolytic Medication Timing[1]	11	64%	56%	54%
Heart Failure Care				
ACE Inhibitor or ARB for LVSD	48	79%	90%	94%
Discharge Instructions	114	89%	85%	88%
Evaluation of LVS Function	139	99%	97%	98%
Smoking Cessation Advice[1]	24	100%	97%	98%
Pneumonia Care				
Appropriate Initial Antibiotic	120	92%	89%	92%
Blood Culture Timing	196	94%	95%	96%
Influenza Vaccine	164	96%	90%	91%
Initial Antibiotic Timing	198	97%	94%	95%
Pneumococcal Vaccine	205	99%	91%	93%
Smoking Cessation Advice	116	97%	96%	97%
Surgical Care Improvement Project				
Appropriate VTP Within 24 Hours	93	98%	91%	92%
Appropriate Hair Removal	199	100%	99%	99%
Appropriate Beta Blocker Usage	60	93%	93%	93%
Controlled Postoperative Blood Glucose	0	-	91%	93%
Prophylactic Antibiotic Timing	127	98%	97%	97%
Prophylactic Antibiotic Timing (Outpatient)	127	97%	90%	92%
Prophylactic Antibiotic Selection	130	99%	97%	97%
Prophylactic Antibiotic Select. (Outpatient)	124	98%	91%	94%
Prophylactic Antibiotic Stopped	121	93%	94%	94%
Recommended VTP Ordered	93	98%	92%	94%
Urinary Catheter Removal	38	79%	90%	90%
Children's Asthma Care				
Received Systemic Corticosteroids	-	-	-	100%
Received Home Management Plan	-	-	-	71%
Received Reliever Medication	-	-	-	100%
Use of Medical Imaging				
Combination Abdominal CT Scan	757	0.145	0.304	0.191
Combination Chest CT Scan	561	0.002	0.063	0.054
Follow-up Mammogram/Ultrasound	488	12.7%	8.8%	8.4%
MRI for Low Back Pain	202	35.1%	38.5%	32.7%
Survey of Patients' Hospital Experiences				
Area Around Room 'Always' Quiet at Night	300+	51%	-	58%
Doctors 'Always' Communicated Well	300+	81%	-	80%
Home Recovery Information Given	300+	80%	-	82%
Hospital Given 9 or 10 on 10 Point Scale	300+	60%	-	67%
Meds 'Always' Explained Before Given	300+	55%	-	60%
Nurses 'Always' Communicated Well	300+	73%	-	76%
Pain 'Always' Well Controlled	300+	68%	-	69%
Room and Bathroom 'Always' Clean	300+	62%	-	71%
Timely Help 'Always' Received	300+	57%	-	64%
Would Definitely Recommend Hospital	300+	59%	-	69%

Sistersville General Hospital

314 South Wells Street Phone: 304-652-2611
Sistersville, WV 26175 Fax: 304-652-1448
E-mail: sisgen@ovis.net
URL: www.sistersvillegeneral.com
Type: Critical Access Hospitals Emergency Services: Yes
Ownership: Government - Local Beds: 12

Key Personnel:
CEO/President. . . . . Brian Lowther
Chief of Medical Staff. . . . . Ramon Fagundo
Radiology. . . . . Anna Carson
Emergency Room . . . . Jason Enoch

Measure	Cases	This Hosp.	State Avg.	U.S. Avg.
Heart Attack Care				
ACE Inhibitor or ARB for LVSD[5]	0	-	94%	96%
Aspirin at Arrival[5]	0	-	97%	99%
Aspirin at Discharge[5]	0	-	98%	98%
Beta Blocker at Discharge[5]	0	-	98%	98%
Fibrinolytic Medication Timing[5]	0	-	29%	55%
PCI Within 90 Minutes of Arrival[5]	0	-	85%	90%
Smoking Cessation Advice[5]	0	-	99%	99%
Chest Pain/Possible Heart Attack Care				
Aspirin at Arrival	-	-	95%	95%
Median Time to ECG (minutes)	-	-	12	8
Median Time to Transfer (minutes)	-	-	77	61
Fibrinolytic Medication Timing	-	-	56%	54%
Heart Failure Care				
ACE Inhibitor or ARB for LVSD[3]	0	-	90%	94%
Discharge Instructions[1,3]	2	0%	85%	88%
Evaluation of LVS Function[1,3]	3	0%	97%	98%
Smoking Cessation Advice[3]	0	-	97%	98%
Pneumonia Care				
Appropriate Initial Antibiotic[1,3]	8	88%	89%	92%
Blood Culture Timing[1,3]	9	100%	95%	96%
Influenza Vaccine[1]	10	60%	90%	91%
Initial Antibiotic Timing[1,3]	8	88%	94%	95%
Pneumococcal Vaccine[1,3]	8	62%	91%	93%
Smoking Cessation Advice[1,3]	3	67%	96%	97%
Surgical Care Improvement Project				
Appropriate VTP Within 24 Hours[5]	0	-	91%	92%
Appropriate Hair Removal[5]	0	-	99%	99%
Appropriate Beta Blocker Usage[5]	0	-	93%	93%
Controlled Postoperative Blood Glucose[5]	0	-	91%	93%
Prophylactic Antibiotic Timing[5]	0	-	97%	97%
Prophylactic Antibiotic Timing (Outpatient)	-	-	90%	92%
Prophylactic Antibiotic Selection[5]	0	-	97%	97%
Prophylactic Antibiotic Select. (Outpatient)	-	-	91%	94%
Prophylactic Antibiotic Stopped[5]	0	-	94%	94%
Recommended VTP Ordered[5]	0	-	92%	94%
Urinary Catheter Removal[5]	0	-	90%	90%
Children's Asthma Care				
Received Systemic Corticosteroids	-	-	-	100%
Received Home Management Plan	-	-	-	71%
Received Reliever Medication	-	-	-	100%
Use of Medical Imaging				
Combination Abdominal CT Scan	-	-	0.304	0.191
Combination Chest CT Scan	-	-	0.063	0.054
Follow-up Mammogram/Ultrasound	-	-	8.8%	8.4%
MRI for Low Back Pain	-	-	38.5%	32.7%
Survey of Patients' Hospital Experiences				
Area Around Room 'Always' Quiet at Night[8]	-	-	-	58%
Doctors 'Always' Communicated Well[8]	-	-	-	80%
Home Recovery Information Given[8]	-	-	-	82%
Hospital Given 9 or 10 on 10 Point Scale[8]	-	-	-	67%
Meds 'Always' Explained Before Given[8]	-	-	-	60%
Nurses 'Always' Communicated Well[8]	-	-	-	76%
Pain 'Always' Well Controlled[8]	-	-	-	69%
Room and Bathroom 'Always' Clean[8]	-	-	-	71%
Timely Help 'Always' Received[8]	-	-	-	64%
Would Definitely Recommend Hospital[8]	-	-	-	69%

NOTE: Hospital profiles are in alphabetical order by state, then city, then hospital within the city; Rankings exclude hospitals with less than 25 cases except for patient surveys which excludes hospitals with less than 100 cases; (a) 100–299 cases; (1) The number of cases is too small to be sure how well a hospital is performing; (2) The hospital indicated that the data submitted for this measure were based on a sample of cases; (3) Data was collected during a shorter time period (fewer quarters) than the maximum possible time for this measure; (4) Suppressed for one or more quarters by CMS; (5) No data is available from the hospital for this measure; (6) Fewer than 100 patients completed the HCAHPS survey. Use these rates with caution, as the number of surveys may be too low to reliably assess hospital performance; (7) Survey results are based on less than 12 months of data; (8) Survey results are not available for this reporting period; (9) No or very few patients were eligible for the HCAHPS survey. The scores shown, if any, reflect a very small number of surveys; (10) A state average was not calculated because too few hospitals in the state submitted data; (11) There were discrepancies in the data collection process; Please refer to the User's Guide for a full explanation of data.

Thomas Memorial Hospital

4605 Maccorkle Ave SW
South Charleston, WV 25309
URL: www.thomaswv.org
Type: Acute Care Hospitals
Ownership: Government - Local
Phone: 304-766-3600
Fax: 304-766-3477
Emergency Services: Yes
Beds: 296

Key Personnel:
CEO/President. . . . . Stephen P Dexter
Chief of Medical Staff. . . . . James Mears, MD
Coronary Care . . . . Lynn Storrick
Infection Control. . . . . Sara K Spencer
Operating Room. . . . . Rudy Mancuso
Pediatric Ambulatory Care . . . . . Sandy Young
Quality Assurance . . . . Renee Amend
Radiology. . . . . Mark Wilcox

Measure	Cases	This Hosp.	State Avg.	U.S. Avg.
Heart Attack Care				
ACE Inhibitor or ARB for LVSD[1,2]	23	70%	94%	96%
Aspirin at Arrival[2]	114	90%	97%	99%
Aspirin at Discharge[2]	80	94%	98%	98%
Beta Blocker at Discharge[2]	82	91%	98%	98%
Fibrinolytic Medication Timing[1,2]	1	0%	29%	55%
PCI Within 90 Minutes of Arrival[1,2]	11	64%	85%	90%
Smoking Cessation Advice[2]	30	100%	99%	99%
Chest Pain/Possible Heart Attack Care				
Aspirin at Arrival[1,3]	17	88%	95%	95%
Median Time to ECG (minutes)[1,3]	17	25	12	8
Median Time to Transfer (minutes)[3]	0	-	77	61
Fibrinolytic Medication Timing[1,3]	1	100%	56%	54%
Heart Failure Care				
ACE Inhibitor or ARB for LVSD[2]	52	90%	90%	94%
Discharge Instructions[2]	163	85%	85%	88%
Evaluation of LVS Function[2]	207	95%	97%	98%
Smoking Cessation Advice[2]	27	96%	97%	98%
Pneumonia Care				
Appropriate Initial Antibiotic[2]	189	88%	89%	92%
Blood Culture Timing[2]	282	94%	95%	96%
Influenza Vaccine	198	72%	90%	91%
Initial Antibiotic Timing[2]	288	92%	94%	95%
Pneumococcal Vaccine[2]	242	70%	91%	93%
Smoking Cessation Advice[2]	114	98%	96%	97%
Surgical Care Improvement Project				
Appropriate VTP Within 24 Hours[2]	235	71%	91%	92%
Appropriate Hair Removal[2]	683	96%	99%	99%
Appropriate Beta Blocker Usage[2]	215	84%	93%	93%
Controlled Postoperative Blood Glucose[2]	0	-	91%	93%
Prophylactic Antibiotic Timing[2]	454	97%	97%	97%
Prophylactic Antibiotic Timing (Outpatient)	156	90%	90%	92%
Prophylactic Antibiotic Selection[2]	456	97%	97%	97%
Prophylactic Antibiotic Select. (Outpatient)	144	96%	91%	94%
Prophylactic Antibiotic Stopped[2]	433	87%	94%	94%
Recommended VTP Ordered[2]	237	78%	92%	94%
Urinary Catheter Removal	78	85%	90%	90%
Children's Asthma Care				
Received Systemic Corticosteroids	-	-	-	100%
Received Home Management Plan	-	-	-	71%
Received Reliever Medication	-	-	-	100%
Use of Medical Imaging				
Combination Abdominal CT Scan	876	0.030	0.304	0.191
Combination Chest CT Scan	580	0.000	0.063	0.054
Follow-up Mammogram/Ultrasound	1,121	7.4%	8.8%	8.4%
MRI for Low Back Pain	406	35.7%	38.5%	32.7%
Survey of Patients' Hospital Experiences				
Area Around Room 'Always' Quiet at Night	300+	43%	-	58%
Doctors 'Always' Communicated Well	300+	79%	-	80%
Home Recovery Information Given	300+	82%	-	82%
Hospital Given 9 or 10 on 10 Point Scale	300+	60%	-	67%
Meds 'Always' Explained Before Given	300+	52%	-	60%
Nurses 'Always' Communicated Well	300+	71%	-	76%
Pain 'Always' Well Controlled	300+	65%	-	69%
Room and Bathroom 'Always' Clean	300+	60%	-	71%
Timely Help 'Always' Received	300+	58%	-	64%
Would Definitely Recommend Hospital	300+	63%	-	69%

Roane General Hospital

200 Hospital Drive
Spencer, WV 25276
URL: www.roanegeneralhospital.com
Type: Critical Access Hospitals
Ownership: Voluntary Non-Profit - Private
Phone: 304-927-4444
Fax: 304-927-6390
Emergency Services: Yes
Beds: 60

Key Personnel:
CEO/President. . . . . Doug Bentz
Chief of Medical Staff . . . . Ken Seen
Operating Room. . . . . Robin Miller, RN
Quality Assurance . . . . Martha Hardman
Radiology. . . . . George Wilson
Anesthesiology. . . . . Gerald Princesa, MD
Emergency Room . . . . Julie Carr
Patient Relations . . . . Louise Ward

Measure	Cases	This Hosp.	State Avg.	U.S. Avg.
Heart Attack Care				
ACE Inhibitor or ARB for LVSD[1]	1	100%	94%	96%
Aspirin at Arrival[1]	9	89%	97%	99%
Aspirin at Discharge[1]	4	100%	98%	98%
Beta Blocker at Discharge[1]	6	100%	98%	98%
Fibrinolytic Medication Timing	0	-	29%	55%
PCI Within 90 Minutes of Arrival	0	-	85%	90%
Smoking Cessation Advice[1]	1	100%	99%	99%
Chest Pain/Possible Heart Attack Care				
Aspirin at Arrival	38	97%	95%	95%
Median Time to ECG (minutes)	40	0	12	8
Median Time to Transfer (minutes)[3]	0	-	77	61
Fibrinolytic Medication Timing[1]	3	100%	56%	54%
Heart Failure Care				
ACE Inhibitor or ARB for LVSD[3]	0	-	90%	94%
Discharge Instructions[1,3]	6	67%	85%	88%
Evaluation of LVS Function[1,3]	8	100%	97%	98%
Smoking Cessation Advice[3]	0	-	97%	98%
Pneumonia Care				
Appropriate Initial Antibiotic[1]	21	95%	89%	92%
Blood Culture Timing[1]	16	100%	95%	96%
Influenza Vaccine[1]	22	91%	90%	91%
Initial Antibiotic Timing	25	92%	94%	95%
Pneumococcal Vaccine	30	93%	91%	93%
Smoking Cessation Advice[1]	8	75%	96%	97%
Surgical Care Improvement Project				
Appropriate VTP Within 24 Hours[1]	11	91%	91%	92%
Appropriate Hair Removal[1]	19	100%	99%	99%
Appropriate Beta Blocker Usage[1]	4	100%	93%	93%
Controlled Postoperative Blood Glucose	0	-	91%	93%
Prophylactic Antibiotic Timing[1]	5	100%	97%	97%
Prophylactic Antibiotic Timing (Outpatient)[1,3]	2	100%	90%	92%
Prophylactic Antibiotic Selection[1]	5	100%	97%	97%
Prophylactic Antibiotic Select. (Outpatient)[1,3]	2	100%	91%	94%
Prophylactic Antibiotic Stopped[1]	5	100%	94%	94%
Recommended VTP Ordered[1]	11	91%	92%	94%
Urinary Catheter Removal[1]	2	100%	90%	90%
Children's Asthma Care				
Received Systemic Corticosteroids	-	-	-	100%
Received Home Management Plan	-	-	-	71%
Received Reliever Medication	-	-	-	100%
Use of Medical Imaging				
Combination Abdominal CT Scan	132	0.523	0.304	0.191
Combination Chest CT Scan	83	0.000	0.063	0.054
Follow-up Mammogram/Ultrasound	235	23.0%	8.8%	8.4%
MRI for Low Back Pain[1]	13	69.2%	38.5%	32.7%
Survey of Patients' Hospital Experiences				
Area Around Room 'Always' Quiet at Night	(a)	56%	-	58%
Doctors 'Always' Communicated Well	(a)	84%	-	80%
Home Recovery Information Given	(a)	85%	-	82%
Hospital Given 9 or 10 on 10 Point Scale	(a)	77%	-	67%
Meds 'Always' Explained Before Given	(a)	60%	-	60%
Nurses 'Always' Communicated Well	(a)	79%	-	76%
Pain 'Always' Well Controlled	(a)	71%	-	69%
Room and Bathroom 'Always' Clean	(a)	78%	-	71%
Timely Help 'Always' Received	(a)	74%	-	64%
Would Definitely Recommend Hospital	(a)	65%	-	69%

Summersville Regional Medical Center

400 Fairview Heights Road
Summersville, WV 26651
E-mail: susies@wirefire.com
URL: www.summersvillememorial.org
Type: Acute Care Hospitals
Ownership: Government - Local
Phone: 304-872-2891
Fax: 304-872-4546
Emergency Services: Yes
Beds: 109

Key Personnel:
CEO/President. . . . . Debra Hill
Chief of Medical Staff . . . . Mark Wanez
Infection Control. . . . . Paula Fields, RN
Operating Room. . . . . Betty O'Neil, RN
Quality Assurance . . . . Susie Keaton, RN
Anesthesiology. . . . . Cecil Graham, MD
Emergency Room . . . . Robert Fleer, MD

Measure	Cases	This Hosp.	State Avg.	U.S. Avg.
Heart Attack Care				
ACE Inhibitor or ARB for LVSD[1]	5	80%	94%	96%
Aspirin at Arrival[1]	17	88%	97%	99%
Aspirin at Discharge[1]	10	90%	98%	98%
Beta Blocker at Discharge[1]	9	100%	98%	98%
Fibrinolytic Medication Timing	0	-	29%	55%
PCI Within 90 Minutes of Arrival	0	-	85%	90%
Smoking Cessation Advice[1]	1	100%	99%	99%
Chest Pain/Possible Heart Attack Care				
Aspirin at Arrival	81	94%	95%	95%
Median Time to ECG (minutes)	86	14	12	8
Median Time to Transfer (minutes)[1,3]	2	310	77	61
Fibrinolytic Medication Timing[1]	13	69%	56%	54%
Heart Failure Care				
ACE Inhibitor or ARB for LVSD[1,2]	17	88%	90%	94%
Discharge Instructions[2]	35	37%	85%	88%
Evaluation of LVS Function[2]	53	94%	97%	98%
Smoking Cessation Advice[1,2]	9	78%	97%	98%
Pneumonia Care				
Appropriate Initial Antibiotic	43	91%	89%	92%
Blood Culture Timing	101	78%	95%	96%
Influenza Vaccine	59	80%	90%	91%
Initial Antibiotic Timing	120	95%	94%	95%
Pneumococcal Vaccine	86	79%	91%	93%
Smoking Cessation Advice	30	67%	96%	97%
Surgical Care Improvement Project				
Appropriate VTP Within 24 Hours[2]	64	95%	91%	92%
Appropriate Hair Removal[2]	101	100%	99%	99%
Appropriate Beta Blocker Usage[2]	32	100%	93%	93%
Controlled Postoperative Blood Glucose[2]	0	-	91%	93%
Prophylactic Antibiotic Timing[2]	58	93%	97%	97%
Prophylactic Antibiotic Timing (Outpatient)	56	80%	90%	92%
Prophylactic Antibiotic Selection[2]	57	82%	97%	97%
Prophylactic Antibiotic Select. (Outpatient)	45	78%	91%	94%
Prophylactic Antibiotic Stopped[2]	55	80%	94%	94%
Recommended VTP Ordered[2]	64	97%	92%	94%
Urinary Catheter Removal[1]	19	89%	90%	90%
Children's Asthma Care				
Received Systemic Corticosteroids	-	-	-	100%
Received Home Management Plan	-	-	-	71%
Received Reliever Medication	-	-	-	100%
Use of Medical Imaging				
Combination Abdominal CT Scan	502	0.046	0.304	0.191
Combination Chest CT Scan	261	0.050	0.063	0.054
Follow-up Mammogram/Ultrasound	236	9.7%	8.8%	8.4%
MRI for Low Back Pain	113	37.2%	38.5%	32.7%
Survey of Patients' Hospital Experiences				
Area Around Room 'Always' Quiet at Night	300+	44%	-	58%
Doctors 'Always' Communicated Well	300+	84%	-	80%
Home Recovery Information Given	300+	75%	-	82%
Hospital Given 9 or 10 on 10 Point Scale	300+	60%	-	67%
Meds 'Always' Explained Before Given	300+	62%	-	60%
Nurses 'Always' Communicated Well	300+	74%	-	76%
Pain 'Always' Well Controlled	300+	69%	-	69%
Room and Bathroom 'Always' Clean	300+	69%	-	71%
Timely Help 'Always' Received	300+	61%	-	64%
Would Definitely Recommend Hospital	300+	64%	-	69%

NOTE: Hospital profiles are in alphabetical order by state, then city, then hospital within the city; Rankings exclude hospitals with less than 25 cases except for patient surveys which excludes hospitals with less than 100 cases; (a) 100–299 cases; (1) The number of cases is too small to be sure how well a hospital is performing; (2) The hospital indicated that the data submitted for this measure were based on a sample of cases; (3) Data was collected during a shorter time period (fewer quarters) than the maximum possible time for this measure; (4) Suppressed for one or more quarters by CMS; (5) No data is available from the hospital for this measure; (6) Fewer than 100 patients completed the HCAHPS survey. Use these rates with caution, as the number of surveys may be too low to reliably assess hospital performance; (7) Survey results are based on less than 12 months of data; (8) Survey results are not available for this reporting period; (9) No or very few patients were eligible for the HCAHPS survey. The scores shown, if any, reflect a very small number of surveys; (10) A state average was not calculated because too few hospitals in the state submitted data; (11) There were discrepancies in the data collection process; Please refer to the User's Guide for a full explanation of data.

Webster County Memorial Hospital

162 Goldenwood Dr Phone: 304-847-5682
Webster Springs, WV 26288 Fax: 304-847-7660
E-mail: admin@wcmhwv.com
URL: www.wcmhwv.com
Type: Critical Access Hospitals Emergency Services: Yes
Ownership: Government - Local Beds: 25

Key Personnel:

Chief of Medical Staff.......... Robert Mace, MD
Infection Control............. Mary Leonard
Pediatric Ambulatory Care ...... Mark Hardway, MD
Quality Assurance .... Betty Skidmore
Emergency Room .... Larry Clevenger, MD
Patient Relations .... Betty Skidmore

Measure	Cases	This Hosp.	State Avg.	U.S. Avg.
Heart Attack Care				
ACE Inhibitor or ARB for LVSD[5]	0	-	94%	96%
Aspirin at Arrival[5]	0	-	97%	99%
Aspirin at Discharge[5]	0	-	98%	98%
Beta Blocker at Discharge[5]	0	-	98%	98%
Fibrinolytic Medication Timing[5]	0	-	29%	55%
PCI Within 90 Minutes of Arrival[5]	0	-	85%	90%
Smoking Cessation Advice[5]	0	-	99%	99%
Chest Pain/Possible Heart Attack Care				
Aspirin at Arrival	-	-	95%	95%
Median Time to ECG (minutes)	-	-	12	8
Median Time to Transfer (minutes)	-	-	77	61
Fibrinolytic Medication Timing	-	-	56%	54%
Heart Failure Care				
ACE Inhibitor or ARB for LVSD[3]	0	-	90%	94%
Discharge Instructions[1,3]	8	88%	85%	88%
Evaluation of LVS Function[1,3]	8	0%	97%	98%
Smoking Cessation Advice[1,3]	1	100%	97%	98%
Pneumonia Care				
Appropriate Initial Antibiotic[1,3]	17	76%	89%	92%
Blood Culture Timing[1,3]	7	57%	95%	96%
Influenza Vaccine[5]	0	-	90%	91%
Initial Antibiotic Timing[1,3]	21	76%	94%	95%
Pneumococcal Vaccine[1,3]	11	55%	91%	93%
Smoking Cessation Advice[1,3]	8	100%	96%	97%
Surgical Care Improvement Project				
Appropriate VTP Within 24 Hours[5]	0	-	91%	92%
Appropriate Hair Removal[5]	0	-	99%	99%
Appropriate Beta Blocker Usage[5]	0	-	93%	93%
Controlled Postoperative Blood Glucose[5]	0	-	91%	93%
Prophylactic Antibiotic Timing[5]	0	-	97%	97%
Prophylactic Antibiotic Timing (Outpatient)	-	-	90%	92%
Prophylactic Antibiotic Selection[5]	0	-	97%	97%
Prophylactic Antibiotic Select. (Outpatient)	-	-	91%	94%
Prophylactic Antibiotic Stopped[5]	0	-	94%	94%
Recommended VTP Ordered[5]	0	-	92%	94%
Urinary Catheter Removal[5]	0	-	90%	90%
Children's Asthma Care				
Received Systemic Corticosteroids	-	-	-	100%
Received Home Management Plan	-	-	-	71%
Received Reliever Medication	-	-	-	100%
Use of Medical Imaging				
Combination Abdominal CT Scan	-	-	0.304	0.191
Combination Chest CT Scan	-	-	0.063	0.054
Follow-up Mammogram/Ultrasound	-	-	8.8%	8.4%
MRI for Low Back Pain	-	-	38.5%	32.7%
Survey of Patients' Hospital Experiences				
Area Around Room 'Always' Quiet at Night[8]	-	-	-	58%
Doctors 'Always' Communicated Well[8]	-	-	-	80%
Home Recovery Information Given[8]	-	-	-	82%
Hospital Given 9 or 10 on 10 Point Scale[8]	-	-	-	67%
Meds 'Always' Explained Before Given[8]	-	-	-	60%
Nurses 'Always' Communicated Well[8]	-	-	-	76%
Pain 'Always' Well Controlled[8]	-	-	-	69%
Room and Bathroom 'Always' Clean[8]	-	-	-	71%
Timely Help 'Always' Received[8]	-	-	-	64%
Would Definitely Recommend Hospital[8]	-	-	-	69%

Weirton Medical Center

601 Colliers Way Phone: 304-797-6000
Weirton, WV 26062 Fax: 304-797-6449
URL: www.weirtonmedical.com
Type: Acute Care Hospitals Emergency Services: Yes
Ownership: Government - Local Beds: 240

Key Personnel:

CEO/President................ Joseph P Endrich, MD
Cardiac Laboratory............ Carletta Williams
Chief of Medical Staff.......... Garry Hanson
Operating Room.............. Adnan Abla, RN
Quality Assurance .... R Nolan
Radiology................... Peter Aragones
Emergency Room .... Neal Aulick

Measure	Cases	This Hosp.	State Avg.	U.S. Avg.
Heart Attack Care				
ACE Inhibitor or ARB for LVSD[1]	9	100%	94%	96%
Aspirin at Arrival	68	94%	97%	99%
Aspirin at Discharge	57	82%	98%	98%
Beta Blocker at Discharge	58	90%	98%	98%
Fibrinolytic Medication Timing	0	-	29%	55%
PCI Within 90 Minutes of Arrival[1]	23	65%	85%	90%
Smoking Cessation Advice[1]	23	96%	99%	99%
Chest Pain/Possible Heart Attack Care				
Aspirin at Arrival[1]	17	94%	95%	95%
Median Time to ECG (minutes)[1]	16	8	12	8
Median Time to Transfer (minutes)[5]	0	-	77	61
Fibrinolytic Medication Timing[3]	0	-	56%	54%
Heart Failure Care				
ACE Inhibitor or ARB for LVSD	63	97%	90%	94%
Discharge Instructions	171	86%	85%	88%
Evaluation of LVS Function	212	99%	97%	98%
Smoking Cessation Advice	35	100%	97%	98%
Pneumonia Care				
Appropriate Initial Antibiotic	232	92%	89%	92%
Blood Culture Timing	321	99%	95%	96%
Influenza Vaccine	210	97%	90%	91%
Initial Antibiotic Timing	313	98%	94%	95%
Pneumococcal Vaccine	286	95%	91%	93%
Smoking Cessation Advice	139	100%	96%	97%
Surgical Care Improvement Project				
Appropriate VTP Within 24 Hours[2]	118	86%	91%	92%
Appropriate Hair Removal[2]	329	98%	99%	99%
Appropriate Beta Blocker Usage[2]	79	97%	93%	93%
Controlled Postoperative Blood Glucose[2]	0	-	91%	93%
Prophylactic Antibiotic Timing[2]	245	97%	97%	97%
Prophylactic Antibiotic Timing (Outpatient)	85	80%	90%	92%
Prophylactic Antibiotic Selection[2]	245	95%	97%	97%
Prophylactic Antibiotic Select. (Outpatient)	82	68%	91%	94%
Prophylactic Antibiotic Stopped[2]	236	89%	94%	94%
Recommended VTP Ordered[2]	118	89%	92%	94%
Urinary Catheter Removal	88	70%	90%	90%
Children's Asthma Care				
Received Systemic Corticosteroids	-	-	-	100%
Received Home Management Plan	-	-	-	71%
Received Reliever Medication	-	-	-	100%
Use of Medical Imaging				
Combination Abdominal CT Scan	524	0.149	0.304	0.191
Combination Chest CT Scan	352	0.037	0.063	0.054
Follow-up Mammogram/Ultrasound	552	9.4%	8.8%	8.4%
MRI for Low Back Pain	142	31.7%	38.5%	32.7%
Survey of Patients' Hospital Experiences				
Area Around Room 'Always' Quiet at Night	300+	36%	-	58%
Doctors 'Always' Communicated Well	300+	73%	-	80%
Home Recovery Information Given	300+	76%	-	82%
Hospital Given 9 or 10 on 10 Point Scale	300+	44%	-	67%
Meds 'Always' Explained Before Given	300+	51%	-	60%
Nurses 'Always' Communicated Well	300+	62%	-	76%
Pain 'Always' Well Controlled	300+	61%	-	69%
Room and Bathroom 'Always' Clean	300+	51%	-	71%
Timely Help 'Always' Received	300+	40%	-	64%
Would Definitely Recommend Hospital	300+	41%	-	69%

Welch Community Hospital

454 Mcdowell Street Phone: 304-436-8461
Welch, WV 24801 Fax: 304-436-6380
Type: Acute Care Hospitals Emergency Services: Yes
Ownership: Government - State Beds: 124

Key Personnel:

CEO/President............... Walter J Garrett
Infection Control............. Peggy Miller, RN
Operating Room.............. Debbie Myers, RN
Anesthesiology............... Bill Shrewsberry
Emergency Room .... Barbara Dalton, RN
Intensive Care Unit............ Janice Hagy, RN

Measure	Cases	This Hosp.	State Avg.	U.S. Avg.
Heart Attack Care				
ACE Inhibitor or ARB for LVSD[3]	0	-	94%	96%
Aspirin at Arrival[1,3]	1	0%	97%	99%
Aspirin at Discharge[3]	0	-	98%	98%
Beta Blocker at Discharge[3]	0	-	98%	98%
Fibrinolytic Medication Timing[3]	0	-	29%	55%
PCI Within 90 Minutes of Arrival[3]	0	-	85%	90%
Smoking Cessation Advice[3]	0	-	99%	99%
Chest Pain/Possible Heart Attack Care				
Aspirin at Arrival	140	90%	95%	95%
Median Time to ECG (minutes)	142	41	12	8
Median Time to Transfer (minutes)[5]	0	-	77	61
Fibrinolytic Medication Timing[1]	11	18%	56%	54%
Heart Failure Care				
ACE Inhibitor or ARB for LVSD[1]	2	50%	90%	94%
Discharge Instructions[1]	12	8%	85%	88%
Evaluation of LVS Function[1]	13	38%	97%	98%
Smoking Cessation Advice[1]	2	50%	97%	98%
Pneumonia Care				
Appropriate Initial Antibiotic	45	93%	89%	92%
Blood Culture Timing[1]	7	29%	95%	96%
Influenza Vaccine	29	34%	90%	91%
Initial Antibiotic Timing	45	89%	94%	95%
Pneumococcal Vaccine	34	50%	91%	93%
Smoking Cessation Advice	25	68%	96%	97%
Surgical Care Improvement Project				
Appropriate VTP Within 24 Hours[1]	16	69%	91%	92%
Appropriate Hair Removal	26	85%	99%	99%
Appropriate Beta Blocker Usage[1]	7	29%	93%	93%
Controlled Postoperative Blood Glucose	0	-	91%	93%
Prophylactic Antibiotic Timing[1]	8	50%	97%	97%
Prophylactic Antibiotic Timing (Outpatient)[5]	0	-	90%	92%
Prophylactic Antibiotic Selection[1]	8	62%	97%	97%
Prophylactic Antibiotic Select. (Outpatient)[5]	0	-	91%	94%
Prophylactic Antibiotic Stopped[1]	8	50%	94%	94%
Recommended VTP Ordered[1]	17	82%	92%	94%
Urinary Catheter Removal[1]	3	67%	90%	90%
Children's Asthma Care				
Received Systemic Corticosteroids	-	-	-	100%
Received Home Management Plan	-	-	-	71%
Received Reliever Medication	-	-	-	100%
Use of Medical Imaging				
Combination Abdominal CT Scan	62	0.258	0.304	0.191
Combination Chest CT Scan[1]	24	0.292	0.063	0.054
Follow-up Mammogram/Ultrasound	106	4.7%	8.8%	8.4%
MRI for Low Back Pain[5]	0	-	38.5%	32.7%
Survey of Patients' Hospital Experiences				
Area Around Room 'Always' Quiet at Night	(a)	72%	-	58%
Doctors 'Always' Communicated Well	(a)	85%	-	80%
Home Recovery Information Given	(a)	82%	-	82%
Hospital Given 9 or 10 on 10 Point Scale	(a)	74%	-	67%
Meds 'Always' Explained Before Given	(a)	69%	-	60%
Nurses 'Always' Communicated Well	(a)	86%	-	76%
Pain 'Always' Well Controlled	(a)	75%	-	69%
Room and Bathroom 'Always' Clean	(a)	81%	-	71%
Timely Help 'Always' Received	(a)	78%	-	64%
Would Definitely Recommend Hospital	(a)	66%	-	69%

NOTE: Hospital profiles are in alphabetical order by state, then city, then hospital within the city; Rankings exclude hospitals with less than 25 cases except for patient surveys which excludes hospitals with less than 100 cases; (a) 100–299 cases; (1) The number of cases is too small to be sure how well a hospital is performing; (2) The hospital indicated that the data submitted for this measure were based on a sample of cases; (3) Data was collected during a shorter time period (fewer quarters) than the maximum possible time for this measure; (4) Suppressed for one or more quarters by CMS; (5) No data is available from the hospital for this measure; (6) Fewer than 100 patients completed the HCAHPS survey. Use these rates with caution, as the number of surveys may be too low to reliably assess hospital performance; (7) Survey results are based on less than 12 months of data; (8) Survey results are not available for this reporting period; (9) No or very few patients were eligible for the HCAHPS survey. The scores shown, if any, reflect a very small number of surveys; (10) A state average was not calculated because too few hospitals in the state submitted data; (11) There were discrepancies in the data collection process; Please refer to the User's Guide for a full explanation of data.

Stonewall Jackson Memorial Hospital

230 Hospital Plaza
Weston, WV 26452
Phone: 304-269-8080
Fax: 304-269-8090
E-mail: hospital@stonewallhospital.com
URL: www.stonewallhospital.com
Type: Acute Care Hospitals
Emergency Services: Yes
Ownership: Voluntary Non-Profit - Private
Beds: 70

Key Personnel:
CEO/President. . . . . David D Shaffer
Chief of Medical Staff. . . . . K Mahmoud, MD
Infection Control. . . . . Diane Bennett, RN
Operating Room. . . . . Mark Casto, RN
Quality Assurance . . . . Debbie Corder
Emergency Room . . . . Carla Hamner, RN
Intensive Care Unit. . . . . Lisa Henry, RN
Patient Relations . . . . Julia Spelsburg

Measure	Cases	This Hosp.	State Avg.	U.S. Avg.
Heart Attack Care				
ACE Inhibitor or ARB for LVSD[1]	6	100%	94%	96%
Aspirin at Arrival[1]	24	96%	97%	99%
Aspirin at Discharge[1]	13	100%	98%	98%
Beta Blocker at Discharge[1]	12	100%	98%	98%
Fibrinolytic Medication Timing[1]	5	20%	29%	55%
PCI Within 90 Minutes of Arrival	0	-	85%	90%
Smoking Cessation Advice	0	-	99%	99%
Chest Pain/Possible Heart Attack Care				
Aspirin at Arrival	45	96%	95%	95%
Median Time to ECG (minutes)	48	7	12	8
Median Time to Transfer (minutes)[1]	5	21	77	61
Fibrinolytic Medication Timing[1]	1	0%	56%	54%
Heart Failure Care				
ACE Inhibitor or ARB for LVSD	25	100%	90%	94%
Discharge Instructions	69	100%	85%	88%
Evaluation of LVS Function	76	100%	97%	98%
Smoking Cessation Advice[1]	6	83%	97%	98%
Pneumonia Care				
Appropriate Initial Antibiotic	93	87%	89%	92%
Blood Culture Timing	82	99%	95%	96%
Influenza Vaccine	92	92%	90%	91%
Initial Antibiotic Timing	149	97%	94%	95%
Pneumococcal Vaccine	127	93%	91%	93%
Smoking Cessation Advice	53	100%	96%	97%
Surgical Care Improvement Project				
Appropriate VTP Within 24 Hours	62	87%	91%	92%
Appropriate Hair Removal	148	100%	99%	99%
Appropriate Beta Blocker Usage	28	89%	93%	93%
Controlled Postoperative Blood Glucose	0	-	91%	93%
Prophylactic Antibiotic Timing	95	100%	97%	97%
Prophylactic Antibiotic Timing (Outpatient)	53	92%	90%	92%
Prophylactic Antibiotic Selection	96	96%	97%	97%
Prophylactic Antibiotic Select. (Outpatient)	72	99%	91%	94%
Prophylactic Antibiotic Stopped	93	90%	94%	94%
Recommended VTP Ordered	64	89%	92%	94%
Urinary Catheter Removal[1]	23	96%	90%	90%
Children's Asthma Care				
Received Systemic Corticosteroids	-	-	-	100%
Received Home Management Plan	-	-	-	71%
Received Reliever Medication	-	-	-	100%
Use of Medical Imaging				
Combination Abdominal CT Scan	213	0.648	0.304	0.191
Combination Chest CT Scan	103	0.000	0.063	0.054
Follow-up Mammogram/Ultrasound	288	10.1%	8.8%	8.4%
MRI for Low Back Pain[1]	23	30.4%	38.5%	32.7%
Survey of Patients' Hospital Experiences				
Area Around Room 'Always' Quiet at Night	300+	52%	-	58%
Doctors 'Always' Communicated Well	300+	83%	-	80%
Home Recovery Information Given	300+	74%	-	82%
Hospital Given 9 or 10 on 10 Point Scale	300+	67%	-	67%
Meds 'Always' Explained Before Given	300+	63%	-	60%
Nurses 'Always' Communicated Well	300+	79%	-	76%
Pain 'Always' Well Controlled	300+	70%	-	69%
Room and Bathroom 'Always' Clean	300+	77%	-	71%
Timely Help 'Always' Received	300+	67%	-	64%
Would Definitely Recommend Hospital	300+	68%	-	69%

Ohio Valley Medical Center

2000 Eoff Street
Wheeling, WV 26003
Phone: 304-234-0123
Fax: 304-234-1830
URL: www.ohiovalleymedicalcenter.com
Type: Acute Care Hospitals
Emergency Services: Yes
Ownership: Voluntary Non-Profit - Private
Beds: 200

Key Personnel:
CEO/President. . . . . Brian K Felici
Chief of Medical Staff. . . . . Satinder Bhullar
Radiology. . . . . Vicente P Almario

Measure	Cases	This Hosp.	State Avg.	U.S. Avg.
Heart Attack Care				
ACE Inhibitor or ARB for LVSD[1]	11	73%	94%	96%
Aspirin at Arrival	66	95%	97%	99%
Aspirin at Discharge	38	100%	98%	98%
Beta Blocker at Discharge	41	98%	98%	98%
Fibrinolytic Medication Timing	0	-	29%	55%
PCI Within 90 Minutes of Arrival	0	-	85%	90%
Smoking Cessation Advice[1]	12	100%	99%	99%
Chest Pain/Possible Heart Attack Care				
Aspirin at Arrival	33	88%	95%	95%
Median Time to ECG (minutes)	34	8	12	8
Median Time to Transfer (minutes)[1]	15	56	77	61
Fibrinolytic Medication Timing	0	-	56%	54%
Heart Failure Care				
ACE Inhibitor or ARB for LVSD	49	90%	90%	94%
Discharge Instructions	127	96%	85%	88%
Evaluation of LVS Function	177	98%	97%	98%
Smoking Cessation Advice	27	100%	97%	98%
Pneumonia Care				
Appropriate Initial Antibiotic	88	82%	89%	92%
Blood Culture Timing	133	97%	95%	96%
Influenza Vaccine	109	81%	90%	91%
Initial Antibiotic Timing	167	94%	94%	95%
Pneumococcal Vaccine	130	92%	91%	93%
Smoking Cessation Advice	65	100%	96%	97%
Surgical Care Improvement Project				
Appropriate VTP Within 24 Hours	146	85%	91%	92%
Appropriate Hair Removal	363	97%	99%	99%
Appropriate Beta Blocker Usage	109	76%	93%	93%
Controlled Postoperative Blood Glucose	0	-	91%	93%
Prophylactic Antibiotic Timing	239	95%	97%	97%
Prophylactic Antibiotic Timing (Outpatient)	80	84%	90%	92%
Prophylactic Antibiotic Selection	238	96%	97%	97%
Prophylactic Antibiotic Select. (Outpatient)	70	100%	91%	94%
Prophylactic Antibiotic Stopped	235	93%	94%	94%
Recommended VTP Ordered	149	87%	92%	94%
Urinary Catheter Removal	78	53%	90%	90%
Children's Asthma Care				
Received Systemic Corticosteroids	-	-	-	100%
Received Home Management Plan	-	-	-	71%
Received Reliever Medication	-	-	-	100%
Use of Medical Imaging				
Combination Abdominal CT Scan	344	0.640	0.304	0.191
Combination Chest CT Scan	374	0.000	0.063	0.054
Follow-up Mammogram/Ultrasound	474	13.3%	8.8%	8.4%
MRI for Low Back Pain	90	31.1%	38.5%	32.7%
Survey of Patients' Hospital Experiences				
Area Around Room 'Always' Quiet at Night	300+	56%	-	58%
Doctors 'Always' Communicated Well	300+	76%	-	80%
Home Recovery Information Given	300+	76%	-	82%
Hospital Given 9 or 10 on 10 Point Scale	300+	63%	-	67%
Meds 'Always' Explained Before Given	300+	57%	-	60%
Nurses 'Always' Communicated Well	300+	73%	-	76%
Pain 'Always' Well Controlled	300+	67%	-	69%
Room and Bathroom 'Always' Clean	300+	73%	-	71%
Timely Help 'Always' Received	300+	55%	-	64%
Would Definitely Recommend Hospital	300+	70%	-	69%

Wheeling Hospital

1 Medical Park
Wheeling, WV 26003
Phone: 304-243-3000
Fax: 304-243-3060
E-mail: webmaster@wheelinghospital.com
URL: www.wheelinghospital.com
Type: Acute Care Hospitals
Emergency Services: Yes
Ownership: Voluntary Non-Profit - Church
Beds: 277

Key Personnel:
CEO/President. . . . . Donald H Hofreuter, MD

Measure	Cases	This Hosp.	State Avg.	U.S. Avg.
Heart Attack Care				
ACE Inhibitor or ARB for LVSD	91	95%	94%	96%
Aspirin at Arrival	245	98%	97%	99%
Aspirin at Discharge	402	98%	98%	98%
Beta Blocker at Discharge	404	99%	98%	98%
Fibrinolytic Medication Timing	0	-	29%	55%
PCI Within 90 Minutes of Arrival	60	98%	85%	90%
Smoking Cessation Advice	164	100%	99%	99%
Chest Pain/Possible Heart Attack Care				
Aspirin at Arrival[1]	7	86%	95%	95%
Median Time to ECG (minutes)[1]	10	7	12	8
Median Time to Transfer (minutes)[5]	0	-	77	61
Fibrinolytic Medication Timing[5]	0	-	56%	54%
Heart Failure Care				
ACE Inhibitor or ARB for LVSD	123	92%	90%	94%
Discharge Instructions	239	95%	85%	88%
Evaluation of LVS Function	312	99%	97%	98%
Smoking Cessation Advice	35	100%	97%	98%
Pneumonia Care				
Appropriate Initial Antibiotic[2]	107	88%	89%	92%
Blood Culture Timing[2]	155	95%	95%	96%
Influenza Vaccine[2]	140	87%	90%	91%
Initial Antibiotic Timing[2]	182	94%	94%	95%
Pneumococcal Vaccine[2]	206	87%	91%	93%
Smoking Cessation Advice[2]	66	88%	96%	97%
Surgical Care Improvement Project				
Appropriate VTP Within 24 Hours	243	97%	91%	92%
Appropriate Hair Removal	1,191	98%	99%	99%
Appropriate Beta Blocker Usage	412	92%	93%	93%
Controlled Postoperative Blood Glucose	243	82%	91%	93%
Prophylactic Antibiotic Timing	910	96%	97%	97%
Prophylactic Antibiotic Timing (Outpatient)	207	90%	90%	92%
Prophylactic Antibiotic Selection	934	98%	97%	97%
Prophylactic Antibiotic Select. (Outpatient)	217	88%	91%	94%
Prophylactic Antibiotic Stopped	850	93%	94%	94%
Recommended VTP Ordered	244	97%	92%	94%
Urinary Catheter Removal	141	73%	90%	90%
Children's Asthma Care				
Received Systemic Corticosteroids	-	-	-	100%
Received Home Management Plan	-	-	-	71%
Received Reliever Medication	-	-	-	100%
Use of Medical Imaging				
Combination Abdominal CT Scan	752	0.165	0.304	0.191
Combination Chest CT Scan	894	0.013	0.063	0.054
Follow-up Mammogram/Ultrasound	1,056	13.4%	8.8%	8.4%
MRI for Low Back Pain	131	34.4%	38.5%	32.7%
Survey of Patients' Hospital Experiences				
Area Around Room 'Always' Quiet at Night	300+	49%	-	58%
Doctors 'Always' Communicated Well	300+	78%	-	80%
Home Recovery Information Given	300+	86%	-	82%
Hospital Given 9 or 10 on 10 Point Scale	300+	67%	-	67%
Meds 'Always' Explained Before Given	300+	58%	-	60%
Nurses 'Always' Communicated Well	300+	74%	-	76%
Pain 'Always' Well Controlled	300+	69%	-	69%
Room and Bathroom 'Always' Clean	300+	70%	-	71%
Timely Help 'Always' Received	300+	60%	-	64%
Would Definitely Recommend Hospital	300+	70%	-	69%

NOTE: Hospital profiles are in alphabetical order by state, then city, then hospital within the city; Rankings exclude hospitals with less than 25 cases except for patient surveys which excludes hospitals with less than 100 cases; (a) 100–299 cases; (1) The number of cases is too small to be sure how well a hospital is performing; (2) The hospital indicated that the data submitted for this measure were based on a sample of cases; (3) Data was collected during a shorter time period (fewer quarters) than the maximum possible time for this measure; (4) Suppressed for one or more quarters by CMS; (5) No data is available from the hospital for this measure; (6) Fewer than 100 patients completed the HCAHPS survey. Use these rates with caution, as the number of surveys may be too low to reliably assess hospital performance; (7) Survey results are based on less than 12 months of data; (8) Survey results are not available for this reporting period; (9) No or very few patients were eligible for the HCAHPS survey. The scores shown, if any, reflect a very small number of surveys; (10) A state average was not calculated because too few hospitals in the state submitted data; (11) There were discrepancies in the data collection process; Please refer to the User's Guide for a full explanation of data.

Williamson Memorial Hospital

859 Alderson Street   Phone: 304-235-2500
Williamson, WV 25661   Fax: 304-235-0538
URL: www.hmawmh.com
Type: Acute Care Hospitals   Emergency Services: Yes
Ownership: Voluntary Non-Profit - Private   Beds: 76
Key Personnel:
CEO/President. . . . . Stephen Young
Cardiac Laboratory. . . . . Ashik Patnaik, MD
Chief of Medical Staff . . . . Manuel Angco, MD
Infection Control. . . . . Sandy Loew
Operating Room. . . . . Nyoka Farley
Anesthesiology. . . . . Jhansi Rani Lanka, MD

Measure	Cases	This Hosp.	State Avg.	U.S. Avg.
Heart Attack Care				
ACE Inhibitor or ARB for LVSD[1]	3	100%	94%	96%
Aspirin at Arrival[1]	16	94%	97%	99%
Aspirin at Discharge[1]	10	100%	98%	98%
Beta Blocker at Discharge[1]	12	100%	98%	98%
Fibrinolytic Medication Timing[1]	2	50%	29%	55%
PCI Within 90 Minutes of Arrival	0	-	85%	90%
Smoking Cessation Advice[1]	4	100%	99%	99%
Chest Pain/Possible Heart Attack Care				
Aspirin at Arrival	46	98%	95%	95%
Median Time to ECG (minutes)	59	7	12	8
Median Time to Transfer (minutes)[1]	11	165	77	61
Fibrinolytic Medication Timing[1]	2	50%	56%	54%
Heart Failure Care				
ACE Inhibitor or ARB for LVSD[1]	10	90%	90%	94%
Discharge Instructions	83	100%	85%	88%
Evaluation of LVS Function	92	97%	97%	98%
Smoking Cessation Advice[1]	24	100%	97%	98%
Pneumonia Care				
Appropriate Initial Antibiotic	57	98%	89%	92%
Blood Culture Timing	71	97%	95%	96%
Influenza Vaccine	42	100%	90%	91%
Initial Antibiotic Timing[1]	2	100%	94%	95%
Pneumococcal Vaccine	37	100%	91%	93%
Smoking Cessation Advice	32	100%	96%	97%
Surgical Care Improvement Project				
Appropriate VTP Within 24 Hours[1]	11	100%	91%	92%
Appropriate Hair Removal	27	100%	99%	99%
Appropriate Beta Blocker Usage[1]	6	100%	93%	93%
Controlled Postoperative Blood Glucose	0	-	91%	93%
Prophylactic Antibiotic Timing	0	-	97%	97%
Prophylactic Antibiotic Timing (Outpatient)	46	96%	90%	92%
Prophylactic Antibiotic Selection	0	-	97%	97%
Prophylactic Antibiotic Select. (Outpatient)	44	100%	91%	94%
Prophylactic Antibiotic Stopped	0	-	94%	94%
Recommended VTP Ordered[1]	11	100%	92%	94%
Urinary Catheter Removal[1]	1	100%	90%	90%
Children's Asthma Care				
Received Systemic Corticosteroids	34	97%	-	100%
Received Home Management Plan	33	100%	-	71%
Received Reliever Medication	34	100%	-	100%
Use of Medical Imaging				
Combination Abdominal CT Scan	249	0.088	0.304	0.191
Combination Chest CT Scan	78	0.090	0.063	0.054
Follow-up Mammogram/Ultrasound	98	7.1%	8.8%	8.4%
MRI for Low Back Pain[1]	19	26.3%	38.5%	32.7%
Survey of Patients' Hospital Experiences				
Area Around Room 'Always' Quiet at Night	300+	53%	-	58%
Doctors 'Always' Communicated Well	300+	83%	-	80%
Home Recovery Information Given	300+	77%	-	82%
Hospital Given 9 or 10 on 10 Point Scale	300+	62%	-	67%
Meds 'Always' Explained Before Given	300+	59%	-	60%
Nurses 'Always' Communicated Well	300+	78%	-	76%
Pain 'Always' Well Controlled	300+	63%	-	69%
Room and Bathroom 'Always' Clean	300+	73%	-	71%
Timely Help 'Always' Received	300+	62%	-	64%
Would Definitely Recommend Hospital	300+	65%	-	69%

NOTE: Hospital profiles are in alphabetical order by state, then city, then hospital within the city; Rankings exclude hospitals with less than 25 cases except for patient surveys which excludes hospitals with less than 100 cases; (a) 100–299 cases; (1) The number of cases is too small to be sure how well a hospital is performing; (2) The hospital indicated that the data submitted for this measure were based on a sample of cases; (3) Data was collected during a shorter time period (fewer quarters) than the maximum possible time for this measure; (4) Suppressed for one or more quarters by CMS; (5) No data is available from the hospital for this measure; (6) Fewer than 100 patients completed the HCAHPS survey. Use these rates with caution, as the number of surveys may be too low to reliably assess hospital performance; (7) Survey results are based on less than 12 months of data; (8) Survey results are not available for this reporting period; (9) No or very few patients were eligible for the HCAHPS survey. The scores shown, if any, reflect a very small number of surveys; (10) A state average was not calculated because too few hospitals in the state submitted data; (11) There were discrepancies in the data collection process; Please refer to the User's Guide for a full explanation of data.

Hospital	Heart Attack Care							Chest Pain/Possible Heart Attack Care				Heart Failure Care			
	1	2	3	4	5	6	7	8	9	10	11	12	13	14	15
CONNECTICUT															
Bridgeport Hospital, Bridgeport, CT	88 60	99 225	96 253	95 258	- 0	91 22	100 46	- 0	- 0	- 0	- 0	90 84	82 195	100 291	100 41
Bristol Hospital, Bristol, CT	100 5	100 35	100 24	100 23	- 0	- 0	88 8	96 57	9 57	57 25	- 0	100 58	76 125	97 187	88 17
Charlotte Hungerford Hospital, Torrington, CT	100 3	100 47	100 36	100 38	- 0	- 0	100 3	96 118	12 118	80 10	9 11	88 32	90 73	98 129	100 9
Connecticut Childrens Medical Center, Hartford, CT	-	-	-	-	-	-	-	-	-	-	-	-	-	-	-
Danbury Hospital, Danbury, CT	85 66	99 303	99 356	98 333	- 0	91 56	100 82	100 1	18 1	- 0	- 0	95 131	80 346	100 516	90 39
Day Kimball Hospital, Putnam, CT	100 5	94 33	90 20	89 19	- 0	- 0	100 1	96 115	8 120	44 13	- 0	96 47	81 78	97 114	87 15
Greenwich Hospital Association, Greenwich, CT	82 11	99 74	100 49	100 49	- 0	89 18	100 4	- 0	- 0	- 0	- 0	90 83	91 183	98 256	100 13
Griffin Hospital, Derby, CT	100 7	99 92	96 53	100 51	- 0	- 0	100 6	100 47	9 47	56 26	- 0	98 42	99 165	100 257	100 23
Hartford Hospital, Hartford, CT	98 140	99 337	99 788	99 781	50 4	84 56	100 219	0 1	16 1	- 0	- 0	94 327	85 656	100 925	100 117
Hebrew Home and Hospital, West Hartford, CT	- 0	- 0	- 0	- 0	- 0	- 0	- 0	- 0	- 0	- 0	- 0	50 2	0 1	94 17	0 2
The Hospital of Central Connecticut, New Britain, CT	88 41	97 247	93 175	98 185	- 0	97 39	100 52	95 40	11 41	44 9	- 0	89 186	91 501	100 689	100 117
Hospital of St Raphael, New Haven, CT	100 55	98 227	99 351	99 334	- 0	60 53	100 93	- 0	- 0	- 0	- 0	94 77	95 228	98 333	100 42
John Dempsey Hospital, Farmington, CT	95 21	100 116	99 134	99 138	- 0	83 18	100 26	- 0	- 0	- 0	- 0	98 64	96 156	100 218	100 15
Johnson Memorial Hospital, Stafford Springs, CT	67 3	82 11	80 5	83 6	- 0	- 0	- 0	97 65	12 68	328 2	67 9	92 26	99 77	97 120	100 6
Lawrence & Memorial Hospital, New London, CT	100 18	98 133	99 117	100 109	- 0	84 31	100 39	100 26	8 28	122 2	- 0	91 53	79 194	97 287	100 28
Manchester Memorial Hospital, Manchester, CT	100 7	100 44	97 31	100 31	- 0	- 0	100 7	96 50	14 50	88 4	0 1	98 42	87 140	100 195	100 21
Masonic Home and Hospital, Wallingford, CT	- 0	- 0	- 0	- 0	- 0	- 0	- 0	- 0	- 0	- 0	- 0	50 6	25 8	80 40	- 0
Middlesex Hospital, Middletown, CT	94 31	100 59	100 70	100 77	- 0	- 0	100 6	99 311	9 321	76 43	0 3	97 126	91 197	100 329	97 31
Midstate Medical Center, Meriden, CT	100 6	98 56	97 38	97 35	- 0	- 0	100 3	97 123	6 120	74 18	50 16	90 61	72 166	96 245	97 30
Milford Hospital, Milford, CT	100 1	100 34	100 14	93 14	- 0	- 0	100 6	100 6	2 6	34 2	- 0	97 37	93 123	99 187	95 19
New Milford Hospital, New Milford, CT	100 2	100 11	100 8	88 8	- 0	- 0	- 0	98 42	10 41	84 12	- 0	90 21	83 41	99 75	100 9
Norwalk Hospital Association, Norwalk, CT	100 21	99 161	100 94	99 98	- 0	94 33	100 26	100 15	12 16	- 0	- 0	96 82	72 220	100 330	97 37
Rockville General Hospital, Rockville, CT	100 5	100 26	100 17	100 21	- 0	- 0	- 0	88 40	5 42	84 15	- 0	100 20	88 58	100 93	100 2
Saint Francis Hospital & Medical Center, Hartford, CT	93 112	99 317	99 546	98 527	- 0	96 73	100 166	100 2	16 2	- 0	- 0	94 123	64 225	100 317	100 37
Saint Marys Hospital, Waterbury, CT	100 31	100 168	100 164	100 155	- 0	98 42	96 54	100 1	4 1	- 0	- 0	100 83	100 204	100 301	100 27
Saint Vincent's Medical Center, Bridgeport, CT	96 74	99 261	99 309	98 307	- 0	88 59	98 61	- 0	- 0	- 0	- 0	90 186	92 391	99 577	100 57
Sharon Hospital, Sharon, CT	0 1	100 15	100 7	91 11	- 0	- 0	100 1	98 40	8 43	160 13	25 4	100 8	90 21	95 43	100 2
Stamford Hospital, Stamford, CT	92 39	98 195	98 180	98 179	- 0	81 27	100 36	- 0	- 0	- 0	- 0	93 149	88 216	98 328	100 33
Waterbury Hospital, Waterbury, CT	91 34	100 227	100 219	100 215	- 0	89 38	100 64	- 0	- 0	- 0	- 0	84 93	77 203	98 321	100 48
West Haven VA Medical Center, West Haven, CT	- 0	- 0	- 0	- 0	- 0	- 0	- 0	-	-	-	-	100 43	100 161	99 184	100 25
William W Backus Hospital, Norwich, CT	100 9	97 61	92 39	100 37	100 1	- 0	100 7	99 220	5 224	86 52	40 5	96 85	84 226	100 305	100 57
Windham Hospital, Willimantic, CT	0 2	96 27	89 19	95 20	0 1	- 0	100 3	100 46	10 48	54 8	40 5	79 43	80 91	100 138	100 10
Yale-New Haven Hospital, New Haven, CT	97 29	100 127	99 282	98 264	- 0	76 21	100 82	- 0	- 0	- 0	- 0	93 84	90 223	100 287	100 48
DELAWARE															
Bayhealth - Kent General Hospital, Dover, DE	94 49	99 329	100 341	99 335	- 0	91 53	99 139	100 31	6 32	72 5	- 0	99 171	95 416	100 506	100 123
Beebe Medical Center, Lewes, DE	97 39	100 264	100 261	97 258	- 0	92 40	100 85	100 4	2 5	- 0	- 0	95 104	97 276	98 353	98 59
Christiana Care Health Services, Newark, DE	94 114	99 484	99 632	99 609	0 1	89 140	100 220	- 0	- 0	- 0	- 0	89 284	86 616	99 802	100 121
Nanticoke Memorial Hospital, Seaford, DE	100 11	100 97	99 81	99 83	100 2	100 19	100 27	100 15	7 15	- 0	- 0	100 37	98 166	99 202	100 39
Saint Francis Hospital, Wilmington, DE	94 33	97 116	99 109	99 102	- 0	73 11	100 49	- 0	- 0	- 0	- 0	97 102	94 205	96 234	100 54
Wilmington VA Medical Center, Wilmington, DE	- 0	- 0	- 0	- 0	- 0	- 0	- 0	-	-	-	-	100 21	90 49	100 52	89 9
DISTRICT OF COLUMBIA															
Children's Hospital NMC, Washington, DC	-	-	-	-	-	-	-	-	-	-	-	-	-	-	-
George Washington Univ Hospital, Washington, DC	91 33	99 191	98 259	97 232	- 0	88 34	100 73	50 2	228 2	- 0	- 0	95 167	100 331	98 372	100 67
Georgetown University Hospital, Washington, DC	100 1	100 5	100 3	100 3	- 0	- 0	100 3	- 0	14 53	84 6	- 0	100 37	89 73	99 90	100 22
Howard University Hospital, Washington, DC	100 9	91 45	100 45	96 45	- 0	0 4	100 26	86 5	26 9	- 0	- 0	97 154	99 268	98 286	100 94
Providence Hospital, Washington, DC	82 17	95 60	89 45	81 43	- 0	0 1	93 14	75 12	33 12	1131 1	- 0	83 255	24 504	92 588	95 101
Sibley Memorial Hospital, Washington, DC	100 4	97 32	100 19	100 18	- 0	- 0	100 2	98 47	10 49	101 13	- 0	97 35	83 102	99 124	100 6
United Medical Center, Washington, DC	0 1	57 7	75 4	50 4	- 0	- 0	0 1	100 9	19 10	- 0	- 0	81 122	60 235	91 270	97 116
Washington DC VA Medical Center, Washington, DC	100 6	100 25	100 31	100 29	- 0	80 5	100 12	-	-	-	-	94 160	96 224	99 234	100 74
Washington Hospital Center, Washington, DC	97 78	98 263	99 282	99 269	- 0	100 5	100 79	100 1	4 1	- 0	- 0	97 193	93 355	98 393	100 72
KENTUCKY															
Baptist Hospital East, Louisville, KY	96 80	100 443	99 474	100 448	- 0	89 89	100 142	80 5	0 5	- 0	- 0	88 255	76 654	100 913	100 112
Baptist Hospital Northeast, La Grange, KY	100 3	97 33	100 11	100 10	0 1	- 0	100 1	100 29	5 31	48 5	100 3	80 15	92 79	100 107	93 14
Baptist Regional Medical Center, Corbin, KY	100 4	100 53	100 20	100 22	- 0	- 0	100 5	98 144	7 150	58 10	0 2	100 41	99 136	100 179	100 30
Bluegrass Community Hospital, Versailles, KY	- 0	- 0	- 0	- 0	- 0	- 0	- 0	- 0	- 0	- 0	- 0	100 3	100 11	100 13	100 3
Bourbon Community Hospital, Paris, KY	- 0	75 4	100 2	100 1	- 0	- 0	- 0	98 84	4 87	119 4	100 1	71 7	94 34	98 46	100 4
Breckinridge Memorial Hospital, Hardinsburg, KY	- 0	- 0	- 0	- 0	- 0	- 0	- 0	- 0	- 0	- 0	- 0	100 2	94 31	44 41	71 7
Caldwell Medical Center, Princeton, KY	- 0	- 0	- 0	- 0	- 0	- 0	- 0	- 0	- 0	- 0	- 0	83 6	100 15	86 21	100 5
Carroll County Hospital, Carrollton, KY	- 0	100 4	67 3	50 2	- 0	- 0	- 0	- 0	- 0	- 0	- 0	50 6	100 17	81 27	80 5
Casey County Hospital, Liberty, KY	- 0	- 0	- 0	100 1	- 0	- 0	- 0	- 0	- 0	- 0	- 0	0 1	70 10	50 16	75 4
Caverna Memorial Hospital, Horse Cave, KY	- 0	75 4	50 2	50 2	- 0	- 0	- 0	0 1	- 0	- 0	- 0	75 4	42 26	55 38	75 8
Central Baptist Hospital, Lexington, KY	100 95	99 146	100 671	100 625	- 0	100 47	100 269	100 2	2 2	- 0	- 0	99 137	92 297	99 331	100 56
Clark Regional Medical Center, Winchester, KY	50 4	91 11	100 7	100 7	- 0	- 0	100 2	89 331	7 346	76 4	0 1	58 19	76 45	94 51	100 11
Clinton County Hospital, Albany, KY	- 0	100 5	67 3	67 3	- 0	- 0	- 0	89 28	5 34	125 2	67 3	62 37	75 67	76 72	100 15
Crittenden Health System, Marion, KY	- 0	91 11	67 6	86 7	- 0	- 0	100 3	91 33	3 35	88 2	80 5	82 11	100 37	89 61	100 11
Cumberland County Hospital, Burkesville, KY	- 0	100 1	100 5	100 3	- 0	- 0	- 0	- 0	- 0	- 0	- 0	50 2	37 38	32 53	45 7

NOTE: The first number in each column (boldface) is the score, the second number is the number of patients; Please refer to the main entry for footnotes; (a) 100-299
MEASURES: **Heart Attack Care:** 1. ACE Inhibitor or ARB for LVSD; 2. Aspirin at Arrival; 3. Aspirin at Discharge; 4. Beta Blocker at Discharge; 5. Fibrinolytic Medication Timing; 6. PCI Within 90 Minutes of Arrival; 7. Smoking Cessation Advice; **Chest Pain/Possible Heart Attack Care:** 8. Aspirin at Arrival; 9. Median Time to ECG (minutes); 10. Median Time to Transfer (minutes); 11. Fibrinolytic Medication Timing; **Heart Failure Care:** 12. ACE Inhibitor or ARB for LVSD; 13. Discharge Instructions; 14. Evaluation of LVS Function; 15. Smoking Cessation Advice

Hospital	Heart Attack Care 1	2	3	4	5	6	7	Chest Pain/Possible Heart Attack Care 8	9	10	11	Heart Failure Care 12	13	14	15
Ephraim Mcdowell Fort Logan Hospital, Stanford, KY	- 0	86 7	100 2	100 2	- 0	- 0	100 1					89 9	96 27	100 36	100 7
Ephraim Mcdowell Regional Medical Center, Danville, KY	100 12	98 102	99 79	96 78	- 0	78 9	100 22	96 101	2 104	65 15	- 0	95 61	98 187	100 228	98 44
Flaget Memorial Hospital, Bardstown, KY	- 0	95 19	83 12	100 11	- 0	- 0	100 1	95 225	12 228	132 1	77 13	81 16	84 43	98 52	100 13
Fleming County Hospital, Flemingsburg, KY	- 0	67 3	0 1	100 1	- 0	- 0	- 0	88 51	13 51	266 3	67 12	61 18	78 78	81 98	100 12
Frankfort Regional Medical Center, Frankfort, KY	100 5	100 30	100 16	100 16	- 0	- 0	100 4	100 151	5 156	51 22	50 2	100 33	98 121	100 137	100 23
Georgetown Community Hospital, Georgetown, KY	100 2	100 5	100 3	100 3	- 0	- 0	- 0	99 82	7 84	82 6	50 2	92 13	82 34	100 42	100 7
Greenview Regional Hospital, Bowling Green, KY	- 0	100 29	100 20	95 22	- 0	100 1	100 9	100 13	5 13	65 3	- 0	100 20	100 67	100 96	100 11
Hardin Memorial Hospital, Elizabethtown, KY	98 47	98 293	98 291	100 294	67 36	12 8	100 116	92 12	14 12	- 0	- 0	92 144	83 379	99 487	99 123
Harlan Appalachian Regional Healthcare Hospital, Harlan, KY	- 0	71 7	100 1	100 1	- 0	- 0	- 0	98 98	15 108	83 1	83 6	100 33	99 153	100 187	100 33
Harrison Memorial Hospital, Cynthiana, KY	- 0	100 3	100 2	100 2	- 0	- 0	- 0	99 101	9 101	109 2	60 10	85 13	82 34	100 49	100 10
Hazard Arh Regional Medical Center, Hazard, KY	81 52	93 111	92 167	89 170	- 0	60 15	98 86	84 25	9 24	- 0	- 0	83 63	67 276	98 306	100 53
Highlands Regional Medical Center, Prestonsburg, KY	100 4	97 30	100 20	95 20	- 0	- 0	100 5	88 258	8 268	183 11	50 4	85 60	97 162	97 201	100 33
Jackson Purchase Medical Center, Mayfield, KY	- 0	95 20	100 13	100 13	- 0	- 0	100 4	90 10	4 12	185 1	- 0	97 29	100 77	98 103	100 27
The James B Haggin Memorial Hospital, Harrodsburg, KY	- 0	- 0	- 0	- 0	- 0	- 0	- 0					83 12	79 24	75 40	73 11
Jane Todd Crawford Hospital, Greensburg, KY	- 0	100 2	50 2	100 1	- 0	- 0	100 1					100 1	80 5	17 6	33 3
Jennie Stuart Medical Center, Hopkinsville, KY	100 4	90 20	87 15	100 15	- 0	- 0	100 5	96 214	8 231	164 14	37 19	94 81	73 141	84 181	91 55
Jewish Hospital & St Mary's Healthcare, Louisville, KY	96 165	100 402	99 965	97 921	- 0	73 22	100 411	97 385	4 393	63 38	0 2	86 438	66 1079	99 1301	99 312
Jewish Hospital - Shelbyville, Shelbyville, KY	100 1	100 29	100 12	91 11	- 0	- 0	- 0	96 100	4 104	125 1	54 13	75 16	80 70	99 102	100 24
Kentucky River Medical Center, Jackson, KY	100 3	100 24	100 13	89 9	- 0	- 0	100 6	94 78	8 82	72 4	78 9	95 22	82 78	100 99	100 24
King's Daughters' Medical Center, Ashland, KY	97 103	98 452	100 732	99 712	- 0	92 84	100 351	- 0	- 0	- 0	- 0	98 209	91 783	100 901	100 185
Knox County Hospital, Barbourville, KY	- 0	100 11	100 6	88 8	- 0	- 0	50 2					75 12	58 43	73 49	100 10
Lake Cumberland Regional Hospital, Somerset, KY	97 30	99 178	98 193	99 177	- 0	86 49	100 93	87 23	6 23	- 0	- 0	90 84	84 202	99 235	100 59
Lexington-Leestown VA Medical Center, Lexington, KY	100 17	98 128	99 121	99 113	- 0	42 12	100 42					93 82	99 255	100 270	100 50
Livingston Hospital and Healthcare, Salem, KY	- 0	33 6	83 6	83 6	- 0	- 0	0 1					50 4	0 45	39 56	100 10
Logan Memorial Hospital, Russellville, KY	- 0	75 4	100 2	100 2	- 0	- 0	100 1	96 128	5 135	92 2	90 10	86 22	84 80	97 97	100 29
Louisville VA Medical Center, Louisville, KY	100 10	96 80	100 65	100 61	- 0	60 5	96 25					100 95	99 193	100 213	98 57
Lourdes Hospital, Paducah, KY	98 52	100 129	100 178	99 173	- 0	90 20	100 84	100 2	13 2	- 0	- 0	92 132	88 209	100 272	100 45
Marcum and Wallace Memorial Hospital, Irvine, KY	- 0	- 0	- 0	- 0	- 0	- 0	- 0					100 2	80 10	70 10	- 0
Marshall County Hospital, Benton, KY	- 0	60 5	50 2	33 3	- 0	- 0	- 0					33 3	44 25	54 41	57 7
Mary Breckinridge Hospital, Hyden, KY	- 0	100 1	100 1	0 1	- 0	- 0	- 0					100 8	83 42	92 52	100 7
McDowell Arh Hospital, McDowell, KY	- 0	- 0	- 0	- 0	- 0	- 0	- 0					94 16	100 51	100 52	100 15
Meadowview Regional Medical Center, Maysville, KY	100 10	100 82	100 78	100 71	- 0	94 17	100 37	100 46	2 45	116 2	- 0	100 22	100 55	100 67	100 11
The Medical Center at Bowling Green, Bowling Green, KY	82 55	96 218	97 297	95 281	- 0	86 49	99 149	79 19	10 20	- 0	- 0	77 183	64 490	95 593	100 138
The Medical Center at Franklin, Franklin, KY	0 1	50 2	100 1	100 2	- 0	- 0	100 1					78 9	68 31	55 47	100 3
The Medical Center at Scottsville, Scottsville, KY	- 0	- 0	- 0	- 0	- 0	- 0	- 0					75 4	30 20	75 32	100 6
Memorial Hospital, Manchester, KY	100 2	100 13	100 6	100 4	- 0	- 0	100 2	91 11	12 11	- 0	- 0	94 17	100 88	100 102	100 20
Methodist Hospital, Henderson, KY	100 9	91 23	76 17	84 19	0 1	- 0	67 6	94 101	4 104	66 8	- 0	89 53	84 165	98 210	100 39
Methodist Hospital Union County, Morganfield, KY	100 1	100 1	100 1	100 1	- 0	- 0	- 0	88 73	8 80	- 0	- 0	80 10	100 24	78 27	100 4
Middlesboro Appalachian Reg Healthcare Hosp, Middlesboro, KY	80 5	100 6	100 5	100 7	- 0	- 0	- 0	95 126	7 130	60 9	- 0	94 36	96 92	99 129	100 18
Monroe County Medical Center, Tompkinsville, KY	67 3	78 9	75 4	60 5	- 0	- 0	100 2	100 79	6 83	182 1	80 5	71 21	67 86	79 112	77 35
Morgan County Arh Hospital, West Liberty, KY	- 0	- 0	- 0	- 0	- 0	- 0	- 0					67 6	100 28	91 32	100 6
Muhlenberg Community Hospital, Greenville, KY	- 0	80 5	100 2	100 1	- 0	- 0	100 2	95 179	8 190	66 18	33 3	100 19	85 39	84 62	92 12
Murray-Calloway County Hospital, Murray, KY	67 3	83 18	100 11	92 12	- 0	- 0	50 2	98 125	9 124	55 5	20 5	67 21	65 101	91 116	92 13
New Horizons Medical Center, Owenton, KY	- 0	- 0	- 0	- 0	- 0	- 0	- 0					100 6	54 13	83 18	75 4
Nicholas County Hospital, Carlisle, KY	- 0	- 0	- 0	- 0	- 0	- 0	- 0					0 2	40 5	100 7	100 1
Norton Hospitals, Louisville, KY	96 140	98 458	100 724	100 705	- 0	84 70	100 319	92 36	5 36	56 8	- 0	95 386	73 1003	99 1290	100 311
Ohio County Hospital, Hartford, KY	- 0	- 0	- 0	- 0	- 0	- 0	- 0					86 7	86 28	85 34	100 5
Our Lady of Bellefonte Hospital, Ashland, KY	100 4	96 54	97 29	100 30	- 0	- 0	100 9	98 65	20 65	- 0	0 1	100 37	90 220	98 250	100 46
Owensboro Medical Health System, Owensboro, KY	87 82	99 282	99 292	98 283	- 0	85 34	100 137	100 1	- 0	- 0	- 0	88 219	91 462	100 553	100 92
Parkway Regional Hospital, Fulton, KY	- 0	100 2	100 1	100 1	- 0	- 0	- 0	100 40	4 43	- 0	67 3	100 10	100 19	100 27	100 4
Pattie A Clay Regional Medical Center, Richmond, KY	100 7	95 22	100 13	100 16	- 0	- 0	100 4	95 141	4 142	69 35	0 4	92 25	98 47	97 66	100 9
Paul B Hall Regional Medical Center, Paintsville, KY	100 1	100 5	100 3	100 3	- 0	- 0	100 1	98 125	2 133	165 1	80 5	96 25	90 87	99 105	100 25
Pikeville Medical Center, Pikeville, KY	97 33	99 163	100 224	98 216	- 0	80 25	100 115	- 0	- 0	- 0	- 0	90 105	98 279	99 308	100 62
Pineville Community Hospital, Pineville, KY	0 1	75 8	75 4	50 4	- 0	- 0	0 2	89 46	13 49	102 6	0 3	77 56	53 214	90 241	86 51
Regional Medical Center of Hopkins County, Madisonville, KY	94 65	99 180	97 218	97 202	- 0	97 32	99 107	83 6	3 7	- 0	- 0	89 134	78 191	98 238	100 64
Rockcastle Reg Hosp & Resp Care Ctr, Mount Vernon, KY	100 1	100 4	100 3	100 3	- 0	- 0	- 0	94 85	12 87	72 10	- 0	92 12	88 32	100 41	100 6
Russell County Hospital, Russell Springs, KY	100 1	62 8	62 8	62 8	- 0	- 0	- 0	87 38	14 40	140 3	0 1	60 5	92 24	74 31	100 8
Saint Claire Regional Medical Center, Morehead, KY	79 14	100 84	96 72	99 73	- 0	100 10	97 36	99 85	1 95	54 4	33 3	96 49	88 104	97 129	97 30
Saint Elizabeth Florence, Florence, KY	100 15	100 104	100 64	100 59	- 0	- 0	100 2	97 37	11 38	55 23	- 0	100 68	88 149	100 200	100 42
Saint Elizabeth Ft Thomas, Fort Thomas, KY	100 12	100 129	100 66	100 67	- 0	- 0	100 2	100 37	11 40	48 14	- 0	100 44	92 173	100 234	100 35
Saint Elizabeth Grant, Williamstown, KY	- 0	100 1	- 0	- 0	- 0	- 0	- 0					100 4	88 33	100 34	100 8
Saint Elizabeth Medical Center North, Covington, KY	100 47	100 211	100 303	100 283	- 0	95 42	100 117	92 24	10 26	- 0	- 0	100 90	96 273	100 320	100 67
Saint Joseph Berea, Berea, KY	100 2	100 6	100 3	100 5	- 0	- 0	100 3					100 14	80 30	97 38	100 11
Saint Joseph East, Lexington, KY	97 39	97 75	99 203	97 184	- 0	100 18	100 100	100 18	15 18	- 0	- 0	89 45	82 101	98 108	100 30
Saint Joseph Hospital, Lexington, KY	92 83	98 172	99 437	98 414	- 0	86 22	100 205	96 28	7 31	- 0	- 0	95 112	82 268	99 300	100 62
Saint Joseph Hospital London, London, KY	100 40	99 171	100 296	99 275	- 0	98 42	100 165	98 80	8 94	- 0	- 0	100 90	93 266	100 295	100 79
Saint Joseph Martin, Martin, KY	- 0	- 0	- 0	- 0	- 0	- 0	- 0					81 16	100 49	98 52	100 7

NOTE: The first number in each column (boldface) is the score, the second number is the number of patients; Please refer to the main entry for footnotes; (a) 100-299

MEASURES: **Heart Attack Care:** 1. ACE Inhibitor or ARB for LVSD; 2. Aspirin at Arrival; 3. Aspirin at Discharge; 4. Beta Blocker at Discharge; 5. Fibrinolytic Medication Timing; 6. PCI Within 90 Minutes of Arrival; 7. Smoking Cessation Advice; **Chest Pain/Possible Heart Attack Care:** 8. Aspirin at Arrival; 9. Median Time to ECG (minutes); 10. Median Time to Transfer (minutes); 11. Fibrinolytic Medication Timing; **Heart Failure Care:** 12. ACE Inhibitor or ARB for LVSD; 13. Discharge Instructions; 14. Evaluation of LVS Function; 15. Smoking Cessation Advice

Hospital	Heart Attack Care							Chest Pain/Possible Heart Attack Care				Heart Failure Care			
	1	2	3	4	5	6	7	8	9	10	11	12	13	14	15
Saint Joseph Mount Sterling, Mount Sterling, KY	0 1	100 5	100 3	100 3	- 0	- 0	- 0	97 218	6 221	52 1	53 15	100 7	90 30	92 38	100 12
Spring View Hospital, Lebanon, KY	100 2	100 7	100 6	100 6	- 0	- 0	- 0	98 121	7 124	- 0	100 4	94 18	100 53	100 75	100 11
T J Samson Community Hospital, Glasgow, KY	74 27	93 165	94 148	96 154	33 6	86 21	100 63	88 24	2 25	42 1	75 4	77 57	69 154	99 184	100 40
Taylor Regional Hospital, Campbellsville, KY	67 3	86 21	88 8	64 11	- 0	- 0	100 4	94 143	11 147	105 3	62 21	88 16	75 53	92 64	100 15
Three Rivers Medical Center, Louisa, KY	- 0	100 6	100 2	100 2	- 0	- 0	- 0	100 142	5 144	50 6	100 1	97 35	99 89	100 98	100 25
Trigg County Hospital, Cadiz, KY	- 0	- 0	- 0	- 0	- 0	- 0	- 0					50 2	100 13	29 24	100 5
Twin Lakes Regional Medical Center, Leitchfield, KY	- 0	67 3	100 2	100 2	- 0	- 0	- 0	95 101	8 110	130 2	92 13	100 1	84 38	91 44	100 14
University of Kentucky Hospital, Lexington, KY	96 71	99 127	99 280	98 269	- 0	83 23	99 135	- 0	- 0	- 0	- 0	97 159	74 314	97 356	97 115
University of Louisville Hospital, Louisville, KY	94 16	97 107	95 107	97 97	- 0	91 22	99 73	- 0	- 0	- 0	- 0	95 111	75 186	98 200	100 115
Wayne County Hospital, Monticello, KY	- 0	100 1	- 0	- 0	- 0	- 0	- 0					67 6	73 15	68 19	100 2
Western Baptist Hospital, Paducah, KY	100 62	98 237	100 395	100 374	- 0	86 36	100 170	100 1	0 1	- 0	- 0	100 171	95 390	100 462	100 112
Westlake Regional Hospital, Columbia, KY	- 0	100 5	100 4	100 4	- 0	- 0	100 1	90 105	10 110	128 2	67 6	88 42	93 170	92 221	87 38
Whitesburg ARH Hospital, Whitesburg, KY	100 1	100 7	100 4	100 3	100 1	- 0	100 2	99 124	17 116	- 0	100 3	96 28	92 177	95 201	100 41
Williamson ARH Hospital, South Williamson, KY	- 0	90 10	100 4	100 6	- 0	- 0	100 2	98 45	10 43	- 0	100 1	100 17	94 110	98 123	100 31
MAINE															
Aroostook Medical Center, Presque Isle, ME	80 5	96 49	97 36	95 37	- 0	- 0	100 3	98 50	3 50	- 0	67 6	100 17	81 58	99 67	100 7
Blue Hill Memorial Hospital, Blue Hill, ME	100 3	100 10	88 8	100 8	- 0	- 0	100 1					100 5	100 16	94 18	100 2
Bridgton Hospital, Bridgton, ME	- 0	- 0	- 0	- 0	- 0	- 0	- 0					100 2	90 30	94 31	100 5
Calais Regional Hospital, Calais, ME	100 4	100 15	100 11	90 10	- 0	- 0	100 1	- 0	- 0	- 0	- 0	100 2	94 16	100 22	75 4
Cary Medical Center, Caribou, ME	100 2	100 28	100 18	100 19	- 0	- 0	100 1	100 8	0 9	- 0	50 4	100 9	98 52	100 69	100 4
Central Maine Medical Center, Lewiston, ME	97 31	99 176	100 289	97 278	- 0	100 23	100 109	100 4	3 5	- 0	0 1	99 79	99 194	100 258	100 42
Charles A Dean Memorial Hospital, Greenville, ME	- 0	- 0	- 0	- 0	- 0	- 0	- 0						100 2	100 4	- 0
Down East Community Hospital, Machias, ME	100 1	94 17	81 16	94 16	- 0	- 0	100 1	100 81	10 85	- 0	67 3	100 9	100 29	100 39	100 6
Eastern Maine Medical Center, Bangor, ME	99 110	100 247	99 921	100 880	- 0	95 38	100 310	100 6	16 6	- 0	- 0	100 118	90 301	100 375	99 73
Franklin Memorial Hospital, Farmington, ME	100 4	100 18	100 12	100 13	- 0	- 0	50 2	92 39	8 39	- 0	50 2	83 23	99 67	95 91	100 4
Henrietta D Goodall Hospital, Sanford, ME	100 5	94 36	95 21	100 26	- 0	- 0	100 1	96 50	3 50	48 2	64 14	100 6	86 65	99 90	100 13
Houlton Regional Hospital, Houlton, ME	100 1	89 9	67 3	100 2	0 1	- 0	- 0					100 5	100 26	98 50	100 8
Inland Hospital, Waterville, ME	- 0	100 6	100 1	100 1	- 0	- 0	- 0	100 74	5 77	135 2	67 3	75 8	83 29	100 56	92 12
Maine Coast Memorial Hospital, Ellsworth, ME	100 2	100 47	96 27	96 24	100 1	- 0	100 4	96 47	10 47	85 1	44 9	89 19	79 43	100 63	100 3
Maine General Medical Center, Augusta, ME	94 17	99 166	98 89	100 100	- 0	- 0	100 10	99 113	5 118	165 3	88 43	96 68	92 167	100 215	100 28
Maine Medical Center, Portland, ME	99 100	99 372	100 988	99 979	50 2	92 76	99 286	- 0	- 0	- 0	- 0	96 160	86 477	99 619	93 67
Mayo Regional Hospital, Dover Foxcroft, ME	100 2	100 19	100 12	100 11	100 1	- 0	100 1					100 6	88 16	100 21	100 3
Mercy Hospital, Portland, ME	100 4	100 55	100 32	97 31	- 0	- 0	100 7	100 23	17 22	94 9	- 0	96 24	99 98	100 166	93 30
Mid Coast Hospital, Brunswick, ME	100 11	100 49	100 31	100 31	- 0	- 0	100 5	98 60	4 61	- 0	80 20	100 42	100 75	100 95	100 15
Miles Memorial Hospital, Damariscotta, ME	- 0	100 5	100 2	100 2	- 0	- 0	- 0	96 77	6 78	193 1	100 6	89 18	91 54	100 68	100 7
Millinocket Regional Hospital, Millinocket, ME	- 0	100 8	100 7	100 7	- 0	- 0	- 0					100 8	81 27	97 35	100 5
Mount Desert Island Hospital, Bar Harbor, ME	100 1	100 12	100 6	80 5	- 0	- 0	100 1	- 0	- 0	- 0	- 0	88 8	100 14	97 29	100 1
Northern Maine Medical Center, Fort Kent, ME	100 1	100 9	100 4	100 4	0 1	- 0	- 0	100 19	6 18	- 0	100 4	100 11	90 21	100 32	100 4
Parkview Adventist Medical Center, Brunswick, ME	86 7	78 9	83 6	100 7	- 0	- 0	100 1	100 22	12 22	55 4	100 1	94 16	87 38	92 48	100 3
Penobscot Bay Medical Center, Rockport, ME	100 1	100 38	100 25	100 23	- 0	- 0	100 3	100 49	6 51	- 0	69 13	100 20	96 80	99 116	90 10
Penobscot Valley Hospital, Lincoln, ME	- 0	100 6	100 2	100 2	- 0	- 0	- 0					100 4	78 9	100 12	- 0
Redington Fairview General Hospital, Skowhegan, ME	100 1	100 21	100 11	100 11	- 0	- 0	100 2	93 29	5 33	440 2	67 6	100 10	84 38	98 52	100 3
Rumford Hospital, Rumford, ME	100 1	100 2	100 4	100 4	- 0	- 0	- 0					83 6	96 24	97 35	100 1
Saint Andrews Hospital, Boothbay Harbor, ME	- 0	100 1	- 0	100 1	- 0	- 0	- 0	100 49	7 49	- 0	67 3	100 2	75 4	89 9	100 1
Saint Joseph Hospital, Bangor, ME	100 8	100 78	98 51	100 50	- 0	- 0	100 8	100 23	20 24	55 9	- 0	100 35	98 109	100 144	100 22
Saint Marys Regional Medical Center, Lewiston, ME	100 4	98 51	100 37	94 35	- 0	- 0	100 7	95 21	8 22	56 7	0 1	90 21	93 68	99 133	100 14
Sebasticook Valley Hospital, Pittsfield, ME	100 1	100 7	100 7	100 6	- 0	- 0	- 0					100 4	100 38	93 44	100 5
Southern Maine Medical Center, Biddeford, ME	100 12	99 99	99 67	100 70	- 0	- 0	100 10	100 73	11 73	26 32	100 1	98 40	90 141	100 207	100 16
Stephens Memorial Hospital, Norway, ME	50 2	100 12	100 12	91 11	0 1	- 0	- 0	98 58	8 58	35 4	71 7	100 8	91 54	86 35	100 2
Togus VA Medical Center, Augusta, ME	- 0	- 0	- 0	- 0	- 0	- 0	- 0					85 20	88 64	100 78	82 17
Waldo County General Hospital, Belfast, ME	100 6	95 19	100 15	100 15	- 0	- 0	100 2					100 4	86 22	93 30	100 6
York Hospital, York, ME	100 9	100 71	98 60	100 59	- 0	90 10	100 13	100 6	10 6	- 0	- 0	95 22	96 93	98 122	100 6
MARYLAND															
Anne Arundel Medical Center, Annapolis, MD	100 24	98 208	99 153	99 153	- 0	80 70	100 53					87 171	79 418	97 535	100 69
Atlantic General Hospital, Berlin, MD	- 0	100 7	100 4	100 5	- 0	- 0	- 0					97 38	99 100	98 125	100 29
Baltimore Washington Medical Center, Glen Burnie, MD	91 11	99 202	98 124	96 127	- 0	84 83	100 35					94 196	84 608	99 715	100 96
Bon Secours Hospital, Baltimore, MD	80 5	93 29	95 19	95 20	- 0	- 0	100 8					88 113	95 313	92 376	97 128
Calvert Memorial Hospital, Prince Frederick, MD	100 4	95 43	96 27	100 27	- 0	- 0	100 2					100 67	96 174	100 233	100 21
Carroll Hospital Center, Westminster, MD	100 20	98 150	99 93	97 89	100 1	88 48	100 25					89 80	92 205	95 269	100 39
Chester River Hospital Center, Chestertown, MD	67 3	83 12	88 8	89 9	- 0	- 0	100 1					85 41	76 97	90 126	95 24
Civista Medical Center, La Plata, MD	100 6	100 36	100 14	89 18	- 0	- 0	100 6					90 79	94 226	99 270	100 42
Doctors' Community Hospital, Lanham, MD	100 8	90 50	85 20	86 22	- 0	- 0	100 1					90 195	79 440	95 495	100 86
Edward Mccready Memorial Hospital, Crisfield, MD	- 0	100 2	100 2	100 2	- 0	- 0	- 0					100 9	79 14	100 20	100 5
Fort Washington Hospital, Fort Washington, MD	- 0	100 4	50 2	33 3	- 0	- 0	- 0					86 66	95 150	94 170	100 21
Franklin Square Hospital Center, Baltimore, MD	100 20	99 203	100 123	99 121	- 0	84 56	95 44					97 218	79 594	100 753	93 121
Frederick Memorial Hospital, Frederick, MD	96 27	97 164	98 134	97 135	- 0	98 63	100 4					93 153	76 378	100 489	100 45
Garrett County Memorial Hospital, Oakland, MD	100 1	92 13	86 7	88 8	- 0	- 0	100 3					89 27	75 64	97 89	100 9

NOTE: The first number in each column (boldface) is the score, the second number is the number of patients; Please refer to the main entry for footnotes; (a) 100-299

MEASURES: **Heart Attack Care**: 1. ACE Inhibitor or ARB for LVSD; 2. Aspirin at Arrival; 3. Aspirin at Discharge; 4. Beta Blocker at Discharge; 5. Fibrinolytic Medication Timing; 6. PCI Within 90 Minutes of Arrival; 7. Smoking Cessation Advice; **Chest Pain/Possible Heart Attack Care**: 8. Aspirin at Arrival; 9. Median Time to ECG (minutes); 10. Median Time to Transfer (minutes); 11. Fibrinolytic Medication Timing; **Heart Failure Care**: 12. ACE Inhibitor or ARB for LVSD; 13. Discharge Instructions; 14. Evaluation of LVS Function; 15. Smoking Cessation Advice

Hospital	Heart Attack Care							Chest Pain/Possible Heart Attack Care				Heart Failure Care			
	1	2	3	4	5	6	7	8	9	10	11	12	13	14	15
Good Samaritan Hospital, Baltimore, MD	100 23	96 103	95 81	100 81	- 0	- 0	100 13	- -	- -	- -	- -	93 264	88 624	97 829	97 123
Greater Baltimore Medical Center, Baltimore, MD	100 2	93 15	100 7	100 6	- 0	- 0	100 1	- -	- -	- -	- -	92 62	97 173	97 261	100 19
Harbor Hospital, Brooklyn, MD	100 4	100 42	100 13	100 14	- 0	- 0	100 3	- -	- -	- -	- -	91 129	79 309	99 343	98 114
Harford Memorial Hospital, Havre De Grace, MD	100 4	97 36	95 19	95 21	- 0	- 0	100 3	- -	- -	- -	- -	98 58	98 183	100 223	100 30
Holy Cross Hospital, Silver Spring, MD	95 21	100 188	100 110	99 114	- 0	89 38	100 15	- 0	- 0	- 0	- 0	99 134	89 316	99 414	100 43
Howard County General Hospital, Columbia, MD	100 10	98 129	100 90	99 90	- 0	78 64	100 30	- -	- -	- -	- -	96 77	94 217	99 281	100 21
Johns Hopkins Bayview Medical Center, Baltimore, MD	96 28	100 172	98 129	98 127	- 0	93 27	100 55	- -	- -	- -	- -	96 234	77 509	99 671	99 197
The Johns Hopkins Hospital, Baltimore, MD	100 44	100 90	99 301	99 284	- 0	55 11	100 110	- -	- -	- -	- -	98 200	88 361	99 404	97 109
Laurel Regional Medical Center, Laurel, MD	100 4	96 55	81 27	93 29	0 1	- 0	100 2	- -	- -	- -	- -	98 50	96 112	96 160	96 28
Maryland General Hospital, Baltimore, MD	60 5	100 24	88 17	83 18	- 0	- 0	100 5	- -	- -	- -	- -	80 123	99 242	94 300	96 139
Memorial Hospital & Med Ctr of Cumberland, Cumberland, MD	100 1	92 12	100 8	100 9	- 0	- 0	- 0	- 0	- 0	- 0	- 0	83 18	82 34	96 50	100 7
Memorial Hospital at Easton, Easton, MD	91 11	100 84	100 47	98 46	42 12	- 0	100 13	- -	- -	- -	- -	94 154	75 420	98 516	100 90
Mercy Medical Center, Baltimore, MD	100 3	100 18	100 14	100 13	- 0	- 0	100 5	- -	- -	- -	- -	95 153	96 339	99 369	99 111
Meritus Medical Center, Hagerstown, MD	100 20	100 156	100 129	99 128	- 0	89 46	100 49	- -	- -	- -	- -	99 101	96 281	100 344	100 53
Montgomery General Hospital, Olney, MD	100 7	100 48	100 22	100 6	40 5	- 0	100 1	- -	- -	- -	- -	96 77	89 152	99 215	100 16
Northwest Hospital Center, Randallstown, MD	75 12	96 93	95 56	96 57	- 0	- 0	100 1	- -	- -	- -	- -	98 185	84 344	99 470	100 58
Peninsula Regional Medical Center, Salisbury, MD	95 100	97 403	99 540	99 536	- 0	80 91	99 172	- -	- -	- -	- -	98 265	88 727	96 932	98 151
Prince Georges Hospital Center, Cheverly, MD	87 30	91 171	86 170	90 165	- 0	42 31	98 64	- -	- -	- -	- -	89 105	85 276	89 304	98 99
Saint Agnes Hospital, Baltimore, MD	100 27	95 133	99 105	99 105	0 2	80 50	95 40	- -	- -	- -	- -	91 285	76 492	95 635	98 124
Saint Joseph Medical Center, Towson, MD	100 54	100 172	99 323	99 321	- 0	75 20	100 87	- -	- -	- -	- -	99 94	94 252	100 325	100 38
Saint Mary's Hospital, Leonardtown, MD	100 3	97 38	100 16	100 15	- 0	- 0	100 1	- -	- -	- -	- -	97 68	94 215	100 254	100 40
Shady Grove Adventist Hospital, Rockville, MD	96 27	100 180	99 159	99 156	- 0	87 71	98 59	- -	- -	- -	- -	100 140	96 284	100 377	100 39
Sinai Hospital of Baltimore, Baltimore, MD	86 71	100 210	98 379	97 372	- 0	82 51	100 129	- -	- -	- -	- -	93 249	67 587	97 708	99 139
Southern Maryland Hospital Center, Clinton, MD	85 34	96 159	98 123	97 118	100 2	87 38	100 43	- -	- -	- -	- -	94 277	94 661	98 752	100 123
Suburban Hospital, Bethesda, MD	95 44	99 177	99 241	98 240	- 0	72 36	100 38	- -	- -	- -	- -	90 108	99 198	98 288	100 7
Union Hospital of Cecil County, Elkton, MD	100 5	100 55	100 14	94 16	- 0	- 0	100 3	- -	- -	- -	- -	96 68	93 161	98 199	89 45
Union Memorial Hospital, Baltimore, MD	94 108	96 116	99 696	96 674	- 0	83 18	93 252	- -	- -	- -	- -	92 311	93 620	95 739	94 196
University of Maryland Medical Center, Baltimore, MD	92 77	99 83	98 471	97 444	- 0	60 15	99 166	- -	- -	- -	- -	94 251	78 391	98 429	100 115
Upper Chesapeake Medical Center, Bel Air, MD	100 30	99 202	97 145	99 145	- 0	86 79	100 54	- -	- -	- -	- -	96 78	97 301	100 374	100 46
VA Maryland Healthcare System - Baltimore, Baltimore, MD	100 3	100 36	93 29	97 29	- 0	0 2	100 12	- -	- -	- -	- -	93 117	98 252	100 252	100 57
Washington Adventist Hospital, Takoma Park, MD	96 71	99 83	98 292	98 282	0 1	95 20	100 81	- -	- -	- -	- -	95 182	77 311	96 398	100 50
Western Maryland Regional Medical Center, Cumberland, MD	83 46	97 193	98 219	91 213	- 0	86 7	99 86	- 0	- 0	- 0	- 0	93 183	84 361	99 472	98 51
MASSACHUSETTS															
Adcare Hospital of Worcester, Worcester, MA	- 0	- 0	- 0	- 0	- 0	- 0	- 0	- 0	- 0	- 0	- 0	- 0	- 0	- 0	- 0
Anna Jaques Hospital, Newburyport, MA	86 7	96 54	96 24	100 26	- 0	- 0	100 3	98 57	7 56	77 24	- 0	88 51	93 138	96 204	100 18
Athol Memorial Hospital, Athol, MA	- 0	80 5	100 5	100 6	- 0	- 0	- 0	- -	- -	- -	- -	100 9	94 31	88 48	100 2
Baystate Franklin Medical Center, Greenfield, MA	100 3	97 29	93 15	100 17	50 2	- 0	100 1	98 45	7 48	70 6	73 11	100 23	95 99	97 143	100 20
Baystate Mary Lane Hospital, Ware, MA	100 3	100 13	100 4	100 6	0 1	- 0	100 1	95 43	17 45	118 6	100 4	100 10	100 37	100 50	100 3
Baystate Medical Center, Springfield, MA	93 193	100 500	100 1055	99 1015	100 1	96 138	100 311	100 1	8 2	- -	- -	96 311	97 750	98 967	97 166
Bedford VA Medical Center, Bedford, MA	- 0	- 0	- 0	- 0	- 0	- 0	- 0	- 0	- 0	- 0	- 0	- 0	- 0	- 0	- 0
Berkshire Medical Center, Pittsfield, MA	100 9	100 88	100 58	100 64	0 1	- 0	100 7	100 109	8 109	55 1	81 31	100 55	100 201	100 284	100 29
Beth Israel Deaconess Hospital - Needham, Needham, MA	100 2	100 13	100 9	100 9	- 0	- 0	- 0	94 85	4 89	66 14	- 0	96 24	81 72	98 128	78 9
Beth Israel Deaconess Medical Center, Boston, MA	92 88	100 170	100 529	100 503	- 0	100 27	100 107	- 0	- -	- -	- -	91 138	95 433	100 431	100 61
Beverly Hospital Corporation, Beverly, MA	93 27	100 188	100 123	100 127	- 0	- 0	100 14	99 144	10 149	56 44	- 0	97 94	89 251	100 396	100 34
Boston Medical Center Corporation, Boston, MA	93 67	100 159	100 456	100 430	- 0	96 28	100 161	100 6	18 6	- 0	- -	95 325	99 697	100 831	100 216
Brigham and Women's Hosptial, Boston, MA	92 98	100 270	100 598	98 575	- 0	86 42	98 139	- 0	- -	- -	- -	95 96	99 244	99 281	98 43
Cambridge Health Alliance, Cambridge, MA	100 11	97 70	100 52	98 50	- 0	- 0	100 11	94 86	5 90	56 13	- 0	98 48	93 191	100 276	89 45
Cape Cod Hospital, Hyannis, MA	82 38	99 256	99 289	98 276	- 0	100 37	92 65	94 18	5 19	- 0	- -	79 87	73 192	100 295	84 31
Carney Hospital, Boston, MA	100 5	100 13	100 9	100 7	- 0	- 0	- 0	91 22	13 24	65 7	- 0	99 73	88 144	99 195	100 32
Children's Hospital Boston, Boston, MA	-	-	-	-	-	-	-	-	-	-	-	-	-	-	-
Clinton Hospital Association, Clinton, MA	100 1	100 9	88 8	100 7	- 0	- 0	100 1	92 13	3 13	60 3	100 1	100 5	100 31	98 44	100 6
The Cooley Dickinson Hospital, Northampton, MA	88 8	100 47	97 39	97 34	- 0	- 0	100 2	98 83	8 82	55 33	- 0	98 53	94 122	99 163	100 13
Dana-Farber Cancer Institute, Boston, MA	- 0	- 0	- 0	- 0	- 0	- 0	- 0	- 0	- 0	- 0	- 0	- 0	- 0	- 0	- 0
Emerson Hospital, West Concord, MA	100 6	97 60	100 33	97 33	- 0	- 0	80 5	99 70	7 71	70 22	- 0	98 45	78 127	99 193	100 10
Fairview Hospital, Great Barrington, MA	100 2	100 8	100 7	100 9	- 0	- 0	- 0	- -	- -	- -	- -	100 17	91 44	100 56	100 6
Falmouth Hospital, Falmouth, MA	100 10	100 94	100 68	98 61	- 0	- 0	100 3	95 38	8 39	- 0	- -	100 46	90 177	100 261	95 19
Faulkner Hospital, Boston, MA	100 1	100 22	100 18	100 18	- 0	- 0	100 2	96 49	15 51	58 11	- 0	100 38	100 151	100 211	100 12
Good Samaritan Medical Center, Brockton, MA	85 27	100 173	100 127	100 120	- 0	83 63	100 34	100 61	3 69	- 0	- -	95 87	83 243	100 387	96 48
Hallmark Health System, Melrose, MA	93 15	100 112	100 79	97 79	- 0	76 17	100 21	100 104	12 116	72 10	- 0	96 70	98 211	99 298	100 33
Harrington Memorial Hospital, Southbridge, MA	100 3	96 27	100 20	95 21	- 0	- 0	100 3	88 146	18 152	117 17	- 0	89 36	61 90	97 128	100 9
Healthalliance Hospitals, Leominster, MA	100 5	100 96	99 69	99 74	- 0	- 0	100 18	97 159	7 159	57 29	- 0	95 41	87 205	99 271	100 26
Heywood Hospital, Gardner, MA	83 12	100 49	89 28	97 35	- 0	- 0	100 1	98 160	18 173	95 12	- 0	88 25	76 86	93 116	100 10
Holy Family Hospital, Methuen, MA	90 10	97 79	100 50	95 57	- 0	88 26	100 16	91 64	8 69	56 2	- 0	96 56	86 160	100 242	90 21
Holyoke Medical Center, Holyoke, MA	93 14	95 110	94 69	96 71	- 0	- 0	83 6	94 49	13 50	65 21	- 0	87 53	85 123	100 191	92 26
Jordan Hospital, Plymouth, MA	100 11	100 82	94 48	100 56	- 0	- 0	67 3	98 165	22 174	- 0	- -	98 56	82 194	97 268	100 20
Lahey Clinic Hospital, Burlington, MA	96 139	100 298	100 703	99 687	100 1	93 69	99 156	83 6	9 6	- 0	- -	88 66	93 217	99 278	100 22
Lawrence General Hospital, Lawrence, MA	93 14	99 102	100 59	100 75	- 0	92 36	92 13	61 71	1 61	71 1	- 0	79 119	70 282	92 408	100 41

NOTE: The first number in each column (boldface) is the score, the second number is the number of patients; Please refer to the main entry for footnotes; (a) 100-299
MEASURES: **Heart Attack Care:** 1. ACE Inhibitor or ARB for LVSD; 2. Aspirin at Arrival; 3. Aspirin at Discharge; 4. Beta Blocker at Discharge; 5. Fibrinolytic Medication Timing; 6. PCI Within 90 Minutes of Arrival; 7. Smoking Cessation Advice; **Chest Pain/Possible Heart Attack Care:** 8. Aspirin at Arrival; 9. Median Time to ECG (minutes); 10. Median Time to Transfer (minutes); 11. Fibrinolytic Medication Timing; **Heart Failure Care:** 12. ACE Inhibitor or ARB for LVSD; 13. Discharge Instructions; 14. Evaluation of LVS Function; 15. Smoking Cessation Advice

Hospital	Heart Attack Care							Chest Pain/Possible Heart Attack Care				Heart Failure Care			
	1	2	3	4	5	6	7	8	9	10	11	12	13	14	15
Lowell General Hospital, Lowell, MA	100 20	100 137	100 115	100 121	- 0	98 43	100 27	88 8	6 8	- 0	- 0	93 59	76 249	97 329	83 30
Marlborough Hospital, Marlborough, MA	100 8	100 36	100 24	100 23	- 0	- 0	100 3	100 79	5 81	36 22	- 0	96 28	83 75	100 130	100 11
Martha's Vineyard Hospital, Oak Bluffs, MA	- 0	- 0	- 0	- 0	- 0	- 0	- 0	- 0	- 0	- 0	- 0	88 8	90 21	84 32	67 3
Massachusetts Eye and Ear Infirmary, Boston, MA	- 0	- 0	- 0	- 0	- 0	- 0	- 0	33 3	- 0	- 0	- 0	- 0	- 0	- 0	- 0
Massachusetts General Hospital, Boston, MA	99 79	100 273	100 758	99 727	- 0	95 57	100 197	100 12	9 13	- 0	- 0	96 72	91 217	99 270	100 41
Mercy Medical Center, Springfield, MA	83 6	98 87	98 55	98 60	- 0	- 0	100 5	93 46	7 49	71 15	- 0	97 79	77 249	99 321	98 61
Merrimack Valley Hospital, Haverhill, MA	67 3	95 41	97 31	100 29	- 0	- 0	100 5	98 46	7 49	51 17	- 0	92 36	98 122	99 193	100 26
Metrowest Medical Center, Framingham, MA	100 30	100 121	100 107	100 104	- 0	95 42	100 25	98 55	2 56	84 2	- 0	96 154	97 320	99 459	98 41
Milford Regional Medical Center, Milford, MA	100 10	100 72	96 56	98 53	- 0	- 0	75 4	95 48	15 91	76 31	- 0	98 59	91 178	99 276	83 18
Milton Hospital, Milton, MA	100 7	98 60	100 42	95 41	- 0	- 0	100 3	99 73	8 76	89 17	- 0	95 38	99 133	97 175	100 7
Morton Hospital & Medical Center, Taunton, MA	100 8	98 52	97 34	100 35	- 0	- 0	100 1	99 89	16 95	113 17	- 0	93 73	91 166	100 245	100 26
Mount Auburn Hospital, Cambridge, MA	100 38	99 191	100 228	100 225	- 0	92 36	100 39	100 2	30 2	- 0	- 0	100 82	100 264	100 347	100 30
Nantucket Cottage Hospital, Nantucket, MA	- 0	- 0	- 0	- 0	- 0	- 0	- 0	88 25	4 26	- 0	- 0	0 1	78 9	45 11	- 0
Nashoba Valley Medical Center, Ayer, MA	100 4	100 18	100 12	100 14	- 0	- 0	100 1	98 96	11 100	45 9	- 0	100 22	88 64	96 95	71 7
New England Baptist Hospital, Boston, MA	- 0	100 3	0 1	100 1	- 0	- 0	- 0	- 0	- 0	- 0	- 0	100 8	100 29	100 38	100 3
Newton-Wellesley Hospital, Newton, MA	100 8	100 59	100 38	100 41	- 0	- 0	100 3	95 56	0 58	65 3	- 0	96 54	95 193	100 264	100 16
Noble Hospital, Westfield, MA	100 2	100 26	100 20	100 22	- 0	- 0	100 5	98 40	6 41	34 17	- 0	100 30	93 82	91 104	100 8
North Adams Regional Hospital, North Adams, MA	100 8	100 37	100 27	100 26	- 0	- 0	100 5	96 48	6 52	- 0	80 15	91 22	95 75	100 101	100 13
North Shore Medical Center, Salem, MA	100 46	100 298	100 301	100 304	- 0	98 91	100 106	100 3	9 3	- 0	- 0	98 108	95 425	100 596	100 54
Northampton VA Medical Center, Leeds, MA	- 0	- 0	- 0	- 0	- 0	- 0	- 0	- 0	- 0	- 0	- 0	- 0	- 0	- 0	- 0
Norwood Hospital, Norwood, MA	100 18	100 142	98 101	100 96	- 0	100 40	100 23	100 54	8 57	47 1	- 0	97 58	90 164	99 271	100 25
Quincy Medical Center, Quincy, MA	100 10	100 70	100 51	98 50	- 0	- 0	83 6	100 59	17 63	91 22	- 0	98 61	96 164	99 246	100 30
Saint Anne's Hospital, Fall River, MA	100 6	100 54	97 31	100 30	- 0	- 0	100 6	92 25	11 27	54 13	- 0	100 24	78 144	100 185	100 25
Saint Elizabeth's Medical Center, Brighton, MA	83 71	99 107	96 326	96 307	- 0	75 16	99 96	100 1	21 1	- 0	- 0	84 101	93 303	98 404	98 57
Saint Vincent Hospital, Worcester, MA	97 73	100 368	100 446	99 434	- 0	98 44	100 127	100 1	9 7	- 0	- 0	98 138	97 396	100 592	100 53
Saints Medical Center, Lowell, MA	100 11	99 137	99 110	97 105	- 0	84 32	100 39	88 17	6 17	- 0	- 0	86 64	88 217	99 321	100 40
Signature Healthcare Brockton Hospital, Brockton, MA	100 22	100 188	99 145	100 144	- 0	98 44	100 54	100 18	6 20	- 0	- 0	99 96	97 206	100 290	100 60
Soldiers Home in Massachusetts, Chelsea, MA	-	-	-	-	-	-	-	- 0	- 0	- 0	- 0	-	-	-	-
South Shore Hospital, South Weymouth, MA	89 38	100 281	99 240	100 233	- 0	94 89	99 70	90 51	9 54	188 2	- 0	84 176	64 540	99 858	96 82
Southcoast Hospital Group, Fall River, MA	84 148	98 640	99 687	98 706	- 0	84 58	92 195	94 128	6 133	69 45	0 1	89 362	66 872	95 1287	81 139
Sturdy Memorial Hospital, Attleboro, MA	100 6	97 30	100 20	100 20	- 0	- 0	100 3	96 141	10 144	45 23	- 0	100 54	98 140	95 202	100 30
Tufts Medical Center, Boston, MA	100 90	100 73	100 398	99 376	- 0	100 8	99 103	100 2	16 2	- 0	- 0	99 193	97 348	100 417	100 59
UMass Memorial Medical Center, Worcester, MA	98 151	99 353	100 825	100 793	- 0	96 81	100 261	- 0	- 0	- 0	- 0	93 247	91 553	100 799	100 103
VA Boston Healthcare System - Jamaica Plain, Jamaica Plain, MA	- 0	- 0	- 0	- 0	- 0	- 0	- 0	-	-	-	-	88 97	100 236	100 289	100 27
Winchester Hospital, Winchester, MA	100 13	98 94	100 67	99 74	- 0	- 0	100 8	93 122	11 127	66 22	- 0	96 51	90 175	99 262	100 18
Wing Memorial Hospital and Medical Center, Palmer, MA	83 6	100 17	100 11	100 11	- 0	- 0	100 2	85 41	12 46	48 10	0 1	90 21	96 103	100 143	100 15
NEW HAMPSHIRE															
Alice Peck Day Memorial Hospital, Lebanon, NH	- 0	- 0	- 0	- 0	- 0	- 0	- 0	-	-	-	-	100 3	50 4	100 6	100 2
Androscoggin Valley Hospital, Berlin, NH	100 2	100 11	100 8	100 9	- 0	- 0	- 0	-	-	-	-	100 13	70 27	98 41	100 2
Catholic Medical Center, Manchester, NH	100 76	100 213	100 460	100 451	- 0	95 43	100 148	25 4	6 4	- 0	- 0	100 102	97 208	100 260	100 40
Cheshire Medical Center, Keene, NH	100 3	100 31	100 19	100 17	- 0	- 0	100 3	99 98	5 99	181 2	57	95 21	90 70	100 97	100 14
Concord Hospital, Concord, NH	100 29	100 165	100 228	100 226	- 0	96 48	100 69	100 1	4 2	- 0	- 0	99 86	96 261	100 343	100 53
Cottage Hospital, Woodsville, NH	- 0	100 3	100 2	100 2	- 0	- 0	- 0	-	-	-	- 0	92 12	93 15	- 0	- 0
Elliot Hospital, Manchester, NH	100 20	100 139	100 118	100 104	100 1	75 16	100 37	90 20	10 21	- 0	- 0	98 56	91 135	99 195	100 21
Exeter Hospital, Exeter, NH	100 8	100 118	99 96	100 88	- 0	94 32	100 29	100 5	15 5	48 3	- 0	92 39	100 137	100 185	100 10
Franklin Regional Hospital, Franklin, NH	- 0	100 9	100 6	100 5	- 0	- 0	- 0	100 31	7 31	62 10	- 0	83 6	60 10	87 30	100 2
Frisbie Memorial Hospital, Rochester, NH	- 0	100 18	100 4	100 3	- 0	- 0	100 2	89 37	5 37	43 12	- 0	94 17	95 81	99 108	100 11
Huggins Hospital, Wolfeboro, NH	100 3	100 15	100 10	100 11	- 0	- 0	- 0	-	-	-	-	75 20	57 21	98 41	100 4
Lakes Region General Hospital, Laconia, NH	83 6	98 44	100 26	100 24	- 0	- 0	50 2	97 135	7 137	36 34	- 0	83 24	65 62	97 90	100 19
Littleton Regional Hospital, Littleton, NH	100 1	100 6	100 6	100 6	- 0	- 0	- 0	-	-	-	-	100 4	53 15	75 20	80 5
Mary Hitchcock Memorial Hospital, Lebanon, NH	94 51	100 88	99 510	99 498	- 0	86 21	95 152	- 0	- 0	- 0	- 0	93 104	84 239	100 281	98 46
The Memorial Hospital, North Conway, NH	0 1	100 10	100 6	83 6	- 0	- 0	100 1	-	-	-	-	87 15	97 30	88 43	100 7
Monadnock Community Hospital, Peterborough, NH	100 5	100 10	100 8	100 8	- 0	- 0	- 0	94 33	11 35	66 2	33 3	100 4	89 18	97 29	100 5
New London Hospital, New London, NH	100 1	88 8	100 5	80 5	- 0	- 0	- 0	95 37	10 38	78 6	0 1	100 4	92 32	100 38	100 3
Parkland Medical Center, Derry, NH	100 15	100 85	100 73	100 74	- 0	100 23	100 25	100 4	2 4	- 0	- 0	100 27	98 104	100 109	100 7
Portsmouth Regional Hospital, Portsmouth, NH	100 35	100 150	100 278	100 267	- 0	93 28	100 81	100 2	- 0	- 0	- 0	100 59	90 78	100 169	100 7
Saint Joseph Hospital, Nashua, NH	100 8	100 65	100 46	100 44	- 0	- 0	- 0	50 2	8 32	37 14	- 0	100 59	84 123	100 201	100 6
Southern Nh Medical Center, Nashua, NH	96 28	100 148	98 123	100 122	- 0	72 18	100 34	100 13	11 12	- 0	- 0	98 42	99 189	100 227	100 37
Speare Memorial Hospital, Plymouth, NH	- 0	100 4	100 2	100 2	- 0	- 0	100 1	100 40	14 40	- 0	67 6	100 6	100 30	100 33	100 1
Upper Connecticut Valley Hospital, Colebrook, NH	- 0	100 6	75 4	100 5	- 0	- 0	- 0	97 38	10 38	- 0	25 4	100 5	100 15	91 23	100 1
Valley Regional Hospital, Claremont, NH	100 2	100 9	86 7	100 6	- 0	- 0	- 0	-	-	-	-	100 2	91 11	100 20	100 3
Weeks Medical Center, Lancaster, NH	100 4	100 14	100 13	91 11	- 0	- 0	100 4	98 60	11 65	- 0	- 0	93 14	83 6	100 34	100 1
Wentworth-Douglass Hospital, Dover, NH	100 5	100 77	97 74	100 72	- 0	71 21	100 26	100 4	12 12	- 0	- 0	100 48	99 165	99 203	100 18
NEW JERSEY															
Atlanticare Regional Medical Center - City Division, Atlantic City, NJ	98 66	100 238	100 330	100 325	- 0	83 60	100 114	67 6	29 7	- 0	- 0	100 229	100 468	100 618	100 138
Bayonne Hospital Center, Bayonne, NJ	100 29	100 139	100 100	100 109	- 0	83 18	100 37	100 1	3 1	- 0	- 0	93 60	99 156	99 259	100 19
Bayshore Community Hospital, Holmdel, NJ	100 11	100 152	100 59	100 67	- 0	- 0	100 16	100 40	8 38	- 0	83 6	100 67	100 162	100 284	100 26

NOTE: The first number in each column (boldface) is the score, the second number is the number of patients; Please refer to the main entry for footnotes; (a) 100–299
MEASURES: **Heart Attack Care:** 1. ACE Inhibitor or ARB for LVSD; 2. Aspirin at Arrival; 3. Aspirin at Discharge; 4. Beta Blocker at Discharge; 5. Fibrinolytic Medication Timing; 6. PCI Within 90 Minutes of Arrival; 7. Smoking Cessation Advice; **Chest Pain/Possible Heart Attack Care:** 8. Aspirin at Arrival; 9. Median Time to ECG (minutes); 10. Median Time to Transfer (minutes); 11. Fibrinolytic Medication Timing; **Heart Failure Care:** 12. ACE Inhibitor or ARB for LVSD; 13. Discharge Instructions; 14. Evaluation of LVS Function; 15. Smoking Cessation Advice

Hospital	Heart Attack Care							Chest Pain/Possible Heart Attack Care				Heart Failure Care			
	1	2	3	4	5	6	7	8	9	10	11	12	13	14	15
Bergen Regional Medical Center, Paramus, NJ	**100** 4	**100** 10	**100** 11	**89** 9	- 0	- 0	**100** 2	**100** 2	**6** 2	- 0	- 0	**100** 12	**100** 10	**100** 23	**100** 6
Cape Regional Medical Center, Cape May Ct Hse, NJ	**100** 3	**100** 50	**94** 16	**100** 18	- 0	- 0	**100** 2	**98** 83	**8** 85	**78** 9	**53** 17	**95** 82	**86** 230	**100** 302	**100** 46
Capital Health System - Mercer Campus, Trenton, NJ	**100** 15	**97** 61	**98** 46	**100** 46	- 0	**79** 14	**100** 19	**100** 4	**2** 4	- 0	- 0	**90** 83	**95** 197	**95** 235	**100** 51
Capital Health System-Fuld Campus, Trenton, NJ	**67** 3	**92** 37	**100** 14	**100** 14	- 0	- 0	**100** 2	**90** 21	**2** 22	**64** 10	- 0	**92** 87	**96** 197	**99** 242	**100** 56
Centrastate Medical Center, Freehold, NJ	**88** 8	**100** 111	**100** 38	**100** 38	**100** 2	- 0	**100** 3	**96** 81	**5** 83	**98** 6	**62** 16	**93** 90	**83** 230	**99** 356	**100** 22
Chilton Hospital, Pompton Plains, NJ	**100** 29	**99** 172	**98** 102	**98** 106	- 0	**90** 49	**100** 19	**100** 1	**4** 1	- 0	- 0	**96** 81	**92** 200	**99** 328	**100** 38
Christ Hospital, Jersey City, NJ	**100** 18	**96** 161	**98** 81	**98** 87	- 0	**94** 31	**100** 18	**100** 3	**9** 3	**160** 1	**0** 1	**98** 124	**100** 312	**99** 430	**100** 62
Clara Maass Medical Center, Belleville, NJ	**100** 28	**100** 240	**100** 123	**100** 121	- 0	**100** 24	**100** 29	**100** 9	**11** 9	- 0	- 0	**100** 91	**100** 245	**100** 329	**100** 37
Community Medical Center, Toms River, NJ	**100** 41	**100** 467	**100** 251	**100** 264	**100** 1	**100** 72	**100** 57	**100** 46	**9** 46	**110** 6	- 0	**100** 78	**100** 190	**100** 325	**100** 28
Cooper University Hospital, Camden, NJ	**98** 100	**99** 151	**99** 437	**100** 422	- 0	**77** 30	**100** 198	**100** 1	**4** 1	- 0	- 0	**99** 200	**99** 422	**100** 491	**100** 140
Deborah Heart and Lung Center, Browns Mills, NJ	**98** 55	**100** 17	**100** 355	**100** 343	- 0	- 0	**100** 100	- 0	- 0	- 0	- 0	**94** 68	**99** 170	**100** 195	**100** 36
East Orange General Hospital, East Orange, NJ	**100** 4	**100** 70	**100** 42	**100** 48	- 0	- 0	**100** 8	- 0	- 0	- 0	- 0	**97** 71	**99** 176	**100** 276	**100** 44
Englewood Hospital and Medical Center, Englewood, NJ	**98** 55	**100** 248	**100** 268	**98** 261	- 0	**87** 39	**100** 42	**100** 1	**0** 1	- 0	- 0	**98** 166	**94** 363	**99** 498	**100** 40
Hackensack University Medical Center, Hackensack, NJ	**100** 165	**100** 524	**100** 741	**100** 731	- 0	**98** 88	**100** 165	**94** 33	**6** 37	- 0	- 0	**94** 372	**87** 794	**100** 1086	**100** 100
Hackettstown Regional Medical Center, Hackettstown, NJ	**100** 8	**100** 61	**100** 32	**100** 35	- 0	- 0	**100** 5	**100** 33	**15** 37	- 0	**71** 7	**100** 34	**96** 117	**100** 204	**100** 13
Hoboken University Medical Center, Hoboken, NJ	**100** 2	**95** 43	**100** 17	**100** 16	**0** 1	- 0	**100** 1	**100** 4	**6** 4	- 0	**0** 1	**100** 95	**100** 176	**100** 215	**100** 37
Holy Name Medical Center, Teaneck, NJ	**100** 27	**100** 200	**100** 140	**100** 146	- 0	**100** 29	**100** 33	**100** 1	**14** 1	- 0	- 0	**100** 79	**100** 238	**100** 335	**100** 26
Hunterdon Medical Center, Flemington, NJ	**100** 17	**100** 117	**100** 75	**100** 75	- 0	**95** 42	**100** 25	**91** 11	**9** 11	**184** 1	- 0	**100** 57	**93** 107	**99** 146	**100** 14
Jersey Shore University Medical Center, Neptune, NJ	**97** 60	**99** 159	**99** 486	**98** 465	- 0	**88** 41	**100** 161	**100** 1	**21** 1	- 0	- 0	**99** 133	**91** 268	**99** 362	**100** 52
JFK Medical Center, Edison, NJ	**87** 39	**97** 263	**98** 163	**97** 172	- 0	**75** 61	**100** 26	**57** 7	**18** 8	- 0	- 0	**90** 178	**74** 436	**99** 650	**98** 59
Kennedy University Hospital, Stratford, NJ	**100** 14	**96** 238	**96** 120	**96** 113	**33** 3	- 0	**100** 14	**97** 179	**9** 183	**108** 22	**56** 18	**88** 170	**85** 672	**99** 905	**99** 141
Kimball Medical Center, Lakewood, NJ	**90** 10	**99** 149	**98** 58	**100** 60	**100** 5	- 0	**100** 3	**100** 27	**10** 27	- 0	**100** 2	**99** 90	**85** 199	**99** 329	**100** 34
Libertyhealth-Jersey City Medical Center Campus, Jersey City, NJ	**100** 49	**100** 189	**99** 220	**99** 219	- 0	**92** 37	**100** 67	**100** 4	**30** 6	- 0	- 0	**99** 168	**99** 284	**100** 338	**99** 78
Lourdes Medical Center of Burlington County, Willingboro, NJ	**100** 8	**99** 71	**92** 39	**95** 44	- 0	- 0	**100** 4	**95** 306	**9** 309	**73** 9	**100** 4	**92** 116	**99** 276	**98** 340	**100** 41
Meadowlands Hospital Medical Center, Secaucus, NJ	**100** 4	**100** 29	**100** 10	**100** 9	- 0	- 0	- 0	**100** 5	**10** 5	- 0	**100** 1	**97** 39	**98** 83	**99** 118	**100** 9
Memorial Hospital of Salem County, Salem, NJ	**100** 5	**100** 30	**100** 10	**100** 13	- 0	- 0	**100** 3	**95** 19	**8** 21	**68** 1	**100** 7	**100** 50	**99** 151	**100** 186	**100** 36
Monmouth Medical Center, Long Branch, NJ	**100** 8	**99** 127	**99** 70	**98** 65	- 0	**100** 14	**100** 14	**88** 8	**4** 9	**75** 2	- 0	**100** 53	**100** 182	**100** 268	**100** 31
Morristown Memorial Hospital, Morristown, NJ	**92** 52	**96** 161	**99** 334	**99** 324	- 0	**89** 35	**100** 84	- 0	- 0	- 0	- 0	**94** 128	**99** 249	**98** 338	**100** 36
Mountainside Hospital, Montclair, NJ	**100** 19	**100** 165	**100** 97	**100** 105	- 0	**85** 40	**100** 13	- 0	- 0	- 0	- 0	**100** 121	**96** 255	**100** 385	**100** 19
Newark Beth Israel Medical Center, Newark, NJ	**100** 69	**100** 200	**100** 284	**100** 276	- 0	**100** 24	**100** 81	**100** 1	**24** 3	- 0	- 0	**100** 175	**100** 304	**100** 359	**100** 59
Newton Memorial Hospital, Newton, NJ	**100** 5	**100** 66	**100** 26	**100** 32	**0** 1	- 0	**100** 5	**100** 31	**5** 34	**90** 5	**75** 4	**98** 61	**100** 151	**100** 251	**100** 23
Ocean Medical Center, Brick, NJ	**90** 10	**100** 215	**98** 111	**100** 110	**100** 1	**90** 42	**100** 17	**93** 14	**9** 14	**57** 3	**0** 1	**99** 68	**96** 223	**98** 351	**100** 23
Our Lady of Lourdes Medical Center, Camden, NJ	**98** 51	**99** 116	**100** 293	**98** 278	- 0	**86** 22	**100** 79	**100** 2	**11** 2	- 0	- 0	**100** 90	**98** 245	**100** 307	**100** 61
Overlook Hospital, Summit, NJ	**91** 32	**97** 192	**97** 151	**98** 151	- 0	**78** 41	**80** 15	- 0	- 0	- 0	- 0	**89** 99	**92** 247	**97** 360	**96** 24
Palisades Medical Center, North Bergen, NJ	**100** 10	**97** 88	**100** 33	**100** 35	**0** 1	- 0	**100** 2	- 0	- 0	- 0	- 0	**100** 79	**100** 169	**99** 255	**100** 17
Raritan Bay Medical Center, Perth Amboy, NJ	**100** 30	**98** 204	**96** 134	**98** 132	- 0	**87** 31	**100** 42	**100** 7	**12** 7	- 0	- 0	**99** 193	**96** 370	**100** 542	**100** 54
Riverview Medical Center, Red Bank, NJ	**100** 9	**100** 187	**100** 113	**100** 116	- 0	**95** 39	**100** 25	**100** 10	**11** 11	**103** 1	**100** 1	**100** 46	**100** 229	**100** 320	**100** 31
Robert Wood Johnson University Hospital, New Brunswick, NJ	**99** 108	**99** 419	**100** 859	**100** 814	- 0	**80** 103	**100** 199	- 0	- 0	- 0	- 0	**99** 378	**87** 771	**100** 1029	**100** 117
Robert Wood Johnson University Hospital at Rahway, Rahway, NJ	**100** 12	**100** 106	**100** 38	**100** 44	**44** 9	- 0	**100** 4	**95** 20	**7** 21	**136** 2	**67** 3	**99** 131	**83** 259	**100** 430	**100** 41
Robert Wood Johnson University Hospital Hamilton, Hamilton, NJ	**91** 11	**94** 161	**93** 89	**98** 86	- 0	**61** 36	**100** 26	- 0	- 0	- 0	- 0	**94** 102	**92** 314	**100** 413	**100** 41
Saint Barnabas Medical Center, Livingston, NJ	**100** 64	**100** 271	**100** 351	**100** 350	- 0	**97** 29	**100** 73	**100** 1	**9** 1	- 0	- 0	**99** 113	**100** 268	**100** 332	**100** 21
Saint Clare's Hospital, Denville, NJ	**100** 16	**100** 169	**100** 123	**100** 121	- 0	**98** 43	**100** 30	**100** 26	**11** 26	**60** 5	**67** 3	**99** 129	**90** 381	**100** 560	**100** 51
Saint Clare's Hospital - Sussex, Sussex, NJ	**100** 1	**100** 8	**100** 3	**100** 3	- 0	- 0	**100** 1	**100** 10	**10** 10	**74** 1	**100** 1	**100** 8	**89** 46	**98** 53	**100** 6
Saint Francis Medical Center, Trenton, NJ	**100** 48	**100** 118	**100** 291	**99** 270	- 0	**59** 34	**100** 99	- 0	- 0	- 0	- 0	**98** 110	**94** 244	**100** 297	**100** 65
Saint Joseph's Regional Medical Center, Paterson, NJ	**94** 64	**99** 379	**97** 377	**96** 358	**100** 4	**97** 79	**100** 115	- 0	- 0	- 0	- 0	**98** 335	**98** 754	**98** 1003	**100** 175
Saint Joseph's Wayne Hospital, Wayne, NJ	- -	- -	- -	- -	- -	- -	- -	- -	- -	- -	- -	- -	- -	- -	- -
Saint Mary's Hospital - Passaic, Passaic, NJ	**100** 18	**99** 84	**97** 73	**99** 78	- 0	**65** 23	**100** 26	- 0	- 0	- 0	- 0	**94** 98	**88** 247	**100** 335	**100** 33
Saint Michael's Medical Center, Newark, NJ	**95** 78	**99** 97	**96** 315	**97** 317	- 0	**80** 10	**100** 93	- 0	- 0	- 0	- 0	**95** 174	**87** 243	**100** 342	**99** 67
Saint Peter's University Hospital, New Brunswick, NJ	**100** 11	**100** 103	**98** 56	**100** 59	- 0	**79** 19	**100** 16	**100** 3	**46** 3	- 0	- 0	**96** 70	**67** 246	**99** 328	**100** 39
Shore Memorial Hospital, Somers Point, NJ	**100** 11	**99** 89	**100** 43	**100** 49	- 0	- 0	**100** 8	**100** 68	**8** 70	**82** 20	- 0	**97** 64	**96** 200	**100** 268	**100** 32
Somerset Medical Center, Somerville, NJ	**96** 25	**100** 252	**99** 175	**99** 175	- 0	**86** 64	**100** 50	**0** 1	**14** 4	- 0	- 0	**100** 78	**100** 209	**99** 327	**97** 34
South Jersey Healthcare Regional Med Ctr, Vineland, NJ	**100** 13	**99** 125	**100** 56	**100** 57	**100** 2	- 0	**100** 11	**98** 96	**5** 99	**71** 19	**75** 28	**100** 107	**100** 253	**100** 322	**100** 47
South Jersey Healthcare-Elmer Hospital, Elmer, NJ	**83** 6	**100** 39	**94** 17	**100** 19	- 0	- 0	**100** 1	**100** 22	**10** 21	**140** 1	**60** 5	**92** 36	**100** 98	**100** 122	**100** 10
Southern Ocean Medical Center, Manahawkin, NJ	**100** 17	**99** 95	**100** 53	**100** 54	- 0	- 0	**100** 8	**100** 134	**7** 136	**89** 13	**20** 10	**94** 86	**85** 142	**99** 234	**100** 48
Trinitas Regional Medical Center, Elizabeth, NJ	**100** 35	**96** 163	**95** 109	**96** 114	- 0	**80** 35	**100** 35	**100** 2	**4** 2	- 0	- 0	**85** 127	**91** 235	**98** 299	**100** 57
UMDNJ University Hospital, Newark, NJ	**100** 29	**100** 97	**100** 112	**100** 105	- 0	**82** 28	**100** 49	- 0	- 0	- 0	- 0	**100** 269	**100** 371	**100** 412	**100** 164
Underwood Memorial Hospital, Woodbury, NJ	**95** 20	**99** 228	**98** 142	**99** 144	- 0	**92** 64	**100** 55	**100** 12	**15** 13	**90** 1	- 0	**98** 133	**100** 356	**100** 470	**100** 70
University Medical Center at Princeton, Princeton, NJ	**100** 16	**100** 129	**100** 80	**100** 85	- 0	**100** 20	**100** 8	**100** 7	**0** 7	**167** 1	- 0	**100** 60	**100** 164	**100** 255	**100** 19
VA New Jersey Health Care System, East Orange, NJ	- 0	- 0	- 0	- 0	- 0	- 0	- 0	- -	- -	- -	- -	**100** 60	**87** 103	**100** 115	**100** 29
Valley Hospital, Ridgewood, NJ	**93** 46	**98** 289	**100** 291	**99** 296	- 0	**96** 46	**100** 56	**100** 1	**9** 1	- 0	- 0	**92** 59	**77** 244	**99** 321	**100** 24
Virtua Memorial Hospital of Burlington County, Mount Holly, NJ	**97** 29	**100** 247	**97** 146	**99** 155	- 0	**45** 20	**100** 28	**99** 143	**11** 149	**49** 30	**100** 1	**92** 110	**83** 336	**98** 486	**100** 71
Virtua West Jersey Hospitals Berlin, Berlin, NJ	**100** 45	**100** 356	**100** 277	**99** 271	**50** 4	**80** 45	**100** 67	**97** 119	**10** 124	**124** 11	**50** 2	**99** 172	**87** 588	**100** 859	**100** 113
Warren Hospital, Phillipsburg, NJ	**100** 7	**97** 29	**100** 20	**96** 23	- 0	- 0	**100** 3	**100** 34	**6** 36	**50** 13	- 0	**100** 38	**98** 111	**100** 176	**100** 25
NEW YORK															
Adirondack Medical Center, Saranac Lake, NY	**100** 4	**91** 22	**86** 14	**88** 16	- 0	- 0	**100** 3	**100** 51	**5** 50	- 0	**20** 5	**80** 25	**90** 62	**91** 69	**100** 9
Albany Medical Center - South Clinical Campus, Albany, NY	- 0	- 0	- 0	- 0	- 0	- 0	- 0	- 0	- 0	- 0	- 0	- 0	- 0	- 0	- 0
Albany Medical Center Hospital, Albany, NY	**99** 82	**100** 188	**100** 484	**100** 480	**0** 1	**96** 49	**100** 204	- 0	- 0	- 0	- 0	**95** 172	**91** 324	**100** 386	**100** 64

NOTE: The first number in each column (boldface) is the score, the second number is the number of patients; Please refer to the main entry for footnotes; (a) 100-299
*MEASURES: **Heart Attack Care:** 1. ACE Inhibitor or ARB for LVSD; 2. Aspirin at Arrival; 3. Aspirin at Discharge; 4. Beta Blocker at Discharge; 5. Fibrinolytic Medication Timing; 6. PCI Within 90 Minutes of Arrival; 7. Smoking Cessation Advice; **Chest Pain/Possible Heart Attack Care:** 8. Aspirin at Arrival; 9. Median Time to ECG (minutes); 10. Median Time to Transfer (minutes); 11. Fibrinolytic Medication Timing; **Heart Failure Care:** 12. ACE Inhibitor or ARB for LVSD; 13. Discharge Instructions; 14. Evaluation of LVS Function; 15. Smoking Cessation Advice*

Hospital	Heart Attack Care							Chest Pain/Possible Heart Attack Care				Heart Failure Care			
	1	2	3	4	5	6	7	8	9	10	11	12	13	14	15
Albany Memorial Hospital, Albany, NY	100 5	94 33	96 23	92 25	- 0	- 0	100 2	95 22	12 22	55 10	- 0	100 22	83 102	96 135	91 22
Albany VA Medical Center, Albany, NY	100 2	100 21	100 16	100 15	- 0	- 0	100 1	-	-	-	-	100 22	100 62	100 71	100 13
Alice Hyde Medical Center, Malone, NY	100 2	100 9	100 6	100 6	- 0	- 0	- 0	98 84	13 89	106 2	60 10	100 16	90 50	97 59	100 6
Arnot Ogden Medical Center, Elmira, NY	99 94	100 193	100 293	99 313	- 0	90 40	100 119	- 0	- 0	- 0	- 0	95 74	81 188	100 225	100 38
Auburn Memorial Hospital, Auburn, NY	83 6	100 34	100 20	100 22	- 0	- 0	- 0	95 137	9 140	60 27	- 0	91 54	79 155	96 196	83 18
Aurelia Osborn Fox Memorial Hospital, Oneonta, NY	100 4	94 51	85 39	93 42	- 0	- 0	57 7	93 46	10 47	75 13	0 1	93 44	84 138	94 170	100 20
Bath VA Medical Center, Bath, NY	- 0	- 0	- 0	- 0	- 0	- 0	- 0	-	-	-	-	100 7	95 21	100 23	100 5
Bellevue Hospital Center, New York, NY	99 137	100 188	100 520	99 491	- 0	96 24	100 183	- 0	- 0	- 0	- 0	100 313	100 471	100 539	100 129
Benedictine Hospital, Kingston, NY	100 5	97 38	95 22	100 25	43 7	- 0	100 9	89 18	8 21	- 0	43 7	97 61	99 186	98 239	100 40
Bertrand Chaffee Hospital, Springville, NY	40 5	88 17	86 7	80 10	- 0	- 0	- 0	84 93	18 97	228 1	67 6	83 12	91 32	100 53	100 6
Beth Israel Medical Center, New York, NY	95 66	96 257	98 263	98 258	- 0	71 24	100 53	- 0	- 0	- 0	- 0	95 91	64 260	98 307	97 33
Bon Secours Community Hospital, Port Jervis, NY	100 4	94 31	100 19	95 22	- 0	- 0	100 4	100 55	12 57	68 8	50 6	100 23	84 77	99 97	100 23
Bronx VA Medical Center, Bronx, NY	100 1	100 11	100 5	100 5	- 0	- 0	100 2	-	-	-	-	93 82	99 138	100 149	100 22
Bronx-Lebanon Hospital Center, Bronx, NY	100 23	100 194	99 137	99 124	- 0	88 33	100 55	100 1	1354 1	- 0	- 0	97 159	99 327	99 371	99 80
Brookdale Hospital Medical Center, Brooklyn, NY	100 40	99 245	99 185	99 187	- 0	81 36	98 53	- 0	- 0	- 0	- 0	96 126	93 286	99 327	97 61
Brookhaven Memorial Hospital Medical Center, Patchogue, NY	94 18	99 185	100 79	100 94	- 0	- 0	100 12	99 105	16 110	125 1	- 0	95 106	88 302	99 457	100 48
Brooklyn Hospital Center at Downtown Campus, Brooklyn, NY	89 9	97 120	100 45	96 50	- 0	- 0	100 2	100 26	31 23	208 3	- 0	96 145	91 361	98 426	100 61
Brooks Memorial Hospital, Dunkirk, NY	67 3	91 11	86 7	89 9	- 0	- 0	100 4	96 147	17 151	78 1	67 9	89 18	82 50	97 76	75 12
Canandaigua VA Medical Center, Canandaigua, NY	- 0	- 0	- 0	- 0	- 0	- 0	- 0	-	-	-	-	- 0	- 0	- 0	- 0
Canton-Potsdam Hospital, Potsdam, NY	- 0	100 11	100 4	80 5	- 0	- 0	- 0	97 65	6 67	255 1	62 21	97 34	87 85	97 99	95 20
Carthage Area Hospital, Carthage, NY	- 0	100 7	50 2	100 2	- 0	- 0	0 1	92 40	7 41	320 3	- 0	80 15	70 54	97 61	86 7
Catskill Regional Medical Center, Harris, NY	100 2	90 41	100 14	100 13	- 0	- 0	100 2	96 51	21 54	95 5	- 0	93 27	85 55	100 80	100 19
Cayuga Medical Center at Ithaca, Ithaca, NY	50 6	98 40	90 29	93 30	25 4	- 0	100 5	96 72	9 74	- 0	79 24	79 38	75 103	96 130	100 17
Champlain Valley Physicians Hospital Med Ctr, Plattsburgh, NY	97 38	99 185	99 257	97 269	- 0	93 28	98 92	100 11	15 11	- 0	- 0	83 78	86 286	100 356	97 62
Chenango Memorial Hospital, Norwich, NY	50 2	100 32	100 19	100 17	- 0	- 0	100 2	94 71	8 72	82 5	100 1	90 10	95 58	96 71	100 2
Claxton-Hepburn Medical Center, Ogdensburg, NY	100 5	100 32	95 22	100 18	100 1	- 0	100 6	97 59	8 62	196 5	33 12	100 11	91 45	100 57	100 6
Clifton Springs Hospital and Clinic, Clifton Springs, NY	100 3	100 15	100 6	100 9	- 0	- 0	- 0	97 63	13 64	80 6	0 2	100 25	97 72	100 81	100 7
Cobleskill Regional Hospital, Cobleskill, NY	100 2	100 4	100 4	100 4	- 0	- 0	100 2	99 114	9 118	73 10	- 0	100 11	94 33	95 42	100 5
Columbia Memorial Hospital, Hudson, NY	100 10	92 86	100 57	96 56	- 0	- 0	89 9	95 40	10 44	120 4	0 3	85 48	90 164	95 226	100 34
Community Memorial Hospital, Hamilton, NY	100 1	100 7	100 4	100 4	- 0	- 0	100 1	100 28	4 30	49 1	- 0	100 12	87 30	91 44	100 1
Community-General Hospital of Greater Syracuse, Syracuse, NY	86 7	93 43	90 30	96 28	0 2	- 0	100 3	82 17	19 17	86 6	33 3	86 43	73 121	96 189	100 15
Coney Island Hospital, Brooklyn, NY	94 17	99 115	100 60	98 62	50 14	- 0	100 8	100 5	14 5	- 0	- 0	93 153	93 406	99 498	100 96
Corning Hospital, Corning, NY	100 2	100 13	100 8	100 8	- 0	- 0	100 1	97 79	19 82	52 6	100 1	95 42	92 96	100 137	87 15
Cortland Regional Medical Center, Cortland, NY	100 1	100 21	100 9	100 7	- 0	- 0	100 1	93 174	13 179	- 0	0 2	66 38	88 88	92 118	95 19
Crouse Hospital, Syracuse, NY	96 25	98 146	99 143	97 135	- 0	98 46	100 51	100 1	8 2	- 0	- 0	96 97	71 331	99 409	98 56
Delaware Valley Hospital, Walton, NY	100 1	100 2	100 2	100 2	- 0	- 0	- 0	100 23	7 24	155 1	- 0	86 7	95 21	89 27	100 4
Eastern Long Island Hospital, Greenport, NY	100 1	100 12	100 9	100 11	- 0	- 0	- 0	100 20	9 19	82 1	100 1	91 11	81 36	100 47	100 3
Eastern Niagara Hospital, Lockport, NY	0 1	92 37	74 23	78 27	- 0	- 0	100 4	94 151	15 154	413 1	33 15	74 38	71 128	90 181	83 18
Edward John Noble Hospital of Gouverneur, Gouverneur, NY	- 0	100 4	100 1	100 1	- 0	- 0	- 0	95 20	7 20	255 1	33 3	83 7	42 40	79 53	86 7
Elizabethtown Community Hospital, Elizabethtown, NY	100 1	100 2	50 2	100 3	- 0	- 0	- 0	- 0	-	-	-	100 2	86 7	92 12	100 1
Ellenville Regional Hospital, Ellenville, NY	- 0	- 0	- 0	- 0	- 0	- 0	- 0	-	-	-	-	100 1	75 8	100 9	- 0
Ellis Hospital, Schenectady, NY	100 71	98 409	99 510	100 506	- 0	94 65	100 151	100 1	5 1	- 0	- 0	99 99	99 440	98 572	100 73
Elmhurst Hospital Center, Elmhurst, NY	95 61	100 267	100 268	100 262	- 0	67 90	100 91	100 192	0 198	- 0	- 0	94 141	100 315	100 339	100 61
Erie County Medical Center, Buffalo, NY	95 44	96 131	98 214	99 204	- 0	80 35	100 100	- 0	- 0	- 0	- 0	88 133	97 254	99 311	100 90
F F Thompson Hospital, Canandaigua, NY	100 5	89 35	92 24	93 30	- 0	- 0	100 3	96 123	10 124	44 28	- 0	82 33	66 123	99 145	100 4
Faxton-St Luke's Healthcare, Utica, NY	91 32	95 119	95 110	97 115	- 0	58 12	93 27	100 1	0 1	- 0	- 0	85 103	81 208	93 309	97 34
Flushing Hospital Medical Center, Flushing, NY	93 15	89 105	86 64	90 70	- 0	- 0	86 7	100 23	13 23	139 5	100 2	81 68	89 124	98 255	86 14
Forest Hills Hospital, Forest Hills, NY	100 12	95 111	97 61	97 67	- 0	- 0	100 6	98 60	11 62	80 19	- 0	91 65	91 191	100 267	100 22
Franklin Hospital, Valley Stream, NY	80 5	95 56	95 20	90 20	- 0	- 0	- 0	99 110	16 111	94 46	- 0	95 87	95 204	100 273	100 29
Geneva General Hospital, Geneva, NY	100 4	100 31	100 20	90 20	- 0	- 0	100 1	98 61	20 64	74 3	75 4	100 20	77 109	94 148	100 16
Glen Cove Hospital, Glen Cove, NY	100 7	100 47	96 28	100 24	- 0	- 0	100 2	100 36	8 37	78 18	- 0	96 28	96 170	100 249	100 7
Glens Falls Hospital, Glens Falls, NY	98 43	100 268	100 229	100 235	- 0	96 47	100 73	100 3	5 3	- 0	- 0	98 112	75 268	100 338	100 40
Good Samaritan Hospital Medical Center, West Islip, NY	100 23	100 248	100 202	100 200	- 0	100 35	100 61	100 6	3 7	- 0	- 0	100 78	100 259	100 344	100 34
Good Samaritan Hospital of Suffern, Suffern, NY	94 87	99 251	100 421	100 418	- 0	87 69	99 120	100 2	8 1	- 0	- 0	99 145	98 263	99 375	100 52
Harlem Hospital Center, New York, NY	100 9	100 38	100 20	100 19	0 1	- 0	100 7	100 6	26 6	- 0	0 1	93 76	78 206	99 219	100 69
Helen Hayes Hospital, West Haverstraw, NY	- 0	- 0	- 0	- 0	- 0	- 0	- 0	-	-	-	-	- 0	- 0	- 0	- 0
Highland Hospital, Rochester, NY	92 13	97 68	100 52	100 49	- 0	- 0	100 7	96 24	22 25	45 5	- 0	98 59	97 215	99 309	100 43
Hospital for Special Surgery, New York, NY	- 0	- 0	- 0	- 0	- 0	- 0	- 0	-	-	-	-	- 0	- 0	- 0	- 0
Hudson Valley Hospital Center, Cortlandt Manor, NY	100 12	98 113	100 65	100 68	83 6	- 0	100 4	98 62	7 67	99 8	83 6	97 63	90 157	100 257	100 32
Huntington Hospital, Huntington, NY	100 15	100 159	100 103	100 102	- 0	91 47	100 24	100 25	4 26	61 1	- 0	98 65	100 220	100 292	100 21
Interfaith Medical Center, Brooklyn, NY	100 8	95 57	91 22	92 26	0 1	- 0	90 10	-	-	-	-	97 88	82 188	100 209	91 82
Ira Davenport Memorial Hospital, Bath, NY	100 2	100 6	83 6	100 5	- 0	- 0	50 2	100 19	14 19	- 0	100 1	89 9	100 31	100 38	75 4
Jacobi Medical Center, Bronx, NY	94 18	99 116	96 70	95 64	- 0	- 0	100 16	100 18	4 19	85 7	- 0	98 93	99 232	99 276	100 64
Jamaica Hospital Medical Center, Jamaica, NY	100 44	100 262	100 169	100 169	- 0	96 71	100 58	95 19	16 20	176 1	- 0	100 132	100 271	100 310	100 45
J T Mather Mem Hosp of Port Jefferson, Port Jefferson, NY	100 10	100 147	100 68	99 73	- 0	- 0	100 2	100 118	10 120	84 28	- 0	98 63	98 250	100 389	100 29
Jones Memorial Hospital, Wellsville, NY	100 2	92 13	71 7	100 8	- 0	- 0	100 1	98 58	6 63	181 1	75 8	87 15	74 54	94 63	100 14
Kaleida Health, Buffalo, NY	93 116	99 448	97 854	98 873	83 6	83 36	100 250	78 9	11 10	- 0	- 0	96 489	84 1265	99 1555	100 274

NOTE: The first number in each column (boldface) is the score, the second number is the number of patients; Please refer to the main entry for footnotes. (a) 100-299
MEASURES: **Heart Attack Care:** 1. ACE Inhibitor or ARB for LVSD; 2. Aspirin at Arrival; 3. Aspirin at Discharge; 4. Beta Blocker at Discharge; 5. Fibrinolytic Medication Timing; 6. PCI Within 90 Minutes of Arrival; 7. Smoking Cessation Advice; **Chest Pain/Possible Heart Attack Care:** 8. Aspirin at Arrival; 9. Median Time to ECG (minutes); 10. Median Time to Transfer (minutes); 11. Fibrinolytic Medication Timing; **Heart Failure Care:** 12. ACE Inhibitor or ARB for LVSD; 13. Discharge Instructions; 14. Evaluation of LVS Function; 15. Smoking Cessation Advice

Hospital	Heart Attack Care							Chest Pain/Possible Heart Attack Care				Heart Failure Care			
	1	2	3	4	5	6	7	8	9	10	11	12	13	14	15
Kenmore Mercy Hospital, Kenmore, NY	100 19	97 91	98 58	98 60	- 0	- 0	100 9	97 36	13 36	55 2	80 5	96 69	86 197	99 274	100 22
Kings County Hospital Center, Brooklyn, NY	89 9	98 97	100 58	98 53	- 0	- 0	100 8	100 3	12 3	129 3	- 0	98 306	69 577	100 602	96 105
Kingsbrook Jewish Medical Center, Brooklyn, NY	100 3	98 42	100 15	100 17	- 0	- 0	100 2	100 20	12 20	200 1	- 0	99 107	90 174	100 265	100 21
Kingston Hospital, Kingston, NY	100 14	100 56	100 41	100 40	50 4	- 0	100 8	95 37	5 39	94 1	79 14	88 69	95 167	99 208	100 37
Lakeside Memorial Hospital, Brockport, NY	100 3	100 28	100 20	100 21	- 0	- 0	- 0	95 106	10 108	81 23	- 0	100 22	98 96	98 124	100 11
Lawrence Hospital Center, Bronxville, NY	100 5	95 38	86 14	95 19	0 2	- 0	100 2	96 55	17 59	82 3	35 20	99 77	98 195	99 256	89 9
Lenox Hill Hospital, New York, NY	97 75	99 136	100 331	99 321	- 0	100 15	99 70	- 0	- 0	- 0	- 0	96 192	88 365	100 444	91 54
Lewis County General Hospital, Lowville, NY	100 2	100 8	71 7	100 1	100 1	- 0	100 1	100 20	10 19	- 0	33 3	67 15	48 29	93 42	50 6
Lincoln Medical & Mental Health Center, Bronx, NY	100 14	100 129	100 63	100 64	69 13	- 0	100 16	100 7	5 7	- 0	100 5	99 122	100 366	100 396	100 69
Little Falls Hospital, Little Falls, NY	0 1	90 10	100 9	100 8	- 0	- 0	- 0	96 51	11 52	74 5	- 0	60 5	77 13	96 24	0 2
Long Beach Medical Center, Long Beach, NY	100 1	100 8	100 8	80 5	- 0	- 0	- 0	98 86	10 95	99 9	- 0	90 21	89 61	95 103	100 10
Long Island College Hospital, Brooklyn, NY	85 41	97 227	94 176	94 177	0 1	62 13	100 42	80 5	28 5	- 0	- 0	91 114	97 272	96 311	100 43
Long Island Jewish Medical Center, New Hyde Park, NY	100 75	98 159	99 301	99 294	- 0	100 33	100 82	- 0	14 1	- 0	- 0	95 142	89 243	99 306	97 39
Lutheran Medical Center, Brooklyn, NY	91 32	98 256	97 173	97 177	- 0	97 39	100 33	88 17	8 17	109 3	- 0	84 79	97 296	98 402	95 21
Maimonides Medical Center, Brooklyn, NY	91 87	95 284	96 302	95 307	100 1	69 29	99 77	- 0	- 0	- 0	- 0	96 114	86 300	100 359	100 29
Margaretville Memorial Hospital, Margaretville, NY	- 0	- 0	- 0	- 0	- 0	- 0	- 0	- 0	- 0	- 0	- 0	100 2	88 8	88 8	100 1
Mary Imogene Bassett Hospital, Cooperstown, NY	86 37	96 114	100 234	100 233	- 0	76 21	100 78	- 0	- 0	- 0	- 0	91 78	83 185	100 216	100 35
Massena Memorial Hospital, Massena, NY	- 0	91 11	100 3	100 3	100 1	- 0	100 1	98 49	19 50	- 0	95 21	95 19	97 75	99 103	85 13
Medina Memorial Hospital, Medina, NY	33 3	93 27	85 20	82 22	0 1	- 0	100 7	95 60	6 62	60 3	67 6	73 37	81 63	96 102	100 12
Mercy Hospital, Buffalo, NY	98 43	99 201	98 320	98 319	67 3	88 26	100 112	84 19	20 19	80 1	- 0	96 69	90 244	100 334	95 37
Mercy Medical Center, Rockville Centre, NY	80 5	100 59	96 25	100 24	- 0	- 0	100 2	100 53	8 56	45 21	- 0	97 78	92 160	99 226	100 18
Metropolitan Hospital Center, New York, NY	100 6	97 39	100 18	100 17	- 0	- 0	100 3	100 1	82 2	- 0	- 0	100 49	83 128	99 142	100 9
Monroe Community Hospital, Rochester, NY	- 0	- 0	- 0	- 0	- 0	- 0	- 0								
Montefiore Medical Center, Bronx, NY	71 63	95 281	96 373	96 366	- 0	84 51	99 116	100 2	10 2	- 0	- 0	81 251	86 544	98 679	100 103
Moses-Ludington Hospital, Ticonderoga, NY	- 0	100 1	- 0	- 0	- 0	- 0	- 0	- 0	- 0	- 0	-	100 2	75 4	88 8	100 1
Mount Sinai Hospital, New York, NY	89 57	97 188	98 327	96 319	- 0	100 11	100 80	97 61	12 64	120 28	- 0	95 215	81 441	97 555	97 72
Mount St Mary's Hospital and Health Center, Lewiston, NY	100 13	100 100	100 62	100 69	33 3	- 0	100 12	92 13	15 13	- 0	- 0	100 55	89 190	100 241	100 15
Mount Vernon Hospital, Mount Vernon, NY	80 5	89 45	96 26	80 25	0 1	- 0	100 4	100 5	58 5	- 0	0 1	92 38	88 84	88 122	100 27
Nassau University Medical Center, East Meadow, NY	100 10	100 50	100 31	100 33	- 0	- 0	100 6	100 4	22 4	- 0	- 0	100 86	97 198	100 245	100 54
Nathan Littauer Hospital, Gloversville, NY	100 1	95 43	92 24	100 28	- 0	- 0	75 4	94 54	8 56	56 10	- 0	100 36	96 78	87 93	71 17
New York Community Hospital of Brooklyn, Brooklyn, NY	100 5	99 85	100 42	100 49	100 1	- 0	100 1	- 0	- 0	- 0	- 0	100 38	95 233	100 266	100 12
New York Downtown Hospital, New York, NY	100 2	97 36	100 8	100 7	- 0	- 0	100 1	92 38	14 35	120 3	0 1	95 39	97 119	100 133	100 23
New York Hospital Medical Center of Queens, Flushing, NY	88 60	98 320	95 292	97 289	100 1	100 39	100 71	- 0	- 0	- 0	- 0	88 107	93 257	100 337	100 34
New York Methodist Hospital, Brooklyn, NY	91 66	99 203	99 241	98 244	- 0	78 32	100 65	- 0	- 0	- 0	- 0	93 148	90 277	100 340	100 32
New York Westchester Square Medical Center, Bronx, NY	100 3	100 43	100 14	95 20	- 0	- 0	100 1	100 32	13 32	353 1	40 5	100 54	80 159	100 257	100 33
New York-Presbyterian Hospital, New York, NY	94 158	99 353	98 744	95 718	- 0	96 46	99 152	- 0	- 0	- 0	- 0	87 452	70 883	97 1062	97 87
Newark-Wayne Community Hospital, Newark, NY	100 3	98 43	94 32	100 30	- 0	- 0	100 5	94 145	10 147	93 18	- 0	96 26	87 78	99 108	100 13
Niagara Falls Memorial Medical Center, Niagara Falls, NY	100 2	100 49	100 27	100 30	- 0	- 0	100 6	96 46	6 47	68 1	42 12	100 49	93 121	98 145	100 35
Nicholas H Noyes Memorial Hospital, Dansville, NY	67 3	92 13	88 7	88 8	- 0	- 0	100 2	89 45	5 45	77 3	50 8	71 51	82 115	91 148	83 18
North Central Bronx Hospital, Bronx, NY	100 7	97 39	100 20	100 19	- 0	- 0	100 7	100 8	6 7	67 4	- 0	98 61	99 131	100 139	100 40
North General Hospital, New York, NY	-	-	-	-	-	-	-	-	-	-	-	-	-	-	-
North Shore University Hospital, Manhasset, NY	98 53	99 109	100 311	100 294	- 0	90 21	100 67	100 4	16 4	48 1	- 0	99 131	98 313	100 398	100 26
Northern Dutchess Hospital, Rhinebeck, NY	100 4	89 28	100 16	100 17	- 0	- 0	100 1	100 17	14 19	70 4	- 0	95 22	80 51	100 77	43 7
Northern Westchester Hospital, Mount Kisco, NY	100 4	100 26	100 12	100 16	0 1	- 0	- 0	100 108	5 112	72 12	100 4	98 49	95 156	100 198	92 12
Northport VA Medical Center, Northport, NY	- 0	- 0	- 0	- 0	- 0	- 0	- 0	- 0	- 0	- 0	-	97 39	98 115	100 131	100 15
NY Eye and Ear Infirmary, New York, NY	- 0	- 0	- 0	- 0	- 0	- 0	- 0	- 0	- 0	- 0	- 0	- 0	- 0	- 0	- 0
Nyack Hospital, Nyack, NY	100 11	99 67	100 41	100 39	- 0	- 0	100 1	100 57	6 58	53 17	- 0	96 80	90 176	99 249	100 14
NYU Hospitals Center, New York, NY	100 47	100 223	100 254	99 248	- 0	90 29	100 48	- 0	- 0	- 0	- 0	100 83	97 217	100 283	100 23
O'Connor Hospital, Delhi, NY	- 0	- 0	- 0	- 0	- 0	- 0	- 0	- 0	- 0	- 0	- 0	100 4	75 12	93 15	- 0
Olean General Hospital, Olean, NY	100 16	99 80	98 43	98 52	- 0	- 0	100 3	97 348	19 359	- 0	38 13	97 78	87 171	100 261	100 32
Oneida Healthcare Center, Oneida, NY	100 1	100 8	100 3	100 3	- 0	- 0	- 0	95 59	5 65	54 7	0 3	73 11	90 20	87 30	- 0
Orange Regional Medical Center, Goshen, NY	100 28	100 211	100 176	100 179	- 0	100 45	100 52	92 13	10 14	81 1	- 0	98 129	88 360	99 485	100 52
Oswego Hospital, Oswego, NY	83 6	94 63	96 23	94 31	- 0	- 0	100 8	85 66	17 69	80 19	- 0	81 37	81 99	94 160	85 20
Our Lady of Lourdes Memorial Hospital, Binghamton, NY	100 10	100 101	100 73	99 76	0 1	- 0	100 7	100 42	6 41	54 15	0 1	98 55	87 163	98 226	100 24
Peconic Bay Medical Center, Riverhead, NY	80 5	98 49	100 25	100 29	- 0	- 0	100 3	100 121	10 126	50 18	100 2	98 54	98 177	96 234	100 13
Peninsula Hospital Center, Far Rockaway, NY	100 1	100 14	75 4	100 6	0 2	- 0	- 0	100 5	21 5	- 0	50 2	97 61	96 114	99 157	100 26
Phelps Memorial Hospital Assn, Sleepy Hollow, NY	100 8	100 57	100 47	100 46	100 2	- 0	100 5	100 10	12 10	130 1	- 0	100 39	94 98	99 152	100 10
Plainview Hospital, Plainview, NY	100 12	98 109	95 62	100 61	- 0	- 0	100 3	98 110	9 112	58 32	- 0	98 51	95 192	100 270	100 12
Putnam Hospital Center, Carmel, NY	83 6	98 43	100 25	100 24	- 0	- 0	100 3	96 67	12 67	198 3	43 14	90 62	91 159	99 225	100 20
Queens Hospital Center, Jamaica, NY	80 5	100 44	100 13	100 9	- 0	- 0	- 0	97 89	11 92	66 23	- 0	94 100	96 246	100 269	94 35
Richmond University Medical Center, Staten Island, NY	88 8	98 90	100 34	95 37	- 0	- 0	100 16	100 19	25 20	71 7	- 0	89 57	99 105	99 158	100 31
River Hospital, Alexandria Bay, NY	- 0	- 0	- 0	- 0	- 0	- 0	- 0	- 0	- 0	- 0	- 0	- 0	- 0	0 1	- 0
Rochester General Hospital, Rochester, NY	100 42	98 213	100 308	100 309	- 0	76 33	100 113	82 11	27 11	- 0	- 0	97 109	92 259	99 315	100 48
Rome Memorial Hospital, Rome, NY	100 6	94 36	95 20	95 19	- 0	- 0	100 2	98 50	6 52	70 4	100 1	93 55	89 126	96 204	91 23
Saint Anthony Community Hospital, Warwick, NY	100 4	100 23	100 12	100 11	- 0	- 0	100 2	95 21	5 19	332 1	- 0	95 21	100 73	99 92	100 11
Saint Barnabas Hospital, Bronx, NY	88 8	98 66	100 34	94 34	- 0	- 0	100 9	- 0	- 0	- 0	- 0	97 175	93 324	100 354	99 123
Saint Catherine of Siena Hospital, Smithtown, NY	79 14	97 120	96 92	98 97	- 0	62 37	100 18	86 22	14 24	137 2	- 0	95 58	99 195	95 326	100 11

NOTE: The first number in each column (boldface) is the score, the second number is the number of patients; Please refer to the main entry for footnotes; (a) 100-299

MEASURES: **Heart Attack Care:** 1. ACE Inhibitor or ARB for LVSD; 2. Aspirin at Arrival; 3. Aspirin at Discharge; 4. Beta Blocker at Discharge; 5. Fibrinolytic Medication Timing; 6. PCI Within 90 Minutes of Arrival; 7. Smoking Cessation Advice; **Chest Pain/Possible Heart Attack Care:** 8. Aspirin at Arrival; 9. Median Time to ECG (minutes); 10. Median Time to Transfer (minutes); 11. Fibrinolytic Medication Timing; **Heart Failure Care:** 12. ACE Inhibitor or ARB for LVSD; 13. Discharge Instructions; 14. Evaluation of LVS Function; 15. Smoking Cessation Advice

Hospital	Heart Attack Care 1	2	3	4	5	6	7	Chest Pain/Possible Heart Attack Care 8	9	10	11	Heart Failure Care 12	13	14	15
Saint Charles Hospital, Port Jefferson, NY	100 1	100 21	100 7	100 8	- 0	- 0	100 1	100 10	9 11	80 5	- 0	100 16	100 67	99 80	100 10
Saint Elizabeth Medical Center, Utica, NY	92 107	99 194	99 316	98 309	- 0	85 65	100 125	- 0	- 0	- 0	- 0	84 262	88 465	96 607	99 89
Saint Francis Hospital, Poughkeepsie, NY	100 1	100 25	100 17	100 15	- 0	- 0	100 6	100 10	16 10	48 5	- 0	100 20	100 42	100 79	100 15
Saint Francis Hospital - Roslyn, Roslyn, NY	96 79	98 132	99 337	99 342	- 0	89 9	100 73	- 0	- 0	- 0	- 0	90 146	86 310	100 357	100 30
Saint James Mercy Hospital, Hornell, NY	- 0	93 15	91 11	100 12	- 0	- 0	100 2	100 86	9 88	72 2	17 6	100 2	95 22	93 29	100 2
Saint John's Episcopal Hospital at South Shore, Far Rockaway, NY	100 6	100 40	100 23	100 22	- 0	- 0	100 1	100 12	10 12	- 0	- 0	92 61	100 110	96 186	100 39
Saint John's Riverside Hospital, Yonkers, NY	100 2	96 53	91 23	92 24	0 1	- 0	100 1	98 41	14 41	152 8	50 4	93 70	86 191	93 260	74 19
Saint Joseph Hospital, Bethpage, NY	50 2	100 47	100 16	100 17	0 1	- 0	100 1	99 138	7 139	45 51	100 6	100 34	97 200	100 251	100 16
Saint Joseph's Hospital, Elmira, NY	100 5	95 19	100 15	100 17	- 0	- 0	100 4	88 17	13 18	42 3	- 0	96 45	94 69	100 93	100 20
Saint Joseph's Hospital Health Center, Syracuse, NY	81 114	99 507	99 945	98 913	- 0	95 126	100 397	- 0	174 1	- 0	- 0	87 254	89 561	98 697	99 163
Saint Joseph's Medical Center, Yonkers, NY	100 5	92 37	84 19	90 20	- 0	- 0	100 4	97 32	12 35	115 6	- 0	92 51	91 135	100 200	100 26
Saint Luke's Cornwall Hospital, Newburgh, NY	100 28	99 190	99 168	100 164	- 0	90 30	100 45	96 54	1 55	- 0	- 0	93 119	80 337	100 429	100 50
Saint Luke's Roosevelt Hospital, New York, NY	95 88	99 312	98 294	96 290	- 0	70 46	100 98	- 0	- 0	- 0	- 0	94 166	96 282	97 324	100 70
Saint Mary's Hospital at Amsterdam, Amsterdam, NY	100 6	100 57	100 30	100 39	- 0	- 0	100 7	90 70	11 68	66 22	- 0	100 53	92 195	100 244	100 30
Saint Peter's Hospital, Albany, NY	99 85	100 383	99 635	99 646	- 0	81 48	100 180	- 0	- 0	- 0	- 0	95 132	92 399	97 490	100 61
Samaritan Hospital, Troy, NY	80 5	100 51	94 33	100 38	- 0	- 0	100 8	94 34	14 36	86 13	- 0	97 58	80 143	99 183	100 29
Samaritan Medical Center, Watertown, NY	100 2	95 43	96 23	95 21	0 1	- 0	100 2	94 101	6 107	130 5	44 16	96 28	81 188	98 216	100 23
Saratoga Hospital, Saratoga Springs, NY	80 10	100 62	95 37	98 45	50 2	- 0	100 7	96 27	8 27	199 2	36 14	98 43	95 239	100 280	100 40
Schuyler Hospital, Montour Falls, NY	100 1	100 4	100 3	75 4	- 0	- 0	- 0	-	-	-	-	80 5	100 18	100 33	100 2
Seton Health System-St Mary's Campus, Troy, NY	100 3	100 36	92 25	100 25	- 0	- 0	100 8	- 0	- 0	- 0	- 0	97 32	90 139	98 172	100 25
Sheehan Memorial Hospital, Buffalo, NY	- 0	- 0	- 0	- 0	- 0	- 0	- 0	- 0	- 0	- 0	- 0	- 0	- 0	- 0	- 0
Sisters of Charity Hospital, Buffalo, NY	93 15	97 146	95 79	99 84	100 1	- 0	100 11	100 61	14 64	108 5	67 3	92 118	77 393	100 516	97 61
Soldiers and Sailors Memorial Hospital of Yates, Penn Yan, NY	100 1	100 11	100 6	100 6	- 0	- 0	- 0	91 44	12 44	- 0	75 4	100 7	97 29	88 34	100 2
Sound Shore Medical Center of Westchester, New Rochelle, NY	100 12	100 108	98 62	99 69	29 7	- 0	100 5	98 54	18 55	- 0	67 9	97 87	98 177	99 291	100 30
South Nassau Communities Hospital, Oceanside, NY	89 38	96 313	96 262	97 263	- 0	92 40	100 59	92 13	5 12	- 0	- 0	93 179	98 382	99 502	100 34
Southampton Hospital, Southampton, NY	100 1	100 12	100 6	100 7	- 0	- 0	- 0	95 65	17 65	75 7	80 10	100 20	99 88	99 113	100 14
Southside Hospital, Bay Shore, NY	100 19	100 187	100 157	100 155	0 1	93 41	100 50	100 8	11 9	- 0	- 0	100 90	98 228	100 287	100 47
Staten Island University Hospital, Staten Island, NY	100 42	100 260	100 280	100 249	- 0	98 45	100 71	100 1	11 1	- 0	- 0	100 95	98 241	100 301	100 35
Strong Memorial Hospital, Rochester, NY	99 207	100 350	100 684	100 663	- 0	96 77	100 226	- 0	- 0	- 0	- 0	100 232	98 647	99 738	99 124
Sunnyview Hospital and Rehabilitation Center, Schenectady, NY	- 0	- 0	- 0	- 0	- 0	- 0	- 0	- 0	- 0	- 0	- 0	- 0	- 0	- 0	- 0
Syracuse VA Medical Center, Syracuse, NY	100 7	100 37	100 24	95 22	- 0	0 2	100 8	-	-	-	-	100 47	93 152	99 167	100 25
TLC Health Network, Gowanda, NY	100 1	94 16	88 8	100 9	- 0	- 0	- 0	83 82	10 79	315 1	56 9	72 18	90 42	88 72	89 9
United Health Services Hospitals, Johnson City, NY	97 113	99 334	100 463	99 473	- 0	85 60	100 155	- 0	- 0	- 0	- 0	95 141	87 343	99 451	100 51
United Memorial Medical Center, Batavia, NY	80 5	92 26	93 15	100 16	- 0	- 0	- 0	99 134	13 139	127 7	38 13	94 36	91 114	99 158	68 19
Unity Hospital of Rochester, Rochester, NY	100 39	97 242	99 202	100 207	- 0	94 47	100 55	96 23	12 24	- 0	- 0	98 87	97 253	100 322	100 35
University Hospital - Stony Brook, Stony Brook, NY	96 92	100 224	98 532	98 523	- 0	86 57	100 149	- 0	- 0	- 0	- 0	89 107	91 213	99 275	100 50
University Hospital of Brooklyn - Downstate, Brooklyn, NY	99 81	100 196	99 237	96 239	- 0	95 37	97 67	93 15	28 16	- 0	- 0	95 165	94 282	98 292	92 36
University Hospital S U N Y Health Science Center, Syracuse, NY	98 53	100 91	99 183	99 179	- 0	88 24	100 83	- 0	- 0	- 0	- 0	96 100	85 212	100 266	100 66
Upstate New York VA Healthcare System, Buffalo, NY	71 14	100 46	100 46	100 45	0 1	83 6	100 15	- 0	- 0	- 0	- 0	82 91	95 154	100 184	100 27
VA Hudson Valley Healthcare System, Montrose, NY	- 0	- 0	- 0	- 0	- 0	- 0	- 0	- 0	- 0	- 0	- 0	100 5	100 21	100 26	- 0
VA New York Harbor Healthcare System, New York, NY	96 23	100 86	99 117	99 107	75 4	60 5	100 31	- 0	- 0	- 0	- 0	93 167	98 353	100 364	98 61
Vassar Brothers Medical Center, Poughkeepsie, NY	100 62	100 292	100 378	100 394	0 1	90 67	100 121	- 0	- 0	- 0	- 0	96 176	98 466	100 632	100 78
Westchester Medical Center, Valhalla, NY	100 73	100 57	99 311	99 305	- 0	94 17	99 81	- 0	- 0	- 0	- 0	99 135	91 257	100 293	100 47
Westfield Memorial Hospital, Westfield, NY	- 0	- 0	- 0	- 0	- 0	- 0	- 0	99 128	5 130	- 0	- 0	- 0	- 0	100 1	- 0
White Plains Hospital Center, White Plains, NY	100 16	96 81	100 60	95 63	0 1	82 11	100 12	97 70	11 71	98 13	42 12	93 84	90 208	100 277	96 25
Winifred Masterson Burke Rehab Hospital, White Plains, NY	- 0	- 0	- 0	- 0	- 0	- 0	- 0	- 0	- 0	- 0	- 0	- 0	- 0	- 0	- 0
Winthrop-University Hospital, Mineola, NY	98 96	97 282	99 387	100 378	- 0	83 58	100 90	- 0	- 0	- 0	- 0	98 130	87 284	100 337	100 39
Woman's Christian Association, Jamestown, NY	100 15	98 94	100 59	98 66	- 0	- 0	100 7	96 77	12 79	121 2	67 3	98 65	81 224	100 273	100 39
Woodhull Medical and Mental Health Center, Brooklyn, NY	100 4	98 52	71 7	75 8	100 2	- 0	100 2	100 9	13 10	340 1	25 4	100 186	85 287	100 317	100 132
Wyckoff Heights Medical Center, Brooklyn, NY	70 10	96 106	95 62	93 60	- 0	- 0	86 7	100 31	32 30	179 1	25 4	97 132	97 249	100 297	100 44
Wyoming County Community Hospital, Warsaw, NY	100 1	92 12	80 5	100 5	100 1	- 0	- 0	99 95	13 100	- 0	38 8	97 29	81 57	100 85	82 17
NORTH CAROLINA															
Alamance Regional Medical Center, Burlington, NC	94 32	99 196	99 154	94 151	- 0	92 25	100 55	88 73	6 74	32 23	- 0	95 112	86 294	99 365	100 86
Albemarle Hospital Authority, Elizabeth City, NC	75 8	95 38	100 27	97 32	- 0	- 0	100 8	94 69	17 72	118 15	20 10	91 86	80 163	97 197	98 40
Alleghany County Memorial Hospital, Sparta, NC	- 0	83 12	89 9	100 9	- 0	- 0	- 0	91 11	46 12	- 0	0 4	100 3	100 27	91 33	50 2
Angel Medical Center, Franklin, NC	100 1	100 6	100 5	100 4	- 0	- 0	- 0	98 99	10 102	105 7	67 3	95 20	86 49	87 54	73 11
Anson Community Hospital, Wadesboro, NC	100 1	100 1	100 1	- 0	0 1	- 0	- 0	88 210	6 221	52 2	67 3	100 20	92 39	100 52	100 6
Ashe Memorial Hospital, Jefferson, NC	0 1	100 7	100 5	60 5	- 0	- 0	- 0	97 90	9 97	43 1	100 6	44 9	93 28	89 35	75 4
Asheville-Oteen VA Medical Center, Asheville, NC	90 10	100 46	95 41	98 41	- 0	25 4	100 16	- 0	- 0	- 0	- 0	86 51	85 96	98 117	100 25
Beaufort County Medical Center, Washington, NC	100 4	94 16	93 14	100 14	- 0	- 0	100 4	94 173	6 176	45 1	67 15	92 24	81 91	93 98	100 17
Bertie Memorial Hospital, Windsor, NC	- 0	- 0	- 0	- 0	- 0	- 0	- 0	- 0	- 0	- 0	- 0	100 14	87 30	100 39	100 5
Betsy Johnson Regional Hospital, Dunn, NC	100 1	79 14	86 7	100 7	- 0	- 0	- 0	91 261	9 275	61 1	33 6	100 44	63 150	93 201	96 26
Blowing Rock Hospital, Blowing Rock, NC	- 0	- 0	- 0	- 0	- 0	- 0	- 0	- 0	- 0	- 0	- 0	- 0	- 0	- 0	- 0
Brunswick Community Hospital, Supply, NC	100 1	100 12	3 100	100 3	- 0	- 0	- 0	97 87	3 86	32 15	100 1	100 4	98 92	100 117	100 26
C J Harris Community Hospital, Sylva, NC	- 0	100 8	100 2	100 1	- 0	- 0	- 0	97 34	10 33	103 5	- 0	98 42	78 73	97 87	100 15
Caldwell Memorial Hospital, Lenoir, NC	0 1	92 25	92 12	100 12	- 0	- 0	100 5	96 54	8 56	35 13	- 0	81 31	65 95	99 117	95 21
Cape Fear Valley Medical Center, Fayetteville, NC	96 102	99 499	100 542	97 517	- 0	84 92	100 235	92 63	18 69	44 1	- 0	97 396	91 899	100 1036	100 220

NOTE: The first number in each column (boldface) is the score, the second number is the number of patients; Please refer to the main entry for footnotes; (a) 100-299

MEASURES: **Heart Attack Care:** 1. ACE Inhibitor or ARB for LVSD; 2. Aspirin at Arrival; 3. Aspirin at Discharge; 4. Beta Blocker at Discharge; 5. Fibrinolytic Medication Timing; 6. PCI Within 90 Minutes of Arrival; 7. Smoking Cessation Advice; **Chest Pain/Possible Heart Attack Care:** 8. Aspirin at Arrival; 9. Median Time to ECG (minutes); 10. Median Time to Transfer (minutes); 11. Fibrinolytic Medication Timing; **Heart Failure Care:** 12. ACE Inhibitor or ARB for LVSD; 13. Discharge Instructions; 14. Evaluation of LVS Function; 15. Smoking Cessation Advice

Hospital	Heart Attack Care							Chest Pain/Possible Heart Attack Care				Heart Failure Care			
	1	2	3	4	5	6	7	8	9	10	11	12	13	14	15
Cape Fear Valley-Bladen County Hospital, Elizabethtown, NC	- 0	- 0	- 0	- 0	- 0	- 0	- 0	- 0	- 0	- 0	- 0	100 10	80 15	88 26	75 4
Carolina East Medical Center, New Bern, NC	93 83	99 315	99 399	96 365	- 0	93 75	100 146	90 10	6 11	447 1	- 0	86 173	59 483	98 529	100 102
Carolinas Medical Center-Behavioral Health, Charlotte, NC	98 220	99 319	98 1058	99 1010	- 0	97 88	100 423	100 1	10 1	- 0	- 0	99 383	98 681	100 766	100 196
Carolinas Medical Center-Lincoln, Lincolnton, NC	100 2	100 16	100 3	100 5	- 0	- 0	100 1	96 89	2 89	35 28	- 0	100 28	99 101	100 120	100 23
Carolinas Medical Center-Mercy, Charlotte, NC	100 51	100 85	98 213	97 201	- 0	100 24	100 74	99 118	6 117	40 13	- 0	98 133	94 327	99 398	100 65
Carolinas Medical Center-Northeast, Concord, NC	99 105	98 439	99 483	100 479	- 0	95 85	99 184	75 4	14 4	- 0	- 0	94 233	88 559	100 635	100 130
Carolinas Medical Center-Union, Monroe, NC	100 6	100 70	100 40	100 42	- 0	- 0	100 10	96 147	9 145	41 43	- 0	98 133	98 323	100 356	100 68
Carolinas Medical Center-University, Charlotte, NC	100 7	100 29	100 19	100 19	- 0	- 0	100 8	100 106	9 106	42 22	- 0	100 77	97 150	98 169	100 46
Carteret General Hospital, Morehead City, NC	100 12	99 117	93 55	91 53	0 1	- 0	100 13	97 111	11 113	169 5	32 19	91 74	89 193	99 251	100 40
Catawba Valley Medical Center, Hickory, NC	100 15	98 95	100 73	97 70	- 0	50 4	100 32	90 48	11 48	79 15	- 0	91 46	84 107	99 141	100 36
Central Carolina Hospital, Sanford, NC	100 2	100 33	100 12	100 14	- 0	- 0	100 2	99 99	6 102	37 7	- 0	100 73	100 225	99 266	100 62
Charles A Cannon Jr Memorial Hospital, Linville, NC	- 0	- 0	- 0	- 0	- 0	- 0	- 0	- 0	- 0	- 0	- 0	100 5	100 52	93 76	100 10
Chatham Hospital, Siler City, NC	- 0	100 8	80 5	80 5	- 0	- 0	100 1	- 0	- 0	- 0	- 0	100 8	67 27	97 30	89 9
Cherokee Indian Hospital Authority, Cherokee, NC	- 0	- 0	- 0	- 0	- 0	- 0	- 0	- 0	- 0	- 0	- 0	100 3	50 4	80 5	- 0
Chowan Hospital, Edenton, NC	100 1	100 4	100 1	67 3	- 0	- 0	100 1	- 0	- 0	- 0	- 0	95 20	96 49	97 65	100 13
Cleveland Regional Medical Center, Shelby, NC	100 7	99 79	95 42	90 41	- 0	- 0	100 8	100 127	3 129	- 0	60 5	90 63	87 211	100 263	100 66
Columbus Regional Healthcare System, Whiteville, NC	100 1	88 8	100 6	100 6	- 0	- 0	- 0	95 118	11 123	63 7	29 7	83 30	91 121	96 157	100 21
Davie County Hospital, Mocksville, NC	- 0	- 0	- 0	- 0	- 0	- 0	- 0	- 0	- 0	- 0	- 0	- 0	100 4	17 6	- 0
Davis Regional Medical Center, Statesville, NC	100 1	100 8	100 4	100 5	- 0	- 0	100 2	100 40	3 40	24 7	67 3	100 31	100 159	100 180	100 71
Duke Health Raleigh Hospital, Raleigh, NC	100 6	100 71	100 63	100 62	- 0	100 3	100 14	95 20	16 18	49 5	- 0	100 64	98 134	99 158	100 30
Duke University Hospital, Durham, NC	100 127	99 338	100 622	100 583	50 2	94 79	100 237	- 0	- 0	- 0	- 0	98 362	98 776	100 853	100 135
Duplin General Hospital, Kenansville, NC	- 0	100 9	86 7	100 8	- 0	- 0	- 0	100 82	8 87	364 2	0 4	100 23	97 59	100 66	100 14
Durham Regional Hospital, Durham, NC	98 52	100 247	100 228	99 219	- 0	83 30	100 85	100 2	34 4	- 0	- 0	95 166	92 317	100 394	100 84
Durham VA Medical Center, Durham, NC	90 10	98 43	98 45	100 45	- 0	50 4	100 16	- 0	- 0	- 0	- 0	96 68	99 160	100 173	96 24
Fayetteville North Carolina VA Medical Center, Fayetteville, NC	- 0	- 0	- 0	- 0	- 0	- 0	- 0	- 0	- 0	- 0	- 0	98 47	100 116	100 118	100 31
Firsthealth Montgomery Memorial Hospital, Troy, NC	- 0	100 3	100 2	100 2	- 0	- 0	- 0	- 0	- 0	- 0	- 0	100 3	94 16	100 18	100 5
Firsthealth Moore Regional Hospital, Pinehurst, NC	96 94	99 309	100 467	97 451	- 0	95 38	100 163	100 3	10 6	- 0	- 0	94 221	82 511	99 583	100 101
Firsthealth Richmond Memorial Hospital, Rockingham, NC	-	-	-	-	-	-	-	-	-	-	-	-	-	-	-
Forsyth Memorial Hospital, Winston-Salem, NC	100 120	100 608	100 834	100 792	- 0	99 151	100 337	100 1	29 1	- 0	- 0	100 254	100 814	100 989	100 142
Franklin Regional Medical Center, Louisburg, NC	- 0	100 2	- 0	- 0	- 0	- 0	- 0	99 95	5 96	50 15	- 0	91 22	86 58	100 73	100 17
Frye Regional Medical Center, Hickory, NC	93 57	99 308	98 487	99 481	- 0	97 134	100 218	86 7	1 7	- 0	- 0	91 79	93 251	98 294	100 57
Gaston Memorial Hospital, Gastonia, NC	100 96	100 523	100 503	100 467	100 1	100 107	100 211	- 0	- 0	- 0	- 0	99 236	94 654	100 735	100 152
Grace Hospital, Morganton, NC	100 8	98 51	100 34	100 37	- 0	- 0	100 12	94 72	12 78	46 29	- 0	93 44	97 97	97 124	100 30
Granville Medical Center, Oxford, NC	- 0	94 17	100 11	100 10	- 0	- 0	100 1	100 79	6 86	29 3	- 0	91 35	99 99	98 122	100 17
Halifax Regional Medical Center, Roanoke Rapids, NC	83 6	90 52	91 22	100 24	- 0	- 0	100 2	95 186	6 194	57 1	75 12	90 91	90 263	97 303	100 61
Haywood Regional Medical Center, Clyde, NC	100 2	100 21	100 10	100 8	- 0	- 0	50 2	85 75	8 78	64 16	- 0	80 25	79 77	96 99	91 11
Heritage Hospital, Tarboro, NC	100 1	100 17	88 8	100 10	- 0	- 0	- 0	100 51	9 51	- 0	100 2	99 75	98 151	100 196	100 36
High Point Regional Hospital, High Point, NC	98 91	100 368	99 516	100 521	- 0	99 88	100 205	100 2	1 3	- 0	- 0	99 155	93 384	98 460	100 110
Highlands Cashiers Hospital, Highlands, NC	- 0	- 0	- 0	- 0	- 0	- 0	- 0	- 0	- 0	- 0	- 0	100 1	0 4	40 5	50 2
Hugh Chatham Memorial Hospital, Elkin, NC	100 7	100 63	98 45	94 47	- 0	- 0	100 10	99 152	5 157	46 4	60 5	95 21	85 142	100 175	100 30
Iredell Memorial Hospital, Statesville, NC	100 2	100 59	100 39	97 37	- 0	100 5	100 9	99 88	7 89	58 33	67 3	100 62	94 250	100 316	100 70
J Arthur Dosher Memorial Hospital, Southport, NC	-	-	-	-	-	-	-	92 72	17 73	- 0	- 0	-	-	-	-
Johnston Memorial Hospital, Smithfield, NC	100 2	97 109	88 33	94 33	25 4	- 0	100 8	92 257	13 268	80 12	75 4	67 85	86 253	100 310	100 54
Kings Mountain Hospital, Kings Mountain, NC	100 1	93 15	83 6	86 7	- 0	- 0	100 4	97 87	4 89	64 4	0 1	79 14	90 40	100 50	100 18
Lake Norman Regional Medical Center, Mooresville, NC	100 14	100 76	100 55	100 54	100 1	- 0	100 17	100 61	4 62	26 23	- 0	100 41	92 115	99 161	100 27
Lenoir Memorial Hospital, Kinston, NC	92 13	94 133	93 82	91 85	- 0	- 0	100 11	94 94	8 97	101 5	60 20	87 143	76 404	96 479	100 86
Lexington Memorial Hospital, Lexington, NC	83 6	94 50	79 29	97 30	- 0	- 0	100 4	97 64	9 65	46 21	- 0	95 37	98 117	98 142	100 30
Margaret R Pardee Memorial Hospital, Hendersonville, NC	100 6	100 58	97 32	97 32	- 0	- 0	100 5	99 89	8 92	55 35	- 0	96 67	73 144	98 195	100 25
Maria Parham Hospital, Henderson, NC	92 13	98 45	97 31	89 35	- 0	- 0	100 7	94 145	12 143	49 15	- 0	88 88	76 150	97 180	100 21
Martin General Hospital, Williamston, NC	100 3	95 20	88 16	94 17	- 0	- 0	100 5	95 40	8 39	168 4	33 3	92 36	85 82	97 108	100 21
The Mcdowell Hospital, Marion, NC	50 2	100 6	100 3	100 3	- 0	- 0	100 1	96 84	7 87	32 9	- 0	96 24	94 47	100 52	100 11
Medical Park Hospital, Winston-Salem, NC	- 0	- 0	- 0	- 0	- 0	- 0	- 0	- 0	- 0	- 0	- 0	- 0	- 0	- 0	- 0
Memorial Mission Hosp/Asheville Surgery Ctr, Asheville, NC	100 310	100 696	100 1297	100 1273	- 0	95 109	100 455	100 4	18 4	- 0	- 0	98 314	91 665	100 791	100 131
Morehead Memorial Hospital, Eden, NC	80 5	92 38	79 29	90 29	- 0	- 0	75 4	98 103	9 95	47 21	- 0	80 66	70 209	84 258	88 43
The Moses H Cone Memorial Hospital, Greensboro, NC	100 38	99 200	99 288	99 266	- 0	86 37	100 119	99 76	10 78	- 0	- 0	95 132	84 330	100 390	100 108
Murphy Medical Center, Murphy, NC	50 2	100 20	100 8	83 6	100 1	- 0	100 1	94 127	9 133	- 0	50 14	88 25	70 54	97 78	100 5
Nash General Hospital, Rocky Mount, NC	90 50	95 309	90 210	92 215	- 0	- 0	100 66	89 264	9 268	90 1	33 21	91 156	97 387	99 447	100 114
New Hanover Regional Medical Center, Wilmington, NC	84 55	99 160	100 283	97 275	0 1	85 39	97 107	100 1	4 1	- 0	- 0	95 198	79 542	97 652	94 134
North Carolina Baptist Hospital, Winston-Salem, NC	97 119	100 239	99 571	100 541	- 0	100 49	100 268	- 0	- 0	- 0	- 0	97 257	96 602	100 652	100 161
North Carolina Specialty Hospital, Durham, NC	- 0	- 0	- 0	- 0	- 0	- 0	- 0	- 0	- 0	- 0	- 0	- 0	- 0	- 0	- 0
Northern Hospital of Surry County, Mount Airy, NC	100 6	100 15	100 8	100 12	- 0	- 0	100 4	98 255	12 264	40 4	100 1	95 40	97 145	99 167	96 28
Onslow Memorial Hospital, Jacksonville, NC	- 0	87 23	87 15	87 15	- 0	- 0	100 2	87 173	13 172	363 1	44 16	98 55	82 166	99 202	100 40
The Outer Banks Hospital, Nags Head, NC	- 0	- 0	- 0	- 0	- 0	- 0	- 0	- 0	- 0	- 0	- 0	100 4	100 7	100 11	100 2
Park Ridge Hospital, Fletcher, NC	100 1	95 21	100 11	92 12	- 0	- 0	100 1	89 18	23 19	- 0	- 0	78 9	85 39	98 52	100 5
Pender Memorial Hospital, Burgaw, NC	- 0	- 0	- 0	- 0	- 0	- 0	- 0	- 0	- 0	- 0	- 0	100 3	100 11	92 13	83 6
Person Memorial Hospital, Roxboro, NC	- 0	100 7	100 4	33 3	- 0	- 0	- 0	92 132	7 139	32 15	- 0	86 21	96 71	99 88	86 7
Pitt County Memorial Hospital, Greenville, NC	95 276	98 400	98 1326	100 1293	- 0	92 39	100 581	- 0	- 0	- 0	- 0	94 537	80 941	99 1057	100 247

NOTE: The first number in each column (boldface) is the score, the second number is the number of patients; Please refer to the main entry for footnotes; (a) 100-299
MEASURES: **Heart Attack Care**: 1. ACE Inhibitor or ARB for LVSD; 2. Aspirin at Arrival; 3. Aspirin at Discharge; 4. Beta Blocker at Discharge; 5. Fibrinolytic Medication Timing; 6. PCI Within 90 Minutes of Arrival; 7. Smoking Cessation Advice; **Chest Pain/Possible Heart Attack Care**: 8. Aspirin at Arrival; 9. Median Time to ECG (minutes); 10. Median Time to Transfer (minutes); 11. Fibrinolytic Medication Timing; **Heart Failure Care**: 12. ACE Inhibitor or ARB for LVSD; 13. Discharge Instructions; 14. Evaluation of LVS Function; 15. Smoking Cessation Advice.

Hospital	Heart Attack Care							Chest Pain/Possible Heart Attack Care				Heart Failure Care			
	1	2	3	4	5	6	7	8	9	10	11	12	13	14	15
Presbyterian Hospital, Charlotte, NC	100 115	100 295	100 593	100 583	- 0	98 88	100 186	- 0	- 0	- 0	- 0	100 207	99 491	100 584	100 106
Presbyterian Hospital Huntersville, Huntersville, NC	100 4	100 22	100 10	100 9	- 0	- 0	- 0	99 87	6 91	32 25	- 0	100 36	97 97	100 110	100 12
Presbyterian Hospital Matthews, Matthews, NC	100 4	100 57	100 36	100 37	- 0	- 0	100 8	100 73	4 77	34 36	- 0	100 43	96 142	100 180	100 16
Presbyterian-Orthopaedic Hospital, Charlotte, NC	- 0	- 0	- 0	- 0	- 0	- 0	- 0	- 0	- 0	- 0	- 0	- 0	- 0	- 0	- 0
Pungo District Hospital, Belhaven, NC	- 0	- 0	- 0	- 0	- 0	- 0	- 0	-	-	-	-	100 7	96 26	100 24	100 5
Randolph Hospital, Asheboro, NC	100 6	97 59	88 32	100 36	- 0	- 0	100 7	94 178	8 185	58 40	- 0	81 59	66 219	97 284	100 59
Rex Hospital, Raleigh, NC	100 42	100 298	100 312	99 297	- 0	93 67	100 67	- 0	- 0	- 0	- 0	92 106	83 257	98 325	100 46
Roanoke Chowan Hospital, Ahoskie, NC	100 2	100 19	100 18	94 18	- 0	- 0	100 9	100 61	8 64	- 0	67 3	96 50	97 155	100 175	100 36
Rowan Regional Medical Center, Salisbury, NC	100 21	99 141	100 104	100 87	- 0	88 8	100 32	99 88	6 92	42 42	- 0	100 114	97 237	100 289	100 75
Rutherford Hospital, Rutherfordton, NC	100 3	97 35	100 17	100 22	- 0	- 0	100 5	95 165	12 168	73 18	15 13	89 37	90 126	100 168	100 32
Saint Lukes Hospital, Columbus, NC	- 0	- 0	- 0	- 0	- 0	- 0	- 0	- 0	- 0	- 0	- 0	100 7	95 21	90 49	60 5
Sampson Regional Medical Center, Clinton, NC	100 3	100 13	100 6	83 6	- 0	- 0	- 0	90 418	10 442	118 6	67 21	86 72	89 139	99 196	100 38
Sandhills Regional Medical Center, Hamlet, NC	100 4	97 36	95 22	95 22	- 0	- 0	100 10	83 12	11 12	67 1	- 0	97 78	97 174	99 188	100 69
Scotland Memorial Hospital, Laurinburg, NC	100 9	97 72	100 41	100 39	- 0	- 0	100 13	98 46	10 46	84 19	50 2	87 116	82 320	99 345	100 96
Southeastern Regional Medical Center, Lumberton, NC	92 26	97 207	98 171	99 171	- 0	60 10	100 84	83 36	23 35	185 4	17 6	95 155	85 525	100 572	100 138
Spruce Pine Community Hospital, Spruce Pine, NC	100 1	100 10	60 5	100 5	- 0	- 0	- 0	91 58	8 61	108 5	0 2	88 16	94 48	78 64	82 11
Stanly Regional Medical Center, Albemarle, NC	92 13	95 41	100 26	89 27	0 1	- 0	100 3	97 92	6 90	42 2	67 6	94 54	70 135	95 184	100 29
Stokes-Reynolds Memorial Hospital, Danbury, NC	- 0	- 0	- 0	- 0	- 0	- 0	- 0	-	-	-	-	100 1	75 4	33 3	100 2
Thomasville Medical Center, Thomasville, NC	100 6	100 32	100 15	100 19	- 0	- 0	100 5	100 52	4 52	38 5	67 3	100 32	97 90	100 101	100 19
Transylvania Regional Hospital, Brevard, NC	- 0	86 7	100 5	100 5	- 0	- 0	- 0	-	-	-	-	100 16	71 28	100 42	100 10
University of North Carolina Hospital, Chapel Hill, NC	98 42	100 165	99 236	100 219	- 0	93 29	100 84	- 0	- 0	- 0	- 0	99 118	91 242	100 272	100 65
Valdese General Hospital, Valdese, NC	67 3	100 16	100 8	100 7	- 0	- 0	100 2	91 35	9 37	27 15	- 0	79 19	91 54	99 81	100 24
W G (Bill) Hefner Salisbury VA Medical Center, Salisbury, NC	- 0	- 0	- 0	- 0	- 0	- 0	- 0	- 0	- 0	- 0	- 0	94 17	92 48	100 53	100 5
Wakemed - Cary Hospital, Cary, NC	100 2	100 62	100 35	100 34	- 0	- 0	100 6	97 31	6 32	31 5	- 0	93 57	82 209	100 265	100 51
Wakemed - Raleigh Campus, Raleigh, NC	95 234	100 530	99 1539	99 1432	- 0	100 105	100 622	97 32	2 33	- 0	- 0	98 123	83 278	100 328	100 86
Washington County Hospital, Plymouth, NC	100 2	100 3	100 3	100 3	- 0	- 0	- 0	100 25	5 28	139 3	100 2	100 19	84 31	92 39	70 10
Watauga Medical Center, Boone, NC	100 4	98 61	89 38	94 33	- 0	- 0	100 5	100 77	12 79	81 1	67 9	100 36	94 102	100 127	100 10
Wayne Memorial Hospital, Goldsboro, NC	100 12	100 50	100 28	100 35	- 0	- 0	100 5	99 295	7 304	46 1	71 34	96 176	90 389	99 456	99 98
Wilkes Regional Medical Center, North Wilkesboro, NC	- 0	93 14	100 8	100 6	- 0	- 0	100 1	99 284	6 291	31 2	75 4	97 32	92 86	99 117	100 18
Wilson Medical Center, Wilson, NC	91 11	94 63	95 37	94 34	- 0	- 0	100 5	97 96	15 88	415 4	67 9	87 94	94 222	96 275	100 65
Yadkin Valley Community Hospital, Yadkinville, NC	- 0	- 0	- 0	- 0	- 0	- 0	- 0	-	-	-	-	100 2	100 1	100 3	- 0
OHIO															
Adams County Regional Medical Center, Seaman, OH	100 1	- 0	100 1	100 1	- 0	- 0	- 0	-	-	-	-	83 6	53 19	100 26	100 8
Adena Regional Medical Center, Chillicothe, OH	96 118	98 347	98 442	98 453	- 0	74 47	100 175	99 118	6 121	51 3	- 0	93 134	84 271	99 344	98 62
Affinity Medical Center, Massillon, OH	92 12	98 82	98 85	96 90	- 0	85 27	100 35	100 8	4 8	- 0	- 0	94 50	87 119	100 174	100 24
Akron General Medical Center, Akron, OH	94 71	99 216	97 284	99 270	- 0	87 47	100 104	100 2	0 2	- 0	- 0	91 102	77 244	99 302	96 46
Allen Community Hospital, Oberlin, OH	- 0	- 0	100 1	- 0	- 0	- 0	- 0	-	-	-	-	100 4	100 16	100 18	100 4
Alliance Community Hospital, Alliance, OH	100 7	93 30	91 23	96 23	- 0	- 0	100 2	100 101	9 107	46 14	- 0	87 45	90 99	98 132	89 27
Amherst Hospital, Amherst, OH	- 0	- 0	- 0	- 0	- 0	- 0	- 0	84 121	10 131	29 0	- 0	100 4	50 8	83 12	100 1
Ashtabula County Medical Center, Ashtabula, OH	- 0	100 26	100 11	86 14	- 0	- 0	100 5	98 137	2 146	75 9	- 0	98 53	86 142	99 187	100 32
Atrium Medical Center, Franklin, OH	100 42	100 280	100 251	100 240	- 0	85 54	100 98	100 31	7 31	54 2	- 0	98 64	81 290	100 358	100 86
Aultman Hospital, Canton, OH	99 105	99 394	100 619	100 603	- 0	92 90	100 213	82 17	6 18	- 0	- 0	99 163	87 445	100 593	100 99
Barnesville Hospital Association, Barnesville, OH	100 5	100 19	93 14	94 17	- 0	- 0	100 1	- 0	- 0	- 0	- 0	95 20	97 74	99 90	100 10
Bay Park Community Hospital, Oregon, OH	- 0	100 20	100 14	100 14	- 0	- 0	100 2	100 46	4 46	70 4	- 0	100 25	100 100	100 139	100 21
Bellevue Hospital, Bellevue, OH	- 0	100 10	100 6	100 9	- 0	- 0	100 1	93 72	3 74	67 9	25 4	81 21	85 27	95 39	100 4
Belmont Community Hospital, Bellaire, OH	- 0	82 11	60 5	100 4	- 0	- 0	- 0	100 3	3 3	- 0	0 1	83 6	23 43	98 48	91 11
Berger Hospital, Circleville, OH	- 0	100 11	100 8	100 9	- 0	- 0	- 0	99 179	7 180	66 13	80 10	92 13	100 84	100 108	100 22
Bethesda North Hospital, Cincinnati, OH	97 87	98 357	100 471	99 433	- 0	97 75	100 153	94 48	5 52	193 1	0 1	97 251	96 601	100 742	100 101
Blanchard Valley Hospital, Findlay, OH	100 19	100 124	100 128	100 117	- 0	94 50	98 45	100 3	8 4	- 0	- 0	100 47	96 70	100 105	100 23
Bluffton Hospital, Bluffton, OH	- 0	100 1	0 1	0 1	- 0	- 0	- 0	96 24	11 26	54 3	- 0	- 0	- 0	100 2	- 0
Brown County Hospital, Georgetown, OH	- 0	100 4	100 2	100 2	- 0	- 0	0 1	99 87	6 94	- 0	- 0	100 16	87 39	100 62	92 12
Bucyrus Community Hospital, Bucyrus, OH	100 2	100 1	100 1	100 1	- 0	- 0	- 0	- 0	- 0	- 0	- 0	83 6	85 13	100 25	100 3
Butler County Medical Center, Hamilton, OH	- 0	- 0	- 0	- 0	- 0	- 0	- 0	-	-	-	-	- 0	- 0	- 0	- 0
Chillicothe VA Medical Center, Chillicothe, OH	- 0	- 0	- 0	- 0	- 0	- 0	- 0	-	-	-	-	96 23	94 99	99 105	92 38
Christ Hospital, Cincinnati, OH	100 101	100 196	100 509	100 486	- 0	100 33	100 200	- 0	- 0	- 0	- 0	99 396	99 826	100 996	100 194
Cincinnati VA Medical Center, Cincinnati, OH	100 7	100 52	100 37	100 34	- 0	100 1	100 18	- 0	- 0	- 0	- 0	99 93	95 191	100 207	100 64
Cleveland Clinic, Cleveland, OH	99 180	100 156	100 839	100 804	- 0	87 15	100 288	100 4	2 4	- 0	- 0	98 487	93 1009	100 1206	100 220
Cleveland-Wade Park VA Medical Center, Cleveland, OH	100 4	97 36	100 35	100 35	- 0	100 3	100 11	- 0	- 0	- 0	- 0	98 174	100 391	100 417	100 95
CMH Regional Health System, Wilmington, OH	100 4	100 18	100 12	100 13	- 0	- 0	100 1	98 97	10 110	102 21	0 1	100 40	100 130	99 160	100 25
Community Hospitals and Wellness Centers, Bryan, OH	77 13	100 52	99 72	97 68	- 0	69 16	100 25	96 46	6 48	57 3	- 0	92 52	96 92	100 115	100 7
Community Regional Medical Center, Lorain, OH	100 43	100 228	100 228	100 228	- 0	88 50	98 98	100 11	6 13	- 0	- 0	98 121	96 317	100 402	100 62
Coshocton County Memorial Hospital, Coshocton, OH	- 0	100 2	100 2	100 2	- 0	- 0	- 0	94 228	12 236	78 6	25 4	67 9	75 36	96 48	100 6
Crystal Clinic Orthopaedic Center, Akron, OH	- 0	- 0	- 0	- 0	- 0	- 0	- 0	- 0	- 0	- 0	- 0	- 0	- 0	- 0	- 0
Dayton VA Medical Center, Dayton, OH	100 1	100 21	100 20	100 19	- 0	- 0	100 9	- 0	- 0	- 0	- 0	96 70	89 150	100 174	94 49
Deaconess Hospital, Cincinnati, OH	- 0	100 4	100 2	100 2	- 0	- 0	100 1	100 3	1 3	- 0	- 0	83 18	12 33	87 39	40 10
Defiance Regional Medical Center, Defiance, OH	25 4	100 15	100 12	92 12	- 0	- 0	67 3	- 0	- 0	- 0	- 0	100 7	96 27	100 37	100 6
Diley Ridge Medical Center, Canal Winchester, OH	- 0	- 0	- 0	- 0	- 0	- 0	- 0	-	-	-	-	- 0	- 0	- 0	- 0

NOTE: The first number in each column (boldface) is the score, the second number is the number of patients; Please refer to the main entry for footnotes; (a) 100-299
MEASURES: **Heart Attack Care:** 1. ACE Inhibitor or ARB for LVSD; 2. Aspirin at Arrival; 3. Aspirin at Discharge; 4. Beta Blocker at Discharge; 5. Fibrinolytic Medication Timing; 6. PCI Within 90 Minutes of Arrival; 7. Smoking Cessation Advice; **Chest Pain/Possible Heart Attack Care:** 8. Aspirin at Arrival; 9. Median Time to ECG (minutes); 10. Median Time to Transfer (minutes); 11. Fibrinolytic Medication Timing; **Heart Failure Care:** 12. ACE Inhibitor or ARB for LVSD; 13. Discharge Instructions; 14. Evaluation of LVS Function; 15. Smoking Cessation Advice

Hospital	Heart Attack Care							Chest Pain/Possible Heart Attack Care				Heart Failure Care			
	1	2	3	4	5	6	7	8	9	10	11	12	13	14	15
Doctors Hospital, Columbus, OH	97 32	100 175	99 195	100 192	- 0	97 37	100 98	81 21	3 21	- 0	- 0	97 89	98 180	100 158	100 44
Doctors Hospital of Nelsonville, Nelsonville, OH	- 0	- 0	- 0	- 0	- 0	- 0	- 0	-	-	-	-	100 5	93 15	100 18	100 5
Dublin Methodist Hospital, Dublin, OH	100 1	100 4	100 2	100 2	- 0	- 0	- 0	91 120	9 123	80 18	- 0	100 7	100 35	98 46	100 6
Dunlap Memorial Hospital, Orrville, OH	- 0	- 0	- 0	- 0	- 0	- 0	- 0	-	-	-	-	100 4	47 15	50 18	100 1
East Liverpool City Hospital, East Liverpool, OH	100 2	85 13	86 7	86 7	- 0	- 0	- 0	85 124	20 126	77 28	0 2	96 48	95 162	95 193	90 41
East Ohio Regional Hospital, Martins Ferry, OH	75 4	82 51	95 20	95 21	- 0	- 0	100 1	94 47	14 52	54 12	- 0	90 39	72 137	100 204	100 23
Edwin Shaw Rehabilitation Institute, Cuyahoga Falls, OH	- 0	- 0	- 0	- 0	- 0	- 0	- 0	-	-	-	-	- 0	- 0	- 0	- 0
Emh Regional Medical Center, Elyria, OH	91 58	97 244	100 291	99 292	- 0	98 40	100 106	85 110	9 120	- 0	- 0	87 108	72 229	98 287	96 49
Euclid Hospital, Euclid, OH	100 2	97 29	100 23	100 21	- 0	- 0	100 11	98 84	5 91	55 11	- 0	98 84	91 222	100 309	100 84
Evendale Medical Center, Cincinnati, OH	- 0	- 0	- 0	- 0	- 0	- 0	- 0	-	-	-	-	- 0	- 0	- 0	- 0
Fairfield Medical Center, Lancaster, OH	98 53	99 243	97 252	100 240	- 0	81 52	99 93	97 33	11 37	86 1	- 0	98 92	99 298	100 362	100 73
Fairview Hospital, Cleveland, OH	96 28	99 225	98 269	97 268	- 0	92 49	100 87	98 47	7 48	- 0	- 0	86 200	95 578	93 805	100 109
Fayette County Memorial Hospital, Washington CH, OH	- 0	- 0	- 0	- 0	- 0	- 0	- 0	97 143	6 153	58 8	25 4	93 15	74 39	93 45	100 10
Firelands Regional Medical Center, Sandusky, OH	100 28	100 89	100 129	98 125	- 0	95 19	100 45	96 24	5 25	62 9	- 0	100 81	96 183	98 255	98 42
Fisher Titus Memorial Hospital, Norwalk, OH	100 4	100 12	100 6	100 8	- 0	- 0	100 1	95 74	6 76	74 25	- 0	87 39	90 80	99 109	100 13
Flower Hospital, Sylvania, OH	75 4	100 61	95 38	100 41	- 0	- 0	100 7	96 53	5 57	66 16	- 0	100 41	87 146	97 210	100 21
Fort Hamilton Hughes Memorial Hospital, Hamilton, OH	100 7	98 40	96 26	100 25	- 0	100 1	100 7	100 36	4 38	95 2	- 0	99 69	98 211	100 269	100 54
Fostoria Community Hospital, Fostoria, OH	100 1	100 14	100 6	89 9	- 0	- 0	- 0	-	-	-	-	100 8	97 29	100 32	100 9
Fulton County Health Center, Wauseon, OH	100 1	80 5	100 4	100 5	- 0	- 0	100 1	74 107	15 114	143 3	- 0	79 14	69 26	81 37	100 2
Galion Community Hospital, Galion, OH	- 0	83 6	50 4	100 4	- 0	- 0	- 0	-	-	-	-	78 9	92 13	95 21	75 4
Genesis Healthcare System, Zanesville, OH	98 63	98 281	99 388	99 379	- 0	91 58	99 149	100 6	5 6	- 0	- 0	90 100	96 331	100 392	100 64
Glenbeigh, Rock Creek, OH	- 0	- 0	- 0	- 0	- 0	- 0	- 0	- 0	- 0	- 0	- 0	-	-	-	-
Good Samaritan Hospital, Dayton, OH	95 74	100 324	98 493	99 474	- 0	91 66	99 175	100 6	9 7	- 0	- 0	92 100	91 248	100 290	100 54
Good Samaritan Hospital, Cincinnati, OH	98 49	99 221	100 372	100 364	- 0	98 43	100 160	100 1	36 1	- 0	- 0	93 202	94 472	100 555	100 127
Grady Memorial Hospital, Delaware, OH	100 1	100 17	100 5	100 7	- 0	- 0	- 0	99 123	4 133	58 10	50 2	94 35	98 95	98 115	100 15
Grandview Hospital & Medical Center, Dayton, OH	100 28	98 132	99 177	99 175	- 0	85 34	100 74	75 8	4 8	- 0	- 0	100 93	97 315	100 410	100 74
Grant Medical Center, Columbus, OH	100 41	100 179	100 306	99 306	- 0	93 42	100 138	100 1	10 1	- 0	- 0	99 129	100 266	100 306	100 76
Greene Memorial Hospital, Xenia, OH	100 3	100 29	94 16	94 18	- 0	- 0	100 1	98 56	6 58	85 21	- 0	88 32	98 127	100 157	100 25
Greenfield Area Medical Center, Greenfield, OH	- 0	- 0	- 0	- 0	- 0	- 0	- 0	- 0	- 0	- 0	- 0	-	-	-	-
H B Magruder Memorial Hospital, Port Clinton, OH	- 0	- 0	- 0	- 0	- 0	- 0	- 0	-	-	-	-	88 16	69 26	100 33	57 7
Hardin Memorial Hospital, Kenton, OH	100 1	- 0	- 0	100 1	- 0	- 0	- 0	-	-	-	-	88 8	100 29	100 42	100 7
Harrison Community Hospital, Cadiz, OH	- 0	- 0	- 0	- 0	- 0	- 0	- 0	-	-	-	-	50 2	67 3	90 10	100 3
Henry County Hospital, Napoleon, OH	100 1	100 1	100 1	100 1	- 0	- 0	- 0	-	-	-	-	86 7	92 25	92 39	100 2
Highland District Hospital, Hillsboro, OH	- 0	100 1	100 1	100 1	- 0	- 0	- 0	100 19	6 20	- 0	- 0	86 21	66 53	81 70	100 7
Hillcrest Hospital, Mayfield Heights, OH	100 68	100 250	100 311	100 306	- 0	92 49	100 81	92 48	0 52	- 0	- 0	99 167	86 398	99 598	100 51
Hocking Valley Community Hospital, Logan, OH	- 0	- 0	- 0	- 0	- 0	- 0	- 0	-	-	-	-	100 8	38 16	86 21	50 4
Holzer Medical Center, Gallipolis, OH	86 14	96 95	92 95	95 98	- 0	73 11	97 30	82 33	5 31	125 1	0 1	86 84	85 253	97 309	93 43
Holzer Medical Center Jackson, Jackson, OH	- 0	75 8	75 4	100 5	- 0	- 0	- 0	- 0	- 0	- 0	- 0	84 19	80 74	81 108	100 11
Huron Hospital, Cleveland, OH	- 0	100 13	100 7	100 9	- 0	- 0	100 5	94 63	10 62	68 8	100 1	98 97	99 192	100 223	100 76
Institute for Orthopedic Surgery, Lima, OH	- 0	- 0	- 0	- 0	- 0	- 0	- 0	-	-	-	-	- 0	- 0	- 0	- 0
Jewish Hospital, Cincinnati, OH	98 41	100 165	96 165	99 153	- 0	89 28	100 57	100 3	1 3	- 0	- 0	95 139	96 302	100 405	100 65
Joel Pomerene Memorial Hospital, Millersburg, OH	- 0	100 2	100 1	100 1	- 0	- 0	- 0	96 140	4 142	28 2	- 0	100 9	97 38	98 52	100 8
Joint Township District Memorial Hospital, Saint Marys, OH	91 11	96 24	100 18	100 20	- 0	- 0	100 1	94 136	7 150	53 5	- 0	94 48	79 79	99 121	100 13
Kettering Medical Center, Kettering, OH	99 86	100 260	99 372	99 365	- 0	92 60	100 100	67 3	11 3	- 0	- 0	99 195	95 387	100 500	100 61
Kettering Medical Center - Sycamore, Miamisburg, OH	100 2	100 22	100 15	100 15	- 0	- 0	100 4	99 97	6 99	44 25	- 0	100 24	98 96	100 127	100 15
Knox Community Hospital, Mount Vernon, OH	78 18	98 51	98 40	95 42	- 0	- 0	75 4	94 48	5 50	128 2	- 0	98 55	71 132	98 184	83 18
Lake Health, Concord, OH	100 51	98 259	99 271	100 280	- 0	90 50	98 97	94 48	6 49	79 2	- 0	91 119	85 371	98 511	99 82
Lakewood Hospital, Lakewood, OH	94 16	97 96	98 87	99 89	- 0	82 28	100 38	93 29	5 29	- 0	- 0	99 67	98 187	99 306	100 58
Licking Memorial Hospital, Newark, OH	100 4	100 40	91 33	100 32	- 0	- 0	100 10	95 64	3 65	76 3	50 4	97 73	92 188	99 239	100 58
Life Line Hospital, Wintersville, OH	- 0	- 0	- 0	- 0	- 0	- 0	- 0	-	-	-	-	- 0	- 0	- 0	- 0
Lima Memorial Health System, Lima, OH	100 29	100 136	100 232	99 210	0 3	100 14	100 81	67 3	4 4	- 0	- 0	98 63	92 158	100 191	100 26
Lodi Community Hospital, Lodi, OH	- 0	- 0	- 0	- 0	- 0	- 0	- 0	99 134	7 138	58 4	- 0	- 0	- 0	- 0	- 0
Lutheran Hospital, Cleveland, OH	- 0	100 17	100 9	100 5	- 0	- 0	100 1	91 44	4 48	56 2	- 0	92 38	98 84	99 108	100 23
Madison County Hospital, London, OH	0 1	100 4	100 1	100 1	- 0	- 0	- 0	97 115	4 117	187 2	20 5	100 15	74 57	85 67	93 15
Marietta Memorial Hospital, Marietta, OH	100 24	99 95	100 81	100 88	- 0	92 12	100 27	94 50	10 51	51 2	- 0	99 74	85 217	100 278	100 45
Marion General Hospital, Marion, OH	97 35	100 164	100 169	99 169	- 0	98 53	100 72	99 134	3 135	- 0	- 0	96 126	96 256	100 339	100 59
Mary Rutan Hospital, Bellefontaine, OH	100 10	100 46	100 38	97 39	- 0	- 0	100 4	97 126	6 132	40 35	100 3	96 28	83 47	96 70	100 9
Marymount Hospital, Garfield Heights, OH	100 5	100 62	100 37	100 38	- 0	- 0	100 6	96 134	7 137	55 33	- 0	95 178	92 439	99 623	97 98
McCullough-Hyde Memorial Hospital, Oxford, OH	100 1	100 10	100 2	50 2	- 0	- 0	- 0	100 64	3 65	82 7	100 2	94 34	99 70	99 113	100 8
Medcentral Health System, Mansfield, OH	96 50	98 266	94 377	97 397	- 0	79 39	100 165	91 55	7 63	122 4	- 0	92 86	100 254	98 330	98 60
Medcentral Health System Shelby Hospital, Shelby, OH	- 0	- 0	- 0	- 0	- 0	- 0	- 0	-	-	-	-	- 0	- 0	- 0	- 0
Medical Center at Elizabeth Place, Dayton, OH	- 0	- 0	- 0	- 0	- 0	- 0	- 0	-	-	-	-	100 1	67 3	75 4	0 1
Medical Center of Newark, Newark, OH	- 0	- 0	- 0	- 0	- 0	- 0	- 0	-	-	-	-	50 2	12 8	38 13	0 1
Medina Hospital, Medina, OH	100 5	85 34	74 19	84 19	- 0	- 0	100 4	91 123	2 122	68 25	- 0	82 51	87 163	99 225	91 22
Memorial Hospital, Fremont, OH	100 1	100 12	88 8	88 8	0 1	- 0	- 0	89 98	14 108	90 6	50 2	93 14	79 34	95 44	100 8
Memorial Hospital of Union County, Marysville, OH	- 0	100 5	100 4	100 4	0 1	- 0	- 0	96 196	4 205	47 12	33 3	94 16	100 37	100 51	100 8
Mercer County Joint Twp Community Hospital, Coldwater, OH	- 0	100 5	75 4	100 4	- 0	- 0	100 1	100 83	8 84	75 9	75 4	97 29	100 33	100 54	75 4

NOTE: The first number in each column (boldface) is the score, the second number is the number of patients; Please refer to the main entry for footnotes; (a) 100-299

MEASURES: **Heart Attack Care:** 1. ACE Inhibitor or ARB for LVSD; 2. Aspirin at Arrival; 3. Aspirin at Discharge; 4. Beta Blocker at Discharge; 5. Fibrinolytic Medication Timing; 6. PCI Within 90 Minutes of Arrival; 7. Smoking Cessation Advice; **Chest Pain/Possible Heart Attack Care:** 8. Aspirin at Arrival; 9. Median Time to ECG (minutes); 10. Median Time to Transfer (minutes); 11. Fibrinolytic Medication Timing; **Heart Failure Care:** 12. ACE Inhibitor or ARB for LVSD; 13. Discharge Instructions; 14. Evaluation of LVS Function; 15. Smoking Cessation Advice

Hospital	Heart Attack Care							Chest Pain/Possible Heart Attack Care				Heart Failure Care			
	1	2	3	4	5	6	7	8	9	10	11	12	13	14	15
Mercy Franciscan Hospital - Mt Airy, Cincinnati, OH	100 5	98 64	100 27	100 31	- 0	- 0	100 6	100 41	11 42	63 15	- 0	100 69	87 205	100 254	100 44
Mercy Franciscan Hospital Western Hills, Cincinnati, OH	100 8	99 71	100 34	100 38	- 0	- 0	100 9	96 132	8 139	60 24	0 1	100 47	96 160	98 212	97 35
Mercy Hospital Anderson, Cincinnati, OH	98 63	99 235	100 255	99 240	- 0	94 51	100 105	100 8	6 10	- 0	- 0	98 90	93 262	98 328	97 30
Mercy Hospital Clermont, Batavia, OH	100 3	100 47	100 23	100 19	- 0	- 0	100 4	96 106	11 114	128 29	- 0	100 32	95 76	100 90	100 25
Mercy Hospital Fairfield, Fairfield, OH	100 54	99 268	100 291	99 273	- 0	94 48	100 110	100 7	10 8	- 0	- 0	99 138	96 347	99 411	100 68
Mercy Hospital of Defiance, Defiance, OH	- 0	100 2	100 1	100 1	- 0	- 0	- 0	98 62	4 66	115 8	- 0	100 10	96 26	100 36	100 4
Mercy Hospital of Willard, Willard, OH	- 0	- 0	- 0	- 0	- 0	- 0	- 0	- 0	- 0	- 0	- 0	90 10	100 20	100 23	100 6
Mercy Medical Center, Canton, OH	90 61	96 317	97 352	98 350	- 0	94 70	100 130	100 21	7 21	- 0	- 0	98 146	86 333	100 431	97 76
Mercy Memorial Hospital, Urbana, OH	100 1	100 6	100 4	100 3	- 0	- 0	100 2					91 23	100 52	100 64	100 12
Mercy St Anne Hospital, Toledo, OH	100 3	95 37	96 23	100 21	- 0	- 0	100 5	100 71	21 75	69 11	- 0	91 47	97 157	99 195	98 43
Mercy St Charles Hospital, Oregon, OH	100 7	92 40	91 22	88 24	- 0	- 0	100 5	100 83	4 85	63 14	0 1	90 67	98 172	100 217	100 41
Mercy St Vincent Medical Center, Toledo, OH	97 149	99 331	100 645	100 632	- 0	93 82	100 283	85 13	5 13	173 1	- 0	97 324	100 565	100 657	100 190
Mercy Tiffin Hospital, Tiffin, OH	100 1	100 14	100 9	100 8	- 0	- 0	- 0	91 100	6 105	110 14	0 3	100 20	97 66	99 103	100 8
Metro Health Medical Center, Cleveland, OH	93 27	100 236	99 226	100 227	- 0	91 44	100 126	93 15	12 16	- 0	- 0	95 261	63 589	100 660	98 225
Miami Valley Hospital, Dayton, OH	92 59	100 263	100 321	99 318	- 0	92 60	100 149	90 20	12 21	- 0	- 0	95 106	85 253	100 317	100 84
Morrow County Hospital, Mount Gilead, OH	- 0	- 0	- 0	- 0	- 0	- 0	- 0	90 60	13 63	113 8	0 1	86 7	86 21	89 37	80 5
Mount Carmel Health, Columbus, OH	100 133	100 688	100 855	100 819	- 0	96 170	100 355	100 5	0 6	- 0	- 0	100 411	86 956	100 1208	100 194
Mount Carmel New Albany Surgical Hospital, New Albany, OH	- 0	- 0	- 0	- 0	- 0	- 0	- 0	- 0	- 0	- 0	- 0	- 0	- 0	- 0	- 0
Mount Carmel St Ann's Hospital, Westerville, OH	100 10	100 118	100 88	99 83	- 0	97 33	100 23	93 30	4 30	- 0	- 0	100 97	91 247	100 337	100 44
Northside Medical Center, Youngstown, OH	100 21	100 101	100 153	100 154	- 0	62 16	100 51	- 0	- 0	- 0	- 0	99 71	96 238	99 293	100 51
O'Bleness Memorial Hospital, Athens, OH	100 4	73 15	90 10	80 10	- 0	- 0	100 5	93 312	7 315	166 5	53 15	69 29	64 72	100 90	100 21
Ohio State University Hospitals, Columbus, OH	97 66	99 120	99 279	100 284	- 0	83 12	100 110	- 0	- 0	- 0	- 0	99 139	100 260	100 295	100 76
Ohio Valley Medical Center, Springfield, OH	- 0	- 0	- 0	- 0	- 0	- 0	- 0	- 0	- 0	- 0	- 0	- 0	- 0	- 0	- 0
Parma Community General Hospital, Parma, OH	93 72	98 303	99 313	96 305	- 0	93 61	99 85	95 43	2 43	- 0	- 0	87 208	81 418	99 625	91 46
Paulding County Hospital, Paulding, OH	- 0	100 2	100 1	100 1	- 0	- 0	- 0					100 1	67 12	94 16	100 1
Physician's Choice Hospital - Fremont, Fremont, OH	- 0	50 2	100 1	100 1	- 0	- 0	- 0					0 1	0 3	67 3	- 0
Pike Community Hospital, Waverly, OH	- 0	- 0	- 0	- 0	- 0	- 0	- 0					82 11	91 23	44 39	100 1
Riverside Methodist Hospital, Columbus, OH	97 125	98 296	99 581	98 572	- 0	98 87	100 209	100 2	2 2	- 0	- 0	98 252	100 487	100 648	100 100
Robinson Memorial Hospital, Ravenna, OH	93 15	96 81	98 55	98 56	- 0	- 0	100 14	98 115	7 117	50 40	- 0	94 78	100 267	99 336	100 52
Saint Elizabeth Boardman Health Center, Youngstown, OH	100 9	100 42	100 25	100 30	- 0	- 0	100 5	97 119	6 125	48 56	- 0	93 58	100 153	99 224	100 25
Saint Elizabeth Health Center, Youngstown, OH	97 79	100 274	100 490	100 487	- 0	95 62	99 190	97 63	6 64	- 0	- 0	100 85	100 221	100 301	100 55
Saint John Medical Center, Westlake, OH	100 20	100 214	100 190	100 194	- 0	100 44	100 70	97 36	5 38	- 0	- 0	90 40	100 143	100 206	100 17
Saint Joseph Health Center, Warren, OH	100 5	100 46	100 11	100 15	- 0	- 0	100 5	99 134	5 139	62 46	0 1	97 71	100 209	100 254	100 61
Saint Luke's Hospital, Maumee, OH	100 41	98 143	99 157	99 156	- 0	88 42	98 55	86 7	8 7	- 0	- 0	98 97	96 254	99 317	94 32
Saint Rita's Medical Center, Lima, OH	99 71	100 252	100 301	100 302	- 0	100 49	100 121	100 58	9 66	28 1	- 0	97 152	97 267	99 343	100 62
Saint Vincent Charity Medical Center, Cleveland, OH	93 14	98 66	100 66	97 67	- 0	90 10	100 28	97 159	8 159	31 1	- 0	95 118	94 236	100 287	99 86
Salem Community Hospital, Salem, OH	88 8	95 44	86 21	87 23	- 0	- 0	75 4	93 75	4 75	62 21	100 1	93 27	91 122	99 165	93 15
Samaritan Hospital - Peoples Hospital, Ashland, OH	100 2	100 15	100 9	100 9	- 0	- 0	100 2	96 159	6 172	70 19	67 3	100 23	97 69	99 85	100 6
Selby General Hospital, Marietta, OH	- 0	100 1	100 1	100 1	- 0	- 0	100 1	- 0				75 4	60 25	75 32	100 4
South Pointe Hospital, Warrensville Hgts, OH	100 7	100 52	100 28	100 36	- 0	- 0	100 7	98 398	7 411	60 29	- 0	99 137	99 301	100 399	100 98
Southeastern Ohio Regional Medical Center, Cambridge, OH	100 1	100 9	100 4	100 4	- 0	- 0	100 1	97 276	8 275	50 14	60 3	89 28	91 102	95 128	100 26
Southern Ohio Medical Center, Portsmouth, OH	97 39	100 203	100 181	100 189	- 0	98 46	100 86	97 104	5 113	- 0	- 0	99 123	100 334	100 419	100 71
Southwest General Health Center, Middleburg Hgts, OH	95 73	98 424	96 410	95 409	- 0	98 61	98 105	89 84	8 84	- 0	- 0	100 141	98 374	100 527	96 52
Springfield Regional Medical Center, Springfield, OH	96 71	97 310	98 348	97 339	- 0	88 49	100 126	67 9	10 11	- 0	- 0	97 180	92 261	100 477	99 88
Summa Barberton Hospital, Barberton, OH	100 16	100 88	100 83	100 79	- 0	100 17	100 25	100 25	6 25	35 2	- 0	100 54	100 260	100 337	100 64
Summa Health Systems Hospitals, Akron, OH	100 56	100 198	99 314	100 292	- 0	100 59	99 123	100 9	16 9	- 0	- 0	97 110	92 266	98 308	100 70
Summa Wadsworth-Rittman Hospital, Wadsworth, OH	- 0	100 9	100 7	100 5	- 0	- 0	- 0	99 99	4 102	44 16	- 0	100 22	93 69	99 87	100 5
Summa Western Reserve Hospital, Cuyahoga Falls, OH	100 1	100 15	90 10	100 7	- 0	- 0	100 3	92 40	11 43	48 11	- 0	100 27	84 80	94 95	100 6
Surgical Hospital at Southwoods, Youngstown, OH	- 0	- 0	- 0	- 0	- 0	- 0	- 0	- 0	- 0	- 0	- 0	- 0	- 0	- 0	- 0
Three Gables Surgery Center, Proctorville, OH	- 0	- 0	- 0	- 0	- 0	- 0	- 0	- 0	- 0	- 0	- 0	- 0	- 0	- 0	- 0
The Toledo Hospital, Toledo, OH	97 60	99 125	99 300	100 303	- 0	100 17	99 123	100 1	8 2	- 0	- 0	95 75	64 224	98 286	100 44
Trinity Medical Center East & TMC West, Steubenville, OH	93 89	96 251	98 317	97 324	- 0	73 33	100 105	100 3	12 4	- 0	- 0	84 205	92 406	99 579	100 85
Trumbull Memorial Hospital, Warren, OH	100 35	100 194	100 180	100 177	0 1	76 42	100 61	60 5	4 6	- 0	- 0	100 117	74 408	100 519	100 84
Twin City Hospital, Dennison, OH	- 0	- 0	- 0	- 0	- 0	- 0	- 0	- 0	- 0	- 0	- 0	100 3	21 14	93 15	50 2
UH Geauga Medical Center, Chardon, OH	100 13	100 73	100 59	100 66	- 0	71 7	100 23	100 68	2 68	40 10	- 0	100 49	100 123	100 175	100 22
UHHS Bedford Medical Center, Bedford, OH	100 1	94 35	96 23	100 28	- 0	- 0	100 6	96 94	4 103	42 18	- 0	100 59	97 146	100 200	100 39
UHHS Memorial Hospital of Geneva, Geneva, OH	- 0	100 4	100 1	100 1	- 0	- 0	- 0	100 222	5 235	49 21	- 0	100 19	96 24	100 44	100 26
UHHS Richmond Heights Hospital, Richmond Heights, OH	100 5	100 31	100 22	100 25	- 0	- 0	100 5	94 63	6 68	45 12	- 0	92 63	93 148	100 215	100 26
Union Hospital, Dover, OH	100 7	100 63	100 42	98 44	- 0	- 0	100 5	97 185	11 195	48 42	- 0	100 72	98 210	100 301	100 38
University Hospital, Cincinnati, OH	89 44	99 182	98 217	99 202	- 0	88 40	100 114	100 3	14 3	- 0	- 0	98 332	76 489	99 559	99 202
University Hospitals Conneaut Medical Center, Conneaut, OH	- 0	100 2	100 1	100 3	- 0	- 0	100 1	100 56	7 60	145 2	50 2	100 6	100 25	100 38	100 2
University Hospitals of Cleveland, Cleveland, OH	94 97	100 181	99 439	100 424	- 0	86 28	100 154	100 5	0 5	- 0	- 0	97 308	93 667	100 795	100 143
University of Toledo Medical Center, Toledo, OH	100 32	99 100	99 178	100 172	- 0	92 25	100 75	- 0	- 0	- 0	- 0	99 85	93 212	100 244	100 43
University Pointe Surgical Hospital, West Chester, OH	- 0	- 0	- 0	- 0	- 0	- 0	- 0	- 0	- 0	- 0	- 0	- 0	- 0	- 0	- 0
Upper Valley Medical Center, Troy, OH	100 13	99 85	98 59	98 58	- 0	- 0	83 6	96 124	8 126	65 57	100 1	100 44	92 173	100 221	100 15
Van Wert County Hospital, Van Wert, OH	0 1	100 10	100 5	100 6	- 0	- 0	100 6	95 172	13 176	85 5	29 7	93 14	79 28	98 53	86 7
Wayne Hospital, Greenville, OH	- 0	- 0	- 0	- 0	- 0	- 0	- 0	93 134	22 150	85 9	67 3	100 15	51 84	86 120	83 15

NOTE: The first number in each column (boldface) is the score, the second number is the number of patients; Please refer to the main entry for footnotes; (a) 100–299
MEASURES: **Heart Attack Care:** 1. ACE Inhibitor or ARB for LVSD; 2. Aspirin at Arrival; 3. Aspirin at Discharge; 4. Beta Blocker at Discharge; 5. Fibrinolytic Medication Timing; 6. PCI Within 90 Minutes of Arrival; 7. Smoking Cessation Advice; **Chest Pain/Possible Heart Attack Care:** 8. Aspirin at Arrival; 9. Median Time to ECG (minutes); 10. Median Time to Transfer (minutes); 11. Fibrinolytic Medication Timing; **Heart Failure Care:** 12. ACE Inhibitor or ARB for LVSD; 13. Discharge Instructions; 14. Evaluation of LVS Function; 15. Smoking Cessation Advice

Hospital	Heart Attack Care							Chest Pain/Possible Heart Attack Care				Heart Failure Care			
	1	2	3	4	5	6	7	8	9	10	11	12	13	14	15
West Chester Medical Center, West Chester, OH	100 2	100 15	100 10	89 9	100 1	- 0	100 3	98 46	11 47	65 9	0 2	98 40	95 64	99 102	100 10
Wilson Memorial Hospital, Sidney, OH	0 1	100 7	75 4	75 4	- 0	- 0	100 1	99 99	12 100	90 4	46 13	81 21	88 41	95 73	100 7
Wood County Hospital, Bowling Green, OH	100 3	100 11	100 7	100 7	- 0	- 0	- 0	96 91	10 94	72 8	33 3	96 23	83 58	90 73	100 10
The Woods at Parkside, Columbus, OH	- 0	- 0	- 0	- 0	- 0	- 0	- 0	- 0	- 0	- 0	- 0	- 0	- 0	- 0	- 0
Wooster Community Hospital, Wooster, OH	100 2	88 34	95 20	100 20	- 0	- 0	- 0	98 218	5 229	44 23	- 0	89 27	85 81	92 104	93 15
Wyandot Memorial Hospital, Upper Sandusky, OH	- 0	100 3	- 0	- 0	- 0	- 0	- 0	- 0	- -	- -	- -	100 6	78 23	96 26	100 1
PENNSYLVANIA															
Abington Memorial Hospital, Abington, PA	96 73	99 358	99 393	97 393	- 0	86 65	100 96	- 0	- 0	- 0	- 0	98 335	88 701	100 923	100 91
ACMH Hospital, Kittanning, PA	100 7	91 55	81 32	86 37	- 0	- 0	100 2	94 135	6 140	54 27	- 0	91 35	87 111	100 151	100 17
Advanced Surgical Hospital, Washington, PA	- 0	- 0	- 0	- 0	- 0	- 0	- 0	- 0	- 0	- 0	- 0	- 0	- 0	- 0	- 0
Albert Einstein Medical Center, Philadelphia, PA	97 68	99 243	99 301	98 292	100 1	95 42	100 114	100 2	8 2	- 0	- 0	93 142	96 221	99 305	100 96
Alle Kiski Medical Center, Natrona, PA	100 16	98 167	100 103	100 104	- 0	- 0	100 11	96 158	10 165	55 27	- 0	96 96	84 370	100 469	100 55
Allegheny General Hospital, Pittsburgh, PA	100 110	100 310	100 581	99 523	- 0	93 55	100 193	96 23	14 22	68 2	- 0	99 285	95 571	100 674	100 109
Altoona Regional Health System, Altoona, PA	86 141	98 362	97 522	97 515	- 0	90 70	100 172	- 0	- 0	- 0	- 0	88 165	89 402	99 542	100 57
Aria Health, Philadelphia, PA	100 63	99 460	100 465	99 451	0 1	88 52	100 172	82 17	7 18	- 0	- 0	96 333	94 765	100 953	100 201
Berwick Hospital Center, Berwick, PA	100 2	96 27	100 19	100 24	- 0	- 0	100 4	96 51	6 52	46 18	- 0	100 24	89 113	99 160	100 21
Bloomsburg Hospital, Bloomsburg, PA	100 3	100 16	80 10	80 10	- 0	- 0	0 1	92 101	0 106	65 33	- 0	85 26	87 67	89 91	75 8
Bradford Regional Medical Center, Bradford, PA	100 11	100 48	96 26	91 35	- 0	- 0	86 7	100 30	7 31	198 2	50 4	100 43	87 62	95 86	80 5
Brandywine Hospital, Coatesville, PA	90 10	98 137	93 122	95 121	- 0	93 29	98 56	100 5	4 5	50 1	- 0	81 70	94 157	100 231	100 36
Brookville Hospital, Brookville, PA	100 1	86 7	100 3	86 7	- 0	- 0	- 0	- -	- -	- -	- 0	100 17	83 53	97 63	100 6
Bucks County Specialty Hospital, Bensalem, PA	- 0	- 0	- 0	- 0	- 0	- 0	- 0	- 0	- 0	- 0	- 0	- 0	- 0	- 0	- 0
Butler Memorial Hospital, Butler, PA	100 62	100 201	100 261	100 246	- 0	93 30	100 99	- 0	- 0	- 0	- 0	99 121	97 304	100 387	100 49
Cancer Treatment Centers of America, Philadelphia, PA	- 0	100 1	100 1	100 1	- 0	- 0	- 0	- 0	- 0	- 0	- 0	100 1	100 1	100 1	- 0
Canonsburg General Hospital, Canonsburg, PA	100 4	95 41	93 15	92 13	- 0	- 0	100 2	99 83	12 86	83 10	- 0	92 40	65 105	99 152	100 15
Carlisle Regional Medical Center, Carlisle, PA	67 9	96 52	91 22	100 25	- 0	- 0	100 2	97 116	5 119	51 14	- 0	90 61	89 165	99 245	100 33
Chambersburg Hospital, Chambersburg, PA	96 70	98 292	98 329	97 338	- 0	85 46	99 102	90 31	12 34	- 0	- 0	94 95	88 314	97 394	97 61
Charles Cole Memorial Hospital, Coudersport, PA	100 2	92 12	100 10	100 8	- 0	- 0	100 2	92 39	6 42	91 9	0 1	100 12	87 47	87 70	100 6
Chester County Hospital, West Chester, PA	100 34	100 189	99 181	99 181	- 0	91 34	98 46	100 7	10 7	44 1	- 0	98 98	88 265	100 351	100 55
Chestnut Hill Hospital, Philadelphia, PA	100 8	100 40	91 23	95 22	- 0	- 0	100 3	90 59	16 62	64 28	100 1	99 99	97 171	97 296	100 29
Children's Hospital of Philadelphia, Philadelphia, PA	- -	- -	- -	- -	- -	- -	- -	- -	- -	- -	- -	- -	- -	- -	- -
Children's Hospital of Pittsburgh of UPMC, Pittsburgh, PA	- -	- -	- -	- -	- -	- -	- -	- -	- -	- -	- -	- -	- -	- -	- -
Clarion Hospital, Clarion, PA	100 6	90 20	92 13	100 13	100 1	- 0	100 1	95 63	21 65	71 4	0 3	73 30	67 86	88 112	50 6
Clearfield Hospital, Clearfield, PA	100 2	100 17	100 7	86 7	- 0	- 0	- 0	93 128	2 138	58 8	25 4	89 37	67 114	99 159	100 17
Coatesville VA Medical Center, Coatesville, PA	- 0	- 0	- 0	- 0	- 0	- 0	- 0	- 0	- 0	- 0	- 0	- 0	- 0	- 0	- 0
Community Medical Center, Scranton, PA	96 50	99 171	99 223	100 230	- 0	84 31	100 83	- 0	- 0	- 0	- 0	90 110	90 225	99 304	100 37
Conemaugh Valley Memorial Hospital, Johnstown, PA	81 136	98 452	99 590	96 588	- 0	89 64	98 170	80 5	13 5	- 0	- 0	83 222	78 614	96 803	100 94
Coordinated Health Orthopedic Hospital, Bethlehem, PA	- 0	- 0	- 0	- 0	- 0	- 0	- 0	- 0	- 0	- 0	- 0	- 0	- 0	- 0	- 0
Corry Memorial Hospital, Corry, PA	- 0	100 1	- 0	- 0	- 0	- 0	- 0	- 0	- 0	- 0	- 0	87 15	95 58	86 76	100 7
Crozer Chester Medical Center, Upland, PA	98 65	99 275	99 354	99 351	0 2	94 31	100 114	80 5	16 6	300 1	- 0	90 345	97 801	98 927	100 203
Delaware County Memorial Hospital, Drexel Hill, PA	100 2	98 65	100 34	100 32	- 0	- 0	100 8	95 44	8 45	72 12	- 0	95 87	97 279	99 342	100 50
Doylestown Hospital, Doylestown, PA	100 37	100 240	100 301	100 281	- 0	94 53	100 62	- 0	- 0	- 0	- 0	98 133	92 357	100 462	97 31
Dubois Regional Medical Center, Dubois, PA	100 66	100 126	99 323	100 321	- 0	87 23	100 112	- 0	- 0	- 0	- 0	94 89	87 226	100 263	100 36
Eagleville Hospital, Eagleville, PA	- 0	- 0	- 0	- 0	- 0	- 0	- 0	- 0	- 0	- 0	- 0	- 0	- 0	- 0	- 0
Easton Hospital, Easton, PA	100 48	99 171	99 202	99 204	- 0	100 40	100 80	100 1	6 1	- 0	- 0	98 126	92 312	100 428	100 49
Edgewood Surgical Hospital, Transfer, PA	- 0	- 0	- 0	- 0	- 0	- 0	- 0	- 0	- 0	- 0	- 0	- 0	- 0	- 0	- 0
Elk Regional Health Center, Saint Marys, PA	67 3	79 24	50 12	87 15	- 0	- 0	100 2	93 90	4 91	57 10	38 8	86 44	58 122	90 178	100 17
Ellwood City Hospital, Ellwood City, PA	100 1	100 14	100 6	67 6	- 0	- 0	- 0	97 68	15 72	86 22	- 0	98 42	98 99	100 130	100 14
Ephrata Community Hospital, Ephrata, PA	100 1	98 49	95 21	82 22	- 0	- 0	83 6	95 38	4 39	38 8	- 0	91 46	82 131	100 183	62 16
Erie VA Medical Center, Erie, PA	- 0	- 0	- 0	- 0	- 0	- 0	- 0	- 0	- 0	- 0	- 0	75 8	89 28	100 34	86 7
Evangelical Community Hospital, Lewisburg, PA	87 15	99 149	97 122	98 129	- 0	- 0	89 9	96 150	6 153	58 24	- 0	89 27	95 106	99 143	100 9
Excela Health Frick Hospital, Mount Pleasant, PA	0 1	87 30	92 13	93 14	- 0	- 0	- 0	99 106	6 110	56 20	- 0	91 46	97 197	100 223	100 37
Excela Health Latrobe Hospital, Latrobe, PA	100 17	97 61	91 35	97 36	- 0	- 0	100 5	97 173	11 176	70 35	- 0	91 76	91 223	100 293	100 26
Excela Health Westmoreland Regional Hospital, Greensburg, PA	86 79	99 328	99 451	96 420	- 0	81 64	99 137	81 32	14 30	67 1	- 0	86 170	90 536	100 758	100 54
Fulton County Medical Center, Mcconnellsburg, PA	- 0	- 0	- 0	- 0	- 0	- 0	- 0	- 0	- 0	- 0	- 0	100 6	71 14	90 20	0 1
Geisinger Medical Center, Danville, PA	99 102	99 260	100 679	100 660	- 0	96 52	100 226	- 0	- 0	- 0	- 0	100 103	96 304	100 402	100 68
Geisinger Wyoming Valley Medical Center, Wilkes-Barre, PA	95 40	99 182	99 189	100 186	- 0	76 42	100 61	67 3	1 4	- 0	- 0	83 94	83 193	100 255	100 34
Gettysburg Hospital, Gettysburg, PA	83 6	100 43	97 31	100 30	- 0	- 0	100 6	99 74	9 76	74 11	67 3	98 42	96 90	100 131	100 9
Gnaden Huetten Memorial Hospital, Lehighton, PA	100 1	85 13	100 8	100 8	- 0	- 0	100 1	95 94	6 101	60 24	- 0	95 20	99 99	99 127	80 15
Good Samaritan Hospital, Lebanon, PA	100 36	100 200	100 192	100 193	- 0	88 48	100 68	100 1	10 1	- 0	- 0	99 67	92 160	99 223	100 18
Grand View Hospital, Sellersville, PA	100 10	99 69	100 49	100 46	- 0	75 4	100 4	99 67	5 67	38 23	- 0	100 58	91 245	100 310	100 13
Grove City Medical Center, Grove City, PA	75 4	92 13	85 13	91 11	- 0	- 0	50 2	98 158	6 164	60 15	- 0	85 27	94 51	97 98	100 6
Hahnemann University Hospital, Philadelphia, PA	100 43	98 103	99 195	100 192	- 0	88 8	100 72	100 1	40 1	- 0	- 0	99 389	97 642	100 699	98 193
Hamot Medical Center, Erie, PA	99 148	99 278	99 713	99 703	- 0	91 64	100 275	100 1	5 1	- 0	- 0	95 171	91 422	100 538	100 91
Hanover Hospital, Hanover, PA	79 29	97 174	88 114	90 112	20 5	- 0	94 16	93 59	5 63	76 8	71 7	81 62	94 156	76 197	100 23
Hazleton General Hospital, Hazleton, PA	100 3	97 61	97 39	100 48	- 0	- 0	100 5	92 321	14 333	52 44	- 0	98 53	95 183	100 282	100 32
Heart of Lancaster Regional Medical Center, Lititz, PA	- 0	100 10	100 5	100 4	- 0	- 0	- 0	100 17	4 18	68 4	- 0	94 16	96 24	98 46	100 4
Heritage Valley Beaver, PA	98 63	97 336	98 412	100 367	- 0	82 66	100 135	100 9	12 10	- 0	- 0	100 184	93 638	99 787	100 83

NOTE: The first number in each column (boldface) is the score, the second number is the number of patients; Please refer to the main entry for footnotes; (a) 100-299
MEASURES: **Heart Attack Care:** *1. ACE Inhibitor or ARB for LVSD; 2. Aspirin at Arrival; 3. Aspirin at Discharge; 4. Beta Blocker at Discharge; 5. Fibrinolytic Medication Timing; 6. PCI Within 90 Minutes of Arrival; 7. Smoking Cessation Advice;* **Chest Pain/Possible Heart Attack Care:** *8. Aspirin at Arrival; 9. Median Time to ECG (minutes); 10. Median Time to Transfer (minutes); 11. Fibrinolytic Medication Timing;* **Heart Failure Care:** *12. ACE Inhibitor or ARB for LVSD; 13. Discharge Instructions; 14. Evaluation of LVS Function; 15. Smoking Cessation Advice*

Hospital	Heart Attack Care							Chest Pain/Possible Heart Attack Care				Heart Failure Care			
	1	2	3	4	5	6	7	8	9	10	11	12	13	14	15
Heritage Valley Sewickley, Sewickley, PA	100 4	98 43	90 21	95 20	- 0	- 0	100 1	96 70	12 72	- 0	- 0	100 74	93 241	99 312	98 41
Highlands Hospital, Connellsville, PA	0 1	100 5	100 4	100 4	- 0	- 0	- 0	81 98	12 102	75 15	- 0	85 13	85 59	100 61	100 3
Holy Redeemer Hospital and Medical Center, Meadowbrook, PA	92 26	97 176	97 139	98 141	- 0	85 33	100 30	100 1	308178 1	- 0	- 0	98 63	100 232	99 339	100 21
Holy Spirit Hospital, Camp Hill, PA	98 66	98 308	100 334	100 324	- 0	97 68	100 100	- 0	- 0	- 0	- 0	97 117	96 339	100 468	100 52
Hospital of Univ of Pennsylvania, Philadelphia, PA	98 40	100 112	100 204	98 198	- 0	72 29	99 70	- 0	- 0	- 0	- 0	98 402	88 708	100 781	99 174
Indiana Regional Medical Center, Indiana, PA	81 16	95 80	97 59	98 62	100 1	- 0	100 4	97 212	14 217	82 49	- 0	85 151	85 260	97 333	94 35
J C Blair Memorial Hospital, Huntingdon, PA	- 0	83 6	100 2	100 2	- 0	- 0	- 0	90 151	12 158	86 12	100 1	88 17	79 57	92 75	100 12
James E. Van Zandt VA Medical Center - Altoona, Altoona, PA	100 1	100 11	100 5	100 5	- 0	- 0	100 1	-	-	-	-	100 17	97 35	100 37	100 3
Jameson Memorial Hospital, New Castle, PA	75 12	97 137	96 98	99 95	- 0	43 7	100 27	100 23	9 24	68 8	- 0	83 94	91 285	96 365	100 35
Jeanes Hospital, Philadelphia, PA	97 30	98 164	99 146	98 164	- 0	45 20	100 42	100 3	11 3	- 0	- 0	92 115	94 278	98 355	100 39
Jefferson Regional Medical Center, Pittsburgh, PA	90 60	99 271	100 309	99 300	- 0	81 64	99 104	89 9	4 10	- 0	- 0	85 217	90 605	99 744	100 74
Jennersville Regional Hospital, West Grove, PA	100 5	100 26	100 14	100 14	- 0	- 0	100 3	100 29	7 31	132 12	0 2	100 11	100 53	100 95	100 9
Jersey Shore Hospital, Jersey Shore, PA	- 0	100 5	100 4	71 7	- 0	- 0	- 0	- 0	- 0	- 0	- 0	100 12	100 72	100 86	100 4
Kane Community Hospital, Kane, PA	100 2	75 4	100 4	67 3	- 0	- 0	- 0	100 11	6 12	227 3	0 1	100 17	18 74	82 95	43 7
Kensington Hospital, Philadelphia, PA	- 0	- 0	- 0	- 0	- 0	- 0	- 0	- 0	- 0	- 0	- 0	- 0	- 0	- 0	- 0
Lancaster General Hospital, Lancaster, PA	91 117	98 717	100 749	98 733	- 0	79 122	100 211	100 1	0 1	- 0	- 0	93 284	74 794	99 1005	100 126
Lancaster Regional Medical Center, Lancaster, PA	100 10	98 40	100 52	100 48	- 0	86 7	100 17	100 1	0 1	- 0	- 0	98 47	95 87	100 112	100 31
Lansdale Hospital, Lansdale, PA	100 12	100 60	100 33	100 33	0 1	- 0	100 2	94 48	11 50	58 4	- 0	95 61	77 146	99 222	100 22
Lebanon VA Medical Center, Lebanon, PA	- 0	- 0	- 0	- 0	- 0	- 0	- 0	-	-	-	-	100 32	98 57	100 76	100 16
Lehigh Valley Hospital, Allentown, PA	96 149	100 648	99 976	99 951	- 0	96 118	100 247	75 4	12 5	- 0	- 0	99 308	95 879	99 1112	100 115
Lehigh Valley Hospital - Muhlenberg, Bethlehem, PA	97 33	100 288	99 281	100 283	- 0	89 71	100 78	89 9	9 9	- 0	- 0	100 106	98 366	100 466	100 41
Lewistown Hospital, Lewistown, PA	86 22	97 123	93 76	99 86	0 1	- 0	88 8	96 47	7 47	45 5	100 1	85 54	89 178	100 274	85 20
Lock Haven Hospital, Lock Haven, PA	100 1	89 9	71 7	100 7	- 0	- 0	100 4	94 34	9 37	44 3	- 0	100 14	97 60	99 79	100 14
Lower Bucks Hospital, Bristol, PA	87 15	98 124	96 114	97 119	- 0	60 5	92 49	- 0	- 0	- 0	- 0	89 88	71 215	98 262	90 39
Magee Womens Hospital of UPMC Health System, Pittsburgh, PA	- 0	100 3	100 3	100 3	- 0	- 0	- 0	- 0	- 0	- 0	- 0	100 21	100 59	100 83	100 12
Main Line Hospital Bryn Mawr Campus, Bryn Mawr, PA	100 27	100 206	100 232	100 212	- 0	100 30	100 47	100 1	11 1	- 0	- 0	99 143	98 339	100 491	100 22
Main Line Hospital Lankenau, Wynnewood, PA	100 52	100 216	100 298	100 293	100 1	98 42	100 58	67 3	20 3	- 0	- 0	99 331	94 666	100 857	100 139
Main Line Hospital Paoli, Paoli, PA	100 10	99 153	100 136	99 131	- 0	88 25	100 19	67 9	5 9	- 0	- 0	100 68	99 181	100 246	100 20
Marian Community Hospital, Carbondale, PA	100 1	100 16	50 6	100 5	- 0	- 0	- 0	98 48	8 49	43 11	- 0	95 20	95 65	98 93	100 5
Meadville Medical Center, Meadville, PA	100 1	100 21	78 9	88 8	- 0	- 0	50 2	98 152	9 156	70 11	40 5	94 31	77 91	97 129	100 14
Memorial Hospital - Towanda, Towanda, PA	100 2	100 6	100 3	100 3	- 0	- 0	100 1	93 42	6 47	92 5	- 0	80 10	100 42	92 52	100 5
Memorial Hospital York, York, PA	100 6	98 62	100 38	97 34	- 0	75 4	90 10	100 50	7 51	81 18	- 0	89 37	96 114	99 144	100 17
Mercy Fitzgerald Hospital, Darby, PA	98 48	100 183	99 179	99 177	- 0	86 21	100 65	88 8	16 8	- 0	- 0	99 487	98 842	99 973	100 305
Mercy Hospital Scranton, Scranton, PA	100 59	98 204	99 287	100 274	0 1	93 45	100 110	- 0	- 0	- 0	- 0	100 84	100 202	99 303	100 46
Mercy Suburban Hospital, Norristown, PA	100 1	100 35	94 16	100 20	- 0	- 0	100 1	97 30	11 30	- 0	- 0	100 62	98 137	100 193	100 25
Mercy Tyler Hospital, Tunkhannock, PA	0 1	100 4	100 1	100 1	- 0	- 0	0 1	92 60	12 62	94 9	- 0	70 10	26 39	94 50	67 6
Mid-Valley Hospital, Peckville, PA	0 1	83 6	0 1	100 2	- 0	- 0	- 0	-	-	-	-	100 7	95 22	100 33	100 2
Millcreek Community Hospital, Erie, PA	0 1	100 3	0 1	- 0	- 0	- 0	- 0	100 12	18 12	- 0	- 0	90 20	80 46	98 80	100 11
Milton S Hershey Medical Center, Hershey, PA	97 35	100 234	99 349	99 340	100 1	88 41	100 89	- 0	- 0	- 0	- 0	99 113	89 399	99 462	98 54
Miners Medical Center, Hastings, PA	100 1	100 12	100 8	86 7	- 0	- 0	- 0	92 117	16 123	62 8	- 0	67 12	41 27	85 34	83 6
Monongahela Valley Hospital, Monongahela, PA	100 8	96 107	92 63	96 72	- 0	20 5	100 11	99 86	10 91	86 14	- 0	92 96	91 191	99 399	100 47
Montgomery Hospital, Norristown, PA	94 32	98 128	98 131	98 133	- 0	100 25	100 44	- 0	- 0	- 0	- 0	88 69	91 191	99 234	100 39
Montrose General Hospital, Montrose, PA	100 1	100 3	100 1	100 2	100 1	- 0	- 0	-	-	-	-	91 11	70 20	70 27	100 4
Moses Taylor Hospital, Scranton, PA	83 6	100 42	100 20	100 25	- 0	- 0	100 3	97 37	14 37	125 11	- 0	95 41	90 125	99 197	100 34
Mount Nittany Medical Center, State College, PA	94 18	99 139	98 120	98 121	- 0	85 39	100 27	100 14	16 14	51 1	- 0	92 60	86 235	99 298	100 41
Muncy Valley Hospital, Muncy, PA	- 0	100 3	100 3	100 3	- 0	- 0	- 0	-	-	-	-	91 11	73 26	100 35	100 4
Nason Hospital, Roaring Spring, PA	- 0	100 22	100 3	100 3	- 0	- 0	- 0	94 34	7 35	- 0	100 4	100 21	97 62	100 82	100 4
Nazareth Hospital, Philadelphia, PA	100 6	100 109	97 60	98 63	- 0	- 0	100 3	97 61	9 66	72 26	0 2	100 50	99 230	100 398	100 37
Ohio Valley General Hospital, Mckees Rocks, PA	- 0	100 18	100 9	100 10	- 0	- 0	100 1	98 47	21 47	75 12	- 0	80 70	67 151	100 212	92 25
Palmerton Hospital, Palmerton, PA	50 2	93 15	100 9	100 8	- 0	- 0	100 2	90 40	4 42	58 7	- 0	83 30	89 90	94 115	86 7
Penn Presbyterian Medical Center, Philadelphia, PA	95 140	100 408	100 696	99 692	- 0	100 2	100 208	- 0	- 0	- 0	- 0	98 350	89 691	99 804	100 160
Penn Hospital of the U of Penn Health Sys, Philadelphia, PA	93 45	100 132	99 186	97 172	100 1	48 23	100 79	- 0	- 0	- 0	- 0	92 132	97 384	100 433	100 66
Philadelphia VA Medical Center, Philadelphia, PA	- 0	- 0	- 0	- 0	- 0	- 0	- 0	-	-	-	-	93 135	81 272	98 282	99 107
Phoenixville Hospital, Phoenixville, PA	92 40	99 157	100 217	100 215	- 0	86 22	98 64	100 3	5 3	- 0	- 0	99 102	95 207	96 257	96 28
Pinnacle Health Hospitals, Harrisburg, PA	97 149	99 545	99 637	99 633	- 0	97 90	100 183	100 2	1 2	- 0	- 0	100 256	89 605	100 769	100 113
Pocono Medical Center, East Stroudsburg, PA	97 66	98 297	99 283	99 258	- 0	96 83	100 112	100 3	6 4	- 0	- 0	93 136	68 367	99 433	98 83
Pottstown Memorial Medical Center, Pottstown, PA	100 7	100 48	100 26	100 25	- 0	- 0	100 3	99 70	10 73	62 14	- 0	93 104	95 183	99 253	100 27
Punxsutawney Area Hospital, Punxsutawney, PA	100 2	100 9	100 3	100 3	- 0	- 0	- 0	100 22	8 22	88 3	- 0	100 12	75 48	93 57	100 1
Reading Hospital Medical Center, Reading, PA	98 51	99 399	100 397	100 392	- 0	92 112	100 115	100 1	0 1	- 0	- 0	100 193	98 582	100 789	100 87
Riddle Memorial Hospital, Media, PA	100 25	98 130	100 100	100 99	- 0	88 32	100 29	100 1	68 1	- 0	- 0	97 66	88 192	99 286	96 23
Robert Packer Hospital, Sayre, PA	97 94	99 161	99 345	99 330	- 0	78 23	100 112	- 0	- 0	- 0	- 0	95 208	87 303	100 370	100 31
Roxborough Memorial Hospital, Phila, PA	50 2	95 41	90 21	100 21	- 0	- 0	100 6	- 0	- 0	- 0	- 0	87 69	93 131	99 206	100 51
Sacred Heart Hospital, Allentown, PA	50 4	97 31	100 21	100 19	- 0	- 0	100 3	100 8	9 8	67 4	- 0	96 24	90 93	95 130	93 13
Saint Catherine Medical Center Fountain Springs, Ashland, PA	75 4	100 12	100 6	88 8	- 0	- 0	- 0	96 46	14 44	69 8	0 1	94 16	92 64	84 87	100 18
Saint Clair Memorial Hospital, Pittsburgh, PA	76 34	97 269	100 257	97 240	- 0	94 71	100 68	92 12	2 12	- 0	- 0	84 152	79 454	98 614	100 39
Saint Joseph Medical Center, Reading, PA	100 21	99 144	99 159	100 157	- 0	100 43	98 51	- 0	- 0	- 0	- 0	100 109	96 301	100 368	98 55
Saint Joseph's Hospital, Philadelphia, PA	50 4	89 56	82 17	68 19	0 1	- 0	60 5	100 5	8 3	- 0	- 0	76 80	23 213	79 257	61 112

NOTE: The first number in each column (boldface) is the score, the second number is the number of patients; Please refer to the main entry for footnotes; (a) 100-299
MEASURES: *Heart Attack Care:* 1. ACE Inhibitor or ARB for LVSD; 2. Aspirin at Arrival; 3. Aspirin at Discharge; 4. Beta Blocker at Discharge; 5. Fibrinolytic Medication Timing; 6. PCI Within 90 Minutes of Arrival; 7. Smoking Cessation Advice; *Chest Pain/Possible Heart Attack Care:* 8. Aspirin at Arrival; 9. Median Time to ECG (minutes); 10. Median Time to Transfer (minutes); 11. Fibrinolytic Medication Timing; *Heart Failure Care:* 12. ACE Inhibitor or ARB for LVSD; 13. Discharge Instructions; 14. Evaluation of LVS Function; 15. Smoking Cessation Advice

Hospital	Heart Attack Care							Chest Pain/Possible Heart Attack Care				Heart Failure Care			
	1	2	3	4	5	6	7	8	9	10	11	12	13	14	15
Saint Luke's Hospital Bethlehem, Bethlehem, PA	100 62	98 367	99 445	99 434	- 0	87 46	100 128	- 0	- 0	- 0	- 0	98 247	92 770	99 992	99 110
Saint Luke's Miners Memorial Hospital, Coaldale, PA	100 1	80 20	71 14	92 13	- 0	- 0	- 0	- 0	- 0	- 0	- 0	89 18	100 55	97 74	100 7
Saint Luke's Quakertown Hospital, Quakertown, PA	100 3	91 23	92 13	100 12	- 0	- 0	- 0	- 0	- 0	- 0	- 0	100 23	93 55	99 93	100 14
Saint Mary Medical Center, Langhorne, PA	100 51	100 416	100 407	100 383	- 0	95 55	100 105	100 4	12 4	- 0	- 0	100 149	100 458	100 598	100 51
Saint Vincent Health Center, Erie, PA	98 80	100 240	100 461	99 457	0 1	82 49	100 173	- 0	- 0	- 0	- 0	90 147	95 390	100 539	100 58
Schuylkill Medical Center - East Norwegian Street, Pottsville, PA	33 3	95 61	95 38	91 45	- 0	- 0	100 5	94 48	8 47	55 7	0 1	84 63	90 186	95 297	100 15
Schuylkill Medical Center - South Jackson Street, Pottsville, PA	100 7	96 45	91 23	97 29	- 0	- 0	100 4	98 85	6 87	56 14	100 1	79 39	88 152	79 218	96 23
Shamokin Area Community Hospital, Coal Township, PA	100 12	99 100	96 76	97 91	- 0	- 0	94 17	95 88	2 92	50 14	- 0	100 16	72 102	99 174	86 7
Sharon Regional Health System, Sharon, PA	100 18	100 157	100 145	100 136	- 0	100 22	97 35	67 9	12 9	- 0	- 0	90 48	94 153	99 202	87 23
Soldiers and Sailors Memorial Hospital, Wellsboro, PA	- 0	83 6	100 4	100 5	- 0	- 0	100 2	99 84	6 85	86 12	40 5	100 28	97 77	98 94	100 11
Somerset Hospital, Somerset, PA	100 6	99 76	98 62	100 62	- 0	58 12	92 12	100 19	12 19	70 2	- 0	97 38	99 92	100 114	92 12
Southwest Regional Medical Center, Waynesburg, PA	- 0	92 13	73 11	89 9	- 0	- 0	- 0	94 107	10 110	67 11	- 0	90 40	83 156	96 198	92 37
Sunbury Community Hospital, Sunbury, PA	67 3	100 17	100 6	100 7	- 0	- 0	100 1	90 42	11 46	49 11	- 0	81 16	83 65	98 106	94 16
Surgical Institute of Reading, Wyomissing, PA	- 0	- 0	- 0	- 0	- 0	- 0	- 0	- 0	- 0	- 0	- 0	- 0	- 0	- 0	- 0
Surgical Specialty Center at Coordinated Health, Allentown, PA	- 0	- 0	- 0	- 0	- 0	- 0	- 0	- 0	- 0	- 0	- 0	- 0	- 0	- 0	- 0
Temple University Hospital, Philadelphia, PA	97 90	99 235	99 297	100 277	- 0	74 23	100 122	100 9	14 10	- 0	- 0	96 692	96 1216	99 1294	100 428
Thomas Jefferson University Hospital, Philadelphia, PA	100 60	99 184	99 263	100 250	- 0	86 7	100 88	- 0	- 0	- 0	- 0	99 412	98 853	99 985	100 229
Titusville Hospital, Titusville, PA	100 1	100 3	100 4	100 4	- 0	- 0	- 0	98 116	8 119	65 1	50 2	76 17	89 46	97 63	57 7
Troy Community Hospital, Troy, PA	- 0	100 2	100 1	100 1	- 0	- 0	- 0	100 30	7 32	155 11	- 0	78 9	86 7	93 14	33 3
Uniontown Hospital, Uniontown, PA	86 22	99 128	100 98	94 94	- 0	88 25	97 32	97 68	22 71	92 8	- 0	87 100	76 309	98 410	94 63
UPMC Bedford, Everett, PA	- 0	100 4	100 4	100 5	- 0	- 0	- 0	97 118	9 126	74 14	50 2	81 21	80 45	100 63	100 9
UPMC Horizon, Greenville, PA	100 12	98 61	100 42	100 44	- 0	- 0	100 5	99 130	12 138	62 22	40 5	100 55	99 165	100 224	100 31
UPMC Mckeesport, McKeesport, PA	100 19	100 108	100 78	100 85	- 0	- 0	100 21	97 30	12 32	- 0	- 0	100 107	99 305	100 442	100 52
UPMC Mercy, Pittsburgh, PA	99 73	98 259	100 374	100 353	- 0	80 45	100 149	- 0	- 0	- 0	- 0	99 168	87 366	100 487	100 96
UPMC Northwest, Seneca, PA	80 5	100 38	100 20	100 17	- 0	- 0	100 3	99 141	5 148	125 3	70 10	100 49	92 138	100 201	100 28
UPMC Passavant, Pittsburgh, PA	98 61	100 316	100 449	100 440	- 0	97 30	100 123	98 48	9 51	92 1	- 0	100 144	97 347	100 508	100 37
UPMC Presbyterian Shadyside, Pittsburgh, PA	100 189	100 456	100 1034	100 998	- 0	94 85	100 374	95 217	9 226	- 0	- 0	100 515	98 1113	100 1383	100 260
UPMC Saint Margaret, Pittsburgh, PA	100 9	96 102	100 49	100 61	- 0	- 0	100 4	98 132	12 138	92 34	0 1	96 113	91 389	100 573	100 60
VA Pittsburgh Healthcare System, Pittsburgh, PA	100 3	100 41	100 46	100 47	- 0	73 11	100 16	- 0	- 0	- 0	- 0	99 72	96 217	100 237	100 51
Valley Forge Medical Center and Hospital, Norristown, PA	- 0	- 0	- 0	- 0	- 0	- 0	- 0	- 0	- 0	- 0	- 0	- 0	- 0	- 0	- 0
Warren General Hospital, Warren, PA	- 0	83 12	86 7	80 10	- 0	- 0	- 0	98 167	6 173	218 5	40 5	81 32	60 78	93 111	88 8
The Washington Hospital, Washington, PA	98 65	100 285	99 359	99 349	- 0	94 50	100 117	100 9	13 10	- 0	- 0	99 190	93 528	100 666	100 105
Wayne Memorial Hospital, Honesdale, PA	100 5	93 46	92 25	96 25	- 0	- 0	100 7	95 38	4 38	53 9	- 0	96 26	94 83	98 102	100 18
Waynesboro Hospital, Waynesboro, PA	100 6	97 34	100 17	95 22	- 0	- 0	100 2	96 47	4 56	48 11	- 0	97 31	85 87	99 106	100 7
Western Pennsylvania Hospital, Pittsburgh, PA	97 37	99 110	100 215	99 205	- 0	87 15	100 72	100 1	12 1	- 0	- 0	94 141	90 288	99 334	100 64
Western Penn Hosp-Forbes Reg Campus, Monroeville, PA	91 32	100 230	96 222	99 218	- 0	79 42	100 64	86 86	7 92	75 1	- 0	96 173	85 470	99 667	100 77
Westfield Hospital, Allentown, PA	- 0	0 1	- 0	- 0	- 0	- 0	- 0	- 0	- 0	- 0	- 0	- 0	0 2	0 4	- 0
Wilkes-Barre General Hospital, Wilkes-Barre, PA	89 70	97 341	97 329	96 337	- 0	73 41	100 104	100 7	8 8	18 1	- 0	80 135	88 395	94 579	98 55
Wilkes-Barre VA Medical Center, Wilkes-Barre, PA	- 0	- 0	- 0	- 0	- 0	- 0	- 0	- 0	- 0	- 0	- 0	100 39	99 109	100 129	100 22
Williamsport Hospital & Medical Center, Williamsport, PA	91 43	99 185	100 265	98 260	- 0	83 42	100 91	88 8	7 8	- 0	- 0	97 89	90 198	99 253	94 35
Windber Hospital, Windber, PA	100 1	91 33	94 18	94 16	- 0	- 0	- 0	98 62	12 66	71 9	- 0	93 29	88 92	98 118	89 9
York Hospital, York, PA	95 125	98 437	99 531	99 538	- 0	90 102	100 200	- 0	- 0	- 0	- 0	93 203	82 617	99 756	97 126
RHODE ISLAND															
Kent County Memorial Hospital, Warwick, RI	100 11	97 184	98 123	99 122	- 0	96 23	- 0	95 104	5 109	57 43	- 0	94 98	78 348	99 529	91 67
Landmark Medical Center, Woonsocket, RI	100 20	99 143	98 111	97 112	- 0	100 23	97 31	97 30	4 31	37 1	- 0	99 79	92 206	99 319	100 50
Memorial Hospital of Rhode Island, Pawtucket, RI	86 7	96 51	100 25	100 25	- 0	- 0	100 7	97 39	18 45	98 24	- 0	85 62	93 175	98 242	100 37
Miriam Hospital, Providence, RI	98 115	99 344	100 629	99 610	- 0	85 66	100 187	100 4	10 4	- 0	- 0	95 165	91 421	99 541	100 67
Newport Hospital, Newport, RI	100 4	90 21	100 13	100 9	- 0	- 0	100 1	97 78	8 76	90 12	- 0	94 51	97 119	99 162	100 9
Providence VA Medical Center, Providence, RI	- 0	- 0	- 0	- 0	- 0	- 0	- 0	- 0	- 0	- 0	- 0	96 57	92 131	99 169	85 27
Rhode Island Hospital, Providence, RI	99 83	100 407	100 643	100 616	0 1	94 80	100 212	100 2	8 2	- 0	- 0	94 130	87 267	99 346	100 54
Roger Williams Medical Center, Providence, RI	89 9	98 66	92 50	100 50	- 0	- 0	100 7	100 13	9 13	72 5	- 0	85 34	67 109	96 162	100 14
Saint Joseph Health Services of RI, North Providence, RI	100 10	97 60	97 37	98 41	- 0	- 0	67 3	97 32	0 32	58 8	- 0	93 44	72 155	97 261	96 23
South County Hospital, Wakefield, RI	100 3	100 29	100 15	94 12	- 0	- 0	100 1	94 35	10 35	52 8	50 2	100 31	97 88	100 111	100 8
Westerly Hospital, Westerly, RI	100 2	90 21	93 15	100 12	- 0	- 0	83 6	98 51	10 51	80 9	100 6	92 51	72 122	96 180	96 25
Women and Infants Hospital of Rhode Island, Providence, RI	- 0	- 0	- 0	- 0	- 0	- 0	- 0	65 43	14 38	- 0	- 0	- 0	0 1	0 1	- 0
TENNESSEE															
Athens Regional Medical Center, Athens, TN	- 0	100 4	100 2	100 2	- 0	- 0	- 0	99 203	5 210	59 17	40 5	81 32	93 82	99 101	100 23
Baptist Hospital, Nashville, TN	96 51	99 199	99 235	100 237	- 0	100 25	100 87	100 2	9 2	- 0	- 0	95 193	85 503	98 574	100 109
Baptist Hospital of Cocke County, Newport, TN	- 0	100 8	100 4	100 6	- 0	- 0	- 0	96 315	17 334	95 5	0 2	93 27	69 59	99 69	95 22
Baptist Hospital West, Knoxville, TN	- 0	- 0	- 0	- 0	- 0	- 0	- 0	- 0	- 0	- 0	- 0	- 0	- 0	- 0	- 0
Baptist Memorial Hospital, Memphis, TN	99 117	98 519	98 692	98 654	- 0	80 44	100 214	91 22	23 21	- 0	- 0	96 448	84 1171	100 1294	100 229
Baptist Memorial Hospital Huntingdon, Huntingdon, TN	- 0	100 3	100 1	100 1	- 0	- 0	- 0	92 104	7 113	258 2	0 4	100 13	98 40	98 58	100 15
Baptist Memorial Hospital Tipton, Covington, TN	- 0	75 4	50 2	100 1	- 0	- 0	- 0	90 185	20 198	170 12	20 5	88 17	80 45	95 62	100 10
Baptist Memorial Hospital Union City, Union City, TN	100 1	100 12	100 7	100 8	- 0	- 0	100 2	98 157	4 164	118 3	60 10	100 20	93 61	100 84	100 15
Baptist Rehabilitation Germantown, Germantown, TN	- 0	- 0	- 0	- 0	- 0	- 0	- 0	- 0	- 0	- 0	- 0	- 0	- 0	- 0	- 0
Blount Memorial Hospital, Maryville, TN	94 32	99 191	99 177	100 170	- 0	93 43	100 62	82 11	8 12	- 0	- 0	99 78	88 205	99 267	100 30
Bolivar General Hospital, Bolivar, TN	- 0	- 0	- 0	- 0	- 0	- 0	- 0	97 86	15 102	453 4	0 2	100 8	68 25	59 29	100 5

NOTE: The first number in each column (boldface) is the score, the second number is the number of patients; Please refer to the main entry for footnotes; (a) 100-299
MEASURES: **Heart Attack Care:** 1. ACE Inhibitor or ARB for LVSD; 2. Aspirin at Arrival; 3. Aspirin at Discharge; 4. Beta Blocker at Discharge; 5. Fibrinolytic Medication Timing; 6. PCI Within 90 Minutes of Arrival; 7. Smoking Cessation Advice; **Chest Pain/Possible Heart Attack Care:** 8. Aspirin at Arrival; 9. Median Time to ECG (minutes); 10. Median Time to Transfer (minutes); 11. Fibrinolytic Medication Timing; **Heart Failure Care:** 12. ACE Inhibitor or ARB for LVSD; 13. Discharge Instructions; 14. Evaluation of LVS Function; 15. Smoking Cessation Advice

Hospital		Heart Attack Care							Chest Pain/Possible Heart Attack Care				Heart Failure Care			
	1	2	3	4	5	6	7	8	9	10	11	12	13	14	15
Camden General Hospital, Camden, TN	- 0	- 0	- 0	- 0	- 0	- 0	- 0	-	-	-	-	- 0	- 0	- 0	- 0
Centennial Medical Center, Nashville, TN	100 104	100 141	100 555	100 528	- 0	100 18	100 250	100 5	9 5	- 0	- 0	95 221	94 482	100 537	100 123
Centennial Medical Center of Ashland City, Ashland City, TN	- 0	- 0	- 0	- 0	- 0	- 0	- 0	100 107	8 120	40 10	50 2	- 0	- 0	- 0	- 0
The Center for Spinal Surgery, Nashville, TN	- 0	- 0	- 0	- 0	- 0	- 0	- 0	- 0	- 0	- 0	- 0	- 0	- 0	- 0	- 0
Claiborne County Hospital, Tazewell, TN	100 1	80 10	75 8	60 10	- 0	- 0	100 1	90 130	10 137	65 13	0 2	47 15	87 135	37 175	100 39
Cookeville Regional Medical Center, Cookeville, TN	96 143	99 320	99 522	99 514	- 0	89 82	100 219	96 27	5 25	- 0	- 0	86 138	71 300	98 350	98 61
Copper Basin Medical Center, Copperhill, TN	0 1	100 1	100 1	50 2	- 0	- 0	- 0	83 75	21 77	170 3	0 3	89 9	96 27	97 29	75 4
Crockett Hospital, Lawrenceburg, TN	- 0	100 2	100 1	100 1	- 0	- 0	- 0	98 240	5 250	122 13	60 10	94 17	91 58	96 77	100 6
Cumberland Medical Center, Crossville, TN	88 8	95 40	100 30	97 31	- 0	- 0	100 5	99 123	13 122	- 0	53 19	82 60	88 258	97 293	100 54
Cumberland River Hospital, Celina, TN	- 0	100 2	100 1	100 1	- 0	- 0	- 0	64 11	16 12	200 1	0 1	100 12	96 25	86 36	100 4
Decatur County General Hospital, Parsons, TN	- 0	100 3	100 2	100 2	- 0	- 0	- 0	97 124	6 137	117 3	40 5	67 3	95 21	97 31	100 2
Delta Medical Center, Memphis, TN	100 1	100 11	80 5	80 5	- 0	- 0	100 3	- 0	- 0	- 0	- 0	91 56	94 149	96 161	96 46
Dyersburg Regional Medical Center, Dyersburg, TN	100 4	91 22	86 14	100 14	- 0	- 0	100 1	100 207	1 218	- 0	83 12	98 51	95 197	100 252	100 46
Erlanger Medical Center, Chattanooga, TN	100 52	99 234	100 391	100 354	- 0	92 72	100 208	91 23	12 24	58 3	- 0	97 133	88 304	99 341	100 117
Fort Loudoun Medical Center, Lenoir City, TN	100 4	100 17	100 10	100 11	- 0	- 0	100 1	100 56	8 58	56 8	- 0	100 18	96 81	100 92	100 12
Fort Sanders Regional Medical Center, Knoxville, TN	100 53	100 166	100 302	100 287	- 0	98 57	100 120	0 1	0 1	- 0	- 0	100 123	98 353	100 424	100 73
Franklin Woods Community Hospital, Johnson City, TN	- 0	- 0	- 0	- 0	- 0	- 0	- 0	87 135	4 145	52 3	- 0	100 4	84 19	100 26	100 6
Gateway Medical Center, Clarksville, TN	95 37	99 180	94 188	94 194	- 0	76 45	100 104	98 124	4 129	53 5	0 1	96 108	96 286	88 322	99 79
Gibson General Hospital, Trenton, TN	100 1	100 3	100 3	67 3	- 0	- 0	0 1	94 70	21 73	685 1	20 5	70 10	67 12	81 27	50 2
Grandview Medical Center, Jasper, TN	100 2	100 3	100 3	100 3	- 0	- 0	- 0	97 210	12 229	54 13	60 5	91 11	64 28	100 33	91 11
Hardin Medical Center, Savannah, TN	- 0	100 3	67 3	50 2	- 0	- 0	- 0	97 324	9 345	- 0	62 16	94 17	93 43	98 64	100 13
Harton Regional Medical Center, Tullahoma, TN	100 4	100 59	100 52	100 51	100 3	91 11	100 23	94 65	6 66	52 4	67 6	100 51	95 164	100 194	100 34
Haywood Park Community Hospital, Brownsville, TN	- 0	100 1	- 0	- 0	- 0	- 0	- 0	96 105	4 108	- 0	50 2	80 10	100 35	100 44	100 7
Healthsouth Chattanooga Rehab Hospital, Chattanooga, TN	- 0	- 0	- 0	- 0	- 0	- 0	- 0	-	-	-	-	- 0	- 0	- 0	- 0
Henderson County Community Hospital, Lexington, TN	100 1	100 5	100 4	100 4	- 0	- 0	100 1	100 116	2 130	- 0	100 3	100 12	100 46	100 64	100 16
Hendersonville Medical Center, Hendersonville, TN	100 10	100 42	100 48	100 47	- 0	100 10	100 22	100 40	5 45	- 0	- 0	100 32	99 97	100 121	100 25
Henry County Medical Center, Paris, TN	100 4	96 24	88 17	100 15	- 0	- 0	100 3	96 219	6 217	67 1	59 17	100 38	78 76	99 97	100 19
Heritage Medical Center, Shelbyville, TN	100 3	100 13	80 5	100 5	- 0	- 0	- 0	97 155	4 162	42 5	50 2	86 29	79 67	98 86	100 16
Hickman Community Health Services, Centerville, TN	- 0	- 0	- 0	- 0	- 0	- 0	- 0	-	-	-	-	- 0	- 0	- 0	- 0
Hillside Hospital, Pulaski, TN	- 0	100 1	0 1	100 1	- 0	- 0	- 0	94 281	5 292	79 3	50 4	67 6	95 19	100 25	100 7
Horizon Medical Center, Dickson, TN	100 8	98 48	100 37	100 34	- 0	100 4	100 14	97 159	6 170	34 20	100 1	96 45	90 140	100 178	97 33
Humboldt General Hospital, Humboldt, TN	- 0	100 2	50 2	50 2	- 0	- 0	- 0	86 90	33 93	135 3	0 3	85 13	96 25	91 33	100 9
Indian Path Medical Center, Kingsport, TN	93 14	100 46	100 42	100 45	- 0	100 3	100 13	94 34	4 35	48 8	- 0	100 37	85 130	99 164	100 34
Jackson-Madison County General Hospital, Jackson, TN	91 194	95 553	96 994	95 967	0 1	85 72	99 436	50 1	18 5	- 0	- 0	90 369	62 720	98 882	100 201
Jamestown Regional Medical Center, Jamestown, TN	- 0	100 5	100 2	100 4	- 0	- 0	100 1	100 92	5 99	- 0	100 1	100 24	99 83	100 96	100 23
Jellico Community Hospital, Jellico, TN	- 0	100 9	100 1	100 2	- 0	- 0	- 0	92 71	10 73	93 7	33 3	92 13	98 48	100 54	100 16
Johnson City Medical Center, Johnson City, TN	92 51	98 140	99 284	97 280	- 0	89 27	100 112	80 5	3 5	- 0	- 0	87 109	79 231	99 298	100 53
Johnson City Specialty Hospital, Johnson City, TN	- 0	- 0	- 0	- 0	- 0	- 0	- 0	- 0	- 0	- 0	- 0	- 0	- 0	- 0	- 0
Johnson County Community Hospital, Mountain City, TN	-	-	-	-	-	-	-	94 138	13 149	- 0	- 1	-	-	-	-
Lakeway Regional Hospital, Morristown, TN	67 3	75 12	79 14	92 13	- 0	- 0	100 3	94 18	6 18	79 3	- 0	100 8	96 57	98 66	100 11
Lauderdale Community Hospital, Ripley, TN	- 0	100 1	0 1	100 3	- 0	- 0	- 0	94 81	9 81	- 0	33 1	100 10	46 28	88 40	100 2
Laughlin Memorial Hospital, Greeneville, TN	100 1	100 9	100 6	100 5	- 0	- 0	- 0	97 299	10 316	54 25	50 2	100 34	100 113	99 163	100 18
Leconte Medical Center, Sevierville, TN	100 3	100 23	95 19	100 20	- 0	- 0	100 4	98 194	9 198	55 31	- 0	96 25	94 121	100 133	100 19
Lincoln Medical Center, Fayetteville, TN	- 0	100 2	100 2	100 2	- 0	- 0	- 0	96 322	5 334	66 1	38 8	78 18	74 42	91 58	100 4
Livingston Regional Hospital, Livingston, TN	100 1	88 8	100 4	100 4	- 0	- 0	100 3	100 69	4 81	70 7	0 1	89 18	100 67	100 103	100 2
Macon County General Hospital, Lafayette, TN	-	-	-	-	-	-	-	93 71	10 72	- 0	0 1	-	-	-	-
Marshall Medical Center, Lewisburg, TN	- 0	- 0	- 0	- 0	- 0	- 0	- 0	-	-	-	-	80 5	100 20	87 23	100 7
Maury Regional Hospital, Columbia, TN	93 88	98 199	99 267	98 254	- 0	94 36	100 124	92 48	5 53	- 0	- 0	95 174	93 333	100 422	100 105
McKenzie Regional Hospital, McKenzie, TN	- 0	100 2	100 1	100 1	- 0	- 0	- 0	99 142	8 154	- 0	67 6	100 2	100 16	100 23	100 2
McNairy Regional Hospital, Selmer, TN	67 3	100 11	86 7	100 9	- 0	- 0	- 0	97 140	6 150	- 0	0 1	80 15	93 44	98 63	100 10
Medical Center of Manchester, Manchester, TN	- 0	- 0	- 0	- 0	- 0	- 0	- 0	84 81	14 84	82 6	50 2	100 4	67 18	14 29	0 5
Memorial Healthcare System, Chattanooga, TN	100 122	99 530	100 746	100 705	- 0	85 104	100 240	94 33	2 31	57 11	- 0	98 249	84 663	99 785	98 129
Memphis VA Medical Center, Memphis, TN	94 17	100 68	100 65	100 61	- 0	100 5	100 28	- 0	- 0	- 0	- 0	98 126	99 246	99 255	100 79
Mercy Medical Center, Knoxville, TN	95 111	99 337	99 559	99 554	- 0	81 48	100 255	74 19	11 17	262876 2	- 0	99 171	87 487	100 589	99 128
Methodist Healthcare Fayette Hospital, Somerville, TN	- 0	- 0	- 0	- 0	- 0	- 0	- 0	97 97	0 100	103 1	100 2	100 4	92 13	100 17	100 4
Methodist Healthcare Memphis Hospitals, Memphis, TN	99 182	100 741	100 950	100 941	- 0	99 155	100 435	80 20	8 23	- 0	- 0	99 531	94 1084	100 1215	100 268
Methodist Medical Center of Oak Ridge, Oak Ridge, TN	100 64	99 191	98 281	99 269	0 1	100 51	100 118	90 10	8 12	- 0	- 0	100 91	94 287	99 344	100 57
Metro Nashville General Hospital, Nashville, TN	100 20	93 90	95 87	99 82	- 0	67 3	100 48	100 8	24 9	281 4	- 0	100 91	77 174	100 172	100 92
Middle Tennessee Medical Center, Murfreesboro, TN	94 34	97 212	99 190	98 178	- 0	82 49	100 90	84 75	10 60	298 6	- 0	88 137	96 308	99 397	100 71
Milan General Hospital, Milan, TN	- 0	- 0	- 0	- 0	- 0	- 0	- 0	93 123	12 138	- 0	58 12	100 2	100 4	100 6	- 0
Morristown Hamblen Hospital Association, Morristown, TN	93 14	99 195	98 202	97 209	- 0	96 51	99 95	95 20	11 25	- 0	- 0	98 63	88 245	99 270	97 69
Mountain Home VA Medical Center, Mountain Home, TN	100 14	100 79	100 62	100 61	- 0	31 13	100 24	-	-	-	-	98 53	100 156	100 172	100 37
Northcrest Medical Center, Springfield, TN	100 4	100 56	100 42	100 43	- 0	27 11	100 20	91 34	7 36	114 1	0 1	98 53	96 117	99 140	100 30
Parkridge Medical Center, Chattanooga, TN	100 24	100 111	100 230	100 218	100 2	100 14	100 117	98 65	6 71	28 8	- 0	99 98	97 258	100 323	100 85
Parkwest Medical Center, Knoxville, TN	95 84	99 333	100 506	99 505	- 0	92 78	100 212	72 18	10 19	- 0	- 0	94 86	93 318	99 396	100 71
Patients' Choice Medical Center of Erin, Erin, TN	- 0	- 0	- 0	100 1	- 0	- 0	- 0	-	-	-	-	100 3	73 15	62 50	67 6
Perry Community Hospital, Linden, TN	- 0	- 0	- 0	100 1	- 0	- 0	- 0	85 41	9 55	96 2	50 4	100 1	10 39	2 85	30 10

NOTE: The first number in each column (boldface) is the score, the second number is the number of patients; Please refer to the main entry for footnotes; (a) 100-299
MEASURES: **Heart Attack Care:** 1. ACE Inhibitor or ARB for LVSD; 2. Aspirin at Arrival; 3. Aspirin at Discharge; 4. Beta Blocker at Discharge; 5. Fibrinolytic Medication Timing; 6. PCI Within 90 Minutes of Arrival; 7. Smoking Cessation Advice; **Chest Pain/Possible Heart Attack Care:** 8. Aspirin at Arrival; 9. Median Time to ECG (minutes); 10. Median Time to Transfer (minutes); 11. Fibrinolytic Medication Timing; **Heart Failure Care:** 12. ACE Inhibitor or ARB for LVSD; 13. Discharge Instructions; 14. Evaluation of LVS Function; 15. Smoking Cessation Advice

Hospital	Heart Attack Care 1	2	3	4	5	6	7	Chest Pain/Possible Heart Attack Care 8	9	10	11	Heart Failure Care 12	13	14	15
Regional Hospital of Jackson, Jackson, TN	97 34	96 52	95 164	96 152	- 0	57 7	100 76	100 9	6 10	- 0	- 0	95 60	90 162	99 181	100 39
Regional Medical Center at Memphis, Memphis, TN	100 9	91 46	98 43	95 40	0 2	20 5	100 32	- 0	- 0	- 0	- 0	100 151	79 241	100 254	100 118
Rhea Medical Center, Dayton, TN	- 0	100 3	100 2	100 2	- 0	- 0	100 1	86 159	7 167	72 6	25 8	100 6	53 19	96 27	80 5
River Park Hospital, McMinnville, TN	100 4	93 14	100 10	83 12	- 0	- 0	100 4	95 163	4 173	140 4	43 21	93 29	83 127	99 161	98 42
Riverview Regional Medical Center North, Carthage, TN	- 0	100 1	100 1	100 1	- 0	- 0	- 0	98 125	8 138	165 1	50 2	86 7	97 36	90 50	100 8
Riverview Regional Medical Center South, Carthage, TN	- 0	- 0	- 0	- 0	- 0	- 0	- 0	- -	- -	- -	- -	- 0	- 0	- 0	- 0
Roane Medical Center, Harriman, TN	100 1	100 10	100 3	100 2	- 0	- 0	100 1	96 180	7 190	125 8	50 6	91 22	87 67	99 88	94 17
Saint Francis Bartlett Medical Center, Bartlett, TN	100 3	100 26	100 15	95 19	- 0	- 0	100 6	100 60	14 63	63 5	100 1	100 45	100 138	99 162	100 27
Saint Francis Hospital, Memphis, TN	100 39	98 248	98 292	100 289	- 0	86 44	100 96	- 0	- 0	- 0	- 0	98 293	95 660	100 763	100 117
Saint Mary's Jefferson Memorial Hospital, Jefferson City, TN	100 6	100 14	100 11	100 12	- 0	- 0	- 0	97 191	14 195	81 4	0 1	92 51	87 109	97 137	100 22
Saint Mary's Med Ctr of Campbell County, La Follette, TN	100 2	100 18	100 13	100 16	- 0	- 0	100 4	95 136	6 152	100 13	67 3	100 19	98 129	99 163	100 31
Saint Thomas Hospital, Nashville, TN	95 283	99 423	99 1322	98 1283	- 0	98 65	100 472	100 3	4 4	- 0	- 0	94 399	86 925	99 1049	100 149
Scott County Hospital, Oneida, TN	100 1	100 3	100 4	100 5	- 0	- 0	100 2	100 120	6 131	48 2	50 6	95 21	93 70	91 69	100 12
Skyline Medical Center, Nashville, TN	100 13	100 152	99 127	100 124	- 0	100 33	100 52	99 72	4 118	- 0	- 0	99 94	100 246	99 285	100 79
Skyridge Medical Center, Cleveland, TN	92 12	98 94	100 47	98 52	- 0	- 0	100 14	98 91	10 95	73 54	- 0	95 61	92 205	99 241	100 53
Southern Hills Medical Center, Nashville, TN	89 9	99 78	95 58	96 69	100 3	100 23	100 36	100 31	7 33	- 0	- 0	100 32	99 109	98 122	100 32
Southern Tennessee Medical Center, Winchester, TN	100 8	89 28	72 18	82 22	100 1	- 0	100 3	97 213	7 225	36 1	88 8	95 38	93 125	97 154	100 19
Stonecrest Medical Center, Smyrna, TN	100 3	100 27	94 16	100 20	- 0	- 0	100 12	99 109	5 119	42 28	- 0	100 20	98 66	98 84	100 21
Stones River Hosp & Dekalb Comm Hosp, Woodbury, TN	- 0	100 3	100 2	100 2	- 0	- 0	100 1	94 48	7 51	- 0	0 2	100 3	92 12	100 16	- 0
Stones River Hosp & Dekalb Comm Hosp, Smithville, TN	- 0	100 4	100 2	100 4	- 0	- 0	- 0	94 99	8 105	- 0	0 4	100 10	61 51	100 74	100 6
Summit Medical Center, Hermitage, TN	100 12	100 112	100 95	98 97	100 1	100 25	100 32	100 70	4 72	51 23	- 0	100 64	100 171	98 212	100 35
Sumner Regional Medical Center, Gallatin, TN	89 19	98 111	94 101	95 99	- 0	82 11	100 44	96 48	4 52	- 0	- 0	91 55	87 154	93 194	97 32
Sweetwater Hospital Association, Sweetwater, TN	- 0	78 18	82 11	64 11	- 0	- 0	100 5	97 144	6 152	41 5	50 2	88 17	53 73	89 91	86 21
Sycamore Shoals Hospital, Elizabethton, TN	100 1	86 7	80 5	100 4	- 0	- 0	100 1	87 157	21 165	55 7	- 0	97 31	93 56	100 78	100 17
Takoma Regional Hospital, Greeneville, TN	100 2	100 8	100 5	100 4	- 0	- 0	100 1	98 65	10 71	158 1	80 5	96 23	94 49	100 64	100 5
Trousdale Medical Center, Hartsville, TN	- 0	- 0	- 0	- 0	- 0	- 0	- 0	- -	- -	- -	- -	78 9	97 33	77 61	93 27
Unicoi County Memorial Hospital, Erwin, TN	- 0	0 1	100 1	100 1	- 0	- 0	- 0	99 153	8 165	53 1	- 0	67 6	58 26	80 35	100 4
United Regional Medical Center, Manchester, TN	100 1	83 18	53 17	41 17	- 0	- 0	50 6	55 51	22 52	96 3	0 1	100 4	3 33	42 40	60 5
University Medical Center, Lebanon, TN	100 7	97 37	100 16	94 18	- 0	- 0	100 7	96 95	7 99	62 22	43 7	96 25	90 122	99 144	100 24
University of Tennessee Memorial Hospital, Knoxville, TN	98 62	100 212	99 316	99 321	- 0	89 61	100 156	100 1	23 1	- 0	- 0	89 115	86 276	100 323	100 64
VA Middle Tennessee Healthcare System, Nashville, TN	100 40	99 142	99 136	100 139	- 0	39 23	100 57	- 0	- 0	- 0	- 0	93 160	98 347	99 361	99 96
Vanderbilt University Hospital, Nashville, TN	100 53	99 148	100 359	99 349	- 0	96 24	100 144	100 2	8 2	- 0	- 0	93 150	92 333	99 367	100 70
Volunteer Community Hospital, Martin, TN	- 0	100 3	100 2	100 4	- 0	- 0	- 0	97 276	12 294	- 0	0 1	87 23	85 33	96 67	100 6
Wayne Medical Center, Waynesboro, TN	- 0	- 0	- 0	- 0	- 0	- 0	- 0	91 53	13 57	- 0	100 1	100 10	69 26	85 34	100 3
Wellmont Bristol Regional Medical Center, Bristol, TN	92 49	98 183	100 267	100 262	- 0	100 26	100 117	75 4	4 4	- 0	- 0	90 83	94 229	97 274	100 46
Wellmont Hancock County Hospital, Sneedville, TN	- 0	100 1	100 1	100 1	- 0	- 0	100 1	- -	- -	- -	- -	100 3	100 16	89 18	100 5
Wellmont Hawkins County Memorial Hospital, Rogersville, TN	100 1	90 10	100 5	100 6	- 0	- 0	100 1	91 121	12 122	180 0	0 1	96 25	83 84	99 94	100 9
Wellmont Holston Valley Medical Center, Kingsport, TN	98 60	98 124	100 259	100 257	0 1	96 24	100 104	75 4	8 4	- 0	- 0	98 109	99 231	97 272	98 57
White County Community Hospital, Sparta, TN	- 0	100 15	100 9	90 10	- 0	- 0	100 1	96 47	10 47	223 4	100 1	100 7	89 36	91 45	100 6
Williamson Medical Center, Franklin, TN	100 18	98 137	98 133	99 128	- 0	86 44	100 47	97 33	6 36	44 3	- 0	98 58	87 167	100 213	100 21
Woods Memorial Hospital, Etowah, TN	100 2	100 5	100 3	100 2	- 0	- 0	100 1	98 43	11 45	94 0	- 0	93 44	96 48	87 55	100 12
VERMONT															
Brattleboro Memorial Hospital, Brattleboro, VT	100 3	100 13	100 9	100 10	- 0	- 0	100 1	86 7	4 7	328 2	- 0	88 8	96 23	100 31	100 3
Central Vermont Medical Center, Barre, VT	100 2	100 7	100 3	100 5	- 0	- 0	- 0	99 156	6 159	31 17	100 1	93 15	82 51	97 65	100 11
Copley Hospital, Morrisville, VT	100 3	100 7	100 6	100 3	- 0	- 0	100 1	- -	- -	- -	- -	100 2	95 22	96 28	100 1
Fletcher Allen Hospital of Vermont, Burlington, VT	97 116	100 242	99 631	99 627	- 0	- 0	100 212	- 0	- 0	- 0	- 0	94 117	91 247	98 316	100 55
Gifford Medical Center, Randolph, VT	100 2	100 7	100 6	100 5	- 0	- 0	100 2	- -	- -	- -	- -	100 5	100 44	84 56	100 4
Grace Cottage Hospital, Townshend, VT	- 0	- 0	- 0	- 0	- 0	- 0	- 0	- -	- -	- -	- -	100 1	75 4	80 5	100 1
Mount Ascutney Hospital, Windsor, VT	- 0	100 1	- 0	- 0	- 0	- 0	- 0	- -	- -	- -	- -	75 4	75 12	100 24	100 1
North Country Hospital and Health Center, Newport, VT	- 0	100 9	100 7	100 6	- 0	- 0	100 1	- -	- -	- -	- -	100 13	91 35	100 53	100 4
Northeastern Vermont Regional Hospital, Saint Johnsbury, VT	50 2	100 12	90 10	100 11	- 0	- 0	- 0	- -	- -	- -	- -	100 13	52 33	100 41	100 2
Northwestern Medical Center, Saint Albans, VT	100 5	100 22	94 17	100 16	- 0	- 0	100 1	99 127	4 133	31 17	- 0	100 3	78 32	100 39	100 12
Porter Hospital, Middlebury, VT	- 0	67 3	50 2	100 2	- 0	- 0	- 0	- -	- -	- -	- -	100 6	83 23	89 27	100 4
Rutland Regional Medical Center, Rutland, VT	100 7	97 61	96 45	100 44	0 2	- 0	100 9	98 96	6 98	193 3	74 19	87 38	83 109	100 144	92 13
Southwestern Vermont Medical Center, Bennington, VT	100 3	100 36	100 23	100 25	- 0	- 0	100 7	99 110	7 120	96 4	50 4	100 26	89 89	99 130	100 10
Springfield Hospital, Springfield, VT	100 1	100 11	100 9	100 8	- 0	- 0	- 0	- -	- -	- -	- -	94 18	100 45	100 62	100 2
White River Junction VA Medical Center, White River Junction, VT	100 2	100 6	100 4	100 4	- 0	- 0	- 0	- -	- -	- -	- -	100 29	100 81	100 88	100 17
VIRGINIA															
Alleghany Regional Hospital, Low Moor, VA	100 2	93 14	100 8	100 10	- 0	- 0	100 2	100 74	6 76	- 0	100 6	95 21	100 94	100 120	100 19
Augusta Health, Fishersville, VA	95 21	100 129	94 115	97 105	- 0	100 10	100 100	99 108	8 109	74 33	67 3	96 112	91 260	100 332	100 53
Bath County Community Hospital, Hot Springs, VA	- 0	- 0	- 0	- 0	- 0	- 0	- 0	- -	- -	- -	- -	100 6	62 13	94 16	75 4
Bedford Memorial Hospital, Bedford, VA	100 3	93 14	100 10	100 11	- 0	- 0	100 3	83 64	10 66	40 16	- 0	95 19	98 55	93 67	100 16
Bon Secours - Depaul Medical Center, Norfolk, VA	94 16	97 143	98 127	89 129	- 0	82 28	100 51	86 14	0 15	- 0	- 0	96 70	95 190	99 252	98 56
Bon Secours - Maryview Medical Center, Portsmouth, VA	100 43	100 207	100 227	100 220	- 0	90 30	100 81	95 21	11 22	57 3	- 0	100 144	98 374	99 429	100 89
Bon Secours - Memorial Regional Medical, Mechanicsville, VA	100 88	100 323	100 319	100 308	- 0	95 60	100 96	100 4	4 4	- 0	- 0	100 120	100 293	100 353	100 54
Bon Secours - Richmond Community Hospital, Richmond, VA	- 0	100 5	100 1	100 1	- 0	- 0	- 0	100 15	13 15	58 2	- 0	100 15	75 51	98 57	100 25
Bon Secours - St Francis Medical Center, Midlothian, VA	100 29	99 116	100 98	97 94	- 0	86 22	100 30	89 9	9 9	- 0	- 0	100 58	100 176	99 211	100 26

NOTE: The first number in each column (boldface) is the score, the second number is the number of patients; Please refer to the main entry for footnotes; (a) 100-299
MEASURES: **Heart Attack Care:** 1. ACE Inhibitor or ARB for LVSD; 2. Aspirin at Arrival; 3. Aspirin at Discharge; 4. Beta Blocker at Discharge; 5. Fibrinolytic Medication Timing; 6. PCI Within 90 Minutes of Arrival; 7. Smoking Cessation Advice; **Chest Pain/Possible Heart Attack Care:** 8. Aspirin at Arrival; 9. Median Time to ECG (minutes); 10. Median Time to Transfer (minutes); 11. Fibrinolytic Medication Timing; **Heart Failure Care:** 12. ACE Inhibitor or ARB for LVSD; 13. Discharge Instructions; 14. Evaluation of LVS Function; 15. Smoking Cessation Advice

Hospital	Heart Attack Care							Chest Pain/Possible Heart Attack Care				Heart Failure Care			
	1	2	3	4	5	6	7	8	9	10	11	12	13	14	15
Bon Secours - St Marys Hospital of Richmond, Richmond, VA	**100** 58	**99** 195	**100** 225	**100** 220	- 0	**100** 46	**100** 71	**67** 3	**230** 3	- 0	- 0	**95** 107	**98** 324	**100** 423	**100** 56
Buchanan General Hospital, Grundy, VA	- 0	**94** 17	**91** 11	**91** 11	- 0	- 0	**100** 1	**100** 61	**7** 62	- 0	**100** 1	**90** 20	**96** 76	**100** 84	**100** 5
Carilion Franklin Memorial Hospital, Rocky Mount, VA	**100** 2	**100** 11	**100** 8	**100** 6	- 0	- 0	- 0	**94** 204	**31** 221	**86** 4	- 0	**100** 9	**91** 53	**96** 76	**100** 11
Carilion Giles Memorial Hospital, Pearisburg, VA	**100** 2	**100** 17	**100** 13	**100** 12	- 0	- 0	**100** 3	**100** 48	**18** 53	**60** 1	**0** 1	**91** 11	**85** 53	**86** 65	**100** 11
Carilion Medical Center, Roanoke, VA	**95** 228	**99** 560	**99** 1249	**98** 1264	- 0	**88** 104	**100** 509	- 0	**91** 1	- 0	- 0	**87** 300	**92** 636	**96** 780	**98** 200
Carilion New River Valley Medical Center, Christiansburg, VA	**100** 2	**100** 23	**100** 11	**100** 11	- 0	- 0	**100** 2	**95** 39	**25** 27	**50** 4	- 0	**88** 34	**88** 100	**99** 123	**100** 22
Carilion Stonewall Jackson Hospital, Lexington, VA	**100** 5	**95** 20	**100** 14	**100** 14	- 0	- 0	**100** 2	- -	- -	- -	- -	**95** 19	**90** 49	**100** 61	**100** 7
Carilion Tazewell Community Hospital, Tazewell, VA	**100** 1	**90** 10	**100** 8	**100** 8	- 0	- 0	**100** 2	**91** 23	**27** 24	**204** 1	**0** 1	**80** 15	**77** 44	**87** 55	**100** 21
Centra Health, Lynchburg, VA	**97** 72	**100** 479	**100** 572	**99** 563	- 0	**97** 79	**100** 222	**100** 1	**61** 1	- 0	- 0	**96** 219	**100** 616	**99** 818	**100** 168
Chesapeake General Hospital, Chesapeake, VA	**100** 46	**98** 267	**100** 229	**100** 227	- 0	**85** 52	**100** 88	- 0	- 0	- 0	- 0	**94** 220	**91** 475	**100** 548	**100** 112
CJW Medical Center, Richmond, VA	**100** 93	**100** 376	**100** 435	**100** 401	- 0	**98** 62	**100** 166	**100** 4	**4** 4	- 0	- 0	**100** 224	**99** 596	**100** 734	**100** 141
Clinch Valley Medical Center, Richlands, VA	**100** 5	**100** 33	**100** 22	**100** 28	- 0	- 0	**100** 5	**97** 63	**12** 70	**86** 1	**82** 22	**100** 32	**99** 150	**99** 165	**100** 28
Community Memorial Healthcenter, South Hill, VA	**100** 11	**100** 54	**100** 42	**100** 44	**67** 3	- 0	**100** 6	**94** 97	**8** 95	- 0	**50** 4	**100** 51	**100** 158	**100** 190	**100** 37
Culpeper Regional Hospital, Culpeper, VA	**100** 3	**100** 15	**100** 14	**100** 14	- 0	- 0	**100** 3	**100** 64	**16** 68	**60** 9	- 0	**97** 29	**82** 84	**94** 107	**100** 12
Danville Regional Medical Center, Danville, VA	**95** 19	**99** 166	**98** 132	**99** 132	**88** 8	**94** 17	**100** 55	**97** 35	**9** 37	- 0	**86** 7	**96** 130	**76** 264	**97** 343	**100** 86
Dickenson Community Hospital, Clintwood, VA	- 0	- 0	- 0	- 0	- 0	- 0	- 0	**95** 111	**6** 117	- 0	**25** 4	- 0	- 0	- 0	- 0
Eastern State Hospital, Williamsburg, VA	- 0	- 0	- 0	- 0	- 0	- 0	- 0	- 0	- 0	- 0	- 0	- 0	- 0	- 0	- 0
The Fauquier Hospital, Warrenton, VA	**100** 5	**100** 28	**100** 11	**100** 11	- 0	- 0	**100** 1	**98** 83	**8** 87	**79** 19	**50** 2	**100** 55	**93** 146	**100** 174	**100** 34
Halifax Regional Hospital, Halifax, VA	**100** 7	**100** 58	**100** 41	**100** 39	- 0	- 0	**100** 11	**91** 34	**4** 35	**69** 1	**100** 6	**98** 57	**94** 178	**100** 205	**98** 42
Hampton VA Medical Center, Hampton, VA	- 0	- 0	- 0	- 0	- 0	- 0	- 0	- -	- -	- -	- -	**95** 22	**100** 78	**100** 79	**100** 22
Henrico Doctors' Hospital, Richmond, VA	**100** 53	**100** 180	**100** 276	**100** 259	- 0	**100** 34	**100** 114	**100** 5	**8** 6	**47** 1	- 0	**100** 144	**93** 330	**100** 432	**100** 52
Inova Alexandria Hospital, Alexandria, VA	**94** 34	**97** 204	**99** 228	**99** 222	- 0	**94** 32	**97** 61	**89** 9	**0** 10	- 0	- 0	**98** 112	**67** 231	**95** 283	**95** 56
Inova Fair Oaks Hospital, Fairfax, VA	**100** 5	**97** 31	**89** 19	**95** 19	- 0	- 0	**100** 3	**91** 123	**10** 133	**60** 20	- 0	**97** 33	**89** 160	**98** 187	**94** 16
Inova Fairfax Hospital, Falls Church, VA	**100** 31	**100** 150	**99** 280	**99** 228	- 0	**100** 33	**100** 63	**94** 207	**6** 213	**36** 6	- 0	**92** 95	**88** 238	**99** 290	**100** 27
Inova Loudoun Hospital, Leesburg, VA	**88** 8	**100** 95	**98** 85	**100** 86	- 0	**83** 24	**100** 27	**90** 91	**7** 98	**72** 20	- 0	**98** 51	**95** 173	**99** 209	**100** 25
Inova Mount Vernon Hospital, Alexandria, VA	**80** 5	**100** 44	**94** 18	**100** 19	- 0	- 0	**100** 2	**96** 48	**7** 47	**76** 6	- 0	**98** 49	**91** 172	**99** 216	**100** 25
John Randolph Medical Center, Hopewell, VA	**100** 10	**100** 43	**100** 27	**100** 28	- 0	- 0	**100** 8	**100** 26	**8** 27	**49** 11	- 0	**100** 81	**97** 153	**100** 190	**100** 52
Johnston Memorial Hospital, Abingdon, VA	**75** 4	**93** 55	**91** 33	**92** 36	**100** 1	- 0	**83** 6	**97** 206	**4** 212	**35** 34	**100** 1	**68** 31	**82** 125	**94** 155	**62** 24
Lee Regional Medical Center, Pennington Gap, VA	- 0	**91** 23	**86** 14	**100** 12	- 0	- 0	**100** 1	**97** 29	**10** 34	- 0	**67** 3	**91** 22	**38** 80	**71** 91	**77** 13
Lewis-Gale Medical Center, Salem, VA	**100** 55	**100** 203	**100** 355	**100** 356	- 0	**98** 41	**100** 139	**100** 4	**9** 3	- 0	- 0	**100** 121	**98** 284	**100** 393	**100** 48
Martha Jefferson Hospital, Charlottesville, VA	**100** 36	**98** 164	**99** 155	**99** 142	- 0	**91** 43	**100** 32	**100** 3	**11** 3	- 0	- 0	**93** 129	**75** 273	**100** 321	**95** 55
Mary Immaculate Hospital, Newport News, VA	**90** 21	**100** 93	**98** 85	**98** 81	- 0	**94** 17	**100** 29	**83** 6	**46** 6	- 0	- 0	**99** 74	**94** 142	**99** 173	**100** 27
Mary Washington Hospital, Fredericksburg, VA	**99** 75	**100** 473	**98** 515	**99** 495	- 0	**96** 55	**100** 197	**100** 39	**12** 40	- 0	- 0	**100** 176	**89** 560	**100** 669	**100** 126
Memorial Hospital of Martinsville & Henry County, Martinsville, VA	**100** 8	**96** 68	**100** 50	**98** 52	- 0	**80** 10	**100** 22	**95** 174	**11** 179	**158** 13	**36** 11	**97** 93	**78** 195	**100** 253	**100** 56
Montgomery Regional Hospital, Blacksburg, VA	**100** 6	**100** 61	**100** 42	**100** 40	- 0	**100** 18	**100** 22	**100** 22	**10** 22	- 0	- 0	**100** 25	**98** 56	**100** 79	**100** 8
Mountain View Regional Medical Center, Norton, VA	**100** 3	**100** 17	**100** 10	**100** 12	- 0	- 0	**100** 1	**86** 21	**2** 24	- 0	**38** 8	**100** 24	**100** 84	**100** 101	**100** 15
Norton Community Hospital, Norton, VA	- 0	**100** 3	**100** 3	**100** 3	- 0	- 0	- 0	**93** 140	**14** 151	- 0	**0** 3	**100** 15	**94** 84	**98** 94	**100** 25
Page Memorial Hospital, Luray, VA	- 0	**100** 8	**100** 6	**100** 7	- 0	- 0	- 0	- -	- -	- -	- -	**77** 22	**89** 27	**100** 50	**100** 1
Piedmont Geriatric Hospital, Burkeville, VA	- 0	- 0	- 0	- 0	- 0	- 0	- 0	- -	- -	- -	- -	- 0	- 0	- 0	- 0
Pioneer Health Services of Patrick County, Stuart, VA	- 0	- 0	- 0	- 0	- 0	- 0	- 0	- -	- -	- -	- -	- 0	- 0	- 0	- 0
Potomac Hospital, Woodbridge, VA	**96** 23	**99** 108	**96** 55	**96** 47	- 0	- 0	**100** 9	**99** 157	**9** 164	**77** 4	- 0	**100** 65	**83** 240	**93** 260	**98** 46
Prince William Hospital, Manassas, VA	**91** 11	**96** 84	**100** 29	**100** 33	**0** 1	- 0	**90** 10	**96** 153	**5** 161	**43** 33	**100** 1	**94** 48	**80** 112	**99** 133	**100** 25
Pulaski Community Hospital, Pulaski, VA	**100** 21	**100** 53	**100** 37	**100** 45	- 0	- 0	**100** 8	**100** 59	**1** 66	**59** 5	- 0	**100** 23	**100** 65	**100** 88	**100** 5
Rappahannock General Hospital, Kilmarnock, VA	- 0	**100** 8	**100** 4	**100** 2	- 0	- 0	**100** 1	**97** 92	**8** 96	**63** 7	**33** 9	**100** 16	**100** 43	**98** 51	**100** 8
Reston Hospital Center, Reston, VA	**100** 13	**100** 103	**100** 79	**100** 77	- 0	**88** 25	**100** 20	**100** 24	**9** 25	- 0	- 0	**100** 29	**100** 144	**99** 172	**100** 12
Richmond VA Medical Center, Richmond, VA	**85** 13	**98** 50	**98** 54	**96** 51	- 0	**50** 2	**100** 15	- -	- -	- -	- -	**97** 137	**95** 262	**100** 273	**97** 58
Riverside Regional Medical Center, Newport News, VA	**100** 52	**100** 241	**100** 350	**100** 342	- 0	**92** 36	**100** 129	**100** 2	**5** 2	- 0	- 0	**100** 166	**94** 361	**100** 442	**100** 89
Riverside Shore Memorial Hospital, Nassawadox, VA	**100** 3	**100** 23	**100** 12	**100** 14	- 0	- 0	**100** 2	**86** 36	**15** 36	**206** 1	- 0	**100** 53	**95** 112	**100** 134	**100** 26
Riverside Tappahannock Hospital, Tappahannock, VA	**75** 4	**100** 24	**100** 13	**100** 14	- 0	- 0	**100** 5	**96** 46	**2** 45	**89** 5	**0** 1	**100** 33	**99** 76	**100** 93	**100** 15
Riverside Walter Reed Hospital, Gloucester, VA	**100** 3	**97** 39	**93** 14	**88** 16	- 0	- 0	**100** 2	**94** 48	**0** 51	**92** 13	- 0	**95** 41	**96** 91	**100** 128	**100** 15
Rockingham Memorial Hospital, Harrisonburg, VA	**98** 44	**99** 349	**99** 344	**99** 341	- 0	**100** 59	**100** 105	**100** 7	**12** 7	- 0	- 0	**97** 101	**91** 304	**100** 388	**100** 59
Russell County Medical Center, Lebanon, VA	- 0	**100** 10	**80** 5	**100** 3	- 0	- 0	**100** 1	**78** 59	**5** 58	- 0	**100** 2	**95** 20	**84** 79	**90** 89	**100** 20
Salem VA Medical Center, Salem, VA	**80** 5	**100** 43	**100** 32	**100** 32	- 0	**67** 3	**90** 10	- -	- -	- -	- -	**100** 66	**87** 121	**100** 143	**100** 35
Sentara Bayside Hospital, Virginia Beach, VA	**89** 9	**100** 80	**100** 70	**100** 70	**0** 1	**93** 14	**100** 22	**97** 226	**8** 225	**54** 13	- 0	**100** 66	**98** 186	**100** 219	**100** 36
Sentara Careplex Hospital, Hampton, VA	**100** 13	**100** 150	**100** 125	**99** 119	- 0	**97** 33	**100** 49	**100** 39	**6** 47	**53** 5	- 0	**100** 113	**97** 338	**100** 392	**100** 96
Sentara Leigh Hospital, Norfolk, VA	**88** 16	**99** 110	**99** 83	**100** 80	- 0	**94** 33	**100** 29	**100** 16	**10** 16	- 0	- 0	**95** 147	**99** 345	**100** 425	**99** 75
Sentara Norfolk General Hospital, Norfolk, VA	**99** 87	**100** 133	**99** 458	**99** 448	- 0	**87** 23	**100** 165	**100** 1	**20** 1	- 0	- 0	**100** 345	**95** 788	**100** 886	**100** 193
Sentara Obici Hospital, Suffolk, VA	**86** 14	**98** 125	**98** 88	**96** 82	- 0	**88** 26	**100** 35	**97** 78	**5** 78	**70** 13	- 0	**96** 145	**86** 331	**100** 416	**98** 80
Sentara Virginia Beach General Hospital, Virginia Beach, VA	**100** 63	**100** 196	**100** 241	**100** 252	- 0	**100** 42	**98** 93	**100** 7	**11** 7	- 0	- 0	**98** 118	**92** 360	**100** 453	**100** 75
Sentara Williamsburg Regional Medical Center, Williamsburg, VA	**100** 22	**100** 120	**100** 101	**99** 108	- 0	**97** 30	**100** 20	**91** 11	**7** 12	**44800** 1	- 0	**97** 77	**94** 225	**100** 275	**100** 62
Shenandoah Memorial Hospital, Woodstock, VA	- 0	**100** 6	**100** 2	**50** 2	- 0	- 0	**100** 1	- -	- -	- -	- -	**100** 8	**68** 31	**100** 41	**100** 4
Smyth County Community Hospital, Marion, VA	**83** 6	**100** 15	**100** 10	**100** 11	- 0	- 0	**100** 1	**95** 39	**21** 41	- 0	**20** 5	**90** 20	**78** 50	**99** 68	**82** 11
Southampton Memorial Hospital, Franklin, VA	**80** 5	**100** 12	**86** 7	**100** 7	- 0	- 0	**100** 1	**95** 55	**3** 55	**155** 8	- 0	**98** 61	**88** 108	**99** 133	**100** 28
Southern Virginia Regional Medical Center, Emporia, VA	**100** 8	**96** 51	**100** 26	**100** 28	- 0	- 0	**100** 7	**98** 44	**5** 47	**57** 7	- 0	**100** 62	**96** 197	**100** 219	**100** 43
Southside Community Hospital, Farmville, VA	**100** 2	**100** 10	**100** 7	**100** 8	- 0	- 0	**100** 1	**89** 93	**6** 96	**42** 3	**100** 1	**97** 58	**66** 118	**97** 149	**100** 32
Southside Regional Medical Center, Petersburg, VA	**95** 42	**98** 213	**94** 200	**96** 199	**100** 1	**94** 48	**99** 92	**93** 15	**1** 15	**154** 1	- 0	**92** 203	**97** 376	**99** 468	**100** 110
Southwestern Virginia Mental Health Institute, Marion, VA	- 0	- 0	- 0	- 0	- 0	- 0	- 0	- -	- -	- -	- -	- 0	- 0	- 0	- 0

NOTE: The first number in each column (boldface) is the score, the second number is the number of patients; Please refer to the main entry for footnotes; (a) 100-299
*MEASURES: **Heart Attack Care:** 1. ACE Inhibitor or ARB for LVSD; 2. Aspirin at Arrival; 3. Aspirin at Discharge; 4. Beta Blocker at Discharge; 5. Fibrinolytic Medication Timing; 6. PCI Within 90 Minutes of Arrival; 7. Smoking Cessation Advice; **Chest Pain/Possible Heart Attack Care:** 8. Aspirin at Arrival; 9. Median Time to ECG (minutes); 10. Median Time to Transfer (minutes); 11. Fibrinolytic Medication Timing; **Heart Failure Care:** 12. ACE Inhibitor or ARB for LVSD; 13. Discharge Instructions; 14. Evaluation of LVS Function; 15. Smoking Cessation Advice*

Hospital	Heart Attack Care 1	2	3	4	5	6	7	Chest Pain/Possible Heart Attack Care 8	9	10	11	Heart Failure Care 12	13	14	15
Spotsylvania Regional Medical Center, Fredericksburg, VA	- 0	- 0	- 0	- 0	- 0	- 0	- 0					- 0	- 0	- 0	- 0
Stafford Hospital Center, Stafford, VA	- 0	100 23	92 12	91 11	- 0	- 0	- 0	99 67	12 68	58 5	- 0	100 15	83 88	100 99	100 19
Twin County Regional Hospital, Galax, VA	- 0	93 14	100 7	100 10	- 0	- 0	100 1	98 104	9 117	190 4	64 14	100 37	97 88	100 122	100 15
University of Virginia Medical Center, Charlottesville, VA	98 65	99 161	99 322	98 289	100 1	80 30	100 126	- 0	- 0	- 0	- 0	98 131	80 240	99 282	99 74
Virginia Commonwealth University Health System, Richmond, VA	90 93	99 255	98 358	99 328	- 0	98 57	100 160	- 0	- 0	- 0	- 0	95 338	97 659	100 709	100 219
Virginia Hospital Center - Arlington, Arlington, VA	96 28	100 185	100 202	99 199	- 0	83 41	100 43	100 3	0 4	- 0	- 0	99 93	79 225	96 292	100 29
Warren Memorial Hospital, Front Royal, VA	- 0	100 8	75 4	100 5	- 0	- 0	100 1	100 33	10 33	- 0	- 0	91 23	83 47	100 55	100 8
Wellmont Lonesome Pine Hospital, Big Stone Gap, VA	86 7	93 44	88 32	92 37	- 0	- 0	100 1	92 63	17 66	65 1	0 6	96 28	72 86	99 108	100 22
Western State Hospital, Staunton, VA	- 0	- 0	- 0	- 0	- 0	- 0	- 0					- 0	- 0	- 0	- 0
Winchester Medical Center, Winchester, VA	100 67	100 157	99 333	99 316	- 0	93 30	100 137	- 0	- 0	- 0	- 0	99 208	90 573	100 660	100 129
Wythe County Community Hospital, Wytheville, VA	100 1	100 21	94 18	100 17	- 0	- 0	100 1	100 159	6 165	51 1	73 15	100 24	91 75	100 99	100 11
WEST VIRGINIA															
Beckley Arh Hospital, Beckley, WV	50 2	81 27	88 8	100 8	- 0	- 0	100 1	90 48	11 51	55 3	60 10	64 33	72 124	91 152	97 34
Beckley VA Medical Center, Beckley, WV	100 1	100 4	100 1	100 1	- 0	- 0	- 0					92 25	100 49	100 56	100 10
Bluefield Regional Medical Center, Bluefield, WV	100 3	95 42	88 25	94 31	0 1	- 0	100 6	93 121	16 123	155 4	29 17	82 62	72 178	98 193	76 33
Boone Memorial Hospital, Madison, WV	- 0	- 0	- 0	- 0	- 0	- 0	- 0					100 2	69 13	46 13	0 1
Braxton County Memorial Hospital, Gassaway, WV	- 0	- 0	- 0	- 0	- 0	- 0	- 0					47 17	55 31	71 35	100 3
Broaddus Hospital Association, Philippi, WV	- 0	- 0	- 0	- 0	- 0	- 0	- 0					- 0	62 8	100 9	- 0
Cabell-Huntington Hospital, Huntington, WV	100 7	97 32	100 18	95 19	- 0	- 0	100 3	97 34	11 36	112 13	- 0	96 45	87 121	99 150	100 36
Camc Teays Valley Hospital, Hurricane, WV	0 1	87 15	100 6	100 6	- 0	- 0	100 1	83 24	30 26	- 0	- 0	89 36	70 47	100 60	100 8
Camden Clark Memorial Hospital, Parkersburg, WV	100 15	98 172	98 108	99 104	- 0	50 2	100 24	91 56	14 55	69 13	- 0	99 76	89 255	100 362	100 42
Charleston Area Medical Center, Charleston, WV	94 218	98 469	99 997	99 996	0 1	67 73	100 410	100 1	53 1	- 0	- 0	92 259	67 610	99 684	98 133
Charleston Surgical Hospital, Charleston, WV	- 0	- 0	- 0	- 0	- 0	- 0	- 0					- 0	- 0	- 0	- 0
City Hospital, Martinsburg, WV	100 6	100 108	80 54	81 52	100 2	- 0	93 14	93 110	6 108	254 3	43 21	77 43	71 142	89 157	84 25
Clarksburg VA Medical Center, Clarksburg, WV	100 2	100 26	93 15	100 16	- 0	- 0	100 1					96 25	100 88	98 91	100 15
Davis Memorial Hospital, Elkins, WV	100 7	90 30	100 18	95 20	- 0	- 0	100 5	97 216	7 229	200 7	75 12	100 45	94 126	100 138	100 21
Fairmont General Hospital, Fairmont, WV	100 10	98 61	100 40	100 44	- 0	- 0	100 10	98 156	9 160	48 6	67 9	98 45	87 161	100 213	100 23
Grafton City Hospital, Grafton, WV	- 0	- 0	- 0	- 0	- 0	- 0	- 0					100 5	100 14	100 18	100 2
Grant Memorial Hospital, Petersburg, WV	- 0	75 4	100 4	75 4	- 0	- 0	- 0					83 18	77 35	81 68	67 3
Greenbrier Valley Medical Center, Ronceverte, WV	100 1	100 19	100 8	86 7	- 0	- 0	100 2	97 76	3 83	130 2	64 11	79 48	89 114	99 139	100 24
Hampshire Memorial Hospital, Romney, WV	- 0	- 0	- 0	- 0	- 0	- 0	- 0					- 0	- 0	- 0	- 0
Huntington VA Medical Center, Huntington, WV	100 3	100 23	100 12	100 12	- 0	- 0	100 6					94 66	100 157	100 168	100 43
Jackson General Hospital, Ripley, WV	0 1	91 11	75 4	100 4	- 0	- 0	- 0	97 104	10 107	- 0	81 16	100 20	78 83	99 103	100 12
Jefferson Memorial Hospital, Ranson, WV	- 0	67 3	- 0	- 0	- 0	- 0	- 0					100 5	84 19	100 28	100 4
Logan Regional Medical Center, Logan, WV	- 0	93 15	100 5	100 5	- 0	- 0	100 2	98 239	18 253	104 6	45 11	100 40	98 178	100 213	100 30
Martinsburg VA Medical Center, Martinsburg, WV	100 3	100 13	100 8	100 8	- 0	- 0	100 5					93 46	72 78	100 97	100 29
Minnie Hamilton Health Care Center, Grantsville, WV	- 0	- 0	- 0	- 0	- 0	- 0	- 0					- 0	- 0	- 0	- 0
Monongalia County General Hospital, Morgantown, WV	100 71	99 138	100 264	99 266	- 0	91 35	100 90	100 2	7 2	- 0	- 0	83 92	87 229	98 276	100 39
Montgomery General Hospital, Montgomery, WV	0 1	92 13	73 11	100 10	- 0	- 0	- 0					54 13	79 29	78 37	100 3
Morgan County War Memorial, Berkeley Springs, WV	- 0	- 0	- 0	- 0	0 1	- 0	- 0					50 4	62 8	80 15	0 1
Ohio Valley Medical Center, Wheeling, WV	73 11	95 66	100 38	98 41	- 0	- 0	100 12	88 33	8 34	56 15	- 0	90 49	96 127	98 177	100 27
Plateau Medical Center, Oak Hill, WV	100 1	100 12	100 9	86 7	- 0	- 0	100 2	98 131	12 139	50 1	40 5	85 13	83 54	99 78	100 14
Pleasant Valley Hospital, Point Pleasant, WV	100 2	91 22	69 13	77 13	- 0	- 0	100 1	89 76	10 78	66 10	100 1	58 36	92 87	98 116	94 16
Pocahontas Memorial Hospital, Buckeye, WV	- 0	- 0	- 0	- 0	- 0	- 0	- 0					- 0	- 0	- 0	- 0
Potomac Valley Hospital, Keyser, WV	100 1	86 7	80 5	100 5	- 0	- 0	- 0					91 11	76 34	92 38	75 4
Preston Memorial Hospital, Kingwood, WV	0 1	100 2	100 2	100 2	- 0	- 0	- 0	95 55	23 55	112 1	0 1	67 9	76 21	83 23	0 1
Princeton Community Hospital, Princeton, WV	88 8	93 60	87 38	100 36	- 0	- 0	100 3	95 187	9 201	244 4	71 17	97 68	98 248	96 282	100 35
Raleigh General Hospital, Beckley, WV	100 26	100 159	96 185	96 171	0 1	62 29	100 78	100 88	20 94	131 2	33 12	97 79	86 311	100 365	100 86
Reynolds Memorial Hospital, Glen Dale, WV	50 6	86 37	90 20	86 22	- 0	- 0	100 3	100 12	8 12	33 6	100 1	72 43	92 87	94 130	100 23
Roane General Hospital, Spencer, WV	100 1	89 9	100 4	100 6	- 0	- 0	100 1	97 38	0 40	- 0	100 3	- 0	67 6	100 8	- 0
Saint Francis Hospital, Charleston, WV	100 15	97 37	93 60	97 60	- 0	60 5	100 29	- 0	- 0	- 0	- 0	100 52	98 88	100 100	100 28
Saint Joseph Hospital, Buckhannon, WV	0 1	100 7	100 4	100 5	- 0	- 0	50 2	100 40	16 44	218 1	100 3	83 6	75 20	91 23	60 5
Saint Josephs Healthcare System, Parkersburg, WV	92 36	96 151	98 234	99 230	- 0	90 30	100 80	83 6	15 7	- 0	- 0	78 85	73 268	95 323	100 48
Saint Mary's Medical Center, Huntington, WV	94 77	98 357	100 576	99 560	- 0	97 64	100 257	- 0	- 0	- 0	- 0	92 136	90 451	100 525	100 102
Sistersville General Hospital, Sistersville, WV	- 0	- 0	- 0	- 0	- 0	- 0	- 0					- 0	100 2	0 3	- 0
Stonewall Jackson Memorial Hospital, Weston, WV	100 6	96 24	100 13	100 12	20 5	- 0	- 0	96 45	7 48	21 5	- 0	100 25	100 69	100 76	83 6
Summers County ARH Hospital, Hinton, WV	- 0	100 2	- 0	- 0	- 0	- 0	- 0					92 13	93 29	100 43	90 10
Summersville Regional Medical Center, Summersville, WV	80 5	88 17	90 10	100 9	- 0	- 0	100 1	94 81	14 86	310 2	69 13	88 17	37 35	94 53	78 9
Thomas Memorial Hospital, South Charleston, WV	70 23	90 114	94 80	91 82	0 1	64 11	100 30	88 17	25 17	- 0	100 1	90 52	85 163	95 207	96 27
United Hospital Center, Bridgeport, WV	100 54	100 192	100 195	100 189	- 0	100 33	100 91	97 33	13 31	- 0	- 0	100 126	95 212	100 258	100 46
Webster County Memorial Hospital, Webster Springs, WV	- 0	- 0	- 0	- 0	- 0	- 0	- 0					- 0	88 8	0 8	100 1
Weirton Medical Center, Weirton, WV	100 9	94 68	82 57	90 58	- 0	65 23	96 23	94 17	8 16	- 0	- 0	97 63	86 171	99 212	100 35
Welch Community Hospital, Welch, WV	- 0	0 1	- 0	- 0	- 0	- 0	- 0	90 140	41 142	- 0	18 11	50 2	8 12	38 13	50 2
West Virginia University Hospitals, Morgantown, WV	96 85	100 196	100 461	99 453	- 0	97 31	97 173	100 2	46 2	- 0	- 0	98 111	97 266	99 315	99 69
Wetzel County Hospital, New Martinsville, WV	100 2	92 25	64 14	80 15	- 0	- 0	100 1	92 72	13 83	59 8	100 4	72 18	80 40	88 58	100 3
Wheeling Hospital, Wheeling, WV	95 91	98 245	98 402	99 404	- 0	98 60	100 164	86 7	7 10	- 0	- 0	92 123	95 239	99 312	100 35
Williamson Memorial Hospital, Williamson, WV	- 0	94 16	100 12	100 12	- 0	- 0	100 4	98 46	7 59	165 11	50 2	90 10	100 83	97 92	100 24

NOTE: The first number in each column (boldface) is the score, the second number is the number of patients; Please refer to the main entry for footnotes; (a) 100-299

MEASURES: **Heart Attack Care:** 1. ACE Inhibitor or ARB for LVSD; 2. Aspirin at Arrival; 3. Aspirin at Discharge; 4. Beta Blocker at Discharge; 5. Fibrinolytic Medication Timing; 6. PCI Within 90 Minutes of Arrival; 7. Smoking Cessation Advice; **Chest Pain/Possible Heart Attack Care:** 8. Aspirin at Arrival; 9. Median Time to ECG (minutes); 10. Median Time to Transfer (minutes); 11. Fibrinolytic Medication Timing; **Heart Failure Care:** 12. ACE Inhibitor or ARB for LVSD; 13. Discharge Instructions; 14. Evaluation of LVS Function; 15. Smoking Cessation Advice

Hospital	Pneumonia Care						Surgical Care Improvement Project										
	16	17	18	19	20	21	22	23	24	25	26	27	28	29	30	31	32
CONNECTICUT																	
Bridgeport Hospital, Bridgeport, CT	**91** 67	**96** 106	**81** 81	**85** 102	**90** 123	**100** 31	**97** 117	**98** 468	**90** 184	**96** 76	**97** 303	**85** 467	**99** 307	**87** 427	**91** 267	**97** 117	**92** 95
Bristol Hospital, Bristol, CT	**97** 118	**87** 236	**96** 142	**100** 225	**96** 196	**97** 65	**98** 144	**99** 351	**100** 74	- 0	**97** 189	**100** 114	**95** 187	**96** 114	**97** 180	**99** 144	**100** 52
Charlotte Hungerford Hospital, Torrington, CT	**90** 68	**98** 101	**97** 117	**95** 123	**96** 169	**100** 44	**95** 101	**100** 312	**93** 104	- 0	**91** 199	**88** 160	**96** 199	**95** 151	**94** 190	**97** 101	**54** 26
Connecticut Childrens Medical Center, Hartford, CT	- -	- -	- -	- -	- -	- -	- -	- -	- -	- -	- -	- -	- -	- -	- -	- -	- -
Danbury Hospital, Danbury, CT	**97** 266	**95** 373	**89** 338	**98** 444	**88** 496	**89** 82	**85** 188	**100** 794	**97** 301	**95** 135	**98** 563	**92** 577	**98** 564	**97** 558	**95** 538	**91** 188	**96** 198
Day Kimball Hospital, Putnam, CT	**97** 86	**96** 155	**79** 76	**96** 155	**88** 121	**100** 35	**90** 99	**100** 328	**90** 100	- 0	**95** 258	**90** 110	**98** 256	**94** 101	**93** 249	**93** 100	**100** 11
Greenwich Hospital Association, Greenwich, CT	**90** 72	**93** 151	**85** 91	**98** 120	**91** 159	**100** 11	**88** 137	**100** 295	**92** 97	- 0	**96** 228	**96** 349	**98** 229	**97** 347	**94** 214	**88** 138	**89** 37
Griffin Hospital, Derby, CT	**98** 80	**98** 164	**95** 91	**99** 165	**98** 180	**100** 41	**98** 130	**100** 286	**92** 96	- 0	**97** 166	**94** 64	**95** 172	**97** 73	**97** 148	**98** 130	**93** 60
Hartford Hospital, Hartford, CT	**95** 185	**96** 397	**100** 255	**95** 349	**98** 384	**100** 130	**97** 175	**100** 759	**91** 263	**92** 155	**95** 451	**92** 610	**97** 464	**98** 604	**94** 437	**98** 175	**91** 186
Hebrew Home and Hospital, West Hartford, CT	- 0	- 0	**86** 7	**100** 8	**86** 14	**0** 3	- 0	- 0	- 0	- 0	- 0	- 0	- 0	- 0	- 0	- 0	- 0
The Hospital of Central Connecticut, New Britain, CT	**98** 290	**99** 518	**96** 318	**99** 442	**98** 405	**100** 153	**98** 355	**100** 975	**97** 322	- 0	**95** 723	**82** 236	**97** 723	**92** 201	**97** 691	**99** 355	**93** 265
Hospital of St Raphael, New Haven, CT	**95** 106	**91** 163	**85** 118	**95** 205	**94** 221	**100** 48	**97** 178	**100** 888	**92** 333	**85** 205	**96** 668	**89** 510	**96** 675	**84** 482	**97** 638	**97** 178	**92** 216
John Dempsey Hospital, Farmington, CT	**92** 76	**89** 151	**99** 77	**97** 130	**99** 132	**100** 18	**100** 85	**100** 302	**100** 83	**100** 16	**96** 196	**99** 202	**96** 199	**91** 200	**98** 189	**100** 85	**97** 95
Johnson Memorial Hospital, Stafford Springs, CT	**95** 74	**97** 142	**96** 77	**94** 108	**98** 125	**100** 39	**94** 96	**97** 182	**96** 48	- 0	**98** 115	**96** 113	**93** 114	**90** 110	**93** 110	**96** 96	**89** 45
Lawrence & Memorial Hospital, New London, CT	**81** 73	**95** 123	**93** 82	**94** 122	**93** 133	**100** 52	**92** 156	**99** 426	**94** 150	- 0	**98** 301	**96** 211	**97** 302	**96** 205	**96** 296	**94** 156	**92** 85
Manchester Memorial Hospital, Manchester, CT	**92** 133	**98** 233	**96** 150	**98** 201	**99** 230	**100** 63	**94** 234	**100** 507	**97** 153	- 0	**97** 301	**95** 184	**96** 304	**92** 177	**98** 283	**98** 234	**93** 75
Masonic Home and Hospital, Wallingford, CT	- 0	- 0	**91** 22	**33** 3	**94** 48	**100** 1	- 0	- 0	- 0	- 0	- 0	- 0	- 0	- 0	- 0	- 0	- 0
Middlesex Hospital, Middletown, CT	**96** 130	**100** 215	**95** 210	**96** 223	**99** 352	**99** 102	**94** 431	**100** 1160	**92** 343	- 0	**98** 700	**92** 164	**97** 702	**94** 160	**98** 683	**96** 431	**92** 254
Midstate Medical Center, Meriden, CT	**92** 127	**96** 197	**92** 120	**90** 204	**90** 199	**93** 55	**99** 212	**99** 601	**90** 177	- 0	**96** 402	**89** 158	**95** 404	**93** 157	**98** 369	**98** 214	**90** 113
Milford Hospital, Milford, CT	**96** 95	**94** 179	**95** 106	**97** 151	**98** 175	**97** 37	**89** 114	**100** 449	**97** 125	- 0	**98** 298	**95** 39	**100** 300	**100** 37	**95** 289	**92** 114	**98** 149
New Milford Hospital, New Milford, CT	**93** 44	**92** 53	**77** 35	**100** 57	**81** 57	**100** 16	**99** 76	**100** 252	**100** 73	- 0	**97** 187	**91** 77	**97** 189	**99** 70	**96** 185	**99** 76	**76** 17
Norwalk Hospital Association, Norwalk, CT	**98** 100	**100** 156	**85** 96	**96** 182	**88** 208	**100** 49	**94** 341	**100** 765	**91** 207	**100** 2	**99** 448	**96** 247	**98** 450	**88** 242	**97** 412	**94** 341	**70** 80
Rockville General Hospital, Rockville, CT	**84** 74	**99** 128	**96** 92	**99** 106	**97** 117	**100** 43	**89** 72	**100** 210	**89** 57	- 0	**99** 144	**96** 97	**100** 145	**98** 94	**99** 137	**96** 72	**79** 28
Saint Francis Hospital & Medical Center, Hartford, CT	**92** 71	**94** 210	**87** 109	**90** 176	**94** 181	**100** 61	**95** 180	**99** 850	**92** 320	**89** 166	**97** 603	**94** 756	**98** 616	**99** 777	**96** 587	**97** 180	**93** 227
Saint Marys Hospital, Waterbury, CT	**90** 111	**95** 175	**97** 72	**87** 169	**83** 144	**97** 39	**94** 173	**98** 615	**95** 193	**96** 101	**93** 437	**77** 123	**96** 443	**93** 104	**92** 431	**94** 173	**80** 66
Saint Vincent's Medical Center, Bridgeport, CT	**96** 180	**98** 325	**86** 198	**99** 317	**96** 292	**99** 82	**98** 149	**100** 520	**95** 184	**97** 125	**97** 357	**91** 229	**97** 364	**89** 211	**92** 330	**99** 149	**91** 117
Sharon Hospital, Sharon, CT	**87** 45	**96** 77	**100** 39	**100** 79	**100** 68	**80** 15	**85** 52	**100** 138	**100** 30	- 0	**98** 91	**96** 23	**95** 91	**100** 22	**95** 87	**87** 53	**82** 22
Stamford Hospital, Stamford, CT	**92** 136	**100** 208	**92** 133	**96** 196	**96** 195	**100** 48	**99** 152	**100** 439	**95** 130	**100** 36	**99** 297	**96** 428	**99** 302	**96** 422	**98** 287	**97** 154	**95** 61
Waterbury Hospital, Waterbury, CT	**86** 88	**94** 199	**79** 117	**93** 198	**90** 195	**100** 79	**98** 155	**100** 635	**90** 185	**83** 87	**94** 449	**91** 140	**97** 450	**94** 137	**91** 438	**99** 155	**95** 66
West Haven VA Medical Center, West Haven, CT	**93** 46	**98** 90	**95** 65	**77** 74	**99** 97	**100** 33	**100** 142	**100** 288	**100** 165	**98** 60	**98** 189	- -	**99** 203	- -	**92** 178	**100** 142	**100** 118
William W Backus Hospital, Norwich, CT	**92** 99	**92** 161	**81** 120	**97** 195	**87** 181	**100** 83	**92** 219	**99** 481	**92** 143	- 0	**92** 323	**92** 291	**97** 320	**93** 290	**96** 307	**96** 219	**92** 87
Windham Hospital, Willimantic, CT	**95** 80	**98** 131	**87** 68	**100** 126	**88** 97	**100** 41	**100** 88	**99** 155	**86** 49	- 0	**99** 90	**90** 63	**97** 90	**78** 58	**99** 85	**100** 88	**85** 39
Yale-New Haven Hospital, New Haven, CT	**75** 36	**93** 85	**67** 73	**95** 86	**74** 114	**100** 47	**93** 180	**99** 608	**87** 218	**90** 120	**96** 389	**87** 514	**98** 395	**65** 493	**96** 344	**94** 181	**82** 160
DELAWARE																	
Bayhealth - Kent General Hospital, Dover, DE	**90** 303	**95** 488	**93** 357	**93** 497	**95** 449	**99** 261	**88** 329	**100** 1203	**88** 414	**99** 158	**96** 886	**83** 211	**98** 893	**84** 200	**95** 808	**95** 329	**93** 220
Beebe Medical Center, Lewes, DE	**95** 190	**99** 290	**98** 165	**97** 273	**97** 260	**99** 99	**96** 264	**100** 1279	**99** 462	**96** 138	**98** 982	**95** 294	**99** 988	**97** 288	**100** 981	**96** 264	**98** 471
Christiana Care Health Services, Newark, DE	**85** 310	**87** 450	**73** 284	**92** 492	**80** 411	**100** 171	**95** 278	**100** 1096	**97** 321	**91** 195	**97** 716	**89** 903	**100** 725	**83** 872	**98** 682	**98** 278	**94** 249
Nanticoke Memorial Hospital, Seaford, DE	**97** 103	**100** 158	**89** 136	**98** 168	**98** 170	**100** 94	**91** 86	**100** 170	**100** 50	- 0	**97** 69	**93** 103	**97** 70	**80** 98	**90** 62	**95** 86	**89** 18
Saint Francis Hospital, Wilmington, DE	**92** 85	**93** 122	**92** 52	**96** 112	**90** 68	**100** 48	**94** 125	**100** 551	**94** 136	**85** 82	**93** 333	**95** 310	**98** 336	**94** 304	**94** 301	**96** 125	**90** 48
Wilmington VA Medical Center, Wilmington, DE	**81** 21	**97** 34	**100** 21	**83** 36	**100** 19	**88** 16	**93** 46	**100** 59	**100** 23	- 0	**95** 20	- -	**95** 20	- -	**100** 20	**93** 46	**100** 20
DISTRICT OF COLUMBIA																	
Children's Hospital NMC, Washington, DC	- -	- -	- -	- -	- -	- -	- -	- -	- -	- -	- -	- -	- -	- -	- -	- -	- -
George Washington Univ Hospital, Washington, DC	**71** 55	**94** 47	**95** 43	**97** 69	**88** 51	**97** 32	**98** 215	**98** 714	**93** 191	**96** 160	**97** 536	**97** 410	**95** 543	**93** 404	**92** 450	**99** 215	**82** 205
Georgetown University Hospital, Washington, DC	**95** 38	**87** 60	**85** 66	**96** 75	**93** 60	**100** 27	**99** 231	**100** 415	**95** 113	- 0	**96** 273	**94** 356	**97** 279	**96** 352	**95** 257	**99** 232	**92** 119
Howard University Hospital, Washington, DC	**92** 64	**92** 90	**89** 57	**75** 113	**73** 45	**99** 84	**88** 165	**95** 248	**82** 45	**62** 8	**77** 165	**23** 147	**94** 166	**73** 52	**84** 160	**88** 165	**88** 64
Providence Hospital, Washington, DC	**85** 120	**82** 170	**40** 149	**80** 188	**50** 158	**96** 85	**89** 175	**100** 364	**82** 67	- 0	**92** 249	**73** 281	**83** 250	**85** 231	**80** 237	**91** 175	**78** 93
Sibley Memorial Hospital, Washington, DC	**92** 87	**98** 135	**92** 74	**98** 105	**90** 120	**100** 22	**96** 269	**100** 635	**93** 135	- 0	**96** 466	**91** 265	**96** 468	**88** 264	**94** 454	**97** 269	**94** 146
United Medical Center, Washington, DC	**98** 87	**79** 115	**33** 79	**67** 153	**27** 73	**86** 105	**83** 65	**99** 110	**50** 24	- 0	**93** 27	**40** 25	**96** 27	**80** 20	**68** 25	**85** 66	**75** 20
Washington DC VA Medical Center, Washington, DC	**97** 33	**97** 60	**90** 50	**88** 57	**96** 49	**100** 17	**93** 96	**100** 227	**100** 99	**92** 106	**100** 144	- -	**99** 145	- -	**96** 140	**92** 97	**99** 87
Washington Hospital Center, Washington, DC	**98** 58	**86** 56	**93** 75	**98** 111	**94** 87	**100** 52	**99** 299	**100** 808	**98** 306	**98** 209	**97** 564	**95** 526	**98** 580	**96** 523	**96** 553	**99** 299	**92** 220
KENTUCKY																	
Baptist Hospital East, Louisville, KY	**87** 385	**94** 620	**96** 492	**96** 628	**95** 689	**99** 195	**90** 1105	**98** 4190	**92** 1285	**93** 266	**98** 2912	**96** 1548	**97** 2935	**95** 1554	**96** 2791	**95** 1106	**91** 479
Baptist Hospital Northeast, La Grange, KY	**82** 84	**98** 108	**99** 80	**98** 113	**99** 106	**98** 44	**94** 98	**100** 210	**95** 57	- 0	**97** 146	**86** 50	**99** 146	**98** 45	**97** 141	**95** 98	**60** 15
Baptist Regional Medical Center, Corbin, KY	**95** 214	**96** 225	**100** 188	**98** 253	**100** 256	**100** 151	**97** 130	**100** 316	**99** 106	- 0	**98** 222	**98** 215	**99** 223	**98** 210	**98** 210	**97** 130	**100** 55
Bluegrass Community Hospital, Versailles, KY	**96** 26	**100** 30	**100** 24	**100** 37	**100** 24	**100** 18	**92** 12	**100** 40	**100** 8	- 0	**100** 30	- -	**100** 30	- -	**93** 29	**92** 12	**100** 10
Bourbon Community Hospital, Paris, KY	**88** 33	**91** 53	**87** 38	**100** 51	**89** 46	**100** 18	**78** 9	**100** 13	**80** 5	- 0	**100** 6	**80** 5	**83** 6	**100** 4	**100** 6	**89** 9	- 0
Breckinridge Memorial Hospital, Hardinsburg, KY	**69** 26	**64** 11	**57** 21	**82** 38	**73** 30	**89** 19	- 0	- 0	- 0	- 0	- 0	- -	- 0	- -	- 0	- 0	- 0
Caldwell Medical Center, Princeton, KY	**79** 28	**87** 23	**86** 14	**91** 34	**83** 23	**100** 4	- 0	- 0	- 0	- 0	- 0	- -	- 0	- -	- 0	- 0	- 0
Carroll County Hospital, Carrollton, KY	**82** 22	**98** 41	**93** 29	**93** 56	**94** 35	**93** 30	- 0	- 0	- 0	- 0	- 0	- -	- 0	- -	- 0	- 0	- 0
Casey County Hospital, Liberty, KY	**83** 59	**100** 1	**66** 61	**96** 91	**77** 78	**96** 25	- 0	- 0	- 0	- 0	- 0	- -	- 0	- -	- 0	- 0	- 0
Caverna Memorial Hospital, Horse Cave, KY	**100** 14	**100** 17	**79** 19	**0** 1	**70** 27	**86** 7	- 0	- 0	- 0	- 0	- 0	- -	- 0	- -	- 0	- 0	- 0
Central Baptist Hospital, Lexington, KY	**95** 150	**98** 219	**99** 170	**98** 216	**99** 248	**100** 130	**95** 587	**100** 2109	**97** 709	**97** 379	**100** 1292	**99** 1921	**99** 1313	**99** 1907	**98** 1234	**96** 590	**88** 433
Clark Regional Medical Center, Winchester, KY	**83** 154	**92** 155	**95** 86	**96** 182	**97** 116	**98** 91	**84** 50	**100** 189	**76** 45	- 0	**94** 158	**76** 46	**97** 158	**95** 41	**88** 153	**92** 50	**84** 43
Clinton County Hospital, Albany, KY	**76** 78	**74** 19	**96** 48	**93** 57	**91** 58	**100** 39	**100** 1	**93** 14	**0** 2	- 0	**75** 8	**0** 2	**100** 7	- 0	**100** 7	**100** 1	- 0
Crittenden Health System, Marion, KY	**60** 45	**94** 31	**89** 53	**95** 59	**72** 69	**100** 33	**50** 2	**60** 5	**0** 1	- 0	**50** 4	**0** 5	**0** 4	- 0	**25** 4	**50** 2	**0** 1
Cumberland County Hospital, Burkesville, KY	**71** 14	**100** 6	**87** 31	**76** 45	**80** 40	**68** 34	- 0	- 0	- 0	- 0	- 0	- -	- 0	- -	- 0	- 0	- 0
Ephraim Mcdowell Fort Logan Hospital, Stanford, KY	**100** 48	**98** 66	**98** 59	**98** 93	**100** 83	**100** 47	**100** 1	**100** 30	**75** 4	- 0	**97** 32	- -	**97** 32	- -	**100** 31	**100** 1	- 0

NOTE: The first number in each column (boldface) is the score, the second number is the number of patients; Please refer to the main entry for footnotes; (a) 100-299
*MEASURES: **Pneumonia Care:** 16. Appropriate Initial Antibiotic; 17. Blood Culture Timing; 18. Influenza Vaccine; 19. Initial Antibiotic Timing; 20. Pneumococcal Vaccine; 21. Smoking Cessation Advice; **Surgical Care Improvement Project:** 22. Appropriate VTP Within 24 Hours; 23. Appropriate Hair Removal; 24. Appropriate Beta Blocker Usage; 25. Controlled Postoperative Blood Glucose; 26. Prophylactic Antibiotic Timing; 27. Prophylactic Antibiotic Timing (Outpatient); 28. Prophylactic Antibiotic Selection; 29. Prophylactic Antibiotic Selection (Outpatient); 30. Prophylactic Antibiotic Stopped; 31. Recommended VTP Ordered; 32. Urinary Catheter Removal*

Hospital	Pneumonia Care						Surgical Care Improvement Project										
	16	17	18	19	20	21	22	23	24	25	26	27	28	29	30	31	32
Ephraim Mcdowell Regional Medical Center, Danville, KY	**88** 138	**97** 180	**97** 220	**96** 285	**97** 273	**100** 156	**98** 189	**100** 514	**98** 146	**-** 0	**99** 337	**78** 267	**100** 337	**92** 231	**99** 321	**99** 189	**100** 102
Flaget Memorial Hospital, Bardstown, KY	**96** 85	**92** 106	**94** 66	**100** 100	**95** 83	**100** 54	**95** 74	**100** 301	**87** 98	**-** 0	**97** 223	**94** 95	**99** 223	**87** 91	**97** 220	**97** 74	**97** 90
Fleming County Hospital, Flemingsburg, KY	**81** 117	**91** 101	**92** 66	**94** 94	**86** 98	**84** 58	**89** 9	**100** 14	**33** 6	**-** 0	**70** 10	**81** 21	**100** 10	**90** 21	**80** 10	**89** 9	**100** 7
Frankfort Regional Medical Center, Frankfort, KY	**97** 68	**100** 121	**100** 82	**98** 121	**100** 114	**98** 54	**94** 144	**100** 253	**99** 75	**-** 0	**98** 132	**95** 241	**99** 134	**97** 234	**94** 127	**98** 144	**98** 51
Georgetown Community Hospital, Georgetown, KY	**96** 45	**96** 75	**96** 49	**100** 75	**95** 59	**100** 34	**81** 43	**100** 88	**96** 24	**-** 0	**98** 42	**99** 185	**100** 41	**99** 185	**85** 39	**84** 43	**69** 13
Greenview Regional Hospital, Bowling Green, KY	**99** 76	**98** 100	**100** 67	**97** 117	**100** 86	**100** 68	**96** 156	**100** 450	**98** 160	**-** 0	**100** 355	**96** 168	**99** 356	**98** 166	**98** 342	**99** 156	**98** 180
Hardin Memorial Hospital, Elizabethtown, KY	**92** 98	**83** 103	**92** 91	**93** 136	**94** 133	**94** 69	**87** 191	**100** 556	**90** 186	**95** 76	**97** 387	**96** 514	**94** 393	**91** 502	**77** 374	**86** 194	**87** 142
Harlan Appalachian Regional Healthcare Hospital, Harlan, KY	**92** 149	**95** 164	**100** 104	**97** 232	**100** 125	**100** 98	**100** 25	**100** 65	**100** 11	**-** 0	**97** 39	**94** 49	**100** 39	**94** 54	**100** 38	**100** 25	**100** 4
Harrison Memorial Hospital, Cynthiana, KY	**94** 115	**95** 123	**90** 69	**99** 136	**96** 121	**100** 53	**97** 38	**99** 77	**95** 20	**-** 0	**92** 40	**95** 38	**93** 41	**86** 37	**92** 39	**100** 38	**100** 9
Hazard Arh Regional Medical Center, Hazard, KY	**83** 75	**100** 32	**68** 82	**88** 116	**78** 88	**99** 70	**89** 128	**100** 354	**94** 152	**98** 84	**99** 210	**71** 127	**89** 212	**93** 126	**95** 196	**92** 128	**88** 66
Highlands Regional Medical Center, Prestonsburg, KY	**84** 144	**93** 153	**95** 132	**95** 240	**89** 173	**100** 98	**100** 41	**100** 85	**100** 16	**-** 0	**97** 31	**94** 141	**97** 31	**93** 134	**97** 30	**100** 41	**88** 16
Jackson Purchase Medical Center, Mayfield, KY	**89** 97	**98** 128	**90** 142	**98** 161	**94** 212	**100** 93	**99** 185	**100** 318	**99** 95	**-** 0	**100** 253	**99** 92	**100** 254	**100** 91	**98** 235	**99** 186	**97** 105
The James B Haggin Memorial Hospital, Harrodsburg, KY	**89** 36	**80** 50	**85** 53	**95** 44	**82** 71	**61** 41	**-** 0	**-** 0	**-** 0	**-** 0	**-** 0	**-** -	**-** 0	**-** -	**-** 0	**-** 0	**-** 0
Jane Todd Crawford Hospital, Greensburg, KY	**82** 22	**-** 0	**42** 19	**92** 25	**62** 24	**94** 16	**-** 0	**-** 0	**-** 0	**-** 0	**-** 0	**-** -	**-** 0	**-** -	**-** 0	**-** 0	**-** 0
Jennie Stuart Medical Center, Hopkinsville, KY	**90** 170	**92** 179	**92** 143	**92** 238	**89** 186	**95** 101	**96** 126	**93** 421	**85** 85	**-** 0	**93** 315	**87** 166	**97** 318	**92** 165	**87** 307	**90** 134	**75** 101
Jewish Hospital & St Mary's Healthcare, Louisville, KY	**93** 442	**96** 735	**87** 617	**94** 712	**92** 724	**100** 475	**88** 352	**99** 1108	**94** 409	**90** 181	**96** 705	**95** 1033	**97** 710	**97** 1011	**93** 650	**92** 354	**87** 218
Jewish Hospital - Shelbyville, Shelbyville, KY	**89** 81	**90** 92	**95** 73	**96** 116	**92** 88	**100** 55	**83** 66	**100** 138	**97** 35	**-** 0	**92** 65	**82** 33	**91** 68	**93** 27	**98** 64	**82** 67	**83** 24
Kentucky River Medical Center, Jackson, KY	**94** 64	**96** 72	**95** 58	**100** 116	**100** 79	**100** 65	**100** 12	**100** 21	**83** 6	**-** 0	**100** 9	**100** 75	**90** 10	**99** 75	**67** 9	**100** 12	**100** 3
King's Daughters' Medical Center, Ashland, KY	**94** 358	**96** 318	**95** 421	**96** 493	**95** 536	**99** 368	**91** 171	**100** 732	**97** 264	**100** 124	**97** 516	**81** 343	**99** 522	**87** 319	**97** 505	**95** 172	**87** 189
Knox County Hospital, Barbourville, KY	**70** 63	**94** 54	**100** 48	**94** 78	**97** 60	**89** 37	**67** 3	**60** 5	**0** 1	**-** 0	**50** 2	**-** -	**50** 2	**-** -	**50** 2	**67** 3	**100** 1
Lake Cumberland Regional Hospital, Somerset, KY	**93** 236	**96** 196	**97** 235	**98** 339	**100** 285	**99** 166	**95** 275	**100** 722	**97** 229	**96** 83	**98** 363	**99** 468	**97** 371	**96** 468	**93** 342	**97** 275	**85** 131
Lexington-Leestown VA Medical Center, Lexington, KY	**96** 94	**98** 179	**92** 103	**93** 162	**98** 151	**100** 43	**-** 0	**-** 0	**-** 0	**-** 0	**-** 0	**-** -	**-** 0	**-** -	**-** 0	**-** 0	**-** 0
Livingston Hospital and Healthcare, Salem, KY	**68** 25	**67** 3	**13** 15	**92** 26	**29** 21	**86** 14	**-** 0	**-** 0	**-** 0	**-** 0	**-** 0	**-** -	**-** 0	**-** -	**-** 0	**-** 0	**-** 0
Logan Memorial Hospital, Russellville, KY	**99** 145	**97** 99	**95** 131	**99** 170	**97** 151	**100** 82	**94** 16	**100** 23	**78** 9	**-** 0	**92** 12	**94** 18	**100** 12	**89** 18	**100** 11	**94** 16	**100** 4
Louisville VA Medical Center, Louisville, KY	**95** 87	**98** 151	**95** 101	**94** 147	**98** 117	**100** 81	**-** 0	**-** 0	**-** 0	**-** 0	**-** 0	**-** -	**-** 0	**-** -	**-** 0	**-** 0	**-** 0
Lourdes Hospital, Paducah, KY	**97** 148	**97** 183	**100** 169	**96** 205	**100** 194	**100** 94	**93** 401	**100** 955	**95** 347	**95** 164	**98** 761	**95** 276	**99** 773	**93** 272	**93** 710	**98** 404	**90** 173
Marcum and Wallace Memorial Hospital, Irvine, KY	**92** 38	**95** 42	**92** 40	**96** 51	**90** 59	**95** 21	**-** 0	**-** 0	**-** 0	**-** 0	**-** 0	**-** -	**-** 0	**-** -	**-** 0	**-** 0	**-** 0
Marshall County Hospital, Benton, KY	**74** 19	**70** 20	**60** 15	**82** 22	**55** 22	**44** 9	**-** 0	**-** 0	**-** 0	**-** 0	**-** 0	**-** -	**-** 0	**-** -	**-** 0	**-** 0	**-** 0
Mary Breckinridge Hospital, Hyden, KY	**88** 52	**97** 69	**88** 51	**99** 71	**96** 55	**97** 29	**-** 0	**-** 0	**-** 0	**-** 0	**-** 0	**-** -	**-** 0	**-** -	**-** 0	**-** 0	**-** 0
McDowell Arh Hospital, McDowell, KY	**66** 85	**83** 65	**85** 39	**83** 106	**93** 45	**100** 39	**-** 0	**-** 0	**-** 0	**-** 0	**-** 0	**-** 0	**-** 0	**-** 0	**-** 0	**-** 0	**-** 0
Meadowview Regional Medical Center, Maysville, KY	**99** 85	**100** 103	**94** 79	**100** 104	**100** 99	**100** 37	**100** 34	**100** 74	**100** 19	**-** 0	**100** 53	**97** 135	**100** 53	**95** 132	**100** 53	**100** 34	**100** 20
The Medical Center at Bowling Green, Bowling Green, KY	**86** 217	**95** 258	**93** 316	**93** 338	**96** 380	**100** 199	**84** 402	**100** 1480	**79** 461	**92** 245	**96** 979	**82** 540	**97** 987	**92** 483	**96** 957	**85** 405	**94** 377
The Medical Center at Franklin, Franklin, KY	**94** 70	**97** 31	**85** 62	**94** 88	**89** 80	**100** 35	**-** 0	**-** 0	**-** 0	**-** 0	**-** 0	**-** -	**-** 0	**-** -	**-** 0	**-** 0	**-** 0
The Medical Center at Scottsville, Scottsville, KY	**80** 30	**100** 8	**84** 19	**91** 35	**96** 28	**100** 9	**-** 0	**-** 0	**-** 0	**-** 0	**-** 0	**-** -	**-** 0	**-** -	**-** 0	**-** 0	**-** 0
Memorial Hospital, Manchester, KY	**89** 173	**94** 152	**97** 115	**93** 194	**96** 113	**100** 123	**63** 19	**100** 24	**100** 5	**-** 0	**100** 3	**79** 24	**100** 3	**79** 19	**67** 3	**68** 19	**67** 3
Methodist Hospital, Henderson, KY	**77** 150	**99** 154	**85** 143	**95** 231	**91** 191	**92** 105	**95** 75	**93** 218	**93** 56	**-** 0	**97** 138	**94** 225	**99** 139	**91** 220	**90** 135	**96** 76	**85** 52
Methodist Hospital Union County, Morganfield, KY	**88** 32	**78** 23	**90** 29	**89** 37	**89** 37	**100** 14	**-** 0	**-** 0	**-** 0	**-** 0	**-** 0	**-** 0	**-** 0	**-** 0	**-** 0	**-** 0	**-** 0
Middlesboro Appalachian Reg Healthcare Hosp, Middlesboro, KY	**95** 130	**99** 162	**96** 98	**97** 170	**97** 110	**100** 75	**89** 28	**100** 51	**90** 10	**-** 0	**100** 25	**93** 43	**96** 26	**100** 40	**92** 25	**93** 28	**75** 4
Monroe County Medical Center, Tompkinsville, KY	**86** 59	**70** 54	**77** 64	**94** 96	**81** 86	**83** 46	**-** 0	**-** 0	**-** 0	**-** 0	**-** 0	**-** 0	**-** 0	**-** 0	**-** 0	**-** 0	**-** 0
Morgan County Arh Hospital, West Liberty, KY	**89** 72	**92** 61	**100** 45	**97** 78	**100** 62	**100** 21	**-** 0	**-** 0	**-** 0	**-** 0	**-** 0	**-** 0	**-** 0	**-** 0	**-** 0	**-** 0	**-** 0
Muhlenberg Community Hospital, Greenville, KY	**90** 116	**100** 51	**88** 93	**99** 144	**88** 110	**93** 75	**100** 55	**100** 120	**87** 23	**-** 0	**97** 67	**17** 6	**95** 66	**100** 1	**91** 64	**100** 55	**91** 11
Murray-Calloway County Hospital, Murray, KY	**71** 114	**96** 105	**55** 118	**92** 161	**68** 139	**94** 67	**81** 109	**99** 268	**93** 69	**-** 0	**93** 167	**82** 187	**91** 169	**90** 168	**83** 163	**82** 109	**94** 52
New Horizons Medical Center, Owenton, KY	**87** 15	**93** 14	**80** 15	**96** 28	**62** 26	**71** 7	**-** 0	**-** 0	**-** 0	**-** 0	**-** 0	**-** -	**-** 0	**-** -	**-** 0	**-** 0	**-** 0
Nicholas County Hospital, Carlisle, KY	**59** 29	**71** 24	**87** 23	**94** 36	**68** 19	**100** 21	**-** 0	**-** 0	**-** 0	**-** 0	**-** 0	**-** -	**-** 0	**-** -	**-** 0	**-** 0	**-** 0
Norton Hospitals, Louisville, KY	**93** 538	**97** 935	**95** 671	**95** 892	**96** 779	**100** 475	**89** 969	**100** 3536	**93** 1186	**96** 516	**96** 2460	**90** 1238	**98** 2490	**87** 1190	**89** 2227	**93** 977	**92** 853
Ohio County Hospital, Hartford, KY	**85** 33	**94** 32	**62** 34	**97** 38	**69** 39	**89** 18	**91** 11	**100** 24	**-** 0	**-** 0	**90** 20	**-** -	**50** 20	**-** -	**89** 19	**91** 11	**100** 2
Our Lady of Bellefonte Hospital, Ashland, KY	**90** 170	**97** 223	**99** 217	**96** 275	**99** 256	**100** 161	**85** 148	**100** 544	**100** 144	**-** 0	**98** 380	**95** 203	**99** 379	**97** 197	**99** 341	**89** 148	**93** 158
Owensboro Medical Health System, Owensboro, KY	**91** 128	**96** 253	**100** 191	**93** 364	**97** 312	**99** 180	**92** 266	**99** 1045	**99** 394	**96** 219	**98** 791	**92** 890	**99** 799	**86** 901	**99** 771	**94** 270	**95** 195
Parkway Regional Hospital, Fulton, KY	**93** 45	**100** 47	**100** 28	**100** 63	**100** 53	**100** 26	**86** 7	**100** 26	**100** 4	**-** 0	**100** 14	**100** 1	**100** 14	**0** 1	**100** 14	**86** 7	**-** 0
Pattie A Clay Regional Medical Center, Richmond, KY	**95** 114	**87** 127	**100** 94	**99** 140	**98** 120	**100** 57	**92** 89	**100** 490	**100** 82	**-** 0	**98** 372	**97** 116	**98** 370	**99** 117	**95** 363	**92** 89	**94** 54
Paul B Hall Regional Medical Center, Paintsville, KY	**98** 122	**99** 195	**98** 128	**99** 212	**99** 174	**100** 143	**100** 27	**100** 33	**100** 6	**-** 0	**100** 11	**50** 2	**100** 11	**100** 1	**67** 3	**100** 27	**-** 0
Pikeville Medical Center, Pikeville, KY	**90** 190	**95** 252	**93** 235	**95** 316	**97** 308	**100** 195	**89** 274	**100** 856	**92** 334	**85** 124	**95** 623	**74** 144	**99** 627	**94** 108	**91** 597	**94** 276	**88** 257
Pineville Community Hospital, Pineville, KY	**79** 97	**86** 79	**83** 94	**88** 125	**88** 107	**77** 62	**94** 33	**100** 74	**73** 11	**-** 0	**93** 56	**-** 0	**93** 56	**-** 0	**74** 54	**94** 33	**33** 3
Regional Medical Center of Hopkins County, Madisonville, KY	**91** 105	**99** 187	**91** 168	**92** 271	**97** 220	**99** 158	**88** 253	**100** 789	**95** 256	**89** 123	**97** 550	**91** 140	**98** 557	**91** 138	**95** 518	**90** 255	**95** 172
Rockcastle Reg Hosp & Resp Care Ctr, Mount Vernon, KY	**89** 35	**100** 35	**95** 42	**97** 64	**100** 66	**100** 34	**100** 1	**100** 1	**-** 0	**-** 0	**0** 1	**50** 2	**100** 1	**100** 1	**100** 1	**100** 1	**100** 1
Russell County Hospital, Russell Springs, KY	**85** 68	**77** 65	**70** 47	**94** 89	**75** 61	**85** 41	**-** 0	**-** 0	**-** 0	**-** 0	**-** 0	**-** 0	**-** 0	**-** 0	**-** 0	**-** 0	**-** 0
Saint Claire Regional Medical Center, Morehead, KY	**92** 106	**92** 216	**96** 113	**97** 196	**91** 183	**97** 108	**96** 92	**99** 196	**92** 78	**-** 0	**88** 118	**91** 80	**97** 119	**91** 117	**90** 116	**98** 92	**71** 42
Saint Elizabeth Florence, Florence, KY	**88** 85	**96** 112	**97** 118	**93** 134	**96** 164	**100** 76	**90** 102	**100** 252	**95** 41	**-** 0	**98** 119	**88** 25	**99** 120	**72** 25	**94** 112	**92** 103	**56** 18
Saint Elizabeth Ft Thomas, Fort Thomas, KY	**94** 157	**97** 116	**95** 133	**98** 161	**97** 174	**100** 82	**97** 123	**100** 215	**100** 42	**-** 0	**100** 92	**63** 19	**98** 92	**81** 16	**97** 79	**98** 123	**75** 24
Saint Elizabeth Grant, Williamstown, KY	**100** 32	**100** 12	**100** 18	**100** 37	**100** 28	**100** 12	**-** 0	**-** 0	**-** 0	**-** 0	**-** 0	**-** 0	**-** 0	**-** 0	**-** 0	**-** 0	**-** 0
Saint Elizabeth Medical Center North, Covington, KY	**91** 68	**100** 62	**98** 90	**99** 122	**99** 115	**100** 81	**95** 166	**100** 712	**97** 226	**92** 156	**99** 487	**97** 593	**98** 493	**96** 592	**98** 460	**97** 166	**84** 88
Saint Joseph Berea, Berea, KY	**87** 39	**100** 33	**98** 42	**100** 56	**100** 46	**100** 38	**92** 26	**100** 41	**100** 10	**-** 0	**100** 27	**-** -	**100** 27	**-** -	**96** 26	**100** 26	**100** 5
Saint Joseph East, Lexington, KY	**96** 68	**92** 79	**96** 72	**89** 83	**96** 89	**100** 69	**91** 176	**100** 548	**95** 157	**-** 0	**99** 398	**98** 307	**97** 400	**96** 303	**96** 390	**94** 177	**86** 91
Saint Joseph Hospital, Lexington, KY	**93** 95	**99** 145	**97** 164	**96** 153	**99** 220	**100** 105	**94** 418	**100** 1230	**94** 496	**95** 439	**98** 685	**83** 878	**98** 706	**92** 868	**96** 638	**97** 418	**79** 247
Saint Joseph Hospital London, London, KY	**90** 121	**98** 178	**98** 85	**98** 152	**98** 148	**100** 114	**99** 98	**100** 401	**98** 176	**97** 124	**99** 272	**96** 291	**99** 279	**98** 283	**98** 221	**99** 99	**93** 59
Saint Joseph Martin, Martin, KY	**85** 60	**97** 66	**96** 25	**100** 70	**94** 33	**100** 37	**-** 0	**-** 0	**-** 0	**-** 0	**-** 0	**-** -	**-** 0	**-** -	**-** 0	**-** 0	**-** 0
Saint Joseph Mount Sterling, Mount Sterling, KY	**94** 83	**95** 103	**91** 54	**99** 89	**87** 83	**96** 46	**100** 51	**100** 219	**96** 80	**-** 0	**98** 185	**91** 35	**100** 185	**100** 34	**95** 183	**100** 51	**100** 86
Spring View Hospital, Lebanon, KY	**95** 41	**97** 67	**95** 38	**97** 73	**96** 55	**100** 13	**98** 80	**100** 238	**98** 51	**-** 0	**99** 187	**100** 24	**100** 189	**100** 24	**100** 185	**96** 81	**78** 46

NOTE: The first number in each column (boldface) is the score, the second number is the number of patients; Please refer to the main entry for footnotes; (a) 100-299

*MEASURES: **Pneumonia Care:** 16. Appropriate Initial Antibiotic; 17. Blood Culture Timing; 18. Influenza Vaccine; 19. Initial Antibiotic Timing; 20. Pneumococcal Vaccine; 21. Smoking Cessation Advice; **Surgical Care Improvement Project:** 22. Appropriate VTP Within 24 Hours; 23. Appropriate Hair Removal; 24. Appropriate Beta Blocker Usage; 25. Controlled Postoperative Blood Glucose; 26. Prophylactic Antibiotic Timing; 27. Prophylactic Antibiotic Timing (Outpatient); 28. Prophylactic Antibiotic Selection; 29. Prophylactic Antibiotic Selection (Outpatient); 30. Prophylactic Antibiotic Stopped; 31. Recommended VTP Ordered; 32. Urinary Catheter Removal*

Hospital	Pneumonia Care						Surgical Care Improvement Project										
	16	17	18	19	20	21	22	23	24	25	26	27	28	29	30	31	32
T J Samson Community Hospital, Glasgow, KY	95 101	98 60	98 95	97 154	99 153	100 95	79 128	89 292	93 107	- 0	83 260	75 173	92 261	89 142	80 260	78 129	80 81
Taylor Regional Hospital, Campbellsville, KY	81 98	97 103	68 107	87 128	76 134	84 67	89 97	94 223	80 45	- 0	95 135	87 77	96 134	97 73	89 133	90 98	75 16
Three Rivers Medical Center, Louisa, KY	99 94	100 84	100 73	100 122	100 72	100 71	100 17	99 81	100 12	- 0	100 71	93 15	100 73	87 15	99 68	100 17	- 0
Trigg County Hospital, Cadiz, KY	91 32	82 11	93 15	97 36	92 26	100 10	- 0	- 0	- 0	- 0	- 0	- -	- 0	- -	- 0	- 0	- 0
Twin Lakes Regional Medical Center, Leitchfield, KY	91 99	94 110	93 83	98 114	92 115	100 57	92 80	100 189	93 46	- 0	98 117	90 41	98 119	100 37	96 114	95 80	100 42
University of Kentucky Hospital, Lexington, KY	74 58	88 119	85 109	84 123	85 104	97 119	91 287	99 761	85 248	90 100	94 487	87 796	95 486	93 727	91 465	92 291	85 143
University of Louisville Hospital, Louisville, KY	88 67	83 103	69 75	82 121	79 52	99 109	84 160	96 421	64 107	98 58	94 271	79 277	95 279	90 238	90 246	86 160	76 71
Wayne County Hospital, Monticello, KY	86 37	94 36	76 33	100 48	91 55	81 16	- 0	- 0	- 0	- 0	- 0	- -	- 0	- -	- 0	- 0	- 0
Western Baptist Hospital, Paducah, KY	94 206	99 250	97 241	99 270	99 267	100 162	92 473	100 1128	84 372	90 244	95 713	94 628	98 724	89 619	89 665	95 484	83 279
Westlake Regional Hospital, Columbia, KY	93 91	- 0	71 68	98 121	78 96	89 63	- 0	- 0	- 0	- 0	- 0	83 12	- 0	80 10	- 0	- 0	- 0
Whitesburg ARH Hospital, Whitesburg, KY	93 150	92 108	79 105	98 181	86 113	100 89	100 20	100 63	92 12	- 0	96 46	96 121	91 47	93 118	91 44	100 20	100 2
Williamson ARH Hospital, South Williamson, KY	88 95	75 65	100 65	94 108	99 82	100 55	97 33	100 70	95 22	- 0	100 42	81 26	100 42	100 27	92 39	97 33	80 10
MAINE																	
Aroostook Medical Center, Presque Isle, ME	89 44	95 83	100 33	96 72	96 74	96 28	99 127	100 182	100 58	- 0	98 135	92 78	99 135	96 73	98 129	99 127	96 50
Blue Hill Memorial Hospital, Blue Hill, ME	92 24	94 31	89 18	100 23	85 27	100 6	93 15	100 51	90 10	- 0	95 20	- -	95 21	- -	95 20	93 15	100 1
Bridgton Hospital, Bridgton, ME	91 46	97 58	94 36	95 59	92 53	100 16	90 10	100 27	- 0	- 0	95 20	- -	100 21	- -	90 20	100 10	100 1
Calais Regional Hospital, Calais, ME	96 45	- 0	100 26	100 53	100 43	93 15	100 19	100 51	100 13	- 0	97 39	- 0	97 39	- 0	97 38	100 19	100 19
Cary Medical Center, Caribou, ME	97 32	100 39	100 22	100 41	100 39	89 9	96 47	100 107	94 36	- 0	99 67	54 28	97 67	90 70	97 65	98 47	94 18
Central Maine Medical Center, Lewiston, ME	97 69	91 139	91 90	100 137	95 120	100 60	95 171	100 655	88 199	95 121	96 477	96 502	98 485	94 600	95 452	96 172	84 92
Charles A Dean Memorial Hospital, Greenville, ME	100 1	91 11	100 4	100 11	100 8	100 2	- 0	100 2	- 0	- 0	100 2	- -	50 2	- -	100 2	- 0	- 0
Down East Community Hospital, Machias, ME	81 26	94 47	89 18	90 42	93 43	100 10	100 6	100 15	100 2	- 0	100 10	94 49	100 10	92 49	100 10	100 6	- 0
Eastern Maine Medical Center, Bangor, ME	91 108	98 220	98 191	98 201	98 212	100 144	98 403	100 1492	99 592	97 386	99 1031	95 820	99 1058	95 960	98 974	99 403	93 409
Franklin Memorial Hospital, Farmington, ME	97 30	94 71	100 46	94 88	96 68	100 17	88 73	100 222	94 66	- 0	98 167	92 50	98 167	92 59	95 165	92 73	93 45
Henrietta D Goodall Hospital, Sanford, ME	96 71	100 103	100 82	99 105	100 106	100 37	100 55	100 151	100 41	- 0	100 127	93 45	99 127	95 42	97 123	100 55	100 52
Houlton Regional Hospital, Houlton, ME	95 62	100 78	98 51	97 74	99 77	100 21	100 12	100 30	100 7	- 0	92 26	- -	100 26	- -	96 23	100 12	80 5
Inland Hospital, Waterville, ME	89 27	100 52	97 32	100 43	100 51	100 14	100 70	100 125	70 20	- 0	98 87	98 166	98 87	95 165	92 86	100 70	81 47
Maine Coast Memorial Hospital, Ellsworth, ME	95 44	87 55	59 51	97 74	99 94	100 42	99 177	100 240	89 73	- 0	96 159	85 34	100 159	94 79	94 151	99 177	86 73
Maine General Medical Center, Augusta, ME	97 154	97 235	99 167	96 248	99 216	98 84	96 222	100 751	91 222	- 0	98 598	97 398	99 600	99 393	96 586	96 222	94 227
Maine Medical Center, Portland, ME	93 111	89 338	97 207	97 303	96 302	100 91	99 208	97 818	96 316	96 174	99 606	93 883	99 615	98 858	98 599	100 208	94 164
Mayo Regional Hospital, Dover Foxcroft, ME	91 35	93 46	100 29	95 55	100 48	92 13	90 42	100 148	94 47	- 0	99 134	- -	99 134	- -	100 134	90 42	100 45
Mercy Hospital, Portland, ME	88 115	92 149	95 103	97 155	97 144	100 50	90 126	100 447	100 113	- 0	97 318	86 629	98 316	90 587	98 312	92 127	92 131
Mid Coast Hospital, Brunswick, ME	99 83	89 66	100 78	99 104	99 120	100 25	96 90	100 227	100 45	- 0	99 175	99 151	99 175	96 167	99 168	98 90	92 13
Miles Memorial Hospital, Damariscotta, ME	94 49	99 75	100 43	99 73	98 65	100 21	97 64	100 146	88 41	- 0	94 127	93 30	99 127	97 36	97 121	97 64	97 38
Millinocket Regional Hospital, Millinocket, ME	95 20	100 30	100 15	96 27	100 28	100 5	100 23	98 44	100 11	- 0	100 42	- -	100 43	- -	98 40	100 23	94 18
Mount Desert Island Hospital, Bar Harbor, ME	88 17	100 31	100 14	100 27	100 30	100 1	95 22	100 56	86 7	- 0	95 41	- 0	100 42	- 0	100 41	91 23	95 20
Northern Maine Medical Center, Fort Kent, ME	92 38	98 45	94 34	98 58	96 49	90 10	87 23	100 39	100 9	- 0	94 33	76 29	100 33	97 34	82 33	100 23	100 21
Parkview Adventist Medical Center, Brunswick, ME	82 39	91 46	97 33	98 53	96 48	100 10	98 44	100 68	100 21	- 0	93 43	48 33	91 43	94 16	95 42	98 44	60 5
Penobscot Bay Medical Center, Rockport, ME	94 64	97 92	98 65	98 88	97 90	100 37	92 74	100 270	96 76	- 0	98 210	86 59	98 211	96 84	96 208	95 74	80 10
Penobscot Valley Hospital, Lincoln, ME	100 27	100 36	100 17	100 38	100 35	90 10	100 6	100 8	100 3	- 0	100 7	- -	100 7	- -	100 7	100 6	100 1
Redington Fairview General Hospital, Skowhegan, ME	100 72	98 105	100 92	99 124	100 117	97 29	100 48	100 70	- 0	- 0	100 45	100 9	100 45	100 9	98 43	100 48	90 20
Rumford Hospital, Rumford, ME	91 23	86 44	100 28	100 42	93 42	100 13	- 0	- 0	- 0	- 0	- 0	- -	- 0	- -	- 0	- 0	- 0
Saint Andrews Hospital, Boothbay Harbor, ME	100 5	100 4	100 7	100 9	90 10	100 1	- 0	- 0	- 0	- 0	- 0	- 0	- 0	- 0	- 0	- 0	- 0
Saint Joseph Hospital, Bangor, ME	99 121	96 162	100 116	97 184	98 177	100 66	98 199	100 507	97 134	- 0	100 380	98 328	99 381	99 325	100 376	99 199	86 28
Saint Marys Regional Medical Center, Lewiston, ME	93 58	95 44	82 62	95 79	95 82	100 31	94 136	100 532	97 162	- 0	99 403	92 140	100 405	91 137	97 394	96 136	78 58
Sebasticook Valley Hospital, Pittsfield, ME	93 41	98 47	100 18	100 43	92 40	100 14	96 28	100 43	- 0	- 0	100 35	- -	100 35	- -	100 35	100 28	92 13
Southern Maine Medical Center, Biddeford, ME	96 80	89 81	98 91	99 125	99 121	97 38	94 101	100 304	90 102	- 0	97 194	93 61	97 194	91 58	100 190	94 102	96 57
Stephens Memorial Hospital, Norway, ME	91 45	97 71	98 49	98 94	98 85	100 17	92 50	100 172	96 45	- 0	98 118	96 93	97 118	94 90	97 118	96 50	93 56
Togus VA Medical Center, Augusta, ME	92 36	88 41	95 43	93 43	96 49	96 28	94 86	100 155	95 55	- 0	95 105	- -	95 104	- -	94 103	94 87	79 28
Waldo County General Hospital, Belfast, ME	96 56	100 34	100 46	100 76	99 79	100 18	88 51	99 154	96 49	- 0	97 112	- -	98 112	- -	96 105	88 51	93 43
York Hospital, York, ME	97 65	97 67	100 66	99 95	95 95	96 25	98 117	100 275	99 85	- 0	98 164	96 98	98 165	99 97	97 163	98 117	96 50
MARYLAND																	
Anne Arundel Medical Center, Annapolis, MD	90 252	88 423	83 271	91 371	93 407	100 130	86 290	100 1356	91 318	- 0	90 1050	- -	94 1046	- -	95 1006	89 291	92 309
Atlantic General Hospital, Berlin, MD	94 83	97 118	99 76	98 116	98 126	94 33	93 153	99 304	99 95	- 0	97 197	- -	98 198	- -	94 188	93 153	87 93
Baltimore Washington Medical Center, Glen Burnie, MD	92 452	93 653	93 389	96 581	98 493	100 220	80 322	99 958	86 326	- 0	95 659	- -	97 668	- -	89 628	81 323	82 156
Bon Secours Hospital, Baltimore, MD	98 94	91 183	64 102	89 167	68 78	97 150	83 83	99 130	82 22	- 0	83 42	- -	86 44	- -	65 40	85 87	80 25
Calvert Memorial Hospital, Prince Frederick, MD	96 116	92 168	92 88	98 172	96 141	100 59	92 72	100 326	96 54	- 0	96 258	- -	97 260	- -	95 254	99 72	97 64
Carroll Hospital Center, Westminster, MD	99 105	98 184	95 100	98 171	96 146	100 38	86 145	100 506	88 122	- 0	93 334	- -	97 335	- -	94 328	94 145	74 43
Chester River Hospital Center, Chestertown, MD	100 29	89 37	92 50	95 41	96 54	93 14	61 54	99 135	100 39	- 0	84 95	- -	93 95	- -	88 91	61 54	73 33
Civista Medical Center, La Plata, MD	97 124	99 203	95 99	96 204	98 160	100 63	93 153	100 394	84 77	- 0	96 240	- -	99 239	- -	96 206	94 153	85 88
Doctors' Community Hospital, Lanham, MD	95 219	87 343	64 177	95 301	85 226	100 82	87 233	100 482	- 0	- 0	97 353	- -	99 356	- -	89 339	92 233	87 122
Edward Mccready Memorial Hospital, Crisfield, MD	79 14	100 16	100 15	100 21	94 17	100 3	100 4	100 4	100 2	- 0	100 2	- -	100 2	- -	100 2	100 4	100 2
Fort Washington Hospital, Fort Washington, MD	61 18	91 106	95 38	91 106	96 56	100 25	92 75	100 203	85 20	- 0	92 130	- -	92 133	- -	92 130	92 75	65 17
Franklin Square Hospital Center, Baltimore, MD	91 306	94 391	96 299	97 474	97 399	89 199	93 335	99 1077	90 348	- 0	98 797	- -	95 809	- -	99 746	97 335	94 232
Frederick Memorial Hospital, Frederick, MD	97 250	90 216	93 236	96 411	96 415	99 150	91 172	100 730	93 241	- 0	98 590	- -	99 589	- -	93 569	92 172	95 288
Garrett County Memorial Hospital, Oakland, MD	74 27	100 38	100 26	98 43	100 33	91 11	94 70	100 202	89 61	- 0	93 155	- -	93 156	- -	88 151	93 71	36 64
Good Samaritan Hospital, Baltimore, MD	92 181	90 271	91 173	93 302	96 183	92 103	94 324	100 977	97 276	- 0	96 635	- -	99 643	- -	98 608	96 324	93 329
Greater Baltimore Medical Center, Baltimore, MD	94 156	86 249	91 203	92 236	92 298	98 48	89 336	100 1220	83 334	- 0	91 703	- -	96 712	- -	92 683	89 336	85 310
Harbor Hospital, Brooklyn, MD	89 254	93 356	91 191	97 341	91 215	99 218	91 199	99 820	91 194	- 0	97 665	- -	94 669	- -	92 653	93 199	86 141

NOTE: The first number in each column (boldface) is the score, the second number is the number of patients; Please refer to the main entry for footnotes; (a) 100-299
*MEASURES: **Pneumonia Care:** 16. Appropriate Initial Antibiotic; 17. Blood Culture Timing; 18. Influenza Vaccine; 19. Initial Antibiotic Timing; 20. Pneumococcal Vaccine; 21. Smoking Cessation Advice; **Surgical Care Improvement Project:** 22. Appropriate VTP Within 24 Hours; 23. Appropriate Hair Removal; 24. Appropriate Beta Blocker Usage; 25. Controlled Postoperative Blood Glucose; 26. Prophylactic Antibiotic Timing; 27. Prophylactic Antibiotic Timing (Outpatient); 28. Prophylactic Antibiotic Selection; 29. Prophylactic Antibiotic Selection (Outpatient); 30. Prophylactic Antibiotic Stopped; 31. Recommended VTP Ordered; 32. Urinary Catheter Removal*

Hospital	Pneumonia Care						Surgical Care Improvement Project										
	16	17	18	19	20	21	22	23	24	25	26	27	28	29	30	31	32
Harford Memorial Hospital, Havre De Grace, MD	**95** 132	**92** 211	**93** 104	**94** 183	**96** 125	**100** 82	**93** 75	**100** 220	**100** 64	**-** 0	**94** 146	**-** -	**98** 152	**-** -	**98** 139	**93** 75	**97** 68
Holy Cross Hospital, Silver Spring, MD	**94** 168	**96** 175	**98** 176	**96** 241	**99** 262	**100** 50	**96** 234	**100** 680	**99** 146	**-** 0	**96** 396	**-** 0	**96** 395	**-** 0	**97** 381	**96** 234	**99** 71
Howard County General Hospital, Columbia, MD	**95** 84	**84** 110	**91** 79	**97** 95	**91** 122	**100** 35	**93** 144	**100** 440	**88** 88	**-** 0	**99** 265	**-** -	**98** 266	**-** -	**91** 246	**97** 144	**92** 80
Johns Hopkins Bayview Medical Center, Baltimore, MD	**89** 183	**94** 273	**68** 241	**89** 342	**77** 304	**96** 187	**99** 259	**100** 743	**97** 233	**-** 0	**98** 579	**-** -	**98** 578	**-** -	**94** 567	**99** 259	**99** 284
The Johns Hopkins Hospital, Baltimore, MD	**93** 69	**98** 65	**75** 109	**97** 142	**76** 71	**100** 117	**98** 238	**100** 877	**92** 320	**94** 330	**99** 567	**-** -	**98** 581	**-** -	**95** 541	**98** 238	**75** 190
Laurel Regional Medical Center, Laurel, MD	**88** 98	**93** 175	**79** 110	**91** 159	**77** 135	**100** 35	**82** 50	**100** 167	**89** 37	**-** 0	**97** 112	**-** -	**94** 112	**-** -	**89** 108	**84** 51	**87** 23
Maryland General Hospital, Baltimore, MD	**84** 69	**87** 189	**58** 125	**86** 190	**85** 110	**96** 163	**78** 102	**100** 219	**75** 44	**-** 0	**94** 120	**-** -	**94** 117	**-** -	**87** 116	**76** 106	**62** 39
Memorial Hospital & Med Ctr of Cumberland, Cumberland, MD	**81** 31	**92** 26	**76** 21	**83** 46	**68** 28	**90** 21	**83** 48	**100** 245	**80** 90	**-** 0	**91** 190	**-** 0	**99** 194	**-** 0	**89** 189	**84** 50	**-** 0
Memorial Hospital at Easton, Easton, MD	**94** 216	**95** 306	**86** 162	**97** 293	**91** 260	**100** 96	**83** 222	**100** 881	**89** 253	**-** 0	**98** 609	**-** -	**99** 614	**-** -	**98** 601	**89** 224	**91** 217
Mercy Medical Center, Baltimore, MD	**96** 110	**95** 136	**92** 77	**98** 170	**94** 81	**98** 100	**96** 248	**99** 1112	**90** 250	**-** 0	**97** 910	**-** -	**99** 917	**-** -	**95** 884	**98** 248	**97** 411
Meritus Medical Center, Hagerstown, MD	**90** 320	**94** 346	**100** 218	**90** 517	**98** 429	**100** 211	**96** 350	**100** 1338	**95** 375	**-** 0	**98** 916	**-** -	**99** 917	**-** -	**97** 867	**99** 350	**90** 173
Montgomery General Hospital, Olney, MD	**99** 151	**97** 212	**94** 152	**99** 190	**98** 211	**98** 41	**93** 182	**100** 478	**95** 110	**-** 0	**97** 305	**-** -	**98** 314	**-** -	**92** 292	**93** 182	**93** 166
Northwest Hospital Center, Randallstown, MD	**96** 220	**93** 311	**97** 210	**95** 410	**98** 287	**100** 100	**89** 177	**100** 460	**89** 113	**100** 1	**95** 280	**-** -	**98** 281	**-** -	**97** 260	**89** 177	**94** 34
Peninsula Regional Medical Center, Salisbury, MD	**91** 186	**94** 264	**87** 191	**95** 343	**86** 354	**95** 104	**72** 133	**100** 566	**88** 209	**89** 129	**95** 411	**-** -	**95** 419	**-** -	**95** 396	**74** 133	**89** 142
Prince Georges Hospital Center, Cheverly, MD	**84** 63	**87** 84	**47** 73	**85** 46	**47** 88	**90** 60	**45** 105	**99** 250	**-** 0	**86** 14	**91** 135	**-** -	**93** 137	**-** -	**75** 126	**50** 105	**65** 48
Saint Agnes Hospital, Baltimore, MD	**93** 72	**87** 166	**94** 79	**93** 162	**94** 108	**92** 62	**99** 177	**99** 686	**98** 161	**-** 0	**97** 519	**-** -	**98** 521	**-** -	**94** 489	**98** 178	**95** 129
Saint Joseph Medical Center, Towson, MD	**92** 95	**96** 135	**87** 54	**95** 148	**96** 164	**100** 38	**97** 102	**99** 568	**95** 224	**96** 118	**97** 369	**-** -	**98** 384	**-** -	**97** 340	**98** 102	**88** 74
Saint Mary's Hospital, Leonardtown, MD	**97** 73	**97** 111	**95** 85	**98** 125	**98** 102	**100** 40	**95** 66	**100** 369	**100** 86	**-** 0	**99** 302	**-** -	**98** 304	**-** -	**97** 297	**95** 66	**98** 118
Shady Grove Adventist Hospital, Rockville, MD	**93** 90	**94** 101	**78** 80	**97** 121	**73** 133	**94** 36	**91** 152	**100** 464	**94** 123	**-** 0	**96** 325	**-** -	**97** 323	**-** -	**91** 310	**94** 152	**99** 118
Sinai Hospital of Baltimore, Baltimore, MD	**89** 158	**90** 296	**93** 190	**94** 290	**93** 251	**100** 112	**88** 299	**100** 985	**95** 274	**91** 233	**97** 677	**-** -	**97** 685	**-** -	**95** 626	**89** 299	**92** 276
Southern Maryland Hospital Center, Clinton, MD	**89** 123	**85** 160	**95** 95	**93** 182	**96** 131	**100** 66	**94** 208	**100** 682	**93** 153	**-** 0	**99** 476	**-** -	**95** 481	**-** -	**95** 460	**97** 208	**91** 69
Suburban Hospital, Bethesda, MD	**88** 146	**86** 241	**80** 133	**96** 209	**73** 224	**100** 21	**92** 258	**100** 1268	**98** 384	**93** 205	**95** 1065	**-** -	**97** 1067	**-** -	**94** 1058	**91** 261	**99** 337
Union Hospital of Cecil County, Elkton, MD	**92** 116	**98** 196	**100** 115	**94** 202	**96** 165	**92** 143	**89** 142	**100** 429	**88** 92	**-** 0	**98** 272	**-** -	**95** 276	**-** -	**94** 261	**90** 142	**91** 98
Union Memorial Hospital, Baltimore, MD	**91** 118	**88** 185	**94** 138	**96** 219	**96** 159	**91** 86	**97** 250	**99** 1727	**96** 506	**88** 173	**96** 1511	**-** -	**99** 1512	**-** -	**97** 1487	**97** 250	**91** 116
University of Maryland Medical Center, Baltimore, MD	**91** 98	**88** 229	**91** 150	**93** 223	**92** 131	**99** 190	**96** 669	**97** 1727	**78** 603	**93** 510	**95** 823	**-** -	**98** 857	**-** -	**93** 780	**97** 673	**80** 455
Upper Chesapeake Medical Center, Bel Air, MD	**98** 249	**99** 446	**93** 199	**96** 387	**98** 278	**100** 113	**98** 181	**100** 607	**92** 181	**-** 0	**95** 421	**-** -	**94** 435	**-** -	**94** 407	**98** 181	**91** 140
VA Maryland Healthcare System - Baltimore, Baltimore, MD	**96** 100	**99** 157	**91** 81	**92** 159	**100** 103	**100** 70	**95** 113	**100** 140	**98** 51	**-** 0	**98** 66	**-** -	**98** 66	**-** -	**97** 63	**96** 113	**88** 49
Washington Adventist Hospital, Takoma Park, MD	**96** 55	**98** 112	**72** 67	**97** 117	**81** 119	**100** 18	**89** 123	**100** 492	**79** 169	**86** 137	**97** 344	**-** -	**98** 351	**-** -	**94** 334	**94** 123	**90** 125
Western Maryland Regional Medical Center, Cumberland, MD	**84** 183	**91** 180	**82** 196	**85** 267	**87** 260	**90** 87	**79** 214	**100** 768	**83** 263	**88** 206	**91** 503	**-** 0	**98** 512	**-** 0	**88** 488	**80** 216	**63** 76
MASSACHUSETTS																	
Adcare Hospital of Worcester, Worcester, MA	**-** 0	**-** 0	**-** 0	**-** 0	**-** 0	**-** 0	**-** 0	**-** 0	**-** 0	**-** 0	**-** 0	**-** 0	**-** 0	**-** 0	**-** 0	**-** 0	**-** 0
Anna Jaques Hospital, Newburyport, MA	**95** 124	**99** 136	**98** 112	**97** 181	**98** 171	**100** 55	**95** 204	**100** 346	**93** 115	**-** 0	**99** 220	**93** 133	**97** 222	**91** 131	**95** 213	**95** 204	**78** 41
Athol Memorial Hospital, Athol, MA	**79** 24	**93** 45	**91** 34	**98** 45	**98** 43	**100** 9	**100** 11	**100** 19	**67** 6	**-** 0	**100** 15	**-** -	**93** 15	**-** -	**93** 15	**92** 12	**100** 8
Baystate Franklin Medical Center, Greenfield, MA	**95** 78	**96** 137	**93** 76	**94** 133	**94** 133	**100** 29	**96** 141	**100** 205	**94** 64	**-** 0	**98** 119	**98** 85	**99** 119	**93** 84	**94** 115	**99** 141	**69** 32
Baystate Mary Lane Hospital, Ware, MA	**92** 37	**98** 47	**100** 23	**95** 38	**97** 34	**100** 15	**100** 13	**100** 45	**100** 10	**-** 0	**94** 35	**100** 1	**97** 34	**100** 1	**97** 34	**100** 13	**100** 4
Baystate Medical Center, Springfield, MA	**91** 268	**84** 410	**86** 301	**91** 503	**89** 386	**95** 158	**99** 320	**100** 1670	**97** 580	**97** 341	**99** 1436	**92** 669	**100** 1446	**98** 645	**99** 1380	**100** 320	**100** 687
Bedford VA Medical Center, Bedford, MA	**-** 0	**-** 0	**-** 0	**-** 0	**-** 0	**-** 0	**-** 0	**-** 0	**-** 0	**-** 0	**-** 0	**-** 0	**-** 0	**-** 0	**-** 0	**-** 0	**-** 0
Berkshire Medical Center, Pittsfield, MA	**99** 148	**99** 283	**95** 195	**98** 250	**98** 282	**100** 69	**98** 335	**100** 721	**100** 236	**-** 0	**98** 441	**98** 279	**98** 441	**98** 276	**98** 432	**98** 335	**93** 166
Beth Israel Deaconess Hospital - Needham, Needham, MA	**95** 61	**95** 84	**95** 64	**97** 78	**87** 100	**89** 9	**100** 60	**99** 127	**93** 43	**-** 0	**94** 84	**96** 70	**99** 85	**94** 70	**99** 81	**100** 60	**97** 33
Beth Israel Deaconess Medical Center, Boston, MA	**93** 113	**96** 248	**91** 75	**97** 210	**84** 245	**100** 75	**99** 417	**99** 1243	**100** 482	**95** 242	**99** 632	**85** 480	**98** 707	**89** 448	**98** 614	**99** 417	**91** 264
Beverly Hospital Corporation, Beverly, MA	**97** 229	**97** 373	**89** 211	**99** 362	**92** 322	**100** 88	**98** 448	**100** 1136	**97** 339	**-** 0	**99** 838	**97** 280	**99** 841	**96** 278	**99** 803	**98** 448	**95** 344
Boston Medical Center Corporation, Boston, MA	**93** 144	**96** 136	**80** 230	**96** 230	**85** 231	**97** 260	**100** 551	**100** 1127	**92** 462	**96** 247	**98** 884	**89** 298	**99** 895	**93** 297	**87** 865	**100** 551	**98** 266
Brigham and Women's Hospital, Boston, MA	**100** 23	**98** 65	**92** 73	**99** 68	**98** 86	**96** 25	**98** 252	**100** 691	**93** 256	**97** 147	**99** 427	**91** 364	**98** 435	**93** 352	**94** 415	**98** 254	**87** 167
Cambridge Health Alliance, Cambridge, MA	**96** 156	**95** 278	**95** 159	**98** 248	**97** 206	**93** 117	**97** 172	**100** 289	**96** 70	**-** 0	**95** 185	**90** 71	**97** 189	**99** 71	**98** 180	**98** 173	**97** 87
Cape Cod Hospital, Hyannis, MA	**92** 214	**91** 251	**95** 173	**98** 284	**93** 301	**92** 80	**99** 360	**100** 1174	**95** 404	**93** 184	**99** 969	**96** 470	**98** 979	**95** 465	**97** 943	**99** 360	**94** 321
Carney Hospital, Boston, MA	**89** 62	**93** 69	**92** 61	**97** 86	**97** 88	**100** 42	**98** 142	**100** 208	**98** 62	**-** 0	**98** 127	**65** 34	**94** 126	**88** 26	**90** 116	**98** 142	**83** 30
Children's Hospital Boston, Boston, MA	**-** -	**-** -	**-** -	**-** -	**-** -	**-** -	**-** -	**-** -	**-** -	**-** -	**-** -	**-** -	**-** -	**-** -	**-** -	**-** -	**-** -
Clinton Hospital Association, Clinton, MA	**100** 31	**83** 36	**92** 24	**97** 39	**82** 50	**100** 7	**75** 4	**100** 5	**100** 3	**-** 0	**100** 1	**-** 0	**0** 1	**-** 0	**100** 1	**75** 4	**-** 0
The Cooley Dickinson Hospital, Northampton, MA	**96** 124	**96** 194	**95** 131	**96** 196	**95** 168	**94** 66	**89** 145	**100** 456	**98** 109	**-** 0	**98** 292	**99** 149	**98** 293	**100** 148	**100** 284	**92** 147	**94** 162
Dana-Farber Cancer Institute, Boston, MA	**100** 2	**100** 14	**87** 15	**100** 7	**93** 14	**100** 4	**-** 0	**-** 0	**-** 0	**-** 0	**-** 0	**-** -	**-** 0	**-** -	**-** 0	**-** 0	**-** 0
Emerson Hospital, West Concord, MA	**94** 87	**97** 171	**95** 113	**97** 172	**95** 188	**96** 24	**91** 217	**100** 529	**91** 139	**-** 0	**92** 361	**94** 278	**99** 361	**96** 272	**98** 345	**96** 217	**88** 176
Fairview Hospital, Great Barrington, MA	**100** 38	**98** 63	**100** 42	**100** 59	**98** 65	**100** 16	**97** 33	**100** 80	**96** 27	**-** 0	**100** 55	**-** -	**100** 56	**-** -	**100** 55	**97** 33	**100** 7
Falmouth Hospital, Falmouth, MA	**99** 106	**99** 197	**94** 124	**98** 181	**97** 177	**100** 40	**95** 202	**100** 644	**100** 143	**-** 0	**99** 506	**100** 80	**98** 509	**96** 80	**99** 490	**95** 202	**98** 225
Faulkner Hospital, Boston, MA	**90** 86	**97** 143	**98** 91	**97** 148	**99** 142	**100** 25	**99** 84	**98** 242	**100** 49	**-** 0	**99** 134	**97** 224	**98** 137	**96** 224	**98** 131	**99** 84	**96** 45
Good Samaritan Medical Center, Brockton, MA	**98** 233	**97** 233	**96** 255	**94** 375	**91** 348	**96** 109	**99** 247	**100** 706	**98** 215	**-** 0	**98** 559	**92** 219	**98** 560	**95** 202	**94** 534	**99** 247	**76** 34
Hallmark Health System, Melrose, MA	**92** 117	**94** 187	**91** 133	**97** 188	**95** 204	**98** 45	**90** 193	**100** 389	**92** 133	**0** 1	**98** 249	**94** 117	**95** 250	**94** 113	**96** 240	**91** 194	**89** 98
Harrington Memorial Hospital, Southbridge, MA	**85** 107	**89** 113	**82** 84	**97** 130	**86** 138	**83** 42	**85** 66	**99** 139	**100** 35	**-** 0	**88** 83	**85** 125	**95** 83	**87** 122	**94** 78	**85** 66	**97** 36
Healthalliance Hospitals, Leominster, MA	**90** 143	**97** 275	**99** 148	**97** 241	**98** 206	**95** 75	**95** 186	**100** 404	**94** 124	**-** 0	**97** 283	**88** 86	**100** 283	**91** 89	**97** 272	**97** 186	**96** 98
Heywood Hospital, Gardner, MA	**89** 95	**96** 111	**95** 76	**97** 134	**94** 125	**90** 58	**85** 96	**98** 282	**92** 87	**-** 0	**99** 232	**48** 81	**98** 232	**94** 66	**99** 226	**90** 96	**82** 94
Holy Family Hospital, Methuen, MA	**92** 111	**96** 98	**96** 107	**96** 155	**92** 154	**94** 63	**86** 123	**100** 529	**97** 182	**-** 0	**98** 411	**87** 112	**97** 413	**93** 100	**96** 402	**87** 123	**84** 167
Holyoke Medical Center, Holyoke, MA	**87** 108	**91** 201	**98** 121	**93** 188	**99** 159	**83** 66	**85** 114	**100** 234	**91** 69	**-** 0	**96** 147	**96** 84	**100** 146	**98** 82	**95** 138	**88** 114	**76** 46
Jordan Hospital, Plymouth, MA	**94** 203	**96** 277	**92** 220	**97** 372	**93** 301	**98** 94	**99** 159	**100** 579	**91** 174	**-** 0	**96** 428	**95** 77	**98** 429	**97** 76	**99** 420	**99** 160	**91** 77
Lahey Clinic Hospital, Burlington, MA	**95** 55	**99** 81	**90** 78	**87** 95	**90** 133	**77** 26	**100** 231	**100** 641	**100** 262	**88** 126	**99** 396	**86** 370	**100** 398	**96** 596	**95** 376	**100** 231	**80** 95
Lawrence General Hospital, Lawrence, MA	**86** 127	**94** 160	**78** 125	**93** 220	**95** 205	**85** 61	**79** 145	**95** 301	**93** 86	**-** 0	**98** 137	**71** 85	**88** 146	**93** 81	**90** 131	**83** 145	**58** 50
Lowell General Hospital, Lowell, MA	**97** 146	**92** 143	**94** 78	**96** 187	**87** 157	**93** 60	**92** 172	**100** 606	**94** 201	**-** 0	**97** 428	**93** 290	**98** 429	**98** 283	**93** 404	**93** 172	**98** 107
Marlborough Hospital, Marlborough, MA	**96** 81	**94** 157	**100** 99	**97** 148	**98** 148	**100** 41	**96** 93	**98** 208	**92** 64	**-** 0	**95** 155	**94** 52	**99** 155	**92** 49	**95** 152	**96** 93	**81** 68
Martha's Vineyard Hospital, Oak Bluffs, MA	**88** 24	**91** 23	**50** 18	**100** 38	**42** 40	**100** 3	**-** 0	**-** 0	**-** 0	**-** 0	**-** 0	**-** -	**-** 0	**-** -	**-** 0	**-** 0	**-** 0
Massachusetts Eye and Ear Infirmary, Boston, MA	**-** 0	**-** 0	**-** 0	**-** 0	**-** 0	**-** 0	**100** 2	**100** 7	**-** 0	**-** 0	**-** 0	**42** 12	**-** 0	**36** 11	**-** 0	**100** 2	**100** 3

NOTE: The first number in each column (boldface) is the score, the second number is the number of patients; Please refer to the main entry for footnotes; (a) 100-299
*MEASURES: **Pneumonia Care:** 16. Appropriate Initial Antibiotic; 17. Blood Culture Timing; 18. Influenza Vaccine; 19. Initial Antibiotic Timing; 20. Pneumococcal Vaccine; 21. Smoking Cessation Advice; **Surgical Care Improvement Project:** 22. Appropriate VTP Within 24 Hours; 23. Appropriate Hair Removal; 24. Appropriate Beta Blocker Usage; 25. Controlled Postoperative Blood Glucose; 26. Prophylactic Antibiotic Timing; 27. Prophylactic Antibiotic Timing (Outpatient); 28. Prophylactic Antibiotic Selection; 29. Prophylactic Antibiotic Selection (Outpatient); 30. Prophylactic Antibiotic Stopped; 31. Recommended VTP Ordered; 32. Urinary Catheter Removal*

Hospital	Pneumonia Care							Surgical Care Improvement Project									
	16	17	18	19	20	21	22	23	24	25	26	27	28	29	30	31	32
Massachusetts General Hospital, Boston, MA	**94** 63	**94** 82	**95** 61	**98** 101	**91** 161	**100** 39	**96** 267	**96** 752	**94** 279	**93** 129	**98** 440	**74** 479	**96** 446	**90** 477	**94** 377	**100** 268	**88** 179
Mercy Medical Center, Springfield, MA	**97** 146	**96** 213	**96** 140	**99** 211	**94** 190	**97** 75	**98** 482	**100** 977	**93** 256	- 0	**95** 532	**96** 658	**97** 537	**98** 654	**96** 497	**99** 482	**86** 216
Merrimack Valley Hospital, Haverhill, MA	**90** 105	**94** 168	**93** 87	**99** 152	**91** 140	**100** 47	**94** 82	**100** 191	**100** 62	- 0	**96** 124	**87** 31	**98** 124	**79** 28	**98** 122	**94** 82	**88** 41
Metrowest Medical Center, Framingham, MA	**96** 231	**98** 209	**95** 204	**98** 327	**95** 303	**99** 83	**94** 259	**100** 626	**98** 220	- 0	**94** 371	**84** 325	**98** 371	**93** 290	**97** 359	**94** 259	**92** 156
Milford Regional Medical Center, Milford, MA	**95** 170	**96** 283	**90** 174	**98** 253	**93** 246	**85** 61	**94** 118	**99** 388	**98** 128	- 0	**100** 231	**95** 168	**95** 231	**88** 161	**95** 227	**95** 118	**100** 101
Milton Hospital, Milton, MA	**91** 89	**88** 89	**96** 76	**96** 139	**95** 130	**96** 28	**95** 199	**100** 313	**89** 106	- 0	**96** 210	**99** 77	**100** 208	**88** 77	**94** 200	**96** 199	**87** 92
Morton Hospital & Medical Center, Taunton, MA	**94** 125	**95** 177	**100** 6	**97** 197	**97** 146	**100** 39	**92** 181	**100** 437	**89** 151	- 0	**98** 298	**99** 92	**97** 301	**92** 93	**96** 290	**94** 182	**92** 93
Mount Auburn Hospital, Cambridge, MA	**99** 175	**97** 280	**93** 193	**100** 254	**97** 254	**100** 60	**98** 432	**100** 1018	**92** 358	**94** 181	**98** 727	**98** 406	**97** 732	**97** 405	**99** 712	**99** 432	**73** 311
Nantucket Cottage Hospital, Nantucket, MA	**100** 5	**100** 5	**100** 2	**100** 2	**100** 5	**100** 1	- 0	**100** 1	- 0	- 0	- 0	**0** 1	- 0	**100** 1	- 0	**0** 1	**0** 1
Nashoba Valley Medical Center, Ayer, MA	**95** 76	**93** 107	**99** 73	**97** 92	**98** 102	**92** 24	**92** 71	**100** 101	**100** 40	- 0	**97** 65	**89** 47	**100** 65	**96** 46	**92** 63	**97** 71	**76** 29
New England Baptist Hospital, Boston, MA	**100** 17	- 0	**100** 26	**100** 18	**100** 28	**100** 3	**97** 1849	**100** 4252	**99** 1125	- 0	**97** 3872	**96** 549	**100** 3874	**100** 547	**96** 3864	**97** 1855	**92** 1771
Newton-Wellesley Hospital, Newton, MA	**99** 72	**99** 139	**99** 85	**100** 116	**99** 148	**96** 23	**91** 92	**99** 326	**95** 74	- 0	**97** 217	**96** 254	**98** 217	**98** 251	**96** 213	**92** 92	**89** 54
Noble Hospital, Westfield, MA	**88** 85	**91** 131	**100** 91	**96** 126	**100** 119	**100** 26	**100** 40	**100** 73	**100** 23	- 0	**96** 49	**96** 23	**96** 49	**96** 23	**100** 46	**100** 40	**89** 9
North Adams Regional Hospital, North Adams, MA	**98** 65	**97** 124	**97** 64	**98** 116	**99** 113	**97** 37	**99** 74	**100** 214	**95** 55	- 0	**100** 146	**96** 56	**96** 146	**100** 55	**99** 141	**100** 74	**91** 23
North Shore Medical Center, Salem, MA	**97** 334	**94** 526	**95** 352	**94** 493	**90** 502	**98** 150	**97** 157	**100** 525	**97** 222	**100** 114	**98** 388	**99** 505	**98** 399	**99** 501	**97** 365	**98** 159	**78** 122
Northampton VA Medical Center, Leeds, MA	- 0	- 0	- 0	- 0	- 0	- 0	- 0	- 0	- 0	- 0	- 0	- -	- 0	- -	- 0	- 0	- 0
Norwood Hospital, Norwood, MA	**95** 133	**97** 146	**89** 113	**98** 189	**91** 154	**100** 57	**100** 256	**100** 378	**96** 157	- 0	**95** 205	**89** 127	**98** 207	**89** 123	**95** 191	**100** 256	**66** 89
Quincy Medical Center, Quincy, MA	**96** 138	**90** 163	**88** 104	**96** 176	**90** 155	**100** 72	**98** 210	**99** 395	**91** 119	- 0	**81** 97	**85** 75	**95** 95	**81** 67	**89** 87	**100** 210	**54** 46
Saint Anne's Hospital, Fall River, MA	**91** 128	**96** 103	**92** 156	**99** 224	**96** 226	**100** 81	**97** 112	**100** 193	**97** 74	- 0	**98** 120	**90** 49	**98** 120	**94** 49	**95** 110	**99** 112	**84** 51
Saint Elizabeth's Medical Center, Brighton, MA	**90** 106	**94** 128	**83** 129	**96** 169	**90** 184	**89** 47	**97** 190	**100** 631	**97** 228	**98** 178	**99** 491	**94** 138	**99** 492	**92** 133	**95** 480	**98** 190	**86** 157
Saint Vincent Hospital, Worcester, MA	**95** 236	**98** 348	**98** 317	**96** 436	**98** 451	**98** 142	**100** 445	**100** 1593	**100** 585	**93** 165	**96** 954	**96** 781	**98** 959	**95** 780	**97** 828	**100** 445	**99** 411
Saints Medical Center, Lowell, MA	**95** 129	**94** 189	**84** 149	**96** 230	**91** 203	**100** 87	**89** 148	**100** 435	**94** 133	- 0	**98** 297	**96** 165	**99** 297	**92** 163	**98** 292	**91** 148	**78** 58
Signature Healthcare Brockton Hospital, Brockton, MA	**98** 114	**99** 83	**91** 105	**99** 176	**95** 178	**100** 95	**99** 186	**100** 447	**99** 144	- 0	**100** 261	**92** 87	**98** 264	**91** 82	**98** 248	**99** 186	**87** 52
Soldiers Home in Massachusetts, Chelsea, MA	- -	- -	- -	- -	- -	- -	- -	- -	- -	- -	- 0	- 0	- 0	- 0	- -	- -	- -
South Shore Hospital, South Weymouth, MA	**97** 251	**90** 263	**98** 283	**96** 492	**98** 481	**99** 101	**98** 479	**97** 1123	**89** 371	- 0	**98** 725	**94** 356	**98** 725	**93** 345	**96** 712	**98** 481	**75** 159
Southcoast Hospital Group, Fall River, MA	**85** 684	**90** 853	**91** 621	**89** 1053	**93** 921	**88** 317	**87** 1022	**100** 2258	**96** 670	**95** 283	**97** 1488	**91** 834	**96** 1507	**94** 799	**97** 1443	**91** 1025	**73** 501
Sturdy Memorial Hospital, Attleboro, MA	**93** 196	**99** 280	**90** 200	**96** 321	**93** 261	**98** 100	**94** 337	**99** 609	**96** 183	- 0	**93** 374	**92** 160	**97** 376	**92** 154	**94** 368	**96** 337	**81** 174
Tufts Medical Center, Boston, MA	**95** 96	**97** 167	**94** 174	**95** 193	**93** 218	**95** 102	**96** 245	**98** 923	**89** 414	**92** 336	**98** 714	**92** 237	**99** 727	**96** 381	**93** 690	**98** 245	**94** 197
UMass Memorial Medical Center, Worcester, MA	**91** 174	**92** 310	**79** 289	**93** 329	**89** 413	**100** 144	**98** 169	**100** 607	**97** 237	**99** 121	**97** 398	**99** 451	**97** 409	**96** 449	**95** 377	**99** 169	**79** 104
VA Boston Healthcare System - Jamaica Plain, Jamaica Plain, MA	**97** 87	**96** 112	**99** 135	**94** 124	**99** 143	**100** 45	**100** 239	**100** 510	**100** 272	**86** 151	**100** 397	- -	**98** 402	- -	**100** 397	**100** 239	**100** 185
Winchester Hospital, Winchester, MA	**91** 208	**92** 240	**79** 204	**96** 276	**88** 301	**100** 69	**95** 333	**100** 903	**98** 322	- 0	**95** 602	**88** 241	**97** 604	**94** 231	**97** 592	**95** 333	**91** 239
Wing Memorial Hospital and Medical Center, Palmer, MA	**92** 64	**99** 119	**97** 100	**97** 117	**98** 124	**98** 48	**100** 25	**100** 46	**100** 20	- 0	**100** 28	**83** 23	**100** 28	**100** 19	**100** 26	**100** 25	**100** 1
NEW HAMPSHIRE																	
Alice Peck Day Memorial Hospital, Lebanon, NH	**94** 18	**90** 20	**100** 10	**100** 20	**100** 11	**100** 7	**89** 27	**90** 62	- 0	- 0	**98** 48	- -	**96** 48	- -	**100** 48	**89** 27	**89** 19
Androscoggin Valley Hospital, Berlin, NH	**100** 21	**100** 37	**100** 20	**100** 36	**95** 44	**100** 10	**95** 19	**100** 44	- 0	- 0	**94** 35	- -	**91** 35	- -	**88** 32	**95** 19	- 0
Catholic Medical Center, Manchester, NH	**100** 80	**98** 139	**99** 93	**99** 125	**100** 130	**100** 50	**96** 81	**100** 524	**94** 226	**98** 131	**98** 376	**95** 316	**98** 383	**98** 320	**97** 362	**98** 81	**95** 140
Cheshire Medical Center, Keene, NH	**95** 87	**97** 144	**98** 81	**97** 146	**99** 123	**98** 50	**95** 110	**100** 263	**99** 69	- 0	**98** 194	**96** 110	**99** 194	**96** 109	**99** 191	**97** 110	**98** 82
Concord Hospital, Concord, NH	**95** 196	**96** 285	**97** 186	**97** 284	**95** 273	**97** 104	**92** 122	**100** 464	**99** 172	**95** 106	**96** 360	**98** 406	**97** 369	**96** 402	**95** 355	**92** 122	**84** 111
Cottage Hospital, Woodsville, NH	**93** 14	**97** 30	**100** 19	**100** 32	**100** 32	**83** 6	**92** 13	**100** 58	- 0	- 0	**93** 42	- -	**98** 42	- -	**90** 42	**92** 13	**100** 20
Elliot Hospital, Manchester, NH	**93** 88	**90** 127	**84** 77	**99** 135	**99** 119	**93** 42	**100** 131	**100** 377	**86** 86	- 0	**98** 255	**96** 466	**99** 257	**98** 463	**96** 244	**100** 131	**89** 76
Exeter Hospital, Exeter, NH	**94** 123	**96** 166	**95** 111	**95** 182	**94** 165	**100** 59	**94** 141	**100** 543	**93** 212	- 0	**99** 395	**99** 195	**98** 399	**96** 194	**97** 386	**97** 141	**98** 142
Franklin Regional Hospital, Franklin, NH	**98** 44	**98** 64	**91** 53	**93** 68	**100** 80	**94** 17	**100** 9	**100** 28	- 0	- 0	**100** 16	**88** 17	**100** 17	**100** 16	**94** 16	**100** 9	**75** 4
Frisbie Memorial Hospital, Rochester, NH	**92** 97	**96** 122	**88** 95	**98** 100	**96** 112	**100** 59	**92** 80	**100** 258	**100** 92	- 0	**97** 174	**94** 78	**99** 177	**89** 73	**99** 169	**92** 80	**97** 79
Huggins Hospital, Wolfeboro, NH	**94** 34	**96** 55	**89** 18	**98** 54	**100** 44	**100** 10	**100** 41	**99** 91	**100** 30	- 0	**98** 56	- -	**91** 56	- -	**98** 55	**100** 41	**95** 19
Lakes Region General Hospital, Laconia, NH	**91** 79	**97** 87	**87** 78	**98** 120	**93** 107	**97** 36	**94** 199	**100** 448	**94** 133	- 0	**96** 311	**93** 182	**97** 314	**95** 175	**95** 301	**95** 199	**78** 134
Littleton Regional Hospital, Littleton, NH	**75** 16	**96** 24	**95** 20	**94** 33	**64** 36	**83** 6	**87** 61	**100** 204	**87** 45	- 0	**96** 150	- -	**98** 150	- -	**95** 150	**90** 61	**80** 65
Mary Hitchcock Memorial Hospital, Lebanon, NH	**88** 74	**95** 128	**98** 147	**92** 133	**96** 159	**87** 77	**99** 269	**100** 871	**89** 348	**96** 207	**97** 633	**97** 608	**99** 647	**98** 640	**96** 615	**99** 270	**84** 230
The Memorial Hospital, North Conway, NH	**89** 27	**93** 29	**67** 18	**97** 29	**97** 29	**78** 9	**100** 29	**100** 62	- 0	- 0	**95** 59	- -	**98** 58	- -	**86** 57	**100** 29	**100** 21
Monadnock Community Hospital, Peterborough, NH	**96** 52	**99** 96	**94** 52	**99** 84	**97** 71	**92** 26	**97** 36	**100** 128	- 0	- 0	**97** 111	**98** 45	**96** 115	**96** 45	**98** 107	**100** 36	**50** 8
New London Hospital, New London, NH	**97** 29	**97** 36	**97** 31	**97** 33	**98** 46	**67** 3	**91** 35	**100** 112	**100** 27	- 0	**76** 97	**75** 83	**99** 98	**99** 81	**99** 96	**91** 35	**87** 30
Parkland Medical Center, Derry, NH	**98** 58	**99** 96	**98** 63	**100** 76	**99** 93	**100** 33	**94** 70	**100** 161	**100** 41	- 0	**98** 56	**100** 80	**100** 55	**94** 116	**98** 52	**100** 70	**80** 15
Portsmouth Regional Hospital, Portsmouth, NH	**100** 59	**98** 111	**100** 59	**100** 101	**100** 101	**100** 23	**97** 166	**100** 595	**100** 256	**92** 170	**100** 373	**99** 259	**100** 407	**99** 258	**98** 348	**99** 166	**100** 121
Saint Joseph Hospital, Nashua, NH	**89** 84	**100** 114	**99** 78	**92** 131	**97** 125	**100** 27	**99** 151	**100** 312	**98** 82	- 0	**96** 218	**94** 140	**99** 219	**96** 139	**96** 211	**99** 151	**83** 63
Southern Nh Medical Center, Nashua, NH	**99** 86	**98** 167	**97** 116	**97** 174	**95** 144	**100** 67	**94** 215	**100** 589	**98** 137	- 0	**100** 422	**96** 224	**99** 428	**99** 216	**98** 419	**94** 217	**86** 136
Speare Memorial Hospital, Plymouth, NH	**100** 27	**100** 30	**100** 20	**100** 43	**100** 38	**100** 13	**100** 22	**100** 73	**95** 22	- 0	**98** 60	**100** 59	**100** 59	**97** 59	**95** 57	**100** 22	**100** 31
Upper Connecticut Valley Hospital, Colebrook, NH	**100** 17	**100** 10	**80** 10	**100** 21	**75** 20	**90** 10	- 0	**100** 2	**100** 2	- 0	**100** 2	- 0	**100** 2	- 0	**100** 2	- 0	- 0
Valley Regional Hospital, Claremont, NH	**100** 26	**92** 36	**89** 27	**100** 31	**88** 32	**100** 11	**100** 49	**100** 94	- 0	- 0	**98** 82	- -	**98** 81	- -	**99** 79	**100** 49	**82** 34
Weeks Medical Center, Lancaster, NH	**100** 28	**98** 46	**100** 34	**98** 55	**98** 49	**100** 10	**100** 18	**100** 29	- 0	- 0	**92** 26	- 0	**100** 26	- 0	**96** 25	**100** 18	**55** 11
Wentworth-Douglass Hospital, Dover, NH	**98** 99	**99** 135	**94** 82	**96** 139	**93** 116	**97** 38	**93** 152	**100** 448	**92** 119	- 0	**100** 307	**99** 346	**99** 310	**98** 345	**99** 302	**95** 152	**88** 127
NEW JERSEY																	
Atlanticare Regional Medical Center - City Division, Atlantic City, NJ	**95** 195	**99** 358	**100** 166	**95** 313	**100** 234	**100** 138	**94** 285	**100** 1054	**88** 361	**97** 143	**97** 546	**92** 293	**98** 560	**95** 293	**92** 502	**97** 285	**94** 217
Bayonne Hospital Center, Bayonne, NJ	**92** 86	**98** 151	**97** 72	**98** 135	**95** 138	**100** 49	**93** 97	**100** 141	**84** 38	- 0	**97** 35	**91** 22	**100** 36	**95** 20	**82** 28	**96** 97	**100** 7
Bayshore Community Hospital, Holmdel, NJ	**95** 133	**100** 228	**99** 159	**99** 229	**100** 222	**100** 97	**99** 123	**100** 216	**100** 53	- 0	**100** 117	**95** 59	**98** 117	**98** 57	**97** 106	**100** 123	**97** 39
Bergen Regional Medical Center, Paramus, NJ	**92** 38	**96** 78	**95** 42	**96** 46	**99** 68	**100** 14	**96** 25	**100** 33	**50** 2	- 0	**96** 26	**50** 4	**92** 26	**50** 2	**100** 26	**96** 25	**100** 7
Cape Regional Medical Center, Cape May Ct Hse, NJ	**96** 289	**94** 482	**87** 253	**98** 454	**91** 375	**99** 155	**89** 161	**100** 427	**93** 135	- 0	**99** 272	**86** 73	**96** 274	**96** 69	**95** 262	**91** 164	**94** 77
Capital Health System - Mercer Campus, Trenton, NJ	**93** 95	**94** 144	**96** 70	**98** 129	**91** 81	**100** 59	**81** 157	**100** 498	**95** 139	- 0	**99** 344	**85** 95	**96** 345	**95** 83	**93** 331	**84** 158	**76** 93
Capital Health System-Fuld Campus, Trenton, NJ	**93** 88	**91** 162	**92** 77	**93** 153	**90** 98	**100** 65	**95** 116	**100** 253	**99** 77	- 0	**98** 130	**92** 92	**95** 127	**87** 91	**90** 124	**94** 117	**80** 51
Centrastate Medical Center, Freehold, NJ	**93** 193	**97** 356	**95** 214	**97** 339	**96** 352	**100** 71	**80** 284	**99** 716	**74** 200	- 0	**97** 415	**89** 65	**93** 418	**94** 192	**92** 402	**81** 284	**87** 130

NOTE: The first number in each column (boldface) is the score, the second number is the number of patients; Please refer to the main entry for footnotes; (a) 100-299
*MEASURES: **Pneumonia Care:** 16. Appropriate Initial Antibiotic; 17. Blood Culture Timing; 18. Influenza Vaccine; 19. Initial Antibiotic Timing; 20. Pneumococcal Vaccine; 21. Smoking Cessation Advice; **Surgical Care Improvement Project:** 22. Appropriate VTP Within 24 Hours; 23. Appropriate Hair Removal; 24. Appropriate Beta Blocker Usage; 25. Controlled Postoperative Blood Glucose; 26. Prophylactic Antibiotic Timing; 27. Prophylactic Antibiotic Timing (Outpatient); 28. Prophylactic Antibiotic Selection; 29. Prophylactic Antibiotic Selection (Outpatient); 30. Prophylactic Antibiotic Stopped; 31. Recommended VTP Ordered; 32. Urinary Catheter Removal*

Hospital	Pneumonia Care 16	17	18	19	20	21	Surgical Care Improvement Project 22	23	24	25	26	27	28	29	30	31	32
Chilton Hospital, Pompton Plains, NJ	**89** 84	**97** 154	**91** 92	**96** 139	**95** 157	**100** 37	**89** 186	**100** 438	**93** 122	**-** 0	**99** 256	**93** 174	**97** 257	**91** 164	**95** 229	**93** 186	**90** 86
Christ Hospital, Jersey City, NJ	**95** 173	**98** 234	**88** 124	**97** 184	**89** 166	**100** 33	**82** 191	**100** 400	**84** 75	**-** 0	**94** 224	**77** 204	**96** 226	**82** 206	**91** 210	**83** 192	**96** 57
Clara Maass Medical Center, Belleville, NJ	**100** 124	**100** 241	**100** 125	**99** 203	**100** 189	**100** 61	**100** 259	**100** 659	**100** 141	**100** 1	**99** 386	**91** 138	**98** 386	**97** 127	**98** 363	**100** 259	**97** 115
Community Medical Center, Toms River, NJ	**97** 124	**100** 216	**100** 120	**99** 193	**100** 202	**100** 55	**100** 230	**100** 601	**100** 178	**100** 1	**99** 325	**97** 418	**99** 323	**98** 417	**98** 300	**100** 230	**91** 23
Cooper University Hospital, Camden, NJ	**96** 113	**95** 183	**100** 23	**96** 160	**85** 110	**100** 88	**98** 374	**100** 1414	**95** 460	**94** 394	**96** 1148	**94** 407	**96** 1174	**95** 425	**98** 1112	**99** 374	**94** 318
Deborah Heart and Lung Center, Browns Mills, NJ	**-** 0	**-** 0	**100** 6	**83** 6	**83** 12	**100** 11	**83** 29	**100** 440	**97** 267	**86** 325	**98** 342	**88** 260	**100** 354	**100** 254	**100** 317	**83** 29	**99** 91
East Orange General Hospital, East Orange, NJ	**85** 41	**98** 184	**92** 92	**99** 168	**99** 141	**100** 34	**98** 82	**100** 131	**92** 25	**-** 0	**98** 49	**84** 63	**98** 51	**95** 58	**93** 44	**99** 82	**91** 22
Englewood Hospital and Medical Center, Englewood, NJ	**99** 119	**97** 197	**96** 170	**99** 185	**97** 264	**100** 32	**94** 311	**100** 1154	**100** 429	**97** 259	**99** 869	**96** 334	**99** 871	**90** 338	**98** 839	**96** 313	**96** 297
Hackensack University Medical Center, Hackensack, NJ	**99** 270	**98** 258	**96** 339	**97** 384	**96** 482	**100** 103	**86** 148	**100** 658	**93** 247	**95** 136	**99** 454	**96** 668	**97** 462	**94** 662	**95** 433	**87** 149	**96** 187
Hackettstown Regional Medical Center, Hackettstown, NJ	**98** 66	**98** 102	**96** 51	**100** 82	**100** 85	**95** 21	**95** 76	**100** 257	**99** 75	**-** 0	**99** 176	**96** 52	**95** 177	**94** 52	**96** 168	**94** 77	**100** 41
Hoboken University Medical Center, Hoboken, NJ	**85** 86	**90** 112	**82** 80	**89** 132	**93** 120	**100** 24	**90** 89	**100** 187	**82** 44	**-** 0	**99** 110	**90** 143	**98** 113	**96** 137	**93** 104	**95** 91	**80** 40
Holy Name Medical Center, Teaneck, NJ	**95** 96	**98** 188	**100** 94	**96** 198	**100** 175	**100** 30	**98** 238	**100** 518	**96** 151	**-** 0	**100** 290	**87** 193	**99** 296	**98** 181	**99** 270	**98** 238	**99** 102
Hunterdon Medical Center, Flemington, NJ	**97** 90	**98** 197	**97** 94	**98** 149	**97** 138	**96** 23	**92** 139	**100** 418	**93** 100	**-** 0	**98** 291	**87** 180	**99** 289	**86** 176	**97** 286	**96** 139	**87** 90
Jersey Shore University Medical Center, Neptune, NJ	**95** 146	**99** 209	**93** 180	**97** 206	**94** 246	**99** 93	**95** 254	**100** 1179	**98** 496	**95** 402	**99** 826	**98** 703	**98** 846	**100** 692	**96** 774	**96** 254	**98** 260
JFK Medical Center, Edison, NJ	**93** 262	**98** 384	**91** 250	**91** 418	**94** 346	**99** 90	**90** 408	**98** 959	**84** 276	**-** 0	**96** 762	**87** 400	**96** 763	**94** 373	**92** 747	**91** 413	**65** 118
Kennedy University Hospital, Stratford, NJ	**97** 520	**97** 1002	**93** 417	**97** 860	**96** 662	**100** 307	**98** 383	**99** 969	**96** 283	**-** 0	**99** 562	**91** 267	**99** 565	**92** 251	**99** 549	**99** 383	**95** 164
Kimball Medical Center, Lakewood, NJ	**99** 156	**100** 306	**97** 202	**99** 274	**100** 309	**100** 80	**97** 87	**100** 172	**95** 41	**-** 0	**99** 77	**99** 136	**99** 77	**97** 135	**99** 67	**98** 87	**85** 13
Libertyhealth-Jersey City Medical Center Campus, Jersey City, NJ	**98** 59	**96** 74	**96** 75	**100** 73	**93** 69	**100** 49	**98** 163	**100** 472	**100** 96	**100** 79	**100** 211	**70** 43	**98** 214	**91** 34	**97** 201	**99** 163	**100** 63
Lourdes Medical Center of Burlington County, Willingboro, NJ	**99** 87	**97** 155	**86** 87	**99** 147	**89** 124	**100** 55	**96** 138	**100** 287	**95** 74	**-** 0	**97** 159	**93** 92	**96** 159	**98** 88	**96** 156	**99** 138	**82** 61
Meadowlands Hospital Medical Center, Secaucus, NJ	**95** 75	**98** 120	**93** 60	**98** 103	**95** 78	**100** 18	**62** 47	**100** 165	**100** 18	**-** 0	**97** 89	**98** 90	**91** 90	**97** 89	**86** 86	**62** 47	**100** 7
Memorial Hospital of Salem County, Salem, NJ	**91** 110	**98** 105	**91** 125	**100** 180	**96** 132	**100** 91	**98** 62	**100** 169	**82** 38	**-** 0	**97** 89	**89** 38	**98** 90	**91** 34	**95** 82	**98** 62	**87** 23
Monmouth Medical Center, Long Branch, NJ	**96** 116	**99** 175	**92** 93	**98** 157	**94** 131	**100** 49	**97** 192	**100** 523	**99** 120	**-** 0	**99** 326	**96** 294	**97** 328	**97** 295	**97** 312	**98** 192	**96** 130
Morristown Memorial Hospital, Morristown, NJ	**96** 78	**98** 168	**89** 93	**93** 148	**93** 149	**100** 34	**97** 209	**100** 840	**91** 287	**95** 168	**93** 566	**93** 531	**98** 582	**98** 524	**97** 521	**97** 209	**95** 168
Mountainside Hospital, Montclair, NJ	**100** 138	**99** 243	**92** 142	**97** 215	**91** 233	**95** 61	**85** 206	**100** 522	**92** 113	**0** 1	**98** 249	**90** 192	**96** 255	**89** 178	**91** 233	**90** 207	**91** 97
Newark Beth Israel Medical Center, Newark, NJ	**100** 70	**99** 131	**100** 88	**100** 110	**100** 98	**100** 45	**97** 169	**100** 624	**100** 192	**96** 180	**100** 452	**99** 371	**100** 466	**98** 368	**100** 430	**98** 169	**98** 60
Newton Memorial Hospital, Newton, NJ	**93** 84	**99** 187	**90** 105	**100** 169	**96** 178	**100** 44	**94** 152	**100** 272	**95** 93	**-** 0	**98** 164	**98** 50	**95** 165	**98** 52	**88** 143	**94** 153	**86** 56
Ocean Medical Center, Brick, NJ	**96** 95	**99** 169	**99** 91	**99** 154	**98** 165	**100** 46	**99** 222	**100** 558	**94** 154	**-** 0	**99** 301	**92** 195	**98** 301	**96** 181	**97** 283	**99** 222	**93** 130
Our Lady of Lourdes Medical Center, Camden, NJ	**99** 87	**98** 140	**99** 85	**98** 122	**98** 118	**100** 54	**100** 152	**100** 516	**95** 207	**98** 173	**99** 317	**100** 446	**98** 324	**100** 445	**94** 292	**100** 152	**89** 94
Overlook Hospital, Summit, NJ	**88** 162	**96** 213	**98** 133	**99** 174	**97** 228	**92** 37	**98** 208	**100** 577	**96** 124	**-** 0	**99** 371	**98** 462	**97** 378	**94** 459	**96** 364	**99** 209	**96** 95
Palisades Medical Center, North Bergen, NJ	**95** 80	**93** 110	**97** 65	**100** 100	**100** 134	**100** 15	**100** 83	**100** 192	**97** 64	**-** 0	**98** 103	**70** 37	**93** 105	**96** 26	**97** 88	**100** 83	**86** 35
Raritan Bay Medical Center, Perth Amboy, NJ	**96** 183	**97** 343	**95** 156	**95** 306	**98** 261	**99** 92	**93** 164	**100** 330	**92** 106	**-** 0	**99** 164	**89** 130	**94** 164	**97** 117	**97** 151	**95** 165	**90** 31
Riverview Medical Center, Red Bank, NJ	**95** 142	**99** 219	**100** 133	**97** 183	**99** 204	**100** 59	**95** 317	**100** 990	**99** 240	**100** 1	**100** 689	**98** 200	**98** 693	**98** 199	**97** 658	**96** 317	**97** 278
Robert Wood Johnson University Hospital, New Brunswick, NJ	**91** 185	**92** 431	**87** 279	**97** 377	**96** 411	**100** 82	**99** 494	**100** 2018	**99** 746	**88** 728	**96** 1494	**88** 793	**98** 1520	**91** 777	**94** 1447	**99** 495	**89** 497
Robert Wood Johnson University Hospital at Rahway, Rahway, NJ	**96** 141	**96** 254	**98** 157	**96** 230	**98** 241	**95** 42	**96** 145	**100** 321	**95** 110	**-** 0	**100** 161	**98** 121	**99** 162	**98** 120	**99** 154	**97** 145	**97** 32
Robert Wood Johnson University Hospital Hamilton, Hamilton, NJ	**90** 203	**98** 367	**93** 195	**97** 322	**94** 268	**99** 88	**89** 312	**100** 782	**92** 289	**-** 0	**97** 515	**77** 131	**96** 520	**89** 109	**94** 484	**93** 312	**93** 242
Saint Barnabas Medical Center, Livingston, NJ	**94** 87	**97** 94	**97** 95	**99** 132	**95** 130	**100** 29	**91** 199	**100** 805	**100** 258	**99** 168	**99** 537	**94** 780	**97** 550	**96** 762	**95** 515	**93** 199	**93** 95
Saint Clare's Hospital, Denville, NJ	**99** 176	**100** 278	**99** 160	**99** 237	**100** 243	**100** 71	**96** 376	**100** 872	**95** 217	**0** 1	**100** 475	**98** 230	**97** 478	**93** 229	**96** 465	**97** 376	**90** 168
Saint Clare's Hospital - Sussex, Sussex, NJ	**95** 40	**98** 53	**100** 30	**100** 49	**100** 40	**100** 27	**96** 24	**100** 29	**67** 9	**-** 0	**100** 3	**100** 3	**67** 3	**100** 3	**100** 3	**100** 24	**100** 4
Saint Francis Medical Center, Trenton, NJ	**99** 91	**98** 132	**88** 75	**94** 134	**93** 99	**100** 60	**98** 117	**100** 332	**98** 158	**80** 139	**96** 167	**94** 306	**98** 175	**98** 291	**87** 152	**98** 117	**99** 68
Saint Joseph's Regional Medical Center, Paterson, NJ	**86** 321	**97** 521	**85** 344	**95** 540	**87** 444	**100** 103	**91** 339	**100** 1127	**99** 365	**95** 253	**97** 878	**87** 144	**97** 878	**80** 128	**96** 848	**94** 341	**94** 307
Saint Joseph's Wayne Hospital, Wayne, NJ	-	-	-	-	-	-	-	-	-	-	-	-	-	-	-	-	-
Saint Mary's Hospital - Passaic, Passaic, NJ	**93** 95	**97** 180	**99** 112	**97** 159	**97** 186	**100** 41	**81** 171	**99** 499	**91** 155	**80** 96	**99** 271	**91** 275	**95** 280	**91** 263	**84** 250	**83** 172	**91** 86
Saint Michael's Medical Center, Newark, NJ	**92** 62	**98** 124	**88** 67	**87** 128	**88** 112	**98** 42	**87** 135	**100** 563	**98** 216	**97** 166	**100** 367	**100** 150	**98** 377	**98** 150	**99** 346	**90** 135	**95** 80
Saint Peter's University Hospital, New Brunswick, NJ	**79** 179	**80** 204	**93** 151	**82** 215	**94** 209	**100** 67	**95** 190	**81** 549	**91** 173	**-** 0	**99** 338	**79** 91	**98** 339	**75** 81	**95** 312	**96** 190	**93** 60
Shore Memorial Hospital, Somers Point, NJ	**97** 120	**99** 168	**99** 77	**97** 136	**99** 114	**100** 56	**97** 198	**100** 577	**97** 206	**-** 0	**100** 359	**99** 146	**99** 360	**100** 145	**99** 334	**98** 199	**98** 47
Somerset Medical Center, Somerville, NJ	**93** 100	**99** 126	**98** 83	**99** 139	**98** 164	**100** 26	**97** 220	**100** 541	**93** 161	**-** 0	**100** 338	**92** 106	**98** 339	**96** 97	**96** 322	**99** 220	**85** 71
South Jersey Healthcare Regional Med Ctr, Vineland, NJ	**99** 93	**97** 123	**100** 65	**92** 177	**100** 108	**100** 59	**84** 202	**99** 515	**89** 117	**-** 0	**95** 290	**98** 240	**94** 290	**93** 237	**95** 281	**83** 204	**94** 113
South Jersey Healthcare-Elmer Hospital, Elmer, NJ	**97** 79	**99** 99	**98** 66	**95** 110	**99** 98	**100** 34	**91** 67	**100** 216	**95** 73	**-** 0	**99** 140	**96** 49	**98** 140	**98** 47	**95** 139	**91** 67	**89** 84
Southern Ocean Medical Center, Manahawkin, NJ	**93** 103	**90** 248	**91** 121	**95** 210	**89** 225	**100** 55	**88** 163	**100** 313	**88** 110	**-** 0	**98** 173	**86** 69	**95** 172	**98** 64	**93** 161	**96** 163	**97** 65
Trinitas Regional Medical Center, Elizabeth, NJ	**84** 94	**98** 131	**94** 89	**91** 172	**98** 126	**100** 57	**82** 186	**99** 454	**98** 129	**-** 0	**99** 210	**98** 274	**95** 211	**96** 271	**94** 205	**83** 189	**90** 48
UMDNJ University Hospital, Newark, NJ	**92** 100	**89** 250	**96** 101	**88** 239	**95** 60	**97** 173	**94** 194	**100** 435	**100** 91	**95** 74	**98** 300	**84** 160	**97** 320	**81** 139	**95** 284	**96** 194	**95** 75
Underwood Memorial Hospital, Woodbury, NJ	**92** 181	**99** 267	**92** 167	**95** 255	**97** 249	**100** 105	**96** 290	**100** 637	**94** 141	**-** 0	**94** 373	**86** 105	**96** 376	**92** 98	**94** 359	**98** 290	**89** 44
University Medical Center at Princeton, Princeton, NJ	**97** 102	**97** 68	**99** 97	**99** 138	**98** 142	**100** 29	**98** 180	**99** 507	**99** 126	**0** 1	**99** 265	**91** 246	**98** 266	**96** 228	**98** 261	**98** 180	**98** 133
VA New Jersey Health Care System, East Orange, NJ	**93** 29	**95** 56	**97** 30	**96** 55	**91** 35	**100** 22	**91** 119	**100** 154	**98** 45	**100** 1	**91** 93	**-** -	**96** 92	**-** -	**92** 89	**95** 120	**84** 57
Valley Hospital, Ridgewood, NJ	**94** 96	**99** 163	**100** 92	**98** 158	**99** 172	**100** 22	**87** 219	**100** 807	**90** 286	**97** 169	**98** 538	**92** 458	**97** 549	**95** 441	**95** 519	**94** 219	**93** 209
Virtua Memorial Hospital of Burlington County, Mount Holly, NJ	**93** 241	**95** 351	**90** 156	**99** 319	**88** 290	**100** 95	**98** 427	**100** 1517	**94** 506	**-** 0	**97** 1155	**95** 210	**98** 1155	**76** 209	**99** 1098	**99** 427	**96** 457
Virtua West Jersey Hospitals Berlin, Berlin, NJ	**95** 490	**99** 818	**96** 363	**99** 741	**98** 677	**100** 222	**96** 778	**100** 1856	**96** 507	**-** 0	**98** 1248	**94** 361	**98** 1268	**94** 355	**97** 1208	**97** 780	**93** 401
Warren Hospital, Phillipsburg, NJ	**98** 100	**99** 155	**97** 130	**98** 153	**98** 192	**100** 71	**97** 93	**100** 270	**96** 76	**-** 0	**99** 151	**95** 107	**99** 151	**96** 105	**94** 145	**98** 93	**94** 71
NEW YORK																	
Adirondack Medical Center, Saranac Lake, NY	**78** 27	**82** 34	**87** 45	**92** 49	**93** 60	**92** 13	**50** 150	**100** 250	**90** 69	**-** 0	**87** 157	**87** 99	**96** 157	**91** 90	**68** 155	**49** 154	**90** 88
Albany Medical Center - South Clinical Campus, Albany, NY	**-** 0	**-** 0	**-** 0	**-** 0	**-** 0	**-** 0	**-** 0	**100** 7	**-** 0	**-** 0	**100** 4	**90** 154	**100** 4	**96** 146	**100** 4	**-** 0	**-** 0
Albany Medical Center Hospital, Albany, NY	**88** 123	**94** 218	**96** 105	**91** 166	**94** 129	**96** 80	**97** 135	**98** 527	**97** 195	**85** 103	**98** 333	**96** 594	**97** 352	**94** 577	**94** 326	**99** 135	**99** 79
Albany Memorial Hospital, Albany, NY	**96** 75	**96** 177	**93** 92	**96** 158	**91** 137	**100** 45	**90** 194	**98** 449	**84** 133	**-** 0	**93** 300	**91** 190	**89** 298	**96** 181	**85** 296	**92** 194	**75** 73
Albany VA Medical Center, Albany, NY	**93** 27	**100** 60	**100** 41	**93** 61	**100** 52	**100** 31	**100** 62	**100** 122	**100** 51	**-** 0	**100** 68	**-** -	**100** 69	**-** -	**98** 66	**100** 62	**100** 47
Alice Hyde Medical Center, Malone, NY	**93** 75	**97** 90	**91** 53	**93** 97	**93** 67	**100** 32	**87** 97	**100** 159	**93** 42	**-** 0	**95** 98	**96** 82	**96** 98	**72** 81	**98** 93	**90** 97	**92** 40
Arnot Ogden Medical Center, Elmira, NY	**93** 122	**95** 260	**97** 179	**96** 226	**98** 255	**99** 67	**97** 149	**98** 732	**100** 293	**89** 114	**99** 572	**97** 439	**99** 578	**98** 436	**97** 547	**98** 149	**97** 100
Auburn Memorial Hospital, Auburn, NY	**88** 205	**91** 233	**85** 149	**94** 247	**87** 208	**88** 73	**92** 127	**99** 255	**89** 71	**-** 0	**88** 166	**93** 116	**89** 161	**88** 110	**94** 152	**94** 129	**79** 38
Aurelia Osborn Fox Memorial Hospital, Oneonta, NY	**91** 74	**95** 127	**93** 69	**95** 132	**97** 103	**100** 41	**93** 102	**99** 191	**84** 44	**-** 0	**93** 89	**100** 1	**98** 89	**100** 1	**99** 88	**96** 102	**95** 37

NOTE: The first number in each column (boldface) is the score, the second number is the number of patients; Please refer to the main entry for footnotes; (a) 100-299
*MEASURES: **Pneumonia Care:** 16. Appropriate Initial Antibiotic; 17. Blood Culture Timing; 18. Influenza Vaccine; 19. Initial Antibiotic Timing; 20. Pneumococcal Vaccine; 21. Smoking Cessation Advice; **Surgical Care Improvement Project:** 22. Appropriate VTP Within 24 Hours; 23. Appropriate Hair Removal; 24. Appropriate Beta Blocker Usage; 25. Controlled Postoperative Blood Glucose; 26. Prophylactic Antibiotic Timing; 27. Prophylactic Antibiotic Timing (Outpatient); 28. Prophylactic Antibiotic Selection; 29. Prophylactic Antibiotic Selection (Outpatient); 30. Prophylactic Antibiotic Stopped; 31. Recommended VTP Ordered; 32. Urinary Catheter Removal*

Hospital	Pneumonia Care						Surgical Care Improvement Project										
	16	17	18	19	20	21	22	23	24	25	26	27	28	29	30	31	32
Bath VA Medical Center, Bath, NY	**100** 41	**100** 71	**100** 24	**98** 56	**100** 41	**94** 17	- 0	- 0	- 0	- 0	- 0	- -	- 0	- -	- 0	- 0	- 0
Bellevue Hospital Center, New York, NY	**87** 134	**88** 195	**90** 127	**87** 214	**97** 121	**96** 96	**97** 298	**100** 747	**99** 190	**97** 192	**97** 410	**98** 47	**98** 418	**99** 164	**99** 401	**97** 298	**92** 109
Benedictine Hospital, Kingston, NY	**94** 79	**98** 125	**91** 87	**100** 117	**96** 113	**100** 40	**86** 138	**99** 373	**92** 124	- 0	**95** 230	**88** 115	**100** 236	**97** 110	**95** 227	**91** 138	**97** 132
Bertrand Chaffee Hospital, Springville, NY	**95** 88	**97** 116	**92** 65	**96** 105	**91** 102	**100** 25	**71** 7	**88** 8	**0** 1	- 0	**50** 2	**93** 14	**100** 2	**64** 14	**100** 2	**71** 7	**100** 1
Beth Israel Medical Center, New York, NY	**93** 108	**99** 172	**85** 98	**92** 170	**78** 165	**100** 53	**98** 229	**99** 690	**78** 222	**88** 141	**99** 490	**95** 642	**96** 490	**96** 649	**91** 474	**98** 229	**80** 196
Bon Secours Community Hospital, Port Jervis, NY	**95** 75	**97** 107	**100** 62	**97** 93	**94** 90	**100** 37	**97** 62	**100** 109	**95** 40	- 0	**100** 53	**88** 16	**96** 55	**94** 16	**92** 50	**98** 62	**64** 14
Bronx VA Medical Center, Bronx, NY	**93** 58	**98** 83	**88** 51	**99** 79	**95** 63	**100** 28	**99** 118	**100** 151	**100** 41	- 0	**99** 81	- -	**96** 81	- -	**95** 79	**98** 120	**100** 49
Bronx-Lebanon Hospital Center, Bronx, NY	**74** 121	**76** 139	**99** 92	**81** 233	**99** 128	**100** 80	**96** 185	**100** 289	**53** 58	- 0	**91** 176	**81** 53	**96** 176	**98** 46	**90** 162	**96** 185	**57** 14
Brookdale Hospital Medical Center, Brooklyn, NY	**91** 79	**90** 178	**79** 70	**91** 161	**78** 85	**97** 69	**87** 189	**99** 308	**86** 71	- 0	**91** 111	**76** 157	**95** 109	**79** 135	**70** 107	**87** 189	**42** 33
Brookhaven Memorial Hospital Medical Center, Patchogue, NY	**89** 240	**94** 454	**93** 283	**89** 428	**91** 429	**100** 163	**87** 236	**100** 392	**88** 121	- 0	**91** 237	**81** 79	**96** 238	**94** 65	**94** 228	**95** 237	**82** 121
Brooklyn Hospital Center at Downtown Campus, Brooklyn, NY	**98** 96	**89** 303	**80** 149	**92** 305	**82** 201	**100** 62	**87** 254	**99** 438	**89** 107	- 0	**87** 178	**51** 164	**94** 179	**84** 179	**72** 164	**87** 254	**83** 52
Brooks Memorial Hospital, Dunkirk, NY	**89** 62	**86** 114	**81** 57	**94** 118	**88** 95	**75** 24	**99** 153	**99** 358	**97** 111	- 0	**98** 313	**88** 34	**99** 313	**100** 31	**97** 313	**99** 154	**94** 101
Canandaigua VA Medical Center, Canandaigua, NY	- 0	- 0	- 0	- 0	- 0	- 0	- 0	- 0	- 0	- 0	- 0	- -	- 0	- -	- 0	- 0	- 0
Canton-Potsdam Hospital, Potsdam, NY	**86** 74	**94** 100	**88** 69	**95** 122	**95** 103	**95** 42	**99** 139	**100** 318	**94** 86	- 0	**99** 220	**99** 83	**96** 221	**67** 83	**100** 220	**99** 139	**98** 55
Carthage Area Hospital, Carthage, NY	**77** 26	**79** 29	**79** 24	**91** 34	**88** 33	**100** 12	**40** 10	**100** 45	**75** 4	- 0	**86** 29	**55** 38	**97** 29	**45** 31	**90** 29	**50** 10	**100** 1
Catskill Regional Medical Center, Harris, NY	**93** 83	**95** 133	**98** 84	**92** 126	**100** 100	**100** 58	**93** 119	**100** 235	**83** 54	- 0	**98** 157	**93** 41	**85** 158	**88** 40	**95** 151	**97** 119	**92** 24
Cayuga Medical Center at Ithaca, Ithaca, NY	**78** 107	**92** 192	**82** 91	**91** 196	**79** 151	**98** 52	**91** 153	**99** 324	**94** 80	- 0	**95** 212	**85** 109	**98** 213	**99** 99	**93** 210	**90** 155	**87** 82
Champlain Valley Physicians Hospital Med Ctr, Plattsburgh, NY	**85** 187	**92** 322	**92** 184	**89** 326	**95** 302	**96** 140	**88** 320	**100** 845	**94** 290	**99** 127	**91** 589	**82** 311	**95** 591	**92** 283	**92** 581	**91** 320	**92** 234
Chenango Memorial Hospital, Norwich, NY	**85** 66	**97** 117	**96** 53	**96** 111	**100** 64	**93** 28	**92** 89	**100** 183	**96** 47	- 0	**94** 142	**83** 6	**91** 141	**100** 6	**94** 137	**93** 89	**98** 62
Claxton-Hepburn Medical Center, Ogdensburg, NY	**98** 48	**97** 92	**91** 67	**98** 92	**94** 88	**100** 20	**84** 44	**98** 100	**88** 24	- 0	**95** 59	**87** 45	**97** 60	**95** 42	**100** 56	**87** 45	**91** 11
Clifton Springs Hospital and Clinic, Clifton Springs, NY	**100** 85	**99** 114	**96** 68	**94** 108	**90** 94	**100** 29	**100** 52	**100** 331	**100** 111	- 0	**99** 255	**96** 71	**100** 259	**97** 71	**100** 254	**100** 52	**100** 136
Cobleskill Regional Hospital, Cobleskill, NY	**100** 61	**100** 55	**91** 43	**96** 71	**92** 63	**95** 21	- 0	- 0	- 0	- 0	- 0	**100** 4	- 0	**94** 18	- 0	- 0	- 0
Columbia Memorial Hospital, Hudson, NY	**90** 126	**94** 266	**87** 146	**93** 246	**85** 225	**94** 64	**90** 163	**100** 253	**93** 83	- 0	**89** 125	**90** 97	**100** 124	**80** 93	**89** 121	**91** 163	**89** 65
Community Memorial Hospital, Hamilton, NY	**94** 70	**98** 96	**96** 57	**99** 97	**94** 78	**91** 11	**100** 183	**100** 521	**100** 180	- 0	**100** 490	**100** 98	**100** 489	**100** 98	**99** 486	**100** 183	**97** 39
Community-General Hospital of Greater Syracuse, Syracuse, NY	**97** 91	**93** 164	**85** 97	**80** 155	**79** 150	**100** 31	**96** 164	**100** 412	**78** 118	- 0	**91** 267	**90** 591	**97** 270	**96** 581	**96** 261	**98** 164	**81** 145
Coney Island Hospital, Brooklyn, NY	**88** 108	**91** 202	**89** 157	**96** 186	**94** 260	**96** 45	**100** 145	**100** 240	**100** 53	- 0	**99** 88	**94** 50	**95** 88	**97** 99	**98** 82	**100** 145	**98** 44
Corning Hospital, Corning, NY	**95** 81	**99** 150	**94** 116	**91** 137	**96** 155	**91** 54	**88** 98	**99** 264	**86** 74	- 0	**97** 184	**85** 52	**96** 186	**88** 48	**96** 177	**88** 98	**100** 46
Cortland Regional Medical Center, Cortland, NY	**84** 170	**89** 259	**88** 136	**93** 223	**82** 192	**98** 58	**91** 74	**98** 153	**93** 30	- 0	**94** 63	**82** 60	**97** 63	**84** 56	**87** 63	**91** 74	**69** 36
Crouse Hospital, Syracuse, NY	**93** 180	**96** 310	**86** 182	**94** 307	**97** 259	**100** 90	**95** 141	**98** 530	**100** 143	- 0	**96** 370	**96** 870	**93** 368	**92** 862	**95** 361	**94** 142	**94** 115
Delaware Valley Hospital, Walton, NY	**91** 47	**98** 56	**100** 22	**100** 49	**94** 32	**88** 8	- 0	- 0	- 0	- 0	- 0	- 0	- 0	- 0	- 0	- 0	- 0
Eastern Long Island Hospital, Greenport, NY	**82** 39	**98** 58	**100** 26	**100** 49	**100** 43	**100** 5	**94** 36	**100** 45	**100** 13	- 0	**100** 24	**89** 46	**100** 24	**95** 43	**88** 24	**94** 36	**50** 2
Eastern Niagara Hospital, Lockport, NY	**92** 129	**99** 155	**92** 116	**99** 203	**95** 185	**91** 78	**83** 89	**100** 231	**70** 50	- 0	**98** 169	**91** 68	**94** 169	**91** 64	**90** 169	**87** 89	**58** 19
Edward John Noble Hospital of Gouverneur, Gouverneur, NY	**93** 15	**100** 23	**73** 15	**89** 28	**58** 19	**100** 7	**33** 3	**90** 21	**67** 3	- 0	**67** 18	**40** 5	**94** 18	**100** 5	**83** 18	**33** 3	**100** 2
Elizabethtown Community Hospital, Elizabethtown, NY	**91** 22	**91** 23	**94** 16	**96** 23	**87** 23	**100** 2	- 0	- 0	- 0	- 0	- 0	- -	- 0	- -	- 0	- 0	- 0
Ellenville Regional Hospital, Ellenville, NY	**33** 3	**100** 7	**50** 2	**100** 3	**86** 7	**100** 1	- 0	- 0	- 0	- 0	- 0	- -	- 0	- -	- 0	- 0	- 0
Ellis Hospital, Schenectady, NY	**96** 171	**99** 371	**95** 249	**95** 309	**97** 323	**98** 108	**97** 225	**99** 874	**93** 343	**96** 192	**100** 668	**92** 538	**97** 680	**96** 515	**98** 647	**100** 225	**90** 106
Elmhurst Hospital Center, Elmhurst, NY	**93** 225	**89** 228	**82** 165	**93** 252	**87** 251	**100** 95	**98** 323	**97** 436	**100** 74	**100** 1	**99** 127	**86** 21	**98** 129	**95** 84	**92** 125	**98** 323	**91** 70
Erie County Medical Center, Buffalo, NY	**88** 93	**94** 219	**71** 109	**82** 217	**74** 109	**95** 98	**92** 335	**99** 741	**79** 240	**91** 127	**97** 364	**94** 583	**98** 372	**98** 598	**92** 345	**97** 339	**85** 155
F F Thompson Hospital, Canandaigua, NY	**87** 163	**97** 221	**90** 124	**97** 215	**91** 194	**100** 63	**90** 146	**100** 464	**86** 125	- 0	**98** 401	**96** 84	**96** 401	**99** 83	**98** 388	**90** 146	**93** 135
Faxton-St Luke's Healthcare, Utica, NY	**76** 169	**92** 266	**83** 211	**85** 311	**85** 301	**99** 75	**89** 183	**100** 499	**99** 146	- 0	**91** 333	**80** 181	**93** 332	**78** 156	**75** 325	**90** 183	**92** 85
Flushing Hospital Medical Center, Flushing, NY	**93** 42	**99** 160	**76** 100	**98** 130	**84** 161	**92** 13	**96** 229	**100** 616	**96** 112	**100** 1	**99** 402	**92** 166	**95** 404	**90** 162	**90** 391	**96** 231	**75** 56
Forest Hills Hospital, Forest Hills, NY	**87** 77	**97** 141	**96** 89	**93** 122	**96** 162	**95** 21	**97** 191	**100** 411	**98** 110	- 0	**99** 269	**96** 122	**98** 270	**88** 118	**92** 257	**99** 191	**99** 106
Franklin Hospital, Valley Stream, NY	**95** 94	**99** 154	**97** 89	**97** 151	**96** 135	**100** 17	**98** 205	**100** 328	**95** 87	- 0	**98** 209	**96** 112	**94** 209	**96** 113	**98** 197	**99** 205	**98** 103
Geneva General Hospital, Geneva, NY	**85** 73	**91** 138	**79** 96	**86** 116	**87** 122	**88** 32	**85** 116	**100** 238	**95** 55	- 0	**96** 166	**92** 72	**94** 153	**98** 101	**97** 150	**97** 116	**84** 67
Glen Cove Hospital, Glen Cove, NY	**96** 71	**100** 126	**94** 72	**99** 119	**92** 142	**100** 15	**98** 183	**100** 299	**97** 95	- 0	**97** 194	**93** 44	**100** 194	**100** 41	**98** 189	**99** 183	**92** 105
Glens Falls Hospital, Glens Falls, NY	**90** 132	**89** 170	**92** 129	**95** 197	**97** 205	**100** 75	**91** 268	**100** 655	**93** 202	- 0	**97** 442	**95** 424	**95** 447	**94** 413	**96** 428	**92** 268	**90** 60
Good Samaritan Hospital Medical Center, West Islip, NY	**100** 73	**100** 135	**100** 100	**100** 126	**100** 158	**100** 36	**96** 281	**100** 500	**97** 190	- 0	**98** 296	**99** 352	**99** 298	**99** 351	**96** 277	**97** 281	**99** 109
Good Samaritan Hospital of Suffern, Suffern, NY	**85** 184	**94** 278	**92** 220	**94** 267	**93** 317	**100** 67	**70** 158	**100** 540	**100** 221	**99** 155	**94** 338	**92** 247	**94** 375	**95** 231	**88** 329	**74** 159	**88** 110
Harlem Hospital Center, New York, NY	**98** 47	**96** 147	**80** 65	**94** 144	**99** 72	**99** 72	**95** 77	**94** 120	**83** 12	- 0	**94** 34	**88** 26	**100** 34	**98** 43	**89** 28	**97** 77	**100** 3
Helen Hayes Hospital, West Haverstraw, NY	- 0	- 0	- 0	- 0	- 0	- 0	- 0	- 0	- 0	- 0	- 0	- 0	- 0	- 0	- 0	- 0	- 0
Highland Hospital, Rochester, NY	**98** 167	**98** 277	**96** 173	**99** 218	**98** 249	**100** 77	**98** 231	**100** 992	**86** 304	- 0	**96** 781	**95** 203	**97** 777	**96** 202	**99** 765	**99** 231	**95** 287
Hospital for Special Surgery, New York, NY	- 0	- 0	- 0	- 0	- 0	- 0	**96** 310	**100** 566	**97** 147	- 0	**97** 367	**97** 270	**100** 369	**100** 270	**94** 365	**96** 310	**88** 42
Hudson Valley Hospital Center, Cortlandt Manor, NY	**98** 96	**96** 186	**97** 121	**97** 197	**97** 246	**100** 63	**93** 239	**98** 389	**78** 101	- 0	**100** 224	**97** 97	**95** 224	**95** 95	**96** 223	**96** 239	**89** 110
Huntington Hospital, Huntington, NY	**96** 82	**95** 149	**99** 93	**96** 132	**95** 152	**100** 24	**98** 175	**100** 397	**96** 137	- 0	**98** 249	**95** 363	**98** 249	**94** 355	**97** 234	**99** 175	**80** 30
Interfaith Medical Center, Brooklyn, NY	**96** 81	**76** 129	**75** 65	**77** 147	**85** 84	**94** 65	**99** 82	**99** 113	**44** 9	- 0	**91** 47	**76** 21	**93** 46	**100** 17	**76** 45	**99** 82	**88** 8
Ira Davenport Memorial Hospital, Bath, NY	**80** 41	**100** 49	**91** 32	**100** 52	**96** 53	**95** 19	**100** 3	**100** 5	**100** 2	- 0	**100** 4	**92** 25	**100** 4	**100** 23	**100** 4	**100** 3	- 0
Jacobi Medical Center, Bronx, NY	**92** 86	**92** 174	**90** 120	**81** 186	**92** 133	**99** 69	**95** 284	**98** 447	**95** 101	**50** 2	**90** 160	**71** 31	**99** 159	**97** 88	**89** 155	**96** 285	**76** 67
Jamaica Hospital Medical Center, Jamaica, NY	**99** 95	**97** 115	**100** 63	**96** 112	**100** 86	**100** 43	**97** 199	**100** 412	**83** 75	**0** 1	**95** 188	**74** 101	**96** 190	**92** 87	**92** 178	**95** 206	**92** 39
J T Mather Mem Hosp of Port Jefferson, Port Jefferson, NY	**98** 193	**99** 352	**97** 197	**98** 281	**99** 262	**100** 110	**94** 304	**100** 536	**97** 191	- 0	**100** 276	**97** 165	**98** 282	**94** 178	**97** 266	**95** 304	**92** 74
Jones Memorial Hospital, Wellsville, NY	**88** 52	**94** 93	**79** 47	**95** 80	**93** 86	**83** 29	**88** 34	**99** 114	**96** 27	- 0	**97** 76	**98** 43	**99** 77	**98** 43	**100** 75	**88** 34	**86** 7
Kaleida Health, Buffalo, NY	**95** 623	**96** 951	**93** 551	**92** 943	**87** 830	**100** 240	**95** 454	**100** 1365	**91** 431	**92** 240	**94** 907	**89** 1163	**97** 922	**91** 1122	**94** 863	**97** 454	**84** 321
Kenmore Mercy Hospital, Kenmore, NY	**94** 93	**94** 157	**97** 100	**95** 150	**97** 154	**97** 38	**97** 126	**100** 384	**88** 129	- 0	**93** 250	**97** 705	**97** 253	**99** 697	**91** 240	**96** 127	**67** 30
Kings County Hospital Center, Brooklyn, NY	**97** 117	**92** 238	**86** 126	**91** 213	**91** 132	**96** 101	**97** 219	**100** 330	**91** 44	**100** 1	**99** 115	**100** 45	**98** 117	**99** 126	**88** 114	**97** 219	**68** 31
Kingsbrook Jewish Medical Center, Brooklyn, NY	**100** 105	**98** 299	**85** 244	**95** 280	**97** 385	**92** 49	**97** 126	**100** 170	**95** 43	- 0	**99** 78	**93** 61	**98** 81	**86** 58	**95** 65	**98** 127	**89** 36
Kingston Hospital, Kingston, NY	**96** 135	**97** 232	**94** 123	**99** 206	**96** 157	**100** 76	**87** 171	**99** 319	**92** 83	- 0	**97** 177	**91** 126	**97** 178	**96** 122	**87** 174	**90** 174	**84** 19
Lakeside Memorial Hospital, Brockport, NY	**83** 98	**97** 143	**100** 83	**100** 148	**98** 123	**100** 45	**100** 71	**100** 113	**97** 33	- 0	**100** 69	**88** 51	**94** 69	**98** 45	**88** 66	**100** 71	**85** 13
Lawrence Hospital Center, Bronxville, NY	**93** 105	**97** 88	**93** 96	**91** 163	**96** 160	**100** 28	**86** 141	**100** 295	**92** 77	- 0	**97** 183	**95** 110	**98** 184	**91** 106	**80** 180	**89** 142	**86** 42
Lenox Hill Hospital, New York, NY	**100** 88	**98** 171	**93** 94	**98** 133	**93** 141	**100** 22	**98** 245	**99** 741	**98** 266	**93** 166	**98** 521	**89** 606	**99** 540	**95** 577	**98** 503	**98** 247	**92** 118

NOTE: The first number in each column (boldface) is the score, the second number is the number of patients; Please refer to the main entry for footnotes; (a) 100-299
*MEASURES: **Pneumonia Care:** 16. Appropriate Initial Antibiotic; 17. Blood Culture Timing; 18. Influenza Vaccine; 19. Initial Antibiotic Timing; 20. Pneumococcal Vaccine; 21. Smoking Cessation Advice; **Surgical Care Improvement Project:** 22. Appropriate VTP Within 24 Hours; 23. Appropriate Hair Removal; 24. Appropriate Beta Blocker Usage; 25. Controlled Postoperative Blood Glucose; 26. Prophylactic Antibiotic Timing; 27. Prophylactic Antibiotic Timing (Outpatient); 28. Prophylactic Antibiotic Selection; 29. Prophylactic Antibiotic Selection (Outpatient); 30. Prophylactic Antibiotic Stopped; 31. Recommended VTP Ordered; 32. Urinary Catheter Removal*

Hospital	Pneumonia Care						Surgical Care Improvement Project										
	16	17	18	19	20	21	22	23	24	25	26	27	28	29	30	31	32
Lewis County General Hospital, Lowville, NY	**77** 43	**95** 60	**93** 30	**94** 67	**96** 52	**80** 10	**95** 58	**100** 132	**73** 26	**-** 0	**91** 103	**50** 2	**93** 102	**100** 2	**97** 98	**95** 58	**97** 32
Lincoln Medical & Mental Health Center, Bronx, NY	**95** 257	**97** 510	**89** 179	**91** 464	**96** 159	**100** 156	**98** 166	**100** 276	**98** 54	**-** 0	**97** 133	**88** 127	**99** 136	**89** 133	**91** 128	**99** 166	**83** 58
Little Falls Hospital, Little Falls, NY	**81** 42	**86** 51	**77** 48	**93** 59	**66** 56	**75** 12	**-** 0	**-** 0	**-** 0	**-** 0	**-** 0	**56** 25	**-** 0	**77** 22	**-** 0	**-** 0	**-** 0
Long Beach Medical Center, Long Beach, NY	**91** 58	**95** 163	**95** 80	**99** 143	**93** 140	**88** 24	**90** 39	**100** 61	**94** 16	**-** 0	**100** 28	**95** 20	**82** 28	**100** 19	**85** 27	**97** 39	**86** 7
Long Island College Hospital, Brooklyn, NY	**91** 77	**99** 139	**83** 75	**89** 142	**67** 102	**98** 40	**97** 233	**99** 436	**93** 100	**-** 0	**93** 312	**86** 176	**94** 307	**92** 162	**86** 300	**97** 233	**91** 101
Long Island Jewish Medical Center, New Hyde Park, NY	**90** 92	**99** 157	**100** 85	**95** 151	**96** 119	**100** 23	**99** 169	**100** 671	**88** 221	**99** 154	**98** 473	**87** 145	**94** 482	**85** 131	**96** 453	**98** 171	**92** 153
Lutheran Medical Center, Brooklyn, NY	**97** 219	**96** 382	**96** 246	**95** 335	**90** 344	**93** 60	**98** 482	**99** 959	**86** 292	**-** 0	**99** 665	**87** 118	**98** 665	**83** 103	**94** 645	**99** 482	**88** 165
Maimonides Medical Center, Brooklyn, NY	**96** 74	**96** 160	**57** 96	**90** 134	**84** 174	**100** 19	**94** 314	**100** 1231	**89** 496	**93** 373	**93** 933	**85** 176	**97** 945	**88** 158	**91** 904	**97** 321	**90** 256
Margaretville Memorial Hospital, Margaretville, NY	**83** 12	**84** 19	**100** 8	**-** 0	**100** 18	**100** 1	**-** 0	**-** 0	**-** 0	**-** 0	**-** 0	**-** 0	**-** 0	**-** 0	**-** 0	**-** 0	**-** 0
Mary Imogene Bassett Hospital, Cooperstown, NY	**95** 57	**97** 98	**82** 102	**91** 104	**97** 134	**92** 63	**97** 237	**100** 610	**94** 263	**89** 109	**96** 449	**89** 283	**98** 455	**91** 362	**92** 418	**97** 237	**86** 170
Massena Memorial Hospital, Massena, NY	**87** 61	**95** 116	**96** 54	**99** 125	**97** 77	**97** 35	**95** 39	**100** 105	**96** 24	**-** 0	**93** 89	**84** 43	**81** 86	**85** 40	**87** 85	**95** 39	**100** 25
Medina Memorial Hospital, Medina, NY	**86** 73	**96** 107	**91** 67	**95** 116	**90** 100	**100** 21	**85** 34	**100** 63	**83** 24	**-** 0	**100** 30	**53** 15	**93** 30	**75** 32	**93** 27	**94** 34	**75** 8
Mercy Hospital, Buffalo, NY	**95** 97	**98** 133	**90** 79	**94** 129	**95** 124	**100** 56	**95** 152	**100** 701	**93** 265	**95** 170	**94** 486	**97** 560	**97** 506	**98** 548	**97** 459	**99** 152	**94** 156
Mercy Medical Center, Rockville Centre, NY	**91** 113	**94** 207	**91** 118	**94** 203	**85** 215	**100** 34	**91** 274	**100** 497	**100** 216	**100** 1	**97** 316	**95** 99	**97** 317	**86** 96	**95** 298	**97** 274	**99** 137
Metropolitan Hospital Center, New York, NY	**100** 70	**92** 112	**98** 54	**96** 104	**92** 59	**100** 39	**99** 128	**100** 257	**94** 48	**-** 0	**96** 163	**94** 65	**94** 163	**97** 63	**95** 149	**99** 128	**100** 46
Monroe Community Hospital, Rochester, NY	**-** 0	**-** 0	**-** 0	**-** 0	**-** 0	**-** 0	**-** 0	**-** 0	**-** 0	**-** 0	**-** 0	**-** -	**-** 0	**-** -	**-** 0	**-** 0	**-** 0
Montefiore Medical Center, Bronx, NY	**81** 190	**82** 374	**77** 232	**79** 413	**89** 340	**100** 91	**88** 411	**96** 1163	**77** 415	**83** 212	**85** 750	**73** 681	**97** 749	**66** 624	**90** 711	**91** 416	**76** 210
Moses-Ludington Hospital, Ticonderoga, NY	**79** 24	**88** 33	**87** 23	**50** 2	**93** 30	**100** 6	**-** 0	**-** 0	**-** 0	**-** 0	**-** 0	**-** -	**-** 0	**-** -	**-** 0	**-** 0	**-** 0
Mount Sinai Hospital, New York, NY	**91** 129	**95** 204	**83** 154	**92** 237	**79** 220	**99** 68	**93** 526	**99** 1156	**96** 369	**91** 174	**97** 710	**89** 557	**98** 721	**95** 539	**93** 675	**97** 526	**80** 257
Mount St Mary's Hospital and Health Center, Lewiston, NY	**93** 140	**98** 222	**97** 117	**98** 214	**95** 188	**89** 56	**96** 121	**100** 385	**99** 101	**-** 0	**96** 289	**82** 196	**97** 289	**70** 186	**93** 289	**97** 121	**98** 86
Mount Vernon Hospital, Mount Vernon, NY	**94** 52	**100** 107	**71** 45	**92** 91	**92** 59	**100** 31	**68** 62	**100** 92	**63** 19	**-** 0	**91** 34	**94** 53	**85** 34	**86** 51	**78** 32	**76** 63	**91** 23
Nassau University Medical Center, East Meadow, NY	**85** 93	**79** 92	**100** 115	**92** 142	**93** 142	**100** 55	**99** 178	**100** 326	**100** 56	**-** 0	**97** 165	**93** 59	**91** 164	**78** 90	**96** 161	**99** 178	**100** 39
Nathan Littauer Hospital, Gloversville, NY	**89** 66	**80** 104	**95** 73	**93** 114	**65** 108	**97** 33	**83** 63	**99** 148	**100** 47	**-** 0	**76** 46	**80** 59	**91** 46	**85** 52	**87** 45	**90** 63	**100** 3
New York Community Hospital of Brooklyn, Brooklyn, NY	**100** 81	**95** 110	**96** 70	**99** 89	**98** 115	**100** 14	**100** 85	**100** 141	**100** 53	**100** 1	**94** 63	**100** 22	**94** 63	**82** 22	**94** 50	**100** 85	**94** 16
New York Downtown Hospital, New York, NY	**96** 107	**99** 155	**93** 84	**96** 139	**91** 159	**100** 35	**94** 144	**100** 316	**92** 65	**-** 0	**100** 214	**89** 76	**98** 213	**100** 69	**95** 208	**96** 144	**94** 36
New York Hospital Medical Center of Queens, Flushing, NY	**93** 90	**98** 187	**90** 105	**90** 173	**85** 181	**100** 26	**98** 326	**100** 771	**96** 230	**99** 107	**100** 496	**93** 312	**97** 501	**94** 298	**96** 451	**98** 326	**94** 156
New York Methodist Hospital, Brooklyn, NY	**93** 90	**69** 111	**89** 94	**88** 171	**98** 165	**100** 39	**99** 334	**100** 791	**86** 251	**97** 118	**98** 521	**95** 186	**97** 528	**96** 182	**85** 479	**99** 334	**91** 180
New York Westchester Square Medical Center, Bronx, NY	**93** 114	**98** 236	**96** 108	**99** 229	**95** 187	**100** 40	**98** 200	**100** 321	**98** 53	**-** 0	**98** 189	**96** 81	**98** 190	**96** 79	**90** 186	**99** 200	**65** 78
New York-Presbyterian Hospital, New York, NY	**94** 210	**91** 549	**91** 410	**83** 465	**90** 590	**95** 109	**100** 633	**100** 1737	**99** 539	**87** 339	**95** 811	**90** 1187	**97** 954	**90** 1154	**93** 776	**100** 635	**91** 234
Newark-Wayne Community Hospital, Newark, NY	**85** 91	**96** 121	**97** 75	**98** 136	**96** 105	**100** 53	**96** 95	**100** 259	**79** 77	**-** 0	**97** 192	**86** 76	**99** 191	**97** 67	**91** 188	**97** 95	**100** 18
Niagara Falls Memorial Medical Center, Niagara Falls, NY	**97** 96	**99** 150	**92** 106	**98** 106	**94** 111	**100** 83	**94** 72	**100** 134	**93** 29	**-** 0	**100** 65	**93** 89	**92** 65	**94** 90	**85** 61	**94** 72	**100** 11
Nicholas H Noyes Memorial Hospital, Dansville, NY	**93** 91	**98** 103	**86** 81	**93** 123	**92** 120	**95** 21	**82** 44	**100** 150	**81** 54	**-** 0	**93** 98	**88** 40	**92** 96	**61** 36	**91** 96	**82** 44	**98** 53
North Central Bronx Hospital, Bronx, NY	**98** 55	**97** 97	**65** 49	**98** 95	**89** 37	**97** 35	**83** 30	**96** 72	**100** 6	**-** 0	**94** 35	**69** 13	**85** 34	**100** 24	**76** 34	**87** 30	**25** 4
North General Hospital, New York, NY	**-** -	**-** -	**-** -	**-** -	**-** -	**-** -	**-** -	**-** -	**-** -	**-** -	**-** -	**-** -	**-** -	**-** -	**-** -	**-** -	**-** -
North Shore University Hospital, Manhasset, NY	**95** 154	**99** 286	**99** 148	**99** 253	**98** 266	**100** 39	**99** 352	**100** 982	**96** 297	**97** 159	**98** 594	**91** 291	**98** 603	**98** 281	**96** 575	**99** 352	**80** 189
Northern Dutchess Hospital, Rhinebeck, NY	**84** 38	**92** 71	**84** 56	**96** 70	**86** 73	**72** 18	**89** 101	**100** 320	**84** 90	**-** 0	**95** 206	**86** 110	**98** 207	**98** 103	**98** 203	**94** 101	**86** 123
Northern Westchester Hospital, Mount Kisco, NY	**94** 71	**96** 175	**93** 95	**100** 159	**93** 169	**95** 21	**94** 140	**100** 371	**94** 83	**-** 0	**97** 231	**97** 336	**97** 245	**97** 333	**96** 226	**96** 141	**97** 108
Northport VA Medical Center, Northport, NY	**98** 43	**92** 93	**94** 47	**91** 87	**97** 77	**100** 23	**99** 99	**100** 126	**88** 43	**-** 0	**98** 61	**-** -	**95** 63	**-** -	**90** 60	**100** 99	**85** 53
NY Eye and Ear Infirmary, New York, NY	**-** 0	**-** 0	**-** 0	**-** 0	**-** 0	**-** 0	**-** 0	**-** 0	**-** 0	**-** 0	**-** 0	**-** 0	**-** 0	**-** 0	**-** 0	**-** 0	**-** 0
Nyack Hospital, Nyack, NY	**96** 105	**98** 173	**99** 108	**97** 165	**99** 160	**100** 29	**98** 255	**100** 664	**99** 138	**-** 0	**100** 411	**98** 121	**99** 412	**93** 119	**98** 394	**98** 255	**99** 168
NYU Hospitals Center, New York, NY	**100** 74	**96** 140	**98** 84	**98** 129	**98** 138	**100** 25	**98** 274	**100** 710	**98** 214	**98** 131	**98** 485	**99** 422	**98** 490	**96** 422	**98** 462	**100** 274	**93** 169
O'Connor Hospital, Delhi, NY	**100** 6	**100** 4	**100** 3	**100** 3	**100** 8	**-** 0	**-** 0	**-** 0	**-** 0	**-** 0	**-** 0	**-** -	**-** 0	**-** -	**-** 0	**-** 0	**-** 0
Olean General Hospital, Olean, NY	**88** 138	**97** 232	**91** 166	**96** 221	**96** 227	**100** 78	**99** 181	**100** 399	**94** 97	**-** 0	**100** 275	**89** 151	**97** 276	**85** 139	**97** 248	**98** 183	**83** 48
Oneida Healthcare Center, Oneida, NY	**94** 65	**97** 70	**86** 50	**97** 76	**92** 64	**97** 34	**99** 174	**98** 275	**86** 69	**-** 0	**94** 181	**95** 219	**97** 181	**92** 216	**97** 179	**99** 174	**70** 20
Orange Regional Medical Center, Goshen, NY	**91** 284	**96** 547	**96** 302	**96** 524	**95** 490	**99** 153	**94** 409	**100** 930	**93** 304	**100** 1	**98** 682	**92** 314	**98** 687	**88** 297	**97** 666	**96** 409	**98** 265
Oswego Hospital, Oswego, NY	**93** 130	**97** 218	**88** 142	**89** 223	**88** 224	**97** 96	**92** 97	**100** 190	**81** 36	**-** 0	**92** 109	**97** 156	**89** 112	**95** 155	**78** 102	**92** 97	**91** 11
Our Lady of Lourdes Memorial Hospital, Binghamton, NY	**93** 200	**90** 383	**87** 222	**97** 330	**86** 335	**100** 100	**98** 122	**100** 349	**100** 77	**-** 0	**95** 229	**94** 422	**96** 230	**92** 452	**97** 225	**98** 122	**100** 24
Peconic Bay Medical Center, Riverhead, NY	**89** 82	**85** 124	**73** 70	**95** 115	**70** 105	**100** 35	**92** 229	**100** 463	**90** 146	**-** 0	**95** 308	**93** 67	**93** 308	**97** 62	**92** 298	**97** 229	**96** 159
Peninsula Hospital Center, Far Rockaway, NY	**88** 84	**84** 171	**83** 112	**83** 195	**86** 192	**100** 43	**59** 54	**100** 88	**90** 20	**100** 1	**92** 36	**93** 60	**94** 36	**73** 56	**87** 30	**61** 54	**82** 11
Phelps Memorial Hospital Assn, Sleepy Hollow, NY	**92** 73	**97** 136	**97** 92	**96** 114	**95** 115	**100** 23	**99** 272	**100** 486	**98** 174	**-** 0	**97** 340	**92** 73	**97** 341	**94** 104	**91** 327	**100** 272	**99** 159
Plainview Hospital, Plainview, NY	**95** 96	**99** 150	**99** 93	**99** 141	**98** 164	**100** 30	**99** 227	**100** 434	**100** 159	**100** 1	**98** 265	**89** 153	**98** 265	**79** 155	**96** 252	**100** 228	**98** 52
Putnam Hospital Center, Carmel, NY	**94** 107	**98** 157	**98** 97	**99** 148	**97** 142	**100** 38	**93** 424	**100** 708	**96** 224	**-** 0	**98** 538	**94** 150	**98** 537	**92** 148	**98** 535	**95** 424	**95** 289
Queens Hospital Center, Jamaica, NY	**95** 103	**84** 124	**98** 88	**78** 161	**97** 94	**94** 32	**98** 195	**100** 319	**67** 52	**-** 0	**95** 133	**82** 38	**95** 132	**98** 93	**88** 125	**98** 195	**92** 13
Richmond University Medical Center, Staten Island, NY	**90** 51	**94** 157	**96** 76	**97** 130	**98** 122	**100** 38	**98** 183	**100** 434	**97** 122	**100** 1	**99** 293	**91** 207	**93** 295	**96** 199	**95** 285	**98** 183	**78** 40
River Hospital, Alexandria Bay, NY	**0** 1	**-** 0	**-** 0	**100** 2	**67** 6	**0** 1	**-** 0	**-** 0	**-** 0	**-** 0	**-** 0	**-** 0	**-** 0	**-** 0	**-** 0	**-** 0	**-** 0
Rochester General Hospital, Rochester, NY	**95** 369	**98** 514	**89** 348	**88** 557	**85** 491	**100** 186	**96** 553	**100** 2308	**93** 1057	**98** 634	**99** 1832	**92** 690	**99** 1874	**90** 650	**99** 1774	**96** 553	**97** 327
Rome Memorial Hospital, Rome, NY	**88** 100	**99** 207	**94** 123	**96** 192	**96** 162	**92** 53	**93** 112	**100** 239	**89** 35	**-** 0	**91** 116	**79** 53	**89** 115	**85** 46	**94** 108	**94** 112	**95** 20
Saint Anthony Community Hospital, Warwick, NY	**86** 49	**97** 88	**78** 60	**98** 83	**84** 91	**100** 22	**92** 76	**100** 233	**90** 50	**-** 0	**96** 155	**96** 49	**88** 155	**84** 49	**97** 149	**95** 76	**85** 27
Saint Barnabas Hospital, Bronx, NY	**97** 150	**95** 261	**83** 125	**95** 214	**95** 122	**97** 110	**95** 132	**99** 196	**95** 40	**-** 0	**94** 100	**87** 139	**96** 98	**95** 155	**88** 91	**97** 132	**94** 17
Saint Catherine of Siena Hospital, Smithtown, NY	**81** 110	**94** 35	**99** 139	**89** 228	**100** 219	**100** 36	**98** 232	**100** 445	**100** 151	**-** 0	**99** 250	**98** 387	**96** 252	**84** 383	**98** 237	**99** 232	**100** 89
Saint Charles Hospital, Port Jefferson, NY	**96** 73	**100** 130	**100** 56	**100** 98	**100** 62	**97** 30	**99** 269	**100** 691	**100** 204	**-** 0	**100** 488	**98** 46	**100** 490	**96** 45	**100** 483	**99** 269	**100** 248
Saint Elizabeth Medical Center, Utica, NY	**91** 103	**93** 117	**86** 168	**96** 176	**90** 236	**97** 74	**75** 173	**99** 1070	**89** 514	**95** 350	**92** 834	**77** 183	**98** 851	**94** 150	**96** 818	**86** 173	**62** 90
Saint Francis Hospital, Poughkeepsie, NY	**99** 67	**99** 120	**99** 94	**97** 118	**99** 115	**100** 56	**96** 136	**100** 367	**98** 115	**-** 0	**100** 233	**94** 181	**99** 231	**95** 176	**99** 227	**99** 136	**100** 32
Saint Francis Hospital - Roslyn, Roslyn, NY	**86** 110	**95** 173	**100** 113	**88** 154	**99** 203	**100** 21	**97** 188	**100** 650	**97** 331	**97** 234	**97** 399	**95** 340	**99** 416	**96** 341	**97** 381	**98** 188	**90** 141
Saint James Mercy Hospital, Hornell, NY	**94** 71	**97** 106	**98** 61	**99** 100	**100** 87	**87** 23	**87** 60	**100** 117	**100** 29	**-** 0	**97** 76	**100** 15	**90** 78	**93** 15	**88** 69	**88** 60	**100** 19
Saint John's Episcopal Hospital at South Shore, Far Rockaway, NY	**92** 24	**98** 124	**93** 75	**90** 129	**94** 132	**100** 18	**88** 88	**100** 148	**100** 38	**-** 0	**93** 61	**87** 69	**89** 63	**90** 62	**95** 57	**88** 88	**94** 17
Saint John's Riverside Hospital, Yonkers, NY	**87** 75	**86** 165	**87** 69	**91** 142	**91** 134	**86** 29	**77** 208	**99** 354	**93** 100	**-** 0	**89** 218	**83** 83	**95** 220	**92** 78	**84** 214	**85** 208	**71** 48
Saint Joseph Hospital, Bethpage, NY	**93** 120	**93** 163	**93** 73	**92** 131	**94** 112	**100** 38	**88** 154	**100** 262	**99** 85	**-** 0	**97** 162	**91** 58	**96** 162	**95** 55	**98** 152	**97** 154	**86** 28

NOTE: The first number in each column (boldface) is the score, the second number is the number of patients; Please refer to the main entry for footnotes; (a) 100-299
*MEASURES: **Pneumonia Care:** 16. Appropriate Initial Antibiotic; 17. Blood Culture Timing; 18. Influenza Vaccine; 19. Initial Antibiotic Timing; 20. Pneumococcal Vaccine; 21. Smoking Cessation Advice; **Surgical Care Improvement Project:** 22. Appropriate VTP Within 24 Hours; 23. Appropriate Hair Removal; 24. Appropriate Beta Blocker Usage; 25. Controlled Postoperative Blood Glucose; 26. Prophylactic Antibiotic Timing; 27. Prophylactic Antibiotic Timing (Outpatient); 28. Prophylactic Antibiotic Selection; 29. Prophylactic Antibiotic Selection (Outpatient); 30. Prophylactic Antibiotic Stopped; 31. Recommended VTP Ordered; 32. Urinary Catheter Removal*

Hospital	Pneumonia Care							Surgical Care Improvement Project									
	16	17	18	19	20	21	22	23	24	25	26	27	28	29	30	31	32
Saint Joseph's Hospital, Elmira, NY	98 95	95 158	95 119	95 156	93 179	100 56	100 49	100 203	92 59	- 0	98 173	100 94	99 174	98 94	99 168	100 49	95 21
Saint Joseph's Hospital Health Center, Syracuse, NY	91 387	96 615	95 418	82 568	94 696	100 314	98 170	100 752	91 292	87 180	94 536	94 794	98 541	98 789	89 497	99 170	77 73
Saint Joseph's Medical Center, Yonkers, NY	94 84	95 192	92 116	97 190	92 162	97 35	93 85	100 132	95 40	- 0	88 69	96 83	90 71	76 82	83 60	93 85	50 6
Saint Luke's Cornwall Hospital, Newburgh, NY	86 115	92 157	85 106	89 169	88 153	96 49	90 123	100 360	98 95	100 1	100 228	97 152	100 228	93 149	100 226	93 123	96 23
Saint Luke's Roosevelt Hospital, New York, NY	91 115	97 176	52 93	93 178	66 129	100 58	92 322	99 768	86 181	96 144	94 571	92 341	96 579	93 323	94 549	92 322	93 178
Saint Mary's Hospital at Amsterdam, Amsterdam, NY	94 81	97 125	97 79	94 148	99 116	100 33	93 122	100 297	100 100	- 0	99 178	81 91	98 179	97 116	99 174	94 122	76 78
Saint Peter's Hospital, Albany, NY	92 91	92 131	89 100	90 147	93 150	100 30	97 252	98 737	71 210	98 183	95 547	90 971	97 548	89 952	93 536	99 252	82 112
Samaritan Hospital, Troy, NY	93 94	94 171	77 92	97 171	89 155	93 58	74 152	96 380	89 109	- 0	92 229	64 85	90 231	93 67	90 221	84 154	76 87
Samaritan Medical Center, Watertown, NY	94 101	99 189	95 120	92 176	92 168	96 57	93 189	100 468	83 143	- 0	95 343	84 443	98 348	96 453	92 340	94 189	86 149
Saratoga Hospital, Saratoga Springs, NY	94 162	96 258	99 167	94 246	98 229	99 90	93 345	100 713	80 205	- 0	98 489	88 238	97 488	96 214	85 472	93 349	91 225
Schuyler Hospital, Montour Falls, NY	90 41	97 71	98 54	96 76	96 70	100 15	- 0	100 60	- 0	- 0	- 0	- -	- 0	- -	- 0	- 0	100 7
Seton Health System-St Mary's Campus, Troy, NY	90 94	94 108	94 88	97 140	89 121	100 39	96 203	100 383	96 104	- 0	97 259	96 258	97 258	97 256	98 248	97 203	97 129
Sheehan Memorial Hospital, Buffalo, NY	- 0	- 0	- 0	- 0	- 0	- 0	- 0	- 0	- 0	- 0	- 0	- 0	- 0	- 0	- 0	- 0	- 0
Sisters of Charity Hospital, Buffalo, NY	91 216	96 263	89 168	94 285	92 248	98 104	91 257	100 873	90 284	- 0	96 567	91 614	95 571	97 596	92 545	93 258	88 215
Soldiers and Sailors Memorial Hospital of Yates, Penn Yan, NY	81 36	94 54	81 32	98 41	83 47	86 7	- 0	- 0	- 0	- 0	- 0	- 0	- 0	- 0	- 0	- 0	- 0
Sound Shore Medical Center of Westschester, New Rochelle, NY	91 117	98 130	96 122	98 156	97 183	100 39	88 282	100 473	85 153	- 0	97 298	89 97	99 324	91 88	98 291	94 282	95 152
South Nassau Communities Hospital, Oceanside, NY	93 211	98 364	97 219	98 314	97 344	100 69	96 343	100 969	95 333	- 0	100 707	98 378	97 708	94 379	95 687	99 343	96 290
Southampton Hospital, Southampton, NY	95 118	92 194	99 108	94 172	98 181	100 34	84 70	100 168	93 42	- 0	98 85	88 50	86 85	87 47	90 79	86 70	82 11
Southside Hospital, Bay Shore, NY	97 104	99 139	100 84	99 160	98 125	100 53	97 236	100 419	99 131	- 0	98 264	99 164	99 266	99 163	98 251	97 236	100 103
Staten Island University Hospital, Staten Island, NY	96 89	99 209	96 80	96 120	98 117	100 40	99 188	100 536	95 175	92 128	98 381	84 233	97 387	90 253	97 353	99 188	99 98
Strong Memorial Hospital, Rochester, NY	82 74	88 157	86 66	81 136	87 77	93 61	100 306	100 1282	97 532	92 428	99 847	98 572	99 868	99 572	99 818	100 306	98 327
Sunnyview Hospital and Rehabilitation Center, Schenectady, NY	- 0	- 0	- 0	- 0	- 0	- 0	- 0	- 0	- 0	- 0	- 0	- 0	- 0	- 0	- 0	- 0	- 0
Syracuse VA Medical Center, Syracuse, NY	99 82	99 132	99 76	94 121	98 115	100 43	100 107	100 135	85 62	- 0	96 72	- -	90 72	- -	92 72	99 108	100 66
TLC Health Network, Gowanda, NY	95 63	96 72	92 61	94 89	97 78	86 29	100 111	100 159	73 51	- 0	94 126	89 19	94 126	100 19	90 122	100 111	50 12
United Health Services Hospitals, Johnson City, NY	96 200	96 386	95 232	92 350	94 345	100 144	96 470	100 1500	95 503	95 285	98 967	98 1362	97 975	97 1361	95 933	97 470	92 406
United Memorial Medical Center, Batavia, NY	93 83	89 183	93 103	98 167	93 163	88 59	92 150	100 268	100 102	- 0	94 217	90 60	98 215	84 61	79 211	95 150	66 68
Unity Hospital of Rochester, Rochester, NY	97 114	98 200	93 105	91 190	93 168	100 52	99 170	98 561	81 254	- 0	93 393	93 423	94 391	98 414	93 387	99 170	90 161
University Hospital - Stony Brook, Stony Brook, NY	88 69	90 132	62 65	91 135	80 94	100 55	99 175	100 542	82 176	92 119	99 358	88 384	98 367	96 399	93 347	99 176	87 134
University Hospital of Brooklyn - Downstate, Brooklyn, NY	86 76	85 124	82 71	80 137	68 95	81 31	98 184	100 382	99 110	90 60	93 256	94 108	98 261	91 103	92 244	98 184	98 90
University Hospital S U N Y Health Science Center, Syracuse, NY	96 78	96 168	85 134	94 145	84 126	100 90	99 171	100 588	98 235	97 198	97 421	86 269	99 427	98 337	91 365	99 172	78 124
Upstate New York VA Healthcare System, Buffalo, NY	91 57	99 107	88 59	91 95	95 92	100 26	94 116	100 282	96 129	96 67	96 156	- -	98 163	- -	94 151	94 116	63 86
VA Hudson Valley Healthcare System, Montrose, NY	100 8	100 21	100 26	100 25	100 29	100 9	- 0	- 0	- 0	- 0	- 0	- -	- 0	- -	- 0	- 0	- 0
VA New York Harbor Healthcare System, New York, NY	95 88	97 157	80 98	94 143	97 131	100 48	99 108	100 243	99 128	91 75	100 140	- -	100 149	- -	93 136	98 109	100 55
Vassar Brothers Medical Center, Poughkeepsie, NY	92 142	100 247	98 204	98 251	97 302	100 64	92 187	99 642	95 274	96 171	97 442	95 637	98 446	95 632	97 409	98 187	96 55
Westchester Medical Center, Valhalla, NY	78 32	90 61	73 59	97 59	80 79	100 27	95 348	100 1026	92 475	96 335	94 588	94 377	99 614	97 366	95 537	96 348	86 186
Westfield Memorial Hospital, Westfield, NY	60 5	100 3	100 3	100 3	100 4	100 2	- 0	100 9	100 1	- 0	100 8	- 0	100 8	- 0	100 8	- 0	- 0
White Plains Hospital Center, White Plains, NY	88 108	98 115	82 98	95 163	85 168	89 28	90 225	100 429	97 97	- 0	99 296	97 354	97 297	99 351	83 288	92 225	72 46
Winifred Masterson Burke Rehab Hospital, White Plains, NY	- 0	- 0	- 0	- 0	- 0	- 0	- 0	- 0	- 0	- 0	- 0	- 0	- 0	- 0	- 0	- 0	- 0
Winthrop-University Hospital, Mineola, NY	94 107	99 187	97 101	96 157	97 164	100 32	98 279	100 902	95 398	89 212	95 642	96 477	98 648	94 475	99 605	99 279	91 211
Woman's Christian Association, Jamestown, NY	91 105	98 180	83 115	97 187	90 176	98 62	83 126	99 429	89 154	- 0	98 298	79 124	98 299	96 112	92 283	85 126	50 18
Woodhull Medical and Mental Health Center, Brooklyn, NY	96 124	87 231	81 101	87 193	90 117	97 108	97 145	100 257	86 28	- 0	97 94	84 38	97 93	98 117	97 89	97 145	73 22
Wyckoff Heights Medical Center, Brooklyn, NY	88 117	89 107	86 90	83 173	89 142	100 36	94 210	99 329	87 79	- 0	95 143	77 132	92 146	93 161	80 132	96 210	57 42
Wyoming County Community Hospital, Warsaw, NY	81 54	89 75	77 56	95 82	86 70	91 22	73 82	100 157	93 46	- 0	94 119	78 23	97 120	74 19	87 119	73 82	100 6
NORTH CAROLINA																	
Alamance Regional Medical Center, Burlington, NC	87 115	93 149	94 130	93 166	95 173	100 59	95 427	100 755	90 208	- 0	97 519	93 283	94 520	95 273	93 506	95 431	84 199
Albemarle Hospital Authority, Elizabeth City, NC	83 66	88 94	82 88	88 101	95 112	97 39	96 124	100 232	95 62	- 0	100 141	97 256	98 146	92 252	97 128	98 124	68 37
Alleghany County Memorial Hospital, Sparta, NC	86 51	91 55	90 48	92 65	95 61	96 23	- 0	- 0	- 0	- 0	- 0	67 3	- 0	100 2	- 0	- 0	- 0
Angel Medical Center, Franklin, NC	88 50	91 47	85 41	98 64	91 67	100 15	91 45	97 69	100 15	- 0	98 47	95 19	100 47	95 19	85 46	93 45	91 11
Anson Community Hospital, Wadesboro, NC	94 47	94 89	100 56	99 88	100 88	100 21	100 8	100 20	50 2	- 0	100 9	88 8	100 9	67 9	100 8	100 8	50 2
Ashe Memorial Hospital, Jefferson, NC	96 99	98 53	73 85	95 111	88 136	95 42	100 22	100 29	60 5	- 0	100 8	100 9	88 8	100 9	100 8	100 22	100 2
Asheville-Oteen VA Medical Center, Asheville, NC	82 106	99 127	90 87	93 129	92 126	100 40	97 87	100 477	100 263	97 194	99 387	- -	100 389	- -	99 369	97 87	100 297
Beaufort County Medical Center, Washington, NC	82 49	88 67	91 54	93 76	90 61	96 26	85 106	100 275	81 53	- 0	99 181	91 160	95 182	99 163	98 173	83 108	88 93
Bertie Memorial Hospital, Windsor, NC	100 15	100 22	90 10	100 23	95 19	100 2	- 0	- 0	- 0	- 0	- 0	- -	- 0	- -	- 0	- 0	- 0
Betsy Johnson Regional Hospital, Dunn, NC	87 159	93 188	87 162	95 206	96 173	99 78	75 102	99 206	71 51	- 0	95 125	86 157	98 125	96 142	91 121	82 102	82 50
Blowing Rock Hospital, Blowing Rock, NC	- 0	- 0	- 0	- 0	- 0	- 0	- 0	- 0	- 0	- 0	- 0	- -	- 0	- -	- 0	- 0	- 0
Brunswick Community Hospital, Supply, NC	93 74	99 106	100 68	100 105	99 94	100 56	99 134	100 307	100 73	- 0	100 233	96 98	100 233	88 95	98 220	99 134	95 82
C J Harris Community Hospital, Sylva, NC	94 141	96 158	96 130	94 179	99 193	100 81	85 152	100 274	100 47	- 0	95 212	90 144	98 214	91 139	96 193	95 152	92 74
Caldwell Memorial Hospital, Lenoir, NC	82 74	98 140	81 97	91 125	93 120	97 72	89 113	100 308	96 56	- 0	95 199	94 105	99 202	95 104	90 187	91 113	89 73
Cape Fear Valley Medical Center, Fayetteville, NC	95 377	97 634	95 447	94 593	97 512	100 296	90 199	100 615	98 187	94 101	98 444	92 486	97 451	83 471	91 434	94 199	87 127
Cape Fear Valley-Bladen County Hospital, Elizabethtown, NC	92 24	85 34	92 24	87 23	87 30	71 7	67 6	100 24	- 0	- 0	88 17	- 0	100 17	- 0	100 16	67 6	- 0
Carolina East Medical Center, New Bern, NC	93 147	95 300	78 204	95 283	82 258	99 142	93 665	100 1419	83 383	74 198	96 1028	92 589	97 1031	94 571	88 1004	93 667	76 422
Carolinas Medical Center-Behavioral Health, Charlotte, NC	90 145	94 174	98 204	92 236	98 244	98 178	95 571	100 2153	96 650	92 520	98 1653	87 1148	97 1675	96 1168	97 1581	98 572	65 337
Carolinas Medical Center-Lincoln, Lincolnton, NC	98 109	98 139	99 82	96 135	98 80	100 82	95 39	100 113	100 19	- 0	98 81	89 19	99 83	100 17	96 68	92 40	75 8
Carolinas Medical Center-Mercy, Charlotte, NC	95 177	96 235	97 184	94 266	98 217	100 99	98 725	100 2101	97 483	83 30	97 1774	92 1223	99 1780	98 1174	97 1747	98 726	96 829
Carolinas Medical Center-Northeast, Concord, NC	98 431	100 635	98 392	97 606	96 483	100 245	93 455	100 1225	96 398	91 190	99 965	99 565	100 978	97 563	98 921	96 455	90 398
Carolinas Medical Center-Union, Monroe, NC	94 89	98 137	95 83	98 128	96 109	100 75	97 212	100 359	96 69	- 0	100 235	95 170	99 235	96 166	97 216	98 212	89 71
Carolinas Medical Center-University, Charlotte, NC	95 112	98 158	99 85	99 155	98 86	100 73	95 154	100 328	98 59	- 0	99 239	98 362	98 239	96 362	97 227	98 154	76 17
Carteret General Hospital, Morehead City, NC	88 95	97 129	94 94	92 142	96 110	98 54	72 155	100 497	94 118	- 0	98 306	99 152	100 306	95 152	98 297	77 155	60 30

NOTE: The first number in each column (boldface) is the score, the second number is the number of patients; Please refer to the main entry for footnotes; (a) 100-299
*MEASURES: **Pneumonia Care:** 16. Appropriate Initial Antibiotic; 17. Blood Culture Timing; 18. Influenza Vaccine; 19. Initial Antibiotic Timing; 20. Pneumococcal Vaccine; 21. Smoking Cessation Advice; **Surgical Care Improvement Project:** 22. Appropriate VTP Within 24 Hours; 23. Appropriate Hair Removal; 24. Appropriate Beta Blocker Usage; 25. Controlled Postoperative Blood Glucose; 26. Prophylactic Antibiotic Timing; 27. Prophylactic Antibiotic Timing (Outpatient); 28. Prophylactic Antibiotic Selection; 29. Prophylactic Antibiotic Selection (Outpatient); 30. Prophylactic Antibiotic Stopped; 31. Recommended VTP Ordered; 32. Urinary Catheter Removal*

Hospital	Pneumonia Care						Surgical Care Improvement Project										
	16	**17**	**18**	**19**	**20**	**21**	**22**	**23**	**24**	**25**	**26**	**27**	**28**	**29**	**30**	**31**	**32**
Catawba Valley Medical Center, Hickory, NC	**90** 156	**92** 253	**86** 108	**94** 217	**91** 154	**99** 74	**94** 263	**100** 671	**99** 164	- 0	**96** 472	**97** 649	**99** 476	**98** 638	**95** 463	**95** 263	**96** 197
Central Carolina Hospital, Sanford, NC	**98** 123	**97** 157	**98** 111	**100** 157	**98** 133	**100** 53	**91** 123	**100** 201	**100** 45	- 0	**99** 101	**94** 200	**90** 101	**89** 194	**94** 97	**92** 123	**85** 34
Charles A Cannon Jr Memorial Hospital, Linville, NC	**73** 37	**98** 46	**97** 34	**94** 72	**98** 61	**100** 14	- 0	- 0	- 0	- 0	- 0	- -	- 0	- -	- 0	- 0	- 0
Chatham Hospital, Siler City, NC	**88** 42	**98** 51	**98** 47	**88** 49	**96** 54	**94** 16	**55** 11	**100** 13	- 0	- 0	**100** 4	- -	**100** 4	- -	**100** 4	**55** 11	**100** 5
Cherokee Indian Hospital Authority, Cherokee, NC	**65** 26	**80** 15	**80** 20	**83** 6	**100** 20	**88** 17	- 0	- 0	- 0	- 0	- 0	- -	- 0	- -	- 0	- 0	- 0
Chowan Hospital, Edenton, NC	**90** 31	**95** 41	**92** 25	**100** 39	**95** 37	**100** 19	**98** 65	**98** 177	**98** 52	- 0	**98** 140	- -	**100** 139	- -	**99** 136	**98** 65	**94** 69
Cleveland Regional Medical Center, Shelby, NC	**85** 169	**90** 202	**95** 169	**93** 214	**97** 188	**99** 109	**94** 170	**100** 587	**95** 130	- 0	**98** 438	**100** 249	**94** 441	**91** 249	**93** 432	**95** 170	**81** 91
Columbus Regional Healthcare System, Whiteville, NC	**99** 68	**98** 137	**99** 76	**88** 136	**96** 108	**100** 53	**90** 170	**100** 256	**93** 73	- 0	**97** 138	**80** 40	**96** 138	**84** 32	**93** 128	**91** 170	**92** 39
Davie County Hospital, Mocksville, NC	**71** 21	**95** 22	**71** 14	**85** 27	**92** 25	**62** 8	- 0	- 0	- 0	- 0	- 0	- -	- 0	- -	- 0	- 0	- 0
Davis Regional Medical Center, Statesville, NC	**95** 78	**97** 116	**100** 62	**98** 94	**100** 68	**100** 59	**99** 135	**100** 192	**100** 48	- 0	**98** 119	**100** 308	**98** 120	**99** 308	**93** 114	**99** 135	**98** 48
Duke Health Raleigh Hospital, Raleigh, NC	**93** 103	**98** 148	**99** 90	**100** 125	**96** 121	**98** 42	**91** 414	**99** 1098	**88** 294	- 0	**93** 799	**87** 515	**98** 801	**98** 508	**98** 789	**93** 414	**91** 447
Duke University Hospital, Durham, NC	**98** 90	**98** 240	**98** 232	**91** 233	**99** 251	**100** 78	**100** 202	**98** 634	**97** 160	**98** 126	**97** 396	**88** 749	**97** 405	**87** 832	**99** 371	**100** 202	**92** 160
Duplin General Hospital, Kenansville, NC	**98** 65	**99** 102	**98** 51	**100** 85	**97** 70	**100** 29	**70** 10	**100** 47	**100** 7	- 0	**100** 34	**71** 7	**100** 35	**86** 7	**94** 31	**80** 10	**100** 2
Durham Regional Hospital, Durham, NC	**95** 195	**98** 321	**98** 199	**94** 297	**97** 274	**99** 145	**95** 196	**100** 935	**95** 253	**94** 51	**99** 781	**97** 560	**99** 781	**99** 556	**97** 747	**98** 196	**95** 357
Durham VA Medical Center, Durham, NC	**85** 26	**96** 57	**97** 60	**88** 60	**98** 59	**100** 29	**92** 111	**100** 276	**100** 80	**95** 111	**99** 176	- -	**98** 180	- -	**92** 174	**91** 112	**95** 97
Fayetteville North Carolina VA Medical Center, Fayetteville, NC	**89** 46	**100** 52	**97** 32	**75** 4	**100** 33	**100** 23	- 0	- 0	- 0	- 0	- 0	- -	- 0	- -	- 0	- 0	- 0
Firsthealth Montgomery Memorial Hospital, Troy, NC	**90** 10	**100** 16	**100** 17	**100** 17	**95** 19	**100** 11	- 0	- 0	- 0	- 0	- 0	- -	- 0	- -	- 0	- 0	- 0
Firsthealth Moore Regional Hospital, Pinehurst, NC	**93** 180	**97** 262	**97** 268	**96** 281	**97** 300	**100** 142	**92** 376	**99** 1626	**97** 579	**96** 306	**98** 1129	**84** 614	**98** 1140	**96** 599	**98** 1095	**95** 380	**92** 244
Firsthealth Richmond Memorial Hospital, Rockingham, NC	- -	- -	- -	- -	- -	- -	- -	- -	- -	- -	- -	- -	- -	- -	- -	- -	- -
Forsyth Memorial Hospital, Winston-Salem, NC	**98** 418	**100** 694	**100** 531	**100** 624	**100** 710	**100** 323	**97** 1018	**100** 2869	**97** 1006	**99** 483	**100** 2078	**98** 1706	**100** 2095	**99** 1702	**100** 1984	**98** 1018	**98** 921
Franklin Regional Medical Center, Louisburg, NC	**95** 37	**96** 68	**98** 48	**95** 59	**97** 63	**100** 26	**75** 12	**100** 14	**100** 4	- 0	**100** 5	**100** 1	**100** 5	**100** 1	**100** 4	**75** 12	**40** 5
Frye Regional Medical Center, Hickory, NC	**95** 221	**96** 335	**96** 209	**98** 291	**95** 276	**98** 100	**91** 149	**100** 662	**93** 215	**86** 261	**96** 517	**97** 693	**99** 522	**98** 684	**91** 495	**91** 149	**91** 187
Gaston Memorial Hospital, Gastonia, NC	**100** 359	**100** 842	**100** 555	**99** 706	**100** 603	**100** 375	**99** 393	**100** 1384	**100** 404	**97** 142	**99** 897	**99** 750	**99** 902	**97** 749	**100** 846	**99** 394	**100** 358
Grace Hospital, Morganton, NC	**87** 112	**98** 204	**99** 129	**97** 181	**99** 162	**99** 84	**76** 136	**100** 240	**89** 47	- 0	**95** 129	**96** 333	**98** 128	**92** 324	**92** 117	**77** 139	**96** 50
Granville Medical Center, Oxford, NC	**90** 59	**95** 66	**100** 56	**95** 76	**100** 52	**100** 35	**99** 88	**100** 218	**94** 50	- 0	**95** 147	**93** 43	**99** 148	**95** 42	**94** 133	**99** 88	**94** 68
Halifax Regional Medical Center, Roanoke Rapids, NC	**85** 104	**92** 132	**91** 111	**92** 155	**91** 134	**100** 66	**72** 74	**100** 423	**86** 129	- 0	**97** 285	**92** 135	**99** 290	**95** 129	**98** 274	**76** 76	**67** 9
Haywood Regional Medical Center, Clyde, NC	**83** 135	**96** 159	**89** 146	**87** 191	**92** 182	**92** 103	**93** 110	**100** 472	**92** 123	- 0	**94** 341	**86** 266	**98** 340	**96** 266	**98** 329	**95** 111	**94** 18
Heritage Hospital, Tarboro, NC	**93** 44	**97** 76	**91** 53	**100** 72	**95** 58	**100** 24	**93** 75	**100** 130	**96** 24	- 0	**100** 64	**99** 154	**98** 64	**93** 153	**95** 62	**92** 76	**95** 22
High Point Regional Hospital, High Point, NC	**91** 220	**93** 397	**73** 249	**96** 421	**87** 347	**100** 196	**99** 131	**100** 506	**81** 167	**95** 102	**98** 344	**90** 489	**97** 348	**68** 470	**96** 288	**99** 131	**92** 106
Highlands Cashiers Hospital, Highlands, NC	**75** 4	**83** 6	**80** 5	**0** 1	**46** 13	**100** 1	- 0	- 0	- 0	- 0	- 0	- -	- 0	- -	- 0	- 0	- 0
Hugh Chatham Memorial Hospital, Elkin, NC	**98** 127	**98** 155	**93** 112	**98** 155	**92** 130	**100** 87	**99** 118	**100** 344	**100** 112	- 0	**100** 313	**100** 99	**98** 312	**99** 100	**98** 299	**99** 118	**84** 19
Iredell Memorial Hospital, Statesville, NC	**90** 175	**97** 200	**99** 142	**99** 253	**99** 238	**100** 93	**94** 242	**100** 389	**96** 117	- 0	**98** 238	**92** 200	**96** 240	**93** 192	**95** 228	**96** 245	**95** 61
J Arthur Dosher Memorial Hospital, Southport, NC	- -	- -	- -	- -	- -	- -	- -	- -	- -	- -	- 0	- 0	- 0	- 0	- -	- -	- -
Johnston Memorial Hospital, Smithfield, NC	**84** 171	**91** 213	**67** 163	**91** 253	**70** 222	**100** 82	**77** 195	**100** 450	**89** 160	- 0	**98** 285	**96** 252	**89** 287	**88** 247	**88** 277	**81** 200	**80** 110
Kings Mountain Hospital, Kings Mountain, NC	**92** 51	**98** 51	**98** 43	**99** 68	**100** 46	**100** 35	**86** 28	**100** 37	**67** 9	- 0	**93** 15	**100** 4	**75** 16	**75** 4	**92** 13	**89** 28	**89** 9
Lake Norman Regional Medical Center, Mooresville, NC	**99** 69	**100** 97	**100** 68	**96** 103	**100** 87	**100** 50	**96** 171	**100** 377	**99** 74	- 0	**99** 225	**100** 469	**98** 227	**97** 468	**99** 201	**97** 172	**99** 70
Lenoir Memorial Hospital, Kinston, NC	**93** 136	**97** 206	**74** 151	**96** 241	**97** 229	**100** 68	**66** 217	**100** 461	**58** 125	- 0	**97** 317	**73** 142	**95** 320	**91** 112	**92** 305	**70** 221	**73** 62
Lexington Memorial Hospital, Lexington, NC	**87** 126	**97** 185	**95** 105	**99** 175	**98** 158	**100** 55	**89** 80	**98** 298	**97** 70	- 0	**95** 236	**91** 205	**98** 235	**91** 201	**98** 229	**87** 82	**96** 81
Margaret R Pardee Memorial Hospital, Hendersonville, NC	**95** 139	**96** 186	**87** 126	**97** 184	**91** 162	**98** 63	**90** 245	**100** 408	**98** 102	- 0	**98** 284	**94** 223	**98** 285	**95** 214	**98** 273	**95** 245	**91** 85
Maria Parham Hospital, Henderson, NC	**92** 85	**90** 102	**89** 82	**89** 121	**93** 103	**100** 47	**92** 77	**100** 180	**82** 40	- 0	**97** 95	**95** 81	**94** 96	**94** 81	**93** 91	**95** 77	**94** 32
Martin General Hospital, Williamston, NC	**80** 55	**100** 58	**93** 44	**100** 70	**94** 66	**100** 21	**86** 50	**100** 97	**90** 20	- 0	**99** 91	**98** 54	**100** 91	**96** 55	**100** 91	**92** 50	**62** 8
The Mcdowell Hospital, Marion, NC	**94** 31	**100** 64	**94** 54	**100** 65	**98** 65	**100** 36	**92** 63	**100** 111	**75** 20	- 0	**95** 64	**95** 57	**91** 64	**96** 54	**89** 57	**94** 63	**81** 16
Medical Park Hospital, Winston-Salem, NC	- 0	- 0	- 0	- 0	- 0	- 0	**96** 179	**100** 412	**99** 85	- 0	**100** 230	**99** 434	**100** 230	**99** 434	**100** 220	**98** 179	**88** 60
Memorial Mission Hosp/Asheville Surgery Ctr, Asheville, NC	**86** 146	**94** 256	**87** 416	**92** 275	**94** 532	**100** 244	**97** 906	**100** 3005	**98** 999	**99** 611	**98** 2378	**97** 1003	**100** 2405	**98** 1003	**97** 2258	**98** 906	**95** 544
Morehead Memorial Hospital, Eden, NC	**87** 182	**96** 129	**91** 149	**94** 227	**90** 197	**89** 89	**86** 103	**100** 176	**78** 40	- 0	**95** 112	**89** 72	**98** 109	**93** 68	**78** 99	**88** 104	**73** 26
The Moses H Cone Memorial Hospital, Greensboro, NC	**94** 141	**95** 131	**97** 163	**97** 244	**97** 228	**100** 106	**87** 415	**100** 1088	**87** 337	**94** 160	**96** 753	**96** 969	**99** 754	**96** 948	**97** 712	**92** 416	**88** 280
Murphy Medical Center, Murphy, NC	**89** 88	**95** 129	**93** 83	**93** 138	**87** 116	**98** 51	**84** 64	**100** 168	**85** 40	- 0	**97** 117	**89** 27	**93** 119	**92** 25	**96** 116	**84** 64	**91** 33
Nash General Hospital, Rocky Mount, NC	**86** 114	**92** 259	**92** 194	**94** 233	**95** 213	**98** 128	**90** 146	**100** 698	**96** 180	- 0	**96** 564	**94** 400	**99** 565	**94** 409	**95** 550	**95** 146	**94** 180
New Hanover Regional Medical Center, Wilmington, NC	**88** 75	**86** 81	**83** 87	**88** 104	**88** 113	**91** 66	**95** 345	**98** 961	**89** 317	**95** 134	**95** 622	**93** 751	**96** 633	**93** 733	**93** 579	**97** 347	**90** 211
North Carolina Baptist Hospital, Winston-Salem, NC	**94** 171	**97** 453	**92** 142	**98** 413	**92** 283	**100** 264	**97** 363	**100** 954	**96** 328	**96** 187	**99** 619	**97** 672	**99** 633	**98** 680	**97** 599	**97** 363	**88** 229
North Carolina Specialty Hospital, Durham, NC	- 0	- 0	- 0	- 0	- 0	- 0	**100** 47	**100** 265	**100** 57	- 0	**99** 187	**97** 95	**100** 187	**97** 95	**99** 186	**100** 47	**97** 118
Northern Hospital of Surry County, Mount Airy, NC	**94** 119	**96** 216	**92** 146	**95** 203	**88** 190	**99** 92	**92** 126	**100** 337	**78** 101	- 0	**96** 235	**89** 70	**99** 235	**88** 68	**98** 231	**99** 126	**68** 25
Onslow Memorial Hospital, Jacksonville, NC	**90** 126	**93** 176	**98** 126	**83** 180	**99** 142	**100** 82	**88** 136	**100** 294	**80** 74	- 0	**97** 194	**91** 233	**96** 197	**94** 228	**94** 186	**88** 137	**87** 45
The Outer Banks Hospital, Nags Head, NC	**95** 39	**94** 48	**100** 18	**100** 32	**100** 39	**100** 18	**100** 37	**100** 109	**81** 21	- 0	**98** 85	- -	**99** 85	- -	**100** 80	**100** 37	**100** 48
Park Ridge Hospital, Fletcher, NC	**88** 73	**94** 101	**93** 58	**97** 94	**95** 83	**100** 42	**92** 112	**100** 231	**100** 42	- 0	**97** 141	**95** 126	**95** 148	**95** 131	**95** 125	**96** 112	**92** 49
Pender Memorial Hospital, Burgaw, NC	- 0	**100** 17	**86** 7	**96** 23	**80** 15	**100** 7	**0** 1	**100** 4	- 0	- 0	**100** 1	- -	**100** 1	- -	**100** 1	**0** 1	- 0
Person Memorial Hospital, Roxboro, NC	**84** 61	**95** 95	**95** 61	**98** 85	**98** 82	**100** 28	**90** 105	**100** 200	**92** 77	- 0	**96** 144	**75** 16	**99** 146	**100** 14	**99** 143	**89** 108	**93** 74
Pitt County Memorial Hospital, Greenville, NC	**82** 181	**92** 272	**95** 312	**87** 271	**94** 371	**100** 200	**95** 700	**98** 2790	**93** 1105	**90** 786	**97** 1919	**93** 1400	**98** 1950	**94** 1374	**94** 1822	**97** 701	**87** 438
Presbyterian Hospital, Charlotte, NC	**99** 202	**100** 277	**98** 225	**99** 314	**99** 268	**100** 149	**97** 499	**100** 1515	**100** 430	**100** 408	**100** 1096	**97** 1140	**99** 1124	**98** 1141	**99** 1037	**98** 499	**88** 263
Presbyterian Hospital Huntersville, Huntersville, NC	**98** 129	**100** 167	**98** 89	**98** 156	**98** 129	**100** 46	**93** 201	**100** 540	**95** 128	- 0	**99** 396	**97** 162	**100** 396	**94** 161	**98** 387	**94** 201	**95** 143
Presbyterian Hospital Matthews, Matthews, NC	**97** 193	**100** 258	**99** 160	**99** 236	**99** 197	**100** 70	**96** 216	**100** 468	**98** 85	- 0	**98** 303	**98** 336	**99** 303	**98** 336	**98** 290	**97** 216	**97** 119
Presbyterian-Orthopaedic Hospital, Charlotte, NC	- 0	- 0	- 0	- 0	- 0	- 0	**100** 616	**100** 1497	**97** 384	- 0	**100** 1255	**99** 692	**100** 1256	**100** 687	**99** 1234	**100** 616	**96** 604
Pungo District Hospital, Belhaven, NC	**61** 18	**74** 19	**100** 16	**86** 22	**100** 25	**100** 7	- 0	- 0	- 0	- 0	- 0	- -	- 0	- -	- 0	- 0	- 0
Randolph Hospital, Asheboro, NC	**89** 116	**95** 140	**92** 89	**94** 108	**85** 109	**100** 75	**83** 125	**99** 229	**79** 70	- 0	**95** 125	**95** 193	**97** 126	**91** 191	**91** 116	**88** 125	**100** 25
Rex Hospital, Raleigh, NC	**96** 129	**96** 227	**91** 127	**93** 189	**96** 213	**98** 43	**89** 287	**99** 947	**94** 329	**94** 176	**98** 674	**94** 1091	**97** 675	**92** 1060	**95** 654	**89** 288	**89** 245
Roanoke Chowan Hospital, Ahoskie, NC	**87** 62	**95** 99	**97** 66	**98** 94	**98** 80	**100** 30	**100** 66	**100** 189	**100** 39	- 0	**97** 143	**84** 37	**97** 143	**95** 43	**97** 136	**100** 66	**100** 23
Rowan Regional Medical Center, Salisbury, NC	**98** 206	**100** 303	**100** 236	**99** 348	**100** 276	**100** 143	**97** 241	**100** 779	**100** 204	- 0	**100** 582	**99** 526	**99** 585	**99** 526	**99** 553	**100** 241	**99** 166
Rutherford Hospital, Rutherfordton, NC	**81** 116	**94** 183	**86** 118	**93** 168	**91** 167	**100** 60	**95** 113	**100** 340	**96** 71	- 0	**99** 244	**90** 117	**98** 245	**92** 111	**96** 233	**98** 113	**79** 19

NOTE: The first number in each column (boldface) is the score, the second number is the number of patients; Please refer to the main entry for footnotes; (a) 100-299

*MEASURES: **Pneumonia Care:** 16. Appropriate Initial Antibiotic; 17. Blood Culture Timing; 18. Influenza Vaccine; 19. Initial Antibiotic Timing; 20. Pneumococcal Vaccine; 21. Smoking Cessation Advice; **Surgical Care Improvement Project:** 22. Appropriate VTP Within 24 Hours; 23. Appropriate Hair Removal; 24. Appropriate Beta Blocker Usage; 25. Controlled Postoperative Blood Glucose; 26. Prophylactic Antibiotic Timing; 27. Prophylactic Antibiotic Timing (Outpatient); 28. Prophylactic Antibiotic Selection; 29. Prophylactic Antibiotic Selection (Outpatient); 30. Prophylactic Antibiotic Stopped; 31. Recommended VTP Ordered; 32. Urinary Catheter Removal*

Hospital	Pneumonia Care						Surgical Care Improvement Project										
	16	17	18	19	20	21	22	23	24	25	26	27	28	29	30	31	32
Saint Lukes Hospital, Columbus, NC	**96** 47	**93** 76	**97** 38	**97** 59	**91** 58	**100** 12	**86** 36	**100** 174	**92** 52	- 0	**99** 136	- 0	**100** 137	- 0	**98** 129	**86** 36	**91** 44
Sampson Regional Medical Center, Clinton, NC	**90** 86	**90** 133	**88** 85	**96** 113	**94** 143	**100** 36	**62** 60	**100** 146	**92** 40	- 0	**91** 79	**77** 13	**97** 79	**73** 11	**87** 75	**68** 60	**82** 40
Sandhills Regional Medical Center, Hamlet, NC	**92** 48	**93** 60	**100** 29	**96** 54	**100** 28	**100** 33	**95** 22	**100** 52	**83** 12	- 0	**100** 37	**97** 37	**100** 39	**92** 37	**91** 35	**91** 23	**100** 1
Scotland Memorial Hospital, Laurinburg, NC	**90** 72	**99** 121	**100** 77	**98** 113	**100** 107	**100** 63	**98** 195	**100** 318	**98** 102	- 0	**98** 204	**95** 153	**98** 205	**88** 153	**98** 198	**99** 195	**97** 93
Southeastern Regional Medical Center, Lumberton, NC	**91** 242	**93** 307	**92** 220	**94** 314	**96** 253	**99** 174	**90** 185	**100** 389	**92** 110	**100** 33	**99** 251	**95** 357	**97** 251	**95** 344	**96** 239	**97** 185	**96** 97
Spruce Pine Community Hospital, Spruce Pine, NC	**80** 112	**82** 114	**88** 74	**85** 139	**94** 129	**74** 46	**89** 57	**100** 137	**88** 33	- 0	**95** 104	**100** 25	**99** 103	**92** 25	**96** 100	**96** 57	- 0
Stanly Regional Medical Center, Albemarle, NC	**87** 124	**95** 203	**91** 137	**95** 191	**93** 191	**98** 81	**88** 90	**99** 222	**93** 59	- 0	**97** 121	**80** 127	**97** 121	**88** 129	**94** 108	**90** 91	**81** 27
Stokes-Reynolds Memorial Hospital, Danbury, NC	- 0	**100** 6	**50** 2	**100** 10	**50** 6	**100** 4	- 0	- 0	- 0	- 0	- 0	- -	- 0	- -	- 0	- 0	- 0
Thomasville Medical Center, Thomasville, NC	**96** 75	**100** 135	**96** 51	**99** 110	**99** 90	**100** 45	**93** 90	**100** 178	**97** 29	- 0	**100** 97	**96** 211	**98** 99	**93** 204	**99** 81	**94** 90	**85** 20
Transylvania Regional Hospital, Brevard, NC	**95** 57	**99** 70	**97** 37	**97** 67	**100** 59	**92** 24	**97** 58	**100** 126	**100** 30	- 0	**100** 84	- -	**100** 87	- -	**99** 83	**95** 59	**88** 25
University of North Carolina Hospital, Chapel Hill, NC	**88** 49	**95** 99	**99** 68	**96** 93	**99** 89	**100** 48	**95** 286	**100** 568	**94** 174	**96** 71	**98** 309	**94** 688	**98** 313	**94** 685	**94** 294	**97** 287	**92** 138
Valdese General Hospital, Valdese, NC	**87** 55	**98** 97	**99** 76	**88** 90	**98** 107	**100** 50	**95** 66	**100** 148	**98** 48	- 0	**99** 108	**92** 87	**99** 108	**90** 82	**93** 103	**96** 68	**98** 45
W G (Bill) Hefner Salisbury VA Medical Center, Salisbury, NC	**94** 35	**100** 61	**100** 35	**98** 49	**100** 40	**93** 27	**88** 40	**100** 77	**93** 14	- 0	**98** 44	- -	**98** 43	- -	**100** 42	**93** 40	**86** 14
Wakemed - Cary Hospital, Cary, NC	**97** 74	**97** 134	**95** 122	**98** 122	**94** 144	**100** 55	**94** 145	**100** 383	**95** 78	- 0	**96** 208	**97** 366	**97** 212	**95** 365	**93** 198	**97** 145	**97** 78
Wakemed - Raleigh Campus, Raleigh, NC	**95** 152	**99** 276	**93** 274	**93** 204	**96** 315	**99** 206	**92** 241	**100** 751	**96** 268	**99** 170	**98** 511	**96** 955	**98** 523	**99** 933	**98** 484	**93** 242	**98** 130
Washington County Hospital, Plymouth, NC	**80** 20	**89** 27	**92** 12	**100** 30	**95** 21	**50** 2	- 0	- 0	- 0	- 0	- 0	- 0	- 0	- 0	- 0	- 0	- 0
Watauga Medical Center, Boone, NC	**94** 88	**97** 137	**85** 153	**97** 145	**96** 200	**97** 66	**82** 136	**100** 308	**97** 75	- 0	**98** 224	**93** 128	**96** 226	**79** 123	**90** 212	**85** 136	**84** 25
Wayne Memorial Hospital, Goldsboro, NC	**97** 96	**96** 112	**57** 155	**90** 160	**81** 180	**100** 105	**93** 299	**99** 571	**88** 162	- 0	**97** 386	**92** 344	**97** 386	**98** 333	**93** 378	**94** 303	**84** 122
Wilkes Regional Medical Center, North Wilkesboro, NC	**89** 139	**98** 217	**94** 126	**99** 195	**97** 198	**95** 77	**89** 83	**100** 168	**100** 35	- 0	**98** 111	**80** 20	**88** 110	**88** 16	**92** 102	**90** 83	**91** 43
Wilson Medical Center, Wilson, NC	**79** 121	**82** 191	**83** 162	**89** 230	**81** 203	**96** 89	**78** 167	**99** 539	**96** 136	- 0	**97** 397	**96** 93	**99** 421	**98** 93	**89** 394	**88** 169	**96** 186
Yadkin Valley Community Hospital, Yadkinville, NC	**83** 6	**100** 8	**50** 4	**100** 7	**88** 8	**67** 3	- 0	- 0	- 0	- 0	- 0	- -	- 0	- -	- 0	- 0	- 0
OHIO																	
Adams County Regional Medical Center, Seaman, OH	**91** 58	**96** 74	**98** 42	**98** 53	**100** 48	**100** 33	**100** 1	**100** 3	- 0	- 0	**67** 3	- -	**67** 3	- -	**67** 3	**100** 1	- 0
Adena Regional Medical Center, Chillicothe, OH	**96** 162	**93** 120	**98** 250	**96** 249	**95** 318	**98** 187	**88** 266	**100** 850	**94** 348	**88** 109	**97** 736	**96** 314	**99** 744	**99** 307	**97** 704	**91** 268	**97** 240
Affinity Medical Center, Massillon, OH	**97** 119	**93** 198	**95** 136	**97** 197	**95** 180	**100** 80	**99** 134	**100** 492	**94** 177	**93** 88	**99** 378	**90** 144	**100** 384	**89** 140	**97** 355	**100** 134	**99** 147
Akron General Medical Center, Akron, OH	**94** 69	**99** 81	**85** 92	**76** 108	**87** 127	**93** 59	**93** 248	**100** 614	**92** 180	**97** 116	**97** 442	**95** 698	**98** 448	**93** 687	**99** 422	**98** 248	**82** 105
Allen Community Hospital, Oberlin, OH	**91** 35	**100** 35	**100** 17	**100** 42	**100** 25	**100** 13	**100** 16	**100** 118	- 0	- 0	**100** 99	- -	**99** 101	- -	**100** 99	**100** 16	**100** 49
Alliance Community Hospital, Alliance, OH	**93** 92	**90** 156	**94** 126	**98** 144	**97** 156	**90** 67	**76** 119	**96** 344	**92** 101	- 0	**97** 221	**85** 82	**100** 220	**100** 70	**84** 206	**76** 120	**64** 56
Amherst Hospital, Amherst, OH	**76** 25	**94** 16	**79** 19	**82** 28	**85** 26	**92** 12	**96** 26	**100** 217	**90** 62	- 0	**98** 178	**62** 29	**100** 178	**83** 23	**90** 173	**93** 27	**88** 91
Ashtabula County Medical Center, Ashtabula, OH	**93** 87	**96** 164	**98** 80	**97** 145	**95** 109	**100** 72	**94** 77	**100** 225	**97** 63	- 0	**99** 149	**92** 154	**99** 149	**94** 195	**91** 135	**95** 77	**83** 18
Atrium Medical Center, Franklin, OH	**93** 182	**97** 286	**98** 201	**97** 268	**98** 264	**100** 181	**97** 312	**100** 894	**100** 256	**96** 97	**99** 508	**91** 255	**99** 512	**95** 238	**98** 483	**99** 312	**98** 167
Aultman Hospital, Canton, OH	**95** 370	**97** 632	**94** 499	**96** 609	**97** 627	**97** 240	**89** 205	**100** 739	**96** 289	**94** 182	**96** 554	**92** 1067	**98** 563	**96** 1296	**96** 538	**94** 206	**94** 168
Barnesville Hospital Association, Barnesville, OH	**88** 91	**98** 53	**88** 59	**97** 100	**88** 101	**100** 30	- 0	- 0	- 0	- 0	- 0	- 0	- 0	- 0	- 0	- 0	- 0
Bay Park Community Hospital, Oregon, OH	**93** 94	**98** 121	**99** 91	**99** 138	**98** 123	**100** 46	**92** 114	**100** 348	**94** 121	- 0	**97** 263	**92** 78	**97** 264	**99** 73	**94** 252	**97** 114	**87** 127
Bellevue Hospital, Bellevue, OH	**77** 69	**99** 73	**88** 51	**91** 74	**100** 71	**93** 46	**78** 69	**100** 201	**91** 35	- 0	**94** 138	**74** 73	**94** 140	**71** 63	**91** 137	**84** 69	**86** 36
Belmont Community Hospital, Bellaire, OH	**75** 32	**96** 27	**79** 34	**95** 39	**92** 39	**100** 16	- 0	**100** 3	- 0	- 0	**100** 3	**0** 5	**100** 3	**100** 1	**67** 3	- 0	- 0
Berger Hospital, Circleville, OH	**95** 74	**95** 130	**99** 84	**100** 117	**100** 98	**100** 55	**88** 84	**100** 377	**99** 103	- 0	**99** 281	**100** 40	**99** 284	**85** 40	**95** 274	**95** 84	**100** 103
Bethesda North Hospital, Cincinnati, OH	**94** 363	**98** 643	**93** 469	**94** 564	**94** 595	**100** 231	**92** 173	**100** 628	**96** 198	**100** 137	**96** 440	**93** 655	**98** 438	**97** 634	**96** 412	**95** 173	**83** 135
Blanchard Valley Hospital, Findlay, OH	**89** 95	**98** 120	**99** 90	**97** 118	**100** 127	**93** 44	**86** 183	**100** 754	**87** 216	**96** 69	**98** 604	**98** 545	**98** 614	**97** 538	**97** 585	**88** 184	**82** 131
Bluffton Hospital, Bluffton, OH	**100** 6	**100** 12	**100** 9	**100** 12	**100** 13	**100** 2	**100** 1	**100** 23	**100** 3	- 0	**73** 22	**91** 106	**100** 22	**96** 104	**100** 22	**100** 1	- 0
Brown County Hospital, Georgetown, OH	**98** 44	**94** 112	**94** 65	**99** 107	**97** 93	**98** 43	**100** 10	**100** 39	**100** 8	- 0	**79** 19	**84** 38	**86** 21	**92** 36	**89** 19	**100** 10	**100** 4
Bucyrus Community Hospital, Bucyrus, OH	**100** 31	**100** 49	**96** 28	**100** 42	**100** 30	**100** 13	**97** 33	**99** 113	- 0	- 0	**99** 94	- -	**99** 94	- -	**98** 93	**97** 33	**100** 30
Butler County Medical Center, Hamilton, OH	- 0	- 0	- 0	- 0	- 0	- 0	**86** 7	**100** 209	**61** 41	- 0	**93** 190	**82** 90	**95** 186	**93** 75	**95** 180	**86** 7	**86** 14
Chillicothe VA Medical Center, Chillicothe, OH	**92** 59	**92** 13	**94** 54	**94** 54	**100** 39	**95** 64	- 0	- 0	- 0	- 0	- 0	- -	- 0	- -	- 0	- 0	- 0
Christ Hospital, Cincinnati, OH	**100** 40	**94** 84	**98** 87	**92** 74	**100** 113	**98** 48	**98** 148	**100** 734	**98** 229	**92** 152	**95** 492	**94** 815	**98** 504	**96** 825	**96** 456	**98** 148	**90** 156
Cincinnati VA Medical Center, Cincinnati, OH	**100** 57	**99** 97	**91** 81	**99** 96	**96** 79	**100** 59	**99** 139	**100** 238	**98** 83	- 0	**99** 152	- -	**97** 152	- -	**99** 150	**99** 139	**58** 19
Cleveland Clinic, Cleveland, OH	**92** 71	**96** 106	**100** 189	**92** 142	**98** 225	**95** 110	**96** 461	**91** 1487	**95** 538	**92** 407	**98** 1019	**83** 826	**97** 1050	**88** 1336	**92** 989	**96** 462	**89** 313
Cleveland-Wade Park VA Medical Center, Cleveland, OH	**95** 56	**98** 91	**89** 118	**91** 93	**99** 104	**100** 83	**94** 254	**100** 559	**99** 298	**96** 157	**98** 401	- -	**100** 403	- -	**97** 379	**94** 254	**93** 215
CMH Regional Health System, Wilmington, OH	**87** 82	**97** 130	**96** 95	**97** 121	**99** 115	**96** 26	**97** 66	**100** 254	**97** 69	- 0	**96** 190	**90** 134	**96** 188	**89** 122	**97** 187	**97** 66	**100** 76
Community Hospitals and Wellness Centers, Bryan, OH	**91** 68	**100** 61	**94** 66	**99** 83	**97** 69	**100** 28	**90** 101	**100** 237	**93** 94	- 0	**96** 180	**92** 85	**99** 180	**96** 79	**97** 175	**97** 101	**97** 35
Community Regional Medical Center, Lorain, OH	**94** 221	**98** 386	**96** 225	**97** 348	**97** 290	**99** 152	**97** 258	**100** 621	**98** 264	**95** 42	**100** 481	**98** 307	**97** 485	**94** 307	**99** 453	**97** 260	**99** 156
Coshocton County Memorial Hospital, Coshocton, OH	**73** 30	**92** 37	**87** 31	**93** 42	**94** 36	**93** 15	**72** 29	**99** 74	**94** 16	- 0	**98** 43	**74** 19	**93** 43	**80** 15	**81** 42	**81** 31	**75** 4
Crystal Clinic Orthopaedic Center, Akron, OH	- 0	- 0	- 0	- 0	- 0	- 0	**100** 24	**100** 139	**85** 41	- 0	**95** 98	**98** 324	**100** 98	**100** 324	**100** 98	**100** 24	**73** 11
Dayton VA Medical Center, Dayton, OH	**91** 79	**98** 113	**95** 92	**91** 119	**98** 93	**98** 53	**95** 40	**100** 156	**98** 64	- 0	**98** 111	- -	**100** 111	- -	**99** 109	**95** 40	**94** 17
Deaconess Hospital, Cincinnati, OH	**61** 18	**86** 22	**46** 13	**88** 33	**52** 29	**33** 6	**90** 21	**98** 125	**88** 60	**88** 80	**97** 34	**67** 3	**94** 34	**50** 2	**91** 33	**90** 21	**98** 41
Defiance Regional Medical Center, Defiance, OH	**96** 52	**97** 68	**98** 53	**100** 75	**98** 62	**97** 37	**88** 48	**99** 162	- 0	- 0	**98** 125	- -	**96** 126	- -	**95** 114	**94** 48	**89** 18
Diley Ridge Medical Center, Canal Winchester, OH	**100** 2	**100** 4	- 0	**100** 2	**50** 2	**50** 2	- 0	- 0	- 0	- 0	- 0	- -	- 0	- -	- 0	- 0	- 0
Doctors Hospital, Columbus, OH	**97** 182	**97** 183	**90** 176	**98** 277	**97** 177	**100** 155	**99** 137	**100** 523	**97** 146	**99** 94	**99** 387	**92** 201	**98** 391	**98** 189	**99** 375	**99** 137	**98** 122
Doctors Hospital of Nelsonville, Nelsonville, OH	**100** 26	**100** 14	**100** 10	**100** 28	**100** 16	**91** 11	**50** 2	**100** 3	**100** 2	- 0	- 0	- -	- 0	- -	- 0	**50** 2	- 0
Dublin Methodist Hospital, Dublin, OH	**95** 87	**98** 109	**89** 56	**100** 110	**96** 67	**100** 29	**95** 75	**100** 166	**100** 26	- 0	**100** 95	**98** 541	**93** 95	**100** 536	**98** 94	**97** 75	**61** 23
Dunlap Memorial Hospital, Orrville, OH	**93** 14	**100** 11	**100** 10	**100** 15	**94** 18	**75** 4	**57** 7	**91** 23	- 0	- 0	**80** 10	- -	**100** 9	- -	**100** 9	**57** 7	**67** 3
East Liverpool City Hospital, East Liverpool, OH	**72** 114	**88** 103	**65** 78	**92** 141	**96** 90	**92** 66	**77** 53	**100** 141	**60** 42	- 0	**87** 94	**67** 18	**93** 94	**75** 12	**85** 88	**83** 53	**79** 14
East Ohio Regional Hospital, Martins Ferry, OH	**87** 110	**92** 149	**64** 78	**95** 167	**81** 104	**98** 48	**77** 90	**100** 353	**94** 144	- 0	**97** 296	**82** 66	**99** 297	**95** 58	**94** 293	**77** 90	**90** 113
Edwin Shaw Rehabilitation Institute, Cuyahoga Falls, OH	- 0	- 0	- 0	- 0	- 0	- 0	- 0	- 0	- 0	- 0	- 0	- 0	- 0	- 0	- 0	- 0	- 0
Emh Regional Medical Center, Elyria, OH	**89** 79	**99** 70	**58** 100	**91** 116	**81** 143	**100** 58	**94** 193	**100** 620	**90** 249	**77** 117	**98** 449	**94** 459	**98** 453	**95** 448	**79** 442	**93** 199	**76** 142
Euclid Hospital, Euclid, OH	**99** 73	**97** 132	**93** 76	**98** 144	**93** 125	**100** 69	**97** 214	**100** 948	**94** 264	- 0	**96** 765	**92** 90	**100** 768	**98** 86	**99** 744	**98** 214	**93** 369
Evendale Medical Center, Cincinnati, OH	- 0	- 0	- 0	- 0	- 0	- 0	**100** 8	**100** 287	**90** 61	- 0	**89** 208	**69** 232	**100** 208	**98** 165	**97** 206	**100** 8	**97** 110
Fairfield Medical Center, Lancaster, OH	**88** 140	**95** 289	**93** 259	**92** 285	**95** 339	**100** 155	**97** 209	**99** 990	**86** 312	**78** 154	**94** 761	**87** 427	**98** 769	**92** 388	**96** 722	**95** 214	**87** 234

NOTE: The first number in each column (boldface) is the score, the second number is the number of patients; Please refer to the main entry for footnotes; (a) 100-299
*MEASURES: **Pneumonia Care:** 16. Appropriate Initial Antibiotic; 17. Blood Culture Timing; 18. Influenza Vaccine; 19. Initial Antibiotic Timing; 20. Pneumococcal Vaccine; 21. Smoking Cessation Advice; **Surgical Care Improvement Project:** 22. Appropriate VTP Within 24 Hours; 23. Appropriate Hair Removal; 24. Appropriate Beta Blocker Usage; 25. Controlled Postoperative Blood Glucose; 26. Prophylactic Antibiotic Timing; 27. Prophylactic Antibiotic Timing (Outpatient); 28. Prophylactic Antibiotic Selection; 29. Prophylactic Antibiotic Selection (Outpatient); 30. Prophylactic Antibiotic Stopped; 31. Recommended VTP Ordered; 32. Urinary Catheter Removal*

Hospital	Pneumonia Care							Surgical Care Improvement Project									
	16	17	18	19	20	21	22	23	24	25	26	27	28	29	30	31	32
Fairview Hospital, Cleveland, OH	94 250	99 339	91 207	98 322	96 296	100 104	91 285	100 616	94 226	90 119	99 450	92 626	93 454	94 666	97 439	95 286	89 142
Fayette County Memorial Hospital, Washington CH, OH	92 37	88 59	76 21	96 51	84 37	100 17	100 12	100 28	90 10	- 0	100 15	92 61	100 15	98 58	93 15	100 12	100 2
Firelands Regional Medical Center, Sandusky, OH	90 99	97 152	99 100	98 166	99 135	98 53	90 144	99 517	89 184	90 31	95 353	88 281	91 352	90 254	93 342	92 145	89 135
Fisher Titus Memorial Hospital, Norwalk, OH	95 110	97 167	90 101	99 158	97 147	98 51	82 82	100 298	90 121	- 0	96 211	86 93	98 210	91 88	92 200	90 82	95 113
Flower Hospital, Sylvania, OH	93 120	97 199	92 146	98 188	94 181	97 65	93 202	99 473	96 152	- 0	97 314	89 179	98 316	94 174	98 295	94 202	94 100
Fort Hamilton Hughes Memorial Hospital, Hamilton, OH	96 73	97 113	99 97	95 126	100 134	100 72	99 147	100 353	95 81	- 0	98 185	92 78	93 184	97 78	96 155	99 147	96 48
Fostoria Community Hospital, Fostoria, OH	97 38	100 36	88 25	100 46	97 35	100 17	100 12	100 141	- 0	- 0	100 135	- -	99 135	- -	100 132	100 12	- 0
Fulton County Health Center, Wauseon, OH	100 40	85 39	91 34	98 51	94 48	92 13	66 50	100 263	79 92	- 0	96 208	70 141	98 208	74 121	98 206	82 50	67 6
Galion Community Hospital, Galion, OH	95 19	86 21	85 13	100 23	100 13	89 9	96 24	100 123	80 40	- 0	94 112	- -	96 114	- -	96 112	96 24	72 18
Genesis Healthcare System, Zanesville, OH	97 261	95 392	87 282	96 396	87 343	99 172	94 107	100 518	97 193	98 97	93 368	69 188	99 374	91 182	97 359	94 108	60 52
Glenbeigh, Rock Creek, OH	- 0	- 0	- 0	- 0	- 0	- 0	- 0	- 0	- 0	- 0	- 0	- 0	- 0	- 0	- 0	- 0	- 0
Good Samaritan Hospital, Dayton, OH	99 78	85 131	93 59	97 123	92 100	98 63	89 122	100 650	95 220	95 162	96 488	85 609	98 500	97 593	92 464	92 123	95 148
Good Samaritan Hospital, Cincinnati, OH	98 218	99 407	94 277	96 394	94 297	100 181	95 119	99 621	95 185	96 126	96 436	92 603	97 446	92 586	96 417	95 119	99 87
Grady Memorial Hospital, Delaware, OH	88 77	97 68	98 62	100 104	98 85	100 37	98 96	100 221	92 64	- 0	99 142	92 113	100 142	94 110	99 137	99 96	93 60
Grandview Hospital & Medical Center, Dayton, OH	98 165	99 280	99 175	97 236	100 215	100 115	96 276	100 1007	97 316	89 126	99 780	95 559	97 786	96 547	96 737	97 277	92 95
Grant Medical Center, Columbus, OH	98 91	99 105	96 68	97 151	100 75	100 102	98 188	100 886	100 265	97 180	100 693	97 627	99 699	97 616	99 676	100 188	98 218
Greene Memorial Hospital, Xenia, OH	93 151	98 239	97 167	99 173	96 208	100 83	89 83	100 239	95 74	- 0	99 155	93 72	97 155	99 70	95 150	96 83	98 63
Greenfield Area Medical Center, Greenfield, OH	- -	- -	- -	- -	- -	- -	- -	- -	- -	- -	- 0	- 0	- 0	- 0	- -	- -	- -
H B Magruder Memorial Hospital, Port Clinton, OH	81 26	92 40	97 30	100 39	91 35	100 10	79 24	100 57	- 0	- 0	98 41	- -	100 41	- -	92 38	79 24	70 10
Hardin Memorial Hospital, Kenton, OH	93 41	93 41	100 21	95 39	96 25	100 19	- 0	- 0	- 0	- 0	- 0	- -	- 0	- -	- 0	- 0	- 0
Harrison Community Hospital, Cadiz, OH	100 12	100 4	100 3	93 14	88 8	100 4	67 3	100 7	- 0	- 0	86 7	- -	86 7	- -	100 7	67 3	- 0
Henry County Hospital, Napoleon, OH	100 23	100 20	84 19	97 30	96 24	100 9	91 23	100 48	83 12	- 0	97 39	- -	97 39	- -	85 39	91 23	100 14
Highland District Hospital, Hillsboro, OH	80 90	83 98	83 60	94 68	87 68	92 26	- 0	- 0	- 0	- 0	92 26	58 19	88 25	91 11	100 25	- 0	- 0
Hillcrest Hospital, Mayfield Heights, OH	94 204	98 248	96 208	94 316	92 368	100 95	95 307	100 837	93 297	96 185	97 593	90 648	98 597	94 619	92 580	96 307	79 160
Hocking Valley Community Hospital, Logan, OH	83 58	84 43	93 28	96 52	97 31	56 18	96 25	100 57	- 0	- 0	94 51	- -	96 51	- -	94 51	96 25	100 18
Holzer Medical Center, Gallipolis, OH	85 115	90 115	86 91	95 136	98 122	95 76	86 94	99 302	87 117	91 35	97 179	90 59	95 179	98 54	87 175	86 98	80 44
Holzer Medical Center Jackson, Jackson, OH	85 108	93 117	86 49	96 113	86 78	100 38	79 34	99 171	- 0	- 0	84 158	- 0	99 156	- 0	92 158	79 34	97 29
Huron Hospital, Cleveland, OH	97 39	93 83	85 55	94 98	97 72	97 62	97 127	100 208	97 35	- 0	100 73	84 32	96 75	54 28	98 64	98 127	96 23
Institute for Orthopedic Surgery, Lima, OH	- 0	- 0	- 0	- 0	- 0	- 0	100 9	99 214	97 64	- 0	100 191	100 83	100 191	98 83	98 189	100 9	100 16
Jewish Hospital, Cincinnati, OH	98 63	99 123	100 84	94 127	95 119	100 44	93 132	100 523	95 164	95 88	98 338	86 324	99 342	93 296	98 325	94 132	91 35
Joel Pomerene Memorial Hospital, Millersburg, OH	100 29	100 78	100 41	100 64	98 56	100 15	91 45	100 113	84 25	- 0	98 64	91 23	97 64	77 22	93 61	96 45	100 13
Joint Township District Memorial Hospital, Saint Marys, OH	100 73	96 67	88 51	100 84	95 84	100 25	88 68	97 189	80 60	- 0	92 146	87 31	97 146	96 28	92 142	89 70	75 40
Kettering Medical Center, Kettering, OH	97 189	100 320	96 231	99 287	99 260	99 111	100 617	100 2599	98 892	97 355	100 2258	95 622	100 2280	97 615	99 2191	100 617	99 683
Kettering Medical Center - Sycamore, Miamisburg, OH	99 114	99 171	99 143	100 165	99 173	100 61	99 215	100 447	99 164	- 0	99 304	92 145	100 305	99 169	99 294	100 215	96 50
Knox Community Hospital, Mount Vernon, OH	94 107	84 153	84 87	97 114	91 122	85 41	87 86	100 447	89 117	- 0	98 382	76 85	100 383	89 73	95 373	93 86	99 115
Lake Health, Concord, OH	88 284	91 333	97 273	92 394	95 388	93 147	68 146	99 530	81 201	91 99	92 377	85 377	96 381	96 354	82 355	72 146	76 97
Lakewood Hospital, Lakewood, OH	89 89	97 164	97 88	95 158	99 110	99 68	96 245	100 564	96 191	- 0	96 363	88 151	99 364	94 138	99 342	97 245	99 175
Licking Memorial Hospital, Newark, OH	85 166	98 207	95 174	98 229	98 180	99 136	80 121	99 444	90 140	- 0	95 279	79 89	99 278	92 105	97 266	87 121	89 85
Life Line Hospital, Wintersville, OH	- 0	- 0	- 0	- 0	- 0	- 0	- 0	- 0	- 0	- 0	- 0	- -	- 0	- -	- 0	- 0	- 0
Lima Memorial Health System, Lima, OH	93 120	99 160	98 132	96 140	98 151	100 66	91 140	100 580	95 185	96 240	95 406	87 370	99 410	99 359	93 382	96 141	64 78
Lodi Community Hospital, Lodi, OH	100 15	100 15	100 5	100 15	100 8	80 5	- 0	- 0	- 0	- 0	- 0	- 0	- 0	- 0	- 0	- 0	- 0
Lutheran Hospital, Cleveland, OH	96 83	97 123	100 83	95 152	100 82	100 79	98 130	100 343	99 115	- 0	98 216	98 226	99 217	96 222	99 213	98 130	98 126
Madison County Hospital, London, OH	93 60	98 43	88 43	95 62	90 50	100 20	84 31	100 105	50 22	- 0	94 62	40 40	98 62	89 19	93 59	84 32	95 22
Marietta Memorial Hospital, Marietta, OH	92 40	100 81	98 58	95 110	95 100	100 41	96 214	100 610	90 188	- 0	92 473	71 162	99 476	93 126	96 451	97 215	92 131
Marion General Hospital, Marion, OH	97 156	98 200	99 145	99 220	99 171	100 87	98 195	100 486	100 217	100 59	99 406	97 198	98 409	99 197	98 397	98 195	79 156
Mary Rutan Hospital, Bellefontaine, OH	90 78	95 79	100 65	97 99	98 90	100 27	96 82	99 264	90 80	- 0	95 207	90 68	97 208	95 63	98 202	96 83	81 67
Marymount Hospital, Garfield Heights, OH	94 140	97 293	93 249	96 280	94 324	100 125	87 182	100 526	91 173	- 0	99 363	97 254	97 367	94 297	97 351	87 182	89 139
McCullough-Hyde Memorial Hospital, Oxford, OH	89 84	96 98	91 69	98 101	88 90	96 48	97 120	100 265	93 54	- 0	96 207	95 42	98 208	92 40	98 204	96 121	92 77
Medcentral Health System, Mansfield, OH	91 195	94 328	92 284	91 371	95 342	99 135	88 288	97 930	96 380	96 304	97 639	84 319	96 647	87 275	92 624	90 289	74 213
Medcentral Health System Shelby Hospital, Shelby, OH	- 0	- 0	- 0	- 0	- 0	- 0	- 0	- 0	- 0	- 0	- 0	- -	- 0	- -	- 0	- 0	- 0
Medical Center at Elizabeth Place, Dayton, OH	- 0	- 0	100 2	100 1	- 0	100 1	80 10	100 160	100 27	- 0	97 63	94 111	85 65	84 109	92 63	80 10	100 5
Medical Center of Newark, Newark, OH	81 26	- 0	9 11	89 27	20 20	25 8	71 42	98 104	61 23	- 0	90 72	63 43	94 72	85 27	76 71	70 43	84 32
Medina Hospital, Medina, OH	84 176	97 228	91 173	92 238	96 222	94 66	88 152	100 426	90 127	- 0	99 303	90 214	100 305	93 203	97 299	92 152	79 123
Memorial Hospital, Fremont, OH	82 40	93 73	78 46	92 71	88 56	89 28	81 62	99 220	85 62	- 0	83 173	65 79	97 174	93 54	71 171	80 64	94 62
Memorial Hospital of Union County, Marysville, OH	89 64	97 75	96 51	95 84	98 62	91 33	82 33	99 122	88 25	- 0	92 93	90 62	98 93	95 61	93 90	82 33	88 17
Mercer County Joint Twp Community Hospital, Coldwater, OH	93 67	94 78	98 54	100 80	96 74	88 17	92 50	99 131	93 28	- 0	91 96	71 35	94 96	85 27	94 95	92 50	89 28
Mercy Franciscan Hospital - Mt Airy, Cincinnati, OH	98 144	99 234	98 132	98 202	99 179	97 104	97 130	100 493	98 156	- 0	97 331	95 104	100 331	99 102	97 314	98 130	83 36
Mercy Franciscan Hospital Western Hills, Cincinnati, OH	95 188	99 272	95 166	96 257	96 221	100 108	97 156	100 331	99 146	- 0	99 194	92 59	99 194	90 58	99 190	98 156	100 26
Mercy Hospital Anderson, Cincinnati, OH	96 216	97 327	96 228	95 381	98 325	98 162	90 207	100 908	95 283	98 85	98 673	96 261	99 695	96 255	99 622	100 207	96 204
Mercy Hospital Clermont, Batavia, OH	93 151	99 230	98 185	98 257	100 216	100 170	99 158	100 388	95 112	- 0	100 267	91 65	99 269	86 74	98 254	99 158	84 89
Mercy Hospital Fairfield, Fairfield, OH	92 237	99 388	99 210	98 340	98 255	100 127	91 260	100 963	92 268	96 187	96 716	89 159	97 716	90 181	95 691	94 260	91 249
Mercy Hospital of Defiance, Defiance, OH	98 64	99 83	100 46	99 84	100 72	100 13	98 62	100 113	94 34	- 0	98 84	100 12	99 85	83 12	96 83	98 62	100 35
Mercy Hospital of Willard, Willard, OH	89 18	100 19	100 16	100 20	100 19	100 6	92 12	100 42	- 0	- 0	94 35	- 0	97 36	- 0	100 33	92 12	100 5
Mercy Medical Center, Canton, OH	89 243	98 305	95 231	93 341	96 264	99 148	89 205	100 788	86 258	96 145	96 610	92 810	97 617	98 767	91 594	94 205	88 159
Mercy Memorial Hospital, Urbana, OH	100 57	99 83	100 48	99 79	98 59	100 20	100 16	100 20	- 0	- 0	88 8	- -	88 8	- -	100 7	100 16	100 2
Mercy St Anne Hospital, Toledo, OH	95 107	98 166	96 80	99 140	97 94	100 75	96 170	100 412	98 143	- 0	95 284	97 101	98 285	97 99	94 267	97 170	99 103
Mercy St Charles Hospital, Oregon, OH	90 112	99 174	98 120	94 180	95 154	99 96	89 170	100 489	98 171	- 0	99 331	93 108	99 345	98 102	97 322	92 170	98 142
Mercy St Vincent Medical Center, Toledo, OH	92 97	95 212	96 160	97 183	96 167	100 154	90 175	100 872	95 319	100 314	98 672	97 474	99 681	90 474	98 647	97 175	98 172

NOTE: The first number in each column (boldface) is the score, the second number is the number of patients; Please refer to the main entry for footnotes; (a) 100-299

*MEASURES: **Pneumonia Care:** 16. Appropriate Initial Antibiotic; 17. Blood Culture Timing; 18. Influenza Vaccine; 19. Initial Antibiotic Timing; 20. Pneumococcal Vaccine; 21. Smoking Cessation Advice; **Surgical Care Improvement Project:** 22. Appropriate VTP Within 24 Hours; 23. Appropriate Hair Removal; 24. Appropriate Beta Blocker Usage; 25. Controlled Postoperative Blood Glucose; 26. Prophylactic Antibiotic Timing; 27. Prophylactic Antibiotic Timing (Outpatient); 28. Prophylactic Antibiotic Selection; 29. Prophylactic Antibiotic Selection (Outpatient); 30. Prophylactic Antibiotic Stopped; 31. Recommended VTP Ordered; 32. Urinary Catheter Removal*

Hospital	Pneumonia Care							Surgical Care Improvement Project									
	16	17	18	19	20	21	22	23	24	25	26	27	28	29	30	31	32
Mercy Tiffin Hospital, Tiffin, OH	94 62	99 82	94 65	100 84	93 88	97 37	80 50	100 166	94 52	- 0	99 136	60 43	98 136	69 62	98 134	98 50	100 10
Metro Health Medical Center, Cleveland, OH	95 113	86 97	59 186	95 241	88 161	98 236	98 219	100 662	90 244	94 95	98 483	95 599	98 492	97 687	94 466	98 219	93 163
Miami Valley Hospital, Dayton, OH	87 104	94 174	86 102	96 159	87 156	98 91	87 206	100 729	90 239	99 135	96 492	97 912	99 499	96 913	90 465	92 206	89 137
Morrow County Hospital, Mount Gilead, OH	96 54	96 75	66 41	99 71	80 54	96 24	50 6	100 19	- 0	- 0	100 19	- 0	100 19	- 0	95 19	50 6	88 8
Mount Carmel Health, Columbus, OH	95 240	96 383	85 218	95 344	89 306	99 150	92 208	100 1104	93 427	96 206	98 839	97 758	98 851	93 746	98 818	96 209	95 344
Mount Carmel New Albany Surgical Hospital, New Albany, OH	- 0	- 0	- 0	- 0	- 0	- 0	100 31	100 596	90 178	- 0	99 466	100 503	100 469	100 502	99 462	100 31	100 183
Mount Carmel St Ann's Hospital, Westerville, OH	96 173	97 243	81 111	97 231	89 160	99 96	97 150	100 553	96 193	- 0	99 380	61 240	98 380	91 149	96 364	99 150	92 104
Northside Medical Center, Youngstown, OH	86 100	92 189	97 130	93 199	97 190	96 77	94 269	100 1070	95 352	92 98	97 829	93 260	98 836	94 252	94 816	96 269	92 177
O'Bleness Memorial Hospital, Athens, OH	81 67	88 120	85 65	93 118	88 78	100 44	83 52	100 89	67 21	- 0	96 71	97 199	96 71	87 197	83 71	94 52	87 30
Ohio State University Hospitals, Columbus, OH	96 51	94 95	90 42	95 97	93 56	100 86	95 184	100 607	92 206	98 129	99 385	97 377	98 396	97 370	98 371	96 184	91 145
Ohio Valley Medical Center, Springfield, OH	- 0	- 0	- 0	- 0	- 0	- 0	100 26	100 230	81 43	- 0	100 202	94 31	99 202	97 31	99 200	100 26	91 68
Parma Community General Hospital, Parma, OH	87 276	99 409	87 334	95 438	96 467	99 114	92 320	100 1136	94 423	92 97	96 819	74 263	99 822	70 211	98 790	94 321	97 325
Paulding County Hospital, Paulding, OH	95 21	100 14	50 8	100 18	88 16	100 5	100 2	100 9	- 0	- 0	44 9	- -	100 9	- -	100 9	100 2	100 3
Physician's Choice Hospital - Fremont, Fremont, OH	- 0	50 2	- 0	100 1	100 1	- 0	- 0	- 0	- 0	- 0	- 0	- -	- 0	- -	- 0	- 0	- 0
Pike Community Hospital, Waverly, OH	85 40	95 58	95 21	95 61	68 41	86 7	- 0	- 0	- 0	- 0	- 0	- -	- 0	- -	- 0	- 0	- 0
Riverside Methodist Hospital, Columbus, OH	95 212	99 322	93 181	97 288	95 307	100 153	98 880	100 3209	97 1072	95 527	99 2123	95 806	99 2151	98 780	97 2064	99 881	93 1408
Robinson Memorial Hospital, Ravenna, OH	95 134	89 157	100 77	97 193	97 151	100 65	86 175	100 451	96 139	- 0	99 296	94 264	96 297	95 273	95 279	91 176	84 89
Saint Elizabeth Boardman Health Center, Youngstown, OH	93 76	100 98	100 82	96 126	99 126	100 33	92 157	100 363	95 105	- 0	99 226	78 135	99 226	91 119	98 219	94 157	98 103
Saint Elizabeth Health Center, Youngstown, OH	97 58	98 52	86 78	91 90	97 94	100 51	97 174	100 660	97 249	92 144	98 463	89 528	96 467	95 511	97 445	97 175	99 143
Saint John Medical Center, Westlake, OH	96 98	96 137	95 62	98 142	98 110	100 41	87 160	100 417	97 148	96 51	95 285	96 276	99 289	88 269	94 265	87 160	92 114
Saint Joseph Health Center, Warren, OH	94 90	99 80	95 83	96 126	96 103	100 67	93 151	100 417	95 111	- 0	98 269	83 249	96 269	92 226	98 253	95 151	97 63
Saint Luke's Hospital, Maumee, OH	94 137	99 160	94 128	97 182	95 155	100 56	92 203	99 893	94 295	100 121	98 632	95 262	96 636	96 254	97 609	97 203	91 57
Saint Rita's Medical Center, Lima, OH	98 157	96 321	100 133	98 217	99 229	100 132	92 388	99 1164	97 436	100 163	98 693	91 275	98 703	96 266	92 669	95 388	82 171
Saint Vincent Charity Medical Center, Cleveland, OH	92 53	95 83	91 65	90 99	94 79	100 42	96 120	100 352	86 123	86 50	97 248	97 145	96 248	91 145	91 238	97 120	85 143
Salem Community Hospital, Salem, OH	93 123	96 147	92 119	95 188	89 164	80 46	76 135	100 351	95 100	- 0	96 228	83 98	95 228	94 82	97 222	76 135	84 91
Samaritan Hospital - Peoples Hospital, Ashland, OH	93 70	91 90	98 51	95 87	97 74	95 21	92 60	100 535	99 169	- 0	98 473	84 88	99 473	96 78	99 472	98 60	99 164
Selby General Hospital, Marietta, OH	53 19	83 6	87 15	67 12	100 8	93 15	100 32	98 82	- 0	- 0	89 70	- 0	96 69	- 0	91 67	100 32	93 14
South Pointe Hospital, Warrensville Hgts, OH	95 118	99 137	97 146	98 244	98 200	100 114	93 141	100 305	98 102	- 0	93 176	69 167	95 176	82 134	96 169	96 141	84 76
Southeastern Ohio Regional Medical Center, Cambridge, OH	89 112	99 144	98 91	96 150	96 136	100 72	87 90	100 183	97 63	- 0	99 141	93 155	94 143	91 145	95 131	87 90	93 44
Southern Ohio Medical Center, Portsmouth, OH	87 252	93 293	94 103	96 311	97 262	99 134	90 237	100 867	93 275	95 137	96 600	94 161	98 610	95 155	96 565	92 238	99 214
Southwest General Health Center, Middleburg Hgts, OH	92 255	97 456	83 236	96 427	85 358	76 89	86 160	100 1092	95 429	97 71	97 890	89 371	98 895	89 349	95 879	91 160	90 317
Springfield Regional Medical Center, Springfield, OH	95 304	98 455	98 277	95 469	98 344	98 179	86 384	100 1068	98 386	98 172	98 635	87 197	98 647	91 174	98 615	91 386	86 99
Summa Barberton Hospital, Barberton, OH	97 120	100 239	100 174	99 212	100 184	100 90	97 279	100 553	100 146	81 37	100 333	99 114	99 334	98 113	99 305	97 279	88 42
Summa Health Systems Hospitals, Akron, OH	94 71	92 106	81 107	98 153	73 128	100 63	95 150	99 495	62 178	81 149	92 343	95 529	95 349	92 530	88 329	95 150	72 90
Summa Wadsworth-Rittman Hospital, Wadsworth, OH	93 103	98 136	96 70	97 118	98 87	100 49	95 57	100 172	98 53	- 0	98 127	99 81	99 127	99 80	96 124	95 57	92 13
Summa Western Reserve Hospital, Cuyahoga Falls, OH	94 111	95 128	94 93	100 149	87 132	100 40	81 84	100 261	82 55	- 0	95 172	97 122	100 172	94 118	93 165	88 84	89 53
Surgical Hospital at Southwoods, Youngstown, OH	- 0	- 0	- 0	- 0	- 0	- 0	95 21	100 289	98 47	- 0	91 267	66 218	94 269	87 182	97 265	95 21	99 68
Three Gables Surgery Center, Proctorville, OH	- 0	- 0	- 0	- 0	- 0	- 0	- 0	- 0	- 0	- 0	- 0	95 57	- 0	22 54	- 0	- 0	- 0
The Toledo Hospital, Toledo, OH	86 65	96 106	90 73	96 103	91 97	90 49	89 152	100 674	97 268	90 151	96 486	97 588	97 495	93 581	91 468	91 152	88 153
Trinity Medical Center East & TMC West, Steubenville, OH	93 212	97 309	90 208	98 311	90 261	100 111	90 138	100 547	88 206	90 109	97 410	93 270	98 415	95 262	91 400	91 139	87 110
Trumbull Memorial Hospital, Warren, OH	89 232	99 236	95 196	91 280	96 292	98 101	85 196	99 699	89 201	84 86	95 475	94 304	97 477	85 303	97 463	89 197	79 57
Twin City Hospital, Dennison, OH	100 9	100 12	100 6	100 12	100 10	100 3	- 0	- 0	- 0	- 0	- 0	- -	- 0	- -	- 0	- 0	- 0
UH Geauga Medical Center, Chardon, OH	86 113	92 153	100 121	93 156	100 168	100 31	92 155	100 491	88 163	- 0	95 363	83 249	99 365	85 229	92 350	94 156	87 140
UHHS Bedford Medical Center, Bedford, OH	98 52	98 107	87 76	95 110	92 109	94 35	91 94	100 187	100 50	- 0	99 109	87 79	99 110	97 70	99 100	91 94	81 21
UHHS Memorial Hospital of Geneva, Geneva, OH	94 49	99 90	93 41	100 69	100 48	100 28	100 5	100 25	100 6	- 0	100 19	100 51	100 19	100 51	100 18	100 5	100 2
UHHS Richmond Heights Hospital, Richmond Heights, OH	96 46	97 73	95 60	96 89	95 79	100 24	93 75	100 218	97 67	- 0	98 146	90 87	99 147	93 90	96 142	97 75	94 71
Union Hospital, Dover, OH	95 184	97 231	98 220	98 302	98 303	97 98	93 114	100 404	97 109	- 0	99 266	93 143	99 268	99 139	98 254	99 114	96 69
University Hospital, Cincinnati, OH	92 49	98 123	82 72	86 115	82 55	98 83	97 211	100 645	92 181	95 106	97 418	84 395	95 435	93 375	93 409	98 214	79 131
University Hospitals Conneaut Medical Center, Conneaut, OH	93 28	100 31	100 20	100 30	100 24	90 10	100 5	99 92	100 26	- 0	99 76	83 6	100 76	100 5	100 75	100 5	100 74
University Hospitals of Cleveland, Cleveland, OH	95 135	96 246	82 193	88 284	91 257	99 138	99 251	99 785	99 281	95 162	99 518	94 678	98 524	88 670	93 502	99 251	87 210
University of Toledo Medical Center, Toledo, OH	75 53	94 83	82 78	96 76	78 87	100 55	96 152	100 477	96 200	90 94	96 337	97 196	98 345	95 210	97 295	100 152	98 102
University Pointe Surgical Hospital, West Chester, OH	- 0	- 0	- 0	- 0	- 0	- 0	- 0	100 5	- 0	- 0	100 4	100 8	25 4	88 8	100 4	- 0	- 0
Upper Valley Medical Center, Troy, OH	94 188	96 301	91 141	99 263	93 246	98 87	95 185	100 420	93 105	- 0	96 264	95 100	96 266	91 96	90 250	98 185	94 34
Van Wert County Hospital, Van Wert, OH	92 65	89 54	88 32	98 64	87 52	92 13	81 62	100 157	100 56	- 0	93 113	97 88	89 114	93 88	91 107	81 62	94 17
Wayne Hospital, Greenville, OH	81 62	91 97	96 67	98 91	92 86	89 28	90 82	96 207	94 48	- 0	99 140	62 21	88 141	89 36	82 137	96 82	65 37
West Chester Medical Center, West Chester, OH	86 77	97 128	93 60	94 85	94 96	92 39	92 130	100 402	89 111	- 0	98 297	94 67	98 300	100 65	98 288	95 130	97 145
Wilson Memorial Hospital, Sidney, OH	82 78	99 124	94 79	97 93	96 108	77 22	96 54	100 165	89 47	- 0	95 110	91 115	97 108	89 113	87 108	98 54	96 25
Wood County Hospital, Bowling Green, OH	67 114	89 105	86 63	88 114	91 69	100 28	92 112	99 225	84 69	- 0	92 178	86 110	96 178	54 104	88 171	88 118	53 70
The Woods at Parkside, Columbus, OH	- 0	- 0	- 0	- 0	- 0	- 0	- 0	- 0	- 0	- 0	- 0	- 0	- 0	- 0	- 0	- 0	- 0
Wooster Community Hospital, Wooster, OH	90 120	98 169	98 154	97 212	99 216	99 67	68 75	99 465	80 122	- 0	94 387	87 191	95 387	95 170	95 385	75 75	89 19
Wyandot Memorial Hospital, Upper Sandusky, OH	100 12	100 13	83 6	87 15	100 12	83 6	100 14	100 31	- 0	- 0	79 29	- -	97 29	- -	90 29	100 14	78 9
PENNSYLVANIA																	
Abington Memorial Hospital, Abington, PA	96 249	95 558	92 336	97 565	96 487	100 140	98 138	99 651	86 217	96 150	96 494	97 412	99 498	96 411	95 478	98 139	96 166
ACMH Hospital, Kittanning, PA	97 91	96 109	91 104	98 129	95 133	100 46	97 159	100 480	95 108	- 0	97 378	98 82	98 378	94 81	97 369	97 159	90 78
Advanced Surgical Hospital, Washington, PA	- 0	- 0	- 0	- 0	- 0	- 0	- 0	- 0	- 0	- 0	- 0	- -	- 0	- -	- 0	- 0	- 0
Albert Einstein Medical Center, Philadelphia, PA	98 99	94 203	83 138	98 241	92 176	100 155	99 308	100 738	98 200	93 89	98 498	93 252	98 511	92 240	99 481	99 308	95 222
Alle Kiski Medical Center, Natrona, PA	91 148	99 69	95 191	99 244	97 292	100 112	100 220	100 509	84 148	- 0	97 344	88 210	97 344	94 217	94 327	100 220	94 141
Allegheny General Hospital, Pittsburgh, PA	96 109	95 206	99 201	98 247	98 264	97 160	98 1416	100 2957	95 875	94 383	99 1377	97 541	99 1417	60 537	95 1265	99 1416	97 651

NOTE: The first number in each column (boldface) is the score, the second number is the number of patients; Please refer to the main entry for footnotes; (a) 100-299

*MEASURES: **Pneumonia Care:** 16. Appropriate Initial Antibiotic; 17. Blood Culture Timing; 18. Influenza Vaccine; 19. Initial Antibiotic Timing; 20. Pneumococcal Vaccine; 21. Smoking Cessation Advice; **Surgical Care Improvement Project:** 22. Appropriate VTP Within 24 Hours; 23. Appropriate Hair Removal; 24. Appropriate Beta Blocker Usage; 25. Controlled Postoperative Blood Glucose; 26. Prophylactic Antibiotic Timing; 27. Prophylactic Antibiotic Timing (Outpatient); 28. Prophylactic Antibiotic Selection; 29. Prophylactic Antibiotic Selection (Outpatient); 30. Prophylactic Antibiotic Stopped; 31. Recommended VTP Ordered; 32. Urinary Catheter Removal*

Hospital	Pneumonia Care						Surgical Care Improvement Project										
	16	17	18	19	20	21	22	23	24	25	26	27	28	29	30	31	32
Altoona Regional Health System, Altoona, PA	**90** 198	**97** 323	**99** 221	**96** 317	**98** 326	**100** 127	**94** 488	**100** 2077	**87** 634	**94** 256	**97** 1524	**89** 694	**97** 1559	**98** 646	**93** 1491	**93** 494	**87** 173
Aria Health, Philadelphia, PA	**97** 505	**98** 829	**100** 465	**95** 819	**99** 518	**100** 367	**98** 311	**100** 710	**95** 236	**97** 88	**96** 353	**94** 293	**97** 357	**98** 276	**96** 308	**99** 311	**97** 147
Berwick Hospital Center, Berwick, PA	**87** 53	**96** 76	**100** 56	**96** 78	**94** 71	**100** 22	**86** 42	**100** 169	**94** 32	- 0	**98** 129	**100** 36	**95** 131	**92** 36	**90** 126	**86** 43	**83** 6
Bloomsburg Hospital, Bloomsburg, PA	**95** 91	**85** 136	**90** 84	**98** 137	**90** 101	**85** 34	**80** 60	**100** 274	**75** 75	- 0	**97** 213	**45** 113	**99** 215	**98** 51	**97** 208	**80** 60	**98** 54
Bradford Regional Medical Center, Bradford, PA	**92** 59	**94** 88	**85** 78	**95** 111	**94** 99	**94** 31	**89** 57	**99** 137	**83** 35	- 0	**93** 90	**88** 42	**89** 89	**88** 40	**87** 85	**93** 57	**73** 15
Brandywine Hospital, Coatesville, PA	**92** 129	**97** 166	**95** 126	**92** 197	**98** 167	**100** 72	**83** 106	**100** 300	**89** 114	**95** 21	**97** 169	**94** 105	**93** 169	**97** 100	**95** 152	**88** 107	**94** 71
Brookville Hospital, Brookville, PA	**94** 31	**100** 37	**92** 38	**98** 43	**94** 50	**95** 21	**100** 29	**100** 54	- 0	- 0	**100** 34	- -	**91** 34	- -	**93** 30	**100** 29	**100** 12
Bucks County Specialty Hospital, Bensalem, PA	- 0	- 0	- 0	- 0	- 0	- 0	- 0	**100** 99	**93** 27	- 0	**97** 99	- -	**100** 99	- -	**100** 99	- 0	**92** 39
Butler Memorial Hospital, Butler, PA	**97** 188	**100** 217	**98** 143	**98** 233	**98** 232	**99** 107	**97** 271	**100** 1315	**92** 420	**99** 326	**99** 990	**95** 220	**99** 999	**94** 217	**94** 953	**99** 271	**94** 227
Cancer Treatment Centers of America, Philadelphia, PA	- 0	- 0	**25** 4	**64** 14	**0** 1	**0** 1	**91** 76	**43** 82	**56** 9	- 0	**81** 21	**100** 5	**86** 22	**100** 5	**86** 21	**97** 76	**70** 10
Canonsburg General Hospital, Canonsburg, PA	**93** 72	**100** 143	**69** 106	**96** 128	**88** 138	**100** 39	**97** 152	**100** 479	**83** 133	- 0	**97** 339	**72** 36	**96** 340	**97** 31	**97** 336	**98** 152	**72** 29
Carlisle Regional Medical Center, Carlisle, PA	**97** 93	**95** 175	**98** 106	**96** 154	**99** 145	**100** 40	**94** 187	**100** 561	**93** 179	- 0	**99** 394	**87** 137	**97** 395	**91** 120	**97** 375	**99** 187	**98** 59
Chambersburg Hospital, Chambersburg, PA	**89** 152	**98** 223	**96** 139	**96** 221	**97** 219	**94** 85	**95** 344	**100** 921	**95** 301	- 0	**98** 798	**92** 71	**97** 800	**74** 69	**94** 764	**96** 344	**82** 56
Charles Cole Memorial Hospital, Coudersport, PA	**98** 44	**94** 71	**86** 36	**94** 66	**94** 70	**100** 13	**95** 57	**98** 239	**100** 19	- 0	**87** 195	**71** 34	**97** 192	**92** 26	**95** 186	**92** 59	**99** 81
Chester County Hospital, West Chester, PA	**90** 156	**96** 251	**90** 167	**92** 256	**95** 245	**100** 76	**96** 371	**100** 1081	**94** 328	**99** 90	**99** 730	**93** 248	**99** 734	**94** 237	**96** 680	**97** 371	**91** 220
Chestnut Hill Hospital, Philadelphia, PA	**96** 77	**98** 184	**94** 108	**96** 183	**96** 166	**100** 46	**92** 133	**100** 309	**95** 76	- 0	**100** 203	**93** 110	**99** 206	**98** 104	**99** 189	**98** 133	**92** 49
Children's Hospital of Philadelphia, Philadelphia, PA	-	-	-	-	-	-	-	-	-	-	-	-	-	-	-	-	-
Children's Hospital of Pittsburgh of UPMC, Pittsburgh, PA	-	-	-	-	-	-	-	-	-	-	-	-	-	-	-	-	-
Clarion Hospital, Clarion, PA	**89** 94	**90** 125	**93** 72	**97** 144	**80** 112	**71** 45	**86** 43	**100** 238	**79** 48	- 0	**96** 186	**83** 30	**98** 185	**71** 28	**93** 184	**86** 43	**90** 52
Clearfield Hospital, Clearfield, PA	**92** 118	**92** 211	**91** 105	**99** 203	**94** 176	**100** 35	**94** 156	**99** 273	**90** 93	- 0	**91** 203	**96** 99	**95** 203	**97** 97	**91** 195	**95** 156	**61** 28
Coatesville VA Medical Center, Coatesville, PA	**0** 1	**100** 1	**100** 3	**100** 2	**100** 1	**100** 1	- 0	- 0	- 0	- 0	- 0	- -	- 0	- -	- 0	- 0	- 0
Community Medical Center, Scranton, PA	**97** 175	**99** 211	**84** 143	**96** 269	**90** 183	**96** 77	**97** 381	**100** 1141	**95** 424	**100** 226	**99** 781	**97** 461	**99** 795	**98** 451	**97** 768	**97** 383	**91** 203
Conemaugh Valley Memorial Hospital, Johnstown, PA	**93** 209	**98** 343	**90** 346	**94** 453	**93** 475	**96** 170	**95** 584	**99** 1837	**94** 712	**95** 201	**99** 1157	**90** 628	**99** 1164	**93** 586	**97** 1124	**97** 584	**93** 292
Coordinated Health Orthopedic Hospital, Bethlehem, PA	- 0	- 0	- 0	- 0	- 0	- 0	**100** 26	**100** 202	**92** 12	- 0	**98** 180	**100** 33	**98** 180	**100** 33	**93** 180	**100** 26	**100** 72
Corry Memorial Hospital, Corry, PA	**94** 52	**100** 46	**95** 42	**99** 72	**99** 71	**100** 20	- 0	- 0	- 0	- 0	- 0	- -	- 0	- -	- 0	- 0	- 0
Crozer Chester Medical Center, Upland, PA	**95** 352	**98** 466	**94** 362	**95** 588	**95** 444	**100** 254	**97** 343	**100** 1128	**95** 302	**96** 130	**98** 845	**98** 177	**96** 850	**97** 174	**97** 814	**98** 343	**94** 302
Delaware County Memorial Hospital, Drexel Hill, PA	**95** 111	**96** 184	**92** 117	**96** 192	**92** 144	**100** 62	**100** 348	**100** 551	**91** 140	- 0	**97** 379	**100** 69	**97** 382	**97** 69	**97** 354	**100** 349	**92** 165
Doylestown Hospital, Doylestown, PA	**87** 183	**95** 295	**95** 210	**97** 291	**95** 326	**96** 78	**96** 315	**100** 944	**93** 302	**99** 192	**94** 644	**88** 196	**98** 648	**51** 190	**92** 605	**97** 315	**96** 277
Dubois Regional Medical Center, Dubois, PA	**89** 70	**99** 109	**95** 73	**97** 114	**98** 120	**100** 52	**94** 112	**99** 554	**95** 224	**99** 148	**96** 443	**95** 319	**96** 449	**97** 409	**98** 409	**96** 112	**96** 133
Eagleville Hospital, Eagleville, PA	- 0	- 0	- 0	- 0	- 0	- 0	- 0	- 0	- 0	- 0	- 0	- 0	- 0	- 0	- 0	- 0	- 0
Easton Hospital, Easton, PA	**84** 123	**95** 201	**97** 153	**91** 224	**98** 252	**100** 56	**97** 225	**100** 741	**91** 277	**98** 121	**94** 458	**90** 84	**98** 462	**92** 83	**96** 444	**98** 225	**96** 136
Edgewood Surgical Hospital, Transfer, PA	- 0	- 0	- 0	- 0	- 0	- 0	**100** 7	**100** 127	**100** 24	- 0	**99** 119	- 0	**100** 119	- 0	**100** 119	**100** 7	**100** 15
Elk Regional Health Center, Saint Marys, PA	**85** 111	**94** 187	**85** 114	**95** 171	**96** 155	**94** 52	**78** 76	**100** 248	**79** 70	- 0	**87** 167	**91** 141	**92** 167	**91** 135	**87** 167	**79** 78	**90** 50
Ellwood City Hospital, Ellwood City, PA	**90** 42	**92** 38	**93** 44	**98** 64	**97** 62	**95** 20	**93** 56	**99** 96	**86** 29	- 0	**94** 32	**89** 35	**78** 32	**88** 32	**87** 31	**93** 56	**33** 6
Ephrata Community Hospital, Ephrata, PA	**90** 144	**96** 196	**97** 111	**86** 188	**99** 183	**85** 53	**98** 239	**100** 597	**96** 161	- 0	**94** 431	**92** 304	**98** 432	**97** 286	**93** 410	**98** 239	**98** 195
Erie VA Medical Center, Erie, PA	**91** 33	**98** 55	**97** 38	**98** 51	**98** 53	**81** 21	**100** 14	**100** 45	**100** 19	- 0	**98** 41	- -	**95** 41	- -	**95** 39	**100** 14	**100** 1
Evangelical Community Hospital, Lewisburg, PA	**95** 117	**97** 199	**95** 123	**97** 183	**95** 208	**93** 44	**85** 131	**100** 466	**98** 131	- 0	**95** 321	**93** 402	**99** 322	**98** 393	**95** 315	**86** 131	**97** 144
Excela Health Frick Hospital, Mount Pleasant, PA	**90** 73	**100** 97	**99** 81	**99** 109	**100** 105	**100** 29	**97** 64	**99** 82	**93** 27	- 0	**97** 39	**95** 43	**100** 39	**91** 43	**90** 39	**97** 64	**100** 14
Excela Health Latrobe Hospital, Latrobe, PA	**96** 124	**98** 200	**91** 159	**95** 186	**97** 238	**99** 70	**92** 276	**100** 610	**95** 150	- 0	**98** 400	**92** 191	**98** 402	**90** 188	**98** 377	**96** 276	**88** 68
Excela Health Westmoreland Regional Hospital, Greensburg, PA	**92** 185	**99** 284	**95** 220	**97** 319	**98** 336	**94** 105	**97** 507	**99** 1561	**96** 490	**98** 348	**99** 1095	**91** 245	**99** 1109	**95** 240	**96** 1039	**98** 507	**90** 353
Fulton County Medical Center, Mcconnellsburg, PA	**96** 24	**93** 15	**90** 20	**92** 25	**83** 24	**10** 10	- 0	- 0	- 0	- 0	- 0	- -	- 0	- -	- 0	- 0	- 0
Geisinger Medical Center, Danville, PA	**97** 102	**88** 187	**90** 207	**98** 195	**95** 254	**100** 107	**95** 176	**100** 767	**90** 322	**99** 167	**97** 471	**93** 820	**99** 480	**97** 1064	**98** 445	**97** 176	**98** 131
Geisinger Wyoming Valley Medical Center, Wilkes-Barre, PA	**96** 129	**90** 194	**87** 174	**93** 193	**94** 272	**100** 99	**92** 167	**100** 713	**83** 314	**98** 123	**96** 454	**92** 531	**97** 465	**97** 596	**96** 438	**94** 167	**96** 188
Gettysburg Hospital, Gettysburg, PA	**99** 71	**94** 158	**98** 116	**98** 131	**95** 143	**100** 40	**96** 161	**100** 409	**99** 110	- 0	**100** 297	**97** 104	**97** 301	**99** 101	**96** 291	**98** 161	**94** 32
Gnaden Huetten Memorial Hospital, Lehighton, PA	**83** 48	**94** 67	**94** 48	**94** 69	**98** 57	**100** 29	**96** 72	**100** 161	**100** 33	- 0	**100** 96	**86** 71	**95** 96	**87** 70	**89** 90	**96** 72	**90** 41
Good Samaritan Hospital, Lebanon, PA	**91** 160	**93** 202	**82** 136	**93** 208	**87** 186	**97** 61	**94** 170	**100** 509	**92** 230	**95** 131	**91** 383	**90** 338	**97** 389	**95** 320	**88** 364	**94** 171	**92** 124
Grand View Hospital, Sellersville, PA	**99** 146	**99** 229	**99** 159	**99** 211	**99** 234	**100** 55	**99** 165	**100** 454	**96** 114	- 0	**99** 312	**94** 121	**98** 313	**98** 124	**98** 296	**99** 165	**100** 27
Grove City Medical Center, Grove City, PA	**98** 65	**100** 80	**90** 49	**98** 88	**97** 69	**88** 17	**77** 35	**100** 152	**97** 37	- 0	**99** 113	**95** 88	**100** 113	**89** 84	**95** 113	**80** 35	**89** 19
Hahnemann University Hospital, Philadelphia, PA	**97** 99	**98** 200	**94** 117	**97** 192	**94** 109	**96** 120	**89** 294	**98** 686	**95** 214	**94** 137	**96** 468	**95** 416	**97** 473	**97** 419	**92** 455	**89** 295	**97** 143
Hamot Medical Center, Erie, PA	**95** 180	**94** 288	**93** 235	**95** 347	**96** 356	**100** 178	**97** 613	**100** 1832	**96** 688	**91** 375	**98** 1107	**96** 421	**99** 1126	**97** 424	**96** 1076	**98** 613	**96** 538
Hanover Hospital, Hanover, PA	**85** 93	**91** 141	**81** 113	**96** 127	**93** 136	**96** 27	**87** 163	**100** 750	**95** 207	- 0	**97** 628	**91** 194	**98** 624	**96** 183	**88** 619	**88** 164	**95** 262
Hazleton General Hospital, Hazleton, PA	**93** 141	**97** 171	**98** 198	**97** 257	**99** 276	**99** 90	**94** 153	**100** 323	**94** 94	- 0	**97** 178	**92** 78	**98** 179	**85** 75	**95** 169	**97** 153	**100** 54
Heart of Lancaster Regional Medical Center, Lititz, PA	**100** 28	**100** 50	**100** 29	**100** 48	**100** 42	**100** 16	**98** 83	**100** 184	**97** 32	- 0	**99** 91	**99** 77	**100** 93	**97** 76	**99** 88	**98** 83	**100** 22
Heritage Valley Beaver, Beaver, PA	**92** 211	**98** 361	**100** 229	**99** 327	**99** 281	**100** 132	**85** 358	**100** 1303	**80** 363	**95** 243	**98** 911	**87** 196	**96** 924	**92** 186	**96** 879	**89** 359	**93** 279
Heritage Valley Sewickley, Sewickley, PA	**93** 150	**99** 240	**99** 148	**97** 234	**100** 202	**100** 65	**91** 259	**100** 1182	**90** 331	- 0	**98** 889	**87** 119	**99** 893	**89** 114	**97** 836	**92** 260	**93** 374
Highlands Hospital, Connellsville, PA	**82** 60	**98** 61	**79** 33	**97** 67	**94** 51	**100** 24	**84** 45	**99** 70	**94** 16	- 0	**75** 32	**62** 8	**94** 32	**83** 6	**84** 31	**89** 45	**80** 20
Holy Redeemer Hospital and Medical Center, Meadowbrook, PA	**91** 109	**96** 228	**98** 163	**97** 236	**98** 244	**98** 42	**98** 254	**100** 829	**89** 228	- 0	**99** 601	**74** 58	**98** 601	**86** 44	**97** 577	**98** 254	**100** 191
Holy Spirit Hospital, Camp Hill, PA	**99** 256	**99** 369	**96** 258	**96** 348	**97** 348	**100** 88	**89** 279	**100** 1007	**89** 387	**99** 272	**97** 842	**94** 588	**98** 854	**95** 564	**96** 811	**92** 279	**98** 170
Hospital of Univ of Pennsylvania, Philadelphia, PA	**88** 96	**66** 161	**89** 84	**92** 174	**92** 160	**95** 96	**99** 384	**100** 982	**77** 293	**98** 278	**99** 580	**51** 690	**96** 598	**77** 538	**76** 557	**100** 384	**87** 175
Indiana Regional Medical Center, Indiana, PA	**92** 126	**98** 204	**85** 134	**96** 190	**91** 185	**88** 56	**91** 159	**100** 394	**97** 117	- 0	**98** 287	**96** 177	**99** 287	**97** 213	**94** 271	**94** 161	**92** 109
J C Blair Memorial Hospital, Huntingdon, PA	**93** 44	**98** 51	**93** 42	**97** 59	**91** 55	**94** 17	**94** 33	**100** 58	**78** 9	- 0	**88** 33	**76** 17	**79** 33	**100** 15	**69** 29	**94** 34	**0** 7
James E. Van Zandt VA Medical Center - Altoona, Altoona, PA	**92** 36	**97** 38	**100** 35	**97** 37	**100** 32	**100** 17	- 0	- 0	- 0	- 0	- 0	- -	- 0	- -	- 0	- 0	- 0
Jameson Memorial Hospital, New Castle, PA	**93** 162	**100** 248	**84** 210	**98** 269	**89** 299	**100** 122	**96** 299	**100** 561	**92** 146	- 0	**98** 377	**88** 77	**94** 379	**86** 70	**97** 355	**97** 301	**82** 65
Jeanes Hospital, Philadelphia, PA	**98** 122	**97** 188	**99** 97	**94** 175	**94** 158	**100** 48	**98** 235	**95** 658	**99** 196	**94** 87	**98** 456	**94** 48	**98** 459	**98** 49	**94** 441	**97** 239	**100** 1
Jefferson Regional Medical Center, Pittsburgh, PA	**90** 232	**97** 229	**96** 250	**96** 357	**94** 323	**95** 95	**95** 700	**100** 1780	**99** 643	**98** 363	**99** 1174	**94** 268	**99** 1197	**80** 258	**94** 1150	**96** 703	**97** 583
Jennersville Regional Hospital, West Grove, PA	**94** 151	**97** 233	**100** 130	**97** 222	**100** 194	**100** 72	**100** 64	**100** 144	**94** 33	- 0	**100** 91	**98** 47	**99** 90	**98** 98	**100** 90	**100** 64	**100** 18
Jersey Shore Hospital, Jersey Shore, PA	**88** 60	**96** 56	**88** 42	**93** 76	**91** 65	**100** 15	**45** 53	**100** 84	- 0	- 0	**78** 37	- 0	**71** 35	- 0	**71** 35	**47** 53	**95** 21
Kane Community Hospital, Kane, PA	**84** 44	**89** 54	**27** 52	**92** 74	**22** 85	**67** 21	**69** 16	**69** 26	**0** 6	- 0	**67** 9	**50** 4	**100** 9	**100** 2	**78** 9	**75** 16	**50** 4

NOTE: The first number in each column (boldface) is the score, the second number is the number of patients; Please refer to the main entry for footnotes; (a) 100-299
*MEASURES: **Pneumonia Care:** 16. Appropriate Initial Antibiotic; 17. Blood Culture Timing; 18. Influenza Vaccine; 19. Initial Antibiotic Timing; 20. Pneumococcal Vaccine; 21. Smoking Cessation Advice; **Surgical Care Improvement Project:** 22. Appropriate VTP Within 24 Hours; 23. Appropriate Hair Removal; 24. Appropriate Beta Blocker Usage; 25. Controlled Postoperative Blood Glucose; 26. Prophylactic Antibiotic Timing; 27. Prophylactic Antibiotic Timing (Outpatient); 28. Prophylactic Antibiotic Selection; 29. Prophylactic Antibiotic Selection (Outpatient); 30. Prophylactic Antibiotic Stopped; 31. Recommended VTP Ordered; 32. Urinary Catheter Removal*

Hospital	Pneumonia Care							Surgical Care Improvement Project										
	16	17	18	19	20	21	22	23	24	25	26	27	28	29	30	31	32
Kensington Hospital, Philadelphia, PA	- 0	- 0	- 0	- 0	- 0	- 0	- 0	- 0	- 0	- 0	- 0	- 0	- 0	- 0	- 0	- 0	- 0
Lancaster General Hospital, Lancaster, PA	95 243	97 356	96 342	95 384	95 434	100 145	94 679	96 2163	89 764	96 278	95 1457	91 1616	98 1477	97 1535	96 1401	95 681	95 591
Lancaster Regional Medical Center, Lancaster, PA	94 70	95 86	100 35	96 92	99 67	100 40	99 177	100 498	100 146	93 54	99 269	100 305	97 275	99 305	95 255	99 177	97 146
Lansdale Hospital, Lansdale, PA	96 78	90 132	92 80	98 123	86 132	100 17	94 141	100 213	98 60	- 0	96 112	98 50	98 113	100 50	94 111	94 141	98 43
Lebanon VA Medical Center, Lebanon, PA	87 23	93 29	100 25	87 31	100 19	100 20	90 58	100 234	97 95	- 0	99 187	- -	99 190	- -	98 186	91 58	97 87
Lehigh Valley Hospital, Allentown, PA	94 257	98 489	98 353	95 519	96 499	100 149	98 1432	100 4121	99 1325	98 581	97 2490	98 1177	99 2523	96 1169	98 2407	99 1433	95 975
Lehigh Valley Hospital - Muhlenberg, Bethlehem, PA	96 158	97 312	98 200	98 323	99 308	100 92	96 352	100 802	96 248	97 119	96 495	96 277	97 499	96 270	96 475	97 355	89 135
Lewistown Hospital, Lewistown, PA	92 128	99 224	86 139	97 189	91 188	88 60	81 100	100 267	94 78	- 0	98 176	95 119	95 176	97 117	97 166	82 102	100 11
Lock Haven Hospital, Lock Haven, PA	96 50	100 59	97 31	98 59	92 40	100 13	84 19	100 63	77 13	- 0	96 25	89 9	92 24	94 35	83 24	85 20	100 6
Lower Bucks Hospital, Bristol, PA	84 90	97 125	57 51	96 113	67 70	97 36	80 102	100 293	90 89	92 38	96 190	88 83	91 189	90 80	86 186	82 102	86 42
Magee Womens Hospital of UPMC Health System, Pittsburgh, PA	94 34	100 32	91 45	100 40	92 51	100 33	97 549	100 2291	95 436	- 0	98 1880	91 330	97 1878	94 309	96 1854	98 550	100 525
Main Line Hospital Bryn Mawr Campus, Bryn Mawr, PA	99 145	100 271	100 177	99 224	99 273	100 44	100 224	100 1526	98 427	98 89	99 1296	93 238	99 1307	88 224	100 1262	100 224	100 134
Main Line Hospital Lankenau, Wynnewood, PA	97 124	99 278	91 134	98 240	97 209	100 75	97 300	100 1423	97 505	99 456	99 1161	93 348	98 1183	97 341	99 1116	99 300	99 343
Main Line Hospital Paoli, Paoli, PA	97 127	100 164	96 132	96 168	99 186	100 34	98 234	100 912	99 237	95 82	99 715	95 197	98 720	92 193	99 660	99 235	100 241
Marian Community Hospital, Carbondale, PA	90 108	96 160	96 81	99 158	99 125	100 31	94 33	100 108	89 45	- 0	99 93	84 19	93 95	94 17	98 91	97 33	96 23
Meadville Medical Center, Meadville, PA	97 92	98 129	92 85	98 139	99 114	100 50	95 182	100 824	96 262	- 0	98 631	93 178	99 633	85 219	96 617	95 186	87 31
Memorial Hospital - Towanda, Towanda, PA	74 61	91 66	68 40	94 68	70 50	100 22	93 14	100 26	75 4	- 0	86 14	97 30	79 14	90 30	77 13	93 14	100 2
Memorial Hospital York, York, PA	94 127	97 197	87 99	94 177	91 138	100 47	91 133	100 554	98 111	- 0	96 447	94 96	97 447	81 94	92 438	92 133	100 39
Mercy Fitzgerald Hospital, Darby, PA	95 186	97 392	93 133	98 359	96 185	99 187	100 272	100 525	92 142	96 72	98 264	91 151	97 272	93 155	94 248	100 272	93 84
Mercy Hospital Scranton, Scranton, PA	90 71	99 99	100 81	98 135	98 146	92 37	96 147	100 581	99 212	92 179	99 423	82 281	99 436	93 250	96 385	97 147	98 58
Mercy Suburban Hospital, Norristown, PA	97 63	98 146	98 64	95 133	99 87	100 45	97 123	100 316	96 89	- 0	100 184	98 58	97 185	96 57	96 179	98 123	94 32
Mercy Tyler Hospital, Tunkhannock, PA	82 68	93 72	67 63	99 92	93 102	76 29	79 28	100 40	80 15	- 0	71 31	69 16	90 30	80 15	83 29	79 28	80 10
Mid-Valley Hospital, Peckville, PA	95 19	90 31	100 14	93 30	100 32	100 5	- 0	- 0	- 0	- 0	- 0	- -	- 0	- -	- 0	- 0	- 0
Millcreek Community Hospital, Erie, PA	83 24	95 40	100 33	96 47	100 46	100 22	95 43	99 126	73 30	- 0	93 85	97 30	95 87	86 29	85 81	93 44	83 18
Milton S Hershey Medical Center, Hershey, PA	95 129	89 275	78 188	95 237	82 285	99 93	95 426	98 1642	86 534	92 333	93 1275	93 710	98 1287	94 702	94 1205	95 428	92 349
Miners Medical Center, Hastings, PA	79 43	74 35	38 37	96 53	36 50	62 21	47 19	79 24	12 8	- 0	79 14	33 3	93 14	50 2	100 13	47 19	50 2
Monongahela Valley Hospital, Monongahela, PA	94 170	98 130	95 162	94 249	93 210	96 91	95 333	100 665	98 162	- 0	97 425	95 94	97 425	89 90	94 398	95 333	84 64
Montgomery Hospital, Norristown, PA	90 82	97 66	91 68	93 105	92 90	100 29	68 60	100 291	87 106	- 0	92 197	95 59	98 194	93 58	100 192	78 60	84 19
Montrose General Hospital, Montrose, PA	57 21	80 5	93 14	97 30	97 37	83 6	- 0	- 0	- 0	- 0	59 97	- -	100 97	- -	46 97	- 0	- 0
Moses Taylor Hospital, Scranton, PA	85 121	100 184	95 129	98 171	98 180	100 78	99 254	100 613	97 161	100 1	99 400	95 58	96 400	93 56	93 388	99 254	81 125
Mount Nittany Medical Center, State College, PA	95 134	94 209	93 179	92 226	98 251	100 62	94 373	98 1632	89 482	- 0	97 1229	95 221	99 1232	96 215	99 1201	95 373	94 228
Muncy Valley Hospital, Muncy, PA	95 38	94 31	85 27	94 34	98 44	100 6	85 13	86 14	100 3	- 0	62 8	- -	88 8	- -	88 8	85 13	100 2
Nason Hospital, Roaring Spring, PA	94 63	100 76	100 53	99 77	100 72	94 18	100 76	99 155	100 43	- 0	100 91	91 58	99 91	82 55	98 89	100 76	79 19
Nazareth Hospital, Philadelphia, PA	97 143	98 303	82 152	97 279	95 202	98 66	97 236	100 643	95 190	- 0	99 479	100 73	99 480	97 73	99 465	98 236	93 213
Ohio Valley General Hospital, Mckees Rocks, PA	84 98	87 93	76 75	91 134	86 106	96 54	93 163	100 307	81 78	- 0	92 210	80 45	95 213	82 38	87 198	94 164	78 23
Palmerton Hospital, Palmerton, PA	76 41	96 55	89 35	91 56	98 54	93 15	88 58	100 106	94 31	- 0	93 55	69 78	98 55	91 64	87 54	88 58	88 25
Penn Presbyterian Medical Center, Philadelphia, PA	91 76	95 155	61 95	97 139	97 110	100 71	94 576	100 2635	100 787	98 394	97 1482	90 343	98 1485	91 313	86 1440	99 576	99 734
Penn Hospital of the U of Penn Health Sys, Philadelphia, PA	90 99	96 147	79 66	90 154	91 103	100 62	96 245	100 689	87 218	84 106	98 483	98 572	97 494	96 571	79 464	97 247	92 199
Philadelphia VA Medical Center, Philadelphia, PA	86 58	97 88	88 58	85 72	98 50	100 33	96 67	100 90	100 24	- 0	88 32	- -	94 31	- -	77 26	97 67	61 33
Phoenixville Hospital, Phoenixville, PA	90 105	93 140	85 131	95 172	92 195	98 43	93 224	100 550	99 189	96 99	97 325	98 114	98 328	93 115	92 304	96 224	90 126
Pinnacle Health Hospitals, Harrisburg, PA	97 229	96 333	94 321	96 342	98 380	99 140	95 746	100 3582	94 1087	99 497	99 2975	96 1109	97 3010	87 1086	95 2912	99 746	98 624
Pocono Medical Center, East Stroudsburg, PA	94 207	92 253	92 207	96 322	89 316	97 157	90 230	100 659	96 214	96 165	99 379	97 192	97 380	95 186	97 355	91 234	91 156
Pottstown Memorial Medical Center, Pottstown, PA	97 195	98 327	95 193	98 318	96 271	100 112	89 244	100 491	76 102	- 0	95 287	89 146	93 289	90 143	87 275	93 245	94 129
Punxsutawney Area Hospital, Punxsutawney, PA	95 61	90 62	95 41	96 74	100 64	88 25	91 58	100 146	97 33	- 0	97 102	96 70	100 103	95 98	98 99	92 59	91 32
Reading Hospital Medical Center, Reading, PA	95 331	95 633	99 420	97 555	100 586	100 154	97 521	100 1981	94 730	98 213	98 1568	89 747	98 1580	95 724	94 1462	98 522	96 433
Riddle Memorial Hospital, Media, PA	96 150	93 204	97 149	98 261	99 242	95 64	92 272	99 1284	94 308	- 0	100 996	97 238	98 1002	97 234	97 980	93 272	99 460
Robert Packer Hospital, Sayre, PA	96 95	96 147	97 141	89 144	97 223	100 68	97 500	100 1482	84 529	95 187	96 878	95 618	99 887	96 605	97 844	98 502	83 185
Roxborough Memorial Hospital, Phila, PA	98 43	90 92	90 49	98 104	91 98	100 37	95 81	100 144	100 40	- 0	98 66	100 52	96 70	98 52	91 64	96 81	97 39
Sacred Heart Hospital, Allentown, PA	80 51	96 67	80 54	95 76	78 73	96 25	85 155	99 397	87 99	0 1	93 280	91 85	94 280	88 80	82 276	91 162	84 45
Saint Catherine Medical Center Fountain Springs, Ashland, PA	78 32	93 43	79 39	89 53	80 51	100 20	100 20	100 53	100 10	- 0	92 25	56 9	72 25	100 5	79 24	95 21	71 7
Saint Clair Memorial Hospital, Pittsburgh, PA	96 360	98 401	91 389	96 540	93 554	100 131	93 569	99 1508	92 438	96 204	94 1086	76 336	97 1098	93 287	97 1046	96 569	92 167
Saint Joseph Medical Center, Reading, PA	89 124	93 188	98 145	93 178	97 193	100 59	99 183	100 613	100 232	93 121	98 456	92 201	96 468	96 187	97 445	100 183	96 156
Saint Joseph's Hospital, Philadelphia, PA	68 37	81 75	30 37	77 79	52 48	40 25	84 38	87 63	70 10	- 0	38 13	62 16	69 13	100 13	38 13	85 41	83 6
Saint Luke's Hospital Bethlehem, Bethlehem, PA	95 300	97 470	92 313	96 493	93 414	100 161	94 430	100 1622	87 550	97 227	99 1242	89 700	98 1266	92 639	97 1203	95 432	98 457
Saint Luke's Miners Memorial Hospital, Coaldale, PA	90 39	100 57	100 39	97 58	100 62	100 16	98 58	100 188	67 52	- 0	99 158	84 19	99 159	94 16	95 153	100 58	84 74
Saint Luke's Quakertown Hospital, Quakertown, PA	97 78	98 92	97 65	98 99	99 92	100 35	93 45	100 106	92 38	- 0	99 68	86 29	99 68	88 25	96 57	96 45	100 28
Saint Mary Medical Center, Langhorne, PA	95 256	99 435	100 246	100 437	100 328	100 116	91 158	100 701	97 261	97 155	99 517	97 273	99 523	93 264	96 483	94 158	98 182
Saint Vincent Health Center, Erie, PA	93 154	94 224	89 189	97 253	96 268	100 99	95 498	100 1898	95 621	96 423	97 1319	97 333	97 1336	93 338	96 1297	96 499	89 476
Schuylkill Medical Center - East Norwegian Street, Pottsville, PA	92 64	94 122	89 117	96 162	94 164	100 31	95 159	99 265	87 101	- 0	93 149	92 12	97 148	67 12	71 140	97 159	78 41
Schuylkill Medical Center - South Jackson Street, Pottsville, PA	85 99	92 170	85 134	95 208	88 186	98 64	98 146	100 413	98 113	- 0	96 302	68 122	91 301	84 90	89 290	97 148	90 29
Shamokin Area Community Hospital, Coal Township, PA	89 37	94 86	100 103	97 135	100 142	93 30	88 41	100 128	88 56	- 0	95 92	85 20	98 92	84 19	85 89	90 41	98 50
Sharon Regional Health System, Sharon, PA	87 94	98 126	92 99	94 140	98 129	95 44	99 244	100 621	99 204	93 84	98 472	98 157	99 477	98 155	96 467	98 247	95 112
Soldiers and Sailors Memorial Hospital, Wellsboro, PA	96 72	93 98	98 55	97 103	98 91	88 26	90 77	99 195	98 51	- 0	95 127	83 48	94 127	99 109	99 126	90 77	89 36
Somerset Hospital, Somerset, PA	89 76	87 124	98 62	94 114	95 94	72 32	94 97	100 293	99 82	- 0	92 212	94 77	86 214	82 76	84 210	94 97	98 43
Southwest Regional Medical Center, Waynesburg, PA	98 111	100 120	73 116	99 154	79 131	93 59	89 47	100 114	82 34	- 0	88 64	88 33	95 64	91 33	92 61	92 48	94 16
Sunbury Community Hospital, Sunbury, PA	94 67	97 128	94 85	94 125	90 109	84 19	80 44	100 102	91 35	- 0	100 71	72 32	99 71	95 38	80 65	80 44	94 35
Surgical Institute of Reading, Wyomissing, PA	- 0	- 0	- 0	- 0	- 0	- 0	84 49	99 418	88 112	- 0	94 395	98 204	96 395	95 202	100 393	84 49	99 189
Surgical Specialty Center at Coordinated Health, Allentown, PA	- 0	- 0	- 0	- 0	- 0	- 0	100 4	100 71	29 7	- 0	97 65	- 0	100 65	- 0	100 65	100 4	100 66

NOTE: The first number in each column (boldface) is the score, the second number is the number of patients; Please refer to the main entry for footnotes; (a) 100-299

*MEASURES: **Pneumonia Care:** 16. Appropriate Initial Antibiotic; 17. Blood Culture Timing; 18. Influenza Vaccine; 19. Initial Antibiotic Timing; 20. Pneumococcal Vaccine; 21. Smoking Cessation Advice; **Surgical Care Improvement Project:** 22. Appropriate VTP Within 24 Hours; 23. Appropriate Hair Removal; 24. Appropriate Beta Blocker Usage; 25. Controlled Postoperative Blood Glucose; 26. Prophylactic Antibiotic Timing; 27. Prophylactic Antibiotic Timing (Outpatient); 28. Prophylactic Antibiotic Selection; 29. Prophylactic Antibiotic Selection (Outpatient); 30. Prophylactic Antibiotic Stopped; 31. Recommended VTP Ordered; 32. Urinary Catheter Removal*

Hospital	Pneumonia Care							Surgical Care Improvement Project									
	16	17	18	19	20	21	22	23	24	25	26	27	28	29	30	31	32
Temple University Hospital, Philadelphia, PA	**94** 218	**95** 298	**92** 240	**90** 360	**86** 226	**100** 274	**97** 394	**100** 1112	**86** 289	**87** 141	**97** 789	**93** 402	**95** 804	**91** 394	**99** 618	**99** 394	**81** 159
Thomas Jefferson University Hospital, Philadelphia, PA	**92** 264	**86** 435	**90** 241	**88** 400	**93** 289	**99** 177	**98** 814	**100** 3104	**96** 763	**87** 184	**99** 2538	**84** 487	**98** 2558	**99** 485	**98** 2489	**99** 816	**97** 978
Titusville Hospital, Titusville, PA	**87** 47	**96** 55	**87** 46	**90** 71	**83** 72	**80** 30	**54** 37	**99** 118	**91** 33	**-** 0	**85** 85	**58** 38	**73** 84	**61** 31	**85** 78	**62** 37	**33** 3
Troy Community Hospital, Troy, PA	**96** 26	**94** 34	**94** 17	**100** 2	**78** 27	**100** 4	**-** 0	**-** 0	**-** 0	**-** 0	**-** 0	**-** 0	**-** 0	**-** 0	**-** 0	**-** 0	**-** 0
Uniontown Hospital, Uniontown, PA	**91** 183	**96** 115	**83** 163	**93** 231	**86** 212	**91** 85	**95** 308	**100** 910	**95** 220	**-** 0	**97** 640	**84** 141	**95** 644	**88** 128	**95** 620	**98** 308	**96** 109
UPMC Bedford, Everett, PA	**97** 59	**98** 87	**100** 45	**99** 74	**99** 72	**86** 14	**100** 64	**100** 157	**91** 44	**-** 0	**98** 114	**83** 36	**98** 114	**82** 33	**94** 109	**100** 64	**95** 20
UPMC Horizon, Greenville, PA	**95** 147	**99** 179	**99** 155	**98** 188	**100** 201	**100** 59	**98** 384	**100** 778	**96** 254	**-** 0	**97** 537	**91** 201	**97** 539	**91** 195	**97** 506	**98** 384	**98** 43
UPMC Mckeesport, McKeesport, PA	**98** 103	**100** 252	**97** 199	**98** 251	**100** 253	**100** 96	**100** 209	**100** 377	**99** 114	**-** 0	**99** 195	**97** 95	**97** 197	**90** 93	**100** 191	**100** 209	**97** 39
UPMC Mercy, Pittsburgh, PA	**92** 212	**98** 242	**90** 205	**96** 329	**94** 274	**100** 197	**98** 227	**100** 617	**98** 197	**96** 132	**95** 425	**93** 441	**98** 436	**95** 419	**94** 393	**99** 227	**91** 118
UPMC Northwest, Seneca, PA	**94** 107	**99** 160	**99** 120	**99** 164	**98** 184	**100** 58	**98** 129	**100** 369	**98** 94	**100** 1	**100** 251	**95** 139	**100** 252	**99** 242	**100** 240	**98** 129	**100** 40
UPMC Passavant, Pittsburgh, PA	**88** 263	**98** 387	**98** 288	**95** 413	**99** 408	**99** 111	**98** 970	**100** 1951	**98** 627	**95** 392	**97** 1232	**93** 519	**98** 1248	**91** 519	**98** 1190	**99** 971	**90** 397
UPMC Presbyterian Shadyside, Pittsburgh, PA	**100** 240	**100** 447	**99** 421	**99** 545	**100** 488	**100** 326	**99** 3593	**100** 7812	**98** 2600	**96** 894	**99** 2801	**97** 970	**99** 2889	**97** 973	**99** 2516	**99** 3593	**95** 1697
UPMC Saint Margaret, Pittsburgh, PA	**95** 221	**99** 259	**99** 207	**96** 327	**98** 279	**100** 93	**99** 849	**100** 1600	**99** 531	**100** 1	**96** 1095	**96** 357	**99** 1100	**99** 350	**96** 1056	**100** 849	**96** 549
VA Pittsburgh Healthcare System, Pittsburgh, PA	**89** 56	**99** 121	**95** 61	**93** 136	**99** 72	**100** 36	**98** 176	**100** 457	**98** 236	**94** 156	**99** 366	**-** -	**99** 372	**-** -	**91** 358	**98** 176	**86** 220
Valley Forge Medical Center and Hospital, Norristown, PA	**-** 0	**-** 0	**-** 0	**-** 0	**-** 0	**-** 0	**-** 0	**-** 0	**-** 0	**-** 0	**-** 0	**-** -	**-** 0	**-** -	**-** 0	**-** 0	**-** 0
Warren General Hospital, Warren, PA	**87** 67	**94** 95	**85** 47	**97** 95	**89** 79	**96** 26	**72** 50	**100** 231	**69** 61	**-** 0	**93** 228	**71** 35	**94** 229	**63** 27	**90** 221	**64** 58	**78** 55
The Washington Hospital, Washington, PA	**94** 244	**100** 301	**98** 274	**96** 360	**97** 364	**99** 134	**95** 218	**100** 835	**94** 258	**98** 162	**99** 625	**92** 216	**97** 630	**93** 244	**96** 604	**97** 218	**96** 121
Wayne Memorial Hospital, Honesdale, PA	**92** 83	**97** 102	**94** 66	**96** 104	**96** 97	**100** 36	**96** 109	**100** 255	**76** 54	**-** 0	**97** 162	**89** 47	**95** 162	**88** 49	**96** 158	**96** 109	**79** 63
Waynesboro Hospital, Waynesboro, PA	**99** 71	**96** 84	**98** 52	**96** 108	**99** 107	**100** 26	**89** 81	**100** 192	**93** 43	**-** 0	**96** 134	**77** 26	**99** 132	**86** 22	**98** 129	**89** 81	**93** 14
Western Pennsylvania Hospital, Pittsburgh, PA	**93** 104	**96** 134	**86** 122	**94** 152	**80** 127	**100** 87	**100** 218	**100** 1030	**99** 273	**98** 206	**100** 870	**98** 350	**96** 886	**97** 347	**97** 844	**98** 221	**98** 207
Western Penn Hosp-Forbes Reg Campus, Monroeville, PA	**94** 215	**98** 180	**86** 229	**92** 303	**93** 311	**100** 97	**97** 299	**99** 969	**98** 341	**97** 180	**100** 703	**83** 281	**98** 712	**85** 242	**98** 682	**98** 300	**97** 285
Westfield Hospital, Allentown, PA	**92** 12	**75** 8	**75** 4	**100** 4	**43** 7	**67** 3	**40** 5	**97** 29	**25** 4	**-** 0	**37** 19	**-** 0	**87** 15	**-** 0	**87** 15	**40** 5	**100** 1
Wilkes-Barre General Hospital, Wilkes-Barre, PA	**91** 260	**96** 394	**88** 290	**94** 432	**88** 406	**99** 146	**90** 616	**100** 1668	**90** 600	**100** 264	**98** 1114	**91** 423	**97** 1127	**91** 402	**95** 1079	**91** 617	**100** 404
Wilkes-Barre VA Medical Center, Wilkes-Barre, PA	**100** 42	**99** 77	**98** 41	**96** 70	**100** 63	**96** 24	**94** 34	**100** 48	**83** 18	**-** 0	**97** 32	**-** -	**97** 32	**-** -	**82** 28	**94** 34	**86** 22
Williamsport Hospital & Medical Center, Williamsport, PA	**94** 149	**98** 152	**90** 156	**97** 193	**97** 220	**98** 89	**97** 536	**99** 1184	**97** 425	**100** 119	**96** 917	**93** 396	**98** 926	**99** 386	**96** 902	**98** 537	**97** 311
Windber Hospital, Windber, PA	**93** 59	**100** 72	**88** 50	**99** 87	**99** 72	**75** 12	**95** 38	**99** 138	**94** 34	**-** 0	**96** 94	**91** 44	**96** 94	**100** 41	**92** 92	**97** 38	**91** 23
York Hospital, York, PA	**100** 223	**84** 608	**97** 245	**92** 559	**96** 463	**100** 162	**93** 611	**100** 2258	**92** 775	**90** 366	**96** 1723	**96** 832	**96** 1760	**96** 831	**95** 1668	**96** 617	**92** 424
RHODE ISLAND																	
Kent County Memorial Hospital, Warwick, RI	**86** 158	**89** 273	**67** 150	**94** 236	**85** 243	**93** 99	**93** 436	**99** 721	**90** 230	**-** 0	**93** 460	**90** 262	**98** 464	**95** 255	**92** 445	**94** 437	**82** 184
Landmark Medical Center, Woonsocket, RI	**96** 116	**98** 168	**92** 133	**98** 199	**87** 172	**97** 66	**94** 137	**100** 283	**90** 86	**-** 0	**98** 179	**94** 155	**96** 182	**94** 153	**96** 161	**97** 138	**69** 32
Memorial Hospital of Rhode Island, Pawtucket, RI	**92** 92	**96** 105	**94** 100	**91** 172	**88** 160	**99** 72	**95** 149	**98** 322	**88** 81	**-** 0	**98** 187	**98** 208	**96** 187	**93** 207	**99** 172	**92** 156	**90** 51
Miriam Hospital, Providence, RI	**96** 98	**98** 167	**96** 105	**97** 176	**91** 162	**100** 46	**93** 442	**100** 1111	**96** 455	**94** 195	**98** 728	**95** 289	**99** 729	**99** 280	**97** 704	**94** 442	**85** 330
Newport Hospital, Newport, RI	**97** 118	**98** 193	**96** 85	**97** 185	**96** 148	**100** 33	**93** 186	**100** 287	**97** 77	**-** 0	**97** 180	**92** 80	**96** 180	**99** 77	**94** 171	**95** 186	**93** 28
Providence VA Medical Center, Providence, RI	**92** 25	**97** 73	**93** 40	**95** 76	**99** 74	**100** 16	**99** 90	**100** 140	**92** 53	**-** 0	**95** 74	**-** -	**96** 75	**-** -	**90** 71	**99** 90	**96** 53
Rhode Island Hospital, Providence, RI	**97** 59	**97** 129	**82** 78	**94** 138	**85** 115	**100** 52	**99** 221	**100** 687	**97** 255	**94** 160	**97** 447	**93** 479	**99** 449	**96** 531	**98** 408	**99** 221	**88** 164
Roger Williams Medical Center, Providence, RI	**88** 78	**92** 109	**74** 69	**92** 146	**72** 125	**100** 33	**97** 181	**100** 377	**98** 112	**100** 1	**100** 255	**90** 138	**97** 256	**98** 130	**97** 247	**99** 181	**86** 140
Saint Joseph Health Services of RI, North Providence, RI	**95** 108	**94** 195	**75** 99	**98** 153	**85** 183	**96** 49	**89** 206	**100** 467	**99** 163	**-** 0	**98** 280	**96** 476	**98** 280	**96** 464	**93** 275	**91** 206	**72** 79
South County Hospital, Wakefield, RI	**92** 99	**98** 156	**100** 104	**96** 156	**99** 148	**97** 33	**94** 140	**100** 431	**97** 110	**-** 0	**98** 285	**94** 109	**99** 288	**98** 106	**94** 278	**94** 140	**93** 127
Westerly Hospital, Westerly, RI	**88** 99	**98** 91	**79** 77	**95** 151	**69** 139	**96** 27	**85** 114	**99** 338	**83** 117	**-** 0	**97** 232	**99** 80	**97** 232	**100** 80	**96** 227	**91** 114	**94** 93
Women and Infants Hospital of Rhode Island, Providence, RI	**0** 1	**100** 3	**57** 7	**80** 10	**33** 6	**100** 2	**99** 86	**99** 328	**96** 52	**-** 0	**92** 237	**88** 189	**98** 234	**91** 186	**98** 231	**100** 86	**100** 4
TENNESSEE																	
Athens Regional Medical Center, Athens, TN	**98** 126	**100** 116	**100** 89	**99** 162	**98** 130	**99** 74	**92** 98	**100** 149	**93** 43	**-** 0	**89** 90	**96** 104	**98** 91	**92** 108	**91** 80	**95** 98	**80** 30
Baptist Hospital, Nashville, TN	**91** 159	**100** 247	**98** 211	**94** 254	**96** 269	**100** 141	**90** 211	**100** 749	**93** 206	**99** 118	**98** 514	**97** 697	**99** 525	**95** 693	**93** 490	**94** 211	**89** 183
Baptist Hospital of Cocke County, Newport, TN	**89** 142	**97** 195	**99** 121	**99** 182	**99** 143	**100** 84	**33** 6	**100** 6	**100** 1	**-** 0	**50** 4	**0** 1	**100** 4	**-** 0	**100** 3	**33** 6	**-** 0
Baptist Hospital West, Knoxville, TN	**-** -	**-** -	**-** -	**-** -	**-** -	**-** -	**-** -	**-** -	**-** -	**-** -	**-** -	**-** -	**-** -	**-** -	**-** -	**-** -	**-** -
Baptist Memorial Hospital, Memphis, TN	**92** 451	**98** 530	**96** 480	**96** 617	**96** 584	**100** 226	**90** 362	**100** 1112	**89** 338	**86** 149	**96** 701	**94** 1372	**97** 707	**95** 1359	**90** 659	**93** 366	**85** 128
Baptist Memorial Hospital Huntingdon, Huntingdon, TN	**86** 28	**98** 41	**100** 18	**94** 32	**100** 29	**100** 17	**100** 21	**100** 37	**100** 6	**-** 0	**92** 24	**86** 7	**100** 25	**100** 6	**86** 22	**100** 21	**40** 5
Baptist Memorial Hospital Tipton, Covington, TN	**91** 47	**97** 66	**95** 41	**91** 53	**98** 41	**96** 24	**57** 7	**94** 31	**0** 1	**-** 0	**95** 20	**85** 13	**95** 21	**92** 12	**90** 20	**57** 7	**-** 0
Baptist Memorial Hospital Union City, Union City, TN	**100** 56	**100** 55	**96** 50	**100** 76	**94** 52	**100** 30	**84** 57	**100** 149	**100** 29	**-** 0	**98** 99	**100** 98	**100** 99	**90** 99	**94** 93	**86** 57	**93** 14
Baptist Rehabilitation Germantown, Germantown, TN	**-** 0	**-** 0	**-** 0	**-** 0	**-** 0	**-** 0	**-** 0	**-** 0	**-** 0	**-** 0	**-** 0	**-** 0	**-** 0	**-** 0	**-** 0	**-** 0	**-** 0
Blount Memorial Hospital, Maryville, TN	**94** 79	**95** 161	**97** 102	**95** 140	**99** 146	**99** 74	**92** 178	**100** 454	**100** 130	**-** 0	**94** 294	**82** 278	**98** 296	**94** 255	**95** 279	**93** 178	**80** 99
Bolivar General Hospital, Bolivar, TN	**76** 17	**81** 26	**61** 18	**93** 27	**65** 26	**89** 9	**-** 0	**-** 0	**-** 0	**-** 0	**-** 0	**0** 5	**-** 0	**-** 0	**-** 0	**-** 0	**-** 0
Camden General Hospital, Camden, TN	**100** 4	**100** 6	**100** 1	**100** 7	**100** 1	**100** 2	**-** 0	**-** 0	**-** 0	**-** 0	**-** 0	**-** -	**-** 0	**-** -	**-** 0	**-** 0	**-** 0
Centennial Medical Center, Nashville, TN	**95** 88	**98** 105	**99** 207	**99** 155	**100** 246	**99** 181	**98** 276	**100** 924	**98** 346	**92** 224	**99** 622	**98** 788	**99** 634	**98** 782	**95** 557	**99** 276	**94** 218
Centennial Medical Center of Ashland City, Ashland City, TN	**100** 2	**-** 0	**100** 3	**100** 1	**100** 2	**100** 2	**-** 0	**-** 0	**-** 0	**-** 0	**-** 0	**-** 0	**-** 0	**-** 0	**-** 0	**-** 0	**-** 0
The Center for Spinal Surgery, Nashville, TN	**-** 0	**-** 0	**-** 0	**-** 0	**-** 0	**-** 0	**-** 0	**-** 0	**-** 0	**-** 0	**-** 0	**100** 913	**-** 0	**100** 913	**-** 0	**-** 0	**-** 0
Claiborne County Hospital, Tazewell, TN	**89** 28	**97** 73	**95** 57	**94** 114	**90** 89	**100** 38	**69** 32	**100** 42	**75** 8	**-** 0	**74** 19	**50** 34	**85** 20	**84** 19	**67** 18	**65** 34	**45** 11
Cookeville Regional Medical Center, Cookeville, TN	**85** 243	**96** 314	**78** 250	**97** 356	**87** 330	**98** 205	**89** 377	**100** 1288	**88** 508	**94** 216	**95** 870	**97** 714	**96** 877	**94** 710	**93** 831	**90** 377	**84** 347
Copper Basin Medical Center, Copperhill, TN	**92** 13	**71** 7	**80** 10	**100** 2	**88** 16	**80** 5	**-** 0	**-** 0	**-** 0	**-** 0	**-** 0	**-** 0	**-** 0	**-** 0	**-** 0	**-** 0	**-** 0
Crockett Hospital, Lawrenceburg, TN	**95** 115	**92** 108	**97** 79	**95** 132	**95** 116	**100** 48	**94** 17	**100** 41	**100** 10	**-** 0	**100** 26	**79** 19	**100** 26	**94** 17	**100** 26	**100** 17	**100** 3
Cumberland Medical Center, Crossville, TN	**82** 272	**96** 289	**61** 221	**95** 343	**89** 316	**99** 140	**73** 125	**99** 200	**100** 71	**-** 0	**77** 112	**71** 194	**76** 112	**90** 181	**85** 110	**72** 129	**72** 36
Cumberland River Hospital, Celina, TN	**100** 26	**100** 44	**80** 44	**94** 72	**69** 61	**100** 23	**-** 0	**-** 0	**-** 0	**-** 0	**-** 0	**-** 0	**-** 0	**-** 0	**-** 0	**-** 0	**-** 0
Decatur County General Hospital, Parsons, TN	**89** 44	**94** 50	**96** 45	**97** 68	**99** 74	**100** 11	**-** 0	**-** 0	**-** 0	**-** 0	**-** 0	**-** 0	**-** 0	**-** 0	**-** 0	**-** 0	**-** 0
Delta Medical Center, Memphis, TN	**98** 40	**97** 59	**87** 23	**90** 52	**100** 15	**97** 35	**85** 40	**100** 131	**82** 17	**-** 0	**96** 77	**89** 9	**99** 79	**100** 9	**92** 73	**74** 46	**70** 10
Dyersburg Regional Medical Center, Dyersburg, TN	**92** 75	**98** 100	**98** 62	**99** 113	**98** 80	**100** 50	**91** 68	**100** 114	**100** 17	**-** 0	**96** 53	**95** 109	**100** 53	**94** 126	**96** 49	**96** 68	**94** 17
Erlanger Medical Center, Chattanooga, TN	**91** 113	**95** 175	**96** 163	**96** 195	**98** 164	**99** 179	**97** 156	**100** 518	**91** 140	**91** 102	**97** 339	**94** 539	**98** 351	**95** 525	**93** 321	**99** 156	**80** 64
Fort Loudoun Medical Center, Lenoir City, TN	**93** 86	**100** 127	**99** 69	**98** 116	**98** 95	**100** 44	**90** 30	**100** 38	**71** 14	**-** 0	**90** 10	**95** 44	**80** 10	**98** 43	**100** 9	**93** 30	**67** 6
Fort Sanders Regional Medical Center, Knoxville, TN	**94** 198	**99** 357	**100** 244	**99** 329	**100** 346	**100** 239	**94** 310	**100** 1004	**98** 201	**97** 153	**98** 772	**95** 719	**99** 773	**97** 708	**99** 742	**95** 311	**95** 205

NOTE: The first number in each column (boldface) is the score, the second number is the number of patients; Please refer to the main entry for footnotes; (a) 100-299
*MEASURES: **Pneumonia Care:** 16. Appropriate Initial Antibiotic; 17. Blood Culture Timing; 18. Influenza Vaccine; 19. Initial Antibiotic Timing; 20. Pneumococcal Vaccine; 21. Smoking Cessation Advice; **Surgical Care Improvement Project:** 22. Appropriate VTP Within 24 Hours; 23. Appropriate Hair Removal; 24. Appropriate Beta Blocker Usage; 25. Controlled Postoperative Blood Glucose; 26. Prophylactic Antibiotic Timing; 27. Prophylactic Antibiotic Timing (Outpatient); 28. Prophylactic Antibiotic Selection; 29. Prophylactic Antibiotic Selection (Outpatient); 30. Prophylactic Antibiotic Stopped; 31. Recommended VTP Ordered; 32. Urinary Catheter Removal*

Hospital	Pneumonia Care						Surgical Care Improvement Project										
	16	17	18	19	20	21	22	23	24	25	26	27	28	29	30	31	32
Franklin Woods Community Hospital, Johnson City, TN	**92** 83	**98** 93	**97** 62	**99** 96	**100** 69	**100** 62	- 0	- 0	- 0	- 0	- 0	- 0	- 0	- 0	- 0	- 0	- 0
Gateway Medical Center, Clarksville, TN	**94** 204	**95** 327	**94** 218	**96** 315	**96** 252	**100** 116	**92** 279	**95** 767	**97** 215	**96** 80	**98** 535	**94** 174	**98** 542	**97** 173	**90** 512	**96** 279	**89** 185
Gibson General Hospital, Trenton, TN	**75** 12	**95** 21	**86** 7	**100** 22	**71** 17	**100** 4	**80** 5	**83** 6	**50** 2	- 0	**67** 6	**38** 8	**0** 5	**100** 3	**33** 6	**80** 5	- 0
Grandview Medical Center, Jasper, TN	**97** 117	**97** 99	**100** 90	**98** 157	**100** 121	**99** 104	**80** 20	**100** 24	**80** 5	- 0	**100** 6	**90** 29	**100** 7	**85** 27	**100** 6	**90** 20	**100** 4
Hardin Medical Center, Savannah, TN	**93** 87	**93** 100	**87** 61	**95** 103	**94** 90	**94** 32	**87** 23	**100** 64	**82** 11	- 0	**97** 39	**79** 28	**100** 39	**96** 23	**89** 36	**91** 23	**89** 9
Harton Regional Medical Center, Tullahoma, TN	**91** 94	**98** 127	**99** 109	**97** 123	**99** 136	**100** 55	**88** 86	**100** 272	**100** 64	- 0	**99** 170	**99** 433	**99** 172	**98** 435	**98** 134	**92** 87	**96** 28
Haywood Park Community Hospital, Brownsville, TN	**100** 16	**100** 8	**88** 17	**100** 22	**100** 16	**100** 10	- 0	- 0	- 0	- 0	- 0	**50** 2	- 0	**100** 1	- 0	- 0	- 0
Healthsouth Chattanooga Rehab Hospital, Chattanooga, TN	- 0	- 0	- 0	- 0	- 0	- 0	- 0	- 0	- 0	- 0	- 0	- -	- 0	- -	- 0	- 0	- 0
Henderson County Community Hospital, Lexington, TN	**100** 26	**100** 28	**100** 27	**100** 36	**100** 35	**100** 17	**100** 5	**100** 9	**100** 3	- 0	**100** 1	**100** 2	**100** 1	**100** 2	**100** 1	**100** 5	- 0
Hendersonville Medical Center, Hendersonville, TN	**95** 60	**99** 79	**99** 85	**96** 83	**100** 97	**100** 65	**94** 125	**100** 314	**100** 78	- 0	**95** 189	**94** 178	**98** 190	**98** 177	**99** 177	**97** 125	**100** 65
Henry County Medical Center, Paris, TN	**95** 111	**95** 88	**85** 95	**94** 125	**95** 124	**100** 50	**94** 199	**100** 524	**97** 138	- 0	**99** 395	**78** 46	**99** 403	**92** 37	**97** 369	**95** 199	**88** 67
Heritage Medical Center, Shelbyville, TN	**94** 101	**98** 93	**91** 88	**98** 120	**94** 89	**100** 57	**98** 43	**98** 82	**93** 15	- 0	**98** 50	**100** 8	**98** 50	**88** 8	**85** 48	**100** 43	**84** 19
Hickman Community Health Services, Centerville, TN	**81** 16	**95** 20	**14** 21	**88** 16	**16** 25	**100** 2	- 0	- 0	- 0	- 0	- 0	- -	- 0	- -	- 0	- 0	- 0
Hillside Hospital, Pulaski, TN	**93** 60	**100** 54	**93** 57	**98** 84	**99** 71	**97** 35	**100** 21	**99** 72	**79** 14	- 0	**96** 56	**82** 11	**98** 56	**60** 10	**96** 54	**100** 21	**91** 11
Horizon Medical Center, Dickson, TN	**95** 133	**99** 179	**100** 106	**99** 176	**99** 153	**98** 102	**90** 103	**100** 156	**100** 40	- 0	**99** 91	**97** 76	**97** 91	**97** 75	**94** 88	**92** 103	**88** 43
Humboldt General Hospital, Humboldt, TN	**84** 19	**93** 15	**100** 11	**92** 24	**77** 22	**100** 8	- 0	- 0	- 0	- 0	- 0	**0** 3	- 0	- 0	- 0	- 0	- 0
Indian Path Medical Center, Kingsport, TN	**93** 76	**96** 110	**95** 85	**95** 109	**96** 140	**100** 68	**97** 185	**98** 394	**94** 103	- 0	**100** 273	**92** 225	**99** 275	**91** 239	**96** 256	**98** 186	**94** 35
Jackson-Madison County General Hospital, Jackson, TN	**94** 80	**91** 87	**86** 170	**92** 149	**83** 194	**99** 122	**93** 635	**99** 1625	**79** 497	**93** 372	**87** 1267	**83** 1600	**93** 1272	**87** 1551	**84** 1197	**97** 635	**82** 419
Jamestown Regional Medical Center, Jamestown, TN	**96** 68	**100** 73	**100** 67	**97** 129	**99** 78	**100** 55	**60** 5	**100** 19	**100** 2	- 0	**100** 15	**0** 2	**85** 13	- 0	**91** 11	**60** 5	**100** 3
Jellico Community Hospital, Jellico, TN	**89** 73	**96** 113	**93** 73	**97** 112	**98** 98	**99** 88	**67** 15	**100** 56	**100** 13	- 0	**89** 37	**79** 24	**97** 33	**100** 21	**90** 30	**67** 15	**50** 2
Johnson City Medical Center, Johnson City, TN	**92** 72	**87** 99	**89** 106	**90** 123	**95** 119	**100** 71	**78** 172	**100** 634	**96** 239	**88** 139	**98** 443	**83** 681	**99** 452	**86** 674	**81** 421	**83** 173	**89** 158
Johnson City Specialty Hospital, Johnson City, TN	- 0	- 0	- 0	- 0	- 0	- 0	**100** 3	**100** 33	**80** 5	- 0	**100** 26	**99** 280	**88** 26	**94** 280	**84** 25	**100** 3	- 0
Johnson County Community Hospital, Mountain City, TN	- -	- -	- -	- -	- -	- -	- -	- -	- -	- -	- 0	- 0	- 0	- 0	- -	- -	- -
Lakeway Regional Hospital, Morristown, TN	**98** 51	**100** 58	**85** 41	**98** 90	**85** 52	**100** 42	**82** 51	**99** 149	**93** 45	- 0	**98** 123	**95** 168	**99** 126	**90** 166	**93** 122	**85** 52	**89** 44
Lauderdale Community Hospital, Ripley, TN	**81** 32	**96** 28	**100** 20	**89** 46	**79** 28	**100** 17	- 0	- 0	- 0	- 0	- 0	- 0	- 0	- 0	- 0	- 0	- 0
Laughlin Memorial Hospital, Greeneville, TN	**89** 161	**97** 233	**91** 170	**100** 254	**97** 233	**100** 77	**95** 139	**100** 302	**99** 98	- 0	**97** 207	**97** 133	**98** 208	**93** 132	**95** 190	**95** 139	**97** 79
Leconte Medical Center, Sevierville, TN	**96** 137	**94** 199	**96** 77	**96** 185	**98** 115	**100** 63	**89** 83	**100** 249	**99** 69	- 0	**99** 196	**98** 117	**99** 198	**97** 116	**97** 192	**94** 83	**100** 4
Lincoln Medical Center, Fayetteville, TN	**92** 80	**95** 106	**93** 58	**98** 111	**96** 92	**98** 40	**69** 13	**96** 27	**83** 6	- 0	**94** 17	**90** 31	**100** 17	**90** 30	**94** 16	**85** 13	**0** 2
Livingston Regional Hospital, Livingston, TN	**94** 98	**100** 128	**100** 94	**99** 164	**98** 144	**100** 66	**85** 39	**100** 78	**83** 18	- 0	**100** 52	**97** 30	**94** 52	**97** 29	**96** 48	**92** 39	**94** 16
Macon County General Hospital, Lafayette, TN	- -	- -	- -	- -	- -	- -	- -	- -	- -	- -	- 0	- 0	- 0	- 0	- -	- -	- -
Marshall Medical Center, Lewisburg, TN	**95** 21	**83** 29	**68** 19	**100** 28	**95** 21	**100** 16	- 0	- 0	- 0	- 0	- 0	- -	- 0	- -	- 0	- 0	- 0
Maury Regional Hospital, Columbia, TN	**85** 66	**96** 112	**95** 97	**96** 106	**93** 140	**100** 66	**87** 162	**100** 655	**94** 170	**99** 74	**98** 474	**91** 453	**96** 483	**94** 424	**95** 446	**91** 162	**90** 119
McKenzie Regional Hospital, McKenzie, TN	**100** 40	**100** 49	**98** 51	**100** 64	**100** 57	**100** 26	**100** 3	**97** 59	**100** 7	- 0	**98** 57	**100** 2	**93** 57	**100** 2	**100** 57	**100** 3	**100** 2
McNairy Regional Hospital, Selmer, TN	**89** 38	**100** 23	**100** 33	**100** 58	**100** 40	**100** 19	**100** 1	**100** 14	**100** 3	- 0	**92** 13	**94** 16	**92** 13	**100** 16	**100** 13	**100** 1	- 0
Medical Center of Manchester, Manchester, TN	**94** 18	**71** 7	**71** 14	**80** 15	**82** 17	**22** 9	- 0	- 0	- 0	- 0	- 0	- 0	- 0	- 0	- 0	- 0	- 0
Memorial Healthcare System, Chattanooga, TN	**100** 411	**99** 724	**99** 488	**96** 815	**99** 706	**100** 231	**90** 657	**100** 2756	**91** 888	**89** 702	**97** 2048	**95** 522	**100** 2064	**99** 545	**97** 2005	**93** 658	**90** 754
Memphis VA Medical Center, Memphis, TN	**99** 99	**99** 154	**85** 108	**94** 146	**94** 107	**100** 62	- 0	- 0	- 0	- 0	- 0	- -	- 0	- -	- 0	- 0	- 0
Mercy Medical Center, Knoxville, TN	**93** 469	**96** 649	**98** 474	**95** 628	**98** 595	**100** 403	**91** 611	**100** 2647	**95** 867	**94** 388	**99** 2001	**94** 1180	**99** 2023	**92** 1164	**98** 1934	**92** 613	**97** 870
Methodist Healthcare Fayette Hospital, Somerville, TN	**97** 29	**100** 33	**91** 23	**95** 42	**100** 36	**92** 13	**100** 4	**100** 4	**100** 1	- 0	**100** 1	- 0	**100** 1	**0** 1	**100** 1	**100** 4	- 0
Methodist Healthcare Memphis Hospitals, Memphis, TN	**93** 289	**98** 453	**100** 219	**98** 424	**100** 294	**100** 235	**95** 1309	**100** 3589	**95** 988	**97** 478	**99** 2254	**96** 1189	**97** 2277	**95** 1177	**95** 2142	**96** 1318	**90** 452
Methodist Medical Center of Oak Ridge, Oak Ridge, TN	**98** 276	**98** 525	**96** 382	**98** 444	**97** 510	**100** 252	**99** 224	**100** 1253	**96** 193	**97** 184	**99** 1019	**98** 502	**98** 1017	**96** 503	**98** 963	**99** 224	**89** 217
Metro Nashville General Hospital, Nashville, TN	**93** 54	**92** 80	**100** 19	**88** 78	**63** 19	**100** 58	**84** 135	**99** 233	**91** 32	- 0	**71** 139	**58** 88	**90** 127	**59** 86	**88** 117	**83** 138	**83** 52
Middle Tennessee Medical Center, Murfreesboro, TN	**91** 254	**98** 376	**100** 309	**96** 477	**99** 377	**100** 196	**90** 215	**100** 888	**92** 207	- 0	**99** 671	**98** 505	**97** 675	**98** 502	**91** 649	**93** 215	**88** 111
Milan General Hospital, Milan, TN	**75** 16	**100** 16	**100** 7	**94** 16	**100** 12	**100** 4	**100** 11	**100** 21	**100** 3	- 0	**100** 4	**67** 12	**75** 4	**62** 8	**75** 4	**100** 11	**100** 1
Morristown Hamblen Hospital Association, Morristown, TN	**87** 203	**99** 288	**99** 162	**98** 300	**95** 216	**100** 139	**93** 130	**100** 387	**91** 122	- 0	**97** 274	**88** 271	**99** 278	**91** 252	**95** 262	**97** 130	**96** 102
Mountain Home VA Medical Center, Mountain Home, TN	**97** 91	**98** 143	**97** 115	**95** 150	**100** 136	**100** 67	- 0	- 0	- 0	- 0	- 0	- -	- 0	- -	- 0	- 0	- 0
Northcrest Medical Center, Springfield, TN	**97** 149	**98** 270	**96** 166	**97** 225	**99** 195	**100** 98	**98** 85	**100** 196	**100** 46	- 0	**99** 110	**90** 100	**95** 110	**89** 98	**95** 104	**98** 85	**95** 44
Parkridge Medical Center, Chattanooga, TN	**97** 171	**99** 171	**100** 153	**100** 226	**100** 183	**100** 149	**96** 198	**100** 696	**98** 212	**95** 157	**99** 460	**99** 695	**98** 470	**98** 693	**97** 419	**97** 198	**90** 109
Parkwest Medical Center, Knoxville, TN	**92** 298	**96** 413	**93** 280	**96** 400	**97** 368	**100** 141	**92** 408	**100** 1918	**96** 570	**89** 341	**99** 1671	**95** 1443	**100** 1686	**97** 1424	**98** 1610	**93** 410	**89** 466
Patients' Choice Medical Center of Erin, Erin, TN	**88** 33	**90** 21	**68** 31	**100** 45	**72** 40	**64** 11	- 0	- 0	- 0	- 0	- 0	- -	- 0	- -	- 0	- 0	- 0
Perry Community Hospital, Linden, TN	**35** 48	**80** 5	**0** 50	**92** 75	**1** 72	**21** 19	- 0	- 0	- 0	- 0	- 0	- 0	- 0	- 0	- 0	- 0	- 0
Regional Hospital of Jackson, Jackson, TN	**92** 62	**100** 89	**94** 98	**98** 95	**93** 105	**99** 95	**96** 197	**100** 359	**99** 70	- 0	**97** 218	**96** 79	**100** 218	**97** 79	**96** 199	**98** 199	**90** 78
Regional Medical Center at Memphis, Memphis, TN	**98** 46	**86** 73	**92** 12	**82** 80	**100** 18	**100** 67	**93** 318	**100** 486	**84** 50	**100** 4	**93** 119	**96** 45	**95** 123	**95** 44	**93** 116	**96** 318	**73** 41
Rhea Medical Center, Dayton, TN	**90** 107	**96** 106	**90** 72	**96** 135	**84** 90	**100** 54	**100** 5	**100** 9	**100** 3	- 0	**100** 3	**100** 1	**67** 3	**100** 1	**100** 2	**100** 5	**100** 2
River Park Hospital, McMinnville, TN	**88** 149	**95** 210	**95** 154	**91** 229	**92** 194	**100** 127	**96** 57	**100** 86	**95** 22	- 0	**97** 61	**86** 183	**97** 63	**92** 192	**93** 55	**96** 57	**83** 24
Riverview Regional Medical Center North, Carthage, TN	**100** 58	**99** 86	**89** 56	**100** 92	**98** 58	**98** 48	**91** 11	**100** 21	**100** 3	- 0	**75** 12	**67** 3	**92** 12	**100** 2	**91** 11	**100** 11	**80** 5
Riverview Regional Medical Center South, Carthage, TN	- 0	- 0	- 0	- 0	- 0	- 0	- 0	- 0	- 0	- 0	- 0	- -	- 0	- -	- 0	- 0	- 0
Roane Medical Center, Harriman, TN	**96** 133	**97** 160	**95** 100	**95** 164	**98** 115	**99** 76	**97** 34	**100** 55	**100** 6	- 0	**100** 20	**100** 3	**95** 20	**67** 3	**100** 16	**97** 34	**75** 8
Saint Francis Bartlett Medical Center, Bartlett, TN	**97** 206	**99** 308	**99** 152	**100** 270	**100** 168	**100** 81	**91** 114	**100** 290	**84** 51	- 0	**99** 189	**96** 92	**83** 191	**90** 89	**99** 188	**93** 115	**86** 22
Saint Francis Hospital, Memphis, TN	**88** 108	**95** 172	**95** 142	**92** 209	**97** 192	**100** 79	**88** 236	**99** 599	**91** 208	**96** 166	**95** 418	**93** 461	**95** 425	**91** 449	**92** 396	**92** 236	**80** 101
Saint Mary's Jefferson Memorial Hospital, Jefferson City, TN	**94** 123	**99** 153	**97** 88	**92** 171	**97** 141	**97** 65	**82** 28	**100** 61	**90** 21	- 0	**97** 63	**81** 27	**98** 63	**88** 25	**97** 61	**82** 28	**97** 36
Saint Mary's Med Ctr of Campbell County, La Follette, TN	**94** 185	**98** 291	**96** 190	**99** 300	**95** 251	**100** 143	**67** 6	**100** 9	**75** 4	- 0	**100** 2	**82** 28	**100** 3	**96** 23	**100** 2	**57** 7	**100** 1
Saint Thomas Hospital, Nashville, TN	**91** 206	**96** 348	**98** 301	**94** 320	**97** 410	**99** 196	**99** 187	**100** 806	**95** 258	**93** 174	**99** 542	**97** 526	**99** 552	**92** 525	**94** 525	**99** 187	**89** 179
Scott County Hospital, Oneida, TN	**86** 102	**98** 98	**94** 51	**99** 103	**96** 76	**100** 35	**0** 6	**100** 9	**100** 2	- 0	**75** 4	**100** 1	**25** 4	**100** 1	**100** 4	**0** 6	- 0
Skyline Medical Center, Nashville, TN	**94** 102	**98** 201	**98** 102	**99** 163	**100** 144	**100** 84	**92** 208	**100** 481	**93** 136	- 0	**98** 277	**97** 302	**99** 278	**98** 299	**96** 244	**97** 209	**99** 94
Skyridge Medical Center, Cleveland, TN	**89** 253	**98** 280	**95** 249	**97** 349	**98** 320	**100** 186	**98** 242	**99** 427	**87** 92	- 0	**90** 241	**84** 316	**94** 240	**97** 294	**91** 220	**98** 243	**73** 55
Southern Hills Medical Center, Nashville, TN	**97** 118	**100** 172	**99** 78	**99** 165	**100** 90	**100** 79	**98** 118	**100** 293	**100** 68	- 0	**100** 169	**99** 113	**97** 172	**97** 112	**98** 154	**98** 118	**98** 61
Southern Tennessee Medical Center, Winchester, TN	**91** 97	**96** 102	**86** 113	**96** 159	**96** 142	**100** 70	**96** 103	**100** 271	**99** 68	- 0	**98** 186	**92** 140	**98** 187	**95** 132	**94** 174	**99** 103	**96** 84

NOTE: The first number in each column (boldface) is the score, the second number is the number of patients; Please refer to the main entry for footnotes; (a) 100-299

*MEASURES: **Pneumonia Care:** 16. Appropriate Initial Antibiotic; 17. Blood Culture Timing; 18. Influenza Vaccine; 19. Initial Antibiotic Timing; 20. Pneumococcal Vaccine; 21. Smoking Cessation Advice; **Surgical Care Improvement Project:** 22. Appropriate VTP Within 24 Hours; 23. Appropriate Hair Removal; 24. Appropriate Beta Blocker Usage; 25. Controlled Postoperative Blood Glucose; 26. Prophylactic Antibiotic Timing; 27. Prophylactic Antibiotic Timing (Outpatient); 28. Prophylactic Antibiotic Selection; 29. Prophylactic Antibiotic Selection (Outpatient); 30. Prophylactic Antibiotic Stopped; 31. Recommended VTP Ordered; 32. Urinary Catheter Removal*

Hospital	Pneumonia Care 16	17	18	19	20	21	Surgical Care Improvement Project 22	23	24	25	26	27	28	29	30	31	32
Stonecrest Medical Center, Smyrna, TN	**92** 111	**99** 163	**96** 78	**99** 140	**97** 113	**100** 64	**96** 116	**100** 316	**98** 58	- 0	**98** 202	**98** 204	**98** 204	**98** 212	**96** 184	**97** 116	**97** 58
Stones River Hosp & Dekalb Comm Hosp, Woodbury, TN	**95** 39	**93** 27	**70** 27	**100** 34	**81** 36	**100** 24	**100** 12	**100** 44	**100** 13	- 0	**100** 41	**100** 5	**100** 41	**100** 5	**100** 40	**100** 12	**100** 17
Stones River Hosp & Dekalb Comm Hosp, Smithville, TN	**94** 121	**94** 84	**68** 94	**94** 149	**86** 132	**95** 63	**88** 24	**100** 68	**100** 22	- 0	**98** 50	**97** 30	**96** 50	**94** 31	**87** 46	**88** 24	**88** 16
Summit Medical Center, Hermitage, TN	**93** 233	**98** 290	**99** 212	**96** 291	**100** 263	**100** 121	**96** 224	**100** 440	**100** 99	- 0	**97** 241	**99** 493	**99** 242	**97** 489	**96** 223	**98** 224	**99** 87
Sumner Regional Medical Center, Gallatin, TN	**89** 135	**95** 187	**78** 153	**98** 164	**86** 185	**95** 97	**84** 115	**100** 385	**93** 104	**0** 1	**97** 280	**83** 115	**100** 276	**90** 107	**97** 271	**93** 115	**93** 106
Sweetwater Hospital Association, Sweetwater, TN	**93** 88	**94** 131	**89** 117	**91** 174	**95** 163	**94** 86	**81** 59	**99** 97	**75** 20	- 0	**90** 42	**77** 48	**77** 43	**95** 39	**83** 35	**90** 61	**83** 6
Sycamore Shoals Hospital, Elizabethton, TN	**96** 73	**97** 89	**100** 71	**92** 115	**100** 114	**100** 74	**91** 80	**100** 183	**88** 32	- 0	**98** 124	**88** 66	**96** 128	**95** 62	**97** 120	**92** 80	**86** 29
Takoma Regional Hospital, Greeneville, TN	**95** 96	**97** 169	**100** 90	**100** 152	**99** 111	**100** 82	**83** 36	**100** 83	**79** 14	- 0	**100** 49	**94** 62	**94** 50	**98** 59	**96** 46	**86** 36	**100** 13
Trousdale Medical Center, Hartsville, TN	**100** 25	**92** 12	**100** 30	**91** 35	**100** 32	**100** 14	- 0	- 0	- 0	- 0	- 0	- 0	- 0	- 0	- 0	- 0	- 0
Unicoi County Memorial Hospital, Erwin, TN	**89** 57	**89** 66	**55** 44	**97** 92	**68** 73	**97** 29	**90** 40	**99** 91	**96** 23	- 0	**100** 70	**92** 12	**100** 70	**83** 12	**93** 68	**95** 40	**100** 25
United Regional Medical Center, Manchester, TN	**77** 115	**75** 28	**59** 107	**84** 170	**54** 148	**79** 97	- 0	- 0	- 0	- 0	- 0	- 0	- 0	- 0	- 0	- 0	- 0
University Medical Center, Lebanon, TN	**90** 137	**96** 166	**97** 115	**97** 180	**99** 140	**100** 110	**95** 240	**100** 456	**98** 126	- 0	**99** 318	**97** 218	**98** 321	**93** 215	**93** 296	**96** 241	**91** 85
University of Tennessee Memorial Hospital, Knoxville, TN	**93** 69	**95** 136	**92** 83	**97** 143	**93** 100	**100** 90	**99** 207	**100** 658	**100** 225	**95** 150	**96** 469	**94** 852	**97** 479	**94** 832	**92** 441	**99** 207	**97** 174
VA Middle Tennessee Healthcare System, Nashville, TN	**92** 118	**99** 190	**98** 177	**96** 179	**99** 183	**100** 107	**98** 81	**100** 222	**92** 104	**96** 105	**93** 138	- -	**99** 139	- -	**91** 126	**96** 82	**84** 44
Vanderbilt University Hospital, Nashville, TN	**97** 39	**92** 100	**84** 81	**94** 106	**83** 87	**100** 66	**99** 198	**99** 682	**91** 186	**92** 109	**99** 421	**94** 779	**98** 434	**96** 911	**97** 401	**99** 198	**96** 151
Volunteer Community Hospital, Martin, TN	**89** 53	**100** 60	**95** 75	**96** 84	**95** 97	**100** 35	**92** 52	**100** 74	**81** 21	- 0	**98** 47	**98** 111	**94** 47	**95** 110	**93** 45	**92** 52	**86** 7
Wayne Medical Center, Waynesboro, TN	**91** 34	**100** 21	**49** 35	**100** 66	**94** 67	**53** 15	- 0	- 0	- 0	- 0	- 0	- 0	- 0	- 0	- 0	- 0	- 0
Wellmont Bristol Regional Medical Center, Bristol, TN	**92** 61	**98** 46	**99** 70	**95** 109	**98** 105	**100** 68	**71** 144	**98** 493	**66** 164	**80** 88	**98** 317	**96** 363	**97** 323	**96** 362	**93** 309	**74** 145	**77** 97
Wellmont Hancock County Hospital, Sneedville, TN	**95** 19	**96** 26	**100** 13	**100** 24	**100** 20	**100** 11	- 0	- 0	- 0	- 0	- 0	- 0	- 0	- 0	- 0	- 0	- 0
Wellmont Hawkins County Memorial Hospital, Rogersville, TN	**90** 129	**92** 114	**97** 98	**96** 163	**98** 129	**100** 99	**75** 16	**100** 22	**67** 6	- 0	**80** 5	**100** 5	**100** 5	**80** 5	**75** 4	**75** 16	**100** 2
Wellmont Holston Valley Medical Center, Kingsport, TN	**88** 57	**91** 94	**83** 76	**93** 88	**87** 109	**98** 51	**97** 151	**100** 557	**91** 225	**98** 130	**98** 400	**95** 561	**98** 401	**88** 561	**97** 377	**99** 151	**85** 130
White County Community Hospital, Sparta, TN	**92** 73	**99** 101	**88** 66	**99** 104	**89** 91	**100** 41	**75** 12	**97** 66	**100** 14	- 0	**90** 42	**79** 24	**84** 43	**100** 19	**73** 41	**69** 13	**67** 3
Williamson Medical Center, Franklin, TN	**94** 111	**98** 156	**96** 108	**95** 164	**95** 153	**96** 55	**91** 154	**100** 373	**96** 106	- 0	**99** 257	**99** 353	**94** 262	**97** 353	**89** 241	**90** 155	**92** 89
Woods Memorial Hospital, Etowah, TN	**92** 37	**95** 92	**69** 74	**98** 108	**76** 113	**96** 54	**83** 35	**100** 75	**70** 23	- 0	**88** 52	**100** 16	**98** 52	**94** 16	**88** 50	**83** 35	**95** 20
VERMONT																	
Brattleboro Memorial Hospital, Brattleboro, VT	**93** 42	**98** 58	**94** 36	**97** 66	**91** 57	**100** 15	**95** 99	**100** 251	**95** 82	- 0	**98** 183	**96** 73	**99** 183	**93** 72	**98** 181	**99** 99	**99** 76
Central Vermont Medical Center, Barre, VT	**99** 84	**92** 52	**99** 88	**99** 129	**100** 126	**100** 45	**94** 70	**100** 186	**90** 51	- 0	**97** 123	**78** 101	**99** 122	**96** 98	**97** 117	**96** 70	**94** 49
Copley Hospital, Morrisville, VT	**96** 49	**81** 37	**81** 32	**96** 55	**91** 56	**100** 14	**98** 44	**100** 140	**100** 23	- 0	**90** 115	- -	**100** 115	- -	**91** 114	**98** 44	**100** 49
Fletcher Allen Hospital of Vermont, Burlington, VT	**97** 138	**92** 227	**92** 174	**96** 229	**94** 265	**100** 131	**97** 148	**100** 469	**95** 193	**90** 127	**95** 432	**95** 863	**97** 439	**97** 844	**99** 418	**97** 148	**100** 135
Gifford Medical Center, Randolph, VT	**97** 36	**100** 42	**84** 38	**98** 58	**92** 52	**100** 13	**100** 20	**100** 80	**100** 5	- 0	**91** 77	- -	**100** 77	- -	**96** 75	**100** 20	**100** 31
Grace Cottage Hospital, Townshend, VT	**93** 15	**100** 7	**100** 14	**88** 17	**100** 20	**100** 4	- 0	- 0	- 0	- 0	- 0	- -	- 0	- -	- 0	- 0	- 0
Mount Ascutney Hospital, Windsor, VT	**100** 27	**100** 29	**88** 16	**94** 33	**92** 39	**40** 5	**95** 21	**100** 32	**71** 14	- 0	**97** 29	- -	**97** 29	- -	**96** 28	**95** 21	**100** 10
North Country Hospital and Health Center, Newport, VT	**96** 23	**95** 19	**89** 19	**100** 24	**100** 26	**100** 7	**100** 30	**100** 59	**94** 18	- 0	**100** 55	- -	**95** 55	- -	**74** 54	**100** 30	**91** 22
Northeastern Vermont Regional Hospital, Saint Johnsbury, VT	**87** 53	**95** 62	**100** 36	**97** 70	**100** 59	**93** 14	**86** 103	**100** 126	**91** 33	- 0	**100** 97	- -	**99** 97	- -	**98** 97	**88** 103	**97** 39
Northwestern Medical Center, Saint Albans, VT	**96** 85	**98** 115	**96** 67	**100** 109	**97** 98	**93** 27	**92** 38	**100** 183	**96** 46	- 0	**99** 144	**96** 144	**99** 144	**96** 138	**96** 140	**90** 39	**100** 32
Porter Hospital, Middlebury, VT	**95** 76	**97** 63	**94** 54	**99** 108	**99** 102	**95** 21	**100** 41	**100** 168	**95** 40	- 0	**99** 135	- -	**100** 135	- -	**99** 134	**100** 41	**98** 60
Rutland Regional Medical Center, Rutland, VT	**92** 123	**94** 194	**89** 112	**94** 203	**94** 201	**93** 71	**94** 161	**100** 601	**81** 202	- 0	**98** 449	**91** 169	**99** 450	**98** 161	**97** 439	**95** 161	**90** 111
Southwestern Vermont Medical Center, Bennington, VT	**96** 101	**97** 193	**92** 118	**98** 178	**92** 195	**98** 48	**99** 136	**100** 273	**94** 79	- 0	**100** 167	**99** 161	**99** 168	**99** 161	**100** 163	**99** 136	**98** 62
Springfield Hospital, Springfield, VT	**96** 112	**100** 150	**100** 91	**100** 145	**100** 124	**100** 41	**100** 35	**100** 100	**100** 38	- 0	**99** 73	- -	**100** 73	- -	**100** 73	**100** 35	**100** 38
White River Junction VA Medical Center, White River Junction, VT	**89** 37	**96** 52	**97** 38	**92** 25	**100** 60	**100** 14	**100** 91	**100** 127	**97** 66	- 0	**100** 63	- -	**94** 64	- -	**98** 60	**100** 91	**98** 48
VIRGINIA																	
Alleghany Regional Hospital, Low Moor, VA	**95** 106	**100** 131	**100** 91	**96** 114	**100** 111	**100** 48	**97** 109	**100** 233	**100** 35	- 0	**100** 198	**97** 34	**98** 198	**100** 33	**98** 196	**97** 109	**83** 12
Augusta Health, Fishersville, VA	**94** 204	**96** 329	**94** 203	**96** 314	**96** 299	**99** 105	**89** 227	**100** 867	**91** 247	- 0	**98** 696	**91** 216	**99** 697	**96** 205	**98** 684	**92** 227	**88** 42
Bath County Community Hospital, Hot Springs, VA	**80** 15	**92** 13	**75** 12	**95** 22	**68** 19	**83** 6	- 0	- 0	- 0	- 0	- 0	- -	- 0	- -	- 0	- 0	- 0
Bedford Memorial Hospital, Bedford, VA	**75** 61	**97** 96	**87** 31	**88** 26	**75** 61	**100** 21	**62** 13	**100** 29	**60** 5	- 0	**100** 18	**60** 5	**95** 19	**100** 3	**100** 18	**69** 13	**75** 4
Bon Secours - Depaul Medical Center, Norfolk, VA	**86** 78	**98** 129	**100** 85	**97** 131	**97** 111	**100** 49	**94** 152	**100** 406	**92** 87	- 0	**99** 280	**97** 358	**96** 280	**98** 353	**95** 265	**95** 153	**90** 39
Bon Secours - Maryview Medical Center, Portsmouth, VA	**94** 85	**98** 171	**89** 132	**95** 157	**91** 175	**100** 73	**98** 192	**100** 828	**99** 229	**96** 124	**94** 654	**95** 279	**95** 657	**93** 276	**95** 641	**98** 192	**98** 258
Bon Secours - Memorial Regional Medical, Mechanicsville, VA	**100** 162	**98** 244	**96** 118	**100** 230	**98** 178	**100** 72	**97** 308	**100** 1049	**100** 326	**98** 177	**99** 764	**94** 460	**99** 763	**97** 455	**98** 733	**98** 308	**97** 347
Bon Secours - Richmond Community Hospital, Richmond, VA	**79** 47	**100** 57	**100** 14	**97** 61	**94** 18	**100** 35	**80** 10	**100** 13	**50** 2	- 0	**67** 6	**63** 27	**83** 6	**95** 22	**83** 6	**82** 11	**80** 5
Bon Secours - St Francis Medical Center, Midlothian, VA	**92** 129	**95** 183	**93** 76	**98** 163	**97** 118	**100** 38	**96** 288	**100** 1020	**96** 228	- 0	**97** 721	**94** 392	**98** 722	**97** 385	**97** 699	**97** 288	**85** 52
Bon Secours - St Marys Hospital of Richmond, Richmond, VA	**97** 126	**97** 249	**97** 198	**96** 227	**97** 243	**100** 57	**99** 524	**100** 2049	**98** 514	**100** 257	**99** 1769	**96** 606	**99** 1777	**97** 593	**98** 1725	**99** 524	**97** 651
Buchanan General Hospital, Grundy, VA	**94** 63	**99** 86	**97** 61	**98** 100	**100** 74	**100** 41	**54** 24	**100** 34	**83** 6	- 0	**100** 8	- 0	**100** 8	- 0	**71** 7	**54** 24	**100** 7
Carilion Franklin Memorial Hospital, Rocky Mount, VA	**93** 68	**96** 120	**92** 63	**97** 108	**94** 93	**100** 38	**94** 16	**100** 59	**62** 8	- 0	**86** 36	**56** 16	**92** 36	**100** 10	**97** 35	**94** 16	**100** 5
Carilion Giles Memorial Hospital, Pearisburg, VA	**89** 36	**95** 57	**97** 33	**95** 55	**96** 57	**94** 17	**0** 2	**100** 2	**100** 1	- 0	**100** 1	**0** 1	**100** 1	- 0	**100** 1	**0** 2	- 0
Carilion Medical Center, Roanoke, VA	**84** 288	**88** 398	**89** 270	**87** 485	**92** 366	**99** 232	**96** 447	**100** 2675	**88** 815	**96** 570	**95** 2261	**91** 598	**98** 2269	**96** 575	**95** 2203	**96** 448	**94** 325
Carilion New River Valley Medical Center, Christiansburg, VA	**85** 132	**93** 163	**94** 94	**90** 154	**96** 120	**100** 57	**92** 124	**99** 347	**80** 111	- 0	**97** 238	**90** 203	**99** 240	**83** 212	**95** 231	**97** 124	**95** 73
Carilion Stonewall Jackson Hospital, Lexington, VA	**87** 31	**95** 41	**94** 35	**88** 43	**98** 40	**100** 12	**91** 32	**100** 64	**74** 19	- 0	**100** 51	- -	**100** 52	- -	**98** 51	**97** 32	**95** 19
Carilion Tazewell Community Hospital, Tazewell, VA	**74** 38	**81** 58	**95** 39	**79** 73	**87** 53	**89** 27	**25** 4	**83** 6	**0** 1	- 0	**75** 4	**71** 7	**100** 4	**100** 5	**100** 4	**20** 5	**0** 3
Centra Health, Lynchburg, VA	**88** 209	**95** 318	**95** 220	**95** 382	**98** 337	**99** 177	**98** 408	**100** 1548	**100** 528	**100** 289	**100** 1075	**92** 444	**98** 1090	**98** 432	**100** 1016	**99** 408	**97** 135
Chesapeake General Hospital, Chesapeake, VA	**93** 227	**99** 364	**96** 251	**93** 352	**94** 357	**100** 122	**95** 177	**99** 395	**93** 107	- 0	**96** 265	**96** 464	**97** 265	**96** 450	**94** 250	**97** 177	**79** 91
CJW Medical Center, Richmond, VA	**96** 200	**100** 400	**98** 246	**98** 338	**100** 296	**100** 135	**97** 270	**99** 843	**98** 281	**99** 155	**100** 531	**94** 690	**98** 543	**97** 680	**95** 491	**97** 271	**95** 195
Clinch Valley Medical Center, Richlands, VA	**95** 77	**97** 109	**97** 60	**97** 116	**97** 75	**100** 43	**82** 33	**100** 155	**93** 27	- 0	**97** 110	**95** 62	**88** 112	**98** 95	**99** 107	**91** 33	**100** 2
Community Memorial Healthcenter, South Hill, VA	**95** 65	**99** 82	**100** 50	**97** 93	**96** 76	**100** 31	**71** 49	**100** 85	**80** 20	- 0	**97** 33	**74** 50	**97** 35	**73** 37	**97** 32	**80** 49	**100** 8
Culpeper Regional Hospital, Culpeper, VA	**92** 77	**96** 156	**82** 89	**97** 134	**86** 126	**92** 36	**89** 108	**100** 322	**92** 76	- 0	**96** 246	**94** 65	**99** 243	**89** 65	**88** 239	**97** 108	**93** 107
Danville Regional Medical Center, Danville, VA	**96** 78	**96** 123	**76** 89	**88** 132	**86** 139	**100** 72	**90** 176	**100** 452	**86** 154	**99** 68	**96** 309	**83** 119	**97** 310	**84** 113	**98** 298	**93** 178	**60** 43
Dickenson Community Hospital, Clintwood, VA	- 0	- 0	- 0	- 0	- 0	- 0	- 0	- 0	- 0	- 0	- 0	- 0	- 0	- 0	- 0	- 0	- 0
Eastern State Hospital, Williamsburg, VA	- 0	- 0	**100** 6	**100** 9	**100** 1	- 0	- 0	- 0	- 0	- 0	- 0	- 0	- 0	- 0	- 0	- 0	- 0
The Fauquier Hospital, Warrenton, VA	**97** 108	**96** 202	**96** 102	**95** 169	**99** 142	**96** 57	**98** 168	**100** 342	**99** 68	- 0	**95** 240	**92** 88	**98** 240	**98** 86	**96** 226	**99** 168	**94** 100

NOTE: The first number in each column (boldface) is the score, the second number is the number of patients; Please refer to the main entry for footnotes; (a) 100-299
*MEASURES: **Pneumonia Care:** 16. Appropriate Initial Antibiotic; 17. Blood Culture Timing; 18. Influenza Vaccine; 19. Initial Antibiotic Timing; 20. Pneumococcal Vaccine; 21. Smoking Cessation Advice; **Surgical Care Improvement Project:** 22. Appropriate VTP Within 24 Hours; 23. Appropriate Hair Removal; 24. Appropriate Beta Blocker Usage; 25. Controlled Postoperative Blood Glucose; 26. Prophylactic Antibiotic Timing; 27. Prophylactic Antibiotic Timing (Outpatient); 28. Prophylactic Antibiotic Selection; 29. Prophylactic Antibiotic Selection (Outpatient); 30. Prophylactic Antibiotic Stopped; 31. Recommended VTP Ordered; 32. Urinary Catheter Removal*

Hospital	Pneumonia Care						Surgical Care Improvement Project										
	16	17	18	19	20	21	22	23	24	25	26	27	28	29	30	31	32
Halifax Regional Hospital, Halifax, VA	97 69	97 89	69 112	88 126	83 140	94 64	71 120	97 275	96 96	- 0	90 186	94 93	96 181	99 89	89 171	75 124	55 38
Hampton VA Medical Center, Hampton, VA	96 28	98 46	68 31	95 40	94 18	100 21	100 18	100 71	100 17	- 0	100 56	- -	98 57	- -	91 56	100 18	100 4
Henrico Doctors' Hospital, Richmond, VA	92 119	96 153	97 147	95 208	98 235	99 72	95 208	99 875	98 261	98 172	98 599	97 662	97 606	98 649	95 574	96 208	88 195
Inova Alexandria Hospital, Alexandria, VA	97 90	99 143	94 69	99 139	91 105	100 27	90 146	100 467	98 128	98 87	98 325	93 309	98 331	96 300	89 316	94 146	93 114
Inova Fair Oaks Hospital, Fairfax, VA	92 84	96 135	96 73	99 130	98 117	81 27	96 76	100 337	99 89	- 0	100 226	99 656	99 229	96 655	96 219	96 76	100 61
Inova Fairfax Hospital, Falls Church, VA	89 57	99 90	87 79	99 90	92 102	96 27	98 184	100 620	96 114	98 114	95 415	94 984	97 422	94 937	94 407	98 184	93 163
Inova Loudoun Hospital, Leesburg, VA	93 111	92 141	94 127	97 143	98 158	98 60	86 156	100 449	95 102	- 0	95 270	96 342	97 272	91 348	89 260	91 156	88 48
Inova Mount Vernon Hospital, Alexandria, VA	95 63	98 90	91 58	100 86	92 84	100 24	95 94	100 329	96 92	- 0	99 214	93 70	99 214	97 70	96 207	96 95	94 133
John Randolph Medical Center, Hopewell, VA	96 73	100 120	100 62	98 103	100 78	100 43	100 66	100 93	100 18	- 0	100 41	98 58	100 41	97 58	100 35	100 66	100 12
Johnston Memorial Hospital, Abingdon, VA	91 111	97 156	89 88	97 150	93 128	84 62	87 132	100 429	88 129	- 0	95 293	76 125	98 293	92 111	96 263	87 133	86 92
Lee Regional Medical Center, Pennington Gap, VA	91 127	98 150	76 102	98 166	81 124	65 68	54 24	100 30	78 9	- 0	57 7	33 3	43 7	0 1	57 7	54 24	67 3
Lewis-Gale Medical Center, Salem, VA	98 248	99 370	100 252	98 354	100 378	99 115	98 219	100 724	99 278	99 139	99 538	99 618	99 545	99 620	99 521	98 219	88 100
Martha Jefferson Hospital, Charlottesville, VA	91 85	93 103	78 96	94 129	77 149	97 31	91 127	100 473	88 126	- 0	97 325	92 204	97 326	96 201	98 314	93 127	89 66
Mary Immaculate Hospital, Newport News, VA	90 84	98 160	99 79	96 163	98 103	100 30	89 159	100 1451	99 332	- 0	96 1292	85 283	99 1295	93 273	96 1263	91 159	100 57
Mary Washington Hospital, Fredericksburg, VA	95 275	96 401	90 211	97 372	94 325	100 150	90 249	100 1000	92 318	91 188	94 664	96 588	99 673	97 583	95 630	95 249	92 185
Memorial Hospital of Martinsville & Henry County, Martinsville, VA	94 109	96 184	99 111	96 158	99 164	100 93	81 124	100 299	99 78	- 0	94 179	93 175	96 182	97 168	95 160	80 130	91 44
Montgomery Regional Hospital, Blacksburg, VA	95 78	98 119	100 92	100 118	100 110	100 53	99 108	100 416	99 115	- 0	100 312	99 92	99 317	98 98	99 298	99 108	99 79
Mountain View Regional Medical Center, Norton, VA	86 51	100 73	98 54	96 75	100 74	100 36	91 23	99 73	89 19	- 0	96 56	67 54	98 55	98 42	81 53	96 23	81 16
Norton Community Hospital, Norton, VA	92 89	93 153	97 86	94 142	96 119	97 67	95 37	100 74	85 13	- 0	95 41	85 27	95 41	95 41	95 39	95 37	86 7
Page Memorial Hospital, Luray, VA	88 25	96 27	89 19	94 33	96 28	89 9	- 0	- 0	- 0	- 0	- 0	- -	- 0	- -	- 0	- 0	- 0
Piedmont Geriatric Hospital, Burkeville, VA	- 0	- 0	- 0	- 0	- 0	- 0	- 0	- 0	- 0	- 0	- 0	- -	- 0	- -	- 0	- 0	- 0
Pioneer Health Services of Patrick County, Stuart, VA	- 0	- 0	- 0	- 0	- 0	- 0	- 0	- 0	- 0	- 0	- 0	- -	- 0	- -	- 0	- 0	- 0
Potomac Hospital, Woodbridge, VA	91 98	89 143	79 73	91 132	77 84	80 50	97 101	100 320	96 55	- 0	96 194	98 214	98 196	91 220	86 186	97 101	100 61
Prince William Hospital, Manassas, VA	92 130	97 223	89 122	98 187	96 167	90 70	87 117	100 536	95 118	- 0	98 373	93 439	98 376	97 421	96 367	92 118	99 123
Pulaski Community Hospital, Pulaski, VA	95 73	99 104	99 88	97 59	99 109	100 41	100 43	100 82	100 26	- 0	100 38	100 39	97 39	98 40	100 33	100 43	90 10
Rappahannock General Hospital, Kilmarnock, VA	89 44	100 68	94 17	100 70	94 62	87 15	92 80	100 127	90 41	- 0	97 79	95 44	98 80	98 43	93 75	95 80	88 33
Reston Hospital Center, Reston, VA	96 111	99 179	100 111	99 137	100 144	100 32	94 157	100 477	96 105	- 0	98 312	98 948	99 321	99 945	93 296	95 157	94 130
Richmond VA Medical Center, Richmond, VA	93 85	99 150	94 110	97 157	99 105	98 57	98 163	100 351	100 150	96 95	96 253	- -	98 257	- -	94 232	98 163	95 131
Riverside Regional Medical Center, Newport News, VA	95 119	97 231	98 135	95 209	99 185	100 80	94 189	100 577	95 175	97 97	99 405	98 588	99 409	97 583	97 392	94 189	97 118
Riverside Shore Memorial Hospital, Nassawadox, VA	95 59	99 119	95 75	95 125	94 97	100 33	83 30	100 85	100 20	- 0	91 57	90 31	90 59	94 62	100 56	83 30	60 15
Riverside Tappahannock Hospital, Tappahannock, VA	96 49	98 49	100 32	91 34	100 42	100 15	96 77	100 112	97 31	- 0	99 87	96 25	97 87	99 75	99 85	96 77	100 7
Riverside Walter Reed Hospital, Gloucester, VA	97 121	99 195	100 108	98 179	99 148	100 52	97 78	100 187	89 55	- 0	99 134	83 35	99 134	97 33	98 125	97 79	100 69
Rockingham Memorial Hospital, Harrisonburg, VA	97 123	99 170	90 140	97 175	91 204	100 76	98 181	100 563	95 190	98 85	90 385	93 257	95 386	97 249	94 351	99 182	93 108
Russell County Medical Center, Lebanon, VA	90 103	100 98	99 94	99 143	100 122	96 70	- 0	- 0	- 0	- 0	- 0	100 1	- 0	0 1	- 0	- 0	- 0
Salem VA Medical Center, Salem, VA	95 62	98 96	97 78	95 83	98 90	94 36	100 114	100 214	98 66	- 0	97 141	- -	99 144	- -	99 140	100 114	93 85
Sentara Bayside Hospital, Virginia Beach, VA	93 96	99 161	96 136	99 165	99 162	100 81	99 104	100 226	100 45	- 0	98 129	85 147	98 130	92 256	94 124	99 104	100 37
Sentara Careplex Hospital, Hampton, VA	99 151	97 294	98 176	99 271	98 228	100 99	98 126	100 540	100 145	- 0	99 384	93 307	99 385	96 508	98 378	99 126	100 100
Sentara Leigh Hospital, Norfolk, VA	96 141	98 284	93 205	96 272	95 247	99 105	99 818	99 1879	91 452	- 0	98 1673	97 363	97 1674	95 354	98 1655	99 820	98 674
Sentara Norfolk General Hospital, Norfolk, VA	98 107	97 211	97 151	98 241	95 175	99 121	97 187	99 1401	94 645	96 781	98 1043	89 655	99 1087	97 621	95 974	96 188	92 331
Sentara Obici Hospital, Suffolk, VA	92 119	97 174	97 137	97 196	95 177	99 85	94 215	100 746	95 207	- 0	98 586	96 141	98 589	94 140	95 554	95 216	89 135
Sentara Virginia Beach General Hospital, Virginia Beach, VA	94 173	96 290	99 239	94 299	96 361	98 125	98 365	100 947	91 233	88 101	99 721	94 490	99 730	96 480	96 692	99 365	97 220
Sentara Williamsburg Regional Medical Center, Williamsburg, VA	98 124	98 169	98 112	97 191	98 165	100 50	97 172	100 445	100 111	- 0	97 302	90 266	99 304	88 286	97 289	97 172	95 112
Shenandoah Memorial Hospital, Woodstock, VA	85 61	95 83	84 50	97 75	96 78	96 23	97 88	100 261	89 89	- 0	90 178	- -	100 179	- -	95 170	97 88	85 48
Smyth County Community Hospital, Marion, VA	91 81	99 76	100 73	98 116	100 89	92 48	88 66	100 175	97 33	- 0	98 126	82 49	99 126	95 40	94 123	88 66	95 22
Southampton Memorial Hospital, Franklin, VA	84 56	96 83	94 63	96 84	96 98	100 34	89 36	100 126	100 27	- 0	100 101	65 43	97 101	97 59	98 95	97 36	100 7
Southern Virginia Regional Medical Center, Emporia, VA	97 115	99 76	97 86	99 150	100 89	100 50	97 32	100 48	90 10	- 0	100 27	71 7	100 27	100 20	100 26	100 32	87 15
Southside Community Hospital, Farmville, VA	91 91	96 123	93 69	95 127	91 103	100 39	95 66	99 142	70 37	- 0	89 79	41 17	97 79	100 7	90 71	96 67	50 26
Southside Regional Medical Center, Petersburg, VA	93 139	97 175	93 130	95 213	94 167	100 93	90 177	100 520	96 114	100 1	99 374	92 181	97 375	97 177	94 361	93 178	85 81
Southwestern Virginia Mental Health Institute, Marion, VA	- 0	- 0	- 0	- 0	- 0	- 0	- 0	- 0	- 0	- 0	- 0	- -	- 0	- -	- 0	- 0	- 0
Spotsylvania Regional Medical Center, Fredericksburg, VA	- 0	- 0	- 0	- 0	- 0	- 0	- 0	- 0	- 0	- 0	- 0	- -	- 0	- -	- 0	- 0	- 0
Stafford Hospital Center, Stafford, VA	96 72	95 80	80 55	98 64	86 56	100 25	79 52	100 142	95 20	- 0	92 88	86 88	99 88	95 80	92 85	81 52	98 40
Twin County Regional Hospital, Galax, VA	99 118	100 221	100 125	99 190	99 198	100 61	98 90	100 173	100 34	- 0	100 100	90 20	98 105	100 18	98 86	99 90	100 24
University of Virginia Medical Center, Charlottesville, VA	93 54	95 81	88 67	87 93	91 92	98 56	90 193	96 636	86 218	85 120	96 402	95 367	97 409	97 362	93 387	94 193	59 121
Virginia Commonwealth University Health System, Richmond, VA	90 86	86 206	84 146	91 226	83 113	99 183	97 259	98 741	93 211	93 140	93 445	86 866	97 456	93 839	87 423	98 259	85 161
Virginia Hospital Center - Arlington, Arlington, VA	100 74	99 125	93 126	99 108	95 184	100 37	97 210	100 632	96 171	93 110	100 465	95 439	97 469	98 435	97 434	97 210	95 106
Warren Memorial Hospital, Front Royal, VA	94 49	95 63	100 35	95 63	96 52	100 24	96 46	99 92	100 21	- 0	100 55	89 35	96 56	94 35	98 49	98 46	100 5
Wellmont Lonesome Pine Hospital, Big Stone Gap, VA	84 73	95 92	97 76	95 106	96 84	100 58	82 22	100 64	69 13	- 0	90 49	40 15	98 49	50 6	89 45	95 22	88 16
Western State Hospital, Staunton, VA	- 0	- 0	- 0	- 0	- 0	- 0	- 0	- 0	- 0	- 0	- 0	- 0	- 0	- 0	- 0	- 0	- 0
Winchester Medical Center, Winchester, VA	92 158	95 187	92 157	95 222	92 218	100 119	97 274	100 952	95 331	86 194	95 639	81 642	99 647	97 631	95 603	97 274	79 141
Wythe County Community Hospital, Wytheville, VA	98 103	99 107	100 121	99 147	100 125	100 63	82 33	100 247	92 61	- 0	99 204	94 51	100 204	96 49	97 203	91 33	97 69
WEST VIRGINIA																	
Beckley Arh Hospital, Beckley, WV	84 64	86 105	75 69	92 107	83 81	95 59	75 80	99 152	83 41	- 0	88 42	54 84	79 43	91 53	90 40	72 85	75 16
Beckley VA Medical Center, Beckley, WV	93 107	96 158	100 104	98 160	99 162	100 64	- 0	- 0	- 0	- 0	- 0	- -	- 0	- -	- 0	- 0	- 0
Bluefield Regional Medical Center, Bluefield, WV	75 121	93 169	80 90	88 172	84 136	95 62	76 79	99 285	86 90	- 0	97 260	88 133	93 259	94 121	90 257	89 83	62 16
Boone Memorial Hospital, Madison, WV	69 29	86 49	79 24	91 11	82 28	83 18	- 0	- 0	- 0	- 0	- 0	- -	- 0	- -	- 0	- 0	- 0
Braxton County Memorial Hospital, Gassaway, WV	93 30	72 39	43 35	89 44	34 41	75 8	- 0	- 0	- 0	- 0	- 0	- -	- 0	- -	- 0	- 0	- 0
Broaddus Hospital Association, Philippi, WV	0 3	100 3	67 3	80 5	50 4	- 0	- 0	- 0	- 0	- 0	- 0	- 0	- 0	- 0	- 0	- 0	- 0
Cabell-Huntington Hospital, Huntington, WV	98 61	97 193	93 128	95 192	97 142	100 155	97 141	100 441	94 120	- 0	96 295	84 186	95 297	96 255	93 283	99 141	89 36

NOTE: The first number in each column (boldface) is the score, the second number is the number of patients; Please refer to the main entry for footnotes; (a) 100-299
*MEASURES: **Pneumonia Care:** 16. Appropriate Initial Antibiotic; 17. Blood Culture Timing; 18. Influenza Vaccine; 19. Initial Antibiotic Timing; 20. Pneumococcal Vaccine; 21. Smoking Cessation Advice; **Surgical Care Improvement Project:** 22. Appropriate VTP Within 24 Hours; 23. Appropriate Hair Removal; 24. Appropriate Beta Blocker Usage; 25. Controlled Postoperative Blood Glucose; 26. Prophylactic Antibiotic Timing; 27. Prophylactic Antibiotic Timing (Outpatient); 28. Prophylactic Antibiotic Selection; 29. Prophylactic Antibiotic Selection (Outpatient); 30. Prophylactic Antibiotic Stopped; 31. Recommended VTP Ordered; 32. Urinary Catheter Removal*

Hospital	Pneumonia Care							Surgical Care Improvement Project									
	16	17	18	19	20	21	22	23	24	25	26	27	28	29	30	31	32
Camc Teays Valley Hospital, Hurricane, WV	89 70	91 95	82 68	92 88	86 83	98 43	80 70	99 155	85 52	- 0	91 85	96 48	95 88	83 47	90 83	89 70	94 47
Camden Clark Memorial Hospital, Parkersburg, WV	91 199	99 294	97 233	97 325	99 349	95 113	90 233	100 756	97 198	- 0	97 532	80 175	97 536	81 144	97 492	92 234	89 83
Charleston Area Medical Center, Charleston, WV	85 340	94 541	85 378	89 494	92 487	97 375	95 465	100 2464	96 928	91 960	99 1885	97 903	99 1943	91 892	95 1639	95 470	93 418
Charleston Surgical Hospital, Charleston, WV	- 0	- 0	- 0	- 0	- 0	- 0	- 0	- 0	- 0	- 0	100 4	- 0	100 4	- 0	- 0	- 0	- 0
City Hospital, Martinsburg, WV	91 176	90 208	88 113	97 210	92 149	84 96	96 252	100 573	100 145	- 0	94 214	90 112	95 220	88 104	96 190	96 252	98 138
Clarksburg VA Medical Center, Clarksburg, WV	90 59	99 93	99 68	97 103	99 93	100 29	- 0	- 0	- 0	- 0	- 0	- 0	- 0	- 0	- 0	- 0	- 0
Davis Memorial Hospital, Elkins, WV	89 92	99 118	91 81	97 107	94 102	100 38	94 120	100 322	92 85	- 0	95 230	93 170	97 230	98 162	96 222	95 120	90 50
Fairmont General Hospital, Fairmont, WV	95 105	96 121	98 116	99 138	99 161	100 79	99 117	100 216	97 67	- 0	99 139	98 89	100 139	94 87	100 124	99 117	97 32
Grafton City Hospital, Grafton, WV	50 12	92 12	94 16	88 25	85 20	33 9	- 0	- 0	- 0	- 0	- 0	- 0	- 0	- 0	- 0	- 0	- 0
Grant Memorial Hospital, Petersburg, WV	84 38	95 20	72 29	90 48	67 42	77 13	88 25	100 124	85 27	- 0	97 114	- -	97 114	- -	93 112	88 25	90 21
Greenbrier Valley Medical Center, Ronceverte, WV	92 120	94 196	96 164	97 198	99 205	97 116	98 93	100 199	93 60	- 0	98 127	97 127	99 130	98 124	93 121	98 93	79 38
Hampshire Memorial Hospital, Romney, WV	- 0	- 0	- 0	- 0	- 0	- 0	- 0	- 0	- 0	- 0	- 0	- 0	- 0	- 0	- 0	- 0	- 0
Huntington VA Medical Center, Huntington, WV	96 77	99 178	95 119	99 113	98 168	100 88	98 94	99 182	100 75	- 0	99 121	- -	100 122	- -	100 116	99 94	100 103
Jackson General Hospital, Ripley, WV	92 49	98 97	98 56	96 103	97 94	95 22	83 12	100 18	20 5	- 0	100 2	100 5	100 2	100 5	100 2	92 12	67 3
Jefferson Memorial Hospital, Ranson, WV	86 28	88 52	90 10	87 54	71 34	100 14	82 34	100 55	100 6	- 0	71 24	- -	83 24	- -	61 18	82 34	100 1
Logan Regional Medical Center, Logan, WV	88 227	95 323	100 232	93 348	100 235	99 162	95 132	100 268	94 64	- 0	97 165	87 61	95 166	84 57	93 94	95 132	79 28
Martinsburg VA Medical Center, Martinsburg, WV	94 67	96 82	97 67	93 95	100 86	98 47	- 0	- 0	- 0	- 0	- 0	- 0	- 0	- 0	- 0	- 0	- 0
Minnie Hamilton Health Care Center, Grantsville, WV	- 0	- 0	- 0	- 0	- 0	- 0	- 0	- 0	- 0	- 0	- 0	- 0	- 0	- 0	- 0	- 0	- 0
Monongalia County General Hospital, Morgantown, WV	88 103	98 125	95 96	97 115	98 121	93 46	97 388	100 1210	90 426	93 211	97 1020	85 361	98 1030	98 316	97 1003	97 392	80 103
Montgomery General Hospital, Montgomery, WV	88 75	98 82	88 42	100 93	84 69	97 29	- 0	- 0	- 0	- 0	- 0	- 0	- 0	- 0	- 0	- 0	- 0
Morgan County War Memorial, Berkeley Springs, WV	89 9	75 12	100 4	93 14	90 10	75 4	- 0	- 0	- 0	- 0	- 0	- 0	- 0	- 0	- 0	- 0	- 0
Ohio Valley Medical Center, Wheeling, WV	82 88	97 133	81 109	94 167	92 130	100 65	85 146	97 363	76 109	- -	95 239	84 80	96 238	100 70	93 235	87 149	53 78
Plateau Medical Center, Oak Hill, WV	83 64	95 88	98 60	95 94	94 71	96 28	94 48	100 186	97 61	- 0	97 130	75 12	98 150	92 12	98 129	94 48	98 57
Pleasant Valley Hospital, Point Pleasant, WV	81 64	94 66	93 60	94 105	98 48	98 48	71 70	98 109	76 29	- 0	90 73	63 54	92 73	75 53	83 71	74 70	43 7
Pocahontas Memorial Hospital, Buckeye, WV	- 0	- 0	- 0	- 0	- 0	- 0	- 0	- 0	- 0	- 0	- 0	- 0	- 0	- 0	- 0	- 0	- 0
Potomac Valley Hospital, Keyser, WV	100 30	96 28	68 19	90 31	86 21	100 9	80 5	100 16	- 0	- 0	77 13	- -	85 13	- -	85 13	80 5	89 9
Preston Memorial Hospital, Kingwood, WV	75 8	80 25	72 18	85 20	83 24	50 8	- 0	- 0	- 0	- 0	- 0	- 0	- 0	- 0	- 0	- 0	100 1
Princeton Community Hospital, Princeton, WV	80 210	97 224	97 218	89 332	96 275	100 143	93 179	100 618	94 168	- 0	98 498	83 147	96 499	83 145	96 471	94 181	83 35
Raleigh General Hospital, Beckley, WV	97 213	92 323	90 218	98 319	97 249	100 171	94 159	100 496	97 92	- 0	98 309	97 179	96 311	98 176	95 301	98 160	96 50
Reynolds Memorial Hospital, Glen Dale, WV	83 64	88 48	90 61	93 84	95 87	97 33	82 44	100 95	90 29	- 0	96 72	94 31	93 73	100 29	95 65	82 44	95 19
Roane General Hospital, Spencer, WV	95 21	100 16	91 22	92 25	93 30	75 8	91 11	100 19	100 4	- 0	100 5	100 2	100 5	100 2	100 5	91 11	100 2
Saint Francis Hospital, Charleston, WV	93 61	93 88	89 61	90 93	78 76	89 53	81 140	99 598	82 174	- 0	96 482	84 213	92 483	77 197	91 482	80 147	90 205
Saint Joseph Hospital, Buckhannon, WV	90 29	89 36	94 18	98 42	88 26	83 18	60 25	100 66	100 12	- 0	91 44	94 16	98 45	100 15	81 42	62 26	92 13
Saint Josephs Healthcare System, Parkersburg, WV	94 104	96 173	91 117	91 165	92 167	100 65	87 157	99 551	97 181	97 72	99 349	82 155	98 351	99 136	92 333	88 161	93 190
Saint Mary's Medical Center, Huntington, WV	95 317	97 590	88 285	93 580	91 445	99 260	88 237	100 1204	96 453	98 312	98 965	91 448	98 981	89 422	96 904	94 237	95 383
Sistersville General Hospital, Sistersville, WV	88 8	100 9	60 10	88 6	62 8	67 3	- 0	- 0	- 0	- 0	- 0	- 0	- 0	- 0	- 0	- 0	- 0
Stonewall Jackson Memorial Hospital, Weston, WV	87 93	99 82	92 92	97 149	93 127	100 53	87 62	100 148	89 28	- 0	100 95	92 53	96 96	99 72	90 93	89 64	96 23
Summers County ARH Hospital, Hinton, WV	94 32	97 34	90 29	100 41	86 37	100 20	- 0	- 0	- 0	- 0	- 0	- 0	- 0	- 0	- 0	- 0	- 0
Summersville Regional Medical Center, Summersville, WV	91 43	78 101	80 59	95 120	79 86	67 30	95 64	100 101	100 32	- 0	93 58	80 56	82 57	78 45	80 55	97 64	89 19
Thomas Memorial Hospital, South Charleston, WV	88 189	94 282	72 198	92 288	70 242	98 114	71 235	96 683	84 215	- 0	97 454	90 156	97 456	96 144	87 433	78 237	85 78
United Hospital Center, Bridgeport, WV	98 205	99 255	96 257	97 116	97 319	100 149	97 254	100 739	100 214	- 0	99 552	95 109	100 561	94 107	97 519	98 254	99 186
Webster County Memorial Hospital, Webster Springs, WV	76 17	57 7	- 0	76 21	55 11	100 8	- 0	- 0	- 0	- 0	- 0	- 0	- 0	- 0	- 0	- 0	- 0
Weirton Medical Center, Weirton, WV	92 232	99 321	97 210	98 313	95 286	100 139	86 118	98 329	97 79	- 0	97 245	80 85	95 245	68 63	89 236	89 118	70 88
Welch Community Hospital, Welch, WV	93 45	29 7	34 29	89 45	50 34	68 25	69 16	85 26	29 7	- 0	50 8	- 0	62 8	- 0	50 8	82 17	67 3
West Virginia University Hospitals, Morgantown, WV	97 99	94 199	94 189	90 225	96 199	97 131	99 287	100 1153	100 362	86 313	99 926	94 285	99 945	94 279	98 900	99 287	100 284
Wetzel County Hospital, New Martinsville, WV	86 70	93 55	93 58	95 82	79 90	97 34	91 11	93 15	75 4	- 0	86 7	67 6	86 7	100 5	100 7	91 11	75 4
Wheeling Hospital, Wheeling, WV	88 107	95 155	87 140	94 182	87 206	88 66	97 243	98 1191	92 412	82 243	96 910	90 207	98 934	88 217	93 850	97 244	73 141
Williamson Memorial Hospital, Williamson, WV	98 57	97 71	100 42	100 2	100 37	100 32	100 11	100 27	100 6	- 0	- 0	96 46	- 0	100 44	- 0	100 11	100 1

NOTE: The first number in each column (boldface) is the score, the second number is the number of patients; Please refer to the main entry for footnotes; (a) 100-299
MEASURES: **Pneumonia Care:** 16. Appropriate Initial Antibiotic; 17. Blood Culture Timing; 18. Influenza Vaccine; 19. Initial Antibiotic Timing; 20. Pneumococcal Vaccine; 21. Smoking Cessation Advice; **Surgical Care Improvement Project:** 22. Appropriate VTP Within 24 Hours; 23. Appropriate Hair Removal; 24. Appropriate Beta Blocker Usage; 25. Controlled Postoperative Blood Glucose; 26. Prophylactic Antibiotic Timing; 27. Prophylactic Antibiotic Timing (Outpatient); 28. Prophylactic Antibiotic Selection; 29. Prophylactic Antibiotic Selection (Outpatient); 30. Prophylactic Antibiotic Stopped; 31. Recommended VTP Ordered; 32. Urinary Catheter Removal

Hospital	Children's Asthma Care 33	34	35	Use of Medical Imaging 36	37	38	39	Survey of Patients' Hospital Experiences 40	41	42	43	44	45	46	47	48	49
CONNECTICUT																	
Bridgeport Hospital, Bridgeport, CT	- -	- -	- -	**0.464** 308	**0.009** 106	**14.9** 87	- 0	**41** 300+	**76** 300+	**77** 300+	**56** 300+	**56** 300+	**72** 300+	**66** 300+	**57** 300+	**54** 300+	**64** 300+
Bristol Hospital, Bristol, CT	- -	- -	- -	**0.010** 781	**0.002** 537	**8.3** 169	**27.3** 77	**50** 300+	**81** 300+	**85** 300+	**63** 300+	**66** 300+	**80** 300+	**72** 300+	**67** 300+	**62** 300+	**66** 300+
Charlotte Hungerford Hospital, Torrington, CT	- -	- -	- -	**0.101** 663	**0.075** 562	**10.3** 2202	**57.1** 7	**48** 300+	**79** 300+	**84** 300+	**66** 300+	**59** 300+	**78** 300+	**71** 300+	**72** 300+	**64** 300+	**62** 300+
Connecticut Childrens Medical Center, Hartford, CT	**100** 365	**90** 365	**100** 365	- -	- -	- -	- -	- -	- -	- -	- -	- -	- -	- -	- -	- -	- -
Danbury Hospital, Danbury, CT	- -	- -	- -	**0.065** 1360	**0.002** 1454	**4.9** 1377	**27.8** 198	**47** 300+	**80** 300+	**79** 300+	**70** 300+	**58** 300+	**80** 300+	**74** 300+	**68** 300+	**65** 300+	**81** 300+
Day Kimball Hospital, Putnam, CT	- -	- -	- -	**0.052** 556	**0.004** 513	**5.5** 1339	**26.2** 84	**52** 300+	**82** 300+	**81** 300+	**64** 300+	**60** 300+	**79** 300+	**67** 300+	**80** 300+	**67** 300+	**67** 300+
Greenwich Hospital Association, Greenwich, CT	- -	- -	- -	**0.050** 1070	**0.034** 935	**8.9** 1309	**24.3** 263	**58** 300+	**82** 300+	**80** 300+	**79** 300+	**61** 300+	**77** 300+	**68** 300+	**76** 300+	**62** 300+	**83** 300+
Griffin Hospital, Derby, CT	- -	- -	- -	**0.040** 545	**0.003** 631	**10.5** 637	**28.6** 119	**56** 300+	**78** 300+	**84** 300+	**71** 300+	**62** 300+	**77** 300+	**69** 300+	**74** 300+	**63** 300+	**76** 300+
Hartford Hospital, Hartford, CT	- -	- -	- -	**0.043** 490	**0.232** 211	**14.0** 285	**29.4** 51	**44** 300+	**76** 300+	**86** 300+	**60** 300+	**54** 300+	**71** 300+	**64** 300+	**63** 300+	**50** 300+	**71** 300+
Hebrew Home and Hospital, West Hartford, CT	- -	- -	- -	- 0	- 0	- 0	- 0	**54** <100	**72** <100	**81** <100	**71** <100	**29** <100	**68** <100	**55** <100	**79** <100	**51** <100	**65** <100
The Hospital of Central Connecticut, New Britain, CT	- -	- -	- -	**0.066** 1586	**0.012** 1171	**13.1** 2652	**21.5** 191	**46** 300+	**76** 300+	**82** 300+	**65** 300+	**60** 300+	**75** 300+	**69** 300+	**72** 300+	**60** 300+	**69** 300+
Hospital of St Raphael, New Haven, CT	- -	- -	- -	**0.093** 1177	**0.009** 1250	**8.1** 529	**0.0** 1	**42** 300+	**75** 300+	**82** 300+	**65** 300+	**58** 300+	**75** 300+	**68** 300+	**68** 300+	**62** 300+	**71** 300+
John Dempsey Hospital, Farmington, CT	- -	- -	- -	**0.724** 721	**0.480** 638	**8.5** 704	**23.6** 216	**37** 300+	**75** 300+	**85** 300+	**62** 300+	**58** 300+	**73** 300+	**67** 300+	**68** 300+	**52** 300+	**67** 300+
Johnson Memorial Hospital, Stafford Springs, CT	- -	- -	- -	**0.024** 372	**0.000** 276	**6.4** 500	**31.0** 58	**57** 300+	**76** 300+	**84** 300+	**61** 300+	**55** 300+	**73** 300+	**67** 300+	**69** 300+	**55** 300+	**66** 300+
Lawrence & Memorial Hospital, New London, CT	- -	- -	- -	**0.088** 1370	**0.000** 1183	**5.6** 3080	**32.0** 228	**46** 300+	**75** 300+	**80** 300+	**60** 300+	**56** 300+	**75** 300+	**69** 300+	**65** 300+	**58** 300+	**69** 300+
Manchester Memorial Hospital, Manchester, CT	- -	- -	- -	**0.081** 1081	**0.009** 974	**10.1** 543	**22.7** 154	**48** 300+	**77** 300+	**81** 300+	**59** 300+	**59** 300+	**74** 300+	**69** 300+	**62** 300+	**57** 300+	**66** 300+
Masonic Home and Hospital, Wallingford, CT	- -	- -	- -	- 0	- 0	- 0	- 0	**43** (a)	**60** (a)	**77** (a)	**57** (a)	**40** (a)	**64** (a)	**65** (a)	**69** (a)	**42** (a)	**65** (a)
Middlesex Hospital, Middletown, CT	- -	- -	- -	**0.064** 2046	**0.023** 1295	**9.0** 2828	**25.1** 323	**53** 300+	**79** 300+	**85** 300+	**75** 300+	**63** 300+	**78** 300+	**71** 300+	**79** 300+	**66** 300+	**79** 300+
Midstate Medical Center, Meriden, CT	- -	- -	- -	**0.613** 917	**0.002** 419	**8.8** 712	**29.0** 169	**56** 300+	**81** 300+	**82** 300+	**71** 300+	**66** 300+	**81** 300+	**73** 300+	**73** 300+	**67** 300+	**74** 300+
Milford Hospital, Milford, CT	- -	- -	- -	**0.127** 425	**0.054** 186	**23.5** 51	**19.7** 71	**61** 300+	**81** 300+	**81** 300+	**71** 300+	**57** 300+	**78** 300+	**70** 300+	**81** 300+	**69** 300+	**75** 300+
New Milford Hospital, New Milford, CT	- -	- -	- -	**0.057** 628	**0.005** 618	**4.7** 709	**34.5** 84	**56** 300+	**81** 300+	**82** 300+	**70** 300+	**57** 300+	**78** 300+	**71** 300+	**74** 300+	**64** 300+	**75** 300+
Norwalk Hospital Association, Norwalk, CT	- -	- -	- -	**0.066** 758	**0.059** 590	**14.3** 294	**24.7** 397	**38** 300+	**80** 300+	**79** 300+	**67** 300+	**60** 300+	**74** 300+	**72** 300+	**73** 300+	**62** 300+	**75** 300+
Rockville General Hospital, Rockville, CT	- -	- -	- -	**0.081** 546	**0.023** 431	**6.5** 415	**32.6** 95	**55** 300+	**75** 300+	**81** 300+	**65** 300+	**57** 300+	**77** 300+	**70** 300+	**69** 300+	**63** 300+	**69** 300+
Saint Francis Hospital & Medical Center, Hartford, CT	- -	- -	- -	**0.058** 1474	**0.007** 1265	**15.9** 1175	**31.1** 312	**47** 300+	**77** 300+	**82** 300+	**62** 300+	**54** 300+	**72** 300+	**66** 300+	**66** 300+	**55** 300+	**71** 300+
Saint Marys Hospital, Waterbury, CT	- -	- -	- -	**0.061** 846	**0.003** 700	**11.5** 489	**37.8** 37	**48** 300+	**78** 300+	**85** 300+	**63** 300+	**57** 300+	**73** 300+	**67** 300+	**71** 300+	**57** 300+	**69** 300+
Saint Vincent's Medical Center, Bridgeport, CT	- -	- -	- -	**0.195** 527	**0.014** 218	**11.0** 317	**16.0** 50	**49** 300+	**80** 300+	**78** 300+	**67** 300+	**58** 300+	**76** 300+	**67** 300+	**63** 300+	**61** 300+	**73** 300+
Sharon Hospital, Sharon, CT	- -	- -	- -	**0.694** 363	**0.017** 290	**8.5** 887	**32.7** 98	**60** 300+	**85** 300+	**84** 300+	**74** 300+	**61** 300+	**78** 300+	**73** 300+	**72** 300+	**63** 300+	**75** 300+
Stamford Hospital, Stamford, CT	- -	- -	- -	**0.040** 1708	**0.002** 1200	**16.5** 2159	**31.3** 176	**53** 300+	**78** 300+	**74** 300+	**65** 300+	**58** 300+	**75** 300+	**70** 300+	**63** 300+	**56** 300+	**70** 300+
Waterbury Hospital, Waterbury, CT	- -	- -	- -	**0.028** 825	**0.000** 634	**10.4** 298	**42.9** 7	**44** 300+	**81** 300+	**88** 300+	**64** 300+	**58** 300+	**77** 300+	**69** 300+	**61** 300+	**59** 300+	**70** 300+
West Haven VA Medical Center, West Haven, CT	- -	- -	- -	- -	- -	- -	- -	- -	- -	- -	- -	- -	- -	- -	- -	- -	- -
William W Backus Hospital, Norwich, CT	- -	- -	- -	**0.061** 1563	**0.006** 1444	**6.2** 2020	**25.2** 278	**48** 300+	**74** 300+	**82** 300+	**67** 300+	**55** 300+	**74** 300+	**64** 300+	**74** 300+	**60** 300+	**71** 300+
Windham Hospital, Willimantic, CT	- -	- -	- -	**0.079** 554	**0.021** 434	**9.6** 1222	**33.1** 127	**43** 300+	**79** 300+	**81** 300+	**66** 300+	**64** 300+	**77** 300+	**68** 300+	**72** 300+	**64** 300+	**69** 300+
Yale-New Haven Hospital, New Haven, CT	**100** 322	**73** 324	**100** 323	**0.135** 2598	**0.003** 2902	**7.8** 4522	**23.3** 460	**47** 300+	**75** 300+	**82** 300+	**64** 300+	**59** 300+	**73** 300+	**65** 300+	**61** 300+	**55** 300+	**71** 300+
DELAWARE																	
Bayhealth - Kent General Hospital, Dover, DE	- -	- -	- -	**0.688** 2515	**0.113** 1602	**9.4** 3440	**23.7** 257	**54** 300+	**80** 300+	**84** 300+	**65** 300+	**60** 300+	**76** 300+	**69** 300+	**65** 300+	**59** 300+	**66** 300+
Beebe Medical Center, Lewes, DE	- -	- -	- -	**0.076** 2079	**0.040** 1296	**5.7** 3147	**23.5** 293	**47** 300+	**79** 300+	**83** 300+	**70** 300+	**63** 300+	**79** 300+	**72** 300+	**68** 300+	**68** 300+	**70** 300+
Christiana Care Health Services, Newark, DE	- -	- -	- -	**0.029** 2682	**0.000** 2929	**7.8** 2424	**32.5** 252	**49** 300+	**78** 300+	**79** 300+	**67** 300+	**61** 300+	**76** 300+	**70** 300+	**69** 300+	**66** 300+	**76** 300+
Nanticoke Memorial Hospital, Seaford, DE	- -	- -	- -	**0.268** 694	**0.021** 521	**6.9** 1178	**21.7** 92	**44** 300+	**81** 300+	**84** 300+	**61** 300+	**62** 300+	**76** 300+	**68** 300+	**70** 300+	**59** 300+	**62** 300+
Saint Francis Hospital, Wilmington, DE	- -	- -	- -	**0.022** 410	**0.003** 295	**3.5** 864	**21.6** 37	**57** 300+	**78** 300+	**74** 300+	**60** 300+	**54** 300+	**71** 300+	**63** 300+	**59** 300+	**59** 300+	**60** 300+
Wilmington VA Medical Center, Wilmington, DE	- -	- -	- -	- -	- -	- -	- -	- -	- -	- -	- -	- -	- -	- -	- -	- -	- -
DISTRICT OF COLUMBIA																	
Children's Hospital NMC, Washington, DC	**100** 419	**71** 417	**100** 420	- -	- -	- -	- -	- -	- -	- -	- -	- -	- -	- -	- -	- -	- -
George Washington Univ Hospital, Washington, DC	- -	- -	- -	**0.179** 697	**0.058** 635	**5.4** 575	**26.7** 101	**59** 300+	**76** 300+	**80** 300+	**62** 300+	**54** 300+	**66** 300+	**59** 300+	**60** 300+	**48** 300+	**67** 300+
Georgetown University Hospital, Washington, DC	**97** 39	**53** 40	**100** 40	**0.081** 1367	**0.012** 1455	**10.4** 867	**30.3** 109	**55** 300+	**77** 300+	**87** 300+	**68** 300+	**61** 300+	**75** 300+	**67** 300+	**63** 300+	**55** 300+	**75** 300+
Howard University Hospital, Washington, DC	**97** 34	**0** 34	**100** 34	**0.061** 244	**0.027** 187	**9.2** 541	**50.0** 38	**68** 300+	**77** 300+	**74** 300+	**57** 300+	**55** 300+	**68** 300+	**63** 300+	**64** 300+	**55** 300+	**57** 300+
Providence Hospital, Washington, DC	- -	- -	- -	**0.574** 810	**0.484** 409	**5.7** 1909	**36.5** 115	**62** 300+	**77** 300+	**74** 300+	**61** 300+	**54** 300+	**70** 300+	**64** 300+	**67** 300+	**54** 300+	**63** 300+
Sibley Memorial Hospital, Washington, DC	- -	- -	- -	**0.039** 1095	**0.003** 966	**8.6** 2076	**30.8** 263	**48** 300+	**77** 300+	**75** 300+	**62** 300+	**54** 300+	**69** 300+	**69** 300+	**67** 300+	**52** 300+	**72** 300+
United Medical Center, Washington, DC	- -	- -	- -	**0.016** 123	**0.011** 90	**5.7** 348	- 0	**55** 300+	**68** 300+	**64** 300+	**41** 300+	**51** 300+	**61** 300+	**58** 300+	**63** 300+	**45** 300+	**36** 300+
Washington DC VA Medical Center, Washington, DC	- -	- -	- -	- -	- -	- -	- -	- -	- -	- -	- -	- -	- -	- -	- -	- -	- -
Washington Hospital Center, Washington, DC	- -	- -	- -	**0.009** 1843	**0.002** 1377	**4.0** 1845	**31.0** 245	**53** 300+	**79** 300+	**83** 300+	**61** 300+	**53** 300+	**67** 300+	**64** 300+	**61** 300+	**47** 300+	**66** 300+
KENTUCKY																	
Baptist Hospital East, Louisville, KY	- -	- -	- -	**0.072** 2433	**0.001** 1748	**9.1** 2907	**33.9** 584	**58** 300+	**80** 300+	**88** 300+	**75** 300+	**57** 300+	**79** 300+	**71** 300+	**66** 300+	**64** 300+	**81** 300+
Baptist Hospital Northeast, La Grange, KY	- -	- -	- -	**0.101** 288	**0.005** 222	**5.0** 555	**23.9** 88	**48** 300+	**77** 300+	**84** 300+	**64** 300+	**53** 300+	**76** 300+	**65** 300+	**62** 300+	**56** 300+	**67** 300+
Baptist Regional Medical Center, Corbin, KY	- -	- -	- -	**0.063** 667	**0.019** 480	**7.2** 945	**50.0** 208	**48** 300+	**84** 300+	**82** 300+	**64** 300+	**58** 300+	**77** 300+	**67** 300+	**66** 300+	**67** 300+	**64** 300+
Bluegrass Community Hospital, Versailles, KY	- -	- -	- -	- -	- -	- -	- -	**65** <100	**82** <100	**83** <100	**81** <100	**51** <100	**78** <100	**66** <100	**77** <100	**69** <100	**66** <100
Bourbon Community Hospital, Paris, KY	- -	- -	- -	**0.110** 264	**0.008** 121	**8.1** 371	**40.0** 40	**67** (a)	**85** (a)	**87** (a)	**71** (a)	**62** (a)	**81** (a)	**76** (a)	**72** (a)	**71** (a)	**74** (a)
Breckinridge Memorial Hospital, Hardinsburg, KY	- -	- -	- -	- -	- -	- -	- -	- -	- -	- -	- -	- -	- -	- -	- -	- -	- -
Caldwell Medical Center, Princeton, KY	- -	- -	- -	- -	- -	- -	- -	- -	- -	- -	- -	- -	- -	- -	- -	- -	- -
Carroll County Hospital, Carrollton, KY	- -	- -	- -	- -	- -	- -	- -	- -	- -	- -	- -	- -	- -	- -	- -	- -	- -
Casey County Hospital, Liberty, KY	- -	- -	- -	- -	- -	- -	- -	- -	- -	- -	- -	- -	- -	- -	- -	- -	- -
Caverna Memorial Hospital, Horse Cave, KY	- -	- -	- -	- -	- -	- -	- -	- -	- -	- -	- -	- -	- -	- -	- -	- -	- -
Central Baptist Hospital, Lexington, KY	- -	- -	- -	**0.035** 1358	**0.014** 1233	**19.0** 2541	**32.5** 157	**53** 300+	**81** 300+	**81** 300+	**74** 300+	**64** 300+	**80** 300+	**72** 300+	**62** 300+	**65** 300+	**82** 300+
Clark Regional Medical Center, Winchester, KY	- -	- -	- -	**0.515** 443	**0.429** 282	**3.3** 480	**39.7** 73	**58** 300+	**90** 300+	**88** 300+	**74** 300+	**74** 300+	**85** 300+	**78** 300+	**84** 300+	**76** 300+	**75** 300+
Clinton County Hospital, Albany, KY	- -	- -	- -	**0.171** 152	**0.298** 94	**4.0** 175	- 0	**79** 300+	**92** 300+	**76** 300+	**81** 300+	**62** 300+	**83** 300+	**71** 300+	**89** 300+	**69** 300+	**85** 300+
Crittenden Health System, Marion, KY	- -	- -	- -	**0.043** 93	**0.016** 63	**7.4** 135	**28.9** 45	**57** (a)	**87** (a)	**69** (a)	**58** (a)	**64** (a)	**79** (a)	**68** (a)	**79** (a)	**66** (a)	**63** (a)
Cumberland County Hospital, Burkesville, KY	- -	- -	- -	- -	- -	- -	- -	- -	- -	- -	- -	- -	- -	- -	- -	- -	- -

NOTE: The first number in each column (boldface) is the score, the second number is the number of patients; Please refer to the main entry for footnotes; (a) 100-299

*MEASURES: **Children's Asthma Care:** 33. Received Systemic Corticosteroids; 34. Received Home Management Plan of Care; 35. Received Reliever Medication; **Use of Medical Imaging:** 36. Combination Abdominal CT Scan; 37. Combination Chest CT Scan; 38. Follow-up Mammogram/Ultrasound; 39. MRI for Low Back Pain; **Survey of Patients' Hospital Experiences:** 40. Area Around Room 'Always' Quiet at Night; 41. Doctors 'Always' Communicated Well; 42. Home Recovery Information Given; 43. Hospital Given 9 or 10 on 10 Point Scale; 44. Meds 'Always' Explained Before Given; 45. Nurses 'Always' Communicated Well; 46. Pain 'Always' Well Controlled; 47. Room and Bathroom 'Always' Clean; 48. Timely Help 'Always' Received; 49. Would Definitely Recommend Hospital*

Hospital	Children's Asthma Care			Use of Medical Imaging				Survey of Patients' Hospital Experiences									
	33	34	35	36	37	38	39	40	41	42	43	44	45	46	47	48	49
Ephraim Mcdowell Fort Logan Hospital, Stanford, KY	- -	- -	- -	- -	- -	- -	- -	61 (a)	77 (a)	84 (a)	71 (a)	65 (a)	78 (a)	65 (a)	77 (a)	69 (a)	72 (a)
Ephraim Mcdowell Regional Medical Center, Danville, KY	- -	- -	- -	0.107 797	0.000 403	5.0 1364	34.2 316	54 300+	77 300+	78 300+	59 300+	52 300+	71 300+	64 300+	67 300+	55 300+	62 300+
Flaget Memorial Hospital, Bardstown, KY	- -	- -	- -	0.047 407	0.000 290	8.8 464	42.7 117	59 300+	82 300+	86 300+	74 300+	67 300+	78 300+	74 300+	75 300+	72 300+	73 300+
Fleming County Hospital, Flemingsburg, KY	- -	- -	- -	0.581 191	0.012 167	13.5 237	46.7 30	64 (a)	78 (a)	82 (a)	76 (a)	64 (a)	79 (a)	70 (a)	87 (a)	64 (a)	75 (a)
Frankfort Regional Medical Center, Frankfort, KY	- -	- -	- -	0.024 533	0.000 311	1.9 775	32.6 43	64 300+	84 300+	87 300+	69 300+	65 300+	78 300+	73 300+	70 300+	65 300+	64 300+
Georgetown Community Hospital, Georgetown, KY	- -	- -	- -	0.058 345	0.024 167	5.9 354	44.8 58	62 300+	87 300+	86 300+	70 300+	63 300+	77 300+	71 300+	64 300+	64 300+	71 300+
Greenview Regional Hospital, Bowling Green, KY	- -	- -	- -	0.436 514	0.086 186	10.8 287	27.4 73	65 300+	84 300+	85 300+	73 300+	66 300+	79 300+	71 300+	74 300+	62 300+	76 300+
Hardin Memorial Hospital, Elizabethtown, KY	- -	- -	- -	0.092 1344	0.001 960	14.6 1804	31.0 187	44 300+	83 300+	79 300+	64 300+	63 300+	77 300+	67 300+	69 300+	58 300+	65 300+
Harlan Appalachian Regional Healthcare Hospital, Harlan, KY	- -	- -	- -	0.424 420	0.235 196	8.9 359	42.3 104	63 300+	79 300+	80 300+	66 300+	61 300+	77 300+	68 300+	72 300+	70 300+	62 300+
Harrison Memorial Hospital, Cynthiana, KY	- -	- -	- -	0.063 272	0.006 167	11.9 329	- 0	55 300+	88 300+	83 300+	71 300+	65 300+	80 300+	71 300+	78 300+	63 300+	67 300+
Hazard Arh Regional Medical Center, Hazard, KY	- -	- -	- -	0.006 542	0.017 233	6.1 360	44.0 25	62 300+	83 300+	78 300+	67 300+	59 300+	77 300+	70 300+	73 300+	64 300+	63 300+
Highlands Regional Medical Center, Prestonsburg, KY	- -	- -	- -	0.372 1015	0.002 502	1.6 962	35.3 156	55 300+	83 300+	70 300+	58 300+	56 300+	75 300+	63 300+	69 300+	64 300+	59 300+
Jackson Purchase Medical Center, Mayfield, KY	- -	- -	- -	0.343 335	0.000 289	7.4 610	42.2 64	66 300+	84 300+	83 300+	70 300+	62 300+	76 300+	68 300+	69 300+	60 300+	68 300+
The James B Haggin Memorial Hospital, Harrodsburg, KY	- -	- -	- -	- -	- -	- -	- -	- -	- -	- -	- -	- -	- -	- -	- -	- -	- -
Jane Todd Crawford Hospital, Greensburg, KY	- -	- -	- -	- -	- -	- -	- -	- -	- -	- -	- -	- -	- -	- -	- -	- -	- -
Jennie Stuart Medical Center, Hopkinsville, KY	- -	- -	- -	0.032 587	0.003 308	5.6 1059	32.6 132	57 300+	75 300+	80 300+	54 300+	54 300+	67 300+	63 300+	66 300+	56 300+	50 300+
Jewish Hospital & St Mary's Healthcare, Louisville, KY	- -	- -	- -	0.091 3041	0.002 3085	4.7 3462	36.9 718	53 300+	73 300+	77 300+	60 300+	54 300+	70 300+	61 300+	57 300+	52 300+	63 300+
Jewish Hospital - Shelbyville, Shelbyville, KY	- -	- -	- -	0.072 349	0.007 290	5.6 663	30.4 69	47 300+	77 300+	73 300+	60 300+	53 300+	72 300+	64 300+	67 300+	58 300+	57 300+
Kentucky River Medical Center, Jackson, KY	- -	- -	- -	0.157 166	0.139 115	8.6 174	48.4 64	61 300+	80 300+	79 300+	63 300+	58 300+	76 300+	68 300+	69 300+	62 300+	59 300+
King's Daughters' Medical Center, Ashland, KY	- -	- -	- -	0.050 2364	0.013 2154	7.6 2425	28.0 632	63 300+	82 300+	82 300+	77 300+	65 300+	83 300+	74 300+	74 300+	68 300+	82 300+
Knox County Hospital, Barbourville, KY	- -	- -	- -	- -	- -	- -	- -	- -	- -	- -	- -	- -	- -	- -	- -	- -	- -
Lake Cumberland Regional Hospital, Somerset, KY	- -	- -	- -	0.150 1074	0.069 765	6.1 1498	41.5 258	61 300+	84 300+	82 300+	65 300+	61 300+	76 300+	73 300+	71 300+	64 300+	65 300+
Lexington-Leestown VA Medical Center, Lexington, KY	- -	- -	- -	- -	- -	- -	- -	- -	- -	- -	- -	- -	- -	- -	- -	- -	- -
Livingston Hospital and Healthcare, Salem, KY	- -	- -	- -	- -	- -	- -	- -	- -	- -	- -	- -	- -	- -	- -	- -	- -	- -
Logan Memorial Hospital, Russellville, KY	100 5	83 6	100 6	0.069 218	0.013 160	13.1 480	38.5 26	64 300+	84 300+	80 300+	66 300+	58 300+	78 300+	74 300+	65 300+	69 300+	61 300+
Louisville VA Medical Center, Louisville, KY	- -	- -	- -	- -	- -	- -	- -	- -	- -	- -	- -	- -	- -	- -	- -	- -	- -
Lourdes Hospital, Paducah, KY	- -	- -	- -	0.312 650	0.036 496	9.6 353	36.4 154	54 300+	81 300+	79 300+	66 300+	54 300+	74 300+	65 300+	61 300+	60 300+	70 300+
Marcum and Wallace Memorial Hospital, Irvine, KY	- -	- -	- -	- -	- -	- -	- -	74 (a)	87 (a)	81 (a)	78 (a)	74 (a)	91 (a)	78 (a)	93 (a)	82 (a)	76 (a)
Marshall County Hospital, Benton, KY	- -	- -	- -	- -	- -	- -	- -	- -	- -	- -	- -	- -	- -	- -	- -	- -	- -
Mary Breckinridge Hospital, Hyden, KY	- -	- -	- -	- -	- -	- -	- -	- -	- -	- -	- -	- -	- -	- -	- -	- -	- -
McDowell Arh Hospital, McDowell, KY	- -	- -	- -	0.006 180	0.037 81	12.4 137	72.7 33	76 (a)	88 (a)	88 (a)	75 (a)	68 (a)	83 (a)	74 (a)	85 (a)	80 (a)	76 (a)
Meadowview Regional Medical Center, Maysville, KY	- -	- -	- -	0.649 288	0.000 239	9.9 436	66.7 6	63 300+	82 300+	82 300+	64 300+	57 300+	77 300+	72 300+	74 300+	61 300+	65 300+
The Medical Center at Bowling Green, Bowling Green, KY	- -	- -	- -	0.064 897	0.175 417	5.1 803	34.7 150	60 300+	81 300+	85 300+	69 300+	60 300+	77 300+	70 300+	69 300+	65 300+	74 300+
The Medical Center at Franklin, Franklin, KY	- -	- -	- -	- -	- -	- -	- -	- -	- -	- -	- -	- -	- -	- -	- -	- -	- -
The Medical Center at Scottsville, Scottsville, KY	- -	- -	- -	- -	- -	- -	- -	- -	- -	- -	- -	- -	- -	- -	- -	- -	- -
Memorial Hospital, Manchester, KY	- -	- -	- -	0.135 282	0.145 138	5.5 256	32.1 81	45 (a)	75 (a)	83 (a)	54 (a)	52 (a)	72 (a)	63 (a)	66 (a)	56 (a)	49 (a)
Methodist Hospital, Henderson, KY	- -	- -	- -	0.177 492	0.018 331	3.8 785	42.6 122	58 300+	84 300+	79 300+	61 300+	58 300+	77 300+	71 300+	73 300+	61 300+	60 300+
Methodist Hospital Union County, Morganfield, KY	- -	- -	- -	0.134 142	0.185 81	5.4 279	- 0	69 (a)	92 (a)	78 (a)	76 (a)	62 (a)	87 (a)	75 (a)	84 (a)	77 (a)	78 (a)
Middlesboro Appalachian Reg Healthcare Hosp, Middlesboro, KY	- -	- -	- -	0.467 377	0.045 222	7.2 390	37.5 136	69 300+	88 300+	84 300+	70 300+	61 300+	80 300+	70 300+	74 300+	70 300+	65 300+
Monroe County Medical Center, Tompkinsville, KY	- -	- -	- -	0.459 196	0.338 145	5.7 106	29.3 58	62 300+	85 300+	73 300+	65 300+	57 300+	77 300+	70 300+	82 300+	56 300+	61 300+
Morgan County Arh Hospital, West Liberty, KY	- -	- -	- -	0.022 185	0.026 77	4.7 86	44.1 34	76 (a)	92 (a)	91 (a)	79 (a)	79 (a)	81 (a)	76 (a)	86 (a)	81 (a)	82 (a)
Muhlenberg Community Hospital, Greenville, KY	- -	- -	- -	0.419 191	0.075 67	5.8 172	51.8 83	61 300+	89 300+	85 300+	64 300+	67 300+	81 300+	77 300+	75 300+	68 300+	63 300+
Murray-Calloway County Hospital, Murray, KY	- -	- -	- -	0.182 533	0.011 274	4.6 1007	39.0 118	55 300+	83 300+	81 300+	60 300+	56 300+	74 300+	65 300+	67 300+	61 300+	60 300+
New Horizons Medical Center, Owenton, KY	- -	- -	- -	- -	- -	- -	- -	- -	- -	- -	- -	- -	- -	- -	- -	- -	- -
Nicholas County Hospital, Carlisle, KY	- -	- -	- -	- -	- -	- -	- -	- -	- -	- -	- -	- -	- -	- -	- -	- -	- -
Norton Hospitals, Louisville, KY	100 795	89 792	100 795	0.184 3316	0.233 2506	9.6 4166	29.1 873	58 300+	78 300+	83 300+	69 300+	61 300+	77 300+	70 300+	70 300+	64 300+	72 300+
Ohio County Hospital, Hartford, KY	- -	- -	- -	- -	- -	- -	- -	60 (a)	83 (a)	83 (a)	59 (a)	48 (a)	79 (a)	74 (a)	79 (a)	69 (a)	66 (a)
Our Lady of Bellefonte Hospital, Ashland, KY	- -	- -	- -	0.083 929	0.080 522	8.4 1149	40.3 268	73 300+	86 300+	83 300+	78 300+	67 300+	84 300+	76 300+	78 300+	70 300+	79 300+
Owensboro Medical Health System, Owensboro, KY	- -	- -	- -	0.433 1695	0.020 1282	5.9 2576	33.2 416	56 300+	82 300+	85 300+	71 300+	56 300+	78 300+	71 300+	71 300+	64 300+	71 300+
Parkway Regional Hospital, Fulton, KY	- -	- -	- -	0.577 104	0.044 45	4.1 196	47.1 17	73 (a)	88 (a)	83 (a)	74 (a)	64 (a)	82 (a)	77 (a)	78 (a)	74 (a)	67 (a)
Pattie A Clay Regional Medical Center, Richmond, KY	- -	- -	- -	0.015 588	0.020 345	3.5 739	31.5 149	56 300+	78 300+	82 300+	59 300+	55 300+	71 300+	66 300+	69 300+	61 300+	61 300+
Paul B Hall Regional Medical Center, Paintsville, KY	99 85	99 86	100 88	0.216 328	0.248 218	18.1 127	35.1 57	60 300+	79 300+	78 300+	58 300+	57 300+	71 300+	62 300+	68 300+	57 300+	58 300+
Pikeville Medical Center, Pikeville, KY	- -	- -	- -	0.040 1272	0.038 797	7.9 1225	36.0 397	61 300+	87 300+	86 300+	76 300+	65 300+	81 300+	77 300+	72 300+	68 300+	78 300+
Pineville Community Hospital, Pineville, KY	- -	- -	- -	0.294 265	0.322 90	6.6 318	- 0	57 300+	86 300+	77 300+	62 300+	56 300+	76 300+	66 300+	78 300+	59 300+	68 300+
Regional Medical Center of Hopkins County, Madisonville, KY	- -	- -	- -	0.078 637	0.005 367	- 0	39.2 130	58 300+	83 300+	84 300+	70 300+	66 300+	80 300+	73 300+	69 300+	59 300+	71 300+
Rockcastle Reg Hosp & Resp Care Ctr, Mount Vernon, KY	- -	- -	- -	0.000 254	0.127 173	5.9 256	30.1 93	59 (a)	89 (a)	77 (a)	75 (a)	63 (a)	82 (a)	72 (a)	81 (a)	65 (a)	73 (a)
Russell County Hospital, Russell Springs, KY	- -	- -	- -	0.710 248	0.013 151	4.6 326	- 0	- -	- -	- -	- -	- -	- -	- -	- -	- -	- -
Saint Claire Regional Medical Center, Morehead, KY	100 4	80 5	100 5	0.616 700	0.039 463	7.9 756	43.4 143	49 300+	85 300+	83 300+	62 300+	64 300+	80 300+	71 300+	71 300+	64 300+	66 300+
Saint Elizabeth Florence, Florence, KY	- -	- -	- -	0.056 413	0.000 185	7.6 514	25.8 31	57 300+	75 300+	83 300+	61 300+	59 300+	74 300+	68 300+	67 300+	59 300+	63 300+
Saint Elizabeth Ft Thomas, Fort Thomas, KY	- -	- -	- -	0.025 523	0.000 342	7.9 611	30.4 46	52 300+	76 300+	85 300+	59 300+	61 300+	75 300+	69 300+	71 300+	60 300+	63 300+
Saint Elizabeth Grant, Williamstown, KY	- -	- -	- -	0.062 369	0.000 144	6.8 235	44.4 90	67 (a)	84 (a)	88 (a)	80 (a)	66 (a)	83 (a)	75 (a)	78 (a)	83 (a)	74 (a)
Saint Elizabeth Medical Center North, Covington, KY	- -	- -	- -	0.061 2226	0.002 1311	7.2 3448	36.6 145	60 300+	79 300+	86 300+	74 300+	63 300+	78 300+	70 300+	70 300+	65 300+	79 300+
Saint Joseph Berea, Berea, KY	- -	- -	- -	- -	- -	- -	- -	67 300+	86 300+	84 300+	76 300+	64 300+	82 300+	72 300+	73 300+	70 300+	79 300+
Saint Joseph East, Lexington, KY	- -	- -	- -	0.012 257	0.000 33	3.1 739	37.5 32	60 300+	81 300+	85 300+	70 300+	58 300+	75 300+	70 300+	64 300+	61 300+	74 300+
Saint Joseph Hospital, Lexington, KY	- -	- -	- -	0.016 565	0.009 115	4.9 759	33.7 98	62 300+	81 300+	83 300+	71 300+	60 300+	78 300+	71 300+	66 300+	63 300+	77 300+
Saint Joseph Hospital London, London, KY	- -	- -	- -	0.052 698	0.011 380	6.3 525	35.2 128	52 300+	79 300+	81 300+	70 300+	62 300+	80 300+	73 300+	72 300+	72 300+	73 300+
Saint Joseph Martin, Martin, KY	- -	- -	- -	- -	- -	- -	- -	61 300+	86 300+	80 300+	76 300+	72 300+	86 300+	73 300+	82 300+	79 300+	79 300+

NOTE: The first number in each column (boldface) is the score, the second number is the number of patients; Please refer to the main entry for footnotes; (a) 100-299
*MEASURES: **Children's Asthma Care:** 33. Received Systemic Corticosteroids; 34. Received Home Management Plan of Care; 35. Received Reliever Medication; **Use of Medical Imaging:** 36. Combination Abdominal CT Scan; 37. Combination Chest CT Scan; 38. Follow-up Mammogram/Ultrasound; 39. MRI for Low Back Pain; **Survey of Patients' Hospital Experiences:** 40. Area Around Room 'Always' Quiet at Night; 41. Doctors 'Always' Communicated Well; 42. Home Recovery Information Given; 43. Hospital Given 9 or 10 on 10 Point Scale; 44. Meds 'Always' Explained Before Given; 45. Nurses 'Always' Communicated Well; 46. Pain 'Always' Well Controlled; 47. Room and Bathroom 'Always' Clean; 48. Timely Help 'Always' Received; 49. Would Definitely Recommend Hospital*

Hospital	Children's Asthma Care			Use of Medical Imaging				Survey of Patients' Hospital Experiences									
	33	34	35	36	37	38	39	40	41	42	43	44	45	46	47	48	49
Saint Joseph Mount Sterling, Mount Sterling, KY	-	-	-	0.057 477	0.009 330	11.5 304	- 0	61 (a)	82 (a)	84 (a)	66 (a)	66 (a)	78 (a)	72 (a)	73 (a)	66 (a)	66 (a)
Spring View Hospital, Lebanon, KY	-	-	-	0.241 224	0.198 131	2.1 419	46.3 54	65 300+	81 300+	79 300+	61 300+	54 300+	75 300+	69 300+	66 300+	61 300+	60 300+
T J Samson Community Hospital, Glasgow, KY	-	-	-	0.256 841	0.175 605	8.0 1292	38.5 130	68 300+	84 300+	84 300+	70 300+	66 300+	81 300+	73 300+	86 300+	74 300+	70 300+
Taylor Regional Hospital, Campbellsville, KY	-	-	-	0.414 694	0.006 537	17.0 911	23.9 159	58 300+	84 300+	79 300+	67 300+	59 300+	77 300+	69 300+	73 300+	66 300+	66 300+
Three Rivers Medical Center, Louisa, KY	-	-	-	0.046 241	0.061 132	18.1 149	43.9 57	62 300+	88 300+	81 300+	67 300+	69 300+	80 300+	72 300+	74 300+	68 300+	65 300+
Trigg County Hospital, Cadiz, KY	-	-	-	-	-	-	-	60 <100	81 <100	67 <100	60 <100	66 <100	80 <100	68 <100	75 <100	67 <100	64 <100
Twin Lakes Regional Medical Center, Leitchfield, KY	-	-	-	0.034 296	0.000 278	6.8 428	36.0 86	53 300+	77 300+	77 300+	57 300+	58 300+	74 300+	67 300+	67 300+	64 300+	59 300+
University of Kentucky Hospital, Lexington, KY	97 127	61 127	100 127	0.020 1583	0.005 1979	3.4 357	28.9 197	52 300+	76 300+	86 300+	61 300+	58 300+	74 300+	65 300+	60 300+	61 300+	67 300+
University of Louisville Hospital, Louisville, KY	-	-	-	0.063 702	0.006 844	7.8 1378	50.9 57	48 300+	73 300+	81 300+	63 300+	57 300+	71 300+	63 300+	61 300+	52 300+	65 300+
Wayne County Hospital, Monticello, KY	-	-	-	-	-	-	-	-	-	-	-	-	-	-	-	-	-
Western Baptist Hospital, Paducah, KY	-	-	-	0.113 1835	0.058 1178	11.6 982	33.8 275	65 300+	79 300+	86 300+	72 300+	59 300+	79 300+	68 300+	73 300+	62 300+	79 300+
Westlake Regional Hospital, Columbia, KY	-	-	-	0.462 195	0.225 102	11.6 190	- 0	87 300+	100 300+	99 300+	80 300+	87 300+	99 300+	99 300+	96 300+	97 300+	98 300+
Whitesburg ARH Hospital, Whitesburg, KY	-	-	-	0.030 265	0.020 101	7.7 260	26.0 73	62 300+	87 300+	84 300+	72 300+	64 300+	82 300+	71 300+	75 300+	74 300+	71 300+
Williamson ARH Hospital, South Williamson, KY	-	-	-	0.006 179	0.011 92	9.3 216	50.9 57	64 300+	84 300+	83 300+	74 300+	66 300+	79 300+	74 300+	72 300+	68 300+	73 300+
MAINE																	
Aroostook Medical Center, Presque Isle, ME	-	-	-	0.475 577	0.290 486	10.1 999	- 0	46 300+	74 300+	76 300+	61 300+	53 300+	75 300+	63 300+	79 300+	66 300+	56 300+
Blue Hill Memorial Hospital, Blue Hill, ME	-	-	-	-	-	-	-	57 (a)	79 (a)	80 (a)	64 (a)	64 (a)	75 (a)	65 (a)	78 (a)	70 (a)	63 (a)
Bridgton Hospital, Bridgton, ME	-	-	-	-	-	-	-	61 300+	86 300+	90 300+	76 300+	69 300+	79 300+	75 300+	79 300+	74 300+	75 300+
Calais Regional Hospital, Calais, ME	-	-	-	0.391 230	0.461 152	4.5 397	52.2 23	71 (a)	81 (a)	82 (a)	66 (a)	68 (a)	80 (a)	78 (a)	79 (a)	78 (a)	66 (a)
Cary Medical Center, Caribou, ME	-	-	-	0.558 403	0.400 443	14.2 773	44.3 70	60 300+	87 300+	88 300+	69 300+	61 300+	81 300+	72 300+	73 300+	72 300+	72 300+
Central Maine Medical Center, Lewiston, ME	-	-	-	0.084 1073	0.001 873	4.8 1410	- 0	50 300+	77 300+	85 300+	67 300+	59 300+	75 300+	68 300+	69 300+	64 300+	77 300+
Charles A Dean Memorial Hospital, Greenville, ME	-	-	-	-	-	-	-	63 <100	92 <100	88 <100	81 <100	76 <100	92 <100	82 <100	82 <100	91 <100	88 <100
Down East Community Hospital, Machias, ME	-	-	-	0.233 283	0.176 255	11.9 571	- 0	65 (a)	86 (a)	83 (a)	71 (a)	68 (a)	85 (a)	82 (a)	86 (a)	77 (a)	69 (a)
Eastern Maine Medical Center, Bangor, ME	-	-	-	0.029 1584	0.002 1475	5.4 1435	36.9 293	44 300+	77 300+	85 300+	69 300+	59 300+	77 300+	69 300+	73 300+	62 300+	76 300+
Franklin Memorial Hospital, Farmington, ME	-	-	-	0.148 438	0.009 322	7.5 1189	43.7 135	53 300+	80 300+	86 300+	68 300+	62 300+	79 300+	70 300+	81 300+	64 300+	68 300+
Henrietta D Goodall Hospital, Sanford, ME	-	-	-	0.096 457	0.027 369	8.7 967	37.1 105	59 300+	79 300+	88 300+	57 300+	61 300+	73 300+	67 300+	75 300+	64 300+	60 300+
Houlton Regional Hospital, Houlton, ME	-	-	-	-	-	-	-	58 300+	84 300+	86 300+	74 300+	63 300+	83 300+	71 300+	79 300+	80 300+	73 300+
Inland Hospital, Waterville, ME	-	-	-	0.023 308	0.000 125	8.1 419	- 0	69 (a)	79 (a)	85 (a)	70 (a)	60 (a)	83 (a)	72 (a)	77 (a)	72 (a)	78 (a)
Maine Coast Memorial Hospital, Ellsworth, ME	-	-	-	0.080 386	0.000 266	3.0 946	34.8 141	55 300+	86 300+	88 300+	78 300+	73 300+	85 300+	80 300+	86 300+	77 300+	82 300+
Maine General Medical Center, Augusta, ME	-	-	-	0.043 1618	0.006 1388	6.5 3702	50.0 4	45 300+	79 300+	88 300+	63 300+	66 300+	78 300+	71 300+	77 300+	64 300+	70 300+
Maine Medical Center, Portland, ME	-	-	-	0.102 1961	0.004 2037	11.0 2473	33.6 149	49 300+	77 300+	84 300+	70 300+	60 300+	75 300+	70 300+	69 300+	62 300+	77 300+
Mayo Regional Hospital, Dover Foxcroft, ME	-	-	-	-	-	-	-	57 (a)	87 (a)	88 (a)	73 (a)	65 (a)	79 (a)	73 (a)	82 (a)	75 (a)	75 (a)
Mercy Hospital, Portland, ME	-	-	-	0.049 594	0.008 597	5.7 2053	35.5 211	62 300+	78 300+	86 300+	74 300+	64 300+	77 300+	66 300+	71 300+	60 300+	79 300+
Mid Coast Hospital, Brunswick, ME	-	-	-	0.161 639	0.002 499	8.0 1088	29.3 147	52 300+	78 300+	85 300+	70 300+	60 300+	75 300+	70 300+	74 300+	60 300+	78 300+
Miles Memorial Hospital, Damariscotta, ME	-	-	-	0.052 289	0.010 203	5.4 706	- 0	53 300+	84 300+	83 300+	72 300+	66 300+	79 300+	73 300+	76 300+	70 300+	79 300+
Millinocket Regional Hospital, Millinocket, ME	-	-	-	-	-	-	-	66 (a)	87 (a)	87 (a)	79 (a)	74 (a)	87 (a)	76 (a)	91 (a)	85 (a)	81 (a)
Mount Desert Island Hospital, Bar Harbor, ME	-	-	-	0.259 259	0.147 109	4.9 367	- 0	63 (a)	90 (a)	90 (a)	84 (a)	72 (a)	86 (a)	76 (a)	86 (a)	82 (a)	87 (a)
Northern Maine Medical Center, Fort Kent, ME	-	-	-	0.345 203	0.023 215	7.9 692	56.8 74	57 (a)	81 (a)	81 (a)	60 (a)	67 (a)	79 (a)	69 (a)	80 (a)	70 (a)	67 (a)
Parkview Adventist Medical Center, Brunswick, ME	-	-	-	0.078 230	0.025 120	10.7 718	44.1 59	55 300+	84 300+	87 300+	83 300+	65 300+	80 300+	72 300+	86 300+	72 300+	87 300+
Penobscot Bay Medical Center, Rockport, ME	-	-	-	0.080 552	0.002 480	- 0	25.0 4	53 300+	80 300+	88 300+	66 300+	62 300+	76 300+	70 300+	73 300+	67 300+	69 300+
Penobscot Valley Hospital, Lincoln, ME	-	-	-	-	-	-	-	62 (a)	84 (a)	88 (a)	68 (a)	69 (a)	80 (a)	79 (a)	82 (a)	69 (a)	67 (a)
Redington Fairview General Hospital, Skowhegan, ME	-	-	-	0.123 481	0.066 196	8.7 932	- 0	60 300+	85 300+	91 300+	73 300+	70 300+	83 300+	73 300+	83 300+	71 300+	77 300+
Rumford Hospital, Rumford, ME	-	-	-	-	-	-	-	69 (a)	72 (a)	88 (a)	70 (a)	53 (a)	75 (a)	68 (a)	85 (a)	71 (a)	69 (a)
Saint Andrews Hospital, Boothbay Harbor, ME	-	-	-	0.047 85	0.038 53	13.7 190	- 0	47 <100	87 <100	91 <100	69 <100	73 <100	75 <100	65 <100	66 <100	61 <100	78 <100
Saint Joseph Hospital, Bangor, ME	-	-	-	0.058 567	0.000 401	4.9 2577	32.8 262	59 300+	82 300+	89 300+	80 300+	63 300+	81 300+	73 300+	79 300+	65 300+	83 300+
Saint Marys Regional Medical Center, Lewiston, ME	-	-	-	0.071 722	0.008 633	9.3 1273	29.8 208	58 300+	80 300+	87 300+	71 300+	61 300+	79 300+	68 300+	78 300+	61 300+	79 300+
Sebasticook Valley Hospital, Pittsfield, ME	-	-	-	-	-	-	-	46 (a)	76 (a)	88 (a)	67 (a)	65 (a)	77 (a)	59 (a)	84 (a)	62 (a)	68 (a)
Southern Maine Medical Center, Biddeford, ME	-	-	-	0.037 756	0.000 470	7.2 1344	37.1 175	48 300+	81 300+	86 300+	66 300+	62 300+	78 300+	70 300+	73 300+	62 300+	76 300+
Stephens Memorial Hospital, Norway, ME	-	-	-	0.609 330	0.013 380	8.5 1139	49.4 79	56 300+	84 300+	90 300+	74 300+	64 300+	77 300+	71 300+	77 300+	63 300+	76 300+
Togus VA Medical Center, Augusta, ME	-	-	-	-	-	-	-	-	-	-	-	-	-	-	-	-	-
Waldo County General Hospital, Belfast, ME	-	-	-	-	-	-	-	62 (a)	83 (a)	89 (a)	79 (a)	68 (a)	84 (a)	81 (a)	85 (a)	79 (a)	78 (a)
York Hospital, York, ME	-	-	-	0.131 657	0.008 502	10.7 1207	26.2 141	58 300+	87 300+	87 300+	84 300+	67 300+	84 300+	75 300+	77 300+	72 300+	90 300+
MARYLAND																	
Anne Arundel Medical Center, Annapolis, MD	-	-	-	-	-	-	-	61 300+	80 300+	86 300+	74 300+	61 300+	78 300+	70 300+	66 300+	65 300+	81 300+
Atlantic General Hospital, Berlin, MD	-	-	-	-	-	-	-	50 300+	77 300+	84 300+	69 300+	57 300+	76 300+	69 300+	65 300+	63 300+	75 300+
Baltimore Washington Medical Center, Glen Burnie, MD	100 121	84 116	100 121	-	-	-	-	56 300+	77 300+	81 300+	66 300+	54 300+	74 300+	67 300+	66 300+	59 300+	69 300+
Bon Secours Hospital, Baltimore, MD	-	-	-	-	-	-	-	63 300+	77 300+	77 300+	52 300+	52 300+	68 300+	64 300+	65 300+	54 300+	49 300+
Calvert Memorial Hospital, Prince Frederick, MD	-	-	-	-	-	-	-	54 300+	78 300+	83 300+	64 300+	58 300+	72 300+	66 300+	65 300+	59 300+	65 300+
Carroll Hospital Center, Westminster, MD	-	-	-	-	-	-	-	47 300+	76 300+	78 300+	66 300+	63 300+	76 300+	68 300+	64 300+	61 300+	66 300+
Chester River Hospital Center, Chestertown, MD	-	-	-	-	-	-	-	58 300+	78 300+	84 300+	65 300+	61 300+	76 300+	69 300+	73 300+	68 300+	62 300+
Civista Medical Center, La Plata, MD	-	-	-	-	-	-	-	56 300+	73 300+	76 300+	56 300+	57 300+	73 300+	65 300+	65 300+	61 300+	59 300+
Doctors' Community Hospital, Lanham, MD	-	-	-	-	-	-	-	49 300+	74 300+	77 300+	58 300+	50 300+	67 300+	61 300+	71 300+	50 300+	63 300+
Edward Mccready Memorial Hospital, Crisfield, MD	-	-	-	-	-	-	-	61 (a)	86 (a)	87 (a)	73 (a)	68 (a)	86 (a)	80 (a)	78 (a)	80 (a)	74 (a)
Fort Washington Hospital, Fort Washington, MD	-	-	-	-	-	-	-	56 300+	76 300+	75 300+	53 300+	52 300+	70 300+	63 300+	61 300+	57 300+	56 300+
Franklin Square Hospital Center, Baltimore, MD	-	-	-	-	-	-	-	48 300+	77 300+	80 300+	59 300+	51 300+	72 300+	62 300+	53 300+	53 300+	59 300+
Frederick Memorial Hospital, Frederick, MD	-	-	-	-	-	-	-	51 300+	76 300+	80 300+	66 300+	58 300+	78 300+	70 300+	70 300+	57 300+	70 300+
Garrett County Memorial Hospital, Oakland, MD	-	-	-	-	-	-	-	50 300+	85 300+	85 300+	68 300+	63 300+	80 300+	72 300+	71 300+	70 300+	69 300+

NOTE: The first number in each column (boldface) is the score, the second number is the number of patients; Please refer to the main entry for footnotes; (a) 100-299
*MEASURES: **Children's Asthma Care:** 33. Received Systemic Corticosteroids; 34. Received Home Management Plan of Care; 35. Received Reliever Medication; **Use of Medical Imaging:** 36. Combination Abdominal CT Scan; 37. Combination Chest CT Scan; 38. Follow-up Mammogram/Ultrasound; 39. MRI for Low Back Pain; **Survey of Patients' Hospital Experiences:** 40. Area Around Room 'Always' Quiet at Night; 41. Doctors 'Always' Communicated Well; 42. Home Recovery Information Given; 43. Hospital Given 9 or 10 on 10 Point Scale; 44. Meds 'Always' Explained Before Given; 45. Nurses 'Always' Communicated Well; 46. Pain 'Always' Well Controlled; 47. Room and Bathroom 'Always' Clean; 48. Timely Help 'Always' Received; 49. Would Definitely Recommend Hospital*

Hospital	Children's Asthma Care			Use of Medical Imaging				Survey of Patients' Hospital Experiences									
	33	34	35	36	37	38	39	40	41	42	43	44	45	46	47	48	49
Good Samaritan Hospital, Baltimore, MD	- -	- -	- -	- -	- -	- -	- -	62 300+	80 300+	85 300+	70 300+	56 300+	76 300+	69 300+	72 300+	58 300+	76 300+
Greater Baltimore Medical Center, Baltimore, MD	- -	- -	- -	- -	- -	- -	- -	51 300+	81 300+	77 300+	67 300+	58 300+	73 300+	68 300+	59 300+	57 300+	76 300+
Harbor Hospital, Brooklyn, MD	- -	- -	- -	- -	- -	- -	- -	55 300+	78 300+	79 300+	65 300+	56 300+	74 300+	65 300+	58 300+	52 300+	66 300+
Harford Memorial Hospital, Havre De Grace, MD	- -	- -	- -	- -	- -	- -	- -	55 300+	78 300+	81 300+	64 300+	61 300+	76 300+	68 300+	66 300+	57 300+	64 300+
Holy Cross Hospital, Silver Spring, MD	- -	- -	- -	0.026 538	0.004 265	9.9 111	38.6 44	56 300+	75 300+	74 300+	58 300+	50 300+	67 300+	63 300+	59 300+	52 300+	63 300+
Howard County General Hospital, Columbia, MD	- -	- -	- -	- -	- -	- -	- -	53 300+	75 300+	81 300+	64 300+	54 300+	72 300+	66 300+	70 300+	56 300+	71 300+
Johns Hopkins Bayview Medical Center, Baltimore, MD	- -	- -	- -	- -	- -	- -	- -	48 300+	79 300+	84 300+	66 300+	59 300+	74 300+	63 300+	59 300+	58 300+	69 300+
The Johns Hopkins Hospital, Baltimore, MD	- -	- -	- -	- -	- -	- -	- -	56 300+	79 300+	85 300+	76 300+	62 300+	77 300+	70 300+	65 300+	61 300+	82 300+
Laurel Regional Medical Center, Laurel, MD	- -	- -	- -	- -	- -	- -	- -	52 300+	68 300+	70 300+	44 300+	51 300+	62 300+	58 300+	55 300+	45 300+	44 300+
Maryland General Hospital, Baltimore, MD	- -	- -	- -	- -	- -	- -	- -	61 300+	78 300+	79 300+	57 300+	56 300+	72 300+	62 300+	60 300+	58 300+	56 300+
Memorial Hospital & Med Ctr of Cumberland, Cumberland, MD	- -	- -	- -	0.017 476	0.003 377	- 0	0.0 1	- -	- -	- -	- -	- -	- -	- -	- -	- -	- -
Memorial Hospital at Easton, Easton, MD	- -	- -	- -	- -	- -	- -	- -	57 300+	81 300+	86 300+	70 300+	61 300+	79 300+	72 300+	71 300+	68 300+	68 300+
Mercy Medical Center, Baltimore, MD	- -	- -	- -	- -	- -	- -	- -	59 300+	84 300+	87 300+	72 300+	61 300+	78 300+	73 300+	63 300+	57 300+	74 300+
Meritus Medical Center, Hagerstown, MD	- -	- -	- -	- -	- -	- -	- -	39 300+	73 300+	84 300+	55 300+	59 300+	75 300+	66 300+	68 300+	58 300+	58 300+
Montgomery General Hospital, Olney, MD	- -	- -	- -	- -	- -	- -	- -	45 300+	73 300+	84 300+	58 300+	58 300+	69 300+	60 300+	57 300+	54 300+	64 300+
Northwest Hospital Center, Randallstown, MD	- -	- -	- -	- -	- -	- -	- -	55 300+	71 300+	71 300+	61 300+	55 300+	72 300+	62 300+	62 300+	55 300+	62 300+
Peninsula Regional Medical Center, Salisbury, MD	- -	- -	- -	- -	- -	- -	- -	48 300+	74 300+	81 300+	60 300+	50 300+	70 300+	64 300+	63 300+	51 300+	64 300+
Prince Georges Hospital Center, Cheverly, MD	100 7	0 7	100 7	- -	- -	- -	- -	49 300+	69 300+	73 300+	44 300+	49 300+	60 300+	56 300+	59 300+	39 300+	41 300+
Saint Agnes Hospital, Baltimore, MD	- -	- -	- -	- -	- -	- -	- -	54 300+	78 300+	82 300+	61 300+	56 300+	72 300+	67 300+	56 300+	54 300+	65 300+
Saint Joseph Medical Center, Towson, MD	- -	- -	- -	- -	- -	- -	- -	56 300+	80 300+	80 300+	67 300+	53 300+	74 300+	69 300+	59 300+	60 300+	74 300+
Saint Mary's Hospital, Leonardtown, MD	- -	- -	- -	- -	- -	- -	- -	57 300+	80 300+	81 300+	65 300+	64 300+	80 300+	67 300+	72 300+	63 300+	65 300+
Shady Grove Adventist Hospital, Rockville, MD	- -	- -	- -	- -	- -	- -	- -	51 300+	73 300+	75 300+	51 300+	48 300+	62 300+	58 300+	53 300+	39 300+	57 300+
Sinai Hospital of Baltimore, Baltimore, MD	- -	- -	- -	- -	- -	- -	- -	51 300+	73 300+	78 300+	58 300+	56 300+	70 300+	59 300+	59 300+	51 300+	63 300+
Southern Maryland Hospital Center, Clinton, MD	- -	- -	- -	- -	- -	- -	- -	43 300+	72 300+	71 300+	42 300+	52 300+	66 300+	64 300+	53 300+	52 300+	42 300+
Suburban Hospital, Bethesda, MD	- -	- -	- -	- -	- -	- -	- -	51 300+	79 300+	79 300+	62 300+	58 300+	69 300+	65 300+	63 300+	54 300+	73 300+
Union Hospital of Cecil County, Elkton, MD	- -	- -	- -	- -	- -	- -	- -	57 300+	81 300+	82 300+	68 300+	60 300+	76 300+	67 300+	66 300+	57 300+	65 300+
Union Memorial Hospital, Baltimore, MD	- -	- -	- -	- -	- -	- -	- -	63 300+	81 300+	83 300+	72 300+	59 300+	74 300+	67 300+	68 300+	60 300+	77 300+
University of Maryland Medical Center, Baltimore, MD	- -	- -	- -	- -	- -	- -	- -	53 300+	78 300+	86 300+	67 300+	61 300+	74 300+	67 300+	58 300+	59 300+	73 300+
Upper Chesapeake Medical Center, Bel Air, MD	- -	- -	- -	- -	- -	- -	- -	58 300+	75 300+	83 300+	64 300+	57 300+	75 300+	67 300+	64 300+	56 300+	65 300+
VA Maryland Healthcare System - Baltimore, Baltimore, MD	- -	- -	- -	- -	- -	- -	- -	- -	- -	- -	- -	- -	- -	- -	- -	- -	- -
Washington Adventist Hospital, Takoma Park, MD	- -	- -	- -	- -	- -	- -	- -	47 300+	76 300+	77 300+	53 300+	47 300+	64 300+	58 300+	54 300+	44 300+	60 300+
Western Maryland Regional Medical Center, Cumberland, MD	- -	- -	- -	0.062 1176	0.010 1007	7.4 1400	36.1 183	48 300+	75 300+	83 300+	60 300+	53 300+	71 300+	65 300+	69 300+	61 300+	64 300+
MASSACHUSETTS																	
Adcare Hospital of Worcester, Worcester, MA	- -	- -	- -	- 0	- 0	- 0	- 0	- -	- -	- -	- -	- -	- -	- -	- -	- -	- -
Anna Jaques Hospital, Newburyport, MA	- -	- -	- -	0.041 636	0.009 585	9.4 1792	- 0	50 300+	80 300+	87 300+	62 300+	62 300+	79 300+	74 300+	67 300+	68 300+	70 300+
Athol Memorial Hospital, Athol, MA	- -	- -	- -	- -	- -	- -	- -	- -	- -	- -	- -	- -	- -	- -	- -	- -	- -
Baystate Franklin Medical Center, Greenfield, MA	- -	- -	- -	0.132 705	0.002 419	8.2 575	0.0 2	49 300+	76 300+	85 300+	64 300+	60 300+	77 300+	67 300+	66 300+	64 300+	70 300+
Baystate Mary Lane Hospital, Ware, MA	- -	- -	- -	0.035 230	0.000 149	5.4 298	- 0	64 (a)	80 (a)	88 (a)	73 (a)	63 (a)	81 (a)	72 (a)	76 (a)	73 (a)	75 (a)
Baystate Medical Center, Springfield, MA	100 129	75 129	99 129	0.042 1645	0.001 1406	7.2 1662	27.3 121	42 300+	80 300+	85 300+	65 300+	63 300+	77 300+	69 300+	66 300+	57 300+	75 300+
Bedford VA Medical Center, Bedford, MA	- -	- -	- -	- -	- -	- -	- -	- -	- -	- -	- -	- -	- -	- -	- -	- -	- -
Berkshire Medical Center, Pittsfield, MA	- -	- -	- -	0.090 1989	0.059 1860	5.7 2984	29.3 399	43 300+	76 300+	91 300+	66 300+	58 300+	80 300+	72 300+	76 300+	64 300+	69 300+
Beth Israel Deaconess Hospital - Needham, Needham, MA	- -	- -	- -	0.234 291	0.158 203	10.4 473	27.8 79	50 300+	79 300+	83 300+	72 300+	64 300+	78 300+	69 300+	80 300+	66 300+	78 300+
Beth Israel Deaconess Medical Center, Boston, MA	- -	- -	- -	0.247 2159	0.002 2491	5.8 1884	25.9 282	50 300+	78 300+	87 300+	73 300+	63 300+	77 300+	68 300+	70 300+	58 300+	80 300+
Beverly Hospital Corporation, Beverly, MA	- -	- -	- -	0.060 1246	0.001 998	8.1 3148	22.6 221	48 300+	78 300+	85 300+	68 300+	60 300+	78 300+	74 300+	70 300+	63 300+	74 300+
Boston Medical Center Corporation, Boston, MA	- -	- -	- -	0.065 1366	0.023 1070	6.0 2567	28.2 248	49 300+	80 300+	87 300+	67 300+	61 300+	74 300+	66 300+	68 300+	57 300+	72 300+
Brigham and Women's Hospital, Boston, MA	- -	- -	- -	0.083 2296	0.001 3685	9.5 3398	30.2 394	53 300+	79 300+	88 300+	79 300+	61 300+	79 300+	71 300+	70 300+	65 300+	87 300+
Cambridge Health Alliance, Cambridge, MA	- -	- -	- -	0.196 657	0.003 348	8.4 1396	28.6 119	53 300+	78 300+	86 300+	59 300+	62 300+	72 300+	67 300+	67 300+	57 300+	64 300+
Cape Cod Hospital, Hyannis, MA	- -	- -	- -	0.098 2516	0.018 2213	16.8 3645	31.3 587	51 300+	81 300+	84 300+	76 300+	63 300+	80 300+	72 300+	78 300+	64 300+	81 300+
Carney Hospital, Boston, MA	- -	- -	- -	0.139 482	0.012 346	26.8 895	44.6 101	59 300+	83 300+	87 300+	65 300+	66 300+	80 300+	71 300+	76 300+	68 300+	65 300+
Children's Hospital Boston, Boston, MA	100 364	67 364	100 364	- -	- -	- -	- -	- -	- -	- -	- -	- -	- -	- -	- -	- -	- -
Clinton Hospital Association, Clinton, MA	- -	- -	- -	0.024 126	0.000 63	2.9 342	29.4 17	63 (a)	80 (a)	87 (a)	75 (a)	72 (a)	85 (a)	80 (a)	79 (a)	76 (a)	80 (a)
The Cooley Dickinson Hospital, Northampton, MA	- -	- -	- -	0.055 740	0.000 535	6.4 1628	22.2 234	54 300+	78 300+	86 300+	68 300+	59 300+	75 300+	67 300+	76 300+	63 300+	72 300+
Dana-Farber Cancer Institute, Boston, MA	- -	- -	- -	- -	- -	- -	- -	- -	- -	- -	- -	- -	- -	- -	- -	- -	- -
Emerson Hospital, West Concord, MA	- -	- -	- -	0.055 686	0.002 614	14.5 1698	32.2 205	50 300+	82 300+	86 300+	74 300+	66 300+	81 300+	75 300+	68 300+	64 300+	80 300+
Fairview Hospital, Great Barrington, MA	- -	- -	- -	- -	- -	- -	- -	61 300+	84 300+	88 300+	85 300+	76 300+	87 300+	79 300+	86 300+	84 300+	88 300+
Falmouth Hospital, Falmouth, MA	- -	- -	- -	0.079 1145	0.027 1065	7.9 2764	29.4 289	47 300+	77 300+	85 300+	68 300+	58 300+	77 300+	70 300+	73 300+	61 300+	74 300+
Faulkner Hospital, Boston, MA	- -	- -	- -	0.070 812	0.002 950	13.3 5107	29.0 69	54 300+	84 300+	89 300+	78 300+	63 300+	83 300+	76 300+	73 300+	71 300+	79 300+
Good Samaritan Medical Center, Brockton, MA	- -	- -	- -	0.065 1131	0.001 1024	9.5 1342	36.6 112	47 300+	78 300+	84 300+	62 300+	60 300+	78 300+	68 300+	67 300+	56 300+	66 300+
Hallmark Health System, Melrose, MA	- -	- -	- -	0.110 1549	0.025 1219	10.7 3532	30.3 400	51 300+	81 300+	84 300+	65 300+	61 300+	80 300+	75 300+	67 300+	67 300+	70 300+
Harrington Memorial Hospital, Southbridge, MA	- -	- -	- -	0.235 323	0.037 294	10.4 628	38.1 63	50 300+	78 300+	83 300+	67 300+	61 300+	75 300+	71 300+	79 300+	67 300+	71 300+
Healthalliance Hospitals, Leominster, MA	- -	- -	- -	0.042 601	0.004 520	7.2 1107	- 0	50 300+	79 300+	88 300+	60 300+	62 300+	78 300+	71 300+	72 300+	62 300+	65 300+
Heywood Hospital, Gardner, MA	- -	- -	- -	0.020 301	0.000 292	6.9 596	36.0 136	53 300+	80 300+	86 300+	66 300+	64 300+	77 300+	75 300+	70 300+	64 300+	73 300+
Holy Family Hospital, Methuen, MA	- -	- -	- -	0.410 882	0.031 551	6.4 929	- 0	50 300+	79 300+	83 300+	63 300+	63 300+	77 300+	72 300+	67 300+	63 300+	69 300+
Holyoke Medical Center, Holyoke, MA	- -	- -	- -	0.053 865	0.000 315	6.5 1546	36.0 222	53 300+	75 300+	87 300+	60 300+	59 300+	73 300+	67 300+	75 300+	55 300+	68 300+
Jordan Hospital, Plymouth, MA	- -	- -	- -	0.159 1338	0.012 893	9.8 1832	29.0 255	45 300+	78 300+	80 300+	65 300+	60 300+	73 300+	73 300+	64 300+	63 300+	70 300+
Lahey Clinic Hospital, Burlington, MA	- -	- -	- -	0.208 2824	0.001 2722	10.8 3572	30.8 454	44 300+	77 300+	85 300+	68 300+	61 300+	72 300+	63 300+	65 300+	56 300+	74 300+
Lawrence General Hospital, Lawrence, MA	- -	- -	- -	0.072 782	0.032 467	11.4 729	- 0	50 300+	78 300+	81 300+	57 300+	63 300+	75 300+	72 300+	67 300+	60 300+	68 300+

NOTE: The first number in each column (boldface) is the score, the second number is the number of patients; Please refer to the main entry for footnotes; (a) 100-299

*MEASURES: **Children's Asthma Care:** 33. Received Systemic Corticosteroids; 34. Received Home Management Plan of Care; 35. Received Reliever Medication; **Use of Medical Imaging:** 36. Combination Abdominal CT Scan; 37. Combination Chest CT Scan; 38. Follow-up Mammogram/Ultrasound; 39. MRI for Low Back Pain; **Survey of Patients' Hospital Experiences:** 40. Area Around Room 'Always' Quiet at Night; 41. Doctors 'Always' Communicated Well; 42. Home Recovery Information Given; 43. Hospital Given 9 or 10 on 10 Point Scale; 44. Meds 'Always' Explained Before Given; 45. Nurses 'Always' Communicated Well; 46. Pain 'Always' Well Controlled; 47. Room and Bathroom 'Always' Clean; 48. Timely Help 'Always' Received; 49. Would Definitely Recommend Hospital*

Hospital	Children's Asthma Care			Use of Medical Imaging				Survey of Patients' Hospital Experiences									
	33	34	35	36	37	38	39	40	41	42	43	44	45	46	47	48	49
Lowell General Hospital, Lowell, MA	-	-	-	0.048 1021	0.001 683	8.2 1083	29.2 154	52 300+	78 300+	81 300+	65 300+	60 300+	79 300+	69 300+	68 300+	61 300+	74 300+
Marlborough Hospital, Marlborough, MA	-	-	-	0.050 361	0.000 178	3.3 694	- 0	40 300+	77 300+	85 300+	60 300+	63 300+	75 300+	73 300+	70 300+	59 300+	66 300+
Martha's Vineyard Hospital, Oak Bluffs, MA	-	-	-	-	-	-	-	55 (a)	84 (a)	87 (a)	61 (a)	64 (a)	77 (a)	75 (a)	72 (a)	61 (a)	72 (a)
Massachusetts Eye and Ear Infirmary, Boston, MA	-	-	-	0.000 4	0.000 279	- 0	- 0	44 300+	81 300+	85 300+	67 300+	58 300+	71 300+	72 300+	61 300+	59 300+	78 300+
Massachusetts General Hospital, Boston, MA	-	-	-	0.062 3641	0.001 4973	5.6 6012	27.1 439	50 300+	78 300+	87 300+	78 300+	63 300+	78 300+	70 300+	71 300+	62 300+	88 300+
Mercy Medical Center, Springfield, MA	-	-	-	0.087 1387	0.011 760	12.5 1941	- 0	37 300+	77 300+	86 300+	61 300+	57 300+	72 300+	64 300+	67 300+	57 300+	69 300+
Merrimack Valley Hospital, Haverhill, MA	-	-	-	0.064 498	0.016 372	11.5 1126	36.1 119	46 300+	78 300+	87 300+	64 300+	59 300+	74 300+	70 300+	66 300+	62 300+	63 300+
Metrowest Medical Center, Framingham, MA	-	-	-	0.087 1060	0.006 1024	17.8 2148	- 0	54 300+	80 300+	82 300+	66 300+	62 300+	79 300+	72 300+	72 300+	66 300+	72 300+
Milford Regional Medical Center, Milford, MA	-	-	-	0.089 879	0.001 693	7.1 1520	32.4 207	51 300+	83 300+	88 300+	77 300+	65 300+	82 300+	75 300+	79 300+	67 300+	81 300+
Milton Hospital, Milton, MA	-	-	-	0.167 408	0.000 243	5.2 878	30.2 149	52 300+	80 300+	81 300+	66 300+	60 300+	75 300+	67 300+	72 300+	60 300+	72 300+
Morton Hospital & Medical Center, Taunton, MA	-	-	-	0.036 831	0.003 642	6.3 1926	29.6 152	49 300+	78 300+	83 300+	57 300+	60 300+	75 300+	70 300+	72 300+	62 300+	57 300+
Mount Auburn Hospital, Cambridge, MA	-	-	-	0.127 938	0.000 627	6.9 1618	32.4 290	50 300+	80 300+	85 300+	71 300+	64 300+	80 300+	73 300+	72 300+	68 300+	77 300+
Nantucket Cottage Hospital, Nantucket, MA	-	-	-	0.055 110	0.000 73	3.7 134	25.8 31	65 <100	88 <100	74 <100	74 <100	61 <100	84 <100	78 <100	73 <100	87 <100	82 <100
Nashoba Valley Medical Center, Ayer, MA	-	-	-	0.160 338	0.011 186	18.5 351	29.3 58	62 300+	79 300+	87 300+	67 300+	59 300+	78 300+	76 300+	77 300+	59 300+	72 300+
New England Baptist Hospital, Boston, MA	-	-	-	0.040 329	0.021 284	- 0	28.1 484	50 300+	82 300+	93 300+	84 300+	64 300+	84 300+	71 300+	78 300+	70 300+	91 300+
Newton-Wellesley Hospital, Newton, MA	-	-	-	0.097 1181	0.003 1135	11.0 2613	28.9 159	55 300+	82 300+	87 300+	72 300+	63 300+	78 300+	71 300+	76 300+	63 300+	81 300+
Noble Hospital, Westfield, MA	-	-	-	0.018 439	0.000 234	10.9 832	33.3 78	52 300+	80 300+	90 300+	67 300+	63 300+	79 300+	76 300+	78 300+	71 300+	69 300+
North Adams Regional Hospital, North Adams, MA	-	-	-	0.149 609	0.009 555	4.5 1369	36.1 133	56 300+	81 300+	89 300+	65 300+	64 300+	79 300+	73 300+	77 300+	65 300+	70 300+
North Shore Medical Center, Salem, MA	-	-	-	0.091 2380	0.001 2048	8.5 5237	31.5 375	53 300+	76 300+	85 300+	66 300+	60 300+	75 300+	70 300+	69 300+	63 300+	74 300+
Northampton VA Medical Center, Leeds, MA	-	-	-	-	-	-	-	-	-	-	-	-	-	-	-	-	-
Norwood Hospital, Norwood, MA	-	-	-	0.078 605	0.002 444	18.8 704	28.0 25	41 300+	80 300+	83 300+	63 300+	62 300+	79 300+	74 300+	75 300+	65 300+	64 300+
Quincy Medical Center, Quincy, MA	-	-	-	0.067 751	0.016 435	4.7 975	- 0	44 300+	73 300+	85 300+	59 300+	59 300+	74 300+	72 300+	70 300+	59 300+	61 300+
Saint Anne's Hospital, Fall River, MA	-	-	-	0.072 666	0.003 587	8.2 1299	29.8 104	52 300+	78 300+	86 300+	66 300+	61 300+	79 300+	69 300+	75 300+	63 300+	72 300+
Saint Elizabeth's Medical Center, Brighton, MA	-	-	-	0.169 709	0.005 745	9.3 1072	39.1 174	52 300+	81 300+	83 300+	68 300+	65 300+	77 300+	71 300+	73 300+	63 300+	73 300+
Saint Vincent Hospital, Worcester, MA	-	-	-	0.035 606	0.000 431	7.2 377	17.6 74	44 300+	78 300+	84 300+	70 300+	59 300+	73 300+	72 300+	69 300+	59 300+	76 300+
Saints Medical Center, Lowell, MA	-	-	-	0.191 770	0.002 507	9.4 1155	- 0	57 300+	81 300+	87 300+	68 300+	61 300+	78 300+	73 300+	76 300+	65 300+	72 300+
Signature Healthcare Brockton Hospital, Brockton, MA	-	-	-	0.057 714	0.030 535	9.8 860	38.5 104	41 300+	76 300+	85 300+	60 300+	58 300+	76 300+	67 300+	69 300+	63 300+	65 300+
Soldiers Home in Massachusetts, Chelsea, MA	-	-	-	- 0	- 0	- 0	- 0	-	-	-	-	-	-	-	-	-	-
South Shore Hospital, South Weymouth, MA	-	-	-	0.105 1304	0.042 945	9.7 1772	30.2 139	52 300+	79 300+	88 300+	69 300+	65 300+	78 300+	70 300+	73 300+	65 300+	74 300+
Southcoast Hospital Group, Fall River, MA	-	-	-	0.075 2982	0.005 2408	10.0 6895	29.9 298	51 300+	79 300+	86 300+	62 300+	59 300+	75 300+	67 300+	73 300+	58 300+	68 300+
Sturdy Memorial Hospital, Attleboro, MA	-	-	-	0.078 838	0.105 466	8.3 1840	26.6 263	47 300+	78 300+	86 300+	67 300+	60 300+	76 300+	70 300+	78 300+	61 300+	72 300+
Tufts Medical Center, Boston, MA	-	-	-	0.242 829	0.005 971	1.1 1042	23.6 144	55 300+	80 300+	85 300+	70 300+	61 300+	79 300+	67 300+	68 300+	60 300+	77 300+
UMass Memorial Medical Center, Worcester, MA	-	-	-	0.135 2202	0.006 1687	6.8 2418	- 0	45 300+	74 300+	88 300+	66 300+	59 300+	72 300+	65 300+	60 300+	55 300+	75 300+
VA Boston Healthcare System - Jamaica Plain, Jamaica Plain, MA	-	-	-	-	-	-	-	-	-	-	-	-	-	-	-	-	-
Winchester Hospital, Winchester, MA	-	-	-	0.070 1193	0.000 1052	9.4 2478	30.3 228	49 300+	81 300+	84 300+	75 300+	65 300+	80 300+	71 300+	73 300+	67 300+	81 300+
Wing Memorial Hospital and Medical Center, Palmer, MA	-	-	-	0.056 444	0.002 442	5.2 639	- 0	58 300+	83 300+	89 300+	71 300+	62 300+	79 300+	73 300+	75 300+	66 300+	77 300+
NEW HAMPSHIRE																	
Alice Peck Day Memorial Hospital, Lebanon, NH	-	-	-	-	-	-	-	-	-	-	-	-	-	-	-	-	-
Androscoggin Valley Hospital, Berlin, NH	-	-	-	-	-	-	-	49 (a)	81 (a)	83 (a)	61 (a)	63 (a)	78 (a)	64 (a)	79 (a)	72 (a)	58 (a)
Catholic Medical Center, Manchester, NH	-	-	-	0.071 688	0.008 487	11.9 1641	33.0 176	57 300+	79 300+	86 300+	70 300+	64 300+	81 300+	69 300+	70 300+	67 300+	76 300+
Cheshire Medical Center, Keene, NH	-	-	-	0.011 620	0.000 564	3.8 1331	31.6 206	47 300+	80 300+	86 300+	67 300+	62 300+	78 300+	70 300+	79 300+	64 300+	68 300+
Concord Hospital, Concord, NH	-	-	-	0.139 743	0.046 439	8.1 713	27.3 99	62 300+	82 300+	87 300+	78 300+	65 300+	82 300+	71 300+	75 300+	69 300+	82 300+
Cottage Hospital, Woodsville, NH	-	-	-	-	-	-	-	-	-	-	-	-	-	-	-	-	-
Elliot Hospital, Manchester, NH	-	-	-	0.091 950	0.000 701	5.5 1924	32.9 359	50 300+	77 300+	85 300+	68 300+	62 300+	77 300+	72 300+	73 300+	62 300+	76 300+
Exeter Hospital, Exeter, NH	-	-	-	0.068 841	0.016 825	3.8 1950	24.5 192	51 300+	82 300+	89 300+	77 300+	62 300+	81 300+	75 300+	72 300+	71 300+	79 300+
Franklin Regional Hospital, Franklin, NH	-	-	-	0.013 156	0.000 141	6.2 307	24.1 29	57 (a)	71 (a)	79 (a)	63 (a)	61 (a)	71 (a)	65 (a)	79 (a)	63 (a)	60 (a)
Frisbie Memorial Hospital, Rochester, NH	-	-	-	0.054 633	0.000 586	- 0	31.5 92	66 300+	78 300+	87 300+	69 300+	65 300+	79 300+	71 300+	83 300+	74 300+	73 300+
Huggins Hospital, Wolfeboro, NH	-	-	-	-	-	-	-	51 300+	78 300+	84 300+	62 300+	60 300+	77 300+	75 300+	73 300+	63 300+	64 300+
Lakes Region General Hospital, Laconia, NH	-	-	-	0.061 727	0.000 623	6.1 1315	35.6 236	49 300+	76 300+	86 300+	63 300+	55 300+	71 300+	64 300+	69 300+	59 300+	58 300+
Littleton Regional Hospital, Littleton, NH	-	-	-	-	-	-	-	55 (a)	84 (a)	90 (a)	69 (a)	62 (a)	74 (a)	70 (a)	77 (a)	67 (a)	68 (a)
Mary Hitchcock Memorial Hospital, Lebanon, NH	-	-	-	0.052 1772	0.001 1847	7.5 2249	27.5 454	40 300+	80 300+	87 300+	78 300+	63 300+	78 300+	68 300+	71 300+	73 300+	84 300+
The Memorial Hospital, North Conway, NH	-	-	-	-	-	-	-	-	-	-	-	-	-	-	-	-	-
Monadnock Community Hospital, Peterborough, NH	-	-	-	0.057 283	0.004 246	11.8 621	22.4 58	58 300+	87 300+	88 300+	79 300+	71 300+	86 300+	76 300+	82 300+	80 300+	81 300+
New London Hospital, New London, NH	-	-	-	0.095 221	0.000 145	8.8 909	47.2 53	65 (a)	81 (a)	79 (a)	71 (a)	58 (a)	78 (a)	69 (a)	84 (a)	75 (a)	75 (a)
Parkland Medical Center, Derry, NH	-	-	-	0.072 304	0.021 191	8.7 358	21.9 32	60 300+	81 300+	90 300+	71 300+	68 300+	82 300+	75 300+	82 300+	76 300+	71 300+
Portsmouth Regional Hospital, Portsmouth, NH	-	-	-	0.081 595	0.000 392	10.8 1479	24.7 194	55 300+	81 300+	90 300+	68 300+	57 300+	75 300+	69 300+	72 300+	62 300+	72 300+
Saint Joseph Hospital, Nashua, NH	-	-	-	0.078 703	0.000 583	7.8 1620	31.3 144	61 300+	77 300+	86 300+	70 300+	62 300+	81 300+	75 300+	75 300+	64 300+	75 300+
Southern Nh Medical Center, Nashua, NH	-	-	-	0.080 537	0.005 372	6.4 1695	30.1 173	58 300+	80 300+	89 300+	74 300+	66 300+	80 300+	72 300+	70 300+	64 300+	79 300+
Speare Memorial Hospital, Plymouth, NH	-	-	-	0.056 248	0.000 182	7.5 571	49.0 49	56 300+	87 300+	91 300+	75 300+	68 300+	86 300+	77 300+	86 300+	78 300+	80 300+
Upper Connecticut Valley Hospital, Colebrook, NH	-	-	-	0.213 80	0.135 52	2.8 181	- 0	-	-	-	-	-	-	-	-	-	-
Valley Regional Hospital, Claremont, NH	-	-	-	-	-	-	-	-	-	-	-	-	-	-	-	-	-
Weeks Medical Center, Lancaster, NH	-	-	-	0.594 175	0.133 83	3.4 294	65.9 44	-	-	-	-	-	-	-	-	-	-
Wentworth-Douglass Hospital, Dover, NH	-	-	-	0.037 848	0.001 725	- 0	30.9 178	56 300+	79 300+	93 300+	73 300+	64 300+	81 300+	75 300+	81 300+	69 300+	80 300+
NEW JERSEY																	
Atlanticare Regional Medical Center - City Division, Atlantic City, NJ	-	-	-	0.040 805	0.100 329	5.3 891	19.2 73	48 300+	75 300+	89 300+	66 300+	58 300+	75 300+	64 300+	66 300+	59 300+	72 300+
Bayonne Hospital Center, Bayonne, NJ	-	-	-	0.099 779	0.037 813	5.7 795	26.2 141	49 300+	76 300+	79 300+	47 300+	51 300+	67 300+	62 300+	60 300+	52 300+	38 300+
Bayshore Community Hospital, Holmdel, NJ	-	-	-	0.058 866	0.010 629	11.1 948	29.0 100	48 300+	76 300+	79 300+	53 300+	43 300+	69 300+	64 300+	58 300+	50 300+	54 300+

NOTE: The first number in each column (boldface) is the score, the second number is the number of patients; Please refer to the main entry for footnotes; (a) 100-299
*MEASURES: **Children's Asthma Care:** 33. Received Systemic Corticosteroids; 34. Received Home Management Plan of Care; 35. Received Reliever Medication; **Use of Medical Imaging:** 36. Combination Abdominal CT Scan; 37. Combination Chest CT Scan; 38. Follow-up Mammogram/Ultrasound; 39. MRI for Low Back Pain; **Survey of Patients' Hospital Experiences:** 40. Area Around Room 'Always' Quiet at Night; 41. Doctors 'Always' Communicated Well; 42. Home Recovery Information Given; 43. Hospital Given 9 or 10 on 10 Point Scale; 44. Meds 'Always' Explained Before Given; 45. Nurses 'Always' Communicated Well; 46. Pain 'Always' Well Controlled; 47. Room and Bathroom 'Always' Clean; 48. Timely Help 'Always' Received; 49. Would Definitely Recommend Hospital*

Hospital	Children's Asthma Care			Use of Medical Imaging				Survey of Patients' Hospital Experiences									
	33	34	35	36	37	38	39	40	41	42	43	44	45	46	47	48	49
Bergen Regional Medical Center, Paramus, NJ	- -	- -	- -	**0.167** 48	**0.051** 39	**8.0** 87	**42.9** 7	**38** (a)	**55** (a)	**63** (a)	**32** (a)	**43** (a)	**48** (a)	**47** (a)	**50** (a)	**35** (a)	**41** (a)
Cape Regional Medical Center, Cape May Ct Hse, NJ	- -	- -	- -	**0.433** 559	**0.004** 242	**12.9** 326	**31.9** 47	**49** 300+	**77** 300+	**79** 300+	**63** 300+	**62** 300+	**78** 300+	**71** 300+	**70** 300+	**63** 300+	**66** 300+
Capital Health System - Mercer Campus, Trenton, NJ	- -	- -	- -	**0.108** 623	**0.044** 520	**5.9** 1215	**30.8** 26	**61** 300+	**82** 300+	**77** 300+	**63** 300+	**61** 300+	**77** 300+	**66** 300+	**71** 300+	**56** 300+	**65** 300+
Capital Health System-Fuld Campus, Trenton, NJ	- -	- -	- -	**0.079** 430	**0.083** 314	**6.4** 251	**18.2** 66	**45** 300+	**77** 300+	**74** 300+	**58** 300+	**57** 300+	**73** 300+	**65** 300+	**69** 300+	**57** 300+	**62** 300+
Centrastate Medical Center, Freehold, NJ	- -	- -	- -	**0.073** 757	**0.003** 591	**9.8** 784	**0.0** 1	**52** 300+	**76** 300+	**80** 300+	**69** 300+	**60** 300+	**74** 300+	**65** 300+	**72** 300+	**61** 300+	**72** 300+
Chilton Hospital, Pompton Plains, NJ	- -	- -	- -	**0.569** 1053	**0.006** 780	**12.0** 1959	**23.7** 207	**45** 300+	**77** 300+	**76** 300+	**61** 300+	**55** 300+	**76** 300+	**70** 300+	**62** 300+	**63** 300+	**66** 300+
Christ Hospital, Jersey City, NJ	- -	- -	- -	**0.078** 709	**0.003** 343	**12.5** 184	**0.0** 1	**58** (a)	**74** (a)	**72** (a)	**54** (a)	**49** (a)	**66** (a)	**62** (a)	**62** (a)	**53** (a)	**61** (a)
Clara Maass Medical Center, Belleville, NJ	- -	- -	- -	**0.101** 526	**0.034** 232	**13.9** 374	**0.0** 5	**50** 300+	**78** 300+	**72** 300+	**54** 300+	**57** 300+	**72** 300+	**67** 300+	**66** 300+	**58** 300+	**59** 300+
Community Medical Center, Toms River, NJ	- -	- -	- -	**0.036** 1131	**0.005** 635	**7.8** 902	**41.1** 56	**48** 300+	**76** 300+	**80** 300+	**57** 300+	**60** 300+	**75** 300+	**69** 300+	**63** 300+	**61** 300+	**61** 300+
Cooper University Hospital, Camden, NJ	- -	- -	- -	**0.045** 1051	**0.008** 914	**12.1** 1293	**34.6** 127	**53** 300+	**77** 300+	**82** 300+	**65** 300+	**57** 300+	**71** 300+	**64** 300+	**64** 300+	**57** 300+	**70** 300+
Deborah Heart and Lung Center, Browns Mills, NJ	- -	- -	- -	**0.043** 47	**0.013** 635	**-** 0	**-** 0	**62** 300+	**81** 300+	**88** 300+	**82** 300+	**63** 300+	**82** 300+	**73** 300+	**76** 300+	**69** 300+	**87** 300+
East Orange General Hospital, East Orange, NJ	- -	- -	- -	**0.483** 203	**0.033** 121	**8.1** 395	**-** 0	**57** 300+	**76** 300+	**74** 300+	**51** 300+	**54** 300+	**69** 300+	**64** 300+	**65** 300+	**54** 300+	**50** 300+
Englewood Hospital and Medical Center, Englewood, NJ	- -	- -	- -	**0.183** 1560	**0.008** 1105	**13.9** 2429	**23.4** 231	**52** 300+	**79** 300+	**74** 300+	**67** 300+	**56** 300+	**74** 300+	**68** 300+	**74** 300+	**54** 300+	**73** 300+
Hackensack University Medical Center, Hackensack, NJ	- -	- -	- -	**0.088** 2096	**0.051** 2549	**8.4** 2174	**23.2** 95	**49** 300+	**78** 300+	**81** 300+	**72** 300+	**59** 300+	**77** 300+	**69** 300+	**72** 300+	**59** 300+	**80** 300+
Hackettstown Regional Medical Center, Hackettstown, NJ	- -	- -	- -	**0.083** 493	**0.012** 253	**14.5** 512	**25.9** 54	**49** 300+	**78** 300+	**83** 300+	**67** 300+	**53** 300+	**75** 300+	**64** 300+	**67** 300+	**59** 300+	**69** 300+
Hoboken University Medical Center, Hoboken, NJ	- -	- -	- -	**0.101** 367	**0.046** 217	**9.6** 374	**22.2** 36	**47** 300+	**81** 300+	**81** 300+	**61** 300+	**54** 300+	**72** 300+	**68** 300+	**62** 300+	**59** 300+	**66** 300+
Holy Name Medical Center, Teaneck, NJ	- -	- -	- -	**0.110** 1103	**0.059** 828	**26.0** 1067	**25.3** 312	**52** 300+	**80** 300+	**81** 300+	**67** 300+	**55** 300+	**74** 300+	**67** 300+	**67** 300+	**53** 300+	**75** 300+
Hunterdon Medical Center, Flemington, NJ	- -	- -	- -	**0.069** 737	**0.018** 832	**12.5** 576	**-** 0	**47** 300+	**80** 300+	**84** 300+	**71** 300+	**61** 300+	**79** 300+	**72** 300+	**73** 300+	**64** 300+	**75** 300+
Jersey Shore University Medical Center, Neptune, NJ	- -	- -	- -	**0.061** 1271	**0.003** 1053	**10.3** 545	**27.3** 88	**58** 300+	**78** 300+	**77** 300+	**69** 300+	**60** 300+	**79** 300+	**72** 300+	**69** 300+	**64** 300+	**75** 300+
JFK Medical Center, Edison, NJ	- -	- -	- -	**0.618** 1192	**0.002** 1081	**9.6** 1516	**20.4** 147	**43** 300+	**78** 300+	**76** 300+	**54** 300+	**55** 300+	**72** 300+	**66** 300+	**69** 300+	**51** 300+	**56** 300+
Kennedy University Hospital, Stratford, NJ	- -	- -	- -	**0.047** 1770	**0.007** 995	**11.0** 836	**24.4** 90	**45** 300+	**74** 300+	**77** 300+	**56** 300+	**56** 300+	**75** 300+	**66** 300+	**67** 300+	**57** 300+	**59** 300+
Kimball Medical Center, Lakewood, NJ	- -	- -	- -	**0.383** 686	**0.088** 669	**-** 0	**28.3** 106	**50** 300+	**76** 300+	**81** 300+	**54** 300+	**51** 300+	**71** 300+	**69** 300+	**65** 300+	**54** 300+	**52** 300+
Libertyhealth-Jersey City Medical Center Campus, Jersey City, NJ	- -	- -	- -	**0.015** 199	**0.000** 94	**-** 0	**25.0** 24	**57** 300+	**77** 300+	**76** 300+	**62** 300+	**56** 300+	**70** 300+	**65** 300+	**70** 300+	**53** 300+	**67** 300+
Lourdes Medical Center of Burlington County, Willingboro, NJ	- -	- -	- -	**0.014** 576	**0.000** 281	**11.1** 587	**18.2** 22	**49** 300+	**68** 300+	**70** 300+	**46** 300+	**48** 300+	**65** 300+	**63** 300+	**59** 300+	**55** 300+	**47** 300+
Meadowlands Hospital Medical Center, Secaucus, NJ	- -	- -	- -	**0.196** 107	**0.027** 75	**5.6** 125	**-** 0	**62** 300+	**80** 300+	**75** 300+	**62** 300+	**59** 300+	**76** 300+	**74** 300+	**78** 300+	**64** 300+	**68** 300+
Memorial Hospital of Salem County, Salem, NJ	- -	- -	- -	**0.072** 359	**0.012** 258	**7.3** 357	**33.3** 69	**58** 300+	**75** 300+	**79** 300+	**52** 300+	**57** 300+	**70** 300+	**63** 300+	**59** 300+	**53** 300+	**46** 300+
Monmouth Medical Center, Long Branch, NJ	- -	- -	- -	**0.094** 757	**0.047** 770	**7.2** 2020	**29.9** 87	**46** 300+	**75** 300+	**72** 300+	**54** 300+	**55** 300+	**69** 300+	**61** 300+	**58** 300+	**50** 300+	**62** 300+
Morristown Memorial Hospital, Morristown, NJ	- -	- -	- -	**0.020** 1618	**0.030** 1505	**20.1** 648	**21.2** 52	**55** 300+	**77** 300+	**81** 300+	**75** 300+	**59** 300+	**76** 300+	**70** 300+	**73** 300+	**56** 300+	**81** 300+
Mountainside Hospital, Montclair, NJ	- -	- -	- -	**0.109** 724	**0.061** 410	**11.8** 415	**38.3** 47	**51** 300+	**80** 300+	**71** 300+	**60** 300+	**57** 300+	**73** 300+	**66** 300+	**65** 300+	**55** 300+	**62** 300+
Newark Beth Israel Medical Center, Newark, NJ	- -	- -	- -	**0.444** 532	**0.020** 547	**6.7** 741	**41.3** 63	**60** 300+	**81** 300+	**79** 300+	**62** 300+	**59** 300+	**74** 300+	**68** 300+	**65** 300+	**58** 300+	**66** 300+
Newton Memorial Hospital, Newton, NJ	- -	- -	- -	**0.038** 653	**0.010** 419	**10.3** 398	**-** 0	**44** 300+	**72** 300+	**80** 300+	**63** 300+	**52** 300+	**76** 300+	**68** 300+	**76** 300+	**60** 300+	**66** 300+
Ocean Medical Center, Brick, NJ	- -	- -	- -	**0.106** 1172	**0.006** 927	**13.2** 816	**19.5** 82	**52** 300+	**73** 300+	**79** 300+	**66** 300+	**58** 300+	**77** 300+	**72** 300+	**71** 300+	**58** 300+	**68** 300+
Our Lady of Lourdes Medical Center, Camden, NJ	- -	- -	- -	**0.139** 592	**0.098** 224	**19.0** 210	**33.3** 21	**45** 300+	**71** 300+	**75** 300+	**62** 300+	**54** 300+	**71** 300+	**61** 300+	**56** 300+	**50** 300+	**65** 300+
Overlook Hospital, Summit, NJ	- -	- -	- -	**0.079** 1249	**0.055** 1183	**20.0** 828	**25.9** 85	**51** 300+	**77** 300+	**81** 300+	**66** 300+	**54** 300+	**75** 300+	**67** 300+	**66** 300+	**55** 300+	**73** 300+
Palisades Medical Center, North Bergen, NJ	- -	- -	- -	**0.081** 492	**0.000** 291	**9.3** 421	**33.8** 65	**45** 300+	**76** 300+	**74** 300+	**50** 300+	**46** 300+	**60** 300+	**56** 300+	**62** 300+	**44** 300+	**53** 300+
Raritan Bay Medical Center, Perth Amboy, NJ	- -	- -	- -	**0.047** 761	**0.000** 409	**4.1** 880	**35.5** 31	**52** 300+	**76** 300+	**77** 300+	**57** 300+	**54** 300+	**74** 300+	**65** 300+	**65** 300+	**58** 300+	**60** 300+
Riverview Medical Center, Red Bank, NJ	- -	- -	- -	**0.073** 1238	**0.014** 915	**16.2** 582	**19.3** 83	**52** 300+	**79** 300+	**81** 300+	**63** 300+	**61** 300+	**76** 300+	**70** 300+	**70** 300+	**61** 300+	**71** 300+
Robert Wood Johnson University Hospital, New Brunswick, NJ	- -	- -	- -	**0.018** 709	**0.002** 473	**17.7** 379	**33.3** 27	**49** 300+	**78** 300+	**81** 300+	**68** 300+	**59** 300+	**76** 300+	**68** 300+	**65** 300+	**62** 300+	**75** 300+
Robert Wood Johnson University Hospital at Rahway, Rahway, NJ	- -	- -	- -	**0.101** 513	**0.023** 440	**9.4** 266	**14.0** 86	**48** 300+	**75** 300+	**78** 300+	**56** 300+	**56** 300+	**71** 300+	**66** 300+	**69** 300+	**55** 300+	**58** 300+
Robert Wood Johnson University Hospital Hamilton, Hamilton, NJ	- -	- -	- -	**0.042** 983	**0.017** 783	**10.7** 1096	**29.6** 108	**56** 300+	**78** 300+	**83** 300+	**64** 300+	**58** 300+	**74** 300+	**67** 300+	**69** 300+	**59** 300+	**68** 300+
Saint Barnabas Medical Center, Livingston, NJ	- -	- -	- -	**0.071** 764	**0.071** 324	**-** 0	**20.8** 24	**49** 300+	**77** 300+	**76** 300+	**64** 300+	**60** 300+	**74** 300+	**67** 300+	**64** 300+	**54** 300+	**72** 300+
Saint Clare's Hospital, Denville, NJ	- -	- -	- -	**0.087** 1911	**0.011** 1398	**12.5** 2620	**-** 0	**50** 300+	**77** 300+	**78** 300+	**60** 300+	**54** 300+	**73** 300+	**65** 300+	**63** 300+	**56** 300+	**66** 300+
Saint Clare's Hospital - Sussex, Sussex, NJ	- -	- -	- -	**0.018** 166	**0.000** 83	**9.7** 155	**-** 0	**54** (a)	**81** (a)	**77** (a)	**69** (a)	**61** (a)	**77** (a)	**69** (a)	**76** (a)	**67** (a)	**67** (a)
Saint Francis Medical Center, Trenton, NJ	- -	- -	- -	**0.081** 347	**0.022** 225	**6.3** 457	**26.1** 23	**44** 300+	**75** 300+	**77** 300+	**56** 300+	**52** 300+	**72** 300+	**65** 300+	**66** 300+	**56** 300+	**58** 300+
Saint Joseph's Regional Medical Center, Paterson, NJ	- -	- -	- -	**0.105** 1029	**0.041** 582	**5.2** 1132	**27.6** 196	**45** 300+	**73** 300+	**80** 300+	**57** 300+	**52** 300+	**67** 300+	**62** 300+	**65** 300+	**49** 300+	**64** 300+
Saint Joseph's Wayne Hospital, Wayne, NJ	- -	- -	- -	- -	- -	- -	- -	- -	- -	- -	- -	- -	- -	- -	- -	- -	- -
Saint Mary's Hospital - Passaic, Passaic, NJ	- -	- -	- -	**0.107** 626	**0.003** 384	**9.1** 729	**35.2** 54	**48** 300+	**78** 300+	**73** 300+	**47** 300+	**49** 300+	**67** 300+	**65** 300+	**64** 300+	**50** 300+	**49** 300+
Saint Michael's Medical Center, Newark, NJ	- -	- -	- -	**0.060** 500	**0.010** 305	**8.4** 645	**13.6** 44	**55** 300+	**75** 300+	**69** 300+	**53** 300+	**49** 300+	**62** 300+	**56** 300+	**62** 300+	**50** 300+	**54** 300+
Saint Peter's University Hospital, New Brunswick, NJ	- -	- -	- -	**0.017** 348	**0.000** 184	**18.0** 294	**22.2** 18	**55** 300+	**78** 300+	**76** 300+	**68** 300+	**62** 300+	**77** 300+	**70** 300+	**77** 300+	**64** 300+	**76** 300+
Shore Memorial Hospital, Somers Point, NJ	- -	- -	- -	**0.512** 484	**0.043** 278	**16.5** 704	**17.1** 41	**51** 300+	**80** 300+	**82** 300+	**67** 300+	**58** 300+	**75** 300+	**73** 300+	**67** 300+	**61** 300+	**74** 300+
Somerset Medical Center, Somerville, NJ	- -	- -	- -	**0.381** 788	**0.008** 634	**10.8** 800	**28.4** 116	**46** 300+	**77** 300+	**73** 300+	**60** 300+	**56** 300+	**74** 300+	**72** 300+	**71** 300+	**56** 300+	**67** 300+
South Jersey Healthcare Regional Med Ctr, Vineland, NJ	- -	- -	- -	**0.138** 898	**0.041** 559	**6.1** 1487	**33.9** 115	**59** 300+	**77** 300+	**83** 300+	**65** 300+	**57** 300+	**73** 300+	**67** 300+	**71** 300+	**62** 300+	**64** 300+
South Jersey Healthcare-Elmer Hospital, Elmer, NJ	- -	- -	- -	**0.132** 349	**0.017** 299	**6.8** 657	**33.3** 12	**55** 300+	**81** 300+	**86** 300+	**73** 300+	**61** 300+	**80** 300+	**73** 300+	**77** 300+	**69** 300+	**80** 300+
Southern Ocean Medical Center, Manahawkin, NJ	- -	- -	- -	**0.058** 712	**0.055** 343	**12.1** 2049	**32.7** 55	**52** 300+	**80** 300+	**82** 300+	**64** 300+	**63** 300+	**81** 300+	**74** 300+	**70** 300+	**71** 300+	**65** 300+
Trinitas Regional Medical Center, Elizabeth, NJ	- -	- -	- -	**0.032** 563	**0.017** 475	**6.1** 1048	**25.0** 64	**56** 300+	**80** 300+	**74** 300+	**62** 300+	**57** 300+	**75** 300+	**64** 300+	**73** 300+	**59** 300+	**59** 300+
UMDNJ University Hospital, Newark, NJ	- -	- -	- -	**0.332** 617	**0.046** 261	**10.7** 513	**8.9** 56	**55** 300+	**78** 300+	**78** 300+	**58** 300+	**55** 300+	**67** 300+	**65** 300+	**62** 300+	**53** 300+	**61** 300+
Underwood Memorial Hospital, Woodbury, NJ	- -	- -	- -	**0.061** 589	**0.083** 278	**18.6** 161	**-** 0	**51** 300+	**75** 300+	**79** 300+	**60** 300+	**61** 300+	**78** 300+	**68** 300+	**70** 300+	**63** 300+	**59** 300+
University Medical Center at Princeton, Princeton, NJ	- -	- -	- -	**0.140** 769	**0.014** 499	**12.9** 528	**25.5** 55	**48** 300+	**77** 300+	**79** 300+	**60** 300+	**57** 300+	**71** 300+	**67** 300+	**61** 300+	**54** 300+	**67** 300+
VA New Jersey Health Care System, East Orange, NJ	- -	- -	- -	- -	- -	- -	- -	- -	- -	- -	- -	- -	- -	- -	- -	- -	- -
Valley Hospital, Ridgewood, NJ	- -	- -	- -	**0.106** 2036	**0.016** 2050	**8.7** 1605	**28.4** 211	**54** 300+	**80** 300+	**80** 300+	**76** 300+	**58** 300+	**82** 300+	**74** 300+	**80** 300+	**65** 300+	**82** 300+
Virtua Memorial Hospital of Burlington County, Mount Holly, NJ	- -	- -	- -	**0.016** 808	**0.000** 321	**11.2** 322	**28.3** 46	**50** 300+	**78** 300+	**82** 300+	**68** 300+	**61** 300+	**78** 300+	**70** 300+	**64** 300+	**58** 300+	**71** 300+
Virtua West Jersey Hospitals Berlin, Berlin, NJ	- -	- -	- -	**0.050** 966	**0.038** 529	**14.5** 152	**21.3** 61	**47** 300+	**75** 300+	**78** 300+	**66** 300+	**58** 300+	**79** 300+	**71** 300+	**70** 300+	**62** 300+	**72** 300+
Warren Hospital, Phillipsburg, NJ	- -	- -	- -	**0.068** 799	**0.042** 520	**6.7** 1082	**32.9** 143	**50** 300+	**77** 300+	**78** 300+	**57** 300+	**57** 300+	**76** 300+	**70** 300+	**70** 300+	**56** 300+	**55** 300+
NEW YORK																	
Adirondack Medical Center, Saranac Lake, NY	- -	- -	- -	**0.674** 344	**0.677** 303	**18.5** 853	**24.2** 33	**60** 300+	**82** 300+	**82** 300+	**69** 300+	**66** 300+	**77** 300+	**72** 300+	**73** 300+	**72** 300+	**75** 300+
Albany Medical Center - South Clinical Campus, Albany, NY	- -	- -	- -	**0.252** 246	**0.007** 137	**13.0** 693	**36.4** 22	- -	- -	- -	- -	- -	- -	- -	- -	- -	- -
Albany Medical Center Hospital, Albany, NY	- -	- -	- -	**0.124** 707	**0.004** 512	**-** 0	**32.8** 58	**44** 300+	**67** 300+	**81** 300+	**57** 300+	**53** 300+	**67** 300+	**64** 300+	**64** 300+	**53** 300+	**67** 300+

NOTE: The first number in each column (boldface) is the score, the second number is the number of patients; Please refer to the main entry for footnotes; (a) 100-299

*MEASURES: **Children's Asthma Care:** 33. Received Systemic Corticosteroids; 34. Received Home Management Plan of Care; 35. Received Reliever Medication; **Use of Medical Imaging:** 36. Combination Abdominal CT Scan; 37. Combination Chest CT Scan; 38. Follow-up Mammogram/Ultrasound; 39. MRI for Low Back Pain; **Survey of Patients' Hospital Experiences:** 40. Area Around Room 'Always' Quiet at Night; 41. Doctors 'Always' Communicated Well; 42. Home Recovery Information Given; 43. Hospital Given 9 or 10 on 10 Point Scale; 44. Meds 'Always' Explained Before Given; 45. Nurses 'Always' Communicated Well; 46. Pain 'Always' Well Controlled; 47. Room and Bathroom 'Always' Clean; 48. Timely Help 'Always' Received; 49. Would Definitely Recommend Hospital*

Hospital	Children's Asthma Care			Use of Medical Imaging				Survey of Patients' Hospital Experiences									
	33	34	35	36	37	38	39	40	41	42	43	44	45	46	47	48	49
Albany Memorial Hospital, Albany, NY	-	-	-	**0.038** 555	**0.000** 288	**6.2** 1097	**23.2** 95	**53** 300+	**76** 300+	**85** 300+	**66** 300+	**54** 300+	**74** 300+	**70** 300+	**70** 300+	**59** 300+	**71** 300+
Albany VA Medical Center, Albany, NY	-	-	-	-	-	-	-	-	-	-	-	-	-	-	-	-	-
Alice Hyde Medical Center, Malone, NY	-	-	-	**0.043** 421	**0.003** 322	**6.7** 993	**28.8** 80	**42** 300+	**80** 300+	**82** 300+	**59** 300+	**57** 300+	**73** 300+	**66** 300+	**75** 300+	**57** 300+	**59** 300+
Arnot Ogden Medical Center, Elmira, NY	-	-	-	**0.077** 1141	**0.002** 600	**4.3** 1843	**32.9** 143	**45** 300+	**79** 300+	**85** 300+	**67** 300+	**59** 300+	**79** 300+	**71** 300+	**69** 300+	**63** 300+	**75** 300+
Auburn Memorial Hospital, Auburn, NY	-	-	-	**0.082** 625	**0.000** 260	**6.5** 775	- 0	**47** 300+	**79** 300+	**87** 300+	**59** 300+	**61** 300+	**76** 300+	**68** 300+	**67** 300+	**59** 300+	**62** 300+
Aurelia Osborn Fox Memorial Hospital, Oneonta, NY	-	-	-	**0.092** 393	**0.035** 171	**3.7** 938	**45.2** 42	**49** 300+	**75** 300+	**85** 300+	**55** 300+	**56** 300+	**69** 300+	**66** 300+	**70** 300+	**58** 300+	**58** 300+
Bath VA Medical Center, Bath, NY	-	-	-	-	-	-	-	-	-	-	-	-	-	-	-	-	-
Bellevue Hospital Center, New York, NY	-	-	-	**0.118** 245	**0.014** 219	**9.1** 44	**44.4** 9	**42** 300+	**75** 300+	**78** 300+	**52** 300+	**49** 300+	**61** 300+	**58** 300+	**55** 300+	**48** 300+	**62** 300+
Benedictine Hospital, Kingston, NY	-	-	-	**0.062** 601	**0.003** 290	**3.4** 1029	- 0	**48** (a)	**77** (a)	**83** (a)	**67** (a)	**57** (a)	**74** (a)	**70** (a)	**62** (a)	**58** (a)	**71** (a)
Bertrand Chaffee Hospital, Springville, NY	-	-	-	**0.098** 92	**0.056** 36	**5.0** 200	- 0	**52** 300+	**87** 300+	**92** 300+	**74** 300+	**65** 300+	**84** 300+	**74** 300+	**79** 300+	**78** 300+	**74** 300+
Beth Israel Medical Center, New York, NY	-	-	-	**0.165** 872	**0.052** 483	**7.8** 884	**24.0** 96	**50** 300+	**73** 300+	**76** 300+	**56** 300+	**52** 300+	**66** 300+	**61** 300+	**64** 300+	**57** 300+	**61** 300+
Bon Secours Community Hospital, Port Jervis, NY	-	-	-	**0.066** 452	**0.032** 253	**7.1** 603	**28.1** 96	**58** 300+	**77** 300+	**78** 300+	**60** 300+	**59** 300+	**76** 300+	**72** 300+	**70** 300+	**64** 300+	**60** 300+
Bronx VA Medical Center, Bronx, NY	-	-	-	-	-	-	-	-	-	-	-	-	-	-	-	-	-
Bronx-Lebanon Hospital Center, Bronx, NY	-	-	-	**0.279** 183	**0.284** 116	**0.0** 4	**60.0** 5	**49** 300+	**67** 300+	**70** 300+	**43** 300+	**44** 300+	**57** 300+	**50** 300+	**51** 300+	**37** 300+	**44** 300+
Brookdale Hospital Medical Center, Brooklyn, NY	-	-	-	**0.071** 226	**0.000** 117	**4.1** 318	**40.0** 20	**45** 300+	**67** 300+	**66** 300+	**37** 300+	**50** 300+	**57** 300+	**45** 300+	**60** 300+	**36** 300+	**37** 300+
Brookhaven Memorial Hospital Medical Center, Patchogue, NY	-	-	-	**0.061** 759	**0.013** 520	**11.3** 1189	**24.4** 45	**41** 300+	**75** 300+	**81** 300+	**48** 300+	**51** 300+	**67** 300+	**62** 300+	**59** 300+	**49** 300+	**50** 300+
Brooklyn Hospital Center at Downtown Campus, Brooklyn, NY	-	-	-	**0.195** 307	**0.019** 214	**5.6** 286	**14.7** 34	**46** 300+	**72** 300+	**64** 300+	**48** 300+	**49** 300+	**63** 300+	**61** 300+	**61** 300+	**39** 300+	**50** 300+
Brooks Memorial Hospital, Dunkirk, NY	-	-	-	**0.077** 287	**0.045** 134	**4.1** 390	**42.1** 38	**47** 300+	**77** 300+	**80** 300+	**53** 300+	**47** 300+	**69** 300+	**61** 300+	**66** 300+	**52** 300+	**56** 300+
Canandaigua VA Medical Center, Canandaigua, NY	-	-	-	-	-	-	-	-	-	-	-	-	-	-	-	-	-
Canton-Potsdam Hospital, Potsdam, NY	-	-	-	**0.046** 459	**0.003** 294	**5.7** 978	**24.4** 135	**50** 300+	**81** 300+	**88** 300+	**65** 300+	**64** 300+	**75** 300+	**68** 300+	**77** 300+	**64** 300+	**70** 300+
Carthage Area Hospital, Carthage, NY	-	-	-	**0.331** 169	**0.077** 130	**2.3** 213	**26.1** 23	**47** 300+	**74** 300+	**83** 300+	**57** 300+	**59** 300+	**69** 300+	**62** 300+	**72** 300+	**54** 300+	**62** 300+
Catskill Regional Medical Center, Harris, NY	-	-	-	**0.153** 491	**0.032** 282	**6.4** 422	**30.4** 92	**48** 300+	**71** 300+	**79** 300+	**40** 300+	**49** 300+	**64** 300+	**64** 300+	**53** 300+	**55** 300+	**46** 300+
Cayuga Medical Center at Ithaca, Ithaca, NY	-	-	-	**0.025** 998	**0.001** 672	**3.2** 1676	**32.7** 223	**54** 300+	**78** 300+	**83** 300+	**66** 300+	**61** 300+	**74** 300+	**67** 300+	**69** 300+	**64** 300+	**71** 300+
Champlain Valley Physicians Hospital Med Ctr, Plattsburgh, NY	-	-	-	**0.052** 956	**0.056** 694	**9.0** 2543	**46.7** 45	**43** 300+	**77** 300+	**81** 300+	**57** 300+	**59** 300+	**73** 300+	**66** 300+	**67** 300+	**59** 300+	**63** 300+
Chenango Memorial Hospital, Norwich, NY	-	-	-	**0.066** 244	**0.000** 138	**7.9** 304	- 0	**47** 300+	**76** 300+	**81** 300+	**60** 300+	**53** 300+	**70** 300+	**64** 300+	**66** 300+	**61** 300+	**53** 300+
Claxton-Hepburn Medical Center, Ogdensburg, NY	-	-	-	**0.028** 469	**0.018** 330	**9.3** 1085	**30.9** 81	**49** (a)	**85** (a)	**87** (a)	**63** (a)	**66** (a)	**77** (a)	**69** (a)	**73** (a)	**67** (a)	**68** (a)
Clifton Springs Hospital and Clinic, Clifton Springs, NY	-	-	-	**0.304** 316	**0.010** 206	**7.1** 562	**34.5** 29	**50** 300+	**86** 300+	**91** 300+	**79** 300+	**64** 300+	**80** 300+	**72** 300+	**73** 300+	**72** 300+	**84** 300+
Cobleskill Regional Hospital, Cobleskill, NY	-	-	-	**0.103** 312	**0.018** 166	**5.9** 510	**25.0** 60	**54** (a)	**84** (a)	**85** (a)	**70** (a)	**58** (a)	**78** (a)	**69** (a)	**76** (a)	**60** (a)	**67** (a)
Columbia Memorial Hospital, Hudson, NY	-	-	-	**0.406** 581	**0.016** 438	**9.5** 623	**29.3** 41	**38** 300+	**76** 300+	**79** 300+	**47** 300+	**55** 300+	**69** 300+	**64** 300+	**62** 300+	**53** 300+	**51** 300+
Community Memorial Hospital, Hamilton, NY	-	-	-	**0.147** 191	**0.040** 125	**4.1** 266	**38.9** 54	**57** 300+	**83** 300+	**88** 300+	**73** 300+	**66** 300+	**79** 300+	**72** 300+	**77** 300+	**67** 300+	**78** 300+
Community-General Hospital of Greater Syracuse, Syracuse, NY	-	-	-	**0.031** 710	**0.000** 293	**6.8** 1552	- 0	**52** 300+	**80** 300+	**83** 300+	**61** 300+	**59** 300+	**74** 300+	**69** 300+	**57** 300+	**59** 300+	**66** 300+
Coney Island Hospital, Brooklyn, NY	-	-	-	**0.139** 245	**0.043** 92	**2.1** 94	**21.4** 14	**49** 300+	**72** 300+	**77** 300+	**55** 300+	**50** 300+	**64** 300+	**60** 300+	**63** 300+	**54** 300+	**56** 300+
Corning Hospital, Corning, NY	-	-	-	**0.114** 753	**0.005** 546	**14.6** 858	**36.1** 72	**55** 300+	**74** 300+	**82** 300+	**56** 300+	**60** 300+	**74** 300+	**69** 300+	**67** 300+	**59** 300+	**56** 300+
Cortland Regional Medical Center, Cortland, NY	-	-	-	**0.070** 681	**0.022** 315	**13.2** 439	**42.4** 33	**41** 300+	**72** 300+	**83** 300+	**52** 300+	**59** 300+	**71** 300+	**61** 300+	**66** 300+	**54** 300+	**50** 300+
Crouse Hospital, Syracuse, NY	-	-	-	**0.054** 727	**0.006** 524	**2.7** 1161	- 0	**43** 300+	**73** 300+	**86** 300+	**61** 300+	**55** 300+	**72** 300+	**64** 300+	**64** 300+	**53** 300+	**73** 300+
Delaware Valley Hospital, Walton, NY	-	-	-	**0.040** 100	**0.050** 40	**12.1** 206	- 0	**61** (a)	**86** (a)	**86** (a)	**73** (a)	**60** (a)	**85** (a)	**76** (a)	**87** (a)	**77** (a)	**76** (a)
Eastern Long Island Hospital, Greenport, NY	-	-	-	**0.000** 1	- 0	**26.2** 386	**24.5** 49	**53** 300+	**85** 300+	**84** 300+	**78** 300+	**57** 300+	**80** 300+	**78** 300+	**74** 300+	**65** 300+	**84** 300+
Eastern Niagara Hospital, Lockport, NY	-	-	-	**0.316** 244	**0.006** 173	**1.1** 528	**0.0** 7	**43** 300+	**78** 300+	**78** 300+	**59** 300+	**54** 300+	**71** 300+	**65** 300+	**73** 300+	**56** 300+	**62** 300+
Edward John Noble Hospital of Gouverneur, Gouverneur, NY	-	-	-	**0.046** 109	**0.000** 84	**3.2** 250	**21.4** 14	**45** 300+	**82** 300+	**84** 300+	**50** 300+	**61** 300+	**73** 300+	**65** 300+	**70** 300+	**68** 300+	**42** 300+
Elizabethtown Community Hospital, Elizabethtown, NY	-	-	-	-	-	-	-	-	-	-	-	-	-	-	-	-	-
Ellenville Regional Hospital, Ellenville, NY	-	-	-	-	-	-	-	-	-	-	-	-	-	-	-	-	-
Ellis Hospital, Schenectady, NY	-	-	-	**0.026** 1049	**0.000** 926	**6.9** 2387	**26.7** 101	**44** 300+	**72** 300+	**85** 300+	**59** 300+	**53** 300+	**69** 300+	**63** 300+	**62** 300+	**53** 300+	**64** 300+
Elmhurst Hospital Center, Elmhurst, NY	-	-	-	**0.127** 150	**0.011** 87	**4.0** 175	**12.5** 8	**41** 300+	**74** 300+	**81** 300+	**56** 300+	**48** 300+	**65** 300+	**58** 300+	**58** 300+	**51** 300+	**60** 300+
Erie County Medical Center, Buffalo, NY	-	-	-	**0.260** 415	**0.010** 197	**13.6** 360	- 0	**40** 300+	**72** 300+	**79** 300+	**53** 300+	**51** 300+	**66** 300+	**60** 300+	**49** 300+	**44** 300+	**58** 300+
F F Thompson Hospital, Canandaigua, NY	-	-	-	**0.551** 361	**0.014** 212	**4.5** 649	- 0	**47** 300+	**80** 300+	**87** 300+	**69** 300+	**61** 300+	**77** 300+	**68** 300+	**69** 300+	**68** 300+	**76** 300+
Faxton-St Luke's Healthcare, Utica, NY	-	-	-	**0.054** 483	**0.000** 608	**18.4** 1552	- 0	**42** 300+	**74** 300+	**80** 300+	**57** 300+	**53** 300+	**71** 300+	**65** 300+	**52** 300+	**57** 300+	**63** 300+
Flushing Hospital Medical Center, Flushing, NY	-	-	-	**0.000** 3	**0.000** 54	**6.9** 131	**0.0** 1	**38** 300+	**65** 300+	**70** 300+	**43** 300+	**42** 300+	**57** 300+	**50** 300+	**60** 300+	**44** 300+	**47** 300+
Forest Hills Hospital, Forest Hills, NY	-	-	-	**0.022** 228	**0.000** 103	**43.2** 88	**41.7** 12	**44** 300+	**70** 300+	**72** 300+	**51** 300+	**51** 300+	**64** 300+	**61** 300+	**66** 300+	**52** 300+	**58** 300+
Franklin Hospital, Valley Stream, NY	-	-	-	**0.018** 276	**0.000** 112	**13.0** 115	**30.0** 10	**49** 300+	**75** 300+	**73** 300+	**56** 300+	**52** 300+	**69** 300+	**64** 300+	**66** 300+	**53** 300+	**59** 300+
Geneva General Hospital, Geneva, NY	-	-	-	**0.440** 361	**0.017** 173	**9.7** 677	- 0	**55** 300+	**75** 300+	**87** 300+	**57** 300+	**59** 300+	**72** 300+	**65** 300+	**63** 300+	**56** 300+	**61** 300+
Glen Cove Hospital, Glen Cove, NY	-	-	-	**0.455** 365	**0.000** 279	**15.3** 235	- 0	**50** 300+	**79** 300+	**78** 300+	**67** 300+	**59** 300+	**78** 300+	**66** 300+	**74** 300+	**62** 300+	**70** 300+
Glens Falls Hospital, Glens Falls, NY	-	-	-	**0.044** 1653	**0.002** 1383	**8.9** 1655	- 0	**46** 300+	**79** 300+	**85** 300+	**60** 300+	**56** 300+	**70** 300+	**67** 300+	**69** 300+	**57** 300+	**65** 300+
Good Samaritan Hospital Medical Center, West Islip, NY	-	-	-	**0.038** 1058	**0.001** 785	**16.0** 1604	**24.2** 33	**43** 300+	**76** 300+	**83** 300+	**62** 300+	**56** 300+	**73** 300+	**69** 300+	**71** 300+	**56** 300+	**68** 300+
Good Samaritan Hospital of Suffern, Suffern, NY	-	-	-	**0.087** 516	**0.036** 279	**21.0** 362	**7.7** 26	**46** 300+	**75** 300+	**78** 300+	**56** 300+	**54** 300+	**68** 300+	**59** 300+	**58** 300+	**47** 300+	**61** 300+
Harlem Hospital Center, New York, NY	-	-	-	**0.348** 115	**0.242** 62	**8.1** 136	**33.3** 6	**58** 300+	**76** 300+	**78** 300+	**45** 300+	**54** 300+	**61** 300+	**57** 300+	**58** 300+	**47** 300+	**52** 300+
Helen Hayes Hospital, West Haverstraw, NY	-	-	-	- 0	- 0	- 0	- 0	-	-	-	-	-	-	-	-	-	-
Highland Hospital, Rochester, NY	-	-	-	**0.310** 471	**0.337** 338	**10.0** 720	- 0	**48** 300+	**79** 300+	**86** 300+	**69** 300+	**61** 300+	**76** 300+	**68** 300+	**65** 300+	**56** 300+	**76** 300+
Hospital for Special Surgery, New York, NY	-	-	-	**0.237** 38	**0.000** 91	- 0	**22.5** 1071	**51** 300+	**83** 300+	**88** 300+	**85** 300+	**60** 300+	**79** 300+	**74** 300+	**78** 300+	**63** 300+	**89** 300+
Hudson Valley Hospital Center, Cortlandt Manor, NY	-	-	-	**0.146** 670	**0.084** 547	**6.9** 1007	**24.4** 172	**50** 300+	**79** 300+	**80** 300+	**65** 300+	**61** 300+	**76** 300+	**72** 300+	**72** 300+	**62** 300+	**68** 300+
Huntington Hospital, Huntington, NY	-	-	-	**0.066** 527	**0.000** 448	**15.3** 907	**30.0** 20	**46** 300+	**78** 300+	**75** 300+	**60** 300+	**55** 300+	**75** 300+	**70** 300+	**68** 300+	**57** 300+	**68** 300+
Interfaith Medical Center, Brooklyn, NY	-	-	-	**0.024** 41	**0.017** 60	**7.4** 94	**25.0** 4	**56** 300+	**67** 300+	**64** 300+	**45** 300+	**51** 300+	**63** 300+	**53** 300+	**72** 300+	**38** 300+	**45** 300+
Ira Davenport Memorial Hospital, Bath, NY	-	-	-	**0.068** 162	**0.000** 70	**4.5** 243	**29.2** 24	**47** (a)	**74** (a)	**75** (a)	**46** (a)	**58** (a)	**68** (a)	**56** (a)	**64** (a)	**57** (a)	**42** (a)
Jacobi Medical Center, Bronx, NY	-	-	-	**0.150** 240	**0.061** 164	**2.7** 482	**33.3** 12	**50** 300+	**77** 300+	**78** 300+	**55** 300+	**49** 300+	**64** 300+	**57** 300+	**65** 300+	**50** 300+	**60** 300+
Jamaica Hospital Medical Center, Jamaica, NY	-	-	-	**0.000** 200	**0.000** 136	**5.3** 432	**29.4** 17	**40** 300+	**66** 300+	**70** 300+	**43** 300+	**43** 300+	**56** 300+	**51** 300+	**56** 300+	**40** 300+	**49** 300+
J T Mather Mem Hosp of Port Jefferson, Port Jefferson, NY	-	-	-	**0.064** 949	**0.008** 643	**33.7** 1724	**17.0** 53	**49** 300+	**79** 300+	**87** 300+	**70** 300+	**61** 300+	**78** 300+	**72** 300+	**70** 300+	**65** 300+	**76** 300+
Jones Memorial Hospital, Wellsville, NY	-	-	-	**0.119** 218	**0.096** 115	**5.2** 461	**32.4** 37	**49** 300+	**77** 300+	**78** 300+	**55** 300+	**54** 300+	**72** 300+	**62** 300+	**65** 300+	**58** 300+	**56** 300+
Kaleida Health, Buffalo, NY	**98** 550	**16** 552	**100** 553	**0.600** 1233	**0.091** 623	**11.7** 1095	**25.2** 111	**44** 300+	**74** 300+	**82** 300+	**60** 300+	**54** 300+	**71** 300+	**64** 300+	**57** 300+	**54** 300+	**64** 300+

NOTE: The first number in each column (boldface) is the score, the second number is the number of patients; Please refer to the main entry for footnotes; (a) 100-299
*MEASURES: **Children's Asthma Care:** 33. Received Systemic Corticosteroids; 34. Received Home Management Plan of Care; 35. Received Reliever Medication; **Use of Medical Imaging:** 36. Combination Abdominal CT Scan; 37. Combination Chest CT Scan; 38. Follow-up Mammogram/Ultrasound; 39. MRI for Low Back Pain; **Survey of Patients' Hospital Experiences:** 40. Area Around Room 'Always' Quiet at Night; 41. Doctors 'Always' Communicated Well; 42. Home Recovery Information Given; 43. Hospital Given 9 or 10 on 10 Point Scale; 44. Meds 'Always' Explained Before Given; 45. Nurses 'Always' Communicated Well; 46. Pain 'Always' Well Controlled; 47. Room and Bathroom 'Always' Clean; 48. Timely Help 'Always' Received; 49. Would Definitely Recommend Hospital*

Hospital	Children's Asthma Care			Use of Medical Imaging				Survey of Patients' Hospital Experiences									
	33	34	35	36	37	38	39	40	41	42	43	44	45	46	47	48	49
Kenmore Mercy Hospital, Kenmore, NY	- -	- -	- -	**0.392** 459	**0.099** 233	**11.8** 441	**-** 0	**43** 300+	**75** 300+	**85** 300+	**64** 300+	**58** 300+	**73** 300+	**70** 300+	**58** 300+	**56** 300+	**69** 300+
Kings County Hospital Center, Brooklyn, NY	- -	- -	- -	**0.263** 133	**0.256** 43	**0.0** 10	**0.0** 8	**59** 300+	**78** 300+	**79** 300+	**57** 300+	**61** 300+	**67** 300+	**59** 300+	**74** 300+	**45** 300+	**63** 300+
Kingsbrook Jewish Medical Center, Brooklyn, NY	- -	- -	- -	**0.159** 208	**0.015** 136	**19.8** 273	**28.0** 25	**51** 300+	**75** 300+	**76** 300+	**51** 300+	**54** 300+	**69** 300+	**56** 300+	**67** 300+	**45** 300+	**61** 300+
Kingston Hospital, Kingston, NY	- -	- -	- -	**0.089** 541	**0.013** 306	**7.3** 877	**31.9** 113	**39** 300+	**72** 300+	**77** 300+	**53** 300+	**53** 300+	**70** 300+	**61** 300+	**61** 300+	**50** 300+	**58** 300+
Lakeside Memorial Hospital, Brockport, NY	- -	- -	- -	**0.698** 202	**0.047** 107	**15.6** 192	**35.3** 34	**51** 300+	**78** 300+	**89** 300+	**65** 300+	**60** 300+	**76** 300+	**67** 300+	**69** 300+	**58** 300+	**68** 300+
Lawrence Hospital Center, Bronxville, NY	- -	- -	- -	**0.108** 584	**0.017** 476	**13.2** 642	**23.7** 139	**59** 300+	**80** 300+	**73** 300+	**66** 300+	**59** 300+	**75** 300+	**69** 300+	**71** 300+	**60** 300+	**74** 300+
Lenox Hill Hospital, New York, NY	- -	- -	- -	**0.090** 567	**0.009** 434	**36.7** 196	**17.9** 84	**49** 300+	**79** 300+	**75** 300+	**61** 300+	**54** 300+	**70** 300+	**69** 300+	**55** 300+	**53** 300+	**71** 300+
Lewis County General Hospital, Lowville, NY	- -	- -	- -	**0.460** 202	**0.105** 172	**5.7** 522	**22.2** 27	**53** 300+	**84** 300+	**86** 300+	**69** 300+	**67** 300+	**75** 300+	**73** 300+	**76** 300+	**64** 300+	**77** 300+
Lincoln Medical & Mental Health Center, Bronx, NY	- -	- -	- -	**0.095** 262	**0.044** 159	**9.7** 176	**-** 0	**54** 300+	**76** 300+	**73** 300+	**52** 300+	**50** 300+	**64** 300+	**53** 300+	**60** 300+	**49** 300+	**53** 300+
Little Falls Hospital, Little Falls, NY	- -	- -	- -	**0.146** 301	**0.014** 138	**10.3** 300	**-** 0	**49** 300+	**83** 300+	**83** 300+	**64** 300+	**65** 300+	**76** 300+	**71** 300+	**75** 300+	**57** 300+	**61** 300+
Long Beach Medical Center, Long Beach, NY	- -	- -	- -	**0.592** 311	**0.005** 195	**66.7** 3	**26.7** 15	**42** 300+	**71** 300+	**73** 300+	**41** 300+	**49** 300+	**61** 300+	**60** 300+	**61** 300+	**48** 300+	**45** 300+
Long Island College Hospital, Brooklyn, NY	- -	- -	- -	**0.267** 457	**0.008** 239	**5.0** 519	**18.0** 50	**52** 300+	**71** 300+	**66** 300+	**44** 300+	**48** 300+	**59** 300+	**53** 300+	**53** 300+	**45** 300+	**55** 300+
Long Island Jewish Medical Center, New Hyde Park, NY	- -	- -	- -	**0.086** 561	**0.000** 278	**-** 0	**37.5** 24	**46** 300+	**74** 300+	**75** 300+	**58** 300+	**55** 300+	**69** 300+	**61** 300+	**60** 300+	**56** 300+	**66** 300+
Lutheran Medical Center, Brooklyn, NY	- -	- -	- -	**0.023** 400	**0.000** 177	**7.4** 243	**18.2** 11	**34** 300+	**72** 300+	**76** 300+	**49** 300+	**46** 300+	**64** 300+	**59** 300+	**53** 300+	**50** 300+	**54** 300+
Maimonides Medical Center, Brooklyn, NY	- -	- -	- -	**0.021** 751	**0.022** 491	**-** 0	**24.4** 45	**45** 300+	**77** 300+	**77** 300+	**50** 300+	**53** 300+	**66** 300+	**60** 300+	**58** 300+	**53** 300+	**62** 300+
Margaretville Memorial Hospital, Margaretville, NY	- -	- -	- -	**0.052** 97	**0.025** 40	**9.0** 133	**-** 0	**63** <100	**82** <100	**81** <100	**77** <100	**66** <100	**83** <100	**75** <100	**84** <100	**79** <100	**66** <100
Mary Imogene Bassett Hospital, Cooperstown, NY	- -	- -	- -	**0.150** 652	**0.021** 608	**6.4** 1829	**31.7** 123	**44** 300+	**78** 300+	**88** 300+	**64** 300+	**65** 300+	**74** 300+	**67** 300+	**67** 300+	**58** 300+	**75** 300+
Massena Memorial Hospital, Massena, NY	- -	- -	- -	**0.022** 464	**0.000** 307	**11.4** 519	**36.0** 50	**52** 300+	**82** 300+	**82** 300+	**61** 300+	**61** 300+	**77** 300+	**72** 300+	**75** 300+	**67** 300+	**59** 300+
Medina Memorial Hospital, Medina, NY	- -	- -	- -	**0.164** 171	**0.242** 91	**6.5** 245	**-** 0	**46** 300+	**77** 300+	**84** 300+	**61** 300+	**55** 300+	**74** 300+	**64** 300+	**70** 300+	**61** 300+	**64** 300+
Mercy Hospital, Buffalo, NY	- -	- -	- -	**0.084** 692	**0.000** 449	**5.4** 1002	**28.6** 14	**39** 300+	**72** 300+	**80** 300+	**48** 300+	**47** 300+	**68** 300+	**61** 300+	**53** 300+	**47** 300+	**49** 300+
Mercy Medical Center, Rockville Centre, NY	- -	- -	- -	**0.016** 607	**0.008** 492	**9.0** 680	**21.8** 55	**54** 300+	**78** 300+	**81** 300+	**59** 300+	**54** 300+	**71** 300+	**66** 300+	**63** 300+	**55** 300+	**65** 300+
Metropolitan Hospital Center, New York, NY	- -	- -	- -	**0.280** 93	**0.054** 56	**0.0** 17	**-** 0	**48** 300+	**75** 300+	**83** 300+	**62** 300+	**53** 300+	**62** 300+	**52** 300+	**59** 300+	**48** 300+	**60** 300+
Monroe Community Hospital, Rochester, NY	- -	- -	- -	- -	- -	- -	- -	- -	- -	- -	- -	- -	- -	- -	- -	- -	- -
Montefiore Medical Center, Bronx, NY	- -	- -	- -	**0.070** 1769	**0.013** 1222	**3.7** 2215	**29.2** 120	**54** 300+	**77** 300+	**76** 300+	**59** 300+	**57** 300+	**72** 300+	**63** 300+	**68** 300+	**48** 300+	**67** 300+
Moses-Ludington Hospital, Ticonderoga, NY	- -	- -	- -	- -	- -	- -	- -	- -	- -	- -	- -	- -	- -	- -	- -	- -	- -
Mount Sinai Hospital, New York, NY	- -	- -	- -	**0.046** 539	**0.024** 169	**9.1** 165	**27.3** 22	**49** 300+	**78** 300+	**77** 300+	**62** 300+	**53** 300+	**71** 300+	**65** 300+	**62** 300+	**51** 300+	**71** 300+
Mount St Mary's Hospital and Health Center, Lewiston, NY	- -	- -	- -	**0.079** 356	**0.011** 357	**13.7** 736	**37.5** 136	**55** 300+	**78** 300+	**82** 300+	**69** 300+	**57** 300+	**77** 300+	**71** 300+	**75** 300+	**59** 300+	**73** 300+
Mount Vernon Hospital, Mount Vernon, NY	- -	- -	- -	**0.005** 212	**0.006** 173	**9.5** 367	**38.1** 21	**59** 300+	**83** 300+	**82** 300+	**56** 300+	**54** 300+	**73** 300+	**67** 300+	**67** 300+	**61** 300+	**59** 300+
Nassau University Medical Center, East Meadow, NY	- -	- -	- -	**0.007** 147	**0.013** 80	**20.9** 503	**22.2** 18	**42** 300+	**65** 300+	**70** 300+	**43** 300+	**46** 300+	**56** 300+	**56** 300+	**51** 300+	**44** 300+	**42** 300+
Nathan Littauer Hospital, Gloversville, NY	- -	- -	- -	**0.045** 464	**0.026** 309	**6.4** 754	**42.6** 47	**54** 300+	**77** 300+	**83** 300+	**61** 300+	**62** 300+	**75** 300+	**70** 300+	**77** 300+	**63** 300+	**61** 300+
New York Community Hospital of Brooklyn, Brooklyn, NY	- -	- -	- -	**0.009** 110	**0.000** 32	**0.0** 3	**-** 0	**44** 300+	**70** 300+	**76** 300+	**47** 300+	**52** 300+	**65** 300+	**57** 300+	**67** 300+	**51** 300+	**51** 300+
New York Downtown Hospital, New York, NY	- -	- -	- -	**0.088** 194	**0.040** 101	**37.7** 191	**-** 0	**37** 300+	**66** 300+	**73** 300+	**37** 300+	**48** 300+	**57** 300+	**52** 300+	**57** 300+	**46** 300+	**43** 300+
New York Hospital Medical Center of Queens, Flushing, NY	- -	- -	- -	**0.057** 1018	**0.005** 591	**11.9** 1525	**34.1** 91	**42** 300+	**69** 300+	**75** 300+	**52** 300+	**50** 300+	**64** 300+	**55** 300+	**63** 300+	**46** 300+	**61** 300+
New York Methodist Hospital, Brooklyn, NY	- -	- -	- -	**0.065** 570	**0.012** 409	**4.8** 862	**29.7** 74	**45** 300+	**71** 300+	**75** 300+	**52** 300+	**44** 300+	**62** 300+	**56** 300+	**56** 300+	**42** 300+	**61** 300+
New York Westchester Square Medical Center, Bronx, NY	- -	- -	- -	**0.000** 47	**0.000** 3	**50.9** 108	**-** 0	**61** (a)	**74** (a)	**74** (a)	**50** (a)	**39** (a)	**68** (a)	**66** (a)	**74** (a)	**59** (a)	**64** (a)
New York-Presbyterian Hospital, New York, NY	**100** 412	**78** 410	**100** 412	**0.415** 2357	**0.025** 2332	**7.7** 3236	**25.0** 192	**54** 300+	**78** 300+	**78** 300+	**73** 300+	**58** 300+	**72** 300+	**65** 300+	**64** 300+	**55** 300+	**80** 300+
Newark-Wayne Community Hospital, Newark, NY	- -	- -	- -	**0.442** 233	**0.088** 148	**5.5** 346	**31.4** 35	**49** 300+	**80** 300+	**87** 300+	**63** 300+	**62** 300+	**78** 300+	**70** 300+	**69** 300+	**69** 300+	**61** 300+
Niagara Falls Memorial Medical Center, Niagara Falls, NY	- -	- -	- -	**0.070** 328	**0.068** 251	**4.6** 918	**30.5** 118	**50** 300+	**70** 300+	**77** 300+	**53** 300+	**53** 300+	**68** 300+	**63** 300+	**61** 300+	**53** 300+	**57** 300+
Nicholas H Noyes Memorial Hospital, Dansville, NY	- -	- -	- -	**0.683** 243	**0.676** 182	**56.6** 412	**-** 0	**58** 300+	**78** 300+	**81** 300+	**70** 300+	**57** 300+	**77** 300+	**70** 300+	**67** 300+	**68** 300+	**70** 300+
North Central Bronx Hospital, Bronx, NY	- -	- -	- -	**0.102** 49	**0.059** 34	**1.4** 220	**50.0** 4	**58** 300+	**77** 300+	**76** 300+	**62** 300+	**58** 300+	**66** 300+	**63** 300+	**60** 300+	**49** 300+	**63** 300+
North General Hospital, New York, NY	- -	- -	- -	- -	- -	- -	- -	- -	- -	- -	- -	- -	- -	- -	- -	- -	- -
North Shore University Hospital, Manhasset, NY	- -	- -	- -	**0.098** 2232	**0.009** 2012	**10.2** 1496	**14.4** 118	**40** 300+	**75** 300+	**76** 300+	**63** 300+	**56** 300+	**71** 300+	**62** 300+	**66** 300+	**49** 300+	**74** 300+
Northern Dutchess Hospital, Rhinebeck, NY	- -	- -	- -	**0.359** 304	**0.054** 168	**8.8** 605	**31.8** 44	**51** 300+	**80** 300+	**84** 300+	**73** 300+	**64** 300+	**80** 300+	**72** 300+	**67** 300+	**64** 300+	**79** 300+
Northern Westchester Hospital, Mount Kisco, NY	- -	- -	- -	**0.105** 382	**0.000** 244	**28.6** 35	**30.2** 53	**57** 300+	**83** 300+	**78** 300+	**74** 300+	**63** 300+	**82** 300+	**75** 300+	**70** 300+	**66** 300+	**81** 300+
Northport VA Medical Center, Northport, NY	- -	- -	- -	- -	- -	- -	- -	- -	- -	- -	- -	- -	- -	- -	- -	- -	- -
NY Eye and Ear Infirmary, New York, NY	- -	- -	- -	**0.667** 6	**0.000** 16	**-** 0	**-** 0	**63** 300+	**75** 300+	**75** 300+	**60** 300+	**54** 300+	**68** 300+	**62** 300+	**68** 300+	**60** 300+	**72** 300+
Nyack Hospital, Nyack, NY	- -	- -	- -	**0.031** 508	**0.025** 365	**13.5** 579	**-** 0	**47** 300+	**73** 300+	**68** 300+	**53** 300+	**57** 300+	**69** 300+	**64** 300+	**73** 300+	**59** 300+	**59** 300+
NYU Hospitals Center, New York, NY	**100** 19	**0** 19	**100** 19	**0.035** 228	**0.000** 77	**8.8** 1071	**24.1** 87	**43** 300+	**75** 300+	**78** 300+	**61** 300+	**58** 300+	**71** 300+	**64** 300+	**60** 300+	**53** 300+	**71** 300+
O'Connor Hospital, Delhi, NY	- -	- -	- -	- -	- -	- -	- -	- -	- -	- -	- -	- -	- -	- -	- -	- -	- -
Olean General Hospital, Olean, NY	- -	- -	- -	**0.259** 606	**0.398** 259	**15.6** 294	**37.6** 117	**45** 300+	**75** 300+	**81** 300+	**58** 300+	**54** 300+	**73** 300+	**65** 300+	**74** 300+	**60** 300+	**56** 300+
Oneida Healthcare Center, Oneida, NY	- -	- -	- -	**0.259** 464	**0.011** 174	**5.4** 443	**32.4** 37	**52** 300+	**83** 300+	**84** 300+	**66** 300+	**66** 300+	**75** 300+	**71** 300+	**73** 300+	**63** 300+	**69** 300+
Orange Regional Medical Center, Goshen, NY	- -	- -	- -	**0.116** 1430	**0.014** 1410	**6.2** 1909	**22.6** 133	**41** 300+	**72** 300+	**80** 300+	**49** 300+	**52** 300+	**68** 300+	**61** 300+	**60** 300+	**51** 300+	**52** 300+
Oswego Hospital, Oswego, NY	- -	- -	- -	**0.158** 417	**0.020** 344	**3.5** 1327	**30.4** 23	**45** 300+	**76** 300+	**84** 300+	**50** 300+	**57** 300+	**71** 300+	**61** 300+	**66** 300+	**54** 300+	**50** 300+
Our Lady of Lourdes Memorial Hospital, Binghamton, NY	- -	- -	- -	**0.146** 1550	**0.094** 1151	**7.5** 3113	**23.6** 203	**54** 300+	**76** 300+	**86** 300+	**68** 300+	**60** 300+	**75** 300+	**67** 300+	**67** 300+	**63** 300+	**74** 300+
Peconic Bay Medical Center, Riverhead, NY	- -	- -	- -	**0.041** 462	**0.013** 391	**5.1** 59	**19.3** 88	**39** 300+	**73** 300+	**80** 300+	**50** 300+	**52** 300+	**69** 300+	**61** 300+	**58** 300+	**47** 300+	**53** 300+
Peninsula Hospital Center, Far Rockaway, NY	- -	- -	- -	**0.002** 415	**0.000** 291	**18.8** 458	**20.6** 68	**41** 300+	**66** 300+	**70** 300+	**33** 300+	**42** 300+	**54** 300+	**51** 300+	**59** 300+	**39** 300+	**41** 300+
Phelps Memorial Hospital Assn, Sleepy Hollow, NY	- -	- -	- -	**0.216** 1006	**0.000** 967	**8.0** 1436	**33.3** 3	**45** 300+	**78** 300+	**79** 300+	**66** 300+	**59** 300+	**71** 300+	**66** 300+	**70** 300+	**55** 300+	**69** 300+
Plainview Hospital, Plainview, NY	- -	- -	- -	**0.019** 324	**0.000** 64	**-** 0	**66.7** 3	**36** 300+	**74** 300+	**73** 300+	**53** 300+	**53** 300+	**71** 300+	**65** 300+	**62** 300+	**56** 300+	**60** 300+
Putnam Hospital Center, Carmel, NY	- -	- -	- -	**0.120** 566	**0.002** 463	**8.3** 811	**30.2** 129	**55** 300+	**83** 300+	**81** 300+	**74** 300+	**60** 300+	**79** 300+	**73** 300+	**74** 300+	**66** 300+	**76** 300+
Queens Hospital Center, Jamaica, NY	- -	- -	- -	**0.022** 180	**0.009** 109	**4.7** 316	**16.7** 6	**55** 300+	**79** 300+	**78** 300+	**61** 300+	**58** 300+	**66** 300+	**62** 300+	**68** 300+	**56** 300+	**70** 300+
Richmond University Medical Center, Staten Island, NY	- -	- -	- -	**0.041** 49	**0.000** 65	**29.4** 143	**-** 0	**41** 300+	**70** 300+	**70** 300+	**44** 300+	**56** 300+	**69** 300+	**63** 300+	**58** 300+	**56** 300+	**51** 300+
River Hospital, Alexandria Bay, NY	- -	- -	- -	**0.012** 86	**0.000** 58	**9.1** 132	**-** 0	**59** <100	**85** <100	**81** <100	**82** <100	**71** <100	**82** <100	**73** <100	**87** <100	**78** <100	**86** <100
Rochester General Hospital, Rochester, NY	- -	- -	- -	**0.592** 596	**0.317** 328	**7.8** 232	**42.1** 19	**42** 300+	**80** 300+	**91** 300+	**71** 300+	**63** 300+	**79** 300+	**70** 300+	**66** 300+	**62** 300+	**78** 300+
Rome Memorial Hospital, Rome, NY	- -	- -	- -	**0.592** 591	**0.020** 343	**25.6** 425	**-** 0	**45** 300+	**72** 300+	**85** 300+	**55** 300+	**58** 300+	**73** 300+	**68** 300+	**70** 300+	**54** 300+	**58** 300+
Saint Anthony Community Hospital, Warwick, NY	- -	- -	- -	**0.061** 326	**0.000** 227	**14.1** 455	**10.9** 55	**55** 300+	**79** 300+	**85** 300+	**72** 300+	**63** 300+	**80** 300+	**74** 300+	**61** 300+	**66** 300+	**73** 300+
Saint Barnabas Hospital, Bronx, NY	- -	- -	- -	**0.036** 167	**0.014** 74	**6.0** 133	**55.6** 9	**50** 300+	**75** 300+	**70** 300+	**42** 300+	**47** 300+	**61** 300+	**54** 300+	**63** 300+	**42** 300+	**49** 300+
Saint Catherine of Siena Hospital, Smithtown, NY	- -	- -	- -	**0.477** 666	**0.026** 390	**23.2** 155	**20.0** 45	**40** 300+	**77** 300+	**81** 300+	**60** 300+	**53** 300+	**71** 300+	**65** 300+	**68** 300+	**52** 300+	**61** 300+

NOTE: The first number in each column (boldface) is the score, the second number is the number of patients; Please refer to the main entry for footnotes; (a) 100-299
*MEASURES: **Children's Asthma Care:** 33. Received Systemic Corticosteroids; 34. Received Home Management Plan of Care; 35. Received Reliever Medication; **Use of Medical Imaging:** 36. Combination Abdominal CT Scan; 37. Combination Chest CT Scan; 38. Follow-up Mammogram/Ultrasound; 39. MRI for Low Back Pain; **Survey of Patients' Hospital Experiences:** 40. Area Around Room 'Always' Quiet at Night; 41. Doctors 'Always' Communicated Well; 42. Home Recovery Information Given; 43. Hospital Given 9 or 10 on 10 Point Scale; 44. Meds 'Always' Explained Before Given; 45. Nurses 'Always' Communicated Well; 46. Pain 'Always' Well Controlled; 47. Room and Bathroom 'Always' Clean; 48. Timely Help 'Always' Received; 49. Would Definitely Recommend Hospital*

Hospital	Children's Asthma Care			Use of Medical Imaging				Survey of Patients' Hospital Experiences									
	33	34	35	36	37	38	39	40	41	42	43	44	45	46	47	48	49
Saint Charles Hospital, Port Jefferson, NY	- -	- -	- -	0.043 328	0.011 261	24.2 429	10.3 39	50 300+	81 300+	86 300+	70 300+	57 300+	75 300+	67 300+	70 300+	59 300+	75 300+
Saint Elizabeth Medical Center, Utica, NY	- -	- -	- -	0.315 515	0.039 357	5.7 822	- 0	44 300+	74 300+	81 300+	64 300+	53 300+	77 300+	68 300+	71 300+	66 300+	70 300+
Saint Francis Hospital, Poughkeepsie, NY	- -	- -	- -	0.153 444	0.048 312	15.0 452	31.6 38	49 300+	74 300+	85 300+	61 300+	58 300+	72 300+	67 300+	67 300+	63 300+	67 300+
Saint Francis Hospital - Roslyn, Roslyn, NY	- -	- -	- -	0.070 428	0.017 537	35.4 577	27.3 22	53 300+	81 300+	87 300+	82 300+	61 300+	81 300+	71 300+	77 300+	65 300+	86 300+
Saint James Mercy Hospital, Hornell, NY	- -	- -	- -	0.289 301	0.027 257	5.5 309	- 0	59 300+	77 300+	87 300+	51 300+	59 300+	70 300+	63 300+	69 300+	65 300+	51 300+
Saint John's Episcopal Hospital at South Shore, Far Rockaway, NY	- -	- -	- -	0.000 183	0.000 122	11.5 192	0.0 1	53 300+	73 300+	76 300+	48 300+	52 300+	66 300+	60 300+	65 300+	48 300+	49 300+
Saint John's Riverside Hospital, Yonkers, NY	- -	- -	- -	0.090 659	0.000 748	12.0 951	21.3 61	47 300+	79 300+	72 300+	59 300+	53 300+	72 300+	66 300+	76 300+	54 300+	66 300+
Saint Joseph Hospital, Bethpage, NY	- -	- -	- -	0.022 228	0.000 73	46.2 13	- 0	43 300+	73 300+	80 300+	49 300+	53 300+	69 300+	65 300+	61 300+	49 300+	54 300+
Saint Joseph's Hospital, Elmira, NY	- -	- -	- -	0.000 1	- 0	4.7 741	28.9 76	47 300+	74 300+	81 300+	55 300+	53 300+	68 300+	66 300+	62 300+	53 300+	59 300+
Saint Joseph's Hospital Health Center, Syracuse, NY	- -	- -	- -	0.088 774	0.006 320	13.9 187	0.0 1	44 300+	75 300+	88 300+	71 300+	59 300+	75 300+	71 300+	64 300+	59 300+	77 300+
Saint Joseph's Medical Center, Yonkers, NY	- -	- -	- -	0.106 340	0.010 208	4.8 518	22.8 57	51 300+	73 300+	75 300+	48 300+	50 300+	65 300+	58 300+	65 300+	43 300+	52 300+
Saint Luke's Cornwall Hospital, Newburgh, NY	- -	- -	- -	0.092 567	0.031 353	3.7 323	- 0	47 300+	75 300+	81 300+	54 300+	57 300+	69 300+	64 300+	63 300+	51 300+	57 300+
Saint Luke's Roosevelt Hospital, New York, NY	- -	- -	- -	0.081 683	0.012 417	6.5 246	22.8 57	48 300+	73 300+	72 300+	50 300+	51 300+	62 300+	58 300+	54 300+	47 300+	60 300+
Saint Mary's Hospital at Amsterdam, Amsterdam, NY	- -	- -	- -	0.431 800	0.041 437	5.3 904	37.5 80	49 300+	78 300+	87 300+	69 300+	61 300+	80 300+	71 300+	75 300+	66 300+	72 300+
Saint Peter's Hospital, Albany, NY	- -	- -	- -	0.070 1069	0.045 865	5.4 2040	22.6 31	38 300+	72 300+	84 300+	63 300+	57 300+	69 300+	61 300+	63 300+	49 300+	71 300+
Samaritan Hospital, Troy, NY	- -	- -	- -	0.051 548	0.009 325	11.7 538	27.7 65	45 300+	73 300+	82 300+	60 300+	53 300+	69 300+	64 300+	66 300+	56 300+	63 300+
Samaritan Medical Center, Watertown, NY	- -	- -	- -	0.567 735	0.026 680	9.2 1354	24.0 75	46 300+	76 300+	84 300+	51 300+	57 300+	73 300+	65 300+	71 300+	62 300+	54 300+
Saratoga Hospital, Saratoga Springs, NY	- -	- -	- -	0.042 990	0.002 570	5.8 993	32.3 96	39 300+	80 300+	91 300+	66 300+	64 300+	79 300+	72 300+	70 300+	65 300+	71 300+
Schuyler Hospital, Montour Falls, NY	- -	- -	- -	- -	- -	- -	- -	- -	- -	- -	- -	- -	- -	- -	- -	- -	- -
Seton Health System-St Mary's Campus, Troy, NY	- -	- -	- -	0.065 649	0.000 329	7.6 733	43.5 46	53 300+	80 300+	84 300+	68 300+	59 300+	80 300+	68 300+	64 300+	65 300+	67 300+
Sheehan Memorial Hospital, Buffalo, NY	- -	- -	- -	0.000 6	0.000 9	5.9 34	- 0	- -	- -	- -	- -	- -	- -	- -	- -	- -	- -
Sisters of Charity Hospital, Buffalo, NY	- -	- -	- -	0.051 292	0.043 188	8.1 372	18.2 11	47 300+	73 300+	84 300+	64 300+	55 300+	73 300+	66 300+	61 300+	56 300+	68 300+
Soldiers and Sailors Memorial Hospital of Yates, Penn Yan, NY	- -	- -	- -	0.189 122	0.000 54	12.9 357	- 0	65 (a)	75 (a)	86 (a)	66 (a)	55 (a)	76 (a)	60 (a)	72 (a)	64 (a)	70 (a)
Sound Shore Medical Center of Westschester, New Rochelle, NY	- -	- -	- -	0.044 294	0.011 88	5.7 175	- 0	44 300+	74 300+	75 300+	45 300+	51 300+	64 300+	59 300+	53 300+	47 300+	49 300+
South Nassau Communities Hospital, Oceanside, NY	- -	- -	- -	0.181 833	0.002 407	39.4 815	29.4 34	49 300+	76 300+	80 300+	65 300+	57 300+	73 300+	67 300+	66 300+	57 300+	70 300+
Southampton Hospital, Southampton, NY	- -	- -	- -	0.059 768	0.002 618	7.9 1073	24.2 165	49 300+	79 300+	73 300+	60 300+	59 300+	74 300+	66 300+	74 300+	59 300+	63 300+
Southside Hospital, Bay Shore, NY	- -	- -	- -	0.023 443	0.004 253	36.2 58	16.7 30	49 300+	77 300+	79 300+	61 300+	58 300+	77 300+	67 300+	71 300+	56 300+	67 300+
Staten Island University Hospital, Staten Island, NY	- -	- -	- -	0.071 608	0.069 232	7.7 2091	25.9 27	44 300+	72 300+	76 300+	57 300+	55 300+	72 300+	65 300+	64 300+	56 300+	61 300+
Strong Memorial Hospital, Rochester, NY	- -	- -	- -	0.239 952	0.123 788	8.3 169	28.3 53	37 300+	75 300+	87 300+	65 300+	60 300+	75 300+	65 300+	61 300+	56 300+	74 300+
Sunnyview Hospital and Rehabilitation Center, Schenectady, NY	- -	- -	- -	- 0	- 0	- 0	- 0	- -	- -	- -	- -	- -	- -	- -	- -	- -	- -
Syracuse VA Medical Center, Syracuse, NY	- -	- -	- -	- -	- -	- -	- -	- -	- -	- -	- -	- -	- -	- -	- -	- -	- -
TLC Health Network, Gowanda, NY	- -	- -	- -	0.058 206	0.000 99	4.4 364	- 0	41 300+	77 300+	88 300+	58 300+	57 300+	72 300+	67 300+	62 300+	57 300+	62 300+
United Health Services Hospitals, Johnson City, NY	- -	- -	- -	0.055 1770	0.022 1065	11.0 2794	- 0	39 300+	75 300+	85 300+	64 300+	58 300+	75 300+	69 300+	67 300+	63 300+	72 300+
United Memorial Medical Center, Batavia, NY	- -	- -	- -	0.554 294	0.023 175	7.0 458	27.8 18	45 300+	77 300+	86 300+	60 300+	63 300+	78 300+	67 300+	68 300+	63 300+	56 300+
Unity Hospital of Rochester, Rochester, NY	- -	- -	- -	0.608 240	0.205 44	11.3 391	- 0	47 300+	78 300+	88 300+	65 300+	55 300+	75 300+	65 300+	58 300+	56 300+	72 300+
University Hospital - Stony Brook, Stony Brook, NY	95 20	45 20	100 20	0.156 1100	0.012 1186	5.0 1177	25.5 149	44 300+	73 300+	79 300+	63 300+	54 300+	73 300+	67 300+	69 300+	58 300+	70 300+
University Hospital of Brooklyn - Downstate, Brooklyn, NY	- -	- -	- -	0.084 273	0.023 129	1.9 480	17.2 29	51 300+	77 300+	74 300+	47 300+	51 300+	65 300+	61 300+	58 300+	48 300+	57 300+
University Hospital S U N Y Health Science Center, Syracuse, NY	- -	- -	- -	0.115 583	0.048 745	21.7 506	10.3 29	46 300+	73 300+	83 300+	65 300+	59 300+	72 300+	67 300+	67 300+	55 300+	69 300+
Upstate New York VA Healthcare System, Buffalo, NY	- -	- -	- -	- -	- -	- -	- -	- -	- -	- -	- -	- -	- -	- -	- -	- -	- -
VA Hudson Valley Healthcare System, Montrose, NY	- -	- -	- -	- -	- -	- -	- -	- -	- -	- -	- -	- -	- -	- -	- -	- -	- -
VA New York Harbor Healthcare System, New York, NY	- -	- -	- -	- -	- -	- -	- -	- -	- -	- -	- -	- -	- -	- -	- -	- -	- -
Vassar Brothers Medical Center, Poughkeepsie, NY	- -	- -	- -	0.216 709	0.008 357	13.4 679	32.0 25	53 300+	79 300+	83 300+	71 300+	62 300+	81 300+	75 300+	71 300+	63 300+	80 300+
Westchester Medical Center, Valhalla, NY	- -	- -	- -	0.364 689	0.094 479	13.1 359	20.4 54	35 300+	71 300+	74 300+	56 300+	48 300+	64 300+	59 300+	53 300+	54 300+	61 300+
Westfield Memorial Hospital, Westfield, NY	- -	- -	- -	0.206 170	0.154 78	7.2 320	- 0	83 (a)	88 (a)	86 (a)	91 (a)	82 (a)	93 (a)	82 (a)	87 (a)	90 (a)	92 (a)
White Plains Hospital Center, White Plains, NY	- -	- -	- -	0.031 1967	0.000 2229	15.4 1982	- 0	53 300+	79 300+	72 300+	68 300+	62 300+	79 300+	71 300+	68 300+	63 300+	79 300+
Winifred Masterson Burke Rehab Hospital, White Plains, NY	- -	- -	- -	- 0	- 0	- 0	- 0	- -	- -	- -	- -	- -	- -	- -	- -	- -	- -
Winthrop-University Hospital, Mineola, NY	- -	- -	- -	0.014 284	0.000 79	17.0 525	20.0 10	45 300+	77 300+	83 300+	67 300+	57 300+	76 300+	67 300+	70 300+	57 300+	73 300+
Woman's Christian Association, Jamestown, NY	- -	- -	- -	0.144 563	0.003 313	5.2 1350	34.2 79	47 300+	78 300+	87 300+	54 300+	53 300+	71 300+	62 300+	65 300+	55 300+	56 300+
Woodhull Medical and Mental Health Center, Brooklyn, NY	- -	- -	- -	0.034 87	0.029 35	3.8 186	14.3 7	49 300+	74 300+	82 300+	51 300+	52 300+	63 300+	57 300+	63 300+	45 300+	53 300+
Wyckoff Heights Medical Center, Brooklyn, NY	- -	- -	- -	0.034 290	0.013 150	7.7 404	22.7 44	39 300+	66 300+	70 300+	39 300+	45 300+	54 300+	46 300+	55 300+	33 300+	44 300+
Wyoming County Community Hospital, Warsaw, NY	- -	- -	- -	0.568 132	0.096 104	17.8 191	11.1 9	38 300+	74 300+	84 300+	55 300+	55 300+	72 300+	67 300+	72 300+	57 300+	54 300+
NORTH CAROLINA																	
Alamance Regional Medical Center, Burlington, NC	- -	- -	- -	0.090 1037	0.000 942	6.9 2443	33.6 318	51 300+	82 300+	81 300+	62 300+	65 300+	77 300+	69 300+	73 300+	65 300+	62 300+
Albemarle Hospital Authority, Elizabeth City, NC	- -	- -	- -	0.037 730	0.001 679	10.1 1849	35.9 206	60 300+	80 300+	85 300+	66 300+	57 300+	76 300+	70 300+	74 300+	63 300+	65 300+
Alleghany County Memorial Hospital, Sparta, NC	- -	- -	- -	0.469 81	0.000 33	3.0 298	- 0	50 (a)	83 (a)	83 (a)	67 (a)	57 (a)	78 (a)	67 (a)	65 (a)	63 (a)	69 (a)
Angel Medical Center, Franklin, NC	- -	- -	- -	- 0	- 0	- 0	- 0	63 300+	88 300+	82 300+	76 300+	60 300+	82 300+	76 300+	71 300+	74 300+	82 300+
Anson Community Hospital, Wadesboro, NC	- -	- -	- -	0.027 222	0.023 88	10.7 419	40.0 5	67 (a)	86 (a)	79 (a)	70 (a)	74 (a)	79 (a)	70 (a)	69 (a)	67 (a)	59 (a)
Ashe Memorial Hospital, Jefferson, NC	- -	- -	- -	0.710 279	0.050 159	3.6 753	30.8 65	57 300+	86 300+	84 300+	71 300+	66 300+	83 300+	70 300+	80 300+	69 300+	68 300+
Asheville-Oteen VA Medical Center, Asheville, NC	- -	- -	- -	- -	- -	- -	- -	- -	- -	- -	- -	- -	- -	- -	- -	- -	- -
Beaufort County Medical Center, Washington, NC	- -	- -	- -	0.090 633	0.010 492	- 0	38.7 155	55 300+	83 300+	85 300+	64 300+	65 300+	78 300+	67 300+	71 300+	65 300+	67 300+
Bertie Memorial Hospital, Windsor, NC	- -	- -	- -	- -	- -	- -	- -	81 (a)	93 (a)	89 (a)	81 (a)	76 (a)	90 (a)	85 (a)	89 (a)	85 (a)	85 (a)
Betsy Johnson Regional Hospital, Dunn, NC	- -	- -	- -	0.228 707	0.015 327	11.6 715	27.7 155	64 300+	75 300+	75 300+	56 300+	57 300+	72 300+	64 300+	65 300+	54 300+	53 300+
Blowing Rock Hospital, Blowing Rock, NC	- -	- -	- -	- -	- -	- -	- -	- -	- -	- -	- -	- -	- -	- -	- -	- -	- -
Brunswick Community Hospital, Supply, NC	- -	- -	- -	0.050 516	0.018 337	5.5 1086	28.3 106	50 300+	82 300+	84 300+	62 300+	55 300+	76 300+	69 300+	63 300+	70 300+	62 300+
C J Harris Community Hospital, Sylva, NC	- -	- -	- -	0.583 544	0.125 655	12.4 956	28.7 223	61 300+	83 300+	83 300+	74 300+	63 300+	81 300+	73 300+	65 300+	70 300+	76 300+
Caldwell Memorial Hospital, Lenoir, NC	- -	- -	- -	0.059 438	0.000 327	11.1 1333	34.1 132	59 300+	83 300+	85 300+	63 300+	62 300+	76 300+	70 300+	63 300+	62 300+	62 300+
Cape Fear Valley Medical Center, Fayetteville, NC	- -	- -	- -	0.140 1359	0.082 944	6.6 1006	23.6 55	53 300+	76 300+	77 300+	58 300+	60 300+	73 300+	65 300+	66 300+	56 300+	59 300+

NOTE: The first number in each column (boldface) is the score, the second number is the number of patients; Please refer to the main entry for footnotes; (a) 100-299
*MEASURES: **Children's Asthma Care:** 33. Received Systemic Corticosteroids; 34. Received Home Management Plan of Care; 35. Received Reliever Medication; **Use of Medical Imaging:** 36. Combination Abdominal CT Scan; 37. Combination Chest CT Scan; 38. Follow-up Mammogram/Ultrasound; 39. MRI for Low Back Pain; **Survey of Patients' Hospital Experiences:** 40. Area Around Room 'Always' Quiet at Night; 41. Doctors 'Always' Communicated Well; 42. Home Recovery Information Given; 43. Hospital Given 9 or 10 on 10 Point Scale; 44. Meds 'Always' Explained Before Given; 45. Nurses 'Always' Communicated Well; 46. Pain 'Always' Well Controlled; 47. Room and Bathroom 'Always' Clean; 48. Timely Help 'Always' Received; 49. Would Definitely Recommend Hospital*

Hospital	Children's Asthma Care			Use of Medical Imaging				Survey of Patients' Hospital Experiences									
	33	34	35	36	37	38	39	40	41	42	43	44	45	46	47	48	49
Cape Fear Valley-Bladen County Hospital, Elizabethtown, NC	-	-	-	0.025 278	0.013 75	7.6 409	37.8 37	-	-	-	-	-	-	-	-	-	-
Carolina East Medical Center, New Bern, NC	-	-	-	0.069 598	0.029 244	8.9 1119	32.4 176	56 300+	75 300+	82 300+	59 300+	55 300+	73 300+	67 300+	57 300+	63 300+	66 300+
Carolinas Medical Center-Behavioral Health, Charlotte, NC	100 429	87 427	100 430	0.109 1772	0.000 1593	- 0	34.6 188	64 300+	82 300+	85 300+	71 300+	61 300+	76 300+	72 300+	60 300+	65 300+	76 300+
Carolinas Medical Center-Lincoln, Lincolnton, NC	-	-	-	0.030 467	0.020 307	10.8 720	38.2 123	54 300+	81 300+	86 300+	69 300+	58 300+	79 300+	68 300+	72 300+	67 300+	63 300+
Carolinas Medical Center-Mercy, Charlotte, NC	-	-	-	0.081 1763	0.016 1267	- 0	32.5 338	67 300+	84 300+	88 300+	78 300+	64 300+	81 300+	73 300+	64 300+	69 300+	81 300+
Carolinas Medical Center-Northeast, Concord, NC	100 44	82 45	100 45	0.042 2369	0.031 2438	5.4 3964	27.8 837	61 300+	85 300+	86 300+	72 300+	66 300+	80 300+	69 300+	71 300+	66 300+	76 300+
Carolinas Medical Center-Union, Monroe, NC	-	-	-	0.090 1185	0.148 896	0.0 9	28.9 232	63 300+	83 300+	86 300+	72 300+	65 300+	83 300+	73 300+	71 300+	71 300+	70 300+
Carolinas Medical Center-University, Charlotte, NC	-	-	-	0.085 845	0.003 372	- 0	38.3 128	63 300+	84 300+	86 300+	72 300+	67 300+	80 300+	71 300+	69 300+	63 300+	75 300+
Carteret General Hospital, Morehead City, NC	-	-	-	0.059 909	0.000 658	9.6 1516	29.5 166	61 300+	81 300+	79 300+	68 300+	63 300+	80 300+	72 300+	72 300+	72 300+	71 300+
Catawba Valley Medical Center, Hickory, NC	-	-	-	0.055 875	0.016 708	8.3 2280	30.2 305	56 300+	80 300+	84 300+	70 300+	62 300+	77 300+	71 300+	67 300+	64 300+	75 300+
Central Carolina Hospital, Sanford, NC	-	-	-	0.126 525	0.099 333	3.4 1508	27.7 137	56 300+	83 300+	83 300+	60 300+	60 300+	76 300+	70 300+	68 300+	59 300+	59 300+
Charles A Cannon Jr Memorial Hospital, Linville, NC	-	-	-	-	-	-	-	-	-	-	-	-	-	-	-	-	-
Chatham Hospital, Siler City, NC	-	-	-	-	-	-	-	70 (a)	90 (a)	75 (a)	77 (a)	73 (a)	86 (a)	71 (a)	82 (a)	79 (a)	71 (a)
Cherokee Indian Hospital Authority, Cherokee, NC	-	-	-	-	-	-	-	67 (a)	71 (a)	71 (a)	58 (a)	52 (a)	70 (a)	51 (a)	67 (a)	63 (a)	55 (a)
Chowan Hospital, Edenton, NC	-	-	-	-	-	-	-	63 300+	88 300+	88 300+	73 300+	65 300+	84 300+	76 300+	74 300+	73 300+	74 300+
Cleveland Regional Medical Center, Shelby, NC	-	-	-	0.655 1011	0.002 896	12.1 741	35.9 295	72 300+	86 300+	87 300+	76 300+	74 300+	84 300+	79 300+	69 300+	77 300+	77 300+
Columbus Regional Healthcare System, Whiteville, NC	-	-	-	0.098 500	0.013 237	2.9 1328	27.7 141	61 300+	81 300+	85 300+	66 300+	67 300+	79 300+	77 300+	66 300+	65 300+	63 300+
Davie County Hospital, Mocksville, NC	-	-	-	-	-	-	-	68 <100	79 <100	68 <100	54 <100	46 <100	74 <100	62 <100	69 <100	60 <100	60 <100
Davis Regional Medical Center, Statesville, NC	100 29	97 29	100 29	0.070 329	0.011 89	10.7 103	27.7 166	67 300+	82 300+	81 300+	74 300+	64 300+	77 300+	65 300+	76 300+	67 300+	75 300+
Duke Health Raleigh Hospital, Raleigh, NC	-	-	-	0.129 775	0.119 899	13.8 232	26.5 98	62 300+	84 300+	88 300+	71 300+	66 300+	78 300+	74 300+	68 300+	62 300+	77 300+
Duke University Hospital, Durham, NC	-	-	-	0.092 3829	0.034 5860	7.7 2854	32.1 446	55 300+	80 300+	88 300+	74 300+	64 300+	77 300+	65 300+	56 300+	54 300+	80 300+
Duplin General Hospital, Kenansville, NC	-	-	-	0.117 264	0.000 166	4.8 482	50.0 54	69 300+	81 300+	81 300+	69 300+	69 300+	79 300+	67 300+	72 300+	69 300+	62 300+
Durham Regional Hospital, Durham, NC	-	-	-	0.020 744	0.012 432	9.5 526	33.0 100	45 300+	78 300+	77 300+	58 300+	55 300+	70 300+	63 300+	59 300+	55 300+	69 300+
Durham VA Medical Center, Durham, NC	-	-	-	-	-	-	-	-	-	-	-	-	-	-	-	-	-
Fayetteville North Carolina VA Medical Center, Fayetteville, NC	-	-	-	-	-	-	-	-	-	-	-	-	-	-	-	-	-
Firsthealth Montgomery Memorial Hospital, Troy, NC	-	-	-	-	-	-	-	-	-	-	-	-	-	-	-	-	-
Firsthealth Moore Regional Hospital, Pinehurst, NC	100 55	22 54	100 55	0.090 1089	0.026 926	8.8 272	25.5 756	61 300+	85 300+	83 300+	79 300+	64 300+	81 300+	76 300+	74 300+	72 300+	83 300+
Firsthealth Richmond Memorial Hospital, Rockingham, NC	-	-	-	-	-	-	-	-	-	-	-	-	-	-	-	-	-
Forsyth Memorial Hospital, Winston-Salem, NC	-	-	-	0.001 991	0.000 204	- 0	31.0 42	56 300+	83 300+	83 300+	75 300+	64 300+	79 300+	71 300+	65 300+	65 300+	82 300+
Franklin Regional Medical Center, Louisburg, NC	-	-	-	0.075 255	0.070 200	8.8 546	37.1 62	67 (a)	79 (a)	87 (a)	70 (a)	66 (a)	79 (a)	73 (a)	71 (a)	71 (a)	66 (a)
Frye Regional Medical Center, Hickory, NC	-	-	-	0.070 952	0.025 849	7.5 2322	27.3 432	60 300+	84 300+	88 300+	66 300+	64 300+	76 300+	69 300+	62 300+	72 300+	72 300+
Gaston Memorial Hospital, Gastonia, NC	-	-	-	0.046 1769	0.008 1005	9.0 3801	24.6 780	56 300+	82 300+	83 300+	68 300+	62 300+	80 300+	72 300+	68 300+	69 300+	72 300+
Grace Hospital, Morganton, NC	-	-	-	0.116 302	0.011 271	16.2 499	32.1 106	67 300+	83 300+	85 300+	66 300+	65 300+	78 300+	68 300+	72 300+	63 300+	66 300+
Granville Medical Center, Oxford, NC	-	-	-	0.038 286	0.008 126	13.9 525	23.3 116	72 300+	84 300+	80 300+	67 300+	59 300+	79 300+	69 300+	69 300+	67 300+	70 300+
Halifax Regional Medical Center, Roanoke Rapids, NC	-	-	-	0.092 606	0.000 458	11.4 1381	39.4 94	63 300+	81 300+	79 300+	62 300+	62 300+	74 300+	67 300+	62 300+	64 300+	59 300+
Haywood Regional Medical Center, Clyde, NC	-	-	-	0.084 370	0.026 308	7.7 673	27.6 283	55 300+	84 300+	81 300+	61 300+	63 300+	79 300+	71 300+	59 300+	67 300+	67 300+
Heritage Hospital, Tarboro, NC	-	-	-	0.066 304	0.005 201	6.0 1019	24.1 141	67 300+	85 300+	87 300+	77 300+	72 300+	83 300+	75 300+	73 300+	74 300+	75 300+
High Point Regional Hospital, High Point, NC	-	-	-	0.013 748	0.009 223	5.5 289	30.1 186	58 300+	78 300+	80 300+	68 300+	58 300+	76 300+	69 300+	68 300+	63 300+	72 300+
Highlands Cashiers Hospital, Highlands, NC	-	-	-	-	-	-	-	-	-	-	-	-	-	-	-	-	-
Hugh Chatham Memorial Hospital, Elkin, NC	-	-	-	0.093 518	0.010 315	3.3 848	34.2 155	67 300+	85 300+	83 300+	79 300+	66 300+	84 300+	73 300+	82 300+	71 300+	78 300+
Iredell Memorial Hospital, Statesville, NC	-	-	-	0.029 756	0.005 366	3.1 1783	28.6 175	66 300+	86 300+	84 300+	74 300+	68 300+	82 300+	73 300+	73 300+	67 300+	79 300+
J Arthur Dosher Memorial Hospital, Southport, NC	-	-	-	-	-	-	-	-	-	-	-	-	-	-	-	-	-
Johnston Memorial Hospital, Smithfield, NC	-	-	-	0.105 553	0.041 591	9.7 1057	30.2 139	64 300+	81 300+	83 300+	62 300+	64 300+	78 300+	70 300+	68 300+	63 300+	63 300+
Kings Mountain Hospital, Kings Mountain, NC	-	-	-	0.585 205	0.000 92	10.6 378	49.4 81	71 (a)	86 (a)	85 (a)	77 (a)	71 (a)	84 (a)	77 (a)	68 (a)	75 (a)	74 (a)
Lake Norman Regional Medical Center, Mooresville, NC	100 25	100 23	100 25	0.080 858	0.010 620	7.9 1339	25.7 140	58 300+	84 300+	86 300+	70 300+	62 300+	76 300+	71 300+	73 300+	65 300+	72 300+
Lenoir Memorial Hospital, Kinston, NC	-	-	-	0.324 565	0.000 400	- 0	28.7 157	55 300+	77 300+	78 300+	62 300+	56 300+	75 300+	68 300+	70 300+	58 300+	61 300+
Lexington Memorial Hospital, Lexington, NC	-	-	-	0.045 514	0.003 349	7.8 857	29.3 133	58 300+	82 300+	83 300+	66 300+	67 300+	79 300+	71 300+	75 300+	68 300+	63 300+
Margaret R Pardee Memorial Hospital, Hendersonville, NC	-	-	-	0.127 1234	0.043 792	9.4 2610	29.3 451	53 300+	80 300+	81 300+	64 300+	60 300+	75 300+	64 300+	74 300+	62 300+	70 300+
Maria Parham Hospital, Henderson, NC	-	-	-	0.029 653	0.017 468	8.4 1250	36.1 97	68 300+	83 300+	83 300+	63 300+	65 300+	80 300+	74 300+	74 300+	68 300+	64 300+
Martin General Hospital, Williamston, NC	-	-	-	0.689 135	0.000 101	6.4 515	35.9 64	68 300+	83 300+	82 300+	60 300+	61 300+	76 300+	70 300+	58 300+	57 300+	61 300+
The Mcdowell Hospital, Marion, NC	-	-	-	0.028 464	0.003 291	5.0 707	- 0	64 300+	81 300+	84 300+	69 300+	64 300+	80 300+	72 300+	77 300+	70 300+	68 300+
Medical Park Hospital, Winston-Salem, NC	-	-	-	- 0	- 0	- 0	- 0	71 300+	86 300+	82 300+	84 300+	64 300+	83 300+	75 300+	75 300+	76 300+	88 300+
Memorial Mission Hosp/Asheville Surgery Ctr, Asheville, NC	100 36	19 36	100 36	0.013 1109	0.000 407	- 0	36.4 151	60 300+	83 300+	85 300+	71 300+	59 300+	79 300+	72 300+	63 300+	67 300+	84 300+
Morehead Memorial Hospital, Eden, NC	-	-	-	0.127 503	0.094 469	5.4 745	42.0 119	48 300+	84 300+	80 300+	66 300+	60 300+	78 300+	69 300+	76 300+	67 300+	74 300+
The Moses H Cone Memorial Hospital, Greensboro, NC	-	-	-	0.033 1813	0.001 1623	7.1 1837	30.8 312	59 300+	78 300+	80 300+	63 300+	56 300+	72 300+	67 300+	63 300+	58 300+	73 300+
Murphy Medical Center, Murphy, NC	-	-	-	0.366 755	0.006 473	3.1 786	29.1 151	53 300+	83 300+	82 300+	63 300+	58 300+	77 300+	69 300+	72 300+	65 300+	67 300+
Nash General Hospital, Rocky Mount, NC	-	-	-	0.040 970	0.012 490	12.5 1224	32.6 427	54 300+	82 300+	81 300+	60 300+	65 300+	78 300+	71 300+	67 300+	64 300+	57 300+
New Hanover Regional Medical Center, Wilmington, NC	-	-	-	0.053 1836	0.006 1150	9.0 1355	23.7 558	62 300+	82 300+	85 300+	74 300+	64 300+	83 300+	73 300+	75 300+	67 300+	80 300+
North Carolina Baptist Hospital, Winston-Salem, NC	100 72	68 72	100 72	0.293 3253	0.006 3046	8.5 1443	28.3 219	66 300+	80 300+	82 300+	76 300+	61 300+	75 300+	68 300+	69 300+	59 300+	82 300+
North Carolina Specialty Hospital, Durham, NC	-	-	-	- 0	- 0	- 0	- 0	83 300+	91 300+	91 300+	89 300+	73 300+	87 300+	79 300+	88 300+	82 300+	92 300+
Northern Hospital of Surry County, Mount Airy, NC	-	-	-	0.108 986	0.000 786	6.5 1137	31.1 164	58 300+	78 300+	82 300+	61 300+	54 300+	75 300+	68 300+	78 300+	65 300+	60 300+
Onslow Memorial Hospital, Jacksonville, NC	-	-	-	0.107 579	0.008 374	11.9 732	22.8 57	56 300+	77 300+	85 300+	63 300+	60 300+	78 300+	68 300+	66 300+	69 300+	60 300+
The Outer Banks Hospital, Nags Head, NC	-	-	-	-	-	-	-	66 300+	85 300+	88 300+	78 300+	70 300+	81 300+	74 300+	76 300+	79 300+	75 300+
Park Ridge Hospital, Fletcher, NC	-	-	-	0.091 463	0.092 305	10.4 597	26.6 188	58 300+	81 300+	81 300+	71 300+	56 300+	75 300+	68 300+	68 300+	63 300+	73 300+
Pender Memorial Hospital, Burgaw, NC	-	-	-	-	-	-	-	-	-	-	-	-	-	-	-	-	-
Person Memorial Hospital, Roxboro, NC	-	-	-	0.075 227	0.016 187	5.5 685	36.9 65	67 300+	84 300+	78 300+	64 300+	57 300+	77 300+	68 300+	66 300+	60 300+	70 300+
Pitt County Memorial Hospital, Greenville, NC	-	-	-	0.088 1155	0.014 694	11.3 71	30.9 123	60 300+	82 300+	88 300+	78 300+	66 300+	81 300+	73 300+	72 300+	66 300+	82 300+

NOTE: The first number in each column (boldface) is the score, the second number is the number of patients; Please refer to the main entry for footnotes; (a) 100-299

*MEASURES: **Children's Asthma Care:** 33. Received Systemic Corticosteroids; 34. Received Home Management Plan of Care; 35. Received Reliever Medication; **Use of Medical Imaging:** 36. Combination Abdominal CT Scan; 37. Combination Chest CT Scan; 38. Follow-up Mammogram/Ultrasound; 39. MRI for Low Back Pain; **Survey of Patients' Hospital Experiences:** 40. Area Around Room 'Always' Quiet at Night; 41. Doctors 'Always' Communicated Well; 42. Home Recovery Information Given; 43. Hospital Given 9 or 10 on 10 Point Scale; 44. Meds 'Always' Explained Before Given; 45. Nurses 'Always' Communicated Well; 46. Pain 'Always' Well Controlled; 47. Room and Bathroom 'Always' Clean; 48. Timely Help 'Always' Received; 49. Would Definitely Recommend Hospital*

Hospital	Children's Asthma Care			Use of Medical Imaging				Survey of Patients' Hospital Experiences									
	33	34	35	36	37	38	39	40	41	42	43	44	45	46	47	48	49
Presbyterian Hospital, Charlotte, NC	100 173	82 172	100 173	0.024 829	0.003 380	- 0	25.4 71	61 300+	84 300+	83 300+	77 300+	63 300+	82 300+	76 300+	71 300+	68 300+	81 300+
Presbyterian Hospital Huntersville, Huntersville, NC	- -	- -	- -	0.033 850	0.000 695	- 0	30.6 170	61 300+	83 300+	86 300+	77 300+	59 300+	77 300+	72 300+	65 300+	67 300+	82 300+
Presbyterian Hospital Matthews, Matthews, NC	- -	- -	- -	0.051 1365	0.000 907	5.8 1153	26.7 243	62 300+	78 300+	85 300+	70 300+	57 300+	73 300+	67 300+	70 300+	60 300+	77 300+
Presbyterian-Orthopaedic Hospital, Charlotte, NC	- -	- -	- -	0.045 156	0.000 107	- 0	28.1 114	57 300+	84 300+	89 300+	68 300+	61 300+	71 300+	66 300+	65 300+	49 300+	76 300+
Pungo District Hospital, Belhaven, NC	- -	- -	- -	- -	- -	- -	- -	- -	- -	- -	- -	- -	- -	- -	- -	- -	- -
Randolph Hospital, Asheboro, NC	- -	- -	- -	0.032 727	0.130 532	10.0 928	29.3 157	58 300+	80 300+	79 300+	67 300+	62 300+	80 300+	68 300+	73 300+	68 300+	68 300+
Rex Hospital, Raleigh, NC	- -	- -	- -	0.173 1430	0.056 1014	5.8 1895	30.7 316	52 300+	82 300+	87 300+	75 300+	62 300+	77 300+	69 300+	64 300+	64 300+	84 300+
Roanoke Chowan Hospital, Ahoskie, NC	- -	- -	- -	0.094 448	0.005 200	10.6 1225	45.6 57	64 300+	85 300+	84 300+	69 300+	74 300+	82 300+	74 300+	69 300+	71 300+	64 300+
Rowan Regional Medical Center, Salisbury, NC	100 18	100 18	100 18	0.170 949	0.202 575	17.6 771	29.7 438	67 300+	83 300+	85 300+	69 300+	63 300+	80 300+	73 300+	70 300+	68 300+	67 300+
Rutherford Hospital, Rutherfordton, NC	- -	- -	- -	0.039 837	0.002 412	9.5 1637	29.4 211	65 300+	86 300+	82 300+	70 300+	64 300+	80 300+	69 300+	77 300+	73 300+	68 300+
Saint Lukes Hospital, Columbus, NC	- -	- -	- -	0.125 305	0.144 132	9.3 536	27.9 68	62 (a)	82 (a)	84 (a)	74 (a)	59 (a)	79 (a)	71 (a)	73 (a)	75 (a)	77 (a)
Sampson Regional Medical Center, Clinton, NC	- -	- -	- -	0.395 588	0.081 369	4.7 993	41.0 134	69 300+	84 300+	85 300+	65 300+	65 300+	79 300+	71 300+	68 300+	65 300+	61 300+
Sandhills Regional Medical Center, Hamlet, NC	- -	- -	- -	0.545 132	0.371 97	9.7 258	29.7 64	72 300+	81 300+	78 300+	58 300+	59 300+	74 300+	70 300+	66 300+	60 300+	59 300+
Scotland Memorial Hospital, Laurinburg, NC	- -	- -	- -	0.099 1048	0.115 399	6.2 1181	30.5 164	67 300+	84 300+	80 300+	64 300+	65 300+	78 300+	71 300+	63 300+	68 300+	62 300+
Southeastern Regional Medical Center, Lumberton, NC	- -	- -	- -	0.037 970	0.016 708	- 0	31.1 338	72 300+	84 300+	84 300+	67 300+	70 300+	81 300+	70 300+	70 300+	70 300+	64 300+
Spruce Pine Community Hospital, Spruce Pine, NC	- -	- -	- -	0.790 315	0.890 200	3.7 574	40.7 81	68 300+	84 300+	79 300+	76 300+	66 300+	82 300+	75 300+	77 300+	72 300+	75 300+
Stanly Regional Medical Center, Albemarle, NC	- -	- -	- -	0.079 828	0.020 543	5.1 1442	34.6 156	59 300+	81 300+	80 300+	63 300+	60 300+	76 300+	68 300+	71 300+	66 300+	60 300+
Stokes-Reynolds Memorial Hospital, Danbury, NC	- -	- -	- -	- -	- -	- -	- -	- -	- -	- -	- -	- -	- -	- -	- -	- -	- -
Thomasville Medical Center, Thomasville, NC	100 9	33 9	100 9	0.021 387	0.016 190	6.6 588	39.0 77	63 300+	86 300+	85 300+	73 300+	60 300+	80 300+	69 300+	78 300+	71 300+	74 300+
Transylvania Regional Hospital, Brevard, NC	- -	- -	- -	- -	- -	- -	- -	68 300+	80 300+	87 300+	76 300+	62 300+	81 300+	71 300+	78 300+	68 300+	75 300+
University of North Carolina Hospital, Chapel Hill, NC	- -	- -	- -	0.059 1762	0.000 1929	7.5 1715	23.0 200	64 300+	82 300+	88 300+	81 300+	68 300+	80 300+	73 300+	72 300+	65 300+	85 300+
Valdese General Hospital, Valdese, NC	- -	- -	- -	0.137 263	0.000 272	18.0 372	26.2 84	69 300+	85 300+	91 300+	75 300+	65 300+	83 300+	77 300+	76 300+	73 300+	77 300+
W G (Bill) Hefner Salisbury VA Medical Center, Salisbury, NC	- -	- -	- -	- -	- -	- -	- -	- -	- -	- -	- -	- -	- -	- -	- -	- -	- -
Wakemed - Cary Hospital, Cary, NC	- -	- -	- -	0.050 619	0.017 424	4.1 458	27.8 115	57 300+	80 300+	82 300+	68 300+	60 300+	75 300+	67 300+	67 300+	61 300+	75 300+
Wakemed - Raleigh Campus, Raleigh, NC	- -	- -	- -	0.049 835	0.033 599	5.8 1184	38.3 149	60 300+	79 300+	85 300+	74 300+	62 300+	76 300+	71 300+	62 300+	64 300+	75 300+
Washington County Hospital, Plymouth, NC	- -	- -	- -	0.881 67	0.000 35	9.3 225	42.3 26	- -	- -	- -	- -	- -	- -	- -	- -	- -	- -
Watauga Medical Center, Boone, NC	- -	- -	- -	0.210 572	0.041 462	10.6 1171	26.5 170	60 300+	86 300+	83 300+	71 300+	63 300+	79 300+	73 300+	74 300+	64 300+	77 300+
Wayne Memorial Hospital, Goldsboro, NC	- -	- -	- -	0.026 495	0.023 310	5.1 292	37.2 406	64 300+	83 300+	82 300+	69 300+	63 300+	80 300+	70 300+	75 300+	63 300+	67 300+
Wilkes Regional Medical Center, North Wilkesboro, NC	- -	- -	- -	0.105 743	0.063 334	9.3 1388	34.7 176	71 300+	85 300+	81 300+	70 300+	66 300+	82 300+	72 300+	74 300+	74 300+	65 300+
Wilson Medical Center, Wilson, NC	97 30	90 30	97 30	0.126 1007	0.325 787	7.6 1520	38.1 181	68 300+	84 300+	87 300+	70 300+	61 300+	80 300+	75 300+	67 300+	66 300+	67 300+
Yadkin Valley Community Hospital, Yadkinville, NC	- -	- -	- -	- -	- -	- -	- -	- -	- -	- -	- -	- -	- -	- -	- -	- -	- -
OHIO																	
Adams County Regional Medical Center, Seaman, OH	- -	- -	- -	- -	- -	- -	- -	- -	- -	- -	- -	- -	- -	- -	- -	- -	- -
Adena Regional Medical Center, Chillicothe, OH	- -	- -	- -	0.039 1190	0.076 939	8.2 1710	28.7 397	41 300+	81 300+	77 300+	62 300+	58 300+	76 300+	68 300+	60 300+	58 300+	66 300+
Affinity Medical Center, Massillon, OH	- -	- -	- -	0.067 478	0.160 324	11.1 633	25.8 66	46 300+	77 300+	85 300+	64 300+	55 300+	72 300+	69 300+	67 300+	57 300+	65 300+
Akron General Medical Center, Akron, OH	- -	- -	- -	0.105 1703	0.007 1532	6.4 4412	32.5 379	46 300+	76 300+	86 300+	66 300+	59 300+	76 300+	69 300+	61 300+	63 300+	72 300+
Allen Community Hospital, Oberlin, OH	- -	- -	- -	- -	- -	- -	- -	56 300+	84 300+	83 300+	75 300+	66 300+	82 300+	76 300+	79 300+	71 300+	75 300+
Alliance Community Hospital, Alliance, OH	- -	- -	- -	0.678 574	0.016 377	6.5 769	23.3 90	48 300+	75 300+	84 300+	66 300+	56 300+	73 300+	64 300+	75 300+	64 300+	64 300+
Amherst Hospital, Amherst, OH	- -	- -	- -	0.000 97	0.000 47	- 0	- 0	67 300+	77 300+	85 300+	80 300+	63 300+	83 300+	75 300+	84 300+	75 300+	82 300+
Ashtabula County Medical Center, Ashtabula, OH	- -	- -	- -	0.027 634	0.004 560	13.9 677	34.7 95	39 300+	73 300+	75 300+	49 300+	55 300+	72 300+	63 300+	76 300+	58 300+	49 300+
Atrium Medical Center, Franklin, OH	- -	- -	- -	0.062 961	0.016 765	8.9 1455	29.9 147	59 300+	76 300+	82 300+	64 300+	57 300+	73 300+	68 300+	73 300+	55 300+	65 300+
Aultman Hospital, Canton, OH	100 13	62 13	100 14	0.071 1864	0.059 1474	8.6 1705	31.9 389	52 300+	78 300+	79 300+	74 300+	63 300+	77 300+	70 300+	67 300+	64 300+	79 300+
Barnesville Hospital Association, Barnesville, OH	- -	- -	- -	0.181 177	0.101 138	17.6 159	50.0 14	51 300+	82 300+	79 300+	77 300+	67 300+	85 300+	75 300+	80 300+	80 300+	75 300+
Bay Park Community Hospital, Oregon, OH	- -	- -	- -	0.045 246	0.004 254	8.9 484	36.2 58	60 300+	73 300+	86 300+	74 300+	61 300+	78 300+	70 300+	74 300+	66 300+	76 300+
Bellevue Hospital, Bellevue, OH	- -	- -	- -	0.330 306	0.381 202	10.3 390	31.5 73	59 300+	85 300+	85 300+	82 300+	64 300+	79 300+	71 300+	83 300+	67 300+	80 300+
Belmont Community Hospital, Bellaire, OH	- -	- -	- -	0.152 79	0.000 100	14.4 180	30.4 56	49 (a)	77 (a)	79 (a)	64 (a)	59 (a)	70 (a)	69 (a)	70 (a)	63 (a)	64 (a)
Berger Hospital, Circleville, OH	- -	- -	- -	0.049 546	0.011 366	10.5 630	31.2 77	37 300+	74 300+	83 300+	56 300+	53 300+	72 300+	65 300+	63 300+	64 300+	58 300+
Bethesda North Hospital, Cincinnati, OH	- -	- -	- -	0.098 1959	0.010 1878	16.0 2888	29.7 273	52 300+	75 300+	87 300+	72 300+	52 300+	75 300+	66 300+	71 300+	61 300+	78 300+
Blanchard Valley Hospital, Findlay, OH	- -	- -	- -	0.121 1107	0.034 582	9.3 1414	27.1 339	61 300+	83 300+	83 300+	72 300+	62 300+	76 300+	71 300+	82 300+	67 300+	72 300+
Bluffton Hospital, Bluffton, OH	- -	- -	- -	0.061 99	0.022 45	13.0 276	- 0	75 (a)	87 (a)	87 (a)	87 (a)	69 (a)	86 (a)	79 (a)	81 (a)	83 (a)	89 (a)
Brown County Hospital, Georgetown, OH	- -	- -	- -	0.041 241	0.053 132	9.4 299	50.0 60	49 300+	72 300+	80 300+	51 300+	51 300+	71 300+	61 300+	70 300+	59 300+	51 300+
Bucyrus Community Hospital, Bucyrus, OH	- -	- -	- -	- -	- -	- -	- -	62 (a)	80 (a)	90 (a)	69 (a)	65 (a)	77 (a)	72 (a)	68 (a)	76 (a)	64 (a)
Butler County Medical Center, Hamilton, OH	- -	- -	- -	0.087 286	0.004 244	12.7 166	30.4 168	80 (a)	97 (a)	91 (a)	93 (a)	77 (a)	92 (a)	86 (a)	88 (a)	88 (a)	90 (a)
Chillicothe VA Medical Center, Chillicothe, OH	- -	- -	- -	- -	- -	- -	- -	- -	- -	- -	- -	- -	- -	- -	- -	- -	- -
Christ Hospital, Cincinnati, OH	- -	- -	- -	0.069 1411	0.011 1279	5.1 2445	35.7 213	54 300+	82 300+	86 300+	80 300+	62 300+	83 300+	73 300+	64 300+	68 300+	85 300+
Cincinnati VA Medical Center, Cincinnati, OH	- -	- -	- -	- -	- -	- -	- -	- -	- -	- -	- -	- -	- -	- -	- -	- -	- -
Cleveland Clinic, Cleveland, OH	100 30	0 29	100 30	0.311 3773	0.002 3973	12.1 1905	24.9 205	51 300+	76 300+	83 300+	76 300+	59 300+	75 300+	68 300+	68 300+	58 300+	82 300+
Cleveland-Wade Park VA Medical Center, Cleveland, OH	- -	- -	- -	- -	- -	- -	- -	- -	- -	- -	- -	- -	- -	- -	- -	- -	- -
CMH Regional Health System, Wilmington, OH	- -	- -	- -	0.563 528	0.025 447	8.1 980	30.1 113	54 300+	77 300+	87 300+	69 300+	64 300+	78 300+	66 300+	83 300+	69 300+	67 300+
Community Hospitals and Wellness Centers, Bryan, OH	- -	- -	- -	0.049 246	0.073 219	7.3 179	20.7 92	62 300+	79 300+	84 300+	73 300+	63 300+	78 300+	72 300+	82 300+	74 300+	70 300+
Community Regional Medical Center, Lorain, OH	- -	- -	- -	0.051 995	0.269 759	7.4 2206	27.6 246	52 300+	77 300+	85 300+	60 300+	58 300+	73 300+	65 300+	70 300+	57 300+	59 300+
Coshocton County Memorial Hospital, Coshocton, OH	- -	- -	- -	0.098 315	0.024 207	9.2 654	27.9 68	47 300+	76 300+	80 300+	58 300+	55 300+	74 300+	65 300+	72 300+	65 300+	51 300+
Crystal Clinic Orthopaedic Center, Akron, OH	- -	- -	- -	- 0	- 0	- 0	- 0	- -	- -	- -	- -	- -	- -	- -	- -	- -	- -
Dayton VA Medical Center, Dayton, OH	- -	- -	- -	- -	- -	- -	- -	- -	- -	- -	- -	- -	- -	- -	- -	- -	- -
Deaconess Hospital, Cincinnati, OH	- -	- -	- -	0.484 215	0.159 157	5.4 332	18.4 49	55 (a)	86 (a)	90 (a)	79 (a)	66 (a)	78 (a)	73 (a)	62 (a)	68 (a)	74 (a)
Defiance Regional Medical Center, Defiance, OH	- -	- -	- -	- -	- -	- -	- -	63 300+	77 300+	85 300+	75 300+	60 300+	77 300+	68 300+	76 300+	69 300+	77 300+
Diley Ridge Medical Center, Canal Winchester, OH	- -	- -	- -	- -	- -	- -	- -	- -	- -	- -	- -	- -	- -	- -	- -	- -	- -

NOTE: The first number in each column (boldface) is the score, the second number is the number of patients; Please refer to the main entry for footnotes; (a) 100-299
*MEASURES: **Children's Asthma Care:** 33. Received Systemic Corticosteroids; 34. Received Home Management Plan of Care; 35. Received Reliever Medication; **Use of Medical Imaging:** 36. Combination Abdominal CT Scan; 37. Combination Chest CT Scan; 38. Follow-up Mammogram/Ultrasound; 39. MRI for Low Back Pain; **Survey of Patients' Hospital Experiences:** 40. Area Around Room 'Always' Quiet at Night; 41. Doctors 'Always' Communicated Well; 42. Home Recovery Information Given; 43. Hospital Given 9 or 10 on 10 Point Scale; 44. Meds 'Always' Explained Before Given; 45. Nurses 'Always' Communicated Well; 46. Pain 'Always' Well Controlled; 47. Room and Bathroom 'Always' Clean; 48. Timely Help 'Always' Received; 49. Would Definitely Recommend Hospital*

Hospital	Children's Asthma Care			Use of Medical Imaging				Survey of Patients' Hospital Experiences									
	33	34	35	36	37	38	39	40	41	42	43	44	45	46	47	48	49
Doctors Hospital, Columbus, OH	-	-	-	0.074 498	0.013 391	6.7 582	17.7 96	58 300+	79 300+	82 300+	72 300+	64 300+	81 300+	69 300+	68 300+	69 300+	73 300+
Doctors Hospital of Nelsonville, Nelsonville, OH	-	-	-	-	-	-	-	-	-	-	-	-	-	-	-	-	-
Dublin Methodist Hospital, Dublin, OH	-	-	-	0.035 142	0.035 85	0.0 2	42.9 7	78 300+	83 300+	81 300+	82 300+	65 300+	80 300+	71 300+	73 300+	67 300+	86 300+
Dunlap Memorial Hospital, Orrville, OH	-	-	-	-	-	-	-	-	-	-	-	-	-	-	-	-	-
East Liverpool City Hospital, East Liverpool, OH	-	-	-	0.079 390	0.069 274	7.2 446	32.7 98	50 300+	78 300+	76 300+	55 300+	57 300+	70 300+	63 300+	69 300+	60 300+	50 300+
East Ohio Regional Hospital, Martins Ferry, OH	-	-	-	0.632 277	0.006 340	12.3 471	31.3 32	37 300+	70 300+	76 300+	49 300+	51 300+	67 300+	62 300+	60 300+	51 300+	51 300+
Edwin Shaw Rehabilitation Institute, Cuyahoga Falls, OH	-	-	-	-	-	-	-	-	-	-	-	-	-	-	-	-	-
Emh Regional Medical Center, Elyria, OH	-	-	-	0.053 1118	0.001 722	6.1 558	28.2 117	45 300+	71 300+	79 300+	60 300+	55 300+	71 300+	64 300+	62 300+	60 300+	62 300+
Euclid Hospital, Euclid, OH	-	-	-	0.065 291	0.000 248	9.7 422	17.0 47	52 300+	76 300+	84 300+	63 300+	58 300+	75 300+	67 300+	63 300+	56 300+	68 300+
Evendale Medical Center, Cincinnati, OH	-	-	-	- 0	- 0	- 0	- 0	80 300+	91 300+	92 300+	83 300+	71 300+	82 300+	76 300+	84 300+	77 300+	81 300+
Fairfield Medical Center, Lancaster, OH	-	-	-	0.081 853	0.002 550	9.6 655	27.1 96	42 300+	76 300+	83 300+	64 300+	56 300+	76 300+	68 300+	72 300+	64 300+	68 300+
Fairview Hospital, Cleveland, OH	-	-	-	0.073 926	0.003 641	13.9 1415	36.4 55	57 300+	77 300+	81 300+	73 300+	60 300+	74 300+	68 300+	83 300+	62 300+	77 300+
Fayette County Memorial Hospital, Washington CH, OH	-	-	-	0.044 343	0.006 176	10.8 344	37.5 32	53 (a)	75 (a)	81 (a)	59 (a)	61 (a)	76 (a)	61 (a)	74 (a)	70 (a)	54 (a)
Firelands Regional Medical Center, Sandusky, OH	-	-	-	0.150 851	0.032 527	4.4 1373	27.2 173	54 300+	78 300+	83 300+	65 300+	59 300+	77 300+	67 300+	82 300+	63 300+	69 300+
Fisher Titus Memorial Hospital, Norwalk, OH	-	-	-	0.106 395	0.014 281	9.2 661	30.6 85	55 300+	74 300+	86 300+	71 300+	63 300+	74 300+	68 300+	79 300+	61 300+	74 300+
Flower Hospital, Sylvania, OH	-	-	-	0.022 458	0.016 378	8.5 661	32.0 97	50 300+	78 300+	87 300+	70 300+	57 300+	77 300+	67 300+	71 300+	61 300+	73 300+
Fort Hamilton Hughes Memorial Hospital, Hamilton, OH	-	-	-	0.057 645	0.002 441	9.3 983	36.1 119	49 300+	75 300+	75 300+	55 300+	54 300+	74 300+	66 300+	70 300+	60 300+	58 300+
Fostoria Community Hospital, Fostoria, OH	-	-	-	-	-	-	-	59 300+	80 300+	87 300+	70 300+	61 300+	79 300+	72 300+	77 300+	71 300+	74 300+
Fulton County Health Center, Wauseon, OH	-	-	-	0.173 387	0.041 217	3.9 512	25.5 55	50 300+	80 300+	85 300+	73 300+	58 300+	74 300+	72 300+	84 300+	68 300+	72 300+
Galion Community Hospital, Galion, OH	-	-	-	-	-	-	-	55 300+	88 300+	89 300+	73 300+	69 300+	83 300+	77 300+	81 300+	79 300+	73 300+
Genesis Healthcare System, Zanesville, OH	-	-	-	0.085 756	0.000 485	5.0 101	42.1 38	57 300+	78 300+	82 300+	69 300+	61 300+	79 300+	72 300+	72 300+	71 300+	70 300+
Glenbeigh, Rock Creek, OH	-	-	-	- 0	- 0	- 0	- 0	-	-	-	-	-	-	-	-	-	-
Good Samaritan Hospital, Dayton, OH	-	-	-	0.047 1102	0.011 1070	9.7 2531	33.5 200	50 300+	73 300+	85 300+	62 300+	54 300+	71 300+	64 300+	58 300+	53 300+	65 300+
Good Samaritan Hospital, Cincinnati, OH	-	-	-	0.082 939	0.002 919	9.4 1559	28.1 160	53 300+	77 300+	87 300+	73 300+	59 300+	77 300+	71 300+	66 300+	63 300+	76 300+
Grady Memorial Hospital, Delaware, OH	-	-	-	0.040 346	0.010 195	12.1 527	23.4 64	53 300+	81 300+	83 300+	67 300+	59 300+	76 300+	69 300+	72 300+	60 300+	68 300+
Grandview Hospital & Medical Center, Dayton, OH	-	-	-	0.263 1413	0.171 643	5.9 942	29.8 235	51 300+	79 300+	83 300+	68 300+	55 300+	75 300+	66 300+	67 300+	59 300+	71 300+
Grant Medical Center, Columbus, OH	-	-	-	0.032 658	0.009 441	10.1 485	23.0 122	51 300+	79 300+	87 300+	68 300+	61 300+	78 300+	70 300+	70 300+	62 300+	74 300+
Greene Memorial Hospital, Xenia, OH	-	-	-	0.107 467	0.188 287	11.1 704	23.8 63	46 300+	77 300+	81 300+	56 300+	57 300+	72 300+	65 300+	64 300+	56 300+	59 300+
Greenfield Area Medical Center, Greenfield, OH	-	-	-	0.027 110	0.111 63	8.9 112	- 0	-	-	-	-	-	-	-	-	-	-
H B Magruder Memorial Hospital, Port Clinton, OH	-	-	-	-	-	-	-	66 300+	90 300+	82 300+	81 300+	71 300+	88 300+	77 300+	85 300+	83 300+	81 300+
Hardin Memorial Hospital, Kenton, OH	-	-	-	-	-	-	-	61 (a)	78 (a)	76 (a)	67 (a)	62 (a)	78 (a)	68 (a)	79 (a)	69 (a)	59 (a)
Harrison Community Hospital, Cadiz, OH	-	-	-	-	-	-	-	-	-	-	-	-	-	-	-	-	-
Henry County Hospital, Napoleon, OH	-	-	-	-	-	-	-	72 (a)	87 (a)	90 (a)	84 (a)	73 (a)	86 (a)	81 (a)	90 (a)	84 (a)	78 (a)
Highland District Hospital, Hillsboro, OH	-	-	-	0.613 507	0.333 330	11.9 461	33.3 72	-	-	-	-	-	-	-	-	-	-
Hillcrest Hospital, Mayfield Heights, OH	-	-	-	0.403 1485	0.000 1074	10.3 1692	27.6 214	39 300+	73 300+	76 300+	59 300+	52 300+	68 300+	63 300+	63 300+	56 300+	65 300+
Hocking Valley Community Hospital, Logan, OH	-	-	-	-	-	-	-	62 300+	83 300+	88 300+	76 300+	64 300+	81 300+	76 300+	73 300+	71 300+	66 300+
Holzer Medical Center, Gallipolis, OH	-	-	-	0.061 294	0.009 110	- 0	- 0	57 300+	80 300+	85 300+	65 300+	61 300+	79 300+	73 300+	77 300+	68 300+	63 300+
Holzer Medical Center Jackson, Jackson, OH	-	-	-	0.041 416	0.000 107	4.3 70	26.5 34	71 300+	80 300+	85 300+	70 300+	65 300+	84 300+	75 300+	81 300+	77 300+	70 300+
Huron Hospital, Cleveland, OH	-	-	-	0.019 158	0.029 139	8.1 186	25.9 27	56 300+	72 300+	79 300+	50 300+	55 300+	70 300+	62 300+	62 300+	48 300+	48 300+
Institute for Orthopedic Surgery, Lima, OH	-	-	-	- 0	- 0	- 0	- 0	78 300+	90 300+	95 300+	92 300+	78 300+	91 300+	80 300+	82 300+	88 300+	94 300+
Jewish Hospital, Cincinnati, OH	-	-	-	0.087 1196	0.010 955	8.2 3500	34.3 396	51 300+	77 300+	82 300+	68 300+	62 300+	78 300+	69 300+	69 300+	62 300+	75 300+
Joel Pomerene Memorial Hospital, Millersburg, OH	-	-	-	0.101 109	0.000 99	8.2 233	24.0 25	59 300+	80 300+	83 300+	67 300+	57 300+	76 300+	65 300+	78 300+	62 300+	60 300+
Joint Township District Memorial Hospital, Saint Marys, OH	-	-	-	0.582 354	0.074 257	5.4 553	24.4 82	59 300+	81 300+	85 300+	72 300+	68 300+	81 300+	73 300+	82 300+	72 300+	73 300+
Kettering Medical Center, Kettering, OH	-	-	-	0.119 1540	0.028 1350	- 0	32.0 172	44 300+	77 300+	86 300+	68 300+	58 300+	75 300+	67 300+	64 300+	56 300+	75 300+
Kettering Medical Center - Sycamore, Miamisburg, OH	-	-	-	0.088 922	0.014 507	- 0	27.3 99	48 300+	74 300+	86 300+	68 300+	53 300+	73 300+	62 300+	68 300+	53 300+	73 300+
Knox Community Hospital, Mount Vernon, OH	-	-	-	0.540 611	0.101 337	5.4 736	39.8 113	53 300+	76 300+	79 300+	63 300+	57 300+	78 300+	68 300+	70 300+	66 300+	63 300+
Lake Health, Concord, OH	-	-	-	0.045 1628	0.004 1310	7.2 2629	38.0 171	49 300+	74 300+	84 300+	63 300+	57 300+	73 300+	66 300+	70 300+	58 300+	67 300+
Lakewood Hospital, Lakewood, OH	-	-	-	0.047 444	0.015 324	6.8 717	35.5 76	45 300+	73 300+	79 300+	59 300+	56 300+	74 300+	66 300+	68 300+	57 300+	66 300+
Licking Memorial Hospital, Newark, OH	-	-	-	0.019 1257	0.000 666	2.4 2142	32.3 158	58 300+	79 300+	87 300+	66 300+	59 300+	77 300+	67 300+	74 300+	66 300+	61 300+
Life Line Hospital, Wintersville, OH	-	-	-	-	-	-	-	-	-	-	-	-	-	-	-	-	-
Lima Memorial Health System, Lima, OH	-	-	-	0.046 694	0.005 582	12.1 1360	29.5 173	57 300+	78 300+	89 300+	69 300+	57 300+	72 300+	67 300+	74 300+	57 300+	75 300+
Lodi Community Hospital, Lodi, OH	-	-	-	0.076 105	0.045 44	16.4 134	83.3 6	61 (a)	79 (a)	90 (a)	84 (a)	63 (a)	87 (a)	75 (a)	84 (a)	74 (a)	86 (a)
Lutheran Hospital, Cleveland, OH	-	-	-	0.049 243	0.000 123	4.4 321	33.3 54	52 300+	74 300+	81 300+	54 300+	54 300+	68 300+	62 300+	59 300+	51 300+	59 300+
Madison County Hospital, London, OH	-	-	-	0.042 165	0.000 128	6.6 256	13.6 22	56 300+	83 300+	79 300+	66 300+	60 300+	79 300+	74 300+	73 300+	71 300+	66 300+
Marietta Memorial Hospital, Marietta, OH	-	-	-	0.755 783	0.137 942	4.9 1015	37.7 159	40 300+	74 300+	87 300+	62 300+	54 300+	73 300+	68 300+	67 300+	62 300+	64 300+
Marion General Hospital, Marion, OH	-	-	-	0.027 221	0.019 52	- 0	50.0 6	49 300+	81 300+	87 300+	68 300+	66 300+	80 300+	71 300+	75 300+	70 300+	69 300+
Mary Rutan Hospital, Bellefontaine, OH	-	-	-	0.048 504	0.033 305	10.9 787	30.1 83	46 300+	84 300+	82 300+	61 300+	62 300+	79 300+	68 300+	69 300+	71 300+	59 300+
Marymount Hospital, Garfield Heights, OH	-	-	-	0.244 766	0.008 502	8.0 1116	37.1 151	41 300+	72 300+	83 300+	55 300+	52 300+	69 300+	62 300+	65 300+	55 300+	57 300+
McCullough-Hyde Memorial Hospital, Oxford, OH	-	-	-	0.059 358	0.000 273	14.7 421	34.7 98	60 300+	84 300+	82 300+	75 300+	65 300+	81 300+	75 300+	83 300+	70 300+	76 300+
Medcentral Health System, Mansfield, OH	-	-	-	0.035 1143	0.060 833	8.3 1715	25.8 198	39 300+	71 300+	83 300+	62 300+	52 300+	72 300+	64 300+	68 300+	62 300+	61 300+
Medcentral Health System Shelby Hospital, Shelby, OH	-	-	-	-	-	-	-	53 300+	82 300+	88 300+	73 300+	64 300+	84 300+	73 300+	78 300+	77 300+	78 300+
Medical Center at Elizabeth Place, Dayton, OH	-	-	-	0.063 80	0.061 66	- 0	20.9 110	78 (a)	79 (a)	88 (a)	79 (a)	63 (a)	85 (a)	77 (a)	75 (a)	79 (a)	76 (a)
Medical Center of Newark, Newark, OH	-	-	-	0.145 276	0.000 165	- 0	26.7 116	73 300+	81 300+	79 300+	74 300+	60 300+	79 300+	69 300+	77 300+	72 300+	78 300+
Medina Hospital, Medina, OH	-	-	-	0.310 675	0.040 323	8.0 1232	28.9 114	46 300+	78 300+	78 300+	60 300+	56 300+	72 300+	66 300+	66 300+	59 300+	62 300+
Memorial Hospital, Fremont, OH	-	-	-	0.639 468	0.227 392	6.9 807	26.4 125	55 300+	84 300+	87 300+	65 300+	61 300+	78 300+	70 300+	75 300+	68 300+	62 300+
Memorial Hospital of Union County, Marysville, OH	-	-	-	0.088 306	0.018 222	10.1 435	33.3 51	62 300+	83 300+	86 300+	73 300+	67 300+	81 300+	74 300+	76 300+	76 300+	76 300+
Mercer County Joint Twp Community Hospital, Coldwater, OH	-	-	-	0.142 254	0.013 154	14.0 435	35.8 67	50 (a)	80 (a)	82 (a)	71 (a)	60 (a)	81 (a)	73 (a)	79 (a)	75 (a)	75 (a)

NOTE: The first number in each column (boldface) is the score, the second number is the number of patients; Please refer to the main entry for footnotes; (a) 100-299
*MEASURES: **Children's Asthma Care:** 33. Received Systemic Corticosteroids; 34. Received Home Management Plan of Care; 35. Received Reliever Medication; **Use of Medical Imaging:** 36. Combination Abdominal CT Scan; 37. Combination Chest CT Scan; 38. Follow-up Mammogram/Ultrasound; 39. MRI for Low Back Pain; **Survey of Patients' Hospital Experiences:** 40. Area Around Room 'Always' Quiet at Night; 41. Doctors 'Always' Communicated Well; 42. Home Recovery Information Given; 43. Hospital Given 9 or 10 on 10 Point Scale; 44. Meds 'Always' Explained Before Given; 45. Nurses 'Always' Communicated Well; 46. Pain 'Always' Well Controlled; 47. Room and Bathroom 'Always' Clean; 48. Timely Help 'Always' Received; 49. Would Definitely Recommend Hospital*

Hospital	Children's Asthma Care			Use of Medical Imaging				Survey of Patients' Hospital Experiences									
	33	34	35	36	37	38	39	40	41	42	43	44	45	46	47	48	49
Mercy Franciscan Hospital - Mt Airy, Cincinnati, OH	- -	- -	- -	0.148 779	0.000 664	10.2 1033	32.2 174	44 300+	72 300+	79 300+	53 300+	50 300+	69 300+	64 300+	58 300+	54 300+	57 300+
Mercy Franciscan Hospital Western Hills, Cincinnati, OH	- -	- -	- -	0.315 930	0.010 820	10.3 1184	22.9 83	46 300+	77 300+	76 300+	61 300+	54 300+	73 300+	65 300+	62 300+	60 300+	57 300+
Mercy Hospital Anderson, Cincinnati, OH	- -	- -	- -	0.072 1074	0.002 930	7.5 1554	30.9 272	45 300+	74 300+	80 300+	63 300+	55 300+	74 300+	66 300+	63 300+	58 300+	67 300+
Mercy Hospital Clermont, Batavia, OH	- -	- -	- -	0.187 646	0.003 633	8.6 1039	32.2 242	54 300+	76 300+	82 300+	69 300+	61 300+	78 300+	69 300+	71 300+	62 300+	72 300+
Mercy Hospital Fairfield, Fairfield, OH	- -	- -	- -	0.045 1221	0.026 820	3.0 1186	25.1 215	54 300+	76 300+	80 300+	70 300+	60 300+	77 300+	71 300+	68 300+	65 300+	75 300+
Mercy Hospital of Defiance, Defiance, OH	- -	- -	- -	0.046 151	0.013 78	- 0	- 0	62 300+	84 300+	88 300+	77 300+	63 300+	83 300+	80 300+	84 300+	78 300+	78 300+
Mercy Hospital of Willard, Willard, OH	- -	- -	- -	0.281 139	0.056 72	5.7 261	33.3 21	57 (a)	93 (a)	90 (a)	85 (a)	73 (a)	87 (a)	84 (a)	85 (a)	84 (a)	84 (a)
Mercy Medical Center, Canton, OH	- -	- -	- -	0.122 1174	0.001 814	8.3 1712	30.2 159	50 300+	76 300+	81 300+	70 300+	59 300+	77 300+	73 300+	73 300+	62 300+	73 300+
Mercy Memorial Hospital, Urbana, OH	- -	- -	- -	- -	- -	- -	- -	44 300+	77 300+	81 300+	70 300+	62 300+	81 300+	68 300+	83 300+	73 300+	68 300+
Mercy St Anne Hospital, Toledo, OH	- -	- -	- -	0.021 473	0.000 315	6.8 1406	32.9 73	64 300+	75 300+	85 300+	74 300+	59 300+	78 300+	70 300+	78 300+	64 300+	78 300+
Mercy St Charles Hospital, Oregon, OH	- -	- -	- -	0.022 811	0.003 667	12.0 1176	28.7 167	49 300+	72 300+	81 300+	71 300+	55 300+	78 300+	69 300+	80 300+	67 300+	73 300+
Mercy St Vincent Medical Center, Toledo, OH	- -	- -	- -	0.023 436	0.002 410	8.5 471	32.0 75	55 300+	73 300+	85 300+	67 300+	57 300+	76 300+	65 300+	73 300+	63 300+	73 300+
Mercy Tiffin Hospital, Tiffin, OH	- -	- -	- -	0.691 431	0.079 241	6.0 600	24.0 129	62 300+	84 300+	89 300+	73 300+	67 300+	82 300+	71 300+	83 300+	68 300+	69 300+
Metro Health Medical Center, Cleveland, OH	- -	- -	- -	0.054 782	0.024 830	19.1 1611	31.3 147	59 300+	76 300+	83 300+	64 300+	60 300+	72 300+	66 300+	61 300+	59 300+	73 300+
Miami Valley Hospital, Dayton, OH	- -	- -	- -	0.076 2133	0.017 1834	5.6 2588	29.4 350	46 300+	74 300+	88 300+	66 300+	56 300+	74 300+	68 300+	61 300+	55 300+	72 300+
Morrow County Hospital, Mount Gilead, OH	- -	- -	- -	0.256 215	0.325 126	4.9 244	47.8 23	56 (a)	84 (a)	91 (a)	80 (a)	68 (a)	84 (a)	65 (a)	89 (a)	77 (a)	79 (a)
Mount Carmel Health, Columbus, OH	- -	- -	- -	0.050 2279	0.018 1181	6.4 3959	33.7 439	50 300+	80 300+	83 300+	68 300+	57 300+	76 300+	69 300+	64 300+	60 300+	72 300+
Mount Carmel New Albany Surgical Hospital, New Albany, OH	- -	- -	- -	0.182 11	0.167 6	- 0	22.2 63	79 300+	85 300+	90 300+	86 300+	70 300+	84 300+	76 300+	81 300+	72 300+	89 300+
Mount Carmel St Ann's Hospital, Westerville, OH	- -	- -	- -	0.060 815	0.011 354	8.7 1369	33.6 122	49 300+	78 300+	83 300+	68 300+	56 300+	74 300+	68 300+	63 300+	61 300+	71 300+
Northside Medical Center, Youngstown, OH	- -	- -	- -	0.057 530	0.003 333	10.1 566	20.0 5	40 300+	74 300+	80 300+	59 300+	53 300+	71 300+	66 300+	63 300+	55 300+	64 300+
O'Bleness Memorial Hospital, Athens, OH	- -	- -	- -	0.074 350	0.000 161	4.1 736	38.4 73	50 300+	79 300+	81 300+	58 300+	57 300+	75 300+	67 300+	65 300+	61 300+	56 300+
Ohio State University Hospitals, Columbus, OH	- -	- -	- -	0.028 1351	0.048 1010	7.6 382	25.3 198	53 300+	76 300+	84 300+	71 300+	59 300+	77 300+	70 300+	68 300+	62 300+	73 300+
Ohio Valley Medical Center, Springfield, OH	- -	- -	- -	- 0	- 0	- 0	- 0	- -	- -	- -	- -	- -	- -	- -	- -	- -	- -
Parma Community General Hospital, Parma, OH	- -	- -	- -	0.041 1159	0.014 859	5.7 1649	33.9 115	45 300+	77 300+	83 300+	60 300+	53 300+	72 300+	67 300+	65 300+	58 300+	62 300+
Paulding County Hospital, Paulding, OH	- -	- -	- -	- -	- -	- -	- -	- -	- -	- -	- -	- -	- -	- -	- -	- -	- -
Physician's Choice Hospital - Fremont, Fremont, OH	- -	- -	- -	- -	- -	- -	- -	- -	- -	- -	- -	- -	- -	- -	- -	- -	- -
Pike Community Hospital, Waverly, OH	- -	- -	- -	- -	- -	- -	- -	- -	- -	- -	- -	- -	- -	- -	- -	- -	- -
Riverside Methodist Hospital, Columbus, OH	- -	- -	- -	0.113 2908	0.056 2735	8.5 5816	30.5 537	48 300+	79 300+	85 300+	74 300+	62 300+	79 300+	71 300+	66 300+	61 300+	83 300+
Robinson Memorial Hospital, Ravenna, OH	- -	- -	- -	0.148 751	0.000 437	7.6 1328	26.6 154	46 300+	78 300+	78 300+	64 300+	56 300+	76 300+	69 300+	70 300+	59 300+	62 300+
Saint Elizabeth Boardman Health Center, Youngstown, OH	- -	- -	- -	0.028 496	0.034 205	2.9 70	18.8 16	56 300+	77 300+	79 300+	78 300+	60 300+	79 300+	68 300+	72 300+	57 300+	82 300+
Saint Elizabeth Health Center, Youngstown, OH	- -	- -	- -	0.131 883	0.038 524	4.8 584	36.6 71	42 300+	77 300+	78 300+	59 300+	53 300+	69 300+	61 300+	61 300+	53 300+	61 300+
Saint John Medical Center, Westlake, OH	100 28	83 24	100 28	0.057 526	0.000 519	10.2 648	33.9 62	56 300+	78 300+	86 300+	71 300+	56 300+	74 300+	69 300+	65 300+	59 300+	72 300+
Saint Joseph Health Center, Warren, OH	- -	- -	- -	0.662 749	0.015 608	10.4 811	24.2 153	42 300+	78 300+	82 300+	68 300+	57 300+	72 300+	64 300+	64 300+	57 300+	73 300+
Saint Luke's Hospital, Maumee, OH	- -	- -	- -	0.088 826	0.102 420	4.8 482	26.0 123	52 300+	76 300+	82 300+	70 300+	61 300+	77 300+	67 300+	71 300+	65 300+	73 300+
Saint Rita's Medical Center, Lima, OH	- -	- -	- -	0.091 1586	0.015 952	8.2 2427	28.1 288	55 300+	78 300+	85 300+	73 300+	60 300+	78 300+	69 300+	69 300+	69 300+	76 300+
Saint Vincent Charity Medical Center, Cleveland, OH	- -	- -	- -	0.049 288	0.000 189	12.7 314	36.7 60	70 300+	80 300+	85 300+	70 300+	59 300+	76 300+	69 300+	68 300+	61 300+	71 300+
Salem Community Hospital, Salem, OH	- -	- -	- -	0.102 811	0.001 710	7.9 1087	29.8 171	35 300+	77 300+	80 300+	57 300+	53 300+	69 300+	60 300+	63 300+	58 300+	59 300+
Samaritan Hospital - Peoples Hospital, Ashland, OH	- -	- -	- -	0.069 506	0.085 295	6.6 699	27.3 99	55 300+	78 300+	88 300+	67 300+	59 300+	76 300+	64 300+	68 300+	59 300+	63 300+
Selby General Hospital, Marietta, OH	- -	- -	- -	0.727 143	0.000 91	5.9 135	62.5 8	- -	- -	- -	- -	- -	- -	- -	- -	- -	- -
South Pointe Hospital, Warrensville Hgts, OH	- -	- -	- -	0.067 869	0.103 513	5.7 945	31.9 141	50 300+	74 300+	80 300+	60 300+	54 300+	70 300+	66 300+	63 300+	60 300+	59 300+
Southeastern Ohio Regional Medical Center, Cambridge, OH	- -	- -	- -	0.156 598	0.183 436	5.1 901	36.1 36	57 300+	81 300+	83 300+	68 300+	64 300+	81 300+	68 300+	77 300+	68 300+	64 300+
Southern Ohio Medical Center, Portsmouth, OH	- -	- -	- -	0.547 1527	0.110 1359	5.7 1356	37.4 257	65 300+	83 300+	88 300+	75 300+	64 300+	83 300+	81 300+	81 300+	68 300+	73 300+
Southwest General Health Center, Middleburg Hgts, OH	- -	- -	- -	0.057 1359	0.017 1261	5.8 1435	32.7 110	45 300+	78 300+	80 300+	68 300+	61 300+	79 300+	70 300+	66 300+	65 300+	71 300+
Springfield Regional Medical Center, Springfield, OH	- -	- -	- -	0.083 1085	0.035 803	5.9 1449	30.5 177	40 300+	75 300+	74 300+	45 300+	54 300+	66 300+	60 300+	56 300+	49 300+	45 300+
Summa Barberton Hospital, Barberton, OH	- -	- -	- -	0.073 506	0.010 311	16.0 681	31.8 88	46 300+	76 300+	76 300+	65 300+	57 300+	77 300+	69 300+	68 300+	66 300+	67 300+
Summa Health Systems Hospitals, Akron, OH	- -	- -	- -	0.116 1395	0.001 1495	4.3 2614	33.8 361	45 300+	74 300+	82 300+	62 300+	55 300+	73 300+	66 300+	65 300+	61 300+	69 300+
Summa Wadsworth-Rittman Hospital, Wadsworth, OH	- -	- -	- -	0.101 415	0.025 276	2.8 639	31.0 71	40 300+	76 300+	85 300+	64 300+	54 300+	74 300+	67 300+	69 300+	67 300+	67 300+
Summa Western Reserve Hospital, Cuyahoga Falls, OH	- -	- -	- -	0.075 254	0.005 205	- 0	29.7 128	61 300+	77 300+	81 300+	70 300+	57 300+	75 300+	66 300+	69 300+	63 300+	75 300+
Surgical Hospital at Southwoods, Youngstown, OH	- -	- -	- -	- 0	- 0	- 0	- 0	84 (a)	98 (a)	93 (a)	100 (a)	80 (a)	97 (a)	90 (a)	87 (a)	92 (a)	97 (a)
Three Gables Surgery Center, Proctorville, OH	- -	- -	- -	1.000 1	0.200 5	- 0	30.0 10	87 <100	89 <100	83 <100	76 <100	24 <100	79 <100	65 <100	89 <100	80 <100	76 <100
The Toledo Hospital, Toledo, OH	100 201	95 201	100 201	0.049 790	0.017 654	9.0 2091	22.8 193	48 300+	70 300+	85 300+	63 300+	52 300+	68 300+	65 300+	68 300+	56 300+	66 300+
Trinity Medical Center East & TMC West, Steubenville, OH	- -	- -	- -	0.659 543	0.708 411	8.5 982	30.5 128	51 300+	79 300+	86 300+	64 300+	60 300+	75 300+	68 300+	70 300+	62 300+	66 300+
Trumbull Memorial Hospital, Warren, OH	- -	- -	- -	0.648 1081	0.008 846	9.4 2456	26.6 218	41 300+	77 300+	80 300+	54 300+	50 300+	67 300+	59 300+	56 300+	55 300+	57 300+
Twin City Hospital, Dennison, OH	- -	- -	- -	- -	- -	- -	- -	- -	- -	- -	- -	- -	- -	- -	- -	- -	- -
UH Geauga Medical Center, Chardon, OH	- -	- -	- -	0.096 500	0.027 291	7.4 571	37.9 66	46 300+	78 300+	79 300+	65 300+	56 300+	75 300+	67 300+	67 300+	62 300+	67 300+
UHHS Bedford Medical Center, Bedford, OH	- -	- -	- -	0.107 262	0.047 279	7.4 443	40.7 54	45 300+	71 300+	73 300+	55 300+	53 300+	71 300+	64 300+	63 300+	54 300+	55 300+
UHHS Memorial Hospital of Geneva, Geneva, OH	- -	- -	- -	0.142 431	0.004 508	11.2 258	24.2 62	47 300+	83 300+	83 300+	72 300+	63 300+	80 300+	70 300+	82 300+	73 300+	76 300+
UHHS Richmond Heights Hospital, Richmond Heights, OH	- -	- -	- -	0.294 272	0.087 195	3.5 395	34.4 64	43 300+	70 300+	74 300+	54 300+	52 300+	66 300+	62 300+	59 300+	48 300+	56 300+
Union Hospital, Dover, OH	- -	- -	- -	0.101 759	0.005 610	6.6 776	33.1 139	46 300+	80 300+	82 300+	66 300+	57 300+	73 300+	68 300+	71 300+	64 300+	63 300+
University Hospital, Cincinnati, OH	- -	- -	- -	0.078 688	0.020 649	11.4 1540	33.3 183	54 300+	73 300+	83 300+	63 300+	57 300+	72 300+	63 300+	61 300+	55 300+	67 300+
University Hospitals Conneaut Medical Center, Conneaut, OH	- -	- -	- -	0.146 178	0.009 108	4.5 221	12.5 8	64 (a)	87 (a)	86 (a)	83 (a)	74 (a)	87 (a)	75 (a)	89 (a)	85 (a)	82 (a)
University Hospitals of Cleveland, Cleveland, OH	99 378	95 380	100 380	0.604 2483	0.007 2916	15.5 1589	25.8 360	47 300+	75 300+	82 300+	69 300+	59 300+	75 300+	66 300+	62 300+	55 300+	76 300+
University of Toledo Medical Center, Toledo, OH	- -	- -	- -	0.341 505	0.027 366	4.1 536	27.1 181	35 300+	66 300+	80 300+	52 300+	53 300+	63 300+	60 300+	52 300+	51 300+	53 300+
University Pointe Surgical Hospital, West Chester, OH	- -	- -	- -	0.105 267	0.009 326	12.9 139	42.9 56	93 <100	93 <100	92 <100	93 <100	70 <100	95 <100	83 <100	92 <100	92 <100	89 <100
Upper Valley Medical Center, Troy, OH	- -	- -	- -	0.066 869	0.010 711	5.4 1622	22.4 116	47 300+	76 300+	82 300+	59 300+	57 300+	74 300+	66 300+	67 300+	63 300+	60 300+
Van Wert County Hospital, Van Wert, OH	- -	- -	- -	0.672 421	0.065 214	3.0 297	27.1 70	54 300+	81 300+	87 300+	68 300+	65 300+	78 300+	73 300+	79 300+	68 300+	65 300+
Wayne Hospital, Greenville, OH	- -	- -	- -	0.024 458	0.000 308	9.0 846	33.7 98	53 300+	77 300+	80 300+	59 300+	59 300+	74 300+	68 300+	73 300+	68 300+	57 300+

NOTE: The first number in each column (boldface) is the score, the second number is the number of patients; Please refer to the main entry for footnotes; (a) 100-299

*MEASURES: **Children's Asthma Care:** 33. Received Systemic Corticosteroids; 34. Received Home Management Plan of Care; 35. Received Reliever Medication; **Use of Medical Imaging:** 36. Combination Abdominal CT Scan; 37. Combination Chest CT Scan; 38. Follow-up Mammogram/Ultrasound; 39. MRI for Low Back Pain; **Survey of Patients' Hospital Experiences:** 40. Area Around Room 'Always' Quiet at Night; 41. Doctors 'Always' Communicated Well; 42. Home Recovery Information Given; 43. Hospital Given 9 or 10 on 10 Point Scale; 44. Meds 'Always' Explained Before Given; 45. Nurses 'Always' Communicated Well; 46. Pain 'Always' Well Controlled; 47. Room and Bathroom 'Always' Clean; 48. Timely Help 'Always' Received; 49. Would Definitely Recommend Hospital*

Hospital	Children's Asthma Care			Use of Medical Imaging				Survey of Patients' Hospital Experiences									
	33	34	35	36	37	38	39	40	41	42	43	44	45	46	47	48	49
West Chester Medical Center, West Chester, OH	-	-	-	- 0	- 0	- 0	- 0	71 300+	79 300+	85 300+	80 300+	61 300+	81 300+	74 300+	73 300+	65 300+	85 300+
Wilson Memorial Hospital, Sidney, OH	-	-	-	0.236 364	0.158 298	13.5 645	32.5 80	60 300+	84 300+	81 300+	69 300+	62 300+	80 300+	70 300+	80 300+	68 300+	64 300+
Wood County Hospital, Bowling Green, OH	-	-	-	0.077 469	0.130 330	7.7 598	19.5 82	56 300+	78 300+	89 300+	67 300+	61 300+	72 300+	67 300+	76 300+	70 300+	65 300+
The Woods at Parkside, Columbus, OH	-	-	-	- 0	- 0	- 0	- 0	-	-	-	-	-	-	-	-	-	-
Wooster Community Hospital, Wooster, OH	-	-	-	0.124 507	0.131 496	18.1 602	22.9 96	53 300+	80 300+	84 300+	75 300+	60 300+	80 300+	74 300+	77 300+	64 300+	76 300+
Wyandot Memorial Hospital, Upper Sandusky, OH	-	-	-	-	-	-	-	-	-	-	-	-	-	-	-	-	-
PENNSYLVANIA																	
Abington Memorial Hospital, Abington, PA	-	-	-	0.039 2284	0.012 1943	10.3 2769	29.7 370	46 300+	77 300+	80 300+	70 300+	59 300+	77 300+	66 300+	60 300+	62 300+	76 300+
ACMH Hospital, Kittanning, PA	-	-	-	0.147 184	0.020 147	15.2 356	40.0 35	41 300+	83 300+	83 300+	63 300+	61 300+	78 300+	68 300+	64 300+	68 300+	64 300+
Advanced Surgical Hospital, Washington, PA	-	-	-	-	-	-	-	-	-	-	-	-	-	-	-	-	-
Albert Einstein Medical Center, Philadelphia, PA	-	-	-	0.094 838	0.021 533	5.4 2369	29.4 143	50 300+	73 300+	77 300+	55 300+	56 300+	67 300+	64 300+	60 300+	51 300+	55 300+
Alle Kiski Medical Center, Natrona, PA	-	-	-	0.397 536	0.005 412	17.4 700	42.7 82	39 300+	73 300+	81 300+	58 300+	55 300+	72 300+	60 300+	73 300+	58 300+	54 300+
Allegheny General Hospital, Pittsburgh, PA	-	-	-	0.472 1052	0.100 872	8.2 833	39.6 96	47 300+	73 300+	80 300+	61 300+	55 300+	71 300+	60 300+	60 300+	52 300+	65 300+
Altoona Regional Health System, Altoona, PA	-	-	-	0.321 1317	0.036 873	5.0 1148	31.8 148	53 300+	82 300+	84 300+	68 300+	61 300+	81 300+	72 300+	75 300+	67 300+	72 300+
Aria Health, Philadelphia, PA	-	-	-	0.034 1382	0.003 1164	8.6 1126	- 0	49 300+	72 300+	81 300+	65 300+	58 300+	78 300+	71 300+	70 300+	67 300+	67 300+
Berwick Hospital Center, Berwick, PA	-	-	-	0.335 185	0.117 120	11.6 372	17.2 58	55 300+	83 300+	78 300+	59 300+	62 300+	77 300+	68 300+	71 300+	60 300+	59 300+
Bloomsburg Hospital, Bloomsburg, PA	-	-	-	0.340 206	0.484 64	8.2 474	26.0 50	51 300+	77 300+	77 300+	70 300+	57 300+	79 300+	70 300+	71 300+	68 300+	72 300+
Bradford Regional Medical Center, Bradford, PA	-	-	-	0.092 469	0.031 325	8.9 697	45.2 84	43 300+	76 300+	77 300+	54 300+	53 300+	74 300+	69 300+	67 300+	70 300+	53 300+
Brandywine Hospital, Coatesville, PA	-	-	-	0.166 355	0.011 270	15.7 623	31.5 92	44 300+	74 300+	80 300+	57 300+	50 300+	71 300+	64 300+	61 300+	52 300+	55 300+
Brookville Hospital, Brookville, PA	-	-	-	-	-	-	-	-	-	-	-	-	-	-	-	-	-
Bucks County Specialty Hospital, Bensalem, PA	-	-	-	-	-	-	-	-	-	-	-	-	-	-	-	-	-
Butler Memorial Hospital, Butler, PA	-	-	-	0.131 677	0.012 500	9.9 1060	31.4 194	48 300+	77 300+	89 300+	67 300+	60 300+	77 300+	70 300+	64 300+	62 300+	68 300+
Cancer Treatment Centers of America, Philadelphia, PA	-	-	-	0.785 181	0.009 220	- 0	- 0	61 (a)	87 (a)	90 (a)	88 (a)	70 (a)	82 (a)	80 (a)	83 (a)	72 (a)	95 (a)
Canonsburg General Hospital, Canonsburg, PA	-	-	-	0.544 206	0.013 149	13.0 247	45.5 33	52 300+	80 300+	76 300+	68 300+	59 300+	80 300+	69 300+	67 300+	65 300+	73 300+
Carlisle Regional Medical Center, Carlisle, PA	-	-	-	0.178 759	0.164 549	3.9 563	20.8 77	52 300+	76 300+	82 300+	58 300+	53 300+	73 300+	67 300+	75 300+	62 300+	57 300+
Chambersburg Hospital, Chambersburg, PA	-	-	-	0.190 1277	0.046 698	5.5 2854	31.9 367	46 300+	76 300+	81 300+	64 300+	59 300+	77 300+	69 300+	75 300+	65 300+	63 300+
Charles Cole Memorial Hospital, Coudersport, PA	-	-	-	0.025 237	0.007 142	7.4 488	48.2 56	60 300+	83 300+	88 300+	68 300+	66 300+	80 300+	72 300+	76 300+	73 300+	67 300+
Chester County Hospital, West Chester, PA	-	-	-	0.094 981	0.012 864	10.6 1780	30.2 126	47 300+	80 300+	78 300+	71 300+	62 300+	78 300+	71 300+	67 300+	67 300+	77 300+
Chestnut Hill Hospital, Philadelphia, PA	-	-	-	0.094 459	0.024 333	7.2 1295	33.9 62	56 300+	76 300+	80 300+	62 300+	53 300+	73 300+	67 300+	65 300+	52 300+	62 300+
Children's Hospital of Philadelphia, Philadelphia, PA	100 547	47 546	100 548	-	-	-	-	-	-	-	-	-	-	-	-	-	-
Children's Hospital of Pittsburgh of UPMC, Pittsburgh, PA	100 476	57 476	100 478	-	-	-	-	-	-	-	-	-	-	-	-	-	-
Clarion Hospital, Clarion, PA	-	-	-	0.491 379	0.512 207	10.5 561	32.6 86	50 300+	78 300+	81 300+	61 300+	54 300+	71 300+	67 300+	65 300+	65 300+	59 300+
Clearfield Hospital, Clearfield, PA	-	-	-	0.663 854	0.033 303	4.3 769	40.3 77	44 300+	80 300+	84 300+	54 300+	59 300+	71 300+	64 300+	69 300+	59 300+	51 300+
Coatesville VA Medical Center, Coatesville, PA	-	-	-	-	-	-	-	-	-	-	-	-	-	-	-	-	-
Community Medical Center, Scranton, PA	-	-	-	0.109 588	0.100 329	6.3 761	30.6 36	54 300+	79 300+	82 300+	62 300+	56 300+	75 300+	69 300+	69 300+	64 300+	66 300+
Conemaugh Valley Memorial Hospital, Johnstown, PA	-	-	-	0.019 723	0.002 489	5.1 950	22.2 9	47 300+	77 300+	84 300+	65 300+	60 300+	77 300+	69 300+	74 300+	62 300+	67 300+
Coordinated Health Orthopedic Hospital, Bethlehem, PA	-	-	-	- 0	- 0	- 0	- 0	80 300+	87 300+	89 300+	90 300+	73 300+	92 300+	80 300+	85 300+	90 300+	90 300+
Corry Memorial Hospital, Corry, PA	-	-	-	-	-	-	-	37 (a)	81 (a)	81 (a)	50 (a)	61 (a)	73 (a)	62 (a)	71 (a)	60 (a)	45 (a)
Crozer Chester Medical Center, Upland, PA	-	-	-	0.196 1278	0.008 1085	8.6 1887	33.2 292	49 300+	75 300+	78 300+	58 300+	59 300+	73 300+	67 300+	64 300+	57 300+	60 300+
Delaware County Memorial Hospital, Drexel Hill, PA	-	-	-	0.435 706	0.004 539	5.5 566	34.4 64	50 300+	77 300+	83 300+	61 300+	61 300+	75 300+	65 300+	65 300+	57 300+	67 300+
Doylestown Hospital, Doylestown, PA	-	-	-	0.180 899	0.002 928	10.9 2039	26.5 196	51 300+	82 300+	86 300+	79 300+	64 300+	84 300+	78 300+	74 300+	74 300+	85 300+
Dubois Regional Medical Center, Dubois, PA	-	-	-	0.278 1231	0.004 728	6.7 1688	0.0 1	52 300+	79 300+	87 300+	70 300+	66 300+	79 300+	73 300+	67 300+	66 300+	79 300+
Eagleville Hospital, Eagleville, PA	-	-	-	- 0	- 0	- 0	- 0	-	-	-	-	-	-	-	-	-	-
Easton Hospital, Easton, PA	-	-	-	0.137 818	0.030 573	9.7 1525	43.5 46	49 300+	75 300+	82 300+	55 300+	54 300+	71 300+	67 300+	65 300+	49 300+	53 300+
Edgewood Surgical Hospital, Transfer, PA	-	-	-	- 0	- 0	- 0	39.3 117	87 (a)	92 (a)	93 (a)	87 (a)	77 (a)	88 (a)	80 (a)	81 (a)	84 (a)	87 (a)
Elk Regional Health Center, Saint Marys, PA	-	-	-	0.611 707	0.567 305	12.0 897	34.8 164	44 300+	75 300+	82 300+	51 300+	58 300+	72 300+	67 300+	72 300+	63 300+	53 300+
Ellwood City Hospital, Ellwood City, PA	-	-	-	0.081 124	0.010 105	12.4 226	14.3 21	58 300+	77 300+	81 300+	65 300+	60 300+	77 300+	71 300+	76 300+	67 300+	68 300+
Ephrata Community Hospital, Ephrata, PA	-	-	-	0.496 811	0.023 740	15.4 1492	25.3 162	43 300+	75 300+	83 300+	63 300+	57 300+	77 300+	66 300+	69 300+	63 300+	69 300+
Erie VA Medical Center, Erie, PA	-	-	-	-	-	-	-	-	-	-	-	-	-	-	-	-	-
Evangelical Community Hospital, Lewisburg, PA	-	-	-	0.064 1019	0.000 434	6.8 1761	28.4 169	51 300+	80 300+	85 300+	71 300+	60 300+	78 300+	71 300+	74 300+	69 300+	80 300+
Excela Health Frick Hospital, Mount Pleasant, PA	-	-	-	0.007 271	0.005 188	10.1 237	45.9 37	49 300+	84 300+	84 300+	71 300+	64 300+	82 300+	72 300+	76 300+	69 300+	72 300+
Excela Health Latrobe Hospital, Latrobe, PA	-	-	-	0.041 555	0.011 448	10.7 571	32.9 85	45 300+	80 300+	80 300+	62 300+	60 300+	79 300+	68 300+	61 300+	69 300+	65 300+
Excela Health Westmoreland Regional Hospital, Greensburg, PA	-	-	-	0.021 653	0.000 503	8.7 959	35.8 95	44 300+	79 300+	79 300+	58 300+	62 300+	74 300+	69 300+	66 300+	64 300+	63 300+
Fulton County Medical Center, Mcconnellsburg, PA	-	-	-	-	-	-	-	-	-	-	-	-	-	-	-	-	-
Geisinger Medical Center, Danville, PA	-	-	-	0.097 1575	0.011 1407	11.0 1366	26.2 221	43 300+	79 300+	88 300+	76 300+	62 300+	79 300+	68 300+	75 300+	68 300+	81 300+
Geisinger Wyoming Valley Medical Center, Wilkes-Barre, PA	-	-	-	0.624 901	0.020 846	12.9 735	29.3 150	49 300+	81 300+	83 300+	64 300+	56 300+	74 300+	65 300+	67 300+	61 300+	70 300+
Gettysburg Hospital, Gettysburg, PA	-	-	-	0.664 658	0.082 379	14.8 1343	25.4 209	44 300+	78 300+	87 300+	60 300+	61 300+	75 300+	67 300+	66 300+	64 300+	61 300+
Gnaden Huetten Memorial Hospital, Lehighton, PA	-	-	-	0.068 443	0.042 312	12.6 625	33.7 190	47 300+	75 300+	83 300+	57 300+	58 300+	74 300+	67 300+	73 300+	62 300+	57 300+
Good Samaritan Hospital, Lebanon, PA	-	-	-	0.482 1288	0.020 919	4.0 2993	- 0	46 300+	77 300+	83 300+	65 300+	61 300+	77 300+	70 300+	77 300+	63 300+	66 300+
Grand View Hospital, Sellersville, PA	-	-	-	0.059 901	0.007 842	8.1 1568	24.0 146	52 300+	75 300+	86 300+	73 300+	65 300+	78 300+	68 300+	82 300+	69 300+	82 300+
Grove City Medical Center, Grove City, PA	-	-	-	0.211 237	0.006 161	10.0 370	40.8 49	52 300+	83 300+	87 300+	70 300+	68 300+	77 300+	72 300+	78 300+	68 300+	66 300+
Hahnemann University Hospital, Philadelphia, PA	-	-	-	0.079 302	0.008 237	10.1 435	30.0 50	59 300+	82 300+	83 300+	66 300+	65 300+	78 300+	72 300+	68 300+	64 300+	71 300+
Hamot Medical Center, Erie, PA	-	-	-	0.052 690	0.008 242	- 0	27.1 133	48 300+	78 300+	83 300+	71 300+	61 300+	79 300+	72 300+	70 300+	66 300+	77 300+
Hanover Hospital, Hanover, PA	-	-	-	0.093 890	0.019 697	12.0 1172	24.2 236	45 300+	79 300+	81 300+	64 300+	52 300+	71 300+	67 300+	74 300+	57 300+	65 300+
Hazleton General Hospital, Hazleton, PA	-	-	-	0.017 579	0.000 410	7.5 345	31.2 109	45 300+	80 300+	74 300+	49 300+	53 300+	71 300+	66 300+	75 300+	62 300+	44 300+
Heart of Lancaster Regional Medical Center, Lititz, PA	100 11	100 11	100 11	0.151 152	0.085 94	3.7 188	23.8 21	57 300+	77 300+	80 300+	65 300+	59 300+	72 300+	65 300+	72 300+	63 300+	68 300+
Heritage Valley Beaver, Beaver, PA	-	-	-	0.136 698	0.002 487	11.3 1183	29.3 92	41 300+	79 300+	76 300+	59 300+	53 300+	74 300+	68 300+	66 300+	62 300+	61 300+

NOTE: The first number in each column (boldface) is the score, the second number is the number of patients; Please refer to the main entry for footnotes; (a) 100-299
*MEASURES: **Children's Asthma Care:** 33. Received Systemic Corticosteroids; 34. Received Home Management Plan of Care; 35. Received Reliever Medication; **Use of Medical Imaging:** 36. Combination Abdominal CT Scan; 37. Combination Chest CT Scan; 38. Follow-up Mammogram/Ultrasound; 39. MRI for Low Back Pain; **Survey of Patients' Hospital Experiences:** 40. Area Around Room 'Always' Quiet at Night; 41. Doctors 'Always' Communicated Well; 42. Home Recovery Information Given; 43. Hospital Given 9 or 10 on 10 Point Scale; 44. Meds 'Always' Explained Before Given; 45. Nurses 'Always' Communicated Well; 46. Pain 'Always' Well Controlled; 47. Room and Bathroom 'Always' Clean; 48. Timely Help 'Always' Received; 49. Would Definitely Recommend Hospital*

Hospital	Children's Asthma Care			Use of Medical Imaging				Survey of Patients' Hospital Experiences									
	33	34	35	36	37	38	39	40	41	42	43	44	45	46	47	48	49
Heritage Valley Sewickley, Sewickley, PA	-	-	-	**0.113** 337	**0.000** 236	**11.3** 247	**42.1** 57	**50** 300+	**82** 300+	**82** 300+	**68** 300+	**62** 300+	**80** 300+	**73** 300+	**67** 300+	**66** 300+	**72** 300+
Highlands Hospital, Connellsville, PA	-	-	-	**0.673** 113	**0.083** 60	**4.3** 184	- 0	**46** 300+	**90** 300+	**86** 300+	**71** 300+	**65** 300+	**82** 300+	**78** 300+	**82** 300+	**75** 300+	**72** 300+
Holy Redeemer Hospital and Medical Center, Meadowbrook, PA	-	-	-	**0.045** 622	**0.000** 563	**8.8** 1264	- 0	**53** 300+	**80** 300+	**80** 300+	**72** 300+	**60** 300+	**78** 300+	**68** 300+	**66** 300+	**63** 300+	**77** 300+
Holy Spirit Hospital, Camp Hill, PA	-	-	-	**0.361** 850	**0.009** 530	**7.7** 728	**40.3** 62	**44** 300+	**72** 300+	**77** 300+	**64** 300+	**55** 300+	**72** 300+	**66** 300+	**66** 300+	**57** 300+	**66** 300+
Hospital of Univ of Pennsylvania, Philadelphia, PA	-	-	-	**0.141** 1579	**0.001** 2172	**6.2** 1136	**33.5** 212	**46** 300+	**80** 300+	**87** 300+	**71** 300+	**63** 300+	**76** 300+	**70** 300+	**55** 300+	**60** 300+	**81** 300+
Indiana Regional Medical Center, Indiana, PA	-	-	-	**0.512** 385	**0.008** 257	**7.7** 674	**32.8** 67	**46** 300+	**82** 300+	**87** 300+	**69** 300+	**62** 300+	**81** 300+	**69** 300+	**75** 300+	**70** 300+	**70** 300+
J C Blair Memorial Hospital, Huntingdon, PA	-	-	-	**0.022** 409	**0.005** 204	**6.0** 804	**46.3** 41	**51** 300+	**83** 300+	**84** 300+	**62** 300+	**58** 300+	**78** 300+	**71** 300+	**77** 300+	**70** 300+	**58** 300+
James E. Van Zandt VA Medical Center - Altoona, Altoona, PA	-	-	-	-	-	-	-	-	-	-	-	-	-	-	-	-	-
Jameson Memorial Hospital, New Castle, PA	-	-	-	**0.063** 458	**0.003** 359	**10.4** 451	**46.2** 52	**44** 300+	**79** 300+	**84** 300+	**53** 300+	**56** 300+	**73** 300+	**67** 300+	**73** 300+	**53** 300+	**47** 300+
Jeanes Hospital, Philadelphia, PA	-	-	-	**0.068** 559	**0.015** 272	**4.6** 828	**24.2** 91	**54** 300+	**81** 300+	**81** 300+	**68** 300+	**59** 300+	**74** 300+	**72** 300+	**67** 300+	**56** 300+	**70** 300+
Jefferson Regional Medical Center, Pittsburgh, PA	-	-	-	**0.134** 625	**0.063** 432	**21.4** 248	**57.1** 14	**49** 300+	**80** 300+	**85** 300+	**71** 300+	**57** 300+	**80** 300+	**72** 300+	**71** 300+	**60** 300+	**76** 300+
Jennersville Regional Hospital, West Grove, PA	-	-	-	**0.157** 261	**0.000** 223	**14.1** 377	**29.5** 78	**53** 300+	**72** 300+	**82** 300+	**57** 300+	**59** 300+	**74** 300+	**67** 300+	**66** 300+	**58** 300+	**55** 300+
Jersey Shore Hospital, Jersey Shore, PA	-	-	-	**0.080** 374	**0.011** 180	**6.0** 399	**31.8** 44	-	-	-	-	-	-	-	-	-	-
Kane Community Hospital, Kane, PA	-	-	-	**0.575** 247	**0.750** 124	**43.6** 236	**19.4** 36	**53** (a)	**83** (a)	**84** (a)	**65** (a)	**64** (a)	**78** (a)	**67** (a)	**77** (a)	**65** (a)	**65** (a)
Kensington Hospital, Philadelphia, PA	-	-	-	- 0	- 0	**0.0** 18	- 0	**47** <100	**47** <100	- <100	- <100	- <100	**46** <100	**47** <100	**100** <100	**22** <100	- <100
Lancaster General Hospital, Lancaster, PA	-	-	-	**0.412** 2670	**0.032** 2583	**7.9** 5423	**0.0** 2	**48** 300+	**74** 300+	**86** 300+	**71** 300+	**56** 300+	**74** 300+	**66** 300+	**70** 300+	**56** 300+	**80** 300+
Lancaster Regional Medical Center, Lancaster, PA	-	-	-	**0.090** 266	**0.020** 255	- 0	**47.8** 23	**57** 300+	**80** 300+	**85** 300+	**70** 300+	**60** 300+	**75** 300+	**69** 300+	**80** 300+	**70** 300+	**71** 300+
Lansdale Hospital, Lansdale, PA	-	-	-	**0.084** 407	**0.016** 244	**4.6** 673	**18.4** 49	**53** 300+	**75** 300+	**74** 300+	**55** 300+	**59** 300+	**73** 300+	**66** 300+	**64** 300+	**58** 300+	**57** 300+
Lebanon VA Medical Center, Lebanon, PA	-	-	-	-	-	-	-	-	-	-	-	-	-	-	-	-	-
Lehigh Valley Hospital, Allentown, PA	-	-	-	**0.017** 779	**0.058** 514	**6.7** 3682	**18.2** 11	**48** 300+	**79** 300+	**85** 300+	**73** 300+	**60** 300+	**79** 300+	**70** 300+	**62** 300+	**61** 300+	**79** 300+
Lehigh Valley Hospital - Muhlenberg, Bethlehem, PA	-	-	-	**0.082** 1040	**0.033** 932	**6.7** 1557	**30.3** 76	**51** 300+	**78** 300+	**85** 300+	**76** 300+	**61** 300+	**79** 300+	**68** 300+	**72** 300+	**61** 300+	**81** 300+
Lewistown Hospital, Lewistown, PA	-	-	-	**0.278** 701	**0.002** 536	**10.4** 895	**36.9** 255	**44** 300+	**75** 300+	**78** 300+	**55** 300+	**51** 300+	**70** 300+	**61** 300+	**74** 300+	**60** 300+	**47** 300+
Lock Haven Hospital, Lock Haven, PA	-	-	-	**0.430** 223	**0.037** 109	**12.9** 271	**35.3** 34	**58** 300+	**77** 300+	**82** 300+	**59** 300+	**57** 300+	**74** 300+	**69** 300+	**68** 300+	**68** 300+	**50** 300+
Lower Bucks Hospital, Bristol, PA	-	-	-	**0.262** 275	**0.011** 266	**7.7** 671	- 0	**51** 300+	**75** 300+	**80** 300+	**55** 300+	**59** 300+	**74** 300+	**71** 300+	**65** 300+	**63** 300+	**55** 300+
Magee Womens Hospital of UPMC Health System, Pittsburgh, PA	-	-	-	**0.156** 545	**0.004** 505	**8.5** 3186	**30.0** 10	**44** 300+	**76** 300+	**79** 300+	**64** 300+	**54** 300+	**70** 300+	**63** 300+	**63** 300+	**56** 300+	**72** 300+
Main Line Hospital Bryn Mawr Campus, Bryn Mawr, PA	-	-	-	**0.228** 1068	**0.023** 972	**6.9** 1404	**0.0** 2	**45** 300+	**76** 300+	**82** 300+	**74** 300+	**60** 300+	**79** 300+	**70** 300+	**65** 300+	**62** 300+	**80** 300+
Main Line Hospital Lankenau, Wynnewood, PA	-	-	-	**0.142** 1174	**0.019** 1079	**8.2** 2031	**28.9** 190	**48** 300+	**80** 300+	**79** 300+	**75** 300+	**60** 300+	**77** 300+	**70** 300+	**65** 300+	**57** 300+	**80** 300+
Main Line Hospital Paoli, Paoli, PA	-	-	-	**0.113** 1237	**0.019** 1044	**7.2** 1544	**50.0** 2	**54** 300+	**79** 300+	**79** 300+	**81** 300+	**61** 300+	**80** 300+	**73** 300+	**73** 300+	**63** 300+	**87** 300+
Marian Community Hospital, Carbondale, PA	-	-	-	**0.394** 297	**0.023** 177	**6.5** 567	**27.5** 51	**45** 300+	**81** 300+	**84** 300+	**61** 300+	**60** 300+	**75** 300+	**66** 300+	**78** 300+	**68** 300+	**57** 300+
Meadville Medical Center, Meadville, PA	-	-	-	**0.048** 702	**0.008** 514	**3.5** 1434	**31.0** 268	**51** 300+	**82** 300+	**82** 300+	**68** 300+	**59** 300+	**77** 300+	**75** 300+	**77** 300+	**67** 300+	**65** 300+
Memorial Hospital - Towanda, Towanda, PA	-	-	-	**0.063** 239	**0.011** 93	**5.9** 337	**37.1** 89	**62** 300+	**83** 300+	**84** 300+	**77** 300+	**63** 300+	**81** 300+	**75** 300+	**84** 300+	**77** 300+	**70** 300+
Memorial Hospital York, York, PA	-	-	-	**0.500** 2	**0.000** 2	**10.6** 795	**28.0** 82	**42** 300+	**71** 300+	**80** 300+	**64** 300+	**56** 300+	**70** 300+	**63** 300+	**68** 300+	**54** 300+	**71** 300+
Mercy Fitzgerald Hospital, Darby, PA	-	-	-	**0.073** 578	**0.028** 578	**5.1** 1236	**31.6** 114	**52** 300+	**73** 300+	**81** 300+	**55** 300+	**52** 300+	**70** 300+	**61** 300+	**62** 300+	**49** 300+	**53** 300+
Mercy Hospital Scranton, Scranton, PA	-	-	-	**0.163** 771	**0.023** 655	**7.3** 731	**37.8** 74	**47** 300+	**78** 300+	**80** 300+	**64** 300+	**54** 300+	**72** 300+	**68** 300+	**57** 300+	**54** 300+	**67** 300+
Mercy Suburban Hospital, Norristown, PA	-	-	-	**0.059** 410	**0.000** 217	**7.7** 363	**36.4** 55	**37** 300+	**76** 300+	**85** 300+	**57** 300+	**58** 300+	**71** 300+	**65** 300+	**57** 300+	**51** 300+	**58** 300+
Mercy Tyler Hospital, Tunkhannock, PA	-	-	-	**0.364** 187	**0.029** 103	**7.1** 239	**36.0** 50	**41** (a)	**84** (a)	**85** (a)	**64** (a)	**64** (a)	**75** (a)	**69** (a)	**76** (a)	**69** (a)	**64** (a)
Mid-Valley Hospital, Peckville, PA	-	-	-	-	-	-	-	-	-	-	-	-	-	-	-	-	-
Millcreek Community Hospital, Erie, PA	-	-	-	**0.030** 100	**0.000** 31	**0.0** 56	**33.3** 24	**51** 300+	**83** 300+	**74** 300+	**61** 300+	**57** 300+	**72** 300+	**64** 300+	**71** 300+	**63** 300+	**60** 300+
Milton S Hershey Medical Center, Hershey, PA	-	-	-	**0.206** 1858	**0.006** 1991	**5.0** 1085	**26.6** 319	**42** 300+	**76** 300+	**89** 300+	**72** 300+	**58** 300+	**74** 300+	**68** 300+	**65** 300+	**59** 300+	**78** 300+
Miners Medical Center, Hastings, PA	-	-	-	**0.024** 254	**0.008** 130	**4.4** 135	**47.7** 44	**67** (a)	**89** (a)	**83** (a)	**77** (a)	**62** (a)	**86** (a)	**79** (a)	**77** (a)	**83** (a)	**74** (a)
Monongahela Valley Hospital, Monongahela, PA	-	-	-	**0.612** 397	**0.000** 185	**4.9** 536	**50.5** 97	**57** 300+	**83** 300+	**79** 300+	**70** 300+	**60** 300+	**80** 300+	**69** 300+	**76** 300+	**67** 300+	**67** 300+
Montgomery Hospital, Norristown, PA	-	-	-	**0.112** 465	**0.006** 348	**6.8** 725	**22.1** 77	**50** 300+	**76** 300+	**79** 300+	**52** 300+	**57** 300+	**75** 300+	**67** 300+	**60** 300+	**64** 300+	**54** 300+
Montrose General Hospital, Montrose, PA	-	-	-	-	-	-	-	-	-	-	-	-	-	-	-	-	-
Moses Taylor Hospital, Scranton, PA	-	-	-	**0.071** 538	**0.000** 325	**12.2** 699	**48.6** 35	**53** 300+	**81** 300+	**81** 300+	**64** 300+	**62** 300+	**76** 300+	**66** 300+	**70** 300+	**59** 300+	**70** 300+
Mount Nittany Medical Center, State College, PA	-	-	-	**0.129** 581	**0.017** 539	**10.2** 1584	**29.3** 82	**41** 300+	**81** 300+	**84** 300+	**65** 300+	**61** 300+	**76** 300+	**73** 300+	**76** 300+	**66** 300+	**67** 300+
Muncy Valley Hospital, Muncy, PA	-	-	-	-	-	-	-	**59** (a)	**86** (a)	**84** (a)	**74** (a)	**64** (a)	**82** (a)	**73** (a)	**81** (a)	**74** (a)	**75** (a)
Nason Hospital, Roaring Spring, PA	-	-	-	**0.049** 185	**0.019** 103	**10.3** 377	**33.3** 24	**56** 300+	**83** 300+	**77** 300+	**76** 300+	**63** 300+	**79** 300+	**74** 300+	**81** 300+	**70** 300+	**77** 300+
Nazareth Hospital, Philadelphia, PA	-	-	-	**0.070** 441	**0.005** 380	**10.5** 418	**27.8** 151	**54** 300+	**74** 300+	**83** 300+	**59** 300+	**56** 300+	**71** 300+	**66** 300+	**70** 300+	**56** 300+	**59** 300+
Ohio Valley General Hospital, Mckees Rocks, PA	-	-	-	**0.083** 157	**0.000** 146	**12.4** 177	**34.3** 35	**56** 300+	**77** 300+	**80** 300+	**63** 300+	**55** 300+	**73** 300+	**64** 300+	**68** 300+	**65** 300+	**69** 300+
Palmerton Hospital, Palmerton, PA	-	-	-	**0.026** 347	**0.004** 268	**15.4** 505	- 0	**52** 300+	**75** 300+	**82** 300+	**61** 300+	**63** 300+	**74** 300+	**71** 300+	**74** 300+	**62** 300+	**56** 300+
Penn Presbyterian Medical Center, Philadelphia, PA	-	-	-	**0.025** 324	**0.024** 255	**10.1** 207	**33.3** 36	**53** 300+	**80** 300+	**84** 300+	**68** 300+	**63** 300+	**77** 300+	**72** 300+	**67** 300+	**61** 300+	**74** 300+
Penn Hospital of the U of Penn Health Sys, Philadelphia, PA	-	-	-	**0.071** 794	**0.013** 716	**11.6** 946	**33.3** 3	**50** 300+	**76** 300+	**80** 300+	**64** 300+	**58** 300+	**70** 300+	**65** 300+	**64** 300+	**55** 300+	**71** 300+
Philadelphia VA Medical Center, Philadelphia, PA	-	-	-	-	-	-	-	-	-	-	-	-	-	-	-	-	-
Phoenixville Hospital, Phoenixville, PA	-	-	-	**0.338** 470	**0.045** 424	**9.2** 841	**36.1** 133	**54** 300+	**73** 300+	**81** 300+	**64** 300+	**57** 300+	**73** 300+	**66** 300+	**62** 300+	**54** 300+	**64** 300+
Pinnacle Health Hospitals, Harrisburg, PA	-	-	-	**0.272** 993	**0.158** 608	**7.7** 1189	**32.2** 118	**46** 300+	**74** 300+	**78** 300+	**59** 300+	**56** 300+	**72** 300+	**67** 300+	**60** 300+	**53** 300+	**68** 300+
Pocono Medical Center, East Stroudsburg, PA	-	-	-	**0.069** 1120	**0.034** 558	**9.0** 357	**20.0** 70	**50** 300+	**78** 300+	**84** 300+	**63** 300+	**61** 300+	**76** 300+	**72** 300+	**71** 300+	**63** 300+	**65** 300+
Pottstown Memorial Medical Center, Pottstown, PA	-	-	-	**0.190** 823	**0.038** 478	**6.7** 1064	**34.3** 210	**45** 300+	**71** 300+	**82** 300+	**55** 300+	**54** 300+	**70** 300+	**65** 300+	**60** 300+	**53** 300+	**53** 300+
Punxsutawney Area Hospital, Punxsutawney, PA	-	-	-	**0.484** 283	**0.000** 142	**7.2** 375	**31.0** 29	**53** 300+	**82** 300+	**92** 300+	**65** 300+	**61** 300+	**78** 300+	**71** 300+	**72** 300+	**70** 300+	**67** 300+
Reading Hospital Medical Center, Reading, PA	-	-	-	**0.067** 2807	**0.061** 2818	**6.5** 5143	**28.9** 602	**47** 300+	**76** 300+	**85** 300+	**64** 300+	**55** 300+	**73** 300+	**67** 300+	**62** 300+	**58** 300+	**67** 300+
Riddle Memorial Hospital, Media, PA	-	-	-	**0.612** 701	**0.018** 507	**0.0** 1	**20.0** 5	**46** 300+	**77** 300+	**81** 300+	**63** 300+	**60** 300+	**77** 300+	**69** 300+	**62** 300+	**65** 300+	**68** 300+
Robert Packer Hospital, Sayre, PA	-	-	-	**0.136** 1657	**0.005** 1324	**13.6** 1612	**34.4** 195	**50** 300+	**78** 300+	**81** 300+	**75** 300+	**63** 300+	**79** 300+	**72** 300+	**75** 300+	**66** 300+	**77** 300+
Roxborough Memorial Hospital, Phila, PA	-	-	-	**0.110** 146	**0.018** 112	**5.2** 327	**44.4** 9	**40** 300+	**74** 300+	**76** 300+	**50** 300+	**54** 300+	**70** 300+	**60** 300+	**56** 300+	**51** 300+	**47** 300+
Sacred Heart Hospital, Allentown, PA	-	-	-	**0.182** 472	**0.029** 375	**23.4** 824	**34.6** 52	**58** 300+	**75** 300+	**82** 300+	**59** 300+	**54** 300+	**71** 300+	**62** 300+	**67** 300+	**55** 300+	**58** 300+
Saint Catherine Medical Center Fountain Springs, Ashland, PA	-	-	-	**0.581** 93	**0.022** 45	**7.6** 131	**23.5** 17	**53** (a)	**85** (a)	**86** (a)	**61** (a)	**61** (a)	**76** (a)	**75** (a)	**83** (a)	**70** (a)	**56** (a)
Saint Clair Memorial Hospital, Pittsburgh, PA	-	-	-	**0.080** 981	**0.000** 672	**11.2** 699	**36.5** 156	**51** 300+	**78** 300+	**81** 300+	**71** 300+	**57** 300+	**79** 300+	**72** 300+	**69** 300+	**64** 300+	**75** 300+
Saint Joseph Medical Center, Reading, PA	-	-	-	**0.700** 543	**0.014** 499	**4.7** 1549	**34.4** 151	**57** 300+	**77** 300+	**85** 300+	**72** 300+	**54** 300+	**75** 300+	**69** 300+	**67** 300+	**62** 300+	**76** 300+
Saint Joseph's Hospital, Philadelphia, PA	-	-	-	**0.133** 15	**0.000** 6	**0.0** 41	- 0	**49** (a)	**70** (a)	**64** (a)	**40** (a)	**45** (a)	**56** (a)	**59** (a)	**61** (a)	**43** (a)	**35** (a)

NOTE: The first number in each column (boldface) is the score, the second number is the number of patients; Please refer to the main entry for footnotes; (a) 100-299

*MEASURES: **Children's Asthma Care:** 33. Received Systemic Corticosteroids; 34. Received Home Management Plan of Care; 35. Received Reliever Medication; **Use of Medical Imaging:** 36. Combination Abdominal CT Scan; 37. Combination Chest CT Scan; 38. Follow-up Mammogram/Ultrasound; 39. MRI for Low Back Pain; **Survey of Patients' Hospital Experiences:** 40. Area Around Room 'Always' Quiet at Night; 41. Doctors 'Always' Communicated Well; 42. Home Recovery Information Given; 43. Hospital Given 9 or 10 on 10 Point Scale; 44. Meds 'Always' Explained Before Given; 45. Nurses 'Always' Communicated Well; 46. Pain 'Always' Well Controlled; 47. Room and Bathroom 'Always' Clean; 48. Timely Help 'Always' Received; 49. Would Definitely Recommend Hospital*

Hospital	Children's Asthma Care			Use of Medical Imaging				Survey of Patients' Hospital Experiences									
	33	34	35	36	37	38	39	40	41	42	43	44	45	46	47	48	49
Saint Luke's Hospital Bethlehem, Bethlehem, PA	**100** 74	**64** 72	**100** 74	**0.254** 2147	**0.004** 1810	**8.4** 3599	**35.1** 239	**51** 300+	**78** 300+	**78** 300+	**73** 300+	**63** 300+	**78** 300+	**71** 300+	**71** 300+	**64** 300+	**78** 300+
Saint Luke's Miners Memorial Hospital, Coaldale, PA	- -	- -	- -	**0.218** 349	**0.084** 239	**3.7** 406	**30.4** 69	**51** 300+	**80** 300+	**82** 300+	**61** 300+	**58** 300+	**77** 300+	**67** 300+	**79** 300+	**58** 300+	**64** 300+
Saint Luke's Quakertown Hospital, Quakertown, PA	- -	- -	- -	**0.130** 354	**0.088** 240	**7.8** 486	**29.2** 89	**50** 300+	**78** 300+	**83** 300+	**68** 300+	**63** 300+	**82** 300+	**71** 300+	**70** 300+	**65** 300+	**71** 300+
Saint Mary Medical Center, Langhorne, PA	- -	- -	- -	**0.059** 1193	**0.020** 836	**7.4** 1535	**25.7** 148	**43** 300+	**74** 300+	**79** 300+	**76** 300+	**59** 300+	**77** 300+	**71** 300+	**71** 300+	**68** 300+	**80** 300+
Saint Vincent Health Center, Erie, PA	- -	- -	- -	**0.111** 946	**0.005** 424	**6.7** 1253	**31.3** 291	**51** 300+	**76** 300+	**84** 300+	**65** 300+	**55** 300+	**73** 300+	**64** 300+	**57** 300+	**59** 300+	**70** 300+
Schuylkill Medical Center - East Norwegian Street, Pottsville, PA	- -	- -	- -	**0.063** 587	**0.006** 341	**10.5** 740	**30.3** 142	**39** 300+	**75** 300+	**77** 300+	**57** 300+	**55** 300+	**73** 300+	**66** 300+	**71** 300+	**56** 300+	**57** 300+
Schuylkill Medical Center - South Jackson Street, Pottsville, PA	- -	- -	- -	**0.030** 778	**0.000** 357	**3.3** 1162	**31.8** 148	**45** 300+	**77** 300+	**73** 300+	**55** 300+	**53** 300+	**71** 300+	**63** 300+	**71** 300+	**64** 300+	**54** 300+
Shamokin Area Community Hospital, Coal Township, PA	- -	- -	- -	**0.626** 321	**0.064** 264	**6.8** 921	**40.4** 94	**54** 300+	**86** 300+	**83** 300+	**82** 300+	**61** 300+	**83** 300+	**72** 300+	**89** 300+	**78** 300+	**83** 300+
Sharon Regional Health System, Sharon, PA	- -	- -	- -	**0.439** 827	**0.008** 712	**8.5** 988	**32.7** 147	**45** 300+	**82** 300+	**80** 300+	**63** 300+	**61** 300+	**76** 300+	**70** 300+	**69** 300+	**67** 300+	**66** 300+
Soldiers and Sailors Memorial Hospital, Wellsboro, PA	- -	- -	- -	**0.571** 464	**0.008** 242	**6.9** 978	**32.8** 122	**52** 300+	**85** 300+	**85** 300+	**73** 300+	**67** 300+	**83** 300+	**75** 300+	**86** 300+	**79** 300+	**70** 300+
Somerset Hospital, Somerset, PA	- -	- -	- -	**0.562** 315	**0.325** 163	**6.1** 363	**37.5** 64	**44** 300+	**75** 300+	**84** 300+	**56** 300+	**55** 300+	**72** 300+	**64** 300+	**73** 300+	**57** 300+	**52** 300+
Southwest Regional Medical Center, Waynesburg, PA	- -	- -	- -	**0.576** 158	**0.157** 115	**11.8** 203	**38.2** 34	**52** 300+	**84** 300+	**84** 300+	**61** 300+	**57** 300+	**77** 300+	**70** 300+	**64** 300+	**64** 300+	**60** 300+
Sunbury Community Hospital, Sunbury, PA	- -	- -	- -	**0.099** 192	**0.042** 143	**2.8** 435	**40.0** 30	**48** 300+	**81** 300+	**82** 300+	**62** 300+	**56** 300+	**75** 300+	**66** 300+	**68** 300+	**66** 300+	**61** 300+
Surgical Institute of Reading, Wyomissing, PA	- -	- -	- -	**0.100** 10	**0.000** 12	- 0	- 0	**74** 300+	**94** 300+	**94** 300+	**93** 300+	**74** 300+	**88** 300+	**80** 300+	**85** 300+	**84** 300+	**94** 300+
Surgical Specialty Center at Coordinated Health, Allentown, PA	- -	- -	- -	- 0	- 0	- 0	- 0	- -	- -	- -	- -	- -	- -	- -	- -	- -	- -
Temple University Hospital, Philadelphia, PA	- -	- -	- -	**0.164** 633	**0.017** 827	**5.7** 888	**40.5** 79	**53** 300+	**77** 300+	**82** 300+	**59** 300+	**56** 300+	**69** 300+	**62** 300+	**64** 300+	**50** 300+	**61** 300+
Thomas Jefferson University Hospital, Philadelphia, PA	- -	- -	- -	**0.195** 1346	**0.011** 1046	**9.0** 3292	**27.4** 201	**50** 300+	**77** 300+	**84** 300+	**70** 300+	**61** 300+	**77** 300+	**70** 300+	**66** 300+	**67** 300+	**75** 300+
Titusville Hospital, Titusville, PA	- -	- -	- -	**0.163** 282	**0.000** 244	**0.4** 538	**28.3** 60	**66** 300+	**87** 300+	**85** 300+	**76** 300+	**61** 300+	**81** 300+	**75** 300+	**83** 300+	**74** 300+	**73** 300+
Troy Community Hospital, Troy, PA	- -	- -	- -	**0.022** 228	**0.008** 129	**12.3** 310	**34.6** 26	- -	- -	- -	- -	- -	- -	- -	- -	- -	- -
Uniontown Hospital, Uniontown, PA	- -	- -	- -	**0.381** 833	**0.002** 471	**4.6** 718	**34.3** 99	**51** 300+	**82** 300+	**88** 300+	**63** 300+	**60** 300+	**76** 300+	**70** 300+	**71** 300+	**63** 300+	**63** 300+
UPMC Bedford, Everett, PA	- -	- -	- -	**0.017** 343	**0.030** 165	**4.5** 420	**34.6** 26	**53** 300+	**78** 300+	**83** 300+	**60** 300+	**61** 300+	**76** 300+	**67** 300+	**78** 300+	**64** 300+	**56** 300+
UPMC Horizon, Greenville, PA	- -	- -	- -	**0.128** 889	**0.002** 553	**7.4** 1168	**32.4** 188	**42** 300+	**80** 300+	**82** 300+	**60** 300+	**56** 300+	**71** 300+	**64** 300+	**68** 300+	**57** 300+	**62** 300+
UPMC Mckeesport, McKeesport, PA	- -	- -	- -	**0.108** 372	**0.051** 293	**3.1** 260	**25.8** 31	**50** 300+	**79** 300+	**79** 300+	**59** 300+	**59** 300+	**74** 300+	**67** 300+	**69** 300+	**60** 300+	**57** 300+
UPMC Mercy, Pittsburgh, PA	- -	- -	- -	**0.093** 301	**0.008** 251	**7.5** 292	**45.7** 35	**48** 300+	**74** 300+	**80** 300+	**53** 300+	**51** 300+	**64** 300+	**58** 300+	**55** 300+	**45** 300+	**57** 300+
UPMC Northwest, Seneca, PA	- -	- -	- -	**0.076** 1032	**0.020** 938	**7.5** 1769	**33.3** 306	**48** 300+	**74** 300+	**77** 300+	**53** 300+	**52** 300+	**69** 300+	**66** 300+	**70** 300+	**60** 300+	**50** 300+
UPMC Passavant, Pittsburgh, PA	- -	- -	- -	**0.593** 958	**0.012** 847	**11.1** 587	**34.0** 150	**43** 300+	**75** 300+	**84** 300+	**60** 300+	**52** 300+	**69** 300+	**65** 300+	**55** 300+	**52** 300+	**64** 300+
UPMC Presbyterian Shadyside, Pittsburgh, PA	- -	- -	- -	**0.256** 3464	**0.014** 3991	- 0	**34.1** 270	**45** 300+	**75** 300+	**85** 300+	**63** 300+	**56** 300+	**73** 300+	**65** 300+	**57** 300+	**56** 300+	**69** 300+
UPMC Saint Margaret, Pittsburgh, PA	- -	- -	- -	**0.221** 810	**0.001** 691	**6.4** 561	**39.0** 159	**45** 300+	**77** 300+	**87** 300+	**66** 300+	**57** 300+	**74** 300+	**66** 300+	**61** 300+	**56** 300+	**73** 300+
VA Pittsburgh Healthcare System, Pittsburgh, PA	- -	- -	- -	- -	- -	- -	- -	- -	- -	- -	- -	- -	- -	- -	- -	- -	- -
Valley Forge Medical Center and Hospital, Norristown, PA	- -	- -	- -	- -	- -	- -	- -	- -	- -	- -	- -	- -	- -	- -	- -	- -	- -
Warren General Hospital, Warren, PA	- -	- -	- -	**0.415** 470	**0.004** 282	**2.0** 816	**32.9** 164	**48** 300+	**77** 300+	**75** 300+	**63** 300+	**61** 300+	**78** 300+	**71** 300+	**72** 300+	**67** 300+	**62** 300+
The Washington Hospital, Washington, PA	- -	- -	- -	**0.153** 393	**0.000** 380	**7.3** 959	**43.1** 116	**48** 300+	**82** 300+	**83** 300+	**64** 300+	**61** 300+	**79** 300+	**70** 300+	**78** 300+	**65** 300+	**66** 300+
Wayne Memorial Hospital, Honesdale, PA	- -	- -	- -	**0.127** 647	**0.045** 581	**5.6** 1071	**44.7** 94	**46** 300+	**78** 300+	**86** 300+	**63** 300+	**59** 300+	**77** 300+	**75** 300+	**73** 300+	**68** 300+	**63** 300+
Waynesboro Hospital, Waynesboro, PA	- -	- -	- -	**0.135** 446	**0.018** 271	**7.6** 1073	**39.5** 81	**52** 300+	**79** 300+	**85** 300+	**73** 300+	**67** 300+	**82** 300+	**74** 300+	**73** 300+	**78** 300+	**76** 300+
Western Pennsylvania Hospital, Pittsburgh, PA	- -	- -	- -	**0.156** 391	**0.003** 363	**9.9** 605	**29.6** 54	**53** 300+	**80** 300+	**81** 300+	**64** 300+	**58** 300+	**75** 300+	**67** 300+	**64** 300+	**61** 300+	**67** 300+
Western Penn Hosp-Forbes Reg Campus, Monroeville, PA	- -	- -	- -	**0.083** 483	**0.020** 345	**17.6** 324	**46.5** 43	**42** 300+	**74** 300+	**79** 300+	**57** 300+	**55** 300+	**71** 300+	**66** 300+	**60** 300+	**63** 300+	**62** 300+
Westfield Hospital, Allentown, PA	- -	- -	- -	**0.061** 49	**0.067** 15	- 0	**33.9** 56	**68** (a)	**79** (a)	**78** (a)	**79** (a)	**66** (a)	**81** (a)	**70** (a)	**81** (a)	**82** (a)	**78** (a)
Wilkes-Barre General Hospital, Wilkes-Barre, PA	- -	- -	- -	**0.311** 1842	**0.008** 1323	**7.2** 2678	**36.7** 139	**45** 300+	**80** 300+	**80** 300+	**59** 300+	**56** 300+	**76** 300+	**68** 300+	**64** 300+	**59** 300+	**60** 300+
Wilkes-Barre VA Medical Center, Wilkes-Barre, PA	- -	- -	- -	- -	- -	- -	- -	- -	- -	- -	- -	- -	- -	- -	- -	- -	- -
Williamsport Hospital & Medical Center, Williamsport, PA	- -	- -	- -	**0.083** 1095	**0.017** 535	- 0	- 0	**48** 300+	**83** 300+	**85** 300+	**71** 300+	**63** 300+	**80** 300+	**71** 300+	**71** 300+	**67** 300+	**69** 300+
Windber Hospital, Windber, PA	- -	- -	- -	**0.014** 278	**0.000** 231	**5.9** 461	**41.5** 53	**56** 300+	**87** 300+	**87** 300+	**76** 300+	**65** 300+	**81** 300+	**71** 300+	**82** 300+	**72** 300+	**79** 300+
York Hospital, York, PA	- -	- -	- -	**0.118** 2450	**0.006** 2749	**9.5** 5709	**34.3** 207	**44** 300+	**76** 300+	**84** 300+	**67** 300+	**59** 300+	**76** 300+	**68** 300+	**56** 300+	**67** 300+	**71** 300+
RHODE ISLAND																	
Kent County Memorial Hospital, Warwick, RI	- -	- -	- -	**0.082** 655	**0.040** 428	**11.5** 1185	**28.3** 106	**46** 300+	**75** 300+	**81** 300+	**58** 300+	**53** 300+	**74** 300+	**69** 300+	**66** 300+	**62** 300+	**60** 300+
Landmark Medical Center, Woonsocket, RI	- -	- -	- -	**0.071** 491	**0.018** 272	**5.1** 746	**37.4** 91	**41** 300+	**75** 300+	**83** 300+	**52** 300+	**54** 300+	**69** 300+	**65** 300+	**65** 300+	**57** 300+	**53** 300+
Memorial Hospital of Rhode Island, Pawtucket, RI	- -	- -	- -	**0.130** 431	**0.025** 324	**9.0** 525	**33.9** 56	**53** 300+	**81** 300+	**82** 300+	**65** 300+	**58** 300+	**76** 300+	**70** 300+	**72** 300+	**63** 300+	**68** 300+
Miriam Hospital, Providence, RI	- -	- -	- -	**0.071** 1293	**0.000** 1071	**12.1** 680	**30.1** 73	**49** 300+	**82** 300+	**84** 300+	**76** 300+	**62** 300+	**81** 300+	**73** 300+	**74** 300+	**62** 300+	**84** 300+
Newport Hospital, Newport, RI	- -	- -	- -	**0.069** 779	**0.005** 432	**5.9** 1128	**32.8** 189	**58** 300+	**78** 300+	**86** 300+	**71** 300+	**63** 300+	**78** 300+	**69** 300+	**74** 300+	**62** 300+	**74** 300+
Providence VA Medical Center, Providence, RI	- -	- -	- -	- -	- -	- -	- -	- -	- -	- -	- -	- -	- -	- -	- -	- -	- -
Rhode Island Hospital, Providence, RI	- -	- -	- -	**0.100** 1687	**0.062** 1377	**6.7** 1163	**29.8** 94	**46** 300+	**77** 300+	**82** 300+	**62** 300+	**55** 300+	**73** 300+	**67** 300+	**70** 300+	**60** 300+	**67** 300+
Roger Williams Medical Center, Providence, RI	- -	- -	- -	**0.085** 399	**0.022** 368	**4.9** 266	**48.3** 29	**48** 300+	**78** 300+	**85** 300+	**58** 300+	**55** 300+	**72** 300+	**65** 300+	**69** 300+	**58** 300+	**62** 300+
Saint Joseph Health Services of RI, North Providence, RI	- -	- -	- -	**0.124** 565	**0.000** 291	**14.0** 414	**33.3** 30	**45** 300+	**76** 300+	**81** 300+	**49** 300+	**52** 300+	**67** 300+	**63** 300+	**61** 300+	**50** 300+	**52** 300+
South County Hospital, Wakefield, RI	- -	- -	- -	**0.160** 470	**0.031** 386	**10.6** 738	**26.0** 104	**60** 300+	**82** 300+	**84** 300+	**77** 300+	**65** 300+	**80** 300+	**75** 300+	**74** 300+	**72** 300+	**80** 300+
Westerly Hospital, Westerly, RI	- -	- -	- -	**0.079** 684	**0.004** 566	**13.5** 1029	**31.2** 141	**54** 300+	**82** 300+	**80** 300+	**68** 300+	**60** 300+	**77** 300+	**76** 300+	**83** 300+	**66** 300+	**73** 300+
Women and Infants Hospital of Rhode Island, Providence, RI	- -	- -	- -	**0.031** 256	**0.000** 244	**9.1** 647	**33.3** 3	**59** 300+	**84** 300+	**83** 300+	**74** 300+	**62** 300+	**79** 300+	**78** 300+	**72** 300+	**68** 300+	**85** 300+
TENNESSEE																	
Athens Regional Medical Center, Athens, TN	- -	- -	- -	**0.353** 481	**0.026** 190	**11.3** 961	**35.5** 138	**67** 300+	**88** 300+	**83** 300+	**68** 300+	**65** 300+	**77** 300+	**75** 300+	**67** 300+	**65** 300+	**68** 300+
Baptist Hospital, Nashville, TN	- -	- -	- -	**0.139** 894	**0.132** 768	**10.1** 1712	**39.6** 144	**62** 300+	**84** 300+	**84** 300+	**71** 300+	**63** 300+	**78** 300+	**72** 300+	**64** 300+	**66** 300+	**77** 300+
Baptist Hospital of Cocke County, Newport, TN	- -	- -	- -	**0.088** 362	**0.090** 266	**11.9** 506	**44.2** 104	**59** 300+	**82** 300+	**79** 300+	**64** 300+	**61** 300+	**81** 300+	**72** 300+	**72** 300+	**69** 300+	**65** 300+
Baptist Hospital West, Knoxville, TN	- -	- -	- -	- -	- -	- -	- -	- -	- -	- -	- -	- -	- -	- -	- -	- -	- -
Baptist Memorial Hospital, Memphis, TN	- -	- -	- -	**0.051** 1699	**0.060** 1306	**10.0** 3419	**35.8** 268	**63** 300+	**81** 300+	**79** 300+	**72** 300+	**61** 300+	**76** 300+	**70** 300+	**72** 300+	**62** 300+	**76** 300+
Baptist Memorial Hospital Huntingdon, Huntingdon, TN	- -	- -	- -	**0.639** 155	**0.649** 94	**12.8** 243	**31.2** 93	**76** (a)	**88** (a)	**82** (a)	**74** (a)	**68** (a)	**87** (a)	**78** (a)	**75** (a)	**74** (a)	**77** (a)
Baptist Memorial Hospital Tipton, Covington, TN	- -	- -	- -	**0.025** 323	**0.005** 213	**7.6** 331	**22.6** 62	**64** (a)	**82** (a)	**75** (a)	**59** (a)	**65** (a)	**77** (a)	**72** (a)	**74** (a)	**65** (a)	**60** (a)
Baptist Memorial Hospital Union City, Union City, TN	- -	- -	- -	**0.052** 480	**0.038** 316	**6.7** 360	**35.1** 111	**68** 300+	**83** 300+	**83** 300+	**71** 300+	**64** 300+	**80** 300+	**71** 300+	**78** 300+	**71** 300+	**68** 300+
Baptist Rehabilitation Germantown, Germantown, TN	- -	- -	- -	- -	- -	- -	- -	- -	- -	- -	- -	- -	- -	- -	- -	- -	- -
Blount Memorial Hospital, Maryville, TN	- -	- -	- -	**0.129** 1077	**0.064** 643	**10.2** 1525	**31.6** 282	**48** 300+	**78** 300+	**84** 300+	**60** 300+	**54** 300+	**73** 300+	**67** 300+	**67** 300+	**59** 300+	**62** 300+
Bolivar General Hospital, Bolivar, TN	- -	- -	- -	**0.013** 153	**0.020** 50	**4.0** 149	- 0	**78** <100	**79** <100	**54** <100	**59** <100	**63** <100	**80** <100	**62** <100	**88** <100	**67** <100	**47** <100

NOTE: The first number in each column (boldface) is the score, the second number is the number of patients; Please refer to the main entry for footnotes; (a) 100-299
*MEASURES: **Children's Asthma Care:** 33. Received Systemic Corticosteroids; 34. Received Home Management Plan of Care; 35. Received Reliever Medication; **Use of Medical Imaging:** 36. Combination Abdominal CT Scan; 37. Combination Chest CT Scan; 38. Follow-up Mammogram/Ultrasound; 39. MRI for Low Back Pain; **Survey of Patients' Hospital Experiences:** 40. Area Around Room 'Always' Quiet at Night; 41. Doctors 'Always' Communicated Well; 42. Home Recovery Information Given; 43. Hospital Given 9 or 10 on 10 Point Scale; 44. Meds 'Always' Explained Before Given; 45. Nurses 'Always' Communicated Well; 46. Pain 'Always' Well Controlled; 47. Room and Bathroom 'Always' Clean; 48. Timely Help 'Always' Received; 49. Would Definitely Recommend Hospital*

Hospital	Children's Asthma Care			Use of Medical Imaging				Survey of Patients' Hospital Experiences									
	33	34	35	36	37	38	39	40	41	42	43	44	45	46	47	48	49
Camden General Hospital, Camden, TN	-	-	-	-	-	-	-	63 <100	79 <100	78 <100	59 <100	45 <100	76 <100	76 <100	74 <100	77 <100	57 <100
Centennial Medical Center, Nashville, TN	-	-	-	0.107 863	0.040 606	7.3 1051	33.3 180	67 300+	85 300+	87 300+	79 300+	67 300+	81 300+	75 300+	74 300+	71 300+	81 300+
Centennial Medical Center of Ashland City, Ashland City, TN	-	-	-	0.076 66	0.029 35	4.3 46	33.3 15	80 <100	92 <100	76 <100	87 <100	67 <100	82 <100	71 <100	74 <100	69 <100	95 <100
The Center for Spinal Surgery, Nashville, TN	-	-	-	- 0	- 0	- 0	- 0	91 300+	93 300+	90 300+	93 300+	74 300+	92 300+	84 300+	83 300+	85 300+	95 300+
Claiborne County Hospital, Tazewell, TN	-	-	-	0.024 376	0.000 288	9.0 299	32.6 86	53 (a)	86 (a)	79 (a)	63 (a)	63 (a)	77 (a)	66 (a)	70 (a)	64 (a)	67 (a)
Cookeville Regional Medical Center, Cookeville, TN	-	-	-	0.057 888	0.078 694	7.0 1003	25.4 331	59 300+	80 300+	81 300+	70 300+	57 300+	77 300+	69 300+	75 300+	67 300+	76 300+
Copper Basin Medical Center, Copperhill, TN	-	-	-	0.229 166	0.189 90	2.9 238	60.0 5	-	-	-	-	-	-	-	-	-	-
Crockett Hospital, Lawrenceburg, TN	-	-	-	0.210 405	0.023 393	10.1 662	36.0 136	64 300+	82 300+	74 300+	63 300+	56 300+	75 300+	68 300+	67 300+	61 300+	60 300+
Cumberland Medical Center, Crossville, TN	-	-	-	0.110 970	0.129 1038	5.3 2102	31.3 415	57 300+	81 300+	76 300+	63 300+	58 300+	77 300+	69 300+	75 300+	64 300+	66 300+
Cumberland River Hospital, Celina, TN	-	-	-	0.674 43	0.739 23	5.3 94	- 0	56 (a)	84 (a)	82 (a)	68 (a)	66 (a)	81 (a)	70 (a)	82 (a)	77 (a)	72 (a)
Decatur County General Hospital, Parsons, TN	-	-	-	0.410 173	0.051 98	17.4 281	55.6 9	59 (a)	81 (a)	77 (a)	63 (a)	58 (a)	82 (a)	72 (a)	77 (a)	72 (a)	58 (a)
Delta Medical Center, Memphis, TN	-	-	-	0.596 47	0.060 50	7.6 119	71.4 14	76 300+	73 300+	72 300+	60 300+	55 300+	71 300+	63 300+	74 300+	51 300+	57 300+
Dyersburg Regional Medical Center, Dyersburg, TN	-	-	-	0.013 454	0.011 280	7.0 672	26.8 142	65 300+	79 300+	78 300+	57 300+	62 300+	75 300+	71 300+	64 300+	65 300+	54 300+
Erlanger Medical Center, Chattanooga, TN	100 39	82 39	100 39	0.296 1071	0.153 940	5.1 2058	36.6 164	62 300+	81 300+	80 300+	66 300+	61 300+	76 300+	69 300+	62 300+	61 300+	74 300+
Fort Loudoun Medical Center, Lenoir City, TN	-	-	-	0.293 256	0.166 290	12.8 337	34.2 79	71 300+	84 300+	85 300+	73 300+	66 300+	80 300+	74 300+	74 300+	69 300+	76 300+
Fort Sanders Regional Medical Center, Knoxville, TN	-	-	-	0.141 740	0.103 692	6.4 593	33.1 248	65 300+	83 300+	83 300+	75 300+	59 300+	80 300+	69 300+	69 300+	64 300+	76 300+
Franklin Woods Community Hospital, Johnson City, TN	-	-	-	0.333 420	0.455 200	- 0	20.5 127	59 (a)	73 (a)	85 (a)	69 (a)	61 (a)	79 (a)	75 (a)	71 (a)	65 (a)	72 (a)
Gateway Medical Center, Clarksville, TN	-	-	-	0.042 954	0.005 768	6.5 1261	28.4 268	58 300+	79 300+	77 300+	60 300+	56 300+	73 300+	70 300+	65 300+	61 300+	60 300+
Gibson General Hospital, Trenton, TN	-	-	-	0.011 89	0.077 26	6.6 228	- 0	75 (a)	90 (a)	77 (a)	68 (a)	66 (a)	84 (a)	86 (a)	69 (a)	79 (a)	60 (a)
Grandview Medical Center, Jasper, TN	-	-	-	0.283 311	0.234 124	6.2 355	25.8 66	65 (a)	79 (a)	78 (a)	63 (a)	53 (a)	75 (a)	65 (a)	71 (a)	60 (a)	57 (a)
Hardin Medical Center, Savannah, TN	-	-	-	0.034 466	0.011 261	19.0 399	39.6 106	74 300+	90 300+	86 300+	71 300+	71 300+	85 300+	82 300+	75 300+	79 300+	71 300+
Harton Regional Medical Center, Tullahoma, TN	95 20	100 20	100 20	0.330 518	0.301 309	11.2 1036	26.4 178	57 300+	78 300+	80 300+	58 300+	55 300+	71 300+	61 300+	68 300+	56 300+	60 300+
Haywood Park Community Hospital, Brownsville, TN	-	-	-	0.069 102	0.018 56	6.0 348	- 0	79 (a)	87 (a)	77 (a)	65 (a)	72 (a)	77 (a)	70 (a)	60 (a)	67 (a)	53 (a)
Healthsouth Chattanooga Rehab Hospital, Chattanooga, TN	-	-	-	-	-	-	-	-	-	-	-	-	-	-	-	-	-
Henderson County Community Hospital, Lexington, TN	-	-	-	0.363 91	0.476 21	8.2 255	21.0 62	71 (a)	80 (a)	80 (a)	61 (a)	61 (a)	79 (a)	65 (a)	65 (a)	67 (a)	59 (a)
Hendersonville Medical Center, Hendersonville, TN	-	-	-	0.174 522	0.017 346	11.2 721	23.6 178	61 300+	82 300+	84 300+	65 300+	58 300+	75 300+	69 300+	66 300+	61 300+	67 300+
Henry County Medical Center, Paris, TN	-	-	-	0.563 710	0.000 436	5.3 836	29.8 181	68 300+	84 300+	82 300+	69 300+	65 300+	76 300+	70 300+	68 300+	61 300+	71 300+
Heritage Medical Center, Shelbyville, TN	-	-	-	0.146 219	0.413 138	5.4 444	32.8 64	61 300+	84 300+	81 300+	66 300+	60 300+	74 300+	68 300+	73 300+	60 300+	63 300+
Hickman Community Health Services, Centerville, TN	-	-	-	-	-	-	-	-	-	-	-	-	-	-	-	-	-
Hillside Hospital, Pulaski, TN	-	-	-	0.156 282	0.006 159	9.4 499	22.8 57	63 (a)	85 (a)	81 (a)	65 (a)	61 (a)	76 (a)	69 (a)	64 (a)	65 (a)	61 (a)
Horizon Medical Center, Dickson, TN	-	-	-	0.136 440	0.012 163	5.2 650	28.7 178	60 300+	83 300+	87 300+	67 300+	60 300+	79 300+	72 300+	71 300+	68 300+	66 300+
Humboldt General Hospital, Humboldt, TN	-	-	-	0.070 86	0.000 49	2.2 268	- 0	73 (a)	93 (a)	67 (a)	72 (a)	63 (a)	85 (a)	80 (a)	76 (a)	79 (a)	76 (a)
Indian Path Medical Center, Kingsport, TN	-	-	-	0.565 391	0.520 177	8.4 598	30.5 105	57 300+	81 300+	83 300+	71 300+	59 300+	78 300+	71 300+	70 300+	65 300+	74 300+
Jackson-Madison County General Hospital, Jackson, TN	-	-	-	0.039 1630	0.008 1313	7.2 1994	30.4 678	67 300+	79 300+	81 300+	66 300+	56 300+	75 300+	66 300+	65 300+	61 300+	70 300+
Jamestown Regional Medical Center, Jamestown, TN	90 10	80 10	100 10	0.079 165	0.022 89	3.7 376	14.0 43	63 300+	83 300+	75 300+	55 300+	63 300+	78 300+	65 300+	71 300+	66 300+	52 300+
Jellico Community Hospital, Jellico, TN	-	-	-	0.588 216	0.754 199	15.9 308	67.9 56	65 (a)	86 (a)	82 (a)	68 (a)	65 (a)	78 (a)	70 (a)	75 (a)	61 (a)	66 (a)
Johnson City Medical Center, Johnson City, TN	97 66	9 66	100 66	0.349 1194	0.418 813	7.6 2602	27.3 414	54 300+	76 300+	81 300+	68 300+	62 300+	77 300+	66 300+	64 300+	64 300+	70 300+
Johnson City Specialty Hospital, Johnson City, TN	-	-	-	- 0	- 0	7.9 114	- 0	75 300+	92 300+	90 300+	90 300+	74 300+	89 300+	85 300+	85 300+	81 300+	94 300+
Johnson County Community Hospital, Mountain City, TN	-	-	-	0.272 162	0.458 83	8.5 176	- 0	-	-	-	-	-	-	-	-	-	-
Lakeway Regional Hospital, Morristown, TN	-	-	-	0.582 220	0.610 82	8.9 157	25.2 107	65 300+	78 300+	81 300+	65 300+	59 300+	74 300+	65 300+	65 300+	59 300+	66 300+
Lauderdale Community Hospital, Ripley, TN	-	-	-	0.050 140	0.009 115	4.1 318	26.3 19	-	-	-	-	-	-	-	-	-	-
Laughlin Memorial Hospital, Greeneville, TN	-	-	-	0.128 897	0.105 459	8.7 969	33.6 214	56 300+	84 300+	74 300+	67 300+	58 300+	74 300+	66 300+	69 300+	64 300+	70 300+
Leconte Medical Center, Sevierville, TN	-	-	-	0.141 802	0.066 711	7.5 933	40.1 172	65 300+	86 300+	89 300+	74 300+	66 300+	79 300+	72 300+	76 300+	66 300+	72 300+
Lincoln Medical Center, Fayetteville, TN	-	-	-	0.635 249	0.434 175	7.2 429	35.1 57	63 300+	78 300+	74 300+	53 300+	61 300+	76 300+	64 300+	68 300+	61 300+	50 300+
Livingston Regional Hospital, Livingston, TN	-	-	-	0.622 246	0.874 111	3.0 337	29.8 84	59 300+	86 300+	75 300+	62 300+	56 300+	75 300+	69 300+	68 300+	64 300+	64 300+
Macon County General Hospital, Lafayette, TN	-	-	-	0.581 105	0.494 85	23.2 155	27.8 36	-	-	-	-	-	-	-	-	-	-
Marshall Medical Center, Lewisburg, TN	-	-	-	-	-	-	-	-	-	-	-	-	-	-	-	-	-
Maury Regional Hospital, Columbia, TN	-	-	-	0.128 1324	0.059 1232	10.7 1690	27.8 230	63 300+	84 300+	83 300+	75 300+	69 300+	83 300+	76 300+	77 300+	74 300+	76 300+
McKenzie Regional Hospital, McKenzie, TN	-	-	-	0.417 60	0.833 30	13.3 264	33.3 6	70 300+	81 300+	80 300+	65 300+	62 300+	73 300+	66 300+	68 300+	61 300+	65 300+
McNairy Regional Hospital, Selmer, TN	-	-	-	0.050 161	0.049 81	4.8 294	37.5 48	74 (a)	85 (a)	78 (a)	65 (a)	64 (a)	78 (a)	74 (a)	70 (a)	67 (a)	66 (a)
Medical Center of Manchester, Manchester, TN	-	-	-	0.333 150	0.469 49	- 0	26.9 26	-	-	-	-	-	-	-	-	-	-
Memorial Healthcare System, Chattanooga, TN	-	-	-	0.390 2724	0.045 1359	4.6 4438	33.3 568	68 300+	84 300+	85 300+	78 300+	63 300+	82 300+	74 300+	71 300+	69 300+	84 300+
Memphis VA Medical Center, Memphis, TN	-	-	-	-	-	-	-	-	-	-	-	-	-	-	-	-	-
Mercy Medical Center, Knoxville, TN	-	-	-	0.066 1189	0.020 841	10.8 742	29.0 383	65 300+	82 300+	83 300+	72 300+	59 300+	77 300+	71 300+	71 300+	65 300+	76 300+
Methodist Healthcare Fayette Hospital, Somerville, TN	-	-	-	0.038 184	0.020 101	8.4 202	45.0 20	87 (a)	95 (a)	84 (a)	75 (a)	79 (a)	89 (a)	87 (a)	83 (a)	79 (a)	86 (a)
Methodist Healthcare Memphis Hospitals, Memphis, TN	-	-	-	0.245 3067	0.150 2231	10.0 4237	33.5 505	63 300+	77 300+	79 300+	68 300+	59 300+	74 300+	68 300+	64 300+	57 300+	72 300+
Methodist Medical Center of Oak Ridge, Oak Ridge, TN	-	-	-	0.059 1105	0.003 738	8.8 2390	24.6 357	65 300+	82 300+	83 300+	66 300+	63 300+	76 300+	66 300+	74 300+	61 300+	76 300+
Metro Nashville General Hospital, Nashville, TN	-	-	-	0.057 70	0.030 33	3.2 124	57.1 7	62 300+	82 300+	81 300+	65 300+	62 300+	73 300+	66 300+	68 300+	57 300+	64 300+
Middle Tennessee Medical Center, Murfreesboro, TN	-	-	-	0.215 608	0.018 111	7.8 729	38.9 36	57 300+	84 300+	84 300+	57 300+	60 300+	74 300+	69 300+	58 300+	57 300+	62 300+
Milan General Hospital, Milan, TN	-	-	-	0.000 166	0.000 71	9.2 271	- 0	81 <100	94 <100	84 <100	79 <100	74 <100	91 <100	88 <100	84 <100	82 <100	79 <100
Morristown Hamblen Hospital Association, Morristown, TN	-	-	-	0.118 619	0.159 389	7.8 541	19.6 189	54 300+	81 300+	88 300+	65 300+	61 300+	79 300+	67 300+	77 300+	66 300+	71 300+
Mountain Home VA Medical Center, Mountain Home, TN	-	-	-	-	-	-	-	-	-	-	-	-	-	-	-	-	-
Northcrest Medical Center, Springfield, TN	-	-	-	0.073 381	0.006 316	13.1 672	33.7 95	59 300+	82 300+	86 300+	70 300+	64 300+	78 300+	71 300+	72 300+	67 300+	68 300+
Parkridge Medical Center, Chattanooga, TN	-	-	-	0.173 819	0.119 311	12.3 625	33.9 118	65 300+	83 300+	83 300+	73 300+	61 300+	78 300+	73 300+	73 300+	65 300+	76 300+
Parkwest Medical Center, Knoxville, TN	-	-	-	0.155 885	0.076 682	6.4 779	24.4 176	69 300+	85 300+	86 300+	82 300+	66 300+	79 300+	74 300+	72 300+	66 300+	86 300+
Patients' Choice Medical Center of Erin, Erin, TN	-	-	-	-	-	-	-	-	-	-	-	-	-	-	-	-	-
Perry Community Hospital, Linden, TN	-	-	-	0.058 104	0.040 75	- 0	- 0	53 <100	64 <100	45 <100	33 <100	8 <100	57 <100	37 <100	74 <100	39 <100	6 <100

NOTE: The first number in each column (boldface) is the score, the second number is the number of patients; Please refer to the main entry for footnotes; (a) 100-299
*MEASURES: **Children's Asthma Care:** 33. Received Systemic Corticosteroids; 34. Received Home Management Plan of Care; 35. Received Reliever Medication; **Use of Medical Imaging:** 36. Combination Abdominal CT Scan; 37. Combination Chest CT Scan; 38. Follow-up Mammogram/Ultrasound; 39. MRI for Low Back Pain; **Survey of Patients' Hospital Experiences:** 40. Area Around Room 'Always' Quiet at Night; 41. Doctors 'Always' Communicated Well; 42. Home Recovery Information Given; 43. Hospital Given 9 or 10 on 10 Point Scale; 44. Meds 'Always' Explained Before Given; 45. Nurses 'Always' Communicated Well; 46. Pain 'Always' Well Controlled; 47. Room and Bathroom 'Always' Clean; 48. Timely Help 'Always' Received; 49. Would Definitely Recommend Hospital*

Hospital	Children's Asthma Care			Use of Medical Imaging				Survey of Patients' Hospital Experiences									
	33	34	35	36	37	38	39	40	41	42	43	44	45	46	47	48	49
Regional Hospital of Jackson, Jackson, TN	- -	- -	- -	0.013 228	0.005 197	8.7 161	26.8 56	67 300+	81 300+	78 300+	71 300+	58 300+	78 300+	71 300+	66 300+	65 300+	74 300+
Regional Medical Center at Memphis, Memphis, TN	- -	- -	- -	0.377 273	0.119 260	7.4 257	37.5 24	58 300+	79 300+	81 300+	55 300+	57 300+	69 300+	60 300+	59 300+	51 300+	63 300+
Rhea Medical Center, Dayton, TN	- -	- -	- -	0.096 384	0.110 200	11.6 380	32.1 53	61 300+	88 300+	77 300+	67 300+	58 300+	78 300+	66 300+	65 300+	63 300+	68 300+
River Park Hospital, McMinnville, TN	- -	- -	- -	0.023 385	0.252 393	4.8 744	17.8 157	63 300+	77 300+	81 300+	59 300+	57 300+	72 300+	65 300+	64 300+	60 300+	57 300+
Riverview Regional Medical Center North, Carthage, TN	- -	- -	- -	0.403 191	0.361 119	- 0	20.0 55	70 (a)	84 (a)	78 (a)	66 (a)	61 (a)	77 (a)	67 (a)	82 (a)	70 (a)	60 (a)
Riverview Regional Medical Center South, Carthage, TN	- -	- -	- -	- -	- -	- -	- -	- -	- -	- -	- -	- -	- -	- -	- -	- -	- -
Roane Medical Center, Harriman, TN	- -	- -	- -	0.162 359	0.164 323	4.1 534	33.3 66	71 300+	81 300+	82 300+	68 300+	62 300+	78 300+	66 300+	75 300+	75 300+	62 300+
Saint Francis Bartlett Medical Center, Bartlett, TN	- -	- -	- -	0.694 369	0.010 208	7.0 314	35.3 68	72 300+	83 300+	83 300+	72 300+	62 300+	78 300+	73 300+	68 300+	66 300+	77 300+
Saint Francis Hospital, Memphis, TN	- -	- -	- -	0.747 770	0.004 525	7.3 1212	31.4 210	67 300+	83 300+	80 300+	65 300+	63 300+	75 300+	69 300+	63 300+	57 300+	69 300+
Saint Mary's Jefferson Memorial Hospital, Jefferson City, TN	- -	- -	- -	0.049 531	0.022 320	10.1 596	35.1 114	56 300+	84 300+	81 300+	67 300+	60 300+	75 300+	63 300+	73 300+	58 300+	71 300+
Saint Mary's Med Ctr of Campbell County, La Follette, TN	- -	- -	- -	0.344 256	0.180 206	2.8 320	47.1 119	57 300+	83 300+	79 300+	58 300+	62 300+	77 300+	71 300+	69 300+	68 300+	58 300+
Saint Thomas Hospital, Nashville, TN	- -	- -	- -	0.055 902	0.017 896	7.8 1619	28.6 147	51 300+	83 300+	84 300+	81 300+	61 300+	79 300+	73 300+	65 300+	61 300+	87 300+
Scott County Hospital, Oneida, TN	- -	- -	- -	- 0	- 0	- 0	- 0	65 (a)	85 (a)	80 (a)	60 (a)	65 (a)	78 (a)	75 (a)	81 (a)	71 (a)	63 (a)
Skyline Medical Center, Nashville, TN	- -	- -	- -	0.277 822	0.003 629	7.9 1095	31.6 244	65 300+	80 300+	84 300+	66 300+	59 300+	75 300+	69 300+	66 300+	62 300+	70 300+
Skyridge Medical Center, Cleveland, TN	- -	- -	- -	0.195 967	0.014 702	5.1 1145	31.5 317	60 300+	78 300+	78 300+	58 300+	53 300+	73 300+	68 300+	63 300+	58 300+	56 300+
Southern Hills Medical Center, Nashville, TN	- -	- -	- -	0.122 395	0.020 246	5.9 656	25.8 62	65 300+	82 300+	85 300+	67 300+	59 300+	75 300+	69 300+	70 300+	60 300+	65 300+
Southern Tennessee Medical Center, Winchester, TN	- -	- -	- -	0.061 396	0.012 167	5.1 891	33.1 142	64 300+	82 300+	80 300+	61 300+	60 300+	75 300+	71 300+	66 300+	59 300+	63 300+
Stonecrest Medical Center, Smyrna, TN	- -	- -	- -	0.064 346	0.032 155	9.0 480	33.8 65	70 300+	82 300+	87 300+	71 300+	61 300+	77 300+	73 300+	74 300+	64 300+	77 300+
Stones River Hosp & Dekalb Comm Hosp, Woodbury, TN	- -	- -	- -	0.000 43	0.000 52	7.8 77	26.8 41	66 (a)	85 (a)	82 (a)	58 (a)	55 (a)	76 (a)	69 (a)	71 (a)	66 (a)	59 (a)
Stones River Hosp & Dekalb Comm Hosp, Smithville, TN	- -	- -	- -	0.327 226	0.057 175	8.4 323	35.5 62	67 300+	90 300+	84 300+	71 300+	58 300+	83 300+	77 300+	75 300+	68 300+	73 300+
Summit Medical Center, Hermitage, TN	- -	- -	- -	0.341 722	0.069 421	10.2 1258	25.7 257	63 300+	82 300+	88 300+	72 300+	59 300+	76 300+	70 300+	71 300+	66 300+	75 300+
Sumner Regional Medical Center, Gallatin, TN	- -	- -	- -	0.552 600	0.422 597	12.5 615	25.5 141	60 300+	81 300+	76 300+	64 300+	57 300+	75 300+	69 300+	76 300+	62 300+	67 300+
Sweetwater Hospital Association, Sweetwater, TN	- -	- -	- -	0.092 392	0.041 295	7.8 257	43.3 90	62 (a)	87 (a)	83 (a)	69 (a)	68 (a)	76 (a)	69 (a)	74 (a)	68 (a)	64 (a)
Sycamore Shoals Hospital, Elizabethton, TN	- -	- -	- -	0.386 541	0.321 293	9.9 708	37.1 210	70 300+	84 300+	81 300+	74 300+	68 300+	82 300+	77 300+	76 300+	72 300+	75 300+
Takoma Regional Hospital, Greeneville, TN	- -	- -	- -	0.457 313	0.367 221	6.9 420	26.3 76	63 (a)	78 (a)	86 (a)	68 (a)	63 (a)	75 (a)	67 (a)	73 (a)	66 (a)	71 (a)
Trousdale Medical Center, Hartsville, TN	- -	- -	- -	- -	- -	- -	- -	67 (a)	89 (a)	85 (a)	70 (a)	72 (a)	85 (a)	76 (a)	92 (a)	67 (a)	71 (a)
Unicoi County Memorial Hospital, Erwin, TN	- -	- -	- -	0.148 209	0.129 139	8.5 342	32.8 58	57 300+	87 300+	77 300+	72 300+	65 300+	75 300+	65 300+	76 300+	65 300+	81 300+
United Regional Medical Center, Manchester, TN	- -	- -	- -	0.106 94	0.122 82	7.4 256	22.8 215	76 300+	91 300+	85 300+	62 300+	63 300+	84 300+	79 300+	80 300+	75 300+	77 300+
University Medical Center, Lebanon, TN	100 7	71 7	100 7	0.180 510	0.150 367	10.4 595	24.4 82	61 300+	80 300+	80 300+	59 300+	54 300+	72 300+	65 300+	70 300+	55 300+	58 300+
University of Tennessee Memorial Hospital, Knoxville, TN	- -	- -	- -	0.080 2016	0.018 2392	6.6 1935	23.2 323	63 300+	83 300+	82 300+	76 300+	61 300+	81 300+	72 300+	75 300+	63 300+	82 300+
VA Middle Tennessee Healthcare System, Nashville, TN	- -	- -	- -	- -	- -	- -	- -	- -	- -	- -	- -	- -	- -	- -	- -	- -	- -
Vanderbilt University Hospital, Nashville, TN	- -	- -	- -	0.212 2684	0.018 2521	11.3 990	28.7 101	55 300+	83 300+	85 300+	74 300+	60 300+	78 300+	70 300+	64 300+	62 300+	81 300+
Volunteer Community Hospital, Martin, TN	- -	- -	- -	0.147 238	0.085 164	4.2 120	30.0 60	62 300+	82 300+	79 300+	66 300+	56 300+	77 300+	72 300+	71 300+	63 300+	64 300+
Wayne Medical Center, Waynesboro, TN	- -	- -	- -	0.615 91	0.731 67	6.8 162	36.2 47	63 (a)	79 (a)	73 (a)	61 (a)	56 (a)	78 (a)	63 (a)	76 (a)	62 (a)	62 (a)
Wellmont Bristol Regional Medical Center, Bristol, TN	- -	- -	- -	0.696 1463	0.167 927	8.5 1183	35.8 439	58 300+	78 300+	79 300+	67 300+	56 300+	77 300+	64 300+	64 300+	57 300+	67 300+
Wellmont Hancock County Hospital, Sneedville, TN	- -	- -	- -	- -	- -	- -	- -	- -	- -	- -	- -	- -	- -	- -	- -	- -	- -
Wellmont Hawkins County Memorial Hospital, Rogersville, TN	- -	- -	- -	0.173 197	0.030 167	13.0 223	39.2 74	75 300+	88 300+	83 300+	73 300+	69 300+	83 300+	76 300+	82 300+	73 300+	75 300+
Wellmont Holston Valley Medical Center, Kingsport, TN	- -	- -	- -	0.256 540	0.024 289	4.0 1696	28.9 45	55 300+	83 300+	79 300+	64 300+	59 300+	76 300+	69 300+	69 300+	62 300+	73 300+
White County Community Hospital, Sparta, TN	- -	- -	- -	0.356 160	0.023 132	9.5 338	28.3 53	72 300+	85 300+	84 300+	68 300+	65 300+	76 300+	72 300+	77 300+	68 300+	63 300+
Williamson Medical Center, Franklin, TN	- -	- -	- -	0.256 632	0.172 344	3.8 996	36.8 68	66 300+	84 300+	84 300+	74 300+	63 300+	78 300+	69 300+	70 300+	65 300+	78 300+
Woods Memorial Hospital, Etowah, TN	- -	- -	- -	0.317 319	0.041 145	12.8 345	35.4 79	70 300+	87 300+	83 300+	73 300+	57 300+	80 300+	74 300+	71 300+	72 300+	76 300+
VERMONT																	
Brattleboro Memorial Hospital, Brattleboro, VT	- -	- -	- -	0.099 312	0.062 162	7.2 1058	25.0 92	52 300+	81 300+	82 300+	67 300+	64 300+	80 300+	71 300+	79 300+	72 300+	73 300+
Central Vermont Medical Center, Barre, VT	- -	- -	- -	0.103 650	0.000 386	12.0 1746	30.6 85	54 300+	76 300+	87 300+	62 300+	59 300+	74 300+	64 300+	79 300+	66 300+	62 300+
Copley Hospital, Morrisville, VT	- -	- -	- -	- -	- -	- -	- -	61 300+	87 300+	88 300+	74 300+	68 300+	81 300+	78 300+	76 300+	76 300+	77 300+
Fletcher Allen Hospital of Vermont, Burlington, VT	- -	- -	- -	0.106 1844	0.002 1878	8.9 4637	19.2 411	43 300+	79 300+	87 300+	71 300+	61 300+	77 300+	69 300+	77 300+	65 300+	77 300+
Gifford Medical Center, Randolph, VT	- -	- -	- -	- -	- -	- -	- -	61 300+	80 300+	87 300+	75 300+	66 300+	79 300+	72 300+	72 300+	70 300+	76 300+
Grace Cottage Hospital, Townshend, VT	- -	- -	- -	- -	- -	- -	- -	61 <100	88 <100	85 <100	83 <100	66 <100	83 <100	73 <100	91 <100	75 <100	93 <100
Mount Ascutney Hospital, Windsor, VT	- -	- -	- -	- -	- -	- -	- -	50 (a)	85 (a)	88 (a)	73 (a)	67 (a)	79 (a)	78 (a)	81 (a)	69 (a)	81 (a)
North Country Hospital and Health Center, Newport, VT	- -	- -	- -	- -	- -	- -	- -	60 300+	88 300+	90 300+	71 300+	66 300+	82 300+	72 300+	82 300+	75 300+	70 300+
Northeastern Vermont Regional Hospital, Saint Johnsbury, VT	- -	- -	- -	- -	- -	- -	- -	57 300+	85 300+	87 300+	69 300+	67 300+	79 300+	72 300+	83 300+	72 300+	73 300+
Northwestern Medical Center, Saint Albans, VT	- -	- -	- -	0.110 538	0.017 346	11.7 920	36.5 63	61 300+	82 300+	88 300+	74 300+	66 300+	82 300+	74 300+	83 300+	70 300+	79 300+
Porter Hospital, Middlebury, VT	- -	- -	- -	- -	- -	- -	- -	55 300+	85 300+	88 300+	69 300+	68 300+	81 300+	73 300+	74 300+	68 300+	74 300+
Rutland Regional Medical Center, Rutland, VT	- -	- -	- -	0.046 677	0.042 501	3.8 1798	29.5 264	49 300+	79 300+	86 300+	64 300+	59 300+	76 300+	74 300+	71 300+	69 300+	63 300+
Southwestern Vermont Medical Center, Bennington, VT	- -	- -	- -	0.107 758	0.016 575	8.0 1331	23.1 134	53 300+	85 300+	86 300+	76 300+	66 300+	82 300+	76 300+	81 300+	71 300+	80 300+
Springfield Hospital, Springfield, VT	- -	- -	- -	- -	- -	- -	- -	52 300+	83 300+	84 300+	65 300+	67 300+	82 300+	72 300+	79 300+	75 300+	65 300+
White River Junction VA Medical Center, White River Junction, VT	- -	- -	- -	- -	- -	- -	- -	- -	- -	- -	- -	- -	- -	- -	- -	- -	- -
VIRGINIA																	
Alleghany Regional Hospital, Low Moor, VA	- -	- -	- -	0.061 443	0.000 346	10.1 833	33.7 92	60 300+	82 300+	83 300+	64 300+	62 300+	78 300+	72 300+	67 300+	61 300+	66 300+
Augusta Health, Fishersville, VA	- -	- -	- -	0.163 1673	0.001 1236	12.5 2916	34.6 503	51 300+	81 300+	85 300+	63 300+	61 300+	74 300+	69 300+	73 300+	66 300+	71 300+
Bath County Community Hospital, Hot Springs, VA	- -	- -	- -	- -	- -	- -	- -	- -	- -	- -	- -	- -	- -	- -	- -	- -	- -
Bedford Memorial Hospital, Bedford, VA	- -	- -	- -	0.230 257	0.000 170	8.5 648	41.3 46	58 300+	86 300+	79 300+	64 300+	61 300+	81 300+	73 300+	70 300+	72 300+	68 300+
Bon Secours - Depaul Medical Center, Norfolk, VA	- -	- -	- -	0.149 793	0.003 718	5.7 1458	28.4 169	61 300+	78 300+	85 300+	63 300+	57 300+	70 300+	68 300+	68 300+	61 300+	66 300+
Bon Secours - Maryview Medical Center, Portsmouth, VA	- -	- -	- -	0.116 1505	0.028 1172	7.3 2111	21.8 404	65 300+	81 300+	85 300+	62 300+	54 300+	73 300+	69 300+	68 300+	60 300+	58 300+
Bon Secours - Memorial Regional Medical, Mechanicsville, VA	- -	- -	- -	0.139 1472	0.006 843	7.4 2636	28.7 362	57 300+	84 300+	86 300+	74 300+	59 300+	80 300+	74 300+	66 300+	69 300+	78 300+
Bon Secours - Richmond Community Hospital, Richmond, VA	- -	- -	- -	0.233 103	0.022 45	10.4 202	44.4 18	77 (a)	88 (a)	86 (a)	67 (a)	69 (a)	78 (a)	74 (a)	73 (a)	62 (a)	60 (a)
Bon Secours - St Francis Medical Center, Midlothian, VA	- -	- -	- -	0.267 647	0.022 369	12.9 457	23.5 51	66 300+	77 300+	86 300+	75 300+	59 300+	76 300+	69 300+	72 300+	58 300+	78 300+

NOTE: The first number in each column (boldface) is the score, the second number is the number of patients; Please refer to the main entry for footnotes; (a) 100-299
*MEASURES: **Children's Asthma Care:** 33. Received Systemic Corticosteroids; 34. Received Home Management Plan of Care; 35. Received Reliever Medication; **Use of Medical Imaging:** 36. Combination Abdominal CT Scan; 37. Combination Chest CT Scan; 38. Follow-up Mammogram/Ultrasound; 39. MRI for Low Back Pain; **Survey of Patients' Hospital Experiences:** 40. Area Around Room 'Always' Quiet at Night; 41. Doctors 'Always' Communicated Well; 42. Home Recovery Information Given; 43. Hospital Given 9 or 10 on 10 Point Scale; 44. Meds 'Always' Explained Before Given; 45. Nurses 'Always' Communicated Well; 46. Pain 'Always' Well Controlled; 47. Room and Bathroom 'Always' Clean; 48. Timely Help 'Always' Received; 49. Would Definitely Recommend Hospital*

Hospital	Children's Asthma Care			Use of Medical Imaging				Survey of Patients' Hospital Experiences									
	33	34	35	36	37	38	39	40	41	42	43	44	45	46	47	48	49
Bon Secours - St Marys Hospital of Richmond, Richmond, VA	- -	- -	- -	0.138 1040	0.012 499	7.9 3046	29.6 422	64 300+	81 300+	83 300+	72 300+	58 300+	76 300+	71 300+	69 300+	62 300+	77 300+
Buchanan General Hospital, Grundy, VA	- -	- -	- -	0.097 278	0.155 181	17.9 246	41.8 79	61 300+	86 300+	76 300+	64 300+	63 300+	78 300+	68 300+	72 300+	67 300+	64 300+
Carilion Franklin Memorial Hospital, Rocky Mount, VA	- -	- -	- -	0.032 408	0.067 163	4.4 681	38.2 89	59 300+	83 300+	83 300+	71 300+	67 300+	82 300+	75 300+	77 300+	71 300+	70 300+
Carilion Giles Memorial Hospital, Pearisburg, VA	- -	- -	- -	0.104 317	0.287 129	4.7 548	33.3 57	62 (a)	86 (a)	82 (a)	72 (a)	64 (a)	83 (a)	76 (a)	75 (a)	74 (a)	68 (a)
Carilion Medical Center, Roanoke, VA	- -	- -	- -	0.027 1721	0.038 1131	4.3 4239	32.7 459	60 300+	78 300+	84 300+	71 300+	67 300+	77 300+	69 300+	60 300+	65 300+	74 300+
Carilion New River Valley Medical Center, Christiansburg, VA	- -	- -	- -	0.086 850	0.041 680	8.6 1497	42.0 200	58 300+	80 300+	87 300+	69 300+	60 300+	78 300+	68 300+	71 300+	74 300+	77 300+
Carilion Stonewall Jackson Hospital, Lexington, VA	- -	- -	- -	- -	- -	- -	- -	61 300+	86 300+	82 300+	65 300+	68 300+	81 300+	74 300+	75 300+	75 300+	63 300+
Carilion Tazewell Community Hospital, Tazewell, VA	- -	- -	- -	0.067 135	0.114 79	4.9 223	48.0 25	69 (a)	81 (a)	80 (a)	67 (a)	63 (a)	79 (a)	71 (a)	72 (a)	76 (a)	67 (a)
Centra Health, Lynchburg, VA	100 74	94 70	100 75	0.097 1628	0.016 1074	33.3 6	28.5 267	60 300+	83 300+	83 300+	74 300+	63 300+	81 300+	72 300+	77 300+	66 300+	81 300+
Chesapeake General Hospital, Chesapeake, VA	- -	- -	- -	0.395 1313	0.007 1249	10.0 1989	32.6 227	55 300+	77 300+	82 300+	63 300+	55 300+	69 300+	67 300+	56 300+	57 300+	68 300+
CJW Medical Center, Richmond, VA	- -	- -	- -	0.324 1776	0.052 897	5.6 2755	30.9 282	58 300+	80 300+	84 300+	67 300+	56 300+	74 300+	69 300+	66 300+	59 300+	70 300+
Clinch Valley Medical Center, Richlands, VA	- -	- -	- -	0.333 708	0.122 615	7.4 135	43.2 111	61 300+	84 300+	83 300+	63 300+	61 300+	76 300+	67 300+	71 300+	63 300+	64 300+
Community Memorial Healthcenter, South Hill, VA	100 12	100 12	100 12	0.409 545	0.059 321	4.6 1230	47.1 70	60 300+	82 300+	83 300+	63 300+	66 300+	76 300+	68 300+	70 300+	60 300+	63 300+
Culpeper Regional Hospital, Culpeper, VA	- -	- -	- -	0.074 537	0.007 304	10.8 702	25.0 128	56 300+	68 300+	79 300+	61 300+	56 300+	72 300+	62 300+	72 300+	58 300+	64 300+
Danville Regional Medical Center, Danville, VA	- -	- -	- -	0.187 327	0.000 301	7.7 117	32.4 37	64 300+	76 300+	76 300+	51 300+	54 300+	70 300+	65 300+	66 300+	52 300+	44 300+
Dickenson Community Hospital, Clintwood, VA	- -	- -	- -	0.402 102	0.338 80	- 0	- 0	-	-	-	-	-	-	-	-	-	-
Eastern State Hospital, Williamsburg, VA	- -	- -	- -	- 0	- 0	- 0	- 0	-	-	-	-	-	-	-	-	-	-
The Fauquier Hospital, Warrenton, VA	- -	- -	- -	0.061 656	0.000 384	10.3 769	33.6 125	61 300+	80 300+	84 300+	70 300+	63 300+	76 300+	71 300+	74 300+	65 300+	76 300+
Halifax Regional Hospital, Halifax, VA	- -	- -	- -	0.371 574	0.011 374	10.4 1288	30.5 128	65 300+	85 300+	85 300+	67 300+	57 300+	78 300+	70 300+	68 300+	67 300+	64 300+
Hampton VA Medical Center, Hampton, VA	- -	- -	- -	- -	- -	- -	- -	-	-	-	-	-	-	-	-	-	-
Henrico Doctors' Hospital, Richmond, VA	- -	- -	- -	0.141 1202	0.012 890	8.0 1467	26.6 214	61 300+	82 300+	84 300+	71 300+	59 300+	76 300+	73 300+	66 300+	65 300+	76 300+
Inova Alexandria Hospital, Alexandria, VA	- -	- -	- -	0.123 819	0.014 655	6.5 417	32.2 295	52 300+	74 300+	82 300+	65 300+	54 300+	71 300+	69 300+	62 300+	59 300+	67 300+
Inova Fair Oaks Hospital, Fairfax, VA	- -	- -	- -	0.054 607	0.019 540	5.6 356	29.6 270	50 300+	78 300+	82 300+	71 300+	61 300+	75 300+	68 300+	70 300+	57 300+	78 300+
Inova Fairfax Hospital, Falls Church, VA	100 309	78 310	100 310	0.026 1485	0.011 1218	8.6 487	34.0 147	49 300+	76 300+	83 300+	68 300+	58 300+	73 300+	67 300+	60 300+	59 300+	75 300+
Inova Loudoun Hospital, Leesburg, VA	- -	- -	- -	0.066 797	0.010 775	10.3 544	26.6 124	45 300+	80 300+	87 300+	72 300+	60 300+	76 300+	67 300+	64 300+	63 300+	74 300+
Inova Mount Vernon Hospital, Alexandria, VA	- -	- -	- -	0.095 613	0.023 559	8.7 756	34.2 190	56 300+	81 300+	82 300+	66 300+	60 300+	71 300+	68 300+	62 300+	57 300+	72 300+
John Randolph Medical Center, Hopewell, VA	- -	- -	- -	0.384 631	0.007 428	4.5 731	40.0 115	61 300+	77 300+	81 300+	59 300+	56 300+	73 300+	70 300+	70 300+	57 300+	58 300+
Johnston Memorial Hospital, Abingdon, VA	- -	- -	- -	0.125 1032	0.095 761	3.8 1565	40.1 324	52 300+	84 300+	80 300+	63 300+	60 300+	76 300+	71 300+	65 300+	66 300+	66 300+
Lee Regional Medical Center, Pennington Gap, VA	- -	- -	- -	0.614 197	0.584 77	10.2 305	20.5 39	54 300+	80 300+	74 300+	58 300+	58 300+	78 300+	62 300+	69 300+	69 300+	54 300+
Lewis-Gale Medical Center, Salem, VA	- -	- -	- -	0.057 1458	0.008 992	8.7 2523	28.0 275	55 300+	82 300+	87 300+	72 300+	58 300+	77 300+	71 300+	67 300+	61 300+	77 300+
Martha Jefferson Hospital, Charlottesville, VA	- -	- -	- -	0.125 1435	0.000 1024	7.8 3457	31.8 330	53 300+	88 300+	85 300+	75 300+	65 300+	80 300+	73 300+	66 300+	64 300+	83 300+
Mary Immaculate Hospital, Newport News, VA	- -	- -	- -	0.060 366	0.048 165	8.2 476	24.3 70	64 300+	79 300+	84 300+	59 300+	56 300+	69 300+	66 300+	56 300+	51 300+	65 300+
Mary Washington Hospital, Fredericksburg, VA	100 47	76 45	100 47	0.013 602	0.009 109	15.4 228	33.3 30	51 300+	74 300+	79 300+	58 300+	54 300+	70 300+	65 300+	60 300+	55 300+	61 300+
Memorial Hospital of Martinsville & Henry County, Martinsville, VA	- -	- -	- -	0.076 719	0.032 440	3.1 2087	42.9 161	53 300+	81 300+	83 300+	58 300+	54 300+	71 300+	65 300+	65 300+	62 300+	53 300+
Montgomery Regional Hospital, Blacksburg, VA	- -	- -	- -	0.075 518	0.030 296	10.9 827	35.0 214	63 300+	84 300+	88 300+	71 300+	60 300+	80 300+	74 300+	76 300+	66 300+	74 300+
Mountain View Regional Medical Center, Norton, VA	- -	- -	- -	0.322 208	0.324 182	5.6 341	50.0 66	50 (a)	81 (a)	82 (a)	56 (a)	55 (a)	74 (a)	61 (a)	77 (a)	54 (a)	60 (a)
Norton Community Hospital, Norton, VA	- -	- -	- -	0.543 468	0.361 410	16.6 500	33.8 65	47 300+	80 300+	76 300+	59 300+	60 300+	76 300+	66 300+	61 300+	65 300+	62 300+
Page Memorial Hospital, Luray, VA	- -	- -	- -	- -	- -	- -	- -	54 (a)	74 (a)	91 (a)	58 (a)	44 (a)	72 (a)	65 (a)	70 (a)	56 (a)	58 (a)
Piedmont Geriatric Hospital, Burkeville, VA	- -	- -	- -	- -	- -	- -	- -	-	-	-	-	-	-	-	-	-	-
Pioneer Health Services of Patrick County, Stuart, VA	- -	- -	- -	- -	- -	- -	- -	-	-	-	-	-	-	-	-	-	-
Potomac Hospital, Woodbridge, VA	- -	- -	- -	0.070 660	0.022 631	13.8 385	22.3 157	67 300+	76 300+	79 300+	59 300+	59 300+	70 300+	65 300+	76 300+	53 300+	62 300+
Prince William Hospital, Manassas, VA	- -	- -	- -	0.074 914	0.014 591	10.3 1023	31.3 195	52 300+	79 300+	84 300+	65 300+	53 300+	74 300+	70 300+	72 300+	59 300+	68 300+
Pulaski Community Hospital, Pulaski, VA	- -	- -	- -	0.031 359	0.010 202	3.8 420	27.5 80	61 300+	86 300+	86 300+	70 300+	64 300+	81 300+	74 300+	69 300+	68 300+	71 300+
Rappahannock General Hospital, Kilmarnock, VA	- -	- -	- -	0.110 474	0.053 320	4.2 891	26.7 161	49 300+	82 300+	80 300+	68 300+	62 300+	81 300+	70 300+	79 300+	74 300+	72 300+
Reston Hospital Center, Reston, VA	- -	- -	- -	0.080 638	0.032 501	9.5 455	60.0 5	62 300+	79 300+	81 300+	63 300+	57 300+	69 300+	65 300+	64 300+	52 300+	69 300+
Richmond VA Medical Center, Richmond, VA	- -	- -	- -	- -	- -	- -	- -	-	-	-	-	-	-	-	-	-	-
Riverside Regional Medical Center, Newport News, VA	- -	- -	- -	0.117 1839	0.023 1627	8.1 2204	26.4 277	45 300+	76 300+	81 300+	60 300+	54 300+	69 300+	66 300+	61 300+	52 300+	63 300+
Riverside Shore Memorial Hospital, Nassawadox, VA	- -	- -	- -	0.076 447	0.009 322	3.6 1034	25.0 32	52 300+	85 300+	81 300+	61 300+	60 300+	74 300+	70 300+	66 300+	61 300+	54 300+
Riverside Tappahannock Hospital, Tappahannock, VA	- -	- -	- -	0.050 459	0.021 375	6.0 651	26.5 34	50 300+	78 300+	79 300+	59 300+	60 300+	75 300+	69 300+	63 300+	59 300+	61 300+
Riverside Walter Reed Hospital, Gloucester, VA	- -	- -	- -	0.086 570	0.004 454	5.3 1037	33.8 145	54 300+	81 300+	80 300+	59 300+	54 300+	74 300+	66 300+	73 300+	65 300+	60 300+
Rockingham Memorial Hospital, Harrisonburg, VA	- -	- -	- -	0.053 1312	0.003 745	6.2 2521	30.7 358	52 300+	77 300+	81 300+	63 300+	56 300+	73 300+	65 300+	68 300+	58 300+	67 300+
Russell County Medical Center, Lebanon, VA	- -	- -	- -	0.027 148	0.240 125	15.3 163	47.4 19	55 300+	82 300+	81 300+	59 300+	61 300+	79 300+	68 300+	74 300+	67 300+	58 300+
Salem VA Medical Center, Salem, VA	- -	- -	- -	- -	- -	- -	- -	-	-	-	-	-	-	-	-	-	-
Sentara Bayside Hospital, Virginia Beach, VA	- -	- -	- -	0.119 1363	0.048 986	7.8 1504	26.7 247	54 300+	75 300+	83 300+	61 300+	60 300+	74 300+	69 300+	64 300+	55 300+	65 300+
Sentara Careplex Hospital, Hampton, VA	- -	- -	- -	0.137 2040	0.002 1253	10.8 2681	31.9 232	60 300+	75 300+	78 300+	62 300+	51 300+	67 300+	60 300+	62 300+	54 300+	64 300+
Sentara Leigh Hospital, Norfolk, VA	- -	- -	- -	0.126 1835	0.007 1671	7.9 2507	27.1 221	45 300+	73 300+	84 300+	65 300+	56 300+	68 300+	63 300+	59 300+	56 300+	70 300+
Sentara Norfolk General Hospital, Norfolk, VA	- -	- -	- -	0.120 1338	0.008 1183	8.4 1752	28.0 125	54 300+	79 300+	84 300+	70 300+	56 300+	75 300+	69 300+	60 300+	64 300+	76 300+
Sentara Obici Hospital, Suffolk, VA	- -	- -	- -	0.184 898	0.000 514	7.0 1260	28.6 220	54 300+	72 300+	84 300+	56 300+	55 300+	70 300+	62 300+	67 300+	56 300+	63 300+
Sentara Virginia Beach General Hospital, Virginia Beach, VA	- -	- -	- -	0.087 1523	0.004 1375	6.3 2093	21.9 187	52 300+	74 300+	84 300+	66 300+	54 300+	71 300+	64 300+	63 300+	54 300+	69 300+
Sentara Williamsburg Regional Medical Center, Williamsburg, VA	- -	- -	- -	0.065 1052	0.005 737	8.9 2860	27.8 237	58 300+	75 300+	83 300+	63 300+	55 300+	70 300+	62 300+	66 300+	50 300+	68 300+
Shenandoah Memorial Hospital, Woodstock, VA	- -	- -	- -	- -	- -	- -	- -	61 300+	80 300+	87 300+	68 300+	60 300+	79 300+	71 300+	80 300+	67 300+	71 300+
Smyth County Community Hospital, Marion, VA	- -	- -	- -	0.560 377	0.004 229	17.1 578	43.0 79	54 300+	75 300+	79 300+	56 300+	62 300+	76 300+	66 300+	72 300+	66 300+	53 300+
Southampton Memorial Hospital, Franklin, VA	- -	- -	- -	0.352 347	0.098 183	4.9 427	55.2 29	65 300+	82 300+	84 300+	65 300+	60 300+	78 300+	70 300+	74 300+	63 300+	57 300+
Southern Virginia Regional Medical Center, Emporia, VA	- -	- -	- -	0.123 243	0.039 129	3.4 470	30.8 13	66 300+	85 300+	82 300+	62 300+	61 300+	73 300+	68 300+	63 300+	59 300+	58 300+
Southside Community Hospital, Farmville, VA	- -	- -	- -	0.093 399	0.288 191	5.7 663	23.8 63	58 300+	79 300+	80 300+	57 300+	61 300+	76 300+	68 300+	73 300+	64 300+	54 300+
Southside Regional Medical Center, Petersburg, VA	- -	- -	- -	0.205 929	0.006 694	8.5 1383	30.4 181	56 300+	79 300+	79 300+	63 300+	55 300+	73 300+	68 300+	62 300+	53 300+	61 300+
Southwestern Virginia Mental Health Institute, Marion, VA	- -	- -	- -	- -	- -	- -	- -	-	-	-	-	-	-	-	-	-	-

NOTE: The first number in each column (boldface) is the score, the second number is the number of patients; Please refer to the main entry for footnotes; (a) 100-299

*MEASURES: **Children's Asthma Care:** 33. Received Systemic Corticosteroids; 34. Received Home Management Plan of Care; 35. Received Reliever Medication; **Use of Medical Imaging:** 36. Combination Abdominal CT Scan; 37. Combination Chest CT Scan; 38. Follow-up Mammogram/Ultrasound; 39. MRI for Low Back Pain; **Survey of Patients' Hospital Experiences:** 40. Area Around Room 'Always' Quiet at Night; 41. Doctors 'Always' Communicated Well; 42. Home Recovery Information Given; 43. Hospital Given 9 or 10 on 10 Point Scale; 44. Meds 'Always' Explained Before Given; 45. Nurses 'Always' Communicated Well; 46. Pain 'Always' Well Controlled; 47. Room and Bathroom 'Always' Clean; 48. Timely Help 'Always' Received; 49. Would Definitely Recommend Hospital*

Hospital	Children's Asthma Care			Use of Medical Imaging				Survey of Patients' Hospital Experiences									
	33	34	35	36	37	38	39	40	41	42	43	44	45	46	47	48	49
Spotsylvania Regional Medical Center, Fredericksburg, VA	-	-	-	-	-	-	-	-	-	-	-	-	-	-	-	-	-
Stafford Hospital Center, Stafford, VA	-	-	-	- 0	- 0	- 0	- 0	54 300+	75 300+	79 300+	71 300+	57 300+	73 300+	64 300+	72 300+	62 300+	76 300+
Twin County Regional Hospital, Galax, VA	-	-	-	0.530 776	0.020 244	4.0 1485	43.5 147	59 300+	82 300+	80 300+	67 300+	59 300+	79 300+	73 300+	82 300+	73 300+	66 300+
University of Virginia Medical Center, Charlottesville, VA	97 38	61 38	100 38	0.056 589	0.003 357	9.6 3221	23.5 17	42 300+	76 300+	86 300+	65 300+	56 300+	74 300+	65 300+	62 300+	53 300+	74 300+
Virginia Commonwealth University Health System, Richmond, VA	-	-	-	0.124 1225	0.040 1549	3.9 1917	28.8 226	59 300+	80 300+	86 300+	68 300+	61 300+	75 300+	69 300+	65 300+	60 300+	71 300+
Virginia Hospital Center - Arlington, Arlington, VA	-	-	-	0.072 1478	0.002 1170	6.0 2248	31.9 329	58 300+	78 300+	76 300+	74 300+	58 300+	74 300+	68 300+	74 300+	61 300+	80 300+
Warren Memorial Hospital, Front Royal, VA	-	-	-	0.010 290	0.008 250	12.5 407	15.8 38	55 300+	77 300+	82 300+	55 300+	54 300+	72 300+	63 300+	66 300+	59 300+	57 300+
Wellmont Lonesome Pine Hospital, Big Stone Gap, VA	-	-	-	0.641 370	0.243 235	8.7 355	47.5 61	59 300+	75 300+	73 300+	58 300+	58 300+	75 300+	66 300+	75 300+	57 300+	59 300+
Western State Hospital, Staunton, VA	-	-	-	- 0	- 0	- 0	- 0	-	-	-	-	-	-	-	-	-	-
Winchester Medical Center, Winchester, VA	-	-	-	0.111 1393	0.010 1384	6.1 2748	30.3 501	53 (a)	80 (a)	82 (a)	74 (a)	61 (a)	75 (a)	70 (a)	72 (a)	64 (a)	82 (a)
Wythe County Community Hospital, Wytheville, VA	-	-	-	0.042 384	0.000 240	7.9 471	39.5 86	60 300+	85 300+	88 300+	68 300+	60 300+	81 300+	71 300+	70 300+	73 300+	65 300+
WEST VIRGINIA																	
Beckley Arh Hospital, Beckley, WV	-	-	-	0.615 356	0.308 224	6.6 332	37.3 110	52 300+	76 300+	76 300+	59 300+	54 300+	71 300+	66 300+	59 300+	53 300+	65 300+
Beckley VA Medical Center, Beckley, WV	-	-	-	-	-	-	-	-	-	-	-	-	-	-	-	-	-
Bluefield Regional Medical Center, Bluefield, WV	-	-	-	0.500 688	0.321 380	9.8 712	44.3 88	54 300+	79 300+	81 300+	56 300+	60 300+	75 300+	66 300+	69 300+	60 300+	57 300+
Boone Memorial Hospital, Madison, WV	-	-	-	-	-	-	-	62 (a)	88 (a)	87 (a)	70 (a)	74 (a)	84 (a)	83 (a)	82 (a)	77 (a)	61 (a)
Braxton County Memorial Hospital, Gassaway, WV	-	-	-	-	-	-	-	56 (a)	89 (a)	83 (a)	76 (a)	64 (a)	85 (a)	73 (a)	77 (a)	74 (a)	72 (a)
Broaddus Hospital Association, Philippi, WV	-	-	-	0.482 114	0.642 67	4.9 162	63.6 22	64 <100	85 <100	89 <100	70 <100	70 <100	87 <100	76 <100	89 <100	78 <100	73 <100
Cabell-Huntington Hospital, Huntington, WV	-	-	-	0.046 988	0.024 581	11.4 1749	35.8 134	68 300+	80 300+	83 300+	75 300+	62 300+	77 300+	72 300+	74 300+	67 300+	76 300+
Camc Teays Valley Hospital, Hurricane, WV	-	-	-	0.055 417	0.004 278	10.6 339	40.0 95	35 300+	78 300+	78 300+	59 300+	59 300+	68 300+	64 300+	65 300+	50 300+	59 300+
Camden Clark Memorial Hospital, Parkersburg, WV	-	-	-	0.595 1643	0.031 1071	7.0 2174	34.4 355	40 300+	76 300+	79 300+	60 300+	51 300+	69 300+	61 300+	64 300+	55 300+	66 300+
Charleston Area Medical Center, Charleston, WV	-	-	-	0.058 1752	0.006 1689	9.8 2401	42.3 333	45 300+	79 300+	78 300+	66 300+	57 300+	72 300+	67 300+	64 300+	59 300+	73 300+
Charleston Surgical Hospital, Charleston, WV	-	-	-	- 0	- 0	- 0	- 0	-	-	-	-	-	-	-	-	-	-
City Hospital, Martinsburg, WV	-	-	-	0.035 1129	0.011 463	2.0 1091	31.9 163	41 300+	79 300+	78 300+	53 300+	59 300+	73 300+	69 300+	71 300+	65 300+	55 300+
Clarksburg VA Medical Center, Clarksburg, WV	-	-	-	-	-	-	-	-	-	-	-	-	-	-	-	-	-
Davis Memorial Hospital, Elkins, WV	-	-	-	0.373 702	0.063 302	5.8 824	33.3 102	52 300+	80 300+	86 300+	63 300+	61 300+	78 300+	70 300+	76 300+	65 300+	62 300+
Fairmont General Hospital, Fairmont, WV	-	-	-	0.673 710	0.002 407	4.2 648	41.3 143	56 300+	83 300+	84 300+	63 300+	65 300+	78 300+	74 300+	74 300+	65 300+	62 300+
Grafton City Hospital, Grafton, WV	-	-	-	-	-	-	-	-	-	-	-	-	-	-	-	-	-
Grant Memorial Hospital, Petersburg, WV	-	-	-	-	-	-	-	47 300+	79 300+	88 300+	59 300+	66 300+	80 300+	68 300+	83 300+	71 300+	59 300+
Greenbrier Valley Medical Center, Ronceverte, WV	-	-	-	0.145 757	0.002 561	12.7 488	35.1 202	51 300+	81 300+	80 300+	60 300+	55 300+	73 300+	68 300+	62 300+	57 300+	59 300+
Hampshire Memorial Hospital, Romney, WV	-	-	-	-	-	-	-	49 <100	88 <100	80 <100	48 <100	64 <100	79 <100	60 <100	80 <100	81 <100	60 <100
Huntington VA Medical Center, Huntington, WV	-	-	-	-	-	-	-	-	-	-	-	-	-	-	-	-	-
Jackson General Hospital, Ripley, WV	-	-	-	0.150 314	0.000 189	6.1 410	41.0 105	50 300+	86 300+	87 300+	67 300+	61 300+	77 300+	72 300+	78 300+	68 300+	67 300+
Jefferson Memorial Hospital, Ranson, WV	-	-	-	-	-	-	-	55 (a)	85 (a)	83 (a)	59 (a)	62 (a)	74 (a)	69 (a)	83 (a)	63 (a)	59 (a)
Logan Regional Medical Center, Logan, WV	-	-	-	0.005 571	0.000 547	19.3 420	45.5 99	52 300+	82 300+	78 300+	55 300+	51 300+	69 300+	63 300+	61 300+	55 300+	53 300+
Martinsburg VA Medical Center, Martinsburg, WV	-	-	-	-	-	-	-	-	-	-	-	-	-	-	-	-	-
Minnie Hamilton Health Care Center, Grantsville, WV	-	-	-	-	-	-	-	-	-	-	-	-	-	-	-	-	-
Monongalia County General Hospital, Morgantown, WV	-	-	-	0.638 939	0.004 737	10.1 835	37.5 104	61 300+	85 300+	78 300+	76 300+	62 300+	80 300+	68 300+	78 300+	67 300+	83 300+
Montgomery General Hospital, Montgomery, WV	-	-	-	-	-	-	-	61 (a)	80 (a)	72 (a)	72 (a)	59 (a)	80 (a)	66 (a)	76 (a)	67 (a)	61 (a)
Morgan County War Memorial, Berkeley Springs, WV	-	-	-	-	-	-	-	54 (a)	74 (a)	83 (a)	61 (a)	57 (a)	69 (a)	61 (a)	79 (a)	64 (a)	62 (a)
Ohio Valley Medical Center, Wheeling, WV	-	-	-	0.640 344	0.000 374	13.3 474	31.1 90	56 300+	76 300+	76 300+	63 300+	57 300+	73 300+	67 300+	73 300+	55 300+	70 300+
Plateau Medical Center, Oak Hill, WV	-	-	-	0.132 182	0.219 105	11.3 106	52.9 34	57 300+	84 300+	79 300+	70 300+	58 300+	79 300+	68 300+	70 300+	71 300+	69 300+
Pleasant Valley Hospital, Point Pleasant, WV	-	-	-	0.041 362	0.033 209	9.6 334	36.3 113	57 300+	81 300+	87 300+	66 300+	60 300+	75 300+	68 300+	78 300+	65 300+	69 300+
Pocahontas Memorial Hospital, Buckeye, WV	-	-	-	-	-	-	-	-	-	-	-	-	-	-	-	-	-
Potomac Valley Hospital, Keyser, WV	-	-	-	-	-	-	-	-	-	-	-	-	-	-	-	-	-
Preston Memorial Hospital, Kingwood, WV	-	-	-	0.146 89	0.071 70	9.8 215	38.5 13	47 (a)	85 (a)	79 (a)	62 (a)	65 (a)	79 (a)	71 (a)	82 (a)	65 (a)	63 (a)
Princeton Community Hospital, Princeton, WV	-	-	-	0.720 1159	0.019 745	5.1 1076	48.2 251	52 300+	82 300+	85 300+	62 300+	64 300+	79 300+	70 300+	65 300+	59 300+	67 300+
Raleigh General Hospital, Beckley, WV	100 30	90 30	100 31	0.838 588	0.716 535	10.9 128	44.2 396	51 300+	77 300+	80 300+	64 300+	57 300+	73 300+	70 300+	64 300+	53 300+	62 300+
Reynolds Memorial Hospital, Glen Dale, WV	-	-	-	0.423 163	0.000 129	11.0 255	28.9 38	51 300+	80 300+	87 300+	66 300+	64 300+	76 300+	66 300+	70 300+	71 300+	67 300+
Roane General Hospital, Spencer, WV	-	-	-	0.523 132	0.000 83	23.0 235	69.2 13	56 (a)	84 (a)	85 (a)	77 (a)	60 (a)	79 (a)	71 (a)	78 (a)	74 (a)	65 (a)
Saint Francis Hospital, Charleston, WV	-	-	-	0.017 241	0.000 111	6.4 1003	38.6 145	64 300+	81 300+	81 300+	75 300+	58 300+	79 300+	75 300+	69 300+	69 300+	77 300+
Saint Joseph Hospital, Buckhannon, WV	-	-	-	0.498 217	0.000 128	8.3 412	33.3 24	56 (a)	85 (a)	85 (a)	75 (a)	65 (a)	81 (a)	74 (a)	70 (a)	76 (a)	73 (a)
Saint Josephs Healthcare System, Parkersburg, WV	-	-	-	0.011 738	0.000 572	4.7 1021	29.9 204	44 300+	81 300+	84 300+	64 300+	54 300+	72 300+	65 300+	62 300+	56 300+	66 300+
Saint Mary's Medical Center, Huntington, WV	-	-	-	0.083 1399	0.001 720	9.7 967	37.3 75	54 300+	79 300+	82 300+	74 300+	60 300+	80 300+	70 300+	80 300+	63 300+	80 300+
Sistersville General Hospital, Sistersville, WV	-	-	-	-	-	-	-	-	-	-	-	-	-	-	-	-	-
Stonewall Jackson Memorial Hospital, Weston, WV	-	-	-	0.648 213	0.000 103	10.1 288	30.4 23	52 300+	83 300+	74 300+	67 300+	63 300+	79 300+	70 300+	77 300+	67 300+	68 300+
Summers County ARH Hospital, Hinton, WV	-	-	-	-	-	-	-	63 (a)	92 (a)	81 (a)	81 (a)	71 (a)	86 (a)	81 (a)	83 (a)	76 (a)	81 (a)
Summersville Regional Medical Center, Summersville, WV	-	-	-	0.046 502	0.050 261	9.7 236	37.2 113	44 300+	84 300+	75 300+	60 300+	62 300+	74 300+	69 300+	69 300+	61 300+	64 300+
Thomas Memorial Hospital, South Charleston, WV	-	-	-	0.030 876	0.000 580	7.4 1121	35.7 406	43 300+	79 300+	82 300+	60 300+	52 300+	71 300+	65 300+	60 300+	58 300+	63 300+
United Hospital Center, Bridgeport, WV	-	-	-	0.750 1314	0.001 886	6.4 1853	39.3 323	43 300+	79 300+	80 300+	51 300+	54 300+	70 300+	61 300+	62 300+	54 300+	54 300+
Webster County Memorial Hospital, Webster Springs, WV	-	-	-	-	-	-	-	-	-	-	-	-	-	-	-	-	-
Weirton Medical Center, Weirton, WV	-	-	-	0.149 524	0.037 352	9.4 552	31.7 142	36 300+	73 300+	76 300+	44 300+	51 300+	62 300+	61 300+	51 300+	40 300+	41 300+
Welch Community Hospital, Welch, WV	-	-	-	0.258 62	0.292 24	4.7 106	- 0	72 (a)	85 (a)	82 (a)	74 (a)	69 (a)	86 (a)	75 (a)	81 (a)	78 (a)	66 (a)
West Virginia University Hospitals, Morgantown, WV	-	-	-	0.189 824	0.120 947	7.7 1132	- 0	47 300+	74 300+	81 300+	64 300+	61 300+	76 300+	65 300+	64 300+	58 300+	69 300+
Wetzel County Hospital, New Martinsville, WV	-	-	-	0.495 204	0.000 170	8.7 343	37.3 59	53 300+	82 300+	74 300+	65 300+	64 300+	81 300+	73 300+	81 300+	72 300+	66 300+
Wheeling Hospital, Wheeling, WV	-	-	-	0.165 752	0.013 894	13.4 1056	34.4 131	49 300+	78 300+	86 300+	67 300+	58 300+	74 300+	69 300+	70 300+	60 300+	70 300+
Williamson Memorial Hospital, Williamson, WV	97 34	100 33	100 34	0.088 249	0.090 78	7.1 98	26.3 19	53 300+	83 300+	77 300+	62 300+	59 300+	78 300+	63 300+	73 300+	62 300+	65 300+

NOTE: The first number in each column (boldface) is the score, the second number is the number of patients; Please refer to the main entry for footnotes; (a) 100-299
*MEASURES: **Children's Asthma Care:** 33. Received Systemic Corticosteroids; 34. Received Home Management Plan of Care; 35. Received Reliever Medication; **Use of Medical Imaging:** 36. Combination Abdominal CT Scan; 37. Combination Chest CT Scan; 38. Follow-up Mammogram/Ultrasound; 39. MRI for Low Back Pain; **Survey of Patients' Hospital Experiences:** 40. Area Around Room 'Always' Quiet at Night; 41. Doctors 'Always' Communicated Well; 42. Home Recovery Information Given; 43. Hospital Given 9 or 10 on 10 Point Scale; 44. Meds 'Always' Explained Before Given; 45. Nurses 'Always' Communicated Well; 46. Pain 'Always' Well Controlled; 47. Room and Bathroom 'Always' Clean; 48. Timely Help 'Always' Received; 49. Would Definitely Recommend Hospital*

Hospitals whose Heart Attack 30-Day Mortality Rate is Better (Lower) than the U.S. National Rate

Hospital	City	State	Phone	Web Site
Advocate Good Shepherd Hospital	Barrington	Illinois	847-381-9600	www.advocatehealth.com
Alameda Hospital	Alameda	California	510-522-3700	www.alamedahospital.org
Arizona Heart Hospital	Phoenix	Arizona	602-532-1000	www.azhearthospital.com
Arkansas Heart Hospital	Little Rock	Arkansas	501-219-7000	www.arheart.com
Aurora St Lukes Medical Center	Milwaukee	Wisconsin	414-649-6000	www.aurorahealthcare.org
Avera Heart Hospital of South Dakota	Sioux Falls	South Dakota	605-977-7000	
Banner Good Samaritan Medical Center	Phoenix	Arizona	602-239-2000	www.bannerhealth.com
Baptist Hospital East	Louisville	Kentucky	502-897-8100	www.baptisteast.com
Barnes Jewish Hospital	Saint Louis	Missouri	314-747-3000	www.barnesjewish.org
Bayhealth - Kent General Hospital	Dover	Delaware	302-744-7001	www.bayhealth.org/about/kent.asp
Baystate Medical Center	Springfield	Massachusetts	413-794-0000	www.baystatehealth.com
Bellin Memorial Hospital	Green Bay	Wisconsin	920-433-3500	www.bellin.org
Beth Israel Deaconess Medical Center	Boston	Massachusetts	617-667-7000	www.bidmc.harvard.edu
Boone Hospital Center	Columbia	Missouri	573-815-8000	
Cape Cod Hospital	Hyannis	Massachusetts	508-771-1800	www.capecodhealth.org
Carolinas Medical Center-Northeast	Concord	North Carolina	704-783-3000	www.northeastmedical.org
Cedars-Sinai Medical Center	Los Angeles	California	310-423-5000	www.cedars-sinai.edu
Christian Hospital Northeast	Saint Louis	Missouri	314-653-5000	www.christianhospital.org
Clear Lake Regional Medical Center	Webster	Texas	281-332-2511	www.clearlakermc.com
Community Regional Medical Center	Lorain	Ohio	440-960-3295	
Conemaugh Valley Memorial Hospital	Johnstown	Pennsylvania	814-534-9000	www.conemaugh.org
Doylestown Hospital	Doylestown	Pennsylvania	215-345-2200	www.dh.org
Durham Regional Hospital	Durham	North Carolina	919-620-1078	durhamregional.org
Edward Hospital	Naperville	Illinois	630-527-3000	www.edward.org
Emh Regional Medical Center	Elyria	Ohio	440-329-7500	
Englewood Hospital and Medical Center	Englewood	New Jersey	201-894-3000	www.englewoodhospital.com
Ephraim Mcdowell Regional Medical Center	Danville	Kentucky	859-239-2409	www.emrmc.com
Evanston Hospital	Evanston	Illinois	847-432-8000	www.enh.org
Franciscan St Margaret Health - Hammond	Hammond	Indiana	219-932-2300	www.smmhc.com
Hackensack University Medical Center	Hackensack	New Jersey	201-996-2000	www.humed.com
Heart Hospital of Austin	Austin	Texas	512-407-7581	www.hearthospitalofaustin.com
Heart Hospital of New Mexico	Albuquerque	New Mexico	505-724-2000	www.hearthospitalnm.com
Henry Ford Hospital	Detroit	Michigan	313-916-2600	www.henryfordhospital.com
Henry Ford Macomb Hospital	Clinton Township	Michigan	586-263-2300	www.stjoe-macomb.com
Holy Name Medical Center	Teaneck	New Jersey	201-833-3000	www.holyname.org
Inova Fairfax Hospital	Falls Church	Virginia	703-776-3332	www.inova.org
John T Mather Memorial Hospital of Port Jefferson	Port Jefferson	New York	631-473-1320	www.matherhospital.com
Lahey Clinic Hospital	Burlington	Massachusetts	781-744-5100	www.lahey.org
Lehigh Valley Hospital	Allentown	Pennsylvania	610-402-2273	www.lvhhn.org
Lenox Hill Hospital	New York	New York	212-439-2345	www.lenoxhillhospital.org
Los Robles Hospital & Medical Center	Thousand Oaks	California	805-497-2727	www.losrobleshospital.com
Maimonides Medical Center	Brooklyn	New York	718-283-6000	www.maimonidesmed.org
Marlborough Hospital	Marlborough	Massachusetts	508-481-5000	
Mary Hitchcock Memorial Hospital	Lebanon	New Hampshire	603-650-5000	www.dhmc.org
Massachusetts General Hospital	Boston	Massachusetts	617-726-2000	www.massgeneral.org
Mayo Clinic - Saint Marys Hospital	Rochester	Minnesota	507-255-5123	www.mayoclinic.org/saintmaryshospital
Memorial Medical Center	Springfield	Illinois	217-788-3000	www.memorialmedical.com
Memorial Mission Hospital and Asheville Surgery Center	Asheville	North Carolina	828-213-1111	www.missionhospitals.org
Meriter Hospital	Madison	Wisconsin	608-417-6210	www.meriter.com
The Methodist Hospital	Houston	Texas	713-790-2221	www.methodisthealth.com
Methodist Medical Center of Oak Ridge	Oak Ridge	Tennessee	865-835-1000	www.mmcoakridge.com
Methodist Willowbrook Hospital	Houston	Texas	281-477-1000	
Middlesex Hospital	Middletown	Connecticut	860-344-6000	www.midhosp.org
Midwest Regional Medical Center	Midwest City	Oklahoma	405-610-4411	www.midwestregional.com
Montefiore Medical Center	Bronx	New York	718-920-4321	www.montefiore.org
Morton Plant Hospital	Clearwater	Florida	727-462-7000	www.measehospitals.com
Mount Sinai Hospital	New York	New York	212-241-7981	www.mountsinai.org
Mount Sinai Medical Center	Miami Beach	Florida	305-674-2121	www.msmc.com
Munson Medical Center	Traverse City	Michigan	231-935-5000	www.munsonhealthcare.org
Naples Community Hospital	Naples	Florida	239-436-5000	www.nchmd.org
New York-Presbyterian Hospital	New York	New York	212-746-4189	www.nyp.org
Newton-Wellesley Hospital	Newton	Massachusetts	617-243-6000	www.nwh.org
Northeast Georgia Medical Center	Gainesville	Georgia	770-535-3553	www.nghs.com
Norwalk Hospital Association	Norwalk	Connecticut	203-852-2000	www.norwalkhosp.org

Hospital	City	State	Phone	Web Site
NYU Hospitals Center	New York	New York	212-263-7300	www.med.nyu.edu
Ohio State University Hospitals	Columbus	Ohio	614-293-9700	www.jamesline.com
Palm Beach Gardens Medical Center	Palm Beach Gardens	Florida	561-622-1411	www.pbgmc.com
Park Nicollet Methodist Hospital	Saint Louis Park	Minnesota	952-993-5000	www.parknicollet.com/methodist
Providence Hospital and Medical Centers	Southfield	Michigan	248-849-3011	www.stjohn.org/Providence
Rochester General Hospital	Rochester	New York	585-922-4000	www.rochestergeneral.org
Saint John's Health Center	Santa Monica	California	310-829-5511	www.stjohns.org
Saint Marys Hospital	Waterbury	Connecticut	203-574-6000	
Sarasota Memorial Hospital	Sarasota	Florida	941-917-9000	www.smh.com
Seton Medical Center Austin	Austin	Texas	512-324-1000	www.seton.net
Sinai Hospital of Baltimore	Baltimore	Maryland	410-601-5131	www.sinai-balt.com
Southcoast Hospital Group	Fall River	Massachusetts	508-679-3131	www.southcoast.org/charlton
Saint Elizabeth Medical Center North	Covington	Kentucky	859-292-2000	www.stelizabeth.com
Saint Francis Hospital and Health Centers-Indianapolis	Indianapolis	Indiana	317-865-5001	www.stfrancishospitals.org
Saint Francis Hospital - Roslyn	Roslyn	New York	516-562-6000	www.stfrancisheartcenter.com
Saint Johns Hospital	Springfield	Illinois	217-544-6464	www.st-johns.org
Saint Joseph Hospital	Bethpage	New York	516-579-6000	www.newislandhospital.org
Saint Joseph Mercy Hospital	Ann Arbor	Michigan	734-712-3791	
Saint Lukes Episcopal Hospital	Houston	Texas	832-355-1000	www.sleh.com
Saint Mary's Hospital	Madison	Wisconsin	608-251-6100	www.stmarysmadison.com
Saint Vincent Heart Center of Indiana	Indianapolis	Indiana	317-583-5000	www.theheartcenter.com
Saint Vincent's Medical Center	Bridgeport	Connecticut	203-576-5551	www.stvincents.org
Stamford Hospital	Stamford	Connecticut	203-276-1000	www.stamhealth.org
Tallahassee Memorial Healthcare	Tallahassee	Florida	850-431-1155	www.tmh.org
Texsan Heart Hospital	San Antonio	Texas	210-736-8013	www.texsanhearthospital.com
The Nebraska Methodist Hospital	Omaha	Nebraska	402-390-4000	www.bestcare.org
UMass Memorial Medical Center	Worcester	Massachusetts	508-334-1000	www.umassmemorial.org
University of Michigan Health System	Ann Arbor	Michigan	734-764-1505	www.med.umich.edu
UPMC Passavant	Pittsburgh	Pennsylvania	412-367-6700	passavant.upmc.com
Waterbury Hospital	Waterbury	Connecticut	203-573-6000	www.waterburyhospital.org
Yale-New Haven Hospital	New Haven	Connecticut	203-688-4242	www.ynhh.org

Note: Table shows hospitals nationwide whose Acute Myocardial Infarction 30-day risk-adjusted mortality rate is better (lower) than U.S. rate of 16.2%

Hospitals whose Heart Attack 30-Day Mortality Rate is Worse (Higher) than the U.S. National Rate

Hospital	City	State	Phone	Web Site
Albemarle Hospital Authority	Elizabeth City	North Carolina	252-335-0531	www.albemarlehealth.org
Arkansas Methodist Medical Center	Paragould	Arkansas	870-239-7000	www.arkansasmethodist.org
Baptist Memorial Hospital Huntingdon	Huntingdon	Tennessee	731-986-4461	www.bmhcc.org
Baxter Regional Medical Center	Mountain Home	Arkansas	870-508-1000	www.baxterregional.org
Brookdale Hospital Medical Center	Brooklyn	New York	718-240-5966	www.brookdalehospital.org
Brooklyn Hospital Center at Downtown Campus	Brooklyn	New York	718-250-8000	www.tbh.org
Cape Coral Hospital	Cape Coral	Florida	239-574-2323	
Catawba Valley Medical Center	Hickory	North Carolina	828-326-3809	www.catawbavalleymc.org
Clearfield Hospital	Clearfield	Pennsylvania	814-765-5341	www.clearfieldhosp.org
Community Regional Medical Center	Fresno	California	559-459-6000	www.communitymedical.org
Danville Regional Medical Center	Danville	Virginia	434-799-2100	www.danvilleregional.org
Dyersburg Regional Medical Center	Dyersburg	Tennessee	731-285-2410	
Edward W Sparrow Hospital	Lansing	Michigan	517-364-5000	www.sparrow.org
Erie County Medical Center	Buffalo	New York	716-898-3936	www.ecmc.edu
Forrest General Hospital	Hattiesburg	Mississippi	601-288-7000	www.forrestgeneral.com
Good Samaritan Hospital & Rehab Center	Puyallup	Washington	253-848-6661	www.multicare.org/goodsam
Great River Medical Center	Blytheville	Arkansas	870-838-7300	www.greatrivermc.com
Hospital Damas	Ponce	Puerto Rico	787-840-8460	
Howard Regional Health System	Kokomo	Indiana	765-453-8371	www.howardcommunity.org
Hurley Medical Center	Flint	Michigan	810-257-9000	www.hurleymc.com
Jefferson Regional Medical Center	Pine Bluff	Arkansas	870-541-7100	www.jrmc.org
Kennewick General Hospital	Kennewick	Washington	509-586-6111	www.kennewickgeneral.com
Kettering Medical Center - Sycamore	Miamisburg	Ohio	937-384-8776	www.khnetwork.org/sycamore
Lafayette General Medical Center	Lafayette	Louisiana	337-289-7991	www.lafayettegeneral.org
Laredo Medical Center	Laredo	Texas	956-796-5000	www.laredomedical.com
Manatee Memorial Hospital	Bradenton	Florida	941-746-5111	www.manateememorial.com
Massena Memorial Hospital	Massena	New York	315-764-1711	www.massenahospital.org
Mena Regional Health System	Mena	Arkansas	479-394-6100	
Mercy Memorial Health Center	Ardmore	Oklahoma	405-223-5400	www.mercyok.com/mmhc
Nassau University Medical Center	East Meadow	New York	516-572-0123	www.numc.edu
Navarro Regional Hospital	Corsicana	Texas	903-654-6800	www.navarrohospital.com
North Broward Medical Center	Pompano Beach	Florida	954-786-6950	www.browardhealth.org
Piedmont Medical Center	Rock Hill	South Carolina	803-329-1234	www.piedmontmedicalcenter.com
Raleigh General Hospital	Beckley	West Virginia	304-256-4100	
Schuylkill Medical Center - South Jackson Street	Pottsville	Pennsylvania	570-621-5000	www.pottsvillehospital.com
Seton Medical Center	Daly City	California	650-992-4000	www.setonmedicalcenter.org
Southwest Mississippi Regional Medical Center	Mccomb	Mississippi	601-249-5500	www.smrmc.com
Saint Francis Hospital	Columbus	Georgia	706-596-4020	wecareforlife.com
Saint Joseph Medical Center	Tacoma	Washington	253-627-4101	www.fhshealth.org
Saint Joseph's Regional Medical Center	Paterson	New Jersey	973-754-2000	www.sjhmc.org
Saint Lucie Medical Center	Port Saint Lucie	Florida	772-335-4000	www.stluciemed.com
Saint Mary's Regional Medical Center	Enid	Oklahoma	580-233-6100	www.stmarysregional.com
University Medical Center	Lubbock	Texas	806-775-8200	www.teamumc.org
Virginia Commonwealth University Health System	Richmond	Virginia	804-828-0938	www.vcuhealth.org
Wheaton Franciscan Healthcare - St Francis	Milwaukee	Wisconsin	414-647-5000	www.mywheaton.org

Note: Table shows hospitals nationwide whose Acute Myocardial Infarction 30-day risk-adjusted mortality rate is worse (higher) than U.S. rate of 16.2%

Hospitals whose Heart Failure 30-Day Mortality Rate is Better (Lower) than the U.S. National Rate

Hospital	City	State	Phone	Web Site
Adventist La Grange Memorial Hospital	La Grange	Illinois	708-352-1200	www.keepingyouwell.com
Advocate Good Samaritan Hospital	Downers Grove	Illinois	630-275-5900	www.advocatehealth.com/gsam
Advocate Good Shepherd Hospital	Barrington	Illinois	847-381-9600	www.advocatehealth.com
Advocate Illinois Masonic Medical Center	Chicago	Illinois	773-975-1600	www.advocatehealth.com/immc
Advocate South Suburban Hospital	Hazel Crest	Illinois	708-799-8000	www.advocatehealth.com
Advocate Trinity Hospital	Chicago	Illinois	773-967-2000	www.advocatehealth.com/trin
Alexian Brothers Medical Center	Elk Grove Village	Illinois	847-437-5500	www.alexian.org
Alle Kiski Medical Center	Natrona	Pennsylvania	412-224-5100	www.wpahs.org
Anna Jaques Hospital	Newburyport	Massachusetts	978-463-1000	www.ajh.org
Ashtabula County Medical Center	Ashtabula	Ohio	440-997-2262	www.acmchealth.org
Audrain Medical Center	Mexico	Missouri	573-582-5000	www.audrainmedicalcenter.com
Aventura Hospital and Medical Center	Aventura	Florida	305-682-7000	www.aventurahospital.com
Baptist Hospital East	Louisville	Kentucky	502-897-8100	www.baptisteast.com
Baptist Medical Center	San Antonio	Texas	210-297-1020	www.baptisthealthsystem.org
Baptist Memorial Hospital	Memphis	Tennessee	901-226-5000	www.bmhcc.org
Barnes Jewish Hospital	Saint Louis	Missouri	314-747-3000	www.barnesjewish.org
Bay Medical Center	Panama City	Florida	850-769-1511	www.baymedical.org
Bay Regional Medical Center	Bay City	Michigan	989-894-3000	www.baymed.org
Baylor Medical Center at Garland	Garland	Texas	972-487-5000	www.baylorhealth.com
Bayonne Hospital Center	Bayonne	New Jersey	201-858-5000	www.bayonnemedicalcenter.org
Beaumont Hospital - Grosse Pointe	Grosse Pointe	Michigan	313-343-1000	www.beaumonthospitals.com
Beth Israel Deaconess Medical Center	Boston	Massachusetts	617-667-7000	www.bidmc.harvard.edu
Beth Israel Medical Center	New York	New York	212-420-2000	www.wehealny.org
Brandon Regional Hospital	Brandon	Florida	813-681-5551	www.brandonregionalhospital.com
Brigham and Women's Hosptial	Boston	Massachusetts	617-732-5500	www.brighamandwomens.org
Bronx-Lebanon Hospital Center	Bronx	New York	212-588-7000	www.bronx-leb.org
Brookwood Medical Center	Birmingham	Alabama	205-877-1000	www.bwmc.com
Cedars-Sinai Medical Center	Los Angeles	California	310-423-5000	www.cedars-sinai.edu
Centinela Hospital Medical Center	Inglewood	California	310-673-4660	www.centinelafreeman.com
Centrastate Medical Center	Freehold	New Jersey	732-431-2000	www.centrastate.com
Charlotte Regional Medical Center	Punta Gorda	Florida	941-639-3131	www.charlotteregional.com
Christus Spohn Hospital Alice	Alice	Texas	361-661-8000	www.christusspohn.org
Citizens Medical Center	Victoria	Texas	361-573-9181	www.citizensmedicalcenter.org
Cleveland Clinic	Cleveland	Ohio	216-444-2200	www.clevelandclinic.org
Cleveland Clinic Hospital	Weston	Florida	954-689-5000	www.clevelandclinic.org
Community Hospital	Munster	Indiana	219-836-1600	www.comhs.org/community
Community Medical Center	Toms River	New Jersey	732-557-8000	www.sbhcs.com
D C H Regional Medical Center	Tuscaloosa	Alabama	205-759-7111	www.dchsystem.com
Deborah Heart and Lung Center	Browns Mills	New Jersey	609-893-6611	
East Orange General Hospital	East Orange	New Jersey	973-266-4401	www.evh.org
Easton Hospital	Easton	Pennsylvania	610-250-4076	www.easton-hospital.com
Elmhurst Memorial Hospital	Elmhurst	Illinois	630-833-1400	www.emhc.org
Emory University Hospital	Atlanta	Georgia	404-686-8500	www.emoryhealthcare.org
Englewood Hospital and Medical Center	Englewood	New Jersey	201-894-3000	www.englewoodhospital.com
Evanston Hospital	Evanston	Illinois	847-432-8000	www.enh.org
Fairview Hospital	Cleveland	Ohio	216-476-7000	www.fairviewhospital.org
Fairview Southdale Hospital	Edina	Minnesota	952-924-5000	www.fairview.org
Faulkner Hospital	Boston	Massachusetts	617-983-7000	
Firsthealth Moore Regional Hospital	Pinehurst	North Carolina	910-715-1000	www.firsthealth.org
Flagler Hospital	Saint Augustine	Florida	904-819-4426	www.flaglerhospital.com
Florida Hospital	Orlando	Florida	407-303-1976	www.floridahospital.com
Florida Hospital Fish Memorial	Orange City	Florida	386-917-5000	www.fhfishmemorial.org
Franciscan St Margaret Health - Hammond	Hammond	Indiana	219-932-2300	www.smmhc.com
Franklin Square Hospital Center	Baltimore	Maryland	443-777-7850	www.franklinsquare.org
Froedtert Memorial Lutheran Hospital	Milwaukee	Wisconsin	414-805-3000	www.froedtert.com
Garfield Medical Center	Monterey Park	California	626-573-2222	www.garfieldmedicalcenter.com
Genesys Regional Medical Center - Health Park	Grand Blanc	Michigan	810-606-5000	www.genesys.org
Glendale Adventist Medical Center	Glendale	California	818-409-8202	www.glendaleadventist.com
Glendale Memorial Hospital & Health Center	Glendale	California	818-502-1900	www.glendalememorialhospital.org
Good Samaritan Hospital	Baltimore	Maryland	443-444-3902	www.goodsam-md.org
Good Samaritan Hospital	Dayton	Ohio	937-278-2612	
Grand View Hospital	Sellersville	Pennsylvania	215-453-4615	www.gvh.org
Grandview Hospital & Medical Center	Dayton	Ohio	937-723-4988	www.kmcnetwork.org
Griffin Hospital	Derby	Connecticut	203-732-7500	www.griffinhealth.org

Hospital	City	State	Phone	Web Site
Hackensack University Medical Center	Hackensack	New Jersey	201-996-2000	www.humed.com
Hahnemann University Hospital	Philadelphia	Pennsylvania	215-762-7000	www.hahnemannhospital.com
Hamilton General Hospital	Hamilton	Texas	254-386-3151	www.hamiltonhospital.org
Hamot Medical Center	Erie	Pennsylvania	814-877-6000	www.hamot.org
Harper University Hospital	Detroit	Michigan	313-745-6211	www.harperhospital.org
Hazleton General Hospital	Hazleton	Pennsylvania	570-501-4000	www.ghha.org
Henry Ford Hospital	Detroit	Michigan	313-916-2600	www.henryfordhospital.com
Highlands Regional Medical Center	Sebring	Florida	863-385-6101	www.highlandsregional.com
Hillcrest Hospital	Mayfield Heights	Ohio	440-312-4500	www.hillcresthospital.org
Holy Name Medical Center	Teaneck	New Jersey	201-833-3000	www.holyname.org
Holy Redeemer Hospital and Medical Center	Meadowbrook	Pennsylvania	215-947-3000	www.holyredeemer.com
Hospital of St Raphael	New Haven	Connecticut	203-789-3000	www.srhs.org
Houston Medical Center	Warner Robins	Georgia	478-922-4281	www.hhc.org
Huntington Memorial Hospital	Pasadena	California	626-397-5000	www.huntingtonhospital.com
Huron Hospital	Cleveland	Ohio	216-761-3300	
Huron Valley-Sinai Hospital	Commerce Township	Michigan	248-937-3370	www.hvsh.org
Ingalls Memorial Hospital	Harvey	Illinois	708-333-2300	www.ingalls.org
Inova Alexandria Hospital	Alexandria	Virginia	703-504-3000	www.inova.com/inovapublic.srt/iah/index.jsp
Jeanes Hospital	Philadelphia	Pennsylvania	215-728-2000	www.jeanes.com
Jersey Shore University Medical Center	Neptune	New Jersey	732-775-5500	www.meridianhealth.com
Jewish Hospital & St Mary's Healthcare	Louisville	Kentucky	502-587-4011	www.jhhs.org
Johns Hopkins Bayview Medical Center	Baltimore	Maryland	410-550-0123	www.hopkinsbayview.org
Kingsbrook Jewish Medical Center	Brooklyn	New York	718-604-5789	www.kingsbrook.org
Lake Region Healthcare Corporation	Fergus Falls	Minnesota	218-736-8000	www.lrhc.org
Lakewood Hospital	Lakewood	Ohio	216-529-4200	www.lakewoodhospital.org
Lehigh Valley Hospital	Allentown	Pennsylvania	610-402-2273	www.lvhhn.org
Lehigh Valley Hospital - Muhlenberg	Bethlehem	Pennsylvania	610-402-2273	www.lvhn.org
Lenox Hill Hospital	New York	New York	212-439-2345	www.lenoxhillhospital.org
Liberty Hospital	Liberty	Missouri	816-781-7200	www.libertyhospital.org
Little Company of Mary Hospital	Evergreen Park	Illinois	708-422-6200	www.lcmh.org
Loyola University Medical Center	Maywood	Illinois	708-216-9000	www.lumc.edu
Maimonides Medical Center	Brooklyn	New York	718-283-6000	www.maimonidesmed.org
Main Line Hospital Bryn Mawr Campus	Bryn Mawr	Pennsylvania	610-526-3000	www.mainlinehealth.org
Main Line Hospital Lankenau	Wynnewood	Pennsylvania	610-645-2000	www.mainlinehealth.org/lh
Maryland General Hospital	Baltimore	Maryland	410-225-8996	www.marylandgeneral.org
Marymount Hospital	Garfield Heights	Ohio	216-581-0500	www.marymount.org
Massachusetts General Hospital	Boston	Massachusetts	617-726-2000	www.massgeneral.org
Mayo Clinic - Saint Marys Hospital	Rochester	Minnesota	507-255-5123	www.mayoclinic.org/saintmaryshospital
Mclaren Regional Medical Center	Flint	Michigan	810-342-2000	www.mclaren.org
Memorial Health University Medical Center	Savannah	Georgia	912-350-8000	www.memorialhealth.com
Memorial Hermann Hospital System	Houston	Texas	713-448-6796	www.memorialhermann.org
Memorial Hospital	Manchester	Kentucky	606-598-5104	www.manchestermemorial.com
Mercy Hospital	Miami	Florida	305-285-2121	www.mercymiami.com
Meriter Hospital	Madison	Wisconsin	608-417-6210	www.meriter.com
The Methodist Hospital	Houston	Texas	713-790-2221	www.methodisthealth.com
Methodist Hospitals	Gary	Indiana	219-886-4601	www.methodisthospital.org
Metrosouth Medical Center	Blue Island	Illinois	708-597-2000	www.stfrancisblueisland.com
Miami Valley Hospital	Dayton	Ohio	937-208-8000	www.miamivalleyhospital.com
Missouri Baptist Medical Center	Town and Country	Missouri	314-996-5000	www.missouribaptistmedicalcenter.org
Montefiore Medical Center	Bronx	New York	718-920-4321	www.montefiore.org
Mount Auburn Hospital	Cambridge	Massachusetts	617-492-3500	
Mount Sinai Hospital	New York	New York	212-241-7981	www.mountsinai.org
Mount Sinai Medical Center	Miami Beach	Florida	305-674-2121	www.msmc.com
Natchitoches Regional Medical Center	Natchitoches	Louisiana	318-352-1200	www.natchitocheshospital.org
Nebraska Heart Hospital	Lincoln	Nebraska	402-328-3000	www.neheart.com
New York Methodist Hospital	Brooklyn	New York	718-780-3000	www.nym.org
New York-Presbyterian Hospital	New York	New York	212-746-4189	www.nyp.org
Newton-Wellesley Hospital	Newton	Massachusetts	617-243-6000	www.nwh.org
North Kansas City Hospital	North Kansas City	Missouri	816-691-2000	www.nkch.org
North Shore Medical Center	Salem	Massachusetts	978-741-1215	
Northeast Georgia Medical Center	Gainesville	Georgia	770-535-3553	www.nghs.com
Northwestern Memorial Hospital	Chicago	Illinois	312-926-2000	www.nmh.org
Norwood Hospital	Norwood	Massachusetts	508-772-1000	www.caritasnorwood.org
NYU Hospitals Center	New York	New York	212-263-7300	www.med.nyu.edu
Oakwood Annapolis Hospital	Wayne	Michigan	734-467-4175	www.oakwood.org
Oakwood Hospital and Medical Center	Dearborn	Michigan	313-593-7125	www.oakwood.org
Oklahoma Heart Hospital	Oklahoma City	Oklahoma	405-608-3200	www.okheart.com

Hospital	City	State	Phone	Web Site
Olympia Medical Center	Los Angeles	California	310-657-5900	www.olympiamc.com
Orange Regional Medical Center	Goshen	New York	845-343-2424	
Our Lady of Bellefonte Hospital	Ashland	Kentucky	606-833-3600	www.olbh.com
Pacific Alliance Medical Center	Los Angeles	California	213-624-8411	www.pamc.net
Piedmont Hospital	Atlanta	Georgia	404-605-5000	www.piedmonthospital.org
Princeton Community Hospital	Princeton	West Virginia	304-487-7260	www.pchonline.org
Provena St Joseph Medical Center	Joliet	Illinois	815-725-7133	www.provena.org/stjoes
Providence Hospital	Washington	District of Columbia	202-269-7000	www.provhosp.org
Providence Hospital and Medical Centers	Southfield	Michigan	248-849-3011	www.stjohn.org/Providence
RHC St Francis Hospital	Evanston	Illinois	847-316-4000	www.reshealth.org
Rio Grande Regional Hospital	Mcallen	Texas	956-632-6000	www.riohealth.com
Rush University Medical Center	Chicago	Illinois	312-942-5000	www.ruch.edu
Saint Anne's Hospital	Fall River	Massachusetts	508-674-5600	www.saintanneshospital.org
Saint Barnabas Medical Center	Livingston	New Jersey	973-322-5000	www.saintbarnabas.com
Saint Joseph Hospital	Chicago	Illinois	773-665-3000	www.res-health.org
Saint Michael's Medical Center	Newark	New Jersey	973-877-5350	www.cathedralhealth.org
Saint Vincent Health Center	Erie	Pennsylvania	814-452-5000	www.svhs.org
Saint Vincent Medical Center	Los Angeles	California	213-484-7111	
Scripps Mercy Hospital	San Diego	California	619-294-8111	www.scrippshealth.org
Sharp Chula Vista Medical Center	Chula Vista	California	619-502-5800	www.sharp.com
Sherman Oaks Hospital	Sherman Oaks	California	818-981-7111	www.shermanoakshospital.com
Sinai-Grace Hospital	Detroit	Michigan	313-966-3300	www.sinaigrace.org
Southcoast Hospital Group	Fall River	Massachusetts	508-679-3131	www.southcoast.org/charlton
Southeast Alabama Medical Center	Dothan	Alabama	334-793-8701	www.samc.org
Southwest General Health Center	Middleburg Heights	Ohio	440-816-8000	www.swgeneral.com
Saint Alexius Medical Center	Hoffman Estates	Illinois	847-843-2000	www.alexianbrothershealth.org
Saint Catherine Hospital	East Chicago	Indiana	219-392-7004	www.comhs.org/stcatherine
Saint Elizabeth Ft Thomas	Fort Thomas	Kentucky	859-572-3100	www.cardinalhill.org
Saint Elizabeth's Medical Center	Brighton	Massachusetts	617-789-3000	www.semc.org
Saint Francis Hospital & Medical Center	Hartford	Connecticut	860-714-4000	www.saintfranciscare.com
Saint Francis Hospital - Roslyn	Roslyn	New York	516-562-6000	www.stfrancisheartcenter.com
Saint James Hospital & Health Center-Olympia Fields	Olympia Fields	Illinois	708-747-4000	
Saint John Hospital and Medical Center	Detroit	Michigan	313-343-4000	www.stjohnprovidence.org
Saint John Macomb-Oakland Hospital-Macomb Center	Warren	Michigan	586-573-5000	www.stjohn.org
Saint John Medical Center	Westlake	Ohio	440-835-8000	www.sjws.net
Saint John's Riverside Hospital	Yonkers	New York	914-964-4444	www.riversidehealth.org
Saint Joseph Hospital	Bethpage	New York	516-579-6000	www.newislandhospital.org
Saint Josephs Hospital	Marshfield	Wisconsin	715-387-7850	www.stjosephs-marshfield.org
Saint Luke's Cornwall Hospital	Newburgh	New York	845-561-4400	www.stlukeshospital.org
Saint Luke's Roosevelt Hospital	New York	New York	212-523-4000	www.wehealny.org
Saint Lukes Episcopal Hospital	Houston	Texas	832-355-1000	www.sleh.com
Saint Vincent Charity Medical Center	Cleveland	Ohio	216-861-6200	
Saint Vincent Hospital & Health Services	Indianapolis	Indiana	317-338-7000	www.indianapolis.stvincent.org
Suburban Hospital	Bethesda	Maryland	301-896-2576	www.suburbanhospital.org
Swedish Covenant Hospital	Chicago	Illinois	773-878-8200	
Thomas Jefferson University Hospital	Philadelphia	Pennsylvania	215-955-6000	www.jeffersonhospital.org
Tomball Regional Hospital	Tomball	Texas	281-351-1623	www.tomballhospital.org
Trumbull Memorial Hospital	Warren	Ohio	330-841-9820	www.trumhosp.org
Union Hospital	Dover	Ohio	330-343-3311	www.unionhospital.org
University Hospital - Stony Brook	Stony Brook	New York	631-444-4000	www.stonybrookmedicalcenter.org
UPMC Mckeesport	McKeesport	Pennsylvania	412-664-2000	www.selectmedicalcorp.com
UPMC Presbyterian Shadyside	Pittsburgh	Pennsylvania	412-647-8788	www.upmc.edu
Upper Valley Medical Center	Troy	Ohio	937-440-7853	www.uvmc.com
Valley Baptist Medical Center	Harlingen	Texas	956-389-1100	www.vbmc.org
Valley Hospital	Ridgewood	New Jersey	201-447-8000	www.valleyhealth.com
Virtua West Jersey Hospitals Berlin	Berlin	New Jersey	856-322-3200	
Washington Hospital Center	Washington	District of Columbia	202-877-7000	www.whcenter.org
Wellstar Kennestone Hospital	Marietta	Georgia	770-793-5000	www.wellstar.org
West Hills Hospital & Medical Center	West Hills	California	818-676-4100	www.westhillshospital.com
Western Pennsylvania Hospital - Forbes Regional Campus	Monroeville	Pennsylvania	412-858-2000	www.wpahs.org
Wheaton Franciscan - St Joseph	Milwaukee	Wisconsin	414-447-2000	www.wfhealthcare.org
William Beaumont Hospital-Troy	Troy	Michigan	248-964-8800	www.beaumonthospitals.com
Willis Knighton Medical Center	Shreveport	Louisiana	318-632-4000	www.wkhs.com//Locations/MedicalCenter.aspx
Wyckoff Heights Medical Center	Brooklyn	New York	718-963-7272	www.wyckoffhospital.org
Yale-New Haven Hospital	New Haven	Connecticut	203-688-4242	www.ynhh.org

Note: Table shows hospitals nationwide whose Heart Failure 30-day risk-adjusted mortality rate is better (lower) than U.S. rate of 11.2%.

Hospitals whose Heart Failure 30-Day Mortality Rate is Worse (Higher) than the U.S. National Rate

Hospital	City	State	Phone	Web Site
Adventist Medical Center	Portland	Oregon	503-257-2500	www.adventisthealth.com
Aiken Regional Medical Center	Aiken	South Carolina	803-641-5900	www.aikenregional.com
Alamance Regional Medical Center	Burlington	North Carolina	336-538-7000	www.armc.com
Albany Memorial Hospital	Albany	New York	518-471-3221	www.nehealth.com
American Legion Hospital	Crowley	Louisiana	337-788-6400	
Athens Regional Medical Center	Athens	Tennessee	423-745-1411	www.athensrmc.com
Auburn Regional Medical Center	Auburn	Washington	253-833-7711	www.armcuhs.com/p1.html
Aurora Sheboygan Memorial Medical Center	Sheboygan	Wisconsin	920-451-5000	www.aurorahealthcare.org/facilities
Bay Area Hospital	Coos Bay	Oregon	541-269-8111	www.bayareahospital.org
Beloit Memorial Hospital	Beloit	Wisconsin	608-364-5011	
Blake Medical Center	Bradenton	Florida	941-792-6611	www.blakemedicalcenter.com
Blanchard Valley Hospital	Findlay	Ohio	419-423-4500	www.bvha.org
Blessing Hospital	Quincy	Illinois	217-223-5811	www.blessinghealthsystem.org
Bromenn Healthcare	Normal	Illinois	309-454-1400	
Camden Clark Memorial Hospital	Parkersburg	West Virginia	304-424-2111	www.ccmh.org
Capital Region Medical Center	Jefferson City	Missouri	573-632-5000	www.crmc.org
Centerpoint Medical Center of Independence	Independence	Missouri	816-698-7000	
Central Washington Hospital	Wenatchee	Washington	509-662-1511	www.cwhs.com
Clarion Hospital	Clarion	Pennsylvania	814-226-9500	www.clarionhospital.org
Columbia St Mary's Hospital Ozaukee	Mequon	Wisconsin	262-243-7300	
Community Health Center of Branch County	Coldwater	Michigan	517-279-5400	www.chcbc.com
Community Hospitals and Wellness Centers	Bryan	Ohio	419-636-1131	www.chwchospital.com
Conway Regional Medical Center	Conway	Arkansas	501-329-3831	www.conwayregional.org
Cox Medical Center	Springfield	Missouri	417-269-6000	www.coxhealth.com
Danville Regional Medical Center	Danville	Virginia	434-799-2100	www.danvilleregional.com
Decatur County General Hospital	Parsons	Tennessee	731-847-3031	www.dcgh.org
Decatur Memorial Hospital	Decatur	Illinois	217-877-8121	www.dmhcares.org
Desert Regional Medical Center	Palm Springs	California	760-323-6511	www.desertmedctr.com
Dixie Regional Medical Center	Saint George	Utah	435-251-1000	intermountainhealthcare.org
El Centro Regional Medical Center	El Centro	California	760-339-7100	www.ecrmc.org
Fayette Regional Health System	Connersville	Indiana	765-825-5131	www.fayettememorial.org
Ferrell Hospital Community Foundations	Eldorado	Illinois	618-273-3361	
Fhn Memorial Hospital	Freeport	Illinois	815-235-4131	www.fhn.org
Fletcher Allen Hospital of Vermont	Burlington	Vermont	802-847-0000	www.fletcherallen.org
Forrest General Hospital	Hattiesburg	Mississippi	601-288-7000	www.forrestgeneral.com
Geisinger Medical Center	Danville	Pennsylvania	570-271-6211	www.geisinger.org
Good Samaritan Hospital	Kearney	Nebraska	308-865-7900	www.gshs.org
Good Samaritan Hospital	Lebanon	Pennsylvania	717-270-7500	www.gshleb.org
Grossmont Hospital	La Mesa	California	619-465-0711	www.sharp.com
Halifax Health Medical Center	Daytona Beach	Florida	386-254-4000	www.halifax.org
Harrison Medical Center	Bremerton	Washington	360-377-3911	www.harrisonmedical.org
Harton Regional Medical Center	Tullahoma	Tennessee	931-393-3000	www.hartonmedicalcenter.com
Hendrick Medical Center	Abilene	Texas	325-670-2000	www.ehendrick.org
Henry County Medical Center	Paris	Tennessee	731-642-1220	www.hcmc-tn.org
Highland Hospital	Rochester	New York	585-473-2200	www.urmc.rochester.edu
Holzer Medical Center	Gallipolis	Ohio	740-446-5000	www.holzer.org
Indian River Medical Center	Vero Beach	Florida	772-567-4311	www.irmh.com
Integris Grove Hospital	Grove	Oklahoma	918-786-2243	www.integris-health.com
Kadlec Regional Medical Center	Richland	Washington	509-946-4611	www.kadlecmed.org
Kenmore Mercy Hospital	Kenmore	New York	716-447-6100	www.chsbuffalo.org
Kennewick General Hospital	Kennewick	Washington	509-586-6111	www.kennewickgeneral.com
Lafayette General Medical Center	Lafayette	Louisiana	337-289-7991	www.lafayettegeneral.org
Lake Charles Memorial Hospital	Lake Charles	Louisiana	337-494-3200	www.lcmh.com
Lake Granbury Medical Center	Granbury	Texas	817-573-2683	www.lakegranburymedicalcenter.com
Laporte Hospital and Health Services	La Porte	Indiana	219-326-1234	www.laportehealth.org
Lodi Memorial Hospital	Lodi	California	209-334-3411	www.lodihealth.org
Manatee Memorial Hospital	Bradenton	Florida	941-746-5111	www.manateememorial.com
Marian Medical Center	Santa Maria	California	805-739-3000	www.marinmedicalcenter.org
Marietta Memorial Hospital	Marietta	Ohio	740-374-1400	www.mmhospital.org
Marion General Hospital	Columbia	Mississippi	601-736-6303	
McNairy Regional Hospital	Selmer	Tennessee	731-645-3221	www.mcnairyregionalhospital.com
Memorial Healthcare	Owosso	Michigan	989-723-5211	www.memorialhealthcare.org
Memorial Hospital of Martinsville & Henry County	Martinsville	Virginia	276-666-7200	www.martinsvillehospital.com
Memorial Medical Center	Las Cruces	New Mexico	575-522-8641	www.mmclc.org

Hospital	City	State	Phone	Web Site
Mercy Medical Center Redding	Redding	California	530-225-6102	www.redding.mercy.org
Mercy Medical Center-North Iowa	Mason City	Iowa	641-422-7000	www.mercynorthiowa.com
Metro Health Hospital	Wyoming	Michigan	616-252-7200	www.metrohealth.net
Mid-Columbia Medical Center	The Dalles	Oregon	541-296-1111	www.mcmc.net
Midland Memorial Hospital	Midland	Texas	432-685-1111	www.midland-memorial.com
Mississippi Baptist Medical Center	Jackson	Mississippi	601-968-1000	www.mbmc.org
Missouri Delta Medical Center	Sikeston	Missouri	573-471-1600	www.missouridelta.com
Mount Nittany Medical Center	State College	Pennsylvania	814-231-7000	www.mountnittany.org
Munroe Regional Medical Center	Ocala	Florida	352-351-7200	www.munroeregional.com
National Park Medical Center	Hot Springs	Arkansas	501-321-1000	www.nationalparkmedical.com
NEA Baptist Memorial Hospital	Jonesboro	Arkansas	870-972-7000	www.baptistonline.com
North Mississippi Medical Center	Tupelo	Mississippi	662-377-7176	www.nmhs.net/nmmc
Northwest Hospital	Seattle	Washington	206-364-0500	www.nwhospital.org
Northwestern Medical Center	Saint Albans	Vermont	802-524-1231	www.northwesternmedicalcenter.org
Ogden Regional Medical Center	Ogden	Utah	801-479-2111	
Oneida Healthcare Center	Oneida	New York	315-363-6000	www.oneidahealthcare.org
Otto Kaiser Memorial Hospital	Kenedy	Texas	830-583-3401	www.okmh.net
Our Lady of the Lake Regional Medical Center	Baton Rouge	Louisiana	225-765-8902	www.ololrmc.com
Peacehealth St Joseph Medical Center	Bellingham	Washington	360-734-5400	www.peacehealth.org
Piedmont Medical Center	Rock Hill	South Carolina	803-329-1234	www.piedmontmedicalcenter.com
Pikeville Medical Center	Pikeville	Kentucky	606-437-3500	www.pikevillehospital.org
Providence St Peter Hospital	Olympia	Washington	360-491-9480	www.providence.org/swsa
Putnam Community Medical Center	Palatka	Florida	386-326-8500	www.pcmcfl.com
Rideout Memorial Hospital	Marysville	California	530-749-4300	www.frhg.org
Riverside Medical Center	Waupaca	Wisconsin	715-258-1000	www.riversidemedical.org
Riverview Hospital	Noblesville	Indiana	317-776-7108	www.riverviewhospital.org
Saint Clare Hospital	Lakewood	Washington	253-588-1711	www.fhshealth.org
Saint Francis Medical Center	Peoria	Illinois	309-655-2000	www.osfsaintfrancis.org
Salem Hospital	Salem	Oregon	503-561-2278	www.salemhospital.org
Salina Regional Health Center	Salina	Kansas	785-452-7000	www.srhc.com
Saline Memorial Hospital	Benton	Arkansas	501-776-6000	www.salinememorial.org
Samaritan Hospital	Troy	New York	518-271-3225	www.nehealth.com
Samaritan North Lincoln Hospital	Lincoln City	Oregon	541-994-3661	www.samhealth.org/shs_facilities
Self Regional Healthcare	Greenwood	South Carolina	864-227-4111	www.selfregional.org
Sentara Leigh Hospital	Norfolk	Virginia	757-261-6601	www.sentara.com
Sheridan Memorial Hospital	Sheridan	Wyoming	307-672-1000	www.sheridanhospital.org
Sierra View District Hospital	Porterville	California	559-784-1110	www.sierra-view.com
Skyridge Medical Center	Cleveland	Tennessee	423-339-4132	www.skyridgemedcenter.com
South County Hospital	Wakefield	Rhode Island	401-782-8000	www.schospital.com
South Georgia Medical Center	Valdosta	Georgia	229-333-1020	www.sgmc.org
Southampton Hospital	Southampton	New York	516-726-8200	www.southamptonhospital.org
Southwestern Medical Center	Lawton	Oklahoma	580-531-4700	www.swmconline.com
Southwestern Vermont Medical Center	Bennington	Vermont	802-442-6361	www.svhealthcare.org
Sparks Regional Medical Center	Fort Smith	Arkansas	501-441-4000	www.sparks.org
Saint Agnes Hospital	Fond Du Lac	Wisconsin	920-926-5408	www.agnesian.com
Saint Anthony's Healthcare Center	Morrilton	Arkansas	501-977-2300	stvincenthealth.com
Saint Bernards Medical Center	Jonesboro	Arkansas	870-972-4100	www.sbrmc.com
Saint Francis Hospital	Litchfield	Illinois	217-324-2191	www.stfrancis-litchfield.org
Saint Francis Hospital	Columbus	Georgia	706-596-4020	wecareforlife.com
Saint Francis Medical Center	Cape Girardeau	Missouri	573-331-3000	www.sfmc.net
Saint Joseph Hospital	Eureka	California	707-443-8051	www.stjosepheureka.org
Saint Joseph Hospital	Nashua	New Hampshire	603-882-3000	www.stjosephhospital.com
Saint Joseph Medical Center	Tacoma	Washington	253-627-4101	www.fhshealth.org
Saint Josephs Medical Center of Stockton	Stockton	California	209-943-2000	www.stjospehscares.org
Saint Josephs Mercy Health Center	Hot Springs	Arkansas	501-622-1000	www.saintjosephs.com
Saint Lucie Medical Center	Port Saint Lucie	Florida	772-335-4000	www.stluciemed.com
Saint Mary Medical Center	Langhorne	Pennsylvania	215-750-2003	stmaryhealthcare.org
Saint Mary's Medical Center	Huntington	West Virginia	304-526-1234	www.st-marys.org
Saint Peter's Hospital	Helena	Montana	406-442-2100	www.stpetes.org
Summa Health Systems Hospitals	Akron	Ohio	330-375-3000	www.summahealth.org
Summit Medical Center	Hermitage	Tennessee	615-316-3000	www.summitmedctr.com
Sutter Auburn Faith Hospital	Auburn	California	530-888-4500	www.sutterauburnfaith.org
Sycamore Shoals Hospital	Elizabethton	Tennessee	423-542-1300	www.msha.com
Tacoma General Allenmore Hospital	Tacoma	Washington	253-403-1000	www.multicare.org
Tallahassee Memorial Healthcare	Tallahassee	Florida	850-431-1155	www.tmh.org
Thibodaux Regional Medical Center	Thibodaux	Louisiana	985-447-5500	www.thibodaux.com
Three Rivers Community Hospital	Grants Pass	Oregon	541-472-7000	www.asante.org

Hospital	City	State	Phone	Web Site
Trident Medical Center	Charleston	South Carolina	843-797-8800	www.tridenthealthsystem.com
Trinity Medical Center East & Trinity Medical Center West	Steubenville	Ohio	740-264-7212	www.trinityhealth.com
United Memorial Medical Center	Batavia	New York	585-343-6030	www.ummc.org
United Regional Health Care System	Wichita Falls	Texas	940-764-3055	www.urhcs.org
Upson Regional Medical Center	Thomaston	Georgia	706-647-8111	www.urmc.org
Virtua Memorial Hospital of Burlington County	Mount Holly	New Jersey	609-914-6200	www.virtua.org
White County Medical Center	Searcy	Arkansas	501-278-3100	www.centralarkhospital.com
Wilkes-Barre General Hospital	Wilkes-Barre	Pennsylvania	570-829-8111	www.wvhcs.org

Note: Table shows hospitals nationwide whose Heart Failure 30-day risk-adjusted mortality rate is worse (higher) than U.S. rate of 11.2%

Hospitals whose Pneumonia 30-Day Mortality Rate is Better (Lower) than the U.S. National Rate

Hospital	City	State	Phone	Web Site
Abbott Northwestern Hospital	Minneapolis	Minnesota	612-863-4000	www.abbottnorthwestern.com
Advocate Good Samaritan Hospital	Downers Grove	Illinois	630-275-5900	www.advocatehealth.com/gsam
Advocate South Suburban Hospital	Hazel Crest	Illinois	708-799-8000	www.advocatehealth.com
Akron General Medical Center	Akron	Ohio	330-344-6000	www.akrongeneral.org
Alexian Brothers Medical Center	Elk Grove Village	Illinois	847-437-5500	www.alexian.org
Alhambra Hospital Medical Center	Alhambra	California	626-570-1606	www.alhambrahospital.com
Alle Kiski Medical Center	Natrona	Pennsylvania	412-224-5100	www.wpahs.org
Anmed Health	Anderson	South Carolina	864-261-1109	www.anmed.com
Aultman Hospital	Canton	Ohio	330-452-9911	www.aultman.com
Aurelia Osborn Fox Memorial Hospital	Oneonta	New York	607-423-2000	www.foxcarenetwork.com
Aurora West Allis Medical Center	West Allis	Wisconsin	414-328-6000	www.aurorahealthcare.org
Austin Medical Center	Austin	Minnesota	507-433-7351	www.mayohealthsystem.org
Aventura Hospital and Medical Center	Aventura	Florida	305-682-7000	www.aventurahospital.com
Baptist Medical Center	San Antonio	Texas	210-297-1020	www.baptisthealthsystem.org
Bay Medical Center	Panama City	Florida	850-769-1511	www.baymedical.org
Bayshore Community Hospital	Holmdel	New Jersey	732-739-5900	www.bchs.com
Bayshore Medical Center	Pasadena	Texas	713-359-2000	www.bayshoremedical.com
Berkshire Medical Center	Pittsfield	Massachusetts	413-447-2000	www.berkshirehealthsystems.org
Beth Israel Deaconess Medical Center	Boston	Massachusetts	617-667-7000	www.bidmc.harvard.edu
Beth Israel Medical Center	New York	New York	212-420-2000	www.wehealny.org
Betsy Johnson Regional Hospital	Dunn	North Carolina	910-892-7161	www.bjrh.org
Boca Raton Regional Hospital	Boca Raton	Florida	561-362-5002	
Bon Secours - St Francis Xavier Hospital	Charleston	South Carolina	843-402-1000	www.stfrancishealth.org
Boston Medical Center Corporation	Boston	Massachusetts	617-638-8000	www.bmc.org
Bronx-Lebanon Hospital Center	Bronx	New York	212-588-7000	www.bronx-leb.org
Calvert Memorial Hospital	Prince Frederick	Maryland	410-535-8239	www.calverthospital.com
Candler Hospital	Savannah	Georgia	912-819-6000	
Cape Regional Medical Center	Cape May Court House	New Jersey	609-463-2000	www.caperegional.com
Cedars-Sinai Medical Center	Los Angeles	California	310-423-5000	www.cedars-sinai.edu
Centura Health-Penrose St Francis Health Services	Colorado Springs	Colorado	719-776-5000	www.centurahealth.com
Centura Health-Porter Adventist Hospital	Denver	Colorado	303-778-1955	www.centura.org
Christ Hospital	Cincinnati	Ohio	513-585-2771	www.thechristhospital.com
Christus St Michael Health System	Texarkana	Texas	903-614-1000	www.christusstmichael.org
Clark Regional Medical Center	Winchester	Kentucky	859-745-3500	www.clarkregional.org
Coffeyville Regional Medical Center	Coffeyville	Kansas	620-252-1200	www.crmcinc.com
Community Hospital	Munster	Indiana	219-836-1600	www.comhs.org/community
Community Medical Center	Toms River	New Jersey	732-557-8000	www.sbhcs.com
The Cooley Dickinson Hospital	Northampton	Massachusetts	413-582-2000	www.cooley-dickinson.org
Coral Gables Hospital	Coral Gables	Florida	305-445-8461	www.coralgableshospital.com
Covenant Medical Center	Lubbock	Texas	806-725-6000	www.covenanthealth.org
Crittenden Health System	Marion	Kentucky	270-965-5281	www.crittenden-health.org
Cumberland River Hospital	Celina	Tennessee	931-243-3581	
D C H Regional Medical Center	Tuscaloosa	Alabama	205-759-7111	www.dchsystem.com
Danbury Hospital	Danbury	Connecticut	203-797-7000	www.danburyhospital.com
Delray Medical Center	Delray Beach	Florida	561-498-4440	www.delraymedicalctr.com
Doctors Hospital	Dallas	Texas	214-324-6100	www.doctorshospitaldallas.com
Doctors Hospital	Coral Gables	Florida	305-666-2111	www.baptisthealth.net
East Valley Hospital Medical Center	Glendora	California	626-335-0231	www.eastvalleyhospital.org
Easton Hospital	Easton	Pennsylvania	610-250-4076	www.easton-hospital.com
Elmhurst Memorial Hospital	Elmhurst	Illinois	630-833-1400	www.emhc.org
Emh Regional Medical Center	Elyria	Ohio	440-329-7500	
Encino Hospital Medical Center	Encino	California	818-995-5000	www.encino-tarzana.com
Essentia Health St Joseph's Medical Center	Brainerd	Minnesota	218-829-2861	www.sjmcmn.org
Evanston Hospital	Evanston	Illinois	847-432-8000	www.enh.org
Evergreen Hospital Medical Center	Kirkland	Washington	425-899-1000	www.evergreenhospital.org
Exeter Hospital	Exeter	New Hampshire	603-778-7311	
Fairview Hospital	Cleveland	Ohio	216-476-7000	www.fairviewhospital.org
Falmouth Hospital	Falmouth	Massachusetts	508-548-5300	www.capecodhealth.com
Faxton-St Luke's Healthcare	Utica	New York	315-798-6000	
Flagler Hospital	Saint Augustine	Florida	904-819-4426	www.flaglerhospital.com
Florida Hospital	Orlando	Florida	407-303-1976	www.floridahospital.com
Franciscan St Margaret Health - Hammond	Hammond	Indiana	219-932-2300	www.smmhc.com
Franklin Square Hospital Center	Baltimore	Maryland	443-777-7850	www.franklinsquare.org
Frederick Memorial Hospital	Frederick	Maryland	240-566-3300	www.fmh.org

Hospital	City	State	Phone	Web Site
Genesys Regional Medical Center - Health Park	Grand Blanc	Michigan	810-606-5000	www.genesys.org
Good Samaritan Hospital	Baltimore	Maryland	443-444-3902	www.goodsam-md.org
Good Samaritan Medical Center	West Palm Beach	Florida	561-655-5511	www.goodsamartianmc.com
Greater Baltimore Medical Center	Baltimore	Maryland	443-849-2121	www.gbmc.org
Gulf Coast Medical Center	Panama City	Florida	850-747-7926	www.egulfcoastmedical.com
Hackensack University Medical Center	Hackensack	New Jersey	201-996-2000	www.humed.com
Hackettstown Regional Medical Center	Hackettstown	New Jersey	908-852-5100	www.hrmcnj.org
Hallmark Health System	Melrose	Massachusetts	781-979-3000	www.hallmarkhealth.org
Hamilton General Hospital	Hamilton	Texas	254-386-3151	www.hamiltonhospital.org
Hamot Medical Center	Erie	Pennsylvania	814-877-6000	www.hamot.org
Harmon Memorial Hospital	Hollis	Oklahoma	580-688-3363	
Harper University Hospital	Detroit	Michigan	313-745-6211	www.harperhospital.org
Hazleton General Hospital	Hazleton	Pennsylvania	570-501-4000	www.ghha.org
Henry Ford Macomb Hospital	Clinton Township	Michigan	586-263-2300	www.stjoe-macomb.com
Hillcrest Hospital	Mayfield Heights	Ohio	440-312-4500	www.hillcresthospital.org
Homestead Hospital	Homestead	Florida	786-243-8000	www.baptisthealth.net
The Hospital of Central Connecticut	New Britain	Connecticut	860-224-5011	www.thocc.org
Hospital of St Raphael	New Haven	Connecticut	203-789-3000	www.srhs.org
Houston Medical Center	Warner Robins	Georgia	478-922-4281	www.hhc.org
Howard Regional Health System	Kokomo	Indiana	765-453-8371	www.howardcommunity.org
Huntington Hospital	Huntington	New York	631-351-2000	www.hunthosp.org
Huntington Memorial Hospital	Pasadena	California	626-397-5000	www.huntingtonhospital.com
Ingalls Memorial Hospital	Harvey	Illinois	708-333-2300	www.ingalls.org
Inland Hospital	Waterville	Maine	207-861-3000	www.inlandhospital.org
Integris Clinton Regional Hospital	Clinton	Oklahoma	580-323-2363	www.integris-health.com
Integris Southwest Medical Center	Oklahoma City	Oklahoma	405-636-7777	www.integris-health.com
J C Blair Memorial Hospital	Huntingdon	Pennsylvania	814-643-2290	www.jcblair.org
John Muir Medical Center - Walnut Creek Campus	Walnut Creek	California	925-939-3000	www.jmmdhs.com
Jupiter Medical Center	Jupiter	Florida	561-747-2234	www.jupitermed.com
Kingsbrook Jewish Medical Center	Brooklyn	New York	718-604-5789	www.kingsbrook.org
Lake Forest Hospital	Lake Forest	Illinois	847-234-5600	www.lakeforesthospital.com
Lakewood Hospital	Lakewood	Ohio	216-529-4200	www.lakewoodhospital.org
Laredo Medical Center	Laredo	Texas	956-796-5000	www.laredomedical.com
Larkin Community Hospital	South Miami	Florida	305-284-7500	www.larkinhospital.com
Lawrence General Hospital	Lawrence	Massachusetts	978-683-4000	www.lawrencegeneral.org
Lehigh Valley Hospital	Allentown	Pennsylvania	610-402-2273	www.lvhhn.org
Lehigh Valley Hospital - Muhlenberg	Bethlehem	Pennsylvania	610-402-2273	www.lvhn.org
Liberty Hospital	Liberty	Missouri	816-781-7200	www.libertyhospital.org
Lutheran Medical Center	Brooklyn	New York	718-630-8000	www.lmcmc.com
Maimonides Medical Center	Brooklyn	New York	718-283-6000	www.maimonidesmed.org
Main Line Hospital Lankenau	Wynnewood	Pennsylvania	610-645-2000	www.mainlinehealth.org/lh
Mainland Medical Center	Texas City	Texas	409-938-5000	www.mainlandmedical.com
Marshall Medical Center (1-Rh)	Placerville	California	530-622-1441	www.marshallmedical.org
Mary Greeley Medical Center	Ames	Iowa	515-239-2011	www.mgmc.org
Massachusetts General Hospital	Boston	Massachusetts	617-726-2000	www.massgeneral.org
Mayo Clinic Hospital	Phoenix	Arizona	480-515-6296	www.mayoclinic.org
Mclaren Regional Medical Center	Flint	Michigan	810-342-2000	www.mclaren.org
Memorial Hospital York	York	Pennsylvania	717-843-8623	www.mhyork.org
Mercy Health Partners - Hackley Campus	Muskegon	Michigan	231-726-3511	www.hackley.org
Mercy Hospital	Iowa City	Iowa	319-339-0300	www.mercyiowacity.org
Mercy Hospital - Grayling	Grayling	Michigan	989-348-5461	www.mercygrayling.munsonhealthcare.org
Mercy Hospital	Miami	Florida	305-285-2121	www.mercymiami.com
Methodist Hospital	San Antonio	Texas	210-575-4000	www.mh.sahealth.com
Methodist Hospital of Chicago	Chicago	Illinois	773-271-9040	www.methodistchicago.org
The Methodist Hospital	Houston	Texas	713-790-2221	www.methodisthealth.com
Metrosouth Medical Center	Blue Island	Illinois	708-597-2000	www.stfrancisblueisland.com
Miami Valley Hospital	Dayton	Ohio	937-208-8000	www.miamivalleyhospital.com
Mission Regional Medical Center	Mission	Texas	956-323-9000	www.missionhospital.org
Missouri Baptist Medical Center	Town and Country	Missouri	314-996-5000	www.missouribaptistmedicalcenter.org
Monmouth Medical Center	Long Branch	New Jersey	732-222-5200	www.sbhcs.com
Montgomery General Hospital	Olney	Maryland	301-774-8771	www.montgomerygeneral.com
Mount Auburn Hospital	Cambridge	Massachusetts	617-492-3500	
Mount Sinai Hospital	New York	New York	212-241-7981	www.mountsinai.org
Mount Sinai Medical Center	Miami Beach	Florida	305-674-2121	www.msmc.com
Munson Medical Center	Traverse City	Michigan	231-935-5000	www.munsonhealthcare.org
Natchitoches Regional Medical Center	Natchitoches	Louisiana	318-352-1200	www.natchitocheshospital.org
New York-Presbyterian Hospital	New York	New York	212-746-4189	www.nyp.org

Hospital	City	State	Phone	Web Site
Newton-Wellesley Hospital	Newton	Massachusetts	617-243-6000	www.nwh.org
North Kansas City Hospital	North Kansas City	Missouri	816-691-2000	www.nkch.org
North Shore Medical Center	Salem	Massachusetts	978-741-1215	
Norwood Hospital	Norwood	Massachusetts	508-772-1000	www.caritasnorwood.org
NYU Hospitals Center	New York	New York	212-263-7300	www.med.nyu.edu
O'Bleness Memorial Hospital	Athens	Ohio	740-593-5551	www.obleness.org
Ocean Medical Center	Brick	New Jersey	732-840-2200	www.meridianhealth.com/mcoc.cfm/ind
Ouachita County Medical Center	Camden	Arkansas	870-836-1000	www.ouachitamedcenter.com
Pacific Alliance Medical Center	Los Angeles	California	213-624-8411	www.pamc.net
Palos Community Hospital	Palos Heights	Illinois	708-923-4000	www.paloshospital.org
Park Nicollet Methodist Hospital	Saint Louis Park	Minnesota	952-993-5000	www.parknicollet.com/methodist
Parkview Adventist Medical Center	Brunswick	Maine	207-373-2000	www.parkviewamc.org
Parkview Medical Center	Pueblo	Colorado	719-584-4000	www.parkviewmc.com
Peninsula Regional Medical Center	Salisbury	Maryland	410-543-7116	www.peninsula.org
Perry Hospital	Perry	Georgia	478-987-3600	www.hhc.org
Piedmont Fayette Hospital	Fayetteville	Georgia	770-719-7071	www.fayettehospital.org
Piedmont Hospital	Atlanta	Georgia	404-605-5000	www.piedmonthospital.org
Presbyterian Intercommunity Hospital	Whittier	California	526-698-0811	www.whittierpres.com
Provena-Saint Joseph Hospital	Elgin	Illinois	847-695-3200	www.provenasaintjoeph.com
Provena St Joseph Medical Center	Joliet	Illinois	815-725-7133	www.provena.org/stjoes
Providence Hospital and Medical Centers	Southfield	Michigan	248-849-3011	www.stjohn.org/Providence
Providence Medical Center	Kansas City	Kansas	913-596-3930	www.providence-health.org
Putnam Hospital Center	Carmel	New York	914-279-5711	www.putnamhospital.org
Raritan Bay Medical Center	Perth Amboy	New Jersey	732-442-3700	
Rex Hospital	Raleigh	North Carolina	919-784-3100	www.rexhealth.com
Richland Parish Hospital-Delhi	Delhi	Louisiana	318-878-5171	www.delhihospital.com
Rogue Valley Medical Center	Medford	Oregon	541-789-7000	www.asante.org
Saint John's Health Center	Santa Monica	California	310-829-5511	www.stjohns.org
Saint John's Health System	Anderson	Indiana	765-649-2511	www.stjohnshealthsystem.org
Saint Joseph Hospital	Chicago	Illinois	773-665-3000	www.res-health.org
Saint Joseph Hospital London	London	Kentucky	606-330-6000	www.sjhlex.org
Saint Marys Hospital	Waterbury	Connecticut	203-574-6000	
Saint Vincent Medical Center	Los Angeles	California	213-484-7111	
San Gabriel Valley Medical Center	San Gabriel	California	626-289-5454	www.sangabrielvalleymedctr.org
San Luis Valley Regional Medical Center	Alamosa	Colorado	719-589-2511	www.slvrmc.org
Scripps Mercy Hospital	San Diego	California	619-294-8111	www.scrippshealth.org
Seton Northwest Hospital	Austin	Texas	512-324-6000	www.seton.net
Seton Medical Center Austin	Austin	Texas	512-324-1000	www.seton.net
Shore Memorial Hospital	Somers Point	New Jersey	609-653-3545	www.shorememorial.org
Skaggs Community Health Center	Branson	Missouri	417-335-7000	www.skaggs.net
Skokie Hospital	Skokie	Illinois	847-677-9600	
South Pointe Hospital	Warrensville Heights	Ohio	216-491-6000	www.southpointehospital.org
Southampton Hospital	Southampton	New York	516-726-8200	www.southamptonhospital.org
Southeast Alabama Medical Center	Dothan	Alabama	334-793-8701	www.samc.org
Southern Ohio Medical Center	Portsmouth	Ohio	740-354-5000	www.somc.org
Southwest General Health Center	Middleburg Heights	Ohio	440-816-8000	www.swgeneral.com
SSM St Joseph Hospital West	Lake Saint Louis	Missouri	636-625-5200	
Saint Alexius Medical Center	Hoffman Estates	Illinois	847-843-2000	www.alexianbrothershealth.org
Saint Cloud Hospital	Saint Cloud	Minnesota	320-251-2700	www.centracare.com
Saint Francis Health Center	Topeka	Kansas	785-295-8000	www.stfrancistopeka.org
Saint Francis Hospital and Health Centers-Indianapolis	Indianapolis	Indiana	317-865-5001	www.stfrancishospitals.org
Saint Francis Hospital - Roslyn	Roslyn	New York	516-562-6000	www.stfrancisheartcenter.com
Saint John Medical Center	Westlake	Ohio	440-835-8000	www.sjws.net
Saint John's Episcopal Hospital at South Shore	Far Rockaway	New York	718-869-7000	
Saint John's Riverside Hospital	Yonkers	New York	914-964-4444	www.riversidehealth.org
Saint Joseph Health Center	Warren	Ohio	330-841-4000	
Saint Luke's Hospital Bethlehem	Bethlehem	Pennsylvania	610-954-4000	www.slhn-lehighvalley.org
Saint Lukes Hospital	Cedar Rapids	Iowa	319-369-7211	www.crstlukes.com
Saint Lukes Hospital	Chesterfield	Missouri	314-434-1500	www.goodhealthmatters.com
Saint Mary & Elizabeth Medical Center-Division Campus	Chicago	Illinois	312-633-5896	www.reshealth.org
Saint Mary Medical Center	Long Beach	California	562-491-9000	www.stmarymedicalcenter.org
Saint Mary Medical Center	Hobart	Indiana	219-942-0551	
Saint Marys Hospital	Centralia	Illinois	618-436-8000	www.stmarys-goodsamaritan.com
Saint Vincent Hospital & Health Services	Indianapolis	Indiana	317-338-7000	www.indianapolis.stvincent.org
Suburban Hospital	Bethesda	Maryland	301-896-2576	www.suburbanhospital.org
Swedish Covenant Hospital	Chicago	Illinois	773-878-8200	
Texas Health Harris Methodist Hospital - SW Fort Worth	Fort Worth	Texas	817-433-5000	www.texahealth.org

Hospital	City	State	Phone	Web Site
Tomball Regional Hospital	Tomball	Texas	281-351-1623	www.tomballhospital.org
Tri-City Regional Medical Center	Hawaiian Gardens	California	562-860-0401	www.tri-cityrmc.org
Tuba City Regional Health Care Corporation	Tuba City	Arizona	928-283-2501	www.tcrhcc.org
Unicoi County Memorial Hospital	Erwin	Tennessee	423-743-3141	
United Hospital Center	Bridgeport	West Virginia	681-342-1000	www.uhcwv.org
University of Michigan Health System	Ann Arbor	Michigan	734-764-1505	www.med.umich.edu
UPMC Presbyterian Shadyside	Pittsburgh	Pennsylvania	412-647-8788	www.upmc.edu
Valley Baptist Medical Center	Harlingen	Texas	956-389-1100	www.vbmc.org
Valley Baptist Medical Center - Brownsville	Brownsville	Texas	956-544-1400	www.brownsvillemedical.com
Valley Hospital	Ridgewood	New Jersey	201-447-8000	www.valleyhealth.com
Via Christi Hospitals Wichita	Wichita	Kansas	316-268-5000	www.via-christi.org
Virginia Mason Medical Center	Seattle	Washington	206-223-6600	www.vmmc.org
Wadley Regional Medical Center	Texarkana	Texas	903-798-8000	www.wadleyhealth.com
Western Pennsylvania Hospital - Forbes Regional Campus	Monroeville	Pennsylvania	412-858-2000	www.wpahs.org
Westlake Regional Hospital	Columbia	Kentucky	270-384-4753	www.westlake-healthcare.org
William Beaumont Hospital	Royal Oak	Michigan	248-898-5000	www.beaumonthospitals.com
William Beaumont Hospital-Troy	Troy	Michigan	248-964-8800	www.beaumonthospitals.com
Willis Knighton Bossier Health Center	Bossier City	Louisiana	318-212-7000	www.wkhs.com/Locations/Bossier.aspx
Willis Knighton Medical Center	Shreveport	Louisiana	318-632-4000	www.wkhs.com//Locations/MedicalCenter.aspx
Winchester Hospital	Winchester	Massachusetts	781-729-9000	www.winchesterhospital.org
Yale-New Haven Hospital	New Haven	Connecticut	203-688-4242	www.ynhh.org

Note: Table shows hospitals nationwide whose Pneumonia 30-day risk-adjusted mortality rate is better (lower) than U.S. rate of 11.6%

Hospitals whose Pneumonia 30-Day Mortality Rate is Worse (Higher) than the U.S. National Rate

Hospital	City	State	Phone	Web Site
Abilene Regional Medical Center	Abilene	Texas	325-428-1000	www.abileneregional.com
Adventist Medical Center	Portland	Oregon	503-257-2500	www.adventisthealth.com
Aiken Regional Medical Center	Aiken	South Carolina	803-641-5900	www.aikenregional.com
Athens Regional Medical Center	Athens	Tennessee	423-745-1411	www.athensrmc.com
Aurora Lakeland Medical Center	Elkhorn	Wisconsin	262-741-2000	www.aurorahealthcare.org/facilities
Baptist Memorial Hospital Golden Triangle	Columbus	Mississippi	662-244-1500	www.bmhcc.org/facilities/goldentriangle
Baylor Medical Center at Waxahachie	Waxahachie	Texas	972-923-7000	www.bhcs.com/locations/waxahachie
Beloit Memorial Hospital	Beloit	Wisconsin	608-364-5011	
Blanchard Valley Hospital	Findlay	Ohio	419-423-4500	www.bvha.org
Blessing Hospital	Quincy	Illinois	217-223-5811	www.blessinghealthsystem.org
Boulder City Hospital	Boulder City	Nevada	702-293-4111	www.bouldercityhospital.org
Bromenn Healthcare	Normal	Illinois	309-454-1400	
Cabell-Huntington Hospital	Huntington	West Virginia	304-526-2000	www.cabellhuntington.org
Cameron Regional Medical Center	Cameron	Missouri	816-632-2101	www.cameronregional.org
Cannon Memorial Hospital	Pickens	South Carolina	864-878-4791	www.cannonhospital.org
Canton-Potsdam Hospital	Potsdam	New York	315-265-3300	www.cphospital.org
Capital Region Medical Center	Jefferson City	Missouri	573-632-5000	www.crmc.org
Carilion Medical Center	Roanoke	Virginia	540-981-7000	www.carilion.com/crmh
Carlisle Regional Medical Center	Carlisle	Pennsylvania	717-249-1212	www.carlislermc.com
Carolina East Medical Center	New Bern	North Carolina	252-633-8640	www.cravenhealthcare.org
Carson Tahoe Regional Medical Center	Carson City	Nevada	775-445-8000	www.carsontahoehospital.com
Carteret General Hospital	Morehead City	North Carolina	252-808-6000	www.ccgh.org
Cass Medical Center	Harrisonville	Missouri	816-380-5888	www.cassregional.org
Catawba Valley Medical Center	Hickory	North Carolina	828-326-3809	www.catawbavalleymc.org
Chadron Community Hospital and Health Services	Chadron	Nebraska	308-432-5586	www.chadronhospital.com
Citrus Memorial Hospital	Inverness	Florida	352-726-1551	www.citrusmh.com
Clarinda Regional Health Center	Clarinda	Iowa	712-542-2176	www.clarindahealth.com
Coleman County Medical Center	Coleman	Texas	325-625-2135	
Community-General Hospital of Greater Syracuse	Syracuse	New York	315-492-5011	www.cgh.org
Concord Hospital	Concord	New Hampshire	603-225-2711	www.concordhospital.org
Conway Regional Medical Center	Conway	Arkansas	501-329-3831	www.conwayregional.org
Corona Regional Medical Center	Corona	California	951-737-4343	www.coronaregional.com
Covenant Hospital Plainview	Plainview	Texas	806-296-5531	www.covenantplainview.org
Covington County Hospital	Collins	Mississippi	601-765-6711	
Dameron Hospital	Stockton	California	209-944-5550	www.dameronhospital.org
Danville Regional Medical Center	Danville	Virginia	434-799-2100	www.danvilleregional.org
Decatur County General Hospital	Parsons	Tennessee	731-847-3031	www.dcgh.org
Delano Regional Medical Center	Delano	California	661-725-4800	www.drmc.com
Dyersburg Regional Medical Center	Dyersburg	Tennessee	731-285-2410	
Eastern Niagara Hospital	Lockport	New York	716-514-5700	
Elliot Hospital	Manchester	New Hampshire	603-669-5300	www.elliothospital.org
Elmhurst Hospital Center	Elmhurst	New York	718-334-1141	nyc.gov
Emanuel Medical Center	Turlock	California	209-667-4200	www.emanuelmedicalcenter.org
Fairchild Medical Center	Yreka	California	530-842-4121	www.fairchildmed.org
Fairview Park Hospital	Dublin	Georgia	478-274-3100	www.fairviewparkhospital.com
Firelands Regional Medical Center	Sandusky	Ohio	419-557-7400	www.firelands.com
Fletcher Allen Hospital of Vermont	Burlington	Vermont	802-847-0000	www.fletcherallen.org
Flushing Hospital Medical Center	Flushing	New York	718-670-5000	www.flushinghospital.org
Frye Regional Medical Center	Hickory	North Carolina	828-322-6070	www.fryemedctr.com
Gateway Medical Center	Clarksville	Tennessee	931-502-1000	www.todaysgateway.com
Good Samaritan Hospital	San Jose	California	408-559-2011	www.goodsamsj.org
Good Samaritan Hospital	Lebanon	Pennsylvania	717-270-7500	www.gshleb.org
Greater Regional Medical Center	Creston	Iowa	641-782-7091	
Guadalupe Regional Medical Center	Seguin	Texas	830-379-2411	www.gvh.com
Hammond Henry Hospital	Geneseo	Illinois	309-944-6431	www.hammondhenry.com
Hanford Community Medical Center	Hanford	California	559-582-9000	www.hanfordhealth.com
Hardin Medical Center	Savannah	Tennessee	731-926-8121	
Hardin Memorial Hospital	Kenton	Ohio	419-673-0761	www.hardinmemorial.org
Harrison County Hospital	Corydon	Indiana	812-738-4251	www.hchin.org
Harrison Memorial Hospital	Cynthiana	Kentucky	859-234-2300	www.harrisonmemhosp.com
Hart County Hospital	Hartwell	Georgia	706-856-6113	www.tycobbhealthcaresystem.org
Hawaii Medical Center East	Honolulu	Hawaii	808-547-6011	www.hawaiimedcent.com
Hemet Valley Medical Center	Hemet	California	951-652-2811	www.valleyhealthsystem.com/hemmain
Herrin Hospital	Herrin	Illinois	618-942-2171	www.sih.net

Hospital	City	State	Phone	Web Site
Hi-Desert Medical Center	Joshua Tree	California	760-366-6285	www.hdmc.org
Holdenville General Hospital	Holdenville	Oklahoma	405-379-4200	
Holland Community Hospital	Holland	Michigan	616-392-5141	www.hoho.org
Hospital De La Concepcion	San German	Puerto Rico	787-892-1860	www.hospitalconcepcion.org
Hospital Dr Cayetano Coll y Toste	Arecibo	Puerto Rico	787-650-7272	
Hospital Hima-San Pablo Bayamon	Bayamon	Puerto Rico	787-620-4747	
Hospital Dr Federico Trilla	Carolina	Puerto Rico	787-757-1800	
Iberia General Hospital and Medical Center	New Iberia	Louisiana	337-374-7104	www.iberiamedicalcenter.com
Indian River Medical Center	Vero Beach	Florida	772-567-4311	www.irmh.com
Integris Grove Hospital	Grove	Oklahoma	918-786-2243	www.integris-health.com
IU Health Goshen Hospital	Goshen	Indiana	574-533-2141	www.goshenhosp.com
Jane Phillips Medical Center	Bartlesville	Oklahoma	918-333-7200	www.jpmc.org
Jefferson County Health Center	Fairfield	Iowa	641-472-4111	www.jchospital.org
Jefferson Regional Medical Center	Pine Bluff	Arkansas	870-541-7100	www.jrmc.org
Jennie Edmundson Hospital	Council Bluffs	Iowa	712-396-6000	www.bestcare.org
Jennie Stuart Medical Center	Hopkinsville	Kentucky	270-887-0100	www.jsmc.org
Johnston Memorial Hospital	Abingdon	Virginia	276-676-7000	www.jmh.org
Kaweah Delta Medical Center	Visalia	California	559-624-2000	www.kaweahdelta.org
Lake Pointe Medical Center	Rowlett	Texas	972-412-2273	www.lakepointemedical.com
Laurens County Healthcare System	Clinton	South Carolina	864-833-9100	www.lchcs.org
Leesburg Regional Medical Center	Leesburg	Florida	352-323-5762	www.leesburgregional.org
Limestone Medical Center	Groesbeck	Texas	254-729-3281	lmchospital.com
Litzenberg Memorial County Hospital	Central City	Nebraska	308-946-3015	www.lmchealth.com
Lodi Memorial Hospital	Lodi	California	209-334-3411	www.lodihealth.org
Lompoc Valley Medical Center	Lompoc	California	805-737-3300	lompochospital.org
Madera Community Hospital	Madera	California	559-675-5555	www.maderahospital.org
Madison St Joseph Health Center	Madisonville	Texas	936-348-2631	www.st-joseph.org/madison
Manatee Memorial Hospital	Bradenton	Florida	941-746-5111	www.manateememorial.com
Manati Medical Center Dr Otero Lopez	Manati	Puerto Rico	787-621-3700	www.mmcaol.com
Margaret Mary Community Hospital	Batesville	Indiana	812-934-6624	www.mmch.org
Maria Parham Hospital	Henderson	North Carolina	252-438-4143	www.mphosp.org
Marshall County Hospital	Benton	Kentucky	270-527-4800	
Mary Hitchcock Memorial Hospital	Lebanon	New Hampshire	603-650-5000	www.dhmc.org
Massena Memorial Hospital	Massena	New York	315-764-1711	www.massenahospital.org
Maury Regional Hospital	Columbia	Tennessee	931-381-1111	www.maurgregional.com
McDuffie Regional Medical Center	Thomson	Georgia	706-595-1411	
Medical Center of Central Georgia	Macon	Georgia	478-633-6805	www.mccg.org
Medical Center South Arkansas	El Dorado	Arkansas	870-863-2000	www.themedcenter.net
Medical College of Georgia Hospitals and Clinics	Augusta	Georgia	706-721-6569	www.mcghealth.org
Memorial Community Hospital	Blair	Nebraska	402-426-2182	www.mchhs.org
Memorial Health System of East Texas - Lufkin	Lufkin	Texas	936-634-8111	www.mymemorialhealth.org
Memorial Healthcare	Owosso	Michigan	989-723-5211	www.memorialhealthcare.org
Memorial Hermann Baptist Beaumont Hospital	Beaumont	Texas	409-212-5012	www.mhbh.org
Memorial Medical Center	Springfield	Illinois	217-788-3000	www.memorialmedical.com
Mena Regional Health System	Mena	Arkansas	479-394-6100	
Menifee Valley Medical Center	Sun City	California	951-679-8888	www.valleyhealthsystem.com
Mercy Health Center	Oklahoma City	Oklahoma	405-755-1515	www.mercyok.net/mhc
Mercy Hospital of Defiance	Defiance	Ohio	419-782-8444	
Mercy Hospital of Kansas Independence	Independence	Kansas	620-331-2200	
Mercy Medical Center-North Iowa	Mason City	Iowa	641-422-7000	www.mercynorthiowa.com
Mercy Memorial Health Center	Ardmore	Oklahoma	405-223-5400	www.mercyok.com/mmhc
Methodist Healthcare Memphis Hospitals	Memphis	Tennessee	901-516-8274	www.methodisthealth.org
Midland Memorial Hospital	Midland	Texas	432-685-1111	www.midland-memorial.com
Milton S Hershey Medical Center	Hershey	Pennsylvania	717-531-8521	www.hmc.psu.edu
Morehead Memorial Hospital	Eden	North Carolina	336-623-9711	www.morehead.org
Morrow County Hospital	Mount Gilead	Ohio	419-949-3180	www.morrowcountyhospital.com
The Moses H Cone Memorial Hospital	Greensboro	North Carolina	336-832-7000	www.mosescone.com
Natchez Regional Medical Center	Natchez	Mississippi	601-443-2100	
Nemaha County Hospital	Auburn	Nebraska	402-274-4366	www.nchnet.org
North Carolina Baptist Hospital	Winston-Salem	North Carolina	336-716-2011	www.wfubmc.edu
Olympic Medical Center	Port Angeles	Washington	360-417-7000	www.olympicmedical.org
Oneida Healthcare Center	Oneida	New York	315-363-6000	www.oneidahealthcare.org
Oswego Hospital	Oswego	New York	315-349-5511	www.oswegohealth.org
Our Lady of the Lake Regional Medical Center	Baton Rouge	Louisiana	225-765-8902	www.ololrmc.com
Paris Regional Medical Center	Paris	Texas	903-785-4521	www.parisregional.com
Passavant Area Hospital	Jacksonville	Illinois	217-245-9551	www.passavanthospital.com
Penobscot Valley Hospital	Lincoln	Maine	207-794-3321	www.pvhhealthcare.org

Hospital	City	State	Phone	Web Site
Perry Memorial Hospital	Princeton	Illinois	815-875-2811	www.perry-memorial.org
Phelps County Regional Medical Center	Rolla	Missouri	573-458-8899	www.rollanet.org/~pcrmc
Phoebe Putney Memorial Hospital	Albany	Georgia	229-312-4053	www.phoebeputney.com
Phoenixville Hospital	Phoenixville	Pennsylvania	610-983-1000	www.pennhealth.com
Piedmont Medical Center	Rock Hill	South Carolina	803-329-1234	www.piedmontmedicalcenter.com
Pike Community Hospital	Waverly	Ohio	740-947-2186	
Pikeville Medical Center	Pikeville	Kentucky	606-437-3500	www.pikevillehospital.org
Pioneer Health Services of Patrick County	Stuart	Virginia	276-694-8678	www.rjrhospital.com
Pomerado Hospital	Poway	California	858-485-6511	www.pph.org
Ponca City Medical Center	Ponca City	Oklahoma	580-765-3321	www.poncamedcenter.com
Poplar Bluff Regional Medical Center	Poplar Bluff	Missouri	573-686-5313	www.poplarbluffregional.com
Pottstown Memorial Medical Center	Pottstown	Pennsylvania	610-327-7000	www.pmmctr.org
Proctor Hospital	Peoria	Illinois	309-691-1000	www.proctor.org
Putnam County Hospital	Greencastle	Indiana	765-655-2620	
Regional West Medical Center	Scottsbluff	Nebraska	308-635-3711	www.rwmc.net
River Parishes Hospital	Laplace	Louisiana	985-652-7000	www.riverparisheshospital.com
River Region Health System	Vicksburg	Mississippi	601-883-5000	www.riverregion.com
Riverside Medical Center	Waupaca	Wisconsin	715-258-1000	www.riversidemedical.org
Roane General Hospital	Spencer	West Virginia	304-927-4444	www.roanegeneralhospital.com
Rockcastle Regional Hospital & Respiratory Care Center	Mount Vernon	Kentucky	606-256-2195	www.rockcastlehospital.com
Rockdale Medical Center	Conyers	Georgia	770-918-3000	www.rockdalehospital.org
Russell County Medical Center	Lebanon	Virginia	276-883-8000	
Ryder Memorial Hospital	Humacao	Puerto Rico	787-852-0768	
Saint Agnes Medical Center	Fresno	California	559-450-3000	www.samc.com
Saint Mary's Regional Medical Center	Reno	Nevada	775-770-3000	www.saintmarysreno.com
Samaritan Hospital	Moses Lake	Washington	509-765-5606	www.samaritanhealthcare.com
Samaritan Medical Center	Watertown	New York	315-785-4121	www.samaritanhealth.com
San Gorgonio Memorial Hospital	Banning	California	951-769-2101	www.sgmh.org
San Luke's Memorial Hospital	Ponce	Puerto Rico	787-844-2080	www.ssepr.com/hospital_sanlucas.html
Scenic Mountain Medical Center	Big Spring	Texas	432-263-1211	www.smmccares.com
Selby General Hospital	Marietta	Ohio	740-568-2000	www.selbygeneralhospital.con
Self Regional Healthcare	Greenwood	South Carolina	864-227-4111	www.selfregional.org
Sentara Obici Hospital	Suffolk	Virginia	757-934-4000	www.sentara.com
Seven Rivers Regional Medical Center	Crystal River	Florida	352-795-6560	www.srrmc.com
Shands Live Oak Regional Medical Center	Live Oak	Florida	904-362-1413	www.shands.org
Sharp Memorial Hospital	San Diego	California	858-939-3400	www.sharp.com/memorial
Sierra View District Hospital	Porterville	California	559-784-1110	www.sierra-view.com
Simpson General Hospital	Mendenhall	Mississippi	601-847-2221	www.simpsongeneralhospital.com
Skagit Valley Hospital	Mount Vernon	Washington	360-424-4111	www.skagitvalleyhospital.org
Skyridge Medical Center	Cleveland	Tennessee	423-339-4132	www.skyridgemedcenter.com
South Central Regional Medical Center	Laurel	Mississippi	601-649-4000	www.scrmc.com
South Jersey Healthcare Regional Medical Center	Vineland	New Jersey	856-641-8000	www.sjhs.com
Southeast Georgia Health System - Brunswick Campus	Brunswick	Georgia	912-466-7000	www.sghs.org
Saint Bernards Medical Center	Jonesboro	Arkansas	870-972-4100	www.sbrmc.com
Saint Francis Hospital	Columbus	Georgia	706-596-4020	wecareforlife.com
Saint Francis Medical Center	Cape Girardeau	Missouri	573-331-3000	www.sfmc.net
Saint Helena Hosptial-Clearlake	Clearlake	California	707-994-6486	www.redbudhospital.org
Saint Johns Hospital	Springfield	Illinois	217-544-6464	www.st-johns.org
Saint Joseph Hospital	Orange	California	714-633-9111	www.sjo.org
Saint Joseph Regional Medical Center	Lewiston	Idaho	208-743-2511	www.sjrmc.org
Saint Josephs Medical Center of Stockton	Stockton	California	209-943-2000	www.stjospehscares.org
Saint Mary's Community Hospital	Nebraska City	Nebraska	402-873-3321	www.stmaryshospitalnecity.com
Saint Mary's Hospital - Passaic	Passaic	New Jersey	973-365-4300	www.smh-nj.com
Saint Mary's Medical Center	West Palm Beach	Florida	561-840-6202	www.stmarysmc.com
Saint Marys Regional Medical Center	Russellville	Arkansas	479-968-2841	www.saintmarysregional.com
Saint Peter's Hospital	Helena	Montana	406-442-2100	www.stpetes.org
Strong Memorial Hospital	Rochester	New York	585-275-2121	www.urmc.rochester.edu
Sturdy Memorial Hospital	Attleboro	Massachusetts	508-222-5200	
Sumner Regional Medical Center	Gallatin	Tennessee	615-452-4210	
Tanner Medical Center - Carrollton	Carrollton	Georgia	770-836-9580	www.tanner.org
Terrebonne General Medical Center	Houma	Louisiana	985-873-4141	www.tgmc.com
TLC Health Network	Gowanda	New York	716-532-3377	
Tri-City Medical Center	Oceanside	California	760-724-8411	www.tricitymed.org
Trinity Rock Island	Rock Island	Illinois	309-779-5000	www.trinityqc.com
Tulare Regional Medical Center	Tulare	California	559-688-0821	www.tdhs.org
United Hospital System	Kenosha	Wisconsin	262-656-2368	
Unity Health Center	Shawnee	Oklahoma	405-273-2270	www.unityhealthcenter.com

Hospital	City	State	Phone	Web Site
University Hospital	Augusta	Georgia	706-722-9011	www.universityhealth.org
University Hospital S U N Y Health Science Center	Syracuse	New York	315-473-4240	www.upstate.edu
University of Louisville Hospital	Louisville	Kentucky	502-562-3000	www.uoflhealthcare.org
Venice Regional Medical Center	Venice	Florida	941-485-7711	www.veniceregional.com
Washington County Hospital	Plymouth	North Carolina	252-793-4135	www.wchonline.com
Washington County Hospital	Washington	Iowa	319-653-5481	www.wchc.org
West Branch Regional Medical Center	West Branch	Michigan	989-345-6366	www.wbrmc.org
Western Plains Medical Complex	Dodge City	Kansas	620-225-8400	www.westernplainsmc.com
Wheeling Hospital	Wheeling	West Virginia	304-243-3000	www.wheelinghospital.com
Williamsburg Regional Hospital	Kingstree	South Carolina	843-355-0167	www.w-rh.org
Wilson Medical Center	Wilson	North Carolina	252-399-8040	www.wilmed.org/contact.asp
Yakima Valley Memorial Hospital	Yakima	Washington	509-575-8000	www.yakimamemorialhospital.org

Note: Table shows hospitals nationwide whose Pneumonia 30-day risk-adjusted mortality rate is worse (higher) than U.S. rate of 11.6%

Hospital Mortality from Heart Attack: State and National Summary

Area	Number of Hospitals			
	Better than U.S. National Rate[1]	Worse than U.S. National Rate[2]	No Different than U.S. National Rate[3]	Number of Cases Too Small[4]
U.S. and Territories	95	45	2744	1685
Alabama	0	0	60	40
Alaska	0	0	5	13
American Samoa	0	0	0	0
Arizona	2	0	43	26
Arkansas	1	5	37	32
California	4	2	228	99
Colorado	0	0	33	31
Connecticut	7	0	22	3
Delaware	1	0	4	0
District of Columbia	0	0	5	2
Florida	6	4	147	26
Georgia	1	1	84	58
Guam	0	0	1	0
Hawaii	0	0	12	4
Idaho	0	0	9	27
Illinois	5	0	121	56
Indiana	3	1	74	39
Iowa	0	0	41	70
Kansas	0	0	31	84
Kentucky	3	0	56	38
Louisiana	0	1	59	48
Maine	0	0	32	4
Maryland	1	0	42	2
Massachusetts	9	0	51	5
Michigan	6	2	83	38
Minnesota	2	0	42	81
Mississippi	0	2	36	49
Missouri	3	0	62	46
Montana	0	0	9	38
N. Mariana Islands	0	0	0	1
Nebraska	1	0	18	61
Nevada	0	0	17	13
New Hampshire	1	0	20	5
New Jersey	3	1	67	3
New Mexico	1	0	17	23
New York	10	5	154	19
North Carolina	3	2	82	22
North Dakota	0	0	11	30
Ohio	3	1	121	34
Oklahoma	1	2	37	69
Oregon	0	0	39	17
Pennsylvania	4	2	136	20
Puerto Rico	0	1	29	16
Rhode Island	0	0	10	0
South Carolina	0	1	43	13
South Dakota	1	0	10	36
Tennessee	1	2	70	43
Texas	7	3	200	134
Utah	0	0	13	24
Vermont	0	0	12	2
Virgin Islands	0	0	1	1
Virginia	1	2	71	5
Washington	0	3	41	41
West Virginia	0	1	34	16
Wisconsin	4	1	60	54
Wyoming	0	0	2	24

Note: (1) 30-day risk-adjusted mortality rate is better (lower) than U.S. rate of 16.2%; (2) 30-day risk-adjusted mortality rate is worse (higher) than U.S. rate of 16.2%; (3) 30-day risk-adjusted mortality rate is about the same as U.S. rate of 16.2%; (4) The number of cases is too small to classify the hospital

Hospital Mortality from Heart Failure: State and National Summary

Area	Number of Hospitals			
	Better than U.S. National Rate[1]	Worse than U.S. National Rate[2]	No Different than U.S. National Rate[3]	Number of Cases Too Small[4]
U.S. and Territories	199	140	3801	603
Alabama	3	0	93	5
Alaska	0	0	10	11
American Samoa	0	0	0	1
Arizona	0	0	61	17
Arkansas	0	10	62	4
California	13	11	267	55
Colorado	0	0	55	17
Connecticut	4	0	28	0
Delaware	0	0	5	0
District of Columbia	2	0	5	0
Florida	11	8	157	7
Georgia	6	3	122	15
Guam	0	0	1	0
Hawaii	0	0	13	5
Idaho	0	0	26	10
Illinois	21	7	150	5
Indiana	5	3	107	3
Iowa	0	1	101	14
Kansas	0	1	92	33
Kentucky	5	1	88	3
Louisiana	2	5	87	25
Maine	0	0	34	2
Maryland	5	0	40	1
Massachusetts	12	0	50	3
Michigan	14	3	107	8
Minnesota	3	0	94	33
Mississippi	0	4	82	8
Missouri	5	5	100	3
Montana	0	1	30	28
N. Mariana Islands	0	0	0	1
Nebraska	1	1	53	29
Nevada	0	0	26	7
New Hampshire	0	1	24	1
New Jersey	14	1	59	0
New Mexico	0	1	34	7
New York	19	7	158	6
North Carolina	1	1	100	8
North Dakota	0	0	28	14
Ohio	16	6	134	6
Oklahoma	1	2	81	33
Oregon	0	6	46	6
Pennsylvania	17	6	135	6
Puerto Rico	0	0	35	14
Rhode Island	0	1	9	0
South Carolina	0	4	53	2
South Dakota	0	0	29	25
Tennessee	1	8	104	4
Texas	12	5	296	58
Utah	0	2	23	15
Vermont	0	3	10	1
Virgin Islands	0	0	2	0
Virginia	1	3	74	4
Washington	0	11	55	20
West Virginia	1	2	45	4
Wisconsin	4	5	105	7
Wyoming	0	1	16	9

Note: (1) 30-day risk-adjusted mortality rate is better (lower) than U.S. rate of 11.2%; (2) 30-day risk-adjusted mortality rate is worse (higher) than U.S. rate of 11.2%; (3) 30-day risk-adjusted mortality rate is about the same as U.S. rate of 11.2%; (4) The number of cases is too small to classify the hospital

Hospital Mortality from Pneumonia: State and National Summary

Area	Number of Hospitals			
	Better than U.S. National Rate[1]	Worse than U.S. National Rate[2]	No Different than U.S. National Rate[3]	Number of Cases Too Small[4]
U.S. and Territories	222	221	3988	357
Alabama	2	0	95	4
Alaska	0	0	16	6
American Samoa	0	0	1	0
Arizona	2	0	65	11
Arkansas	1	7	67	1
California	16	26	258	53
Colorado	4	0	59	11
Connecticut	5	0	26	1
Delaware	0	0	5	0
District of Columbia	0	0	7	0
Florida	15	9	155	7
Georgia	5	12	121	6
Guam	0	1	0	0
Hawaii	0	1	13	6
Idaho	0	2	31	4
Illinois	18	10	149	6
Indiana	7	4	104	3
Iowa	3	6	104	3
Kansas	4	2	109	13
Kentucky	4	6	85	2
Louisiana	5	4	88	24
Maine	2	1	33	0
Maryland	8	0	37	1
Massachusetts	13	1	49	3
Michigan	11	3	114	4
Minnesota	5	0	113	13
Mississippi	0	6	81	8
Missouri	6	6	100	3
Montana	0	1	41	18
N. Mariana Islands	0	0	1	0
Nebraska	0	6	72	7
Nevada	0	3	27	3
New Hampshire	1	3	22	0
New Jersey	10	2	61	1
New Mexico	0	0	40	3
New York	17	14	155	6
North Carolina	2	10	96	2
North Dakota	0	0	41	3
Ohio	14	7	138	3
Oklahoma	3	7	97	10
Oregon	1	1	53	3
Pennsylvania	12	5	143	5
Puerto Rico	0	7	29	15
Rhode Island	0	0	10	0
South Carolina	2	6	50	1
South Dakota	0	0	47	8
Tennessee	2	10	101	5
Texas	18	14	300	43
Utah	0	0	36	4
Vermont	0	1	13	0
Virgin Islands	0	0	2	0
Virginia	0	6	73	6
Washington	2	4	71	11
West Virginia	1	3	48	0
Wisconsin	1	4	113	3
Wyoming	0	0	23	4

Note: (1) 30-day risk-adjusted mortality rate is better (lower) than U.S. rate of 11.6%; (2) 30-day risk-adjusted mortality rate is worse (higher) than U.S. rate of 11.6%; (3) 30-day risk-adjusted mortality rate is about the same as U.S. rate of 11.6%; (4) The number of cases is too small to classify the hospital

What Do These Mortality Categories Show?

These categories show how hospitals' risk-adjusted 30-Day Death (mortality) rates compare to the rate across the U.S., after making adjustments for how sick patients were before they were admitted to the hospital and taking into account differences in death rates that might be due to chance.

Hospitals are shown to be Better or Worse Than U.S. National Rate only if we can be 95% certain that the difference between their risk-adjusted death (mortality) rates and the U.S. National rate is not due to chance. All others are shown in the No Different Than U.S. National Rate and Number of Cases Too Small categories.

Better than U.S. National Rate. Hospitals in the Better Than U.S. National Rate category have risk-adjusted 30-day death (mortality) rates that are lower than the U.S. National rate, and we can be 95% certain that this difference is not due to chance.

No Different than U.S. National Rate. Many hospitals in the No Different Than U.S. National Rate category have risk-adjusted 30-day death (mortality) rates that are about the same as the U.S. National rate. Other hospitals in this category have rates that are higher or lower than the U.S. National rate, but we cannot be 95% certain that these differences are not due to chance.

Worse than U.S. National Rate. Hospitals in the Worse Than U.S. National Rate category have risk-adjusted 30-day death (mortality) rates that are higher than the U.S. National rate, and we can be 95% certain that this difference is not due to chance.

Number of Cases Too Small. The number of cases is too small to classify the hospital. One cannot be certain about differences when a hospital has very few relevant patients.

Why are Death Rates for Individual Hospitals Not Shown?

Comparisons based on estimated death (mortality) rates alone can be misleading. Risk-adjusted death (mortality) rates are estimated for individual hospitals based on information taken from a particular time period. If a slightly different time period had been chosen, chances are that each hospital's results would have been somewhat different.

Researchers almost always report a range ("confidence interval" or in this case an "interval estimate") around their estimates, to show how much variation might be due to this kind of chance. A confidence interval or interval estimate tells us we can be reasonably "confident" (in this case, 95% confident) that a hospital's death (mortality) rate fell somewhere within this specified range. The smaller the range, the more precise the estimate.

When hospitals treat a very large number of patients, chance differences will not have much effect on the overall rates. The range will be small, and the estimated death (mortality) rates will be more precise. In hospitals that treat smaller numbers of patients, however, even small chance differences could have a big impact on death (mortality) rates. The 95% confidence interval, or range, will be large, and the estimated death (mortality) rates will be much less precise.

Because the number of patients treated at U.S. hospitals varies widely, the precision of hospitals' estimated death (mortality) rates also varies.

Calculation of 30-Day Risk-Standardized Mortality Rates

The 30-day risk-standardized mortality measures for heart attack, heart failure, and pneumonia are produced from Medicare claims and enrollment data using sophisticated statistical modeling techniques that adjust for patient-level risk factors and account for the clustering of patients within hospitals.

The three mortality models estimate hospital-specific, risk-standardized, all-cause 30-day mortality rates for patients hospitalized with a principal diagnosis of heart attack, heart failure, and pneumonia. All-cause mortality is defined as death from any cause within 30 days after the add link here index admission date, regardless of whether the patient dies while still in the hospital or after discharge. For each condition, the risk-standardized ("adjusted" or "risk-adjusted") hospital mortality rate can be used to compare performance across hospitals. The mortality measures for heart attack, heart failure, and pneumonia have been endorsed by the National Quality Forum (NQF), the non-profit public-private partnership organization that endorses national healthcare performance measures.

Data Collection Methods

Cases Included in the Model. All admissions for people with Medicare aged 65 or over who were enrolled in Original Medicare (traditional fee-for-service Medicare) for the entire 12 months prior to their hospital admission for heart attack or heart failure or pneumonia, and for whom complete administrative data for that 12-month period are available, are included in the model. The model identifies (1) all short-stay acute-care hospital discharges for heart attack or heart failure or pneumonia in the reference year based on a principal discharge diagnosis on the Medicare beneficiary's inpatient claim, and (2) all deaths (for all causes) within 30 days of admission. Hospital stays that lasted one day or less are excluded, provided the patient was discharged alive and not against medical advice. The measure now excludes admissions for patients who enrolled into the Medicare Hospice program on the first day of the admission and continue to exclude patients enrolled any time in the 12 months prior to admission. Discharges for patients who left against medical advice (AMA) are excluded beginning in 2009. If a beneficiary had multiple admissions during a year, one admission is chosen randomly for inclusion in the model from each year. (For the publication of the rates in June 2009, the reference period used for calculating mortality rates is July 2005 through June 2008. Subsequent updates to the rates are expected to use the same July/June three-year reference period.)

Hospital mortality rates for heart attack are calculated based on all admissions for heart attack, even if an individual Medicare beneficiary was hospitalized more than once for this condition during the 12-month period. However, for purposes of calculating heart failure mortality rates, if a beneficiary had multiple admissions during the 12-month period, one admission is chosen randomly for inclusion in the model.

Use of a 30-Day Period to Assess Mortality

The model tracks deaths that occur within 30 days of a hospital admission, rather than inpatient mortality only, or mortality over some other post-discharge period. Thirty-day mortality was chosen over inpatient mortality because variability across hospitals in lengths of stay can make differences in inpatient mortality hard to interpret. For example, a heart attack patient hospitalized for 12 days may have a higher chance of dying during the hospital stay than a patient hospitalized for only 7 days, merely because the first patient's outcome is tracked for 5 days longer than the second patient's. Thirty-day mortality was chosen over longer windows (such as 90 days or one year), because mortality over longer periods may have less to do with the care received in the hospital and more to do with other complicating illnesses, patients' own behavior, or the care they received after discharge.

Use of Administrative Claims Data

Administrative claims data, rather than medical records data, are used to predict 30-day mortality. These data are widely available for Original Medicare (traditional fee-for-service) beneficiaries, are relatively inexpensive to acquire, and are timely. Using administrative data makes it possible to calculate mortality without having to do chart reviews or requiring hospitals to report additional data. Research conducted when the measures were being developed demonstrated that the administrative claims-based models perform well in predicting mortality compared with models based on chart reviews.

Risk-Adjustment and Covariates Included in the Model

Risk-Adjustment. The model adjusts for differences in patients' risks unrelated to their hospital care (risk-adjustment). The characteristics that Medicare patients bring with them when they arrive at a hospital with a heart attack or heart failure or pneumonia are not under the control of the hospital. However, some patient characteristics may make death more likely (increase the "risk" of death), no matter where the patient is treated or how good the care is. Moreover, some hospitals may treat people with a history of more severe disease. Therefore, when mortality rates are calculated for each hospital for a 12-month period, they are adjusted based on the unique mix of patients that hospital treated during that period. Factors included in the risk-adjustment model include age, gender, past medical history, and other diseases or conditions (comorbidities) that patients had when they arrived at the hospital that are known to increase their risk.

Past medical history and comorbidities are included in the model using CMS's condition categories (CCs) and a history of certain procedures. Medicare patients are assigned to one or more CCs based on diagnoses (ICD-9 codes) obtained from the patient's discharge claim, and from the hospital inpatient, hospital outpatient, and physician Medicare claims submitted for the patient one year prior to the admission. Secondary diagnoses from the patient's hospital discharge claim that might represent complications that occurred while the patient was in the hospital, rather than conditions that were present on admission, are not included in assigning the patient's CC. Research has shown that coding differences among providers affect CCs only slightly. Diagnoses from unreliable sources (such as laboratory or other claims that were not based on face-to-face encounters) are not included when assigning the CCs in the model.

To "risk-adjust" mortality rates for patient characteristics, the statistical model estimates the independent effects of age, gender, comorbidities, and a hospital-specific component of quality on mortality of patients within 30 days of hospital admission (the dependent variable). Using these estimates, the model calculates an adjusted mortality rate for each hospital that can be compared with those of other hospitals with different case mixes.

Covariates in 30-Day Mortality Risk-Adjustment Models		
Heart Attack	Heart Failure	Pneumonia
Age-65	Age-65	Age-65
Gender (male)	Gender (male)	Gender (male)
History of PTCA	History of PTCA	History of PTCA
History of CABG	History of CABG	History of CABG
History of heart failure	History of heart failure	History of heart failure
History of MI	History of MI	History of MI
AMI location (Group 1): anterior, anterolateral		
AMI location (Group 2): inferolateral, inferior, inferoposterior, other lateral, and true posterior		
Unstable angina	Unstable angina	Unstable angina
Chronic atherosclerosis	Chronic atherosclerosis	Chronic atherosclerosis
Cardiopulmonary-respiratory failure and shock	Cardiopulmonary-respiratory failure and shock	
Valvular heart disease	Valvular heart disease	Valvular heart disease
Hypertension	Hypertension	Hypertension
Stroke	Stroke	Stroke
Cerebrovascular disease		
Renal failure	Renal failure	Renal failure
COPD	COPD	COPD
Pneumonia	Pneumonia	Pneumonia
Diabetes	Diabetes	Diabetes
Protein-calorie malnutrition	Protein-calorie malnutrition	Protein-calorie malnutrition
Dementia	Dementia	Dementia
Functional disability	Functional disability	Functional disability
Peripheral vascular disease	Peripheral vascular disease	Peripheral vascular disease
Metastatic cancer	Metastatic cancer	Metastatic cancer
Trauma in last year	Trauma in last year	Trauma in last year
Major psych disorder	Major psych disorder	Major psych disorder
Chronic liver disease	Chronic liver disease	Chronic liver disease
		Severe hematological disorders
		Depression
		Seizure disorders/ convulsions
		Asthma
		Iron deficiency/anemias
		Parkinson's/Huntington's
		Lung fibrosis/chronic lung disorders
		Vertebral fractures

Statistical Methods Used to Calculate Mortality Rates

Hierarchical Regression Model. The statistical model for computing 30-day risk-adjusted mortality rate measures is a "hierarchical regression model." This type of model is based on the assumption that any heart attack or heart failure patients treated at a particular hospital will experience a level of quality of care that applies to all patients treated for the same condition in that hospital. In other words, the expected risk of death for two similar heart attack or heart failure patients treated in the same hospital would be more alike than the risk of death for the same two patients treated in two different hospitals. The likelihood that an individual patient will die is therefore a combination of (1) his or her individual risk characteristics (for example, gender, comorbidities, and past medical history) and 2) the hospital's unique quality of care for all patients treated for that condition in that hospital. The model estimates the effects of both of these components on mortality.

Calculating Mortality Rates. Each hospital's "30-day risk-adjusted mortality rate" (also called the "Risk Standardized Mortality Rate" or RSMR) is computed in several steps. First, the predicted 30-day mortality for a particular hospital obtained from the hierarchical regression model is divided by the expected mortality for that hospital, which is also obtained from the regression model. Predicted mortality is the rate of deaths from heart attack or heart failure that would be anticipated in the particular hospital during the 12-month period, given the patient case mix and the hospital's unique quality of care effect on mortality. Expected mortality is the rate of deaths from heart attack or heart failure that would be expected if the same patients with the same characteristics had

instead been treated at an "average" hospital, given the "average" hospital's quality of care effect on mortality for patients with that condition. This ratio is then multiplied by the national unadjusted mortality rate for the condition for all hospitals to compute a "risk-adjusted mortality rate" for the hospital. So, the higher a hospital's predicted 30-day mortality rate, relative to expected mortality for the hospital's particular case mix of patients, the higher its adjusted mortality rate will be. Hospitals with better quality will have lower rates.

(Predicted 30-day mortality/Expected mortality) * U.S. National mortality rate = RSMR

For example, suppose the model predicts that 10 percent of Hospital A's heart attack patients would die within 30 days of admission in a given year, based on their ages, gender mix, and pre-existing health conditions, and based on the estimate of the hospital's specific quality of care. Then, suppose that the expected rate of 30-day deaths for those same patients were higher – say, 15 percent – if they had instead been treated at an "average" U.S. hospital. If the actual mortality rate for the 12-month period for all heart attack patients in all hospitals in the U.S. is 12 percent, then the hospital's risk-adjusted 30-day mortality rate would be 8 percent.

(10%/15%)* 12% = RSMR for Hospital A 8%

If, instead, 9 percent of these patients would be expected to have died if treated at the average hospital, then the hospital's mortality rate would be 13.3 percent.

(10%/9%)* 12% = RSMR for Hospital A 13.3%

In the first case, the hospital performed better than the average hospital and had a relatively low risk-adjusted mortality rate (8 percent); in the second case it performed worse and had a relatively high rate (13.3 percent).

Hospitals with relatively low-risk patients whose predicted mortality rate is the same as the expected mortality rate for the average hospital for the same group of low-risk patients would have an adjusted mortality rate equal to the national rate (12 percent in this example). Similarly, hospitals with high-risk patients whose predicted mortality rate is the same as the expected mortality rate for the average hospital for the same group of high-risk patients would also have an adjusted mortality rate equal to the national rate of 12 percent. Thus, each hospital's case mix should not affect the adjusted mortality rates used to compare hospitals.

Adjusting for Small Hospitals or a Small Number of Cases. The hierarchical regression model also adjusts mortality rates results for small hospitals or hospitals with few heart attack or heart failure cases in a given year. This reduces the chance that such hospitals' performance will fluctuate wildly from year to year or that they will be wrongly classified as either a worse or better performer. For these hospitals, the model not only considers deaths among patients treated for the condition in the small sample size of cases, but pools together patients from all hospitals treated for the given condition, to make the result more reliable. In essence, the predicted mortality rate for a hospital with a small number of cases is moved toward the overall U.S. National mortality rate for all hospitals. The estimates of mortality for hospitals with few patients will rely considerably on the pooled data for all hospitals, making it less likely that small hospitals will fall into either of the outlier categories. This pooling affords a "borrowing of statistical strength" that provides more confidence in the results.

Significance Testing, Interval Estimates, and Comparing Rates Among Hospitals

Significance Testing and Interval Estimates. The model also calculates how precise the estimates of the adjusted mortality rate are, and determines upper and lower bounds (Interval Estimates) for each hospital's risk-adjusted rate. Interval estimates, which are like confidence intervals, describe how much uncertainty there is around the rate—how much bigger or smaller the rate might really be. Larger hospitals typically have more precise estimates and smaller interval estimates, since more data are available to estimate mortality. The smaller the sample size, the greater the difference in mortality rates between a hospital and the national rate must be in order for that difference to be statistically meaningful.

Comparing Mortality Rates Among Hospitals. The risk-adjusted hospital rate with its interval estimate can be compared to the U.S. National crude mortality rate. If the interval estimate includes (overlaps with) the national crude mortality rate, the hospital's performance is in the "no different than U.S. National rate" category. If the entire interval estimate is below the national crude mortality rate, then the hospital is performing "better than U.S. National rate." If the entire interval estimate is above the national crude mortality rate, it is "worse than U.S. National rate."

Hospitals whose Heart Attack 30-Day Readmission Rate is Better (Lower) than the U.S. National Rate

Hospital	City	State	Phone	Web Site
Anmed Health	Anderson	South Carolina	864-261-1109	www.anmed.com
Avera Heart Hospital of South Dakota	Sioux Falls	South Dakota	605-977-7000	
Ball Memorial Hospital	Muncie	Indiana	765-747-3111	www.accesschs.org/baal-memorial-l
Boca Raton Regional Hospital	Boca Raton	Florida	561-362-5002	
Carilion Medical Center	Roanoke	Virginia	540-981-7000	www.carilion.com/crmh
Cox Medical Center	Springfield	Missouri	417-269-6000	www.coxhealth.com
Greenville Memorial Hospital	Greenville	South Carolina	864-455-7000	www.ghs.org
Indiana University Health	Indianapolis	Indiana	317-962-5900	
Lancaster General Hospital	Lancaster	Pennsylvania	717-299-5511	www.lancastergeneral.org
Lutheran Hospital of Indiana	Fort Wayne	Indiana	260-435-7001	www.lutheranhospital.com
Memorial Mission Hospital and Asheville Surgery Center	Asheville	North Carolina	828-213-1111	www.missionhospitals.org
Munson Medical Center	Traverse City	Michigan	231-935-5000	www.munsonhealthcare.org
Naples Community Hospital	Naples	Florida	239-436-5000	www.nchmd.org
Northeast Georgia Medical Center	Gainesville	Georgia	770-535-3553	www.nghs.com
Piedmont Hospital	Atlanta	Georgia	404-605-5000	www.piedmonthospital.org
Rogue Valley Medical Center	Medford	Oregon	541-789-7000	www.asante.org
Santa Barbara Cottage Hospital	Santa Barbara	California	805-682-7111	www.cottagehealthsystem.org
Santa Rosa Memorial Hospital	Santa Rosa	California	707-525-5300	www.stjosephhealth.org
Sarasota Memorial Hospital	Sarasota	Florida	941-917-9000	www.smh.com
Shannon Medical Center	San Angelo	Texas	325-653-6741	www.shannonhealth.com
Sisters of Charity Providence Hospitals	Columbia	South Carolina	803-256-5300	www.providencehospitals.com
Spectrum Health - Butterworth Campus	Grand Rapids	Michigan	616-391-1774	www.spectrum-health.org
Saint John's Regional Health Center	Springfield	Missouri	417-820-2000	www.stjohns.com
Saint Mary's Medical Center	Huntington	West Virginia	304-526-1234	www.st-marys.org
Saint Vincent Heart Center of Indiana	Indianapolis	Indiana	317-583-5000	www.theheartcenter.com
Stanford Hospital	Stanford	California	650-723-5708	www.stanfordhospital.com
Tri-City Medical Center	Oceanside	California	760-724-8411	www.tricitymed.org
Venice Regional Medical Center	Venice	Florida	941-485-7711	www.veniceregional.com
York Hospital	York	Pennsylvania	717-851-2345	www.wellspan.org

Note: Table shows hospitals nationwide whose Acute Myocardial Infarction 30-day readmission rate is better (lower) than U.S. rate of 19.9%

Hospitals whose Heart Attack 30-Day Readmission Rate is Worse (Higher) than the U.S. National Rate

Hospital	City	State	Phone	Web Site
Abington Memorial Hospital	Abington	Pennsylvania	215-481-2000	www.amh.org
Advocate South Suburban Hospital	Hazel Crest	Illinois	708-799-8000	www.advocatehealth.com
Albert Einstein Medical Center	Philadelphia	Pennsylvania	215-456-6090	www.einstein.edu
Banner Boswell Medical Center	Sun City	Arizona	623-977-7211	www.bannerhealth.com
Barnes Jewish Hospital	Saint Louis	Missouri	314-747-3000	www.barnesjewish.org
Beth Israel Deaconess Medical Center	Boston	Massachusetts	617-667-7000	www.bidmc.harvard.edu
Christian Hospital Northeast	Saint Louis	Missouri	314-653-5000	www.christianhospital.org
Cleveland Clinic	Cleveland	Ohio	216-444-2200	www.clevelandclinic.org
Duke University Hospital	Durham	North Carolina	919-684-8111	www.dukehealth.org
Easton Hospital	Easton	Pennsylvania	610-250-4076	www.easton-hospital.com
Fairfield Medical Center	Lancaster	Ohio	740-687-8009	www.fmchealth.org
Florida Hospital	Orlando	Florida	407-303-1976	www.floridahospital.com
Floyd Memorial Hospital and Health Services	New Albany	Indiana	812-949-5500	www.floydmedical.org
Franciscan St Margaret Health - Hammond	Hammond	Indiana	219-932-2300	www.smmhc.com
Hallmark Health System	Melrose	Massachusetts	781-979-3000	www.hallmarkhealth.org
Jacobi Medical Center	Bronx	New York	718-918-5000	www.ci.nyc.ny.us/html/hhc
Jamaica Hospital Medical Center	Jamaica	New York	718-262-6000	www.jamaicahospital.org
Johnson City Medical Center	Johnson City	Tennessee	423-431-6111	www.msha.com
Libertyhealth-Jersey City Medical Center Campus	Jersey City	New Jersey	201-915-2000	www.libertyhcs.org
Lutheran Medical Center	Brooklyn	New York	718-630-8000	www.lmcmc.com
Maimonides Medical Center	Brooklyn	New York	718-283-6000	www.maimonidesmed.org
Mary Washington Hospital	Fredericksburg	Virginia	540-741-1100	www.medicorp.org
Metrosouth Medical Center	Blue Island	Illinois	708-597-2000	www.stfrancisblueisland.com
Mount Sinai Hospital	New York	New York	212-241-7981	www.mountsinai.org
Nassau University Medical Center	East Meadow	New York	516-572-0123	www.numc.edu
New York Methodist Hospital	Brooklyn	New York	718-780-3000	www.nym.org
North Carolina Baptist Hospital	Winston-Salem	North Carolina	336-716-2011	www.wfubmc.edu
North Shore University Hospital	Manhasset	New York	516-562-0100	www.northshorelij.com
Our Lady of the Resurrection Medical Center	Chicago	Illinois	773-282-7000	www.reshealth.org
Raritan Bay Medical Center	Perth Amboy	New Jersey	732-442-3700	
Rochester General Hospital	Rochester	New York	585-922-4000	www.rochestergeneral.org
Saint Michael's Medical Center	Newark	New Jersey	973-877-5350	www.cathedralhealth.org
South Shore Hospital	South Weymouth	Massachusetts	781-340-8000	www.southshorehospital.org
Saint Elizabeth's Medical Center	Brighton	Massachusetts	617-789-3000	www.semc.org
Saint Francis Medical Center	Monroe	Louisiana	318-966-4141	www.stfran.com
Saint John Hospital and Medical Center	Detroit	Michigan	313-343-4000	www.stjohnprovidence.org
Trinity Medical Center East & Trinity Medical Center West	Steubenville	Ohio	740-264-7212	www.trinityhealth.com
Trinity Rock Island	Rock Island	Illinois	309-779-5000	www.trinityqc.com
Union Memorial Hospital	Baltimore	Maryland	410-554-2227	www.unionmemorial.org
University Hospital	Cincinnati	Ohio	513-584-1000	www.universityhospitalcincinnati.com
University of Iowa Hospital & Clinics	Iowa City	Iowa	319-356-1616	www.uihealthcare.com
Waterbury Hospital	Waterbury	Connecticut	203-573-6000	www.waterburyhospital.org
Wyckoff Heights Medical Center	Brooklyn	New York	718-963-7272	www.wyckoffhospital.org

Note: Table shows hospitals nationwide whose Acute Myocardial Infarction 30-day readmission rate is worse (higher) than U.S. rate of 19.9%.

Hospitals whose Heart Failure 30-Day Readmission Rate is Better (Lower) than the U.S. National Rate

Hospital	City	State	Phone	Web Site
Allegiance Health	Jackson	Michigan	517-788-4800	www.footehealth.org
Allen Memorial Hospital	Waterloo	Iowa	319-235-3941	www.allenhospital.org
Alpena Regional Medical Center	Alpena	Michigan	989-356-7390	www.agh.org
Athens Regional Medical Center	Athens	Georgia	706-475-7000	www.armc.org
Aultman Hospital	Canton	Ohio	330-452-9911	www.aultman.com
Aurora St Lukes Medical Center	Milwaukee	Wisconsin	414-649-6000	www.aurorahealthcare.org
Ball Memorial Hospital	Muncie	Indiana	765-747-3111	www.accesschs.org/baal-memorial-l
Baptist Health Medical Center-Little Rock	Little Rock	Arkansas	501-202-2000	www.baptist-health.com
Baptist St Anthonys Health System-Baptist Campus	Amarillo	Texas	806-212-2000	www.bsahs.com
Bay Medical Center	Panama City	Florida	850-769-1511	www.baymedical.org
Baylor Heart and Vascular Hospital	Dallas	Texas	214-820-0670	
Baylor University Medical Center	Dallas	Texas	214-820-0111	www.baylorhealth.com
Bellin Memorial Hospital	Green Bay	Wisconsin	920-433-3500	www.bellin.org
Bethesda Memorial Hospital	Boynton Beach	Florida	561-737-7733	www.bethesdahealthcare.com
Bon Secours - Depaul Medical Center	Norfolk	Virginia	757-889-5000	www.bonsecourshamptonroads.com
Borgess Medical Center	Kalamazoo	Michigan	269-226-7000	www.borgess.com
Bromenn Healthcare	Normal	Illinois	309-454-1400	
Cape Coral Hospital	Cape Coral	Florida	239-574-2323	
Capital Regional Medical Center	Tallahassee	Florida	850-656-5000	www.capitalregionalmedicalcenter.com
Carolinas Medical Center-Behavioral Health	Charlotte	North Carolina	704-355-2000	www.carolinasmedicalcenter.org
Catholic Medical Center	Manchester	New Hampshire	603-668-3545	www.catholicmedicalcenter.org
Central Baptist Hospital	Lexington	Kentucky	859-260-6100	www.centralbap.com
Central Vermont Medical Center	Barre	Vermont	802-371-4100	www.cvmc.hitchcock.org
Central Washington Hospital	Wenatchee	Washington	509-662-1511	www.cwhs.com
Christus Schumpert Health System	Shreveport	Louisiana	318-681-4215	www.christusschumpert.org
Citrus Memorial Hospital	Inverness	Florida	352-726-1551	www.citrusmh.com
Citrus Valley Medical Center-IC Campus	Covina	California	626-814-2468	www.cvhp.org
Community Hospital of the Monterey Peninsula	Monterey	California	831-624-5311	www.chomp.org
Cookeville Regional Medical Center	Cookeville	Tennessee	931-646-2000	www.crmchealth.org
The Cooley Dickinson Hospital	Northampton	Massachusetts	413-582-2000	www.cooley-dickinson.org
The Corpus Christi Medical Center	Corpus Christi	Texas	361-761-1000	
Cox Medical Center	Springfield	Missouri	417-269-6000	www.coxhealth.com
Deborah Heart and Lung Center	Browns Mills	New Jersey	609-893-6611	
Dixie Regional Medical Center	Saint George	Utah	435-251-1000	intermountainhealthcare.org
Doctors Hospital at Renaissance	Edinburg	Texas	956-666-7100	www.dhr-rgv.com
Door County Memorial Hospital	Sturgeon Bay	Wisconsin	920-743-5566	www.doorcountymemorial.org
East Jefferson General Hospital	Metairie	Louisiana	504-454-4000	www.EastJeffHospital.org
Ephrata Community Hospital	Ephrata	Pennsylvania	717-733-0311	www.ephratahospital.org
Exempla Lutheran Medical Center	Wheat Ridge	Colorado	303-425-4500	www.exemlpa.org
Florida Hospital Waterman	Tavares	Florida	352-253-3300	www.fhwat.org
Flower Hospital	Sylvania	Ohio	419-824-1444	www.promedica.org
Flowers Hospital	Dothan	Alabama	334-793-5000	www.flowershospital.com
Gaston Memorial Hospital	Gastonia	North Carolina	704-834-2000	www.caromont.org
Geisinger Medical Center	Danville	Pennsylvania	570-271-6211	www.geisinger.org
Genesis Healthcare System	Zanesville	Ohio	740-454-5000	www.genesishcs.org
Greenville Memorial Hospital	Greenville	South Carolina	864-455-7000	www.ghs.org
Hamilton Medical Center	Dalton	Georgia	706-272-6105	www.hamiltonhealth.com
Hamot Medical Center	Erie	Pennsylvania	814-877-6000	www.hamot.org
Heart Hospital of Austin	Austin	Texas	512-407-7581	www.hearthospitalofaustin.com
Hendrick Medical Center	Abilene	Texas	325-670-2000	www.ehendrick.org
Hendricks Regional Health	Danville	Indiana	317-745-4451	www.hendricksregional.org
Henrico Doctors' Hospital	Richmond	Virginia	804-289-4500	www.henricodoctors.com
Immanuel-St Josephs-Mayo Health System	Mankato	Minnesota	507-625-4031	www.isj-mhs.org
Intermountain Medical Center	Murray	Utah	801-507-7000	intermountainhealthcare.org
Iowa Lutheran Hospital	Des Moines	Iowa	515-263-5612	ihsdesmoines.org
Johnston Memorial Hospital	Smithfield	North Carolina	919-934-8171	www.johnstanmemorial.org
Kadlec Regional Medical Center	Richland	Washington	509-946-4611	www.kadlecmed.org
Kalispell Regional Medical Center	Kalispell	Montana	406-752-1774	www.krmc.org
Kaweah Delta Medical Center	Visalia	California	559-624-2000	www.kaweahdelta.org
Lancaster General Hospital	Lancaster	Pennsylvania	717-299-5511	www.lancastergeneral.org
Lawrence & Memorial Hospital	New London	Connecticut	860-442-0711	www.lmhospital.org
Lee Memorial Hospital	Fort Myers	Florida	239-332-1111	www.leememorial.org
Manatee Memorial Hospital	Bradenton	Florida	941-746-5111	www.manateememorial.com
Martin Memorial Medical Center	Stuart	Florida	772-287-5200	www.mmhs.com

Hospital	City	State	Phone	Web Site
Mary Hitchcock Memorial Hospital	Lebanon	New Hampshire	603-650-5000	www.dhmc.org
Massachusetts General Hospital	Boston	Massachusetts	617-726-2000	www.massgeneral.org
McKay-Dee Hospital Center	Ogden	Utah	801-387-2800	intermountainhealthcare.org
Memorial Healthcare System	Chattanooga	Tennessee	423-495-2525	www.memorial.org
Memorial Hermann Hospital System	Houston	Texas	713-448-6796	www.memorialhermann.org
Memorial Hospital and Health Care Center	Jasper	Indiana	812-482-2345	www.mhhcc.org
Memorial Hospital of South Bend	South Bend	Indiana	574-647-3632	www.qualityoflife.org
Memorial Medical Center of West Michigan	Ludington	Michigan	231-843-2591	www.mmcwm.com
Memorial Mission Hospital and Asheville Surgery Center	Asheville	North Carolina	828-213-1111	www.missionhospitals.org
Mercy Health Partners - Mercy Campus	Muskegon	Michigan	231-672-3901	www.mghp.com
Mercy Medical Center-Cedar Rapids	Cedar Rapids	Iowa	319-398-6011	www.mercycare.org
Mercy Medical Center Redding	Redding	California	530-225-6102	www.redding.mercy.org
Methodist Hospital	San Antonio	Texas	210-575-4000	www.mh.sahealth.com
Mount Carmel Health	Columbus	Ohio	614-546-4533	www.mountcarmelhealth.com
Naples Community Hospital	Naples	Florida	239-436-5000	www.nchmd.org
Nebraska Heart Hospital	Lincoln	Nebraska	402-328-3000	www.neheart.com
North Kansas City Hospital	North Kansas City	Missouri	816-691-2000	www.nkch.org
Northeast Georgia Medical Center	Gainesville	Georgia	770-535-3553	www.nghs.com
Northern Michigan Regional Hospital	Petoskey	Michigan	231-487-4000	www.northernhealth.org
Our Lady of the Lake Regional Medical Center	Baton Rouge	Louisiana	225-765-8902	www.ololrmc.com
Park Nicollet Methodist Hospital	Saint Louis Park	Minnesota	952-993-5000	www.parknicollet.com/methodist
Parkview Hospital	Fort Wayne	Indiana	260-373-4000	www.parkview.com
Parkview Medical Center	Pueblo	Colorado	719-584-4000	www.parkviewmc.com
Peacehealth St Joseph Medical Center	Bellingham	Washington	360-734-5400	www.peacehealth.org
Peninsula Medical Center	Burlingame	California	650-696-5270	www.mills-peninsula.org
Peninsula Regional Medical Center	Salisbury	Maryland	410-543-7116	www.peninsula.org
Piedmont Hospital	Atlanta	Georgia	404-605-5000	www.piedmonthospital.org
Portneuf Medical Center	Pocatello	Idaho	208-239-1000	www.portmed.org
Presbyterian Hospital	Albuquerque	New Mexico	505-724-7281	www.phs.org
Providence Alaska Medical Center	Anchorage	Alaska	907-261-3675	www.providence.org
Providence Hospital	Mobile	Alabama	251-633-1000	www.providencehospital.org
Providence Regional Medical Center Everett	Everett	Washington	425-261-2000	www.providence.org
Providence Sacred Heart Medical Center	Spokane	Washington	509-474-3040	www.shmc.org
Providence St Vincent Medical Center	Portland	Oregon	503-216-1234	www.providence.org
Rapid City Regional Hospital	Rapid City	South Dakota	605-719-1000	www.rcrh.org
Reading Hospital Medical Center	Reading	Pennsylvania	610-988-8000	www.readinghospital.org
Redmond Regional Medical Center	Rome	Georgia	706-802-3012	
Regional Medical Center Bayonet Point	Hudson	Florida	727-819-2929	www.mchealth.com or www.heartoftampa.com
Riverside Regional Medical Center	Newport News	Virginia	757-594-2000	www.riversideonline.com
Rogue Valley Medical Center	Medford	Oregon	541-789-7000	www.asante.org
Rowan Regional Medical Center	Salisbury	North Carolina	704-210-5000	www.rowan.org
Sacred Heart Medical Center - University District	Eugene	Oregon	541-686-7274	www.peacehealth.org
Saint Joseph Regional Medical Center	Mishawaka	Indiana	574-335-5000	www.sjmed.com
Saint Joseph's Hospital of Atlanta	Atlanta	Georgia	678-843-5720	www.stjosephsatlanta.org
Saint Vincent Health Center	Erie	Pennsylvania	814-452-5000	www.svhs.org
Santa Barbara Cottage Hospital	Santa Barbara	California	805-682-7111	www.cottagehealthsystem.org
Santa Rosa Memorial Hospital	Santa Rosa	California	707-525-5300	www.stjosephhealth.org
Sarasota Memorial Hospital	Sarasota	Florida	941-917-9000	www.smh.com
Scott & White Memorial Hospital	Temple	Texas	254-724-2111	www.sw.org
Sentara Leigh Hospital	Norfolk	Virginia	757-261-6601	www.sentara.com
Sequoia Hospital	Redwood City	California	650-367-5551	www.sequoiahospital.org
Sisters of Charity Providence Hospitals	Columbia	South Carolina	803-256-5300	www.providencehospitals.com
Saint Clare Medical Center	Crawfordsville	Indiana	765-362-2800	www.stclaremedical.org
Saint Dominic-Jackson Memorial Hospital	Jackson	Mississippi	601-200-2000	stdom.com
Saint Francis Health Center	Topeka	Kansas	785-295-8000	www.stfrancistopeka.org
Saint Francis Hospital	Columbus	Georgia	706-596-4020	wecareforlife.com
Saint Francis-Downtown	Greenville	South Carolina	864-255-1000	www.stfrancishealth.org
Saint John's Regional Health Center	Springfield	Missouri	417-820-2000	www.stjohns.com
Saint Lukes Episcopal Hospital	Houston	Texas	832-355-1000	www.sleh.com
Saint Lukes Regional Medical Center	Boise	Idaho	208-381-2222	www.slrmc.org
Saint Marks Hospital	Salt Lake City	Utah	801-268-7700	www.stmarkshospital.com
Saint Patrick Hospital and Health Sciences Center	Missoula	Montana	406-543-7271	www.saintpatrick.org
Saint Vincent Heart Center of Indiana	Indianapolis	Indiana	317-583-5000	www.theheartcenter.com
Sutter Medical Center of Santa Rosa	Santa Rosa	California	707-576-4000	www.suttersantarosa.org
Tallahassee Memorial Healthcare	Tallahassee	Florida	850-431-1155	www.tmh.org
The Toledo Hospital	Toledo	Ohio	419-291-7463	www.promedica.org
Tucson Medical Center	Tucson	Arizona	520-327-5461	www.tmcaz.com

Hospital	City	State	Phone	Web Site
United Regional Health Care System	Wichita Falls	Texas	940-764-3055	www.urhcs.org
University Health Care - University Hospitals and Clinics	Salt Lake City	Utah	801-581-2121	www.healthcare.utah.edu
University Hospital	Augusta	Georgia	706-722-9011	www.universityhealth.org
UPMC Horizon	Greenville	Pennsylvania	724-588-2100	www.upmc.com
Upper Valley Medical Center	Troy	Ohio	937-440-7853	www.uvmc.com
Via Christi Hospitals Wichita	Wichita	Kansas	316-268-5000	www.via-christi.org
Virtua Memorial Hospital of Burlington County	Mount Holly	New Jersey	609-914-6200	www.virtua.org
Warren General Hospital	Warren	Pennsylvania	814-723-3300	
Wentworth-Douglass Hospital	Dover	New Hampshire	603-740-2580	
Wesley Medical Center	Wichita	Kansas	316-962-2000	www.wesleymc.com
Westerly Hospital	Westerly	Rhode Island	401-596-6000	
Wilkes-Barre General Hospital	Wilkes-Barre	Pennsylvania	570-829-8111	www.wvhcs.org
Williamsport Hospital & Medical Center	Williamsport	Pennsylvania	570-321-1000	www.susquehannahealth.org
Willis Knighton Bossier Health Center	Bossier City	Louisiana	318-212-7000	www.wkhs.com/Locations/Bossier.aspx
Woman's Christian Association	Jamestown	New York	716-487-0141	www.wcahospital.org
Yakima Valley Memorial Hospital	Yakima	Washington	509-575-8000	www.yakimamemorialhospital.org

Note: Table shows hospitals nationwide whose Heart Failure 30-day readmission rate is better (lower) than U.S. rate of 24.7%.

Hospitals whose Heart Failure 30-Day Readmission Rate is Worse (Higher) than the U.S. National Rate

Hospital	City	State	Phone	Web Site
Advocate Trinity Hospital	Chicago	Illinois	773-967-2000	www.advocatehealth.com/trin
Albert Einstein Medical Center	Philadelphia	Pennsylvania	215-456-6090	www.einstein.edu
Alegent Health Midlands Hospital	Papillion	Nebraska	402-593-3000	www.alegent.com
Aria Health	Philadelphia	Pennsylvania	215-612-4129	www.ariahealth.com
Avoyelles Hospital	Marksville	Louisiana	318-240-6000	www.avoyelleshospital.com
Barnes Jewish Hospital	Saint Louis	Missouri	314-747-3000	www.barnesjewish.org
Bates County Memorial Hospital	Butler	Missouri	660-200-7000	www.bcmhospital.com
Bayshore Community Hospital	Holmdel	New Jersey	732-739-5900	www.bchs.com
Bellevue Hospital Center	New York	New York	212-561-4132	www.nyc.gov/html/hhc/html/facilities/bellevue.shtml
Beth Israel Deaconess Medical Center	Boston	Massachusetts	617-667-7000	www.bidmc.harvard.edu
Beth Israel Medical Center	New York	New York	212-420-2000	www.wehealny.org
Biloxi Regional Medical Center	Biloxi	Mississippi	228-436-1104	www.hmabrmc.com
Bolivar Medical Center	Cleveland	Mississippi	662-846-2551	www.bolivarmedical.com
Bronx-Lebanon Hospital Center	Bronx	New York	212-588-7000	www.bronx-leb.org
Brookdale Hospital Medical Center	Brooklyn	New York	718-240-5966	www.brookdalehospital.org
Caldwell Memorial Hospital	Columbia	Louisiana	318-649-6111	
Cambridge Health Alliance	Cambridge	Massachusetts	617-665-2300	
Carolina Pines Regional Medical Center	Hartsville	South Carolina	864-339-2100	www.cprmc.com
Centegra Health System - McHenry Hospital	Mchenry	Illinois	815-344-5000	www.centegra.org
Centrastate Medical Center	Freehold	New Jersey	732-431-2000	www.centrastate.com
Chicot Memorial Medical Center	Lake Village	Arkansas	870-265-5351	www.chicotmemorial.com
Christian Hospital Northeast	Saint Louis	Missouri	314-653-5000	www.christianhospital.org
Civista Medical Center	La Plata	Maryland	301-609-4265	www.civista.org
Cleveland Clinic	Cleveland	Ohio	216-444-2200	www.clevelandclinic.org
Cleveland Regional Medical Center	Cleveland	Texas	281-593-1811	www.clevelandregionalmedical.com
Coffee Regional Medical Center	Douglas	Georgia	229-384-1900	www.coffeeregional.org
Community Regional Medical Center	Fresno	California	559-459-6000	www.communitymedical.org
Community Regional Medical Center	Lorain	Ohio	440-960-3295	
Coney Island Hospital	Brooklyn	New York	718-616-3000	
Cooper University Hospital	Camden	New Jersey	856-342-2000	www.cooperhealth.org
Davis Regional Medical Center	Statesville	North Carolina	704-873-0281	
Detroit Receiving Hospital & Univ Health Center	Detroit	Michigan	313-745-3104	www.drhuhc.org
Doctors' Community Hospital	Lanham	Maryland	301-552-8085	www.DCHweb.org
East Orange General Hospital	East Orange	New Jersey	973-266-4401	www.evh.org
Eastern Oklahoma Medical Center	Poteau	Oklahoma	918-647-8161	www.eomchospital.com
Fleming County Hospital	Flemingsburg	Kentucky	606-849-2351	www.flemingcountyhospital.org
Flushing Hospital Medical Center	Flushing	New York	718-670-5000	www.flushinghospital.org
Forest Hills Hospital	Forest Hills	New York	718-830-4000	www.northshorelij.com
Forrest General Hospital	Hattiesburg	Mississippi	601-288-7000	www.forrestgeneral.com
Franklin Square Hospital Center	Baltimore	Maryland	443-777-7850	www.franklinsquare.org
Galichia Heart Hospital	Wichita	Kansas	316-858-2610	www.ghhospital.com
George Washington Univ Hospital	Washington	District of Columbia	202-716-4605	www.gwhospital.com
Georgiana Hospital	Georgiana	Alabama	334-376-2205	
Hackensack University Medical Center	Hackensack	New Jersey	201-996-2000	www.humed.com
Halifax Regional Medical Center	Roanoke Rapids	North Carolina	252-535-8005	www.halifaxmedicalcenter.org
Hallmark Health System	Melrose	Massachusetts	781-979-3000	www.hallmarkhealth.org
Harbor Hospital	Brooklyn	Maryland	410-350-3201	www.harborhospital.org
Harlan Appalachian Regional Healthcare Hospital	Harlan	Kentucky	606-573-8100	www.arh.org
Harris Hospital	Newport	Arkansas	870-523-8911	www.harrishospital.com
Hawaii Medical Center West	Ewa Beach	Hawaii	808-678-7000	
Henry Ford Hospital	Detroit	Michigan	313-916-2600	www.henryfordhospital.com
Highlands Medical Center	Scottsboro	Alabama	256-259-4444	www.highlandsmedcenter.com
Highlands Regional Medical Center	Prestonsburg	Kentucky	606-886-8511	www.hrmc.org
Hollywood Presbyterian Medical Center	Los Angeles	California	213-413-3000	www.qahpmc.com
Holy Cross Hospital	Chicago	Illinois	773-471-8000	www.holycrosshospital.org
Holy Name Medical Center	Teaneck	New Jersey	201-833-3000	www.holyname.org
Holy Redeemer Hospital and Medical Center	Meadowbrook	Pennsylvania	215-947-3000	www.holyredeemer.com
Holzer Medical Center	Gallipolis	Ohio	740-446-5000	www.holzer.org
Howard University Hospital	Washington	District of Columbia	202-745-6100	www.huhosp.org
Hugh Chatham Memorial Hospital	Elkin	North Carolina	336-527-7000	www.hughchatham.org
Ingalls Memorial Hospital	Harvey	Illinois	708-333-2300	www.ingalls.org
Integris Baptist Regional Health Center	Miami	Oklahoma	918-542-6611	www.integris-health.com
Jackson Health System	Miami	Florida	305-585-1111	www.jhsmiami.org
Jameson Memorial Hospital	New Castle	Pennsylvania	724-658-9001	

Hospital	City	State	Phone	Web Site
Jefferson Regional Medical Center	Crystal City	Missouri	636-933-1000	www.jeffersonmemorial.org
Jennersville Regional Hospital	West Grove	Pennsylvania	610-869-1000	www.jennersville.com
JFK Medical Center	Edison	New Jersey	732-321-7000	www.jfkmc.org
Johnson City Medical Center	Johnson City	Tennessee	423-431-6111	www.msha.com
Johnson Memorial Hospital	Stafford Springs	Connecticut	860-684-4251	www.johnsonhealthnetwork.com
Kennedy University Hospital	Stratford	New Jersey	856-346-6000	www.kennedyhealth.org
Kimball Medical Center	Lakewood	New Jersey	732-363-1900	www.sbhcs.com
King's Daughters' Medical Center	Ashland	Kentucky	606-327-4000	www.kdmc.com
Kings County Hospital Center	Brooklyn	New York	718-245-3901	www.nyc.gov/html/hhc/html/facilities/kings.shtml
Lake Wales Medical Center	Lake Wales	Florida	863-676-1433	www.lakewalesmedicalcenter.com
Lakeway Regional Hospital	Morristown	Tennessee	423-522-6000	
Lane Regional Medical Center	Zachary	Louisiana	225-658-4303	www.lanehospital.org
Lenox Hill Hospital	New York	New York	212-439-2345	www.lenoxhillhospital.org
Libertyhealth-Jersey City Medical Center Campus	Jersey City	New Jersey	201-915-2000	www.libertyhcs.org
Lincoln Medical & Mental Health Center	Bronx	New York	718-579-5000	
Livingston Regional Hospital	Livingston	Tennessee	931-823-5611	www.livingstonregionalhospital.com
Long Beach Medical Center	Long Beach	New York	516-897-1000	www.lbmc.org
Long Island College Hospital	Brooklyn	New York	718-780-4651	www.wehealny.org
Lower Bucks Hospital	Bristol	Pennsylvania	215-785-9200	www.lowerbuckshospital.org
Lutheran Medical Center	Brooklyn	New York	718-630-8000	www.lmcmc.com
Magee General Hospital	Magee	Mississippi	601-849-5070	www.mghosp.org
Magnolia Regional Health Center	Corinth	Mississippi	662-293-7660	www.mrhc.org
Mary Washington Hospital	Fredericksburg	Virginia	540-741-1100	www.medicorp.org
Medical Center of Southeastern Oklahoma	Durant	Oklahoma	405-924-3080	www.mcsohealth.com
Memorial Hermann Katy Hospital	Katy	Texas	281-392-1111	www.memorialhermann.org
Memorial Hospital	Manchester	Kentucky	606-598-5104	www.manchestermemorial.com
Memorial Hospital	Nacogdoches	Texas	936-564-4611	www.nacmem.org
Memorial Hospital of Rhode Island	Pawtucket	Rhode Island	401-729-2000	mhriweb.org
Memorial Hospital of Salem County	Salem	New Jersey	856-935-1000	www.mhshealth.com
Memorial Hospital of Stilwell	Stilwell	Oklahoma	918-696-3101	
Mercy Fitzgerald Hospital	Darby	Pennsylvania	215-237-4000	www.mercyhealth.org
Mercy Regional Medical Center	Ville Platte	Louisiana	337-363-5684	www.vpmc.com
Methodist Hospital	Henderson	Kentucky	270-827-7700	www.methodisthospital.net
Methodist Hospitals	Gary	Indiana	219-886-4601	www.methodisthospital.org
Metrosouth Medical Center	Blue Island	Illinois	708-597-2000	www.stfrancisblueisland.com
Monongahela Valley Hospital	Monongahela	Pennsylvania	724-258-1000	www.monvalleyhospital.com
Monroe County Medical Center	Tompkinsville	Kentucky	270-487-9231	www.mcmccares.com
Montefiore Medical Center	Bronx	New York	718-920-4321	www.montefiore.org
Montgomery General Hospital	Olney	Maryland	301-774-8771	www.montgomerygeneral.com
Mount Sinai Hospital	New York	New York	212-241-7981	www.mountsinai.org
New York Hospital Medical Center of Queens	Flushing	New York	718-670-1231	www.nyhq.org
New York Methodist Hospital	Brooklyn	New York	718-780-3000	www.nym.org
New York Westchester Square Medical Center	Bronx	New York	718-430-7300	www.nywsmc.org
New York-Presbyterian Hospital	New York	New York	212-746-4189	www.nyp.org
Newark Beth Israel Medical Center	Newark	New Jersey	973-926-7850	www.sbhcs.com
North Carolina Baptist Hospital	Winston-Salem	North Carolina	336-716-2011	www.wfubmc.edu
North Oaks Medical Center	Hammond	Louisiana	985-345-2700	www.northoaks.org
North Shore University Hospital	Manhasset	New York	516-562-0100	www.northshorelij.com
Northwest Community Hospital	Arlington Heights	Illinois	847-618-1000	www.nch.org
Northwestern Memorial Hospital	Chicago	Illinois	312-926-2000	www.nmh.org
NW Mississippi Regional Medical Center	Clarksdale	Mississippi	662-627-3211	www.nwmsregionalmedcenter.com
O'Connor Hospital	San Jose	California	408-947-2500	www.oconnorhospital.org
Oakdale Community Hospital	Oakdale	Louisiana	318-335-3700	www.oakdalecommunityhospital.com
Oakwood Annapolis Hospital	Wayne	Michigan	734-467-4175	www.oakwood.org
Oakwood Hospital and Medical Center	Dearborn	Michigan	313-593-7125	www.oakwood.org
Ocean Medical Center	Brick	New Jersey	732-840-2200	www.meridianhealth.com/mcoc.cfm/ind
Olympia Medical Center	Los Angeles	California	310-657-5900	www.olympiamc.com
Oroville Hospital	Oroville	California	530-533-8500	www.orovillehospital.com
Our Lady of the Resurrection Medical Center	Chicago	Illinois	773-282-7000	www.reshealth.org
Palisades Medical Center - NY Presbyterian Healthcare System	North Bergen	New Jersey	201-854-5000	www.palisadesmedical.org
Palos Community Hospital	Palos Heights	Illinois	708-923-4000	www.paloshospital.org
Paul B Hall Regional Medical Center	Paintsville	Kentucky	606-789-3511	www.pbhrmc.com
Perry Community Hospital	Linden	Tennessee	931-589-2121	
Pineville Community Hospital	Pineville	Kentucky	606-337-3051	
Pitt County Memorial Hospital	Greenville	North Carolina	252-847-4100	www.uhseast.com
Plainview Hospital	Plainview	New York	516-719-3000	www.nslij.com
Pleasant Valley Hospital	Point Pleasant	West Virginia	304-675-4340	

Hospital	City	State	Phone	Web Site
Prince Georges Hospital Center	Cheverly	Maryland	301-618-2000	www.princegeorgeshospital.org
Raleigh General Hospital	Beckley	West Virginia	304-256-4100	
Raritan Bay Medical Center	Perth Amboy	New Jersey	732-442-3700	
Regional Medical Center of San Jose	San Jose	California	408-259-5000	www.regionalmedicalsanjose.com
RHC St Francis Hospital	Evanston	Illinois	847-316-4000	www.reshealth.org
Ripley County Memorial Hospital	Doniphan	Missouri	573-996-2141	
Robert Packer Hospital	Sayre	Pennsylvania	570-888-6666	www.guthrie.org
Robert Wood Johnson University Hospital at Rahway	Rahway	New Jersey	732-381-4200	www.rwjuhr.com/about/history.html
Robert Wood Johnson University Hospital Hamilton	Hamilton	New Jersey	609-586-7900	www.rwjhamilton.org
Rush University Medical Center	Chicago	Illinois	312-942-5000	www.ruch.edu
Russell County Medical Center	Lebanon	Virginia	276-883-8000	
Saint Peter's University Hospital	New Brunswick	New Jersey	732-745-7944	www.saintpetersuh.com
San Gabriel Valley Medical Center	San Gabriel	California	626-289-5454	www.sangabrielvalleymedctr.org
Sandhills Regional Medical Center	Hamlet	North Carolina	910-958-2361	www.hma-corp.com
Seton Health System-St Mary's Campus	Troy	New York	518-272-5000	www.setonhealth.org
Silver Cross Hospital	Joliet	Illinois	815-740-1100	www.silvercross.org
Sinai Hospital of Baltimore	Baltimore	Maryland	410-601-5131	www.sinai-balt.com
Sinai-Grace Hospital	Detroit	Michigan	313-966-3300	www.sinaigrace.org
Somerset Medical Center	Somerville	New Jersey	908-685-2200	www.somersetmedicalcenter.com
South Bay Hospital	Sun City Center	Florida	813-634-3301	www.southbayhospital.com
Southern Tennessee Medical Center	Winchester	Tennessee	931-967-8295	www.southerntennessee.com
Southwest General Health Center	Middleburg Heights	Ohio	440-816-8000	www.swgeneral.com
Southwest Mississippi Regional Medical Center	Mccomb	Mississippi	601-249-5500	www.smrmc.com
SSM Depaul Health Center	Bridgeton	Missouri	314-344-6000	www.ssmdepaul.com
SSM St Marys Health Center	Richmond Heights	Missouri	314-768-8000	
Saint Barnabas Hospital	Bronx	New York	212-960-9000	www.stbarnabashospital.org
Saint Bernard Hospital	Chicago	Illinois	773-962-3900	www.stbernardhospital.com
Saint Catherine Hospital	East Chicago	Indiana	219-392-7004	www.comhs.org/stcatherine
Saint Clair Memorial Hospital	Pittsburgh	Pennsylvania	412-561-4900	www.stclair.org
Saint James Hospital & Health Center-Olympia Fields	Olympia Fields	Illinois	708-747-4000	
Saint John Hospital and Medical Center	Detroit	Michigan	313-343-4000	www.stjohnprovidence.org
Saint Joseph's Regional Medical Center	Paterson	New Jersey	973-754-2000	www.sjhmc.org
Saint Luke's Roosevelt Hospital	New York	New York	212-523-4000	www.wehealny.org
Saint Mary Mercy Hospital	Livonia	Michigan	734-655-4800	www.stmarymercy.org
Saint Mary's Hospital - Passaic	Passaic	New Jersey	973-365-4300	www.smh-nj.com
Saint Marys Hospital	Centralia	Illinois	618-436-8000	www.stmarys-goodsamaritan.com
Saint Tammany Parish Hospital	Covington	Louisiana	985-898-4000	www.stph.org
Staten Island University Hospital	Staten Island	New York	718-226-9000	www.siuh.edu
Swedish American Hospital	Rockford	Illinois	815-968-4400	www.swedishamerican.org
Teche Regional Medical Center	Morgan City	Louisiana	504-384-2200	www.techeregional.com
The Regional Medical Center of Acadiana	Lafayette	Louisiana	337-989-6700	www.medicalcentersw.com
Thomas Jefferson University Hospital	Philadelphia	Pennsylvania	215-955-6000	www.jeffersonhospital.org
Trinitas Regional Medical Center	Elizabeth	New Jersey	908-994-5000	www.trinitashospital.org
Trinity Medical Center East & Trinity Medical Center West	Steubenville	Ohio	740-264-7212	www.trinityhealth.com
Tufts Medical Center	Boston	Massachusetts	617-636-5000	www.tuftsmedicalcenter.org
UHHS Bedford Medical Center	Bedford	Ohio	440-735-3628	www.uhhsbmc.com
Unity Hospital	Fridley	Minnesota	763-236-5000	www.mercyunity.com
University Hospital	Cincinnati	Ohio	513-584-1000	www.universityhospitalcincinnati.com
University of Illinois Hospital	Chicago	Illinois	312-996-3900	www.uic.edu
Valley Baptist Medical Center	Harlingen	Texas	956-389-1100	www.vbmc.org
Valley Baptist Medical Center - Brownsville	Brownsville	Texas	956-544-1400	www.brownsvillemedical.com
Vassar Brothers Medical Center	Poughkeepsie	New York	845-454-8500	www.vasserbrothers.org
Western Pennsylvania Hospital - Forbes Regional Campus	Monroeville	Pennsylvania	412-858-2000	www.wpahs.org
Westlake Regional Hospital	Columbia	Kentucky	270-384-4753	www.westlake-healthcare.org
White County Medical Center	Searcy	Arkansas	501-278-3100	www.centralarkhospital.com
Williamson ARH Hospital	South Williamson	Kentucky	606-237-1700	www.arh.org
Williamson Memorial Hospital	Williamson	West Virginia	304-235-2500	www.hmawmh.com
Woodhull Medical and Mental Health Center	Brooklyn	New York	718-963-8100	www.ci.nyc.ny.us
Yakima Regional Medical and Cardiac Center	Yakima	Washington	509-575-5102	www.yakimaregional.org
Yale-New Haven Hospital	New Haven	Connecticut	203-688-4242	www.ynhh.org

Note: Table shows hospitals nationwide whose Heart Failure 30-day readmission rate is worse (higher) than U.S. rate of 24.7%

Hospitals whose Pneumonia 30-Day Readmission Rate is Better (Lower) than the U.S. National Rate

Hospital	City	State	Phone	Web Site
Alpena Regional Medical Center	Alpena	Michigan	989-356-7390	www.agh.org
Augusta Health	Fishersville	Virginia	540-932-4000	www.augustamed.com
Ball Memorial Hospital	Muncie	Indiana	765-747-3111	www.accesschs.org/baal-memorial-l
Bayfront Medical Center	Saint Petersburg	Florida	727-823-1234	www.bayfront.org
Bloomington Hospital	Bloomington	Indiana	812-353-9555	bloomingtonhospital.org
Boca Raton Regional Hospital	Boca Raton	Florida	561-362-5002	
Central Washington Hospital	Wenatchee	Washington	509-662-1511	www.cwhs.com
Cherokee Regional Medical Center	Cherokee	Iowa	712-225-5101	www.cherokeermc.org
Christus Santa Rosa Hospital	San Antonio	Texas	210-794-3336	www.christussantarosa.org
Christus Spohn Hospital Corpus Christi	Corpus Christi	Texas	361-902-4103	www.christusspohn.org
Citrus Memorial Hospital	Inverness	Florida	352-726-1551	www.citrusmh.com
Conroe Regional Medical Center	Conroe	Texas	936-539-1111	www.conroeregional.com
The Corpus Christi Medical Center	Corpus Christi	Texas	361-761-1000	
East Jefferson General Hospital	Metairie	Louisiana	504-454-4000	www.EastJeffHospital.org
Elmhurst Memorial Hospital	Elmhurst	Illinois	630-833-1400	www.emhc.org
Georgetown Memorial Hospital	Georgetown	South Carolina	843-527-7000	www.gmhsc.com
Gulf Breeze Hospital	Gulf Breeze	Florida	850-934-2000	www.ebaptisthealthcare.org/GulfBreezeHospital/Default
Hamot Medical Center	Erie	Pennsylvania	814-877-6000	www.hamot.org
Howard Regional Health System	Kokomo	Indiana	765-453-8371	www.howardcommunity.org
Intermountain Medical Center	Murray	Utah	801-507-7000	intermountainhealthcare.org
Kootenai Medical Center	Coeur D'alene	Idaho	208-666-2003	www.kootenaihealth.org
Lancaster General Hospital	Lancaster	Pennsylvania	717-299-5511	www.lancastergeneral.org
Logan Regional Hospital	Logan	Utah	435-716-1000	intermountainhealthcare.org
Marshalltown Medical & Surgical Center	Marshalltown	Iowa	641-754-5151	www.everydaychampions.org
McDonough District Hospital	Macomb	Illinois	309-833-4101	www.mdh.org
McAlester Regional Health Center	Mcalester	Oklahoma	918-426-1800	www.mrhcok.com
McKay-Dee Hospital Center	Ogden	Utah	801-387-2800	intermountainhealthcare.org
Memorial Healthcare System	Chattanooga	Tennessee	423-495-2525	www.memorial.org
Memorial Hermann Hospital System	Houston	Texas	713-448-6796	www.memorialhermann.org
Memorial Hermann Memorial City Medical Center	Houston	Texas	713-242-3000	www.mhhs.org
Mercy Medical Center-Cedar Rapids	Cedar Rapids	Iowa	319-398-6011	www.mercycare.org
Methodist Hospital	San Antonio	Texas	210-575-4000	www.mh.sahealth.com
Midmichigan Medical Center-Midland	Midland	Michigan	989-839-3000	www.midmichigan.org
Munson Medical Center	Traverse City	Michigan	231-935-5000	www.munsonhealthcare.org
Naples Community Hospital	Naples	Florida	239-436-5000	www.nchmd.org
National Park Medical Center	Hot Springs	Arkansas	501-321-1000	www.nationalparkmedical.com
Nor Lea General Hospital	Lovington	New Mexico	575-396-6611	www.nlgh.org
Northwest Hospital	Seattle	Washington	206-364-0500	www.nwhospital.org
Olympic Medical Center	Port Angeles	Washington	360-417-7000	www.olympicmedical.org
Parkview Hospital	Fort Wayne	Indiana	260-373-4000	www.parkview.com
Peacehealth St Joseph Medical Center	Bellingham	Washington	360-734-5400	www.peacehealth.org
Presbyterian Hospital	Albuquerque	New Mexico	505-724-7281	www.phs.org
Providence Hospital	Mobile	Alabama	251-633-1000	www.providencehospital.org
Providence Portland Medical Center	Portland	Oregon	503-215-1111	www.providence.org/oregon
Rapid City Regional Hospital	Rapid City	South Dakota	605-719-1000	www.rcrh.org
Reading Hospital Medical Center	Reading	Pennsylvania	610-988-8000	www.readinghospital.org
Salinas Valley Memorial Hospital	Salinas	California	831-757-4333	www.svmh.com
San Juan Regional Medical Center	Farmington	New Mexico	505-609-2000	www.sanjuanregional.com
Santa Barbara Cottage Hospital	Santa Barbara	California	805-682-7111	www.cottagehealthsystem.org
Sarasota Memorial Hospital	Sarasota	Florida	941-917-9000	www.smh.com
Shenandoah Memorial Hospital	Woodstock	Virginia	540-459-1100	www.valleyhealthlink.com
Skaggs Community Health Center	Branson	Missouri	417-335-7000	www.skaggs.net
Spartanburg Regional Medical Center	Spartanburg	South Carolina	864-560-6000	www.srhs.com
Saint Edward Mercy Medical Center	Fort Smith	Arkansas	479-314-6000	www.stedwardmercy.com
Saint Elizabeth East	Lafayette	Indiana	765-502-4000	www.ste.org
Saint John Medical Center	Tulsa	Oklahoma	918-744-2345	www.sjmc.org
Saint John's Regional Health Center	Springfield	Missouri	417-820-2000	www.stjohns.com
Saint Lukes Magic Valley RMC	Twin Falls	Idaho	208-737-2103	www.stlukesonline.org/magic_valley
Waverly Health Center	Waverly	Iowa	319-352-4120	www.waverlyhealthcenter.org
Wesley Medical Center	Wichita	Kansas	316-962-2000	www.wesleymc.com
Wheaton Franciscan Healthcare - Elmbrook Memorial	Brookfield	Wisconsin	262-785-2000	www.mywheaton.org
Williamsport Hospital & Medical Center	Williamsport	Pennsylvania	570-321-1000	www.susquehannahealth.org
Willis Knighton Medical Center	Shreveport	Louisiana	318-632-4000	www.wkhs.com//Locations/MedicalCenter.aspx
Wooster Community Hospital	Wooster	Ohio	330-263-8100	www.woosterhospital.org

Note: Table shows hospitals nationwide whose Pneumonia 30-day readmission rate is better (lower) than U.S. rate of 18.3%

Hospitals whose Pneumonia 30-Day Readmission Rate is Worse (Higher) than the U.S. National Rate

Hospital	City	State	Phone	Web Site
Adena Regional Medical Center	Chillicothe	Ohio	740-779-7778	www.adena.org
Advocate Christ Hospital & Medical Center	Oak Lawn	Illinois	708-684-8000	www.advocatehealth.com
Advocate Lutheran General Hospital	Park Ridge	Illinois	847-723-2210	www.advocatehealth.com
Allegheny General Hospital	Pittsburgh	Pennsylvania	412-359-3131	www.allhealth.edu
Aurora St Lukes Medical Center	Milwaukee	Wisconsin	414-649-6000	www.aurorahealthcare.org
Baptist Medical Center South	Montgomery	Alabama	334-288-2100	www.baptistfirst.org/south
Barnes Jewish Hospital	Saint Louis	Missouri	314-747-3000	www.barnesjewish.com
Baxter Regional Medical Center	Mountain Home	Arkansas	870-508-1000	www.baxterregional.org
Bayshore Community Hospital	Holmdel	New Jersey	732-739-5900	www.bchs.com
Beth Israel Deaconess Medical Center	Boston	Massachusetts	617-667-7000	www.bidmc.harvard.edu
Beth Israel Medical Center	New York	New York	212-420-2000	www.wehealny.org
Botsford Hospital	Farmington Hills	Michigan	248-471-8000	www.botsfordsystem.org
Bronx-Lebanon Hospital Center	Bronx	New York	212-588-7000	www.bronx-leb.org
Brookhaven Memorial Hospital Medical Center	Patchogue	New York	631-654-7100	www.brookhavenhospitalorg
Brooklyn Hospital Center at Downtown Campus	Brooklyn	New York	718-250-8000	www.tbh.org
Cameron Regional Medical Center	Cameron	Missouri	816-632-2101	www.cameronregional.org
Carolina Pines Regional Medical Center	Hartsville	South Carolina	864-339-2100	www.cprmc.com
Centegra Health System - McHenry Hospital	Mchenry	Illinois	815-344-5000	www.centegra.org
Centegra Health System - Woodstock Hospital	Woodstock	Illinois	815-788-5823	
Centinela Hospital Medical Center	Inglewood	California	310-673-4660	www.centinelafreeman.com
Centrastate Medical Center	Freehold	New Jersey	732-431-2000	www.centrastate.com
Choctaw Memorial Hospital	Hugo	Oklahoma	580-317-9500	
Christ Hospital	Jersey City	New Jersey	201-795-8200	www.christhospital.org
Crockett Hospital	Lawrenceburg	Tennessee	931-762-6571	www.crocketthospital.com
Crossroads Community Hospital	Mount Vernon	Illinois	618-244-5500	www.crossroadscommnityhospital.com
Doctors Memorial Hospital	Bonifay	Florida	850-547-1120	www.pahn.org/dmh.cfm
Dyersburg Regional Medical Center	Dyersburg	Tennessee	731-285-2410	
East Orange General Hospital	East Orange	New Jersey	973-266-4401	www.evh.org
Elmhurst Hospital Center	Elmhurst	New York	718-334-1141	nyc.gov
Enloe Medical Center	Chico	California	530-332-7300	www.enloe.org
Fairmont General Hospital	Fairmont	West Virginia	304-367-7100	www.fghi.com
Faxton-St Luke's Healthcare	Utica	New York	315-798-6000	
Fayette County Hospital	Vandalia	Illinois	618-283-1231	
Fleming County Hospital	Flemingsburg	Kentucky	606-849-2351	www.flemingcountyhospital.org
Forest Hills Hospital	Forest Hills	New York	718-830-4000	www.northshorelij.com
Forrest General Hospital	Hattiesburg	Mississippi	601-288-7000	www.forrestgeneral.com
Galesburg Cottage Hospital	Galesburg	Illinois	309-345-4555	www.cottagehospital.com
Garden City Hospital	Garden City	Michigan	734-421-3300	www.gchosp.org
Georgiana Hospital	Georgiana	Alabama	334-376-2205	
Harlan Appalachian Regional Healthcare Hospital	Harlan	Kentucky	606-573-8100	www.arh.org
Hazard Arh Regional Medical Center	Hazard	Kentucky	606-439-6600	www.arh.org/hazard
Henry Ford Hospital	Detroit	Michigan	313-916-2600	www.henryfordhospital.com
Highlands Regional Medical Center	Sebring	Florida	863-385-6101	www.highlandsregional.com
Highlands Regional Medical Center	Prestonsburg	Kentucky	606-886-8511	www.hrmc.org
Hoboken University Medical Center	Hoboken	New Jersey	201-418-1004	www.bonsecoursnj.com
Holy Cross Hospital	Silver Spring	Maryland	301-754-7010	www.holycrosshealth.org
Holzer Medical Center	Gallipolis	Ohio	740-446-5000	www.holzer.org
Hospital of St Raphael	New Haven	Connecticut	203-789-3000	www.srhs.org
Jennersville Regional Hospital	West Grove	Pennsylvania	610-869-1000	www.jennersville.com
Jennie Stuart Medical Center	Hopkinsville	Kentucky	270-887-0100	www.jsmc.org
Jewish Hospital	Cincinnati	Ohio	513-686-3003	www.jewishhospitalcincinnati.com
John Ed Chambers Memorial Hospital	Danville	Arkansas	479-495-2241	
Johns Hopkins Bayview Medical Center	Baltimore	Maryland	410-550-0123	www.hopkinsbayview.org
Jordan Hospital	Plymouth	Massachusetts	508-746-2000	www.jordanhospital.org
Kennedy University Hospital	Stratford	New Jersey	856-346-6000	www.kennedyhealth.org
Kimball Medical Center	Lakewood	New Jersey	732-363-1900	www.sbhcs.com
Kings County Hospital Center	Brooklyn	New York	718-245-3901	www.nyc.gov/html/hhc/html/facilities/kings.shtml
Kingston Hospital	Kingston	New York	914-331-3131	www.kingstonregionalhealth.org
Lake Cumberland Regional Hospital	Somerset	Kentucky	606-679-7441	
Laughlin Memorial Hospital	Greeneville	Tennessee	423-787-5000	
Lee Regional Medical Center	Pennington Gap	Virginia	276-546-1440	www.leeregional.com
Liberty Hospital	Liberty	Missouri	816-781-7200	www.libertyhospital.org
Little Company of Mary Hospital	Evergreen Park	Illinois	708-422-6200	www.lcmh.org
Magee General Hospital	Magee	Mississippi	601-849-5070	www.mghosp.org

Hospital	City	State	Phone	Web Site
Magnolia Regional Health Center	Corinth	Mississippi	662-293-7660	www.mrhc.org
Mary Washington Hospital	Fredericksburg	Virginia	540-741-1100	www.medicorp.org
Maryland General Hospital	Baltimore	Maryland	410-225-8996	www.marylandgeneral.org
Marymount Hospital	Garfield Heights	Ohio	216-581-0500	www.marymount.org
Massena Memorial Hospital	Massena	New York	315-764-1711	www.massenahospital.org
Medical Center of Southeastern Oklahoma	Durant	Oklahoma	405-924-3080	www.mcsohealth.com
Medical Park Hospital	Hope	Arkansas	870-777-2323	www.medicalparkhospitals.com
Memorial Hermann Baptist Beaumont Hospital	Beaumont	Texas	409-212-5012	www.mhbh.org
Memorial Hospital at Easton	Easton	Maryland	410-822-1000	www.shorehealth.org
Memorial Hospital of Rhode Island	Pawtucket	Rhode Island	401-729-2000	mhriweb.org
Memorial Hospital of Salem County	Salem	New Jersey	856-935-1000	www.mhshealth.com
Mercy Fitzgerald Hospital	Darby	Pennsylvania	215-237-4000	www.mercyhealth.org
Mercy Memorial Health Center	Ardmore	Oklahoma	405-223-5400	www.mercyok.com/mmhc
Mercy Regional Medical Center	Ville Platte	Louisiana	337-363-5684	www.vpmc.com
Methodist Hospital	Henderson	Kentucky	270-827-7700	www.methodisthospital.net
Methodist Hospital of Chicago	Chicago	Illinois	773-271-9040	www.methodistchicago.org
Metro Health Medical Center	Cleveland	Ohio	216-778-5700	www.metrohealth.org
Midstate Medical Center	Meriden	Connecticut	203-694-8200	www.midstatemedical.org
Montefiore Medical Center	Bronx	New York	718-920-4321	www.montefiore.org
Mount Sinai Hospital	New York	New York	212-241-7981	www.mountsinai.org
Nassau University Medical Center	East Meadow	New York	516-572-0123	www.numc.edu
New York Community Hospital of Brooklyn	Brooklyn	New York	718-692-5302	www.nych.com
New York Downtown Hospital	New York	New York	212-312-5000	www.downtownhospital.org
New York Hospital Medical Center of Queens	Flushing	New York	718-670-1231	www.nyhq.org
New York Westchester Square Medical Center	Bronx	New York	718-430-7300	www.nywsmc.org
North Arkansas Regional Medical Center	Harrison	Arkansas	870-414-4000	www.narmc.com
North Carolina Baptist Hospital	Winston-Salem	North Carolina	336-716-2011	www.wfubmc.edu
North Central Bronx Hospital	Bronx	New York	212-519-5000	www.nyc.gov/html/hhc/ncbh/home.html
Northside Medical Center	Youngstown	Ohio	330-884-1000	
Northwest Community Hospital	Arlington Heights	Illinois	847-618-1000	www.nch.org
Northwestern Memorial Hospital	Chicago	Illinois	312-926-2000	www.nmh.org
Norwegian-American Hospital	Chicago	Illinois	773-292-8200	www.nahospital.org
O'Bleness Memorial Hospital	Athens	Ohio	740-593-5551	www.obleness.org
Oakdale Community Hospital	Oakdale	Louisiana	318-335-3700	www.oakdalecommunityhospital.com
Orange Regional Medical Center	Goshen	New York	845-343-2424	
Oroville Hospital	Oroville	California	530-533-8500	www.orovillehospital.com
Our Lady of the Resurrection Medical Center	Chicago	Illinois	773-282-7000	www.reshealth.org
Palos Community Hospital	Palos Heights	Illinois	708-923-4000	www.paloshospital.org
Parkview Regional Hospital	Mexia	Texas	254-562-5332	www.parkviewregional.com
Paul B Hall Regional Medical Center	Paintsville	Kentucky	606-789-3511	www.pbhrmc.com
Pottstown Memorial Medical Center	Pottstown	Pennsylvania	610-327-7000	www.pmmctr.org
Presbyterian Hospital	Charlotte	North Carolina	704-384-4000	www.presbyterian.org
Princeton Community Hospital	Princeton	West Virginia	304-487-7260	www.pchonline.org
Raritan Bay Medical Center	Perth Amboy	New Jersey	732-442-3700	
Regional Hospital of Jackson	Jackson	Tennessee	731-661-2000	www.regionalhospitaljackson.com
RHC St Francis Hospital	Evanston	Illinois	847-316-4000	www.reshealth.org
Rhode Island Hospital	Providence	Rhode Island	401-444-4000	www.rhodeislandhospital.org
River Park Hospital	McMinnville	Tennessee	931-815-4101	www.riverparkhospital.com
Riverview Regional Medical Center	Gadsden	Alabama	256-543-5200	www.riverviewregional.com
Robert Packer Hospital	Sayre	Pennsylvania	570-888-6666	www.guthrie.org
Robert Wood Johnson University Hospital	New Brunswick	New Jersey	732-828-3000	www.rwjuh.edu
Robert Wood Johnson University Hospital Hamilton	Hamilton	New Jersey	609-586-7900	www.rwjhamilton.org
Russell County Medical Center	Lebanon	Virginia	276-883-8000	
Russellville Hospital	Russellville	Alabama	256-332-1611	
Saint Francis Hospital	Tulsa	Oklahoma	918-494-2200	www.saintfrancis.com
Schuylkill Medical Center - South Jackson Street	Pottsville	Pennsylvania	570-621-5000	www.pottsvillehospital.com
Sinai-Grace Hospital	Detroit	Michigan	313-966-3300	www.sinaigrace.org
South Nassau Communities Hospital	Oceanside	New York	516-632-3000	www.southnassau.org
Southeastern Ohio Regional Medical Center	Cambridge	Ohio	740-439-8111	www.seormc.org
Southern Maryland Hospital Center	Clinton	Maryland	301-877-4530	www.smhcealth.org
SSM Depaul Health Center	Bridgeton	Missouri	314-344-6000	www.ssmdepaul.com
Saint Barnabas Hospital	Bronx	New York	212-960-9000	www.stbarnabashospital.org
Saint Bernard Hospital	Chicago	Illinois	773-962-3900	www.stbernardhospital.com
Saint Elizabeth's Medical Center	Brighton	Massachusetts	617-789-3000	www.semc.org
Saint Francis Hospital & Medical Center	Hartford	Connecticut	860-714-4000	www.saintfranciscare.com
Saint James Hospital & Health Center-Olympia Fields	Olympia Fields	Illinois	708-747-4000	
Saint John's Episcopal Hospital at South Shore	Far Rockaway	New York	718-869-7000	

Hospital	City	State	Phone	Web Site
Saint Joseph's Regional Medical Center	Paterson	New Jersey	973-754-2000	www.sjhmc.org
Saint Luke's Cornwall Hospital	Newburgh	New York	845-561-4400	www.stlukeshospital.org
Saint Lukes Hospital	Chesterfield	Missouri	314-434-1500	www.goodhealthmatters.com
Saint Mary Mercy Hospital	Livonia	Michigan	734-655-4800	www.stmarymercy.org
Saint Mary's Medical Center of Campbell County	La Follette	Tennessee	423-907-1200	www.stmaryshealth.com
Saint Marys Hospital	Centralia	Illinois	618-436-8000	www.stmarys-goodsamaritan.com
Saint Vincent Hospital	Worcester	Massachusetts	508-363-5000	www.stvincenthospital.com
Saint Vincent's Medical Center	Jacksonville	Florida	904-308-7300	www.jaxhealth.com
Stonewall Jackson Memorial Hospital	Weston	West Virginia	304-269-8080	www.stonewallhospital.com
Sweetwater Hospital Association	Sweetwater	Tennessee	865-213-8200	www.sweetwaterhospital.org
The Medical Center at Bowling Green	Bowling Green	Kentucky	270-745-1000	www.mcbg.org
Three Rivers Medical Center	Louisa	Kentucky	606-638-9451	www.threeriversmedicalcenter.com
Trego County Lemke Memorial Hospital	Wa Keeney	Kansas	785-743-2182	
UHHS Bedford Medical Center	Bedford	Ohio	440-735-3628	www.uhhsbmc.com
Unity Hospital of Rochester	Rochester	New York	585-723-7000	www.unityhealth.org
University Hospital	Cincinnati	Ohio	513-584-1000	www.universityhospitalcincinnati.com
University of Kansas Hospital	Kansas City	Kansas	913-588-7332	www.kumc.edu
Valley Medical Center	Renton	Washington	425-228-3450	www.valleymed.org
Vanderbilt University Hospital	Nashville	Tennessee	615-322-3454	www.mc.vanderbilt.edu
Vassar Brothers Medical Center	Poughkeepsie	New York	845-454-8500	www.vasserbrothers.org
The Washington Hospital	Washington	Pennsylvania	724-225-7000	www.washingtonhospital.org
Webster General Hospital	Eupora	Mississippi	662-258-6221	
Westlake Regional Hospital	Columbia	Kentucky	270-384-4753	www.westlake-healthcare.org
White County Medical Center	Searcy	Arkansas	501-278-3100	www.centralarkhospital.com
Wyckoff Heights Medical Center	Brooklyn	New York	718-963-7272	www.wyckoffhospital.org
Yale-New Haven Hospital	New Haven	Connecticut	203-688-4242	www.ynhh.org

Note: Table shows hospitals nationwide whose Pneumonia 30-day readmission rate is worse (higher) than U.S. rate of 18.3%

Hospital Heart Attack Readmission Rates: State and National Summary

Area	Number of Hospitals			
	Better than U.S. National Rate[1]	Worse than U.S. National Rate[2]	No Different than U.S. National Rate[3]	Number of Cases Too Small[4]
U.S. and Territories	29	45	2403	1999
Alabama	0	0	44	56
Alaska	0	0	4	13
American Samoa	0	0	0	0
Arizona	0	1	43	25
Arkansas	0	0	30	44
California	4	0	200	122
Colorado	0	0	29	36
Connecticut	0	1	28	2
Delaware	0	0	5	0
District of Columbia	0	0	5	2
Florida	4	1	140	37
Georgia	2	0	63	75
Guam	0	0	1	0
Hawaii	0	0	10	6
Idaho	0	0	9	24
Illinois	0	4	103	73
Indiana	4	2	61	50
Iowa	0	1	26	82
Kansas	0	0	25	84
Kentucky	0	0	43	53
Louisiana	0	1	49	55
Maine	0	0	25	11
Maryland	0	1	39	5
Massachusetts	0	4	53	7
Michigan	2	1	76	49
Minnesota	0	0	30	91
Mississippi	0	0	28	54
Missouri	2	2	51	55
Montana	0	0	9	37
N. Mariana Islands	0	0	0	1
Nebraska	0	0	18	55
Nevada	0	0	16	13
New Hampshire	0	0	18	8
New Jersey	0	3	67	4
New Mexico	0	0	11	24
New York	0	12	139	35
North Carolina	1	2	69	36
North Dakota	0	0	7	33
Ohio	0	4	104	50
Oklahoma	0	0	33	72
Oregon	1	0	27	28
Pennsylvania	2	3	125	32
Puerto Rico	0	0	26	21
Rhode Island	0	0	10	0
South Carolina	3	0	33	21
South Dakota	1	0	8	33
Tennessee	0	1	61	54
Texas	1	0	185	151
Utah	0	0	14	20
Vermont	0	0	10	4
Virgin Islands	0	0	1	1
Virginia	1	1	65	12
Washington	0	0	42	38
West Virginia	1	0	25	24
Wisconsin	0	0	58	59
Wyoming	0	0	2	22

Note: (1) 30-day readmission rate is better (lower) than U.S. rate of 19.9%; (2) 30-day readmission rate is worse (higher) than U.S. rate of 19.9%; (3) 30-day readmission rate is about the same as U.S. rate of 19.9%; (4) The number of cases is too small to classify the hospital

Hospital Heart Failure Readmission Rates: State and National Summary

Area	Number of Hospitals			
	Better than U.S. National Rate[1]	Worse than U.S. National Rate[2]	No Different than U.S. National Rate[3]	Number of Cases Too Small[4]
U.S. and Territories	147	193	3869	550
Alabama	2	2	93	4
Alaska	1	0	9	12
American Samoa	0	0	0	1
Arizona	1	0	60	17
Arkansas	1	3	69	4
California	9	7	280	51
Colorado	2	0	53	16
Connecticut	1	2	29	0
Delaware	0	0	5	0
District of Columbia	0	2	5	0
Florida	13	3	162	6
Georgia	8	1	126	11
Guam	0	0	1	0
Hawaii	0	1	12	6
Idaho	2	0	24	10
Illinois	1	18	160	4
Indiana	8	2	105	3
Iowa	3	0	101	12
Kansas	3	1	90	32
Kentucky	1	11	83	2
Louisiana	4	9	85	21
Maine	0	0	35	1
Maryland	1	7	37	1
Massachusetts	2	4	56	3
Michigan	6	7	112	8
Minnesota	2	1	102	25
Mississippi	1	7	78	8
Missouri	3	7	100	4
Montana	2	0	29	28
N. Mariana Islands	0	0	1	0
Nebraska	1	1	54	28
Nevada	0	0	27	6
New Hampshire	3	0	22	1
New Jersey	2	22	50	0
New Mexico	1	0	33	8
New York	1	28	155	6
North Carolina	5	6	92	6
North Dakota	0	0	31	11
Ohio	6	7	145	4
Oklahoma	0	4	87	27
Oregon	3	0	50	5
Pennsylvania	10	12	138	5
Puerto Rico	0	0	35	13
Rhode Island	1	1	8	0
South Carolina	3	1	53	2
South Dakota	1	0	28	25
Tennessee	2	5	107	3
Texas	12	5	303	59
Utah	5	0	23	12
Vermont	1	0	12	1
Virgin Islands	0	0	2	0
Virginia	4	2	73	4
Washington	6	1	63	17
West Virginia	0	3	46	3
Wisconsin	3	0	112	6
Wyoming	0	0	18	8

Note: (1) 30-day readmission rate is better (lower) than U.S. rate of 24.7%; (2) 30-day readmission rate is worse (higher) than U.S. rate of 24.7%; (3) 30-day readmission rate is about the same as U.S. rate of 24.7%; (4) The number of cases is too small to classify the hospital

Hospital Pneumonia Readmission Rates: State and National Summary

Area	Number of Hospitals			
	Better than U.S. National Rate[1]	Worse than U.S. National Rate[2]	No Different than U.S. National Rate[3]	Number of Cases Too Small[4]
U.S. and Territories	64	163	4223	363
Alabama	1	4	92	4
Alaska	0	0	16	6
American Samoa	0	0	0	0
Arizona	0	0	68	10
Arkansas	2	5	69	2
California	2	3	296	54
Colorado	0	0	63	12
Connecticut	0	4	27	1
Delaware	0	0	5	0
District of Columbia	0	0	7	0
Florida	6	3	170	9
Georgia	0	0	140	5
Guam	0	0	1	0
Hawaii	0	0	15	6
Idaho	2	0	31	4
Illinois	2	18	158	5
Indiana	5	0	111	2
Iowa	4	0	109	3
Kansas	1	2	113	12
Kentucky	0	11	84	2
Louisiana	2	2	93	23
Maine	0	0	36	0
Maryland	0	5	40	1
Massachusetts	0	4	59	3
Michigan	3	5	120	4
Minnesota	0	0	118	13
Mississippi	0	4	84	8
Missouri	2	5	105	5
Montana	0	0	44	16
N. Mariana Islands	0	0	1	0
Nebraska	0	0	78	7
Nevada	0	0	30	3
New Hampshire	0	0	26	1
New Jersey	0	12	62	0
New Mexico	3	0	37	3
New York	0	30	156	5
North Carolina	0	2	105	3
North Dakota	0	0	42	2
Ohio	1	10	148	4
Oklahoma	2	4	102	11
Oregon	1	0	55	2
Pennsylvania	4	7	149	6
Puerto Rico	0	0	36	13
Rhode Island	0	2	8	1
South Carolina	2	1	55	1
South Dakota	1	0	48	6
Tennessee	1	8	103	6
Texas	7	4	322	52
Utah	3	0	33	4
Vermont	0	0	14	0
Virgin Islands	0	0	2	0
Virginia	2	3	74	7
Washington	4	1	74	9
West Virginia	0	3	49	1
Wisconsin	1	1	116	3
Wyoming	0	0	23	4

Note: (1) 30-day readmission rate is better (lower) than U.S. rate of 18.3%; (2) 30-day readmission rate is worse (higher) than U.S. rate of 18.3%; (3) 30-day readmission rate is about the same as U.S. rate of 18.3%; (4) The number of cases is too small to classify the hospital

What Do These Readmission Categories Show?

"Readmission" is when patients who have had a recent stay in the hospital go back into a hospital again. The information shows how often patients are readmitted within 30 days of discharge from a previous hospital stay for heart attack, heart failure, or pneumonia. Patients may have been readmitted back to the same hospital or to a different hospital or acute care facility. They may have been readmitted for the same condition as their recent hospital stay, or for a different reason.

This appendix shows how different hospitals' rates of readmission for heart attack, heart failure, and pneumonia patients compared to the U.S. National Rate. You can see whether the 30-day risk-adjusted rate of readmission for a hospital is lower (better) than the national rate, no different than the national rate, or higher (worse) than the national rate, given how sick patients were when they were admitted to the hospital. For some hospitals, the number of cases is too small (fewer than 25) to reliably tell how well the hospital is performing, so no comparison to the national rate is shown.

Better than U.S. National Rate. Hospitals in the Better Than U.S. National Rate category have risk-adjusted 30-day readmission rates that are lower than the U.S. National rate, and we can be 95% certain that this difference is not due to chance.

No Different than U.S. National Rate. Many hospitals in the No Different Than U.S. National Rate category have risk-adjusted 30-day readmission rates that are about the same as the U.S. National rate. Other hospitals in this category have rates that are higher or lower than the U.S. National rate, but we cannot be 95% certain that these differences are not due to chance.

Worse than U.S. National Rate. Hospitals in the Worse Than U.S. National Rate category have risk-adjusted 30-day readmission rates that are higher than the U.S. National rate, and we can be 95% certain that this difference is not due to chance.

Number of Cases Too Small. The number of cases is too small to classify the hospital. One cannot be certain about differences when a hospital has very few relevant patients.

Why are Readmission Rates for Individual Hospitals Not Shown?

Comparisons based on estimated readmission rates alone can be misleading. Risk-adjusted readmission rates are estimated for individual hospitals based on information taken from a particular time period. If a slightly different time period had been chosen, chances are that each hospital's results would have been somewhat different.

Researchers almost always report a range ("confidence interval" or in this case an "interval estimate") around their estimates, to show how much variation might be due to this kind of chance. A confidence interval or interval estimate tells us we can be reasonably "confident" (in this case, 95% confident) that a hospital's readmission rate fell somewhere within this specified range. The smaller the range, the more precise the estimate.

When hospitals treat a very large number of patients, chance differences will not have much effect on the overall rates. The range will be small, and the estimated readmission rates will be more precise. In hospitals that treat smaller numbers of patients, however, even small chance differences could have a big impact on readmission rates. The 95% confidence interval, or range, will be large, and the estimated readmission rates will be much less precise.

Because the number of patients treated at U.S. hospitals varies widely, the precision of hospitals' estimated readmission rates also varies.

Calculation of 30-Day Risk-Standardized Rates of Readmission

The three readmission models estimate hospital-specific, risk-standardized, all-cause 30-day readmission rates for patients discharged alive to a non-acute care setting with a principal diagnosis of heart attack, heart failure, and pneumonia. For each condition, the risk-standardized ("adjusted" or "risk-adjusted") hospital readmission rate can be used to compare performance across hospitals. The readmission measures for heart attack, heart failure, and pneumonia have been endorsed by the National Quality Forum (NQF).

Because of the way hospitals are paid under Medicare in Maryland, readmissions to hospital-owned rehabilitation and psychiatric facilities were counted as readmissions to acute care hospitals. This adversely impacted the 30-day readmission rates for some Maryland hospitals. CMS suppressed the readmission measures results for Maryland Hospitals in June 2009 due to these coding issues unique to Maryland.

CMS has resolved this coding issue to accurately reflect readmissions in Maryland for the June 2010 (and beyond) updates of the readmission data for Maryland hospitals and will no longer suppress readmission measures results for Maryland Hospitals.

Data Collection Methods

Cases Included in the Model. For each of the three principal discharge diagnoses (heart attack, heart failure, and pneumonia), the model includes admissions to all short-stay acute-care hospitals for people age 65 years or older who are enrolled in Original Medicare (traditional fee-for-service Medicare) and who have a complete claims history for 12 months prior to admission.

Excluded Admissions. For the heart attack, heart failure, and pneumonia readmission measures, admissions are excluded if they meet any of the following criteria:

- Admissions for patients with an in-hospital death are excluded because they are not eligible for readmission.

- Admissions for patients subsequently transferred to another acute care facility are excluded because we are focusing on discharges to non-acute care settings.

- Admissions for patients who are discharged against medical advice (AMA) are excluded because providers did not have the opportunity to deliver full care and prepare the patient for discharge.

- Admissions for patients without at least 30 days post-discharge enrollment in fee-for-service Medicare are excluded because the 30-day readmission outcome cannot be assessed in this group.

- If a patient has one or more additional admissions for the given condition (heart attack, heart failure, or pneumonia) within 30 days of discharge from an index admission- Opens in a new window, we do not consider the additional admissions as index admissions- Opens in a new window (they are considered as readmissions). Thus, any admission is either an index admission- Opens in a new window or a readmission, but not both.

For the heart attack readmission measure only, the following exclusion criterion also applies:

- Admissions are excluded for patients who are discharged alive on the same day that they are admitted because these patients are unlikely to have had a heart attack.

Admissions Not Counted As Readmissions

The measure does not count as readmissions claims for same-day readmissions to the same hospital for the same condition. This is done to put all hospitals on an even playing field, as CMS rules already require Prospective Payment System (PPS) acute-care hospitals to combine same-day, same condition readmissions into one claim (so the readmission would appear as part of the initial stay in the administrative data).

For the heart attack readmission measure only, readmissions within 30 days for percutaneous transluminal coronary angioplasty (PTCA) or coronary artery bypass graft (CABG) procedures are not counted as readmissions if they likely represent planned readmissions that are part of the same episode of care as the index admission.

Use of a 30-Day Period to Assess Readmissions

The model tracks readmissions that occur within 30 days of a hospital discharge, rather than readmission over some other post-discharge period. Thirty-day readmission was chosen over longer windows (such as 90 days), because readmission over longer periods may have less to do with the care received in the hospital and more to do with other complicating illnesses, patients' own behavior, or the care they received after discharge.

Use of Administrative Claims Data

Administrative claims data, rather than medical record data, are used to predict 30-day readmission. These data are widely available for people with Original Medicare (traditional fee-for-service), are relatively inexpensive to acquire, and are timely. Using administrative data makes it possible to calculate readmission without having to do chart reviews or requiring hospitals to report additional data. Research conducted when the measures were being developed demonstrated that the administrative claims-based models perform well in predicting readmission compared with models based on chart reviews.

Risk-Adjustment and Covariates Included in the Model

Risk-Adjustment. For each of the three principal discharge diagnoses (heart attack, heart failure, and pneumonia), the model adjusts for differences in patients' risks unrelated to their hospital care (risk-adjustment). The characteristics that Medicare patients bring with them when they arrive at a hospital with a heart attack, heart failure, or pneumonia are not under the control of the hospital. However, some patient characteristics may make readmission more likely (increase the "risk" of readmission), no

matter where the patient is treated or how good the care is. Moreover, some hospitals may treat people with a history of more severe disease. Therefore, when readmission rates are calculated for each hospital, they are adjusted based on the unique mix of patients that the hospital treated during the study period. Factors included in the risk-adjustment model include age, gender, past medical history, and other diseases or conditions (comorbidities) that patients had when they arrived at the hospital and increase their risk of readmission.

Past medical history and comorbidities are included in the model using CMS's Condition Categories (CCs) and a history of certain procedures. Medicare patients are assigned to one or more CCs based on diagnoses (ICD-9 codes) obtained from the patient's discharge claim, and from the hospital inpatient, hospital outpatient, and physician Medicare claims submitted for the patient up to 12 months prior to the admission. Secondary diagnoses from the patient's hospital discharge claim that might represent complications that occurred while the patient was in the hospital, rather than conditions that were present on admission, are not included in assigning the patient's CCs. Research has shown that coding differences among providers affect CCs only slightly. Diagnoses from unreliable sources (such as laboratory or other claims that were not based on face-to-face encounters) are not included when assigning the CCs in the model.

To "risk-adjust" readmission rates for patient characteristics, the statistical model estimates the independent effects of age, gender, past medical history, comorbidities, and a hospital-specific component of quality on readmission of patients within 30 days of hospital discharge (the dependent variable). Using these estimates, the model calculates an adjusted readmission rate for each hospital that can be compared with those of other hospitals with different case mixes.

Statistical Methods Used to Calculate Readmission Rates

Hierarchical Regression Model. The statistical model for computing the 30-day risk-standardized readmission rates is a "hierarchical regression model." This type of model is based on the assumption that any heart attack, heart failure, or pneumonia patient treated at a particular hospital will experience a level of quality of care that applies to all patients treated for the same condition in that hospital. In other words, the expected risk of readmission for two similar heart attack, heart failure, or pneumonia patients treated in the same hospital would be more alike than the risk of readmission for the same two patients treated in two different hospitals. The likelihood that an individual patient will be readmitted is therefore a combination of:

- his or her individual risk characteristics (for example, gender, comorbidities, and past medical history) and

- the hospital's unique quality of care for all patients treated for that condition in that hospital.

The model estimates the effects of both of these components on on risk of readmission.

Calculating Readmission Rates. Each hospital's 30-day risk-standardized readmission rate (RSRR) is computed in several steps. First, the predicted 30-day readmission for a particular hospital obtained from the hierarchical regression model is divided by the expected readmission for that hospital, which is also obtained from the regression model. Predicted readmission is the number of readmissions (following discharge for heart attack, heart failure, or pneumonia) that would be anticipated in the particular hospital during the study period, given the patient case mix and the hospital's unique quality of

Covariates in 30-Day Risk-Standardized Readmission Models		
Heart Attack	Heart Failure	Pneumonia
Age, years over 65	Age, years over 65	Age, years over 65
Males	Males	Males
History of percutaneous transluminal coronary angioplasty (PTCA)		
History of coronary artery bypass graft (CABG) surgery	History of coronary artery bypass graft (CABG) surgery	History of coronary artery bypass graft (CABG) surgery
Anterior myocardial infarction		
Other location of myocardial infarction		
	Cardio-respiratory failure or shock	Cardio-respiratory failure or shock
History of congestive heart failure	History of congestive heart failure	History of congestive heart failure
Acute coronary syndrome	Acute coronary syndrome	Acute coronary syndrome
Angina pectoris/old myocardial infarction		
Coronary atherosclerosis		
	Coronary atherosclerosis or angina	Coronary atherosclerosis or angina
Valvular or rheumatic heart disease	Valvular or rheumatic heart disease	Valvular or rheumatic heart disease
Arrhythmias	Arrhythmias	Arrhythmias
	Other heart disorders	
Stroke	Stroke	Stroke
Cerebrovascular disease		
Hemiplegia, paraplegia, paralysis, functional disability	Hemiplegia, paraplegia, paralysis, functional disability	Hemiplegia, paraplegia, paralysis, functional disability
Vascular or circulatory disease	Vascular or circulatory disease	Vascular or circulatory disease
Diabetes or DM complications	Diabetes or DM complications	Diabetes or DM complications
Renal failure	Renal failure	Renal failure
End-stage renal disease or dialysis	End-stage renal disease or dialysis	End-stage renal disease or dialysis
Chronic obstructive pulmonary disease (COPD)	Chronic obstructive pulmonary disease (COPD)	Chronic obstructive pulmonary disease (COPD)
History of pneumonia	History of pneumonia	History of pneumonia
	Lung fibrosis or other chronic lung disorders	Lung fibrosis or other chronic lung disorders
Asthma	Asthma	Asthma
	Pleural effusion/pneumothorax	Pleural effusion/pneumothorax
	Other lung disorders	Other lung disorders
	Severe hematological disorders	Severe hematological disorders
Iron deficiency or other unspecified anemias and blood disease	Iron deficiency or other unspecified anemias and blood disease	Iron deficiency or other unspecified anemias and blood disease
Dementia or other specified brain disorders	Dementia or other specified brain disorders	Dementia or other specified brain disorders
	Drug/alcohol abuse/dependence/psychosis	Drug/alcohol abuse/dependence/psychosis
	Major psychiatric disorders	Major psychiatric disorders
	Depression	
	Other psychiatric disorders	Other psychiatric disorders
Metastatic cancer or acute leukemia	Metastatic cancer or acute leukemia	Metastatic cancer or acute leukemia
Cancer	Cancer	
		Lung or other severe cancers
		Other major cancers
Protein-calorie malnutrition	Protein-calorie malnutrition	Protein-calorie malnutrition
Disorders of fluid/electrolyte/acid-base	Disorders of fluid/electrolyte/acid-base	Disorders of fluid/electrolyte/acid-base
	End stage liver disease	
	Peptic ulcer, hemorrhage, other specified gastrointestinal disorders	
	Other gastrointestinal disorders	Other gastrointestinal disorders
History of infection	History of infection	History of infection
		Septicemia/shock
	Nephritis	
		Urinary tract infection
Other urinary tract disorders	Other urinary tract disorders	Other urinary tract disorders
Decubitus ulcer or chronic skin ulcer	Decubitus ulcer or chronic skin ulcer	Decubitus ulcer or chronic skin ulcer
		Vertebral fractures
		Other injuries

care effect on readmission. Expected readmission is the number of readmissions (following discharge for heart attack, heart failure, or pneumonia) that would be expected if the same patients with the same characteristics had instead been treated at an "average" hospital, given the "average" hospital's quality of care effect on readmission for patients with that condition. This ratio is then multiplied by the national unadjusted readmission rate for the condition for all hospitals to compute an RSRR for the hospital. So, the higher a hospital's predicted 30-day readmission rate, relative to expected readmission for the hospital's particular case mix of patients, the higher its adjusted readmission rate will be. Hospitals with better quality will have lower rates.

(Predicted 30-day readmission/Expected readmission) * U.S. National readmission rate = RSRR

For example, suppose the model predicts that 10 of Hospital A's heart attack admissions would be readmitted within 30 days of discharge in a given year, based on their age, gender, and pre-existing health conditions, and based on the estimate of the hospital's specific quality of care. Then, suppose that the expected number of 30-day readmissions for those same patients were higher – say, 15 – if they had instead been treated at an "average" U.S. hospital. If the actual readmission rate for the study period for all heart attack admissions in all hospitals in the U.S. is 12 percent, then the hospital's 30-day risk-standardized readmission rate would be 8 percent.

RSRR for Hospital A = (10/15)* 12% = 8%

If, instead, 9 of these patients would be expected to have been readmitted if treated at the "average" hospital, then the hospital's readmission rate would be 13.3 percent.

RSRR for Hospital A = (10/9)* 12% = 13.3%

In the first case, the hospital performed better than the national average and had a relatively low risk-standardized readmission rate (8 percent); in the second case, it performed worse and had a relatively high rate (13.3 percent).

Hospitals with relatively low-risk patients whose predicted readmission is the same as the expected readmission for the average hospital for the same group of low-risk patients would have an adjusted readmission rate equal to the national rate (12 percent in this example). Similarly, hospitals with high-risk patients whose predicted readmission is the same as the expected readmission for the average hospital for the same group of high-risk patients would also have an adjusted readmission rate equal to the national rate of 12 percent. Thus, each hospital's case mix should not affect the adjusted readmission rates used to compare hospitals.

Adjusting for Small Hospitals or a Small Number of Cases. The hierarchical regression model also adjusts readmission rate results for small hospitals or hospitals with few heart attack, heart failure, or pneumonia cases in a given reference period. This reduces the chance that such hospitals' performance will fluctuate wildly from year to year or that they will be wrongly classified as either a worse or a better performer. For these hospitals, the model not only considers readmissions among patients treated for the condition in the small sample size of cases, but pools together patients from all hospitals treated for the given condition, to make the result more reliable. In essence, the predicted readmission rate for a hospital with a small number of cases is moved toward the overall U.S. National readmission rate for all hospitals. The estimates of readmission for hospitals with few patients will rely considerably on the pooled data for all hospitals, making it less likely that small hospitals will fall into either of the outlier categories. This pooling affords a "borrowing of statistical strength" that provides more confidence in the results.

Significance Testing and Interval Estimates

The model also calculates how precise the estimates of the adjusted readmission rate are, and determines upper and lower bounds (Interval Estimates) for each hospital's risk-standardized readmission rate. Interval estimates, which are like confidence intervals, describe how much uncertainty there is around the rate—how much bigger or smaller the rate might really be. Larger hospitals typically have more precise estimates and smaller interval estimates, since more data are available to estimate readmission. The smaller the sample size, the greater the difference in readmission rates between a hospital and the national rate must be in order for that difference to be statistically meaningful.

Comparing Readmission Rates Among Hospitals

The risk-standardized hospital rate with its interval estimate can be compared to the U.S. National crude readmission rate. If the interval estimate includes (overlaps with) the national crude readmission rate, the hospital's performance is in the "no different than U.S. National rate" category. If the entire interval estimate is below the national crude readmission rate, then the hospital is performing "better than U.S. National rate." If the entire interval estimate is above the national crude readmission rate, it is "worse than U.S. National rate." Hospitals with extremely few cases—those with fewer than 25 qualifying cases in the 3-year period—will be reported separately as: "number of cases too small (fewer than 25) to reliably tell how the hospital is performing."

Glossary of Terms

Accreditation
An evaluative process in which a healthcare organization undergoes an examination of its policies, procedures and performance by an external private sector organization ("accrediting body") to ensure that it is meeting predetermined criteria. It usually involves both on- and off-site surveys. Also see the terms AOA, The Joint Commission, and Medicare-Certified Hospitals.

Acute Care Hospital
A hospital that provides inpatient medical care and other related services for surgery, acute medical conditions or injuries (usually for a short term illness or condition).

Acute Myocardial Infarction (AMI)
A condition (also called a heart attack) that occurs when the arteries leading to the heart become blocked and the blood supply is slowed or stopped. When the heart muscle can't get the oxygen and nutrients it needs, the part of the heart tissue that is affected may die.

American Hospital Association (AHA)
The national organization that represents and serves all types of hospitals, health care networks, and their patients and communities. AHA takes part in national health policy development, legislative and regulatory debates, and legal matters. AHA provides education for health care leaders and is a source of information on health care issues and trends.

American Osteopathic Association (AOA)
A member association representing approximately 52,000 osteopathic physicians (D.O.s). The AOA serves as the primary certifying body for D.O.s, and is the accrediting agency for all osteopathic medical colleges and health care facilities. The AOA writes a performance report on each hospital that it checks. You can call or write to AOA to find out a hospital's level of accreditation.

Angioplasty
In angioplasty, a catheter is used to insert a balloon that is inflated to open a blocked blood vessel. Percutaneous transluminal coronary angioplasty (PTCA) is one of several procedures used to open a blocked blood vessel, known collectively as a percutaneous coronary intervention or PCI.

Angiotensin Converting Enzyme (ACE) Inhibitor
A medicine used to treat heart attacks, heart failure, or a decreased function of the left heart. They stop production of a hormone that can narrow blood vessels. This helps reduce the pressure in the heart and lower blood pressure.

Angiotensin Receptor Blocker (ARB)
A medicine used to treat patients with heart failure and a decreased function of the left heart. ARBs block the action of a hormone that can narrow blood vessels. This helps reduce the pressure in the heart and lower blood pressure.

Antibiotic
Medicine used to fight bacteria in the body.

Atherectomy
A procedure where a blade or laser on a catheter cuts through and removes blockages in blood vessels. It is one of several procedures used to open a blocked blood vessel (known as a Percutaneous Coronary Intervention or PCI).

Beta Blocker
A type of medicine that is used to lower blood pressure, treat chest pain (angina) and heart failure, and to help prevent a heart attack. Beta blockers relieve the stress on the heart by slowing the heart rate and reducing the force with which the heart muscles contract to pump blood. They also help keep blood vessels from constricting in the heart, brain, and body.

Blood Culture
A blood test that shows if there are bacteria in the blood, and what type of bacteria it is. It helps your doctor decide which antibiotic to use to treat a bacterial infection.

Centers for Medicare & Medicaid Services (CMS)
The federal agency that runs the Medicare program for the elderly aged and disabled. In addition, CMS works with the states to run the Medicaid program for low-income individuals. CMS works to make sure that the people in these programs are able to get high quality health care. Also see the term DHHS.

Certification (Medicare-Certified)
State government agencies inspect health care providers, including hospitals, nursing homes, dialysis facilities and home health agencies, as well as other health care providers. These providers are certified if they pass inspection. Being certified is not the same as being accredited. Medicare or Medicaid only pays for care provided by certified or accredited providers.

Critical Access Hospital (CAH)
A small, generally geographically remote facility that provides outpatient and inpatient hospital services to people in rural areas. The designation was established by law, for special payments under the Medicare program. To be designated as a CAH, a hospital must be located in a rural area, provide 24-hour emergency services; have an average length-of-stay for its patients of 96 hours or less; be located more than 35 miles (or more than 15 miles in areas with mountainous terrain) from the nearest hospital or be designated by its State as a "necessary provider". Hospitals may have no more than 25 beds.

Department of Health and Human Services (DHHS)
A division of the U.S. government that administers many of the social programs at the Federal level dealing with the health and welfare of the citizens of the United States. CMS is an agency within DHHS.

Diastolic Pressure
The lowest pressure in the artery when the heart is filling with blood. In a blood pressure reading, the diastolic pressure is the second number recorded.

Do hospitals that treat sicker patients have worse death rates? (Risk-adjustment)
Hospitals that treat sicker patients do not necessarily have worse death rates. The hospital-specific 30-day death (mortality) rates used in this report have been adjusted to account for differences in patients' health before their hospital admission.

Sicker patients or patients with more health-related risks may be more likely to die than healthier patients. Moreover, patients who are sicker may be more likely to be treated at particular hospitals while patients who are healthier may be more likely to be treated at other hospitals.

To compare hospitals fairly (and to avoid penalizing those that treat sicker patients) it is therefore important to consider differences in patients' health before they were admitted to the hospital. The statistical process of accounting for differences in patients' sickness before they were admitted to the hospital is called risk-adjustment. This statistical process aims to 'level the playing field' by accounting for health risks that patients have before they enter the hospital.

Fibrinolysis, Fibrinolytic Drugs
Fibrinolytic drugs are "clot-busting" medicines that can help dissolve blood clots in blood vessels and improve blood flow to your heart. They are important for treating heart attacks. If you have a heart attack, your doctor may give you a fibrinolytic drug, perform a percutaneous coronary intervention (PCI), or both.

Hospital Quality Alliance (HQA): Improving Care Through Information
In December 2002, the American Hospital Association (AHA), Federation of American Hospitals (FAH), and Association of American Medical Colleges (AAMC) launched the Hospital Quality Alliance (HQA), a national public-private collaboration to encourage hospitals to voluntarily collect and report hospital quality performance information. This effort is intended to make important information about hospital performance accessible to the public and to inform and invigorate efforts to improve quality. CMS and the Joint Commission participate in the HQA, along with the AHA, the FAH, the AAMC, the American Medical Association, the American Nurses Association, the National Association of Children's Hospitals and Related Organizations, American Association of Retired People, American Federation of Labor and Council of Industrial Organizations, the Consumer-Purchaser Disclosure Project, the Agency for Healthcare Research and Quality, the National Quality Forum, the Blue Cross and Blue Shield Association, the National Business Coalition on Health, General Electric, and the U.S. Chamber of Commerce.

Influenza
Influenza is a serious and sometimes deadly lung infection that can spread quickly in a community. Symptoms include fever-often a high temperature of more than 102° Fahrenheit (38.9° Celsius), headache, muscle aches and pains, chills, cough and chest pain when you take a breath ("pleuritic chest pain"). Although most people recover from the illness, the Centers for Disease Control and Prevention (the CDC) estimates that in the United States more than 200,000 people are hospitalized and about 36,000 people die from the flu and its complications every year.

Influenza Vaccination ("Flu Shot")
The main way to keep from getting flu is to get a yearly flu vaccination. Scientists make a different vaccine every year because the strains of flu viruses change from year to year. Nine to 10 months before the flu season begins, they prepare a new vaccine made from inactivated (killed) flu viruses. Because the viruses have been killed, they cannot cause infection. The vaccine preparation is based on the strains of the flu viruses that are in circulation at the time.

Hospitals should check to make sure that pneumonia patients get a flu shot during flu season to protect them from another lung infection and to help prevent the spread of

influenza in the community. You can also get the vaccine at your doctor's office or a local clinic, and in many communities at workplaces, supermarkets, and drugstores. You must get the vaccine every year because it changes.

Inpatient Hospital Services
Services provided to patients admitted to a hospital that include bed and board, nursing services, diagnostic or therapeutic services, and medical or surgical services.

Left Ventricular Function Assessment
A test to check how well the heart is pumping.

Long-term Care Hospital
A facility, like a nursing home, that provides a variety of services that help people with health or personal needs and activities of daily living (like walking, eating, and going to the bathroom) over a period of time. Most long-term care is custodial care, for which Medicare does not pay.

Measurement
The process of collecting data to assess performance conducted at a single point in time or repeated over time.

Medicaid
A joint federal and state program that helps with medical costs for some people with low incomes and limited resources. Medicaid programs vary from state to state, but most health care costs are covered if you qualify for both Medicare and Medicaid.

Medicare-Certified Hospital
In order to receive any payment from either the Medicare or Medicaid programs, a hospital must meet a set of basic standards for quality of care, called "conditions of participation". Medicare-certified hospitals are reviewed periodically (every three years) to assure that they are continuing to provide services of acceptable quality.

Medicare also considers or "deems" hospitals as Medicare-certified that meet the accreditation requirements of the The Joint Commission or the American Osteopathic Association. Most short-term acute care hospitals in the United States choose to be Medicare-certified, either directly or through accreditation.

Medicare Provider Number
Medicare identifies the hospitals with which it works using a unique number. These numbers were used to identify the facilities that reported data for Hospital Compare. If hospitals share a Medicare Provider Number (for example, they bill Medicare for services as a single legal entity), the performance data for those hospitals are, in effect, combined into an aggregate rate representing all of the hospitals represented by the Medicare Provider Number. If you are interested in a hospital that is part of a system or network, you may not be able to find your specific hospital.

Medigap Policy
A Medicare supplement insurance policy sold by private insurance companies to fill "gaps" in Original Medicare Plan coverage. Except in Massachusetts, Minnesota and Wisconsin, there are 10 standardized plans labeled Plan A through Plan J. Medigap policies only work with the Original Medicare Plan.

Original Medicare Plan
A pay-per-visit health plan that lets you go to any doctor, hospital, or other health care supplier who accepts Medicare and is accepting new Medicare patients. You must pay the deductible. Medicare pays its share of the Medicare-approved amount, and you pay your share (coinsurance). In some cases you may be charged more than the Medicare-approved amount. The Original Medicare Plan has two parts: Part A (Hospital Insurance) and Part B (Medical Insurance).

Osteopathic Doctor
A licensed physician who can do surgery and prescribe drugs who has training in manipulative therapy. Also called a Doctor of Osteopathy or DO.

Outcome Measures
Measures designed to reflect the results of care, rather than how frequently a specific treatment or intervention was performed.

Oxygenation Assessment
Test that measures the amount of oxygen in your blood to see if you need oxygen therapy.

Percutaneous Coronary Interventions (PCI)
The procedures called Percutaneous Coronary Interventions (PCI), such as angioplasty and atherectomy are among those that are the most effective for opening blocked blood vessels that cause heart attacks. Doctors may perform a PCI, or give medicine to open the blockage, and in some cases, may do both.

Plan of Care
A written plan of care created with your physician and hospital staff. It tells what services you will get to reach and keep your best physical, mental, and social well being. The hospital staff keeps your doctor up-to-date on how you are doing and updates your care plan as needed.

Pneumonia
An inflammation of the lungs caused by a viral or bacterial infection. This fills your lungs with mucus and lowers the oxygen level in your blood. Symptoms can include fever, fatigue, difficulty breathing, chills, a "wet" cough, and chest pain.

Pneumonia (pneumococcal) Vaccination
Vaccine given to prevent pneumonia, estimated to protect against 80% of bacteria causing pneumonia.

Process of Care Measures
Measures that show, in percentage form or as a rate, how often a health care provider gives recommended care; that is, the treatment known to give the best results for most patients with a particular condition.

Provider
A doctor, hospital, health care professional, or health care facility.

Psychiatric Hospital
A facility that provides inpatient psychiatric services for the diagnosis and treatment of mental illness on a 24-hour basis, by or under the supervision of a physician.

Quality
Quality health care is how well a doctor, hospital, health plan, or other provider of health care, keeps its members healthy or treats them when they are sick. Good quality health care means doing the right thing at the right time, in the right way, for the right person and getting the best possible results.

Quality Assurance
The process of looking at how well a medical service is provided. The process may include formally reviewing health care given to a person, or group of persons, locating the problem, correcting the problem, and then checking to see if what you did worked.

Quality Improvement Organizations (QIOs)
Groups of practicing doctors and other health care experts who are paid by the federal government to check and improve the care given to Medicare patients. They must review your complaints about the quality of care given by: inpatient hospitals, hospital outpatient departments, hospital emergency rooms, skilled nursing facilities, home health agencies, Private Fee-for-Service plans, and ambulatory surgical centers.

Rehabilitation Hospital
A hospital that specializes in improving or restoring a patient's functional ability through therapies. Sometimes called a post-acute hospital.

Risk-Adjusted 30-Day Death (Mortality) Rates
The 30-day Risk-Adjusted Death (Mortality) Rates are produced using a complex statistical model, that relies on Medicare claims and enrollment information. The model predicts patient deaths for any cause within 30 days of hospital admission for heart attack or heart failure, whether the patients die while still in the hospital or after discharge. Thirty-day mortality is used because this is the time period when deaths are most likely to be related to the care patients received in the hospital. Deaths that occur outside the hospital within 30 days are included along with deaths that occur in the hospital, because some hospitals discharge patients sooner than others.

Stent
A small wire tube inserted in a blood vessel by a catheter to hold open a blocked blood vessel. One of several procedures to open a blocked blood vessel called a percutaneous coronary intervention (PCI).

The Joint Commission
An organization that evaluates and accredits health care organizations and programs in the United States. The Joint Commission is an independent, not-for-profit organization. The Joint Commission looks at how well a hospital treats patients and how good a hospital's staff and equipment are. A hospital is accredited by The Joint Commission if it meets certain quality standards. These checks are done at least every 3 years. Most hospitals take part in these accreditations.

The Joint Commission writes a "performance report" on each hospital that it checks. You can order these reports free of charge.

Thirty-Day Mortality Model Information
See Krumholtz, H., et al. "An Administrative Claims Model Suitable for Profiling Hospital Performance Based on 30-Day Mortality Rates Among Patients with an Acute Myocardial Infarction." Circulation. Vol. 113: 1683-1692, 2006, for details on the development of the AMI model. An accompanying article in the same volume discusses the heart failure model.

Treatment
Something done to help with a health problem. For example, medicine and surgery are treatments.

Treatment Options
The choices you have when there is more than one way to treat your health problem.

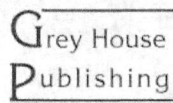

General Reference

American Environmental Leaders: From Colonial Times to the Present
An African Biographical Dictionary
An Encyclopedia of Human Rights in the United States
Encyclopedia of African-American Writing
Encyclopedia of Gun Control & Gun Rights
Encyclopedia of Invasions & Conquests
Encyclopedia of Prisoners of War & Internment
Encyclopedia of Religion & Law in America
Encyclopedia of Rural America
Encyclopedia of the United States Cabinet, 1789-2010
Encyclopedia of War Journalism
Encyclopedia of Warrior Peoples & Fighting Groups
From Suffrage to the Senate: America's Political Women
Nations of the World
Political Corruption in America
Speakers of the House of Representatives, 1789-2009
The Environmental Debate: A Documentary History
The Evolution Wars: A Guide to the Debates
The Religious Right: A Reference Handbook
The Value of a Dollar: 1860-2009
The Value of a Dollar: Colonial Era
University & College Museums, Galleries & Related Facilities
US Land & Natural Resource Policy
Weather America
Working Americans 1770-1869 Vol. IX: Revol. War to the Civil War
Working Americans 1880-1999 Vol. I: The Working Class
Working Americans 1880-1999 Vol. II: The Middle Class
Working Americans 1880-1999 Vol. III: The Upper Class
Working Americans 1880-1999 Vol. IV: Their Children
Working Americans 1880-2003 Vol. V: At War
Working Americans 1880-2005 Vol. VI: Women at Work
Working Americans 1880-2006 Vol. VII: Social Movements
Working Americans 1880-2007 Vol. VIII: Immigrants
Working Americans 1880-2009 Vol. X: Sports & Recreation
Working Americans 1880-2010 Vol. XI: Inventors & Entrepreneurs
Working Americans 1880-2011 Vol. XII: Musicians
World Cultural Leaders of the 20th & 21st Centuries

Business Information

Directory of Business Information Resources
Directory of Mail Order Catalogs
Directory of Venture Capital & Private Equity Firms
Environmental Resource Handbook
Food & Beverage Market Place
Grey House Homeland Security Directory
Grey House Performing Arts Directory
Hudson's Washington News Media Contacts Directory
New York State Directory
Sports Market Place Directory
The Rauch Guides – Industry Market Research Reports

Statistics & Demographics

America's Top-Rated Cities
America's Top-Rated Small Towns & Cities
America's Top-Rated Smaller Cities
Comparative Guide to American Hospitals
Comparative Guide to American Suburbs
Comparative Guide to Health in America
Profiles of... Series – State Handbooks

Health Information

Comparative Guide to American Hospitals
Comparative Guide to Health in America
Complete Directory for Pediatric Disorders
Complete Directory for People with Chronic Illness
Complete Directory for People with Disabilities
Complete Mental Health Directory
Directory of Health Care Group Purchasing Organizations
Directory of Hospital Personnel
HMO/PPO Directory
Medical Device Register
Older Americans Information Directory

Education Information

Charter School Movement
Comparative Guide to American Elementary & Secondary Schools
Complete Learning Disabilities Directory
Educators Resource Directory
Special Education

Financial Ratings Series

TheStreet.com Ratings Guide to Bond & Money Market Mutual Funds
TheStreet.com Ratings Guide to Common Stocks
TheStreet.com Ratings Guide to Exchange-Traded Funds
TheStreet.com Ratings Guide to Stock Mutual Funds
TheStreet.com Ratings Ultimate Guided Tour of Stock Investing
Weiss Ratings Consumer Box Set
Weiss Ratings Guide to Banks & Thrifts
Weiss Ratings Guide to Credit Unions
Weiss Ratings Guide to Health Insurers
Weiss Ratings Guide to Life & Annuity Insurers
Weiss Ratings Guide to Property & Casualty Insurers

Bowker's Books In Print® Titles

Books In Print®
Books In Print® Supplement
American Book Publishing Record® Annual
American Book Publishing Record® Monthly
Books Out Loud™
Bowker's Complete Video Directory™
Children's Books In Print®
Complete Directory of Large Print Books & Serials™
El-Hi Textbooks & Serials In Print®
Forthcoming Books®
Law Books & Serials In Print™
Medical & Health Care Books In Print™
Publishers, Distributors & Wholesalers of the US™
Subject Guide to Books In Print®
Subject Guide to Children's Books In Print®

Canadian General Reference

Associations Canada
Canadian Almanac & Directory
Canadian Environmental Resource Guide
Canadian Parliamentary Guide
Financial Services Canada
Governments Canada
Libraries Canada
The History of Canada

Grey House Publishing

4919 Route 22, PO Box 56, Amenia NY 12501-0056 | (800) 562-2139 | www.greyhouse.com | books@greyhouse.com